CRITICAL CARE NURSING

John M. Clochesy, PhD, RN, CS, FAAN, FCCM
Associate Professor and Assistant Dean for Clinical Affairs
School of Nursing
University of Pittsburgh
Pittsburgh, Pennsylvania

Christine Breu, RN, MN, CNAA, FAAN
Director of Operations
Hospice of Louisville
Louisville, Kentucky

Suzette Cardin, RN, DNSc, CNAA
Unit Director
Cardiac Care Unit/Cardiac Observation Unit
UCLA Medical Center
Los Angeles, California

Alice A. Whittaker, RN, MS
Assistant Professor
Creighton University School of Nursing
Mary Lanning Campus
Hastings, Nebraska

Ellen B. Rudy, RN, PhD, FAAN
Dean, School of Nursing
University of Pittsburgh
Pittsburgh, Pennsylvania

CRITICAL CARE NURSING

SECOND EDITION

W. B. SAUNDERS COMPANY
A Division of Harcourt Brace & Company
Philadelphia London Toronto Montreal Sydney Tokyo

W. B. SAUNDERS COMPANY
A Division of Harcourt Brace & Company

The Curtis Center
Independence Square West
Philadelphia, Pennsylvania 19106

Library of Congress Cataloging-in-Publication Data

Critical care nursing / [edited by] John M. Clochesy, Christine Breu, Suzette Cardin, Alice A. Whittaker, Ellen B. Rudy. — 2nd ed.
p. cm.
Includes bibliographical references and index.
ISBN 0-7216-5674-9
1. Intensive care nursing. I. Clochesy, John M. II. Breu, Christine. III. Cardin, Suzette. IV. Whittaker, Alice A. V. Rudy, Ellen B.
[DNLM: 1. Critical Care—nurses' instruction. WY 154 C93332 1966]
RT120.T5C743 1996
810.73'61—dc20
DNLM/DLC 95-42806

NOTICE

Critical Care Nursing is an ever-changing field. Standard safety precautions must be followed, but as new research and clinical experience broaden our knowledge, changes in treatment and drug therapy become necessary or appropriate. The editors of this work have carefully checked the generic and trade drug names and verified drug dosages to ensure that the dosage information in this work is accurate and in accord with the standards accepted at the time of publication. Readers are advised, however, to check the product information currently provided by the manufacturer of each drug to be administered to be certain that changes have not been made in the recommended dose or in the contraindications for administration. This is of particular importance in regard to new or infrequently used drugs. It is the responsibility of the treating physician, relying on experience and knowledge of the patient, to determine dosages and the best treatment for the patient. The editors cannot be responsible for misuse or misapplication of the material in this work.

The Publisher

CRITICAL CARE NURSING ISBN 0-7216-5674-9

Printed in the United States of America.

Last digit is the print number: 9 8 7 6 5 4 3 2 1

CONTRIBUTORS

Thomas S. Ahrens, RN, DNS, CCRN
Assistant Professor, Southern Illinois University; Clinical Specialist, Critical Care, Barnes Hospital, St. Louis, Missouri
Chapter 15, Respiratory Monitoring

Barbara Albee, RN, BSN, MS
Director of Nursing, Hastings Peritoneal Center, Hastings, Nebraska
Chapter 45, Patients With End-Stage Renal Disease

Carol F. Baker, RN, PhD
Director of Nursing Research and Education, General Clinical Research Center, School of Medicine; Clinical Assistant Professor, School of Nursing, University of North Carolina, Chapel Hill, North Carolina
Chapter 28, Acid–Base Physiology

Rita M. Barden, RN, MSN, CCRN
Clinical Nurse, Post-Anesthesia Care Unit, UCSD Medical Center, San Diego, California
Chapter 25, Patients With Hypertension

Marilyn Rossman Bartucci, RN, MSN, CS, CCTC
Clinical Instructor, Case Western Reserve University; Kent State University School of Nursing, Kent, Ohio; Head Nurse Manager, Transplant Center, University Hospitals of Cleveland, Cleveland, Ohio
Chapter 56, Organ Donation

Kim Rutherford Basham, RN, MSN, CCRN
Adjunct Faculty, University of Louisville School of Nursing, Critical Care Nurse Specialist, Baptist Hospital East, Louisville, Kentucky
Editor, Multidisciplinary Care Guides

Nancy J. Beckman, MSN
Assistant Nurse Manager, Kidney Transplant Unit, Medical Center, University of California, San Francisco, San Francisco, California
Chapter 45, Patients With End-Stage Renal Disease

Deanna Bevans, RN, MS, CCRN
Adjunct Faculty, Samaritan College of Nursing, Grand Canyon University; Adult-Pediatric Flight Nurse, Samaritan Air Evac, Phoenix, Arizona
Chapter 66, Chemical and Drug Overdose

Teresa Britt, RN, MS
Research Analyst, Carle's Health Systems Research Center, Carle Clinic Association, Urbana, Illinois
Chapter 71, Elderly Patients

Danni Brown, BS, MS
Manager, Hypothermia Project, University of Pittsburgh Medical Center, Pittsburgh, Pennsylvania
Chapter 52, Patients With Disorders of the Neurohypophysis, Thyroid, and Adrenals

Randy M. Caine, EdD, RN, CS, CCRN, ANP-C
Professor of Nursing, California State University, Long Beach, California
Chapter 60, Patients With Burns

Vic Campbell, PhD, RN
Assistant Professor, Ohio State University, Columbus, Ohio
Chapter 34, Neurophysiology

Mary M. Canobbio, RN, MN
Clinical Researcher, Adult Congenital Heart Disease, Assistant Clinical Professor, UCLA School of Nursing, Los Angeles, California
Chapter 22, Adults With Congenital Heart Defects

Suzette Cardin, RN, DNSc, CNAA
Unit Director, Cardiac Care Unit/Cardiac Observation Unit, UCLA Medical Center; Los Angeles, California
Chapter 21, Heart Failure

Kathleen McMahon Casey, RN, MEd, MA
Associate, Columbia University School of Nursing, New York, New York; Medical Consultant, Rhinebeck, New York
Chapter 58, Patients With HIV Disease

Suzanne Clark, RN, MSN, MA, CS, RNP
Assistant Clinical Professor, UCLA School of Nursing; Clinical Nurse Specialist, Department of Psychiatry, Kaiser Permanente, Los Angeles, California
Chapter 5, Psychosocial Needs of Critically Ill Patients

John M. Clochesy, PhD, RN, CS, FAAN, FCCM
Associate Professor, Acute and Tertiary Care, University of Pittsburgh School of Nursing, Pittsburgh, Pennsylvania
Chapter 34, Neurophysiology; Chapter 36, Patients With Cerebral Vascular Disorders; Chapter 40, Craniotomy; Chapter 63, Patients With Systemic Inflammatory Response Syndrome

Bernice Coleman, RN, MSN, CCRN
Clinical Nurse Specialist, Cardiovascular Surgery and Thoracic Transplant Services, Cedars-Sinai Medical Center, Los Angeles, California
Chapter 24, Patients Undergoing Cardiothoracic Surgery and Transplants

Barbara J. Daly, RN, PhD, FAAN
Assistant Professor, Frances Payne Bolton School of Nursing, Case Western Reserve University; Co-Director, Clinical Ethics Service, University Hospitals of Cleveland, Cleveland, Ohio
Chapter 2, Ethics in Critical Care

Joanne M. Disch, RN, PhD, FAAN
Senior Associate Director/Director of Patient-Family Services, University of Minnesota Hospital and Clinic; Adjunct Associate Professor, School of Nursing, University of Minnesota, Minneapolis, Minnesota
Chapter 1, Practice Within the Current Health Care Environment

Peter R. Doyle, BS, RRT
Product Manager, Puritan-Bennett Corp., Vista, California
Chapter 16, Mechanical Ventilation: Current Uses and Advances

Diane K. Dressler, RN, MSN, CCTC
Senior Transplant Coordinator, St. Luke's Medical Center, Milwaukee, Wisconsin
Chapter 53, Hematologic Physiology; Chapter 54, Patients With Coagulopathies

Elaine L. Enger, RN, MS
Director, Midwest Heart Research Foundation, Lombard, Illinois
Chapter 32, Patients With Adult Respiratory Distress Syndrome

DeAnn Englert, BSN, MSN
Independent Nursing Consultant, Houston, Texas
Chapter 48, Patients With Gastrointestinal Bleeding

Carol M. Flavell, RN, MS, CCRN
Clinician Nurse Specialist, Cardiac Transplantation, Brigham & Women's Hospital, Boston, Massachusetts
Chapter 24, Patients Undergoing Cardiothoracic Surgery and Transplants

Julie Fleury, RN, PhD
Assistant Professor, Department of Adult and Geriatric Health, University of North Carolina, Chapel Hill, North Carolina
Chapter 19, Patients With Coronary Artery Disease

Dorrie K. Fontaine, RN, DNSc, FAAN
Clinical Associate Professor, School of Nursing, Georgetown University; Clinical Nurse Researcher, Critical Care, Georgetown University Hospital, Washington, District of Columbia
Chapter 8, Effect of Sensory Alterations

Kathy Goff, RNC, MS
Patient Care Manager, University Medical Center, Tucson, Arizona
Chapter 69, Patients With Obstetric Crises

Stacey B. Gross, RN, MS, CS, ANP
Adult Nurse Practitioner, East Boston Neighborhood Health Center, Boston, Massachusetts
Chapter 24, Patients Undergoing Cardiothoracic Surgery and Transplants

Ginny Wacker Guido, RN, JD, MSN
Professor and Chair, Department of Nursing, Eastern New Mexico University, Portales, New Mexico
Chapter 3, Legal Issues in Critical Care

Diana W. Guthrie, PhD, FAAN, ARNP
Professor, Department of Pediatrics, University of Kansas; Professor, Department of Psychiatry and Nursing, University of Kansas; Adjunct Professor, Wichita State University, School of Nursing; Allied Health Professional, St. Joseph Medical Center; St. Francis Regional Medical Center; Wesley Medical Center, Wichita, Kansas
Chapter 51, Patients With Disorders of Glucose Metabolism

Jan L. Hawthorne, RN, MSN, OCN
Clinical Faculty, Frances Payne Bolton School of Nursing, Case Western Reserve University; Clinical Nurse Specialist, Women's Surgical Oncology, University Hospitals of Cleveland, Cleveland, Ohio
Chapter 57, Immunocompromised Patients

Margaret Heitkemper, BSN, MN, PhD
Professor, Department of Biobehavioral Nursing and Health Systems, University of Washington, Seattle, Washington
Chapter 46, Gastrointestinal Physiology

Richard Henker, RN, PhD, CCRN
Assistant Professor, University of Pittsburgh School of Nursing, Pittsburgh, Pennsylvania
Chapter 67, Alterations in Thermoregulation

Elizabeth A. Henneman, RN, MS, CCRN
Assistant Clinical Professor, UCLA School of Nursing; Clinical Nurse Specialist, Medical Intensive Care Unit, UCLA Medical Center, Los Angeles, California
Chapter 31, Patients With Acute Respiratory Failure

Kathryn A. Hennessy, RN, MS, CNSN
Manager, Nursing Services, Professional Services, Clintec Nutrition Company, Deerfield, Illinois
Chapter 50, Patients With Acute Pancreatitis

Mairead Hickey, RN, PhD
Director, Patient Care Services Research, Evaluation and Outcomes Measurement, Director, Quality Measurement, Brigham and Women's Hospital, Boston, Massachusetts
Chapter 6, Psychosocial Needs of Families

Becky Hull, MS
Director, Nursing Information Systems, University Medical Center, Tucson, Arizona
Chapter 69, Patients With Obstetric Crises

Connie A. (Walleck) Jastremski, RN, MS, CNAA, FCCM
Adjunct Associate Professor, SUNY College of Nursing, Syracuse, New York; Consultant, Critical Care Management Consultants, Albany, New York
Chapter 35, Patients With Head Injury and Brain Dysfunction; Chapter 38, Patients With Spinal Cord Injury

Kimmith M. Jones, RN, MS, CCRN
Faculty Associate, University of Maryland; Clinical Nurse Specialist, Critical Care, Franklin Square Hospital Center, Baltimore, Maryland
Chapter 64, Shock

Margaret Catherine Jones, RN, MSN, CCRN
Clinical Instructor, Anna Jaques Hospital, Newburyport, Massachusetts
Chapter 12, Pacemakers

Colleen Keller, RN, PhD
Professor, University of Texas Health Science Center; Family Nurse Practitioner, Ella Austin Community Health Clinic, San Antonio, Texas
Chapter 19, Patients With Coronary Artery Disease

Deborah Goldenberg Klein, BSN, MSN, CCRN, CS
Clinical Instructor, Frances Payne Bolton School of Nursing, Case Western Reserve University; Clinical Nurse Specialist, Trauma/Critical Care Nursing, Metro Health Medical Center, Cleveland, Ohio
Chapter 62, Patients With Trauma

Darlene Averell Lovasik, RN, MN, CCRN, CNRN
Clinical Director, Trauma and Intensive Care Units, University Medical Center, Pittsburgh, Pennsylvania
Chapter 41, Infections of the Central Nervous System

Norma D. McNair, RN, MSN, CS, CCRN, CNRN
Assistant Clinical Professor, UCLA School of Nursing; Former Clinical Nurse Specialist, Neurosurgery/Trauma Intensive Care Units, UCLA Medical Center, Los Angeles, California
Chapter 17, Intracranial Pressure Monitoring

Linda Menzel, RN, PhD, CCRN
Assistant Professor, University of Wisconsin School of Nursing, Milwaukee, Wisconsin
Chapter 11, Electrocardiogram Interpretation

Leanna R. Miller, RN, MN, CCRN, CEN, PNP
Critical Care Clinical Nurse Specialist, Children's Hospital, Medical Center of Central Georgia, Macon, Georgia
Chapter 13, Hemodynamic Monitoring; Chapter 43, Patients With Fluid and Electrolyte Disturbances

Vickie A. Miracle, RN, EdD, CCRN
Adjunct Faculty, University of Louisville School of Nursing; Clinical Coordinator, Jewish Hospital, Heart and Lung Institute, Louisville, Kentucky
Editor, Multidisciplinary Care Guides

Debra K. Moser, RN, DNSc
Assistant Professor, Ohio State University College of Nursing, Columbus, Ohio
Chapter 21, Heart Failure

Carolyn Murdaugh, RN, PhD
Director of Research, University of Arizona College of Nursing; Director of Clinical Research Services, University Medical Center, Tucson, Arizona
Chapter 19, Patients With Coronary Artery Disease

Susan C. Nolt, RN, BS, MBA
Coordinator of Field Management Development, First American Home Care, Lancaster, Pennsylvania
Chapter 10, Preparing the Patient and Family for Home Care

Jane Parthum, RN, MS
Clinical Nurse Specialist, St. Luke's Medical Center, Milwaukee, Wisconsin
Chapter 26, Vascular Emergencies

Patricia Peschman, MS
Geriatric Nurse Practitioner, Evercare, Minneapolis, Minnesota
Chapter 42, Renal Physiology

Carol Rauen, RN, MS, CCRN
Nursing Coordinator and Clinical Nurse Specialist, Cardiovascular Intensive Care Unit and Stepdown, Georgetown University Medical Center, Washington, District of Columbia
Chapter 71, Elderly Patients

Sara J. Reeder, BSN, MSN, PhD
Assistant Professor, University of Pittsburgh School of Nursing, Pittsburgh, Pennsylvania
Chapter 65, Patients With Pain

Barbara Riegel, RN, DNSc, CS
Associate Professor, San Diego State University School of Nursing; Clinical Researcher, Sharp HealthCare, San Diego, California
Chapter 20, Myocardial Infarction

Marcia Rostad, RN, MS, NS, OCN
Adjunct Clinical Assistant Professor, University of Arizona; Pediatric Oncology Clinical Nurse Specialist, University Medical Center, Tucson, Arizona
Chapter 70, Patients With Oncologic Emergencies

Ellen B. Rudy, RN, PhD, FAAN
Dean, School of Nursing, University of Pittsburgh, Pittsburgh, Pennsylvania
Chapter 37, Brain Death

Susan D. Ruppert, RN, PhD, CCRN, FNP
Associate Professor, University of Texas Health Science Center School of Nursing, Houston, Texas
Chapter 48, Patients With Gastrointestinal Bleeding

Shelley Ruzevich, RN
Clinical Heart/Lung Transplant Coordinator, Nurse Clinician Circulatory Support, UCLA Medical Center, Los Angeles, California
Chapter 14, Cardiac Assist Devices

Catherine J. Ryan, RN, MS, CCRN
Clinical Nurse Specialist, Critical Care, Alexian Brothers Medical Center, Elk Grove Village, Illinois
Chapter 30, Pulmonary Infections

Johanna Salamandra, RN
Administrative Transplant Coordinator, Cardiothoracic Transplant Programs, UCLA Medical Center, Los Angeles, California
Chapter 24, Patients Undergoing Cardiothoracic Surgery and Transplants

Michael A. Salatka, JD, MPH
Blue Cross and Blue Shield of Ohio, Cleveland, Ohio
Chapter 4, Occupational Health Hazards in Critical Care

Linda H. Schakenbach, RN, MSN, CCRN, CETN, CS
Adjunct Associate Professor, Catholic University of America School of Nursing, Washington, DC; Clinical Lecturer, School of Nursing, George Mason University, Clinical Nurse Specialist, Surgical Nursing, Fairfax Hospital, Falls Church, Virginia
Chapter 23, Patients With Valvular Disease

Hildy M. Schell, RN, MS, CCRN
Assistant Clinical Professor, University of California School of Nursing; Clinical Nurse Specialist, Critical Care, University of California Medical Center, San Francisco, California
Chapter 45, Patients With End-Stage Renal Disease

Melanie H. Shuster, RN, BSN, MSN
Adjunct Instructor, University of Pittsburgh School of Nursing; Nutritional Clinical Nurse Specialist, Department of Veterans Affairs, VA Medical Center, Pittsburgh, Pennsylvania
Chapter 47, Nutrition in the Critically Ill

Verna A. Sitzer, RN, MN, CCRN
Senior Clinical Nurse Specialist; Critical Care, Sharp HealthCare, San Diego, California
Chapter 7, Enhancing Communication With Critically Ill Patients and Families

Susan L. Smith, RN, PhD
Clinical Nurse Specialist, Transplant Services, Emory University Hospital, Atlanta, Georgia
Chapter 49, Patients With Liver Dysfunction

Kathleen S. Stone, RN, PhD, FANN
Professor, College of Nursing, Ohio State University, Columbus, Ohio
Chapter 27, Respiratory Physiology

Nancy A. Stotts, MN, EdD
Associate Professor, University of California School of Nursing, San Francisco, California
Chapter 59, Wound Healing

Nancy L. Szaflarski, RN, PhD, CVS, FCCM
Adjunct Clinical Lecturer, University of Pennsylvania School of Nursing, Philadelphia, Pennsylvania
Chapter 61, Immobility Phenomena in Critically Ill Adults

Julie N. Tackenberg, RN, MA, MADM, CNRN
Clinical Specialist, Arizona Health Sciences Center, Tucson, Arizona
Chapter 40, Craniotomy

Frederick J. Tasota, RN, MSN, CCRN
Research Project Director, University of Pittsburgh School of Nursing; Staff Nurse, University of Pittsburgh Medical Center, Pittsburgh, Pennsylvania
Chapter 29, Patients With Chronic Obstructive Pulmonary Diseases

Kathy Sabo Thompson, RN, MSN
Head Nurse, Special Care Unit and Surgical Intensive Care Unit, University Hospitals of Cleveland, Cleveland, Ohio
Chapter 39, Patients With Guillain-Barré Syndrome

Marita G. Titler, RN, PhD, FAAN
Adjunct Assistant Professor, University of Iowa College of Nursing; Associate Director, Research, and Senior Associate Director, Office of Outcomes Evaluation and Management, University of Iowa Hospitals and Clinics, Iowa City, Iowa
Chapter 9, Chronic Illness and Critical Care Practice

Patricia L. Vaska, RN, MSN, CNP, CCRN
Cardiovascular Surgery Clinical Nurse Specialist and Nurse Practitioner, Sioux Falls, South Dakota
Chapter 18, Cardiovascular Anatomy and Physiology

Una E. Westfall, RN, PhD, MSN
Associate Professor, School of Nursing, Oregon Health Sciences University, Portland, Oregon
Chapter 46, Gastrointestinal Physiology

Marjorie B. Wheeler, RN, MS
Assistant Clinical Professor, University of California; Nurse Surveyor, Joint Commission on Accreditation of Healthcare Organizations, San Francisco, California; Nurse Consultant, Stetson Associates, Mill Valley, California
Chapter 10, Preparing the Patient and Family for Home Care

Jill M. White, RN, MSN
Doctoral Candidate, University of Wisconsin School of Nursing, Milwaukee, Wisconsin
Chapter 11, Electrocardiogram Interpretation

JoAnne D. Whitney, PhD, MS, BSN
Assistant Professor, University of Washington, Seattle, Washington
Chapter 59, Wound Healing

Alice A. Whittaker, RN, MS
Assistant Professor, Creighton University School of Nursing, Mary Lanning Campus, Hastings, Nebraska
Chapter 44, Patients With Acute Renal Failure

Donna J. Wilson, RN, MSN, RRT
Pulmonary Clinical Nurse Specialist, Memorial Sloan-Kettering Cancer Center, New York, New York
Chapter 33, Care of the Chronic Mechanically Ventilated Patient

Ginger S. Wlody, RN, EdD, FCCM
Assistant Clinical Professor, UCLA School of Nursing, Los Angeles, California
Chapter 68, Preventing Postanesthesia Complications

M. Linda Workman, RN, PhD, RN, FAAN
Associate Professor, Frances Payne Bolton School of Nursing, Case Western Reserve University, Cleveland, Ohio
Chapter 55, Physiologic Response to Infection

John W. Wright, MBA, BS, RRT
Assistant Director, Respiratory Therapy Department, UCLA Medical Center, Los Angeles, California
Chapter 16, Mechanical Ventilation: Current Uses and Advances

Gary Yoshihara, BA, RRT, RCP
Clinical Supervisor, UCLA Medical Center, Los Angeles, California
Chapter 16, Mechanical Ventilation: Current Uses and Advances

FOREWORD

In the brief time that has passed since the publication of the first edition of *Critical Care Nursing* the health care system has undergone a profound transformation. The financial basis of intensive care has altered dramatically, and with this alteration patients stay an even shorter length of time in the intensive care unit setting and are more likely to be in severe physiological crisis than the patients of just a few years ago.

We do not know what the changes of the next ten years will bring, but clearly nurses will be responsible for complex clinical judgments requiring expert knowledge. Even more importantly, they will have to coordinate the care patients receive with a variety of individuals from various disciplines and skill levels. The revisions incorporated in this text are exactly what nurses need in this new environment. The editors and authors provide the latest theory and science on a variety of clinical conditions and treatments. They have emphasized multidisciplinary care guides or care maps that can help coordinate patient care at the bedside and provide a framework for planning for each patient from admission to discharge.

This test is a unique and important contribution to our discipline and is essential for every practicing critical care nurse. The editors and authors are to be congratulated on their achievement.

Kathleen Dracup
Professor and L.W. Hassenplug Chair of Nursing
University of California, Los Angeles

PREFACE

The second edition of *Critical Care Nursing* continues to emphasize the editors' belief in the essential elements of critical care nursing practice. The first of these is skilled and competent staff who have a solid understanding of the body of knowledge of critical care nursing and of pertinent information from other disciplines. Other elements essential to critical care nursing practice include patient and family centered care, multidisciplinary collaboration, the critical care environment, and smooth coordinated transitions between all phases of the patient and family illness experience. The editors and contributors have addressed each of these essential elements in this revision, integrating each component as described below.

This text is written from the perspective that critical care nurses require a *thorough understanding of the physiologic basis of critical care illness* and its treatment. This text provides an in-depth physiologic basis for each body system and has individual chapters addressing various critical illnesses and treatments. These authors also recognize the complexities of patient responses and *the reciprocal relationship between the physiologic, psychological, social, and spiritual dimensions of the patient* by integrating all of these domains in this text.

The *critical care environment* in which critical care nursing is practiced strongly influences the outcomes of the care provided to the patient and the family. This environment includes collaborative relationships, continuous learning, innovation, and shared expertise. It also includes the effectiveness of support systems and resources, and the philosophy and leadership that exists within the hospital milieu. Comprehensive information is contained in this text on the environment and its impact on practice (Chapter 1), the ethical domain in which critical care nurses practice (Chapter 2), and legal aspects of critical care nursing practice (Chapter 3). In addition, occupational safety issues are discussed in detail (Chapter 4).

Patient and family centered care is a core theme within this text. Critical care nurses provide care to patients who are experiencing life-threatening or potentially life-threatening illness or injury. These critically ill patients are particularly vulnerable because of the disease states that put them at physiologic and psychological risk. This vulnerability is compounded by the fast-paced, labor-intensive environment in which care is delivered. Although the technology and vigilance in this environment are lifesaving, constant and deliberate effort is required to keep the patient and family as the center focus of this environment. The stresses inherent within the intensive care unit require critical care nurses to create a compassionate, humanistic, and flexible approach to care. In-depth information is provided on psychosocial needs of patients (Chapter 5), psychosocial needs of families (Chapter 6), and enhancing communication with patients and families (Chapter 7). Patient and family decision making is stressed throughout this text.

To achieve successful outcomes in patient and family centered care, *collaboration with other disciplines* in the planning, delivering, and evaluating of care is required. In today's evolving critical care world, collaboration includes recognizing the value and rights of each individual care provider and respecting each team member's expertise and contribution. Collaboration also means assuring the full involvement of all disciplines required to meet the patient's needs by integrating activities of all care providers and thus decreasing the fragmentation of care that occurs when disciplines work parallel to but not with each other.

One way to enhance this collaboration and full integration of disciplines into a single plan of care is through the use of team-developed care guides. A new addition to this text is *multidisciplinary care guides* that have been included for many of the major critical illnesses. These care guides stress the role of the patient and family in all decision making and the inclusiveness required of all disciplines for both the development and revisions of the plan of care. The care guides include both basic and advanced information for use by a variety of levels of care providers. They address the physiologic, psychological, and self-determination needs of the patient and family unit as well as patient and family education. The care guides are organized into three phases of care: diagnosis/stabilization, acute management, and recovery. These phases are not defined specifically because the activities identified in each phase may occur in different care delivery settings, depending on the type of resources available at a facility. The multidisciplinary care guides are meant to be used as a resource in the development of facility-specific care guides.

The goal for health care today is to have *smooth transitions in care* provided throughout all phases of the patient's illness. In today's health care environment, significant emphasis is placed on the integration of patient and family needs across all care delivery settings. Within the first few hours of admission of a patient, critical care nurses begin to identify the resources that will be needed as the patient moves through various phases of illness and the various care settings. Comprehensive information on chronic illness recovery process and *the illness continuum* (Chapter 9) is provided in this edition; in-depth information on home care and the critical care nurses's role in mobilizing resources for ongoing patient care (Chapter 10) is also provided.

To help critical care nurses meet the needs of patients and families, the editors have *added chapters* on nutrition, CNS infections, pacemakers, thermoregulation, chronic illness and patient recovery, and the transition to home care.

Critical care nursing practice remains challenging not only because of the efforts required to achieve quality patient and family outcomes but also because of the constantly changing hospital and health care environments. For successful practice in today's environment, critical care nurses need to continually expand their knowledge base, seek practice innovations, understand the environment in which practice occurs, and promote integrated, patient-centered care with other disciplines. Because this text contains all of these aspects of practice, the editors of this edition feel that this text is an excellent resource for critical care nurses as they face the challenges in today's practice environment.

CONTENTS

UNIT 1
THE PRACTICE ENVIRONMENT 1

CHAPTER 1
Practice Within the Current Health Care Environment 3
Joanne M. Disch
Background for Change 3
The New Direction for Health Care Reform 6
Strategies for Competing in a Managed Care Environment 7
Implications for Critical Care 9
Implications for Critical Care Nursing 9
Strategies for Success 10
Summary 12

CHAPTER 2
Ethics in Critical Care 15
Barbara J. Daly
Nursing Ethics 15
Ethical Reasoning 16
Myths and Handicaps in Ethical Reasoning 20
Making Ethical Decision Making Operational 21
The Ethical Agenda of Critical Care Nursing for the Future 22
Summary 23

CHAPTER 3
Legal Issues in Critical Care 25
Ginny Wacker Guido
Standards of Care 25
Negligence and Malpractice 26
Intentional Torts 28
Quasi-Intentional Torts 28
Liability and the Critical Care Nurse 29
Specific Legal Concerns in Critical Care 32
Summary 35

CHAPTER 4
Occupational Health Hazards in Critical Care 36
Michael A. Salatka
Infectious Hazards 36
Musculoskeletal Injuries 37
Chemical Hazards 40
Radiation Hazards 40
Noise 41
Chemical Dependency 42
Conclusion 44

UNIT 2
PATIENT AND FAMILY CARE 47

CHAPTER 5
Psychosocial Needs of Critically Ill Patients 49
Suzanne Clark
Meeting Psychosocial Needs in Critical Care: The Challenge 49
Holistic Nursing in a Technical Environment 49
Stress–Coping Framework 50
Stress–Coping Framework: Planning Nursing Care 52
Assessments and Interventions Related to Cognitive Appraisal 56
Assessment of and Interventions for Affective or Physiologic Arousal 57
Supporting Adaptive Coping Responses and Defense Mechanisms 59
Prerequisite for Nursing Interventions: A Caring Relationship 61
Summary 62

CHAPTER 6
Psychosocial Needs of Families 65
Mairead Hickey
Contemporary Families 65
Critical Illness—A Crisis for the Family 65
Common Responses of Families to Critical Illness 66
Needs of Families of Critically Ill Patients 68
Interventions for Families of Critically Ill Patients 68
Summary 72

CHAPTER 7
Enhancing Communication With Critically Ill Patients and Families 74
Verna A. Sitzer
Communication Process 74
Communication Channels 75
Essential Elements for Effective Communication 77
Communication Barriers 79
Interventions That Improve Communication 81
Summary 87

CHAPTER 8
Effect of Sensory Alterations 89
Dorrie K. Fontaine
Psychophysical Environment of Critical Care Units 89
Impact of the Critical Care Environment 90
The Nature of Sensory Perception 91
Alterations in Sensory Perceptions due to Critical Illness 92
Nursing Diagnosis: Sensory–Perceptual Alterations 92
Sensory Deprivation 93
Sensory Overload 96
Nursing Therapeutics for Sensory–Perceptual Alterations 98
Sleep and Rest Disturbances in the Critical Care Unit 100
Nursing Therapeutics for Sleep Pattern Disturbance 103
Summary 104

CHAPTER 9
Chronic Illness and Critical Care Practice 107
Marita G. Titler
The Nature of Chronic Illness 107
Responses to Chronic Illness 109
Resources 110
Summary 115

CHAPTER 10
Preparing the Patient and Family for Home Care 117
Marjorie B. Wheeler and Susan C. Nolt
Background 117
Selecting Patients for Home Care 118
The ICU–Home Care Team 118
Comprehensive Assessment 120
Transition: Critical Care to Home 122
Evaluation of the Transition to Home Care 123
Summary 124

UNIT 3
MONITORING AND TECHNOLOGY 125

CHAPTER 11
Electrocardiogram Interpretation 127
Linda K. Menzel and Jill M. White
Anatomy and Physiology 127
Electrophysiology 131
Interpretation of the ECG 135
Electrocardiographic Changes With Coronary Artery Disease 143
Impulse Conduction 150
Wide QRS Complexes: Differentiating Supraventricular and Ventricular Rhythms 152
Preexcitation Syndromes 157
Ventricular Dysrhythmias 162
Paradysrhythmias: Parasystole and AV Dissociation 164
Summary 165

CHAPTER 12
Pacemakers 167
Margaret Catherine Jones
Permanent Pacing 167
Physiologic Pacing 174
Temporary Pacing 177
ECG Interpretation of Pacemaker Function 191
Implantable Devices for Cardioversion, Defibrillation, and Pacing 196
Summary 200

CHAPTER 13
Hemodynamic Monitoring 203
Leanna R. Miller
Hemodynamic Monitoring Systems 203
Central Venous Pressure Monitoring 204

Intraarterial Pressure Monitoring 205
Pulmonary Artery Pressure Monitoring 208
Cardiac Output Measurements 222
Clinical Application of Hemodynamic Monitoring 227
Summary 231

CHAPTER 14
Cardiac Assist Devices **235**
Shelley Ruzevich
Centrifugal Assist Devices 235
External Pulsatile Devices 236
Implantable Assist Devices 237
Extracorporeal Membrane Oxygenation 238
Cannulation 238
Nursing Care 241
Summary 243

CHAPTER 15
Respiratory Monitoring **245**
Tom Ahrens
Oxygenation Components 245
Assessment of Oxygen Transport and Consumption 249
Pa_{O_2} and Intrapulmonary Shunting 253
VD/VT Application 256
Summary 259

CHAPTER 16
Mechanical Ventilation: Current Uses and Advances **262**
John Wright, Peter Doyle, and Gary Yoshihara
Historical Overview 262
General Ventilatory Concepts 262
Volume Ventilation 266
Pressure Ventilation 268
Weaning Models 270
Informational Feedback Features 276
Noninvasive Ventilation: BiPAP 277
Prolonged Inspiration Ventilation 277
High-Frequency Ventilation 279
Differential Lung Ventilation 282
Mechanical Ventilation With Unconventional Gases 283
Gas Exchange Devices 285
Routine Care of Patients on Mechanical Ventilation 286
Ventilator Troubleshooting 287

CHAPTER 17
Intracranial Pressure Monitoring **289**
Norma D. McNair
Physiology of Intracranial Pressure 289
Etiology of Increased Intracranial Pressure 293
Neurologic Assessment 294
Intracranial Pressure Monitoring 295
Management of Intracranial Hypertension 303
Clinical Management 303
Summary 306

UNIT 4
CARDIOVASCULAR SYSTEM 309

CHAPTER 18
Cardiovascular Anatomy and Physiology **311**
Patricia L. Vaska
Overview 311
Electrical Activity of the Heart 317
Cardiac Pumping 319
Systemic Circulation 324
Integration of Central and Peripheral Factors in Cardiac Output Control 332
Summary 334

CHAPTER 19
Patients With Coronary Artery Disease **336**
Julie Fleury, Colleen Keller, and Carolyn Murdaugh
Atherosclerosis: The Lesion of Coronary Artery Disease 336
Myocardial Ischemia 337
Noninvasive Diagnosis 338
Invasive Diagnosis 340
Angina Pectoris 342
Invasive Management 346
Sudden Death 349
Summary 352

CHAPTER 20
Myocardial Infarction **354**
Barbara Riegel
Pathophysiology 354
Clinical Presentation 357
Physical Assessment 358
Laboratory Findings 360
Diagnostic Procedures 361
Clinical Management 364
Pharmaceutical Agents 364
Therapeutic Interventions 367
Summary 370

CHAPTER 21
Heart Failure 380
Debra K. Moser and Suzette Cardin
Pathophysiology of Heart Failure 380
Clinical Manifestations and Diagnostic Testing 387
Treatment 390
Summary 403

CHAPTER 22
Adults With Congenital Heart Defects 413
Mary M. Canobbio
Etiology 413
Incidence and Prevalence 413
Factors Influencing Long-Term Survival 416
Complications Associated With Long-Term Survival of CHD 421
Collaborative Management 425
Summary 426

CHAPTER 23
Patients With Valvular Disease 428
Linda H. Schakenbach
Pathophysiology: Overview 428
Mitral Regurgitation 429
Mitral Valve Prolapse 436
Mitral Stenosis 439
Aortic Regurgitation 442
Aortic Stenosis 446
Tricuspid Regurgitation 449
Tricuspid Stenosis 452
Pulmonic Regurgitation 453
Pulmonic Stenosis 455
Summary 456

CHAPTER 24
Patients Undergoing Cardiothoracic Surgery and Transplants 458
Stacey Gross, Bernice Coleman, Carol Flavell, and Johanna Salamandra
Coronary Artery Bypass Graft Surgery 458
Preoperative Care 471
Intraoperative Management 473
Thoracic Transplants 494
Summary 504

CHAPTER 25
Patients With Hypertension 519
Rita M. Barden
Regulation of Arterial Blood Pressure 519
Definition and Prevalence of Hypertension 521
Classification of Hypertension 522
Primary (Essential) Hypertension 523
Secondary Hypertension 525
Evaluation and Diagnosis of Hypertensive Emergencies 528
Treatment of Hypertensive Emergencies 530
Management of Secondary Hypertension 531
Clinical Management 533
Summary 533

CHAPTER 26
Vascular Emergencies 535
Jane Parthum
Aortic Aneurysm 535
Acute Aortic Dissection 539
Acute Arterial Occlusion 543
Vascular Trauma 547
Summary 550

UNIT 5
PULMONARY SYSTEM 559

CHAPTER 27
Respiratory Physiology 561
Kathleen S. Stone
Anatomy of the Respiratory Tract 561
Anatomy of the Respiratory Gas Exchange Unit 565
Pulmonary Circulation 565
Mechanics of Pulmonary Ventilation 567
Pulmonary Function Measurements 571
Diffusion of Respiratory Gases 574
Transport of Respiratory Gases 576
Control of Respiration 579
Summary 581

CHAPTER 28
Acid–Base Physiology 583
Carol F. Baker
Key Definitions 583
Sources of Acids and Bases in the Body 584
pH of Normal Body Fluids 585
Defense Against Changes in Acid–Base Balance 585
Assessment of Acid–Base Balance and Imbalance 590
Clinical Alterations in Acid–Base Balance 593
Summary 600

CHAPTER 29
Patients With Chronic Obstructive Pulmonary Diseases 601
Frederick J. Tasota
Epidemiology 601
Etiology 602
Chronic Bronchitis 603
Emphysema 606
Acute Management of the Patient With COPD 608
Asthma 612
Summary 618

CHAPTER 30
Pulmonary Infections 620
Catherine J. Ryan
Incidence 620
Tuberculosis 626
Aspiration Pneumonitis 627
Summary 628

CHAPTER 31
Patients With Acute Respiratory Failure 630
Elizabeth A. Henneman
Pathophysiology 630
Clinical Assessment 635
Psychosocial Assessment 636
Diagnostic Tests 636
Management of Acute Respiratory Failure 639
Managing Complications of Acute Respiratory Failure 644
Weaning From Mechanical Ventilation 645
Providing Psychosocial Support to the Patient and Family 646
Summary 647

CHAPTER 32
Patients With Adult Respiratory Distress Syndrome 656
Elaine L. Enger
Structure of the Alveolar-Capillary Membrane 656
Physiologic Basis of Fluid Movement 657
General Pathogenesis of Pulmonary Edema 659
Predisposing Factors for ARDS 660
Mechanisms and Mediators of Acute Lung Injury: The Role of Polymorphonuclear Leukocytes 661
The Clinical and Pathologic Phases of ARDS 665
The Clinical Diagnosis of ARDS 667
Medical Treatment 668
Primary Outcome Pathway: Adequacy of Oxygenation/Ventilation 674
Prognosis 676

CHAPTER 33
Care of the Chronic Mechanically Ventilated Patient 689
Donna J. Wilson
Respiratory Decompensation 689
Weaning 692
Airway Management 697
Summary 703

UNIT 6
NERVOUS SYSTEM 715

CHAPTER 34
Neurophysiology 717
Victor G. Campbell and John M. Clochesy
Neuroglia Cells 717
The Neuron 717
The Nerve 719
Central Nervous System 723

CHAPTER 35
Patients With Head Injury and Brain Dysfunction 749
Connie (Walleck) Jastremski
Traumatic Brain Injury 749
Ischemic Brain Injury 764
Seizures 770
Summary 772

CHAPTER 36
Patients With Cerebral Vascular Disorders 781
John M. Clochesy
Cerebrovascular System 781
Nonhemorrhagic Stroke 782
Hemorrhagic Stroke 791
Nursing Care of the Patient With an Acute Cerebrovascular Event 799

CHAPTER 37
Brain Death 803
Ellen B. Rudy
Statutory Recognition of Brain Death 804
Criteria for Determining Brain Death 804
Management of Patients Who Meet Brain Death Criteria 807

Problems in Determining Brain Death 807
Brain Death in Children 809
Summary 810

CHAPTER 38
Patients With Spinal Cord Injury 812
Connie (Walleck) Jastremski
Epidemiology 812
Types of Spinal Cord Injury 813
Pathophysiology of Spinal Cord Injury 814
Spinal Shock 815
Clinical Presentation 816
Medical Management 819
Nursing Management 824
Summary 829

CHAPTER 39
Patients With Guillain-Barré Syndrome 831
Kathryn Sabo Thompson
Etiology 831
Clinical Presentation 832
Clinical Management 833
Summary 838

CHAPTER 40
Craniotomy 846
Julie Tackenberg and John M. Clochesy
Intracranial Tumors 846
Epilepsies 849
Craniotomy 850
Specific Surgeries 855
General Clinical Care After Craniotomy 855
Summary 860

CHAPTER 41
Infections of the Central Nervous System 862
Darlene Averell Lovasik
Meningitis 862
Encephalitis 864
Brain Abscess 865
Subdural Empyema 865
Intracranial Epidural Abscess 866
Spinal Epidural Abscess 866
Bacterial Ventriculitis 866
Creutzfeldt-Jakob Disease 866
Human Immunodeficiency Virus 866
Uncommon Viral Diseases Targeting the CNS 867
Isolation 867

UNIT 7
RENAL SYSTEM 869

CHAPTER 42
Renal Physiology 871
Patricia Peschman
Renal Anatomy 871
Renal Hemodynamics 875
Physiologic Functions Performed by the Kidney 879
Summary 890

CHAPTER 43
Patients With Fluid and Electrolyte Disturbances 892
Leanna R. Miller
Body Fluid Compartments 892
Fluid Volume and Osmolality 894
Electrolyte Regulation and Balance 906
Summary 924

CHAPTER 44
Patients With Acute Renal Failure 926
Alice (Ali) Whittaker
Pathophysiology 926
Clinical Presentation 930
Clinical Management 933
Dialysis Therapy 936
Discharge Preparation 939
Summary 940

CHAPTER 45
Patients With End-Stage Renal Disease 949
Barbara Albee, Nancy J. Beckman, and Hildegarde M. Schell
Historical Perspective on ESRD and Dialysis 949
Pathophysiology of ESRD 949
Renal Replacement Therapy 950
Clinical Management 953
Renal Transplantation 961
Summary 966

UNIT 8

GASTROINTESTINAL SYSTEM 977

CHAPTER 46
***Gastrointestinal Physiology* 979**
Una E. Westfall and Margaret Heitkemper
Anatomy of the Gut Wall 979
Neural Innervation 980
Hormonal Control 981
Blood Supply 982
Major Functions of the GI Tract 984
Physiologic Adaptation to Pathology 990
Accessory Gastrointestinal Organs 991

CHAPTER 47
***Nutrition in the Critically Ill* 994**
Melanie H. Shuster
Nutrition and Metabolism 994
Provision of Nutrition 1000
Disease-Specific Nutritional Therapy in the Critically Ill 1017
Summary 1019

CHAPTER 48
***Patients With Gastrointestinal Bleeding* 1022**
Susan D. Ruppert and DeAnn M. Englert
Pathophysiology 1022
Causes of Gastrointestinal Hemorrhage 1024
Clinical Assessment 1029
Clinical Management of Gastrointestinal Bleeding 1031
Nasogastric Intubation or Lavage 1032
Discharge Planning 1040
Summary 1040

CHAPTER 49
***Patients With Liver Dysfunction* 1048**
Susan L. Smith
Anatomy of the Liver and Hepatobiliary System 1048
Physiology of the Liver and Hepatobiliary System 1051
Assessment of Liver Function 1053
Acute Fulminant Hepatic Failure 1056
Hepatitis 1059
Alcoholic Liver Disease 1062
Cirrhosis 1063
Ascites 1070
Hepatorenal Syndrome 1072
Hepatic Encephalopathy 1073
Splenomegaly 1075
Surgical Treatment of Portal Hypertension 1077
Liver Transplantation 1081
Social Aspects of Liver Disease 1082
Summary 1083

CHAPTER 50
***Patients With Acute Pancreatitis* 1091**
Kathryn Hennessy
Pathophysiology 1091
Clinical Presentation 1092
Diagnostic Studies 1094
Prognostic Assessment 1097
Clinical Management 1099
Summary 1103

UNIT 9

ENDOCRINE SYSTEM 1105

CHAPTER 51
***Patients With Disorders of Glucose Metabolism* 1107**
Diana W. Guthrie
Diabetic Ketoacidosis 1107
Hyperglycemic Hyperosmolar Nonketotic Syndrome 1111
Severe Hypoglycemia 1112
Surgery and Trauma 1113
Illness 1113
Pancreas Transplants 1113
Diabetes Monitoring 1114
Summary 1114

CHAPTER 52
***Patients With Disorders of the Neurohypophysis, Thyroid, and Adrenals* 1122**
Danni Brown
Pituitary Gland 1122
Disorders of the Neurohypophysis 1122
Thyroid Gland 1125
Sick Euthyroid Syndrome 1125
Thyroid Disorders 1125
Adrenal Glands 1128
Summary 1130

UNIT 10

HEMATOLOGIC SYSTEM 1137

CHAPTER 53

Hematologic Physiology 1139

Diane K. Dressler

The Composition of Blood 1139
The Normal Hemostatic Mechanism 1141
Summary 1146

CHAPTER 54

Patients With Coagulopathies 1147

Diane K. Dressler

Disseminated Intravascular Coagulation 1147
Other Acquired Coagulation Disorders 1153
Clinical Management of the Patient With Coagulopathy 1157
Prevention of Coagulopathies 1160
Summary 1161

UNIT 11

IMMUNE SYSTEM 1163

CHAPTER 55

Physiologic Response to Infection 1165

M. Linda Workman

Basic Concepts of Immunology 1165
The Basic Functions of the Immune System 1168
Tissues of the Immune System 1168
Cells of the Immune System 1170
Nonspecific Immunity 1178
Specific Immunity 1183
Immunocompetence 1186
Summary 1189

CHAPTER 56

Organ Donation 1192

Marilyn Rossman Bartucci

Overview of Transplantation 1192
Shortage of Donor Organs 1192
Alternative Organ Sources 1193
Methods of Obtaining Consent 1194
Role of Nursing in Donation Process 1195
Donor Family Support 1196
Donor Management 1199
Bereavement 1200
Psychosocial Implications 1200
Surgical Retrieval 1202
Summary 1204

CHAPTER 57

Immunocompromised Patients 1205

Jan L. Hawthorne

Nursing Assessment 1205
Collaborative Management 1207
Bone Marrow Transplantation 1210
Drugs Used in Transplantation 1217
Summary 1223

CHAPTER 58

Patients With HIV Disease 1224

Kathleen McMahon Casey

Historical Development 1224
Epidemiology 1224
International Statistics 1226
Human Immunodeficiency Virus 1227
Classification of HIV Infection 1233
Natural History 1233
Definition of AIDS 1234
Opportunistic Illnesses Frequently Associated With AIDS 1235
HIV-Related Conditions 1240
Patient Care Planning 1250
Summary 1250

UNIT 12

INTEGUMENTARY SYSTEM 1257

CHAPTER 59

Wound Healing 1259

Nancy A. Stotts and JoAnne D. Whitney

Physiology of Wound Healing 1259
Determinants of Healing 1261
Clinical Presentation of Impaired Tissue 1265
Dressings 1267
Topical Solutions and Ointments 1272
Debridement 1273
Nursing Patients With Wounds 1274
Collaboration 1275

CHAPTER 60

Patients With Burns 1279

Randy M. Caine

Types of Burn Injuries 1279
Pathophysiology 1280
Phases of Burn Physiology and Patient Care Management 1283
Relevant Research 1301
Summary 1301

UNIT 13

MULTISYSTEM DISORDERS 1311

CHAPTER 61

Immobility Phenomena in Critically Ill Adults 1313

Nancy L. Szaflarski

Physiologic and Pathophysiologic Effects of Immobility 1314
Clinical Management of Major Complications Resulting From Immobility 1322
Summary 1332

CHAPTER 62

Patients With Trauma 1335

Deborah Goldenberg Klein

What Makes the Trauma Patient Unique 1335
Epidemiology of Trauma 1335
Systems Approach to Trauma Care 1335
Mechanism of Injury 1340
Prehospital Care and Transport 1341
Emergency Care Phase 1342
Critical Care Phase 1350
Continuing Care 1356

CHAPTER 63

Patients With Systemic Inflammatory Response Syndrome 1359

John M. Clochesy

Significance 1359
Susceptibility 1359
Stimulus-Response Systems Precipitating Septic Shock 1360
Chemical Mediators 1360
Pathophysiology 1364
Signs and Symptoms 1365
Management 1367
Summary 1370

CHAPTER 64

Shock 1371

Kimmith Jones

Definition of Shock 1371
Pathophysiology 1371
Compensatory Mechanisms 1373
Classification of Shock 1375
General Assessment 1379
Summary 1379

CHAPTER 65

Patients With Pain 1381

Sara Reeder

Historical Events of Pain in the Critically Ill 1381
Theories of Pain 1386
Pathophysiology of Pain 1389
Assessment of Pain 1395
Management of Pain 1399
Ethical Issues in Pain Management 1409

CHAPTER 66

Chemical and Drug Overdose 1413

Deanna Bevans

Initial Stabilization 1413
Diagnosis 1414
Decontamination 1414
Specific Drugs 1417
Summary 1427

UNIT 14

CLINICAL SITUATIONS 1429

CHAPTER 67

Alterations in Thermoregulation 1431

Richard Henker

Anatomy and Physiology of Thermoregulation 1431

Regulated Changes in Body Temperature: Fever 1433

Nonregulated Changes in Body Temperature 1435

Summary 1440

CHAPTER 68

Preventing Postanesthesia Complications 1442

Ginger Schafer Wlody

Identifying Preoperative Risk Factors 1442

Intraoperative Factors 1445

Preventing Postanesthesia Complications 1449

Central Nervous System Complications 1455

Summary 1456

CHAPTER 69

Patients With Obstetric Crises 1458

Kathy Goff and Becky Hull

Pregnancy-Induced Hypertension (Severe Preeclampsia) 1458

Amniotic Fluid Embolism 1466

Summary 1468

CHAPTER 70

Patients With Oncologic Emergencies 1476

Marcia Rostad

Pathophysiology of Cancer 1476

Spinal Cord Compression 1478

Superior Vena Cava Syndrome 1483

Pathophysiology 1483

Hypercalcemia 1487

Discharge Planning for the Patient With Cancer 1491

Summary 1492

CHAPTER 71

Elderly Patients 1493

Carol A. Rauen and Teresa L. Britt

Systems Overview of Age-Related Changes 1493

Cardiovascular System 1493

Respiratory System 1497

Nervous System 1498

Gastrointestinal System 1500

Renal System 1501

Endocrine System 1502

Immune System 1503

Musculoskeletal System 1504

Integumentary System 1505

Pharmacologic Considerations in the Elderly 1506

Summary 1508

Index 1511

UNIT 1

THE PRACTICE ENVIRONMENT

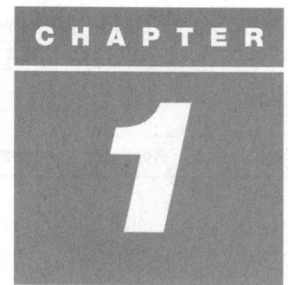

Practice Within the Current Health Care Environment

Joanne M. Disch

"Mr. Johnson, I'm Dr. Keene. We've reviewed your wife's case and, unfortunately, she isn't making the progress we had hoped she would. We've tried just about everything and nothing seems to be doing the trick. We'd like to move her out of the ICU tomorrow."

"Dr. Nathan. I see that you've ordered daily blood gases on this child. Do you mind telling me and the rest of the rounding team why you feel that's indicated, especially given the cost of each individual blood gas?"

"I've scheduled this staff meeting so that we can discuss how we're going to be using nursing assistants here in the unit to help with patient care."

"Have you set up a meeting yet with home health? They're going to need to begin learning her dressing changes, ventilator care, antibiotic regimen and TPN schedule."

The scenarios above embody only some of the changes occurring within the critical care environment. Are these changes good or bad? Are they preventable? Would we want to prevent them if we could? What is behind these new ways of deciding what care is needed, and where care should be given, and what resources should be used? What are the implications of these changes for critical care nurses as they try to meet the needs of their patients and families in this new environment?

This chapter provides a framework for understanding some of the changes being experienced by critical care nurses throughout the country. It reviews the impetus for change within the health care environment, the trends evolving from health care reform, the impact on critical care nurses, and implications for practice.

BACKGROUND FOR CHANGE

What has happened to cause such drastic, pervasive change within the health care environment? In the 1980s, the health care industry shifted to prospective reimbursement. Using Diagnosis-Related Groups (DRGs) as tools, the sole intent of this health care reform was to redirect care delivery away from costly, inpatient-based care. The results have been mixed. Although growth in inpatient costs has been slowed, the total costs of health care continue to spiral upward. Consequently, a new focus for health care reform is emerging and promises to be equally as revolutionary, but with different incentives and strategies.

THE INSTITUTION OF DRGs. In the early 1980s, the United States experienced a paradox within health care: the country faced increasing costs, decreasing access, and variable outcomes of care. Examples of these realities include: health care costs had risen from \$27.1 billion/year in 1960 to \$250 billion/year in 1980 (Prospective Payment Assessment Commission [PROPAC] 1994); one in eight Americans had serious difficulty in obtaining medical treatment, and one in nine had no regular source of health care (Aday et al., 1984); and the United States ranked 22nd overall in infant mortality rates (*State of America's Children Yearbook,* 1994).

In short, with the increasing cost of health care came the realization that neither quality of care nor access to care was improving accordingly. Perceptions about realistic health goals and capabilities were challenged. Financial pressures forced changes in the basic assumptions underlying health care and new ones emerged, a primary one being that the goal for health care reform was cost containment. Moreover, the market for health care was purposefully redirected toward a competitive market.

A competitive market is one in which there are many buyers and sellers of a service or product. Both buyers and sellers are involved in a transaction, and negotiation centers around the price or cost of the service. Although quality is certainly considered in the decision-making, usually as a factor in weighing alternative choices, the key factor in a competitive market is that both buyers and sellers have some sensitivity to the cost. There is some financial stake or benefit in the decisions made by each (i.e., what an individual chooses has financial implications to him).

Finally, in a competitive market, buyers are actively involved in choosing among alternatives, which

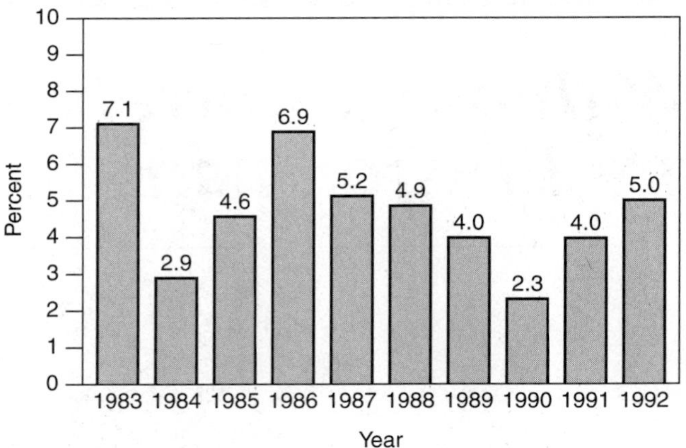

FIGURE 1–1. Real change in hospital total expenses per adjusted admission, 1983–1992 (in percent). (From the American Hospital Association. [1993]. *Hospital statistics: 1980–1993.* Chicago: American Hospital Association Publications.)

TABLE 1–1. **National Health Spending, Selected Years**

Year	Total Spending (In Billions) Nominal	Total Spending (In Billions) Real*	Per Capita Spending Nominal	Per Capita Spending Real*
1960	$ 27.1	$ 121.9	$ 143	$ 641
1965	41.6	176.0	204	862
1970	74.4	260.4	346	1,213
1975	132.9	342.1	592	1,523
1980	250.1	439.5	1,064	1,869
1985	422.6	567.9	1,712	2,301
1990	675.0	746.8	2,604	2,880
1993†	898.4	898.4	3,358	3,358
1995†	1,069.1	1,010.4	3,921	3,706
2000†	1,613.3	1,309.1	5,675	4,605
Average annual change				
1960–1993	11.2%	6.2%	10.0%	5.1%
1993–2000	8.7%	5.5%	7.8%	4.6%

*Adjusted by a variant of the consumer price index for all urban consumers (CPI-U-X1) and expressed in 1993 dollars.

†Projection.

From the Health Care Financing Administration, Office of the Actuary (1994); and the Congressional Budget Office (for projections).

implies that there are alternatives from which to choose. For this to happen, barriers to pratice must be eliminated, and qualified providers must have equal access to the system.

Prospective reimbursement through the use of DRGs provided an incentive and a mechanism by which hospitals and other providers were encouraged to control the costs of health care. With DRGs, hospitals were paid a standardized amount according to patient diagnosis and other selected variables. If the hospital spent less on a patient's hospitalization, it essentially kept the balance. If costs exceeded the standardized amount, the hospital incurred a debt. Consequently, there was great incentive to:

- Decrease the length of patient stay
- Increase the hospital's mix of patients for whom reimbursement was profitable
- Increase the turnover of patients
- Decrease the costs of providing care.

THE IMPACT OF DRGs. The institution of DRGs produced mixed results. In general, although the growth in the cost of inpatient care slowed, the total costs of health care continued to climb. Figure 1–1 shows the change in hospital total expenses for the period between 1983 and 1992 (American Hospital Association [AHA] 1993). Additional data for the first three quarters of 1993 indicate that real costs increased by approximately only 2%. Although this downward trend is good, the pattern is certainly not definitive and indicates only a temporary reaction to national discussion about further cost control.

National health spending for periods between 1960 and 2000 (projected) is presented in Table 1–1 (HCFA, 1994). Of particular interest is the change in real per capita spending increased from $641 to $3358. Whereas health expenditures totalled 5.3% of the gross national product in 1960, they totaled 14.1% in 1993. Many health care analysts project that the total cost of health care will soon exceed $1 trillion. Clearly, total health care costs have not been curbed.

Many other changes occurred that warrant attention:

1. As would be expected, there were shifts in the site of care delivery to the ambulatory and home setting. Table 1–2 reflects the change in the proportion of

TABLE 1–2. **Change in Hospital Revenue and Proportion of Revenue, by Source, 1980–1993 (in Percent)**

Year	Change in Revenue: Inpatient Revenue per Admission	Change in Revenue: Outpatient Revenue per Visit	Proportion of Revenue: Inpatient	Proportion of Revenue: Outpatient	Proportion of Revenue: Other
1980	14.5	15.8	83.2	12.5	4.3
1981	17.3	19.2	82.7	12.7	4.5
1982	16.2	16.8	82.7	12.9	4.4
1983	10.4	11.5	82.4	13.4	4.2
1984	8.6	12.4	81.3	14.4	4.3
1985	8.9	13.2	79.3	16.1	4.6
1986	8.5	8.3	78.0	17.5	4.5
1987	8.9	10.7	76.8	18.6	4.6
1988	8.5	11.4	75.2	20.0	4.8
1989	9.4	11.5	74.0	21.1	4.9
1990	9.2	11.7	72.5	22.5	5.0
1991	9.3	12.0	71.1	24.0	4.8
1992	8.2	8.6	69.8	25.4	4.9
1993	4.9	3.8	68.9	26.2	5.0
Averages					
1980–1983	14.6	15.8			
1984–1993	8.4	10.3			

From the American Hospital Association. (1993). *Hospital statistics: 1980–1993.* Chicago: American Hospital Association Publications.

TABLE 1–3. **National Health Spending, by Source of Payment, 1965 and 1991 (in Percent)**

Payment Source	1965	1991
Medicare	0.0	16.3
Medicaid	0.0	13.4
Other government programs*	24.7	14.2
Private	75.3	56.1
Health insurance	24.0	32.5
Out of pocket	45.7	19.2
Other†	5.5	4.4

*Includes Department of Defense, Department of Veterans Affairs, Public Health Service, Federal research, Federal and state and local workers' compensation, subsidies to hospitals, and public health activities.

†Includes industrial in-plant health services, provider nonpatient revenues, private donations, and privately financed construction.

From the Health Care Financing Administration, Office of the Actuary (1994).

revenue gained between inpatient and outpatient care (AHA, 1993). A major cause of this change is the growth in outpatient surgical centers, now representing 54% of all hospital-provided surgeries, up from 21% in 1982. It is predicted that in 1995, more than 75% of all surgical procedures will be done in these centers (PROPAC, 1994). Interestingly, although costs are lower when surgery is done in these centers, the increased number of procedures may result in increased total costs.

Another area of growth is home health. In 1974, 16 Medicare enrollees per 1000 received home health care, compared to 80/1000 enrollees in 1992 (PROPAC, 1994). Moreover, the number of visits per user increased as well, from 21 in 1974 to 53 in 1992. Hospice programs also multiplied, from 1529 programs in 1989 to 1935 programs in 1992 (PROPAC, 1994). Many of these changes can be attributed to the shortened length of inpatient stay and the increased acuity of the patients at discharge.

2. Financing for health care has shifted from the private sector to the public. Table 1–3 shows that about 75% of total spending for health care was financed from private sources in 1965, the year before implementation of Medicare, compared to 56% in 1991 (HCFA, 1994). Concurrently, governmental programs have increased coverage from 24% to 44%. Furthermore, in 1993, 37 million people (15% of the population) had no health insurance (CBO, 1993). And although some of the uninsured do receive health services from various sources, research suggests that they get less care than those with insurance (Hadley et al., 1991).

3. Admission rates and length of stay have declined since 1980, as has the number of hospital beds. As a result of these changes, numerous hospitals have closed across the country. Figure 1–2 highlights the Minneapolis/St. Paul market and demonstrates the extent to which hospitals changed from being freestanding and independent to members of health systems. Even with the extensive downsizing that has occurred there, common wisdom has it that this area still has 30% to 40% more inpatient beds than needed.

4. Remarkably, hospital financial performance has stayed stable. Although the yearly profit from operating the hospital is smaller, the overall profit, which includes gains from investment income, is holding steady and actually growing in some sectors. Moreover, although losses have occurred because Medicare and Medicaid are controlling their payment rates more tightly, hospitals have recouped these losses by receiving increased revenue from private payers. In addition, the revenue obtained per outpatient visit has grown rapidly, averaging 10% between 1984 and 1993 (PROPAC, 1994).

5. The number of physicians providing patient care has increased to 19.5 per 10,000 population in 1990, compared with 13.5 per 10,000 in 1975 (PROPAC, 1994). Predictably, this increase occurred among specialists. This is a focus for current health care reform in that the goal is to expand access to primary care, not specialty services.

Over the past 30 years, the percentage of actively practicing physicians who are generalists has declined to less than 30% of the total (Colwill, 1992). This has happened for several reasons: (1) medical education is expensive and repayment of loan burdens is difficult within a generalist practice; (2) most medical students are taught in acute care facilities by subspecialists; and (3) society rewards generalist practice with lower compensation, longer working hours, significant administrative burden, and less respect. Moreover, a recent study contends that managed care will create a surplus of 165,000 physicians and a "deluge of specialists" ("Overflow," 1994).

6. The nature of services provided has also changed. Between 1982 and 1991, the percentage of hospitals offering the following procedures increased as listed: open heart surgery (11% to 17%); cardiac catheterization (16% to 29%); and computed tomography (31% to 73%); (AHA, 1993). For the elderly, some of these changes are particularly striking. Of 1000 men older than 65 years of age, 5 underwent cardiac catheterization in 1980 versus 18.4 in 1991; for women, it was 2.1 versus 11.1 (U.S. Department of Health and Human Services, 1993).

In summary, DRGs have precipitated a number of changes. They have shifted the focus of care from inpatient to outpatient, altered the utilization rates for many procedures, and stimulated the development of new therapies and sites of care. However, their impact on reducing the overall costs of health care has been disappointing.

Of particular concern are the continuing lack of health care for millions of Americans and the absence of high-quality outcomes, especially considering the money that has been spent on health care. Actually, for many economists, the key issue is not the absolute money spent; many would say that 13% to 14% of the total gross national product is not excessive for a nation concerned with its people and their health. However, there is a problem when 37 million people do not

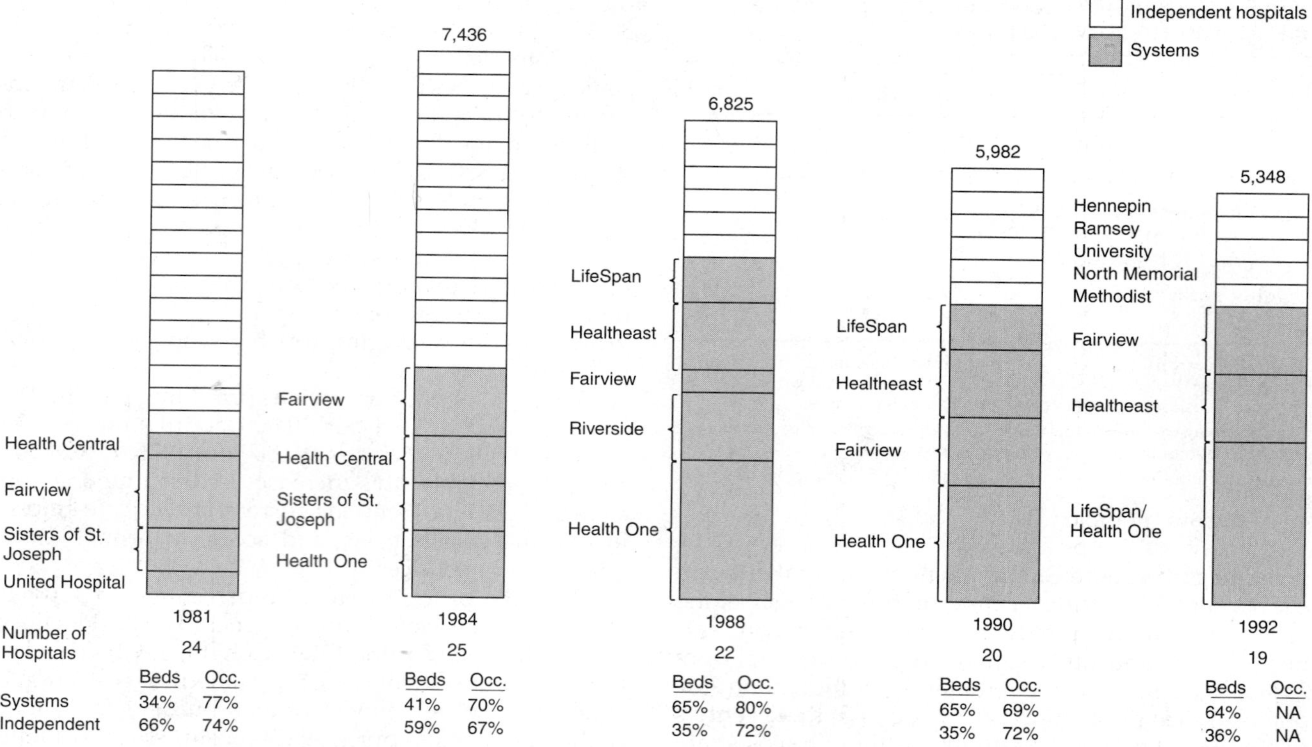

FIGURE 1–2. Changes in number of hospitals, number of beds, and number of hospital systems, Minneapolis-St. Paul, 1981–1992. (From the University Hospital Consortium. [1993]. Oakbrook, IL: University Hospital Consortium Publications.)

have coverage; when the United States ranks so poorly compared to other nations in indicators such as infant mortality and immunization rates; and when total costs of health care continue to climb. Although some progress had been made, it is clear that further reform was necessary.

THE NEW DIRECTION FOR HEALTH CARE REFORM

Just as DRGs were never intended to be an end in themselves, neither was it sufficient to solve health care problems by focusing only on cost containment within hospitals. Specifically, the earlier efforts failed because of three factors:

1. The focus for reform was on hospitals alone.
2. Incentives for physician behavior were different than those for hospitals. Physicians continued to be reimbursed for procedures and patient days in the hospital, whereas hospitals were rewarded for shortened lengths of stay.
3. Health care delivery continued to be illness oriented.

Health care reform in the 1990s seeks to address the shortcomings of earlier efforts through three primary strategies. These are instituting incentives for primary care, expanding the use of certain providers, and incorporating the concept of capitation.

The first strategy, instituting incentives for primary care, seeks to redirect attention toward wellness, health promotion, and disease prevention. In the belief that preventing illness is less costly than treating it, efforts are underway to reward providers for increasing primary care services, patients for using them, and educators for training more practitioners skilled in primary care.

The second strategy, expanding the use of certain providers, stems from the first strategy. In addition to increasing the use of generalist physicians, this strategy seeks to expand opportunities for providing primary care not only to physicians, but to others who have demonstrated competence in this level of care, such as nurse practitioners. Furthermore, even within the hospital setting, this strategy would promote the use of alternatives such as nurse practitioners, nurse-midwives and nurse-anesthetists for some of the costly inpatient care.

Elements of the third strategy, capitation, were present with DRGs, but are being expanded within the new health care reform initiatives. Capitation is a system of payment in which a health care provider receives a fixed amount for each person served, regardless of the extent of services used. Thus, providers have tremendous incentive to keep patients away from costly inpatient care, use effective yet less costly sites of care and caregivers, and prevent serious illness in the people being covered. Although DRGs represented a form of capitation, payment for services covered only inpatient care. With the new capitation strategy, the intent is to cover *all* care within the capitation payment, including physician charges.

To accomplish this capitation, networks or systems within which all care will be provided are being established. Two key concepts for achieving health care reform are integrated service networks and managed care.

INTEGRATED SERVICE NETWORKS. A cornerstone of current health care reform is the use of capitated health networks. These are relationships in which providers and insurers join together as partners to provide care across a variety of settings to a captive group of beneficiaries. Their goals are to achieve economies of scale, to eliminate inefficiency and duplication, and to have an effective mix of providers and facilities so that a full array of care can be delivered efficiently. These goals are accomplished through the use of standardized protocols and clinical pathways, case management, precertification, and utilization review.

MANAGED CARE. Managed care is a system of health care that seeks to regulate the use of various services, procedures, and treatment modalities through a combination of prepayment arrangements, negotiated discounts, agreements for prior authorization, and audits of performance. Its purpose is to modify the behavior of providers and consumers so that the efficiency of the entire health care system is enhanced. The goal is to have decision-makers carefully consider the relative efficacy and efficiency of alternative therapies, and to make judicious decisions regarding their use.

Evidence of the changes within health care can already be seen in the degree of evolution of managed care markets. In communities across the country, predictable events are unfolding:

- Health Maintenance Organizations (HMOs) are forming. These are comprehensive health care systems that, for a monthly or annual fee, provide an individual with all of his or her health care. The choice of providers is somewhat limited; however, there are usually minimal deductibles or copayments.
- Preferred Provider Organizations (PPOs) are also forming and consolidating. These are networks or groupings of physicians that provide care for a set payment and agree to participate in resource management activities as they relate to the provision of patient care.
- Independent Practice Associations (IPAs) are being established at a rapid pace. These are groups of physicians set up as separate entities for contracting in a capitated system.
- Multi-Hospital Systems are developing, aggressively competing for primary care physician practices.
- Large employer groups are coming together to form coalitions and negotiate with providers as to the best price for the provision of services to their employees.
- Hospitals are increasingly having to accept a capitated price as payment for services, regardless of what the services cost to provide.
- Hospitals are closing.

Although the changes listed above reflect the extension of managed care, communities vary as to the degree to which they have embraced managed care. For example, some communities have a long history of experience with HMOs (e.g., California with the Kaiser-Permanente plan), whereas other communities have no HMOs.

The University Hospital Consortium (UHC), a membership organization of more than 60 academic medical centers, has developed a model for tracking the evolution of managed care within health care markets. The market stages have been defined as Unstructured, Loose Framework, Consolidation, and Managed Competition. Table 1–4 describes the different characteristics associated with each market, and Table 1–5 indicates which communities are in each stage. The numbers alongside each community respresent assigned scores reflecting the degree to which various market factors were present (e.g., percentage of HMOs, extent to which physician group practices had developed, extent of capitation, number of hospital beds within systems). Although not all markets will proceed to stage IV, most markets do proceed along this continuum, sometimes very rapidly.

STRATEGIES FOR COMPETING IN A MANAGED CARE ENVIRONMENT

In addition to developing the Model for Managed Care Market Evolution, UHC identified six objectives with key strategies for effectively competing within managed care markets. Although their implementation may vary in different settings, achieving these objectives would appear to be critical for success, if not survival, for all facilities in health care today.

BUILD A STRONG PRIMARY CARE BASE. To strengthen the delivery of primary care, health care institutions are acquiring and setting up primary care practices. The purpose of these practices is to provide needed primary care services and to serve as a referral base for inpatient care. The goal is to build a geographically dominant ambulatory clinic system in targeted markets. In addition, efforts are being directed toward creating training environments conducive to increased generalist practice. In 1994, the Council on Graduate Medical Education recommended that 50% of new physicians go into primary care, and also asked Congress to develop a policing mechanism to assure this would happen (“Overflow,” 1994).

TABLE 1–4. **Four Stages of Market Evolution**

Stages	Characteristics	Pricing	Basis for Health Care Purchasing
Stage I (unstructured)	Independent hospitals, physicians, employers, and HMOs	Fee for service	Encounter, cost of claim Volume
Stage II (loose framework)	Lead HMOs or PPOs emerge, loose provider networks and weak hospital affiliations form Excess inpatient capacity develops Hospital discounts widen	Discount, per diem	Encounter, cost of claim
Stage III (consolidation)	Lead HMOs/PPOs achieve critical mass, begin to consolidate; hospital systems form; all aggressively recruit/compete for primary care group practices Selective contracting by major purchasers Development of large multispecialty, primary care, and IPA groups Specialist practices underutilized; discounts increase Beds close, hospital profits increase	Per diem, per case, physician capitation	Cost per covered life per health plan Integration
Stage IV (managed competition)	Purchasers contract with integrated hospital/physician systems to provide comprehensive services to their beneficiaries Financial risk shifts to primary medical groups/provider networks Beneficiaries have strong incentives to use contract network (extensive channeling) Capitation model becomes prevalent	Stage III plus capitation	Beneficiary health status, total health care costs

Abbreviations: HMO, health maintenance organization; PPO, preferred provider organization; IPA, independent practice association. From the University Hospital Consortium. (1993). Oakbrook, IL: University Hospital Consortium Publications.

ORGANIZE THE INTERNAL CLINICAL DELIVERY SYSTEM. Within organizations, leaders are establishing multispecialty group practices to deliver care to people covered by the system (referred to as *covered lives*) on a prepaid basis. Although these group practices are largely composed of physicians, innovative organizations incorporate a wide array of nonphysician care providers. Regardless of membership, the goal is to organize the specialties to work on a comprehensive and coordinated basis across departments.

As a related effort, institutions are creating new ways to reward clinicians. Particularly in academic medical centers, physicians have historically been rewarded for conducting research and teaching students. In today's health care environment, the caregiver component of their role is increasingly valued. Therefore, in many institutions, criteria are being rewritten for tenure review so that credit for clinical practice is included; the payment structure for specialists is being reevaluated; and incentives are being developed to increase physicians' clinical practice.

ACHIEVE A COMPETITIVE COST POSITION. Most health care organizations are undergoing extensive cost reduction and efficiency enhancement efforts. Patient care delivery systems are being restructured and, in academic medical centers, the goal is to approach community hospital costs. The research agenda is increasingly being focused on clinical effectiveness and resource utilization. Quality improvement programs are being established to track utilization and efficiency patterns, not only of employees, but of physicians in particular. Physician profiles are being developed that reflect outcomes achieved and resources utilized. To accomplish these objectives, institutions are increasingly investing in information systems for managing clinical and financial outcomes.

ACHIEVE A HIGH SERVICE POSITION. In a similar vein, health care organizations are establishing and enforcing service standards, again not only for employees but for physicians as well. Not only is patient satisfaction tracked, but waiting times, scheduling of appointment times, delay of surgeries, response times to the referring physician, and so forth. The achievement and measurement of clinical outcomes are increasingly being examined, not only as they relate to the absence of complications, but to the presence of a quality of life, functional status, and return to and maintaining work status. A commitment to the continuous pursuit of excellence is fostered.

CREATE MULTIPLE MANAGED CARE PRODUCTS. Another major effort within health care organizations is the integrating, pricing, and managing of physician and hospital services for specific patient conditions or populations, which can then be sold as a "package deal" to buyers of health care. For example, one institution may package its bone marrow transplant services for a capitated fee, covering all pretransplant and posttransplant care, as well as physician services. Another institution might package its intensive care services so that for a given price per year, the enrollees of a health care plan could receive all required intensive care unit (ICU) care from that organization. After the care has been packaged, direct contracts need to be established with groups such as employers, business coalitions, and government programs.

CREATE AN INTEGRATED DELIVERY SYSTEM. Finally, efforts must be targeted toward creating a community-based delivery system that can enroll and manage a large number of covered lives. An infrastructure must be established by which systems and processes are developed to support these initiatives. For the most part, the traditional, hierarchical, department-based hospital structure is ill-equipped to handle the complexities of these kinds of activities, so a new organizational structure is often warranted. New roles are also needed to create, manage, and represent the new delivery and marketing systems.

In summary, using capitation and managed care, the objectives of health care reform are (1) to redirect care delivery toward primary care, wellness, and prevention; and (2) to enhance the efficiency of the system to achieve important outcomes, such as access, cost-effectiveness, and quality of care, among others.

IMPLICATIONS FOR CRITICAL CARE

Eighty percent of Americans will experience a critical illness or injury through the role of patient, family member, or friend (Society of Critical Care Medicine, 1992). Although critical care beds represent roughly 8% of licensed hospital beds nationally, the total cost of critical care in the United States is estimated at $47 billion, or 28% of total hospital costs for acute care (Groeger et al., 1992). From all perspectives, critical care consumes many resources.

However, several studies do reflect the positive outcomes associated with critical care intervention (Knaus et al., 1986; Reynolds et al., 1988; Shoemaker et al., 1988; Brown & Sullivan, 1989; Berlauk et al., 1991; Zimmerman et al., 1993). Millions of lives have been saved, and the quality of life for many has been enhanced, regardless of whether the ultimate goal of restoring health was achieved.

As with all of health care, critical care is also undergoing change. Critically ill patients are cared for not only in ICUs, but in trauma bays, in helicopters, in hyperbaric chambers, in transport vehicles, and in other acute care locations. Technology that previously was restricted to ICUs is commonly found on general care units, in surgical centers, and in the home. Care is overseen by critical care nurses, but may be provided by assistive personnel, depending on the condition and needs of the patient. A constant, however, is that the team continues to be a vital component of a patient's successful critical care experience.

Although the focus of health care reform is shifting toward primary care, many patients will still require intensive care, with its sophisticated technology and experienced practitioners. The challenges for the critical care team are to ensure that clinical outcomes are clearly defined, measured, and attained; that resources are used judiciously; and that accountability and continuity across settings is achieved.

IMPLICATIONS FOR CRITICAL CARE NURSING

Several trends are emerging that have dramatic implications for nursing in general, but critical care nursing in particular.

TABLE 1–5. **University Hospital Consortium Member Markets Market Classification**

Unstructured (Stage I)		Loose Framework (Stage II)		Consolidation (Stage III)		Managed Competition (Stage IV)	
Nashville	1.5	Chicago	2.3	Los Angeles	3.2	Minneapolis/St. Paul	3.4
New Orleans	1.5	Salt Lake City	2.3	Orange	3.1		
Newark	1.5	Tucson	2.3	San Diego	3.1		
Oklahoma City	1.5	Houston	2.2	Worcester	3.0		
Toledo	1.5	Cincinnati	2.2	Portland	3.0		
Nassau	1.4	Dallas	2.2	Sacramento	3.0		
Galveston	1.4	Madison	2.2	San Francisco/Oakland	2.8		
Harrisburg	1.4	Cleveland	2.1	Denver	2.7		
Little Rock	1.3	Washington, DC	2.1	Seattle	2.4		
Chapel Hill (Triangle)	1.3	Baltimore	2.0				
Pittsburgh	1.3	Columbus	2.0				
Syracuse	1.3	Philadelphia	2.0				
Augusta	1.2	Albany	1.9				
Lexington	1.2	St. Louis	1.9				
Omaha	1.2	Gainesville	1.9				
Columbia	1.1	Richmond	1.8				
Charlottesville	1.0	Atlanta	1.8				
Morgantown	1.0	Indianapolis	1.7				
		Hartford	1.7				
		Birmingham	1.7				
		New York City	1.6				
		Middlesex	1.6				

From the University Hospital Consortium. (1993). Oakbrook, IL: University Hospital Consortium Publications.

- The emphasis in health care is on wellness, prevention, and primary care. Efforts will be focused on keeping patients out of hospitals and critical care environments.
- As networks, systems, and partnerships evolve, the hospital will increasingly be seen as only one of many sites of care delivery. Places such as the home, short-stay centers, ambulatory surgery clinics, hospices, schools, clinics, and churches will gain prominence as alternative areas for care delivery. Hospitals and critical care units will continue to exist and provide a much-needed level of care, but attention will increasingly by paid toward getting patients to the right level of care.
- Attention will also be paid toward getting patients to the right care provider. Health care reform should provide incentives for using advanced practice nurses in a variety of roles (e.g., expert clinician, case manager, acute care nurse practitioner, nurse manager, or patient care unit director). Nurses who are experienced and possess expertise in the care of their patients will continue to be highly valued.
- On the other hand, attention also needs to be paid toward ensuring that nurses are doing nursing, not spending time unnecessarily on secretarial work or on tasks that other, less-prepared workers can perform. Efforts toward work redesign are important to make sure that personnel are being appropriately utilized, while still preserving required nursing expertise to meet patients' needs.
- Continuity among care providers will be increasingly important. Nurses in one area will need to have effective communication and practice linkages with nurses in other units and care sites who provide care to the same patient population. Nursing staff who function within one area will need effectively to partner, negotiate, and collaborate with others to see that patient care needs are met. The days of one nurse functioning as though he or she were an island, doing all things alone, and meeting all needs for the patient, are gone.
- The outcomes movement has been called "the third revolution in medical care" (Relman, 1990), and has gained momentum as a major force in health care reform. In addition to monitoring traditional outcomes such as morbidity and mortality, practitioners, payors, and policymakers are tracking other outcomes: functional status, emotional health, consumer satisfaction, cognitive functioning, and quality of life. Differences among physicians are being tracked in terms of their patients' performance on these indicators, as well as on length of stay and use of other hospital resources. In Minnesota, base salaries for physicians within one health system will be increased in 1995 only if "the company meets targeted levels of performance in customer service, care outcome, member satisfaction and profit" (Borger, 1994).
- Employers will value those individuals who embrace change, deliver high-quality care with a responsible use of resources, and collaborate well with a variety of individuals. In the new order of things, information is power but relationships are the key.
- Organizations are going to look very different from how they have in the past or how they look today. The organizational structures will be flatter, with fewer managers. Performance outcomes will be tracked to the team and to the individual level. In the hospital, departments and systems will be organized more according to patient focus (e.g., transplant, oncology, pediatrics). Individuals will function within work teams and relate across departments, rather than in hierarchical, bureaucratic turfdoms.

STRATEGIES FOR SUCCESS

The objectives in health care reform are twofold: (1) redirect care delivery toward primary care, health promotion, and illness prevention; and (2) establish systems of health care delivery that are cost-effective, provide continuity, and enable a variety of outcomes to be achieved. Table 1–6 reflects the paradigm shift that is occurring in health care.

To operate successfully within health care today, critical care nurses must analyze their settings and develop a plan of action for addressing each trend. Because change is inevitable, critical care nurses must take the lead and determine what changes are needed and how to accomplish them.

EVALUATE PRACTICES WITHIN THE ICU. Rather than waiting for administrators to dictate change in the critical care unit, critical care nurses should begin the process of evaluating practice and instituting warranted change proactively. Listed here are a number of questions that could be used. What are the characteristics of the patient population in this ICU? What are the particular needs of these patients? What care is essential for nurses to provide? What care or tasks could be delegated to or partnered with other caregivers, both within nursing and in other departments? What care

TABLE 1–6. **Paradigm Shift Associated With Health Care Delivery Today**

From	To
Managing sickness	Managing health
Treating patients	Covering lives
Discharges	Transitions
Rigid organizational structures	Flexible structures
Investment in clinical technologies	Investment in information systems
Entitled staff	Empowered staff

could be eliminated or reduced in frequency? In doing this evaluation, seek the perspective of nurses from other ICUs, or nurses who are reassigned to the ICU, because they will be less vested in the traditions and routines of the unit. Clinical specialists can also offer a helpful perspective regarding what care requires the specialized expertise of the critical care nurse.

As part of the evaluation, review the utilization of supplies and equipment. Evaluate whether standard set-ups or practices are necessary, such as routinely changing all intravenous tubing when a patient is received in the unit. What equipment can be safely reused? Are there systems in place to return equipment for proper crediting as soon as the patient no longer needs it?

A final area for evaluation relates to the appropriateness of the critical care unit as the site for care delivery. Which patients within the unit could be safely cared for in another, less resource-intensive area of the hospital? Which patients might be better cared for in a less acute setting, and are plans being developed to transfer patients to other institutions when their care requirements change? Enlist physician support to determine appropriate patient placement and safe transition of care delivery. Chapter 10 contains additional information on the evaluation of long-term patients for home care.

TABLE 1–7. **Cost-Reduction Ideas for Critical Care Areas**

Minimize use of standing orders/protocols
Reduce and limit inventory of catheters
Eliminate rewrite of orders for patients moving out of the ICU but on same service
Replace only needed intravenous tubing and solutions when patient transferred in or out of ICU
Switch from disposable to reusable oximeter sensors
Institute needleless system
Replace disposable resuscitator bags with reusable
Eliminate paraprofessional shift overlap
Examine and revise role of charge nurse
Expand role of unit secretary to encompass some care responsibilities
Institute daily patient flow rounds to promote patient discharge from the ICU
Reduce number of blood draws
Establish dual appointments of staff to critical care and partner stepdown unit
Establish a critical care float role, available for sudden, short-term staffing assistance

GATHER DATA ON RESOURCE UTILIZATION AND PRACTICES WITHIN OTHER ICUs. Information and data should be gathered from other resources. Find out why other ICUs use fewer resources for comparable patient populations. Review the literature to see whether or how other critical care nurses have addressed this issue. Call or visit other ICUs. Network with other critical care nurses at professional meetings. Contact resources at the American Association of Critical-Care Nurses. Even within the institution, opportunities for data collection can be found by floating to other ICUs or gaining insight from supervisors and float nurses who routinely work in other areas.

INITIATE EFFORTS TO IMPROVE EFFICIENCY AND SERVICE. Select a few practice changes and test their effectiveness. Table 1–7 lists several strategies that have been identified as best practice opportunities associated with high-quality care and efficient use of resources. After instituting changes, reevaluate and make adjustments; then select new changes to trial.

DEVELOP MECHANISMS FOR PATIENT AND FAMILY PARTICIPATION AND FEEDBACK. Over the past 20 years, multiple studies have been conducted in which the benefits of patient and family participation have been identified (Gerteis et al., 1993; Lathrop, 1992; Weber, 1991). A strong cornerstone of health care reform is a knowledgeable and involved patient and family. To accomplish this in your setting:

- Establish individualized visiting hours
- Develop a sibling visitation policy
- Institute visits by nurses with families in the waiting rooms
- Develop patient satisfaction surveys specific to the ICU
- Recruit previous patients and family members to form a Patient Advisory Board.

In an ongoing manner, seek and incorporate the input of patients and families in all endeavors.

DEVELOP OR STRENGTHEN CARE DELIVERY SYSTEMS, SUCH AS PRIMARY NURSING, THAT SPECIFY ACCOUNTABILITY FOR NURSING CARE. The likelihood of fragmented care is increased with shortened lengths of stay, staff who work part-time, and the multitude of disciplines involved in the care of critically ill patients. Thus, models of care are needed that clearly identify who is responsible for the plan of nursing care and the resultant patient outcomes. This is important to ensure coordination of care, foster continuity across settings, and provide a consistent nursing resource for the patient. Although it may be increasingly difficult in today's ICU, it is correspondingly important.

ESTABLISH EFFECTIVE LINKAGES ACROSS DEPARTMENTS, DISCIPLINES, AND SETTINGS. The accountability for ensuring patient outcomes has extended beyond the critical care unit to the organization and into the home. Rather than focusing only on the patient's acute care episode, critical care nurses must coordinate care with preadmission personnel, as well as with those caregivers who will be responsible for addressing the more chronic aspects of care. Increasingly, payors want to negotiate for the care of specific subsets of patients across the entire spectrum (e.g., patients with psychiatric problems, patients undergoing transplantation) to achieve the best level of care for a given price. Clusters of caregivers associated with the care of particular patient populations will need to work together to ensure that care across the continuum is planned, coordinated, delivered, and evaluated. Chapters 9 and 10 offer further information on these areas.

GATHER DATA TO CLEARLY IDENTIFY NURSING'S IMPACT. Nursing's influence on a number of key variables has been well demonstrated (Brooten et al., 1986; Ethridge & Lamb, 1989; McCorkle & Benoliel, 1990; Padilla et al., 1990). But within individual ICUs, similar demonstrations are necessary. Nursing staff must gather data to indicate how nursing staff can shorten lengths of stay, prevent complications, minimize loss of functional status, enhance patient satisfaction, and decrease supply costs. In collaboration with physicians and other caregivers, nurses can be leaders in developing clinical pathways, practice protocols, admission/discharge criteria, interdisciplinary databases, and integrated charts.

CREATE A HEALTHY WORK ENVIRONMENT FOR EMPLOYEES. Although the focus of health care reform is understandably on the patient, attention also must be paid to the caregivers. Establishing an environment of mutual respect, trust, open communication, and teamwork is essential if efforts at improving patient care are to be successful. Developing a culture in which employees are recognized, valued, and encouraged to participate is a critical first step. Another step is to identify the characteristics that are desirable within a healthy work environment. Figure 1–3 depicts the framework developed at the University of Minnesota Hospital and Clinic.

DEVELOP THE NECESSARY SKILLS. Critical care nurses have already developed skills in a number of areas to enable them to thrive in the current health care environment: functioning as a team member; understanding how organizations work and how to get things done; conducting quick, accurate assessments and responding rapidly; relating effectively with a wide variety of people; helping patients and families learn to cope during a particularly difficult time; and making the most of scarce resources. Moreover, maintaining highly refined clinical skills in the care of the critically ill patient has always been a hallmark of the practice of critical care nurses.

However, there are other skills or qualities that may need attention as well. The first is *flexibility.* Because of the rapid changes occurring within the health care system, individuals who are able to anticipate system changes, act quickly, and adapt readily are particularly valued. Those who bemoan change, struggle to maintain the status quo, or resist the inevitable are not.

A second quality is *optimism.* Individuals who can accept that change must occur and who have a "can-do" spirit will survive. Coupled with this quality is a sense of balance. Change is associated with loss, but it can also lead to satisfying experiences. If a nurse is hopeful, and can see possibilities inherent in the changes occurring, then that nurse will be valued and fit into today's environment.

A third quality is the *ability to tolerate ambiguity.* Few things in life or health care are absolute, or black and white. Issues are complex, and solutions are rarely clear-cut. Just as critical care nurses must often make a clinical judgment based on only a few pieces of data, so too administrative decisions must occasionally be made without all of the facts. To work effectively within the tumultuous health care environment, critical care nurses must stay informed of changes that are occurring, be proactive in anticipating changes, and initiate efforts to ensure that the right changes are being made.

Critical care nurses must also *be involved.* With so much change occurring, the critical care nurse needs to stay current with certain elements of the big picture—community trends in health care, hospital goals and initiatives, and hospital financial performance and status or market share within the community. Moreover, involvement in decision-making through formal and informal mechanisms is crucial. Because of the critical care nurses' background, knowledge, and commitment, their potential for impact is significant in many arenas (i.e., unit committees and councils, hospital work groups, interdisciplinary quality improvement teams, ethics committees, product evaluation). Although the organization certainly benefits from this participation, so too do the critical care nurse and critically ill patient. Given that change is inevitable, the critical care nurse can help ensure that the changes made will incorporate concern for patient needs.

Finally, few characteristics or qualities are more important than the *ability to develop effective interpersonal relationships.* The history of critical care strongly reflects a tradition of teamwork, yet today's health care environment requires that collaboration be stronger than ever before, and with new partners as well as the old. Diversity must be valued, cooperation sought, and conflicts resolved. Effective interdisciplinary teams within critical care must continue to be nurtured, but new relationships must be developed across the institution. Linkages must be developed with caregivers who provide care to the patients in other settings across the continuum to ensure communication, consistency, and a coordinated plan of care. Partnerships must be fostered with individuals from other departments, including administration, so that patient care objectives are met and staff experience a feeling of satisfaction and accomplishment.

SUMMARY

Health care continues to change dramatically. Whereas earlier reform efforts sought to curb health care costs, current efforts seek to redefine the total

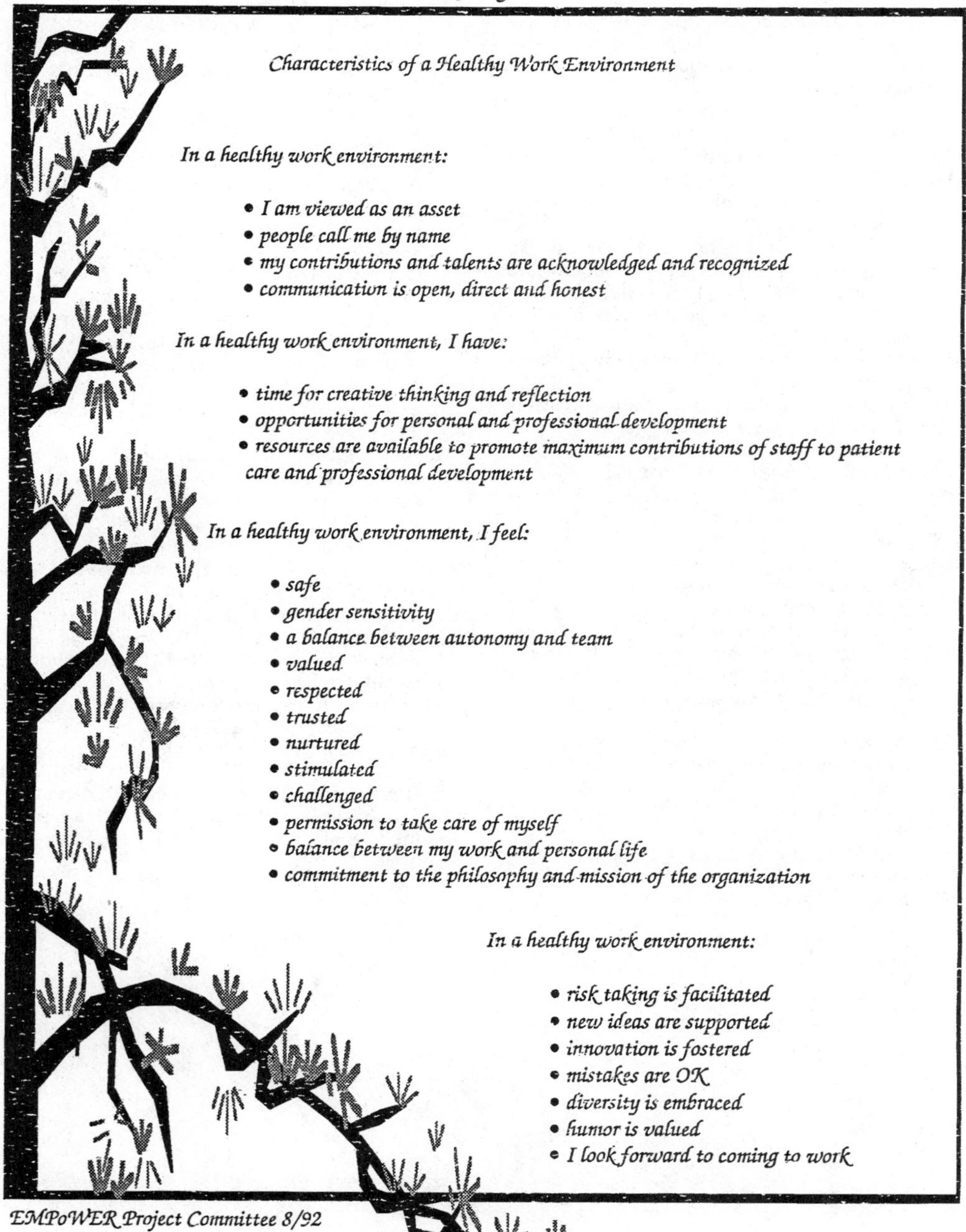
University of Minnesota Hospital & Clinic
Nursing

Characteristics of a Healthy Work Environment

In a healthy work environment:

- I am viewed as an asset
- people call me by name
- my contributions and talents are acknowledged and recognized
- communication is open, direct and honest

In a healthy work environment, I have:

- time for creative thinking and reflection
- opportunities for personal and professional development
- resources are available to promote maximum contributions of staff to patient care and professional development

In a healthy work environment, I feel:

- safe
- gender sensitivity
- a balance between autonomy and team
- valued
- respected
- trusted
- nurtured
- stimulated
- challenged
- permission to take care of myself
- balance between my work and personal life
- commitment to the philosophy and mission of the organization

In a healthy work environment:

- risk taking is facilitated
- new ideas are supported
- innovation is fostered
- mistakes are OK
- diversity is embraced
- humor is valued
- I look forward to coming to work

EMPoWER Project Committee 8/92

FIGURE 1–3. Characteristics of a healthy work environment. (From the Empower Project Committee. [1992]. Nursing, University of Minnesota Hospital and Clinic.)

health care system. The major objectives are (1) to redirect care delivery toward primary care, wellness, and prevention; (2) to achieve cost-effectiveness throughout the system; and (3) to achieve a broad array of outcomes reflecting morbidity and mortality, but also access to care, quality of care, functional status, and patient satisfaction.

Critical care will be a major focus for attention, because the costs associated with delivering critical care services are significant. In this regard, critical care nurses are well placed to take a leadership role in identifying needed changes and in defining preferred courses of action. Employing the recommended strategies will enable critical care nurses to tackle health care challenges effectively for their patients and families, and themselves.

REFERENCES

Aday, L. A., Fleming, G. V., & Andersen, R. (1984). *Access to medical care in the U.S.: Who has it? Who doesn't?* Chicago: Pluribus Press.

American Hospital Association. (1993). *Hospital statistics: 1980–1993.* Chicago: AHA Publications.

Berlauk, J. F., Abrams, J. A., Gilmour, I. J., O'Connor, S. R., Knighton, D. R., & Cerra, F. B. (1991). Preoperative optimization of cardiovascular hemodynamics improves outcome in peripheral vascular surgery. *Annals of Surgery, 214*(3), 289–299.

Borger, J. Y. (1994). HealthPartners ties doctors' pay to patients' satisfaction, profit. *Pioneer Press,* July 19.

Brooten, D., Kuman, S., Brown, L. P., Butts, P., Finkler, S. A., Bakewell-Sachs, S., Gibbons, A., & Delivoria-Papadopoulos, M. (1986). A randomized clinical trial of early hospital discharge and home follow-up of very-low-birth-weight infants. *New England Journal of Medicine, 315,* 934–939.

Brown, J. J., & Sullivan, G. (1989). Effect on ICU mortality of a full-time critical care specialist. *Chest, 96,* 127.

Colwill, J. M. (1992). Where have all the primary care applicants gone? *New England Journal of Medicine, 326,* 387–409.

Epstein, A. M. (1990). The outcomes movement: Will it get us where we want to go? *New England Journal of Medicine, 323,* 266–269.

Ethridge, P., & Lamb, G. S. (1989). Professional nursing case management improves quality, access and costs. *Nursing Management, 20*(3), 30–35.

Gerteis, M., Edgman-Levitan, S., Daley, J., Delbanco, T. L. (1993). *Through the patient's eyes.* San Francisco: Jossey-Bass.

Groeger, J. S., Strosberg, M. A., Halpern, N. A., Raphaely, R. C., Kaye, W. E., Guntupalli, K. K., Bertram, D. L., Greenbaum, D. M., Clemmer, T. P., Gallagher, T. J., Nelson, L. D., Thompson, A. E., Cerra, F. B., & Davis, W. R. (1992). Descriptive analysis of critical care units in the United States. *Critical Care Medicine, 20,* 846–863.

Hadley, J., Steinberg, E. P., & Feder, J. (1991). Comparison of uninsured and privately insured hospital patients. *Journal of the American Medical Association, 265,* 374–379.

Health Care Financing Administration. (1994). Office of Actuary, National Health Statistics, Washington, DC.

Knaus, W. A., Wagner, D. P., & Zimmerman, J. E. (1986). An evaluation of outcome from intensive care in major medical centers. *Annals of Internal Medicine, 104,* 410–418.

Lathrop, J. P. (1992). The patient-focused hospital. *Healthcare Forum Journal,* May/June, 76–79.

McCorkle, R., & Benoliel, J. Q. (1990). The effects of home care on patients' functional status. In S. G. Funk, E. M. Tornquist, M. T. Champagne, L. A. Copp, & R. A. Wiese (Eds.), *Key aspects of recovery: Improving nutrition, rest and mobility.* New York: Springer-Verlag.

Overflow of specialists predicted by year 2000. (1994). *Modern Healthcare, 24*(30), 10.

Padilla, G., Ferrell, B., Grant, M. M., & Rhiner, M. (1990). Defining the content domain of quality of life for cancer patients with pain. *Cancer Nursing, 13*(2), 108–115.

Prospective Payment Assessment Commission (PROPAC). (1994). *Medicare and the American health care system: Report to the Congress.* Washington, DC: U. S. Government Printing Office.

Relman, A. S. (1990). Is rationing inevitable? *New England Journal of Medicine, 322,* 1809–1810.

Reynolds, H. N., Haupt, M. T., Thill-Baharozian, M. D., & Carlson, R. W. (1988). Impact of critical care physician staffing on patients with septic shock in a university hospital medical intensive care unit. *Journal of the American Medical Association, 260,* 3446–3450.

Shoemaker, W. C., Appel, P. L., Kra, H. B., Waxman, K., & Lee, T. (1988). Prospective trial of supranormal values of survivors as therapeutic goals in high-risk surgical patients. *Chest, 94,* 1176–1186.

Society of Critical Care Medicine. (1992). *Critical care in the United States.* Anaheim, CA: Author.

State of America's Children Yearbook. (1994). Washington, DC: Children's Defense Fund.

U.S. Department of Health and Human Services, National Center for Health Statistics. (1993). *Health, United States, 1992.* DHHS Publication No. (PHS) 93-1232. Hyattsville, MD: U. S. Public Health Service.

Weber, D. (1991). Six models of patient-focused care. *Healthcare Forum Journal,* Jul/Aug, 23–31.

Zimmerman, J. E., Shortell, S. M., Rousseau, D. M., Duffy, J., Gillies, R. R., Knaus, W. A., Devers, K., Wagner, D. P., & Draper, E. A. (1993). Improving intensive care: Observations based on organizational case studies in nine intensive care units: A prospective multicenter study. *Critical Care Medicine, 21,* 1443–1451.

Ethics in Critical Care

Barbara J. Daly

Critical care has become a well recognized and respected specialty within modern health care. Paralleling the growth of this specialty, new problems have developed related to the decisions involved in providing care to critically ill individuals. Bioethics has emerged as a growing field of inquiry that seeks to answer questions about the appropriateness of what we can do, the proper way of distributing scarce resources, and the meaning of what is being done in health care.

NURSING ETHICS

Ethics is a branch of moral philosophy that attempts to address questions about right conduct. In clinical practice, ethical study generally focuses on specific rules, principles, and approaches that can be used to guide decision making. As shown in Figure 2–1, it rests on a broader philosophical base that examines the fundamental meaning of such terms as right, goodness, moral, and duty. Bioethics may be defined as the study of the "moral and conceptual problems associated with health care and the biomedical sciences" (Engelhardt, 1986). Nursing ethics is a branch of bioethics and is different and distinct from other branches, such as medical ethics or research ethics, only in the sense that the responsibilities, constraints, and particular questions nurses face are inextricably related to the role of the nurse in modern health care. The term "nursing ethics" should not be interpreted to mean that there are necessarily different principles or moral rules that apply only to nurses.

Critical care nursing is, first and foremost, the actual provision of care to critically ill patients. It is based on a body of knowledge established through ongoing investigation. As a specialty within a practice discipline, the primary concern of critical care nurses is effectiveness. That is, the chief responsibility of the critical care nurse is to deliver care that assists the patient in achieving health-related goals. These goals usually entail regaining and maintaining biologic and psychological wellness, but may also include ensuring a peaceful death. Ethical principles and beliefs serve as one framework within which the nurse practices, providing guidelines that assist in determining which goals are worthwhile and which methods are acceptable. With this as an assumption, the purpose of this chapter is *not* to provide an in-depth analysis of the many theories and principles that may underlie moral responsibility. Rather, this chapter will assist the reader in developing an understanding of broad moral concepts and fundamental steps of moral analysis, as well as in increasing knowledge of practical issues in resolution of moral dilemmas.

A further assumption is that most nurses have some degree of moral intuition. Benner and Tanner, in their extensive studies of expert nurses, described nurses' clinical intuition as "understanding without a rationale" (Benner & Tanner, 1987). Experienced practitioners are often able to respond to cues in an ethical dilemma, identify the situation as similar or dissimilar to others, and attain a commonsense grasp of the whole. Yet, at the same time, they may be unable to articulate the elements and provide a rationale that convinces others of the validity and "rightness" of their views. Just as intuitive clinical judgment actually

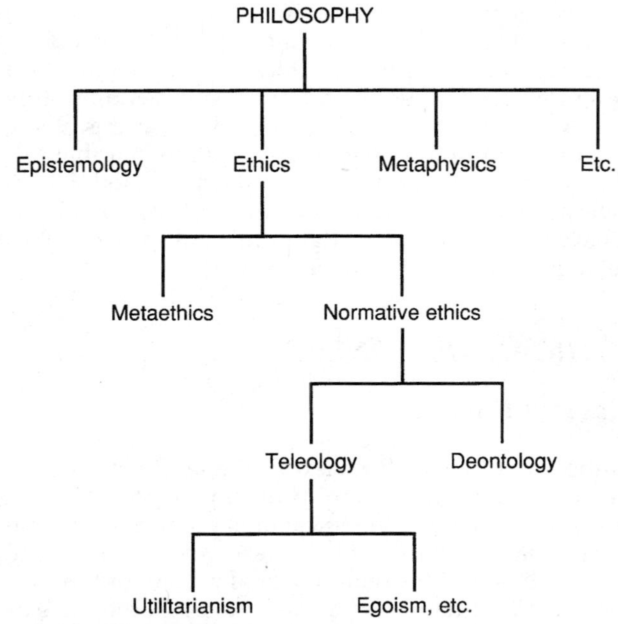

FIGURE 2–1. Derivation of the study of ethics.

ETHICAL REASONING PROCESS

1. Review facts and assumptions
   a. Clinical data related to prognosis, treatment options, etc.
   b. Relevant law
   c. Preferences and beliefs of patients, families, and health care team
   d. Goals of treatment
2. Define the problem in specific terms
3. List the choices
4. Choose an action, considering
   a. Patient goals
   b. Professional norms
   c. Relevant law
   d. Personal values and principles
5. Evaluate the choice
   a. Is this decision consistent with other decisions made in similar cases?
   b. Does this decision stem from reasoned principles?
   c. What are the consequences of this decision?
   d. Is this decision coherent with the values of the people involved?

FIGURE 2–2. Steps in ethical problem solving.

represents the acquisition of knowledge and use of complex analysis drawing on past experience, moral intuition also stems from assumptions, learned beliefs, experience, and reliance on fundamental principles. Both kinds of intuitive thinking can be subjected to critical inquiry to improve the practitioner's judgment and abilities.

In the acquisition of most skills, the initial stages involve learning steps in a process using certain facts and principles as tools. In the case of ethics, many authors recommend a multistep process of ethical reasoning that can be used by the novice in learning (Krekeler, 1987; Fowler, 1987; Curtin, 1982). Although there is some variation in the exact components and number of steps, the processes recommended are very similar. A five-step process, described in Figure 2–2, will be used as the organizing framework for the rest of this chapter. It is important for the reader to keep in mind that this process is most helpful when one is first beginning to pursue ethical inquiry seriously. It is less helpful as the practitioner becomes more fully involved in analyzing ethical dilemmas and is able to use moral intuition. Regan (1986) points out that, like the scientific method, any standard method for answering moral questions will not *in itself* contain the answer to the problem. Rather, it may prove to be a reliable way to get to the answer.

ETHICAL REASONING

Review the Facts

Although a thorough review of the facts may seem to be an obvious step in any problem-solving situation, the importance of it in ethical deliberation is often underestimated. There are two reasons why it is helpful to start this process with a formal review of the exact facts of the situation. First, we often assume the existence of more unanimity about the facts of a case than is actually warranted. This is particularly true of data and opinion regarding prognosis or patient and family wishes. What seems to be an ethical dispute may be a difference in assessment or in data base. This situation very often occurs with issues related to the withdrawal of life support, involving appraisal of the usefulness or futility of treatment, the probable outcome, and the choice the patient would make in light of these predictions. When caregivers disagree with each other about the proper course of action because they differ in their assessments of the likely benefits, the disagreement is one of fact, not morals. The following case study illustrates how these different data bases may lead to apparently different ethical choices.

CASE HISTORY

Mr. T is a 54-year-old widower with two sons. He was diagnosed 10 months ago with small cell carcinoma of the lung and underwent a lobectomy, followed by a course of radiation therapy that he did not complete. Several weeks ago he began complaining of memory loss, headaches, and bouts of confusion that were becoming worse. He was readmitted to the hospital, and a series of diagnostic tests was ordered. A large space-occupying mass was found in the temporal area. The neurosurgeon recommended a craniotomy and resection of the tumor, which was thought to be a metastatic lesion. Mr. T has refused the surgery. His son is supporting this decision. The medical and nursing staff disagree about the best course of action.

The neurosurgeon believes that the patient is not competent to make an informed choice because, on examination, the patient could not consistently state the correct date or where he was. He was not able to solve the standard number or sentence interpretation tests (e.g., performing serial 7s). The neurosurgeon believes that the surgical procedure presents a relatively low risk, could relieve the patient's symptoms of lethargy and confusion, and could extend his life at least 6 months to 1 year. He has never spoken to the patient's son but feels that the son does not have the right to make a decision for an incompetent parent unless he has been declared Mr. T's guardian by the courts. He believes that the best course of action is to petition the court to appoint a legal guardian, who may be willing to consent to what is clearly the "best medical care."

The patient's primary nurse has had several conversations with Mr. T's son. He has consistently stated that his father did not want aggressive treatment and that he had not finished the radiation therapy because he did not like the side effects and just "didn't see any reason to put himself through that." He is aware that his father is not now competent, but believes that if he were, he would definitely not agree to the surgery. Both of Mr. T's sons are concerned about their father's welfare and have asked the nurse for advice. Both are unmarried and do not feel they would be able to care for their father in their homes, but are willing to pay jointly for whatever kind of nursing home or extended care he may need. The nurse feels that, given the circumstances, the best option is to arrange for hospice care for Mr. T.

The patient's internist also agrees that Mr. T is not now competent to make his own decisions. However, she remembers several conversations she had in the past with Mr. T after his lobectomy. He repeatedly stated that he regretted having the surgery, that it was terribly painful, and that he would never go through that again. She thinks that Mr. T might agree to treatment but not if it involved surgery. Consequently, she would like to keep Mr. T in the hospital and explore the possibility of enrolling him in an experimental chemotherapy protocol.

This case illustrates how several caregivers may come to very different conclusions about the best course of action. The differences arise not from any disagreement about important ethical principles or values but from different responses to different facts. At this point, the disagreement does not yet constitute an ethical problem. It may be possible to resolve the apparent disagreement by sharing all of the facts and then discussing the ethical components.

The second reason that it is useful to start with a formal review of the facts is that such a review identifies to which of the many immediate elements of the situation the players are responding. As opposed to a philosophical problem, ethical dilemmas are significantly affected by the details of the situation. Jonsen and Toulmin (1988) point out that the biomedical sciences have a tradition of relying on the rules and formal principles of the biologic sciences, even though the aesthetic components of the art of medicine are also recognized. This is especially true in areas of health care where technology is heavily used. Critical care is one such area. To match principles to cases, one must not forget that these principles are "general rules involved to support *practical* decisions that require *specific* actions affecting *personal* circumstances of *individual* human beings" (Jonsen & Toulmin, 1988). Starting the process by a review of these personal, individual facts grounds the deliberations in the here and now and guards against making a sterile and unrealistic although "principled" decision.

Explicitly reviewing facts and assumptions also provides an opportunity to clarify misunderstandings. For example, the neurosurgeon in this case believes that the patient's son is not entitled to make decisions regarding his father's care unless he is appointed guardian by the courts. However, in many states family members do have legal authority to make health care decisions. If the surgeon's belief about the best course of action is founded on incorrect information about the statutes in that state, the disagreement among caregivers may be easily resolved by obtaining consultation from hospital attorneys. This also illustrates the value of collaborating with other disciplines when faced with ethical problems.

Define the Problem

The next step in the process is to define the problem. An ethical dilemma is a situation in which a choice must be made between various courses of action, and the conflict between these choices involves fundamental concepts of right and wrong. Ethical choices are not matters of different appraisals of facts or a difference in opinion about the most effective care or treatment approach. Ethical dilemmas almost always involve the concepts of rights, duties, and responsibilities, as they apply to specific clinical situations.

The purpose of defining the problem, using one or two clear sentences, is to focus one's own attention on the specific aspect or choice of action that must be addressed to resolve the dilemma. In some situations, this step also brings to light different dilemmas faced by other caregivers. For example, in the case described earlier, suppose that, after sharing all of the facts and discussing the options, some caregivers still felt that it would be wrong to allow Mr. T to be discharged without treatment, whereas others felt that it would be wrong to initiate treatment against his previous wishes to refuse it. In this situation, the problem might be described as follows: "This adult patient, who is not now fully competent, is, with his family's agreement, refusing therapy that has been deemed the preferred medical therapy. The question is, what course of action at this point is indicated?" Stating the problem in this way leads naturally to consideration of how to address the problem by specifying the issues involved. Is there any justification for violating this person's expressed wishes, such as a serious doubt about the validity of those wishes or the likelihood that he will change his mind if given a better explanation of facts or more time to think about it? Conversely, are the health care professionals justified in refraining from providing the indicated therapy for this patient's health problem? That is, is it certain that a valid indication of patient choice exists? Have the benefits and risks of the offered therapy been clearly described? Has the situation been explored on several different occasions with all interested parties?

List the Choices

The third step in ethical reasoning is to list all of the possible options. This step ensures that some options are not eliminated because of invalid assumptions. Options in Mr. T's case might include: (1) Discharge the patient home; (2) discharge the patient to a hospice or other facility; (3) keep the patient in the hospital and reevaluate the situation in another few days, continuing discussions with him and his sons; or (4) begin legal proceedings to have a guardian appointed. Performing this step also ensures that an action is chosen in an ethical dilemma, rather than a principle or a theory.

Decide on the Action

The next step is to make a choice from the list of possible options, using theories, principles, and intuitions for reference or direction. There is a tendency to jump to this step first rather than waiting until the earlier steps have been completed. It is this step that is sometimes considered the most formal aspect of ethical analysis.

THEORIES AND PRINCIPLES. There are several levels of analysis in ethics. On the most general level are theories that direct our method or criteria for determining right actions. The two theories most widely discussed are utilitarianism (also called the consequentialist or teleological approach) and deontology.

Utilitarianism looks to the consequences of an action in judging its goodness. The best action is that which results in the greatest benefit with the least harm for the greatest number of people. In making a choice between conflicting actions, the utilitarian would attempt to compute a kind of moral calculus in comparing the net effects, both short- and long-term, of one action with the net effects of another. Act utilitarians limit their analysis to the effects of the specific acts in question, whereas rule utilitarians examine the effects of acting according to one rule versus another.

Deontologists analyze possible courses of action in terms of their adherence to moral imperatives or rules. This theory is also referred to as a duty-based theory (Benjamin & Curtis, 1992). Assessment of the particular consequences of an act plays no part in the analysis. The rules may take various forms, ranging from the most general prescriptions to more specific provisions such as those found in modern professional codes of ethics. Some philosophers, like Immanuel Kant, believe that there is only one guiding principle or rule. Others are pluralists, identifying several principles such as beneficence and justice that should in all cases direct our actions (Frankena, 1973).

The major difference between these two theories lies in the justification for the methods and rules employed in making decisions regarding right action. As can be seen, both involve the use of rules and principles. Although it is helpful to have some familiarity with the major forms of utilitarianism and deontology, these theories do not in themselves provide useful direction without further discussion of the specific values and principles they utilize. A value may be defined simply as something of worth or importance to us. Values include both nonmoral goods, such as a nice house, job, or leisure time, and moral goods, such as freedom and justice. Values are, however, closely linked to principles that delineate fundamental laws or codes of conduct and entail obligation or an "ought" clause (e.g., we are obligated to [ought to] respect all persons). As can be seen, principles usually reflect the things—beings, objects, or concepts—we value and equate with "the good."

Many values and principles underlie the moral traditions of nursing. Several clearly have such an important influence on daily practice that they warrant more discussion. These are the principles of autonomy, beneficence, and justice (Table 2–1).

Autonomy refers to the right of self-determination. It is grounded in one's status as a rational human being and closely allied to the concepts of liberty and freedom. In western culture, we believe that all people have the right to make their own decisions, to choose freely, and to act on that choice, limited only by the restriction that we do not infringe on the rights of others. Respect for the individual's autonomy is a prima facie principle; that is, we must act according to the dictates of this principle unless another, overriding principle, such as beneficence, intervenes.

TABLE 2–1. **Major Ethical Principles in Health Care**

Autonomy: The principle of self-determination; the fundamental human right to make one's own decisions

Beneficence: The duty to do good or maximize good over harm

Nonmaleficence: The duty to refrain from harm

Justice: The principle of fairness; the duty to treat equals equally, to refrain from discrimination

The principle of autonomy has generated many specific rules regarding conduct in health care settings. The requirement that we obtain informed consent before intervening stems from recognition of the individual's right to make decisions about what is done to him. The principle of veracity, or the obligation to tell the truth, also derives in part from the right of individuals to have access to information needed to make informed decisions. More recently, passage of the Patient Self-Determination Act, requiring health care facilities to inform patients of their right to utilize advance directives, including the living will and durable power of attorney for health care, also represents a strong commitment to the principle of autonomy (Marsden, 1992; Sabatino, 1993).

Beneficence is the obligation to do good or to prevent or minimize harm. Closely related is the principle of nonmaleficence, which imposes the duty to avoid or refrain from inflicting harm. Beneficence and nonmaleficence are probably the strongest principles underlying professional ethics in health care. The Hippocratic oath, the oldest of all codes, specifies: "I will apply dietetic measures for the *benefit* of the sick according to my ability and judgment: I will keep them from *harm and injustice*" (emphases added) (Beauchamp & Walters, 1978). The first sentence in the International Council of Nurses Code for Nurses states, "The fundamental responsibility of the nurse is fourfold: to promote health, to prevent illness, to restore health and to alleviate suffering" (Benjamin & Curtis, 1992, p. 216). In the most recent revision of the American Nurses Association Code for Nurses (1984), the preamble reads:

> *Nursing encompasses the protection, promotion, and restoration of health; the prevention of illness; and the alleviation of suffering in the care of clients. . . . When making clinical judgments, nurses base their decisions on consequences and universal moral principles. . . . The most fundamental of these principles is respect for persons. Other principles stemming from this basic principle are autonomy, beneficence, nonmaleficence, veracity, confidentiality, fidelity, and justice.*

Both the medical and nursing codes utilize the concept of benefit, referring to the good toward which our professional activities are directed. This statement raises the question of what that good is—how we determine it and how we resolve conflicts between opposing goods. The conflicting directions we receive from these two crucial principles, autonomy and beneficence, illustrates that merely having a clear idea of important principles does not always solve dilemmas.

When a patient wishes to make a choice that is in agreement with our assessment of what is "good" or beneficial or in his best interests, we find it easy to believe in autonomy. Likewise, when a patient wishes us to administer the treatment or service that is in her best interests, we find it easy to believe that beneficence is of primary importance in meeting our professional obligations. The difficulty arises when a patient does not choose what we believe to be clearly and definitely in her own interests. Similarly, a conflict arises when we seem to be in a situation in which the only way to help a patient, and thus meet our obligations, is to go against her wishes.

Although any two principles may conflict in this way, this particular struggle, between autonomy and beneficence, is very common in health care and is at the heart of the problem of paternalism. Paternalism is an action deemed to be in the client's or patient's best interest without or regardless of that person's completely voluntary and informed consent (Bayles, 1981). Some authors use the term weak or justified paternalism to refer to situations in which informed consent is impossible (Veatch, 1981), such as emergency situations or when a patient is incompetent. Those who defend some limited forms of paternalism cite the impossibility of ensuring that lay people possess the meaningful understanding needed to meet the requirements of true informed consent. Also cited is the conscious willingness of many patients to give decision-making responsibility to trusted professionals. Opponents warn against the dangers of chipping away at respect for individual autonomy. They point to the inconsistency of any form of paternalism with the principle of liberty.

Pelligrino (1985), discussing ethics in critical care medicine, suggests an approach that may be helpful in sorting out these conflicting obligations. He believes that acting for the patient's good is, indeed, the central principle of medical ethics. However, there are several possible components of "good":

- The ultimate good as defined by the patient's most considered, enduring judgment
- The good of the patient as a person
- The patient's perception of the good at that moment
- The biomedical or technical good of the patient

Although all four are appropriate aims of the practitioner and serve as the reference standard for choices, in situations of conflict we can order them by rank. They are presented in the order of their importance, with the first "good" being the good of last resort, or the one to which we must look in final decisions.

For example, in our case study there are several "goods" that might be achievable. Reducing the tumor mass would be a biologic good; it would extend Mr. T's life. Avoiding the pain and suffering associated with surgery is a good in Mr. T's perception. Respecting Mr. T's wishes, and thus treating him as an autonomous individual with the right to have his wishes followed, recognizes his worth and value as a person. Desire for each of these goods seems to direct us to pursue different courses of actions. In conflicts like this we can respond to the dictates of beneficence by seeking to determine which of these goods represents Mr. T's most authentic choice, the good that provides the greatest benefit to him as a person, not just as a patient.

Justice is a complex principle that is particularly important in this age of health care reform. In its most basic form, the principle of justice requires us to treat others fairly and to treat equals equally. This means that differences in how we treat others, particularly in how we distribute scarce resources like health care, must be based on criteria that can be shown to be morally relevant. For example, many would say that income, wealth, or the ability to purchase insurance should be irrelevant in determining access to basic health care. Health care resources, it is argued, should be distributed according to need alone. The principle of justice also places demands on the nurse in clinical practice. The frequent situation of having too few intensive care beds for the number of patients who seem to need care in the unit could be viewed a justice problem.

At this time, the most important responsibility of the nurse in addressing the justice of our health care system is to be an active participant in the debate over reform legislation. The decisions made regarding the health care system of the future will affect all patients, particularly those who require the expensive resources of critical care. Nurses must become knowledgeable about reform initiatives and contribute their knowledge and experience in addressing this very challenging problem, either as individual voters, through participation in professional nursing associations, or through direct communication with their legislators.

Evaluation of Choice

As can be seen from this brief discussion of theories and principles, a mere understanding of the meaning of the terms does not automatically provide direction in moral debate. To use these tools, one must have some individual system of morality that orders these principles and provides guidelines for applying them in real-life situations. The fifth step in the process of ethical reasoning provides a check on the degree to which one's decision is consistent with other similar decisions and coherent with one's overall moral scheme.

A very practical problem faced by all of us in dealing with moral dilemmas is the sorting out of the conflicting feelings or emotions that inevitably arise. The pace, the demands, and the stresses of critical care generate strong emotions in most nurses. These can easily influence decision making. We may have very valid desires to see a patient's suffering end, to have fewer patients admitted, to not have to deal with a noncompliant patient who keeps returning to the intensive care unit (ICU) for treatment, and to avoid conflicts with physicians, administrators, or coworkers. It can be difficult to separate the influences of these forces from stringent moral considerations. One way to make this more likely, however, is to examine our choices in terms of their consistency and coherence.

Consistency refers to the criterion of universalizability. A valid moral decision should reflect principles and values that are consistently important guides in all similar situations. That is, if in a particular case we believe we are making a decision to refrain from providing a certain treatment for a patient because the patient has made a competent choice to refuse the treatment and we must respect his autonomy, then we should expect to apply this principle consistently in all similar cases. Most important, we should apply this principle even when we do not agree with the patient's choice.

Coherence refers to the degree to which our moral principles fit together in an overall pattern. For example, it is unlikely that we could regard the principle of autonomy as very important if, in addition, we did not have a clear belief in the worth and dignity of all human beings. As part of our ongoing development as moral agents, we must assess how a given choice reflects basic principles and if we would be willing, or have been willing in the past, to adhere to this same principle in other similar situations. We must ask if the most important of our principles and beliefs fit together into a logical, compatible whole.

In addition, because we are making decisions about real situations rather than abstract or hypothetical problems, we must examine the consequences of our decisions. Regardless of whether we are using a deontological or consequential approach to answering moral questions, the effect of our decision on all participants must play a role in the evaluation of the soundness of the decision.

MYTHS AND HANDICAPS IN ETHICAL REASONING

Use of the process just outlined can be helpful in approaching ethical dilemmas in a rational, orderly fashion. However, the process does not ensure that the outcome will be the right or best decision because a number of myths and handicaps play a part in constraining our ability to make reasoned ethical decisions.

The term "myth," as used here, indicates beliefs that, although untrue, persist in the minds of many. They may stem simply from misunderstanding, or they may reflect a less conscious bias. The most profound of these is the belief that there is no right or wrong in ethics, that ethics are a matter of personal choice, and one person's ethical beliefs are just as valid and sound as another's. There are actually two components to this belief: an acceptance of ethical relativism and an assumption that there can be no changes in ethical belief systems based on considered review of facts and principles. Ethical relativism is the belief that whatever customs, actions, and mores are believed to be right by any one culture or society are right, and that there are no basic, fundamental, or absolute moral principles that apply to all peoples. This is not just the recognition that different people *think* different acts are right, but the belief that, because the acts are thought right, they in fact *are* right.

The variations in both practice and moral systems that exist in the world and even within one hospital unit may seem, on first consideration, to support the idea of relativism. In addition, it is very difficult and requires considerable study to find and support a foundation on which absolute morality can rest. On the other hand, most philosophers recognize that we do in fact have a very strong *intuitive* belief that there are some absolute rights and wrongs. More important, if we were to accept the belief that ethical relativism is true, then there would be no reason for any ethical inquiry at all. In fact, concepts such as right and wrong and good and evil would have no meaning outside of the individual.

Another myth or misunderstanding is the belief that establishing the legality or illegality of an action answers the moral question. Although laws are assumed to represent the will and mores of the people, many acts that are quite legal, such as violating confidentiality or breaking promises between friends, are quite immoral. The legal system is designed, in theory, first and foremost to uphold the principle of justice. Although this may be a relevant principle in many situations, it is inadequate for determining the moral action in *all* cases.

For example, there is no actual law against deceiving a patient, yet most of us clearly view this as morally wrong. The case study described earlier also presented a dilemma that, although influenced by laws regarding decision-making authority, could not be solved entirely by referring to these laws. It might be the case that, although Mr. T's son had a legal right to make a decision for his father, the nurse or physician sincerely believed that the son was not acting in his father's best interest. Obeying the law in such situations does not relieve the caregiver of any further moral responsibility.

A similar error in moral reasoning is to mistake expertise in one area for expertise in moral debate. This is a particular danger in critical care units, where medical and nursing professionals are accustomed to acting decisively and to being deferred to and treated by others as experts. Knowledge of the biomedical sciences, obviously important in its own right, is unrelated to the ability to make sound ethical judgments. The most accomplished professional is no more capable, by virtue of clincal expertise, of sound moral reasoning than the least prepossessing of lay people.

The last common myth or handicap in resolving eithical dilemmas is one that is particularly relevant to nurses. Perhaps the most important practical constraint on moral inquiry by a nurse is the belief that nurses are powerless to affect the outcome of a moral dilemma because they lack formal authority in the health care system. There are many factors that contribute to the perception that nurses cannot affect moral decisions. These include unfamiliarity with the process of ethical reasoning, which leads to a lack of confidence in their own decisions and intuitions. In addition, many people, not just nurses, are confused about the distinction between legal and moral issues. This leads to a perception of constraints where none exists. Last, there are very real institutional and personal constraints imposed on nurses by virtue of their status as employees. Many people still hold the traditional view of nurses as "order followers" rather than professionals who have an independent code of conduct that takes precedence over institutional policies and procedures (Pence, 1994).

Nurses, by virtue of their primary accountability to the patient and their constant presence at the bedside, are always participants in dilemmas concerning treatment decisions. In addition, because patients and families often choose to discuss their questions, doubts, and preferences with nurses before voicing them to physicians, the nurse may be the individual who first identifies a moral issue. It is particularly important in critical care, where end-of-life decisions are frequently a source of conflict, that nurses become adept at overcoming obstacles to careful moral analysis and participate in the resolution of ethical dilemmas (Marsden, 1993).

The existence of bureaucratic constraints does pose barriers. The nurse who chooses to implement a moral decision that is in conflict with either institutional policy or the wishes or decisions of others, particularly supervisors or physicians, may encounter very real consequences. However, the reality of nonmoral consequences, such as conflict, censure, or disciplinary action, do not make the nurse powerless. They do present the need to add to the moral equation the evaluation of whether the principle or issue at hand is important enough for the nurse to risk the consequences.

MAKING ETHICAL DECISION MAKING OPERATIONAL

Because there are very real constraints against moral inquiry by nurses, it is equally important to consider how we can facilitate this process and use available resources (Table 2–2). The making of an isolated decision by a nurse, regardless of how valid or sound it is, is of limited value unless nurses are empowered to implement it.

TABLE 2–2. **Resources for Addressing Ethical Dilemmas**

Formal education programs
Staff ethicist/philosopher
Interdisciplinary meetings
Ethics committees
Ethics consultation service
Policies related to ethical issues

Education is, of course, the first step. This should include both learning about the actual process of moral reasoning and learning about resources and methods for addressing issues of concern. The popularity of continuing education offerings in the area of ethics attests to both the recognized importance of this area and the willingness of practitioners to engage in active study. The effectiveness of educational programs in the hospital setting depends on a planned, well designed ethics curriculum. The curriculum should begin with basic orientation classes and proceed throughout the professional development program, regardless of whether it is provided on a centralized or unit-based basis. Sporadic, single classes that are not integrated within the entire educational plan are less likely to have a lasting impact on the development of moral reasoning skills.

A number of pragmatic considerations can be helpful to nurses in the practice setting. Even before the nurse has developed clear ideas on an issue, it is helpful to discuss the situation with colleagues. It is very difficult, if not impossible, to resolve these thorny issues and sort through the many considerations without help from others, even if it is just in the form of listening and validating the data base or the logic of the process. Although it may be ideal to have an ethicist or nurse philosopher help the staff in these investigations, it is not necessary. It is more important for some dialogue and exchange of views to take place among coworkers.

Interdisciplinary meetings serve as an excellent forum for discussions of ethical views and concerns. Problems are best analyzed through application of the varying perspectives of several disciplines. All individuals involved in a specfic patient situation need the opportunity to contribute ideas, and the beliefs of all must be taken into account in coming to consensus. If interdisciplinary meetings are not a regular part of unit operations, the nurse can be instrumental in problem resolution by arranging for a collaborative discussion with all those involved.

Ethics committees can be of great assistance to all caregivers when ethical dilemmas occur. These are multidisciplinary groups that serve an advisory function. They generally meet at the request of a caregiver and review the facts of the case, discuss the relevant ethical considerations, and provide recommendations about possible courses of action (Cohen 1988a, b). Such meetings provide caregivers with a chance to talk with other clinicians who are knowledgeable about clinical ethics and often provide the support necessary to implement a difficult decision. Although many hospitals have implemented ethics committees within the past few years, they are still underutilized, particularly by nurses.

Partly in response to this general underutilization of ethics committees, some hospitals have developed ethics consultation services (Simpson, 1992). These services provide on-call consultation by individuals, academically prepared in ethics, who can go to the patient unit and meet with the staff, patient, and family. The consultants are able to offer guidance and can actually participate in decision making or family meetings. Consultants are often able to respond in a more timely fashion and are easier for staff to utilize than requesting a formal committee meeting.

Situations that are most difficult for nurses are those in which there is disagreement among caregivers about what action is proper or those in which the nurse perceives an improper action on the part of another caregiver. Under these circumstances formal administrative support for intervention and resolution is essential. This can take many forms. Formal policies outlining the chain of command to be used in addressing ethical issues provide nurses with guidance as to procedure. A formal policy is also a tangible sign of the appropriateness and importance attached by the administration to the right and the responsibility of every caregiver to address ethical concerns. Ethics grand rounds and ethics nursing care conferences serve the same function in an even more public fashion.

When formal administrative support is absent, there are still some guidelines that can be helpful to individual nurses facing ethical dilemmas. In addition to discussing the issue with colleagues, it is usually more effective to pursue the desired course of action with at least one other person, if not a small group. Groups provide support, and it is less likely that the concerns of a group will be ignored. Paying attention to the chain of command is always important, especially when issues of proper performance are concerned. Gaining the support of at least one person in the administrative or management hierarchy is useful. Putting concerns in writing at some stage can be helpful, both in assisting the nurse to lay out the issue in a clear, concise, and logical format and in beginning a process of documentation that may be needed if the concerns are not addressed.

In critical care, unfortunately, some issues arise that need to be dealt with immediately, and the options discussed above cannot be utilized. In these cases, it is obviously important for nurses to have the knowledge needed to analyze complex situations and come to decisions quickly. It is vital for them to know that the nursing department, if not the hospital bureaucracy as a whole, will support them in these endeavors. For this reason, it is important that staff members keep the nurse manager informed of persistent issues and dilemmas. The manager of the unit is in a pivotal position both to reinforce to nurses and others that registered nurses have the right and responsibility to address ethical concerns, and to obtain resources to assist staff in fulfilling their moral obligations.

THE ETHICAL AGENDA OF CRITICAL CARE NURSING FOR THE FUTURE

In addition to the preceding discussion of theoretical issues and practical guidelines, the future direction or agenda for critical care nursing as a practice discipline needs to be considered. Three items are significant enough to warrant special consideration.

Help the Patient to "Own" His or Her Care

If we accept autonomy as one of the primary values, if not the most important, then we must take active steps to ensure that patients are capable of acting autonomously. This is particularly important in the very foreign environment of the critical care unit. We must routinely talk with patients about their goals for health care, the measures we can offer, the priorities that we recommend. Obviously, this cannot be done in emergency situations, with patients who are incompetent by virtue of their physical condition, or abruptly in the midst of an ICU admission. Because there are so many practical limitations on these kinds of discussions, it is all the more imperative to take advantage of the opportunities we do have to move away from the rigid care practices so common in critical care.

In considering how we can help the patient to own his care, the concept of advocacy is relevant. Given the highly complex nature of most hospitals today, it is easy to see why the patient may need someone to speak for him, to represent his interests, and to safeguard his rights. Nowhere does this seem more necessary than in the very technical, foreign environment of the intensive care unit. Nurses are, in many ways, uniquely qualified for the role of advocate because of their continual presence at the bedside and their special relationship to and knowledge of patients and their families. However, there are two considerations that may limit the usefulness of the advocate role for nurses.

First, by definition, the first duty of the person whose goal is to protect patients' rights is to promote informed consent. This includes and may even start with enabling the patient to choose his or her own advocate. Patients may or may not choose a nurse. It is unlikely that patients will see nurses as candidates for this role in environments where a different nurse is assigned to the patient each day and no attempt is made by the nurse to involve the patient and family in discussions about care routines and options. All caregivers—physicians, social workers, respiratory therapists, nurses—would insist that their actions are guided by a concern for patient welfare and that their role is to benefit the patient. If we believe that nurses have an additional role as patient advocates, then we must pay attention to the characteristics of the environment and the health care delivery system that foster or hinder this role.

The second limit on the advocacy role for nurses lies in focusing too narrowly on the role of advocate. Patients may always need a member of the health care team to act as a guide through the bureaucratic maze and as a counselor in decision making. It may be far more valuable, however, for nurses to concentrate some of their energies on changing at least some small part of the system to minimize the need for an advocate in the first place.

As part of this process, nurses can actively evaluate the routine practices used in critical care nursing, which they accept without question, in terms of their effect on patient autonomy. For example, is it really necessary to limit visiting hours, to restrict the family's access to the patient? Most individuals are certainly more at ease in discussing their concerns with their friends and family, yet the restrictive visiting policies of many ICUs may have the unintended effect of making it more difficult for the patient to express his wishes. Similarly, would it really be impossible to let the patient choose the routine for the day, such as when to have a bath, when to get out of bed, when to eat? The actual practice is less important than the nurse's willingness to provide opportunities for the patient to have choices, or, at the very least, to make explicit which routines are negotiable and which must be prescribed.

Avoid Having to Solve Ethical Dilemmas in Crisis Situations

As with any problem, the best approach is prevention. Although we cannot hope to prevent ethical dilemmas from arising, we can be alert to the beginnings of situations that herald a dilemma. We can intervene before we are in a forced-choice situation. For example, when a patient with a clearly poor prognosis is admitted to the ICU, that is the time to clarify with all caregivers involved which discussions about aggressive treatment and resuscitation have taken place—not when the patient develops a cardiopulmonary arrest. If there are practice issues that are repeatedly problematic, such as do not resuscitate (DNR) orders, allocation of scarce ICU beds, or utilization of experimental protocols, these should be addressed proactively, not in the heat of a specific patient problem.

Participate in Policy-Making Decisions

This item refers to activities that do not usually take place at the bedside yet affect each nurse's practice. As mentioned earlier, one of the important ways in which we can support and foster ethical inquiry is in establishing formal policies governing the procedure to be used for ethical debate and guidelines for managing problematic issues such as DNR orders. Engelhardt (1985) pointed out the importance of the joint decision making that is used in today's pluralistic society to reach mutual agreement on moral issues. We can no longer rely on a predominant religious view or a predominant social value system; therefore, "if authority cannot be derived from the grace of God or from a successful rational argument, it can be derived from . . . the consent of all involved . . . in a project" (Engelhardt, 1985). Nurses, as the primary implementers of many of the decisions affecting patient care, must be among those involved in reaching a consensus. Most hospitals use either standing committees or ad hoc groups to develop practice policies. These groups provide excellent opportunities for staff nurses to make contributions and develop skill in moral debate.

On another level, nurses must be active participants in social policy development that affects the health care of individuals and groups. We will continue to face new and puzzling dilemmas as technology continues to expand the limits of our knowledge. Mandatory testing for AIDS, reconsideration of the meaning of brain death (Veatch, 1993), use of information from genetic testing (Murray, 1993), justification for refusing to provide futile treatments (Morreim, 1994), and the ethics of health care reform (Wolf, 1994) are just a few of the new issues we face in this decade. Nurses can play a crucial role in developing consensus, but only if they are willing to become involved. The most essential factor in fulfilling our moral obligations is recognizing that, as critical care nurses, we bring a unique knowledge and perspective to these complex human problems and we must invest ourselves in working toward solutions (Corley et al., 1993).

SUMMARY

This chapter has reviewed selected principles and concepts that are relevant to the practice of critical care nursing. A process for addressing ethical dilemmas was suggested, recommending the following steps: review the facts, define the problem, list the choices, decide on the proper action, and evaluate the choice.

Although many principles are relevant to ethical inquiry in nursing, autonomy and beneficence were selected as illustrative of these principles. Respect for autonomy reflects a fundamental value placed on human beings and requires us to respect each individual's right of self-determination. As a prima facie duty, it obligates us to ensure that patients have the necessary information and the opportunity to give informed consent before we act on them. Beneficence directs us to aim for the good and further requires us to evaluate and define the meaning of this good, giving priority to the patient's own conception of good.

Practical considerations were also discussed. Because the ethics of nursing as a practice discipline must involve the active engagement of nurses in addressing moral questions, an agenda for the future was offered. This agenda includes helping the patient to own her own care, avoiding the need to solve ethical dilemmas in crisis situations, and participating in policy-making decisions. These steps were suggested as a means both of developing a more effective ethical practice and improving the moral environment in which this practice takes place.

REFERENCES

American Nurses Association. (1984). *Code for nurses with interpretive statements.* Kansas City, MO: American Nurses Association.

Bayles, M. D. (1981). *Professional ethics.* Belmont, CA: Wadsworth Publishing.

Beauchamp, T. L., & Walters, L. (Eds.). (1978). *Contemporary issues in bioethics* (p. 138). Encino, CA: Dickenson Publishing.

Benjamin, M., & Curtis, J. (1992). *Ethics in nursing* (3rd ed.). New York: Oxford University Press.

Benner, P., & Tanner, C. (1987). Clinical judgment: How expert nurses use intuition. *American Journal of Nursing, 87*(1), 23–31.

Cohen, C. B. (Ed.). (1988a). Birth of a network. *Hastings Center Report, 18*(1), 11–13.

Cohen, C. B. (Ed.). (1988b). Is case consultation in retreat? *Hastings Center Report, 18*(4), 23–24.

Corley, M. C., Selig, P., & Ferguson, C. (1993). Critical care nurse participation in ethical and work decisions. *Critical Care Nurse, 13*(3), 120–125.

Curtin, L. (1982). No rush to judgment. In L. Curtin & M. J. Flaherty (Eds.), *Nursing ethics—theories and pragmatics* (pp. 57–66). Bowie, MD: Robert J. Brady Company.

Engelhardt, H. T. (1985). Moral tensions in critical care medicine: "Absurdities" as indications of finititude. In J. C. Moskop & L. Kopelman (Eds.), *Ethics and critical care medicine* (pp. 23–34). Boston: D. Reidel Publishing.

Engelhardt, H. T. (1986). *The foundations of bioethics.* New York: Oxford University Press.

Fowler, M. D. (1987). Piecing together the ethical puzzle: Operationalizing nursing's ethics in critical care. In M. D. Fowler & J. Levine-Ariff (Eds.), *Ethics at the bedside* (pp. 182–212). Philadelphia: J. B. Lippincott.

Frankena, W. K. (1973). *Ethics* (2nd ed.). Englewood Cliffs, NJ: Prentice-Hall.

Jonsen, A., & Toulmin, S. (1988). *The abuse of casuistry.* Berkeley: University of California Press.

Krekeler, K. (1987). Critical care nursing and moral development. *Critical Care Nursing Quarterly, 10*(2), 1–8.

Marsden, C. (1992). Making patient self determination a reality in critical care. *American Journal of Critical Care, 1*(1), 122–124.

Marsden, C. (1993). Do not resuscitate orders and end of life care planning. *American Journal of Critical Care, 2*(2), 177–179.

Morreim, E. H. (1994). Profoundly diminished life: The casualties of coercion. *Hastings Center Report, 24*(1), 33–41.

Murray, T. H. (1993). Genetics and just health care: A genome task force report. *Kennedy Institute of Ethics Journal, 3,* 327–332.

Pence, T. (1994). Nursing's most pressing problem. *Bioethics Forum, 10*(1), 3–9.

Pelligrino, E. D. (1985). Moral choice, the good of the patient, and the patient's good. In J. C. Moskop & L. Kopelman (Eds.), *Ethics and critical care medicine* (pp. 117–138). Boston: D. Reidel Publishing.

Regan, T. (Ed.) (1986). *Matters of life and death* (2nd ed.) (pp. 3–34). New York: Random House.

Sabatino, C. P. (1993). Surely the wizard will help us, Toto? Implementing the patient self determination act. *Hastings Center Report, 23*(1), 12–16.

Simpson, K. H. (1992). The development of a clinical ethics consultation service in a community hospital. *Journal of Clinical Ethics, 3,* 124–130.

Veatch, R. M. (1981). *A theory of medical ethics.* New York: Basic Books.

Veatch, R. M. (1993). The impending collapse of the whole-brain definition of death. *Hastings Center Report, 23*(4), 18–24.

Wolff, S. M. (1994). Health care reform and the future of physician ethics. *Hastings Center Report, 24*(2), 28–40.

Legal Issues in Critical Care

Ginny Wacker Guido

As society has become more litigious, increasing numbers of nurses are being named as defendants in medical malpractice lawsuits. Understanding and applying a few legal principles will help critical care nurses to protect themselves against these growing numbers of lawsuits. Legal issues, though extremely important, should not be totally separated from ethics and ethical principles. Clinical issues often involve both legal and ethical components. Therefore the reader is cautioned to view this chapter in light of the chapter on ethics in nursing (Chapter 2).

Until the present time, few lawsuits originated within critical care settings. Several factors may account for this phenomenon: (1) the competency and accountability of critical care nurses; (2) the advanced technologic skills required in all aspects of critical care medicine and nursing; and (3) the relatively low nurse–patient ratios in critical care areas. Perhaps the single most significant factor is the open communication that occurs in the critical care setting between health care givers and patients and family members. Patients and families are much less apt to file lawsuits when they perceive the potential defendants as open, honest, and caring (Bernzweig, 1990).

Despite the factors mitigating the risk of lawsuits against health care providers in critical care settings, increasing consumer knowledge and "malpractice fever" in general mean that the possibility of lawsuits cannot be ignored. Two factors that may help to keep the numbers of lawsuits low are the increased education of consumers about the limitations of medicine and realistic ideas about the benefits that can be expected from medical care, and the increased involvement of patients and their families in the decision-making process. Perhaps the best means of reducing the risk of a potential lawsuit is for nurses to gain a working knowledge of the basic principles of law underlying their professional practice. Tort law involves compensation to individuals wrongly injured by others' actions; this area of law is frequently referred to as personal injury law. Table 3–1 summarizes the various torts discussed in this chapter.

STANDARDS OF CARE

From a legal perspective, standards of care or standards of practice define the minimum level of care provided by a given profession that is considered adequate. In other words, the law views standards of care as the skills and knowledge commonly possessed by members of a given profession. Standards of care are used daily in all aspects of health care delivery. Standards form the basis for care and serve as the criteria for determining whether less-than-adequate care was delivered to a specific patient. Thus, the concept of standards of care is a basic legal issue that critical care nurses must understand and deal with in their everyday practice.

Standards of care are derived from various sources and may be classified into two broad categories: internal and external. Internal standards are those established by the nurse's background and role and include the nurse's specific job description as well as the institution's policies and procedures. An important internal standard is the standard of care set by a particular nurse's education and experience. The more education a nurse has and the greater the nurse's professional skills, the more potentially liable the nurse becomes for failure to perform at an acceptable level of care. Thus, to a certain degree, the definition of "acceptable care" changes as the nurse gains education and experience. Another important internal standard today is the unit-based standard of care. These standards are specific to the care of the patient within a given setting, and should be reviewed and updated as needed to continually reflect the quality of care delivered to patients.

External standards are established by professional nursing organizations, the state nurse practice act, federal guidelines and policies, precedent court decisions, current textbooks and journal articles, and certification standards.

The legal system views standards of care as the pivotal point in a malpractice action. Nurses have a duty to use reasonable care in interactions with patients. The minimum or reasonable level of care that should be given is the care that would be given by a prudent critical care nurse under similar circumstances. The question to be asked is, "How would a reasonably prudent critical care nurse with the same skills, experience, and educational level as the defendant critical care nurse have acted under the same or similar circumstances?" If the reasonable, prudent critical care nurse would have acted in the same manner as the defendant nurse did, then the defendant nurse may not be legally liable to the injured patient.

TABLE 3–1. **Negligent, Intentional, and Quasi-Intentional Torts**

Elements of the Tort	Nursing Examples
Negligence	
1. Duty owed the patient 2. Breach of duty owed 3. Foreseeability 4. Causation 5. Injury 6. Damages a. General b. Specific c. Emotional d. Punitive or exemplary	Failure to monitor the patient as ordered Failure to communicate a change in the patient's status Failure to prevent the patient from falling Failure to provide patient education Failure to provide safety for the patient
Intentional Torts	
Shared elements of all intentional torts 1. There must be a volitional action by the defendant 2. The person so acting must intend to bring about the consequences 3. There must be causation: The act must be a substantial factor in bringing about the consequences	
Assault 1. Shared elements plus: 2. Placing another person in apprehension of being touched in an offensive or insulting manner	Threatening the patient with an injection or an intravenous line
Battery 1. Shared elements plus: 2. Actual contact with another person without his or her consent	Forcing a patient to ambulate
False Imprisonment 1. Shared elements plus: 2. Unjustifiable detention or confinement of a person	Refusing to allow a patient to leave against medical advice
Quasi-Intentional Torts	
Invasion of Privacy 1. An act that intrudes or pries into another's seclusion 2. The intrusion must be objectionable to a reasonable person 3. The intrusion must concern private facts 4. There must be public disclosure of private information	Taking unauthorized pictures of a patient Releasing confidential information to others without consent Allowing unauthorized people to witness patient procedures
Defamation 1. Use of language that adversely affects one's reputation 2. Use of false language about or concerning a living person 3. Publication of false information to a third person 4. Damage to one's reputation	Making false chart entries about the patient's lifestyle Falsely accusing staff members in front of other staff or patients

Perhaps standards of care become most crucial whenever there is the potential that a lawsuit will be filed or when the nurse or institution is notified of a newly filed lawsuit by an injured patient. Standards of care determine much of what will be presented in an ensuing lawsuit and actually form the basis for negligence and malpractice.

In the legal system, standards of care are established during court trials by the use of expert witnesses. The expert witness aids the judge and jury in determining the acceptable standard of care in a given case. The expert witness explains the actual care that was given and describes what the acceptable level of care should have been. The judge and jury then decide whether the defendant acted according to the appropriate standard of care. Thus, an expert witness testifying in a lawsuit that involves a critical care nurse's performance must have a thorough understanding of the skills and clinical expertise needed at the time of the alleged malpractice. The expert would then establish, for the court, the standard of care for which the defendant nurse is accountable.

NEGLIGENCE AND MALPRACTICE

Most of the lawsuits or potential lawsuits encountered in clinical practice involve negligence or malpractice. Although frequently used interchangeably, these two terms are not synonymous. Negligence is either an act or a failure to act that leads to the injury of another. In its simplest definition, negligence is carelessness. Negligence may be attributed to either a professional or a nonprofessional person. Anyone who fails to perform to the standard of care that a reasonable person would meet in a particular set of circumstances may be liable for negligence. Malpractice is a specific type of negligence that includes the status of the care giver as well as the standard of care owed. Courts have defined malpractice as any professional misconduct, unreasonable lack of skill or fidelity in professional duties, or illegal and immoral conduct (*Napier v. Greenzweig*, 1919; *Forthofer v. Arnold*, 1938). In a more modern definition, malpractice is the failure of a professional person to act in accordance with prevailing professional standards or a failure to foresee consequences that a professional person, who has the necessary skills and education, should foresee.

The most common areas of negligence or malpractice in critical care settings include medication errors, patient falls, failing to assess the patient for changes in clinical status, and failing to notify the primary health care provider of changes in patient status.

In accusations of either malpractice or negligence, the person bringing the lawsuit (plaintiff) must prove to the court that the health care professional or health care institution was truly at fault. To do so, the plaintiff must establish six legal elements: the duty owed the patient, breach of the duty owed the patient, foreseeability, causation, injury, and damages. Each of these six elements is discussed in the following pages.

Duty Owed the Patient

Establishing that a duty was owed the patient requires the plaintiff to demonstrate that a professional relationship existed between the nurse and the plaintiff and that the nurse owed the patient a specific standard of care. Historically, the relationship between a nurse and a patient is the easiest element to prove in a court of law. This is certainly true of critical care nurses who work in hospital settings. Because the nurse works for the hospital and the patient is the hospital's patient, a nurse–patient relationship is readily established. Some courts also refer to this relationship as a reliance relationship because the patient is relying on the nurse for his or her professional expertise.

The second step under duty owed the patient is establishment of the standard of care that was owed. This is accomplished through the use of expert witnesses and through the use of hospital and unit-based standards.

Breach of Duty Owed the Patient

This legal element involves showing a deviation from the standard of care owed the patient. For example, if the acceptable standard of care involves taking and recording vital signs every 5 to 15 minutes, then recording vital signs every 30 minutes is below the acceptable standard of care. The nurse has breached the duty owed the patient.

Usually a deviation from a standard of care is called ordinary or mere negligence, implying professional negligence either in performing an action or in omitting a required action. However, a nurse may be liable for gross negligence if he or she willingly or consciously ignores a risk known to be significantly harmful to a given patient. For example, if the nurse assesses vital signs every 30 minutes in a patient who has just been placed on potent vasopressors and the patient then suffers a stroke, the nurse may be considered grossly negligent.

Foreseeability

The third element of malpractice that must be shown by the plaintiff is foreseeability, defined as the recognition that certain events are expected to cause certain outcomes. In the previous example, it is foreseeable that an elevated blood pressure might result in a stroke and that infusion of potent vasopressors could cause a significantly elevated blood pressure.

Foreseeability is judged on the facts known at the time of the occurrence or happening, not at the time the case finally comes to court. The question asked is, "Could the reasonable, prudent critical care nurse have foreseen a particular result based on the level of medical knowledge available to practitioners at the time of the occurrence?" Journal articles and textbooks aid in establishing the level of medical and nursing knowledge available to professionals at the time of the happening.

Causation

Demonstration of causation requires proof that the injury resulted directly from a negligent action or omission of a required action. The injury itself is not sufficient proof. Nor does the failure to meet appropriate standards of care result in liability. The injury must be a direct outcome of the negligence.

The legal system uses two different approaches in establishing cause. If a single defendant is involved in the lawsuit, the court asks the "but for" question: "Would this injury have resulted but for the action or omission of the defendant?" "Would the patient have fallen and broken his hip but for the nurse's negligence in failing to put the side rail in its up position?" When two or more defendants are involved in the lawsuit, the court uses the substantial factor test. Each defendant's action is examined to see if it was a substantial factor in the resultant injury. For example, "Was the failure of a nurse to verify the physician's order a substantial factor in the overdosing of the patient with a given medication?" If the answer is yes to the substantial factor question, then causation has been established.

Injury

The plaintiff must demonstrate that some type of physical, financial, or emotional injury resulted from the breach of duty owed the patient. For example, a critical care nurse may be at fault for failing to raise the side rails on the bed of a combative, disoriented patient, but unless some injury results (e.g., the patient falls and sustains a broken hip), there is no liability in a court of law for the negligent care.

Generally speaking, the courts do not allow damages for emotional injuries unless they are accompanied by physical injuries. For example, damages for pain and suffering are allowed when there is physical injury but not when no physical injury can be shown.

Damages

Damages compensate the injured person for the cost of medical care for injuries sustained and for restoring the patient to his or her original state, as far as financially possible. Damages are not necessarily meant to punish the wrongdoer for the negligent action. For example, the awarded damages are greater if the patient requires prolonged hospitalization and future medical care than if the patient has failed to survive the negligent act.

Damages are grouped into four categories: general, special, emotional, and punitive or exemplary. General damages are those inherent to the injury itself. Included in this category are pain and suffering and any permanent disability or disfigurement. Special damages include all losses and expenses incurred as a result of the injury. These include medical bills, lost wages, and expenses incurred for hiring medical personnel at home or for mechanical alterations needed at home (e.g., wheelchair ramps, safety rails for bathtubs, and so on). Emotional damages are those allowed for counseling and for pain and suffering of the spouse. Punitive damages are allowed only if the action has been willful or conscious and if gross negligence has been found by the court. Punitive damages are meant to punish the wrongdoer and set an example for the remainder of the profession, thus deterring future misconduct.

INTENTIONAL TORTS

A tort is a civil wrong committed against a person or a person's property. Civil law, the body of law dealing with the rights of private citizens, is based on fault. The accountable person has either failed to meet his or her responsibility or has performed an action below acceptable standards. Once fault has been shown, the person harmed may be awarded compensation.

Intentional torts committed by nurses differ from negligence and malpractice in several ways. Intent is necessary for an intentional tort. The nurse must intend to do a particular action or appear to intend a particular action that brings about a consequence. For example, the nurse must *intend* to hold or restrain a patient to give the patient an injection. Likewise, an action must take place for an intentional tort to occur. An omitted action can never be an intentional tort. In the previous example, the nurse *held* the patient to administer the injection. An intentional tort need not involve actual injury. That is, the plaintiff must show that the tort occurred, not that an injury or damage occurred. Using the same example, the patient would need to show that the nurse held him or her against his or her will, not that the injection caused any physical injury. Intentional torts most commonly seen in critical care settings include assault, battery, and false imprisonment.

Assault and Battery

Although commonly pled together, assault and battery are two separate torts. An assault is any action by one person that makes another person fear that he or she will be touched without consent in an offensive, insulting, or physically injurious manner. Actual touching is not required; the action or motion alone creates the fear. For example, if a nurse approaches a patient with a syringe as if to administer an injection without the patient's consent, no contact has occurred, yet the patient could successfully show that an assault has taken place.

Battery is harmful or unwarranted contact with a person without his permission. The person need not be injured by the contact, nor does he need to be aware that the contact has taken place. For example, a battery occurs when a patient is restrained for the purpose of giving some type of necessary nursing care, regardless of whether the patient knows about the contact. It is the contact, not the knowledge of the contact or the manner of the contact, that results in the commission of a battery.

In most situations, assault and battery are averted because the health care provider has the prior consent of the patient to proceed with the treatment or therapy. Also, self-defense may be a valid defense in a lawsuit brought by a patient for assault and battery. The health care provider may use necessary force to prevent patients from harming either themselves or others in their immediate area.

False Imprisonment

False imprisonment is the unjustifiable detention of a person without a legal right to detain that person. A nurse falsely imprisons a patient when she or he confines or restrains the patient within a confined, bounded area with the intent of limiting the patient's freedom. Refusing to return the patient's clothing, car keys, or other personal belongings may also be considered false imprisonment.

To prove liability of the health care provider for this action, the patient must show that he or she was aware of the confinement. Confused and disoriented people who are restrained for their own or other people's protection will not be successful in bringing a lawsuit for false imprisonment. Care, caution, and reasonableness are prerequisites in the use of restraints.

QUASI-INTENTIONAL TORTS

Quasi-intentional torts are those that lack the intent that is so crucial to intentional torts. Because action and causation must be shown, these torts involve more than mere negligence. The two quasi-intentional torts seen most frequently in critical care settings are invasion of privacy and defamation of character.

Invasion of Privacy

The right of protection against unreasonable and unwarranted interference with one's solitude is well recognized in the legal system. This tort is frequently encountered in critical care settings when confidential information is given to people not entitled to it. For example, pictures may be taken of a patient with a particularly interesting diagnosis and used without the patient's consent. More commonly, information about a patient's diagnosis and status may be given over the telephone to interested callers without the patient's permission.

Nurses must be cautious when releasing information about patients. Even family members do not have a right to information about the adult patient without the patient's permission. Before releasing information over the telephone, the nurse should verify that the patient has consented to the release of the information and that the caller is entitled to receive the information. A simple notation on the Kardex listing who is authorized to receive information should be made at the time of the patient's admission. If the caller is not entitled to the information, the caller should be referred to the patient's spouse or other family member.

Invasion of patient privacy rights may also occur during shift reports, particularly if the institution utilizes walking reports or walking rounds. Frequently, nurses relay information about patients to other health care providers at the patient's bedside or in a central location. Because other patients and family members may overhear such reports, the potential for invasion of privacy is great. Nurses should either ask family members to leave during reports or give the reports in a more secluded area.

Defamation

Defamation is a tort of wrongful injury to a living person's reputation. Such wrongful injury may consist of either written or oral communication to someone other than the defamed person. A claim of defamation may arise from the release of inaccurate or inappropriate medical information or from untruthful statements made about a patient.

Caution is the key advice in preventing this tort. Nurses must be careful about making comments about patients, especially when making entries in the patient's chart or medical record. For example, writing in the chart that a patient is "crazy" may be defamation; describing the actual behaviors or statements of the patient is not.

LIABILITY AND THE CRITICAL CARE NURSE

The hospital or employing institution may incur liability for the actions of its employees under the doctrine of respondeat superior, or "let the master respond." According to this legal doctrine, the employer has the right to both hire and fire the individual employee and thus becomes accountable for negligence occurring during the employee's work day. In other words, the nurse would not have been in a position to allow harm to come to a patient if the hospital had not hired the nurse and allowed the patient to come into contact with that nurse. For the hospital to be liable for the negligent action, the nurse must be acting within the course and scope of employment at the time of the incident. For example, if a nurse allows a patient to fall, the employing hospital as well as the nurse may be found liable in a subsequent lawsuit. If the nurse is acting outside of his or her job description or against hospital policy and procedure, the hospital may escape liability. For example, a hospital may have a policy that forbids nurses to remove invasive lines (e.g., pulmonary artery balloon catheters, external pacemaker wires) from patients. If a nurse harms a patient by negligently removing an external pacemaker wire, the hospital will argue that the nurse was acting outside the course and scope of his or her employment. The nurse, thus, remains liable but the hospital is not.

The hospital and the supervising physician may jointly be liable for a nurse's actions. Termed dual servant role, this type of situation is most often encountered in critical care settings during cardiopulmonary resuscitation. Because one person is directly in charge of the resuscitation efforts, the nurse may be said to be acting as an employee of the directing physician as well as an employee of the institution. In this type of situation, a negligent action on the part of the nurse could potentially make the nurse, the physician, and the hospital liable to the injured party.

Always to be remembered is that the person directly responsible for a negligent action will retain accountability for that action. The law may make others liable for a given employee's actions, but the employee always retains some individual liability.

Supervisor Liability

If a staff nurse in a critical care setting performs a required nursing action negligently or fails to assess a given patient accurately and the patient sustains an injury, the staff nurse may be liable for that injury. But what about the charge nurse and the supervising nurse? Is the charge nurse or supervisor potentially liable merely because he or she assigned the staff nurse to care for that particular patient? What is the potential liability of the manager or supervisor who assigned the staff nurse to that unit?

The answers to these questions depend on several factors. If the staff nurse is consistently competent and has the necessary education and experience required to care for critically ill patients, then the supervisor and charge nurse would incur no liability merely by assigning the staff nurse to work in the unit and care for the patient. Also, if the staff nurse does nothing, either in words or actions, to alert the supervisor or charge nurse that he or she is not competent to care for the patient, then the supervisor and charge nurse are not liable. For example, suppose the supervisor and charge nurse have frequently observed a staff nurse caring for critically ill patients in a competent manner, and the staff nurse has said nothing to either of them about personal problems or about feeling unable to care for a specific patient. Should an untoward occurrence happen and the patient be injured, there is no vicarious liability on the part of either the supervisor or the charge nurse.

The situation is different, however, if at the beginning of the shift, the staff nurse had talked with the supervisor about a personal crisis at home and asked to be assigned only to stable patients. Or, perhaps the supervisor and charge nurse had noted that the staff nurse was consistently giving care below the accepted standard of care and had said nothing to the staff nurse. In these cases, the supervisor and charge nurse would incur some liability for the untoward happening that injured the patient. They knew or should have known that there was a problem and did nothing to protect the patient from harm. A supervisor may also incur liability if he or she continues to employ a nurse who does not meet the requirements of the unit. Any incompetent action by that nurse that results in harm to a patient could then be imputed to the supervisor.

An issue that frequently arises is that of the nurse who is temporarily assigned (float nurse) to a critical care setting. What is the standard of care required of the float nurse, who typically works in other areas of the hospital and who is unfamiliar with the policies and procedures of the unit? Generally speaking, the float nurse is held to the same standard of care required of all critical care nurses if the float nurse accepts responsibility for patients within this very specialized setting. Some points that will help protect the float nurse from liability in these settings include the following. The float nurse's expertise and general nursing skills must be ascertained before the nurse is assigned to a specific patient. Patient assignments should always be made on the basis of the type of care the float nurse is capable of giving. The charge nurse serves as a resource person to answer questions and reassign the float nurse if it becomes apparent that his or her expertise has been exceeded. It is often helpful to "buddy" a float nurse with a regular unit nurse. Implementation of classes to cross-educate nurses to the critical care unit will assist the float nurse to give the same standard of care that is required of all nurses working within the setting.

Sometimes, a pressing issue is the understaffing of patient care units, which potentially creates issues of liability for both administration as well as the individual professional nurse. For administration and supervising nursing personnel, the issue is addressed by the Joint Commission for the Accreditation of Health Organizations (JCAHO), which mandates that hospitals provide qualified practitioners in sufficient numbers to provide patients with optimal nursing care at all times. For individual practitioners, many of the malpractice suits arising from understaffing are filed for failure to adequately monitor patients or for failure to report significant changes in the patient's condition.

Before refusing to accept an assignment because staffing is inadequate or appears to be inadequate at the start of the work shift, remember that the individual nurse will be viewed based on what is reasonable given the circumstances. In other words, a court would first determine what the reasonable, prudent nurse would have done in similar circumstances. For most nurses, this comprises accepting the assignment, taking report, and appraising the nursing supervisor about additional needs for staffing.

The most important factor that courts assess in a staffing situation concerns the nurse's decision-making process, not the possible understaffing issue. For example, in the often-quoted case of *Horton v. Niagara Falls Memorial Medical Center* (1976), the final decision of the court was based on what the staff did to protect the suicidal patient and on how decisions were made, not on whether there was adequate staffing. In that case, a confused patient, trying to jump from a balcony, had first been spotted by construction workers, thus alerting the staff to the seriousness of the patient's mental condition. At the time of his fatal fall from the balcony, staff were busy performing routine duties, one staff member was at supper, and the patient had not been moved to a vacant room nearer to the nurses' station. Thus, the court concluded that it was the nurses and their judgment that was at fault because professional judgment had not been exercised.

Steps can be taken to increase protection from potential liability related to staffing resources. They include:

- Complete a thorough and accurate assessment of all patients, identifying their actual and potential needs and staff skills that are required to meet these needs.
- Assess any additional requirements that are projected (i.e., patients waiting in the emergency room or in the recovery room, and their expected needs).
- Evaluate the available staff's experience, competencies, and education as it relates to the needs of the patients.
- Pool ideas and recommendations from other staff members related to meeting patients' needs.
- Communicate this information to the nursing supervisor, identifying the needs for staff as related to the needs of patients. Consult with the supervisor as to what types of personnel will be needed and at what times to adequately meet the needs of these patients.
- Keep a list of decisions that were made, staff qualifications and assignments, and tasks that were delegated to meet patients' needs.

It is also helpful for staff to be actively involved in the unit's decision-making processes (i.e., committees and task forces). This ensures expert staff input into staffing policies, competency requirements, recruitment of qualified staff, and general unit policies and procedures.

Expanded Roles in Nursing

As the scopes of nursing and of medicine become more intertwined, the question is raised whether critical care nurses are indeed practicing medicine rather than nursing. This question is especially pertinent in situations that require expert clinical skills and immediate action. For example, a patient in the coronary care unit may begin to have frequent paired multifocal premature ventricular contractions (PVCs) and short bursts of ventricular tachycardia. Lidocaine is readily available in its intravenous form. If the coronary care nurse acts on this medical diagnosis by administering 100 mg of lidocaine through a previously ordered and placed intravenous line, is that nurse practicing medicine? Or, as Roth and Daze (1984) contend, is the nurse, who has accepted an increased level of responsibility through advanced education and experience, merely practicing good nursing?

To answer this question, several factors must be addressed. First, the courts have long recognized the duty of a nurse to use individual judgment when caring for patients, and have held nurses accountable for using this independent judgment (*Fraijo v. Hartland Hospital*, 1979; *Cooper v. National Motor Bearing Company*, 1955). This type of court interpretation provides the basis for interpreting the legal liability of expanded nursing roles.

The state nurse practice acts also provide guidance for interpreting acceptable nursing roles and practices. Several of these practice acts now allow nurses to make nursing diagnoses and to treat patients based on these diagnoses. If the acceptable standard, according to the state nurse practice act, is that intensive care nurses may institute appropriate measures to alleviate a patient's presenting symptoms in emergency situations, then to take such measures is considered the practice of nursing, not medicine. A nurse so acting may be said to be making a nursing assessment of the patient and responding accordingly.

Hospital policies and protocols may also give guidance to nurses. If the protocol of the unit is to act on presenting symptoms in emergency situations, then the coronary care nurse is acting within the scope of nursing when he or she administers lidocaine to a patient with multiple PVCs and short runs of ventricular tachycardia. Such hospital protocols should be established by a joint committee representing both nursing and medicine. The joint committee must take the state nurse and medical practice acts into consideration when establishing the protocols. The guidelines for standards of care published by JCAHO should also be reviewed. These published standards are nationally based, and provide evidence of reasonable nursing care. Unit and hospital protocols should be reviewed and updated regularly to allow their recommendations to remain current in the light of changing technology and standards of care and to ensure that they are within the guidelines of the state practice acts for both professions.

The presence of an emergency may give the experienced critical care nurse legal standing to initiate immediate therapy. It is important for the nurse to ensure that the situation is an appropriate emergency based on the following criteria: (1) the patient's life or physical well-being is imminently threatened; (2) the nurse's level of expertise and skill is not exceeded by taking the appropriate actions; and (3) there is no one more qualified in the immediate situation to take control and initiate therapy. A judgment on what is allowable under a true emergency situation is usually based on whether the nurse acted in a reasonable manner and whether sound nursing practices were followed.

In the example cited earlier, the nurse giving lidocaine to a patient with multiple PVCs should document in the patient's record how the patient's life or physical well-being was threatened. In this case, rhythm strips can be permanent documentation of the life-threatening nature of the event. Before proceeding, the nurse must ensure that his or her skills and level of expertise will not be exceeded by taking the actions required. In this example, the nurse was well versed in the effects of lidocaine, the proper dosage, and the rate of administration. Suppose, however, that the patient required immediate oral intubation and the critical care nurse was the only health care provider available. Unless the nurse had received training and had experience in intubating patients, proceeding with the emergent intubation would exceed the nurse's level of expertise.

Another criterion of the emergency situation is that no one more qualified is present to take control and initiate therapy. This means that the nurse may not proceed if a person with more authority under the medical practice act is present. In the lidocaine example, suppose that a medical resident had walked into the coronary care unit just as the nurse was deciding to give the lidocaine, and, when asked, had said to give an alternative drug instead of the lidocaine. If the nurse had proceeded to administer the lidocaine in that situation, he or she could be liable to the charge of practicing medicine without a license. The nurse could be liable even if the patient responded in the desired manner.

Suppose, on the other hand, that no physician was available and the nurse had administered the intravenous lidocaine. Despite the nursing action, the patient experienced cardiac arrest and could not be resuscitated. Does the unfavorable outcome increase the nurse's liability? No. Liability is not increased if the nurse met the three criteria previously stated and acted reasonably and in accordance with sound nursing judgment.

What if the nurse has the necessary skills and expertise but fails to respond to an emergency situation, and the patient dies because immediate action was not taken? Does the failure of the nurse to respond in accordance with his or her education and experience result in liability to the patient's family? Recent literature suggests that such a failure to act might be the basis of a successful malpractice lawsuit against the nonresponding nurse. A California lawsuit indicated that the nurse in such a situation was not acting as a patient advocate and would be held liable for the result (*Bardenilla v. Kaiser Foundation Hospital*, 1988).

Certification is the process of granting recognition to individuals who have attained a specific level of knowledge and expertise in a given field of a profession. Certification may aid nurses in showing that they have the necessary skills and expertise to proceed in an emergency situation. Such advanced credentials may weigh favorably in the event of a subsequent lawsuit.

SPECIFIC LEGAL CONCERNS IN CRITICAL CARE

Critical care nurses face several specific legal concerns in their day-to-day clinical practice. Some of the more commonly encountered concerns include issues relating to patient consent, do-not-resuscitate orders, life support, withdrawal of "ordinary" care, and documentation.

Informed Consent

All patients have the right to be consulted and to give consent before health care providers proceed with ordered treatments and interventions. Once the patient or his or her legal representative gives informed consent, the health care provider may proceed without fear that a lawsuit for battery will be filed.

Informed consent, a concept of the late 1950s, ensures that the patient or his or her legal representative has been given sufficient information on which to base an informed choice. This means that the person has been told about the nature of the proposed therapy or procedure, the risks inherent in the procedure or therapy, any alternatives to the therapy or procedure, and the complications that might arise with the proposed therapy or procedure. Table 3–2 summarizes the criteria that are necessary to establish informed consent. The patient or legal representative, once aware of these facts, may refuse to give consent. At law, such refusal is termed "informed refusal" because the person is fully aware of what is being refused.

Informed consent is usually obtained from the patient or legal representative as a signature on a consent form. Other valid legal means of obtaining consent include oral consent, apparent consent, and implied consent. Oral consent is consent given freely by word of mouth. Unless the institution has a policy that no verbal consent will be accepted, verbal consent is just as valid as written consent. It differs in that verbal consent is more difficult to prove.

Apparent consent is inferred by the patient's conduct. The foundation for apparent consent is an 1899 lawsuit, *O'Brien v. Cunard Steamship Company.* In that case, a female passenger joined a line of people receiving vaccinations. She neither questioned nor refused the vaccination but merely held out her arm for the injection. Examples of apparent consent may be found in most critical care settings today. The reasonable practitioner infers by the patient's actions that the patient both understands and consents to the therapy or intervention.

Implied consent normally is involved in true emergency situations. The patient is unable to make his or her consent known, is incapable of refusing the procedure or therapy, and a delay in providing care would result in loss of life or permanent injury to the patient. The law of implied consent allows the health care provider to proceed in emergency situations as if valid consent had been obtained. Areas of the hospital where implied consent is most often relied on include the emergency department and the critical care unit.

The duty to see that informed consent is obtained before initiating therapy or interventions usually falls on the physician or primary health care practitioner. The nurse's role in this area of the law is still evolving. Some hospitals by policy make the nurse accountable for seeing that the patient or legal representative signs the informed consent form. Other hospitals have policies mandating that valid informed consent forms be obtained by the primary health care provider and that the nurse may sign only as a witness to the patient's signature. Some institutions require a separate signed form for each procedure and therapy, whereas others rely on documentation of the patient's consent in the medical record.

Generally, the nurse is responsible for informing the physician and hospital administration if there is a problem with informed consent. For example, the patient may ask a nurse about the surgical procedure scheduled for the next day. It then becomes clear to the nurse that the patient has not been informed by the physician, the information given was incomplete, or that it was not comprehended by the patient. The nurse now has a duty to see that valid consent is obtained before the scheduled surgery. This may be done by talking with the primary physician, notifying the nursing supervisor, or alerting the operating room staff.

Just as important as conveying necessary information on which to base informed consent is the acquisition of the proper signature on the informed consent form. The competent adult patient presents no problem in this area of the law. For minors and people who are incompetent to sign a consent form, the various states' statutes mandate who may legally sign for the

TABLE 3–2. **Elements of Informed Consent**

The Person(s) Giving Consent Must Fully Comprehend

The procedure or therapy to be performed
The risks involved in the procedure or therapy
The expected or desired outcomes of the procedure or therapy
Any complications or undesired side effects
Alternative therapies, including no therapy at all

The Consent Is Given by One Who Has the Legal Capacity for Giving the Consent

Competent adult
Legal guardian or representative for the incompetent adult
Emancipated, married minor
Mature minor (if applicable)
Parent or legal guardian of a minor
Minor (for diagnosis and treatment of specific disease states or conditions)
Court order

patient and when a court-appointed guardian is necessary.

Durable Power of Attorney for Health Care

A newer concept in substituted decision-making authority is the power of attorney for health care. Legally, this concept allows patients to give valid authorization for informed consent or informed refusal to a person of their choosing. The authorization must be made while the patient is still competent and capable of authorizing a substitute decision maker.

Durable power of attorney for health care has become a popular concept in states that do not recognize family consent laws. Under the current informed consent doctrines, the competent adult is the proper person who either gives or refuses informed consent. What happens, though, if that competent adult sustains a severe head injury in an accident or becomes comatose due to metabolic derangements? Under current law in most states, a relative or friend would be required to obtain the court's permission to become guardian for the now incompetent adult. Using the durable power of attorney for health care doctrine, the competent adult signs a document declaring that a certain named person has his or her authorization to provide informed consent should the adult in question not be able to give consent because of injury, disease, or disability.

Use of the durable power of attorney is common in three situations. Individuals use this method to allow a family member or a significant other to make end-of-life decisions if they should become incompetent. Many nonmarried couples use the durable power of attorney for health care to ensure that if anything should happen to one partner, the other partner would be able to give valid informed consent for necessary medical care. The durable power of attorney for health care is also used by elderly widows or widowers to ensure that one of their children can give valid consent for medical care. In these cases, the durable power of attorney for health care is often used when there are several children and the mother or father desires that a prenamed child serve as his or her substituted decision maker. This designation avoids the chance that family members will be unable to agree on what medical care the parent would have wanted.

To protect health care providers from liability, all durable power of attorney documents should be verified with the hospital's legal department before implementation. This procedure simply verifies the fact that the document is in accordance with state laws. Once a person holding a valid power of attorney for health care is identified, health care providers can avoid allegations of invasion of privacy, breach of confidentiality, and negligence based on lack of informed consent.

Do-Not-Resuscitate Issues

Since the mid-1960s, the use of cardiopulmonary resuscitation has been fairly standard for all hospitalized patients unless other orders exist. The problem at issue for nursing generally has not been whether one could or should obtain a "no code" order for a given patient, but rather whether a verbal order is sufficient and whether the manner in which the code is implemented is correct. In considering the manner in which a "no code" order is obtained, the nurse should first consider the wishes and requests of the competent patient. As with any other consent issue, the competent patient has the right either to accept or refuse resuscitative care should his or her condition deteriorate and such care becomes necessary. Also remember to validate if the incompetent patient initiated other written documentation to indicate whether he or she would accept resuscitative care; such written documentation includes the Durable Power of Attorney for Health Care and Living Wills forms.

It has always been the best course of action for nurses to obtain a written and documented "do-not-resuscitate" order. Most hospital policies require the attending or primary physician to write such an order before resuscitation efforts will be withheld. In the absence of policy or state statute, a verbal "no code" order is legally enforceable, although it may be more difficult to prove the existence of such in a court of law. It is also recommended that written or verbal orders be reevaluated and revalidated every 24 to 72 hours. This measure is thought to ensure that the patient's status will be closely followed by the primary health care provider.

If cardiopulmonary resuscitation is to be initiated, a "slow" or "partial" code, in which the nurses move slowly or fail to respond in a timely manner, should never be permitted. Such actions always fall below the minimum standard of care and open the nursing staff to liability. The patient should either be resuscitated in a competent manner, or a valid "no code" order should be obtained so that no resuscitation efforts need be initiated.

A newer concept, the "chemical" code, is sometimes ordered. This order may be carried out by nurses without fear of liability if this concept is clearly defined in hospital policies and procedures and if the specifics related to the order are clarified when it is written. This type of code involves the use of drug interventions only. If the patient has a respiratory or cardiac arrest, he or she is allowed to die without chest compressions or intubation. Many families feel that this type of intervention prevents unnecessary suffering in their loved one, yet allows the person to die with some dignity.

Living Wills and Natural Death Acts

To ensure that a patient's wishes in regard to life-support measures are respected, living wills and natural death acts have become popular. A living will is a document made by a competent individual and directed to medical personnel and family members regarding the type of treatment the individual wishes to receive if a diagnosis of terminal illness is made. The living will is not necessary if the person, once diagnosed, remains competent, but becomes valid if the person has become incompetent at the time of the terminal diagnosis. Natural death acts, also called medical treatment decision acts, are in reality statutory enactments of living wills.

The great majority of states in the United States have enacted natural death acts. The statutory provisions of these acts vary greatly from state to state. All ensure that practitioners who, in good faith, follow the dictates of the natural death act will be immune from civil and criminal lawsuits. Specific requirements for the living will, for example, witness and signature requirements, and the consequences of noncompliance with the act, vary according to the state or territory. Critical care nurses should become familiar with their state requirements and have these incorporated into their hospital policies and procedures.

Withdrawal of Ordinary Care Measures

Perhaps one of the only areas in medicine in which the state courts have concurred in their opinions is the withdrawal of ordinary care measures. These ordinary care measures include supplemental oxygen therapy, tube feedings, and nutritional and hydration support. The question of removing such ordinary care devices usually arises in the patient who is terminally ill or who is in a persistent vegetative state. Although agreeing that there should be strict guidelines for decision making in this area, all courts have allowed the removal of such devices in the terminally ill and in patients who remain in a persistent vegetative state. Even the President's Commission in 1983 concluded that "no particular treatments—including such ordinary hospital intervention as parenteral nutrition or hydration, antibiotics, and transfusions—are universally warranted and thus obligatory for a patient to accept" (President's Commission, 1983).

When confronted with withdrawal of ordinary care measures, the nurse must ensure that such action concurs with the patient's oral or written requests. For the competent patient, withdrawal of ordinary care measures is governed by the doctrine of informed consent, and the law recognizes the right of the competent patient to refuse or request withdrawal of ordinary care measures (Emanuel & Emanuel, 1993).

The more difficult situations occur with the incompetent patient when the family or significant other requests the withdrawal of ordinary care measures. In these situations, written directives, either a durable power of attorney for health care or living will, will help determine if the requesting individual has the authority to make such a request. Remember, if the incompetent patient has no written directives and there are inconsistencies in the perception of the patient's expressed wishes, or if the directives as written are not valid under state law, then the court may be requested to appoint a legal guardian for the patient and that legal guardian will have the legal power to validly refuse or request removal of ordinary care measures. Courts have also responded by appointing a guardian-ad-litem, whose function is to determine what is best for the patient given the specific circumstances and diagnosis, and then either to give or refuse consent for the removal of ordinary care measures.

Documentation

A major responsibility of all health care providers is the keeping of accurate and complete records of both the care provided and the progress of the patient. A complete and accurate record may be very instrumental in the prevention of successful malpractice suits by a patient against health care providers and their employing institutions. Lawsuits (*Engle v. Clarke,* 1961; *Sheppard v. Kimbrough,* 1984) have been successful for defendants (nurses, physicians, and institutions) when the medical record was introduced to prove exactly what was done for the patient, responses to therapy, and noncompliance with medical and nursing therapies and treatments.

When charting, the critical care nurse should adhere to the following guidelines.

- Document any and all information that is necessary to communicate the patient's status and progress. This documentation should include: initial and subsequent assessment data; descriptions of actual and potential problems; all procedures, treatments, medications, and care given to the patient; all health teaching provided to the patient and family; complete descriptions of the patient's reactions to treatments, procedures, medications, and teaching; and actions taken and person contacted. The information must be presented in such a way that it communicates the patient's progress.
- Document all intermediate steps that were taken—for example, steps taken to clarify an order or to alert a physician about a potential problem. In addition, record all routine assessments and nursing care. The legal system usually believes that if it was not documented, it probably was not done or not observed. Likewise, if something is documented, it was observed or completed and is accurately reflected in the documentation.
- Documentation should be done at the time or immediately after the event that is being recorded. It needs to be correctly dated and timed. It is advisable to place these notes in a chronologic order, remembering that late entries are far superior to no entry at all. Late entries must be timed when entered, but a notation is needed to indicate when the observation or event actually occurred.
- The documentation needs to be written in a legible manner, and be neat and orderly. Documentation that is sloppy or incomplete brings into question the manner of nursing care. If the documentation is haphazard, the inference could be made in court that the nursing care was also haphazard.

Documentation should be printed if needed for legibility.

- Entries into the patient's record should be concise, unambiguous, and accurate. All entries should be free of bias, subjectivity, and personal opinions. The information must be presented in such a way that it communicates the patient's progress. Never allow inaccuracies to be documented. Such inaccuracies place the veracity and character of the documenting nurse in question should the patient subsequently bring a lawsuit. Once placed in question, all actions by that nurse could become suspect.
- It is recommended that nurses use institution-approved abbreviations sparingly because there may be abbreviations that are similar or the same. For instance, MI may stand for both myocardial infarction and mitral insufficiency in the same institution. Never coin new abbreviations, because other personnel may be confused as to the meaning and sometimes, at a later date, the nurse cannot remember what the abbreviation meant.
- Refrain from using medical terminology unless certain that the term is correct. It is better to document in lay terms and be certain that the next health care provider will comprehend the meaning of the documentation and the current patient status.
- Never allow any part of the record to be obliterated. Draw a single line through mistakes, misspellings, and the like. If the documentation is obliterated, it raises the question that there is something to hide. The same question will be asked if parts of the record are recopied. Leave the original documentation on the record, even if stained with blood, vomit, or other fluid.

SUMMARY

This chapter has explored various legal doctrines applicable to critical care, the legal definition of standards of care, the basis for nursing liability, and some specific concerns of critical care nurses. Because individual state laws may vary, the nurse is cautioned to read this chapter in conjunction with his or her individual nurse practice act and to explore the state statutes, particularly in the areas of informed consent, living wills and natural death acts, and personal injury actions. Knowledge of the interplay between nursing and the law not only helps to prevent the nurse from becoming involved in a potential lawsuit, but ensures professional growth and improved clinical practice.

REFERENCES

Bardenilla v. Kaiser Foundation Hospital, Cal-LA Superior Court, (1988).

Bernzweig, E. P. (1990). *The nurse's liability for malpractice: A programmed course* (5th ed.). St Louis: C. V. Mosby.

Cooper v. National Bearing Motor Company, 288 F 2d 581 (California, 1955).

Emanuel, L. L., & Emanuel, E. J. (1993). Decisions at the end of life. *Hastings Center Report, 23*(5), 6–13.

Engle v. Clarke, 346 S.W. 2d.13 (KY, 1961).

Forthofer v. Arnold, 60 Ohio App 436, 21 NE 2d 869 (1938).

Fraijo v. Hartland Hospital, 160 Cal Rept 246, 99 Cal App 3d 331 (1979).

Horton v. Niagara Falls Memorial Medical Center, 51 AD 2d 152, 380 NYS 2d 116 (1976).

Joint Commission for the Accreditation of Health Organizations (JCAHO). (1995). *Accreditation manual.* Chicago: Author.

Napier v. Greenzweig, 256 F 196 (2d Cir, 1919).

President's Commission. (1983). *Deciding to forego life-sustaining treatment.* Washington, DC: Author.

Roth, M. D., & Daze, A. M. (1984). Are nurses practicing medicine in the ICU? *Dimensions of Critical Care Nursing, 3*(4), 230–237.

Sheppard v. Kimbrough, 318 SE 2d 573 (SC App., 1984).

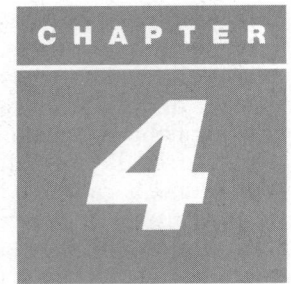

Occupational Health Hazards in Critical Care

Michael A. Salatka

Critical care nurses are exposed to a variety of biologic, physical, chemical, ergonomic, and psychosocial hazards in the hospital environment. There is increasing concern among all health care professionals about the transmission of blood- and air-borne pathogens, musculoskeletal injury, toxic chemicals, radiation, noise, and chemical dependency. This chapter addresses the potential hazards that critical care nurses face and provides recommendations for effective strategies.

INFECTIOUS HAZARDS

There is a potentially high risk of acquiring infectious diseases in the critical care unit. Potential infections may be transmitted by blood or body fluids, by droplets in the air, or by direct contact. Blood-borne pathogens of major concern include human immunodeficiency virus (HIV) and the five identified types of viral hepatitis. Infections transmitted by air-borne particles include cytomegalovirus (CMV), tuberculosis (TB), and meningococcal disease. Direct contact with secretions infected with herpes simplex virus produces herpetic whitlow. There is also potential for exposure to additional pathogens from direct contact with other infected material. Adherence to strict procedures involving body substance isolation (BSI) minimizes the risk of occupational exposure to infectious agents.

HIV Exposure

In a recent study among 860 health care workers who were exposed to the blood of HIV-infected patients from needle-stick injuries or cuts with a sharp object, only 3 were subsequently shown to convert from seronegative to seropositive (Brookmeyer & Gail, 1994). The risk of acquiring HIV infection from a needle-stick injury is less than 1% (Brookmeyer and Gail, 1994; Tokars et al., 1993; Bowden et al., 1993; Gurevich, 1989). Of 103 health care workers exposed to infected blood by contact with mucous membranes or nonintact skin, none was observed to seroconvert (Brookmeyer & Gail, 1994).

Viral Hepatitis Exposure

Several distinct infections are grouped under viral hepatitis. The five identified types include hepatitis A (infectious hepatitis), hepatitis B (serum hepatitis), hepatitis C (posttransfusion non-A, non-B hepatitis), hepatitis D (delta virus), and hepatitis E (enteric non-A, non-B hepatitis).

Both hepatitis A and hepatitis E are transmitted through the oral / fecal route, usually by food and water contaminated with feces. Up to 50% of all people in the United States become infected with hepatitis A by the time they reach adulthood (Marx, 1993). Most people are either asymptomatic or exhibit minimal symptoms and recover in 6 to 10 weeks with lifetime immunity.

Hepatitis B, on the other hand, has a high mortality rate and often progresses to cirrhosis, chronic hepatitis, and liver cancer. The virus is transmitted perinatally and through needle-stick injuries, sexual activity, intravenous drug use, dialysis, and transfusions. Over 300,000 new cases are reported each year. Nearly 200 health care workers die from occupationally acquired hepatitis B each year (Marx, 1993). It is estimated that health care professionals who have not received a hepatitis B vaccination have a 6% to 30% chance of becoming infected with hepatitis B after a needle-stick injury (Lesniak & Parpart, 1994; Gerberding & Henderson, 1992).

Hepatitis D always develops as a coinfection with hepatitis B and may occur either simultaneously during an acute phase of hepatitis B infection or superimposed on a carrier state. The routes of transmission are identical to hepatitis B. Hepatitis D frequently leads to cirrhosis, chronic active hepatitis, and death. The mortality rate is high. Immunity to hepatitis B will provide immunity to hepatitis D.

Hepatitis C is transmitted through needle-stick injuries, blood transfusions, intravenous drug use, parenterally, and by other unidentified means. Studies show that health care workers have a 2% to 3% chance of becoming infected with hepatitis C after a needle-stick injury (Forseter et al., 1993; Marx, 1993; Kiyosawa et al., 1991; Stevens et al., 1990). Approximately 170,000 new cases of hepatitis C are reported each year (Forseter et al., 1993; Marx, 1993). Patients can become chronic carriers. Fifty percent of all cases progress to chronic hepatitis, and 20% of all chronic cases progress to cirrhosis. Hepatitis E has a 10% mortality rate in pregnant women, but is rare in the United States.

Protection From Infections

According to the Occupational Safety and Health Administration (OSHA) standards and Centers for Disease Control and Prevention (CDC) recommendations, employers and employees are responsible for minimizing exposure to all blood and body fluids.

Methods of minimizing exposure to blood and body fluids are known as universal precautions or BSI. Because the infection status of patients is usually unknown, all patients should be considered potential carriers of HIV, viral hepatitis, and other blood-borne pathogens. Recommendations from the OSHA and CDC for health care professionals who are likely to have percutaneous or mucous membrane exposure to blood or body fluids include:

1. Proper handling and disposal of needles or other sharp instruments
2. Use of gloves, masks, gowns, or eyewear when direct contact, aerosolization, or splashing of blood and body fluids is likely
3. Immediate washing of hands and other skin surfaces after contamination with blood or body fluids
4. Removal of personal protective equipment immediately after leaving the patient's room
5. Discarding infectious waste in color-coded, leakproof containers before handling, storing, or transporting
6. Use of effective germicides for cleaning spills of blood or body fluids (1:10 dilution of household bleach)
7. Refraining from rendering patient care or handling equipment when the care provider has open lesions or dermatitis

Special attention should be given to proper handling and disposal of needles because the incidence of needle-stick injury remains high among nurses (Jackson et al., 1986; Bowden et al., 1993; Jenner & Bourke, 1993; Marcus, 1988). Table 4–1 lists situations during which potential needle-stick injuries occur most frequently. Needles should never be recapped, bent, or separated from the syringe. Impervious receptacles for needle disposal should be conveniently placed as close to the bedside as possible.

OSHA has proposed a standard to protect health care workers from exposure to blood-borne pathogens (OSHA, 1992; Gurevich, 1993a; Goldstein & Johnson, 1991). The OSHA blood-borne standard is based almost entirely on procedures for BSI from the CDC (CDC, 1989). Gloves should be worn when handling body fluids or substances such as stool, urine, and vomitus. Hands should be washed, even when gloves are worn, after the gloves are removed (Turner, 1993; Gurevich, 1993a).

TABLE 4–1. **Potential Situations for Needle-Stick Injury**

Carelessness
Inattentiveness or distractions
Fatigue
Stress
Recapping needles after use
Disposal of used needles or receptacles
Administration of parenteral medications
Drawing blood
Failure to ensure adequate restraint of uncooperative patients
Drawing medications from ampules or vials
Cleaning trays after procedures
Working in minimally lighted areas
Inadequate staffing
Handling linens or trash containing uncapped needles
Lack of experience or technique with needles and syringes

Hepatitis B is the only form of viral hepatitis for which a vaccine is available (CDC, 1990). Preexposure vaccination is recommended for all health care and public health workers because of their risk of exposure to blood and body fluids (CDC, 1990). Hospitals and other health care employers are required by law to provide free preexposure hepatitis B vaccinations as a precautionary measure for workers who are exposed to blood (OSHA, 1992; Gurevich, 1993b). The vaccine protects the worker for 5 years or longer. The CDC recommends having an antibody test 5 years after the vaccination (CDC, 1991a). A booster should be given if the antibody level is low. Postexposure management should include a confidential medical evaluation, baseline testing for HIV and hepatitis B, source case testing (if known), serial testing (if appropriate), and posttest counseling sessions (Lesniak & Parpart, 1994).

The benefits of chemoprophylaxis for health care workers exposed to HIV in clinical settings is uncertain. There is no evidence to substantiate the efficacy or safety of postexposure treatment with antiretrovirals such as zidovudine, dideoxytidine, and dideoxyinosine (CDC, 1991b; Tokars et al., 1993; Lesniak & Parpart, 1994; Henderson & Gerberding, 1990; Sachs & Rose, 1990).

The potential risk of acquiring infectious diseases in the critical care unit is high; however, the risk can be reduced to a minimum when the recommended protection procedures are followed. Complying with these guidelines promotes the highest degree of protection for critical care nurses and their patients.

MUSCULOSKELETAL INJURIES

Back pain occurs frequently among nurses despite their training and experience. The frustration and discomfort of back pain decreases patient care efficiency. Determining the cause in individual cases is complex because nurses perform many activities that lead to musculoskeletal strain. Because the continuum of symptoms ranges from minor to severe pain, it is difficult to characterize back injury. Most injuries involve the lumbar muscle group.

Occupational back injury is the second leading injury and illness problem in the United States (National Institute for Occupational Safety and Health [NIOSH], 1985a). Strains and sprains of the lower back account for 50% of all musculoskeletal disorders among American workers (Williamson et al., 1988). Musculoskeletal injuries cost approximately $20 billion per year in lost productivity, employee turnover, workers' compensation, disability, and insurance premiums (McAbee, 1988; McAbee & Wilkinson, 1988). In addition, other hidden factors that inflate the cost of back injury include training and salary for temporary replacement personnel, overtime, repair or replacement of damaged property, legal fees, and claims processing (Charney et al., 1991). The true expense to an individual and organization cannot be assessed easily because other, less tangible costs include psychological trauma from physical pain, fear of recurring back injury, and anxiety about the financial obligations due to loss of work.

Each year, 40,000 nurses report problems with back pain, and over 764,000 working days are lost annually as a result (Garrett et al., 1992). Results from occupational back injury studies conducted over the past 15 years show that low back pain continues to pose a significant problem for nurses. (Garrett et al., 1992; Feldstein et al., 1990; Videman, 1989; Harber et al., 1988; McAbee, 1988; McAbee & Wilkinson, 1988; Arad & Ryan, 1986). Back injuries result in more lost time and wages among nurses who provide bedside care than any other single injury.

Nursing is unique because the occupation involves lilfting and transferring human beings rather than inanimate objects. As Harber and associates (1985) point out, the human body is not a compact mass, and patients are unpredictable. Sudden resisting movements are common in critical care. The proper technique for lifting or transferring a patient may depend on patient size, available staffing, or accessible lifting equipment (Feldstein et al., 1990). Lifting and transferring patients is widely recognized as a risk for back injury, but the incidence and prevalence of patient handling is poorly documented (Charney et al., 1991; Strobbe et al., 1988). Nurses must assess each individual patient separately to minimize the risk of back injury, especially during patient transfers.

Conditions that predispose nurses to musculoskeletal injury can be classified into two major categories: nurse characteristics and hospital environment (Feldman, 1986). Table 4–2 summarizes the factors in these

TABLE 4–2. **Nurse, Patient, and Hospital Environment Factors That Increase the Risk of Back Injury**

Nurse	Patient	Hospital Environment
Physical		
Weak abdominal or lumbar muscles	Mental status	Inadequate staffing
Poor posture	Level of cooperation	Absence of lifting devices
Static actions	Obesity	Stressful environment
Previous or recurrent back problems	Number of catheters, tubes, and lines connected to patient	Inadequate storage space for equipment and furniture
Unequal leg length		Obstacles to patient transfer
Decreased proprioception		Inadequate leg, head, and elbow clearances
Hereditary back problems		Poor workstation design
Headache		Poor equipment design
Fatigue		Heavy "portable" equipment
Obesity		Inadequate work surface height
Poor nutrition		Slippery floor surfaces
Lifestyle		
Smoking, drug use, inadequate exercise		
Emotional		
Stress		
Lack of motivation		
Job dissatisfaction		
Preferential		
Ignoring physical limitations		
Not soliciting assistance from patient or coworkers		
Lack of training and experience with lifting and transfer techniques and devices		
Carelessness		
Restrictive clothing		
Risk-taking behavior		

two categories that increase the risk of back injury. Nurse characteristics are divided into three subgroups: physical, emotional, and preferential. Preferential characteristics include activities that nurses perform on their own volition. The categories and subgroups are not mutually exclusive. For example, stress caused by extremely busy shifts may cause fatigue, which in turn may produce carelessness when lifting or transferring patients.

Physical characteristics such as leg length or heredity cannot be changed. However, emotional and preferential characteristics of nurses can be modified or alleviated to reduce the risk of back injury. Characteristics of the work environment cannot always be altered as effectively as the personal characteristics of the nurse. For example, the height of the bed influences the working posture of the nurse. The optimal bed height for a nurse's performance of routine procedures is usually higher than the desired height for the patient (Pheasant, 1987). Patient comfort and safety may be compromised if a nurse adjusts the bed height to provide protection from back strain. Bed height will be different for each nurse depending on the procedure to be performed and the height of the nurse. Maintaining ergonomically correct equipment for each nurse at any given time is problematic, especially when more than one nurse is assigned to a patient.

Patient contact activities in critical care frequently require nurses to maintain an awkward, stressful posture for an extended period of time. These actions may be particularly stressful on the lower back because the same muscle groups are involved throughout the activity (Haber et al., 1987a, 1987b).

TABLE 4–3. **Methods for Minimizing Back Injury**

Personal

Strengthen abdominal and lumbar muscles through regular exercise
Perform stretching exercises before shift
Maintain good posture
Maintain proper nutrition
Solicit assistance from coworkers and patients
Use mechanical devices for lifting
Review knowledge of proper lifting techniques
Alleviate risk-taking behaviors
Wear nonrestrictive clothing
Lift no more than 35% of your body weight
Raise or lower beds to facilitate good posture
Minimize stress

Environmental

Design workplace layout using ergonomic principles
Provide adequate staffing
Conduct preemployment strength testing and evaluation
Keep lifting devices accessible
Conduct regular in-service training (include techniques for use of transfer boards, bed scales, back supports)
Consult or hire a nursing ergonomic specialist
Redesign storage areas
Maintain clear paths for walking and moving furniture or equipment
Install nonslippery floor surfaces

Minimizing Back Injury

It is important to recognize and develop ways to minimize stressful postures. Methods for minimizing back pain are listed in Table 4–3. A combination of personal and environmental modifications should be implemented to be effective (Addington, 1994; Steinbrecher, 1994; Feldstein et al., 1993; Glazner et al., 1993; Karwowski, 1993; Charney et al., 1991; Jensen, 1991; Triolo, 1989). No single method will completely prevent or control low back pain.

Nurses are not selected by physical ability, and job strength requirements are rarely addressed in critical care. Conducting preemployment strength tests to determine whether the nurse can perform strenuous nursing tasks is feasible (Keyserling et al., 1980). Patient assignments could then be matched according to the physical strength of the nurse.

Because the number of low back injuries among nurses has not shown any appreciable decline, researchers question the effectiveness of training programs that focus on safe lifting procedures (Harber et al., 1985, 1987a, b). As Cato and colleagues (1989) point out, perhaps training programs are more effective when used in conjunction with ergonomic job analysis and job-specific training.

Traditional techniques for lifting may not be best for all nurses because they do not use the lumbar muscle group and completely ignore the principles of leverage with balance. Consistent use of the lumbar muscles in synchronization with other muscle groups increases strength and reduces the risk of injury. Training programs should provide information on correct postures to minimize muscle strain, exercises to strengthen the back, and proper lifting techniques. A well trained "nursing ergonomic consultant" who is sensitive to each nurse's physical ability could provide services and assistance to individuals who are at risk of low back injury (Harbor et al., 1985).

The use of lifting devices and back supports is important for minimizing back injury. The most commonly used devices in critical care are bed scales, transfer boards, and draw sheets. When lifting devices and back supports are used in conjunction with proper lifting techniques and procedures, there may be a corresponding reduction in lost time due to back injury (Charney et al., 1991).

Although patient comfort and safety are the highest priorities in hospital care, nurses should be encouraged to develop an understanding of basic ergonomic concepts and to analyze their own safety at the bedside and work station. Personal habits are not easily modified, but an awareness and effort to maintain a safe environment in the workplace is important. Efforts should be made to minimize back injury away from the workplace as well. Application of these principles will reduce musculoskeletal injury, increase productivity, improve health and safety, and provide a higher quality of patient care.

CHEMICAL HAZARDS

There are a variety of chemicals, including many therapeutic agents, in the critical care setting that pose a hazard to nurses. There are at least 179 known skin and eye irritants and 135 carcinogenic, mutagenic and teratogenic agents used by hospital workers (NIOSH, 1985b).

Critical care nurses occasionally handle antineoplastic agents. This class of pharmaceuticals inhibits tumor growth by disrupting cell division and killing actively growing cells. Antineoplastic drugs that may be dispensed in critical care include cerubidine, methotrexate, adriamycin, cyclophosphamide, doxorubicin, vincristine, and ribavirin. Nurses may be exposed to antineoplastics while mixing or administering the drug, cleaning spills, or discarding excreta of patients who have received chemotherapy during the previous 48 hours.

The potential for mutagenic, carcinogenic, or teratogenic effects from exposure to antineoplastics is well documented (McDevitt et al., 1993; Valanis et al., 1992; Stucker et al., 1986, 1990; McDiarmid & Egan, 1988; Selevan et al., 1985; Hemminki et al., 1985). There are three primary routes of exposure: inhalation of an aerosolized drug; direct contact with eyes, mucous membranes, or skin; and accidental oral ingestion. Nurses must be aware of the possibility of low-level dermal exposure from contaminated work surfaces (McDevitt et al., 1993).

Given that most nurses are women and the major effects from exposure to antineoplastic drugs involve reproductive outcomes (menstrual cycle changes, fetal loss, and congenital malformations) (Valanis et al., 1992), the importance of complying with the guidelines set forth by OSHA is crucial. The guidelines recommend the use of laminar airflow biologic safety cabinets (BSC) during drug preparation (OSHA, 1986; Yodaiken, 1986). Research studies indicate that nurses who prepare antineoplastics in large hospitals are significantly less likely to use laminar flow hoods than pharmacists in the same setting (Valanis et al., 1992; McDevitt et al., 1993). If access to a BSC is limited, nurses who prepare antineoplastics should insist that the hospital provide convenient access to a BSC. Gowns and double pairs of latex gloves should be worn during preparation and administration. Intravenous bags should be spiked and lines should be purged in the preparation area or BSC. Contaminated articles, including needles, gloves, gowns, alcohol swabs, or any other materials that may become contaminated during preparation, should be placed in leak-proof containers within the BSC.

Mechanisms for identifying potentially hazardous chemicals in the critical care unit are needed (McDiarmed et al., 1991). Health care facilities that prepare, administer, or dispose of antineoplastic agents should provide education and training on proper handling procedures. Surveillance programs to ensure compliance with hospital policies are recommended.

RADIATION HAZARDS

Portable radiography and fluoroscopy are routine bedside procedures in critical care. Radiation exposure carries the potential for both short-term and long-term biologic effects. Familiarity with the types and sources of radiation, the maximum permissible doses for occupational exposure, and ways in which the risk of exposure to ionizing radiation can be minimized will protect nurses from harmful biologic effects.

When atoms and molecules undergo change, energy is released in the form of heat or light. This energy is referred to as radiation. The three common forms of radiation used in hospitals are alpha particles, beta particles, and gamma rays (x-rays). Alpha particles travel only inches in the air and are stopped by healthy skin tissue. Beta particles may travel several feet before they are absorbed by a thin piece of metal or wood. Gamma rays travel hundreds of feet and have great penetrating power (Fig. 4–1).

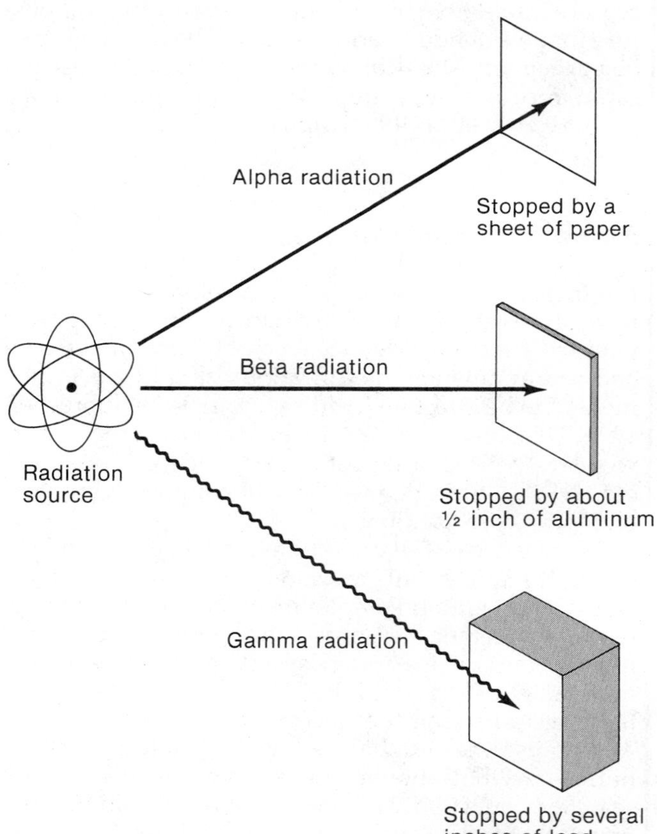

FIGURE 4–1. Relative penetrating power of alpha, beta, and gamma radiation.

The penetrating ability of each type of radiation varies. Harmful effects to human tissue result largely from the energy absorbed by the cells (Bomberger & Dannenfelser, 1984). The amount of energy absorbed or deposited in human tissue determines the total biologic effect. The rem (roentgen equivalent man or mammal) is the unit that represents the biologic dose used to estimate potential damage caused by radiation.

There are three potential sources of scattered radiation in the critical care environment: portable x-ray equipment, fluoroscopic equipment, and diagnostic or therapeutic radionuclides. Scattered or "secondary" radiation occurs after the primary radiation beam or application passes through matter. All x-ray and fluoroscopic examinations generate some scattered radiation. Alpha, beta, and gamma rays exist in the isotopes used for external and internal radiation treatments. The amount of secondary radiation emitted by patients receiving radionuclide therapy depends on the organ in which it is localized, the dosage, the elapsed time after injection, patient size, and the distance from the patient (Jankowski, 1984). Critical care nurses should pay particular attention to the levels of secondary radiation received from patients who receive radionuclides because the number of hours they spend in contact with individual patients is greater than the contact with individual patients in other types of nursing units. The body fluids of patients who have received injections of radioactive substances contain significant amounts of radioactivity (Huda et al., 1989). Compliance with BSI procedures, as described earlier, is crucial.

The National Council on Radiation Protection and Measurements (NCRPM) establishes maximum permissible dose levels of radiation for occupational exposure. The current recommendation is 5000 mrem per year for employees who are likely to be exposed to ionizing radiation during the course of their work (NCRPM, 1980). According to the Code of Federal Regulations, radiation dosimetry badges are required when nurses receive doses in excess of 1250 mrem every 3 months.

Actively proliferating cells, such as the reproductive organs, are highly sensitive to radiation. Teratogenic or carcinogenic effects may occur when an embryo, fetus, or male germ cell is irradiated. Studies show that ionizing radiation damages the gonads, alters genetic material, reduces fertility, and induces spontaneous abortion (Hunt, 1978).

Female nurses represent the largest number of potentially pregnant women exposed to low-level radiation (Burks et al., 1982). Nurses of childbearing age must be aware of the hazards of radiation because there is increased potential for damage to a developing embryo during the first month of pregnancy. This is especially important because women generally do not realize they are pregnant at this stage of fetal development. The Nuclear Regulatory Commission standards recommend that pregnant women do not receive more than 500 mrem of radiation during gestation.

Exposure to scattered radiation can be minimized in three ways: by *time,* by *distance,* and by *shielding.* Protection from secondary radiation can be enhanced by completing nursing procedures in the shortest possible time without compromising good clinical practice. Penetrating radiation rapidly decreases as the distance from the source increases. For example, a single film taken by a portable x-ray machine at 1 meter will produce approximately 0.06 mrem of scattered radiation. At 2 meters, the amount is indistinguishable from background radiation existing in the natural environment (Herman et al., 1980).

The third method of minimizing exposure to secondary radiation is the use of protective shielding. Lead screens or aprons 5 mm in lead-equivalent thickness should be used during x-rays and fluoroscopy to protect the reproductive organs. Protective shielding is particularly important when working with patients who have received radiopharmaceuticals. Leaded glasses and a thyroid shield are recommended during procedures involving elevated levels of radiation, such as angioplasty (Patterson et al., 1985).

Further epidemiologic studies on the effects of long-term occupational exposure to ionizing radiation are needed (Dowd, 1990). Until more data are available, pocket dosimeters and film badges for monitoring exposure to radiation should be used by nurses who are likely to receive more than 1250 mrem in a 3-month period. Radiation safety committees should periodically monitor nurses for proper radiation safety techniques. Radiation safety instruction should be included in hospital orientation programs for new staff and repeated annually for all new employees. Finally, hospital policies regarding the use of radioactive substances and equipment should be reviewed and revised to include methods for minimizing radiologic hazards to staff.

NOISE

Noise pollution and occupational hearing loss is a significant problem in the United States. Approximately 15 million Americans are currently exposed to hazardous noise levels on the job (Harrison, 1989). More than 8 million workers suffer from some degree of noise-induced hearing loss (Tortora, 1987). No studies have been conducted to determine whether critical care nurses experience a higher rate of hearing loss than the general population.

Prolonged exposure to noise of great intensity can be distracting and can prohibit mental concentration. Psychological responses to noise include increased annoyance and irritability, impaired judgment, and altered perception (Hilton, 1987; Gasaway, 1985). Factors that influence the impact of noise on nurses include the intensity or loudness of the sound, type of sound, distance from the source, frequency and duration of exposure, individual perception of sound, stress level, and age.

The decibel (dB) is used to express the sound level

associated with noise measurement. The OSHA standard states that an employer shall administer a hearing conservation program whenever employee noise levels are equal to or exceed an 8-hour, time-weighted average of 85 dB (Code of Federal Regulations, 1985). The International Noise Council recommends that sound levels in patient care areas not exceed 45 dB during the day and 20 dB at night (Hansell, 1984).

Background noise occurs in most work environments. Critical care areas, however, are remarkably loud. One study reported that sound levels in four critical care units were as high as 77 dB, which is comparable to a hospital cafeteria at noon (Redding et al., 1977). Other studies have reported sound levels greater than 50 dB over a 24-hour period, with a number of noises exceeding 70 dB (Hilton, 1987; Hansell, 1984). Noise levels of this magnitude increase the tendency for nurses to become densensitized to noise levels in the critical care environment. Table 4–4 lists the most frequent sources of noise in critical care units.

Elimination or reduction of unnecessary sources of noise is essential. Controlling noise in the critical care environment is beneficial for patients (Topf & Davis, 1993), and may help minimize staff fatigue and reduce errors. Increasing nurses' sensitivity to the level of noise on the unit will assist in developing appropriate interventions to decrease or control unwanted sound. Education about the effect of noise on the ear is key for developing successful hearing conservation programs.

TABLE 4–4. **Sources of Noise in the Critical Care Unit**

Equipment or Alarms

Ventilators
Monitor alarms
Chest drainage systems
Special therapy beds
Infusion pumps
Intraaortic balloon pumps
Suction machines
Cooling blankets
Cooling fans in computers and monitoring equipment
Personnel beepers
Computer printers

Extraneous Sound

Telephones
Televisions and radios
Doors
Intercoms and pagers
Sinks and toilets
Refrigerators
Ice machines
Bedrails
Squeaking equipment (chairs, drawers, carts)
Personnel activity (rustling papers, binders)

People

Staff conversations
Patients
Visitors

Hearing loss usually occurs over a long period of time, without pain, and cannot be corrected by medical or surgical treatments (Harrison, 1989).

Everyone should be encouraged to speak softly. Patients report that staff conversations and activity are the most disturbing noise (Hansell, 1984). Discussions among nurses and other hospital staff can generate sound levels as high as 90 dB (Hilton, 1987). Normal conversational tones measure between 56 and 60 dB. As Hilton (1987) points out, whispering may be appropriate at night. Conversations between staff should be limited to patient care concerns, especially at the bedside. A system of constant reminders, such as signs near areas of concentrated noise, may be helpful (Lindenmuth et al., 1980).

Nurses must take an active role in developing effective strategies to reduce noise. Strict compliance with the standards of occupational exposure to noise will enhance awareness of noise reduction among the staff. Nurses should be responsible for evaluating and purchasing equipment such as ventilators, monitors, and balloon pumps. Equipment that produces excess noise can be modified by the manufacturer to meet noise reduction standards. Nursing consultants should assist in the development of plans for construction or remodeling of critical care units (Dracup, 1988).

Noise can also be reduced by introducing sound-absorbing materials into the architectural design of the unit. Carpeted walls and floors in the nursing station and patient care areas will have a dramatic effect on reducing noise. Each unit should have a soundproof section in which nurses and physicians can confer or spend break periods without disturbing patients (Dracup, 1988). Utility rooms with sinks, refrigerators, and ice machines should be partitioned separately from patient care areas. Alarm parameters should be set appropriately to avoid false alarms.

Suppression of noise is an important element of occupational safety and health in the critical care environment. Nurses and other hospital staff must develop an appreciation for a quiet working environment. Keeping the noise level as low as reasonably possible is advantageous to nurses and beneficial to patients.

CHEMICAL DEPENDENCY

Chemical dependency occurs among workers in every occupation. Alcohol and drug abuse is the third leading health problem in the United States. Over one-half of the 13 million people who are addicted to alcohol or drugs are employed (National Institute of Alcohol Abuse and Alcoholism, 1990). Until recently, information about chemical dependency as a disease among health care workers was scarce. Although there are still no reliable estimates of the number of nurses who suffer from chemical dependency, the problem continues to surface nationwide (Scanlon, 1991; Floyd, 1991; Sullivan et al., 1988).

Chemical dependency is a chronic, permanent, and progressive disease. The symptoms are predictable and can be fatal if left untreated (Catanzarite, 1992). This disease is characterized by individuals with a physical or psychological dependency on drugs or alcohol that affects their personal, social, economic, and employment situations.

Nurses are exposed to constant stress and human suffering in the critical care environment. Many factors may influence the amount and types of stress felt by the critical care nurse. In addition to patient care issues, inadequate staffing, difficult patient assignments, high patient acuity, excessive overtime, and difficult relationships with peers, management, or physicians may cause work overload and insomnia. When these factors are coupled with personal situations at home, feelings of low self-esteem, or chronic tension, fatigue, and anxiety, nurses may initiate chemical use to relax or sleep.

Without healthy coping skills, a nurse may secretly turn to drugs or alcohol for emotional and spiritual support. Drugs that are commonly abused include cocaine, marijuana, alcohol, narcotics, amphetamines, and tranquilizers. It is not uncommon for critical care nurses who are chemically dependent to use drugs that are frequently found in the unit. For example, meperidal hydrochloride (Demerol) is often abused by impaired nurses who work in critical care settings (Selbach, 1990).

Nurses should be observant of colleagues who display signs of impairment or chemical dependency. Table 4–5 lists personal and professional indicators of chemical dependency in the workplace (Clemmer, 1990; Hyman et al., 1991). Personal indicators include changes in physical appearance, personality, and behavior. Professional indicators include changes in work performance. Supervisors and coworkers should be particularly attentive to the nurse who exhibits a combination of personal and professional indicators. Occasionally, supervisors and coworkers deny that a colleague is chemically dependent by making excuses, tolerating abusive behavior, or completing assignments for the impaired nurse (Selbach, 1990). It is the duty of coworkers to confront the impaired nurse or bring the matter to the attention of a peer counseling program or Employee Assistance Program (EAP) at the hospital (Baywood, 1990). An impaired nurse may cause harm to patients by working while under the influence of drugs or by diverting prescribed medication intended for the patient. Taking action to prevent a nurse from harming a patient or from inflicting further self-harm is crucial.

TABLE 4–5. **Indicators of Chemical Dependency**

Personal Indicators

Increased irritability, suspicion or paranoia
Increased nervousness, anxiety, or depression
Frequent symptoms of "hangover" including
- Red or watery eyes
- Alcohol breath
- Tremors
- Flushed skin color

Sudden changes in dress (towards sloppiness or neatness)
Forgetfulness
Feigning illness

Professional Indicators

Excessive use of sick leave, disability, or workers' compensation
Avoidance of supervisors or co-workers
Lessened quality or quantity of work
Increased incident reports
Increased tardiness or early departures
Extended lunch hours
Frequent trips off the unit
Increased accidents
Disruptive conduct
Increased use of employee health services
Failure to adhere to hospital policies or procedures

From Clemmer, J. (1990). Dealing with chemical dependency. *Nursing Management, 21*(3), 90; and Hyman, Z., Haughey, B. P., Dittmar, S. S., et al. (1991). Chemical impairment in colleagues: Perceptions of western New York nurses. *Journal of the New York State Nurses Association, 22,* 6–10.

The professional, emotional, and economic costs of chemical dependency to the critical care unit, the health care facility, and to society are enormous. These costs include increased use of health insurance benefits, decreased productivity, increased absenteeism, poor patient relations, increased overtime, reduced staff morale, poor judgment, and increased mistakes and accidents. Mistakes or accidents can lead to expensive litigation and damage to the reputations of both the organization and the nurse. If a patient is injured in some way by an intoxicated nurse, a case can be made for negligence. When an impaired nurse diverts medication from the patient for personal consumption, the nurse is stealing from both the patient and the institution that purchased the drugs (Ensor, 1991). Tampering or falsifying patient records to obtain drugs may result in malpractice awards (American College of Legal Medicine, 1990).

Effective treatment for the impaired nurse must be flexible and individualized. Many factors affect the nurse's treatment plan, including his or her physiologic state, family situation, motivation, gender, religious background, ethnicity, and available resources (Selbach, 1990). In addition, a nurse must have continuous access to appropriate support and recovery mechanisms (Sisney, 1993). The supportive role of peers and the assistance they can provide during recovery cannot be understated. Peers are important for helping the impaired nurse into treatment and preventing recidivism (Catanzarite, 1992).

Interventions should be initiated through confidential conversations and include referrals for treatment. Initial treatment includes therapy and education. Membership in a 12-step recovery program is beneficial as a self-care mechanism and as a support group. In addition, participation in aftercare programs and regular meetings with a recovery counselor are highly recommended. Employee Assistance Programs (EAPs) are being incorporated into more hospitals. An EAP is a system designed to provide professional care to employees whose job performance is affected by personal problems (Callery, 1994; Lachman, 1988).

The ultimate goal of intervention and treatment is the nurse's reentry into practice. Understanding the relapse process and developing effective relapse prevention plans is essential (Gorski, 1987). The vast majority of chemically dependent health care workers who undergo a treatment program have a successful recovery, and most of those who seek treatment return to work as productive employees (Lachman, 1988).

CONCLUSION

Nurses must examine the potential hazards in the critical care work environment. An awareness of hazards, their causes, and solutions sets the stage for developing appropriate occupational safety programs. Nurses with research skills and a familiarity with the tasks, procedures, and physical environment of the critical care unit have an opportunity to study and contribute to the understanding of occupational hazards and ways to prevent them. Nurses should become more involved in ensuring that policies and procedures on the unit and in the hospital are consistent with nationally recommended standards. It is the role of critical care nurses to promote and develop occupational safety programs for their own benefit and for the benefit of their colleagues and patients.

REFERENCES

Addington, C. (1994). All the right moves: A program to reduce back injuries in OR nurses. *Association of Operating Room Nurses Journal, 59,* 483–488.

American College of Legal Medicine. (1990). *Legal medicine: Legal dynamics of medical encounters* (pp. 218–231). St. Louis: C. V. Mosby.

Arad, D., & Ryan, M. D. (1986). The incidence and prevalence in nurses of low back pain: A definitive survey exposes the hazards. *Australian Nursing Journal, 16,* 44–48.

Baywood, T. (1990). Substance abuse and obligations to colleagues. *Nursing Management, 21,* 40–41.

Bomberger, A. S., & Dannenfelser, B. A. (1984). *Radiation and health.* Rockville, MD: Aspen Publishers.

Bowden, F. J., Pollett, B., Birrell, F., & Dax, E. M. (1993). Occupational exposure to the human immunodeficiency virus and other blood-borne pathogens. *Medical Journal of Australia, 158,* 810–812.

Brookmeyer, R., & Gail, M. H. (1994). *AIDS epidemiology: A quantitative approach.* New York: Oxford University Press.

Burks, J., Griffith, P., McCormick, K., et al. (1982). Radiation exposure to nursing personnel from patients receiving diagnostic radionuclides. *Heart and Lung, 11,* 217–220.

Callery, Y. C. (1994). Chemical abuse rehabilitation for hospital employees: Examination of benefit usage when referred by an employee assistance professional. *American Association of Occupational Health Nursing Journal, 42,* 67–75.

Catanzarite, A. M. (1992). *Managing the chemically dependent nurse: A guide to identification, intervention & retention.* Chicago: American Hospital Publishing.

Cato, C., Olson, D. K., & Studer, M. (1989). Incidence, prevalence, and variables associated with low back pain in staff nurses. *American Association of Occupational Health Nursing Journal, 37,* 321–327.

Centers for Disease Control and Prevention (CDC). (1989). Guidelines for prevention of transmission of human immunodeficiency virus and hepatitis B virus to health-care and public safety workers. *Morbidity and Mortality Weekly Report, 38,* 3–37.

Centers for Disease Control and Prevention (CDC). (1990). Protection against viral hepatitis. Recommendations of the Immunization Practices Advisory Committee (ACIP). *Morbidity and Mortality Weekly Report, 39* (RR-2), 10–16.

Centers for Disease Control and Prevention (CDC). (1991a). Hepatitis B virus: A comprehensive strategy for eliminating transmission in the United States through universal childhood vaccination. *Morbidity and Mortality Weekly Report, 40,* 1–25.

Centers for Disease Control and Prevention (CDC). (1991b). Public Health Service statement on management of occupational exposure to human immunodeficiency virus, including considerations regarding zidovudine postexposure use. *Morbidity and Mortality Weekly Report, 39,* 1–11.

Charney, W., Zimmerman, K., & Walara, E. (1991). The lifting team: A design method to reduce lost time back injury in nursing. *American Association of Occupational Health Nursing Journal, 39,* 231–234.

Clemmer, J. (1990). Dealing with chemical dependency. *Nursing Management, 21*(3), 90.

Code of Federal Regulations. (1985). *Hearing standard and amendments.* Vol. 29, Part 19-10.95.

Dowd, S. B. (1990). Radiation safety and the nurse. *The Journal of Practical Nursing, 40,* 31–33.

Dracup, K. (1988). Are critical care units hazardous to health? *Applied Nursing Research, 1,* 14–21.

Ensor, J., & Giovinco, G. (1991). Ethical issues related to chemical dependency. *Imprint, 38,* 85–87.

Feldman, R. (1986). Hospital injuries. *Occupational Health and Safety, 55,* 12–17.

Feldstein, A., Valanis, B., Vollmer, W., et al. (1993). The back injury prevention project pilot study: Assessing the effectiveness of back attack, an injury prevention program among nurses, aides, and orderlies. *Journal of Occupational Medicine, 35,* 114–120.

Feldstein, A., Vollmer, W., and Valanis, B. (1990). Evaluating the patient-handling tasks of nurses. *Journal of Occupational Medicine, 32,* 1009–1013.

Floyd, J. A. (1991). Nursing students' stress levels, attitude toward drugs, and drug use. *Archives of Psychiatric Nursing, 5,* 46–53.

Forseter, G., Wormser, G. P., Adler, S., et al. (1993). Hepatitis C in the health care setting: II. Seroprevalence among hemodialysis staff and patients in suburban New York City. *American Journal of Infection Control, 21,* 5–8.

Garrett, B., Singiser, D., & Banks, S. M. (1992). Back injuries among nursing personnel: The relationship of personal characteristics, risk factors, and nursing practices. *American Association of Occupational Health Nursing Journal, 40,* 510–516.

Gasaway, D. C. (1985). Hearing loss compensation: Stemming the tide with conservation programs. *National Safety and Health News, 132,* 1.

Gerberding, J. L., & Henderson, D. K. (1992). Management of occupational exposures to bloodborne pathogens: Hepatitis B virus, hepatitis C virus, and human immunodeficiency virus. *Clinical Infectious Diseases, 14,* 1179–1185.

Glazner, J. K., Yaloff, F., Forsyth, M., et al. (1993). Back health: Development of a risk assessment tool. *American Association of Occupational Health Nursing Journal, 41,* 289–292.

Goldstein, L., & Johnson, S. (1991). OSHA Bloodborne Pathogens Standard. *American Association of Occupational Health Nursing Journal, 39,* 182–188.

Gorski, T., & Miller, M. (1987). *Staying sober: A guide for relapse prevention.* Independence, MO: Herald House / Independent Press.

Gurevich, I. (1989). Acquired immunodeficiency syndrome: Realistic concerns and appropriate precautions. *Heart and Lung, 18,* 107–112.

Gurevich, I. (1993a). Enterically transmitted viral hepatitis: Etiology, epidemiology, and prevention. *Heart and Lung, 22,* 370–372.

Gurevich, I. (1993b). Hepatitis part II: Viral hepatitis B, C, and D. *Heart and Lung, 22,* 450–456.

Hansell, H. N. (1984). The behavioral effects of noise on man: The patient with intensive care unit psychosis. *Heart and Lung, 13,* 59–65.

Harber, P., Billet, E., Gutowski, M., et al. (1985). Occupational low-back pain in hospital nurses. *Journal of Occupational Medicine, 27,* 518–524.

Harber, P., Billet, E., Lew, M., et al. (1987a). Importance of non-patient transfer activities in nursing-related back pain: I. Questionnaire survey. *Journal of Occupational Medicine, 29,* 967–970.

Harber, P., Billet, E., Shimozaki, S., et al. (1988). Occupational back pain of nurses: Special problems and prevention. *Applied Ergonomics, 19,* 219–224.

Harber, P., Shimozaki, S., Gardner, G., et al. (1987b). Importance of non-patient transfer activities in nursing-related back pain: II. Observational study and implications. *Journal of Occupational Medicine, 29,* 971–974.

Harrison, R. K. (1989). Hearing conservation: Implementing and evaluating a program. *American Association of Occupational Health Nursing Journal, 37,* 107–111.

Hemminki, K., Kyyronen, P., & Lindbohm, M. L. (1985). Spontaneous abortion and malformations in the offspring of nurses exposed to anaesthetic gases, cytostatic drugs, and other potential hazards in hospitals, based on registered information of outcome. *Journal of Epidemiology and Community Health, 39,* 141–147.

Henderson, D., & Gerberding, J. (1990). Prophylactic zidovudine after occupational exposure to the human immunodeficiency virus: An interim analysis. *Journal of Infectious Diseases, 160,* 321–327.

Herman, M. W., Patrick, J., & Tabrisky, J. (1980). A comparative study of scattered radiation levels from 80-kVp and 240-kVp x-rays in the surgical intensive care unit. *Radiology, 137,* 552–553.

Hilton, A. (1987). The hospital racket: How noisy is your unit? *American Journal of Nursing, 87,* 59–61.

Huda, W., Bews, J., & Sourkes, A. M. (1989). Occupational doses in radiation oncology in Manitoba—1980 to 1986. *Health Physics, 57,* 521–527.

Hunt, V. (1978). Occupational radiation exposure of woman workers. *Preventive Medicine, 7,* 294–310.

Hyman, Z., Haughey, B. P., Dittmar, S. S., et al. (1991). Chemical impairment in colleagues: Perceptions of western New York nurses. *Journal of the New York State Nurses Association, 22,* 6–10.

Jackson, M. M., Dechairo, D. C., & Gardner, D. F. (1986). Perceptions and beliefs of nursing and medical personnel about needle-stick handling practices and needle-stick injuries. *American Journal of Infection Control, 14,* 1–10.

Jankowski, C. (1984). Radiation exposure of nurses in a coronary care unit. *Heart and Lung, 13,* 55–58.

Jenner, R. K., & Bourke, M. K. (1993). Needlesticks, infection control and nurse liability. *National Medical Legal Journal, 4,* 6–7.

Jensen, R. C. (1991). Prevention of back injuries among nursing staff. In W. Charney & J. Schirmer (Eds.), *Essentials of modern hospital safety* (Vol. 2) (pp. 237–258). Chelsea, MI: Lewis Publishers.

Karwowski, W. (1993). Back injury at work: A new beginning for prevention. *Ergonomics, 26,* 747–748.

Keyserling, W. M., Herrin, G. D., & Chaffin, D. B. (1980). Isometric strength testing as a means to controlling medical incidents on strenuous jobs. *Journal of Occupational Medicine, 22,* 332–336.

Kiyosawa K., Sodeyama, T., Tanaka, E., et al. (1991). Hepatitis C in hospital employees with needlestick injuries. *Annals of Internal Medicine, 115,* 367–369.

Lachman, V. D. (1988). The chemically dependent nurse. *Holistic Nursing Practice, 2,* 41.

Lesniak, L. P., & Parpart, C. F. (1994). Postexposure requirements and counseling issues resulting from the bloodborne pathogens standard. *American Association of Occupational Health Nursing Journal, 42,* 130–134.

Lindenmuth, J. E., Breu, C. S., & Malooley, J. A. (1980). Sensory overload. *American Journal of Nursing, 8,* 1456–1458.

Marcus, R. (1988). CDC Cooperative Needlestick Surveillance Group: Surveillance of health care workers exposed to blood from patients with the human immunodeficiency virus. *New England Journal of Medicine, 319,* 1118.

Marx, J. F. (1993). Viral hepatitis: Unscrambling the alphabet. *Nursing 93, 23,* 34–41.

McAbee, R. R. (1988). Nurses and back injuries. *American Association of Occupational Health Nursing Journal, 36,* 200–209.

McAbee, R. R., & Wilkinson, W. E. (1988). Back injuries and registered nurses. *American Association of Occupational Health Nursing Journal, 36,* 106–112.

McDevitt, J. J., Lees, P. S. J., & McDiarmed, M. A. (1993). Exposure of hospital pharmacists and nurses to antineoplastic agents. *Journal of Occupational Medicine, 35,* 57–60.

McDiarmed, M. A., & Egan, T. (1988). Acute occupational exposure to antineoplastic agents. *Journal of Occupational Medicine, 30,* 984–987.

McDiarmed, M. A., Gurley, H. T., & Arrington, D. (1991). Pharmaceuticals as hospital hazards: Managing the risks. *Journal of Occupational Medicine, 33,* 155–158.

National Council on Radiation Protection and Measurements (NCRPM). (1980). *Basic radiation protection criteria.* NCRP Report No. 39. Washington DC: Government Printing Office.

National Institute for Occupational Safety and Health (NIOSH). (1985a). *Program of the National Institute for Occupational Safety and Health, FY 1985 program plan.* Publication No. 85-109. Atlanta, GA: Centers for Disease Control and Prevention.

National Institute for Occupational Safety and Health (NIOSH). (1985b). *Report of the Division of Surveillance, Health Evaluations and Field Studies Task Force on hospital worker health.* Cincinnati, OH: Centers for Disease Control and Prevention.

National Institute of Alcohol Abuse and Alcoholism. (1990). *Seventh special report to the U.S. Congress on alcohol and health.* Rockville, MD: U.S. Department of Health and Human Services.

Occupational Safety and Health Administration (OSHA). (1992). Occupational exposure to bloodborne pathogens: Final rule. *Federal Register, 56,* 64175–64182.

Occupational Safety and Health Administration (OSHA), Office of Occupational Medicine. (1986). *Work practice guidelines for personnel dealing with cytotoxic (antineoplastic) drugs.* Washington, DC: Department of Labor.

Patterson, W. B., Craven, D. E., Schwartz, D. A., et al. (1985). Occupational hazards to hospital personnel. *Annals of Internal Medicine, 102,* 658–680.

Pheasant, S. (1987). Some anthropometric aspects of workstation design. *International Journal of Nursing Studies, 24,* 291–298.

Redding, J. S., Hargest, T. S., & Minsky, S. H. (1977). How noisy is intensive care? *Critical Care Medicine, 5,* 275–276.

Sachs, H., & Rose, D. (1990). Zidovudine prophylaxis for needlestick exposure to human immunodeficiency virus: A decision analysis. *Journal of General Internal Medicine, 5,* 132–137.

Scanlon, W. (1991). *Alcoholism and drug abuse in the workplace.* New York: Praeger.

Selbach, K. H. (1990). Chemical dependency in nursing: Identifying and helping the troubled nurse. *Association of Operating Room Nurses Journal, 52,* 531–542.

Selevan, S. G., Lindbohm, M. L., Hornung, R. W., & Hemminki, K. (1985). A study of occupational exposure to antineoplastic drugs and fetal loss in nurses. *New England Journal of Medicine, 313,* 1173–1178.

Sisney, K. F. (1993). The relationship between social support and depression in recovering chemically dependent nurses. *Image, 25,* 107–112.

Steinbrecher, S. M. (1994). The revised NIOSH lifting guidelines: Application in a hospital setting. *American Association of Occupational Health Nursing Journal, 42,* 62–66.

Stevens, C., Taylor, P. E., Pindyck, J., et al. (1990). Epidemiology of hepatitis C virus: A preliminary study in volunteer blood donors. *Journal of the American Medical Association, 263,* 49–53.

Strobbe, T., Plummer, R., Jensen, R., & Attfield, M. (1988). Incidence of low back injury among personnel as a function of patient lifting frequency. *Journal of Safety Research, 19,* 21–25.

Stucker, I., Caillard, J. F., Collier, R., et al. (1990). Risk of spontaneous abortion among nurses handling antineoplastic drugs. *Scandinavian Journal of Work Environment, and Health, 16,* 102–107.

Stucker, I., Hirsch, A., Bastoe-Sigeac, I., et al. (1986). Urine mutagenicity, chromosomal abnormalities and sister chromatid exchanges in lymphocytes of nurses handling cytotoxic drugs. *International Archives of Occupational and Environmental Health, 57,* 195–205.

Sullivan, E., Bissell, L., & Williams, E. (1988). *Chemical dependency in nursing: The deadly diversion.* Menlo Park, CA: Addison-Wesley Publishing.

Topf, M., & Davis, J. E. (1993). Critical care unit noise and rapid eye movement (REM) sleep. *Heart and Lung, 22,* 252–258.

Tokars, J. I., Marcus, R., Culver, D. H., et al. (1993). Surveillance of HIV infection and zidovudine use among health care workers after occupational exposure to HIV-infected blood. *Annals of Internal Medicine, 118,* 913–919.

Tortora, M. L. (1987). Noise induced hearing loss: Prevention in the workplace. *American Association of Occupational Health Nursing Journal, 35,* 271–273.

Triolo, P. K. (1989). Occupational health hazards of hospital staff nurses: Part II: Physical, chemical and biological stressors. *American Association of Occupational Health Nursing Journal, 37,* 274–279.

Turner, J. (1993). Hand-washing behavior versus hand-washing guidelines in the ICU. *Heart and Lung, 22,* 275–277.

Valanis, B., Vollmer, W. M., Labuhn, K., et al. (1992). Antineoplastic drug handling protection after OSHA guidelines: Comparison by profession, handling activity, and work site. *Journal of Occupational Medicine, 34,* 149–155.

Videman, T. (1989). Patient handling skill, back injuries, and back pain: An intervention study in nursing. *Spine, 14,* 148–156.

Williamson, K., Turner, J., Brown, K., et al. (1988). Occupational health hazards for nurses: Part II. *Image, 20,* 162–168.

Yodaiken, R. E. (1986). OSHA work practice guidelines for personnel dealing with cytotoxic drugs. *American Journal of Hospital Pharmacy, 43,* 1193–1204.

UNIT

2

PATIENT AND FAMILY CARE

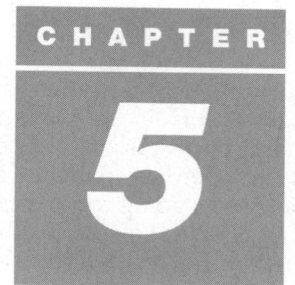

Psychosocial Needs of Critically Ill Patients

Suzanne Clark

The Critical Care Nurse shall gather pertinent physical, social, psychological, and spiritual data from the patient, significant others, and other health team members.

AMERICAN ASSOCIATION OF CRITICAL-CARE NURSES
Standards for Nursing Care of the Critically Ill

MEETING PSYCHOSOCIAL NEEDS IN CRTICIAL CARE: THE CHALLENGE

Patients with diseases or traumatic injuries that lead to admission to a critical care unit almost always face severe disruptions in a previously balanced existence. The patient responds to the challenges created by the illness, the treatment, and the environment to regain some sense of equilibrium. Nurses interact with patients and their situations in ways that assist them to regain control and to integrate the experience into their lives.

The *Standards for Nursing Care* developed by the American Association of Critical-Care Nurses (1989) clearly support a holistic approach to the care of the critically ill patient. A holistic approach is based on the premise that disease is never the result of one causative agent or condition but rather the result of a complex interplay between people and their physical, emotional, cultural, social, and spiritual situations. To care optimally for patients, nurses must assess all aspects of the patient's response to his or her illness and hospitalization, identify the physiologic and psychosocial concerns that may influence the patient's course, and use a variety of interventions targeted to the specific problems identified.

This chapter discusses a framework for critical care nurses to use in identifying psychosocial needs and specific interventions to meet those needs. The nursing diagnosis, Ineffective Coping, is addressed throughout the chapter.

HOLISTIC NURSING IN A TECHNICAL ENVIRONMENT

The most important relationships in the critical care setting are between nurses and patients. Nurses spend more time with the patient than any other caregiver. They are responsible for the environment in which the patient is cared for, identifying and mitigating unsafe and harmful stimuli. They carefully assess physiologic parameters to maintain or achieve homeostasis. They implement plans of care and alert physicians to rapidly changing situations that need their attention. They anticipate problems and respond as first-line defenses in life-threatening emergencies.

At the same time, to optimize patient care, nurses must practice in a holistic way, considering data from the psychological, cultural, and spiritual realm to formulate successful nursing interventions. However, multiple forces in health care and the critical care environment work together to deter nurses from attending to the psychosocial needs of patients.

Traditional views of health and medicine developed in the seventeenth and eighteenth centuries separated the mind and the body and defined disease as a malfunction at the molecular level (Benner & Wrubel, 1989, p. 30). This view opposes nursing's holistic vision and does not provide solutions to the illness experience that engulfs individuals and has far-reaching effects on their lives.

Second, the explosion in computerized and automated monitoring systems that provide minute-to-minute data on multiple physiologic responses, although freeing nurses from former repetitive tasks, has created significant challenges for nurses, who must now manage both patients and machines (Sinclair, 1988). The plethora of equipment may not only create a mechanistic, dehumanizing atmosphere, but build a physical barrier that prevents meaningful patient–nurse contact (Halm & Alpen, 1993).

Finally, hospitals are adapting to the current uncertainty in the health care delivery system by restructuring the work environment. This redesign has sometimes included changes in skill mix or replacing registered nurses with unlicensed ancillary personnel (Ketter, 1994). In some cases, nurses in the critical care setting may have limited direct patient contact, but work through others who provide a portion of direct patient care (Dracup & Bryan-Brown, 1993).

Counteracting the multiple forces that could inhibit

nurses from attending to the psychosocial needs of patients is the recent interest in the relationships of genetic, biologic, psychological, sociocultural, and ecologic factors to physical health and disease. Increasing numbers of researchers in the fields of neurophysiology, neuropsychology, and neuroimmunology strive to find the connective links between psychological and biologic responses (Reichlin, 1993; Solomon, 1993).

Research linking psychosocial factors has taken many directions: the impact of sociocultural factors on disease etiology; personality and behavior patterns and their impact on disease onset and outcomes; the effect of exposure to stress and disease onset; the impact of stress on the immune system; the individual resources that mediate the stress–illness connection; and behavioral interventions that influence a person's response to illness and treatment (Berkman & Syme, 1979; Fawzy et al., 1990; Holmes & Rahe, 1967; House et al., 1988; Quinn & Strelkauskas, 1993). These directions have been influenced by, among other things, researchers being unable to explain in a conclusive way why some people become ill and others remain well even when they have been exposed to the same pathogens. These studies formalize and add credence to what any experienced nurse already knows: that the course of illness is heavily influenced by the individual's psychological and social milieu. Each nurse, working with each patient, must find a way through the maze of equipment and the stress of nursing in today's environment to develop a therapeutic relationship that combines technical proficiency with caring. This process is a complex interplay of rational and intuitive thinking that often takes years to refine (Benner, 1984).

How can nurses develop the level of expertise that allows them to practice holistically and intuitively, almost effortlessly combining technical proficiency and caring? In terms of understanding and meeting psychosocial needs, this means having a model that charts the territory of human responses to illness and directs the nurse's attention to specific patient behaviors. There are a variety of models that attempt to simplify the complexities of the human response to severe illness. A model based on the concepts of adaptation and stress–coping research is a practical starting point for critical care nurses (Lazarus, 1966; Selye, 1956).

STRESS–COPING FRAMEWORK (Fig. 5–1)

Stressors

Stressors are situational demands that disrupt smooth functioning and interfere with understood meanings in one's life. Noise, lack of sleep, social isolation, enforced immobility, pain from procedures, and poor communication with staff are recognized as stressful almost universally by critically ill patients (Dracup, 1987). Other conditions are interpreted as stressful only by people whose personal meanings of the situation are disrupted.

Cognitive Appraisal

Richard Lazarus has been a contributor to stress and coping theory. Central to his theory is the cognitive process of appraisal. With regard to stressors that confront them in the critical care setting, patients ask themselves, "What is happening or going to happen?" and "How bad (or good) can it be?" (Lazarus & Folkman, 1984). These questions are not necessarily clear and deliberate but rather automatic and rapid, and may be outside the patient's awareness. This evaluation of the situation is primary to the concept of stress when stress is defined as an interaction between person and environment. Variation in responses to situations of apparently objective danger, such as an earthquake or admission to a critical care unit, is explained by an individual's unique appraisal of the circumstances.

How critically ill patients appraise the stressors associated with admission to a critical care unit is influenced by their past experiences with illness, disfigurement, death, and dependency; cognitive and emotional development; personal traits; philosophy of life; and the type of coping responses available.

Appraisal of threat also depends on how much is at risk for the person. The perception of a stressor as threatening depends on how dangerous the threat appears to be in relationship to a patient's feeling of competence to intervene. The relationship between the size of the threat and the person's perception of resources is known as the threat:resource ratio (Lazarus & Folkman, 1984).

Affective or Physiologic Response

If the answer to the question, conscious or subconscious "How bad can this be?" confirms that something terrible is happening or about to happen, the patient usually experiences feelings of threat or vulnerability (the affective response) as well as some physiologic response (Breier et al., 1987). This mind–body connection is the "fight or flight" response. In this context, stress is defined as a response. Seyle used the term general adaptation syndrome (GAS) to describe the body's stress response to a variety of stressors (Selye, 1956).

The body's response can be activated by a variety of sources, including biologic sources, such as infection, trauma, and drugs; environmental sources, such as noise, heat, and cold; and psychological sources, such as fear, anxiety, loss, and change in life circumstances. The response to these stressors, all common to critically ill patients, is a complex interaction between hormonal and neurologic factors that influences the function of specific organs. For example, an increase in circulating epinephrine and norepinephrine, as well as the release of mineralocorticoids, triggers major cardiovascular effects. The resulting increase in heart rate, vasoconstriction, myocardial contractility, and sodium

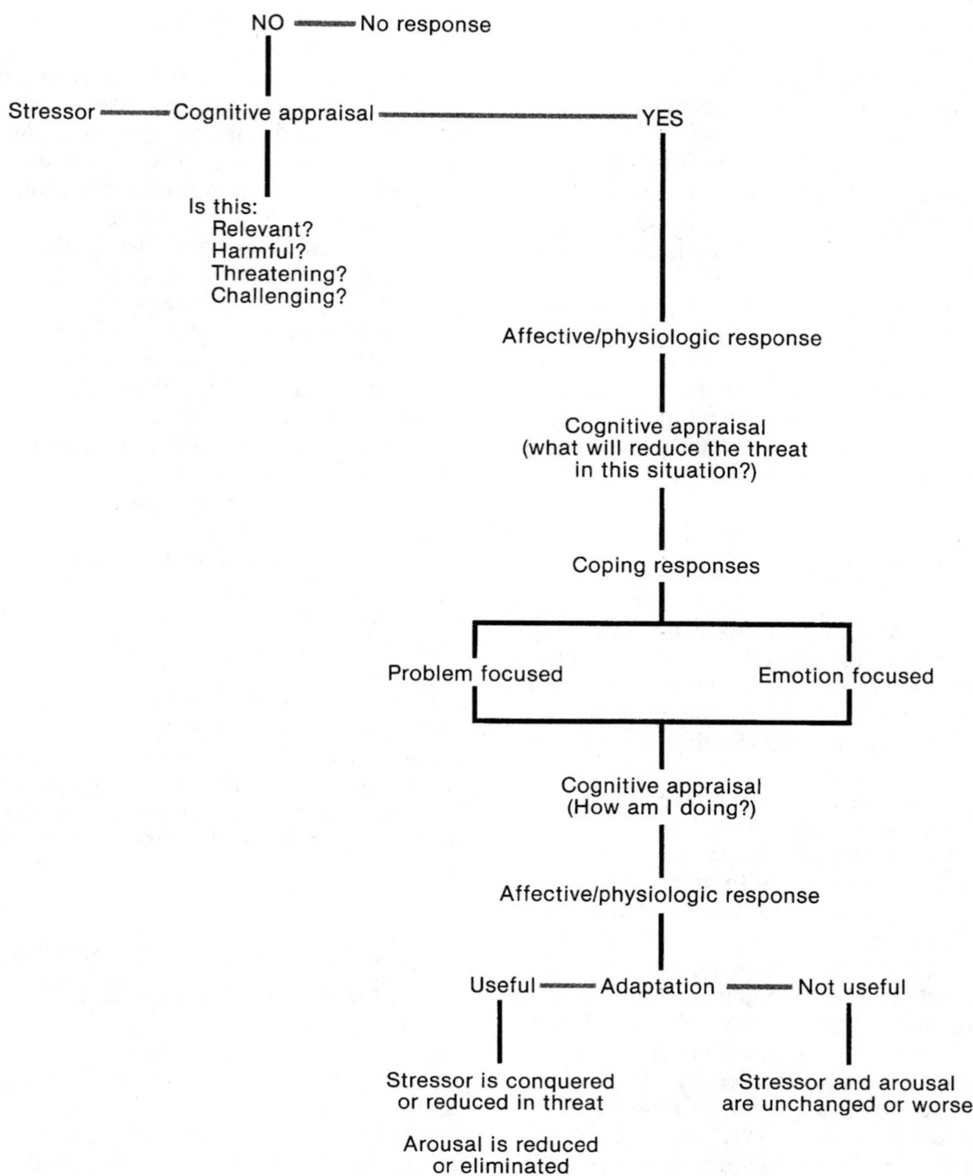

FIGURE 5–1. Stress–coping framework. (From Lazarus, R. S. (1966) *Psychological stress and the coping process.* New York: McGraw-Hill, Inc. Reproduced with permission of McGraw-Hill, Inc.)

and water retention all serve to increase myocardial oxygen consumption and the work of the heart. These responses are relevant to any critically ill patient because of the link between emotional reactions, physiologic response, and significant cardiac dysrhythmias. Emotional stress has also been implicated in platelet aggregation in the small vessels of the heart, suggesting a relationship between acute myocardial infarction and severe stress that results from catecholamine release (Patterson et al., 1994).

Other potentially deleterious effects of the stress response are related to immunologic changes (Reichlin, 1993). Although current thinking about the relationship between behavior and the immune system is far from definitive, research demonstrates a causal relationship between stress and susceptibility to disease. Behavioral factors can affect both cell-mediated and hormonal immunity through the release of corticosteroids and catecholamines, which in turn inhibit immune responses (Nguyen, 1991; Houldin et al., 1991).

There is some evidence that exposure to severe stressors that overpower an individual's coping ability can lead to immunosuppressive changes (Calbrese et al., 1987; Bartrop et al., 1977; Stein, 1989; Kiecolt-Glaser & Glaser, 1992). Also, the direct effects of the cortisol that is released during the stress response can retard wound healing. The inflammatory response can be blocked, granulation response and antibody formation are inhibited, and the supply of oxygen and nutrients to the wound site is limited by peripheral vasoconstriction (McCarthy et al., 1991). Inhibited wound healing can increase the length of the recovery period and hospital stay, contributing to feelings of hopelessness in the patient, which may further inhibit the immune response.

Emotional disturbance may be experienced in a variety of ways. Feelings of turmoil, agitation, anxiety, fear, depression, helplessness, hopelessness, worthlessness, or frustration are common responses (Weisman, 1987).

Nurses cannot directly experience a person's perceptual and appraisal processes. Rather, nurses see the affective and physiologic responses in their patients and recognize them as the end result of a response to a threat. The oberved physiologic responses and dysphoric feelings are clues to the fact that something is wrong and needs to be assessed further.

Coping and Adaptive Responses

Most people who perceive conditions as threatening to their psychological equilbrium will attempt to restore some sort of balance in their lives. Feelings of vulnerability and physiologic responses lead the involved person to question what will reduce the threat, given the circumstances and known resources. Again, this question is not necessarily conscious but occurs almost automatically and instantaneously in stressful circumstances. People evaluate the threat–resource ratio and make their best attempt to cope with or master the demands that are felt to be straining or overtaking their usual resources. Coping is an ongoing process of cognitive and behavioral efforts to manage internal or external demands that are seen to be taxing or exceeding one's personal resources (Lazarus & Folkman, 1984).

Coping behaviors can be problem-focused, directed toward the stressor in some way, or emotion-focused, directed toward mitigating or altering one's emotional response (Benner & Wrubel, 1989, p. 62; Lazarus, 1966, pp. 258–319; Weisman, 1987, p. 287). Problem-focused options include:

- Gathering more information
- Identifying alternative solutions
- Letting someone else solve the problem
- Talking the problem over with others who have had the same problem
- Consciously deciding to do nothing

Some types of emotion-focused coping are:

- Practicing relaxation techniques
- Altering the way one thinks about a situation
- Making light of a situation
- Putting the problem out of one's mind
- Using drugs and food
- Becoming angry or depressed

Some forms of coping have elements of both approaches. Gathering information can be a way to solve problems as well as a way to support a decision already made or add to feelings of control (Lazarus & Folkman, 1984, p. 285).

The use of defense mechanisms, which are primarily unconscious mental processes, is also a way to control anxiety and internal conflict, and is a form of emotion-focused adaptation (Lazarus, 1993). The use of defenses is an attempt to avoid direct confrontation with a stressor. In trying to maintain a sense of balance and limited vulnerability, patients using defense mechanisms distort and deny the full impact of stressors or painful emotions.

In summary, as coping and adaptative responses are initiated, the patient has an opportunity to reappraise the situation. Cognitive appraisal should not be mistaken for an entirely conscious process because it often takes place below the patient's level of awareness. Affective and physiologic responses are reevaluated to see if further response is needed. Coping and adaptive responses occur over time, with ongoing reappraisal of the situation and personal responses, until adaptation or neutralization of the stressor occurs. Adaptation can be defined as useful when patients experience reduced feelings of threat and vulnerability and physiologic arousal is reduced or eliminated. Adaptation using harmful strategies can occur, however, and not be useful to the patient. For example, some patients use withdrawal to protect themselves from feeling overwhelmed. Although this response may reduce anxiety, the stressors remain unchanged, and the patient has cut himself or herself off from available support.

STRESS–COPING FRAMEWORK: PLANNING NURSING CARE

The stress–coping model provides a unified way of approaching the challenge of meeting the psychosocial needs of critically ill patients. Nurses can identify appropriate interventions and approaches by understanding the relationships of the model's components to each other and how they combine to influence a patient's ability to cope (Clark, 1988, p. 293).

Identifying and Reducing Known Stressors for Critically Ill Patients

One of the ways in which nurses can make an impact on patients' responses to being sick is to identify stressors inherent in the critical care setting and the illness experience, and either remove them when possible or lessen their impact if complete elimination is not realistic.

A critical illness involving hospitalization in a critical care unit by itself creates predictable stressors (Moos & Tsu, 1979; Wilson, 1987). Pain, separation from support systems, fear, and anxiety related to death are all aspects of an illness that can lead to feelings of vulnerability. The critical care environment itself can lead to decompensation and ineffective coping.

UNIVERSAL STRESSORS

Pain

A major stressor for critically ill patients is the experience of or the threat of pain. In Wilson's study of patients in a surgical intensive care unit, pain was ranked as the number-one stressor (Wilson, 1987). Because of the physiologic and psychological ramifications of pain, it is an important stressor for nurses to attend to.

Autonomic nervous system responses to acute pain include increased heart rate, blood pressure, and depth and rate of respirations (Puntillo, 1988). These responses can result in pulmonary and cardiovascular complications. Intolerable pain may lead to depression or suicidal ideation. Pain contributes to feelings of powerlessness and increases susceptibility of other stressors that might otherwise be tolerated.

Aside from the careful administration of appropriate analgesics, there are three major independent nursing approaches that are important in the control of pain: relaxation techniques, information sharing, and a commitment to pain relief.

RELAXATION TECHNIQUES. The relaxation response provides opposition to the sympathetic nervous response. It includes a decrease in heart rate, oxygen consumption, respiratory rate, and muscle tension (Benson, 1975). In one early study, a very simple relaxation technique was used: The patient was instructed to lower the jaw, keep the tongue quiet in the bottom of the mouth, relax the lips, breathe slowly and rhythmically in an inhale, exhale, and rest pattern, and refrain mentally from forming words. The experimental group used the technique during postoperative ambulation. This group reported less pain and used less narcotics in the first 24-hour period after surgery (Flaherty & Fitzpatrick, 1978).

This and similar relaxation techniques are relatively easy to explain and use. They are not meant to replace analgesia administration, but rather serve as an adjunct to pharmacologic interventions. These techniques not only reduce pain but increase feelings of personal control. Increased feelings of personal control were found to reduce stress in a study of male patients admitted to a critical care unit (Lindquist et al., 1985). Helping patients cope with pain is an example of a combined problem-focused and emotion-focused intervention.

INFORMATION SHARING. Radwin (1987), in a summary article on patients with acute pain, cites several studies demonstrating that patients who learn about the potential pain and discomfort of upcoming procedures as well as methods to reduce pain experience less subjective pain. In some cases, patients have been able to decrease the amount of analgesia used and even the length of the hospital stay. Teaching patients about the procedural and sensory components of upcoming treatments can reduce pain as well as increase feelings of self-control, and is an example of facilitating problem-focused coping.

HOLISTIC APPROACH. Patients who have been cared for by nurses who approach patients holistically have also experienced more pain relief than control group patients who were given only routine pain medications (Radwin, 1987). Interventions employed in the holistic approach included

- Identifying pain relief as a mutual goal
- Addressing all physical and psychological factors that might be contributing to the pain
- Offering alternatives for pain control such as analgesia, relaxation, or distraction
- Allowing the patient to choose among alternatives whenever possible

Despite growing attention to pain management, recent studies have shown that, in many cases, pain is still inadequately managed. MaCaffery and Ferrell identified several misconceptions that have resulted in inadequate pain management by nurses (McCaffery & Ferrell, 1991a, 1991b, 1992a, 1992b, 1992c). Gujol (1994), in a survey of pain assessment and management practices among critical care nurses, found that nurses' skepticism regarding patients' reports of pain led to poor judgment in management of pain. She also found that unrealistic concerns and inadequate knowledge regarding addiction, respiratory depression, and physical dependence adversely affected nurses' pain relief interventions. Puntillo (1994), in a study of pain related to endotracheal suctioning and chest tube removal in critically ill surgical patients, concluded that the related pain was not well managed by nursing staff.

Attending to pain addresses several points in the stress–coping cycle. It decreases the size of the threat while at the same time increasing feelings of control and confidence in one's ability to cope. It provides a problem-oriented coping strategy that may at the same time increase feelings of self-esteem and confidence. It may decrease the sympathetic nervous system response to pain, thus influencing the physiologic response to stress. It may make other stressors more tolerable. Although life-threatening events or hemodynamic instability may compete with nurses' attention, helping patients cope with pain can have far-reaching implications for patient care outcomes. Attending to pain relief is a powerful strategy whereby nurses have to address both the physiologic and psychological needs of their patients.

Separation from Support Systems

Admission to a critical care unit forces separation between patients and their families, interrupting an important source of support. This separation may cause emotional distress, but growing evidence demonstrates that disrupted social networks may contribute to disease processes. For example, patients who had a myocardial infarction and lived alone had a significantly higher rate of recurrent cardiac events in the first 6 months after discharge than those who lived with others (Case et al., 1992). In another study of 194 patients with myocardial infarctions, lack of emotional support was significantly associated with a higher death rate at 6 months (Berkman et al., 1992). Emotional support has also been shown to influence immune function by enhancing natural killer cell activity in breast cancer patients (Levy et al., 1990).

The connection between social networks and illness is not entirely clear, but support systems may, in some way, serve as buffers between risk factors and disease (Syme, 1984). It is possible that disrupted social connections affect resistance to disease, increasing vulnerability to a wide range of pathologic processes.

Family members, too, believe that it is important to spend time with patients. In numerous studies with families of critically ill patients, a consistently identified need is to have freedom of access to the patient (Molter, 1979; Leske, 1992; Kleinpell & Powers, 1992; Ward et al., 1990). Despite the potential positive impact of social support on health, as well as the importance that families place on being with patients, nurses have been reluctant to include families in patient care (Hickey, 1988).

Researchers have found that nurses and families differ in their attitudes and beliefs about visiting. Visiting practices are not always in concert with visiting policies. Nurses make independent decisions about visiting based on their beliefs about the harm or benefit patients might receive from the visit, on the disruption the visitors might cause to the smooth functioning of the unit, and on the harm or benefit the visit might have on the family (Kirchoff et al., 1993). Often the needs of patients and families seem to be in conflict with the needs of the nursing staff. However, the current pressures to reduce health care costs often mean earlier transfers out of the critical care setting and earlier hospital discharges. It is essential that families become more involved with visiting and learning aspects of care.

Nurses need to find ways to maintain the important connections in patients' lives. Open visiting policies may be one such intervention. Henneman and Cardin (1989) studied the effect of open visiting hours on nursing staff. Most nurses polled felt that an open visiting policy was beneficial for both patients and families, and they did not feel that the flexible visiting interfered with patient care.

Ward and colleagues (1990) developed a formal intervention program for the families of cardiac surgery patients. The program included an educational program for the nursing staff as well as giving information and support to the family member visiting in the intensive care unit. The nurses followed an intervention checklist of behaviors (Table 5–1). Family members who received the intervention program reported higher levels of need satisfaction and lower anxiety levels than those family members who did not receive the intervention.

TABLE 5–1. **Visiting Intervention Checklist**

Patient: ______ Date ______ Shift: ______

Please complete for each visitation period:

______ Introduce yourself to each family member
______ Ask or confirm relationship of family member to patient
______ Give some specific facts in understandable terms about patient's condition, including specific changes since last visit
______ Ask the family member if he or she has any questions.
______ Indicate concern for the patient
______ Ask about the family member's condition, i.e., "How are you doing? Are you getting any sleep? Did you find the cafeteria? Do you have a place to stay tonight?"
______ Give or confirm the phone number for the family to call the ICU
______ Reassure the family member that it is okay to call and inquire about the patient's condition
______ Take or confirm the family's phone number where they can be reached. Show family members where the phone number is written on the Kardex
______ Reassure family member that he/she would be called at home in the event of a major change in the patient's condition
______ Discuss transfer plans, whether possible or known
______ Ask about plans for next visit
______ Allow family member to visit as frequently as possible
______ Give family member ICU visiting policies
______ Give family member booklet on critical care

From Ward, C. R., Constancia, R. E., & Kern, L. (1990). Nursing interventions for families of cardiac surgery patients. *Journal of Cardiovascular Nursing*, 5(1), 34–42.

Incorporating families in the plan of care may have an impact on the disease process, the patient's feelings of self-esteem, and the family's ability to cope, which may, in turn, positively affect the nurse's stress level and the smooth functioning of the unit. Promoting family support for patients is a way to increase the resource aspect of the threat : resource ratio.

Anxiety and Fear Related to Death

When facing a life-threatening illness, patients confront the reality of death and characteristically experience intense anxiety, which triggers profound defensive behavior. Interventions that are appropriate to help the patient adapt to this threat include giving information, providing hope, helping to maintain relationships with family, and allowing the patient to talk about his or her feelings. The type of intervention and support needed depends on the type of dying pattern: uncertain death at an uncertain time, certain death at an unknown time, or certain death at a known time (Glaser & Straus, 1968).

For some patients, such as those with uncomplicated myocardial infarctions, the possibility of death is present but not certain. In these cases, rehabilitative interventions are usually emphasized. Patients, families, and staff use education about postdischarge lifestyle changes as a way of coping with the uncertain prognosis.

There is a greater possibility of death for patients who are experiencing acute exacerbations of a chronic illness. Nurses are often uncertain as to whether interventions should be directed toward plans for living or for dying. It is helpful for patients to talk about the full range of their feelings, both the possibility of death and the potential for survival. This helps them to talk about their fears while at the same time supporting their hope for recovery.

For patients for whom there is no hope for survival, death will occur within a specified period of time. Some patients will be too exhausted to share their feelings at this time. Others may need to find meaning and purpose in their experience. Nurses can assess a patient's readiness to talk about his or her feelings by asking open-ended questions such as: "What is your understanding of what is happening to you?" or, "How are you feeling about what is happening to you?" Patients' responses will reflect their readiness to grieve actively.

ENVIRONMENTAL STRESSORS: NOISE

Acute care settings are particularly stressful because of, among other things, excess noise (Zimmerman, 1988) (see Chapter 8). Noise is an important stressor because it is related to a startle response that elicits increases in heart rate, metabolism, and overall oxygen consumption. Both lymphocyte and granulocyte functions are reduced during sleep deprivation (Palmblad et al., 1979; McCarthy et al., 1991). Noise is also an important factor in sleep disruption and consequent episodes of delirium (Hansell, 1984; Easton & MacKenzie, 1988). In a study conducted by Helton and colleagues (1980) a 33% increase in mental status changes occurred in patients who were rated as severely sleep deprived.

In studies done in acute care settings, the noise levels were consistently above the limits set by the International Noise Council (Bentley et al., 1977; Aitkin, 1982). Noise comes from two primary sources—equipment and staff. One study showed that noise levels in the critical care unit were comparable to the hospital's cafeteria at noon and slightly less noisy than the boiler room (Redding et al., 1977). Another study concluded that the noise levels produced by conversations between nursing and medical personnel were louder than those made by equipment (Woods & Falk, 1974). Staff communication was found to be loud and unrelated to patient care (Hilton, 1987; Griffin, 1992).

Noise is an important environmental stressor that can interfere with sleep, rest, and healing. Sleep disturbance can lead to perceptual alterations that contribute to increased anxiety and physiologic response. It is also a stressor that can be easily attended to and altered by nursing personnel.

DISEASE-SPECIFIC STRESSORS

One of the most important questions to ask when assessing a patient's coping response is, What is it that the patient must cope with? Each disease poses unique threats, follows a relatively predictable course, makes certain demands on patient and family, and creates particular limitations and possibilities.

The behavioral responses and coping strategies used by the patient depend in large part on the situational demands created by this illness trajectory. A person coping with the acute onset of an illness for the first time will respond differently than a patient who has an acute exacerbation of a chronic illness. For example, the symptoms may be more frightening because the patient already understands their implications, or they may be less frightening because the patient is familiar with them. Different phases of an illness present different challenges. The period between the appearance of symptoms and the diagnosis presents multiple ambiguities. During the treatment phase, patients may have more knowledge of the implications and potential outcomes of the illness. At first, patients must cope with uncertainty, whereas later they must cope with the reality of the illness. If the illness has remissions and exacerbations or downward spirals, patients must learn to balance wellness with illness, hope with despair.

Recent trends in nursing research demonstrate an interest in identifying those aspects of specific situations that patients rate as stressors. One study looked at the incidence and severity of stressors associated with coronary artery bypass surgery (Carr & Powers, 1986). Results showed that there were significant differences between nurse and patient perceptions of stress. Stress for both hospital- and illness-related items was rated significantly higher by the nurse than the patient. The situations that were ranked as more stressful by the patients than the nurses are listed in Table 5–2. The situations that were ranked more stressful by the nurses than the patients are listed in Table 5–3. This study not only identifies illness-specific stressors but emphasizes the point that if nurses make assumptions about patients' experiences and base their interactions on inaccurate information, patient concerns will not be addressed. For example,

TABLE 5–2. **Cardiac Surgery Stressors Ranked Greater by Patients than Nurses***

Stressor	Patient Ranking	Nurse Ranking
Resuming previous lifestyle	2.0	7.0
Absence from home/business	5.0	14.0
Increasing activity	7.0	20.0
Sharing room with another patient	9.0	18.5
Needing pain medications	10.0	26.0

*1 = Highest stressor.

Data from Carr, J. A., & Powers, M. J. (1986). Stressors associated with coronary bypass surgery. *Nursing Research, 35,* 243–246.

TABLE 5–3. **Cardiac Surgery Stressors Ranked Greater by Nurses than Patients***

Stressor	Patient Ranking	Nurse Ranking
Monitors/other equipment	23.5	15.5
Call light not being answered	20.0	4.5
Explanations of hospital procedures	28.0	17.0
Loss of income	13.0	9.0

*1 = Highest stressor.

Data from Carr, J. A., & Powers, M. J. (1986). Stressors associated with coronary bypass surgery. *Nursing Research, 35,* 243–246.

TABLE 5–4. **Assessment Questions to Identify a Patient's Perception**

What do you think is the matter with you?
What does it mean to you that you have a __________ (valve replacement)?
What does it feel like to use the word __________ (tumor)?
What do you think may have caused this to happen?
Do you think you are making progress?
Are you worried about any long-term effects?

Data from Bilodeau, C. B. (1981). Psychologic aspects. In C. V. Kenner, C. E. Guggetta, & B. M. Dossey (Eds.), *Critical care nursing: Body–mind–spirit.* Boston: Little, Brown.

the patients in this study were quite concerned about increasing their activities after cardiac surgery, whereas the nurses ranked these activities as less stressful. Patients who are reluctant to increase their independence and take longer than the care givers think they should are often labeled as dependent and unwilling to do what they have to do to get well. These patients would be helped by the opportunity to discuss their fears in relation to the likelihood of another cardiac event, distinguishing between postoperative pain and cardiac-related pain, and the suspicion that activity may cause their incision to reopen.

Using interviews with patients who had been mechanically ventilated, another study revealed the specific stressors associated with that experience (Gries & Fernsler 1988). Immobility, positive pressure ventilation, insufficient explanations, suctioning, and extubation were some of the situations that were identified by patients as stressful.

Helping to prepare patients by giving simple, clear preprocedural information to reduce the impact of specific stressors is one important intervention that can be used by nurses. Interestingly, however, in the study just mentioned of patients undergoing mechanical ventilation, most patients were unable to recall specific nursing interventions that were done. Those that were recalled were reassuring words, just the presence of the nurse, and a caring manner. Studies like these help nurses understand the patient experience and allow them to plan their interventions accordingly.

Expert nurses are aware of the expected and serve as guides for patients, making what is strange and frightening more approachable (Benner & Wrubel, 1989). They can provide a road map for patients to help them anticipate and plan for known stressors. This is one of the many ways in which nurses can incorporate research into their practice.

ASSESSMENTS AND INTERVENTIONS RELATED TO COGNITIVE APPRAISAL

Understanding the Patient's Perspective

An individual's appraisal of a situation is the major determinant of what is and what is not stressful. Nurses demonstrate understanding of the concept of individual appraisal of stressors when they are willing to accept the patient's perception of the threat. For example, alterations in appearance will not be as threatening to an individual in which attractiveness is not a prime source of self-esteem or identity. This is an example of how individual values determine stressors.

A heart transplant candidate who viewed the heart as a repository for the soul found the idea of using another's heart more stressful than another candidate who viewed the heart as a mechanical pump. This is an example of how an individual's belief system determines what is stressful.

A patient who is generally mistrustful of others will experience more stress at having to place himself in the care of strangers than someone who is generally trustful. Some patients who feel that they can and should be able to have some impact on the surrounding circumstances may experience a more stressful response to hospitalization than patients who do not have as high a need for control. This is an example of how an individual's personality style can influence his or her appraisal of the stress inherent in some situations.

The most important intervention that nurses can use in understanding a patient's perspective is empathetic listening, which is the ability to hear the patient's perception of his or her situation completely without offering advice or solutions. Many nurses feel uncomfortable working with a patient's psychosocial needs because they are unsure of what to say. In actuality, it is more important to hear what the patient has to say. The skill that is most important is knowing how to help people express their concerns fully, thus validating their perceptions and reactions. In this way, nurses provide an opportunity for patients to express their fears and concerns, and this by itself may be enough to decrease anxiety and its corresponding physiologic reactivity (Tables 5–4 and 5–5).

Another reason for allowing patients to express their perceptions fully is to identify misconceptions that can be corrected based on the nurse's experience with the specific illness. For example, if a patient with a colostomy expresses concerns about loss of sexual function and vitality, the nurse can assist in redefining the situation based on her or his reality-based expe-

TABLE 5–5. **Therapeutic and Nontherapeutic Communication Techniques**

Therapeutic Techniques	Nontherapeutic Techniques
Develop caring, nondjudgmental relationship that will allow for the expression of feelings	*Passing judgment* on behavior or feelings: "Most patients don't get this anxious."
Open-ended questions: "What is your understanding of what the doctor has told you?"	*Giving advice:* "You should make your husband stop smoking now."
Reflection of thoughts or feelings: "It sounds as if you are really worried"; or, "It sounds as if you've been thinking about hurting yourself."	*Giving false reassurance:* "I'm sure everything will turn out just fine."

Data from Gorman, L .M., Sultan, D., & Luna-Raines, M. (1989). *Psychosocial nursing handbook for the nonpsychiatric nurse* (pp. 8–9). Baltimore: Williams & Wilkins. © 1989, the Williams & Wilkins Co., Baltimore.

rience with other patients (Lindquist, 1986). By assisting the patient to redefine the situation, the nurse can be a source of hope and strength. By helping patients identify the meaning the situation holds for them, nurses can help patients move from generalized concerns that may be overwhelming to specific concerns that may be more manageable.

Alterations in Cognitive Function

The ability to perceive and interpret reality accurately is vital to coping effectively. Neurologic and metabolic changes leading to delirium can distort perception, sensation, and thinking, thus interfering with effective coping responses. This perceptual distortion is known as delirium or "ICU psychosis." At the very least, delirium is anxiety-producing for the patient and the family. Delirium marked by paranoid ideation and hallucinations can be life-threatening if patients pull out important intravenous lines or other equipment and attempt to get out of bed. Anxiety, agitation, and combativeness can induce life-threatening dysrhythmias, wound dehiscence, and orthopedic injuries. Many factors can contribute to this response: metabolic factors such as pain, hemodynamic instability, electrolyte imbalance, sepsis, pharmaceuticals, and history of drug abuse; environmental factors such as noise, sleep deprivation, frightening atmosphere, and absence of windows; psychological factors such as anxiety, fear, and lack of control.

Some of the behavioral changes accompanying delirium can be mistaken for ineffective coping responses. Patients may become restless, listless, irritable, depressed, anxious, combative, and incoherent. They may refuse to answer questions or demonstrate alterations in intellectual capacity and memory. They may become defensive and paranoid. They may experience delusions, illusions, and hallucinations. A case example illustrates the importance of a methodical approach to assessing changes in behavior.

CASE HISTORY

Mr. G. had a long-standing history of restrictive cardiomyopathy resulting in symptoms of right-sided heart failure, severe ascites, liver engorgement, and cardiac cachexia. He was admitted to the hospital for evaluation for a cardiac transplant. The transplant team was uncertain about the patient's medical suitability. They had vacillated, telling the patient at one point that he was a candidate and then withdrawing that decision when new data about him came to light. The patient was placed in the very difficult position of waiting for further evaluation before a third and final decision was made.

One night when the nurse went to administer his routine medication, Mr. G. was lethargic and refused to respond to her questions. The nurse thought that he was becoming depressed about the uncertainty of his situation. Her interventions included explanations and comfort measures, but as the night wore on the patient became angry and uncooperative, trying to get out of bed without assistance. When he fell and was incontinent the nurse restrained him to prevent further incident. She felt frustrated that no intervention had helped to calm him. In the morning, his blood ammonia level was tested and was found to be toxic. Treatment to reduce the blood ammonia was started, and 3 days later the patient's behavior returned to normal. The behavioral changes noted in this patient had been inappropriately ascribed to psychological causes and diagnosed as ineffective coping responses.

An estimated 40% of patients admitted to critical care units experience delirium that may be terrifying to the patient and may be unrecognized by the nurse (Easton & MacKenzie, 1988; Geary, 1994). Assessing delirium is difficult because the most common affects seen are anxiety, fear, and depression, alone or in combination. Also, many patients may be aware that something is wrong and are afraid they are going crazy. They may try to hide the alteration from themselves and others by denying any problem or withdrawing to prevent detection (Murray, 1987). Important symptoms to be noted are disorientation as to time, place, and person; failure to recognize family members; perceptual illusions (mistaking environmental stimuli such as hearing the hissing of the oxygen valve as whispering); paranoid ideation; and hallucinations (perceiving environmental stimuli when there are none) (Geary, 1994).

Patients should be told about the possibility of delirium and given brief explanations and assurances as well as instructions to inform nurses of any unusual sensations or thoughts. The importance of providing adequate rest and sleep and controlling pain as preventive measures has already been discussed.

ASSESSMENT OF AND INTERVENTIONS FOR AFFECTIVE OR PHYSIOLOGIC AROUSAL

As discussed earlier, nurses can intervene in the stress–coping cycle at the point of cognitive appraisal. Nurses can also intervene by working directly to correct the physiologic and emotional arousal states that result when a threat is recognized.

Fight-or-Flight Response

Physiologic arousal can cause increases in oxygen consumption, heart rate, lethal dysrhythmias, blood pressure, respiratory rate, fatigue, and irritability. As discussed in the earlier section on pain, the relaxation response has been shown to counter these effects by producing an opposing response that includes decreases in oxygen consumption, respiratory rate, and heart rate. The relaxation response generally involves four elements: a comfortable position, a quiet environment, concentration on one's breathing, and a passive attitude (Clark, 1988). The use of a physiologic monitoring device to give the patient immediate information about the state of relaxation is called biofeedback. Often, special time is set aside to teach patients these techniques and allow time for practice (Melville, 1987; Miller, 1985; Acosta, 1988). Guided imagery is another technique that has been used in conjunction with relaxation to counter the affective and physiologic stress response. Imagery is an ancient healing technique in which purposeful mental images are used to achieve a desired therapeutic goal. Imagery engages the patient's senses in an attempt to communicate and influence physiologic processes. Imagery has been used for healing, anxiety reduction, acute and chronic pain, stress management , rehabilitation, and problem-solving (Stephens, 1993a). One of the most frequent types of imagery is mental rehearsal, which can prepare patients for painful or fearful situations, diagnostic tests, and difficult treatments. Guidelines for the use of imagery and scripts for the beginning practitioner can be found in the nursing literature (Stephens, 1993b).

The critical care unit is not the ideal atmosphere for helping patients to achieve a state of relaxation. But the following example illustrates how an expert nurse was able to incorporate this technique into her care.

CASE HISTORY

A patient who had been admitted to the critical care unit with acute chest pain started to have ventricular irritability. He had multifocal premature ventricular contractions and runs of ventricular tachycardia. Eventually, despite maximum doses of lidocaine, his heart rhythm deteriorated to the point of ventricular fibrillation. A "code" was called, and he was successfully resuscitated. However, his monitor continued to show extreme ventricular irritability. The patient lay awake and alert in his bed, surrounded by nurses and doctors nervously eyeing his monitor and talking about what to do next. A nurse went to the patient's side, took his hand, got his attention, and helped him to concentrate on his breathing, guiding him to inhale through his nose and exhale slowly through his mouth. He visibly relaxed, his body became less tense, he focused his attention on the nurse and participated in the rhythmic breathing. While this was taking place, another nurse had hung a different intravenous antiarrhythmic medication. After several minutes, the patient's rhythm returned to a regular sinus pattern, and the physicians thought that they had made the right treatment decision regarding the medication. By using a holistic model, the nurse also played an important role in this successful ending. Her attention to the patient as a biopsychosocial being prompted her intervention and allowed the patient to participate in his own treatment. Even in highly charged situations, nurses who have a commitment to holistic care will find ways to practice it.

Anxiety and Fear

Although patients can respond to threats to their physical safety in a variety of ways, a common response is one of fear and anxiety. These are closely linked emotions that differ only in terms of cause. Fear is a response to an identified stressor such as impending surgery, possible death, pain, and diagnostic procedures. Anxiety is characterized by feelings of dread, worry, and apprehension that cannot be specifically linked to an external cause. For example, a patient who has never acknowledged dependency needs may feel extremely uncomfortable at the prospect of placing himself in the care of others, but will be unaware that this is the issue that is causing distress. Anxiety can range from vague feelings of edginess to feelings of uncontrolled terror and panic.

MILD ANXIETY

Some anxiety is an expected response to illness and in its more mild form may actually stimulate a coping response by increasing alertness and motivating learning or change. Signs and symptoms may include statements from the patient that he or she is worried, anxious, nervous, and so on; increases in pulse, blood pressure, and respirations; and narrowed focus of attention. Nursing interventions for patients experiencing this level of anxiety include encouraging the patient to talk about specific concerns and providing realistic information to assist with problem-solving.

MODERATE ANXIETY

Anxiety at a moderate level may decrease a patient's ability to take in information and communicate needs. Patients may ask the same questions repeatedly. Providing more information at this time may contribute to the feeling of being overwhelmed. The patient may be acutely aware of the uncomfortable physiologic response that can occur with anxiety. Certainly, medication with a mild anxiolytic would be appropriate to assist the patient to regain control. Staying with the patient and providing reassurance may also help him or her to regain control.

SEVERE ANXIETY

Severe anxiety or panic resists efforts to change it made by either the individual or through the environment. Patients have little ability to withstand the level of discomfort they are experiencing. They have an extremely narrow focus of attention, are unable to take in information or solve problems, may have difficulty in concentrating, and may have distorted perceptions. This level of anxiety impairs the ability to cope, may lead to extremes of withdrawal or avoidance, and disrupts all normal functioning.

Although pharmacologic intervention with short-acting benzodiazepines is appropriate in these situations, the approach to the patient is also critical. Patients experiencing extreme anxiety usually cannot respond to rational explanations and information because cognitive function is seriously impaired. A more helpful approach is to speak softly and simply and to indicate a willingness to be with the patient. These patients should not be left alone because they may harm themselves either purposefully or inadvertently. It is important to transmit feelings of calm and being in control of the situation so that the patient feels that someone is in charge while he or she cannot be. Do not attempt to engage the patient in problem-solving behavior until you know that he or she is certain that you fully understand his or her fears and concerns, and the ability to attend to explanations has returned.

Hopelessness

Feelings of helplessness and lowered self-esteem that seem to be a natural response to the threats posed by a critical illness can contribute to feelings of hopelessness. It is important to help patients combat these feelings because they can contribute to a lack of participation in treatment and therefore to increased complications. A major contributor to feelings of hopelessness is the patient's perception that her or his condition is at a standstill and that there is nothing she or he can do to get well. Nurses can provide hope by normalizing the experience by assuring patients that much of the weakness and fatigue they are experiencing is a normal response to illness and prolonged bed rest. It is also important to anticipate setbacks and let the patient know that progress is rarely a steady uphill climb.

Nurses can assist patients to set small goals that are realistic and attainable. Many patients want to leap past the day-to-day discomfort of gradually regaining strength and function; they have unrealistic expectations about what they can actually do. By setting small goals in consultation with the patient and then pointing out the small steps that are achieved, the nurse can provide hope that things are in fact improving. By helping patients recognize the signs of progress, nurses instill hope while at the same time increasing the patient's feelings of control and self-esteem.

SUPPORTING ADAPTIVE COPING RESPONSES AND DEFENSE MECHANISMS

Another goal of nursing interventions is to support effective coping responses. More research is being done to identify exactly what patients do in certain situations to help them manage their uncomfortable reactions, and which of these responses are most effective.

Problem-Focused and Emotion-Focused Coping

Studies have been conducted to identify exactly what patients do to cope in specific situations (Nyamathi, 1987; King, 1985; Sutherland, 1988), and several broad generalizations about coping can be made:

- Most people in complex situations use a combination of problem-focused and emotion-focused coping responses.
- Coping responses can change from one encounter to another and over time.
- Coping behaviors that work well in one phase of the illness may not be useful in another phase.
- Coping depends on the stake that the individual has in the stressor.
- The coping process depends on the patient's appraisal of what can and cannot be done; if an individual believes that something can be done, problem-focused coping will be used, but if he or she feels that nothing can be done, emotion-focused coping predominates.

This information supports the idea that there may not be a "right" way to cope and that nurses must see the patient's attempts to cope as the best he or she can do at a given point in time. Attempts to change a particular coping behavior must be made carefully and with the knowledge that behavior change takes time and a commitment to change on the part of the patient.

As nurses try to evaluate the effectiveness of coping responses of critically ill patients who are responding to often overwhelming threats to body, ego, and social situation, the most important question to ask is: Does this behavior work for this person, at this time, in this context? Coping can be judged only in terms of its consequences for an individual in terms of his or her ability to maintain adequate social relationships, keep feelings of anxiety at a manageable level, and minimize the effects of the stressor on physical well-being (Lazarus & Folkman, 1984).

For example, patients who experience symptoms but deny them and delay seeking treatment are coping ineffectively because the behavior has implications for their physical well-being. One patient experiencing crushing chest pain while riding his bicycle turned around and rode back home rather than seeking help. On the other hand, patients who use denial to control their anxiety about the meaning of their symptoms but seek out and participate in treatment are still coping effectively even though they are not able to face the problem directly. Patients who get angry to avoid feelings of powerlessness but are able to talk about their feelings with caregivers are coping effectively. Patients who direct their anger toward caregivers as if they rather than the situation were the source of the stress cut themselves off from support and are coping ineffectively. However, the need to defend oneself against the painful feelings initiated by the stressors of illness is universal, and people make do with whatever tools they have to achieve the greatest level of peace and functioning during the crisis (Groves & Kucharski, 1987).

Sometimes coping involves the use of defense mechanisms that are unconscious psychological processes used to control feelings of intense anxiety. They are not directed toward problem-solving but instead help to deceive the person about the actual threat. Defense mechanisms permit a person to take in only as much reality as he feels equipped to handle and serve to keep anxiety at tolerable levels.

Some defenses are more costly than others in terms of effects on well-being, social interaction, and morale. Vaillant (1976) constructed a theoretical hierarchy of ego defenses that may help caregivers understand the degree of threat a person may be experiencing. The more primitive or regressive the defense mechanism, the higher the degree of threat (Groves & Kucharski, 1987).

Primitive Defenses

The least effective mechanisms are those that alter reality for the person using them but seem "crazy" to others. Distortion involving delusions and hallucinations to reshape reality to meet internal needs is an example of this level of defense. These defenses are very difficult to change and respond best to medication and removal of the stressor rather than to therapeutic interactions. Although the patient who is using this level of defense may be frightening to work with because his behavior is so bizarre, nurses can see that the behavior is not directed at them, and they usually do not get caught in defensive responses to such patients.

Immature Defenses

Immature mechanisms are used by normal children or adults who have regressed to earlier behavior patterns. These mechanisms may decrease anxiety for the person using them but generally create feelings of annoyance and irritation in the people around them. Three examples of this level of defense are (1) projection, attributing one's own unacceptable feelings to others; (2) passive–aggressive behavior, covertly expressing hostility while appearing to be compliant; and (3) acting-out, the direct expression of impulses. These behaviors are often deeply ingrained and inflexible but are amenable to change by prolonged relationships with caring and mature individuals who are willing to develop a therapeutic relationship.

Patients using immature defense mechanisms are often the most frustrating to work with because their affect and behavior cause negative reactions in the people who care for them. For example, one of the most difficult patients to care for is the one who uses acting-out and anger to gain control. This angry response is not the same as rational anger, which is a response to the external situation and is expressed directly to create constructive change. Rather, this type of anger is characterized by verbal threats, physical aggression, and hostility and is connected more to internal threats than to external reality. This type of behavior often sets up an automatic defensive reaction in the nurse that, although understandable, escalates the patient's anger and usually leads to a no-win power struggle (Minarik & Leavitt, 1988).

Interventions that are most likely to succeed in these cases include a nondefensive acceptance of the situation from the patient's point of view and a sincere effort to discover what can be done to alleviate the situation. Allowing the patient to express anger fully without offering resistance eliminates the patient's need to continue escalating her or his behavior to make sure he or she is understood.

Different approaches are appropriate for the different ways people express anger. When anger is expressed passively, as when patients pull out lines or deliberately spill food or water, an attempt should be made to look for the underlying intention so that the concerns can be expressed more directly. If anger is expressed directly, it is better to focus on the factor in the situation that caused the anger rather than on the anger itself. If anger is expressed in a destructive and hostile manner, the nurse should calmly set limits on the unacceptable behavior without cutting off the anger. Setting limits makes the environment safe but should not be a way for the nurse to express his or her own anger.

The most important approach for nurses to take with all patients using immature defense mechanisms is first to recognize their own reactions and accept them as normal rather than as an indication of personal inadequacy. Once nurses can monitor their own reactions, they can begin to work with the patient's behavior in a problem-solving way. These patients are troublesome to the whole staff and generate feelings of frustration and of wanting to flee. Often, a consultant not directly involved in the situation is necessary to help sort through the various feelings and develop a reasonable plan.

Neurotic Defenses

Neurotic defenses are common and can be seen in most healthy adults, especially at times of acute stress. Examples of this type of defense mechanism are (1) displacement, the focusing on less threatening aspects of a situation, and (2) intellectualization, the avoidance of the emotional components of the situation.

Patients who use neurotic defenses can be very rewarding to work with. If their behavior is the result of regression due to the immediate situation rather than to rigidly held beliefs, it is amenable to dramatic change with even brief therapeutic interactions that help them identify the underlying source of the anxiety. For example, some patients who have had spinal cord injuries begin to make sexual jokes and treat the nursing staff as sexual objects. If nurses understand that this behavior is a response to an underlying anxiety related to sexual performance they can help the patient by acknowledging the behavior and wondering out loud if he is having some concerns about this area. This type of confrontation must be done within the context of a therapeutic relationship based on trust, which permits the patient to acknowledge the underlying anxiety that the defensive behavior was intended to mask.

It is important for nurses to remember that defense mechanisms are neither "bad" nor "good" but are the person's best available method for containing feelings of anxiety. They serve a useful purpose and should be left in place unless they can be replaced by something else that will be useful to the patient. Also, defense mechanisms are unconscious and may not be specifically intended to create negative reactions in others, although that is often the end result (Clark, 1988). Approaching patients with these concepts in mind helps nurses to cope more effectively with patients' upsetting affects and behaviors (Table 5–6).

TABLE 5–6. **Patient Care Plan for Ineffective Coping**

Defining Characteristics	Interventions
Patient states that he or she is unable to cope Stressor appears greater than available resources Behaviors that are destructive to self or others: aggression; suicide; use of alcohol or drugs Unable to solve problems Use of defense mechanisms that interfere with getting treatment or support	Identify potential organic causes of behavior 1. Assess orientation to time/place/person 2. Assess memory for recent events and immediate recall 3. Observe for altered perceptions 4. Assess thought processes 5. Confer with physician regarding diagnostic tests During high levels of anxiety, give short, simple explanations Develop caring, nonjudgmental relationship through use of effective communication skills that will 1. Encourage expression of feelings 2. Allow development of alternative perceptions of the event that promote evaluation of the stressor in manageable terms 3. Allow reassessment of the situation without making patient feel discounted Set limits on unacceptable behavior Develop support system 1. Involve mental health professional to assess and treat acute confusional states, major depression, suicide risk 2. If present and helpful, involve significant others 3. Develop own support system to help cope with own reactions to difficult patients

Reprinted from Clark, S. (1989). Transplantation. In B. Reigel & D. Ehrenreich (Eds.), *Psychological aspects of critical care nursing* (p. 202). Rockville, MD: Aspen. With permission of Aspen Publishers, Inc., © 1989.

PREREQUISITE FOR NURSING INTERVENTIONS: A CARING RELATIONSHIP

The relationship that is formed between the patient and the nurse is the vehicle through which all other interventions take place and is based on caring. Caring is essential for effective nursing practice. It causes the nurse to notice subtle changes in the patient's condition and identify what needs to be done. Caring makes the nurse notice which interventions work and which do not. Caring sets up the conditions of trust that allow the one cared for to use the help that is offered (Benner & Wrubel, 1989).

How do nurses convey that they care about patients? Caring is demonstrated by interventions that meet the treatment needs of patients (instrumental activities) as well as by those that are more psychologically oriented (expressive functions). A recent small study explored critically ill patients' perceptions of caring. Important caring behaviors identified by these patients included attentiveness, highly skilled practice, life-saving behaviors, and energy-freeing acts. This study highlighted that caring nurses combine technical skill with behaviors that are identified with kindness and nurturing (Burfitt et al., 1993).

Patients and family members rank instrumental activities as most important to feeling cared for, whereas nurses rank meeting expressive needs as most important to caring. Patients perceive that nurses who know what they are doing, know how to give shots, know when to call the physician, give treatments on time, are well organized, answer questions clearly, and provide information are demonstrating caring (Brown, 1986; Cronin & Harrison, 1988). However, nurses ranked the following behaviors as important caring activities: allowing expression of feelings, realizing that the patient knows himself best, listening to the patient, touching the patient for comfort, and perceiving patient needs as important (Larson, 1987; Mayer, 1986).

What accounts for this discrepancy? Caring is always understood within the context of the situation. When a swift and accurate intervention is necessary, that is what the patient will perceive as caring. When technical actions are *not* called for, psychologically directed activities will be perceived as caring (Benner & Wrubel, 1989).

One implication of these differences in perception is that patients must first feel safe and have confidence in the nurses caring for them. Once that goal is achieved, the expressive nursing activities become more prominent in the patient's awareness. Another important implication is that nurses cannot assume that their well intentioned acts of what they consider caring will be experienced as such by patients expecting something else (Brown, 1986).

However, just as one cannot split the mind–body connection, neither can instrumental and expressive nursing functions be considered separately. Nursing care, even technical functions, delivered in a noncaring manner has important implications for patients and health. Nursing care that was perceived as distancing was described in the following terms: too casual an attitude; the nurse just doing a job; not using eye contact; treating patients as objects; being rough and in a hurry; not listening; not responding; being stiff, starchy, insensitive, irritated, or defensive. As a result of these noncaring behaviors, patients felt humiliated, out of control, and frightened. Patients felt that being cared for by nurses with these behaviors could slow the process of recovery and leave patients feeling hopeless. Others felt that noncaring relationships added to their stress and depleted energy that could be used for healing (Drew, 1986; Reimaen, 1986).

On the other hand, nurses who were perceived as caring were described as concerned about what happened, liking their work, using eye contact, physically relaxed, matter-of-fact about messes, and not in a hurry. Almost any action was seen as caring if it was not done in a hurry. Patients who received care from these nurses felt more confident, more in control, and more relaxed. They felt that some form of energy was passed from the caregiver to them and that this energy contributed to their healing and recovery (Drew, 1986). As one patient explained, "The nurses came in and they talked to me and hugged me because they knew about my problem. And it seemed like I started getting better right away, right then" (Brown, 1986).

SUMMARY

The stress–coping model seeks to identify aspects of the patient care situation that need to be attended to. Expert nurses learn to assess the different components of the model almost automatically and decide intuitively what intervention would best serve the patient. They weave technical activities into an intricate pattern with expressive actions. Every contact with the patient is purposeful and goal-directed in terms of understanding the stressors affecting the patient, the patient's cognitive appraisal process, the affective and physiologic responses, and the effectiveness of the coping strategies used by the patient.

Meeting the psychosocial needs of critically ill patients is not something that nurses do when they have a few extra minutes, but rather it is a consistent commitment to a holistic approach to patient care. Nurses who learn to integrate these components into an intuitive whole and meet both the physical and psychosocial needs of their patients are the expert nurses who exemplify the goals, values, and beliefs of the profession.

REFERENCES

Acosta, F. (1988). Biofeedback and progressive relaxation in weaning the anxious patient from the ventilator: A brief report. *Heart and Lung, 17,* 299–301.

Aitkin, R. J. (1982). Quantitative noise analysis in a modern hospital. *Archives of Environmental Health, 37,* 361–364.

American Association of Critical-Care Nurses. (1989). *Standards for nursing care of the critically ill* (p. 64). 2nd ed. Aliso Viejo, CA: American Association of Critical-Care Nurses.

Bartrop, R. W., Luckhurst, E., Lazarus, L., Kiloh, L. G., & Penny, R. (1977). Depressed lymphocyte function after bereavement. *Lancet, 1,* 834.

Benner, P. (1984). *From novice to expert: Excellence and power in clinical nursing practice.* Menlo Park, CA: Addison-Wesley.

Benner, P., & Wrubel, J. (1989). *The primacy of caring: Stress and coping in health and illness.* Menlo Park, CA: Addison-Wesley.

Benson, H. (1975). *The relaxation response.* New York: Avon Books.

Bentley, S., Murphy, F., & Dudley, H. (1977). Perceived noise in surgical wards and in intensive care areas: An objective analysis. *British Medical Journal, 2,* 1503.

Berkman, L. F., & Syme, S. (1979). Social networks, host resistance and mortality: A nine year follow-up study of Alameda County residents. *American Journal of Epidemiology, 102,* 186–204.

Berkman, L. F., Leo-Summers, L., & Horowitz, R. I. (1992). Emotional support and survival after myocardial infarction. *Annals of Internal Medicine, 117,* 1003–1009.

Breier, A., Albus, M., Pickar, D., Zahn, T. P., Wolkowitz, O. M., & Paul, S. M. (1987). Controllable and uncontrollable stress in humans: Alterations in mood and neuroendocrine and psychophysiological function. *American Journal of Psychiatry, 144,* 1419–1425.

Brown, L. (1986). The experience of care: Patient perspectives. *Topics in Clinical Nursing, 8*(2), 56–62.

Burfitt, S. N., Greiner, D. S., Miers, L. J., & Kinney, M. R. (1993). Professional nurse caring as perceived by critically ill patients: A phenomenologic study. *American Journal of Critical Care, 2,* 489–499.

Calabrese, J. R., King, M. A., & Gold, P. W. (1987). Alterations in immunocompetence during stress, bereavement and depression: Focus on neuroendocrine regulation. *American Journal of Psychiatry, 144,* 1123–1134.

Carr, J. A., & Powers, M. J. (1986). Stressors associated with coronary bypass surgery. *Nursing Research, 35,* 243–246.

Case, R. B., Moss, A. J., Case, N., McDermott, M., & Eberly, S. (1992). Living alone after myocardial infarction: Impact on prognosis. *Journal of the American Medical Association, 267,* 515–519.

Clark, S. (1988). Ineffective coping: Patient and family. In L. Kern (Ed.), *Cardiac critical care nursing* (p. 293). Rockville, MD: Aspen Press.

Cronin, S. N., & Harrison, B. (1988). Importance of nurse caring behaviors as perceived by patients after myocardial infarction. *Heart and Lung, 17,* 374–380.

Dracup, K., & Bryan-Brown, C. (1993). Critical care and healthcare reform. *American Journal of Critical Care, 2,* 351–353.

Dracup, K. (1987). Critical care nursing. *Annual Review of Nursing Research, 5,* 107–133.

Drew, N. (1986). Exclusion and confirmation: A phenomenology of patients' experiences with caregivers. *Image, 18*(2), 39–43.

Easton, C., & MacKenzie, F. (1988). Sensory-perceptual alterations: Delirium in the intensive care unit. *Heart and Lung, 17,* 229–235.

Fawzy, F. I., Kemeny, M. E., Fawzy, N. W., Elashoff, R., Morton, D., Cousins, N., & Fahey, J. L. (1990). A structured psychiatric intervention for cancer patients: Changes over time in immunological measures. *Archives of Psychiatry, 47,* 729–735.

Flaherty, G. G., & Fitzpatrick, J. J. (1978). Relaxation techniques to increase comfort level in postoperative patients: A preliminary study. *Nursing Research, 27,* 352.

Geary, S. M. (1994). Intensive care unit psychosis revisited: Understanding and managing delirium in the critical care setting. *Critical Care Nurse Quarterly, 17*(1), 51–63.

Glaser, B. G., & Straus, A. L. (1968). *A time for dying.* Chicago: Adeline.

Gries, M. L., & Fernsler, J. (1988). Patient perceptions of the mechanical ventilation experience. *Focus on Critical Care, 15*(2), 52–59.

Griffin, J. P. (1992). The impact of noise on critically ill people. *Holistic Nursing Practice, 6*(4), 53–56.

Groves, J. E., & Kucharski, A. (1987). Brief psychotherapy. In T. P. Hackett & N. H. Cassem (Eds.), *Massachusetts General Hospital handbook of general hospital psychiatry* (p. 322). Littleton, MA: PSG Publishing.

Gujol, M. C. (1994). A survey of pain assessment and management practices among critical care nurses. *American Journal of Critical Care, 3*(2), 123–128.

Halm, M. A., & Alpen, M. A. (1993). The impact of technology on patients and families. *Nursing Clinics of North America, 28,* 443–457.

Hansell, H. N. (1984). The behavioral effects of noise on man: The patient with "intensive care unit psychosis." *Heart and Lung, 13,* 59–65.

Helton, M. C., Gordon, S. H., & Nunnery, S. L. (1980). The correlation between sleep deprivation and the intensive care unit syndrome. *Heart and Lung, 9,* 464.

Henneman, E. A., & Cardin, S. (1989). Open visiting hours in the critical care setting: Effect on nursing staff. *Heart and Lung, 18,* 291–292.

Hickey, M. L. (1988). What are the needs of families of critically ill patients? A review of the literature since 1976. *Heart and Lung, 17,* 670–676.

Hilton, A. (1987). The hospital racket: How noisy is your unit? *American Journal of Nursing, 87*(1), 59–61.

Holmes, T. H., & Rahe, R. H. (1967). The social readjustment rating scale. *Journal of Psychosomatic Research, 11,* 213–218.

Houldin, A. D., Lev, E., Prystowsky, M. B., Redei, E., & Lowrey, B. J. (1991). Psychoneuroimmunology: A review of literature. *Holistic Nursing Practice, 5*(4), 10–21.

House, J. S., Landis, K. R., & Umberson, D. (1988). Social relationships and health. *Science, 241,* 540–544.

Ketter, J. (1994). ANA: Protecting nurses and patient care in the face of restructuring. *The American Nurse, 26*(5), 1.

Kiecolt-Glaser, J. K., & Glaser, R. (1992). Psychoneuroimmunology: Can psychological interventions modulate immunity? *Journal of Consulting and Clinical Psychology, 60,* 569–575.

King, K. B. (1985). Measurement of coping strategies, concerns, and emotional response in patients undergoing coronary bypass grafting. *Heart and Lung, 14,* 579–586.

Kirchhoff, K. T., Pugh, E., Calame, R. M., & Reynolds, N. (1993). Nurses' beliefs and attitudes toward visiting in adult critical care settings. *American Journal of Critical Care, 2,* 238–245.

Kleinpell, R. M., & Powers, M. J. (1992). Needs of family members of intensive care unit patients. *Applied Nursing Research, 5*(1), 2–8.

Larson, P. J. (1987). Comparison of cancer patients' and professional nurses' perceptions of important nurse caring behaviors. *Heart and Lung, 16,* 187–192.

Lazarus, R. S. (1966). *Psychological stress and the coping process.* New York: McGraw-Hill.

Lazarus, R. (1993). Coping theory and research: Past, present, and future. *Psychosomatic Medicine, 55,* 234–247.

Lazarus, R. S., & Folkman, S. (1984). Coping and adaptation. In W. D. Gentry (Ed.), *Handbook of behavioral medicine* (p. 291). New York: Guilford Press.

Leske, J. S. (1992). Comparison rating of need importance after critical illness from family members with varied demographic characteristics. *Critical Care Clinics of North America, 4,* 597.

Levy, S. M., Herberman, R. B., Whiteside, T., Sanzo, K., Lee, J., & Kirkwood, J. (1990). Perceived social support and tumor estrogen/progesterone receptor status as predictors of natural killer cell activity in breast cancer patients. *Psychosomatic Medicine, 52,* 73–85.

Lindquist, R. D. (1986). Providing patient opportunities to increase control. *Dimensions of Critical Care Nursing, 5,* 304–309.

Lindquist, R. D., Jeffrey, R. W., Johnson, A., & Haus, E. (1985). The stress of patient adjustment to the coronary care unit as related to perceptions of personal control and control preferences. *Heart and Lung, 14,* 297–298.

Mayer, D. K. (1986). Cancer patients' and families' perceptions of nursing care behaviors. *Topics in Clinical Nursing, 8*(2), 63–69.

McCaffery, M., & Ferrell, B. (1991a). How would you respond to these patients in pain? *Nursing91, 21*(6), 34–37.

McCaffery, M., & Ferrell, B. (1991b). Patient age: Does it affect your pain control decisions? *Nursing91, 21*(9), 44–48.

McCaffery, M., & Ferrell, B. (1992a). Does life-style affect your pain control decisions? *Nursing92, 22*(4), 58–61.

McCaffery, M., & Ferrell, B. (1992b). Does the gender gap affect your pain control decisions? *Nursing92, 22*(8), 48–51.

McCaffery, M., & Ferrell, B. (1992c). How vital are vital signs? *Nursing92, 22*(1), 42–46.

McCarthy, D. O., Ouimet, M. E., & Daun, J. M. (1991). Shades of Florence Nightingale: Potential impact of noise stress on wound healing. *Holistic Nursing Practice, 5*(4), 39–48.

Melville, S. B. (1987). Relaxation techniques in acute myocardial infarction: The theoretic rationale. *Focus on Critical Care, 14*(1), 9–11.

Miller, B. K. (1985). Teaching biofeedback techniques in critical care. *Dimensions of Critical Care Nursing, 4,* 314–318.

Minarik, P., & Leavitt, M. (1988). The angry, demanding, hostile response. In B. Reigel & D. Ehrenreich (Eds.), *Psychological aspects of critical care nursing.* Rockville, MD: Aspen Press.

Molter, N. C. (1979). Needs of relatives of critically ill patients: A descriptive study. *Heart and Lung, 8,* 332–339.

Moos, R. H., & Tsu, V. S. (1979). The crisis of physical illness: An overview. In R. Moos (Ed.), *Coping with physical illness.* New York: Plenum Medical Books.

Murray, G. B. (1987). Confusion, delirium, and dementia. In T. P. Hackett & N. H. Cassem (Eds.), *Massachusetts General Hospital handbook of general hospital psychiatry.* Littleton, MA: PSG Publishing.

Nguyen, T. V. (1991). Mind, brain and immunity: A critical review. *Holistic Nursing Practice, 5*(4), 1–9.

Nyamathi, A. (1987). Coping response of spouses of MI patients and of hemodialysis patients as measured by the Jalowiec Coping Scale. *Journal of Cardiovascular Nursing, 2,* 67–74.

Palmblad, J., Petrini, B., Wasserman, J., & Akerstedt, T. (1979). Lymphocyte and granulocyte reactions during sleep deprivation. *Psychosomatic Medicine 41,* 273–277.

Patterson, S. M., Zakowski, S. G., Hall, M. H., Cohen, L., Wollman, K., & Baum, A. (1994). Psychological stress and platelet activation: Differences in platelet reactivity in healthy men during active and passive stressors. *Health Psychology, 13*(1), 34–38.

Puntillo, K. A. (1988). The phenomenon of pain and critical care nursing. *Heart and Lung, 17,* 262–271.

Puntillo, K. A. (1994). Dimensions of procedural pain and its analgesic management in critically ill surgical patients. *American Journal of Critical Care, 3,* 116–122.

Quinn, J. F., & Strelkauskas, A. J. (1993). Psychoneuroimmunologic effects of therapeutic touch on practitioners and recently bereaved recipients: A pilot study. *Advances in Nursing Science, 15*(4), 13–26.

Radwin, L. E. (1987). Autonomous nursing interventions for treating the patient in acute pain: A standard. *Heart and Lung, 16,* 258–265.

Redding, J. S., Hargest, T. S., & Minsky, S. H. (1977). How noisy is intensive care? *Critical Care Medicine, 5,* 275.

Reichlin, S. (1993). Mechanisms of disease: Neuroendocrine interactions. *New England Journal of Medicine, 329,* 1246–1253.

Reimaen, D. J. (1986). Noncaring and caring in the clinical setting: Patients' descriptions. *Topics in Clinical Nursing, 8*(2), 30–36.

Selye, H. (1956). *The stress of life.* New York: McGraw-Hill.

Sinclair, V. (1988). High technology in critical care: Implications for nursing's role and practice. *Focus on Critical Care, 15*(4), 36–41.

Solomon, G. F. (1993). Whither psychoneuroimmunology? A new era of immunology, of psychosomatic medicine, and of neuroscience. *Brain, Behavior, and Immunity, 7,* 352–366.

Stein, M. (1989). Stress, depression, and the immune systerm. *Journal of Clinical Psychiatry, 50*(5), 35–40.

Stephens, R. (1993a). Imagery: A strategic intervention to empower clients. Part I: Review of research literature. *Clinical Nurse Specialist, 7,* 170–174.

Stephens, R. (1993b). Imagery: A strategic intervention to empower clients. Part II: A practical guide. *Clinical Nurse Specialist, 7,* 235–240.

Sutherland, S. (1988). Burned adolescents' descriptions of their coping strategies. *Heart and Lung, 17,* 150–157.

Syme, S. L. (1984). Sociocultural factors in disease etiology. In W. D. Gentry (Ed.), *Handbook of behavioral medicine* (pp. 13–37). New York: Guilford Press.

Vaillant, G. E. (1976). Theoretical hierarchy of adaptive ego mechanisms. *Archives of General Psychiatry, 24,* 535–545.

Ward, C. R., Constancia, P. E., & Kern, L. (1990). Nursing interventions for families of cardiac surgery patients. *Journal of Cardiovascular Nursing, 5*(1), 34–42.

Weisman, A. D. (1987). Coping with illness. In T. P. Hackett & N. H. Cassem (Eds.), *Massachusetts General Hospital handbook of general hospital psychiatry.* Littleton, MA: PSG Publishing Co.

Wilson, V. S. (1987). Identification of stressors related to patients' psychologic responses to the surgical intensive care unit. *Heart and Lung, 16,* 267–273.

Woods, N. F., & Falk, S. A. (1974). Noise stimuli in the acute care area. *Nursing Research, 23,* 144.

Zimmerman, L. M., Pierson, M. A., & Marker, J. (1988). Effects of music on patient anxiety in coronary care units. *Heart and Lung, 17,* 560–566.

Psychosocial Needs of Families

Mairead Hickey

Health care is rapidly changing, and nowhere is this more evident than in critical care. The advanced technologies and therapies used in critical care not only have the ability to preserve and save lives, but to dehumanize the environment and cause moral and ethical dilemmas for health care practitioners, policy makers, and society as a whole.

In light of this highly technical environment, whether it be in the hospital or in the home, the importance of a supportive, stabilizing, and caring family cannot be underestimated. Typically, families function to provide an environment that supports and meets the needs of its members. Bound by affection, loyalty, caring, and trust, family members have the capacity to assume new roles and adjust the basic family structure as necessary to meet the needs of its members.

Because the family unit is the sum of its members, when one member becomes critically ill, the whole family is affected. Critical illness threatens the family's most basic function—the support of its members' survival and developmental needs. When a member experiences a crisis, the family actively helps the member in need, and thus, when a family member is critically ill, the family feels responsible for helping that person. In light of the family's sense of responsibility, it is ironic that during a critically ill patient's hospitalization, families are usually physically separated from their sick relative. During such hospitalization families may be ambivalent; on the one hand, they are relieved that their loved one is receiving the best care possible, but on the other hand, they sense a loss of control over what is happening to their sick family member.

The family's ability to provide support to the critically ill patient depends on many factors and needs. Often, critical illness affects the family's basic function and needs, and they must rely on their supports and resources to maintain or restore their equilibrium. The health care system provides supports and resources to help critically ill patients meet their needs, but who helps the family meet its needs during the crisis of critical illness?

This chapter examines how contemporary families experience the critical illness of a hospitalized family member. (Chapter 10 presents an overview of families' experiences with critically ill patients who are being cared for at home.) Specifically, it describes how the crisis of critical illness affects families, and provides an overview of the research that has been conducted on the needs of families of critically ill patients, from which intervention plans for these families can be developed.

CONTEMPORARY FAMILIES

The institution known as the *family* has changed. Although the traditional image of a family as a heterosexual married couple with two or three children related by marriage, birth, or adoption still exists, most Americans have broadened their definition of the family to include any group of people who love and care for each other (McCool et al., 1992). Although the profile of the contemporary family is continuously changing, its function remains constant—to adjust and change as necessary to support the survival and developmental needs of its members (Woolley, 1990).

Critical illness often causes family members to change and modify their roles and responsibilities. As families change and adjust during critical illness, however, they are vulnerable to crisis states. During the crisis of critical illness, the family's ability to function depends on how well it is able to use its repertoire of coping mechanisms and employ its available supports.

CRITICAL ILLNESS—A CRISIS FOR THE FAMILY

Individuals and families normally exist in a state of equilibrium—they are able to "manage" or function despite daily upsets and turmoils. They maintain this state and meet their needs by using their coping behaviors and problem-solving techniques. In states of crisis, however, people face obstacles that threaten their equilibrium and life goals. These obstacles may be insurmountable through use of their customary coping mechanisms and problem-solving techniques, and the family may not be able to maintain its equilibrium (Aguilera, 1990).

Critical illness almost inevitably induces a crisis state in families, regardless of their coping skills (Woolley, 1990). Critical illness can be sudden or expected, and may or may not include periods of exacerbations and remissions. In either case, critical illnesses have the same potential to disrupt the structure and function of the family. A critical illness with a sudden onset gives the family little or no time to prepare for the crisis. Families often experience shock and disbelief on hearing the news of a sudden illness, and disorganization in family structure and function may follow. Expected and long-term critical illnesses, on the other hand, usually contribute to fewer feelings of shock and disbelief and more to emotional and physical exhaustion among family members. Both types of critical illness pose threats to the family. Therefore, regardless of whether critical illness is sudden or expected, it is disruptive to families and often forces them to make major adjustments and rely on their coping behaviors to restore or maintain their equilibrium.

Factors Affecting the Family's Response to the Crisis of Critical Illness

Not all individuals or families, when faced with the same stressful event, will be in crisis. However, some events that typically precipitate crisis states for most people are death, critical illness, or other situations that trigger grief and bereavement. Aguilera (1990) suggests that a family's vulnerability to crisis is influenced by many factors, including the family's perception of the event, their available situational supports, and the type and availability of their coping mechanisms.

Perception of the Event

Individuals respond differently to similar situations because of the way they perceive the situation. Their perceptions of an event will certainly influence both their responses to the event and their susceptibility to crisis. For example, whether they perceive an event as serious, important, or irrelevant will influence their reaction to the event and whether they need to use coping strategies or seek support. During critical illness, families have a high potential for cognitive confusion and inaccurate perceptions. Thus, ensuring their accurate and realistic perceptions is a very important, yet an often difficult task for staff.

Available Situational Supports

Families' abilities to cope during the crisis of critical illness are often influenced not only by the availability and quality of situational supports, but by the manner in which individuals use them. Families use a variety of situational supports to maintain or restore their equilibrium. Situational supports refer to those people, places, or things in the environment that assist individuals or families to solve the problems at hand. Support may be provided by professional staff, such as nurses, social workers, chaplains, or therapists; other family members or friends; or by the individual's own internal support resources, such as relaxation techniques or exercise. Often, the family's response to critical illness is related to how much support is available to them at the time and what they feel comfortable drawing on. An important role of the critical care team is to assist family members to find and use appropriate supports and coping behaviors during critical illness.

Coping Mechanisms

Families also respond to the critical illness of a loved one by relying on their past coping mechanisms and behaviors. Although in some cases their behavioral patterns may seem unusual to an unrelated observer, these behaviors are usually essential to the family's success in maintaining or restoring equilibrium. For example, some families are exceedingly vigilant, appearing to be overly focused on the care staff are providing to the patient, and resist leaving the patient's bedside. Other families may withdraw from the crisis and avoid visiting the patient altogether, whereas others may demonstrate their reaction to the crisis through emotional outbursts that the staff may believe are disruptive, but the patient may view as "normal." In general, coping behaviors allow the family to repress the excessive threats of the critical illness situation and focus on what they can actually deal with (Leavitt, 1989).

COMMON RESPONSES OF FAMILIES TO CRITICAL ILLNESS

Although critical illnesses vary in intensity, they are usually a burden for the family. Even as they use a variety of coping behaviors to alleviate the crisis, families have many unmet needs. They often feel helpless, hopeless, and powerless; and they are easily confused and unable to concentrate on details. Their perceptions of reality and normal daily events may be distorted (Leavitt, 1989). In addition to the critical illness itself, the hospital environment is stressful for the entire family. The critical care environment with its sights, smells, and sounds is often a major source of discomfort for the family. Also, the sight of a critically ill family member, perhaps unresponsive and connected to many tubes and machines, may be overwhelming for families (Hickey & Rykerson, 1992). Fear of death, emotional turmoil, role changes, disruption of family activities, along with the fact that families must depend on strangers to care for their loved ones, are sources of stress for families (Titler & Walsh, 1992).

Although families may react differently to the stress and discomforts associated with critical illness,

TABLE 6–1. **Families' Common Responses to Critical Illness**

Decreased ability to concentrate
Decreased ability to use incoming information
Reduced ability to make decisions and solve problems
Decreased sense of personal effectiveness
Decreased sensitivity to or awareness of the environment
Stress related to changes in structure and roles in the family

there are patterns of responses and behaviors that are frequently seen (Table 6–1). Families' common responses to critical illness are described in the following sections.

Decreased Ability to Concentrate and Use Incoming Information

During crises, people have difficulty hearing and comprehending information. Ironically, it is during this time of cognitive confusion that families are inundated with information about the patient, the critical care unit, and upcoming tests and procedures. In fact, studies have shown that families of critically ill patients are adamant about receiving information about their loved ones (Hickey, 1990). Their need for information, coupled with their difficulty in processing information, may explain why families often repeat the same questions to many care providers. The inability of families to comprehend information, along with their desire to be kept informed about their loved one's condition, presents a challenge to the critical care team as they try to keep families informed.

Decreased Ability to Make Decisions and Solve Problems

Just as in the previous example, although families of critically ill patients have difficulty processing and understanding highly technical and important information, they frequently need to make decisions that may seriously affect the lives of both the patient and themselves (Henneman & Cardin, 1992). During critical illness, families may be asked to make decisions about the extent of treatment for the patient, whether they are willing to grant permission for surgery, or, perhaps, whether treatments should be terminated. In addition to making difficult decisions about the care and treatment of their critically ill loved one, families may also have trouble making decisions about their daily routines. For example, they may need guidance about whether they should leave the patient and go home to rest. Or, they may wonder if they should go to work or stay at the patient's bedside. In any of these cases, it is important that staff be aware of families' cognitive limitations and be patient with families as they try to deal with and make decisions for themselves and their family members.

Decreased Sensitivity to or Awareness of the Environment

Another response that is related to families' cognitive confusion is their apparent lack of awareness of and insight into their surroundings, which is often the critical care unit. Perhaps this explains why families may be found standing in the hallway and blocking the normal traffic flow in the critical care unit, or why they may "camp out" in the waiting room, apparently insensitive to the needs of other families who are also waiting there. Often, they may need sensitive direction about where to rest or wait so they will be more comfortable and, at the same time, not impede the critical care unit's activities.

Decreased Sense of Personal Effectiveness

Families report feeling less than helpful during the hospitalization of a family member (Leske, 1991). Typically, because critically ill patients' conditions are so complex and labile, critical care nurses and other team members almost exclusively provide care to these patients. Although this practice is certainly understandable and necessary, it is important for staff to understand that many families have the strong need to feel helpful. In some cases, a family's sense of helpfulness may be enhanced if they can assist in the care of their critically ill family member (Artinian, 1991; Molter, 1976; Titler & Walsh, 1992). In other cases, just knowing how important their presence is to the patient or just holding the patient's hand may make the family feel more helpful.

Stress Related to the Changes in Structure and Roles in the Family

Families may experience stress as a result of the way critical illness and hospitalization affect their ability to function. During the acute crisis of critical illness, when the family's energies and efforts are almost exclusively directed toward the patient, critical illness can disrupt the family's structure and function. Even reassignment of the most routine tasks, such as defrosting food for dinner or washing clothes, may cause stress on the family. As Breu and Dracup (1978) described in the early study of interventions to help spouses of critically ill patients, and Nyamathi and colleagues (1992) have recently described, drastic role reversals by wives of myocardial infarction patients contribute to an intense sense of loss and stress for family members. Again, the extent to which family function is disrupted during these stressful times depends greatly on the support and coping behaviors available to and used by individual family members and the family as a whole.

These common responses to critical illness provide insight into why families of critically ill patients behave the way they do during acute events. It is important that the critical care team understand these behaviors rather than judge them as appropriate or inappropriate, because it is usually these coping behaviors and responses to stress that help families restore equilibrium during critical illness. Only if a behavior is obviously detrimental to the patient, family, or other patients and their families should it be modified with the help and support of the nursing staff.

NEEDS OF FAMILIES OF CRITICALLY ILL PATIENTS

As families attempt to cope with and adjust to the crisis of critical illness, they have many needs that the critical care team can help them meet. Historically, many investigators have explored the needs of families of critically ill patients (Bernstein, 1990; Bouman, 1984; Breu & Dracup, 1978; Chavez & Faber, 1987; Daley, 1984; Dracup & Breu, 1978; Freichels, 1991; Gilliss, 1984; Kleinpell & Powers, 1992; Kahn, 1992; Koller, 1991; Leske, 1992; Molter, 1979; Norris & Grove, 1986; Nyamathi et al., 1992; Pelletier, 1993; Pike, 1984; Price et al., 1991; Rodgers, 1983; Simpson, 1989; Stillwell, 1984; Warren, 1993). They sampled the needs of families from a wide variety of critically ill patients, ranging across such spectra as diagnosis, age, geographic locale, type of hospital, and ethnicity. Although, for the most part, these studies are limited by small sample size, their findings consistently underscore similarities in the needs of families of critically ill patients. Specifically, families rate information about their loved one's condition as their most important need, followed by their needs to be reassured that their loved ones are comfortable and receiving the best possible care, to be able to visit the patient, and to be able to have conveniences such as a telephone and waiting area available to them.

This apparent consistency in findings has been validated by integrative and statistical reviews, which have been conducted on the reports of the needs of families of critically ill patients (Hickey, 1990; Leske, 1991; Simpson, 1989). On secondary analyses, these reviews suggest that family members place a great deal of importance on the following set of needs: *receiving assurance* about the treatments and prognosis of the critically ill patient, being able to *remain near* the critically ill patient, *receiving information* about the critically ill patient's condition, having environmental *comforts* available to them, and *receiving support* (Table 6–2). In addition, on more extensive secondary analysis, Leske (1992) found that family needs remained the same across families, regardless of the patient's age, gender, relationship to family members, prior critical care experience, and diagnosis.

TABLE 6–2. **Needs That Are Ranked Most Important by Families of Critically Ill Patients**

Assurance	Support
Proximity	Comfort
Information	

This wide body of evidence about the needs of families during the stress and crisis of critical illness provides a substantial foundation for designing interventions for patients and families. In the next section, the needs listed in Table 6–2 will be presented, with a discussion of interventions to meet these needs.

INTERVENTIONS FOR FAMILIES OF CRITICALLY ILL PATIENTS

Although the major focus of the critical care team is to support the needs of critically ill patients, these same patients require support from their families. As members of families, patients act and react not only as individuals but also as family members. Thus, when designing care for critically ill patients, actions should be taken to ensure that families' needs are met so that families can provide a supportive environment for the patient's recovery (Table 6–3).

Consideration of the following points about families and how they respond to critical illness will assist staff in planning care for critically ill patients and their families:

- Families function primarily to support their members.
- Many aspects of critical illness—the illness itself, the hospitalization, the intensive care unit environment, and the related demands placed on the structure and function of families—are stressful and may potentiate crises for families of critically ill patients.
- Families respond to the crisis of critical illness by employing a variety of coping mechanisms to restore their equilibrium.
- Family members have specific needs of their own during the critical illness of a loved one.

In light of these major points, the goal of care for families of critically ill patients is to provide them with resources so they can employ coping behaviors to restore and maintain their equilibrium during critical illness. It is only when families are dealing adequately with the stress of critical illness that they can support the recovery of their critically ill family member.

Family Assessment

To plan care for families, a comprehensive family assessment is necessary. The structure and function of the family, including its religious affiliations, previous coping behaviors, prior experiences with critical illness, beliefs and values with regard to health and disease, and needs must be identified and examined. Because of the crisis nature of critical illness, families are often unable to provide family assessment infor-

TABLE 6–3. **Interventions Related to Families' Needs**

Provide Assurance

- Establish an environment that is patient focused and sensitive to family needs
- Convey the staff's caring attitude to the family
- Demonstrate sensitivity, caring, and respect for the patient's needs
- Explain how the patient will be monitored closely and will receive highly skilled care
- Reassure the family that every measure will be taken to make the patient as comfortable as possible
- Provide realistic hope to the family
- Convey to family members the advocacy role that nurses have for patients
- Stress improvements in the patient's condition as appropriate

Facilitate Proximity (the Need to Be with the Patient)

- Create unit policies that facilitate individualized family visiting based on patient and family needs
- Assess patient's preference for visiting (who, when, length)
- Assess the family's need to be with the patient
- Establish a visitation plan that meets the patient's and family's needs
- Encourage family members to get adequate rest, nutrition, and exercise
- Prepare family members for visits
- Accompany family members as needed (assist them to be near or to touch the patient if they wish; encourage them to talk with the patient)
- Teach family members how to assist with patient care as appropriate and as desired

Provide Information

- Conduct frequent assessments to determine the amount and kind of information the family is able to receive and understand
- Provide information based on the family's needs and interests
- Provide information that is concrete, simple, and nontechnical
- Discuss realistic long-term goals (predict, with family, the difficulties or probable events that may be encountered in the future)
- Provide written information to supplement verbal information

Provide Support

- Assess the family's structure, function, and usual coping mechanisms
- Respect the coping behaviors of the family and intervene only if the behavior is detrimental to the family or patient
- Provide consistent staff contact
- Assess family–staff communication patterns
- Allow families to ventilate emotions
- Foster acceptance, comfort, and support from all health care providers
- Provide families with needed information
- Point out how the family is being helpful to the patient
- Guide the family to make well informed decisions
- Use other support staff as needed
- Inform family of available resources (e.g., financial, social, group)

Provide Comfort

- Evaluate environmental conveniences near the unit
- Provide for comfort needs near the unit
- Provide information on resources and facilities that may be needed near the hospital

mation during a single interview. It may be necessary to collect family history and assessment data over an extended period of time, perhaps during the first 48 hours after the patient's admission to the critical care unit. After these initial data are collected, periodic follow-up assessments should be done throughout hospitalization to evaluate how well the family is functioning.

Data from the family assessment, coupled with empiric knowledge about the role of the family and the needs of families of critically ill patients, provide the basis for individualized family care. In the following sections, each family need category is described, along with a set of generic interventions that should be assessed and individualized to meet the specific needs of patients and families.

The Need for Asssurance

Families report that their need for assurance and hope is very important. They want to be assured that the patient is receiving the best possible care from staff who actually care about the patient. They also need to have a sense of hope about the condition and prognosis of their family member. During critical illness and hospitalization, family members are forced to relinquish their caring and supportive role vìs-à-vìs the patient. It is difficult for them to give up their caring responsibilities to the "strangers" on the critical care team. When a family member is hospitalized, they often sense a loss of control over the situation. If families believe that staff are genuinely concerned about their family member and that staff will keep them informed about the patient's condition, their need for assurance may be met.

During critical illness, families also place a great deal of importance on their need to hope for a certain outcome. Initially, they may hope for survival, without knowledge or consideration of the patient's quality of life (Danis et al., 1988). By providing families with thoughtful and sensitive information, the critical care team can assist families to perceive realistically the critically ill patient's condition and prognosis. In some situations, hope for recovery may be redirected to hope for a peaceful death (Leske, 1992).

In general, by establishing an environment that is patient-focused and sensitive to families' needs, staff can create relationships with families that will support families' needs for assurance about the care being provided to the critically ill patient. Staff who demonstrate sensitivity and caring and who respect the patients' best interests provide assurance to families. Although most staff pride themselves on the way they care and assume an advocacy role for patients, they may need to convey this message to families to put them more at ease during the hospitalization of their critically ill family member.

The Need for Information

Families repeatedly identify the importance of receiving information about their family member's condition. They do not want to be surprised by a change in their relative's condition when they visit, nor do they want to fear that information is being withheld. By keeping families informed about the patient's condition, staff are able to assume an advocacy role for the patient and other family members. Research reports suggest that family members want honest, current information (Hickey, 1990; Leskey, 1992; Simpson, 1989). Families have a fundamental need to receive information about their sick family member; however, they are not necessarily selective in the information they seek about their loved one. They may solicit information about the patient from anyone who will provide it, and may actively seek information from many sources until they receive indications that realistically or unrealistically suggest that the patient is improving.

At a time when families feel isolated from their sick relative and quite helpless to care for the person, information may provide them with a sense of control that may relieve some of their anxieties. Information and communication also contribute to the accuracy with which familes perceive the illness of their family member. Realistic perceptions of their family member's condition allow them to use the coping behaviors necessary to maintain their equilibrium and functional ability.

Providing information to families may be challenging to the team. Families' interests and needs for information are diverse, ranging from information about the diagnosis and prognosis, to what may be interpreted by the "busy" critical care team as trivial information about how the patient ate or slept. In addition, although family members frequently seek and may even demand information, their ability to comprehend and process information usually is impaired during the crisis of critical illness. Owing to this cognitive confusion, it is important to do frequent assessments to determine the amount and kind of information the family is able to receive and understand.

To ensure communication and help meet the information needs of families, the critical care team may find it helpful to establish family representatives who can be contacted at least daily with information about the patient. The representative can then communicate with the rest of the family, thereby decreasing the number of family members inquiring about the patient's general condition. In addition to having a family contact person for the staff, families also identify the importance of having a contact person for them to call with questions and concerns. By identifying such team and family contacts and by establishing a system of communication and information exchange, many information needs of families can be met (Henneman & Cardin, 1992). In addition, this relationship-building process is an essential component of preparing families to assume patient care responsibilities after discharge. (See Chapter 10 on preparing families for home care.)

Usually it is best to provide information that is concrete, simple, and nontechnical. In addition, the same information may need to be reviewed with the family over and over again before they can actually understand it. Written information about routine hospital services and unit policies is an appropriate method of communication because family members can read this information when they are emotionally and cognitively ready to do so. A study by Chavez and Faber (1987) supports the idea that written information is an effective way to provide families with information.

The Need to Be With the Patient (Proximity)

Family members also report the need to be with the patient, especially during the very acute and unstable periods of critical illness (Hickey, 1990; Leske, 1992). Because it is difficult and often logistically impossible to prepare families adequately for the emergency nature of a family member's critical illness and hospitalization, families receive more comfort by actually *seeing* their relative than by relying on reports from staff. Also, families who are able to spend time with their family member will be more likely to have an accurate perception of the critically ill patient's condition.

Given that the basic function of families is to support their members, it is not surprising that they have a heightened need not only to be with, but also helpful to, the patient during critical illness. As already mentioned, during a crisis family members come to the aid of family members in need. However, during the hospitalization of a critically ill family member, they are usually unable to offer and provide the help they believe to be an important part of their role. This feeling of helplessness adds to their sense of ineffectiveness during crisis.

Research suggests that in terms of visitation, families prefer visiting hours that are not restricted to any specific time, with families and patients both preferring flexible visiting policies (Boykoff, 1986; Halm & Titler, 1990; Simpson, 1991). Visiting policies that restrict the frequency and length of time can contribute to the stressfulness of the event for the family. When family members are not permitted to see their sick relative, they may imagine a scenario far worse than what actually exists. Limited or infrequent visiting policies, such as 10 minutes per hour and two to three visits per day, may lead to more anxiety and confusion within the family. With visitation policies that facilitate, rather than restrict, individualized family visiting based on patient and family needs, families may have a more realistic perception of the patient and may be more likely to employ coping behaviors that address their needs.

It is important to assess individual patient and family responses to family visits to determine the relative benefit of family visits for both the patient and family. Whenever possible, both on admission and periodically thereafter, staff should ask patients about their preferences for visiting, including who should visit, how long visits should be, best time of day for visits, and so forth. Their emotional and physiologic reactions to visiting should be examined. Studies suggest that when considering changes in hemodynamic parameters as criteria for modifying visiting policies for individual patients, hemodynamic assessments should be made only after the first 10 minutes of the visit (Zetterlund, 1971). Typically, families believe that their visits calm a patient's fears and improve his or her spirits (Halm & Titler, 1990). Although this is often true, extensive family vigils may not be good for the family or the patient. When appropriate, staff need to be aware of the impact of critical illness on the family and need to encourage the family to get adequate sleep, nutrition, and exercise (Titler & Walsh, 1992).

Another important aspect of family visiting is related to the preparation families need about what to expect before they visit their critically ill relative. To ensure family preparation and also to ensure that the patient is ready for visitors, information explaining the procedure for contacting the patient's nurse before entering the patient's room should be available to families. Despite efforts to prepare family members, they often need additional support and gentle direction when they first enter the patient's room. A comfortable place to sit near the patient and simple instructions about how to touch and talk to the patient are most helpful to the family. Although the staff often regard themselves as advocates for patients, it is important for staff to remember that patients usually receive comfort from family visits, no matter how atypical the family's behavior may seem.

As hospitals become more patient and family focused, many different types of visiting policies have emerged. Although today most critical care units still employ some type of structured–restrictive visiting policies, more lenient alternative practices are being introduced (Stockdale & Hughes, 1988). Open visiting policies, for example, place no restriction on length, frequency, or time of visit. Individualized, flexible visiting practices in which the nurse, patient, and family members mutually agree on the time, length, and frequency of visits, along with the number, ages, and relationship of visitors, are described by Woellner (1988). Other researchers describe contract visiting, in which the above parties not only mutually agree to the conditions of time, length, and frequency of visits, but they sign a contract that outlines the specific characteristics of the patient's visitation (Ziemann & Dracup, 1990). Any of these visiting practices offers the forum for individualized discussion and negotiation among families, patients, and staff, and "opens the door" for relationships to be built between families and staff.

Associated with their need to be near the patient, families also report the need to help their critically ill relative. This is especially true in parents of critically ill children or family members who have been long-term caregivers for the patient (Hickey & Rykerson, 1992). Although families often want to help in the care of their critically ill relative, some may have difficulty mastering new or difficult care-related tasks. Therefore, when families wish to participate in care, they can be taught to assist with simple, yet important tasks for the patient. Families can learn to assist with feeding patients, washing their face, or turning their pillow. If the patient's condition stabilizes and if family members are interested in mastering more difficult tasks, the feasibility of teaching family members how to give backrubs, record hourly drainage, or change the patient's position can be explored. Also, if the family member(s) will provide care at home, they may need to become involved in the more complex aspects of the patient's care (See Chapter 10, Preparing Families for Home Care.)

In addition to providing physical care to the patient, staff can remind family members that they are also contributing to the care of the patient by taking care of matters at home, coordinating attendance at family–staff meetings, and meeting with resources such as social services or chaplain services. All of these contributions will assist the family to meet their need to be helpful and near the patient, and may actually help the family cope during critical illness.

Support Needs

Family members also need emotional support during the critical illness of a family member. Although during this time families are concerned with issues associated with whether their relative will live or die, there are many other factors that contribute to families' stress and need for support (Halm, 1992). Hospitalization and the host of unfamiliar people, sights, and sounds; changes in family roles and function; geographic distance from the critically ill relative; or geographic distance from customary family supports contribute to the family's need for support.

Interestingly, families of critically ill patients do not perceive staff as being responsible for helping them meet support needs—they believe the critical care team should direct their time and energies toward the care of patients (Kleinpell & Powers, 1992). However, as Norbeck (1981) suggests, because individuals are more receptive to outside influence during crisis, critical care staff have an important opportunity to support families during crisis. Unfortunately, critical care nurses may not feel prepared to provide families with support (Hickey & Lewandowski, 1988; Rodgers, 1983). This inconsistency underscores the importance of critical care staff being prepared to assume responsibility for assessing the family's ability to function during the crisis and for providing or coordinating the necessary services to help families restore their equilibrium.

Little research has been conducted to examine how interventions actually affect families' need for support. Reports from a few studies describe support-enhancing interventions as those that provide the family with information, allow for flexible visitation, support families' needs to ventilate their emotions, and provide environmental comfort (Chavez & Faber, 1987; Dracup & Breu, 1978; Forrester et al., 1990; McHale & Bellinger, 1988; Nyamathi et al., 1992).

In one experimental study, Halm (1990) reported that educational and psychological support groups for families of critically ill patients alleviated the stress experienced by families of these patients. Support for the family can also be provided by a variety of hospital services and staff. For example, chaplains, clinical nurse specialists, and social workers may be valuable resources for families during this time of crisis and associated stress.

Comfort Needs

It is not surprising that families need environmental comforts and conveniences during the critical illness of a family member. Nearby bathrooms and telephones, comfortable furniture, and information on nearby restaurants, hotels, or rest areas in the hospital, are examples of the environmental comforts families need. Although research has not been conducted to study the effect of such environmental comforts on families of critically ill patients, whenever possible it seems reasonable that basic conveniences such as telephones and waiting areas should be located near the critical care area. Critical care staff can provide valuable insight into family needs during building and renovation programs. Also, staff can evaluate environmental conveniences at the local unit level and make recommendations as appropriate to meet families' needs.

SUMMARY

Nursing has made great strides during the past 15 years in acknowledging the role of families and their needs during the critical illness of a family member. Research reports about the needs of families during critical illness provide a body of knowledge from which interventions for families of critically ill patients can be developed and further evaluated. In addition, anecdotal accounts about how contemporary families respond to critical illness give reason to incorporate families into care.

Today's families are not content passively to sit by and gratefully wait for information and caring gestures from the critical care team (Hickey & Leske, 1992). Instead, families expect to participate in care decisions and be provided the information necessary to do so. More than ever, it is essential that staff expand their concept of the patient from an individual in a bed to that of a member of a family. This is especially important when we consider that the family is with the patient not only during the critical phase of illness, but through the often long recovery process. Their physical presence and support of the patient during highly unstable times as well as their active participation in care as the patient becomes more stable is important to the overall recovery of both the patient and family. As critically ill patients are cared for outside the confines of a critical care unit (in the home, for example), staff will not only acknowledge the importance of the family in care, but will grow to depend on the family to assist with care. By supporting families and meeting their needs during critical illness, staff assist in developing the foundation from which families can support patients throughout their recovery from critical illness.

REFERENCES

Aguilera, D. C. (1990). *Crisis intervention, theory and methods* (6th ed.). St. Louis: C. V. Mosby.

Artinian, N. (1991). Strengthening nurse–family relationships in critical care. *Clinical Issues in Critical Care Nursing, 2,* 269–275.

Bernstein, L. P. (1990). Family-centered care of the critically ill neurological patient. *Critical Care Nursing Clinics of North America, 2,* 41–50.

Bouman, C. C. (1984). Identifying priority concerns of families of ill patients. *Dimensions of Critical Care Nursing, 3*(5), 313–319.

Boykoff, S. (1986). Visitation needs reported by patients with cardiac disease and their families. *Heart and Lung, 15*(5), 573–577.

Breu, C., & Dracup, K. (1978). Helping the spouses of critically ill patients. *American Journal of Nursing, 78*(1), 50–53.

Chavez, C. W., & Faber, L. (1987). Effect of an education–orientation program on family members who visit their significant other in the intensive care unit. *Heart and Lung, 16*(1), 92–99.

Daley, L. (1984). The perceived immediate needs of families with relatives in the intensive care setting. *Heart and Lung, 13*(2), 231–237.

Danis, M., Jarr, S., Southerland, L. I., et al. (1987). A comparison of patient, family, and nurse evaluation of the usefulness of intensive care. *Critical Care Medicine, 15*(2), 138–143.

Danis, M., Patrick, D. L., Southerland, L. I., et al. (1988). Patients' and families' preferences for medical intensive care. *Journal of the American Medical Association, 260*(5), 797–802.

Dracup, K. A., & Breu, C. S. (1978). Using nursing research findings to meet the needs of grieving spouses. *Nursing Research, 27*(4), 212–216.

Forrester, D., Murphy, P., Price, D., & Monaghan, J. (1990). Critical care family needs: Nurse–family member confederate pairs. *Heart and Lung, 19,* 655–661.

Freichels, T. A. (1991). Needs of family members of patients in the intensive care unit over time. *Critical Care Nursing Quarterly, 14,* 16–29.

Gilliss, C. L. (1984). Reducing family stress during and after coronary artery bypass surgery. *Nursing Clinics of North America, 19*(1), 103–112.

Halm, M. (1990). The effect of support groups on anxiety of family members during critical illness. *Heart and Lung, 19*(1), 62–71.

Halm, M. A. (1992). Support and reassurance needs: Strategies for practice. *Critical Care Nursing Clinics of North America, 4,* 633–643.

Halm, M. A., & Titler, M. G. (1990). Appropriateness of critical care visitation: Perceptions of patients, families, nurses, and physicians. *Journal of Nursing Quality Assurance, 5,* 25–37.

Henneman, E. A., and Cardin, S. (1992). Need for information: Interventions for practice. *Critical Care Nursing Clinics of North America, 4*(4), 615–622.

Hickey, M. (1990). What are the needs of families of critically ill patients? A review of the literature since 1976. *Heart and Lung, 19,* 401–415.

Hickey, M., & Leske, J. S. (1992). Needs of families of critically ill patients. *Critical Care Nursing Clinics of North America, 4,* 645–649.

Hickey, M., & Lewandoski, L. (1988). Critical care nurses' role with families: A descriptive study. *Heart and Lung, 17,* 670–676.

Hickey, P. A., & Rykerson, S. (1992). Caring for parents of critically ill infants and children. *Critical Care Nursing Clinics of North America, 4,* 565–571.

Kahn, E. (1992). A comparison of family needs based on the presence of DNR orders. *Dimensions of Critical Care Nursing, 11*(5), 286–292.

Kleinpell, R. M., & Powers, M. J. (1992). Needs of family members of intensive unit patients. *Applied Nursing Research, 5,* 2–8.

Koller, P. (1991). Family needs and coping strategies during illness crisis. *AACN Clinical Issues in Critical Care Nursing, 2,* 338–345.

Leavitt, M. B. (1989). Transition to illness: The family in the hospital. In C. L. Gilliss, B. L. Highley, & B. M. Roberts, et al. (Eds.), *Toward a science of family nursing.* Menlo Park, CA: Addison-Wesley.

Leske, J. S. (1991). Internal psychometric properties of the Critical Care Family Needs Inventory. *Heart and Lung, 20*(3), 236–244.

Leske, J. S. (1992). Needs of adult family members after critical illness. *Critical Care Nursing Clinics of North America, 4,* 587–596.

McCool, W., Tuttle, J., & Crowley, A. (1992). Overview of contemporary families. *Critical Care Nursing Clinics of North America, 4,* 549–558.

McHale, D., & Bellinger, A. (1988). Need satisfaction levels of family members of critical care patients and accuracy of nurses' perceptions. *Heart and Lung, 17,* 447–453.

Molter, N. C. (1979). Needs of relatives of critically ill patients: A descriptive study. *Heart and Lung, 8*(2), 332–339.

Norbeck, J. (1981). Social support: A model for clinical research and applications. *Advances in Nursing Science, 3,* 43–59.

Norris, L. O., & Grove, S. K. (1986). Investigation of selected psychosocial needs of family members of critically ill adult patients. *Heart and Lung, 15*(2), 194–199.

Nyamathi, A. M., Jacoby, A., Constancia, P., & Ruvevich, S. (1992). Coping and adjustment of spouses of critically ill patients with cardiac disease. *Heart and Lung, 21,* 160–166.

Pelletier, M. (1993). The needs of family members of organ and tissue donors. *Heart and Lung, 22,* 151–157.

Pike, A. W. (1984). The effects of information about the intensive care environment on the distress levels of families of critically ill patients. Unpublished master's thesis, Yale University School of Nursing, New Haven, CT.

Price, D. M., Forrester, A., Murphy, P. A., & Monaghan, J. F. (1991). Critical care family needs in an urban teaching center. *Heart and Lung, 20,* 183–188.

Rodgers, C. D. (1983). Needs of relatives of cardiac surgery patients during the critical care phase. *Focus on Critical Care, 10*(5), 50–55.

Simpson, T. (1989). Needs and concerns of families of critically ill adults. *Focus on Critical Care, 16,* 388–397.

Simpson, T. (1990). Cardiovascular responses to family visits in coronary unit patients. *Heart and Lung, 19,* 344–351.

Simpson, T. (1991). The family as a source of support for the critically ill adult. *AACN Issues in Critical Care Nursing, 2,* 229–235.

Stillwell, S. B. (1984). Importance of visiting needs as perceived by family members of patients in the intensive care unit. *Heart and Lung, 13*(3), 238–242.

Stockdale, L., & Hughes, J. (1988). Critical care unit visiting policies: A survey. *Focus on Critical Care, 15,* 45–51.

Titler, M. G., and Walsh, S. M. (1992). Visiting critically ill patients—Strategies for practice. *Critical Care Nursing Clinics of North America, 4*(4), 623–632.

Warren, N. (1993). Perceived needs of the family members in the critical care waiting room. *Critical Care Nursing Quarterly, 16,* 56–63.

Woellner, D. S. (1988). Flexible visiting hours in the adult critical care unit. *Focus on Critical Care, 15,* 66.

Wooley, N. (1990). Crisis theory: A paradigm of effective intervention with families of critically ill people. *Journal of Advanced Nursing, 15,* 1402–1408.

Zetterlund, J. (1971). An evaluation of visiting policies for intensive and coronary care units. In M. Puffy, M. Anderson, & B. Bergerson (Eds.), *Current concepts in clinical nursing.* St. Louis: C. V. Mosby, 1971.

Ziemann, K. M., & Dracup, K. (1990). Patient–nurse contracts in critical care: A controlled trial. *Progress in Cardiovascular Nursing, 5,* 98.

Chapter 7 Enhancing Communication With Critically Ill Patients and Families

Verna A. Sitzer

The critical care setting is an environment that necessitates effective communication between health care providers and hospitalized patients. Effective communication implies that both verbal and nonverbal messages are understood and that the interaction results in a positive experience or outcome. Communication interactions within the hospital are aimed toward improving patient outcomes. Patients must be assisted in understanding and interpreting the meaning of their illness, communicating their needs, communicating with support systems, and in assuming self-care on discharge. Usual communication patterns may be altered because of role changes associated with hospitalization, illness, medications, and therapeutic adjuncts. Communication may be impaired secondary to stroke, mechanical ventilation, or therapeutic paralysis. In addition to these physical limitations, environmental, sociocultural, and psychological factors may influence communication interactions as well. This chapter presents a review of the communication process, elements that enhance and interfere with effective communication, and strategies to overcome common communication difficulties encountered in the critical care setting.

COMMUNICATION PROCESS

Interpersonal communication involves the transfer of information between two or more people. It is the concurrent process of sending messages, receiving messages, and obtaining immediate feedback (DeVito, 1980). The roles of sender and receiver are both assumed by each individual. In the communication interaction the sender generates and delivers information in the form of a code (a process referred to as *encoding*). The receiver accepts and interprets the information (a process referred to as *decoding*). For communication to occur, messages must be sent and received, or encoded and decoded. Messages conveyed by the sender serve as stimuli for the receiver. Messages may be verbal, nonverbal, or written. In response to the stimulus or message, the receiver generates and delivers a message back to the sender. Thus, the receiver becomes the sender and the sender becomes the receiver. Participants in the communication process both send and receive messages at the same time. Messages received in response to information conveyed are called feedback. Feedback may be verbal or nonverbal cues and may be positive or negative. Feedback enables individuals to judge the effectiveness of their communication interactions and to adjust their messages and behavior accordingly. Communication is a continuous process whereby every message is influenced by the messages preceding it (Fig. 7–1).

The communication interaction is affected by attitudes, feelings, beliefs, and values of both sender and receiver and by the context in which the interaction occurs. These elements constantly interact during the communication process and serve as reference points for interpretation of messages. The sender and the receiver are influenced by each other, and both are influenced by the context in which the interaction takes place. For example, communication that occurs between the nurse and a patient in the hectic critical care environment will certainly be different from communication that occurs between a patient and his or her family in the home.

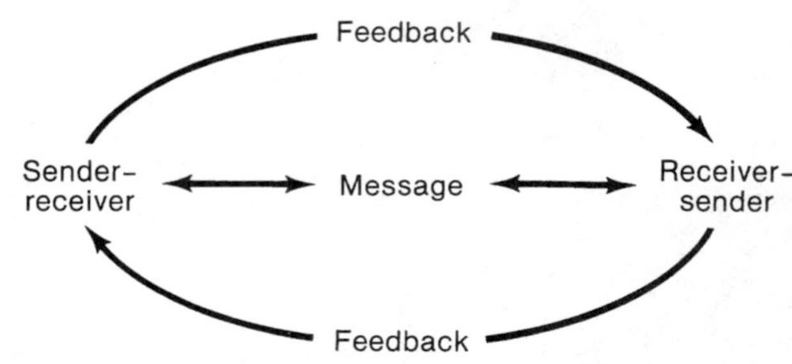

FIGURE 7–1. Communication process within a context.

An important aspect of communication is that one cannot choose not to communicate. Although one may not be aware of it, body positioning, facial expressions, gestures, silence, and even body odors communicate a message. Choosing not to respond in a communication interaction is itself a response. Another aspect of communication is that it is irreversible. Once a message is conveyed it cannot be retrieved.

COMMUNICATION CHANNELS

Communication can occur through one or more channels or routes. Messages are received through visual, auditory, kinesthetic, olfactory, and gustatory routes. Messages are conveyed through verbal and written language and nonverbal language such as gestures, facial expressions, and body positioning. Communication interactions usually involve a combination of these channels. The more channels that are used, the clearer the message transmission and reception. The aim is to send or receive messages in the hope that they are understood as intended.

VISUAL CHANNEL. Vision is one of the most important senses used in communication. Observing a person's eyes, lips, facial expressions, body movements, and other facets in a communication interaction can provide significant information about that person's behavior and attitude. When communicating with patients in the critical care unit, nurses frequently focus on nonverbal messages to provide clues to their patients' feelings. For example, facial expressions and guarding movements can alert the nurse to the patient's pain or distress. In addition, much of the physiologic information obtained from the patient (e.g., vital signs, cardiac rhythm, urine output) is observed and interpreted through the visual channel.

The visual pathway begins with light rays entering each eye and striking the retina. Light rays entering from the peripheral or temporal field hit the nasal region of the retina, and those entering from the nasal field strike the temporal region of the retina (Fig. 7–2). From each retina, visual impulses are transmitted by nerve fibers in the optic nerve within the brain. Nerve fibers from the nasal region of both retinas cross at the optic chiasm and continue with nerve fibers from the temporal regions (which do not cross), forming optic tracts. The optic tracts terminate in the thalamic areas of the brain, at which point visual impulses are carried by optic radiations to the visual center in the occipital cortex.

The crossing of nerve fibers in the optic chiasm results in transmission of visual impulses from the same half of each retina along one side of the pathway to the visual cortex. Lesions or injury affecting the visual pathway can result in blindness of specific visual fields (see Fig. 7–2). Injury to the retina or optic nerve on one side of the pathway will result in total blindness of the eye on the same side of the lesion (unilateral blindness). Injury to the optic chiasm will result in partial blindness affecting only the temporal fields of both eyes (bitemporal hemianopsia). Injury to the optic tract or radiation on one side of the visual pathway will result in partial blindness affecting the temporal field of the same side and the nasal field of the opposite side

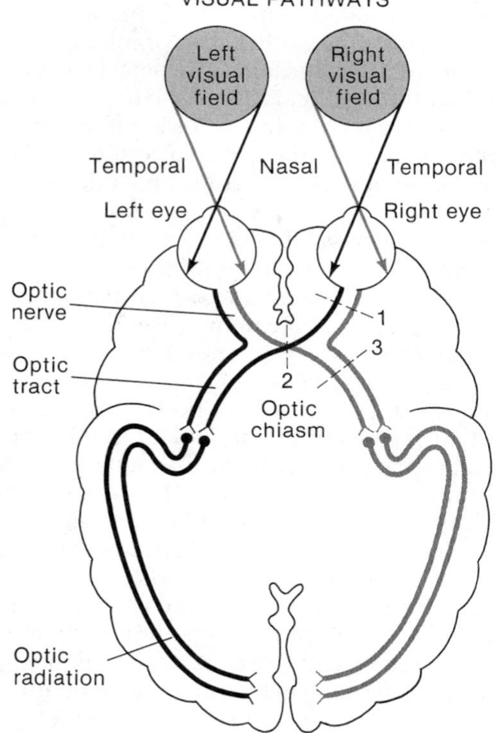

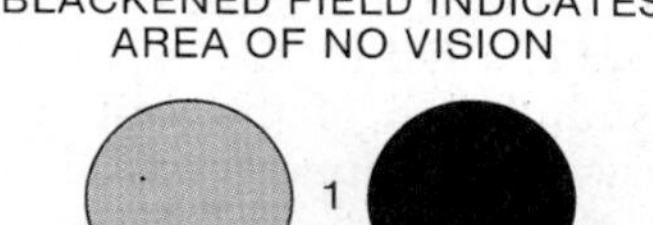

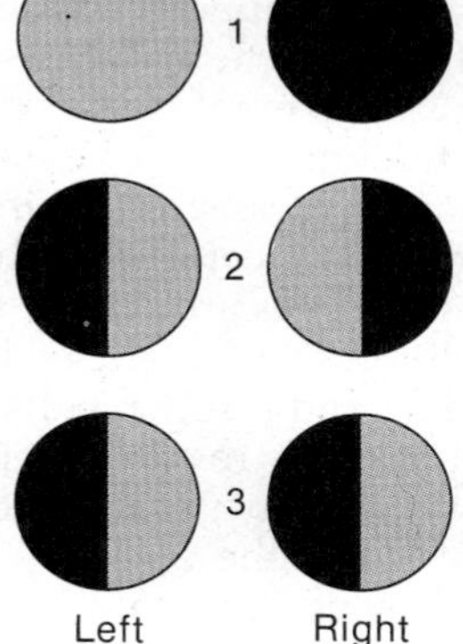

FIGURE 7–2. Visual field defects. 1, Unilateral blindness—injury to retina or optic nerve on one side of pathway results in total blindness of eye on same side of lesion; 2, bitemporal hemianopsia—injury to optic chiasm results in partial blindness of temporal fields of both eyes; 3, homonymous hemianopsia—injury to optic tract on one side of pathway results in partial blindness affecting temporal field of same side and nasal field of opposite side. (Redrawn from Bates, B. [1991]. *A guide to physical examination* [5th ed., p. 198]. Philadelphia: J. B. Lippincott.)

(homonymous hemianopsia). These visual defects are commonly associated with visual pathway injuries. However, depending on the area of injury and extent of involvement, other visual field defects can occur. It is essential for the critical care nurse to possess knowledge of the visual pathway and the effects of various lesions to detect potential or actual visual field defects and to develop appropriate communication strategies.

AUDITORY CHANNEL. Listening is another important component of communication. Messages sent verbally must be accurately received or heard before the receiver can assign true meaning. True meaning is congruent with the sender's intended message. Listening is an active process that necessitates attention, concentration, and supportive use of body language to hear what is being said and to understand it. It is important to hear all aspects of speech such as tone, pitch, speed, and volume, not just the words. By careful listening, critical care nurses can not only obtain important and useful information about the patient but detect hidden concerns, fears, anxieties, and needs.

Sounds in the environment are conducted inward toward auditory receptors in the inner ear by sound waves, vibrations, and pressure waves. Sound waves traverse the external ear to reach the tympanic membrane, where they are converted to vibrations. These vibrations are then relayed to the inner ear, where they are converted to pressure waves. In the cochlea, pressure waves stimulate the sensory receptors (hair cells), which are innervated by the vestibulocochlear nerve. With the stimulation of the vestibulocochlear nerve (cranial nerve VIII), sound impulses are carried to the auditory center in the temporal lobes.

A hearing impairment exists when sounds are unable to reach the inner ear or when the neural mechanism responsible for transmitting impulses to the brain has been damaged. A conductive hearing loss is present when sound waves are unable to reach the middle ear. This condition may be caused by trauma, obstruction, or infection, and rarely results in deafness. A sensorineural hearing loss results when the inner ear (hair cells) or neural pathway is damaged, in which case impulses do not reach the auditory center. Conditions that can cause a sensorineural loss include trauma, anoxia, and toxic medications such as aminoglycosides and loop diuretics. Damage to the hair cells and nerve tissue of the inner ear usually produces permanent deafness. Another type of hearing loss occurs with aging. Presbycusis is the gradual hearing loss that results from degenerative processes.

KINESTHETIC CHANNEL. Significant information can be obtained and communicated through touch. Touch is an important aspect of nursing practice. Critical care nurses and other health care professionals use casual touch to administer care and needed therapeutic procedures to their patients. This privilege is granted to nurses and physicians by virtue of their role in the institution. However, touch can also be used as a channel for communicating feelings of concern, support, and empathy and for developing a therapeutic relationship.

Touch receptors are located superficially on the skin surface. Sensory information such as touch, temperature, pain, and pressure are conveyed to the thalamus and cerebral cortex through either the spinothalamic or dorsal tract in the spinal cord. Lesions that interfere with the conduction of sensory impulses to the brain may result in an inability to experience sensations such as touch.

OUTPUT CHANNELS. Messages received through each of the above channels are processed in specific areas of the brain. After messages have been integrated, ideas are generated and a response is made. There are two important speech centers in the brain, Broca's area and Wernicke's area. The left hemisphere of the brain is usually dominant for speech functions. Broca's area, located in the frontal lobe, is the motor speech area and controls movement of the tongue, lips, and vocal cords responsible for speech. It also directs and coordinates the muscles involved in writing. Wernicke's area, located in the temporal lobe, is important for the comprehension of spoken or written language.

Injury to these areas can have a profound impact on a person's ability to communicate. Aphasia is the loss or impairment of the ability to communicate through speech by expression or comprehension or both (Louis & Povse, 1980; Pimental, 1986; Boss, 1991). Focal brain injury such as a cerebrovascular accident or a hemorrhage affecting Broca's area can result in loss of speech, and is termed expressive aphasia. Language comprehension remains intact; however, speech is usually slow and unintelligible. Receptive aphasia, or loss of language comprehension, occurs with injury to Wernicke's area. Speech may be fluent, but the content is usually unorganized. Global aphasia may occur when several areas in the dominant hemisphere are damaged. Both comprehension and speech are impaired. Dysarthria is a group of speech disorders resulting from damage to or poor coordination of the speech muscles. Comprehension is unaffected, but the resulting speech pattern is slow and slurred. The ability to swallow may also be affected. Damage to Broca's or Wernicke's area and other areas of the brain significantly affects a patient's ability to communicate through speech, writing, and gestures.

NONVERBAL COMMUNICATION. Nonverbal communication involves gestures, facial expressions, touch, and body language. Body language refers to the way a person uses body position or movements to communicate. Nonverbal communication often accompanies verbal messages. For example, saying "yes" is often accompanied by nodding the head up and down. However, nonverbal communication may also contradict what is said. For example, a patient may claim he is feeling fine, but his body language may indicate anxiety and restlessness. Body posture can help determine a patient's feelings as well. A slouched position may indicate lack of energy or motivation, whereas a rigid or tense posture may indicate pain or fear. Nonverbal messages are generally good indicators of how a person feels.

Eye contact and physical appearance are other forms of nonverbal communication that play a role in the communication process. The use and interpretation of eye contact is a cultural variable that must be explored before appropriate meaning can be assigned. Avoidance of eye contact during a communication interaction may indicate feelings of shame, fear, or low self-worth. It can be used to maintain distance, prevent an interaction from occurring, or halt a present interaction. Appearance also provides clues to the patient's feelings. An unkempt appearance may suggest lack of energy and motivation, or even depression. It is important to note when nonverbal communication is incongruent with spoken words. Critical care nurses must skillfully interpret and validate the patient's nonverbal communication to understand its intended meaning.

ESSENTIAL ELEMENTS FOR EFFECTIVE COMMUNICATION

Equally important in the communication process are elements that can enhance communication interactions. These include trust, active listening, empathy, and the use of touch.

TRUST. The communication interaction between a patient or his or her family and the nurse is enhanced when a trusting relationship is established. Trust is reliance on, belief in, and confidence in another individual without any doubt (Bradley & Edinberg, 1990). In the critical care unit, patients are bombarded with new information and requests to make decisions about their illness and treatment options. Without a trusting relationship, the patient may be faced with uncertainty, fear, and inability to make decisions. The patient may also manifest anger and withdrawal. A common misconception of health care professionals is that patients and their families trust immediately and automatically when a relationship is begun. Trust develops over time. It occurs when repeated interactions have a positive or significant impact on the patient. The development of trust is also affected by past experiences (Sundeen et al., 1994).

The critical care nurse must develop trust through open and honest communication. Establishing a trusting relationship in the critical care setting is often difficult because of the numerous and varying kinds of personnel involved in a patient's care. A nurse's work schedule and shift rotation can interfere with progression through the orientation, working, and termination phases of developing a relationship with patients and their families. In the orientation phase, the relationship is superficial. Rapport is developed as the nurse gathers important information about the patient and plans his or her nursing care. Information is also gathered from and given to the patient's family about the patient's illness, prognosis, and treatment plan. It is during the working phase that the critical care nurse and the patient feel enough comfort with each other to share their feelings. Focus is placed on the patient's needs and concerns. The nurse intervenes to help the patient and his or her family cope, adapt, or achieve comfort. To enhance this phase, as much as possible, continuity of the same caregiver should be maintained. If this is not possible, extra efforts must be made to maintain follow-through and communication of patient needs from one caregiver to the next. In most instances, the critical care nurse is unable to terminate his or her relationship with the patient properly. This may be because of staffing arrangements or the sudden transfer of the patient to surgery or another service. A rapid, unexpected end to a therapeutic, trusting relationship may affect a patient's sense of trust in future relationships. The nurse who possesses a trusting attitude is likely to foster trust in the patient (Sundeen et al., 1994). Characteristics of trust that foster effective communication are listed in Table 7–1. Establishing trust will help the patient to communicate concerns and feelings more openly. This in turn will enable the nurse to intervene more specifically to meet individual patient needs.

TABLE 7–1. **Characteristics of Trust**

Caring attitude	Consistency
Honesty	Credibility
Genuineness	Professionalism
Dependability	Competence
Reliability	

ACTIVE LISTENING. Listening is usually considered a passive rather than an active process. Listening passively does not ensure that the message delivered was understood as intended (Smith, 1992). On the contrary, active listening requires concentration and attention to both verbal and nonverbal messages. It involves letting the patient know that he or she has been understood. To listen with understanding implies placing one's self in another person's frame of mind. The critical care nurse is actively listening when he or she is able to hear and derive meaning from what is said.

The nature of the critical care environment makes active listening difficult and challenging for the nurse. Active listening is facilitated by making time to listen, removing barriers to listening, and paying attention to and analyzing nonverbal cues (Table 7–2). The nurse in the critical care setting must allocate time for active listening to meet the needs of the patient. Barriers to listening must also be eliminated. These include judgments, biases, and environmental noise.

Wallston and Wallston (1975) identified other factors that influence listening behaviors of nurses, such as patient's medical diagnosis and style of responding. Listening that is therapeutic and effective involves the use of all senses. It involves empathizing, maintaining

TABLE 7–2. **Guidelines for Active Listening**

Evaluate own listening skills
Plan time for active listening
Clear mind of personal thoughts and biases, concentrate, and interpret the patient's verbal and nonverbal messages
Remove distractions as much as possible (i.e., noise, interruptions, conversation of others)
Pay attention to patient's verbal and nonverbal messages
Augment listening with body language: maintain eye contact, use facial expressions, nod head, use expressive touch
Ask relevant questions and summarize key points using patient's words
Evaluate outcome of active listening

eye contact, attending to verbal and nonverbal messages, attending to body posture and distance, responding with facial expressions, gestures, words, and touch, asking relevant questions, and summarizing messages using the patient's words (Kemper, 1992). When a patient has a communication impairment, the nurse should be persistent in listening even if listening must take place over several sessions (Lekander et al., 1993). Pettigrew (1990) describes the phenomenon of presence or the act of being available wholeheartedly and listening to another person with all of one's self. Presence counteracts the negative effects of hospitalization in an intensive care unit by allowing the patient to be comforted, experience caring, and to be heard.

EMPATHY. Empathy is a process whereby an individual attempts to think and feel like another individual (Northouse, 1979). The critical care nurse who practices empathy places himself or herself in the patient's shoes and experiences that patient's situation from the patient's point of view rather than his or her own. This is done to accept, understand, and validate what the patient is experiencing. To practice empathy is to maintain one's identity while feeling with another, to be objective while at the same time offering support and understanding. Empathy differs from sympathy in that the latter involves relinquishing one's identity. To sympathize is to be subjective and feel sorry for the other (Bradley & Edinberg, 1990; Smith, 1992).

For the critical care nurse to use empathy to improve communication, three elements must exist: the nurse must be able to understand and experience what the patient is feeling, empathy must be communicated genuinely to the patient, and the empathy must be perceived by the patient (Bradley & Edinberg, 1990; Smith, 1992). Smith (1992) outlined six steps that are necessary to communicate with empathy (Table 7–3). The use of empathy promotes effective communication by enabling the patient to know he or she is understood.

TOUCH. Touch is a form of communication that can significantly improve communication interactions. In an interpersonal interaction, touch is given meaning by its quality. In the highly technical arena of intensive care, critical care nurses and physicians are constantly touching patients. The nature of health care delivery necessitates access to a patient's body for examination, treatment, and provision of hygienic measures. Touch in these situations is usually task-oriented or procedural. Procedural touch occurs during most nursing procedures.

Another form of touch, expressive or caring touch, is used outside routine nursing procedures. Expressive touch is spontaneously directed toward improving communication (Pearce, 1988). It is used to establish rapport and convey acceptance, empathy, and closeness. It is also employed to comfort, support, and reassure patients in physical or psychological pain. For the unconscious or blind patient, expressive touch increases awareness that someone is present and links them to the environment. For the patient or family in distress, it facilitates expression of feelings.

The use and interpretation of touch is influenced by variables such as culture, past experiences, personality, emotions, environment, and patient factors (such as age and gender). Some nurses may be hesitant or uncomfortable using touch with their patients, fearing that it might be misinterpreted. Others may use touch without regard to its impact on the patient. It is important to recognize factors that influence touch, evaluate one's own feelings regarding touch, and assess the patient's desire for and response to touch. For touch to be effective, its meaning must be accurately conveyed and received.

In examining touch used among nurses in the intensive care unit, Estabrooks (1989) confirmed the use of caring and procedural touch and described protective touch, a type not previously identified. Caring touch is used to communicate caring, procedural touch is used to accomplish a task, and protective touch is used to protect the patient physically or to protect the nurse physically or emotionally. Restraining patients to prevent self-extubation or inadvertent discontinuance of an invasive catheter is an example of touch used to protect the patient. Preventing a patient from harming the nurse or protecting against infection are

TABLE 7–3. **Guidelines for Communicating With Empathy**

Free mind of distractions
Focus on the patient
Pay attention to patient's verbal and nonverbal messages: listen and observe
Cue in on central message patient is communicating
Convey an empathetic response: verbally reflect the patient's feelings, ensure your nonverbal messages are congruent with acceptance and understanding
Evaluate patient's response to empathy (e.g., patient feels interaction was positive)

TABLE 7–4. **Guidelines for Using Touch to Improve Communication**

Be familiar with the use, effects, and applications of the different forms of touch (i.e., procedural, expressive, and therapeutic)
Evaluate own feelings and comfort regarding touch
Assess the patient's desire for and response to touch
Use touch for a purpose
Be aware of cultural, familial, and gender-related factors
Be sensitive to the setting and timing in which touch is delivered
Use expressive touch to communicate caring, comfort, and encouragement (i.e., hold the patient's hand, stroke the arm or forehead, place hand on or squeeze shoulder)
Incorporate expressive touch when delivering procedural touch
Evaluate use of touch and patient's response

examples of touch used to protect the nurse. Withdrawal of touch or cold touch are examples of protective touch used by the nurse to distance herself from emotional pain. Touch that is delivered in a harsh or severe manner and imparts a negative feeling to the patient is a form of protective touch used by the nurse to release emotional tension. Protective touch is not advocated for effective communication. Awareness of this form of touch is important so that the nurse can modify factors that lead to its use.

Schoenhofer (1989), in a study of factors involved in the use of touch by critical care nurses, found that the use of expressive touch was infrequent. In observing 1-hour segments of nurse–patient interactions with 30 patients, there were 181 instances where nurses were at patients' bedsides but did not use touch. In instances when it was used, it was of short duration and low intensity.

These few studies demonstrate that how the nurse uses touch will influence communication interactions. Strategies to consider when using touch to communicate are presented in Table 7–4. The critical care environment, with all its technical wonders, diverts the nurse's time and attention away from the patient. Critical care nurses can counterbalance this highly technical environment by providing personalized care through the use of touch (Sinclair, 1988).

COMMUNICATION BARRIERS

The continuous nature of the communication process is theoretical. In reality, a breakdown in communication can occur at any point. Anything that interferes with message transmission forms a barrier. For communication to be effective in the critical care setting, barriers must be recognized and overcome. These include physical limitations, environmental factors, sociocultural factors, and psychosocial factors.

PHYSICAL LIMITATIONS. Communication deficits resulting from injury to the speech centers in the brain have previously been discussed. Transitory alterations in communication can occur when mentation is affected by medications, hypoxia, and electrolyte imbalances. Endotracheal intubation, however, is the most common cause of impaired communication in the ICU.

Endotracheal intubation is established to provide a patient with an airway and to facilitate mechanical ventilation. The presence of an artificial airway interferes with the patient's ability to communicate by affecting the vocal cords. This inability to communicate creates stress in mechanically ventilated patients. In an exploratory study conducted by Johnson and Sexton (1990) to identify distressing factors associated with mechanical ventilation, patients identified inability to speak and use former methods of communication as most distressing. In another exploratory study conducted by Gries and Fernsler (1988), communication problems such as insufficient explanations and inability to communicate were cited as major sources of stress by mechanically ventilated patients. Patients' perceptions of impaired communication related to mechanical ventilation have been categorized by Connolly and Shekleton (1991) as inability to communicate, insufficient explanations, inadequate understanding, fears and dangers of not being able to speak, and difficulty with communication methods.

Several other factors contribute to a patient's inability to communicate. These include restricted body movements secondary to wrist restraints, ventilator tubing, or presence of invasive lines; changes in mentation due to medications, sleep disturbances, and sensory overload; and therapeutic paralysis. Communication difficulties are also influenced by interactions with the nurse. Salyer and Stuart (1985), in examining communication interactions between intubated patients and nurses, found a lack of patient-initiated interactions. In one-third of positive interactions initiated by the patient, nurses tended to respond negatively. Few nurses attempted to clarify what was observed or said by the patient. Silence by the nurse was the most common action or reaction that elicited a negative patient response. In another study, patients had difficulty communicating their message to the nurse, and therefore restricted communication to essential information only (Gries & Fernsler, 1988). Stovsky et al. (1988), in a study comparing communication methods in intubated patients after cardiac surgery, found that nurses and patients use different methods of communication. These studies highlight the need for effective communication interactions between the intubated patient and the nurse.

The challenge of communicating effectively with mechanically ventilated patients is heightened when patients are paralyzed to achieve adequate ventilation and oxygenation. In this situation, the patient is unable to communicate at all. Furthermore, patients are usually sedated to blunt their perceptions and to decrease the fear and anxiety of not being able to move. Although the patient is paralyzed, he or she may remain conscious with intact auditory and kinesthetic abilities (Parker et al., 1984; Vitello-Cicciu, 1984). It is especially important that nurses maintain and enhance communication with these patients (see Interventions section).

ENVIRONMENTAL FACTORS. The special characteristics of the critical care unit often create communication barriers. Specifically, these include lack of privacy, high noise levels, use of technical language, and rigid routines.

The patient's privacy is often violated in the critical care setting. The patient's body is subjected to numerous examinations and procedures by health care workers who may or may not have an established relationship with the patient. A patient's disease, treatment, and prognosis are sometimes discussed with other members of the health care team around the unit, in elevators, and in cafeterias, often without sensitivity to the presence of patients, visitors, and other personnel. Careless treatment of privileged information and poor regard for patient privacy can lead to misinterpretation by the patient and reluctance to disclose information to health care providers. Respect for a patient's physical privacy and confidentiality will significantly influence communication interactions.

Noise is another environmental factor that affects communication. A considerable amount of information exists on the effect of noise on patients (Hansell, 1984; Baker, 1984; Green, 1992; Grumet, 1993) (see Chapter 8). Noise is anything that interferes with effective transmission of messages. Visual distractions, unintelligible writing, offensive odors, and biases all constitute "noise." In the critical care unit, noise is generated by sounds of beeping monitors, alarms, ventilators, and staff conversations. These sounds not only contribute to the physiologic stress experienced by critically ill patients, but can lead to sensory–perceptual alterations or "ICU psychosis." The contribution of noise to sensory alterations is described further in Chapter 8.

Critical care nurses have become accustomed to unit noises and may not recognize them as potential barriers to communication. Developing an awareness of "noise" in the critical care unit can assist a nurse in controlling or reducing its impact on critically ill patients. To start with, nurses can lower the tone of their voices and limit their personal conversations around the bedside. If possible, the door to a patient's room should be closed. The volume of telephones, cardiac monitors, and other monitoring equipment must be kept low but discernible. Attention to noises generated by hurried conversations (e.g., yelling across the room) and treatment of supplies (e.g., slamming cabinets or drawers) is crucial. Selecting equipment with noise reduction features such as waterless chest tube drainage systems is also helpful. The unit can supply and offer ear plugs to patients. Minimizing noise is beneficial for the patient as well as for effective communication.

Another environmental factor that affects communication is technical language. Language that is specific to a particular field, such as medicine, is referred to as "jargon." For the health care professional, jargon is part of everyday language and conversation. For the patient, highly technical language is perceived as foreign and serves to distance him or her and his family from the communication interaction. Without appropriate explanations in "lay" terms, words the patient and family can understand clearly, communication may be fraught with misinterpretations and misconceptions. Critical care nurses should consciously examine their communication with patients and families and eliminate the use of jargon. They should be astute in noting a patient's or family's nonverbal cues indicating a lack of understanding and quick to adjust their level of communication. Most importantly, nurses should encourage patients and their families to ask questions.

The patient and his or her visitors are frequently reminded of the hospital's policies and routines. The monitoring of vital signs, provision of hygienic measures, scheduling of procedures, and maintenance of visiting hours are parts of the hospital routine that are often inflexible and interfere with effective communication. As much as possible, traditional practices should be arranged to promote effective communication interactions. Environmental barriers must be prevented from interfering with the communication process. A proper climate for clear transmission of messages, careful listening, and thoughtful discussion should be established.

SOCIOCULTURAL FACTORS. Sociocultural barriers that can influence communication between patients and the health care team include differences in culture, language, and behaviors. Culture is the sum of all experiences past and present that provide criteria against which choices and decisions are made. Each patient is a unique individual, possessing a different value system and cultural background. Cultural differences result in various patient behaviors and communication styles. In an interpersonal interaction, culture influences the display of emotions, the use and interpretation of eye contact and touch, and who in the family should be spoken to for proper respect. Variables such as these must be explored by the culturally sensitive nurse to facilitate communication.

The cultural needs of a patient and his or her family must be identified for effective communication to occur. Routinely, these include language spoken, food preferences, religious affiliation, and cultural rituals. It is also important to assess the patient's family structure, role relationships, decision-making practices, beliefs about health and illness, and expectations of hospitalization. In exploring nurses' experiences in caring for culturally diverse patients, Murphy and Clark (1993) found that communication problems and a lack of knowledge regarding cultural differences were common problems nurses encountered in the clinical setting. Other problems included difficulty establishing relationships with patients and their relatives and feelings of frustration, stress, and helplessness. Nurses in the study cited that communication difficulties—the inability to talk with the patient, explain aspects of care, and know what was acceptable to the patient—

affected the care delivered. It is essential that critical care nurses not only assess their patients' cultural beliefs, values, and attitudes, but develop cultural awareness to meet the needs of each patient.

Cultural needs are determined in order to avoid ethnocentrism and stereotyping (Parfitt, 1988). Ethnocentrism is the belief that one's own culture is superior to another's. The nurse who conveys such a belief is unaccepting of a patient's individuality. The patient who perceives this attitude may be unwilling or reluctant to share meaningful and useful information. It is essential that the nurse demonstrate an attitude of acceptance and the belief that no one culture is superior to another to facilitate effective communication.

The possession of preconceived ideas about a patient's cultural pattern or group can severely affect communication and can lead to misguided interventions. Stereotyping occurs when a person believes that all members of a particular group are the same. The tendency to label ethnic groups based on frequently observed reactions to certain situations is not uncommon and impairs effective communication. Because of past or present experiences or beliefs, the nurse may possess a certain attitude toward a particular group that surfaces on contact with a member of that group. This tendency is evident in nurses' labeling of hospitalized patients in terms of "good" or "difficult" patients. "Good" patients tend to be quiet, nondemanding, and cooperative. "Difficult" patients, defined in a survey of nurses, are "demanding, complaining, frustrating, time-consuming, requesting, frequently calling, manipulative, female, impolite, unreasonable or uncooperative" (Podrasky & Sexton, 1988). The nurse's reaction and response to these types of patients may be based on such false assumptions. Critical care nurses should consciously treat every patient as an individual with a set of unique characteristics and experiences.

PSYCHOLOGICAL FACTORS. Anxiety, fear, and loneliness are feelings of patients and families that can affect the communication interaction. Such feelings arise when patients experience unexpected illnesses and sensations, life-threatening conditions, environmental changes, and role changes. Ironically, critically ill patients and families must attempt to cope with these feelings when they are least capable of doing so. The critical care nurse can do much to alleviate or reduce these feelings by providing patients and families with information and assisting them to interpret the environment.

Anxiety and fear are feelings that arise when a perceived threat is present. Anxiety differs from fear in that the latter is more tangible and easier to identify. Anxiety is a state of mind that exists when one's sense of well-being is threatened. There are various levels of anxiety that can significantly affect a person's ability to communicate effectively. Mild anxiety is experienced frequently in day-to-day life. It improves one's functioning by motivating, preparing, and sharpening the senses and perceptions. An individual experiencing mild anxiety tends to solve problems more effectively. Moderate anxiety limits one's perceptual field to a degree that one's problem-solving ability is lessened. Severe anxiety occurs when stress is intense. A person in this state can focus on only one detail (relieving anxiety) due to limited attention and perception. Panic, the most destructive level of anxiety, impairs an individual's perceptual ability to a point where effective communication and functioning are disabled.

Critical illness and hospitalization can precipitate feelings of loneliness in a patient. Loneliness should not be confused with social isolation because the former is not an imposed condition; rather, it is a disheartened awareness of being alone. Loneliness creates physical and psychological pain and anxiety for the patient (Buchda, 1987). This pain may be caused by the threat of illness on life or by separation from loved ones and familiar surroundings. A patient experiencing loneliness may appear quiet and withdrawn or may display tearfulness or restlessness. Feelings of anxiety may be present, arising from a fear of being lonely.

Anxiety, fear, and loneliness are feelings that may be felt alone or in combination with each other. The critical care nurse should recognize situations and behaviors that can precipitate or indicate the presence of such feelings in order to plan and develop proper strategies to alleviate them. Whenever possible, the precipitating stressor should be identified and either reduced or eliminated. Understanding the different levels of anxiety and their effects on communication can allow the nurse to intervene at an early stage. Patients should be encouraged to express their concerns to decrease their feelings of anxiety, fear, or loneliness. Nurses should attempt to reduce these feelings by providing time, support, reassurance, and personalized care. The family should be encouraged to visit and participate in the patient's care. Minimizing and controlling the stressful feelings of a patient can facilitate effective communication interactions. (Refer to Chapters 5 and 6.)

INTERVENTIONS THAT IMPROVE COMMUNICATION

Communicating effectively in an ICU is a challenge faced by critical care nurses on a daily basis. The presence of physical, environmental, sociocultural, and psychological barriers affect the quality of messages exchanged. Nurses must possess the necessary skills to promote an environment conducive to the mutual sharing of information. Strategies for commonly encountered situations are presented to assist in achieving this environment.

COMMUNICATING WITH THE VISUALLY IMPAIRED PATIENT. Patients who have had a stroke or intracerebral hemorrhage may have a visual impairment if the visual pathway is affected. Other factors that may cause a visual impairment include aging, glaucoma, cataract, diabetes, and direct trauma. The stroke patient who has a visual defect may or not may be aware of his or her visual impairment. By observing the patient's activities and reactions to movement around him or her, the nurse can detect if an impairment exists. For example, the patient may eat from only one side of the plate or respond to the nurse or visitor on only one side of the bed. A patient with homonymous hemianopsia (loss of half of visual field affecting the same side of each eye) should be taught to compensate for the visual defect by turning his or her head. This allows the patient to use the intact visual fields of each eye. The nurse and other personnel should be taught to announce their presence and approach the patient on the unaffected side. Essential objects, such as a clock or calendar, should be placed in the field of vision that is unaffected. When visual perception is affected, the patient may not see or deny seeing objects on a particular side. In this case, the nurse must provide the patient with step-by-step verbal guidance during an activity. Detailed explanations may be necessary, especially if the patient is completely blind.

For effective communication to occur between the nurse and patient, it is important to identify the degree of visual impairment and the patient's adaptation. In a study conducted by Waterman and Webb (1992), stressors experienced by visually impaired patients and methods of coping were found to be specific to individual patients. Patients in this study generally felt that their physical needs were met by nurses; however, communication was reported to be a problematic area. Table 7–5 summarizes general strategies for patients with partial or complete blindness. When communicating with visually impaired patients, the critical care nurse should maximize the use of auditory and kinesthetic channels.

COMMUNICATING WITH THE HEARING-IMPAIRED PATIENT. Hospitalization in an ICU is a frightening experience that may be exacerbated in patients who have a hearing impairment. Unless the hearing impairment is an obvious complication of injury or treatment (i.e., medications that affect hearing in high doses), an assessment of the patient's hearing must be made. Otherwise, a lack of awareness will lead to poor communication. In assessing for a hearing impairment, the nurse should also assess the patient's ability to read, write, and understand as well as the ability to lip-read or use sign language. It should be determined whether the patient has a hearing aid and if it is working properly. The presence of ear wax or cerumen should be assessed and removed if present according to hospital protocols. The presence of a hearing aid in the ear canal increases cerumen accumulation that can lead to conductive hearing loss (Palumbo, 1990). The hearing aid should be worn by the patient and not removed or stored while in the hospital, unless contraindicated. Because these devices amplify sound, they do not distinguish between background noise and verbal speech. To maximize transmission of verbal messages, it is essential that background noise be reduced or eliminated.

Sounds usually help to orient people to their environment. Without the aid of an assistive hearing device, the patient will rely heavily on visual cues. Characteristics of a critical care unit can be overwhelming to the patient. It is imperative that the nurse maintain effective communication with the patient (see Table 7–5) and assist with interpretation of the environment.

Awareness of one's nonverbal messages is important because tone, pitch, and volume of speech are not perceived by the patient. The critical care nurse must use nonverbal messages to convey caring and concern. Patients who have a hearing impairment should be clearly identified so other members of the interdisciplinary team can be alerted and prepared. A sign placed at the room, at the bedside, and on the patient care plan can facilitate awareness.

COMMUNICATING WITH THE APHASIC PATIENT. Aphasia, often resulting from a stroke, poses a significant communication challenge to the critical care nurse. These patients not only have impaired comprehension, speech, or both, but they often exhibit frustration, anger, and depression because of it (Keller et al., 1989). Patients must cope with the communication difficulties as well as the precipitating event. The critical care nurse can assist the aphasic patient by establishing effective communication strategies. Interventions that assist with communication disorders have been identified by Boss (1991) as follows: manipulate the environment, show supportive behaviors, institute measures that enhance communication, and educate the patient, family, and significant others.

Before effective strategies can be planned, it is important that the nurse first assess the patient's ability to speak and comprehend language. The nurse should engage the patient in conversation to determine his or her speech and language skills such as fluency, difficulty in finding words, and difficulty in building grammatically correct sentences (Boykin, 1984). Comprehension can be assessed by asking the patient to answer simple questions, repeat words and sentences, and to carry out motor commands. It is also important to assess the patient's ability to read and understand written language. Some aphasic patients are unable to understand words but do well with pictures and diagrams. To facilitate communication with these patients, nurses must create an environment of concern and support. When the type of aphasia is known, more appropriate strategies can be used to facilitate communication (Table 7–6).

Patients who have extreme difficulty with verbal expression may find writing more manageable. For these patients, writing materials should be readily available. When both verbal and written expression are impaired, having the patient read may be a way to communicate. Patients who have difficulty reading can be taught later on how to recognize words (Loughrey, 1992). When the patient is asked to read, it is important to use words that contribute directly

TABLE 7–5. **Communication Strategies for Specific Clinical Situations**

Communication Strategies for the Visually Impaired

Announce presence, introduce self
Approach patient on unaffected side
Teach patient to compensate for deficit by turning head
Place objects in patient's field of vision
Have adequate lighting in room
Ensure written material is clear and large enough to see
Provide detailed explanations through verbal guidance
Use qualities of speech and touch to augment communication

Communication Strategies for the Hearing Impaired

Assess presence and functioning of hearing aid
Establish a quiet environment, decrease background noise
Face patient so patient can see lips
Speak slowly, use simple words and short phrases
Use nonverbal messages to enhance communication
Avoid anything that distracts or obscures mouth (e.g., eating, chewing gum)
Use illustrations, written material, communication board
Signal patient toward person who is speaking
Use trained interpreter for sign language, when applicable

Communicating With Mechanically Ventilated Patients

Intubated Patient
Establish communication method before intubation (if possible)
Assess ability to communicate: mentation, motor strength, coordination, and endurance
Reduce stressors to communication (e.g., restraints, environmental stimuli, sleep deprivation)
Use communication methods appropriate for patient's abilities (e.g., pencil and paper, letter and/or picture board, magic slate, lip reading)
Use multiple methods of communication to match patient's abilities, desires, and needs
Facilitate communication (i.e., eyeglasses, hearing aid, accessibility and visibility of communication aids, positioning of patient)
Have call bell within reach at all times
Pay attention to and interpret patient's nonverbal cues
Convey interest, acceptance, patience, understanding with own nonverbal behaviors (e.g., facial expressions, eye contact, touch)
Communicate effective methods to others by incorporating strategies in care plan
Investigate other methods (e.g., electronic devices, specialized tracheostomy tubes, computer)
Provide frequent explanations in lay terms and repeat as needed; offer support and encouragement
Evaluate effectiveness of methods and restrategize if necessary

Pharmacologically Paralyzed Patient
Introduce self
Provide patient with frequent orientation to time, place, environment
Explain all interventions
Use expressive touch to comfort and reassure

to the intended meaning or convey specific images such as chair, bed, orange.

Patients with receptive aphasia may understand and express themselves better in writing than through speech. Only pertinent information should be provided to avoid overstimulating and fatiguing the patient. Communicating with patients who have global aphasia is more difficult. Both comprehension and speech are impaired. The patient's ability to read, write, or speak is severely limited. The nurse must rely on nonverbal messages to communicate acceptance, trust, and reassurance.

COMMUNICATING WITH THE MECHANICALLY VENTILATED PATIENT. Effective communication with patients who are mechanically ventilated remains a significant challenge to critical care nurses. Impaired communication can lead to anxiety, fear, and frustration in patients requiring such support. Knowing and understanding the factors that influence communication interactions in the mechanically ventilated patient can assist the nurse in planning communication strategies. Communication strategies and nursing interventions that are effective and mutually satisfying to the patient and nurse have yet to be identified and validated (Funk, 1989; Menzel, 1994). Strategies commonly used and perceived as helpful by intubated patients and nurses are identified in Table 7–5 and include gestures, writing, asking questions, and lip-reading (Johnson & Sexton, 1990). Connolly and Shekleton (1991), in surveying communication methods used with intubated patients, found that pencil and paper, picture boards, and lip-reading were the most often used forms of communication. Sign language is another method that was found to be commonly used (Gries & Fernsler, 1988).

In selecting a method of communication to use with mechanically ventilated patients, the nurse must

TABLE 7–6. **Communication Strategies When Type of Aphasia Is Known**

Type of Aphasia	Characteristics	Interventions
Expressive aphasia (Broca's aphasia)	Comprehension intact Speech impaired: nonfluent and telegraphic (short sentences and phrases with omission of words) Impaired ability to write, name objects, and repeat words Patient is aware of communication deficit	Acknowledge patient's difficulties Be patient, allow time for patient to respond Allow patient to speak for himself—don't interrupt, interpret, or finish what is being said May rephrase statement and have patient fill in word Encourage patient to use simple words Have patient use pictures, written material, and gestures
Receptive aphasia (Wernicke's aphasia)	Comprehension impaired Speech intact: fluent but meaningless (without content) Impaired ability to read, write, name objects, and repeat words Patient is not aware of communication deficit	Speak clearly and slowly Use simple words and phrases Repeat or reword instructions and questions as necessary Ask only pertinent questions to avoid patient fatigue Avoid compound commands (series of commands simultaneously) Delineate each task step by step, one at a time Use nonverbal messages to facilitate communication
Global aphasia	Comprehension and speech impaired	Use and encourage use of nonverbal communication such as gestures, pantomime, pointing, and facial expressions

consider patient- and technique-related factors (Williams, 1992). Patient factors to consider include cognitive ability; presence of weakness, fatigue, or activity restrictions; effects of medications and fluid and electrolyte imbalances; and neurologic or sensory impairments (visual, auditory, or kinesthetic). Communication technique factors include availability, ease of use, visibility, readability, motor requirements of the patient, cost, and time requirements. After assessing these factors, the nurse should select the most appropriate communication method. It is important to keep in mind that various methods should be used because patients' needs and abilities may change. Connolly and Shekleton (1991) recommend using methods that are least frustrating and most satisfying for the patient and the nurse. Once a method is selected, the nurse should facilitate the communication interaction by ensuring that eyeglasses or a hearing aid is worn when indicated, placing the communication aid or one's body in an optimal position for the patient to see, and including family and significant others.

Writing material, picture and alphabet boards, or magic slates should be used by the patient if and when he or she is able to do so. A communication board with illustrations, words, and letters of the alphabet can facilitate communication and reduce frustration associated with spelling out words (Fig. 7–3).

Every attempt must be made by the nurse to interpret the patient's verbal and nonverbal messages. Establishing a communication plan with the patient and sharing it with the interdisciplinary team and family can enhance the communication process. Stovsky et al. (1988) found that including a method of communication with preoperative instructions increased patient satisfaction in postoperative cardiac surgical patients. In their study, a communication board was used.

Communication with patients who have been pharmacologically paralyzed must be ongoing. Families and members of the interdisciplinary team must be reminded that the patient is awake and can hear. A constant reminder that has been used consists of placing a sign over the patient's bed indicating the patient's situation and essential communication points (Barton, 1993). Because consciousness, hearing, and feeling remain intact in these patients, critical care nurses must continue to provide sensitive and caring communication (see Table 7–5). The patient should be provided with explanations about his or her care and with frequent orientation to the surroundings. The patient must be reassured about his or her situation and the nature of his or her paralysis. Expressive touch should be used to link him or her to the environment. The family should be encouraged to touch and communicate with their loved one.

COMMUNICATING WITH CULTURALLY DIVERSE PATIENTS. Communicating with culturally diverse patients in the critical care setting is a challenging responsibility for nurses and other health care providers. Critical care nurses must promote an environment in which the patient's cultural beliefs, values, and attitudes are accepted and respected. Communication is further challenged when a language barrier exists. Patients who are unable to speak the dominant language may not effectively communicate their needs. Interactions between the patient and the nurse may be fraught with anxiety and frustration. It is often through nonverbal communication that needs are ascertained. However, the nurse must recognize that the use and meaning of nonverbal messages is culturally influenced. Likewise, culture will affect how the patient interprets the nurse's nonverbal communication.

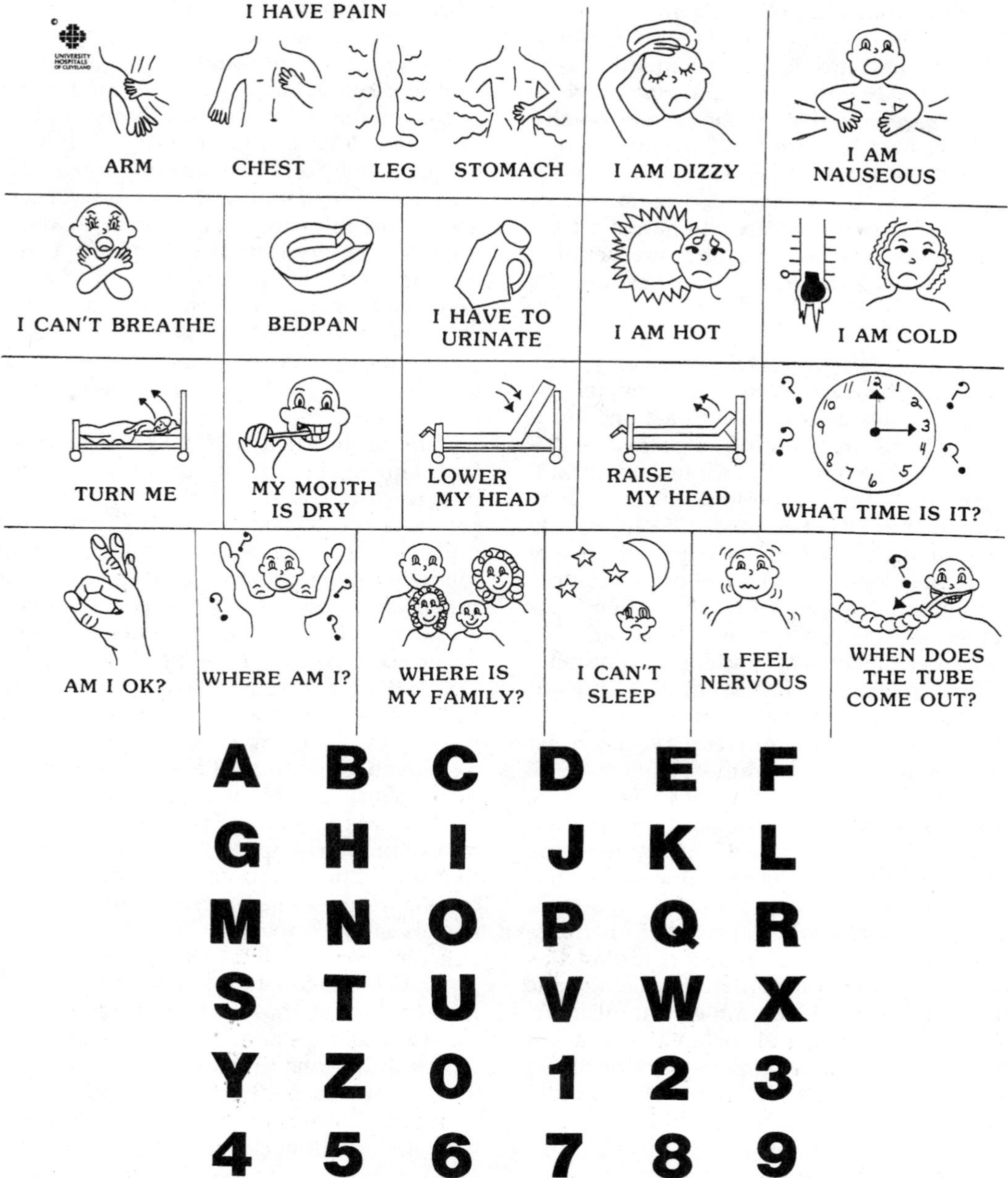
I HAVE PAIN
ARM
CHEST
LEG
STOMACH
I AM DIZZY
I AM NAUSEOUS
I CAN'T BREATHE
BEDPAN
I HAVE TO URINATE
I AM HOT
I AM COLD
TURN ME
MY MOUTH IS DRY
LOWER MY HEAD
RAISE MY HEAD
WHAT TIME IS IT?
AM I OK?
WHERE AM I?
WHERE IS MY FAMILY?
I CAN'T SLEEP
I FEEL NERVOUS
WHEN DOES THE TUBE COME OUT?
A B C D E F
G H I J K L
M N O P Q R
S T U V W X
Y Z 0 1 2 3
4 5 6 7 8 9

FIGURE 7–3. Communication board. (Courtesy of the University Hospitals of Cleveland.)

When a language barrier is present, the nurse should begin with an assessment of the patient's ability to speak and understand English. This can be done by assessing the patient's response to questions or commands and observing nonverbal cues. The nurse should attempt to establish a relationship by spending time with the patient, using nonverbal communication, being with the patient, and involving family in the patient's care (Murphy & Clark, 1993). An attempt should be made to learn a few words or phrases of the patient's language (Diaz-Gilbert, 1993). The nurse can convey respect for the patient by taking the time to do this. Dictionaries and other translation aids should be used if available. It is important that communication with the patient continue despite the language barrier. The nurse should schedule extra time to communicate, speak slowly, and repeat information as necessary. Trained interpreters within the hospital, facility, or community should be used to facilitate communication. Family members or employees of the hospital may be used when necessary, but with caution, because the potential for translation errors and misinterpretation exists. When an interpreter is not available, the nurse must be creative. Gestures, demonstrations, pictures, and written material in the patient's language can be helpful. Communication boards with common patient complaints and needs are frequently used when there is impaired communication. Having communication boards in several languages can be a valuable tool in any critical care unit, especially in areas where there are culturally diverse populations. A translation booklet has been suggested as an aid in communicating with culturally diverse patients (Anthonypillai, 1993). As with any nursing intervention, the effectiveness of communication strategies must be evaluated.

COMMUNICATING WITH THE PATIENT'S FAMILY. It is important for the critical care nurse to consider the patient's family in communication interactions. Sudden or unexpected hospitalization of a patient is distressing not only for the patient, but for his or her family. Family members may experience fear, worry, anger, and exhaustion (Kleiber et al., 1994). Family structure, roles of family members, and patterns of functioning may be altered because of hospitalization. Families have a significant impact on the patient's response to illness and hospitalization. However, they may also be a source of stress for patients and nursing personnel if their needs are not identified and addressed. The needs of family members of critically ill patients and interventions for nurses have been extensively documented in the literature (Molter, 1979; Halm, 1992; Henneman & Cardin, 1992; Hickey & Leske, 1992; Leske, 1992). The need for information and reassurance about the patient's condition was commonly identified as a high need. Information and communication are also crucial in reducing anxiety in family members, especially when the patient is transferred from the ICU to a less intensive area (Bokinskie, 1992). Critical care nurses must identify the specific needs of family members, develop meaningful interventions, and demonstrate caring behaviors to assist families to cope. The needs of families of critically ill patients and nursing interventions are presented in detail in Chapter 6.

COMMUNICATING WITH HEALTH CARE TEAM MEMBERS. The critical care setting is a stressful environment for both the patient and the nurse. The stress of caring for a critically ill patient is compounded by factors related to personnel interactions, staffing patterns, compensation, problems with supplies and equipment, job expectations, and relationships with peers, administrators, physicians, and other health care workers. In addition, the current health care environment is changing dramatically and rapidly. New roles, changing roles, partnerships, and health care networks are developing, all of which affect communication among health care providers and within the critical care unit (see Chapter 1). Critical care nurses need to establish new and, in some cases, better relationships with all health care team members to influence patient care delivery. Effective communication with all members of the health care team is now more important than ever to meet patient needs and achieve desired patient outcomes.

Much of the information presented on barriers to communication also pertains to communication between members of the health care team. For example, noise levels, unit routines, cultural differences, language barriers, and anxiety can influence the effectiveness of communication between a nurse and another health care team member. Other factors that impede communication with health care team members include different views on role expectations, perceived or real power and authority of various members, past communications, interdepartmental communication barriers, fatigue level, efficiency of interdepartmental systems, and the urgency of a situation or need.

Communication with all team members is important. However, communication is particularly crucial between the nurse and the physician to accomplish collaborative efforts toward patient outcomes. For a nurse and physician to communicate effectively, the following must be present: open communication; mutual trust, respect, and support; willingness to cooperate; and professional competence in one's work (Bradley & Edinberg, 1990; Lappe, 1993; Bushnell & Dean, 1993). Bushnell and Dean (1993) identified five key building blocks for achieving collaboration in an ICU: clinical competence, credibility, consistency, assertiveness, and a collaborative management structure. When nurses and physicians work collaboratively, unit functioning, patient care, and staff satisfaction improve (Lappe, 1993). Knaus et al. (1988) found that interactions and communication between physicians and nurses can directly affect patient outcomes. In this study, mortality rates decreased when there was collaboration between physicians and nurses.

To achieve collaboration with other team members, it is important that each discipline communicate its role expectations and recognize the unique and essential contributions that are made by all team members to the care of patients. The same factors discussed above apply to communication with other team members. In addition, collaboration can be enhanced by eliminating the traditional fragmented methods of documentation and instituting a multidisciplinary progress note. Patient rounds should be expanded to include not only the physician and nurse but other members of the interdisciplinary team (e.g., pharmacist, dietitian, respiratory therapist, social worker). Increased use of multidisciplinary patient care conferences, self-directed care teams, and multidisciplinary care guides also promote collaboration.

Effective communication with all team members can assist in reducing stress, which can lead to greater job satisfaction for the nurse. Blegen (1993), in a meta-analysis of studies on nurses' job satisfaction, linked job satisfaction to communication with supervisors and peers. Therefore, to increase job satisfaction and maximally affect patient outcomes, it is critical that nurses possess skills to communicate effectively with all health care team members.

SUMMARY

Communication is an interactive process that involves sensory channels to transmit or receive messages. The communication interaction is enhanced through trust, active listening, empathy, and touch and by overcoming physical, psychological, environmental, and sociocultural barriers. Specific interventions to improve communication with commonly encountered patient situations, families, and health care workers are presented. This information can serve as a foundation for critical care nurses to sensitively and creatively plan meaningful communication interactions in the critical care setting.

REFERENCES

Anthonypillai, F. (1993). Cross-cultural communication in an intensive therapy unit. *Intensive and Critical Care Nursing, 9*(4), 263–268.

Baker, C. F. (1984). Sensory overload and noise in the ICU: Sources of environmental stress. *Critical Care Quarterly, 6*, 66–80.

Barton, C. R. (1993). *Management and monitoring of neuromuscular blocking agents in critically ill patients requiring long-term ventilatory support.* Syllabus, KS: MidAmerica Education Resources.

Blegen, M. A. (1993). Nurses' job satisfaction: A meta-analysis of related variables. *Nursing Research, 42*(1), 36–41.

Bokinskie, J. C. (1992). Family conferences: A method to diminish transfer anxiety. *Journal of Neuroscience Nursing, 24*(3), 129–133.

Boss, B. J. (1991). Managing communication disorders in stroke. *Nursing Clinics of North America, 26*(4), 985–991.

Boykin, G. V. (1984). Strategies for increasing communication with the dysphagic patient. *Dimensions of Critical Care Nursing, 3*(5), 279–287.

Bradley, J. C., & Edinberg, M. A. (1990). *Communicating in the nursing context* (3rd ed.). Norwalk, CT: Appleton & Lange.

Buchda, V. L. (1987). Loneliness in critically ill adults. *Dimensions of Critical Care Nursing, 6*(6), 335–340.

Bushnell, M. S., & Dean, J. M. (1993). Managing the intensive care unit: Physician–nurse collaboration. *Critical Care Medicine, 21*(9 Suppl), S389–S390.

Clement, J. M. (1986). Caring and touching as nursing interventions. In C. Hudak et al. (Eds.), *Critical care nursing: A holistic approach* (4th ed.) (pp. 33–42). Philadelphia: J. B. Lippincott.

Connolly, M. A., & Shekleton, M. E. (1991). Communicating with ventilator dependent patients. *Dimensions of Critical Care Nursing, 10*(2), 115–122.

DeVito, J. A. (1980). *The interpersonal communication book* (2nd ed.). New York: Harper & Row.

Diaz-Gilbert, M. (1993). Caring for culturally diverse patients. *Nursing, 23*(10), 44–45.

Easton, J. (1988). Alternative communication for patients in intensive care. *Intensive Care Nursing, 4*, 47–55.

Estabrooks, C. A. (1989). Touch: A nursing strategy in the intensive care unit. *Heart and Lung, 18*(4), 392–401.

Funk, M. (1989). Research priorities in critical care nursing. *Focus on Critical Care, 16*(2), 135–138.

Green, A. (1992). How nurses can ensure the sounds patients hear have a positive rather than a negative effect upon recovery and quality of life. *Intensive and Critical Care Nursing, 8*(4), 245–248.

Gries, M. L., & Fernsler, J. (1988). Patient perception of the mechanical ventilation experience. *Focus on Critical Care, 15*(2), 52–59.

Grumet, G. W. (1993). Pandemonium in the modern hospital. *The New England Journal of Medicine, 328*(6), 433–437.

Halm, M. A. (1992). Support and reassurance needs: Strategies for practice. *Critical Care Clinics of North America, 4*(4), 633–643.

Hansell, H. N. (1984). The behavioral effects of noise on man: The patient with "intensive care unit psychosis." *Heart and Lung, 13*, 59–65.

Heidt, P. (1981). Effect of therapeutic touch on anxiety level of hospitalized patients. *Nursing Research, 30*(1), 32–37.

Heidt, P. R. (1990). Openness: A qualitative analysis of nurses' and patients' experiences of therapeutic touch. *Image: Journal of Nursing Scholarship, 22*(3), 180–186.

Heidt, P. R. (1991). Helping patients to rest: Clinical studies in therapeutic touch. *Holistic Nursing Practice, 5*(4), 57–66.

Henneman, E. A., & Cardin, S. (1992). Need for information: Interventions for practice. *Critical Care Clinics of North America, 4*(4), 615–621.

Hickey, M. L., & Leske, J. S. (1992). Needs of families of critically ill patients: State of the science and future directions. *Critical Care Clinics of North America, 4*(4), 645–649.

Johnson, M. M., & Sexton, D. L. (1990). Distress during mechanical ventilation: Patients' perceptions. *Critical Care Nurse, 10*(7), 48–57.

Keller, E., & Bzdek, V. (1986). Effects of therapeutic touch on tension headache pain. *Nursing Research, 35*(2), 101–105.

Keller, C., Tanner, D., & Urbenia, C. M. (1989). Psychological responses in aphasia: Theoretical considerations and nursing implications. *Journal of Neuroscience Nursing, 21*, 290–294.

Kemper, B. J. (1992). Therapeutic listening. *Journal of Psychosocial Nursing and Mental Health Services, 30*(7), 21–23.

Kleiber, C., et al. (1994). Emotional responses of family members during a critical care hospitalization. *American Journal of Critical Care, 3*(1), 70–76.

Knaus, W. A., et al. (1988). An evaluation of outcome from intensive care in major medical centers. *Annals of Internal Medicine, 104*, 410–418.

Kreiger, D. (1975). Therapeutic touch: The imprimatur of nursing. *American Journal of Nursing, 5*, 784–787.

Kreiger, D., Peper, E., & Ancoli, S. (1979). Physiologic indices of therapeutic touch. *American Journal of Nursing, 4*, 660–662.

Kreiger, D. (1990). Therapeutic touch: Two decades of research, teaching and clinical practice. *Imprint, 37*(3), 83, 86–88.

Lappe, D. G. (1993). Managing the intensive care unit: Nurse/physician collaboration. *Critical Care Medicine, 21*(9 Suppl), S388.

Lekander, B. J., Lehmann, S., & Lindquist, R. (1993). Therapeutic listening: Key interventions for several nursing diagnoses. *Dimensions of Critical Care Nursing, 12*(1), 24–30.

Leske, J. S. (1992). Needs of adult family members after critical illness: Prescriptions for interventions. *Critical Care Nursing Clinics of North America, 4*(4), 587–596.

Loughrey, L. (1992). The effects of two teaching techniques on recognition and use of function words by aphasic stroke patients. *Rehabilitation Nursing, 17*(3), 134–137.

Louis, M., & Povse, S. (1980). Aphasia and endurance: Considerations in assessment and care of the stroke patient. *Nursing Clinics of North America, 15*(2), 265–283.

MacRae, J. (1990). *Therapeutic touch: A practical guide.* New York: Knopf.

Menzel, L. (1994). Need for communication-related research in mechanically ventilated patients. *American Journal of Critical Care, 3*(3), 165–167.

Molter, N. C. (1979). Needs of relatives of critically ill patients: A descriptive study. *Heart and Lung, 8*(2), 332–339.

Morse, J. M., et al. (1992a). Exploring empathy: A conceptual fit for nursing practice? *Image: Journal of Nursing Scholarship, 24*(4), 273–280.

Morse, J. M., et al. (1992b). Beyond empathy: Expanding expressions of caring. *Journal of Advanced Nursing, 17*, 809–821.

Murphy, M., & Clark, J. M. (1993). Nurses' experiences of caring for ethnic-minority clients. *Journal of Advanced Nursing, 18*(3), 442–450.

Northouse, P. G. (1979). Interpersonal trust and empathy in nurse-nurse relationships. *Nursing Research, 28*(6), 365–368.

Palumbo, M. V. (1990). Hearing access 2000: Increasing awareness of the hearing impaired. *Journal of Gerontological Nursing, 16*(9), 26–31.

Parfitt, B. A. (1988). Cultural assessment in the intensive care unit. *Intensive Care Nursing, 4*(3), 124–127.

Parker, M. M., Schubert, W., & Schelhamer, J. H. (1984). Perceptions of a critically ill patient experiencing paralysis in an ICU. *Critical Care Medicine, 12*(1), 69–71.

Pearce, J. (1988). The power of touch. *Nursing Times, 15*(84), 26–29.

Pettigrew, J. (1990). Intensive nursing care: The ministry of presence. *Critical Care Nursing Clinics of North America, 2*(3), 503–508.

Pimental, P. (1986). Alterations in communication. *Nursing Clinics of North America, 21*(2), 321–337.

Podrasky, D. L., & Sexton, D. L. (1988). Nurses' reactions to difficult patients. *Image: Journal of Nursing Scholarship, 20*(1), 16–21.

Quinn, J. F. (1984). Therapeutic touch as energy exchange: Testing the theory. *Advances in Nursing Science, 6,* 42–49.

Quinn, J. F. (1992). The senior's therapeutic touch education program. *Holistic Nursing Practice, 7*(1), 32–37.

Randolph, G. L. (1984). Therapeutic and physical touch: Physiological response to stressful stimuli. *Nursing Research, 33*(1), 33–36.

Salyer, J., & Stuart, B. J. (1985). Nurse–patient interaction in the intensive care unit. *Heart and Lung, 14*(1), 20–24.

Samarel, N. (1992). The experience of receiving therapeutic touch. *Journal of Advanced Nursing, 17*(6), 651–657.

Schoenfofer, S. O. (1989). Affectional touch in critical care nursing: A descriptive study. *Heart and Lung, 18*(2), 146–154.

Sinclair, V. (1988). High technology in critical care: Implications for nursing's role and practice. *Focus on Critical Care, 15*(4), 36–41.

Smith, S. (1992). *Communications in nursing.* St. Louis: Mosby Year Book.

Stovsky, B., Rudy, E., & Dragonette, P. (1988). Comparison of two types of communication methods used after cardiac surgery with patients with endotracheal tubes. *Heart and Lung, 17,* 281–289.

Sundeen, S. J., et al. (1994). *Nurse–client interaction: Implementing the nursing process* (5th ed.). St. Louis: Mosby Year Book.

Vitello-Cicciu, J. M. (1984). Recalled perceptions of patients administered pancuronium bromide. *Focus on Critical Care, 11*(1), 30–35.

Wallston, B. S., & Wallston, K. A. (1975). Nurses' decisions to listen to patients. *Nursing Research, 24,* 16–22.

Waterman, H., & Webb, C. (1992). Visually impaired patients' perceptions of their needs in hospital. *Nursing Practice, 5*(3), 6–9.

Williams, M. L. (1992). An algorithm for selecting a communication technique with intubated patients. *Dimensions of Critical Care Nursing, 11*(4), 222–229.

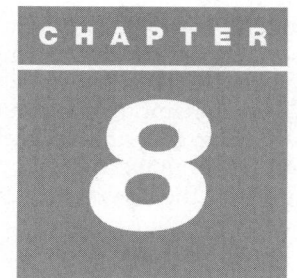

Effect of Sensory Alterations

Dorrie K. Fontaine

The technologic critical care environment offers numerous benefits to the critically ill patient, including increased survival, rapid identification of complications, and prompt intervention, which often achieve dramatic results. These well recognized benefits are attended by several physical and psychosocial burdens imposed by the environment that have been of interest to many researchers in a variety of disciplines. The sensory alterations accompanying immobility, pain, and noise are well documented. Indeed, despite modern advances, the intensive care unit (ICU) has been referred to as ''both psychologically and physically a very unkind environment'' (Bryan-Brown, 1986). To maximize patient benefit and minimize physical and psychosocial distress, the critical care nurse manipulates and controls the environment. This can optimally be accomplished only if the nurse has a keen awareness of the impact of the sensory technical environment on the critically ill patient.

Critical care units are characterized by a triumph of life-saving high technology, which lends a space-age appearance to even the smallest ICU. Brightly lit, frequently windowless units are often noticed by infrequent vistors to appear noisy, hustling, crowded, and tense. In fact, ICUs are noisy (Hilton, 1985; Woods & Falk, 1974) and communication is not always therapeutic (Noble, 1979). Sleep deprivation caused by the environment may be detrimental to recovery and is often not diagnosed by the health care team.

The purpose of this chapter is to describe the sensory–perceptual alterations common to patients in critical care settings. Environmental stressors that create excessive stimuli such as noise or reduced stimuli such as immobility are examined. Research evidence suggesting that various stressors are detrimental to patient outcomes is explored. A common consequence of multiple sensory–perceptual alterations is sleep pattern disturbance, and this is reviewed in depth. Nursing therapies directed toward minimizing the psychophysiologic effects of the critical care setting are reviewed, with recommendations for practice and further research.

PSYCHOPHYSICAL ENVIRONMENT OF CRITICAL CARE UNITS

A central theme throughout the nursing literature is the impact of the person–environment interaction on health and illness (Meleis, 1985). The environment as a key concept in critical care nursing is depicted in the model shown in Figure 8–1 (American Association of Critical-Care Nurses, 1986). Three levels are depicted in this model: (1) the direct interactive nurse–patient environment, (2) the resource environment in terms of supplies and patient safety, and (3) the institutional administrative setting. These levels suggest the dynamic interaction of the critical care environment as the nurse strives to meet patients' needs in more humane ways. The psychophysical environment within the dashed lines demonstrates the continuous inter-

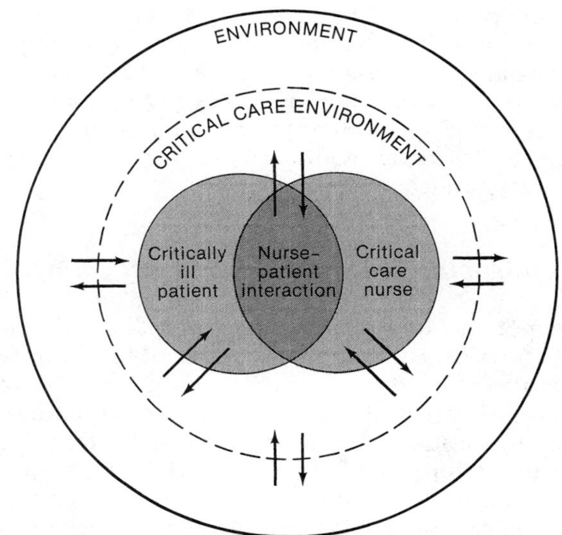

FIGURE 8–1. The critical care environment. (Redrawn from American Association of Critical-Care Nurses. [1986]. *Scope of critical care nursing practice.* AACN Position Statement, Aliso Viejo, CA.)

change between the nurse and the patient, including the totality of sensory stimuli received by the critically ill patient. It is the immediate sensory environment, depicted as the first and second levels in the model, that is the focus of this chapter.

An encompassing definition of environment includes the myriad aspects that surround an individual or a group, with emphasis on continuous interaction between the person and the environment. The critical care environment contains noise, drugs, communication patterns, temperature, and potentially unknown factors affecting how a patient ultimately perceives and responds to the clinical setting.

Nursing therapeutics that promote, maintain, or change the environment for the benefit of the patient are the focus of increasing attention (McCarthy et al., 1991; Meleis, 1985). Evidence is accumulating that the therapeutic environment provided by the nurse brings about positive patient outcomes through competent caring (Cooper, 1993). Critical care nurses who are simultaneously attuned to the environment, the technology, and, most of all, the patient will encourage more rapid recovery.

Physical Features of the Environment

The central features of the critical care units that make up the physical environment are related primarily to the surveillance function for which critical care units were first developed. Beds may be close together, creating little privacy but permitting ready observation of more than one patient by the nurse. Monitoring equipment and ventilators surround the critically ill patient with the unique tones and intensity of various continuous or intermittent alarms. Typically, these generate dissonance when sounding together. Noises from equipment are accompanied by often tense, shouted conversation, hurried footsteps, or the sound of running water. Visually, the continuous lighting, which produces an absence of time cues, accompanied by the distortion of viewing all caregivers by gazing upward 2 or more feet, contributes to altered time and space perceptions by the patient. The physical environment thus created may be perceived by the individual in varying ways ranging from reassurance to terror.

Psychosocial Features of the Environment

The emotional tone of a critical care unit is determined by its physical configuration, degree of family access, and, to a great extent, the communication patterns of the critical care team. The physical configuration of most units leads to limited personal space for the patient and frequent loss of control over all space owing to health team spatial invasions. Territorial dominance struggles can occur and create tension between nurses, physicians, patients, and families. This factor is typified by the restricted access of the family and significant others to the patient, a traditionally central feature of the psychosocial environment in all critical care settings that is undergoing serious review and change (Moseley & Jones, 1991; Simpson, 1991; Hickey, 1990). Perhaps Viner (1985) identified the emotional climate of critical care best when stating that the critically ill patient lives in a narrowly circumscribed world acutely aware and at the mercy of the mood and tone set by all caregivers.

IMPACT OF THE CRITICAL CARE ENVIRONMENT

The impact of the critical care environment on the patient is best considered in terms of a psychophysiologic framework that considers the interaction among physiologic, personal, and cognitive patient responses. Physiologic responses are those characteristic biologic actions common to all individuals; the metabolism of nutrients and the sympathoadrenal stress reaction are examples. Personal responses include the affective, feeling aspects of the person and account for his or her unique value system. Patterns of thinking and communicating characterize the cognitive responses of individuals. The complex pattern of patient responses to the environment is inherently integrated, with sensation and perception playing fundamental roles. Patient response to noise demonstrates this integration. Perception of sound as noise causes personal discomfort and may lead to physiologic vasoconstriction and elevated blood pressure (Kryter, 1985).

The environment may be perceived by the patient as frightening because of the physical and psychosocial features described. In the critical care setting, psychological factors such as fear or anxiety can worsen physiologic instability through stimulation of neurohormonal messengers in the brain (Dossey et al., 1988). Although psychological turmoil may not always be revealed by the critically ill (Easton & MacKenzie, 1988), researchers have identified multiple stressors reported by ICU patients. Many of these are related to sensory alterations, and are described in the next section.

Environmental Stressors in the Critical Care Unit

The combination of a painful, life-threatening illness, an uncertain outcome, and the closeness of strangers caring for intimate bodily processes creates the context in which environmental stressors must be viewed. It is not surprising that since the advent of critical care units, patients report a variety of noxious stimuli during their stay in an ICU (Dracup, 1988). Nonetheless, it is useful to consider the following paradox: Although the patient and family are often reassured by the close surveillance opportunities allowed by the ICU, the environment also creates numerous stressful phenomena. Indeeed, patients and their families are known to experience "transfer anxiety" when recov-

TABLE 8–1. **Environmental Stressors Reported by Patients in Critical Care Units**

Being tied down by tubes/not being able to move freely
Being in pain
Being thirsty
Being on a ventilator/having to wear an oxygen mask
Frequent interruptions of sleep
Missing your spouse
Seeing family and friends for only a few minutes each day
Not being able to sleep
Having too many tubes
Not knowing when to expect things will be done to you
Losing track of time
Having doctors and nurses talk about you rather than to you
Too much noise
Having no privacy
Too much light
Inability to communicate

Data from Ballard (1981), Wilson (1987), Bergbom-Engberg and Haljame (1989), and Simpson et al. (1989).

ery necessitates a less intense level of care despite the adverse effects reported by patients during the critical care stay (Urban, 1993). These stressors are important because many could be better anticipated and controlled by the critical care team.

Table 8–1 identifies major environmental stressors reported by critically ill patients in several studies in the 1980s (Ballard, 1981; Bergbom-Engberg & Haljamae, 1989; Simpson et al., 1989; Wilson, 1987). Sensory alterations caused by inability to communicate, pain, immobility, and sleeplessness were common in all studies. Bright lighting and high noise levels remain environmental stressors in the 1990s (Meyer et al., 1994) despite recommendations for more humane critical care settings (Harvey et al., 1993).

THE NATURE OF SENSORY PERCEPTION

The degree to which an environmental feature causes arousal and discomfort to the patient, resulting in psychophysiologic effects, is determined by the processes of sensation and perception. An interesting example is conversation at the patient's bedside, considered a potential stressor in critical care (Mitchell & Mauss, 1978; Noble, 1979; Johnson et al., 1989). Johnson and colleagues (1989) reexamined the finding of Mitchell and Mauss (1978) that conversation about a neurologically impaired patient's condition at his bedside elevated intracranial pressure (ICP). Johnson and colleagues reported the effects on ICP of two types of conversation between nurses at the bedside of the head-injured patient—one a social conversation and the other a discussion of the patient's condition. Results demonstrated no significant difference between conversations; however, individual differences in response to conversation were noted, and ICP was significantly lower during the social conversation compared with the patient's baseline ICP. The researchers recommended careful scrutiny of all bedside conversations and further examination of the effects of conversation and other environmental factors on ICP.

The critical care patient has a driving need to make sense of and order the environment in an attempt to adapt to it. This is demonstrated by the patient who strives to touch and examine his or her endotracheal tube, pulmonary artery catheter, or dressings. Critically ill patients interpret the environment based on the raw data of sensory exposure. These data come from the sensory modalities: visual, auditory, tactile, gustatory, and kinesthetic. Defining reality to make sense of the surrounding stimuli is the purpose of perception. However, many patients have alterations in their sensory–perceptual equipment that endanger their ability to understand the environment fully. In addition, the cues in the sensory environment itself may serve to confuse and cloud even the patient who is cognitively intact. The nature of sensory perception itself is first briefly considered.

Critical attributes for receiving and processing sensory information include a stimulus, intact sensory receptors, intact neural pathways, and adequate processing by the brain to assign meaning to the stimuli (DiMinno & Ozuna, 1987). The neural pathways involve the reticular formation (RF), a network of neurons extending from the lower brain to the thalamus in the diencephalon. The reticular activating system (RAS) is an area within the RF that has a neurophysiologic role in cortical arousal. The RF, along with the thalamus and hypothalamus, collects sensory information. A stimulus of a given intensity is necessary to stimulate a healthy RAS; without adequate individual stimulation, boredom, restlessness, or drowsiness may occur (DiMinno & Ozuna, 1987).

Perception occurs when the sensory input is received, decoded, and analyzed by the cerebral cortex. Characteristics of perception can be summarized as follows: Perception is a universal and individual process; it is interactive and continuous and has maturational and developmental features (Thompson et al., 1993). The critically ill patient has a unique view of the world of the ICU depending on age, previous experience, and severity of illness. The nurse strives to understand individual impressions of the critical care environment from the patient's psychophysiologic responses.

An optimal sensory stimulation level for each individual is unknown. At what precise point adequacy of sensory stimuli moves toward monotony, a condition of sensory deprivation, or noise, a condition of sensory overload, is also an unknown. Sensory alterations in critical care typically span the continuum from deprivation to overload. Of interest to the clinician is the fact that both conditions demonstrate psychophysiologic effects (Kryter, 1985; Zubek, 1969).

ALTERATIONS IN SENSORY PERCEPTIONS DUE TO CRITICAL ILLNESS

Critically ill patients may experience a wide range of potential alterations in sensory perception. Some are the result of the nature of the critical illness, whereas others arise from the therapeutically and socially restricted environment. In the first category, injury to the sense organs themselves may occur, as in a patient with multiple traumatic injuries creating blindness or with massive facial fractures causing altered smell and taste. The patient who survives a traumatic ruptured aorta may experience paraplegia and an altered kinesthetic sense. Obviously, any damage to the brain, such as occurs with head injury or a cerebrovascular accident, will lead to altered reception of stimuli. All patients with endotracheal tubes used for mechanical ventilation experience unpleasant stimuli such as gagging and frustration with communication (Gries & Fernsler, 1988).

The therapeutic critical care environment, with its varying degrees of overload and deprivation of stimuli, presents a sensory challenge to the patient. Social isolation and immobility alone can create perceptual distortions. Externally, noise, odors, and lack of space all bombard the senses. Internally, the polypharmacy of critical care, experienced by most patients, and potential electrolyte imbalances all tend to promote sensory distortion. The environment itself, with its monotonous though loud sounds, as well as the lack of a usual pattern of stimulation from family, friends, work, and recreation, adds to the reduced sensory input. Patients with restricted movement due to pain, traction, equipment, or the injury itself experience a positional deprivation due to immobility.

In summary, an alteration in sensory perception may occur owing to an unfamiliar environment, altered sensory reception, immobility, injury to the sensing organ, chemical alterations such as electrolyte imbalance or drugs, and extreme anxiety or panic, which will narrow perceptual fields (Thompson et al., 1993). Anxiety, as a defining characteristic of sensory–perceptual alterations, is an important area for creative calming nursing interventions. In this regard, the concept of patient control has been investigated in terms of sensory input. A focus on patient control has several implications in critical care, especially for mediating the sensory stimuli of noise and pain.

Patient Control of Sensory Stimuli

Patients interact with the environment, responding to stimuli and attempting to seek or avoid that which is pleasurable or noxious, respectively. Such interaction may be difficult in the critical care setting, where patient control is uncommon. Patients lose situational control over many impinging stimuli, of which noise and pain are paramount.

Topf (1984) described a framework suggesting that perceived control and exercised control over an aversive environmental effect such as noise could decrease reactivity and the damaging psychophysiologic response to this stimulus. Exercised control is the ability to regulate intended outcomes, whereas perceived control refers to an expectation of having the ability to make decisions to achieve desirable outcomes (Topf, 1984). A similar hypothesis of control has been used to investigate patient-controlled analgesia in several patient populations (Giuffre et al., 1988). Many nursing therapeutics addressing sensory alterations are currently based on the concept of patient control and should promote recovery in the critically ill (Riegel, 1989).

Using personal control devices such as taped sound or music has been investigated. Topf (1992) was unable to demonstrate improved sleep using a sound conditioner as a personal control intervention. Healthy volunteers listened to taped critical care sounds at night in a sleep laboratory with continuous polysomnographic sleep monitoring. Subjects were taught to use the sound conditioner, which simulated ocean or rainfall sounds to block out the unit noise. In contrast, Williamson (1992) determined that critically ill patients' perceptions of sleep quality and quantity were greatly improved compared to a control group using taped sounds to mask noise after cardiac surgery.

NURSING DIAGNOSIS: SENSORY–PERCEPTUAL ALTERATIONS

Sensory–perceptual alterations, as defined by the North American Nursing Diagnosis Association (NANDA), are considered a "state in which the individual/group experiences or is at risk of experiencing a change in the amount, pattern, or interpretation of incoming stimuli" (Carpenito, 1993). Alterations may be of a visual, auditory, kinesthetic, gustatory, tactile, or olfactory nature. Table 8–2 lists

TABLE 8–2. **Defining Characteristics of the Nursing Diagnosis: Sensory–Perceptual Alterations**

Major Defining Characteristics

Inaccurate interpretation of environmental stimuli and/or negative change in amount or pattern of incoming stimuli

Minor Defining Characteristics

Disoriented in time or place
Disoriented about people
Altered ability to problem-solve
Altered behavior or communication pattern
Sleep pattern disturbances
Restlessness
Reports auditory or visual hallucinations
Fear
Anxiety
Apathy

From Carpenito, L. J. (1993). *Nursing diagnoses: Application to clinical practice* (5th ed., p. 695). Philadelphia: J. B. Lippincott.

the major and minor defining characteristics approved for clinical testing.

Sensory–Perceptual Alterations in the Critically Ill: Overview of Research

Patients undergoing open heart surgery were one of the first critical care groups believed to experience transient sensory–perceptual alterations. Findings of studies of these patients suggest that multiple factors may be involved, including unit design, cardiac bypass pump time, 24-hour nursing care interruptions, and drugs. Little conclusive evidence points to one stressor over another in precipitating the unique psychological disturbance that has become known as "ICU psychosis." Nursing research has continued to identify several perceptual distortions that may be experienced by more than 50% of critically ill patients.

In interviewing 38 patients in a surgical ICU, Wilson (1987) identified a 58% incidence of transient delirium or impaired psychological response (IPR). The instrument used to measure psychological status examined orientation, cognitive function and memory, hallucinations, illusions, and delusions and had been used in previous research. Patient perception of stressors was also examined. Patients who had an IPR were more likely to state that noise, losing track of time, being talked about rather than to, and multiple examinations were highly stressful. This finding supports the concept that sensory impingement in critical care situations can have adverse psychological effects. Patients often hesitate to mention sensory changes to the nurse because they believe that they would be labeled "crazy" and that no one else experiences bizarre dreams.

Easton and MacKenzie (1988) interviewed 10 surgical ICU patients using a semistructured interview guide to elicit specific information about the nature and incidence of the illusions, hallucinations, or delusions they experienced. Patients were interviewed after transfer from the unit. As in the study by Wilson (1987), 50% of the patients experienced psychological reactions such as delusions and nightmares. Patients experienced distorted perceptions related to space ships, buildings rotating, feelings of persecution, and a fear of falling.

Medical research in the form of case reports has also supported the existence of transient sensory–perceptual changes during critical care. Dreams and fantasies were related to the lack of privacy and the fear that werewolves would eat the blood stains on the sheet.

When critical care patients demonstrate any abnormal behavior, the label frequently applied to the condition is "ICU psychosis." Cassem (1989) cautions that often this diagnosis is one of convenience and fixing the blame on the sensory environment may limit a thorough search for other causative factors. The etiology of delirium in patients with ICU psychosis is typically unknown, and external and internal stressors must be examined. Drugs, lack of sleep, and sensory monotony are all potential contributing factors, especially drugs.

The polypharmacy of critical care is life-saving in many instances. However, the critically ill patient may pay a psychological price for the therapeutic effects of many needed drugs. Table 8–3 identifies the medications that have been previously linked to delirium in patient care.

As the research demonstrates, not all patients experience psychological disruptions while in the critical care setting. Why some experience perceptual alterations and others escape them is an important question. Factors associated with ICU psychosis include sleep deprivation (Helton et al., 1980), unit design without windows (Keep, 1977), and multiple other variables. Figure 8–2 shows numerous environmental and individual patient factors that together create patient anxiety. The nurse needs to be cognizant that the level of anxiety alway depends on the meaning of the environmental stressor and the patient's unique set of coping skills. In-depth knowledge of the individual behind the critical illness is essential to maximize the patient's recovery.

Before suggesting specific therapeutic interventions for mediating sensory–perceptual alterations, the two common categories of sensory alteration will be reviewed. Sensory deprivation of some senses (visual, auditory, and tactile) often accompanies sensory bombardment of others. An example is the immobilized, elderly, multiple trauma patient with a pelvic external fixator device who is forced to listen to loud rock music from the nurse's station. Although the distinction between deprivation and overload is often arbitrary, the important factor remains patient perception. In this example, sensory deprivation results from immobility and overload occurs secondary to the undesirable noise.

SENSORY DEPRIVATION

Sensory deprivation refers to a reduction in the amount or intensity of sensory stimulation (Jackson & Ellis, 1971; Goldberger, 1966). Perceptual isolation, in contrast, refers to a severe reduction in the patterning or meaningfulness of sensory stimuli. Some relate sensory deprivation to the uniqueness of each individual by defining it as a reduction in sensory stimulation below the individual's tolerance level (DiMinno & Ozuna, 1987).

Jackson and Ellis (1971) categorized the phenomena associated with the majority of experimental and clinical sensory deprivation reports as follows: (1) perceptual—mild images to hallucinations; (2) cognitive—difficulty thinking or paying attention; (3) emotional—fear, depression, or anxiety; (4) motor—impaired fine or gross coordination; (5) somatic—galvanic skin response or catecholamine changes; and (6) other behaviors, such as noncompliance. Of these, the first two categories of experience are most frequently

TABLE 8–3. **Drugs Associated With Delirium and Other Psychiatric Symptoms**

Antiarrhythmics	Cimetidine, ranitidine
Diisopropamide	Digitalis preparations
Lidocaine	Disulfiram, metronidazole
Mexilitine	Dopamine agonists (central)
Procainamide	Amantadine
Quinidine	Bromocriptine
Tocainide	Levodopa
Antibiotics	Ergotamine
Aminoglycosides	GABA agonists
Amodioquin	Benzodiazepines
Amphotericin	Baclofen
Cephalosporins	Immunosuppressives
Chloramphenicol	Procarbazine
Chloroquine	L-Asparaginase
Colistin	Methotrexate (high dose)
Ethambutol	5-Azacytidine
Gentamicin	Cytosine arabinoside (high dose)
Isoniazid	Vincristine
Rifampin	Vinblastine
Sulfonamides	5-Fluorouracil
Tetracyclines	Hexamethylmelamine
Ticarcillin	DTIC
Vancomycin	Aminoglutethimide
Anticholinergics	Tamoxifen
Atropine	Lithium
Scopolamine	Metrizamide
Tricyclic antidepressants:	Monoamine oxidase inhibitors
amitriptyline	Isoniazid
protriptyline	Phenelzine
imipramine	Procarbazine
desipramine	Narcotic analgesics
notriptyline	Meperidine (Normeperidine)
trimipramine	Pentazocine
maprotiline	Nonsteroidal antiinflammatory drugs
Trihexyphenidyl	Ibuprofen
Benztropine	Indomethacin
Diphenhydramine	Naproxen
Thioridazine	Sulindac
Eye and nose drops	Podophyllin (topical)
Anticonvulsants	Steroids, ACTH
Phenytoin	Sympathomimetics
Antihypertensives	Amphetamine
Captopril	Cocaine
Clonidine	Ephedrine
Methyldopa	Phenylephrine
Reserpine	Phenylpropanolamine
Antiviral agents	Aminophylline
Acyclovir	Theophylline
Interferon	
Barbiturates	
Benzodiazepines	
Beta-blockers	
Propranolol	
Timolol	

Abbreviations: GABA = gamma-aminobutyric acid; DTIC = dacarbazine; ACTH = adrenocorticotropic hormone.

From Cassem, N. H. (1989). Psychiatric problems of the critically ill patient. In W. C. Shoemaker, S. Ayres, A. Grenvik, et al. (Eds.), *Textbook of critical care* (2nd ed., p. 1406). Philadelphia: W. B. Saunders.

reported. However, individual responses to the deprivation experience are emphasized.

Clinical sensory deprivation has been less systematically studied than experimental deprivation. The difficulty in interpreting clinical sensory deprivation studies is that they rarely encompass deprivation alone but may include sensory overload as well. For example, the surgical patient may experience sensory deprivation due to immobility and sensory overload due to intense pain. Methodical identification of variables for the clinical study of sensory deprivation has been a challenge.

Immobility and Sensory Deprivation

Alterations in mobility produce sensory–perceptual changes even in healthy individuals. The recumbent position alters perception, and when forced because of critical illness or injury, free movement is restricted, leading to dependence and loss of control (Barry, 1979). Individuals restricted to bed rest, even for brief periods of time, may experience sensory–perceptual alterations (Downs, 1974). In Downs' (1974) classic research, 20% of 180 healthy adults who experienced bed rest for nearly 3 hours in a laboratory simulation of a hospital room reported sensory distortions. Various audiotapes were used to simulate half-heard hospital conversations. Sensory distortions included hallucinations, mini-dreams, and altered time perception. The subjects described various sensations: visual, auditory, olfactory, kinesthetic, and tactile. These have been referred to as "indeterminate sensory experiences." Minimal human contact causing social isolation may have enhanced the sensory alterations.

In a clinical, noncritical care setting, Bolin (1974) identified sleep and dream pattern changes in a small group of immobilized orthopedic patients. An immobilized patient experiences minimal and restricted visual input and may be unable to receive the necessary feedback that would help to orient his or her body and its parts in relation to the environment (Scanlon, 1994) (see Chapter 61). The spinal cord–injured patient on a Stryker frame is an example of a person whose perceptual world may be limited to the floor, the ceiling, and whatever peripheral vision provides. Most critically ill patients begin their ICU stay on bed rest and thus experience the sensory restrictions of that position. Sensory perceptions of critical care patients who are cared for in an increasing variety of specialty beds, such as the Kinetic Roto Rest, the Mediscus low air loss beds, and others are unknown.

Neuromuscular Blocking Agents and Sensory Deprivation

Perhaps the ultimate example of sensory deprivation in a critical care setting is the patient who is receiving neuromuscular blocking agents. These commonly

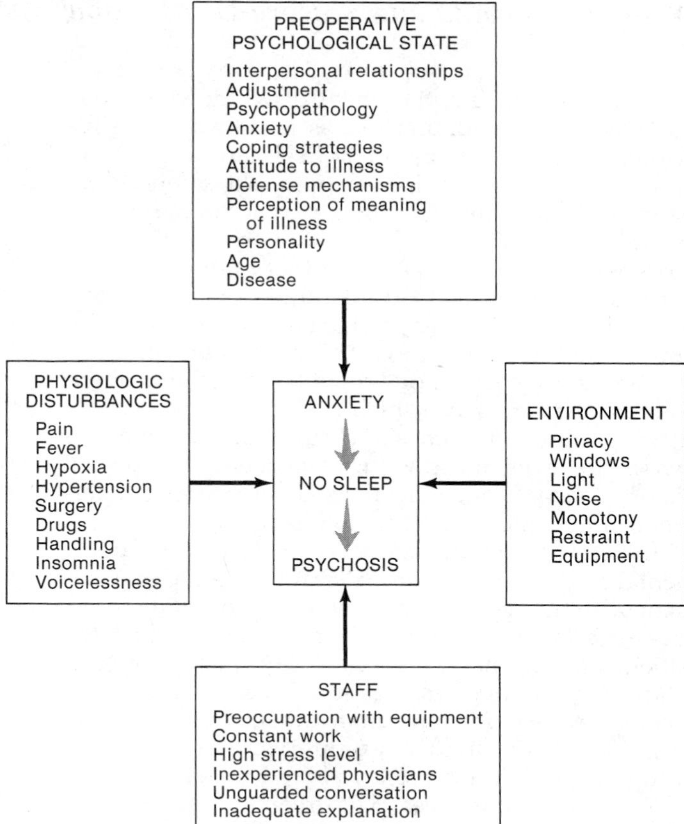

FIGURE 8–2. Intrinsic and extrinsic factors combine to cause sleeplessness and anxiety in the ICU patient. (Redrawn from Cousins, M. J., & Phillips, G. D. [1984]. Sleep, pain, and sedation. In W. C. Shoemaker, W. L. Thompson, & P. R. Holbrook (Eds.), *Textbook of critical care.* Philadelphia: W. B. Saunders, p. 798.)

used drugs (pancuronium bromide [Pavulon], metocurine iodide [Metubine Iodide], or vecuronium bromide [Norcuron]) create widespread systemic paralysis without accompanying central nervous system depression. Sedatives and narcotics are thus required. Neuromuscular blocking agents are increasingly used in the management of acute respiratory insufficiency in critical care settings to better control ventilation (Topulos, 1993).

Several reports indicate that patients receiving this type of drug therapy remember feeling isolated and alone, not sure if they were alive or dead (Parker et al., 1984; Schapner, 1975; Vitello-Cicciu, 1984). Patients report a desire to be touched and to be called by name. Contact with reality would seem to assist in counteracting the severe sensory deprivation and perceptual monotony reported by this patient group. Conversations of staff at the bedside are recalled by these patients and can be a major source of anxiety. One patient vividly recalled hearing a nurse remark on the futility of further treatment for the patient because she was going to "die anyway" (Schnaper, 1975). Examples such as this provide the reason for all caregivers to engage in therapeutic bedside conversation.

Time Alteration and Sensory Deprivation

Critically ill patients lose track of time because the constant fluorescent lights create a confused day–night orientation (Kleck, 1984). Time is an important component of the environment because it allows individuals to make adjustments and establish contact with and ultimately control their environment (Snyder, 1985). Research has determined that the perception of time passing can be affected by emotions, temperature, or immobility (Snyder, 1985). Patients in critical care settings may have a greatly distorted sense of time because of fever, medications, or continuous bed rest.

Individuals are equipped with a biologic clock that sets a unique pattern for endocrine, temperature, and sleep–wake cycles, among others. In the altered hospital environment, numerous internal rhythms shift out of phase with external cues, or zeitgebers, that normally assist in synchronizing circadian rhythms (Felton, 1987). To judge time accurately, a constant source of invariable stimuli such as physiologic body rhythms and interaction with the environment is needed (Felton, 1987). The environment should be consistent and familiar, which is not possible in typical hospital settings. Nurses can use a knowledge of chronobiology (analysis of how biologic phenomena, such as temperature, fluctuate over time in a given patient) to help synchronize the patients' unique biologic rhythms (Snyder, 1985; Westfall, 1992). Timing of drug administration and independent nursing activities such as scheduling of relaxation techniques may have superior outcomes when patient rhythms are taken into account.

Windowless Units and Sensory Deprivation

Environmental designers in critical care units often recommend strategic placement of windows (Ulrich, 1984), a recommendation that is not always feasible in older recovery rooms or critical care units. Windowless units may result in memory alterations, delusions, and hallucinations. In a study comparing the mental status of 72 former patients in an ICU with windows with that of 78 patients in a windowless unit, Keep and associates (1980) identified twice the presence of delusions and hallucinations in the windowless unit group. Nearly 25% of the patients without windows could not remember anything about their critical care stay, which is similar to Schnaper's (1975) finding of amnesia in multiple trauma patients. However, those with intact memory reported distorted visual images, feelings of persecution, depersonalization, and "out of body" experiences.

Increasing evidence supports the existence of detrimental sensory–perceptual alterations in an environment with no view to the outside. Although the presence of a hospital window helps to ensure that the patient at least has a sense of day and night, one unique report suggests that some scenery may have greater healing potential than others. A total of 46 surgical patients in two groups were studied, one group facing a brown brick wall and the other with a view of deciduous trees. The tree-view patients received significantly less postoperative narcotic than the wall-view group. Being able to look out a window at a natural scene rather than a more monotonous one may decrease patient requirements for medication and length of hospital stay (Ulrich, 1984). Further research on the effects of other potentially therapeutic views such as posters or paintings in windowless units is needed.

SENSORY OVERLOAD

Sensory overload is defined as a marked increase in the intensity of stimuli at greater than normal levels or simultaneous multisensory experiences (Baker, 1984). At its most damaging, sensory overload promotes patient hypervigilance in the critical care setting because of continuous arousal. Escape from fear, anxiety, or pain through sleep is often not possible. Noise is implicated most often and has been extensively studied. However, pain is probably the best known stressor causing sensory overload in the critical care patient. The combination of pain and a noisy environment serves only to increase patient perception of pain.

In the critical care setting, sensory overload is the most important immediate perception of the infrequent visitor and the patient. Health care professionals may become desensitized over time so that the impinging multisensory stimuli are not cognitively processed but become background. However, patients remain in the unit 24 hours a day, whereas the health care team and visitors come and go.

Noise and Sensory Overload

Noise or unwanted sound can be considered as an audible acoustic energy that adversely affects physiologic or psychological well-being (Kryter, 1985). Individual perceptions of a sound constitute the uniqueness of noise. Noise pollution in the hospital environment, especially critical care areas, has been well documented (Hilton, 1985; Meyer et al., 1994; Redding et al., 1977; Woods & Falk, 1974).

A model of the relationship of noise and human response is depicted in Figure 8–3. The physiologic response approximates the stress response initiated when sound is perceived as annoying (Baker, 1984). The physical effects of noise consist of general physiologic overarousal, demonstrated by increased respiratory rate, peripheral blood vessel vasoconstriction, minimum heart rate change, adrenal gland secretions, and elevated levels of blood cortisol and cholesterol (Kryter, 1985). A startle effect may initiate the autonomic and endocrine response. Noise is an important sensory stressor for critically ill patients because exposure to noise alters normal responses to wound healing (McCarthy et al., 1991) and suppresses rapid eye movement sleep (Topf & Davis, 1993).

Cognitive functioning may be affected when noise competes with nonauditory stimuli in the environment (Kryter, 1985). As decibel levels rise, noise in the environment affects the cognitive and perceptual ability of healthy individuals (Hansell, 1984).

The meaningfulness of the sound is a critical variable for the patient. Stress occurs when the sound is annoying or its meaning uncertain. Critical care patients often struggle cognitively to make sense of the sounds they hear. Smith (1986) determined that it was more restful to listen to patterned audio input, such as music or taped stories, than to experience ambient environmental sounds. The experiment was conducted with 120 healthy subjects confined to bed in a laboratory setting. Examination of an intervention such as patterned sound in severely ill patients needs investigation.

Although hospitalized patients complain of noise as a stressor, little is known about the precise psychophysiologic response of the severely ill patient to noise. Baker (1992) investigated effects of noise on the heart rate of 28 critically ill patients and found elevations of heart rate during talking in the patient's room. The rise in heart rate could be attributed not only to sound levels but to the meaning of the bedside conversation to the patient.

Sound has frequency and intensity. Frequency is measured in cycles per second (Hz), and normal hearing covers the 20- to 2000-Hz range. Intensity is the loudness of a sound (Woods & Falk, 1974). Sound is measured in decibel (dB) units on the A scale to ap-

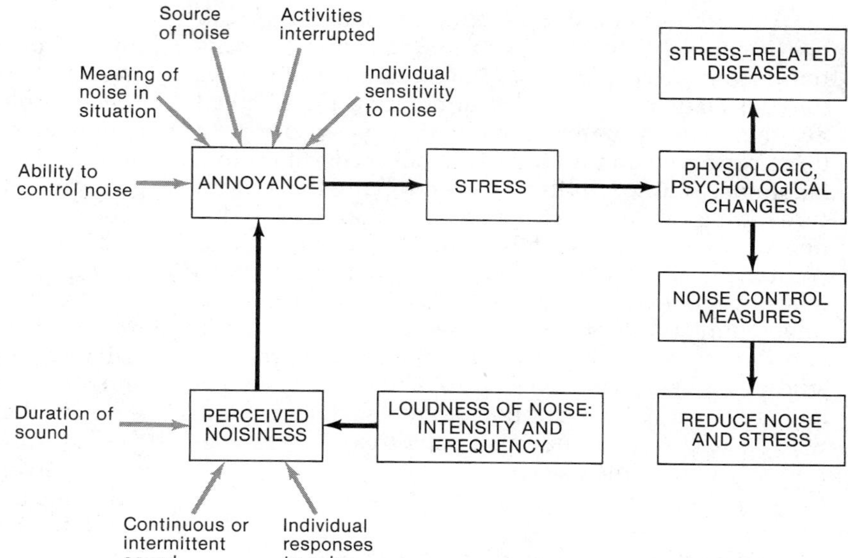

FIGURE 8–3. Relationship between characteristics of noise and human response. (Reprinted from Baker, C. [1984]. Sensory overload and noise in the ICU: Sources of environmental stress. *Critical Care Quarterly, 6* [4], 72, with permission of Aspen Publishers, Inc., © 1984.)

proximate closely frequencies of the human ear. Decibels are one-tenth of a bel and increase exponentially. For example, a 10-dB(A) noise sounds twice as loud as a 1-dB(A) noise (Baker 1984; Kryter, 1985).

Sound Levels in Critical Care Units

Researchers have identified the high levels of noise in critical care settings. Table 8–4 summarizes data obtained from the work of several researchers on clinical noise. Most equipment produces noise close to 70 db(A), which is the level at which annoyance occurs (Baker, 1984). Sleep occurs best at levels below 35 dB(A). To gain perspective on these noise levels, normal ambient living room noise is 30 to 40 dB(A), conversational voices are heard at 60 dB(A), heavy traffic or a noisy restaurant produces sound in the 70- to 80-dB(A) range (Baker, 1984), and a pneumatic drill at a distance of 50 feet has a decibel level of 80 dB(A) (Redding et al., 1977).

Hilton (1985) compared the level of sound in four ICUs and two general care units. Continuous dB(A) level recordings were made for 24 hours, and observations of the sources of sound were made for briefer periods. Continuous sound recorded in the open heart recovery room and ICU in the larger hospital ranged between 48.5 and 68.5 dB(A), even at night. Although some patients were not concerned about the noise level, others were highly upset. Communication by staff at the bedside was loud. This finding supports other research suggesting that staff communication is not only noisy but often nontherapeutic as well (Noble, 1979). Importantly, Hilton noted that several sounds can be greatly diminished. Turning the bell down on telephones decreases the noise level from 70 to 60 dB(A), whereas closing a patient's door in the ICU can decrease noise by 15 dB(A).

TABLE 8–4. **Noise Levels in the Critical Care Setting**

Noise Source	Intensity in dB(A)
Equipment	
Ventilator (at HOB)	60–65
Ventilator alarm at 20 feet	71–76
Cardiac alarm (at HOB)	71
Ice machine dispensing ice	62–64
Radio (at HOB)	64–68
Oxygen by mask	63
Treatments	
Chest percussion	83
Patient weighed	60–64
Putting HOB up	68–78
Endotracheal suction	70
Obtaining vital signs	60–68
Environment	
Garbage cans moved	48–83
Things thrown into garbage can	67–80
Water running	44–70
Voice over intercom	60–70
Toilet flushed	44–60
Telephone ringing (at 6 feet)	60–65
Squeaking chair	76
Telephone ringing (at 10 feet)	67
Staff conversation at bedside	63
Rattling side rails	80
Computer printer	70–72
Patient crying out	80

Abbreviation: HOB = head of bed.

Adapted from Baker (1984); Hilton (1985); Redding et al. (1977); Woods & Falk (1974).

Although several studies report that noise from staff is particularly disturbing (Noble, 1982), others identify noise from mechanical equipment as most annoying (Snyder-Halpern, 1985). The latter study investigated healthy subjects' perceptions of their sleep during a quiet condition and a taped ICU noise condition in a laboratory setting. Undisputed is the claim that critical care settings are noisy 24 hours a day, and much of the noise can be controlled through staff behavior and equipment adjustments. Meyer and colleagues (1994) investigated noise and light levels for 7 days in ICU settings. Sound peaks greater than 80 dB(A) were common and were consistently higher than reported in previous studies. Light levels showed normal rhythmicity for day and night. Patient interruptions were also documented, with no ICU area permitting greater than a 4-hour period of uninterrupted sleep.

NURSING THERAPEUTICS FOR SENSORY–PERCEPTUAL ALTERATIONS

Numerous nursing therapies addressing sensory alterations in the critically ill have been described in the literature. Several of these can be considered collaborative interventions with medicine; many more are in the realm of independent nursing strategy. All of the therapies suggested can be usefully categorized as: (1) surveillance, (2) shielding, or (3) modification.

Surveillance

Monitoring of the patient–environment interface is an initial nursing strategy. The critically ill patient and the environment are assessed separately at least twice each day or with changes, and the quality of the interaction is determined based on these findings. Critical care nurses are known to become desensitized to environmental stimuli. Lindenmuth and colleagues (1980) investigated the effects of environmental stimuli on critical care nurses acting as patients in an ICU bed for 1½ hours. Perceptions were similar to those reported by patients, with noise from alarms on monitors and ventilators found to be bothersome. Feelings of loneliness and immobility were experienced, along with the perception of time as slowing down. These authors advocated a plan to sensitize critical care nurses to environmental stimuli, a concept that may be especially important with the widespread institution of 12-hour shifts.

Function of all sensory modalities needs to be carefully assessed along with the ability to process information (Scanlon, 1994). This information needs to be communicated to all health care providers in an accessible, written plan of care. Patient perception of the environment is evaluated by means of direct questions related to the stressors previously identified by researchers (see Table 8–1). How stressful is immobility in this patient? How supportive is the family, and what is the patient's psychophysiologic response when family members visit? (Bay et al., 1988). Patient characteristics obtained from the patient or family and recorded on the data base are useful in suggesting avenues for further assessment. For example, patients with significant drug histories may have problems with forced dependency and loss of control in the critical care unit. They may also experience perceptual distortions and loss of reality due to the effects of withdrawal.

Knowledge of a usual coping pattern for any critically ill patient is useful in planning therapy to mediate sensory alterations. Dealing with special populations such as children or elderly people in critical care units requires a knowledge of the developmental level and stressors unique to that age group in critical care.

Surveillance for environmental effects ensures that the critical care nurse question the patient about noise perception, time perception, and distracting or annoying environmental factors that can potentially be manipulated. The view that the patient has of the critical care setting should be identified and analyzed in terms of lighting, privacy, and monotony.

Surveillance of the sensory environment to sensitize the nurse to potential negative effects is recommended. One technique that assists the critical care staff in increasing sensitivity to environmental overload is to place a tape recorder close to the patient's ear to record environmental sounds for 1 to 2 hours. This allows a close approximation to the reality of noise in the ICU as the patient receives it. Reviewing the taped sounds of the critical care unit later at a staff meeting is a good learning opportunity whether the nurse is a novice, an advanced beginner, or an expert in critical care practice.

Dossey and colleagues (1988) recommended the following environmental excercise for nurses to deal with our increasing technologic environment:

> *At different times during the day, close your eyes and take a few moments to listen carefully to all sounds in your environment. Jot down the many different sounds you hear, noting which are distracting or disturbing noises. Become aware of all the sounds that you ordinarily hear, such as the air conditioner, radios and televisions, the hum of fluorescent lights, the beeping and buzzing of hospital machinery, or the incessant MUSAK that some institutions play over the speaker system. Notice new smells, feelings or temperature, etc. There will be many sounds, smells, and sensations of which you may not have previously been aware.*

Orienting patients to these same sounds may be especially helpful to calm fears from unexplained and potentially frightening noises. This exercise may be suggested to nurses when they are introduced to a new critical care practice setting and repeated at intervals of weeks to months.

Patients should be asked about any dreams or altered feelings. They should be encouraged in a nonjudgmental way to identify unusual sensations. Wakeful patients may confess to a fear of falling asleep and experiencing nightmares. Critical care patients need to be assured that these are common transient experiences and encouraged to discuss them; ICU patients may erroneously believe they have become psychologically ill (Easton & MacKenzie, 1988). Multiple trauma patients need to be assessed for hyperalertness, survivor guilt, and other behaviors classified as the posttraumatic stress disorder (Scanlon, 1994). Wilson (1987) advocates frequent use of a mental status examination to document disorientation, hallucinations, illusions, delusions, or paranoia.

Shielding

The nursing therapy of shielding refers to protection of the critically ill patient from the aversive effects of the critical care environment. Shielding the patient physically through noise abatement and psychologically from nontherapeutic bedside conversation are good examples. Recommendations for protection of the patient from noise range from simply closing the patient's door when possible (Hilton, 1985) to developing strict guidelines on new equipment noise. The critical care nurse who successfully uses shielding has a keen awareness of the environment and sensitively screens out potentially harmful elements based on knowledge of unique patient characteristics. Some patients are more sensitive to cold, to odors, or to a loud radio.

Providing orientation to reality is a protective nursing therapy. Addressing the patient by name, interpreting stimuli in the environment, and assisting in clarifying reality are useful in restoring or maintaining sensory-perceptual function (Thompson et al., 1993).

Modification

Modification involves numerous independent interventions to restructure the patient's external and internal environment. Family visiting, use of earphones or television, dim lighting at night, possibly a window, use of calendars, clocks, and radios, music, or tapes are all examples of modifying the external environment to overcome the damaging effects of sensory alterations. The nurse manipulates the sensory environment by altering the patient's position at frequent intervals and moving him or her to a chair or instituting ambulation as early as possible. Music therapy has the potential to mask noise, decrease anxiety, reduce pain, create positive emotions, and promote sleep in critically ill patients (Guzzetta, 1988). Several studies suggest the power of music in decreasing patient stress from the illness and the sensory environment (Guzzetta, 1989; Updike, 1990; White, 1992). Patients should select their own music.

Establishing an effective communication link between the patient and the nurse is essential. Patients claim that they experience much stress because of an inability to communicate (Menzel, 1994) (see Chapter 7). The work of Stovsky and associates (1988) in investigating patient and nurse satisfaction with different methods of communication needs to be continued in examining several populations in critical care settings.

Barriers to flexible visiting policies in critical care settings need to be removed as evidence mounts that less restrictive visiting for patients may lead to improved orientation, decreased anxiety, and increased sleep (Titler & Walsh, 1992). Nurses still attempt to justify restricting visiting hours for critically ill patients for a variety of reasons, including the potential for causing adverse consequences and exhausting the family, as well as concern regarding the inability to complete nursing tasks (Kirchhoff et al., 1993). In an investigation of critically ill patients' perceptions, it was found that the sicker the patient, the more visitors were wanted, with visits viewed as helpful and not tiring (Simpson, 1991). Preferences for length and timing of visits for older patients are also becoming known (Simpson, 1993). It is increasingly recommended that nurses tailor a flexible visiting policy for the individual patient and family (Moseley & Jones, 1991; Simpson, 1993).

Modification of the physical environment to limit noise can be accomplished in many ways, ranging from turning equipment alarms away from the patient's ear to making complete structural changes in a new unit (Hilton, 1987; Hansell, 1984; Harvey et al., 1993). Brewer (1985) recommended several features for an "ideal" critical care unit. Many recently constructed or renovated critical care units have taken at least some of these design features into account. Such features include (1) spacious, attractively decorated private rooms with outside windows and window coverings, variable lighting, adequate storage, a clock and calendar easily visible from the patient's bed, adjustable bedside monitors, accurate, individually controlled thermostats, and television or radio; (2) nursing work stations separate from but convenient to patient rooms; (3) utility rooms separate from the general unit for noise and odor control; (4) separate but convenient conference rooms for staff reports, breaks, and family conferences; and (5) volume control for equipment and dimmers for lighting. In addition, nurses could carry a silent pager, to decrease the annoyance of overhead paging (Harvey et al., 1993). Private rooms and outside windows have been shown to mediate the environmental load on the patient and promote more timely recovery. It is essential that critical care nurses collaborate early with other disciplines when any blueprint designs for new units are generated.

Critical care nurses should ask questions related to noise as follows: How subjectively loud is the unit? Does the patient have specific complaints of disturbing noises that can be removed or explained? Are alarms turned away from the patient, and are all alarms on the unit answered promptly? Can the door to the patient's room be closed?

Last, but just as important, manipulation and modification of the patient's internal psychophysiologic environment is a priority. Nursing therapies range from collaborative ones, such as the administration of various medications that may ease pain and promote rest, to independent actions such as the judicious use of nontraditional approaches to helping the patient cope in a stressful environment. These include relaxation techniques, guided imagery, music therapy, and others (Dossey et al., 1988). Research investigating patient outcomes in critical care settings needs to be undertaken. Paradoxic reactions to drugs intended to relax and calm patients need to be quickly identified. Evaluation and documentation of the effectiveness of all therapies directed at mediating the patient's internal environment are needed.

SLEEP AND REST DISTURBANCES IN THE CRITICAL CARE UNIT

The strongest impact of the environment, whether sensory overload or sensory deprivation, is exerted on the normal sleep pattern of a critically ill patient. Sleep disturbance has intrigued researchers since the inception of ICUs, with the discipline of nursing providing much of the widely cited research literature. This chapter on sensory alterations concludes with a discussion of the nursing diagnosis of Sleep Pattern Disturbance and nursing interventions for this universal phenomenon.

Critically ill patients have difficulty meeting their need for sleep and rest in the intensive care environment. Although the precise psychophysiologic effects of sleep deprivation are controversial, there is no dispute about the severe sleep disruption that routinely occurs in the hospital setting, especially in critical care units (Aurell & Elmqvist, 1985; Helton et al., 1980; Hilton, 1976; Meyer et al., 1994). Beginning with the classic work of Dlin and colleagues in 1971, sleep problems of the critically ill have often been noted. Studies that critically examine activities that promote sleep and rest that would benefit the critically ill, as recommended by an AACN Delphi Study of research priorities in critical care nursing (Lewandowski & Kositsky, 1983) have been recently reported (Richards, 1994; Ryan et al., 1992; Williamson, 1992).

Complicating the sleep and rest problem is the fact that the critical care team may view sleep disruption as an expected and uncontrollable aspect of patient care and therefore place a low priority on sleep promotion activities. According to Walker (1993), patients have serious complaints about the low priority of sleep, as reported by the following patient's comment: "Of all things, they would wake me up about 4:30 in the morning and get me on the scale and weigh me." This attitude directly conflicts with the nurse's accepted role of manipulating the environment to promote healing. Despite controversies over the consequences of sleep deprivation (Naitoh et al., 1990; Parkes, 1985), increasing support for the possibility of patient harm due to sleep pattern disturbance cannot be ignored.

Evidence suggests that sleep disruption may lead to depressed ventilation (White et al., 1983), decreased immunocompetence (Palmblad et al., 1979), increased pain perception (Phillips & Cousins, 1986), and the confusional syndrome of ICU psychosis (Helton et al., 1980). In addition to patients' own complaints that sleep disturbance is a major stressor during their ICU stay, many of the potential problems of sleep pattern disturbance may worsen patient psychophysiologic status. For example, weaning the patient from a ventilator, healing difficult wounds, and limiting confusion in the critically ill patient may all be greatly assisted by a rested patient, one who is at least achieving some complete sleep cycles.

Physiology of Sleep

Sleep is referred to as a "soft area" in physiologic research, owing to the many gaps in our present knowledge of sleep mechanisms and other biochemical aspects of sleep (Karnofsky, 1986). Much of what is known about sleep is less than 40 years old, and even the question of the function of sleep remains elusive. Sleep researchers have identified the stages of sleep and several neurochemical regulators of sleep, and have proposed sleep factors, hypnogenic areas, and immune modulators for sleep (Gaillard, 1990; Institute of Medicine, 1990; Parkes, 1985).

The field of sleep research is flourishing. Sleep is a complex, multidimensional process that is cyclical, reversible, and characterized by a comparative decrease in the levels of cortical vigilance (Hartman, 1973; Koella, 1978). Sleep can be measured by behavioral observation, subjective reports, and physiologic monitoring. However, the only method that accurately detects specific sleep stages is polysomnography (PSG), in which simultaneous electroencephalograms (EEGs), electrooculograms (EOGs), and electromyograms (EMGs) are made. These cortical tracings emerge from intense brain activity during sleep, which is not the passive state previously assumed.

STRUCTURES OF SLEEP AND NEUROTRANSMITTERS

Primary brain areas implicated in sleep and wakefulness include the locus ceruleus, the raphe nuclei, and the hippocampus (Robinson, 1986). Numerous neurotransmitters have been implicated in the regulation of vigilance (Wauquier et al., 1985). Those most examined are serotonin, norepinephrine, and acetylcholine, although researchers continue to identify biologic substances with potential sleep generation capabilities (Gaillard, 1990). The importance of neurotransmitter interaction in the sleep-organizing apparatus is well recognized, but the patterns of integration continue to be investigated.

Specific neurotransmitters that are more easily measured have been linked to anatomic sites within the brain. These substances can be characterized as vigilance enhancers, which promote wakefulness, or vigilance suppressors, which elicit sleep (Koella, 1985). Nonrapid eye movement (NREM) sleep stages 1 through 4 were purportedly under the control of serotonin, but this theory has been abandoned (Institute of Medicine, 1990). According to Gaillard (1990), serotonin may be important throughout the sleep–wake cycle for the synthesis and use of unknown sleep-promoting factors. Rapid eye movement (REM) sleep, characterized by intense activation of the central nervous system, is mediated by acetylcholine from the hippocampus. During REM sleep, acetylcholine is released by the caudate nucleus at the same level as during the awake state. The vigilant awake state is under the control of the norepinephrine adrenergic system, which discharges from the locus ceruleus. It is the interaction among and modulation of these neurotransmitters that permits the well established progression of sleep and waking stages.

Descent into the various stages of sleep is more complex than this brief review of neurotransmitters permits. Researchers are beginning to discover the integral network of many hypnogenic systems, and specific sleep factors such as factor S or delta sleep-inducing peptides have been isolated in animals (Gaillard, 1990). Other substances under study include gamma-aminobutyric acid, dopamine, and various hypnogenic peptides.

SLEEP ARCHITECTURE

Sleep is categorized into five stages based on the PSG criteria of the EEG, EOG, and EMG: stages 1 through 4 NREM sleep, and REM sleep. An individual progresses from the drowsy state of stage 1 sleep through the slow-wave sleep of stages 3 and 4. The REM stage of sleep is reached by recycling through stage 2, in which the young adult spends 50% of the night. Table 8–5 depicts the characteristics of each sleep stage as developed by a consensus of sleep researchers. The mean time percentage spent by young adults in each stage is also presented, based on normative data from the University of Florida (Williams et al., 1974).

TABLE 8–5. **Sleep Characteristics and Percentage of Time Spent in Each Sleep Stage in Young Adulthood**

Stage	Sleep Characteristics	Percentage of Sleep Time for Men Aged 20 to 29 Years
Awake	Alpha activity 8–13 Hz or mixed-frequency EEG; high tonic EMG; eye blinks on EOG	1.26
1	Low-voltage, mixed-frequency EEG; EOG shows slow rolling eye movements	4.44
2	Sleep spindles on EEG (12–14 Hz) and K complexes	45.54
3	At least 20% to 50% of the sleep record (30-second epoch) contains delta waves of 2–4 Hz and 75 microvolts	6.21
4	Greater than 50% of the sleep record contains delta waves of 75 microvolts	14.55
REM	Low-voltage, mixed-frequency EEG; episodic eye movements on EOG; low-amplitude EMG	28.00

Abbreviations: EEG = electroencephalography; EMG = electromyography; EOG = electrooculography; Hz = hertz; REM = rapid eye movement.

Data from Rechtschaffen, A., & Kales, A. (Eds.). (1968). *A manual of standardized terminology, techniques, and scoring system for sleep stages of human subjects.* Bethesda, MD: U.S. Department of Health, Education, and Welfare; and Williams, R. L., Karacan, I., & Hursch, C. J. (1974). *Electroencephalography (EEG) of human sleep: Clinical applications.* New York: John Wiley & Sons.

Sleep Measurement

Because nurses make decisions about sleep promotion acitivities based on their assessment of the quality and quantity of a patient's sleep, it is important to consider the components of sleep measurement. Nurses often represent a patient's sleep with the ubiquitous comment "Patient appears to be sleeping" documented in the patient record. The measurement of sleep patterns reflects the complexity of sleep. To show the multidimensionality of sleep clearly, sleep measurement instruments can be categorized as follows: physiologic, objective, and subjective (Beck, 1988; Johns, 1971; Richards, 1987). When possible, sleep assessment measures should provide a sense of the quality of sleep, and not quantity alone.

Physiologic sleep measurement instruments include the PSG, in which EEG, EOG, and EMG tracings are recorded simultaneously. This is the only scientific measure of sleep in which precise sleep stages can be discerned, and is primarily a research or diagnostic tool. Objective sleep measures include the nurse's estimate of a patient's sleep through observation of a combination of the following: (1) respiratory pattern, (2) movement, (3) possibly monitored heart rate and blood pressure changes, and (4) lack of arousal to environmental stimuli. Several researchers have used a sleep estimate form to document observable behaviors (Aurell & Elmqvist, 1985; McFadden & Giblin, 1971; Woods, 1972; Edwards & Schuring, 1993a). The frequency of observation is a concern because infrequent observations may miss either awakenings or a return to sleep. These instruments have been used solely for research purposes. Other physiologic and observable measures are critiqued by Johns (1971) and Richards (1987).

A third category of sleep measures is the subjective one, in which patients examine their own perceptions of sleep quality. Patients assess the quality of their sleep based on sleep latency, or the time it takes to fall asleep; the number of awakenings experienced or disrupted sleep; and the total sleep time. Delayed sleep onset is often cited by patients as contributing to poor-quality sleep. A patient may be lying awake with eyes closed but feeling anxious, fearful, or in pain. Robinson (1986) pointed out that insomnia can be induced through stress by shunting tryptophan away from the serotonin pathway. This would create long sleep latencies or difficulty in returning to sleep once interrupted.

Several subjective instruments use either a questionnaire approach (Parsons & Ver Beek, 1982) or a visual analogue scale. The Richards-Campbell Sleep Questionnaire (Richards, 1987) and the Verran/Snyder-Halpern Sleep Tool (Snyder-Halpern & Verran,

TABLE 8–6. **Overview of Sleep Research in Critical Care**

Year	Author/Topic	Subjects	Selected Results/Implications
1971	McFadden & Giblin. Sleep deprivation in patients having open heart surgery	4 open heart surgery patients	All patients were sleep-deprived during their first 6 postoperative nights; 3 of 4 patients demonstrated behavior changes. Patients require more periods of uninterrupted rest.
1972	Woods. Patterns of sleep in postcardiotomy patients	4 open heart surgery patients	Potential sleep cycles were low, indicating sleep deprivation. Sleep–wakefulness rhythms should be promoted through nursing control of the environment.
1972	Walker. Amount of uninterrupted time for sleep and rest during the first, second, and third postoperative days in a teaching hospital	4 open heart surgery patients	Frequency of patient interactions (up to 56 in 8 hours) prevents adequate time for sleep. Nurses need to make sleep a priority by distinguishing between essential and nonessential tasks.
1976	Hilton. Quantity and quality of patients' sleep and sleep-disturbing factors in a respiratory ICU	10 respiratory ICU patients	Patients slept little, but half of the sleep time occurred during the day. No complete sleep cycles were experienced. Noise from equipment and discomfort kept patients awake. Nurses should use more judgment in deciding when to disturb a patient.
1978	Broughton & Baron. Sleep patterns in the intensive care unit and on the ward after acute myocardial infarction	12 myocardial infarction patients	Nocturnal sleep is very disturbed after a myocardial infarction. Stress of illness and not the unusual environment may be the cause of the sleep disturbance.
1979	Dohno et al. Some aspects of sleep disturbance in coronary patients	42 coronary care patients	All patients experienced sleep disturbance. The more severely ill patients had more awakenings.
1980	Helton et al. Correlation between sleep deprivation and the intensive care unit syndrome	62 critical care patients	One-third of patients with severe sleep deprivation had mental status changes. Nurses should control the environment by decreasing noise and light to promote sleep.
1985	Aurell & Elmqvist. Sleep in the surgical ICU: Continuous polygraphic recording of sleep in nine patients receiving postoperative care	9 surgical ICU patients	Patients were severely sleep-deprived. Sleep time was greatly decreased, with little REM sleep. Surgery may cause a fundamental disorder of the sleep–wake regulating mechanism.
1988	Richards & Bairnsfather. Night sleep patterns in the critical care unit	10 medical ICU patients	Patients experienced severely altered sleep with a decreased total sleep time while in an open critical care unit. Nurses should limit noise and patient interruptions.
1989	Fontaine. Measurement of nocturnal sleep patterns in trauma patients	20 multisystem trauma patients	Patients experienced a mean of 32 awakenings at night and severely disrupted sleep. Nursing observation of sleep is valid when compared to polysomnography. Patient perceptions of awakenings lasting longer than 4 minutes is valid. Nursing observation of sleep can be used to test sleep-promoting interventions.
1992	Knapp-Spooner & Yarcheski. Sleep patterns and stress in patients having coronary bypass	24 CABG patients	Postoperative sleep disturbance increased and sleep effectiveness decreased based on patient perceptions. Illness-related stress did not correlate with the degree of sleep disturbance.
1992	Ryan et al. Effect of nitropaste administration times on sleep and nocturnal angina	33 patients with coronary artery disease	Collaboratively revising nocturnal nitropaste administration times enhanced patients' sleep quality and quantity without increasing angina. Nurses should consider medication administration times that promote optimal sleep.
1992	Williamson. The effects of ocean sounds on sleep after coronary artery bypass graft surgery	60 CABG patients	Patients who listened to taped ocean sounds reported they slept more deeply and were awake less often than a control group. White noise may be useful in promoting sleep.

TABLE 8–6. **Overview of Sleep Research in Critical Care** *Continued*

Year	Author/Topic	Subjects	Selected Results/Implications
1993	Edwards & Schuring. Pilot study: Validating staff nurses' observations of sleep and wake states among critically ill patients, using polysomnography	21 medical ICU patients	Nurses' assessments of sleep–wake state were correct 82% of the time. This supports nursing observation as a valid and reliable method to assess sleep.
1994	Richards. The effect of a muscle relaxation, imagery, and relaxing intervention and a back massage on the sleep and psychophysiological arousal of elderly males hospitalized in the critical care environment	69 patients with CV disease	The group receiving back massage had a higher sleep efficiency index, greater REM sleep, and slept 1 hour longer than the control group. Providing patients a back massage may be a powerful intervention for promoting sleep.

Abbreviations: ICU = intensive care unit; CABG = coronary artery bypass graft; CV = cardiovascular; REM = rapid eye movement.

1987) are examples of visual analogue scales that have been tested in critical care settings (Fontaine, 1989). At present, there is no one instrument that will reliably and validly assess a critical care patient's sleep that is feasible in all settings and with all patients.

Comparison of nursing observations and PSG data reveals inconsistent findings. Nurses consistently overestimated the sleep time of ICU patients in a study comparing all-night PSG recordings of sleep stages and nursing observations made at 5-minute intervals (Aurell & Elmqvist, 1985). The reliability and validity of the sleep observation measure were not reported. Other research using a reliable sleep observation tool with specific criteria demonstrated good correlation with PSG data for waking after sleep onset in 20 trauma patients in an ICU setting (Fontaine, 1989). Edwards and Schuring (1993a) determined that nurses observed sleep–wake states correctly 82% of the time compared with PSG data in 21 patients in a critical care setting. Because of the difficulty of observing sleep accurately, several researchers examined "potential sleep cycles" by noting periods when patients were undisturbed (Helton et al., 1980).

Measuring sleep in an accurate, noninvasive, and unobtrusive manner in critical care patients can be problematic. It is a mistake to assume that just leaving the patient undisturbed will guarantee sleep. Therefore, when an opportunity to sleep is provided, it is essential to examine what the patient does with the chance to sleep. A combination of nursing observation of sleep and eliciting the patient's perception of his or her sleep quality should be used.

Sleep Research in Critical Care

The sleep patterns of a variety of cardiac and other patients in critical care have been studied in critical care settings with the same general findings. Table 8–6 lists most of the sleep research studies that have been done in critical care for the past two decades. Greatly disturbed sleep occurred in patients in all studies, whether measured by PSG recordings, nursing observations, or patient perception.

Sleep fragmentation leading to altered sleep architecture is noted in any study using PSG monitoring in the critical care unit. Sleep cycles are rarely completed, and there is a noted absence of REM sleep. Even when patients do fall asleep, they may awaken as often as a mean of 50 times per night (Richards & Bairnsfather, 1988). Of interest were two reports that at least 40% to 60% of sleep time was found to occur during the day (Aurell & Elmqvist, 1985; Hilton, 1976). Sleeping during the day may be explained by the widespread occurrence of sleep deprivation. Noise, the stress of injury, frequent interruptions, and pain were believed to contribute to sleep disruption. Noise levels often demonstrate little difference between day and night (Hilton, 1985).

In addition to environmental stimuli, numerous medications are known to disrupt sleep in the critically ill. Many patients in the studies listed in Table 8–6 probably received sleep-altering drugs. Narcotic analgesics often head the list, with morphine quantitatively decreasing stages 3 and 4 sleep and REM sleep (Thorpy, 1990). Various barbiturates and hypnotics may also depress certain sleep stages. Hypnotics in critical care settings require further evaluation. The polypharmacy of critical care makes it increasingly difficult to examine any one drug's effects on sleep pattern. Patient perception thus becomes of great importance in evaluating sleep promotion using pharmacotherapy.

Although the literature contains numerous prescriptions for promoting sleep, few have been tested in the critical care setting. An interesting multidisciplinary sleep protocol identifies an excellent method for leaving selected patients undisturbed for sleep (Edwards & Schuring, 1993). The protocol specifically prohibits middle-of-the-night bathing unless requested by the patient.

NURSING THERAPEUTICS FOR SLEEP PATTERN DISTURBANCE

Sleep probably holds unknown healing powers that critical care nurses should strive to harness. Of interest is the substantial number of independent nursing interventions for the nursing diagnosis of Sleep Pattern

Disturbance. Sleep promotion in critical care is very much a nursing role. Selected strategies for sleep promotion are identified in Table 8–7. The therapeutic intervention categories are designed to assist in keeping the goal and patient outcomes clearly in mind.

Surveillance activities are designed to assess specific patient characteristics or behaviors and to make the nursing diagnosis. Obtaining a sleep history and documenting sleep–wake times on the flow sheet are important surveillance activities. Patients who will spend days to weeks in the critical care unit are at greatest risk of experiencing sleep deprivation and are the primary patients for whom sleep time documentation should be a priority.

Shielding interventions attempt to protect the patient from the aversive effects of the environment. Finally, modification as a nursing therapeutic strategy focuses on two areas, changing the external environment through activities such as noise abatement and realigning the internal environment through the use of independent actions such as relaxation techniques or collaborative approaches using medications. These overlap with activities suggested for modification of sensory alterations.

TABLE 8–7. **Strategies to Promote Sleep**

Surveillance

Obtain and use sleep history to plan care.
Assess quality and quantity of sleep using appropriate methods.
Document sleep/wake time for all high-risk patients.
Monitor patient for psychophysiologic signs of sleep deprivation.
Determine if sleep occurs during the limited opportunity provided.

Shielding

Increase nurses' sensitivity to sounds and lights in the intensive care unit.
Prevent excessive lights and noise from alarms and limit staff conversation.
Evaluate the need for nursing care interruptions.
Use a nursing care plan to individualize and block sleep times.
Allow an opportunity for uninterrupted sleep time during day and night.
Promote comfortable positioning of the patient for sleep.
Explain environmental sounds and provide other information to lower patient anxiety.

Modification

Provide adequate pain relief and evaluate continuous analgesia or epidural anesthesia for promoting effective sleep.
Include backrubs and patient's own presleep routine.
Use relaxation techniques and imagery or music therapy.
Administer hypnotics according to patient protocol and evaluate their effectiveness.
Maximize patient privacy through the use of curtains and doors.
Post sign at designated sleep times—**Patient Sleeping.**
Provide large clocks and natural lighting.
Evaluate bed for comfort and sleep quality.
Ease visitor restrictions if this encourages patient to sleep.

From Fontaine, D. K. (1987). Sleep deprivation in the critical care unit. *Critical Care Nursing Currents, 5*(4), p. 22. Reprinted with permission from Ross Laboratories.

Whether to interfere with a patient's sleep to change wound dressings or initiate chest physiotherapy is at times a collaborative nursing decision with the medical team. More likely, the nursing care plan reflects the priority the nurse places on sleep promotion by giving sleep and rest a prominent role alongside physiologic interventions. The nurse uses clinical decision-making skills to determine if a 5 A.M. bath is in the patient's best interests or the interests of the nursing staff. Novice nurses who are socialized into a critical care unit need to identify quickly the priority of rest and sleep along with continuous surveillance. In the future, increasing sophistication of monitoring equipment will permit even further physiologic assessment without disturbing the patient.

All sleep-promoting interventions need to be studied to determine the effectiveness of each for the different critical care populations. Of special interest is the investigation of pain control and sleep quality in critically ill patients. With advances in pain management, such as patient-controlled analgesia, studies examining the effect of pain management on sleep patterns are a high priority. Exploration of sleep patterns is needed in patients with differing environmental configurations, in various specialty beds, and after independent nursing interventions for relaxation. Richards (1994) investigated the effects of a back massage and a combination of muscle relaxation, mental imagery, and music on the sleep of 69 older men with cardiac disease in a critical care setting. Patients were randomly assigned to the back massage, the combination intervention, or routine nursing care. The patients receiving the back massage had a significantly greater sleep quantity as measured by PSG than the control group. Back massages are likely very useful in promoting patient sleep in a critical care setting.

SUMMARY

The common sensory alterations identified in the critically ill were the focus of this chapter. Immobility, altered time perception, and the use of neuromuscular blocking agents are several areas in which patients are at risk for experiencing sensory deprivation. The consistently high noise levels in critical care settings make noise a universal sensory overload phenomenon. Collaborative and independent nursing therapeutics addressing the sensory–perceptual alterations were recommended. In addition, sleep pattern disturbances, the ultimate consequence of environmental intrusion in critical care, was reviewed, with suggestions for independent nursing strategies and further needed research. The uniqueness of these patient problems in critical care settings centers not only on their universal nature in critical care but on the importance of independent nursing therapies in mediating the effects of an aversive critical care environment. The critically ill patient requires a nurse who can truly "tame the technology" (Jennett, 1984) in the critical care setting and create the necessary healing environment.

REFERENCES

American Association of Critical-Care Nurses (1986). *Scope of critical care nursing practice* (AACN Position Statement, Newport Beach, CA).

Aurell, J., & Elmqvist, D. (1985). Sleep in the surgical intensive care unit: Continuous polygraphic recording of sleep in nine patients receiving postoperative care. *British Medical Journal, 290,* 1029–1032.

Baker, C. (1984). Sensory overload and noise in the ICU: Sources of environmental stress. *Critical Care Quarterly, 6*(4), 66–80.

Baker, C. F. (1992). Discomfort to environmental noise: Heart rate responses of SICU patients. *Critical Care Nursing Quarterly, 15*(2), 75–90.

Ballard, K. S. (1981). Identification of environmental stressors for patients in a surgical intensive care unit. *Issues in Mental Health Nursing, 3,* 89–108.

Barry, M. J. (1979). Sensory alterations, overload, and underload: Making a nursing diagnosis. In M. S. Kennedy & G. M. Pfeifer (Eds.), *Current practice in nursing care of the adult: Issues and concepts* (pp. 33–45). St. Louis: C. V. Mosby.

Bay, E. J., Kupferschmidt, B., Opperwal, B. J., et al. (1988). Effect of the family visit on the patient's mental status. *Focus on Critical Care, 15*(1), 10–16.

Beck, S. L. (1988). Measuring sleep. In M. Frank-Stromborg (Ed.), *Instruments for clinical nursing research* (pp. 255–267). Norwalk, CT: Appleton & Lange.

Bergbom-Engberg, I., & Haljame, H. (1989). Assessment of patients' experience of discomforts during respirator therapy. *Critical Care Medicine, 17,* 1068–1072.

Bolin, R. H. (1974). Sensory deprivation: An overview. *Nursing Forum, 13,* 240–258.

Broughton, R., & Baron, R. (1978). Sleep patterns in the intensive care unit and on the ward after acute myocardial infarction. *Electroencephalography and Clinical Neurophysiology, 45,* 348–360.

Bryan-Brown, C. W. (1986). Development of pain management in critical care. In M. J. Cousins & G. D. Phillips (Eds.), *Acute pain management* (pp. 1–19). New York: Churchill-Livingstone.

Carpenito, L. J. (1993). *Nursing diagnoses: Application to clinical practice* (5th ed.). Philadelphia: J. B. Lippincott.

Cassem, N. H. (1989). Psychiatric problems of the critically ill patient. In W. C. Shoemaker, S. Ayres, A. Grenvik, et al. (Eds.), *Textbook of critical care* (2nd ed., pp. 1404–1414). Philadelphia: W. B. Saunders.

Cooper, M. C. (1993). The intersection of technology and care in the ICU. *Advances in Nursing Science, 15*(3), 23–32.

DiMinno, M., & Ozuna, J. H. (1987). Sensory overload and sensory deprivation. In W. J. Phipps, B. C. Long, & N. F. Woods (Eds.), *Medical-surgical nursing concepts and clinical practice* (3rd ed., pp. 397–407). St. Louis: C. V. Mosby.

Dlin, B. M., Rosen, H., Dickstein, K., et al. (1971). The problems of sleep and rest in the intensive care unit. *Psychosomatics, 12*(3), 155–163.

Dohno, S., Paskewitz, D. A., Lynch, J. J., et al. (1979). Some aspects of sleep disturbance in coronary patients. *Perceptual and Motor Skills, 48,* 199–205.

Dossey, B. M., Keegan, L., Guzzetta, C. E., et al. (1988). *Holistic nursing: A handbook for practice.* Rockville, MD: Aspen Publishers.

Downs, F. (1974). Bedrest and sensory disturbances. *American Journal of Nursing, 74,* 434–438.

Dracup, K. (1988). Are critical care units hazardous to health? *Applied Nursing Research, 1,* 14–21.

Easton, C., and MacKenzie, F. (1988). Sensory–perceptual alterations: Delirium in the intensive care unit. *Heart and Lung, 17,* 229–235.

Edwards, G. B., & Schuring, L. M. (1993a). Pilot study: Validating staff nurses' observations of sleep and wake states among critically ill patients, using polysomnography. *American Journal of Critical Care, 2,* 125–131.

Edwards, G. B., & Schuring, L. M. (1993b). Sleep protocol: A research-based practice change. *Critical Care Nurse, 13,* 84–88.

Felton, G. (1987). Human biologic rhythms. In J. J. Fitzpatrick & R. L. Taunton (Eds.), *Annual review of nursing research* (pp. 45–77). New York: Springer.

Fontaine, D. K. (1989). Measurement of nocturnal sleep patterns in trauma patients. *Heart and Lung, 18,* 402–410.

Gaillard, J. M. (1990). Neurotransmitters and sleep pharmacology. In M. J. Thorpy (Ed.), *Handbook of sleep disorders* (pp. 55–76). New York: Marcel Dekker.

Giuffre, M., Keane, A., Hatfield, S. M., et al. (1988). Patient controlled analgesia in clinical pain research management. *Nursing Research, 37,* 254–255.

Gries, M. L., & Fernsler, J. (1988). Patient perceptions of the mechanical ventilation experience. *Focus on Critical Care, 15*(2), 52–59.

Guzzetta, C. E. (1988). Music therapy: Hearing the melody of the soul. In B. M. Dossey, L. Keegan, C. E. Guzzetta, et al. (Eds.), *Holistic nursing: A handbook for practice* (pp. 263–287). Gaithersburg, MD: Aspen.

Guzzetta, C. E. (1989). Effects of music therapy on patients in a coronary care unit with presumptive acute myocardial infarction. *Heart and Lung, 18,* 609–616.

Hansell, H. N. (1984). The behavior effects of noise on man: The patient with "intensive care unit psychosis." *Heart and Lung, 13,* 59–65.

Hartman, E. (1973). *The functions of sleep.* New Haven, CT: Yale University Press.

Harvey, M. A., Ninos, N. P., Adler, D. C., et al. (1993). Results of the consensus conference on fostering more humane critical care: Creating a healing environment. *AACN Clinical Issues in Critical Care Nursing, 4,* 484–507.

Helton, M. C., Gordon, S. H., & Nunnery, S. L. (1980). The correlation between sleep deprivation and the intensive care unit syndrome. *Heart and Lung, 9,* 464–468.

Hickey, M. (1990). What are the needs of families of critically ill patients? A review. *Heart and Lung, 19,* 401–415.

Hilton, B. A. (1976). Quantity and quality of patients' sleep and sleep-disturbing factors in a respiratory intensive care unit. *Journal of Advanced Nursing, 1,* 453–468.

Hilton, B. A. (1985). Noise in acute patient care areas. *Research in Nursing and Health, 8,* 283–291.

Hilton, B. A. (1987). The hospital racket: How noisy is your unit? *American Journal of Nursing, 87,* 59–61.

Institute of Medicine. (1990). *Basic sleep research.* Washington, DC: National Academy Press.

Jennett, B. (1984). *High technology medicine: Benefits and burdens.* London: The Nuffield Provincial Hospitals Trust.

Johns, M. W. (1971). Methods for assessing human sleep. *Archives of Internal Medicine, 127,* 484–492.

Johnson, S. M., Omery, A., & Nikas, D. (1989). Effects of conversation on intracranial pressure in comatose patients. *Heart and Lung, 18,* 56–63.

Karnofsky, M. L. (1986). Progress in sleep. *New England Journal of Medicine, 315,* 1026–1028.

Keep, P. J. (1977). Stimulus deprivation in windowless rooms. *Anaesthesia 32,* 598–602.

Keep, P. J., James, J., & Inman, M. (1980). Windows in the intensive therapy unit. *Anaesthesia, 35,* 256–262.

Kirchhoff, K. T., Pugh, E., Calame, R. M., et al. (1993). Nurses' beliefs and attitudes toward visiting in adult critical care settings. *American Journal of Critical Care, 2,* 238–245.

Kleck, H. G. (1984). ICU syndrome: Onset, manifestations, treatment, stressors, and prevention. *Critical Care Quarterly, 6,* 21–28.

Knapp-Spooner, C., & Yarcheski, A. (1992). Sleep patterns and stress in patients having coronary bypass. *Heart and Lung, 21,* 342–349.

Koella, W. P. (1978). Vigilance: A concept and its neurophysiological and biochemical implications. In P. Passouant & I. Oswald (Eds.), *Pharmacology of the states of alertness* (pp. 171–178). Oxford, England: Pergamon Press.

Koella, W. P. (1985). Organization of sleep. In D. J. McGinty, R.

Drucker-Colin, A. Morrison, et al. (Eds.), *Brain mechanisms of sleep.* New York: Raven Press.
Kryter, K. D. (1985). *The effects of noise on man* (2nd ed.). Menlo Park, CA: Academic Press.
Lewandowski, L. A., & Kositsky, A. M. (1983). Research priorities for critical care nursing. *Heart and Lung, 12,* 35–44.
Lindenmuth, J. E., Breu, C. S., & Malooley, J. A. (1980). Sensory overload. *American Journal of Nursing, 80,* 1456–1458.
McCarthy, D. O., Ouimet, M. E., & Daun, J. M. (1991). Shades of Florence Nightingale: Potential impact of noise stress on wound healing. *Holistic Nursing Practice, 5,* 39–48.
McFadden, E. H., & Giblin, E. C. (1971). Sleep deprivation in patients having open heart surgery. *Nursing Research, 20,* 249–254.
Meleis, A. I. (1985). *Theoretical nursing: Development and progress.* Philadelphia: J. B. Lippincott.
Menzel, L. (1994). Need for communication-related research in mechanically ventilated patients. *American Journal of Critical Care, 3,* 165–167.
Meyer, T. J., Eveloff, S. E., Bauer, M. S., Schwartz, W. A., Hill, N. S., & Millman, R. P. (1994). Adverse environmental conditions in the respiratory and medical ICU settings. *Chest, 105,* 1211–1216.
Mitchell, P., & Mauss, N. (1978). Relationships of patient/nurse activity to intracranial pressure variations: A pilot study. *Nursing Research, 27,* 4–10.
Moseley, M. J., & Jones, A. M. (1991). Contracting for visitation with families. *Dimensions of Critical Care Nursing, 10,* 364–371.
Naitoh, P., Kelly, T. L., & Englund, C. (1990). Health effects of sleep deprivation. *Occupational Medicine, 5,* 209–237.
Nightingale, F. (1859). *Notes on nursing.* London: Harrison & Sons.
Noble, M. A. (1979). Communication in the ICU: Therapeutic or disturbing? *Nursing Outlook, 27,* 195–198.
Noble, M. A. (Ed.). (1982). *The ICU environment: Directions for nursing.* Reston, VA: Reston Publishing.
Palmblad, J., Petrini, B., Wasserman, J., et al. (1979). Lymphocyte and granulocyte reactions during sleep deprivation. *Psychosomatic Medicine, 41,* 273–277.
Parker, M. M., Schubert, W., Shelhamer, J. H., et al. (1984). Perceptions of a critically ill patient experiencing paralysis in an ICU. *Critical Care Medicine, 12,* 69–71.
Parkes, J. D. (1985). *Sleep and its disorders.* Philadelphia: W. B. Saunders.
Parsons, L. C., & Ver Beek, D. (1982). Sleep–awake patterns following cerebral concussion. *Nursing Research, 31,* 260–264.
Phillips, G. D., & Cousins, M. J. (1986). Neurological mechanisms of pain and the relationship of pain, anxiety, and sleep. In M. J. Cousins & G. D. Phillips (Eds.), *Acute pain management* (pp. 21–48). New York: Churchill-Livingstone.
Redding, J. S., Hargest, T. S., & Minsky, S. H. (1977). How noisy is intensive care? *Critical Care Medicine, 5,* 275–276.
Richards, K. C. (1987). Techniques for measurement of sleep in critical care. *Focus on Critical Care, 14,* 34–40.
Richards, K. C. (1994). Sleep promotion in the critical care unit. *AACN Clinical Issues in Critical Care Nursing, 5,* 152–158.
Richards, K. C., and Bairnsfather, L. (1988). A description of night sleep patterns in the critical care unit. *Heart and Lung, 17,* 35–42.
Robinson, C. (1986). Impaired sleep. In V. K. Carrieri, A. M. Lindsey, & C. M. West (Eds.), *Pathophysiological phenomena in nursing: Human responses to illness* (pp. 390–417). Philadelphia: W. B. Saunders.
Ryan, M., Gallagher, S., & Wandel, J. C. (1992). Effect of nitropaste administration times on sleep and nocturnal angina. *Applied Nursing Research, 5*(2), 84–85.
Scanlon, A. M. (1994). Psychosocial responses of the human spirit: The journey of trauma. In V. D. Cardona, P. D. Hurn, P. J. B. Mason, et al. (Eds.), *Trauma nursing from resuscitation through rehabilitation* (2nd ed., pp. 179–198). Philadelphia: W. B. Saunders.
Schnaper, N. (1975). The psychological implications of severe trauma—emotional sequelae to unconsciousness. *Journal of Trauma, 15,* 94–98.
Simpson, T. (1991). Critical care patient's perceptions of visits. *Heart and Lung, 20,* 681–688.
Simpson, T. (1993). Visit preferences of middle aged vs older critically ill patients. *American Journal of Critical Care, 2,* 339–345.
Simpson, T. F., Armstrong, S., & Mitchell, P. (1989). American Association of Critical-Care Nurses Demonstration Project: Patients' recollections of critical care. *Heart and Lung, 18,* 325–332.
Smith, M. J. (1986). Human-environment process: A test of Rogers' principle of integrality. *Advances in Nursing Science, 9*(1), 21–28.
Snyder, M. (1985). *Independent nursing interventions.* New York: John Wiley & Sons.
Snyder-Halpern, R. (1985). The effect of critical care unit noise on patient sleep cycles. *Critical Care Quarterly, 7*(4), 41–50.
Snyder-Halpern, R., & Verran, J. (1987). Instrumentation to describe subjective sleep characteristics in healthy subjects. *Research in Nursing and Health, 10,* 155–163.
Thompson, J. M., McFarland, G. K., Hirsch, J. E., et al. (1993). *Clinical nursing* (3rd ed.). St. Louis: C. V. Mosby.
Thorpy, M. J. (Ed.). (1990). *Handbook of sleep disorders.* New York: Marcel Dekker.
Titler, M. G., & Walsh, S. M. (1992). Visiting critically ill adults: Strategies for practice. *Critical Care Nursing Clinics of North America, 4,* 623–632.
Topf, M. (1984). A framework for research on aversive physical aspects of the environment. *Research in Nursing and Health, 7,* 35–42.
Topf, M. (1992). Effects of personal control over hospital noise and sleep. *Research in Nursing and Health, 15,* 19–28.
Topf, M., & Davis, J. E. (1993). Critical care unit noise and rapid eye movement (REM) sleep. *Heart and Lung, 22,* 252–258.
Topulos, G. P. (1993). Neuromuscular blockade in adult intensive care. *New Horizons, 1,* 447–462.
Ulrich, R. S. (1984). View through a window may influence recovery from surgery. *Science, 224,* 420–421.
Updike, P. (1990). Music therapy results for ICU patients. *Dimensions of Critical Care Nursing, 9,* 39–45.
Urban, N. (1993). Patient responses to the environment. In M. R. Kinney, D. R. Packa, & S. B. Dunbar (Eds.), *AACN's clinical reference for critical-care nursing* (3rd ed., pp. 117–128). St. Louis: C. V. Mosby.
Vitello-Cicciu, J. M. (1984). Recalled perceptions of patients administered pancuronium bromide. *Focus on Critical Care, 11*(1), 30–35.
Walker, B. B. (1972). The postsurgery heart patient: Amount of uninterrupted time for sleep and rest during the first, second, and third postoperative days in a teaching hospital. *Nursing Research, 21,* 164–169.
Walker, J. D. (1993). Enhancing patient comfort. In M. Gerteis, S. Edgman-Levitan, J. Daley, et al. (Eds.), *Through the patient's eyes: Understanding and promoting patient-centered care* (pp. 119–153). San Francisco: Jossey-Bass.
Wauquier, A., Monti, J. M., Gaillard, J. M., et al. (1985). *Sleep neurotransmitters and neuromodulators.* New York: Raven Press.
Westfall, U. E. (1992). Nursing chronotherapeutics: A conceptual framework. *Image: The Journal of Nursing Scholarship, 24,* 307–312.
White, D. P., Douglas, N. J., Pickett, C. K., et al. (1983). Sleep deprivation and the control of ventilation. *American Review of Respiratory Diseases, 128,* 984–986.
White, J. M. (1992). Music therapy: An intervention to reduce anxiety in the myocardial infarction patient. *Clinical Nurse Specialist, 6,* 58–63.
Williams, R. L., Karacan, I., & Hursch, C. J. (1974). *Electroencephalography (EEG) of human sleep. Clinical applications.* New York: John Wiley & Sons.
Williamson, J. W. (1992). The effects of ocean sounds on sleep after coronary artery bypass graft surgery. *American Journal of Critical Care, 1,* 91–97.
Wilson, V. S. (1987). Identification of stressors related to patients' psychologic responses to the surgical intensive care unit. *Heart and Lung, 16,* 267–273.
Woods, N. F. (1972). Patterns of sleep in postcardiotomy patients. *Nursing Research, 21,* 347–352.

Chronic Illness and Critical Care Practice

Marita G. Titler

Chronic illness represents a major health problem for many Americans. Factors that contribute to the increased incidence of chronicity in the United States include use of life-saving technology, eradication of life-threatening infections, and an increasing proportion of older Americans (Hanson & Danis, 1991; Larkin, 1987). About 50% of the American population has one or more chronic health conditions, with nearly 32.4 million people being limited in normal activities of daily living (Lambert & Lambert, 1987; Strauss & Corbin, 1988). Consequences of chronic illness can range from relatively minor inconveniences to catastrophic consequences in which a person's existence and accustomed way of life are radically altered (Dimond, 1983).

Neither the incidence nor prevalence of chronic illness is a sufficient indication of the magnitude of the problem. The real measure of effective outcomes of chronic illness management is the extent to which individuals with chronic illness and their families are functioning at levels that are acceptable to them (Dimond, 1983).

Most patients admitted to an intensive care unit (ICU) have some sort of underlying chronic health problem (Oye & Bellamy, 1991). Patients who receive intensive care services tend to have higher chronic disease scores than those who do not receive these services (Hanson & Danis, 1991). There is some evidence, however, that intensive care services are limited for the chronically ill elderly who are older than 75 years of age and suffering from advanced malignancy, pneumonia, and acute stroke (Hanson & Danis, 1991).

Various studies have shown that there is an increased mortality in ICU patients who have a preexisting chronic illness. The most common of these are cardiac and pulmonary disease, resulting in some of the highest mortality rates (Milzman et al., 1993). More and more, ongoing care of chronically critically ill patients in the critical care setting is creating a financial crisis for hospitals (Daly et al., 1991). In addition, the high-cost group of ICU patients differs significantly from the low-cost group by having a greater proportion of chronic illnesses (Oye & Bellamy, 1991).

Similarly, successful treatment of acute life-threatening illnesses in critical care settings has resulted in an increase in the numbers of individuals with residual limitations and chronic physical and emotional problems. The difficulties accompanying many chronic conditions continue long after the acute stage of the illness has been successfully managed (Dimond, 1983).

THE NATURE OF CHRONIC ILLNESS

Chronic illness refers to a large number of diseases characterized by a slow, progressive decline in functioning. Although there is not consensus about what chronic illness means, a definition frequently cited in the literature is the 1956 definition of chronic disease by the Commission of Chronic Illness:

All impairments or deviations from normal which have one or more of the following characteristics: are permanent; leave residual disability; are caused by nonreversible pathological alterations; require special training of the patient for rehabilitation; may be expected to require a long period of supervision, observation or care. This definition focuses on physiological abnormalities and gives little consideration to the psychological and social component of chronic illness (Strauss et al., 1984, p. 1).

Terms such as sickness, illness, and disease are often used when describing chronic illness (Dimond, 1983). Disease refers to the objective phenomenon or state in which the body is suffering from malfunctioning of one or more parts. In contrast, illness denotes the phenomena that are apparent only to the ill person, such as pain, nausea, and dyspnea. Illness becomes sickness when it becomes a social phenomenon, that is, when it becomes visible to others or is communicated to others. Once the illness becomes social, interactions of the ill person with those around him or her are modified (Dimond, 1983). Although each chronic illness presents unique demands on the patient and family, two generalizations can be made: (1) the person with a chronic illness experiences impaired functioning in one or more systems, and (2) the illness-related demands on the individual and family are never completely eliminated (Miller, 1983).

Common problems faced by the chronically ill are (1) prevention of medical crisis, (2) control of symptoms, (3) carrying out prescribed treatment regimens and concomitant challenges inherent in those regimens, (4) adjusting social interactions and leisure activities, (5) attempting to normalize interactions with others and their lifestyle, (6) adjusting to changes in the course of the disease, (7) finding the necessary monetary resources to pay for treatment or to survive despite partial or complete loss of employment, and (8) dealing with accompanying psychological, marital, and family problems (Corbin & Strauss, 1988; Strauss et al., 1984; Strauss & Corbin, 1988).

The Phases and Trajectory of Chronic Illness

Several phases follow the diagnosis of a chronic illness. These include the acute phase, the comeback or recovery phase, the stability phase, the instability phase, the phase of deterioration, and the phase of dying (Table 9–1) (Corbin & Strauss, 1988, 1992; Strauss & Corbin, 1988). These phases are not necessarily neatly distinguishable from one another, and can appear in combination or in rapid alternation (Corbin & Strauss, 1988). For example, some people living with coronary artery disease may experience stability most of the time but rapidly become unstable, deteriorate, and die.

Based on the trajectory model of chronic illness described by Strauss, Corbin, and colleagues (1984, 1988, 1992), people play an active role in shaping the course of their illness. Ultimately, it is the ill person and his or her family that carry out the work of chronic illness management. Trajectory captures the temporal phase of the chronic illness, the work of managing it, the interplay of the workers, and the medical and nonmedical features of chronic illness management (Strauss & Corbin, 1988).

Chronic illness trajectories take different paths and thus assume various shapes. What gives a trajectory its shape are the phases the patient passes through (Strauss & Corbin, 1988). For example, the trajectory shape of someone with a history of chest pain and a new myocardial infarct is likely to be multiphased, as

TABLE 9–1. **Phases of Chronic Illness**

Phase	Characteristics
Acute phase	1. Affected to a degree that necessitates immediate medical attention and hospitalization; may be life-threatening 2. Work to be directed at promoting stabilization and promoting recovery 3. Psychological work may be held "in check" until the acute episode has passed
Comeback or recovery phase	1. Physical and emotional recovery after acute phase 2. Upward course 3. Management is directed at getting physically well, regaining functional ability, and coming to terms with the illness and any residual disability 4. Questions include: "Will I come back?" "How far will I come back?" "How long will it take?"
Stable phase	1. Little change in the cause of the illness, either upward or downward 2. Management is aimed at maintaining stability 3. Only minor complications experienced 4. Questions asked include: "How long will this last?" "How do I keep it this way?" "How will I know if a change begins?" 5. Hope that the present is unending
Unstable phase	1. Not acute but persistently out of control 2. Management is aimed at discovering the source of the instability and finding tactics that will bring and keep the conditions under some degree of control 3. Normal living may be seriously hampered 4. May be hospitalized, but often remain at home 5. Questions include: "Will they ever find out why this is happening?" "Why is this happening?" "What does this mean in terms of my life?" "How much longer can I go on living this way?"
Deterioration (downward) phase	1. Course of an illness is slowly or rapidly descending 2. Progressive deterioration in physical and/or mental status 3. Characterized by increasing disability or worsening symptoms 4. Exact state of the future is unknown 5. Management is aimed at controlling rate and extent of the descent and reprioritizing activities and social relationships 6. Questions include: "How fast?" "How far?"
Dying phase	1. Immediate weeks, days, hours preceding death 2. Questions include: "When will it happen?" "How will I physically die?" "How will I know I am actually dying?" "Where will it happen?"

Data from Corbin, J. M., & Strauss, A. (1988). *Unending work and care.* San Francisco: Jossey-Bass; and Corbin, J. M., & Strauss, A. (1992). A nursing model for chronic illness management based upon the trajectory framework. In P. Woog (Ed.), *The chronic illness trajectory framework* (pp. 9–28). New York: Springer. Used by permission of Springer Publishing Company, Inc., New York 10012.

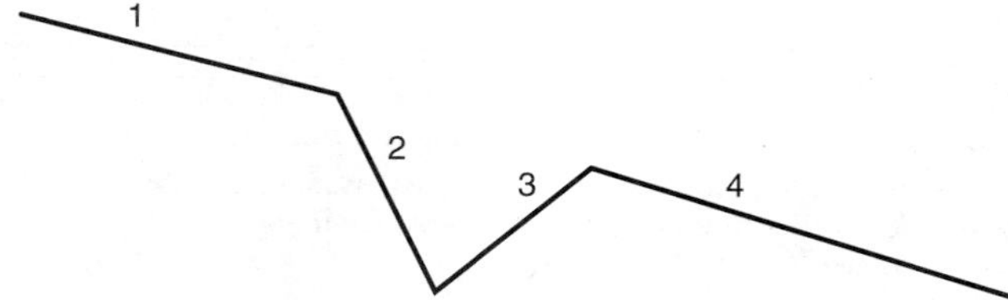

FIGURE 9–1. Example of a chronic illness trajectory—myocardial infarct. 1 = Stabilization phase; 2 = acute phase; 3 = comeback phase; 4 = deterioration phase.

illustrated in Figure 9–1. Care of the patient in the critical care unit is most likely to occur in the acute phase, the deterioration phase, and the dying phase of chronic illness.

Resources are necessary to carry out the work of the various phases of chronic illness (Corbin & Strauss, 1988; Dimond, 1983). When the biologic processes are no longer able to provide the appropriate internal homeostatic resources, then adequate substitute resources must be obtained. Although this may appear rather simplistic, arrangements are needed to find and use these substitute resources. This process is quite complex once one considers the cost of finding and using the resources, determining under what conditions they will be available, and appraising the consequences of using the resources, both positive and negative. Acquiring and using these resources can in turn affect the psychological and social resources of those with chronic illness and their family members. Possible challenges that face those dealing with chronic illnesses include personal and family suffering in relation to a changing home environment, loss of jobs, changing family roles, and diminished psychological energy for problem-solving. Sustaining the work and resources used in living daily with a chronic illness may be a relatively unobservable process in some cases, until the management mechanisms go awry. Thus, living with a chronic illness is a complex interaction of demand for and supply of resources.

Chronic Illness and Critical Care

Patients enter critical care units for acute care and stabilization of physiologic processes. Traditionally, little attention has been given to the underlying chronicity of patients cared for in these settings other than as a component of severity scoring. The special needs of patients with chronic illnesses cared for in critical care settings is rarely addressed, and little research is available to guide nursing practice (Daly et al., 1991; Jillings, 1987).

Some patients, such as those with chronic lung disease, are recipients of care during the acute phase of their chronic illness trajectory. In contrast, others may have only recently become very acutely ill, and are dealing for the first time with the possibility of an ongoing chronic illness (e.g., spinal cord trauma; coronary artery disease with no previous history). Therefore, it is important to acknowledge where patients and their families are in the trajectory of chronic illness, as well as their unique needs, when providing critical care services for them during this relatively brief time of their total chronic illness experience.

Furthermore, management of the critical care patient with an underlying chronic illness should encompass much more than achieving physical stabilization and relieving symptoms. It should also include the chronically ill patient and his or her family as key members in care delivery, along with the health professionals. The challenge is to mesh the health professionals' "expected" shape of the chronic illness trajectory with those trajectories *experienced* by the patient and family. This can be achieved only through open and honest exchange of information on the part of all the participants (Strauss & Corbin, 1988; Corbin & Strauss, 1988).

RESPONSES TO CHRONIC ILLNESS

Responses to chronic illness can be viewed as a group of management or adaptive tasks, most of which have to do less with the chronic illness itself and more with the consequences of managing symptoms and changed social relationships that result from the chronic illness (Dimond, 1983). The impact of chronic illness on any patient depends on the individual's appraisal of the meaning associated with the chronicity of the illness and the phase they are experiencing in the chronic illness trajectory. The meaning of chronic illness is viewed by some patients as a series of losses, whereas others view their chronic illness as an opportunity to change their lifestyle and experience a "new lease on life" (Cousins, 1989; Dimond, 1983).

Once this appraisal of the chronic illness and its meaning is achieved, various biologic, psychological, and sociocultural adaptive or management tasks are used to deal and live with the chronic illness. An important part of this adaptive process is known as secondary appraisal—the ongoing assessment and selection by patients of the coping behaviors they will use to complete these adaptive tasks and manage their chronic illness. For example, a middle-aged, overweight, sedentary woman diagnosed for the first time with hypertension may view this diagnosis as an opportunity to change some of her health habits, or as a loss of those high-fat foods she enjoys. To adapt to this diagnosis and manage her chronic illness, she will assess what resources she has available to her to make some lifestyle changes, such as losing weight, learning how to select and prepare a low-fat diet, and exercising. She may continue in her current lifestyle and not make any changes, particularly if she views this diagnosis as minor, without symptomatology. In contrast, she may view this diagnosis as particularly threatening to her overall health and select the adaptive tasks of exercise and changing her eating habits, especially if she has the resources to participate in a group exercise

TABLE 9–2. **Coping Strategies in Chronic Illness Management**

Coping Strategy	Considerations
I. Information seeking	Assess for type and amount of information being sought. Not acquiring information is a choice. Usually focus on what they see as problematic. Most receptive to information that enables them to make sound decisions. Want individualized information. Allow / facilitate patients prioritizing information they want.
II. Direct action	Noncognitive actions / behaviors aimed at self or environment intended to reduce stressful situation. Examples: altering home environment; adhering to medical regimen; taking one's own life. Patient views direct action to be beneficial in some way. Not all direct actions are congruent with views of professionals. Assist patients and families to assess consequences and intentions of their actions with regard to short- and long-term outcomes.
III. Inhibition of action	Avoiding actions that have potential for doing harm. Balance avoiding actions with participating in activities that increase self-esteem. Ask: "Is the action or lack of action resulting in an adaptive outcome for the patient?"
IV. Intrapsychic processes	What people say to themselves to regulate emotions. Defense mechanisms of denial, intellectualization, avoidance, detachment; relaxation; biofeedback; cognitive transformation. Includes reappraising situations, refocusing attention, seeking alternative methods of gratification. When misperceptions and distorted beliefs are a major problem, cognitive restructuring can modify emotional reactions.
V. Turning to others	Turning to others for support buffers the impact of the event, changes interpretation of the event and the emotional response. Assist patients and families in finding community-based supports, either formal or informal.

Data from Burckhardt, C. S. (1987). Coping strategies of the chronically ill. *Nursing Clinics of North America, 22,* 543–550.

program, has family members participating with her in an exercise program, and receives encouragement from her family to make these changes.

Coping is interpreted as effective or ineffective in meeting the adaptive tasks. Corbin and Strauss (1992) caution, however, that before labeling someone with a chronic illness as not coping or coping ineffectively, it is important to step back and determine whether the individual indeed is not coping or if he or she is in a transitional period in which new conditions are being struggled with and being worked out emotionally and physically. "The key factors of adaptation are a hopeful perspective; a sense of being needed, and the maintenance of self-esteem, personal worth and human dignity in the face of impaired functioning" (Craig, 1983, p. 402).

Coping strategies are central in chronic illness management (Burckhardt, 1987; Dimond, 1983; Foxall et al., 1985; Lazarus & Folkman, 1984; Lyon & Werner, 1987). Patients find that they must adjust not only to new physical expectations but to new roles in their families and social networks (Burkhardt, 1987). To make these adjustments, five major coping strategies are used in chronic illness management. These include information-seeking, direct action, inhibition of action, intrapsychic processes, and turning to others (Table 9–2).

Adapting to chronic illness is a dynamic process of continuous negotiation between the individual and the environment. Dimond (1983) notes that flexibility (the ability to plan multiple approaches) and farsightedness (anticipating how the environment will respond to a given strategy) are two characteristics that enter into most coping strategies resulting in positive adaptation.

Coming to terms with the realities of a chronic illness is a long-term process. Surviving the initial shock, assessing the remaining capabilities, and planning strategies to cope with limitations takes time. Because of the uncertainty that surrounds many chronic conditions, it is often necessary periodically to reassess and reorganize one's life to meet the requirements of the changing situation. For example, the social network most appropriate at the onset of a chronic illness may not be as appropriate in later stages, when the individual begins to negotiate and renegotiate lifestyle changes to meet the demands of the illness (Dimond, 1983).

RESOURCES

Work is required to manage chronic illness. In the hospital and particularly in the ICU environment, the work is traditionally done by health care personnel (Dimond, 1983; Hawthorne, 1992). In the home and community, the work of chronic illness management is done by the chronically ill person and those around him or her.

Resources commonly cited to accomplish the work of chronic illness management are (1) the internal resources of energy, hardiness and control, hope, self-efficacy, and information; and (2) the external resource of social support. This resource perspective of chronic illness management is used as a framework for describing the unique needs of critically ill patients with chronic illnesses.

Internal Resources and Physiologic Needs

ENERGY NEEDS

Energy is a major resource used in adaptation, mobility, and growth. An important part of energy production and storage relies on the ability of the body to process and distribute ingested food, oxygen, and water. Interference with the biophysical processes of digestion, absorption, circulation, respiration, fluid balance, and cellular metabolism disrupts energy production and depletes this valuable resource that is an integral part of physiologic, psychological, and social adaptation.

The first priority of energy expenditure is for life-sustaining activities, including both physiologic functioning and protective psychosocial processes such as withdrawal or denial. If there is energy remaining after these compensatory behaviors, it can then be used for more active problem-solving strategies such as seeking information.

The onset of the acute phase of chronic illness requires additional energy expenditure for healing, fighting infection, tissue repair, and coping with disruptions in normal patterns of behavior. As described by Strauss and Corbin (1988), the trajectory of chronic illness requires work and varying amounts of energy, depending on the phase in the trajectory. For example, during a medical crisis, much energy is used to re-establish physiologic stability. There may be little energy for use of problem-solving coping strategies such as information seeking, and the affective processes of detachment, avoidance, or denial will be more prominent. Thus, energy is a crucial resource in adaptation to chronic illness, particularly during the acute phase of the trajectory.

Critically ill patients with an underlying chronic illness have limited energy to use in achieving some sort of stabilization. With this in mind, the physiologic needs of critically ill patients with chronic illness can be seen to have some special considerations beyond those traditionally viewed in critical care practice. The first consideration is determining or redefining physiologic normality for these patients. For example, patients and family members who have managed chronic lung disease at home will perceive the level of dyspnea differently from the health care provider (DeVito, 1990). The nurse needs to assess the level of dyspnea with regard to the usual level experienced by such patients at home, rather than assuming absence of dyspnea as normal. Likewise, applying high-technology equipment to individuals with chronic illness makes physiologic data available that may be viewed as abnormal but must be interpreted in light of what is "normal" for that patient.

ENERGY RESTORATION: ASSESSMENT AND INTERVENTIONS

Nurses and physicians alike must have an appreciation for the baseline functioning of the patient before the critical illness event. Use of a standardized functional health status instrument such as the MOS SF-36 (Medical Outcomes Study Short Form, 36 questions) is one way to assess the level of functioning before admission (Ware, 1993). This tool can be completed by the patient as a self-report, by the nurse as part of admission assessment, or by a family member or caregiver who knows the patient well. Information from this tool can then be used to determine levels of physical functioning, role functioning, social functioning, bodily pain, mental health, vitality, and general health perception of the patient, all of which can then be used to set realistic expected outcomes.

Many patients with chronic illness have developed compensatory mechanisms that permit adequate functioning at home with less than optimal physiologic laboratory values (e.g., oxygen saturation). Patients may be unaware of the compromised value until they enter an acute care setting and are connected to high-tech physiologic monitoring equipment. These compensatory mechanisms must be supported to maximize the energy expenditure for stabilization.

Other people with chronic illness are tuned in to their physiologic processes and may perceive subtle symptom changes before observed changes in physiologic parameters take place. Therefore, the nurse must learn from the patient and family what is normal physiologic functioning for this patient, and be sensitive to cues offered by the patient that may be early warning signs of a decline in physiologic functioning. The nurse must also work with the patient and family in conserving energy for use in healing rather than dealing with unnecessary stressors such as pain and noise.

Furthermore, the nurse must view trends in changing physiologic data from both an acute and chronic illness perspective, considering the type of underlying chronic condition the patient has, and the superimposed acute illness. For example, a patient with hypertension admitted for possible stroke may be viewed as normovolemic with a blood pressure of 150/92 after being in the ICU for 24 hours. However, if this patient usually has a blood pressure between 180 and 190 systolic, the nurse should question if a decline of 30 to 40 mm Hg is a normal trend for this patient, possibly putting him at risk for adverse occurrences such as deep venous thrombosis. Are there other acute treatments he has received that may explain this decline in blood pressure over the last 24 hours?

In addition, it is important to consider where the patient is with regard to disease progression. If the patient is in a rapid deterioration or dying phase of the trajectory (e.g., end-stage lung disease), focusing on decision-making support with the patient and family and keeping the patient comfortable may be of higher priority than frequent monitoring of ongoing physiologic data.

Several treatments should be considered for facilitating energy restoration and conservation in these patients. Examples of these interventions and their definitions are listed in Table 9–3. Continuous surveillance and management of technology are important treatments. Physiologic normality is redefined and data are trended and interpreted to make clinical decisions about the patient's response to medical and nursing treatments. Circulatory care, and nutrition, fluid, electrolyte, and airway management are needed to promote energy production at the cellular level. Enhanc-

TABLE 9–3. **Interventions to Support Internal Resources of Energy**

Intervention	Definition
Surveillance	Purposeful and ongoing acquisition, interpretation, and synthesis of patient data for clinical decision-making
Technology management	Use of technical equipment and devices to monitor patient condition or sustain life
Circulatory care	Promotion of arterial and venous circulation
Nutrition management	Assisting with or providing a balanced dietary intake of foods and fluids
Fluid and electrolyte management	Regulation and prevention of complications from altered fluid and electrolyte levels
Airway management	Facilitation of patency of air passages
Sleep enhancement	Facilitation of regular sleep–wake cycles
Pain management	Alleviation of pain or a reduction in pain to a level of comfort that is acceptable to the patient
Therapeutic touch	Directing one's own interpersonal energy to flow through the hands to help or heal another

From McCloskey, J. C., & Bulechek, G. M. (1992). *Nursing interventions classification (NIC)*. St. Louis: Mosby Year Book.

ing sleep, managing pain, and using therapeutic touch are three interventions the nurse can use to facilitate energy production and healing.

Internal Resources and Psychosocial Needs

Critically ill patients with an underlying chronic illness have special psychosocial needs that must be addressed in care delivery. Patients and their families use coping strategies they have developed by drawing on internal resources. A number of personal internal resources are thought to be related to an individual's ability to meet his or her psychosocial needs and cope effectively. These resources include hardiness and control, hope, self-efficacy, and information.

The role of nurses is to understand and support the coping strategies of patients. Critical care nurses see these patients for a short time period in their entire chronic illness trajectory, usually during the acute or rapid deterioration phase. Nurses should expect that coping strategies may change depending on the type of underlying chronic illness, the perception of control patients have over the situation, the phase of the chronic illness trajectory patients are in (e.g., newly diagnosed versus medical crisis of a long-standing chronic condition), and the type of information and method by which it is conveyed.

HARDINESS AND CONTROL

Hardiness has received considerable attention in recent years as an important resource in coping with and adapting to chronic illness (Kobasa, 1979; Kobasa et al., 1982, 1983; Norwack, 1989; Pollock, 1986, 1989). Hardiness is a personality resource related to how a person perceives stressors. Three perspectives on life function as a buffer to stressors: viewing work and life as a commitment, rather than succumbing to alienation; having personal control over individual outcomes; and viewing life as a challenge rather than a threat. Hardiness seems to have a direct positive effect on use of adaptive behaviors in people with chronic illness. Hardiness may also have an indirect effect on adaptation by influencing the person's perception of chronic illness, the coping strategies chosen, and the social resources used (Pollock, 1986, 1989; Pollock & Duffy, 1990).

Control, an integral part of hardiness, is an important resource in adaptation to chronic illness (Dimond, 1983; Lewis, 1982; Miller, 1983; Pollock, 1987). Perceived control is positively correlated with increased physical and psychological well-being, increased self-esteem, decreased anxiety, and increased quality of life (Lewis, 1982; Padilla & Grant, 1985). In one study, for example, the process of adjustment after myocardial infarction varied, but all patients spent much time and energy trying to regain a sense of control and mastery as they moved into the stabilization phase of their chronic illness trajectory (Johnson & Morse, 1990). Therefore, patients who are chronically ill must have the power to be managers of their care and must be made to feel like they do not have to forfeit this role to health care professionals, as is often the case in the critical care setting.

Critical care nurses need to assess the internal psychological resource of hardiness, which includes the characteristic of control. The 34-item Health Related Hardiness Scale could be completed by the patient or by a family member on the patient's behalf (Pollock & Duffy, 1990). Selected items from the scale could be incorporated into the nursing admission assessment to determine the patient's perspective regarding control, commitment, and challenge.

Armed with information from this assessment, critical care nurses can verbally acknowledge the patient's need for control and discuss with the patient how to adjust the critical care environment to meet their needs (Pollock, 1984). Those who have a high degree of hardiness can be given some sense of control over their care by being provided with options regarding interactions with family members, timing of treatments, and access to personal possessions in the environment. Providing these patients with some sense of control over the environment in the ICU should result in a conservation of energy because they no longer have to struggle to gain control. Those who have a high degree of hardiness and control will also have a greater need to participate in their treatment decisions, and are more likely to use direct actions to cope (Burckhardt, 1987).

One must acknowledge, however, that not all direct actions initiated by the patient will be congruent with the wishes, desires, or treatment recommendations of the health care professionals, particularly in the critical care setting, where it is customary for the members of the health care delivery system to be "in charge and in control" (Strauss & Corbin, 1988; Thorne, 1993). Furthermore, patients in the deterioration or dying phase of their chronic illness trajectory may perceive a critical care hospitalization as the final battle, and have great difficulty "letting go" in the face of life-saving technology. In such cases, the emphasis must be in facilitating control and decision-making by patients and their families.

HOPE

Hope is another important resource to consider in adapting to chronic illness. It has been demonstrated that hope plays a central part in the patient's coping ability, and that maintaining hope is a primary response in patients dealing with a chronic illness (Cousins, 1989; Forsyth et al., 1984; Hamberg & Hamberg, 1953; O'Malley & Menke, 1988). Hope is perceived as a basic part of human existence that transcends grief, suffering, and pain and provides life-sustaining energy (Menniger, 1959).

Maintaining some degree of hope during the critical care experience in the face of chronic illness is extremely important for patients and their family members. This hope may range from hope for stabilization and a return home, to hope for a peaceful death. The nature of the hope is highly influenced by the meaning patients give to their acute exacerbation and their phase within the chronic illness trajectory (Corbin & Strauss, 1988). Supporting the hope patients and family members have is extremely important because that is often the major factor keeping the patient and family going.

SELF-EFFICACY

Self-efficacy, another important internal resource, is an individual's conviction that he or she can successfully execute or master a particular task or behavior to produce a specific outcome. People tend to execute tasks that fall within their perceived range of self-efficacy, but avoid tasks that exceed their perceived efficacy expectations. Acting on misjudgment of personal self-efficacy can have adverse consequences such as unnecessary avoidance (Bandura, 1977, 1982, 1983).

How a person perceives self-efficacy acts as a basis for action but differs from outcome expectations, in which a person perceives that participating in a particular behavior will lead to a certain outcome. For example, a person who has chronic obstructive lung disease may believe that she is unable to walk five blocks without becoming severely short of breath (perceived self-efficacy) and therefore not participate in activities that require walking a distance of about five blocks. The basis for her not participating in activities that require this amount of walking is her belief that she cannot participate in the activity without becoming severely short of breath. Likewise, this same person may believe that participating in a pulmonary rehabilitation program will lead to an *expected outcome* of decreased severity of dyspnea experienced with walking. Therefore, she may participate in a pulmonary rehabilitation program. Judgments about personal efficacy, whether accurate or faulty, influence the choice of behavior.

A person uses two major sources to develop self-efficacy: information sources and cognitive appraisal. These two components interact to formulate the strength, magnitude, and generality of self-efficacy perception. The four major sources of information that contribute to self-efficacy are (1) performance accomplishments, (2) vicarious experiences, (3) verbal persuasion, and (4) emotional arousal (Bandura, 1982).

Self-efficacy has been demonstrated to affect how a person manages his or her chronic illness. It was found to be a major predictor of functional health status in patients 6 months after coronary artery bypass grafting (Allen et al., 1990). In this study, self-efficacy independently explained 24% of the variance in social and leisure function, and 20% of the variance in intermediate activities of daily living. Self-efficacy explained more of the variance in functional outcomes than did measures of disease severity, functional capacity, comorbidity, or preoperative functioning. Similar findings have been documented by other investigators (Ewart et al., 1983; Jenkins, 1986; Kaplan & Atkins, 1984, 1988; Taylor et al., 1985).

To assess the level of self-efficacy of critically ill patients with a chronic illness, the critical care nurse needs to determine the patients' beliefs regarding their ability to improve or stabilize physiologically, their ability to learn new self-care skills, and their ability to return to their previous level of functioning. Positive self-efficacy expectations serve as a motivating force for critically ill patients dealing with a new chronic illness to redefine normality and to return to the community with positive self-esteem. In turn, families who have been caring for their loved one at home may have a high degree of self-efficacy regarding provision of physical care to the patient, and thus may expect to participate as equal partners in delivery of care, and to stay at the bedside for extended periods of time.

NEED FOR INFORMATION

Evidence suggests that the need for diagnostic and treatment information is consistently high across the various phases of chronic illness. Patients also have a need to be understood relative to services they believe are required to control their illness (e.g., decision-making exploration, collaborative relationships, use of problem-solving strategies, availability of service). Although these needs ranked high in a hierarchy of needs across all phases of chronic illness (Salmond, 1987), it is unknown if these needs continue during a crisis requiring critical care hospitalization.

Therefore, critical care nurses must assess what, if any, information patients and families are asking for. The belief that more information is always best for all patients under all circumstances is not documented by current research (Burckhardt, 1987). The nurse must look for cues that the patient is seeking information, and the type of information requested. People with chronic illnesses want information that has direct utility in solving their current problems, they prefer individualized information, and they prefer it be prioritized according to *their* needs rather than those of the health care provider (Burckhardt, 1987). Patients at times need to be allowed *not* to acquire information because some degree of the unknown may facilitate hope.

Treatments aimed at supporting the internal resources of hardiness, control, hope, self-efficacy, and information are summarized in Table 9–4. Patients who desire a high degree of control in managing their chronic illness may benefit from mutual goal setting, management of the environment, milieu therapy, and support in decision-making. Clarifying values, enhancing communication, and protecting the rights of patients are important interventions to use in gaining understanding and providing the type and amount of information the patient and family desires.

Providing emotional support and instilling hope are essential as the patient and family try to make sense of the meaning this episode of critical illness has in the overall chronic illness trajectory. Enhancing positive coping, using cognitive restructuring, and involving families in the care of the critically ill patient are important interventions to consider in light of the coping strategies used by patients and families during this phase of chronic illness. Because patients come from a community and will return to a community unless the outcome is death, discharge planning and referral should be initiated early in their critical care hospitalization.

TABLE 9–4. **Interventions to Support Internal Resources of Hardiness, Control, Hope, Information, and Self-Efficacy**

Intervention	Definition
Mutual goal setting	Collaborating with patient to identify and prioritize care goals, then developing a plan for achieving those goals through the construction and use of goal attainment scaling
Decision-making support	Providing information and support for a patient who is making a decision regarding health care
Environmental management	Manipulation of the patient's surroundings for therapeutic benefit
Milieu therapy	Use of people, resources, and events in the patient's immediate environment to promote optimal psychosocial functioning
Values clarification	Assisting another to clarify her or his own values to facilitate effective decision-making
Patient rights protection	Protection of health care rights of a patient, especially a minor, incapacitated, or incompetent patient unable to make decisions
Communication enhancement	Facilitating interaction with a patient who has difficulty delivering or receiving verbal or nonverbal messages
Emotional support	Provision of reassurance, acceptance, and encouragement during times of stress
Hope instillation	Facilitation of the development of a positive outlook in a given situation
Coping enhancement	Assisting a patient to adapt to perceived stressors, changes, or threats that interfere with meeting life demands and roles
Cognitive restructuring	Challenging a patient to alter distorted thought patterns and view self and the world more realistically
Family involvement	Facilitating family participation in the emotional and physical care of the patient
Discharge planning	Preparation for moving a patient from one level of care to another within or outside the current health care agency
Referral	Arrangement for services by another care provider or agency

From McCloskey, J. C., & Bulechek, G. M. (1992). *Nursing interventions classification (NIC)*. St. Louis: Mosby Year Book.

External Resources: Social Support

Social support is an external resource that influences how people manage their chronic illness. Social support, which has received widespread attention in the chronic illness literature, refers to the psychosocial and tangible aid provided by the social network to the person (Stewart, 1989; Tilden & Weinert, 1987). The functional component of social support is the type of support that is exchanged: (1) emotional—concern, trust, caring; (2) appraisal—feedback that affirms self-worth; (3) informational—advice, suggestions, directives; and (4) instrumental—aid in kind, money, labor, time, modification of the environment. By its essential nature, social support is informal, noncontractual, and reciprocal (Stewart, 1989; Tilden & Weinert, 1987).

Research suggests that social support buffers the effect of stress on health outcomes (Flynn, 1984; Larkin, 1987; McNett, 1987; Norbeck, 1988; Norbeck et al., 1981; Yates, 1990). The exact mechanisms by which social support works have not been clearly identified. There is some evidence, however, that social support (1) may enhance feelings of personal control, which leads to problem-focused coping strategies; (2) may prevent stressors from occurring (e.g., loneliness); or (3) may have a direct positive effect on health outcomes without mediating the stress response (Flynn, 1984; Johnson & Morse, 1990; McNett, 1987; Schlenk & Hart, 1984; Tilden & Weinert, 1987).

Traditionally, people with chronic illness who are

admitted to the intensive care unit leave their social support at the doorway of the ICU because of visiting restrictions. Research findings demonstrate that such restrictions are not healthy for the family members or the patient. Interventions that facilitate the presence of family members at the bedside of their loved one while in the ICU have positive patient outcomes, including improved orientation, decreased anxiety, and increased sleep (Titler & Walsh, 1992) (see Chapter 6).

In turn, families of critically ill patients have unique needs for social support because of the uncertainty surrounding this acute phase in the chronic illness trajectory. The patient and family alike may wonder how life may change in the future, or if the patient will have a future outside of the ICU. Physical separation from the patient, geographic distance from home, a foreign critical care environment, and changing family roles and responsibilities are but a few of the challenges faced by the family and patient (Halm, 1992). The family's social network may not be available to provide the type of support that once was provided in the home or community.

Just as social support is an important component of chronic illness management, it is also important during critical care hospitalization. It is a resource that can facilitate family adaptation during the critical illness and during the transition home.

It is important to incorporate a family assessment into critical care practice and to promote the provision of family-centered care. Doing a family assessment is a form of social support that promotes a sense of belonging during this crisis. This assessment provides an opportunity to determine how the family has been assisting the patient to manage his or her chronic illness at home, and what strategies work best for the patient. It is also a time to determine what the family's economic resources are, what financial needs they have, what support systems are available to them now, and which ones were available in the past (Halm, 1992).

Interventions aimed at promoting the external resources of social support are outlined in Table 9–5. Use of support groups, enhancing the patient's and family's support system, promoting the integrity of the family as much as possible, and facilitating visiting in the critical care setting are important interventions to consider to maintain existing supports and establish new support networks for the critically ill patient and family. Helping the patient and family navigate the health care system is another important consideration often overlooked during the critical care phase of the chronic illness trajectory.

TABLE 9–5. **Interventions to Provide External Resource of Social Support**

Intervention	Definition
Support group	Use of a group environment to provide emotional support and health-related information to members
Support system enhancement	Facilitation of support to patient by family, friends, and community
Visitation facilitation	Promoting beneficial visits by family and friends
Family integrity promotion	Promotion of family cohesion and unity
Health system guidance	Facilitating a patient's location and use of appropriate health services

From McCloskey, J. C., & Bulechek, G. M. (1992). *Nursing interventions classification (NIC).* St. Louis: Mosby Year Book.

SUMMARY

Interventions for critically ill patients with a chronic illness are aimed at supporting and restoring the internal and external resources needed in chronic illness management. It is acknowledged that the nursing treatments used in care of these patients will depend on the nature of the acute illness and the phase of the patient's chronic illness trajectory. The interventions discussed herein are not exhaustive but are meant to exemplify the special needs of the critically ill patient with a chronic illness, keeping in mind that critical care is but one phase of the chronic illness trajectory.

Providing care for critically ill patients with a chronic illness must begin with viewing such care as only a small part of the entire chronic illness experience. If critical care practice is to be driven by the needs of the patient, then we must listen carefully to the patient and family with regard to what strategies they have used in managing their chronic illness. Closing the doors of the ICU can no longer mean shutting out the major support systems of the patient, nor can it mean giving over completely the control of chronic illness management to the health care provider. It is essential to view patients and their family members as partners in health care delivery, and facilitate involvement of family members in the care of the critically ill patient when they so desire. Only when we internalize and value critical care practice as a small window in the entire chronic illness trajectory, will we be able to begin meeting the unique needs of these patients and their families.

REFERENCES

Allen, J. K., Becker, D. M., & Swank, R. T. (1990). Factors related to functional status after coronary artery bypass surgery. *Heart and Lung, 19,* 337–343.

Bandura, A. (1977). Self-efficacy: Toward a unifying theory of behavioral change. *Psychological Review, 84,* 191–215.

Bandura, A. (1982). Self-efficacy mechanism in human agency. *American Psychologist, 37,* 122–147.

Bandura, A. (1983). Self-efficacy determinants of anticipated fears and calamities. *Journal of Personality and Social Psychology, 45,* 464–469.

Burckhardt, C. S. (1987). Coping strategies of the chronically ill. *Nursing Clinics of North America, 22,* 543–550.

Corbin, J. M., & Strauss, A. (1988). *Unending work and care.* San Francisco: Jossey-Bass.

Corbin, J. M., & Strauss, A. (1992). A nursing model for chronic illness management based upon the trajectory framework. In P.

Woog (Ed.), *The chronic illness trajectory framework* (pp. 9–28). New York: Springer.

Cousins, N. (1989). *Head first: The biology of hope and the healing of the human spirit.* New York: Penguin Books.

Craig, H. M. (1983). Adaptation in chronic illness: An eclectic model for nurses. *Journal of Advanced Nursing, 8,* 397–404.

Daly, B. J., Rudy, E. B., Thompson, K. S., & Happ, M. B. (1991). Development of a special care unit for chronically critically ill patients. *Heart and Lung, 20,* 45–52.

DeVito, A. J. (1990). Dyspnea during hospitalization for acute phase of illness as recalled by patients with chronic obstructive pulmonary disease. *Heart and Lung, 19,* 186–191.

Dimond, M. (1983). Social adaptation of the chronically ill. In D. Mechanic (Ed.), *Handbook of health, health care and the health professions* (pp. 636–654). New York: Macmillian.

Ewart, C., Taylor, C., Reese, L., & DeBusk, F. (1983). Effects of early postmyocardial infarction exercise testing in self-perception and subsequent physical activity. *American Journal of Cardiology, 51,* 1076–1080.

Flynn, M. K. (1984). *Quality of life of coronary artery bypass patients during early convalescence.* Master's thesis, University of Iowa, College of Nursing, Iowa City, Iowa.

Forsyth, G. L., Delaney, K. D., & Grisham, M. L. (1984). Vying for a winning position: Management style of the chronically ill. *Research in Nursing and Health, 7,* 181–188.

Foxall, M. J., Ekberg, J. Y., & Griffith, N. (1985). Adjustment patterns of chronically ill middle-aged persons and spouses. *Western Journal of Nursing Research, 7,* 425–444.

Halm, M. (1992). Support and reassurance needs: Strategies for practice. *Critical Care Clinics of North America, 4,* 633–643.

Hamberg, D., & Hamberg, B. (1953). Adaptive problems and mechanisms in severely burned patients. *Psychiatry, 16,* 1–7.

Hanson, L. C., & Danis, M. (1991). Use of life-sustaining care for the elderly. *Journal of the American Geriatric Society, 39,* 772–777.

Hawthorne, M. H. (1992). Using the trajectory framework: Reconceptualizing cardiac illness. In P. Woog (Ed.), *The chronic illness trajectory framework* (pp. 39–50). New York: Springer.

Jenkins, L. (1986). Self-efficacy: New perspectives in caring for patients recovering from myocardial infarction. *Progress in Cardiovascular Nursing, 2,* 32–35.

Jillings, C. (1987). Is chronic illness a relevant topic for the critical care nurse? *Critical Care Nurse, 7*(3), 14–17.

Johnson, J. L., & Morse, J. M. (1990). Regaining control: The process of adjustment after myocardial infarction. *Heart and Lung, 19,* 126–135.

Kaplan, R. M., & Atkins, C. J. (1984). Specific efficacy expectations mediate exercise compliance in patients with COPD. *Health Psychology, 3,* 223–242.

Kaplan, R. M., & Atkins, C. J. (1988). Behavioral interventions for patients with COPD. In A. J. McSweeny & I. Grant (Eds.), *Chronic obstructive pulmonary disease: A behavioral perspective* (pp. 123–161). New York: Marcel Dekker.

Kobasa, S. C. (1979). Stressful life events, personality and health: An inquiry into hardiness. *Journal of Personality and Social Psychology, 37,* 1–11.

Kobasa, S. C., Maddi, S. R., & Kahn, S. (1982). Hardiness and health: A prospective study. *Journal of Behavioral Medicine, 6,* 41–51.

Kobasa, S. C., Maddi, S. R., & Zola, M. D. (1983). Type A and hardiness. *Journal of Behavioral Medicine, 7,* 41–51.

Lambert, C. E., & Lambert, V. A. (1987). Psychosocial impacts created by chronic illness. *Nursing Clinics of North America, 22,* 527–533.

Larkin, J. (1987). Factors influencing one's ability to adapt to chronic illness. *Nursing Clinics of North America, 22,* 535–542.

Lazarus, R. S., & Folkman, S. (1984). *Stress, appraisal, and coping.* New York: Springer.

Lewis, F. M. (1982). Experienced personal control and quality of life in late stage cancer patients. *Nursing Research, 31,* 113–118.

Lyon, B. L., & Werner, J. S. (1987). Stress. *Annual Review of Nursing Research, 6,* 3–22.

McNett, S. C. (1987). Social support, threat, and coping responses and effectiveness in the functionally disabled. *Nursing Research, 36,* 98–103.

Menninger, K. (1959). Hope. *American Journal of Psychology, 116,* 6–17.

Miller, J. F. (1983). *Coping with chronic illness: Overcoming powerlessness.* Philadelphia: F. A. Davis.

Milzman, D. P., Hinson, D., & Magnant, C. M. (1993). Trauma and pre-existing disease: Part 1. Critical considerations. *Critical Care Clinics, 9,* 633–656.

Norbeck, J. S. (1988). Social support. *Annual Review of Nursing Research, 6,* 85–109.

Norbeck, J. S., Lindsey, A. M., & Carrieri, V. L. (1981). The development of an instrument to measure social support. *Nursing Research, 30,* 264–269.

Norwack, K. M. (1989). Coping style, cognitive hardiness, and health status. *Journal of Behavioral Medicine, 12*(2), 145–158.

O'Malley, P. A., & Menke, E. (1988). Relationship of hope and stress after myocardial infarction. *Heart and Lung, 17,* 184–190.

Oye, R. K., & Bellamy, P. E. (1991). Patterns of resource consumption in medical intensive care. *Chest, 99,* 685–689.

Padilla, G. V., & Grant, M. M. (1985). Quality of life as a cancer nursing outcome variable. *Advances in Nursing Science, 8,* 45–60.

Pollock, S. E. (1984). The stress response. *Critical Care Quarterly, 6*(4), 1–13.

Pollock, S. E. (1986). Human responses to chronic illness: Physiologic and psychosocial adaptation. *Nursing Research, 35,* 90–95.

Pollock, S. E. (1987). Adaptation to chronic illness. *Nursing Clinics of North America, 22,* 631–643.

Pollock, S. E. (1989). The hardiness characteristic: A motivating factor in adaptation. *Advances in Nursing Science, 11*(2), 53–62.

Pollock, S. E., & Duffy, M. E. (1990). The health-related hardiness scale: Development and psychometric analysis. *Nursing Research, 39,* 218–222.

Salmond, S. W. (1987). Health care needs of the chronically ill. *Orthopaedic Nursing, 6*(6), 39–45.

Schlenk, E. A., & Hart, L. K. (1984). Relationship between health locus of control, health value, and social support, and the compliance of persons with diabetes mellitus. *Diabetes Care, 7,* 565–574.

Stewart, M. J. (1989). Social support instruments created by nurse investigators. *Nursing Research, 38,* 268–275.

Strauss, A., & Corbin, J. M. (1988). *Shaping a new health care system.* San Francisco: Jossey-Bass.

Strauss, A., Corbin, J. M., Fagerhaugh, S., Glaser, B., Maines, D., Suzeck, B., & Weiner, C. (1984). *Chronic illness and the quality of life* (2nd ed.). St. Louis: C. V. Mosby.

Taylor, C. B., Bandura, A., Ewart, C. K., Miller, N. H., & DeBusk, R. F. (1985). Raising spouse's and patient's perception of his cardiac capabilities following a myocardial infarction. *American Journal of Cardiology, 55,* 635–638.

Thorne, S. E. (1993). *Negotiating health care: The social context of chronic illness.* Newbury Park, CA: Sage Publications.

Tilden, V. P., & Weinert, C. (1987). Social support and the chronically ill individual. *Nursing Clinics of North America, 22,* 613–620.

Titler, M. G., & Walsh, S. M. (1992). Visiting critically ill adults: Strategies for practice. *Critical Care Clinics of North America, 4,* 623–632.

Ware, J. E. (1993). *SF-36 health survey: Manual and interpretation guide.* Boston: The Health Institute, New England Medical Center.

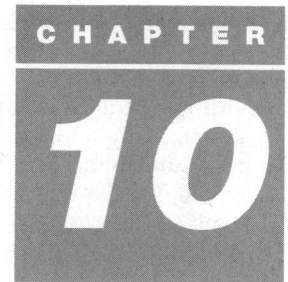

Preparing the Patient and Family for Home Care

Marjorie B. Wheeler and Susan C. Nolt

The radically changing health care system is moving forward into a new century, and the nurse's approach to patient care must keep pace. Home care, although not new, has become an equal partner in the scheme of medicine and needs to be considered for the stable ICU patient. This chapter discusses the transition of the critically ill to the home, including selection of appropriate patients, assessing the home needs, and preparing the patient, caregivers, and family for home care.

BACKGROUND

History

Historically, home care dates back to the late 1700s, when the wealthy were treated at home while the poor were treated in hospitals. To decrease the welfare stigma, the Boston Dispensary began to treat all people at home. During the late 1800s, other home nursing services were organized and run by lay people. These organizations evolved into the traditional visiting nurse organizations. All care at the chronic or maintenance level was provided by nurses. Throughout the 1900s, however, hospitals became the setting for acute care. High technology and increasingly sophisticated medical equipment contributed to the public expectation that most medical and nursing care would occur in the acute care hospital.

During the 1960s, the Medicare program was enacted by Congress, broadening the scope of service for home care agencies. Agencies could now provide nurses, aides, social workers, and therapists on an intermittent basis. In the late 1970s and 1980s, health care experienced a sudden growth in the number of agencies, with a broadening of the scope of services provided—intravenous (IV) therapy, continuous care, and fetal monitoring, for example. Today, almost any stable patient could be a serious candidate for home care as long as the transfer to home is well planned and coordinated with all appropriate parties.

Practice Setting Trends

Critical care financing will change considerably as the health care reforms of the 1990s continue to unfold. More health care will move from costly acute care settings into community facilities, such as skilled nursing facilities with special care units, board and care facilities, and the home (Fields et al., 1991; Ventafridda et al., 1989). Many patients do not require admission to intensive care, acute care, or special subacute skilled nursing units to receive certain medications that would resolve critical medical episodes. Such patients do not necessarily require hospitalization when treated aggressively in the home with appropriate nursing observations and actions.

For example, patients who are in the end stages of their illness could be seen by a critical care nurse who works for a home health agency. The nurse can start an infusion, administer intravenous medication, observe responses, report findings to the physician, and return later in the day or the next day to assess progress. Thus, the patient has received appropriate care from a nurse trained in acute life-threatening episodes and assessments. The patient has been saved a costly trip to the hospital, and has saved precious energy by staying on bed rest, at home, with services brought to the home. Another example is selected ventilator-dependent patients whose care has moved from the costly critical care unit into the home setting (Ryan, 1992; Plummer et al., 1989).

It is likely that the present trend to move to less costly settings for patient care will continue during the rest of the 1990s and into the twenty-first century. This will cause critical care units and critical care nurses to scrutinize closely alternative methods and settings as a way of cost reduction. This group of patients may well be termed "extended critical care" (Alspach, 1990; Hutchings & McPherson, 1991).

Home health can be an appropriate setting for patients requiring high-technological support. Critical care nurses are responding to challenges to identify appropriate patients, assess their needs, plan and implement their care and equipment needs, and, in some cases, deliver that care in the patients' homes. Critical care nurses have proven to be highly successful in assisting patients, families, and support systems to facilitate the transition from intensive care to the home environment (Rose, 1989).

Differences in Practice Settings

Home care nursing offers unique opportunities to practice the nursing skills developed in the critical care unit. There are similarities between the two environments in the areas of patient assessment, planning and evaluation, and in reporting observations. Further similarities include patient teaching needs, a one-to-one relationship with the patient, and the need for independent critical thinking. Both environments require that the professional have confidence in his or her assessment skills, and the ability to take appropriate action based on those assessments. Both settings demand an ability to act as a patient advocate.

There are several differences between critical care in the hospital and at home. First, home-based patients have the ability to make final decisions about most aspects of their care, including whether to open their front door to let the nurse in their home. Second, patients decide where equipment and furniture will be placed, not necessarily for the convenience of the nurse. Third, the type of equipment and supplies found in critical care units may not be readily available in the home. (However, home health nurses quickly learn to use their clinical judgment and become very creative at finding alternatives until a more appropriate supply or piece of equipment can be obtained.) Fourth, unlike in the ICU, with its readily available peer resources, the nurse is most often alone in the home setting. Therefore, a home care nurse has to be able to identify when another nursing opinion is needed. The nurse may then need to arrange for an in-home consultation by another nurse. Fifth, it is the nurse who decides when to request an increase or decrease in nursing visits or time, therapy consultations, and additional equipment and supplies. Further, the nurse may identify additional needs for a physician visit, or may recommend a trip to the emergency room. The nurse is also responsible for communicating with the physician and following up on all clinical problems. Finally, the critical care nurse often spends time ensuring that the unit and hospital systems are functioning properly. The home health nurse spends more nursing time and energy focusing on the patient and community support systems, often with the assistance of a clinical social worker (Neary, 1993).

Understanding these differences helps the critical care nurse effectively assess critical care patients for their home care potential and effectively collaborate with home health colleagues.

SELECTING PATIENTS FOR HOME CARE

Several types of critical care patients, who are now successfully cared for in their own homes, previously would not have left the intensive care unit or the acute care setting. Examples include patients with the following care needs and therapies: implanted infusion devices providing intrathecal and epidural medication; major open, draining abdominal wounds; total parenteral nutrition; multiple IV antibiotic therapies; oral suctioning; ventilator dependency; quadriplegia; chemotherapy; tocolytic therapy; home uterine monitoring; apnea monitoring; phototherapy (bililights) for neonatal hyperbilirubinemia; and dopamine therapy for end-stage cardiac disease (Hanly, 1989). Today, key questions to ask are: Should my patients remain in the ICU? Is home care a viable alternative?

Patient selection for home care is not limited to the above. Technology is advancing rapidly; equipment is becoming more portable, more user-friendly, and possesses a high degree of accuracy and dependability. Telephone modems are used to transmit patient data from the home to medical centers. The range of possibilities for home care is changing at an explosive rate. Because of these rapid changes, patient selection for home care is accomplished through team discussions and a comprehensive assessment by experts from a variety of disciplines.

THE ICU–HOME CARE TEAM

A well coordinated ICU–home care team is essential (Kersten & Hachenitz, 1991). The team should consist of the patient, appropriate family member representative(s), primary physician, ICU nurse, social worker, discharge planner, physical or occupational therapists, home care primary nurse, and home care agency liaison nurse. The team's responsibility is to assess the patient's current health care needs; the home care needs, resources, equipment, supplies, and cost factors; and training needs of the patient and family or caregivers. It is the team's challenge to develop creative ways to meet the patient's needs in the home, to make the community support systems effective for the home environment, and to minimize the need for emergency room or in-hospital intensive care.

THE PATIENT AND FAMILY. The patient and family are critical members of the team, and need to be involved early on, beginning with the initial discussions with the physician regarding prognosis and options available for ongoing care needs. Thereafter, the patient and family are involved in every step as ongoing care needs are addressed. It is the patient and family who will ultimately take over the responsibility for continuing care needs in the home setting, with appropriate support systems in place. Although the critical care nurse's role is highlighted throughout this chapter, it is very clear that it is the comprehensive team, beginning with the physician's and nurse's assessment, and the involvement of patient

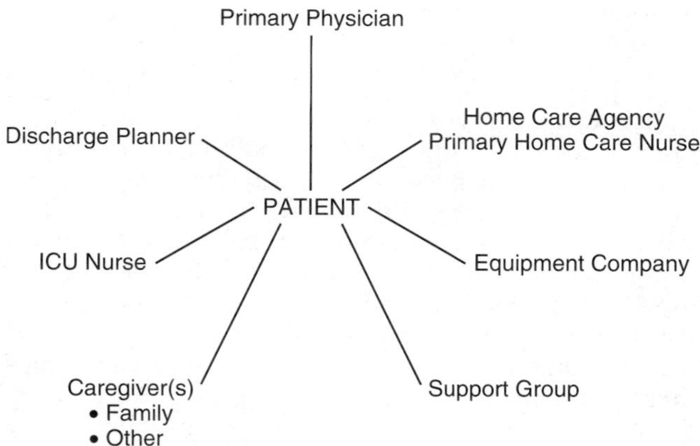

FIGURE 10–1. The ICU-home care team.

and family, that drives the successful home care plan (Fig. 10–1).

THE CRITICAL CARE NURSE. The role of the primary ICU nurse is to assess potential patients for home care with the primary physician. The ICU nurse is also instrumental in supporting patients and families who are beginning to think about home care. Nurses should involve the patient, family, and significant others in the care while in the ICU, to the level of involvement that is practical and desired by the patient and family. Assisting with care in the ICU helps to build a foundation for a successful transition to home care. As a member of the home care transition team, the ICU nurse plays an essential role in teaching caregivers, verifying skills and knowledge required in the patient's care, and in building confidence in the patient and caregivers (Handy et al., 1989; Miller, 1991).

THE PHYSICIAN. The physician provides the medical assessment as to the patient's overall medical condition, medical stability, and overall medical prognosis (Goldberg & Monahan, 1989). The physician predicts what tests and medical support are needed and functions as the medical manager of the case in the home. Often, the physician has followed the patient and family members for long periods of time prior to the patient's need for intensive care. The physician insights into family and patient strengths and limitations become a part of the team's information base.

THE HOSPITAL DISCHARGE PLANNER. When the patient is identified as a potential home care patient, the ICU nurse refers the patient to the discharge planner. The discharge planner possesses knowledge of appropriate available community resources and sets the stage for a smooth transition to home (O'Brien & Boisvert, 1989). This team member reviews the ICU nurse's assessment as well as the rest of the team's assessment, and provides input regarding any additional information. Once there is agreement that the patient is a candidate for home care, referrals are made to the home care agency and other appropriate services, such as equipment companies, support groups, and other resources.

For patients who require continuous nursing coverage, advance notice needs to be given to the home health agency. There may be as many as 12 home health staff involved, because many home health staff work part-time. It is important that the patient and family caregivers have an opportunity to meet and interview the home care staff because the patient will be opening his or her home to someone who is, at first, a stranger.

ADVANCE PRACTICE NURSE. Advance practice nurses are being used in some settings and should be considered members of the team in those settings. Their role is evolving rapidly. Advance practice roles include assisting patients with their health difficulties, regardless of the setting. The nurse may be employed by a health maintenance organization or another care management company. There may be an advance practice nurse based in the acute care hospital whose role is to help move the patient through the health care system (Nugent, 1992; Goodwin, 1992). The advance practice nurse's role on the transition to home care team could involve facilitating care needs with the hospital discharge planner, the ICU nurse, the liaison nurse, and the home care nurse.

THE HOME CARE LIAISON NURSE. The home care liaison nurse accesses the various therapists, equipment representatives, and suppliers as needed (Smith, 1993). Each of these specific disciplines makes an assessment and contributes to the patient's plan.

The occupational and physical therapists conduct assessments for safety and home adaptive devices and equipment. They will be responsible for assessing activities of daily living needs as well as mobility needs.

The patient's primary home care nurse assesses the patient needs, physician orders, and the need for any nursing supplies and equipment. In addition, the nurse assesses the need for assistance with activities of daily living and identifies the appropriate skill level required of the other nursing personnel, such as RN, LVN, and home health aide.

THE CLINICAL SOCIAL WORKER. The clinical social worker becomes involved in assessing the patient's financial and medical insurance coverage, in collaboration with the efforts of the hospital discharge planner. This team member will assess: Who will pay for care at home? Will the insurance pay for all services? Will supplies and equipment be reimbursed? How much will the patient have to pay out-of-pocket? When referring the patient to a home health agency, what will happen to the patient if funding is no longer available? The medical social worker becomes involved in assessing support systems, long-range financial needs, and community resources.

The ICU–home care team is essential in helping the patient and family make a successful transition to the home setting (Alspach, 1990). Through the team's efforts in assessing, planning, finding resources, and identifying appropriate home care candidates, the patient and family stand an excellent chance of receiving health care in a less costly setting—in their own home.

COMPREHENSIVE ASSESSMENT

Patient Assessment

The patient assessment for home care begins with an understanding of the range of home care services possible in the geographic area in which the patient lives. In rural areas, back-up systems for equipment such as ventilators and specific infusion pumps may not be readily available. In other areas, the patient may be snowed in for days at a time during the winter. Furthermore, some patients, such as high-risk obstetric patients, may live too far from the acute care hospital to arrive in time if a life-threatening emergency occurs.

The critical care nurse should not necessarily be limited by current practice. A thorough and comprehensive assessment of the patient and family needs may reveal areas in which new resources are needed. The nurse and planning team should then look for creative ways to meet those needs (Rapp, 1993). The comprehensive assessment should include the following areas: medical condition, patient attitude, support systems, ability to learn required care, ability to provide care, home environment, and community resources. In addition, as the assessment moves forward, other areas may also need to be evaluated and addressed.

MEDICAL CONDITION. It is recommended that the patient's medical condition be stable before discharge. Additional medical questions include: What was the patient's prior level of functioning? What progression or regression is expected in this medical condition? What are the medical emergencies associated with this condition? Can the anticipated emergencies be handled or prevented in the home setting? What equipment will be needed? If there are complex multiple infusions anticipated, are there infusion pumps available capable of multiple infusions, with flushing capabilities? How close does the patient live to medical facilities when needed? An integral part of the medical condition includes the patient's functional status. Will the patient be bedridden or have limited mobility? What functional limitations will exist? What level of self-care might the patient achieve?

It is also important to assess what medications, routes of administration, and timing and frequency of administration the patient will need in the home. After discharge from the hospital, changes in medication and treatment regimes will need to be able to be carried out by the patient, family, caregivers, or home care staff. Therefore, the patient and family will often need to be able to administer medication, and be capable of learning to do so.

In sum, the medical questions to be assessed are multiple and complex. Of these, the key questions involve the areas of medical stability, access to necessary equipment and support systems, and the patient's own attitude toward going home.

PATIENT ATTITUDE. The patient must want to go home and, most important, be willing to accept responsibility for aspects of care. If the patient depends on IV therapy or a ventilator, he or she will need to work through the associated fears and anxieties, in addition to mastering the actual care skills required. For example, the patient and family caregivers need to learn how to provide the necessary care, how to maintain equipment, and when and how to report equipment problems. The patient must also be able to identify emergencies, know what to do about them, know when to call the doctor, and when to call their vendors for medical supplies. In sum, the patient or caregivers must assume responsibility for many aspects of the ongoing care.

Such responsibility means that the patient and family become "the experts" in the patient's care; they do not wait for others to tell them what to do. Patients and families who assume care responsibilities can be truly remarkable in their ability to know all aspects of care in the home and effectively to communicate their needs to others. This responsibility may also require the ability to solicit life-long, continuous caregiving behaviors from family, friends, and the community.

SUPPORT SYSTEMS. The importance of the family to the critically ill patient has been documented in the recent literature and cannot be overemphasized (Artinian, 1991; Hickey, 1993; Krumberger, 1991; Lynn-McHale & Smith, 1991; Miller, 1991; O'Brien & Boisvert, 1989; Simpson, 1991; Titler et al., 1991). It is the family that provides the context for nursing care. Completing a thorough family assessment and asking relevant questions are essential (Lynn-McHale & Smith, 1991; Miles et al., 1991; Reeder, 1991). In considering a transition to home, family members or significant others must want the patient to come home. Likewise, they must be willing and able to participate in the patient's care. The family needs to know that even though there is involvement of an outside home care agency, it is the family who accepts the 24-hour responsibility for the patient's care. This treatment may include dressing changes, suctioning, administering intravenous medications and solutions, coordinating visits of home care staff, or even providing care in the event the agency is unable to supply supplemental staff.

It should also be emphasized that the role of the caregiver does not stop with an 8-hour shift, and can be very exhausting. The support system for the caregivers must be developed from the beginning of the home care planning, using community, family, and friends as resources. Often, a home health agency may be used to provide the needed respite services. These issues should be addressed early, as the caregiver begins participating in the patient's care while the patient still is in the critical care unit (Thomas et al., 1992).

ABILITY TO LEARN REQUIRED CARE. Another factor to assess in the ICU is the willingness and ability of the patient, family, and potential caregiver(s) to learn the required aspects of care. Some patients and family members find it impossible to accept the idea of giving themselves or family members care such as insulin injections, let alone ventilator or IV care. It may be unrealistic for the patient to learn much of her or his own care while in the ICU due to the critical physiologic problems. Therefore, it may be more realistic to teach the family or caregivers initially and leave most, if not all, of the patient teaching for the home care staff. This aspect of patient learning in the ICU must be individually assessed and planned for accordingly. The family member's ability to learn required care is not always a simple issue. It is one thing for the family to want the patient to be at home; it may be quite another thing for the family to learn the necessary care or arrange for someone to learn the care. This factor can be a sensitive area. Some family members do not see themselves in a caregiver role (Jorm et al., 1993). However, denial of this supportive role is socially unacceptable in many circumstances, depending on the potential caregiver's cultural and socioeconomic background, age, and sex. This factor alone may be a substantial roadblock to learning complex care.

ABILITY TO PROVIDE CARE. Once the willingness and ability to learn the required care has been assessed, the caregiver must be assessed for the ability to actually provide care. Such care can include operation of life support systems and mechanical equipment. In some cases, family members themselves have medical or emotional limitations to their abilities to provide aspects of the care. Patients may have family members who have neurologic, learning, coordination, memory, or endurance limitations that prevent them from being able to carry out care procedures accurately and consistently (Engelke et al., 1992).

These five areas are assessed by the critical care nurse and discussed with the home health nurse, who will complete the assessment.

HOME ENVIRONMENT. The assessment for home care includes a thorough assessment of the home environment. This assessment is often completed by the home health agency's liaison nurse, along with physical and occupational therapists and a medical social worker. Patient-specific requirements are first outlined by the hospital-based intensive care nurse. The agency's home care liaison staff then conducts a home assessment with the family. Such an assessment includes the following areas:

1. *Space.* Depending on the complexity of the patient's required care, an entire room may be needed. This may mean that the care is provided in a room previously used as a family room, living room, or dining room. It is important to consider how privacy will be provided for the patient for rest, treatments, and care if the patient is in a heavily trafficked area. It is also necessary to find space for equipment and supplies. The nurse should make an inventory of potential equipment and supplies so that the family can evaluate whether there is sufficient storage space. Consideration must also be given to whether necessary equipment such as a hospital bed, electric wheelchair, Hoyer lift, suction machine, IV equipment, oxygen, and back-up emergency supplies can be safely accommodated in the home.
2. *Facilities.* Is there enough electrical power and outlets to support the needed equipment, such as a ventilator? Is refrigeration available for storing medication and IV therapy solutions? Is a telephone available? Are plumbing facilities adequate to maintain hygiene, cleanliness, and laundry?
3. *Safety.* Are there steps into the house? If so, how many? Where are the bathroom facilities? Are these facilities accessible to the handicapped? How wide are the doorways throughout the house? Will a wheelchair pass through the doorways? Have caregivers been taught body mechanics for lifting or turning the patient either from a regular home low bed or hospital bed? What will be the emergency evacuation plan from the home?

Ultimately, many disciplines and service vendors become involved in the fine details of planning the set-up for home care. The major areas listed above highlight the importance of the ICU nurse in identifying the patient's current and predictable needs that might occur in transferring the patient to the home. The

Item	Yes	No	Comments
1. Patient Room			
2. Electricity			
3. Phone			
4. Description of Home			
Number of Floors			
Bathrooms			
Number			
Location(s)			
Steps			
Number outside			
Number inside			
Where?			
5. Finances			
Insurance			
Nurses			
Intermittent			
Shifts			
Medical Equipment (identify)			
Supplies (identify)			

FIGURE 10–2. Predischarge home assessment checklist.

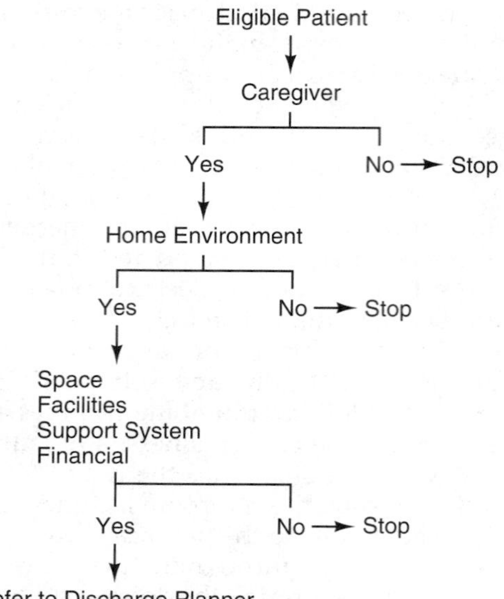

FIGURE 10–3. Discharge planning needs assessment flow chart.

home environment assessment also highlights the coordination and responsibility of the home care agency staff in continuing to meet the needs in the home environment.

COMMUNITY RESOURCES. The medical social worker and the agency home care nurse typically become involved in the community resources assessment. A predischarge checklist can be developed to use as an outline for assessing the needs for community resources (Fig. 10–2).

In summary, the assessment phase of planning for discharge to home care is crucial because of the complexity of care needs. The Assessment Flow Sheet shows one method for beginning this process of discharge planning from the ICU (Fig. 10–3).

TRANSITION: CRITICAL CARE TO HOME

Successful Transition to the Home Setting

Setting the stage for home care begins with the patient's admission to intensive care. Throughout the course of care in the ICU, the nurse must use every possible opportunity, given the patient's condition, to find ways to have the family or potential caregivers participate in the patient's care. Thus, the family learns during the patient's stay in the ICU about patient needs that family members can potentially address in the home.

It is most important to develop a comprehensive teaching plan for the patient and family. The teaching plan needs to be a coordinated plan that is communicated and followed through on from shift to shift. Implementation of the teaching plan needs to start early on as part of the patient's preparation for discharge, so there will be many opportunities for reinforcement. In addition to verbal information and observation of skills, written information is also part of the teaching plan. To be effective and helpful, all information must be in language easily understood by the patient and family.

Teaching family members in the ICU can be highly effective, despite the high level of anxiety and stress that characterizes the ICU stay. Relief of anxiety and stress can begin with step-by-step instruction in simple terms, unhurried instruction, and much reinforcement and encouragement. The ICU can be an excellent learning place for the family. By explaining what is happening to the patient, the nurse puts the family in a much better position to recognize signs of impending problems that the patient may encounter at home. The family members' ability to retain information learned in the intensive care setting varies, but the instruction, reinforcement, the observation of skills, and validation of the family members' information does, in fact, carry over to the home setting (Leske, 1991; Lynn-McHale & Smith, 1991; O'Brien & Boisvert, 1989; Thomas et al., 1992).

The learning that has taken place in the hospital sets the stage for performance of required care tasks in the home. When the patient or their family member(s) have had infusion care explained during the course of care in the ICU, they can perform skills such as starting, maintaining, and stopping their infusions; flushing their infusion lines with saline and Heparin; giving multiple IV antibiotics, total parenteral nutrition, and lipids; and solving pump problems with much greater speed, accuracy, and confidence. Confidence-building begins in the ICU with even the simplest of tasks. Patients and family members can understand fairly complex concepts when they relate directly to their own care or that of the family member. For example, an understanding of how to operate a ventilator, suction machine, or oxygen equipment becomes the patient's lifeline. A step-by-step approach to learning all aspects of relevant care, moving from the simple steps to the more complex concepts, with reinforcement, makes such learning realistic and achievable. The ability of the patient and family to assume responsibility for complex care procedures is much greater than they have been given credit for.

Involving the Supplemental Home Staff

The transition to the home may require home care agency staff to supplement the care provided by family caregivers. The goal for the agency is to obtain a core staff who can meet or supplement the patient's medical needs, as well as have compatible personalities with the patient and family. The primary home care nurse must emphasize to the patient and caregiver that the patient may, after a reasonable trial period, request a change in staff without any negative effects. If at all possible, the home care staff may want to spend time in the unit getting to know the patient, the care involved, and the patient's routine. If there is medical equipment involved, such as a ventilator, the durable medical equipment company may want to initiate use of the specific ventilator that will be used at home while the patient is still in the hospital. This process may assist in the patient's adjustment while in a supervised setting. Likewise, the home care nurse may have the opportunity to work with the patient and equipment before the move to a seemingly less controlled setting. The ICU and primary home care nurses may also suggest that the patient go home for a trial weekend once the essential systems are in place.

Throughout the entire transition process, there must be team meetings that include the patient, caregiver, family, home care representatives, inpatient staff, and the physician. Lines of communication must remain open to allow the patient and family to express their desires, expectations, and concerns.

CASE HISTORY

Mr. S was a 70-year-old man, a retired coal miner, who was admitted to the ICU in acute respiratory distress, intubated and mechanically ventilated. The original goal was eventually to wean Mr. S from the ventilator before sending him home. However, efforts to wean the patient proved unsuccessful due to the extent of the black lung disease, which left Mr. S with about a third of one lung functioning. He remained stable on the ventilator with a tracheostomy, but was unable to be weaned. Long-term plans for ongoing care were initiated. The physician informed the patient and family that Mr. S needed to be placed in an extended care facility.

Mrs. S, who was in her sixties, had been married to Mr. S for their entire adult life. She told the physician and staff that placing her husband in an extended care facility wasn't going to work. The extended care facility was 100 miles from her home and she did not drive. She stated that she would never see him and she knew he would die if he had to go to an extended care facility. In addition, the patient did not want to go to an extended care facility. Mrs. S was very determined and insistent that she be allowed to take him home and care for him at home. The physician response was that she had no idea how much work that care would involve. Mrs. S's response was "do you know how much care he has always been?" Before admission to the ICU, Mr. S had such severely limited respiratory function that he was unable to do much of any activities of daily living for himself and was homebound.

Mrs. S persisted. She insisted she be allowed at least a 2-week trial period to see if she could manage his care at home. At that point, the physician, nurses, social services, and home care agency began the home care planning process.

Mrs. S was taught all aspects of Mr. S's care in the ICU by the intensive care staff. This care included: operation of the Bennett LP-4 portable ventilator, tracheostomy care, suctioning, oxygen therapy, changing and cleaning the tubing, trouble-shooting the ventilator, operation on battery mode, turning, bathing, transferring to and from the bed to the chair, medication administration, and home safety.

Preparation at the home included building a short ramp for wheelchair access, setting aside a specific room devoted to Mr. S and his equipment and supplies, developing a schedule of home care RNs to work from 11 P.M. to 7 A.M. and provide respite care as needed, installing a call system at the bedside, purchasing a hospital bed, and renting the ventilator and suction equipment. The family bought a second portable dishwasher so that Mrs. S could use that dishwasher exclusively for cleaning the ventilator tubing. The physician agreed to make home visits as needed.

Two of the ICU nurses worked some of the night shifts in the home, which eased the transition and provided long-term continuity. The ICU nurses updated the care plan and home routines tailored to Mr. S's needs.

Mrs. S and their four adult children took Mr. S home, which was 10 blocks from the hospital. He did not return to the hospital for 3 years. His children all learned how to take care of his needs, including the ventilator and suctioning needs. His grandchildren knew when he needed to be suctioned and would run to get an adult to suction him. Mr. S was able to go out in his backyard for the first time in years and to play cards with his grandchildren. Before his ICU experience, he lacked the energy and endurance to go down the three steps to his backyard, and slept most of the time.

Mrs. S became "the expert" in her husband's care, in addition to giving up smoking because of the oxygen in the home. She prepared breakfast for the night RN and was known to make special "kolachy" that she shared with only one other person—a special nurse. Mrs. S also was known to call the home care agency and request that a nurse not return to the home. When the nurse tried to tell Mrs. S how to give care to Mr. S, Mrs. S stated, "I've been doing this for two and a half years, so don't tell me how to do things." Mrs. S was correct. She had learned all aspects of care with the support of the physician and ICU nurses, who were still occasionally covering the night shift. Mrs. S had these nurses validate her skills and would make any needed modifications.

Mr. S died at home in his sleep with his children around him 7 years after he left the ICU. His ventilator and all the concomitant equipment and care needs provided Mr. S the opportunity to do the activities he enjoyed with his wife, children, and grandchildren. Mrs. S more than surpassed the original 2 weeks' trial of taking care of Mr. S in their own home, and consequently had several more years with her husband.

EVALUATION OF THE TRANSITION TO HOME CARE

Evaluation of the ICU to home care transition includes assessing the patient's medical and nursing outcomes, patient and family satisfaction, and provision of supplies and equipment, including maintenance. In addition, there must be consistent demonstration of accurate provision of care by the caregivers, ongoing physician satisfaction with the patient's medical treatment plan, and decrease in, or absence of, hospitalizations. Program evaluation will also include the degree to which the goals and objectives set at the discharge planning meetings in the hospital have been realized (Leimnetzer et al., 1993). Finally, there must be evidence of continuous clinical problem-solving once the patient is in the home.

It is usually the home care team that is in the position to do this evaluation and has the long-range responsibility for evaluating the continued progress and status at home. This component of the evaluation process consists of quarterly utilization reviews and patient care conferences to assess the patient and family status. In addition, patient, family, and physician satisfaction surveys, equipment and supplier surveys, analysis of rehospitalizations, and supervisory visits to the patient's home are used to evaluate the multiple aspects of the complex patient care being given (Bobnet et al., 1993).

An increasingly essential component of the evaluation process is the financial savings to the health care system. Financial analysis of savings needs to include costs saved through earlier discharge from the ICU as well as the costs incurred in purchasing equipment and services for home care.

Equally important, if not more so, to the patients and their families is the degree to which they experience a higher quality of life (Chelluri et al., 1992). In the case of Mr. and Mrs. S, the combination of intensive care followed by meticulous planning for transition to home care resulted in a higher quality of life for the patient and family.

SUMMARY

The era of health care reform is explosive and chaotic. Health care that has in the past been provided only in ICUs is now being given at a maintenance level in the home setting. The challenge for critical care nurses in the late 1990s and into the twenty-first century includes redefining how we can make an optimal impact on those changes by focusing on patient and family needs. Critical care nurses are the experts in the use of the high technology required for life support and life-sustaining care. Critical care nurses must extend that knowledge into the community to nontraditional settings, including the home. They need to be a part of generating new ideas for technology that could be used in a less costly setting. Critical care nurses can be active participants, now and in the future, in extending their expertise beyond traditional settings and in ensuring successful transitions to the home setting.

REFERENCES

Alspach, J. G. (1990). Preparing critical care patients for discharge home. *Critical Care Nurse, 10*(7), 11–13.

Artinian, N. T. (1991). Strengthening nurse–family relationships in critical care. *AACN Clinical Issues, 2,* 269–275.

Bobnet, N. L., Ilcyn, J., Milanovich, P. S., Ream, M. A., & Wright, K. (1993). Continuous quality improvement: Improving quality in your home care organization. *JONA, 23*(2), 42–48.

Chelluri, L., Pinsky, M. R., & Grenvik, A. N. A. (1992). Outcome of intensive care of the "oldest-old" critically ill patients. *Critical Care Medicine, 20*(6), 757–761.

Engelke, M. K., & Engelke, S. C. (1992). Predictors of the home environment of high-risk infants. *Journal of Community Health Nursing, 9,* 171–181.

Fields, A. I., Rosenblatt, A., Pollack, M. M., & Kaufman, J. (1991). Home care cost-effectiveness for respiratory technology-dependent children. *ADJC, 145,* 729–733.

Goldberg, A. I., & Monahan, C. A. (1989). Home health care for children assisted by mechanical ventilation: The physician's perspective. *The Journal of Pediatrics, 114*(3), 378–383.

Goodwin, D. R. (1992). Critical pathways in home healthcare. *JONA, 22*(2), 35–40.

Handy, C. M. (1989). Patient-centered high-technology home care. *Holistic Nursing Practice, 3*(2), 46–53.

Hickey, M. (1993). Psychosocial needs of families. In J. M. Clochesy, C. Breu, S. Cardin et al. (Eds.). *Critical care nursing* (pp. 91–100). Philadelphia: W. B. Saunders.

Hutchins, V. L., & McPherson, M. (1991). National agenda for children with special health needs: Social policy for the 1990s through the 21st century. *American Psychologist, 46*(2), 141–143.

Jorm, A. F., Henderson, S., Scott, R., Mackinnon, A. J., Korten, A. E., & Christensen, H. (1993). The disabled elderly living in the community: Care received from family and formal services. *The Medical Journal of Australia, 158,* 383–388.

Kersten, D., & Hackenitz, E. (1991). How to bridge the gap between hospital and home? *Journal of Advanced Nursing, 16,* 4–14.

Krumberger, J. M. (1991). Linking critical care family research to quality assurance. *AACN Clinical Issues, 2,* 321–328.

Leimnetzer, M. J., Ryan, D. A., & Niemann, V. G. (1993). The Hospital-Visiting Nurse Association partnership: A continuous quality improvement program. *JONA, 23*(11), 20–23.

Leske, J. S. (1991). Overview of family needs after critical illness: From assessment to intervention. *AACN Clinical Issues, 2,* 220–226.

Lynn-McHale, D. J., & Smith, A. (1991). Comprehensive assessment of families of the critically ill. *AACN Clinical Issues, 2,* 195–209.

Miles, M. S., Funk, S. G., & Kasper, M. A. (1991). The neonatal intensive care unit environment: Sources of stress for parents. *AACN Clinical Issues, 2,* 346–354.

Miller, J. F. (1991). Developing and maintaining hope in families of the critically ill. *AACN Clinical Issues, 2,* 307–315.

Molter, N. C. (1979). Needs of relatives of critically ill patients: A descriptive study. *Heart and Lung, 8*(2), 332–339.

Neary, M. A. (1993). Community services in the 1990's: Are they meeting the needs of caregivers? *Journal of Community Health Nursing, 10,* 105–111.

Nugent, K. E. (1992). The clinical nurse specialist as case manager in a collaborative practice model: Bridging the gap between quality and cost of care. *Clinical Nurse Specialist, 6*(2), 106–111.

O'Brien, P., & Boisvert, J. T. (1989). Discharge planning for children with heart disease. *Critical Care Nursing Clinics of North America, 1,* 297–305.

Plummer, A. L., O'Donohue, W. J., & Petty, T. L. (1989). Conference Report: Consensus Conference on Problems in Home Mechanical Ventilation. *AM REV Respir Dis, 140,* 555–560.

Rapp, J. (1993). Discharge of a ventilator-dependent quadriplegic patient from a critical care unit to home. *Rehabilitation Nursing, 18,* 185–188.

Reeder, J. M. (1991). Family perception: A key to intervention. *AACN Clinical Issues, 2,* 188–194.

Rose, M. A. (1989). Home care nursing practice: The new frontier. *Holistic Nursing Practice, 3*(2), 1–8.

Ryan, D. (1992). Case reports: High tech home care: A look at a success story. *Military Medicine, 157*(5), 266–268.

Simpson, T. (1991). The family as a source of support for the critically ill adult. *AACN Clinical Issues, 2,* 229–235.

Smith, B. A. (1993). A TQM model for home care coordination and provider partnering. *Caring, 12*(9), 54–61.

Thomas, V. M., Ellison, K., Howell, E. V., & Winters, K. (1992). Caring for the person receiving ventilatory support at home: Caregiver's needs and involvement. *Heart and Lung, 21,* 180–186.

Titler, M. G., Cohen, M. Z., & Craft, M. J. (1991). Impact of adult critical care hospitalization: Perceptions of patients, spouses, children, and nurses. *Heart and Lung, 20,* 174–182.

Ventafridda, V., DeConno, F., Vigano, A., Ripamonti, C., Gallucci, M., & Gamba, A. (1989). Comparison of home and hospital care of advanced cancer patients. *Tumori, 75,* 619–625.

UNIT 3

MONITORING AND TECHNOLOGY

Electrocardiogram Interpretation

Linda K. Menzel and Jill M. White

The last decade has provided great insight into electrophysiologic phenomena relating to the conduction system of the heart and dysrhythmias. This information, along with new methods of evaluating cardiac cell function, has made the study of electrocardiography increasingly interesting and complex. With this heightened understanding has come additional responsibility for critical care nurses. No longer limited to accountability for interpretation of simple dysrhythmias, nursing duties now include monitoring S-T segment changes, axis deviations, and identification of complex rhythm disturbances. Choosing an appropriate lead or leads with which to monitor a patient's cardiac status must be based on the patient's underlying clinical problem. The decision must be based on a thorough understanding of which leads have the greatest sensitivity and diagnostic accuracy for detecting anticipated dysrhythmias and ischemic events. The twenty-first century will be an exciting time for critical care nurses as they work collaboratively with their medical colleagues in the recognition and diagnoses of complex electrocardiographic phenomena.

This chapter focuses on interpretation of the electrocardiogram (ECG) as it relates to axis deviation, coronary artery disease, and complex dysrhythmias. An understanding of basic electrocardiography is assumed. The chapter begins with a discussion of the conduction system and normal cardiac electrophysiology, and continues on to the interpretation of the 12-lead ECG and dysrhythmias.

ANATOMY AND PHYSIOLOGY

The conduction system of the heart is composed of the sinus node, the atrioventricular (AV) node, and the His-Purkinje system, which is in turn composed of the bundle of His, the right and left bundle branches, and the Purkinje fibers (Fig. 11–1).

The normal cardiac cycle begins with an impulse propagated in the sinus node. The impulse is conducted rapidly through the atria by internodal pathways to the AV node. On entering the AV node, the impulse is slowed to allow time for the atria to empty their contents into the ventricles before ventricular contraction begins (Guyton, 1991). The impulse continues down through the bundle of His, spreading rapidly through the bundle branches to the Purkinje fibers and ventricular myocardium (Fig. 11–2).

SINUS NODE

The sinus node (SA node), first identified by Keith and Flack in 1907, is located in the posterior aspect of the right atrium at the junction of the superior vena cava and the body of the right atrium (Hurst, 1993). The SA node is elliptically shaped, with a cross-section of 0.6 by 1.6 mm and a length that varies from 5 to 8 mm (James, 1977; Mirvis, 1993). Its blood supply arises from the right coronary artery in 55% of people and from the left circumflex coronary artery in the remaining population (Schlant et al., 1994). The SA node is the normal pacemaker of the heart, with an intrinsic rate of approximately 60 to 100 beats per minute.

INTERNODAL TRACTS

The impulse from the SA node passes to the AV node by means of three pathways: the anterior, middle, and posterior tracts. The anterior internodal pathway begins at the anterior margin of the SA node. It then curves anteriorly around the superior vena cava to enter the anterior interatrial band, called Bachmann's bundle. This bundle is the preferential pathway to the left atrium. The middle internodal tract begins at the superior and posterior margins of the SA node. From there, impulses travel behind the superior vena cava to the crest of the interatrial septum. At this location a few strands continue to the left atrium, whereas the bulk of fibers descend in the interatrial septum to the superior margin of the AV node. The posterior internodal tract begins at the posterior margin of the sinus node. It then travels posteriorly around the superior vena cava into the interatrial septum above the coronary sinus and joins the posterior portion of the AV node (Braunwald, 1992). Destruction of one or more of these pathways during surgery has been associated with a higher incidence of postoperative dysrhyth-

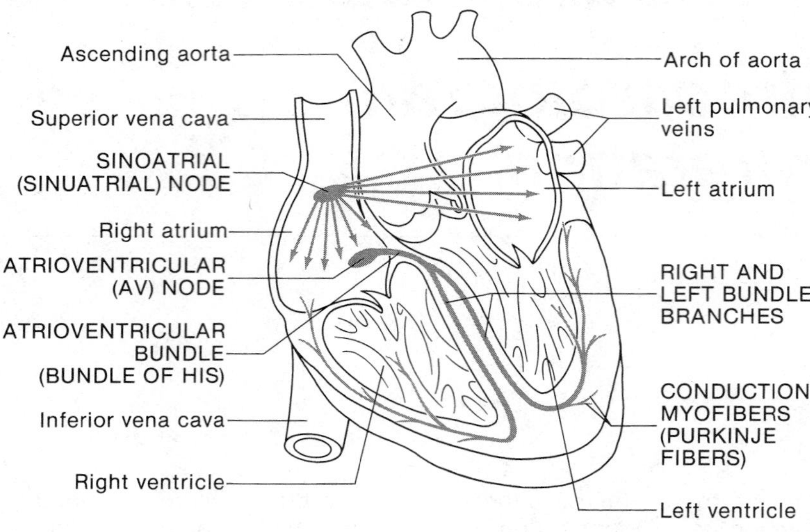

FIGURE 11–1. The sinus node and the Purkinje system of the heart, showing also the AV node, the atrial internodal pathways, and the ventricular bundle branches. (From Guyton, A. C. and Hall, J. E. [1996]. *Textbook of medical physiology* [9th ed.]. Philadelphia: W. B. Saunders.)

mias. There is evidence to suggest that these pathways could form important components of the route taken by the circus movements of atrial flutter (Waldo, 1991).

AV NODE

The AV node is located in the lower atrial septum, bordering the annulus of the mitral valve. It rests above the septal leaflet of the tricuspid valve and anterior to the ostium of the coronary sinus (Abedin & Conner, 1989). The node is about 3 mm wide and 6 mm long, and is a flat, elliptical structure (Schlant et al., 1994).

The AV node may be divided electrophysiologically into three sections according to their respective action potentials and responses to electrical and chemical stimulation: (1) the upper junctional area (atrionodal [AN] region), (2) the middle nodal area (nodal [N] region), and (3) the lower junctional area (nodal-His [NH] region) (Hoffman & Cranefield, 1960) (Fig. 11–3). The upper and lower junctional areas contain cells that depolarize rapidly and demonstrate automaticity. The middle nodal area contains cells that depolarize slowly, conduct slowly, lack automaticity, and are difficult to stimulate electrically. The artery supplying the AV node arises from the right coronary artery in about 85% to 90% of people, whereas the remainder receive their blood supply from the left circumflex coronary artery, or from both (Schlant et al., 1994).

The AV node has two separate conduction pathways, specified as alpha and beta. Each pathway has its own distinct electrophysiologic features. The alpha tract has slower conduction and a shorter refractory period; the beta pathway has faster conduction and a longer refractory period. Impulses originating from the SA node normally travel the beta pathway because of its faster conduction (Fig. 11–4).

BUNDLE OF HIS

The distal end of the AV node continues as the bundle of His and is approximately 2 cm long in the adult. The bundle penetrates the tough, central fibrous body. It lies within the thin, membranous interventricular septum and descends anteriorly into the thick, muscular interventricular septum. In this region, the bundle of His divides into the right and left bundle branches, and finally the Purkinje system. Therefore, the bundle of His is located in the center of the heart, close to the annulus of the aortic valve, the right atrium, the crest of the left ventricle, and the superior extent of the tricuspid valve. Consequently, the bundle of His is vulnerable to injury from disorders affecting any of these structures because of its nearness (Kay & Bubien, 1992).

Impulses entering the His bundle are conducted

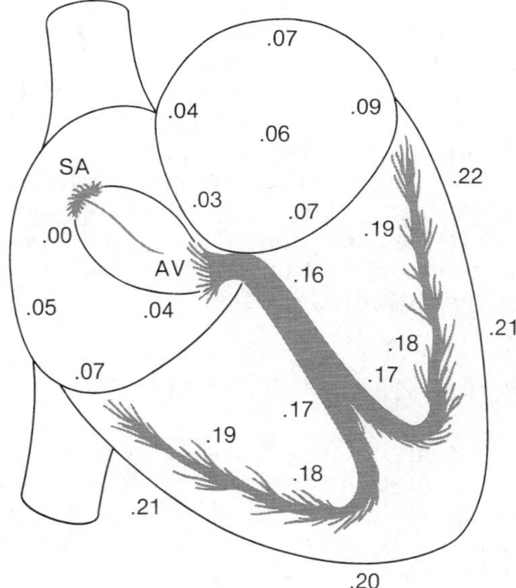

FIGURE 11–2. Transmission of the cardiac impulse through the heart, showing the time of appearance (in fractions of a second) of the impulse in different parts of the heart. (Redrawn from Guyton, A. C. and Hall, J. E. [1996]. *Textbook of medical physiology* [9th ed.]. Philadelphia: W. B. Saunders.)

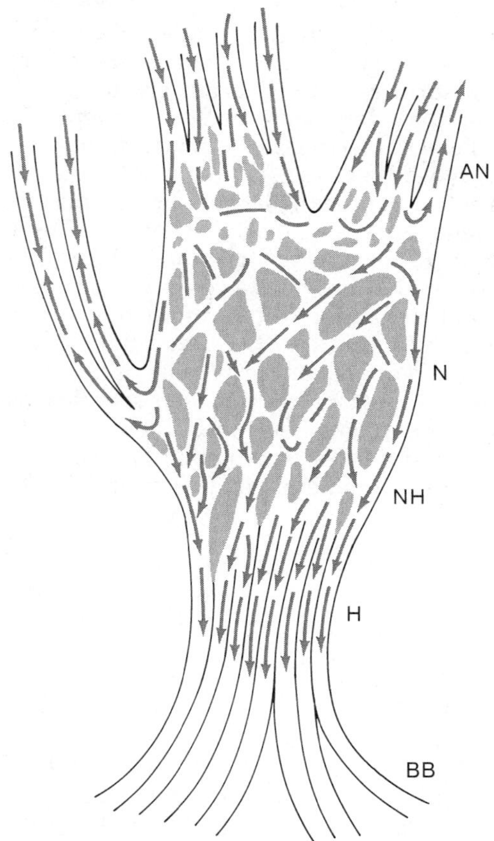

FIGURE 11–3. The AV junction. *Abbreviations:* AN = atrio-nodal; N = nodal; NH = nodal–His; H = bundle of His; BB = bundle branches. (Redrawn from Sherf, L., & James, T. N. [1972]. *American Journal of Cardiology, 29,* 529.)

rapidly—six times faster than through myocardial tissue. In healthy hearts, the bundle of His is the sole muscle connection between atria and ventricles. Pathologic problems of the central fibrous body or of the tricuspid, mitral, or aortic valves may affect the AV node or common bundle. Any dysfunction of this portion of the conducting system may have an impact on the coordinated functioning of the atria and ventricles.

THE BUNDLE BRANCHES AND PURKINJE SYSTEM

The bundle of His divides into the right and left bundle branches. The right bundle branch (RBB) is a thin stalk of fibers, only 1 to 2 mm thick, that extends down the right side of the ventricular septum until it reaches the anterior papillary muscle at the apex of the right ventricle (Kay & Bubien, 1992). There it divides into smaller branches, joining the Purkinje system and spreading out over the free right ventricular wall and adjacent septum. Along two-thirds of its length (proximal third and distal third), the RBB is close to the endocardial surface and is therefore vulnerable to slight pressure changes on the intracavitary portion of the right side of the ventricular septum. Because of its extended length, small diameter, location, and single blood supply, the RBB is more frequently involved in conduction delays or block.

The main trunk of the left bundle branch (LBB) is a short, wide band of conductive fibers. It extends approximately 1 to 2 cm before branching into the anterior (superior) and posterior (inferior) divisions. The anterior fascicle is long and thin and lies below the aortic valve in the left ventricular outflow tract. Its size and location, as well as its single blood supply, make it the next most vulnerable branch after the RBB.

The posterior division of the LBB is much thicker and shorter, and it extends along the septum toward the inferior and posterior surfaces of the left ventricle. This division has a double blood supply from the left anterior descending coronary artery and posterior branch of the right coronary artery, making it much less vulnerable to disease. Hence, a block affecting the posterior division has greater prognostic significance.

Many people have an additional fascicle of the left bundle branch that supplies the septum (Marriott, 1988). This little known fascicle was depicted by Tawara as early as 1906 and has been found to originate either from the common left bundle or from the anterior or posterior fascicle (Marriott & Conover, 1989). Histopathologic studies have noted this midseptal addition in 33 of 49 healthy hearts (Demoulin & Kulbertus, 1972).

As the RBB and LBB spread distally, the Purkinje fibers become evident. They are composed of a specialized interlocking network of cells that are recognized for their ability to rapidly conduct impulses. The Purkinje fibers are broader and shorter than conventional working myocardial cells. An important function of the Purkinje system is the nearly homogeneous depolarization and repolarization it provides for both the right and left ventricles (Kay & Bubien, 1992).

The normal process of depolarization and repolarization occur in opposite directions. Therefore, repolarization proceeds from the base of the heart to the apex, and from epicardium to endocardium. Con-

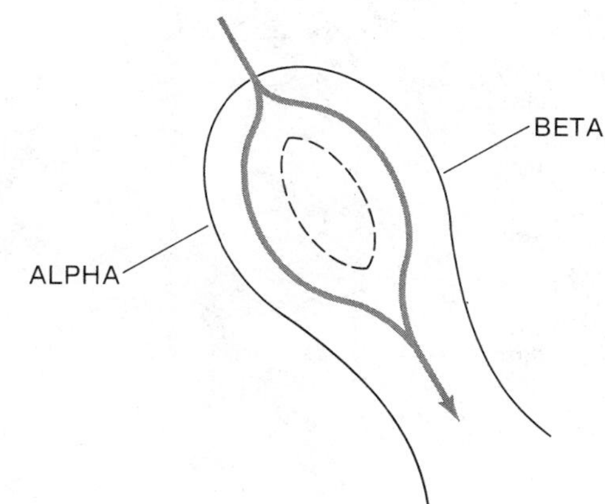

FIGURE 11–4. Normal conduction through fast (beta) and slow (alpha) pathways of the AV node.

versely, during depolarization the progression is from apex to base. This reversed sequence of ventricular depolarization and repolarization allows both ventricles to be repolarized relatively homogeneously, thereby decreasing the risk of dysrhythmias that might be induced by the situation in which some areas are refractory and others are fully recovered.

BLOOD SUPPLY TO CONDUCTING TISSUES

Blood supply to the conduction system comes from the coronary arteries, which are located behind the cusps of the aortic valve. The right coronary artery (RCA) leaves the right aortic sinus and descends in the right atrioventricular groove, curving posteriorly at the acute margin of the right ventricle. The main left coronary artery (LCA) arises from the upper portion of the left aortic sinus, passing behind the right ventricular outflow tract before bifurcating into the left anterior descending (LAD) and circumflex (LCX) branches. Figure 11–5 illustrates circulation to the anterior and posterior surfaces of the heart in greater detail.

The terms "dominant" or "preponderant" are often used when referring to the coronary arteries. These terms relate to the vessel, either the RCA or LCA (usually the left circumflex), that supplies the posterior diaphragmatic surface of the left ventricle. The RCA is dominant in 80% to 90% of human hearts (Guyton, 1991). Table 11–1 provides a comprehensive list of the patterns of circulation to the conduction system.

Frink and James (1973) studied the blood supply to the bundle of His and proximal conduction system in 10 healthy hearts. Although their sample was small, useful information about the blood supply to the conduction system was provided. These researchers found that the bundle of His was supplied by the AV

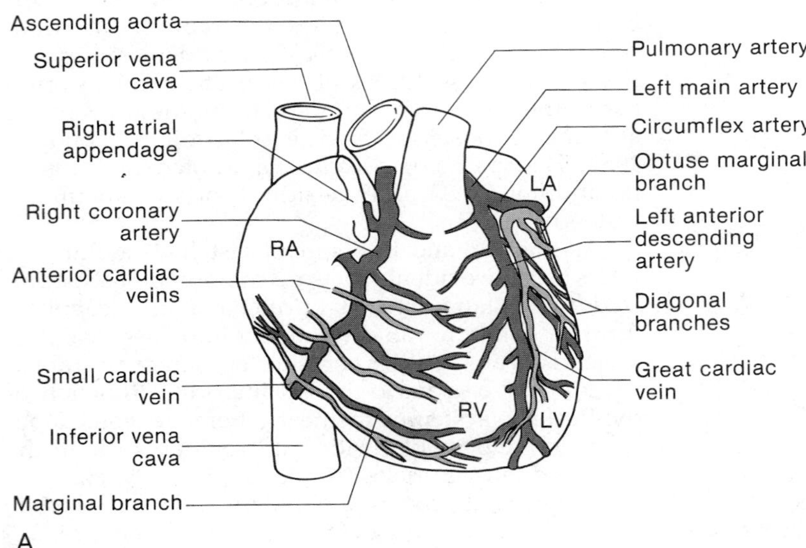

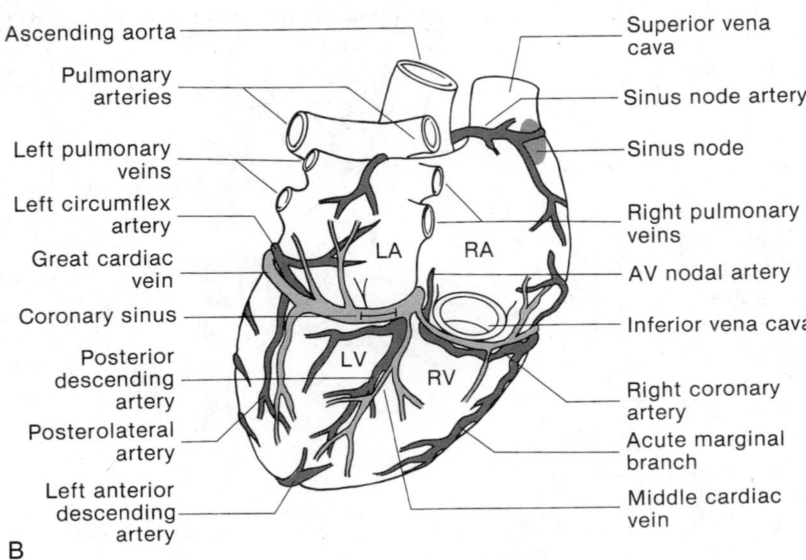

FIGURE 11–5. *A*, Principal arteries and veins on the anterior surface of the heart. Part of the right atrial appendage has been resected. The left coronary artery arises from the left coronary aortic sinus behind the pulmonary trunk. *B*, Principal arteries and veins on the inferior–posterior surfaces of the heart. This schematic drawing illustrates the heart tilted upward at a nonphysiologic angle; normally, little of the inferior cardiac surface is visible posteriorly. The right coronary artery is shown to cross the crux and to supply the atrioventricular node. The artery to the sinus node in this figure arises from the right coronary artery. *Abbreviations:* RA = right atrium; RV = right ventricle; LA = left atrium; LV = left ventricle. (Redrawn from Halpenny, J. [1989]. Functional clinical anatomy. In S. Underhill, S. Woods, E. Sivarajan, & C. Halpenny [Eds.], *Cardiac nursing* [2nd ed., p. 22]. Philadelphia: J. B. Lippincott. Previously adapted from Walmsley, R., & Watson, H. (1978). *Clinical anatomy of the heart* [p. 205]. New York: Churchill-Livingstone.)

TABLE 11–1. **Circulation to the Conduction System**

Structure	RCA	LAD	LCA
SA node	55%	—	45%
Right atrium	55%	—	45%
Left atrium	—	—	Predominantly
AV node	90%	—	10%
Bundle of His	90%	—	10%
Septum	—	Predominantly	Occasionally
RBB	Occasionally	Predominantly	—
Left anterior fascicle	Occasionally	Predominantly	—
Left posterior fascicle			
Right ventricle			
Anterior wall	Predominantly	Occasionally	—
Posterior wall	90%	—	10%
Left ventricle			
inferior	Predominantly	—	—
anterior	—	Predominantly	—
lateral	—	—	Predominantly
posterior	Predominantly	Occasionally	Predominantly
apex	Occasionally	Predominantly	Occasionally

Abbreviations: RCA = right coronary artery; LAD = left anterior descending artery; LCA = left coronary artery; RBB = right bundle branch; AV node = atrioventricular node; SA node = sinus node.

nodal artery in all ten hearts, as well as the septal branch of the LAD in nine cases. The RBB and anterior fascicle of the LBB were supplied by the septal branch of the LAD in nine cases, five of which also received some blood from the AV nodal artery. The posterior fascicle of the LBB was supplied by the septal branch of the LAD in five cases, four of which also received some blood supply from the AV nodal artery. The AV nodal artery alone supplied the RBB in one case, the anterior fascicle in one case, and the posterior fascicle in five cases. The reader is referred to Braunwald (1992) for a comprehensive discussion on the subject.

INNERVATION OF CONDUCTING TISSUES

The heart is supplied with both sympathetic and parasympathetic nerves (Fig. 11–6). Parasympathetic innervation of the heart is transmitted via the vagus nerve. The parasympathetic system has its greatest influence on the SA and AV nodes, as well as the atrial muscle. These areas represent the primary distribution of parasympathetic fibers within the heart (Guyton, 1991). Stimulation of the parasympathetic system causes acetylcholine to be released from vagal nerve endings, with a resulting decrease in heart rate and decrease in rate of conduction through the AV node. In addition, respiratory sinus dysrhythmia, also referred to as heart rate variability, increases in response to increased secretion of acetylcholine.

Sympathetic nerves originate in the spinal cord between the first thoracic and second lumbar vertebrae. Sympathetic nerves are distributed to the same areas as parasympathetic fibers. Their representation is particularly strong in the ventricular muscle, as well as other parts of the heart. With sympathetic stimulation, norepinephrine is released from nerve endings, resulting in increases in heart rate, force of contraction, and speed of conduction through the AV node.

ELECTROPHYSIOLOGY

The fundamental feature of excitable tissue is the existence of an unequal number of positive and negative charges on the inside of the cell membrane compared to the outside. Nerves and muscles are examples of this type of excitable tissue. Various cardiac cells are electrically negative inside the cell compared to outside, with a membrane potential of −60 to −90 milli-

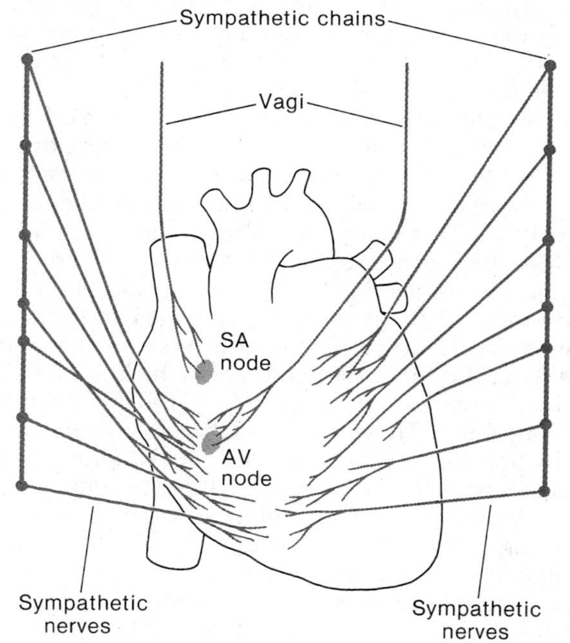

FIGURE 11–6. The cardiac nerves. (Redrawn from Guyton, A. C. [1991]. *Textbook of medical physiology* [8th ed., p. 107]. Philadelphia: W. B. Saunders.)

volts (mV) (Kay & Bubien, 1992). An excess of sodium ions on the outside of the cell is responsible for this separation of charges across the membrane. The voltage created by the separation of charges across the cell membrane is a measure of the electrical energy required to separate the positive and negative charges. This voltage is also the force that would be necessary for charged ions to flow across the membrane if ion movement were not restricted. However, charged sodium ions are unable to flow into the resting cardiac cell because of the normally high resistance to ion movement inherent to the cell membrane.

Electrical activity in the heart precedes and initiates mechanical contraction and relaxation. Electrophysiologic events are regulated by the sarcolemma, the cell membrane of the muscle fiber. The sarcolemma functions as an insulator, thereby preventing leakage of electrical charge. Gates in this membrane open in response to changes in electrical current, allowing movement of ions. These gates are composed of protein or protein–lipid complexes positioned within the phospholipid sarcolemma. Other proteins within the sarcolemma have special pumping functions. The sodium (Na^+)-potassium (K^+) ATPase pump activates adenosine triphosphate (ATP) and moves sodium out of the cell and potassium into the cell against concentration gradients (Berne & Levy, 1993). In addition to the Na^+-K^+ pump, cardiac cells also regulate the concentration of sodium and calcium inside the cell by an active pump that exchanges sodium inside the cell for calcium outside the cell.

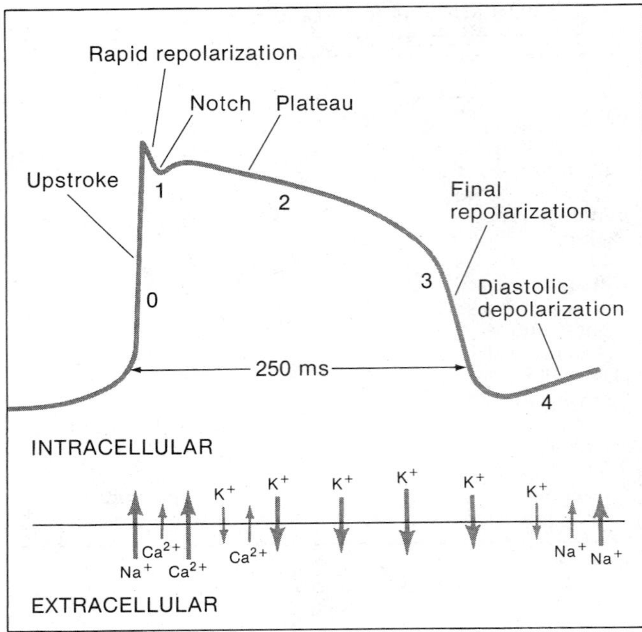

FIGURE 11–7. Schematic illustration of major ionic movements during a Purkinje cell action potential. (Redrawn from Ten Eick, R. E., et al. [1981]. Ventricular dysrhythmia: Membrane basis. *Progress in Cardiovascular Disease, 24*(2), 159; Fozzard, J. A., & Gibbons, W. R. [1973]. Action potential and contraction of heart muscle. *American Journal of Cardiology, 31,* 183; Underhill, S., Woods, S., Sivarajan Froelicher, E., & Halpenny, C. [1989]. *Cardiac nursing* [2nd ed.]. Philadelphia: J. B. Lippincott.)

An action potential is the change in electrical activity that initiates muscular contraction. Action potentials result from changes occurring in the ionic permeability of the cell membrane to such ions as Na^+, K^+, and calcium (Ca^{2+}). The concentration gradient of these ions across the semipermeable membrane of the cardiac cell provides an electrochemical basis for the development of cardiac action potentials.

The interval between action potentials is called the transmembrane resting potential and is approximately −85 to −95 mV in normal cardiac muscle, and approximately −90 to −100 mV in the Purkinje fibers (Guyton, 1991). This is accounted for by intracellular and extracellular concentration differences, whereby potassium levels are 30 times greater inside the cell and sodium is 30 times more prevalent outside the cell. This concentration difference is actively maintained by the outer limiting cell membrane, which possesses an active ion exchange pump: the ATP-dependent Na^+-K^+ ion pump. The enzyme ATPase is responsible for activating this mechanism. The Na^+-K^+ pump is partially responsible for preserving the intracellular negativity by moving three sodium ions out of the cell in exchange for two potassium ions (Katz, 1992). The sarcolemma is not a perfect insulator, and there is a passive leak of positively charged sodium ions into the cardiac cell. Therefore, the Na^+-K^+ ATPase pump is necessary to maintain the resting membrane potential.

The resting cell membrane is relatively permeable to potassium but much less so to sodium and calcium (Fig. 11–7). Many of the remaining anions, such as proteins and phosphates, are unable to diffuse out with potassium. This accumulation of intracellular anions further establishes the intracellular electronegativity, while the extracellular environment remains positive. Furthermore, by sustaining this concentration gradient, the cell remains able to act as a capacitor and store electrical energy.

The action potential of pacemaker cells consists of five phases:

- Phase 0—rapid depolarization
- Phase 1—a brief, rapid period of repolarization
- Phase 2—the plateau phase of repolarization
- Phase 3—the end of repolarization, where the membrane potential returns to resting potential
- Phase 4—resting membrane potential.

Cell membrane permeability changes when the cell receives a sufficiently strong stimulus. The stimulus may be electrical, chemical (as in hypoxia), or mechanical (as in chamber dilation) (Guyton, 1991). With the change in membrane permeability, an influx of sodium occurs through "fast channels" in the cell membrane (also known as "fast-response" action potential). The inside of the cell changes from approximately −90 mV, to a slightly positive value of about +20 mV. This reversal of the membrane polarity is called the overshoot of the cardiac action potential. This rapid depolarization comprises phase 0 and is responsible for the QRS

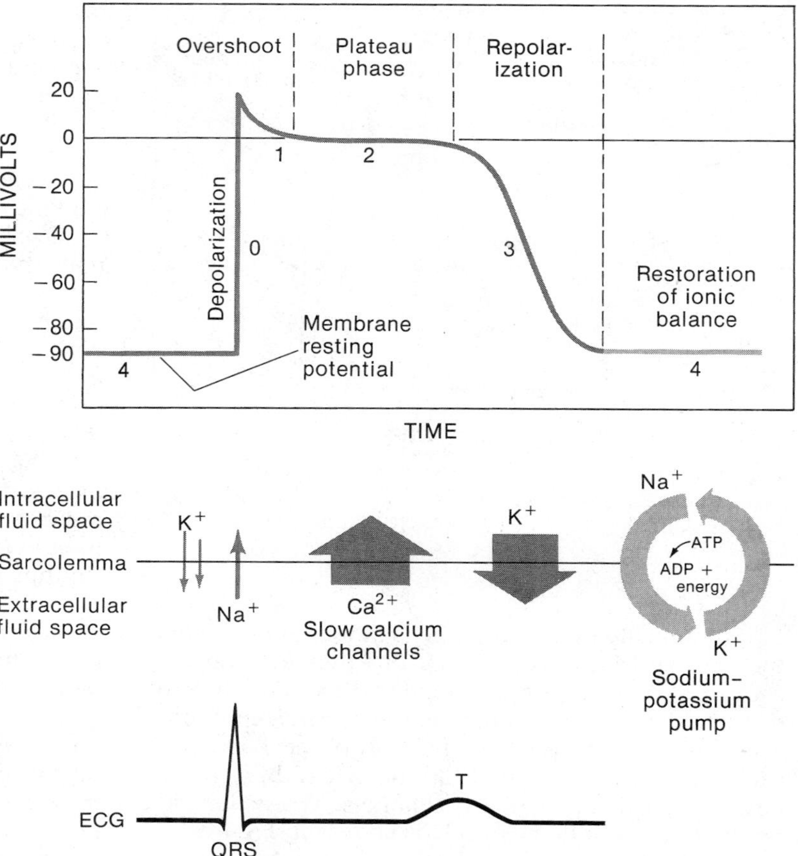

FIGURE 11–8. Transmembrane potential in the resting, depolarized, and repolarized states. (Redrawn from Lipman, B. S., Dunn, M., & Massie, E. [1984]. *Clinical electrocardiography* [7th ed., p. 35]. Chicago: Year Book Medical Publishers.)

complex on the ECG. Because the ionic balance has been disturbed, an attempt to balance the charges occurs. Potassium moves out of the cell, thereby completing the terminal phase of depolarization. Also during phase 0, the threshold potential for calcium is reached and calcium begins flowing into the cell through "calcium–sodium channels" (also called "slow channels") (Guyton, 1991), and will continue to do so until the end of phase 2. The overshoot is immediately followed by repolarization, which occurs in three rapid stages as the transmembrane potential returns to the resting state (Fig. 11–8).

Phase 1 signifies inactivation of the fast sodium channels. The fast sodium channels close and potassium begins to move out of the cell. The slight downward trend is thought to be caused by the influx of a small amount of negatively charged chloride ions and efflux of potassium ions (Braunwald, 1992). During phase 2, the plateau phase, there is primarily an influx of calcium, but sodium also diffuses into the cell through slow channels. This influx maintains a prolonged period of depolarization. Calcium ions entering the muscle during this action potential play an important role in the contractile process. The plateau phase is represented on the ECG by the ST segment. During phase 3, the slow channels close, and the influx of calcium and sodium ceases. The cell membrane becomes more permeable to potassium, which then diffuses out of the cell, reestablishing the cell's electronegative state. Phase 3 correlates with the T wave on the ECG. By the end of phase 3, distribution of sodium and potassium ions is reversed from the normal resting state. Therefore during phase 4, the Na^+-K^+ pump is activated; sodium is actively moved out of the cell, and potassium is transported back into the cell.

Automaticity

Automaticity is the repetitive, spontaneous production of action potentials (Kay & Bubien, 1992). Stimuli are not required for automatic cells to generate action potentials, although the speed of the process may be altered by such factors as catecholamines, hormones, and medications.

The action potential of the pacemaker cell differs from that of the myofibril, the muscle cell. In the myofibril, the potential remains in phase 4 until the membrane is reactivated by another stimulus. In contrast, automaticity is present in pacemaker cells. They are unstable and show an upward drifting of phase 4 that results in spontaneous depolarization when the level of electrical activity falls to a certain critical point. The pacemaker cells located in the SA node, distal part of the AV node, and His–Purkinje network are capable of spontaneous depolarization and are responsible for

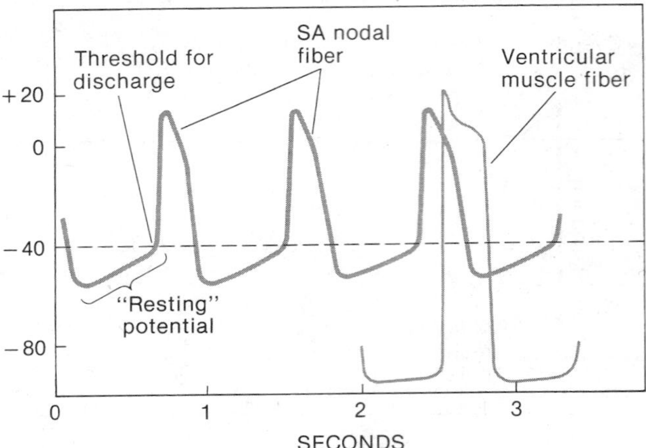

FIGURE 11–9. Action potential of SA nodal fiber and ventricular muscle fiber. (Redrawn from Guyton, A. C. [1991]. *Textbook of medical physiology* [8th ed., p. 112]. Philadelphia: W. B. Saunders.)

the rhythmicity of the heart. Cells in the SA node have the fastest intrinsic rate (60–100) and therefore the fastest rate of rise in phase 4, followed by cells directly distal to the AV node in the bundle of His. Ventricular cells have the slowest rate of rise in phase 4 and produce a slower rate (< 40). Both the SA and AV nodes have slow calcium–sodium channels. The action potential of cells in the SA node is shown in Figure 11–9. The maximum resting potential of −55 to −60 mV for the SA node is substantially less than the −85 to −90 mV characteristic of the ventricular fiber (Guyton, 1991). As the potential reaches approximately −40 mV, sodium ions rapidly enter the cell through specialized membrane protein channels, resulting in the upstroke of the action potential, or rapid and full depolarization (phase 0). Thus, the sinus cell displays automaticity, which is thought to be the result of the inherent leakiness of the SA nodal fibers to sodium ions. Phase 0 is slower, and the phase 2 plateau is absent as phase 2 merges gradually into phase 3. Phase 4 is again established, completing the process of repolarization.

The automatic firing of all pacemaker cells is controlled primarily by the autonomic nervous system. With sympathetic stimulation, the fiber membrane becomes more permeable to sodium and calcium, which increases the slope of phase 4, which in turn results in an increase in heart rate. Parasympathetic stimulation decreases the "resting" membrane potential of the SA nodal fibers to a level more negative than the normal value. This level may be as low as −65 to −75 mV, compared to the normal level of −55 to −60 mV (Guyton, 1991). Thus, the upward drift of the resting membrane potential caused by sodium leakage requires more time to reach the threshold potential for excitation.

Cellular environmental changes with regard to K^+, Ca^{2+}, Cl^-, PO_2, and pH have been shown to exert a secondary effect on the rate of automatic fibers. For example, an elevated serum potassium level requires higher levels of acetylcholine (vagal stimulation) to produce slowing or arrest of the SA node. It has been shown that the presence of acetylcholine increases the permeability of potassium in the SA node. Therefore, it is believed that the increased permeability of potassium in the presence of acetylcholine in the nodal fibers is at least in some part responsible for the vagal slowing (Rardon & Pressler, 1991).

Overdrive suppression is a concept related to automaticity. The SA node with its faster intrinsic rate normally suppresses the automaticity of other potential pacemaker cells, such as those in the AV node and Purkinje system. The automaticity of the pacemaker cells in these areas becomes depressed after a period of exposure to excitation at the higher frequency. Therefore, if the SA node should fail, a new pacemaker in the Purkinje system may take over. However, as a result of overdrive suppression, the Purkinje network may not begin to transmit impulses for 5 to 30 seconds (Guyton, 1991). This delayed resurgence of cardiac rhythm is known as Stokes-Adams syndrome. Likewise, if an ectopic atrial focus takes over the rhythm for a certain time period and then suddenly terminates, the SA node might remain quiescent for a short period of time because of overdrive suppression.

The mechanism for overdrive suppression is uncertain. A reasonable hypothesis is based on the performance of the membrane pump, which actively extrudes sodium from the cell in partial exchange for potassium (Berne & Levy, 1993). Sodium enters the cell during depolarization. The influx of sodium is directly related to heart rate. Therefore, the amount of sodium entering the cell increases as heart rates become faster. Under conditions of overdrive, the sodium pump becomes more active while extruding this larger quantity of sodium from the cell interior. The quantity of sodium expelled by the pump exceeds the quantity of potassium entering the cell. This enhanced activity of the pump results in hyperpolarization of the cell because there is a net loss of positive ions from inside the cell. Because of the hyperpolarization of the cell, the pacemaker potential requires more time to reach threshold. It has been proposed that when overdrive suppression suddenly ceases, the sodium pump continues to operate at an accelerated rate for some time. This extended operation results in an excessive extrusion of sodium, which opposes the gradual depolarization of the pacemaker cell during phase 4 and temporarily suppresses the intrinsic automaticity.

Refractory Periods

Cardiac muscle, like all excitable tissue, is refractory to restimulation during the action potential. Specifically, the heart is refractory from phase 0 until nearly the end of phase 3 of the action potential. The total refractory period is divided into two smaller periods: absolute and relative. From the beginning of depolarization at phase 0, and continuing to approximately the midpoint of phase 3, the heart is in a state of abso-

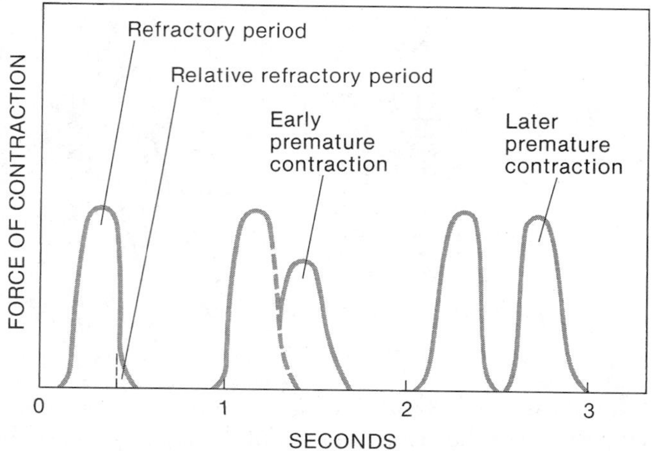

FIGURE 11–10. Contraction of the heart with durations of the refractory period and the relative refractory period, the effect of an early premature contraction, and the effect of a later premature contraction. (Redrawn from Guyton, A. C. [1991]. *Textbook of medical physiology* [8th ed., p. 100]. Philadelphia: W. B. Saunders.)

lute refractoriness. With the onset of depolarization, the cell cannot respond to another stimulus, regardless of its magnitude, until it is repolarized to a value of approximately −50 mV. The absolute refractory period correlates with the beginning of the QRS complex, includes most of the ST segment, and terminates in the early portion of the T wave on the ECG. The relative refractory period extends from the midpoint of phase 3 until the beginning of phase 4. During this time, the cell returns to a transmembrane potential of approximately −60 mV to −85 mV. Phase 3 correlates with the T wave on the ECG. During this period, a relatively strong stimulus may evoke a response, but impulse conduction will be slower than in fully repolarized fibers. If an ectopic focus fires during this vulnerable period (R-on-T phenomenon), lethal dysrhythmias may occur. Figure 11–10 illustrates the durations of the refractory period and the relative refractory period, the effect of an early premature contraction, and the effect of a later premature contraction.

The supernormal period comprises the terminal portion of phase 3, the period immediately preceding the point at which the cell returns to its resting potential (Fig. 11–11). During this period, the cell is capable of responding to a weaker stimulus than normal. Although the membrane potential is closer to threshold than if the cell had achieved repolarization, the cell has recovered sufficiently, and an adequate number of fast sodium channels is available to respond to the incoming stimulus. This period corresponds to the terminal portion of the T and U waves.

INTERPRETATION OF THE ECG

The ECG is a simple, inexpensive, and noninvasive graphic recording of the electrical activity of the heart that is invaluable in the diagnosis of many cardiovascular diseases. It only records activity of the myocardial cells, the muscle cells of the heart. Pacemaker cells (such as those in the SA node) and conducting cells (such as those in Bachmann's bundle in the atrium) conduct impulses too rapidly to be picked up by the ECG.

The ECG records the direction and magnitude of the electrical current produced by the heart. During depolarization and repolarization, current flows in many directions at once. The ECG records the resultant forces at each moment in time by averaging these individual forces into a single vector. If all of the instantaneous resultant vectors occurring during one cycle were added together, their sum would represent the average magnitude and direction of ventricular depolarization. The mean QRS axis that is determined on the standard ECG is the average direction of this sum.

A current develops when electrical activity is transmitted from one cell to the next along a myofibril. This electrical current is transmitted to the body surface and can be recorded and measured by surface ECG. The ECG is made up of 12 leads, each viewing the heart from a different perspective. Each lead is made up of two electrodes, one designated as positive and the other negative (as is the case with the bipolar leads: I, II, and III) or with one designated as positive and the other designated as a reference point (as is the case with the unipolar leads, aVR, aVL, and aVF). This is done automatically by the ECG machine. When the generated electrical current proceeds along or parallel to the lead line, the lead records the current. If an imaginary line were drawn from negative to positive lead, or reference point to positive lead, this line would represent the axis of the lead. To interpret the ECG correctly, it is necessary to know which electrode is positive and which is negative.

Leads are joined by wires that pass through the galvanometer of the electrocardiograph. These electrodes are placed at specific locations on the body, and the leads named according to these body sites. Currents

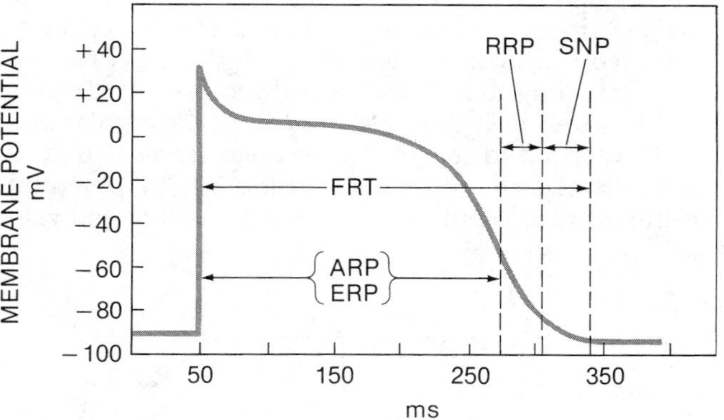

FIGURE 11–11. The various refractory periods during an action potential. *Abbreviations:* ARP = absolute refractory period; ERP = effective refractory period; RRP = relative refractory period; SNP = supernormal refractory period; FRT = full recovery time. (Redrawn from Hoffman, B. F., & Cranefield, P. F. [1960]. *Electrophysiology of the heart.* New York: McGraw-Hill.)

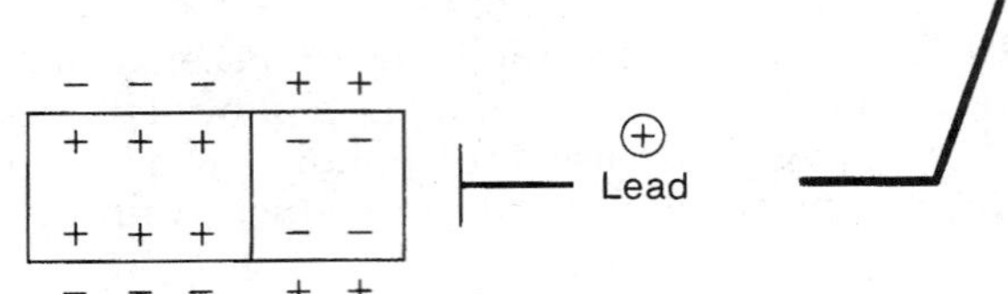

FIGURE 11–12. Depolarization wave toward a positive lead.

generated by the heart cause certain deflections on the ECG according to how they relate to the axis of the lead. A depolarization wave moving toward a positive electrode creates an upright, positive deflection on the ECG (Fig. 11–12). A downward, negative complex on ECG indicates an impulse traveling away from a positive electrode (Fig. 11–13). A depolarization wave that moves toward and then passes the positive lead creates a complex that is biphasic, or half positive and half negative (Fig. 11–14). Absence of current, or a current traveling perpendicular to the lead, results in an isoelectric baseline.

Limb Leads

The limb leads, consisting of three standard (I, II, and III) and three augmented leads (aVR, aVL, and aVF), view the heart in a vertical, or frontal plane. To make up the limb leads, electrodes are placed on the arms and the legs and attached to cables connected to the ECG machine. The electrode at the right leg is consistently the ground, or neutralizing electrode, whereas the left leg leads are consistently positive.

In lead I, the negative electrode is positioned on the right arm and the positive electrode is placed on the left arm. This view records electrical current moving toward the left side of the body as a positive deflection. In lead II, the negative electrode is attached to the right arm and the positive electrode is placed on the left leg. Therefore, current moving downward and toward the left will be recorded as positive deflections. In lead III, the negative electrode is on the left arm and the positive electrode is on the left leg (Fig. 11–15). This lead will record a positive deflection on the ECG for currents traveling in a downward direction.

The same electrodes used to record the bipolar limb leads are used to record the unipolar leads aVR, aVL, and aVF. In each unipolar lead, the electrical potentials of the heart are compared between a designated positive electrode and the zero electrical reference point at the center of the electrical field of the heart. It is possible to achieve this zero potential by summing the electrical potentials of the three bipolar limb leads. Consequently, the axis of each unipolar lead results in a line from the positive electrode to the center of the heart. The electrical forces recorded in the unipolar limb leads are small. By eliminating the negative electrode, it is possible to augment the voltage of these leads. This procedure results in a 50% augmentation of the amplitude of the recording (Conover, 1992). These leads are labeled with an "a," indicating they are augmented, a "V," designating voltage, and the letters "R," "L," or "F," specifying where the positive electrode has been placed—the right arm, left arm, or left leg. Therefore, "aVL" signifies augmented voltage at the left arm (Fig. 11–16).

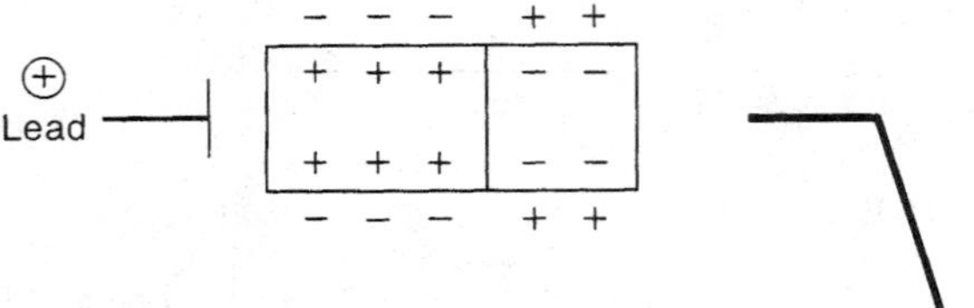

FIGURE 11–13. Depolarization wave moving away from a positive lead.

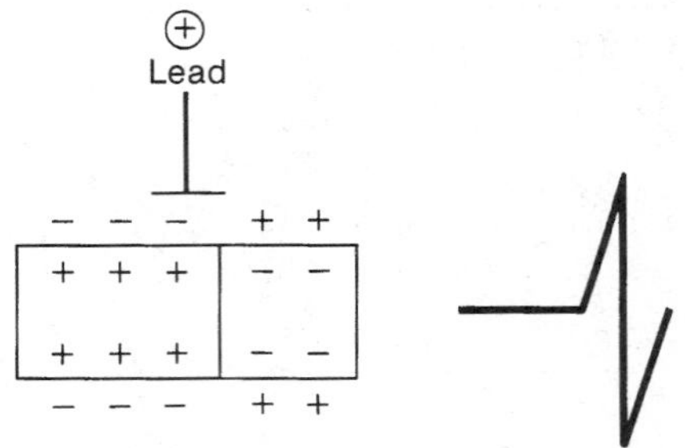

FIGURE 11–14. Biphasic complex.

Willem Einthoven first introduced the three bipolar limb leads in 1902. Einthoven's law states that the complex in lead II is equal to the sum of the complexes in leads I and III. The three leads may be transposed into an equilateral triangle, called the Einthoven triangle (Fig. 11–17*A*). Visualizing the heart in the center of the triangle is helpful in determining its relationship to the directions of current and in visualizing the QRS complex in each lead. The sum of its forces is directed down and toward the left because of the greater mass and electrical force of the left ventricle. The arrows (see Fig. 11–17*B*) show the magnitude and direction of the many vectors, whereas the cone points toward the summation or average orientation of these forces. This summation of forces in the ventricles is called the QRS axis. Although the QRS axis is of primary importance, the axis of the P and T waves can also be calculated.

With the heart in the middle of each of these leads, it is apparent why the QRS appears as it does in each lead in the normal heart (Fig. 11–18). In lead I, the ventricular forces are moving toward the positive electrode, so the QRS complex has a mostly positive deflection. It is important to remember that ventricular depolarization begins with septal depolarization, which occurs from left to right, causing an initial movement toward the negative electrode and resulting in a small Q wave in several leads. This septal Q is seen in leads aVL, I, V_5, V_6, and sometimes in lead III. General characteristics of this nonpathologic Q wave are that the wave must be less than 0.04 second

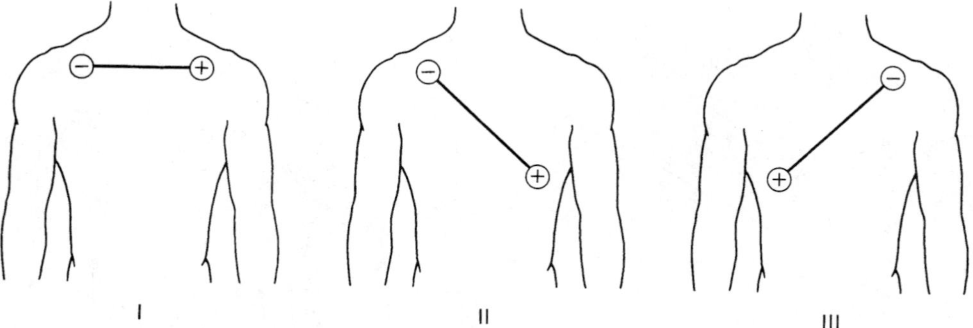

FIGURE 11–15. Three standard limb leads.

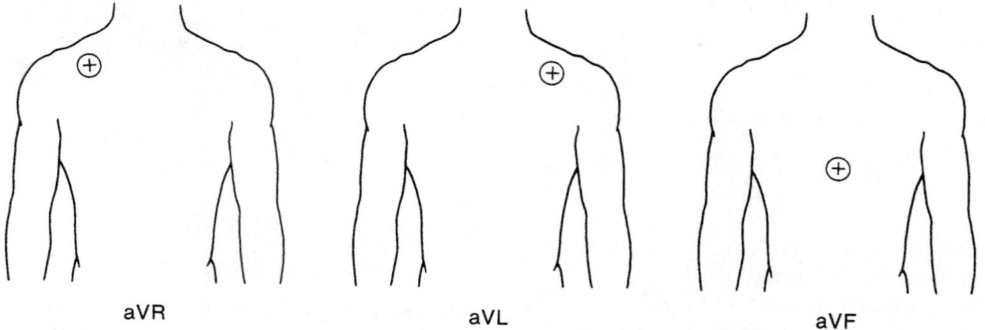

FIGURE 11–16. Three augmented leads.

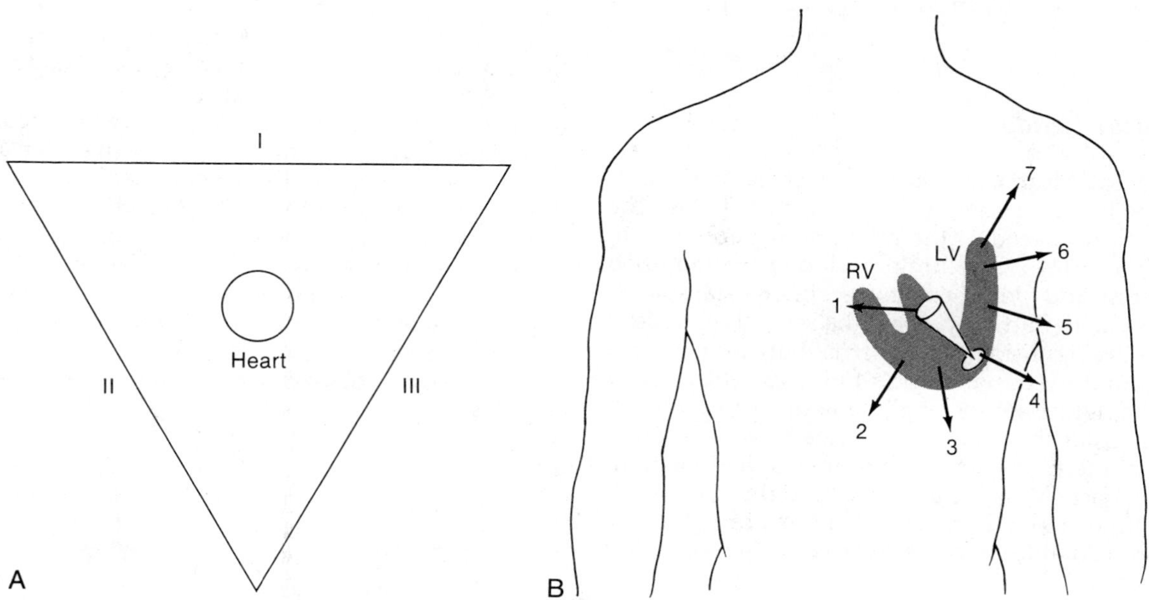

FIGURE 11–17. *A,* Einthoven triangle. *B,* QRS axis.

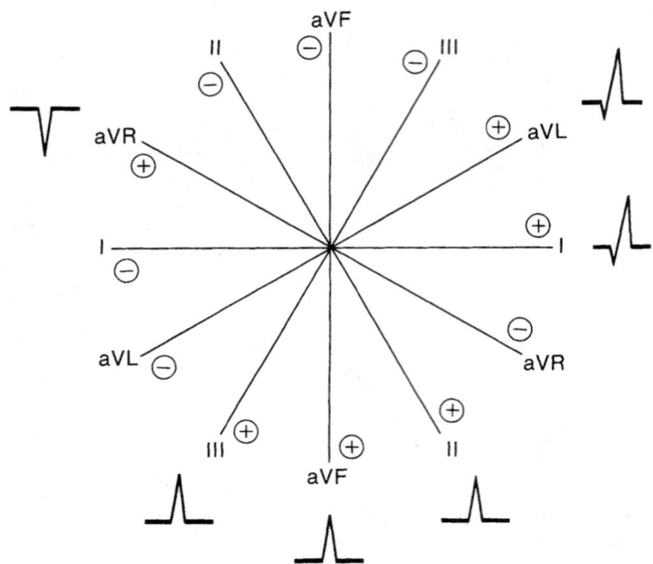

FIGURE 11–18. QRS in each lead.

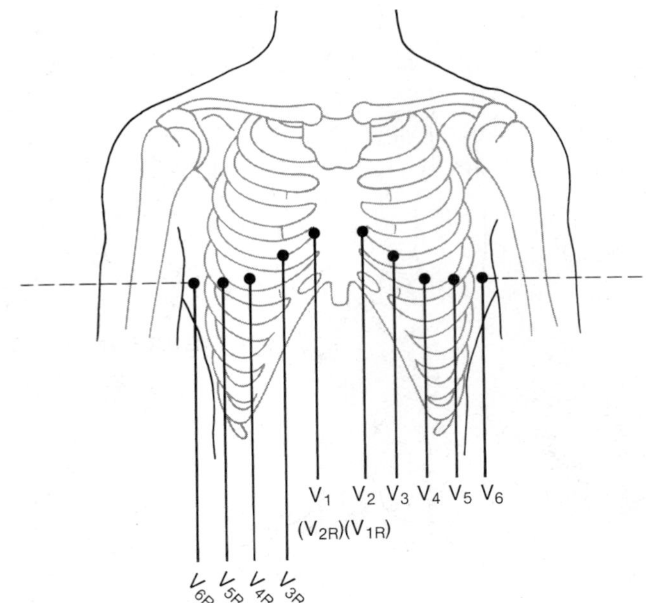

FIGURE 11–19. Precordial leads.

in duration, with a depth of less than 25% of the height of the preceding R wave (Wagner, 1994).

In lead II, the electrical forces travel more directly toward the positive electrode than in all other leads. Because the normal atrial forces also travel toward the positive electrode, the P wave is also upright. In contrast, in aVR, when atrial forces flow directly away from the positive electrode, the P wave is negative, or inverted. Negative P waves in lead II should raise the suspicion that electrodes have been applied incorrectly.

Precordial Leads

The precordial leads, also known as chest or V leads, record the heart's activity in the horizontal plane. The electrodes are placed in the intercostal spaces identified in Figure 11–19. Accurate positions are identified by palpating and identifying correct intercostal spaces. For example, to find V_1, palpate the second intercostal space on the right side of the sternal border. This area can be found by moving one's fingers slightly down and to the right from the angle of Louis. After the second intercostal space has been located, palpate down two more intercostal spaces; this area is the fourth intercostal space. V_1 is located on the right side of the sternum (the sternal border). From this point, the rest of the precordial leads can be placed in the following locations:

V_1, fourth intercostal space (4ICS) at the right sternal border (RSB)
V_2, 4ICS at the left sternal border (LSB)
V_3, midway between V_2 and V_4
V_4, 5ICS at the midclavicular line (MCL)
V_5, 5ICS at anterior axillary line
V_6, 5ICS at midaxillary line.

Occasionally, it may be necessary or advisable to use additional precordial leads, as in patients with congenital heart disease or right ventricular infarction. Leads on the right side of the chest are placed by palpating the right chest wall for the landmarks described earlier. These areas should be marked on the patient's chest on admission to the critical care unit to ensure consistent placement and subsequent accurate interpretation of the ECG. Too often, application of leads is a haphazard procedure, making day-to-day comparison of a patient's ECG a difficult task.

Each of the precordial leads views ventricular depolarization from a different perspective (Fig. 11–20). Lead V_1 lies over the right ventricle. This view provides visualization of the wave of septal depolarization initially coming toward it, before turning and traveling in the opposite direction. Thus, lead V_1 has a small R wave and a deep S wave, and it should have a primarily negative complex. This configuration may be denoted by "rS."

The scenario observed in V_6 is opposite to that pres-

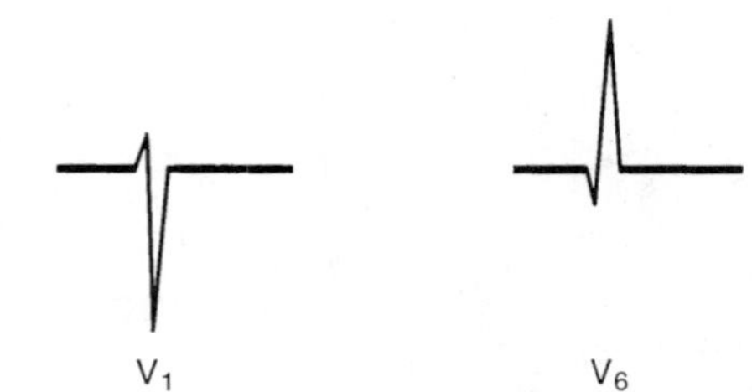

FIGURE 11–20. Ventricular depolarization in the precordial leads.

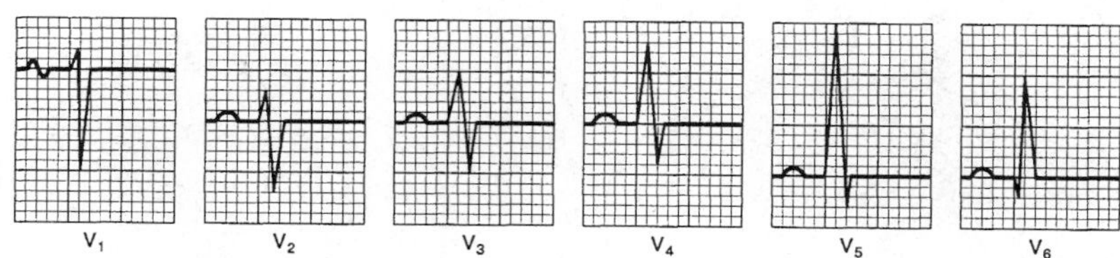

FIGURE 11–21. R-wave progression.

ent in V_1. With V_6, the ventricular depolarization wave (septal depolarization) initially moves away from the positive lead, and then the majority of forces come directly toward the lead as the lateral ventricular wall depolarizes. This progression of electrical impulses creates a QRS with a small Q (a "septal" Q) and a tall R wave. This may be denoted as "qR."

Through applying the preceding information, it is apparent how and why the QRS evolves from V_1 through V_6. This change in QRS complex across the precordium is called "R-wave progression" and is an indication of a healthy myocardium (Fig. 11–21). With normal R-wave progression, the magnitude of the R waves in the precordial leads increases from V_1 to V_3, until a nearly equiphasic RS complex is observed. Leads V_3 and V_4 are usually called the "transition zone." This zone is where one would expect to find the equiphasic RS complex, as is present in V_3 in Figure 11–21. A transition complex (RS) in lead V_1 or V_2 indicates early transition, whereas an equiphasic complex in V_5 or V_6 indicates late transition (Abedin & Connor, 1989).

Monitoring Leads

The goals of continuous bedside cardiac monitoring have shifted from simple heart rate monitoring to identification of ST segment changes, as well as sophisticated dysrhythmia detection, diagnosis, and treatment. A limited number of leads are available for ongoing bedside monitoring of patients in critical care units. Therefore, some patients may require the use of multiple monitors or a single monitor that allows simultaneous examination of multiple leads. Diagnostic criteria for many dysrhythmias may be identified from any monitoring lead. However, some of the most important criteria are "lead specific." Therefore, it is extremely important that the correct monitoring lead or leads are chosen, to maximize the potential for accurately detecting anticipated dysrhythmias and ischemic events on the basis of the patient's underlying clinical problem.

In the past, lead II has frequently been the lead of choice because of the easy visibility of P waves. However, there is good evidence that V_1 and V_6 provide more information. Modified versions of these leads are commonly used for monitoring purposes and are known as MCL_1 and MCL_6, respectively. Lead placement for MCL_1 requires the positive electrode to be placed in the V_1 position, and the negative electrode on the left arm (or left shoulder area). The ground lead may be located anywhere, but is usually placed at the right shoulder. To obtain an MCL_6 lead, the positive electrode is positioned at the V_6 position, with the negative lead at the left shoulder and the ground at the right shoulder. MCL_1 and MCL_6 are useful in detecting bundle branch blocks, differentiating right and left ventricular premature beats, and distinguishing ventricular beats from aberrantly conducted beats (Fig. 11–22). See Table 11–2 for a summary of clinical phenomena and recommended ECG monitoring leads.

Leads V_1 and V_6 are unipolar leads that require placement of five electrodes on the patient's body. One lead is placed on each limb, and the fifth is positioned on the appropriate precordial site. The limb leads may be applied to the shoulder and abdominal areas in place of the actual limbs.

There are three fundamental priorities to consider when continuous bedside cardiac monitoring is implemented. These priorities include differentiation of wide QRS complex tachycardias, diagnosis of acute bundle branch block during acute myocardial infarction, and ST segment monitoring of patients at risk for ischemic events. V_1 is the monitoring lead of choice when only one monitoring lead is possible and the

TABLE 11–2. **Recommended ECG Monitoring Leads for Specific Clinical Phenomena**

Clinical Phenomena	Recommended Monitoring Leads
Atrial flutter	II, III, aVF
Axis deviation	I, aVF
New-onset bundle branch blocks	V_1, V_6, MCL_1, MCL_6
New-onset hemiblocks	I, II, aVF, aVL
Ischemia after angioplasty	III, aVF
Digitalis toxicity	II, V_1
Dysrhythmias	V_1
Broad QRS tachycardia	V_1, V_2, V_6
Paroxysmal supraventricular tachycardia	I, II, III, V_1, V_6
Unstable angina	V_2, V_3 (without pain); 12-lead ECG (with pain)
Inferior wall MI	II, III, aVF
Anterior wall MI	Lead with maximum ST deviation on 12-lead ECG
Complications of acute MI	I, II, V_1, V_{4R}

Abbreviations: ECG = electrocardiogram; MI = myocardial infarction.

Data from Conover, M. (1992). *Understanding electrocardiography.* St. Louis: Mosby–Year Book; Drew, B. J. (1991). Bedside electrocardiographic monitoring: State of the art for the 1990s. *Heart and Lung, 20,* 610–623; and Drew, B. J. (1993). Bedside electrocardiogram monitoring. *AACN Clinical Issues in Critical Care Nursing, 4,* 25–33.

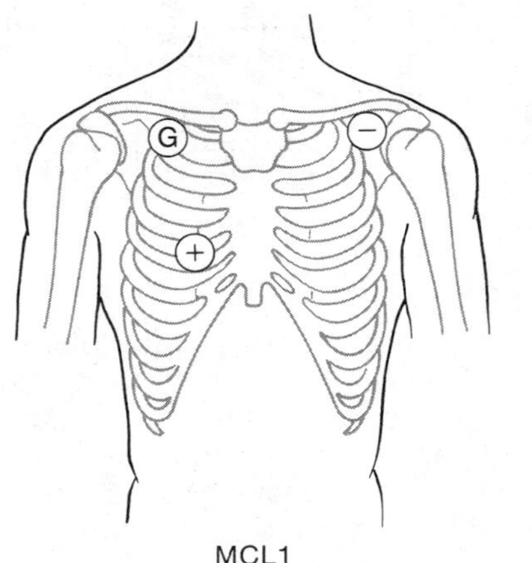

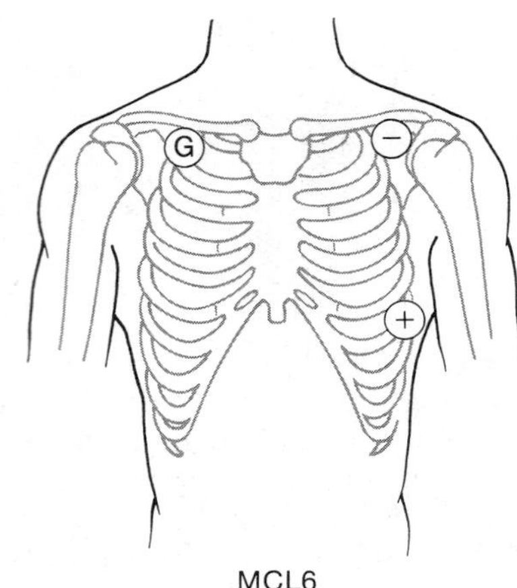

FIGURE 11–22. Monitoring leads of MCL_1 and MCL_6.

monitor has the proper capabilities (Drew, 1993; Drew & Scheinman, 1991; Wagner, 1994). The use of lead V_6 would be a good alternative when a patient cannot have an electrode placed at the sternal border. However, MCL_1 is an acceptable bipolar alternative when only three lead wires are available for the monitoring lead. The next choice for a single bipolar lead would be MCL_6 (Drew, 1991). When dual-lead monitoring is possible, V_1 is the recommended first lead, with the second lead to be determined by the patient's clinical problem. An alternative to this option is an MCL_1–MCL_6 lead combination. This alternative may be an optimal choice for patients for whom there is uncertainty regarding the supraventricular versus ventricular origin of frequent, wide complex ectopic beats and tachycardias (Drew, 1991).

Axis Determination

If the three unipolar and bipolar limb leads were plotted out, it would become apparent that each bipolar lead axis is perpendicular to one of the bipolar leads (see Fig. 11–18). The ECG records the mean vector, which is the sum of electrical potentials, as well as mean magnitude, direction, and polarity. A vector can be drawn for the P wave, QRS complex, and T wave. Each vector is constantly changing and precise calculation is complicated, requiring the use of frequent plotting with a vectorcardiogram. The normal electrical axis of the heart is between −30° and +120°. Some might consider an electrical axis greater than +90° to represent right axis deviation, or less than 0° to be indicative of left axis deviation. Technically speaking, these represent some degree of axis deviation, but they are not considered abnormal.

For most patients, the ECG is sufficient for determining the general orientation of the electrical axis of the heart. This vector normally points leftward and inferiorly, somewhere between the left shoulder and right hip. The ability to determine the axis of QRS complexes is an important tool for the critical care nurse, because it is useful in differentiating between ventricular ectopy and ventricular aberrancy, and in diagnosing hemiblocks.

The QRS axis changes normally with age and may vary with chest size (Hurst, 1993). During infancy and childhood, the axis is more rightward or inferior, and it becomes more leftward or horizontal throughout the lifespan. Individuals with a long, thin chest tend to have a QRS that is more vertical or rightward, whereas those with a thick, wide chest have a leftward, more horizontal axis. The QRS axis may be altered abnormally by pathology, as shown in Table 11–3.

The hexaxial reference system is used for discussing and determining axis. It is enclosed within a circle, with the positive and negative ends of each of the frontal leads labeled, and the degrees of a 360° circle identified (Fig. 11–23). The end of each lead corresponds to a particular degree on the hexaxial reference system.

A quadrant method has been used in an effort to simplify the procedure. Using this method, normal axis includes the region between 0° and +90°. Left axis deviation encompasses the area between 0° and −90°, whereas right axis deviation involves the section between +90° and +180°. The area between −90° and

TABLE 11–3. **Causes of Axis Deviation**

Left	Right
Normal variation	Normal variation
Extensive inferior MI	Lateral MI
Left anterior hemiblock	Left posterior hemiblock
WPW syndrome	Right bundle branch block
Hyperkalemia	Emphysema
Emphysema	Right ventricular hypertrophy
Mechanical shifts—ascites, pregnancy, tumors	WPW syndrome
	Ventricular ectopic rhythms
Left bundle branch block	Left ventricular pacing
Left ventricular hypertrophy	
Older age	
Ventricular ectopic rhythms	

Abbreviations: MI = myocardial infarction; WPW = Wolff-Parkinson-White.

±180° is called indeterminate, extreme right, or extreme left axis deviation, and it must be resolved by methods to be discussed.

The QRS vector is determined from the ECG by projecting the magnitude, direction, and polarity of the QRS deflection in the ECG lead onto its axis lead in the hexaxial reference system. If most of the QRS deflection in a particular lead is positive (above the baseline), the vector points toward the positive end of that axis lead in the hexaxial reference system. If most of the deflection is negative, the vector points toward the negative end of that axis lead. If the QRS is biphasic (equally positive and negative), the vector will be perpendicular to that axis lead in the reference system.

Several principles are useful in axis determination. First, the largest deflection in an ECG lead projects a vector that is parallel to its corresponding axis lead. Conversely, the smallest or most biphasic QRS deflection in a lead projects a vector that is perpendicular to its corresponding axis lead.

There are several ways to determine axis. One of the simplest involves examination of leads I and aVF. If the QRS complex is positive in leads I and aVF, the QRS axis must be normal, because the positive poles of these axis leads outline the quadrant corresponding to normal QRS axis. The positive end of lead I is at 0° in the hexaxial reference system. A complex is positive in lead I if the wave of depolarization is coming toward the positive pole of lead I. A positive deflection in lead I indicates that the vector is between −90° and +90°. The positive pole of aVF is at +90°. The complex will be positive in lead aVF if the wave of depolarization is coming toward it, indicating that the mean vector for the lead is between 0° and 180°. Therefore, if the QRS complex is positive in both leads I and aVF, the mean QRS vector is in the normal quadrant, somewhere between 0° and +90°. Figure 11–24 illustrates the way in which the QRS deflections might appear in leads I and aVF with normal axis and axis deviations.

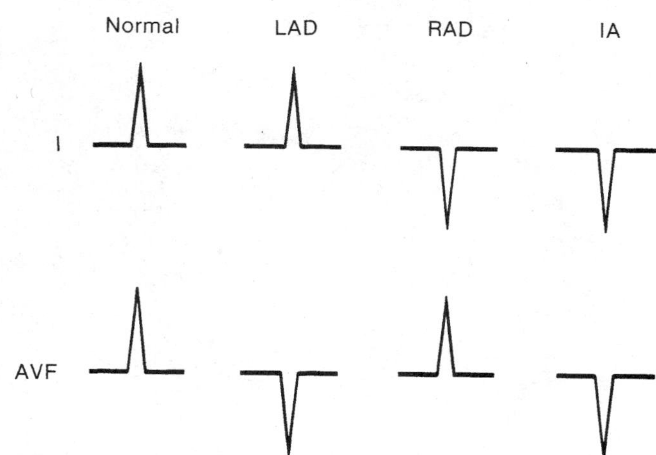

FIGURE 11–24. Normal axis and axis deviation in leads I and aVF. *Abbreviations:* LAD = left axis deviation; RAD = right axis deviation; IA = indeterminate axis.

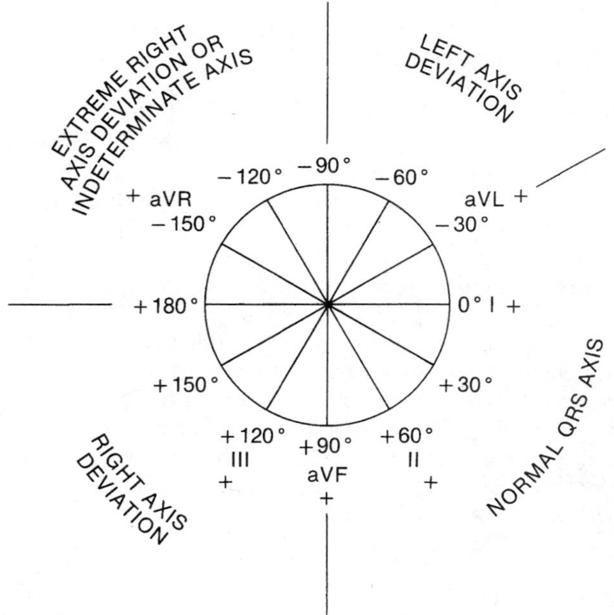

FIGURE 11–23. Hexaxial reference system.

Rotation

The preceding discussion of axis relates exclusively to the QRS vector in the frontal plane. When the vector is determined in the horizontal plane, it is called rotation. Cardiac rotation is conventionally expressed as if one were looking up at the heart from the pelvis. It is determined by looking at the precordial leads and noting the location of the transitional zone (where the R and S waves are approximately equal in size). As discussed earlier, this transition generally occurs in the vicinity of V_3 and V_4. Normally, the interventricular septum is positioned under the center of the sternum, such that lead V_1 is to the right of the septum and is located over the right ventricle. Lead V_2 is located over the interventricular septum and may reflect either the right ventricle or the left ventricle. If the transition occurs early, in V_1 or V_2, the rotation is said to be counterclockwise. If it occurs later, in V_5 or V_6, the rotation is considered clockwise (Fig. 11–25). The top figure in Figure 11–25 shows an observer lying on the ground, viewing someone's heart. The six V leads show normal R-wave progression. In the bottom figure, the V leads show a delayed transition occurring in the area of V_5 and V_6. Clockwise rotation describes a delayed transition zone, and counterclockwise rotation an early transition.

Left Ventricular Hypertrophy

An understanding of axis determination is useful in determining hypertrophy on the ECG. With left ventricular hypertrophy (LVH), left axis deviation may oc-

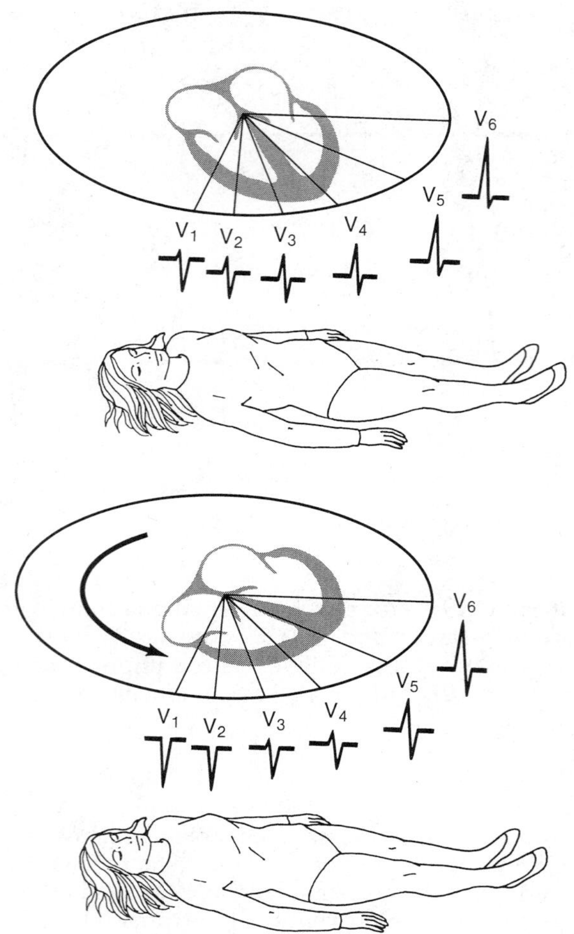

FIGURE 11–25. Cardiac rotation. The top figure shows an observer lying on the ground, viewing someone's heart. The six V leads are illustrated, showing normal R-wave progression. In the bottom figure, the six V leads show a delayed transition zone occurring at V_5/V_6. This situation is created by keeping the V leads where they are but rotating the heart clockwise (as perceived by our supine figure). Clockwise rotation moves the septum, where transition occurs, into the territory of leads V_5 and V_6. Similarly, counterclockwise rotation would move the transition zone into the territory of V_1/V_2. (Redrawn from Thaler, M. S. [1988]. *The only EKG book you'll ever need* [p. 73]. Philadelphia: J. B. Lippincott.)

cur because the mean vector is pulled more to the left than usual. Left axis deviation beyond −15° is often seen. However, the predominant feature of LVH is an increased R-wave amplitude in leads overlying the left ventricle and an increased S-wave amplitude in leads overlying the right ventricle (Fig. 11–26). The increased amplitude in the R wave over the hypertrophied ventricle is an expected occurrence because the increased muscle mass produces an excess of electrical potential. When examining the ECG, the following features may be indicative of left ventricular hypertrophy:

- The R-wave amplitude in lead V_5 or V_6 exceeds 26 mm
- The R-wave amplitude in V_5 or V_6 plus the S-wave amplitude in V_1 exceeds 35 mm
- The largest R wave plus the largest S wave in the precordial leads exceeds 45 mm
- R wave in lead I plus S wave in lead III exceeds 25 mm
- R wave in aVL exceeds 11 mm
- R wave in aVF exceeds 20 mm
- S wave in aVR exceeds 14 mm (Chou, 1991)

The more positive criteria are found, the greater the likelihood that the patient has LVH (Fig. 11–26). Generally, with LVH, the normal dominance of the left ventricle is exaggerated, and tall R waves become taller, and deep S waves become deeper (Wagner, 1994). Patients should be observed for evidence of LVH when there is evidence of hypertension, aortic valvular disorders, mitral valve insufficiency, or any other conditions that lead to pressure or volume overload of the left ventricle.

Right Ventricular Hypertrophy

In patients with right ventricular hypertrophy (RVH), the normal dominance of the left ventricle is upset, and changes occur in the normal precordial pattern (Fig. 11–27). These changes include:

- Reversal of precordial pattern with tall R waves over the right precordium (V_1 and V_2) and deep S over the left precordium (V_5 and V_6); or RS across the precordium
- QRS interval within normal limits
- Late intrinsicoid deflection* in leads V_1 and V_2
- Right axis deviation (Marriott, 1988)

RVH can be caused by abnormalities of the pulmonary valve, conditions causing pulmonary hypertension, and congenital lesions that overload the right ventricle.

Atrial Hypertrophy

The normal P wave is gently rounded, less than 0.12 second in duration, and should not exceed 2.5 mm in amplitude in any lead. The first part of the P wave represents right atrial depolarization, whereas the second part of it reflects left atrial depolarization.

In right atrial hypertrophy, the first portion of the P wave increases in amplitude to 3 mm or greater. This is usually more prominent in leads II, III, and aVF, where P waves are most pronounced. The P wave may be peaked, biphasic, or inverted in lead V_1. In addition, the axis of the P wave may swing rightward of +90° (Fig. 11–28*A*). The duration of the P wave usually remains normal. Right atrial hypertrophy is sometimes referred to as "P pulmonale" because of its association with pulmonary disease.

**A "late intrinsicoid deflection" refers to a downstroke (or S wave) recorded on a clinical lead, rather than direct epicardial, that is delayed longer than 0.02 second in V_1 and 0.04 second in V_6 (Marriott, 1988).*

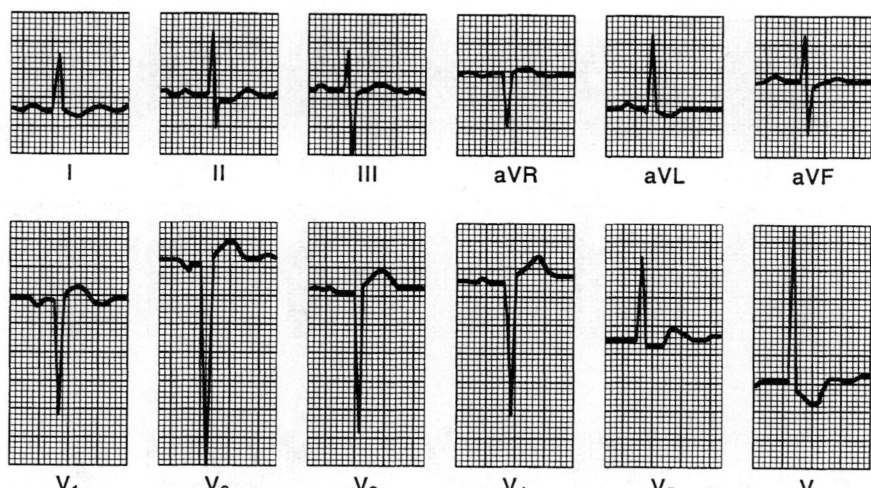

FIGURE 11–26. Left ventricular hypertrophy. (Redrawn from Goldman, M. J. [1986]. *Principles of clinical electrocardiography* [p. 194]. Los Altos, CA: Lange Medical Publications.)

In left atrial hypertrophy, the P wave is often widened to 0.12 second and is notched, and the second portion of the P wave may increase in amplitude (see Fig. 11–28*B*). These changes usually are seen best in leads I and II. The P wave in V_1 is often biphasic, and the large negative portion represents the depolarization forces traveling posteriorly in the larger left atrium (Goldschlager & Goldman, 1989). Left atrial hypertrophy is often referred to as "P mitrale" because it is associated with mitral valve disease.

ELECTROCARDIOGRAPHIC CHANGES WITH CORONARY ARTERY DISEASE

Myocardial Infarction

Myocardial infarction (MI) causes permanent damage to the myocardium, and there are characteristic ECG changes in the T wave, ST segment, and QRS complex. T-wave changes are the first to occur, and indicate myocardial ischemia. Within minutes after the initial decrease in blood supply to the myocardium, T waves become peaked, or hyperacute, indicating severe subendocardial ischemia (Fig. 11–29). The probable etiology of these changes is the leakage of intracellular potassium from damaged muscle cells into the extracellular spaces (Hurst, 1993). The changes in T-wave morphology are frequently missed because they usually last for a period of a few minutes to several hours, and therefore have disappeared by the time the first ECG is recorded.

If ischemia persists, ST segment elevation occurs, representing myocardial injury (Fig. 11–30). ST segment elevation is often the first ECG change noted (Hurst, 1993). During evolution of the MI, the ST segments return to baseline, and an inverted T wave becomes evident. The T waves of myocardial ischemia invert symmetrically, with a gentle downslope and rapid upstroke. This inverted T wave may remain on the ECG for an indefinite period of time during the healing process. Normal ST segments are isoelectric, beginning at the end of the QRS complex, at the J point (the junction between the end of the QRS complex and

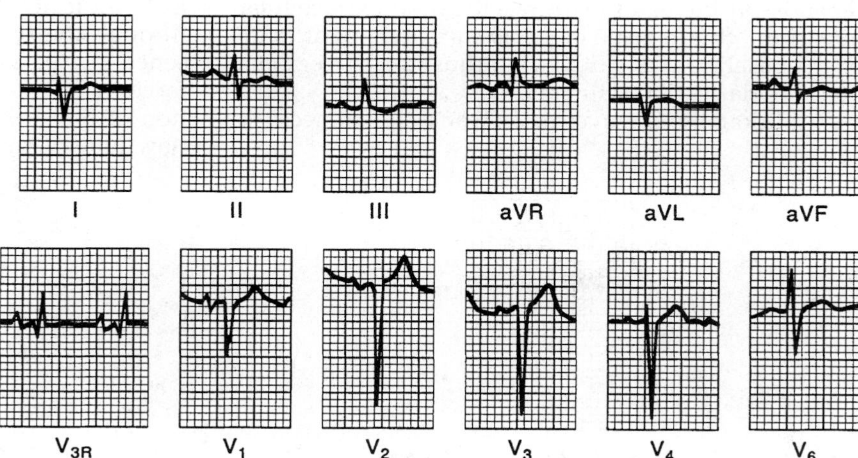

FIGURE 11–27. Right ventricular hypertrophy. (Redrawn from Goldman, M. J. [1986]. *Principles of clinical electrocardiography* [p. 103]. Los Altos, CA: Lange Medical Publications.)

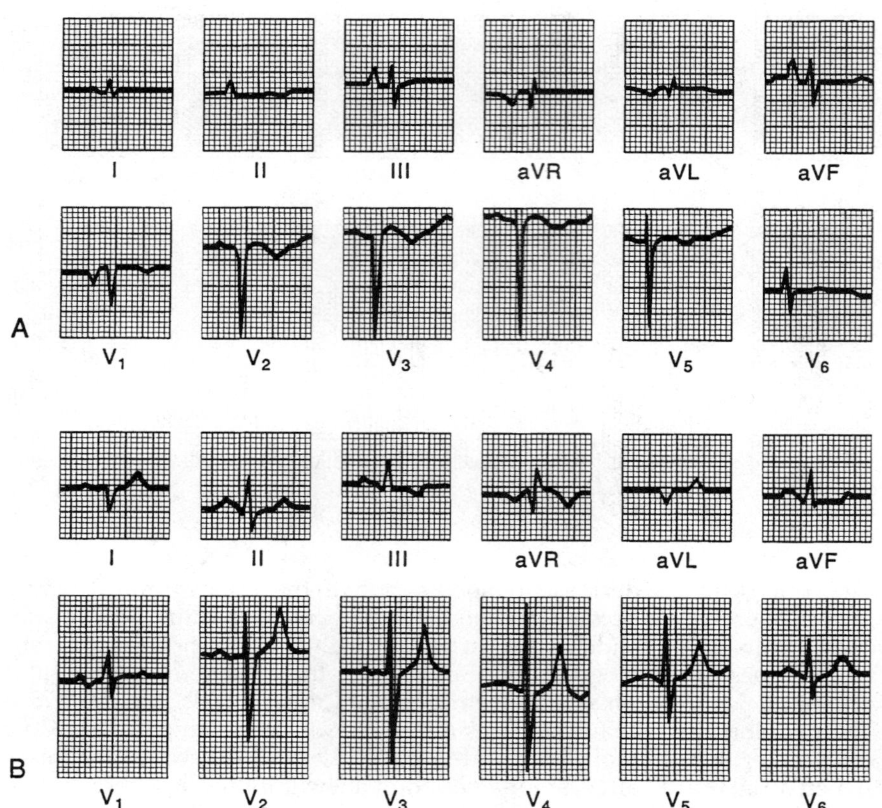

FIGURE 11–28. *A*, Right atrial enlargement. *B*, Left atrial enlargement. (Redrawn from Goldman, M. J. [1986]. *Principles of clinical electrocardiography* [pp. 87 and 88]. Los Altos, CA: Lange Medical Publications.)

beginning of the S-T segment). They may be normally elevated 1 mm in the frontal leads and up to 2 mm in the horizontal leads. ST elevation with MI may be confused with J point elevation of "early repolarization" that occurs in young, healthy people and has no pathologic implications. In J point elevation, the T wave maintains its independent waveform (Mirvis, 1993). With myocardial disease, ST segments are bowed upward and tend to merge imperceptibly with the T wave. Although there is uncertainty regarding the pathophysiology of ST segment elevation, it is known that intracellular potassium leaks from injured tissue. Because the resting potential of myocardial cells depends on the ratio of intracellular to extracellular potassium, this leakage of potassium is thought to alter the baseline of the ECG and, thus, the ST segment after depolarization (Hurst, 1993).

Traditionally, Q waves have been a sign of necrosis associated with transmural MIs, and have been explained using the "electrical window" concept (Fig. 11–31). When an area of myocardium is severely damaged and becomes necrotic, it is unable to depolarize and repolarize normally. This necrotic area provides a "window" for the electrode placed over it, allowing visualization of the electromotive forces moving away from it through the rest of the heart. These forces produce a negative deflection, a Q wave, in this electrode. These Q waves should be 0.03 second or more in duration, compared to normal "septal" Q waves, as previously described.

Until recently, it was believed that Q waves on the ECG indicated a transmural infarction, an infarction through the full thickness of the muscle, and an absence of Q waves indicated a subendocardial infarction, an infarction of only the subendocardial portion of the muscle. Based on pathology reports, it is now known that transmural infarctions can occur in

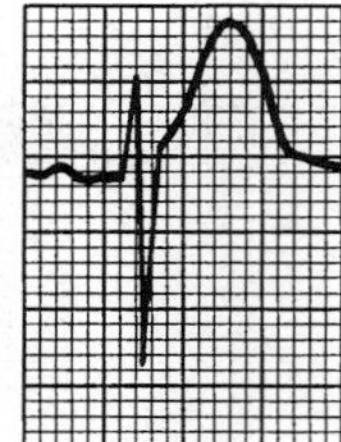

FIGURE 11–29. Peaked T wave.

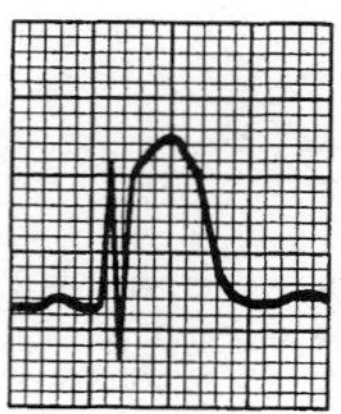

FIGURE 11–30. ST segment elevation.

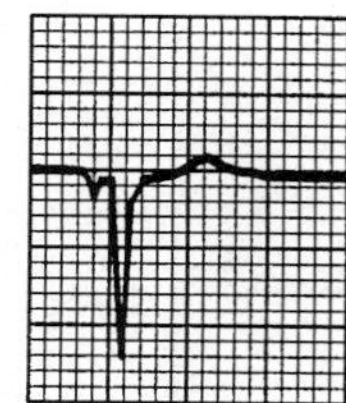

FIGURE 11–31. Q wave.

the absence of Q waves on the ECG, and that nontransmural MIs may be associated with the appearance of new Q waves (Cohn, 1993; Hurst, 1993). Table 11–4 illustrates the frequency of Q waves in transmural and subendocardial MIs in a series of 100 patients. Subsequently, infarctions should be described as either Q wave or non-Q wave on the basis of serial ECG evaluations (Goldberger, 1991; Schlant et al., 1994). In most patients with the presence of Q waves, the MI will probably, although not necessarily, be transmural.

The ECG changes just described are indicative of damage in specific leads overlying the areas of ischemia or infarction. Changes also are recorded on the ECG in leads overlying the opposite side of the heart. These variations are called reciprocal changes. Just as there is an absence of electromotive forces during depolarization and repolarization in the damaged part of the myocardium, there is a concomitant relative gain in forces directed away from the inert area (Goldberger, 1991; Wagner, 1994). These irregularities are assessed by other electrodes. Reciprocal leads will record a mirror image of the damaged area. For example, reciprocal changes that would be recorded opposite a Q wave, elevated ST segments, and inverted T waves would be an increase in the R wave, depressed ST segments, and tall, upright T waves. Table 11–5 indicates where indicative and reciprocal changes occur with different types of MIs.

ANTERIOR WALL MYOCARDIAL INFARCTION. In an anterior wall MI, damage results from the occlusion of the LCA. The left main coronary artery branches into the LAD artery, which supplies the anteroseptal portion of the left circumflex artery, which in turn provides the blood supply for the lateral wall of the left ventricle. ECG changes associated with anterior wall MIs occur in the precordial leads and leads I and aVL, whereas reciprocal changes develop in leads II, III, and aVF (Fig. 11–32). Changes involving all the precordial leads, and leads I and aVL, indicate an extensive anterior wall MI or an anterolateral infarction. Variations seen in leads V_1 to V_4 suggest an anteroseptal MI.

Problems with pump failure and the conduction system can be anticipated because the LCA supplies large areas of left ventricular musculature, as well as the RBB and LBB and the anterior two-thirds of the ventricular septum. If conduction disturbances occur, they represent an extensive loss of myocardium and may indicate a poor prognosis. Mobitz type II and complete heart block are the most frequently seen conduction disturbances in patients with anterior wall MIs. Cardiac pacing is frequently used to improve cardiac performance. Patients who are most likely to require temporary pacing are those who have a combination of a new RBB block with a left hemiblock, or a pattern in which LBB and RBB blocks alternate (Schlant, 1994). Because of the extensive myocardial damage and concomitant pump failure, there is a high rate of mortality in this type of patient.

TABLE 11–4. **Incidence of Q Waves in 100 Infarctions**

	Transmural	Subendocardial
Number	55	45
Q waves	67%	30%
ST–T changes	33%	70%

From Antaloczy, A. (1987). *Journal of Electrocardiology, 20,* 72. © 1987, Churchill-Livingstone, New York.

TABLE 11–5. **Indicative and Reciprocal Changes With Myocardial Infarctions (MIs)**

Site	Indicative	Reciprocal
Inferior	II, III, aVF	I, aVL, V leads
Anteroseptal	V_1–V_3	II, III, AVF
Anterolateral	I, aVL, V_4–V_6	II, III, aVF
Extensive anterior	I, aVL, V_1–V_6	II, III, aVF, posterior chest
Posterior	V_7–V_9*	V_1 (tall R)

*These are leads placed directly over the left posterior chest in the fifth intercostal space beginning at the left posterior axillary line.

INFERIOR WALL MYOCARDIAL INFARCTIONS. Acute inferior wall MI is caused by occlusion of the right coronary artery in 50% to 70% of the cases, whereas most of the remaining cases are a result of occlusion of a dominant left circumflex coronary artery (Shah, 1991). Less commonly, it may be caused by blockage of a very long descending anterior coronary artery supplying the distal aspect of the left ventricular apex and distal part of the inferior wall. Indicative changes occur in leads II, III, and aVF (Fig. 11–33). When the infarction results from involvement of the left circumflex artery, ST elevation is usually evident in at least one of the lateral leads (aVL, V_5, or V_6) with concomitant isoelectric or elevated ST in lead I (Bairey et al., 1987; Shah, 1991). Goldberger (1991) suggested that the presence of Q waves exceeding 0.03 second in lead aVF might provide a useful indicator of inferior wall MI. In addition, a prominent Q wave in lead III is found in inferior wall MIs, but must be differentiated from normal Q waves that may occur in that lead. Deep inspiration will usually cause a positional Q wave to disappear or diminish, whereas pathologic Q waves occurring with an MI will generally remain unchanged (Goldberger, 1991). That is, a large Q wave in leads III and aVF, with

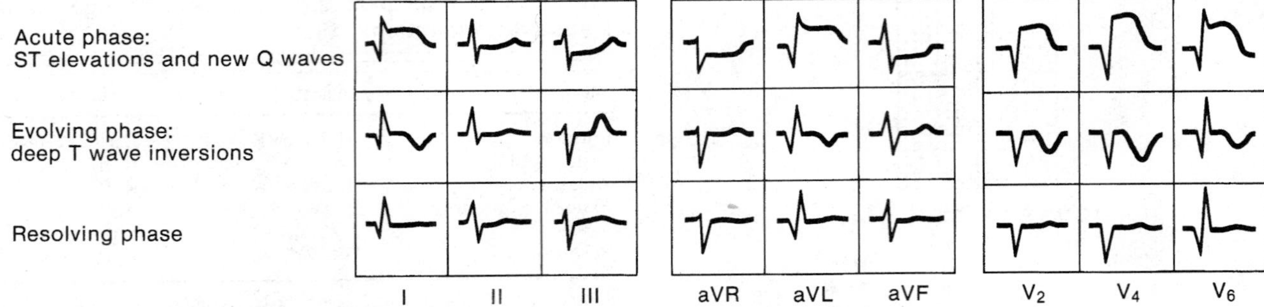

FIGURE 11–32. Anterior wall MI. (Reproduced by permission from: Goldberger, A. L., & Goldberger, E. [1981]. *Clinical electrocardiography* [p. 90]. St. Louis: C. V. Mosby.)

a concomitant rS (or RS) in aVR, is usually indicative of infarction. In contrast, prominent Q waves in leads III and aVF, in the presence of a QR in lead aVR, typically signify normal variant Q waves. However, because leads III and aVF are so sensitive to respiratory and positional changes, they may not be reliable for differentiating normal and pathologic Q waves.

Although most Q waves that develop during an infarction persist for a lifetime, this is not true with inferior wall MIs. In as many as 50% of patients with inferior wall MIs, the criteria for detection of significant Q waves are lost as the MI evolves (Mirvis, 1993).

As discussed earlier, the RCA generally supplies the SA and AV nodes, the bundle of His, the posterior third of the septum, as well as a portion of the posteroinferior division of the left bundle. Occlusion of this artery causes ischemia of the SA and AV nodes and is commonly associated with sinus bradycardia and Mobitz type I (Wenckebach) block (Alpert, 1991). The timing of AV blocks in inferior wall MIs has significance. AV blocks occurring very early after the onset of chest pain are caused by increased vagal tone rather than ischemia and are accompanied by sinus bradycardia. When blocks develop later in the course of the MI, they are caused by ischemia, and atropine does not affect the conduction disturbance (Brugada & Wellens, 1986).

Generally speaking, pacing is not recommended in patients with inferior wall MIs (Kastor, 1994). However, it may become necessary when the escape rhythm is slow or is associated with symptoms, or when an AV block worsens the patient's hemodynamic condition.

POSTERIOR WALL MYOCARDIAL INFARCTIONS. A posterior wall MI involves the dorsal surface of the heart and often occurs in association with inferior or lateral wall MIs. Posterior wall infarction results from occlusion of the posterior descending coronary artery, a branch of the RCA, or less frequently, of the circumflex artery. AV block may occur because, in most cases, a branch of the posterior descending artery also supplies the AV node. In the normal 12-lead ECG, no leads are placed directly over the posterior wall. Diagnosis depends on detecting reciprocal changes in leads V_1 and V_2, which include tall R waves and ST segment depression (Fig. 11–34). A marked loss of R-wave amplitude in the left precordial leads, V_5 and V_6, may occur as well. Tall symmetric T waves will appear later in leads V_1 and V_2. In an adult, an abnormally tall R wave in V_1 or V_2 is defined as an R:S ratio greater than 1, or an R duration of 0.04 second or more (Goldberger, 1991). It is necessary to differentiate a posterior infarction from RVH, which also has a large R wave in V_1. The presence or absence of right axis deviation is the distinguishing characteristic, because a right axis deviation is not present in the posterior leads.

RIGHT VENTRICULAR MYOCARDIAL INFARCTIONS. Approximately one-third of all patients with inferior wall

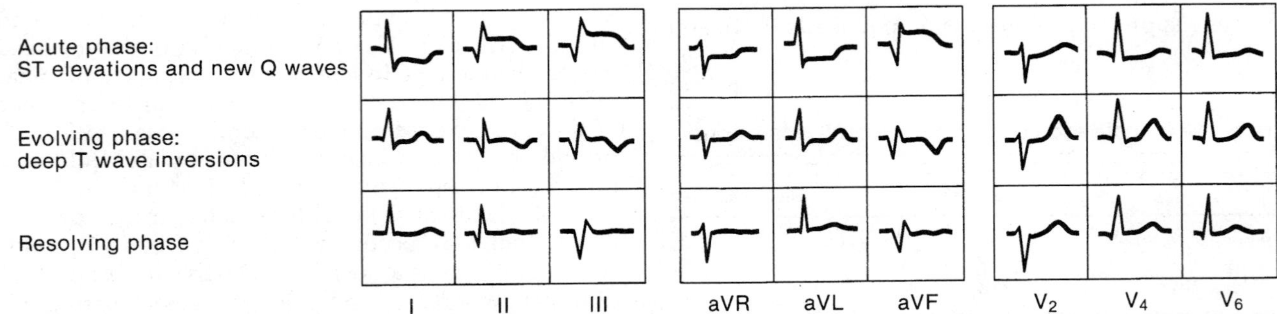

FIGURE 11–33. Inferior wall MI. (Reproduced by permission from: Goldberger, A. L., & Goldberger, E. [1981]. *Clinical electrocardiography* [p. 90]. St. Louis: C. V. Mosby.)

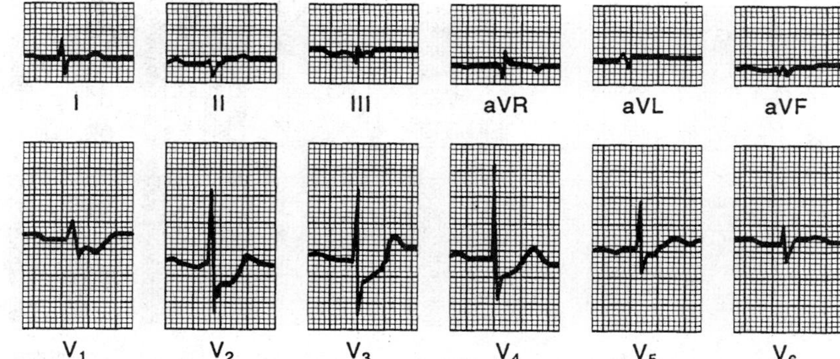

FIGURE 11–34. Posterior wall MI. (Redrawn from Marriott, H. J. L. [1988]. *Practical electrocardiography* [p. 442]. © 1988, The Williams & Wilkins Co., Baltimore.)

MIs have concomitant right ventricular MIs (RVMIs) (Setaro & Cabin, 1992). This occurs as a result of proximal occlusion of the RCA before the take-off of the major right ventricular branch. RVMIs are manifested by ST segment elevation of at least 1 mm in the right precordial leads V_{4R} and V_{5R}. This 1-mm elevation requires 25% or more necrosis of the right ventricle (Setaro & Cabin, 1992). The chance of observing ST segment elevation in the right precordial leads sharply decreases 10 hours or more after onset of chest pain. It is therefore important to record a right chest lead (V_{4R}) on admission to the critical care unit and with daily ECGs. When an RVMI occurs in conjunction with an inferior wall MI, there is increased possibility of AV nodal conduction disturbance (48% versus 13% in patients without RVMI) (Braat et al., 1984). Therefore, the recording of right precordial leads is helpful not only in identifying right ventricular involvement during acute inferior wall MI, but in predicting the development of conduction disturbances and identifying the coronary artery responsible for the acute inferior wall MI (Fig. 11–35). Other complications associated with RVMI include hypotension, atrial tachydysrhythmia, aneurysm, thrombus formation, tricuspid regurgitation, pulmonary embolus, hypoxemia, pleural effusion, and RBB block (Setaro & Cabin, 1992).

ATRIAL INFARCTIONS. Atrial infarctions may accompany ventricular MIs, or they can occur as isolated events. The right atrium is more commonly involved than the left. Regardless of the extent of coronary artery narrowing, pulmonary hypertension is the major contributing factor leading to isolated atrial infarction. The most frequent complications of atrial infarction are congestive heart failure, thromboembolic pneumonia, and supraventricular dysrhythmias (Ventura et al., 1991).

Atrial infarctions should be suspected when atrial dysrhythmias occur with any ventricular MI (Chou, 1992). The ECG findings are often nonspecific. Some indicators of atrial infarction include abnormal P-wave contour, PR segment depression with atrial dysrhythmias, elevation of the PR segment in left chest leads with reciprocal depression in right chest leads, and elevation of the PR segment in lead I with reciprocal depression in lead III (Chou, 1992; Ventura et al., 1991).

Myocardial Ischemia

Myocardial ischemia (angina, coronary insufficiency) refers to reversible changes in the myocardium resulting from a temporary decrease in blood supply.

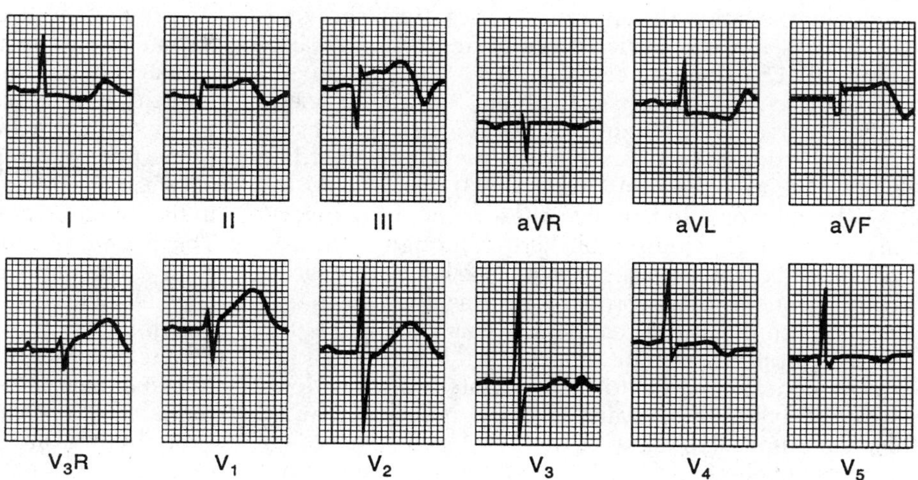

FIGURE 11–35. Right ventricular MI. (Reproduced by permission from: Goldberger, A. L. [1984]. *Myocardial infarction* [p. 316]. St. Louis: C. V. Mosby.)

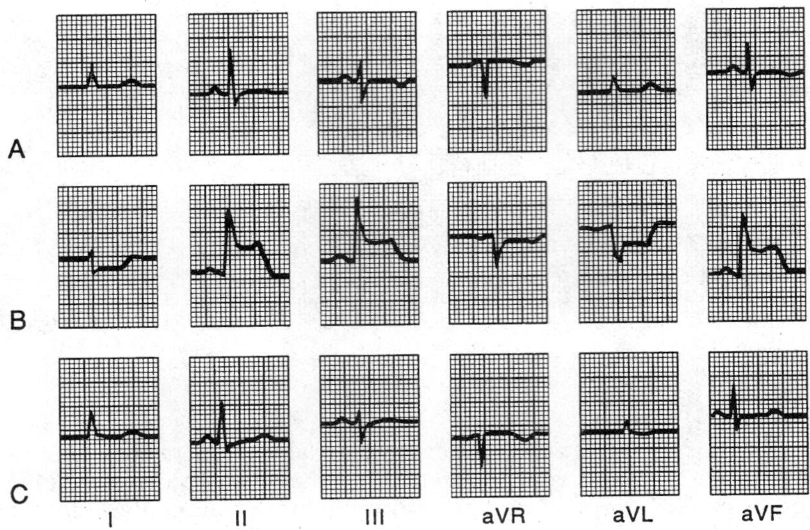

FIGURE 11–36. Prinzmetal angina. *A,* The baseline ECG shows nonspecific inferior ST–T changes. *B,* With chest pain, the marked ST segment elevations occur in leads II, III, and aVF, and there are reciprocal ST depressions in leads I and aVL. *C,* Return of ST segments to baseline. (Reproduced by permission from: Goldberger, A. L. [1989]. *Myocardial infarction* [p. 151]. St. Louis: C. V. Mosby.)

On the ECG, these changes produce ST segment deviations and changes in T-wave morphology. ST segments may be elevated or depressed. As a practical rule, an ECG tracing taken directly over the injured myocardium will record ST segment elevations, whereas ST segment depression results if healthy muscle lies between the injured muscle and the electrode (Hurst, 1993; Schlant et al., 1994). ST segment depression is the most typical pattern. T waves may be peaked or inverted, owing to a delay in phase 3 repolarization in the affected area of the heart. The mean vector is directed away from the ischemic area. Therefore, leads over the surface of the ischemic area generally will exhibit inverted T waves, whereas leads oriented to the opposite or healthy surface will reveal upright T waves. The T wave of myocardial ischemia is characterized by symmetry and increased narrowness.

Prinzmetal angina is a variant form of angina characterized by chest pain that ordinarily occurs at rest and is accompanied by ST segment elevation. Prinzmetal and associates (1959) demonstrated that the chemical behavior of the myocardial areas showing ST segment elevation differs from that of areas showing ST depression with other types of angina. They also found that ST segment elevation represents a more severe degree of oxygen deprivation than does ST segment depression. ST segments are elevated as a result of a reduction in coronary blood flow in the epicardial half of the myocardium (Hurst, 1993) (Fig. 11–36).

The relationship between chest pain and coronary artery spasm is well established. Although some patients with coronary artery spasm also have atherosclerotic lesions in their coronary arteries, the spasm appears to be the critical element that is responsible for their symptoms (Schlant et al., 1994). It is more likely in Prinzmetal angina to be associated with various types of dysrhythmias and conduction defects than in typical angina (Sokolow & McIlroy, 1993). There is a well established relationship with torsades de pointes as well (Horowitz, 1994). For these reasons, it may be useful to monitor these patients in a lead that displays ST elevation, such that changes can be quickly observed and interventions initiated.

Dysrhythmogenesis

Dysrhythmias are abnormalities in heart rate, regularity, or site of origin of cardiac impulses, or disturbances in the conduction of those impulses. Thus, the basic mechanisms of cardiac dysrhythmias are abnormalities of impulse generation, conduction, or a combination of both (Table 11–6).

Abnormal impulse formation occurs as a result of localized changes in ionic currents that flow across the membranes of single cells or groups of cells (Rardon & Pressler, 1991). These deviant impulses arise from normal or enhanced automaticity and triggered activity.

Altered Automaticity

As previously discussed, automaticity is the ability to initiate spontaneous action potentials and is a normal property of pacemaker cells. The basis of normal automaticity is a slow fall in membrane potential during phase 4 of the action potential. This decrease in membrane potential reflects a gradual shift in the balance between the inward and outward current components in the direction of net inward current (Surawicz, 1991). The SA node, normally the controlling pacemaker, both excites and inhibits other potentially automatic cells elsewhere in the heart. When impulses are not generated by the SA node because of sick sinus syndrome or ischemia, pacemaker cells in the AV node or Purkinje network will eventually reach threshold potential and discharge themselves. These secondary escape rhythms are labeled junctional, ventricular, or accelerated idioventricular, depending on the origin of impulse.

TABLE 11–6. **Mechanisms for Dysrhythmias**

I Abnormal Impulse Generation	II Abnormal Impulse Conduction	III Simultaneous Abnormalities of Impulse Generation and Conduction
A. Normal automatic mechanism 1. Abnormal rate a. Tachycardia b. Bradycardia 2. Abnormal rhythm a. Premature impulses b. Delayed impulses c. Absent impulses B. Abnormal automatic mechanism 1. Phase 4 depolarization at low membrane potential 2. Oscillatory depolarizations at low membrane potential preceding upstroke C. Triggered activity 1. Early afterdepolarizations 2. Delayed afterdepolarizations 3. Oscillatory depolarizations at low membrane potentials after action potential upstroke	A. Slowing and block 1. Sinoatrial block 2. Atrioventricular block 3. His bundle block 4. Bundle branch block B. Unidirectional block and reentry 1. Random reentry a. Atrial muscle b. Ventricular muscle 2. Ordered reentry a. Sinoatrial node and junction b. AV node and junction c. His–Purkinje system d. Purkinje fiber–muscle junction e. Abnormal AV connection (WPW) 3. Summation and inhibition C. Conduction block and reflection	A. Phase 4 depolarization and impaired conduction 1. Specialized cardiac fibers B. Parasystole

Abbreviations: AV = atrioventricular; WPW = Wolff-Parkinson-White syndrome.
From Hoffman, B. F., & Rosen, M. R. (1981). *Circulation Research, 49,* 2. By permission of the American Heart Association, Inc.

Altered automaticity may be a product of either enhanced normal automaticity in the Purkinje fibers with high membrane potential or of abnormal automaticity in severely depressed Purkinje or myocardial tissue (Marriott & Conover, 1989; Kay & Bubien, 1992). Enhanced normal automaticity exhibits an acceleration or steepening of phase 4 depolarization in pacemaker cells and may result in dysrhythmias in the Purkinje fibers with high membrane potentials. This situation may occur over a broad range of membrane potentials, from approximately −90 to −50 mV in the Purkinje cells and −60 mV in most myocardial cells. In these instances, automaticity may be readily suppressed by overdrive pacing. Ectopic beats or rhythms occur when the threshold potential of the cell is attained prematurely.

Dysrhythmias may occur because of abnormal automaticity outside the sinus node as well. Working atrial and ventricular myocardial cells do not normally show spontaneous diastolic depolarization. If, however, the resting potential of these cells is increased to approximately −60 mV, spontaneous diastolic depolarization may occur, causing repetitive impulse initiation (Marriott & Conover, 1989; Surawicz, 1991). Such a reduction in membrane potential may be the result of hypocalcemia, cardiomyopathy, ischemia, hypoxia, chamber enlargement, digitalis intoxication, increased extracellular or intracellular potassium, increased sodium permeability, or decreased potassium permeability (Marriott & Conover, 1989). The dysrhythmia gradually accelerates after initiation and gradually decelerates before termination (Surawicz, 1991). Examples of abnormal automaticity are multifocal atrial tachycardia, paroxysmal atrial tachycardia with block secondary to digitalis toxicity, accelerated idioventricular rhythm, and ventricular tachycardia (Kay & Bubien, 1992; Wagner, 1994). Conditions that promote abnormal automaticity include hypoxia, acidosis, alkalosis, hypokalemia, hypocalcemia, and catecholamine administration. Dysrhythmias resulting from abnormal automaticity are spontaneous, persistent, and resistant to cardioversion or overdrive pacing techniques (Kay & Bubien, 1992; Marriott & Conover, 1989). These rhythms do not respond to overdrive suppression because depressed fibers are unable to hyperpolarize like fibers with high membrane potentials.

Distinguishing between enhanced and abnormal automaticity is often a challenge. Ventricular tachycardia in patients who have recently suffered an acute MI with depressed myocardial cells is usually a result of abnormal automaticity. This situation will not respond to lidocaine administration or overdrive pacing. A better treatment would be calcium channel blockers. In contrast, an idioventricular rhythm in a patient who has a complete AV block is probably a result of enhanced automaticity. This scenario calls for withholding administration of lidocaine, which would suppress the life-saving ventricular focus. Overdrive pacing may be an effective treatment modality in this instance (Marriott & Conover, 1989).

Triggered Activity

The concept of triggered activity came from studies of abnormal electrical activity of Purkinje fibers, fibers in the AV valves, and coronary sinus. Triggered activity requires an initiating action potential before one or

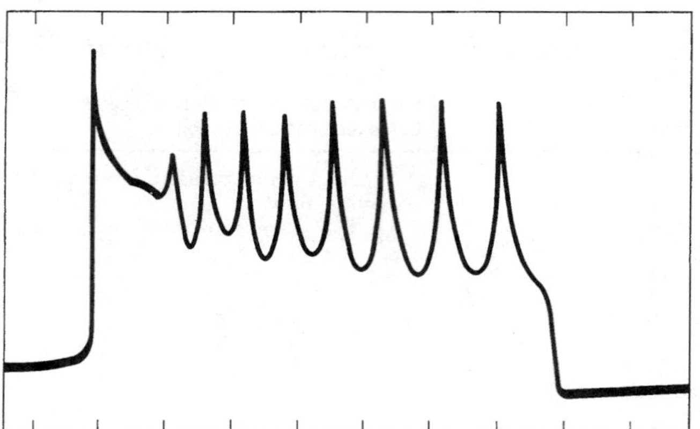

FIGURE 11–37. Early afterdepolarization and repetitive activity in canine cardiac Purkinje fiber. The maximum diastolic potential was −87 mV. A "burst" of rhythmic activity arising from a low level of membrane potential occurred during repolarization of the action potential. The slow responses during this burst peaked near 0 mV. Time marks occur at 1-second intervals. (Redrawn from Wit, A. L., Cranefield, P. R., & Gadsby, D. C. [1980]. Triggered activity. In D. P. Zipes, J. C. Bailey, & V. Elharrar [Eds.], *The slow inward current cardiac arrhythmias.* The Hague: Martinus Nijhoff.)

more additional abnormal impulses are generated. These impulses are called afterdepolarizations. Only if the afterdepolarization achieves threshold potential does triggered activity result. Therefore, triggered action potentials require the presence of a preceding action potential, and this requirement distinguishes triggered activity from automaticity (Kay & Bubien, 1992). Cells that exhibit this mechanism, once excited, give rise to two or more action potentials or a long run of repetitive responses (Schlant et al., 1994).

Depolarizing afterpotentials causing triggered activity can be either early or delayed. Early afterdepolarizations usually occur during phase 3 of the action potential, or the repolarization phase, and have been initiated from a high level of membrane potential, usually between −75 and −90 mV (Josephson & Wellens, 1993) (Fig. 11–37). These early afterdepolarizations are more likely to occur during bradycardia than tachycardia. A number of drugs have been shown experimentally to prolong the action potential duration, and therefore increase the likelihood of early afterdepolarizations. They include aconitine, quinidine, procainamide, and cesium (Kay & Bubien, 1992). In addition, hypokalemia or hypomagnesemia may induce early afterdepolarizations. The prevailing cardiac dysrhythmia associated with early afterdepolarization is torsades de pointes, a form of ventricular tachycardia. Because a prolonged action potential seems to play a crucial role in the development of early afterdepolarization, treatment for drug-induced torsades de pointes should be aimed at shortening the QT interval.

Delayed afterdepolarizations occur after completion of phase 3 of the action potential (i.e., they occur after the membrane is fully repolarized). When afterdepolarizations are of sufficient amplitude to bring the membrane potential to threshold, a triggered impulse arises, which is followed by an afterdepolarization. Delayed afterdepolarizations occur under conditions in which there are large increases in intracellular calcium (Bigger, Jr., 1994; Rosen & Anyukhovsky, 1991). The classic example of delayed afterdepolarization and triggered activity is digitalis toxicity. Digitalis inhibits the Na^+-K^+ pump, leading to an increase in intracellular sodium, which is then exchanged for calcium by a sodium–calcium exchange mechanism (Josephson & Wellens, 1993). Delayed afterdepolarizations are also exaggerated by hypokalemia, hypercalcemia, and toxic concentrations of cardiac glycosides. In contrast to early afterdepolarizations, this situation is more likely to occur with rapid heart rates. Possible dysrhythmias associated with delayed afterdepolarizations and triggered activity include atrial tachycardia with AV block, junctional tachycardia, multifocal atrial tachycardia, and exercise-induced ventricular tachycardia (Kay & Bubien, 1992). Treatment options include beta-blockers or verapamil, whereas beta agonists or theophylline should be avoided.

IMPULSE CONDUCTION

Abnormalities of impulse conduction are probably more common bases for dysrhythmias than abnormal impulse formation. Abnormalities of conduction are caused by conduction block, reentry, or reflection.

Decremental Conduction

Decremental conduction is the slowing of conduction velocity of an impulse by the AV node as it travels from the atria to the ventricles. In the AV fibers, the amplitude of the action potential and the rate of depolarization decrease progressively from cell to cell such that the resulting stimulus becomes weaker as it is propagated (Schlant et al., 1994). The impulse may completely fade out when the strength of the proximal stimulus becomes insufficient to elicit a response in the distal fibers, even if they are still excitable. Decremental conduction normally occurs in areas of the heart where resting potentials are low and upstroke of the action potential depends on slow calcium channels, as in the SA and AV nodes. It also can occur in areas where opening of fast sodium channels is impaired by ischemia, disease, or drugs. These areas are partially depolarized, resulting in inactivation of some sodium channels. This partial depolarization reduces the amplitude of the action potential and the rate of rise of phase 0, thereby decreasing conduction velocity (Gettes, 1990).

Decremental conduction is responsible not only for normal slowing of the impulse in the AV node but for the prolonged AV conduction time of early atrial premature beats. An accentuation of normal decremental conduction through the AV node is the probable explanation of first-degree AV block. Mobitz type I block (Wenkebach phenomenon) has been attributed to decremental conduction in the AV node. In Mobitz type II block, the conduction disturbance is situated in a more peripheral portion of the AV conduction system. The

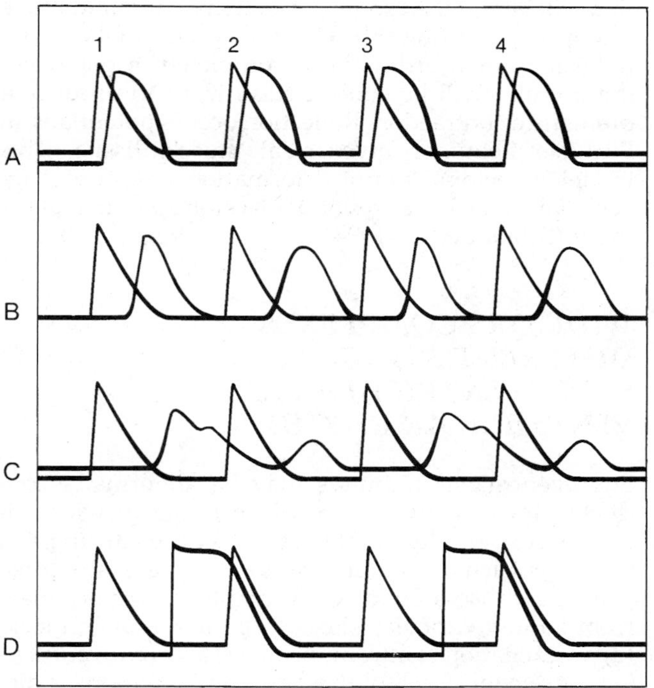

FIGURE 11–38. Tracings of transmembrane action potentials recorded from a single fiber of the atrium and from fibers of the AV node and His bundle, showing decremental conduction during a sustained supraventricular tachycardia. *A,* Atrium and atrial margin of the node. *B,* Atrium and middle node. *C,* Atrium and lower node. *D,* Atrium and His bundle. The same atrial fiber was employed in all records. Note that during the second and fourth beats, the abortive responses in the lower node fail to produce a His bundle response. This is 2:1 AV heart block resulting from complete decrement of beats 2 and 4 within the node. Beats 2 and 4 also are concealed responses. Note the relative loss of resting membrane potential from the fibers in the middle and lower nodal areas, panels *B* and *C*. The resting potential of fibers in the His bundle, panel *D*, is normal. (Redrawn from Hoffman, B., Cranefield, P., & Wallace, A. G. [1966]. Physiological basis of cardiac arrhythmias [II]. *Modern Concepts of Cardiovascular Disease, 35,* 108. By permission of the American Heart Association, Inc.)

mechanism is probably a transient but complete decrement of conduction in both bundle branches, or in one bundle branch if the other is already blocked (Schlant et al., 1994) (Fig. 11–38).

Reentry

Reentry occurs when an impulse continues to excite the atria or ventricles after the refractory period, rather than dying out after the refractory period. In other words, the impulse depolarizes an area of the myocardium and then is able to reenter the same area to depolarize it again. Because the impulse cannot double back on its original route because the tissue is refractory, a separate return pathway must be used. For an impulse to complete a circuit and continue to propagate, at each point in the reentrant loop, the myocardium must have had sufficient time to recover the capability to respond to a depolarizing signal (Conover, 1992; Moser & Woo, 1994).

Reentry has been subdivided into random and ordered reentry (Conover, 1992; Mirvis, 1993). Random reentry is most often associated with atrial or ventricular fibrillation, whereas ordered reentry causes most other types of dysrhythmias. The main distinction between the two is that during random reentry, impulse propagation occurs over reentrant pathways that continuously change their size and location with time, whereas ordered reentry implies a relatively fixed reentrant pathway. Ordered reentry has been divided into microreentry and macroreentry (Conover, 1992). With microreentry, the tissue involved in the reentrant circuit is localized to a small area of the heart, such as the AV node or distal Purkinje network. When large portions of myocardium are involved, as in atrial flutter or Wolff-Parkinson-White (WPW) syndrome, the level is macroreentry.

Several conditions are necessary for the occurrence of reentrant rhythms (Kellen & Ramadan, 1994). First, it is essential that there be a difference in the conduction and refractoriness of at least two distinct pathways that connect proximally and distally. Second, there must be a unidirectional block in one of the pathways that allows the impulse to be conducted in only one direction through an area. Such areas of depressed conduction can occur in ischemic fibers with low threshold resting potentials, where sodium channels are partly or completely inactivated and depolarization depends on slow calcium channels (Mirvis, 1993). Conduction must be slow in the pathway that is not blocked, allowing time for the blocked pathway to recover excitability. If the refractory period of the previously stimulated tissue is long or the conduction is too fast, the impulse will cease. Last, there must be reexcitation of the initially blocked pathway to complete the loop of activation (Fig. 11–39).

Reentry may occur anywhere in the conduction system. A decreased rate of conduction frequently results from blockage of the Purkinje system, ischemia of the myocardium, or high serum potassium levels, among many other factors. A shortened refractory period may occur in response to various drugs, such as epinephrine. Reentry is the cause of many tachydysrhythmias, including various kinds of supraventricular and ventricular tachycardias, flutter, and fibrillation (Braunwald, 1992). Most ventricular dysrhythmias that occur after an acute MI are caused by reentry (Bandari & Rahimtoola, 1991). However, ventricular tachycardia occurring 24 hours after the incident is thought to be caused by abnormal automaticity secondary to ischemia (Conover, 1992). Reentry is the mechanism for supraventricular dysrhythmias due to WPW syndrome involving the normal conducting and accessory pathways.

Tachydysrhythmias due to reentry require an initiating beat. In the case of ventricular tachycardia, the initiating beat may be a sinus or supraventricular impulse that is conducted normally until it reaches a bifurcation, which is usually located in ventricular Purkinje tissue. The impulse activates the ventricles and then reenters the ventricular conduction system to reactivate them. It may or may not be conducted in a

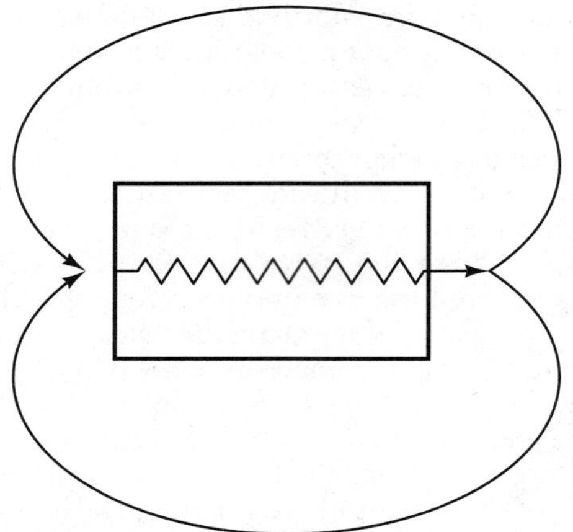

FIGURE 11–39. Anatomic model of reentry. The rectangular area in the center of the figure signifies a region of slow conduction in cardiac tissue. A wavefront of depolarization enters the proximal portion of this area of slow conduction and slowly traverses it to arrive at the distal end. Next, the wavefront of activation spreads in two directions through more normal myocardium to arrive back at the proximal portion of the region of slow conduction, to complete the reentrant circuit. Because more time is required to traverse the area of slow conduction, there is a gap of excitability in the circuit during which portions of the reentrant circuits are not refractory to stimulation. (From Kay, G. N., & Bubien, R. S. [1992]. *Clinical management of cardiac arrhythmias* [p. 18]. Gaithersburg, MD: Aspen. Copyright © 1992 Aspen Publishers, Inc.)

retrograde fashion to activate the atria. The initiating beat is normal in appearance, whereas the following "reentered" beat is wide and bizarre-looking because the reentry process has taken place entirely within the ventricle. This phenomenon is known as a "fixed coupling interval" (Mirvis, 1993).

Reflection

Reflection is a form of reentry in which the two potential conducting circuits are parallel, rather than branching off of a single conduction pathway (Fig. 11–40). Although both circuits may be depressed, an impulse can be conducted through one. This conduction will be slow. At some point, it may turn and move retrogradely through the other fiber back to its origin. If healthy myocardium has completely repolarized, the impulse will be conducted onward to produce a premature contraction. Reflection occurs potentially in Purkinje fibers or myocardial muscle tissue. This model of ectopic impulse formation has been suggested in some instances of parasystolic pacemaker activity (Schlant et al., 1994).

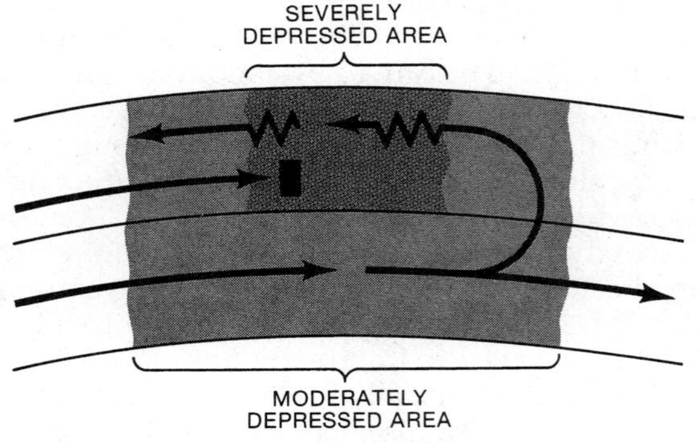

FIGURE 11–40. Reflection.

WIDE QRS COMPLEXES: DIFFERENTIATING SUPRAVENTRICULAR AND VENTRICULAR RHYTHMS

Supraventricular impulses may be abnormally conducted through the ventricles, resulting in wide, bizarre QRS complexes that are difficult to distinguish from ventricular ectopic impulses. There are three principal causes of wide QRS complexes that originate from supraventricular sites: (1) bundle branch block, (2) preexcitation syndromes, and (3) aberrant ventricular conduction. Each of these rhythm variations is discussed in this section.

Bundle Branch Blocks

Conduction defects or intraventricular block may occur in the ventricular conducting system below the bundle of His as the result of ischemia or degeneration of conducting tissue. A block may occur in the RBB, LBB, the left anterior fascicle, or left posterior fascicle, causing abnormal ventricular depolarization. A block in the bundle branches causes the QRS to be prolonged, whereas a block in one of the fascicles of the left bundle causes a QRS shift in axis while maintaining a normal duration. When an intraventricular block is indicated by a wide QRS complex but lacks specific features of either RBB or LBB block, it is called an intraventricular conduction defect.

Normally, impulses from the SA node, atria, and AV node proceed through the common bundle of His and then down both the LBB and RBB to the Purkinje fibers, causing simultaneous ventricular depolarization. Conduction is rapid owing to the character of the action potential of their specialized cells, their large size, their more-or-less parallel alignment, and their relatively sparse branching. Bundle branch blocks alter this normal progression of depolarization, causing the ventricles to depolarize one after the other because the impulses must travel through muscle tissue rather than through specialized conductile tissue. This delayed conduction lengthens the QRS duration to 0.12 second or greater. Leads V_1 and V_6 are the best leads for diagnosing bundle branch blocks and recording ventricular activation time because of their placement over the right (V_1) and left (V_6) ventricles.

Because depolarization is abnormal in bundle

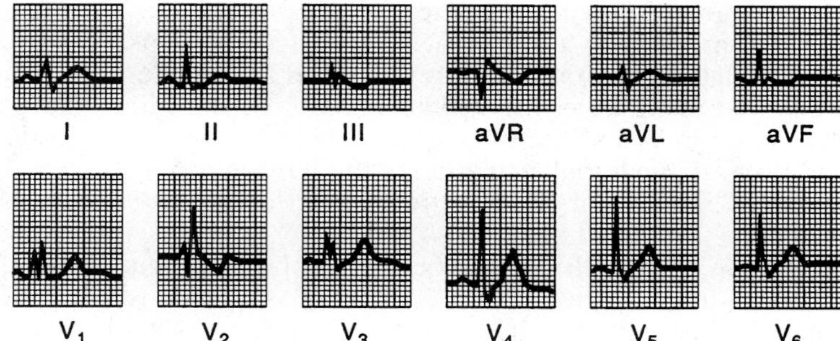

FIGURE 11–41. Right bundle branch block. (Redrawn from Marriott, H. J. L. [1988]. *Practical electrocardiography* [p. 68]. © 1988, The Williams & Wilkins Co., Baltimore.)

branch blocks, it follows that repolarization is altered as well. The terminal component of the QRS complex is opposite in polarity to the resultant T wave. This is a normal consequence of bundle branch blocks. Myocardial disease should be suspected when the T-wave deflection is in the same direction as the terminal component of the QRS complex (Conover, 1992).

Right Bundle Branch Block

The RBB is a long, thin stem, descending along the right ventricular surface of the septum to the right ventricular apex, and then sweeping upward along the lateral endocardial wall. The RBB has a longer refractory period than the LBB, and because of its thin structure, it is more vulnerable to pathologic factors. Blood supply to the RBB comes from the septal perforating branches of the LAD coronary artery, which supplies the anterior surface of the left ventricle.

RBB block (RBBB) is most commonly caused by ischemic heart disease in the anterior septum and degeneration of the conduction system, causing fibrosis and interruption of the conduction fibers. It may be accompanied by rapid heart rates because of its longer refractory period, and it also frequently accompanies supraventricular premature contractions, as is discussed later.

ELECTROCARDIOGRAPHIC FEATURES OF RBBB. V_1 is the best diagnostic lead for the determination of RBBB (Fig. 11–41). V_1 normally shows a small R wave, indicative of septal depolarization, followed by a deep S wave, reflecting the depolarization of the left ventricle. Left ventricular depolarization, because of its magnitude, normally obscures right ventricular depolarization. In RBBB, septal depolarization proceeds normally through the septum and left ventricle, and the right ventricle is depolarized by forces coming from the left ventricle through cells in the intraventricular septum. Figure 11–42 shows the sequence of ventricular activation in RBBB and left bundle branch blocks (LBBB). In V_1, normal septal depolarization causes the normal small r from septal depolarization to be present, followed by an S wave from left ventricular depolarization, and an R′ caused by late right ventricular depolarization. This unopposed right ventricular de-

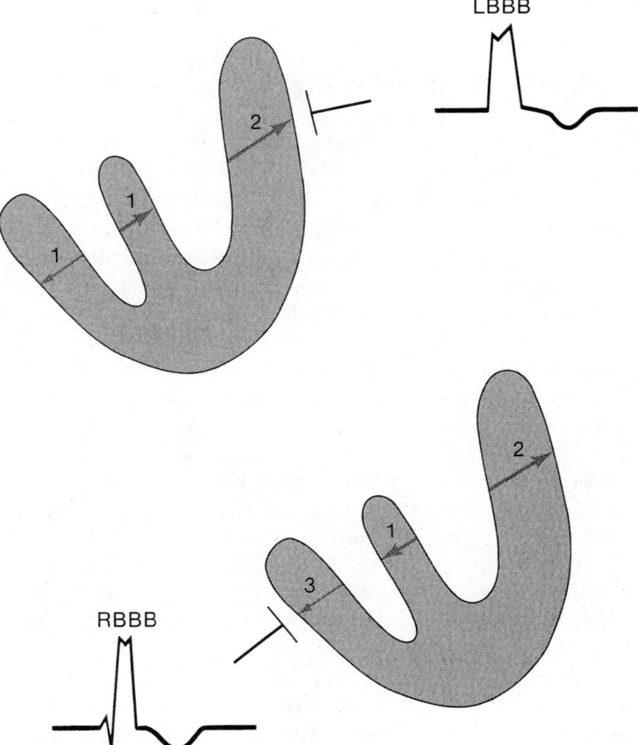

FIGURE 11–42. Sequence of ventricular activation in bundle branch block (BBB). In left bundle branch block (LBBB) (*upper diagram*), the septum is activated (1) exclusively from the right side at the same time that the free wall of the right ventricle (1) is activated. The meager forces of the free wall are overshadowed by the much stronger septal forces. Once the septum and the right ventricle have been depolarized, the left ventricle alone remains and the direction of its activation (2) is similar to that of the septum; hence the complex of LBBB tends to be monophasic and is upright in V_6. In right BBB (*lower diagram*), the septum is first activated, as in the normal heart, from the left side (1); a moment later, activation begins in the left ventricular free wall (2) but, because septal forces are simultaneously spreading in the opposite direction, the free wall deflection (S wave in V_1) is dwarfed. Once the septum and left ventricular free wall have been depolarized, all that is left is the right ventricular free wall. Its feeble forces now are unopposed, and so write the largest deflection of the ventricular complex (R′ in V_1). (Redrawn from Marriott, H. J. L. (1988). *Practical electrocardiography* [p. 67]. © 1988, The Williams & Wilkins Co., Baltimore.)

polarization causes the electrical axis of current to swing sharply back to the right. In V_6, late right ventricular depolarization inscribes reciprocal late deep S waves. If septal forces are lost, as in anteroseptal MI, the small r in V_1 and the small q in V_6 will not be present. Because the initial activation of the septum is normal, RBBB does not obscure the pattern of anterior wall MI.

An rSr′ with a QRS of 0.10 or 0.11 second has been called an incomplete RBBB in the past. It is questionable whether anatomically there is such a thing as an incomplete block. Terms such as "borderline" or "incomplete" may be used within quotation marks to indicate that the diagnosis is merely a description of the ECG.

Left Bundle Branch Block

The LBB arises nearly perpendicularly from the common bundle, and the RBB is a more direct extension of the His bundle. It almost immediately subdivides into the left anterior and posterior fascicles.

Idiopathic bundle branch fibrosis is the most common cause of LBBB. The next most common causes are hypertension, anteroseptal MI, and aortic stenosis. It also may be encountered in patients with cardiomyopathy, myocarditis, and other congenital heart diseases (Mirvis, 1993). When LBBB occurs acutely, it is almost always the result of an acute anteroseptal MI.

The consequences of complete LBBB are similar but opposite to those of RBBB. In LBBB, right ventricular depolarization occurs normally, followed by activation of the septum from right to left, and subsequent activation of the left ventricle. The normal initial activation of the septum is disturbed, and the first part of the QRS is altered, causing normal septal q waves in the left chest leads to disappear.

The QRS complex in LBBB has the same general orientation as in normal depolarization, although it is wide and bizarre in appearance (see Fig. 11–42 for the sequence of ventricular activation in bundle branch blocks). Thus, the main current is directed leftward, away from lead V_1 (causing a deep S wave in that lead) and toward lead V_6 (causing a tall R wave in that lead) (Fig. 11–43). There are many variations in the shape of the QRS complex: unusually high voltage, either deep S waves in lead V_1, V_2, and V_3, or tall R waves in leads I, aVL, V_5, and V_6. There may be very small r waves in leads V_1 through V_3. In addition, there may be some delay in the time elapsing from onset of the QRS to its peak amplitude in leads I, aVL, V_5, and V_6, manifested as a less steep upstroke (or downstroke in negatively deflecting complexes) of the initial portion of the QRS (Mirvis, 1993). This initial upstroke has been called the "intrinsicoid deflection." A delayed intrinsicoid deflection in lead V_5 or V_6 of 0.06 second or more is a feature of LBBB.

LEFT BUNDLE BRANCH BLOCK AND MYOCARDIAL INFARCTION. In the presence of LBBB, an MI cannot usually be diagnosed. LBBB is capable of masking Q waves of infarction because the initial septal vector is directed from right to left, and the infarct is inscribed during the latter part of the QRS complex after septal activation is complete. Consequently, a Q wave cannot be registered except when there is extensive septal infarction (Braunwald, 1992). According to Marriott (1988), "The reputation for difficulty resides in the fact that myocardial infarction and LBBB have opposing designs on the QRS complex—they produce a tug-of-war on the QRS-writing stylus, and sometimes one and sometimes the other wins." In the presence of LBBB, one must look for disproportionate ST-T elevation or depression and loss of the normal ST segment concavity or convexity. An infarction will cause more exaggerated ST elevation than could be explained solely by an LBBB. The evolution of ECG changes accompanying an MI provides further evidence that the changes are the result of an MI and not merely LBBB. By concentrating on the ST-T segment displacement, approximately two-thirds of infarctions can be recognized (Marriott, 1988).

Hemiblocks

Block may occur in the left main bundle before it separates into the fascicles, or it may be present in one or all

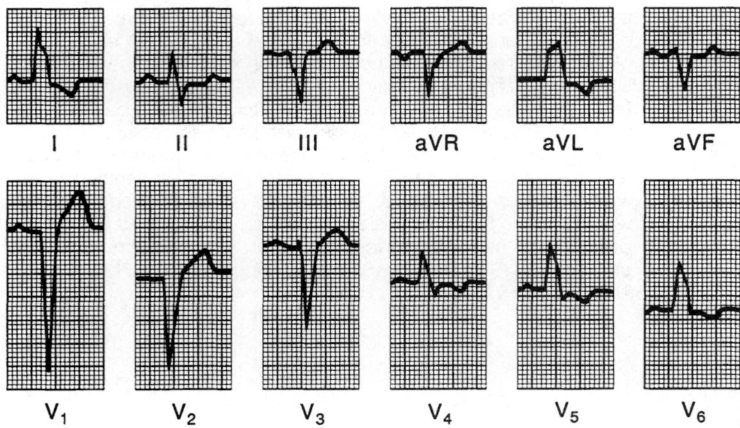

FIGURE 11–43. Left bundle branch block. (Redrawn from Marriott, H. J. L. [1988]. *Practical electrocardiography* [p. 68]. © 1988, The Williams & Wilkins Co., Baltimore.)

of the three major divisions. Although there are three major fascicles of the LBB, the centriseptal branch exerts little influence on the frontal plane axis. Therefore, for the purposes of ECG interpretation, the fascicles usually are discussed as if there were only the anterior and posterior divisions. Consequently, a block of one of these two branches of the left bundle is commonly referred to as a hemiblock. Monofascicular, bifascicular, or trifascicular block refers to block in one, two, or all of the major tributaries of the right bundle branch, the left anterior branch (also called left anterosuperior branch), and the left posterior branch (also called left posteroinferior branch).

Hemiblocks do not cause a prolonged QRS complex because of the rapid spread of electrical activity into the blocked areas. The QRS usually is of normal shape, without unusual notching, delayed upstroke, ST segment changes, or T-wave abnormalities. The major effect that hemiblocks have on the ECG is axis deviation.

LEFT ANTERIOR HEMIBLOCK. The anterior fascicle of the LBB is relatively long and thin and supplies the anterior and superior portions of the left ventricle. It lies superiorly and laterally to the left posterior fascicle. Blood supply to the anterior fascicle comes from the LAD coronary artery, which also supplies the right bundle. This branch lies close to the RBB, and consequently these two fascicles are often injured simultaneously. The anterior fascicle is considered the most vulnerable structure of the conduction system because of its anatomic location in the hemodynamically turbulent aortic area, its size and length, and its single blood supply. A block of the anterosuperior division of the left bundle is called a left anterior hemiblock. With left anterior hemiblock, conduction down the left anterior fascicle is blocked. As a result, the impulse rushes down the left posterior fascicle to the inferior surface of the heart. The signal is conducted superiorly and to the left, causing left axis deviation, inscribing tall positive R waves in the left lateral leads (lead I), and deep S waves in inferior leads II and aVF (Fig. 11–44).

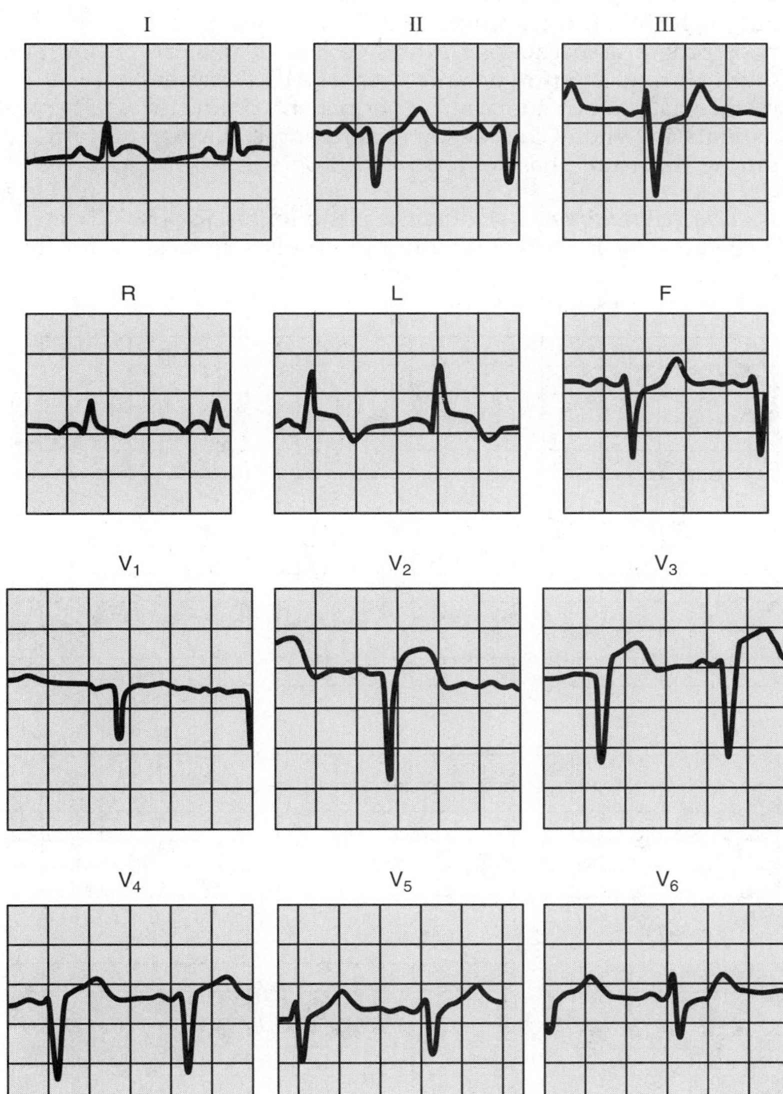

FIGURE 11–44. Anterior hemiblock in a patient with acute anterior wall myocardial infarction. Note the abnormal left axis deviation (greater than −30°), the normal QRS duration, and the q waves in leads I and aVL. (Reproduced by permission from Conover, M. [1992]. *Understanding electrocardiography* [6th ed., p. 332]. St. Louis: Mosby–Year Book.)

These alterations in the ECG complexes result in left axis deviation of −30° or greater. As was discussed earlier, the simplest method to determine axis is to examine the QRS complexes in leads I and aVF. With left axis deviation, the QRS complex is positive in lead I and negative in aVF.

The LAD artery supplies the RBB and the left anterior fascicle. Therefore, RBBB and left anterior hemiblock are commonly associated with extensive anteroseptal infarction. The development of RBBB in patients with anterior or anteroseptal MIs has prognostic significance. In a study of 1,200 patients (Lie et al., 1976), 612 patients had anterior MIs. Of these 612 patients, RBBB developed in 70, LBBB developed in 8, and 13 had preexisting bundle branch blocks. Inpatient mortality rates for these patients were 71%, 21%, and 28%, respectively. The mortality rate for patients without conduction disturbances was 14%.

More recently, Ricou and associates (1991) found that patients who had an RBBB after an anterior MI had increased incidence of left ventricular failure, longer length of stay, and increased mortality 1 year after discharge compared with similar patients without an RBBB. Thus, acquired RBBB indicates a very poor prognosis because of extensive loss of myocardium during anterior or anteroseptal MI. Disagreement exists about the use of permanent pacing in patients in whom conduction disturbances develop during the acute phase of anterior MI.

LEFT POSTERIOR HEMIBLOCK. The posterior fascicle of the left bundle is short and wide and supplies the posterior and inferior portions of the left ventricle through a fan-like array of conducting fibers. The blood supply to the posterior fascicle is provided by the RCA and LCA. It is the least vulnerable fascicle because of its size and dual blood supply. In left posterior hemiblock, the impulse travels down the left anterior fascicle, causing ventricular myocardial depolarization to occur in a superior-to-inferior and left-to-right direction. The axis of depolarization is directed downward and rightward, inscribing tall R waves in II and aVF and deep S waves in aVL. The result is right axis deviation (or an electrical axis of between +90° and +180°).

Left posterior hemiblock is seen in diseased hearts, usually in combination with RBBB (Fig. 11–45), whereas left anterior hemiblock may be seen in healthy as well as diseased hearts. Other potential causes of axis deviation (e.g., chronic lung disease, ventricular hypertrophy) must be ruled out before the diagnoses of right or left hemiblock are determined by means of the ECG.

Monitoring Implications With Conduction Defects

The preceding information has implications for monitoring patients in critical care units. The patient who has an RBBB should be monitored in lead II to observe for left anterior hemiblock. If a left anterior or posterior hemiblock is present, the patient should be monitored for the development of RBBB in lead V_1 or MCL_1. Pa-

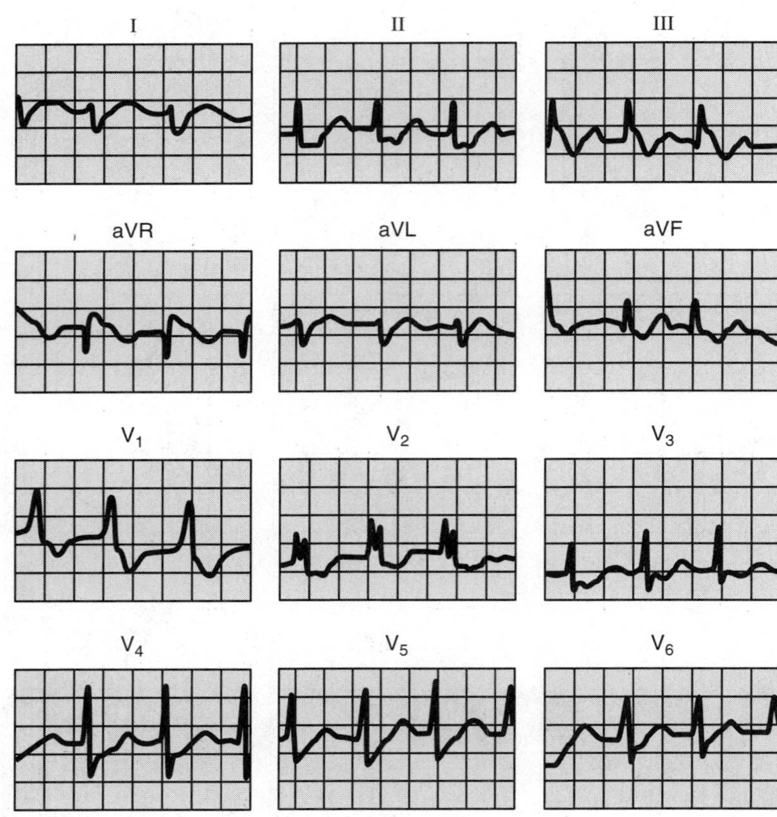

FIGURE 11–45. Bifascicular block (right bundle branch block + posterior hemiblock) in a patient with an old inferior wall and evolving anterior wall myocardial infarction. Note the abnormal right axis deviation. (Reproduced by permission from Conover, M. [1996]. *Understanding electrocardiography* [7th ed., p. 381]. St. Louis: Mosby–Year Book.)

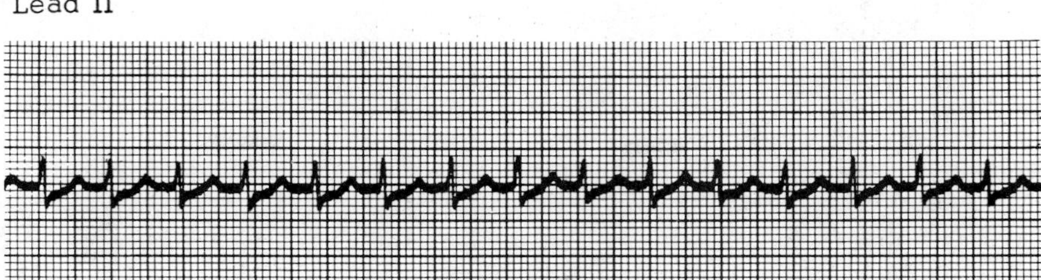

FIGURE 11–46. Lown-Ganong-Levine syndrome. (From Chou, T. [1991]. *Electrocardiography in clinical practice* [3rd ed., p. 449]. Philadelphia: W. B. Saunders.)

tients who have had a recent MI should be monitored in lead V_1 or MCL_1 as well. This strategy will practically guarantee that a new bundle branch block will be detected because both RBBB and LBBB bring about dramatic changes from the normal QRS pattern in both of these leads (Drew, 1991). If for some reason these leads are impractical, V_6 or MCL_6 can be used; however, RBBB will be less obvious in these two leads. When a bifascicular block is present (i.e., RBBB plus left anterior hemiblock or left posterior hemiblock), the patient should be monitored closely for other conduction disturbances (AV block) in the lead that shows the most obvious P waves and QRS complexes.

PREEXCITATION SYNDROMES

"Preexcitation" is a name given to syndromes that permit the ventricles to depolarize earlier than would be possible if an impulse had been conducted through the normal AV conduction system. A number of different accessory pathways have been discovered that allow impulses to bypass the AV node and arrive in the ventricles precipitously. In addition, special pathways have been identified that allow signals to be conducted through the AV node in an accelerated fashion. These tracts are remnants of embryonic stages of development when the atria and ventricles formed an anatomic and electrical continuum across the length of the primitive heart. At 33 to 37 days postconception, these fibers should merge into the AV node with its specialized properties. These accessory pathways may persist in otherwise healthy hearts, or they may be associated with mitral valve prolapse or various congenital disorders.

There are four types of accessory pathways or syndromes discussed in the literature. They include Lown-Ganong-Levine (LGL) syndrome, Mahaim fibers, concealed unidirectional retrograde accessory pathway (CURAP), and Wolff-Parkinson-White (WPW) syndrome.

In LGL syndrome, the accessory pathway is called the James bundle. The pathway originates in the atrial myocardium, inserting into the bundle of His, or the RBB or LBB, thereby bypassing the AV node. ECG features include a short PR interval, absence of a delta wave, and a normal QRS complex (Fig. 11–46). It also is characterized by a paroxysmal tachycardia. When a history of tachycardia is uncertain and ECG findings exhibit a PR interval of less than 0.12 second and a normal QRS complex, the label "accelerated AV conduction" may be more appropriate than LGL syndrome (Chou, 1991). Another name that is frequently used to refer to LGL syndrome is the "short-PR-normal-QRS syndrome" (Marriott & Conover, 1989).

Another preexcitation syndrome, although unnamed, involves the Mahaim fibers. These fibers are muscular bridges that attach proximally at the lower portion of the AV node and distally in the area of the interventricular septum (Chou, 1991) (Fig. 11–47). Conduction through Mahaim fibers generates a normal P-R interval, a delta wave, and possibly a wide QRS complex. The QRS complex associated with this syndrome is not as wide as the one seen with WPW syndrome. The significance of Mahaim fibers is that they may potentially provide one arm of an AV reentry circuit that may result in paroxysmal supraventricular tachycardia (SVT).

The most recent accessory tract to be identified is the CURAP, so called because it does not produce a characteristic pattern at normal sinus rates (Fig. 11–48). This pathway is embedded in the left free wall

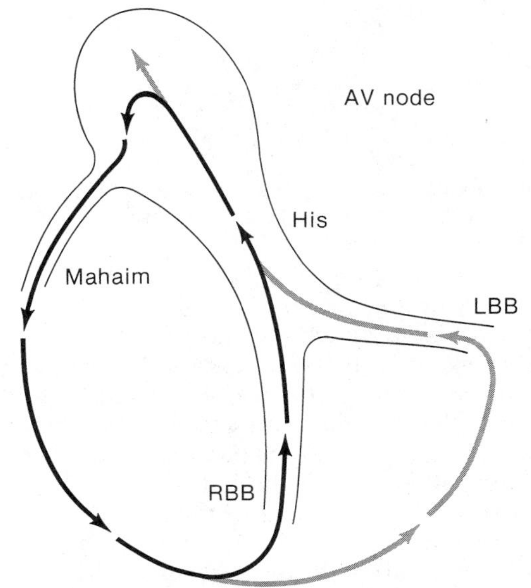

FIGURE 11–47. Mahaim fibers. (Redrawn from Gallagher, J. J., Smith, W. M., Kasall, J. H., et al. [1989]. Role of Mahaim fibers in cardiac arrhythmias in man. *Circulation, 64,* 176. By permission of the American Heart Association, Inc.)

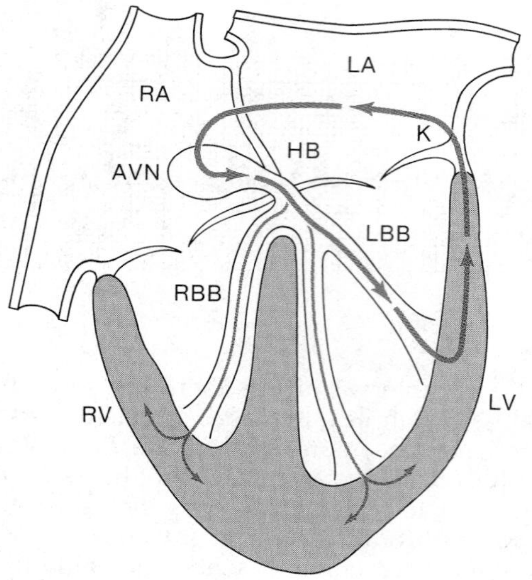

FIGURE 11–48. Concealed unidirectional retrograde accessory pathway. (Redrawn from Horowitz, L. N., & Josephson, M. E. [1980]. *Practical Cardiology, 6*[3], 129–141.)

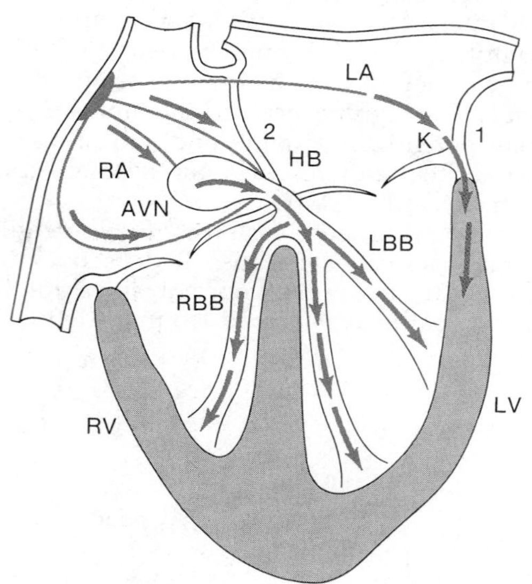

FIGURE 11–49. Wolff-Parkinson-White syndrome conduction pathway. (Redrawn from Horowitz, L. N., & Josephson, M. E. [1980]. *Practical Cardiology, 6*[3], 129–141.)

of the heart, is unidirectional, and, in 95% of the cases, conducts exclusively in a retrograde fashion (Ross, 1984). Its most preferred concealed reentrant circuit consists of the AV node, the His bundle, the LBB (or RBB when the left bundle is blocked), a unidirectional accessory pathway, and the left atrium. Clues to the diagnosis of CURAP include rates greater than 200 beats per minute, inverted P waves after QRS complexes in lead I, atrial flutter or atrial fibrillation during paroxysmal SVT, and a decrease in the tachycardia rate with LBBB. CURAP has been shown to be the second most common cause of reentrant SVT (Ross, 1984).

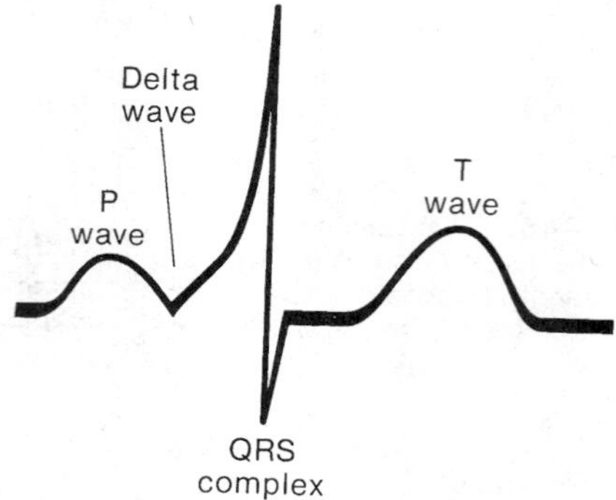

FIGURE 11–50. Slurred upstroke of the QRS (delta wave).

The remainder of this section is devoted to a discussion of WPW syndrome because it is the most commonly occurring preexcitation syndrome.

Wolff-Parkinson-White Syndrome

In WPW syndrome, the bypass pathway is the bundle of Kent. It connects the right or left atria and ventricles (Fig. 11–49). These connections were described by Kent as early as 1893, but it was not until the early 1940s that the accessory AV connections were confirmed on autopsy. The actual prevalence of WPW syndrome is unknown. However, approximately 0.1% to 0.3% of all ECGs performed will exhibit the WPW syndrome pattern (Cain et al., 1992; Oren et al., 1993). Of those patients who manifest the ECG pattern of WPW syndrome, approximately half have true WPW syndrome or a history of paroxysmal atrial dysrhythmias (Berry, 1994).

WPW syndrome is characterized by a bypass pathway between the right atrium and right ventricle or left atrium and left ventricle. The anomalous fibers may be inserted either on the intraventricular septum or on the outer (or parietal) wall of the ventricle (Phillips & Feeney, 1990). WPW syndrome typically causes several changes on the ECG. First, the PR interval is shortened to less than 0.12 second, because the impulse has bypassed the AV node. Second, the QRS is usually wider than normal because of the premature activation of the ventricles. Actually, the QRS complex in WPW syndrome represents a fusion beat, because most of the ventricle is activated via the normal conducting pathways and only a small portion is depolarized early by means of the bundle of Kent. This small portion that depolarizes early causes a characteristic initial upstroke on the ECG called a delta wave (Fig. 11–50). This wave may be present in only a few leads.

There are two types of WPW syndrome, types A and B (Chou, 1991). In type A, the accessory pathway connects the free wall of the left atrium to the left ventricle. Lead V_1 usually has a wide QRS that is upright, inverted T waves, and depressed ST segments, somewhat resembling an RBBB or right ventricular hyper-

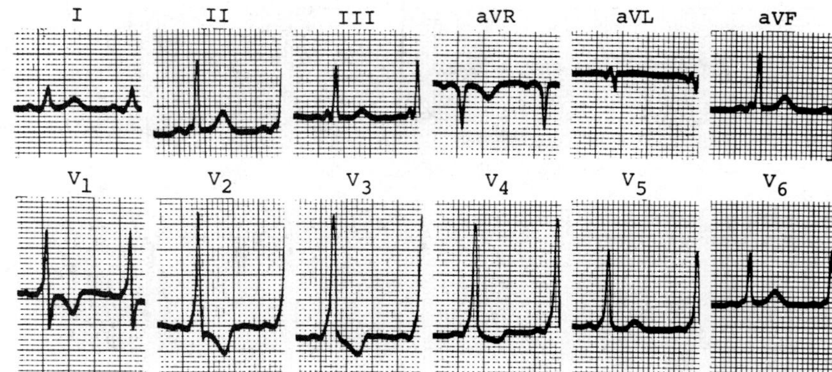

FIGURE 11–51. Type A Wolff-Parkinson-White syndrome. (From Chou, T. [1991]. *Electrocardiography in clinical practice* [3rd ed., p. 434]. Philadelphia: W. B. Saunders.)

trophy (RVH) (Fig. 11–51). Such a pattern can be anticipated because the left ventricle depolarizes first and then the impulse spreads anteriorly to the right ventricle. Type B involves an accessory pathway connecting the right atrium to the right ventricle. It is recognized by a negative delta wave and QRS complex in V_1, resulting from ventricular depolarization that is anterior to posterior, thereby resembling an LBBB (Fig. 11–52).

The most prevalent dysrhythmias associated with WPW syndrome are AV reciprocating tachycardia and atrial fibrillation (Berry, 1994). AV reciprocating tachycardia is a reentrant dysrhythmia. Reentrant dysrhythmias require the existence of two pathways, each with distinct conduction characteristics. With this syndrome, these two pathways include the normal AV node–His–Purkinje system and the accessory pathway. The accessory pathway is composed of muscle tissue and is therefore electrophysiologically different from the AV nodal tissue. These differences include the conduction velocity, the refractory period, and the response the tissue exhibits to medications.

A premature beat usually initiates AV reciprocating tachycardia. When a premature beat occurs, one of the pathways may be refractory to conduction. The impulse then travels across the other nonrefractory pathway and stimulates the atrial or ventricular muscle. As the wave of depolarization extends across the myocardium, it may find the alternate pathway has now sufficiently recovered and is capable of conducting the impulse back to the initiating chamber. With proper conditions, a reentrant tachycardia will begin and persist until it is interrupted chemically or electrically, or the tissue preceding the impulse becomes refractory and is no longer capable of depolarization.

Atrial fibrillation presents in approximately 30% to 40% of patients with WPW syndrome (Berry, 1994), which is greater than the frequency observed in the general population. The etiology of this is unclear, but it is linked to the presence of the accessory pathway. Atrial fibrillation may have life-threatening consequences by precipitating ventricular fibrillation in patients with rapid conduction due to an accessory pathway with short anterograde refractory period (<250 milliseconds) (Brembilla-Perrot & Ghawi, 1993; Duckeck & Kuck, 1993).

Aberrancy

Aberrant ventricular conduction is transient bundle branch block or hemiblock resulting from phase 3

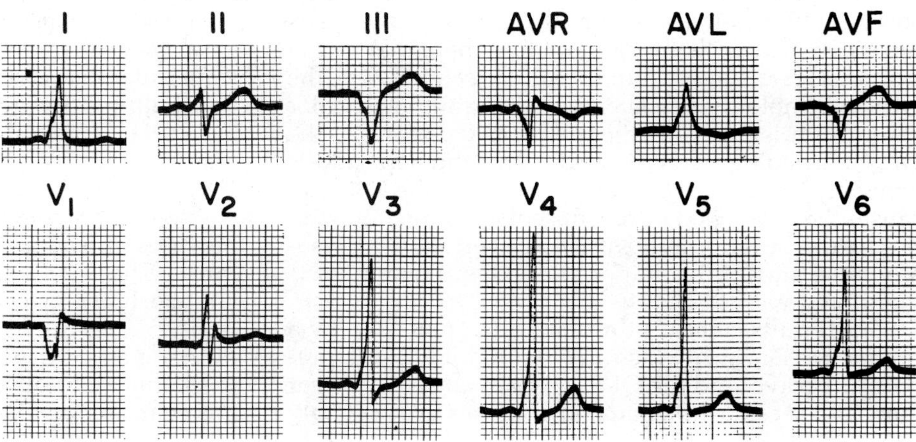

FIGURE 11–52. Type B Wolff-Parkinson-White syndrome. (From Chou, T. [1991]. *Electrocardiography in clinical practice* [3rd ed., p. 434]. Philadelphia: W. B. Saunders.)

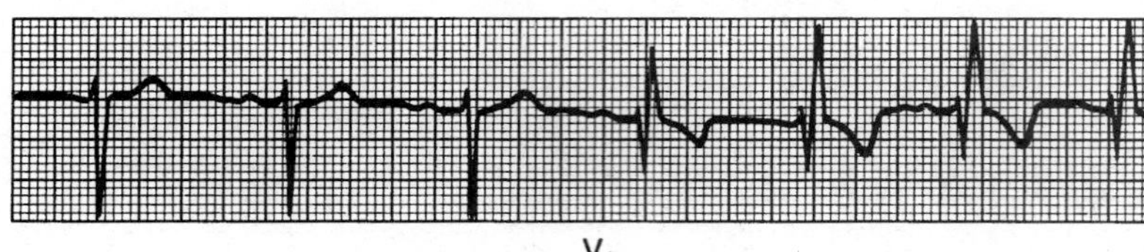

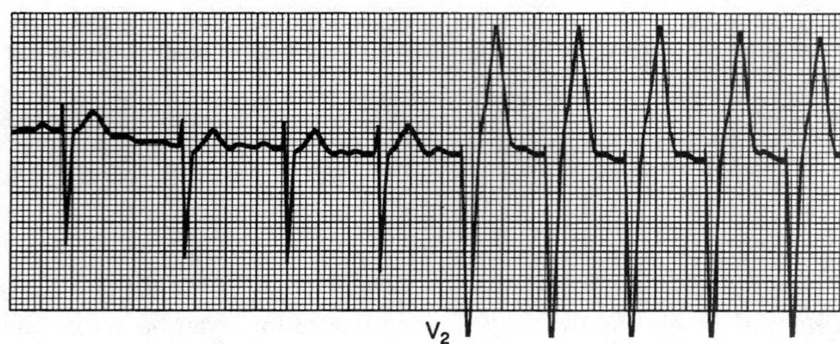

FIGURE 11–53. Aberrant ventricular conduction in two different leads. (Reproduced by permission from Marriott, H. J. L., & Conover, M. [1989]. *Advanced concepts in arrhythmias.* St. Louis: C. V. Mosby.)

block, phase 4 block, or retrograde concealed conduction (Conover, 1992). The outcome of each of these phenomena is activation of a bundle branch when the cells of that bundle have not completely repolarized from the previous depolarization. Aberrant ventricular conduction is characterized by prolonged spread of a supraventricular impulse through the ventricles. The length of the refractory period is directly related to the length of the preceding cycle (RR interval) (Bigger, Jr., 1994). The LBB depolarizes slightly faster than the right. Therefore, the RBB is more commonly the cause of an aberrantly conducted impulse. His bundle studies have shown that a wide rSR′ complex without previous RBBB is aberrant and is rarely caused by ventricular ectopy (Wellens et al., 1978).

Correct interpretation of the ECG is essential. The following criteria can be used to determine the source of wide, bizarre QRS complexes. Ventricular rhythms originate in the ventricle and thus are not preceded by a premature P wave. If a P wave is present, it will occur on time or may be fused with the premature ventricular complex. The QRS duration is usually wide (0.12 second or greater), and the impulse is usually followed by a compensatory pause (Fig. 11–53). Wellens and associates (1978) suggested that the QRS has a left axis deviation greater than $-30°$ and that there may be fusion beats and sinus capture beats. In V_1 (or MCL_1), the QRS morphology associated with aberrant ventricular conduction is a triphasic pattern (rSR′), whereas the QRS morphology in V_6 is a qRS and the R:S ratio is generally less than 1. Because it is usually the RBB that causes the prolonged intraventricular conduction with premature beats, supraventricular aberrant beats usually have an RBBB configuration when the patient is monitored with MCL_1.

Supraventricular rhythms are often preceded by a premature P wave, which may be hidden in the preceding T wave, and the QRS complex can be narrower than 0.12 second. Junctional aberrancies are probably the most difficult complexes to differentiate from ventricular premature beats because they may not be preceded by P waves.

Electrophysiologic studies (EPS) may be performed to differentiate between supraventricular and ventricular dysrhythmias. The EPS provides an intracardiac recording of the electrical activity of the heart. This procedure can differentiate the origin of dysrhythmias, identify characteristics of those dysrhythmias, and evaluate the efficacy of antidysrhythmic therapies such as drugs, pacing, and surgical interventions. The EPS is performed in a cardiac catheterization laboratory and involves introducing catheters into the heart by means of the venous system (usually the femoral, subclavian, internal jugular, or antecubital vein). The catheter tips are positioned at specific sites along the conduction pathway or chamber wall, usually the high right atrium, the bundle of His, the coronary sinus, and the right ventricular apex (Darling, 1994). Sometimes the electrode may be positioned at a reentrant pathway within the ventricle. Recordings are made of intervals of the surface ECG (PR, QRS, QT, and RR) and on the intracardiac ECG (atrial potential, atrium to His, and His to ventricle).

Ventricular tachycardia may be induced by rapid atrial or ventricular pacing or by delivering atrial or ventricular extrasystoles during a paced or spontaneous rhythm. Each extrasystole is delivered slightly earlier in the refractory period in an attempt to find the crucial point of stimulating tachycardia (Darling, 1994). When tachycardia is induced, its characteristics are noted and compared with ECGs recorded during previous episodes of spontaneous ventricular tachycardia. The bundle of His ECG also is inspected for the relationship between atrial and ventricular depolarization.

Ashman's phenomenon, commonly seen in atrial fibrillation, is another example of aberrant conduction. It is characterized by a wide, aberrantly conducted su-

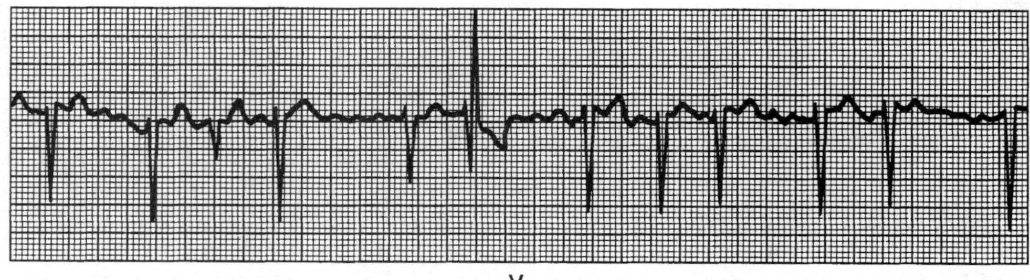

FIGURE 11–54. Ashman's phenomenon. (Reproduced by permission from Marriott, H. J. L., & Conover, M. [1989]. *Advanced concepts in arrhythmias.* St. Louis: C. V. Mosby.)

praventricular beat occurring after a QRS complex that is preceded by a long pause (Fig. 11–54). The bundle branches reset their rate of repolarization according to the length of the preceding beat. If the preceding beat occurred a relatively long time ago, repolarization is slower. If a supraventricular impulse passes through the AV node before repolarization is complete, that beat will be conducted aberrantly, producing a wide, bizarre QRS complex. In Figure 11–54, the sixth beat looks like a premature ventricular contraction but is probably an aberrant beat because it occurred after a long–short cycle.

The value of Ashman's phenomenon in atrial fibrillation is controversial, however. According to Marriott and Conover (1989), because there is concealed conduction (rampant electrical activity of the atria incompletely penetrates the bundle of His and bundle branches), the exact time the bundle branch is activated cannot be ascertained from the surface ECG. This concealed conduction results in an irregular ventricular response and pauses that are longer than the actual refractory period of the AV conduction network. Therefore, if an aberrant beat ends a long–short cycle sequence during atrial fibrillation, it may be the result of refractoriness of a bundle branch secondary to concealed conduction, rather than because of changes in the length of the ventricular cycle.

Treatment of tachydysrhythmias associated with WPW syndrome depends on the patient's hemodynamic status and the mechanism of the dysrhythmia. If the patient is unstable, immediate electrical cardioversion is indicated. However, there are several options available if the patient is stable. These alternatives include antidysrhythmic drug therapy, Valsalva maneuver, carotid sinus massage, antitachycardia pacemakers, and ablation of the accessory pathway (Berry, 1994).

Ablation, the localized destruction, isolation, or excision of cardiac tissue that is considered to be dysrhythmogenic, is the most definitive treatment available. Ablative therapy can be accomplished by means of surgical transection or serial application of radiofrequency waves via intracardiac catheters (Berry, 1994; Finkelmeier, 1994).

Catheter techniques are the preferred method of ablation for most reentrant dysrhythmias, and they are the most widely used nonpharmacologic intervention for treatment of drug-resistant tachydysrhythmias (Finkelmeier, 1994; Scheinman et al., 1991). Among the supraventricular dysrhythmias most commonly treated with catheter ablation techniques are those resulting from anomalous atrial–ventricular conduction or AV nodal reentrant pathways. Surgical ablation techniques are most commonly used for ventricular tachydysrhythmias and for SVTs that were not successfully eradicated by catheter procedures (Finkelmeier, 1994).

Catheter ablation therapy consists of destroying localized areas of tissue with energy delivered by means of an intracardiac catheter. To date, the safest and most effective approach used to perform catheter ablation is the use of radiofrequency as the energy source (Finkelmeier, 1994). This procedure usually involves percutaneous insertion of four catheters by way of the femoral or brachial veins. These catheters are advanced in retrograde fashion into the right side of the heart. Once the catheters are in place, radiofrequency energy is delivered. This radiofrequency is obtained from low-power, high-frequency alternating current, and can be delivered in graded quantities of energy to a specific area of tissue (Scheinman et al., 1991). The resultant lesions are smaller and more controllable than those produced by direct-current electrical energy (Craney, 1993). Application of the radiofrequency energy usually is not felt by the patient, although it has been reported that up to 40% of patients may experience some mild chest discomfort during ablation (Borgrefe et al., 1990). After the procedure, the patient requires 4 to 6 hours of bed rest. Vital signs, insertion site, and the limb distal to the catheter insertion site must be monitored as well. This treatment usually requires that the patient be hospitalized for 24 to 48 hours (Finkelmeier, 1994). Although complications resulting from this procedure are rare, they include arterial injury related to catheter insertion, AV block, and cardiac tamponade.

Surgical ablation is a less frequently performed alternative treatment of tachydysrhythmias. This procedure is performed during a cardiac surgery. It includes incision of tissue, resection of endocardial tissue, and cryoablation (Finkelmeier, 1994). Cryoablation consists of direct application of an extremely cold probe to dysrhythmogenic cardiac tissue to obliterate it. This technique is usually used adjunctively during cardiac surgeries.

VENTRICULAR DYSRHYTHMIAS

More than 400,000 Americans die suddenly each year, most from ventricular tachycardia or fibrillation (Kay & Bubien, 1992), making this a serious concern for critical care nurses. Ventricular dysrhythmias are known to affect adversely the prognosis of patients who have sustained acute MIs, but ventricular premature depolarizations (VPDs) in individuals with no evidence of heart disease do not necessarily predict an unfavorable clinical course. Recurrent ventricular tachycardia most commonly occurs in patients with chronic coronary artery disease and a history of MI.

Historically, critical care nurses have been aware of the need to monitor closely for ventricular dysrhythmias and to treat patients either prophylactically during the first few days of an MI or when the following usual criteria are observed: more than five VPDs per minute, multiformed VPDs, repetitive VPDs (three or more in a row), or when VPDs occur early in the cardiac cycle (R-on-T phenomenon). It was thought that these criteria warned of ventricular fibrillation. More recently, doubts have been cast on the significance of "warning dysrhythmias" (Tisdale, 1991; Wesley et al., 1991). Investigations have demonstrated that as many as 50% of patients with ventricular fibrillation during an acute MI may not exhibit such warning VPDs. Warning dysrhythmias may occur relatively infrequently in a given patient, or may occur only seconds before fibrillation is observed. Conversely, warning dysrhythmias may develop in as many as 50% of patients who do not go on to ventricular fibrillation (Antman & Rutherford, 1986).

There is increasing concern about the benefit of prophylactic lidocaine. With the evolution of more sophisticated coronary care practices, fewer patients experience serious ventricular dysrhythmias. Meta-analytic findings from randomized control studies spanning the years 1969 to 1988 showed that the incidence of primary ventricular fibrillation in MI patients decreased from 4.51% in 1970 to 0.35% in 1990 (Antman & Berlin, 1992). Results of this meta-analysis further revealed that 400 patients would have needed prophylactic lidocaine to prevent one episode of ventricular fibrillation. In addition, prophylactic lidocaine has not been shown to have a beneficial effect on mortality, and it may actually increase mortality by reducing countershock efficacy (Tisdale, 1991; Wesley et al., 1991). Thirty-five percent of the population experience adverse effects from lidocaine (Tisdale, 1991). Consequently, cautious administration of prophylactic lidocaine is advised, and it should be used particularly carefully in patients who have a higher risk for ventricular fibrillation. These include patients who are 40 to 50 years of age, who have no previous history of congestive heart failure or acute MI, and who are admitted early after the onset of chest pain (Antman & Rutherford, 1986).

The ECG leads used to monitor for ventricular tachycardia must be chosen with caution. Recently, Drew and Scheinman (1991) found that 38% of patients with confirmed ventricular tachycardia displayed different QRS morphology when both leads V_1 and MCL_1 were recorded simultaneously. This phenomenon was observed even though the complexes were identical in normal sinus rhythm. Therefore, when applying the morphologic criteria for diagnosing ventricular tachycardia, V_1 is the monitoring lead of choice (Drew, 1993; Drew & Scheinman, 1991).

Torsades de Pointes

Torsades de pointes, a form of polymorphic paroxysmal ventricular tachycardia, occurs in the presence of QT prolongation (Fig. 11–55). It is frequently prefibrillatory and appears to be transitional between conventional ventricular tachycardia and ventricular fibrillation (Horowitz, 1994). Its mechanism may be a form of reentry or triggered activity. The pathogenesis is related to reduction in the normal outward flow of potassium during repolarization, hypokalemia, hypocalcemia, or abnormal sympathetic innervation of the heart (Conover, 1992; Kay & Bubien, 1992).

Characteristics of torsades de pointes include:

- Prominent U wave in the conducted sinus beats
- Initiation depends on a characteristic pause
- Irregular rhythm
- Wide QRS complex
- Prolonged QT interval
- Polymorphism
- QRS configuration twists about the isoelectric point, changing axis every 5 to 20 beats (i.e., QRS changing from an upright complex to isoelectric to downward)
- Heart rate may vary from 150 to 400 beats per minute

In many cases, the twisting of the QRS configuration is apparent only in certain ECG leads. Therefore, a 12-lead ECG should be used to record the dysrhythmia.

Torsades de pointes is caused by acquired or congenital conditions and is associated with a prolonged QT interval during periods of normal sinus rhythm. In acquired torsades de pointes, the QT interval may be prolonged by type I and type III antidysrhythmic drugs (quinidine, procainamide, disopyramide, N-acetyl procainamide, sotalol, amiodarone), phenothiazine drugs, antidepressants, erythromycin, electrolyte abnormalities (hypomagnesemia, hypokalemia, hypocalcemia), arsenic poisoning, increased intracranial pressure, and liquid protein diets (Chou, 1991; Conover, 1992; Kay & Bubien, 1992). It is often associated

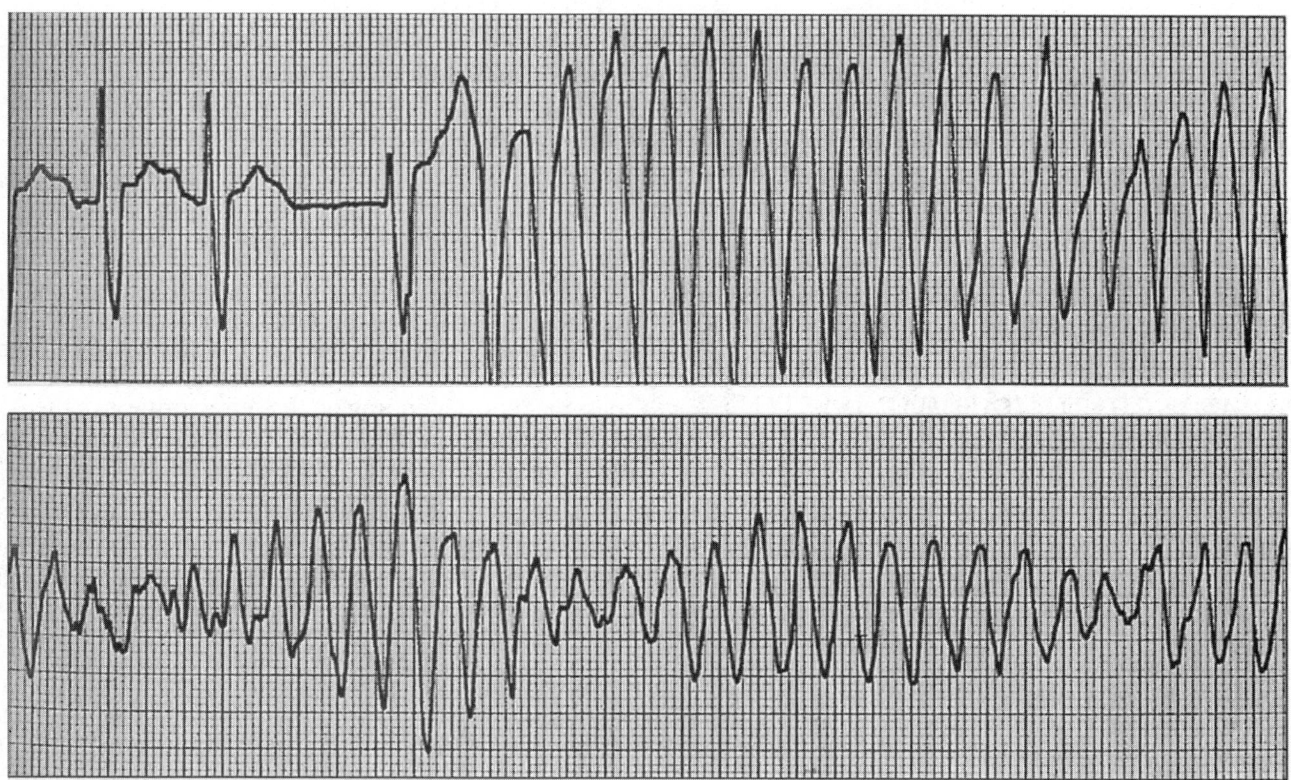

FIGURE 11–55. Torsades de pointes. Note the distortion of the long QT interval as a result of the U wave, the pause before the onset of the tachycardia, and the typical undulating spindle appearance of the pattern. (From the Dr. Alan Lindsay collection.) (Reproduced by permission from Conover, M. B. [1992]. *Understanding electrocardiography* [6th ed., p. 199]. St. Louis: Mosby–Year Book.)

with bradycardia, especially when caused by AV block, and it has been associated with Prinzmetal angina (Chou, 1991). Congenital conditions associated with torsades de pointes include the autosomal recessive Jervell and Lange-Nielsen syndrome with accompanying deafness and the autosomal dominant Romano-Ward syndrome without deafness (Kay & Bubien, 1992).

Treatment of torsades de pointes includes removal of the predisposing cause as well as the use of isoproterenol to increase heart rate and shorten the QT interval, propranolol, phenytoin, and a pacemaker. Some patients with recurrent uncontrolled episodes may require a left stellate ganglionectomy, as well as an implantable cardioverter–defibrillator (Kay & Bubien, 1992).

Monitoring the QT Interval

The QT interval is an important measurement in the routine monitoring of patients in critical care units. The normal value for the QT interval depends on heart rate. As heart rate increases, the QT interval shortens. Conversely, as heart rate decreases, the QT interval lengthens. The normal upper limit for the QT interval in heart rates from 60 to 100 beats per minute ranges between 0.34 to 0.40 second for men and 0.34 to 0.44 second for women (Braunwald, 1992). The formula used to correct the QT interval for heart rate is:

$$QTc = QT/RR$$

where QT is the QT interval measured from the beginning of the QRS complex to the end of the T wave. The RR interval is the time measured between two successive R waves. Generally, a QTc exceeding 0.44 second is prolonged and should be reported, especially in a patient who is receiving antidysrhythmic medications.

The nurse should suspect potential torsades de pointes when the usual treatments, lidocaine and procainamide, are not effective in treating ventricular dysrhythmias. A family and personal history should be obtained from the patient, with a focus on history of syncope or transient palpitations, medication use, and exposure to insecticides.

Correct diagnosis of this form of ventricular tachycardia is critical. If the rhythm is torsades de pointes and the patient receives the usual medications (lidocaine, procainamide, quinidine), the condition will worsen. Similarly, if torsades de pointes is mistaken for SVT with aberrancy, verapamil may be given. Verapamil has been associated with profound hypo-

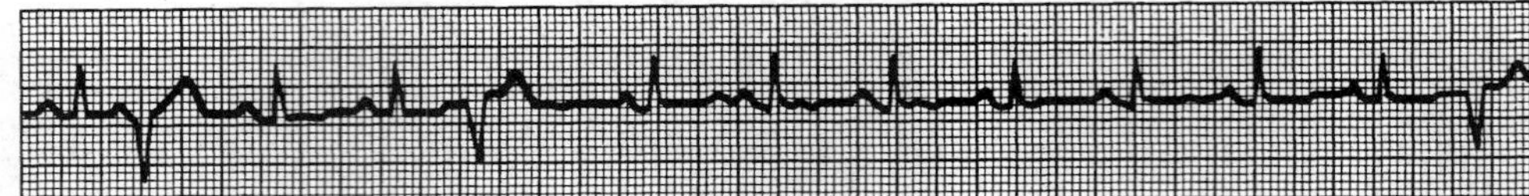

FIGURE 11–56. Parasystole. (Redrawn from Phillips, R., & Feeney, M. [1990]. *The cardiac rhythms* [3rd ed.]. Philadelphia: W. B. Saunders.)

tension and increased mortality when used in the setting of ventricular tachycardia (Steward et al., 1986).

PARADYSRHYTHMIAS: PARASYSTOLE AND AV DISSOCIATION

A paradysrhythmia is an abnormal rhythm in which two pacemakers discharge independently of one another (Mirvis, 1993). One pacemaker is usually the SA node, and the activity of the other pacemaker does not disturb the conduction of the normal sinus impulse. Therefore, complete AV block is not an example of a pardysrhythmia because the conduction of the sinus impulse is blocked through the AV node.

The mechanism seen in paradysrhythmias, with two independent pacemakers activating the heart, could not exist unless the faster rhythm were somehow prevented from taking complete control of the heart. The mechanism that prevents this occurrence is called a "protective" or "entrance" block (Mirvis, 1993). Therefore, entrance blocks impede the invasion and resetting of the ectopic focus by impulses originating from the primary pacemaker (i.e., the SA node). Parasystole and AV dissociation are two forms of paradysrhythmia.

Parasystole

Parasystole is an uncommon dysrhythmia. It is characterized by a primary and secondary pacemaker. The SA node usually is the primary pacemaker and the second is an ectopic site (Mirvis, 1993). It is the result of an abnormality of both automaticity and impulse conduction (Conover, 1992). The parasystolic impulses may originate in the atria, AV junction, ventricles, or the SA node. There is a random relationship between the parasystolic complexes and the underlying rhythm on the ECG recording, and they may or may not appear regularly (Marriott & Conover, 1989).

The most common type of parasystole is one in which the secondary pacemaker competes with the more rapid SA node for control of the heart (Mirvis, 1993). The ventricles may be activated by either of the pacemakers, depending on the refractoriness of the AV node and the ventricles at any point in time. The slower ectopic site will produce an ECG complex with the appearance of an ectopic beat.

A less commonly observed form of parasystole is one in which the rate of impulse discharge from the ectopic site is more rapid than that of the SA node. The probable reason this secondary ectopic focus does not assume complete control of the heart and produce an exclusively ectopic rhythm is that some of the impulses originating in the ectopic site are blocked. At that given point in time, the normal SA node is capable of activating the heart. This phenomenon, called an "exit block" (Mirvis, 1993), limits the number of impulses propagated from the regularly firing ectopic pacemaker. This protection around the ectopic site may be absolute, intermittent, or modulated (Marriott & Conover, 1989). Absolute protection does not allow the underlying rhythm to determine whether the parasystolic focus fires. Intermittent parasystole may have absolute protection, or the protection may be early portions of the cycle (phase 3). In its modulated form, the parasystolic focus is protected from being reset but does not necessarily preserve fixed-cycle intervals.

This dysrhythmia is most commonly seen in association with organic heart disease and has been found to be relatively benign. Atrial parasystoles have been observed in patients who have had heart transplants, as a result of SA node impulse formation and atrial activation from the donor heart and the recipient's residual SA node and atria. Obviously, the P waves that result from depolarization of the recipient's own residual atria never bring about ventricular capture. Patients with implanted asynchronous pacemakers may display an iatrogenic form of parasystole (Goldman, 1989).

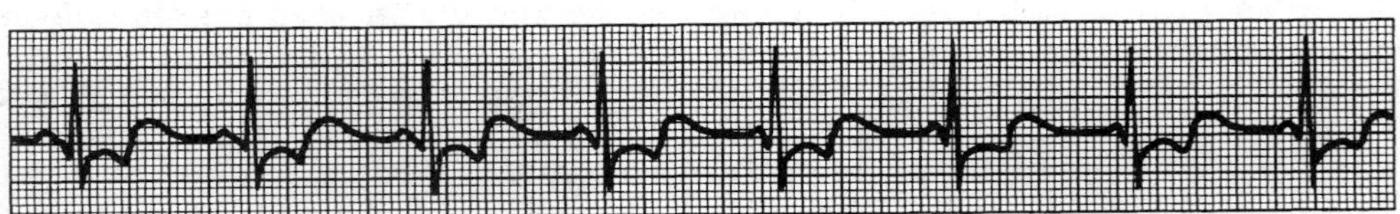

FIGURE 11–57. AV dissociation. (Redrawn from Phillips, R., & Feeney, M. [1990]. *The cardiac rhythms* [3rd ed.]. Philadelphia: W. B. Saunders.)

ECG criteria for parasystole are:

- No constant relationship between the sinus beat and the ectopic beat
- The time interval between ectopic beats may or may not be constant (in its classic form they will be regular, representing the actual rate of discharge from the ectopic site)
- Fusion beats representing depolarization from both sites are commonly seen
- The QRS configuration of the parasystolic beat is unchanging (Fig. 11–56)

Recognizing parasystole requires a long rhythm strip to calculate the interectopic intervals and absence of fixed coupling. For a more in-depth discussion of parasystole, the reader is referred to Marriott and Conover (1989).

AV Dissociation

AV dissociation is a pardysrhythmia in which the atria and ventricles beat independently, that is, they are dissociated (Fig. 11–57). It is a generic term that may be applied to any rhythm, such as ventricular tachycardia, where the atria and ventricles are activated independently. Ventricular activation is controlled by the dominant pacemaker in the AV junction or below, whereas atrial stimulation is caused by another pacemaker in either the SA node or the atria. This occurs because of suppression of the SA node, or it may result from vagal stimulation, drug therapy, or increased automaticity of the junctional tissue.

AV dissociation may be complete or incomplete. If it is incomplete, impulses from the SA node periodically arrive at the AV junction when it is nonrefractory, and the impulses are conducted through to the ventricles. In complete AV dissociation, the AV node is refractory from the dominant junctional pacemaker, and impulses from the SA node cannot be conducted. The major criterion for differentiating complete AV dissociation from complete AV block is that in complete heart block the atrial rate exceeds the AV junctional or idioventricular rate. In contrast, in AV dissociation, the junctional or idioventricular rate is faster than the atrial rate.

With AV dissociation on the ECG, the P waves bear no relationship to the QRS complexes. Because the atrial rhythm is slower than the ventricular rhythm, the P-to-P intervals are longer than the R-to-R intervals. As the result, the P waves overtake the QRS complexes and the PR interval becomes progressively shorter. The P wave then becomes superimposed on the QRS complex, and eventually occurs after the QRS complex. When the P wave falls sufficiently far beyond the QRS complex, the atrial impulse will be conducted to the ventricles, resulting in a captured ventricular beat. This conducted beat is sometimes referred to as "interference" (Chou, 1991).

SUMMARY

This chapter has discussed the interpretation of the ECG as it relates to coronary artery disease, axis deviation, and complex dysrhythmias. Our knowledge base of the conduction system and dysrhythmias has grown considerably over the last 20 years. This knowledge has increased the complexity of critical care nursing as well as nurses' responsibility for the early detection and recognition of alterations in normal cardiac rhythms. The importance of understanding and using proper monitoring leads to assess anticipated rhythm disturbances is paramount. Whether employed in large medical centers or small community hospitals, nurses must be able to combine rapid ECG interpretation with astute assessment skills in anticipating and forestalling life-threatening situations in their patients.

REFERENCES

Abedin, Z., & Connor, R. P. (1989). *12 lead ECG interpretation: The self assessment approach.* Philadelphia: W. B. Saunders.

Alpert, J. S. (1991). Conduction disturbances: Temporary and permanent pacing. In B. J. Gersh & S. H. Rahimtoola (Eds.), *Acute myocardial infarction* (pp. 249–258). New York: Elsevier Science Publishing.

Antman, E. M., & Berlin, J. (1992). Declining incidence of ventricular fibrillation in myocardial infarction. *Circulation, 86,* 764–773.

Antman, E. M., & Rutherford, J. D. (1986). *Coronary care medicine: A practical approach.* Boston: Martinus Nijhoff.

Bairey, C. N., Shah, P. K., Lew, A. S., et al. (1987). Electrocardiographic differentiation of occlusion of the left circumflex versus the right coronary artery as a cause of acute inferior myocardial infarction. *American Journal of Cardiology, 60,* 456–459.

Bandari, A. K., & Rahimtoola, S. H. (1991). Invasive electrophysiologic testing and Holter monitoring in infarct survivors. In B. J. Gersh & S. H. Rahimtoola (Eds.), *Acute myocardial infarction* (pp. 409–422). New York: Elsevier Science Publishing.

Berne, R. M., & Levy, M. N. (1993). *Physiology* (3rd ed.). St. Louis: C. V. Mosby.

Berry, V. A. (1994). The patient with Wolff-Parkinson-White syndrome. *Critical Care Nursing Clinics of North America, 6,* 27–39.

Bigger, Jr., J. T. (1994). Ventricular premature complexes. In J. A. Kastor (Ed.), *Arrhythmias* (pp. 310–325). Philadelphia: W. B. Saunders.

Borgrefe, M., Hindriks, G., Haverkamp, W., et al. (1990). Catheter ablation using radiofrequency energy. *Clinical Cardiology, 13,* 801–824.

Braat, S. H., de Zwaan, C., Brugada, P., et al. (1984). Right ventricular involvement with acute inferior wall infarction identifies high risk of developing atrioventricular nodal conduction disturbances. *American Heart Journal, 107,* 1183.

Braunwald, E. (1992). *Heart disease: A textbook of cardiovascular medicine* (4th ed.). Philadelphia: W. B. Saunders.

Brembilla-Perrot, B., & Ghawi, R. (1993). Electrophysiological characteristics of asymptomatic Wolff-Parkinson-White. *European Heart Journal, 14,* 511–515.

Brugada, P., & Wellens, H. J. J. (1986). How to approach conduction disturbances. In E. Andries & R. Stroobandt (Eds.), *Clinical arrhythmias for the clinical cardiologist* (pp. 95–137). New York: Excerpta Medica.

Cain, M., Luke, R., & Lindsay, B. (1992). Diagnosis and localization of accessory pathway. *Pace—Pacing and Clinical Electrocardiography, 15,* 801–824.

Chou, T. (1991). *Electrocardiography in clinical practice* (3rd ed.). Philadelphia: W. B. Saunders.

Cohn, P. F. (1993). *Silent myocardial ischemia and infarction* (3rd ed.). New York: Mercel Dekker.

Conover, M. (1992). *Understanding electrocardiography.* St. Louis: Mosby–Year Book.

Craney, J. M. (1993). Radiofrequency catheter ablation of supraventricular tachycardias: Clinical considerations and nursing care. *Journal of Cardiovascular Nursing, 7,* 26.

Darling, E. J. (1994). Overview of cardiac electrophysiologic testing. *Critical Care Nursing Clinics of North America, 6,* 1–13.

Demoulin, J. C., & Kulbertus, H. E. (1972). Histopathological examination of concept of left hemiblock. *British Heart Journal, 34,* 809.

Drew, B. J. (1991). Bedside electrocardiographic monitoring: State of the art for the 1990s. *Heart and Lung, 20,* 610–623.

Drew, B. J. (1993). Bedside electrocardiogram monitoring. *AACN Clinical Issues in Critical Care Nursing, 4,* 25–33.

Drew, B. J., & Scheinman, M. M. (1991). Value of electrocardiographic leads in MCL_1, MCL_6 and other selected leads in the diagnosis of wide QRS complex tachycardia. *Journal of the American College of Cardiology, 18,* 1025–1033.

Duckeck, W., & Kuck, K. (1993). Atrial fibrillation in Wolff-Parkinson-White syndrome. *Herz, 18,* 60–66.

Finkelmeier, B. A. (1994). Ablative therapy in the treatment of tachyarrhythmias. *Critical Care Nursing Clinics of North America, 6,* 103–110.

Frink, R. J., & James, T. N. (1973). Normal blood supply to the His bundle and proximal bundle branches. *Circulation, 47,* 8–18.

Gettes, L. S. (1990). Effects of ionic changes on impulse propagation. In M. R. Rosen, M. J. Janse, & A. L. Wit (Eds.), *Cardiac electrophysiology: A textbook* (pp. 459–479). Mount Kisco, NY: Futura.

Goldberger, A. L. (1991). Myocardial infarction: Electrocardiographic differential diagnosis (4th ed.). St. Louis: Mosby–Year Book.

Goldman, M. J. (1989). *Principles of clinical electrocardiography* (13th ed.). Los Altos, CA: Lange Medical Publications.

Goldschlager, N., & Goldman, M. J. (1989). *Principles of clinical electrocardiography.* Norwalk, CT: Appleton & Lange.

Guyton, A. (1991). *Textbook of medical physiology* (8th ed.). Philadelphia: W. B. Saunders.

Hoffman, B. F., & Cranefield, P. F. (1960). *Electrophysiology of the heart.* New York: McGraw-Hill.

Horowitz, L. N. (1994). Polymorphic ventricular tachycardia, including torsades de pointes. In J. A. Kastor (Ed.), *Arrhythmias* (pp. 376–394). Philadelphia: W. B. Saunders.

Hurst, J. W. (1993). *Cardiovascular diagnosis: The initial examination.* St. Louis: C. V. Mosby.

James, T. N. (1977). The sinus node. *American Journal of Cardiology, 40,* 965.

Josephson, M. E., & Wellens, H. J. J. (1993). *Tachycardias: Mechanisms and management.* Mount Kisco, NY: Futura.

Kastor, J. A. (1994). Atrioventricular block. In J. A. Kastor (Ed.), *Arrhythmias* (pp. 145–200). Philadelphia: W. B. Saunders.

Katz, A. M. (1992). *Physiology of the heart* (Vol. 2). New York: Raven Press.

Kay, G. N., & Bubien, R. S. (1992). *Clinical management of cardiac arrhythmias.* Gaithersburg, MD: Aspen.

Kellen, J. C., & Ramadan, D. (1994). The patient with recurrent atrioventricular nodal reentrant tachycardia or chronic atrial fibrillation or atrial flutter. *Critical Care Nursing Clinics of North America, 6,* 41–53.

Lie, K. I., Wellens, H. J. J., & Schuilenburg, R. M. (1976). Bundle branch block in acute myocardial infarction. In H. J. J. Wellens, K. I. Lie, & M. J. Janse (Eds.), *The conduction system of the heart.* Philadelphia: Lea & Febiger.

Lipman, B. C., & Lipman, B. S. (1987). *ECG pocket guide.* Chicago: Year Book Medical Publishers.

Marriott, H. J. L. (1988). *Practical electrocardiography* (8th ed.). Baltimore: Williams & Wilkins.

Marriott, H. J. L., & Conover, M. B. (1989). *Advanced concepts in arrhythmias* (2nd ed.). St. Louis: C. V. Mosby.

Mirvis, D. M. (1993). *Electrocardiography: A physiologic approach.* St. Louis: Mosby–Year Book.

Moser, D., & Woo, M. (1994). Recurrent ventricular tachycardia. *Critical Care Nursing Clinics of North America, 6,* 15–26.

Oren, J. W., Beckman, K. J., McClelland, J. H., et al. (1993). A functional approach to the preexcitation syndromes. *Cardiology Clinics, 11,* 121–149.

Phillips, R., & Feeney, M. (1990). *The cardiac rhythms* (3rd ed.). Philadelphia: W. B. Saunders.

Prinzmetal, M., Ekmekci, A., Toyoshima, H., et al. (1959). Angina pectoris: III. Demonstration of a chemical origin of ST deviation in classic angina pectoris, its variant form, early myocardial infarction, and some noncardiac conditions. *American Journal of Cardiology, 3,* 276.

Rardon, D. P., & Pressler, M. L. (1991). Cardiac resting and action potentials: Current concepts. In C. Fisch & B. Surawicz (Eds.), *Cardiac electrophysiology and arrhythmias* (pp. 3–12). New York: Elsevier Science Publishing.

Ricou, R., Nicod, P., Gilpin, E., et al. (1991). Influence of right bundle branch block on short and long term survival after acute anterior myocardial infarction. *American Journal of Cardiology, 17,* 858–863.

Rosen, M. R., & Anyukhovsky, E. P. (1991). Arrhythmias triggered by afterdepolarizations. In C. Fisch & B. Surawicz (Eds.), *Cardiac electrophysiology and arrhythmias* (pp. 67–75). New York: Elsevier Science Publishing.

Ross, J. H. (1984). Embryonic myocardial remnants and dual pathway conduction: Management of related reentrant supraventricular tachycardia. *Critical Care Nurse, 4*(2), 78–85.

Scheinman, M. M., Laks, M. M., DiMarco, J., et al. (1991). Current role of catheter ablative procedures in patients with cardiac arrhythmias. *Circulation, 83,* 2146.

Schlant, R. C., Alexander, R. W., O'Rourke, R. A., et al. (1994). *Hurst's The heart: Arteries & veins* (8th ed.). New York: McGraw-Hill.

Setaro, J. F., & Cabin, H. S. (1992). Right ventricular infarction. *Cardiology Clinics of North America, 10*(1), 69–90.

Shah, P. K. (1991). New insights into the electrocardiogram. In B. J. Gersh & S. H. Rahimtoola (Eds.), *Acute myocardial infarction* (pp. 128–143). New York: Elsevier Science Publishing.

Sokolow, M., & McIlroy, M. B. (1993). *Clinical cardiology* (6th ed.). Los Altos, CA: Lange Medical Publications.

Steward, R. B., Bardy, G. H., & Green, H. L. (1986). Wide complex tachycardia: Misdiagnosis and outcome after emergent therapy. *Annals of Internal Medicine, 104,* 766–771.

Surawicz, B. (1991). Automaticity. In C. Fisch & B. Surawicz (Eds.), *Cardiac electrophysiology and arrhythmias* (pp. 51–66). New York: Elsevier Science Publishing.

Thalen, H. J. (1981). Anatomy of the conduction system of the human heart. In J. Nieveen (Ed.), *Arrhythmias of the heart.* Oxford: Excerpta Medica.

Tisdale, J. (1991). Lidocaine prophylaxis in acute myocardial infarction. *Henry Ford Hospital Medical Journal, 39*(3–4), 217–225.

Ventura, T., Colantonio, D., Leocata, P., et al. (1991). Isolated atrial myocardial infarction: Pathological and clinical features in ten cases. *Cardiology, 36,* 345–350.

Wagner, G. S. (1994). *Marriott's practical electrocardiography* (9th ed.). Baltimore: Williams & Wilkins.

Waldo, A. L. (1991). What's new in atrial flutter. In C. Fisch & B. Surawicz (Eds.), *Cardiac electrophysiology and arrhythmias* (pp. 176–185). New York: Elsevier Science Publishing.

Wellens, H. J. J., et al. (1978). The value of the electrocardiogram in the differential diagnosis of a tachycardia with a widened QRS complex. *American Journal of Medicine, 64,* 27.

Wesley, R., Resk, W., & Zimmerman, D. (1991). Reconsiderations of the routine and preferential use of lidocaine in the emergent treatment of ventricular arrhythmias. *Critical Care Medicine, 19,* 1439–1444.

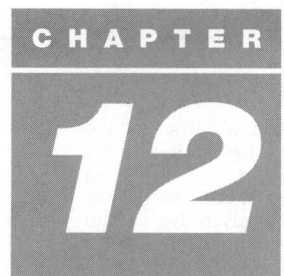

Pacemakers

Margaret Catherine Jones

Efforts at cardiac electrostimulation date back to the eighteenth century when the Italian investigator Galvani experimented with the application of electrical current to frogs' hearts to produce myocardial contraction (Senning, 1983; Bocka, 1989). Extensive research by many talented scientists, namely, Chardack, Furman, Senning, Elmquist, and others, led to the implantation of the first permanent pacemakers around 1960 (Furman & Schwedel, 1959; Chardack et al., 1960). Since then, advances in cardiac pacing have occurred at an astoundingly rapid rate.

During the 1960s, emphasis was on improving both transvenous techniques and pacing leads, and inhibition was the primary mode of response (Hayes, 1992). It was in the 1970s that atrioventricular sequential pacing and basic programmability were introduced (Hayes, 1992). At this point in time, the technological pace quickened. The 1980s saw the introduction of the universal (DDD) pacemaker and rate responsiveness as new pieces to the puzzle of optimal physiologic pacing. Through the efforts of Paul Zoll, transcutaneous pacing resurfaced and became a standard of care in situations requiring emergency cardiac pacing.

Within each decade pacemaker technology accelerates; during the 1990s, the focus is on the following: multiple sensors within a single pacemaker to improve rate modulation, new low-threshold lead designs, increased memory functions, and improved autoprogramming techniques (Hayes, 1992). Implantable cardioverter defibrillators introduced in the 1980s now incorporate pacing therapy as a part of the therapeutic algorithm.

PERMANENT PACING

Indications

In the past 30 years, indications for permanent pacing have expanded. A study of cardiac pacing practices conducted in 1989 at 3,400 centers by Bernstein and Parsonnet (1992) documented 89,445 primary pacemaker implantations and 21,055 pulse generator replacements. Bernstein and Parsonnet (1992) found that 70% of initial implants are ventricular demand pacing systems, and approximately 30% are dual-chamber pacing systems. Since the last survey of pacing practices done in 1985, the proportion of rate-adaptive pacemakers has increased from 1% to 40% of primary implants (Bernstein & Parsonnet, 1992).

Owing to the vast number of pacing systems available, their complexity and their expense, a task force of the American College of Cardiology and The American Heart Association (AHA) developed a written set of "Guidelines for the Implantation of Pacemakers" in which the indications for pacing are divided according to three classifications (Dreifus et al., 1991): (1) those situations in which there is general agreement about the necessity for implantation; (2) those situations in which pacemakers are frequently implanted, but there is divided opinion; and (3) those situations in which there is general agreement that pacemakers are unnecessary. Table 12–1 lists the guidelines according to major categories of indications and according to these three classifications.

Pacemaker Code

ICHD CODE

A three-position pacemaker code was published in 1974 by the pacemaker committee of the Inter-Society Commission for Heart Disease Resources (ICHD) (Furman, 1993b). Its purpose was to establish a standard so that the model or manufacturer of any given pacemaker's mode of operation would be known. The code has been widely used, and although it has undergone two revisions the basic content of the original code remains unchanged. The latest revision was completed in 1987 by the North American Society of Pacing and Electrophysiology (NASPE) and the British Pacing and Electrophysiology Group (BPEG) (Furman, 1993b). It is referred to as the NASPE/BPEG code or simply, the NBG code.

NASPE/BPEG (NBG) CODE

The NBG code has accommodated the rapid changes that have occurred in bradycardia and tachycardia pacing as well as in the evolution of rate responsiveness. The code is a five-position code, of which the first three positions are solely for antibradydysrhyth-

TABLE 12–1. **American College of Cardiology/American Heart Association Guidelines for Permanent Cardiac Pacemaker Implantation**

1. Pacing in Acquired AV Block in Adults

Class 1

A. Complete heart block, permanent or intermittent, at any anatomic level associated with (1) symptomatic tachycardia, (2) congestive heart failure, (3) conditions requiring therapy with drugs which suppress automaticity of escape foci, (4) asystole of 3 seconds or longer or an escape rate of less than 40 beats/minute in asymptomatic patients.
B. Second-degree AV block, permanent or intermittent, regardless of type of site of block, with symptomatic bradycardia.
C. Atrial fibrillation, atrial flutter, or supraventricular tachycardia with complete or advanced AV block, bradycardia, and any condition described under A above. (Bradycardia must be unrelated to drugs that impair AV conduction.)

Class 2

A. Asymptomatic complete AV block, permanent or intermittent, at any anatomic site with ventricular rate of 40 beats/minute.
B. Asymptomatic type II second degree AV block (permanent or intermittent).
C. Asymptomatic type I second degree AV block at intra-His or infra-His level.

Class 3

A. First-degree AV block.
B. Asymptomatic type I second-degree AV block at the supra-His level.

2. Pacing After Myocardial Infarction

Class 1

Persistent advanced second-degree or complete AV block after acute myocardial infarction (almost always in anterior myocardial infarction).

Class 2

A. Persistent first-degree AV block with bundle branch block not documented previously.
B. Transient advanced AV block associated with bundle branch block.

Class 3

A. Transient AV conduction disturbances without intraventricular conduction defects.
B. Transient AV block in presence of isolated left anterior hemiblock.
C. Acquired left anterior hemiblock in the absence of AV block.

3. Pacing in Chronic Bifascicular and Trifascicular Block

Class 1

A. Bifascicular block with intermittent complete heart block associated with symptomatic bradycardia.
B. Bifascicular block with intermittent type II second-degree AV block with symptoms.

Class 2

A. Bifascicular or trifascicular block with intermittent type II second-degree AV block without symptoms.
B. Bifascicular or trifascicular block with syncope not proven to be due to AV block but other possible causes of syncope are not identifiable.

Class 3

A. Fascicular blocks without AV block or symptoms.
B. Fascicular blocks with first-degree AV block without symptoms.

4. Pacing in Sinus Node Dysfunction

Class 1

Sinus node dysfunction with symptomatic bradycardia. (In some patients, this will occur as a consequence of long-term essential drug therapy of a type and dose for which there is no acceptable alternative.)

Class 2

Sinus node dysfunction occurring spontaneously or as a result of necessary drug therapy with heart rates below 40 beats/minute when a clear association between significant symptoms consistent with bradycardia and the actual presence of bradycardia has not been documented.

Class 3

A. Sinus node dysfunction in asymptomatic patients.
B. Sinus node dysfunction when symptoms suggestive of bradycardia are clearly documented not to be associated with a slow rate.

5. Pacing in the Hypersensitive Carotid Syndrome

Class 1

Recurrent syncope associated with spontaneous events provoked by carotid sinus stimulation in patients having a 3-second or greater period of asystole in response to minimal carotid sinus pressure (in the absence of any medication that depresses the sinus node or AV conduction).

Class 2

Recurrent syncope without clear provocative events and with a hypersensitive cardioinhibitory response.

Class 3

A. Asymptomatic patients with hyperactive cardioinhibitory response to carotid stimulation.
B. Vague symptoms (dizziness, lightheadedness) and a hyperactive cardioinhibitory response to carotid sinus stimulation.
C. Symptomatic patients in whom the vasodepressor response to carotid sinus stimulation is the cause for symptoms.

Adapted from Frye, R. L., et al. (1984). Guidelines for permanent cardiac pacemaker implantation, May, 1984: A report of the Joint American College of Cardiology/American Heart Association Task Force on Assessment of Cardiovascular Procedures (Subcommittee on Pacemaker Implantation). Reprinted with permission of The American College of Cardiology. *Journal of the American College of Cardiology, 4,* 434; and Dreifus, L. S., et al. (1991). Guidelines for implantation of cardiac pacemakers and antiarrhythmia devices. *Journal of the American College of Cardiology, 18,* 1.

Abbreviation: AV, atrioventricular.

TABLE 12–2. **The NASPE/BPEG Generic (NBG) Code**

Position				
I	*II*	*III*	*IV*	*V*
Category				
Chamber(s) paced	Chamber(s) sensed	Response to sensing	Programmability, rate modulation	Antitachyarrhythmia function(s)
O = None	O = None	O = None	O = None	O = None
A = Atrium	A = Atrium	T = Triggered	P = Simple programmable	P = Pacing
V = Ventricle	V = Ventricle	I = Inhibited	M = Multiprogrammable	S = Shock
D = Dual (A + V)	D = Dual (A + V)	D = Dual (T + I)	C = Communicating	D = Dual (P + S)
			R = Rate modulation	
Manufacturers' Designation Only				
S = Single (A or V)	S = Single (A or V)			

Note: Positions I through III are used exclusively for antibradyarrhythmia function.

From Bernstein, A. D., et al. (1987). The NASPE/BPEG generic pacemaker code for antibradyarrhythmic and adaptive-rate pacing and antitachyarrhythmia devices. *PACE, 10,* 794–799.

mic function. Each of the five categories designates a specific but standard function of the pacemaker (Table 12–2).

POSITION I. This letter designates the chamber(s) paced. In this category, there are five possibilities: "A" indicates pacing in the atrium alone, "V" indicates pacing in the ventricle alone, "D" indicates pacing in both the atrium and the ventricle, and "O" indicates that no pacing is to occur. The letter "S" is a manufacturer's designation indicating that the device paces a single chamber, either the atrium or the ventricle.

POSITION II. The chamber sensed is designated by this position. Again, there are five possible options: "A" indicates sensing in the atrium alone, "V" indicates sensing in the ventricle alone, "D" indicates sensing in both the atrium and the ventricle, and "O" indicates that there is no sensing of intrinsic cardiac activity by the pacemaker. As in position I, the manufacturer may designate the letter "S," indicating that the device has sensing capability in a single chamber, either the atrium or the ventricle.

POSITION III. The third letter indicates the manner in which the pacemaker responds to a sensed event. In this position, four possibilities exist: "I" indicates that the pacemaker is inhibited in response to a sensed event, whereas the letter "T" indicates that a stimulus is actually triggered by a sensed event. The letter "D" indicates that the pacemaker is inhibited in response to a sensed event and also triggered by a sensed event. "O" indicates no mode of response by the pacemaker.

POSITION IV. Programmability and rate modulation are addressed in this position. The letters are arranged in a hierarchy from absence of function to complex operation, the next higher level incorporating features of the previous levels (Furman, 1993b). Within this position are five levels. "O" indicates that the device has neither programmability nor rate modulation, a rare event in this technological age. The letter "P" indicates simple programmability, where up to two programmable features can be altered. Most commonly, they are rate and output (Furman, 1993b). An "M," designating multiprogrammability, is used with more than two programmable features. The use of the letter "C" for communicating indicates that the device has telemetry capability. Rate modulation is designated by the letter "R," and denotes that the variation of the antibradycardia escape interval is sensor-driven in response to at least one physiologic variable. Activity, respiration, central venous temperature, and QT interval are examples of sensor applications that can directly modulate pacing rate.

POSITION V. The use of this position indicates that one or more antitachycardia functions are programmed into the pacemaker. If so designated, a pacing stimulus ("P"), a synchronized or unsynchronized shock ("S"), or both ("D") can be used on detection of a tachydysrhythmia.

Equipment

PULSE GENERATOR. Once the pacemaker lead (atrial or ventricular) or leads (atrial and ventricular) are inserted, the connection to the pulse generator is made with set screws at the connector block, which is at the top of the pulse generator. Over the years the pulse generator has undergone major changes. Early models of the 1970s weighed approximately 250 g, whereas contemporary units weigh anywhere from 25 to 40 g. There are two components of the pulse generator: the power source (battery) and the electronic circuitry. Both are hermetically sealed in a titanium container, commonly referred to as "the can" (Fig. 12–1).

POWER SOURCE. Permanent pacemakers are powered by battery. The earliest permanent pacemakers in the 1960s and 1970s were powered by mercury–zinc

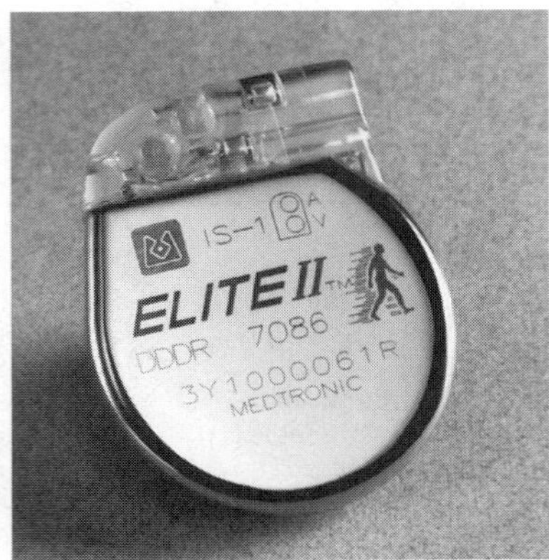

FIGURE 12–1. Permanent pulse generator. (Elite, DDDR; Courtesy of Medtronic, Inc., Minneapolis, MN.)

batteries. They were effective but had two major drawbacks: they had a short life expectancy of 3 to 5 years (Furman, 1993a) with battery depletion occurring rapidly, and they were heavy.

In the 1970s, nuclear batteries were developed; they were powered by plutonium and promethium, with a predicted life expectancy of 20 to 40 years (Furman, 1993a). It is estimated that, worldwide, 3,000 nuclear-powered pacemakers have been implanted. Currently, all promethium units have been removed, but many plutonium implants are still operational (Furman, 1993a). Cost and environmental issues prevented the nuclear power source from gaining popularity. Among current-technology pacemakers, nuclear units are no longer available.

Today, the lithium iodide battery is the power source for essentially all permanent pacemakers. Although there are about five different lithium chemistries that have been used with pacemakers, lithium iodide is the current favorite, providing a life expectancy of anywhere from 4 to 15 years (Furman, 1993a). Depending on the current output to which the pacemaker is programmed and the degree to which the pacemaker is used, the actual longevity will vary from one implant to the next. Today's pacemakers have built-in "end-of-life" (EOL) indicators or elective replacement indicators, where the magnet rate of the pacemaker designates elective battery replacement time. Because the battery and electronic circuitry are housed in one sealed container, a battery change is accomplished through the insertion of an entire new pulse generator. Some pacemakers today are able to estimate the remaining life of the battery and to transmit this information by telemetry.

ELECTRONIC CIRCUITRY. Special electrical circuits, each designed to perform a function for that pacing mode, are combined into an integrated circuit, usually within a single-chip microcomputer. In addition to the pacing and sensing functions, the circuitry allows multiple programmable parameters to be adjusted according to patient need. Today's pacemakers also have the ability to transmit real-time telemetry data that include such information as battery voltage and current, lead impedance and current, pulse amplitude and width, and output energy per paced beat. Other diagnostic features of modern pacemakers include electrograms (EGMs), which provide atrial or ventricular intracardiac waveforms, event counters that can track sensed events, and marker channel telemetry that can mark cardiac events as either sensed or paced, and in some cases provide ladder diagrams of the same.

LEAD/ELECTRODE SYSTEM. The lead/electrode system can be connected to the epicardial or endocardial surface of the heart. It is said that 95% of implantations are endocardial (Furman, 1993a). The lead attached to the pulse generator at the connector block carries current to the electrode. The electrode is the bare metal tip of the lead that is in contact with cardiac tissue. Current exiting this tip stimulates the myocardium to contract. In pacing modes where sensing function is programmed, information regarding the patient's intrinsic cardiac activity is transmitted from cardiac tissue back through the lead to the pulse generator.

Insertion

The epicardial approach to permanent pacemaker implantation is extremely rare in adults, and is used only in children or when the endocardial approach in an adult has failed. Failure of the endocardial approach can be the result of scar tissue on the endocardial surface making lead fixation impossible. The discussion that follows describes permanent pacemaker implantation using a transvenous endocardial approach.

Implantation is done under local anesthesia, and the length of the procedure is less than an hour. Difficulties encountered in venous access as well as lead placement with satisfactory lead thresholds can lengthen the procedure. The subclavian, cephalic, or external jugular veins can be used for lead introduction, the subclavian being the most frequently used approach. In a subclavian approach, the skin incision is made just below the inferior border of the clavicle. The pacemaker pocket lies inferior to the incision. The subclavian vein is entered with a needle, and a guidewire is inserted through the needle, advanced, and the needle withdrawn. The dilator–introducer sheath combination is then inserted over the guidewire and into the vessel, after which the dilator is removed and the pacing lead introduced. Most of the sheaths are designed to be peeled away once their purpose has been served. A ventricular lead is advanced through the right atrium, across the tricuspid valve and into place in the right venticular apex. An atrial J-shaped lead is positioned in the right atrial appendage. Patients who have had coronary bypass surgery no longer have an atrial appendage. An active fixation lead is used to secure the lead to the smooth wall of the right atrium, which is usually the lateral wall. The lead(s) are attached to the connector block on top of the pulse generator with set screws. The pulse generator is then placed in a

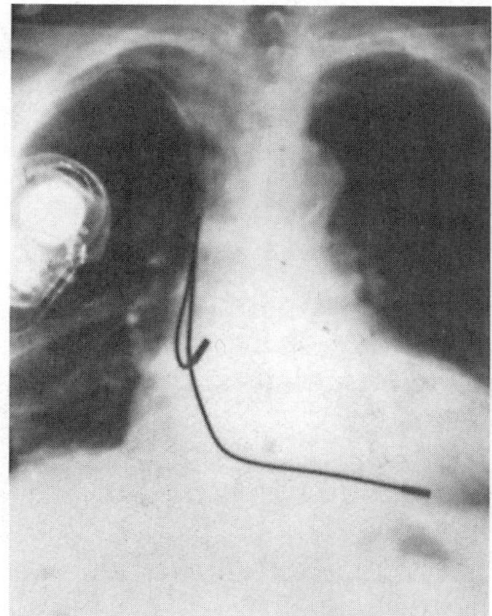
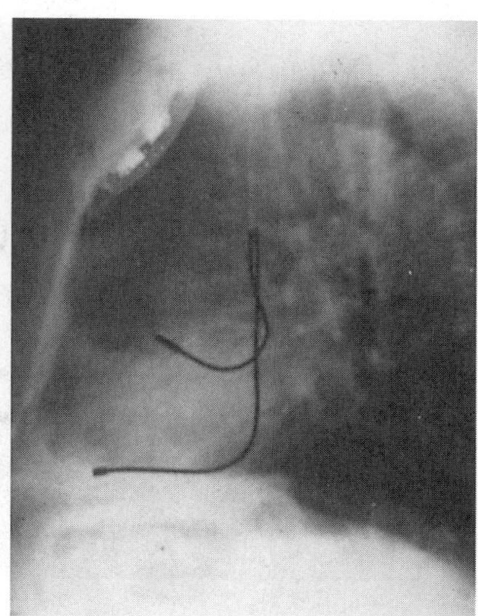

FIGURE 12–2. Anteroposterior and lateral x-ray views of a ventricular endocardial lead lodged in the right ventricular apex, and an atrial J-lead in the atrial appendage. (Courtesy of Medtronic, Inc., Minneapolis, MN.)

Dacron pouch in the subcutaneous pocket, the incision is closed, and a sterile dressing is applied. The Dacron pouch adheres to the subcutaneous pocket with time. After permanent pacemaker implantation, a chest x-ray will confirm placement of the lead(s). Figure 12–2 illustrates the chest x-ray of a dual-lead implantation.

Before attaching the leads to the pulse generator, the implanted lead(s) are attached to a pacing systems analyzer (Fig. 12–3), and external testing is conducted to determine the appropriate settings for the pulse generator in this individual patient. The following settings are now determined: (1) the pacing threshold, (2) lead impedance, and (3) pulse amplitude.

PACING THRESHOLD

The pacing threshold is the amount of voltage, measured in volts (V), at a given pulse width or pulse duration (how long the impulse remains at the electrode tip for the myocardium to respond) that results in constant pacing with capture. The patient's pacing or stimulation threshold has two phases (Fig. 12–4). The acute phase starts at implant, peaks at 10 to 20 days postimplant, and stabilizes at approximately 1 to 2 months (Barold & Zipes, 1992). The chronic phase follows for the lifetime of the lead. Steroid-eluting leads have played a major role in decreasing the stimulation threshold. Edema, inflammation, and the development of fibrous tissue at the electrode tissue interface cause the threshold to rise during the acute phase. To provide a safety margin for the patient, it is necessary to program higher-voltage output for the acute phase. After the acute phase, the pacing threshold is reassessed and the voltage programmed accordingly.

LEAD IMPEDANCE

The resistance to current being delivered is referred to as lead impedance, and is measured in ohms. Normal lead impedance is in the range of 250 to 1,000 ohms.

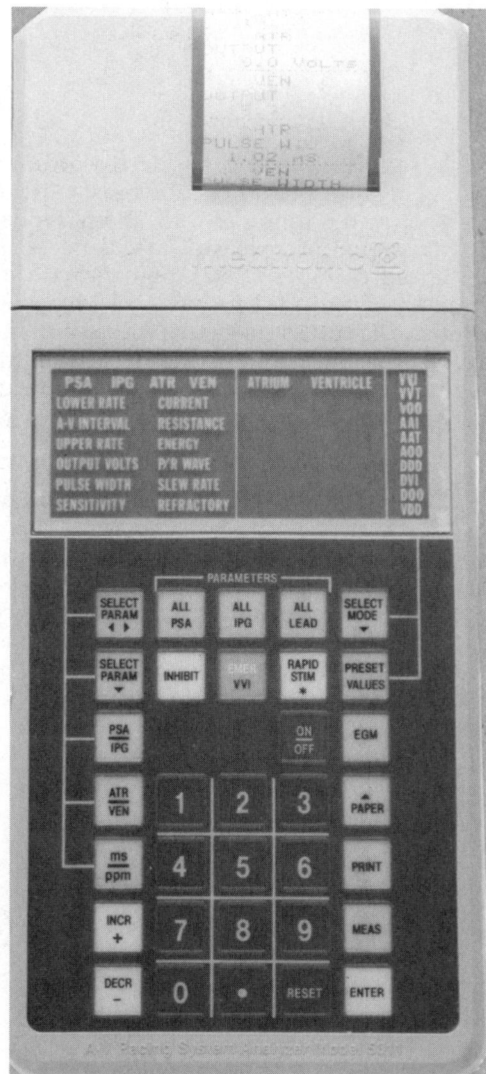

FIGURE 12–3. A pacing systems analyzer. (Courtesy of Medtronic, Inc., Minneapolis, MN.)

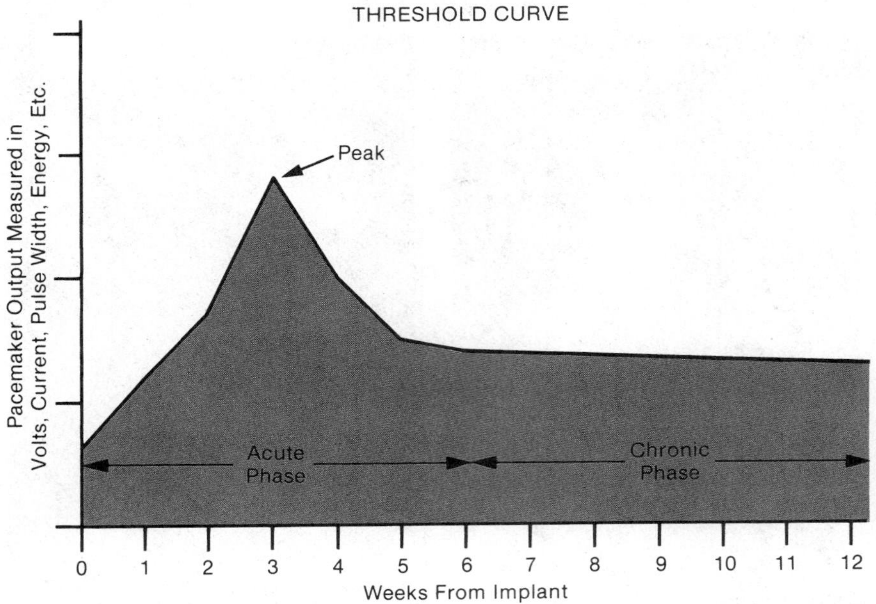

FIGURE 12–4. Threshold margin curve for the acute and chronic phase after pacemaker implantation. (Courtesy of Medtronic, Inc., Minneapolis, MN.)

PULSE AMPLITUDE

For reliable sensing to occur, an electrocardiographic (ECG) signal of sufficient amplitude must exist. A ventricular signal in the range of 6 to 15 millivolts (mV) and an atrial signal of at least 2 mV is necessary for sensing (Barold & Zipes, 1992). Signals with a more gradual upstroke are said to have a lower slew rate and are more difficult to sense than those with a sharp upstroke. Repositioning of the lead may be required to attain higher-voltage signals, resulting in appropriate sensing by the pacemaker.

Unipolar Versus Bipolar Lead Systems

With a unipolar system, there is one insulated pacing wire, the cathode (negative pole) is at the electrode tip, and the anode (positive pole) is a distance away in soft tissue at the pulse generator (Fig. 12–5). Because of the distance between poles, a larger, more easily identified pacing artifact is seen on ECG. However, a unipolar system is more subject to sensing problems related to interference from electromagnetic interference and skeletal myopotentials. A bipolar lead system has two thin coil wires intertwined inside a single insulation covering, one a cathode and one an anode, and both travel from the generator to the heart (Figure 12–5). Both poles are located in the heart, with the cathode at the very distal part of the lead and the anode proximal to it by approximately 2 cm (Furman, 1993a). The current thus travels in a very short circuit between these two poles, creating a very small artifact on ECG. Bipolar leads have fewer sensing problems related to electromagnetic interference and skeletal myopotentials than the unipolar systems. However, with two wires intertwined inside one lead system, the potential exists for more lead problems than with the unipolar system. Among physicians surveyed (Bernstein & Parsonnet, 1992), bipolar leads are used more often.

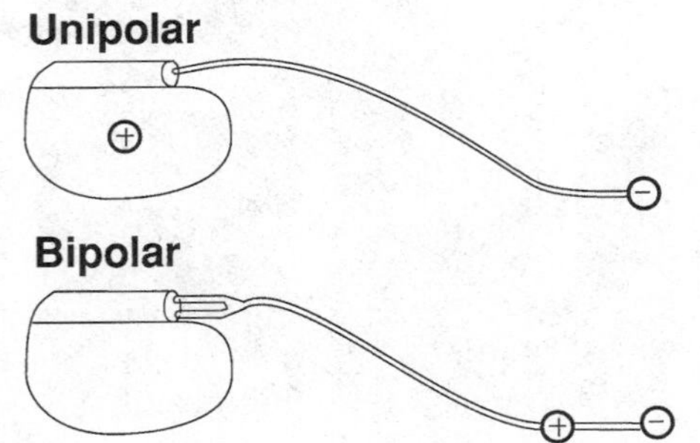

FIGURE 12–5. Schematic of unipolar and bipolar pacing systems. (Courtesy of Medtronic, Inc., Minneapolis, MN.)

Active Versus Passive Fixation

Transvenous leads that are placed in the atrium or the ventricle can be actively or passively fixated (Figs. 12–6 and 12–7). There is more than one type of passive fixation lead, the most common of which is the tined tip. Several short protuberances (tines) that are proximal to the electrode tip catch in the trabeculae of the heart and help to hold the lead in place, whether it be in the atrium or the ventricle. Atrial tined tip leads are "J"-tipped for placement in the atrial appendage (see Fig. 12–6*B*). Active fixation devices provide immediate fixation of the lead, most commonly by a screw-in mechanism. The small retractable screw is at the end

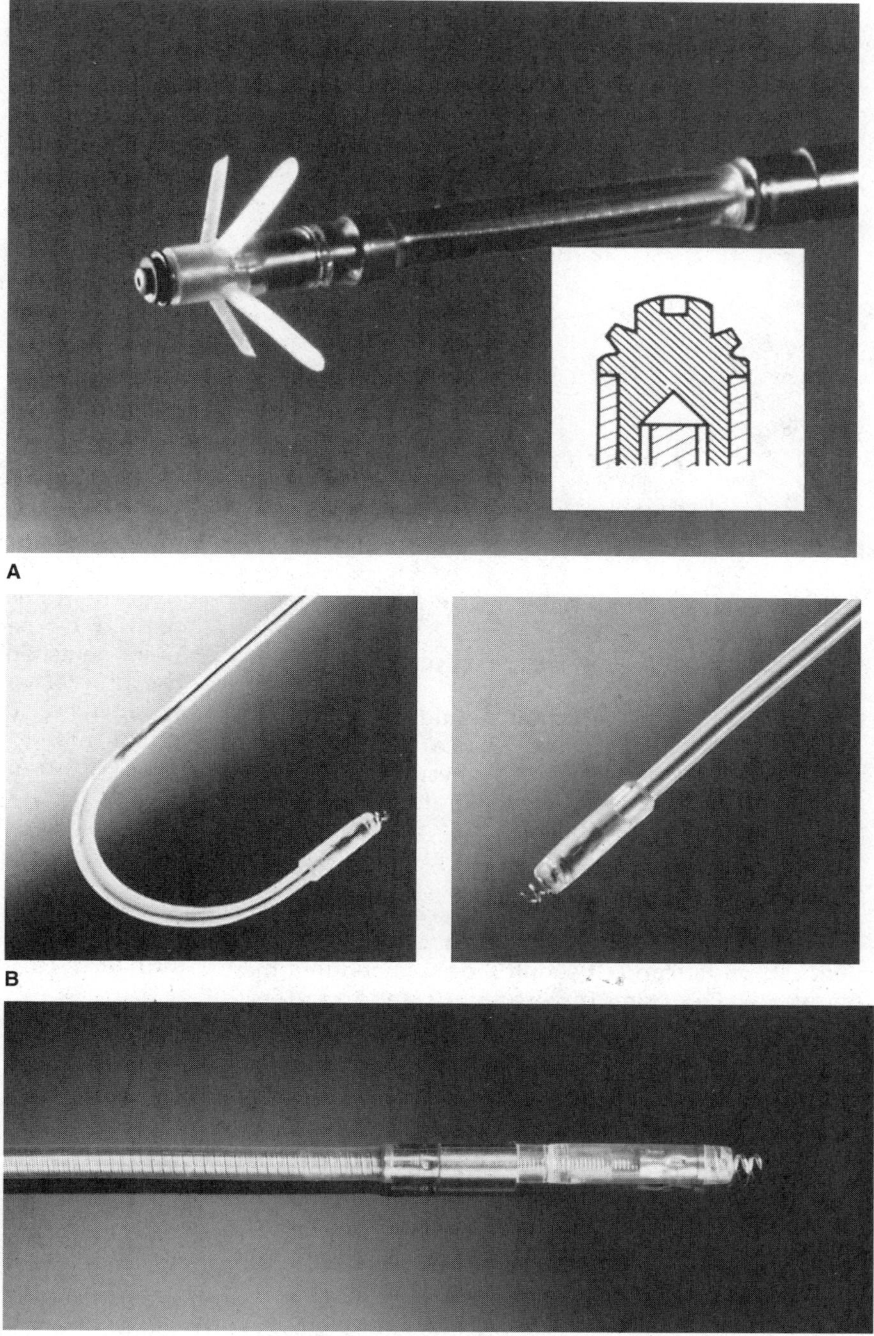

FIGURE 12–6. Types of endocardial pacing leads. *A*, Bipolar ventricular target tip lead with flexible tines attached for passive fixation. *B*, A "J"-shaped screw-in atrial lead and a screw-in atrial or ventricular lead for active fixation. *C*, The screw-in lead as seen in its extended position. (Courtesy of Medtronic, Inc., Minneapolis, MN.)

of the lead. In some cases it functions as the electrode, and in other cases it is simply the fixation device (Furman, 1993a). These devices can also be used in either the atrium or the ventricle.

Steroid-Eluting Leads

When permanent pacing leads are first implanted, inflammation at the electrode tissue interface occurs, resulting in a rise in stimulation threshold. Much research has focused on decreasing this rise in stimulation threshold. The steroid-eluting lead has been a major development in this area (Mond & Stokes, 1992). A silicone rubber reservoir at the tip of the lead contains a small amount of steroid, usually 1 mg of dexamethasone, which is gradually eluted over the expected life of the pacemaker (Furman, 1993a; Hayes, 1992). This feature is now standard on most pacing leads.

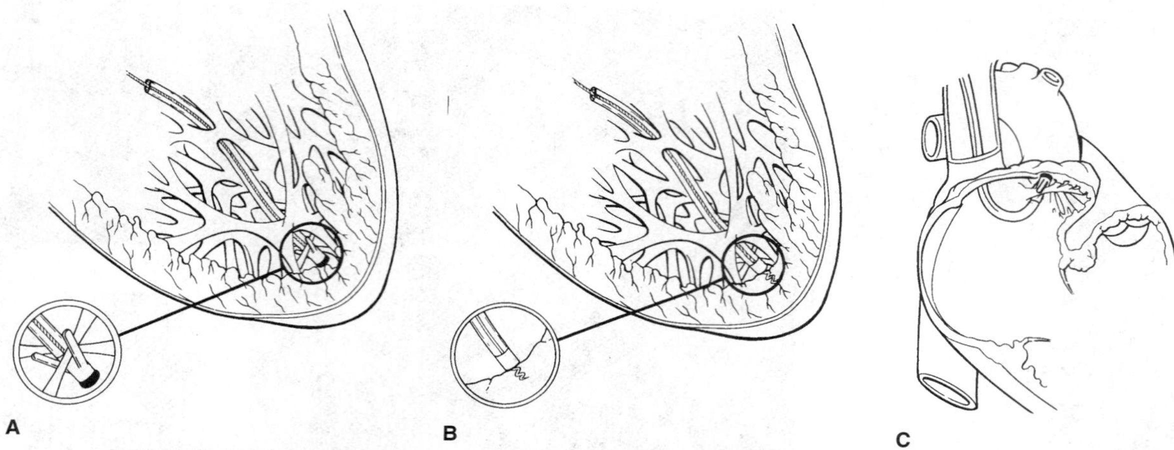

FIGURE 12–7. Lead-tip fixation. *A*, Passive fixation in the ventricle with a tined tip lead. *B*, Active fixation in the ventricle with a screw-in lead. *C*, Passive fixation in the atrial appendage with a J-shaped tined tip lead. (Courtesy of Medtronic, Inc., Minneapolis, MN.)

Clinical Management

Once the need for a permanent pacemaker is identified, preparation involving both the patient and his or her family or significant others should begin. Once the present knowledge and experience level related to pacemaker therapy is assessed, a specific plan of teaching starts. Visual aids that demonstrate how the device will improve cardiac function and what the device looks like, including its size, will give the patient a clearer picture of the entire process. An actual sample pulse generator and lead can be especially helpful. The operative procedure is explained in terms that the patient can understand. It should be explained that they will be awake during the procedure, and to test lead positioning they may be asked to do some specific things, such as coughing and deep breathing. Any pain that the patient experiences during the operative procedure should be reported so that additional local anesthetic may be administered.

Permanent pacemaker postimplant clinical management is geared toward: (1) assessment, through cardiac monitoring of appropriate sensing and pacing by the device; (2) early recognition of complications at the incisional site, such as hematoma and infection; and (3) prevention of lead dislodgment, especially during the initial 24 hours. In some facilities restricted movement in the form of bed rest and adduction of the arm on the side of the implant is either ordered by the physician or is part of the protocol for the care of this patient for the first several hours or longer.

Important written information comes with the pacemaker and should be given to the patient. A temporary pacemaker identification card is included, and should be completed and carried by the patients until they receive their permanent card in the mail from the pacemaker manufacturer. Warranty information also comes with the pacemaker. In addition, there is educational information that can reinforce teaching that has already been done. By the time of discharge, the patient should be able to demonstrate an understanding of his or her pacemaker follow-up and any specific appointments. Follow-up includes both office visits with the physician as well as routine monitoring of the pacemaker, done either in the office or by transtelephonic monitoring. If transtelephonic monitoring is to be used, a trial run before discharge demonstrates the patient's ability to complete the procedure and decreases his or her anxiety related to it.

PHYSIOLOGIC PACING

Normal Physiologic Pacing

The "gold standard" against which developing pacemakers are compared rests within the normal conduction system. The best physiologic pacing exists with normal sinus rhythm and an intact sinoatrial and atrioventricular (AV) conduction. AV synchrony and rate responsiveness are consistently provided, and with increased rate the PR interval is adjusted (shortened) accordingly. In response to either physiologic or nonphysiologic demands such as exercise or emotional stress, cardiac output increases accordingly. Because cardiac output is a product of heart rate and stroke volume, increases in heart rate and stroke volume occur to meet these demands (Hayes & Holmes, 1993a). Heart rate variability is a more critical factor in patients with left ventricular failure whose ability to increase stroke volume is compromised (Hayes & Holmes, 1993a).

Hemodynamics of Single-Chamber Pacing

Single-chamber demand pacing (VVI) provides the patient with reliable ventricular response in the absence of intrinsic activity, but is unable to provide either AV synchrony or rate variation. With the loss of AV synchrony, ventriculoatrial conduction can occur, in which the ventricles contract against AV valves that are open, resulting in decreased stroke volume and decreased cardiac output (Hayes & Holmes, 1993a; Nathan & Davies, 1992). Without AV synchrony, the atria contract against closed valves, activating nearby receptors and resulting in peripheral vasodilation and a consequent decrease in blood pressure (Hayes & Holmes, 1993a).

Pacemaker Syndrome

Many patients have described a variety of symptoms, any of which can result from the physiologic events described earlier. Pacemaker syndrome can be described as adverse hemodynamic effects in the setting of proper pacemaker function that result in symptoms that limit the patient's everyday functioning. Initially, pacemaker syndrome was described as occurring with VVI pacing, but it can occur in any mode of pacing where there is AV dissociation. Common symptoms include fatigue, weakness or dizziness, near or full syncope, cough, chest pain, hypotension, dyspnea, congestive heart failure, and jugular venous pulsations (Hayes & Holmes, 1993a). In the patient with pacemaker syndrome, the arterial blood pressure is often lower during pacing. In a study of pacemaker syndrome, Heldman and associates (1990) took a group of patients with DDD pacemakers and randomized them to either DDD or VVI pacing. After 1 week the participants were paced in the alternate mode. Questionnaires eliciting symptoms experienced were completed by the participants. It was estimated that symptoms related to pacemaker syndrome were present in 83% of patients when they were VVI paced (Heldman et al., 1990).

Rate-Adaptive Pacemakers

RATE VARIATION. Rate variation is a key factor in cardiac output computation. Studies have compared the hemodynamic effects of pacing with rate responsiveness to pacing with rate responsiveness and AV synchrony, and to pacing with neither rate responsiveness nor AV synchrony. Results show that heart rate provides the most important contribution to cardiac output during exercise (Hayes & Holmes, 1993a).

THE CONCEPT OF RATE RESPONSIVENESS. The evolution of dual-chamber pacemakers has enabled patients to achieve AV synchrony through a unique timing mechanism. In those people with normal sinus node function, the ventricular rate will vary according to the sensed atrial depolarization rate, governed by the sinoatrial (SA) node. In SA node disease, the natural physiologic pacemaker is unable to appropriately vary its rate in response to physical and nonphysical stressors; the SA node is said to be chronotropically incompetent. The predictable rate increases normally seen with increased metabolic demands do not occur. In the person with a dual-chamber pacemaker and chronotropic incompetence of the SA node, the benefit of the pacemaker is limited to AV synchrony. Data indicate that in the ventricular rate range of 50 to 100 beats per minute (bpm), AV synchrony is a more critical factor, but in the ventricular rate range of 120 to 180 bpm, heart rate becomes a more significant factor in determining cardiac output (Furman, 1993c). Rate-responsive pacing uses a substitute sensor for those patients who lack normal atrial sensing capability and the ability to vary appropriately their heart rate through SA node functioning.

A sensor detects a physiologic or physical change and produces a signal that is then sensed by the pacemaker circuit to produce a rate change. The rate change produced by a particular sensor is referred to as rate adaptive, rate modulated, or rate responsive. An ideal sensor responds to physiologic and nonphysical needs the same way the normal physiologic mechanism would respond. It would respond to emotions as well as to physical activity, and the rate increase or decrease would mimic the healthy cardiac response. This response would occur reliably each time the need arose, and would be appropriate for the level of demand (Furman, 1993c). After a rate response the decline in heart rate would be gradual. In summary, the ideal sensor is one that would simulate sensing of normal atrial depolarization. Patients with chronic atrial fibrillation, a contraindication to dual-chamber pacing, might benefit from single-chamber, rate-responsive pacing (VVIR). Patients with sick sinus syndrome and bradydysrhythmias might benefit from dual-chamber, rate-responsive pacing (DDDR) (Futterman et al., 1993). Programming rate-modulated pacemakers involves setting upper and lower rate limits, designating the responsiveness of the system on a scale of 1 to 10 to indicate the degree of rate response that will occur, and adjusting the response time, or how quickly the rate response will occur.

RATE-ADAPTIVE SENSORS

ATRIAL DEPOLARIZATION SENSING. Sensing of atrial depolarization is done through a separate atrial lead that makes contact through active or passive fixation with the atrial wall. Alternatively, an atrial electrode can be part of a single ventricular pacing lead so that the atrial electrode is located within the atrium, but not in contact with the atrial wall. Ventricular rate response is determined by the sensing of atrial depolarizations.

ACTIVITY SENSOR. The activity sensor was the first physiologic pacer to be used in the United States (Fabiszewski & Volosin, 1991). The development of dual-chambered pacemakers advanced rapidly in the 1980s, and in one of the VDD devices, atrial sensing was designed to take place at the pulse generator through a piezoelectric crystal (Furman, 1993c). This was the beginning of the activity sensor, in which motion, vibration, or activity is the physiologic event sensed and the pacing rate is adapted accordingly. Ninety percent of all implanted rate-modulated pacemakers are now based on the activity sensor (Furman, 1993c).

A conventional lead–electrode system is used for this pacemaker. Activity, motion, or vibration is sensed by a piezoelectric crystal that is bonded to the inside back surface of the pulse generator. The frequency and amplitude of these signals sensed are computed by a microprocessor, which in turn produces a rise in heart rate. The primary advantage of this sensor is its rapid response to activity. Owing to the sensor's ability to respond to vibration, some undesirable or unnecessary heart rate increases can occur; for example, driving over rough roads can be sensed as vibration or motion by the pacemaker, and the heart rate would increase. A drawback of the activity sensor is its inability to respond to nonphysical activity such as an emotionally stressful situation. The accelerometer, a new development in activity sensing, attempts to make the piezoelectric crystal more sensitive to forward motion by moving the crystal differently within the hermetically sealed container; instead of being mounted against the back of the can, it is mounted to the circuit board (Furman, 1993c). Another version of the motion sensor is referred to as "magnetic ball inductance," in which a magnetic ball housed in plastic and located inside the pulse generator moves in response to motion detected, creating current that is then translated into a rate response (Furman, 1993c).

ENDOCARDIAL EVOKED POTENTIAL

QT INTERVAL OR STIMULUS-T INTERVAL. The QT interval, or stimulus-t interval, represents ventricular depolarization and repolarization on the ECG and varies according to heart rate. The concept of this sensor is that the duration of the QT interval provides an indication of metabolic need and can be used to drive the pacemaker rate. The QT interval shortens in response to increased heart rate, the effect of changing sympathetic tone, and resulting levels of circulating catecholamines during physical exercise and emotional stress (Fabiszewski & Volosin, 1991; Lau, 1992). The QT sensor, first developed in 1981, senses changes in QT intervals and varies pacemaker rate accordingly. An increase in sympathetic tone resulting in QT interval shortening would be detected by the pacemaker and result in an increase in pacemaker rate.

Unlike the activity sensor, the QT sensor is able to respond to emotional activity or stress as well as physical activity. The QT sensor can also be responsive to isometric exercise. Limitations of the QT sensor include its slow initial response time, because it takes some time for the QT interval to shorten in response to metabolic needs and then drive the rate of the pacemaker. The QT interval can be altered by drugs such as the class IA antidysryhthmics and β-adrenergic blocking agents, as well as by ischemia and electrolyte imbalance. Some patients will have a normal catecholamine response, but no change in the QT interval results and therefore no rate modulation occurs (Lau, 1992). Sensing of the T-wave portion of the QT interval has not always been reliable when using this sensor (Stephenson & Coombs, 1991). The QT sensor's ability to respond to emotional activity and stress has been combined with the activity sensor's quick response time to improve overall quality of rate modulation.

PACED DEPOLARIZATION INTEGRAL. Another measurement of endocardial evoked potential is called the paced depolarization integral. The paced depolarization integral is the measurement of the paced ventricular gradient. The measurement of the gradient can be accomplished through a standard bipolar pacing electrode, and thus no additional or special leads are required. The pacemaker adjusts the rate in an attempt to maintain a normal gradient (Furman, 1993c). Exercise and emotional stress will decrease the gradient, resulting in an increase in the pacing rate. An increase in pacing rate increases the gradient, bringing the rate back to its resting level (Lau, 1992). This pacemaker has demonstrated its ability to provide a rapid rate of response to exercise and is also responsive to emotional stress. One major drawback is that a peak heart rate is achieved after 2 to 3 minutes of exercise, and that despite longer and more strenuous exercise, the pacing rate then tends to decline (Lau, 1992).

BODY TEMPERATURE. Central body temperature is a very sensitive barometer of the body's metabolic state. Body metabolism converts energy into heat, with increased muscular activity resulting in an increase in core temperature. Vigorous activity can result in a central venous temperature increase of as much as 1.5°C (Furman, 1993c). Thus it was determined that a thermistor could be used to detect such temperature changes, and that those changes could be used to modulate pacemaker rate. Currently there is one single-chamber, temperature-regulated rate-responsive device commercially available. No extra lead is required because the thermistor is located on the pacing lead itself. The temperature changes are transmitted to a microprocessor in the pulse generator, which translates the temperature change into a rate response. Some limitations with this sensor have been identified. Blood initially returning to the heart is cool in relation to the blood that is already there, and it is therefore possible to have rate slowing during the onset of activity. Because the rate response with this sensor has a slow onset, a brief activity, such as running to catch a train, may result in no rate response or a rate response that occurs too late (Furman, 1993c). The pacemaker also is unable to distinguish between an increase in temperature that results from exercise and one that results from illness. Fever results in a rate change, but after a period of time the pacemaker reverts back to a lower rate setting until it senses another change in temperature. Drinking hot and cold fluids, or taking a hot shower or bath can produce a change in body temperature that is detected by the thermistor and results in unecessary rate modulation (Lau, 1992; Furman, 1993c).

RESPIRATION. There is an increase in oxygen consumption during exercise and an increase in both respiratory rate and tidal volume, the latter two being determinants of minute ventilation. Two separate respiration sensors have been developed to detect increased physiologic need and provide rate modulation accordingly: a respiratory rate sensor and a minute ventilation sensor.

RESPIRATORY RATE. The initial respiratory sensor required the placement of a right ventricular pacing lead and an auxiliary lead that was tunneled into subcutaneous tissue on the thorax, approximately 8 to 10 cm away from the pulse generator pocket (Lau, 1992). A sensing level and resting cardiac rate are programmed at implant (Furman, 1993c). Variations in thoracic impedance between the thoracic electrode and the pulse generator (indifferent electrode) are sensed by the pacemaker as increasing depth or rate of respiration, and the rate is modulated accordingly (Furman, 1993c). Improvements in lead design have resulted in the auxiliary electrode being located on the ventricular pacing lead, eliminating the need for the subcutaneous thoracic electrode (Furman, 1993c). Impedance is thus measured between the electrode and the pulse generator, producing less battery current drain (Furman, 1993c).

MINUTE VENTILATION. The minute ventilation sensor measures changes in transthoracic electrical impedance between the pacing electrode and the pulse generator, and the pacing rate is adapted accordingly (Fabiszewski & Volosin, 1991). Electrical impedance varies with the volume of air in the lungs, increasing during inhalation and decreasing during exhalation (Fabiszewski & Volosin, 1991; Morton, 1991; Furman, 1993c). The amplitude of these changes is proportional to the tidal volume and can be used to calculate the minute ventilation volume (Furman, 1993c; Morton, 1991).

The improved speed of response with the minute ventilation sensor is one of its major advantages; it can provide rapid rate modulation in response to exercise. After exercise there is a reasonable and gradual decline in pacing rate. Minute ventilation sensors are also responsive to emotional stress and fever because both of these usually result in impedance changes.

There are some disadvantages to this particular sensor. In addition to measuring electrical impedance, the sensor can respond to certain actions, such as arm waving, and produce a rate change (Stephenson & Coombs, 1991). Electrocautery can be detected by the sensor as an impedance change, leading to an increase in pacing rate. Lau (1992) states that the rate-adaptive mode should be turned off when electrocautery is in use. This sensor would not be useful in the patient with a high baseline respiratory rate, such as in chronic pulmonary disease. When a patient with a minute ventilation sensor is being mechanically ventilated, the proper functioning of the rate-adaptive sensor may be thrown off, and the rate-adaptive function should be programmed off during this time (Fabiszewski & Volosin, 1991).

RIGHT VENTRICULAR PRESSURE. With an increase in metabolic demand there is stimulation of the sympathetic nervous system, and the resulting catecholamine release results in myocardial muscle contraction. Shortening of the myocardial muscle fibers leads to an increase in ventricular pressure (Morton, 1991). Right ventricular pressure correlates well with increased metabolic demands, and has been developed as a sensor for rate modulation. Although the rate-responsive pacemaker using a right ventricular pressure sensor is implanted in the conventional manner, a special lead is required because the sensor is part of the lead itself. The sensor is a piezoelectric crystal bonded to a titanium diaphragm on a unipolar ventricular lead, and is set 3 cm proximal to the electrode (Furman, 1993c). Right ventricular pressure changes alter the diaphragm, which puts pressure on the piezoelectric crystal and results in rate changes by the pulse generator (Morton, 1991; Furman, 1993c). The advantages of this sensor are that it can respond rapidly to changes, and that it is able to respond to changes in physical activity as well as emotion.

Dual Sensors

Dual-sensor pacemakers attempt to combine the beneficial features of two sensors into one pulse generator's electronic circuitry. The contribution of each sensor to the overall rate response, referred to as "sensor blending," is programmable. In August 1991, a single-chamber pacemaker that uses two sensors, activity and AV interval, became available for clinical evaluation. Connelly (1993) reported on 90 such implants in 21 centers, finding that the dual-sensor mode provided immediate response but a more gradual increase in pacing rate, such that 72 of the 90 patients remained in the dual-chamber mode. Research is being conducted in the effectiveness of dual-sensor, rate-adaptive pacemakers. Other combinations being evaluated include activity and minute ventilation, and minute ventilation and paced depolarization integral (Furman, 1993c).

TEMPORARY PACING

Temporary cardiac pacing is a lifesaving treatment for many patients who experience sudden, either temporary or permanent, alterations in their cardiac rate and rhythm. This modality provides patients with a consistent rhythm as their own conduction system recovers, or as a bridge to permanent pacing. Noninvasive transcutaneous pacing (TCP; temporary external pacing) today reflects a number of changes that have occurred since its introduction by Zoll in 1952. External pacing can be used in a number of situations in which an invasive procedure such as insertion of a temporary transvenous pacemaker is either contraindicated or not clearly warranted. Temporary epicardial pacing is initiated intraoperatively in those patients undergoing open heart surgery. Temporary transvenous pacing, originally designated primarily for the patient in complete heart block, is now used in bradydysrhythmias as well as for specific tachydysrhythmias, and single- as well as dual-chamber temporary pacing is possible. This section discusses the indications for temporary pacing, and reviews noninvasive TCP, temporary epicardial pacing, and temporary transvenous pacing.

Indications

The indications for temporary cardiac pacing fall into three main categories:

1. Bradycardia with symptoms / asystole
2. Tachycardias
3. Asymptomatic bradycardia

BRADYCARDIA WITH SYMPTOMS/ASYSTOLE. The use of temporary transcutaneous or transvenous pacing for this category of patients is generally undisputed. Transcutaneous pacemakers are now a standard piece of equipment in hospital emergency departments and intensive care units. The application of temporary TCP can be almost immediate in patients with serious symptoms. Temporary transvenous pacing, unless contraindicated, can then follow. In the patient with an acute myocardial infarction, AV block is a potentially serious complication. In patients experiencing an acute inferior wall myocardial infarction, conduction abnormalities are usually seen proximal to the bundle of His, and are relatively benign. It is not uncommon to see second-degree AV block type I (Wenckebach) in these patients. In the symptomatic patient this rhythm usually responds to the intravenous administration of atropine sulfate (AHA, 1992). Prophylactic temporary pacing is usually not indicated in this situation (Hayes & Holmes, 1993b; Hickey & Baas, 1991). Conduction abnormalities distal to the bundle of His (type II second-degree AV block or third-degree AV block) are considered less stable, are associated with low rates and wide QRS complexes, and are more likely to progress rapidly to complete heart block (Hayes & Holmes, 1993b). This particular situation can be seen in the patient experiencing an anterior wall myocardial infarction, and prophylactic pacing is recommended (Hayes & Holmes, 1993b; Hickey & Baas, 1991). Prophylactic pacing is also usually recommended in the patient experiencing a myocardial infarction who develops new right bundle branch block (BBB) with left axis deviation (left anterior hemiblock), right BBB with right axis deviation (left posterior hemiblock), left BBB with first-degree AV block, and alternating left and right BBB (Barold & Zipes, 1992). Other situations in which a hemodynamically significant bradydysrhythmia or an asystolic episode could result, and thus require temporary pacing, include chronic conduction system disease, drug intoxication, serious electrolyte imbalance, and failure of a permanent pacemaker (Hayes & Holmes, 1993b; Hickey & Baas, 1991; Jafri & Kruse, 1992; Martinez, 1988).

TACHYCARDIAS. The use of electrical stimulation for the treatment of tachycardias is a relatively new role for temporary pacemaker therapy. Overdrive pacing (atrial or ventricular) is used in the treatment of recurrent ventricular tachycardia and is the treatment of choice in torsades de pointes (Hayes & Holmes, 1993b; Jafri & Kruse, 1992). Overdrive pacing or burst pacing can be used to terminate reentrant atrial or ventricular tachydysrhythmias (Hayes & Holmes, 1993b). Atrial overdrive pacing can be used to terminate atrial flutter and AV nodal reentry (Jafri & Kruse, 1992; Silver & Goldschlager, 1988). Depending on the specific clinical situation, other measures such as pharmacologic therapy and electrical cardioversion may be tried first.

ASYMPTOMATIC BRADYCARDIA. For patients who are at significant risk for development of advanced degrees of AV block or other conduction abnormalities where serious symptoms would present, temporary pacing is indicated (Silver & Goldschlager, 1988). With external temporary pacing readily available and easily applied in almost any situation, the decision to use a noninvasive therapy in a standby mode is a common occurrence.

Transcutaneous Pacing

Transcutaneous pacing was first introduced by Zoll in 1952, when he reported the successful use of external electrical stimulation via subcutaneous needle electrodes in two patients experiencing prolonged episodes of ventricular standstill. The heart was artificially stimulated for 25 minutes in one patient and for 5 days in the other patient (Zoll, 1952). Thus, an effective means of stimulating the ventricles to beat in an emergency situation was demonstrated to be easily applicable, readily responsive, and replicable. The problems encountered with this early pacing technique were painful stimulation, extensive muscle contractions, and soft tissue burns (Beeler, 1993; Persons, 1987; Peters, 1986). The technique was temporarily abandoned with the advent of transvenous pacing.

The Zoll external temporary pacemaker / monitor / defibrillator was introduced in 1981, and is the type that is used today (Fig. 12–8). The transcutaneous pacemakers function primarily in a VVI mode, although there are models where either a fixed rate (VOO) or a demand mode (VVI) may be chosen. The advantages over the initial piece of equipment are the following: (1) the electrodes are much larger, measuring 80 to 100 cm^2; (2) pregelled surface patch electrodes are used; and (3) in comparison to the first TCP introduced by Zoll in 1952, less current for capture is required, thus decreasing painful stimulation. Since

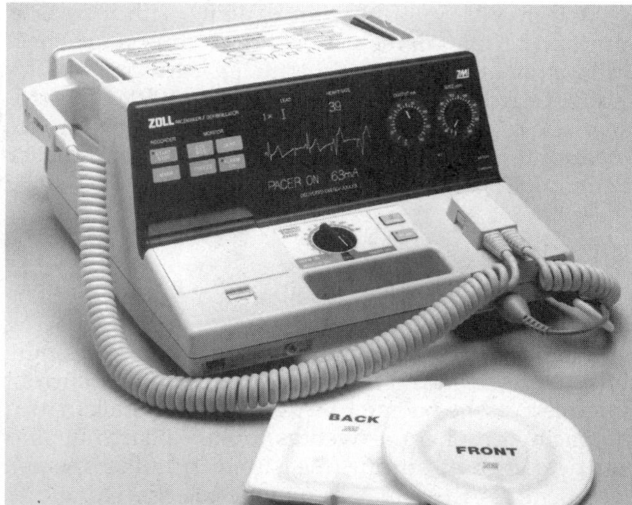

FIGURE 12–8. Photograph of an external pacemaker shows controls for adjustment of rate in pulses per minute (ppm) and output in milliamperes. (Courtesy of ZOLL Medical Inc., Burlington, MA.)

1985, the AHA has included the use of the TCP as a treatment for symptomatic bradycardia and for consideration in the treatment of asystole (AHA, 1992).

EXPANDED INDICATIONS FOR EXTERNAL PACING

Transcutaneous pacing is now used in a number of settings that might previously have been considered "gray areas" for the insertion of a temporary transvenous pacemaker. In addition to the indications listed earlier, some of the clinical situations where a temporary transcutaneous pacemaker might be used, either on standby or for prophylactic use, include but are not limited to patient transport, cardioversion, electrophysiologic studies, administration of thrombolytic therapy, angioplasty, and anesthesia-related bradydysrhythmias (Hickey & Baas, 1991; Jafri & Kruse, 1992; Martinez, 1988; Zoll et al., 1985). In addition, there are certain situations in which a temporary transvenous pacemaker would be relatively or absolutely contraindicated, or associated with a high degree of risk for complications (Table 12–3). Transvenous pacing in the setting of a right ventricular myocardial infarction is associated with frequent episodes of ventricular tachydysrhythmias and difficulty in obtaining acceptable stimulation thresholds (Mittal et al., 1992), thus making TCP a possible option in this situation.

TABLE 12–3. **Temporary Transvenous Pacing: Relative Contraindications**

Coagulopathy, real or potential (e.g., thrombolytic therapy)
Tricuspid valve prosthesis
Digitalis toxicity
Sepsis
Right ventricular infarct

From Pierce, 1989; Teplitz, 1991; Waggoner, 1991; Vukmir, 1993; and Zoll, 1985.

ADVANTAGES

Transcutaneous pacing has several advantages over other pacing techniques (Table 12–4). The effect of TCP on the myocardium and the risk of TCP producing repetitive rhythms such as ventricular tachycardia and ventricular fibrillation have been studied. In a study of canines with induced chronic heart block (Syverud et al., 1986), the hemodynamic effects of TCP and transvenous pacing were compared. Researchers found both techniques to be equally effective. Madsen and colleagues (1988b) conducted TCP on 10 healthy volunteers for 30 minutes at a pacing rate of 85 to 115 pulses per minute at a median current level of 59 milliamperes (mA). Frequent blood sample analyses of myoglobin and enzymes were unchanged from baseline values, and therefore it was concluded that no muscular or myocardial injury occurs from 30 minutes of TCP (Madsen et al., 1988b). The safety and efficacy of TCP using defibrillation-type, low-impedance, self-adhesive polymer electrode pads was validated by 30 healthy volunteers who underwent brief periods of TCP in a study by Chapman and associates (1992). In a series of clinical trials involving TCP of 134 patients in 5 different hospitals (Zoll et al., 1985), no repetitive dysrhythmias were observed. In another study of TCP in 33 patients, no dysrhythmias were induced in any patient (Madsen et al., 1988a).

TCP's noninvasiveness is particularly advantageous in the setting of emergency cardiac pacing. In a cardiac arrest, access for transvenous pacing can be difficult to accomplish and can interfere with resuscitative measures. In a study of temporary pacing over 5 years (Hynes et al., 1983), 13.7% of patients requiring transvenous pacing experienced complications. The advantages of TCP are: (1) it can be initiated almost immediately; (2) it does not interfere with resuscitation; (3) it is not associated with the risks and complications of transvenous pacing; and (4) it can be applied in the prehospital or hospital setting by a paramedic, a nurse, or a physician, but in most facilities it does

TABLE 12–4. **Advantages of Transcutaneous Pacing**

Safe
Noninvasive
Rapid, easy application
Requires no other equipment to implement
Electrocardiographic response is clearly identified
Requires minimal training to implement, and can be used in prehospital settings
Less expensive than other pacing methods
Can be used prophylactically when indications for temporary pacing are borderline
Well tolerated by most conscious patients

From AHA, 1992; Pierce, 1989; Waggoner, 1991; and Zoll, 1985.

TABLE 12–5. **Disadvantages of Transcutaneous Pacing**

Discomfort
Prominent contractions can create difficulty monitoring vital signs
Contraindicated in patients with suspected cervical spine injury or flail chest
May be ineffective in the following situations:
- Patients with increased anteroposterior diameter
- Patients with a very muscular chest wall
- Patients with dilated cardiomyopathy, pericardial effusion

Cannot be used with electrocautery or devices that emit electromagnetic or radiofrequency interference.

From AHA, 1992; Pierce, 1989; Waggoner, 1991; and Zoll, 1985.

not require the presence of a physician. In a study by Dunn and Gregory (1989) of 37 patients who had TCP initiated in the emergency department, intensive care unit, critical care unit, telemetry unit, or recovery room, 51% of pacing interventions were done by nurses, and 49% by physicians.

TCP is less expensive than other pacing techniques and does not require additional specialized equipment such as fluoroscopy. When the indications for temporary pacing are not clearly black or white, standby TCP provides a cost-effective, safe alternative for the patient.

DISADVANTAGES

The disadvantages of TCP are listed in Table 12–5. The major disadvantage is patient discomfort. The discomfort of TCP results from stimulation of cutaneous nerves and contraction of local skeletal muscles, and is also related to the patient's apprehension. The amount of stimulation current (measured in milliamperes) directly affects patient comfort. In a study by Madsen and colleagues (1988a) of TCP in 33 patients, typical findings were that 20 mA created a prickly sensation, 40 mA created a definite thumping sensation on the chest, and 80 mA was considered painful by the patients. Sedation was required for 55% of these patients, and in general seems to be necessary at current outputs greater than 50 mA (Madsen et al., 1988a). In a study by Zoll and colleagues (1985) of 134 patients receiving TCP, the stimulation threshold ranged from 20 to 140 mA, with the usual range being 40 to 70 mA. The researchers reported stimulation to be well tolerated by 73 of 82 conscious patients (Zoll et al., 1985). Careful explanations to the patient and the use of a pharmacologic agent such as morphine sulfate are useful in decreasing discomfort and apprehension. Appropriate placement of electrodes is important to minimize the stimulation threshold. Elderly patients with thin chest walls and decreased muscle mass have lower stimulation thresholds and experience less discomfort, whereas patients with more muscle mass have a higher stimulation threshold, heightened muscle contractions, and thus more discomfort (Dunn & Gregory, 1989; Teplitz, 1991). Prominent muscle contractions can create difficulty in assessing vital signs. TCP is contraindicated in a cervical spine injury or flail chest.

TCP may be ineffective in patients with increased anteroposterior diameter or large muscular chest walls, and in patients with dilated cardiomyopathy and pericardial effusion (Waggoner, 1991). Electromagnetic or radio frequency interference may also alter appropriate function of the external pacemaker (Peters, 1986).

EQUIPMENT

Modern TCP units (Fig. 12–8) are part of a complete resuscitation unit that combines synchronous pacing with defibrillation and cardioversion, all using a single set of large-surface electrodes through which current is delivered. The pacing function includes dials to turn the pacing on or off as well as to vary heart rate and electrical current output (measured in milliamperes). In some units, there may be a mode selection for either demand (synchronous) or nondemand (asynchronous, fixed rate), pacing, and there may be a means to vary the pulse width (the duration of the impulse in milliseconds). A defibrillator–cardioverter is now a standard feature of most units. Electrical wires carry current from the pacing unit to the large patient electrodes.

INITIATION OF NONINVASIVE TCP

In the patient who experiences either a hemodynamically significant bradydysrhythmia or an asystolic event, the simultaneous administration of basic and advanced cardiac life support measures should occur. In the patient with serious signs and symptoms, TCP should not be delayed while waiting for intravenous access or for intravenous atropine sulfate to take effect (AHA, 1992). During the initiation of TCP therapy in the conscious patient, the nurse provides a simple explanation of the procedure and its temporary nature in an effort to decrease the patient's anxiety and provide supportive care.

Steps in Initiating TCP (Table 12–6)

1. Ensure a strong QRS signal in the lead by which the patient is being monitored. In some units the oper-

TABLE 12–6. **Steps in Initiating Transcutaneous Pacing**

1. Ensure a strong QRS signal in the lead that the patient is being monitored in
2. Apply pacing electrodes in the appropriate position
3. Connect the pacing electrodes to the pacemaker cable and its generator unit, and turn the unit on
4. Set the pacing rate
5. Determine the threshold for pacing
6. Ensure effective transcutaneous pacing is occurring
7. Document established pacing parameters and clinical assessment of the patient

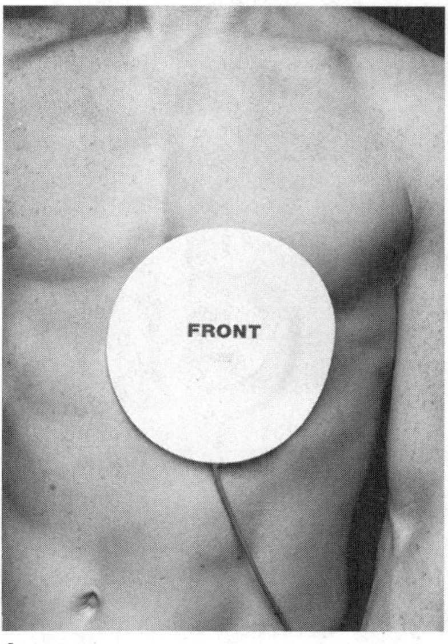

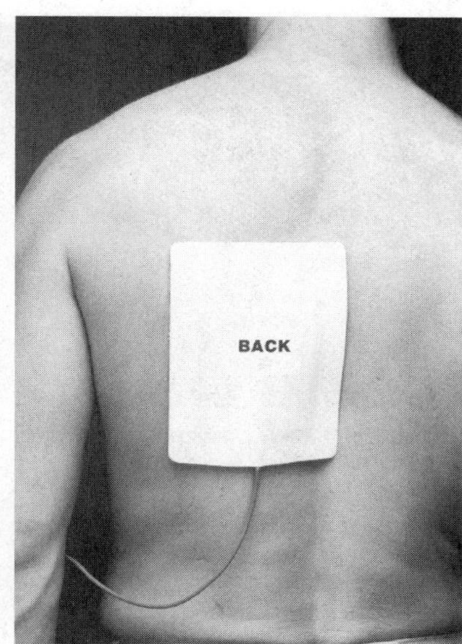

A B

FIGURE 12–9. *A*, Photograph of anterior electrode placement for TCP. *B*, Photograph of posterior electrode placement for TCP. (Courtesy of ZOLL Medical Inc., Burlington, MA.)

ator must choose between the nondemand or demand mode of pacing. The nondemand or fixed-rate mode can be used when the patient has no intrinsic cardiac rhythm. The demand mode of pacing can be used in any situation because the unit senses the presence or absence of the patient's intrinsic rhythm. It responds by inhibiting in the presence of intrinsic beats and pacing in the absence of the patient's own cardiac rhythm. When the unit is accurately identifying the intrinsic beats, each sensed QRS is marked both on the unit's monitor screen and its hard copy. Lead II is often recommended because it provides a strong positive QRS for detection. Most TCP units are able to sense both a positive and a negative QRS deflection. In monitoring the patient, ECG electrodes should be kept away from areas used for defibrillation and external pacing.

2. Apply pacing electrodes in the appropriate position. The electrodes are placed in an anterior–posterior position on the patient's chest wall. The electrodes should be placed on intact skin, away from large bones such as the sternum and scapula, and away from large muscle groups. The negative or anterior electrode is placed on the left chest wall in the V_2–V_3 position or at the V_5 position. The positive or posterior electrode is commonly placed at the level of the heart between the spine and left scapula (Pierce, 1989; Teplitz, 1991). Figure 12–9 depicts this anterior–posterior placement. A study of healthy subjects by Falk and Ngai (1986) compared pacing thresholds with three different electrode positions, and studied the effect that reversing electrode polarity would have on the pacing threshold. The study showed that electrode position was not critical because there was no significant difference in the pacing threshold among the three positions. However, reversing polarity caused an increase in pacing threshold. The study concluded that the positioning of the electrodes is not critical as long as the anterior or apical electrode is of negative polarity (Falk & Ngai, 1986).

Before application of the electrodes, there are some factors to consider regarding skin preparation of the chest wall. To maximize electrode contact, the patient's skin should be clean and dry (Teplitz, 1991; Waggoner, 1991). Lotions, skin oils, and chest hair can increase resistance to pacing current (Teplitz, 1991; Waggoner, 1991). In nonemergent situations chest hair can be clipped (Teplitz, 1991). Current entering small nicks in the skin produced by shaving will result in severe, stinging pain during pacing (Zoll et al., 1985). Because benzoin and alcohol can alter skin resistance, raising the risk of skin irritation, they should not be used in the skin preparation (Teplitz, 1991; Waggoner, 1991).

Once applied, electrode pads should be checked for adherence every 2 to 4 hours and changed every 24 hours (Mickus et al., 1986), or as necessary. Diaphoretic patients will require more frequent assessment. The patient's skin should be assessed for erythematous changes caused by vasodilation during pacing (Mickus et al., 1986). Electrode pads should be replaced over intact skin with any sign of skin breakdown.

3. Connect the pacing electrodes to the pacemaker cable and its generator unit, and turn the unit on. Some units provide a separate start–stop button that actually initiates the pacing function as well as terminates the function when that becomes necessary.

4. Set the pacing rate. In general, the pacing rate is set approximately 10 beats higher than the patient's intrinsic rate (Teplitz, 1991). In most cases, TCP is initiated for a bradydsyrhythmia with symptoms or asystole. Grubb and colleagues (1992) reported that successful use of overdrive pacing (pacing rate of 200, at 120 mA) in six patients presenting to the emergency department in hemodynamically stable ventricular tachycardia.

5. Determine the threshold for pacing. The stimulation threshold, or minimum current required to

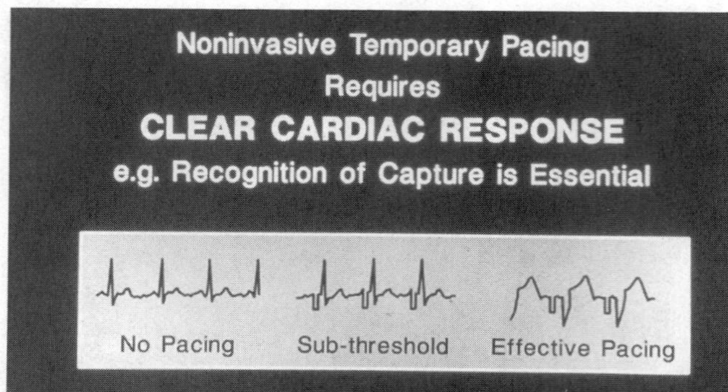

FIGURE 12–10. Nonpacing, suboptimal and effective pacing. (Courtesy of ZOLL Medical Inc., Burlington, MA.)

achieve electrical and mechanical capture, will be primarily effected by the duration of ischemia and the condition of the myocardium (AHA, 1992). In an emergent situation, the current level is rapidly increased until capture is achieved. In less urgent situations, the current can be increased by 10-mA increments until capture is observed. In most patients, stimulation thresholds are in the range of 40 to 70 mA (Zoll et al., 1985). Most instruments are capable of giving up to 200 mA of current, with each current impulse being delivered over a period of 20 to 40 milliseconds.

6. Ensure effective TCP is occurring. Electrical capture is evidenced by the presence of a pacing artifact with each paced beat, a QRS complex greater than 0.14 seconds or 140 milliseconds, and a tall, broad T wave following each paced QRT (Persons, 1987) (Fig. 12–10). Position changes that result in a loosening or buckling of electrode pads may result in loss of capture. Mechanical capture results in the presence of a peripheral pulse that corresponds to the electrical paced beats. Palpation of pulses related to the skeletal contractions produced by pacing, especially on the patient's left side, is often better evaluated by Doppler. Effective mechanical capture will result in improved hemodynamics for the patient.

7. Document established pacing parameters. An ECG or monitor strip is obtained during the initiation of external pacing, documenting the patient's baseline cardiac rhythm as well as the patient's response to external pacing. Table 12–7 lists critical data that should be documented in the patient's record.

Epicardial Pacing

Temporary epicardial wires are routinely placed in patients undergoing cardiac surgery (Baas & Schneider, 1986; Manion, 1993). Implanted epicardial wires in the postoperative cardiac surgical patient are used for the following purposes: (1) to maintain adequate cardiac output through single- or dual-chambered pacing, thus affecting heart rate or AV synchrony; (2) to document and analyze dysrhythmias; and (3) to suppress dysrhythmias that compromise patient hemodynamics, specifically atrial dysrhythmias with rapid atrial pacing (Baas & Schneider, 1986; Manion, 1993; Vitello-Cicciu et al., 1987). The incidence of postoperative dysrhythmias is much higher in patients undergoing valvular surgery (Lynn-McHale et al., 1992). In a study of 3,983 patients who underwent cardiac surgery and who were in normal sinus rhythm before surgery, the incidence of postoperative atrial dysrhythmias was 31.9% in patients who had coronary artery bypass grafting (CABG), 63.6% in those having CABG and mitral valve replacement, and 48.8% in those having CABG and aortic valve replacement (Creswell et al., 1993). Etiologic factors include inflammation and edema at the surgical site, which is in close proximity to the AV junction and bundle of His, effects of cardioplegia, fluid and electrolyte imbalance, acid–base imbalance, hypoxia, and drug effects (Dziadulewicz & Lang, 1992; Lynn-McHale et al., 1992).

APPLICATION OF EPICARDIAL PACING WIRES

Made of stainless steel and coated with Teflon, with the exception of the electrode tips, epicardial pacing wires are implanted during cardiac surgery. The uninsulated tips serve to provide electrical monitoring, deliver electrical impulses, or both (Baas & Schneider, 1987). Usually, four wires are implanted. Because a loose epicardial wire can result in diaphragmatic pacing (Manion, 1993), the distal ends of these wires are held in place on the epicardium by suture or staple, and the proximal ends are brought outside the chest wall through subcutaneous tissue (Baas & Schneider, 1986). Two wires are implanted on the right atrium, and the proximal ends of those wires are brought out through the chest wall at the right subcostal area (Spyrou, 1981; Lynn-McHale et al., 1992). Two additional wires are implanted on the anterior surface of the right ventricle, and their proximal ends exit the chest wall at the left subcostal area (Spyrou, 1981; Lynn-McHale et al., 1992). The location of the atrial wires on the right side of the chest and the ventricular

TABLE 12–7. **Documentation of Transcutaneous Pacing**

1. Electrocardiogram strip of patient's baseline intrinsic rhythm
2. Location of pacing electrodes on patient
3. Pacing mode (demand vs. non-demand)
4. Stimulation threshold in milliamperes of current and actual current setting
5. Pacing rate
6. Electrocardiogram strip documentation of pacing
7. Percentage of time patient is paced with electrical and mechanical capture
8. Patient comfort level during pacing, measures taken to improve comfort
9. Skin condition under electrode pads when changed

From Appel-Hardin, 1992; Beeler, 1993; Daddio-Pierce, 1989; Persons, 1987; Teplitz, 1991; and Waggoner, 1991.

wires on the left side is universal. These four pacing lead wires are attached to an AV sequential pulse generator. The positive pole is always the ground, and the negative pole is the pacing electrode. Before the end of the case, a trial of pacing is conducted to evaluate the integrity of the pacing system (Manion, 1993). Epicardial pacing often requires up to 10 mA of current for capture. Alternatively, but not commonly, a single atrial and ventricular lead are placed (Baas & Schneider, 1986), and a ground wire may be placed under the skin.

PACING MODES

Most commonly, four potential pacing modes are possible with epicardial pacing wires (Table 12–8). Epicardial pacing is frequently in the AOO or DVI mode (Lavieri, 1994). Pacing can be initiated during surgery and can be used anywhere from 12 to 24 hours after open heart surgery. Occasionally, epicardial lead wires remain in place for up to 2 to 3 weeks. With regard to valvular surgery, the operative site is close to the AV node and the bundle of His, making the incidence of AV block higher in this subset of patients. These patients may be paced for longer periods of time after surgery before the hemodynamics of their own spontaneous rhythms are actually assessed (Manion, 1993). In thes patients, the pacemaker is set in the VVI mode as a backup mechanism. If a patient experiences a hemodynamically significant bradydysrhythmia, VVI pacing will occur and subsequently either AOO or DVI pacing can be initated, depending on the integrity of AV conduction (Lavieri, 1994). Some patients will require permanent pacing until the patient reaches his or her preoperative weight or at approximately 2 weeks postcardiac surgery (Lavieri, 1994).

THE ATRIAL ELECTROGRAM

The diagnosis of atrial dysrhythmias by surface 12-lead ECG is sometimes unclear. An atrial electrogram (AEG), also commonly referred to as an atrial wire trace, provides a tracing of electrical atrial activity obtained directly from the epicardial electrode(s). An AEG is obtained via the bedside monitor or ECG, and lead configuration can be unipolar or bipolar. Insulated alligator clips are used to connect the atrial epicardial wires to the right arm and left arm ECG leads. The lower limb leads (left leg and right leg) are attached to the ECG machine in the usual manner. Table 12–9 details the steps of taking an AEG. By attaching the atrial electrodes to both arms, lead I is a bipolar tracing because it is recording electrical activity from two atrial poles, both of which are in contact with the heart (Dziadulewicz & Lang, 1992). Leads II and III are unipolar tracings because they record electrical activity from one pole. Lead II records electrical activity between the atrial wire attached to the right arm and the left leg, and lead III records electrical activity between the atrial wire attached to the left arm and the right leg. Leads II and III are examined for the one with the largest atrial complex because the wire used in that particular lead is the best for pacing and capture, and would be the wire used for rapid atrial pacing should the need arise.

A baseline AEG is obtained in the cardiac surgical patient against which later tracings can be compared. Figure 12–11 depicts an AEG of a patient in normal sinus rhythm. If a rapid atrial rhythm develops in the patient, the nurse uses the AEG to determine whether the rhythm is atrial tachycardia (or an AV nodal reentry tachydysrhythmia), type I atrial flutter, type II atrial flutter, or atrial fibrillation. Waldo and associates (1977) identified two types of atrial flutter: (1) type I, in which the atrial rate is less than 340 bpm, and (2) Type II, in which the atrial rate is greater than 340 bpm. Today, type I flutter is characterized by an atrial rate between 250 and 350 bpm and a regular rhythm. An AEG of type I flutter is depicted in Figure 12–12. Type II flutter is characterized by an atrial rate between 350 and 450 bpm, and the rhythm may be irregular (Fig. 12–13). An atrial

TABLE 12–8. **Epicardial Pacing Modes**

Pacing Mode	Description
AOO	Asynchronous atrial pacing
DOO	Asynchronous atrial and ventricular pacing
VVI	Synchronous ventricular pacing
DVI	Atrioventricular sequential pacing

From Manion, 1993, and Lynn-McHale et al., 1992.

TABLE 12–9. **Taking an Atrial Electrogram/Atrial Wire Trace**

Both atrial wires are labeled so as to distinguish one from another.
One atrial wire is attached by insulated clip to the right arm lead of the ECG machine or bedside monitor. Note which atrial wire is attached where.
The other atrial wire is attached by insulated alligator clip to the left arm lead of the ECG machine or bedside monitor. Note which atrial wire is attached to this lead.
The left leg and right leg leads of the ECG machine or bedside monitor are attached in the usual way.

	Use
Bipolar AEG	
A lead I recording is obtained	Best recording of atrial depolarization Shows large-amplitude P waves Ventricular depolarization is minimally visible
Unipolar AEG	
A lead II or III recording is obtained	Shows both atrial and ventricular depolarization The P wave is amplified

Abbreviations: AEG, atrial electrogram; ECG, electrocardiogram.
From Dziadulewicz, 1992; Lavieri, 1994.

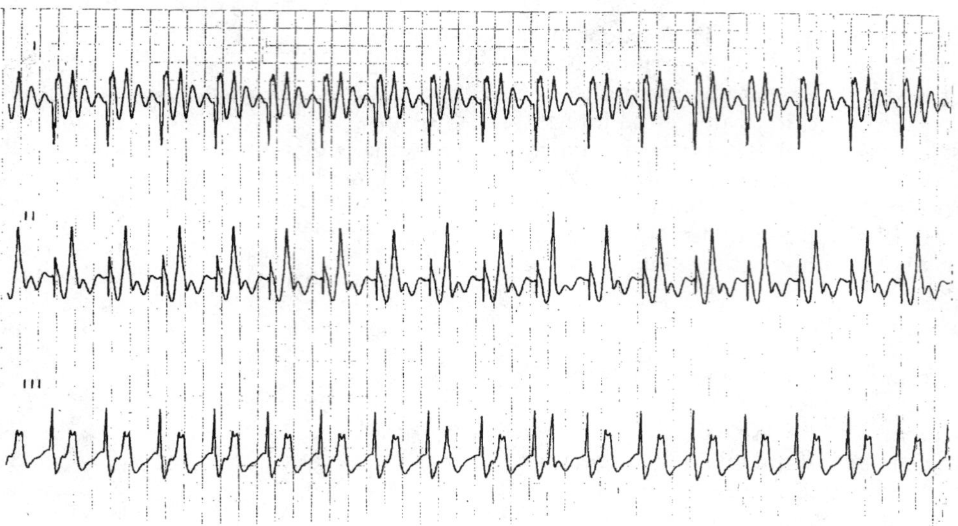

FIGURE 12–11. Atrial electrogram of normal sinus rhythm. (Courtesy of Mary Coughlan Lavieri, RN, MS, CCRN, Beth Israel Hospital, Boston, MA.)

rate greater than 400 bpm and a rhythm that is grossly irregular characterizes atrial fibrillation. Figure 12–14 depicts atrial fibrillation on an AEG. Atrial fibrillation is common after cardiac surgery on day 3, when third-space fluid is mobilizing, increasing preload and right atrial pressures. It commonly resolves when postoperative fluid weight has decreased.

RAPID ATRIAL PACING

Rapid atrial pacing, stimulating the atria at a rate greater than the patient's intrinsic rate, has been a successful treatment for type I atrial flutter (Baas & Schneider, 1986) as well as for atrial tachycardia (Lavieri, 1994). With a backup VVI pacemaker attached to the patient at ordered settings but turned off, the atrial epicardial wires are attached to a high-rate pacemaker box (Lavieri, 1994). The atrial pacemaker is tested to ensure that in fact it does pace the atria, after which a burst technique of rapid atrial pacing is employed. The atrial pacing rate is increased 15% to 25% above the patient's intrinsic atrial rate and maintained for 30 seconds, after which rapid atrial pacing is abruptly discontinued (Lavieri, 1994).

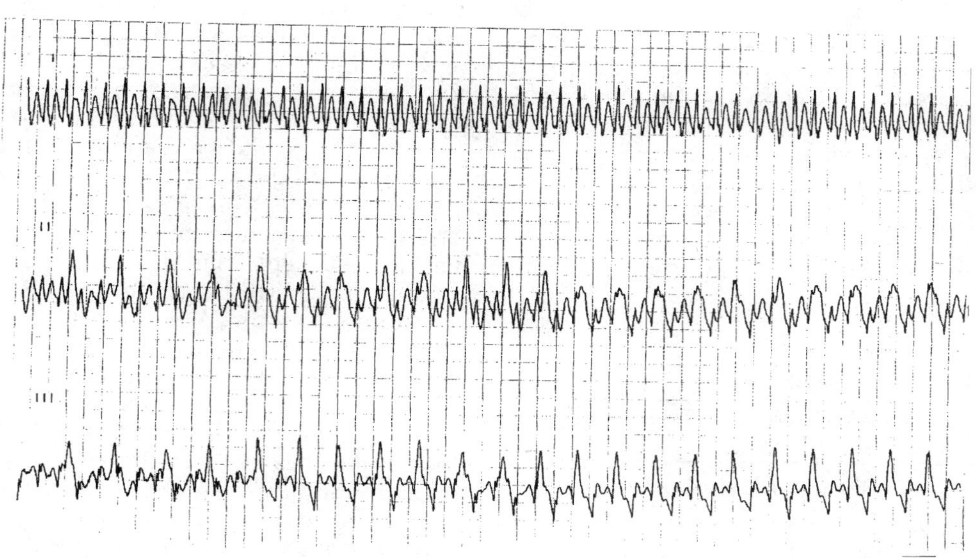

FIGURE 12–12. Atrial electrogram of type I atrial flutter. (Courtesy of Mary Coughlan Lavieri, RN, MS, CCRN, Beth Israel Hospital, Boston, MA.)

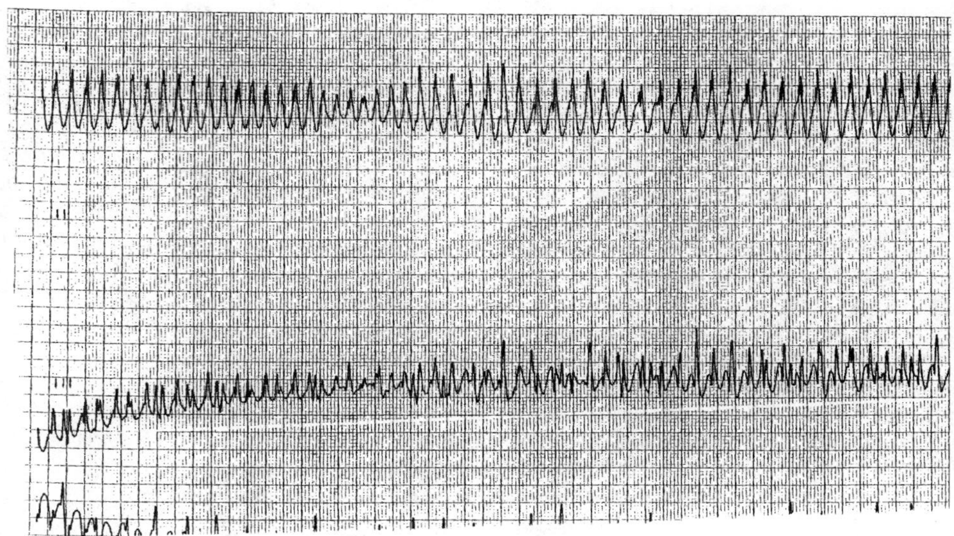

FIGURE 12–13. Atrial electrogram of type II atrial flutter. (Courtesy of Mary Coughlan Lavieri, RN, MS, CCRN, Beth Israel Hospital, Boston, MA.)

EPICARDIAL PACING WIRE REMOVAL

On the fourth or fifth postoperative day, the epicardial wires are removed by gently pulling through the chest wall (Manion, 1993), and examined to ensure full removal (Baas & Schneider, 1986). After the removal of epicardial wires, the patient is monitored for potential complications such as bleeding and pericardial tamponade (Johnson et al., 1993). Wires that are not easily removed are snipped while traction is applied, and the patient is monitored for ventricular dysrhythmias, wire fragment migration, and infection related to retained wire fragment (Johnson et al., 1993; Manion, 1993).

ELECTRICAL SAFETY CONSIDERATIONS

Epicardial pacing wires present a potential electrical hazard. Nurses should guard against static electricity (e.g., slider boards), and gloves should be worn when manipulating any part of the electrical circuit. Any wires not in use should be wrapped and insulated in rubber. Gloves and finger cots have been used for this purpose.

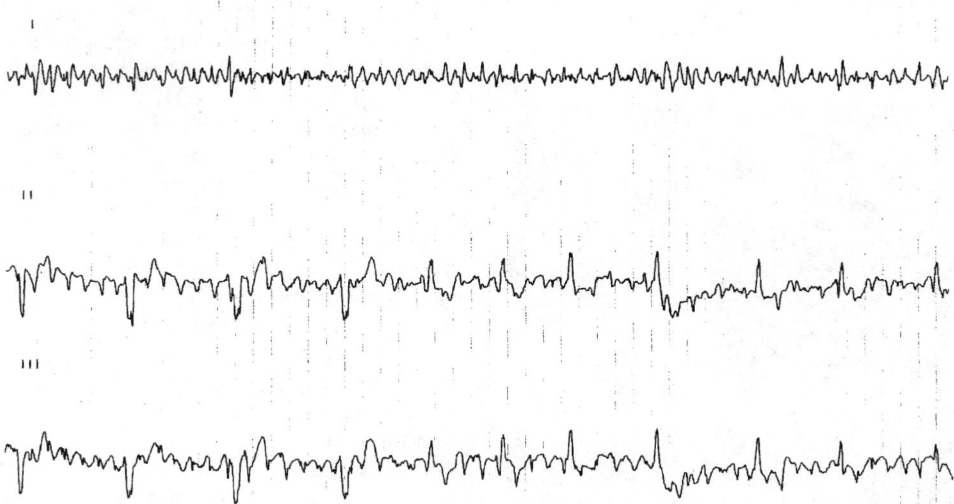

FIGURE 12–14. Atrial electrogram of atrial fibrillation. (Courtesy of Mary Coughlan Lavieri, RN, MS, CCRN, Beth Israel Hospital, Boston, MA.)

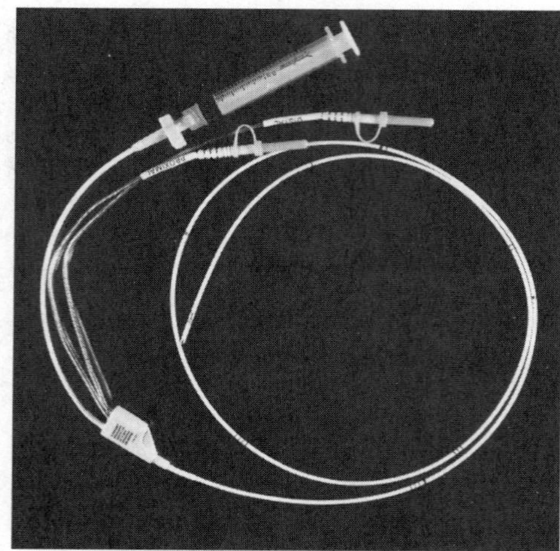

FIGURE 12–15. Photograph of a Baxter bipolar balloon-tipped pacing catheter.

Temporary Transvenous Pacing

TYPES OF CATHETERS

There are several catheters available for both atrial and ventricular temporary pacing. There are primarily two types of bipolar pacing catheters used for single-chamber ventricular pacing (Figs. 12–15 and 12–16). The more commonly used balloon-tipped pacing catheter is a softer, more flexible catheter that is floated into position in the right ventricular apex under either fluoroscopic or ECG guidance (Jafri & Kruse, 1992). Insertion of balloon flotation catheters does not require fluoroscopy, making it preferable in emergency situations. The stiff wire catheter, which is the second type of pacing lead, is easier to position, but also has an increased potential for perforation (Hayes & Holmes, 1993b; Jafri & Kruse, 1992). The stiff wire catheters require placement under fluoroscopy for safe and proper positioning (Hayes & Holmes, 1993b).

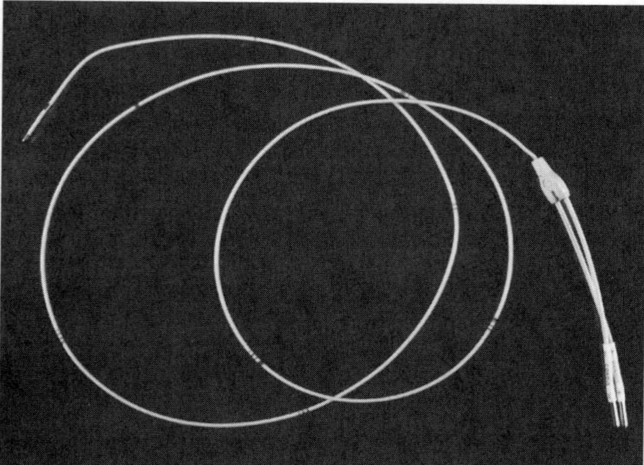

FIGURE 12–16. Photograph of a Cordis stiff wire bipolar pacing catheter.

For atrial pacing, a bipolar "J" lead is available for temporary placement in the right atrial appendage. For AV sequential pacing, the atrial "J" lead and a balloon-tipped ventricular lead are commonly used (Jafri & Kruse, 1992). Some multipurpose pulmonary arterial (PA) catheters have a ventricular pacing port or have both an atrial and ventricular pacing port. The pacing wire is passed via the atrial or ventricular port and positioned for pacing. Dislodgment of the pacing electrode is a potential problem when pacing through the PA catheter, and hence the use of these catheters is usually reserved for prophylactic pacing (Jafri & Kruse, 1992).

GENERATORS

Three types of temporary generators exist: (1) single-chamber (Fig. 12–17*A*), (2) dual-chamber or AV sequential (Fig. 12–17*B*), and (3) dual-chamber of DDD (Fig. 12–17*C*). Most conventional generators have a battery test device. It is recommended that a new battery be used for each patient. Many generators operate on a 9-V alkaline battery; the nurse at the bedside must be knowledgeable regarding the power source for the specific pulse generator being used. Older-model pulse generators with exposed metal require covering with insulated material, such as a rubber glove.

INSERTION

FLUOROSCOPY. When the patient's clinical situation is relatively stable, fluoroscopy is often used to assist in placement of the temporary lead. Sites of venous access include the internal and external jugular veins, the subclavian vein, the brachial vein, and the femoral vein. In a 5-year study of over 1,000 patients who received temporary transvenous pacemakers, the right internal jugular approach was associated with the lowest complication rate (Hynes et al., 1983). Most often the jugular or subclavian vein is used because it provides a more stable site with less risk of dislodgment (Hayes & Holmes, 1993b). If it is likely that a permanent pacemaker will be implanted, the internal or external jugular vein is used. A percutaneous technique is used to insert a temporary lead into either the right atrium or right ventricle. Once the vein is entered with a needle, a guidewire is advanced into the vein and the needle is withdrawn. A dilator and sheath are advanced over the wire. Once the sheath is in place, the pacing lead is inserted via the sheath into the central vein, through the right atrium, across the tricuspid valve, and into place at the right ventricular apex. An atrial pacing lead is positioned in the right atrial appendage. When placement has been achieved, the positive and negative electrodes of the pacing catheter are connected to the corresponding poles of the pulse generator, and pacing is initiated. Verification of lead placement is done by chest x-ray. The patient is monitored for dysrhythmias, especially when the pacing lead is being positioned in the right ventricle, because

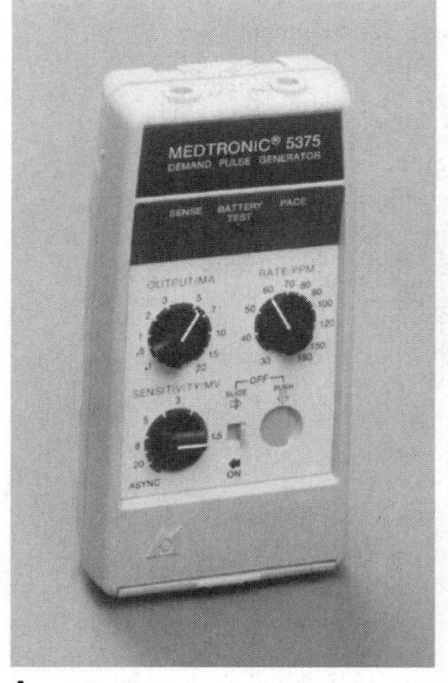

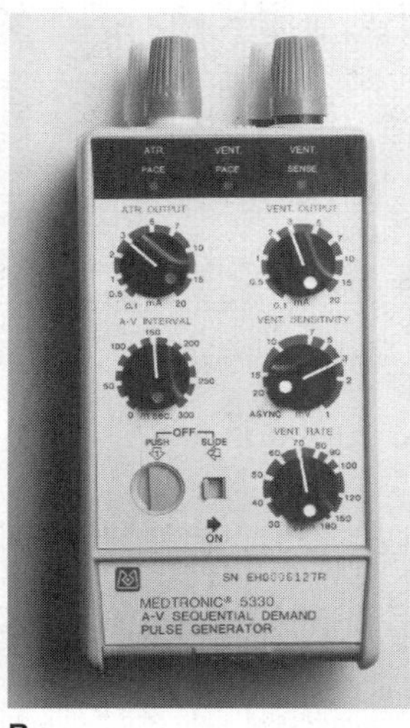

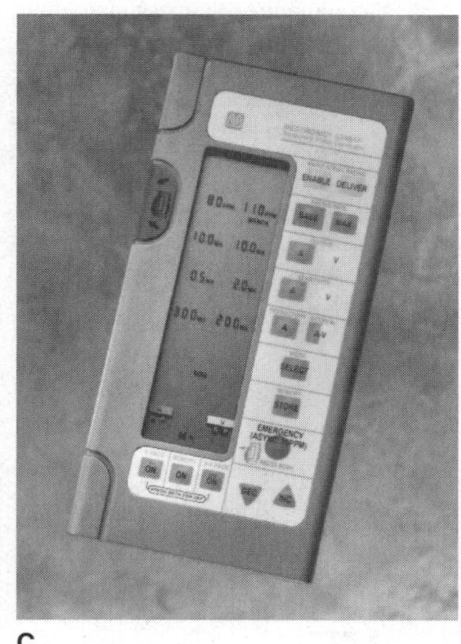

A B C

FIGURE 12–17. Temporary pulse generators: *A*, VVI pulse generator. *B*, DVI pulse generator. *C*, DDD pulse generator. (Courtesy of Medtronic, Inc., Minneapolis, MN.)

ventricular dysrhythmias are common. The nurse also continually assesses the patient's clinical status and tolerance of the procedure, and medicates the patient for discomfort.

INTRACARDIAC ECG. The placement of a temporary pacing catheter can be done using the intracardiac ECG. This is sometimes useful in emergency situations. The patient is attached to the limb leads of the ECG machine. When the bipolar pacing catheter has been placed into the central circulation, an alligator clamp is used to connect the distal (negative) pole of the pacing catheter to the chest or V lead of the ECG machine. Some manufacturers provide a special connector with their pacemaker kits that achieves the same purpose. As the pacing catheter moves from the right atrium to the right ventricle and up against the wall of the right ventricle, certain characteristic ECG changes are seen (Fig. 12–18). As the catheter enters the right ventricle, the amplitude of the QRS increases markedly, and when the catheter makes contact with the endocardial surface, ST segment elevation (current of injury) is seen (Bing et al., 1972; Hayes & Holmes, 1993b). Inadvertent entry into the coronary sinus is signified by the presence of large P waves and large QRS complexes (Jafri & Kruse, 1992). Verification of lead placement is by chest x-ray.

BLIND INSERTION. The insertion of pacing catheters without fluoroscopic or ECG guidance is done in emergency situations (Jafri & Kruse, 1992). The patient is attached to a surface ECG. The pacing catheter, with electrode leads hooked up to the generator, is inserted into the vein, and the only immediate evidence of placement is through electrical capture on the ECG. Verification of lead placement is by chest x-ray.

DETERMINATION OF SENSING AND STIMULATION THRESHOLDS

STIMULATION THRESHOLD DETERMINATION. Once pacing has been initiated, thresholds can be tested. The stimulation or pacing threshold is the minimum current, measured in milliamperes (mA), required to achieve consistent capture. The ideal stimulation threshold for ventricular pacing is less than 1 mA (Hayes & Holmes, 1993b), and for atrial pacing is less than 2 mA (Jafri & Kruse, 1992). Testing stimulation threshold is detailed in Table 12–10. These thresholds can increase postinsertion, and hence should be checked and documented daily. Factors that can increase the stimulation threshold include inflammation at the pacing catheter site, serious electrolyte imbalances, myocardial ischemia, and acidosis.

SENSITIVITY THRESHOLD DETERMINATION. The sensitivity or sensing threshold is the minimum setting, measured in millivolts, that is required to achieve consistent and appropriate sensing of the patient's intrinsic cardiac rhythm. If the sensitivity level is too high, the pacemaker may be oversensing by sensing T waves, artifact, or myopotentials, and thus may inappropriately inhibit pacing (Jafri & Kruse, 1992). Ideally, the sensing level ends up to be about midway between the sensing threshold and the level at which oversensing occurs (Jafri & Kruse, 1992). Sensing levels are depicted in Figure 12–19, and the steps to determining the sensitivity threshold are detailed in Table 12–11.

MODES OF TEMPORARY TRANSVENOUS PACING

The goal of temporary transvenous pacing is to improve cardiac output. With single-chamber pacing,

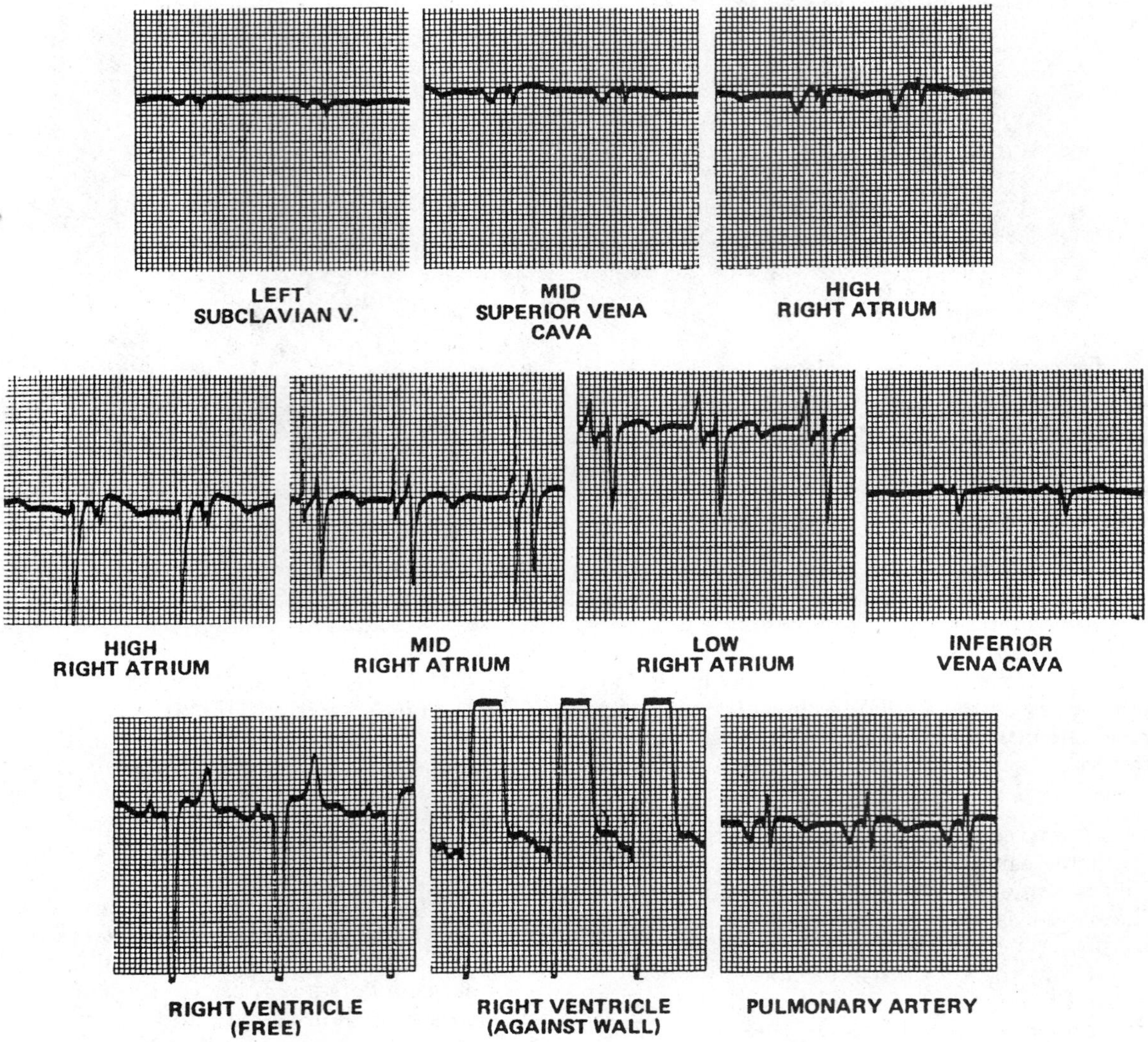

LEFT SUBCLAVIAN V.

MID SUPERIOR VENA CAVA

HIGH RIGHT ATRIUM

HIGH RIGHT ATRIUM

MID RIGHT ATRIUM

LOW RIGHT ATRIUM

INFERIOR VENA CAVA

RIGHT VENTRICLE (FREE)

RIGHT VENTRICLE (AGAINST WALL)

PULMONARY ARTERY

FIGURE 12–18. Temporary pacemaker placement by ECG monitoring. Note the current of injury pattern as the catheter contacts the ventricular endocardium. (From Bing, O. H. et al. (1972). Pacemaker placement by electrocardiographic monitoring. Reprinted by permission of *The New England Journal of Medicine, 287,* 651.)

TABLE 12–10. **Determination of the Stimulation Threshold**

1. The pacing rate is increased as necessary to approximately 10 pulses per minute above the patient's intrinsic rate.
2. With the monitor or electrocardiogram demonstrating 100% capture, the current is decreased gradually until capture is lost.
3. The current is then increased just until capture is returned, and this current level is documented as the stimulation threshold.
4. The current is then increased to at least twice the threshold value to provide a safety margin.

From Hayes and Holmes, 1993b; Jafri and Kruse, 1992; Hickey and Baas, 1991.

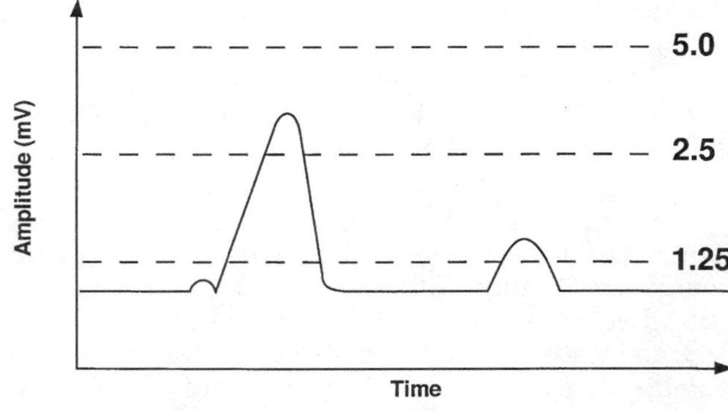

FIGURE 12–19. Sensitivity threshold levels. (Courtesy of Medtronic, Inc., Minneapolis, MN.)

TABLE 12–11. **Determination of the Sensing Threshold**

1. The pacing rate is adjusted so that it is at least 10 pulses per minute less than the patient's intrinsic rate.
2. The sensitivity dial is then rotated fully clockwise to the most sensitive position (approximately 1–1.5 mV).
3. The sensitivity dial should be rotated counterclockwise as necessary until the pacemaker begins to emit pulses during the patient's intrinsic rhythm.
4. The sensitivity dial is then rotated clockwise until (1) flashing of the sensing indicator corresponding to the patient's intrinsic P waves or QRS complexes occurs on a consistent basis, and (2) no pacemaker activity is seen in the presence of the patient's intrinsic rhythm. This millivoltage level is documented as the sensing threshold.
5. The sensitivity level is then set at one-half to one-third of the identified threshold.

From Jafri and Kruse, 1992; Hickey and Baas, 1991.

this is done primarily by increasing heart rate. Dual-chamber pacing not only improves heart rate, but provides AV synchrony, and in some modes has the ability to provide rate responsiveness.

A single-chamber pacemaker can provide asynchronous pacing in the ventricle or in the atrium. This type of pacemaker can also provide synchronous, demand pacing in either chamber. Ventricular demand pacing is an extremely common mode of temporary pacing when correction of a bradycardia is needed. The major drawback of the VVI (demand) mode is that it cannot provide AV synchrony or rate responsiveness.

With a properly timed atrial contraction contributing 25% to 30% of ventricular end-diastolic volume, cardiac output is improved with dual-chamber pacing. Those patients with normal sinus node activity benefit from rate responsiveness. There are two pulse generators available for dual-chamber pacing. The AV sequential pulse generator can provide temporary pacing in either the DOO mode or the DVI mode, the latter being most common. The DDD pulse generator, in addition to the DDD pacing mode, can operate in the VVI, AAI, DVI, or VDD pacing modes. Table 12–12 provides a description of each of the eight temporary pacing modes.

COMPLICATIONS: PREVENTION AND EARLY DETECTION

Complications of temporary pacing can occur related to venous access and placement of the catheter, or related to the pacing system itself. Complications related to central venous access include pneumothorax, air embolus, thrombosis, bleeding, vascular or nerve damage, inadvertent arterial entry or trauma, and thrombophlebitis (Hayes & Holmes, 1993b; Silver & Goldschlager, 1988). During placement of the catheter, perforation of the right ventricle or interventricular septum is a rare but known complication of temporary transvenous pacing, the incidence being slightly higher with the use of the stiff wire type catheter (Hayes & Holmes, 1993b). Clinical signs of perforation may include chest discomfort that is pericardial in nature and associated with a pericardial friction rub, a change in the paced QRS complex to a right bundle branch pattern, and loss of pacing or sensing. Pericardial tamponade is rarely seen. In the event perforation is suspected, the lead is withdrawn and repositioned and the patient is monitored carefully for complications. The placement of a temporary pacing catheter may result in dysrhythmias. The placement of a ventricular catheter can result in mechanically induced ventricular dysrhythmias, a situation that is resolved by pulling the lead away from the ventricular wall and relocating it in a more stable position. Intravenous xylocaine should be available at the bedside. In the case of a temporary catheter with sensing abnormalities, the concern is that a pacemaker stimulus occurring during the vulnerable repolarization period of an intrinsic QRS could induce ventricular tachycardia or ventricular fibrillation (Hayes & Holmes, 1993b). Myocardial ischemia will also increase the potential for ventricular irritability.

During or after placement of the temporary pacing catheter, lead dislodgment may occur, the most common complication of temporary transvenous pacing. Silver and Goldschlager (1988) estimate that lead dislodgment occurs in up to 25% of cases. Clinical signs include intermittent or complete loss of pacing or sensing. Chest x-ray confirms dislodgment, and the lead is repositioned.

Problems within the pacing system itself relate to its ability to pace and to sense. Failure to pace includes both the stimulus to pace as well as ventricular capture. Absence of the pacing stimulus can be caused by loose connections, complete lead fracture, or battery depletion. More commonly, the pacing stimulus is delivered but the chamber "fails to capture" on an intermittent or, less commonly, a continuous basis. Causes for this include increased stimulation threshold, lead dislodgment or fracture, or perforation.

Failure to appropriately sense the intrinsic rhythm can be of two types: oversensing or undersensing. Oversensing occurs when the pacemaker senses more than the intrinsic rhythm, and can result in inappropriate inhibition of the pacemaker. Myopotentials and skeletal muscle electrical potentials can be sensed by the pacemaker as cardiac events, causing inhibition and lack of pacing. Sensing of myopotentials is more common in unipolar lead systems. T-wave sensing is another example of oversensing and results in the pacemaker inhibiting longer than it should. To make the pacemaker less sensitive, the sensitivity threshold must be turned to a higher millivoltage setting (Fig. 12–19). Undersensing occurs when the pacemaker fails to sense an intrinsic P wave or QRS complex, which results in pacing when there should be inhibition. In this case, the pacemaker needs to be made more sensitive, and to accomplish this, the sensitivity threshold is adjusted to a lower millivoltage setting.

TABLE 12–12. **Temporary Pacing Modes**

NBG Code	Previous Terminology	Characteristics	Clinical Applications
AOO	Atrial fixed rate Atrial asynchronous	Paces in the atrium at a continuous set rate; there is no sensing mode; competition with the intrinsic atrial rhythm can result in atrial ectopy, atrial tachycardia, or atrial fibrillation	Used to increase the atrial rate when the remaining conduction system is intact; not indicated with atrial fibrillation or atrial flutter
VOO	Ventricular fixed rate Ventricular asynchronous	Paces in the ventricle at a set rate; there is no sensing mode; competition with the intrinsic ventricular rhythm can result in ventricular tachycardia or ventricular fibrillation	Used to increase the ventricular rate
AAI	Atrial demand Atrial inhibited Atrial synchronous	Paces and senses in the atrium; sensed atrial activity inhibits pacing	Used to increase the atrial rate; sensing prevents competition with the intrinsic rhythm
VVI	Ventricular demand Ventricular inhibited Ventricular synchronous	Paces and senses in the ventricle; sensed ventricular activity inhibits pacing	Used to increase the ventricular rate; sensing prevents competition with the intrinsic rhythm
DOO	Atrial and ventricular fixed rate Dual-chamber fixed rate	Paces in the atrium at a fixed rate, then paces the ventricle at the same fixed rate, following a set AV interval; competition with either the atrial or ventricular intrinsic rhythms can result in dysrhythmias	Used to increase the heart rate in the case of a bradycardia or severe conduction disorder; to maintain AV synchrony
DVI	AV sequential AV sequential with fixed rate	Paces in the atrium and the ventricle; sensing occurs only in the ventricle; a sensed ventricular beat occurring before the end of a set AV interval inhibits ventricular pacing; competition can result if there is intrinsic atrial activity	Used to increase the heart rate in the case of a bradycardia or a severe conduction disturbance; AV synchrony is maintained as long as sinus node function is absent or falls below the pacing rate
VDD	Ventricular paced with dual-chamber sensing	Paces in the ventricle only; sensing occurs in both the atrium and the ventricle; sensed P waves initiate an AV interval; ventricular pacing occurs at the end of the AV interval; a sensed ventricular beat occurring before the end of a set AV interval inhibits ventricular pacing; VVI pacing occurs if the intrinsic atrial rate falls below the lower rate limit	Used to increase the heart rate in the case of a bradycardia or severe conduction disorder; provides rate responsiveness when intrinsic sinus activity exceeds the preset pacing rate
DDD	Dual-chamber demand pacing Universal pacing	Paces and senses, both in the atrium and the ventricle; timing begins with the VA interval: 1. A sensed atrial event occurring before the end of this interval will inhibit the atrial pacing and begin the AV interval 2. Sensing no atrial activity during the VA interval, a paced atrial beat begins the AV interval 3. A sensed ventricular event occurring within the AV interval inhibits the ventricular pacer and restarts the VA interval 4. Sensing no ventricular activity during the AV interval, the ventricle is paced and the VA interval is restarted	Provides increased heart rate and AV synchrony; provides rate responsiveness when sinus activity exceeds the preset pacing rate; contraindicated in atrial flutter and atrial fibrillation; can be altered to AAI, VVI, DVI, or VDD pacing modes

Abbreviations: AV, atrioventricular; VA, ventriculoatrial.

Adapted from Baas, L., & Schneider, C. L. (1986). Temporary epicardial electrodes: Critical care techniques. *Dimensions of Critical Care Nursing, 5*, 90–91.

ECG INTERPRETATION OF PACEMAKER FUNCTION

Single-Chamber Pacing

Some of the common terminology used in ECG interpretation of pacemaker function is listed and defined in Table 12–13. In single-chamber pacing, only one pacing artifact will be seen in each paced cardiac cycle. If the patient's intrinsic atrial or ventricular rate falls below the lower rate limit, the atrium or ventricle will be paced. Monitoring the ECG of a patient with an AAI pacemaker would show the presence of a pacing artifact followed by a P wave in the absence of intrinsic atrial activity, and the appropriate inhibition of the pacemaker in the presence of intrinsic atrial activity. There should be no atrial pacing stimulus visible when the ECG shows intrinsic P waves. With AAI pacing, there should be no pacing stimulus visible within the QRS complex.

In the patient with a VVI pacemaker, the absence of QRS complexes would result in ventricular pacing artifact with ventricular capture. In the presence of intrinsic ventricular activity, the pacemaker is inhibited and no ventricular pacing artifact should be seen (Fig. 12–20). In the VVI mode of pacing, no spikes should be seen during intrinsic atrial activity.

Dual-Chamber Pacing

Electrocardiographic interpretation of dual-chamber pacing is similar in principle to single-chamber pacing. The assessment of pacing and sensing applies to both an atrial lead and a ventricular lead. The following discussion focuses on ECG interpretation of DDD pacing.

TIMING INTERVALS

Three timing intervals in dual-chamber pacemakers are determined at the time of implant, are set according to ventricular and atrial events, and are measured in milliseconds. The first timing interval, the V–A interval, starts at a ventricular event, either intrinsic or paced, and ends at the atrial event, also either intrinsic or paced. The atrial event begins the A–V interval, which ends at the onset of the ventricular event. The V–A interval and the A–V interval combined equal the V–V interval. Figure 12–21 depicts these three timing intervals.

FOUR NORMAL MODES OF DDD OPERATION

ATRIAL PACING, VENTRICULAR PACING. In this mode, the atrial lead senses no intrinsic atrial activity during

TABLE 12–13. **Glossary of Terms**

Pacing artifact	Also referred to as the spike or pacing stimulus; it represents only the electrical stimulation to the myocardium with the expectation that depolarization will follow. An atrial spike should be followed by a P wave and a ventricular spike should be followed by a QRS.
Capture	The depolarization of the atrial or ventricular myocardium after a pacing artifact is referred to as atrial or ventricular capture. Right ventricular pacing produces a left bundle branch block pattern on the electrocardiogram.
Automatic pacing interval	The amount of time, usually expressed in milliseconds (0.20 seconds = 200 milliseconds), that exists between the pacing artifacts of two consecutively paced beats.
Escape interval	The amount of time expressed in milliseconds between a patient's intrinsic beat and the next paced beat. The time is equal to the automatic pacing interval, except when hysteresis has been programmed into the pacemaker.
Hysteresis	This allows for one longer escape interval after any intrinsic beat, thus allowing more opportunity for intrinsic rhythm to occur and decreasing battery use.
Refractory period	A period of time during which the pacemaker is programmed to be insensitive.
Magnet mode	Application of a magnet over the pacemaker results in fixed-rate or asychronous pacing in all single-chamber and most dual-chamber pacemakers (Hayes, 1993). In some dual-chamber pacemakers, the magnet mode can be programmed to OFF, and in some, ventricular sensing is maintained while in magnet mode (Hayes, 1993).
Fusion beat	An intrinsic cardiac beat occurring coincidentally with a paced beat. The result is a complex that looks somewhat like the intrinsic beat and somewhat like that paced beat including the pacing artifact.

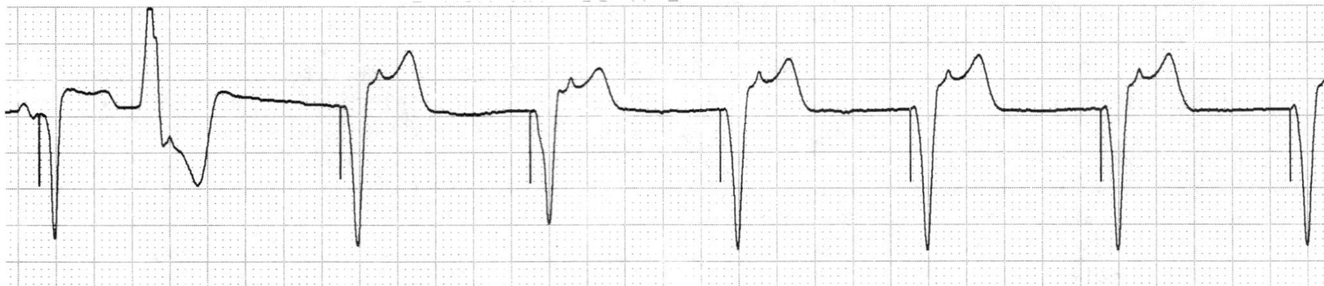

FIGURE 12–20. VVI pacing with appropriate sensing of an intrinsic beat.

the V–A interval. At the completion of that timing interval the atrium is paced, beginning the A–V interval. At the end of the A–V interval the ventricular lead, having sensed no intrinsic QRS complex, paces the ventricle. This mode of pacing is at the lower rate limit set for the pacemaker because both chambers are paced (Fig. 12–22).

ATRIAL SENSING, VENTRICULAR PACING. Intrinsic atrial activity is sensed by the atrial pacing lead. The intrinsic atrial beat starts the A–V interval. If there is no ventricular activity sensed by the ventricular lead, the ventricles will be paced in synchrony with the sensed atrial events. This is referred to as "atrial tracking," and is shown in Figure 12–23. In the patient who has an AV conduction abnormality requiring a pacemaker but has intact sinus node function, a DDD or VDD pacemaker can provide rate variability through atrial tracking. For the patient with chronotropic incompetence, the use of a dual-chamber, sensor-driven, rate-responsive pacemaker will allow rate variability (Fig. 12–24).

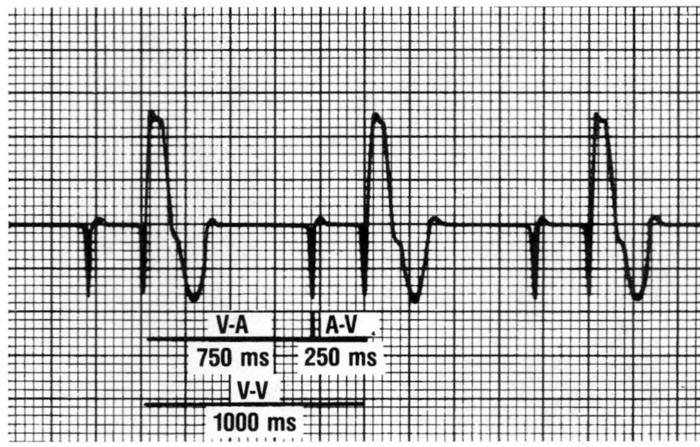

FIGURE 12–21. Dual-chamber pacing mode: atrial pace, ventricular pace. Timing in milliseconds. (Courtesy of Medtronic, Inc., Minneapolis, MN.)

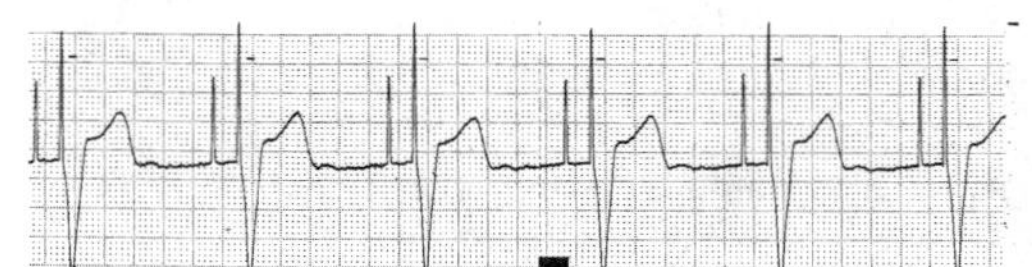

FIGURE 12–22. DDD pacing in the atrial pacing ventricular pacing mode. This is the lower rate limit of the pacemaker.

ATRIAL PACING, VENTRICULAR SENSING. There is no intrinsic atrial activity, so the atria are consistently paced, and the atrially paced beats start the A–V interval. Sensed ventricular beats result in inhibition by the venticular pacing lead, and the ECG shows the patient's intrinsic rhythm. This mode of pacing is uncommon in the DDD pacemaker. Figure 12–25 depicts this mode of pacing.

ATRIAL SENSING, VENTRICULAR SENSING. The fourth mode of normal operation is seen as a completely intrinsic cardiac rhythm. On the atrial lead, sensed atrial depolarizations result in inhibition of atrial pacing, and on the ventricular lead sensed QRS complexes result in inhibition of ventricular pacing. In this mode of operation, one would not be able to identify the presence of pacemaker activity on ECG.

Programmable Features of a DDD Pacemaker

The features of a DDD pacemaker that are programmable are listed in Table 12–14. They are set at implant and can be altered as needed with a programmer for the life of the pacemaker. The lower rate is the rate at which both the atria and the ventricles will be paced. An upper rate limit is programmed as well to allow rate variability with an atrial tracking rhythm. A programmed A–V interval usually is set a little longer than the patient's intrinsic PR interval so that the patient's intrinsic rhythm can surface as much as possible. This prolongs battery life as well. In rate-adaptive DDD pacemakers, a sensed A–V interval can be programmed, so that when the heart rate increases to a certain point the A–V interval will be decreased in an attempt to simulate normal conduction physiology. The postventricular atrial refractory period (PVARP) is the period of time after the ventricular event when the pacing system is not sensitive to atrial activity. The PVARP prevents depolarizations during the vulnerable period of the QT interval and prevents pacemaker-

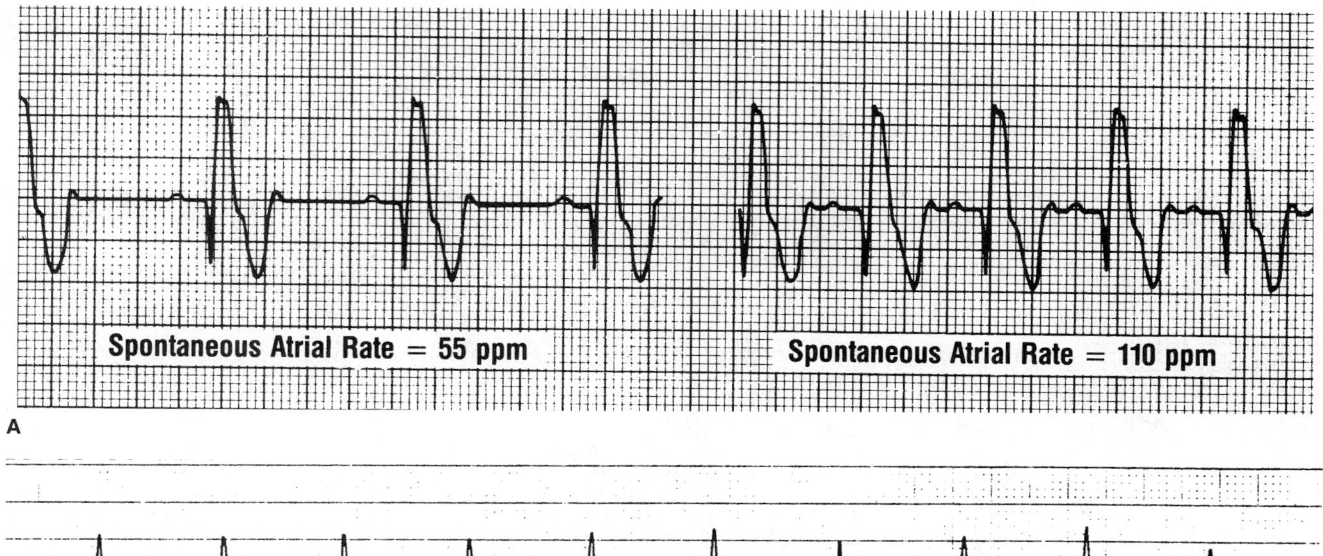

FIGURE 12–23. *A*, Dual-chamber pacing mode: atrial sense, ventricular pace. Atrial tracking occurs in this mode. (Courtesy of Medtronic, Inc., Minneapolis, MN.) *B*, DDD pacing in the atrial tracking mode.

mediated tachycardia (discussed later in this section). During the A–V interval the system is also refractory to atrial activity to prevent the ventricular lead from inadvertently sensing atrial activity at this time. Together the PVARP and the A–V interval make up the total atrial refractory period (TARP). A blanking period, a brief interval in the first part of the A–V interval during which the pacemaker cannot sense any events (atrial or ventricular), is usually set in demand pacemakers. The amplitude refers to the highest value of the electrical waveform and is measured in volts. The pulse width (pulse duration) refers to the duration of the pacing pulse itself and is measured in milliseconds.

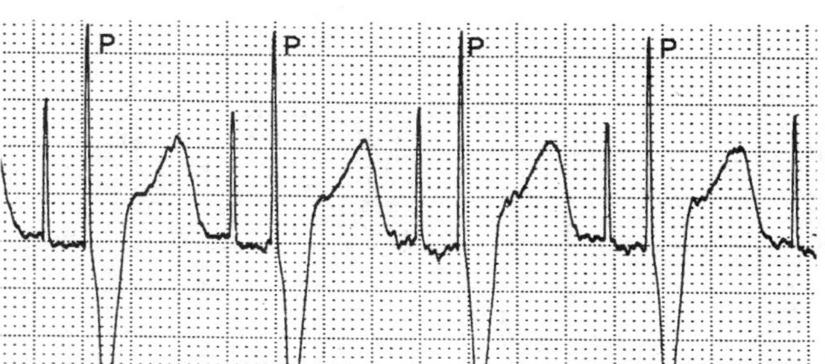

FIGURE 12–24. DDDR pacing. With chronotropic incompetence, rate is increased through a rate-responsive sensor, in this case an activity sensor.

Sensitivity, or how well the pacemaker senses the intrinsic cardiac electrical activity, is measured in millivolts. It is increased to raise the threshold, making the pacemaker less sensitive, and decreased to lower the threshold, making the pacemaker more sensitive. This concept is depicted in Figure 12–19.

Upper Rate Operation

When the pacemaker is operating in the atrial tracking mode (atrial sense, ventricular sense or pace), and the sensed atrial rate reaches the upper rate limit, pacing systems use different methods of preventing the rate from going above the upper rate limit. These methods include fixed-ratio block, Wenckebach, fallback, and rate smoothing.

FIXED-RATIO BLOCK

The sensed atrial rate becomes increasingly rapid and there will be a point at which the cycle length between P waves is shorter than the TARP. When this occurs, the P wave that begins the A–V interval will be tracked, but the subsequent P wave will fall into the refractory period and therefore will not be sensed (Fig. 12–26). The result is usually a 2:1 block that continues as long as the P-to-P cycle length is less than the TARP.

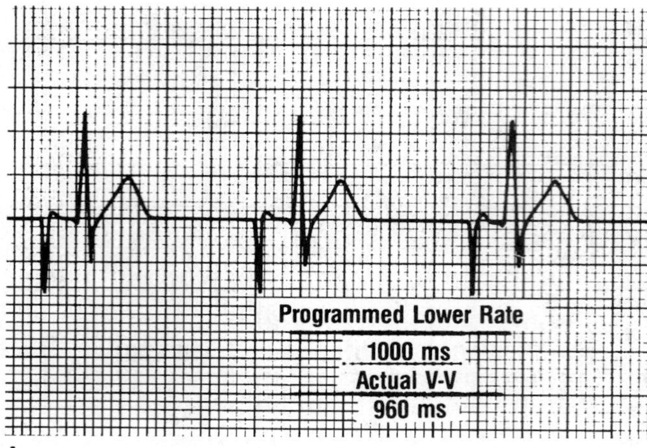

A

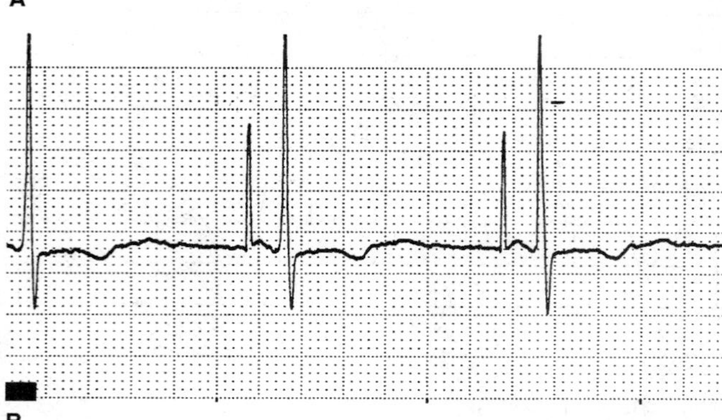

B

FIGURE 12–25. *A,* Dual-chamber pacing mode: atrial pace, ventricular sense. (Courtesy of Medtronic, Inc., Minneapolis, MN.) *B,* DDD pacing: atrial pace, ventricular sense.

The following formula is used to identify the heart rate at which a fixed-ratio block will occur:

$$\text{Block rate} = 60{,}000 \div \text{TARP}$$

The danger of a fixed-ratio A–V block is that the patient with a DDD pacemaker can begin to exercise and in the atrial tracking mode increase the pacing rate substantially, only to have a sudden drop in rate through the fixed ratio A–V block. This type of operation at the upper rate limit is not desirable, and thus some of the other methods of upper rate operation attempt to provide more gradual rate modifications.

TABLE 12–14. **Programmable Features of DDD Pacemaker**

Lower rate
A-V interval
Upper rate
Refractory period (PVARP)
Amplitude
Pulse width
Sensitivity

WENCKEBACH

If the upper rate limit is less than the 2:1 block rate, then the Wenckebach mode of opertion will come into effect before the fixed-ratio block, resulting in a more gradual reduction to the 2:1 ratio (Conover, 1992). Once the atrial rate is above the upper rate limit, Wenckebach rate of operation begins. As the atrial rate advances, the ventricular rate is kept to the upper rate limit. Lengthening A–V intervals occur as the atrially sensed beats fall closer and closer to the PVARP. A "dropped beat" occurs when the sensed P falls into the PVARP and is ignored by the pacemaker. Figure 12–27 illustrates this mode of upper rate operation.

FALLBACK

When the atrial rate exceeds the upper rate limits, the fallback mechanism lowers the ventricular pacing rate in gradual decrements to a predetermined value, temporarily eliminating AV synchrony. AV synchrony is resumed when the predetermined fallback rate is reached (Conover, 1992; Hayes, 1993).

RATE SMOOTHING

Similar in principle to fallback, the rate-smoothing mechanism keeps track of the R-to-R intervals and only allows the rate to change by a certain percentage of the previous R-to-R interval (Conover, 1992; Hayes, 1993). This percentage is a programmable option offered by one of the pacemaker manufacturers (Car-

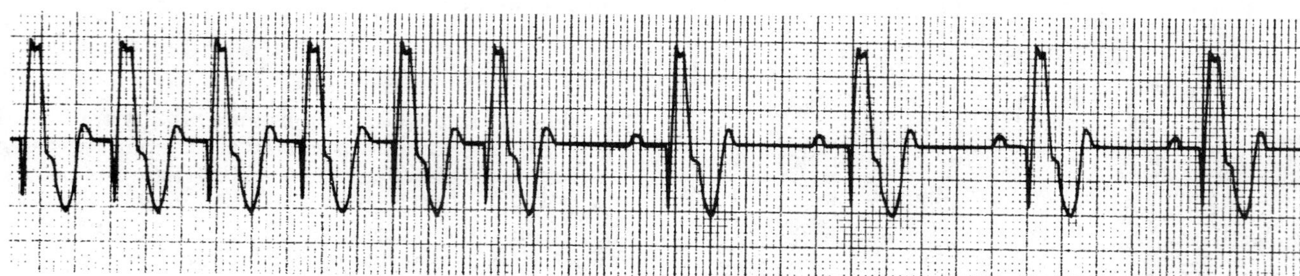

FIGURE 12–26. Upper rate operation: 2:1 fixed ratio block. (Courtesy of Medtronic, Inc., Minneapolis, MN.)

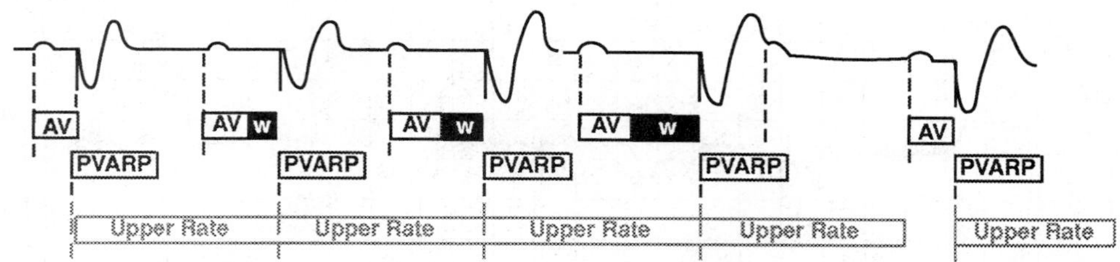

FIGURE 12–27. Upper rate operation. Wenckebach: lengthening of the AV interval until an atrial beat falls into the refractory period and is unsensed by the pacemaker. (Courtesy of Medtronic, Inc., Minneapolis, MN.)

diac Pacemakers, Inc., St. Paul, MN). In a study of 10 exercising patients with DDD pacemakers, Azara and colleagues (1992) compared the effect of the rate-smoothing operation in the on and off setting and found the incidence of dizziness, dyspnea, and discomfort to be less and the exercise ability and duration increased when the rate-smoothing option was turned on.

Single-Chamber and Dual-Chamber Pacing Abnormalities

FAILURE TO OUTPUT A PULSE

Failure to output a pulse is evidenced on the ECG as absence of a pacing artifact. This results in long intervals where there may be absence of an underlying rhythm for that chamber (Fig. 12–28), absence of pacing, or, in the case of a ventricular pacemaker, the presence of escape beats or escape rhythm as compensation. Causes of absent pacing artifacts include oversensing and some type of component failure in the pacing circuit itself. Specific causes within this circuit include total battery failure, lead fracture, lead disconnection, or failure of components within the electronic circuitry. Oversensing is the most common (Hayes, 1993), and is described later in this section.

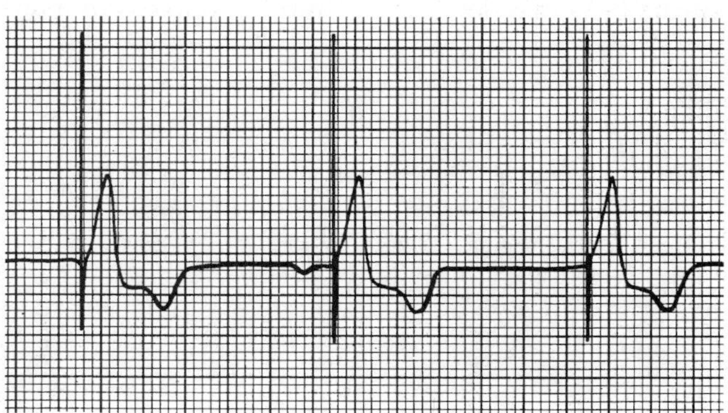

FIGURE 12–28. DDD pacemaker with no atrial output on the ECG and no noted intrinsic atrial activity. (Courtesy of Medtronic, Inc., Minneapolis, MN.)

FAILURE TO CAPTURE

The pacing artifact is present, but there is absence of accompanying depolarization for that chamber. Common causes include lead dislodgment and lead insulation break. Another common cause is related to the current output of the pulse generator, and can include battery depletion or exit block. An increase in the stimulation threshold above the current setting of the pacemaker can result in exit block. Because atrial capture is sometimes difficult to discern on the ECG, viewing several different leads may be necessary to verify atrial pacing with capture. Failure to capture on the ventricular lead is illustrated in Figure 12–29.

FAILURE TO SENSE

UNDERSENSING. When the pacemaker fails to sense a P wave of a QRS that is present on ECG, this is referred to as "undersensing," and often results in the pacemaker emitting an artifact when it should not (Fig. 12–30). If the amplitude of the intrinsic cardiac signal is too low, the pacemaker may be unable to sense it. Problems with the pacing lead can result in undersensing. In the case of lead dislodgment, undersensing and failure to capture can occur at the same time. Poor lead position and a defect in the lead insulation can also result in undersensing (Hayes, 1993).

OVERSENSING. Events other than a P wave or QRS complex cause inhibition of the pacemaker (Fig. 12–31). T-wave sensing is one example. A ventricular pacemaker sensing the T wave would inhibit, resulting in a longer than expected pause before the next paced event. Electromagnetic interference, myopotentials, and cross-talk are examples of other events that, if sensed by the pacemaker, can result in inappropriate pacemaker inhibition. Programmed hysteresis in a pacemaker can be misinterpreted as oversensing because there is a longer programmed interval after any intrinsic ventricular beat (Fig. 12–32).

Dual-Chamber Pacing Abnormalities

PACEMAKER-MEDIATED TACHYCARDIA

A potential complication of dual-chamber pacing, pacemaker-mediated tachycardia (PMT), also known

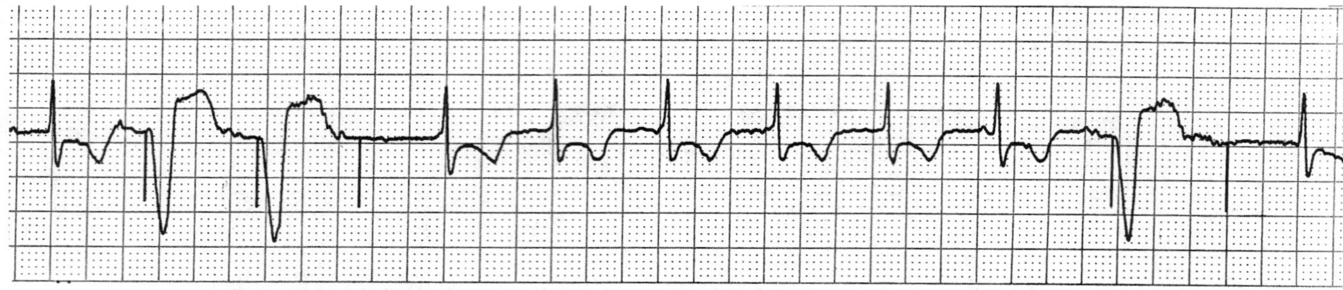

FIGURE 12–29. DDD pacing with appropriate atrial sensing but intermittent failure to capture on the ventricular lead. Supraventricular escape beats maintain an intrinsic rhythm for the patient.

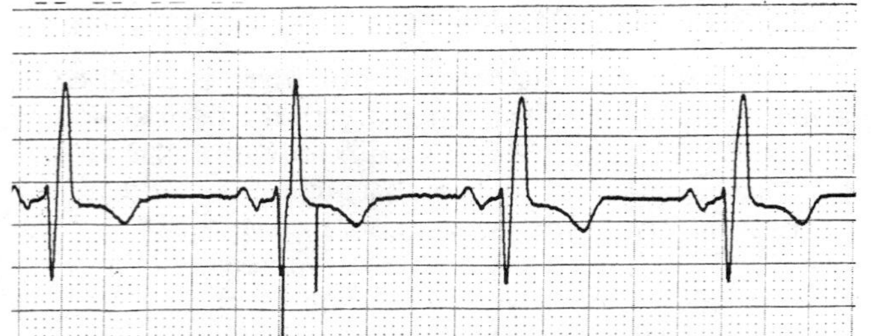

FIGURE 12–30. Undersensing on the atrial lead. In the second PQRST complex, atrial lead fails to sense intrinsic atrial beat. Atrial output occurs within the QRS and begins the AV interval. The ventricular output falls safely in the refractory period.

as endless loop tachycardia and pacemaker reentrant tachycardia (Furman, 1993a), can be initiated by a ventricular premature beat that conducts in a retrograde fashion to the atria. This atrial-conducted beat falls outside of the PVARP and is thus sensed by the pacemaker, which triggers ventricular pacing. Continued retrograde conduction to the atria results in repetition of this circuit—a reentrant, endless loop tachycardia—which can last for several beats or persist for a longer period of time (Futterman et al., 1993). Any situation in which ventriculoatrial conduction can occur and the atrial activity can be sensed has the potential to initiate PMT. The management of this tachycardia consists of making the pacemaker insensitive to atrial stimuli that could initiate a reentry circuit. Lengthening the total refractory period is a successful way of preventing the sensing of retrograde P waves, and thus prevents further occurrences of PMT (Futterman et al., 1993). An automatic extension of the refractory period after any ventricular premature beat can be programmed into the pacemaker.

CROSSTALK

In dual-chamber pacing, it is possible for a stimulus from the atrial lead to be sensed by the ventricular lead as a ventricular event, resulting in inappropriate pacemaker inhibition. Programming the blanking period is one way to prevent this. Ventricular safety pacing is a programmable feature in many pacemakers (Hayes, 1993). This function can be used to help avoid inappropriate pacemaker inhibition. After atrial pacing, if there is ventricular sensing in the initial portion of the A–V interval, the pacemaker will trigger a ventricular pacing output. Therefore, if the event sensed is interference, ventricular pacing will still occur (Fig. 12–33).

IMPLANTABLE DEVICES FOR CARDIOVERSION, DEFIBRILLATION, AND PACING

In the United States, the incidence of sudden cardiac death (SCD) is estimated to be 250,000 annually (AHA, 1993). Researchers believe that SCD results primarily from ventricular fibrillation (VF) or ventricular tachycardia (VT) that degenerates into VF. Successful man-

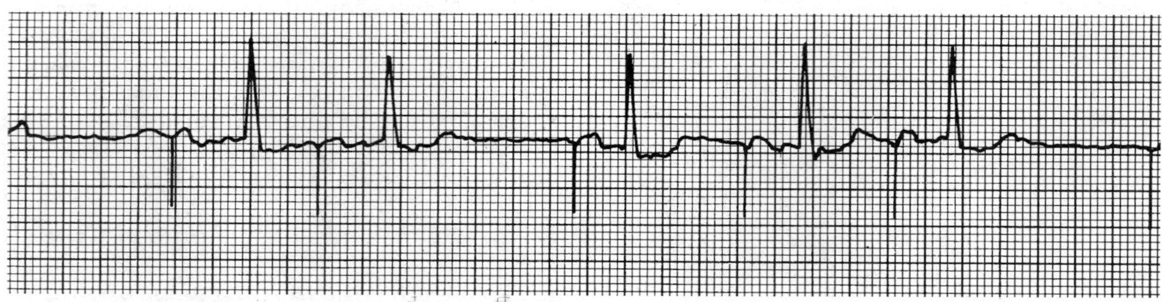

FIGURE 12–31. Ventricular oversensing. After a programmed AV interval of 150 milliseconds, the ventricular lead fails to output a pulse. Use of a programmer indicates that ventricular oversensing is occurring, thus inhibiting ventricular output. (Courtesy of Medtronic, Inc., Minneapolis, MN.)

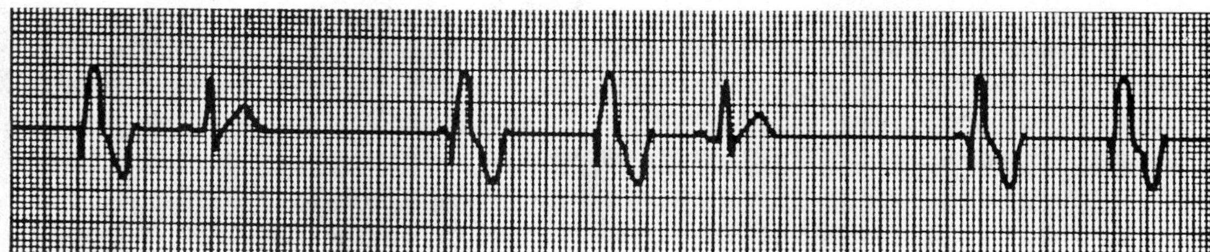

FIGURE 12–32. Hysteresis.

agement of these lethal dysrhythmias depends partly on the setting that the patient is in; time to defibrillation is a key determinant of outcome. The development and use of the implantable cardioverter defibrillator (ICD) in high-risk patients has had a dramatic impact on the incidence of SCD in these patients. It is estimated that 8,000 to 10,000 new devices were implanted in the United States in 1991, at an estimated implant cost of approximately 50,000 dollars per implant (Goldsmith, 1991). Newer technology permits antitachycardia pacing as well as low-energy shocks. Indications for the device can include hemodynamically stable VT (Moser et al., 1993).

Indications

There are two main categories for an ICD. The first include survivors of cardiac arrest events that are not associated with an acute myocardial infarction and in whom electrophysiologic study (EPS) demonstrates no inducible dysrhythmias (Arteaga & Drew, 1991; Mason & McPherson, 1992). The second indication category includes patients with sustained VT or VF, or both, that is inducible at EPS but refractory to drug therapy, and the patient is experiencing syncope (Arteaga & Drew, 1991; Mason & McPherson, 1992). Studies are currently evaluating whether prophylactic ICD implantation is warranted for high risk patients (Mason & McPherson, 1992).

Equipment

PULSE GENERATORS

The newest-model pulse generators are capable of antitachycardia pacing, cardioversion, defibrillation, and antibradycardia pacing. Several devices are currently U.S. Food and Drug Administration (FDA) approved and in clinical use. Medtronic, Inc., manufactures the PCD, and Cardiac Pacemakers, Inc. (CPI), manufactures the Ventak AICD and the Ventak. The pulse generator is about the size of a pack of cards (Goldsmith, 1991) and is implanted in a subcutaneous pocket in the left abdomen (Fig. 12–34). The Ventak PRX AICD (Fig. 12–35) was approved for use by the FDA in May 1995 and is 30% smaller than previous models. The device is powered by a lithium battery and has a current life expectancy of 4 to 5 years.

LEAD SYSTEMS

EPICARDIAL SYSTEM. There are two patches made of a titanium mesh with a Silicone rubber coating that are placed epicardially and deliver the shocks to the myocardium (Arteaga & Drew, 1991). Epicardial leads

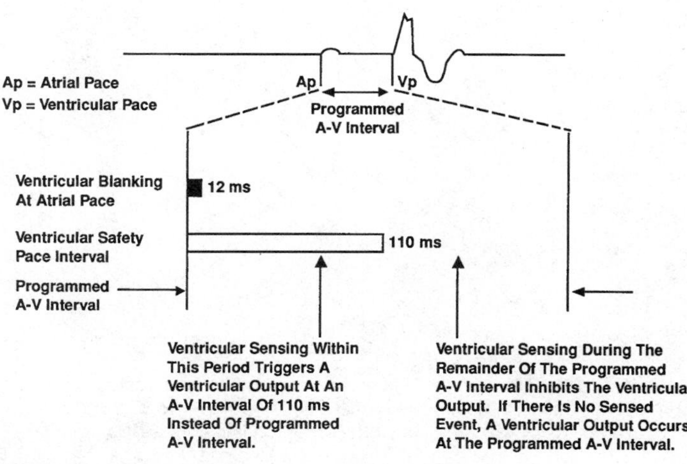

FIGURE 12–33. Ventricular safety pacing. (Courtesy of Medtronic, Inc., Minneapolis, MN.)

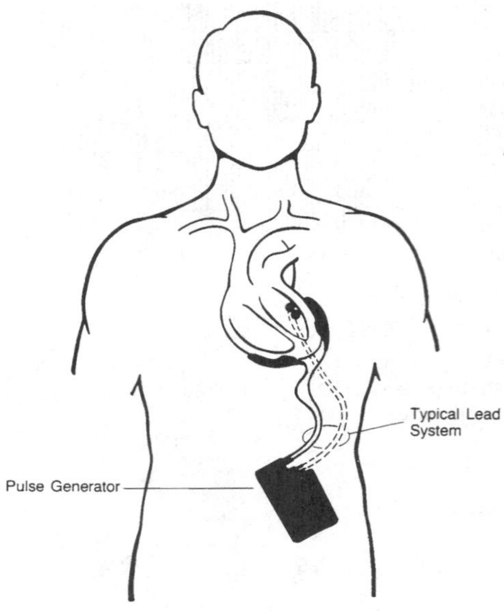

FIGURE 12–34. Implantation of an AICD pulse generator is in the subcutaneous pocket of the left abdomen. (Courtesy of Cardiac Pacemakers, Inc., St. Paul, MN.)

are shown in Figure 12–36. Two rate-sensing leads are placed on the epicardium, to be used for dysrhythmia detection and R-wave synchronization; this can also be accomplished via a transvenous pacing lead placed at the right ventricular apex (Mason & McPherson, 1992).

The surgical approaches for implantation of the pulse generator and its lead system include left lateral thoracotomy, median sternotomy, and subcostal and subxyphoid approaches. Thoracotomy is a common surgical approach. Complications associated with this approach include atelectasis, pleural effusion, hemorrhage, and pericarditis associated with the development of atrial dysrhythmias (McCowan et al., 1991).

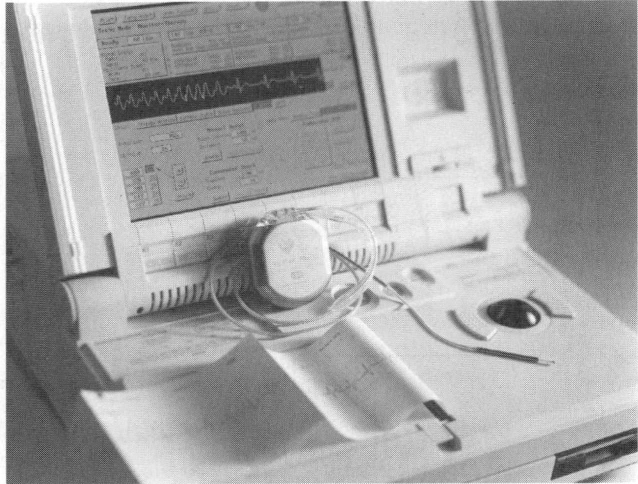

FIGURE 12–35. Ventak PRX III AICD automatic implantable cardioverter defibrillator with the Model 2950 Programmer and Endotak 70 series lead. (Courtesy of Cardiac Pacemakers, Inc., St. Paul, MN.)

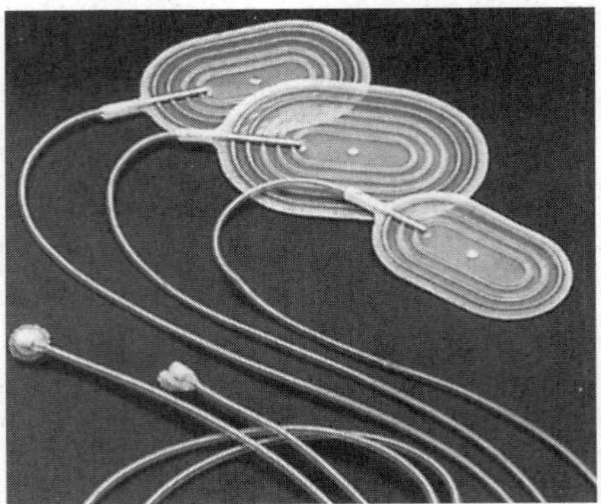

FIGURE 12–36. Epicardial patch electrodes. (Courtesy of Medtronic, Inc., Minneapolis, MN.)

ENDOCARDIAL OR NONEPICARDIAL SYSTEM. The endocardial approach to ICD lead implantation avoids many of the complications associated with thoracotomy, median sternotomy, or the subxyphoid approach. In general, patients undergoing a nonepicardial implant are ambulatory on the first postoperative day and have a hospital stay of 2 to 3 days, significantly shorter than with the epicardial approach (Goldsmith, 1991; McCowan et al., 1991).

The lead system can vary somewhat from one manufacturer to the next. The Endotak lead system (CPI) consists of a tripolar endocardial tined tip catheter. Proximal and distal spring electrodes on this catheter are used for configuration sensing and for delivery of a shock (McCowan et al., 1991). Bipolar sensing of heart rate is accomplished through the catheter tip and distal spring electrodes (McCowan et al., 1991). When necessary, a single patch electrode used for defibrillation is implanted in a submuscular plane of the left midauxiliary region and actually sutured to muscle (McCowan et al., 1991). Currently, the use of an endocardial catheter alone without the patch electrode for defibrillation is possible in most patients.

The implantation is done under general anesthesia. Using the left subclavian vein, the tripolar endocardial catheter is passed into the right venticular apex. Stimulation and sensing thresholds are measured using a pacing systems analyzer. Malignant dysrhythmias are induced and the defibrillation threshold (DFT) is measured. The criteria for establishing the DFT have not yet been clearly defined, but with the ICD, more than one lead configuration and current pathway can be tested in an effort to identify the lowest energy that successfully converts the dysrhythmia on two or more occasions (McCowan et al., 1991). Repositioning of the endocardial lead is necessary in some cases; and in other cases, a patch electrode may need to be implanted to achieve successful rhythm conversion. The output of the ICD is set above the DFT, giving the patient a margin of safety. A margin of 10 joules is advocated by many investigators (Cannom & Winkle, 1986;

McCowan et al., 1991). Once this is accomplished, the lead tails can be tunneled to the pulse generator pocket and the leads attached to the pulse generator. Ventricular fibrillation is again induced to test the performance of the assembled device before placing the pulse generator in its subcutaneous pocket. Often the device is left inactive in the immediate postoperative period (24–72 hours) because of the transient dysrhythmias, especially atrial, that can occur at this time. Atrial fibrillation, a rhythm that is difficult for the device to identify, may falsely trigger a shock. Routine emergency measures are implemented as needed during this time.

Device Function

TACHYCARDIA RECOGNITION

Two basic detection criteria have been used since the inception of the ICD: rate and probable density function (PDF). The device senses a rapid heart rate and can be activated by this criterion alone, or in combination with PDF, thus becoming a dual detection device. PDF looks at the isoelectric activity of the ECG, or how much time the cardiac rhythm spends on the baseline. In sinus rhythm, the PR interval, ST segment, and TP interval are all isoelectric. In VF, much of this malignant dysrhythmia is off the baseline, thereby raising the PDF (time off the isoelectric line, measured in milliseconds) (Arteaga & Drew, 1991). Satisfying the criteria results in the device charging and delivering a shock to terminate the dysrhythmia. Sometimes narrow complex tachydysrhythmias such as atrial fibrillation or sinus tachycardia can satisfy the criteria as well, and an inappropriate shock results.

The rate and PDF criteria have not proved totally satisfactory. Newer devices have other detection features to diagnose dysrhythmias more accurately and avoid inappropriate shocks. To differentiate between sinus tachycardia, where the rate gradually increases, and VT / VF, where the rate suddenly increases, the onset of the dysrhythmia is a newer detection criterion being used. In addition to detecting gradual versus sudden onset, newer-model devices are able to distinguish a regular rhythm from an irregular rhythm in an attempt to distinguish more accurately atrial fibrillation from malignant dysrhythmias. The prematurity of the first beat of the tachycardia is another criterion (Mason & McPherson, 1992). In newer-model devices, a first-shock delay can be programmed to avoid a shock in a nonsustained ventricular tachycardia (Moser et al., 1993).

TACHYCARDIA TERMINATION

Once the criteria for detection are satisfied, the device will generate an electrical charge and deliver a shock. For earlier, nonprogrammable models of ICDs, the initial shock is approximately 25 to 30 joules, usually delivered between 10 to 35 seconds of dysrhythmia onset (Mason & McPherson, 1992), followed by up to four further shocks at approximately 30 joules (Arteaga & Drew, 1991). After five consecutive shocks, the ICD needs to sense at least 35 seconds of a rhythm that does not meet detection criteria before it will shock again (Arteaga & Drew, 1991). In general, patients describe the shock as a moderate blow or shot to the chest, a thump, or a semiexplosion (Cooper et al., 1986; Mirowski, 1985).

Third-generation ICDs offer what is referred to as "tiered therapy," in that tailored treatment for each dysrhythmia can be programmed into the device. Treatments can include antitachycardia pacing, cardioversion, and defibrillation. Often the resulting rhythm after a shock is bradycardic, for which these devices offer ventricular demand pacing (Fromer et al., 1992). These devices have memory capability for sensed events as well as for successful and unsuccessful therapies, and different current pathway options can be selected for shocks (Fromer et al., 1992). Lower tachycardia rates are treated with overdrive pacing or cardioversion, or both, and higher tachycardia rates receive defibrillation (Fromer et al., 1992). Fromer and colleagues (1992) studied 102 patients with third-generation ICDs to evaluate the effectiveness of tiered therapy, and found that of 1,235 spontaneous VT episodes, 1,204 were treated with antitachycardia pacing by the device, with a success rate of 91%. This therapy is painless to the patient.

The Medtronic PCD has two tachycardia detection zones, one for detecting VT and one for detecting VF. In detecting VT, two basic treatments are available (Fromer et al., 1992), overdrive pacing and synchronized cardioversion. Cardioversion is programmable according to energy from 0.2 to 34 joules, pulse width, and current pathway (Fromer et al., 1992). Each of these treatments can be individually tailored to the patient. VF is detected by rate alone and the patient can receive up to four shocks per occurrence, each programmable according to energy, pulse width, and current pathway (Fromer et al., 1992). Figure 12–37 depicts an ECG schematic of an ICD (Model Ventak P 1600) algorithm.

DEVICE ACTIVATION AND DEACTIVATION

To activate an ICD, a doughnut magnet is placed over the right upper corner of the pulse generator, at which point a constant tone is emitted for approximately 30 seconds. A single pulsed tone, synchronous with each R wave, will be heard, indicating the device is now active and the magnet should be removed. Two audible beeps for each QRS indicates that the device is double sensing and could result in administration of an inappropriate shock (Arteaga & Drew, 1991). Deactivation of the device is the same process in reverse. If a magnet is applied to an active device or the patient comes too close to a magnet or magnetic field, pulsing tones will be heard for 30 seconds, than a constant tone. This indicates that the device is now inactive (Moser et al., 1993). It is important to know the specific activation and deactiva-

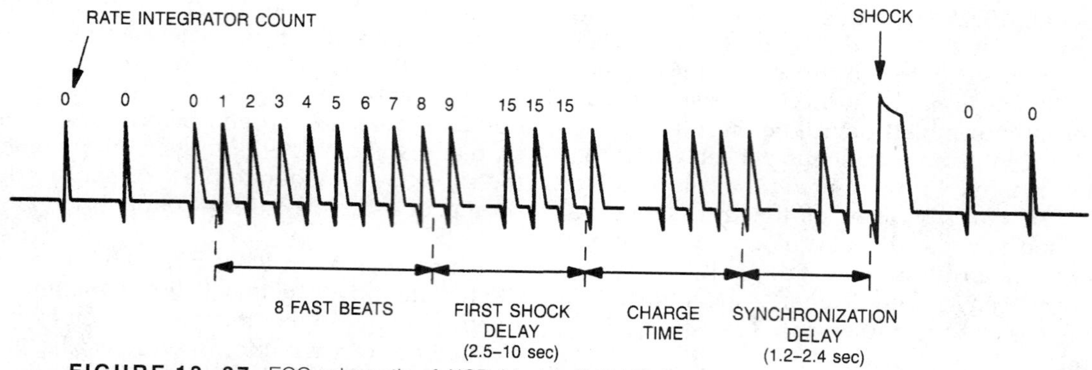

FIGURE 12–37. ECG schematic of AICD (Ventak P 1600) algorithm. (Courtesy of Cardiac Pacemakers, Inc., Minneapolis, MN.)

tion procedure recommended by the manufacturer of the particular ICD that the patient has.

Unrecognized deactivation of ICDs can occur with a person's unknowing exposure to magnets found in everyday life. Exposure to magnets can not only inactivate the device after warning beeps, but can in some models jam the device without any warning to the patient (Arteaga & Drew, 1991; Vlay et al., 1990). Bonnet and colleagues (1990) report on six cases of ICD deactivation in which the tones emitted from the device were not heard by four of the six patients. Deactivation of the device in two of the six cases involved a magnetic bingo wand, in one case a stereo speaker, and in another case a 12-volt starter (Bonnet et al., 1990). Magnetic resonance imaging is contraindicated in a patient with an ICD because either component failure or tissue damage may result (Schuster, 1990). The device must be deactivated for the patient to have a computed tomography scan or for electrocautery to be used, but ultrasound testing requires no special precautions (Moser, 1993; Schuster, 1990). ECG monitoring should be instituted when the device is deactivated.

PREDISCHARGE CLINICAL MANAGEMENT

The patient with a newly implanted ICD should have a specific discharge teaching plan implemented that covers the following areas: care of the implant site; documentation of device-associated events, including action to take if the device discharges; and identification to be carried, including a wallet identification card for the device as well as a medical alert identification bracelet; activity, including proximity to magnets or magnetic field and their potential effect on the device; and a discussion of CPR classes for family members or significant others (Moser et al., 1993).

SUMMARY

Technological advances in the rapidly developing field of electrical stimulation of the heart make the care of the patient with an implanted pacemaker more complex than ever. The nurse must assess the physiologic effects of pacing therapy in each individual patient. The nurse caring for these patients must understand the normal functioning of single- and dual-chamber pacemakers with and without rate response to identify ECG abnormalities. Dual-chamber pacemakers have become a mainstay of pacing therapy. The number of sensors available to provide rate response for the chronotropically incompetent patient continues to grow. Troubleshooting the various types of pacemakers is a constant challenge for nursing.

The impact of the implantable defibrillator on SCD is impressive. A defibrillator at first, these devices are now capable of pacing, cardioversion, and defibrillation. The role of teaching and supportive care is critical for this patient population.

REFERENCES

American Heart Association (AHA), Emergency Cardiac Care Committee and Subcommittees. (1992). Guidelines for cardiopulmonary resuscitation and emergency cardiac care: III. Adult advanced cardiac life support. *Journal of the American Medical Association, 268,* 2213–2214.

American Heart Association (AHA). (1993). *Heart and stroke facts* (55-0514 COM). Dallas, TX: American Heart Association.

Appel-Hardin, S. (1992). The role of the critical care nurse in noninvasive temporary pacing. *Critical Care Nurse, 12*(3), 10–19.

Arteaga, W. J., & Drew, B. J. (1991). Device therapy for ventricular tachycardia or fibrillation: The implantable cardioverter–defibrillator and antitachycardia pacing. *Critical Care Nursing Quarterly, 14*(2), 60–71.

Azara, D. H., Girardi, C. A., Ruffa, H. G., et al. (1992). Assessment of rate smoothing in dual-chamber pacemakers. *American Journal of Cardiology, 70,* 548–550.

Baas, L., & Schneider, C. L. (1986). Temporary epicardial electrodes: Critical care techniques. *Dimensions of Critical Care Nursing, 5,* 80–92.

Barold, S., & Zipes, D. P. (1992). Cardiac pacemakers and antiarrhythmic devices. In E. Braunwald (Ed.), *Heart disease: A textbook of cardiovascular medicine* (Vol. 1, pp. 726–755). Philadelphia: W. B. Saunders.

Beeler, L. (1993). Noninvasive temporary cardiac pacing in the emergency department: A review and update. *Journal of Emergency Nursing, 19,* 202–205.

Bernstein, A. D., & Parsonnet, V. (1992). Survey of cardiac pacing in the United States in 1989. *American Journal of Cardiology, 69,* 331–338.

Bing, O. H., McDowell, J. W., Hantman, J., et al. (1972). Pacemaker placement by electrocardiographic monitoring. *New England Journal of Medicine, 287,* 651.

Bocka, J. J. (1989). External transcutaneous pacemakers. *Annals of Emergency Medicine, 18,* 1280–1286.

Bonnet, C. A., Elson, J. J., & Fogoros, R. N. (1990). Accidental deactivation of the automatic implantable cardioverter defibrillator. *American Heart Journal, 120,* 696–697.

Cannom, D. A., & Winkle, R. A. (1986). Implantation of the automatic implantable cardioverter defibrillator (AICD): Practical aspects. *PACE, 9,* 793–809.

Chapman, P. D., Stratbucker, R. A., Schlageter, D. P., et al. (1992). Efficacy and safety of transcutaneous low impedance cardiac pacing in human volunteers using conventional polymeric defibrillation pads. *Annals of Emergency Medicine, 21,* 1451–1453.

Chardac, W. M., Gage, A. A., & Greatbach, W. (1960). A transistorized self contained implantable pacemaker for long term correction of heart block. *Journal of Surgery, 48,* 643–645.

Connelly, D. T. (1993). Initial experience with a new single chamber dual sensor rate responsive pacemaker: The Topaz Study Group. *PACE, 16,* 1833–1841.

Conover, M. (1992). *Understanding electrocardiography* (6th ed.). St. Louis: C. V. Mosby.

Cooper, D. K., Luceri, R. M., Thurer, R. J., et al. (1986). The impact of the automatic implantable cardioverter defibrillator on quality of life. *Clinical Progress in Electrophysiological Pacing, 4,* 306–309.

Creswell, L. L., Schuessler, R. B., Rosenbloom, M., et al. (1993). Hazards of postoperative atrial arrhythmias. *Annals of Thoracic Surgery, 56,* 539–549.

Daddio-Pierce, C. (1989). Transcutaneous cardiac pacing: Expanding clinical applications. *Critical Care Nursing Clinics of North America, 1*(2), 423–435.

Dreifus, L. S., Fisch, C., Griffin, J. C., et al. (1991). Guidelines for implantation of cardiac pacemakers and antiarrhythmia devices. *Journal of the American College of Cardiology, 18,* 1–13.

Dunn, D. L., & Gregory, J. J. (1989). Noninvasive temporary pacing: Experience in a community hospital. *Heart and Lung, 18,* 23–28.

Dziadulewicz, L., & Lang, R. (1992). The use of atrial electrograms in the diagnosis of supraventricular dysrhythmias. *AACN Clinical Issues in Critical Care Nursing, 3,* 203–207.

Fabiszewski, R., & Volosin, K. J. (1991). Rate modulated pacemakers. *Journal of Cardiovascular Nursing, 5*(3), 21–31.

Falk, R. H., & Ngai, S. ST. (1986). External cardiac pacing: Influence of electrode placement on pacing threshold. *Critical Care Medicine, 14,* 931–932.

Fromer, M., Brachmann, J., Block, M., et al. (1992). Effect of multimodal device therapy for ventricular tachyarrhythmias as delivered by a new implantable cardioverter–defibrillator. *Circulation, 86,* 363–374.

Furman, S. (1993a). Basic concepts. In S. Furman, D. L. Hayes, & D. R. Holmes (Eds.), *A practice of cardiac pacing* (pp. 29–88). Mount Kisco, NY: Futura.

Furman, S. (1993b). Pacemaker codes. In S. Furman, D. L. Hayes, & D. R. Holmes (Eds.), *A practice of pacing* (pp. 219–230). Mount Kisco, NY: Futura.

Furman, S. (1993c). Rate modulated pacing. In S. Furman, D. L. Hayes, & D. R. Holmes (Eds.), *A practice of pacing* (pp. 401–464). Mount Kisco, NY: Futura.

Furman, S., & Schwedel, J. B. (1959). An intracardiac pacemaker for Stokes Adams seizures. *New England Journal of Medicine, 261,* 943–947.

Futterman, L. G., Rhymes-Johnson, P. W., & Lemberg, L. (1993). Pacemaker update: Part III. Pacemaker induced tachycardia. *American Journal of Critical Care, 2,* 180–182.

Goldsmith, M. F. (1991). Implanted defibrillators slash sudden death rate in study, thousands more may get them in future. *Journal of the American Medical Association, 266,* 3400–3402.

Grubb, B. P., Temesy-Amos, P., Hahn, H., et al. (1992). The use of external noninvasive pacing for the termination of ventricular tachycardia in the emergency department setting. *Annals of Emergency Medicine, 21,* 174–176.

Hayes, D. L. (1992). The next five years in cardiac pacemakers: A preview. *Mayo Clinic Proceedings, 67,* 379–384.

Hayes, D. L. (1993). Pacemaker electrocardiography. In S. Furman, D. L. Hayes, & D. R. Holmes (Eds.), *A practice of cardiac pacing* (pp. 309–360). Mount Kisco, NY: Futura.

Hayes, D. L., & Holmes, D. R. (1993a). Hemodynamics of cardiac pacing. In S. Furman, D. L. Hayes, & D. R. Holmes (Eds.), *A practice of cardiac pacing* (pp. 195–218). Mount Kisco, NY: Futura.

Hayes, D. L., & Holmes, D. R. (1993b). Temporary cardiac pacing. In S. Furman, D. L. Hayes, & D. R. Holmes (Eds.), *A practice of cardiac pacing* (pp. 231–260). Mount Kisco, NY: Futura.

Heldman, D., Mulvihill, D., Nguyen, H., et al. (1990). True incidence of pacemaker syndrome. *PACE, 13,* 1742–1750.

Hickey, C. S., & Baas, L. S. (1991). Temporary cardiac pacing. *AACN Clinical Issues in Critical Care Nursing, 2,* 107–117.

Hynes, J. K., Holmes, D. R., & Harrison, C. E. (1983). Five year experience with temporary pacemaker therapy in the coronary care unit. *Mayo Clinic Proceedings, 58,* 122–126.

Jafri, S. M., & Kruse, J. A. (1992). Temporary transvenous cardiac pacing. *Critical Care Clinics, 8,* 713–725.

Johnson, L. G., Brown, O. F., & Alligood, M. R. (1993). Complications of epicardial pacing wire removal. *Journal of Cardiovascular Nursing, 7*(2), 32–40.

Lau, C. (1992). The range of sensors and algorithms used in rate adaptive cardiac pacing. *PACE, 15,* 1177–1211.

Lavieri, M. C. (1994). Personal communication. Beth Israel Hospital, Boston, Massachusetts.

Lynn-McHale, D., Riggs, K. L., & Thurman, L. (1992). Epicardial pacing after cardiac surgery. *Critical Care Nurse, 11*(8), 62–77.

Madsen, J. K., Meiborn, J., Videbak, R., et al. (1988a). Transcutaneous pacing: Experience with the Zoll noninvasive temporary pacemaker. *American Heart Journal, 116,* 7–10.

Madsen, J. K., Pederson, P. G., & Meibom, J. (1988b). Normal myocardial enzymes and normal echocardiographic findings during NTP. *PACE, 11,* 1188–1193.

Manion, P. A. (1993). Temporary epicardial pacing in the postoperative cardiac surgical patient. *Critical Care Nurse, 13*(2), 30–38.

Martinez, R. (1988). Emergency cardiac pacing. *Topics in Emergency Medicine, 10*(1), 81–89.

Mason, P., & McPherson, C. (1992). Implantable cardioverter defibrillator: A review. *Heart and Lung, 21,* 141–147.

McCowan, R., Maloney, J., Wilkoff, B., et al. (1991). Automatic implantable cardioverter–defibrillator implantation without thoracotomy using an endocardial and submuscular patch system. *Journal of the American College of Cardiology, 17,* 415–421.

Mickus, D., Monahan, K. J., & Brown, C. (1986). Exciting external pacemakers. *American Journal of Nursing, 86,* 403–405.

Mirowski, M. (1985). The automatic implantable defibrillator: An overview. *Journal of the American College of Cardiology, 6,* 451–466.

Mittal, S. R., Mahar, M. S., & Gokhroo, R. K. (1992). Transvenous pacing in the presence of acute right ventricular infarction. *International Journal of Cardiology, 34,* 100–101.

Mond, H. G., & Stokes, K. B. (1992). The electrode–tissue interface: The revolutionary role of steroid elution. *PACE, 15,* 95–107.

Morton, P. G. (1991). Rate responsive cardiac pacemakers. *AACN Clinical Issues in Critical Care Nursing, 2,* 140–149.

Moser, S. A., Crawford, D., & Thomas, A. (1993). Updated care guidelines for patients with automatic implantable cardioverter defibrillators. *Critical Care Nurse, 13*(2), 62–71.

Nathan, A. W., & Davies, D. W. (1992). Is VVI pacing outmoded? *British Heart Journal, 67*(4), 285–288.

Persons, C. B. (1987). Transcutaneous pacing: Meeting the challenge. *Focus, 14*(1), 13–19.

Peters, R. W. (1986). Temporary transcutaneous pacing. *AORN Journal, 44,* 245–249.

Pierce, C. D. (1989). Trancutaneous cardiac pacing: Expanding clinical applications. *Critical Care Nursing Clinics of North America, 1,* 423–435.

Schuster, D. M. (1990). Patients with an implanted cardioverter defibrillator: A new challenge. *Journal of Emergency Nursing, 16,* 219–225.

Senning, A. (1983). Cardiac pacing in retrospect. *American Journal of Surgery, 145,* 733–739.

Silver, M. C., & Goldschlager, M. D. (1988). Temporary transvenous cardiac pacing in the critical care setting. *Chest, 93,* 607–613.

Spyrou, P. G. (1981). A simple technique of placing temporary atrial pacemaker electrodes. *Annals of Thoracic Surgery, 31,* 377–378.

Stephenson, N. L., & Coombs, W. (1991). Artificial cardiac pacemakers and implantable cardioverter defibrillators. In M. R. Kinney, et al. (Eds.), *Comprehensive cardiac care* (pp. 398–424). St. Louis: C. V. Mosby.

Syverud, S., et al. (1986). Hemodynamics of transcutaneous pacing. *American Journal of Emergency Medicine, 4,* 17–20.

Teplitz, L. (1991). Transcutaneous pacemakers. *Journal of Cardiovascular Nursing, 5*(3), 44–57.

Vitello-Cicciu, J. M., Brown, M. M., Lazar, H. L., et al. (1987). Profile of patients requiring the use of epicardial pacing wires after coronary artery bypass surgery. *Heart and Lung, 16,* 301–305.

Vlay, S. C., Olson, L. C., & Burger, L. (1990). Automatic internal cardioverter defibrillator lockout. *American Heart Journal, 120,* 697–698.

Vukmir, R. B. (1993). Emergency cardiac pacing. *American Journal of Emergency Medicine, 11*(2), 166–176.

Waggoner, P. C. (1991). Transcutaneous cardiac pacing. *AACN Clinical Issues in Critical Care Nursing, 2,* 118–125.

Waldo, A. L., MacLean, W. A., Karp, R. B., et al. (1977). Entrainment and interruption of atrial flutter and atrial pacing. *Circulation, 56,* 737–745.

Zoll, P. M. (1952). Resuscitation of the heart in ventricular standstill by external electric stimulation. *New England Journal of Medicine, 247,* 768–771.

Zoll, P. M., Zoll, R. H., Falk, R. H., et al. (1985). External noninvasive temporary cardiac pacing: Clinical trials. *Circulation, 71,* 937–944.

CHAPTER 13

Hemodynamic Monitoring

Leanna R. Miller

One of the major differences between a general nursing unit and a critical care nursing unit is the presence of physiologic instrumentation that allows a more extensive assessment of patient conditions. The technology continues to become more sophisticated, requiring the bedside nurse to analyze complex physiologic measurements and, in collaboration with other health care professionals, assess, plan, implement, and evaluate patient care. This chapter discusses the hemodynamic monitoring systems and the principles of central venous pressure, intraarterial pressure, pulmonary artery pressure, and cardiac output monitoring, and concludes with the clinical applications of hemodynamic parameters.

HEMODYNAMIC MONITORING SYSTEMS

The three basic components of a hemodynamic monitoring system are (1) a transducer to detect pressure changes; (2) an amplifier to increase the magnitude of the transducer signals; and (3) a system monitor with a recorder or oscilloscope to display the signal. A transducer detects pressure changes and transmits these signals to the system monitor, which converts the signals into electrical energy. The recorder then displays the signals in digital and graphic form.

Most hemodynamic monitors have the capacity to present hemodynamic pressures by digital display, graphic form on the oscilloscope, and by graphic form on a paper printout. There are different protocols for recording hemodynamic pressures. The key factor is consistent application among clinicians for whatever protocol is used for the interpretation of the waveforms. Changes in pressures can then be attributed to actual changes in the patient's condition, either as a result of therapy or as a consequence of the underlying disease process, and not to different measurement methods. This is particularly important because of the variation in waveforms caused by the respiratory cycle, dysrhythmias, valvular insufficiency, mechanical ventilation, and catheter fling.

The transducer is positioned at the phlebostatic axis to negate the effect of hydrostatic forces on the observed hemodynamic pressures. The phlebostatic axis is located at the intersection of the transverse plane through the fourth intercostal space adjacent to the sternum and the frontal plane midway between the posterior surface of the body and the base of the xiphoid process (Fig. 13–1). As the patient moves from flat to the upright position, the phlebostatic level rotates on the axis and remains horizontal. The use of different reference levels can result in pressure differences of up to 6 mm Hg (Bartz et al., 1988; Windsor & Burch, 1945). The phlebostatic axis should be marked on the patient with a washable felt pen and a level used to ensure consistent measurement technique. Falsely high pressures will result if the transducer is below the phlebostatic axis, and, conversely, falsely low pressures will result if the transducer is above the phlebostatic axis.

The zero-reference is set to negate the force (approximately 760 mm Hg) exerted by the atmosphere so that only the pressures within the heart or vessel are recorded. Pressure transducers are affected by changes in temperature that result in a drift away from the zero baseline. Electrical calibration yields a known pressure value within the monitor, and in some monitors electrical calibration is done by simply pressing the calibration button on the system monitor. Performance of the zero-reference and calibration procedure at least two to three times per day can correct baseline drift.

Performance of the above three procedures may occasionally result in pressures that are markedly different from the last readings recorded by the nurse on the previous shift. The pressure difference may be caused by repositioning of the transducer at the phlebostatic axis, zeroing, recalibration, a different method of measuring the waveform, or an actual change in the patient's condition. A standard protocol will minimize differences due to the way waveforms are measured. A dual-channel tracing (electrocardiogram and pulmonary artery, pulmonary artery wedge, or right atrial pressure) may facilitate identification of atypical waveforms because waveform morphology is more easily identified when timed with the electrocardiogram.

Mounting a paper printout on the chart during each shift with the date, time, scale, and exact location of the part of the waveform where the measurement

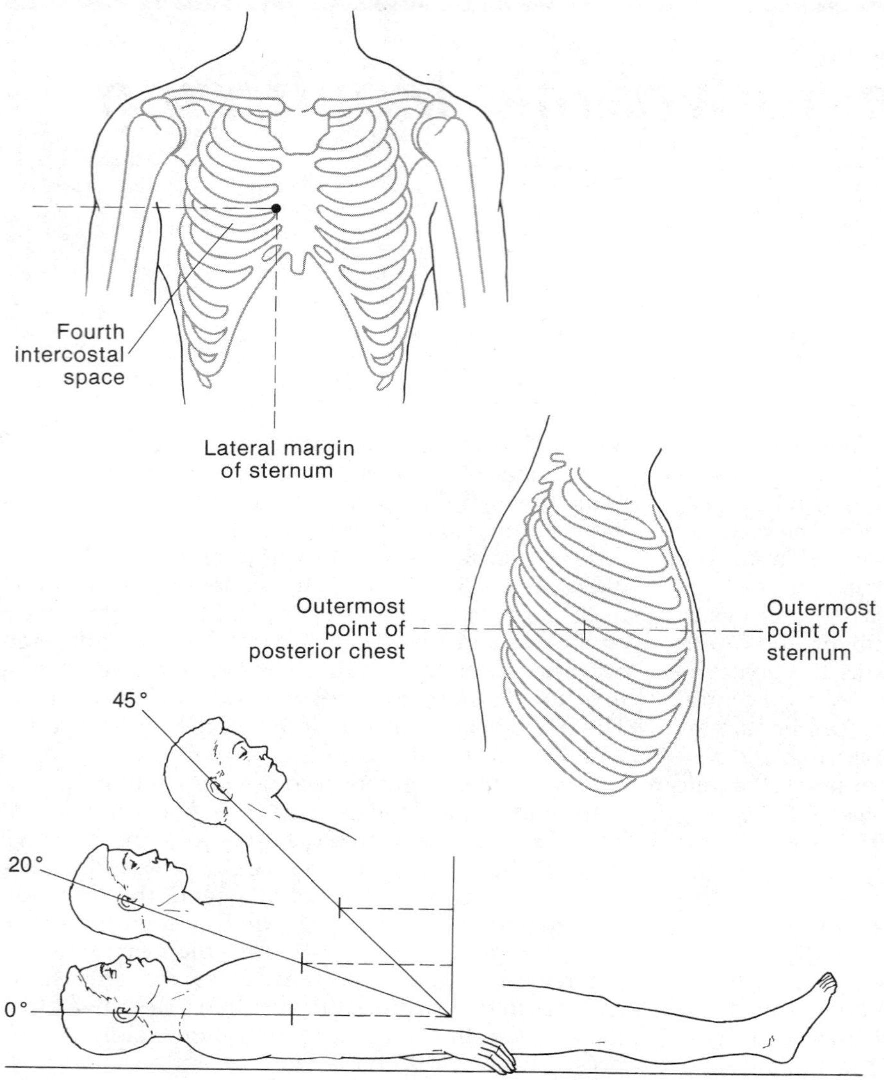

FIGURE 13–1. Phlebostatic axis. The phlebostatic axis is located at the intersection of the transverse plane through the fourth intercostal space adjacent to the sternum and the frontal plane midway between the posterior surface of the body and the base of the xiphoid process. (Redrawn from Shinn, J. A., et al. [1979]. Effect of position changes upon pulmonary artery and pulmonary artery wedge pressures in acutely ill patients. *Heart and Lung, 8,* 322–327; Gardner, P. E., & Woods, S. L. [1989]. Hemodynamic monitoring. In S. L. Underhill, S. L. Woods, E. S. S. Froelicher, et al. [Eds.], *Cardiac nursing* [2nd ed., p. 452]. Philadelphia: J. B. Lippincott.)

was taken can help to maintain consistency, particularly when one is faced with unusual waveforms. The paper printout should include waveforms recorded during at least three respiratory cycles to document clearly the variability resulting from inspiration and expiration (Fig. 13–2).

CENTRAL VENOUS PRESSURE MONITORING

The central venous pressure (CVP) corresponds to the right atrial pressure and reflects the end-diastolic pressure in the right ventricle when the tricuspid valve is open. The CVP is equivalent to the right atrial pressure measured by the pulmonary artery catheter. The mean right atrial pressure is recorded. The determinants of the CVP are blood volume, vascular tone, and right ventricular function.

Insertion sites include the antecubital veins (medial basilic or lateral cephalic), the internal or external jugular vein, or the subclavian vein. Catheter insertion is a sterile procedure, and a mask should be worn (Corona et al., 1990). The insertion site is cleaned, and lidocaine is used for local anesthesia. The catheter is inserted into the vein with the catheter tip in the right atrium or in the superior vena cava just above the right atrium, and the proximal end of the catheter is attached to a manometer or pressure transducer monitoring system. The catheter is then sutured to the skin and a sterile occlusive dressing applied according to institutional protocol. Catheter patency is maintained with a pressurized tubing system that delivers approximately 3 mL of flush solution (1 unit of heparin / mL 5% dextrose or 0.9% saline) or another type of intravenous solution. Intravenous fluids should be kept at a low "to keep vein open" rate (approximately 5 to 10 mL / hour) until catheter placement is confirmed by fluoroscopy or chest x-ray. Details of equipment, inser-

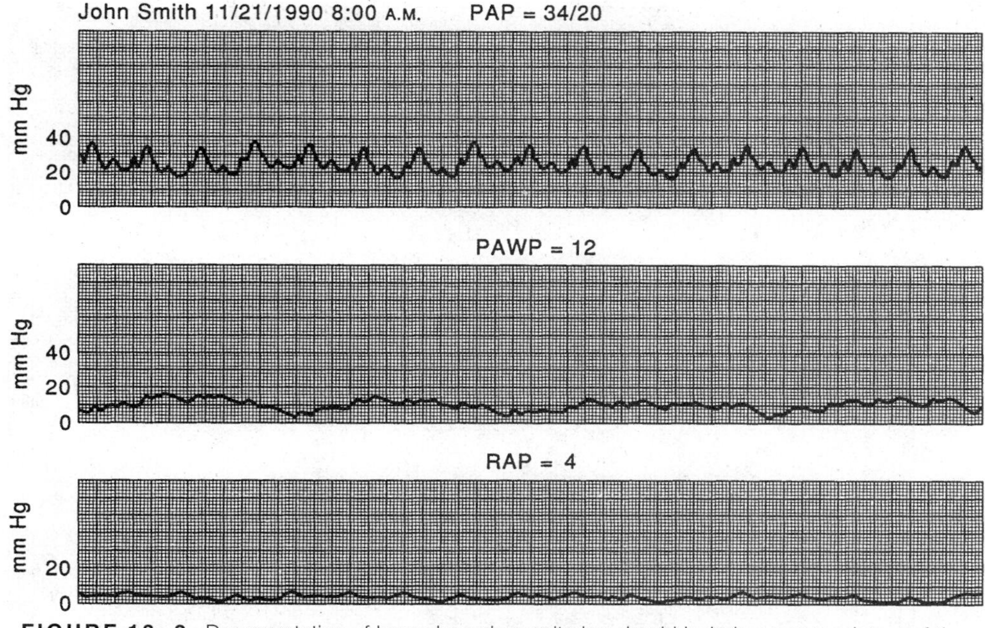

FIGURE 13-2. Documentation of hemodynamic monitoring should include a paper printout of the waveforms recorded over at least three respiratory cycles to display the variability due to inspiration and expiration. The printout should include the patient's name, date, time of measurement, scale, and exact location on the waveform where the measurement was taken.

tion technique, maintenance, and troubleshooting that may be helpful for critical care orientation have been published (Daily & Schroeder, 1989; Kern, 1993; Millar et al., 1980; Yacone, 1987).

The potential complications of CVP monitoring are laceration of the vein, pneumothorax (with subclavian or jugular vein insertion), hydrothorax, hemothorax, brachial plexus injury, dysrhythmias, right ventricular perforation, emboli, thrombosis, thrombophlebitis, or infection (Daly et al., 1975; Kern, 1993; Millar et al., 1980; Thielen, 1990; Thielen & Nyquist, 1990; Yacone, 1987).

Measurement Guidelines

Although it is preferable to measure the CVP with the patient in the same position to minimize sources of variability, reproducible measurements may be obtained with the patient lying supine or sitting with the head rest elevated (Daily, 1972; Driver, 1972; Eckstein, 1972; Windsor & Burch, 1945). The transducer must have its zero-reference point at the patient's phlebostatic axis. At least 5 minutes should elapse after a patient changes position before measurements are performed.

Clinical Interpretation

The normal range of CVP is 4 to 7 cm of water (−1 to 7 mm Hg). A CVP waveform with fluctuations due to respiratory variation is presented in Figure 13–3.

The possible clinical implications of normal, elevated, and low CVP are presented in Table 13–1.

The CVP is one measurement of right heart hemodynamics. Although measurement of CVP is valuable in determining right ventricular preload, in evaluating right ventricular dysfunction in right ventricular infarcts and pulmonary diseases, and as a clue to the diagnosis of cardiac tamponade, it is of limited value in assessing left ventricular hemodynamics. The CVP must be interpreted with caution in patients with coronary atherosclerosis, elevated pulmonary vascular resistance, and valvular disease because normal right and left ventricular function should not be assumed. In these situations, CVP monitoring yields accurate information only about the right heart, and may be seriously misleading if the measurements are extrapolated for the evaluation of left heart hemodynamics (Forrester et al., 1971).

Blood Sampling

The CVP catheter can be used to obtain blood samples for laboratory tests. Reliable plasma glucose, sodium, and potassium levels have been obtained from a multiple-lumen central venous catheter (Anderson et al., 1988).

INTRAARTERIAL PRESSURE MONITORING

Intraarterial monitoring permits direct measurement of the systemic blood pressure and is the standard

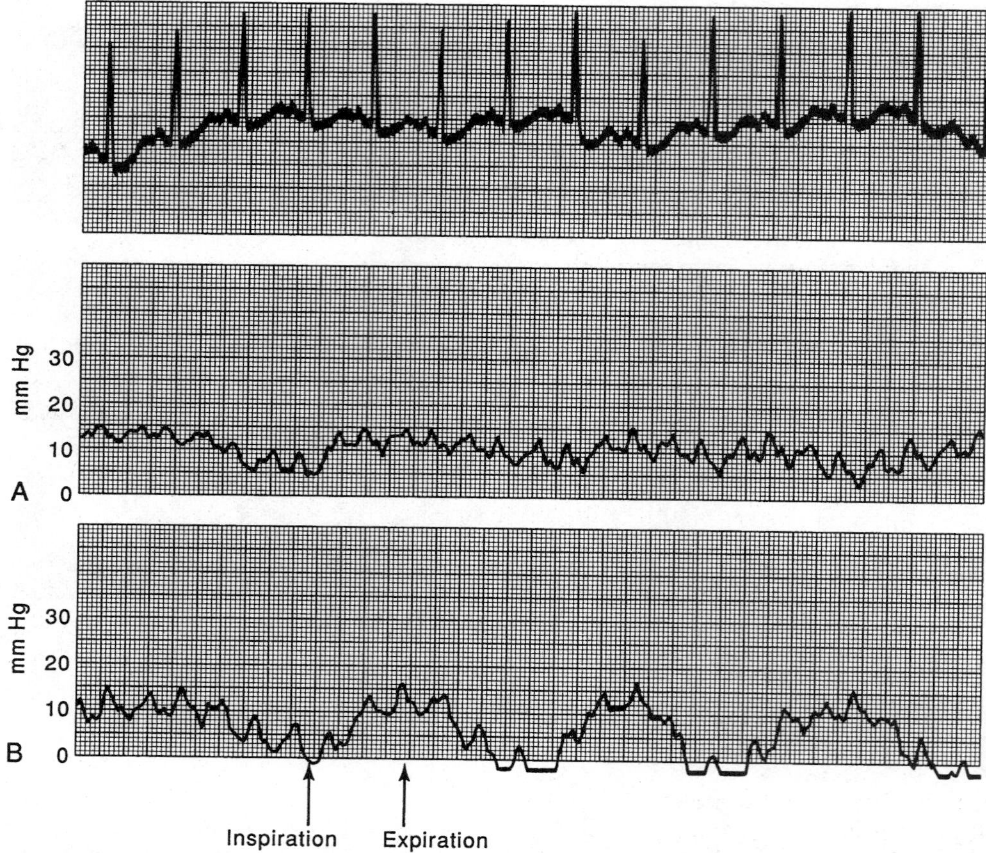

FIGURE 13–3. Central venous pressure waveform. *A*, Central venous pressure waveform with simultaneous electrocardiogram. *B*, Central venous pressure waveform with marked respiratory variation in the same patient.

against which indirect methods of measurement are compared (Gorny, 1993; Ramsey, 1991). Clinically significant differences may occur when blood pressure measurements obtained by palpation or auscultation are compared with intraarterial blood pressure measurements (Rebenson-Piano et al., 1987), particularly in hemodynamically unstable patients and patients with vascular disease. In general, the intraarterial pressure will be more accurate than blood pressures obtained by palpation or auscultation (Joseph & Larrivee, 1992). One exception may occur if the catheter is in a relatively small vessel like the radial artery in patients with marked peripheral vasoconstriction (Bedford & Wollman, 1973; Downs et al., 1973). For these patients, cannulation of more central locations such as the brachial artery or femoral artery may provide more accurate pressure readings (Chatterjee, 1985). Another exception occurs if a clot forms at the catheter tip and results in a dampened waveform. The indications for intraarterial monitoring are hemodynamic instability, need to obtain frequent arterial blood gas samples, and the need to avoid traumatizing vessels for repeated blood samples.

The radial artery is a common site for cannulation because of the good collateral circulation provided by the ulnar artery (in most patients) and its accessibility and ease of maintenance. Alternate sites for intraarterial monitoring are the brachial, axillary, femoral, and dorsalis pedis arteries (Brown et al., 1969; VanRiper & VanRiper, 1987).

The modified Allen test (Allen, 1929; Gelberman & Blasingame, 1981; Millam, 1988) is performed to assess the adequacy of circulation to the hand before cannulation of the radial artery. The radial and ulnar arteries are compressed simultaneously with the clinician's thumbs or fingers. The patient is instructed to open and close his or her fist several times; the patient's hand should appear blanched. The pressure over the ulnar artery is released and the patient's hand observed for reactive hyperemia, which should be completed within 6 seconds if there is adequate circulation.

During insertion, some physicians prefer to stabilize the wrist with an armboard so that the wrist is slightly hyperextended. The insertion site is then cleaned. The over-the-needle catheter (usually 20-gauge for the radial artery) is inserted at a 15- to 45-degree angle (Millam, 1988). When there is a blood return, the inner stylet is removed, and the pressure tubing is attached to the catheter hub. Aspiration of the dead space volume between the catheter tip and the

TABLE 13–1. **Clinical Implications of Normal, Elevated, and Low Central Venous Pressures**

Normal central venous pressure (−1 to 7 mm Hg)
- Normovolemic
- Acute left ventricular failure

High central venous pressure (>7 mm Hg)
- Normovolemia
  - Right-sided heart failure
  - Chronic biventricular failure
  - Left-to-right shunt
  - Pericardial disease
  - Vasopressor medications
  - Restless patient
  - Tachypnea
  - Chronic obstructive pulmonary disease
  - Superior vena cava compression
  - Pulmonic stenosis
  - Pulmonary embolus
  - Positive pressure ventilation
  - Pneumothorax
- Hypervolemia
  - Fluid overload
- Hypovolemia with severe cardiac decompensation

Low central venous pressure (<−1 mm Hg)
- Hypovolemia
  - Dehydration
  - Hemorrhage
  - Diarrhea
  - Peritonitis
- Hypervolemia with profound vasodilation
- Vasodilation
  - Sepsis
  - Vasodilator medications

Data from Daily, E. K., & Schroeder, J. S. (1989). *Techniques in bedside hemodynamic monitoring* (4th ed.). St. Louis: C. V. Mosby.

hub may be done to remove any air bubbles before flushing the catheter. Visualization of the arterial waveform on the oscilloscope will confirm proper placement (Fig. 13–4).

The pressurized transducer tubing system will deliver 3 to 5 mL of heparinized flush solution per hour to maintain catheter patency. If the waveform is dampened, the catheter tip may be lodged against the artery wall. Retracting the catheter slightly usually resolves this problem. If the waveform remains dampened, attempt dynamic response and maximize the natural frequency and damping coefficient with the steps discussed previously. The catheter is then secured to the skin, and a sterile dressing is applied. The cannulation site should be inspected daily for erythema, drainage, bruising, or increasing radial girth, and neurovascular checks should be made to the hand. The assessment should involve comparison of the cannulated extremity with the opposite extremity.

Cannulation of the femoral artery may be done in patients with severe hypotension, peripheral vasoconstriction, cardiac failure, or upper extremity trauma, or in those requiring intraarterial pressure monitoring after percutaneous transluminal coronary angioplasty. A higher risk of contamination is associated with femoral artery cannulation (Spaccavento & Hawley, 1982). Detection and control of bleeding is relatively more difficult with bleeding into the groin than in the arms. The patient must keep his or her hip in straight alignment, and the head of the bed should not be elevated more than 30 degrees. When turning the patient, the patient's entire body should be kept in straight alignment, with the nurse supporting the patient's back and hip. Circulation to the lower extremities is monitored by assessing skin color and temperature, observing patient discomfort (pain, tingling, or numbness), and palpating the dorsalis pedis and posterior tibialis pulses.

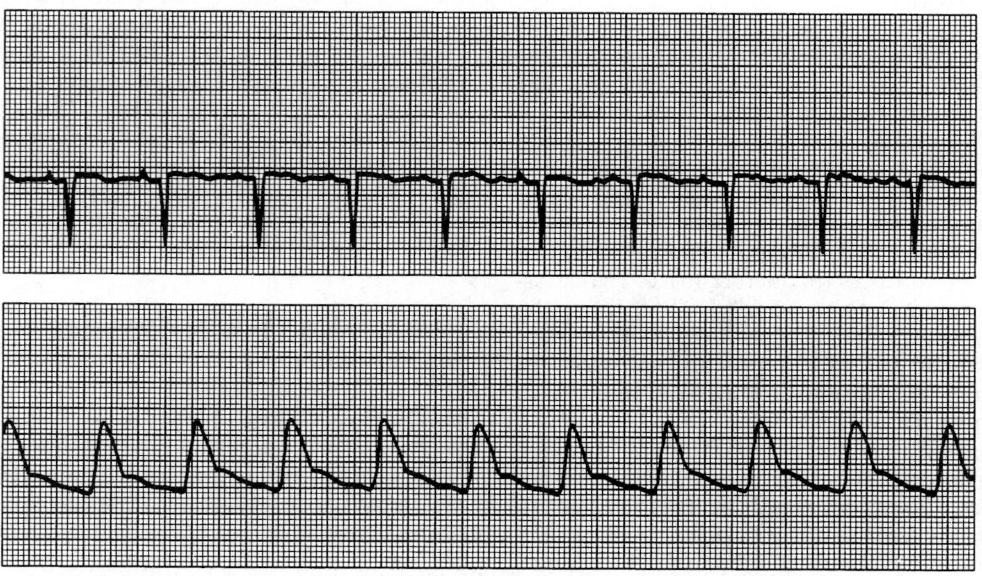

FIGURE 13–4. Intraarterial pressure waveform with simultaneous electrocardiogram.

TABLE 13–2. **Potential Complications of Intraarterial Pressure Monitoring**

Hematoma	Infection
Ecchymosis	Peripheral embolization
Purpura	Ischemia
Bleeding	Distal vascular insufficiency
Sclerosis	Arterial occlusion
Thrombosis	

The potential complications of intraarterial pressure monitoring are listed in Table 13–2.

Measurement Guidelines

The blood pressure obtained from the arterial catheter should be compared to the blood pressure obtained by sphygmomanometer at least two to three times a day, or more often as needed. In stable cardiac patients with radial or pedal artery catheters, the mean arterial pressure can be obtained with the patient in the supine or semi-Fowler's position using either the right atrium or the tip of the intraarterial catheter site as the reference point for calibration. However, in unstable patients or in situations where therapy is based on the mean arterial pressure, the same position and reference point should be used. In such patients, use of the supine position and the right atrium as the reference point may be more convenient for the nurse and more comfortable for the patient because these patients often have both an arterial catheter as well as a pulmonary artery catheter (Rebenson-Piano & Kirchhoff, 1983).

Blood Sampling

The arterial catheter makes it possible to obtain blood specimens without further traumatizing the patient. The need for arterial blood gas tests in patients with ventilatory problems makes the indwelling catheter invaluable. Traditionally, a blood gas sample is obtained 10 to 30 minutes after making a change in ventilator settings. Preliminary research suggests that homeostasis occurs sooner and that it may not be necessary to wait as long as 30 minutes (Schuch & Price, 1987). Aspiration of approximately two and one half times the dead space volume of the arterial tubing between the indwelling catheter and the first stopcock provides blood gas results comparable to those obtained from direct arterial puncture (Molter, 1983).

The use of arterial catheters for obtaining samples for coagulation studies is controversial because contamination of the laboratory specimen by the heparinized flush solution can result in falsely high partial thromboplastin (PTT) and thrombin time (TT) values (Cannon et al., 1985; Gregersen et al., 1987; Kajs, 1986; Molyneaux et al., 1987; Pryor, 1983; Rakowski et al., 1987). Studies indicate that accurate prothrombin time (PT), TT, and PTT results can be obtained from samples taken from arterial catheters in some patients. However, it has not been established how many milliliters of fluid should be withdrawn to clear the heparinized flush solution adequately from the dead space between the arterial catheter tip and the syringe port where the blood specimen is collected (Cannon et al., 1985; Gregersen et al., 1987; Pryor, 1983). The actual volume discarded depends on the distance of the stopcock from the indwelling catheter. Approximately 5 to 10 times the dead space volume (3.3–4.8 mL) (Merenstein, 1971; Molyneaux et al., 1987; Rakowski et al., 1987) seems to be an adequate volume to discard, although one study (Cannon et al., 1985) showed good correlation after discarding only 2 mL from an arterial line with a dead space volume of 1 mL between the catheter tip and syringe port.

Of great concern are abnormally high PTT and TT values in a minority of patients due to contamination of the specimen with heparin from the flush solution (Gregersen et al., 1987; Pryor, 1983). The consequence of an abnormally high PTT value on a sample drawn from a heparinized catheter is that the PTT would have to be redone on a fresh sample because one would not know if the result was caused by heparin contamination or excessive heparin therapy. The delay in making clinical decisions and the cost of repeating laboratory tests may, in the opinion of some clinicians, not be in the patient's best interests compared to the discomfort caused by venipuncture. The reality of the patient's experience in the intensive care unit, however, is one of pain and bruising due to multiple venipunctures and arterial blood samplings.

Venipuncture remains the standard method against which other methods of blood draws for coagulation studies are compared (Kajs, 1986). One potential alternative in patients requiring short-term (less than 72 hours) intraarterial monitoring is the use of nonheparinized flush solutions (Hook et al., 1987). Another alternative may be to obtain the blood sample for the PT, PTT, and TT last when multiple blood tests are done. This would result in 10 to 20 mL of blood being withdrawn before the blood samples for coagulation studies are obtained. This area of research needs further investigation, particularly in patients receiving continuous intravenous infusions of heparin.

PULMONARY ARTERY PRESSURE MONITORING

The landmark paper by Swan and Ganz and their colleagues (1970) described a 5-French balloon-tipped polyvinyl chloride catheter that could be safely used to catheterize the heart in humans. The subsequent addition of pacing capabilities, continuous mixed venous oxygen saturation (Svo_2) monitoring (Martin et al., 1973), and an extra proximal port for drug infusion

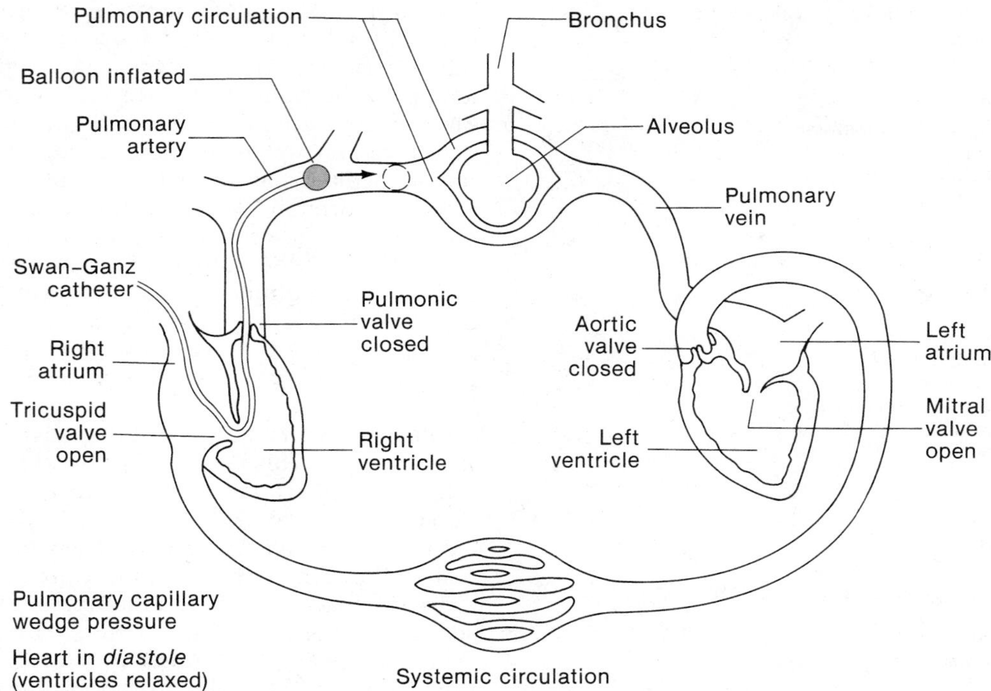

FIGURE 13–5. The pulmonary artery diastolic pressure and the pulmonary artery wedge pressure reflect left ventricular end-diastolic pressure during diastole because there are no closed valves between the pulmonary vascular bed, left atrium, and left ventricle. (Redrawn from Baxter Healthcare Corporation. *Understanding hemodynamic measurements made with the Swan-Ganz catheter.* © 1982 Baxter Healthcare Corporation. All rights reserved. Swan-Ganz® catheter manufactured by the Edwards Critical-Care Division of Baxter Healthcare Corporation; trademarks are registered trademarks of Baxter.)

expanded the utility of the pulmonary artery catheter (Bridges & Woods, 1993; Waite & Parsons, 1991).

The purpose of hemodynamic monitoring is to aid in the establishment of a diagnosis, guide and optimize therapy, and provide prognostic information (Gore et al., 1985; Matthay & Chatterjee, 1988; Bridges & Woods, 1993). The value of pulmonary artery catheter monitoring is that a single catheter placed in the right heart can measure pressures directly in the right heart and indirectly from the left heart. The physiologic basis for this is that during diastole, the valves are open between the pulmonary vascular bed, left atrium, and left ventricle. These form a common chamber, and in patients with normal pulmonary vasculature and normal mitral valve and left ventricular function, the pulmonary artery diastolic pressure (PAD) and the pulmonary artery wedge pressure (PAWP) reflect the left ventricular end-diastolic pressure (Fig. 13–5) (Falicov & Resnekov, 1970; Forrester et al., 1976; Jenkins et al., 1970; Scheinman et al., 1973; Kaltman et al., 1966). The left ventricular end-diastolic pressure is an important measure for evaluating left ventricular function and prognosis, which in turn have a major role in determining which therapy (usually pharmacologic) will best help the patient (American Society of Anesthesiologists, 1993). In patients with coronary artery disease, equal right and left ventricular function cannot be assumed because the amount of function depends on the area that is diseased. The indications for pulmonary artery catheter monitoring are presented in Table 13–3.

Catheter Models

Several catheter models are in use today and are described in the following sections. Three catheter models are illustrated in Figure 13–6. An introducer with sideport can be used for infusing medications and obtaining blood samples, and is placed by the physician at time of insertion.

TRIPLE-LUMEN THERMODILUTION CATHETER. This 7-French catheter has a thermistor near its tip. One lumen terminates in the right atrium and is used for measuring right atrial pressure (RAP) and cardiac output. The second lumen terminates in the pulmonary artery and is used for measuring pulmonary artery pressure (PAP). The third lumen also terminates in the pulmonary artery and is used to measure the PAWP. The PAWP is obtained by using a syringe to inflate the balloon-tipped port with up to 1.5 mL of air.

QUADRUPLE-LUMEN THERMODILUTION CATHETER. This 7.5-French catheter has the features of the triple-

TABLE 13–3. **Indications for Pulmonary Artery Catheter Monitoring**

Medical
- Complicated acute myocardial infarction
- Right ventricular infarction
- Perforated ventricular septum
- Mitral regurgitation
- Cardiac tamponade
- Dilated cardiomyopathy
- End-stage cardiac failure
- Constrictive pericarditis
- Acute pulmonary edema
- Intraaortic balloon support
- Pulmonary embolus
- Pulmonary hypertension
- Cor pulmonale with pneumonia
- Acute respiratory distress syndrome
- Shock
  - Hypovolemic
  - Cardiogenic
  - Septic
- Acute renal failure
- Dialysis
- Complex fluid management (severe burns and sepsis)
- Drug intoxication
- High-risk obstetric patients
  - Preexisting cardiac disease
  - Toxemia
  - Abruptio placentae

Surgical
- Cardiac surgery
  - Valve replacement (multiple, elderly)
  - Severe associated pulmonary disease (mitral stenosis)
- Coronary artery bypass grafting
  - Ventricular aneurysm resection
  - Preoperative congestive heart failure
- High-risk patients
  - Elderly with preexisting cardiac disease
  - Extensive intraabdominal operations

lumen catheter with an additional proximal port that may be used to administer fluids and medication.

PACING THERMODILUTION CATHETER. One model has three ring electrodes for atrial pacing and two ring electrodes for bipolar right ventricular pacing. Some clinicians may prefer not to inflate the balloon to obtain the PAWP to minimize the risk of either the ring electrodes or the pacing wire losing contact with the endocardium.

Another model has an additional lumen through which a 2-French bipolar pacing wire can be inserted into the right ventricle. If this model is used but the pacing wire is not inserted, lumen patency can be maintained with standard intravenous solutions (5% dextrose of 0.9% sodium chloride). The pulmonary artery catheter with pacing capability is indicated as a temporary measure until a more reliable pacing catheter can be inserted (Guzy, 1986).

MIXED VENOUS OXYGEN SATURATION THERMODILUTION CATHETER. This catheter includes the features of the triple-lumen model with an additional lumen for the fiberoptic filaments and an optical connector. Mixed venous oxygen saturation monitoring uses reflection spectrophotometry. A fiberoptic filament transmits light of selected wavelengths through the pulmonary artery catheter and out through the catheter tip in the pulmonary artery. A second fiberoptic filament transmits the reflected light back to a photodetector in the optical module, and the venous saturation is displayed at a bedside module (Baxter Healthcare Corporation, 1987; White, 1987a, 1987b). The blood sample for calibrating the $S\bar{v}O_2$ catheter is obtained through the pulmonary artery port. Indications for use of the pulmonary artery catheter with continuous $S\bar{v}O_2$ monitoring capability are the need to evaluate the response to therapy and the need to check the adequacy of tissue oxygenation.

RIGHT VENTRICULAR EJECTION FRACTION/VOLUMETRIC CATHETER. This catheter is a modified pulmonary artery catheter that permits measurement of traditional parameters, and monitoring of right ventricular ejection fraction and right ventricular volumes (Fig. 13–7). The catheter has two intracardiac electrodes to sense R-wave activity and a thermistor that potentiates sensing of changes in temperature (Vincent, 1986; Vincent et al., 1990). A multihole injectate lumen found in the region of the right atrium facilitates mixing of blood and injectate. Ejection fraction depends on beat-to-beat changes in temperature. The catheter senses these temperature changes and produces a thermodilution curve (Fig. 13–8).

Contraindications and Cautions

Although there are no known absolute contraindications, relative contraindications are recurrent sepsis (Caruthers et al., 1979) or a hypercoagulable state. The electrocardiogram (ECG) should be closely monitored in patients with complete left bundle branch block because of the increased risk of complete heart block; some of these patients may need a pacemaker inserted before insertion of the pulmonary artery catheter. Patients with Wolff-Parkinson-White syndrome and Ebstein malformation are at risk for tachydysrhythmias (Baxter Healthcare Corporation, 1982).

The choice of insertion site depends on the clinical needs of the patient and the skill of the physician. The internal jugular vein is a common site, particularly for patients undergoing cardiothoracic surgery. Alternative sites include the subclavian, brachial, basilic, and femoral veins. Patients undergoing cardiac catheterization or percutaneous transluminal coronary angioplasty sometimes have a pulmonary artery catheter inserted through the femoral vein for short-term monitoring. Catheter position should be confirmed by fluoroscopy or by a chest x-ray.

Measurement Guidelines

The physician advances the pulmonary artery catheter until the RAP waveform appears on the oscilloscope. The balloon is then inflated with air up to the maximum

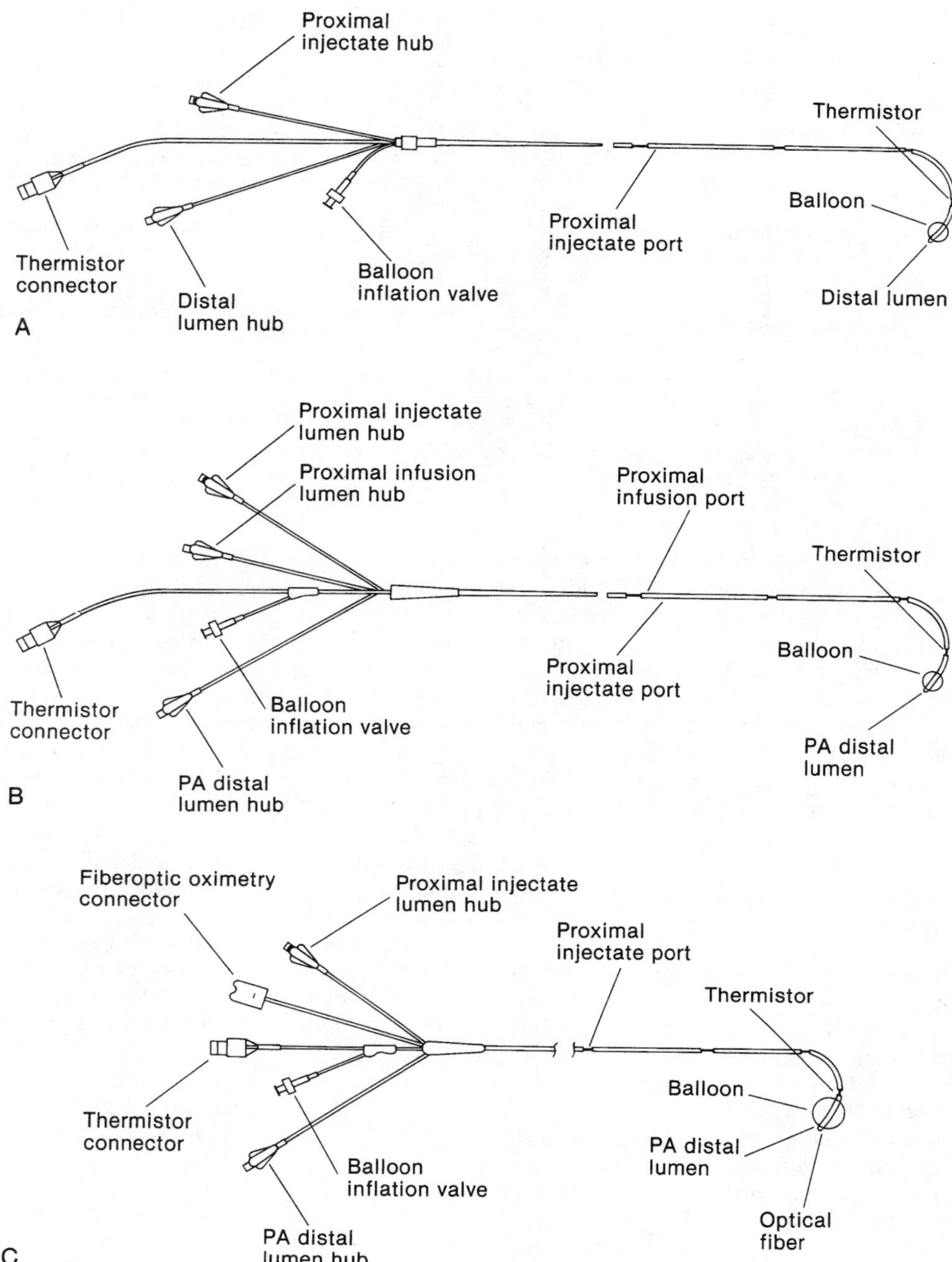

FIGURE 13–6. Types of pulmonary artery catheters. *A*, Triple lumen catheter. *B*, Quadruple lumen catheter. *C*, Oximetry catheter. (Redrawn from Baxter Healthcare Corporation. All rights reserved.)

volume recommended by the manufacturer (1.5 mL in one model). The distinct waveforms (Fig. 13–9) that appear during passage through the right atrium, right ventricle, pulmonary artery, and finally into the pulmonary artery wedge position make it possible to insert the catheter at the bedside without fluoroscopy. The patient should be monitored closely for premature ventricular contractions and ventricular tachycardia during passage of the catheter tip through the right ventricle.

The PAP waveform should remain visible on the oscilloscope because the catheter may become wedged in the pulmonary artery or slip back into the right ventricle, leaving the patient at risk for pulmonary infarction or ventricular dysrhythmias. An attempt to dislodge the catheter should be made by having the patient cough, breathe deeply, or change position (supine to lateral or vice versa). If these interventions do not dislodge the catheter, the physician should be notified to withdraw the catheter to dislodge the catheter tip (Boyd et al., 1983).

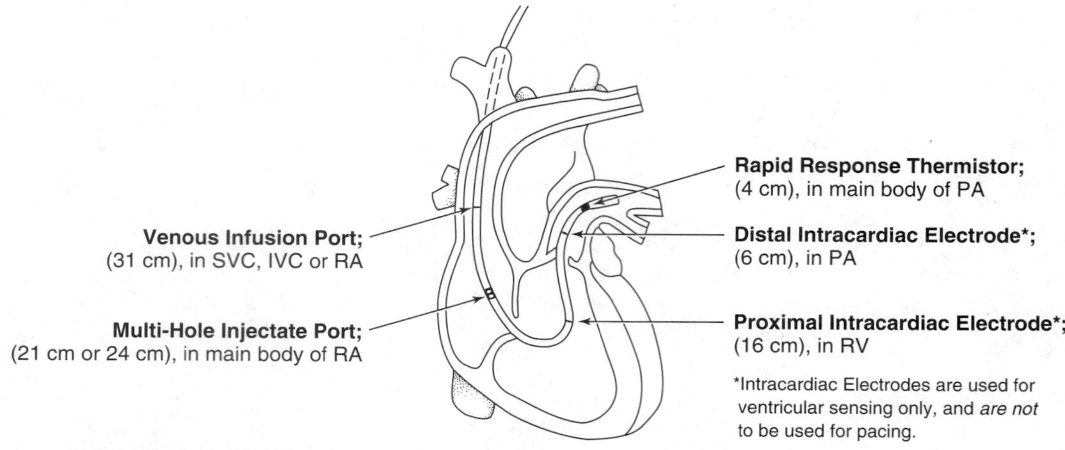

FIGURE 13–7. Swan-Ganz ejection fraction/volumetric catheter characteristics and positioning. (Redrawn with permission from Baxter Healthcare, Edwards Critical-Care Division, Irvine, California.)

The catheter insertion site should be inspected daily for erythema, drainage, or swelling. Swelling is sometimes seen in the arm when the brachial or basilic vein is used because of reduced venous return caused by the presence of the catheter. The insertion site should be cleaned and a sterile occlusive dressing applied. Table 13–4 presents the potential problems and intervention strategies applicable to pulmonary artery catheter monitoring. The potential complications of the pulmonary artery catheter are listed in Table 13–5.

ENSURING ACCURACY OF HEMODYNAMIC MEASUREMENTS

PATIENT POSITION. One of the major concerns in achieving accurate pressure readings is patient position. Supine posturing may be required in your institution, although it may cause pain, discomfort, sleep disturbance, intracranial pressure elevations, or respiratory compromise in the critically ill patient (Dobbin et al., 1992). Turning has many benefits, including positive effects on circulation and ventilation, but it also increases blood pressure and heart rate, both factors that can affect the pressures.

In the lateral position after surgery with the unoperated side dependent, PaO_2 was significantly higher and alveolar–arterial oxygen difference (A-a gradient) and shunt (Qs / Qt) were significantly lower than in the supine position. When turning patients while monitoring SvO_2, most patients had an immediate decrease in SvO_2 after turning but returned to baseline values within 5 minutes; therefore, allowing time for pressure to stabilize is recommended (Pena, 1989).

Recent research has supported the assumption that pulmonary artery pressures can be measured accurately with the patient supine and the head of the bed elevated to angles of 10, 20, 30, and 45 degrees in critically ill patients who have normal pulmonary artery pressures (Cason & Lambert, 1993; Groom et al., 1990; Nelson & Anderson, 1989; Woods & Mansfield, 1976; Woods et al., 1980). Also, backrest elevation to 20, 30, and 45 degrees did not affect pulmonary artery pressures, SvO_2, or mean arterial pressure (MAP) measurements in cardiac surgical patients who had abnormally elevated pulmonary artery pressures. However, hemodynamic pressures measured with the patient in a lateral position should not be used to make therapeutic decisions (Kennedy et al., 1984).

In normotensive patients, the head-down tilt increased preload of both ventricles, increased cardiac output, decreased systemic vascular resistance (SVR), and had no effect on MAP. In hypotensives, the downward tilt had no effect on MAP or preload, slightly increased afterload, and decreased cardiac output (Sibbald et al., 1979).

Prone position may result in higher PaO_2 values in patients with acute respiratory distress syndrome (ARDS). It has also been shown to facilitate weaning to lower levels of supplemental oxygen in mechanically

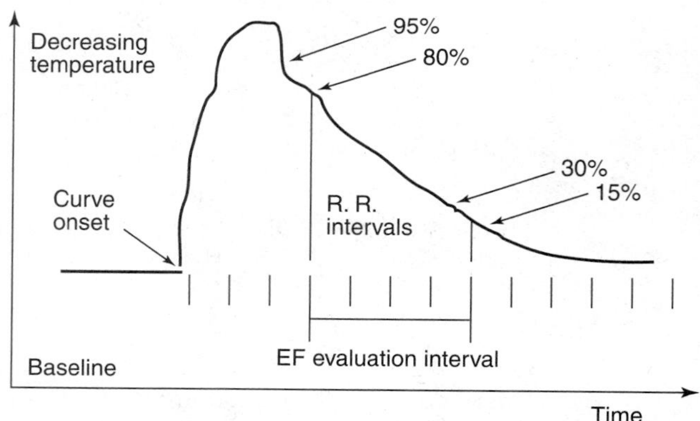

FIGURE 13–8. Determination of ejection fraction (EF). Two reference points at the downslope of the thermodilution curve, one point between 15% and 30% and one between 80% and 95%, correspond to R waves. A curve is fit through these points. Using an exponential method, the slope of the curve is then divided by the number of RR intervals, providing the residual fraction. This value provides the percentage of injectate not ejected; therefore, this value is subtracted from one to determine the percentage ejected or EF (1 residual fraction = EF). (Redrawn with permission from Baxter Healthcare, Edwards Critical-Care Division, Irvine, California.)

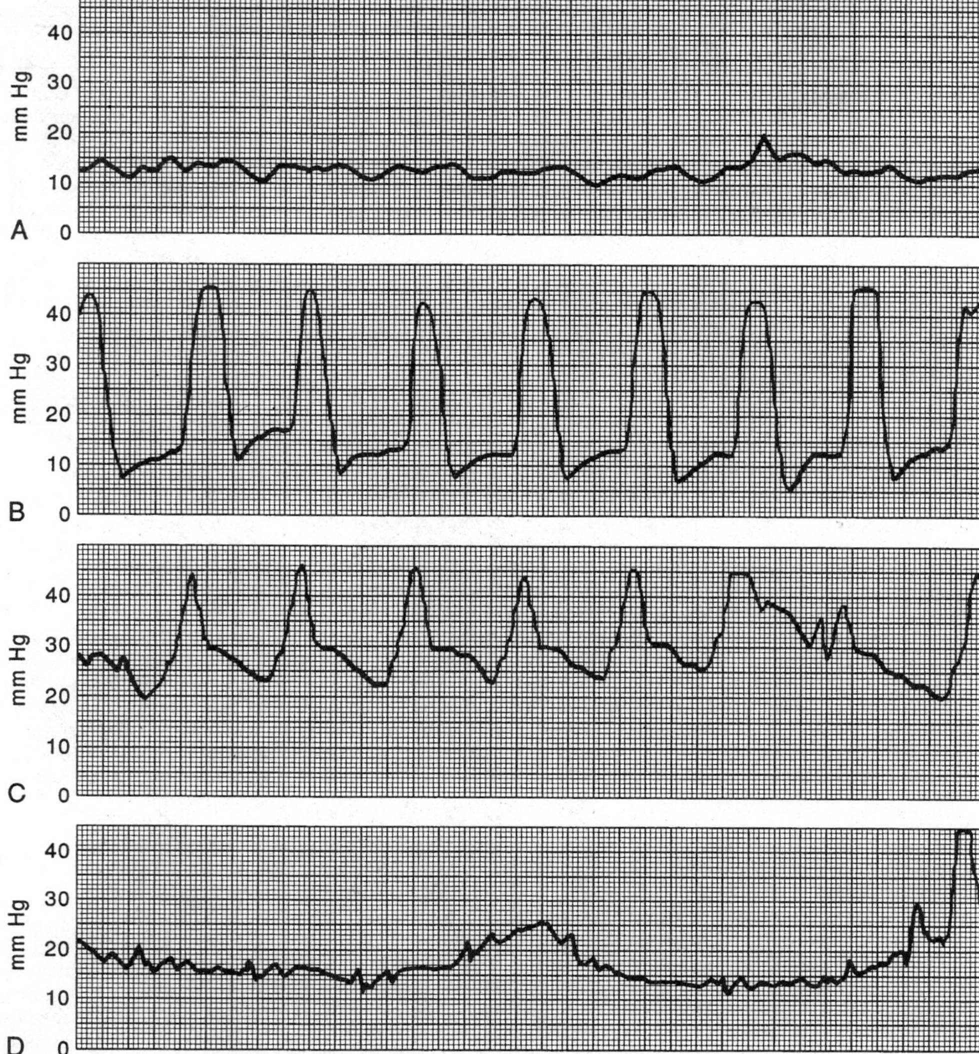

FIGURE 13–9. Waveforms observed during insertion of a pulmonary artery catheter. *A*, Right atrial pressure. *B*, Right ventricular pressure. *C*, Pulmonary artery pressure. *D*, Pulmonary artery wedge pressure.

ventilated patients with diffuse bilateral disease (Langer et al., 1988); however, no studies have determined the effect of prone position on hemodynamic parameters.

Therefore, pulmonary artery pressures can be accurately measured with the head of the bed elevated. The practice of repositioning the bed so that the patient is lying flat before pressure measurement is not necessary and may result in increased patient discomfort or respiratory compromise. However, with any position change, the transducer must be leveled to the phlebostatic axis to avoid errors in hemodynamic pressure measurement. If the transducer is below the level of the right atrium, pressures will be erroneously high; if the transducer is above the level of the right atrium, pressures will be erroneously low. The transducer can be taped on the chest wall of the patient at the phlebostatic axis, saving time during frequent position changes and eliminating PA pressure measurement errors related to inappropriate transducer placement (Dobbin et al., 1992).

In conclusion, backrest elevations up to 60 degrees do not affect measurement of intracardiac pressures or cardiac output, but PaO_2 may diminish in sitting positions after surgical procedures. In lateral positions, measurement of intracardiac pressures and cardiac output is not recommended. In patients with unilateral lung disease, PaO_2 increases with the unaffected lung in the dependent position. Trendelenburg position has not been shown consistently to provide any beneficial effects. Prone positioning may be beneficial in ARDS and in weaning of mechanically ventilated patients (Doering, 1993).

The studies also suggest pulmonary artery pressure readings should be obtained from a graphic recording obtained at the end-expiratory phase of the re-

TABLE 13–4. **Potential Problems and Intervention Strategies for Pulmonary Artery Catheter Monitoring**

Problem	Cause	Intervention
No waveform appears on oscilloscope	Cable disconnected	Secure all cable connections
	Stopcock turned off to the patient	Turn stopcock to open the catheter to the transducer
	Kink in catheter	Check for kinks in the exposed portion of the catheter, particularly near the introducer, and straighten catheter
	Clot in catheter	Aspirate catheter and irrigate; do not irrigate catheter if no fluid is aspirated May need to replace catheter Use continuous flush with heparin in 0.9% sodium chloride 1 units/mL
	Faulty transducer	Replace transducer
Dampened waveform		
All pressures dampened	Insufficient inflation of pressure bag	Inflate pressure bag to 300 mm Hg
	Leak in pressure bag due to faulty valve or defective bladder	Replace pressure bag
	Air bubble in pressure monitoring set	Thoroughly prime pressure monitoring set
	Incorrect calibration or gain control	Recalibrate and adjust gain
Dampened RA waveform only	Gradual clotting of proximal lumen due to stopcock not being returned to the proper position after performing cardiac output measurement, administering medication, or withdrawing blood	Position stopcock to keep the flush system open to the catheter
Dampened PA and PAWP waveform only	Gradual clotting of distal lumen	Use continuous flush system with heparin in 0.9% sodium chloride 1 unit/mL Rapidly flush lumen after obtaining blood
	Catheter tip occluded by balloon or lodged against the wall of the pulmonary artery	Deflate balloon and slowly flush lumen with heparinized solution Chest x-ray can confirm catheter position Physician may need to withdraw the catheter 1–2 cm
Marked change in all pressures	Incorrect calibration. This may occur when patients are moved from one area to another	Recalibrate
	Recalibration; for example, at the change of shift when a different nurse commences monitoring of the patient Baseline drift	The oncoming nurse may take the first set of readings before the zeroing and recalibration procedure and compare these to the last readings taken by the outgoing nurse. The oncoming nurse may then zero and calibrate the equipment and compare readings obtained after this procedure to the first set of readings obtained. This will permit comparison of readings between nurses and by the same nurse before and after zeroing and recalibration
	Different method of measuring waveforms	Establish standard protocol to be used by all personnel involved in hemodynamic monitoring Mount a paper printout in the patient's medical record of the RA, PA, and PAWP waveforms over three respiratory cycles. Label the printout with the patient's name, date, time, scale, and mark the location where the measurements were taken
Right ventricular waveform appears on the oscilloscope	Catheter drifted back into the right ventricle	Notify the physician to advance the catheter. Observe closely for ventricular dysrhythmias and have lidocaine available
Increased frequency of premature ventricular contractions	Catheter may be flipping in and out of the right ventricle or may have drifted back and remained in the right ventricle	Notify the physician to reposition the catheter; keep lidocaine available
Noise or fling in pressure waveform	Excessive catheter movement (fling), particularly in the pulmonary artery	Notify physician because catheter may need to be repositioned; avoid excessive catheter length in the ventricle
Unable to obtain PAWP	Catheter not advanced far enough into the pulmonary artery	Notify physician to advance the catheter

TABLE 13–4. **Potential Problems and Intervention Strategies for Pulmonary Artery Catheter Monitoring** *Continued*

Problem	Cause	Intervention
No resistance to injection of air into the balloon port. Syringe plunger does not spontaneously slide back after attempted inflation	Ruptured balloon	Slide lock on the balloon port to the closed position; do not attempt further inflations
Volume of air needed to inflate balloon is less than was needed for initial flotation	Catheter migrated to a distal pulmonary vessel close to the wedge position	Notify physician because catheter may need to be withdrawn
PAWP waveform remains on the oscilloscope	Catheter migrated distally and lodged in a vessel	Attempt to dislodge catheter by having the patient cough, breathe deeply, or change position; notify physician to withdraw catheter to dislodge the catheter tip; observe chest x-ray for pulmonary infiltrates
	Balloon left inflated	Let balloon deflate spontaneously after each PAWP measurement by disconnecting the syringe or by letting the syringe plunger slide back; do not pull back on plunger
Bleeding from catheter or pressure tubing	Leak in the pressure monitoring set	Tighten all connections Check inflation pressure of pressure bag Flush system
Bleeding from insertion site	Improper anchor or vessel trauma	Inspect insertion site Notify physician Anchor catheter Apply pressure to site until bleeding stops
Pain at insertion site	Pain during the first few hours after insertion may be caused by the local anesthetic wearing off	Analgesia as prescribed
	Local inflammation or infection	Use aseptic technique for insertion and removal Perform daily inspection of insertion site with application of topical antibiotic and sterile dressing May need to remove catheter Exudate and catheter tip may be sent for culture, particularly if patient is febrile
	Excessive motion due to inadequate anchoring of catheter	Anchor catheter
Infection	Contamination during insertion or through stopcocks	Use sterile technique Physician may remove catheter and prescribe antibiotics Cap all stopcock ports Change flush solution every 24 hours Change tubing every 24 to 48 hours

Abbreviations: RA, right atrium, PA, pulmonary artery; PAWP, pulmonary artery wedge pressure.

Data from Armstrong, P. W., & Baigrie, R. S. (1980). Strategy for troubleshooting problems in hemodynamic monitoring. In P. W. Armstrong & R. S. Baigrie (Eds.), *Hemodynamic monitoring in the critically ill.* Hagerstown, MD: Harper & Row; Daily, E. K., & Schroeder, J. S. (1989). *Techniques in bedside hemodynamic monitoring* (4th ed.). St. Louis: C. V. Mosby; and Gardner, P. E., & Woods, S. L. (1989). Hemodynamic monitoring. In S. L. Underhill, S. L. Woods, E. S. S. Froelicher, et al. (Eds.), *Cardiac nursing* (2nd ed.). Philadelphia: J. B. Lippincott.

spiratory cycle. This recommendation is designed to eliminate changes in pulmonary artery pressures induced by intrathoracic pressure fluctuations during respiration (Daily & Schroeder, 1989; Cengiz et al., 1983). During mechanical ventilation, PA pressures measured by the bedside monitor's digital display were similar to measurements obtained from the recording at end-expiration. During normal breathing after extubation, pulmonary artery systolic (PAS) pressures were similar for the two methods of measurement, but PAD/PAWP pressures measured by the bedside monitor's digital display were significantly lower than those obtained from the graphic recording at end expiration (Dobbin et al., 1992).

MEASURING DYNAMIC RESPONSE. To ensure the accuracy of pressure measurements, a dynamic response measurement should be performed. This test reflects the system's ability to reproduce a pressure waveform. Because of the variability of catheter–transducer system set-ups, and even differences in characteristics with identical set-ups, it is necessary to test and optimize each individual monitoring system.

An easy way to measure dynamic response at the bedside is to perform a fast flush test, also known as a square wave test. Flush the hemodynamic line and observe the response or return of the waveform on the monitor. A properly functioning system and an optimum flush, results in one undershoot followed by a

TABLE 13–5. **Potential Complications of the Pulmonary Artery Catheter**

Complications Associated With Insertion and Advancement
Vascular damage (venous and arterial)
Hematoma
Infection
Local thrombus
Premature atrial contractions
Premature ventricular contractions
Ventricular fibrillation
Complete heart block
Right bundle branch block
Complications Associated With an Indwelling Pulmonary Artery Catheter
Thrombosis
Bacteremia
Endocarditis
Valve rupture
Pneumothorax
Pulmonary embolus
Pulmonary infarction
Pulmonary artery rupture and hemorrhage
Pulmonary infiltrates

small overshoot (minimal ringing), then it settles down to the patient's waveform. An overdamped system is sluggish and appears artificially rounded and blunted. It will cause the systolic pressure to be erroneously low and the diastolic reading to be erroneously high. The response to the fast flush test shows no ringing. An underdamped system is overresponsive and produces a hemodynamic waveform that is artificially spiked and exaggerated. The systolic pressure measured on this system is erroneously high, whereas the diastolic pressure is erroneously low (Fig. 13–10).

There are four steps to be taken to correct dynamic response, also known as maximizing natural frequency and damping coefficient. First, be sure all air bubbles are removed from the system. They are often found around the transducer and stopcocks. Make sure that the tubing is primed before the pressure bag is applied. Tap gently to remove the air. Second, long tubing or the addition of extension tubing can have a detrimental effect, similar to that of air bubbles. The length of the tubing should be 4 feet or shorter, and the stiffer pressure tubing should never be substituted. Third, check for loose connections. Stopcocks should have luer-lock adapter and should be snug. Fourth, use a damping device that is available commercially. The damping device affects the damping coefficient without altering natural frequency.

WEST LUNG ZONES. Hemodynamic pressures can be altered by pulmonary artery catheter tip location, an increase in positive end-expiratory pressure (PEEP) in the airway, and hypovolemia. There is a gravity-dependent difference between ventilation and perfusion in the lung, a relationship between arterial pressure (Pa), alveolar pressure (PA), and venous pressure (Pv). In zone I, PA exceeds Pa and Pv. In zone II, PA is greater than Pv but less than Pa. In zone III, Pa and Pv are greater than PA, and blood flow is uninterrupted, allowing the pulmonary artery catheter tip to communicate continuously with distal vascular pressure (Fig. 13–11). Pressures recorded in zones I and II reflect alveolar more than vascular pressure. With increasing alveolar pressure (PEEP), change in position, or decreased intravascular volume, zone III areas can revert to zone II or I. Pulmonary artery catheter tip position in zone III is essential for reliable PAWP monitoring. Cathethers are flow directed; they tend to advance to areas of higher or continuous blood flow, which usually occur in a dependent area of the lung (zone III).

The following characteristics suggest that the catheter tip may be outside zone III: (1) a smooth-appearing PAWP tracing, (2) a PAD that is less than the PAWP, (3) an increase in PAWP greater than 50% of the change in alveolar pressure, and (4) a decrease in PAWP greater than 50% of the reduction in PEEP. A lateral chest radiograph can help confirm the catheter tip location relative to the left atrium. Increasing intravascular volume or decreasing alveolar pressure can convert zones I or II to zone III (Enger, 1989).

PULMONARY ARTERY CATHETER MEASUREMENTS

RIGHT ATRIAL PRESSURE. RAP reflects right ventricular diastolic pressure because the open tricuspid valve permits direct communication between both chambers. The normal RAP is −1 to 7 mm Hg. The RAP has a, c, and v waves and an x and y descent (Fig. 13–12, *I*). The a wave reflects atrial systole and corresponds to the ECG P-R interval.The x descent occurs as atrial pressure drops after atrial systole. The c wave reflects the tricuspid valve bulging into the right atrium with ventricular systole, and is found within the R-S-T interval. The v wave represents right atrial filling and corresponds to the T-P interval on the ECG. The y descent reflects the drop in atrial pressure as the blood flows through the tricuspid valve. The mean RAP is recorded.

Right atrial pressure is elevated in the presence of right ventricular failure, tricuspid regurgitation and stenosis, pericardial tamponade and other constrictive pericardial diseases, chronic left ventricular failure, pulmonary stenosis, pulmonary hypertension, and fluid overload (Forrester et al., 1976), and reduced in the presence of hypovolemia or vasodilation. Right atrial pressure does not reflect right ventricular filling pressure when there is elevated intrapericardial pressure or acute right ventricular dilation (Chatterjee, 1985).

RIGHT VENTRICULAR PRESSURE. The six components of the right ventricular pressure (RVP) are isovolumetric contraction, rapid ejection, reduced ejection, volumetric relaxation, early diastole, and atrial systole (Fig. 13–12, *II*). The normal RVP is 15 to 25 systole/0 to 8

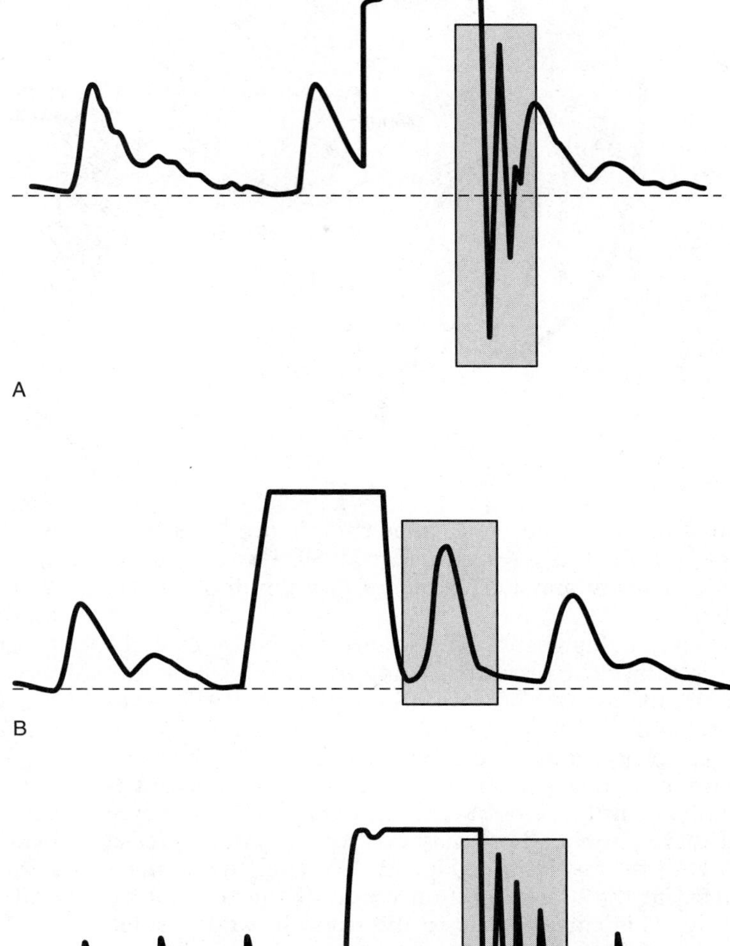

FIGURE 13–10. Square wave testing using the fast-flush feature on the hemodynamic fluid line. *A*, Accurate waveform; *B*, overdamped; *C*, underdamped. (Redrawn by permission from Baxter Healthcare Corporation. All rights reserved.)

mm Hg diastole. If the catheter slips back into the right ventricle, the physician should be notified immediately to reposition the catheter. The balloon should be inflated to flow-direct the catheter back into the pulmonary artery due to risk of ventricular ectopy and trauma.

PULMONARY ARTERY PRESSURE. The components of the PAP are peak systolic pressure, dicrotic notch, and diastole (Fig. 13–12, *III*). The normal PAP is 15 to 25 systole/8 to 15 mm Hg diastole. The PAS is usually equal to the right ventricular systolic pressure. However, the PAD is higher than the right ventricular diastolic pressure because of the closure of the pulmonic valve. The dicrotic notch reflects closure of the pulmonic valve. The pulmonary artery end-diastolic pressure usually correlates with the PAWP when the pulmonary vascular resistance (PVR) is normal. In these patients, the pulmonary artery diastolic pressure may be substituted for the PAWP when the catheter cannot be wedged. However, when the PVR is elevated, the pulmonary artery diastolic pressure will be higher than the PAWP; this may occur in patients with pulmonary hypertension and ARDS. The PAD may not reflect left ventricular end-diastolic pressure when there is left ventricular dysfunction such as mitral ste-

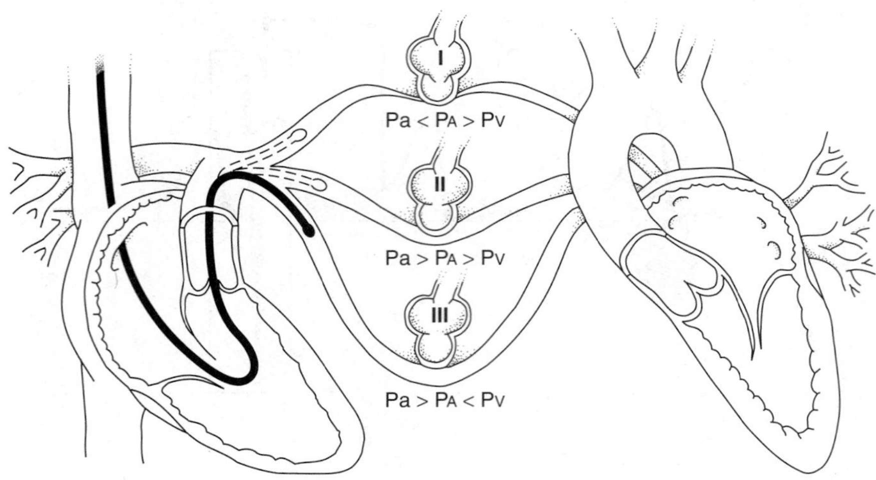

FIGURE 13–11. West lung zones. PAWP estimates Pv only under zone III conditions that allow for a continuous column of blood to exist from the catheter tip to the left heart. (Redrawn with permission from O'Quin, R., & Marini, J. J. [1983]. Pulmonary artery occlusion pressure: Clinical physiology, measurement and interpretation. *American Review of Respiratory Diseases, 128,* 319–326.)

nosis or decreased ventricular compliance (Bouchard et al., 1971; Daily & Schroeder, 1989; Dawson et al., 1993; Falicov and Resnekov, 1970; Rahimtoola et al., 1972).

Cyclic changes in the PAP are caused by changes in intrathoracic pressure during the respiratory cycle. In spontaneously breathing patients, the PAP waveform will dip to its lowest point during inspiration. These changes may become more marked in patients with pulmonary disease, heart failure, or hypovolemia, or in those on mechanical ventilation. In some of these patients there may be a paradoxical increase in PAP on inspiration (Fig. 13–13). The PAP is measured at the end-expiration phase of the respiratory cycle. This corresponds to the diastolic and systolic pressure that exists immediately preceding the lowest point in the tracing during one respiratory cycle (or the highest point if inspiration results in a paradoxical increase in pressure) (Fig. 13–14). The patient's breathing pattern should be observed simultaneously with the tracing on the monitor or paper printout.

Catheter fling (Fig. 13–15) will result in artifact, making it difficult to determine the PAP accurately. The catheter should be repositioned; one possible cause is excessive catheter length in the right ventricle. If the problem cannot be corrected, one possible solution is to use the digital output to obtain a mean pressure.

PULMONARY ARTERY WEDGE PRESSURE. The PAWP reflects the left ventricular filling pressure because during diastole, the pulmonary venous bed and left ventricle are in direct communication (see Fig. 13–7) (Forrester et al., 1976; Gardner, 1993). The normal PAWP is 6 to 12 mm Hg. The PAWP is obtained by slowly inflating the balloon (approximately 1.25–1.5 mL) until a wedge tracing appears on the recorder or until the maximum volume recommended by the manufacturer has been injected.

The a wave reflects atrial contraction and corresponds to the QRS complex on the ECG (see Fig. 13–12, *IV*). The x descent reflects a pressure drop during late diastole when the atria are relaxed and the ventricles are filling. No c wave is generally seen on PAWP recording because the pressure dissipates before reaching the catheter tip. The v wave represents passive atrial filling and will occur during the T-P interval on the ECG. The y descent reflects the drop in atrial pressure when the mitral valve opens and blood moves from the atria to the ventricle.

Elevated a waves on the PAWP recording occur in patients with mitral stenosis and left ventricular failure. The v wave elevates in patients with mitral insufficiency, and both the a and v waves elevate in patients with cardiac tamponade, severe constrictive pericardial disease, and hypervolemia.

There are certain diseases in which the PAWP does not reflect left ventricular filling pressure. These diseases include mitral stenosis and regurgitation, left atrial myxoma, ball valve thrombus, cor triatriatum, pulmonary venoocclusive disease, total anomalous pulmonary venous drainage, cardiac tamponade, and acute right ventricular dilation resulting from right ventricular infarction, massive pulmonary embolism, and acute severe tricuspid regurgitation (Cason & Lambert, 1993; Chatterjee, 1985). In the presence of decreased left ventricular compliance or marked atrial contribution to ventricular filling, the left ventricular end-diastolic pressure may be as much as 20 mm Hg higher than the PAWP or the mean left ventricular diastolic pressure (Enger, 1989; Forrester et al., 1976; Gardner, 1993).

In most patients, the average PAWP is recorded. The value of the average PAWP is usually similar to the PAD . However, if a patient has mitral regurgitation, the v wave will be prominent, and two pressures should be recorded: the PAWP measured without the v wave and the PAWP measured with the v wave (Fig. 13–16). Although the volume of air used for lung inflation in patients receiving mechanical ventilation can affect pulmonary blood flow and PAWP (Murao & Rodbard, 1971), the difference in PAWP measured with patients on and off intermittent positive pressure ventilation is not clinically significant (Shinn et al.,

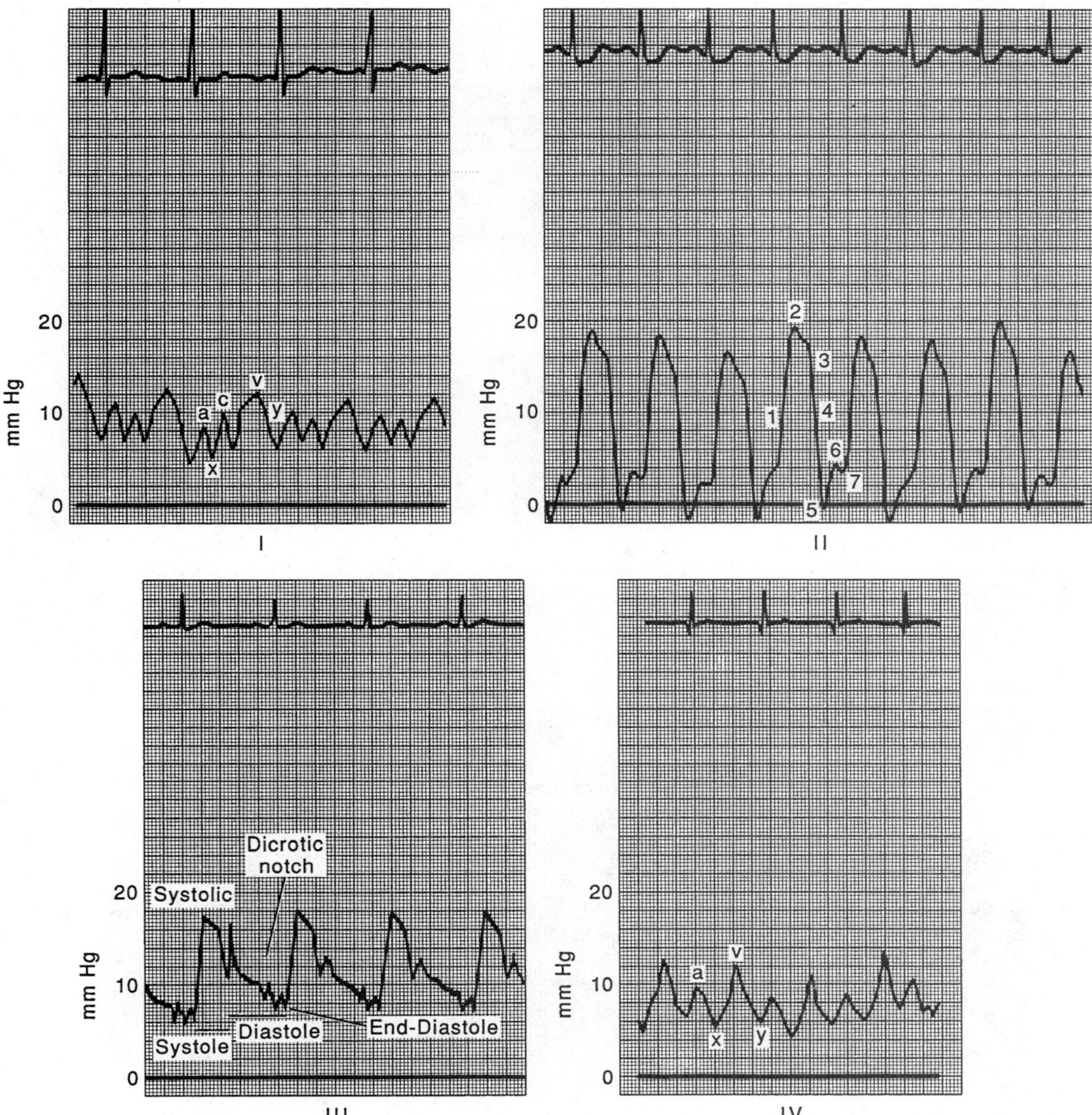

FIGURE 13–12. Right atrial pressure waveform. *II,* Right ventricular waveform (1 = isovolumetric contraction; 2 = rapid ejection; 3 = reduced ejection; 4 = volumetric relaxation; 5 = early diastole; 6 = atrial systole; 7 = end-diastole). *III,* Pulmonary artery waveform. *IV,* Pulmonary artery wedge pressure waveform. a, a wave indicates atrial systole; c, c wave represents the movement of the atrioventricular (AV) valve toward the atrium during valve closure; v, v wave represents filling of the right atrium during ventricular systole with bulging of the AV valve into the atrium; x, the descent after the a wave represents the decline in pressure during atrial relaxation; y, the descent after the v wave represents the opening of the AV valve, allowing blood flow into the ventricle. (Redrawn by permission from Daily, E. K., & Schroeder, J. S. [1989]. *Techniques in bedside hemodynamic monitoring* [4th ed.]. St. Louis: C. V. Mosby.)

1979). It is not necessary to disconnect patients from ventilators during the measurement of the PAWP.

The PAWP may be used as an index of left ventricular volume because of its direct relationship to diastolic myocardial fiber stretch. Starling's law of the heart states that the energy of contraction is a function of the length of the muscle fiber (Forrester et al., 1976; Starling, 1918). When the PAWP is between 6 and 20 mm Hg, it usually correlates closely with the mean left atrial and left ventricular diastolic pressures. However, the PAWP may not equal left ventricular end-diastolic pressure because the mitral valve begins to close before the start of ventricular systole.

During balloon inflation, the injection of 1.25 to 1.50 mL of air should be adequate to obtain a PAWP. The waveform on the oscilloscope should be observed so

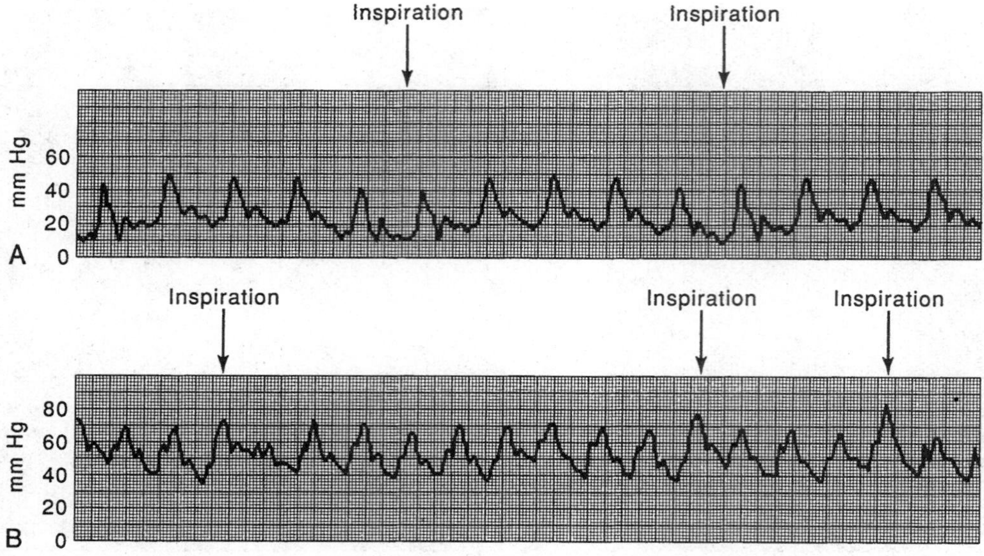

FIGURE 13–13. Pulmonary artery pressure waveform with respiratory variation. *A,* Patient with spontaneous respiration shows typical decrease in pressure during inspiration. *B,* Patient receiving mechanical ventilation shows increase in pressure during inspiration.

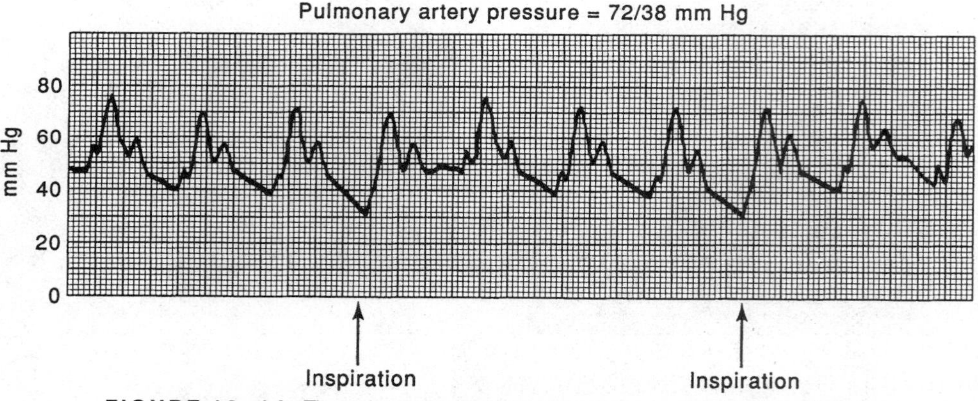

FIGURE 13–14. The pulmonary artery pressure is measured at end-expiration.

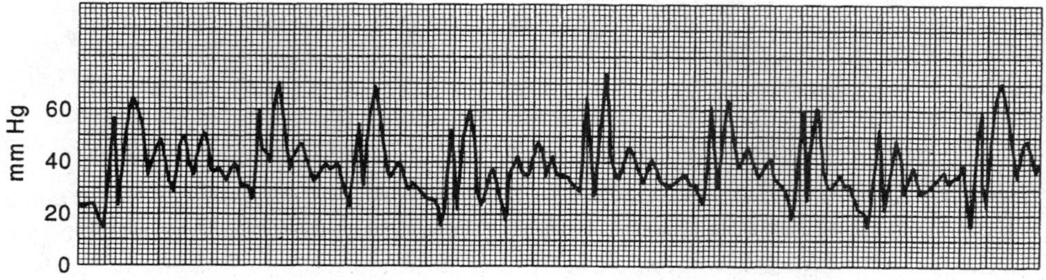

FIGURE 13–15. Pulmonary artery pressure waveform with catheter fling.

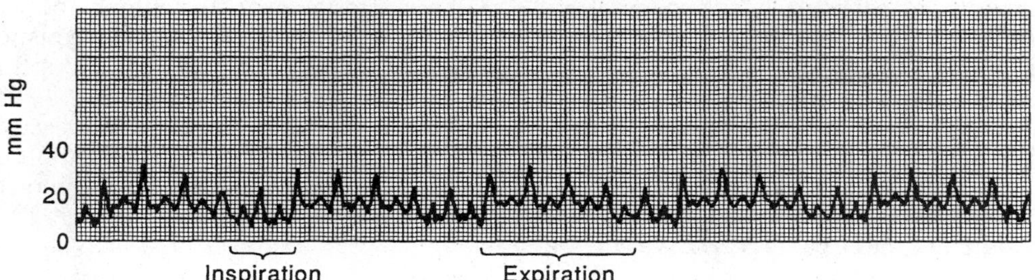

FIGURE 13–16. Pulmonary artery wedge pressure showing the v wave in a patient with mitral regurgitation.

that the minimum volume of air needed to wedge the balloon is used. If the PAWP waveform continues to rise while the balloon is inflated and the tracing dampens, overwedging has occurred (Fig. 13–17). This falsely high pressure may be caused by the pressure from an overinflated balloon (Baxter Healthcare Corporation, 1982). The balloon should be deflated. Reinflation may be attempted after the PAP is visualized on the oscilloscope. Overinflation will increase the risk of balloon rupture, air emboli, and loss of PAWP monitoring capability. If the catheter remains in the wedge position after deflating the balloon, the patient should be asked to cough and breathe deeply, or change position. The physician must be notified immediately if the catheter remains wedged, because the physician will need to pull back on the catheter to dislodge it, thus preventing pulmonary infarction. The catheter should be withdrawn 2 to 3 cm at a time until a pulmonary artery tracing is visualized. When the balloon is reinflated with near-maximum balloon volume, the PAWP waveform should appear. If the balloon volume needed to obtain the PAWP is much less than near the maximum, the tip of the catheter is too far into the pulmonary artery. The balloon should be deflated and the catheter pulled back.

Blood Sampling

The pulmonary artery catheter can be used for obtaining blood for laboratory tests (American Society of Anesthesiologists, 1993; Bodai & Holcroft, 1983). The proximal port (right atrial port) should be used instead of the distal port (pulmonary artery port) to minimize the risk of falsely high results if saline, dextrose, potassium, or other electrolytes are being centrally infused. However, if aspiration from the proximal port is not possible, samples may be obtained from the distal port. If a mixed venous sample is required, the sample must be drawn from the distal port to ensure adequate mixing. It is usually necessary to stop fluids infusing through the side port of the catheter introducer during aspiration because this fluid is entering the right atrium. However, great caution must be taken if vasoactive drugs such as nitroprusside, nitroglycerin, and dopamine are being centrally infused. Patients on such medications often have an intraarterial catheter, and it is preferable to obtain blood specimens from the arterial catheter if the vasoactive drugs are being centrally infused.

Approximately 3 mL of infusate should be aspirated and discarded before the blood sample is drawn.

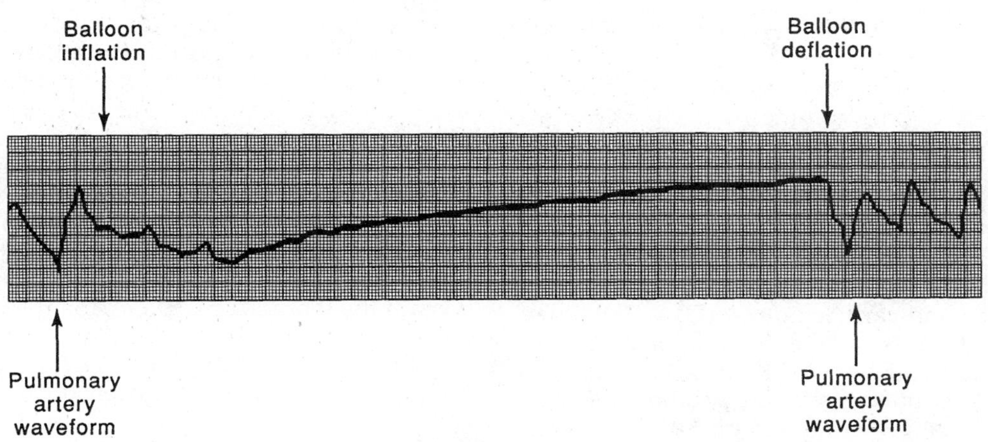

FIGURE 13–17. Overwedging of the pulmonary artery catheter during balloon inflation.

Because existing research is inconclusive, more research is needed to determine the optimal discard volume for laboratory tests, particularly for coagulation studies. The blood should be aspirated slowly to prevent hemolysis. Slow and steady aspiration is also important when obtaining a mixed venous oxygen sample from the distal port to avoid withdrawing arterialized blood (Bodai & Holcroft, 1983).

CARDIAC OUTPUT MEASUREMENTS

Investigators in the mid-1800s broadly estimated the stroke volume in humans to range from 45 to 200 mL per beat (Fick, 1870; Hoff & Scott, 1948; Stewart, 1897). Fick, Stewart, Hamilton, Fegler, and Ganz developed the theoretical framework and instrumentation that laid the foundation for the accurate determination of cardiac output and stroke volume in humans by the thermodilution method (Fegler, 1954, 1957; Fick, 1870; Ganz et al., 1971; Hamilton et al., 1928, 1932, 1948; Stewart, 1893, 1897, 1921; Swan et al., 1970). The accuracy, validity, and reliability of the thermodilution method has been established during the past 35 years (Kadota, 1985).

The theory on which the validity of the thermodilution method is based is the law of conservation of mass. The Fick principle, an application of the law of conservation of mass, is the hypothesis on which the direct Fick method and the dye dilution method are based, and these in turn are the standards against which the thermodilution method is compared. The Fick principle states that flow, measured per unit of time, is equal to the amount of an indicator substance introduced to the flow in that same unit of time divided by the difference in the concentration of the indicator substance before and after the point of entry (Fick, 1870).

Direct Fick Method

Current application of the Fick principle involves calculation of the cardiac output (Berne & Levy, 1986):

$$Q = Vo_2/Cpvo_2 - Cpao_2$$

where Q = cardiac output in liters/minute; Vo_2 = oxygen consumption (mL/minute); $Cpvo_2$ = oxygen content (O_2/mL blood) in the pulmonary vein; $Cpao_2$ = oxygen content (O_2/mL blood) in the pulmonary artery. The amount of substance taken up or released by an organ is equal to the organ's blood flow rate and its arterial–mixed venous oxygen difference. The direct Fick method uses the lung as the organ, oxygen as the substrate, and cardiac output (Q) as the blood flow rate: Q (L/min) is equal to the oxygen consumption (mL/min) divided by the difference between pulmonary venous O_2 content (mL/mL of blood) and pulmonary artery O_2 content (mL/mL of blood). In clinical practice, the direct Fick method involves taking blood samples from a peripheral artery and the right ventricle or pulmonary artery to obtain the values for arterial oxgyen content and venous oxygen content, respectively. The oxygen consumption is measured by having the patient breathe through a valve system that allows the separate collection of expired air. The oxygen concentration in the expired air is subtracted from the oxygen concentration in the inspired air to obtain the value for the oxygen consumption.

Dye Method

The dye dilution method involves the injection of a known quantity and concentration of indocyanine green into the bloodstream. Flow and volume are calculated by measuring the dye concentration at a point downstream at selected time intervals. The cardiac output is equal to the area under the exponential indicator dilution curve. Although the dye dilution method is less cumbersome than the direct Fick method in the clinical setting, this method does involve the problem of dye recirculation, which may cause inaccuracies in subsequent measurements and requires arterial blood sampling.

Thermodilution Method*

Fegler (1954) published the first study using the thermodilution method to measure cardiac output. Ganz and associates (1971) stated the principle of thermodilution cardiac output measurement:

> *A known amount of a cold indicator is injected into the superior vena cava or upper right atrium, and the resultant change in blood temperature detected in the pulmonary artery. The cardiac output is inversely proportional to the fall in temperature.*

Assumptions are made when using the thermodilution method to determine cardiac output. Controlling for these variables will alleviate erroneous measurements. There must be forward flow of blood and adequate mixing of blood and injectate (iced or room temperature). Certain conditions prevent appropriate mixing or directional flow of the indicator solution. Intracardiac shunts, tricuspid regurgitation, and cardiac dysrhythmias—which affect beat-to-beat cardiac injection—can all affect the accuracy of thermodilution cardiac output measurements.

The catheter must be properly placed with the proximal port in the right atrium and the distal port in the pulmonary artery. The catheter thermistor must be positioned freely in the lumen of the pulmonary artery. Falsely elevated cardiac output readings will occur if the thermistor impinges on the vessel wall, insulating it from the "cool" thermal indicator.

The nurse must use proper technique and observe the cardiac output curve to ensure accuracy of the

* *From Kadota, L. T. (1985).* Heart and Lung, 14, *605.*

measurement. Irregular cardiac output curves are caused by poor injectate–balloon mixing, thermistor–vessel wall contact, changes in heart rate or blood pressure, faulty technique, and abnormal respiratory patterns, and can produce inaccurate cardiac output results. Therefore, an important nursing function is interpretation of the thermodilution curve. The curve should be assessed for abnormal inflections in its contour due to catheter wedging or faulty injection technique, oscillations of baseline (more than 15% of pulmonary artery temperature) due to hemodynamic and respiratory effects, prolonged baseline drift due to recirculation of thermal indicator (low-output states), low amplitude of the curve due to small temperature difference (<10°C) between injectate and blood, or thermistor lying against vessel wall (Fig. 13–18).

Injectate

Ten milliliters of iced (0–5°C) 5% dextrose is commonly used as the injectate. An alternative solution is 0.9% saline. The rationale for using iced injectate is to increase the signal-to-noise ratio (Ganz & Swan, 1972). Studies have demonstrated that room temperature injectate correlates well with the dye dilution method (Evonuk et al., 1961) and with iced injectate (Daily & Mersch, 1987; Elkayam et al., 1981; Hruby & Woods, 1983; Killpack et al., 1981; Larson & Woods, 1982; Medley et al., 1992; Shellock & Riedinger, 1983; Swinney et al., 1981; Sawyer-Sommers et al., 1993). Iced injectate may be preferable to room temperature injectate in patients with poor forward blood flow, such as those with right ventricular failure, tricuspid stenosis, or tricuspid regurgitation. These conditions make it difficult to get accurate cardiac output measurements, but the larger signal-to-noise ratio obtained with iced injectate may improve the estimates obtained with the thermodilution method. Hypothermic patients (cardiac surgery, trauma) may also require iced injectate to achieve greater accuracy and precision of measurement. There should be at least 10°C gradient between injectate temperature and patient's blood temperature. Injectate volumes of 1 to 5 mL may be used in infants and children (Freed & Keane, 1978; Headrick, 1992; Mathur et al., 1976; Wyse et al., 1975), and volumes of 5 to 10 mL may be used in adults (Enghoff & Sjogren, 1973). The smaller volume should be considered in fluid-restricted patients. If the actual volume of the delivered injectate is less than it should be, or if the injectate temperature is warmer than the temperature recorded by the temperature probe, falsely high cardiac output measurements will result (Baxter Healthcare Corporation, 1983; Reininger & Troy, 1976; Woods & Osguthorpe, 1993; Yelderman et al., 1992).

The closed system injectate delivery system eliminates the need to uncap the stopcock on the pulmonary artery catheter, thus minimizing the risk of contamination. Although no difference in contamination rates between the closed system and prefilled capped syringes was found in one study, the closed system seemed to be more convenient for nurses to use (Bridges & Woods, 1993; Yonkman & Hamory, 1988).

Measurement Guidelines

At the present time, insufficient data exist to determine whether trends in a patient's hemodynamics or response to therapeutic interventions can be accurately monitored if cardiac output measurements are done with the patient in a sidelying or elevated backrest position instead of in the standard supine position. One study found that accurate measurements using 10 mL of room temperature 5% dextrose injectate may be obtained with the patient in either a supine position or in 45-degree backrest elevation (Shenkman & Kasprow, 1988). Four other studies (Cason et al., 1990; Doering & Dracup, 1988; Grose et al., 1981; Whitman et al., 1982), however, noted clinically significant changes in some of the subjects. More research is needed because these patients are often sleep deprived, due in part to frequent awakenings for respositioning when hemodynamic measurements are done (Doering, 1993).

One factor often forgotten in measurement of cardiac output is setting the cardiac output computer with the correct computation constant. The computation constant is selected based on the cathether size and model, the type of injectate delivery system, and the volume and temperature of the injectate. This constant, along with the patient's pulmonary artery blood temperature, is incorporated into the cardiac output calculation by the computer to account for many of the variables that affect the measurement. When the computation constants are not changed according to these parameters, incorrect measurements are made.

Electronic averaging of the blood temperature before injection and rapid delivery of the injectate minimizes variability caused by the physiologic responses to dysrhythmias, emotional stimuli, and changes in venous return caused by positional changes and the respiratory cycle. Accurate measurements are obtained when the bolus is delivered within 4 seconds with firm, steady pressure. Measurements are unreliable when the bolus lasts 8 seconds or longer (Enghoff & Sjogren, 1973), and falsely low cardiac output measurements will result. Although some studies (Dizon et al., 1977; Nelson & Houtchens, 1982) have demonstrated improved reproducibility of sequential cardiac output measurements when automatic injectors were used instead of manual injections, a clinically significant improvement has not yet been adequately demonstrated to justify the additional equipment (Manifold, 1984; Riedinger & Shellock, 1984). The manual injection method remains acceptable for clinical practice.

Proper measurement technique is important to minimize thermal loss. When measurements are taken with iced injectate, approximately 45 to 60 minutes should be allowed for the prefilled syringes to equilibrate with the ice bath (Levett & Replogle, 1979); less than 10 to 15 minutes are needed for the closed in-

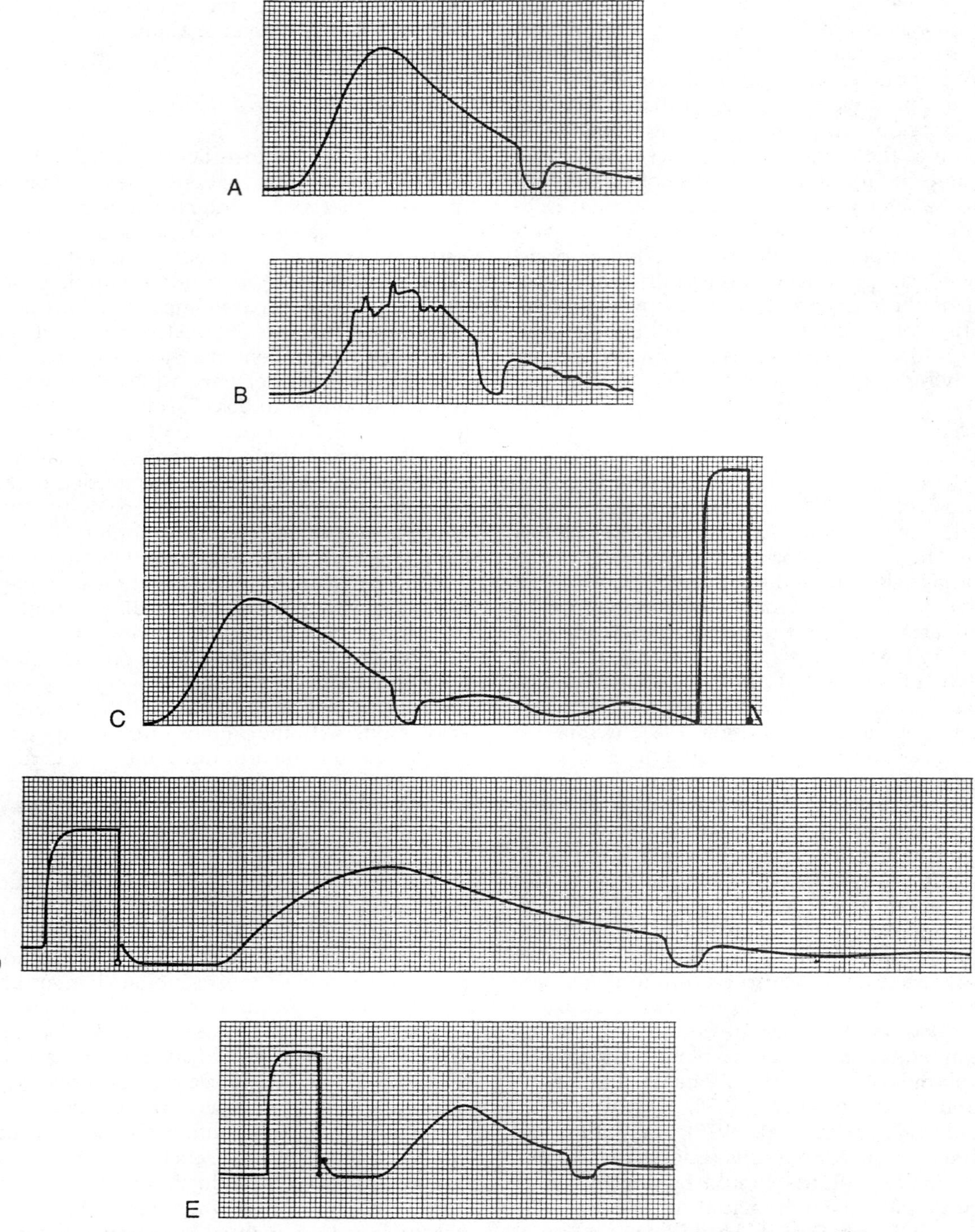

FIGURE 13–18. Thermodilution curves obtained with cardiac output measurement. *A,* Normal thermodilution curve. *B,* Abnormal inflections in curve contour due to catheter wedging or faulty injection technique. *C,* Oscillations of the baseline due to hemodynamic or respiratory effects. *D,* Prolonged baseline drift due to low output states. *E,* Low amplitude of curve due to small temperature difference (<10°C) between injectate and blood or thermistor lying against the vessel wall. (Redrawn with permission from Gardner, P. E., & Woods, S. L. [1989]. Hemodynamic monitoring. In S. L. Underhill, S. L. Woods, E. Froelicher, et al. [Eds.], *Cardiac nursing* [2nd ed., p. 465]. Philadelphia: J. B. Lippincott.)

jectate system. Thermal indicator loss begins from the time the injectate is removed from the ice bath and continues as the injectate flows past the pulmonary artery thermistor. It is estimated that 17% of thermal indicator in 10 mL of 0°C 5% dextrose is lost before the injectate enters the central circulation (Sorensen et al., 1976). Loss of thermal indicator is demonstrated by the tendency of the first in a series of injections to produce the highest cardiac output measurement (Kadota, 1986; Wong et al., 1978). Falsely high cardiac output measurements are avoided when there is minimal handling of the syringe barrel (Levett & Replogle, 1979; Powner, 1975). There is disagreement over whether injection of the bolus should be timed with a particular phase of the respiratory cycle (Armengol et al., 1982; Baxter Healthcare Corporation, 1983; Jansen et al., 1981; Levett & Replogle, 1979; Riedinger & Shellock, 1984; Snyder & Powner, 1982; Wise et al., 1981; Woods et al., 1976). Jansen and coworkers (1981) mapped out the cyclic variations in cardiac output through the respiratory cycle and concluded that end-expiration is the best time to inject the bolus for the left side of the heart; the authors concluded that the data did not reveal a satisfactory moment for timing bolus delivery for the right side of the heart when different levels of positive end-expiratory pressure were used. The cyclic variations in cardiac output for both the left and right sides of the heart are similar to the cyclic variations seen in pulmonary artery pressure waveforms measured at end-expiration. It is important to consider a method that will be consistent and sensitive in detecting trends in a patient's hemodynamic status to permit evaluation of therapeutic interventions. Armengol and coworkers (1982) reported that the standard error of cardiac output measurements taken at random points during the respiratory cycle is 9.8%, compared to 5.1% when measurements are timed at end-expiration. Timing injection with the respiratory cycle (end-expiration) can improve the reproducibility of cardiac output measurements. Cardiac output measurements appear to have the most reproducibility at end-expiration, but they have the most accuracy when spaced throughout the respiratory cycle (Jansen et al., 1990). The recommendation to time the injection of the bolus at the end-expiratory phase of the respiratory cycle appears to be the method that is best suited for the clinical setting (Armengol et al., 1982; Levett & Replogle, 1979; Stevens et al., 1985).

Cardiac output decreases with intermittent positive pressure ventilation, continuous positive pressure ventilation, and PEEP because of the increase in airway and intrapleural pressure (Grenvik, 1966; Jardin et al., 1981; Lamy et al., 1973; Qvist et al., 1975; Rankin et al., 1981), although some patients may have a paradoxical increase (Powers et al., 1973). The patient should not be disconnected from the ventilator for cardiac output measurements. Hemodynamic monitoring and serial arterial blood gases can guide the clinician in optimizing the patient's cardiovascular and pulmonary status.

The thermodilution method has been shown to provide accurate measurements in the presence of pulmonary insufficiency due to pulmonary stenosis or atresia (Beyer et al., 1977). Prosthetic cardiac valves yield a dilution curve with a steep downslope. In patients with enlarged hearts and a low stroke volume or those in cardiogenic shock, the injectate may sometimes take more than 20 seconds to travel from the right atrium to the pulmonary artery thermistor. The cardiac output computer may not be able to process the delay in the onset of the thermodilution curve and the delay in the termination of the curve. In this instance, the "delay START" injection technique may be necessary to measure cardiac output. The details of this technique are described in the cardiac output computer operations manual (Baxter Healthcare Corporation, 1983).

On rare occasions, the proximal port of the pulmonary artery catheter, which is used to deliver the injectate, may no longer be patent because of a blood clot. Reasonably accurate cardiac output measurements using iced 5% dextrose may be made by using the side port of the catheter introducer (Lee & Stevens, 1985). It may also be possible to make accurate meaurements through the venous infusion port of one type of pulmonary artery catheter (Model 93A–831–7.5F, Baxter Healthcare Corportion, Santa Ana, CA) if the proximal port is no longer patent. Critically ill patients often have multiple central infusions, particularly since the development of catheter introducers that have a side port that provides an additional access site. Research is needed to determine the maximum central infusion rate that will still permit clinicians to obtain accurate cardiac output measurements because large volumes of room temperature solutions infusing through or alongside the pulmonary artery thermodilution catheter will lead to an overestimation of cardiac output. Changes were noted in pulmonary artery temperatures with concomitant cold fluids infusing through the proximal port of pulmonary artery catheters. Decreases in cardiac output were noted during concomitant infusions through the distal port of the pulmonary artery catheter or through the sideport. Unless a medication is needed to prevent serious pathophysiologic consequence, concomitant infusion should be turned off during cardiac output measurement. The infusion should be discontinued for 30 seconds before cardiac output measurement (Wetzel et al., 1985). Unstable patients, however, must be closely observed if the central infusions are momentarily stopped, particularly if vasopressor or vasodilator medications are infusing through these ports.

The standard protocol for measuring cardiac output by the thermodilution method involves taking the average of three sequential measurements (Millar et al., 1980). The rationale for averaging multiple measurements is based on the dynamic biologic factors and technical limitations of the thermodilution method that influence reproducibility. Technical and biologic variance accounts for approximately 4% to 10% of the variability among sequential measurements (Singh et al., 1970; Swan, 1990; Weil, 1977). Variations of 10% or more from previous measurements, assuming proper technique and steady-state conditions, indicate a change in cardiac output (Swan, 1990). The data from the study by Wong and associates (1978) suggested that the standard protocol should be modified so that the first in a series of measurements be discarded as a falsely high reading because of thermal loss. It is not recommended that single cardiac output measurements be used to interpret trends in a patient's hemodynamic status because variations of 15% to 25% may occur (Bilfinger et al., 1982; Stetz et al., 1982). Triplicate determinations provide clinically acceptable data (Forrester et al., 1972). Although quadruplicate measurements may reduce the error further, such a protocol may be best reserved for use in research (Rubin et al., 1982) because the volume of injectate may become a significant factor in the fluid status of unstable patients in renal failure who are undergoing simultaneous preload and afterload reduction.

The final step in cardiac output measurement is to calculate the cardiac index using the Dubois body surface area nomogram (Fig. 13–19) to standardize the cardiac output to the size of the patient. Computerized cardiac profiles will automatically calculate this index using the patient's height and weight.

One of the most important factors involved in hemodynamic monitoring is ensuring accuracy of the measured values. Three steps are performed throughout the day—positioning of the transducer at the phlebostatic axis, setting the zero reference, and electrical calibration. These procedures are performed every 4 to 12 hours and as necessary.

In patients with acute myocardial infarction, a cardiac index of 2.7 to 4.3 liters/minute/m^2 is normal, 2.2 to 2.7 liters/minute/m^2 indicates subclinical depression, 1.8 to 2.2 liters/minute/m^2 reflects the onset of clinical hypoperfusion, and less than 1.8 liters/minute/m^2 reflects cardiogenic shock (Forrester et al., 1976). A high cardiac output is seen in patients with septic shock, anemia, or hyperthyroidism and in some with acute myocardial infarction (Swan & Ganz, 1975).

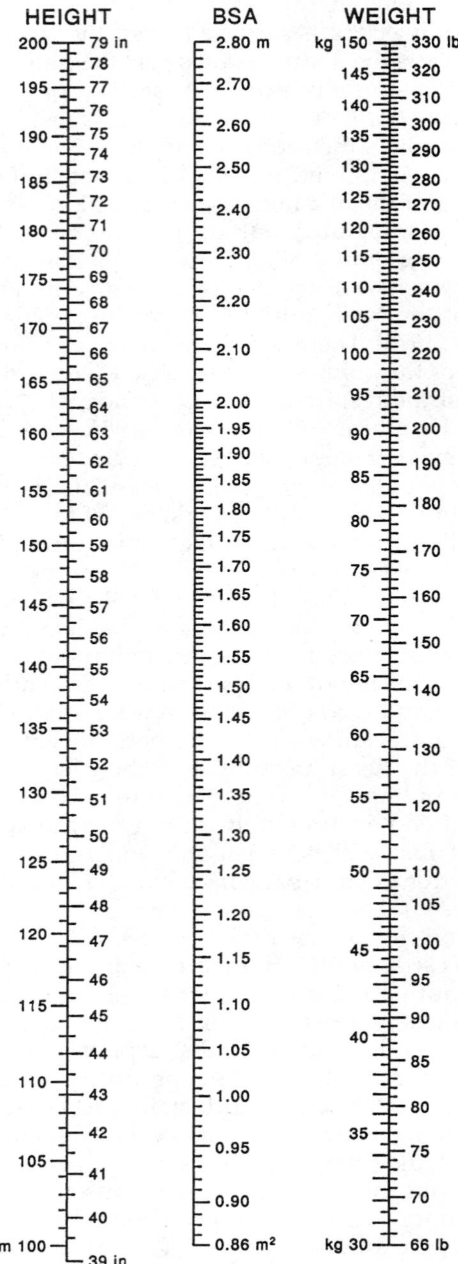

FIGURE 13–19. Body surface area nomogram from the formula of Dubois. Calculating the body surface area: 1. Find the height (in inches or centimeters) of the individual on the scale on the left. 2. Find the weight (in pounds or kilograms) of the individual on the scale on the right. 3. Connect these points with a ruler. 4. The body surface area is at the point where the ruler crosses the scale in the middle. (Redrawn from Grossman, W. [Ed.]. [1986]. *Cardiac catheterization and angiography* [3rd ed.]. Philadelphia: Lea & Febiger.)

Continuous and Noninvasive Measurement of Cardiac Output

One promising method of continuously measuring cardiac output is with a pulse thermodilution catheter. It is a modified pulmonary artery catheter with a heating filament at the injection port (right ventricle) that continuously cycles on and off, alternately warming the blood. A distal thermistor detects the response to blood warming and sends data to a computer, which analyzes the input. This process permits the estimation of continuous cardiac output by analysis of the statistical properties of the input and output signals (Yelderman et al., 1992).

Doppler echocardiography uses ultrasound to determine cardiac output. Cardiac output is determined based on measurement of blood velocity in the ascending aorta and the cross-sectional area of the ascending aorta. Several methods are being explored, including a flow-directed, Doppler pulmonary artery catheter, extractable Doppler probes implanted during surgery, and esophageal Doppler cardiac output measurement (Abrams et al., 1989).

Thoracic electrical bioimpedance cardiac output monitoring is a noninvasive technique for determining cardiac output. Electrodes are placed on the patient's neck and chest that monitor impedance changes with each heartbeat. This method uses the change in potential difference between the sensing and current electrodes to calculate the stroke volume, which is then multiplied by heart rate to determine cardiac output (Pepke-Zaba et al., 1990).

The newest noninvasive technique is thoracocardiography, which uses three plethysmographic transducers to measure cardiac oscillations on the surface of the thorax. A combination of beat-to-beat cardiac oscillations is taken from the respiratory signal during breathing and a volume curve is generated that is used to calculate stroke volume and cardiac output (Sackner et al., 1991).

CLINICAL APPLICATION OF HEMODYNAMIC MONITORING

The hemodynamic data obtained from the pulmonary artery catheter and cardiac output measurements aid in the diagnosis, evaluation, and estimation of prognosis in patients with heart disease. The data from the pulmonary artery catheter should always be used in conjunction with the medical history and physical assessment of the patient to treat the patient as a whole. Remember, one of the most important nursing responsibilities during hemodynamic monitoring is observation of trends in measurements, not treating the absolute number.

Diagnosis

The relationship between intracardiac pressures and characteristic changes in waveform morphology permits the diagnosis of certain cardiac diseases. Tricuspid insufficiency may be diagnosed by the presence of large v waves in the right atrial pressure waveform. Mitral regurgitation may result in large v waves in the pulmonary artery wedge pressure waveform because of the backflow of blood through the incompetent valve during systole.

Pericardial tamponade may be diagnosed when the right atrial pressure is elevated and equal diastolic measurements are obtained from the right atrium, right ventricle, pulmonary artery, and pulmonary artery wedge pressure (Forrester et al., 1976). The PAP is elevated when the pulmonary vascular resistance is high (chronic lung disease, pulmonary embolism, or pulmonary hypertension) or when pulmonary blood flow is increased (ventricular septal defect) (Dawson et al., 1993; Forrester et al., 1976).

Evaluation

Heart function is optimal when there is a balance between myocardial oxygen demand and myocardial oxygen supply. The determinants of cardiac output are preload, afterload, contractility, and heart rate. Therapy can be implemented to affect each of the determinants of cardiac output to achieve optimum heart function. The following discussion examines each of the determinants of cardiac output and the specific therapies used for hemodynamically compromised patients.

PRELOAD. Preload is defined as the volume or pressure generated at end-diastole. In the clinical setting, left-sided preload is measured by PAWP, and right-sided preload is measured by RAP/CVP. RAP/CVP can provide adequate data for appropriate fluid management in most young patients with normal cardiac function. As a general rule, the preload in acutely injured patients should be adjusted to a CVP between 7 to 12 mm Hg. If the fluid state of a patient is still in doubt, a pulmonary artery catheter should be inserted (Domsky & Wilson, 1993).

The PAWP can be used to monitor the relative extent of pulmonary congestion, from no congestion (PAWP = 6–12 mm Hg), mild pulmonary congestion (PAWP = 18–20 mm Hg), to acute pulmonary edema (PAWP > 30 mm Hg). The PAWP is elevated when there is an increased blood volume in the left ventricle, which reflects a reduced ejection fraction. This may be the result of decreased left ventricular compliance or acute mitral insufficiency. The PAWP can also be used to evaluate the effectiveness of interventions to relieve pulmonary congestion. Medications that decrease preload include diuretics, nitroglycerin, morphine sulfate, diphosphoesterase inhibitors (e.g., amrinone, milrinone), and, to a lesser extent, nitroprusside. A diuretic such as furosemide can reduce the PAWP within minutes by venous dilation. A further reduction in the PAWP and RAP occurs within an hour when diuresis commences. The PAWP may be low (PAWP < 6 mm Hg) when there is a fluid deficit due to dehydration, excessive diuresing, third-spacing, or bleeding. The mechanism used to increase preload is to increase the circulating blood volume, which may be accomplished by administering crystalloids or colloids. Support of tissue perfusion is the primary goal of fluid therapy. It is essential to follow changes in PAWP, cardiac output, and tissue perfusion in response to rapid fluid administration.

Inadequate tissue perfusion, the response of PAWP to a "fluid challenge," can be used to assess and guide therapy. Fluid is rapidly administered (10 minutes) in predetermined increments (50–200 mL), and the change in PAWP is monitored. The magnitude of the change in PAWP is determined by the patient's individual ventricular compliance curve. A large increase in wedge (>7 mm Hg) or the development of pulmonary edema suggests an excessive left ventricular end-diastolic pressure (preload) and a position on the steep portion of the ventricular function curve. Further volume administration increases left ventricular end-diastolic pressure, heightens the risk of hydrostatic pulmonary edema, and increases myocardial oxygen consumption with improving cardiac output. Moderate increases in wedge are not too dangerous if pressure decreases within 10 minutes to within 3 mm Hg of the original value. If the wedge does not increase at least 3 mm Hg and perfusion remains inadequate, additional "challenges" are necessary until systemic perfusion returns. If volume has been optimized and tissue perfusion remains inadequate, further intervention is required. Augmentation of stroke volume may be accomplished by inotropic support, afterload reduction, and chronotropic modification. Measurement of cardiac output and calculation of systemic vascular resistance and stroke work index can help assess the effectiveness of these therapies.

Patients with severe pulmonary dysfunction may have elevated systolic and diastolic pulmonary pressures, yet the PAWP may be low, normal, or high. A fluid challenge in such patients often results in increased cardiac output and left ventricular stroke work index without a signficant increase in PAWP, indicating that further fluid administration may be beneficial. A PAWP of 15 to 18 mm Hg generally indicates an adequate preload and allows for a trial of afterload reduction with a vasodilator.

AFTERLOAD. Afterload is defined as the impedance to the ejection of blood from ventricle. It is the resistance that the ventricle must overcome to eject blood in a forward direction. The two determinants of afterload are (1) the volume and mass of blood ejected from the ventricle, and (2) the compliance and total cross-sectional area of the vascular space into which the blood is ejected. In the clinical setting, right ventricular afterload is measured by the PVR, and left ventricular afterload is measured by the SVR.

The normal value of PVR is 150 to 250 dynes/sec/cm^{-5}. The PVR is calculated by the formula:

$$\text{PVR (dynes/sec/cm}^{-5}) = \frac{\text{PAM} - \text{PAWP}}{\text{CO}} \times 80$$

where PAM = pulmonary artery mean (mm Hg); PAWP = pulmonary artery wedge pressure (mm Hg); and CO = cardiac output (L/min).

The PAM is calculated by the formula:

$$\text{PAM} = \frac{[(\text{PAD})(2)] + \text{PAS}}{3}$$

where PAD = pulmonary artery diastolic pressure and PAS = pulmonary artery systolic pressure. A better indicator of right-sided afterload is the pulmonary vascular resistance index (PVRI), calculated by the formula:

$$\text{PVRI (dynes/sec/cm}^{-5}\text{-m}^2) = \frac{\text{PAM} - \text{PAWP}}{\text{CI}} \times 80$$

where CI = cardiac index. The normal value for PVRI is 160 to 280 dynes/sec/cm^{-5}-m^2.

Pulmonary hypertension, reflected by an elevated PVR, occurs when disease alters the determinants of pulmonary vascular pressure. Primary pulmonary hypertension is the diagnosis given when the etiology of the elevated PVR is unknown. Secondary pulmonary hypertension is the diagnosis given when the overall etiology is known. Cardiac diseases that may result in an elevated PVR are (1) increased left atrial pressure due to left ventricular failure, and (2) increased pulmonary blood flow due to an atrial or ventricular septal defect. Pulmonary diseases that may result in an elevated PVR are (1) obstruction that occurs in patients with massive pulmonary emboli or thrombosis, (2) obliteration that occurs in severe emphysema, (3) vasoconstriction that occurs in the pulmonary arterioles in response to alveolar hypoxia. The pulmonary vasculature reacts less to neural and pharmacologic stimuli than the systemic vasculature. This makes it difficult to develop effective therapy for pulmonary hypertension. One medication that may reduce the pulmonary vascular resistance through vasodilation is a prostaglandin, alprostadil. Alprostadil is administered as a continuous intravenous infusion at 0.05 to 0.10 μg/kg/min in adult patients. Patients should be monitored for hypotension and flushing.

The normal value for the SVR is 800 to 1,500 dynes/sec/cm^{-5}. The SVR is calculated by the formula:

$$\text{SVR (dynes/sec/cm}^{-5}) = \frac{\text{MAP} - \text{RAP}}{\text{CO}} \times 80$$

where MAP = mean arterial pressure (mm Hg); RAP = right atrial pressure (mm Hg); and CO = cardiac output (L/min). The MAP is calculated by the formula:

$$\text{MAP} = \frac{[(2)(\text{DP})] + (\text{SP})}{3}$$

where DP = diastolic pressure; and SP = systolic pressure. A better indicator of left-sided afterload is the systemic vascular resistance index (SVRI), calculated by the formula:

$$\text{SVRI (dynes/sec/cm}^{-5}\text{-m}^2) = \frac{\text{MAP} - \text{CVP}}{\text{CI}} \times 80$$

The normal value for SVRI is 1,970 to 2,390 dynes/sec/cm^{-5}-m^2.

A high SVR (>1,500 dynes/sec/cm^{-5} may reflect physiologic stress or left ventricular failure. A low SVR (<600 dynes/sec/cm^{-5}) may reflect septic shock or excessive administration of afterload reduction medications. Medications that decrease the SVR include nitroprusside, hydralazine, and captopril. Dobutamine may also be used to decrease the SVR by increasing the cardiac output. Medications that increase the SVR include dopamine, epinephrine, norepinephrine, and phenylephrine.

In patients with a high PAWP and a low cardiac output, vasodilators such as nitroprusside can improve ventricular function (Chatterjee et al., 1973; Domsky & Wilson, 1993) by reducing the force that the left ventricle has to generate to eject blood. This is reflected in an increased cardiac output, increased systemic blood pressure in hypotensive patients, and a reduction of an abnormally high SVR. In the failing heart, cardiac output may be agumented with dobutamine or dopamine and nitroprusside. The rationale for combining dopamine and nitroprusside is to increase cardiac output by the positive inotropic effect of dopamine and the afterload reduction effect of nitroprusside (Dracup et al., 1981). In contrast, patients with right ventricular infarction require elevated right filling pressures to maintain an adequate cardiac output.

CONTRACTILITY. Contractility is the third determinant of cardiac output. Contractility is defined as the ability to shorten and develop tension. It is not possible at the present time to measure contractility directly in the clinical setting. Positive inotropic agents include caffeine, digitalis, dobutamine, dopamine, epinephrine, isoproterenol, and norepinephrine. Negative inotropic agents include hypoxia, hypercapnia, acidosis, esmolol, propranolol, quinidine, procainamide, and barbiturates.

HEART RATE. The fourth determinant of cardiac output is heart rate. The normal heart rate in an adult at rest is 60 to 100 beats/minute. An elevated heart rate increases myocardial demand and reduces the diastolic phase of the cardiac cycle when the coronary arteries are being filled. Treatment includes resolving the underlying cause of the elevated heart rate (for example, antibiotics and antipyretics for sepsis and sedation for excessive anxiety). The heart rate may also be decreased in patients with heart disease by medications such as digitalis, propranolol, and verapamil. Lower heart rates usually result in a compensatory increase in stroke volume. An extremely low heart rate that causes hemodynamic instability may be increased by administering atropine or isoproternol, or by inserting a pacemaker.

STROKE VOLUME. The stroke volume is the average volume of blood ejected per cardiac contraction. The normal stroke volume depends on the patient's size and level of activity. In an adult at rest, the normal stroke volume is 60 to 130 mL/contraction. The stroke volume is calculated by the formula:

$$SV = \frac{CO}{HR}$$

where SV = stroke volume; HR = heart rate.

STROKE VOLUME INDEX. This is calculated to permit the comparison of the stroke volume in people of different sizes. The normal stroke volume index in an adult at rest is 40 to 50 mL/contraction/m^2 body surface area. The stroke volume index is calculated by the formula:

$$SI = \frac{SV}{BSA}$$

where SI = stroke index; BSA = body surface area (square meters).

LEFT VENTRICULAR STROKE WORK. This value is used to estimate the functional capability of the left ventricle. The normal left ventricular stroke work (LVSW) is 60 to 80 g. An elevated LVSW is seen in patients with hypervolemia or hypertension. A low LVSW is seen in patients with left ventricular failure, acute myocardial infarction, aortic stenosis, septic shock, or cardiogenic shock. The LVSW is calculated by the formula:

$$(SV)(MAP - PAWP)(0.0136)$$

where 0.0136 = constant that converts stroke work units into grams. Again, to compare size to function, stroke work parameters should be indexed. The formula to calculate left ventricular stroke work index (LVSWI) is:

$$LVSWI = SVI\ (MAP - PAWP) \times 0.0136$$

Normal values for LVSWI are 45 to 65 g/beat/m^2.

RIGHT VENTRICULAR STROKE WORK. This value is used to estimate the functional capability of the right ventricle. The normal right ventricular stroke work (RVSW) is 10 to 15 g. An elevated RVSW is seen in patients with hypervolemia and pulmonary embolism with cor pulmonale. A decreased RVSW is seen in patients with right ventricular failure, severe cor pulmonale, ventricular septal defect, or right ventricular infarction. The formula for the RVSW is:

$$(SV)(MPAP = CVP)(0.0136)$$

where CVP = central venous pressure. The right atrial pressure may be substituted for the CVP. The formula to calculate right ventricular stroke work index (RVSWI) is:

$$RVSWI = SVI\ (PAM - CVP) \times 0.0136$$

Normal values for LVSWI are 5 to 10 g/beat/m^2.

MIXED VENOUS OXYGEN SATURATION. Mixed venous oxygen saturation (SVO_2) reflects the adequacy of the oxygen supply relative to the oxygen demand at the tissue level. The normal value for SVO_2 is 60% to 80%. A normal value may indicate that the tissues are being adequately perfused but does not indicate whether compensatory mechanisms are being used to maintain perfusion. For example, a patient may have a normal SvO_2 because an increased cardiac output is compensating for an inadequate blood supply. Table 13–6 presents the possible causes of abnormally high or low

TABLE 13–6. **Interpretation of Svo_2 Monitoring Values**

High Svo_2 (>80%)			
↑ *Oxygen Delivery*	↓ *Oxygen Demand*	*Interference in Oxygen Diffusion*	*Technical Problem*
↑ FIO_2	Hypothermia	Cyanide toxicity	Wedged PA catheter
Hyperoxia	Anesthesia		
Low Svo_2 (<80%)			
↓ *Oxygen Delivery*		↑ *Oxygen Demand*	
↓ Hemoglobin due to anemia, hemorrhage		Hyperthermia	
↓ Sao_2 due to hypoxia, suctioning		Pain	
↓ Cardiac output due to hypovolemia, shock		Shivering	
		Seizures	
		Stress	

Adapted from Baxter Healthcare Corporation. (1987). *Understanding continuous mixed venous oxygen saturation (Svo_2) monitoring with the Swan-Ganz Oximetry TD System.* Santa Ana, CA:

Svo_2 values. A decrease in Svo_2 would indicate the need to assess the effectiveness of the patient's oxygen supply mechanisms (Sao_2, hemoglobin, cardiac output). There may be adjustments to therapy in respiratory treatment, in correcting anemic states, or maximizing cardiac output. An increase in oxygen demand or a decrease in arterial oxygen content is compensated initially by an acute increase in cardiac output or oxygen extraction. In critically ill patients, cardiac reserves can be limited. If oxygen extraction increases, the Svo_2 falls, at a critical level of oxygen delivery, extraction of oxygen decreases, the Svo_2 reaches a plateau, and oxygen consumption (Vo_2) is delivery dependent. When the Svo_2 is 50% or less, tissue oxygen balance is compromised and there is an increased potential for anaerobic metabolism and lactic acidosis. A decrease in Svo_2 often occurs before other clinical signs of hemodynamic instability develop, allowing this measurement to serve as an "early warning system." Multiple indices have been suggested to reflect the adequacy of tissue oxygenation (Pvo_2, Svo_2, oxygen extraction ratio, lactic acid, arteriovenous oxygen content). At present, Svo_2 is the only index clinically available on a continuous, real-time basis.

The range of normal values for hemodynamic parameters is summarized in Table 13–7.

TABLE 13–7. **Range of Normal Values for Hemodynamic Parameters**

Parameter	Normal Values
Mean right atrial pressure	−1–7 mm Hg 4–7 cm H_2O
Right ventricle pressure	
Systolic	15–25 mm Hg
Diastolic	0–8 mm Hg
Pulmonary artery pressure	
Systolic	15–25 mm Hg
Diastolic	8–15 mm Hg
Mean	10–20 mm Hg
Mean pulmonary artery wedge pressure	6–12 mm Hg
Mean arterial pressure	70–105 mm Hg
Systemic vascular resistance	800–1500 dynes/sec/cm^{-5}
Systemic vascular resistance index	1970–2390 dynes/sec/cm^{-5}-m^2
Pulmonary vascular resistance	150–250 dynes/sec/cm^{-5}
Pulmonary vascular resistance index	160–280 dynes/sec/cm^{-5}-m^2
Cardiac output	4.0–8.0 L/min
Cardiac index	2.5–4.5 L/min/m^2
Stroke volume	60–130 mL/beat
Stroke volume index	40–50 mL/beat/m^2
Left ventricular stroke work	60–80 g/beat
Left ventricular stroke work index	45–65 g/beat/m^2
Right ventricular stroke work	10–15 g/beat
Right ventricular stroke work index	5–10 g/beat/m^2
Mixed venous oxygen saturation	60%–80%

Classification of Patients Based on Hemodynamic Data

Forrester and colleagues (1976) developed a classification for estimating short-term mortality in patients with acute myocardial infarction based on clinical and hemodynamic data (Table 13–8). The underlying pathophysiology of subsets II, III, and IV reflect the increasing severity of left ventricular failure that may occur after an acute myocardial infarction. This type of prognostic classification can provide guidance in making medical and nursing decisions about therapy and for providing patient and family support.

TABLE 13–8. **Clinical and Hemodynamic Subsets in Patients With Acute Myocardial Infarction**

Subset	Pulmonary Congestion (PAWP = >18 mm Hg)	Peripheral Hypoperfusion (Cardiac Index <2.2 L/min/m^2BSA)	% Mortality
I	−	−	3
II	+	−	9
III	−	+	23
IV	+	+	51

Abbreviations: PAWP = pulmonary artery wedge pressure; BSA = body surface area; − = No; + = Yes.

Reprinted, by permission, from the *New England Journal of Medicine,* 295, 1356–1362, 1976.

SUMMARY

During the past 25 years, hemodynamic monitoring has become an important aid in the diagnosis, evaluation, and estimation of prognosis in critically ill patients. Expansion of the capabilities of the pulmonary artery catheter to include pacing, continuous Svo_2 and cardiac output monitoring, right ventricular ejection fraction and volume monitoring, and additional access for administration of medications through central infusions has broadened the nursing responsibilities for these patients. One of the research challenges facing clinicians is the refinement of measurement protocols to maximize patient comfort while maintaining a high level of accuracy. These catheters provide an invaluable means of evaluating nursing and medical interventions to provide optimal patient care.

REFERENCES

Hemodynamic Monitoring Systems

Bartz, B., Maroun, C., & Underhill, S. (1988). Differences in mid-anteroposterior level and midaxillary level in patients with a range of chest configurations (Abstract). *Heart and Lung, 17,* 308.

Windsor, T., & Burch, G. E. (1945). Phlebostatic axis and phlebostatic level, reference levels for venous pressure measurements in man. *Proceedings of the Society for Experimental Biology and Medicine, 58*(2), 165–169.

Central Venous Pressure Monitoring

Anderson, H. L., Underhill, S. L., Fine, J. S., et al. (1988). Reliable plasma glucose, sodium, and potassium measurement from a multiple-lumen central venous catheter with concurrent infusion of total parenteral nutrition solution (Abstract). *Heart and Lung, 17,* 302.

Corona, M. L., Peters, S. G., Narr, B. J., et al. (1990). Infections related to central venous catheters. *Mayo Clinic Proceedings, 65,* 979–986.

Daily, E. K., & Schroeder, J. S. (1989). *Techniques in bedside hemodynamic monitoring* (4th ed.). St. Louis: C. V. Mosby.

Daily, P. O. (1972). Position of patient for central venous pressure measurements. *Journal of the American Medical Association, 219,* 1233.

Daly, J. M., Ziegler, B., & Dudrick, S. J. (1975). Central venous catheterization. *American Journal of Nursing, 5,* 820–824.

Driver, C. E. (1972). The effect of elevating the head of the patient's bed while obtaining the central venous pressure measurement. *Circulation, 46* (4, Suppl. II), II–241.

Eckstein, J. W. (1972). Position of patient for central venous pressure measurements. *Journal of the American Medical Association, 219,* 1223.

Forrester, J. S., Diamond, G., McHugh, T. J., et al. (1971). Filling pressures in the right and left sides of the heart in acute myocardial infarction. *New England Journal of Medicine, 285,* 190–193.

Gowen, G. F. (1973). Interpretation of central venous pressure. *Surgical Clinics of North America, 53,* 649–656.

Kern, L. (1993). Hemodynamic monitoring. In R. L. Boggs & M. Wooldridge-King (Eds.), *AACN procedure manual for critical care.* Philadelphia: W. B. Saunders.

Millar, S., Sampson, L. K., Soukup, M., et al. (Eds.). (1980). *Methods in critical care.* Philadelphia: W. B. Saunders.

Thielen, J. B. (1990). Air emboli: A potentially lethal complication of central venous lines. *Focus on Critical Care, 17,* 374–383.

Thielen, J. B., & Nyquist, J. (1991). Subclavian catheter removal: Nursing implications to prevent air emboli. *Journal of Intravenous Nursing, 14*(2), 114–118.

Yacone, L. A. (1987). Monitoring central venous pressure. In G. O. Darovic (Ed.), *Hemodynamic monitoring: Invasive and noninvasive clinical application.* Philadelphia: W. B. Saunders.

Windsor, T., & Burch, G. E. (1945). Phlebostatic axis and phlebostatic level, reference levels for venous pressure measurements in man. *Proceedings of the Society for Experimental Biology and Medicine, 58,* 165–169.

Intraarterial Pressure Monitoring

Allen, E. V. (1929). Thromboangiitis obliterans: Methods of diagnosis of chronic occlusive arterial lesions distal to the wrist with illustrative cases. *American Journal of the Medical Sciences, 178,* 237–244.

Bedford, R. F., & Wollman, H. (1973). Complications of percutaneous radial artery cannulation: An objective prospective study in man. *Anesthesiology, 38,* 228–236.

Brown, A. E., Sweeney, D. B., & Lumley, J. (1969). Percutaneous radial artery cannulation. *Anaesthesia, 24,* 532–536.

Cannon, K., Mitchell, K. A., & Fabian, T. C. (1985). Prospective randomized evaluation of two methods of drawing coagulation studies from heparinized arterial lines. *Heart and Lung, 14,* 392–395.

Chatterjee, K. (1985). Bedside hemodynamic monitoring in the cardiac care unit. In A. N. Brest (Ed.), *Cardiovascular clinics.* Philadelphia: F. A. Davis.

Downs, J. B., Rackstein, A. D., Klein, E. F., Jr., et al. (1973). Hazards of radial-artery catheterization. *Anesthesiology, 38,* 283–286.

Gelberman, R. H., & Blasingame, J. P. (1981). The timed Allen test. *The Journal of Trauma, 21,* 477–479.

Gorny, D. A. (1993). Arterial blood pressure measurement technique. *AACN Clinical Issues, 4*(1), 66–80.

Gregersen, R. A., Underhill, S. L., Detter, J. C., et al. (1987). Accurate coagulation studies from heparinized radial artery catheters. *Heart and Lung, 16,* 686–693.

Hook, M. L., Reuling, J., Luettgen, M. L., et al. (1987). Comparison of the patency of arterial lines maintained with heparinized and nonheparinized solutions. *Heart and Lung, 16,* 693–699.

Joseph, D. H., & Larrivee, C. (1992). A decision-making algorithm for blood pressure measurements. *Dimensions of Critical Care Nursing, 11,* 145–150.

Kajs, M. (1986). Comparison of coagulation values obtained by traditional venipuncture and intra-arterial line methods. *Heart and Lung, 15,* 622–627.

Merenstein, G. B. (1971). Heparinized catheters and coagulation studies. *Journal of Pediatrics, 79,* 117–119.

Millam, D. A. (1988). Mastering arterial punctures. *American Journal of Nursing, 88,* 1213–1224.

Molter, N. (1983). Arterial blood gas analysis: A study of sampling techniques from indwelling arterial catheter systems (Abstract). *Heart and Lung, 12,* 428.

Molyneaux, R. D., Jr., Papciak, B., & Rorem, D. A. (1987). Coagulation studies and the indwelling heparinized catheter. *Heart and Lung, 16,* 20–23.

Pryor, A. C. (1983). The intra-arterial line: A site for obtaining coagulation studies. *Heart and Lung, 12,* 586–590.

Rakowski, A. C., Tonneson, A. S., Bracey, A., et al. (1987). Minimum discard volume from arterial catheters to obtain coagulation studies free of heparin effect. *Heart and Lung, 16,* 699–705.

Ramsey, M. (1991). Blood pressure monitoring: Automated oscillometric devices. *Journal of Clinical Monitoring, 7,* 56–76.

Rebenson-Piano, M., Holm, K., & Powers, M. (1987). An examination of the differences that occur between direct and indirect blood pressure measurement. *Heart and Lung, 16,* 285–294.

Rebenson-Piano, M., & Kirchhoff, K. T. (1983). Mean arterial pressure: Readings in two positions and with two reference points (Abstract). *Heart and Lung, 12,* 431.

Schuch, C. S., & Price, J. G. (1987). Determination of time required for blood gas homeostasis in the intubated post-open-heart surgery adult after a ventilator change. *Heart and Lung, 16,* 364–370.

Spaccavento, L. J., & Hawley, H. B. (1982). Infections associated with intra-arterial lines. *Heart and Lung, 11,* 118–122.

VanRiper, J., & VanRiper, S. (1987). Arterial pressure monitoring. In

G. O. Darovic (Ed.), *Hemodynamic monitoring: Invasive and noninvasive clinical application.* Philadelphia: W. B. Saunders.

Waite, R. M., & Parsons, D. (1991). Measurement of SvO_2, HR, and MAP in myocardial revascularization patients upon initial postoperative activity. *Critical Care Nursing, 5,* 87–91.

Pulmonary Artery Pressure Monitoring

American Society of Anesthesiologists: Task Force on Pulmonary Artery Catheterization. (1993). Practice guidelines for pulmonary artery catheterization. *Anesthesiology, 78,* 380–391.

Baxter Healthcare Corporation. (1982). *Understanding hemodynamic measurements made with the Swan-Ganz catheter.* Santa Ana, CA: Baxter Healthcare Corporation.

Baxter Healthcare Corporation. (1987). *Understanding continuous mixed venous oxygen saturation (SvO_2) monitoring with the Swan-Ganz oximetry TD system.* Santa Ana, CA: Baxter Healthcare Corporation.

Bodai, B. I., & Holcroft, J. W. (1983). (Letter to the editor.) *Heart and Lung, 12,* 329.

Bouchard, R. J., Gault, J. H., & Ross, J., Jr. (1971). Evaluation of pulmonary arterial end-diastolic pressure as an estimate of left ventricular end-diastolic pressure in patients with normal and abnormal left ventricular performance. *Circulation, 46,* 1072–1079.

Boyd, K. D., Thomas, S. J., Gold, J., et al. (1983). A prospective study of complications of pulmonary artery catheterizations in 500 consecutive patients. *Chest, 84,* 245–249.

Bridges, E. J., & Woods, S. L. (1993). Pulmonary artery pressure measurements: State of the art. *Heart and Lung, 22,* 99–111.

Caruthers, T. E., Reno, D. J., & Civetta, J. M. (1979). Implications of positive blood cultures associated with Swan-Ganz catheters. (Abstract). *Critical Care Medicine, 7,* 135.

Cason, C. L., & Lambert, C. W. (1993). Positioning during hemodynamic monitoring: Evaluating the research. *Dimensions of Critical Care Nursing, 12,* 226–233.

Cengiz, M., Crapo, R. O., & Gardner, R. (1983). The effect of ventilation on the accuracy on pulmonary artery and wedge pressure measurements. *Critical Care Medicine, 11,* 502–507.

Chatterjee, K. (1985). Bedside hemodynamic monitoring in the cardiac care unit. In A. N. Brest (Ed.), *Cardiovascular clinics* (pp. 253–268). Philadelphia: F. A. Davis.

Daily, E. K., & Schroeder, J. S. (1989). *Techniques in bedside hemodynamic monitoring* (4th ed.). St. Louis: C. V. Mosby.

Dawson, N. V., Connors, A. F., Speroff, T., et al. (1993). Hemodynamic assessment in managing the critically ill. *Medical Decision Making, 13,* 258–266.

Dobbin, K., Wallace, S., Ahlberg, J., et al. (1992). Pulmonary artery pressure measurement in patients with elevated pressures: Effect of backrest elevation and method of measurement. *American Journal of Critical Care, 1,* 61–69.

Doering, L. V. (1993). The effect of positioning on hemodynamics and gas exchange in the critically ill: A review. *American Journal of Critical Care, 2,* 208–216.

Enger, E. L. (1989). Pulmonary artery wedge pressure: When it's valid, when it's not. *Critical Care Nursing Clinics of North America, 1,* 603–618.

Falicov, R. E., & Resnekov, L. (1970). Relationship of the pulmonary artery end-diastolic pressure to the left ventricular end-diastolic and mean filling pressures in patients with and without left ventricular dysfunction. *Circulation, 42,* 65–73.

Forrester, J. S., Diamond, G., Chatterjee, K., et al. (1976). Medical therapy of acute myocardial infarction by application of hemodynamic subsets (Pt. 1). *New England Journal of Medicine, 295,* 1356–1362.

Gardner, P. E. (1993). Pulmonary artery pressure monitoring. *AACN Clinical Issues, 4*(1), 98–119.

Gore, J. M., Alpert, J. S., Benotti, J. R., et al. (1985). *Handbook of hemodynamic monitoring.* Boston: Little, Brown.

Groom, L., Frisch, S. R., & Elliott, M. (1990). Reproducibility and accuracy of pulmonary artery pressure measurement in supine and lateral positions. *Heart and Lung, 19,* 147–151.

Guzy, P. M. (1986). Emergency cardiac pacing. *Emergency Medicine Clinics of North America, 4,* 745–759.

Jenkins, B. S., Bradley, R. D., & Branthwaite, M. A. (1970). Evaluation of pulmonary arterial end-diastolic pressure as an indirect estimate of left atrial mean pressure. *Circulation, 42,* 75–78.

Kaltman, A. J., Herbert, W. H., Conroy, R. J., et al. (1966). The gradient in pressure across the pulmonary vascular bed during diastole. *Circulation, 34,* 377–384.

Kennedy, G. T., Bryant, A., & Crawford, M. H. (1984). The effect of lateral body positioning measurements of pulmonary artery and pulmonary artery wedge pressures. *Heart and Lung, 13,* 155–158.

Langer, M., Mascheroni, D., Marcolin, R., et al. (1988). The prone position in ARDS patients: A clinical study. *Chest, 94,* 103–107.

Matthay, M. A., & Chatterjee, K. (1988). Bedside catheterization of the pulmonary artery: Risks compared with benefits. *Annals of Internal Medicine, 109,* 826–834.

Martin, W. E., Cheung, P. W., Johnson, C. C., et al. (1973). Continuous monitoring of mixed venous oxygen saturation in man. *Anesthesia and Analgesia, 52,* 784–793.

Murao, H., & Rodbard, S. (1971). Effects of ventilation on pulmonary arterial flow and vascular conductance. *American Heart Journal, 81,* 69–79.

Nelson, L. D., & Anderson, H. B. (1989). Physiologic effects of steep positioning in the surgical intensive care unit. *Archives of Surgery, 125,* 352–355.

Pena, M. A. (1989). The effect of position change on mixed venous oxygen saturation measurements in open heart surgery patients during the immediate postoperative period. *Heart and Lung, 18,* 305.

Rahimtoola, S. H., Loeb, H. S., Ehsani, A., et al. (1972). Relationship of pulmonary artery to left ventricular diastolic pressures in acute myocardial infarction. *Circulation, 46,* 283–290.

Scheinman, M., Evans, G. T., Weiss, A., et al. (1973). Relationship between pulmonary artery end-diastolic pressure and left ventricular filling pressure in patients in shock. *Circulation, 47,* 317–324.

Shinn, J. A., Woods, S. L., & Huseby, J. S. (1979). Effect of intermittent positive pressure ventilation upon pulmonary artery and pulmonary capillary wedge pressures in acutely ill patients. *Heart and Lung, 8,* 322–327.

Sibbald, W. J., Paterson, N. A., Holliday, R. L., et al. (1979). The Trendelenburg position: Hemodynamic effects in hypotensive and normotensive patients. *Critical Care Medicine, 7,* 218–224.

Starling, E. H. (1918). *Th Linacre lecture on the law of the heart.* London: Longmans, Green.

Swan, H. J. C., & Ganz, W. (1982). Measurement of right atrial and pulmonary arterial pressures and cardiac output: Clinical application of hemodynamic monitoring. *Advances in Internal Medicine, 27,* 453–473.

Swan, H. J. C., Ganz, W., Forrester, J., et al. (1970). Catheterization of the heart in man with use of a flow-directed balloon-tipped catheter. *New England Journal of Medicine, 283,* 447–451.

Vincent, J. L. (1990). The measurement of right ventricular ejection fraction. *Intensive Care World, 7*(3), 133–136.

Vincent, J. L., Thirion, M., Brimioulle, S., et al. (1986). Thermodilution measurement of right ventricular ejection fraction with a modified pulmonary artery catheter. *Intensive Care Medicine, 12,* 33–38.

White, K. M. (1987a). Continuous monitoring of mixed venous oxygen saturation (Svo_2): A new assessment tool in critical care nursing (Part I). *Cardiovascular Nursing, 23*(1), 1–6.

White, K. M. (1987b). Continuous monitoring of mixed venous oxygen saturation (Svo_2): A new assessment tool in critical care nursing (Part II). *Cardiovascular Nursing, 23*(2), 7–12.

Woods, S. L., Laurent, D. J., Grose, B. L., et al. (1980). Effect of backrest position on pulmonary artery pressures in acutely ill patients (Abstract). *Circulation, 62,* III–184.

Woods, S. L., & Mansfield, L. W. (1976). Effect of body position upon pulmonary artery and pulmonary capillary wedge pressures in noncritically ill patients. *Heart and Lung, 5,* 83–90.

Cardiac Output Measurements

Abrams, J. H., Weber, R. E., & Holmen, K. D. (1989). Continuous cardiac output determination using transtracheal Doppler: Initial results in humans. *Anesthesiology, 71,* 11–15.

Armengol, J., Man, G. C. W., Balsys, A. J., et al. (1982). Effects of the respiratory cycle on cardiac output measurements: Reproducibility of data enhanced by timing the thermodilution injections in dogs. *Critical Care Medicine, 9,* 852–854.

Baxter Healthcare Corporation. (1983). *Model 9520 and 9520A cardiac output computer operations and troubleshooting manual.* Santa Ana, CA: Baxter Healthcare Corporation.

Berne, R. M., & Levy, M. H. (1986). *Cardiovascular physiology* (5th ed.). St. Louis: C. V. Mosby.

Beyer, J., Lamberti, J. J., & Replogle, R. L. (1977). Validity of thermodilution cardiac output determination in the presence of pulmonary insufficiency. *Thoraxchirurgie Vaskulaere Chirurgie, 35*(1), 40–44.

Bilfinger, T. V., Lin, C., & Anagnostopoulos, C. E. (1982). In vitro determination of accuracy of cardiac output measurements by thermal dilution. *Journal of Surgical Research, 33,* 409–414.

Bridges, E. J., & Woods, S. L. (1993). Pulmonary artery pressure measurements: State of the art. *Heart and Lung, 22,* 99–111.

Cason, C. L., Lambert, C. W., Holland, C. L., et al. (1990). Effect of backrest elevation and position on pulmonary artery pressures. *Cardiovascular Nursing, 26,* 1–5.

Daily, E. K., & Mersch, J. (1987). Thermodilution cardiac outputs using room and ice temperature injectate: Comparison with the fick method. *Heart and Lung, 16,* 294–300.

Dizon, C. T., Gezari, W. A., Barash, P. G., et al. (1977). Hand held thermodilution cardiac output injector. *Critical Care Medicine, 5,* 210–212.

Doering, L. V. (1993). The effect of positioning on hemodynamics and gas exchange in the critically ill: A review. *American Journal of Critical Care, 2,* 208–216.

Doering, L., & Dracup, K. (1988). Comparisons of cardiac output in supine and lateral positions. *Nursing Research, 37,* 114–118.

Elkayam, U., Mumford, M., Tobis, J., et al. (1981). Thermodilution cardiac output determination: The effect of injectate volume and temperature on accuracy and reproducibility (Abstract). *Clinical Research, 29,* 188A.

Enghof, E., & Sjogren, S. (1973). Thermal dilution for measurement of cardiac output in the pulmonary artery in man in relation to choice of indicator volume and injection time. *Uppsala Journal of Medical Sciences, 78*(1), 33–37.

Evonuk, E., Imig, C. J., Greenfield, W., et al. (1961). Cardiac output measured by thermal dilution of room temperature injectate. *Journal of Applied Physiology, 16,* 271–275.

Fegler, G. (1954). Measurement of cardiac output in anaesthetized animals by a thermo-dilution method. *Quarterly Journal of Experimental Physiology and Cognate Medical Sciences, 39*(3), 153–164.

Fegler, G. (1957). The reliability of the thermodilution method for determination of the cardiac output and the blood flow in central veins. *Quarterly Journal of Experimental Physiology and Cognate Medical Sciences, 42*(3), 254–266.

Fick, A. (1870). Über die Messung des Blutquantums in der Herzventrikeln. Verhandl d phys-med Ges zu Wurzberg, 2, 16. In H. E. Hoff and H. J. Scott (Eds) (1948), Physiology. *New England Journal of Medicine, 239,* 120–126.

Forrester, J. S., Diamond, G., Chatterjee, K., et al. (1976). Medical therapy of acute myocardial infarction by application of hemodynamic subsets (Pt. 1). *New England Journal of Medicine, 295,* 1356–1362.

Forrester, J. S., Ganz, W., Diamond, G., et al. (1972). Thermodilution cardiac output determination with a single flow-directed catheter. *American Heart Journal, 83,* 306–311.

Freed, M. D., & Keane, J. F. (1978). Cardiac output measured by thermodilution in infants and children. *Journal of Pediatrics, 92,* 39–42.

Ganz, W., Donoso, R., Marcus, H., et al. (1971). A new technique for measurement of cardiac output by thermodilution in man. *American Journal of Cardiology, 27,* 392–396.

Ganz, W., & Swan, H. J. C. (1972). Measurement of blood flow by thermodilution. *American Journal of Cardiology, 29,* 241–246.

Grenvik, A. (1966). Respiratory, circulatory and metabolic effects of respirator treatment. *Acta Anaesthesiologica Scandinavica, Supplement 19,* 7–152.

Grose, B. L., Woods, S. L., & Laurent, D. J. (1981). Effect of backrest position on cardiac output measured by thermodilution method in acutely ill patients. *Heart and Lung, 10,* 661–665.

Grossman, W. (Ed.). (1986). *Cardiac catheterization and angiography* (3rd ed.). Philadelphia: Lea & Febiger.

Hamilton, W. F., Moore, J. W., Kinsman, J. M., et al. (1928). Simultaneous determination of the pulmonary and systemic circulation times in man and of a figure related to the cardiac output. *American Journal of Physiology, 84,* 338–344.

Hamilton, W. F., Moore, J. W., Kinsman, J. M., et al. (1932). Studies on the circulation: IV. Further analysis of the injection method and of changes in hemodynamics under physiological and pathological conditions. *American Journal of Physiology, 99,* 534–551.

Hamilton, W. F., Riley, R. L., Attyah, A. M., et al. (1948). Comparison of the Fick and dye injection methods of measuring cardiac output in man. *American Journal of Physiology, 153,* 309–311.

Headrick, C. L. (1992). Hemodynamic monitoring of the critically ill neonate. *Journal of Perinatal and Neonatal Nursing, 5*(4), 58–67.

Hoff, H. E., & Scott, H. J. (1948). Physiology. *New England Journal of Medicine, 239,* 120–126.

Hruby, I. M., & Woods, S. L. (1983). Effect of injectate temperature on measurement of thermodilution cardiac output in cardiac surgical patients (Abstract). *Circulation, 68* (Suppl. III), III–222.

Jansen, J. R. C., Schreuder, J. J., Bogard, J. M., et al. (1981). Thermodilution technique for measurement of cardiac output during artificial ventilation. *Journal of Applied Physiology, 50,* 584–591.

Jansen, J. R. C., Schreuder, J. J., Settels, J. J., et al. (1990). An adequate strategy for the thermodilution technique in patients during mechanical ventilation. *Intensive Care Medicine, 16,* 422–425.

Jardin, F., Farcot, J., Boisante, L., et al. (1981). Influence of positive end-expiratory pressure on left ventricular performance. *New England Journal of Medicine, 304,* 387–392.

Kadota, L. T. (1985). Theory and application of thermodilution cardiac output measurement: A review. *Heart and Lung, 14,* 605–614.

Kadota, L. T. (1986). Reproducibility of thermodilution cardiac output measurements. *Heart and Lung, 15,* 618–622.

Killpack, A. K., Davidson, L. J., Woods, S. L., et al. (1981). Effect of injectate volume and temperature on measurement of thermodilution cardiac output in acutely ill patients (Abstract). *Circulation, 64* (Suppl. IV), IV–165.

Lamy, M., Deghislage, J., Lamalle, D., et al. (1973). Hemodynamic effects of intermittent or continuous positive-pressure breathing in man. *Acta Anaesthesiologica Belgica, 24,* 270–287.

Larson, C. A., & Woods, S. L. (1982). Effect of injectate volume and temperature on thermodilution cardiac output measurements in acutely ill adults (Abstract). *Circulation, 66* (Suppl. II), II–98.

Lee, D. W., & Stevens, G. H. (1985). Comparison of thermodilution measurement by injection of the proximal lumen versus side port of the Swan-Ganz catheter. *Heart and Lung, 14,* 126–127.

Levett, J. M., & Replogle, R. L. (1979). Thermodilution cardiac output: A critical analysis and review of the literature. *Journal of Surgical Research, 27,* 392–404.

Manifold, S. (1984). A comparison of two alternate methods for the determination of cardiac output by thermodilution: Automatic vs. manual injections (Abstract). *Heart and Lung, 13,* 304–305.

Mathur, M., Harris, E. A., Yarrow, S., et al. (1976). Measurement of cardiac output by thermodilution in infants and children after open-heart operations. *Journal of Thoracic and Cardiovascular Surgery, 72,* 221–225.

Medley, R. S., DeLapp, T. D., & Fisher, D. G. (1992). Comparability of thermodilution cardiac output method: proximal injectate versus proximal infusion lumens. *Heart and Lung, 21,* 12–17.

Millar, S., Sampson, L. K., Soukup, M., et al. (Eds.). (1980). *Methods in critical care.* Philadelphia: W. B. Saunders.

Nelson, L. D., & Houtchens, B. A. (1982). Automatic versus manual injections for thermodilution cardiac output measurements. *Critical Care Medicine, 10,* 190–192.

Pepke-Zaba, J., Higenbottam, T. W., Dinh Xuan, A. T., et al. (1990). Validation of impedance cardiography measurements of cardiac output during limited exercise in heart transplant recipients. *Transplant International, 3*(2), 108–112.

Powers, S. R., Jr., Mannal, R., Neclerio, M., et al. (1973). Physiologic consequences of positive end expiratory pressure (PEEP) ventilation. *Annals of Surgery, 178,* 265–271.

Powner, D. J. (1975). Thermodilution technic for cardiac output (Letter). *New England Journal of Medicine, 293,* 1210–1211.

Qvist, J., Pontoppidan, H., Wilson, R. S., et al. (1975). Hemodynamic responses to mechanical ventilation with PEEP. *Anesthesiology, 42,* 45–55.

Rankin, J. S., Olsen, C. O., Tyson, G. S., et al. (1981). Effects of airway pressure on cardiac function in intact dogs and man (Abstract). *Circulation, 64* (Suppl. IV), IV–251.

Reininger, E. J., & Troy, B. L. (1976). Error in thermodilution cardiac output caused by variation in syringe volume. *Catheterization and Cardiovascular Diagnosis, 2,* 415–417.

Riedinger, M. S., & Shellock, F. G. (1984). Technical aspects of the thermodilution method for measuring cardiac output. *Heart and Lung, 13,* 215–221.

Rubin, S. A., Siemienczuk, D., Prause, J., et al. (1982). Accuracy of cardiac output, oxygen uptake, and arteriovenous oxygen difference at rest, during exercise, and after vasodilator therapy in patients with severe, chronic heart failure. *American Journal of Cardiology, 50,* 973–978.

Sackner, M. A., Hoffman, R. A., Stroh, D., et al. (1991). Thoracocardiography: Part I. Noninvasive measurement of changes in stroke volume comparison to thermodilution. *Chest, 99,* 613–622.

Sawyer-Sommers, M., Woods, S. L., & Courtade, M. A. (1993). Issues in methods and measurement of thermodilution cardiac output. *Nursing Research, 42,* 228–233.

Shellock, F., & Riedinger, M. S. (1983). Reproducibility and accuracy of using room temperature versus ice temperature injectate for thermodilution cardiac output determination. *Heart and Lung, 12,* 175–176.

Shenkman, E., & Kasprow, M. (1988). Effect of backrest position on cardiac output determinations (Abstract). *Heart and Lung, 17,* 308–309.

Singh, R., Ranieri, A. J., Jr., Vest, H. R., et al. (1970). Simultaneous determinations of cardiac output by thermal dilution, fiberoptic and dye dilution methods. *American Journal of Cardiology, 25,* 579–587.

Snyder, J. V., & Powner, D. J. (1982). Effects of mechanical ventilation on the measurement of cardiac output by thermodilution. *Critical Care Medicine, 10,* 677–682.

Sorensen, M. B., Bille-Brahe, N. E., & Engell, H. C. (1976). Cardiac output measurement by thermal dilution. *Annals of Surgery, 183,* 67–71.

Stetz, C. W., Miller, R. G., Kelly, G. E., et al. (1982). Reliability of the thermodilution method in the determination of cardiac output in clinical practice. *American Review of Respiratory Disease, 126,* 1001–1004.

Stevens, J. H., Raffin, T. A., Mihm, F. G., et al. (1985). Thermodilution cardiac output measurement: Effect of the respiratory cycle on its reproducibility. *Journal of the American Medical Association, 253,* 2240–2242.

Stewart, G. N. (1893). Researches on the circulation time in organs and on the influences which affect it: I. Preliminary paper. *Journal of Physiology, 15*(4), 1–89.

Stewart, G. N. (1897). Researches on the circulation time in organs and the influences which affect it: IV. The output of the heart. *Journal of Physiology, 22*(3), 158–183.

Stewart, G. N. (1921). The output of the heart in dogs. *American Journal of Physiology, 57*(1), 27–50.

Swan, H. J. C. (1990). Techniques of monitoring the seriously ill patient with heart disease (including use of Swan-Ganz catheter). In J. W. Hurst, R. C. Schlant, C. E. Rackley, et al. (Eds.), *The heart, arteries and veins* (7th ed.). New York: McGraw-Hill.

Swan, H. J. C., and Ganz, W. (1975). Use of balloon flotation catheters in critically ill patients. *Surgical Clinics of North America, 55,* 501–520.

Swan, H. J. C., Ganz, W., Forrester, J., et al. (1970). Catheterization of the heart in man with use of a flow-directed balloon-tipped catheter. *New England Journal of Medicine, 283,* 447–451.

Swinney, R. S., Davenport, M. W., Wagers, P. W., et al. (1981). Iced versus room temperature injectate for thermal dilution cardiac output (Abstract). *Critical Care Medicine, 8,* 265.

Weil, M. H. (1977). Measurement of cardiac output (Editorial). *Critical Care Medicine, 5,* 117–119.

Wetzel, R. C., & Latson, T. W. (1985). Major errors in thermodilution cardiac output measurement during rapid volume infusion. *Anesthesiology, 62,* 684–687.

Whitman, G. R., Howaniak, D. L., & Verga, T. S. (1982). Comparison of cardiac output measurements in 20-degree supine and 20-degree right and left lateral recumbent positions (Abstract). *Heart and Lung, 11,* 256–257.

Wise, R. A., Robotham, J. L., Bromberger-Barnea, B., et al. (1981). Effect of PEEP on left ventricular function in right heart-bypassed dogs. *Journal of Applied Physiology, 51,* 541–546.

Wong, M., Skulsky, A., and Moon, E. (1978). Loss of indicator in the thermodilution technique. *Catheterization and Cardiovascular Diagnosis, 4,* 103–109.

Woods, M., Scott, R. N., & Harken, A. H. (1976). Practical considerations for the use of a pulmonary artery thermistor catheter. *Surgery, 79,* 469–475.

Woods, S. L., & Osguthorpe, S. (1993). Cardiac output determination. *AACN Clinical Issues in Critical Care Nursing, 4,* 81–97.

Wyse, S. D., Pfitzner, J., Rees, A., et al. (1975). Measurement of cardiac output by thermal dilution in infants and children. *Thorax, 30,* 262–265.

Yelderman, M. L., Quinn, M. D., & McKown, R. C. (1992). Continuous thermodilution cardiac output measurement in intensive care unit patients. *Journal of Cardiothoracic and Vascular Anesthesia, 6,* 270–274.

Yonkman, C. A., & Hamory, B. H. (1988). Sterility and efficiency of two methods of cardiac output determination: Closed loop and capped syringe methods. *Heart and Lung, 17,* 121–128.

Clinical Application

Chatterjee, K., Parmley, W. W., Ganz, W., et al. (1973). Hemodynamic and metabolic responses to vasodilator therapy in acute myocardial infarction. *Circulation, 48,* 1183–1193.

Daily, E. K., & Schroeder, J. S. (1989). *Techniques in bedside hemodynamic monitoring* (4th ed.). St. Louis: C. V. Mosby.

Dawson, N. V., Connors, A. F., Speroff, T., et al. (1993). Hemodynamic assessment in managing the critically ill. *Medical Decision Making, 13,* 258–266.

Domksy, M. F., & Wilson, R. F. (1993). Hemodynamic resuscitation. *Critical Care Clinics, 10,* 715–726.

Dracup, K. A., Breu, C. S., & Tillisch, J. H. (1981). The physiologic basis for combined nitroprusside–dopamine therapy in post-myocardial infarction heart failure. *Heart and Lung, 10,* 114–120.

Forrester, J. S., Diamond, G., Chatterjee, K., et al. (1976). Medical therapy of acute myocardial infarction by application of hemodynamic subsets (Pt. 1). *New England Journal of Medicine, 295,* 1356–1362.

Cardiac Assist Devices

Shelley Ruzevich

The first effort at mechanical support of the circulation was made in the 1950s with the development of cardiopulmonary bypass (Gibbon, 1954; Kirklin et al., 1955). This initial discovery led to further attempts to support the circulation for extended periods of time, which proved to be generally unsuccessful (Zapoh et al., 1979; Cooley et al., 1969). The development of the intraaortic balloon pump (IABP) aided in the reduction of postcardiotomy mortality (Baldwin et al., 1992; Kantrowitz et al., 1969; Naunhein et al., 1992). Since that time, the IABP has gained widespread recognition in the treatment of patients with low cardiac output conditions. However, many patients with severe cardiogenic shock remained unresponsive to IABP therapy because it is only capable of supplying a limited amount of support. The need for a more complete form of assistance was recognized. Subsequently, several groups began using ventricular assist devices (VAD), which could be implanted for extended periods of time (Farrar et al., 1993; Pennington et al., 1994; Portner et al., 1983). By the mid-1980s, the majority of experience with VADs was with the postcardiotomy population (Farrar et al., 1993; Magovern, 1993; Ruzevich et al., 1987). Recently, the scarcity of donor hearts has led many groups to recognize the role of VADs as a bridge to cardiac transplantation (Farrar et al., 1993; Pennington et al., 1994; Portner et al., 1983). VADs offer the luxury of buying time until a donor heart can be located.

To date, several types of mechanical assistance are available depending on the extent of support that is required. These devices include the IABP, VADs (centrifugal, pneumatic, pulsatile, and electrical pulsatile), and extracorporeal membrane oxygenation (ECMO). Device selection depends on the patient's clinical status, device availability to the institution, type of ventricular failure, and expected outcome. Categories of patients requiring the devices include postcardiotomy patients, patients suffering from acute cardiogenic shock, and patients who are being bridged to cardiac transplantation. This chapter is designed to acquaint the nurse with the different types of support available and the nursing care of patients requiring this support.

CENTRIFUGAL ASSIST DEVICES

Low cost and easy insertion have made centrifugal pumps popular in the field of circulatory support (Table 14–1). One type is the Biomedicus (Eden Prairie, MN) vortex pump, which allows right atrial to pulmonary artery (right ventricular [RV]) assist and left atrium to aorta or left ventricular apex to aorta (left ventricular [LV]) assist (Fig. 14–1). Biopump heads are available in either a 50-mL pediatric or 80-mL adult size. A series of rotating cones speeds up and spins the blood during its course between the inlet and outlet points of the pump head, where rotational energy is recovered in the form of pressure-slow work (Fig. 14–2). The pressure created by the pump facilitates blood movement. While operating at a given steady speed, the biopump generates a nearly constant pressure over a wide range of flow rates. Magnets within the pump head housing approximate magnets in the drive console. When these magnets revolve, the ones within the pump head housing begin to rotate. Most investigators use standard cardiopulmonary bypass cannulas for connection to the device (Magovern, 1993).

Most institutions using a centrifugal pump use

TABLE 14–1. **Centrifugal Pumps**

Advantages
Readily available
Inexpensive
No size limitations
Easy insertion
Capable of biventricular support
Allows for either atrial or ventricular apex cannulation
Not viewed as investigational
Disadvantages
Limited mobility
Increased incidence of thrombus formation
Anticoagulation usually required
Does not provide pulsatile flow
Requires constant surveillance

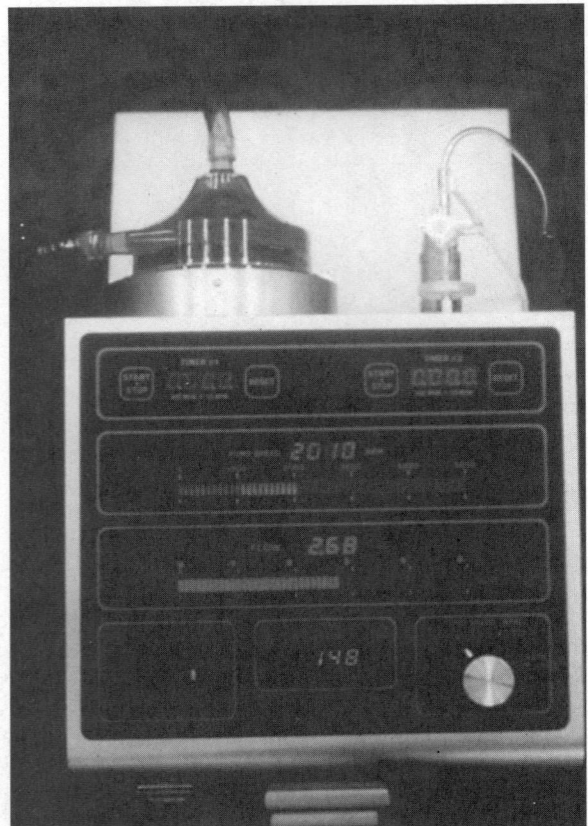

FIGURE 14–1. Biomedicus centrifugal vortex pump and console.

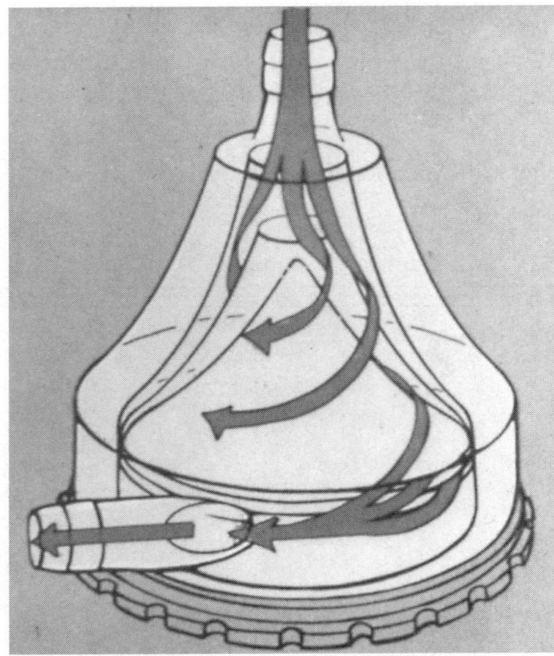

FIGURE 14–2. Biomedicus cone showing direction of blood flow.

some form of anticoagulation therapy (Pennington et al., 1982). However, it has been demonstrated that there is safety against thrombus formation without the need for anticoagulation (Magovern et al., 1985), but there is limited information about long-term support (greater than 14 days) with this type of pump. Frequently, pump heads need to be changed in the event of thrombus. The current standard is to check the pump head every 8 hours for signs of thrombus. This is accomplished by clamping the inflow and outflow lines and turning the pump off. The head can then be removed from the magnet and inspected; the entire procedure can be done in less than 2 to 3 minutes. Also at this time, the flow probe may be recalibrated for better accuracy. This type of procedure is done only by perfusionists or those trained in device management.

EXTERNAL PULSATILE DEVICES

The Pierce-Donachy Ventricular Assist Pump (Thoratec Incorporated, Berkeley, CA) is an external pulsatile device (Fig. 14–3). This system is composed of cannulas, a pump, and a drive and control console. The cannulas provide communication between the patient's own heart and the mechanical device. Cannulation sites include right atrium to pulmonary artery for right ventricular assistance, and left atrium to aorta or left ventricular apex to aorta for left ventricular assistance. The pump is a sac-type pneumatic device with four components:

1. A polysulfone housing, which is the covering of the device
2. The polyurethane blood sac, which provides a highly smooth antithrombolytic surface to inhibit blood coagulation; the sac has a stroke volume of 65 mL with an ejection fraction of 75%
3. Inflow and outflow mechanical valves
4. A sensing instrument (Hall effect switch), which provides information to the pump for regulation of flow (Gaines et al., 1985; Pennington et al., 1994).

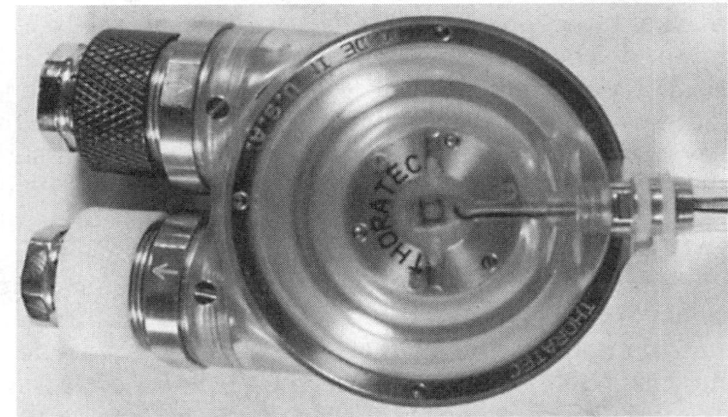

FIGURE 14–3. Pierce-Donachy Ventricular Assist Pump.

TABLE 14–2. **External Pulsatile Pump**

Advantages
Is capable of providing biventricular support
Critical care unit nurse can be trained to manage pump
Allows for either atrial or apex cannulation
Has a proven safety record for long-term support
Moderate expense
Smaller size requirements than the implantable devices
Disadvantages
Requires an investigational device evaluation
Moderate cost
Need to implant a second device in the event of biventricular failure

The control console is electrically powered and is capable of three different modes of operation: fixed-rate mode, fill-to-empty volume mode, and an electrocardiograph (ECG)-synchronized mode (Farrar et al., 1986).

The three different modes of operation are as follows:

1. Fixed-rate mode. This mode operates independent from the heart. The pumps are set at a fixed number of beats per minute. This type of control is often used for initiation to and weaning from the device.
2. Fill-to-empty volume mode. This mode allows the pump to empty as soon as the blood sac is filled. The speed with which the pump is filled with blood determines the rate at which it will operate. This mode also operates independent of the heart.
3. ECG-synchronized mode. The device is synchronized to the natural heart by detecting the R wave of the QRS complex and emptying at the occurrence of each QRS complex. This mode does not ensure full filling and emptying of the assist device.

The Pierce-Donachy pump has been used in the clinical setting for several years by various institutions (Farrar et al., 1993; Pennington et al., 1994). It has proved to be safe and successful in the treatment of patients experiencing cardiogenic shock (Farrar et al., 1993; Pennington et al., 1994; Pae et al., 1990). It has also been used successfully in the treatment of postcardiotomy patients and as a bridge to transplantation. It allows patients to be ambulatory and has successfully supported them for periods of more than 80 days (Reedy et al., 1992). The advantages and disadvantages of this type of device are listed in Table 14–2.

IMPLANTABLE ASSIST DEVICES

Some advantages in the use of implantable systems are the decreased chance for infection, improved mobility, and more intact body image. Disadvantages are the need for left ventricular apical cannulation and the limitation on left ventricular support (Table 14–3). This type of cannulation usually limits the patient to cardiac transplantation because a part of the myocardium is removed during left ventricular placement. A second device must be implanted or pharmacologic support used if right ventricular failure occurs. There are two implantable systems available today, the Heartmate 1000 IP and the Novacor Left Ventricular Assist System.

TABLE 14–3. **Implantable Pump**

Advantages
Implantable, lower infection rate
Proven low risk of thrombus formation
Allows increased mobility
Disadvantages
Expensive
Provides only univentricular support
Can be more difficult to insert than external devices
Apex cannulation only

The Heartmate pump (Thermo Cardiosystems, Inc., Woburn, MA) is designed to provide either pneumatic or electrical action (Fig. 14–4). The device contains a pusher plate design incorporating a biomer diaphragm. Twenty-millimeter Dacron grafts form the outflow conduit, whereas the inlet conduit is 19 mm. Twenty-five–millimeter porcine xenograft tissue valves are positioned in both inlet and outlet conduits. The pump is capable of an 80-mL stroke volume. A Dacron-covered pneumatic driveline connects the pump to a small console. The blood pump is implanted in the abdomen with left ventricular apex (inflow to pump) and ascending aorta (outflow from pump) cannulation. The drive console allows for three modes of operation: fixed-rate nonsynchronous mode, automatic pump on full mode; various pump rates with

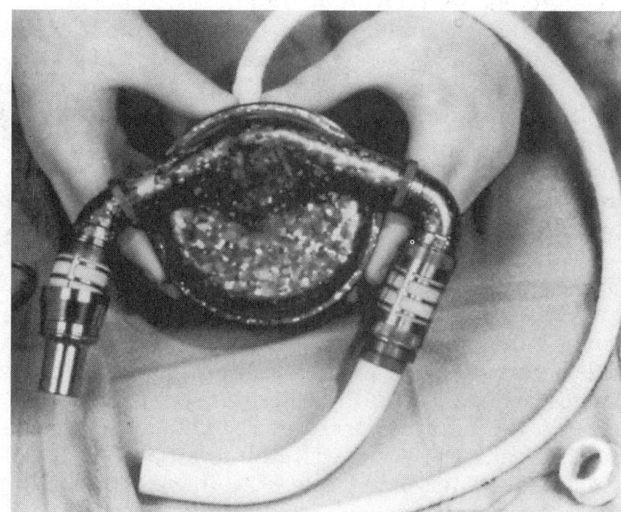

FIGURE 14–4. Heartmate 1000 IP Implantable System.

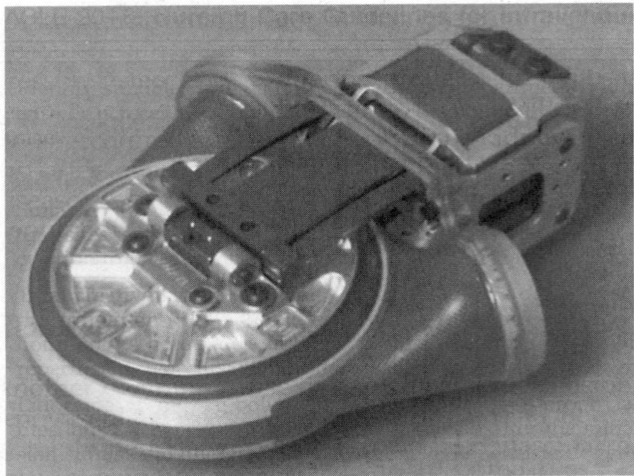

FIGURE 14–5. Novacor Left Ventricular Assist System. (Courtesy of Novacor Division, Baxter Healthcare Corporation, Oakland, CA.)

patient's cardiac output; and external mode, in which pumping is synchronized with an external trigger, such as an R wave on the ECG or a defibrillator synchronization pulse (Nakatani et al., 1989). These types of control modes were also explained in the previous section. The Heartmate 1000 has recently received approval from the FDA for commercial sale. Approximately 400 patients have already benefited from the use of this device and it has proven to be safe without anticoagulation (Frazier et al., 1992).

The Novacor Model 100 Left Ventricular Assist System (Baxter Corporation, Oakland, CA) consists of a balanced solenoid energy converter, dual pusher-plate, sac-type blood pump, and a microprocessor-based control and monitoring console. The energy converter and blood pump are encapsulated in a fiberglass/epoxy resin shell (Fig. 14–5), with Dacron conduits connecting the pump to the left ventricular apex (inflow to pump) and the ascending aorta (outflow from pump). A percutaneous extension cable connects the energy converter to the extracorporeal control console. All tissue- or blood-contacting surfaces are biocompatible. The blood pump consists of a seamless, smooth-surfaced polyurethane sac bonded to dual, symmetrically opposed pusher plates and to a light-weight housing that incorporates the valve fittings. The blood pump is designed to provide optimal flow patterns to reduce blood flow stasis, risk of thrombus formation, and hemolysis. The use of two pusher plates instead of one results in reduced sac deformation and improved flex life as well as improved flow characteristics throughout the pumping cycle. Twenty-one–millimeter Carpentier-Edwards pericardial bioprosthetic valves with modified mounting flanges are used to allow unidirectional blood flow through the pump (Starnes et al., 1988). The console has three modes of operation: fill-to-empty, ECG synchronization, and fixed rate. The longest period for which a patient has been successfully bridged is 370 days.

EXTRACORPOREAL MEMBRANE OXYGENATION

The first multicenter evaluation of ECMO in the 1970s was generally unfavorable (Zapoh et al., 1979). This study involved using ECMO for the treatment of respiratory failure. However, there were documented reports of its success in the treatment of pediatric cardiac failure (Bartlett et al., 1974; Hill et al., 1972; Soeter et al., 1973). Since that time, ECMO has become an acceptable means of supporting pediatric patients in postcardiotomy shock. Unfortunately, it is one of the few types of support available to children (Kanter et al., 1987a; Pennington et al., 1989; Pennington & Swartz, 1993). On the other hand, ECMO in adults is poorly tolerated over long periods of time, but is effective when used as a resuscitative device (Dembitsky et al., 1993) (Table 14–4).

The ECMO perfusion circuit in Figure 14–6 resembles the one developed by Bartlett (Bartlett & Gazzaniga, 1978). It consists of a Scimed Membrane Lung (Scimed, Inc., Minneapolis, MN), a Biopump (Biomedicus, Inc.), and a heat exchange connected together by polyvinyl chloride tubing. Ninety-five percent of the institutions using ECMO use Roller pumps, and the remaining 5% use a Biopump (Rudis & Drinkwater, in press). The membrane lung is connected to gas sources (oxygen and carbon dioxide) through a gas mixer, which allows appropriate changes in gas flow. The heat exchanger is connected to a circulating water heater, usually set at 38°C. Line pressures are continuously monitored before and after the membrane lung (Kanter et al., 1987a). Cannulation can be performed through the femoral vessels (Fig. 14–7) or chest for cardiac support.

CANNULATION

The type of cannulation is decided by the surgeon at the time of implantation of the device. This decision depends on the type of support required, the expected treatment outcome of the patient (recovery versus transplantation), and the condition of the patient's heart at the time of implantation. It is important to con-

TABLE 14–4. **Extracorporeal Membrane Oxygenation**

Advantages
Rapid resuscitation
Biventricular support
Allows time for further evaluation
Provides respiratory support
Disadvantages
Continuous anticoagulation
Increased rate of complications (thrombus, infection, bleeding)
Poorly tolerated for longer than 24 hours in adults
Nonpulsatile flow

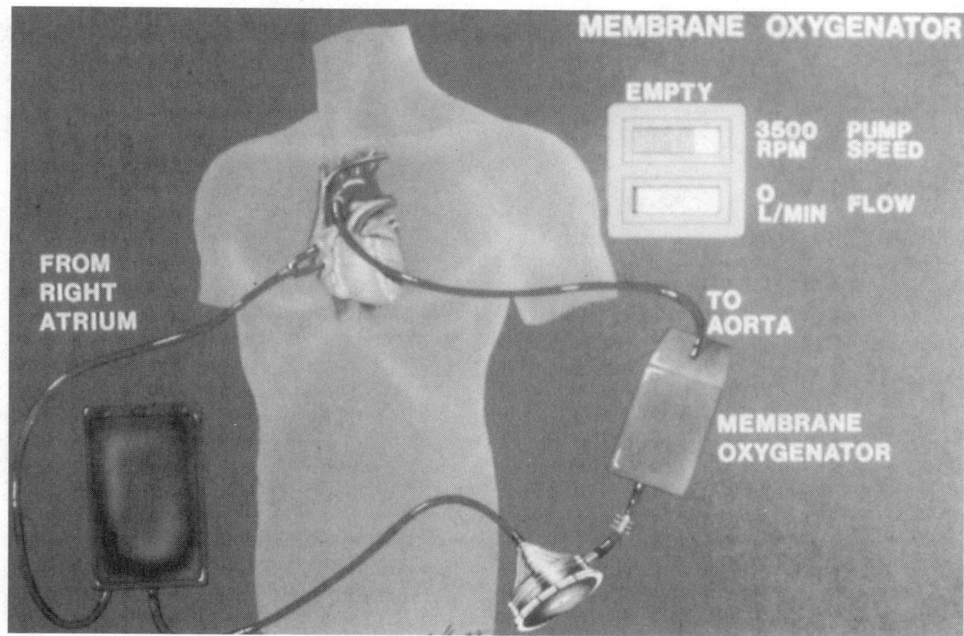

FIGURE 14–6. Extracorporeal membrane oxygenation (ECMO) perfusion circuit showing chest cannulation.

sider separate exit sites for the cannulas to enable closing of the sternum. This procedure allows the patient to be extubated and mobile.

Atrial

With atrial cannulation, the inflow cannula is placed in the atrium to provide removal of blood from the heart to the assist device. The outflow cannula is sutured to the side of the aorta in left ventricular assist (Fig. 14–8) or to the pulmonary artery in right ventricular assist (Fig. 14–9) to facilitate return of the blood to the body. This type of support is preferred if the heart is expected to recover because it is easier technically and less injurious to the myocardium (LaForge et al., 1985; Swartz & Pennington, 1985). The disadvantage is that the left atrium may not be acces-

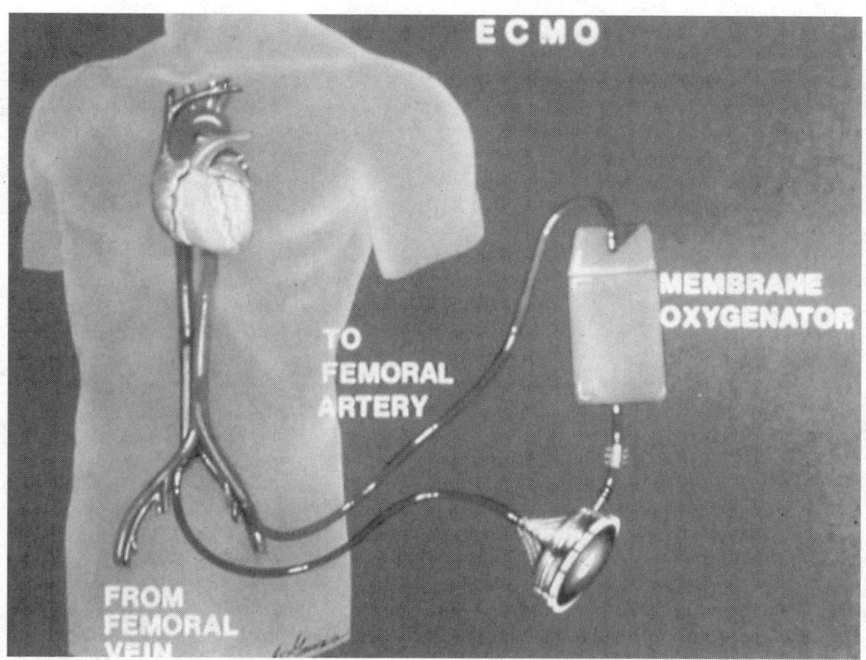

FIGURE 14–7. Extracorporeal membrane oxygenation (ECMO) perfusion circuit showing femoral cannulation.

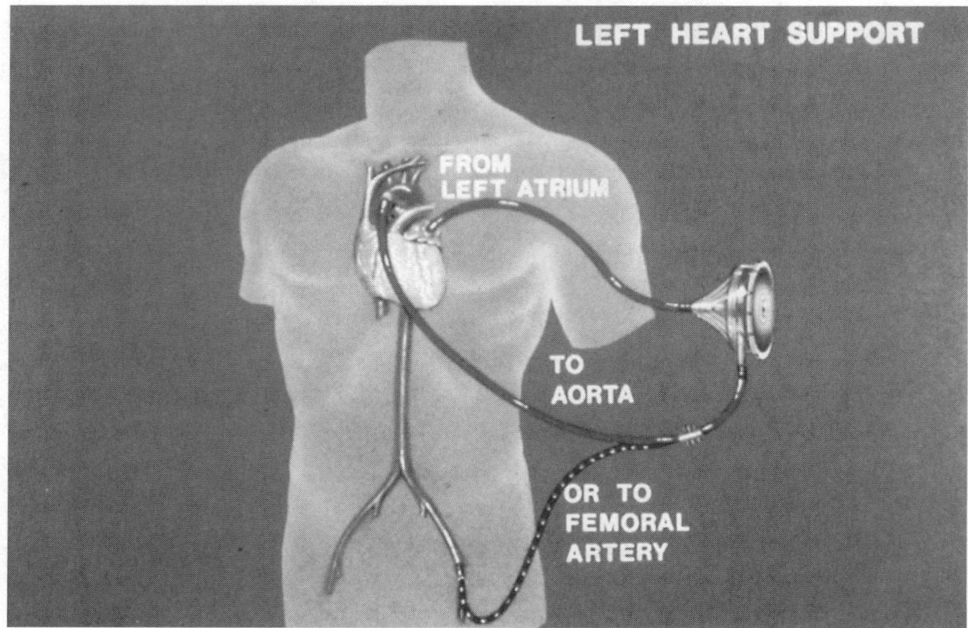

FIGURE 14–8. Left ventricular support using left atrial to aorta cannulation.

sible because of scarring from previous surgeries or the danger of compressing saphenous vein grafts. Figure 14–10 shows biventricular support using atrial cannulation.

Ventricular

In patients being bridged to transplantation, left ventricular cannulation is the method of choice. This allows for total decompression of the ventricle while preserving the atria for attachment during transplantation (LaForge et al., 1985; Swartz & Pennington, 1985). When biventricular assistance is required, a right ventricular assist device (RVAD) is placed with cannulation to the right atrium and pulmonary artery. The right ventricle is not used for cannulation due to its size. The disadvantages of ventricular cannulation include (1) it requires multiple sutures for fixation, (2) it damages an already impaired ventricle, and (3) it

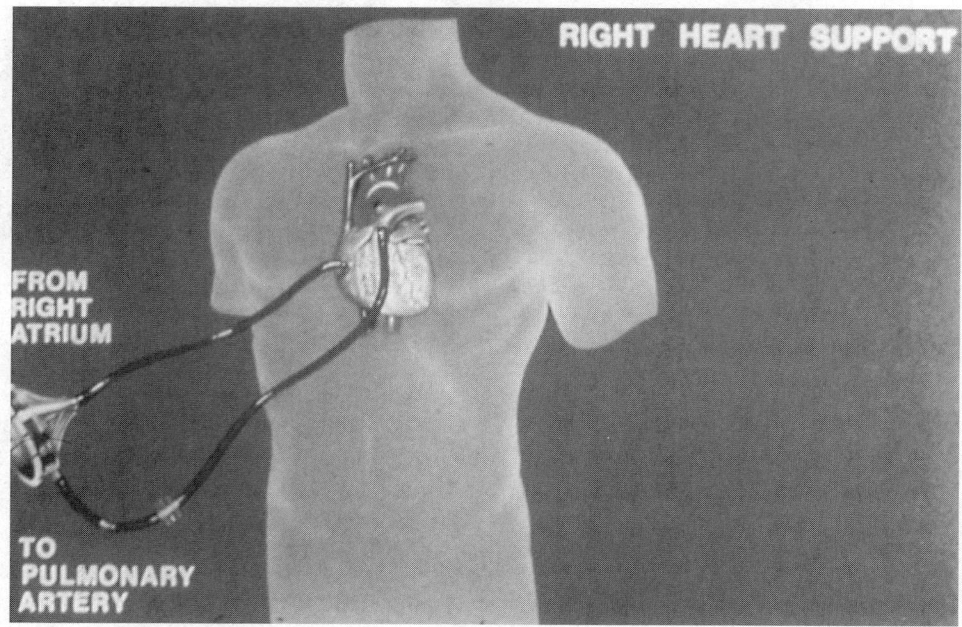

FIGURE 14–9. Right ventricular support using right atrial to pulmonary artery cannulation.

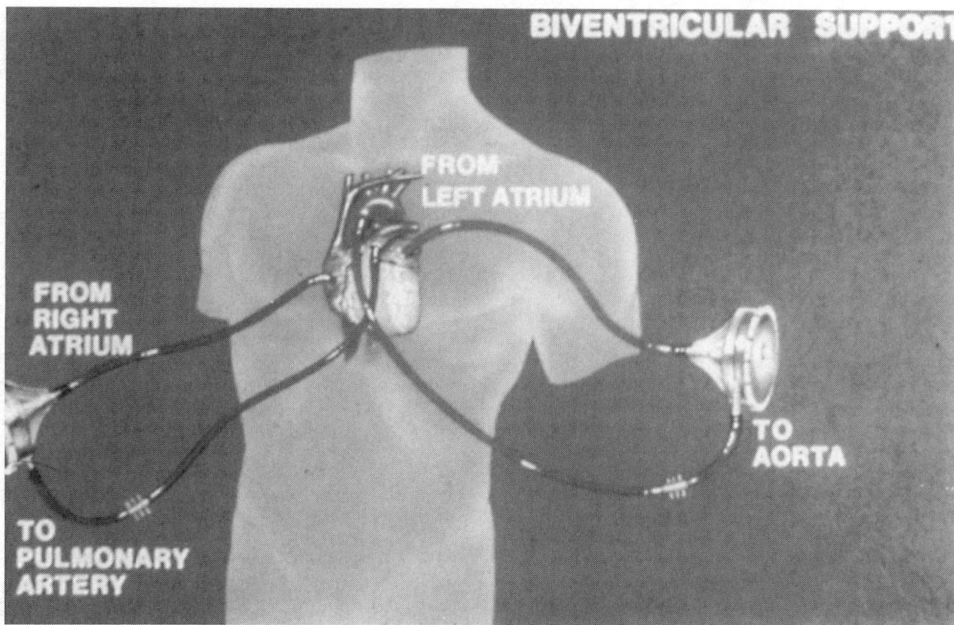

FIGURE 14–10. Biventricular support using atrial cannulation.

places the heart in a position that does not allow for exposure of the posterior surface (LaForge et al., 1985; Swartz & Pennington, 1985).

NURSING CARE

Many institutions use perfusionists or a team consisting of nurses, perfusionists, engineers, and doctors to monitor the devices while in use (Swartz et al., 1989). Limitations in staffing or case loads that require perfusionists to be elsewhere frequently leave management of these patients to the bedside critical care nurse. The nurse should be familiar with the device, acquire a knowledge of its function and safety requirements, and be able to recognize complications associated with its use. There are two categories of complications: device-related complications and complications related to the patient.

Device-Related Complications

HEMOLYSIS. Hemolysis is the destruction of red blood cells, which may be detected by blood in the urine or hemolyzed blood specimens. Hemolysis may also be accompanied by bleeding and hyperkalemia, which are late indicators. It should be determined whether the hemolysis is related to cardiopulmonary bypass, blood transfusions, or the VAD itself. Frequently, patients requiring a VAD have already undergone long bypass times for surgical repair and device implantation. Because bleeding is the most common patient complication, multiple blood transfusions may have been given. If the hemolysis occurs during the immediate postoperative period, it is most likely the result of cardiopulmonary bypass, and should clear. Hemolysis that occurs 3 to 4 days after surgery or has not cleared is usually associated with the device. In this case, drive pressures or the revolutions per minute of the device should be decreased. One way of detecting hemolysis is to measure daily serum hemoglobin. An elevated serum hemoglobin may be indicative of hemolysis. Urine output and change in urine color should be documented by the nurse. Mannitol often can be used to aid in the removal of destroyed red blood cells from the kidneys.

THROMBOEMBOLISM. The presence of artificial surfaces, mechanical valves, and pumping chambers may potentiate thrombus formation. High flows, maintenance of a high-pressure system, and complete emptying of the VAD may assist in preventing thrombus formation. The nurse should observe the cannulas for kinks or disconnections. ECMO requires anticoagulation with heparin. Hourly activated clotting times (ACT) should be performed to allow timely manipulation of the dosage. The nurse should be aware of the ACT limits and the amount of heparin being administered. Overanticoagulation may result in bleeding, whereas inadequate anticoagulation may result in thrombus formation. If there is an increase in the mediastinal chest tube drainage or a noticeable oozing from the cannulation sites and incisions, the ACT may need to be set at a lower limit until the bleeding is controlled. An antithrombolytic agent such as dextran can be started until heparin can be used safely. Once the patient has been extubated, he or she may be switched to a regimen of warfarin (maintaining the partial thromboplastin time at one and one half times normal) and dipyridamole, 75 mg three times a day (Reedy et al., 1989).

MECHANICAL FAILURE. Backup equipment should be available at all times, and the nurse should be aware of its location in case of an emergency. If mechanical failure of the external components of the device occurs, the device should to be switched immediately to the reserve console. Physicians and circulatory team members should be notified to ensure proper connection and adjustment. Mechanical failure can and does occur, but with proper safety techniques complications to the patient may be avoided.

Patient Complications

BIVENTRICULAR FAILURE. Biventricular failure is described as an increase in the atrial pressure of the unassisted ventricle with a corresponding decrease in cardiac output. This results in poor pump filling and low output of the assist device. Biventricular failure occurs because the unassisted ventricle has to handle the output from the mechanical device as well as any cardiac output from the patient's natural heart. This may occur in the operating room on implantation of the device, or later during the postoperative period. In either case, the problem cannot be treated lightly. Inotropic support with dopamine, amnirone, isoproterenol, or prostaglandin E has proved to be beneficial (Pennington et al., 1985; Pierce, 1979). If the failing ventricle does not improve, a second device should be implanted to assist that ventricle as well. In the event of left ventricular failure in a patient with an RVAD, pulmonary congestion and increased left atrial pressure develop, possibly leading to pulmonary edema and lengthening the amount of time the patient is intubated. During implantation of an RVAD, an intraaortic balloon pump may be inserted to assist the left ventricle and, ideally, deter any further development of failure. The critical care unit nurse needs to be able to recognize right ventricular failure when it occurs. Replacement fluids should be administered slowly to avoid overdistending the heart and to prevent the occurrence of right ventricular failure.

BLEEDING. Owing to the prolonged bypass times and multiple insertion sites required for implantation of the VAD, postoperative bleeding is common. The current standard is to have six units of packed red blood cells available while the device is implanted. Coagulation studies (including partial thromboplastin time, prothrombin time, thrombin time, fibrinogen, and platelet count) are checked every 6 hours while the patient is actively bleeding, and then daily. Hourly ACTs are obtained in those patients receiving heparin. Any abnormalities in these results should be treated immediately. A platelet count below 100,000/mm^3 should be corrected by the administration of platelets. Fresh frozen plasma can be given to correct coagulation abnormalities. Administration of anticoagulation agents such as heparin should be avoided until the bleeding has subsided. Washed red blood cells are preferred instead of directly infused, shed mediastinal blood. At the termination of cardiopulmonary bypass, heparin is reversed with protamine. Hemostatic agents such as Surgi-cel, bone wax, and fibrin glue have proved to be beneficial for persistent oozing before closing the chest. The use of cryoprecipitate and vitamin K should be discouraged because of the high risk of clot formation in the device itself (Ruzevich, 1991). A skin closure is used for patients who are bleeding excessively to avoid a cardiac tamponade situation. The sternum can then be closed when the device is removed or when the bleeding has stabilized. If the patient is to be supported for long periods of time, it is ideal to close the sternum so that extubation may be accomplished.

RENAL FAILURE. If the patient has experienced prolonged hypotension and decreased blood flow to the kidneys, acute tubular necrosis, a form of renal failure, may occur. The renal failure may result from the preoperative cardiogenic shock state or decreased perfusion after surgery (Kanter et al., 1987b). A urine output of 1 mL/kg/hour is the goal. Serum electrolytes, blood urea nitrogen, and creatinine values should be obtained and compared daily. Daily weight and accurate intake and output values should be recorded. Daily chest x-rays are advisable to aid in the diagnosis of fluid overload. Progressive renal failure may be treated with dialysis or hemofiltration but can prove to be irreversible. Patients in whom renal failure develops during assistance can be at higher risk for secondary complications such as infection (Ruzevich et al., 1988).

INFECTION. Prevention is the key to minimizing infection. Therefore, aseptic technique should always be observed by all health care personnel. Patients with a VAD may be potential candidates for systemic and local infections because of their preoperative and postoperative debility. Invasion with multiple intravascular monitoring lines and device-related conduits crosses the skin barrier and increases the risk of infection. Strict aseptic technique in handwashing and dressing changes should be observed. Some institutions prefer the use of povidone–iodine spray for insertion sites and avoid the use of ointment because it is harder to remove with each dressing change (Reedy et al., 1989; Ruzevich et al., 1991). Prophylactic antibiotic coverage is recommended, but should be discontinued after 4 days if there is no clinical evidence of infection. Fever and leukocytosis are good indicators of infection. Blood, urine, sputum, and wounds are routinely cultured if the patient has a temperature greater than 38.3°C. Antifungal oral solutions such as nystatin are advisable to prevent fungal infections in the mouth. Such treatment can be advantageous because it is believed that some degree of immunosuppression develops in these patients as soon as 48 hours after VAD placement (Termuhlen et al., 1989).

RESPIRATORY FAILURE. In the past, prolonged intubation of patients with a VAD led to respiratory complications (Hill et al., 1983). Today, patients are being extubated sooner, decreasing their chances of experiencing these complications. It is advisable to suction these patients every 1 to 2 hours if they are intubated, and perform chest physical therapy every 4 hours. Daily chest x-rays aid in the prevention and treatment of future complications. Vigorous pulmonary toilet needs to be continued to prevent the need for reintubation. Extubation allows greater freedom and enables the patient to ambulate.

SUPPORT MEASURES. Initiation of total parenteral nutritional support is recommended within 48 hours of VAD insertion, and administration of at least 3,000 calories a day should be attempted (Reedy et al., 1989; Ruzevich et al., 1988). If the patient can be extubated, the diet can be advanced as tolerated. Proper nutrition can aid in decreasing the risk of infection and assist in wound healing. Air mattresses are advisable because the patient may remain in bed for a prolonged period of time. Once vital signs are stable, turning every 2 hours is initiated. Passive range of motion exercises can be performed at the bedside. Once the patient is awake and hemodynamically stable, sitting in a chair is feasible without harm to the device. Thereafter, ambulation can be encouraged and has been demonstrated to be safe without presenting a risk to function of the device (Reedy et al., 1990, 1992).

The physical and mechanical side effects and implications of the presence of VADs were found to be greater than the emotional complications in a recent psychological study conducted on VAD patients (Ruzevich et al., 1990). Patient comfort may be maintained through the use of pain medications as needed. One important finding from this study is the benefit gained from patient and family teaching. It is important that the family be kept up to date daily on the patient's condition and care. It is also important to recognize each patient's individuality and to ensure that their emotional needs are met as well as their physical needs. Lenient visiting hours that encourage family interaction are advisable and beneficial. These patients may require support for long periods of time, and their psychological outlook can greatly influence their clinical course. A team approach has been found to be very successful in covering all aspects of the patient's care (Swartz et al., 1989). This approach will allow input from various staff members, including critical care nurses, dietitians, physical and occupational therapists, social workers, psychiatric liaison, and pastoral care. This study further revealed that 80% of those surveyed would recommend an assist device to someone who needed one, and 67% of the patients would agree to a second implant if it were necessary. These results demonstrate that despite the fact that patients were connected to mechanical support, they viewed their experience as a positive one. Many patients see this device as a second chance at life and feel fortunate to have this technology available to them.

SUMMARY

Temporary mechanical support of the circulation has proven to be successful in the treatment of reversible cardiac damage (Gaines et al., 1985; Swartz & Pennington 1985). The ability of an injured myocardium to recover is much better than was once thought. Long-term survivors can now return to a New York Heart Association class I cardiac status (Ruzevich et al., 1987). For this reason, more institutions are becoming interested in the use of mechanical support. Several centers already have more than one device in use. This expansion will require intensive care unit nurses to take on a new role. Many institutions rely on one nurse to monitor the device's function and a second nurse to administer patient care. Increased interest has led to advances in the treatment or prevention of complications associated with mechanical assist devices. Major complications such as biventricular failure, bleeding, and infection are being treated more effectively and with lower morbidity and mortality as experience grows. Irreversible cardiac damage remains a major cause of death, but can be avoided if the patient qualifies for cardiac transplantation. It is hoped that with more patients, improved protocols, and multiinstitutional studies, the remaining problems can be solved. Mechanical support has become an acceptable and successful means of supporting patients experiencing cardiac failure that is refractory to other forms of therapy.

REFERENCES

Baldwin, R. T., Slogoff, S., Noon, G. P., et al. (1992). A model to predict survival at the time of postcardiotomy intra-aortic balloon pump insertion. *Annals of Thoracic Surgery, 55,* 908–913.

Bartlett, R. H., & Gazzaniga, A. B. (1978). Extracorporeal circulation for cardiopulmonary failure. In R. H. Bartlett (Ed.), *Current problems in surgery.* (Vol. 15). Chicago: Year Book Medical Publishers.

Bartlett, R. H., Gazzaniga, A. B., Fong, S. W., et al. (1974). Prolonged extracorporeal membrane cardiopulmonary support in man. *Journal of Thoracic and Cardiovascular Surgery, 68,* 918–932.

Cooley, D. A., Liotta, D., Hallman, G. L., et al. (1969). Orthotopic cardiac prosthesis for two-staged cardiac replacement. *American Journal of Cardiology, 24,* 723–730.

Dembitsky, W. P., Moreno-Cabral, R. J., Adamson, R. M., & Daily, P. O. (1993). Emergency resuscitation using portable extracorporeal membrane oxygenation. *Annals of Thoracic Surgery, 55,* 305–309.

Farrar, D. J., Compton, P. G., Lawson, J. H., et al. (1986). Control modes of a clinical assist device. *Engineering and Biology IEEEP,* 19–25.

Farrar, D. J., & Hill, J. D. (1993). Univentricular and biventricular thoracic VAD support as a bridge to transplantation. *Annals of Thoracic Surgery, 55,* 276–282.

Frazier, O. H., Rose, E. A., Macmanus, Q., et al. (1992). Multicenter clinical evaluation of the Heartmate 1000 IP Left Ventricular Assist Device. *Annals of Thoracic Surgery, 53,* 1080–1090.

Gaines, W. E., Pierce W. S., Donachy, J. H., et al. (1985). The Pennsylvania State University paracorporeal ventricular assist pump: Optimal methods of use. *World Journal of Surgery, 9,* 47–54.

Gibbon, J. H., Jr. (1954). Application for a mechanical heart and lung apparatus to cardiac surgery. *Minneapolis Medicine, 37,* 171.

Hill, J. D., De Leval, M. R., & Fallat, R. J. (1972). Acute respiratory insufficiency: Treatment with prolonged extracorporeal membrane oxygenation. *Journal of Thoracic and Cardiovascular Surgery, 64,* 551–662.

Hill, J. D., Farrar, D. J., Compton, P., et al. (1983). Present and future of ventricular support systems for acute and chronic end-stage heart disease. *Journal of Heart Transplantation, 3,* 30–37.

Kanter, K. R., Pennington, D. G., Weber, T. R., et al. (1987a). Extracorporeal membrane oxygenation for post-operative cardiac support in children. *Journal of Thoracic and Cardiovascular Surgery, 93,* 27–35.

Kanter, K. R., Swartz, M. T., Pennington, D. G., et al. (1987b). Renal failure in patients with ventricular assist devices. *ASAIO Journal, 10,* 426–428.

Kantrowitz, A., Krakauer, J. S., Rosenbaum, A., et al. (1969). Phase-shift balloon pumping in medically refractory cardiogenic shock: Results in 27 patients. *Archives of Surgery, 99,* 739–743.

Kirklin, J. W., Dushane, J. W., Patrick, R. T., et al. (1955). Intracardiac surgery with the aid of a mechanical pumpoxygenator (Gibbon type): Report of eight cases. *Proceedings of the Staff Meetings, Mayo Clinic, 30,* 201–206.

LaForge, C. G., Schoen, F. J., Monreld, R. G., et al. (1985). Left-atrium-to-aorta versus left ventricular-to-aorta bypass: The Lewis and anrep effects. *ASAIO Journal, 8,* 191–204.

Magovern, G. J. (1993). The Biopump and postoperative circulatory support. *Annals of Thoracic Surgery, 55,* 245–249.

Magovern, G. J., Park, S. B., & Maher, T. D. (1985). Use of a centrifugal pump without anticoagulation for post-op LV assist. *World Journal of Surgery, 9,* 25–36.

Nakataki, T., Frazier, O. H., & McGee, M. G. (1989). Extended support prior to cardiac transplant: Using a left ventricular assist device with textured blood-contracting surfaces. Paper presented at the Meeting of the International Society for Artificial Organs, Sapporo, Japan.

Naunheim, K. S., Swartz, M. T., Pennington, D. G., et al. (1992). Intra-aortic balloon pumping in patients requiring cardiac operations. *Journal of Thoracic and Cardiovascular Surgery, 106,* 1654–1661.

Pae, W. E., Rosenberg, G., Donachy, J. H., et al. (1990). Mechanical circulatory assistance for postoperative cardiogenic shock: A three year experience. *ASAIO Transactions, 26,* 256–260.

Pennington, D. G., McBride, L. R., Miller, L. M., & Swartz, M. T. (1994, in press). Eleven years experience with Pierce-Donachy ventricular assist device. *Journal of Heart and Lung Transplantation. 5,* 803–810.

Pennington, D. G., Merjavy, J. P., Swartz, M. T., et al. (1982). Clinical experience with a centrifugal pump ventricular assist device. *ASAIO Transactions, 28,* 9395.

Pennington, D. G., Merjavy, S. P., Swartz, M. T., et al. (1985). The importance of biventricular failure in patients with post-operative cardiogenic shock. *Annals of Thoracic Surgery, 39,* 16–21.

Pennington, D. G., & Swartz, M. T. (1993). Circulatory support in infants and children. *Annals of Thoracic Surgery, 55,* 233–237.

Pennington, D. G., Swartz, M. T., Ruzevich, S. A., et al. (1989). In R. H. Anderson (Ed.), *Perspectives in pediatric cardiology* (Vol. 2, pp. 296–301). Mt. Kisco, NY: Futura.

Pierce, W. S. (1979). Clinical left ventricular bypass: Problems of pump inflow obstruction and right ventricular failure. *ASAIO Journal, 1,* 1–9.

Portner, P. M., Oyer, P. E., Jassawatta, J. S., et al. (1983). An alternative in end-stage heart disease: Long term ventricular assistance. *Journal of Heart Transplantation, 3,* 4759.

Reedy, J. E., Ruzevich, S. A., Swartz, M. T., et al. (1989). Nursing care of a patient requiring prolonged mechanical circulatory support. *Progress in Cardiovascular Nursing, 4,* 1–9.

Reedy, J. E., Ruzevich, S. A., Vitali, L. J., et al. (1990). Nursing care of the ambulatory patient with a mechanical assist device. *Journal of Heart Transplantation, 9,* 97–105.

Reedy, J. E., Swartz, M. T., Lohmann, D., et al. (1992). Importance of patient mobility with ventricular assist support. *ASAIO Journal, 38,* 151–153.

Rudis, E., & Drinkwater, D. C. (In press). Circulatory support in children. *Glenn's Thoracic and Cardiovascular Surgery* (6th ed.).

Ruzevich, S. A. (1991). Heart assist devices: State of the art. *Critical Care Nursing Clinics of North America, 3,* 723–732.

Ruzevich, S. A., Pennington, D. G., Kanter, K. R., et al. (1987). Long-term follow-up study of survivors of post-cardiotomy circulatory support. *ASAIO Journal, 10,* 177–181.

Ruzevich, S. A., Swartz, M. T., & Pennington, D. G. (1988). Nursing care of the patient with a pneumatic ventricular assist device. *Heart and Lung, 17,* 399–406.

Ruzevich, S. A., Swartz, M. T., & Reedy, J. E. (1990). Retrospective analysis of the psychological effects of mechanical circulatory support. *Journal of Heart Transplantation, 9,* 209–212.

Soeter, J. R., Mamiya, R. T., Sprague, A. Y., et al. (1973). Prolonged extracorporeal oxygenation for cardiorespiratory failure after tetralogy correction. *Journal of Thoracic and Cardiovascular Surgery, 66,* 214.

Starnes, V. A., Oyer, P. E., Portner, P. M., et al. (1988). Isolated left ventricular assist as bridge to cardiac transplantation. *Journal of Thoracic and Cardiovascular Surgery, 96,* 62–71.

Swartz, M. T., & Pennington, D. G. (1985). Use of a ventricular assist device in postcardiotomy shock. *Journal of Clinical Engineering, 10,* 241–249.

Swartz, M. T., Ruzevich, S. A., Reedy, J. E., et al. (1989). Team approach to circulatory support. *Critical Care Nursing Clinics of North America, 1,* 479–484.

Termuhlen, D. F., Pennington, D. G., Roodman, S. T., et al. (1989). T-cells in ventricular assist device patients. *Circulation, 80,* 174–182.

Zapoh, W. M., Snider, M. T., Hill, J. D., et al. (1979). Extracorporeal membrane oxygenation in severe respiratory failure: A randomized prospective study. *Journal of the American Medical Association, 242,* 2193–2196.

Respiratory Monitoring

Tom Ahrens

Concepts in pulmonary critical care are at the center of much of the assessment and treatments administered in current intensive care units (ICUs). Although it is unrealistic to discuss all aspects of pulmonary critical care in one chapter, the major aspects that are encountered on a daily basis are presented. The key aspects of pulmonary critical care involve concepts relating to oxygenation and gas exchange. The goal of this chapter is to present the fundamentals of oxygenation and gas exchange while simultaneously exploring more advanced applications of these concepts. Blood gas and hemodynamic analysis will be emphasized as the mechanism through which more advanced aspects of pulmonary critical care are applied.

Two features are included in the presentation of oxygenation and gas exchange: first, the separation of oxygenation from gas exchange is emphasized, and second, the influence of other organ systems on oxygenation and gas exchange is recognized. Through analysis of more advanced aspects of oxygenation and gas exchange, critical care nurses can increase their ability to make more sophisticated assessments and interventions in the patient with acute pulmonary disturbances. Practical examples are included to assist the nurse with the interpretation of clinical data.

OXYGENATION COMPONENTS

Cellular oxygenation is a combination of adequate oxygen transport relative to cellular oxygen consumption. Assessment of oxygenation must account for each facet of oxygenation. Using each component also helps to avoid the use of components that are not as important. For example, the partial pressure of arterial oxygen ($Pa{O_2}$) plays a role in oxygenation by aiding oxygen transport. This role is not as important, however, as the other factors in oxygenation. Clinically, the $Pa{O_2}$ has a tendency to be inappropriately applied in the assessment of oxygenation. Some clinicians believe that if the $Pa{O_2}$ is adequate, oxygen transport is adequate. Actually, the $Pa{O_2}$ is poorly correlated with cellular oxygenation. The role of the $Pa{O_2}$ and other components of oxygenation must be clearly understood to apply each component appropriately in oxygenation assessment.

Determinants of Oxygenation

Oxygenation is determined by several factors, four of which are involved in oxygen transport. To determine how important any one parameter is in an oxygenation assessment, the factors in oxygen transport ($D{O_2}$) must be considered. The main factors in oxygen transport, in order of importance, are cardiac output, hemoglobin (Hgb), hemoglobin saturation ($Sa{O_2}$), and $Pa{O_2}$ (Ahrens & Rutherford, 1993). Another factor in oxygenation that has been considered only recently is the cellular utilization of oxygen. Disturbance in cell utilization of oxygen, including mitochondrial dysfunction or breakdown in oxidative phosphorylation (cellular dysoxia) is a likely factor in several conditions, ranging from sepsis to cyanide poisoning. Unfortunately, direct measures of cell utilization of oxygen are not readily available to the ICU clinician. Normal values for oxygenation are listed in Table 15–1.

Oxygen transport is measured by the following equation:

$$O_2 \text{ transport} = \text{cardiac output} \times \text{oxygen content } (Ca{O_2}) \times 10$$

where 10 is a conversion factor to change $Ca{O_2}$ measurement from deciliters to liters. Cardiac output, as seen by this equation, accounts for at least 50% of oxygen transport; $Ca{O_2}$ accounts for the other 50%. Three factors comprise $Ca{O_2}$—Hgb, $Sa{O_2}$, and $Pa{O_2}$. $Ca{O_2}$ is

TABLE 15–1. **Normal Components of Oxygenation**

Oxygen transport	600–1000 cc/minute 500–600 mL/minute/m^2
Oxygen consumption	120–160 mL/minute/m^2 3–4 cc/minute/kg
Oxygen extraction	0.25%–0.35%
Cardiac output	4–8 L/minute 2.5–4 L/minute/m^2
Hemoglobin	12–16 g/dL
$Sa{O_2}$	>0.90
$Pa{O_2}$	60–100 mm Hg

calculated by the following equation:

$$Cao_2 = Hgb \times 1.34 \times Sao_2 + (0.003 \times Pao_2)$$

The 1.34 is the amount of oxygen maximally carried by Hgb if all oxygen sites of Hgb are occupied (Bunn & Forget, 1986). The 0.003 is the oxygen solubility coefficient. The oxygen solubility coefficient is used to determine how much oxygen is being transported by the Pao_2. Hgb accounts for the majority of Cao_2, with Sao_2 and Pao_2 playing smaller roles. Two case examples illustrate the different roles of Hgb, Sao_2, and Pao_2 in determination of Cao_2.

CASE HISTORIES

Case 1. An 80-year-old male patient was admitted to the ICU with pneumonia. The initial blood gas determination was listed at 8 A.M. The fraction of inspired oxygen (Fio_2) was increased at this time. Later in the morning, the patient had an episode of hematemesis. Repeat blood gas and Hgb measurements demonstrated the values listed at 10 A.M. The Fio_2 was again increased at this time. A second episode of hematemesis occurred at 12:30 P.M. A repeat blood gas and Hgb were obtained at 1 P.M. From these data, at which time did the patient have the best arterial oxygen content?

	8 A.M.	10 A.M.	1 P.M.
Pao_2 mm Hg	56	87	111
Hgb g/dL	15	12	10
Sao_2%	0.88	0.96	0.98
Fio_2	0.21	0.30	0.40

Cao_2 Computation

8 A.M. $Cao_2 = 15 \times 1.34 \times 0.88 + (0.003 \times 56) =$
$17.7 + 0.168 = 17.868$ cc/dL

10 A.M. $Cao_2 = 12 \times 1.34 \times 0.96 + (0.003 \times 87) =$
$15.5 + 0.261 = 15.79$ cc/dL

1 P.M. $Cao_2 = 10 \times 1.34 \times 0.98 + (0.003 \times 111) =$
$13.1 \quad 0.333 = 13.43$ cc/dL

These calculations demonstrate two important points. First is the significance of Hgb in determining Cao_2. Eight o'clock was the point at which the patient had the highest oxygen content, based on the high Hgb level at this time. The second important point is the minimal contribution of Pao_2 levels to oxygen transport. When the Pao_2 was highest, at 1 P.M., the Cao_2 was at its lowest. Pao_2 and Cao_2 are not linearly related. Shoemaker (1989) has demonstrated in several subgroups of patients (i.e., those with sepsis, trauma, or adult respiratory distress syndrome) that the Pao_2 not only has a weak correlation with oxygenation but has little clinical value in identifying survivors as opposed to nonsurvivors. To further illustrate the small contribution of Pao_2 to Cao_2, note the minimal change in Cao_2 that occurs if the contribution of the Pao_2 is removed:

	With Pao_2	Without Pao_2
8 A.M.	17.868 cc/dL	17.7 cc/dL
10 A.M.	15.79 cc/dL	15.5 cc/dL
1 P.M.	13.42 cc/dL	13.1 cc/dL

The clinical implications of the above computations are easy to apply. Pao_2 levels should not be used as a primary tool in the assessment of oxygenation. A common clinical error is to assume that oxygen transport is adequate if the Pao_2 is normal. It is important to avoid this pitfall. The Pao_2 is a minor contributor to oxygen transport; cardiac output and Hgb levels are far more important. The following case illustrates the importance of cardiac output and Hgb compared with Pao_2.

Case 2. Assume that you are the charge nurse and would like to teach a new orientee one aspect of prioritizing important physiologic data, in this case, oxygen transport. The three patients listed below are in your unit. Which of these three patients would be prioritized as being the most threatened with regard to oxygen transport?

	Patient 1	Patient 2	Patient 3
Pao_2 mm Hg	91	53	160
Hgb g/dL	12	12	10
Sao_2	0.96	0.85	0.99
Cardiac output (L/min)	4.5	6	3

Oxygen transport for each patient:

Pt. 1 $4.5 \times 15.7 \times 10 = 707$ cc/minute
Pt. 2 $6 \times 13.8 \times 10 = 830$ cc/minute
Pt. 3 $3 \times 13.7 \times 10 = 412$ cc/minute

If the Pao_2 were the only assessment tool used to assess oxygenation, the third patient would have been assumed to be adequate. Actually, his oxygen transport level is dangerously low. In the second patient, although Pao_2 levels are lower than desirable, oxygen levels are adequate, and the patient is in no immediate danger from hypoxia. In teaching the new orientee, the charge nurse would emphasize that the person most at risk is the third patient. As long as the limitations of the clinical application of Pao_2 are understood, appropriate use of Pao_2 in assessing oxygenation is possible.

The value of the Pao_2 in assessing oxygenation does not rest in how much oxygen is carried by Pao_2. The Pao_2 does have a value, however, in that one can estimate Sao_2 levels from given Pao_2 values. The Sao_2 indicates how much Hgb is carrying oxygen (oxyhemoglobin). An Sao_2 level of 0.90 indicates that Hgb is carrying 90% of all the oxygen it is capable of carrying. Pao_2 levels are related to Sao_2 levels according to the oxyhemoglobin dissociation curve. As seen in Figure 15–1, Pao_2 levels are related to Sao_2 values and can be used to predict Sao_2 values. At Pao_2 levels in excess of 60 mm Hg, Sao_2 values are greater than 0.90. Pao_2 levels higher than this will contribute to a slight but not substantial increase in Sao_2. For example, a Pao_2 value of 100 mm Hg will have an Sao_2 value of 0.98, whereas a Pao_2 of 60 mm Hg has a saturation value of 0.90. Because Sao_2 does not increase substantially after a Pao_2 of 60 mm Hg is reached, Pao_2 levels of 60 mm Hg or higher are clinically acceptable.

On the other hand, if the partial pressure of oxygen (Po_2) falls to less than 60 mm Hg, Hgb rapidly loses its ability to carry oxygen. From Figure 15–1, a Po_2 of 40 mm Hg is associated with an So_2 of 0.75. If the Po_2 falls to 27 mm Hg, So_2 is near 0.50. The rapid decrease in oxygen-carrying capacity of Hgb as the Po_2 drops to less than 60 mm Hg highlights the clinical significance of Po_2 levels. From the point of view of oxygenation, maintaining the Po_2 value in excess of 60 mm Hg will provide satisfactory hemoglobin saturation levels. Levels in excess of 60 mm Hg will generally provide little further improvement in oxygen transport. For example, in a patient who is admitted

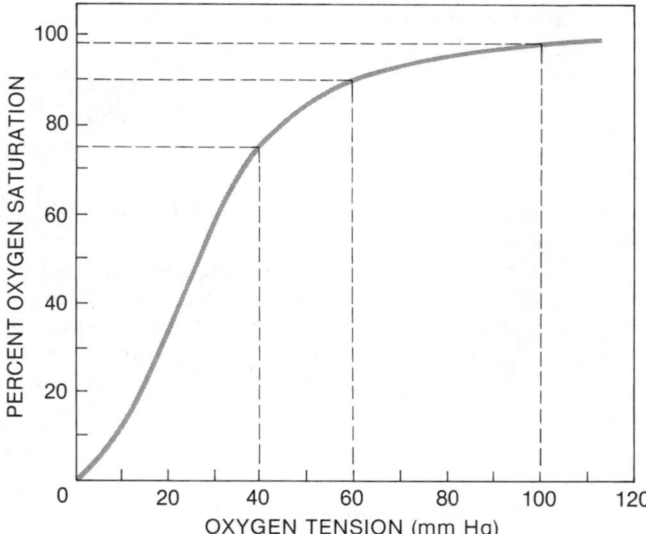

FIGURE 15-1. Oxyhemoglobin dissociation curve.

with a diagnosis of rule out myocardial infarction, who has no evidence of left ventricular failure, and in whom room air blood gases indicate Pa_{O_2} values greater than 60 mm Hg, the addition of oxygen therapy probably will not increase oxygen transport to any substantial degree.

There is one exception to increasing the Pa_{O_2} value when it is higher than 60 mm Hg. When a patient has a low Hgb or a low cardiac output level, improving the Pa_{O_2} value may produce a small improvement in oxygen transport that could be clinically important. In a patient with a low Hgb, oxygen therapy may slightly improve oxygen transport until a transfusion can be initiated. Similarly, in a patient with a low cardiac output, the addition of oxygen therapy may provide a small boost to oxygen transport until the cardiac output can be augmented. The following case example helps to illustrate this point.

Case 3. A 62-year-old woman was admitted with the diagnosis of chronic asthma. Because of a hypotensive episode in the emergency room a few hours earlier, a pulmonary artery catheter was inserted in the ICU. Initial data were listed at 2 A.M. During the night, she developed chest pain, and an electrocardiogram revealed a probable anterior myocardial infarction. Further data were presented at 5 A.M. From these two sets of data, at which time would an increase in oxygen therapy have been most useful?

	2 A.M.	5 A.M.
Pa_{O_2}	63	70
Sa_{O_2}	0.91	0.92
Hgb	13	13
F_{IO_2}	0.21	0.30
Cardiac output	5	3.5

Oxygen transport at 2 A.M.:

$$5 \times (1.34 \times 13 \times 0.91) \times 10 = 793 \text{ cc/minute}$$

Oxygen transport at 5 A.M.:

$$3.5 \times (1.34 \times 13 \times 0.92) \times 10 = 561 \text{ cc/minute}$$

The best time to have administered oxygen therapy would have been at 5 A.M. because of the overall diminished oxygen transport seen at this time. Increasing the F_{IO_2} and therefore the Pa_{O_2} would not address the major problem, but would offer a small improvement in oxygenation until the cardiac output could be improved.

Oximetry

With the advent of pulse oximetry (Sp_{O_2}), the need to use Pa_{O_2} values to estimate Sa_{O_2} levels has markedly diminished. However, understanding how to apply pulse oximetry depends on understanding oxygen transport. Because oximetry estimates Sa_{O_2} values, its use in assessing oxygen transport is limited. Pulse oximetry detects neither Hgb nor cardiac output, and, as such, it reveals little about oxygen transport. Sa_{O_2} levels are very useful in determining changes in lung function (intrapulmonary shunting) and in altering oxygen therapy. Sa_{O_2} values are potentially very useful in appropriate circumstances. A brief review of the principles of pulse oximetry will help to illustrate the basis for the use of Sa_{O_2} values.

Two common clinical applications of oximetry exist: one is invasive and measures venous hemoglobin saturation (Sv_{O_2}), and the other is noninvasive and estimates arterial saturation (Sa_{O_2}). Venous oximetry is related more to oxygenation, and pulse oximetry more to intrapulmonary shunting. In addition, the principles of measurement used in oximetry rely on either an absorptive or a reflectance component. New developments in oximetry are frequently occurring. For example, noninvasive pulse oximetry will shift its focus away from specific locations such as the finger or ear to applications virtually anywhere on the body. Forehead oximetry has already been studied and is an example of a future application of oximetry principles (Cheng et al., 1988).

Oxyhemoglobin

Regardless of the application or of the use of reflectance or absorptive principles, the underlying theory remains the same. The key principle in oximetry is the different properties of absorption of light between oxyhemoglobin and reduced hemoglobin (or deoxyhemoglobin). Two other common types of hemoglobin exist, methemoglobin (MetHgb) and carboxyhemoglobin (COHgb), and although there are instances in which these values are important, the present explanation focuses on oxyhemoglobin. Generally, oxyhemoglobin is the value of interest, with a few clinical exceptions (Severinghaus & Kelleher, 1992). For example, in patients with smoke inhalation, an elevation in COHgb that will decrease the reliability of pulse oximeters in accurately estimating oxyhemoglobin because the pulse oximeter cannot measure COHgb. Because COHgb is assumed to be oxyhemoglobin by the pulse oximeter, the oxyhemoglobin value will be overestimated by the pulse oximeter. High COHgb levels will reduce the oxyhemoglobin value, but the pulse oximeter will not detect the reduction in oxyhemoglobin.

Sao_2 indicates arterial oxyhemoglobin values, and Svo_2 refers to venous oxyhemoglobin. Oxyhemoglobin is identified through oximetry by measuring two lights (red and infrared) emitted by light-emitting diodes. If reflectance oximetry is used, the amount of light reflecting back to the measurement source is measured (e.g., venous oximetry in a pulmonary artery catheter). If absorptive oximetry is used, the amount of light passing through a tissue is measured (e.g., pulse oximetry (Severinghaus & Astrup, 1986).

Two light wavelengths are used to measure oxyhemoglobin and reduced hemoglobin (deoxyhemoglobin). Four wavelengths are required to measure other types of hemoglobins (Barker & Tremper, 1987). Oximetry in the clinical setting uses the two-wavelength system. Failure to measure the other types of hemoglobin can present clinical problems, which are illustrated later.

The two sources of light, red and infrared, are used to measure oxyhemoglobin and reduced hemoglobin have different wavelengths. Red light is emitted at a wavelength of 660 nm, and infrared light is emitted at 940 nm (Alexander et al., 1989; Millikan, 1942). Red light passes through oxyhemoglobin but is absorbed by reduced hemoglobin. Infrared light is absorbed by oxyhemoglobin but passes through reduced hemoglobin. By noting the ratio of the difference in the light that passes through a tissue or is reflected, the amount of oxyhemoglobin and deoxyhemoglobin can be estimated. Red light (660 nm) is considered the numerator of the ratio, infrared light the denominator (940 nm). The ratio is low when oxyhemoglobin values are high (Stasic, 1986). The low ratio results from the fact that more red light reaches the light sensor, indicating a higher oxyhemoglobin level. More infrared light passing through indicates a higher level of deoxyhemoglobin and is reflected in a high red–infrared ratio.

One obvious concern in shining a light through a tissue is the potential for tissue other than hemoglobin to absorb the light. Pulse oximetry circumvents this problem by measuring the red–infrared light ratio only during maximal light absorption, which occurs during pulsation of arterial blood into the tissue. Other tissues that could absorb light (i.e., muscle, fat, connective tissue, and venous and capillary blood) are part of the baseline absorptive components that must be avoided (Fig. 15–2). When the tissue bed expands as a result of arterial pulsation, there is an expansion in the amount of light that passes through the tissue (Tremper & Barker, 1989). By sensing light only during the period of maximal absorption, the influence of other components is reduced.

Clinical Application of Pulse Oximetry

A second point regarding pulse oximetry is helpful in applying the values in the clinical setting. Pulse oximetry measures hemoglobin saturation based on the following equation:

$$\frac{Hgbo_2}{Hgbo_2 + Hb}$$

where $Hgbo_2$ = oxyhemoglobin, and Hb = reduced hemoglobin.

This form of hemoglobin measurement is referred to as functional hemoglobin saturation. Other forms of hemoglobin (i.e., carboxyhemoglobin and methemoglobin) are not measured. To measure other common types of hemoglobins, the following equation would be necessary:

$$\frac{Hgbo_2}{COHgb + MetHgb}$$

The result is that the value displayed on the pulse oximeter is higher than the value of the measurement of all hemoglobins. Measurement of all hemoglobin saturation is referred to as fractional measurement, such as is performed with a laboratory co-oximeter. Clinicians must not compare the Sao_2 values obtained from the oximeter to laboratory oxyhemoglobin values unless the above formula is also applied to the laboratory values. MetHgb and COHgb levels, when combined, usually comprise less than 3% of the total hemoglobin. Based on the combined amounts of MetHgb and CoHgb measuring about 3% of the total, the Spo_2 (pulse oximeter) value usually is about 3% (or more) higher than the actual Sao_2. The only way to validate this estimate is to obtain a fractional hemoglobin saturation and compare the values according to the formulas given earlier. This should be done whenever the accuracy of the pulse oximeter is in question.

Other factors can influence the accuracy of oximetry. In addition to dysfunctional hemoglobins, increased skin pigmentation, anemia, and low perfusion states can interfere with the accuracy of the Spo_2 reading (Ralston et al., 1991; Ramsing & Rosenberg, 1992; Zeballos & Weisman, 1991). The typical error is again an overestimation of the true Sao_2 value by the Spo_2.

The value of measuring Sao_2 from pulse oximetry data centers around two key components, the continuous measurement of Sao_2 and the assessment of intrapulmonary shunting, Qs/Qt. As noted earlier, Sao_2 does not reveal as much about oxygen transport as does hemoglobin or cardiac output. Maintaining Spo_2 values in excess of 0.93 usually will mean that Sao_2 values are higher than 0.90, a value that is adequate for most situations involving oxygen transport.

Use of Spo_2 for assessing Qs/Qt is of value either as an assessment tool or to avoid having to measure blood gases while Fio_2 levels are being reduced. When using Spo_2 for assessing Qs/Qt, the clinician watches for changes in Spo_2 while the Fio_2 remains unchanged. If the Spo_2 falls while the Fio_2 is unchanged, Qs/Qt may be worsening. A falling Spo_2 that is not caused by

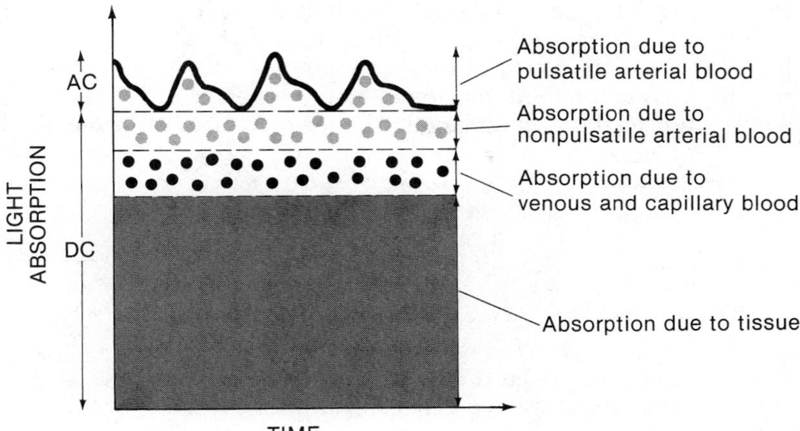

FIGURE 15–2. Factors affecting light transmission through tissue. (Redrawn from Tremper, K. K., & Barker, S. J. [1989]. Pulse oximetry. *Anesthesiology, 70,* 98–101.)

a change in Qs/Qt may occur if the Svo_2 is decreased (Ahrens & Rutherford, 1987).

The most practical use of Spo_2 is in continually monitoring the patient during Fio_2 changes while avoiding the need to measure blood gases (Council on Scientific Affairs, American Medical Association, 1993; Durren, 1992). As a guide, Fio_2 levels can be reduced or increased until a desired Spo_2 (usually 0.93) is reached. The following case study illustrates the use of the Spo_2 in Fio_2 manipulation.

CASE HISTORY

Case 4. A 62-year-old man was admitted to your unit after coronary bypass graft surgery. His initial blood gas values and Spo_2 were as follows:

Pao_2	390
Spo_2	1.00
Fio_2	1.00
$Paco_2$	37
pH	7.41

Your unit has a policy of reducing the Fio_2 by 0.20 and drawing a sample for blood gas determination at each reduction. The Fio_2 is reduced until a Pao_2 value of below 100 but over 80 is reached. This policy usually requires three blood gas samples to reach an Fio_2 value of 0.40. How could obtaining Spo_2 values avoid the need for these blood gas samples?

The answer is to lower the Fio_2 by 0.20 (or another level) until the Spo_2 is 0.93 or higher. Generally, no blood gas samples would need to be obtained during this time to assess Sao_2 or Pao_2, as long as the only change occurred in the Fio_2.

Several research studies have demonstrated the value of Spo_2 in manipulating the Fio_2, particularly in the postoperative setting (Bierman et al., 1992; DiBendetto et al., 1994; Inman et al., 1993; Roberts et al., 1991; Rotello et al., 1992). The use of Spo_2 in tapering Fio_2 values is of clinical value in that the cost of blood gas determinations can be avoided while improving assessment through the continuous monitoring of patients during the manipulation. Also, in the patient without an arterial line, the pain of the arterial puncture is avoided.

ASSESSMENT OF OXYGEN TRANSPORT AND CONSUMPTION

With the exception of the Svo_2, none of the components of oxygen transport presented so far takes into account oxygen consumption. Without understanding the oxygen consumption rates of the cells, the adequacy of oxygen transport can never be known. The concept of comparing oxygen transport with oxygen consumption is at the heart of an accurate assessment of oxygenation.

Oxygen Consumption

Values for oxygen consumption (Vo_2) are not always available unless ready access to exhaled gases or mixed venous oxygen values is present. Two common methods exist to measure Vo_2, neither of which is difficult, but each presents practical problems. The first method is the use of exhaled gas analysis, and the second the use of an indirect application of the Fick equation.

Measurement of Vo_2 through exhaled gas analysis is based on the following simplified formula (several formulas account more accurately for other gases, but this method is simple and relatively accurate):

$$Vo_2 = V_E \times (Fio_2 - Feo_2)$$

where V_E = minute ventilation (liters/minute or cc/minute); Fio_2 = fraction of inspired oxygen; and Feo_2 = fraction of expired oxygen. For example, if the Fio_2 is 0.40, Feo_2 is 0.35, and V_E is 5 L/minute (or 5,000 cc/minute), then:

$$Vo_2 = 5{,}000 \times (0.40 - 0.35) = 250 \text{ cc/minute}$$

The problem with exhaled gas analysis centers mainly on the difficulty of obtaining accurate inspired and expired oxygen levels. Technically, sample collection may be difficult. Evidence also exists that Fio_2 values in excess of 50% may not be accurately used in computing VO_2 (Ultman & Bursztein, 1981). This obviously limits application in critical care settings.

The second method for measuring oxygen consumption uses the Fick equation. The formula is:

$$VO_2 = \text{cardiac output} \times (CaO_2 - CvO_2) \times 10$$

As an example, assume a cardiac output of 5 L/minute, CaO_2 of 15, and CvO_2 of 11. The VO_2 would be:

$$VO_2 = 5 \times (15 - 11) \times 10 = 200 \text{ cc/minute}$$

This method has been demonstrated to correlate closely with measured oxygen consumption by exhaled gas analysis (Liggett et al., 1986).

Nurses in critical care units should be familiar with one of the above methods to make a more complete assessment of oxygenation. The exhaled gas method is more accurate and less invasive but has more technical problems. The indirect Fick equation method requires SvO_2 values and is therefore invasive, yet many patients already have SvO_2 values available if a pulmonary artery catheter is present.

Oxygen Balance

Actual measurement of cellular oxygenation is not possible at this time. To measure the adequacy of oxygenation of the cells, many parameters that are not readily measured at the bedside are necessary. Factors affecting mitochondrial use of oxygen include substrate availability (especially carbohydrates), intercapillary distance, diffusion capabilities of oxygen, tissue PO_2 and oxygen gradients between cells and capillaries, and the adequacy of electron transfer systems. However, instead of measuring these aspects of oxygenation, a more global method of assessment is used clinically. The primary method of assessment involves a comparison of oxygen transport parameters against oxygen consumption. Such a comparison has distinct limitations, but can provide approximate estimates of the adequacy of cellular oxygenation.

Four methods are commonly used to compare oxygen transport with oxygen consumption. None of these methods can be accomplished noninvasively at the present time. These methods include oxygen extraction analysis, SvO_2 monitoring, lactate level measurements, and $FIO_2 - FEO_2$ comparisons.

OXYGEN EXTRACTION. Oxygen extraction (O_{2e}) is obtained by dividing oxygen consumption by oxygen transport. Normal oxygen extraction is approximately 25%. In other words, 25% of all oxygen transported is removed from hemoglobin by the cells. For example, if the oxygen transport was 1,000 cc and the VO_2 250 cc, the extraction rate would be 250/1,000 = 25%.

The following examples help to illustrate the value of oxygen extraction. Note that in the first patient, a normal CaO_2 is present. However, with a low cardiac output and a normal oxygen consumption, cellular oxygenation may be threatened. In the second patient, a low CaO_2 is present with a normal cardiac output and normal VO_2. The low CaO_2 threatens oxygenation. In the third example, normal CaO_2 and cardiac output are present, but a high VO_2 threatens oxygenation.

	Patient 1	Patient 2	Patient 3
PaO_2	75	90	65
SaO_2	0.93	0.96	0.91
Hgb	13	8	14
Cardiac output	3	4.5	5
CaO_2	16.2	10.3	17.1
DO_2	486	463	855
VO_2	245	210	375
Wt (kg)	70	60	70
O_{2e}	0.50	0.45	0.44

Extraction rates become clinically significant as they increase. Although the upper limits tolerated by humans are unknown, empirical evidence suggests that extraction rates in the 40% range may indicate disturbances in cellular oxygenation. The point at which humans reach a dangerous cellular imbalance of oxygen is not clear, although some studies suggest that humans can tolerate oxygen extraction ratios as high as 0.80 (Cain, 1983). It should not be assumed that all patients can achieve extraction rates at this level, however; Shoemaker and Appel (1985) have demonstrated that patients with sepsis have increased mortality at levels as low as the high 0.30s. A more useful way to apply oxygen extraction rates clinically is to note the trend in extraction. As extraction rates increase, cellular oxygenation is being threatened.

Two factors complicate the use of oxygen extraction rates. One is the apparent dependence of VO_2 on DO_2 at critically low levels of adequate oxygen balance. Several studies have indicated that, as DO_2 falls, VO_2 may fall in similar proportions (Appel & Shoemaker, 1992; Inoue et al., 1993; Leach & Treacher, 1992). If this is true, VO_2 falls as DO_2 decreases. The dependence of VO_2 on oxygen delivery emphasizes the need to track oxygen extraction trends rather than noting absolute values of O_{2e}. As O_{2e} increases, the clinician should search for methods of increasing oxygen transport or decreasing VO_2. A stable O_{2e} does not, however, necessarily mean that oxygenation is adequate or stable. The clinician must continue to track all parameters of oxygenation.

The second limiting feature of the assessment of oxygen extraction is the difference between oxygen consumption and oxygen demand. Oxygen consumption of the cells differs from oxygen demand of the cells. In patients with disturbances in cellular utilization of oxygen, oxygen consumption may decrease, although demand for oxygen is high. Unfortunately, measurement of oxygen consumption is easier than that of oxygen demand. When using oxygen extraction rates, simultaneous use of lactate levels may also be helpful to reflect anaerobic metabolism and oxygen demand.

Methods of making lactate measurements are presented later in this chapter. There is considerable debate, however, as to the Vo_2/Do_2 relationship. Several authors claim the apparent Vo_2 dependence on Do_2 is either a measurement error or simply does not exist (Steltzer et al., 1994). The exact Vo_2/Do_2 relationship requires further investigation before it is fully understood. However, it does appear that survivors of hypoxia exhibit higher Do_2 and Vo_2 levels than nonsurvivors (Samsel & Schumaker, 1991; Shoemaker et al., 1993). Therefore, until further information is available, increasing Do_2 levels to supranormal values should be considered in virtually any patient in shock.

Svo_2 MONITORING AND ANALYSIS. With Svo_2 analysis, oxygen extraction can be estimated without performing all the above measurements. Svo_2 analysis applies theoretical principles to estimate the balance between oxygen transport and consumption. Svo_2 values, normally between 0.60 and 0.75, trend oxygen extraction. If, for example, oxygen transport decreases without decreasing oxygen consumption, more oxygen will be extracted from Hgb to maintain cellular oxygen levels. The result of the increased extraction of oxygen from the Hgb is a reduction in hemoglobin saturation. The Svo_2 can therefore be used as an estimate of the adequacy of the balance between oxygen transport and oxygen consumption. Many articles have been written on Svo_2 monitoring, and the reader is referred to these for more introductory material on this subject (Schweiss, 1987; White, 1984). One important point of Svo_2 monitoring that is frequently overlooked is the ability of Svo_2 levels to reflect the adequacy of treatment, as illustrated in the following case study (Ahrens, 1990).

CASE HISTORY

Case 5. A 73-year-old man was admitted with a diagnosis of congestive heart failure. A fiberoptic pulmonary artery catheter was placed to aid in assessment. At 4 P.M., the low cardiac output and high pulmonary capillary wedge pressure (PCWP) were used as the basis for starting dobutamine at 3 μg/kg per minute. Based on the change in cardiac index and PCWP that occurred between 4 P.M. and 5 P.M., was the change in oxygenation adequate?

	4 P.M. (dobutamine started)	5 P.M.
Pao_2	69	72
Sao_2	0.92	0.92
Hgb	12	12
Cardiac output	3.4	4.0
Cardiac index	2.1	2.5
PCWP	21	18
Svo_2	0.52	0.54

Although a subsequent increase in cardiac output was noted, the Svo_2 did not substantially increase. The increase in cardiac output apparently was not enough to change oxygenation substantially.

The Svo_2 can be used in several ways to estimate the adequacy of oxygenation. The most common use is to note trends in Svo_2. If Svo_2 is trending downward, investigation into the components of oxygen transport and consumption to locate a potential disturbance is necessary. If the trend is upward, the patient may be improving, provided no technical problems exist. A second use of Svo_2 monitoring is as a catastrophic warning. Because Svo_2 monitoring can be continuous in patients requiring the use of fiberoptic pulmonary artery catheters, early warnings of severe derangements in oxygenation can be obtained more easily than with any other method of oxygenation monitoring. A third, less common use, was illustrated in Case 5. Svo_2 monitoring can be used as a means of determining the adequacy of therapies in hemodynamics, oxygen, and positive end-expiratory pressure or continuous positive airway pressure therapy and ventilator adjustments. The ability of Svo_2 to aid in treatment assessment is the area of its highest potential.

The disadvantages of Svo_2 monitoring center on the technical problems involved in fiberoptic monitoring and the occurrence of physiologic situations that cause unexpected Svo_2 values. Technically, Svo_2 catheters are reliable, but problems can be experienced in operation. Most of the nursing interventions necessary to correct these problems can be found in the service manuals provided by each manufacturer. Of the three currently available Svo_2 catheters, Abbott's Oximetrix Opticath has been demonstrated to be more clinically reliable (Chulay et al., 1992; Gettinger et al., 1987). Technologic improvements made by the manufacturers are continually reducing the technical problems associated with each catheter, and accuracies associated with each manufacturer need to be assessed frequently. By the time this chapter is published, further changes may have occurred.

Physiologically, Svo_2 monitoring can be misleading in two circumstances. First, in patients with sepsis, precapillary sphincter closure secondary to mechanisms such as endotoxin release cause arterial blood to bypass the cells and empty directly into the veins. The result is high Svo_2 values (generally higher than 75%) that do not reflect cellular oxygenation. Caution in interpreting high Svo_2 values is necessary. If the Svo_2 is higher than 75%, the clinician must decide whether the value is possible, whether a technical problem exists, or whether a potential for pericapillary shunting is present (i.e., the patient may be septic). The second circumstance is again related to the dependence of Vo_2 on Do_2. If Vo_2 is correlated with Do_2, as currently thought, Svo_2 will lose its ability to predict cellular oxygenation as Vo_2 changes with Do_2.

The goal in any Svo_2 evaluation is always to attempt to drive the Svo_2 level back to a normal value (0.60–0.75). If the Svo_2 is low, the goal is to raise it above 0.60. If it is excessively high, the goal is to drive it below 0.75. Svo_2 application has not been studied well enough at this point. Although many nursing studies have investigated the effects of nursing activities on Svo_2, more in-depth studies are needed. For example, do frequent changes in Svo_2 levels predict problems? Or does a decrease in Svo_2 during nursing activities warn of future problems? Svo_2 monitoring is probably underused owing to this lack of research.

One factor that can also be used to assess oxygenation is venous Po_2 values (Pvo_2). Although the arterial Po_2 does not contribute substantially to oxygen transport, venous oxygen tensions can be used to highlight the driving pressure that forces oxygen into the cells. As the Pvo_2 decreases, the pressure driving oxygen into the cells is diminishing. The potential for loss of cellular oxygen will increase as the Pvo_2 falls (Swan et al., 1990). As a guideline, if the Pvo_2 falls less than 35 mm Hg, the potential for cellular hypoxia increases at a faster rate. From a clinical perspective, keeping the Pvo_2 higher than 30 mm Hg may be helpful in protecting cellular oxygenation.

LACTATE LEVELS. A third method of measuring cellular oxygenation is to measure lactic acid levels. Normal lactate levels are between 1 and 2 mmol/L. The potential advantage of using lactate levels is that they reflect a more accurate chemical picture of cellular oxygenation. Normal lactate use can be understood by reviewing substrate metabolism patterns.

To generate energy, carbohydrates must be available to allow fats and proteins to enter the Krebs cycle. Both fats and protein can be catabolized only through the Krebs cycle and oxidative phosphorylation, a process that requires the presence of oxygen to act as the final electron acceptor for the hydrogen electron removed from each substrate. Carbohydrates serve to process fats and proteins through the generation of pyruvate. In the absence of oxygen, pyruvate cannot aid in the processing of other substrates. Without oxygen, carbohydrates form increasing amounts of lactate, an anaerobic method of generating energy, although this process is much less efficient in terms of generating energy (Kruse & Carlson, 1987). Normal lactate/pyruvate levels are about 10:1. In hypoxia, pyruvate will not be produced in quantities as fast as lactate. This results from the lack of oxygen necessary to keep lactate from being preferentially developed during glucose metabolism. Without oxygen, pyruvate cannot combine with acetic acid to form acetyl coenzyme A (CoA). If acetyl CoA is not formed to help fats and proteins into the Krebs cycle, oxidative phosphorylation will not occur, and adenosine triphosphate will not be produced in adequate quantities for cellular work to occur. Because the only substrate capable of producing energy without oxygen is carbohydrates, and normal carbohydrate stores are less than 1,000 Kcal (one-half of 1 day's normal energy requirement), anaerobic metabolism is only a short-term solution to oxygen deprivation.

Lactate levels have a potential clinical use in predicting survival. Since the 1960s, the literature has included references to the correlation of lactate levels with survival (Peretz et al., 1965). These early studies indicated that lactate levels in excess of 4 mmol/L were associated with much higher mortality levels, with only 11% survival in some cases. Lactate levels are not, however, without limitations in predicting outcome. The ability to clear lactate from the blood may be a better indicator of survival than the notation of lactate acid levels alone (Broder & Weil, 1964). The use of lactate levels as a predictor of outcome requires further analysis. Lactate levels may best be used as a means of confirmation of cellular hypoxia in conjunction with other aspects of oxygenation. As lactate levels start to rise over 2 mmol/L, the potential for anaerobic metabolism may be increasing. If the lactate level is rising, the clinician should examine oxygen transport and consumption parameters.

The advantage of measuring lactate is that it reflects cellular oxygenation disturbances with more certainty than other methods. If lactate levels are rising, there is an excellent possibility of an imbalance in cellular oxygenation. Although there are other reasons for lactate increases, the most common and significant reason in the critically ill population is an oxygen deficit.

Lactate levels do not necessarily correlate with other parameters of oxygenation, such as Svo_2 and Do_2 (Astiz et al., 1988). The reasons for this are not well understood, but may be related to variations in individual metabolic needs or regional perfusion problems. The important point is that, in a patient with a threatened oxygenation status, as many variables should be examined as possible to determine whether a trend of worsening oxygenation can be established.

The disadvantage of lactate levels is the lag time between cellular lactate generation and serum values. Levels below 2 mmol/L do not necessarily indicate normal oxygenation because they do not rule out regional or beginning oxygenation imbalances (Mizock, 1987). By the time the cellular lactate level corresponds to the serum level, several minutes (possibly longer in underperfused areas) may have passed. On the other hand, if cellular lactate levels are returning to normal, the serum value will not immediately reflect this change. Although increases in lactate levels indicate that a problem with oxygenation exists, these increases are not as time specific as other parameters of oxygenation. Interpretation of lactate levels is an important part of oxygenation assessments, but should not be used to reflect immediate assessment of oxygenation. When lactate levels change, other factors may be present, such as gluconeogenesis (sepsis) or hepatic dysfunction. These conditions can increase lactate in the absence of hypoxia. Two methods exist for improving the specificity of lactate interpretation. First, measurement of lactate with pyruvate will help distinguish hypoxia from other forms of increased lactate. If hypoxia is present, lactate increases disproportionately to pyruvate. This will distort the normal lactate/pyruvate ratio of 10:1. In hypoxia, the lactate/pyruvate level is greater than 10:1 because pyruvate is not produced at the same rate as lactate.

A second method, although less accurate, is to com-

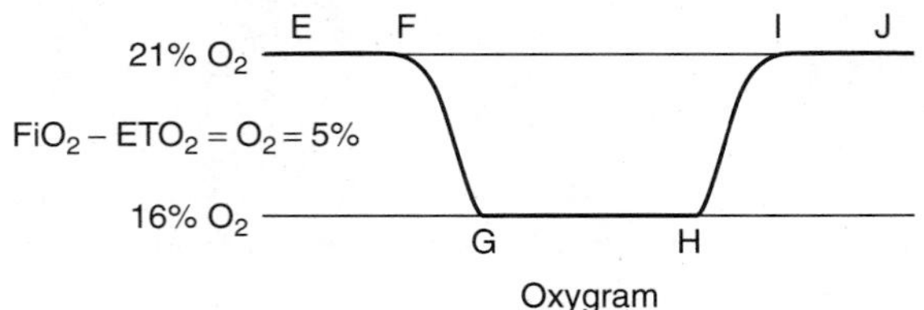

FIGURE 15–3. Oxygram reflecting oxygen extraction through measurement of FIO_2 − FEO_2 difference. (From Weingarten, M., & Wallen, R. D. [1992]. Hewlett-Packard *Advances*, October, 8–13.)

pare lactate with bicarbonate (HCO_3). If hypoxia is present, it should produce a metabolic acidosis, resulting in a decrease in HCO_3 as the lactate increases.

OXYGRAMS. Another method to assess the balance between oxygen delivery and consumption is through the analysis of inspired (FIO_2) and expired (FEO_2) oxygen concentrations. If this assessment is performed continuously, a display of the oxygen concentration can be provided (Fig. 15–3). This display of the inspired and expired oxygen concentrations is referred to as an oxygram (Weingarten, 1990).

The oxygram can be used to display the balance of oxygen delivery and consumption by measuring how great a difference exists between FIO_2 and FEO_2. Normally, the FIO_2 − FEO_2 difference is about 5%. For example, on room air (FIO_2 of 0.21), a healthy person has an FEO_2 of about 0.16. This difference normally holds steady as long as the balance between oxygen delivery and consumption remains adequate. If oxygen delivery falls or oxygen consumption increases faster than oxygen delivery, then the FEO_2 falls. The fall in the FEO_2 reflects a greater extraction of oxygen at the tissue level. Because more oxygen is being extracted at the tissue level, less oxygen is returned to the lungs to be expired. The net result is a drop in the FEO_2.

How much a drop in the FEO_2 must occur before a clinically dangerous situation is present is not clear. What should be noted in observing the oxygram is primarily if the FIO_2 − FEO_2 difference is increasing. If it is increasing, then a threat to oxygenation at the tissue level is potentially present.

The advantage to using the oxygram lies in its noninvasive nature. The measurement of exhaled gases is simple and does not require a pulmonary artery catheter. If a pulmonary artery catheter is not in place, then an oxygram is an appropriate substitute for assessment of tissue oxygenation. The primary disadvantage in the use of the oxygram lies in the imperfect technology available for sampling exhaled air. Measurement of exhaled oxygen requires great precision, precision that is easily altered through technical limitations (such as air leaks in the ventilator circuit and obstructions to aspiration of air for the oxygen analyzer). Although oxygrams are potentially useful, their technical limitations can be problematic.

There is no perfect method of assessing oxygenation at this time. Some advances can be seen in the application of computer technology to the use of simultaneous parameters, such as SpO_2 and SvO_2, to allow more continuous assessment of the components of oxygenation (Rasanen et al., 1987). What is still needed, however, is an easy-to-apply, continuous, and rapid means of reflecting cellular oxygenation. Newer techniques such as positron emission tomography are being developed that should aid in more sophisticated assessment of cellular oxygenation. Until such techniques are fully developed, assessment of oxygenation must depend on combining the components of oxygenation, centering on the aspects of oxygen transport and consumption.

PaO_2 AND INTRAPULMONARY SHUNTING

Although the PaO_2 is of limited use in assessing oxygen transport, it can be used to estimate one of the parameters of lung function. Intrapulmonary shunting (Qs / Qt), the main cause of clinical hypoxemia, can be estimated by noting the discrepancy between alveolar (PAO_2) and arterial (PaO_2) oxygen levels.

Normal intrapulmonary shunts are small, usually less than 5% of the total pulmonary blood flow. Intrapulmonary shunting, defined as blood passing through underventilated alveoli, is illustrated in Figure 15–4. As intrapulmonary shunting increases, the work on the heart and respiratory muscles also increases. Cardiac work increases because an increase in cardiac output is necessary to compensate for the decreased oxygen exchange resulting from reduced alveolar function. Respiratory work increases in an attempt to compensate and to provide increased alveolar ventilation to functioning alveoli.

Clinically, intrapulmonary shunting does not present significant problems until the shunt fraction climbs higher than 15%. Near 15% shunt values, the patient experiences increases in the work of breathing and in myocardial oxygen consumption. At levels higher than 30%, the work of maintaining alveolar ventilation may require mechanical ventilation (West, 1990).

Estimates of Qs / Qt can be useful clinically to track progress or deterioration in clinical situations. Several methods exist that either measure or attempt to estimate intrapulmonary shunting. The key to estimating the size of the intrapulmonary shunt is the concept that alveolar oxygen levels are the primary determinant of arterial levels. Normally, venous blood in the pulmonary circulation is exposed to alveoli with immediate equilibration of alveolar / blood oxygen tensions. Arterial levels should, in theory, equal alveolar levels. The major reason that arterial levels do not equal alveolar levels is that alveoli are not being ventilated. Venous blood passing through nonfunctioning alveoli creates a mixture of venous and arterial blood. The result is a decreased PaO_2.

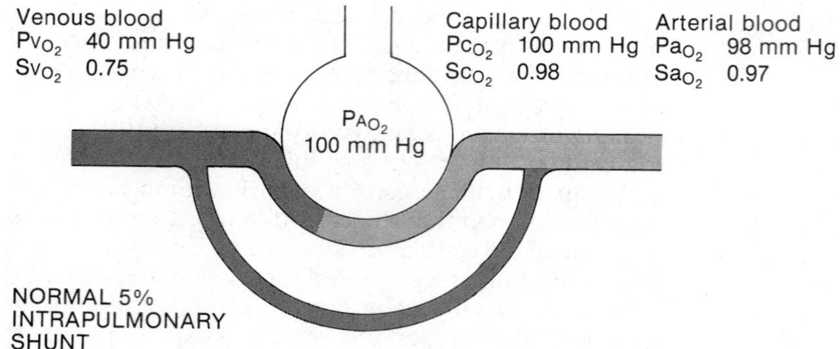

P_{VO_2}—Partial pressure of oxygen in the veins
S_{VO_2}—Hemoglobin saturation with oxygen in the veins
P_{CO_2}—Partial pressure of oxygen in the capillaries
S_{CO_2}—Hemoglobin saturation with oxygen in the capillaries
Pa_{O_2}—Partial pressure of oxygen in the arteries
Sa_{O_2}—Hemoglobin saturation in the arteries
P_{AO_2}—Partial pressure of oxygen in the alveoli

FIGURE 15–4. Normal intrapulmonary shunt. (Copyright 1987, American Journal of Nursing Company. Reprinted from American Journal of Nursing, 1987, 87[3], 337A–340H. Used with permission. All rights reserved.)

Intrapulmonary shunting can be measured by using the shunt formula:

$$Qs/Qt = \frac{Cc_{O_2} - Ca_{O_2}}{Cc_{O_2} - Cv_{O_2}}$$

This formula is the most accurate estimate of Qs/Qt, although it has two obvious drawbacks. The most obvious is the need for a pulmonary artery catheter to obtain the Cv_{O_2} value. The second is the assumption that end-capillary oxygen values for the calculation of Cc_{O_2} will be the same as alveolar oxygen values. The primary problem with the use of the classic shunt equation is its limited practicality in patients without pulmonary artery catheters. Because of this limitation, several other methods of estimating Qs/Qt have been proposed. Included in these estimates are the alveolar/arterial gradient, arterial/alveolar ratio, Pa_{O_2}/F_{IO_2} ratio, and the respiratory index. Each of these has its own strengths and weaknesses. They are all based on a comparison of the difference between alveolar and arterial oxygen values in an attempt to approximate Qs/Qt easily. Table 15–2 presents the formulas and normal values for each of these estimates of Qs/Qt.

Other methods for estimating Qs/Qt exist that attempt to use more data than the oxygen tension indices. The clinical shunt equation, which uses an assumed $Ca_{O_2} - Cv_{O_2}$ value of 3.5 cc/dL, has the potential to be more accurate than the oxygen tension indices (Cane et al., 1988). Another promising technique is possible in patients in whom both Sp_{O_2} and Sv_{O_2} values are available. Through computer integration of simultaneous changes in both Sp_{O_2} and Sv_{O_2}, an improved accuracy in estimating Qs/Qt is possible (Rasanen et al., 1987). If an institution has the technologic ability to integrate data, more accurate assessments are likely. Critical care nurses should learn the capabilities of their institution to explore the potential to calculate more sophisticated estimates of parameters such as Qs/Qt.

The primary advantage of using oxygen tension indices as opposed to the other techniques of measuring Qs/Qt is the ability to apply the indices easily and to use them in all patients with available blood gas values. It is crucial to keep in mind that the oxygen tension indices are guidelines rather than exact values for estimating Qs/Qt. Owing to the ease of use of oxygen tension indices, practical illustrations of Qs/Qt

TABLE 15–2. **Estimates of Intrapulmonary Shunting**

Estimate Measure	Formula	Normal Value
Pa_{O_2}/F_{IO_2} ratio	$\frac{Pa_{O_2}}{F_{IO_2}}$	Greater than 300
Arterial/alveolar ratio	$\frac{Pa_{O_2}}{P_{AO_2}}$	Greater than 60%
Alveolar–arterial gradient	$P_{AO_2} - Pa_{O_2}$	0–20 mm Hg
Respiratory index	$\frac{P_{AO_2} - Pa_{O_2}}{Pa_{O_2}}$	<1
O_2 content index	$\frac{Cc_{O_2} - Ca_{O_2}}{(Cc_{O_2} - Ca_{O_2}) + 3.5}$	<5%

where P_{AO_2} = alveolar oxygen tension; P_{AO_2} is obtained by the following equation

$$F_{IO_2}(Pb - H_2O) - Pa_{CO_2}/RQ$$

where F_{IO_2} = fraction of inspired oxygen
Pb = barometric pressure (approximately 760 mm Hg at sea level)
H_2O = alveolar water vapor pressure (47 mm Hg)
Pa_{CO_2} = partial pressure of arterial carbon dioxide
RQ = respiratory quotient (normally 0.8)

tracking will be explained through common clinical situations.

Clinical Applications of Qs/Qt

Three common methods exist, e.g., the A-a gradient, the PaO_2/FIO_2 ratio, and the a/A ratio. The A-a gradient is the least accurate, the a/A ratio the most accurate, and the PaO_2/FIO_2 ratio the easiest. Either the PaO_2/FIO_2 ratio or the a/A ratio should be used due to their ease of use (PaO_2/FIO_2 ratio) or accuracy (a/A ratio). In this chapter, the a/A ratio will be illustrated although the PaO_2/FIO_2 is a legitimate estimate of Qs/Qt. The arterial-to-alveolar (a/A) ratio is one of the oldest methods of estimating Qs/Qt and has demonstrated clinical utility in several studies (Gilbert & Keighley, 1974). Although the a/A ratio has limitations (Covelli et al., 1983), it can be applied under many conditions (Gilbert et al., 1979). The a/A ratio will be presented here as a satisfactory means of estimating Qs/Qt, with the understanding that other methods can also be used with similar accuracy.

To apply the a/A ratio, the alveolar level must be calculated. Alveolar oxygen levels can be computed by the alveolar air equation:

$$P_AO_2 = FIO_2\ (P_B \times PH_2O) - PaCO_2/r$$

This equation can be simplified by allowing the following assumptions: (1) P_B (barometric pressure) is 760; (2) PH_2O (water vapor pressure) is 47; (3) r (respiratory quotient) is 0.8. These assumptions are generally accurate at sea level. If these assumptions are allowed, then the equation is calculated:

$$P_AO_2 = FIO_2\ (713) - PaCO_2/0.8$$

The alveolar oxygen tension on room air (FIO_2 of 0.21) could be calculated as follows (assume a normal $PaCO_2$ of 40):

$$P_AO_2 = 0.21\ (713) - 40/0.8 = 100 \text{ mm Hg}$$

Normally, arterial levels differ only slightly from alveolar levels. If the acceptable PaO_2 level is 60 to 100 mm Hg, the normal a/A ratio on room air would be between 0.60 and 1.00:

	PaO_2 60	PaO_2 100
P_AO_2	100	100
a/A	0.60	1.00

As long as the a/A ratio is over 0.60, the intrapulmonary shunt is small. If the shunt increases, the a/A ratio decreases. The lower the a/A ratio, the worse the patient's pulmonary status. The following examples illustrate applications of the a/A ratio to clinical settings.

CASE HISTORIES

Case 6. Assume that a patient has returned from the operating room on 100% oxygen. He has the following blood gases: PaO_2, 470; $PaCO_2$, 40. Should his FIO_2 be lowered slowly or quickly? The alveolar oxygen level is: P_AO_2 = 1.00 (713) − 40/0.8 = 663. The patient has an a/A ratio of 0.71 (470/663), which is within the normal range. His intrapulmonary shunt is so small that oxygen therapy is probably unnecessary. For this patient, the oxygen level probably could be reduced markedly and he would still maintain PaO_2 levels higher than 60 mm Hg.

Case 7. A patient with a 40% face mask in place receives a meal. He has a PaO_2 of 88, and a $PaCO_2$ of 35. Can you allow him to remove his mask to eat without replacing it with a nasal cannula? The alveolar oxygen level is: 0.40 (713) − 35/0.8 = 241. The a/A ratio is 0.37 (88/241). The ratio is well below normal limits, indicating substantial intrapulmonary shunting. The patient would therefore require supplemental oxygen even while eating to avoid PaO_2 levels of less than 60 mm Hg.

Case 8. A patient experiences an FIO_2 change from 50% to 30%. His blood gases change as follows:

	FIO_2 0.50	FIO_2 0.30
PaO_2	110	68
$PaCO_2$	39	41

Based on the change in FIO_2, did the lung function change? In the first reading, the a/A ratio is 0.36 (110/307). In the second, the ratio is 0.42 (68/163). Lung function appears to be practically unchanged, although the a/A ratio is slightly improved.

The use of estimates of Qs/Qt can guide assessment of clinical changes relative to lung function. These estimates are not to be assumed to be as accurate as the actual measurement of Qs/Qt. Several limitations of the a/A ratio (and other estimates of Qs/Qt) are present, and the clinician should be aware of these to apply the a/A ratio safely. One limitation is the effect of the SvO_2 on the PaO_2. When Qs/Qt is large, changes in SvO_2 are more likely to change PaO_2 values (Fig. 15–5). Subsequently, the a/A ratio may change without a change in Qs/Qt. If the patient has an unstable oxygenation status with a potential for reductions in SvO_2, a/A ratios should be used more cautiously.

A second limitation is that small changes in the a/A ratio may not have significant meaning. For example, if the a/A ratio changes from 0.35 to 0.39, this change usually does not indicate a substantial change in lung function. The a/A ratio should change by greater than 5% before any assumption of change in Qs/Qt has occurred. How much the a/A ratio should change before it indicates a clinically significant change in Qs/Qt requires further research. In addition, although a normal a/A ratio may be as low as 0.60, a ratio higher than 0.60 should be allowed when using the a/A ratio to estimate what level of FIO_2 support should be used. Because the a/A ratio estimates

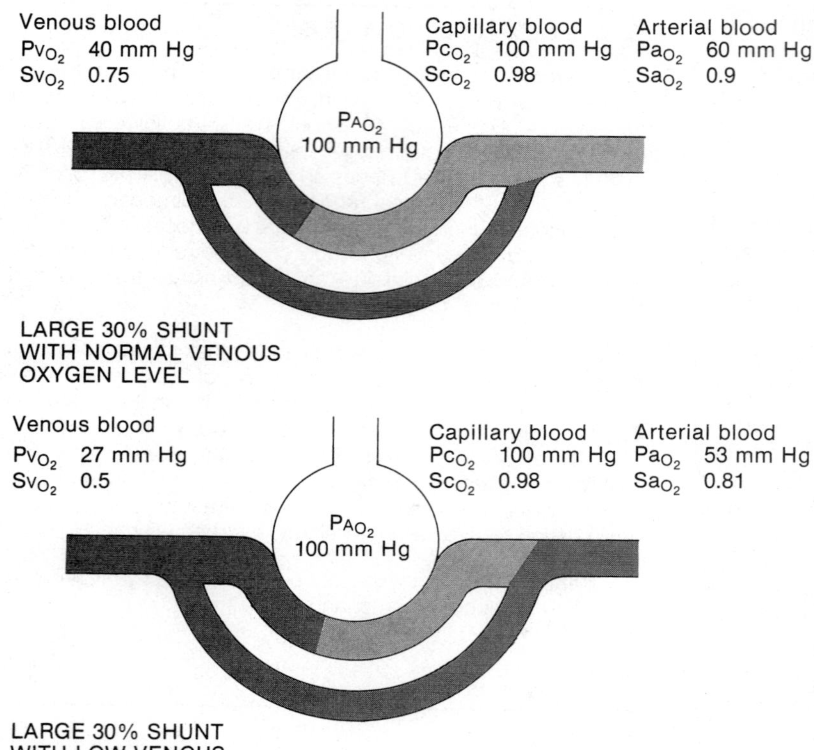

FIGURE 15–5. Effect of Sv_{O_2} on Pa_{O_2}. (Copyright 1987, American Journal of Nursing Company. Reprinted from American Journal of Nursing, 1987, 87[3], 337A–340H. Used with permission. All rights reserved.)

Qs/Qt and is not "rock" stable, a safety margin should be allowed when applying the ratio to change FI_{O_2} support. For example, if the a/A ratio is near 0.60, oxygen support is probably unnecessary. Yet to allow for a safety margin, a reduction in the FI_{O_2} to 0.24 to 0.28 would be more clinically acceptable. This would avoid a situation in which the a/A ratio might change and not predict a fall in the Pa_{O_2} to less than 60 mm Hg.

Another method of estimating the Qs/Qt is the Pa_{O_2}/FI_{O_2} ratio. This value is simpler to calculate than the a/A ratio. Many clinicians prefer this method because it does not require calculation of the alveolar air equation to obtain the PA_{O_2}. A normal Pa_{O_2}/FI_{O_2} ratio is greater than 286. The lower the value, the worse the Qs/Qt. For example, a normal Qs/Qt would have a Pa_{O_2} of 80 on room air (0.21 oxygen). This would result in a Pa_{O_2}/FI_{O_2} ratio of 381 (80/0.21). In another example, if a patient has a Pa_{O_2} of 75 on an FI_{O_2} of 0.40, he or she would have a Pa_{O_2}/FI_{O_2} ratio of 188 (75/0.40). This is abnormally low and would indicate an increased Qs/Qt.

It is important when using estimates of Qs/Qt to acknowledge that they are just estimates, not replacements for Qs/Qt measurements. If one can measure Qs/Qt, as is possible with continuous Sv_{O_2} and Sa_{O_2} monitoring, the actual Qs/Qt should be measured. In the absence of Qs/Qt measurements, techniques such as the a/A and Pa_{O_2}/FI_{O_2} ratios can be used to approximate Qs/Qt.

VD/VT APPLICATION

The Pa_{CO_2} value can be used to estimate a second aspect of lung function in much the same way as Pa_{O_2} is used to estimate Qs/Qt. Pa_{CO_2}, in conjunction with other respiratory parameters, can be used to estimate dead space-to-tidal volume ratio (VD/VT). In addition, actual measurement of dead space can be done if exhaled gases and volumes are present. This section describes the methods used to estimate VD/VT from Pa_{CO_2} values and respiratory parameters, and reviews ways to measure VD/VT from exhaled gases.

The normal amount of dead space (the amount of inspired air not participating in gas exchange) is usually 25% to 35% of each breath or tidal volume (VT). Two types of dead space exist, anatomic and physiologic. Anatomic dead space is the amount of air that will not reach gas-exchanging units owing to the anatomy of the lung. For example, airways as low as the terminal bronchioles contain air that cannot participate in alveolar gas exchange. Physiologic dead space is anatomic dead space plus any increase in inspired volume that cannot participate in gas exchange. For example, if a patient has a pulmonary embolism, no blood will perfuse the affected area of functioning alveoli. The affected area now does not participate in gas exchange and adds to the dead space volume. The dead space volume that is of interest to clinicians is the physiologic dead space.

An understanding of dead space is important because of the impact of increased dead space on respiratory effort. As dead space increases, the work of breathing increases. Increased work of breathing occurs as increased volumes of air are necessary to reach functioning alveoli. If a part of the alveolar area cannot participate in gas exchange, more air must be brought to alveoli that are in contact with functioning pulmonary capillaries. Unfortunately, as a person inspires, part of the air inspired still goes to the lung unit that is not in contact with functioning alveoli. To increase the volume of air to the functioning alveoli, overall ventilation (minute ventilation) must increase. The net result is increased work of breathing proportional to the degree of dead space.

$Paco_2$ is maintained at normal levels as long as adequate alveolar ventilation (VA) is maintained. $Paco_2$ falls if excessive alveolar ventilation occurs relative to carbon dioxide production (Vco_2). $Paco_2$ values rise if alveolar ventilation is inadequate when compared to Vco_2, or if pulmonary blood flow falls. Clinically, a rise in $Paco_2$ has more serious implications because a rise in $Paco_2$ values can bring about an acute respiratory acidosis, producing a simultaneous systematic acidosis. Because of the role of $Paco_2$ in reflecting alveolar ventilation, it can be used to estimate dead space volume.

Under ordinary circumstances, if minute ventilation (VE) is within normal limits (5 to 10 L/minute). $Paco_2$ is also normal provided VD is normal. The combination of normal VD and normal VE will result in adequate alveolar ventilation (VA). Changes in $Paco_2$ levels can usually be traced to the factors affecting VA, such as changes in VD. As a practical aid, VE can be measured by a spirometer or estimated by noting a change in respiratory rate or depth. The following examples of changes in $Paco_2$ values and the influence of VD/VT will aid in identification of the cause of $Paco_2$ changes.

DECREASED $Paco_2$ LEVELS AND VD/VT. When the $Paco_2$ falls below normal levels (less than 35 mm Hg), VA and VE must be increased. In such circumstances, VD is usually normal or minimally increased. It is important to note that when VE is elevated and $Paco_2$ is decreased, pulmonary dysfunction usually is not a problem. The cause of the low $Paco_2$ can usually be narrowed to the following factors:

1. Factors affecting the voluntary control of breathing, such as anxiety or fear, causing an increase in breathing
2. Compensatory response to a metabolic acidosis
3. Excessive ventilation due to inappropriate mechanical ventilation settings
4. Neurologic injury at the brain stem level

Low $Paco_2$ levels are not usually dangerous. They are, however, guides to other problems. Whenever a respiratory alkalosis exists, a search for the problem causing excessive work of breathing should be made. Correction of the problem will correct the abnormal $Paco_2$.

Physical assessment is helpful in the clinical assessment of dead space. VE is the most helpful tool in assessing dead space noninvasively. However, measurement of VE is not always practical. Assessment of respiratory rate and tidal volume (depth of breathing) can be used as a substitute for VE measurement, yet inaccuracies can occur. For example, a patient with a rapid respiratory rate may not have an increased VE if the VT is reduced. Or, a rapid respiratory rate may not lower the $Paco_2$ if the VD/VT has increased. Therefore, if a patient is breathing rapidly or deeply, he or she may or may not be hyperventilating (lowering the $Paco_2$), depending on the VD/VT. If the dead space is large, the patient with a rapid respiratory rate may actually be hypoventilating. Without blood gas measurement to determine $Paco_2$ levels and dead space, a patient breathing rapidly should be identified as tachypneic, not hyperventilating.

INCREASED $Paco_2$ LEVELS. Increased $Paco_2$ levels occur only when alveolar ventilation is inadequate or when decreased pulmonary perfusion occurs. Such a situation could occur in the presence of the following factors:

1. Medication-induced brain stem depression
2. Increased dead space ventilation
   a. Pulmonary emboli
   b. Chronic lung disease
3. Severe hypovolemia
4. Cardiopulmonary resuscitation (CPR; reflecting loss of pulmonary perfusion)

Respiratory acidosis is always significant because it indicates inadequate alveolar air movement. It becomes more serious, however, when the increased $Paco_2$ occurs suddenly without renal compensation. In this situation, the respiratory impairment is of recent origin and implies acute respiratory embarrassment. If the $Paco_2$ rises and produces a pH less than 7.25, intubation should be considered, particularly in light of a decreasing level of consciousness.

Identifying the cause of the increased CO_2 retention involves a search for any reason for respiratory depression or loss of pulmonary blood flow. If respiratory depression or loss of blood flow is not likely, then increased dead space is the likely cause. Even without an identifiable cause of respiratory depression, the reason for an increase in $Paco_2$ level can be determined by a knowledge of the $Paco_2$ level and VE. When both the $Paco_2$ and VE are increased, VD must also be increased, because normally an increased VE would lower the $Paco_2$. In addition, an increased VD can be identified even if the $Paco_2$ is normal, provided the VE is increased.

If the $Paco_2$ is increased but VE is low, VD/VT is probably normal. The cause of the increased $Paco_2$ is respiratory depression. The $Paco_2$ has increased simply because of reduced alveolar ventilation.

CASE HISTORIES

To help illustrate these concepts, the following specific cases are presented.

Case 9. A 42-year-old woman was in your unit postoperatively after a colon resection. She was breathing rapidly and appeared anxious. You obtain a blood gas determination and the following respiratory parameters. From the information presented here, what is the likely cause of the increased work of breathing?

Pa_{CO_2} (mm Hg)	20
Pa_{O_2} (mm Hg)	92
F_{IO_2}	0.21
V_E (L/minute)	15
RR (bpm)	30
V_T (cc)	500

The Pa_{CO_2} is low secondary to an increased V_E. The V_D/V_T is probably normal because the Pa_{CO_2} is expected to decrease with an increase in V_E. One of the reasons listed earlier that increase V_E without pulmonary dysfunction must be present. In this case, anxiety or pain is a potential cause.

Case 10. A 52-year-old man was admitted to your unit after an abdominal aortic aneurysm repair. Shortly after admission to the unit, he was extubated. During your postextubation assessment, you note that he is difficult to wake and responds only to vigorous stimuli. You obtain a set of blood gas levels and respiratory parameters as follows:

Pa_{CO_2} (mm Hg)	55
pH	7.28
Pa_{O_2} (mm Hg)	100
F_{IO_2}	0.30
V_E (L/minute)	3
RR (bpm)	15
V_T (cc)	200

In this patient, the Pa_{CO_2} is high due to a low V_E. The V_D/V_T is probably normal because the Pa_{CO_2} is expected to rise if the V_E is inadequate. The cause of the increased Pa_{CO_2} may be respiratory depression. Perhaps the anesthetic has not been completely eliminated. Reintubation should be considered.

Case 11. A 65-year-old man with a diagnosis of chronic obstructive pulmonary disease is in your unit. He had no immediate distress, although he had complained of shortness of breath in the emergency room. His admitting blood gas levels and respiratory parameters are as follows:

Pa_{CO_2} (mm Hg)	70
pH	7.35
Pa_{O_2} (mm Hg)	67
F_{IO_2}	0.28
V_E (L/minute)	13
RR (bpm)	30
V_T (cc)	433

The Pa_{CO_2} in this patient was increased along with the V_E. The cause is most likely an increased V_D or a reduction in pulmonary blood flow. Because the patient has a compensated respiratory acidosis, the problem is more likely chronic. The chronic nature of the problem probably reflects an increased V_D secondary to the lung disease. Problems of reduced blood flow tend to be short-term in nature.

Case 12. A 32-year-old woman was admitted to the unit complaining of shortness of breath and right-sided chest pain. She had the following blood gas levels and respiratory parameters.

Pa_{CO_2} (mm Hg)	40
pH	7.38
Pa_{O_2} (mm Hg)	89
F_{IO_2}	.40
V_E (L/minute)	16
RR (bpm)	32
V_T (cc)	500

This patient had a normal Pa_{CO_2} with an increased V_E. Either the V_D is increased or the pulmonary perfusion is reduced if the Pa_{CO_2} is normal in the presence of an increased V_E. In this patient, the increased V_E without a corresponding fall in the Pa_{CO_2} is of concern. A problem with pulmonary blood flow (pulmonary embolus) causing a large dead space is likely in this person.

Exhaled Gas Analysis

Estimation of V_D and arterial P_{CO_2} has been made more accurate by the use of exhaled gas analyzers, specifically capnography (carbon dioxide waveform) analysis. Technically, CO_2 is measured by either mass spectrometry or infrared analysis (Stock, 1988). Mass spectrometry requires the aspiration of exhaled gas samples for analysis by a mass spectrometer. Infrared analysis requires a sample chamber and gas analyzer attached to part of the expired circuit (usually the exhalation tubing in the ventilation circuit). Each technique has advantages and limitations, although both can be used with generally accurate results.

The theory of analyzing exhaled CO_2 is based on two factors—first, the CO_2 elimination pattern during exhalation, and second, the total percentage of CO_2 eliminated during exhalation. The CO_2 elimination pattern makes possible the prediction of arterial CO_2 values, and the total percentage of CO_2 exhaled makes dead space analysis feasible. Examples of the clinical application of each of these factors will help to illustrate the theoretical principles of exhaled gas analysis.

END-TIDAL CARBON DIOXIDE (P_{ETCO_2}) ANALYSIS

During exhalation, the initial percentage of CO_2 is minimal. As gas from the alveoli enter the larger airways, the percentage of CO_2 increases until the end of exhalation. At this point, the percentage of CO_2 approximates alveolar levels. An example of the exhaled CO_2 waveform is shown in Figure 15–6. The near-alveolar levels allow a useful clinical application (i.e., prediction of arterial CO_2 values). Because alveolar and arterial CO_2 values are similar, samples of exhaled CO_2 at the end of exhalation can provide approximate Pa_{CO_2} values.

The P_{ETCO_2} is usually lower than Pa_{CO_2} levels. If the P_{ETCO_2} is 30 mm Hg, the Pa_{CO_2} is higher than 30 mm Hg. How much higher depends on several factors, primarily pulmonary blood flow. Under normal circumstances (normal pulmonary blood flow), P_{ETCO_2} does not vary from $Pa{CO_2}$ by more than several millimeters of mercury. Unfortunately, in critical care settings, the assumptions for $P_{ETCO_2}/Pa{CO_2}$ correlations are not always met (Russell & Graybeal, 1994). This means that the clinician needs to apply data from P_{ETCO_2} analysis in conjunction with other clinical data before making judgments based on P_{ETCO_2} changes.

The use of P_{ETCO_2}, despite its limitations, has several clinical applications. The primary benefit of exhaled gas analysis is the continuous evaluation of alveolar ventilation. Reliance on blood gas levels is markedly reduced, providing both an economic (reduction in cost) and patient (reduction in pain) advantage. The value of P_{ETCO_2} analysis centers on assessments that are useful in monitoring $Pa{CO_2}$ changes. P_{ETCO_2} analysis is commonly used for monitoring during spontaneous breathing (weaning) trials, ventilator changes, CPR, endotracheal intubation, and dead space analysis.

During weaning and ventilator changes, the P_{ETCO_2} can be used as a marker for observing acceptable $Pa{CO_2}$ values. If the P_{ETCO_2} increases during weaning, a blood gas determination may be necessary to determine the extent of the developing respiratory acidosis. The value of P_{ETCO_2} lies in its capability for constant monitoring and early identification of problems in alveolar ventilation.

Endotracheal intubation can be confirmed by noting the capnograph waveform. Esophageal intubations do not produce CO_2 waveforms. Avoidance of dangerous situations in which esophageal intubations may occur offers a strong advantage to any unit in which endotracheal intubations are common. P_{ETCO_2} analysis has been so useful in this area that many anesthesia departments are now equipped with mass spectrometers, partly to assess CO_2 waveforms to avoid esophageal intubations (Bhavani-Shankar et al., 1992).

Exhaled CO_2 has been described as useful in determining the adequacy of CPR (Callahan & Barton, 1990; Graver et al., 1991; Weil et al., 1985). The principle applied in CPR is similar to the effect of pulmonary blood flow on P_{ETCO_2} (Boseman et al., 1991; Carroll, 1992; Ornato et al., 1990). Weil and associates (1985) noted that the mixed venous $P{CO_2}$ value increased during CPR, possibly indicating diminished pulmonary blood flow and resulting in inadequate clearance of CO_2. Weil's group postulated that the adequacy of CPR could be determined by noting the capnograph

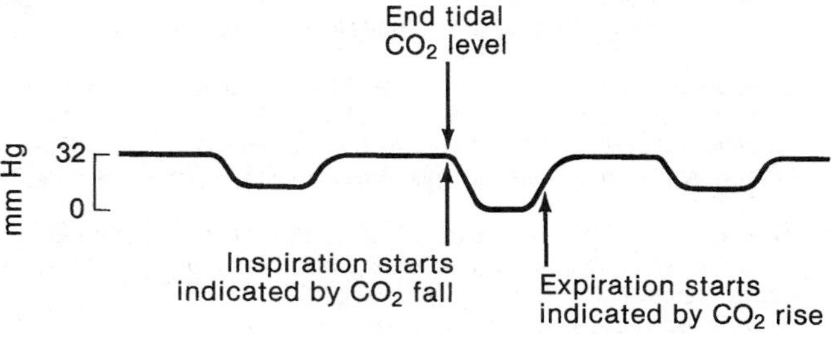

FIGURE 15–6. Tracing of capnogram.

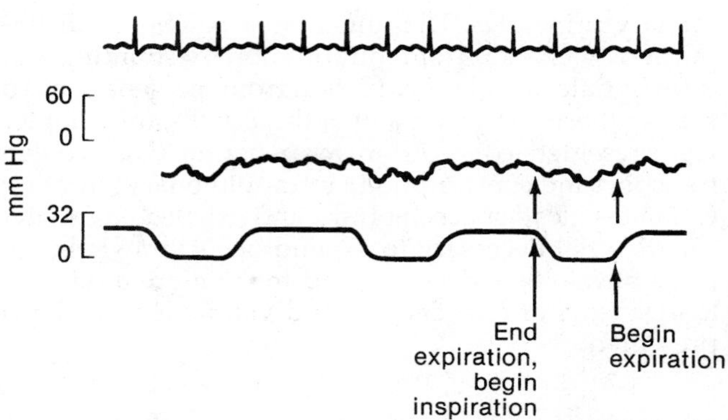

FIGURE 15–7. Use of capnogram in hemodynamic waveform analysis to identify end-exhalation.

results. If blood flow is adequate, a good capnograph is produced. If CPR is inadequate, the capnograph will accurately and quickly illustrate the problem.

Exhaled gas analysis is also helpful in reading end-expiration tracings during hemodynamic waveform analysis. The point at which inspiration begins (end-exhalation) can be noted by a drop in the CO_2 waveform. The point just before the drop in CO_2 level can be used to identify end-exhalation. Through this technique, inspiratory artifact in pulmonary artery tracings can be avoided relatively easily (Fig. 15–7).

DEAD SPACE ANALYSIS WITH EXHALED CARBON DIOXIDE

Dead space data can be obtained using mixed exhaled CO_2 values combined with P_{ETCO_2} values to yield noninvasive assessment of V_D. In practical terms, the mixed exhaled $P{CO_2}$ values are better applied with $Pa{CO_2}$ values, but P_{ETCO_2} can be used as a substitute to provide continuous V_D analysis. If a problem develops in a patient that may change the dead space volume (i.e., a pulmonary embolus), the use of exhaled gas analysis can detect the problem earlier than all other clinical measurements commonly used. The formula for measuring V_D/V_T is:

$$\frac{Pa{CO_2}}{Pa{CO_2} - P_{ETCO_2}}$$

The prime advantage of all exhaled gas analysis methods is the speed with which assessments can be made in regard to pulmonary gas exchange and blood flow. Questions exist about the cost effectiveness of these applications, and these can be answered only through further research. Empirically, exhaled gas analysis appears to have several specific and practical applications.

SUMMARY

Assessment of oxygenation and ventilation requires possession of substantial understanding of cardiopulmonary principles. The nurse must be able to distinguish oxygenation from intrapulmonary shunting and differentiate alveolar ventilation from oxygenation. To further the accomplishment of these skills, this chapter has presented concepts in oxygenation (i.e., oxygen transport and consumption), intrapulmonary shunting estimates, dead space analysis, and exhaled gas analysis. Material necessary to expand one's knowledge of basic physiologic concepts and make more advanced assessments of oxygenation and ventilation has been presented.

REFERENCES

Ahrens, T. S., & Rutherford, K. A. (1993). *Essentials of oxygenation.* Boston: Jones & Bartlett.

Ahrens, T. S., & Rutherford, K. (1987). The new pulmonary math: Applying the a/A ratio. *American Journal of Nursing, 87,* 337A–340H.

Ahrens, T. S. (1990). Svo_2 monitoring: Is it being used appropriately? *Critical Care Nurse, 10,* 70–72.

Alexander, C. M., Teller, L. E., & Gross, J. B. (1989). Principles of oximetry: Theoretical and practical considerations. *Anesthesia and Analgesia, 68,* 368–376.

Appel, P. L., & Shoemaker, W. C. (1992). Relationship of oxygen consumption and oxygen delivery in surgical patients with ARDS. *Chest, 102,* 906–911.

Astiz, M. E., Rachow, E. C., Kaufman, B., et al. (1988). Relationship of oxygen delivery and mixed venous oxygenation to lactic acidosis in patients with sepsis and acute myocardial infarction. *Critical Care Medicine, 16,* 655–658.

Barker, S. J., & Tremper, K. K. (1987). Pulse oximetry: Applications and limitations. *International Anesthesiology Clinics, 25*(3), 155–175.

Bhavani-Shankar, K., Moseley, H., Kumar, A. Y., & Delph, Y. (1992). Capnometry and anaesthesia. *Canadian Journal of Anaesthesia, 39,* 617–632.

Bierman, M. I., Stein, K. L., Snyder, J. V. (1992). Pulse oximetry in the postoperative care of cardiac surgical patients: A randomized controlled trial. *Chest, 102,* 1367–1370.

Boseman, R. J., Stoutenbeek, C. P., & Zandstra, D. F. (1991). Non-invasive pulmonary blood flow measurement by means of CO_2 analysis of expiratory gases. *Intensive Care Medicine, 17,* 98–102.

Broder, G., & Weil, M. H. (1964). Excess lactate: An index of reversibility of shock in human patients. *Science, 143,* 1457–1459.

Bunn, H. F., & Forget, B. G. (1986). *Hemoglobin: Molecular genetics, and clinical aspects.* Philadelphia: W. B. Saunders.

Cain, S. M. (1983). Peripheral oxygen uptake in health and disease. *Clinics in Chest Medicine, 4,* 139–148.

Callaham, M., & Barton, C. (1990). Prediction of outcome of cardiopulmonary resuscitation from end-tidal carbon dioxide concentration. *Critical Care Medicine, 18,* 358–362.

Cane, R. D., Shapiro, B. A., Templin, R., et al. (1988). Unreliability of oxygen derived tension based indices in reflecting intrapulmonary shunting in critically ill patients. *Critical Care Medicine, 16,* 1243–1245.

Carroll, G. C. (1992). Capnographic trend curve monitoring can detect 1 ml pulmonary emboli in humans. *Journal of Clinical Monitoring, 8,* 101–106.

Cheng, E. Y., Hopwood, M. B., & Kay, J. (1988). Forehead pulse oximetry compared with finger pulse oximetry and arterial blood gas measurement. *Journal of Clinical Monitoring, 4,* 223–226.

Chulay, M., Palmer, J., Neblett, J., et al. (1992). Clinical comparison of two and three wavelength systems for continuous measurement of venous oxygen saturation. *American Journal of Critical Care, 1,* 69–75.

Council on Scientific Affairs, American Medical Association. (1993). The use of pulse oximetry during conscious sedation. *Journal of the American Medical Association, 270,* 1463–1468.

Covelli, H. D., Nessan, V. J., & Tuttle, W. K. (1983). Oxygen derived variables in acute respiratory failure. *Critical Care Medicine, 11,* 646–649.

DiBendetto, R. J., Graves, S. A., Gravenstein, N., & Konicek, C. (1994). Pulse oximetry monitoring can change routine oxygen supplementation practices in postanesthesia care unit. *Anesthesia and Analgesia, 78,* 365–368.

Durren, M. (1992). Getting the most from pulse oximetry. *Journal of Emergency Nursing, 18,* 340–342.

Gettinger, A., DeTraglia, M. C., & Glass, P. D. (1987). In vivo comparison of two mixed venous saturation catheters. *Anesthesiology, 66,* 373–375.

Gilbert, R., Auchincloss, J. H., Kuppinger, M., et al. (1979). Stability of the arterial/alveolar oxygen partial pressure ratio. *Critical Care Medicine, 7,* 267–271.

Gilbert, R., & Keighley, J. F. (1974). The arterial/alveolar oxygen tension ratio. *American Review of Respiratory Disease, 109,* 144.

Grauer, K., Cavallaro, D., & Gums, J. (1991). New developments in cardiopulmonary resuscitation. *American Family Physician, 43,* 832–844.

Inman, J. K., Sibbald, W. J., Rutledge, F. S., et al. (1993). Does implementing pulse oximetry in a critical care unit result in substantial arterial blood gas savings? *Chest, 104,* 542–546.

Inoue, T., Marouka, S., Sakai, Y., et al. (1993). Oxygen demand–supply relationship in peripheral tissues as a therapeutic indicator in acute myocardial infarction with advanced heart failure. *Cardiology, 82,* 30–35.

Kruse, J. A., & Carlson, R. W. (1987). Lactate metabolism. *Critical Care Clinics, 5,* 725–746.

Leach, R. M., & Treacher, D. F. (1992). The pulmonary physician and critical care: 6. Oxygen transport: The relation between oxygen delivery and consumption. *Thorax, 47,* 971–978.

Ligget, S. B., St. John, R. E., & Lefrak, S. S. (1986). Determination of resting energy expenditure utilizing the thermodilution pulmonary artery catheter. *Chest, 91,* 562–566.

Millikan, G. A. (1942). The oximeter, an instrument for measuring continuously the oxygen saturation of arterial blood in man. *Review of Scientific Instruments, 13,* 434–444.

Mizock, B. A. (1987). Controversies in lactic acidosis: Implications in critically ill patients. *Journal of the American Medical Association, 258,* 497–501.

Ornato, J. P., Garnett, A. R., & Glauser, F. L. (1990). Relationship between cardiac output and the end-tidal carbon dioxide tension. *Annals of Emergency Medicine, 19,* 1104–1106.

Peretz, D. I., Scott, H. M., Duff, J., et al. (1965). The significance of lactic acidemia in the shock syndrome. *Annals of the New York Academy of Sciences, 119,* 1133–1141.

Ralston, A. C., Ebb, R. K., & Runciman, W. B. (1991). Potential errors in pulse oximetry: I. Pulse oximeter evaluation. *Anesthesia, 46,* 202–206.

Ramsing, T., & Rosenberg, J. (1992). Pulse oximetry in severe anemia. *Intensive Care Medicine, 18,* 125–126.

Rasanen, J., Downs, J. B., Malec, D. J., et al. (1987). Estimation of oxygen utilization by dual oximetry. *Annals of Surgery, 206,* 621.

Roberts, D., Ostryzniuk, P., Lowewen, E., et al. (1991). Control of blood gas measurements in intensive care units. *Lancet, 337,* 1580–1582.

Rotello, L. C., Warren, J., Jastremski, M. S., & Milewski, A. (1992). A nurse directed protocol using pulse oximetry to wean mechanically ventilated patients from toxic oxygen concentrations. *Chest, 102,* 1833–1835.

Russell, G. B., & Graybeal, J. M. (1994). Reliability of the arterial to end-tidal carbon dioxide gradient in mechanically ventilated patients with multisystem trauma. *The Journal of Trauma, 36,* 317–322.

Samsel, R. W., & Schumaker, P. T. (1991). Oxygen delivery to tissues. *European Respiratory Journal, 4,* 1258–1267.

Schweiss, J. F. (1987). Mixed venous hemoglobin saturation: Theory and application. *International Anesthesiology Clinics, 25*(3), 113–136.

Severinghaus, J. W., & Astrup, P. B. (1986). History of blood gas analysis: VI. Oximetry. *Journal of Clinical Monitoring, 2,* 270–288.

Severinghaus, J. W., & Kelleher, J. F. (1992). Recent developments in pulse oximetry. *Anesthesiology, 76,* 1018–1038.

Shoemaker, W. C. (1989). Pathophysiology and fluid management of postoperative and post-traumatic ARDS. In W. C. Shoemaker, et al. (Eds.), *Textbook of critical care* (2nd ed., pp. 615–635). Philadelphia: W. B. Saunders.

Shoemaker, W. C., & Appel, P. L. (1985). Pathophysiology in adult respiratory distress syndrome following sepsis and surgical operations. *Critical Care Medicine, 13,* 166.

Shoemaker, W. C., Appel, P. L., Kram, H. B., et al. (1993). Temporal hemodynamic and oxygen transport patterns in medical patients: Septic shock. *Chest, 104,* 1529–1536.

Stasic, A. F. (1986). Continuous evaluation of oxygenation and ventilation. In D. D. Civetta & D. D. Taylor (Eds.), *Critical care.* Philadelphia: W. B. Saunders.

Steltzer, H., Hiesmayr, M., Mayer, N., et al. (1994). The relationship between oxygen delivery and uptake in the critically ill: Is there a critical or optimal therapeutic value? *Anaesthesia, 49,* 229–236.

Stock, M. C. (1988). Noninvasive carbon dioxide monitoring. *Critical Care Clinics, 4,* 511–526.

Swan, H., Sanchez, M., Tyndall, M., & Koch, C. (1990). Quality control of perfusion: Monitoring venous blood oxygen tension to prevent hypoxic acidosis. *Journal of Thoracic and Cardiovascular Surgery, 99,* 868–872.

Tremper, K. K., & Barker, S. J. (1989). Pulse oximetry. *Anesthesiology, 70,* 98–108.

Ultman, J. S., & Bursztein, S. (1981). Analysis of error in determination of respiratory gas exchange at varying FIO_2. *Journal of Applied Physiology, 50,* 210–216.

Weil, M. H., Bisera, J., & Trevino, R. P., et al. (1985). Cardiac output and end-tidal carbon dioxide. *Critical Care Medicine, 13,* 907.

Weingarten, M. (1990). Respiratory monitoring of carbon dioxide and oxygen: A ten-year perspective. *Journal of Clinical Monitoring, 6,* 217–225.

West, J. B. (1990). *Ventilation—blood flow and gas exchange.* Baltimore: Williams & Wilkins.

White, K. M. (1984). Completing the hemodynamic picture: SvO_2. *Heart and Lung, 14,* 113–136.

Zeballos, R. J., & Weisman, I. M. (1991). Reliability of noninvasive oximetry in black subjects during exercise and hypoxia. *American Review of Respiratory Disease, 144,* 1240–1244.

CHAPTER 16

Mechanical Ventilation: Current Uses and Advances

John Wright, Peter Doyle, and Gary Yoshihara

Mechanical ventilators have been used for decades to support the respiratory function of patients with various degrees of respiratory distress or failure. Patients who have weak or absent spontaneous respiratory efforts usually require mechanical support to assist in ventilation and oxygenation. Neurologic disease or trauma, drug overdose, post-cardiac or respiratory arrest, and postoperative anesthesia are examples of patient conditions that may require ventilatory support. Because the ventilator is an integral and vital piece of life support equipment in the intensive care unit (ICU), it is important for the practitioner to know the basic concepts and applications of mechanical ventilation. In this chapter we review the indications for and the concepts of conventional mechanical ventilation and introduce new modalities currently in clinical use.

HISTORICAL OVERVIEW

For centuries, medical pioneers have experimented with the idea of artificially mimicking the respiratory function of the lungs to sustain human life. Twenty-eight centuries ago, reference to supportive ventilation appeared in the Bible.

And he put his mouth upon his mouth . . . and the flesh of the child became warm.

II Kings 4:34

The biblical story of Elisha, who restored the life of a young boy, recognized the principle that respiratory function could be supported artificially (Burton et al., 1984). In the centuries to follow, many experiments were conducted with animal and human subjects using a variety of mechanical devices to support ventilation. In the sixteenth century Paracelsus placed a tube in the mouth of a patient and used a fireplace bellows to inflate the lungs and assist his ventilation. Similar experiments continued through the seventeenth and eighteenth centuries. In the late 1800s, the first successful use of an endotracheal tube was reported.

Modern mechanical ventilation is a result of the popularity and technology of the iron lung (negative pressure ventilation) developed by Drinker and Shaw in 1929 (Burton et al., 1984; Shapiro et al., 1982). The iron lung, used primarily for polio victims, provided ventilatory support without the use of endotracheal intubation or tracheostomy.

World War II introduced several devices that were later adapted and developed for mechanical ventilation. Continuous positive pressure breathing to increase the altitude tolerance of pilots was used during World War II and later adapted for use in intermittent positive pressure ventilation (Burton et al., 1984). Positive pressure gained support and acceptance during and after World War II because of the questionable effectiveness of the negative pressure ventilators. This acceptance is thought to mark the beginning of the modern era of respiratory care (Burton et al., 1984; Shapiro et al., 1982).

Both types of ventilators, pressure-cycled and volume-cycled, were used in conjunction with cuffless tracheostomy and endotracheal tubes. The dangers of aspiration of gastric contents, the need to deliver consistent tidal volumes, and the desire for allowing inspiratory pressures to be reached for pressure-cycled ventilators led to the development of cuffed endotracheal and tracheostomy tubes.

Significant improvements have been made to mechanical ventilators since the days of the iron lung. Current-generation ventilators incorporate computerized systems to deliver and monitor ventilatory parameters. Newer ventilators are capable of providing a wide range of ventilatory modes and are upgradeable through microprocessor technology.

GENERAL VENTILATORY CONCEPTS

Indications for Mechanical Ventilation

Many factors affect the decision to institute mechanical ventilation, not the least of which is the fact that this invasive procedure has potentially harmful effects. It must also be understood that no mode of mechanical ventilation can or will cure a disease process but merely supports the patient until resolution of his or her symptoms is accomplished. For most patients mechanical ventilation is a relatively short-term support of respiratory function. However, in some circumstances, mechanical ventilation may be perceived as an extraordinary life support measure, prolonging the natural dying process.

Acute respiratory failure is the primary indication for the institution of ventilatory support (Egan et al., 1990). Respiratory failure can be categorized into various types: mechanical failure is the failure of the normal respiratory neuromuscular system, and often requires the institution of mechanical ventilatory support. This includes neuromuscular diseases such as myasthenia gravis, Guillain-Barré syndrome, and poliomyelitis. Respiratory paralysis, whether immediate or gradual, often necessitates ventilatory support to maintain adequate alveolar ventilation. Musculoskeletal abnormalities, such as chest wall trauma (flail chest), may impede the function of respiratory mechanics and thus require ventilatory support. Each of the different disease processes has varying ventilatory requirements, however, and many result in prolonged mechanical ventilatory support.

Abnormalities of pulmonary gas exchange account for most of the patients requiring mechanical ventilatory support. Obstructive lung disease in the form of asthma, chronic bronchitis, or emphysema may result in gas exchange impairment necessitating ventilatory support to oxygenate and ventilate the patient adequately. These patients offer a unique challenge in that they often have abnormal arterial blood gas values as their normal baseline, and must be maintained within these new "normal values." Furthermore, they are at greater risk for respiratory muscle fatigue secondary to diaphragmatic non-use.

Acute respiratory failure requiring mechanical ventilation may also occur from infectious diseases of the lung such as pneumonia, tuberculosis, or pneumocystis. Insufficient gas exchange occurring from conditions such as pulmonary edema, atelectasis, pulmonary fibrosis, or adult respiratory distress syndrome (ARDS) may require mechanical support of the lungs.

Finally, patients who have received general anesthesia as well as postcardiac arrest patients often require ventilatory support until they have recovered from the effects of the anesthesia or the insult of an arrest. In all cases a complete understanding of airway management, use of mechanical ventilators, and the implications of each disease process is required to ensure a successful outcome.

Negative Pressure Ventilation

The Drinker and Shaw tank-type ventilator of 1929 was the first negative pressure ventilator to be widely used for mechanical ventilation (Burton et al., 1984). Better known as the "iron lung," this device used negative pressure applied to the outside of the patient's chest to cause a drop in the intrapulmonary pressure and flow of ambient air into the patient's lungs. On termination of the breath, the negative pressure applied to the chest would drop to zero and the elastic recoil of the chest and lungs would permit passive exhalation. A tight-fitting cylinder completely engulfed the patient up to the neck, allowing for the negative pressure generated by a pump to be exerted on the patient's chest. Although neither a tracheostomy nor endotracheal tube was needed to provide ventilation, patient discomfort and inaccessibility by health care providers made the iron lung a less favorable form of mechanical ventilation. Furthermore, significant negative pressure exerted on the abdomen occasionally resulted in venous blood pooling in the lower torso, with a resultant decrease in cardiac output. Further developments in design led to the production of the "cuirass" or shell unit. This device consisted of a shell and soft bladder combination that covered the patient's chest only.

Although these types of ventilators gave way to the positive pressure devices (because of inability to accurately control tidal volumes, patient inaccessibility, and difficulty in maintaining a tight seal around the chest), a resurgence in their use for specific patient types has recently been seen. Some neuromuscular patients, especially those with residual muscular function, may benefit from nocturnal use of this type of ventilator, while not requiring a tracheostomy with its inherent problems. Furthermore, some home care patients find that even full-time ventilation may be attained using a chest cuirass.

Positive Pressure Ventilation

As mentioned previously, reference can be found as early as biblical times to the use of positive pressure for the purpose of restoring respiration or ventilation. In recent history, advances in the design and function of positive pressure devices have led to today's mechanical ventilators. Although the earlier models terminated the delivered breath when a preset pressure was achieved, the more recent models are most often volume cycled (the breath is terminated after a set volume has been delivered). In either case positive pressure applied at the patient's airway (usually through an endotracheal or tracheostomy tube) causes the flow of gas into the lungs until the ventilator breath is terminated. Passive exhalation occurs as the airway pressure drops to zero, and elastic recoil of the chest then pushes the tidal volume out.

Owing to the improvement of the mechanical ventilator and advances in design of endotracheal and tracheostomy tubes, positive pressure ventilators have become the mainstay of ventilatory support and are used most often in the hospital setting. Clinical uses of positive pressure devices include intermittent positive pressure breathing (IPPB) therapy as well as many modes of sustained mechanical ventilation.

Effects of Positive Pressure

PULMONARY SYSTEM. The effects of positive pressure on the pulmonary system are numerous and often depend on the amount of positive pressure delivered and the patient's lung pathology. Beneficial effects are usually in the form of reversal of atelectatic changes in the lung or regression of pulmonary congestion, resulting in better gas exchange. With improvement in the resting volume (functional residual volume [FRC]) of the lung, positive pressure may in some instances reduce pulmonary vascular resistance and improve arterial oxygenation. The work of breathing is often reduced, and cough effectiveness augmented.

Some of the negative effects include the numerous forms of barotrauma (pressure-induced injury) that can be the result of positive pressure applied to the lungs. These include pneumothorax, pneumomediastinum, pulmonary interstitial emphysema, bronchopulmonary dysplasia, and subcutaneous emphysema. Positive pressure can rupture alveoli, allowing for movement of air into the interstitium, which can then track into the pleural space (pneumothorax), into the pericardium (pneumopericardium), or into the mediastininum (pneumomediastinum). A tension pneumothorax (air in the thorax under pressure) or pneumopericardium can decrease venous blood return as well as reduce left ventricular function. This situation could be life threatening, and emergent decompression of the air is indicated. (Although the presence of subcutaneous emphysema is not in itself dangerous, it may suggest concurrent barotrauma and warrants further investigation.)

One contributory factor in the development of barotrauma is the production of shear forces caused by high initial inspiratory flow rates into the patient's airways. This, together with high peak airway pressure and variances in lung compliance and airway resistance within the lung, lead to the complications of positive pressure collectively known as barotrauma. Therefore, with the use of slower inspiratory flow rates and lower peak airway pressures, the incidence of this type of pulmonary insult may be reduced.

The combination of elevated levels of inspired oxygen, the presence of an endotracheal tube, and positive pressure over time in neonatal patients may result in a chronic form of respiratory distress syndrome termed bronchopulmonary dysplasia. These patients often require long-term ventilatory and oxygen support until their pulmonary disorder regresses.

CARDIOVASCULAR SYSTEM. Positive pressure applied to the lungs can be transmitted to the thorax, reducing cardiac output. Although reduction in venous blood return secondary to positive pressure transmitted to the thoracic space is a potential cause for alterations in cardiac output, other factors may be involved. Ultrasound studies of postcardiac surgery patients undergoing positive pressure ventilation indicate that increased intrapulmonary pressures cause an increase in pulmonary vascular resistance, with the development of right ventricular failure. This, in turn, shifts the ventricular septum into the left ventricular space, thus decreasing left ventricular filling and output. In either case, cardiac output may be impaired. The degree to which this occurs appears to depend on the mean airway pressure, cardiac reserve and function, circulating blood volume, and lung compliance or airway resistance.

RENAL SYSTEM. Any form of circulatory embarrassment may result in hypoperfusion of the kidneys with an alteration in urinary output. Although this phenomenon has been noted during positive pressure ventilation, it may also be secondary to positive pressure effects on antidiuretic hormone secretion. A reduction in venous drainage secondary to increased intrathoracic positive pressure could stimulate osmoreceptors in the hypothalamus to mediate secretion of ADH. This, in turn, results in diminished urinary output. Judicious use of plasma expanders, diuretics, and careful observation of renal function should allow for adequate fluid homeostasis.

Classifications of Positive Pressure Ventilators

Commonly, ventilators are classified by their method of cycling from the inspiratory phase to the expiratory phase (changeover from inspiratory to expiratory phase). The term "cycle" will be used here to indicate a terminating event as opposed to an initiating event.

VOLUME-CYCLED VENTILATOR. A volume-cycled breath is a ventilatory breath that is terminated when a *preset volume* has left the ventilator. This is the most common form of ventilator cycling because it allows a more consistent delivery of volumes. Many ventilators have, as a safety device, a pressure pop-off, or limit, that prevents overpressurization of the pulmonary circuit on any given breath. Depending on the type of pressure-regulating device in use, the breath may be terminated (pressure-cycled) before the entire volume is delivered to the patient. Most volume ventilators have a device that measures exhaled volumes. Therefore, if the entire preset volume is not delivered because of excessive pressure, the exhaled volume will be lower than expected. These devices also serve to monitor for leaks in the patient circuit. Although changes in airway resistance or lung compliance could result in lost ventilation into the ventilator tubing (compressible volume loss), some newer ventilators automatically compensate for this. The Bear 1 or Bear 2 are examples of volume-cycled ventilators (Bear Medical Systems, Inc., Riverside, CA).

PRESSURE-CYCLED VENTILATOR. A pressure-cycled breath is a ventilatory breath that is terminated when a *preset pressure* is reached. Although this will often avoid overpressurization of the pulmonary circuit (above the level set by the operator), the delivered breaths are not as consistent in volume. The size of the tidal volume depends on the patient's airway resistance, lung compliance, inspiratory demand, and the peak pressure that is selected. Thus, changes in the patient's pulmonary status may result in the delivery of inappropriate or inconsistent volumes. Furthermore, large leaks or patient disconnects may not allow for the peak pressure to be reached, with resultant failure of the ventilator to cycle off. Often these types of ventilators do not have the capacity to deliver precisely controlled levels of inspired oxygen. Because of these inconstancies, this type of ventilator is more commonly used only for intermittent treatment modalities (e.g., IPPB). A Bird IPPB machine is an example of a pressure-cycled ventilator (Bird Products Corp., Palm Springs, CA).

TIME-CYCLED VENTILATOR. Time-cycled breaths terminate when a *preset inspiratory time* has elapsed. Often a pressure limit is also incorporated so that the pressure limit is reached and the remainder of the inspiratory phase is in the form of an inspiratory pause. This type of ventilation (breath hold) became the mainstay of neonatal ventilation in the late 1960s and early 1970s, and is currently the mode of choice for neonates and small infants in many medical centers (e.g., the Sechrist IV 100B ventilator Sechrist, Anaheim, CA). Pressure control ventilation is a time-cycled, pressure-limited form of ventilation commonly used in all patient sizes.

Although these types of ventilators do not guarantee a set tidal volume, they do allow for a precise control of inspired fraction of oxygen. There is evidence to suggest that the decelerating flow pattern of this type of breath can improve gas distribution in some disease states. A decelerating flow pattern is the result of a rapid initial flow that quickly raises the pressure to the preset level, followed by degeneration of the flow rate to the baseline pressure level (i.e., positive end-expiratory pressure [PEEP] level). The rate of flow degeneration depends on several factors, including the patient's lung compliance. Also, research suggests that controlling pressures instead of volumes may be more appropriate in the treatment of patients suffering from ARDS.

Some time-cycled ventilators occasionally deliver a constant flow of gas to the patient during the time the exhalation valve is completely closed (inspiration). Thus, the tidal volume is constant (tidal volume = inspiratory flow × time). These types of devices are often used as transport ventilators or in emergency rooms as manual resuscitators (e.g., demand valve).

FLOW-CYCLED VENTILATOR. A flow-cycled ventilator breath is terminated when a predetermined inspiratory flow rate has been achieved. This form of breath termination is common in pressure support ventilation where, during inspiration, a constant pressure is applied to the airway until a variable flow has decelerated to a nominal value, at which point inspiration ends. Flow-cycled breaths tend to deliver more consistent tidal volumes than pressure-cycled breaths, and the variable flow is more likely to match patient inspiratory flow demands.

Triggering Mechanisms

All breaths delivered to patients must be initiated or triggered. Triggering mechanisms used to initiate ventilator breaths operate on the principle of time, pressure, volume, or flow. A manual trigger is also available on many ventilators whereby a mandatory or manual breath can be triggered when a button or key is pressed (Branson, 1994).

TIME TRIGGERED. Patients who are not actively breathing require a backup or preset rate at which the ventilator triggers into inspiration. A timing system is available on most mechanical ventilators that triggers inspiration after the passage of a preset period of time. The time trigger also serves as a backup in the case an actively breathing patient's respiratory rate falls below a preset value on the ventilator.

PRESSURE TRIGGERED. For patients to inspire spontaneously, negative pressure must be generated by the respiratory muscles. This negative pressure is usually transmitted to the ventilator circuit where it can be used as a triggering mechanism. A pressure sensitivity value is set below the preset PEEP. As soon as the patient generates a negative pressure below this level, the ventilator triggers into inspiration. Typical settings for pressure trigger values are 1 to 2 cm H_2O below PEEP. Low pressure sensitivity values reduce the imposed work of breathing required to trigger ventilator breaths; however, pressure fluctuations in the ventilator circuit (e.g., leaks, hiccups) may cause premature triggering (autotriggering) to occur.

FLOW TRIGGERED. Some mechanical ventilators allow patients to trigger the ventilator into inspiration when a measured flow rate (flow sensitivity) has been inspired from the ventilator circuit. A base flow of gas supplied through the ventilator circuit allows the patient to receive flow at the beginning of inspiration. Flow sensors detect the inspiration of the gas flow and, before the base flow of gas is depleted, triggers the ventilator into inspiration. The benefits of this type of triggering include a faster response time of the ventilator and a reduction in the imposed work of breathing required to trigger the ventilator (Sassoon, 1992). Furthermore, PEEP values can be better maintained in the face of leaks provided the base flow and flow sensitivity values exceed the leak rate. Flow-triggering also solves the problem of autotriggering due to leaks.

VOLUME TRIGGERED. A volume trigger initiates breath delivery from the ventilator when a set inspired volume has been detected. A base flow of gas is available before inspiration from which the patient can begin inspiration. When a preset volume has been inspired, the ventilator declares inspiration and the spontaneous or mandatory breath is triggered. A reduction in the imposed work of breathing required to trigger the ventilator should be similar to that seen with flow-triggering systems; however, leaks in patient circuits are more likely to cause autotriggering.

Positive End-Expiratory Pressure

Positive end-expiratory pressure is positive pressure that is applied to the airway at the end of exhalation (after either a mandatory or spontaneous breath). The goal of PEEP therapy is to return the functional residual capacity (FRC) toward normal in patients who have a reduction in FRC. Reduction of the FRC may result in a decrease in lung compliance and an increase in intrapulmonary shunting (lower Pa_{O_2}). Furthermore, as a consequence of lower lung compliance, the overall work of breathing may be increased. Applying continuous positive airway pressure at the end of exhalation causes an increase in alveolar pressure and increases alveolar volume (Craig et al., 1988). This increase in lung volume may improve lung compliance, reduce the work of breathing, and improve ventilation-to-perfusion matching.

Positive end-expiratory pressure therapy is not always beneficial, and can lead to serious consequences. Complications of PEEP include overdistention of alveoli, decreased cardiac output, and barotrauma. Especially in patients with nonuniform lung disease, more compliant areas of the lung will be inflated to a greater degree than those of lower compliance at a constant pressure. This can lead to an increase in ventilation-to-perfusion mismatching and possible alveolar rupture. Overdistention of lung units can also reduce lung compliance and increase work of breathing. Therefore, the patient's lung compliance, arterial blood gases, chest x-rays, hemodynamic status, and peak inflation pressures should be monitored during application of PEEP therapy.

In summary, PEEP therapy is indicated for the treatment of diffuse lung diseases that result in a reduced FRC and an increase in inspired oxygen requirement. In these patients PEEP has the potential to improve compliance, increase FRC, and reduce shunting (Scanlan et al., 1990). The most significant benefit of the use of PEEP is that it may enable the patient to maintain an adequate Pa_{O_2} at a lower concentration of oxygen, thereby reducing the risk of oxygen toxicity.

VOLUME VENTILATION

Control

When a patient is placed on a ventilator in the control mode, the ventilator initiates and controls both the volume delivered and the frequency of the breaths. The tidal volume and frequency of the backup rate are set by the clinician. When used strictly in the control mode, the ventilator will not respond if the patient attempts to initiate a breath. Because the patient is unable to initiate a breath on demand, his or her respiratory pattern and effort may become asynchonous with the ventilator. The failure of the ventilator to respond to the patient's needs may cause the patient to become agitated and to increase his or her work of breathing.

The control mode can be used to override (control) a patient with a high respiratory rate. The patient can be deliberately hyperventilated by increasing his or her minute ventilation with the ventilator. If the patient is not hypoxemic, the resulting hypocapnia often may remove the normal stimulus to breathe, allowing the ventilator to control all inspirations. The control mode can be used in any clinical situation in which the patient is incapable of initiating a ventilator breath and complete ventilatory support is required.

The control mode is rarely used in clinical practice as a stand-alone mode. The assist/control mode is more commonly used, providing the backup support that the control mode offers yet allowing the patient the opportunity to trigger a spontaneous breath. As a result, newer ventilators no longer have separate control and assist modes. The two modes are routinely combined into one assist/control mode.

Volume Assist/Control

This mode of ventilation is a combination of the assist mode and a modified version of the control mode. The assist mode is a mode of ventilation in which the patient is able to initiate inspiration and to control the frequency. The major disadvantage of using this mode is that, in the event of apnea, an inadequate minute ventilation would not be maintained. The control mode was later incorporated with the assist mode (i.e., assist/control) to alleviate this problem. As in the control mode, a tidal volume and rate are preset. However, unlike the control mode, when the patient makes an inspiratory effort, the ventilator responds to the effort and delivers the set volume. Therefore, every breath is supported by the ventilator, with the respiratory pattern varying depending on the timing of the patient efforts. If the patient fails to initiate inspiration, the ventilator will automatically go into the backup mode (control) and deliver the preset rate and volume (i.e., a mandatory breath) until the patient again initiates a ventilator breath. This backup rate ensures a minimum minute ventilation in the event of apnea.

The assist/control mode is indicated in any clinical situation that requires a reduction in the work of breathing—for example, in patients who require a set backup rate but also need an assisted breath on demand to reduce the work of breathing.

A clinical example for using assist/control would be the following: a patient located in a medical unit has worsening respiratory distress as indicated by a respiratory rate of 33 breaths per minute. The patient is intubated, transported to the ICU, and placed on mechanical ventilation. Due to fatigue, the patient initially allows the ventilator to do all the work (i.e., the ventilator initiates all of the breaths at the backup rate of 14 breaths per minute) while the patient's diaphragm rests. After 6 hours, the patient resumes use of his diaphragm and initiates breaths, setting a respiratory rate of 17 breaths per minute.

There are two advantages to the volume assist/control mode. First, this mode ensures a minimum minute ventilation and allows the patient to receive a fully supported breath on demand. The second possible advantage is that cycling the ventilator into the inspiratory phase maintains normal ventilatory activity and therefore prevents atrophy of the respiratory muscles (Burton et al., 1984).

There are also potential disadvantages with the volume assist/control mode. The first is respiratory alkalosis. Because the ventilator delivers the set tidal volume on demand, there is the potential for alveolar hyperventilation, resulting in hypocapnia. The second possible disadvantage is that the patient may "stack" breaths (take several breaths in a row). This may cause ineffective ventilation and asynchronous breathing, requiring the need to sedate or paralyze the patient. A third potential problem may be related to maladjustment of the ventilator settings. Inadequate inspiratory flow rate, tidal volume, or trigger sensitivity can cause excessive work to trigger an assisted breath.

Volume Intermittent Mandatory Ventilation and Synchronized Intermittent Mandatory Ventilation

Intermittent mandatory ventilation (IMV) allows the patient to breath spontaneously in addition to the ventilator providing some mandatory breaths at a predetermined rate and tidal volume. Like the control and assist/control modes, the ventilator provides a minimum minute ventilation in the event of apnea. Between the mandatory ventilator breaths, the patient is able to breath spontaneously, drawing from a source of oxygen of the same concentration, temperature, and humidity as is available for the mandatory breaths. During the spontaneous phase of ventilation the patient determines the respiratory rate and tidal volume. Unfortunately, with this mode of ventilation, asynchronous breathing may be experienced. Because IMV has a controlled rate, the mandatory breath may be imposed on the patient's spontaneous inspiration or exhalation (i.e., "stacking").

Synchronized intermittent mandatory ventilation (SIMV) was developed to prevent the "stacking" effect of IMV. The mandatory breath delivered from the ventilator is synchronized with the beginning of the patient's spontaneous inspiration. With SIMV, four types of breaths are possible:

- Mandatory mechanical ventilation breaths are delivered at the backup rate if the patient effort is absent.
- If the patient makes an inspiratory effort near the time of the next scheduled mandatory breath, the result is the initiation of a preset mandatory breath. Thus, the patient's effort is synchronized with the ventilator, preventing the imposition of the mandatory on top of the spontaneous breaths and providing a more comfortable form of ventilation.
- Like IMV, if the patient makes a spontaneous inspiratory effort that is not within reasonable proximity to the next scheduled mandatory breath, the patient generates an unassisted spontaneous breath.
- The nonmandatory breaths (spontaneous) can be pressure supported. At the onset of a spontaneous inspiration, the pressure rises to the pressure level set by the clinician and plateaus for the duration of the patient's inspiratory effort. The work of breathing during the spontaneous breaths can be reduced using pressure support. The work of breathing is proportional to the pressure support level and is associated with increased tidal volumes, decreased respiratory rates, and improved patient comfort.

A clinical example regarding the use of the SIMV mode is as follows: Mr. S. is 6 hours postoperative coronary artery bypass grafting. He is easily awakened, responds to commands, and is beginning to initiate breaths on his own. He is on SIMV with a rate of 10 with acceptable arterial blood gases (ABGs). The surgeon has directed for the weaning process to begin. Every 2 hours, his SIMV rate is decreased by 2. Six hours later, Mr. S. is on an SIMV rate of 4. His Spo_2 is 96%. He is breathing comfortably at a rate of 15. His respiratory mechanics are acceptable, so he is extubated.

The advantages of SIMV/IMV, compared to the control and assist/control modes already described, include:

- The iatrogenic effects of mechanical ventilation (barotrauma, decreased cardiac output) are minimized because mean airway and intrapleural pressures are lower (Kirby, 1988; Shapiro et al., 1982).
- There is less likelihood of hyperventilation (respiratory alkalosis) (Burton et al., 1984).
- SIMV can be used as a means of weaning the patient from mechanical ventilation because it can provide a variation of mechanical ventilation that ranges from full to minimal support.

The disadvantages of IMV/SIMV include:

- Asynchronous breathing. In the IMV mode, the mandatory breaths may be imposed during the patient's spontaneous inspiration or expiration, which may cause the patient to breathe asynchronously with the ventilator, and not receive adequate ventilation.
- Apnea or hypoventilation. During the weaning process, if the patient is on a low backup rate, and fails to maintain an adequate spontaneous minute ventilation or becomes apneic, respiratory acidosis may occur (alveolar hypoventilation).
- Increased work of breathing. With ventilators that use a demand valve, the patient is required to cause a pressure differential to initiate a spontaneous

breath. The total work required to breathe spontaneously through this system is in addition to the work required to overcome the resistance generated by the endotracheal tube, the ventilator circuit, level of PEEP, and the humidifier.

PRESSURE VENTILATION

DEFINITION. Pressure ventilation differs from volume ventilation in almost every aspect. The most noted and obvious difference is that pressure ventilation involves the delivery of a preset pressure level for a predetermined inspiratory time or inspiration–expiration ratio. For example, every breath given during pressure ventilation may read 25 cm H_2O on the manometer. The independent variable will be the tidal volume. This is in sharp contrast to volume ventilation, whereby the tidal volume is constant and the pressure level varies (Table 16–1).

Until the early 1980s, pressure ventilation was used predominantly in the neonatal and pediatric arenas. With the introduction of pressure ventilation modes on adult ventilators, an alternative therapeutic modality became available.

A few basic concepts and definitions are necessary to fully understand pressure ventilation. The highest level of pressure observed on the manometer during a mechanical ventilation breath is called the peak inspiratory pressure (PIP). As described earlier in this chapter, the baseline pressure level is termed PEEP. The gradient between this baseline pressure and the PIP is called delta P (ΔP). Delta P is the preset pressure that functions as the primary setting of pressure ventilation. In other words, the tidal volume delivered to the patient is a result of the change in pressure from the baseline pressure to the preset PIP. Any ventilator change that results in a change in the PIP or the baseline pressure (PEEP) may cause a change in the tidal volume delivered.

INDICATIONS. Pressure ventilation has been shown to adequately ventilate and oxygenate patients in severe respiratory failure. A recent study showed that it can be used safely and is well tolerated as an initial mode of ventilatory support in patients with acute hypoxic respiratory failure (Rappaport et al., 1994). Pressure ventilation may have a beneficial role when

TABLE 16–1. **Comparison of Volume and Pressure Ventilation**

	Tidal Volume	Peak Inspiratory Pressure	Flow
Volume ventilation	Consistent	Variable	Consistent
Pressure ventilation	Variable	Consistent	Variable, decelerating, influenced by patient

used as the primary ventilatory modality in patients with this clinical condition, because the early initiation of pressure ventilation is associated with lower peak airway pressure and more rapid improvement in static compliance (unit change in volume per unit change in pressure during a condition of no flow) than volume-controlled ventilation. Patients required fewer days of mechanical ventilation than those receiving volume ventilation. No pneumothoraces occurred in any of the study patients. Sedation requirements were equivalent in the two groups.

APPLICATION. A pressure-limited, time-cycled ventilator is used (e.g., Siemens Servo 300 or 900c [Siemens-Elma Life Support Systems Division, Solona, Sweden] or the Puritan-Bennett 7200ae [Puritan-Bennett Corp., Carlsbad, CA]). The clinician sets a specific inspiratory pressure and inspiratory time. The ventilator reaches the preset pressure and maintains that pressure level for the prescribed inspiratory time. Unlike conventional volume ventilation, peak inspiratory flow cannot be adjusted by the clinician. Delta P is usually adjusted to deliver a tidal volume of 5 to 15 mL/kg (Hickling et al., 1990; Kacmarek & Venegas, 1987). In volume ventilation, tidal volumes are also set in this same range.

The preset pressure level (ΔP) selected by the clinician provides a consistent PIP: PEEP + ΔP = PIP. The actual tidal volume, however, fluctuates with the patient's compliance, airway resistance, and length of inspiratory time. Proper airway management is critical to minimizing PIP. Ensure that endotracheal tubes are not kinked, suctioning is performed as needed, etc.

If the patient's compliance is poor, higher levels of ΔP may be required to maintain a tidal volume in the 5 to 15 mL/kg range. A very high pressure level is likely to increase chances of barotrauma. The point where PIP levels become hazardous is unknown. Many would agree that a peak alveolar pressure greater than 35 cm H_2O raises concern regarding the development of barotrauma and increases the chance of ventilator-induced lung injury (Hickling et al., 1990; Marini, 1992).

One potential advantage of using pressure ventilation over volume ventilation is the method by which the flow is delivered. The decelerating flow pattern used in pressure ventilation (Fig. 16–1) enables the ventilator to deliver approximately the same volume as in volume ventilation, but with lower PIP. This is accomplished by adjusting the ΔP, thereby altering the PIP and the tidal volume. The ventilator is time cycled (i.e., inspiration ends at a predetermined time). This enables the clinician to increase the inspiratory time, thus allowing a longer duration to deliver a tidal volume of a size equivalent to the tidal volume delivered on volume ventilation, but at a lower pressure. This longer inspiratory time can optimize the distribution of inspired gas. With short inspiratory times, a bolus of gas has a limited amount of time to inflate all lung units. Because diseased lung units are often less compliant, most of the positive pressure is redistributed to

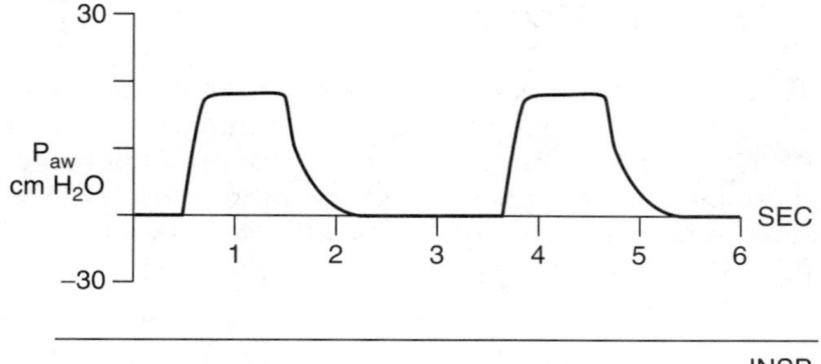

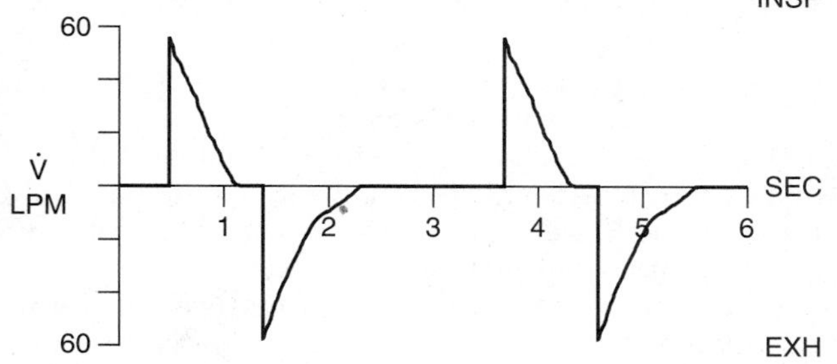

FIGURE 16–1. Pressure and flow curves in pressure control ventilation. The upper wave form shows the rapid rise and plateau in pressure associated with inspiration. Pressure decelerates upon expiration. The lower waveform represents flow during inspiration (above baseline) and expiration (below baseline). P_{aw}, airway pressure; sec, seconds; Insp, inspiration; Exh, exhalation; V̇, flow; LPM, liters per minute. (Used with permission of the Puritan-Bennett Corp., Carlsbad, CA, 1990.)

healthy lung units, which are subsequently prone to overdistention. Longer inspiratory times give the diseased lung units more time to inflate, causing less overdistention in the healthy lung units. A normal inspiratory time for an adult is 0.8 to 1.2 seconds.

Inspiratory time is only part of the overall respiratory cycle. The other major component is expiratory time (which includes the intermittent rests or lulls in respiration). The total time allotted for one respiratory cycle (i.e., one complete inspiration and one complete expiration) is determined by the respiratory rate. For example, a respiratory rate of 20 breaths per minute generates a respiratory cycle time of 3 seconds per breath (60 seconds/minute divided by 20 breaths/minute). If the inspiratory time was set at 1.0 seconds, the expiratory time would have to be the remaining 2.0 seconds. This results in an inspiratory-to-expiratory ratio of 1:2.

During volume ventilation, flow is delivered at a constant level. In pressure ventilation, a very fast initial flow is delivered that overcomes the resistance of the endotracheal tube and upper airways until the predetermined pressure level is reached. Therefore, gas reaches the smaller airways earlier in the inspiratory phase, allowing more time for gas distribution according to regional variations in compliance and resistance. The rapid introduction of gas into the airways may be very uncomfortable for the patient and may require sedation or paralyzation. As the pressure gradient begins to decline, flow decelerates as a function of the back pressure it meets. The flow then decelerates as the lungs fill. Pressure is then maintained until the set inspiratory time has elapsed.

During pressure ventilation, flow is regulated by several factors, including patient demand. Volume ventilation does not allow flow to vary in response to patient demand. Pressure ventilation is therefore useful when the patient has high or fluctuating flows. It is important to distinguish pressure ventilation from the frequently used neonatal version of pressure ventilation in which pressure and inspiratory time are preset, but gas delivery is limited by a preset flow rate.

MONITORING. Alarms are especially important in this type of ventilation. They are essential for alerting the nurse to changes in tidal volume caused by a change in compliance, secretions, and various other factors.

Pressure ventilation can be delivered by several modes. Two of the most commonly used pressure ventilation modes are assist/control and SIMV. All of the aspects of pressure ventilation previously described apply to both of these modes.

Pressure Assist/Control

Pressure assist/control is similar to volume assist/control in many respects. It provides the security, or "fallback," of mandatory breaths if the patient is too weak or otherwise unable to trigger the ventilator. It also allows the patient to set the breathing rhythm, synchronizing with the ventilator, if he or she is making inspiratory efforts. In either case, full support is provided during each breath. Once the ventilator is triggered, the rapid initial flow of gas tends to minimize the chance of excessive work of breathing (see Fig. 16–1).

Disadvantages of using this mode include: excessive work of breathing if the settings are not appropriate, air trapping in patients with chronic obstructive pulmonary disease (COPD), and variable (and sometimes inadequate) tidal volumes due to changes in compliance, the patient's respiratory drive, patient–ventilator dyssynchrony, and secretions.

Pressure Synchronized Intermittent Mandatory Ventilation

Pressure SIMV combines a predetermined number of ventilator-delivered (mandatory) breaths of a preset pressure level with the intermittent possibility of patient-generated spontaneous breaths (Fig. 16–2). The ventilator-delivered breaths can be triggered by the patient. However, if a patient effort is not sensed within a specific period of time, the ventilator delivers a breath at the preset pressure level. Pressure support or volume support may be applied during the intervals between ventilator-delivered breaths.

Advantages of this mode include the ability to provide various levels of respiratory work with the secu-

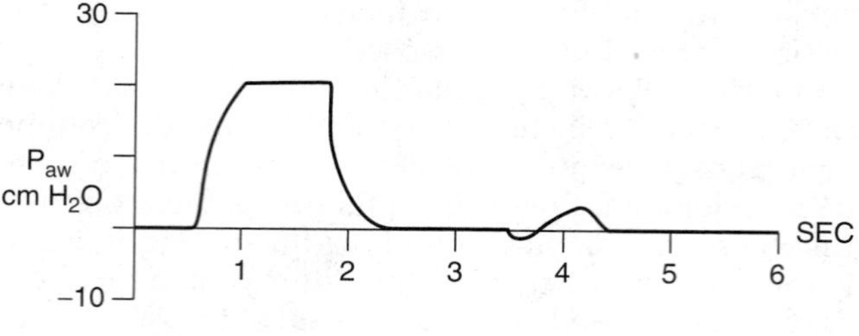

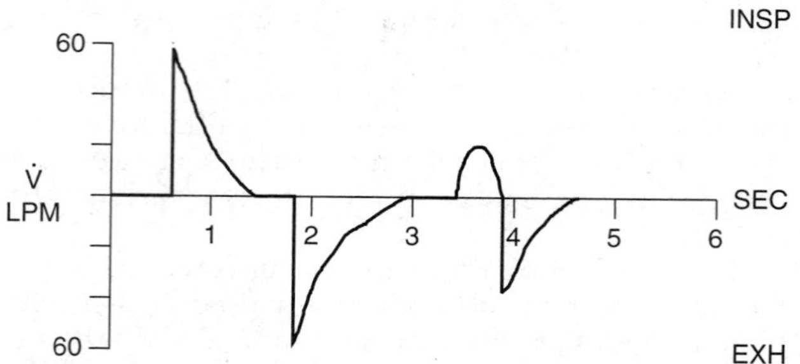

FIGURE 16–2. Synchronized intermittent mandatory ventilation with pressure control ventilation. The larger waveform represents ventilator-initiated breaths. The smaller waveform indicates spontaneous effort. P_{aw}, airway pressure; sec, seconds; Insp, inspiration; Exh, exhalation; V̇, flow; LPM, liters per minute. (Used with permission of the Puritan-Bennett Corp., Carlsbad, CA, 1990.)

rity of a preset level of machine-driven ventilation. It can therefore often be used as a weaning mode.

Disadvantages of using this mode include excessive work of breathing if the settings are not appropriate, and variable (and sometimes inadequate) tidal volumes due to changes in compliance, the patient's respiratory drive, patient–ventilator dyssynchrony, secretions, and patient fatigue.

Pressure-Regulated Volume Control

Pressure regulated volume control (PRVC; Servo 300 [Siemens-Elema Corp.]) is a new mode that combines the benefits of pressure ventilation and volume ventilation. The primary ventilator settings for PRVC are respiratory rate, inspiratory time, and tidal volume/minute volume. The major drawback with the pressure assist/control mode (see section on Pressure Assist/Control) is the possibility of an inconsistent tidal volume based on the mechanical properties of the patient's lungs and resistance of his or her airways. When PRVC is used, the ventilator automatically monitors the patient's lung mechanics and adjusts the pressure level to maintain the targeted tidal volume. Initially, the ventilator calculates a value for compliance based on a "test" breath. The ventilator then monitors the patient's lung mechanics, continuously adjusting the pressure level when necessary to maintain the set tidal volume. Safety features are built in to prevent large pressure changes from occurring.

WEANING MODES

There are three modes of mechanical ventilation that are completely dependent on the spontaneous efforts of the patient for initiation of inspiration. Obviously, these modes are often used for weaning purposes. The three modes are continuous positive airway pressure (CPAP), pressure support, and volume support.

Continuous Positive Airway Pressure

Continuous positive airway pressure has the same physiologic characteristics as PEEP (Table 16–2). The goal of CPAP therapy is to restore or maintain the FRC of a patient who is able to breathe spontaneously. FRC is maintained by elevating the end-expiratory pressure to a level above atmospheric pressure.

Continuous positive airway pressure can be applied via a face or nasal mask, or through an artificial airway. CPAP delivered by mask can often prevent or delay intubation. Mask CPAP can also be used for patients who present with obstructive sleep apnea (see section on BiPAP). Mask CPAP can be delivered with a ventilator, a CPAP machine, or a high-flow oxygen delivery system. CPAP is often used as a primary method of weaning patients from mechanical ventilation. When placed on CPAP, the patient does all the work of breathing without the aid of a backup rate or tidal volume (some ventilators support the patient in the event of apnea).

An example of CPAP via mask is as follows: a 38-year-old patient with acquired immunodeficiency syndrome presents with respiratory failure due to *Pneumocystis carinii* pneumonia. He is in respiratory distress but refuses intubation. A CPAP mask is used to improve his gas exchange and overall respiratory function.

An example of CPAP used for weaning is as follows: a postoperative patient who is awake and alert is placed on SIMV. Her rate has been decreased gradu-

TABLE 16–2. **Comparison of PEEP and CPAP**

PEEP	CPAP
Patient is intubated	Patient is usually intubated (CPAP mask is available)
Used in conjunction with control, assist/control, and SIMV	Not used with other modes of ventilation
Backup rate and tidal volume are provided	No backup rate is set, all breathing is done spontaneously
Goal is to improve or maintain FRC	Goal is to improve FRC Used for weaning patients from mechanical ventilation

Abbreviations: PEEP, positive end-expiratory pressure; CPAP, continuous positive airway pressure; SIMV, synchronized intermittent mandatory ventilation; FRC, functional residual capacity.

ally to 4, with acceptable ABGs. The respiratory therapist suggests 30 minutes of CPAP, then check her ABGs.

Pressure Support Ventilation

Pressure support ventilation (PSV) is a mode that provides augmentation of spontaneously generated breaths with a clinician-selected level of positive pressure. As the patient initiates a breath, the preselected inspiratory pressure level is reached early in the inspiratory phase, and a pressure plateau is sustained for as long as the patient continues to make an inspiratory effort or until a minimum inspiratory flow is reached. Unlike other modes of ventilation, PSV requires the patient to have a continuous spontaneous respiratory drive, because all breaths are patient-initiated.

Pressure support ventilation may help reduce the work of breathing imposed by the resistance to flow through the artificial airway. When PSV is initiated, the peak inspiratory flow, like the PIP, is reached early in the inspiratory phase, filling the ventilator circuit and the patient's airways. Theoretically, the high initial flow overcomes the resistance of the artificial airway, reducing the resistance to flow during the plateau of the positive pressure. Therefore, the ventilator aids in the early phase of the breath, reducing the work of breathing. The level of pressure support determines the level of work done by the ventilator versus the work done by the patient. The patient has control of his or her respiratory rate, tidal volume, inspiratory time, and flow. The volume delivered with each supported breath depends on the pressure support level, the patient's inspiratory effort, the resistance and compliance of the airways, and the system design of the ventilator.

PHYSIOLOGY. The respiratory center in the central nervous system receives input from chemoreceptors (arterial blood gas tensions) and neural pathways that sense the mechanical work of breathing (mechanoreceptors). The respiratory rate and pattern and tidal volume are the result of input from these chemical and mechanical receptors. From this input, the respiratory center of the brain can regulate gas exchange with the minimum amount of work (MacIntyre, 1988). Any variation in the input can cause dyspnea. It is thought that pressure support may interact with the mechanical receptors, and can achieve this balance in a more physiologic fashion in a spontaneously breathing patient (MacIntyre, 1988).

INDICATIONS. The following clinical situations may indicate the possible use of PSV:

1. Patients who are difficult to wean from the mechanical ventilation using conventional means (i.e., T-piece, SIMV, CPAP)
2. Anxious patients, because with PSV they will be able to control their respiratory rate, volume, and inspiratory flow
3. Patients who have less than optimal artificial airways (i.e., too small in diameter); small-diameter airways increase the work of breathing because the patient must overcome the resistance to flow; PSV may help overcome this resistance
4. Patients who have problems synchronizing with other modes of mechanical ventilation
5. Patients with evidence of ventilatory muscle weakness who are unable to trigger a spontaneous SIMV breath on a ventilator that uses a demand valve; or any patient who is unable to maintain an adequate minute ventilation on minimal SIMV settings or on CPAP
6. Any patient in need of a routine method of mechanical ventilation

CONTRAINDICATIONS. Apnea is a contraindication for PSV. When pressure support is used as the primary mode of ventilation, the patient will not receive backup ventilatory support should apnea occur. In addition, patients who fatigue easily may experience alveolar hypoventilation if they are on PSV only, or if they are placed on SIMV with PSV with a low backup rate.

APPLICATION. The patient must be changed to a ventilator that has the capability to deliver pressure support. There are several ways to use PSV as a primary mode of ventilation or as a means to wean the patient from the ventilator. The first application is to incorporate low levels of PSV with SIMV, the PSV being used during the spontaneous breaths. Low levels of PSV, levels maintaining a tidal volume of 5 to 7 cm H_2O, are often used to overcome the resistance of the artificial airway, which may provide improved patient comfort and respiratory muscle function. When weaning, the SIMV support is gradually withdrawn. The second application is to use low levels of PSV for nonventilatory support (patients intubated for airway protection or for airway stabilization using PEEP). The PSV in such situations functions to reduce the work of breathing imposed by the endotracheal tube. The third application is to use PSV alone (PSVmax). When using this method, the pressure support level is set so that the delivered tidal volume is approximately equal to that received during conventional volume ventilation (10–12 mL/kg) (MacIntyre, 1988). It is thought that this method reduces the work of the respiratory muscles and gradually reconditions them. The level of PSV is gradually reduced, allowing the patient to do more of the work of breathing. The patient can be extubated or removed from the ventilator if all other parameters are stable (blood pressure, heart rate, respiratory rate, and so on), all other weaning criteria are met, and a low PSV level maintains a satisfactory tidal volume (volume criteria vary with each institution).

MONITORING. The patient on pressure support should be monitored in the same manner as any pa-

Text continued on page 276

TABLE 16–3. **Ventilation Modalities: Comparative Table**

Mode	Description	Indications	Advantages	Disadvantages
Negative pressure	Negative pressure outside the chest causes a decrease in intrapulmonary pressure and the flow of ambient air into the patient's lungs. Examples include iron lung and cuirass shells.	Neuromuscular diseases Intermittent mechanical ventilation (e.g., nocturnal ventilation).	Artificial airway is not required. Patient/family can initiate. Often used in home setting.	Patient immobility. Inaccessability to health care providers (iron lung). Difficult to maintain chest seal (cuirass). Inconsistent tidal volumes.
Standard Modes				
Control (pressure or volume ventilation)	A predetermined tidal volume or ΔP (depending on whether format is volume or pressure ventilation, respectively) is delivered every breath at a fixed respiratory rate. Patient cannot trigger.	To override patient efforts in order to rest diaphragm. Spinal cord injuries.	Guaranteed minimum minute volume.	Not responsive to patient efforts, causing agitation, anxiety, and asynchrony with ventilator. Can cause distress and increased work of breathing.
Assist/control (pressure or volume ventilation)	A predetermined tidal volume or ΔP (depending on whether format is volume or pressure ventilation, respectively) is delivered every breath. A backup respiratory rate provides a minimum minute ventilation. Patient can initiate breaths and thereby can increase the respiratory rate and minute volume.	Any form of ventilator dependency. Post cardiac/respiratory arrest. Postoperative (postanesthesia). ARDS.	Patient can trigger ventilator and set rate. Guaranteed minimum minute volume via preset tidal volume or ΔP. Patient triggering can prevent muscular atrophy.	Possible hyperventilation. "Stacking" of breaths, causing ineffective ventilation and asynchronous breathing.
IMV (pressure or volume ventilation)	A predetermined tidal volume or ΔP (depending on whether format is volume or pressure ventilation, respectively) is delivered during each of the IMV (mandatory) breaths, providing a minimum minute ventilation. During the period between IMV breaths, the patient can breathe spontaneously. "Stacking" results when spontaneous and mandatory breaths occur simultaneously.	Weaning. Patients who are breathing asynchronously on assist/control. Patients who hyperventilate on assist/control.	Allows spontaneous breathing yet provides mandatory breaths at a predetermined rate. Minimization of barotrauma or decreased cardiac output because of lower mean airway pressure. Can prevent hyperventilation.	Spontaneous and mandatory breaths may be asynchronous ("stacking"). Hypoventilation or bradypnea.
SIMV (pressure or volume ventilation)	Same as IMV except "stacking" is avoided.	Same as IMV.	Eliminates the "stacking" effect. Same as IMV except probably more comfortable.	Same as IMV.
Pressure-regulated volume control	Combines benefits of pressure ventilation (i.e., decelerating waveform and lower PIPs) and volume ventilation (i.e., guaranteed tidal volume).	Refractory hypoxemia that does not respond to volume ventilation.	Tidal volume is maintained. Lower PIPs. Flow varies with patient demand.	Unknown; lack of data as of this writing.

TABLE 16–3. **Ventilation Modalities: Comparative Table** *Continued*

Mode	Description	Indications	Advantages	Disadvantages
Weaning Modes				
CPAP	No mandatory (ventilator-initiated) breaths are delivered in this mode. All ventilation is spontaneously initiated by the patient. A baseline pressure level (CPAP level) is provided constantly with the intent to prevent the collapse of alveoli.	Spontaneously breathing patient who has no need for minimum minute ventilation backup. Weaning.	Allows nurse to observe ability of patient to breathe spontaneously while still on the ventilator. Alarms can notify nurse of patient becoming distressed.	No backup rate (or minimum minute volume). End-expiratory pressure may cause additional work of breathing.
Pressure support	Patient must initiate all pressure support breaths. Patient effort must be maintained throughout inspiration. Patient effort is supported and tidal volume is enhanced.	Patients with small spontaneous tidal volumes. Difficult to wean patients.	High level of patient comfort because patient controls respiratory rate, inspiratory time, tidal volume, and flow.	There is no backup respiratory rate or minimum minute volume (unless used in conjunction with SIMV).
Volume support	Same as pressure support plus tidal volume is guaranteed.	Same as pressure support.	Same as pressure support, plus tidal volume is guaranteed.	Unknown; lack of data as of this writing.
Informational Feedback Modes				
Mandatory minute ventilation	A predetermined minute ventilation is selected. If patient cannot achieve this minute ventilation through spontaneous efforts, additional support is given.	Weaning.	Effective backup system if patient tires or becomes apneic.	Unknown; lack of data as of this writing.
Backup ventilation	Protects microprocessor.	"Brown outs."		
Apnea ventilation	Provides full support to patient in the event of apnea.	Any weaning mode.		
Disconnect ventilation	Ventilates and oxygenates patient at apnea ventilation settings after ventilator senses disconnection or occlusion.	Disconnection from ventilator. Occlusion of circuit.		
Noninvasive Ventilation				
BiPAP (spontaneous)	Respiratory rate is regulated by the patient. Volume will vary with patient effort.	Obstructive sleep apnea. Delay or defer intubation.	Many of the benefits of mechanical ventilation can be obtained without intubation. Benefits similar to pressure support.	Limited capabilities of alarm and monitoring systems (depending on number and type of accessory equipment used).
BiPAP (spontaneous/timed)	Respiratory rate is set by the ventilator and the patient can regulate spontaneous rate. Volume will vary with patient effort.	Obstructive sleep apnea. Delay or defer intubation.	Same as BiPAP (spontaneous) plus the security of a backup respiratory rate and minimum minute volume.	Same as BiPAP (spontaneous/timed).

Table continued on following page

TABLE 16–3. **Ventilation Modalities: Comparative Table** *Continued*

Mode	Description	Indications	Advantages	Disadvantages
Prolonged Inspiratory Ventilation				
Pressure control inverse ratio ventilation	The inspiratory time is longer than expiratory time, creating an unnatural breathing pattern. The prolonged inspiratory time exposes the lung to a longer period of positive pressure, which may cause recruitment of unstable alveoli, thus improving gas exchange. Because less time is provided for gas to expire, air-trapping may occur, causing a PEEP-like effect.	Diffuse pulmonary process. Refractory hypoxemia on conventional mechanical ventilation with high concentrations of O_2 (>60%) and optimized PEEP. Hemodynamic stability.	Possibility of lower PIP. Alternate method for improving oxygenation when conventional methods fail.	Tidal volumes will vary with changes in lung mechanics. Patient must be heavily sedated or paralyzed. Possibility of hemodynamic compromise.
Airway pressure release ventilation	Patient is allowed to breathe spontaneously. This mode augments patient's minute ventilation by alternating between two levels of positive pressure.	Can be used on an intubated or nonintubated patient. Should not be used as sole means of ventilatory support.	Possible reduction of PIPs, barotrauma, and cardiovascular side effects.	Unknown; lack of data as of this writing.
High-Frequency Ventilation				
High-frequency positive pressure ventilation	60–100 bpm (adults). 3–5 mL/kg tidal volume. Conventional ventilator can be used.	Major pulmonary air leak.	Clinicians are likely to be familiar with the equipment.	Driving pressure is often not strong enough, causing inadequate ventilation and oxygenation.
High-frequency jet ventilation	100–150 bpm (adults). Approximately 240–300 bpm (pediatrics). 3–5 mL/kg tidal volume.	Major pulmonary air leaks. Laryngoscopic and bronchoscopic procedures.	Often effective when high-frequency positive pressure ventilation is not (due to stronger driving pressure).	Special equipment is required. Oxygenation may be inadequate when compliance is poor.
High-frequency oscillator	300–3,000 bpm. 1–2 mL/kg tidal volumes.	Pulmonary interstitial emphysema; persistent pulmonary hypertension of the newborn; respiratory distress syndrome; major pulmonary air leaks.	Decreased peak inspiratory pressures.	Air-trapping, lung overdistention.
Differential lung ventilation	Each lung is ventilated by a separate ventilator. Independent ventilation and oxygenation of each lung is possible.	Unilateral lung disease (e.g., trauma, pneumonia, pulmonary hemorrhage, pulmonary contusion, bronchopleural fistula).	All ventilator parameters can be customized for each lung as required.	Difficult intubation process is required.

TABLE 16–3. **Ventilation Modalities: Comparative Table** *Continued*

Mode	Description	Indications	Advantages	Disadvantages
Mechanical Ventilation on Unconventional Gases				
Nitric oxide	Inhaled nitric oxide relaxes smooth muscle, causing reduced pulmonary artery pressure.	Guidelines are not finalized but studies show promise for primary pulmonary hypertension, ARDS, and persistent pulmonary hypertension of the newborn.	Improved oxygenation. Appropriate redirection of blood flow. Lower ventilator pressures.	Nitric oxide can combine with oxygen to form nitrogen dioxide, which can cause pulmonary edema or pneumonia. Nitric oxide and nitrogen dioxide combine to form nitrous or nitric acid, which can damage the patient's lungs, as well as equipment.
Helium	Helium acts as a lower-density carrier of oxygen, carbon dioxide, and medications in the presence of an obstruction.	Obstructions of large airways.	Improved ventilation.	Unknown.
Hypoxic gas mixtures (i.e., nitrogen and carbon dioxide)	By decreasing the FIO_2 to <21%, pulmonary blood flow is decreased and systemic blood flow is increased.	Hypoplastic left heart syndrome.	Redirection of a portion of the pulmonary blood flow.	A very low PaO_2 may indicate inadequately low pulmonary blood flow, requiring an increase in the FIO_2.
Gas Exchange Devices				
ECMO	A circuit and membrane lung remove most of the patient's circulating volume for external oxygenation and ventilation followed by return of the blood to the patient's circulation.	A treatment of last resort. Usually newborns > 2 kg that have not been on ventilator > 7 days, have no intracranial hemorrhage or congenital heart failure. Meconium aspiration, idiopathic respiratory distress syndrome, persistent pulmonary hypertension of the newborn, or sepsis. Common denominator is pulmonary hypertension.	Lung healing is promoted by allowing heart and lung to "rest."	
Extracorporeal carbon dioxide removal	Similar to ECMO (partial cardiopulmonary bypass). Venovenous system is used. Carbon dioxide is removed. Lowered ventilator settings allow lung to "rest." Insufflation of oxygen through a catheter in patient's trachea.	Treatment of last resort. ARDS failing conventional ventilation.	Same as ECMO.	Similar to ECMO.
Intravascular oxygenation	An oxygen and carbon dioxide exchange device is implanted in the inferior vena cava via femoral venotomy.	No specific indications yet. Under clinical investigation. Likely to be used on patients failing conventional ventilation.	Same as ECMO plus possibly less chance of gas embolism. Ease of insertion and simplicity of use reduce costs.	Bleeding, thrombosis formation, infection.

Abbreviations: ARDS, adult respiratory distress syndrome; CPAP, continuous positive airway pressure; ECMO, extracorporeal membrane oxygenation; IMV, intermittent mandatory ventilation; PEEP, positive end-expiratory pressure; PIP, peak inspiratory pressure; SIMV, synchronized intermittent mandatory ventilation.

tient who is being mechanically ventilated or weaned. Hemodynamic parameters such as heart rate and blood pressure are monitored. The patient is also monitored for signs of fatigue. Fatigue may be clinically present as dyspnea, paradoxical abdominal movement, increased respiratory rate and effort, diaphoresis, or a decrease in tidal volume at the same PSV pressure level. ABGs or pulse oximetry are also followed.

CASE HISTORY

Mr. C is a 72-year-old man admitted with acute exacerbation of COPD 4 days ago. He was treated with mechanical ventilation, antibiotics, bronchodilators, and IV aminophyllin. His chest x-ray is improving and his secretions have decreased in volume, and are now thin and white. His physician decides to try to wean Mr. C from the ventilator. Initial weaning attempts of slowly decreasing the SIMV rate have failed. Now Mr. C is placed on an SIMV rate of 8. Pressure support is added to decrease the work of his spontaneous breaths. The amount of pressure support is selected based on the spontaneous tidal volumes. The SIMV rate is decreased, then the pressure support is decreased with successful extubation.

Volume Support Ventilation

The volume support mode (Servo 300) allows the patient to breathe spontaneously, with each breath pressure supported. The difference between volume support and standard PSV is that the patient is guaranteed a minimum minute volume and receives support in the event of apnea. In PSV, as with pressure assist/control, the clinician may be required to adjust the pressure level to maintain adequate ventilation when tidal volumes fluctuate based on changes in the patient's compliance and airway resistance. This mode automatically adjusts the pressure support level on a breath-to-breath basis, maintaining a minimum minute volume. The initial ventilator settings are respiratory rate and minimum tidal volume/minute volume. The initial breath on volume support ventilation is a "test" breath. The ventilator then adjusts the pressure and volume delivery on a breath-to-breath basis based on the changes in the patient's lung mechanics. If the patient fails to meet the criteria for the apnea alarm, the ventilator automatically switches to the PRVC mode (described earlier in this chapter) until reset by the clinician.

INFORMATIONAL FEEDBACK FEATURES

The advent of microprocessors has enabled manufacturers to incorporate informational feedback systems into mechanical ventilation devices. Once informational feedback is received, it can be acted on. Ventilator settings can actually change automatically in response to changes in a patient's clinical status. To a limited degree, the ventilator now has "a mind of its own."

The underlying principle is to monitor and control a specific variable within a limited range. Informational feedback features can be used to ventilate, wean, and ensure safety for the patient and for the equipment itself.

For example, pressure regulated volume control is an informational feedback feature as well as a mode. For details, see the Pressure Ventilation section at the beginning of this chapter. The other informational feedback features are mandatory minute ventilation (MMV), PSV (excluding MMV), backup minute ventilation, apnea ventilation, and disconnect ventilation.

Mandatory Minute Ventilation

The targeted variable in this feature is the minute ventilation. A predetermined minute ventilation is selected for the patient. If the patient cannot achieve this minute ventilation through spontaneous efforts, predetermined tidal volumes are delivered at a respiratory rate that meets the specified minute ventilation.

The SIMV and pressure support modes are commonly used to supplement the minute ventilation. When SIMV is used as an MMV mode, consistent tidal volumes or pressure levels (depending on whether volume ventilation or pressure ventilation is used) are supplied to obtain the specified minute ventilation. When pressure support is used as an MMV mode, pressure support breaths are supplied, usually with incremental increases in the pressure support level until the required minute ventilation is achieved. The incremental increases occur in predetermined amounts and are limited to a certain range of pressure.

Pressure Support Ventilation (Excluding MMV)

In this feature, either the respiratory rate or the tidal volume is the targeted parameter. The theory of operation is similar to that described for pressure support as the MMV mode. See also Volume Support in the section on Weaning Modes.

Backup Ventilation

The ventilator automatically changes to this feature whenever the microprocessor is at risk of being damaged. The most common scenario would be an electrical "brown-out" in which the AC voltage is consistently in a specified voltage range (e.g., 80–95 V) for a specified period of time (e.g., longer than 6 milliseconds). Once the voltage returns to a level sufficiently close to 110 V, the ventilator resumes the previous settings and mode (usually after an electronic systems check). If the ventilator fails the electronic systems check, backup ventilation is resumed at settings fixed at the factory. For example, on the Puritan-Bennett 7200, the settings are Vt = 500 ml, FIO_2 = 100%, respiratory rate = 12 bpm, peak flow = 45 L/minute (personal communication with Don Bogan, Puritan-Bennett Corp., Carlsbad, CA, August 21, 1991).

Apnea Ventilation

The ventilator automatically changes to this feature whenever a preset apnea period is exceeded. Usually the patient can return to the previous settings by means of a manual reset or specified patient effort. For example, on the Puritan-Bennett 7200, a patient can cause the ventilator to return to the previous settings by spontaneously exhaling two breaths that are ≥50% of the set apnea tidal volume (personal communication with Don Bogan, Puritan-Bennett Corp., Carlsbad, CA, August 21, 1991).

Disconnect Ventilation

The ventilator automatically changes to this feature when the apnea period has been exceeded and the ventilator senses a disconnect or occlusion. The sensing process typically involves a comparison of proximal and distal airway pressures. If these pressures vary by more than a specified amount (e.g., 55 cm H_2O), disconnect ventilation is initiated.

On the Puritan-Bennett 7200 ventilator, the patient is ventilated and oxygenated according to the apnea ventilation settings (personal communication with Don Bogan, Puritan-Bennett Corp., Carlsbad, CA, August 21, 1991).

*NONINVASIVE VENTILATION: BiPAP**

BiPAP is a mode of ventilation that can be used noninvasively to assist spontaneous ventilation. BiPAP allows the clinician to set an inspiratory positive airway pressure (IPAP), equivalent to pressure support level, and an expiratory positive airway pressure (EPAP) equivalent to PEEP. BiPAP can be applied via a tightly sealed face or nasal mask, or by an endotracheal tube. The BiPAP system is essentially a CPAP generator that is able to maintain two different levels of pressure. When the patient is breathing spontaneously, the unit cycles from EPAP to IPAP when an inspiratory flow is maintained for a specified time. The unit cycles from IPAP to EPAP when one of the following criteria is met: (1) inspiratory flow decreases to a threshold level, (2) the unit detects an expiratory effort, or (3) inspiration has lasted for longer than threshold time.

There are four methods in which a BiPAP unit can be used: spontaneous, spontaneous/timed, timed, and CPAP.

- Spontaneous: the unit cycles between the IPAP and EPAP in response to the patient's efforts. The tidal volume, flow, and inspiratory time are a function of the patient's effort.
- Spontaneous/timed: the unit cycles in the same manner as in the spontaneous mode. If the patient fails to initiate an inspiration, the unit cycles on, based on the backup rate.
- Timed: the unit cycles between the IPAP and EPAP based only on the set backup rate and percent inspiratory time.
- CPAP: the unit operates as a CPAP generator when the IPAP and EPAP levels are equally set.

Theoretically, like CPAP, BiPAP can alleviate upper airway obstruction experienced with obstructive sleep apnea by splinting open the upper airways, or by increasing the FRC, which in turn maintains the upper airway patency. It has been postulated that if the airway collapse is caused by a subatmospheric pressure in the pharynx, then the IPAP component would be effective in preventing the upper airway obstruction. If the obstruction is caused by the need to maintain FRC, the EPAP component would be essential.

Studies have shown that BiPAP can be used effectively to prevent intubation of acute respiratory distress patients, assist patients who experience nocturnal muscle fatigue, and support postanesthesia and COPD patients. The IPAP component, like pressure support, assists the patient during inspiration, reducing the work of breathing; the EPAP level, similar to PEEP, is used to maintain FRC and improve oxygenation.

PROLONGED INSPIRATION VENTILATION

Pressure Control Inverse Ratio Ventilation

Pressure control inverse ratio ventilation (PCIRV) has been proposed as an alternative method of providing ventilatory support to a group of patients with refractory hypoxemia. With conventional volume ventilation, the expiratory phase of the respiratory cycle is usually longer than the inspiratory phase. In PCIRV, the duration of inspiration exceeds that of expiration. The duration of the inspiratory phase can be reversed to up to 80% of the total cycle time (inspiratory/expiratory ratio of 4:1 vs. the normal ratio of 1:3).

PHYSIOLOGY. PCIRV has been clinically used on patients suffering from ARDS. Although the exact cause of ARDS is unknown (see Chapter 32), the changes in pulmonary lung mechanics of patients with ARDS have been well documented. The primary problem from a ventilatory standpoint is the regional variation in resistance and compliance of the lung. This decrease in compliance, with the resulting increase of elasticity

**BiPAP is the registered trademark of the Respironics Corp., Murraysville, PA.*

of the lung, contributes to the difficulty in ventilating the ARDS patient. The traditional method of treating ARDS is to try to reinflate the areas of collapse with positive pressure on inspiration and stabilize the alveoli during expiration using PEEP. In the past, volume ventilation was the treatment of choice.

There are several problems associated with using volume ventilation on patients with severe ARDS. First, high PIPs are often generated with volume ventilation. Because there are areas of over- and underventilated alveoli, the repeated inflation of the lung at high positive pressures may increase the chances of barotrauma due to shear forces. Second, once the volume is delivered, the pressure within the lung decreases to a baseline pressure. Because the lung is "stiff," as the positive pressure returns to baseline, the lung has a tendency again to collapse. Often, a high level of PEEP is required to splint open the alveoli during expiration. The increased level of PEEP may cause the PIP and the mean airway pressure (MAP) to further increase.

To decrease the chances of barotrauma, the pressure assist/control mode with a prolonged inspiratory time can be used. The pressure assist/control mode is used because of the inspiratory flow characteristics. As the breath is delivered, the pressure and flow rise quickly, filling the ventilator tubing and smaller airways early in the inspiratory phase. As the pressure is sustained, the inspiratory flow declines, allowing distribution of gas between the fast- and slow-filling areas of the lung. Theoretically, the prolonged inspiration time exposes the lung to longer periods of positive pressure, which may cause recruitment of unstable or collapsed alveoli, thus improving gas exchange. It has been suggested that the prolonged inspiration decreases dead space ventilation (V_D/V_T) and improves the matching of ventilation to perfusion (V/Q) in patients who have decreased lung compliance. The MAP is usually higher in the PCIRV mode compared to volume ventilation, despite the lower peak pressures delivered to the patient's lungs. It has been suggested that the increased mean airway pressure (MAP) or the increased total end-expiratory pressure is responsible for the increase in oxygenation. However, physiologically, it is not exactly known why PCIRV improves oxygenation or ventilation.

The significant effects of PEEP are thought to be associated with the increased FRC, which recruits collapsed or unstable alveoli for gas exchange (Cole et al., 1984). Like PEEP, PCIRV can also increase FRC because the shortened expiratory time prevents full expiration. Because inspiration is prolonged and the expiratory phase is short, the lung is reinflated before the expiratory flow from the previous breath reaches zero. This incomplete expiration, or "air trapping," generates what is termed "auto-PEEP." The auto-PEEP therefore can replace the function of set PEEP, which stabilizes the alveoli during the brief release in positive pressure during exhalation.

INDICATIONS. Indications for use of PCIRV include the following:

- Diffuse lung injury demonstrated by chest radiograph
- Refractory hypoxemia on conventional volume ventilation requiring high levels of oxygen (>60%), high levels of PEEP, and high PIPs to deliver the set tidal volume
- Hemodynamic stability
- Decreased lung compliance

CONTRAINDICATIONS. Use of PCIRV in the following conditions may cause severe air trapping and thus result in barotrauma or inadequate ventilation:

- A nondiffuse lung disease process (e.g., lobar pneumonia)
- Obstructive pulmonary disease
- Presence of copious secretions

APPLICATION. A pressure-limited, time-cycled ventilator is placed in the pressure assist/control mode when using PCIRV. Conversion to PCIRV includes the following sequential steps:

1. PEEP should be optimized. In addition, the PIP and static pressure on the volume ventilation settings should be noted.
2. The patient should be heavily sedated or receive neuromuscular paralysis because the prolonged inspiration is seldom tolerated by an alert patient.
3. The patient should be placed on a ventilator that can provide the pressure assist/control mode (e.g., the "pressure control" mode on the Siemens Servo 900C or the "CMV" format of "pressure ventilation" on the Puritan-Bennett 7200) and has the built-in capability to measure auto-PEEP (or a means to measure auto-PEEP).
4. The F_{IO_2} should be set at 1.0 because onset of hypoxemia may occur when the mode of ventilation is changed.
5. The mode of ventilation is changed to pressure assist/control. There are a number of ways to set the initial inspiratory pressure. Whichever method is used, the exhaled tidal volumes should be monitored closely while the adjustments are made. The goal is to try to maintain a consistent tidal volume.
6. The inspiratory time is increased purposely to generate auto-PEEP, which is used partially to replace the set PEEP. The level that the set PEEP is reduced to will vary. The goal is to maintain optimal oxygenation without cardiac compromise. The lowest reversed inspiration–expiration ratio that provides the best oxygenation is recommended.
7. The respiratory rate can be used to "fine tune" the length of expiration, the amount of auto-PEEP, and the minute ventilation. Care should be taken when making a change in the rate to control ventilation. The traditional rules of mechanical ventilation do not always apply when ventilating a patient on PCIRV. Increasing the respiratory rate to increase the minute ventilation may have the opposite effect. As the respiratory rate is increased, the expiratory time is decreased, which may increase the

auto-PEEP level. In pressure assist/control ventilation, the volume that is delivered to the lung is based on the change in pressure from baseline to the PIP (ΔP). If you increase your baseline (set or auto-PEEP), you have decreased the ΔP, and have in effect decreased the delivered volume. This is what occurs when the auto-PEEP level is increased as a result of the increased rate. The opposite is true if you decrease the set PEEP or the auto-PEEP, or increase the PIP. For this reason, it is imperative that an experienced and trained clinician set up and monitor a patient on PCIRV.

8. Oxygenation is primarily regulated by the total end-expiratory pressure (set PEEP plus auto-PEEP). F_{IO_2} can also be adjusted to maintain the level of oxygenation.

MONITORING. The following parameters should be closely monitored when a patient is on PCIRV.

- All hemodynamic parameters, including cardiac output and $S\bar{v}O_2$ monitoring
- Noninvasive parameters such as capnography and oximetry
- Arterial and mixed venous gases
- Airway pressure and flow tracings
- Mean airway, peak pressures, auto-PEEP, and total end-expiratory pressure
- Exhaled tidal volume is extremely important to monitor; as the compliance improves (sometimes referred to as the "grand opening"), the tidal volumes delivered increase; the opposite holds true if the compliance decreases

ADVERSE EFFECTS. Although PCIRV reduces the peak airway pressures needed to ventilate and oxygenate the patient, it may increase the MAP. This increase in pressure due to the prolonged inspiration may affect venous return to the heart, which could result in a decreased cardiac output. For this reason, it is imperative to monitor closely the hemodynamic status of the patient on PCIRV.

In addition, if the ratios are reversed to the maximum level, the resulting increase in MAP exposes the lung to the possible hazard of barotrauma. Chest radiographs, breath sounds, chest rise, and all vital signs should be closely monitored for any signs of barotrauma.

SUMMARY. There is evidence that PCIRV may be beneficial when conventional means of mechanical ventilation have failed to correct or improve hypoxemia due to an acute lung injury. The improvement in gas exchange makes PCIRV an appealing alternative mode to treat ARDS patients.

PCIRV must not be indiscriminately used on any patient. The patient must meet the PCIRV criteria (mentioned earlier), and trained personnel with the proper understanding, technique, and equipment must be used to obtain safely the maximum benefit from this mode of therapy.

HIGH-FREQUENCY VENTILATION

High-frequency ventilation (HFV) should be considered to include any form of mechanical ventilation that functions at a frequency of at least four times the normal respiratory rate, that is, at least 60 breaths/minute (for an adult). This form of ventilation uses ventilator parameters beyond the conventional range, and challenges the traditional theory of ventilation. There are three major categories of HFV: high-frequency positive pressure ventilation (HFPPV), high-frequency jet ventilation (HFJV), and high-frequency oscillatory ventilation (HFOV).

PHYSIOLOGY. All forms of HFV use smaller-than-normal tidal volumes. As tidal volume is lowered, the airways and lungs are exposed to less PIP. This lower airway pressure may decrease the potential for trauma to the pulmonary system, but, as the tidal volume and airway pressure diminish, often so does alveolar ventilation. To make up for this loss, the respiratory rate is increased. Therefore, a normal tidal volume delivered at a normal rate is replaced by a smaller tidal volume delivered at the appropriately chosen higher rate. However, according to the traditional theory of ventilation, if the delivered tidal volume is smaller than the dead space volume (the part of the respiratory tract not involved with gas exchange), logically, this mode should not be successful.

The traditional theory of ventilation and gas exchange centers around the principle that two distinct regions of the lung exist: the dead space region, where gas is carried predominantly by bulk flow, and the alveolar region, which is primarily the area of molecular diffusion (gas exchange). This view, however, does not explain how normal ABG values can be obtained during experiments with HFV in which the tidal volume is much smaller than the dead space volume.

As the respiratory rate and tidal volume are altered from the norm, nontraditional forms of gas transport may come into play at different points and to various degrees. Diffusion plays a major role in gas mixing during HFV with small tidal volumes (Klocke et al., 1990). In other words, it appears that as the respiratory rate increases and the tidal volume decreases, the physiologic dead space diminishes to allow adequate ventilation, or the point at which bulk flow of gas terminates and molecular diffusion commences is repositioned to a location "higher" in the airways (toward the larger airways). Alterations such as this would allow gas to diffuse to the alveoli over a longer distance. This concept is known as augmented diffusion.

High-Frequency Positive Pressure Ventilation

DEFINITION. In general, HFPPV is defined as positive pressure ventilation delivered at a rate of 60 to 100 breaths per minute (bpm) with tidal volumes in the range of 3 to 5 mL/kg through a system that does not involve gas entrainment (i.e., additional gas drawn in from an outside source).

INDICATIONS. HFPPV is primarily used in patients who have major pulmonary air leaks, such as a bronchopleural fistula or a tracheoesophageal fistula, with the intention of minimizing leakage through the fistula by lowering the PIP.

APPLICATION. The cuff on the patient's endotracheal tube (or tracheostomy tube) should be deflated before the patient is connected to the ventilator, especially if the pathologic leak is minimal or intermittent. Placing a patient without a significant air leak on this mode can result in deleterious effects.

The initial ventilator settings may vary according to the functional limits of the type of ventilator being used. The respiratory rate should be set about 90 bpm. The inspiratory time and the preset pressure level should be set to achieve tidal volumes of 3 to 5 mL/kg.

MONITORING. Always keep in mind that HFPPV is delivered through a pressure ventilator, which means that tidal volumes may vary greatly and therefore need to be monitored closely. Decreased lung compliance due to pulmonary edema, fluid overload, and the like can cause a significant drop in tidal volume because of the back-pressure generated. Also, any obstruction of the tubing, such as from water condensation or secretions of the airway, can grossly affect the value of the delivered tidal volume. Therefore, patients on HFPPV need to be routinely suctioned as well as closely monitored for decreased lung compliance.

If the patient starts to retain too much carbon dioxide ($Paco_2 > 45$ mm Hg), the inspiratory time percentage should be increased. This will allow a longer period of inspiration and therefore a larger tidal volume, which will provide better ventilation.

Increasing the respiratory rate does not necessarily result in a decrease in the $Paco_2$, as it does in conventional ventilation. Delivering more breaths per minute will shorten the amount of time allowed for each breath to be delivered, resulting in an even smaller tidal volume and possibly a higher $Paco_2$.

Adequate oxygenation may be maintained by the Fio_2 alone, but another factor involved with determining oxygenation exists, namely, total end-expiratory pressure. Total end-expiratory pressure (the sum of set PEEP plus auto-PEEP, or TEEP) is the actual pressure remaining in the patient's lungs at the end of expiration. This value is not readily observed and therefore must be actively sought. TEEP increases oxygenation in the same way that traditional PEEP does, and, like traditional PEEP, it can cause cardiac compromise if the level is too high.

Traditional PEEP can also be used to improve oxygenation in the usual fashion, but it does not eliminate the need to measure TEEP routinely.

Because HFPPV is used primarily in patients with major pulmonary air leaks, close monitoring of fistula leaks is usually indicated with this mode (for details, see Monitoring in the section on HFJV).

ADVERSE EFFECTS. The major adverse effects seen with HFPPV are associated with hypoventilation. Special concern should always be given to airway management and the monitoring of lung compliance and tidal volume. With proper patient selection and effective monitoring, HFPPV can be a successful mode of ventilation.

High-Frequency Jet Ventilation

DEFINITION. HFJV (otherwise known as jet ventilation) in essence comprises the intermittent delivery of high-pressure gas (usually 2 to 40 psi, which is about 140 to 2,800 cm H_2O) through a small-bore injector cannula placed in the proximal end of the endotracheal tube. Additional gas is drawn in from the outside source (i.e., the negative pressure in the immediate vicinity of the jet "pulls in" or "entrains" extra gas for breathing, usually from a secondary ventilator). Respiratory rates can range from 60 to more than 200 bpm, but rates of 100 to 150 bpm are commonly used for adults.

INDICATIONS AND CONTRAINDICATIONS. HFJV is primarily intended for use in the treatment of large pulmonary air leaks such as bronchopleural fistulas and tracheoesophageal fistulas, and for bronchoscopic and laryngoscopic procedures. It can also be used on children for treatment of respiratory distress syndrome complicated by pulmonary barotrauma (Smith et al., 1993). Another specific clinical situation in which HFJV has been suggested is after lung resection surgery (Lain et al., 1990).

HFJV has been shown to generate lower peak, end-expiratory, and mean airway pressures while maintaining adequate oxygenation. Lower pressure readings, however, did not translate to improved outcomes (Hurst et al., 1990).

Because of the stronger driving pressure in jet ventilators, HFJV might be indicated in patients with large pulmonary air leaks when HFPPV ventilators cannot provide adequate tidal volumes.

APPLICATIONS. The ventilator used for adult HFJV is different from the ventilator used to deliver HFPPV in many respects. Some of its unique features include the following: (1) driving pressures that can be adjusted from 10 to 40 psi (approximately 1,000–2,800 cm H_2O), (2) an injector cannula that protrudes into the most proximal portion of the endotracheal tube, and (3) some types of jet ventilators do not have a built-in humidification system.

Adequate humidification is a persistent problem with most HFJV systems used on adult patients. To provide adequate humidification, a second source of humidification must be integrated into the system. There are reports of hemorrhagic tracheitis (Clevenger et al., 1990) and severe necrotizing tracheobronchitis (Circeo et al., 1991) associated with HFV treatment, and these are believed to have resulted from insufficient humidification of the gas.

To monitor airway pressures adequately, the pressure-monitoring tubing should be advanced through its designated port on the injector cannula system to a point where it is at least 10 cm away from the tip of the injector cannula. If the tubing is any closer to the injector cannula, the subatmospheric pressure created by the jet stream will affect the pressure readings. When it is properly positioned, the pressure monitor tubing will display a value close to alveolar pressure.

A respiratory rate of 100 bpm and an inspiratory time percentage of 30% are often used as initial settings for HFJV on adults. Both the tidal volume and PaO_2 can fall when the respiratory rate is adjusted to a level below 50 bpm (Lin et al., 1990). Rates of 240 to 300 bpm are often used on children (Smith et al., 1990). The FIO_2 is adjusted to achieve adequate oxygenation (O_2 saturation > 90% or PaO_2 > 60 mm Hg). The driving pressure is adjusted to deliver the desired tidal volume (usually 1–4 mL/kg). The patient's response to a change in the driving pressure (or ΔP) will be regulated by his or her compliance. The better the compliance, the greater the change in tidal volume (Pittet et al., 1990b).

MONITORING. Managing a patient on HFJV is similar to the method described for HFPPV.

Regulation of $PaCO_2$ is done primarily by adjusting the driving pressure. Increasing the driving pressure should decrease the $PaCO_2$ level, and vice versa. Tidal volumes correlate directly with the driving pressure.

With respiratory rates of 100 bpm or more, it may be difficult to obtain increased ventilation with increased respiratory rates. As the respiratory rate increases, less time is available for each inspiration, and subsequently ventilation diminishes. Increased respiratory rates as well as increased levels of the inspiratory time percentage (>30%) in this mode usually cause increased auto-PEEP with decreased ventilation.

Oxygenation, of course, can be regulated by the FIO_2 and the PEEP in the traditional fashion. Also, TEEP levels can be regulated by adjusting the respiratory rate and the inspiratory time percentage. An increase or decrease in either parameter usually causes an increase or decrease, respectively, in the level of TEEP.

Because HFJV is primarily used on patients with major pulmonary air leaks, leakage from the fistula should be monitored closely and routinely. A recent study (Roth et al., 1988) indicates that chest tube suction may influence the efficacy of a jet ventilator in the treatment of a bronchopleural fistula. In other words, the suction system creates subatmospheric pressure in the region of the lung adjacent to the chest tube. Therefore, a pressure gradient may exist, flowing from the positive pressure of the ventilator toward the subatmospheric region adjacent to the chest tube. In this study, as suction was increased, the minute volume inspired had to be increased to maintain an equivalent $PaCO_2$. The need for an increase in the minute volume inspired may have been the result of an increase in leakage through the fistula, facilitated by the pressure gradient (Fig. 16–3). Therefore, routine observation of fistula leaks is necessary to monitor the effect of chest tube suction on jet ventilator function as well as to monitor the leak itself.

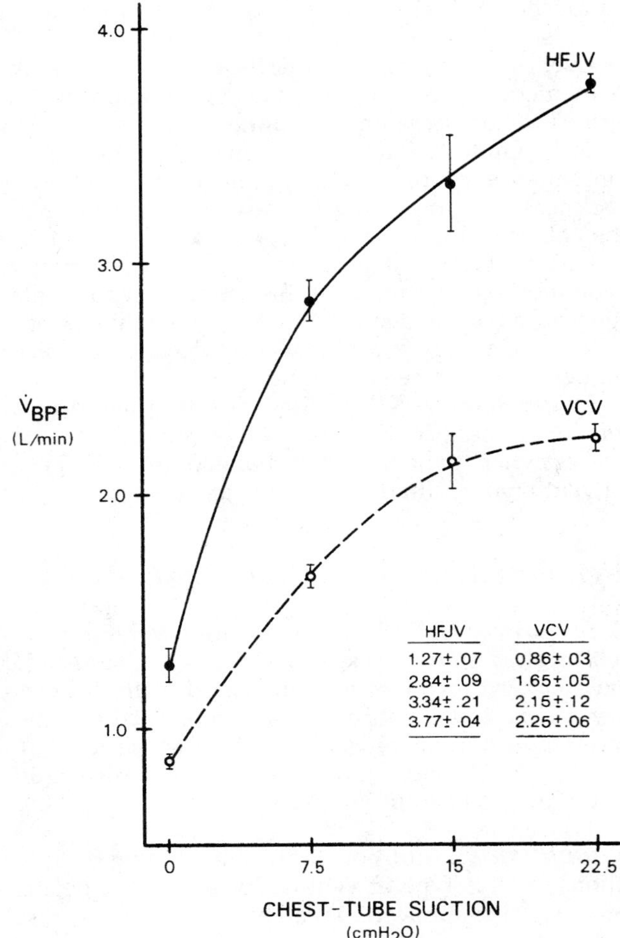

FIGURE 16–3. Flow rates through a bronchopleural fistula ($\dot{V}_{BPF}$) as a function of chest tube suctioning and ventilator type. VCV, volume-cycled ventilation. (From Roth, M. D., Wright, J. W., & Bellamy, P. E. [1988]. Gas flow through a bronchopleural fistula. *Chest, 93,* 210, 213.)

ADVERSE EFFECTS. If water condensation or secretions obstruct the pressure monitoring tubing, the ventilator may sense falsely high airway pressures. When pressures reach the driving pressure limit, the ventilator may stop functioning until the line is cleared. Such a situation may adversely affect the patient. Routine purging of the pressure-sensing line may prevent obstruction of the tubing. Purging is usually accomplished by activating a purge button for 5 to 10 seconds.

Even if a secondary humidification system is implemented, inadequate humidification remains a concern. Thicker secretions are often one of the first clinical manifestations of poor humidification. As a consequence, routine suctioning is a simple yet effective means of preventing the adverse effect of secretions obstructing the airway.

Because HFJV is delivered by a pressure ventilator, a common adverse effect of this mode is hypoventilation caused by a decrease in lung compliance or a build-up of airway secretions. This further emphasizes the need for routine suctioning.

Investigators failed to discover any differences in hemodynamics (Conti et al., 1990) or cerebral vascular indices when patients were changed from HFJV to conventional ventilation (Pittet et al., 1990a).

High-Frequency Oscillatory Ventilation

DEFINITION. HFOV is the application of rapid (300–3,000 cycles/minute) pulsations of gas in a sinusoidal wave pattern (symmetric with regard to the inspiratory and expiratory portions) providing tidal volumes lower than normal physiologic dead space levels to maintain MAP and support ventilation with significantly lower peak airway pressures.

INDICATIONS. Additional research defining the indications for this type of ventilatory support is needed before specific applications can be made. However, recent studies have demonstrated improvement of gas exchange in patients suffering from either infant respiratory distress syndrome or ARDS. It is believed that in these patients the high-frequency technique serves to apply a form of distending pressure (similar to CPAP) while effectively removing carbon dioxide (Froese & Bryan, 1987). Other possible patient groups include those with pulmonary interstitial emphysema, persistent tracheoesophageal fistulas, and persistent pulmonary hypertension of the newborn. The main goal here again would be to allow for adequate oxygenation and ventilation while lowering peak intrapulmonary pressures.

PHYSIOLOGY. Contrary to past accepted respiratory physiologic beliefs, carbon dioxide can be effectively removed (ventilated) with tidal volumes less than the normal anatomic dead space. The mechanism for this phenomenon appears to be multifactorial, and is not totally understood. Although bulk movement of gas still plays a role in gas exchange, other, possibly more dominant effects, contribute. These include (1) molecular diffusion (the normal movement of gas at and below the terminal bronchioles); (2) the pendeluft effect, or the movement of gas from areas of greater airway resistance or lower lung compliance to those of lower airway resistance or higher lung compliance; (3) cardiogenic mixing, which in essence is the rhythmic motion of the heart facilitating gas mixing inside the lungs; and (4) velocity profiles, where inspiratory gas characteristics are unlike those of exhaled gas because of the presence of directional changes (bifurcations of the airway directionally into the lung) (Froese & Bryan, 1987).

Oxygenation appears to be improved by mechanisms resulting in increased MAPs. Specifically, PEEP-like effects are achieved, allowing for recruitment of collapsed alveoli, which in turn reduces the overall shunt fraction. Furthermore, animal research indicates that surfactant secretion from type II alveolar cells is enhanced with HFOV, consequently providing improvement in alveolar stability.

APPLICATION. Oscillatory ventilators vary in their design and function. Some require the augmentation of another ventilator to assist with carbon dioxide removal or to supply bias gas flow. Others operate as a stand-alone ventilator. Instead of relying on passive exhalation, some oscillator ventilators actively pull delivered volumes of gas out of the patient's airway. Often a frequency of approximately 10 to 15 Hz (600–900 cycles/minute) is established, with an inspiration–expiration ratio of 1:2. Alveolar ventilation is accomplished by adjusting tidal volumes (amplitude settings), and arterial oxygenation is managed by adjusting F_{IO_2} and mean airway pressure settings. If the Pa_{CO_2} cannot be managed by increases in amplitude, the frequency is sometimes lowered to allow longer expiratory times and more complete exhalation.

Weaning from HFOV is accomplished by reducing amplitude settings and MAP settings as the patient's compliance improves. Patients are either returned to a conventional mode of ventilation or extubated directly from the oscillator.

MONITORING. Monitoring these patients requires observation of those parameters often associated with other modes of ventilation. These include ABG analysis, hemodynamics monitoring, airway pressures, oximetry, and the like. In addition, the potential for gas trapping is high, and attempts at detecting it are required. This may be achieved by closely following serial chest x-rays.

ADVERSE EFFECTS. Adverse effects include air trapping with overdistention of the lungs, carbon dioxide retention, hypoxemia, hemodynamic compromise, and a transient increase in respiratory secretion production. Sudden increases in arterial oxygenation may indicate recruitment of previously collapsed alveoli. Although this is a desired effect, it may herald lung overdistention. A chest x-ray will confirm concomitant lung overdistention.

DIFFERENTIAL LUNG VENTILATION

DEFINITION. Differential lung ventilation (DLV) is a method of ventilating each lung independently. The patient is mechanically ventilated by two ventilators, one for each lung. In essence, from a pulmonary standpoint, the "lungs are treated as two separate patients." The parameters of each ventilator can be customized optimally to ventilate and oxygenate each lung independently.

INDICATIONS AND CONTRAINDICATIONS. The primary indication for DLV is unilateral lung disease that has failed conventional treatment. It may be advantageous during the course of unilateral lung disease to ventilate the more diseased lung in a manner dissimilar to the method used on the more normal lung. DLV has often been effective in unilateral lung diseases such as pneumonia, pulmonary hemorrhage, pulmonary contusion, bronchopleural fistula, and flail chest. DLV has been shown to improve oxygenation after single-lung transplant in patients with differential lung compliance, and does not adversely affect hemodynamic status (Anton et al., 1993). Differential lung ventilation should not be implemented when personnel are inadequately trained to work with this mode, or when the difficulty of performing bilateral intubations outweighs the benefits of using the mode.

PHYSIOLOGY. Ventilation takes the path of least resistance, often resulting in the underinflation of atelectatic (or diseased) regions and the overinflation of healthy regions. With unilateral lung disease, this phenomenon is often emphasized.

Some pulmonary disorders will only add to the maldistribution problem. What might be useful to one lung might be harmful to another. A possible solution is to attempt to segregate lung regions that are underexpanded from regions that are overdistended. DLV makes such a concept a possibility.

APPLICATION. One major step that must be taken before initiating DLV is to institute the appropriate intubation process. Ventilation can be provided separately to each lung by (1) selectively intubating each mainstem bronchus, (2) selectively intubating one mainstem bronchus and then placing a second endotracheal tube in the trachea, or (3) using a double-lumen endotracheal tube.

After intubation, the endotracheal tube(s) is connected to two ventilators. A technique often used with DLV is to place the patient in a lateral position with the "bad" lung up. PEEP is then selectively adjusted to shift pulmonary perfusion to the relatively hyperinflated lung while simultaneously increasing ventilation to the relatively hyperperfused lung. The result is often increased V/Q matching. Compliance curves are likely to vary with the position of the patient. Appropriate adjustments should be made after repositioning.

The sum of the two delivered tidal volumes should be kept at 7 to 10 mL/kg (Beahrendtz, 1983). A static pressure measurement should be performed for each lung, and PEEP should be optimized according to the individual compliance curves of each lung. PEEP may be added to the more diseased (or traumatized) lung.

MONITORING. The general areas to be monitored are the various airway pressures, hemodynamic parameters, static compliance, and ABG values. During DLV, the healthier lung tends to have PIPs and MAPs that may be lower than those received with conventional ventilation (Beahrendtz, 1983). The more diseased lung should have PIPs and MAPs that are higher than those received with conventional ventilation (Beahrendtz, 1983) because this lung actually experiences more ventilation (and thus more positive pressure). A slight decrease in cardiac output can be observed, possibly the result of decreases in pulmonary vascular resistance and mean intrathoracic pressure (Beahrendtz, 1983).

MECHANICAL VENTILATION WITH UNCONVENTIONAL GASES

A mixture of oxygen and nitrogen is the gas most commonly used to provide mechanical ventilation in the ICU. Recently, nonconventional gases have been delivered through the ventilator for a desired therapeutic effect. These unique gases include nitric oxide (NO) for the treatment of pulmonary hypertension and improvement of V/Q mismatching, heliox (a mixture of helium and oxygen), used to reduce airway pressures and improve ventilation in patients with airway obstruction, and hypoxic gases (room air diluted with carbon dioxide or nitrogen) to reduce pulmonary blood flow in infants with hypoplastic left heart syndrome (HLHS). This section briefly addresses the clinical applications of these nonconventional gases.

Nitric Oxide

Two complications patients may experience while being mechanically ventilated are pulmonary hypertension and V/Q mismatching. These complications are often a consequence of the patient's underlying disease process and not a direct result of mechanical ventilation. Pulmonary hypertension may lead to right ventricular failure and a reduction in cardiac output. Treatment of this condition with infused medications (e.g., prostacyclin) may also cause systemic hypotension because of the inability to selectively direct the therapy to the pulmonary circulation.

Ventilation/perfusion mismatching, a common complication of pulmonary illness, may result in an altered gas exchange capability of the lung; a low V/Q ratio results in a reduction in arterial oxygenation. Infusion of vasodilators to treat pulmonary hypertension may increase pulmonary blood flow to poorly ventilated areas of the lung, worsening V/Q ratios. NO, an endogenous endothelium-derived gas, has been discovered to provide a therapeutic effect of reducing pulmonary hypertension and improving V/Q ratios in some patients with these abnormalities (Rossaint et al., 1993). Inhaled NO has a direct effect of relaxing smooth muscle, and, when inhaled into the lungs, reduces pulmonary artery pressures. Furthermore, the vasodilation (increased pulmonary blood flow) to those areas where NO is delivered (ventilated areas of the lung) reduces pulmonary blood flow to those areas of no or little ventilation (low V/Q). The overall effect is a reduction in pulmonary artery pressures and an increase in arterial oxygenation. Although NO is rapidly absorbed into the bloodstream, it is immediately inactivated by hemoglobin, thus avoiding the problems of peripheral vasodilation (systemic hypotension).

INDICATIONS AND APPLICATIONS. Guidelines for the administration of NO have not been completed; however, clinical studies have suggested possible uses for NO in ARDS, primary pulmonary hypertension, and persistent pulmonary hypertension of the newborn. NO is delivered directly through the ventilator pneumatic system (as a supplement to the supply gas mixture) in concentrations that vary from 8 to 80 ppm (parts per million). Either a chemiluminescence or an electrochemical NO analyzer placed in the delivery side of the ventilator is used to measure the inspired concentration of NO. A scavenging device is added to the expiratory side of the ventilator to prevent exposure of caretakers to the NO gas. Inspired concentrations of NO are adjusted within safe levels to produce the desired effect. The NO concentration is slowly reduced as the patient's condition improves.

HAZARDS. NO can cause serious side effects if not administered in low doses, and patients must be monitored carefully. NO combines with oxygen to form nitrogen dioxide (NO_2). The rate at which NO_2 is formed is accelerated by high levels of F_{IO_2} and NO. NO_2 is known to cause lung damage in the form of pulmonary edema or pneumonia. Together, NO and NO_2 combine to form dinitrogen trioxide, which dissolved in water may form nitrous or nitric acid (Miller & Miller, 1992). These acids are damaging to patients' lungs and to some plastic and metallic components of medical equipment. NO also combines with hemoglobin to form methemoglobin. Methemoglobin cannot combine reversibly with oxygen, reducing the overall carrying capacity of blood for oxygen. Continuous analysis of inspired levels of NO and NO_2 and periodic blood analysis for the presence of methemoglobin (co-oximetry) should be part of the NO therapy monitoring.

Heliox

Although oxygen–nitrogen gas mixtures are sufficient for ventilating most patients in the ICU, some patient conditions warrant the use of a lower-density gas. Specifically, in the case of airway obstruction, the flow of oxygen–nitrogen gas mixtures may become turbulent and thus require high inflation pressures. Helium has a lower density and a higher kinematic viscosity (a ratio of viscosity to density) than oxygen–nitrogen gas mixtures and is able to act as a carrier gas for oxygen and carbon dioxide with less turbulence and lower inflation pressures. This section provides some indications for the use of heliox (helium–oxygen).

INDICATIONS AND APPLICATIONS. Since its discovery as a useful medical gas in 1935, heliox has been applied to numerous patient conditions. Airway obstructions, especially those involving large airways where bulk flow of gas is prevalent, can cause turbulent gas flow and high inflation pressures. Laryngeal tumors, postextubation stridor (Kemper et al., 1991), and status asthmaticus (Gluck et al., 1990) have been described as conditions where heliox has been beneficial in reducing inflation pressures and improving CO_2 removal. A heliox gas source containing at least 20% oxygen (80/20 heliox mixture) is used to supply helium to the gas source of the ventilator. Concentrations of 40% to 60% helium are required to gain the beneficial effects of helium. Helium is substituted for nitrogen, with the remaining oxygen portion adjusted to maintain adequate arterial oxygenation. The helium is weaned as the patient's underlying condition is corrected or improves.

HAZARDS. Helium is an inert gas that has no known adverse effects when inhaled with oxygen or oxygen–nitrogen mixtures. Long-term use of inhaled heliox mixture has not produced any deleterious effects. Adequate oxygen concentrations must be supplied with the helium to maintain arterial oxygenation. Patients requiring high levels of inspired oxygen (F_{IO_2}) are not candidates for heliox because the resultant low percentage of helium is not clinically effective.

Hypoxic Gas Mixtures

Gas mixtures used to ventilate patients contain at least 21% oxygen (room air). There are a few clinical instances in which inhaled gas containing lower than room air concentrations of oxygen (hypoxic gas) have been supplied to patients for a therapeutic purpose. The goal of using hypoxic gas is to reduce pulmonary blood flow and increase systemic blood flow in selected patients with hypoplastic left heart syndrome (HLHS) (Malinowski, 1993). The following section describes the application of hypoxic gas administration.

APPLICATIONS. HLHS is a rare but commonly fatal congenital heart condition in which the neonate has a severely hypoplastic left ventricle and ascending aorta. These patients rely on the patency of the ductus arteriosus to sustain aortic (systemic) blood flow. Prostaglandin E_1 is administered to maintain ductal patency until surgical correction is performed. HLHS is corrected with either cardiac transplantation or through a series of surgeries (Norwood procedures). The stage 1 Norwood procedure results in the redirection of right ventricular blood flow to both the pulmonary and systemic circulation. HLHS patients awaiting cardiac transplantation or who have undergone a stage 1 Norwood procedure may present with increased pulmonary blood flow that is difficult to treat with infused medications owing to the inability selectively to apply vasoactive agents to the pulmonary circulation. Inhaled hypoxic gases (room air diluted with nitrogen or carbon dioxide) cause pulmonary vasoconstriction, with a reduction in pulmonary blood flow. This in turn reduces pulmonary edema and improves systemic blood flow until cardiac transplantation can be performed, or, in the case of a postoperative stage 1 Norwood procedure, until the patient's physiology has adapted and can maintain a balanced pulmonary and systemic blood flow. Patients' Pa_{O_2} values are expected to be maintained in a 35- to 40-mm Hg range with clinical signs of adequate systemic blood flow (blood pressure, urinary output, and acid–base balance). Nitrogen or carbon dioxide gas, or both, is added to the supply gas of the ventilator while continuously monitoring F_{IO_2} and F_{ICO_2} values. The F_{IO_2} is adjusted to maintain adequate oxygenation as well as pulmonary and systemic blood flow.

HAZARDS. Careful attention must be paid to arterial oxygenation. Pa_{O_2} values are expected to be in the 35- to 45-mm Hg range. Too low a Pa_{O_2} may indicate too little pulmonary blood flow, requiring increases in F_{IO_2}.

GAS EXCHANGE DEVICES

Three types of gas exchange devices are discussed. They are extracorporeal membrane oxygenation (ECMO), extracorporeal carbon dioxide removal ($ECCO_2R$), and intravascular oxygenation (IVOX).

Extracorporeal Membrane Oxygenation

The first type of gas exchange device to be discussed is ECMO.

DEFINITION. ECMO is the implementation of a circuit and membrane lung to remove most of a patient's circulating volume for the purpose of oxygenation and ventilation, followed by return of the blood to the patient's circulation. The vast majority of ECMO applications involve full-term neonates. Most neonatal ECMO systems operate as a venoarterial system, draining blood from the venous side of a patient's circulation and returning it to the arterial side (O'Rourke, 1991).

INDICATIONS. ECMO is the treatment of last resort for term infants who would otherwise die because of their decreased lung function. The patient must meet specific criteria before institution of ECMO can be considered. The patient is usually a newborn of at least 2 kg, having been on mechanical ventilatory assist for no more than 7 days, who has no intracranial hemorrhage or congenital heart disease but who does have reversible lung disease, and meets the respiratory failure index indicative of an 80% to 100% predicted mortality. Often these patients suffer from either meconium aspiration syndrome, idiopathic respiratory distress syndrome, persistent pulmonary hypertension, or sepsis. The common denominator in all of these patients is the presence of pulmonary hypertension.

CONTRAINDICATIONS. Failure to meet the above criteria or lack of parental or guardian consent constitutes a contraindication for ECMO.

PHYSIOLOGY. In some newborn infants, pulmonary hypertension develops secondary to various disease processes. As a result, significant right-to-left (cyanotic) shunting can occur, leaving the patient in a state of cyanosis and acidosis. This essentially is a persistence of fetal circulation. In a select group of these patients, reduction of pulmonary and cardiac blood flow for 5 to 7 days allows for return of the pulmonary pressures to near-normal values while the heart and lungs are rested. This can be accomplished by diverting approximately 75% of the cardiac output from the venous side of the patient and circulating it through a membrane lung. This permits oxygenation and ventilation of the blood. A circulating pump returns the "arterialized" blood to the aorta of the patient, where it can supply the body with necessary oxygen and nutrients (Fig. 16–4).

APPLICATION. Once the decision has been made to institute ECMO, the patient is heparinized to prevent embolic events from occurring while on circulatory assist. The right jugular vein is cannulated so that a venous catheter can be inserted into the right atrium. Similarly, an arterial catheter is inserted into the right carotid artery so that the tip is inside the aortic arch.

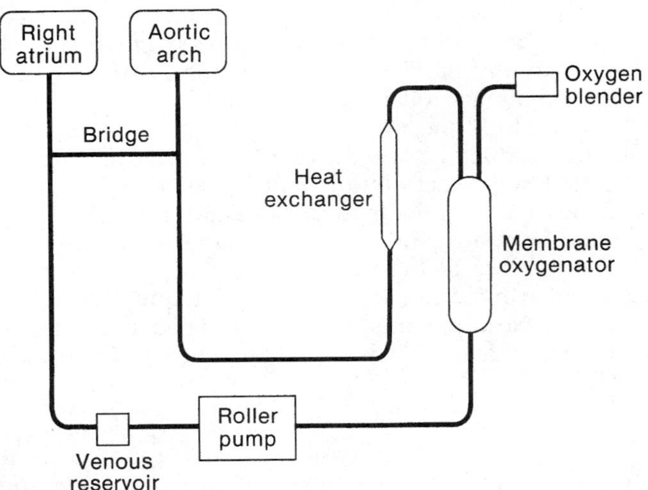

FIGURE 16–4. Extracorporeal membrane oxygenation (ECMO) circuit.

Once attached to the ECMO pump circuit, venous blood can drain by gravity toward a circulating pump. From there it is pumped through a membrane lung. Here, oxygen and carbon dioxide can be exchanged by the same mechanisms that operate in the natural lung (diffusion). By adjusting the flow of oxygen (and occasionally low concentrations of carbon dioxide) through the membrane lung, arterialization of the venous blood is achieved. The blood is rewarmed and then returned to the patient through the arterial catheter located in the arch of the aorta. The blood then can enter the brain through the left carotid artery as well as continue to the body through the normal circulation. The lungs and heart are now able to "rest," and healing of the diseased lungs is promoted. Weaning involves reduction of the extracorporeal blood flow so that the patient's lungs and heart begin to resume their normal function. Once most of the circulatory bypass has been weaned, the patient is removed from the ECMO circuit. The right carotid artery and jugular vein are ligated to prevent cranial embolisms. Note that before the institution of ECMO, these patients require high levels of inspired oxygen and ventilatory support. However, once on ECMO they can be placed on very low ventilatory settings.

MONITORING. The bulk of the monitoring in these patients lies with the close observation of the ECMO circuit, the heparinization of the patient and circuit, adjustments in circulatory flows, stabilization of ABGs, and observation of the patient's hemodynamics. The greatest concern rests with the regulation of coagulation times. These patients are at a greater risk for intracranial bleeding, and thus a combination of overanticoagulation and elevated intracranial blood pressure could be lethal. Adjustments of the sweep gases (gas that provides ventilation and oxygenation in the membrane lung) and pump flows are determined by analyzing the results of arterial, postmembrane lung, and mixed venous blood gases. Routine neurologic assessments are performed to alert the clinician to any possibility of intracranial hemorrhage. Aseptic techniques are strictly adhered to when dealing with any part of the ECMO circuit. Airway care and pulmonary toilet are carried out as per ICU protocols, and full-time, one-to-one nursing care is required. Blood products, especially platelets, are replenished as needed, and electrolyte balances are carefully maintained. These patients, once on ECMO, become very stable from a cardiopulmonary standpoint. Also, despite the loss of the right jugular vein and the right carotid artery, the outcome is usually quite favorable. In fact, these patients, with a predicted mortality of over 85%, have a 90% survival rate with the institution of ECMO.

ADVERSE EFFECTS. Possible complications include the development of an intracranial hemorrhage and sepsis. Other complications include bleeding, failure to wean from ECMO, air embolism, and mechanical failure of the ECMO circuit or pump.

ROUTINE CARE OF PATIENTS ON MECHANICAL VENTILATION

Humanistic Approach

Most, if not all, patients have a resistance to being placed on mechanical ventilation and other technological devices. Often they are the primary means of life support for the patient. At all times, the clinician must recognize the fact that he or she is managing the care of the patient connected to the ventilator, not the ventilator itself. The needs of the patient should be assessed through frequent communication with the patient. The patient can best determine his or her own comfort, and is the source of valuable feedback for the clinician. Individual plans of care can then be developed based on specific patient needs. Communication techniques (see Chapter 7) include letter boards, picture boards, and "common phrase" boards. Speaking devices such as the electrolarynx and the Passy-Muir speaking valve can be very effective in enhancing verbalization. Because of the increased work of breathing, however, these devices should be used only for a brief period (i.e., several minutes based on patient tolerance).

Ventilator Checks and Humidification

The ventilator should be checked regularly for proper functioning, proper parameter settings, appropriate alarm settings, and proper delivery of humidification (American Association for Respiratory Care, 1992b). Patency of the circuit and artificial airway should also be routinely checked. This procedure includes checking the cuff pressure. Inadequate cuff pressure can lead to loss of delivered tidal volume.

Humidification of inspired gas during mechanical ventilation is mandatory when an endotracheal tube or tracheostomy tube is present (American Association for Respiratory Care, 1992a). To maintain adequate humidification, the humidifier reservoir must be filled with water to the level indicating "full," and the water level should not be allowed to descend below the "refill" level. The heating device should be adjusted so that inspired gas is kept between 34°C and 37°C. Higher airway temperatures (up to 39°C) are occasionally used on hypothermic patients. Warmer airway temperatures (approximately 37°C) usually facilitate the mobilization of tenacious secretions. The tenacity of secretions is a clinical manifestation that is often used to determine the efficacy of the current airway temperature setting. Higher airway temperatures increase the ability of gas to hold water vapor. Therefore, condensation or "rain out" also increases as a result. Water should be drained as it accumulates in the tubing of the ventilator circuit. The water condensation problem is significantly minimized by using a heated-wire circuit. This system stabilizes the temperature, preventing condensation.

A physician order should routinely include the mode, FIO_2, the backup respiratory rate, and PEEP. Tidal volumes are commonly set at 10 mL/kg (±5 mL/kg based on other factors).

The nurse should become familiar with the fundamental alarm settings: apnea, low volume, pressure limit, and high respiratory rate. Although the specific technique for setting alarms can vary significantly from one model of ventilator to another, the general concepts are consistent. The apnea alarm is activated when a predetermined time period (usually 10–20 seconds) has elapsed without the ventilator "sensing" a respiration. The apnea alarm can be activated by a disconnected circuit, an obstructed airway or tubing, and the absence of patient effort to breathe. Low-volume alarms respond to exhalations that are smaller than the predetermined level (usually 50–100 mL below the set mandatory volume or the average spontaneous volume). This alarm setting may be difficult to make when exhaled tidal volumes vary considerably (e.g., during SIMV with small spontaneous tidal volumes). On volume ventilators, a pressure limit is used as an alarm as well as a safeguard to prevent overpressurization of the lungs. Pressure limit is usually set at 5 to 10 cm H_2O above the patient's PIP. High respiratory rate alarms alert clinicians to episodes of tachypnea.

Suctioning

Endotracheal suctioning is a component of bronchial hygiene therapy and mechanical ventilation, and involves the mechanical aspiration of pulmonary secretions from a patient with an artificial airway in place (American Association of Respiratory Care, 1993). To maintain a patient airway, suctioning is an essential nursing intervention. Secretion build-up can increase airway pressure readings, diminish ventilation and oxygenation, decrease the patient's comfort, and obstruct the airway. Suctioning pressure is 80 to 120 mm Hg for adults. Suctioning should not exceed 5 to 10 seconds. The patient should be hyperoxygenated before and after suctioning to prevent desaturation. Hyperinflating (i.e., sighing) the patient is sometimes performed in addition to hyperoxygenation to further decrease the chance of desaturation.

Assessment

Mechanical ventilation is a dynamic mode of therapy. The patient's status can change quickly. Breath sounds must be checked routinely for adverse clinical signs, adequacy of ventilation, and endotracheal tube position. Breath sounds are also essential in determining whether bronchodilators are needed or if mucolytics or increased humidification are needed for mucokinesis. Endotracheal tubes must be taped securely, and tracheostomy tubes should be cleaned routinely. Frequent monitoring of hemoynamic parameters, airway pressures, and ABG values is essential.

VENTILATOR TROUBLESHOOTING

The optimal response to problems with ventilators is calm and systematic action. On many occasions, the clinician may become overwhelmed by the amount of technologic equipment found in the ICU setting, and may respond with anxiety to alarms or problems with the performance of the ventilator. To rectify the situation, he or she must quickly assess whether the patient is in immediate danger. If so, the clinician is responsible for ensuring that the fundamentals of ventilation and oxygenation have been implemented.

Whenever a problem occurs with a patient on mechanical ventilation, the basics of ventilation and oxygenation can be provided with a handbag resuscitator connected to an oxygen source. If this equipment and a suctioning set-up are readily available at the bedside (and they must be), the clinician should have confidence that, if all else fails, he or she can maintain ventilation and oxygenation and manage the airway as well. Once the patient is out of danger and stabilized, the problem-solving process can begin. Using the systematic approach, the simplest problems and their potential solutions are sought first, and the more difficult problems and their solutions are then gradually considered.

A quick general surveillance of the immediate area is often the starting point. In other words, the clinician should look for the obvious, such as a disconnected ventilator circuit, crimped ventilator tubing, or a need for suctioning. If this process does not unveil the problem, then the alarm system must be checked. One should determine which alarm or alarms have been triggered and then search for possible causes (e.g., pressure limit alarm for obstruction, low tidal volume due to a loosely fitted section of tubing).

The systematic approach to the ventilator itself begins at the medical gas outlets on the wall and works toward the patient. If the patient is being ventilated by a handbag resuscitator, the tubing can be disconnected at various points along the circuit (that correlate with the flow of gas), and a volume-measuring device such as a Wright's respirometer can be connected to determine the amount of gas delivered. If the volume measured is grossly different from the volume preset on the ventilator, the ventilator itself may be malfunctioning and must be replaced. If the volume measured approximates the preset volume, then the ventilator is probably not the source of the trouble.

The next step in the systematic check is the humidifier. It can be ruled out as a leak source by simply bypassing it. The volume is measured distally (toward the patient). If the volume measures less with the humidifier connected, then it is the source of a leak.

The entire ventilator circuit tubing should be checked for an air-tight fit. Be sure to rule out an endotracheal tube cuff leak. If the circuit has an in-line nebulizer for aerosol treatments, it should be bypassed to rule it out as a leak source. As long as a handbag resuscitator is readily available and connected to an oxygen source, troubleshooting can be done without haste and without harm to the patient.

REFERENCES

American Association for Respiratory Care. (1993). Clinical practice guidelines for endotracheal suctioning of mechanically ventilated adults and children with artificial airways. *Respiratory Care, 38,* 500.

American Association for Respiratory Care. (1992a). Clinical practice guidelines for humidification during mechanical ventilation. *Respiratory Care, 37,* 887.

American Association for Respiratory Care. (1992b). Clinical practice guidelines for patient–ventilator system check. *Respiratory Care, 37,* 882.

Anton, W., Albert, R., Ralph, D., et al. (1993). Independent lung ventilation (ILV) following single lung transplant (SLT). Presented Dec. 11–14, 1993 at the National Convention of the American Association for Respiratory Care. Nashville, TN.

Beahrendtz, S. (1983). Differential ventilation and selective positive end-expiratory pressure: Effects on patients during anesthesia and intensive care. *Opuscula Medica,* Suppl. LXI.

Branson, R. (1994). Flow triggering systems. *Respiratory Care, 39,* 138–144.

Burton, B. G., Hodgkin, J. E., & Gee, G. N. (1984). *Respiratory care: A guide to clinical practice.* Philadelphia: J. B. Lippincott.

Circeo, L. E., Heard, S. O., Griffiths, E., et al. (1991). Overwhelming necrotizing tracheobronchitis due to inadequate humidification during high frequency jet ventilation. *Chest, 100,* 268–269.

Clevenger, F. W., Acosta, J. A., Osler, T. M., et al. (1990). Barotrauma associated with high frequency jet ventilation for hypoxic salvage. *Archives of Surgery, 125,* 1542–1545.

Cole, A. G. H., Weller, S. F., & Sykes, M. K. (1984). Inverse ratio ventilation compared with PEEP in adult respiratory failure. *Intensive Care Medicine, 10,* 227–232.

Conti, G., Bufi, M., Rocco, M., et al. (1990). Auto-PEEP and dynamic hyperinflation in COPD patients during controlled mechanical ventilation and high frequency jet ventilation. *Critical Care Medicine, 16,* 81–84.

Craig, K., Pierson, D., & Carrico, J. (1988). The clinical application of positive end-expiratory pressure (PEEP) in the adult respiratory distress syndrome (ARDS). *Respiratory Care, 30,* 185–201.

Froese, A. B., & Bryan, A. L. (1987). State of art: High frequency ventilation. *American Review of Respiratory Diseases, 135,* 1363–1374.

Gluck, E. H., Onorato, D. J., & Castriota, R. C. (1990). Helium–oxygen mixtures in intubated patients with status asthmaticus and respiratory acidosis. *Chest, 90,* 993–998.

Hickling, K. G., Henderson, S. J., & Jackson, R. (1990). Low mortality associated with low volume, pressure limited ventilation with permissive hypercapnia in severe adult respiratory distress syndrome. *Intensive Care Medicine, 16,* 372–377.

Hurst, J. M., Branson, R., Davis, K., et al. (1990). Comparison of conventional mechanical ventilation and high-frequency ventilation. *Annals of Surgery, 211,* 486–491.

Kacmarek, R. M., & Venegas, J. (1987). Mechanical ventilatory rates and tidal volumes. *Respiratory Care, 32,* 466–478.

Kemper, K. J., Ritz, R. H., Benson, M. S., & Bishop, M. S. (1991). Helium–oxygen mixture in the treatment of postextubation stridor in pediatric trauma patients. *Critical Care Medicine, 19,* 356–359.

Kirby, R. (1988). Modes of mechanical ventilation. In R. M. Kacmarek & J. K. Stoller (Eds.), *Current respiratory care.* Toronto: B. C. Decker.

Klocke, R. A., Saltzman, A. R., Grant, B. J. B., et al. (1990). Role of molecular diffusion in conventional and high frequency ventilation. *American Review of Respiratory Disease, 142,* 802.

Lain, D., Crocker, E. F., Choudhay, B. A., et al. (1990). Reduction of peak inspiratory pressure using high frequency jet ventilation and pressure control ventilation following pneumonectomy. *Chest, 98,* 229–230.

Lin, S., Jones, M. J., Mottram, S. D., et al. (1990). Relationship between resonance and gas exchange during high frequency jet ventilation. *British Journal of Anaesthesiology, 64,* 453–459.

MacIntyre, N. R. (1988). Pressure support: Inspiratory assist. In R. M. Kacmarek & J. K. Stoller (Eds.), *Current respiratory care.* Toronto: B. C. Decker.

Malinowski, C. (1993). Hypoxic gas mixture in the treatment of hypoplastic left heart syndrome: A case study. *Respiratory Care, 38,* 1235.

Marini, J. J. (1992). New approaches to the ventilatory management of the adult respiratory distress syndrome. *Journal of Critical Care, 87,* 256–257.

Miller, C. C., & Miller, W. R. (1992). Pulmonary vascular smooth-muscle regulation: The role of inhaled nitric oxide gas. *Respiratory Care, 37,* 1175–1185.

Morris, A. H., Wallace, C. J., Clemmer, T. P., et al. (1990). Extracorporeal CO_2 therapy for adult respiratory distress syndrome patients. *Respiratory Care, 35,* 224–231.

O'Rourke, P. P. (1991). ECMO: Where have we been? Where are we going? *Respiratory Care, 36,* 683–690.

Pittet, J. F., Forster, A., & Suter, P. M. (1990a). High frequency jet ventilation and intermittent positive pressure ventilation: Effect of cerebral blood flow in patients after open heart surgery. *Chest, 97,* 420–424.

Pittet, J. F., Morel, D. R., Bachmann, M., et al. (1990b). Predictive value of FRC and respiratory compliance on pulmonary gas exchange induced by high frequency jet ventilation in humans. *British Journal of Anaesthesiology, 64,* 460–468.

Rappaport, S., Shpiner, R., Yoshihara, G., et al. (1994). Randomized, prospective trial of pressure-limited versus volume-controlled ventilation in severe respiratory failure. *Critical Care Medicine, 22,* 22–32.

Rossaint, R., Falke, K. J., Lopez, F., et al. (1993). Inhaled nitric oxide for the treatment of the adult respiratory distress syndrome. *New England Journal of Medicine, 328,* 399–405.

Roth, M. D., Wright, J. W., & Bellamy, P. E. (1988). Gas flow through a bronchopleural fistula. *Chest, 93,* 210–213.

Sassoon, C. (1992). Mechanical ventilator design: The trigger variable. *Respiratory Care, 37,* 1056–1069.

Scanlan, C. L., Spearman, C. B., Sheldon, R. L., & Egan, D. F. (1990). *Egan's fundamentals of respiratory care* (5th ed.). St. Louis: C. V. Mosby.

Shapiro, B., Harrison, R., & Trout, C. (1982). *Clinical application of respiratory care* (2nd ed.). Chicago: Year Book.

Smith, D. W., Frankel, L. R., Derish, M. T., et al. (1993). High-frequency jet ventilation in children with the adult respiratory distress syndrome complicated by pulmonary barotrauma. *Pediatric Pulmonology, 15,* 279.

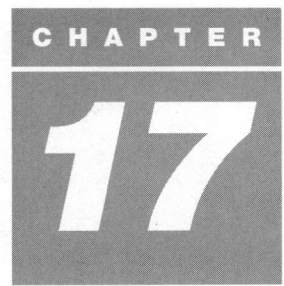

Intracranial Pressure Monitoring

Norma D. McNair

Intracranial pressure (ICP) is a dynamic process influenced by physiologic variables that affect the volume within the intracranial compartment. The major components of intracranial volume include the cerebrospinal fluid, intracranial blood volume, and brain tissue. The equilibrium pressure generated by the total volume within the confines of the intracranial compartment is referred to as the ICP. This pressure can be measured in the ventricles, in the subarachnoid, subdural, or epidural space, or in the brain parenchymal tissue. Normal intracranial pressure is between 0 and 15 mm Hg (Doyle & Mark, 1992; Marshall et al., 1990). ICP values may vary slightly depending on the site of ICP monitoring, the location of the intracranial pathology, and the monitoring equipment used. Continuous ICP monitoring can serve as a guide for the diagnosis and continuing management of patients with increased ICP. The pathophysiologic basis of increased ICP as well as related assessment parameters will be reviewed in this chapter before the techniques of ICP monitoring are described.

PHYSIOLOGY OF INTRACRANIAL PRESSURE

Intracranial Volume Relationships

In a normal adult, the total intracranial volume is approximately 1900 mL (Rosner, 1993). This volume includes the cerebrospinal fluid (CSF; approximately 10%, or 150 mL), brain tissue with its associated intracellular and extracellular fluid (approximately 80%, or 1,500 mL), and the cerebral blood volume (CBV) contained within the venous, capillary, and arterial vessels (approximately 10%, or 150 mL) (Rosner, 1993). Changes in volume of any one of these components, if uncompensated for, will influence the ICP.

Observations relating to the intracranial volume relationships of the brain and blood volume were first reported in the late eighteenth and early nineteenth centuries by Alexander Monro and George Kellie. During the nineteenth and twentieth centuries, the contribution of the CSF to intracranial volume was appreciated, and a greater understanding of the interrelationships among the brain, blood, and CSF volumes and their effects on ICP was achieved. The key principles governing the relationships between these volumes and changes in ICP have been referred to as the modified Monro-Kellie doctrine, and can be summarized by the following points. The intracranial space is nearly constant in volume, with essentially noncompressible contents (Langfitt, 1990). The intracranial components, including the blood, brain matter, and CSF, fill the skull to capacity. If any one of these components increases in volume, there must be a compensatory decrease in another for the overall volume to remain constant; otherwise, there will be an increase in ICP. Pathologic ICP is an estimate of the force required to displace blood and CSF from the intracranial vault in an effort to accommodate new volume that may be added (Rosner, 1993).

These principles apply primarily to rigid, fused skulls. In certain situations the intracranial space has a limited ability to respond to an increased volume by expansion of the skull, for example, in the infant before the sutures of the skull have fused, or in the patient with a skull fracture.

Physiologic Compensatory Response to Volume Changes

The first potential compensatory response to the need to accommodate increased volume is a reduction in the volume of the intracranial CSF. This occurs primarily through displacement or shunting of CSF from the intracranial space to the spinal subarachnoid space. Reduction in total CSF volume may also be achieved by increasing reabsorption of CSF through the arachnoid villi (Marshall et al., 1990; Rosner, 1993). CSF production, in most situations, is not significantly affected by volume or pressure changes except in severe cases, when cerebral blood flow is compromised (Rosner, 1993).

Another method of compensation involves dis-

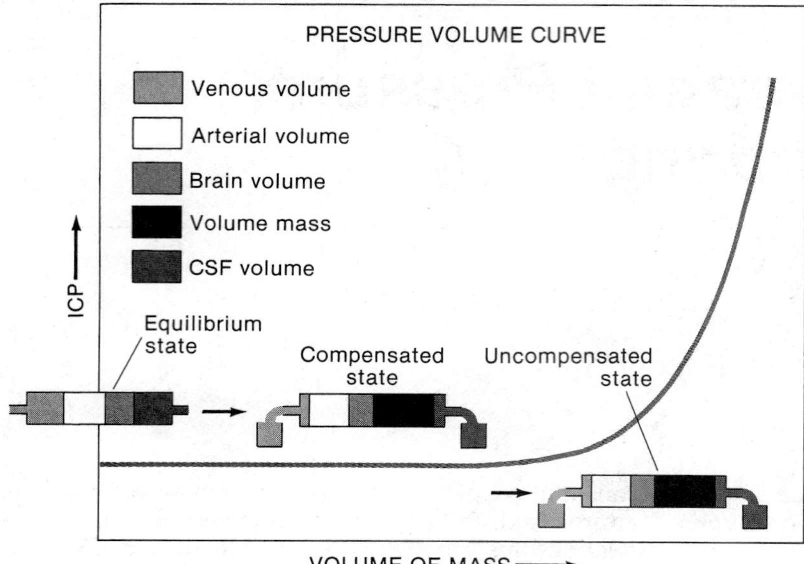

FIGURE 17–1. Physiologic compensatory response to intracranial volume changes. In this figure, "volume mass" indicates any additional volume in the intracranial compartment that is not normally present. This may include additional brain tissue, blood, or CSF volume. (Redrawn from Ward, J. D., et al. [1981]. Intracranial pressure, head injuries, subarachnoid hemorrhage, non-surgical coma, and brain tumors. In W. C. Shoemaker, & W. L. Thompson [Eds.], *Critical care, state of the art* [Vol. II, p. 2]. Fullerton, CA: Society of Critical Care Medicine.)

placement of the low-pressure venous blood volume out of the intracranial compartment (Andrus, 1991; Rosner, 1993). The ability of this response to compensate for an increase in volume is limited, however, by the relatively low volume of venous blood. At some point, the compensatory mechanisms involving CSF and blood volume will be exhausted, and ICP will begin to rise (Fig. 17–1).

FACTORS INFLUENCING ABILITY TO COMPENSATE

Many factors can influence the effectiveness of this intracranial compensation. These factors include the rate of expansion of the mass, the location of the mass or volume in the intracranial compartment, impairment of CSF dynamics, and brain compliance (Marshall et al., 1990; Rosner, 1993).

RATE OF EXPANSION IN INTRACRANIAL VOLUME. An increase in volume that occurs over a long period of time can be compensated for more completely than a rapid increase of the same volume. For example, a patient with an acute epidural hematoma may have markedly increased ICP, whereas a patient with a slowly growing brain tumor of similar size may have a normal or slightly increased ICP.

LOCATION OF MASS OR LESION. The location of the mass or lesion can also influence the ability of the brain to compensate for a change in volume within the intracranial compartment. Intracranial lesions at different sites may result in direct or indirect obstruction of CSF pathways through distortion of brain tissue, limiting the compensatory mechanism of CSF displacement (Langfitt, 1990; Marshall et al., 1990). For example, a large tumor of the third ventricle, in addition to increasing brain volume, may obstruct normal CSF circulation, resulting in increased ICP with minimal compensatory ability.

IMPAIRED CSF DRAINAGE OR REABSORPTION. CSF drainage and reabsorption can also be limited by obstruction or inflammation of the arachnoid villi. This causes resistance to absorption to CSF and contributes to increased ICP. A complication of subarachnoid hemorrhage is hydrocephalus resulting from blood obstructing the arachnoid villi. CNS infections such as meningitis may also result in increased ICP due to inflammation of the meningeal layers and secondary obstruction of the arachnoid villi (Rosner, 1993).

COMPLIANCE

Compliance (C) refers to the ratio of the change (Δ) in volume (V) to the resulting change in pressure (P). It is a measure of the amount of "give" in the system (Langfitt, 1990). When compliance is high, larger volume changes can occur without causing a significant change in ICP. Conversely, when compliance is low, any small increase in intracranial volume results in a marked increase in ICP. The following formula represents this relationship:

$$C = \frac{\Delta V}{\Delta P}$$

In the clinical setting, compliance testing can be performed by a physician using the technique described in Figure 17–2.

Elastance is the inverse of compliance and describes the amount of resistance offered to expansion of the mass (Andrus, 1991; Cammermeyer & Appeldorn, 1990; Langfitt, 1990). A diagrammatic representation of this pressure–volume relationship is included

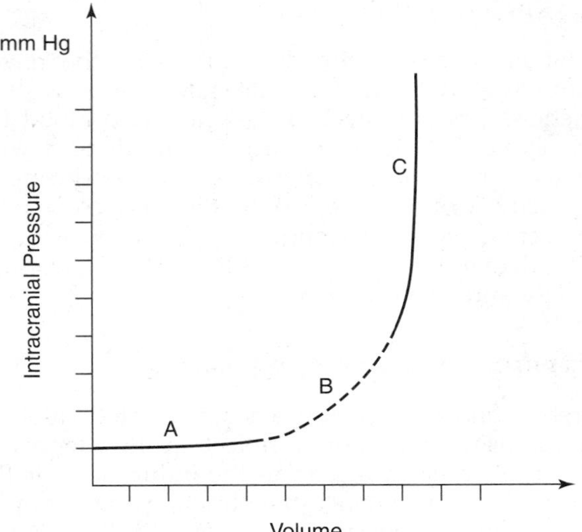

FIGURE 17–2. Compliance testing: (1) A baseline ICP reading is obtained and recorded.* (2) 1 mL of sterile saline is injected into the ventricular catheter within 1 second. (3) ICP readings are then obtained.* (4) Interpretation of data is based on the change in ICP in response to additional 1 mL of volume. If the resulting pressure change is less than or equal to 2 mm Hg (*A*), compliance is high and functional compensatory mechanisms are present. If there is an increase in ICP greater than 2 mm Hg (*B*), this is indicative of low compliance and poor compensatory reserve. Small increases in volume result in tremendous increases in pressure (*C*) (Hickey, 1992). (Redrawn from Germon, K. [1988]. *Journal of Neuroscience Nursing, 20,* 344–351.)

**Note:* It is recommended that a test dose of 0.2 mL of sterile normal saline be injected before the complete 1-mL injection (Hickey, 1992). If there is no change in pressure, the additional 0.8 mL may be quickly injected. This precaution will prevent unnecessary pressure spikes in a patient with very low compliance.

in Figure 17–1. As illustrated in the initial portion of the curve, a small increase in volume does not result in an increase in pressure because compensatory mechanisms are effective and compliance is high. When the compensatory mechanisms are exhausted and compliance decreases, any addition in volume will result in a sharp increase in pressure. The precise shape of the curve and the point at which an additional increase in volume results in a sharp increase in pressure varies with the individual patient and the pathophysiologic condition.

Cerebral Blood Flow

The brain demands a constant supply of oxygen, glucose, and the other metabolic substrates for cellular oxygenation and metabolism in the brain. An understanding of the factors that influence cerebral blood flow (CBF) is essential. CBF and CBV are independent of each other; high CBF does not necessarily mean that there will be a high CBV (Rosner, 1993). Variables that have a significant effect on CBF include the following: metabolic demands of the brain, the influence of ICP reflected in the cerebral perfusion pressure (CPP), and the influence of arterial blood gas parameters and systemic blood pressure on autoregulatory mechanisms. Before these variables are discussed, however, the next section presents various techniques for CBF monitoring.

CEREBRAL BLOOD FLOW MONITORING

Cerebral blood flow monitoring techniques provide additional and valuable information regarding the circulatory status of the brain. Various techniques are available, and each one provides a slightly different emphasis.

TRANSCRANIAL DOPPLER. Doppler ultrasonography is the technique used for measuring the velocity of blood flow in the arteries of the circle of Willis. This technique does not provide information regarding the quantitative flow (mL/100 g/second), nor does it measure flow in the peripheral cerebral blood vessels. Information about velocities in the basal arteries can provide data regarding the integrity of the major cerebral vessels. The arteries that are routinely examined are the middle cerebral arteries, the anterior cerebral arteries, and the posterior communicating arteries. In addition, the posterior circulation (vertebral, basilar, and posterior cerebral arteries) can be examined. Vasospasm, hyperemia, and low or no flow states can be identified and followed over time.

Transcranial Doppler is an important adjunct in the intensive care unit (ICU) because it is noninvasive, can be performed at the bedside, and can be repeated as often as needed. Patients can be monitored outside of the ICU as well for long-term follow-up. The test should be performed by an individual trained and practiced in the use of transcranial Doppler to ensure accurate and consistent results. It is now possible to place a probe with a headband for prolonged monitoring (Newell & Aaslid, 1992; Obana & Andrews, 1993).

THERMAL DILUTION CBF MONITORING. Thermal dilution CBF monitoring allows for localized CBF monitoring. Because it is based on thermal dilution principles, data can be obtained only from a limited area of the brain, such as one gyrus. The probe is placed intraoperatively in the subdural space, where there is continual contact with the brain. The data are recorded in mL/100 g/minute. Data are evaluated based on relative flow changes, which indicate ischemia or hyperemia. This type of monitoring is accurate and reproducible (Carter et al., 1991; Dickman et al., 1991; Meyerson et al., 1991; Obana & Andrews, 1993).

GLOBAL CBF MEASUREMENT. Techniques that measure whole brain blood flow may provide a more accurate representation of global CBF. The most common technique of measurement requires that an inert substance such as xenon-133 be given and its washout measured.

Xenon-133 can be given intravenously or via inhalation. Scintillation counters are placed over both hemispheres and the isotope concentration is measured. Computer analysis then provides an estimate of CBF. Results are reported in mL/100 g/minute. The test requires trained personnel and the use of additional equipment at the bedside. Although repeated tests are possible, time must be allowed between examinations for all of the inert gas to dissipate. In addition, there is exposure to radioactive tracer, but exposure is thought to be minimal (Obana & Andrews, 1993).

STABLE XENON COMPUTED TOMOGRAPHY. The use of stable xenon computed tomography (CT) is relatively new. The advantage of this technique is that it provides CBF information from cortical regions and deep brain structures that cannot be assessed from the xenon-133 examination. The values obtained correlate well with xenon-133 studies. A disadvantage to this technique is that it requires the patient to go to the CT scanner, and thus the test is not easily repeated (Marion & Bouma, 1991). Xenon may cause cerebral vasodilation, leading to an increased ICP and CBF. Studies have shown that 33% stable xenon over 4.5 minutes does not significantly increase ICP (Bouma et al., 1992a; Marion & Bouma, 1991).

JUGULAR VENOUS OXYGEN SATURATION. Metabolism and CBF are closely linked and chemical end products of metabolism can be measured from CSF or from jugular venous blood. Saturated venous jugular oxygen ($SvjO_2$) gives an indication of central nervous system circulatory effectiveness. The range should be 60% to 70%. An oximetric catheter is inserted into the jugular vein and values are recorded continuously. Low and high values indicate alterations in the oxygen delivery and utilization in the brain. Limitations to the use of the catheter include the invasiveness of the catheter and maintaining placement. Some catheters may not remain accurate for a long period of time, limiting the usefulness of the catheter and the results. Placement of the catheter does allow intermittent blood sampling to evaluate the $SvjO_2$, should the catheter malfunction or the saturation drop below 50%.

Advantages of $SvjO_2$ monitoring include detecting episodes of desaturation that might otherwise go unnoticed. Desaturation occurring in patients generally correlates with a higher mortality rate if not corrected. A disadvantage of this monitoring is that the $SvjO_2$ may not decrease until herniation is already observed clinically. In addition, if CBF drops considerably, an accurate $SvjO_2$ may not be obtained because of extracerebral contamination of jugular blood (Obana & Andrews, 1993; Sheinberg et al., 1992).

These various types of CBF monitoring provide useful information to the nurse and to the physician that can assist in promoting optimum management of ICP. These various CBF monitoring systems may not be seen in most institutions; thus, ICP monitoring becomes more important in patient management.

METABOLIC DEMANDS

Metabolic demands are determined by the relative neuronal activity in the brain. CBF varies with the functional activity level of the brain, and blood flow increases as activity increases. In conditions in which metabolic demands are increased, such as during seizure activity or febrile episodes, there is a corresponding increase in CBF. Conditions that decrease metabolic demands and thus CBF include barbiturate therapy and hypothermia.

CEREBRAL PERFUSION PRESSURE

Cerebral perfusion pressure is a calculated value that may be used as a guide in reflecting the adequacy of CBF. This value incorporates the influence of ICP on CBF and is calculated by subtracting the mean ICP from the mean arterial pressure (MAP). For example, a patient with an MAP of 90 and an ICP of 10 would have a CPP of 80. An example of how this calculated value is obtained is shown by this equation:

$$\text{MAP (90)} - \text{ICP (10)} = \text{CPP (80)}$$

A normal range for CPP is approximately 70 to 100 mm Hg (Cammermeyer & Appeldorn, 1990). A CPP of at least 60 to 70 mm Hg is necessary for adequate cerebral perfusion. Ischemia and neuronal death may be seen when CPP falls below 30 to 40 mm Hg (Germon, 1994). A word of caution is in order when assessing the CPP of head-injured patients. These patients may appear to maintain an adequate CPP (>60 mm Hg) by calculations based on MAP and ICP; however, this may not reflect problems with inadequate perfusion to regions of the brain that have been injured. For this reason, in head-injured patients, adequate cerebral perfusion cannot be ensured for all regions of the brain based solely on the calculation of CPP values. These patients may require a higher CPP than previously thought to perfuse all regions of the brain.

AUTOREGULATION

Autoregulation refers to the ability to maintain a relatively constant CBF over a wide range of CPP, arterial blood pressures, and metabolic conditions. Autoregulatory control is achieved by initiating a change in cerebral vascular resistance, which regulates CBF in the absence of severe brain injury. CPP is the stimulus for autoregulation, not the systemic arterial pressure (Rosner, 1993).

METABOLIC AUTOREGULATION. Metabolic autoregulation maintains a relatively constant CBF with PaO_2 greater than 50 mm Hg. Profound hypoxia or PaO_2 less than 50 mm Hg will result in cerebral vasodilation and increased CBF (Rosner, 1993). CBF is very sensitive to changes in PCO_2. From approximately 20 to 80 mm Hg, cerebral vasodilation occurs, and CBV increases with an increasing PCO_2. In contrast, a decreased PCO_2 results in vasoconstriction and decreased CBV. This is the basis for therapeutic hyperventilation of a patient with increased ICP to maintain a P_{CO_2} of between 30 and 35 mm Hg.

PRESSURE AUTOREGULATION. CBF is constant in healthy adults with an MAP ranging from approximately 60 to 160 mm Hg and a CPP of between 50 and 150 mm Hg owing to pressure autoregulatory mechanisms maintained in part through control of arteriolar resistance (Marshall et al., 1990). As perfusion pressure decreases, cerebral vessels dilate to maintain a relatively constant CBF. When perfusion pressure increases, cerebral vasoconstriction occurs, and CBF is maintained within a normal range. With an MAP of less than 60 or greater than 160 mm Hg, or a CPP of less than 50 or greater than 150 mm Hg, autoregulation may cease to function, and CBF may become passively dependent on changes in systemic arterial pressure (Marshall et al., 1990). If this pathologic state begins, an increase in MAP will result in increased CBF, increased CBV, and further increases in ICP. As the MAP falls to less than 60 mm Hg, CBF will continue to decrease, resulting in eventual neuronal hypoxia and cell death.

ETIOLOGY OF INCREASED INTRACRANIAL PRESSURE

Multiple etiologies and pathophysiologic conditions are associated with increased ICP (Table 17–1). Many of these are discussed in detail in Chapters 35, 36, and 40. To facilitate an understanding of the primary mechanisms resulting in increased ICP, the more common etiologies and general conditions associated with increased ICP are reviewed in relation to their potential effects on increases in brain volume, blood volume, or the volume of CSF. Various conditions associated with increased ICP entail more than one mechanism through which the increase in ICP can occur. For example, mechanisms resulting in increased ICP associated with a brain tumor may be the mass effect (increased brain tissue volume), cerebral edema (increased brain tissue volume), obstruction to CSF circulation (increased CSF), and even increased blood volume, varying with the vascularity of the tumor.

TABLE 17–1. **Factors Associated With Increased Intracranial Pressure**

Influence on Intracranial Volume	Associated Factors

Increased total brain volume	Mass lesions
	  Brain tumors
	  Intracranial hematomas
	  Abscesses
	Cerebral edema

Increased intravascular blood volume	Cerebral vasodilation
	  Hypoxia, hypercapnia
	  Increased metabolic demands
	  Drug effect
	Venous outflow obstruction
	  Head position
	    Hyperextension, flexion, rotation
	  Circumferential ties around neck
	  Positive end-expiratory pressure
	  Valsalva maneuver
	Other
	  Endotracheal suctioning

Increased CSF volume	Increased CSF production
	  Choroid plexus papilloma
	Decreased CSF reabsorption
	  Communicating hydrocephalus
	CSF outflow obstruction
	  Obstructive hydrocephalus

Abbreviation: CSF, cerebrospinal fluid.

Increases in Total Brain Tissue Volume

MASS LESIONS. Increases in brain tissue volume can result from a number of conditions. Neoplasms, including primary brain tumors, as well as metastatic tumors, produce a mass effect resulting in an increase in total brain volume. Space-occupying mass lesions may result from any subdural, epidural, or intracerebral hematoma that may occur spontaneously or as a result of head trauma. A cyst, abscess, or any other space-occupying lesion may also result in increased ICP.

CEREBRAL EDEMA. Cerebral edema refers to an abnormal accumulation of water or fluid in the intracellular space or extracellular space that results in an increase in brain tissue volume. This edema can be vasogenic, cytotoxic, or interstitial. The specific types of cerebral edema are further discussed in Chapter 35 of this text.

Increased Intravascular Blood Volume

VENOUS OUTFLOW OBSTRUCTION. Increased intrathoracic or intraabdominal pressures may result in impaired venous return from the intracranial compartment. Because there are no valves in the central venous system, this pressure is transmitted through the great veins, resulting in impaired venous return. The Valsalva maneuver, coughing, vomiting, or positive end-expiratory pressure may cause this phenomenon. Additional research has also demonstrated that hyperextension or hyperflexion of the head may cause compression or extrinsic pressure on the great veins of the neck, resulting in venous engorgement and decreased venous return from the intracranial compartment (Williams & Coyne, 1993).

CEREBRAL VASODILATION. Cerebral vasodilation results in increased CBV and increased ICP. As described previously, hypoventilation leading to increasing P_{CO_2} results in cerebral vasodilation. Hypoxia also results in vasodilation if the Pa_{CO_2} is less than 50 to 60 mm Hg. In addition, certain anesthetic agents such as halothane, ketamine, and nitrous oxide result in cerebral vasodilation and thus should be avoided in patients at risk for increased ICP (Eichelberger, 1985). Nitroprusside also may cause vasodilation and should be used with caution in patients at risk for increased ICP (Nikas, 1991).

Increased Volume of Cerebrospinal Fluid

Conditions that affect CSF production, absorption, and circulation may also result in increased ICP. A choroid plexus papilloma may result in increased CSF production, although this condition is rare. Subarachnoid hemorrhage or inflammatory meningitis may result in obstruction of the arachnoid villi, leading to decreased CSF reabsorption and communicating hydrocephalus. Any condition that obstructs the normal CSF circulation pathway may result in noncommunicating or obstructive hydrocephalus and increased ICP due to increased CSF volume in one location.

NEUROLOGIC ASSESSMENT

In any patient with known or suspected increased ICP, the neurologic examination is an essential component of patient management. Although ICP monitoring is the most precise method of assessing ICP, it is not practical or feasible in all patients. If ICP monitoring is implemented, the data from the neurologic assessment will supplement the data obtained with ICP monitoring. The presenting signs and symptoms vary with the location of the mass or lesion, the degree of intracranial compensation, and the effect of the lesion on CPP or brain tissue distortion. Many of the neurologic signs and symptoms associated with increased ICP are not caused by increased ICP alone but by distortion and shifting of brain tissue in response to the underlying lesion. Signs and symptoms that may be indicative of increasing ICP include decreased level of consciousness, headache, vomiting, papilledema, pupillary dysfunction or visual abnormalities, motor or sensory dysfunction, and alterations in vital signs or respiratory patterns. Although any of these signs and symptoms may alert the caregiver to the possibility of increased ICP, the presence or progression of these signs and symptoms does not always indicate or parallel an increasing ICP.

Potential Signs and Symptoms Associated With Increased Intracranial Pressure

DECREASED LEVEL OF CONSCIOUSNESS. Change in the level of consciousness is considered to be one of the most sensitive, reliable, and earliest indicators of neurologic deterioration (Hickey, 1992). This change may be caused by interference with functioning of the reticular activating system at the level of the diencephalon or high midbrain. Decreased level of consciousness may also be caused by cerebral hypoxia secondary to decreased CBF. Early changes reflecting a decreased level of consciousness may include confusion, restlessness, or lethargy. Disorientation to time, place, and then person may follow (Hickey, 1992). As the patient's condition deteriorates, these symptoms may progress to eventual coma. The Glasgow Coma Scale is an assessment tool that has become widely used to describe and consistently document changes in the level of consciousness. It is essential to identify very subtle changes in the level of consciousness as early as possible.

Other causes of changes in level of consciousness must be ruled out, such as fever, seizures, hypothermia, hypotension, hypertension, hypoxia, infection, or sedatives (Obana & Andrews, 1993).

HEADACHE. Headache has been an associated symptom of increased ICP, but is not a common complaint in the presence of increased ICP. Patients who do have a headache may complain of a vague or slight headache (Hickey, 1992). The pain-sensitive structures within the intracranial compartment include the middle meningeal artery and its branches, the large arteries at the base of the brain, the sinuses and bridging veins, and the dura at the base of the cranial fossae (Langfitt, 1990). Headache that occurs with increased ICP is generally caused by displacement or traction on bridging cerebral vessels, stretching of the arteries, and pressure on the dura at the base of the skull. The headache is usually reported to be most severe on awakening in the morning because ICP increases during rapid eye movement sleep. Metabolism also increases in this phase of sleep, and carbon dioxide is produced as a result. Hypercapnia increases vasodilation, leading to the headache (Hickey, 1992; Langfitt, 1990). Nurses should recognize the request for pain medication by patients with intracranial pathology to be a potential indication of increasing ICP. A careful neurologic assessment should be done when these patients report headache pain.

PUPILLARY CHANGES. Pupillary changes in patients with increased ICP are a reflection of tissue shifts, which may result in compression of the oculomotor nerve (cranial nerve III) or distortion of the midbrain. When pupillary changes occur they are often associated with increased ICP. Pupillary changes may also occur in patients with eye trauma, cranial nerve injuries, or after aneurysm clipping. Atropine and barbiturates may also influence pupil reactivity (Obana & Andrews, 1993). Pupillary changes have been reported in patients with low ICPs, depending on the location of the lesion, and they are especially common in patients with middle fossa or medial temporal lobe lesions, which may cause early midbrain or oculomotor nerve compression (Obana & Andrews, 1993).

MOTOR FUNCTION CHANGES. In the earlier stages of increased ICP, hemiparesis may develop contralateral to the intracranial mass because of pressure on the motor tracts. In the later stages, hemiplegia, decortication, or decerebration may occur as a result of increasing pressure on the brainstem (Hickey, 1992).

PAPILLEDEMA. Papilledema is edema of the optic disc resulting from compression on the optic nerve that may be seen in patients with increased ICP (Langfitt, 1990). It may be detected during the ophthalmoscopic evaluation of the patient. It appears as a blurring of the disc margins due to engorgement and swelling of the disc vessels and elevation of the disc margins. Papilledema is usually a late sign of increased ICP. It is not seen in all patients but may be one of the first signs of increased ICP in patients in whom increased ICP has developed gradually (Hickey, 1992).

VITAL SIGN CHANGES. Abnormalities of respiratory rate and rhythm may be the first change in vital signs in a patient with increased ICP. These respiratory changes may not be evident, however, until several hours after an increase in ICP, and the specific respiratory pattern changes do not correlate consistently with increasing ICP (Hickey, 1992; Obana & Andrews, 1993).

The Cushing response of bradycardia, increasing systolic pressure, and widening pulse pressure has been associated with increasing ICP. This mechanism is thought to be one of the body's final compensatory mechanisms to maintain adequate CBF. Patients may not have the classic symptoms of the Cushing response, and may present only with hypertension or bradycardia. The presence of hypertension or bradycardia requires further investigation. In the final decompensatory stages of increased ICP, hypotension and tachycardia may be observed.

Although the neurologic assessment is very important in the patient with or at risk for increased ICP, it may be unreliable as an early indicator of this condition. These findings support the role of direct ICP monitoring as an important tool in the early detection and management of increased ICP.

INTRACRANIAL PRESSURE MONITORING

In 1960, Lundberg published the results of his experience with ICP monitoring using a ventricular catheter in a series of 143 patients with a variety of neurosurgical problems (Lundberg, 1960). This report has been cited as a major landmark in our understanding of the clinical significance of ICP monitoring as well as in establishing the safety and feasibility of ICP monitoring. Since 1960, many new methods of ICP monitoring have been introduced. The indications for and the various techniques used for ICP monitoring will be reviewed, focusing on the advantages and disadvantages of each technique.

Indications for Intracranial Pressure Monitoring

Many neurologic disorders place patients at risk for development of increased ICP. This, in addition to the fact that neurologic signs and symptoms alone may be unreliable indicators of increased ICP, has warranted consideration of ICP monitoring in patients who have evidence of or are at significant risk for the development of increased ICP. ICP monitoring, however, is not indicated for every patient. Although complications related to ICP monitoring are infrequent, monitoring does carry some degree of risk. Many authorities, therefore, have addressed the question of which patients require ICP monitoring. Consideration should be given to the likelihood of impaired perfusion developing in the patient, and to the patient's prognosis (Germon, 1994). Objective indications include disease processes that are known to be associated with a significant incidence of intracranial hypertension and are amenable to medical therapies. Additional indications include situations in which the neurologic examination is either ineffective, insensitive, or equivocal, as in the chemically paralyzed or physically paralyzed patient. Finally, in patients who exhibit clinical signs of increased ICP, ICP monitoring serves as a method for documenting clinical suspicion and evaluating the effectiveness of therapy and the patient's responses to nursing interventions (Hickey, 1992; Richmond, 1993) (Table 17–2).

Rockoff and Kennedy (1988) suggest that the intracranial dynamics of many of the conditions that can result in increased ICP should be considered in deciding which patients require ICP monitoring. Chronic slow changes in ICP are better tolerated than acute changes. Pressure equilibrium or high but equal pres-

TABLE 17–2. **Generally Accepted Criteria for Monitoring Intracranial Pressure in Critically Ill Patients**

General Criteria	Specific Examples
Pathophysiologic indications	Head injury Intracerebral hematoma Subarachnoid hemorrhage Space-occupying lesions Central nervous system infections Metabolic encephalopathies Cerebral edema Hydrocephalus Near drowning
Neurologic compromise	Glasgow Coma Scale score <8 High potential for neurologic deterioration
Unable to clinically assess	Paralytic agents High-dose barbiturates General anesthesia

From Richmond, T. S. (1993). Intracranial pressure monitoring. *AACN Clinical Issues in Critical Care, 4,* 148–160.

sures on both sides of the tentorium, as in communicating hydrocephalus or pseudotumor cerebri, are better tolerated than unequal transtentorial pressures, as with a mass lesion that can result in herniation. In a young child, open fontanelles and separated sutures may delay some of the deleterious effects of increased ICP (Rockoff & Kennedy, 1988).

Features that are strongly associated with intracranial hypertension in head-injured patients include lesions visible on computed tomography scan at the time of admission as well as two or more of the following features in patients with no visible lesion on admission: age greater than 40 years, systolic blood pressure under 90 mm Hg, and motor posturing (Andrews, 1993).

In summary, the decision to monitor ICP is not based on one set of absolute criteria. It is a subjective decision made by the physician based on the patient's history, clinical diagnosis, presentation, and plan of therapy.

Techniques for Measurement of Intracranial Pressure

Intracranial pressure monitoring systems most commonly used today involve the use of a sensor or transducer to pick up mechanical (pressure) impulses and convert them to electrical impulses. In addition, a monitor or recording device, preferably with an oscilloscopic display, is required to convert these impulses into visible signals. ICP is usually measured in the supratentorial space, with potential sites for ICP monitoring being the lateral ventricles, the subarachnoid, the subdural or epidural spaces, or the brain parenchymal tissue (Fig. 17–3). Ideally, all of these pressures should be approximately the same. However, with certain pathophysiologic conditions, there may be slight variations in values depending on the location of the monitoring device. Normal intracranial pressure varies from 0 to 15 mm Hg.

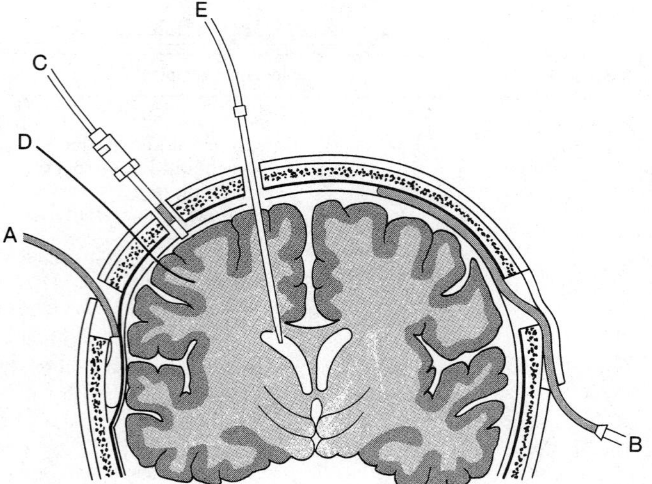

FIGURE 17–3. Coronal section of brain showing potential sites for placement of ICP monitoring devices. *A*, Epidural. *B*, Subdural. *C*, Subarachnoid. *D*, Intraparenchymal. *E*, Intraventricular.

BASIC SYSTEMS FOR INTRACRANIAL PRESSURE MONITORING

Before each of the available ICP monitoring devices is described, it is helpful to understand the two primary categories of ICP monitoring devices. The first group includes those devices that use fluid or hydrostatic coupling to transmit the reflected ICP to an extracranial transducer. This group includes the traditional ventricular catheters, subarachnoid bolts or screws, and the subdural catheters. The second group includes monitoring devices that directly monitor ICP using an intracranial membrane or transducer. These intracranial transducers use such devices of fiberoptics, pneumatic systems, or intracranial strain gauges to transmit pressures. ICP may be monitored in any of the potential intracranial locations according to the specific device used.

PRINCIPLES OF CALIBRATION OF INTRACRANIAL PRESSURE MONITORING SYSTEMS

Intracranial pressure is a relative value, obtained in reference to atmospheric pressure. The point at which the atmospheric reference is made is referred to as the "zero" point. The technique of referencing the transducer to atmospheric pressure is referred to as "zeroing the transducer." For fluid-coupled systems using external transducers, hydrostatic forces dictate that the position of the transducer when the reference is made as well as when readings are obtained must remain constant in relation to a specific point on the patient's head. For ICP monitoring, this reference point is the inferred anatomic level of the foramen of Monro. Some clinicians identify this site as a point lateral to the outer canthus of the eye or the top of the ear, whereas others use the external auditory meatus as a reference point (Cammermeyer & Appeldorn, 1990; Nikas, 1991). Whichever point is used, consistency is essential when fluid-coupled systems are used because a 1.38-cm variation in the reference point can result in a 1-mm Hg change in the measured pressure due to hydrostatic effects. Any change in the height of the patient's head with respect to the transducer requires the transducer to be leveled to the anatomic reference point and, ideally, zeroed to atmospheric pressure before obtaining readings to ensure the highest accuracy.

In ICP monitoring systems using intracranial transducers that do not depend on fluid-coupling effects, the atmospheric reference point is constant at the position of the transducer. Because the transducer is in the catheter tip, repeated leveling to an external site is not necessary. In using intracranial transducers, this zero point may be defined in reference to atmospheric pressure either before insertion of the device, or, with some monitors, "in vivo" calibration may be performed. The ability to reference the transducer to atmosphere in vivo ensures the greatest accuracy over time because the atmospheric reference can be recalibrated periodically during ICP monitoring. If in vivo calibration is not possible, the transducer is referenced once to atmospheric pressure before insertion. In this situation there is, however, no method of assessing for any slight drift or variation of the atmospheric reference after insertion.

EXTERNAL TRANSDUCER SYSTEMS

Devices that couple ICP to an external transducer system through a fluid-filled pressure tubing have been commonly used as ICP monitoring devices. Advantages of this type of a system include simplicity, low cost, familiarity, and compatibility with existing monitoring equipment.

VENTRICULAR CATHETER. The ventricular catheter was the first device used for ICP monitoring (Lundberg, 1960). It has been proved to be clinically reliable and accurate and is the current standard against which other methods are compared (Germon, 1994; Richmond, 1993; Unwin et al., 1991). The intraventricular catheter is a soft catheter made of radiopaque Silastic. A wire stylet is introduced into the catheter while it is being inserted to stiffen the catheter. The stylet is then removed after insertion. The catheter is inserted through a twist drill hole through the skull, usually into the anterior horn of the lateral ventricle in the nondominant hemisphere (Richmond, 1993). Placement of the catheter is guided by anatomic landmarks and is confirmed by the drainage of CSF and the presence of an appropriate ICP waveform on the monitor. Some institutions use a method of tunneling the catheter from the point of exit from the skull to a different point of exit from the scalp in an effort to reduce the incidence of infection (Richmond, 1993). After insertion, the catheter is connected to a closed fluid-filled system. There are many systems available, with similar basic features. These include a proximal stopcock or sampling port and a more distal stopcock that allows communication with either an external transducer for ICP monitoring or a collection system for CSF drainage (Fig. 17–4). Accuracy in ICP readings is ensured by using the shortest possible length of tubing between the catheter and the transducer and eliminating air bubbles in the system.

Advantages of the ventricular catheter include accuracy, reliability, and the capability to therapeutically drain CSF and control ICP. It can also be used for CSF sampling, for insertion of contrast medium in diagnostic studies, for compliance testing, and for the instillation of medications (antibiotics, pain medication, chemotherapeutic agents). An additional advantage is its capability of being zeroed as necessary to avoid inaccurate ICP values due to drift of the zero reference point.

Disadvantages of the ventricular catheter include an increased risk of infection because it is the most invasive method of ICP monitoring. Insertion of the ventricular catheter also carries the risk of intracranial hemorrhage. The catheter may be difficult to insert in a patient with small ventricles or a significant intracranial shift (Hickey, 1992; Richmond, 1993). The sensitivity of this device to changes in position of the patient's head is also a relative disadvantage of this system.

Of particular importance in the care of the patient with an intraventricular catheter is the need to maintain a closed system and the need to use meticulous technique in caring for the system to minimize risk of infection. If CSF specimens are obtained, a well controlled protocol for collection of these specimens is essential. This includes maintaining sterile technique and collecting the specimens by passive flow, preventing negative pressure against the ventricles. Details of the maintenance and monitoring of a ventricular drainage system are discussed later in this chapter.

SUBARACHNOID BOLT OR SCREW. A less invasive technique using a fluid-coupled system is the subarachnoid bolt or screw (Fig. 17–5). There are many variations of this device, most of which use a hollow metal shaft or screw that is threaded at one end (McQuillan, 1991; Richmond, 1993). The insertion site is usually in the frontal area over the nondominant hemisphere. The screw or bolt is inserted through a one-quarter-inch twist drill hole in the skull until it protrudes through the dura into the subarachnoid space (Andrews, 1993; Hickey, 1992). The proximal end of the screw lies in direct communication with the subarachnoid space. After insertion, the hollow screw or bolt is hydrostatically coupled to a fluid-filled tubing, a stopcock, and an external transducer.

The advantages of this device are its simplicity and its relative ease and speed of insertion. This device can be used in patients with small, shifted, or collapsed ventricles. In addition, it is less invasive than the ventricular catheter, and there is no disruption of the brain parenchyma. These factors contribute to a decreased risk of infection and hemorrhage compared with the ventricular catheter.

Disadvantages of the subarachnoid bolt or screw include decreased reliability and accuracy of ICP measurements due to obstruction of the device by blood or edematous brain tissue (Hickey, 1992; Richmond, 1993). Some of these problems can be identified by dampened ICP waveforms. Despite the fact that the risk of infection is decreased compared with the ventricular catheter, some risk still remains. CSF drainage from the bolt or screw is not recommended because this may result in occlusion of the device. In addition, compliance testing cannot be performed with this device. Some previously designed metallic screws, specifically those made of ferrous compounds, were not totally compatible with magnetic resonance (MR) imaging because of the strong magnetic field (Cammermeyer & Appeldorn, 1990; Nikas, 1991; Richmond, 1993). It is, therefore, important to know the composition of the bolt being used and whether it is MR compatible.

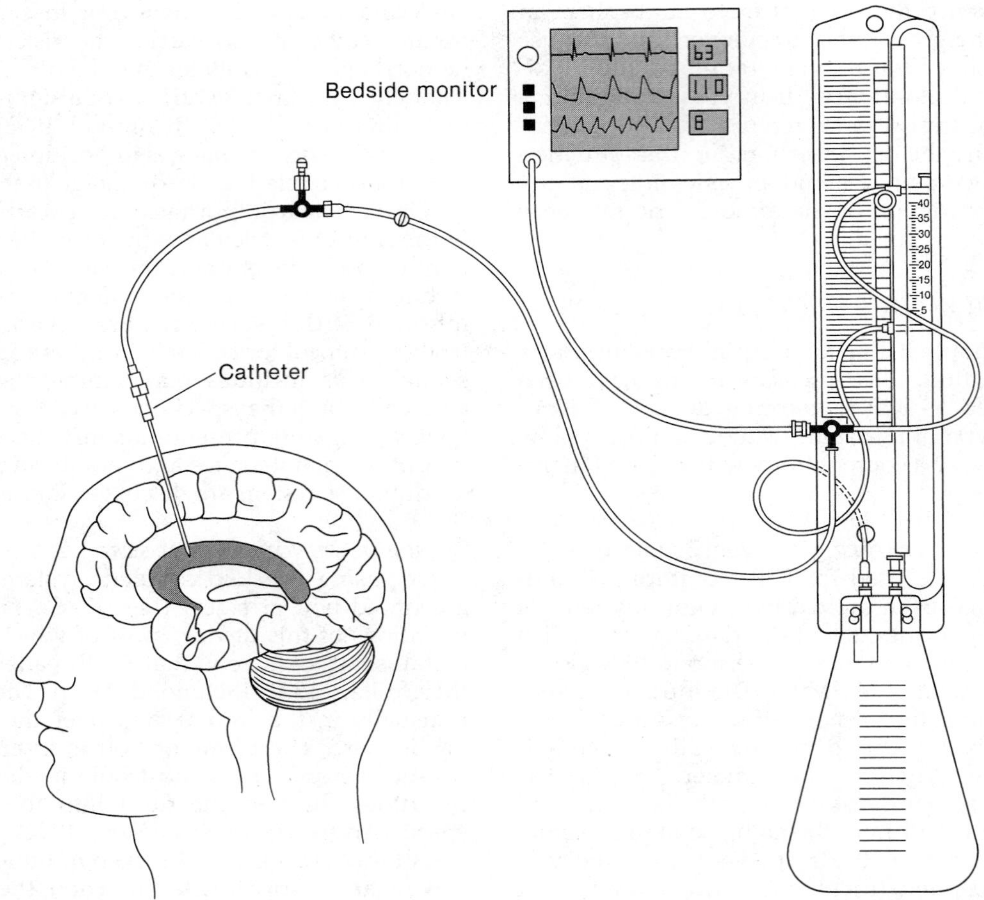

FIGURE 17-4. Intraventricular catheter attached to closed system for ICP monitoring and CSF drainage.

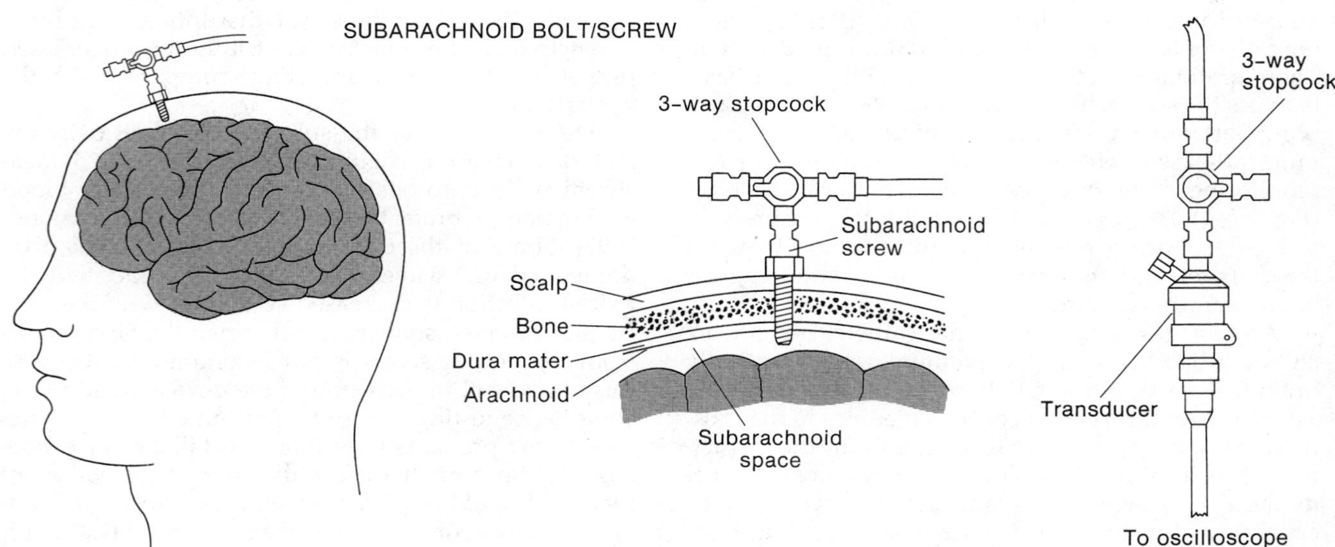

FIGURE 17-5. Subarachnoid bolt pressure monitoring. The subarachnoid bolt is inserted through a burr hole in the skull and is attached to a transducer and oscilloscope for continuous ICP monitoring. (Redrawn by permission from Rudy, E. [1984]. *Advanced neurological and neurosurgical nursing.* St. Louis: The C.V. Mosby Co.)

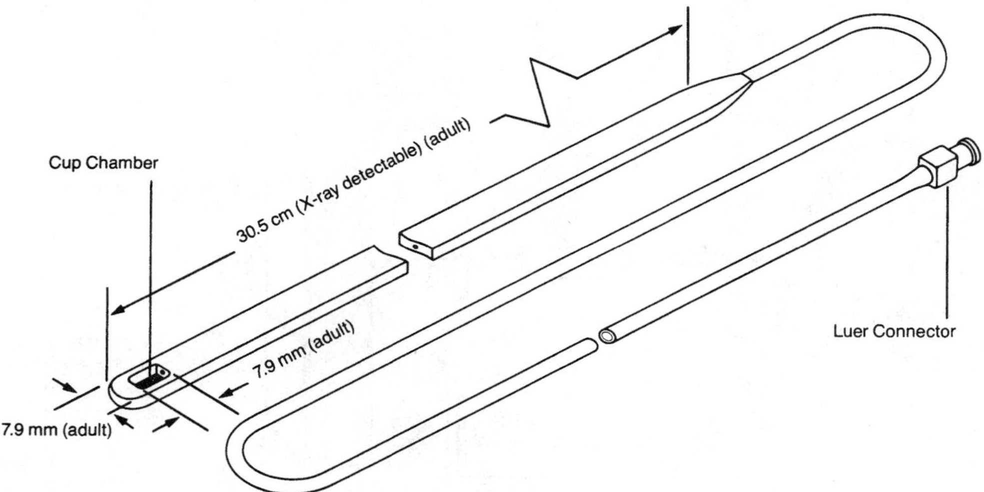

FIGURE 17–6. Subdural cup catheter. This catheter is hydrostatically coupled to an external transducer for use as an ICP monitoring device. The distal portion of the device is ribbon shaped with a central lumen connected to an indented cup near the tip. The proximal tube ends in a Luer connector. When the catheter is in place, the open side of the cup communicates with the arachnoid membrane. (By permission of Cordis Corporation, Miami, FL.)

Troubleshooting of the system includes checking all connections for potential leaks that may contribute to dampened waveforms. Obstructions may be cleared from the system by the physician with intermittent flushes of 0.1 mL of preservative-free saline or other antibiotic flush solution (Doyle & Mark, 1992).

SUBDURAL CATHETERS. Another method of monitoring ICP through an external transducer involves the use of a catheter placed in the subdural space. Various types of catheters have been placed in the subdural space, including red rubber catheters or ventricular catheters, which are then fluid-coupled to a transducer system. Wilkinson (1977) described the use of a ribbon-shaped Silastic catheter with a distal indented cavity or cup on one surface that faces the arachnoid membrane of the brain and communicates with a saline-filled lumen (Fig. 17–6). This catheter is called a subdural cup catheter and has been primarily designed for use after a craniotomy, although it can also be inserted through a burr hole (Wilkinson, 1977). The design of the catheter allows it to be passed through a subcutaneous scalp incision and tunneled to a location away from the point of entry into the subdural space (Wilkinson, 1977). After insertion, this catheter is then connected to fluid-filled pressure tubing and a transducer.

Advantages of this type of catheter include the fact that it is one of the least invasive methods for ICP monitoring and results in a very low incidence of complications of infection or hemorrhage. The device itself is relatively inexpensive and can be used with most currently available electronic pressure transducers in critical care settings.

Disadvantages of this catheter include the fact that small leaks or air in the system or obstruction of the catheter lumen may cause a dampened waveform and inaccurate readings, which are in general lower than the true ICP. In addition, CSF drainage and compliance testing are not possible.

To maintain this system, Wilkinson (1977) recommends that a small amount of sterile solution (0.1–0.25 mL) be injected at 2-hour intervals through a stopcock to replace any fluid leakage from the distal cup. This practice is controversial, and in some institutions may be performed only by a physician. If this practice is followed, a closed system should be maintained to prevent possible contamination. A closed system using a series of stopcocks, an attached reservoir containing flush solution, and a 1-mL Luer lock syringe used for injecting the solution has been recommended by some institutions (Price, 1981; Smith, 1987). To obtain accurate readings, the system should be zeroed and calibrated frequently.

Fiberoptic systems are also available for subdural use, and do not require frequent calibration. The accuracy of the subdural catheter over time has been shown to be poor. Trend data are the most useful information obtained from this type of monitor (Germon, 1994).

INTRACRANIAL TRANSDUCER SYSTEMS

The direct hydrostatic coupling of the intracranial space with an external transducer common to each of the ICP monitoring techniques described so far has some principal disadvantages. These include increased risk of infection through the fluid-filled column and the potential for inaccurate ICP readings because of factors that can interrupt the fluid column. In addition, the need to level the transducer and zero the system with any change in position of the patient's head relative to the transducer is a disadvantage. To avoid these problems, a variety of instruments have

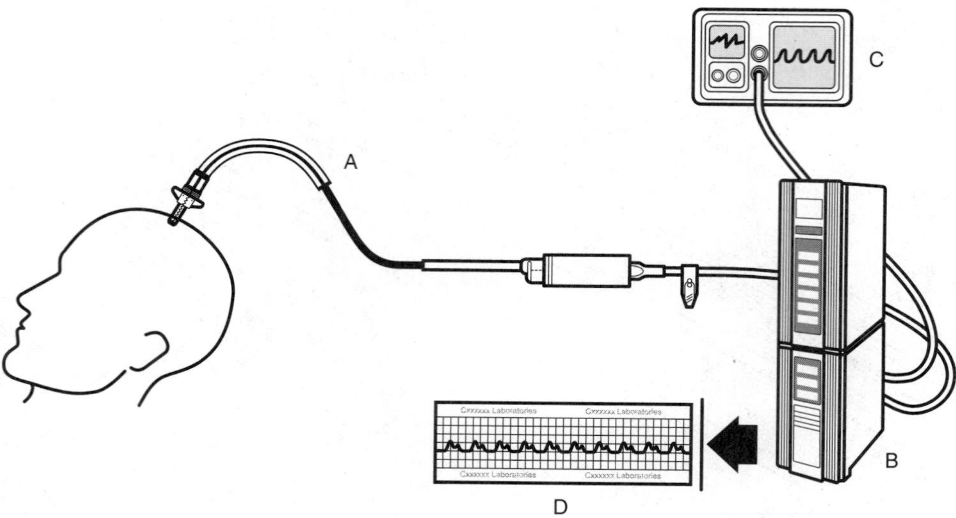

FIGURE 17–7. Fiberoptic transducer system. Catheter (*A*) is connected to a digital monitor (*B*). Monitor interfaces with bedside monitoring system (*C*). Printout of ICP waveform (*D*). (Used with permission. Camino Laboratories, San Diego, CA.)

been designed that use an intracranial transducer system.

FIBEROPTIC MONITORING DEVICES. A fiberoptic transducer-tipped disposable catheter is available for ICP monitoring. This type of catheter uses sophisticated fiberoptic technology, which receives information from a transducer located in the tip of the catheter. Within the transducer, movement of a mirrored diaphragm in response to pressure is sensed by light fibers (Crutchfield et al., 1990). This information is converted into a signal in the amplifier connector, which is based on a precalibrated relationship between the amount of reflected light and the corresponding ICP (Fig. 17–7). The appropriate ICP value is then displayed on a compatible digital monitor. The monitor can "interface with conventional bedside monitoring systems for oscilloscopic display and paper readout of the waveform and pressure value (Crutchfield et al., 1990).

This fiberoptic catheter has been used for ICP monitoring at various locations, including intraventricular, subarachnoid, subdural, and intraparenchymal sites. With intraventricular pressure monitoring, the fiberoptic-tipped catheter is inserted into a ventriculostomy catheter up to the point at which there is a sharp angular bend in the ventricular catheter. A Y-connector at the proximal end of the catheter allows CSF drainage through one port and ICP monitoring through the other (Fig. 17–8).

The fiberoptic transducer-tipped catheter can also be inserted through a subarachnoid bolt with the tip of the catheter extending just slightly beyond the tip of the bolt in the subarachnoid space (Fig. 17–9). The bolt is inserted through a twist drill hole, which is made in either the left or right prefrontal areas. After penetration of the inner table of the skull, the drill is removed, and the hole is irrigated with normal saline. The bolt is then screwed in manually. At this point, a stylet is inserted through the bolt to clear any debris, and the hole is again irrigated with normal saline. The catheter is zeroed, passed through the bolt approximately 1 cm beyond the end of the bolt, and then secured to the bolt by tightening a compression cap.

If brain parenchymal pressure monitoring is to be used, a fiberoptic catheter may be inserted through the meningeal layers and advanced a few centimeters into the brain parenchyma. This type of device can be inserted through a subarachnoid bolt using a technique similar to the one described above.

A transducer-tipped fiberoptic catheter eliminates the problems of dampening waveforms due to catheter

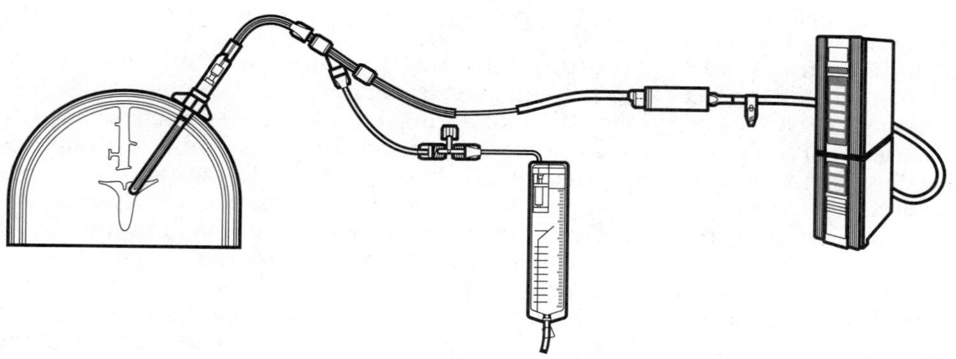

FIGURE 17–8. Fiberoptic transducer system with *Y*-connector for CSF drainage and ICP monitoring. (Used with permission. Camino Laboratories, San Diego, CA.)

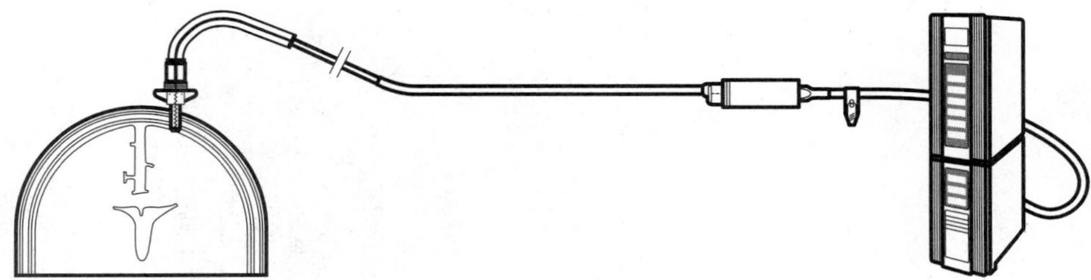

FIGURE 17–9. Fiberoptic transducer system with a subdural bolt. (Used with permission. Camino Laboratories, San Diego, CA.)

occlusion or air bubble entrapment. Because the system is not fluid-coupled, it is not necessary to irrigate the system because of dampening waveforms, and this may reduce the risk of infection (Crutchfield et al., 1990). A more detailed waveform with less artifact has also been reported (McQuillan, 1991). Because the transducer lies in the catheter tip, the zero point relative to atmospheric pressure is independent of the patient's position. Continuous ICP readings may also be obtained during patient transport with a battery-powered monitor. The ability of the fiberoptic catheter to be used in various monitoring locations is an additional advantage.

A specific advantage of the intraventricular monitoring technique is its capability for monitoring ICP and draining CSF. Advantages of the intraparenchymal location include the capability for insertion of this monitor in patients with compressed or distorted ventricles while maintaining accurate readings (Schickner & Young, 1992).

Disadvantages of the fiberoptic transducer-tipped catheter include the expense of the catheters and the initial expense involved in the purchase of the cable and compatible monitor compared to the expense of fluid-coupled monitoring devices. In addition, the catheter is capable of being zeroed to an atmospheric reference only before insertion, and cannot be rezeroed once in place. It is therefore not possible to check for drift, and those who have used the system report that there may be a significant drift over time (Crutchfield et al., 1990) and that there are differences between intraparenchymal and intraventricular measurements (Schickner & Young, 1992; Weinstabl et al., 1992). Another potential disadvantage of the catheter is the risk of fiberoptic breakage due to inadvertent bending of the catheter (Richmond, 1993). If fiberoptic breakage occurs, there is a signal on the monitor that will alert the nurse. However, as those working with the catheters and equipment become increasingly familiar with the equipment, fiberoptic breakage has not been reported to be a significant problem. In addition, if the fiberoptic catheter breaks, it must be replaced for continued monitoring, at an additional cost to the patient (Richmond, 1993).

INTRACRANIAL PRESSURE WAVEFORMS

Oscilloscopic display of ICP waveforms has been considered important in the analysis of ICP. The initial work on ICP monitoring, in which ICP waveforms were described, was done by Lundberg in 1960 using ventricular catheters (Lundberg, 1960). The configuration of the ICP waveform results from the transmission of systolic and diastolic arterial pressures from the cerebrovascular system and choroid plexus (capillaries within the ventricles) to the CSF in the ventricular and subarachnoid spaces. On close analysis, the ICP waveform has three or more peaks (Fig. 17–10). The large initial peak, P_1, the percussion wave, results from transmission of arterial pressure from the choroid plexus (Germon, 1994), has a sharp peak, and is relatively constant in amplitude. The second peak, P_2, generated by venous pressure, is referred to as the tidal wave. It is more variable in shape and amplitude and ends in the dicrotic notch. After the dicrotic notch is the third wave, P_3, the dicrotic wave, which is also thought to be generated by venous pressure (Germon, 1994). After the dicrotic wave, the pressure usually tapers down to its diastolic position, although occasionally a few more peaks may be observed due to retrograde venous pulsations (Germon, 1994). The exact appearance of the waveform and the ability to detect the waveform peaks vary with the type of ICP monitoring device being used.

When caring for a patient with an ICP monitor, it is important to document and compare ICP waveforms to confirm the accuracy of values and to observe for dampening of the waveform. In addition, certain changes in the configuration of the normal ICP waveform have been correlated with actual or future elevations in ICP or decreased compliance (Germon, 1994). When ICP waveforms were studied, it was found that an elevation of the P_2 component of the waveform that was equal to or higher than the P_1 component reflects a state of decreased compliance (Germon, 1994).

Monitors that are capable of providing trends of ICP values over time or that allow slow strip chart recording can also provide valuable information about the patient. The three types of abnormal ICP waveforms that can most readily be identified on a slow strip chart recorder are the A, B, and C waveforms (Fig. 17–11). These waveforms are trend data observed over minutes to hours. These data may be helpful in normal-pressure hydrocephalus and pseudotumor cerebri, but may not identify changes in pressure soon enough for early identification and intervention in acute pathology (Germon, 1994).

A WAVES (PLATEAU WAVES). A waves, also called plateau waves, occur during elevations of ICP from 50 to

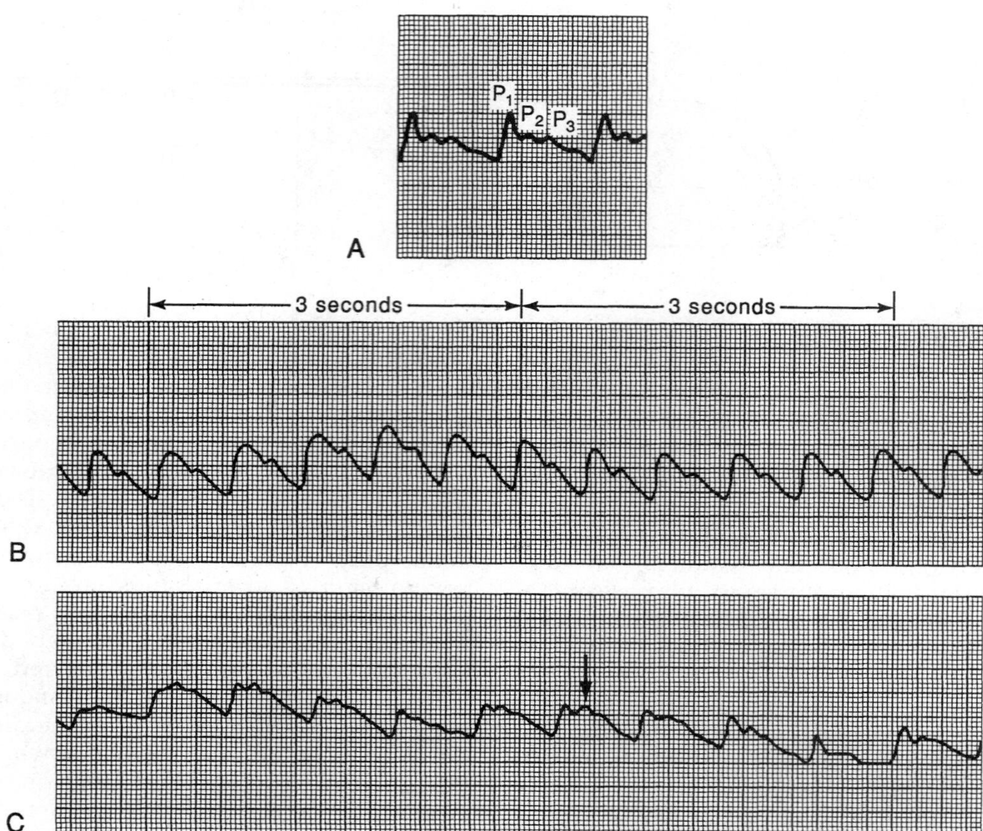

FIGURE 17–10. Normal intracranial pressure waveforms. *A*, ICP pulse wave with three main components: P_1, P_2, and P_3. The clarity of the three distinct waves will vary with the type of ICP monitoring device used and the calibration range of the bedside monitor. *B*, Waveform obtained from fluid-coupled intraventricular catheter. Calibration range is 0–50 mm Hg. *C*, ICP waveform obtained from ventriculostomy catheter. Arrow illustrates elevation of P_2 in relationship to P_1 secondary to increased ICP in a patient with ICP ranging from 20 to 40 mm Hg.

100 mm Hg and last from 5–20 minutes (Lundberg, 1960). These abnormal waveforms have been correlated with falls in CPP due to decreased arterial blood pressure and decreased intracranial compliance, and reflect the occurrence of cerebral ischemia (Germon, 1994; Hickey, 1992). The decrease in perfusion pressure serves as a stimulus for an intact autoregulatory response of cerebral vasodilation, which results in further increases in ICP (Rosner, 1993). Clinical consequences that may result from this marked elevation in ICP include decreased cerebral perfusion and brain cell hypoxia.

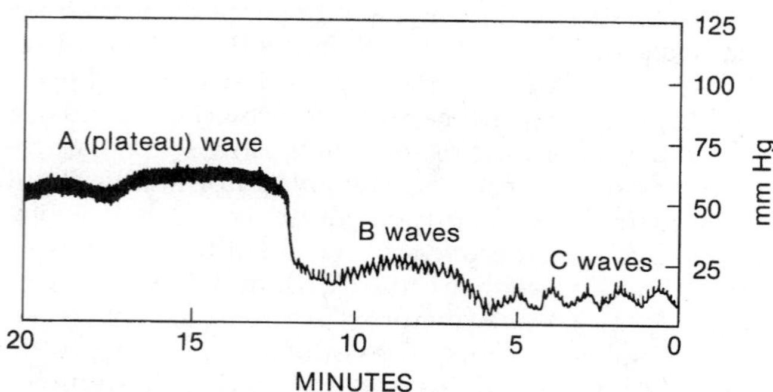

FIGURE 17–11. Abnormal ICP waves. Composite drawing of pressure waves that may be recorded over time with a slow strip chart recorder, including A (plateau) waves, B waves, and C waves. Note that this type of recording is used to illustrate trends in ICP over time. (Redrawn from *Nursing the Critically Ill Adult*, Third Edition, by Nancy Meyer Holloway. Copyright © 1988 by Addison-Wesley Publishing Company. Reprinted by permission.)

B WAVES. B waves are defined as sharp, rhythmic pressure variations occurring at a frequency of 0.5 to 2.0/minute in which the ICP averages 20 to 40 mm Hg but may oscillate to as high as 50 mm Hg. These variations may be caused by variations in cerebrovascular resistance or pressure within the cerebral vasculature bed (Lundberg, 1960), and are influenced by changes in ventilation as well as arterial pressure (Germon, 1994). They indicate a decline in the brain's adaptive capability and may be a warning of impending A waves (McQuillan, 1991).

C WAVES. C waves are transient, rhythmic waves that occur every 4 to 8 minutes and raise ICP to as high as 20 mm Hg (Lundberg, 1960). C waves have been associated with variations in ventilation and arterial pressure (Germon, 1994). The clinical significance of these waves is unknown.

MANAGEMENT OF INTRACRANIAL HYPERTENSION

Intracranial hypertension is defined as a sustained elevation of ICP greater than 15 to 20 mm Hg (Langfitt, 1990). There is, however, no absolute pressure value that indicates a need for treatment. Guidelines provided in the literature state that the decision to initiate treatment should be based on the neurologic condition of the brain, the rapidity with which the ICP is rising, the underlying pathophysiologic condition resulting in increased ICP, and the estimated cerebral perfusion pressure. Results of the neurologic examination also are used as an indicator; however, many patients do not show evidence of neurologic deterioration until ICP has become markedly elevated.

The initial goal for management of patients with increased ICP is to control intracranial hypertension and to maintain a CPP of at least 60 mm Hg. Some believe that keeping a CPP above 70 mm Hg is better for the brain (McQuillan, 1991). Prevention of secondary ischemia is the desired aim. In addition, the underlying cause of intracranial hypertension must be treated and further increases in ICP prevented. Strategies for accomplishment of these goals involve a collaborative effort and include carefully planned medical management and skilled nursing interventions. The major medical interventions in the management of intracranial hypertension vary depending on the underlying condition, but may include the use of mild hyperventilation, osmotic diuretics, other diuretics, fluid restriction, corticosteroids, blood pressure control, and, in extreme situations, barbiturate therapy. Fluid restriction may not be used in some situations because it is important to maintain blood flow and CPP. Corticosteroids are not routinely used in ICP management except in patients with brain tumors. The specific management of conditions associated with increased ICP and possible surgical interventions are presented in Chapter 35 of this text. CSF drainage through a ventriculostomy is a surgical intervention that may be used to control ICP, and is reviewed in the following section.

CEREBROSPINAL FLUID DRAINAGE. As described previously, ICP monitoring with a ventricular catheter has a distinct advantage in that it allows for some control of ICP by providing a capability to drain CSF. This intervention allows for rapid reduction of ICP and is the treatment of choice when increased ICP is caused by hydrocephalus. When CSF drainage is used, the ventricular catheter is connected to an external collecting and measuring system by pressure tubing and a series of stopcocks. One stopcock may be used for intermittent ICP monitoring, if an external transducer is used, by connecting a transducer dome to this port. The other stopcocks may be used for injecting medications, sampling CSF, testing volume pressure response, or intermittently flushing the ventriculostomy if necessary.

Cerebrospinal fluid drainage is regulated or controlled by adjusting the height of the drainage system relative to a reference point on the patient. This reference point is often the inferred anatomic level of the foramen of Monro or the level at the top of the ear, the outer canthus of the eye, or the tragus of the ear. Consistency in use of a reference point is important for consistent measurement of ICP. The height of the fluid column in the pressure tubing above this reference point creates a hydrostatic pressure that opposes the ICP. To increase or decrease this hydrostatic pressure, the height of the highest point of the drainage system may be raised or lowered in relation to the reference point on the patient. If the drainage system is raised, CSF drainage will decrease. In this situation, greater ICP is necessary to overcome the pressure created by the height of the fluid column. When the highest point of the drainage system is lowered, the hydrostatic pressure created by the fluid column is also decreased, and CSF drainage will occur more rapidly.

In an average adult, CSF is normally produced at a rate of 20 to 30 mL/hour, with approximately 90 to 150 mL of CSF circulating between the ventricles and the subarachnoid space at any one time if the normal mechanisms for CSF reabsorption are functional (Marshall et al., 1990). This basic physiologic understanding is important when monitoring CSF drainage. Too rapid drainage of CSF may result in ventricular collapse. Therefore, it is usually recommended that CSF be drained in a controlled manner against a positive back pressure, which corresponds to a predetermined ICP (Cammermeyer & Appeldorn, 1990). Such a procedure can be accomplished by maintaining the drainage system at a specified height (e.g., 10 cm above the top of the ear). To decrease the risk of complications, a pressure-regulated valve may be placed in line with the tubing going to the drainage system. This technique allows close regulation of CSF pressure and decreases the chance of too rapid CSF drainage (Cammermeyer & Appeldorn, 1990). It also retards retrograde travel of bacteria from the closed drainage system.

To minimize the risk of infection, every effort should be made to maintain a closed system. Some preassembled closed drainage systems are available. In addition, sterile technique is essential whenever the system is entered.

CLINICAL MANAGEMENT

Potential for Alteration in Cerebral Tissue Perfusion Related to Increased Intracranial Pressure

In providing nursing care to a patient with or at risk for increased ICP, many nursing interventions can be implemented independently. Defining characteristics for the patient with potential for alteration in cerebral tissue perfusion include an actually measured ICP of greater than 15 mm Hg or signs or symptoms of decreasing cerebral tissue perfusion. These signs or symptoms may include an alteration in the level of consciousness or other changes in the neurologic status of the patient. Nursing goals should be directed toward supporting the patient's functional abilities, which may be compromised as a result of decreased cerebral tissue perfusion, and preventing further increases in ICP. ICP should ideally be maintained between 0 and 15 mm Hg, and CPP should be maintained at greater than or equal to 60 mm Hg.

One limiting factor in this diagnosis is the inability actually to measure cerebral tissue perfusion as well as the lack of correlation between neurologic signs and symptoms and decreasing tissue perfusion. In addition, many nursing interventions are directed toward identifying patients at risk for sharp increases in ICP and preventing these increases before they occur. Mitchell (1986) has proposed the nursing diagnosis "decreased intracranial adaptive capacity" to replace "alteration in cerebral tissue perfusion." In recent research, she has been able to define some characteristics that may be present before these sudden increases in ICP that may help to guide nursing interventions (Rauch et al., 1990).

Several nursing interventions that influence ICP have been reported and are discussed in this section.

PATIENT POSITIONING AND TURNING. Maintaining the head of bed elevation at approximately 30° to 45° in most situations has been found to result in decreased ICP. Some investigators, however, have found that the optimal position for the head of the bed varies between patients and should be determined on an individual basis (March et al., 1990; Rosner & Daughton, 1990). The recommended position is usually ordered by physicians and should be maintained as consistently as possible. Nursing interventions are to continually assess and document changes in ICP in relation to the head of bed elevation.

Turning the head position 90° to the extreme left or right results in increases in ICP ranging from 5 to 20 mm Hg (Lipe & Mitchell, 1980; Williams & Coyne, 1993). This pressure increase is thought to be caused by obstruction of venous outflow, and should be avoided.

Turning the patient in bed may also result in increases in ICP, although this finding is inconsistent. Patients in whom this pattern is identified should be instructed to allow the nurse to turn them passively, avoiding isometric contractions and the Valsalva maneuver, which result in increased ICP (Andrus, 1991; Mitchell, 1980). Hip flexion has been found to produce significant increases in ICP (Andrus, 1991), although others have not seen this result (March et al., 1990).

The use of oscillating beds that rotate from side to side was studied to assess the effect on ICP (Gonzalez-Aries et al., 1983). It was found that changes in bed position from extreme left to right and supine did not result in significant changes in ICP (Gonzalez-Aries et al., 1983). This study supported the finding that raised ICP should not limit the use of oscillating beds in appropriate patients.

SECURING OF ENDOTRACHEAL TUBES. Securing an endotracheal tube with a circumferential tie around the neck can potentially result in increased ICP by obstructing venous outflow. Thus, noncircumferential taping of endotracheal tubes is preferred in patients with or at risk for intracranial hypertension.

ENDOTRACHEAL SUCTIONING. The potential for increased ICP resulting from endotracheal suctioning is a nursing concern because hypoxia or hypercapnia can result in cerebral vasodilation and increased ICP and stimulation may increase ICP. In a literature review of investigations related to endotracheal suctioning and ICP, it was concluded that endotracheal suctioning may produce transient but significant increases in ICP, which quickly return to baseline in patients with a baseline ICP of less than 20 mm Hg (Rudy et al., 1991). In such patients, this transient elevation was of no consequence. In patients with an ICP of greater than 20 mm Hg, however, any further increases in ICP might have significant deleterious effects. Patients with elevated ICP did not return quickly to baseline after suctioning; some patients returned to baseline only after 5 to 10 minutes of rest (Rudy et al., 1991).

Nursing interventions to minimize the negative effects associated with endotracheal suctioning include hyperoxygenating the patient with 100% O_2 for 20 to 30 seconds before suctioning. Hyperventilation should be used with caution because vasoconstriction can cause ischemia (Kerr et al., 1993). In addition, duration of the time of suctioning should be less than 10 seconds with each attempt, and only two attempts should be made because of the cumulative effects of suctioning on ICP (Kerr et al., 1993; Rudy et al., 1991). In additional investigations, intravenous lidocaine administered before suctioning was found to prevent intracranial hypertension effectively during periods of endotracheal suctioning. Studies also have been performed using intratracheal lidocaine, which has also shown effect in blunting the ICP response to suctioning (Brucia et al., 1992). Although this practice is not used routinely, it may be considered in patients at high risk for marked increases in ICP with endotracheal suctioning.

ENVIRONMENTAL STIMULI OR TOUCH. Current research has demonstrated that the effects of certain environmental stimuli may result in either increased or decreased ICP. Conversations about the patient's condition at the bedside may elevate ICP (Boortz-Marx, 1985; Mitchell & Mauss, 1978; Lundberg, 1960; Sisson, 1990). In addition, Bruya (1981) and Mitchell and coworkers (1985) found that the presence of family members and gentle touching or stroking of the patient by family members can produce significant decreases in ICP. Walleck (1987) summarized the findings of studies related to nursing interventions and ICP. She reported that "there appears to be a cumulative effect on ICP when activities are clumped together, but if CPP remains at 50 mm Hg or greater, any nursing activity can be safely performed" (Walleck, 1987).

Infection Related to Intracranial Pressure Monitoring

Although ICP monitoring has been recognized as a valuable tool in the diagnosis and management of intracranial hypertension, the risk of complications associated with such monitoring has been a significant concern with all types of ICP monitoring. A brief summary of some of the variables influencing the incidence of infection and interventions used to decrease the incidence of infection is presented. A review of the literature by Hickman and colleagues (1990) identified the patient who might be at higher risk for an infection associated with an ICP monitor. Risk factors include intracerebral hemorrhage with intraventricular hemorrhage, open head trauma, neurosurgical procedure, ICP of 20 mm Hg or more, older age, burr hole made larger than necessary, placement of device without aseptic technique, device penetrating the meninges, length of monitoring of more than 3 to 5 days, irrigation of ICP system, and an open system.

TYPE OF ICP MONITORING. Ventricular catheters fluid-coupled to external transducers are associated with the overall highest incidence of infection. Research on the incidence of ventriculostomy-related infections has ranged from less than 1% when the catheter is percutaneously tunneled under the scalp to approximately 21.9%, with an average of approximately 9% at 5 days of ICP monitoring (Hickman et al., 1990). The fluid-coupled subarachnoid bolt has been associated with the lowest incidence of infection, ranging from no reported infection to a 7.5% incidence that included the complications of wound infection and osteomyelitis (Hickman et al., 1990).

Intracranial transducer systems and infection rates have not been studied in as much detail; however, it appears that the more invasive monitoring devices are associated with a higher incidence of infection. In addition, because system irrigation is not needed and a static fluid column is not present, it has been suggested that these factors may reduce the risk of infection with internal transducer systems.

LENGTH OF ICP MONITORING. Studies of ICP monitoring have reported a correlation between the incidence of infection and the duration of ICP monitoring. The incidence of infection has been reported to be very low if the monitoring device is in place less than 72 hours. In a study of 255 patients with fluid-coupled ICP monitoring devices, only two cases of infection were reported if the ICP monitoring device was in place for less than 72 hours (Hickman et al., 1990; Schultz et al., 1993). A significantly higher rate of infection was associated with the use of fluid-coupled devices when the ICP monitor remained in place 5 days or longer (Hickman et al., 1990; Schultz et al., 1993).

USE OF PROPHYLACTIC ANTIBIOTICS. Many institutions use prophylactic antibiotic administration in an effort to decrease the incidence of infection during ICP monitoring. The most frequently used prophylactic antibiotics include nafcillin, cephalothin, and gentamicin, although many others are used as well. A decrease in the incidence of infection with the prophylactic use of antibiotics during ICP monitoring has been reported (Schultz et al., 1993); however, data from other studies of infection associated with ICP monitoring have not supported this correlation (Schultz et al., 1993).

USE OF ANTIBIOTIC FLUSH SOLUTION. Many fluid-coupled ICP monitoring systems require the use of a flush solution to maintain patency. Intermittent flushes (every 2–3 hours) with 0.1 to 0.3 ml of sterile saline or an antibiotic flush solution such as bacitracin or gentamicin can prevent occlusion of these devices with blood or brain tissue. An increased incidence of infection, however, has been associated with flushing of ICP monitoring devices (Hickman et al., 1990). One study reported an 18.6% incidence of infection when a bacitracin flush solution was used, in contrast to a 5.7% incidence of infection without the use of a flush solution (Hickman et al., 1990). If the decision is made to use an intermittent flush, the principle of maintaining a closed system is very important.

ADDITIONAL NURSING INTERVENTIONS IN PREVENTION OF INFECTION. In any patient with an ICP monitoring device in place, one of the most important variables influencing the rate of infection is the technique of the nurse working with the system. Strict attention to maintaining aseptic technique in routine use of the system and sterile technique whenever the system is opened cannot be overemphasized. It has been documented that the use of in-line stopcocks in many ICP monitoring methods may increase the incidence of infection (Hickman et al., 1990). To prevent contamination of the stopcock, a T-piece connector or rubber sampling port that is routinely cleaned with bactericidal solution before the system is entered may be used (Hickman et al., 1990).

A consistent recommendation for the frequency of dressing changes over ICP monitoring sites has not been made. In following the recommendations made by individual institutions, sterile technique should be maintained.

CSF SAMPLES. When a patient has a ventriculostomy catheter in place, it is possible to sample CSF specimens daily and to send them for culture and sensitivity testing, for glucose and protein evaluation, and for cell counts to monitor the patient carefully for any evidence of infection. In some institutions CSF sampling is performed by nurses with specialized education, whereas in others it is the responsibility of the physician. CSF samples can be obtained from a ventriculostomy by using a rubber sampling port at a stopcock site. Correct technique for CSF sampling includes first cleaning the sampling port carefully several times with povidone–iodine (Betadine) solution. Specimens may then be obtained by either allowing passive flow through a needle inserted into the sampling port, which drains from the ventricle, or by turning the proximal stopcock to the patient off and withdrawing a small amount (approximately 3 mL) of CSF from the distal tubing using a 25-gauge needle and syringe. In sampling CSF, undue pressure created by aspirating against the ventricles must be avoided because this could result in aspiration of brain tissue or ventricular collapse. The techniques described prevent opening the system and may decrease the incidence of infection. When CSF samples are obtained, the nurse should be aware of the results and should report any evidence of infection immediately. Recent research has shown that CSF lactate increased before the development of ventriculitis. This additional information may be helpful in the early identification and treatment of infection (Schultz et al., 1993).

SUMMARY

This chapter has provided a brief overview of the pathophysiologic basis of increased ICP as well as pertinent assessment parameters in caring for a patient with actual or potential increased ICP. In addition, the importance of ICP monitoring as an adjunctive measure in the assessment and management of increased ICP was presented. The various techniques for ICP monitoring, including the basic principles involved in the use of a fluid-coupled external transducer versus an internal transducer system, were reviewed. Although the advantages and disadvantages of each monitoring technique were presented, no one system that is optimal in every situation has been developed. In 1960, Lundberg presented criteria for an ideal ICP monitoring technique that still serve as standards in the effort to develop an optimal system for ICP monitoring. These criteria include:

1. The technique should cause as little trauma to intracranial structures as possible.
2. It should involve a negligible risk of infection.
3. CSF leakage around the monitor should not be possible.
4. Recording of ICP pressures should be possible during various diagnostic and therapeutic measures without disturbing the care and comfort of the patient.
5. The apparatus should be easy to handle, reliable, and reasonably foolproof.

Although all these standards may not consistently be attained, great progress has been made in the design and maintenance of ICP monitoring systems. The specific techniques used in each situation will vary with the monitoring capabilities of the institution, the pathophysiologic condition of the patient, and the risks and benefits of each technique available in a particular situation. The nurse caring for the patient with an ICP monitoring device must use this information to facilitate an understanding of the basic monitoring techniques and should continue to update and expand his or her knowledge in the highly dynamic area of ICP monitoring.

With increased use of ICP monitoring, there is a great potential to study many of the common interventions used to control intracranial hypertension and their effect on ICP. The generation of nursing research based on observations of response of ICP to various nursing interventions, as well as specific nursing interventions to maintain ICP monitoring devices and prevent infection, are areas with great potential.

REFERENCES

Andrews, B. T. (1993). The intensive care management of patients with head injury. In B. T. Andrews (Ed.), *Neurological intensive care* (pp. 227–242). New York: McGraw-Hill.

Andrus, C. (1991). Intracranial pressure: Dynamics and nursing management. *Journal of Neuroscience Nursing, 23*(2), 85–92.

Boortz-Marx, R. (1985). Factors affecting intracranial pressure: A descriptive study. *Journal of Neurosurgical Nursing, 17*(2), 89–94.

Bouma, G. J., Muizelaar, J. P., Stringer, W. A., et al. (1992a). Ultra-early evaluation of regional cerebral blood flow in severely head injured patients using xenon-enhanced computerized tomography. *Journal of Neurosurgery, 77,* 360–368.

Bouma, G. J., Muizelaar, J. P., Bandoh, K., et al. (1992b). Blood pressure and intracranial pressure–volume dynamics in severe head injury: Relationship with cerebral blood flow. *Journal of Neurosurgery, 77,* 15–19.

Brucia, J. J., Owen, D. C., & Rudy, E. B. (1992). The effects of lidocaine on intracranial hypertension. *Journal of Neuroscience Nursing, 24*(4), 205–214.

Bruya, M. A. (1981). Planned periods of rest in the intensive care unit: Nursing care activities and intracranial pressure. *Journal of Neurosurgical Nursing, 13*(4), 184–193.

Cammermeyer, M., & Appledorn, C. (Eds.). (1990). *Core curriculum for neuroscience nursing.* Chicago: Chicago Press, American Association of Neuroscience Nurses.

Carter, L. P., Grahm, T., Bailes, J. E., et al. (1991). Continuous postoperative monitoring of cortical blood flow and intracranial pressure. *Surgical Neurology, 35,* 36–39.

Crutchfield, J. S., Narayan, R. K., Roberson, C. S., et al. (1990). Evaluation of a fiberoptic intracranial pressure monitor. *Journal of Neurosurgery, 72,* 482–487.

Dickman, C. A., Carter, L. P., Baldwin, H. Z., et al. (1991). Continuous regional cerebral blood flow monitoring in acute craniocerebral trauma. *Neurosurgery, 28,* 467–472.

Doyle, D. J., & Mark, P. W. S. (1992). Analysis of intracranial pressure. *Journal of Clinical Monitoring, 8,* 81–90.

Eichelberger, J. (1985). Clinical monitoring of brain dynamics. *Journal of the American Association of Nurse Anesthetists, 53,* 342–352.

Germon, K. (1994). Intracranial pressure monitoring in the 1990s. *Critical Care Nursing Quarterly, 17*(1), 21–32.

Gonzalez-Aries, S. M., Goldberg, M. L., Baumgartner, R., et al. (1983). Analysis of the effect of kinetic therapy on intracranial pressure in comatose neurosurgical patients. *Neurosurgery, 13*(6), 654–656.

Hickey, J. V. (1992). *The clinical practice of neurological and neurosurgical nursing* (3rd ed.). Philadelphia: J. B. Lippincott.

Hickman, K. M., Mayer, B. L., & Muwaswes, M. (1990). Intracranial pressure monitoring: Review of risk factors associated with infection. *Heart and Lung, 19,* 84–91.

Kerr, M. E., Rudy, E. B., Brucia, J., et al. (1993). Head-injured adults: Recommendations for endotracheal suctioning. *Journal of Neuroscience Nursing, 25,* 86–91.

Langfitt, T. W. (1990). Increased intracranial pressure and the vertebral circulation. In J. R. Youmans (Ed.), *Neurological surgery* (3rd ed.). Philadelphia: W. B. Saunders.

Lipe, H. P., & Mitchell, P. H. (1980). Positioning the patient with intracranial hypertension: How turning and head rotation affect the internal jugular vein. *Heart and Lung, 9,* 1031–1037.

Lundberg, N. (1960). Continuous recording and control of ventricular fluid pressure in neurosurgical practice. *Acta Psychiatrica et Neurologica Scandinavica, 36*(Suppl 149), 1–193.

March, K., Mitchell, P., Grady, S., et al. (1990). Effects of backrest position on intracranial and cerebral perfusion pressures. *Journal of Neuroscience Nursing, 22,* 375–381.

Marion, D. W., & Bouma, G. J. (1991). The use of stable xenon-enhanced computed tomographic studies of cerebral blood flow to define changes in carbon dioxide vasoresponsivity caused by severe head injury. *Neurosurgery, 29,* 869–873.

Marshall, S. B., Marshall, L. F., Vos, H. R., et al. (1990). *Neuroscience critical care: Pathophysiology and patient management.* Philadelphia: W. B. Saunders.

McQuillan, K. A. (1991). Intracranial pressure monitoring: Technical imperatives. *AACN Clinical Issues in Critical Care, 2,* 623–639.

Meyerson, B. A., Gunasekera, L., & Linderoth, B. (1991). Bedside monitoring of regional cortical blood in comatose patients using laser doppler flowmetry. *Neurosurgery, 29,* 750–755.

Mitchell, P. H. (1980). Intracranial hypertension: Implications of research for nursing care. *Journal of Neurosurgical Nursing, 12,* 145–154.

Mitchell, P. H. (1986). Decreased adaptive capacity, intracranial: A proposal for a nursing diagnosis. *Journal of Neuroscience Nursing, 18,* 170–175.

Mitchell, P. H., Habermann-Little, B., Johnson, F., et al. (1985). Critically ill children: The importance of touch in a high-technology environment. *Nursing Administration Quarterly, 9*(4), 38–46.

Mitchell, P. H., & Mauss, N. K. (1978). Relationship of patient–nurse activity to intracranial pressure variations: A pilot study. *Nursing Research, 27,* 4–10.

Muizelaar, J. P., Marmarou, A., Ward, J. D., et al. (1991). Adverse effects of hyperventilation in patients with severe head injury: Randomized clinical trial. *Journal of Neurosurgery, 75,* 731–739.

Newell, D. W., & Aaslid, R. (1992). Transcranial Doppler: Clinical and experimental uses. *Cerebrovascular and Brain Metabolism Reviews, 4,* 122–143.

Nikas, D. L. (1991). The neurological system. In J. G. Alspach (Ed.), *AACN core curriculum for critical care nursing* (4th ed.). Philadelphia: W. B. Saunders.

Obana, W. G., & Andrews, B. T. (1993). The neurologic examination and neurologic monitoring in the intensive care unit. In B. T. Andrews (Ed.), *Neurosurgical intensive care* (pp. 31–42). New York: McGraw-Hill.

Piek, J., & Bock, W. J. (1990). Continuous monitoring of cerebral tissue pressure in neurosurgical practice: Experience with 100 patients. *Intensive Care Medicine, 16,* 184–188.

Price, M. P. (1981). Significance of intracranial pressure waveform. *Journal of Neurosurgical Nursing, 13,* 202–206.

Rauch, M. E., Mitchell, P. H., Tyler, M. L. (1990). Validation of risk factors for the nursing diagnosis decreased intracranial adaptive capacity. *Journal of Neuroscience Nursing, 22,* 173–178.

Richmond, T. S. (1993). Intracranial pressure monitoring. *AACN Clinical Issues in Critical Care, 4,* 148–160.

Rising, C. J. (1993). The relationship of selected nursing activities to ICP. *Journal of Neuroscience Nursing, 25,* 302–308.

Rockoff, M., & Kennedy, S. (1988). Physiology and clinical aspects of raised intracranial pressure. In A. H. Ropper, & S. F. Kennedy (Eds.), *Critical care neurology and neurosurgery.* New York: Praeger Special Studies.

Rosner, M. J., & Daughton, S. (1990). Cerebral perfusion pressure management in head injury. *Journal of Trauma, 30,* 933–941.

Rosner, M. J. (1993). Pathophysiology and management of increased intracranial pressure. In B. T. Andrews (Ed.), *Neurosurgical intensive care* (pp. 57–112). New York: McGraw-Hill.

Rudy, E. B., Turner, B. S., Baun, M., et al. (1991). Endotracheal suctioning in adults with head injury. *Heart and Lung, 20,* 667–674.

Scheinberg, M., Kanter, M. J., Robertson, C. S., et al. (1992). Continuous monitoring of jugular venous oxygen saturation in head-injured patients. *Journal of Neurosurgery, 76,* 212–217.

Schickner, D. J., & Young, R. F. (1992). Intracranial pressure monitoring: Fiberoptic monitor compared with the ventricular catheter. *Surgical Neurology, 37,* 251–254.

Schultz, M., Moore, K., & Foote, A. W. (1993). Bacterial ventriculitis and duration of ventriculostomy catheter insertion. *Journal of Neuroscience Nursing, 25,* 158–164.

Sisson, R. (1990). Effects of auditory stimuli on comatose patients with head injury. *Heart and Lung, 19,* 373–378.

Smith, K. A. (1987). Head trauma: Comparison of infection rates for different methods of intracranial pressure monitoring. *Journal of Neuroscience Nursing, 19,* 310–314.

Unwin, D. H., Giller, C. A., & Kopitnik, T. A. (1991). Central nervous system monitoring: What helps, what does not. *Surgical Clinics of North America, 71,* 733–747.

Walleck, C. A. (1987). Intracranial hypertension: Interventions and outcomes. *Critical Care Quarterly, 10*(1), 45–57.

Weinstabl, C., Richling, B., & Plainer, B. (1992). Comparative analysis between epidural (Gaeltec) and subdural (Camino) intracranial pressure probes. *Journal of Clinical Monitoring, 8,* 116–120.

Wilkinson, H. A. (1977). The intracranial pressure-monitoring cup catheter: Technical note. *Neurosurgery, 1,* 139–141.

Williams, A., & Coyne, S. M. (1993). Effects of neck position on intracranial pressure. *American Journal of Critical Care, 2,* 68–71.

UNIT 4

CARDIOVASCULAR SYSTEM

CHAPTER

18 Cardiovascular Anatomy and Physiology

Patricia L. Vaska

OVERVIEW

The Cardiac Circulation

The purpose of the cardiovascular system is to supply nutrients to cells and remove metabolic waste products. The system is composed of two coordinated pumps—the right side of the heart (the right atrium and ventricle) and the left side of the heart (the left atrium and ventricle)—and two circulations—the pulmonary circulation, between the right side of the heart and the left side of the heart; and the systemic circulation between the left and right sides of the heart (Fig. 18–1).

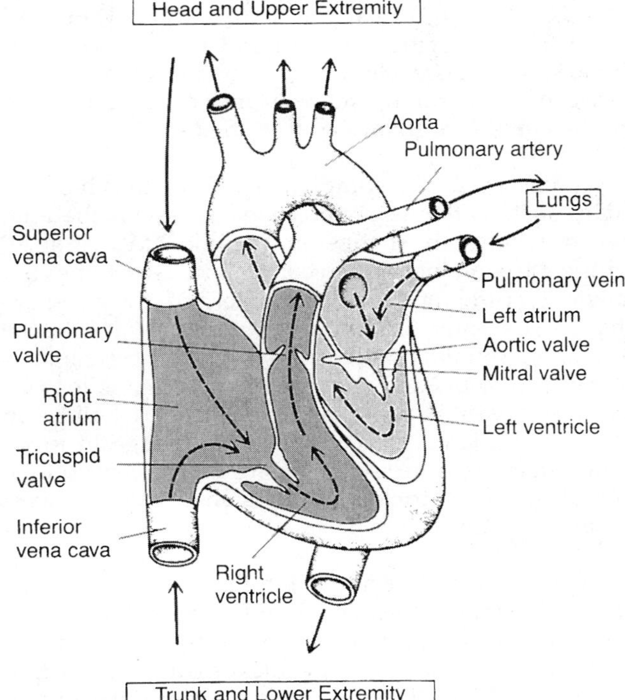

FIGURE 18–1. Structure of the heart and course of blood flow through the heart chambers. (From Guyton, A. C., & Hall, J. E. [1996]. *Textbook of medical physiology* [9th ed., p. 108]. Philadelphia: W. B. Saunders.)

The right and left atria are thin-walled chambers that serve primarily as reservoirs for blood returning to the heart from the systemic and pulmonary circulations (Guyton, 1991). A weak atrial contraction at the end of ventricular diastole provides 10% to 15% of the ventricular end-diastolic volume, the "atrial kick," in healthy hearts. The atria are divided by a septum that continues inferiorly to become the membranous portion of the intraventricular septum that divides the two ventricles. During ventricular diastole (relaxation), blood flows through the atrioventricular valves, the tricuspid valve in the right side of the heart and the mitral valve in the left side of the heart, into the respective ventricles. During ventricular systole (contraction), blood is pumped through the semilunar valves, the pulmonic valve in the right side of the heart and the aortic valve in the left side of the heart, to the pulmonary artery and the aorta.

The pulmonary vasculature is relatively short and broad and has minimal resistance to flow. In contrast to the pulmonary system, the systemic vessels are longer and have a higher resistance. Left-sided pressures are relatively high in comparison with right-sided pressures. The arteries distribute blood to the microcirculation, where exchange of nutrients and waste products occurs. The systemic veins return deoxygenated blood to the right atrium, and the pulmonary veins return oxygenated blood to the left atrium.

Oxygen saturation of blood leaving the left side of the heart is approximately 95%, and oxygen saturation of venous blood returning to the right side of the heart is approximately 75% at rest. Thus, in one circuit, at rest, approximately 25% of available oxygen is extracted by the tissues (Hughes, 1987). Clinically, left-sided cardiac oxygen saturation is measured as arterial oxygen saturation. Right-sided cardiac oxygen saturation is measured as mixed venous oxygen saturation (Svo_2) from a pulmonary artery catheter, or, less accurately, from the right atrium, because total mixing of venous blood occurs in the right ventricle, and right atrial samples may not be homogeneous. Mixed venous oxygen saturation is an overall measure of the adequacy of cardiopulmonary function in relation to tissue demand. In addition, oxygen content, oxygen delivery, and oxygen demand can be calculated (White, 1993).

The circulatory system is composed of arteries, arterioles, capillaries, venules, and veins that branch going away from the heart and coalesce coming toward the heart. As the total cross-sectional area of the system increases, the rate of flow decreases, and conversely, as the cross-sectional area decreases, the rate of flow increases. The aorta and major arteries are conductance vessels, and no nutrient exchange occurs. The arterioles are the primary regulators of resistance. Nutrient exchange occurs at the capillary level. The veins are capacitance vessels and serve as reservoirs for blood volume. In the systemic circuit the total cardiac output is divided among the various organs according to local demand and changes in arteriolar resistance. The pulmonary system receives the total cardiac output (Guyton, 1991).

Physical Properties of the System

Concepts of pressure, resistance, flow, and compliance are essential to an understanding of the cardiovascular system and are briefly reviewed (Table 18–1). These concepts are applied in subsequent discussions.

TABLE 18–1. **Equations Defining Pressure, Flow (Ohm's Law), Resistance (Poiseuille's Law), and Compliance**

Pressure across a vessel:

$$\Delta P = P_1 - P_2$$

where P = Pressure across the vessel
P_1 = Pressure at the proximal end
P_2 = Pressure at the distal end

Ohm's law for calculation of flow through a vessel:

$$\dot{Q} = \frac{\Delta P}{R}$$

where $\dot{Q}$ = Flow
ΔP = Pressure difference between the two ends of the vessel
R = Resistance

Poiseuille's law for the relationship between flow, pressure, and resistance:

$$\dot{Q} = \frac{\pi \Delta P r^4}{8 \eta l}$$

where $\dot{Q}$ = Flow
ΔP = Pressure difference between the ends of the vessel
η = Blood viscosity
r = Radius of the vessel
l = Length of the vessel

Compliance:

$$\text{Compliance} = \frac{\text{Increase in volume}}{\text{Increase in pressure}}$$

PRESSURE. The driving pressure is the difference in pressure between two points in the circuit that drives flow from high pressure to low pressure. For example, the driving pressure for the systemic circuit is the pressure difference (ΔP) between the mean arterial pressure (MAP) and the mean right arterial pressure (RAP). The driving pressure for the pulmonary circuit is the difference between mean pulmonary artery pressure and the mean left atrial pressure, or the pulmonary capillary wedge pressure. The transmural pressure (P_{tm}) is the difference across the wall between the inside of a vessel or a cardiac chamber and the outside.

RESISTANCE. The resistance to flow is directly proportional to the length of the vessel (1) and the viscosity (η) of the fluid and inversely proportional to the fourth power of the radius of the vessel (r^4). The length of the vascular system does not change appreciably in any given individual. The primary determinant of the viscosity of blood is the hematocrit, and within the normal range hematocrit does not significantly alter the viscosity. At hematocrits above 60% viscosity increases, and at hematocrits below 15% viscosity decreases (Fox et al., 1994). The primary determinant of resistance in the body is the radius of the blood vessels, particularly the arterioles (note that the radius is raised to the fourth power in the equation defining Poiseuille's law [see Table 18–1]). Resistance increases as the vessels become more constricted and decreases as vessels dilate (Urban, 1993).

FLOW. Flow ($\dot{Q}$) in the system is directly proportional to the driving pressure and inversely proportional to resistance. Clinically, flow and driving pressure can be measured, and resistance can be calculated by the equations given in Table 18–2.

COMPLIANCE. The compliance of a distensible container such as the heart and blood vessels is the relationship between change in volume (ΔV) and ΔP within the container. When compliance is low, the container is stiffer or less distensible and the pressure change is greater for any given volume put into the container. When compliance is high the container is easily distensible and the pressure change is less for any given volume. For example, in heart failure, in which compliance is decreased, the change in intraventricular pressure is greater for any given volume put into the ventricle than it is in a healthy heart (Goerke & Mines, 1988).

WALL TENSION. Tension (T) in the walls of the heart or blood vessels is described by LaPlace's law, which relates the transmural pressure (P_{tm}) and the radius (r) of the structure to the wall thickness (Th) such that $T = P \times r/2Th$. Wall tension is a major determinant of oxygen consumption. The larger the internal pressure and the larger the radius of the structure in relation to the wall thickness, the greater the oxygen demand. This concept has important implications in relation to cardiac compensatory mechanisms. An in-

TABLE 18–2. **Clinical Equations for Calculation of Pressure and Resistance**

Mean arterial pressure:

$$MAP = \frac{2DP + SP}{3}$$

where MAP = Mean arterial pressure
DP = Diastolic pressure
SP = Systolic pressure

Mean pulmonary artery pressure:

$$PAM = \frac{2PAD + PAS}{3}$$

where PAM = Pulmonary artery mean pressure
PAD = Pulmonary artery diastolic pressure
PS = Pulmonary artery systolic pressure

Systemic vascular resistance:

$$SVR = \frac{MAP - CVP}{CO} \times 80$$

where SVR = Systemic vascular resistance
MAP = Mean arterial pressure
CVP = Central venous pressure
CO = Cardiac output

Pulmonary vascular resistance:

$$PVR = \frac{PAM - PCWP}{CO} \times 80$$

where PVR = Pulmonary vascular resistance
PAM = Pulmonary mean pressure
PCWP = Pulmonary capillary wedge pressure
CO = Cardiac output

creased pressure load on the ventricle, such as occurs with hypertension or aortic stenosis, increases the wall thickness to maintain oxygen consumption at normal levels for the weight of the ventricular muscle. In a failing heart that is dilated, oxygen demand is increased simply by virtue of the increase in ventricular radius and pressure (Goerke & Mines, 1988).

Anatomy of the Heart

The heart hangs in the chest from the great vessels (Fig. 18–2). Anatomically, the right atrium and ventricle are anterior structures, and the left atrium and ventricle are primarily posterior structures. The heart is surrounded by the fibrous pericardium, which protects the heart and, to a degree, limits acute overdistention of the cardiac chambers (Freeman, 1990).

CARDIAC SKELETON AND MUSCULATURE. The cardiac skeleton is a fibrous zone surrounding the valves and separating the atria and the ventricles. Atrial muscle fibers originate and insert on this fibrous skeleton. The atrial muscle fibers are composed of two layers: deep fibers within each atria shorten toward the atrioventricular (AV) valves, propelling blood into the ventricle. Superficial fibers that pass across both atria produce lateral constriction of the atria and coordinated contraction between them (Little & Little, 1985).

The ventricular wall is composed of three layers—the epicardium lying outermost, the myocardium in the middle, and the endocardium, which lines the ventricular chamber. The area next to the myocardium, the subendocardium, is the area at greatest risk for ischemia. Ventricular muscle fibers arise from the fibrous skeleton, the root of the aorta, and the root of the pulmonary artery. Each ventricle is formed from a mass of interlocking, nested fibers that change orientation as they pass from the epicardium through the myocardium to the endocardium. During contraction, this arrangement produces both circumferential and longitudinal compression of the ventricular chamber and propels blood into the great vessels. There are some fibers that surround both ventricles as well (Lee, 1992).

The left ventricle, which is conically shaped, is much thicker than the right ventricle and contracts with a wringing motion that forcefully propels blood into the aorta. The right ventricle wraps around the convex intraventricular septum, is crescent shaped, and contracts with a bellows motion that effectively pumps large volumes of blood into the low-pressure pulmonary circuit. The intraventricular septum is both structurally and functionally more a part of the left ventricle than the right; however, deformation of the septum occurs with abnormal loading conditions in either ventricle, and thus impaired function in one ventricle affects function in the other ventricle (Bond & Halpenny, 1995).

The high-pressure left ventricle is well suited to deliver nutrient-rich blood through the high-resistance peripheral circulation. The left ventricle can provide adequate cardiac output to maintain life in the absence of right ventricular function. In recent years, emphasis has been placed on the right ventricle. Under normal conditions, it serves as a low-pressure reservoir that generates flow through the low-resistance pulmonary circulation. When a disease state exists, such as chronic pulmonary disease, the right ventricle hypertrophies, and it becomes imperative to propagate perfusion through the pulmonary tree and generate adequate cardiac output (Farb et al., 1992; Schulman & Matthay, 1992).

THE VALVES. The valve leaflets are a cartilaginous, avascular matrix with a covering of endothelium. Many mechanisms have been proposed to explain valve motion. Most evidence suggests that the opening and closing motions of the cardiac valves are passive and are caused by differences in pressure between the cardiac chambers or between the chamber and the respective great vessel. The AV valves, the two-leaflet mitral valve, and the three-leaflet tricuspid valve are complicated structures (Fig. 18–3). The atrial wall, the annulus, the papillary muscles, and the chordae ten-

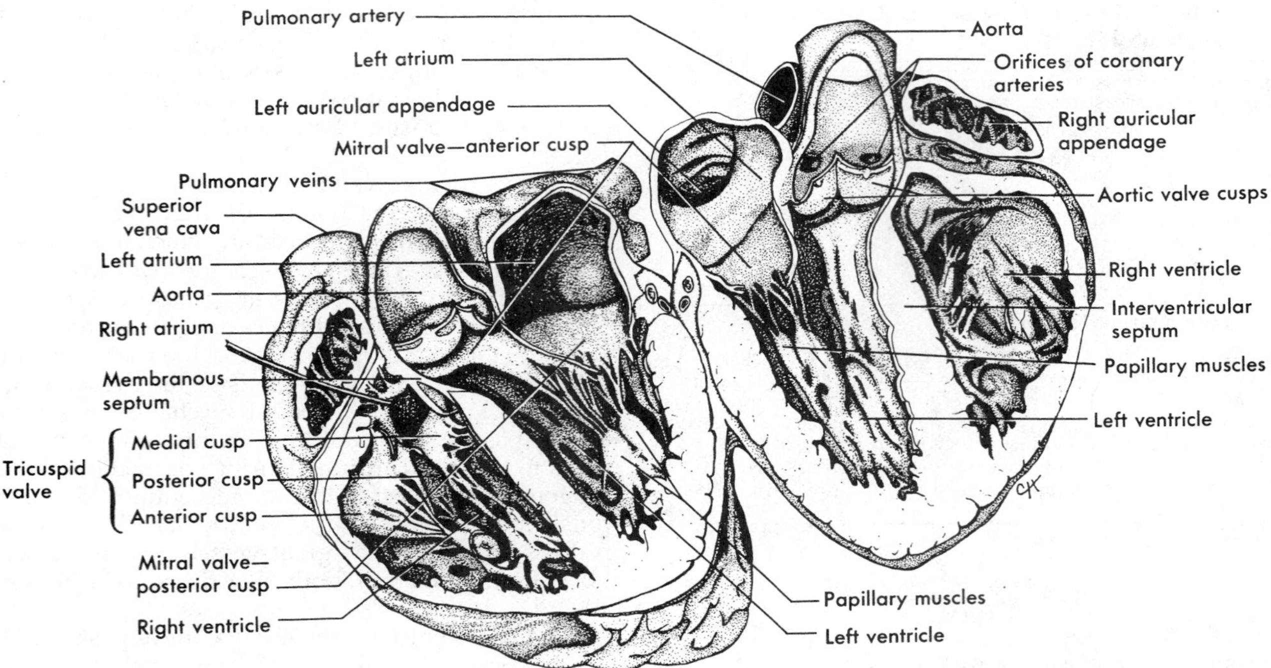

FIGURE 18–2. Drawing of a heart split perpendicular to the interventricular septum to illustrate the anatomic relationship of the leaflets of the atrioventricular (AV) and aortic valves. (Reproduced with permission from Berne, R., & Levy, M. [1986]. *Cardiovascular physiology* [5th ed.]. St. Louis: Mosby Yearbook.)

dineae are all involved in closure and competency of the valve during ventricular systole. As the ventricle contracts and the pressure exceeds that of the atria, the leaflets begin to close. With a long ventricular filling time (P–R interval greater than 0.18), atrial pressure falls below ventricular pressure owing to atrial relaxation, and valve closure may begin before the onset of ventricular systole (Carbello, 1991). Narrowing of the annulus with the decrease in ventricular chamber size assists coaptation of the leaflets. Contraction of the papillary muscles maintains tension on the chordae and prevents eversion of the leaflets into the atria. In addition, chordae from one papillary muscle insert on both leaflets, thus providing some assistance to both leaflets (Zile, 1991).

The semilunar valves, comprising the aortic and pulmonic valves, have three cusps that allow them to open maximally with ventricular ejection. During ejection, the aortic valve leaflets are held away from the aortic wall by turbulent flow in the sinus of Valsalva and do not obstruct the coronary ostia. During ventricular diastole, reversal of flow in the great arteries catches the cusps and closes the valves.

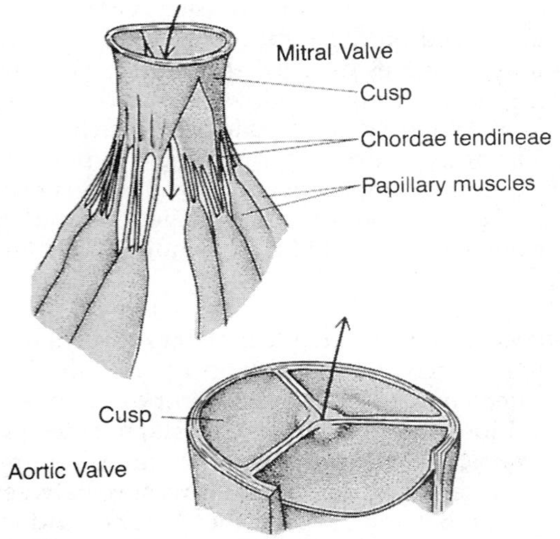

Mitral Valve
Cusp
Chordae tendineae
Papillary muscles
Cusp
Aortic Valve

FIGURE 18–3. Mitral and aortic valves. (From Guyton, A. C., & Hall, J. E. [1996]. *Textbook of medical physiology* [9th ed., p. 112]. Philadelphia: W. B. Saunders.)

THE CORONARY ARTERIES. The coronary arteries arise in the aortic root just above the aortic valve and run in the epicardial layer. They give off penetrating branches that provide blood to the myocardium (Fig. 18–4). Unlike flow in other arteries in the body, most coronary blood flow occurs during ventricular diastole. Thus, the perfusion pressure for the coronary arteries is the aortic diastolic pressure minus the intracavitary diastolic pressure. The subendocardium is most distant from the major epicardial vessels and most affected by intracavitary pressure, and is at greatest risk for ischemia (Fig. 18–5).

The major epicardial vessels (Fig. 18–6) are the right coronary artery and the left main coronary artery, which divides into the left anterior descending branch

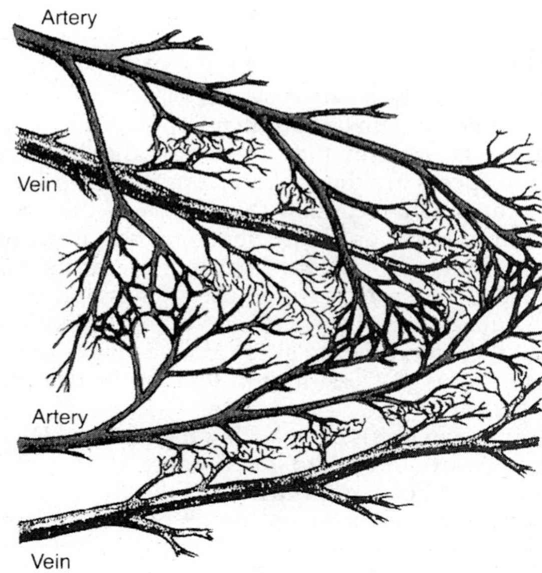

FIGURE 18–4. Minute anastomoses of the coronary arterial system. (From Guyton, A. C., & Hall, J. E. [1996]. *Textbook of medical physiology* [9th ed., p. 260]. Philadelphia: W. B. Saunders.)

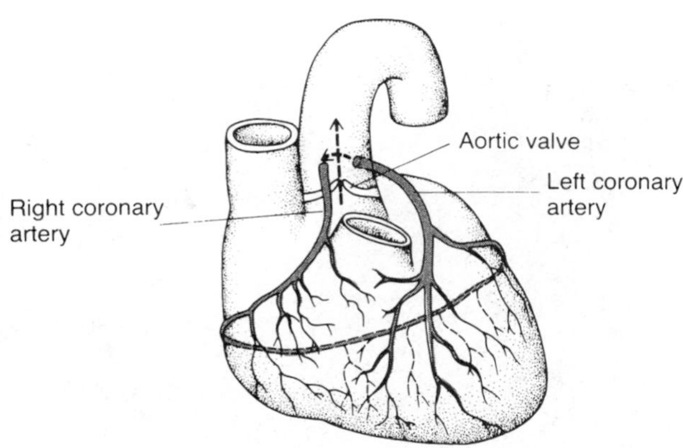

FIGURE 18–6. The coronary vessels. (From Guyton, A. C., & Hall, J. E. [1996]. *Textbook of medical physiology* [9th ed., p. 256]. Philadelphia: W. B. Saunders.)

and the circumflex branch. The right coronary artery runs laterally and posteriorly, in the atrioventricular sulcus between the right atrium and the right ventricle. The acute marginal branches perfuse the right ventricular free wall. Posteriorly, in most of the population, the right coronary artery turns downward in the posterior interventricular sulcus and becomes the posterior descending artery, which perfuses the posterior third of the intraventricular septum and a portion of the posterior left ventricle (Schoen, 1989).

The left main coronary artery is very short and branches into the left anterior descending and the circumflex arteries. The left anterior descending runs inferiorly in the anterior interventricular sulcus and branches into septal perforators that perfuse the anterior two-thirds of the intraventricular septum and most of the conduction system. Diagonal branches perfuse the anterior and lateral walls of the left ventricle. The circumflex turns posteriorly in the atrioventricular sulcus and, with its major branches, the obtuse marginals, perfuses the posterior portion of the left ventricle. Deoxygenated blood from the left ventricle returns via the coronary sinus and from the right ventricle via the anterior cardiac veins. A very small amount of venous blood dumps directly into the cardiac chambers via the thesbian veins (Guyton, 1991; Hurst et al., 1990).

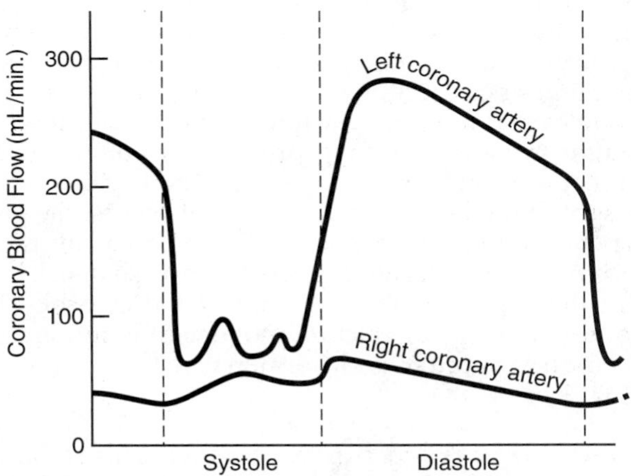

FIGURE 18–5. Phasic flow of blood through the coronary capillaries of the left and right ventricles. (From Guyton, A. C., & Hall, J. E. [1996]. *Textbook of medical physiology* [9th ed., p. 257]. Philadelphia: W. B. Saunders.)

THE CONDUCTION SYSTEM. The conduction system is composed of the sinus (sinoatrial [SA]) node, the atrial internodal tracts, the AV node, the common bundle, the left and right bundle branches, and the Purkinje fibers (Fig. 18–7). Normally, a cell or cells in the SA node reaches threshold first, and this stimulus then spreads to other cells via low-resistance pathways, intercalated discs, and gap junctions. This wave of excitation spreads throughout the atria from cell to cell and to the AV node through specialized conduction pathways. In the AV node the rate of conductance of the impulse is slowed (decremental conduction), allowing time for mechanical contraction in the atria and final filling of the ventricles before ventricular contraction begins. From the AV node, the impulse moves into the common bundle, the only normal conductive pathway between the atria and the ventricles, and then to the left and right bundle branches, the Purkinje fibers, and then from cell to cell (Oren et al., 1993). The ventricle depolarizes from the endocardium to the epicardium. However, unlike other types of cells, it does not repolarize in the same direction. It repolarizes from the epicardium to the endocardium. The reason for this is unclear but is thought to be the result of the stresses placed on the endocardium by the increased intracavitary pressure and decreased blood flow to the endocardium that occurs during ventricular systole (Abraham, 1992).

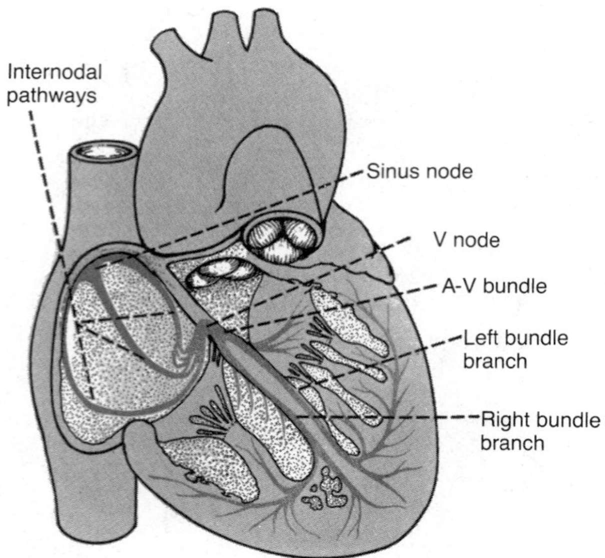

FIGURE 18–7. The sinus node and the Purkinje system of the heart, also showing the AV node, the atrial internodal pathways, and the ventricular bundle branches. (From Guyton, A. C., & Hall, J. E. [1996]. *Textbook of medical physiology* [9th ed., p. 122]. Philadelphia: W. B. Saunders.)

Ultrastructure and Mechanisms of Cardiac Contraction

ULTRASTRUCTURE. Cardiac muscle (Fig. 18–8) is a syncytium multinucleated mass of protoplasm formed by a secondary union of separate cells that acts as a single unit. Cardiac muscle fibers are the cells of the heart. They are joined by a specialized, thickened portion of the cell membrane called the intercalated disc. The intercalated disc allows the contractile force of one cell to be transmitted to the next. In addition, a specialized area within the intercalated disc, called the nexus, is a low-resistance pathway that allows rapid conduction of impulses between adjacent cardiac cells. It is thought that within the nexus there is an area where the membranes of adjoining cells are in extremely close physical proximity, and that some exchange of ions may occur that enhances conduction (Bond, 1989; Cohn, 1985).

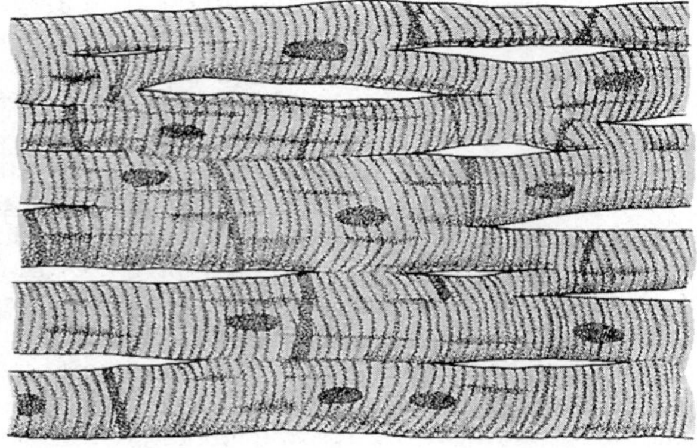

FIGURE 18–8. The "syncytial" interconnecting nature of cardiac muscle. (From Guyton, A. C., & Hall, J. E. [1996]. *Textbook of medical physiology* [9th ed., p. 108]. Philadelphia: W. B. Saunders.)

MOLECULAR BASIS OF CONTRACTION. Each cardiac cell, or fiber, contains multiple myofibrils made up of repeating sarcomeres that are longitudinally joined. The sarcomeres are the functional units of the cardiac muscle fiber. They contain thin bands of the protein actin and thick bands of the protein myosin in an alternating arrangement. Actin filaments are anchored at each end of the sarcomere at the Z-lines and extend toward the center of the sarcomere, but do not meet. At rest, the actin-binding sites for myosin are covered by long chains of tropomyosin that are held in place by troponin.

The myosin fibrils extend from the center of the sarcomere toward, but not to, the Z-lines. After electrical excitation, globular projections on the myosin fibers form cross-bridges between the myosin and actin fibers. There are no globular heads in the middle of the myosin filaments, and therefore connection between myosin and actin cannot occur in the very middle of the sarcomere. The filaments do not shorten themselves but slide past each other, thus shortening the fiber. At very long and very short fiber lengths, the number of cross-bridges that can be attached is reduced, thus limiting the force of contraction (Weisbrodt, 1992).

The T system is composed of the T tubules and the sarcoplasmic reticulum. The T tubules are invaginations of the cell membrane (sarcolemma) that are in direct contact with the extracellular fluid, allowing rapid transmission of the action potential to each of the myofibrils within the cardiac cell so that they contract together. As in other areas of the cell membrane, there are voltage-gated ionic channels and active transport systems as well as receptors for neurotransmitters and hormones (Guyton, 1991; Rhoades & Pflanzer, 1989).

The sarcoplasmic reticulum is an intracellular structure that surrounds the myofibrils and is in close proximity with the T tubules. It is thought to be the primary source of calcium for muscle contraction. The membrane of this organelle is also supplied with active transport systems and receptor sites (Stern et al., 1988).

There is no direct physical connection between the T tubules and the sarcoplasmic reticulum, but there is thought to be a "coupling process," a voltage-gated channel for calcium and possibly other ions. It is thought that when an action potential occurs, the gate is opened, and calcium entering the sarcoplasmic reticulum from the T tubule triggers the release of calcium from the sarcoplasmic reticulum to the cytosol. The quantity and rate of calcium movement is influenced by neurotransmitter and hormonal receptors (Cohn, 1985).

EXCITATION–CONTRACTION COUPLING. This is the sequence of events, initiated by an action potential, that increases the availability of calcium and allows cross-bridging to occur. In the relaxed state, the active binding sites for myosin on the actin chains are covered, or inhibited, by tropomyosin. In the myosin head, the enzyme ATPase splits adenosine triphosphate (ATP) to adenosine diphosphate (ADP) and organic phosphate, providing the energy to be used as soon as the active binding sites on the actin chains become available (Braunwald et al., 1992; Sharaf et al., 1994).

The action potential propagated down the T tubule increases calcium diffusion from the interstitial fluid to the cytosol and also triggers release of calcium from the sarcoplasmic reticulum to the cytosol. The calcium (up to four ions) binds with troponin, which alters the configuration of tropomyosin and exposes the active binding sites on the actin chain. The myosin head attaches to the actin site and swivels toward the center of the sarcomere, pulling the actin filaments past and resulting in fiber shortening. ADP and inorganic phosphate are released from the myosin head, and a binding site for ATP on the myosin head is exposed. The binding of ATP to this site breaks the connection with actin, and the myosin head returns to its original position. Myosin ATPase again splits the ATP, and the myosin head attaches to another binding site. This process is repeated many times during a single contraction and continues as long as ATP and calcium are available and active binding sites on the actin chains are exposed (Byrne & Downey, 1992).

During relaxation, active calcium pumps in the membrane of the sarcoplasmic reticulum and the T tubules remove calcium from the cytosol, and calcium is released by troponin. Tropomyosin returns to its previous configuration, and the active binding sites on the actin chain are covered. In addition, calcium returns to the T tubules through the sodium–calcium exchange mechanism (Ruegg, 1986).

Cytosolic calcium concentration, the rate of calcium exchange, and the resting fiber length determine the number of cross-bridges that can attach, the strength and rate of contraction, and the rate and degree of relaxation. In a healthy person at rest, the cytosolic calcium concentration is relatively low, not all of the troponin molecules are fully activated, and not all of the binding sites on the actin chain are uncovered. In addition, fiber length is relatively short, and the actin and myosin chains are not optimally aligned for the occurrence of maximum cross-bridging. Thus, there is a contractile reserve that can be used to increase the rate and force of contraction when required by metabolic demands (Wright, 1990).

For example, sympathetic stimulation increases both the amount of calcium that enters the cell and the rate of active transport through receptor-mediated channels. Thus, both the strength of the contraction and the rate of contraction and relaxation are increased. Conversely, drugs that block calcium channels produce a negative inotropic effect and slow the rate of fiber shortening and relaxation (White, 1992).

In cardiac failure, fibers are stretched, and the number of cross-bridges that can attach are decreased, and therefore the force of contraction is decreased. In addition, in chronic heart failure the number of beta receptors is reduced (down-regulation), decreasing receptor-mediated calcium transport and further impairing contractile function and the ability to raise cardiac output to meet metabolic demands (Gibson, 1991; Muntz et al., 1994). If cardiac failure is caused by ischemia, the amount of calcium removed from the cytosol is also decreased, which impairs relaxation and decreases ventricular compliance (Rousseau et al., 1994; Wright, 1990).

ELECTRICAL ACTIVITY OF THE HEART

Resting Membrane Potential

In cardiac cells, as in other cells in the body, there is a concentration gradient across the cell membrane for sodium, potassium, calcium, and other ions that is determined by the permeability of the membrane to each ion, its electrical charge, and the functioning of active ionic pumps in the cell membrane. Movement of ions across the cell membrane occurs both passively down the electrochemical gradient and through energy-requiring ionic pumps in the cell membrane that actively transport specific ions against the electrochemical gradients. It must be noted that the ionic exchanges discussed in the following sections involve only a small amount of the total ionic composition of the cell and the extracellular fluid.

MEMBRANE PERMEABILITY. It has been proposed that the permeability of the cell membrane for specific ions is controlled by gates in the cell membrane that open and close in response to electrical stimulation and other factors. These voltage-gated channels open and close within specific voltage ranges. For example, gates that allow rapid sodium influx are activated at about −70 millivolts (mV), whereas slow inward calcium and sodium channels are activated at −40 to −30 mV (Guyton, 1991; Milnor, 1990).

ELECTROCHEMICAL GRADIENTS. In the resting state the cell membrane is permeable to potassium and minimally permeable to sodium. Potassium slowly leaks out of the cell down its concentration gradient, leaving behind negatively charged proteins and other substances. The movement of potassium ions out of the cell is limited by the increasing negativity inside the cell. The diffusion gradient for potassium is counterbalanced by the electrical gradient, and equilibrium is reached when inward and outward movement of potassium is equal. If the membrane were permeable only to potassium, this would establish a resting membrane potential of −95 mV, which is slightly more negative than the actual resting potential in the Purkinje fibers and ventricular cells of about −90 mV (Fig. 18–9). However, the membrane is also slightly permeable to the influx of sodium and calcium, and a true equilibrium is not reached (Goerke & Mines, 1988).

ACTIVE TRANSPORT. In addition to passive movement of ions due to electrochemical gradients, mem-

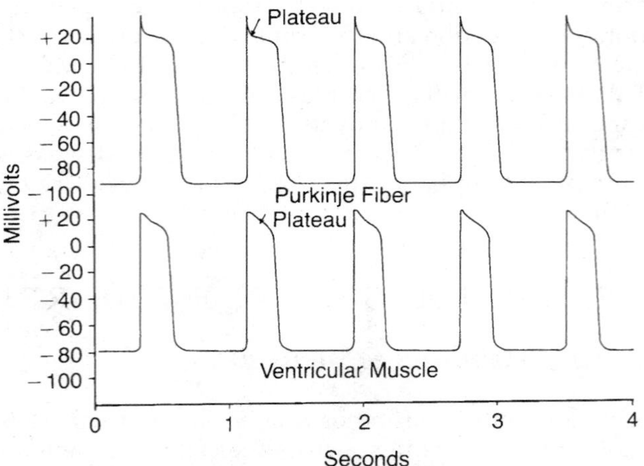

FIGURE 18–9. Rhythmic action potentials from a Purkinje fiber and from a ventricular muscle fiber, recorded by means of microelectrodes. (From Guyton, A. C., & Hall, J. E. [1996]. *Textbook of medical physiology* [9th ed., p. 108]. Philadelphia: W. B. Saunders.)

brane potential is maintained by active transport of ions across the membrane by energy-requiring pumps. The sodium–potassium ATPase pump operates in such a way that two potassium ions are exchanged for three sodium ions, resulting in a net loss of positive ions within the cell and intracellular negativity (Vassalle, 1987). The sodium–calcium exchange system in the cell membrane uses electrochemical energy to transport two sodium ions into the cell for one calcium ion transported out of the cell during the resting phase (McGuigan & Blatter, 1987). The calcium ATPase pump moves calcium out of the cell as well as into the sarcoplasmic reticulum from the cytosol during recovery (McGuigan & Blatter, 1987).

These mechanisms establish and maintain the resting membrane potential. An electrical stimulus or other conditions that alter these mechanisms allows the cell to become more positive until it reaches threshold, when depolarization continues.

Action Potential

VENTRICULAR ACTION POTENTIAL. At rest, potassium channels are open, and potassium is conducted out of the cell, establishing the resting membrane potential. With excitation of the membrane in phase 0, fast sodium channels open, there is a rapid influx of sodium into the cell and a slowing of potassium efflux out of the cell, and the membrane potential rises to +30. In phase 1, the fast inward sodium channels close, and potassium efflux continues at a slower rate, bringing the membrane potential to approximately 0. In phase 2, the plateau phase, slow inward sodium and calcium channels open, the influx of these ions matches the outward flow of potassium, and the membrane remains depolarized. The influx of calcium participates in the cross-bridging of actin and myosin and mechanical contraction and also triggers the release of calcium from the sarcoplasmic reticulum for this process (Hudak & Gallo, 1994). In phase 3, the slow sodium and calcium channels close, and potassium conductance increases to the level of the resting state. The efflux of potassium then returns the membrane to the resting membrane potential, and the sodium–potassium ATPase pump is activated. During phases 0, 1, and 2, the cell is absolutely refractory. It is not polarized and cannot accept another stimulus. As the membrane potential is restored during phase 3, the cell becomes relatively refractory—that is, it can be stimulated but requires a stronger stimulus. At the end of phase 3 there is a supernormal period during which a very small stimulus will elicit an action potential (Fig. 18–10).

SINUS NODE ACTION POTENTIAL. The action potential in the sinus node varies from that of the ventricle and Purkinje fibers in several ways (see Fig. 18–9). The maximum resting potential is only −55 to −60 mV. At this level, fast sodium channels are inactivated, and the rise in phase 0 is slower because of the opening of slow sodium and calcium channels. There is no plateau phase. Sodium and calcium channels become inactivated, and potassium channels open, allowing repolarization to occur.

The spontaneous rise of phase 4 of the sinus node action potential to threshold is the basis of the property of automaticity in the heart. That is, an action potential can be initiated without an outside stimulus. The ionic shifts that produce this spontaneous diastolic depolarization are somewhat controversial. During phase 4 there may be a slow decrease in the rate of outward potassium conductance that limits the amount of negativity that builds up in the cell, allowing the membrane potential to rise to threshold, or creating an increase in inward sodium and calcium flux that would have the same effect, or both (Cohn, 1985; Guyton, 1991). The cell reaches threshold and depolarizes, initiating depolarization for the entire heart, and the cycle starts over.

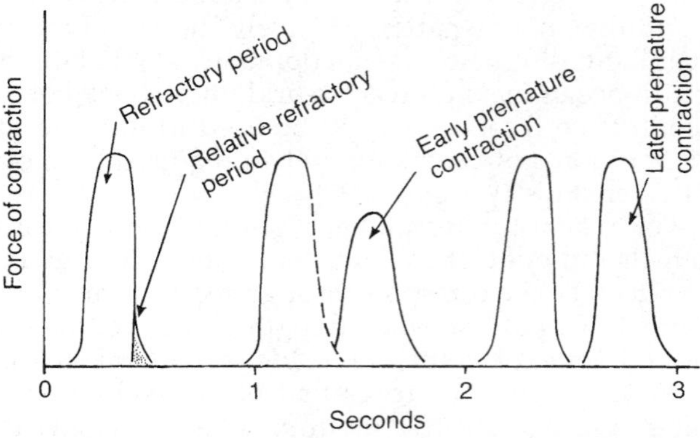

FIGURE 18–10. Contraction of the heart, showing the durations of the refractory period and the relative refractory period, the effect of an early premature contraction, and the effect of a later premature contraction. Note that the premature contractions do not cause wave summation, as occurs in skeletal muscle. (From Guyton, A. C., & Hall, J. E. [1996]. *Textbook of medical physiology* [9th ed., p. 109]. Philadelphia: W. B. Saunders.)

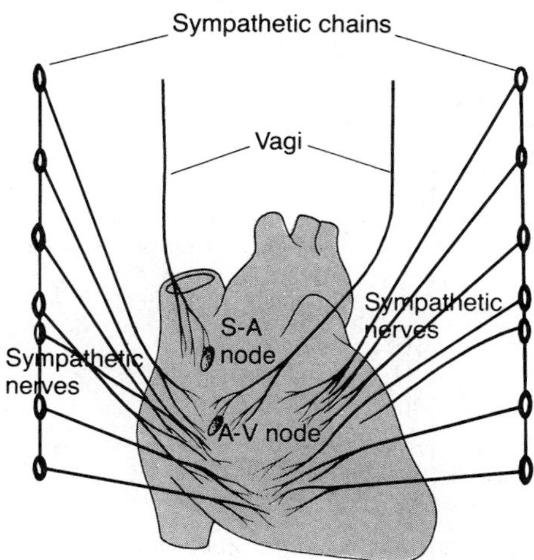

FIGURE 18–11. The cardiac nerves. (From Guyton, A. [1991]. *Textbook of medical physiology* [8th ed.]. Philadelphia: W. B. Saunders.)

The rate of rise of phase 4 in automatic cells is affected by neurotransmitters, thus altering heart rate as well as conduction velocities within the conduction system (Fig. 18–11). Afferent parasympathetic fibers from the vagus nerve innervate primarily the conduction system at the SA and AV nodes. There are few parasympathetic afferents to the ventricle or the ventricular muscle fibers. Parasympathetic stimulation releases the neurotransmitter acetylcholine, causing the resting membrane potential to be more negative, that is, further from threshold, slowing the rate of conduction in the AV node and slowing the rate of spontaneous depolarization in phase 4. It does this by maintaining the rate of potassium conductance and slowing sodium conductance. The effect of this is that it takes longer for the cell to rise to threshold and fire and longer for the stimulus to reach and be conducted through the AV node. Extreme stimulation, such as occurs with carotid sinus massage, may block conduction at the AV node altogether. Normally, parasympathetic tone predominates at rest, and the resting heart rate is 80 beats / minute as opposed to the basic unregulated rate of 100 to 120 beats / minute (Guyton, 1991).

Norepinephrine increases membrane permeability to calcium, increasing the rate of rise of phase 4 to threshold and also increasing the velocity of conduction. It acts along the entire excitation pathway and on contractile muscle cells as well (Guyton, 1991).

CARDIAC PUMPING

The Cardiac Cycle

The relationship of electrical events, mechanical events, and blood flow that occur during each heart beat within the heart itself and in the major vessels is depicted in Figure 18–12. Electrical events are clinically evaluated by the electrocardiogram (ECG) and by electrophysiologic studies.

Arterial and atrial pressures can be monitored at the bedside, and inferences are made about volume and flow. Measurement of ventricular volumes and pressures usually requires diagnostic procedures such as echocardiography or cardiac catheterization; however, a pulmonary artery catheter capable of measuring right ventricular volumes at the bedside is available (Headley & Diethorn, 1993). A clear understanding of the cardiac cycle is essential for clinical assessment of normal and abnormal heart sounds and interpretation of other clinical findings.

The cardiac cycle is divided into two major phases, ventricular systole and ventricular diastole. Atrial systole occurs during late ventricular diastole. Electrical events precede mechanical events because of the time required for the biochemical processes previously described. Mechanical contraction begins in the middle of the QRS complex, and electrical repolarization, the T wave on the ECG, occurs during ventricular ejection. The same events occur on the right side of the heart but at lower pressures owing to the lower resistance of the pulmonary circuit.

VENTRICULAR SYSTOLE. After excitation, the muscle begins to contract. When the ventricular pressure exceeds the pressure in the atria, which occurs almost immediately, the atrioventricular valves close, producing the first heart sound (S_1). At this time, the pressure in the ventricle is less than that in the aorta and the pulmonary artery, and the semilunar valves remain closed. Tension continues to increase in the muscle, increasing the intraventricular pressure. Because all the valves are closed, there is no change in volume, and this is called isovolumetric contraction. During this phase of systole, 90% of myocardial oxygen consumption occurs. The ventricle shortens from base to apex, becoming more spherical, the AV valves bulge into the atria, producing the c wave in the atrial and jugular venous waveforms, and the chordae tendineae tense to prevent eversion of the leaflets into the atria. Continuing increases in ventricular muscle tension pull down on the atrial floor, increasing atrial size and decreasing atrial pressure, as evidenced by the x descent in the atrial and jugular venous waveforms (Gardner, 1993).

When the ventricular pressure exceeds the diastolic pressure in the receiving vessels, the aorta, and the pulmonary artery, the semilunar valves open, and rapid ejection occurs. Peak ejection produces systolic pressure in the receiving vessel. During ejection, ventricular fibers shorten circumferentially as well as longitudinally, wall thickness increases, and chamber size decreases. The atria continue to fill during ventricular ejection, and the increase in pressure produces the v wave in the atrial and jugular venous waveforms (Gardner, 1993).

As the ventricle empties, the volume ejected decreases, and the pressure in the ventricle and the receiving vessels falls. At the end of ejection, reversal of

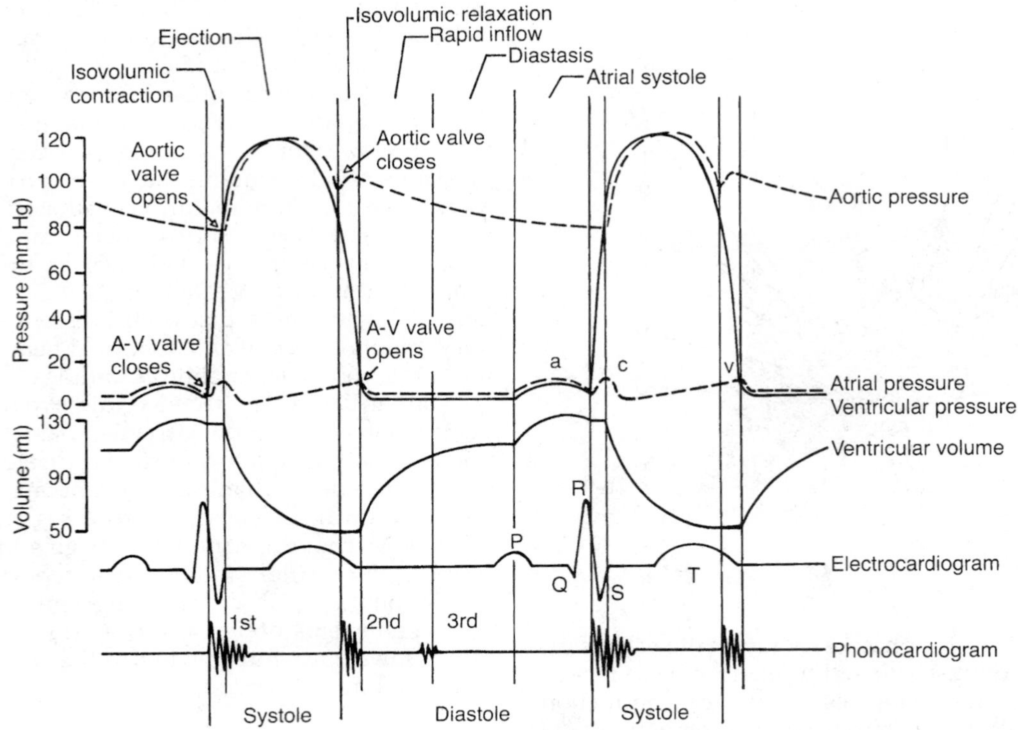

FIGURE 18–12. The events of the cardiac cycle, showing changes in the atrial pressure, left ventricular pressure, aortic pressure, ventricular volume, the electrocardiogram, and the phonocardiogram. (From Guyton, A. C., & Hall, J. E. [1996]. *Textbook of medical physiology* [9th ed., p. 111]. Philadelphia: W. B. Saunders.)

flow catches the cusps of the semilunar valves, closing them and producing the second heart sound (S_2) and the dicrotic notch in the arterial waveforms (Kern & Deligonul, 1993). Aortic pressure declines to the diastolic level as blood runs off into the periphery. Volume left in the ventricle at the end of systole is called the end-systolic volume (ESV) or residual volume and is increased in patients with heart failure. The ESV is a reserve volume that with increased vigor of contraction can be used to increase cardiac output in the healthy heart.

VENTRICULAR DIASTOLE. The ventricle continues to relax with all the valves closed, and there is no change in volume during isovolumetric relaxation. When the pressure in the ventricles falls below that in the atria, the AV valves open, and blood that returned to the atria during ventricular systole rushes into the ventricle during the phase of rapid ventricular filling. This is seen as the y descent in the atrial and jugular venous waveforms. Normally, the ventricle continues to relax during this period, and ventricular pressure continues to decline rapidly despite the inrush of blood. A third heart sound (S_3) may be produced at this time if the heart is already overfilled or poorly compliant. At the end of the rapid filling phase, the ventricle has completed relaxation, and the slow filling phase begins as the ventricle is distended by blood that continues to return to the heart. This is seen as an increase in pressure in the ventricular waveform.

At end-diastole, atrial depolarization (the P wave in the ECG) and subsequent contraction of the atria provide the final component of ventricular filling. This is seen as the a wave in the atrial, jugular venous, and ventricular pressure waveforms. In a healthy heart this atrial kick provides 10% to 15% of the ventricular end-diastolic volume (EDV). However, if ventricular compliance is decreased, as in patients with heart failure, or if the heart rate is rapid, limiting diastolic filling time, the atrial kick may provide 30% to 40% of the ventricular end-diastolic volume. The propulsion of blood into the ventricle by atrial contraction may produce a fourth heart sound (S_4) if the ventricle is poorly compliant.

The amount of blood ejected per beat is the stroke volume and is the EDV minus the ESV. The normal value at rest is about 75 mL. The stroke volume expressed as a percentage of EDV is called the ejection fraction and is a measure of global ventricular function, that is, the percentage of the EDV that is ejected per beat. A normal ejection fraction is between 50% and 70%. Ejection fractions below 40% are considered to represent a clinically significant reduction in myocardial function (Hixon, 1994).

Another way of depicting the changes in pressure and volume that occur during the cardiac cycle is the pressure–volume loop (Fig. 18–13). Ventricular systole begins at the lower right corner, with mitral valve closure producing S_1, followed by isovolumetric contraction. When the pressure in the ventricle exceeds that in the aorta, the aortic valve opens, and the stroke volume is ejected. At end-ejection, the aortic valve closes, producing S_2, and isovolumetric relaxation begins. When the pressure in the relaxing ventricle becomes lower than that in the atria, the mitral valve opens, and rapid filling ensues. Slow filling continues with a gradual rise in ventricular pressure until atrial contraction produces the final EDV, and the cycle starts over. The area enclosed in the diagram in Figure 18–13 is representative of cardiac work during that heartbeat (Yang et al., 1988).

The end-diastolic and end-systolic pressure–volume relationships reflect the interactions between the heart and the circulation. The end-diastolic pressure–volume point is determined by the compliance of the ventricle and the amount of venous return. The end-systolic point is determined by the resistance in the vascular system and the contractile state of the myocardium.

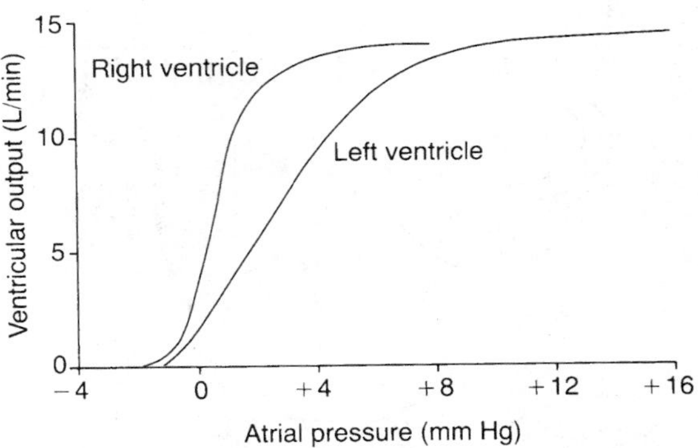

FIGURE 18–14. Approximate normal right and left ventricular output curves for the human heart as extrapolated from data obtained in dogs. (From Guyton, A. C., & Hall, J. E. [1996]. *Textbook of medical physiology* [9th ed.]. Philadelphia: W. B. Saunders.)

Cardiac Output

Cardiac output (CO) is the product of heart rate (HR) and stroke volume (SV) or the amount ejected per beat (CO = HR × SV). The determinants of stroke volume are the end-diastolic fiber tension (preload), the tension developed in the myocardium during ejection (afterload), and the contractile state of the myocardium exclusive of preload (contractility). The ability to contract is a property of muscle and is independent of loading conditions. However, changes in loading conditions or inotropic state will alter the rate and force of contraction.

PRELOAD, THE LENGTH–TENSION RELATIONSHIP. In isolated muscle strips, the force and rate of fiber shortening depend on the resting length of the fiber. The greater the length, within physiologic limits, the more forceful the contraction. Fiber length cannot be directly determined in the intact heart. Starling demonstrated, however, that the same relationship exists between ventricular end-diastolic volume and fiber length. An increase in volume or preload intrinsically increases the force of contraction and the stroke volume, and hence cardiac output, if all other parameters are held constant (Fig. 18–14). Conversely, a decrease in preload decreases the force of contraction and the stroke volume. The major factors that influence preload include venous tone, the pumping action of skeletal muscle, atrial contraction, total blood volume, body position, and intrathoracic and intrapericardial pressure. The preload reserve is the increase in volume that will increase stroke volume and provide a higher cardiac output to meet increases in tissue demand. This mechanism allows the heart to adapt to changes in venous return and maintain equality between the outputs of the right and left sides of the heart. At low and excessively high volumes (short and very long fiber lengths) cross-bridging of myosin and actin filaments is impaired. When the collagen that normally maintains myocardial fiber alignment is disrupted, remodeling occurs. Remodeling is any alteration in the physical structure or biochemical composition of any of the compartments of the heart that are muscular, vascular, or interstitial (McElroy et al., 1989; Weber & Janicki, 1989). Figure 18–15 depicts concentric and eccentric hypertrophy.

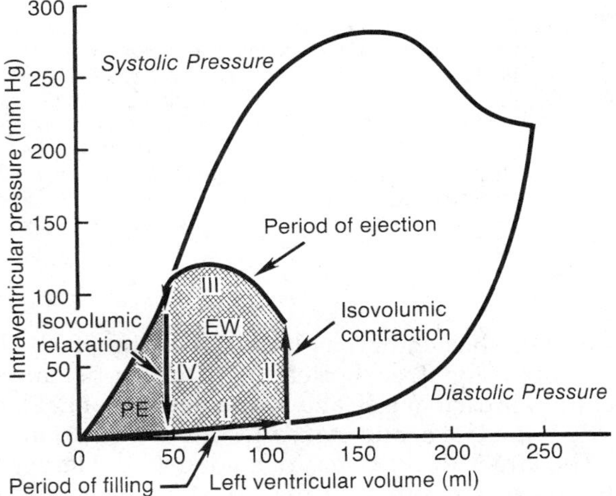

FIGURE 18–13. Relationship between left ventricular volume and intraventricular pressure during diastole and during systole. Also shown by the heavy lines is the "volume–pressure diagram" that illustrates the changes in intraventricular volume and pressure during the cardiac cycle. (From Guyton, A. C., & Hall, J. E. [1996]. *Textbook of medical physiology* [9th ed., p. 114]. Philadelphia: W. B. Saunders.)

At the bedside, pressures are measured rather than volumes. Because the AV valves are open during diastole, the atrial pressures are representative of ventricular diastolic pressures. Thus, the clinical measure of right ventricular preload is the right atrial pressure or central venous pressure, and the measure of left ventricular preload is the left atrial pressure, or pulmonary capillary wedge pressure. In a normal ventricle, a change in pressure reflects a change in volume. However, if ventricular compliance is altered, changes in pressure reflect changes in ventricular volume less

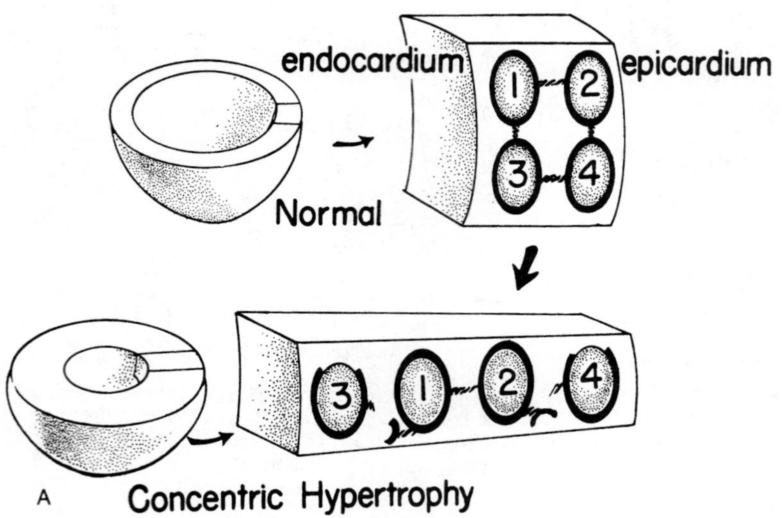

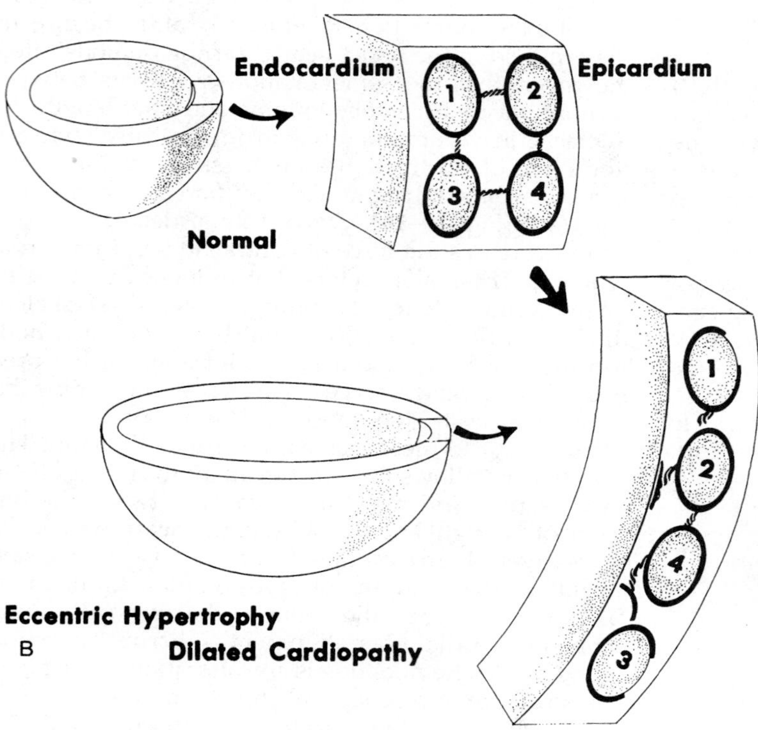

FIGURE 18–15. A slippage of muscle occurs with the concentric or the eccentric remodeling of the hypertrophied myocardium. The anatomic basis that permits this slippage to occur is the disruption of collagen tethers that normally maintain fiber alignment. A slippage of muscle toward or away from the central axis of the chamber is considered a positive (*top*) and negative (*bottom*) slippage, respectively. (From Weber, K., & Janicki, S. [1989]. Pathogenesis of heart failure. *Cardiology Clinics, 7*[1], 15.)

accurately (Fig. 18–16). For example, ischemia or hypertrophy decreases ventricular compliance, and a relatively small change in ventricular volume may produce a large change in pressure.

AFTERLOAD, THE FORCE–VELOCITY RELATIONSHIP. In isolated muscle strips at a fixed length, the force generated by the muscle and the rate of fiber shortening are determined by the load on the muscle. If the load is very heavy, exceptional force is required for the fibers to shorten. If the load is light, less force is required to lift the weight. Afterload in the intact heart is the force per unit of cross-sectional area in the ventricular wall once fiber shortening has begun (Wright, 1990). The forces opposing fiber shortening in the ventricular wall include ventricular size and shape (the law of LaPlace), aortic impedance, and systemic vascular resistance.

The larger the end-diastolic volume, the larger the intraventricular pressure that must be overcome before fiber shortening can actually begin (and hence a longer isovolumetric contraction exists). The larger the radius of the ventricle in relation to wall thickness, the more oxygen is consumed. Thus, the level of preload contributes to the force of the afterload and to the level of myocardial oxygen consumption (Quaal, 1992).

Aortic impedance is the stiffness of the aortic wall

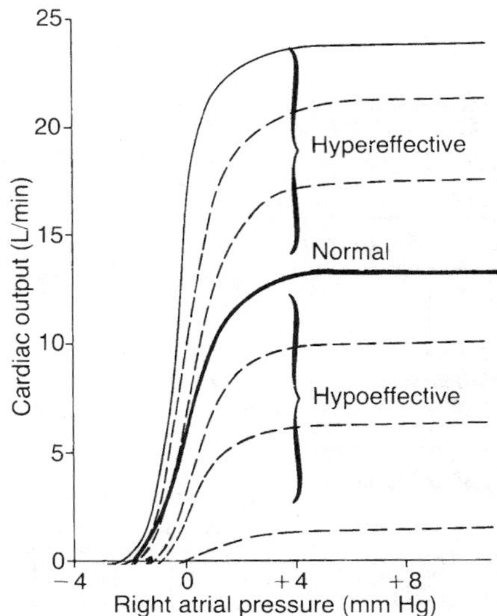

FIGURE 18–16. Cardiac output curves for various degrees of hypoeffective and hypereffective hearts. (From Guyton, A. C., & Hall, J. E. [1996]. *Textbook of medical physiology* [9th ed., p. 241]. Philadelphia: W. B. Saunders.)

and the inertia of the column of blood in the aorta that must be overcome before ejection can begin. The more compliant the aorta, the more easily it will stretch during ventricular ejection and the less force the ventricle must generate.

Systemic vascular resistance (SVR), the degree of constriction (radius) of the arterioles, is the major variable determining afterload and is a function of local tissue demands, the level of autonomic stimulation, and the level of circulating catecholamines. This factor can be calculated clinically if cardiac output, end-diastolic pressure or filling pressure, and output pressure are known (SVR = MAP − RAP/CO × 79.9).

When all other variables are held constant (EDV, contractility, and heart rate), an increase in afterload either increases cardiac work to maintain stroke volume or decreases stroke volume and thus cardiac output. In the healthy heart, a sudden increase in afterload decreases the stroke volume, which increases the end-systolic volume and thus the preload for the next beat. This increases the contractility of subsequent beats through the Starling mechanism and maintains cardiac output in the face of increased afterload, but does so at increased metabolic cost.

An increase in ventricular wall thickness occurs with aging, probably because of the increase in afterload resulting from the structural and functional changes in the aorta, which are discussed later. Capillary growth may not be adequate to supply the increase in muscle mass, and therefore the person may be at risk for ischemia even in the presence of normal coronary vessels.

CONTRACTILITY. Contractility is the effect of extrinsic influences on the rate and force of fiber shortening exclusive of fiber length. Norepinephrine and epinephrine increase the rate of calcium movement into the cytosol during excitation (through cyclic adenosine monophosphate) and back into the sarcoplasmic reticulum, and thus increase both the force and rate of contraction and relaxation. Metabolic imbalances, depressant drugs, and loss of myocardium impair the contractile function of the ventricle (Sitzer, 1991).

HEART RATE. An increase in the heart rate at the same stroke volume increases cardiac output within limits. At rates greater than 160 to 180 beats/minute, the diastolic filling time shortens, decreasing the end-diastolic volume, and this reserve mechanism begins to impair the effectiveness of the preload reserve mechanism. Increased heart rate is the primary mechanism in infants for increasing cardiac output, because the ventricle has more fibrous and fewer contractile elements than the adult heart; it is stiffer and less responsive to increasing preload. Thus, infants are said to be preload limited and heart rate dependent.

Maximum achievable heart rate decreases with age for any given level of exercise, possibly because of diminished adrenergic responsiveness. The balance between catecholamine effect, increased heart rate, and increased rate of contraction and relaxation (Ca^{2+} movement) may become competitive with rather than additive to the preload reserve mechanism (Woo et al., 1994).

Control of the Coronary Circulation

At rest the myocardium extracts most of the available oxygen, so that an increase in oxygen demand can be met only by an increase in coronary flow. The coronary system is autoregulatory between perfusion pressures of approximately 50 and 160 mm Hg. That is, local factors regulating resistance also regulate flow. Below a perfusion pressure of 50 mm Hg, the vessels become maximally dilated, and flow becomes totally pressure dependent. The anatomic relationship of the epicardial, intramuscular, and subendocardial coronary arteries is demonstrated in Figure 18–17.

A variety of factors influence coronary vascular resistance (Fig. 18–18), the most important being local metabolic conditions. A decrease in oxygen delivery such as systemic hypoxia or obstruction of the large epicardial vessels, or an increase in tissue oxygen demand, produces vasodilation either globally or locally. The mechanism for this vasodilation is unclear but is

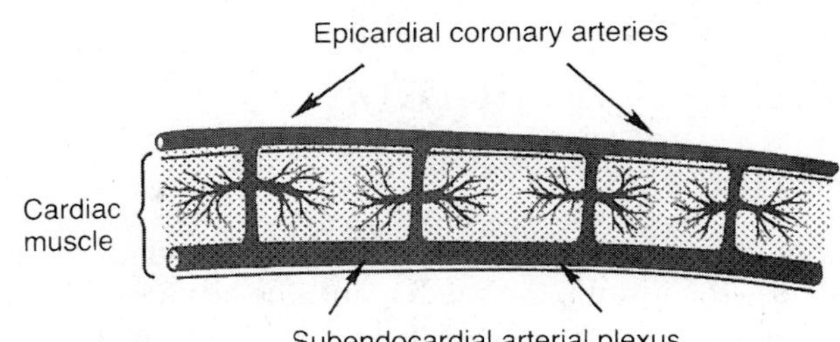

FIGURE 18–17. Diagram of the epicardial, intramuscular, and subendocardial coronary vasculature. (From Guyton, A. C., & Hall, J. E. [1996]. *Textbook of medical physiology* [9th ed., p. 257]. Philadelphia: W. B. Saunders.)

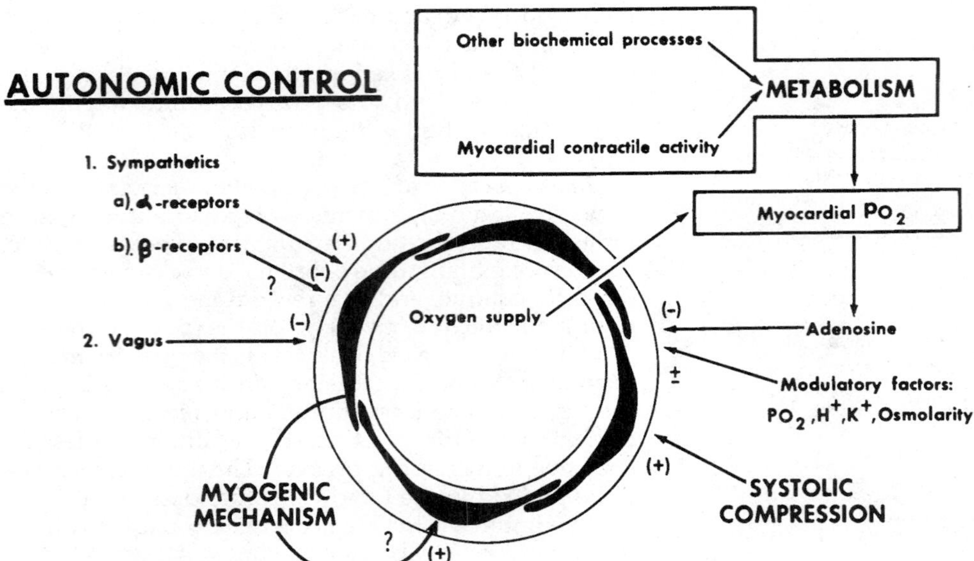

FIGURE 18–18. Factors increasing (+) or decreasing (−) coronary vascular resistance. (From Rubio, R., & Berne, F. M. [1975]. Regulation of coronary blood flow. *Progress in Cardiovascular Diseases, 18,* 120.)

thought to be related to the release of adenosine from the myocardial cells (Milnor, 1990). In addition, parasympathetic stimulation and beta-receptor stimulation may dilate the large epicardial vessels and some of the major branches. It is controversial whether these stimuli have a significant effect on the intramyocardial vessels. Increased resistance occurs primarily from systolic compression and alpha-adrenergic stimulation. It has been demonstrated in the cardiac catheterization laboratory that anger, which increases circulating catecholamine levels, produces vasoconstriction in previously narrowed coronary arteries (Boltwood et al., 1993). The effect of myogenic response and vascular constriction secondary to a large distending pressure remains controversial in the coronary circulation.

DETERMINANTS OF MYOCARDIAL OXYGEN CONSUMPTION. The primary determinants of myocardial oxygen demand are the intramyocardial wall tension, which is related to pressure, volume, and wall thickness (law of LaPlace); the state of myocardial contractility, which is related to adrenergic and cholinergic stimulation; and the heart rate. Minor determinants of oxygen consumption are the resting metabolic rate, myocardial fiber shortening (ejection), and energy available for the activation of contraction (Guyton, 1991).

SYSTEMIC CIRCULATION

Structure

HISTOLOGY. Blood vessels are composed of three layers—the intima, the media, and the adventitia. The intima is composed of a single layer of endothelial cells lining the lumen of the vessels, and a basement membrane. The media is composed of collagen, elastin, and smooth muscle cells. The relative quantities and arrangement of these components influence the compliance, elastic recoil, and resistance of the vessel. The adventitia is the outermost layer of loosely meshed connective tissue. Blood supply to the outer two-thirds of the vessel wall comes from a special network of vessels, the vasa vasorum. The inner third of the vessel wall receives oxygen from diffusion of the blood in the vessels. At the place where these two oxygen supplies meet, the vessel wall is at the greatest risk of ischemia.

THE ARTERIAL SYSTEM. The aorta and major arteries are conduits and pressure reservoirs (Fig. 18–19). No nutrient exchange with tissues occurs in these vessels, which distribute blood throughout the system. The media of the intrathoracic arteries contains more elastin and fewer smooth muscle cells than the media of the more peripheral arteries and the arterioles. Laboratory research has demonstrated that the proliferation and extracellular matrix synthesis of vascular smooth muscle cells are important in atherogenesis, and highly important in the development of restenosis of angioplasted arteries (Lefer, 1993; MacLeod et al., 1994). Volume ejected into the aorta during ventricular systole distends the wall. Elastic recoil of the aorta during ventricular diastole continues to propel blood through the system and maintains diastolic pressure in the system (Windkessel effect) (Fig. 18–20).

Arterial pressures measured clinically reflect two components, aortic compliance and cardiac function. Aortic compliance decreases with age owing to thickening of the intima and media resulting from increasing collagen and smooth muscle cell proliferation. Thus, for any given stroke volume the peak aortic pressure will be higher in the elderly than in the middle-aged adult. Clinically, this result is seen as isolated systolic hypertension in the elderly. Although this is considered part of normal aging, it also increases the risk of cerebral vascular accident. By age 85 years, the

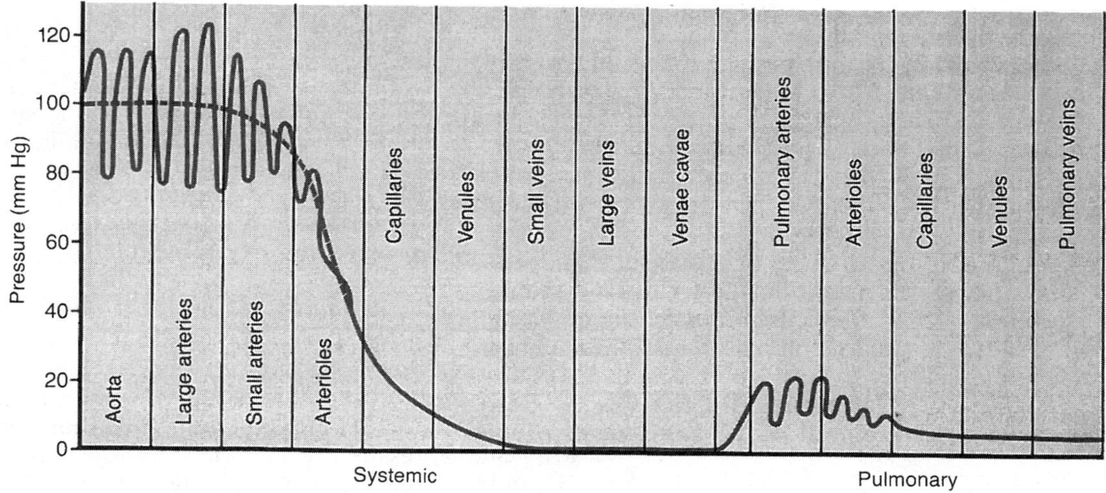

FIGURE 18–19. Blood pressures in the different portions of the circulatory system. (From Guyton, A. C., & Hall, J. E. [1996]. *Textbook of medical physiology* [9th ed.]. Philadelphia: W. B. Saunders.)

occurs as a compensatory response to accommodate the same stroke volume in a more rigid space. Decreased recoil reduces the contribution to forward flow, and the amount of blood in the aorta at end-diastole increases the impedance or afterload to the left ventricle. Similarly, vascular injury imposed by interventional balloon techniques produces an enhanced adrenergic neurotransmission that causes a desensitization to exogenous norepinephrine, with a consequent lack of vasoconstrictor response (Candipan et al., 1994).

THE MICROCIRCULATION. The microcirculation is composed of arterioles, metarterioles, capillaries, and venules. This is the functional unit of the circulation where nutrients are delivered to the tissues and waste products are removed.

Arterioles are resistance vessels. The media contains less collagen and elastin and more smooth muscle cells than does the media of the aorta. Many arterioles branch from each artery and have a smaller radius and a higher resistance. Significant change in the radius of the arteriole is produced by constriction or relaxation of the vascular smooth muscle in response to various stimuli (Fig. 18–21), and thus the arterioles are the primary regulators of changes in resistance. In addition, the increase in total cross-sectional area as a result of branching results in a reduced rate of flow.

Capillaries are the nutrient vessels. Many capillaries branch from each arteriole, and the total cross-sectional area again increases, thus decreasing further the rate of flow (Fig. 18–22). This slow flow rate allows time for exchange of nutrients to occur within the tissues. Capillary walls are one cell thick and contain no smooth muscle cells. Nutrients diffuse through gap junctions or are actively transported to the interstitial fluid and then to the cells from the arterial end of the capillary. Interstitial fluid and waste products reenter the capillary at the venous end or are removed by the lymphatics. Precapillary sphincters control flow through individual capillary beds, depending on tissue demand. During times of low demand, some blood bypasses the true capillaries through the metarterioles and enters the venules directly. Venules contain a small amount of smooth muscle but less than that in the arterioles. As venules coalesce, the cross-sectional area decreases, and the rate of flow begins to increase.

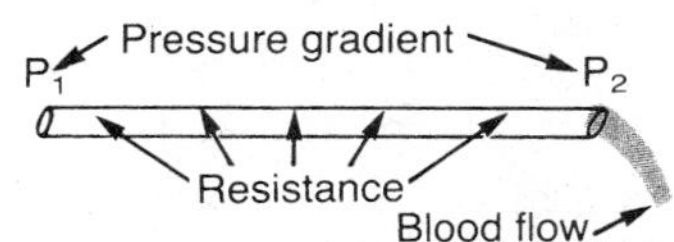

FIGURE 18–20. Relationships among pressure, resistance, and blood flow. (From Guyton, A. C., & Hall, J. E. [1996]. *Textbook of medical physiology* [9th ed.]. Philadelphia: W. B. Saunders.)

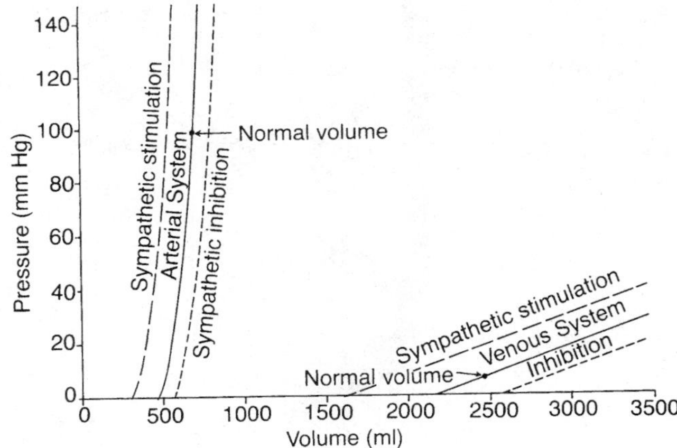

FIGURE 18–21. Volume–pressure curves of the systemic arterial and venous systems, showing also the effects of sympathetic stimulation and sympathetic inhibition. (From Guyton, A. C., & Hall, J. E. [1996]. *Textbook of medical physiology* [9th ed., p. 172]. Philadelphia: W. B. Saunders.)

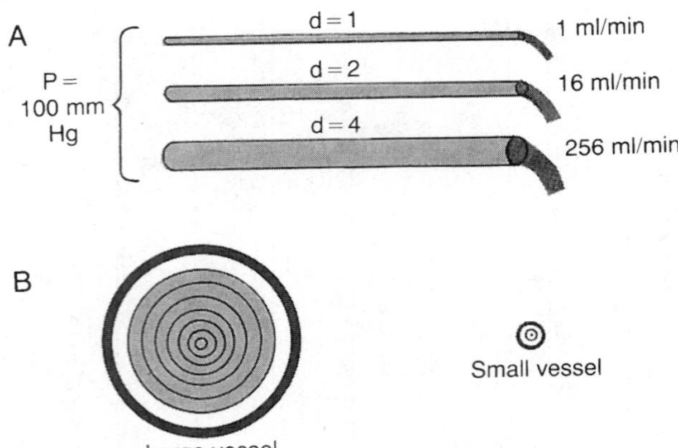

FIGURE 18–22. *A,* Demonstration of the effect of vessel diameter on blood flow. *B,* Concentric rings of blood flowing at different velocities: the farther away from the vessel wall, the faster the flow. (From Guyton, A. C., & Hall, J. E. [1996]. *Textbook of medical physiology* [9th ed., p. 167]. Philadelphia: W. B. Saunders.)

Veins are capacitance vessels. Vein walls have some smooth muscle, but less than that in arteries. They are larger in diameter and therefore have a larger total cross-sectional area. The rate of flow is slower and the pressure is lower because the walls are more compliant. Approximately 64% of the total blood volume is found in the venous circuit at rest (Fig. 18–23). As the veins coalesce at the inferior and superior vena cavae, the rates of flow and pressure increase but remain below aortic rates.

The pulmonary circulation also branches into arteries, arterioles, capillaries, venules, and veins. However, the vessels are shorter and have a larger radius, a relatively high elastin content, a more fragmented arrangement, and fewer smooth muscle cells. The pulmonary artery carries deoxygenated blood, and the pulmonary veins carry oxygenated blood.

Arterial Pressure

SYSTOLIC AND DIASTOLIC BLOOD PRESSURE. The maximum blood pressure at peak ejection is called the systolic pressure. It is a function of the volume ejected and the compliance of the aorta (Fig. 18–24). Only one-third of the stroke volume leaves the arteries during systole, and the rest of the stroke volume must be accommodated by stretching of the aorta and the major arteries.

Diastolic pressure is the minimum pressure just before ejection begins. It is primarily a function of the systemic vascular resistance and elastic recoil. High systolic blood pressure damages endothelial cells in the arteries and now is considered as important as dia-

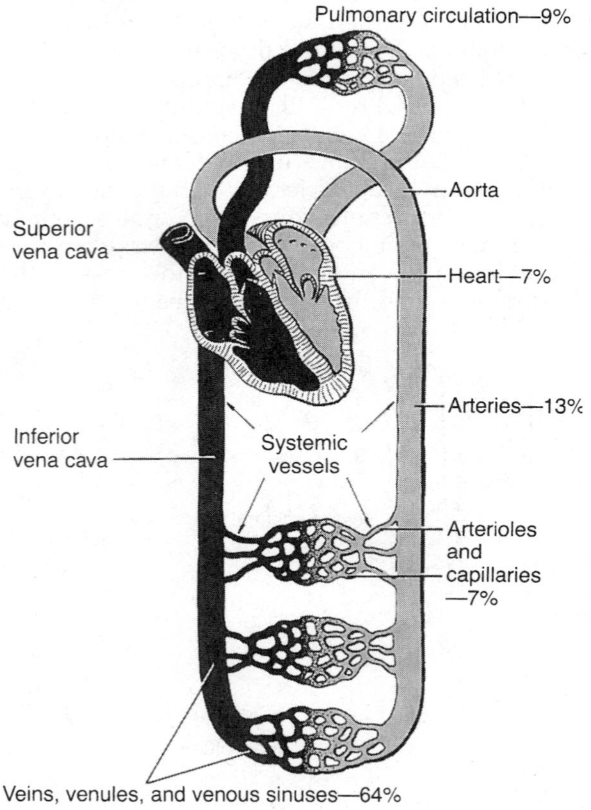

FIGURE 18–23. Distribution of blood volume in the different portions of the circulatory system. (From Guyton, A. C., & Hall. J. E. [1996]. *Textbook of medical physiology* [9th ed.]. Philadelphia: W. B. Saunders.)

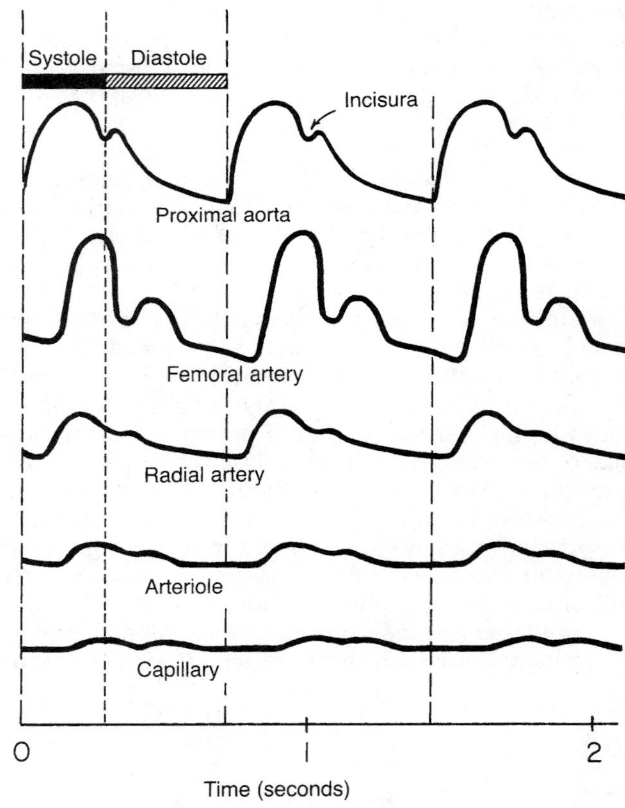

FIGURE 18–24. Changes in the pulse pressure contour as the pulse wave travels toward the smaller vessels. (From Guyton, A. C., & Hall. J. E. [1996]. *Textbook of medical physiology* [9th ed., p. 175]. Philadelphia: W. B. Saunders.)

stolic blood pressure in hypertension control (Felknor, 1994).

MEAN ARTERIAL PRESSURE. The mean perfusion pressure for the tissues is called the MAP. It is a result of the systolic and diastolic blood pressures in the aorta and major arteries during any given cardiac cycle (see Table 18–2). The MAP depends only on the elastic properties of the arterial walls and the mean blood volume in the arterial tree. The arterial volume is contingent on the rate of inflow from the heart into the arteries (cardiac output) and the rate of outflow from the arteries through the capillaries (peripheral runoff). When the rate of inflow exceeds the rate of outflow, the MAP increases as a result of stretch of the arterial walls. When peripheral runoff exceeds cardiac output, the MAP decreases. The MAP remains constant when the rate of arterial inflow equals arterial outflow (cardiac output equals peripheral runoff). Clearly, if the arteries are poorly distensible and cannot accommodate an increased inflow or decreased outflow by stretching, the MAP will rise even further. Therefore, the only factors that determine MAP are cardiac output and peripheral resistance (Hurst et al., 1990).

PULSE PRESSURE. Pulse pressure is the difference between the systolic and diastolic pressures and is a function of stroke volume and the distensibility of the aorta. The speed of systolic ejection also determines the pulse pressure, but is less important than the ratio of stroke volume to aortic compliance (Guyton, 1991).

During systole, a large volume of blood is ejected into the aorta. This volume generally exceeds the peripheral runoff and is called the stroke volume. By introducing the maximum volume into the aorta, a peak pressure is obtained. This is the systolic pressure. As stated earlier, the diastolic pressure depends on the SVR, which is a measure of aortic compliance. Because the pulse pressure is the difference between the systolic and diastolic pressures, it is easy to see why it depends on the stroke volume and aortic compliance.

ARTERIAL PRESSURE CURVES. The transmission of pressure as it is propagated from the aorta to the peripheral arteries produces a characteristic waveform (Fig. 18–24). The stretch of the aorta and its branches is substantially faster than the actual forward movement of blood, and is responsible for the peripheral pulse (Guyton, 1991).

The initial sharp upstroke of the arterial waveform is caused by the rapid ejection period of the heart. It is followed by a slower rise to the peak of the curve, the apex of which is the systolic pressure. The waveform then acutely declines, but the descent is briskly interrupted by a sharp notch, called the incisura in an aortic waveform and the dicrotic notch in a peripheral waveform. The incisura results from the abrupt closure of the aortic valve at the onset of diastole, which causes a temporary rebound of blood into the aorta. After the dicrotic notch, there is an exponential diastolic decline in the waveform that culminates in the diastolic pressure.

The arterial waveform subtly changes as it is propagated from the aortic arch to the distal peripheral arteries (Fig. 18–24). The vascular distensibility varies inversely with the velocity of transmission of the pressure wave. Because vascular capacitance decreases in the distal periphery, the velocity of transmission increases incrementally along the path. There are four changes in the configuration of the arterial waveform associated with distal measurements in the arterial tree: (1) there is a delay in the rapid upslope portion of the waveform; (2) the incisura and other high-frequency portions of the waveform dampen; (3) the peak systolic pressure narrows and culminates at a higher level (systolic pressures can be 25 to 40 mm Hg higher at the dorsalis pedal artery than in the aorta); and (4) a hump may develop at the diastolic portion of the waveform (Gorny, 1993; Guyton, 1991). The magnitude of the changes in waveform from the aorta to the distal periphery is less pronounced in elderly patients, particularly those with atherosclerosis (Kern & Deligonul, 1993). This difference results from (1) backward reflection of the pressure wave; (2) tapering due to progression of the wave from larger to smaller arteries; (3) resonance of the sine waves that compose the waveform; and (4) changes in transmission velocity due to decreased capacitance (Kern & Deligonul, 1993).

Acute Local Control of Blood Pressure

Because there is a finite amount of blood in the body, it is impossible for equal amounts of blood to be circulated to every tissue in the body and still meet the metabolic needs of each tissue. Different tissues have different needs at any given time, and the body is able to deliver increased amounts of nutrients to those tissues based on local needs—hence the concept of autoregulation. Acute local control of the circulation occurs within seconds to minutes and has a limited duration of action.

THE METABOLIC THEORY OF AUTOREGULATION. The metabolic theory of autoregulation simply states that blood flow is controlled by local metabolic needs. When the tissues have increased metabolic needs, vasodilation occurs. Conversely, when metabolic requirements are low, vasoconstriction occurs, thus allowing adequate distribution of the blood volume.

THE VASODILATOR THEORY. The vasodilator theory states that increased metabolic activity causes local formation of vasodilator substances such as adenosine, carbon dioxide, lactic acid, hydrogen ions, and bradykinin (Angelos et al., 1992; Benjamin, 1994). These substances have a direct dilatory effect on the precapillary sphincters, metarterioles, and arterioles. Research suggests that tissue hypoxia is directly responsible for the release of these vasodilating substances (Guyton,

1991). The problem with this theory is that even excessive amounts of any one of these substances do not elicit profound vasodilation in the laboratory (Berne & Levy, 1986).

THE OXYGEN DEMAND THEORY. The oxygen demand theory states that oxygen deficiency in tissues causes vasodilation. This theory is based on the knowledge that oxygen is required to maintain vascular tone (smooth muscle contraction) and that a lack of it, caused by increased metabolic activity, allows the vascular smooth muscle to dilate (Grum, 1993; Guyton, 1991). Contrary to this premise is the result of human research done by Remme and coworkers (1994). They induced myocardial ischemia and discovered that systemic catecholamines and the renin–angiotension system are stimulated by short periods of stress-induced ischemia. The physiologic consequences include increased systemic resistance due to vasoconstriction, increased myocardial oxygen consumption, and decreased myocardial oxygen delivery.

When blood flow to a vascular bed is abruptly obstructed, release of the obstruction causes a surplus blood flow that continues for minutes to hours. This surplus blood flow, called reactive hyperemia, declines to the preocclusion level gradually (Berne & Levy, 1986; Nichols & O'Rourke, 1990). Active hyperemia is the term given to excess blood flow to tissues at the period of increased demand. These phenomena stress the relationship between metabolic requirements and nutrient delivery.

THE MYOGENIC THEORY. The myogenic theory states that vascular smooth muscle contracts and dilates in response to changes in tension. According to this theory, a decrease in MAP reduces arteriolar tone, thus allowing increased flow to the area (Garfein, 1990). Below a MAP of 50 mm Hg, arterioles are maximally dilated and flow is totally pressure dependent. This fact is important in both the coronary and peripheral circulations when obstruction from atherosclerosis or thrombus exists. Conversely, an increase in MAP increases arteriolar tone, decreases radius, and increases resistance. Arterial hypertension is thus minimally transmitted to capillary beds (Nichols & O'Rourke, 1990).

Humoral Regulation of Blood Flow

Humoral factors that affect blood flow include the local substances discussed earlier as well as hormones and other products that are manufactured by the body or absorbed by it. The discussion of humoral factors is based on their effect on the vascular smooth muscle, and is summarized in Figure 18–25.

VASOCONSTRICTORS. Sympathetic stimulation causes direct release of norepinephrine from the nerve fibers. The adrenal medulla secretes epinephrine and norepinephrine, which circulate and cause profound vasoconstriction. Angiotensin II is one of the most powerful vasoconstricting substances known, and causes

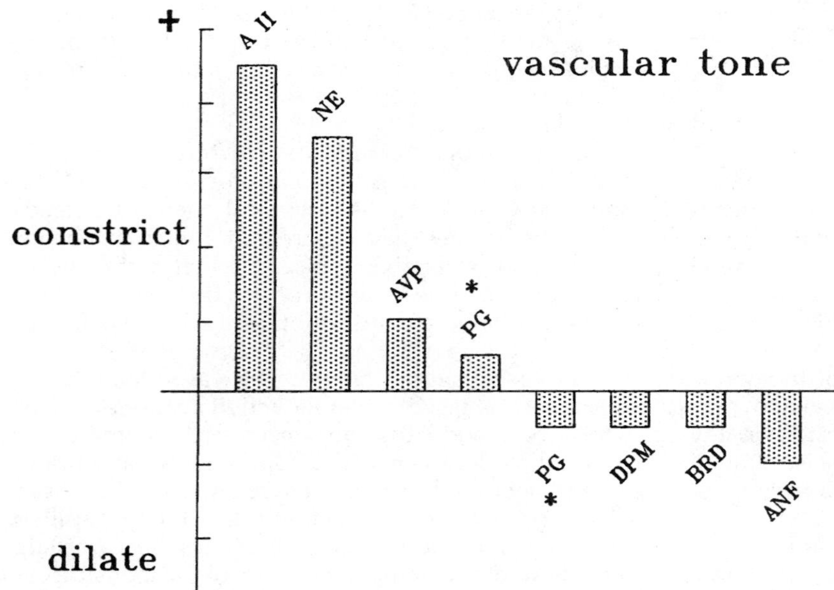

FIGURE 18–25. Relative contributions of neurohormonal systems to the balance of vascular tone. A II, angiotensin II; NE, norepinephrine; AVP, arginine vasopressin; PG, prostaglandin; DPM, dopamine; BRD, bradykinin; ANF, atrial natriuretic factor. Asterisks indicate a different effect for the prostaglandin subgroups. (From Cody, R. [1989]. Neurohormonal influences in the pathogenesis of congestive heart failure. *Cardiology Clinics, 7,* 74.)

a profound increase in the SVR, thus increasing the arterial blood pressure. The role of angiotensin in blood pressure control is discussed in more detail later. Vasopressin, or antidiuretic hormone, is an even more powerful vasoconstrictor than angiotensin. Its release from the posterior pituitary gland, however, occurs in such minute amounts that it has relatively insignificant effects on blood pressure control (Cody, 1989).

VASODILATORS. Bradykinin, a byproduct of kallikrein, produces intense vasodilation and increased capillary permeability. The role of bradykinin is important primarily in the regulation of blood flow to inflamed tissues. Serotonin, which is present in the intestinal tissues and platelets, has both vasodilating and vasoconstricting properties. It has minimal effect on the systemic regulation of blood flow. Histamine, derived from mast cells and released in response to allergy or inflammation, is a powerful vasodilator and also causes capillary leakage. Unlike bradykinin, histamine can produce severe hypotension, such as that resulting from an anaphylactic reaction. Prostaglandins present exciting possibilities for therapeutics because of their potent vasodilatory effects. Prostaglandin E infusions are currently being used to treat refractory pulmonary hypertension (Cody, 1989).

Nervous System Regulation of Blood Pressure

Nervous input to blood pressure regulation operates globally rather than locally. It can redistribute blood flow within the body and affects inotropy and chronotropy of the heart itself. The nervous system exerts extremely rapid control of blood pressure.

AUTONOMIC NERVOUS SYSTEM. The autonomic nervous system (AN) regulates both sympathetic and parasympathetic functions. Parasympathetic stimulation occurs primarily through the vagus nerve and inhibits heart rate and contractility. Its effects on peripheral blood pressure control are negligible.

The sympathetic nervous system (SNS) affects both the heart and the vascular smooth muscle. Cardiac inotropy and chronotropy are increased by SNS stimulation. A myriad of vasoconstrictor fibers and a minimal number of vasodilatory fibers are inherent in the nerves of the SNS (Fig. 18–26). It is through the wide distribution of the vasoconstrictor fibers that the SNS exerts its powerful effects on the systemic blood pressure.

The vasomotor center of the medulla is composed of three major areas (Fig. 18–27). The vasoconstrictor area secretes norepinephrine, which stimulates the vasoconstrictor fibers of the SNS. The vasodilator area of the vasomotor center works by inhibiting vasoconstriction. Sympathetic vasoconstrictor tone is maintained under normal conditions by continuous slow

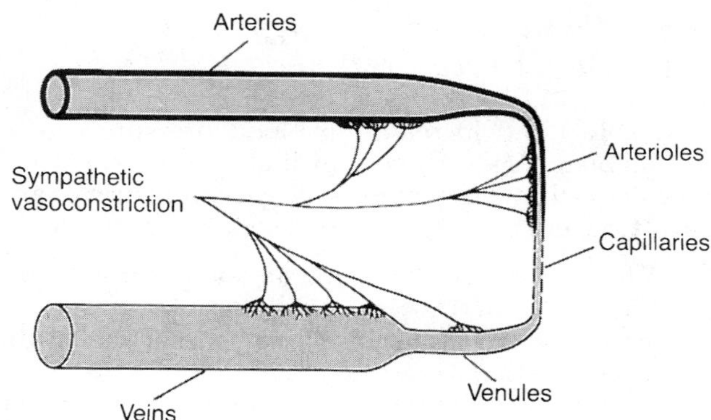

FIGURE 18–26. Sympathetic innervation of the systemic circulation. (From Guyton, A. C., & Hall. J. E. [1996]. *Textbook of medical physiology* [9th ed., p. 210]. Philadelphia: W. B. Saunders.)

firing of the vasoconstrictor area. The sensory area of the vasomotor center is predominantly a reflex center. It receives impulses from the vagus and glossopharyngeal nerves and responds by stimulating the vasoconstrictor or vasodilatory fibers of the SNS according to need (Guyton, 1991; Vander et al., 1990).

The higher centers of the brain also affect vasomotor control (see Fig. 18–27). The pons, mesencephalon, diencephalon, hypothalamus, and regions of the cerebral cortex can stimulate or depress activity of the vasomotor center of the medulla (Guyton, 1991). A vasovagal response that causes hypotension, bradycardia, and fainting can be elicited by emotional upset, thus demonstrating higher nervous controls on the systemic blood flow (Boltwood et al., 1993).

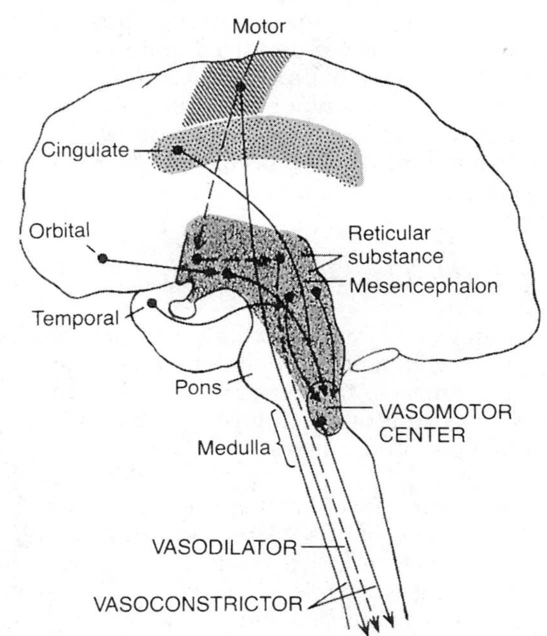

FIGURE 18–27. Areas of the brain that play important roles in the nervous regulation of the circulation. The dashed lines represent inhibitory pathways. (From Guyton, A. C., & Hall. J. E. [1996]. *Textbook of medical physiology* [9th ed., p. 211]. Philadelphia: W. B. Saunders.)

Sympathetic Nervous System Control of the Blood Pressure

Extremely rapid increases in blood pressure can be elicited by the SNS. Three principal responses occur as a result of stimulation of the entire vasoconstrictor and cardioaccelerator areas of the vasomotor centers:

1. SVR is increased by generalized arteriolar constriction.
2. Venous return is increased by constriction of the venous system.
3. Heart rate and strength of contractions are increased (Busch et al., 1992; Guyton, 1991).

BARORECEPTOR CONTROL MECHANISM. Baroreceptors in the aortic arch, atria, large arteries, and veins respond to a decrease in stretch, mean pressure, or pulse pressure by decreasing their rate of firing. The sensory area of the vasomotor center responds by increasing SNS output and decreasing parasympathetic nervous system (PNS) output through the efferent neurons. The immediate response is an increase in venous tone, which increases return to the heart and also increases end-diastolic volume and cardiac output through the Starling mechanism. Increased arteriolar tone maintains central pressure and redistributes blood flow to the most vital organs. Increased heart rate and contractility maintain cardiac output despite increases in resistance (Berne & Levy, 1986).

CENTRAL NERVOUS SYSTEM ISCHEMIC RESPONSE. When ischemia occurs in the vasomotor center, neurons in the medulla itself are stimulated and elicit a powerful vasoconstrictor response. Systemic blood pressure peaks. It is hypothesized that carbon dioxide and other metabolic byproducts accumulate in the local tissues of the vasomotor center and are responsible for the profound excitatory response of the center, much like a local control mechanism that has significant systemic effects (Guyton, 1991).

Long-Term Regulation of Blood Flow

Long-term control of blood flow occurs primarily through activation of the renin–angiotensin system or through changes in tissue vascularity. Pressure diuresis and natriuresis by the kidneys also aid in long-term regulation of blood pressure.

RENIN–ANGIOTENSIN SYSTEM (FIG. 18–28). The juxtaglomerular cells of the kidney produce, store, and secrete a substance called renin. A decrease in renal blood flow causes the release of renin, which enzymatically acts on angiotensinogen to release angiotensin I. The cleft of two amino acids from angiotensin I results in the formation of angiotensin II, the potent vasoconstrictor substance referred to earlier. Angiotensin II has two major effects that cause the arterial pressure to increase. The first and most rapid effect is generalized

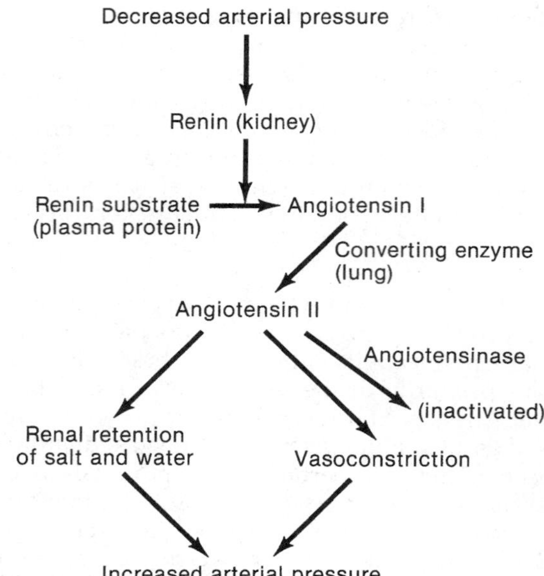

FIGURE 18–28. The renin–angiotensin constrictor mechanisms for arterial pressure control. (From Guyton, A. C., & Hall, J. E. [1996]. *Textbook of medical physiology* [9th ed., p. 228]. Philadelphia: W. B. Saunders.)

vasoconstriction. The second effect is a decrease in sodium and water excretion from the kidneys. Salt and water retention increase the blood volume, thus increasing the blood pressure (Lutterutti et al., 1994). Although the renal action of angiotensin II takes longer to increase the arteriolar pressure, it has longer-term effects than the vasoconstrictor action. Furthermore, animal research has demonstrated that there is an exaggerated norepinephrine-induced vasoconstriction that occurs secondary to endothelial dysfunction, and that the endothelial function can be restored by inhibition of the renin–angiotensin system (Hoshino et al., 1994). This may have major implications in the early treatment of hypertension.

CHANGES IN TISSUE VASCULARITY. Prolonged hypotension (<60 mm Hg) can cause reconstruction of the vasculature in the affected tissues. Reconstruction can take the form of actual changes in the physical structure of the vessels or the development of new vessels (development of collateral circulation). Angiogenesis, the development of new blood vessels, occurs in response to stimulatory factors released from ischemic tissue, rapidly growing tissues, or tissues with an extremely high metabolic activity (Nichols & O'Rourke, 1990).

Specific substances responsible for initiating angiogenesis include endothelial cell growth factor, fibroblast growth factor, and angiogenin. These angiogenic factors cause new vessels to germinate from existing venules and capillaries. Dissolution of the basement membrane of the endothelial cells is followed by brisk multiplication of new endothelial cells that grow out of the originating vessel in cord-like fashion. The cords form a tube that attaches to a tube from another origi-

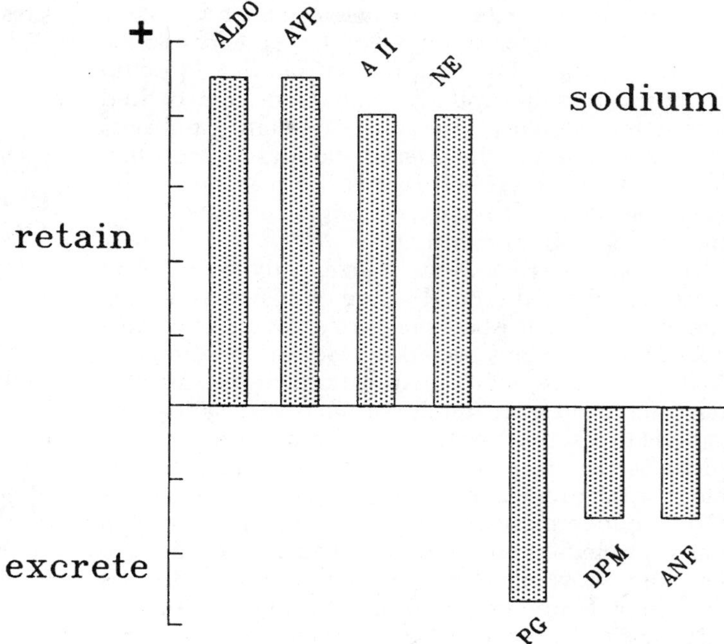

FIGURE 18–29. The relative contribution of neurohormonal systems to sodium homeostasis, as mediated by the kidney. A II, angiotensin II; NE, norepinephrine; AVP, arginine vasopressin; PG, prostaglandin; DPM, dopamine; BRD, bradykinin; ANF, atrial natriuretic factor. (From Cody, R. [1989]. Neurohormal influences in the pathogenesis of congestive heart failure. *Cardiology Clinics, 7,* 76.)

nating vessel, and a capillary loop develops that allows blood to flow through it. Continued blood flow stimulates smooth muscle proliferation inside the tube wall, creating a new arteriole (Guyton, 1991).

VOLUME RETENTION BY THE KIDNEY. Through SNS stimulation and aldosterone secretion from the adrenal medulla, and augmented by atrial receptors, the kidney retains sodium and therefore water (Fig. 18–29). Potassium is excreted. Atrial receptors stimulate antidiuretic hormone release, which results in water retention independently of sodium. This is an effective method of increasing blood volume and is beneficial in hemorrhage. However, if the low-flow state results from pump failure, this additional volume may be detrimental. If cardiac fibers are already stretched beyond their optimum length, additional preload further impairs their contractile function, and heart failure worsens. The normal reserve mechanism now contributes to the pathology.

Atrial stretch, which occurs in congestive heart failure, stimulates the release of atrial natriuretic factor (ANF). ANF stimulates sodium and water excretion and induces systemic vasodilatation (Benedict & Phil, 1994). ANF levels are elevated in chronic congestive heart failure and secondary to other factors that increase the intrathoracic pressure, such as positive end-expiratory pressure (Frass et al., 1993). These high ANF levels may blunt the vasoconstrictive activity of epinephrine (Paradis et al., 1994).

In addition, in cardiac failure there is a chronic elevation of serum catecholamines and ANF. Thus, a portion of the reserves is used to maintain the cardiac output at rest, resulting in less reserve available to increase cardiac output in the presence of increased metabolic requirements. Clinically, the decreased reserve is evidenced as decreased exercise tolerance and impaired functional ability.

Capillary Dynamics

SOLUTE DIFFUSION. Solutes move across the capillary wall down their concentration gradient. Lipid-soluble substances such as oxygen and carbon dioxide are transported through the cells. Other substances move through intercellular junctions, and some are transported through pinocytic vesicles and other passive transport mechanisms. The concentration gradient of the solutes is altered by the rate of blood flow. The faster the flow, the greater the solute washout and the lower the concentration. Large molecules such as proteins, primarily albumin, are too large to filter across the wall and must be actively transported.

FILTRATION OF FLUID. Because the capillary wall is freely permeable to water, the amount of fluid filtered across the wall depends on the balance between the pressure within the capillary and the pressure in the interstitium. The hydrostatic pressure within the capillary is the result of blood pressure at the capillary level, and is about 30 mm Hg. The tissue hydrostatic pressure is very low and in some tissues is negative. The oncotic pressure in the capillary is high and is mostly the result of intravascular albumin. The interstitial oncotic pressure is quite small. Thus, the primary balance is the difference between the hydrostatic pressure favoring filtration out of the capillary and the oncotic pressure favoring reabsorption. A drop in pressure across the capillary results from a loss of fluid within the capillary; therefore, in many capillaries there is filtration at the arterial end and reabsorption at the venous end. Fluid that is not reabsorbed and macromolecules are removed from the interstitium by the lymphatics (Guyton, 1991).

The Starling hypothesis describes the mechanism of transcapillary fluid and solute exchange as a function of (1) the hydrostatic pressure gradient (microvascular pressure minus perimicrovascular pressure) and (2) the protein osmotic pressure gradient (plasma protein osmotic pressure minus perimicrovascular protein osmotic pressure). Normally, the sum of the forces of microvascular pressure, perimicrovascular pressure, and perimicrovascular protein osmotic pressure favoring outward movement is slightly greater than plasma protein osmotic pressure. Thus, there is a slight net fluid movement into the tissue spaces that is equaled by lymph flow returning this fluid to the vascular system. Specific values for each of these factors may vary among tissues. The combination of the net rate of filtration per millimeters of mercury (the hydraulic conductance) and the surface area perfused is called the filtration coefficient. In addition, capillary membranes are not totally impermeable to proteins, as the above relationships suggest. The osmotic reflection coefficient expresses the degree of protein permeability, and is one if the capillary is totally impermeable and zero if the capillary is totally permeable. Thus the Starling equation is:

$$\text{Fluid movement} = k[(P_c + \pi_i) - (P_i + \pi_p)]$$

where P_c = capillary hydrostatic pressure, P_i = interstitial fluid hydrostatic pressure, π_p = plasma protein oncotic pressure, π_i = interstitial fluid oncotic pressure, and K = filtration constant for the capillary membrane. When the algebraic sum is positive, filtration occurs. When the algebraic sum is negative, absorption occurs (Berne & Levy, 1986).

The filtration coefficient and osmotic reflection coefficient for individual tissues and organ system barriers are related to the capillary ultrastructure and its responsiveness to hormonal influences. The presence, type, and number of intercellular junctions, pinocytic vesicles, transendothelial channels, and the structure of the basement membrane affect the rate and degree of edema formation in various tissues. Pinocytic vesicles and transendothelial channels are modes of molecular transport through the cells. Their presence in large numbers increases the filtration coefficient in that tissue. For example, in the hepatic sinusoids, intercellular junctions are quite loose, and the osmotic reflection coefficient approaches zero. Pulmonary capillaries are moderately leaky to proteins, those in skeletal muscle are less so, and in cerebral capillaries the osmotic reflection coefficient approaches one. In general, more sites exist for fluid and solute movement on the venous end of the capillary than on the arterial end.

INTEGRATION OF CENTRAL AND PERIPHERAL FACTORS IN CARDIAC OUTPUT CONTROL

The integration of cardiac output is a function of preload, afterload, heart rate, and contractility. Each of these factors is determined by a myriad of peripheral, central, and intracardiac components that transmit messages to each other on a cellular basis through a process called signal transduction (Fig. 18–30). This intercellular signaling is relayed by a group of polypeptides called endothelins. Endothelins can be responsible for the relay of signals that produce short-term responses (such as increased strength of contraction) or long-term responses (such as cell growth leading to ventricular hypertrophy). Endothelin binding and activity have been demonstrated in cardiac, vascular, adrenal, renal, and nervous tissues, and may be responsible for the development of many cardiovascular diseases (Banasik, 1994; Schwertz & Barry, 1994). This section examines cardiac output as the result of the integration of these influences.

Preload

VENOUS RETURN. Stroke volume is governed by the inotropic ability of the heart and the capability of the peripheral circulation to return blood to the heart. The latter is referred to as venous return. Most alterations in cardiac output in the healthy heart are caused by changes in venous return. In the absence of heart failure, augmentation of contractility (i.e., through pharmaceutical infusions) has a minimal effect on increasing the cardiac output. Modifications of venous return (i.e., through volume or position), however, contribute to relatively large changes in the cardiac output (Garfein, 1990).

Venous constriction has a profound effect on improving venous return and hence cardiac output. Even marked venous constriction has a minimal effect on the total SVR because the venous system is so compliant (Goerke & Mines, 1988). This is important because reduction in total SVR is probably the most influential factor in increasing cardiac output.

TOTAL BLOOD VOLUME. Massive or rapid reduction of the total blood volume causes the stroke volume to decline. However, decreases in cardiac output are barely perceptible with gradual reductions or with loss

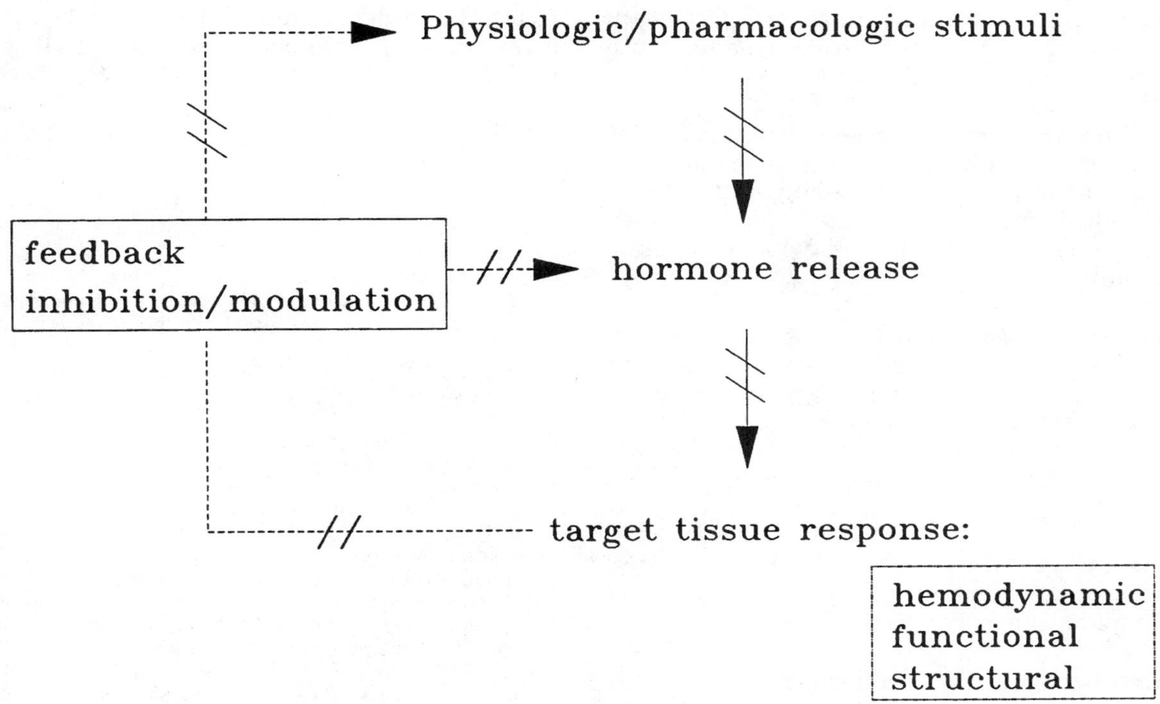

FIGURE 18–30. Characteristic sequence for hormonal activity. *Solid arrows,* path of action; *dashed arrows,* inhibitory, or negative feedback paths; and *double slashes,* potential sites where aberrant or abnormal control of hormonal activity exists in congestive heart failure. (From Cody, R. [1989]. Neurohormal influences in the pathogenesis of congestive heart failure. *Cardiology Clinics, 7,* 82.)

of less than 15% of the total blood volume (Guyton, 1991).

DISTRIBUTION OF BLOOD VOLUME. Distribution of blood volume between the intrathoracic and extrathoracic compartments exerts control over the ventricular end-diastolic volume. Body position affects blood distribution as a result of gravitational forces. While in a supine position, the blood pools in the lower limbs. The Trendelenburg position increases the venous return, thus increasing cardiac output. Military antishock trousers increase venous return through the same mechanism.

Normally, the intrathoracic pressure becomes negative during inspiration. This acts as a vacuum to assist in displacing more blood volume into the intrathoracic cavity. Positive pressure ventilation reverses this phenomenon and can decrease venous return by itself. Combined with positive end-expiratory pressure, cardiac output can be severely embarrassed.

Increased intrapericardial pressure, such as occurs with pericardial effusion, reduces cardiac filling (preload). Complete circulatory collapse can result from significant increases in intrapericardial pressure; cardiac tamponade is the classic clinical condition that results from the increase in pressure.

Venous tone depends on a variety of nervous and humoral factors. The benefits of venoconstriction in augmenting preload were discussed earlier. Venoconstriction can be caused by SNS stimulation, muscular exercise, anxiety, deep respiration, and marked hypotension. Medications that can cause venoconstriction include sympathomimetic agents and cardiac glycosides. Venodilation can be caused by ganglionic blockers and nitrates, and can cause extrathoracic pooling.

Afterload

Stroke volume, a determinant of cardiac output, depends on the degree of ventricular fiber shortening that occurs during systole. It is inversely proportional to afterload. Afterload is chiefly determined by aortic impedance and SVR. Myocardial fiber shortening is reduced with elevations in SVR, and therefore contractility and cardiac output are also decreased (Milnor, 1990).

The key determinants of afterload are SVR, the physical characteristics of the arterial tree (i.e., atherosclerosis), and the volume of blood ejected. SVR is the most easily modified of these factors and is influenced by many diverse humoral, neural, and extrinsic factors. Hypertension, obstruction to ejection (i.e., by aortic stenosis), hypothermia, and SNS stimulation profoundly increase SVR. Acidosis, hyperthermia, aortic incompetence, and many pharmaceutical agents reduce SVR and hence afterload.

Contractility

Contractility, also known as inotropy, influences cardiac output independent of preload or afterload. Inotropy refers to the myocardial force–velocity–length relationship and the level of ventricular performance at end-diastolic volume (Milnor, 1990).

SNS ACTIVITY. Sympathetic stimulation increases cardiac contractility through excitation of the superior, middle, and inferior cardiac nerves and the paravertebral sympathetic chain (Berne & Levy, 1986). Increased inotropy is a result of direct release of norepinephrine into the cardiac tissue.

HUMORAL FACTORS. Circulating catecholamines released by the adrenal medulla, nerve impulses, and extracardiac ganglia augment inotropy. Although circulating catecholamines are slower to stimulate contractility than intracardiac norepinephrine, they are important in chronic conditions (Benedict & Phil, 1994).

EXOGENOUS INOTROPIC AGENTS. Cardiac glycosides, caffeine, sympathomimetic agents, theophylline, and glucagon all have positive inotropic effects.

DEPRESSANTS. Cardiac contractility can be depressed by physiologic and pharmacologic agents. These factors include anoxia, ischemia, acidemia, beta-adrenergic blockade, anesthetics, and barbiturates.

LOSS OF CONTRACTILE MASS. Myocardial infarction results in a loss of functional cardiac muscle. Global ventricular performance (contractility) is thus impaired.

Heart Rate

Alterations in heart rate, called chronotropy, can have positive or negative effects on cardiac output. Because cardiac output is a function of stroke volume times heart rate, it is easy to see how increased heart rate can improve cardiac output. Improved cardiac output can be achieved only as long as the diastolic volume of the heart remains constant (Busch et al., 1992). Extremely rapid or prolonged tachycardia, however, can reduce the diastolic filling time and thus reduce diastolic volume. In this case, cardiac output is reduced by tachycardia.

SUMMARY

This chapter reviews the physical properties of the cardiovascular system and the ultrastructure and mechanisms of contractions. The electrical activity of the heart is described. The mechanical and clinical features of cardiac pumping are delineated. The structure and control of the systemic circulation is discussed. In the discussion of the integration of control of peripheral factors in cardiac output, how the body strives to maintain homeostasis and the mechanisms that it uses to achieve the steady state are reviewed.

REFERENCES

Abraham, T. (1992). Arrhythmogenic mechanisms. *AACN Clinical Issues in Critical Care, 3,* 157–165.

Angelos, M., DeBehnke, D., & Leasure, J. (1992). Arterial pH and carbon dioxide tension as indicators of tissue perfusion during cardiac arrest in a canine model. *Critical Care Medicine, 20,* 1302–1308.

Banasik, J. (1994). Endothelins: New players in cardiovascular physiology and disease. *Journal of Cardiovascular Nursing, 8*(3), 87–104.

Benedict, C., & Phil, D. (1994). Neurohormonal aspects of heart failure. *Cardiology Clinics, 12,* 9–23.

Benjamin, E. (1994). Venous hypercarbia: A nonspecific marker of hypoperfusion. *Critical Care Medicine, 22,* 9–10.

Berne, R., & Levy, M. (1986). *Cardiovascular physiology* (5th ed.). St. Louis: C. V. Mosby.

Boltwood, M., Taylor, C., Burke, M., Grogin, H., & Giacomini, J. (1993). Anger report predicts coronary artery vasomotor response to mental stress in atherosclerotic segments. *American Journal of Cardiology, 72,* 1361–1365.

Bond, E. (1989). Physiology of the heart. In S. Underhill, S. Woods, E. Froelicher, et al. (Eds.), *Cardiac nursing* (pp. 44–56). Philadelphia: J. B. Lippincott.

Bond, E., & Halpenny, C. (1995). Cardiac anatomy. In S. Woods, E. Froelicher, C. Halpenny, et al. (Eds.), *Cardiac nursing* (pp. 11–25). Philadelphia: J. B. Lippincott.

Braunwald, E. B., Sonnenblick, E. H., & Ross, J. (1992). Mechanism of cardiac contraction and relaxation. In E. B. Braunwald (Ed.), *Heart disease: A textbook of cardiovascular medicine* (4th ed.). Philadelphia: W. B. Saunders.

Busch, S., Cowan, M., & Simpson, T. (1992). Heart rate variability in cardiac disease. *Progress in Cardiovascular Nursing, 7*(4), 2–9.

Byrne, J., & Downey, J. (1992). Electrical activity of the heart. In L. Johnson (Ed.), *Essential medical physiology* (pp. 179–188). New York: Raven Press.

Candipan, R., Hsiun, T., Pratt, R., & Cooke, J. (1994). Vascular injury augments adrenergic neurotransmission. *Circulation, 89,* 777–784.

Carbello, B. (1991). Timing of surgery in mitral and aortic stenosis. *Cardiology Clinics, 9,* 229–238.

Cody, R. (1989). Neurohormonal influences in the pathogenesis of congestive heart failure. *Cardiology Clinics, 7,* 73–86.

Cohn, P. (1985). *Clinical cardiovascular physiology.* Philadelphia: W. B. Saunders.

Farb, A., Burke, A., & Virmani, R. (1992). Anatomy and pathology of the right ventricle (including acquired tricuspid and pulmonic valve disease). *Cardiology Clinics, 10*(1), 1–22.

Felknor, R. (1994). New hypertension guidelines stress systolic pressure. *Cardiology World News, 10*(3), 22–23.

Fox, G., Bernsten, A., Lam, C., Neul, A., et al. (1994). Hematocrit modifies the circulatory control of systemic and myocardial oxygen utilization in septic sheep. *Critical Care Medicine, 22,* 470–479.

Frass, M., Watschinger, B., Traindl, O., et al. (1993). Atrial natriuretic peptide release in response to different positive end-expiratory pressure levels. *Critical Care Medicine, 21,* 343–347.

Freeman, G. (1990). The effects of the pericardium on function of normal and enlarged hearts. *Cardiology Clinics, 8,* 579–586.

Gardner, P. (1993). Pulmonary artery pressure monitoring. *AACN Clinical Issues in Critical Care, 4,* 98–119.

Garfein, O. (1990). *Current concepts in cardiovascular physiology.* San Diego: Academic Press.

Gibson, R. (1991). Beta-receptor regulation: Dynamics of density and function throughout the cardiac cycle. *Journal of Cardiovascular Nursing, 5*(4), 49–56.

Goerke, J., & Mines, A. (1988). *Cardiovascular physiology.* New York: Raven Press.

Gorny, D. (1993). Arterial blood pressure measurement technique. *AACN Clinical Issues in Critical Care, 4,* 66–80.

Grum, C. (1993). Tissue oxygenation in low flow states and during hypoxemia. *Critical Care Medicine, 21*(Suppl), 544–549.

Guyton, A. (1991). *Textbook of medical physiology* (8th ed.). Philadelphia: W. B. Saunders.

Headley, J., & Diethorn, M. (1993). Right ventricular volumetric monitoring. *AACN Clinical Issues in Critical Care, 4,* 120–133.

Hixon, M. (1994). Aging and heart failure. *Progress in Cardiovascular Nursing, 9*(1), 4–12.

Hoshino, J., Sakamaki, T., Nakamura, T., et al. (1994). Exaggerated vascular response due to endothelial dysfunction and role of the renin–angiotensin system at early stage of renal hypertension in rats. *Circulation Research, 74,* 130–138.

Hudak, C., & Gallo, B. (1994). *Critical care nursing: A holistic approach* (6th ed.). Philadelphia: J. B. Lippincott.

Hughes, J. M. B. (1987). Pulmonary blood flow and gas exchange: An overview. In J. Will, C. Dawson, E. Weir, & C. Buckner (Eds.). *The pulmonary circulation in health and disease* (pp. 281–287). Orlando, FL: Harcourt Brace Jovanovich.

Hurst, J., Logue, R., & Wenger, N. (1990). *The heart, arteries, and veins* (2nd ed.). New York: McGraw-Hill.

Kern, M., & Deligonul, V. (1993). The stenotic aortic valve. In M. Kern (Ed.), *Hemodynamic rounds* (pp. 7–16). New York: Wiley-Liss.

Lee, F. (1992). Hemodynamics of the right ventricle in normal and disease states. *Cardiology Clinics, 10,* 59–68.

Lefer, A., Ma, X. (1993). Cytokines and growth factors in endothelial dysfunction. *Critical Care Medicine, 21*(Suppl), 59–64.

Little, R., & Little, W. (1985). *Physiology of the heart and circulation.* Chicago: Year Book.

Lutterutti, N., Catanzaro, D., Sealey, J., & Laragh, J. (1994). Renin is synthesized by cardiac and extrarenal vascular tissues: A review of experimental evidence. *Circulation, 89,* 458–470.

MacLeod, D., Strauss, B., DeJong, M., et al. (1994). Proliferation and extracellular matrix synthesis of smooth muscle cells cultured from human coronary atherosclerotic and restentotic lesion. *Journal of the American College of Cardiology, 23,* 59–65.

McElroy, P., Shroff, S., & Weber, K. (1989). Pathophysiology of the failing heart. *Cardiology Clinics, 7,* 25–38.

McGuigan, J., & Blatter, L. (1987). Sodium / calcium exchange in ventricular muscle. *Experientia, 43,* 1140–1145.

Milnor, W. (1990). *Cardiovascular physiology.* New York: Oxford University Press.

Muntz, K., Zhao, M., & Miller, J. (1994). Down regulation of myocardial beta-adrenergic receptors: Receptor subtype selectivity. *Circulation Research, 74,* 369–375.

Nichols, W., & O'Rourke, M. (1990). *McDonald's blood flow in arteries* (3rd ed.). Philadelphia: Lea & Febiger.

Oren, J., Beckman, K., McClelland, J., Wang, X., Lazzara, R., & Jackman, W. (1993). A functional approach to the pre-excitation syndromes. *Cardiology Clinics, 11,* 121–149.

Paradis, N., Wortsman, J., Malarkey, W., et al. (1994). High atrial natriuretic peptide concentrations blunt the presson response during cardiopulmonary resuscitation in humans. *Critical Care Medicine, 22,* 213–218.

Quaal, S. (1992). The person with heart failure and cardiogenic shock. In C. Guzzetta, & E. Dossey (Eds.), *Cardiovascular nursing: Holistic practice,* (pp. 302–356). St. Louis: C. V. Mosby.

Remme, W., Krujssen, D., Look, M., Bootsma, M., & Leeuw, P. (1994). Systemic and cardiac neuroendocrine activation and severity of myocardial ischemia in humans. *Journal of the American College of Cardiology, 23,* 82–91.

Rhoades, R., & Pflanzer, R. (1989). *Human physiology.* Philadelphia: Saunders College Publishing.

Rousseau, M., Konstam, M., Benedict, C., et al. (1994). Progression of left ventricular dysfunction secondary to coronary artery disease, sustained neurohormonal activation and effects of 160 pamine therapy during long-term therapy with angiotensin-converting enzyme inhibitor. *American Journal of Cardiology, 73,* 488–493.

Ruegg, J. (1986). *Calcium in muscle activation.* Berlin: Springer-Verlag.

Schoen, F. (1989). *Interventional and surgical cardiovascular pathology.* Philadelphia: W. B. Saunders.

Schulman, D., & Matthey, R. (1992). The right ventricle in pulmonary disease. *Cardiology Clinics, 10,* 111–136.

Schwertz, D., & Barry, C. (1994). Cellular communication through signal transduction: The background. *Journal of Cardiovascular Nursing, 8*(3), 1–27.

Sharaf, A., Narula, J., Nicol, P., Southern, J., & Khaw, B. (1994). Cardiac sarcoplasmic reticulum calcium ATPase, an autoimmune antigen in experimental cardiomyopathy. *Circulation, 89,* 1217–1228.

Sitzer, V. (1991). Physiologic framework of extrinsic controls. *Journal of Cardiovascular Nursing, 5*(4), 1–9.

Stern, M., Capogrossi, M., & Lakatta, E. (1988). Spontaneous calcium release from the sarcoplasmic reticulum in myocardial cells: Mechanisms and consequences. *Cell Calcium, 9,* 247–256.

Urban, N. (1993). Integrating the hemodynamic profile. *AACN Clinical Issues in Critical Care, 4,* 161–179.

Vander, A., Sherman, J., & Luciano, D. (1990). *Human physiology: The mechanisms of body function* (5th ed.). New York: McGraw-Hill.

Vassalle, M. (1987). Contribution of the Na / K-pump to the membrane potential. *Experientia, 43,* 1135–1140.

Weber, K., & Janicki, J. (1989). Pathogenesis of heart failure. *Cardiology Clinics, 7,* 11–24.

Weisbrodt, N. (1992). Striated muscle. In L. Johnson (Ed.), *Essential medical physiology* (pp. 85–98). New York: Raven Press.

White, K. (1993). Using continuous SVo_2 to assess oxygen supply / demand balance in the critically ill patient. *AACN Clinical Issues in Critical Care, 4,* 134–147.

White, P. (1992). Calcium channel blockers. *AACN Clinical Issues in Critical Care, 3,* 337–446.

Woo, M., Stevenson, W., Moser, D., & Middlekauff, H. (1994). Complex heart rate variability and serum norepinephrine levels in patient with advanced heart failure. *Journal of the American College of Cardiology, 23,* 565–569.

Wright, S. (1990). Pathophysiology of congestive heart failure. *Journal of Cardiovascular Nursing, 4*(3), 1–16.

Yang, S., Bentiuoglio, L., Maranhao, V., & Goldberg, H. (1988). *From cardiac catheterizations data to hemodynamic parameters* (3rd ed.). Philadelphia: F. A. Davis.

Zile, M. (1991). Chronic aortic and mitral regurgitation: Choosing the optimal time for surgical correction. *Cardiology Clinics, 9,* 239–254.

CHAPTER

19 Patients With Coronary Artery Disease

Julie Fleury, Colleen Keller, and Carolyn Murdaugh

ATHEROSCLEROSIS: THE LESION OF CORONARY ARTERY DISEASE

Atherosclerosis is a pathologic condition of the arteries clinically manifested as cardiovascular disease, the major cause of death in the industrialized world. Coronary artery disease (CAD) and cerebrovascular disease, both of which are atherosclerotic diseases, cause more death, disability, and economic loss in the United States than any other disease (American Heart Association, 1992).

Natural History

The lesions of atherosclerosis occur mainly in the intima, the innermost layer of the artery wall. However, secondary changes can be found in the media or middle layer as well. Over a period of years these lesions progress and undergo changes that lead to serious clinical consequences. More precise accounts of the sequential changes that may take place have been difficult owing to the inability to sample human arteries at various time intervals. Until recently, the changes were construed from lesions obtained at autopsies or surgical procedures, or extrapolated from animal studies. In the last few years information on atherosclerotic progression has been obtained through serial imaging of arterial lesions, most commonly by angiography. In addition, ultrasound and magnetic resonance arterial imaging are being used to augment angiography, especially for examination of the aortoiliac and peripheral vessels.

Three characteristic lesions of atherosclerosis have been identified: the fatty streak, the fibrous plaque, and the complicated lesion. The fatty streak, the earliest lesion, begins in early childhood. The fatty streak is a grossly flat, lipid-rich lesion consisting of both macrophages and some smooth muscle. Fatty streaks are found in the aorta shortly after birth and in most children older than 1 year of age in all populations. They increase in number between the ages of 8 and 18 years. Fatty streaks appear in the coronary arteries around age 15 and increase in these vessels through the third decade (Ross, 1990). Fatty streaks are yellowish in appearance as a result of extensive lipid deposits. They cause little or no obstruction and do not produce any clinical effects. By themselves, fatty streaks are considered benign. Whether fatty streaks are the precursors of fibrous plaques and atherosclerosis has not been resolved.

In industrialized nations, such as the United States, more advanced lesions called fibrous plaques begin to develop in the coronary arteries after 20 years of age. They are grossly white in appearance and become elevated so they may protrude into the lumen of the artery. The lesions are composed of increased intimal smooth muscle cells surrounded by connective tissue matrix. The smooth muscle cells may form a fibrous cap because of the accumulation of intracellular and extracellular lipids and deposition of connective tissue. Beneath the fibrous cap, the lesions contain smooth muscle and macrophages that contain lipid droplets surrounded by connective tissue. Beneath these cells there may be an area of necrotic debris, cholesterol crystals, and calcification. Smooth muscle–rich fibrous plaques are often found at the same anatomic sites in coronary and extracranial cerebral arteries where fatty streaks have been found early in life (Braunwald, 1992). This finding suggests that fibrous plaques are derived from fatty streaks that have continued the process of cell proliferation, lipid accumulation, and connective tissue formation.

Advanced or complicated lesions occur over the age of 30 when fibrous plaques undergo complex changes and increase in frequency. The fibrous plaques become vascularized, and the necrotic lipid-rich core increases in size and may become calcified. The initimal surface of the lesion may disintegrate and ulcerate, allowing thrombi to form on the surface of the plaque. The thrombi may further increase the size of the plaque and reduce the lumen of the artery, resulting in a reduction in blood flow (ischemia) or occlusion of an artery (necrosis). Clinical symptoms

The authors wish to acknowledge the assistance of Robert O'Rourke, M.D., in the preparation of this manuscript.

occur as a result of the ischemia or necrosis and are manifested as myocardial infarction, stroke, aortic aneurysm, and gangrene of the extremities.

Pathogenesis

Over the years several theories have been developed to describe the etiology and pathogenesis of atherosclerosis. Two theories that have received the most attention are the response to injury hypothesis and the lipid–lipoprotein hypothesis (Ross, 1990). Four principal cells are involved in both theories: endothelium, smooth muscle, platelets, and monocytes.

RESPONSE TO INJURY HYPOTHESIS. The response to injury hypothesis postulates that injury occurs to the endothelial cells. The injury may be caused by such factors as chronic hypercholesterolemia, increased shear stress from blood flow at bifurcations in arteries, hypertension, and chemical toxins found in cigarette smoke that change the nature of the permeability barrier of the endothelial cells.

Endothelial cells, functionally active components of the intima, perform two vital functions. The cells normally form a permeability barrier that functions to control the passage of molecules from the plasma into the artery wall. Second, the endothelium forms a thromboresistant surface that promotes the continuous flow of blood by producing a heparin-like surface proteoglycan and synthesizing prostacyclin (prostaglandin I_2, PGI_2). Prostacyclin, a potent vasodilator, is also a potent inhibitor of platelet aggregation.

Injury to the endothelium results in an immediate platelet response. Platelets begin to adhere to the subendothelial layer at the site of injury. They aggregate and release their granule contents. Platelets contain several mitogens, one of which is of interest in atherosclerosis: platelet-derived growth factor (PDGF). PDGF can bind to connective tissue at sites of endothelial injury to attract smooth muscle cells from the media into the intima. PDGF induces smooth muscle migration and proliferation. Within 3 to 5 days after platelets release their contents, smooth muscle cells have been shown to migrate from the media into the intima of the artery, inducing proliferation of these smooth muscle cells. According to the hypothesis, if the injury and the tissue response is a self-limited event and the integrity of the endothelium is restored, the lesion may be capable of regressing. For example, endothelial injury occurs when a balloon catheter is placed in an artery. However, endothelial cells regenerate slowly. If the injury is of long standing or is chronically repeated, the lesions may continue to progress to advanced plaques with clinical consequences. An example of a long-standing injury is the chronic elevation of low-density lipoproteins (LDL), also called chronic hypercholesteremia.

LIPOGENIC HYPOTHESIS. The lipogenic hypothesis is associated with elevations of plasma LDL. LDL are the major cholesterol-transporting lipoproteins, and transport cholesterol and phospholipid to the peripheral cells. Elevated levels of LDL may induce injury to the endothelial lining of the artery by infiltrating the intima from the blood.

In its oxidized form, LDL attracts macrophage, which take up the modified LDL via scavenger receptors, turning these into foam cells (Steinberg et al., 1989). The foam cells attract a large number of active substances, including growth factors, oxygen free radicals, collagenase, and lipase. Growth factors function to attract medial smooth muscle cells, and with other active substances, contribute to the process of smooth muscle cell proliferation and collagen matrix synthesis (Vogel, 1994). With the growth of the fibrous collagen matrix as atheroma, the overlying endothelium becomes injured. Endothelial injury occurs both as a result of shear forces and from endothelial cell injury from foam cell secretions. Platelet activation and thrombus formation follow endothelial cell injury and may lead to partial vessel occlusion, total occlusion, or progression of coronary stenosis (Forrester et al., 1987).

In summary, the mechanisms of atherosclerosis are much better understood than they were 15 years ago. Most researchers agree that endothelial injury and dysfunction are key events in the initiation of atherosclerosis. Changes in endothelial function result in a change in the interaction between the artery and the blood cellular elements. Such functional changes promote the entry of monocyte-derived macrophages to the intima, lipid accumulation, and smooth muscle proliferation. Over time, these events produce the vascular lesions of atherosclerosis.

MYOCARDIAL ISCHEMIA

Pathogenesis

Myocardial ischemia stems from an imbalance between myocardial oxygen requirements and oxygen availability. The imbalance can be caused by either a decrease in coronary blood flow (supply) or a disproportionate increase in myocardial oxygen requirements (demand). Decreased coronary blood flow is most commonly caused by atherosclerosis in the coronary arteries. However, myocardial ischemia can also result from nonatherosclerotic disease. For example, congenital anomalies of the coronary arteries, hereditary metabolic disorders, and systemic collagen vascular disease may produce chronic myocardial ischemia (Chatterjee, in press). Increased myocardial oxygen requirements may precipitate myocardial ischemia in valvular heart disease or hypertrophic cardiomyopathy because demand may exceed the capacity to supply oxygen to the myocardium. Recently, vasoconstriction (spasm) of the coronary arteries has also been found to be a cause of myocardial ischemia.

Under normal conditions, myocardial metabolic demands closely parallel coronary blood flow. Ischemia is avoided by a careful matching of blood flow to metabolism. Even in a resting state, the cardiac muscle extracts 65% to 75% of available oxygen. Thus, augmenting coronary blood flow is the principal means of increasing the oxygen supply. In the presence of coronary atherosclerosis, increased demands for blood flow cannot be met, and ischemia results.

Because the major cause of myocardial ischemia is decreased blood flow (supply), emphasis is usually placed on the supply side of the oxygen supply–demand ratio. Under normal hemodynamic conditions, coronary blood flow is distributed uniformly. The amount of coronary blood flow during diastole is usually several times greater than that during systole. Thus, satisfactory regulation of the transmural distribution of coronary blood flow is maintained until the vessels become maximally dilated. However, with progressive obstruction of a large coronary artery with atherosclerotic lesions, adequate flow is maintained in the epicardial (outer myocardial) layers but is insufficient to the subendocardial layers of the heart. Thus, the onset of myocardial ischemia depends on the pathophysiologic mechanisms in the subendocardium.

Several metabolic changes occur in myocardial cells during ischemic episodes. Oxygen diffuses from the capillaries to the mitochondria in the myocardial cells. Ischemia occurs when the concentration of oxygen falls below a critical level in the mitochondria. Within 15 seconds of ischemia there is an acceleration of glycolysis and lactate production from anaerobic metabolic reactions, which leads to a fall in intracellular pH. The altered pH leads to changes in the interaction between calcium and the contractile proteins (actin–myosin), resulting in impaired myocardial contractile function. Ischemia results in cessation of myocardial contraction in the affected zones of the myocardium. Diastolic myocardial function is also impaired because the ischemic cells do not completely relax, as noted by increased ventricular stiffness. This stiffness in turn increases ventricular diastolic pressures.

Left ventricular wall abnormalities occur early in the ischemic episode. These changes are followed by electrocardiographic (ECG) abnormalities and the development of symptoms. The commonly observed ECG changes are ST segment depression or elevation and dysrhythmias due to electrical excitability (Fig. 19–1). Patient symptoms include angina, acute dyspnea, or sudden death.

Investigations have recently focused on the importance of free radicals in the pathophysiology of ischemia. As ischemic tissues are reperfused, molecular oxygen is reintroduced. The oxygen molecule interacts with byproducts of the ischemia to form oxygen-derived free radicals, including the superoxide anion, the hydroxy radical, and hydrogen peroxide. These free radicals can react with various cell components such as unsaturated fatty acids. In turn, loss of membrane permeability and loss of enzyme activity occur, resulting in further damage to the myocardial cells. Enzymes that are present react with the free radicals to prevent further cell damage. These enzymes are termed "free radical scavengers."

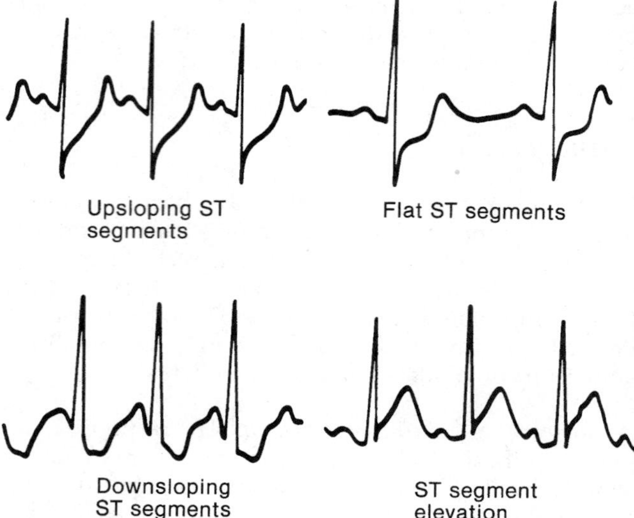

FIGURE 19–1. Family of ST segment changes seen with ischemia. (From Parmley, O., & Chatterjee, K. [1988]. *Cardiology vol. 1: Physiology, pharmacology, diagnoses.* Philadelphia: J. B. Lippincott.)

Clinical, angiographic, and pathologic evidence indicates that an alteration in the integrity of the atherosclerotic plaque is the underlying mechanism of acute coronary ischemia. Endothelial and smooth muscle cells maintain the homeostasis of the vessel wall. Stable states are achieved after injury in that the vessel is able to maintain blood flow. However, injury enables the atherosclerotic plaque to form. Raised plaques consist of a pool of fatty material covered by a cap of fibrous tissue. The fibrous cap may crack, resulting in either rapid plaque progression or hemorrhage into the plaque. These cracks are also referred to as intimal fissures, breaks, tears, ulcers, and ruptures. The clinical manifestations (i.e., angina or infarction) depend on the severity of impaired flow, the presence and extent of impaired flow, and the presence and extent of collateral flow (Cowley et al., 1989; Falk, 1989). The clinical spectrum of ischemic heart disease includes asymptomatic CAD, the anginal syndromes, myocardial infarction, and sudden death.

NONINVASIVE DIAGNOSIS

Recent experimental studies have delineated the sequence of metabolic, mechanical, hemodynamic, and ECG abnormalities resulting from inadequate coronary blood flow to contracting ventricular myocardium. The occurrence of these abnormalities in the presence of myocardial ischemia forms the basis for noninvasive diagnostic testing for CAD.

ELECTROCARDIOGRAPHY

The ECG recorded with the patient at rest may show abnormalities due to a prior myocardial infarction, left ventricular hypertrophy, or other cardiac disease. However, the resting ECG is normal or nonspecific in up to 50% of patients with chronic exertional angina. In patients with angina occurring at rest, ECG abnormalities such as ST-T wave depression, bundle branch block, or dysrhythmias occurring during a painful episode will often lead to the correct diagnosis of CAD. However, rest angina often occurs without ECG changes.

EXERCISE ECG TESTING. ECG monitoring during graded bicycle or treadmill exercise testing is the most commonly used noninvasive method for identifying patients likely to have CAD or likely to be at high risk. High-risk patients are those who have severe myocardial ischemia at a low workload (Froelicher & Pashkow, 1993). Many exercise ECG protocols exist. All are based on increasing the myocardial oxygen demand at 3-minute intervals by altering the workload progressively; the incremental increases in heart rate and systolic blood pressure result in augmented myocardial oxygen demands that eventually cannot be met because of a compromised coronary blood flow reserve.

The sensitivity of exercise ECG recording improves with 12-lead ECG monitoring. The test reaches peak sensitivity for identifying patients with coronary artery stenosis when at least 85% of predicted maximal heart rate is attained during exercise, and is most accurate in patients with a normal resting ECG and no other reasons for ST segment depression during exercise, such as hypokalemia or digitalis therapy.

Exercise ECG testing is generally considered useful for (1) diagnoses of CAD in male patients with atypical symptoms of myocardial ischemia; (2) assessment of the functional capacity and prognosis in patients with known CAD; and (3) evaluation of patients with symptoms consistent with recurrent exercise-induced cardiac dysrhythmias. The specificity of exercise-induced ST segment changes in women with atypical or typical angina has been lower than that in men, producing more false-positive results. Endpoints during exercise testing of importance include ST segment depression, a suboptimal rise or actual fall in the systolic blood pressure, exercise-induced ventricular dysrhythmias, chest pain with or without ECG changes, exercise-induced conduction abnormalities, failure to increase heart rate, and clinical signs of congestive heart failure.

EXERCISE TESTING WITH THALLIUM-201 IMAGING

Myocardial perfusion imaging with thallium-201 (^{201}Tl) has been widely applied in the clinical assessment of patients with known or suspected CAD. The amount of ^{201}Tl extracted by the myocardium depends on regional coronary blood flow (Fig. 19–2). Myocardial uptake in the absence of CAD is relatively homogeneous on assessment by gamma camera imaging.

However, after its initial extraction, ^{201}Tl does not remain fixed within the myocardial cells, and there is a continuous exchange between myocardial thallium and thallium that was initially distributed into the systemic blood pool. Thus, redistribution of ^{201}Tl is defined as the total or partial resolution of myocardial defects that are detected 5 to 20 minutes after intravenous ^{201}Tl. Defect disappearance or partial improvement is determined by obtaining delayed images 3 to 4 hours after the initial injection of ^{201}Tl. Thus, initial thallium defects after intravenous injection of the isotope near the end of exercise that are improved 3 hours later usually indicate reversible ischemia. In contrast, persistent thallium defects during exercise and several hours later usually indicate old or recent irreversible myocardial damage. The use of ^{201}Tl exercise imaging has been beneficial in patients demonstrating nonspecific ST segment depression, left ventricular hypertrophy or preexcitation conduction patterns, or metabolic abnormalities, or in those undergoing digitalis therapy, which may render inconclusive results with standard ECG exercise testing. More recently, tomographic thallium imaging of the heart (single-photon emission computed tomography, or SPECT) has provided increased diagnostic accuracy (Iskandrian et al., 1993; Kahn, 1991).

Using SPECT imaging, the nuclear camera rotates in an arc around the body; reconstruction of the thallium distribution in the heart produces images in three-dimensional slices (Kahn, 1991). SPECT thallium exercise imaging identifies 80% to 90% of patients with CAD, surpassing data obtained from clinical, exercise treadmill, and catheterization (Iskandrian et al., 1993).

RADIONUCLIDE VENTRICULOGRAPHY

This radionuclide technique uses technetium bound to red blood cells for "blood pool" imaging with ECG-gated left ventricular time–activity curves obtained from summed cardiac cycle data at points from end-diastole to end-systole (Froelicher & Pashkow, 1993) (Fig. 19–3). Gamma camera imaging is performed at rest and during the last 2 minutes of exercise, and the global left ventricular ejection fraction is determined from end-diastolic counts minus end-systolic counts divided by end-diastolic counts. Regional wall motion can also be assessed by careful review of the cine-film format of the radionuclide ventriculogram (RVG).

The normal response to exercise has been defined as an absolute increment of at least 5% in the left ventricular ejection fraction without the development of a new wall motion abnormality. An abnormal ejection fraction response occurs in many elderly patients, women without heart disease, patients with depressed cardiac function due to valvular heart disease or cardiomyopathy, and hypertensive patients. The demonstration of a new wall motion abnormality during exercise is less sensitive (65%–76%) but more specific (95%) for a diagnosis of coronary heart disease. Table 19–1 compares the usefulness of ^{201}Tl exercise imaging and exercise RVG in the detection of myocardial ischemia.

EXERCISE ECHOCARDIOGRAPHY

Exercise echocardiography is useful for assessing total and regional left ventricular function to detect abnormalities resulting from myocardial ischemia. Al-

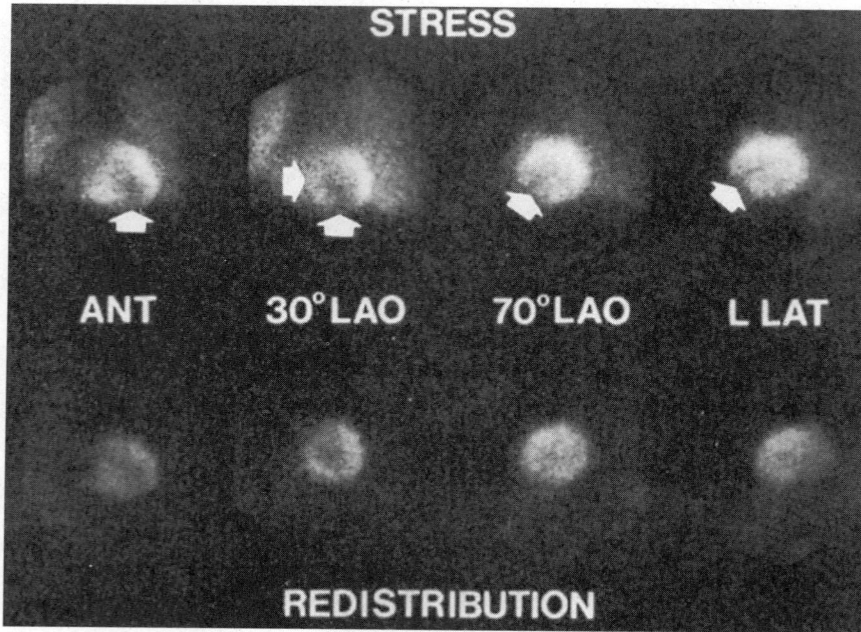

FIGURE 19–2. Myocardial perfusion scintigraphy with thallium-201 in a patient with 90% stenosis of the left anterior descending artery along with less severe stenosis involving the left circumflex system. A large reversible perfusion defect involving the anteroseptal and apical segments of the left ventricle is seen best on the 30-degree LAO immediate postexercise image (*arrows*). The defect is not present on redistribution imaging 4 hours later (*lower panel*) because it is caused by transiently increased lung uptake on the immediate postexercise images (*upper panel*). *Abbreviations:* ANT, anterior; 30 LAO, 30-degree left anterior oblique; 70 LAO, 70-degree left anterior oblique; LLAT, left lateral. (From Braunwald, E. [1988]. *Heart disease: Textbook of cardiovascular medicine* [3rd ed.]. Philadelphia: W. B. Saunders.)

though two-dimensional echocardiography is well established in clinical cardiology, traditional transthoracic approaches are unsatisfactory. Recently, transthoracic esophageal echocardiography (TEE) has provided improved visualization of cardiac structures. With TEE, chest wall interference is eliminated; the close vicinity of the heart and thoracic aorta to the echocardiographic sensor allows the use of high-frequency, near-focused transducers, producing better resolution of cardiac images (Matsuzaki et al., 1990; Seward et al., 1990). The procedure for inserting the transducer is similar to that for inserting a gastrocamera. The patient lies in the left decubitus position, the transducer is advanced, and serial tomographic views of the heart are obtained by tilting and rotating the transducer tip. Obvious contraindications to TEE include esophageal obstruction and upper gastrointestinal bleeding (Fleischer & Goldstein, 1990). Recently, color Doppler imaging from a transesophageal approach has increased clinical diagnostic information.

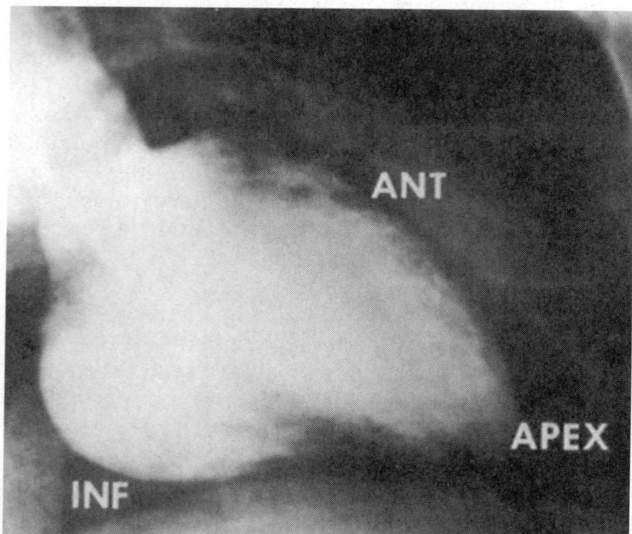

FIGURE 19–3. A 30-degree right anterior oblique projection of the end-diastolic frame of a left ventriculogram. Anterior (*ANT*), apical (*APEX*), and inferior (*INF*) segments of the left ventricle are demonstrated in this view. (From Parmley, O., & Chatterjee, K. [1988]. *Cardiology vol 1: Physiology, pharmacology, diagnoses.* Philadelphia: J. B. Lippincott.)

INVASIVE DIAGNOSIS

CARDIAC CATHETERIZATION

Although noninvasive techniques assume an important role in assessment of cardiovascular disease, car-

TABLE 19–1. **Comparison of Thallium-201 and Exercise Radionuclide Ventriculography**

^{201}Tl is preferable:

1. In the presence of certain dysrhythmias (e.g., atrial fibrillation, frequent premature beats) that may interfere with ability properly to "gate" the blood pool scan
2. When presence of CAD needs to be assessed in a patient who may have exercise-induced LV dysfunction for some other reason (e.g., hypertension)
3. When the LV ejection fraction is severely depressed at rest

Exercise radionuclide ventriculography is preferable:

1. When a measurement of LV ejection fraction is also necessary
2. When extraneous factors could cause the impression of decreased or heterogeneous myocardial uptake (e.g., large breasts, mastectomy, left pleural effusion, pacemaker hardware)
3. When right ventricular function must also be assessed

Abbreviations: CAD, coronary artery disease; LV, left ventricular.

diac catheterization with coronary angiography remains the most definitive procedure for the evaluation and diagnosis of coronary disease. Cardiac catheterization is a combined hemodynamic and angiographic procedure performed for a diagnostic assessment of the presence and extent of CAD. The procedure consists of the introduction of a catheter into the vascular system and heart to obtain hemodynamic measurements, draw blood samples, or inject radiographic indicators. The goals of cardiac catheterization are (1) to define cardiovascular anatomy; (2) document the existence of known or suspected conditions; (3) compare catheterizations to evaluate increased severity of known conditions; (4) explore the possibility of associated conditions that may result from primary cardiac disease; (5) detect intracardiac shunts; and (6) carry out medical or presurgical evaluation. Cardiac catheterization is indicated in preparation for all cardiac surgical procedures. Combined right and left catheterization is now the most widely used approach.

With current levels of safety, there are relatively few contraindications to cardiac catheterization. Acute myocardial infarction, drug toxicities, and controllable dysrhythmias are examples of conditions that need to be managed before catheterization. Cardiac catheterization is contraindicated in patients whose cardiac diagnosis is certain but in whom cardiac surgery must be deferred because of debilitating illness, massive obesity, or severe cardiomegaly. Anticoagulation as a contraindication is debatable. Some investigators have reported an increase in hemorrhages and other complications in patients receiving anticoagulants, whereas others believe that anticoagulants are safe and at times beneficial.

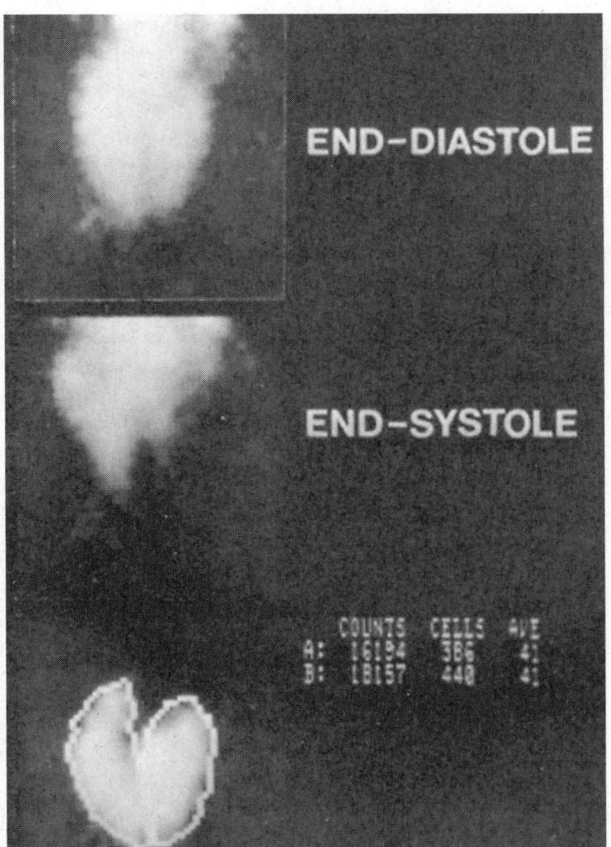

FIGURE 19–4. Equilibrium (gated) radionuclide angiocardiogram of a patient with coronary artery disease and normal ventricular performance at rest. Images were obtained in the 45-degree modified left anterior oblique projection. The end-diastolic image demonstrates vigorous and uniform contraction of the left and right ventricles, which are at the right and left sides of the image, respectively. The stroke volume image (*lower panel*) has uniformly high activity throughout the right and left ventricle, indicating normal ejection of blood from both ventricular cavities. (From Braunwald, E. [1988]. *Heart disease: A textbook of cardiovascular medicine* [3rd ed.]. Philadelphia: W. B. Saunders.)

CORONARY ANGIOGRAPHY

Angiocardiography has played a major role in the clinical assessment of cardiac lesions during the last 25 years. The use of image intensifiers and cineangiography has greatly increased the use of angiography in the diagnosis and evaluation of coronary heart disease. Coronary angiography is an extremely important procedure that is indicated in all patients with CAD in whom surgical treatment is indicated. Specifically, coronary angiography is indicated in those patients who manifest the following:

1. Unstable angina pectoris
2. Prolonged chest pain due to myocardial ischemia without objective signs of myocardial infarction
3. Myocardial infarction with repeated incidence of chest pain
4. Stable angina with stress ECG or thallium myocardial perfusion scan suggesting high-risk CAD
5. Stable angina when revascularization surgery or angioplasty is contemplated
6. Atypical chest pain when diagnostic tests have failed to clarify the diagnosis
7. Angina and valvular heart disease to delineate the coronary anatomy and establish the mechanism of angina
8. Variant angina with ST elevation or depression during angina to determine presence of coronary artery stenosis
9. A diagnosis of variant angina suspected but not documented by noninvasive studies

As a special procedure during cardiac catheterization, coronary angiography allows visualization of cardiac structures through use of contrast agents and x-ray films taken from various projections (Fig. 19–4). The procedure involves inserting a catheter into the femoral artery and passing it under fluoroscopic control to the desired vessel. Coronary angiography can be performed using either the direct brachial approach or the percutaneous femoral approach. Using the direct approach, a single catheter is manipulated to achieve selective catheterization of both the left and right coronary arteries. During passage of the catheter from the subclavian artery to the aortic arch, the patient may be asked to shrug the shoulders, turn the head to the left, or take a deep breath to assist passage of the catheter. With the percutaneous femoral approach, two preformed catheters are used for catheterization of the right and left coronary arteries. The catheters are guided to the distal aortic arch over a Teflon-coated guidewire, the guide is then withdrawn, and the catheter is filled with contrast medium and guided to the appropriate artery.

Assessment of CAD involves evaluation of both the coronary vasculature and left ventricular function. The first step in evaluating the coronary angiogram is determining whether the coronaries are unobstructed and free of lesions. Each major artery is traced along its entire length, and branches and collaterals are noted and evaluated for irregularities or narrowing. When occlusion is present, the degree of disease and the suitability of the artery for revascularization are of primary concern. Lesions are often graded on a percentage basis reflecting the decrease in lumen diameter. Coronary arteriography provides not only an anatomic map of the coronary arteries, including the site and severity of stenotic lesions, but also the characteristics of distal vessels in terms of size, presence of atherosclerotic disease, mass of myocardium served, index of differential coronary flow, identification of collateral vessels, and an estimate of their functional importance.

Left ventriculography provides a visual analysis of wall motion. Ventricular systolic and diastolic volume and ejection fraction can be calculated. Correlation of the coronary arteriogram and left ventriculogram permits identification of stenotic and potentially bypassable arteries that serve viable myocardium. Augmenting left ventricular contraction by the use of nitrates, catecholamines, or post-extrasystolic beats may permit the identification of left ventricular wall segments that have the potential for improved function after revascularization surgery. In patients who have undergone surgery previously, the patency of grafts and the status of native coronary arteries can be ascertained.

Evaluation of myocardial function is an important part of the evaluation of CAD. Patterns of ventricular contraction and the ejection fraction are determined during angiography. Because the ejection fraction represents the ratio of the stroke volume to the end-diastolic volume, a decreasing ejection fraction may represent either a decrease in stroke volume or an increase in end-diastolic volume. The latter situation represents the compensatory mechanism for maintaining cardiac output as myocardial function decreases. Thus, the ejection fraction is a reflection of the degree to which contraction abnormalities have compromised myocardial performance.

In patients with stable angina, the incidence of single-, double-, and triple-vessel CAD is approximately the same. Abnormalities of left ventricular wall motion can be detected by contrast ventriculography in approximately 60% of patients with chronic ischemic heart disease. Intervention ventriculography may be performed in these patients to differentiate between scar tissue and reversibly ischemic myocardial segments. In some patients with chronic ischemic heart disease, a contrast left ventriculogram also reveals mitral regurgitation.

For those patients with unstable angina, single- and multiple-vessel disease also occurs with approximately equal frequency. However, the incidence of single-vessel disease is higher in patients with recent onset of angina. Left main coronary artery stenosis is more frequent in patients with unstable angina, the left anterior descending coronary artery being the most frequently affected vessel. Less developed collateral circulation has been observed in patients with unstable angina than in those with chronic stable angina.

In patients with a diagnosis of variant angina, coronary arteriography reveals fixed proximal stenosis involving at least one major coronary artery in most patients, although in some patients angiographically detectable atherosclerotic lesions are absent. In patients with suspected variant angina, provocation of coronary artery spasm is required to confirm the diagnosis. Ergonovine, methacholine, and hyperventilation have been used to provoke coronary artery spasm. However, unless the provoked coronary artery spasm is accompanied by the patient's usual chest pain, along with ECG changes indicating myocardial ischemia, the diagnosis of variant angina is not established.

ANGINA PECTORIS

Angina pectoris is a symptom of myocardial ischemia resulting from an imbalance between oxygen supply and demand, as previously described. The mechanisms of myocardial ischemia may vary in different circumstances, and, as a result, the clinical manifestations also change. An imbalance between myocardial oxygen supply and demand can occur either from a primary decrease in coronary blood flow or from a disproportionate increase in myocardial oxygen requirements. The capacity to increase coronary blood flow to the increase in myocardial oxygen demand is limited in CAD, resulting in myocardial ischemia whenever this reserve for myocardial perfusion is exceeded. Ischemia also results from a primary decrease in oxygen supply due to coronary artery vasospasm, which may occur at the point of a coronary lesion or in otherwise normal coronary arteries.

Angina can be classified as chronic exertional, variant (Prinzmetal), or unstable. Chronic exertional angina is associated with a characteristic onset, duration, location, radiation, and quality of pain. Variant angina is not typically associated with these characteristic findings. Unstable angina signifies a recent change in frequency, intensity, duration, or character of pain and may signify impending infarction.

Obstructive CAD is the most common cause of chronic ischemic heart disease. In the great majority of patients with chronic exertional angina, resting coronary blood flow is proportional to myocardial oxygen consumption (MVO_2) at rest, indicating that stenotic resistance and the resistance of the distal coronary vascular bed, which promotes coronary blood flow to meet the need for increased MVO_2, are equal. Although vasodilation increases blood flow to potentially ischemic myocardial zones, the increase in flow for a given increase in demand is progressively lessened as the degree of stenosis increases, resulting in relative myocardial ischemia. In patients with stable angina, the level of activity that precipitates angina is usually predictable. The extent of physical activity that precipitates angina appears to be inversely related to the severity but not necessarily to the extent of coronary artery lesions.

Chest discomfort produced by exertion and relieved by rest is most frequently diagnosed as exertional angina by the history alone. Chronic exertional angina may also occur postprandially because of an increase in gastrointestinal oxygen consumption both during and after a large meal. In addition, digestion requires increased cardiac output, which increases myocardial oxygen demands, resulting in anginal pain. Emotional tension has also been identified as a precursor of angina. Chest discomfort due to emotional stress tends to last longer than that produced by physical stress because emotional responses are not as easily limited as activity. For the patient with coronary atherosclerosis who cannot increase coronary blood flow, smoking tobacco will further increase myocardial workload, resulting in angina. This effect may be worsened by the presence of carboxyhemoglobin in the blood due to smoking.

NONPHARMACOLOGIC MANAGEMENT

Management of a patient with ischemic heart disease incorporates modification of risk factors for coronary atherosclerosis with nursing interventions to prevent adverse consequences of myocardial ischemia. Lifestyle changes may provide symptomatic relief or retard or reverse the atherosclerotic process. Thus, treatment of hypertension, hyperlipidemia, obesity, diabetes, and elimination of the use of cigarettes are part of the routine management of patients with ischemic heart disease. Physical exercise has been advocated for select patients with ischemic heart disease to decrease the complications of CAD.

In addition to modification of risk factors for coronary atherosclerosis, the treatment of angina and other manifestations of myocardial ischemia is based on reducing MVO_2 and increasing coronary blood flow to the potentially ischemic myocardium to restore the balance between myocardial oxygen supply and demand.

PHARMACOLOGIC MANAGEMENT

The basic goal in the pharmacologic management of angina is to reduce factors that increase myocardial oxygen demand and improve those that impinge on oxygen supply, depending on the underlying pathologic mechanism. Patients with CAD have relied on the use of pharmacologic agents to prevent and control anginal symptoms. Traditional therapy has centered on the use of nitroglycerin and nitrates for prevention and relief of anginal attacks. Beta-adrenergic blocking agents, calcium channel blockers, and antiplatelet therapies are now used in the treatment of angina.

NITRATES. Nitrates are the most common medications used to treat patients with angina pectoris. Nitroglycerin and nitrates are direct-acting, smooth muscle relaxants and cause vasodilation of the peripheral vascular bed. Peripheral vasodilation with nitrate therapy reduces MVO_2 through a reduction in cardiac preload and afterload. Nitrates dilate venous capacitance vessels, which results in decreased venous return to the heart and decreased left ventricular diastolic volume and pressure or preload. There is a reflex-mediated increase in heart rate and contractility. Arteriolar dilatation reduces systemic vascular resistance, or afterload. This further reduces left ventricular end-diastolic pressure and allows enhanced cardiac output. Decreased arterial pressure and left ventricular volume are associated with decreased left ventricular wall tension and resulting decreased MVO_2.

Nitrate therapy exerts its beneficial effects primarily by decreasing MVO_2 in patients with fixed obstructive CAD and coronary vasospasm. Increases in regional coronary blood flow and myocardial perfusion are associated with relief of angina. However, evidence suggests that it is the systemic vasodilating effects of nitrates that produce relief of anginal symptoms. The combined administration of nitrates and beta-adrenergic blocking drugs may further reduce the frequency of anginal episodes. Beta blockers may also block the reflex tachycardia, which is a potential side effect of nitrate therapy.

Sublingual nitroglycerin is the drug of choice for treatment of acute angina. Sublingual nitroglycerin may be taken prophylactically before activities likely to cause angina. Oral nitrates can increase the activity threshold for anginal symptoms and reduce the incidence of anginal attacks. Topical nitroglycerin allows daily application of medication. Absorption through the skin allows distribution of the medication without inactivation by the liver. Table 19–2 reviews the dosage and effects of the most commonly used nitrates.

BETA-ADRENERGIC BLOCKING AGENTS. Beta blockers inhibit response to adrenergic stimuli by competitively blocking adrenergic receptors. These drugs may selectively block beta-1 adrenergic receptors in the myocardium or both the myocardial beta-1 receptors and beta-2 receptors of bronchial and vascular smooth muscle. Beta blockers are classified as selective or nonselective according to their relative abilities to bind to the different beta receptors. Drugs with an affinity for beta-1 receptors such as atenolol and metoprolol are considered cardioselective because of the predominance of beta-1 receptors in the myocardium. When used in low

TABLE 19–2. **Nitrates for Anginal Therapy: Dosage, Duration, Side Effects**

Drug	Dosage/Formulation	Onset	Duration	Side Effects
Nitrostat	0.3–0.6 mg sublingual tablets	30 seconds	15–30 minutes	Headache Flushing Tachycardia
Nitrobid	2.5 mg 3 times/day sustained release capsules	1 hour	2–4 hours	Dizziness
Nitro-SA	2.5 mg 2 times/day sustained release capsules	1 hour	2–4 hours	Reflex tachycardia
Nitrol ointment	½–2 inches topically	1 hour	6–24 hours	Contact dermatitis
Isosorbid dinitrate (Isordil)	2.5–10 mg every 3 hours sublingual tablets	5 minutes	1–2 hours	Headache Flushing Dizziness Tachycardia

doses, beta-1 selective blocking agents inhibit cardiac beta-1 receptors, but have little influence on bronchial and vascular beta-2 receptors. However, at higher doses beta-1 selective blocking agents will also block beta-2 receptors, leading to increased airway resistance and the potential for bronchospasm.

Beta-blocking drugs are used for the prevention and relief of cardiac ischemia because of their ability to decrease heart rate, blood pressure, and cardiac contractility. Beta blockers, as a class, act by reducing myocardial oxygen utilization. This is accomplished through both negative inotropic and chronotropic actions produced by blockade of the cardiac beta-1 receptors. Thus, beneficial effects are related to a decrease in MVO_2. Reduced heart rate, contractility, and systemic blood pressure at any level of activity account for the reduced oxygen requirements. A decreased frequency of anginal attacks combined with a reduction in nitrate dosage and increased exercise tolerance has been noted.

Some beta-blocking drugs reduce myocardial oxygen demands through differential effects on coronary vascular resistance in both relatively ischemic and nonischemic myocardial segments. Because beta blockers reduce heart rate, diastolic filling time is lengthened, and coronary artery perfusion is improved. Beta blockers have also reduced abnormally increased platelet aggregability in patients with angina pectoris and increased tissue oxygen delivery through a rightward shift of the oxygen–hemoglobin dissociation curve.

Beta-adrenergic blocking drugs may cause fatigue, weakness, depression, gastrointestinal upset, and nightmares. As a result of beta-1 receptor blockade, bradycardia, heart block, heart failure, and hypotension may occur. In patients with impaired left ventricular function, congestive heart failure may occur or may be intensified, a side effect that can be reduced by the use of digitalis or diuretics.

Beta-2 receptor blockade may cause bronchospasm in patients with underlying obstructive lung disease. Inhibition of beta receptors may precipitate vasoconstriction, hyperglycemia, or hypoglycemia in diabetic patients. Coronary vasoconstriction may be intensified by beta-adrenergic blockade with propranolol (Held et al., 1994). Propranolol is contraindicated in patients with Prinzmetal angina because of its role in prolonging episodes of myocardial ischemia. Withdrawal symptoms have been documented when beta-blocker therapy is abruptly discontinued. Beta-blocker therapy should be tapered to avoid acute ischemic episodes.

Eight beta blockers are available for the treatment of angina pectoris. One group of beta blockers with intrinsic stimulating activity causes both blockade and stimulation of beta receptors. These drugs cause less beta antagonism, producing less reduction in resting heart rate and atrioventricular (AV) conduction and contractility at rest while blocking the effects of exercise on these parameters. Thus, a beta blocker with intrinsic stimulating activity is as effective as a beta blocker without this mechanism in reducing the normally increased heart rate and blood pressure response to exercise. Beta blockers with intrinsic stimulating activity may be of value in patients with resting bradycardia, peripheral vascular disease, or obstructive lung disease.

CALCIUM CHANNEL BLOCKERS. Drugs that inhibit the flow of calcium ions across cellular membranes (calcium channel blocking drugs) have emerged as an important addition to the pharmacologic therapy of anginal syndromes. Calcium channel blocking drugs are effective because of their ability to cause direct increases in coronary blood flow and myocardial perfusion as well as decreases in myocardial oxygen requirements. Calcium channel blocking drugs also inhibit calcium entry to the smooth muscles of the peripheral vascular bed. Blockage of calcium inflow in smooth muscle cells by calcium channel blocking agents thus decreases arterial vascular resistance. Heart rate may also decrease with the use of some calcium channel blocking agents. Vasodilation of the coronary arteries provides an increase in coronary blood flow and oxygen supply. Arteriolar vasodilation in peripheral circulation produces a reduction in afterload and reduces myocardial oxygen demand.

Calcium channel blocking agents may also increase coronary blood flow through direct mechanisms. Cal-

TABLE 19–3. **Calcium Channel Blocking Agents: Dosage, Effects**

Drug/Diagnosis	Maintenance Dosage	Metabolism	Side Effects	Contraindications	Drug Interactions
Nifedipine Angina: Prinzmetal Variant Chronic Stable	30–60 mg daily in 3 divided doses	Liver	Cardiovascular: dizziness, headache, flushing, lightheadness, hypotension, peripheral edema Central nervous system: shakiness, mood changes, weakness Gastrointestinal: nausea, diarrhea, constipation Pulmonary: dyspnea, wheeze, cough	Hypersensitivity	Beta blockers: anginal exacerbation, hypotension, congestive heart failure Fentanyl: hypertension Digoxin: increase serum concentrations Hypotensive drugs: potentiate
Verapamil Angina: Prinzmetal Variant chronic Stable	240–480 mg daily in 3–4 divided doses	Liver	Cardiovascular: bradycardia, heart block, congestive heart failure, hypotension Gastrointestinal: nausea, constipation	Left ventricular dysfunction	See under nifedipine Antidysrhythmic drugs: potentiate hypotension

cium channel blocking agents currently in use can cause dilatation of the epicardial coronary arteries, thus preventing and relieving angina due to vasospasm. Thus, coronary blood flow may increase. Three calcium channel blocking agents are approved for the treatment of angina. These agents differ in their effects on peripheral and coronary vasodilation, sinus node automaticity, AV node conduction, and myocardial contractility.

The beneficial effects of calcium channel blocking agents in the treatment of angina result from their ability to reduce myocardial oxygen needs secondary to afterload reduction and to increase coronary blood flow secondary to dilating action on the coronary vascular bed. Nifedipine is the most potent vasodilator among the calcium channel blocking agents.

Both verapamil and diltiazem reduce heart rate and AV node conduction, which may result in sinus bradycardia, sinus arrest, and AV block. Nifedipine does not alter AV node conduction, but may cause an increase in heart rate due to potent peripheral vasodilation (Lichten et al., 1990).

All calcium channel blocking agents depress myocardial contractility to some degree and thus have the potential to precipitate congestive heart failure. Verapamil is the most potent negative inotrope and should be avoided in patients with depressed left ventricular function. Left ventricular function may improve with the use of nifedipine related to its afterload reduction properties. Table 19–3 reviews the calcium channel blocking agents.

COMBINATION DRUG THERAPY. The hemodynamic properties of nitroglycerin and calcium channel blocking drugs suggest that combination therapy might be useful. The choice of pharmacologic therapy is determined by the pathophysiologic mechanism causing the angina, the severity of the angina, concomitant medical conditions, and side effects of medical therapy. Combination therapy may serve to reduce potential side effects of one class of drugs or work to enhance the oxygen supply-and-demand ratio.

The combination of a beta blocker and a calcium channel blocker is superior to either drug used alone for the treatment of angina. However, in combining beta blockers and both verapamil and diltiazem, caution should be used because severe left ventricular dysfunction may result. It is often possible to use low doses of each agent, so that the adverse effects of each drug are diminished (Pearle, 1990).

PLATELET ANTIAGGREGANTS. Platelet aggregation and platelet-derived vasoactive substances have been implicated in the occurrence of ischemic episodes and anginal symptoms. Mechanisms involved include (1) alterations in arterial blood flow due to vasospasm or transient platelet obstruction; (2) release of platelet emboli as an initiating event in sudden cardiac death; and (3) acute arterial thrombotic occlusion (Fuster & Ik-Kyung, 1994).

Currently, the platelet antiaggregants aspirin, nonsteroidal antiinflammatory drugs sulfinpyrazone, dipyridamole, and ticlopidine have been the most

TABLE 19–4. **Platelet Antiaggregants**

Drug	Inhibits Aggregation	Prolongs Bleeding Time	Prolongs Platelet Survival	Duration of Effect
Aspirin	++	++	–	1 week
Calcium channel blockers	++	++	–	24 hours
Dipyridamole	–	–	++	6 hours
Ibuprofen	++	++	–	6 hours
Indomethacin	++	++	–	24 hours
Propranolol	++	–	–	24 hours
Prostacyclin	++	++	++	10 minutes
Sulfinpyrazone	+	–	++	6 hours
Thromboxane A_2 synthesis inhibitors	++	++	++	24 hours
Ticlopidine	++	++	+	12 hours

widely used and evaluated drugs in controlling platelets by pharmacologic therapy. Drugs that modify platelet integrity perform by (1) inhibiting the arachidonic acid pathway; (2) altering platelet cyclic adenosine monophosphate (AMP) levels; (3) inhibiting thrombin formation; and (4) modifying platelet behavior. Table 19–4 describes the varying effects of the most common platelet antiaggregants. Both aspirin and other nonsteroidal antiinflammatory compounds act on the arachidonate pathway by inhibiting its main enzymes. Platelet aggregation is blocked by competitive inactivation of cyclooxygenase, which converts arachidonic acid to indoperoxides. This process leads to the formation of regulatory prostaglandins.

Aspirin acts on platelets by reducing occlusion of small vessels by platelet aggregates. Ingestion of 325 mg of aspirin will inhibit thromboxane A_2 synthesis and platelet aggregation for approximately 48 hours (Clark et al., 1991). Cyclooxygenase is inhibited in 10 days. When administering aspirin in combination with other oral anticoagulants, care should be taken because of the additive effects. In addition, chronic aspirin administration may lead to hyperuricemia or an elevated blood urea nitrogen.

Unlike aspirin, sulfinpyrazone competitively inhibits cyclooxygenase and therefore has reversible side effects. In therapeutic doses of 400 to 800 mg daily, bleeding time is not prolonged, and platelet aggregation is not affected. Sulfinpyrazone has an additive effect when administered with oral anticoagulants, and may produce an increase in hypoglycemia when used with hypoglycemic agents. Because of uricosuric mechanisms, fluid intake must be sufficient to support urinary output and avoid potential uric acid nephropathy. The uricosuric action of sulfinpyrazone is antagonized by aspirin and other salicylates.

Imidazole compounds are selective in platelet inhibition. They inhibit thromboxane synthetase, the enzyme responsible for the synthesis of thromboxane A_2, but not of active prostaglandins. Selective inhibition of thromboxane synthetase may provide an increase in the amount of prostaglandin endoperoxide available for conversion to prostacyclin.

Pharmacologic agents that increase cyclic AMP levels inhibit platelet adhesion and aggregation. Cyclic AMP is increased by stimulation of adenylate cyclase and by blockage of platelet phosphodiesterase, which breaks down cyclic AMP. Dipyridamole is an inhibitor of platelet phosphodiesterase, an enzyme responsible for the conversion of adenosine triphosphate to adenosine diphosphate (ADP). By blocking this conversion, dipyridamole potentiates increased cyclic AMP formation and impairs platelet aggregation. Dipyridamole also lengthens platelet survival and inhibits platelet adhesion to the damaged endothelium, thereby reducing thrombus formation at the sites of injury. Prostacyclin also serves to increase cyclic AMP levels, leading to inhibition of platelet adhesion, release reaction, and aggregation. Dipyridamole is administered in 50-mg doses three times each day. This drug is generally free of toxicity or drug interactions. Potential side effects include gastric distress and headaches.

TICLOPIDINE. Ticlopidine is chemically unrelated to other antithrombotic agents, and its mechanism of action is not completely understood. Ticlopidine appears to alter platelet membrane reactivity, prolongs bleeding time, and normalizes platelet survival. Preliminary evidence suggests that ticlopidine is effective in patients with unstable angina for the prevention of myocardial infarction and cardiovascular death (Balsano et al., 1990), for reducing vein graft closure after coronary bypass surgery (White et al., 1987), and for reducing acute thrombotic occlusion after coronary angioplasty (Limet et al., 1987).

There is no evidence that ticlopidine is superior to aspirin, and therefore its benefits are not clear. Side effects of this agent can be serious. At the present time, ticlopidine is recommended only in patients who cannot take aspirin.

ANTIANGINAL DRUGS AS PLATELET ANTIAGGREGANTS. Nitroglycerin and nitrates inhibit platelet arachidonate metabolism through direct antiplatelet mechanisms and increased prostacyclin synthesis. Both direct antiplatelet effects and prostacyclin synthesis mechanisms are dose dependent. Beta-adrenergic blocking agents such as propranolol have been shown to reduce platelet aggregability in doses sufficient to improve exercise tolerance. Propranolol binds to the platelet membrane and may serve to both inhibit phospholipase and decrease thromboxane A_2 formation and release.

Calcium channel blocking agents function as platelet antiaggregants through a variety of mechanisms. Diltiazem inhibits ADP formation as well as collagen and arachidonate acid-induced platelet aggregation. Nifedipine inhibits epinephrine-induced platelet aggregation through inhibition of thromboxane receptors. Verapamil both inhibits membrane alpha-adrenergic receptors and blocks intraplatelet calcium influx.

INVASIVE MANAGEMENT

CORONARY ARTERY ANGIOPLASTY. Percutaneous transluminal coronary angioplasty (PTCA) has been established as an effective method for both improving symptoms and ameliorating the metabolic, hemodynamic, and functional consequences of myocardial ischemia in selected patients. Angioplasty decreases or eliminates resistance at the site of coronary artery stenosis and enhances blood flow to ischemic myocardial segments. Thus increased coronary perfusion rather than decreased MVO_2 is the mechanism causing the beneficial aspects of angioplasty.

TECHNIQUE. Coronary angioplasty involves the introduction of an outer guiding catheter and a double-lumen dilatation catheter into either the femoral or the brachial artery. The catheter is guided through the ascending aorta and into the ostium of the right or left coronary artery. Advancement of the catheter as well as visualization of the stenotic vessel is enhanced through angiography. When the correct position is ensured, the balloon-tipped dilating catheter is inserted through the guiding catheter and into the artery's stenotic area. Continuous pressure monitoring reveals blockage of the coronary artery ostium and permits measurement of the pressure gradient across the lesion.

The number of balloon inflations, inflation time, and balloon size are relative to the coronary vessel involved, the degree of stenosis, and the occurrence of ischemic symptoms during the procedure. With successful dilation, the balloon catheter is removed after a period of observation, and a repeat angiogram is performed. If residual obstruction is noted, the lesion is recrossed, and additional inflations are performed. When the procedure is completed, the inner cannulas are secured within the femoral sheaths, and the patient is transported to the critical care unit or angioplasty observation unit.

PATIENT SELECTION. Patient eligibility for both initial and repeat PTCA has been established on the basis of clinical and morphologic considerations. Clinical factors associated with reduced procedural risk and successful dilatation include the presence of well defined, limiting ischemic symptoms and ischemic symptoms of short duration. In addition, the eligibility of the patient for potential coronary artery bypass surgery must also be considered.

Isolated, discrete single-vessel disease remains the classic angiographic indication for PTCA (Myler & Stertzer, 1994). In patients with single-vessel disease, PTCA treats fixed, noncalcified lesions in the proximal two-thirds of the coronary circulation that are accessible for dilatation. However, patients with multivessel disease have undergone angioplasty with satisfactory outcome (O'Keefe et al., 1990).

Although repeat PTCA can be performed safely in most patients with restenosis, screening for eligibility in this population is of primary importance. Repeat PTCA should be considered carefully for high-risk patients such as those with left anterior descending artery lesions, a time interval of less than 3 months between the first and second PTCA procedures, diabetes mellitus, and the presence of multiple lesions (Deligonaul et al., 1989).

A subset of patients with double-vessel disease may also be considered as candidates for PTCA. Selection in this group corresponds to the criteria used for single-vessel disease and excludes patients with high-risk lesions at either vessel site.

In selected patients who have undergone coronary artery bypass grafting, PTCA may be used as an alternative to additional surgery. Angiographic indications for PTCA in this population include vessels jeopardized by graft closure, lesions distal to implanted grafts, lesions proximal to patent grafts but compromising collateral flow, and distal anastomoses.

RESULTS. The primary goal of PTCA is the successful dilation of involved coronary arteries as evidenced by angiography. Reduced pressure gradients across the arterial narrowing and the relief of ischemic symptoms are also considered essential (Ellis, 1994). The effectiveness of PTCA in achieving these goals has been documented in patients with both stable and unstable angina pectoris. The long-term efficacy of PTCA in patients with CAD has been established, with follow-up periods of up to 8 years (Myler et al., 1993).

Although most patients continue to demonstrate sustained angiographic and clinical improvement after successful dilatation, a number of patients evidence recurrent stenosis. Occurring in approximately 30% to 50% of patients, restenosis presents an important limitation to the long-term efficacy of coronary angioplasty. Data indicate that patients with multivessel disease and complete revascularization have significantly higher restenosis rates per patient than patients with multivessel disease and incomplete revascularization (Nobuyoshi et al., 1988). In addition, multilesion stenosis has been found to be greater in patients with three-vessel disease than those with two-vessel disease (Deligonaul et al., 1988). The basis for recurrent disease is not known, but may reflect fibrocellular proliferation that exceeds the corrective effects of angioplasty. Restenosis is usually manifested as recurrent angina appearing 2 to 4 months after successful dilatation. Repeat dilatation can be performed in selected patients with a high success rate and a low complication rate (Douglas et al., 1990).

Recurrence rates after successful angioplasty have not been established. Potential reasons are the lack of a standard definition of recurrence as well as the difficulty of achieving angiographic follow-up.

POTENTIAL RISKS. Since 1976, coronary angioplasty has undergone many refinements with resulting reductions in procedural morbidity and mortality. Mortality associated with dilatation in single-vessel disease is approximately 1%. An increased risk of mortality has been identified in women, patients older than 60 years of age, and patients who have had coronary bypass grafting.

The most frequent major complication of PTCA is coronary artery dissection as a result of localized trauma. Reported in approximately 5% of patients, acute reduction in coronary blood flow may be manifested as prolonged angina or coronary occlusion leading to infarction (Holmes et al., 1988). Additional bases for myocardial ischemia include coronary artery spasm, coronary embolization, and intimal trauma.

Associated minor complications include bradycardia, ventricular fibrillation, hypotension, and vascular complications including hematoma formation and retroperitoneal blood loss.

Preangioplasty and postangioplasty nursing interventions are similar to those described for the patient undergoing cardiac catheterization. Nursing interventions specific to PTCA are presented in Table 19–4.

SECOND-GENERATION INTERVENTIONAL DEVICES. The mechanisms of vessel injury and the subsequent healing responses associated with coronary angioplasty suggest a set of specifications for the development and evaluation of second-generation interventional devices. Second-generation interventional devices currently under investigation for the management of CAD include metallic stents, atherectomy, and lasers. Researchers and clinicians are evaluating these devices for their ability to selectively remove atheroma mass or render it more pliable; limit or control intimal or medial injury; minimize elastic recoil of the vessel wall; and limit trauma to normal portions of the vessel wall.

STENTS. As an alternative to repeat dilation after PTCA, Sigwart and associates (1987) developed an intravascular mechanical support with the goal of reducing arterial restenosis and closure after angioplasty. The intravascular stents currently under clinical evaluation consist of a metallic mesh that is implanted deeply into the intima or media and chronically overstretches the vessel wall. Although a number of stent prototypes are available, the principles of deliverability, versatility, and biocompatibility determine the clinical usefulness of the stent.

Several investigators have reported abundant smooth muscle cell proliferation and concentric intimal thickening after stenting normal or atherosclerotic swine vessels. Coronary stenting is associated with more smooth muscle cell proliferation and uniform intimal thickening than balloon injury models. However, the final luminal area by angiographic and histologic analysis is significantly greater in stented vessels.

Data on the incidence of restenosis after stenting are limited. Initial trials indicate an overall incidence of restenosis ranging from 28% in native coronary arteries (Leon et al., 1992) to 21% for de novo native coronary stenosis (Savage et al., 1992). Compared with conventional angioplasty, restenosis rate for stented patients at 3 to 6 months was 10% versus 39% (Kimura et al., 1992). Risk factors for stent restenosis include multiple contiguous stents, final diameter less than or equal to 3.25 mm, stenting restenotic arteries, diabetes, and left anterior descending placement (Carrozza et al., 1992; Fajadet et al., 1992; Strauss et al., 1991).

The precise indications for the use of intravascular stents in the future will be defined only after the completion of additional clinical trials. Current studies are limited because of the exclusion of patients with small or diffusely diseased vessels. In addition, the potential benefits of stenting must be weighed against the risks of subacute thrombosis, bleeding complications, and the costs of prolonged hospital stay (Eigler & Forrester, 1994).

DIRECTIONAL CORONARY ATHERECTOMY. Directional atherectomy, the controlled, transluminal removal of atheroma, was approved for the treatment of coronary atherosclerotic disease in 1990, as a means of addressing the major limitations of PTCA: abrupt closure, primary failure, and restenosis. Directional coronary atherectomy (DCA) has been shown effectively to remove atheromas and increase the pliability of remaining lesions, especially for bulky, noncalcified lesions in large proximal vessels. Multicenter data have documented the safety and efficacy of DCA, with success rates ranging from 86% to 89% (U.S. Directional Coronary Atherectomy Group, 1990).

The large size of the DCA device and its inflexibility make mechanical injury more common than with PTCA. In addition, tissue analysis and intravascular ultrasound imaging have shown that atherectomy frequently removes constituents of the normal vascular wall (Hinohara et al., 1991). Finally, the risk of coronary perforation is greater in DCA compared with conventional balloon angioplasty (Simpson et al., 1989).

Clinical trials document restenosis in 30% to 60% of DCA cases, depending on the patient population (Garratt et al., 1992; Kuntz et al., 1992). Restenosis appears to be lower for de novo lesions in native coronary arteries compared to restenotic lesions (Garratt et al., 1992). Predictors of restenosis after DCA include vessel size less than or equal to 3 mm, post-DCA lesion diameter less than 3 mm, and device size.

Trials have begun in a prospective, randomized fashion to compare DCA with standard balloon angioplasty. The atherectomy procedure will continue to evolve rapidly as design changes are available based on growing experience. Future refinements of the directional atherectomy system will improve flexibility, facilitate excision of calcified tissue, and permit ultrasonic guidance to enhance selective plaque removal (Eigler & Forrester, 1994).

LASER ANGIOPLASTY. The use of laser radiation is an adjunct to PTCA and coronary bypass surgery in the revascularization of occluded vessels. The laser is a monochromatic and coherent light amplification stimulated by the emission of radiation. The suitability of laser radiation for use in opening coronary and peripheral atherosclerotic plaque obstructions is based on the ability to transmit the laser through an optical fiber, to direct it precisely, and to use it for tissue photocoagulation and on its capability for selective absorption.

The total amount of energy delivered by a laser is defined by the pulse duration and strength of the radiation wavelength used. The degree of laser penetration of atherosclerotic plaque depends on the beam focus, the total energy delivered, and the duration of exposure, as well as the density and absorptive characteristics of the atherosclerotic tissue.

When the laser is directed at tissue, the tissue may reflect, absorb, transmit, or scatter the light. Atherosclerotic plaque, which may have a homogeneous or a heterogeneous composition, has an unpredictable absorption pattern. Fibrous areas of plaque or calcified plaque will have different absorption characteristics than primarily lipid-containing lesions.

There are three types of lasers currently used for medical purposes, the carbon dioxide (CO_2) laser, the argon laser, and the neodymium-yttrium-aluminum garnet (Nd:YAG) laser. The infrared wavelength emitted by the CO_2 laser is well absorbed by the water in plasma and in red blood cells. This property makes the CO_2 laser less efficient for vaporizing tissues through a water or blood medium because the majority of laser energy is absorbed by the fluid. Argon laser radiation is poorly absorbed by water but is well absorbed by hemoglobin, making it suitable for use in revascularization. The Nd:YAG laser's wavelength is partially absorbed by water in plasma and in red blood cells, but remains effective in vaporizing tissue through a fluid medium.

Several recent investigations have demonstrated the ability of lasers to penetrate and affect the vaporization of atherosclerotic plaque. Laser recanalization of obstructed vessels can be approached in two ways. In most approaches laser energy is passed through a semiflexible laser fiber using a percutaneous transluminal approach, but some clinicians use direct laser application in laser-assisted endarterectomy.

From the time the laser was shown to be effective in removing coronary atherosclerotic obstruction in cadaver hearts, attempts have been made to apply laser technology to the clinical setting. Clinical trials of laser balloon angioplasty have focused on patients with suboptimal angioplasty results or impending closure after repeated balloon inflations. Directed pulse laser angioplasty has been documented in patients with complex lesions associated with a high incidence of restenosis, chronic total occlusions, and saphenous vein grafts.

Restenosis rates using laser balloon angioplasty have ranged from 56% to over 70% (Reis et al., 1991). Similarly, directed pulsed laser angioplasty has shown a 48% restenosis rate (Bittl et al., 1992). The laser-driven devices may have worsened the extent of vascular injury, compared with standard balloon angioplasty, because of poor temperature control. Studies are now underway that include improvements in delivery catheter design and laser technique to minimize the mechanisms of vascular injury.

The nursing care of the laser angioplasty patient is comparable to that of the patient who has undergone PTCA.

CORONARY ARTERY BYPASS SURGERY. Coronary artery bypass surgery is performed to relieve the symptoms of myocardial ischemia by revascularizing the myocardium. The procedure is not indicated for relief of myocardial ischemia that is not manifested by angina unless a left main coronary lesion has been documented by angiography. (See Chapter 24 for a detailed discussion of surgery.)

SUDDEN DEATH

Sudden cardiac death is defined as an unexpected, witnessed death of an apparently healthy person resulting from cardiac dysfunction and occurring within 6 hours of the onset of new symptoms. This definition does not include people who have had a recent acute onset of heart disease, but does include people with known CAD if their condition is considered stable (Ruskin et al., in press).

More than 300,000 sudden coronary deaths occur each year, representing one-half of the annual coronary mortality. Sudden coronary death occurs in women at only one-fourth the rate seen in men, and the occurrence in women lags behind that of men by 20 years. Sudden death occurs more frequently in men with an average age of 60 years. At any age, in either sex, those who are especially vulnerable can be identified from their coronary risk profile. The presence of CAD is by far the most common indicator of sudden cardiac death. In attempting to define the candidate for sudden death, emphasis must be placed on CAD and its precursors.

Pathophysiology

The atherosclerotic coronary artery plaque is the most frequent pathologic (postmortem) finding in cases of sudden death. Ventricular fibrillation is the leading cause of cardiac arrest in sudden death victims. It is believed to be triggered by ischemia due to coronary vascular changes leading to electrical instability of the myocardium. Most episodes of sudden cardiac death are not initiated by acute myocardial infarction.

The major cardiac risk factors are commonly present in victims of sudden cardiac deaths, namely, hypertension, hypercholesterolemia, or a history of cigarette smoking.

Four major characteristics are associated with an increased risk of sudden death: (1) ventricular electrical instability, (2) extensive coronary artery narrowing, (3) abnormal left ventricular function, and (4) ECG conduction and repolarization abnormalities. Ventricular ectopic activity in people with atherosclerotic heart disease is predictive of sudden cardiac death in 78% to 95% of patients, especially complex ventricular ectopy. It is important to note that ventricular ectopic activity by itself has little prognostic importance in people without atherosclerotic heart disease. Patients who suffer sudden cardiac death typically have severe coronary artery narrowing in two or three coronary arteries. Left ventricular dysfunction and congestive heart failure are associated with ventricular dysrhythmias, indicating a possible interaction between ventricular dysfunction and ventricular dysrhythmias. Impairment of left ventricular function is reflected by the systolic ejection fraction. Last, ECG abnormalities include prolongation of Q–T intervals and ST-T changes.

Data from the Framingham Study indicate a threefold increased risk of sudden death in subjects with ventricular premature contractions compared with those who do not exhibit them on a standard ECG at rest. However, virtually all patients with ventricular premature contractions who died suddenly also had other abnormalities such as left ventricular hypertrophy, ventricular conduction disturbances, or cardiovascular disease history.

Definitive mechanisms of ventricular fibrillation have not been established. However, it is well established that nonuniform cardiac recovery properties reduce the threshold for ventricular fibrillation. A variety of states, including ischemia and sympathetic stimulation, increase the degree of inequality of refractory periods in ventricular muscle.

Ventricular tachycardia can result from several causes, but the predominant theory involves reentry. Reentry is a self-perpetuating tachydysrhythmia frequently associated with hemodynamic collapse and subsequent degeneration to ventricular fibrillation (see Chapter 11). In the reentry mechanism, one of the ventricular pathways may be refractory or may conduct more slowly than an adjacent pathway. The impulse is temporarily slowed but conducts normally through adjacent areas. When the impulse arrives at the previously refractory branch it may find it excitable, thus allowing retrograde conduction. This type of dysrhythmia is frequently found in individuals with a unidirectional block in one limb of the conduction pathway (see Chapter 11). Blocks such as this may occur in individuals with congenitally deformed conduction systems (Braunwald et al., 1992) or diseased, ischemic hearts.

Virtually everyone with premature contractions who dies suddenly has evidence of an ischemic myocardium, usually with other ECG abnormalities. People with overt CAD are at a fourfold increased risk of sudden death, but only because of a greater incidence of coronary attacks.

Ventricular dysrhythmias that are related to myocardial ischemia may be caused by the effects of hypoxia, pH changes, and anaerobic metabolism on the electrical properties of cardiac fibers (see Chapter 11). An abnormal "slow response" action potential of the myocardial cells induced by calcium, potassium, and catecholamine release may be one cause of ventricular fibrillation in sudden cardiac death.

The prevalence of ventricular premature beats is greater in men and increases with age, with the presence of other ECG-demonstrated ischemic abnormalities, and with the severity of the coronary risk profile. Angiographic study in coronary patients indicates that a higher prevalence and a more severe grade of ventricular premature contractions exist in patients with multivessel CAD than in those with only one vessel involved. Thus, ventricular premature contractions, particularly when frequent or complex, often serve as an indicator of severe cardiac disease and left ventricular dysfunction.

Pharmacologic Management

Antidysrhythmic drug therapy is always the first line of defense against recurrent ventricular dysrhythmias. Antidysrhythmic drugs suppress ventricular dysrhythmias by (1) altering the conductivity of myocardial tissue, (2) altering the refractory period of myocardial tissue, and (3) increasing myocardial electrical activity.

Antidysrhythmic drugs are classified according to their effects on cardiac muscle action potential (Table 19–5). Class I drugs interfere directly with depolarization and repolarization of the cardiac muscle. This class of drugs is effective in treating recurrent ventricular dysrhythmias due to abnormal automaticity or reentry mechanisms. Drugs are subclassified according to their effects on action potential duration as follows: IA, prolongation; IB, shortening; IC, no effect. These drugs have little effect on QRS width or QRS interval as seen on ECG. Class II drugs produce antisympathetic effects. Beta-blocking drugs have been shown to control ventricular dysrhythmias associated with exercise or adrenergic stimulation. These drugs are used to treat angina associated with an ischemic myocardium rather than sustained ventricular dysrhythmias. Class III drugs markedly prolong the duration of the action potential. This effect has been successful in treatment of resistant ventricular dysrhythmias. Electrophysiologic effects are QRS widening and Q–T prolongation. Class IV drugs, the calcium antagonists, affect the slow inward depolarizing current in the sinoatrial and AV nodes. These drugs are used in the treatment of angina pectoris as well as supraventricular tachycardias that use the AV node as part of the reentrant circuit. Calcium antagonists are ineffective in treating recurrent ventricular dysrhythmias.

Patients receiving antidysrhythmic drug therapy must be monitored for signs of intolerance, toxicity, increases of intolerance, increases in ventricular ectopic activity, and changes in P–R, QRS, and Q–T intervals. Serum drug levels must also be monitored and toxic or subtherapeutic levels identified.

Nonpharmacologic Management

Occasionally a person will have a dysrhythmia that is resistant to all medications tested. In this event, other treatment modalities are indicated. Intraoperative mapping with endocardial resection of the site of dysrhythmia origination is one possibility. Surgical intervention, intended to excise the focus or interrupt reentrant conduction, is used to abolish dysrhythmias or increase drug manageability.

Currently, antitachycardia pacemakers are being evaluated for efficacy in patients who have had one or more episodes of sustained ventricular tachycardia with hemodynamic collapse and who have failed to respond to antidysrhythmic pharmacologic therapy as evaluated by electrophysiologic testing. The automatic implantable cardioverter defibrillator (AICD) detects and terminates life-threatening ventricular dysrhythmias (see Chapter 12).

Intraoperative mapping is a technique wherein the electrical activity of the epicardial or endocardial surface of the myocardium is recorded with delineation of impulse origination and sequence conduction. In this

TABLE 19–5. **Antidysrhythmic Drugs: Dosage and Effects**

Drug/Class	Maintenance Dosage/ Therapeutic Level	Metabolism	Major Effects	Side Effects
Lidocaine (Class I)	IV bolus: 50–100 mg constant infusion of 2–4 mg/minute. Therapeutic serum level: 1.5–4.0 mg/mL	Liver	↓ Automaticity ↓ Refractory period ↓ Repolarization ECG: No change in QRS or Q–T intervals	Cardiovascular: bradycardia Central nervous system: drowsiness, irritability, tinnitus, focal seizures, weakness, visual disturbances Gastrointestinal: diarrhea, nausea/vomiting
Tocainide (Class I)	PO: 400–600 mg every 8 hours after loading dose	Liver	See under Lidocaine	See under Lidocaine
Quinidine (Class I)	PO: 200–400 mg each 4–6 hours. Therapeutic serum level: 3–6 mg/mL	Liver/Kidney	↓ Automaticity ↓ Conductivity ↑ Repolarization ECG: prolonged Q–T interval; widened QRS interval	Cardiovascular: sinus arrest, sinoatrial block, ventricular fibrillation, hypotension Central nervous system: blurred vision Gastrointestinal: diarrhea, anorexia Hematologic: thrombocytopenia
Procainamide (Class IA)	PO: 1 g initially; 350–500 mg every 4–6 hours. Therapeutic serum level: 4–8 mg/mL	Liver/Kidney	↑ Repolarization ↓ Automaticity ↓ Conductivity ECG: prolonged P–R, Q–T, QRS intervals	Cardiovascular: heart block, ventricular fibrillation, hypotension Central nervous system: insomnia, weakness, depression Gastrointestinal: anorexia, nausea/vomiting Hematologic: agranulocytosis
Flecainide, encainide, lorcainide (Class I)	PO: 100–200 mg twice daily. Therapeutic serum level: 0.2–1 μg/mL	Liver/Kidney	↓ Conductivity ECG: prolonged QRS interval	Cardiovascular: may worsen dysrhythmias Central nervous system: dizziness, blurred vision, headache Gastrointestinal: nausea
Mexilitine (Class I)	PO: 600 mg loading dose; 500–1,000 mg daily	Liver	See under Lidocaine	See under Lidocaine
Disopyramide (Norpace) (Class I)	PO: 200–400 mg loading dose; 100–200 mg every 6 hours		↓ Automaticity ↓ Conductivity ↑ Refractory period ECG: prolonged Q–T interval	Cardiovascular: hypotension, heart block, heart failure Central nervous system: dry mouth, blurred vision, headache, fatigue, aggravation of glaucoma Genitourinary: urinary retention
Propranolol (Class II)	IV: 1 mg/minute to 5–7 mg PO: 10–200 mg 2–3 times a day	Liver	↓ Heart rate ↓ Contractility ↓ Automaticity ↓ Conductivity ↑ AV node ↓ Refractory period ECG: no effect on QRS or Q–T intervals	Cardiovascular: hypotension, bradycardia, congestive heart failure, heart block Central nervous system: dizziness, fatigue, insomnia, depression Gastrointestinal: diarrhea, nausea, cramping, hyperglycemia/hypoglycemia
Amiodarone (Class III)	600–800 mg each day for 1–2 weeks Loading dose: 200–600 mg daily		↑ Refractory period ↑ Repolarization	Cardiovascular: hypotension, AV block, bradycardia Dermatologic: photosensitivity, rash
Bretylium (Class III)	IV: 5–10 mg/kg repeat 1–2 hours; 5 mg/kg every 6–8 hours 1–2 mg/minute drip		↑ Ventricular refractory period ↑ Ventricular fibrillation threshold ECG: prolongation of QRS and Q–T intervals	Cardiovascular: hypotension Gastrointestinal: vomiting/nausea
Verapamil (Class IV)	PO: 480–640 mg/day divided dose	Kidney	↓ AV node conduction ↓ Automaticity ↑ Refractory period	Cardiovascular: hypotension, bradycardia, AV block, asystole Central nervous system: headache, dizziness

Abbreviations: AV, atrioventricular; ECG, electrocardiogram.

way, areas of electrically diseased tissue are identified. Surgical treatment for ventricular dysrhythmias provides elimination of those areas of diseased myocardium that are responsible for recurrent ventricular tachycardia through endocardial resection.

Additional measures that may be used to prevent death or disability from sudden cardiac death episodes include cardiac resuscitation from ventricular fibrillation through community emergency medical aid units and through education of lay persons (including school children) in cardiopulmonary resuscitation. Multifactorial intervention programs that include exercise conditioning and modification of cardiovascular risk factors may also serve to decrease sudden cardiac death by decreasing the incidence of ischemic events due to coronary heart disease.

SUMMARY

Although CAD continues to be the number one cause of disability and death in the western world, a steady decline has been observed over the past 10 to 15 years. The decrease has been attributed to better diagnosis and treatment and primary preventive efforts through elimination or reduction of risk factors. A comprehensive approach to coronary risk management appears most effective for patients with symptomatic CAD. Emphasis must involve avoidance of cigarette smoking, reduction of dietary intake of cholesterol, saturated fat, sodium, and total calories, as well as initiation and maintenance of a program of regular physical activity. Advanced technology and pharmacology for the treatment of CAD mean new responsibilities for the critical care nurse. In addition, the challenge of promoting sustained lifestyle change to reduce or eliminate atherogenic risk factors has not been met. Thus, health care providers in critical care will continue to be faced with new knowledge and the commitment to apply the knowledge to the care of the patient with CAD.

REFERENCES

American Heart Association. (1992). *Heart facts.* Dallas: AHA National Center.

Balsano, R., Rizzon, P., Violi, F., et al. (1990). Antiplatelet treatment with ticlopidine in unstable angina: A controlled multicenter trial. *Circulation, 82,* 17–26.

Bittl, J. A., Kuntz, R. E., Ahmed, W. H., et al. (1992). The effect of acute procedural results on restenosis after excimer laser coronary angioplasty. *Circulation, 86*(Suppl I), I-532.

Bjorntorp, P. (1990). "Portal" adipose tissue as a generator of risk factors for cardiovascular disease and diabetes. *Arteriosclerosis, 10,* 493–496.

Braunwald, E. (1992). *Heart disease: A textbook of cardiovascular medicine* (4th ed.). Philadelphia: W. B. Saunders.

Carrozza, J. P., Kunitz, R. E., Levine, M. J., et al. (1992). Angiographic and clinical outcome of intracoronary stenting: Immediate and long-term results from a large single center experience. *Journal of the American College of Cardiology, 20,* 328.

Chatterjie, K. (1994). Ischemia heart disease. In J. Stein (Ed.), *Internal medicine.* Boston: Little, Brown and Company.

Clark, R. J., Mayo, G., Price, P., & Fitzgerald, G. A. (1991). Suppression of thromboxane A_2 but not systemic prostacycline by controlled-release aspirin. *New England Journal of Medicine, 325,* 1137–1141.

Cowley, M. J., DiSciascio, G., Rehr, G. B., & Vetrovec, G. W. (1989). Angiographic observations and clinical relevance or coronary thrombosis in unstable angina pectoris. *American Journal of Cardiology, 63,* 108E–113E.

Deligonaul, U., Vandormael, M., Kern, M. J., & Galan, K. (1989). Repeat coronary angioplasty for restenosis: Results and predictors for follow-up clinical events. *American Heart Journal, 117,* 997.

Deligonaul, U., Vandormael, M. G., Kern, M. J., et al. (1988). Coronary angioplasty: A therapeutic option for symptomatic patients with two and three vessel coronary disease. *Journal of the American College of Cardiology, 11,* 1173.

Douglas, J. S., King, S. B., & Roubin, G. S. (1990). Technique of percutaneous transluminal angioplasty of the coronary, renal, mesenteric, and peripheral arteries. In W. Hurst, et al. (Eds.), *The heart VII* (pp. 2131–2156). New York: McGraw-Hill.

Eigler, N., & Forrester, J. S. (1994). Nonpharmacologic device prevention of coronary restenosis. In E. J. Topol (Ed.), *Interventional cardiology* (pp. 400–414). Philadelphia: W. B. Saunders.

Ellis, S. (1994). Elective coronary angioplasty: Technique and complications. In E. J. Topol (Ed.), *Interventional cardiology* (pp. 186–206). Philadelphia: W. B. Saunders.

Fajadet, J., Doucet, S., Caillard, J., et al. (1992). Predictors of restenosis after Palmaz-Schatz implantation. *Circulation, 86*(Suppl I), I-531.

Falk, E. (1989). Morphologic features of unstable atherthrombic plaques underlying acute coronary syndromes. *The American Journal of Cardiology, 63,* 114E–120E.

Fleischer, D. E., & Goldstein, S. A. (1990). Transesophageal echocardiology: What the gastroenterologist thinks the cardiologist should know about endoscopy. *Journal of the American Society of Echocardiology, 3,* 428–434.

Forrester, J. S., Litvack, F., Grundfest, W., & Hickey, A. (1987). A perspective of coronary disease seen through the arteries of living man. *Circulation, 75,* 505–513.

Froelicher, V., & Pashkow, F. J. (1993). Exercise electrocardiographic testing. In F. J. Pashkow & W. J. Dafoe (Eds.), *Clinical cardiac rehabilitation* (pp. 49–77). Baltimore: Williams & Wilkins.

Fuster, V., & Ik-Kyung, J. (1994). Role of platelet inhibitor agents in coronary artery disease. In E. J. Topol (Ed.), *Textbook of interventional cardiology* (pp. 3–22). Philadelphia: W. B. Saunders.

Garratt, K. N., Holmes, D. R., Bell, M. R., et al. (1992). Results of directional atherectomy of primary atheromatous and restenosis lesions in coronary arteries and saphenous vein grafts. *American Journal of Cardiology, 70,* 449.

Held, P. H., Teo, K. K., & Yusuf, S. (1994). Effects of beta-blockers, calcium channel blockers, nitrates, and magnesium in acute myocardial infarction and unstable angina pectoris. In E. J. Topol (Ed.), *Interventional cardiology Vol. I.* (pp. 46–59). Philadelphia: W. B. Saunders.

Hinohara, T., Rowe, M. H., Robertson, G. C., et al. (1991). Effect of lesion characteristics on outcome of directional coronary atherectomy. *Journal of the American College of Cardiology, 17,* 1112.

Holmes, D. R., Holbukov, R., & Vliestra, R. E. (1988). Comparison of complications during PTCA in the NHLBI PTCA Registry. *Journal of the American College of Cardiology, 12,* 1149–1155.

Iskandrian, A. S., Chae, S. C., Heo, J., Stanberry, C. D., Wasserleben, V., & Cave, V. (1993). Independent and incremental prognostic value of exercise single-photon emission computed tomographic (SPECT): Thallium imaging in coronary artery disease. *Journal of American College of Cardiology, 22,* 665–670.

Kahn, J. K. (1991). Advances in noninvasive detection of CAD. *Post Graduate Medicine, 89*(5), 149–158.

Kimura, T., Nosaka, H., Nobuyoshi, M., et al. (1992). Serial angiographic follow up after Palmaz-Schatz implantation: Retrospective comparison with conventional balloon angioplasty. *Journal of the American College of Cardiology, 19,* 197A.

King, A. C., Carl, F., Birkel, L., & Haskell, W. L. (1988). Increasing exercise among blue-collar employees: The tailoring of worksite programs to meet specific needs. *Preventive Medicine, 17,* 357–365.

Kuntz, R. E., Safian, R. D., Levine, M. J., et al. (1992). Novel approach to the analysis of restenosis after the use of three new coronary devices. *Journal of the American College of Cardiology, 19,* 1493.

Leon, M. B., Kent, K. M., Baim, D. S., et al. (1992). Comparison of stent implantation in native coronaries and saphenous vein grafts. *Journal of the American College of Cardiology, 19,* 263A.

Lichten, P. R., Hugenholtz, P. G., Rafflenbeul, W., et al. (1990). On behalf of the INTACT group investigators. *Lancet, 335,* 1109–1113.

Limet, R., David, J. L., Magotteaux, P., et al. (1987). Prevention of aortacoronary bypass graft occlusion. *Journal of Thoracic and Vascular Surgery, 94,* 773–783.

Matusuzaki, M., Toma, Y., & Kusukawa, R. (1990). Clinical applications of transesophageal echocardiography. *Circulation, 82,* 709–722.

Myler, R. K., & Stertzer, S. H. (1994). Coronary and peripheral angioplasty: Historic perspective. In E. J. Topol (Ed.), *Interventional cardiology* (pp. 171–185). Philadelphia: W. B. Saunders.

Myler, R. K., Shaw, R. E., Baciewicz, P. A., et al. (1993). Five year comparison of triple vessel revascularization coronary bypass surgery versus balloon angioplasty. *Journal of the American College of Cardiology, 21,* 73A.

Nobuyoshi, M., Kimura, T., & Nosaka, H. (1988). Restenosis after successful percutaneous transluminal coronary angioplasty: Serial angiographic followup of 229 patients. *Journal of the American College of Cardiology, 12,* 616.

O'Keefe, J. H., Rutherford, E. D., McConahay, D. R., et al. (1990). Multivessel coronary angioplasty from 1980 to 1989: Procedural results and long-term outcome. *Journal of the American College of Cardiology, 16,* 1097.

Pearle, D. (1990). Pharmacologic management of ischemic heart disease with β-blockers and calcium channel blockers. *American Heart Journal, 120,* 739.

Reis, G. J., Pomerantz, R. M., Jenkins, R. D., et al. (1991). Laser balloon angioplasty: Clinical, angiographic and histologic results. *Journal of the American College of Cardiology, 18,* 193.

Ross, R. (1990). Factors influencing atherogenesis. In J. W. Hurst, R. C. Schlant, C. E. Rackley, E. H. Sonnenblick, & N. K. Wenger (Eds.), *The Heart, arteries and veins* (7th ed.). New York: McGraw-Hill.

Savage, M., Fischman, D., Leon, M., et al. (1992). Restenosis risk of single Palmar-Schatz stents in native coronaries: Report from the core angiographic laboratory. *Journal of the American College of Cardiology, 19,* 277A.

Seward, I. B., Khandheria, B. K., Edwards, W. D., et al. (1990). Biplanar transesophageal echocardiography: Anatomic correlations, image orientation, and clinical applications. *Mayo Clinic Practice, 65,* 1193–1213.

Sigwart, U., Puel, J., Mirkovitch, V., Joffre, F., & Kappenberger, L. (1987). Intravascular stents to prevent occlusion and restenosis after transluminal angioplasty. *New England Journal of Medicine, 316,* 701–706.

Simpson, J., Hinohara, T., Selmon, M., et al. (1989). Comparison of early and recent experience in percutaneous coronary atherectomy (Abstract). *Journal of the American College of Cardiology, 13,* 108.

Steinberg, D., Parthasarathy, S., Carew, T. E., Khoo, J. C., & Witztum, J. L. (1989). Beyond cholesterol: Modifications of low density lipoprotein that increase its atherogenicity. *New England Journal of Medicine, 320,* 914–924.

Strauss, B. H., Serruys, P. W., Scheerder, I. K., et al. (1991). Relative risk analysis of angiographic predictors of restenosis within the coronary Wallstent. *Circulation, 84,* 1636.

U.S. Directional Coronary Atherectomy Investigator Group. (1990). Complications of directional coronary atherectomy in a multicenter experience. *Circulation, 82*(Suppl 3), 71.

Vogel, R. A. (1994). Hypolipidemic intervention and prospects for regression. In E. J. Topol (Ed.), *Interventional cardiology* (pp. 161–167). Philadelphia: W. B. Saunders.

White, C. W., Chaitman, B., Lasser, T. A., et al. (1987). Antiplatelet agents are effective in reducing the immediate complications of PTCA: Results from the ticlopidine multicenter trial. *Circulation, 76*(Suppl IV), IV-400.

CHAPTER 20

Myocardial Infarction

Barbara Riegel

Acute myocardial infarction (AMI) remains the primary cause of mortality in the United States today. Cardiovascular disease accounts for approximately 43% of all deaths. Over 1.5 million people experience AMI each year, and more than a third of these die. A significant (>250,000) number of deaths occur before patients reach the hospital, a statistic inflated beyond necessity because of denial and delay by the patient (American Heart Association, 1993).

Almost 5 million AMI victims are still living and must learn to cope with chronic coronary artery disease (CAD). Recovery from AMI is difficult; a significant number of patients experience emotional distress and family turmoil after AMI (Malan, 1992). Many patients fail to return to work when physiologically capable of doing so (Shanfield, 1990). Most AMI patients do not return to their previous levels of sexual activity (Razin, 1982). The monetary cost is also high. Cardiovascular disease cost our society over $117 billion in 1993, including fees for professional services, hospital and nursing home facilities, medications, and lost occupational income (American Heart Association, 1993).

The incidence of AMI increases with age. In men, AMI is uncommon before age 40 but 45% of all events occur before age 65. CAD is the leading cause of death in women (Goldberg, 1993); one in three women over age 64 has some form of cardiovascular disease (American Heart Association, 1993). Most acute events occur later in life, perhaps due to a protective effect of estrogen (LaRosa, 1993). This difference in age of onset creates the mistaken impression that CAD is a disease of males.

This chapter describes AMI as an evolving, dynamic event occurring over hours or days. This health crisis has significant physiologic sequelae and long-term psychological implications. Clinical presentation, physical assessment, and diagnostic findings are described following a discussion of the pathophysiology. Clinical management techniques are aimed at early identification of physiologic changes with the goal of limiting infarct size through maintenance of balance between myocardial oxygen supply and demand. Psychological adjustment is facilitated through early mobilization, control of symptoms, and stress reduction techniques such as patient education.

PATHOPHYSIOLOGY

Acute Event

As discussed in Chapter 19, coronary artery disease refers to a progressive accumulation of plaque on the arterial wall or intima. The hemodynamic significance of plaques is not usually apparent until 70% of the arterial cross-sectional area has been compromised. At that time symptoms may result during times of increased myocardial oxygen demand (e.g., exertion, a heavy meal, anxiety) because of inadequate oxygen supply.

Until recently, AMI was thought to occur when the atheromatous plaque grew large enough to totally occlude the coronary artery. It is now recognized that physiologic events cause disruption of the intima covering the plaque (Davies & Thomas, 1985). Thrombosis forms (DeWood et al., 1980), coronary spasm may occur, and blood flow to that area of the heart ceases. Infarction results from the mechanical obstruction caused by thrombosis, plaque rupture, dissection and sometimes spasm (Schwartz & Keller, 1993).

The events triggering plaque disruption and thrombus formation are not yet fully understood, but Tofler and colleagues (1991) propose a theory that integrates their earlier work on triggers with that of other investigators. Tofler and colleagues (1991) propose that coronary thrombosis begins with an atherosclerotic plaque that is vulnerable or susceptible to plaque rupture. Vulnerability typically increases with age. One of three general mechanisms occurs during the stage of vulnerability: (1) physical or mental stress significant enough to produce hemodynamic changes, (2) increases in coagulability, and/or (3) vasoconstriction (Fig. 20–1). If none of these events occurs during the vulnerable period, the plaque may evolve into the non-vulnerable stage. Stress in a person with a vulnerable plaque may cause varying degrees of arterial thrombosis (i.e., minor rupture without symptoms, unstable angina, non–Q wave AMI, Q wave infarct, or sudden cardiac death). Stress may increase coagulability and cause thrombus growth or it may trigger vasoconstriction with complete occlusion of a narrowed lumen. Tofler and colleagues (1991) suggest that an inverse relationship may exist between plaque vulnerability and the amount of stress required to produce rupture.

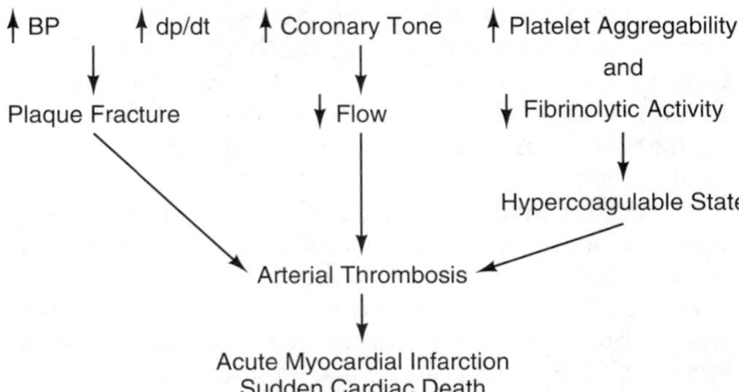

FIGURE 20–1. Hypothetical presentation of the manner in which daily activities may trigger coronary thrombosis. Three triggering mechanisms:—physical or mental stress producing hemodynamic changes leading to plaque rupture, an increase to coagulability, and vasoconstriction—have been added to the well-known scheme depicting the role of coronary thrombosis in unstable angina, myocardial infarction, and sudden cardiac death. (From Tofler, E. H., Koch, M., & Muller, J. E. [1991]. Triggers of onset of acute myocardial infarction. In B. J. Gersh & S. H. Rahimtoola (Eds.), *Acute myocardial infarction* [pp. 78–86]. New York: Elsevier Science Publishing.)

That is, significant mental or physical stress would be required to produce arterial thrombosis in a young man with a plaque just entering the vulnerable phase but little stress could result in thrombosis in an elderly person with a highly vulnerable lesion.

The stresses that stimulate this sequence of events are diverse. Mental stresses include those perceived as stressful by the individual. Physical stresses may include such activities as heavy lifting or snow shoveling. Physiologic stresses include those associated with circadian periodicity. Epidemiologic data demonstrate that AMI occurs more commonly between 6 AM and noon, when systemic arterial pressure, catecholamines, blood viscosity, and platelet aggregability rise with assumption of the upright position. Others have noted that AMI is more common during the winter months when systemic arterial pressure is elevated (Ornato et al., 1990). Cigarette smoking is a physiologic stress that causes vasoconstriction. Mental and physical stresses are additive. Smoking a cigarette may not be sufficient to cause coronary thrombosis in someone with a vulnerable lesion, but smoking immediately on rising during the winter months and while arguing with a loved one may precipitate AMI.

Collateral Circulation

One major factor influencing the incidence and severity of AMI is the presence of collateral coronary circulation. The amount of collateral vessel development determines whether an AMI involves only the subendocardium or the entire transmural area. Collateral circulation decreases wall motion abnormalities, ST segment changes, lactate production, and infarct size (Charney & Cohen, 1993). However Boehrer and associates (1992) demonstrated no differences in long-term outcomes (e.g., recurrent AMI and cardiac death) 12.5 years after AMI between subjects with and without collateral circulation.

Factors influencing collateral vessel development have been a mystery. Previous investigators have suggested that lengthy angina pectoris duration (Juilliere et al., 1990), high-grade stenosis (Araie et al., 1992) and growth factors (Charney & Cohen, 1993) all influence the development of collateral circulation.

These data have important clinical implications. Asymptomatic patients experiencing coronary occlusion who have no collateral support may suffer severe infarction, hemodynamic compromise, and sudden cardiac death. Habib and associates (1991) demonstrated that AMI patients who fail to reperfuse with thrombolytic therapy have a relatively smaller infarct size and better ventricular function at hospital discharge when collateral circulation is present. The time available for beneficial reperfusion following occlusion is also influenced by the presence of collateral vessels. Patients with more than 70% narrowing may tolerate coronary occlusion without transmural infarction and hemodynamic compromise longer than patients with occlusion of a less severe stenosis.

Evolution of Acute Myocardial Infarction

Thus far, AMI has been described as an acute event following chronic atherosclerotic plaque formation involving plaque rupture and thrombus formation that occludes blood flow in the coronary artery. Circadian periodicity data suggest that changes in blood pressure, coronary tone, and coagulability may be associated with sudden occlusion. Collateral circulation, with its potential to protect against dire outcomes, develops in some individuals over time in response to hemodynamically significant narrowing.

Occlusion of a coronary artery may cause a full-thickness, transmural AMI or a non–Q wave, nontransmural (formerly called subendocardial) AMI. Transmural AMI results most frequently from total arterial occlusion. Nontransmural AMI is associated with several factors:

- narrowed but patent coronary arteries
- incomplete occlusion
- early thrombolysis
- illnesses that increase oxygen demand suddenly (e.g., pulmonary embolism)
- collateral circulation

(Pasternak et al., 1992).

Coronary arterial occlusion most frequently results in necrosis of an area of the left ventricle or septum. (See Table 20–1 for the site of AMI typically associated with occlusion of specific coronary arteries.) About 30% to 40% of inferior infarcts also involve the right ventricle (RV) (Setaro & Cabin, 1992). Isolated right ventricular AMI occurs in only 3% to 5% of cases, perhaps because of lower RV oxygen demands, enhanced collateral circulation, and a thinner RV wall, which

TABLE 20–1. **Typical Site of Infarction According to Occluded Coronary Artery**

Left anterior descending coronary artery
Anterior left ventricle
Apical left ventricle
Ventricular septum
Anterolateral left ventricle
Left ventricular papillary muscles
Inferoapical left ventricular wall
Left circumflex artery
Lateral left ventricle
Inferoposterior left ventricle
Right coronary artery
Inferoposterior left ventricle
Inferior septum
Posteromedial left ventricular papillary muscles
Portions of the right ventricle

allows nutrients to be derived from blood in the RV. Situations in which RV oxygen demands are increased, as in chronic lung failure or right ventricular hypertrophy, are associated with right ventricular AMI. Atrial infarction occurs in 7% to 17% of left ventricular (LV) infarcts, usually involving the thin right atrial appendage (Pasternak et al., 1992).

Left ventricular function and prognosis are usually worse after anterior infarcts compared with posterior infarcts of equal size. The poor prognosis after anterior AMI may be due to different involvement of the RV and LV walls. Autopsy data suggest that posterior infarcts typically involve the RV more than anterior infarcts; anterior infarcts involve more of the major pump, the LV. Therefore, anterior infarcts compromise cardiac output and negatively affect prognosis more than posterior infarcts (Anderson et al., 1987).

Total occlusion of a coronary artery does not always result in AMI. Collateral circulation (Charney & Cohen, 1993), level of myocardial metabolism, rate of occlusive development, quantity of myocardium supplied by the vessel (Pasternak et al., 1992), and the presence and location of other stenoses all influence the evolution of AMI. For instance, occlusions of the right coronary artery or the mid or distal left anterior descending (LAD) artery are less likely to cause severe LV dysfunction than occlusions of the proximal LAD (Rentrop et al., 1988). A few (<5%) cases of AMI occur in the absence of any significant atherosclerotic obstruction, perhaps due to embolus or prolonged spasm (Pasternak et al., 1992). Cocaine use has also been shown to cause AMI (House, 1992).

Blockage of a coronary artery produces ischemia immediately. Ischemia is defined as oxygen deprivation accompanied by inadequate removal of metabolites because of inadequate perfusion (Braunwald & Sobel, 1992). Ischemia results from an actual decrease in blood flow (oxygen supply) or an increase in oxygen demand when supply is fixed. When blockage is total, infarction evolves over approximately 3 hours (Ritchie et al., 1988), although the anatomic and hemodynamic factors previously mentioned may slow the process. Edema and color changes in the heart are evident 6 hours after occlusion. A decrease in wall thickness is evident 8 to 10 days after the acute event due to necrotic tissue removal by mononuclear cells (Pasternak et al., 1992).

Systolic function of the LV is altered immediately after the acute event because of abnormal contraction patterns of the damaged myocardium. Ejection fraction is reduced when more than 10% of the LV contracts abnormally. Left ventricular end-diastolic pressure (LVEDP) and volume are elevated when 15% of the LV is involved. When 20% to 25% of the LV contracts abnormally, congestive heart failure results. Cardiogenic shock and often death accompany loss of 40% or more of functional LV (Edwards, 1991). Hypertrophy of the LV is an early compensatory mechanism in patients with left ventricular failure (LVF) (Braunwald, 1992). LV hypertrophy facilitates cardiac emptying initially, conserving myocardial oxygen consumption ($M\dot{V}O_2$) but eventually increases $M\dot{V}O_2$. Some improvement in wall motion occurs with healing because of scarring and stiffness unless infarct extension occurs.

Infarct extension refers to early recurrence and occurs within the first 10 days in approximately 10% of AMI patients and in almost 20% of those treated with thrombolytics. Predictors of infarct extension include obesity, female gender, non–Q wave infarction, diabetes mellitus, previous AMI, early CK-MB peak, and thrombolytic therapy (Pasternak et al., 1992).

Infarct remodeling, a different event, is due to regional expansion and dilation of the ventricle. Ischemia and dyskinesis result in progressive thinning and elongation of muscle fibers that change the size, shape, and thickness of the ventricular wall (Fara, 1993). The pathophysiologic changes of remodeling occur due to a reduction in stroke volume, increases in systolic and diastolic volumes, and resulting ventricular wall stresses. Remodeling occurs in patients who have lost a significant amount of myocardium, especially in the anterior region (Hirose et al., 1993). Remodeling is thought to continue until firm scar forms (over 2 to 3 months), but has been shown to continue over the first year after infarction (Hirose et al., 1993). Antiinflammatory agents (i.e., steroids and nonsteroidal antiinflammatory agents) delay scar formation and exacerbate infarct expansion (Fara, 1993; Pfeffer, 1991). Expansion is assumed to precede aneurysm formation but is a greater risk to patients, because aneurysms are not prone to rupture (Edwards, 1991). Heart failure from ischemic cardiomyopathy is a significant cause of early death.

Limitation of Infarct Size

Data relating the percentage of LV involvement to ejection fraction demonstrate that infarct size is directly associated with prognosis and quality of life. A significant percentage of AMI patients with large infarcts and severe heart failure (ejection fraction <30%) die within 5 years (Shah et al., 1980). Patients with a poor ejection fraction have little energy for the activities of daily living. Therefore, limitation of infarct size, not merely prevention of complications, is the goal of AMI patient care.

Limitation of infarct size is achieved primarily by maintaining a balance of myocardial oxygen supply and demand during the evolution of the acute event. Interventions designed to increase oxygen supply are most effective in limiting infarct size. Minimizing oxygen demand can delay the evolution of the infarct until more definitive interventions can be implemented.

Myocardial oxygen supply is limited by coronary blood flow, oxygen content of arterial blood, and the amount of oxygen extracted from blood by the heart (Stewart, 1992). Coronary blood flow is the most important of these factors because a high percentage of oxygen is normally extracted through the coronary circulation. The myocardium requires a blood flow of 60 to 90 mL/min per 100 g of heart tissue (Braunwald & Sobel, 1992) and consumes 8 to 10 mL of oxygen/min per 100 g of heart tissue under basal conditions, an amount that can increase several times during exercise (Opie, 1991). Little additional oxygen is available for extraction from cardiac venous blood. The oxygen-carrying capacity of the blood cannot be increased significantly unless considerable hypoxemia is present (Enger & Schwertz, 1989).

Myocardial oxygen demand is determined by wall tension, contractility, and heart rate. Ventricular wall tension is influenced by heart size, or preload, and left ventricular systolic pressure, or afterload. Preload is defined as the fiber length at rest (Lakatta, 1987) due to the volume of blood in the ventricles at the end of diastole, immediately prior to systole (Wright, 1990). Afterload is defined as the tension, force, or stress acting on ventricular fibers after the onset of shortening during systole (Braunwald et al., 1992). Afterload is strongly influenced by and often inaccurately thought to be synonymous with arterial pressure or systemic vascular resistance.

The degree of myocardial fiber shortening or contractility influences myocardial oxygen demand to the same extent as wall tension (Braunwald & Sobel, 1992). Lakatta (1987) notes that contractility and preload can no longer theoretically be considered independent determinants of myocardial performance because contraction depends on fiber length and varies throughout contraction as fiber length varies.

Heart rate also influences myocardial oxygen requirements. Heart rate is a function of heart size. The optimum frequency of heart rate at which contraction efficiency is ideal can be estimated for any heart size (Opie, 1991). Increases in heart rate increase $M\dot{V}O_2$ by increasing both the frequency of wall tension development and contractility (Braunwald & Sobel, 1992; Piano, 1994) (Fig. 20–2).

Methods of limiting infarct size focus on increasing the oxygen supply by increasing the flow of well-oxygenated blood through the coronary arteries. Techniques that decrease myocardial oxygen demand include optimizing preload and contractility, and decreasing afterload and heart rate.

CLINICAL PRESENTATION

A significant proportion (20%–60%) of AMI patients experience a prodromal period before infarction. This prodrome is usually characterized by classic angina pectoris that is unrelieved by rest or limitations on activity. According to Pasternak and colleagues (1992), patients experiencing a prodrome can be divided into thirds based on the length of the prodrome:

- One-third have symptoms for 1 to 4 weeks before the AMI.
- One-third have symptoms for a week or less.
- One-third have symptoms for less than 24 hours.

Chest pain of variable intensity is the most common presenting symptom of the AMI patient. Most AMI patients have chest pain, although the pain may be dulled in the elderly. Hofgren and associates (1988) found that patients with larger infarcts required significantly ($P < .01$) more morphine sulfate during the first 3 hours of hospitalization. These data suggest that the severity of pain may predict infarct size and prognosis.

Most AMI patients describe the chest pain as severe and intolerable, lasting more than 30 minutes and sometimes hours. The pain of AMI is thought to be similar in character to that of an individual's preinfarction angina pectoris; therefore, it is helpful to determine what the patient's angina is usually like.

Although the pain of AMI is typically retrosternal, it often involves the entire thorax, particularly the left anterior chest. It may radiate down the ulnar aspect of the left arm, causing tingling or numbness in the wrist, hand, or fingers. Atypical chest pain involves the shoulders, upper extremities, neck, jaw, teeth, and interscapular region.

The pain of angina pectoris and AMI is due to stimulation of nerve endings in ischemic or injured myocardium. Necrotic tissue is not painful; pain indicates that viable myocardium is present. Pain that is referred to the left arm, for instance, probably reflects excitation of afferent sympathetic and vagal fibers (Malliani, 1986).

Many patients describe their discomfort as "indigestion," associating epigastric symptoms with a gastrointestinal (GI) disorder. Approximately 50% of AMI patients experience symptoms of nausea and vomiting along with the pain, probably due to vagal stimulation or bradycardia and hypotension due to activation of the Bezold-Jarisch reflex (Braunwald & Sobel, 1992). Nausea and vomiting are especially common in patients with inferior wall infarction. Other associated symptoms include diaphoresis, pallor, weakness, diarrhea, palpitations, shortness of breath, dizziness, and a sense of impending doom. Inferior infarction is occasionally associated with hiccups, which are thought to

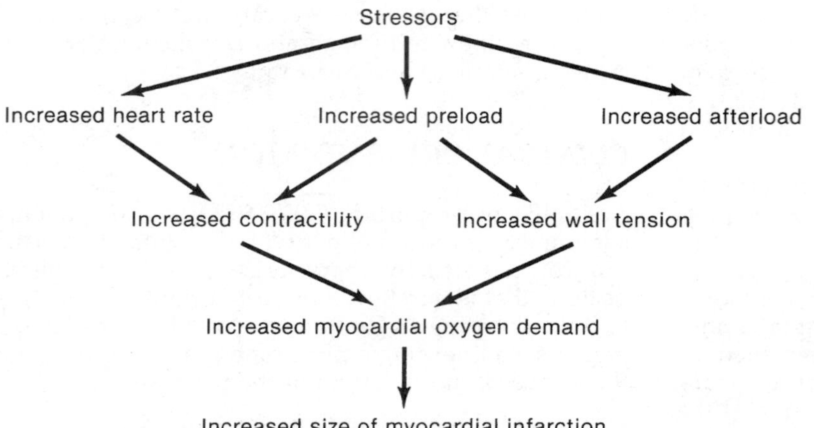

FIGURE 20-2. Effect of physiologic and psychological stressors on myocardial oxygen demand. Myocardial oxygen demand is determined by wall tension—a function of preload and afterload—and by contractility and heart rate.

be due to diaphragmatic irritation. Syncope is reported rarely (Krumholz & Wei, 1991).

Approximately 20% to 60% of infarctions are unrecognized because there are no symptoms ("silent") or because the symptoms are not recognized as infarction. Pasternak and colleagues (1992) suggest that about 30% of infarcts are truly silent and may be more common in patients with diabetes mellitus or hypertension. Deanfield and colleagues (1983) found that 73% of ischemic attacks occurring during activities of daily living were silent. Falcone and coworkers (1988) found that 48% of 108 patients with documented CAD had silent ischemia during exercise testing. Electrical dental stimulation of the same 108 subjects revealed that the majority (71%) of the silent ischemia group did not experience dental pain, even at maximal stimulation, a response significantly different ($P < .0005$) from the subjects in the exercise-induced chest pain group. These data suggest that a generalized hyposensitivity to pain may partly explain the occurrence of silent myocardial ischemia.

PHYSICAL ASSESSMENT

The purpose of a thorough physical assessment is early detection of warning signs of complications and impending decompensation. A significant number of AMI patients die during hospitalization, but mortality is reduced approximately 30% among patients cared for by expert clinicians (American Heart Association, 1993). Physical assessment of the AMI patient includes vital signs and visual inspection of the skin, neck veins, and behavioral patterns. Frequent auscultation of the heart and lungs is essential.

Early Phase

On admission the AMI patient may appear deceivingly well, or will be cool to the touch, clammy, and cyanotic. Severe chest pain or pressure lasting at least 30 minutes or more is typical. AMI patients are commonly anxious, fearful, distressed, and restless. Massaging the chest or placing a closed fist over the chest (Levine's sign) are universal signs of chest pain. Inferior infarction may cause hiccups from diaphragmatic irritation.

Vital signs may be normal, although patients with anterior infarcts often appear obviously ill with hypertension and tachycardia from sympathetic stimulation. Tachycardia may lower stroke volume and cause a slight decrease in systolic blood pressure (BP) and a rise in diastolic BP. Early premature ventricular contractions (PVCs) occur in more than 95% of AMI patients (Pasternak et al., 1992) but usually resolve within the first few days. Hypotension and bradycardia from parasympathetic stimulation are more common among patients with inferior infarction. Hypotension may also be caused by impending cardiogenic shock secondary to extensive myocardial loss in infarcts of any location.

Shortness of breath is common in AMI patients, and the respiratory rate is often elevated initially. Opiates usually mask an elevated respiratory rate due to their depressive effects. Body temperature is normal for the first few hours or days.

Cardiac auscultation often reveals muffled heart sounds early after AMI; heart sounds become clearer as healing progresses. A fourth heart sound (S_4) immediately preceding the first heart sound is also common. An S_4 reflects atrial contraction and is heard best between the left sternal border and the apex. The S_4 is heard because the left atrium is contracting against a noncompliant left ventricle with an elevated LVEDP. An S_3, indicative of the heart's inability to fully empty, is often present in large transmural infarcts with extensive LV dysfunction. An S_3 is heard best at the apex with the patient in the left lateral decubitus position. Coughing accentuates an S_3 by raising pulmonary venous pressure and heart rate. These hemodynamic changes accentuate an S_3 when the ventricle is unable to accommodate the volume of LV inflow occurring during the rapid filling phase of diastole (Walsh &

TABLE 20–2. **Killip Classification of Patients With Acute Myocardial Infarction**

	Definition	Patients with Acute Myocardial Infarction Admitted to CCU in This Category (%)	Approximate Mortality (%)*
Class I	Absence of rales over the lung fields and absence of S_3	30–40	8
Class II	Rales over 50% or less of the lung fields or the presence of an S_3	30–50	30
Class III	Rales over more than 50% of the lung fields (frequently pulmonary edema)	5–10	44
Class IV	Shock	10	80–100

*Estimated mortality in the 1960s. Mortality still rises with increased class, although the values in each class are lower today than in the 1960s.

Adapted from Killip, T., & Kimball, J. T. (1967). *American Journal of Cardiology,* 20, 457; from Braunwald, E. B. (Ed.) (1992). *Heart disease: A textbook of cardiovascular medicine* (4th ed.). Philadelphia: W. B. Saunders.

O'Rourke, 1981). The combination of an S_3 and an S_4, or "gallop" rhythm, is heard best at the apex, and again, may be accentuated by coughing. A third heart sound and a gallop rhythm are prognostic indicators of severe infarction.

A mitral regurgitation murmur is not typically heard in uncomplicated AMI patients. Such a murmur suggests a mechanical problem such as papillary muscle dysfunction or ventricular septal defect. Rapid surgical intervention may be lifesaving; a new mitral regurgitation murmur should be reported immediately. A mitral regurgitation murmur is heard best at the apex, may radiate to the axilla, and may be accompanied by a thrill. A systolic murmur, heard best along the left and right sternal borders, suggests rupture of the interventricular septum due to septal infarction and necrosis.

Auscultation of the lungs may reveal bilateral crackles. Moist crackles suggest LVF or decreased LV compliance. The severity of crackles can be used to estimate prognosis (Table 20–2).

Visual inspection of neck veins may also be helpful, especially if the patient is hypotensive. Hypotension with flat neck veins suggests parasympathetic stimulation associated with inferior infarction or hypovolemia rather than cardiogenic shock. Jugular venous pressure is typically normal in uncomplicated AMI patients, and elevation warns of impending complications. Jugular venous pressure elevation occurs due to right heart diastolic pressure elevation, such as occurs with extensive RV infarction or biventricular failure. A prominent "a" wave in the jugular venous pulse contour is evidence of pulmonary hypertension, which may be due to LVF or decreased LV compliance. A tall "v" wave in the jugular venous pulse indicates tricuspid regurgitation, which may be caused by ischemia or rupture of the RV papillary muscle. Nitroglycerin and furosemide should not be used in AMI patients in whom jugular venous pressure is not normal or elevated.

Examination of the abdomen and extremities is not typically helpful, although hepatomegaly may be present in patients with RV failure due to RV infarct or prolonged LVF. Hepatomegaly indicates a poor prognosis. Pedal edema suggests chronic RV failure because edema occurs in the sacrum and scrotum in individuals on bed rest.

Recovery Phase

Physical assessment remains extremely important during the recovery phase. Fever caused by tissue necrosis occurs 24 to 48 hours after AMI and may reach 101°F to 102° F (38.3°C to 38.8°C) rectally. Transient pericardial friction rubs occur in as many as 20% of transmural infarcts on day two or three. A loud friction rub, heard best along the left sternal border, suggests a large infarct. Heart failure often occurs in large infarcts between days two and five, manifested by an S_3 and crackles. Bronchitis may occur due to the wet environment and cough suppression from narcotic administration.

Iatrogenic complications occur during the recovery phase. A phenomenon of increasing frequency is pericardial tamponade caused by thrombolytic and heparin use. Pericardial tamponade with effusion requires emergent pressure relief by pericardiocentesis. Patients requiring a urinary catheter may develop a urinary tract infection that requires immediate attention because of its potential to increase MVO_2.

Cardiac rupture occurs most commonly between days three and six. In this era of early discharge, this complication may not occur until the patient is home when death is invariable due to the lack of immediate assistance. Venous thrombosis and pulmonary embolism are complications of AMI that have been largely eliminated by early mobilization, antiplatelet therapy, and anticoagulation.

Late complications include postmyocardial infarction syndrome, or Dressler's syndrome. This syndrome is manifested by pleuropericardial chest pain, low-grade fever, a pericardial friction rub, and pericardial and pleural effusions occurring 2 to 10 weeks after AMI. Dressler's syndrome is prone to recurrence and is thought to be due to autoimmune mechanisms or anticoagulant therapy (Edwards, 1991). Interestingly, the incidence of Dressler's syndrome is decreasing. Apical thrombi may occur in patients experiencing large anterior infarction. Such thrombi may be the cause of fatal systemic thromboembolism. Postinfarction angina defines a group of AMI patients in whom both short- and long-term mortality is high. Early cardiac catheterization is appropriate for these patients.

Cardiogenic Shock

Cardiogenic shock occurs in about 10% of AMI patients and is associated with a mortality of 85% to 100% that has not improved during the past 30 years (Killip & Kimball, 1967; Weil et al., 1992). The onset and severity of cardiogenic shock are directly associated with the amount of damaged myocardium. The majority of patients with shock have lost approximately 40% of the left ventricular pump function (Weil et al., 1992).

The physical presentation of AMI patients with cardiogenic shock differs from that of stable AMI patients. These patients usually lie listlessly, moving little because of lack of energy. The face is pale, and the skin is cool and clammy with a bluish, mottled appearance. Peripheral cyanosis of the nailbeds or the perioral area may be evident. The patient may be anxious or fearful. Poor cerebral perfusion may cause confusion or disorientation.

Blood pressure with cardiogenic shock is, by definition, 90 mm Hg systolic or lower. Respiratory rate may be normal or elevated. JVP is elevated. Pulsus alternans may be evident on carotid pulse palpation. Invasive hemodynamic monitoring is essential for these patients. Prognosis can be estimated using arterial blood lactate levels (a byproduct of anaerobic metabolism), cardiac output or stroke work, and arterial pressure, in that order (Weil et al., 1992). According to Afifi and colleagues (1974), the following findings are associated with mortality approaching 100%:

- Lactate levels exceeding 4 mmol/L
- Cardiac index of less than 2.2 L/min/m^2
- Arterial resistance of greater than 2000 dyne/seconds/cm^{-5}
- Left ventricular filling pressure of greater than 18 mm Hg
- Mean arterial pressure of less than 60 mm Hg after fluid challenge

Coronary revascularization with bypass surgery or coronary angioplasty improves survival when performed within 24 hours of onset of cardiogenic shock (Moosvi et al., 1991).

LABORATORY FINDINGS

Three enzymes are released into the blood during AMI: creatine kinase (CK), lactate dehydrogenase (LDH), and (serum) glutamic oxaloacetic transferase (SGOT) now called aspartate aminotransferase (AST). Of these, CK is by far the most specific and useful enzyme. Table 20–3 summarizes the times of initial elevation, peak, return to normal, and conditions causing false-positive elevations of the two most commonly used enzymes.

Creatine kinase, formerly creatinine phosphokinase (CPK), is composed of three isoenzymes: MM, found in both skeletal and cardiac muscle; BB, found in brain and kidney; and MB, found in cardiac muscle. MB-CK is the primary diagnostic enzyme for AMI. It

TABLE 20–3. **Elevation Times and False-Positive Results Associated With Cardiac Enzymes**

Enzyme	Initial	Peak	Return to Baseline	Causes of False-Positive Results
Creatine kinase (CK)	4–8 hr	8–58 hr Average 24 hr	3–4 days	Muscle disease Alcohol intoxication Diabetes mellitus Skeletal muscle trauma Vigorous exercise Convulsions Intramuscular injections Thoracic outlet syndrome Pulmonary embolism Hypothyroidism
Lactate dehydrogenase (LDH)	24–48 hr	3–6 days	8–14 days	Hemolysis Leukemia Liver disease Hepatic congestion Renal disease Neoplasms Pulmonary embolism Myocarditis Skeletal muscle disease Shock

should be noted that small amounts of MB-CK are found in the small intestines, tongue, diaphragm, uterus, and prostate. Therefore, trauma or surgery to any of these organs as well as strenuous exercise or cardiopulmonary resuscitation may cause elevations of MB-CK that do not signify AMI. Total CK values normally range from 40 to 180 IU/L, lower for females. Isoenzyme MB-CK levels should be less than 5% when analyzed by standard methods, or up to 3.7 IU/L using radioimmunoassay (RIA). MB-CK may rise, while CK total remains normal, indicating AMI; minor elevations of MB-CK without subsequent diagnosis of AMI may indicate ischemia or microinfarctions (Pasternak et al., 1992). Peak CK elevations vary greatly and are probably due to dynamic infarct evolution. Thrombolysis causes early enzyme peaking that has complicated efforts to develop a system of sizing infarction based on enzyme release. Cox and colleagues (1987) suggest that early peak MB-CK values indicate a subset of high-risk patients who have residual jeopardized myocardium. Isoforms of MB-CK are available; these isoforms allow diagnosis of AMI within 6 hours. If chest pain is prolonged, MB-CK without isoforms is sufficient to make the diagnosis.

Isoenzymes of LDH (LDH_{1-5}) have also been identified. The heart contains primarily LDH_1; if the LDH_1/LDH_2 ratio is greater than 1.0 in a nonhemolyzed sample, AMI is probably occurring. Troponin T is a new diagnostic marker of AMI that rises earlier than MB-CK. An elevated troponin T on admission in a patient with an acute coronary syndrome has been associated with an increased risk of complications and death.

Other laboratory abnormalities associated with AMI include hyperglycemia and myoglobinemia. Lipid levels are altered by stress, intravenous glucose, and recumbency. Cholesterol and triglyceride analyses should be measured immediately upon admission to the hospital or deferred until approximately 8 weeks after AMI. Lipids should not be measured during hospitalization. Erythrocyte sedimentation rate is frequently elevated, as is the white blood cell (WBC) count. WBC elevations may be due to tissue necrosis or adrenal glucocorticoids released during the stress response. Hematocrit increases due to hemoconcentration.

DIAGNOSTIC PROCEDURES

Electrocardiographic Findings

The electrocardiogram (ECG) can contribute useful information to the diagnosis of AMI. However, a wide variety of conditions mimic infarction (Table 20–4), thereby limiting the specificity of the ECG. Factors such as extent of injury, age and site of the infarction, conduction defects, previous injury, acute pericarditis, electrolyte imbalance, and cardioreactive medications affect the ECG and also limit its usefulness in the diagnosis of AMI (Pasternak et al., 1992). Early diagnosis of AMI is essential if thrombolytics are to be administered. As enzyme elevation is delayed, AMI is best diagnosed using a combination of clinical findings and ECG.

TABLE 20–4. **Conditions Mimicking Infarction on Electrocardiograms**

Ventricular hypertrophy
Conduction disturbances
Wolff-Parkinson-White syndrome
Dilated or hypertrophic cardiomyopathy
Myocarditis
Pneumothorax
Pulmonary embolism
Traumatic heart disease
Intracranial hemorrhage
Hyperkalemia
Pericarditis
Early repolarization
Ventricular aneurysm
Prinzmetal angina

Data from Pasternak, R. C., Braunwald, E., & Sobel, B. E. (1992). Acute myocardial infarction. In E. Braunwald (Ed.), *The heart: A textbook of cardiovascular medicine* (4th ed., pp. 1200–1291). Philadelphia: W. B. Saunders; Fisch, C. (1992). Electrocardiography and vectorcardiography. In E. B. Braunwald (Ed.), *Heart disease: A textbook of cardiovascular medicine* (4th ed., pp. 180–222). Philadelphia: W. B. Saunders.

Electrocardiographic assessment in AMI focuses on three main characteristics: T waves, ST segments, and Q waves; as injury progresses, the changes typically evolve in that order. T wave changes occur with ischemia. With injury to the myocardium, ST segment displacement occurs. Cellular death results in persistent Q waves. Transient Q waves may be caused by angina pectoris or electrolyte imbalance (Pasternak et al., 1992). Serial tracings are diagnostic of AMI in only slightly more than 50% of patients (Fisch, 1992). The first ECGs taken after the onset of symptoms in 40% to 50% of AMI patients may be either normal or have the following nonspecific abnormalities:

- Subtle ST and T wave changes
- Isolated T wave abnormalities
- Transient normalization of T, ST, or QRS changes
- Masking of conduction defects (Fisch, 1992)

The fact that the first ECG observed is often nondiagnostic and thrombolytics are contraindicated when AMI is only suspected and in nontransmural AMI complicates efforts to assess thrombolytic treatment rates. For example, only 39% of AMI patients enrolled in the National Registry of Myocardial Infarction received a thrombolytic agent (Genentech, October 1993). Of the 51,413 patients enrolled in the database, 11.5% lacked diagnostic ECG changes at the time of admission.

The classic ECG pattern of AMI includes abnormalities of the T wave that progress to ST segment elevation in the leads facing the injured area and reciprocal ST depression in the opposite leads. The QRS amplitude decreases and evolves into a QS pattern. Q waves appear immediately, within hours, or perhaps not for days. Q waves are thought to represent electrically in-

TABLE 20–5. **Sites of Infarcts and Corresponding Electrocardiographic Changes**

Septum: V_1, V_2
Anterior wall: V_3, V_4
Anteroseptal surface: V_{1-6}
Lateral wall: I, aV_1, V_6
Anterolateral wall: I, aV_1, V_{3-6}
Extensive anterior infarct: I, aV_1, V_{1-6}
High lateral wall: I, aV_1
Inferior wall: II, III, aVF
Anteroinferior or apical wall: II, III, aV_1, and one or more V_{1-4}
Posterior wall: prominent R wave in V_1 or V_2

Data from Fisch, C. (1992). In E. B. Braunwald (Ed.), *Heart disease: A textbook of cardiovascular medicine* (4th ed.). Philadelphia: W. B. Saunders.

ert myocardium that fails to contribute to the normal electrical forces of contracting myocardium as measured by vector. Q waves had been thought to occur in only transmural infarcts, but approximately 50% of nontransmural infarcts are now known to have Q waves (Fisch, 1992). Non–Q wave patterns suggest that the damage has not involved the entire transmural wall. ECG findings typical of occlusion of specific coronary arteries are listed in Table 20–5.

The site and type (transmural versus nontransmural) of infarct have prognostic significance. Anterior infarcts are typically larger, and are associated with lower LV ejection fractions, a higher incidence of heart failure, and more ectopy, in-hospital deaths, and total cumulative cardiac mortality compared to patients with inferior AMIs. Patients with Q wave patterns typically have larger infarcts, lower ejection fractions, and a higher incidence of heart failure and in-hospital deaths compared to patients with non–Q wave infarcts. Those with anterior infarcts have a poorer prognosis regardless of infarct type (Q wave versus non–Q wave). The better prognosis of patients with inferior AMIs may be due to involvement of the right ventricle and therefore less LV pump impairment.

Right ventricular infarcts are difficult to diagnose because electrical signals of the relatively thin muscle mass are usually dominated by changes in the left ventricle. ST segment elevation in V_1 and the right precordial leads V_{3R} through V_{6R}, especially V_{4R}, may be seen with small inferior infarctions. These ST segment elevations are often only transient, however, lasting only 24 to 48 hours after symptom onset (Dell'Italia & O'Rourke, 1991). Atrial infarctions should be suspected with changes in the PR segment or contour of the P wave. Abnormal atrial rhythms such as atrial flutter, atrial fibrillation, wandering atrial pacemaker, or atrioventricular nodal rhythms also suggest atrial infarction.

Dysrhythmias, especially ventricular ectopy, are extremely common after AMI. The incidence is highest in patients seen early after the onset of symptoms, demonstrating the relationship between ischemia and ectopy. About half of patients with ventricular tachycardia (VT) develop ventricular fibrillation (VF); 40% of those with R-on-T phenomenon develop VF (Norris & Singh, 1982).

Sinus bradycardia is also very common in the early stages of AMI, especially in those with inferior AMI. Sinus tachycardia, although extremely common, is always a symptom, not a primary dysrhythmia. Conditions causing sinus tachycardia, such as pain, anxiety, fever, hypotension, medications, and dehydration should be suspected and treated.

Particular conduction disturbances, dysrhythmias and ischemic patterns should be suspected based on the site of infarction, demonstrating the need for individual monitoring schemes (Drew, 1991). First- and second-degree heart block, type I, are common, transient, and self-limiting effects of inferior infarction. Mobitz type II second-degree heart block is a rare but serious complication of anterior infarcts typically requiring pacing. Bradycardia is more common in inferoposterior infarcts than in anterior ones. Sinus tachycardia is common in patients with anterior AMI. Ventricular tachycardia occurs with equal frequency in inferior and anterior infarcts but is less common in patients with nontransmural AMI.

Clinical lore suggests that AMI patients experience dysrhythmias most commonly during sleep. In a review of the literature, Landis (1988) found that both NREM and REM* sleep states were associated with increased ectopy and angina episodes in cardiac patients. Rhythm disturbances were most common in cardiac patients with neurologic abnormalities and sleep apnea syndromes. No typical pattern of dysrhythmias during sleep has been found.

Radiographic Findings

The chest x-ray is useful in diagnosing heart failure or cardiomegaly in patients with AMI. However, pulmonary vascular markings due to LVF do not appear immediately. Evidence of pulmonary edema on a chest x-ray is found approximately 12 hours after LV filling pressures rise. Further, pulmonary vascular markings may still be found on x-rays after pulmonary edema has been treated successfully because accumulated fluid takes a day or two to be reabsorbed. Cardiomegaly is evidence of impaired ventricular function and suggests a prior AMI or chronic disease causing LV dilation such as aortic or mitral regurgitation or cardiomyopathy.

Cardiac Imaging

A variety of techniques are used to visualize cardiac structures noninvasively. Only the techniques used commonly today and those with great potential for the future are mentioned here.

ECHOCARDIOGRAPHY

M-mode echocardiography is useful for assessing function of the posterior LV wall and the interventric-

**NREM, non–rapid eye movement; REM, rapid eye movement.*

ular septum; small segments of the anterior wall also can be visualized. This type of echocardiography is effective in diagnosing abnormal LV wall motion, LVF, and pericardial effusions.

Two-dimensional echocardiography can be used to visualize a much larger portion of the left ventricle than M-mode. Two-dimensional techniques can be used to diagnose abnormal regional wall motion, especially in patients with transmural infarctions. Estimates of LV wall function obtained from two-dimensional echocardiograms correlate well with those obtained during angiography (Pasternak et al., 1992). AMI diagnostic specificity with two-dimensional echocardiography is poor, however, because both ischemic and infarcted myocardium contract poorly.

Two-dimensional echocardiography is useful in the diagnosis of mechanical complications of AMI, including:

- Left ventricular aneurysm and pseudoaneurysm
- Ventricular septal defect
- Mitral regurgitation
- Myocardial rupture
- Papillary muscle or chordae tendineae rupture
- Pericardial effusion
- Left ventricular thrombus (Pasternak et al., 1992)

The American College of Cardiology/American Heart Association Task Force (1990) recommends that echocardiograms be performed in patients with large infarcts and suspicion of mural thrombus or LV dysfunction due to a surgically correctable lesion. The addition of color Doppler to the two-dimensional echocardiogram can provide quantification of flow, cardiac output, shunts, mitral and tricuspid regurgitation, and ventricular septal defects.

RADIONUCLIDE ANGIOGRAPHY

Technetium-99m pyrophosphate is the substance used to detect a recent AMI using radionuclide scintigraphy. Pyrophosphate binds to free calcium in the necrotic myocardium, resulting in a "hot spot" showing the area of infarct. If the test is performed within a week after AMI it is extremely accurate as a method of diagnosing a transmural infarct. The scan reverts to normal within a week after the event.

PERFUSION SCINTIGRAPHY

First-pass imaging of the LV after injection of technetium-99m allows calculation of the ejection fraction without the need for cardiac catheterization. Subsequent information can be gained during the same or a separate procedure by gated cardiac blood pool imaging. In multiple gated acquisition (MUGA) scanning, motion films are generated that allow evaluation of regional wall motion and ejection fraction. MUGA can also be performed during exercise for evaluation of changes in cardiac function and ejection fraction.

MAGNETIC RESONANCE IMAGING

Magnetic resonance imaging (MRI), formerly called nuclear magnetic resonance, is a noninvasive technique that produces high-resolution three-dimensional tomographic static and cine images. These images provide information about cardiac structure and blood flow in seconds without contrast material (Pettigrew & Cecil, 1993). Although not commonly used for this purpose, MRI can detect, localize, and size an infarct. Future applications of MRI may include judging the severity of ischemia and myocardial perfusion as well as the transition from ischemia to injury (Zerhouni, 1993). MRI can be used to quantify chamber size and identify jeopardized myocardium, evaluate segmental wall motion, and detect abnormalities such as edema, fibrosis, wall thinning, and hypertrophy (Anderson & Brown, 1993; Beache et al., 1993).

POSITRON EMISSION TOMOGRAPHY

Positron emission tomographic (PET) scanning is used to assess regional perfusion and myocardial metabolism noninvasively through direct measurement of fuel uptake and use. Although it is expensive, this procedure has advantages compared to conventional radionuclide studies, which allow assessment of only perfusion and cardiac performance.

Positron emission tomography can distinguish viable myocardium capable of benefiting from revascularization. It can localize and facilitate understanding of ischemia in discrete areas of myocardium resulting from an imbalance of oxygen supply and demand. (Gropler & Bergmann, 1993). During normal aerobic myocardial metabolism, free fatty acids are the energy substrate. The amount of free fatty acids that are metabolized is proportional to increases in MVO_2. Therefore, measures of free fatty acid metabolism can provide information about MVO_2 during ischemia. Glucose is utilized by the heart as an energy substrate during anaerobic metabolism or when high glucose levels are present. Measures of myocardial glucose uptake may allow prediction of ischemic myocardium viability. PET can also provide information about both the size and extent of infarction.

CARDIAC CATHETERIZATION

Cardiac catheterization with angiography is frequently performed after AMI to determine the extent of underlying coronary atherosclerosis that is amenable to definitive intervention. Candidates for percutaneous transluminal coronary angioplasty (PTCA) or surgical intervention require angiographic evidence of the site and severity of plaques in the coronary arteries. The incidence of complications associated with the procedure is extremely low, varying according to patient characteristics such as age, infarct size, hemodynamic profile, time since infarct, and experience of the cardiologist and catheterization laboratory team. Contraindications to the procedure are few; ventricular irritability increases risk and interferes with the quality of the test. A prothrombin time of more than 15 seconds increases the risk of bleeding. Conditions requiring correction before catheterization include digitalis toxicity, severe hypertension, fever, severe LVF,

GI bleeding, anemia, renal failure, and electrolyte imbalance. Allergic reactions to radiographic dye can be prevented by administration of diphenhydramine (Benadryl), cimetidine, or hydroxyzine pamoate (Vistaril). Parents with known dye allergy need pretreatment with methylprednisolone 2 hours before the procedure.

EXERCISE TESTING

Low level submaximal exercise treadmill testing has traditionally been performed within the first 6 to 10 days after AMI. Predischarge exercise testing can be deferred in aggressively treated patients unless the psychological advantage of early testing is evident. Low level treadmill tests use stages zero and one-half until 70% to 75% of the maximum heart rate or effort intolerance is achieved. Stress exercise testing 3 weeks after AMI allows optimal assessment of functional capacity. Results should be evaluated on the basis of ischemia, BP response, dysrhythmias, or symptoms such as exercise tolerance or attainment of adequate workload (Kulick & Rahimtoola, 1991).

CLINICAL MANAGEMENT

Recent Changes in Management of AMI Patients

Treatment of AMI patients has changed radically in the past decade. Historically, patients with CAD were managed primarily with pharmaceutical agents; invasive therapy was unavailable or dangerous. AMI was treated conservatively in the coronary care unit with the goal of preventing complications (Fye, 1991). Today, patients with suspected CAD often undergo diagnostic cardiac catheterization so that definitive therapy such as PTCA, atherectomy, or coronary artery bypass graft (CABG) surgery can be performed before infarction occurs. Patients who present at the hospital within a few hours after the onset of chest pain with an evolving transmural AMI should receive thrombolytic agents. They may undergo PTCA before discharge or bypass surgery within a month (Fremes et al., 1991). Nursing care has also changed. Coronary precautions—enforced, prolonged bedrest, caffeine restriction, assistance with activities of daily living, iced and hot beverage limitations—are no longer practiced. Avoidance of the Valsalva maneuver is the only coronary precaution of universal significance (Porth et al., 1984).

AMI patients are being discharged earlier. In the 1970s AMI patients were typically hospitalized for 2 to 3 weeks. Patients are now discharged in 5 to 7 days. No adverse outcomes have been documented over the past two decades with shorter hospitalization stays.

Changes are also evident in the procedures and medications offered for treatment of uncomplicated AMI. Coronary angiography is recommended for AMI patients at risk for a recurrent event (Kulick & Rahimtoola, 1991). Coronary angiography after an AMI provides information about LAD coronary artery stenoses, ejection fraction, and segments at risk that predicts recurrent coronary events in the subsequent 5 years. These data support the need for intervention to prevent subsequent catastrophes in patients who have experienced AMI.

PHARMACEUTICAL AGENTS

In spite of the recent trend toward aggressive interventional measures, many patients still warrant conservative therapy with purely pharmacologic modalities. Thrombolytics, nitrates, and beta blockers have been shown to limit infarct size effectively, but only when treatment is implemented early, preferably within 4 to 6 hours.

THROMBOLYSIS

The most effective treatment for limiting infarct size is thrombolysis. Because 80% to 90% of AMIs are the result of thrombus (DeWood et al., 1980), early reperfusion of ischemic and jeopardized myocardium can supply needed oxygen to the threatened myocardium if it is implemented early following the onset of symptoms.

The number of large, multisite investigations conducted on thrombolytics since Rentrop and colleagues (1981) first demonstrated the benefits of streptokinase is astounding. More than 50 such studies were found in a recent search of the literature. The advantages of thrombolytics are indisputable but research continues in an attempt to ascertain: (1) the ideal agent, (2) the best dosing regimens, (3) appropriate timing of administration, (4) suitable patient selection criteria (e.g., age, infarct location), and (5) postthrombolytic treatment protocols that reduce reocclusion. At the present time the results can be summarized as follows.

Ideal Agent

Streptokinase and tissue plasminogen activator (t-PA) are the two most commonly used thrombolytics. Results of the recent GUSTO trial (1993) suggest that t-PA opens an occluded artery more quickly than streptokinase. Early opening is a benefit because occlusion time is directly correlated with infarct size. Thirty-day mortality appears to be lower among t-PA treated patients (GUSTO, 1993). However, although statistically significantly different, debate continues about whether or not the differences are clinically important. Further, t-PA is significantly more expensive than streptokinase. Research demonstrating smaller infarct size and better long-term outcomes (e.g., ischemic cardiomyopathy, congestive heart failure) are needed to convince cost-conscious physicians and hospitals to routinely select t-PA over streptokinase.

Dosing Regimen

A trial of streptokinase doses revealed that 3 million IU of streptokinase was superior to higher and lower doses (Six et al., 1990). In 1990 the t-PA dose advocated was 100 mg over 3 hours. Since that time, research on "front loading," in which the majority of the dose is given early, suggests that front-loaded t-PA is superior (Neuhaus et al., 1992; Tanswell et al., 1992; Wall et al., 1992).

Initial recommendations were for thrombolytic administration within 3 to 4 hours. Six hours became acceptable in the late 1980s. Then ISIS-2 (1988) and Grines and DeMaria (1990) demonstrated beneficial effects when thrombolytics were given up to 24 hours after AMI. At this time most clinicians agree that thrombolytics should be administered up to 12 hours after AMI.

Patient Selection

The American College of Cardiology/American Heart Association Task Force (1990) guidelines recommend that thrombolytics be withheld from patients over age 75 although the Cooperative Cardiovascular Project (CCP) revision of those guidelines have expanded the age cutoff to 80. Others argue that age should not be a contraindication at all (Grines & DeMaria, 1990). Infarct location may contribute to success. Bassand et al. (1989) found that streptokinase was most effective in anterior wall infarction, but others have demonstrated success in inferior infarction (Bates et al., 1989; Voth et al., 1990). Anterior infarct results may be more dramatic than those in inferior infarction, but thrombolysis appears to be effective regardless of infarct site. Treatment benefit is evident regardless of gender, heart rate, BP, or history of prior AMI. Benefit is particularly strong in patients with bundle branch block or a history of diabetes mellitus (Table 20–6).

Postthrombolytic Treatment

Maintenance of infarct artery patency is challenging because of coagulation cascade alterations associated with AMI (Webster et al., 1991) and increases in thrombin activity caused by fibrinolytics (Eisenberg et al., 1992). Heparin (Hsia et al., 1990) has been shown not only to facilitate maintenance of patency, but also to increase the incidence of bleeding complications (GISSI-2, 1990; ISIS-3, 1992). Aspirin also is advocated as an adjunct to thrombolytic therapy (Antman et al., 1992; Gunnar et al., 1990; Popma & Topol, 1991). Experimental therapies shown to influence various stages of coagulation cascade include hirudin, argatroban, MCI-9038, glycoprotein IIb/IIIa, prostacyclin, prostaglandin E_1, monoclonal antibodies, thromboxane A_2-receptor antagonists, and a serotonin-receptor antagonist (Webster et al., 1991). Some or all of these drugs may be shown to potentiate thrombolysis with t-PA and heparin in the future.

Reperfusion is not without risk. Even with recanalization, the no-reflow phenomenon may occur when cellular edema from ischemia prevents restoration of flow at the microvascular level. Reperfusion can accentuate this swelling and inhibit oxygenation of ischemic myocardium (Pasternak et al., 1992). Cellular reperfusion injury may also occur due to oxygen-free radicals (Braunwald & Sobel, 1992). It is now recognized that the reintroduction of oxygen to previously anoxic myocardium initiates a series of biochemical reactions resulting in the production of superoxide anion, hydrogen peroxide, and hydroxyl radicals, potent cytotoxic oxygen-free radicals. Oxygen-free radical scavengers are presently being investigated as a means of stopping the cellular destruction associated with reperfusion.

Dysrhythmias are common with reperfusion. PVCs are so common that they are thought to represent markers of successful reperfusion. Other dysrhythmias include sinus bradycardia, especially with inferior AMI, accelerated idioventricular rhythm, and VT. Conversely, ventricular dysrhythmias or heart block secondary to ischemia may improve after reperfusion of ischemic myocardium.

Accelerated idioventricular rhythm or VT may occur without warning. Therefore, prophylactic lidocaine is frequently begun when IV administration of the thrombolytic agent is started. The need for intravenous antidysrhythmic agents complicates patient care, necessitating three IV lines for the thrombolytic agent, heparin, and other agents such as lidocaine. Some centers recommend piggybacking lidocaine, nitroglycerin, and heparin. See Table 20–6 for management guidelines for t-PA administration. Table 20–7 lists current contraindications for thrombolytic administration.

NITRATES

Nitrates are potent vasodilators that act primarily on the capacitance circulation. Venous dilatation occurs at low plasma concentrations; arterial and then arteriolar or resistance vessel dilatation occurs at higher concentrations (Warnica, 1991). Nitrates have been shown to decrease dysrhythmias and death in patients with heart failure, to enhance myocardial perfusion, and to limit infarct size as measured by peak CK levels. These beneficial effects occur, however, only when care is taken to avoid hemodynamic changes that increase myocardial oxygen demand. Hemodynamic effects include decreased pulmonary artery wedge pressure (PAWP) and left ventricular end-diastolic and end-systolic volumes. Decreases in preload lower cardiac output, potentially causing reflex tachycardia. Nitrates also decrease systemic arterial pressure and afterload, which may result in hypotension. Tachycardia and hypotension can both increase infarct size.

In patients with AMI with a systolic BP of greater than 95 mm Hg, nitrates can be used to decrease isch-

TABLE 20–6. **Nursing Care Guidelines for Intravenous Tissue Plasminogen Activator (t-PA)**

1. Identify suitable patients in the emergency department or intensive care unit and contact the attending cardiologist immediately. If no answer is received within 5 minutes, repeat the call. Rationale: Thrombolysis must be administered as soon as possible to limit infarct size.
2. Screen for contraindications to thrombolytic therapy (see Table 20–7). Rationale: This action may avoid a complication.
3. Suitable candidates need three vascular access lines begun with a minimum of excess punctures; adequate hemostasis of unused puncture sites is essential. Rationale: Three lines are needed for t-PA, heparin, and other drugs such as lidocaine. Excess bleeding may occur due to the thrombolytic agent if hemostasis is not adequate.
4. Total creative kinase (CK) and CK-MB should be drawn just before beginning t-PA infusion and every 6 hours for 24 hours. An electrocardiogram (ECG) should be documented before beginning the infusion, at the end of t-PA infusion, 1 hour later, and every 8 hours for 24 hours. Repeat the ECG if chest pain or dysrhythmias recur. Rationale: These diagnostic tests are used to demonstrate reperfusion, reocclusion, and myocardial ischemia or damage.
5. Lidocaine 1.5 mg/kg bolus should be administered prophylactically when t-PA is begun and followed by a 0.75 mg/kg bolus 15 minutes later. A 2 mg/min drip should be started after the initial bolus. Adjust dosages as necessary based on age, liver function, perfusion status, and allergic history. Rationale: Reperfusion dysrhythmias frequently occur without warning.
6. Heparin therapy is begun 1 hour after t-PA is started. Administer a 5000-unit intravenous bolus and infuse heparin at the dose needed to keep the partial thromboplastin time (PTT) between 50 and 80 seconds. Continue heparin infusion for 24 to 48 hours. Although the PTT will be higher during the first 24 hours following t-PA therapy, the heparin should not be discontinued unless frank bleeding occurs. Rationale: t-PA dissolves thrombus; heparin prevents the recurrence of thrombus formation and reocclusion.
7. Monitor for complications during and following t-PA infusion. During infusion, dysrhythmias not prevented by prophylactic lidocaine should be anticipated and treated if serious or symptomatic. Avoid cardiopulmonary resuscitation if possible. After infusion, minor oozing at the venipuncture sites and gingival bleeding are common. Gingival bleeding must be distinguished from gastric hemorrhage. New onset back or leg pain (retroperitoneal bleeding) or a change in mental status (cerebral bleeding) indicates a need to stop t-PA and heparin infusions, draw blood for determination of coagulation parameters, and contact the physician immediately. Reocclusion or reinfarction often occurs in the first few days, suggesting the need for adequate anticoagulation. Monitor PTT closely. Rationale: Serious complications require vigilance.

emia, lessen pain, and facilitate cardiac output by decreasing resistance to ejection or afterload. Nitrates are effective in the treatment of heart failure and pulmonary edema because of their beneficial effects on cardiac output.

Long-acting nitrates should be avoided in acute care of patients with AMI because of the potentially prolonged harmful effects on hemodynamics. One or two tablets of sublingual nitroglycerin should be administered to those with pain and an adequate BP. Patients with an inferior or right ventricular infarct should receive nitroglycerin only with extreme caution because of the potential for sudden and extreme hypotension from inadequate preload. Severe hypotension and tachycardia due to nitrates can be treated with postural changes or reversed with intravenous (IV) atropine.

The American College of Cardiology/American Heart Association Task Force (1990) AMI guidelines recommend that IV nitroglycerin be administered to patients with large anterior AMIs to prevent arterial embolus. IV nitroglycerin also may be administered to decrease ischemia and control symptoms but not preferentially instead of morphine sulfate for pain. One dosing protocol suggests that therapy begin with 10 μg/min followed by stepwise increases of the same dose (Pasternak et al., 1992) until the mean arterial BP is reduced by 10%. Frequent monitoring of vital signs facilitates immediate detection of hypotension or tachycardia. Weaning from nitroglycerin is typically done by decreasing the cost by 10 μg/min every 10 minutes and watching for signs of angina or ST segment changes. Continued administration of IV nitro-

TABLE 20–7. **Contraindications to Thrombolytic Therapy**

Absolute Contraindications

Active internal bleeding
History of hemorrhagic cerebrovascular accident (CVA)
Nonhemorrhagic CVA within 1 year
Major surgery or trauma within 2 weeks
Intracranial neoplasm
Cardiopulmonary resuscitation >10 minutes
Recent head trauma
Suspected aortic dissection
Hemorrhagic ophthalmic condition
Pregnancy
Known allergy
BP > 200/120 mm Hg

Relative Contraindications

Uncontrolled hypertension (BP > 180/110 mm Hg)
History of severe hypertension (controlled or uncontrolled)
Age >80 years
Significant liver dysfunction
Treatment with streptokinase or APSAC within a 6–9 month period
Major surgery or trauma >2 weeks prior
History of CVA
Active peptic ulcer
Known bleeding diathesis or current use of anticoagulants

Sources: American College of Cardiology/American Heart Association Task Force, 1990; Antman, 1994.

glycerin may result in signs of alcohol intoxication because ethanol is a common diluent for commercial preparations (Pasternak et al., 1992). Nitrates can oxidize hemoglobin to methemoglobin, a compound that is ineffective in carrying oxygen. The major symptom of methemoglobinemia is pallor that is unimproved with oxygen therapy. Other nonspecific symptoms include dyspnea, headache, fatigue, and dizziness. A venous blood sample will appear chocolate brown even after being shaken in air (Rosenthal & Braunwald, 1992).

BETA-ADRENORECEPTOR BLOCKERS

Beta blockers have been shown to interrupt evolving infarcts, limit infarct size as measured by CK levels, and decrease the incidence of ventricular dysrhythmias (Warnica, 1991). These agents are effective in reducing ischemic pain, presumably because of changes in cardiac index, stroke index, heart rate, BP, tension-time index, and free fatty acid production, all of which affect $M\dot{V}O_2$. The American College of Cardiology/American Heart Association Task Force (1990) guidelines recommend early IV beta blockers for all AMI patients, including those receiving thrombolytics. Beta blockers are recommended for patients with tachycardia and hypertension because they lower pulse rate and BP. Beta blockers are contraindicated in patients with heart failure, hypotension, bradycardia, heart block, and bronchial asthma.

One protocol recommends metoprolol in three 5-mg IV boluses for AMI. Following each bolus, vital signs must be assessed for 2 to 5 minutes. Any heart rate of less than 60 beats/minute or a BP of less than 100 mm Hg signals the end of the protocol. If, after three boluses, the patient is hemodynamically stable 6 to 8 hours later, 50 mg of metoprolol is given orally. If the patient is still hemodynamically stable a day later, metoprolol 100 mg is given twice a day. Patients treated with beta blockers should be assessed routinely for the following signs, which may warrant drug discontinuation:

- PR interval of greater than 0.24 second
- Second- or third-degree heart block
- Rales in more than one-third of the lung fields
- Wheezes
- Heart rate of less than 50 beats/minute
- Systolic BP of less than 90 mm Hg
- PAWP of more than 20 mm Hg

ASPIRIN

Aspirin is a potent antiplatelet agent that should be administered to all AMI patients except for those with known hypersensitivity and active bleeding. A recent meta-analysis demonstrated that aspirin reduced coronary reocclusion and ischemia following thrombolytic therapy (Roux, 1992). Aspirin alone reduced 35-day mortality 23% (ISIS-2, 1988). AMI patients should be given a low dose aspirin tablet (160–325 mg) immediately after admission to the emergency department. If only enteric coated aspirin is available it should be chewed to facilitate quick absorption. Thereafter, a daily dose of enteric coated aspirin should be incorporated into the course of hospitalization and daily routine after discharge for an indefinite period of time.

OTHER AGENTS

A variety of other agents have been suggested as potentially effective in limiting infarct size. Glucose-insulin-potassium (GIK) has been debated as therapy for AMI for decades. However, little research has been done to document its effectiveness. GIK has been shown to lower plasma concentrations of free fatty acids, which in turn decreases MVO_2 and improves ventricular performance (Pasternak et al., 1992). To date, however, no prospective randomized trials evaluating the effects of GIK on long-term outcomes have been performed.

Glucocorticoids have been studied in treatment of AMI because of their known antiinflammatory effects. However, a series of studies documented that steroids increase infarct size and elevate MB-CK levels. Bulkley and Roberts (1974) found a high incidence of ventricular rupture and mortality thought to be caused by steroid inhibition of healing. Corticosteroids and the nonsteroidal antiinflammatory agents such as ibuprofen and indomethacin are contraindicated after AMI (Fara, 1993). Aspirin is not contraindicated as discussed above.

THERAPEUTIC INTERVENTIONS

Angioplasty in Acute Myocardial Infarction

Since it was first used to dilate coronary stenoses in 1977, PTCA has become one of the most commonly performed procedures in the treatment of CAD. Over 300,000 PTCAs were performed in the United States in 1991 (American Heart Association, 1993).

Direct or primary PTCA is an excellent alternative to thrombolysis when facilities and personnel are available to intervene within the first 6 hours (Bittl, 1991; Tenaglia & Stack, 1993). Controversy remains about the timing of PTCA after thrombolysis. Rescue PTCA, performed immediately after unsuccessful thrombolysis, is also effective (Califf et al., 1991). The controversy arises when thrombolysis is successful and diagnostic angiography indicates that definitive revascularization with PTCA is still indicated. Most authors agree that PTCA should be deferred for at least 3 days (Barbash et al., 1990; Swift, 1991). Waiting approximately 2 weeks is probably ideal (Bittl, 1991; Ellis et al., 1992). Restenosis after PTCA is approximately 25% over the first 6 months.

Patients experiencing a complicated AMI should not be discharged home without further evaluation and intervention if necessary. Postinfarction ischemia and reinfarction are high in patients experiencing complicated hospitalizations. In the low-risk cohort, medical therapy is effective in preventing recurrent events. Patients without evidence of ischemia on stress testing, even if angiography demonstrates significant residual stenosis (Ellis et al., 1992), can be managed with aspirin, beta blockers, and risk factor modification (American College of Cardiology/American Heart Association Task Force, 1990).

Emergent Surgical Revascularization

As with other methods designed to limit infarct size, surgical reperfusion of patients with AMI must be accomplished as rapidly as possible after the onset of symptoms if jeopardized myocardium is to be saved. Early CABG performed after 6 (and preferably 2) hours is contraindicated because it causes hemorrhage into the area of infarct (Pasternak et al., 1992). Transporting the patient to the hospital, performing coronary angiography, administering anesthesia, and getting the patient on cardiopulmonary bypass and surgically revascularized within so few hours is extremely difficult. Widespread use of CABG as a primary treatment for AMI is doubtful.

Appropriate candidates for surgical reperfusion for AMI include hospitalized patients who have been catheterized recently and suffer an infarct. Some stable AMI patients who have received thrombolysis may benefit more from CABG than PTCA before hospital discharge. But ideally bypass surgery should be delayed at least 30 days following AMI (Fremes et al., 1991).

Pain Management

Pain is the most common symptom of AMI. Physiologic response patterns to stressors such as pain depend on the aversiveness, intensity, controllability, novelty, and ambiguity of the situation. Pain of AMI is aversive, uncontrollable, and intense. It is usually a new experience for the patient and has an ambiguous meaning: "Will I die?" This type of situation typically produces a pattern of sympathetic nervous system arousal with increases in BP, heart rate, and cardiac output, skeletal muscle vasodilation, and secretion of both epinephrine and norepinephrine from the adrenal medulla, and cortisol from the adrenal cortex. Zaleska and Ceremuzynski (1980) documented increases in norepinephrine and epinephrine during acute coronary pain lasting an average of 3 hours. Epinephrine levels were higher than those of norepinephrine, suggesting that cardiac pain is associated with anxiety.

Stimulation of the sympathetic nervous system causes physiologic changes that increase myocardial oxygen demand and may extend infarct size. Therefore, pain relief is a primary focus of care for these patients. IV narcotic analgesics should be administered until total pain relief is achieved. After administration of morphine sulfate, the drug of choice for pain of AMI, maximal respiratory depression occurs within 7 minutes and may last for 4 or 5 hours. Hypotension following morphine administration can be treated by placing the patient in the supine position. Elevation of the feet may be necessary if systolic BP declines lower than 100 mm Hg.

Administration of supplemental oxygen may relieve pain in hypoxemic individuals by augmenting the oxygen supply to ischemic tissues but routine, prolonged (greater than 6 hours) oxygen use is unnecessary. Measures potentiating analgesia, such as a confident attitude, a quiet environment (Riegel, 1985), and relaxation techniques (Altice & Jamison, 1989), are appropriate interventions (Guyton-Simmons & Mattoon, 1991).

Patients should be instructed to notify the nurse immediately if discomfort returns. In a study of patients with AMI in the coronary care unit, Schneider (1987) found through interviews that 14 of 19 patients had experienced discomfort that they had not reported. The primary reason for not reporting chest pain was that it was not considered severe enough to report (Schwartz & Keller, 1993). Other reasons included a wish not to bother staff or complain, a desire to see if the pain would subside on its own ("It was nothing I couldn't stand"), and misunderstanding of the need to report chest pain ("They asked me to tell about chest pain; I had a burning in my upper chest and in my arms"). This small study has important implications for practice. When beginning the shift the nurse should question each patient with AMI about the character of his or her discomfort or angina. The patient should then be instructed to inform the nurse of any recurrence of any of those symptoms. Explaining that these symptoms can increase the work of the heart can motivate patients to report symptoms rapidly.

Activity Management

Activity intolerance refers to a state in which the individual is unable to tolerate an increase in activity. Patients with AMI may experience activity intolerance because of pain, alterations in vital signs (i.e., hypotension or tachycardia), or because of short periods of bed rest. Activity intolerance due to pain, medications, or illness states should be noted so that stimulation that accentuates the tachycardia or hypotension is avoided. Activity intolerance due to unnecessary immobility must be avoided by cautious activity as soon as pain is controlled.

Orthostatic intolerance becomes more severe the longer a patient is on bed rest, but tachycardia and narrowed pulse pressure can occur after only 6 hours in the supine position (Chobanian, 1974). These physiologic responses are more pronounced in the elderly and those receiving vasodilators.

Low energy level activities can be used to counteract the physiologic effects of immobility (Winslow et al., 1985). A variety of activities such as bathing, toileting, transfer, bedmaking and positioning have been studied in cardiac and normal subjects (Riegel, 1988a). Most of these studies are one of a kind and use small samples, and generalizations based on these data therefore have limited value. One consistent finding, however, is that none of these activities requires more than a minimal energy expenditure. Thus, typical activities of daily living are appropriate for most AMI patients, even in the early stages.

Most AMI patients can use a bedside commode almost immediately after admission. Appropriate short-term activity goals include assisting with the bath on the first day after admission. On the second day, most patients will be able to sit in the chair and bathe themselves from the sink or basin. On the third day, the patient with an uncomplicated AMI can usually sit in the chair for various periods of time. Most are discharged from the coronary care unit on day two or three. During the fourth day the typical patient is walking in the halls and taking either a shower or a tub bath (Riegel, 1988a).

Factors that influence the response to activity include medications, age, size of the infarct, vital signs, fluid balance, anxiety, body weight, time on bed rest, presence of varicosities, environmental temperature, and time elapsed since other exertion (e.g., meals). Response to activity can be evaluated using the Borg Perceived Exertion Scale (Noble et al., 1983) or the rate pressure product. The product of heart rate multiplied by systolic BP correlates well with $\dot{M}VO_2$ (Gobel et al., 1978). Activity should be terminated for any of the following reasons:

- Complaints of angina
- Generalized fatigue
- Shortness of breath
- Dizziness or lightheadedness
- Unsteady gait
- Heart rate increase greater than 120 beats/minute
- ST segment depression of greater than 1.5 mm
- Drop in systolic BP below the resting level or failure to rise with activity
- Significant dysrhythmias such as PVCs in excess of 10/minute couplets, or R-on-T phenomenon (Alteri, 1984)

Alteration in Cardiac Output

Injured or ischemic myocardium contracts poorly, thereby decreasing cardiac output. Reduced cardiac output results in increases in left ventricular end-systolic volume and pressure, pulmonary vascular congestion, and hypotension (BP equals cardiac output times peripheral resistance). Clinically, the patient may show signs of poor cerebral perfusion, or urine output of less than 30 mL/hr. Direct hemodynamic monitoring reveals decreases in cardiac output and increases in PAWP. Hypotension may be caused by hypovolemia or excess vagotonia. Hypotension from hypovolemia will be accentuated by diuretics.

A variety of pharmacologic agents are typically prescribed during the early stages of AMI to augment cardiac output. Others are avoided because of their effects on heart rate, BP, or contractility (i.e., $\dot{M}VO_2$). Sodium nitroprusside, a potent vasodilator, is commonly prescribed to increase stroke volume and cardiac output in patients with LVF. Any increases in myocardial oxygen demand due to increases in contractility are offset by decreases in arteriolar resistance and afterload, PAWP, and frequency of ectopic beats. IV nitroglycerin is also used to augment cardiac output by decreasing afterload and optimizing preload in patients with heart failure.

Digitalis administration in the early stages of AMI is still debated because: (1) it increases $\dot{M}VO_2$ in normal hearts through enhanced contractility, (2) its beneficial effects are not evident immediately after AMI, and (3) dysrhythmias may be accentuated in hypokalemic patients (Pasternak et al., 1992). However, in failing hearts, digital decreases wall tension, thereby decreasing $\dot{M}VO_2$. At this time, digoxin in patients with AMI is reserved for those with moderate degrees of LVF. Supraventricular dysrhythmias are effectively treated with digoxin.

Dobutamine and dopamine are positive inotropic agents that are useful for patients with decreases in cardiac output. Both drugs are potent inotropic agents; dobutamine has slightly less positive chronotropic effects. Both drugs are administered intravenously and require careful monitoring of systemic arterial pressure, pulmonary artery or pulmonary artery wedge pressure, and cardiac output.

Amrinone is a noncatecholamine, inotropic, and vasodilating agent recommended for decreases in cardiac output. In patients with LVF after AMI, amrinone increases cardiac output and reduces PAWP and afterload.

Angiotensin-converting enzyme (ACE) inhibitors such as captopril are used to increase cardiac output. Ace inhibitors are not direct-acting inotropic agents; rather they decrease afterload by inhibiting vasoconstriction due to angiotensin II. Preload is also decreased through inhibition of sodium retention. Decreases in afterload and preload increase cardiac output and decrease the work of the heart.

Agents that should be avoided in the care of AMI patients include isoproterenol, atropine, norepinephrine, and metaraminol (Pasternak et al., 1992). Routine prophylactic lidocaine is no longer recommended based on a meta-analysis of 14 trials in which the mortality of patients given prophylactic lidocaine was 1.7% and 1.2% in the untreated group (McMahon et al., 1988). Calcium antagonists are not preferred over beta blockers (American College of Cardiology/American Heart Association Task Force, 1990). Isoproterenol is a potent cardiac stimulant that increases $\dot{M}VO_2$ through its effects on contractility. Atropine increases $\dot{M}VO_2$ through augmentation of heart rate. The catecholamine norepinephrine and the stimulant metaraminol are reserved for emergency situations because of their peripheral vasoconstrictor (afterload) and cardiac contractility effects, which increase MVO_2. Atropine should not be administered unless the patient is symptomatic from prolonged bradycardia.

Counterpulsation with the intraaortic balloon pump (IABP) is another intervention used to treat decreases in cardiac output after AMI. Phased pulsations augment coronary perfusion pressure during diastole and deflation throughout systole to facilitate ventricular emptying. In this way, the IABP augments oxygen supply and decreases oxygen demand by minimizing afterload. The IABP is used primarily in treatment of hemodynamically unstable patients, particularly those in cardiogenic shock (Shinn & Joseph, 1994).

Dysrhythmia control is another method of augmenting cardiac output. Tachydysrhythmias decrease cardiac output by limiting the time available for ventricular filling; bradydysrhythmias decrease cardiac output because of the slowed heart rate. Tachydysrhythmias may increase infarct size by increasing heart rate. Although slow rhythms may decrease cardiac output, the slowest rate compatible with cerebral and renal perfusion is recommended. A wide variety of antidysrhythmic agents are available to treat atrial and ventricular dysrhythmias. Dysrhythmias may, however, be a symptom of other treatable conditions such as hypokalemia, hypovolemia, and hypoxemia.

Ineffective Individual and Family Coping

The stressfulness of the critical care environment has been the subject of much research in recent years. Regardless of the type of critically ill patient studied, stressors identified include limited mobility and control necessitated by treatment, pain, sleep interruption, and lack of knowledge and understanding of the illness and its treatment. Patients with AMI specifically fear early death and the impact of serious illness on their finances, family roles, lifestyle, and sexuality (Miller, 1988). Threats to self-identity are common in male patients, who are typically in their late 50s and early 60s.

Patients differ in their ability to cope with critical illness and hospitalization, probably based on differences in cognitive interpretation and perception of events (Lazarus & Folkman, 1984). As noted earlier, situations that are novel, ambiguous, intense, uncontrollable, and aversive cause stimulation of the sympathetic nervous system, producing physiologic effects that increase MVO_2. For this reason as well as for humanitarian, caring concerns, patients at risk for ineffective coping should be identified as soon as possible so that interventions can be implemented early before physiologic and psychological detriment occurs.

Dependable pain relief is one intervention that may build trust and facilitate coping with the stress of admission to the intensive care unit (ICU). Early mobilization can support self-esteem as well as prevent the hazards of immobility. Answering questions and teaching patients what to expect are simple but powerful interventions that may decrease the ambiguity, uncontrollability, and aversiveness of ICU admission.

Families are also at risk for ineffective coping because critical illness in a loved one is a major life stressor. Major stressors facing families of critically ill patients include potential death of a mate, loss of a healthy mate, potential recurrence of the event, financial insecurity, new roles within the family unit, change in one's own life goals or motives, change in responsibility for care of dependents in household, and strange hospital environment.

Family coping can be facilitated by meeting the family's primary needs for hope, information, and the knowledge that hospital personnel really care about the patient (Riegel, 1988b). Nurses can be encouraging, providing honest information that focuses on potential positive outcomes. Information also decreases the novelty, ambiguity, uncontrollability, intensity, and aversiveness of ICU admission. Families can be reassured that they will be contacted immediately if the patient's condition changes. Liberalizing visiting hours, whenever possible, may decrease the novelty, intensity, and uncontrollability of the ICU and relax both patients and their families. Family members should be encouraged to rest, eat well, and exercise to conserve energy and promote relaxation during this stressful time.

SUMMARY

The prognosis for patients experiencing AMI is far better today than it was even a decade ago. A wide variety of diagnostic tools and treatment modalities are now readily available. The problem of widespread practice variability is being addressed nationwide through the adoption of practice guidelines. The American College of Cardiology/American Hospital Association Task Force (1990) guidelines for AMI care are one of the first to be adopted nationwide. Collaborative nursing interventions such as medication administration and independent interventions such as activity management and stress reduction are potent tools for increasing myocardial oxygen supply while minimizing oxygen demand. Nurses who understand these interventions designed to limit infarct size can benefit their patients.

REFERENCES

Afifi, A. A., Chang, P. C., Liu, V. Y., et al. (1974). Prognostic indexes in acute myocardial infarction complicated by shock. *American Journal of Cardiology, 33,* 826.

Alteri, C. A. (1984). The patient with myocardial infarction: Rest prescriptions for activities of daily living. *Heart & Lung, 13,* 355.

Altice, N. L. F., & Jamison, G. B. (1989). Myocardial infarction: Interventions to facilitate pain management. *Journal of Cardiovascular Nursing, 3*(4), 49–56.

American College of Cardiology/American Heart Association Task Force (1990). Guidelines for the early management of patients with acute myocardial infarction. *Journal of the American College of Cardiology, 16*(2), 249–292.

American Heart Association (1993). *Heart and Stroke Facts: 1994 Statistical Supplement.* Dallas: American Heart Association.

Anderson, C. M., & Brown, J. J. (1993). Cardiovascular magnetic resonance imaging: Evaluation of myocardial perfusion. *Coronary Artery Disease, 4*(4), 354–360.

Anderson, H. R., Falk, E., & Nielsen, D. (1987). Right ventricular infarction: Frequency, size and topography in coronary heart disease: A prospective study comprising 107 consecutive autopsies from a coronary care unit. *Journal of the American College of Cardiology, 10*(6), 1223–1232.

Antman, E. M. General hospital management. In Julian, D. & Braunwald, E. (Eds.). *Management of acute myocardial infarction.* London, W. B. Saunders.

Araie, E., Futjita, M., Ohno, A., Ejiri, M., Yamanishi, K., Miwa, K., Nakajima, H., & Sasayama, S. (1992). Relationship between the preexistent coronary collateral circulation and successful intracoronary thrombolysis for acute myocardial infarction. *American Heart Journal, 123*(6), 1452–1455.

Barbash, G. I., Roth, A., Hod, H., Modan, M. Miller, H. I., Rath, S., Zahav, Y. H., Keren, G., Motro, M., Shachar, A., Basan, S., Agranat, O., Rabinowitz, B., Laniado, S., & Kaplinsky, E. (1990). Randomized controlled trial of late in-hospital angiography and angioplasty versus conservative management after treatment with recombinant tissue-type plasminogen activator in acute myocardial infarction. *American Journal of Cardiology, 66,* 538–545.

Bassand, J. P., Machecourt, J., Cassagnes, J., Anguenot, T., Lusson, R., Borel, E., Peycelon, P., Wolf, E., & Ducellier, D., for the APSIM Study Investigators (1989). *Journal of the American College of Cardiology, 13,* 988–997.

Bates, E. R., Califf, R. M., Stack, R. S., Aronson, L., George, B. S., Candela, R. J., Kereiakes, D. J., Abbottsmith, C. W., Anderson, L., Pitt, B., O'Neill, W. W., & Topol, E. J. (1989). The Thrombolysis and Angioplasty in Myocardial Infarction (TAMI) Study Group. *Journal of the American College of Cardiology, 13,* 12–18.

Beache, G. M., Wedeen, V. J., & Dinsmore, R. E. (1993). Magnetic resonance imaging evaluation of left ventricular dimensions and function and pericardial and myocardial disease. *Coronary Artery Disease, 4*(4), 328–333.

Bittl, J. A. (1991). Indications, timing, and optimal technique for diagnostic angiography and angioplasty in acute myocardial infarction. *Chest, 99*(4 Suppl), 150S–156S.

Boehrer, J. D., Lange, R. A., Willard, J. E., & Hillis, L. D. (1992). Influence of collateral filling of the occluded infarct-related coronary artery on prognosis after acute myocardial infarction. *American Journal of Cardiology, 69*(1), 10–12.

Braunwald, E. (1992). Pathophysiology of heart failure. In E. Braunwald (Ed.). *The heart: A textbook of cardiovascular medicine* (4th ed.). Philadelphia: W. B. Saunders.

Braunwald, E. B., & Sobel, B. E. (1992). Coronary blood flow and myocardial ischemia. In E. B. Braunwald (Ed.), *Heart disease: A textbook of cardiovascular medicine* (4th ed.). Philadelphia: W. B. Saunders.

Braunwald, E. B., Sonnenblick, E. H., & Ross, J. (1992). Mechanisms of cardiac contraction and relaxation. In E. B. Braunwald (Ed.), *Heart disease: A textbook of cardiovascular medicine* (4th ed.). Philadelphia: W. B. Saunders.

Bulkey, B. H., & Roberts, W. C. (1974). Steroid therapy during acute myocardial infarction: A cause of delayed healing and of ventricular aneurysm. *American Journal of Medicine, 56,* 244.

Califf, R. M., Topol, E. J., Stack, R. S., Ellis, S. G., George, B. S., Kereiakes, D. J., Samaha, J. K., Worley, S. J., Anderson, J. L., Harrelson-Woodlief, L., et al. for the TAMI Study Group. (1991). Evaluation of combination thrombolytic therapy and timing of cardiac catheterization in acute myocardial infarction. Results of the Thrombolysis and Angiography in Myocardial Infarction–phase 5 randomized trial. *Circulation, 83,* 1543–1556.

Charney, R., & Cohen, M. (1993). The role of the coronary collateral circulation in limiting myocardial ischemia and infarct size. *American Heart Journal, 126*(4), 937–945.

Chobanian, A. (1974). The metabolic and hemodynamic effects of prolonged bed rest in normal subjects. *Circulation, 49,* 551.

Cox, D. A., Stone, P. H., Muller, J. E., et al. (1987). Prognostic implications of an early peak in plasma MB creatine kinase in patients with acute myocardial infarction. *Journal of the American College of Cardiology, 10*(5), 979–990.

Davies, M. J., & Thomas, A. C. (1985). Plaque fissuring—the cause of acute myocardial infarction, sudden ischemic death, and crescendo angina. *British Heart Journal, 53,* 363.

Deanfield, J. E., Selwyn, A. P., & Chierchia, S. (1983). Myocardial ischemia during daily life in patients with stable angina: Its relation to symptoms and heart rate changes. *Lancet, 2,* 753–758.

Dell'Italia, L. J., & O'Rourke, R. A. (1991). Pathophysiology and treatment of right ventricular myocardial infarction. In B. J. Gersh & S. H. Rahimtoola (Eds.), *Acute myocardial infarction* (pp. 205–217). New York: Elsevier Science.

DeWood, M. A., Spores, J., Notske, R., et al. (1980). Prevalence of total coronary occlusion during the early hours of transmural myocardial infarction. *New England Journal of Medicine, 303,* 897.

Drew, B. (1991). Bedside electrocardiographic monitoring: State of the art for the 1990s. *Heart and Lung, 20*(6), 610–623.

Edwards, W. D. (1991). Pathology of myocardial infarction and reperfusion. In B. J. Gersh & S. H. Rahimtoola (Eds.), *Acute myocardial infarction* (pp. 14–48). New York: Elsevier Science.

Eisenberg, P. R., Sobel, B. E., & Jaffe, A. S. (1992). Activation of prothrombin accompanying thrombolysis with recombinant tissue-type plasminogen activator. *Journal of the American College of Cardiology, 19,* 1065–1069.

Ellis, S. G. (1990). Interventions in acute myocardial infarction. *Circulation, 81*(3 Suppl), IV43–IV50.

Ellis, S. G., Mooney, M. R., George, B. S., da Silva, E. E., Talley, J. D., Flanagan, W. H., & Topol, E. J. (1992). Randomized trial of late elective angioplasty versus conservative management for patients with residual stenoses after thrombolytic treatment of myocardial infarction. Treatment of Post-Thrombolytic Stenoses (TOPS) Study Group. *Circulation, 86*(5), 1400–1406.

Enger, E. L., Schwertz, D. W. (1989). Mechanisms of myocardial ischemia. *Journal of Cardiovascular Nursing, 3*(4), 1–16.

Falcone, C., Sconocchia, R., Guasti, L., et al. (1988). Dental pain threshold and angina pectoris in patients with coronary artery disease. *Journal of the American College of Cardiology, 12*(2), 348–352.

Fara, A. (1993). The role of angiotension-converting enzyme inhibitors in reducing ventricular remodeling after myocardial infarction. *Journal of Cardiovascular Nursing, 8*(1), 32–48.

Fisch, C. (1992). Electrocardiography and vectorcardiography. In E. B. Braunwald (Ed.), *Heart disease: A textbook of cardiovascular medicine* (4th ed., pp. 180–222). Philadelphia: W. B. Saunders.

Fremes, S. E., Goldman, B. S., Weisel, R. D., Ivanov, J., Christakis, G. T., Salerno, T. A., & David, T. E. (1991). Recent preoperative myocardial infarction increases the risk of surgery for unstable angina. *Journal of Cardiac Surgery, 6*(1), 2–12.

Fye, W. B. (1991). Acute myocardial infarction: A historical summary. In B. J. Gersh & S. H. Rahimtoola (Eds.), *Acute myocardial infarction* (pp. 3–13). New York: Elsevier Science.

Genentech, Inc. (October 1993). National Registry of Myocardial Infarction.

Gobel, F. L., Nordstrom, L. A., Nelson, R. R., et al. (1978). The rate-pressure-product as an index of myocardial oxygen consumption during exercise in patients with angina pectoris. *Circulation, 57,* 549.

Goldberg, A. C. (1993). Prevention and treatment of coronary artery disease in women, the elderly, and children: Overview. *Coronary Artery Disease 4,* 577–579.

Grines, C. L., & DeMaria, A. N. (1990). Optimal utilization of thrombolytic therapy for acute myocardial infarction: Concepts and controversies. *Journal of the American College of Cardiology, 16,* 223–231.

Gropler, R. J., & Bergmann, S. R. (1993). Flow and metabolic determinants of myocardial viability assessed by positron-emission tomography. *Coronary Artery Disease, 4*(6), 495–504.

Gruppo Italiano per lo Studio della Sopravvivenza nell'Infarto Miocardico (1990) GISSI-2: A factorial randomized trial of alteplase versus streptokinase and heparin versus no heparin among 12,490 patients with acute myocardial infarction. *Lancet 336,* 65–71.

Gunnar, R. M., Bourdillon, P. D., Dixon, D. W., Fuster, V., Karp, R. B., Kennedy, J. W., Klocke, F. J., Passamani, E. R., Pitt, B., Rapaport, E., et al. (1990). ACC/AHA guidelines for the early management of patients with acute myocardial infarction: A report of the American College of Cardiology/American Heart Association Task Force on Assessment of Diagnostic and Therapeutic Cardiovascular Procedures (subcommittee to develop guidelines for the early management of patients wtih acute myocardial infarction). *Circulation, 82*(2): 664–707.

GUSTO Angiographic Investigators. (1993). The effects of tissue plasminogen activator, streptokinase, or both on coronary-artery patency, ventricular function, and survival after acute myocardial infarction. *New England Journal of Medicine, 329,* 1615–1622.

GUSTO Angiographic Investigators. (1993). An international randomized trial comparing four thrombolytic strategies for acute myocardial infarction. *New England Journal of Medicine, 329,* 1673–1682.

Guyton-Simmons, J., & Mattoon, M. (1991). Analysis of strategies in the management of coronary patients' pain. *Dimensions of Critical Care Nursing, 10*(1), 21–27.

Habib, G. H., Heibig, J., Forman, S. A., Brown, B. G., Roberts, R., Terrin, M. L., & Bolli, R. (1991). Influence of coronary collateral vessels on myocardial infarct size in humans. Results of phase I Thrombolysis in Myocardial Infarction (TIMI) trial. *Circulation, 83*(3), 739–746.

Hirose, K., Shu, N. H., Reed, J. E., & Rumberger, J. A. (1993). Right ventricular dilatation and remodeling the first year after an initial transmural wall left ventricular myocardial infarction. *American Journal of Cardiology, 72,* 1126–1130.

Hofgren, K., Bondestam, E., Johansson, F. G., et al. (1988). Initial pain course and delay to hospital admission in relation to myocardial infarct size. *Heart & Lung, 17*(3), 274–280.

House, M. A. (1992). Cardiovascular effects of cocaine. *Journal of Cardiovascular Nursing, 6*(2), 1–11.

Hsia, J., Hamilton, W. P., Kleiman, N., Roberts, R., Chaitman, B. R., & Ross, A. M., for the Heparin Aspirin Reperfusion Trial (HART) Investigators. (1990). A comparison between heparin and low-dose aspirin as adjunctive therapy with tissue plasminogen activator for acute myocardial infarction. *New England Journal of Medicine, 323,* 1433–1437.

ISIS-2 (Second International Study of Infarct Survival) Collaborative Group. (1988). Randomized trial of intravenous streptokinase, oral aspirin, both, or neither among 17,187 cases of suspected acute myocardial infarction: ISIS-2. *Lancet, 2,* 349–360.

ISIS-3 (Third International Study of Infarct Survival) Collaborative Group. (1992). ISIS-3: A randomized comparison of streptokinase vs. tissue plasminogen activator vs. anistreplase and of aspirin plus heparin vs. aspirin alone among 41,299 cases of suspected acute myocardial infarction. *Lancet, 339,* 753–770.

Juilliere, Y., Danchin, N., Grentzinger, A., Suty-Selton, C., Lethor, J. P., Courtalon, T., Pernot, C., & Cherrier, F. (1990). Role of previous angina pectoris and collateral flow to preserve left ventricular function in the presence or absence of myocardial infarction in isolated total occlusion of the left anterior descending coronary artery. *American Journal of Cardiology, 65*(5), 227–281.

Killip, T., & Kimball, J. T. (1967). Treatment of myocardial infarction in a coronary care unit: A 2-year experience with 250 patients. *American Journal of Cardiology, 20,* 457.

Krumholz, H. M., & Wei, J. Y. (1991). Acute myocardial infarction: Clinical presentations and diagnosis. In B. J. Gersh & S. H. Rahimtoola (Eds.), *Acute myocardial infarction* (pp. 101–109). New York: Elsevier Science.

Kulick, D. L., & Rahimtoola, S. H. (1991). Assessment of the survivors of acute myocardial infarction: The case for coronary angiography. In B. J. Gersh & S. H. Rahimtoola (Eds.), *Acute myocardial infarction* (pp. 205–217). New York: Elsevier Science.

Lakatta, E. G. (1987). Starling's law of the heart is explained by an intimate interaction of muscle length and myofilament calcium activation. *Journal of the American College of Cardiology, 10*(5), 1157–1164.

Landis, C. A. (1988). Arrhythmias and sleep pattern disturbances in cardiac patients. *Progress in Cardiovascular Nursing, 3*(3), 73–80.

LaRosa, J. C. (1993). Estrogen: Risk versus benefit for the prevention of coronary artery disease. *Coronary Artery Disease, 4,* 588–594.

Lazarus, R., & Folkman, S. (1984). *Stress appraisal and coping.* New York: Springer.

Levine, H. J. (1987). Optimum heart rate of large failing hearts. *American Journal of Cardiology, 61*(8), 633–636.

MacMahon, S., Collins, R., Petro, R., et al. (1988). Effects of prophylactic lidocaine in suspected acute myocardial infarction. *Journal of the American Medical Association, 260,* 1910–1916.

Malan, S. S. (1992). Psychosocial adjustment following MI: Current views and nursing implications. *Journal of Cardiovascular Nursing, 6*(4), 57–70.

Malliani, A. (1986). The elusive link between transient myocardial ischemia and pain. *Circulation, 73,* 201.

Miller, N. (1988). Acute myocardial infarction. In B. Riegel & D. Ehrenreich (Eds.), *Psychological aspects of critical care nursing.* Rockville, MD: Aspen.

Moosvi, A. R., Gheorghiade, M., Goldstein, S., & Khaja, F. (1991). Management of cardiogenic shock complicating acute myocardial infarction: The Henry Ford Hospital experience and review of the literature. *Henry Ford Hospital Medical Journal, 39*(3–4), 240–244.

Neuhas, K. L., Von Essen, R., Tebbe, U., Vogt, A., Roth, M., Riess, M., Niederer, W., Forycki, F., Wirtzfeld, A., Maeurer, W., et al. (1992). Improved thrombolysis in acute myocardial infarction with front-loaded administration of alteplase: Results of the rt-PA-APSAC Patency Study (TAPS). *Journal of the American College of Cardiology, 19,* 885–891.

Noble, B. J., et al. (1983). A category-ratio perceived exertion scale: Relationship to blood and muscle lactates and heart rate. *Medical Science in Sports and Exercise, 15,* 523.

Norris, R. M., & Singh, B. N. (1982). Arrhythmias in acute myocardial infarction. In R. M. Norris (Ed.), *Myocardial infarction: Its presentation, pathogenesis and treatment.* Edinburgh: Churchill Livingstone.

Opie, L. H. (1991). *The heart: Physiology and metabolism.* New York: Raven Press.

Ornato, J. P., Siegel, L., Craren, E. J., & Nelson, N. (1990). Increased incidence of cardiac death attributed to acute myocardial infarction during winter. *Coronary Artery Disease, 1,* 199–203.

Pasternak, R. C., Braunwald, E., & Sobel, B. E. (1992). Acute myocardial infarction. In E. Braunwald (Ed.), *The heart: A textbook of cardiovascular medicine* (4th ed., pp. 1200–1291). Philadelphia: W. B. Saunders.

Pettigrew, R. I., & Cecil, M. P. (1993). Basic cardiovascular magnetic resonance imaging techniques. *Coronary Artery Disease, 4*(4), 318–327.

Pfeffer, M. A. (1991). Ventricular remodeling and expansion after myocardial infarction. In B. J. Gersh & S. H. Rahimtoola (Eds.), *Acute myocardial infarction* (pp. 438–447). New York: Elsevier Science.

Piano, M. R. (1994). Cellular signaling mechanisms of cardiac hypertrophy. *Journal of Cardiovascular Nursing, 8*(4), 1–27.

Popma, J. J., & Topol, E. J. (1991). Adjuncts to thrombolysis for myocardial reperfusion. *Annals of Internal Medicine, 115,* 34–44.

Porth, C. J., Bamrah, V. S., Tristani, M. F., Smith, J. J. (1984). The Valsalva maneuver: mechanisms and clinical implications. *Heart and Lung, 13,* 507–518.

Razin, A. M. (1982). Psychosocial intervention in coronary artery disease: A review. *Psychosomatic Medicine, 44*(4), 363–387.

Rentrop, K. P., Thornton, J. C., Feit, F., et al. (1988). Determinants and protective potential of coronary arterial collaterals as assessed by an angioplasty model. *American Journal of Cardiology, 61*(10), 677–684.

Riegel, B. (1985). The role of nursing in limiting infarct size. *Heart & Lung, 14*(3), 247–254.

Riegel, B. (1986). History of treatment of coronary artery disease. *Journal of Cardiovascular Nursing, 1*(1), vii–viii.

Riegel, B. (1988a). Acute myocardial infarction: Nursing interventions to optimize oxygen supply and demand. In L. Kern (Ed.), *Cardiac critical care nursing*. Rockville, MD: Aspen.

Riegel, B. (1988b). Family responses to critical illness. In B. Riegel &

D. Ehrenreich (Eds.), *Psychological aspects of critical care nursing.* Rockville, MD: Aspen.

Ritchie J. L., Cerqueira, M., Maynard, C., et al. (1988). Ventricular function and infarct size: The Western Washington Intravenous Streptokinase in Myocardial Infarction trial. *Journal of the American College of Cardiology, 11*(4), 689–697.

Rosenthal, D. S., & Braunwald, E. B. (1992). Hematological-oncological disorders and heart disease. In E. B. Braunwald (Ed.), *Heart disease: A textbook of cardiovascular medicine* (4th ed.). Philadelphia: W. B. Saunders.

Roux, S., Christeller, S., Ludin, E. (1992). Effects of aspirin on coronary reocclusion and recurrent ischemia after thrombolysis: a meta-analysis. *Journal of the American College of Cardiology, 19,* 671–677.

Schneider, A. C. (1987). Unreported chest pain in a coronary care unit. *Focus on Critical Care, 14*(5), 21–25.

Schwartz, C. J., Valente, A. J., Sprague, E. A., Hildenbrandt, E., & Kelley, J. L. (1993). The pathogenesis of atherosclerosis: Current concepts. *American Journal of Cardiology,* special series, 11–18.

Schwartz, J. M., & Keller, C. (1993). Variables affecting the reporting of pain following an acute myocardial infarction. *Applied Nursing Research, 6*(1), 13–18.

Setaro, J. F., & Cabin, H. S. (1992). Right ventricular infarction. *Cardiology Clinics, 10*(1), 69–90.

Shah, P., Pichler, M., Berman, D. S., et al. (1980). Left ventricular ejection fraction determined by radionuclide ventriculography in early stages of first transmural myocardial infarction. *American Journal of Cardiology, 45,* 542.

Shanfield, S. B. (1990). Return to work after an acute myocardial infarction: A review. *Heart and Lung, 19,* 109–117.

Shinn, A. E., & Joseph, D. (1994). Concepts of intraaortic balloon counterpulsation. *Journal of Cardiovascular Nursing, 8*(2), 45–60.

Six, A. J., Louwerenburg, H. W., Braams, R., Mechelse, K., Mosterd, W. L., Bredero, A. C., Dunselman, P. H., van Hemel, N. M. (1990). A double-blind randomized multicenter dose-ranging trial of intravenous streptokinase in acute myocardial infarction. *American Journal of Cardiology, 65,* 119–123.

Stewart, S. L. (1992). Acute MI: A review of pathophysiology, treatment, and complications. *Journal of Cardiovascular Nursing, 6*(4), 1–25.

SWIFT (1991). SWIFT trial of delayed elective intervention vs. conservative treatment after thrombolysis with anistreplase in acute myocardial infarction. *British Medical Journal, 302,* 555–560.

Tanswell, P., Tebbe, U., Neuhaus, K. L., Glasle-Schwarz, L., Wojcik, J., & Siefried, E. Pharmacokinetics and fibrin specificity of alteplase during accelerated infusions in acute myocardial infarction. *Journal of the American College of Cardiology, 19,* 1071–1075.

Tenaglia, A. N., & Stack, R. S. (1993). Angioplasty for acute coronary syndromes. *Annual Review of Medicine, 44,* 465–479.

Tofler, E. H., Koch, M., & Muller, J. E. (1991). Triggers of onset of acute myocardial infarction. In B. J. Gersh & S. H. Rahimtoola (Eds.), *Acute myocardial infarction* (pp. 78–86). New York: Elsevier Science.

Voth, E., Tebbe, U., Schicha, H., Neumann, P., Schroder, R., Neuhaus, K. L., Emrich, D. (1990). Intravenous streptokinase in acute myocardial infarction (ISAM): Assessment by left ventricular function 1 and 7 months after infarction by radionuclide ventriculography. *European Heart Journal, 11,* 885–896.

Wall, T. C., Califf, R. M., George, B. S., Ellis, S. G., Samaha, J. K., Kereiakes, D. J., Worley, S. J., Sigmon, K., & Topol, E. J. for the TAMI-7 Study Group (1992). Accelerated plasminogen activator dose regimens for coronary thrombolysis. *Journal of the American College of Cardiology, 19,* 482–489.

Walsh, R. A., & O'Rourke, R. A. (1981). The physical examination in uncomplicated and complicated myocardial infarction. In J. S. Karliner & G. Gregoratos (Eds.), *Coronary care.* New York: Churchill Livingstone.

Warnica, J. W. (1991). Pharmacologic management of acute myocardial infarction. In B. J. Gersh & S. H. Rahimtoola (Eds.), *Acute myocardial infarction.* (pp. 205–217). New York: Elsevier Science.

Webster, M. W. I., Chesebro, J. H., & Fuster, V. (1991). Antithrombotic therapy in acute myocardial infarction: Enhancement of thrombolysis, reduction of reocclusion, and prevention of thromboembolism. In B. J. Gersh & S. H. Rahimtoola, (Eds.), *Acute myocardial infarction* (pp. 333–348). New York: Elsevier Science.

Weil, M. H., von Planta, M., & Rackow, E. C. (1992). Acute circulatory failure (shock). In E. B. Braunwald (Ed.), *Heart disease: A textbook of cardiovascular medicine* (4th ed.). Philadelphia: W. B. Saunders.

Winslow, E. H., Lane, L., & Gaffney, A. (1985). Oxygen uptake and cardiovascular responses in control adults and acute myocardial infarction patients during bathing. *Nursing Research, 34,* 164.

Wright, S. M. (1990). Pathophysiology of congestive heart failure. *Journal of Cardiovascular Nursing, 4*(3), 1–16.

Zaleska, T., & Ceremuzynski, L. (1980). Metabolic alterations during and after termination of coronary pain in myocardial infarction. *European Journal of Cardiology, 11,* 201–213.

Zerhouni, E. A. (1993). Myocardial tagging by magnetic resonance imaging. *Coronary Artery Disease, 4*(4), 334–339.

MYOCARDIAL INFARCTION MULTIDISCIPLINARY CARE GUIDE

COORDINATION OF CARE

Diagnosis/Stabilization Phase		Acute Management Phase		Recovery Phase	
Outcome	*Intervention*	*Outcome*	*Intervention*	*Outcome*	*Intervention*
All appropriate team members and disciplines will be involved in the plan of care.	Develop the plan of care with the patient, family, primary nurse(s), primary physician(s), cardiologist, social services, chaplain, clinical nurse specialist, other specialists as needed.	All appropriate team members and disciplines will be involved.	Update the plan of care with patient, family, other team members, physical therapist, dietician, discharge planner, cardiac rehabilitation. Initiate planning for anticipated discharge and call home health as indicated. Begin teaching patient/family about care at home.	Patient will understand how to maintain optimal health at home.	Continue cardiac rehabilitation and plan for outpatient cardiac rehabilitation. Provide written guidelines concerning care at home and any necessary follow-up. Provide patient/family with phone number of resources available to answer questions.

FLUID BALANCE

Diagnosis/Stabilization Phase		Acute Management Phase		Recovery Phase	
Outcome	*Intervention*	*Outcome*	*Intervention*	*Outcome*	*Intervention*
Patient will achieve optimal hemodynamic status as evidenced by: • MAP > 70 mm Hg • Hemodynamic parameters WNL • Urine output > 0.5 mL/kg/hr • Free of cardiac dysrhythmias Patient will maintain a normal cardiac output.	Monitor and treat cardiac parameters: • Dysrhythmias • Svo_2 • Blood pressure • Intake and output • PA pressures • PCWP • SV • Left and right ventricular stroke work index • Level of consciousness • Cardiac output • Systemic vascular resistance • Cardiac index • Evidence of tissue perfusion Anticipate need for pacing and/or pharmacologic interventions for dysrhythmias.	Patient will maintain optimal hemodynamic status. Patient will maintain normal cardiac output.	Continue to monitor and treat cardiac parameters. Monitor and treat dysrhythmias. Monitor lab values: PT, PTT, ACT if available, cardiac enzymes, Mg. Monitor ECG for evolutionary changes consistent with MI. Continue to assess for complications associated with acute MI. Assess response to any vasopressors or anticoagulants given. Begin patient/family teaching on cardiac system, current cardiac problems, current treatment, and expected clinical course.	Patient will maintain optimal hemodynamic status.	Same as acute management phase. Teach patient/family signs of fluid overload (edema, shortness of breath, sudden weight gain, rapid heart rate). Continue cardiac teaching. Assess for understanding. Reinforce as needed.

	Intervention (continued)				
	Monitor lab values: electrolytes, Mg, PT, PTT, ACT if available, cardiac enzymes. Monitor for signs of fluid overload or deficit. Anticipate need for vasopressor agents and assess response. Observe for signs of bleeding while patient is receiving thrombolytic and anticoagulation therapy and treat accordingly. Keep antidotes for anticoagulants on unit. Monitor for signs of reperfusion if thrombolytic agents are administered: • Reperfusion dysrhythmias • ST segment return to baseline • Early rise and peak in CK • Relief of pain Monitor for signs of complications that can occur following an acute MI: CHF, cardiogenic shock, ventricular septal defect, mitral regurgitation, papillary muscle dysfunction/rupture, cardiac tamponade, and dysrhythmias. Assess heart sounds q4h and as needed. Assess breath sounds q4h and as needed. Be prepared to initiate counterpulsation if indicated.				

NUTRITION

Diagnosis/Stabilization Phase		Acute Management Phase		Recovery Phase	
Outcome	**Intervention**	**Outcome**	**Intervention**	**Outcome**	**Intervention**
Patient will be adequately nourished.	Clear/full liquids as tolerated first 24 hours. Monitor response to clear/full liquids. Monitor protein and albumin values.	Patient will be adequately nourished.	Advance to heart healthy diet as tolerated (low fat, low cholesterol; low sodium if indicated); monitor response. Monitor daily weight. Arrange dietary consult as needed.	Patient will be adequately nourished.	Teach patient/family about heart healthy diet: • Total fat < 30% of daily intake • Total saturated fat < 10% of daily intake • Total daily cholesterol intake <300 mg • Caloric reduction if indicated • Sodium restriction if indicated

Care Guide continued on following page

MYOCARDIAL INFARCTION MULTIDISCIPLINARY CARE GUIDE continued

MOBILITY

Diagnosis/Stabilization Phase		Acute Management Phase		Recovery Phase	
Outcome	***Intervention***	***Outcome***	***Intervention***	***Outcome***	***Intervention***
Patient will achieve optimal mobility.	Bed rest with bedside commode privileges first 6 hours. Teach patient physiologic basis for rest.	Patient will achieve optimal mobility.	Progress exercise as tolerated: dangle, out of bed for meals, up in chair tid to qid while in critical care environment. Monitor response to increased activity. Decrease activity if adverse events occur (tachycardia, dyspnea, ectopy, syncope, hypotension, chest discomfort). Allow patient to begin light activities of daily living—partial bathing and brushing teeth. Initiate Phase I Cardiac Rehabilitation. Teach patient gradual exercise principles.	Patient will achieve optimal mobility.	Continue to progress exercise as tolerated and monitor response. Walk at least 200 to 300 feet (tid to qid). Walk up and down one flight of stairs. Teach patient/family about home exercise program.

OXYGENATION/VENTILATION

Diagnosis/Stabilization Phase		Acute Management Phase		Recovery Phase	
Outcome	***Intervention***	***Outcome***	***Intervention***	***Outcome***	***Intervention***
Patient will have adequate gas exchange as evidenced by: • Sa_{O_2} >90% • ABGs WNL, Sp_{O_2} > 92% • Clear breath sounds • Respiratory rate, depth, and rhythm WNL • Chest x-ray normal	Apply supplemental oxygen for at least first 4–6 hours. Monitor Sp_{O_2} with pulse oximetry. Assess respiratory functioning, including lung sounds, respiratory rate and depth, and chest x-ray. Encourage coughing and deep breathing while on bed rest. Assess evidence of tissue perfusion. Monitor lab values: hemoglobin, ABGs.	Patient will have adequate gas exchange.	Assess respiratory functioning and intervene as indicated. Assess need for continued supplemental oxygen with use of pulse oximetry. Observe for complications of MI, which may impair oxygenation/ventilation (i.e., CHF, mitral regurgitation, pulmonary embolus, cardiac tamponade, cardiogenic shock).	Same.	Same as acute management phase.

COMFORT

Diagnosis/Stabilization Phase		Acute Management Phase		Recovery Phase	
Outcome	*Intervention*	*Outcome*	*Intervention*	*Outcome*	*Intervention*
Patient will be as comfortable and pain-free as possible as evidenced by: • No objective indicators of discomfort • No complaints of discomfort	Assess quantity and quality of discomfort. Administer narcotics (IV morphine is drug of choice) and monitor response. Initiate nitroglycerin drip and monitor response. Titrate according to hemodynamic parameters and report of pain. Provide a quiet environment to potentiate analgesia. Provide supplemental oxygen. Provide reassurance in a calm, caring, competent manner. Teach patient importance of reporting chest pain and how to quantify. Administer sedatives as needed.	Patient will be relaxed and pain-free.	Same as stabilization phase. Observe for complications of MI that may cause discomfort (i.e., pericarditis, pulmonary embolus, angina, extension of MI). Provide uninterrupted periods of rest. Teach patient/family use of other methods to promote relaxation (i.e., imagery, deep breathing, music therapy, humor therapy).	Patient will be relaxed and pain-free.	Progress analgesics to oral medications as needed, and assess response. Continue alternative methods to promote relaxation as listed above. Teach patient/family alternative methods to promote relaxation at home. Teach patient/family what to do at home if chest discomfort recurs.

SKIN INTEGRITY

Diagnosis/Stabilization Phase		Acute Management Phase		Recovery Phase	
Outcome	*Intervention*	*Outcome*	*Intervention*	*Outcome*	*Intervention*
Patient will have intact skin without abrasions.	Assess all bony prominences at least q4h and treat if needed according to hospital protocol. Assess skin integrity surrounding all invasive sites.	Same.	Same as stabilization phase.	Patient will have intact skin without abrasions.	Teach patient/family proper skin care at home after discharge.

Care Guide continued on following page

MYOCARDIAL INFARCTION MULTIDISCIPLINARY CARE GUIDE continued

PROTECTION/SAFETY

Diagnosis/Stabilization Phase		Acute Management Phase		Recovery Phase	
Outcome	**Intervention**	**Outcome**	**Intervention**	**Outcome**	**Intervention**
Patient will be protected from possible harm.	Assess need for wrist restraints if patient is intubated, has a decreased level of consciousness, is restless or agitated, is unable to follow commands, or has counterpulsation device in place. Explain need for restraints to patient/family. If restrained, assess response to restraints and check q1–2h for skin integrity and impairment to circulation. Follow hospital protocol for use of restraints. Provide sedatives as needed.	Patient will be protected from possible harm.	Provide support when dangling or getting out of bed and monitor response.	Patient will be protected from possible harm.	Provide support with ambulation and climbing stairs. Teach patient/family about any physical limitations in activity after discharge.

PSYCHOSOCIAL/SELF-DETERMINATION

Diagnosis/Stabilization Phase		Acute Management Phase		Recovery Phase	
Outcome	**Intervention**	**Outcome**	**Intervention**	**Outcome**	**Intervention**
Patient will achieve psychophysiologic stability. Patient will demonstrate a decrease in anxiety as evidenced by: • Vital signs WNL • Level of consciousness WNL • Subjective report of decreased anxiety • Objective report of decreased anxiety Patient will begin acceptance process for MI.	Assess physiologic effects of critical care environment on patient (hemodynamic variables, psychological status, signs of increased sympathetic response). Take measures to reduce sensory overload. Provide uninterrupted periods of rest. Use calm, caring, competent, and reassuring approach with patient and family. Allow flexible visiting to meet the needs of the patient and family. Determine coping ability of patient/family and take appropriate measures to meet their needs (i.e., explain condition, equipment, and medications; provide frequent condition reports; use easy to understand terminology; repeat information as needed; answer all questions). Provide sedatives as needed.	Patient will achieve psychophysiologic stability. Patient will demonstrate a decrease in anxiety. Patient will continue acceptance of MI.	Same as stabilization phase. Teach other methods to promote relaxation. Continue to assess coping ability of patient/family and take measures as indicated (family conferences, support services, verbalization of concerns/fears). Initiate cardiac teaching with patient/family: • Risk factor modification • Signs and symptoms of MI • Signs and symptoms of angina • Measures to take should chest pain recur • Diet • Activity • Medications • Cardiac rehabilitation • Signs and symptoms of CHF • Follow-up visits, when to call physician • Phone number of resource person • Pathophysiology of MI	Patient will achieve psychophysiologic stability. Patient will demonstrate a decrease in anxiety. Patient will continue acceptance of MI and implications.	Provide instruction on coping mechanisms. Continue cardiac teaching. Assess understanding. Reinforce as needed. Communicate teaching goals to cardiac rehab. Refer to outside services or agencies as appropriate (chaplain, social services, home health, cardiac rehabilitation).

DIAGNOSTICS

Diagnosis/Stabilization Phase		Acute Management Phase		Recovery Phase	
Outcome	*Intervention*	*Outcome*	*Intervention*	*Outcome*	*Intervention*
Patient will understand any tests or procedures that need to be completed (vital signs, intake and output, hemodynamic monitoring if used, cardiac monitor, chest x-ray, supplemental oxygen, IV lines, pulse oximetry, lab work, and ECGs).	Explain all procedures and tests to patient/family. Be sensitive to individualized needs of patient/family for information.	Patient will understand any tests or procedures that need to be completed (cardiac enzymes, daily ECG, increase in activity, cardiac monitoring, pulse oximetry, supplemental oxygen).	Explain procedures and tests needed to assess recovery from acute MI. Anticipate need for further diagnostic tests such as cardiac catheterization and any interventions that may result from this. Provide information on patient's role concerning diagnostic procedures, such as keeping leg straight after cardiac catheterization and increased fluid intake after cardiac catheterization. Be sensitive to individualized needs of patient/family for information.	Patient will understand meaning of diagnostic tests in relation to continued health (lab tests, ECGs).	Review with patient before discharge results of ECGs and lab tests. Discuss any abnormal values and appropriate measures patient can take at home to help return to normal (i.e., low cholesterol diet for hypercholesterolemia). Anticipate need for any further diagnostic tests such as stress testing or cardiac catheterization and any possible interventions that may result.

REFERENCES

DeAngellis, R. (1991). The cardiovascular system. In J. G. Alspach (Eds.). *Core curriculum for critical care nursing* (4th ed., pp. 132–314). Philadelphia: W. B. Saunders.

Wilson, R. F. (1992). *Critical care manual: Applied physiology and principles of therapy* (2nd ed.). Philadelphia: F. A. Davis.

CHAPTER 21

Heart Failure

Debra K. Moser and Suzette Cardin

Heart failure is a clinical condition in which left ventricular dysfunction results in the characteristic findings of vasoconstriction, fluid retention, activity intolerance, ventricular dysrhythmias, reduced quality of life, and high mortality (Kubo & Cohn, 1994). As one of the few cardiac conditions in which the incidence is increasing, heart failure has become a major public health problem afflicting 2 to 4 million people in the United States. Approximately 400,000 new cases are diagnosed each year. Data from Framingham demonstrate a median survival time once heart failure is diagnosed of 1.7 years for men and 3.2 years for women. With 5-year survival rates of only 25% in men and 38% in women, heart failure can be a more lethal condition than some cancers (Ho et al., 1993).

A significant cause of morbidity, heart failure results in more than 1 million hospitalizations each year. It is the primary or secondary diagnosis in 6% of all hospital discharges and is the most common reason for hospitalization in patients over age 65. Once diagnosed, 35% of patients are rehospitalized each year. An estimated $10 billion annually is spent to care for heart failure patients.

Heart failure also has a significant negative impact on quality of life. Patients often have a markedly decreased quality of life reflected by impaired physical functioning and drastic changes in family, social, and work roles (Walden et al., 1989). Additionally, many factors threaten psychological well-being in heart failure: the looming specter of repeated exacerbations, sudden death, or death from deteriorating heart failure; debilitating symptoms; and complicated medical regimens. It is not surprising that patients with heart failure commonly exhibit poor psychosocial adjustment and mood disturbances such as anxiety, depression, and anger (Dracup et al., 1992; Hawthorne & Hixon, 1994).

The syndrome discussed above, chronic heart failure, is as relevant to critical care nursing practice as acute heart failure. Exacerbation of chronic heart failure is one of the most common reasons for the hospitalization of these patients in the critical care unit. The critical care nurse is uniquely positioned to influence positively both the acute hospital and the postdischarge course of heart failure patients. The purpose of this chapter is to provide the critical care nurse with the information necessary to exert this influence by discussing the pathophysiology, identification, and treatment of heart failure.

PATHOPHYSIOLOGY OF HEART FAILURE

Heart failure is frequently defined as the state in which the heart fails to maintain a cardiac output sufficient to perfuse organ systems adequately and meet the demands of metabolizing tissues. However, many clinicians and researchers contend that this definition fails to describe the condition fully because it does not consider underlying mechanisms. A more complete definition is proposed by Katz:

> *Heart failure is a clinical syndrome in which impaired cardiac pumping decreases ejection and impedes venous return. These hemodynamic abnormalities are generally complicated by depressed myocardial contractility and relaxation, which reflect biochemical and biophysical disorders in the myocardial cells. The latter, in turn, are due partly to molecular abnormalities that not only impair the heart's performance, but also accelerate the deterioration of the myocardium and hasten myocardial cell death.*
>
> ***(Katz, 1992, pp. 638–639)***

The impairment in cardiac pumping ability is usually secondary to left ventricular systolic dysfunction although diastolic dysfunction is often an important additional component. Occasionally diastolic dysfunction is the exclusive cause (Dougherty et al., 1984). Heart failure is the final endpoint of many cardiovascular conditions (Table 21–1). Ischemic heart disease is now the most common cause of heart failure (Garg et al., 1993), but hypertension remains a major contributing factor (Ho et al., 1993).

Ventricular dysfunction is accompanied by an intrinsic decrease in contractility at the level of individual myocardial fibers. The decline in contractility reduces left ventricular ejection fraction, causing stroke volume and cardiac output to fall. To compensate for decreased cardiac output several reflex compensatory mechanisms (Table 21–2) are initiated, which initially improve cardiac output and tissue perfusion, but are

TABLE 21–1. **Conditions Causing Heart Failure**

Cardiovascular Disease

Ischemic heart disease
Toxic cardiomyopathies (e.g., alcohol, chemotherapeutic agents)
Idiopathic cardiomyopathies
- Dilated
- Hypertrophic
- Restrictive

Hypertension
Valvular heart disease
Pericardial disease
Congenital defects
Chronic tachycardia

Noncardiac Disease

Endocrine/metabolic disorders (contractility not usually impaired, rather metabolic demands are in excess of normal cardiac output; volume overload of the left ventricle)
- Thyrotoxicosis
- Anemia
- Pregnancy
- Fever, systemic infection
- Arteriovenous fistulas
- Vitamin B_1 deficiency (beri-beri)

Connective Tissue Diseases

Systemic lupus erythematosus
Polymyositis
Progressive systemic sclerosis (scleroderma)

Pulmonary Diseases

Cor pulmonale secondary to chronic obstructive pulmonary disease
Pulmonary hypertension

ultimately the instruments of cardiac decompensation (Opie, 1990).

Compensatory and Counterregulatory Mechanisms in Heart Failure

The compensatory neuroendocrine systems initially activated in heart failure are those physiologic systems activated under conditions of volume depletion in order to maintain ventricular filling pressure, cardiac output, and blood pressure. Neuroendocrine-activated vasoconstriction and sodium–water retention are hallmarks of the clinical syndrome of heart failure; however, vasodilator, natriuretic, and diuretic systems are also activated (Table 21–3). Although the vasodilator mechanisms known to operate in heart failure appear to be overwhelmed by vasoconstrictor systems, it is apparent that they may operate at some low level that plays a small but important role in maintaining compensation of heart failure over time (Dzau et al., 1984). Vasoconstriction in heart failure is not, however, caused only by activation of these vasoconstrictor systems. Alterations in local endothelial vascular control appear to contribute to abnormalities in vascular tone in heart failure (Hirsch & Creager, 1994). Other local hormonal abnormalities, such as activation of tissue renin–angiotensin systems, also probably contribute to vasoconstriction. Before discussing the systemic and local systems mobilized in heart failure, baroreceptor and cardiac reflex abnormalities instrumental in the development of clinical heart failure will be discussed.

TABLE 21–2. **Compensatory Changes Seen in Heart Failure**

Change	Beneficial Effect	Adverse Effect	Mechanism of Action
Increased heart rate	Increased CO	Increased $M\dot{V}O_2$ Myocardial ischemia Prodysrhythmic effect	SNS → β_1 stimulation
Increased contractility	Increased CO	Increased $M\dot{V}O_2$ β-receptor down-regulation Deterioration of LV function	SNS → β_1 stimulation
Volume expansion	Increased SV secondary to Frank-Starling mechanism	Systemic and pulmonary congestion LV dilation and hypertrophy secondary to increased loading conditions	Renin-angiotensin-aldosterone system → sodium and water retention Arginine vasopression → water retention
Vasoconstriction	Venoconstriction → increased CO secondary to Frank-Starling mechanism Arterial vasoconstriction → increased MAP → increased tissue perfusion	Increased afterload → decreased CO Decreased renal, cerebral, other regional blood flow	Neuroendocrine activation (SNS, renin–angiotensin system, arginine vasopressin) Structural changes in blood vessels Local endothelial changes
LV dilation and hypertrophy	Increased SV secondary to Frank-Starling mechanism Hypertrophy decreases wall stress	Subendocardial ischemia Long-term deterioration of ventricular function	Increased loading conditions Neuroendocrine factors (effect of norepinephrine and angiotensin)

Abbreviations: CO, cardiac output; LV, left ventricular; MAP, mean arterial pressure; $M\dot{V}O_2$, myocardial oxygen consumption; SV, stroke volume; SNS, sympathetic nervous system.

Adapted with permission from Greenberg, B. H. (1994). The medical management of chronic congestive heart failure. In J. D. Hosenpud & B. H. Greenberg (Eds.), *Congestive heart failure: Pathophysiology, diagnosis, and comprehensive approach to management* (p. 629). New York: Springer-Verlag.

TABLE 21–3. **Neuroendocrine Activation in Heart Failure**

Vasoconstrictor Systems
Sympathetic nervous system
Renin–angiotensin system
Arginine vasopressin
Vasodilator Systems
Atrial natriuretic factor
Eicosanoids (prostaglandins and bradykinin)
Dopamine

Baroreceptor and Cardiac Reflex Abnormalities in Heart Failure

Abnormalities of baroreceptor and cardiac reflex control (atrial and ventricular receptor reflexes) of the heart and circulation have been documented in heart failure by a number of investigators (Hirsch et al., 1987; Zucker, 1991). The arterial baroreceptors are stretch receptors located in the carotid sinuses and aortic arch. They sense alterations in arterial pressure and subsequently communicate this information to the central nervous system (Kunze & Andresen, 1991). Baroreceptors are stimulated by increased pressure and inhibited by decreased pressure. Stimulation of the baroreceptor reflex results in stimulation of the parasympathetic nervous system and inhibition of the sympathetic nervous system so that heart rate and systemic vascular resistance (SVR) are reduced. The converse occurs when the receptors are inhibited by decreased arterial pressure. In heart failure, the baroreceptors initially are inhibited appropriately in response to a fall in pressure. The result is sympathetic nervous system activation. However, as heart failure progresses, both baroreceptor discharge and the baroreflex are depressed (Zucker, 1991). A reduction in inhibitory signals from the baroreceptors leads to sympathetic overactivity despite intense vasoconstriction and volume retention.

The cardiac atrial reflexes (i.e., the Henry-Gauer reflex and the Bainbridge reflex) are initiated by stimulation of volume receptors in the atria. When blood volume is increased, increased atrial stretch excites these reflexes to initiate a series of neuroendocrine adjustments designed to return blood volume to normal (Zucker, 1991). These adjustments include the following: (1) a decrease in vasopressin secretion and resulting increase in water excretion, (2) a decrease in renal sympathetic nerve activity with subsequent decrease in renin and aldosterone secretion, (3) an increase in atrial natriuretic factor (ANF) secretion, (4) increased excretion of sodium and water, and (5) increased heart rate and resultant decrease in preload as a result of the Bainbridge reflex. Clearly, stimulation of the atrial reflexes could be beneficial in heart failure by decreasing excess sodium and water retention. However, abnormalities of these reflexes are present in heart failure, and neuroendocrine activation continues unabated by the normally inhibitory influences of these reflexes (Hirsch et al., 1987; Zucker, 1991).

The ventricular receptor reflexes (e.g., the Bezold-Jarisch reflex) are stimulated by both stretch and chemical substances. Decreased heart rate, blood pressure, and peripheral resistance occur in response to stimulation of this reflex. There is evidence that abnormalities of these receptors contribute to abnormalities of vascular resistance seen in heart failure (Zucker, 1991).

To summarize, vasoconstriction and sodium and water excess are characteristic markers of advanced heart failure. Abnormalities of the baroreceptor and cardiac reflexes contribute to this pathophysiology by allowing sympathetic nervous system activation, renin-angiotensin-aldosterone system activation, and vasopressin release to progress relatively unchecked even after intravascular volumes are high and vasoconstriction is apparent.

Neuroendocrine Activation

SYMPATHETIC NERVOUS SYSTEM

In heart failure, loss of effective cardiac muscle results in a decrease in stroke volume and cardiac output. Activation of the sympathetic nervous system compensates for this reduction in stroke volume (Fig. 21–1). Heightened adrenergic activity improves cardiac output by directly stimulating contractility and heart rate through β_1-receptor activation. Increased sympathetic nervous system activity also enhances cardiac output through an α_1-receptor–mediated arteriolar vasoconstriction (especially in the cutaneous, splanchnic, and renal circulatory beds) and venoconstriction. Arterial vasoconstriction maintains blood pressure and tissue perfusion. Venoconstriction improves cardiac output through the Frank-Starling mechanism. Venoconstriction enhances venous return, thereby increasing preload and cardiac output by recruiting volume from the capacitance vessels.

Plasma norepinephrine levels reflect sympathetic nervous system activity. In heart failure, plasma norepinephrine levels are markedly increased (Cohn et al., 1984) due to increased central sympathetic nerve outflow (Ferguson et al., 1990), while myocardial tissue norepinephrine stores are decreased. Patients with the most advanced heart failure have the highest plasma norepinephrine levels (Francis et al., 1990), and the norepinephrine level correlates with the degree of left ventricular dysfunction (Kluger et al., 1982). Higher plasma norepinephrine levels are predictive of mortality in patients with advanced heart failure (Cohn et al., 1984; Swedberg et al., 1990). Cohn and associates (1984) found plasma norepinephrine to be an independent predictor of mortality in heart failure among the indices of plasma norepinephrine, plasma

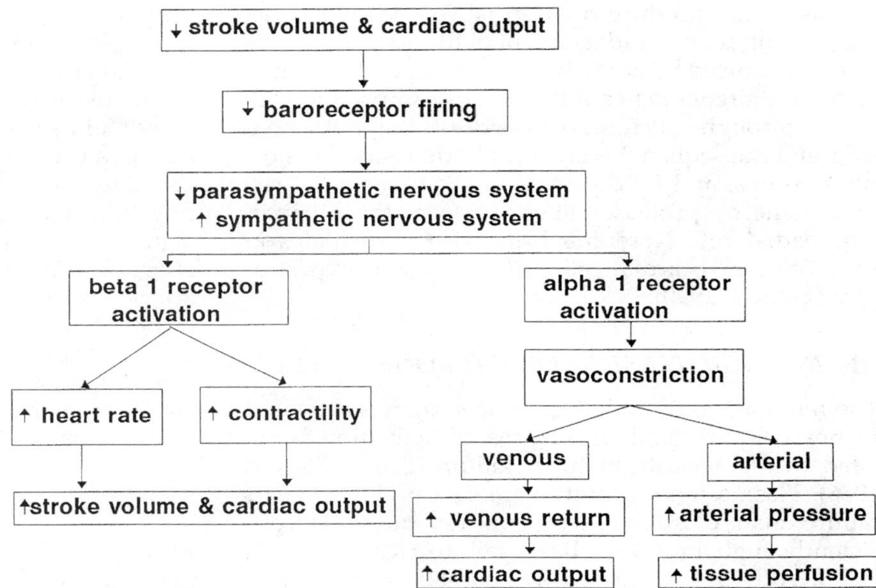

FIGURE 21–1. Sympathetic nervous system activation in response to decreased stroke volume in heart failure.

renin activity, stroke–work index, serum sodium, and heart rate.

Findings that plasma norepinephrine levels are highest in patients with the most severe disease and are predictive of mortality raise questions about the role of norepinephrine as a contributor to morbidity and mortality in heart failure. Whether sustained neuroendocrine activation precedes the development of overt heart failure or occurs as a result of heart failure has long been questioned (Francis, 1990). However, mounting evidence indicates that neuroendocrine activation is related to severity of left ventricular dysfunction (Benedict et al., 1994) and that activation occurs in patients with left ventricular dysfunction before they develop symptoms of heart failure (Francis et al., 1990). It is therefore likely that neuroendocrine activation contributes to the development and progression of heart failure (Francis et al., 1990).

Certainly, the marked vasoconstriction of advanced heart failure adversely affects the loading conditions of the left ventricle, contributing to increased afterload, myocardial wall tension, and myocardial oxygen consumption, thereby hastening the decline in ventricular performance. In addition to inducing pulmonary venous congestion, the increased venous return that accompanies vasoconstriction can also contribute to a decline in ventricular performance by excessively increasing ventricular end-diastolic volume, resulting in increased ventricular wall stress and myocardial oxygen consumption. Sympathetic system-provoked tachycardia can adversely affect myocardial performance by increasing myocardial oxygen consumption and decreasing diastolic filling time and coronary artery perfusion, thereby creating the conditions for an ischemia-induced reduction in contractility (Parmley, 1989). Additionally, diastolic function may be impaired by sinus tachycardia secondary to reduced time for ventricular filling (Daly & Sole, 1990). Finally, ventricular dysrhythmias and sudden death may be induced by high circulating levels of catecholamines (Dargie et al., 1987). A variety of mechanisms related to sympathetic nervous system activation are postulated for ventricular dysrhythmia induction in heart failure, including the following: increased myocardial ischemia (Unverferth et al., 1983), decreased ventricular fibrillation threshold (Daly & Sole, 1990), heterogeneity of sympathetic innervation of the myocardium (Daly & Sole, 1990), and β-receptor–induced hypokalemia.

There is additional evidence that norepinephrine may contribute directly to mortality in heart failure. Exposure of myocardial β-receptors to high circulating catecholamine levels produces decreased density of β-adrenergic receptors and desensitization of remaining β-adrenergic receptors to catecholamine stimulation (Bristow et al., 1982; Bristow, 1984). Additionally, there is uncoupling of β-receptors from adenylate cyclase (Bristow et al., 1982). β-receptor down-regulation occurs regardless of heart failure etiology and correlates with the severity of heart failure (Bristow, 1984). β-receptor down-regulation and desensitization have important implications for myocardial contractility in that the severely failing heart is unable to take advantage of a major inotropic mechanism. However, β-receptor down-regulation is reversible by treatment with β blockers (Heilbrunn et al., 1989), which may partially explain the success of β-blocking agents, especially during long-term treatment, in some heart failure patients (Nemanich et al., 1990).

Norepinephrine also has direct myopathic effects on the myocardium that contribute to deterioration of left ventricular performance (Mann & Cooper, 1989). The myocardium in heart failure is subjected to high levels of circulating catecholamines. Catecholamine profusion can produce myocardial cell death and decrease contractility, independent of the effects of tissue ischemia caused by excessive levels of catecholamines. Excessive circulating catecholamines can produce cell death through calcium overload of the mitochondria and subsequent reduction of adenosine triphosphate stores, and by digestion of the myocardial cell membrane by proteases liberated from the calcium-overloaded cell. Norepinephrine also participates in promoting myocardial cell remodeling and hypertrophy (Francis, 1990).

RENIN-ANGIOTENSIN-ALDOSTERONE SYSTEM

The renin-angiotensin-aldosterone system is activated in heart failure, and the degree of activation is related to the severity of heart failure (Lee & Packer, 1986). Plasma renin activity is more variable in heart failure than plasma norepinephrine, but it is consistently high in severe heart failure (Kluger et al., 1982). Although increased sympathetic nerve traffic through β-adrenergic receptor stimulation to the kidney is, in part, responsible for activation of the renin–angiotensin system, this system may be activated independently of the sympathetic system. Other factors responsible for the activation of the renin–angiotensin system are decreased renal arterial pressure sensed by intrarenal baroreceptors, hyponatremia sensed by the macula densa cells, and diuretic administration (Francis, 1990; Hirsch et al., 1987; Parmley, 1989).

On activation renin is released from the renal juxtaglomerular cells to act upon its circulating substrate, angiotensinogen (formed in the liver) to form angiotensin I. Angiotensin I is, in turn, converted to angiotensin II, a potent vasoconstrictor, by the action of angiotensin-converting enzyme (ACE), which is present in the lungs and vascular endothelium among other locations. Actions of angiotensin II that are initially compensatory and that maintain blood pressure and improve cardiac output in heart failure are arteriolar vasoconstriction, aldosterone release from the adrenal cortex, stimulation of thirst, and a direct renal tubular effect that promotes sodium retention (Fig. 21-2). Aldosterone release promotes sodium and water retention (and potassium excretion) to expand vascular volume. Angiotensin II stimulates norepinephrine synthesis and triggers the release of norepinephrine, potentiating sympathetic system activity.

The intense vasoconstriction, sodium and water retention, and adrenergic potentiation promoted by renin release eventually places the failing myocardium in further jeopardy by excessively increasing preload and afterload and promoting ventricular dysrhythmias, subendocardial ischemia (through coronary artery vasoconstriction), and hyponatremia and hypokalemia. In patients with severe heart failure, the degree of hyponatremia is inversely related to the degree of activation of the renin–angiotensin system, and hyponatremia is an independent predictor of mortality (Lee & Packer, 1986).

In addition to the effects of circulating angiotensin II, ample evidence points to the existence of local or tissue renin–angiotensin systems that do not depend on the release of renin from the kidneys for activation (Lee et al., 1993). Angiotensin II can be locally generated in a variety of tissues and likely influences vascular tone, cardiac contractility, myocardial hypertrophy, and sodium dynamics independent of the effects of the circulating renin–angiotensin system. Cardiac effects of tissue renin–angiotensin include coronary artery vasoconstriction, positive inotropy, and hypertrophy. Local vascular effects include vasoconstriction and changes in vascular structure. The local renin–angiotensin systems also have indirect effects on their target tissue that are mediated by the sympathetic nervous system.

ARGININE VASOPRESSIN

Another vasopressor system active in heart failure is the arginine vasopressin (antidiuretic hormone) system. Although vasopressin is not increased in all heart failure patients, increased levels are seen in patients with severe heart failure, and levels are proportional to severity of disease (Benedict et al., 1994; Creager et al., 1986). The exact stimulus for the release of vasopressin in heart failure is unknown, but evidence points toward the nonosmotic release of vasopressin from the posterior pituitary in response to high levels of angiotensin II and in response to baroreceptor dysfunction (Francis, 1990; Hirsch et al., 1987).

Vasopressin is a potent vasoconstrictor and likely contributes to the vasoconstriction seen in heart failure, but is probably not a chief mechanism (Benedict et al., 1994). Creager and colleagues (1986) characterized the contribution of the three vasoconstrictor systems in heart failure. Vasoconstriction is probably produced mainly by the sympathetic nervous system, next by the renin-angiotensin-aldosterone system, and lastly by the arginine vasopressin system. Vasopressin also has antidiuretic properties and contributes to hyponatremia secondary to excess volume expansion.

ATRIAL NATRIURETIC FACTOR

Atrial natriuretic factor is a peptide released into the circulation from atrial myocytes in response to increased atrial stretch. This hormone attenuates the effects of the vasoconstrictor systems described above, thus acting in an adaptive role to counteract their deleterious effects. ANF is a powerful vasodilator with diuretic and natriuretic properties. This peptide effectively inhibits the renin–angiotensin system, including inhibition of aldosterone release (Fyhrquist & Tikkanen, 1988). ANF also inhibits the release of vasopressin as well as of norepinephrine from its neurotransmitter sites (Packer, 1994). Thus the vasodilatory actions of ANF are a result of active competition with angiotensin II binding sites and inhibition of norepinephrine and vasopressin (Opie, 1991).

Data from the Studies of Left Ventricular Dysfunc-

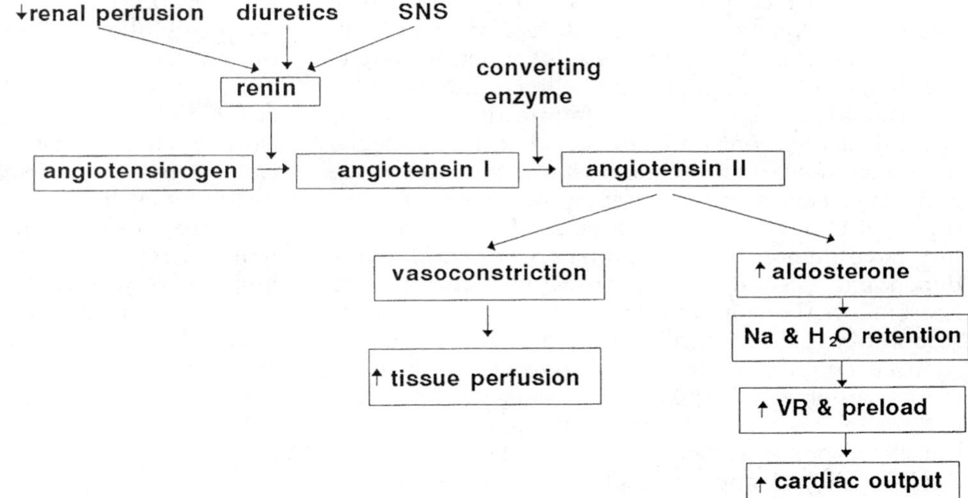

FIGURE 21–2. Renin-angiotensin-aldosterone system activation in heart failure. *Abbreviations:* H_2O, water; Na, sodium; SNS, sympathetic nervous system; VR, venous return.

tion (SOLVD) demonstrate that in patients with left ventricular dysfunction, no overt heart failure, and no diuretic therapy, ANF levels are increased while the renin-angiotensin-aldosterone system is not yet activated (Francis et al., 1990). This suggests that ANF plays a role in suppressing the progression of asymptomatic left ventricular dysfunction to overt congestive heart failure.

Overt chronic heart failure is a potent stimulus to the release of ANF. The release of ANF in heart failure exceeds release rates seen in all other states (Brandt et al., 1993). ANF levels rise as heart failure increases and are highest in those patients with the worst heart failure, correlating inversely with atrial and pulmonary pressures and ejection fraction (Benedict et al., 1994; Fyhrquist & Tikkanen, 1988). Unfortunately, the potential beneficial effects of ANF appear to be overcome by the effects of renin-angiotensin-aldosterone activation in advanced heart failure (Cody, 1989; Parmley, 1989). In chronic heart failure, the function of the atrial stretch receptors responsible for the release of ANF is impaired. In addition, secretion of the peptide may be down-regulated in heart failure and vascular receptors of the peptide desensitized (Opie, 1991). Thus, despite high circulating levels of ANF in advanced chronic heart failure, the effects of this hormone are antagonized by the effects of the renin–angiotensin and sympathetic nervous systems.

EICOSANOIDS

Renal hormones other than renin are released in response to heart failure, including prostaglandins from the arachidonic acid cascade and bradykinin and kallidin from the kallikrein-kinin system (Cannon, 1989). These substances are vasodilators, and the prostaglandins (especially prostaglandin E_2 [PGE_2]) additionally are platelet aggregation inhibitors with natriuretic actions. Prostaglandins are released in heart failure in response to hyponatremia, norepinephrine, and angiotensin II and may be released in proportion to the degree of vasoconstriction. They appear to serve the function of attenuating the renin–angiotensin system of induced vasoconstriction and sodium and water retention (Cannon, 1989; Dzau et al., 1984). As in the case of ANF, the vasodilator effects of prostaglandins are overwhelmed by the vasoconstrictor systems activated in heart failure. However, prostaglandins may maintain renal blood flow in the face of decreased cardiac output in heart failure. Both renal and ventricular function may worsen when nonsteroidal antiinflammatory agents that antagonize prostaglandins are used in patients or animal models with severe heart failure and hyponatremia (Dzau et al., 1984). This finding illustrates that although the natural vasodilator activity appears to be overpowered by vasoconstrictor activity, this activity may serve an unappreciated protective role in the prevention of even more rapid deterioration in heart failure. The roles of bradykinin and kallidin in heart failure are as yet unclear, although both of these substances are inactivated by the enzyme that converts angiotensin I to angiotensin II (Cannon, 1989).

DOPAMINE

Dopamine is a norepinephrine precursor with arterial vasodilator and natriuretic effects. Dopamine levels are frequently elevated in patients with heart failure. However, as is the case with the other vasodilator substances released in heart failure, dopamine appears to be overwhelmed by the vasoconstrictor systems.

ENDOTHELIAL-DERIVED FACTORS

The vascular endothelium has been described as a pharmacologic cornucopia. It is the source of several vasoactive substances that locally promote smooth muscle relaxation and contraction. These substances include the vasodilator endothelium-derived relaxing factor (EDRF) and the extremely potent vasoconstrictor, endothelin. Although research concerning the role of these locally acting substances is in its relative infancy compared to research related to systemic neuroendocrine activation, there is evidence that abnormalities of EDRF and endothelin contribute to the vasoconstriction seen in heart failure (Francis, 1990). Several factors contribute to the abnormal vascular tone seen in heart failure: neuroendocrine factors, salt and water excess in the vascular wall, and local endothelial abnormalities (Katz et al., 1992). Investigators have demonstrated attenuation of endothelium-dependent vasodilator responses in patients with heart failure (Forstermann et al., 1988; Katz et al., 1992; Kubo et al., 1991; Treasure et al., 1990). The cause of reduced endothelial-dependent vasodilation in heart failure is unclear, but abnormalities in the formation and/or release of EDRF and abnormalities in smooth muscle response are possibilities (Katz et al., 1992). Additionally, it appears that endothelin levels are markedly increased in heart failure patients in proportion to the severity of heart failure (Stewart et al., 1992).

Ventricular Remodeling: Dilation and Hypertrophy

Ventricular remodeling is an initially adaptive response to decreased cardiac output and loss of functioning myocardium. Although the course of development of dilation and hypertrophy varies depending on the cause of heart failure (Opie, 1991), an early compensatory mechanism in most cases is ventricular dilation. Dilation results in an increase in ventricular end-diastolic volume. Dilation preserves stroke volume and maintains cardiac output by the Frank-Starling mechanism, and initially stroke volume is maintained at rest. However, ventricular dilation significantly increases wall stress since, according to the law of Laplace, wall stress is equal to the product of ventricular pressure and radius divided by wall thickness. To compensate for an increase in wall stress, ventricular hypertrophy ensues because an increase in wall thickness will decrease wall stress. For a time, the degree of hypertrophy appears to adequately compensate for increased ventricular cavity size. As heart failure progresses and the heart is continually exposed to adverse loading conditions, hypertrophy increases. However, hypertrophy alters myocardial structure such that pumping efficiency is impaired and contractility declines. Ultimately myocardial remodeling progresses to the point that continued ventricular dilation exceeds any compensatory advantage offered by continued hypertrophy (Opie, 1991).

Consideration of the process of ventricular remodeling in heart failure gives rise to two fundamental questions: (1) What is the signal triggering hypertrophy (Katz, 1992)? and (2) What triggers the progression from hypertrophy to failure (Opie, 1991)?

Almost certainly, more than one signal triggers the process of hypertrophy, and presumably several of the hypothesized triggers interact in a complex fashion (Katz, 1992). The cardiac stretch receptors are among the possibilities for the role of initiator of hypertrophy. Several growth factors normally found in the heart are also possible triggers of hypertrophy, in particular the acidic and basic fibroblast growth factors that initiate cardiac cell growth and synthesis of fetal cardiac muscle proteins. Various intracellular second messengers, including cyclic AMP (cAMP) and calcium, also initiate cardiac cell growth and are potentially important in hypertrophy. Particularly prominent candidates for initiators of cell growth in heart failure are the neuroendocrine substances (e.g., norepinephrine and angiotensin II) released in heart failure. Norepinephrine is also capable of inducing hypertrophy and myocardial cell remodeling through the promotion of protooncogene expression, which may be responsible for increasing myocardial cell size. Angiotensin II also can promote gene expression responsible for protein synthesis leading to hypertrophy (Francis, 1990). Recent studies have demonstrated that therapy with the ACE inhibitor captopril improves left ventricular remodeling and function while preventing ventricular enlargement (Bonaduce et al., 1992).

Hypertrophy initially is beneficial in that it increases the number of functioning sarcomeres, thereby reducing the effect of excessive loading conditions on the heart. Hypertrophy also results in a number of structural and biochemical changes that are initially beneficial but that eventually cause myocardial cell death contributing to the progression of heart failure (Katz, 1992; Opie, 1991; Schwartz et al., 1992, 1993). These changes include altered gene expression of both actin and myosin isoforms. What causes the progression from hypertrophy to failure? The basic mechanism is unknown, but numerous pieces of evidence support the belief that an oxygen/supply demand imbalance exists that promotes myocardial cell death (Katz, 1992; Opie, 1991).

Myocardial cell death occurs in the hypertrophied heart for many reasons. The capillary supply to the hypertrophied myocardium does not increase at the same rate as does the growth of muscle tissue (Katz, 1992), thus setting up the conditions for regional necrosis and subsequent fibrosis. Increased intraluminal ventricular pressure promotes subendocardial ischemia (even in the absence of coronary artery disease [CAD]) that results in fibrosis (Unverferth et al., 1983). Fibrosis can also occur as a result of ischemia secondary to subendocardial and coronary artery vasoconstriction from high levels of circulating norepinephrine and angiotensin II. A decrease in mitochondria relative to myofibrils and decreased high-energy phosphate content have been observed in heart failure patients and in rat models of heart failure. The increased collagen deposition seen in hypertrophied hearts initially is beneficial in that it delays ventricular dilation. In later stages, however, increased collagen promotes fibrosis due to ischemia (Jalil et al., 1989). Another finding in heart failure that is presumed to promote cell death and fibrosis is the decrease in myocardial compliance seen in the hypertrophied heart (Opie,

1991). Decreased compliance leads to increased wall stress, which increases oxygen demands, creating a state of "relative hypoxia" that leads to further fibrosis. All of these processes promote cell death, decreasing the number of functional contractile units.

Pathophysiologic Factors Underlying Activity Intolerance

Dyspnea and fatigue with activity are the two characteristic and most common symptoms of heart failure (Poole-Wilson & Buller, 1988). These symptoms are usually severe enough to limit all activities of daily living, not just the more strenuous ativities. Several factors interact to produce these symptoms.

Several abnormalities have been hypothesized to produce the dyspnea seen in heart failure patients (Poole-Wilson, 1993; Wilson & Mancini, 1993). Although increased preload and end-diastolic pressure play a role in producing dyspnea, other factors are equally important, particularly in chronic failure. These additional factors include: (1) an increase in ventilatory requirement, (2) decreased lung compliance, and (3) respiratory muscle underperfusion and diaphragm weakness. The perception of dyspnea may also be greatly influenced by skeletal muscle activation and fatigue.

A major factor contributing to exertional fatigue is a decrease in muscle blood flow (Wilson & Mancini, 1993). An attenuated cardiac output response to exercise occurs in heart failure (Wilson et al., 1984). Further compounding the problem is alteration of the normal vascular tone response to exercise. Normally, vasodilation helps to increase muscle perfusion during activity, but this response is abnormal in heart failure. Adequate vasodilation fails to occur (Sullivan et al., 1989), and multiple possible factors are implicated: (1) fluid and sodium retention, which impairs vasomotor response; (2) acute neuroendocrine activation during exercise; (3) abnormalities of the vascular endothelium and altered responses of EDRF and endothelin; (4) vascular structural changes secondary to angiotensin II; and (5) impaired release of the usual local vasodilator metabolites from active muscle (Wilson & Mancini, 1993).

Another important determinant of muscle fatigue is deconditioning (Wilson & Mancini, 1993). Evidence from exercise rehabilitation (Coats et al., 1992), metabolic, muscle biopsy, and magnetic resonance imaging studies (Wilson & Mancini, 1993) provides strong evidence that muscle deconditioning plays a larger role in the genesis of fatigue in heart failure than originally appreciated.

Summary

The presentation of the patient with heart failure is one in which the compensatory mechanisms that initially improve cardiac output fail, further compromising the patient. The balance between vasoconstrictor and vasodilator systems is tipped in favor of vasoconstriction. In a series of vicious cycles, neuroendocrine activation results in intense vasoconstriction, volume expansion, vascular changes, and ventricular remodeling, exacerbating loading conditions on the failing left ventricle and contributing to a further decrease in myocardial contractility and to the development of overt, symptomatic failure (Fig. 21–3).

CLINICAL MANIFESTATIONS AND DIAGNOSTIC TESTING

Symptoms and Signs

The clinical presentation in heart failure can be quite varied because patients can present at any place on the continuum from asymptomatic left ventricular dysfunction to mild, moderate, or severe heart failure. A significant minority of patients with significant left ventricular dysfunction and low ejection fractions fail to present with signs or symptoms that meet criteria characteristic for the diagnosis of heart failure (Marantz et al., 1988). Typical symptoms and signs of heart failure are presented in Table 21–4. Dyspnea with activity is a common first presenting symptom in heart failure (Wilson & Mancini, 1993). Breathlessness, paroxysmal nocturnal dyspnea, and orthopnea are also highly suggestive of the diagnosis of heart failure (Konstam et al., 1994). Physical signs most suggestive of a diagnosis of heart failure are elevated jugular venous pressure, third heart sound, and laterally displaced apical impulse. In patients with symptoms of heart failure, these signs are "virtually diagnostic" (Konstam et al., 1994).

Diagnostic Evaluation

Diagnostic evaluation for heart failure begins with a thorough history and physical examination to rule out other causes for symptoms and to detect underlying and contributing factors to heart failure. Careful questioning to elicit symptoms as outlined in Table 21–4 is important. Because ischemic heart disease is the most common cause of heart failure, history of chest pain is also important to elicit, as is assessment of other risk factors for CAD. History of CAD, myocardial infarction and/or angina, longstanding hypertension, or other causes of heart failure lends added significance to symptoms of heart failure.

In assessing physical signs, the practitioner must keep in mind that the signs of heart failure are neither highly sensitive nor specific for the diagnosis (Stevenson & Perloff, 1989). Physical findings are often absent even in patients with severe heart failure and pulmonary wedge pressures elevated as high as 35 mm Hg (Stevenson & Perloff, 1989). For this reason, patients

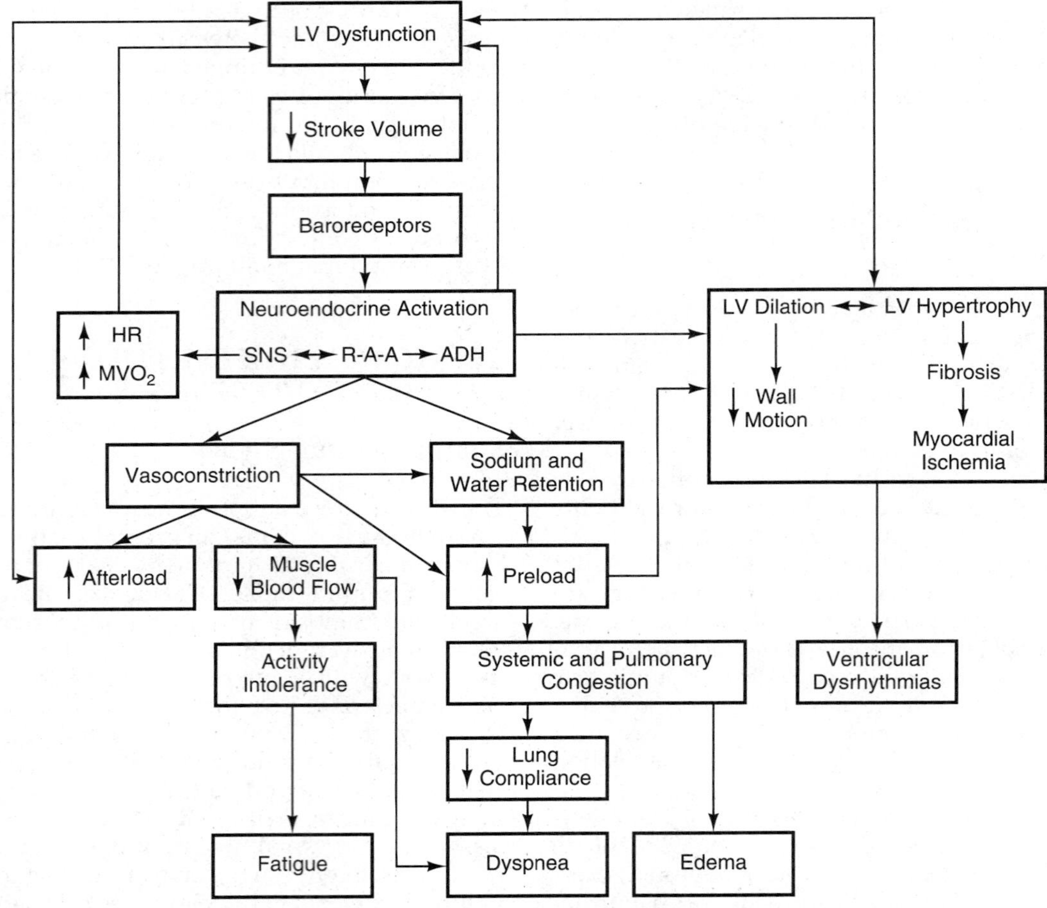

FIGURE 21–3. Pathophysiology of clinical heart failure. (Modified with permission from Cohn, J. N. [1994]. Overview of pathophysiology of heart failure. In J. D. Hosenpud & B. H. Greenberg [Eds.], *Congestive heart failure: Pathophysiology, diagnosis, and comprehensive approach to management* [pp. 11–16]. New York: Springer-Verlag.)

with symptoms suggestive of heart failure require further evaluation even if they do not have supporting signs and symptoms.

CHEST X-RAY

A relatively inexpensive, easily obtained test, the chest x-ray should be done early in the course of evaluation to support the diagnosis of heart failure, rule out pulmonary causes of dyspnea, and help establish degree of pulmonary venous congestion. A common chest x-ray finding in heart failure is cardiomegaly with the cardiothoracic ratio increased >0.50. The chest x-ray provides information about left atrial and right and left ventricular enlargement and the presence of pleural effusion. Early x-ray evidence of pulmonary venous congestion secondary to increased left atrial pressure is interstitial with perivascular pulmonary edema at the lung bases progressing throughout the lung as congestion worsens (Young & Farmer, 1994).

ELECTROCARDIOGRAM

The electrocardiogram (ECG) is nonspecific in heart failure, but provides important information about precipitating or causative factors such as acute ST-T wave change evidence of acute ischemia or Q wave evidence of prior myocardial infarction. When overt failure is present, the underlying rhythm is often sinus tachycardia, but in patients treated with digoxin this sign is often absent. The ECG is rarely normal; there are often nonspecific ST- and T-wave changes, left ventricular hypertrophy, atrial fibrillation, ventricular dysrhythmias, or conduction defects (Unverferth, 1985; Young & Farmer, 1994). In cardiomyopathy patients Q waves may be present when extreme left ventricular fibrosis is present even without discrete myocardial infarction. These Q waves are believed to be due to myonecrosis of the cardiotrophic sinus (Wynne & Braunwald, 1992).

ECHOCARDIOGRAPHY AND RADIONUCLIDE VENTRICULOGRAPHY

Measurement of left ventricular function using echocardiography or radionuclide ventriculography is essential in evaluation of patients with suspected or overt heart failure (Konstam et al., 1994). Assessment of left ventricular function is used to correctly classify

TABLE 21–4. **Clinical Manifestations of Heart Failure**

Symptoms and Signs	Cause
Dyspnea on exertion or at rest	Pulmonary venous congestion, increased ventilatory requirement, decreased lung compliance, possibly respiratory muscle underperfusion
Paroxysmal nocturnal dyspnea, orthopnea	Increased intrathoracic blood volume and left ventricular filling pressures in the supine position
Fatigue, weakness, decreased exercise tolerance	Muscle underperfusion, deconditioning, metabolic factors
Peripheral edema	Right heart failure with systemic venous congestion
Memory loss, confusion	Cerebrovascular underperfusion, drug effects
Cough	Bronchiolar congestion and excessive mucus production
Nocturia	Redistribution of blood flow and increased renal perfusion in supine position
Anorexia, nausea, gastrointestinal complaints	Intestinal, mesenteric, liver, and spleen congestion and edema
Abdominal distention	As above
Elevated jugular venous pressure	Increased ventricular preload and end-diastolic pressure
S_3, S_4, decreased intensity of S_1	Volume overload, reduced ventricular compliance
Laterally displaced apical impulse	Cardiomegaly
Positive hepatojugular reflux	Right heart failure with peripheral venous congestion and systemic venous hypertension producing liver congestion
Tachycardia	Sympathetic nervous system activation
Rales not clearing with cough	Elevated left atrial pressure and pulmonary venous congestion
Pleural effusion	Severe pulmonary congestion
Pulsus alternans	Severe left ventricular dysfunction
Peripheral edema not due to venous insufficiency	Right heart failure with systemic venous congestion
Ascites	Long-standing venous congestion and hypertension
Hepatomegaly	Right heart failure with peripheral venous congestion and systemic venous hypertension producing liver congestion
Left parasternal lift	Cardiomegaly
Systolic regurgitant murmurs	Mitral and tricuspid valve regurgitation secondary to atrioventricular valve insufficiency as ventricles dilate

heart failure as originating from primarily systolic or diastolic dysfunction, valvular dysfunction or noncardiac cause, a distinction that has important treatment implications. Echocardiography is used to assess left ventricular ejection fraction, cardiac chamber size, valve function, wall motion, and pericardial effusion and restriction; to detect the presence of ventricular thrombi; and to estimate the degree of wall stress. Typical findings when left ventricular systolic dysfunction is present include depressed systolic function with ejection fractions less than 35% to 40%, global or regional wall motion abnormalities, atrial and ventricular chamber enlargement, and left ventricular hypertrophy.

Radionuclide ventriculography also assesses left ventricular function and may provide more precise and reliable measurement of ejection fraction. In addition, it allows accurate assessment of ventricular function in the 8% to 18% of patients in whom echocardiography is technically poor (Konstam et al., 1994). Radionuclide studies are useful for quantifying severity of heart failure and degree of contraction and relaxation abnormalities. Additionally, perfusion abnormalities are identified and areas of ischemia and scar formation are delineated (Young & Farmer, 1994).

EXERCISE TESTING

Exercise testing is frequently performed in heart failure patients to determine functional capacity. Functional capacity is often used to determine efficacy of treatment. The results of exercise testing are also used to supply clinicians with prognostic information and to assist in evaluation for cardiac transplantation. Important data obtained from exercise testing include exercise-induced dysrhythmias, metabolic equivalent level reached, oxygen uptake, and ability to increase heart rate and blood pressure appropriately in response to exercise. Patients with severe left ventricular dysfunction have impaired hemodynamic response to exercise. Exercise testing using respiratory gas exchange techniques allows quantification of functional class. Patients in New York Heart Association (NYHA) class IV are capable of only reaching a maximum oxygen consumption ($\dot{V}O_2$ max) of 10 mL O_2/min/kg or less, while normal is greater than 20 mL O_2/min/kg (Young & Farmer, 1994). NYHA class II patients can achieve 16 to 20 mL O_2/min/kg and NYHA class III 10 to 15 mL O_2/min/kg. Recent guidelines from the 24th Bethesda Conference on Cardiac Transplantation (1993) set the following guidelines for cardiac transplantation based on $\dot{V}O_2$ max: transplantation indicated for $\dot{V}O_2$ max $<$ 10 mL O_2/min/kg; aggressive drug therapy and retesting in 90 days indicated for 10 to 14 mL O_2/min/kg; a level of greater than 15 mL O_2/min/kg is an indication for medical therapy with transplantation not indicated.

CARDIAC CATHETERIZATION

Although not indicated for all heart failure patients, cardiac catheterization with coronary angiography is useful for patients with ischemic heart disease to determine whether revascularization with cornary artery

TABLE 21–5. **Hemodynamic Presentation of Heart Failure**

	Normal	Heart Failure
Right atrial pressure	0–8 mm Hg	↑
Systolic pulmonary artery pressure	20–30 mm Hg	↑
Diastolic pulmonary artery pressure	8–12 mm Hg	↑
Pulmonary wedge pressure	5–12 mm Hg	↑
Cardiac output (HR × SV)	4–6 L/min	↓
Cardiac index (CO/BSA)	2.5–4.2 L/min	↓
Pulmonary vascular resistance	100–300 dynes/cm/sec^{-5}	↑
Systemic vascular resistance	800–1200 dynes/cm/sec^{-5}	↑

Abbreviations: HR, heart rate; SV, stroke volume; CO, cardiac output; BSA, body surface area.

bypass grafting is indicated. In addition, when etiology is unclear this test is indicated to rule out coronary artery disease. Cardiac catheterization will usually reveal a hemodynamic profile including elevated cardiac pressures, low cardiac output, and elevated SVR (Table 21–5).

ENDOMYOCARDIAL BIOPSY

Transvenous endomyocardial biopsy (Fig. 21–4) is performed in selected heart failure patients. This test is not indicated for all heart failure patients, but may

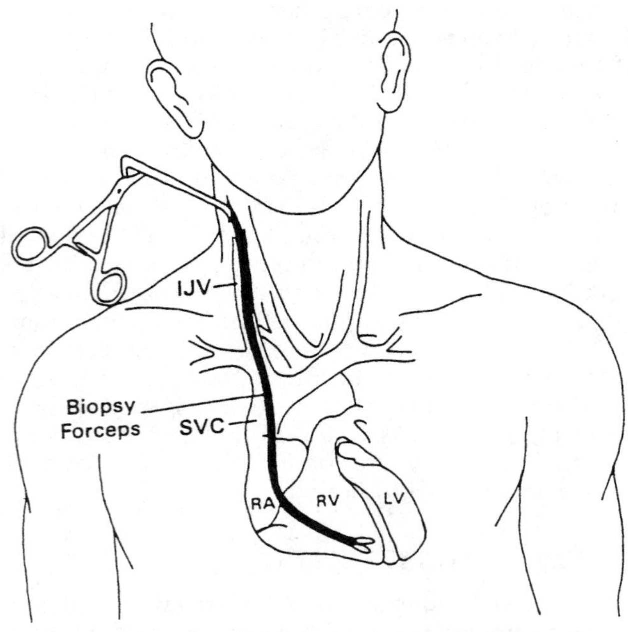

FIGURE 21–4. Transvenous endomyocardial biopsy. *Abbreviations:* IJV, internal jugular vein; SVC, superior vena cava. (From Shoemaker, W. C., et al. [1989]. *Textbook of critical care.* Philadelphia: W. B. Saunders.)

TABLE 21–6. **Indications for Endomyocardial Biopsy**

To differentiate restrictive from constrictive disease
To evaluate cardiac involvement in systemic disease
To evaluate myocarditis
To detect cardiotoxicity due to cardiotoxic agents
To evaluate cardiac transplant rejection
To evaluate cardiac tumors

From Wynne, J., & Braunwald, E. (1992). In E. Braunwald (Ed.), *Heart disease: A textbook of cardiovascular medicine.* Philadelphia: W. B. Saunders.

be useful in detecting myocarditis and distinguishing etiology for some cardiomyopathies (Table 21–6). Endomyocardial biopsy is common in establishing a diagnosis of cardiomyopathy, particularly if there is a viral process component in the patient's history. One drawback of the test is failure to identify an etiology because only small portions of the myocardium are sampled for biopsy, and the problem can be missed. A specific etiology for cardiomyopathy is established in only 20% of cases (Stevenson & Perloff, 1988). Biopsy will show myocardial inflammation, fibrosis, or necrosis, or these processes may go unnoticed depending on where the biopsy is done and where in the myocardium the inflammatory process has occurred.

LABORATORY TESTING

Evaluation of heart failure patients should include a urinalysis and the following blood chemistries: complete blood count (CBC), electrolytes, serum creatinine, blood urea nitrogen (BUN), serum albumin, and liver function studies (Konstam et al., 1994). The CBC is assessed to rule out anemia as a factor aggravating heart failure. Common electrolyte abnormalities, especially in patients with severe heart failure, include hypokalemia and hyponatremia. Both can occur as a result of aggressive diuretic use seen in the treatment of heart failure. In addition, aldosterone production produces these electrolyte abnormalities. Hyponatremia is further aggravated by vasopressin release, which produces a dilutional hyponatremia due to excess water retention. Hyperkalemia can occur in patients treated with ACE inhibitors, especially those with marginal renal blood flow. Another electrolyte disturbance seen in heart failure is hypomagnesemia. Renal function is measured in heart failure to rule out kidney disease as a contributor to failure and to assess the degree of impairment secondary to reduced renal perfusion. Liver function is assessed for similar reasons. Patients with heart failure can have impairment of liver function due to underperfusion, and failure can be intensified by liver dysfunction. Serum albumin is decreased in some heart failure patients secondary to malnutrition, and hypoalbuminemia can aggravate heart failure by stimulating extravascular volume overload.

TREATMENT

The objectives of treatment in heart failure are fourfold: (1) prevention of myocardial damage by pre-

TABLE 21–7. **Medications Used in the Treatment of Chronic Heart Failure**

Drug	Initial Dose (mg)	Target Dose (mg)	Recommended Maximal Dose (mg)	Potential Adverse Reactions
Thiazide Diuretics				
Hydrochlorothiazide	25 QD	As needed	50 QD	Postural hypotension, hypokalemia, hyperglycemia, hyperuricemia, rash
Chlorthalidone	25 QD	As needed	50 QD	
Loop Diuretics				
Furosemide	10–40 QD	As needed	240 BID	Same as thiazide diuretics
Bumetanide	0.5–1.0 QD	As needed	10 QD	
Ethacrynic acid	50 QD	As needed	200 BID	
Potassium-Sparing Diuretics				
Spironolactone	25 QD	As needed	100 BID	Hyperkalemia (especially if given with ACE inhibitor), rash, gynecomastia (spironolactone only)
Triamterene	50 QD	As needed	100 BID	
Amiloride	5 QD	As needed	40 QD	
Thiazide-Related Diuretic				
Metolazone	2.5 as single test dose initially	As needed	10 QD	Same as thiazide diuretics
Angiotensin-Converting Enzyme (ACE) Inhibitors				
Enalapril	2.5 BID	10 BID	20 BID	Hypotension, hyperkalemia, renal insufficiency, cough, rash, angioedema, neutropenia
Captopril	6.25–12.5 TID	50 TID	100 TID	
Lisinopril	5 QD	20 QD	40 QD	
Quinapril	5 BID	20 BID	20 BID	
Digoxin	0.125–0.25 QD	0.125–0.25 QD	0.125–0.25 QD	Cardiotoxicity, confusion, nausea, anorexia, visual disturbances
Hydralazine	10–25 TID	75 TID	100 TID	Headache, nausea, dizziness, tachycardia, lupus-like syndrome
Isosorbide Dinitrate	10 TID	40 TID	80 TID	Headache, hypotension, flushing

Note: Maximal dosages are typical recommendations. In some cases larger doses are given to control symptoms.

From Konstam, M., Dracup, K., Baker, D., et al. (1994). Heart failure: Evaluation and care of patients with left-ventricular systolic dysfunction. Clinical Practice Guideline No. 11. AHCPR Publication No. 94-0612. Rockville, MD: Agency for Health Care Policy and Research, Public Health Services, U.S. Department of Health and Human Services.

venting occurrence or progression of further damaging episodes; (2) prevention of recurrence of clinical failure; (3) relief of symptoms and signs; and (4) improvement in prognosis (Poole-Wilson, 1993). Because morbidity and mortality are so high in heart failure and because the course can be so unrelenting, prevention is vitally important.

Treatment options in heart failure are largely limited to pharmacologic therapy (Table 21–7). Of course, if an underlying correctable cause for heart failure can be found, such as ischemia amenable to revascularization or valvular disease correctable by valve replacement, such intervention should occur. Cardiac transplantation is a viable option for a limited number of patients with end-stage disease. However, pharmacologic intervention, supplemented by nonpharmacologic strategies, remains the mainstay of treatment in heart failure. With therapy tailored to achieve the hemodynamic goals of decreased SVR and ventricular filling pressures, many patients initially referred for cardiac transplantation can be successfully managed with medical therapy (Stevenson et al., 1989).

Nonpharmacologic Therapy

DIET

One of the oldest interventions for the treatment of heart failure is the restriction of dietary sodium, and this intervention is still a fundamental part of treatment. In addition to helping to reduce fluid overload, sodium restriction augments the effectiveness of diuretic therapy (Bousquet, 1990). Although specific level of sodium restriction has not been studied (Konstam et al., 1994), in general the degree of sodium restriction selected depends on the severity of heart failure. For patients with mild to moderate failure a 3-g sodium restriction is usually sufficient. For patients with more severe failure requiring large diuretic doses, a more stringent restriction of 2 G/day is prescribed (Konstam et al., 1994). Both patient and family need thorough instructions about how to achieve the perscribed sodium restriction. Most people are knowledgeable about obvious sources of sodium, but many people are completely unaware of the considerable sodium content of less obvious sources. Dietary sodium indiscretion is a common reason for heart failure exacerbation, and inadequate patient preparation contributes to failure to follow the diet.

Other dietary recommendations include avoidance of alcohol, a myocardial depressant (Jennison & Miller, 1993). For patients who decide to continue to drink, limiting intake to one drink per day is advised. Patients with alcohol-induced cardiomyopathy must be advised to completely refrain from alcohol use.

Although patients should be counseled to refrain from excessive fluid intake, stringent fluid restrictions are not indicated except in selected patients (Konstam et al., 1994). Adequate symptom control with pharmacologic therapy often precludes the need for stringent fluid restriction. However, patients with severe heart failure and difficult to control hyponatremia may benefit from fluid restriction (Bousquet, 1990).

RISK FACTOR MODIFICATION

For heart failure patients with CAD or at risk for developing it, modification of risk factors is vital to prevent further ischemic damage. Patients should be advised to stop smoking and to adopt a prudent, low-fat diet. Elevated lipid levels should be treated, especially in patients with ischemic cardiomyopathy. Guidelines adopted by some institutions include achievement of the following lipid target levels using drug therapy if necessary: total cholesterol < 160 mg/dL, low-density lipoproteins < 100 mg/dL, and high-density lipoproteins > 45 mg/dL. Hypertension should also be controlled because this condition can lead both to further ischemic events stimulating progression of heart failure and to exacerbations of compensated heart failure. Control of even borderline hypertension may have a direct effect on improving heart failure (Konstam et al., 1994).

EXERCISE

Before the advent of effective diuretic therapy, heart failure was commonly treated with bed rest to promote diuresis and activity restriction to decrease myocardial oxygen consumption. Many clinicians still advise activity limitation. However, recent Agency for Health Care Policy and Research (AHCPR) guidelines for the management of patients with left ventricular dysfunction highlight the changing thinking about exercise in heart failure patients. Based on a rapidly expanding body of literature documenting the positive effects and low risk of exercise in heart failure patients, regular exercise (e.g., walking or cycling) is recommended for all stable patients with NYHA functional classification I–III (Konstam et al., 1994). Exercise in these patients improves functional status, exercise tolerance, and symptoms; prevents deconditioning effects; may decrease neuroendocrine activation; corrects impairment of skeletal muscle metabolism; and improves quality of life (Adamopoulos et al., 1993; Sullivan, 1994). Recent evidence demonstrates that even patients with stable severe heart failure (NYHA class IV) can be safely exercised and derive significant benefit (Sullivan, 1994).

Pharmacologic Therapy

TRIPLE THERAPY: ACE INHIBITORS, DIURETICS, DIGITALIS

ACE Inhibitors

Evidence from several recent well-conducted multicenter trials of ACE inhibitors in heart failure has changed the way this condition is treated. ACE inhibition results in substantial clinical improvement of heart failure and offers distinct survival advantages for patients with all classes of failure (Cohn et al., 1991; CONSENSUS Trial Study Group, 1987; Fonarow et al., 1992; SOLVD Investigators, 1991). These effects have prompted the recent recommendation that "the vasodilator of choice in patients with mild, moderate or severe congestive heart failure should be a converting enzyme inhibitor" (Kukin, 1992, p. 1302). ACE inhibitors are also effective in retarding the progression of heart failure, decreasing the incidence of cardiovascular events, and improving survival in patients with left ventricular dysfunction who do not yet have symptoms or signs of overt failure, and thus are recommended in the treatment of these patients (Pfeffer et al., 1992; SOLVD Investigators, 1992).

By blocking angiotensin-converting enzyme, ACE inhibitors suppress the production of angiotensin II. Because cardiac output is highly dependent on afterload in chronic heart failure, the vasodilation produced by ACE inhibition produces a significant increase in cardiac output. Even though arterial pressure may be decreased, tissue perfusion is maintained or is increased due to improvement of cardiac output and redistribution of regional blood flow. ACE inhibitor use is associated with several other favorable hemodynamic effects and has a beneficial impact on other systems in the neurohormonal activation cascade (Table 21–8).

PATIENT OUTCOMES. Angiotensin-converting enzyme inhibitors produce significant sustained hemodynamic and clinical improvement in patients in all classes of heart failure from mild to severe, deterio-

TABLE 21–8. **Effects of Angiotensin-Converting Enzyme Inhibitors**

Suppression of Angiotension II and Aldosterone Production
Vasodilation
Increased cardiac output
Reduced arterial blood pressure with maintenance or improvement in tissue perfusion
Decreased ventricular filling pressures
Improvement in electrolyte (particularly sodium and potassium) balance
Improvement in volume overload state
Reduced left ventricular wall stress
Beneficial impact on the process of ventricular dilation and hypertrophy
Reduced sympathetic nervous system arousal
Attenuation of the direct myopathic effects of angiotensin II
Possible stimulation of prostaglandin production with positive effects on ventricular receptor reflexes
Possible augmentation of bradykinin accumulation

Modified with permission from Moser, D. K. (1993). Pharmacologic management of heart failure: Neurohormonal agents. *Critical Care Nursing Clinics of North America, 5,* 599–608.

rating failure. Cardiac index and stroke index are increased, and left ventricular filling pressures and systemic and pulmonary vascular resistance are decreased by 30% to 40% (Captopril Multicenter Research Group I, 1985; Kramer et al., 1983). Patients report improvement of debilitating symptoms and exercise tolerance. NYHA functional classification is improved and patients experience fewer exacerbations of heart failure (SOLVD Investigators, 1991). Even in patients already on maximal doses of diuretics and digoxin, there is resolution of edema and improvement in and maintenance of electrolyte balance (CONSENSUS Trial Study Group, 1987).

A number of randomized clinical trials have demonstrated the survival benefit of ACE inhibitors over placebo or over therapy with direct-acting vasodilators. Mortality is reduced in all classes of heart failure due to a reduction in deaths from both progressive heart failure and sudden death (Cohn et al., 1991; CONSENSUS Trial Study Group, 1987; Fonarow et al., 1992; SOLVD Investigators, 1991). The overall reduction in mortality is modest, in the range of 16% with long-term follow-up (SOLVD Investigators, 1991).

Among the most interesting outcomes associated with the use of ACE inhibitors are those related to the prevention of the progression of heart failure. Building on a considerable body of animal research demonstrating that ACE inhibitors prevent ventricular remodeling and improve survival (Kubo and Cohn, 1994), human trials in patients with asymptomatic left ventricular dysfunction have been conducted. Most notable of these are the prevention arm of the SOLVD Trial (SOLVD Investigators, 1992) and the Survival and Ventricular Enlargement (SAVE) Trial (Pfeffer et al., 1992). Both trials followed patients for more than 3 years. Outcomes in the SOLVD Prevention Trial included a 36% reduction in first hospitalizations for heart failure and a 37% reduction in the incidence of development of overt heart failure for patients randomized to receive an ACE inhibitor (enalapril). In the SAVE Trial patients randomized to captopril and compared to a placebo group demonstrated a 17% reduction in mortality and a significant reduction in the onset of heart failure and of hospitalizations related to it.

CLINICAL USE. Angiotensin-converting enzyme inhibitors should be used in doses high enough to control symptoms (Table 21–7). A common error in the use of these agents is failure to prescribe adequate doses (Cohn, 1992) because of fear of hypotension, hyperkalemia, and alterations in renal function (Cody, 1992; Konstam et al., 1994). However, in clinical trials the actual incidence of these complications is less than 6% even in patients with severe left ventricular dysfunction and considerably less in patients with less severe failure (CONSENSUS Trial Study Group, 1987; SOLVD Investigators, 1991).

Enalapril, a long-acting agent, is given in daily doses of up to 20 mg, which should be titrated up from an initial dose of 2.5 mg daily. Captopril, with its shorter half-life, is frequently given TID or QID in daily doses of up to 100 mg. Doses of captopril up to 400 mg/day are safely used at some institutions after titration, usually during hemodynamic monitoring (Stevenson & Fonarow, 1992). The dose should be carefully titrated from an initial starting point of 6.25 mg daily, especially in patients at risk for hypotension. All patients at risk for hypotension should be initially tested with a trial of captopril because it is short-acting. At-risk patients include those over age 75, with severe left ventricular dysfunction, resting hemodynamic abnormalities, or hyponatremia (serum sodium < 135 mEq/L).

If hypotension or mild azotemia occur, they are not necessarily indications for withdrawal of therapy. Monitoring of blood pressure and renal function with dosage changes and gradual titration is recommended to reduce problems associated with these effects. Because a decrease in peripheral resistance is usually associated with increased cardiac output and tissue perfusion, asymptomatic hypotension is well tolerated. If hypotension is symptomatic or severe (e.g., less than 90 mm Hg systolic in patients with ischemic heart failure and less than 80 mm Hg systolic in other types of heart failure), the dose should be reduced. Volume status should be assessed and corrected before withdrawal of therapy in patients who develop symptomatic hypotension or renal insufficiency (Konstam et al., 1994; Stevenson, 1993). Excessive volume depletion secondary to diuretic use is a common reason for apparent ACE inhibitor intolerance.

Hyperkalemia may occur during therapy due to inhibited potassium excretion. Therefore, potassium should be monitored when therapy is begun and with dosage changes. Potassium supplements given with diuretics or potassium-sparing diuretic doses may need to be reduced or eliminated (SOLVD Investiga-

TABLE 21–9. **Factors Contributing to Excess Sodium and Water Retention in Heart Failure**

Decreased cardiac output
Decreased glomerular filtration rate secondary to reduced renal blood flow
Redistribution of intrarenal blood flow to salt-conserving medulla
Increased renal sympathetic nerve activity
Increased arginine vasopressin (antidiuretic hormone) levels
Activation of the renin-angiotensin-aldosterone system

tors, 1992). CBC monitoring is usually done because leukopenia is a potential side effect. Other infrequent but troublesome side effects seen include cough and angioedema, which may be related to the accumulation of kinins and prostaglandins occurring with ACE inhibition. Rash and taste disturbances are rarely seen with captopril therapy and may resolve with continued use of captopril or with change to enalapril (Stevenson & Fonarow, 1992).

Specific patient and family education regarding therapy with ACE inhibitors includes basic reasons for the medication, the planned regimen, and the possible adverse consequences of abrupt withdrawal. Patients need to be informed that postural hypotension may occur and how to manage it. With concurrent use of other vasodilators, patients should be taught to stagger dosing so that all vasodilators are not taken at the same time. This information should be reinforced and patient and family understanding of the treatment regimen reassessed at outpatient clinic visits and during rehospitalizations.

Diuretics

Diuretics have long been a primary treatment for heart failure despite the fact that there have been few prospective trials of diuretic use in this condition. Many factors contribute to the sodium and water retention and subsequent volume overload seen in heart failure (Table 21–9). Diuretic agents are effective in reducing volume overload because they block the reabsorption of sodium by cells along the nephron. Water is excreted in proportion to sodium to maintain osmotic balance. By promoting sodium and water excretion, diuretics are particularly effective in relieving the symptoms and signs of systemic and pulmonary congestion seen in heart failure.

Diuretics also may exert hemodynamic effects. Some degree of vasodilation occurs with a resulting decrease in ventricular filling pressures and SVR (Cody, 1993). These effects may be responsible for the sometimes rapid clinical improvement seen in patients before they begin to diurese (Cuny & Enger, 1993). In some studies, however, diuretic use has been associated with vasoconstrictor effects (Cody, 1993). These effects are likely the result of activation of the renin-angiotensin-aldosterone and sympathetic nervous systems. These effects have been seen both acutely and with long-term diuretic therapy although their clinical significance is uncertain and may be negligible with concomitant therapy with ACE inhibitors. Other adverse effects have been associated with diuretic therapy (Table 21–10).

CLINICAL USE. There are many types of diuretic agents classified according to their site of action in the nephron (Fig. 21–5). The choice of which agent to use is frequently based on severity of symptoms and whether the failure is acute or chronic (Cuny & Enger, 1993). Degree of sodium retention also can guide the choice of diuretic agent, and a scheme for directing therapy based on sodium retention has been proposed by Cody (Table 21–11). Patients with mild heart failure are initially usually well-managed on thiazide diuretics (Konstam et al., 1994). In patients in whom systemic and/or pulmonary congestion does not resolve with the use of a thiazide diuretic or who present with symptoms and signs of severe fluid overload or frequent hospitalizations for failure or renal insufficiency, a loop diuretic (e.g., furosemide) is used. Dosages are presented in Table 21–7.

In those patients seemingly refractory to oral diuretics, a combination of therapy with a loop diuretic (e.g., furosemide) and a nonloop diuretic (e.g., metolazone) is often effective (Kubo & Cohn, 1994). Therapy with the second nonloop diuretic is generally required only intermittently. It is important to explore possible causes of seemingly refractory volume overload. Common causes are noncompliance with the medical regimen or failure to follow a low-sodium diet. Diuretic therapy does not take the place of dietary sodium restriction and should always be combined with a sodium-restricted diet (Kubo & Cohn, 1994). Gut edema may limit oral absorption of diuretic agents and patients with severe congestion may require intravenous diuretic therapy to initiate effective diuresis.

The major adverse reaction to diuretic use is electrolyte (particularly potassium and magnesium) depletion. Serum potassium should be checked frequently when beginning or changing diuretic therapy and when adding or changing ACE inhibitor therapy in patients on diuretics. Many patients managed on both drugs have normal potassium levels. In general, potassium-sparing diuretics should not be used in patients on ACE inhibitors to avoid hyperkalemia.

TABLE 21–10. **Adverse Effects of Diuretics in Heart Failure Patients**

Activation of the renin-angiotensin-aldosterone system
Electrolyte imbalance: hypokalemia, hyponatremia, hypomagnesemia
Renal insufficiency
Volume depletion
Hyperuricemia
Hyperlipidemia
Metabolic alkalosis

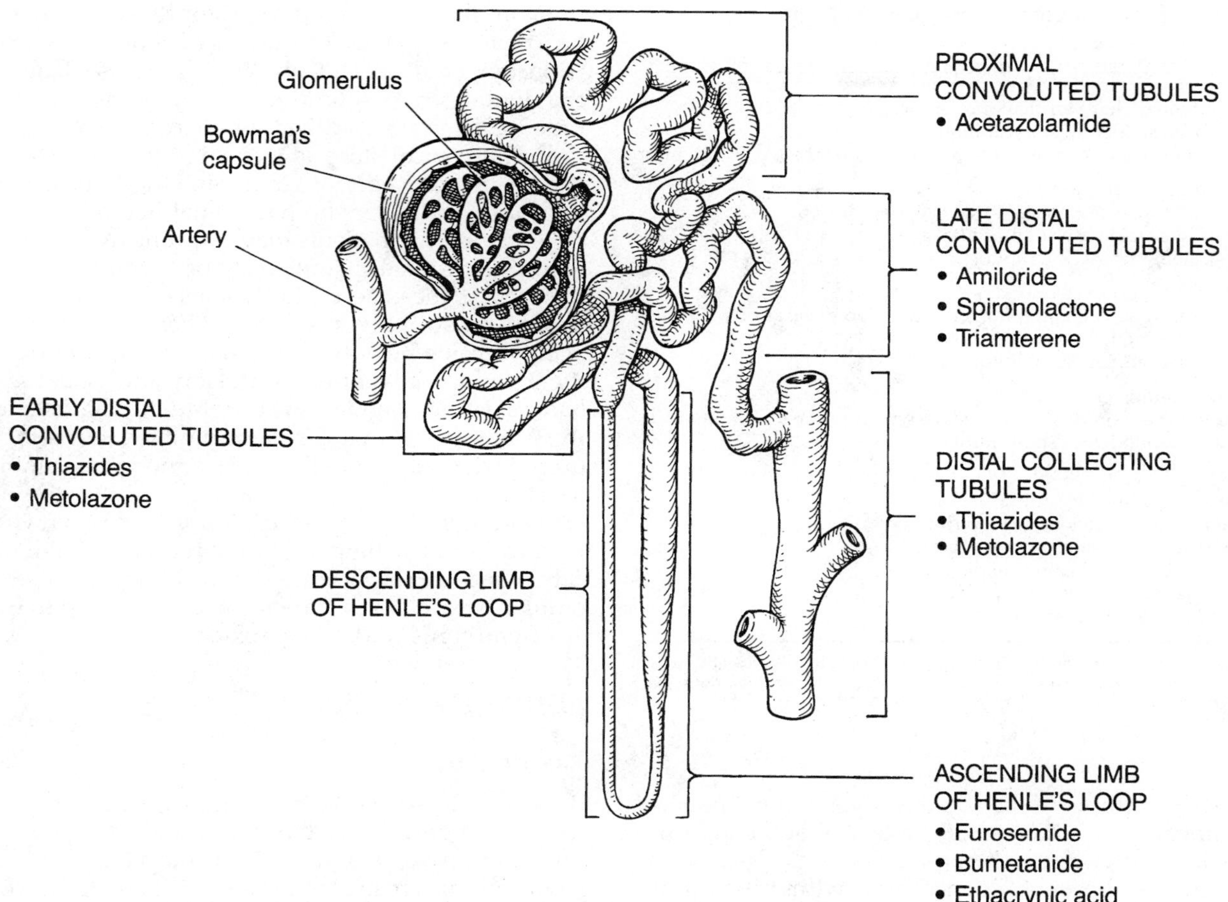

FIGURE 21–5. Site of action of diuretics within the nephron. Blood enters Bowman's capsule from the renal arteries. Sodium and water can continue to be reabsorbed as fluid moves through the tubule, or reabsorption may be blocked by diuretic action. For example, if reabsorption is blocked in the proximal tubules, sodium and water may still be reabsorbed in later segments. This explains why an enhanced diuresis may be achieved by the combination of metolazone and a loop diuretic. (Used with permission from Cuny, J., & Enger, E. L. [1993]. Medical management of chronic heart failure: Direct-acting vasodilators and diuretic agents. *Critical Care Nursing Clinics of North America, 5,* 575–587.)

Patient and family education should include the reasons for the drug regimen and the importance of taking all drugs as prescribed. Every patient must understand that medications are to be taken to keep symptoms to a minimal level and are not to be discontinued or taken erratically just because symptoms appear to be controlled. Patients need to understand the importance of reporting any increase in symptoms so that therapy can be modified before the situation becomes severe (Cuny & Enger, 1993). The importance of restricting dietary sodium intake and of not increasing fluid intake with diuresis should be emphasized. Patients can frequently benefit from counseling about the timing of expected diuresis so they can plan activities appropriately. Elderly patients in particular who may suffer from urinary urgency or incontinence can benefit from such advice (Konstam et al., 1994). In many institutions, patients with advanced chronic heart failure are taught to weigh themselves daily and to increase their diuretic dose if their weight increases by 2 pounds or more. This adds a degree of control and self-management that many patients find gratifying. In addition, such a regimen appears to help maintain a more stable course (Kubo & Cohn, 1994).

Digitalis

Although digitalis is one of the most commonly used drugs in the treatment of heart failure, controversy has surrounded its use for decades (Kelly & Smith, 1993). Some clinicians maintain that digitalis is appropriate only for heart failure patients in atrial fibrillation with a rapid ventricular response because the side effects increase morbidity and mortality. Long-term positive inotropy is harmful in heart failure because it can dangerously increase myocardial oxygen consumption and ventricular dysrhythmias. Others point to the beneficial impact on symptoms demonstrated in some

TABLE 21–11. **Recommended Use of Diuretics in Heart Failure**

Asymptomatic left ventricular dysfunction
- Establish moderate sodium intake
- Consider use of angiotensin-converting enzyme (ACE) inhibitor

Mild sodium retention
- Thiazide-type diuretic or low-dose loop diuretic
- Continue moderate sodium intake
- Combine with ACE inhibitor

Moderate sodium retention
- Loop diuretic, adjusting for renal function as necessary
- Continue moderate sodium intake
- Combine with ACE inhibitor

Severe sodium retention
- Large-dose loop diuretic/thiazide-type diuretic
- Continue moderate sodium intake
- ACE inhibitor

Refractory sodium retention
- Intermittent intravenous loop diuretic
- Short-term infusion of loop diuretic
- Intensified combination therapy
- Intravenous positive inotropic agent
- Ultrafiltration or dialysis

Modified with permission from Cody, R. J. (1993). Clinical trials of diuretic therapy in heart failure: Research directions and clinical considerations. *Journal of the American College of Cardiology, 22,* 165A–171A.

clinical trials as evidence by improvement in ventricular function with the use of digitalis. Conflicting findings in several research reports have heightened the controversy. Recent evidence from withdrawal trials, however, indicates that digitalis effectively improves ventricular function and physical function performance and decreases symptoms and exacerbations of failure (Packer et al., 1993; Uretsky et al., 1993). The effects of digitalis on survival are as yet unknown, but a clinical trial (Digitalis Investigators Group Trial) is currently underway to answer that question.

Digitalis is a positive inotropic agent that exerts its effects by inhibiting the enzyme sodium–potassium ATPase in the cell membrane. Alterations in this enzyme result in inhibition of the sodium–potassium pump with accumulation of intracellular sodium. An increase in intracellular sodium activates the sodium–calcium exchange mechanism to extrude the excess intracellular sodium in exchange for calcium. The end result is an increase in intracellular calcium available for excitation–contraction coupling, producing enhanced contractility. Digitalis also has important electrophysiologic and neuroendocrine effects. It is these effects, particularly normalization of baroreceptor response, inhibition of neuroendocrine activation, and enhancement of the parasympathetic system, that may produce the beneficial effects of digitalis in heart failure (Packer, 1993).

CLINICAL USE. Available evidence suggests that digitalis therapy is appropriate as part of a regimen that includes ACE inhibitors and diuretics for the treatment of symptomatic left ventricular systolic dysfunction, but that it is not indicated for those patients with heart failure primarily due to diastolic dysfunction (Konstam et al., 1994; Kubo & Cohn, 1994). Digoxin is the digitalis glycoside used predominantly in clinical practice. Digitalis loading is not necessary in heart failure. The typical dose is 0.25 mg/day, but the dose should be reduced to 0.125 mg in elderly or small patients and in those who have renal insufficiency.

Heart failure patients may be prone to digitalis toxicity due to renal insufficiency or therapy with other drugs that increase digitalis levels. Digitalis toxicity should be strongly suspected when patients on this agent develop new dysrhythmias. Other signs of toxicity are anorexia, nausea, confusion, and visual disturbances. Hypokalemia can contribute to digitalis toxicity. Medications that can raise digitalis levels include quinidine, verapamil, diltiazem, amiodarone, antibiotics, and anticholinergic agents.

Patient and family education includes, as with all medications, teaching about the reasons for the medication and the importance of not skipping daily doses or taking extra doses. Patients need to be told to report any symptoms of digitalis toxicity.

ADJUNCTIVE THERAPY

Vasodilators

Because intense vasoconstriction is a prominent feature of chronic heart failure, and vasodilation produces improvement in cardiac output, vasodilators have become a mainstay in the treatment of this condition. However, not all vasodilators are created equal. Although often effective in improving symptoms and ventricular performance, use of drugs that produce vasodilation without inhibition of neurohormonal activation frequently results in increased rather than decreased mortality (Packer, 1992). For example, minoxidil, calcium channel blockers such as nifedipine or diltiazem, and phosphodiesterase inhibitors such as milrinone are all potent vasodilators that can exacerbate activation of the neuroendocrine systems, contributing to increased morbidity and mortality. Moreover, some vasodilators such as calcium channel blockers have negative inotropic effects. As such, these classes of vasodilators are not indicated in the long-term treatment of heart failure. Therapy with ACE inhibitors decreases neuroendocrine activation in addition to producing vasodilation. For this reason, ACE inhibition is the vasodilator therapy of choice in heart failure. However, not all patients tolerate therapy with ACE inhibitors. In such cases, vasodilation can be achieved with the combination of hydralazine and isosorbide dinitrate.

In V-HeFT I, the first trial to demonstrate that vasodilators had a positive impact on survival in heart failure, the combination of hydralazine and isosorbide dinitrate was compared to prazosin (an alpha-adrenergic blocker vasodilator) and placebo (Cohn et al., 1986). Both drug regimens acutely improved hemodynamics, but only therapy with hydralazine and isosorbide dinitrate prolonged survival. In direct comparisons, ACE inhibitors appear more effective in enhancing survival than hydralazine and isosorbide dinitrate, but these direct-acting vasodilators are the only other class of drugs to demonstrate a survival advantage (Cohn et al., 1991).

Hydralazine and isosorbide dinitrate are both direct-acting vasodilators. Hydralazine exerts its effects primarily on the arterioles; isosorbide dinitrate acts primarily on the veins. Their use in combination therapy results in an increase in cardiac output secondary to decreased impedance to ventricular ejection. Vasodilation also redistributes blood volume away from the central circulation to the venous capacitance vessels and peripheral circulation effectively, decreasing the signs and symptoms of increased cardiac pressures.

Therapy with hydralazine and isosorbide dinitrate is indicated for patients who do not tolerate ACE inhibitors, and dosage ranges are indicated in Table 21–7 (Konstam et al., 1994). In patients with severe and/or refractory failure, hydralazine and isosorbide dinitrate can be used in addition to ACE inhibitors. In addition, isosorbide dinitrate is often added to the drug regimen in patients with ischemic heart disease.

Beta Blockers

Traditionally contraindicated in heart failure because of their negative inotropic effects, β-blockers improve ventricular function, hemodynamics, functional status, and exercise tolerance, and reduce heart failure exacerbations by decreasing sympathetic stimulation (Bristow, 1993; CIBIS Investigators, 1994; Eichhorn & Hjalmarson, 1994). Assessment of the impact of β-blockers on survival awaits the completion of a large placebo-controlled clinical trial currently underway (Eichhorn & Hjalmarson, 1994). β-adrenergic blocking agents exert their actions by occupying β-adrenergic receptor sites. The result is inability of the neurotransmitters norepinephrine and epinephrine to bind with the receptor and produce their usual effects.

Several mechanisms by which β-blockers exert positive effects in heart failure have been postulated. β blockade decreases heart rate, thereby reducing myocardial oxygen consumption, enhancing coronary artery blood flow, and improving myocardial perfusion and diastolic function. Myocardial energy production also may be improved with the result that both ventricular relaxation and contraction are enhanced. Therapy with β-blockers results in increased density and responsivity of β-receptors (Heilbrunn et al., 1989). Protection from the myopathic effects of norepinephrine may be afforded by a decrease in sympathetic nerve outflow and a reduction in norepinephrine level. Another possible mechanism whereby β-blockers improve heart failure is inhibition of renin release and decreased activation of the renin–angiotensin system (Eichhorn, 1992). The subsequent reduction in angiotension II production can result in attenuation of vasoconstriction and of the myopathic effects of this substance. In addition, β-blocking agents that have a supplementary α_1-receptor blocking or β_2-receptor stimulating properties produce vasodilation that can decrease systemic vascular resistance and increase cardiac output (Bristow, 1993). A final possible positive effect of β-adrenergic receptor blockade is a reduction in incidence of malignant ventricular dysrhythmias.

CLINICAL USE. The use of β-blockers in heart failure is still considered experimental. Nonetheless, because many clinicians currently employ them for adjunctive treatment of this condition, nurses may see these agents used in patients. Metoprolol is commonly used. Recommended therapy begins with low doses followed by careful and gradual titration as tolerated (Bristow, 1993). Therapy with β-blockers should be initiated only after standard therapy, including ACE inhibition, is maximized. Sudden withdrawal of β-blockers after chronic use can result in serious decompensation, and patients should be informed. β-adrenergic blockade is not recommended in patients with bradycardia, heart block, chronic obstructive pulmonary disease, and diabetes.

Antidysrhythmics

As many as 50% of heart failure patients suffer sudden deaths apparently due to malignant ventricular dysrhythmias (Podrid et al., 1992). Given this dismal statistic and the finding that ventricular ectopy and nonsustained ventricular tachycardia are extremely common in heart failure patients, antidysrhythmic therapy seems the intuitive solution. However, traditional antidysrhythmic therapy has not been shown to decrease mortality and may actually increase it. Many antidysrhythmic agents are prodysrhythmic and most can depress ventricular function, exacerbating heart failure. Moreover, data from the Cardiac Arrhythmia Suppression Trial (CAST) demonstrate that therapy with type I antidysrhythmics (i.e., moricizine, encainide, and flecainide) in patients with ejection fractions less than 40% resulted in an *increase* in mortality even though ventricular ectopy was decreased (Cardiac Arrhythmia Suppression Trial Investigators, 1989; Cardiac Arrhythmia Suppression Trial II Investigators, 1992).

Compounding the problem is the fact that the pathogenesis of ventricular dysrhythmias in heart failure is poorly understood. Underlying ischemic heart disease, wall motion abnormalities, overall poor ventricular function, electrolyte imbalances, fibrosis, wall stress, and inotropic therapy may contribute to the high incidence of ventricular dysrhythmias in these patients (Doyle, 1988; Kubo & Cohn, 1994). Ventricular dysrhythmias in patients with dilated cardiomyopathy may be the result of subendocardial ischemia in the presence of normal coronary arteries. The ischemia may be due to reduced cardiac output and coronary artery perfusion or high left ventricular end-diastolic pressures preventing subendocardial coronary filling.

A reasonable approach to treating ventricular dysrhythmias in patients with cardiomyopathy is to limit antiarrhythmic therapy to patients who have inducible ventricular tachycardia or symptomatic dysrhythmias (Stevenson & Perloff, 1988). Low-dose antidysrhythmic therapy is used. Lower doses are required to avoid toxicity, especially if there is renal or liver dysfunction associated with right-sided heart failure (Purcell, 1990). An example of lower dosage might be lidocaine given at 1 to 2 mg/min to minimize liver dysfunction and cerebral side effects.

Treatment of patients who are at high risk of development of a fatal dysrhythmia should probably be guided by the patient's response to programmed electrical stimulation. Drugs with strong negative inotropic effects such as disopyramide and flecainide should be avoided. The most promising drug is amiodarone, which is highly selective in suppressing ventricular dysrhythmias and has a negligible negative inotropic effect (DiMarco, 1989). The adverse effects of amiodarone need to be carefully monitored during therapy. Toxicity noted in the pulmonary system, thyroid gland, corneas, and dermatologic system warrants careful surveillance (DiMarco, 1989).

Anticoagulants

Many clinicians routinely anticoagulate patients with heart failure and dilated cardiomyopathy because of the potential risk of systemic embolism from cardiac thrombus development in the hypokinetic ventricle. Review of evidence from recent multicenter trials suggests that the risk of systemic embolism is far lower than originally thought (Cohn et al., 1991; SOLVD Investigators, 1991). Further evidence suggests that the risk of anticoagulation in heart failure patients may outweigh the benefits in many cases. Given this background and the fact that there are no controlled prospective clinical trials of anticoagulation, current recommendations are to avoid routine anticoagulation in heart failure except in patients at high risk for embolism (Konstam et al., 1994; Kubo & Cohn, 1994). High-risk patients are those with atrial fibrillation, history of emboli, or presence of mobile intracardiac emboli. For high-risk patients, anticoagulation to a prothrombin time ratio of 1.2 to 1.8 times laboratory control with monitoring of levels is recommended (Konstam et al., 1994). Close monitoring of prothrombin time is especially important if heart failure and hepatic congestion worsens because these can alter levels. Patients need to be taught the signs of excess anticoagulation and to report them.

Therapy in Acute Exacerbations and Refractory Failure

Many factors contribute to exacerbations of heart failure (Table 21–12). Additional therapeutic goals in acute or refractory heart failure are: (1) discovering and treating underlying causes of failure, (2) acutely reducing preload, (3) acutely reducing afterload, and (4) acutely increasing contractility.

TABLE 21–12. **Factors Contributing to Heart Failure Exacerbation**

Failure to comply with medical regimen
Patient-related
Failure to follow diet
Failure to take medications as prescribed
Failure to promptly seek treatment for symptoms
Failure of social support system
Health care system–related
Inadequate patient/family education
Inadequate discharge planning
Inadequate follow-up
Inadequately treated, increased, or new ischemia
New or progressive myocardial mechanical defect (e.g., mitral regurgitation)
Inadequate medical therapy
Progressive renal failure
Excess alcohol consumption
New onset of atrial dysrhythmias
Infection
Anemia
Uncontrolled hypertension
Stress
Adverse environmental factors (e.g., excessive heat/humidity or cold)
Inadequately managed pulmonary disease
New medications with cardiac effects (e.g., calcium channel blockers or antidysrhythmics) or systemic effects (e.g., nonsteroidal antiinflammatory agents or steroids)

TREATING UNDERLYING CAUSES

A fundamental tenet in the treatment of heart failure exacerbations and refractory failure is to treat any contributing factors. A careful search to reveal other underlying causes is necessary to avoid another exacerbation once acute decompensation is corrected. The use of invasive hemodynamic monitoring with a pulmonary artery catheter is indicated to define the underlying pathology and to efficiently guide therapy (Vincent, 1994). Reliance on noninvasive clinical evaluation alone can be extremely unreliable (Stevenson & Perloff, 1989).

As can be seen from Table 21–12, noncompliance to the medical regimen and inadequate discharge preparation are major causes of exacerbation. In one study, 64% of cases of readmission for heart failure were due to lack of adherence to the prescribed regimen (Ghali et al., 1988). Factors to improve compliance are discussed in a subsequent section on patient and family education. With any exacerbation special efforts should be made to optimize oral drug therapy. If indicated, hypertension should be treated (Cody, 1992).

For patients with CAD, worsening of ischemia often contributes to decompensation or renders the patient refractory to maximal medical therapy. In such patients, coronary revascularization with coronary artery bypass grafting may be an option (Halfman, 1993). Bypass grafting can be beneficial in ischemic heart failure because still-functioning muscle is preserved, and hibernating cardiac muscle is effectively recruited. Recent reports indicate that heart failure patients with severely depressed left ventricular function (i.e., ejection fraction < 30% with pulmonary edema and/or requiring intraaortic balloon pump support) derive significant benefit without excessive operative mortality from bypass grafting (Elefteriades et al., 1993). Benefits include improvement in ventricular function and decrease in angina and symptoms of heart failure.

REDUCING PRELOAD

In patients with volume overload, reduction of preload results in improvement of symptoms and ventricular performance. It should be emphasized, however, that not all patients with heart failure exacerbation require preload reduction. Careful evaluation of fluid status should be undertaken before vigorous diuretic therapy (Vincent, 1994). Preload reduction is achieved through pharmacologic manipulation and controlled fluid intake. The aim is to decrease intravascular volume, increase venous capacitance, and improve ventricular compliance. Intravenous diuretic and nitrate therapy are utilized to meet these goals. Intravenous diuretic therapy can achieve rapid diuresis even in patients on maximal doses of oral agents because intestinal edema frequently limits oral absorption in patients with severe failure. Multiple diuretic agents acting on different sites in the renal tubule can be used to improve diuresis. In patients in whom the diuretic response is impaired by compromised renal perfusion or intrinsic renal disease, the addition of a distal tubular diuretic such as metolazone increases fluid delivery to the distal site of action to the maintenance diuretic (Stevenson & Perloff, 1988). This has been termed "rescue therapy" for patients with otherwise refractory fluid retention, and intermittent use of metolazone stabilizes many patients so that they do not require frequent hospital readmission for intravenous diuretic therapy.

A concern in acute preload reduction is hypokalemia and hypomagnesemia. A brisk and rapid diuresis is desired to reduce intravascular volume while maintaining surveillance of serum potassium and magnesium levels. The goal is to maintain a potassium level of at least 4.0 mEq/L and a magnesium level of >1.8 mEq/L.

In addition to the traditional methods of diuretic therapy, nitrates are used to achieve further reductions in preload by increasing venous capacitance. Nitrates consistently reduce the left ventricular workload by reducing venous return to the heart, lowering pulmonary capillary wedge pressure (PCWP), and optimizing the Frank-Starling curve (Doyle, 1988). Nitrates also dilate nonstenotic coronary arteries, which can be helpful in patients with ischemic cardiomyopathy.

For intravenous nitrate therapy, doses of less than 1 mcg/kg/min will decrease preload, and doses higher than 1 mcg/kg/min will produce arterial and venous dilation and in some instances will decrease SVR. Topical nitrates are also utilized in patients with acute heart failure, particularly in those who are either edematous or have poor perfusion. Oral preparations seem to be favored over topical agents for long-term maintenance. Doyle (1988) recommends changing the transdermal patch more frequently than every 24 hours as recommended by the manufacturer. Patients with heart failure generally tolerate nitrates quite well. Excessive preload reduction must be guarded against because it can lead to reduced cardiac output, severe hypotension, and syncope.

When pharmacologic therapy, even at maximal doses, fails to reduce preload due to volume overload, dialysis and hemofiltration have been employed in some institutions (Golper, 1994). The use of these aggressive interventions is usually limited to patients with NYHA class III failure and renal failure or NYHA class IV failure refractory to optimal drug therapy. Both patient and physician need to carefully consider the use of such therapy given the risk of complications and the aggressive nature of these interventions when prognosis is poor. In general, use is limited to selected patients as a bridge to transplant (Golper, 1994).

REDUCING AFTERLOAD

Afterload reduction improves the systolic function of the failing ventricle by improving forward cardiac output and decreasing ventricular filling pressures. Afterload reduction is accomplished by agents that reduce SVR, generally through arteriolar vasodilation. The goal of therapy is the achievement of maximal cardiac output. The drug of choice for acute afterload reduction is sodium nitroprusside. The drug's effectiveness in reducing both preload and afterload make it a valuable adjunct in the therapy of low cardiac output syndromes associated with high PCWP and high SVR (Passmore & Goldstein, 1989). Hemodynamically, nitroprusside decreases PCWP and SVR, leading in turn to increases in cardiac output and stroke volume. Nitroprusside acts rapidly, has a duration of 2 to 3 minutes, and can be easily titrated to changing responses in the patient.

Stevenson and Tillisch (1986) advocate use of nitroprusside and diuretics to achieve a PCWP of less than or equal to 15 mm Hg, SVR of less than or equal to 1200 dynes/sec/cm^{-5}, and a systolic blood pressure of greater than or equal to 80 mm Hg. When these goals are achieved, cardiac output is maximal. Nitroprusside is given in a dosage of 100 mg in 250 mL of 5% dextrose and water and started at 20 mcg/kg/min, titrating the dose until acceptable hemodynamics are achieved. This result is usually achieved over a 24- to 48-hour period.

In patients with severe pulmonary hypertension,

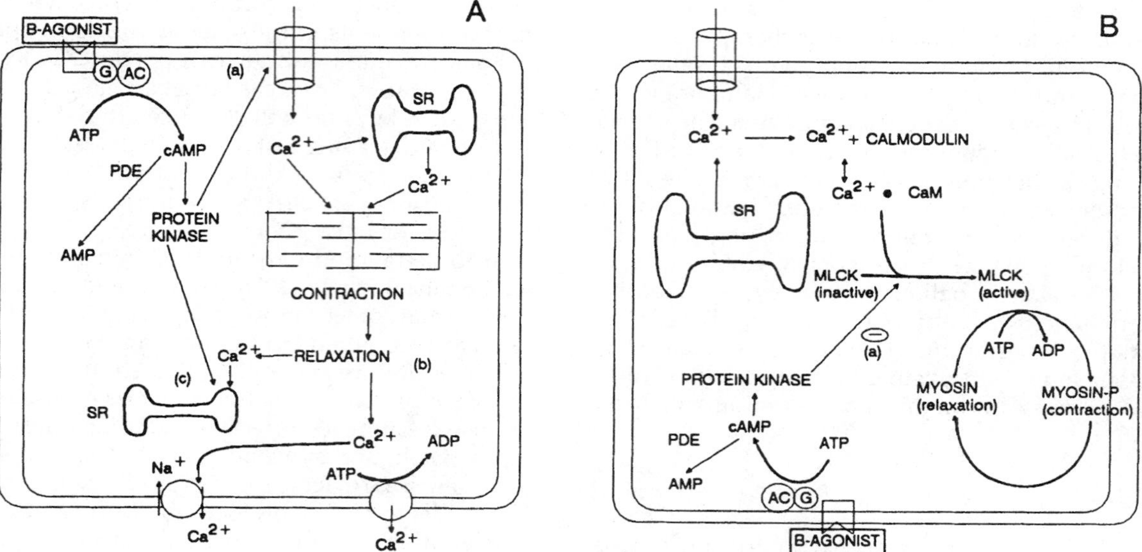

FIGURE 21–6. Influence of cyclic AMP (cAMP) on cardiac contraction and on relaxation (*A*) and smooth muscle contraction (*B*). Agonist binding to β-receptors activates adenylate cyclase (AC), producing cAMP in heart cells. cAMP-dependent protein kinase phosphorylation causes (1) increased influx of Ca^{2+} through cell surface channels (*a*), resulting in enhanced contractile force; and (2) accelerated uptake of Ca^{2+} into sarcoplasmic reticulum (SR), which facilitates relaxation (*b*) and (*c*). In smooth muscle cells, Ca^{2+} calmodulin (CaM) complex activates myosin light chain kinase (MLCK), thus initiating contraction. cAMP-dependent protein kinase phosphorylates MLCK, making it less sensitive to activation (*a*). *Abbreviations:* G, G protein; PDE, phosphodiesterase; AMP, adenosine monophosphate; ADP, adenosine diphosphate; ATP, adenosine triphosphate. (From Schwertz, D. W., & Piano, M. R. [1990]. New inotropic drugs for treatment of congestive heart failure. *Cardiovascular Nursing, 26*[2], 7–12. By permission of the American Heart Association, Inc.)

the vasodilator prostaglandin E_1 (PGE_1) is highly effective in reducing right heart afterload (Vincent, 1994). PGE_1 may also be effective in decreasing both right and left afterload and improving hemodynamics in patients with end-stage heart failure who are receiving dobutamine and dopamine infusions (Pacher et al., 1994).

INCREASING CONTRACTILITY

Although positive inotropic agents are not indicated for the long-term treatment of chronic heart failure because they exert serious negative effects on myocardial dynamics and increase mortality, they do have an important place in the short-term treatment of acute or refractory failure. Improvements in systolic function with increases in stroke volume and cardiac output augment myocardial contractility. Positive inotropic agents improve systolic function by enhancing contractility. These drugs include dobutamine, dopamine, and the phosphodiesterase inhibitor amrinone. The common pathway for augmentation of contractility is enhanced intracellular release and utilization of calcium (Braunwald et al., 1992) (Fig. 21–6). Enhanced use of calcium is accomplished by stimulating the specific β-adrenergic receptor with either dopamine or dobutamine or by blocking cAMP breakdown with amrinone.

Cardiac performance can be improved in heart failure patients with the use of low-dose dopamine. A dosage range of 2 to 5 mcg/kg/min of dopamine stimulates the dopaminergic receptors in the splanchnic and renal vascular beds, producing vasodilation, enhanced blood flow, and diuresis. Cardiac performance is improved by direct stimulation of the β-adrenergic receptors and indirectly by stimulating the release at the nerve endings of norepinephrine. A dosage range higher than 5 mcg/kg/min increases the risk of ischemia and myocardial oxygen consumption (Dasta & Leier, 1989). At higher doses, a greater burden is placed on the myocardial tissue secondary to the rise in myocardial oxygen demand incurred by the increase in mean arterial pressure, PCWP, stroke volume, and heart rate. Dopamine use is therefore restricted to the lower dosage range, especially if heart failure is secondary to advanced ischemic heart disease. As the disease progresses, if either hemodynamic management or renal perfusion is not achieved, drug tolerance develops. Over the long term this becomes a problem because the dosage must be increased to maintain stability, and the patient then is at risk for an increase in myocardial oxygen consumption.

Dobutamine was first used in 1975 to increase cardiac contractility selectively in patients with an altering heart rate or blood pressure (Tuttle & Mills, 1975). In patients with heart failure, the hemodynamic profile of dobutamine use is characterized by consistent increases in cardiac output and stroke volume, decreases in systemic and pulmonary vascular resistance and

PCWP with little effect on heart rate or blood pressure. Dobutamine directly stimulates the β-adrenergic receptors of the heart, which can over time increase heart rate and the force of contraction. This result is achieved with a dosage in the range of 2 to 10 mcg/kg/min. Dobutamine, unlike dopamine, has no direct effect on renal perfusion. Enhancement of cardiac output is improved indirectly with dobutamine therapy and can be measured indirectly by PCWP, the presence of clear lungs, and an increase in urine output.

Both dopamine and dobutamine at doses higher than 15 mcg/kg/min can cause vasoconstriction similar to that seen with stimulation of the α receptors. When such doses are required to sustain the systolic blood pressure, vasodilators (e.g., nitroprusside) may be given to counteract the arterial constriction (Purcell & Holder, 1989). At these doses, Purcell and Holder (1989) also warn of ensuing tachycardia and the development of ectopy. Concurrent use of dopamine or dobutamine with nitroprusside provides optimal pharmacologic support. The following results are achieved when these two drugs are given in coordination: improved cardiac output, maintenance of mean systolic pressure, enhancement of renal function, and decreased arterial vasoconstriction (Purcell & Holder, 1989).

Amrinone, administered intravenously, is useful in the treatment of cardiomyopathy refractory to the combination of vasodilators, diuretics, and digoxin (Braunwald et al., 1992). Amrinone exerts its inotropic and vasodilating action through phosphodiesterase inhibition, thereby indirectly elevating cAMP and increasing calcium availability. Increased cAMP in cardiac tissue activates a protein kinase that enhances the slow inward current and increases the force of myocardial contractions (Dasta & Leier, 1989). In patients with heart failure, amrinone improves exercise tolerance and does not adversely affect myocardial oxygen consumption or coronary blood flow (Colucci et al., 1986). Amrinone has been combined with dobutamine and in heart failure patients can increase the mean cardiac index (Uretsky et al., 1987).

Intravenous amrinone therapy is initiated with a bolus of 0.75 mcg/kg given slowly over 3 to 5 minutes. A maintenance dose is continued at 5 mcg/kg/min, titrated to the desired effect up to 10 mcg/kg/min. The drug must be mixed with saline to avoid a chemical reaction with glucose. Long-term therapy is associated with increased liver function abnormalities such as platelet dysfunction and an increased incidence of dysrhythmias and thrombocytopenia.

Intraaortic Balloon Pump Therapy and Ventricular Assist Devices

In CAD patients who continue to decompensate and cannot be stabilized despite intravenous unloading and inotropic therapy, intraaortic balloon counterpulsation may provide the support necessary to produce improvement (Stevenson, 1993). Intraaortic balloon counterpulsation unloads the left ventricle and increases coronary artery perfusion to reduce myocardial ischemia. Ischemia may be reduced enough to improve ventricular performance. The usual role of intraaortic balloon pump therapy in heart failure patients is for support while awaiting emergent cardiac transplantation.

Ventricular assist devices (e.g., external centrifugal pumps, extracorporeal membrane oxygenation systems, pulsatile short-term pumps, internal mechanical assist devices) temporarily assume ventricular function as a bridge to transplantation (Vargo, 1993). These devices can effectively support cardiac transplant candidates awaiting urgent transplantation (see Chapter 14). Mechanical circulatory support often becomes necessary in urgent candidates awaiting availability of a donor heart who continue to deteriorate such that organ systems are threatened and death appears imminent. Patients in whom ventricular assist devices have been used and who go on to transplantation have long-term survival similar to that of patients who undergo routine transplantation (Stevenson, 1993).

Cardiac Transplantation

Cardiac transplantation has come of age as a reasonable therapeutic option for patients suffering from end-stage heart failure (Cardin & Clark, 1985; Dressler, 1993). Recent advances have made this option possible (Table 21–13). Criteria for patient selection are outlined in Table 21–14. For patients who have severe symptoms for an extended length of time, survival after cardiac transplantation is better than survival on intensive medical therapy. Survival is 80% at 1 year, 70% at 5 years, and 50% at 10 years for patients on current immunosuppressive regimens (Kaye, 1993). For patients with severe symptoms that persist despite intensive medical therapy, the quality of life is also clearly improved by cardiac transplantation (Stevenson & Perloff, 1988). Stevenson and Perloff (1988) emphasize, however, that for patients who have responded well to medical therapy for heart failure, the quality of life may not be significantly improved by transplantation, which requires them to assume constant vigilance for rejection, infection, medications, and repeated biopsies in exchange for functional capacity that is still less than normal.

TABLE 21–13. **Advances in Cardiac Transplantation**

Better organ retrieval
Monitoring for allograft rejection
Use of endomyocardial biopsy
Improvements in surgical technique
More efficient organ preservation
Immunosuppressive drug therapy—cyclosporine
Increase in centers doing transplants
Bridge to transplant devices
Expansion of patient selection criteria

TABLE 21–14. **Criteria for Patient Selection for Heart Transplantation**

1. Severe cardiac disease despite tailored medical therapy:
   Heart failure
   Unacceptable risk of death within the next year
2. No other reasonable surgical options
3. Patient characteristics:
   Over upper age limit of 55–65 years
   Ability to understand and comprehend medical regimen following transplantation
4. Relative contraindications:
   Active infection, particularly respiratory in nature
   Active ulcer disease
   Severe peripheral vascular disease
   Insulin-dependent diabetes with end-organ damage
   Pulmonary vascular resistance over 240 dynes/cm/sec^{-5}
   Pulmonary artery systolic pressure over 60 mm Hg after optimal hemodynamics are reached
   Mean transpulmonary gradient > 15 mm Hg
   Creatinine over 2 mg/dL, creatinine clearance < 50 mL/min
   Bilirubin over 2.5 mg/dL
   AST twice normal
   History of medical noncompliance with prescribed regimen
   History of refractory alcohol or drug abuse
   Inability to make strong, consistent commitment to transplantation program

Adapted from Stevenson, L. W., & Miller, L. W. (1991). Cardiac transplantation as therapy of heart failure. *Current Problems in Cardiology, 16*(4), 219–305.

In spite of recent advances in cardiac transplantation, it is an option only for very few patients due to the limited supply of donor hearts. An estimated 20,000 patients per year could benefit from cardiac transplantation but only 2000 donor hearts are available per year (Evans, 1987). Stevenson, Dracup, & Tillisch (1989) studied 50 patients who were transferred to a tertiary referral center for urgent transplantation and who subsequently received a transplant, and compared them to 40 similar patients who were discharged on oral regimens of vasodilators and diuretics. All were treated with intensive afterload reduction therapy. Both groups reported similar outcomes and an improved quality of life. With new emphasis placed on medical therapy, more effective distribution of limited donor hearts is likely.

Patient and Family Education

More than one-third and possibly up to 50% of rehospitalizations for heart failure are preventable (Vinson et al., 1990). In the study reporting this statistic, major factors contributing to readmissions for heart failure were examined and are as follows: noncompliance with medications or diet (33% of readmissions), failure to seek medical help when appropriate (20% of readmissions), inadequate discharge planning and follow-up (20% of readmissions), and inadequate social support (21% of readmissions). In some cases more than one factor contributed to a readmission. All of these factors are attributable to some degree to failure to properly educate and prepare patients and their families to assume their care.

The vital importance of patient education to the effective management of heart failure is underscored by the following assertion: "patient education is the foundation on which all other therapies for heart failure are built" (Jennison & Miller, 1993). Noncompliance to heart failure treatment regimens is common and appears to increase as the condition progresses (Ghali et al., 1988; SOLVD Investigators, 1991). The number of medications, complexity of dosage schedules, diet restrictions, and the volume of information the patient must retain to adequately participate in his care demands careful patient teaching and an inte-

TABLE 21–15. **Suggested Topics for Patient, Family, and Caregiver Education and Counseling**

General Counseling

Explanation of heart failure and reason for symptoms
Cause of heart failure
Expected symptoms
Symptoms of worsening heart failure and what to do when they occur
What to do it symptoms worsen
Self-monitoring with daily weights
Explanation of treatment/care plan
Clarification of patient responsibilities
Importance of cessation of tobacco use
Role of family members/other caregivers in the treatment/care plan
Availability and value of qualified local support group
Importance of obtaining vaccinations against influenza and pneumococcal disease

Prognosis

Life expectancy
Advance directives
Advice for family members in the event of sudden death

Activity Recommendations

Recreation, leisure, and work activity
Exercise
Sex, sexual difficulties, and coping strategies

Dietary Recommendations

Sodium restriction
Avoidance of excessive fluid intake
Fluid restriction (in selected patients)
Alcohol restriction

Medications

Effects of medications on quality of life and survival
Dosing
Likely side effects and what to do if they occur
Coping mechanisms for complicated medical regimens
Availability of lower cost medications or financial assistance

Importance of Compliance With Treatment/Care Plan

Reprinted from Konstam, M., Dracup, K., Baker, D., et al. (1994). Heart failure: Evaluation and care of patients with left-ventricular systolic dysfunction. Clinical Practice Guideline No. 11. AHCPR Publication No. 94-0612. Rockville, MD: Agency for Health Care Policy and Research, Public Health Services, U.S. Department of Health and Human Services.

grated, multidisciplinary approach. Family involvement in all phases of patient teaching is vital and can improve compliance.

Suggested topics for patient and family education are presented in Table 21–15. The list is extensive, but proper care of these patients requires comprehensive patient preparation from a collaborative perspective. Caring for heart failure patients may place a considerable burden on the family (Karmilovich, 1994). This finding underscores the importance of including and supporting the family in heart failure care.

SUMMARY

Care of the patient with advanced heart failure is a challenge for nurses who work with these patients. The majority of patients usually present with end-stage cardiac failure and require aggressive nursing and medical care considerations. A thorough understanding of hemodynamic monitoring and medication regimens is essential for the collaborative care of these patients. It is only with a continual effort made by all services that these patients are successfully cared for until they have achieved maximal benefit from the medical regimen or have successful transplantation. One does need to remember, however, that not all collaborative efforts are successful, and there are issues that do need to be addressed if the patient does not survive until transplant or is becoming refractory to medical therapy. Collaboration is the key element in the care of these patients and needs to be incorporated into their medical and nursing care.

REFERENCES

Adamopoulos, S., Coats, A. J. S., Brunotte, F., et al. (1993). Physical training improves skeletal muscle metabolism in patients with chronic heart failure. *Journal of the American College of Cardiology, 21,* 1101–1106.

Benedict, C. R., Johnstone, D. E., Weiner, D. H., et al. (1994). Relation of neurohumoral activation to clinical variables and degree of left ventricular dysfunction: A report from the registry of Studies of Left Ventricular Dysfunction. *Journal of the American College of Cardiology, 23,* 1410–1420.

Bonaduce, D., Petretta, M., Arrichiello, P., Conforti, G., Montemurro, M. V., Bianchi, V., & Morgano, G. (1992). Effects of captopril treatment on left ventricular remodeling and function after anterior myocardial infarction: Comparison with digitalis. *Journal of the American College of Cardiology, 19,* 858–863.

Bousquet, G. L. (1990). Congestive heart failure: A review of nonpharmacologic therapy. *The Journal of Cardiovascular Nursing, 4,* 35–46.

Brandt, R. R., Wright, R. S., Redfield, M. M., & Burnett, J. C. (1993). Atrial natriuretic peptide in heart failure. *Circulation, 22*(Suppl A), 86A–92A.

Braunwald, E., Sonnenblick, E. H., & Ross, J. (1992). Mechanisms of cardiac contraction and relaxation. In E. Braunwald (Ed.), *Heart disease: A textbook of cardiovascular medicine* (pp. 383–425). Philadelphia: W. B. Saunders.

Bristow, M. R. (1984). Myocardial β-adrenergic downregulation in heart failure. *International Journal of Cardiology, 5,* 648–652.

Bristow, M. R. (1993). Pathophysiologic and pharmacologic rationales for clinical management of chronic heart failure with beta-blocking agents. *American Journal of Cardiology, 71,* 12C–22C.

Bristow, M. R., Ginsburg, R., Minobe, M., et al. (1982). Decreased catecholamine sensitivity and beta-adrenergic receptor density in failing human hearts. *New England Journal of Medicine, 307,* 205–211.

Cannon, P. J. (1989). Sodium retention in heart failure. *Cardiology Clinics, 7,* 49–62.

Captopril Multicenter Research Group I. (1985). A cooperative multicenter study of captopril in congestive heart failure: Hemodynamic effects and long-term response. *American Heart Journal, 110,* 439–447.

Cardiac Arrhythmia Suppression Trial (CAST) Investigators. (1989). Preliminary report: Effect of encainide and flecainide on mortality in a randomized trial of arrhythmia suppression after myocardial infarction. *New England Journal of Medicine, 321,* 406–412.

Cardiac Arrhythmia Suppression Trial II Investigators. (1992). Effect of the antiarrhythmic agent moricizine on survival after myocardial infarction. *New England Journal of Medicine, 327,* 227–233.

Cardin, S., & Clark, S. (1985). A nursing diagnosis approach to the patient awaiting cardiac transplantation. *Heart & Lung, 14,* 499–504.

CIBIS Investigators and Committees. (1994). A randomized trial of beta-blockade in heart failure: The Cardiac Insufficiency Bisoprolol Study (CIBIS). *Circulation, 90,* 1765–1773.

Coats, A. J. S., Adamopoulos, S., Radealli, A., et al. (1992). Controlled trial of physical training in chronic heart failure: Exercise performance, hemodynamics, ventilation and autonomic function. *Circulation, 85,* 2119–2131.

Cody, R. J. (1989). Neurohormonal influences in the pathogenesis of congestive heart failure. *Cardiology Clinics, 7,* 73–86.

Cody, R. J. (1992). Management of refractory congestive heart failure. *American Journal of Cardiology, 69,* 141G–149G.

Cody, R. J. (1993). Clinical trials of diuretic therapy in heart failure: Research directions and clinical considerations. *Journal of the American College of Cardiology, 22,* 165A–171A.

Cohn, J. N. (1992). The prevention of heart failure: A new agenda. *New England Journal of Medicine, 327,* 725–728.

Cohn, J. N. (1994). Overview of pathophysiology of heart failure. In J. D. Hosenpud & B. H. Greenberg (Eds.), *Congestive heart failure: Pathophysiology, diagnosis, and comprehensive approach to management* (pp. 11–16). New York: Springer-Verlag.

Cohn, J. N., Archibald, D. G., Ziesche, S., et al. (1986). Effect of vasodilator therapy on mortality in chronic congestive heart failure. Results of a Veterans Administration Cooperative Study. *New England Journal of Medicine, 314,* 1547–1552.

Cohn, J. N., Johnson, G., Ziesche S., et al. (1991). A comparison of enalapril with hydralazine-isosorbide dinitrate in the treatment of chronic congestive heart failure. *New England Journal of Medicine, 325,* 303–310.

Cohn, J. N., Levine, T. B., Olivari, M. T., Garberg, V., Lura, D., Francis, G. S., Simon, A. B., & Rector, B. (1984). Plasma norepinephrine as a guide to prognosis in patients with chronic congestive heart failure. *New England Journal of Medicine, 311,* 819–823.

Colucci, W. S., Wright, R. F., & Braunwald, E. (1986). New positive inotropic agents in the treatment of congestive failure. Mechanisms of action and recent clinical developments. *New England Journal of Medicine, 314,* 349–358.

CONSENSUS Trial Study Group. (1987). Effects of enalapril on mortality in severe congestive heart failure: Results of the Cooperative North Scandinavian Enalapril Survival Study (CONSENSUS). *New England Journal of Medicine, 316,* 1429–1435.

Creager, M. A., Faxon, D. P., Cutler, S. S., Kohlmann, O., Ryan, T. J., & Gavras, H. (1986). Contribution of vasopressin to vasoconstriction in patients with congestive heart failure: Comparison with the renin–angiotensin system and the sympathetic nervous system. *Journal of the American College of Cardiology, 7,* 758–765.

Cuny, J., & Enger, E. L. (1993). Medical management of chronic heart failure: Direct-acting vasodilators and diuretic agents. *Critical Care Nursing Clinics of North America, 5,* 575–587.

Daly, P. A., & Sole, M. J. (1990). Myocardial catecholamines and the pathophysiology of heart failure. *Circulation, 82*(Suppl. I), I35–I43.

Dargie, H. J., Cleland, J. G. F., Leckie, V. J., Inglis, C. G., East, B. W., & Ford, I. (1987). Relation of arrhythmias and electrolyte abnormalities to survival in patients with severe chronic heart failure. *Circulation, 75,* 98–107.

Dasta, J. F., & Leier, C. V. (1989). *Perspectives on inotropic therapy: Continuing role of dobutamine.* Springfield, NJ: Scientific Therapeutics Information.

DiMarco, J. P. (1989). Antiarrhythmics. In B. Chernow (Ed.), *Essentials of critical care pharmacology* (pp. 168–206). Baltimore: Williams & Wilkins.

Dougherty, A. H., Naccarelli, G. V., Gray, E. L., Hicks, C. H., & Goldstein, R. A. (1984). Congestive heart failure with normal systolic function. *American Journal of Cardiology, 54,* 778–782.

Doyle, B. (1988). Nursing challenge: The patient with end-stage heart failure. In L. S. Kern (Ed.), *Cardiac critical care nursing* (pp. 311–362). Rockville, MD: Aspen Publishers.

Dracup, K., Walden, J. A., Stevenson, L. W., & Brecht, M. L. (1992). Quality of life in patients with advanced heart failure. *Journal of Heart and Lung Transplantation, 11,* 273–279.

Dressler, D. K. (1993). Transplantation in end-stage heart failure. *Critical Care Nursing Clinics of North America, 5,* 635–648.

Dzau, V. J., Packer, M., Lilly, L. S., Swartz, S. L., Hollenberg, N. K., Williams, G. H. (1984). Prostaglandins in severe heart failure: Relation to activation of the renin–angiotensin system and hyponatremia. *New England Journal of Medicine, 310,* 347–352.

Eichhorn, E. J. (1992). The paradox of β-adrenergic blockade for the management of congestive heart failure. *American Journal of Medicine, 92,* 527.

Eichhorn, E. J., & Hjalmarson, Å. (1994). β-blocker treatment for chronic heart failure. *Circulation, 90,* 2153–2156.

Elefteriades, J. A., Tolis, G., Levi, E., Mills, L. K., & Zaret, B. L. (1993). Coronary artery bypass grafting in severe left ventricular dysfunction: Excellent survival with improved ejection fraction and functional state. *Journal of the American College of Cardiology, 22,* 1411–1417.

Evans, R. W. (1987). The economics of heart transplantation. *Circulation, 75,* 63–75.

Ferguson, D. W., Berg, W. J., Sanders, J. S., & Kempf, J. S. (1990). Clinical and hemodynamic correlates of sympathetic nerve activity in normal humans and patients with heart failure: Evidence from direct microneurographic recordings. *Journal of the American College of Cardiology, 16,* 1125–1134.

Fonarow, G. C., Chelimsky-Fallick, C., Stevenson, L. W., et al. (1992). Effect of direct vasodilation with hydralazine versus angiotensin-converting enzyme inhibition with captopril on mortality in advanced heart failure: The Hy-C trial. *Journal of the American College of Cardiology, 19,* 842.

Forstermann, U., Mugge, A., Alheid, U., Haverich, A., & Frolich, J. C. (1988). Selective attenuation of endothelial-mediated vasodilation in atherosclerotic human coronary arteries. *Circulation Research, 62,* 185–190.

Francis, G. S. (1990). Neuroendocrine activity in congestive heart failure. *American Journal of Cardiology, 66,* 33D–39D.

Francis, G. S., Benedict, C., Johnstone, D. E., et al. (1990). Comparison of neuroendocrine activation in patients with left ventricular dysfunction and without congestive heart failure: A substudy of the Studies of Left Ventricular Dysfunction (SOLVD). *Circulation, 82,* 1724–1729.

Fyhrquist, F., & Tikkanen, I. (1988). Atrial natriuretic peptide in congestive heart failure. *American Journal of Cardiology, 62,* 20A–24A.

Garg, R., Packer, M., Pitt, B., & Yusuf, S. (1993). Heart failure in the 1990s: Evolution of a major public health problem in cardiovascular medicine. *Journal of the American College of Cardiology, 22*(suppl A), 3A–5A.

Ghali, J. K., Kadakia, S., Cooper, R., & Ferlinz, J. (1988). Precipitating factors leading to decompensation of heart failure. *Archives of Internal Medicine, 148,* 2013–2016.

Golper, T. A. (1994). Dialysis and hemofiltration for congestive heart failure. In J. D. Hosenpud & B. H. Greenberg (Eds.), *Congestive heart failure: Pathophysiology, diagnosis, and comprehensive approach to management* (pp. 568–581). New York: Springer-Verlag.

Greenberg, B. H. (1994). The medical management of chronic congestive heart failure. In J. D. Hosenpud & B. H. Greenberg (Eds.), *Congestive heart failure: Pathophysiology, diagnosis, and comprehensive approach to management* (pp. 628–644). New York: Springer-Verlag.

Halfman, M. (1993). Myocardial revascularization in the patient with severe left ventricular dysfunction. *Critical Care Nursing Clinics of North America, 5,* 619–626.

Hawthorne, M. H., & Hixon, M. E. (1994). Functional status, mood disturbance and quality of life in patients with heart failure. *Progress in Cardiovascular Nursing, 9,* 22–32.

Heilbrunn, S. M., Shah, P., Bristow, M. R., Valantine, H. A., Ginsburg, R., & Fowler, M. B. (1989). Increased β-receptor density and improved hemodynamic response to catecholamine stimulation during long-term metoprolol therapy in heart failure from dilated cardiomyopathy. *Circulation, 79,* 483–490.

Hirsch, A. T., & Creager, M. A. (1994). The peripheral circulation in heart failure. In J. D. Hosenpud & B. H. Greenberg (Eds.), *Congestive heart failure: Pathophysiology, diagnosis, and comprehensive approach to management* (pp. 145–160). New York: Springer-Verlag.

Hirsch, A. T., Dzau, V. J., & Creager, M. A. (1987). Baroreceptor function in congestive heart failure: Effect on neurohumoral activation and regional vascular resistance. *Circulation, 75*(Suppl. IV), 36–48.

Ho, K. K. L., Pinsky, J. L., Kannel, W. B., & Levy, D. (1993). The epidemiology of heart failure: The Framingham study. *Journal of the American College of Cardiology, 22*(suppl A), 6A–13A.

Jalil, J. E., Janicki, J. S., Pick, R., Abrahams, C., & Weber, K. T. (1989). Fibrosis-induced reduction of endomyocardium in the rat after isoproterenol treatment. *Circulation Research, 65*(2), 258–264.

Jennison, S. H., & Miller, L. W. (1993). What to try while congestive heart failure patients are still ambulatory. *Postgraduate Medicine, 94,* 66–84.

Karmilovich, S. E. (1994). Burden and stress associated with spousal caregiving for individuals with heart failure. *Progress in Cardiovascular Nursing, 9*(1), 33–38.

Katz, A. M. (1992). *Physiology of the heart.* New York: Raven Press.

Katz, S. D., Biasucci, L., Sabba, C., Strom, J. A., Jondeau, G., Galvao, M., Soloman, S., Nikolic, D., Forman, R., & LeJemtel, T. H. (1992). Impaired endothelium-mediated vasodilation in the peripheral vasculature of patients with congestive heart failure. *Journal of the American College of Cardiology, 19,* 918–925.

Kaye, M. P. (1993). The registry of the International Society for Heart and Lung Transplantation: Tenth official report—1993. *Journal of Heart and Lung Transplantation, 12,* 541–548.

Kelly, R. A., & Smith, T. W. (1993). Digoxin in heart failure: Implications of recent trials. *Journal of the American College of Cardiology, 22*(suppl A), 107A–112A.

Kluger, J., Cody, R. J., & Laragh, J. H. (1982). The contributions of sympathetic tone and the renin–angiotensin system to severe chronic congestive heart failure: Response to specific inhibitors (prazosin and captopril). *American Journal of Cardiology, 49,* 1667–1674.

Konstam, M., Dracup, K., Baker, D., et al. (1994). Heart failure: Evaluation and care of patients with left-ventricular systolic dysfunction. Clinical Practice Guideline No. 11. AHCPR Publication No. 94-0612. Rockville, MD: Agency for Health Care Policy and Research, Public Health Services, U.S. Department of Health and Human Services.

Kramer, B. L., Massie, B. M., & Topic, N. (1983). Controlled trial of captopril in chronic heart failure: A rest and exercise hemodynamic study. *Circulation, 4,* 807–816.

Kubo, S. H., & Cohn, J. N. (1994). Approach to the treatment of the patient with heart failure in 1994. *Advances in Internal Medicine, 39,* 485–515.

Kubo, S. H., Rector, T. S., Bank, A. J., Williams, R. E., & Heifetz, S. M. (1991). Endothelium-dependent vasodilation is attenuated in patients with heart failure. *Circulation, 84,* 1589–1596.

Kukin, M. L. (1992). Vasodilator therapy and survival in chronic congestive heart failure. *Journal of the American College of Cardiology, 19,* 1360–1362.

Kunze, D. L., & Andresen, M. C. (1991). Arterial baroreceptors: Excitation and modulation. In I. H. Zucker & J. P. Gilmore (Eds.), *Reflex control of the circulation* (pp. 165–194). Boca Raton, FL: CRC Press.

Lee, M. A., Böhm, M., Paul, M., & Ganten, D. (1993). Tissue renin–angiotensin systems: Their role in cardiovascular disease. *Circulation, 87*(Suppl IV), IV7–IV13.

Lee, W. H., & Packer, M. (1986). Prognostic importance of serum sodium concentration and its modification by converting-enzyme inhibition in patients with severe heart failure. *Circulation, 73,* 257–267.

Mann, D. L., & Cooper, G. (1989). Neurohumoral activation in congestive heart failure: A double-edged sword? *Clinical Cardiology, 12,* 485–490.

Marantz, P. R., Tobin, J. N., Wassertheil-Smoller, S., et al. (1988). The relationship between left-ventricular systolic function and congestive heart failure diagnosed by clinical criteria. *Circulation, 77,* 607–612.

Nemanich, J. W., Veith, R. C., Abrass, I. B., & Stratton, J. R. (1990). Effects of metoprolol on rest and exercise cardiac function and plasma catecholamines in chronic congestive heart failure secondary to ischemic or idiopathic cardiomyopathy. *American Journal of Cardiology, 66,* 843–848.

Opie, L. H. (1990). Compensation and overcompensation in congestive heart failure. *American Heart Journal, 120,* 1552–1557.

Opie, L. H. (1991). *The heart: Physiology and metabolism.* New York: Raven Press.

Pacher, R., Globitis, S., Wutte, M., et al. (1994). Beneficial hemodynamic effects of prostaglandin E_1 infusion in catecholamine-dependent heart failure: Results of a prospective, randomized, controlled study. *Critical Care Medicine, 22,* 1084–1090.

Packer, M. (1992). The neurohormonal hypothesis: A theory to explain the mechanism of disease progression in heart failure. *Journal of the American College of Cardiology, 20,* 248–254.

Packer, M. (1993). The development of positive inotropic agents for chronic heart failure: How have we gone astray? *Journal of the American College of Cardiology, 22,* 119A–126A.

Packer, M. (1994). Nonadrenergic hormonal alterations in congestive heart failure. In J. D. Hosenpud & B. H. Greenberg (Eds.), *Congestive heart failure: Pathophysiology, diagnosis, and comprehensive approach to management* (pp. 136–144). New York: Springer-Verlag.

Packer, M., Gheorghiade, M., Young, D., et al. (1993). Withdrawal of digoxin from patients with chronic heart failure treated with angiotensin-converting enzyme inhibitors. *New England Journal of Medicine, 329,* 1–7.

Parmley, W. W. (1989). Pathophysiology and current therapy of congestive heart failure. *Journal of the American College of Cardiology, 13,* 771–785.

Passmore, J. M., & Goldstein, R. M. (1989). Acute recognition and management of congestive heart failure. *Critical Care Clinics, 5*(3), 497–532.

Pfeffer, M. A., Braunwald, E., Moyé, L. A., et al. (1992). Effect of captopril on mortality and morbidity in patients with left ventricular dysfunction after myocardial infarction. Results of the Survival and Ventricular Enlargement Trial. *New England Journal of Medicine, 327,* 669–677.

Podrid, P. J., Fogel, R. I., & Fuchs, T. T. (1992). Ventricular arrhythmia in congestive heart failure. *American Journal of Cardiology, 69,* 82G–98G.

Poole-Wilson, P. A. (1993). Relation of pathophysiologic mechanisms to outcome in heart failure. *Circulation, 22*(suppl A), 22A–29A.

Poole-Wilson, P. A., & Buller, N. P. (1988). Causes of symptoms in chronic congestive heart failure and implications for treatment. *American Journal of Cardiology, 62,* 31A–34A.

Purcell, J. A. (1990). Advances in the treatment of dilated cardiomyopathy. *AACN Clinical Issues in Critical Care Nursing, 1*(1), 31–45.

Purcell, J. A., & Holder, C. K. (1989). Cardiomyopathy: Understanding the problem. *American Journal of Nursing, 89*(1), 57–74B.

Schwartz, K., Boheler, K. R., de la Bastie, D., et al. (1992). Switches in cardiac muscle gene expression as a result of pressure and volume overload. *American Journal of Physiology,* 262, R364–R369.

Schwartz, K., Chassagne, C., & Boheler, K. R. (1993). The molecular biology of heart failure. *Journal of the American College of Cardiology, 22*(suppl A), 30A–33A.

SOLVD Investigators. (1991). Effect of enalapril on survival in patients with reduced left ventricular ejection fraction and congestive heart failure. *New England Journal of Medicine, 325,* 293–302.

SOLVD Investigators. (1992). Effect of enalapril on mortality and the development of heart failure in asymptomatic patients with reduced left-ventricular ejection fractions. *New England Journal of Medicine, 327,* 685–691.

Stevenson, L. W. (1993). Advanced heart failure: Inpatient treatment and selection for cardiac transplantation. *Postgraduate Medicine, 94,* 97–116.

Stevenson, L. W., & Fonarow, G. (1992). Vasodilators. A re-evaluation of their role in heart failure. *Drugs, 43,* 15–36.

Stevenson, L. W., & Perloff, J. K. (1988). The dilated cardiomyopathies: Clinical aspects. *Cardiology Clinics, 6,* 187–218.

Stevenson, L. W., & Perloff, J. K. (1989). The limited reliability of physical signs for estimating hemodynamics in chronic heart failure. *Journal of the American Medical Association, 261,* 884–888.

Stevenson, L. W., & Tillisch, J. T. (1986). Maintenance of cardiac output with normal filling pressures in patients with dilated heart failure. *Circulation, 74,* 1303–1308.

Stevenson, L. W., Dracup, K. A., & Tillisch, J. T. (1989). Efficacy of medical therapy tailored for severe congestive heart failure in patients transferred for urgent cardiac transplantation. *American Journal of Cardiology, 63,* 461–464.

Stewart, D. J., Cernacek, P., Costello, K. B., & Rouleau, J. L. (1992). Elevated endothelin-1 in heart failure and loss of normal response to postural change. *Circulation, 85,* 510–517.

Sullivan, M. J. (1994). New trends in cardiac rehabilitation in patients with chronic heart failure. *Progress in Cardiovascular Nursing, 9*(1), 13–21.

Sullivan, M. J., Knight, J. D., Higginbotham, M. B., & Cobb, F. R. (1989). Relation between central and peripheral hemodynamics during exercise in patients with chronic heart failure. *Circulation, 80,* 769–781.

Swedberg, K., Eneroth, P., Kjekshus, J., & Wilhelmson, L. (1990). Hormones regulating cardiovascular function in patients with severe heart failure and their relation to mortality. *Circulation, 82,* 1730–1736.

Treasure, C. B., Vita, J. A., Cox, D. A., et al. (1990). Endothelial-dependent dilation of the coronary microvasculature is impaired in dilated cardiomyopathy. *Circulation, 81,* 772–779.

Tuttle, R. R., & Mills, J. (1975). Dobutamine: Development of a new catecholamine to selectively increase cardiac contractility. *Circulation Research, 36,* 185–196.

24th Bethesda Conference on Cardiac Transplantation (1993). *Journal of the American College of Cardiology, 22*(1), 1–64.

Unverferth, D. V., Magorien, R. D., Lewis, R. P., & Leier, C. V. (1983). The role of subendocardial ischemia in perpetuating myocardial failure in patients with non-ischemic congestive cardiomyopathy. *American Heart Journal, 105,* 176–179.

Uretsky, B. F., Lawless, C. E., Verbalis, J. G., et al. (1987). Combined therapy wtih dobutamine and amrinone in seven heart failure: Improved hemodynamics and increased activation of the renin–angiotensin system with combined intravenous therapy. *Chest, 92,* 657–662.

Uretsky, B. F., Young, J. B., Shahidi, F. E., et al. (1993). Randomized study assessing the effect of digoxin withdrawal in patients with mild to moderate chronic congestive heart failure: Results of the PROVED Trial. *Journal of the American College of Cardiology, 22,* 955–962.

Vargo, R. L. (1993). Bridging to transplant: Mechanical support for heart failure. *Critical Care Nursing Clinics of North America, 5,* 649–659.

Vincent, J.-L. (1994). Hemodynamic monitoring, pharmacologic therapy, and arrhythmia management in acute congestive heart failure. In J. D. Hosenpud & B. H. Greenberg (Eds.), *Congestive heart failure: Pathophysiology, diagnosis, and comprehensive approach to management* (pp. 509–521). New York: Springer-Verlag.

Vinson, J. M., Rich, M. W., Sperry, J. C., Shah, A. S., & McNamara, T. (1990). Early readmission of elderly patients with congestive heart failure. *Journal of the American Geriatric Society, 38,* 1290–1295.

Walden, J. A., Stevenson, L. W., Dracup, K., Wilmarth, J., Kobashigawa, J., & Moriguchi, J. (1989). Heart transplantation may not improve quality of life for patients with stable heart failure. *Heart and Lung, 18,* 497–506.

Wilson, J. R., & Mancini, D. M. (1993). Factors contributing to the exercise limitation of heart failure. *Circulation, 22*(Suppl A), 93A–98A.

Wilson, J. R., Martin, J. L., Schwartz, D., & Ferraro, N. (1984). Exercise intolerance in patients with chronic heart failure: Role of impaired skeletal muscle nutritive flow. *Circulation, 69,* 1079–1087.

Wynne, J., & Braunwald, E. (1992). The cardiomyopathies and myocarditis. In E. Braunwald (Ed.), *Heart disease.* Philadelphia: W. B. Saunders.

Young, J. B., & Farmer, J. A. (1994). The diagnostic evaluation of patients with heart failure. In J. D. Hosenpud & B. H. Greenberg (Eds.), *Congestive heart failure: Pathophysiology, diagnosis, and comprehensive approach to management* (pp. 597–621). New York: Springer-Verlag.

Zucker, I. H. (1991). Baro and cardiac reflex abnormalities in chronic heart failure. In I. H. Zucker & J. P. Gilmore (Eds.), *Reflex control of the circulation* (pp. 849–873). Boca Raton: CRC Press.

HEART FAILURE MULTIDISCIPLINARY CARE GUIDE

COORDINATION OF CARE

Diagnosis/Stabilization Phase		Acute Management Phase		Recovery Phase	
Outcome	**Intervention**	**Outcome**	**Intervention**	**Outcome**	**Intervention**
All appropriate team members and disciplines will be involved in the plan of care.	Develop the plan of care with cardiovascular, and CNS specialists; physical, occupational, and respiratory therapists; and chaplain.	All appropriate team members and disciplines will be involved in the plan of care.	Update the plan of care with the patient/family, other team members, social services, dietician, cardiac rehabilitation (if appropriate), and discharge planner.	All appropriate and team members disciplines will be involved in the plan of care.	Involve the CHF clinic coordinator if available and/or home health for follow-up if needed.

FLUID BALANCE

Diagnosis/Stabilization Phase		Acute Management Phase		Recovery Phase	
Outcome	**Intervention**	**Outcome**	**Intervention**	**Outcome**	**Intervention**
Patient will achieve optimal hemodynamic status as evidenced by: • MAP > 70 mm Hg • Vital signs WNL • Optimal hemodynamic function • Urine output > 0.5 mL/kg/hr • Free from abnormal ECG changes and/or dysrhythmias	Monitor and treat cardiac parameters: • BP • PA pressures • PCWP • C.O./C.I. • Stroke volume • $S\dot{v}O_2$ • SVR/PVR • Left and right ventricular stroke work index • Dysrhythmias • Intake and output • LOC • Evidence of tissue perfusion Monitor effects of medications closely; if patient is on ACE inhibitors, MAP may be as low as 50 mm Hg as long as patient is asymptomatic. Anticipate need for vasopressor agents.	Patient will maintain optimal hemodynamic status.	Monitor hemodynamic parameters and treat patient as needed. Convert vasoactive medications or oral derivatives. Monitor effect on hemodynamics closely. Monitor lab values and treat patient as needed. Evaluate patient for further therapeutic options such as transplant or cardiomyoplasty. Explain risks and benefits clearly to patient/family. Support patient/family physically and psychologically if further therapeutic options are exercised.	Patient will maintain optimal hemodynamics.	Monitor hemodynamic values and treat patient as needed. Monitor lab values and treat patient as needed. Teach patient/family home medication regimen, signs and symptoms of CHF (dyspnea on exertion, shortness of breath, 2–3 pillow orthopnea, weight gain, distended neck veins, peripheral edema) and importance of reporting to physician. Teach patient how to adjust diuretic therapy based on daily weight. Teach patients who are severely hyponatremic *and* unresponsive to diuretics and ACE inhibitors to restrict fluid intake.

Care Guide continued on following page

HEART FAILURE MULTIDISCIPLINARY CARE GUIDE *continued*

FLUID BALANCE *continued*

Diagnosis/Stabilization Phase		Acute Management Phase		Recovery Phase	
Outcome	***Intervention***	***Outcome***	***Intervention***	***Outcome***	***Intervention***
	Assess vital signs, heart sounds, and hemodynamics before and after any vasoactive, diuretic, and/or cardiac drug is given or dosage changed. Anticipate need for pharmacologic interventions for dysrhythmias. Monitor and treat lab values: electrolytes, magnesium, phosphorus, and cardiac enzymes. Monitor for signs of complications that can occur with heart failure, cardiogenic shock, mitral stenosis/regurgitation, dysrhythmias, renal insufficiency or failure, or systemic emboli.				

NUTRITION

Diagnosis/Stabilization Phase		Acute Management Phase		Recovery Phase	
Outcome	***Intervention***	***Outcome***	***Intervention***	***Outcome***	***Intervention***
Patient will be adequately nourished.	Assess nutritional status. Monitor albumin, prealbumin, total protein, cholesterol, and triglycerides.	Patient will be adequately nourished.	Monitor response to low sodium/heart healthy diet. Assess weight daily. Involve dietician. Teach patient/family low sodium/heart healthy diet: • Total fat < 30% of daily intake • Total saturated fat < 10% of daily intake • Total daily cholesterol intake < 300 mg • Total daily sodium intake < 3 g • Caloric reduction if needed • Potassium supplements if on chronic diuretic therapy • Diet supplements for cachectic patients • For patients with alcoholic cardiomyopathy, complete restriction from alcohol; for all other patients, limit alcohol to 8 oz/day of wine/beer or 1 oz/day hard liquor	Patient will be adequately nourished.	Continue diet teaching. Assess understanding. Reinforce as needed.

MOBILITY

Diagnosis/Stabilization Phase		Acute Management Phase		Recovery Phase	
Outcome	Intervention	Outcome	Intervention	Outcome	Intervention
Patient will achieve optimal mobility and participate in spaced activities.	Assess mobility, flexibility, and tone of muscles. Allow frequent rest periods between activities.	Patient will achieve optimal mobility.	Progress exercise as tolerated; monitor response to exercise and increased activity. Decrease activity if adverse events occur (tachycardia, dyspnea, ectopy, syncope, hypotension, chest discomfort). Teach patient pursed-lip breathing techniques and how to coordinate breathing with activity for energy conservation. Involve physical therapy/occupational therapy when indicated.	Patient will achieve optimal mobility.	Same as acute management phase. Assist patient and family in developing home exercise program. Teach patient/family energy-saving techniques.

OXYGENATION/VENTILATION

Diagnosis/Stabilization Phase		Acute Management Phase		Recovery Phase	
Outcome	Intervention	Outcome	Intervention	Outcome	Intervention
Patient will have adequate gas exchange as evidenced by: • $Sao_2 > 90\%$ • ABGs WNL • Clear breath sounds • Respiratory rate, depth, and rhythm WNL • Chest x-ray normal Patient will have adequate tissue oxygenation as evidenced by: • Alert and oriented to person, place, thing • Normal LOC • Urine output >0.5 mL/kg/hr	Monitor and treat oxygenation status per ABGs and/or Sao_2. Monitor and treat ventilatory status per chest assessment, ABGs, adventitious breath sounds, and chest x-ray. Support patient with O_2 therapy and/or mechanical ventilation as indicated. Monitor for signs of fluid overload: intake and output, daily weight, neck vein distension, crackles in lungs, S_3 or S_4, LOC, orientation, and evidence of tissue perfusion to all major organs. Restrict intake when necessary.	Patient will have adequate gas exchange. Patient will maintain adequate tissue perfusion.	Monitor and treat oxygenation/ventilation disturbances. Wean oxygen therapy and/or mechanical ventilation as tolerated. Observe for complications that may impair oxygenation/ventilation (i.e., exacerbation of CHF, mitral stenosis/regurgitation, pulmonary embolus, or cardiogenic shock). Same as stabilization phase.	Patient will have adequate gas exchange. Patient will maintain optimal tissue perfusion.	Teach patient pulmonary signs and symptoms of CHF. Involve home health agency and respiratory therapy if home oxygen indicated. Teach patient hazards of cigarette smoking, secondhand smoke, and environmental factors, which can contribute toward development of atherosclerotic heart disease. Same as acute management phase.

Care Guide continued on following page

HEART FAILURE MULTIDISCIPLINARY CARE GUIDE *continued*

COMFORT

Diagnosis/Stabilization Phase		Acute Management Phase		Recovery Phase	
Outcome	***Intervention***	***Outcome***	***Intervention***	***Outcome***	***Intervention***
Patient will be as comfortable and painfree as possible as evidenced by: • No objective indicators of discomfort • No complaints of discomfort	Provide adequate rest periods between activities. Keep head of bed elevated to enhance breathing comfort. Maintain quiet supportive environment to minimize catecholamine levels. Assess quantity and quality of discomfort. Administer narcotics and/or nitroglycerin for chest pain and monitor response. Provide reassurance in a calm, caring, competent manner.	Patient will be as comfortable as possible.	Provide uninterrupted periods of rest. Teach patient relaxation techniques. Use complementary therapies such as back massage, humor, music therapy, and imagery to promote relaxation. Involve family in strategies.	Patient will be as comfortable as possible.	Teach patient/family relaxation and complementary therapy techniques.

SKIN INTEGRITY

Diagnosis/Stabilization Phase		Acute Management Phase		Recovery Phase	
Outcome	***Intervention***	***Outcome***	***Intervention***	***Outcome***	***Intervention***
Patient will have intact skin without abrasions or pressure ulcers.	Assess skin integrity and all bony prominences q4h and prn. Use preventive pressure-reducing devices if patient is at high-risk for pressure ulcer development. Treat pressure ulcers according to hospital protocol.	Patient will have intact skin without abrasions or pressure ulcers.	Same as stabilization phase.	Patient will have intact skin without abrasions or pressure ulcers.	Teach patient/family proper skin care for at home.

PROTECTION/SAFETY

Diagnosis/Stabilization Phase		Acute Management Phase		Recovery Phase	
Outcome	**Intervention**	**Outcome**	**Intervention**	**Outcome**	**Intervention**
Patient will be protected from possible harm.	Assess need for wrist restraints if patient is intubated, has a decreased LOC, or is unable to follow commands. If restrained, follow hospital protocol for use of restraints. Explain need for restraints to patient and family.	Patient will be protected from possible harm.	Provide support when dangling or beginning progressive exercise program.	Patient will be protected from possible harm.	Provide support with ambulation and progressive exercise. Teach patient/family about any physical limitations the patient might have.

PSYCHOSOCIAL/SELF-DETERMINATION

Diagnosis/Stabilization Phase		Acute Management Phase		Recovery Phase	
Outcome	**Intervention**	**Outcome**	**Intervention**	**Outcome**	**Intervention**
Patient will achieve psychophysiologic stability.	Assess physiologic effect of critical care environment on patient (i.e., physical signs of sympathoadrenal stress response). Assess patient for appropriate level of stress. Assess personal responses (affective and/or feelings) of patient regarding critical illness. Observe the patient's patterns of thinking and communicating. Use calm, competent reassuring approach to interventions. Arrange for flexible visiting to meet needs of patient/family.	Patient will achieve psychophysiologic stability. Patient will demonstrate a decrease in anxiety. Patient will continue acceptance of CHF.	Determine coping ability of patient/family and take appropriate measures to meet their needs (i.e., explain condition, equipment, and medications; provide frequent condition reports; use easy to understand terminology; repeat information as needed; allow family to visit; and answer all questions).	Patient will achieve psychophysiologic stability. Patient will demonstrate a decrease in anxiety. Patient will continue acceptance of CHF.	Continue to assess patient for psychophysiologic stability. Include patient/family in decisions regarding care. Provide support and instructions on coping mechanisms for a chronic illness. Inform patient/family of local support groups. Refer to outpatient counseling if needed postdischarge.
Patient will demonstrate a decreased level of anxiety as evidenced by: • Vital signs WNL • Mental status WNL • Patient reports feeling less anxious • Objective signs of decreased anxiety	Assess and observe factors that make patient/family fearful or anxious. Take measures to reduce the patient's and family's anxiety, fear, and/or sensory overload. (Initiate family conferences, utilize consistent care givers and support services.)				

Care Guide continued on following page

HEART FAILURE MULTIDISCIPLINARY CARE GUIDE *continued*

PSYCHOSOCIAL/SELF-DETERMINATION *continued*

Diagnosis/Stabilization Phase		Acute Management Phase		Recovery Phase	
Outcome	***Intervention***	***Outcome***	***Intervention***	***Outcome***	***Intervention***
Patient will begin acceptance process for CHF.	Use sedatives and anxiolytics as appropriate and monitor response. Provide teaching on care required at home: • Signs and symptoms of CHF • Signs and symptoms of dysrhythmias • Signs and symptoms of angina/MI • Medications • Diet • Activity • When to call physician • Risk factor modification • Energy-saving techniques				

DIAGNOSTICS

Diagnosis/Stabilization Phase		Acute Management Phase		Recovery Phase	
Outcome	***Intervention***	***Outcome***	***Intervention***	***Outcome***	***Intervention***
Patient will understand any tests or procedures that need to be completed, such as hemodynamic assessments, ABGs, echocardiogram, x-ray, ECG.	Explain all procedures and tests to patient. Be sensitive to patient's individual need for information.	Patient will understand any tests or procedures that must be completed.	Explain procedures and tests that must be completed (cardiac enzymes, endomyocardial biopsy, nuclear scans, cardiac angiography and diagnostic workup for cardiac transplant).	Patient will understand the meaning of diagnostic tests in relation to continuing health.	Review with patient before discharge results of ECG, any abnormal lab values, and appropriate measures patient can do to help return to normal. Provide patient with written guidelines concerning follow up care.

Adults With Congenital Heart Defects

Mary M. Canobbio

Contrary to common belief, congenital heart disease (CHD) does not remain static after birth but changes both anatomically and physiologically throughout life. Another serious misconception is that with surgical correction, CHD is "cured." It is now generally accepted that with the possible exception of a ligated patent ductus arteriosus (PDA), there is no cure for CHD; the best one can hope for is a good corrective repair that develops little or no clinical residua. But that is not to say that the patient is categorically assured of a lifetime free of concern for late complications. This concept is important because many defects that are benign or are repaired in infancy and childhood evolve into clinically significant disorders in adulthood. In addition, mild defects may be overlooked or misinterpreted in childhood, setting the stage for serious consequences in early or late adulthood.

This chapter is designed to provide the critical care nurse with an overview of CHD as it currently presents in the adult population. Although an in-depth review of all congenital cardiac defects is beyond the scope of this text, the focus will be on the long-term follow-up of CHD and the issues that influence 10- and 20-year survival.

ETIOLOGY

There is no single cause of congenital heart malformations; rather, they are the result of a complex interaction between genetic and environmental factors. On the genetic side, cardiac malformations are frequently familial. However, the familial recurrence rate due to single gene mutations or chromosomal abnormalities is small. Nora and Nora (1978) found that primary genetic factors accounted for only 8% of all cardiac abnormalities. Of the cardiovascular defects that occur as a result of a genetic disorder, some result from either an autosomal recessive or autosomal dominant pattern, which accounts for 3% of all primary genetic disorders, or by chromosomal transmission, which accounts for 5% of all genetic disorders. Holt-Oram syndrome, Noonan syndrome, and Marfan syndrome are examples of autosomal dominant disorders that have a recurrence rate of 50%; Friedreich ataxia and Duchenne muscular dystrophy are neuromuscular defects associated with myocardiopathy and conduction defects that are transmitted via autosomal recessive genes. Chromosomal abnormalities commonly associated with congenital cardiovascular defects include trisomy 21 (Down syndrome), and XO Turner syndrome. Table 22–1 provides a partial listing of congenital heart malformations that may occur as the result of specific genetic disorders. Because chromosomal and single genetic mutations account for less than 10% of all cardiac anomalies, it is more likely that the etiologic element permitting transmission from one generation to the next is multifactorial, meaning that the interaction of certain genetic patterns with multiple environmental factors is responsible for the familial tendency observed in this group of patients (Goldstein & Brown, 1992).

Environmental factors known to contribute to fetal cardiac embryopathy include a variety of teratogens or exposure by the mother to rubella during the first 8 weeks of pregnancy. Altitude at birth also may be a factor contributing to the occurrence of CHD, particularly PDA. Teratogens, substances used by the mother during gestation, known to cause congenital cardiac defects include thalidomide ingested during the first trimester, trimethadione, hydantoin, and alcohol. Chronic maternal alcohol abuse contributes to the development of fetal alcohol syndrome, which results in a variety of central nervous system defects (e.g., microcephaly) as well as cardiac anomalies. The most frequently seen defects are those involving the ventricular septum, which have been reported to occur in approximately 30% to 45% of affected infants (Nora & Nora, 1978; Friedman, 1992).

INCIDENCE AND PREVALENCE

Precise incidence rates for CHD are not available. It is, however, generally accepted that approximately 0.8% of all live births are complicated by some cardiovascular malformation. Unfortunately, this widely quoted figure underestimates the true incidence of CHD be-

TABLE 22–1. **Partial List of Syndromes Known to Be Associated With Cardiac Malformations**

Syndrome	Cardiac Anomaly	Incidence Rate (Approximate Risk) (%)
Chromosomal Defects		
Trisomy 21 (Down syndrome)	Endocardial cushion defects, ASD, VSD, PDA	50
Trisomy 13 (Patau syndrome)	VSD, PDA, double-outlet right ventricle	90
Trisomy 18 (Edward syndrome)	VSD, PDA, PS	99
XO (Turner syndrome)	Coarctation of aorta, aortic stenosis, ASD	35
Nonchromosomal Disorders		
Autosomal Dominant		
Holt-Oram syndrome	ASD, VSD	50
Noonan (male Turner syndrome)	PS, ASD	50
Ehlers-Danlos syndrome	Dissecting aneurysm, AV valve regurgitation	50
Marfan syndrome	Aortic dilatation and rupture	60–80
Autosomal Recessive		
Cutis laxa	Peripheral pulmonary artery stenosis, pulmonary hypertension	50
Friedreich ataxia	Conduction defects, myocardiomyopathy	50
Laurence-Moon-Biedl syndrome	Tetralogy of Fallot, VSD	30
TAR (thrombocytopenia-absent radius)	ASD, tetralogy of Fallot, dextrocaedia	30
Osteogenesis imperfecta	Aortic insufficiency	5–10
Teratogenic Disorders		
Drugs		
Fetal alcohol syndrome	VSD, ASD, PDA, tetralogy of Fallot	25–30
Fetal hydantoin syndrome	Coarctation of aorta, aortic stenosis, PS, PDA	2–3
Fetal trimethadione syndrome	ASD, tetralogy of Fallot, TGA	15–30
Lithium	Ebstein anomaly, tricuspid atresia, ASD	10
Thalidomide	Tetralogy of Fallot, VSD, ASD, truncus arteriosus	5–10
Infections, Maternal		
Maternal rubella	PDA, pulmonic valvular stenosis, ASD, VSD	35
Other		
Maternal lupus erythematosus	Congenital heart block	?
Maternal diabetes	Coarctation of aorta, TGA, VSD	3–5

Abbreviations: ASD, atrial septal defect; VSD, ventricular septal defect; PDA, patent ductus arteriosus; PS, pulmonic stenosis; TGA, transposition of the great arteries.

Modified from Nora, J. J., & Nora, A. (1978). The evolution of specific genetic and environmental counseling in congenital heart disease. *Circulation, 57,* 205–213. By permission of the American Heart Association, Inc.

cause many defects are undiagnosed at the time of birth. For example, congenital bicuspid aortic valve, which is reported to be the most frequent congenital anomaly of the heart, often goes unnoticed unless it is associated with another defect or becomes dysfunctional later in life (Roberts, 1970). Even less clear is the actual prevalence rate of corrected and uncorrected CHD among adults. Currently in the United States, it is estimated that there are between 500,000 and 600,000 adults with CHD, and an estimated 400,000 have had the defect repaired (McNamara, 1989; Perloff, 1991). Regardless, it is agreed that the rapid advances in surgical interventions have been the primary factor in the increase in life expectancy of patients with defects for which natural survival is common and also permits the survival of a large number of patients with defects that were previously fatal in childhood (Laks et al., 1980; Zuberbuhler, 1983). Today, a life expectancy of 10 to 25 years beyond surgical intervention is not uncommon; therefore, a new population of adult cardiac patients is emerging.

Adults With Congenital Heart Disease

Three categories of adults with CHD are emerging. First and most prevalent are adults with surgically corrected CHD. Although precise numbers are unavailable, it has begun to be evident from the centers that report follow-up studies on large populations of adult patients that the numbers are rising (Schaff & Danielson, 1987; McNamara & Latson, 1982). The recently completed *Second Natural History of Congenital Heart Defects* (O'Fallon & Weidman, 1993) further documents the fact that 20-year survival of individuals with pulmonic stenosis, ventricular septal defect (VSD), and aortic stenosis (with gradients of <50 mm Hg) is now possible after surgical repair.

TABLE 22–2. **Natural Survival of Common and Uncommon Defect Forms of Congenital Heart Disease**

A. Common Congenital Cardiac Defects in Which Adult Survival Is Expected:

Functionally normal bicuspid aortic valve
Congenital valvular aortic stenosis
Coarctation of the aorta
Valvular pulmonic stenosis
Atrial septal defect
Patent ductus arteriosus
Ventricular septal defect with pulmonic stenosis (tetralogy of Fallot)

B. Uncommon Congenital Cardiac Defects in Which Adult Survival Is Expected:

Situs inversus
Dextroversion of the heart
Congenital complete heart block
Congenitally corrected transposition of the great arteries
Idiopathic dilatation of the pulmonary trunk
Subvalvular pulmonic stenosis
Supravalvular pulmonic stenosis
Ebstein anomaly of the tricuspid valve
Congenital pulmonary arteriovenous fistula
Lutembacher syndrome
Common atrium
Congenital coronary arteriovenous fistula
Congenital aneurysms of the sinus of Valsalva
Vena caval to left atrial connection
Congenital pulmonary valve regurgitation
Primary pulmonary hypertension

C. Common Congenital Cardiac Defects in Which Adult Survival Is Exceptional:

Ventricular septal defect
Ventricular septal defect with aortic regurgitation
Atrioventricular canal (endocardial cushion defect)
Tricuspid atresia
Complete transposition of the great arteries

D. Uncommon Congenital Cardiac Defects in Which Adult Survival Is Exceptional:

Anomalous origin of the left coronary artery from pulmonary trunk
Cor triatriatum
Total anomalous pulmonary venous connection
Right ventricular origin of both great arteries (double-outlet right ventricle)
Truncus arteriosus
Single ventricle
Discrete subvalvular aortic stenosis

Adapted from *Critical Care Nursing Quarterly*, Vol. 4, No. 3, p. 41, with permission of Aspen Publishers, Inc., © 1981.

A second group of adults with CHD are those for whom operative correction has been impossible either because their cardiac anomalies have not been amenable to surgical correction or because they have developed pulmonary vascular disease.

The third group of adults with CHD is the small percentage of individuals who have unrecognized or undiagnosed disease. Table 22–2 summarizes both common and uncommon forms of congenital heart defects in which natural survival can be expected or is considered exceptional. Included in this category are patients who may have received palliative treatment in early childhood with the hope of later repair but for a variety of reasons have been lost to follow-up. Larger medical centers have confirmed that a number of cardiac anomalies continue to be detected initially and surgically treated in adulthood (Danielson & McGoon, 1987). To understand what long-term follow-up can be expected, patients can be classified by their functional status rather than by their individual defects (Table 22–3).

Patients in category I are those who either remain unrepaired because their defect is not clinically significant (e.g., bicuspid aortic valve with mild aortic stenosis, small VSD, mild peripheral pulmonary artery stenosis) or have undergone complete repair and have no residual effects. Included in this group are those who have experienced spontaneous closure of a VSD. These patients, who fortunately make up the largest majority of the population of patients with CHD, are asymptomatic and are normal when measured on objective functional tests and evaluation such as exercise tests and echocardiography. Socially, they are able to work, have children, and live well-adjusted lives.

Patients in category II are those with documented residual effects and complications who are either asymptomatic or remain minimally symptomatic for many years and require varying degrees of long-term follow-up care. Conditions characterizing people in this category include residual hypertension following a coarctectomy, residual mitral regurgitation following closure of an ostium primum atrial septal defect (ASD), or a patch leak with residual shunt following

TABLE 22–3. **Four-Category System for Determining Impact on Quality of Life**

Category I: Those who have undergone a complete repair and have no residual effects and are asymptomatic or have had no surgical repair due to clinically insignificant defect. Their clinical course is stable, they have normal functional capacity, are generally less anxious, and lead normal lives.

Category II: Those who have undergone surgical correction but are left with known residual defects or complications, such as the postoperative coarctation patient who is left with residual hypertension. They may remain asymptomatic for years, but over time develop symptoms because of the residual defect. Their level of social adjustment will vary.

Category III: Those who have undergone corrective procedures for complex cardiac defects. They are similar to patients in category I in that they may have had good to excellent repairs and are asymptomatic, but unlike the patient with a common defect the long-term sequelae of these patients remain unknown.

Category IV: Those who may have undergone previous palliative or corrective procedures but remain symptomatic due to a limited cardiac reserve. Their prognosis is usually poor and their social adjustment may have marked limitations.

Adapted with permission from Engle, M. A., & Perloff, J. K. (eds.) (1983). *Congenital heart disease after surgery* (pp. 347–361). Boston: Butterworth.

closure of a VSD. The prognosis for patients in this category is largely dependent on the specific type of lesion and the degree of severity of the residual effects. Their level of social adjustment will vary with the degree of functional limitation. Often, they may live several years before the onset of symptoms and not infrequently will require a repeat operation.

A third category of patients includes those who have undergone successful surgical repair but are subject to unknown residual and long-term sequelae after 10 to 20 years. This group includes patients who have undergone repair for complex congenital defects such as single ventricle, tricuspid atresia, and transposition of the great arteries. By objective measurements, these individuals may have achieved a normal functional capacity and are asymptomatic, but they must be carefully monitored to detect the frequent subtle onset of symptoms.

A fourth category of adult patients includes those whose defects remain unrepaired because they have developed pulmonary hypertension, have an anatomic arrangement not amenable to correction, or have residual effects that have produced complications that are no longer amenable to surgical intervention. Conditions that characterize this last category include: (1) unrepaired defects such as ASDs or VSDs with right to left shunts due to increased pulmonary vascular resistance (commonly referred to as Eisenmenger syndrome—see later discussion), (2) pulmonary atresia with an inadequate supply of pulmonary collaterals for a staged repair, and (3) ventricular failure. The clinical course of this group of patients varies widely. Many patients with Eisenmenger syndrome remain clinically free of symptoms for years and are able to lead relatively normal lives. However, their prognosis is guarded, and they require careful and frequent evaluation. Understandably, the level of social adjustment in this group of patients is hampered by their physical limitations, and they generally require much in the way of emotional support and counseling. They are also the group who may have the greatest difficulty in obtaining health insurance.

FACTORS INFLUENCING LONG-TERM SURVIVAL

In dealing with the adult patient with a congenital heart defect it is important to recognize that survival is influenced by several factors. First, the primary cardiac defect or defects must be considered and the complications, if any, that have developed must be determined. Second, the surgical interventions that may have taken place must be identified. In patients who have undergone previous surgical correction, it is important to consider what postoperative residua and known sequelae are associated with the procedure. Finally, the age at which surgical repair occurred is important.

Primary Defects

Congential heart defects are frequently described in terms of the presence or absence of cyanosis. Although this is clinically correct, for purposes of understanding the hemodynamic consequences of these defects it is preferable to classify congenital heart defects by the direction and magnitude of pulmonary blood flow (Table 22–4) (Morgan, 1978).

Acyanotic Defects

NORMAL PULMONARY BLOOD FLOW

Defects such as coarctation of the aorta, aortic stenosis, and pulmonic stenosis cause impairment or obstruction of ventricular outflow. The result creates an increased pressure load on the ventricle, leading to concentric hypertrophy of the wall of the respective chamber. The anatomic location of the obstruction and the severity of the obstructive gradient together dictate the degree of clinical pathology that results. For example, congenital aortic stenosis can occur at the valvular, subvalvular, or supravalvular level of the aortic ring. The most common type is valvular. If it is stenotic from birth, the valve is usually bicuspid, and the valve tissue becomes progressively thickened and fibrotic during childhood and adolescence. Calcification of the valve that does not usually begin until early adulthood

TABLE 22–4. **Congenital Heart Disease Based on the Direction of Pulmonary Blood Flow**

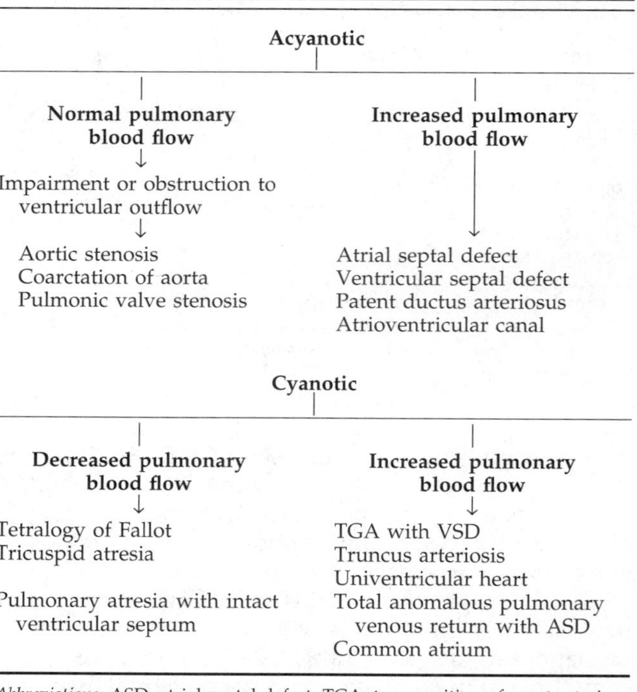

Acyanotic	
Normal pulmonary blood flow ↓ Impairment or obstruction to ventricular outflow ↓	**Increased pulmonary blood flow** ↓
Aortic stenosis Coarctation of aorta Pulmonic valve stenosis	Atrial septal defect Ventricular septal defect Patent ductus arteriosus Atrioventricular canal

Cyanotic	
Decreased pulmonary blood flow ↓	**Increased pulmonary blood flow** ↓
Tetralogy of Fallot Tricuspid atresia Pulmonary atresia with intact ventricular septum	TGA with VSD Truncus arteriosis Univentricular heart Total anomalous pulmonary venous return with ASD Common atrium

Abbreviations: ASD, atrial septal defect; TGA, transposition of great arteries; VSD, ventricular septal defect.

and results in further restriction in valve mobility and obstruction of left ventricular outflow. The clinical manifestations of aortic stenosis, as with other obstructive lesions, are largely determined by the severity of the valve stenosis and the degree of obstruction it presents. In aortic stenosis, the response of the left ventricle to chronic pressure overload is concentric hypertrophy (Friedman, 1992). In severe forms of obstruction of ventricular outflow, the electrocardiogram will show signs of hypertrophy with strain when there is an imbalance between myocardial oxygen supply and demand. As with most cases of persistent increased afterload, dilatation and decompensation occur in the natural progression of the disease process.

INCREASED PULMONARY BLOOD FLOW

Anomalies that redirect the flow of blood from the left heart back to the right side (l → r), as in ASD or VSD, produce an added burden on the right atrium and ventricle and pulmonary vessels. Pathophysiology is largely determined by the size of the defect and the ratio of pulmonary to systemic vascular resistance. For example, a small restrictive VSD may result in little or no increased cardiac or pulmonary workload (Borow & Braunwald, 1992). But when the left to right shunt is large, the additional burden of increased pulmonary blood flow frequently leads to enlargement of the pulmonary artery and thus to pulmonary hypertension. If this situation is left unrepaired, as in the case of a large nonrestrictive VSD, equilibration of systolic pressures in the two ventricles occurs. Pulmonary blood flow is then determined by the ratio of systemic and pulmonary vascular resistance. When pulmonary vascular resistance equals or exceeds systemic vascular resistance, a bidirectional or right to left shunt develops.

Cyanotic Defects

Cyanotic lesions represent a shunting of blood from the right heart to the left. They generally result from an abnormal communication between the two circulations, leading to venoarterial mixing. A variety of cardiac anomalies can result in an abnormal connection between the two circulations. The distinguishing feature, however, is whether the anomaly contributes to a decrease or an increase in pulmonary blood flow, and this then becomes the basis for therapeutic interventions.

DECREASED PULMONARY BLOOD FLOW

Malformations that lead to shunting of blood away from the lungs generally occur because (1) there is a severe pulmonary obstruction, as in tetralogy of Fallot, tricuspid atresia, or pulmonary atresia with intact ventricular septum, or (2) the right ventricle is inadequate as a pumping chamber, as in Ebstein anomaly of the tricuspid valve. Clinically, the patient is deeply cyanotic, hypoxic, and easily fatigued. Rarely do any of these defects go undetected. Because these defects are diagnosed usually in infancy or during early childhood, the majority of adult patients with these defects have undergone definitive intracardiac repair or placement of a surgically created systemic–pulmonary arterial shunt that permits increased pulmonary arterial blood flow with enhanced oxygen saturation. In the latter group of patients, intracardiac repair is still a possibility but only in the absence of pulmonary vascular disease.

INCREASED PULMONARY BLOOD FLOW

Increased pulmonary blood flow is the result of either common mixing of blood in the atrium (common atrium) or ventricles (single ventricle) or an abnormal communication between the great vessels as in transposition of the great arteries with VSD. Excessive pulmonary blood flow generally results in cardiac failure unless a palliative procedure such as pulmonary banding can minimize the amount or unless the patient develops pulmonary vascular disease, which decreases the degree of shunting. Survival to adulthood is possible but generally only with an early palliative procedure followed later by surgical correction.

Surgical Intervention

With few exceptions, surgical intervention is recommended when feasible for the majority of uncorrected congenital heart disorders. But the operative risk and prognosis largely depend on the complexity of the defect, the presence of and severity of associated cardiac symptoms, and the presence or absence of pulmonary hypertension. In the adult patient, surgery for CHD may have been undertaken as a palliative measure or as a method of physiologic intracardiac repair.

PALLIATIVE PROCEDURES

A wide range of palliative procedures has been introduced during the past four decades. These generally serve as a preliminary step toward total intracardiac repair for correctable lesions. For defects that are not reparable, palliative procedures have served as the sole means of survival for patients with defects that would otherwise prove fatal during infancy. Palliative procedures include shunt operations designed to improve pulmonary blood flow (Fig. 22–1) (Table 22–5), surgical operations designed to create arteriovenous mixing at the atrial level (Table 22–6), or pulmonary artery banding to decrease pulmonary blood flow thus protecting the pulmonary vascular bed.

Of the various systemic to pulmonary artery shunting procedures that have been developed to increase pulmonary blood flow, the earliest and perhaps the most widely used is the Blalock-Taussig (BT) or

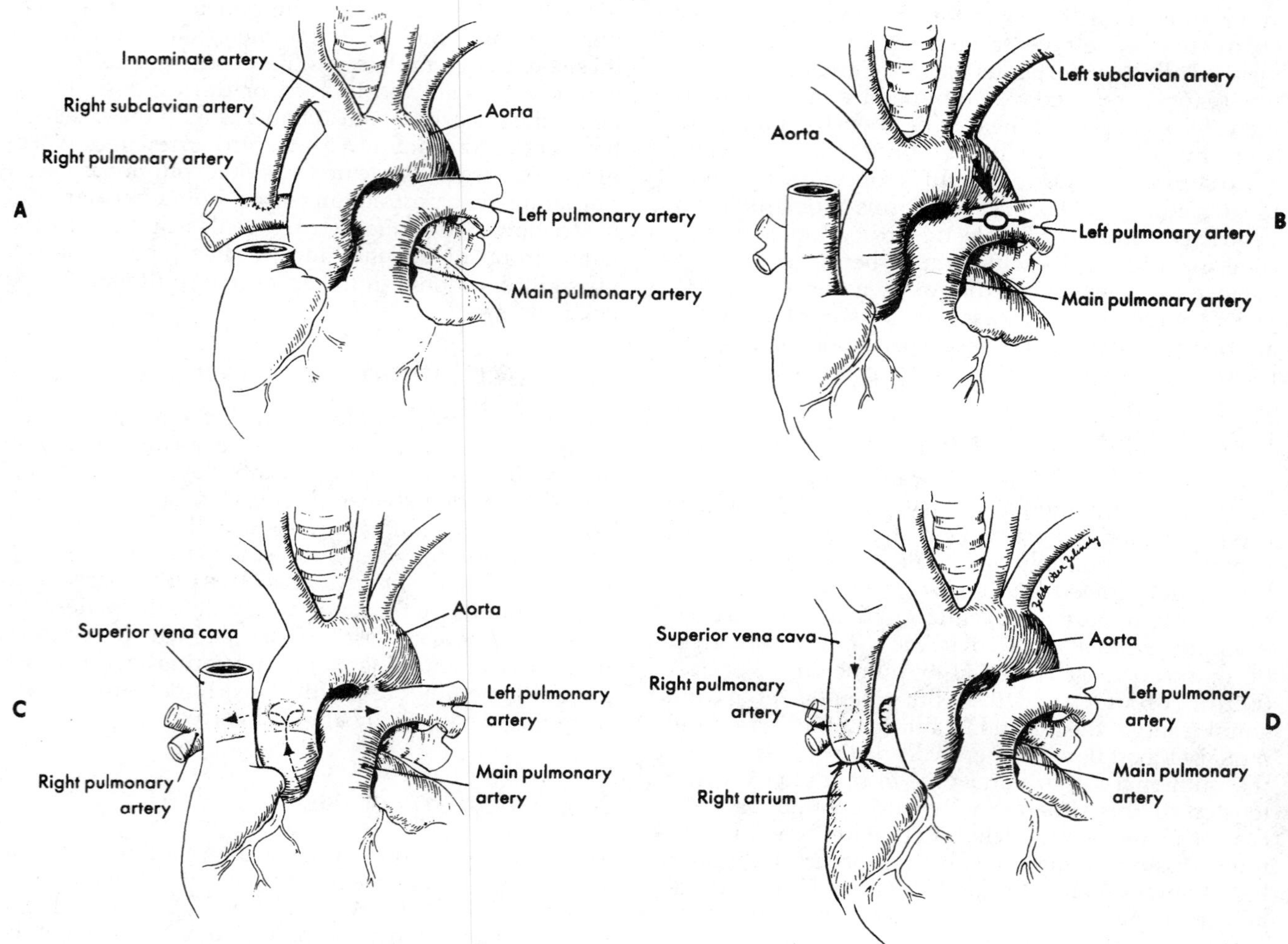

FIGURE 22–1. Shunting procedures used to increase pulmonary artery blood flow. *A*, Blalock-Taussig (BT) shunt. Subclavian artery is divided. The proximal portion is brought down, and the end of the subclavian is anastomosed to the pulmonary artery. *B*, Potts anastomosis. The left pulmonary artery is anastomosed to a portion of the descending aorta. *C*, Waterston-Cooley shunt. A fistula is created between the posterior ascending aorta and the anterior portion of the right pulmonary artery. *D*, Glenn anastomosis. Superior vena cava (SVC) ligated at its junction with right atrium; the SVC is attached to the right pulmonary artery using Gore-Tex graft. SVC blood is directed to the right pulmonary artery. (Reproduced by permission from Hazinski [1984]. *Nursing care of the critically ill child* [p. 195]. St. Louis: C. V. Mosby Co.)

modified BT anastomosis, which connects the subclavian artery to the pulmonary artery. Introduced more than 35 years ago, it has proved to have one of the highest patency rates and lowest complication rates among shunting procedures (complications include heart failure or development of pulmonary vascular disease). Furthermore, it is generally easier to close at the time of definitive repair (Pacifico & Sand, 1987). Over the years additional shunts have been devised, but several, such as the Potts procedure, have been abandoned because they had a tendency toward excessive pulmonary blood flow (von Bermuth et al., 1971).

Other procedures designed to promote mixing of blood by creating an ASD (left to right shunt) include the balloon atrial septostomy (Rashkind procedure) and the atrial septectomy (Blalock-Hanlon technique). These procedures permit a free flow of oxygenated blood to the right atrium, from which it enters the right ventricle and pulmonary circulation (Cooley, 1988). Generally performed during the first two weeks of life, these procedures are used to palliate transposition of the great arteries and tricuspid atresia.

The majority of patients who have undergone these procedures in infancy have later had corrective or definitive repair. However, a small number reach adulthood with no repairs. These patients usually have limited cardiac reserve, and although most have adjusted to their condition, they are functionally limited (Borow & Braunwald, 1992). As adults, some may still be amenable to surgical repair; however, the de-

TABLE 22–5. **Shunting Operations for Congenital Heart Defects: Procedures That Permit Increased Pulmonary Blood Flow by Creating Systemic to Pulmonary Artery Shunt**

Shunt	Year Introduced	Description	Morbidity
Blalock-Taussig	1945	Subclavian artery to pulmonary artery	BA (<6%) IE (<6%) Patency (>50%) PVD (1–5%)
Potts	1946	Descending aorta anastomosed side-to-side to left pulmonary artery	PVD (>15%) IE (15%) CHF (38%)
Glenn	1958	Superior vena cava anastomosed to right pulmonary artery	
Modified Blalock-Taussig	1962	Subclavian artery to pulmonary artery using Gore-Tex graft	
Waterston-Cooley	1962–1966	Ascending aorta anastomosed to right pulmonary artery	PVD (6%) CHF (26%) Kinking of right pulmonary artery

Abbreviations: BA, brain abscess; IE, infective endocarditis; PVD, pulmonary vascular disease; CHF, congestive heart failure.

velopment of pulmonary vascular disease or a failing myocardium in some prohibits further surgical intervention.

CORRECTIVE PROCEDURES

Since the introduction of intracardiac repair for CHD more than 35 years ago, the clinical course of patients in whom congenital cardiac anomalies have been corrected has been carefully scrutinized. It is generally agreed that there are few surgical cures for CHD. In most cases what has been rendered is a definitive repair that has either reestablished anatomic integrity and a normal circulation, or has restored a normal circulation through an artificial inserted conduit or baffle. An example of total correction, which has been available for more than three decades, is the procedure for tetralogy of Fallot. The procedure includes the ligation or takedown of any prior palliative shunts, patch closure of the VSD, and relief of the right ventricular outflow tract obstruction. To accomplish this, one of several techniques is used, infundibular resection, pulmonary valvotomy, insertion of a pulmonary homograft, or transannular patch, depending on the amount of outflow obstruction and the degree of pulmonary valve involvement. Results of long-term survival for tetralogy of Fallot have been very favorable. Today, reports indicate that survival rates of 85% and 95% for up to 20 years after operation are now possible (Pacifico & Sand, 1987; Fuster et al., 1980). Long-term morbidity has been related to dysrhythmias and decreased right and left ventricular function (Higgins & Reed, 1994). Reoperation is reported to occur in 5% of patients (Zaho et al., 1985).

TABLE 22–6. **Palliative Procedures for Congenital Heart Disease: Procedures That Permit Arteriovenous Mixing by Creating Left to Right Shunts**

Procedure	Year Introduced	Description
Blalock-Hanlon (atrial septectomy)	1948	Entering through a left thoracotomy, incisions are made into the right and left atria and interatrial septum is removed
Rashkind (balloon atrial septostomy)	1966	Balloon-tipped catheter passed through inferior vena cava and foramen ovale into left atrium

Another procedure that is now available and typifies the physiologic correction of complex cyanotic defects is the Fontan procedure. Originally described in 1971 (Fontan & Baudet, 1971) for tricuspid atresia, the procedure continues to undergo modifications and is now being used in the treatment of several defects, including single ventricle and double-inlet ventricles (Humes et al., 1988). The procedure involves directing venous blood flow from the right heart directly into the pulmonary arteries.

Of the various operative techniques that have been used in the past two decades, closure of the ASD, if present, and surgical connection of the right atrium to the pulmonary artery or right ventricle by direct anastomosis or by means of a nonvalved conduit were common (Fig. 22–2,A,B). Earlier techniques also included the use of porcine valve conduits, which were abandoned because of development of valvular dysfunction and obstruction. Over time, as data on long-term follow-up has emerged, these procedures have come under debate, particularly with respect to using the right atrium and/or the right ventricle in the primary connection. Concern centers on the potential deleterious effect of making the right atrium a

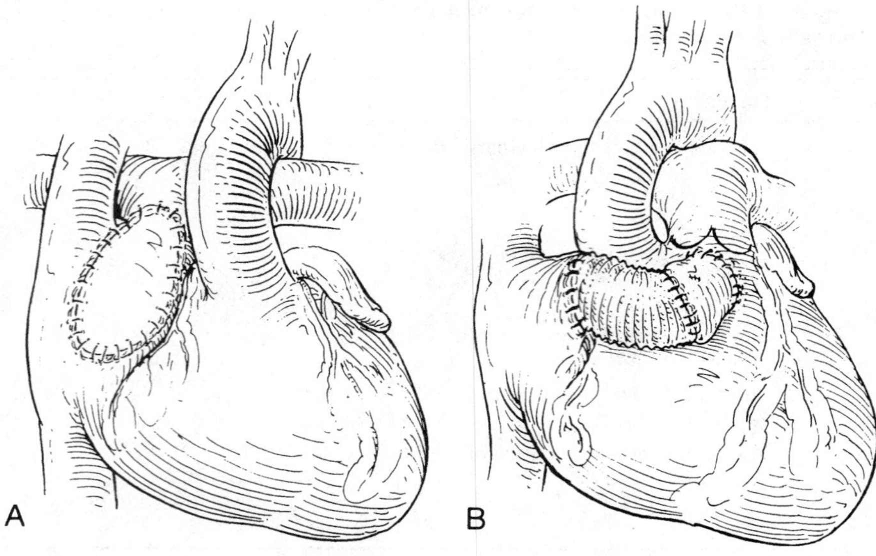

FIGURE 22–2. Fontan procedure. Direct right atrium to pulmonary artery anastomosis. *A,* Direct right atrium to pulmonary artery connection is shown with augmentation of the anastomosis by a pericardial patch. *B,* Right atrium to right ventricle aortic homograft connection. The atrial and ventricular septal defects are closed. (From Barre, A. E., et al. [1991]. *Glenn's thoracic and cardiovascular surgery* [5th ed.]. Norwalk: Appleton & Lange.)

high-pressure systemic venous pathway in the right atrium–pulmonary artery connection. It is believed that chronic exposure to high venous pressure may result in atrial enlargement and thickening, which may contribute to the supraventricular dysrhythmias commonly reported in post-Fontan patients. Similarly, utilization of the hypoplastic right ventricle in the right atrium–right ventricle connection in tricuspid atresia has failed to show any advantage unless the right ventricle has a well-developed trabecular component and is at least one-third to one-half normal size (Kopf, 1993). Furthermore, concern is always raised about possible conduit obstruction.

At present, the procedure being utilized is known as the lateral tunnel and total cavopulmonary anastomosis. This procedure, described by DeLeval (1988), utilizes a method of atrial partitioning called the lateral tunnel to deliver inferior vena cava (IVC) blood to the superior vena cava (SVC) (Fig. 22–3). A total cavopulmonary anastomosis is used to connect the systemic venous pathway to the pulmonary artery. The reported advantages of this procedure include its utility for all types of defects and for use at an early age, its avoidance of valves or conduits, and importantly, its sparing of the right atrium from the high systemic venous pressure. Although survival data is not available for all modifications such as the lateral tunnel, 10- and 15-year survival data for the earlier procedures show the majority of survivors remain in functional class I or II (Fontan et al., 1990). Late morbidity has been related primarily to the persistent elevated right atrial pressure and conduit obstruction associated with earlier techniques that has resulted in supraventricular tachydysrhythmias and protein-losing enteropathy. Hemodynamic results of left ventricular function are critical to the short- and long-term morbidity of the Fontan patient. Ejection factions of $< 45\%$ or ventricular end-diastolic pressure of < 15 mm Hg are necessary if a good clinical result is to occur (Kirklin et al., 1986). Un-

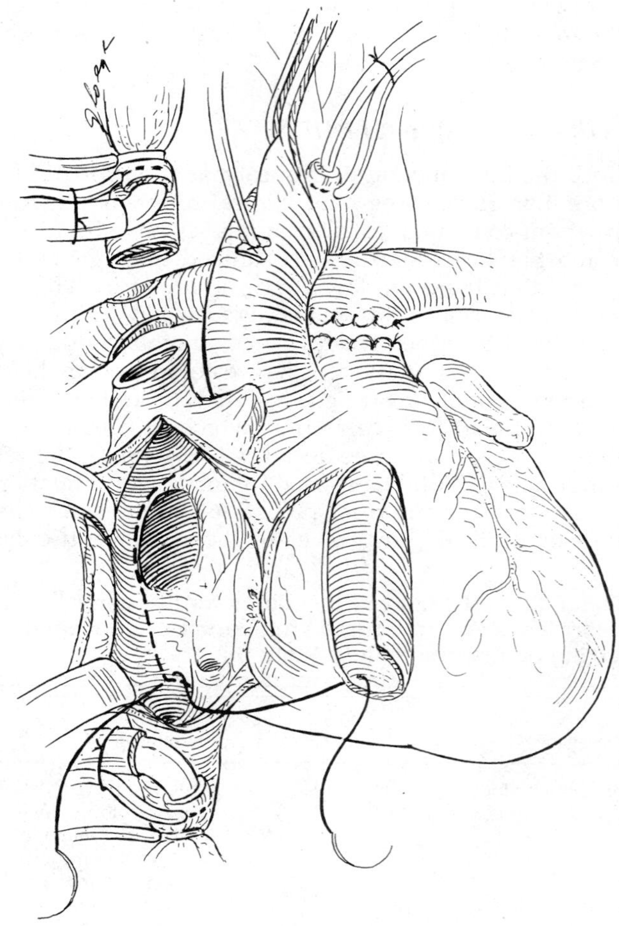

FIGURE 22–3. Creation of the lateral tunnel technique with an 18-mm Gore-Tex tube graft. (From Pearl, J. M., Laks, H., Stein, D. G., et al. [1991]. Total cavopulmonary anastomosis versus conventional modifed Fontan procedure. *Annals of Thoracic Surgery, 52,* 189.)

fortunately, results of studies of the Fontan procedure performed in adults have found that longstanding volume overload is related to poorer outcomes (Humes et al., 1988; Mair et al., 1990). Seliem and colleagues (1989) reported patients with poor outcomes were found to have significantly increased left ventricular muscle mass, showing the need to prevent significant hypertrophy. Earlier repair may minimize this problem in the future.

Thus, despite the favorable results of many surgical interventions for congenital heart defects, over time it has been determined that a wide range of residual effects ranging from mild to severe can exist. These effects may develop as a direct result of the surgical intervention, such as a residual pulmonic stenosis that exists after repair of tetralogy of Fallot, or they may develop separately and demand reoperation, such as a conduit obstruction associated with the Fontan procedure (Laks et al., 1980; Mair et al., 1985). Furthermore, for many complex defects, the long-term natural sequelae of surgical correction remain unknown.

One area of investigation has been the postoperative myocardium. Studies have shown that, regardless of the site of incision (atrium or ventricle), subendocardial fibroelastosis of the left ventricle is likely to develop because of prolonged pump time, and it is this fibrosis that is responsible for the development of late ventricular dysfunction (Henson et al., 1969; Bharati & Levi, 1983). The long-term effects of ventriculotomy and the subsequent development of scar tissue in the myocardium also have been attributed to development of reentry phenomena leading to ventricular tachycardia and sudden death (Bharati & Levi, 1983). Aneurysm formation at the ventriculotomy site is yet another consideration in the development of postoperative ventricular tachycardia. In addition to effects on the myocardium, the bundle of His and its branches also may be damaged by the effects of ventriculotomy, resection of obstructive right ventricular muscle, or development of fibrosis. Sinus node dysfunction is a late concern after complex intraatrial connections such as the Mustard or Senning procedure for transposition of the great arteries, during repair of a sinus venosus ASD, or following the Fontan repair for tricuspid atresia. Similarly, the atrioventricular (AV) node is at risk during repair of AV septal defects, VSDs, or tricuspid valve defects. Consequently, postoperative dysrhythmias pose one of the major challenges to long-term survival.

Additional late complications that have been reported as a direct result of the original surgical procedure include development of true or pseudoaneurysms in the right ventricular outflow tract following the insertion of patches, obstruction of intraatrial baffles or conduits, and valvular incompetence due to suturing.

Although many of the postoperative problems apparent in this first generation of adult patients may be a reflection of early surgical techniques rather than current ones, only time will tell whether improved intraoperative procedures will be able to decrease or eliminate these complications in long-term follow-up.

AGE AT SURGERY

With respect to the clinical outcome, it is becoming increasingly clear that the best surgical results occur when procedures are undertaken in infancy and early childhood rather than in adolescence (McNamara & Latson, 1982). This is true for a wide range of defects, including VSD, tetralogy of Fallot, tricuspid atresia, and single ventricle (Kirklin et al., 1983; Ebert et al., 1984; Mair et al., 1985; Pacifico & Sand, 1987).

In contrast, information about the long-term psychological outcome or emotional adjustment relative to the age at surgery has not been studied as rigorously. To date, the effects of hypothermia, circulatory arrest, and cardiopulmonary bypass (Glasner & Bentovim, 1987) on cognitive and neurologic functioning have been examined. Overall, the clinical findings show that after surgical repair children have intellectual and motor skills normal or equal to those of their age-matched counterparts (Glasner & Bentovim, 1987). Less clear, however, is the issue of age at operation and long-term effects on emotional adjustment. From the limited information available, it appears that individuals on whom surgery was performed in late childhood or preadolescence compared with those who underwent repairs before age 6 are significantly different in terms of personality traits and dependency. As a whole, they tend to display traits similar to those seen in persons who are chronically ill (Baer et al., 1984). Such information suggests that when some state of invalidism is imposed on a child during important periods of cognitive, motor, and emotional development, long-term psychological well-being may be impaired.

COMPLICATIONS ASSOCIATED WITH LONG-TERM SURVIVAL OF CHD

Dysrhythmias

As previously mentioned, dysrhythmias occur frequently as a long-term postoperative complication. But they also are a major cause of morbidity and mortality among patients who have had no repair.

McNamara and Latson (1982), in their 25-year postoperative follow-up of five common congenital heart defects (VSD, ASD, PDA, pulmonary stenosis, and coarctation of the aorta), reported that although most patients were living normal lives, there continued to be a large incidence of residual effects and sequelae—namely, late unexpected dysrhythmias requiring periodic follow-up. The *Second Natural History Study of Congenital Heart Disease* conducted a 20-year follow-up study that included VSD, pulmonic stenosis, and aortic stenosis. The results of this study showed that although patients were generally in good health, individuals with VSD or aortic stenosis with residual gradients were at greater risk of developing late dysrhythmias (O'Fallon & Weidman, 1993).

Dysrhythmias encountered among patients who

have had no repairs are often the result of a complication or electrophysiologic instability associated with the primary congenital defect. For example, patients with Ebstein anomaly may present with rapid heart action resulting from supraventricular tachycardia (SVT). These dysrhythmias, which have been reported in 25% to 30% of patients, represent reentrant SVT, atrial fibrillation, and atrial flutter and are not necessarily related to accelerated or anomalous AV conduction (Ferguson et al., 1986; Perloff, 1987). One variety of Ebstein anomaly is also associated with preexcitation patterns such as Wolff-Parkinson-White syndrome, which usually represents a right bypass tract (Perloff, 1987). Several congenital heart anomalies show evidence of AV conduction abnormalities. For example, first-degree AV block is characteristically seen in patients with endocardial cushion defects (such as ostium primum) and post-Fontan patients. Right bundle branch block is present in 50% to 100% of patients after repair for tetralogy of Fallot (Walsh et al., 1988). Atrial fibrillation and flutter are frequently encountered in patients who develop volume overload. Lesions such as ASD or VSD that produce significant left to right shunting will, over time, lead to atrial tachydysrhythmias. Ventricular dysrhythmias are characteristically seen in the setting of longstanding volume overload or ventricular failure as well as in conditions where there has been chronic pressure overload of the left ventricle as seen in aortic valve disease and palliative systemic–pulmonary shunts (Sloss & Ellison, 1987). Ventricular dysrhythmias also are the most probable cause of sudden death in patients who develop the Eisenmenger syndrome (Wood, 1958; Young & Marks, 1971). Table 22–7 presents a listing of several defects and the dysrhythmias associated with them. Thus, with few exceptions, patients with known CHD should be periodically evaluated for the development of late dysrhythmias.

Infective Endocarditis

Susceptibility to infective endocarditis is an essential concern in the management and long-term follow-up of the adult with CHD. In certain cases, such as patients with a ligated PDA or an ostium secundum defect, the risk of endocarditis may be decreased or eliminated postoperatively. However, all patients must be carefully evaluated for the presence of residual lesions that will necessitate continued preventive measures for prevention of endocarditis. Recommendations from the American Heart Association have stratified risk levels for prevention of endocarditis into a two-dose antibiotic regimen. In general, patients with anomalies associated with jet formation and vortex shedding are considered at greater risk for developing bacteremia than those with low-pressure, high-flow lesions (Dajani et al., 1990). Individuals with prosthetic valves and other prosthesic material such as conduits and shunts should have lifelong prophylaxis. Table 22–8 can be used as a guide in estimating risk for infective endocarditis in patients with CHD (Canobbio, 1987).

Hematologic Disorders

Unique to the population of adult patients with cyanotic CHD are the hematologic abnormalities associated with this chronic disorder. Their special needs, which can include cardiac and noncardiac problems, set these individuals apart from the typical adult patient with acquired cardiac disease.

Erythrocytosis, a direct response to tissue hypoxia, is the adaptive increase in red blood cell (RBC) production designed to compensate for decreased systemic oxygen saturation. The result of erythropoietin production, this increase in circulating whole blood volume increases the oxygen-carrying capacity of the blood and maintains an adequate oxygen supply to metabolizing tissues. As the number of RBCs increases, the position of the oxygen–hemoglobin dissociation curve, one determinant of oxygen transport and delivery, may be slightly shifted to the right (Rosove et al., 1986; Rudolph et al., 1953). This shift permits release of the additional oxygen to the tissues at a higher $Pa{O_2}$. The goal of a compensated erythrocytotic response is to achieve equilibrium conditions at a higher hematocrit level.

The consequences of venoarterial mixing and a higher hematocrit lead to a number of clinical findings that can present a unique challenge to the critical care practitioner (cyanotic patients typically have hematocrits of 45% or greater).

HYPERVISCOSITY

The relationship between RBC volume and blood viscosity, which has been the focus of study, is in the form of a hyperbolic curve, and therefore, minor increases in hematocrits above 65% to 75% may produce marked increase in whole blood viscosity, which can lead to a number of symptoms, including headaches, visual disturbances, paresthesia, myalgia, and muscle weakness.

Whole blood viscosity also can be significantly affected by other variables, including plasma volume (hydration and RBC deformability). The latter may be affected by iron deficiency anemia (Rosenthal et al., 1971; Rosove et al., 1986).

IRON DEFICIENCY ANEMIA

In iron deficiency anemia, the normal flexible biconcave RBC becomes rigid, microcytic, and susceptible to capillary sludging (Hutton, 1979; Rosove et al., 1986), and the red cell indices are low. The presence of iron deficiency in erythrocytotic patients results not only in a reduction in the RBC's oxygen-carrying capacity, but also in the increased viscosity of whole blood. In adults with cyanotic CHD, the usual cause of iron deficiency is the injudicious use of phlebotomy.

TABLE 22–7. **Electrocardiographic Patterns Associated With Congenital Heart Defects**

Cardiac Defect	Atrial Flutter/Fibrillation	Supraventricular Tachycardia	Ventricular Dysrhythmia	Atrioventricular Block	Preexcitation Syndrome	Abnormal P Orientation	Right Atrial Overload	Left Atrial Overload	Left Axis Deviation	Left Bundle Branch Block	Right Bundle Branch Block	Right Ventricular Volume Overload	Right Ventricular Pressure Overload	Left Ventricular Volume Overload	Left Ventricular Pressure Overload	Biventricular Overload	Abnormal Q Waves or Myocardial Infarction Pattern
Atrial septal defect (ostium secundum)	++	+	0	+	0	+	++	+	0	0	+	+++	+	0	0	0	0
Prolapsed mitral valve	+	+	+	0	+	0	0	+	0	0	0	0	0	+	0	0	0
Aortic stenosis	0	0	+	+	0	0	0	+	+	+	0	0	0	0	+++	0	0
Hypertrophic cardiomyopathy	+	0	++	0	+	0	0	++	++	++	0	0	0	0	+++	0	++
Pulmonary stenosis	0	0	0	0	0	0	++	0	0	0	+	+	+++	0	0	0	0
Ventricular septal defect	+	0	0	0	0	0	0	+	+	0	0	0	0	+++	0	+	0
Ductus arteriosus	+	0	0	0	0	0	0	++	+	+	0	0	0	+++	0	+	0
Tetralogy of Fallot	0	0	+	0	0	0	++	0	+	0	+	0	+++	0	0	+	0
Coarctation of aorta	+	0	0	0	0	0	0	+	+	0	0	0	0	0	++	0	0
Eisenmenger syndrome	+	0	+	0	0	0	++	0	0	0	+	0	+++	0	0	+	0
Atrial septal defect (ostium primum)	++	+	0	++	0	0	+	+	+++	0	+	+++	+	+	0	+	0
Corrected transposition*	+	+	0	+++	+	0	+	+	+	0	0	0	0	+	+	+	+++
Ebstein anomaly	++	+++	0	+	++	0	+++	0	+	0	+++	+	0	0	0	0	0
Tricuspid atresia	+	+	+	0	0	0	+++	+	+++	+	0	0	0	+	+	0	+
Coronary artery anomalies	+	0	++	0	0	0	0	++	++	+	0	0	0	+	+	0	+++
Transposition of great arteries (postop)	+	++	0	+	0	0	+	0	0	0	0	0	+++	0	0	0	0

+++, Almost always seen (characteristic of defect)

++, Commonly seen with defect

+, Sometimes seen with defect (especially with associated defects or advancing age)

0, Rarely seen with defect

* The precordial QRS progression in corrected transposition may mimic left ventricular hypertrophy, usually with ST abnormalities. True hypertrophy of the left-sided ventricle can occur in corrected transposition from associated left atrioventricular valvular insufficiency, ventricular septal defect, and so on.

From Sloss, L. J., & Ellison, R. C. (1987). In W. C. Roberts (Ed.), *Adult congenital heart disease* (2nd ed., p. 168). Philadelphia: F. A. Davis.

Severe or recurrent hemoptyses and epistaxes also play an important role.

BLEEDING DIATHESES

Although not clearly understood, patients with cyanotic CHD are at risk for bleeding tendencies characterized by easy bruising, petechial hemorrhages, epistaxis, gingival bleeding, and hemoptysis. Serious and sometimes fatal bleeding can occur with trauma or with surgical procedures. The presence and degree of diathesis seem to be correlated with the degree of erythrocytosis (hematocrit levels > 60%) and the severity of hypoxemia (Territo et al., 1991).

Laboratory studies are directed at monitoring of the erythrocytosis, and include hemoglobin, hematocrit, and mean corpuscular volume (MCV). Because spun hematocrits (microhematocrits) result in plasma trapping and thus falsely elevate hematocrit levels, hematocrits should be done by automated (Coulter)

TABLE 22–8. **Patients at Risk for Infective Endocarditis**

No Risk, Prophylaxis Exempt	Low Risk, Oral Prophylaxis	High Risk,* Injectable
Patent ductus arteriosus (ligated) Repaired ostium secundum atrial septal defect Small ventricular septal defect Trivial pulmonic valve stenosis Repaired ventricular septal defect	Repaired tetralogy of Fallot Tricuspid regurgitation Pulmonic stenosis (moderate to severe) Repaired coarctation of aorta without bicuspid aortic valve Ventricular septal defect, pulmonary hypertension (Eisenmenger syndrome)	Aortic valve stenosis, regurgitation Bicuspid aortic valve Ventricular septal defect Coarctation of aorta Mitral insufficiency Prosthetic valves, conduits Systemic to pulmonary shunts Previous history of endocarditis

* Oral prophylaxis may be used in some high-risk groups (Dajani et al., 1990).

From Canobbio, M. M. (1987). In W. C. Roberts (Ed.), *Adult congenital heart disease* (2nd ed.). Philadelphia: F. A. Davis.

method (Rosove et al., 1986). Iron deficiency is confirmed by MCV or by a low mean corpuscular hemoglobin concentration.

Eisenmenger Syndrome

Eisenmenger syndrome occurs as a result of pulmonary vascular resistence (PVR) greater than 800 dynes/sec/cm^{-5}. It is associated with decreased oxygen saturation in the systemic circulation, cyanosis, and polycythemia (Canobbio, 1984). Originally described as Eisenmenger complex, which referred to a VSD with a reversed or bidirectional shunt (Fig. 22–4), today the term is applied to a number of

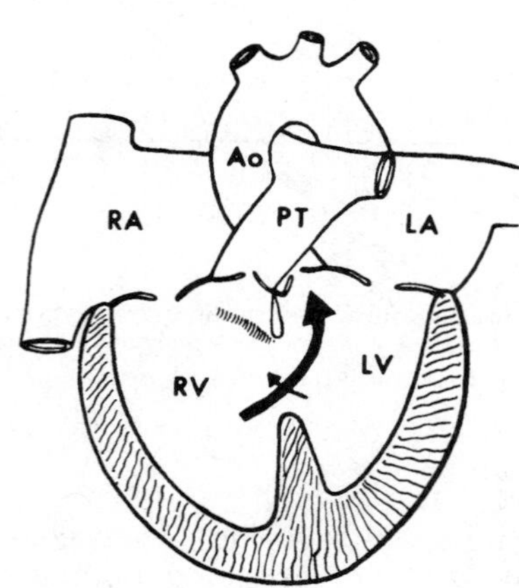

FIGURE 22–4. Schematic illustration of a large ventricular septal defect with high pulmonary vascular resistance and reversed shunt. (Courtesy of J. K. Perloff, M. D., Division of Cardiology, UCLA Medical Center, Los Angeles, Calif. From Canobbio, M. M. [1984]. Eisenmenger syndrome. *Nursing Clinics of North America 19,* 537–545.)

TABLE 22–9. **Physical Findings Common in Patients With Eisenmenger Syndrome**

Central cyanosis
Digital clubbing
Normal jugular venous pressure
Normal arterial pulse volume
Right ventricular thrust
Increased pulmonary closure with variable splitting of S_2
Pulmonary ejection click
Pulmonary ejection murmur
Systolic murmur at the lower sternal border

From Canobbio, M. M. (1984). *Nursing Clinics of North America, 19,* 537–545.

shunting defects occurring at the aorticopulmonary, ventricular, or atrial level. These defects are hemodynamically similar in that they characteristically involve persistent increased pulmonary blood flow that over time will produce pulmonary vascular disease of such severity that a bidirectional or right to left shunt occurs. Eisenmenger syndrome generally develops as a consequence of delayed operation or of failure to detect the lesion until adolescence or adulthood, when surgical repair is of little use. Heart and lung transplantation is the only surgical alternative.

Clinically, the most common complaint is effort intolerance probably related to decreased arterial oxygen saturation and, in the later stages, to ventricular dysfunction. Significant clubbing and polycythemia are usually present. Other clinical findings are summarized in Table 22–9. Medical management is directed by the clinical presentation. Polycythemia, a constant feature of cyanotic CHD, occurs as a compensatory mechanism that maintains adequate oxygen supply to the tissues.

Particular attention must be paid to the use of drugs that lower systemic vascular resistance (SVR). Unloading agents such as nitroglycerin are potentially harmful because they can lead to a sudden drop in SVR, reduced stroke volume, and an increase in the right to left shunt, which leads to further increases in cyanosis and tissue hypoxia.

In the natural course of this disorder the patient becomes increasingly symptomatic after age 30. However, many patients do survive and are able to live reasonably active lives throughout the third, fourth, and fifth decades. Sudden death, presumably from dysrhythmias, is the usual cause of death. Other causes of death include myocardial failure, pulmonary infarction from arterial thrombosis, and complications of cerebral abscesses and cerebrovascular accidents, although the latter are not seen as frequently in older patients (Rosove et al., 1986).

Heart Failure

As in most cases of cardiac failure, heart failure in the adult with CHD occurs as a result of excessive workload imposed on the cardiac muscle, usually by structural defects, or by basic changes in myocardial performance. Excessive workload can occur as a result of volume overload created by a large left to right shunt or by defects that lead to valvular insufficiency. Increased workload also may result from pressure overload of the ventricles, as in lesions causing obstruction to outflow, such as aortic or pulmonic stenosis or coarctation of the aorta. Pressure overload also may occur in lesions causing an obstruction to inflow, such as cor triatriatum or stenosis of the mitral or triscuspid valves (Talner, 1983).

Myocardial performance may be impaired either by changes in the chronotropic state of the heart, as observed with the tachydysrhythmias that can arise as a result of a primary defect, or as a consequence of surgical intervention.

The onset of symptoms of cardiac failure in the adult with CHD is not predictable. Therefore, it is important to continue follow-up on patients who have residual effects, such as volume overload of a ventricle due to patch leak requiring reoperation, if the negative effects of excessive volume and pressure overload are to be avoided.

COLLABORATIVE MANAGEMENT

Although most patients have had surgery in infancy or childhood, there are some who require primary surgical repair as adults. In others, reoperation may be necessary because of a complication or because symptoms are appearing once again. For example, patients who have undergone aortic valvulotomy may again present with clinical signs of severe aortic stenosis. The decision to operate will depend on several factors, beginning with an accurate diagnostic evaluation of the primary defect and its morphology. In addition, careful study of the hemodynamic consequences of many of these disorders is essential. A major concern is the presence of increased pulmonary hypertension, which increases the risk of operation, thereby making it prohibitive. Similarly, evaluation of ventricular function by two-dimensional, Doppler, or color flow echocardiography as well as by angiography offers a basis for determining the feasibility of surgical intervention.

For the patient in whom surgical intervention is not an option, medical therapy is generally directed by the clinical presentation. A brief overview of the most commonly occurring problems observed in this population is presented in this section. For detailed descriptions of therapeutic interventions for the previously described complications of dysrhythmias, heart failure, or endocarditis, the reader is referred to other chapters in this text.

Medical treatment of atrial tachydysrhythmias generally consists of pharmacologic agents or electrical cardioversion to control ventricular response. Symptomatic ventricular dysrhythmias require careful monitoring with or without electrophysiologic testing to determine appropriate use of antidysrhythmic agents to suppress the dysrhythmias (Sloss & Ellison, 1987).

The treatment of cardiac failure begins with digitalization, diuretics, and restriction of sodium. However, as left ventricular dysfunction progresses, it frequently becomes necessary to initiate vasodilator therapy to unload the left ventricle by reducing peripheral vascular resistance or promoting systemic venous pooling.

Clinical management of the adult with cyanotic CHD presents a unique challenge to the critical care practitioner. As mentioned earlier, cyanotic patients, who have increasing erythrocytosis, are bothered by a variety of complaints, including headaches, muscle and joint pain, fatigue, dizziness, and hemoptysis. Isovolumetric phlebotomy for excessive erythrocytosis has been shown to be an effective method of reducing RBC volume (Perloff et al., 1988). Indications for phlebotomy are based on the presence of moderate to severe clinical symptoms of hyperviscosity in conjunction with hematocrits greater than 65%. It must, however, be pointed out that an elevated hematocrit alone is not an appropriate criterion for phlebotomy. Rosove and colleagues (1986) have reported that symptoms of hyperviscosity rarely occur in patients with hematocrits less than 65% unless iron deficiency is present and that reported hematocrits of 69% and 70% have been well tolerated without risk of cerebrovascular events. Measures must also be taken to avoid dehydration. For example, fever, vomiting, and diarrhea may precipitate plasma volume reduction and a rise in hematocrit. Fluid replacement is the treatment of choice. Pharmacologic measures must be managed carefully because indiscriminate use of certain agents can lead to serious complications. For example, diuretics can contribute to hemoconcentration. Drugs such as vasodilating agents, calcium channel blockers, beta blockers, and ACE inhibitors need to be managed closely because they can lower SVR and increase the right to left shunt, which leads to increased cyanosis and tissue hypoxia. In the critical care setting, continuous pulse oximetry is useful in detecting moment-to-moment changes in arterial oxygen saturation. For example, if a patient with Eisenmenger syndrome experiences a sudden drop in oxygen saturation from 85% to 75%, this may be attributed to a drop in blood pressure and pressure of the right to left shunt. Treatment is directed at modifying the shunt by increasing the SVR (Miner & Canobbio, 1994). Finally, because of the right to left shunting present in most of these patients, care must be taken to reduce the risk of air or clot embolization from the venous circulation across a defect into a cerebral or coronary artery. To minimize risk it is advised to use a standard 0.22-μm air / particle filter on all intravenous lines and to avoid using central lines. Special attention must be given to the prevention of venous stasis complications in the bedridden patient. Use of antiembolic support stockings is recommended (Miner & Canobbio, 1994).

If nurses are to carry out collaborative and independent nursing actions in the management of the patient with CHD, they must first understand the basic anatomic defect and be aware of and alert to the potential acute complications associated with the defect, the residual effects of surgical interventions, and any unrepaired defects. For example, failure to recognize the presence of a bicuspid aortic valve increases the risk of the patient developing endocarditis or aortic insufficiency. Similarly, if the nursing staff fails to understand that systemic hypertension may be a long-term postoperative residual finding associated with coarctation of the aorta, this sign may often remain unrecognized. As a consequence, these patients may develop signs and symptoms of heart failure or coronary artery disease (Maron et al., 1973).

Nurses also play an important role in furthering efforts at secondary prevention that must be stressed to patient and family. Nurses must be prepared independently to assess and determine the supportive and health education needs of each patient that will allow him or her to effectively assume responsibility for self-care.

Although each congenital heart defect has its own list of actual and potential nursing problems, the primary problems observed in the critical care unit arise from the complications of dysrhythmias, cardiac failure, excessive erythrocytosis, or endocarditis or from the Eisenmenger syndrome. In addition, many of these patients lack a clear understanding of their clinical problem and need for follow-up care. Frequently, adolescents and adults with CHD are found to be misinformed about their defect and about appropriate activity allowances and limitations. As a result, they may be either limiting their activity inappropriately or engaging in strenuous isometric types of activities. For example, patients with a residual postoperative gradient, such as those with aortic stenosis or coarctation of the aorta, may be engaging in activities that require heavy lifting or participating in competitive sports. Emotionally, the level of individual adjustment may vary greatly. In the adult, the psychological consequences of having CHD may reflect several factors. Among these are the complexity of the primary defect, the surgical repair performed, the age at which repair was undertaken, and the physical restrictions imposed on the individual throughout childhood. The emotional and behavioral reactions of the family also play an important role in the ability of the patient to accept and deal with the consequences of CHD.

SUMMARY

The foregoing discussion has focused on specific issues that influence the long-term survival of adults with CHD. Although the majority of patients do well, there is an increasing awareness that many patients will develop late residual effects from an earlier surgical experience. Consequently, the critical care nurse must be able not only to recognize the most commonly occurring problems, but also have an understanding of their etiology to provide appropriate care and management.

REFERENCES

Baer, P., Freedman, D. A., & Garson, A. (1984). Long-term psychological follow-up of patients after corrective surgery for tetralogy of Fallot. *Journal of American Academy of Child Psychiatry, 23,* 622–625.

Bharati, S., & Levi, M. (1983). The myocardium, the conduction system and general sequelae after surgery for congenital heart. In M. A. Engle & J. K. Perloff (Eds.), *Congenital heart disease after surgery.* New York: Yorke Medical Books.

Borow, K. M., & Braunwald, E. (1992). Congenital heart disease in the adult. In E. Braunwald (Ed.), *Heart disease: A textbook of cardiovascular medicine* (4th ed.). Philadelphia: W. B. Saunders.

Canobbio, M. M. (1984). The Eisenmenger syndrome. *Nursing Clinics of North America, 19,* 537–554.

Canobbio, M. M. (1987). Counseling the adult with congenital heart disease. In W. C. Roberts (Ed.), *Adult congenital heart disease* (2nd ed.) Philadelphia: F. A. Davis.

Cooley, D. A. (1988). Palliative surgery for cyanotic congenital heart disease. *Surgical Clinics of North America, 68,* 474–477.

Dajani, A. S., Bisno, A. L., Chung, K. J., et al. (1990). Prevention of bacterial endocarditis: Recommendations by the American Heart Association. *Journal of the American Medical Association, 264,* 2919–2922.

Danielson, G. K., & McGoon, D. (1987). Surgical therapy and results. In W. C. Roberts (Ed.), *Adult congenital heart disease* (2nd ed.). Philadelphia: F. A. Davis.

DeLeval, M. R., Kilner, P., Gerwillig, M. (1988). Total cavopulmonary connection: A logical alternative to atrial pulmonary connection for complex Fontan operations. *Journal of Thoracic and Cardiovascular Surgery, 96,* 682–688.

Ebert, P. A., Turley, K., Stanger, P., et al. (1984). Surgical treatment of truncus arteriosus in the first 6 months of life. *Annals of Surgery, 200,* 451–454.

Ferguson, T. R., Suping, H., Bland, G., et al. (1986). Four adults with Ebstein's anomaly. *Illinois Medical Journal, 170,* 137–140.

Fontan, F., & Baudet, E. (1971). Surgical repair of tricuspid atresia. *Thorax, 26,* 241–248.

Fontan, F., Kirklin, J. W., Fernandez, G., et al. (1990). Outcome after a "perfect" Fontan operation. *Circulation, 81,* 1520–1536.

Friedman, W. F. (1992). Congenital heart disease in infancy and childhood. In E. Braunwald (Ed.), *Heart disease: A textbook of cardiovascular medicine* (4th ed.). Philadelphia: W. B. Saunders.

Fuster, V., McGoon, D. C., Kennedy, M. A., et al. (1980). Longterm evaluation (12–20 years) of open heart surgery for tetralology of Fallot. *American Journal of Cardiology, 80,* 635–642.

Glasner, D., & Bentovim, A. (1987). Psychological aspects of congenital heart disease. In R. H. Anderson, Macartney, F. J., Shinbone, E., et al. (Eds.), *Paediatric cardiology* (pp. 1373–1383). London: Churchill-Livingstone.

Goldstein, J. L., & Brown, M. S. (1992). Genetics and cardiovascular disease. In E. Braunwald (Ed.), *Heart disease: A textbook of cardiovascular medicine* (4th ed.). Philadelphia: W. B. Saunders.

Henson, D. E., Najafi, R., Callaghan, R., et al. (1969). Myocardial lesions following open-heart surgery. *Archives of Pathology, 88,* 423–430.

Higgins, S. S., & Reed, A. (1994). Common congenital heart defects: Long term follow-up. *Nursing Clinics of North America, 29,* 233–245.

Humes, R. A., Mair, D. D., Poster, C. B., et al. (1988). Results of the modified Fontan operation in adults. *American Journal of Cardiology, 61,* 602–604.

Hutton, R. D. (1979). The effect of iron deficiency on whole blood viscosity for polycythemic patients. *British Journal of Hematology, 43,* 191–199.

Kirklin, J. W., Blackstone, E. H., Dirkin, J. K., et al. (1983). Surgical results and protocols in the spectrum of tetralogy of Fallot. *Annals of Surgery, 198,* 251–265.

Kirklin, J. B., Blackstone, E. H., Kirklin, J. W., et al. (1986). The Fontan operation: Ventricular hypertrophy, age, and date of operation as risk factors. *Journal of Thoracic and Cardiovascular Surgery, 92,* 1049–1064.

Kopf, G. S. (1993). Tricuspid atresia. In C. Mauroudis & C. Backer (Eds.), *Pediatric cardiac surgery* (2nd ed., pp. 379–400). St. Louis: Mosby-Yearbook.

Laks, H., Hellenbrand, W. E., Stansel, H. C., et al. (1980). Repair of complex congenital cardiac defects with the valved conduits. *Surgical Clinics of North America, 60,* 1225–1237.

Mair, D. D., Hagler, D. J., Puga, F. J., et al. (1990). Fontan operation in 176 patients with tricuspid atresia: Results and a proposed new index for patient selection. *Circulation, 82*(Suppl IV), 164–169.

Mair, D. D., Rice, M. J., Hagler, D. J., et al. (1985). Outcome of the Fontan procedure in patients with tricuspid atresia. *Circulation, 72,* Suppl. II, 88–92.

Maron, B. J., Humphries, H. O., Rowe, R. D., et al. (1973). Prognosis of surgically corrected coarctation of the aorta. A 20-year post-operative appraisal. *Circulation, 47,* 19.

McNamara, D. G. (1989). The adult with congenital heart disease. In R. O'Rourke (Ed.), *Current problems in cardiology.* Chicago: Yearbook Medical.

McNamara, D. G., & Latson, L. A. (1982). Long-term follow-up of patients with malformations for which definitive surgical repair has been available for 25 years or more. *American Journal of Cardiology, 50,* 560.

Miner, P. D., & Canobbio, M. C. (1994). Care of the adult with cyanotic congenital heart disease. *Nursing Clinics of North America, 29,* 249–267.

Morgan, B. C. (1978). Incidence, etiology, and classification of congenital heart disease. *Pediatric Clinics of North America, 26,* 700–721.

Nora, J. J., & Nora, A. H. (1978). The evolution of specific genetic and environmental counseling in congenital heart disease. *Circulation, 57,* 205–213.

O'Fallon, W. M., & Weidman, W. H. (1993). Report from the Second Joint Study on the Natural History of Congenital Heart Defects. *Circulation, 87*(Suppl II).

Pacifico, A. D., & Sand, M. E. (1987). Advances in the surgical management of congenital heart disease in infants and children. In D. C. McGoon (Ed.), *Cardiac surgery* (2nd ed., pp. 177–219). Philadelphia: F. A. Davis.

Perloff, J. K. (1987). *The clinical recognition of congenital heart disease* (3rd ed.). Philadelphia: W. B. Saunders.

Perloff, J. K. (1991). Congenital heart disease in adults: A new cardiovascular subspeciality. *Circulation, 84,* 1881–1890.

Perloff, J. K., Rosove, M. H., Child, J. S., et al. (1988). Adults with congenital heart disease: Hematologic management. *Annals of Internal Medicine, 5,* 406–413.

Roberts, W. C. (1970). The congenitally abnormal bicuspid aortic valve—a study of 85 autopsy cases. *American Journal of Cardiology, 26,* 72.

Rosenthal, A., Button, L., Nathan, D. G., et al. (1971). Blood volume changes in cyanotic congenital heart disease. *American Journal of Cardiology, 27,* 162–167.

Rosove, M. H., Perloff, J. K., Hocking, W. G., et al. (1986). Chronic hypoxemia and decompensated erythrocytosis in cyanotic congenital heart disease. *Lancet, 2,* 313–315.

Rudolph, A. M., Nadas, A. S., & Borges, W. H. (1953). Hematologic adjustment to cyanotic congenital heart disease. *Pediatrics, 11,* 454–464.

Schaff, H. V., & Danielson, G. K. (1987). Advances in surgical management of congenital heart disease in adults. In D. C. McGoon (Ed.), *Cardiac Surgery* (2nd ed., pp. 221–238). Philadelphia: F. A. Davis.

Seliem, M., Muster, A. J., Paul, M. H., et al. (1989). Relationship between preoperative left ventricular muscle mass and outcome of the Fontan procedure in patients with tricuspid atresia. *Journal of the American College of Cardiology, 14,* 750–756.

Sloss, L. J., & Ellison, R. C. (1987). Electrocardiographic features. In W. C. Roberts (Ed.), *Adult congenital heart disease* (2nd ed., pp. 167–189). Philadelphia: F. A. Davis.

Talner, N. S. (1983). Heart failure. In F. H. Adams & G. C. Emmanouilides (Eds.), *Heart disease in infants, children and adolescents.* Baltimore: Williams & Wilkins.

Territo, M. C., Rosove, M., & Perloff, J. K. (1991). Cyanotic congenital heart disease: Hematologic management and urate metabolism. In J. K. Perloff & J. K. Child (Eds.), *Congenital heart disease in adults.* Philadelphia: W. B. Saunders.

von Bermuth, G., Ritter, D. G., Frye, R. L., et al. (1971). Evaluation of patients with tetralogy of Fallot and Potts anastomosis. *American Journal of Cardiology, 27,* 259–263.

Walsh, E. P., Rickenmaker, S., Keane, J. F., et al. (1988). Late results in patients with tetralogy of Fallot repair in infancy. *Circulation, 77,* 1062–1068.

Wood, P. (1958). The Eisenmenger syndrome. *British Heart Journal, 2,* 701.

Young, D., & Marks, H. (1971). Fate of the patient with Eisenmenger syndrome. *American Journal of Cardiology, 28,* 658–669.

Zaho, H., Miller, D. C., Reitz, B. A., et al. (1985). Surgical repair of tetralogy of Fallot: Long term follow-up with particular emphasis on late death and reoperation. *Journal of Thoracic and Cardiovascular Surgery, 89,* 204–210.

Zuberbuhler, J. R. (1983). Symposium on results of the Mustard operation for complete transposition of the great arteries. *American Journal of Cardiology, 51,* 1513–1535.

CHAPTER

23 Patients With Valvular Disease

Linda H. Schakenbach

PATHOPHYSIOLOGY: OVERVIEW

The heart moves blood throughout the body via the vascular system. Within the heart, unidirectional blood flow is maintained by valves. Diseases affecting or damaging the cardiac valves impair the heart's ability to maintain an effective cardiac output.

The atrioventricular (AV) valves are located between the atria and the ventricles. The valve on the right side of the heart has three leaflets and is called the tricuspid valve. The valve on the left side of the heart has two leaflets and is called the mitral valve. Both AV valves are complex structures of leaflets with tendinous filaments at the inferior free edges. The other end of these filaments, the chordae tendineae, are attached to the papillary muscles. The papillary muscles arise from the ventricular wall. When pressure in the atrium exceeds ventricular pressure, the AV valve opens and blood flows from the atrium to the ventricle. When pressure in the ventricle exceeds pressure in the atrium, the AV valve closes and blood cannot flow back into the atrium.

A second set of valves, the semilunar valves, are located in the ventricular outflow tracts. The valve between the right ventricle and the pulmonary artery is the pulmonic valve. The valve between the left ventricle and the aorta is the aortic valve. Both semilunar valves have three leaflets called cusps. The semilunar valves do not have chordae tendineae or papillary muscles. The pulmonic and aortic valves also open and close in response to pressure changes. When ventricular pressure exceeds arterial pressure, the valve opens and blood flows from the ventricle to the artery. When arterial pressure is higher than ventricular pressure, the semilunar valve closes and blood cannot flow back into the ventricle.

The pathophysiologic consequence of valvular lesions is loss of unidirectional blood flow. The disorders are categorized into two functional types, regurgitation and stenosis. Regurgitation, also called insufficiency, is blood flowing backward across the valve. Effective forward blood flow may eventually diminish while blood volumes and pressures behind the valve increase. Stenosis is a narrowing of the valve and impedance of forward blood flow. Effective forward blood flow requires greater pressure to open the valve and move the blood volume. Eventually, forward blood flow decreases, and blood volume and pressures behind the valve increase.

Regurgitation and stenosis are not mutually exclusive or limited to a single valve. A valve may not close completely and may also have a narrowed annulus. Regurgitation and stenosis have been reported in all four cardiac valves. Aortic stenosis may cause or be associated with mitral regurgitation or stenosis. Aortic and mitral stenosis are associated with tricuspid stenosis or regurgitation. Aortic regurgitation may precipitate mitral regurgitation. Mitral stenosis or regurgitation may cause or be associated with tricuspid regurgitation. Mitral stenosis has been associated with tricuspid stenosis. Pulmonic stenosis may cause or be associated with tricuspid regurgitation or stenosis. Pulmonic regurgitation may precipitate tricuspid stenosis.

The most characteristic feature of each disease process is the murmur. Murmurs are the result of turbulent blood flow. Turbulence may result from blood flowing in an abnormal direction, such as regurgitation. Blood flow turbulence is also created by abnormal or narrowed blood flow tracts, such as vegetations, calcifications or tears of leaflets, thickened or fused chordae tendineae, and constricted valve orifices. Additionally, turbulence may result from thickened or stiffened leaflets that are unable to open or close completely. The leaflets may create even more turbulence by vibrating.

Historically, rheumatic endocarditis has been the primary etiology of valvular heart disease. The incidence had decreased with better public and medical community awareness and antibiotic therapies. However, in the 1980s a strain of group A streptococci again increased the incidence of rheumatic fever (Markowitz & Kaplan, 1989). Infective endocarditis, myxomatous changes, coronary artery disease (CAD), hypertension, and congenital disorders are some of the other etiologies of cardiac valvular disorders.

Treatment is being prescribed earlier in the course of the lesions. Better, more specific, and frequent monitoring techniques are being used for individuals at risk and for those with murmurs. Surgical interventions are being refined and advances made with prostheses. This chapter will review the specific characteristics of regurgitation and stenosis of each cardiac valve.

MITRAL REGURGITATION

Pathophysiology

Structurally, the mitral valve is the most complex heart valve. The four major components are the leaflets, the annulus, the chordae tendineae, and the papillary muscles. Mitral regurgitation results from a malfunction of one or more of the valve's components and may be either acute or chronic. Barlow (1987) and Braunwald (1992) have summarized the malfunctions of the mitral valve's components. Disorders involving the leaflets are common.

Mitral regurgitation in the United States is most often the result of myxomatous changes in the leaflets. The central layer of the leaflet, the spongiosa, has an overabundance of myxomatous cells. The myxomatous cells spread into the supporting layer of the leaflet, the fibrosa, interfering with the continuity of the layer. The weakened valve thins and stretches, resulting in interchordal hooding and prolapse. Other names for this are "floppy valve," "billowing valve," and "mid-" or "mid-late systolic click" syndromes. As the myxomatous changes progress, the surfaces of the leaflets that make contact with each other fibrose and thicken. Collagenous fibrous tissue develops on the ventricular side of the leaflet in the areas of hooding, thickening the leaflet. Fusion of the commissures and calcification are rare. Regurgitation typically results from severe prolapse causing incompetence of the valve. Myxomatous changes have been identified in the genetic lines of families with both connective tissue disorders, such as Marfan syndrome, and those without connective tissue disorders.

Acute rheumatic endocarditis often results in transient mitral regurgitation. Of more importance is rheumatic myocarditis that leads to chronic mitral regurgitation (Fig. 23–1). In this disease, one or both of the mitral valve leaflets fibrose and shorten as a result of recurrent inflammation. As a leaflet shortens, it becomes incapable of approximation with the other. The shortened leaflet may also calcify, further impairing its movement for valve closure. Rheumatic endocarditis is also known to fuse either the anterolateral or posteromedial commissure and may rarely fuse both. The fusion is unique in that rather than causing stenosis, the fusion prevents complete closure of the leaflets. Rheumatic endocarditis is no longer the leading cause of mitral regurgitation in the United States (Schlant & Alexander, 1994).

Infective endocarditis, usually bacterial but also viral or fungal in origin, erodes, perforates, clefts, or scars the leaflets. Vegetations resulting from infective endocarditis may prevent leaflet approximation acutely or may become fibrous adhesions between the inferior side of the posterior leaflet and the wall of the left ventricle during healing.

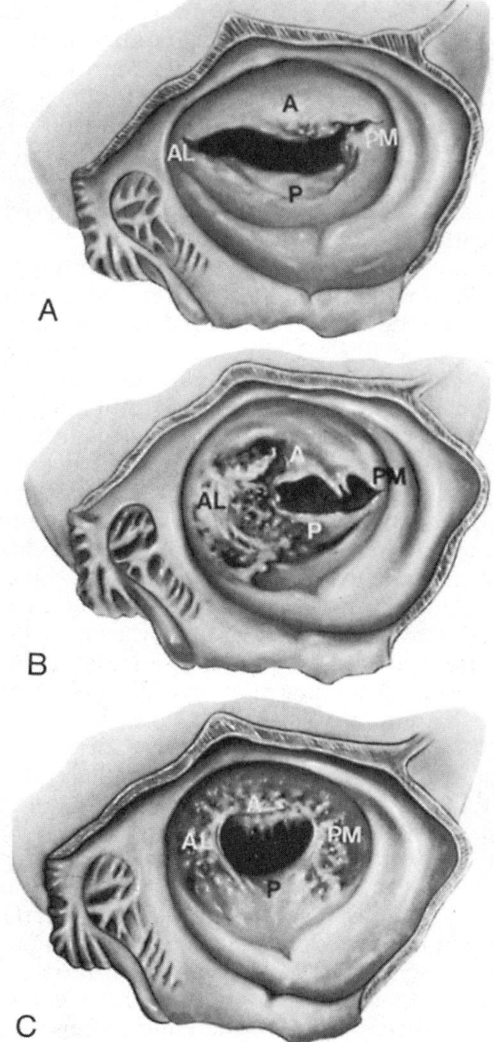

FIGURE 23–1. Anatomic types of rheumatic mitral regurgitation. Each unopened mitral valve viewed from above. In each, A = anterior, P = posterior leaflet of the mitral valve, respectively; AL, PM = anterolateral and posteromedial commissures of the mitral valve. *A,* Intrinsically short leaflets. Commissures essentially unaffected. *B,* Calcification and fusion of anterolateral commissure giving rise to the teardrop type of mitral regurgitation. *C,* Calcification of the leaflets and commissures in continuity, yielding a wedding ring type of mitral regurgitation. Some restriction of the orifice is present, but regurgitation is prominent. (Adapted from Edwards, J. E. [1983]. Pathology of mitral incompetence. In Silver, M. D. [Ed.], *Cardiovascular pathophysiology,* Vol. 1. New York: Churchill Livingstone. By permission.)

The mitral valve leaflets may produce regurgitation by a variety of rarer causes. The posterior leaflet may adhere to the left ventricular wall as a sequela of the hypereosinophilic syndrome (also known as Loeffler syndrome, disseminated eosinophilic collagen disease, and eosinophilic leukemia). The syndrome begins with a myocarditis that progresses through stages of mural thrombosis and fibrosis, the development of collagen fibers, and finally, endocardial thickening and connective tissue development. The inferior aspect of the posterior leaflet is often incorporated in the mural thrombi of the left ventricular endocardium. As the process continues, the leaflet is held to the ventricular wall, rendering it immobile. Hurler syndrome is similar; large balloon cells enter the normal leaflet tissue, thickening and shortening the leaflet. The leaflet becomes less mobile and cannot approximate with the other leaflet of the mitral valve.

Lupus erythematosus also causes mitral regurgitation by immobilizing the posterior mitral leaflet. Vegetations from the inferior surface of the posterior mitral leaflet become fibrous tethers to the left ventricular wall. Left atrial enlargement pulls the posterior mitral leaflet backward and downward until the leaflet is drawn taut across the left ventricular wall. Asymmetric septal hypertrophy, also known as idiopathic hypertrophic subaortic stenosis (IHSS), may result in such high ventricular pressure during systole that the anterior leaflet moves away from the posterior leaflet.

Disorders of the mitral valve annulus also cause mitral regurgitation. Conditions such as cardiomyopathies, left ventricular failure, Marfan syndrome, and Hurler syndrome eventually cause left ventricular dilation. The ventricular dilation pulls the mitral valve annulus wider, and eventually the leaflets cannot cover the broader area, causing regurgitation. The annulus may also calcify. Calcification is known to be idiopathic and may be accelerated by systemic hypertension, aortic stenosis, diabetes, Marfan syndrome, Hurler syndrome, and asymmetric septal hypertrophy. The typical mechanism of regurgitation in calcification is a leaflet, usually the posterior leaflet, that becomes immobilized in the calcification or against the ventricular wall. Atypically, the calcification prevents constriction of the annulus with ventricular systole. Rheumatic disease may thicken and stiffen the annulus, also resulting in immobilization of the annulus. The mitral leaflets are not able to approximate across the orifice.

Disorders of the complex chordae tendineae network cause mitral regurgitation. The myxomatous process discussed previously in regard to leaflet disorders also affects the chordae. In the acute stages, the chordae may weaken and occasionally elongate. As the fibrous changes occur, the chordae may rub on the left ventricular wall, causing fibrous deposits to develop on the endocardium. Eventually, the fibrous deposits can fuse with the chordae. The chordae anchored in the deposits may impair leaflet closure or rupture. If fibrous deposits do not adhere with the chordae, the weakened chordae may rupture from normal strain. Ruptured chordae also occur secondary to rheumatic or bacterial endocarditis and left ventricular dilation. Rupture of the chordae may be caused by friction with the septum in asymmetric septal hypertrophy or secondary to hypoxia from CAD or myocardial infarction (MI). There are also instances of chordae rupture for which the cause is not known. Abnormally elongated or shortened chordae may be caused by prolapsed leaflets, connective tissue disorders such as Marfan syndrome, and unidentified etiologies. Chordae elongation also occurs as the left ventricle dilates, pulling the papillary muscles down and exerting tension on the chordae. Chordae shortening prevents leaflet closure. Chordae elongation and rupture permit the leaflets to move toward the atrium during systole. All three chordae abnormalities may result in mitral regurgitation.

Papillary muscle disorders can cause mitral valve regurgitation. The most common cause of papillary muscle dysfunction is MI. A papillary muscle may become dysfunctional or rupture as a complication of an acute MI. When this complication occurs, the posterior medial papillary muscle is usually involved with inferior or inferolateral MIs and the anterolateral muscle with lateral or anterolateral MIs. Usually rupture of only some of the papillary muscle heads occurs, not the entire muscle. The papillary muscle may not become dysfunctional or rupture as an immediate consequence of MI, but may be pulled out of position as the involved ventricular wall necroses and scars. Myocardial ischemia may impair papillary muscle contraction. Trauma involving the lateral wall or septum of the heart may rupture a papillary muscle.

Mitral regurgitation may also occur in individuals with prosthetic valves. The leaflets, disc, or ball-and-strut components may fail. Tissue valves may experience changes of the annulus as described with native valves. Any of the prostheses may develop regurgitation at the sewing ring when sutures or tissue fail.

Any cause of mitral regurgitation results in bidirectional blood flow. During diastole, blood flows from the left atrium into the left ventricle. During systole, blood flows back from the left ventricle into the left atrium. The pathophysiology depends on how quickly the mitral regurgitation develops. Most commonly, mitral regurgitation develops gradually over a period of time. It is known as chronic mitral regurgitation (Fig. 23–2). Some volume of blood flows retrograde from the left ventricle into the left atrium during isovolumetric contraction or ventricular ejection. Depending on the size of the regurgitation orifice and the ventricular pressures, up to 50% of ventricular volume may enter the atrium during isovolumetric contraction, and more could flow in during ventricular ejection.

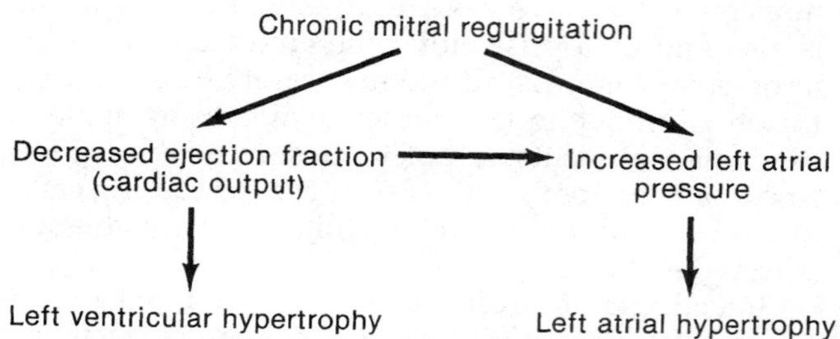

FIGURE 23–2. Pathophysiology of chronic mitral regurgitation. (Adapted from Schakenbach, L. H., Physiologic dynamics of acquired valvular heart disease, *Journal of Cardiovascular Nursing, 1*(3), 1–17, with permission of Aspen Publishers, Inc., © 1987.)

Left atrial pressures rise, leading to left atrial hypertrophy and eventually dilation. As the left atrium dilates, it is displaced caudally and posteriorly. The posterior mitral valve leaflet is then stretched across its annulus, shortening the leaflet and compounding the regurgitation process.

The left ventricle also dilates to accommodate the large diastolic blood volume. It hypertrophies in an attempt to maintain systolic pressures and effective stroke volumes through the aortic valve. In chronic mitral regurgitation, the left ventricular mass to volume ratio (preload) is normal. The wall tension (afterload) is often decreased because regurgitation decreases systolic pressure and systolic ventricular radius (Laplace's law). The myofibril energy is therefore able to be expended as increased velocity of contraction, maintaining cardiac output without increasing heart rate or myocardial oxygen consumption. As the left ventricle dilates, however, papillary muscles and chordae tendineae may become stretched or displaced, worsening the regurgitation.

The dilation of both the left atrium and the left ventricle minimizes pulmonary and right heart symptoms. Eventually, the dilation causes atrial and ventricular dysrhythmias, most commonly atrial fibrillation. As the mitral regurgitation and chamber dilations progress, less blood volume displacement or movement occurs. Stagnated blood leads to thrombus formation, especially common in the left atrium, and the potential for emboli. Progression of left ventricular dilation is evidenced as left ventricular failure.

Mitral regurgitation may also be acute, and the pathophysiology of this condition is quite different from that of chronic mitral regurgitation (Fig. 23–3). The amount of regurgitation, atrial compliance, and ventricular function determine the severity. The atrium and ventricle do not have time to dilate or hypertrophy to compensate for the regurgitation. Blood flows back into the pulmonary and right heart systems. Systemic cardiac output decreases, resulting in increased heart rate and increased systemic vascular resistance. Acute mitral regurgitation may be mild to severe. Mild acute regurgitation may become chronic as the atrium and ventricle begin to dilate and the pathophysiologic events change. Severe acute regurgitation is an emergency situation presenting with acute pulmonary edema of left ventricular failure.

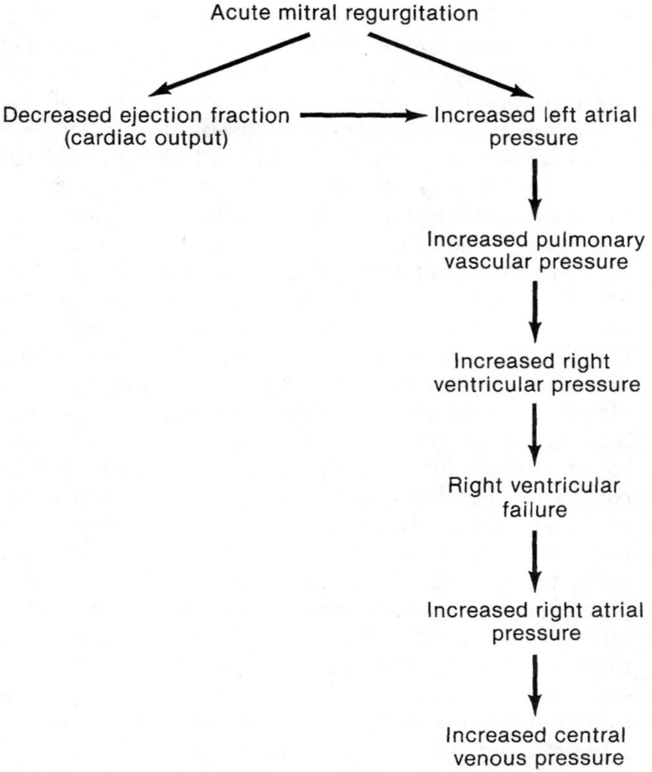

FIGURE 23–3. Pathophysiology of acute mitral regurgitation. (Adapted from Schakenbach, L. H., Physiologic dynamics of acquired valvular heart disease, *Journal of Cardiovascular Nursing, 1*(3), 1–17, with permission of Aspen Publishers, Inc., © 1987.)

Physical Assessment

The signs and symptoms of mitral regurgitation correspond with the pathophysiology. Chronic mitral regurgitation is often asymptomatic, but signs of the disease are usually found on examination. Acute mitral regurgitation is often very symptomatic, and signs supporting the diagnosis are also found on examination.

The presenting symptoms of chronic mitral regurgitation are often those of left ventricular failure—fatigue, weakness, and dyspnea. Other symptoms are palpitations related to dysrhythmias, orthopnea and paroxysmal nocturnal dyspnea related to left ventricular failure, as well as atypical chest pains and dysphagia related to the hypertrophied atrium. Ultimately, right heart failure will result in distended jugular veins, peripheral edema, hepatomegaly, and ascites. Occasionally, the presenting symptom is an embolic phenomenon.

Physical examination may reveal a point of maximal impulse that is brisk, hyperdynamic, and displaced caudally and laterally, related to the left ventricular hypertrophy. The atrial hypertrophy may be evidenced by an impulse in the third intercostal space at the left sternal border during systole. (Atrial contractions are usually weak or absent due to atrial fibrillation; the impulse is the jet of regurgitating blood from the left ventricle.) A brisk upstroke may be palpated in the pulse, and the heart rate may be increased or irregular. The blood pressure and pulse pressures are normal until left ventricular failure occurs.

Auscultation at the point of maximal impulse most often reveals a blowing, high-pitched holosystolic murmur. The murmur may radiate into the left axilla or infrascapular areas. When the posterior leaflet is regurgitant, the murmur may radiate up into the aortic valve auscultation area, the base of the neck, or the spine. The murmur may also be late systolic or may be absent. It is the only murmur that does not change intensity with changes in stroke volume. The grade of the murmur does not correlate with the severity of the regurgitation. The first heart sound may be soft because the mitral component is soft or absent. The second heart sound may be widely split because of the shortened left ventricular ejection time. The dilated left ventricle and large atrial blood volume may result in a third heart sound.

Hemodynamic monitoring often demonstrates left atrial pressures below 20 mm Hg with large *v* waves and steep *y* descents. Left ventricular stroke volumes are high, usually maintaining a normal cardiac output although some of the stroke volume returns to the left atrium. Cardiac output may also be slightly low. Systemic vascular resistance may be normal or elevated to compensate for a decreased cardiac output. Electrocardiographic (ECG) monitoring often demonstrates atrial fibrillation but may also show normal sinus rhythm with premature atrial contractions (PACs), atrial tachycardia, or atrial flutter. The P wave may widen and notch with atrial hypertrophy. Controlled atrial fibrillation is well tolerated if the ventricle is not dependent on the atrial kick. Some ECGs also demonstrate the increased amplitude or wide QRS, ST segment depression, and inverted or wide T wave characteristic of left ventricular hypertrophy (Dubin, 1989; Frankl & Brest, 1993; Marriott, 1993; Schamroth, 1989).

The presenting symptom of acute mitral regurgitation is often pulmonary edema. Other symptoms are severe dyspnea, distended jugular veins, peripheral edema, and shock. Physical examination may reveal a systolic thrill over the left sternal border at the third intercostal space. Blood pressure and pulse pressure are usually low. Tachycardia and tachypnea are typically present. Auscultation of acute mitral regurgitation reveals a harsh decrescendo early systolic murmur. The murmur may radiate across the precordium, left axilla, back, and left sternal border. The third and fourth heart sounds are usually present.

Hemodynamic monitoring demonstrates elevated left atrial pressures and pulmonary artery wedge pressures (PAWP) as high as 25 to 35 mm Hg or more. Left atrial pressures rise as systemic vascular resistance increases and drops as the resistance decreases. There is a prominent *v* wave and steep *y* descent in the atrial tracing. Cardiac output is low. Pulmonary artery pressures, pulmonary vascular resistance, and central venous pressures may be elevated. ECG monitoring usually demonstrates sinus tachycardia but can also demonstrate atrial fibrillation.

Laboratory Findings

Blood samples for oxygen saturation studies may be obtained from pulmonary artery catheters at the bedside or in the cardiac catheterization laboratory. Chronic mitral regurgitation often demonstrates low oxygen saturations, whereas normal oxygen saturation is present in acute mitral regurgitation until the left ventricle fails. As left ventricular failure complicates acute mitral regurgitation, pulmonary artery oxygen saturation falls and indicates a poor prognosis (Table 23–1).

Mitral regurgitation caused by an infectious process often increases the total white blood cell count; increased neutrophils, increased band neutrophils, and increased lymphocytes may also be noted. Mitral regurgitation complicating an MI can be suspected by elevated creatine kinase (CK) enzymes and CK-MB bands, or lactate dehydrogenase$_1$ (LDH_1), greater than LDH_2 within 2 weeks prior to the symptoms of mitral regurgitation.

Diagnostic Procedures

Chest x-rays are commonly performed when diagnosing and monitoring the course of mitral regurgitation. Left ventricular and left atrial enlargement are often seen in chronic mitral regurgitation. Calcification of the annulus may also be seen. The left mainstem bronchus may be elevated by the enlarged left atrium, and Kerley B lines characteristic of interstitial pulmonary edema may be present. Acute mitral regurgitation may or may not demonstrate left ventricular or atrial enlargement but typically presents with pulmonary congestion and edema.

Echocardiograms are another noninvasive technique used to assess patients with mitral regurgitation (Table 23–2). Echocardiograms can diagnose the severity of the lesion and may be used to identify the etiology of the regurgitation and monitor the progression of the pathophysiology. Color and pulsed Doppler echocardiograms are preferred to M-mode and two-dimensional techniques. The best images are obtained by transesophageal echocardiography. Chronic mitral regurgitation will demonstrate enlargement of the left ventricle and atrium as well as increased wall motion of these chambers. The jet of regurgitant blood to the atrium may be identified. Mitral valve leaflet thickening and annulus calcification may also be demonstrated. In patients with acute mitral regurgitation, echocardiography can be used to identify an enlarged left ventricle or atrium when it is present, but is most useful for identifying increased systolic wall motions. The etiology of the acute regurgitation, such as flail or perforated leaflets, vegetations, and ruptured chordae or papillary muscles, may be identified on echocardiography. Prosthetic valves may also be evaluated by echocardiography.

Other noninvasive studies are occasionally used for investigation of mitral regurgitation. Holter monitoring may help to determine the dysrhythmia type, frequency, and duration. Graded exercise studies may be used to evaluate functional cardiac reserve in chronic mitral regurgitation. Radionuclide imaging has been used to identify ejection fractions, diastolic and systolic ventricular volumes, and left ventricular function. Cardiac imaging has been used in patients with chronic mitral regurgitation to help determine the

TABLE 23–1. **Laboratory Findings in Valvular Heart Disease**

Heart Disease	Sao_2	$S\bar{v}o_2$	Pao_2	WBC	RBC	Platelets	Coagulopathies	Liver Enzymes	Blood Cultures	CPK	LDH
MR	Acute: Early: normal Late: decreased Chronic: decreased		Acute: Early: normal Late: decreased	Increased neutrophils,* possibly increased lymphocytes*						If MI, ↑, positive MB bands	If MI, $LDH_1 > LDH_2$
MVP						↓					
MS	↓ **				? ↓			? ↑			
AR	↓ **							↑ ***			
AS	↓ with LVF				? ↓						
TR TS		↓ with low CO					↑ late	↓ albumin	positive****		
PR											
PS											

Abbreviations: Sao_2, oxygen saturation of arterial blood; $S\bar{v}o_2$, oxygen saturation of mixed venous blood; Pao_2, partial pressure of arterial oxygen; MR, mitral regurgitation; MVP, mitral valve prolapse; MS, mitral stenosis; AR, aortic regurgitation; AS, aortic stenosis; TR, tricuspid regurgitation; TS, tricuspid stenosis; PR, pulmonic regurgitation; PS, pulmonic stenosis; LVF, left ventricular failure; WBC, white blood cells; RBC, red blood cells; MI, myocardial infarction; CO, cardiac output; CPK, creatine phosphokinase; LDH, lactic dehydrogenase; *, with an infectious process; **, with pulmonary edema/transudates; ***, with right ventricular failure; ****, with a blood infection; ↑, increased; ↓, decreased.

timing of surgical interventions. Phonocardiography may be used to demonstrate the diminished first heart sound, accentuation of the murmur with increased afterload (Valsalva maneuver, squatting), and diminished intensity with decreased afterload (amyl nitrate). It is also used to graph the murmur. The phonocardiogram of chronic mitral regurgitation shows a high-frequency and holosystolic murmur. There may be a third heart sound and a middiastolic component. Acute mitral regurgitation murmurs are high-frequency, decrescendo sounds that terminate in mid to late systole. Acute mitral regurgitation usually demonstrates third and fourth heart sounds.

The diagnosis and severity of mitral regurgitation is also quantified by cardiac catheterization. Mitral regurgitation is confirmed by a left ventriculogram demonstrating contrast entering the left atrium. The angiogram also provides measurements for determining left ventricular function and left ventricular mass and stress. Cardiac catheterization also provides an opportunity to evaluate the entire cardiac anatomy and identify any other cardiac lesions. In chronic mitral regurgitation, contrast enters the atrium and may not clear for many cardiac cycles. In acute mitral regurgitation, the left atrium and ventricle are often normal in size, and the ventricular contrast medium regurgitates not only to the atrium, but also into the pulmonary veins.

Clinical Management

Chronic mitral regurgitation may not require continuous treatment because there may be no symptoms. Some authorities recommend continuous prophylactic treatment for endocarditis until the patient reaches age 30. Most also recommend specific prophylaxis in these patients for infective endocarditis during dental and surgical procedures (Table 23–3). Symptomatic treatment is used on an individual basis. Atrial fibrillation is usually treated with digoxin to slow the ventricular response, and many clinicians believe that anticoagulation minimizes the risk of embolization. Electrical cardioversion may be used for atrial fibrillation of sudden onset or in cases of mild regurgitation or atrial

TABLE 23–2. **Cardiac Valve Echocardiography**

Valve Disease	M-Mode	Two-Dimensional	Doppler	Color Doppler	Transesophageal
Mitral regurgitation		+	+++	++++	++++
Mitral valve prolapse	+	++	++	+	+++
Mitral stenosis	+	++	+++	+++	+++
Aortic regurgitation	+	++	+++	+++	+
Aortic stenosis	+	++	+++	++	+
Tricuspid regurgitation	+	+	++	++	++
Tricuspid stenosis	++	++	+	+	++
Pulmonic regurgitation	+	+	++	++	+
Pulmonic stenosis	?+	+	++	++	+

Abbreviations: +, somewhat useful; ++, commonly used; +++, examination of choice; ++++, especially recommended.

TABLE 23–3. **Antibiotic Prophylaxis**

For Dental Procedures and Surgery of the Upper Respiratory Tract	
1. For most patients: oral amoxicillin	Adults: 3.0 g orally of amoxicillin 1 hour before procedure and then 1.5 g 6 hours after initial dose.
2. For those *allergic to amoxicillin/penicillin* (may also be selected for those receiving oral penicillin as continuous rheumatic fever prophylaxis): erythromycin or clindamycin	Adults: 1.0 g orally 2 hours before procedure and then 500 mg 6 hours after initial dose.
3. For those patients at *higher risk* of infective endocarditis (especially those with prosthetic heart valves) who are not allergic to penicillin: ampicillin, gentamicin, and amoxicillin	Adults: 2.0 g ampicillin plus 1.5 mg/kg gentamicin IM or IV, both given 30 minutes before procedure; then 1.5 g amoxicillin orally 6 hours after initial dose.
4. For *higher risk* patients (especially those with prosthetic heart valves) who are *allergic to penicillin:* vancomycin	Adults: 1 g IV over 60 minutes begun 60 minutes before procedure; no repeat dose is necessary.
For Gastrointestinal and Genitourinary Tract Surgery and Instrumentation	
1. For most patients: ampicillin, gentamicin, and amoxicillin	Adults: 2.0 g ampicillin IM or IV plus gentamicin 1.5 mg/kg IM or IV given 30 minutes before procedure; followed by 1.5 g amoxicillin orally 6 hours after initial dose. May repeat once 8 hours later.
2. For patients *allergic to penicillin:* vancomycin plus gentamicin	Adults: 1.0 g vancomycin IV given over 60 minutes plus 1.5 mg/kg gentamicin IM or IV, each given 60 minutes before procedure. Doses may be repeated once 8 hours after initial dose.
3. Oral regimen for minor or repetitive procedures in low-risk patients: amoxicillin	Adults: 3.0 g amoxicillin 1 hour before procedure and 1.5 g 6 hours after initial dose.

Note: In patients with compromised renal function, it may be necessary to modify or omit the second dose of antibiotics. Intramuscular injections may be contraindicated in patients receiving anticoagulants.

Adapted from Dajani, A. S., Bisno, A. L., Chung, K. J. et al. (1990) Prevention of bacterial endocarditis. Recommendations by the American Heart Association, *JAMA, 264*(22), 2912–2922. Copyright 1990, American Medical Association.

hypertrophy. With the onset of left ventricular failure, digoxin and diuretics are begun to increase contractility and decrease preload. Dietary sodium, fluid, and activity restrictions are recommended. Decreasing afterload to decrease regurgitation and increase aortic flow combined with decreasing preload to minimize left ventricular volume and the size of the mitral orifice may be accomplished with nitrates, hydralazine, prazosin, or captopril. The comprehensive health care plan should consider all four elements listed in Table 23–4. If the signs and symptoms of left ventricular failure cannot be controlled by these regimens, surgical intervention is considered (see Chapter 24). Some authorities consider performing surgical intervention before the appearance of symptoms of left ventricular failure to secure a better prognosis. (Braunwald, 1992; Baue et al., 1991; Cheitlin et al., 1993; Kirklin & Barratt-Boyes, 1993).

Surgical treatment is based on the underlying pathology as well as the surgeon's opinion and experience. Valvuloplasty (Fig. 23–4) is often a lengthy, complex procedure. When the leaflets have been stretched, such as with prolapse or myxomatous changes, they may be resected. Cleft leaflets may be patched, and retracted leaflets can be extended with prepared pericardium grafts. A dilated or deformed annulus may also be repaired (Fig. 23–5). Annuloplasty with a ring or stent has been used when calcifications are not present (Fig. 23–6).

Short, elongated, or ruptured chordae tendineae may result in mitral regurgitation. Valvuloplasty involves resecting, dividing, or fenestrating shortened or fused chordae. Elongated chordae may be shortened by implanting the superfluous length in its papillary muscle. Ruptured chordae are treated differently depending on which leaflet is involved; however, annuloplasty corrects all procedures to repair ruptured chordae. Ruptured chordae of the posterior leaflet are repaired by resecting the leaflet to eliminate the need for the ruptured chordae. The anterior leaflet is repaired by transposing a section of the posterior leaflet with its chordae to the anterior leaflet. The posterior leaflet is then closed. Ruptured anterior chordae may also be replaced by neochords, synthetic strands (David et al., 1991), or narrow strips of tissue from the leaflet (Gregory et al., 1988). A collagen-type tissue may eventually cover the synthetic strands. Fused or calcified commissures are another cause of chronic mitral regurgitation. A commissurotomy may be used to correct this lesion by splitting the commissures open to within 2 to 3 mm of the annulus.

TABLE 23–4. **Comprehensive Health Care Plan**

Patient, family, and health care professionals are responsible for "having it MADE."	
M—*Medications:*	Antibiotics, antidysrhythmics, afterload reducers, preload reducers, anticoagulants, antifungals, antivirals
A—*Activity:*	Activity (aerobic exercise, avoidance of isometric exercise, cardiac rehabilitation), rest, sleep
D—*Diet:*	Ordered diet (sodium, caffeine, and other restrictions), ordered fluids, routine weights, appropriate weight for height
E—*Etiology:*	Diagnosis, diagnostic/monitoring/treatment regimens (coping, body image), complications, follow-up, genetic factors

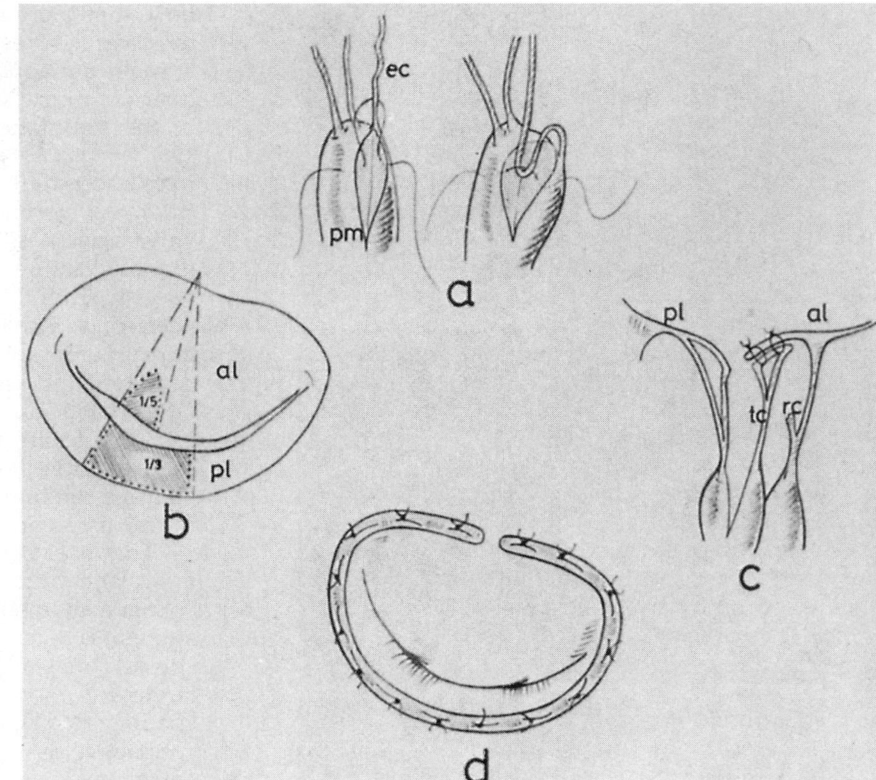

FIGURE 23–4. Techniques of valvuloplasty for correction of mitral regurgitation. *A,* Shortening of elongated chordae tendineae (ec) by burying the excessive length into a trench created in the papillary muscle (pm). *B,* Leaflet resection; the two leaflets are resected following the triangular outline indicated. The anterior leaflet (al) can only tolerate small resections of up to one fifth of its free edge, whereas the posterior leaflet (pl) is amenable to a much wider resection, of up to one third of its substance. *C,* Transposition of the chordae tendineae (tc) from the posterior leaflet (pl) to the anterior leaflet (al) to replace ruptured chordae (rc). *D,* Final result after implantation of a Carpentier ring to consolidate the repair and to reshape the annulus. (From Barlow, J. B. [1987]. *Perspectives on the mitral valve.* Philadelphia: F. A. Davis.)

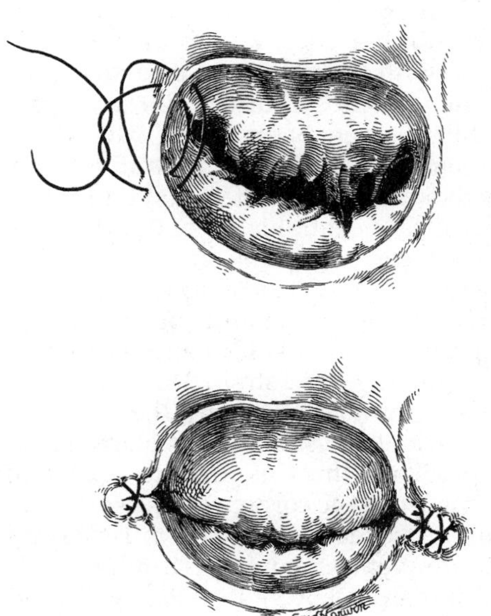

FIGURE 23–5. Commissural plication of the regurgitant mitral valve annulus. (Reproduced by permission from: Starr, A., & Macmanus, Q. [1978]. Acquired valvular heart disease. In D. B. Effler [Ed.]: *Blades' surgical diseases of the chest* [4th ed., p. 513]. St. Louis: C. V. Mosby Co.)

Mitral valve replacement is also a treatment for chronic mitral regurgitation. As with valvuloplasty, the best timing for surgery in the course of the disease is difficult to determine. The surgeon's opinions and experience determine the device utilized, but some general guidelines are commonly agreed upon. Calcified and otherwise immobilized leaflets are indications for valve replacement. Mechanical prostheses, the ball-cage and tilt disc, require lifelong anticoagulation. Porcine and bovine xenografts and homografts do not require anticoagulation for more than 6 weeks postimplantation unless atrial fibrillation or a large left atrium exist. The xenografts and homografts have smaller effective orifices for the size of their sewing rings. Xenograft and homograft prostheses are considered preferable for children, females of childbearing age, patients over age 70, and those with a history of bleeding (Braunwald, 1992) (Fig. 23–7). If possible, surgical replacement should be postponed until 4 to 6 weeks after MI. Management of atrial fibrillation with digoxin and prophylaxis against infective endocarditis should continue postoperatively.

The treatment of acute mitral regurgitation begins with nitroprusside and diuretics to decrease afterload. Ventricular diameter is decreased, minimizing the size of the mitral annulus. An intraaortic balloon may be utilized to further decrease afterload in patients with severe left ventricular failure. In cases of severe regurgitation, surgical intervention is indicated. Less severe regurgitation may be managed medically. A common

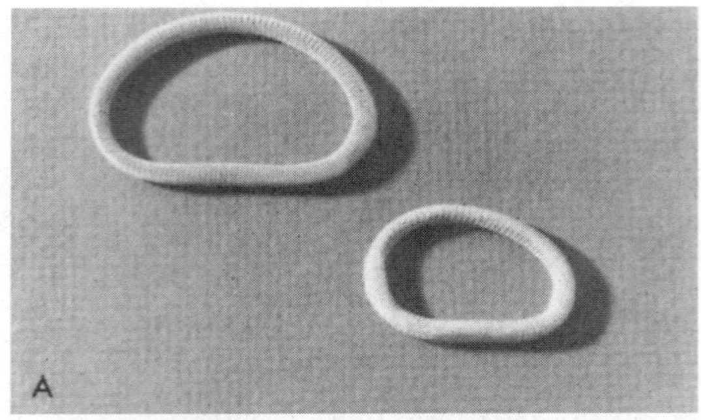

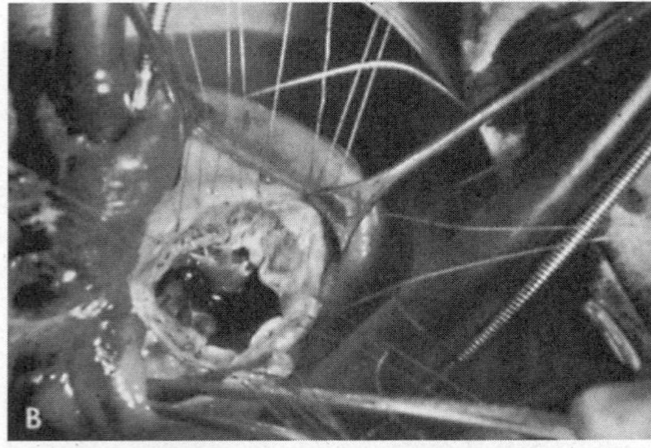

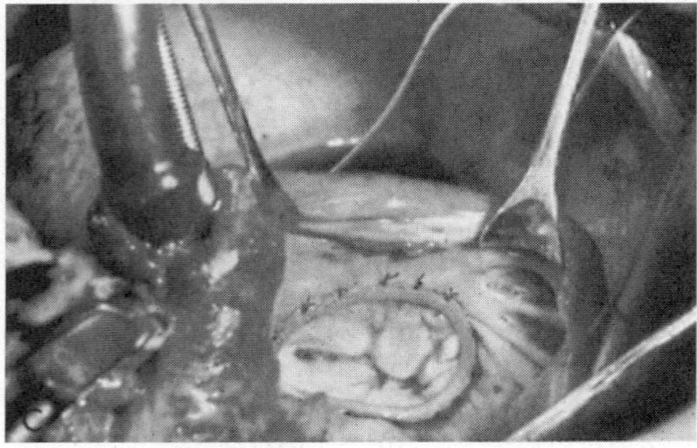

FIGURE 23-6. *A,* Carpentier rings. *B,* Ring being sutured into place. *C,* Completion of Carpentier ring annuloplasty. (From Starr, A. [1976]. Acquired disease of the tricuspid valve. In D. C. Sabiston, Jr., & F. C. Spencer [Eds.]. *Gibbon's surgery of the chest* [p. 1182]. Philadelphia: W. B. Saunders.)

cause of acute mitral regurgitation is elongated or ruptured chordae, which may be repaired as previously described. Mitral valve replacement may also be used to treat acute mitral regurgitation (see Chapter 24).

MITRAL VALVE PROLAPSE

Pathophysiology

Mitral valve prolapse, also called Barlow syndrome, floppy valve, billowing mitral valve, ballooning mitral cusp, midsystolic click-murmur, redundant cusp syndromes, and numerous other names, is usually a benign lesion. Controversy exists as to the definition of mitral valve prolapse. Some state that it is an abnormal or exaggerated movement of a leaflet into the left atrium during ventricular systole, whereas others believe that there must be dissociation of the leaflets at the commissures and the resultant mitral regurgitation to make a diagnosis of mitral valve prolapse. The incidence of mitral valve prolapse ranges from 2% to 21% of the population (Braunwald, 1992; Cheitlin et al., 1993; Frankl & Brest, 1993; Hunt, 1985; Marriott, 1993). In many cases it is inherited as an autosomal dominant trait. Developmentally, the formation of the mitral valve structures, the autonomic nervous system, and the ossification of the thoracic cage occur simultaneously. Individuals with mitral valve prolapse have been found to have a high frequency of dysautonomia, narrow anterior-posterior chest diameters, pectus excavatum, and scoliosis. Barlow (1987) and Braunwald (1992) have summarized the etiologies and conditions associated with mitral valve prolapse. As with mitral regurgitation, disorders of the leaflets, annulus, chordae tendineae, or papillary muscle may result in mitral valve prolapse.

The most common cause of mitral valve prolapse is myxomatous changes of the leaflets. A disorder of collagen metabolism results in a proliferation of the spongiosa layer of the leaflet. As the myxomatous cells spread into the fibrous layer of the leaflet, the leaflet stretches and prolapse occurs. The myxomatous changes may be idiopathic and may be associated with connective tissue disorders such as Marfan syndrome, osteogenesis imperfecta, periarteritis nodosa, Duchenne muscular dystrophy, and cardiomyopathy. Leaflets may also be damaged by left atrial myxomas that rub or fall down onto a leaflet. IHSS often causes anterior leaflet movement, which may in turn precipitate posterior leaflet prolapse. Mitral valve surgery, such as commissurotomies, insufficient leaflet resection, and chordae resection, division, or fenestration, may result in prolapse. Myxomatous changes may also affect the annulus, causing it to dilate, and have been associated with calcification. The distortion of the annulus may result in mitral valve prolapse.

The third element of the mitral valve structure is the chordae tendineae. The degenerative myxomatous changes that affect the leaflets and annulus also affect the chordae. The central layer of the chordae weakens with the collagen disruption, and the chordae elongate and may rupture. CAD and coronary artery spasm may lead to chordae ischemia and rupture. The rheumatic disease process may result in shortened chordae that rupture from prolonged strain. Whatever the cause, the chordae are not able to control the leaflet movement during ventricular systole, and prolapse results.

The papillary muscles are the final mitral valve component. Ischemic coronary disease may cause papillary muscle ischemia, papillary muscle head necrosis and rupture, ventricular hypertrophy, cardiomyopathy, and impaired left ventricular wall motion. Malfunction of the papillary muscle impairs the chordae tendineae, and the leaflets prolapse.

Abnormal movement of the mitral valve leaflets may occur during the patient's lifetime with no pathophysiologic changes. Atrial, junctional, and ventricular dysrhythmias may be precipitated by abnormal leaflet

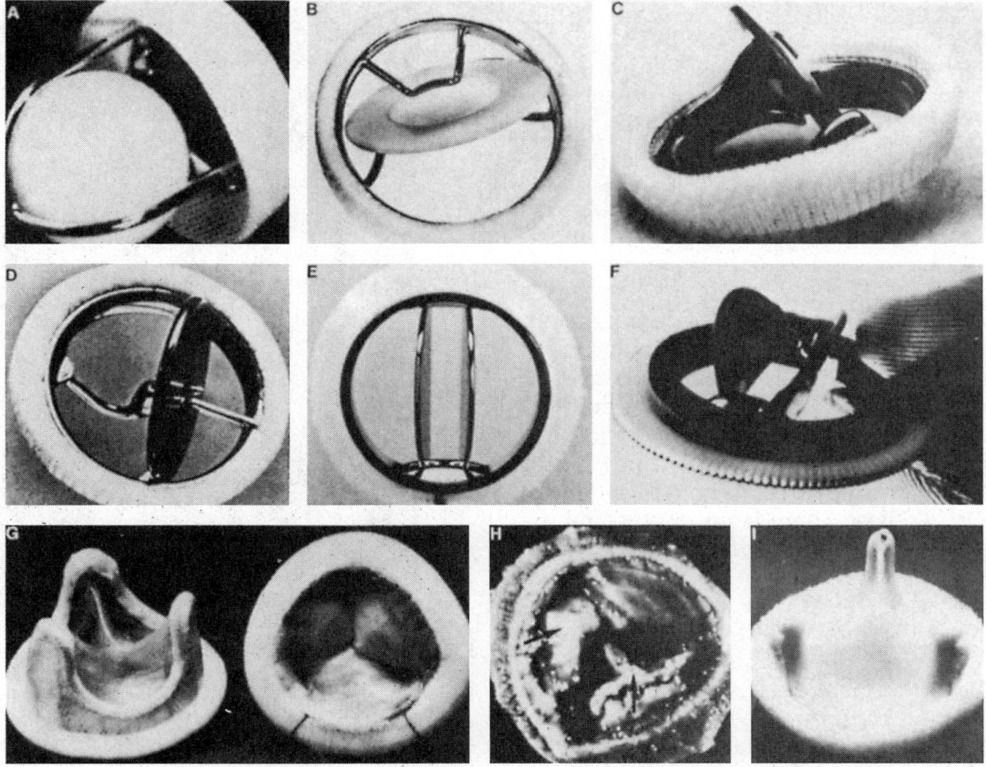

FIGURE 23–7. Prosthetic cardiac valves. *A*, Starr-Edwards ball-cage. *B*, Bjork-Shiley tilting disc. *C*, Omniscience tilting disc. *D*, Medtronic-Hall tilting disc. *E*, St. Jude Medical bileaflet. *F*, Duromedics bileaflet. *G*, Carpentier-Edwards porcine. *H*, Porcine valve removed several years following implantation because of primary valve failure; arrows point to areas of calcification and destruction of leaflets. *I*, Ionescu-Shiley pericardial valve. (Adapted from Braunwald, E. [Ed.]. [1992]. *Heart disease.* [4th ed.]. Philadelphia: W. B. Saunders.)

movement or by the elevated epinephrine or norepinephrine of dysautonomia. The patient may be at increased risk of bacterial endocarditis and cerebral ischemia. Mitral valve prolapse rarely progresses to mitral regurgitation.

Physical Assessment

Many patients with mitral valve prolapse have no signs or symptoms of the disorder. In these individuals prolapse is discovered during examination for another reason or at autopsy. Other patients with mitral valve prolapse may be symptomatic, but there are very few physical signs of the condition.

Inspection of the patient may reveal a narrow anterior-posterior chest diameter, pectus excavatum, or scoliosis. Auscultation is usually the most revealing assessment. Mitral valve prolapse is often characterized by a mid or late systolic click heard best between the apex and the lower left sternal border. The click is often heard after the beginning of the carotid pulsation is felt. The timing of the click or clicks (there may be more than one) can be changed using the usual ventricular size and afterload altering procedures. Standing and administration of amyl nitrate, which decrease ventricular size and afterload, cause the click to occur earlier in the cycle. Squatting, isometric exercise, and lying down, which increase ventricular size and afterload, cause the click to occur later in the cycle. Patients with mitral valve prolapse occurring with or because of left ventricular hypertrophy, mitral regurgitation, or other pathology will demonstrate signs or symptoms of those disorders as well, such as a laterally displaced point of maximal impulse and a systolic murmur.

Although mitral valve prolapse may not provide many physical signs, patients are often quite symptomatic. The presenting symptoms are usually fatigue, shortness of breath, light-headedness, dizziness or syncope, palpitations, chest pain, or anxiety. Fatigue has been attributed to exertion and emotional stress, but the patient is often tired regardless of physical or emotional stress and the amount of rest and sleep. Shortness of breath is not correlated with pulmonary function or graded exercise tests. Dyspnea may be correlated with or contribute to the anxiety associated with mitral valve prolapse. Light-headedness, dizziness, and syncope may be attributed to orthostatic hypotension or dysrhythmias, but this has not always been documented. Palpitations, a frequent complaint, are often correlated with atrial and ventricular dysrhythmias, but not in all cases. Chest pain, which may be typical or atypical, is another common complaint. It responds variably to nitrate treatment in the same patient. The pain is not correlated with physical or emotional stress, is often localized, and diminishes when the patient lies down. The pain may last for seconds to days. The pathogenesis has not been determined. The final symptom of mitral valve prolapse is anxiety. The poor correlation of symptoms with physical signs of pathology has led to other diagnoses, such as neurosis, in many patients. Anxiety may be correlated with dysrhythmias and orthostatic hypotension. Some have correlated all of the symptoms with dysautonomia. When moving from a supine to a standing position, patients with mitral valve prolapse may experience light-headedness, dizziness, syncope, palpitations, chest pains, and anxiety. When returning to the supine position, bradycardias may precipitate fatigue and anxiety. To date, there is no universally accepted explanation for the symptoms.

Electrocardiographic (ECG) monitoring may reveal flattened or inverted T waves in leads II and III and, rarely, a prolonged QT interval. Many dysrhythmias may be observed, among them sinus bradycardia, sinus arrest, PACs, atrial tachycardia, atrial fibrillation, first-degree AV block, right bundle branch block, premature ventricular contractions, ventricular tachycardia, and ventricular fibrillation.

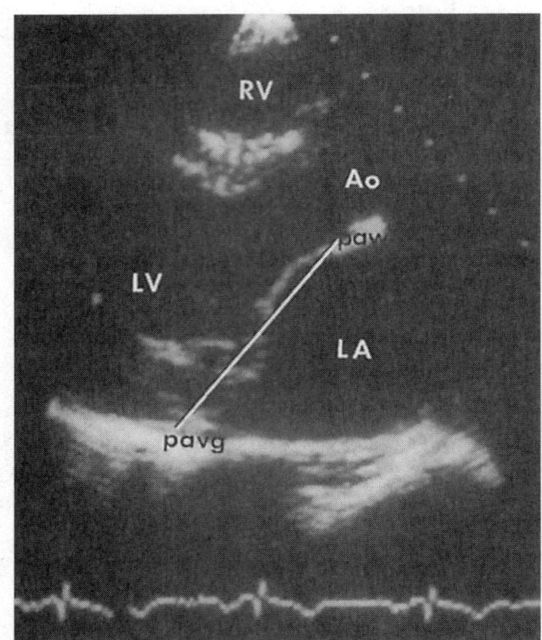

FIGURE 23–8. Two-dimensional echocardiogram from the parasternal long-axis view demonstrates prolapse of the posterior mitral leaflet into the left atrium (LA) during systole. Prolapse is defined as detection of motion of one or both leaflets superior to an imaginary line between the posterior atrioventricular groove (pavg) and the posterior aortic wall (paw). Ao, aorta; LV, left ventricle; RV, right ventricle. (From Marcus, M. L., et al. [1991]. *Cardiac imaging: A companion to Braunwald's heart disease.* [p. 434]. Philadelphia: W. B. Saunders.)

Laboratory Findings

Blood samples from patients with mitral valve prolapse are usually within normal ranges (see Table 23–1). Some patients have been found to have shortened platelet survival times.

Diagnostic Procedures

Electrocardiograms may demonstrate flattening and inversion of the T wave in leads II, III, aVF, V_5, and V_6. Many patients with Wolff-Parkinson-White syndrome also demonstrate mitral valve prolapse. ST segment depression may be noted or accentuated by standing. Graded exercise and Holter monitor studies may be useful for detection of dysrhythmias and ST segment depression. ST segment depression may normalize with peak exertion.

Echocardiograms are the primary diagnostic modality for detecting mitral valve prolapse (see Table 23–2). The pulsed Doppler, transesophageal, and two-dimensional echocardiograms (Fig. 23–8) have been used more frequently than M-mode because of their sensitivity, but many still use M-mode echocardiography successfully. The echocardiographic finding is the posterior movement of a leaflet, usually the posterior leaflet but sometimes the anterior leaflet, or both, into the left atrium.

Radionuclide imaging has been used to identify false-positive graded exercise studies. Phonocardiograms may demonstrate the systolic click at least 0.14 second after the first heart sound and changing timing with the methods discussed in the Physical Assessment section. Cardiac catheterization may demonstrate prolapse of the posterior leaflet but is not as sensitive to the anterior leaflet. One advantage of the ventriculogram is that it may demonstrate mitral regurgitation and assist with differentiation of chest pain by determining the degree of CAD. Cardiac catheterization is not usually necessary for the diagnosis or treatment of mitral valve prolapse.

Clinical Management

Therapy for patients with mitral valve prolapse depends on symptoms and whether or not mitral regurgitation complicates the diagnosis. The comprehensive health care plan should consider all four elements listed in Table 23–4. Antibiotic prophylaxis for bacterial endocarditis is prescribed regardless of whether regurgitation is known or not, and when systolic clicks are auscultated, whether or not echocardiographic prolapse can be demonstrated (see Table 23–3).

Dysautonomia may respond to elimination of caffeine, alcohol, cigarettes, and products containing epinephrine or ephedrine, as well as avoiding competitive sports. These actions will decrease catecholamine levels. Medications may include propranolol or barbiturates. Propranolol may decrease fatigue, lightheadedness, dizziness, syncope, palpitations, supraventricular and ventricular dysrhythmias, chest pain, and anxiety. Dysrhythmias not controlled with propranolol may be treated with quinidine, procainamide, phenytoin, calcium channel blockers, or clonidine. If AV block progresses to Mobitz II or complete heart block, a temporary or permanent pacemaker may be required. Ventricular tachycardia refractory to other therapies may be treated with stellate ganglion blockers.

Chest pain usually decreases with propranolol. Calcium channel blockers may be added when propranolol does not control the chest pain. Nitrates, when used, are used with caution. Nitrates may decrease preload and therefore ventricular size, exaggerating the prolapse and the ischemia.

Systemic emboli may result from fibrin and platelet deposits on the prolapsed leaflet. Prophylaxis for transient ischemic attacks and embolic strokes is accomplished with aspirin or dipyridamole. Some practitioners advise avoiding oral contraceptives.

Mitral valve prolapse rarely requires surgical intervention (see Chapter 24). Mitral valve replacement may be necessitated by refractory dysrhythmias, reduced cardiac reserves, severe mitral regurgitation, or incapacitating pain.

MITRAL STENOSIS

Pathophysiology

The most common etiology of mitral stenosis is rheumatic disease. Rheumatic endocarditis results in an inflammatory process or an abnormal valvular blood flow pattern that initiates progressive changes in the leaflets, annulus, chordae tendineae, or papillary muscles.

Aschoff bodies in the left atrial wall suggest ongoing subclinical rheumatic activity. Other researchers have documented structural valve changes related to abnormal blood flow caused by a limited rheumatic insult. The stenotic process continues for years after the initial insult, and many patients cannot identify a rheumatic episode. Many patients do not develop symptoms for 10 years or more.

The rheumatic inflammatory process causes nodules to develop along the edges of the leaflets at the commissures and within the leaflets themselves. The continuing process may result in fusion of the commissures and thickened, stiff leaflets. Calcification of the leaflets and commissure adhesions are common. The rheumatic process or its sequela may also scar, shorten, or fuse the chordae and shorten or scar the papillary muscles. The fused chordae narrow or obliterate the secondary orifices below the mitral valve leaflets. The rheumatic insult stiffens the mitral valve annulus and may eventually lead to its calcification.

Other causes of mitral stenosis are congenital deformities of shortened, thick chordae tendineae, a decreased number of chordae, or a single papillary muscle. In these conditions, the leaflets may be thickened but are seldom calcified. Infective bacterial endocarditis may result in the development of large vegetations that occlude the mitral valve orifice. Large left atrial ball thrombus or tumors may partially or totally occlude the mitral valve at some time during diastole. Metabolic and enzymatic changes such as mucopolysaccharide deposits, carcinoid heart disease, macrophage collection, and reaction to methysergide treatment may also result in thick, stiff leaflets. Valve prostheses may also become thrombosed (Fig. 23–9) or immobilized by pannus.

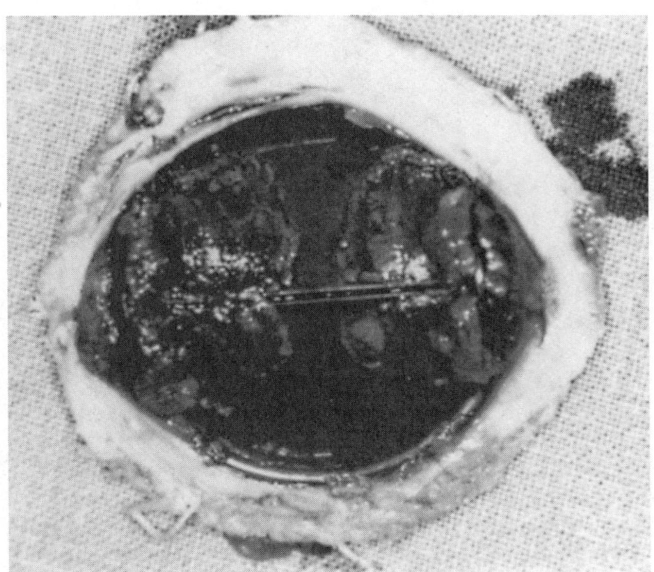

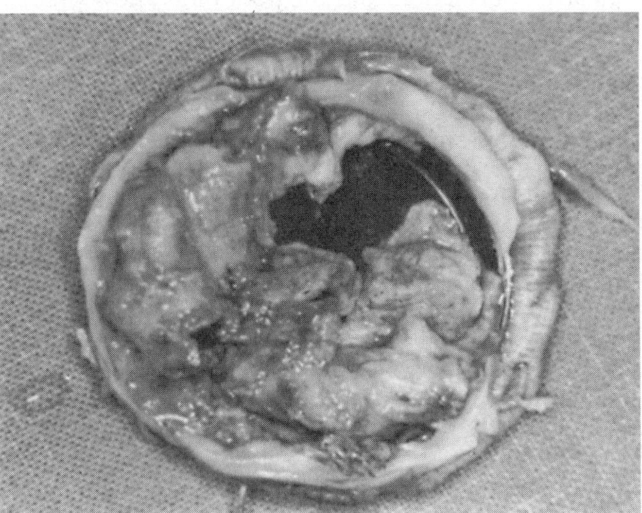

FIGURE 23–9. Thrombosed mechanical prostheses. *Top,* Atrial surface of a St. Jude prosthesis with leaflets immobilized by large clots that appear to originate from the hinge areas. *Bottom,* Thrombosed Medtronic-Hall prosthesis with the disc almost completely covered by a mass of organized blood clot. (From Barlow, J. B. [1987]. *Perspectives on the mitral valve.* Philadelphia: F. A. Davis.)

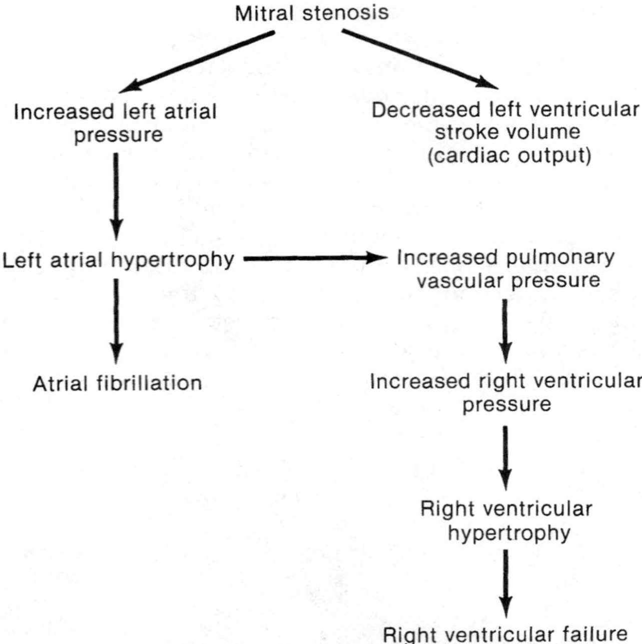

FIGURE 23–10. Pathophysiology of mitral stenosis. (Adapted from Schakenbach, L. H., Physiologic dynamics of acquired valvular heart disease, *Journal of Cardiovascular Nursing, 1*(3), 1–17, with permission of Aspen Publishers, Inc., © 1987.)

Mitral stenosis increases impedance of blood flow from the left atrium to the left ventricle. The ensuing pathophysiology is dependent on the degree of obstruction (Fig. 23–10). The normal mitral orifice is 4 to 6 cm^2, and signs and symptoms may not be noticed until the orifice is 1 to 2 cm^2. The left atrial blood volume and pressures become elevated, resulting in left atrial hypertrophy. The dilated left atrium often develops atrial fibrillation, and the poor blood flow predisposes the patient to the development of atrial thrombus. Elevated atrial blood volume and pressure are referred back into the pulmonary veins, which distend and thin under the stress. Eventually, the blood volume and pressures are referred into the pulmonary capillaries and arteries. Perivascular and perialveolar transudates stiffen the lung and may lead to pulmonary edema. The entire pulmonary vascular system becomes hyperplastic and hypertrophies. Changes in the pulmonary vascular system increase right ventricular afterload. The right ventricle eventually hypertrophies. In severe mitral stenosis, the right ventricle may fail. Mitral stenosis will decrease left ventricular preload and eventually stroke volume. The degree of forward failure is dependent on the ability of the heart rate and systemic vascular resistance to compensate for the decreased stroke volume.

Physical Assessment

Dyspnea is the most common presenting symptom of mitral stenosis. The patient may notice the dyspnea with exertion, anxiety, fever, during pregnancy, or when lying supine. Dyspnea may become more severe with the onset of atrial fibrillation. It is related to the pulmonary transudates, which may also be evidenced by hemoptysis. Progression of pulmonary volumes and pressures may cause pulmonary edema.

A careful history may identify a gradually decreasing exercise tolerance and fatigue related to the dyspnea. As the pulmonary pathology progresses, the patient may develop a chronic cough from the pulmonary congestion. Pulmonary congestion increases the patient's risk of bronchitis, pulmonary embolism, and pulmonary infarction. The distended pulmonary artery has been known to compress the laryngeal nerve against the aorta on rare occasions, causing hoarseness. Pulmonary hypertension has also been manifested as chest pain, associated with dyspnea and responsive to nitroglycerin. No mechanism has been identified for the pain.

Pulmonary symptoms are most common, but there are other symptoms of mitral stenosis. Systemic emboli, especially cerebral emboli, may occur, particularly after the onset of atrial fibrillation. Some patients complain of palpitations. Symptoms of right ventricular failure such as peripheral dependent edema, left upper quadrant fullness (hepatic congestion), abdominal enlargement, and cold extremities may be reported. The enlarged left atrium may cause dysphagia.

Inspection of the patient may reveal flushed cheeks in less pigmented patients, called mitral facies. There may be peripheral cyanosis and jugular vein distention. The respiratory rate is increased. These patients are often thin. Palpation often reveals a normal pulse and point of maximal impulse. The apical impulse may include a tapping vibration of the first heart sound. The left lower sternal and parasternal areas may have a lift if the patient has severe pulmonary hypertension.

Auscultation provides the most revealing assessments. The murmur of mitral stenosis is an early to middiastolic, low-pitched rumbling sound heard best at the apex. The duration of the murmur often correlates with the severity of the stenosis, with longer murmurs indicating more severe stenosis. Turning the patient to the left lateral position facilitates auscultation, as does exhalation exercise, coughing, and amyl nitrate. There is usually an opening snap before the murmur, a high-pitched sound that follows the second heart sound. No opening snap often indicates that both leaflets are immobile. The closer the opening snap to the second heart sound, the more severe the stenosis. The first heart sound is usually loud if the leaflets and chordae are pliable but may be soft if mitral immobility is severe and the sound is produced primarily by the tricuspid valve. Correlating with the pulmonary symptoms, crackles are commonly found in the dependent lung fields, and wheezes may be found if the mitral stenosis has progressed to the stage of chronic coughing.

Hemodynamic monitoring will demonstrate elevated left atrial pressures with an exaggerated *a* wave and a slow *y* descent. Pulmonary artery pressures are elevated in more severe mitral stenosis. If mitral stenosis has caused right ventricular failure, central venous pressure will also be elevated, and large *a* waves and slow *y* descents may be evident. Cardiac output is usually normal until the orifice is less than 1 cm^2.

Electrocardiographic monitoring may demonstrate normal sinus rhythm. In lead II a widened notched P wave (P mitrale) may reflect the left atrial hypertrophy. PACs may occur secondary to atrial dilation. Eventually, most patients with mitral stenosis develop atrial fibrillation from the atrial dilation.

Laboratory Findings

There is seldom any indication of mitral stenosis on laboratory examination of blood (Table 23–1). Red blood cell destruction may be increased across the stenotic valve; after right ventricular failure occurs the liver enzymes may be elevated. Patients with pulmonary edema and possibly those with pulmonary transudates will have decreased oxygen saturation.

Diagnostic Procedures

Electrocardiograms may demonstrate cardiac changes such as the wide (>0.12 second) notched P waves in leads II, III, and aVF or biphasic P waves with the second portion negative in V_1, which is indicative of left atrial hypertrophy. Ultimately atrial fibrillation will occur. Right ventricular hypertrophy may cause a right axis deviation (R wave in V_1).

Chest x-rays may demonstrate left atrial enlargement that may elevate the left mainstem bronchus. Elevated pulmonary pressures cause redistribution of blood flow to the upper lobes of the lung, Kerley B lines in the lung fields, and possibly enlargement of the pulmonary arteries and right ventricle. Calcifications of the mitral valve may be noted. Pulmonary effusions, interstitial edema, and pulmonary edema may also be detected.

Phonocardiograms may be used to clarify the aortic component of the second heart sound and the timing of the opening snap. Serial phonocardiograms demonstrating a narrowing of the interval between the two sounds indicate increasing left atrial pressures. Serial recordings demonstrate increased duration of the murmur as the stenosis increases. Apex cardiograms may be utilized to record or track rapid ventricular filling. As mitral stenosis progresses, the rapid filling wave is lost. The intensity of the mitral component of the first heart sound is usually increased, but as the leaflets become less mobile, this sound may also be lost. As pulmonary hypertension develops, the phonocardiogram can demonstrate the increased intensity of the pulmonic component of the second heart sound.

Echocardiograms can confirm the diagnosis of mitral stenosis (see Table 23–2). M-mode echocardiography can demonstrate the thick leaflets and their limited or abnormal movements. M-mode echocardiography can document the rate of diastolic closure of the mitral valve leaflet or annulus calcification, leaflet vegetations, atrial thrombus or myxoma, and left atrial, left ventricular, and right ventricular size. Two-dimensional echocardiograms offer the advantage of determining the size of the mitral valve orifice as well as all of the information provided by M-mode. Pulsed, color, Doppler, and transesophageal echocardiograms are also used, particularly to measure and trend velocity of blood through the valve.

Contrast and gated pool study radionuclide imaging has been used to calculate ejection fractions. Blood pool studies can determine cardiac chamber and pulmonary artery size. Radionuclide imaging may be used to track left ventricular function but does not play a major role in diagnosing or treating mitral stenosis.

Graded exercise studies can be used to demonstrate a patient's activity tolerance and hemodynamic abnormalities. Exercise studies may be useful to document dysrhythmia control by pharmacologic therapy. However, graded exercise studies are not frequently used for patients with mitral stenosis.

Patients with intermittent symptoms or complaints of palpitations may be evaluated with a Holter monitor. Intermittent atrial fibrillation, PACs, or other dysrhythmias may be identified by this method. Holter monitoring is another diagnostic modality that is seldomly used for mitral stenosis.

Cardiac catheterization is primarily used to measure the gradient across the mitral valve. Angiography may also be used to determine whether CAD, mitral regurgitation, or aortic valve lesions are also present. Ventricular wall motion and size may be determined by angiography. Cardiac catheterization is not considered necessary for diagnosing mitral stenosis, but is often performed before balloon valvuloplasty or cardiac surgery.

Clinical Management

Rheumatic endocarditis is treated with penicillin; alternatively, sulfadiazine or erythromycin is prescribed. Sources differ on the length of time for continued prophylaxis with these antibiotics, ranging from continuing until the patient is age 30 to continuing for life. The second antibiotic regimen is aimed at preventing infective endocarditis. Prophylaxis for dental and surgical procedures consists of amoxicillin, ampicillin, erythromycin, or clindamycin and may be followed or combined with gentamicin or vancomycin. It is typically a two-dose regimen (see Table 23–3). The third antibiotic regimen is short-course, intermittent treatment for infections as they occur.

Dyspnea and other respiratory symptoms are often treated by limiting activity, maintaining appropriate weight for height, eating a sodium-restricted diet, and taking diuretics such as chlorothiazide, chlorthalidone, or furosemide. In severe cases sedation and hospitalization with bed rest are required. Decreased exercise

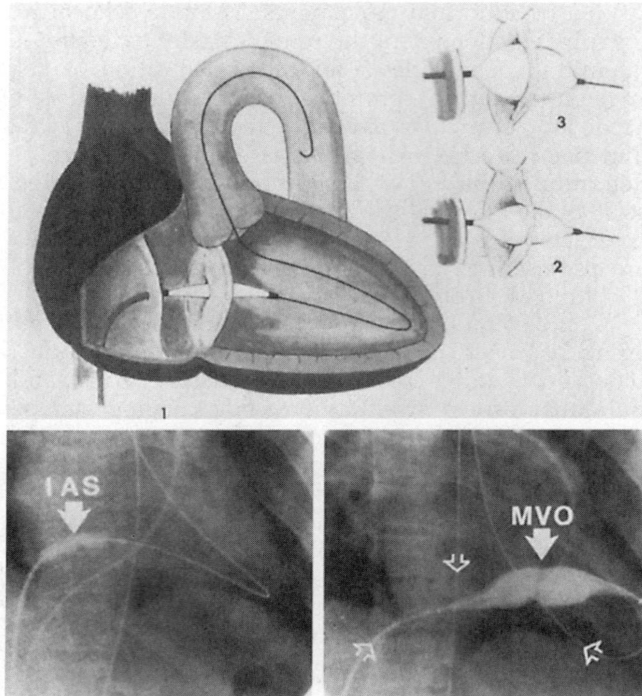

FIGURE 23–11. Mitral balloon valvuloplasty. The top panel shows the transeptal approach to mitral valvuloplasty; the bottom panel shows radiologic frames obtained during an actual procedure. After dilation of the intraatrial septum (IAS) by an 8-mm balloon catheter, a 25-mm dilation catheter is advanced into the mitral valve orifice (MVO) and inflated. Note the appearance of a "waist" corresponding to the impression of the stenotic mitral orifice on the partially inflated dilation catheter. This waist resolved with full inflation of the balloon, associated with an increase in mitral valve area from 0.9–1.6 cm^2. The path of the guidewire from the right atrium to left atrium, to left ventricle, to descending aorta is shown by the open arrows. (From Braunwald, E. [1992]. *Heart disease* [4th ed.]. Philadelphia: W. B. Saunders.)

tolerance and fatigue eventually affect all individuals with mitral stenosis. The limited cardiac reserve usually is the basis for recommending that the patient avoid competitive sports. Many believe that the adrenaline, endorphins, and psychological factors involved in competitive sports may cause the patient to miss or ignore symptoms. Some patients have found nitroglycerin effective in decreasing pulmonary symptoms because it promotes venous dilation. The decreased right ventricular preload and increased pulmonary venous capacitance caused by nitroglycerin reduce pulmonary congestion, transudates, and edema.

Dysrhythmias are usually atrial, and the first signs of cardiac failure usually are those of right ventricular failure. Either of these signs are treated with digoxin. Dysrhythmias may also be treated with propranolol, quinidine, calcium channel blockers, or cardioversion. Anticoagulation is often prescribed for 2 or 3 weeks before attempting cardioversion for longstanding atrial fibrillation. Because of the risk of systemic emboli, the occurrence of left atrial dilation or atrial fibrillation is an indication for anticoagulation with aspirin, warfarin, or dipyridamole. Anemia should be treated by diet, if possible, or transfusions. The comprehensive health care plan should consider all four elements listed in Table 23–4.

Surgical treatment of mitral stenosis is recommended before the occurrence of pulmonary hypertension or right ventricular failure. Valvuloplasty is often attempted. Closed mitral commissurotomy with one or two percutaneous balloons (Vahanian et al., 1989) or a finger or mechanical dilator (Fig. 23–11) may be attempted. Open commissurotomy (Fig. 23–12) provides direct visualization as well as the opportunity to remove the atrial thrombus or amputate or oversew the left atrial appendage to decrease the risk of thrombus formation. Fused chordae may be separated, scarred papillary muscle may be split, and calcium deposits may be removed from the leaflets and annulus. Some patients benefit from two or three different valvuloplasties. Mitral valve replacement is indicated when valvuloplasty is no longer successful or is not possible due to scarring, calcification, or deformity (see earlier discussion of mitral valve replacement in the section on mitral regurgitation, and Chapter 24). Antibiotic prophylaxis, activity restrictions, diet, diuretics, digoxin, other antidysrhythmics, and anticoagulation therapies are usually resumed after surgical intervention.

AORTIC REGURGITATION

Pathophysiology

Aortic regurgitation may result from disorders of the aortic valve leaflets or disorders of the base of the aorta. Connective tissue disorders of the leaflets or aorta are the most common causes of aortic regurgitation. Myxomatous degeneration begins in the central layer of the leaflet, the spongiosa, or in the tunica media of the aorta. The myxomatous cells spread into the supporting layers of the leaflet or aorta, interrupting its continuity and weakening the structure. The aorta often develops cystic medial necrosis secondary to this process. The weakened leaflets prolapse or tear and the aorta dilates, distorting the annulus of the aortic valve. Conditions associated with myxomatous

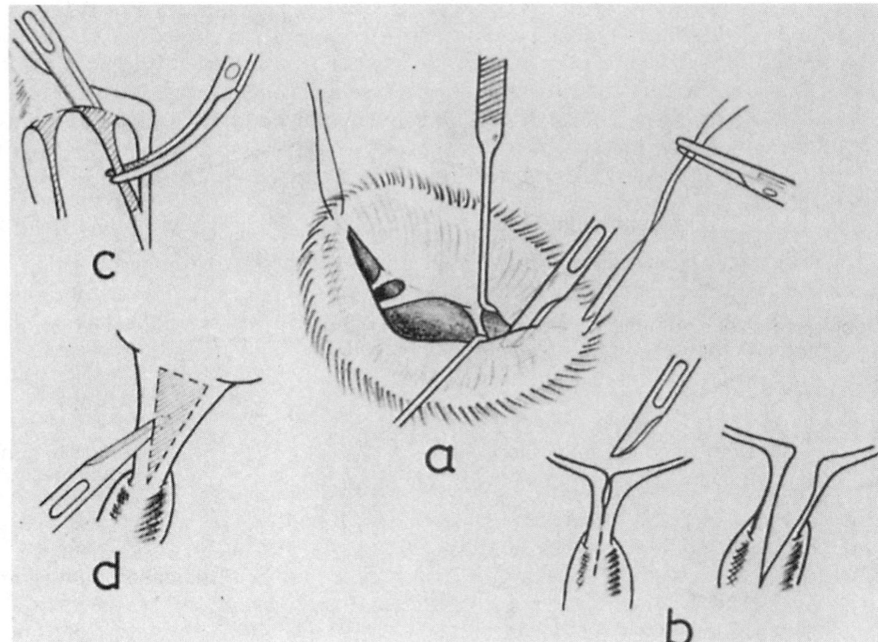

FIGURE 23–12. Technique of open commissurotomy. *a*, Sharp division of the commissures helped by retraction of the free edges of the two leaflets. *b*, When the chordae tendineae and the papillary muscle heads are fused at the commissural level, these are incised longitudinally. *c*, Thickened secondary and basal chordae contribute to the thickening and immobility of the posterior leaflet and are resected thoroughly. *d*, Fused chordae tendineae obstructing the flow of blood are fenestrated by the removal of triangular portions of the fibrosed tissue. (From Barlow, J. B. [1987]. *Perspectives on the mitral valve.* Philadelphia: F. A. Davis.)

changes are Marfan's syndrome and osteogenesis imperfecta.

The rheumatic disease process also affects the aortic valve. The inflammatory reaction causes fibrosis and contracture of the leaflets (Fig. 23–13). One or more of the shortened leaflets, or cusps, cannot approximate with the others, and blood is able to flow back across the valve. The aortic commissures seldom fuse in the rheumatic process.

Infective endocarditis, usually due to *Staphylococcus aureus* or enterococci, may result in aortic regurgitation. The disease process destroys cusp tissue, resulting in perforations of the cusp or tears along the annulus where the cusp attaches to the aorta. Occasionally, vegetations may prevent complete apposition of the cusps. Congenital disorders and atherosclerosis may also distort the leaflets, resulting in regurgitation.

Syphilis (Fig. 23–13) and rheumatoid (ankylosing) spondylitis affect both the aorta and the valve. The aorta dilates, separating the leaflets. As the dilation progresses, tension on the cusps causes them to curl toward their base, further separating the leaflets. Dilation of the aorta may also result from a dissecting aortic aneurysm, hypertension, senile dilation, and hypervolemia (often secondary to renal failure). The annulus may be dilated or distorted from below by a ventricular septal defect. The defect may also weaken the cusp support, distorting the leaflet or permitting prolapse.

Traumatic lesions are another rare cause of aortic regurgitation. Typically, blunt force trauma causes an aortic tear that disrupts the cusp's connection to the aorta. The support of the cusp is weakened and permits prolapse. Direct injury to the valve is rare, but tears in a cusp may occur. Penetrating wounds may lacerate cusps or penetrate the aorta or annulus. Rup-

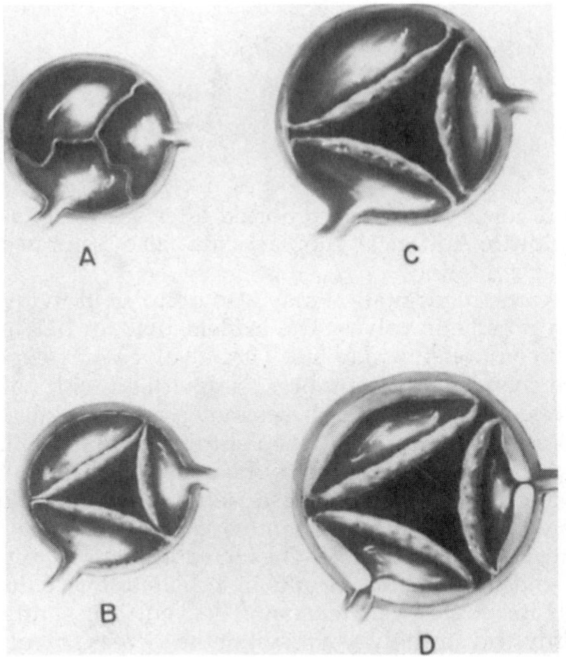

FIGURE 23–13. Variations in the aortic valve. *A*, The normal valve. *B*, Shortening of the cusps characteristic of rheumatic aortic regurgitation. *C*, Dilation of the aorta, as occurs in syphilitic aortitis and other conditions in which dilation is responsible for aortic regurgitation. The main feature results from bowing of the leaflets. Commissural separation is illustrated and may also be present. *D*, In addition to the feature shown in C, there is atherosclerosis of the aorta, as occurs in syphilitic aortitis, with consequent coronary ostial narrowing. (From Roberts, W. C. [1973]. Valvular, subvalvular and supravalvular aortic stenosis: Morphologic features. In J. E. Edwards [Ed.], *Clinical-Pathologic correlations #2* [p. 133]. Philadelphia: F. A. Davis.)

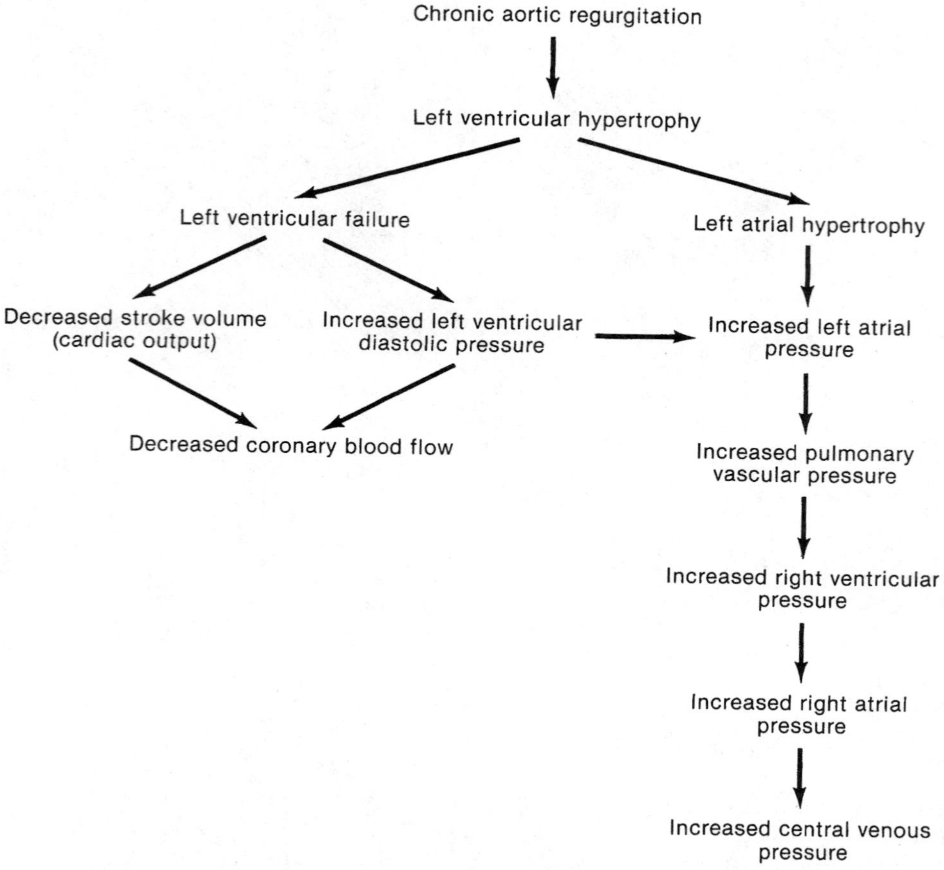

Chronic aortic regurgitation
Left ventricular hypertrophy
Left ventricular failure
Left atrial hypertrophy
Decreased stroke volume (cardiac output)
Increased left ventricular diastolic pressure
Increased left atrial pressure
Decreased coronary blood flow
Increased pulmonary vascular pressure
Increased right ventricular pressure
Increased right atrial pressure
Increased central venous pressure

FIGURE 23–14. Pathophysiology of chronic aortic regurgitation. (Adapted from Schakenbach, L. H., Physiologic dynamics of acquired valvular heart disease, *Journal of Cardiovascular Nursing, 1*(3), 1–17, with permission of Aspen Publishers, Inc., © 1987.)

tured cusps have been reported after straining, as in childbirth. Aortic valvuloplasty may also result in aortic regurgitation.

Aortic regurgitation may also occur in individuals with prosthetic valves. The leaflets, disk, or ball-and-strut components may fail. Tissue valves may experience changes of the annulus as described with native valves. Any of the prostheses may develop regurgitation at the sewing ring when sutures or tissue fail.

Aortic regurgitation may be acute or chronic, but the effect is the same: increased left ventricular volume related to systemic blood flowing back into the left ventricle during diastole. The increased left ventricular end-diastolic volume results in a dilated left ventricle with increased wall tension. The ventricle contracts swiftly and strongly as a result of the increased tension (Starling's law). In chronic aortic regurgitation, the stroke volume increases to maintain the normal forward stroke volume plus the regurgitant volume (Fig. 23–14). The ventricle hypertrophies and thickens, usually maintaining a normal ratio of wall thickness to cavity and size. Eventually, the ventricle fibroses and fails. In acute aortic regurgitation, the ventricle cannot adapt to the increased volume by dilating to the extent required (Fig. 23–15). Ventricular hypertrophy is absent or minimal and the left ventricle fails earlier.

Cardiac output is often maintained in both chronic and acute aortic regurgitation. In the chronic condition, the rapid upstroke and high pressure of systole stimulate the aortic baroreceptors. The reflex dilation of the systemic arteries decreases afterload and minimizes the regurgitant volume. Isotonic exercise causes further vasodilation and an increased heart rate that shortens diastole, thereby decreasing regurgitation. Isometric exercise, cold, and sympathetic stimulation cause vasoconstriction, which may increase the regurgitation. In the acute condition, the heart rate increases rapidly to maintain cardiac output. The hypertrophied ventricle or tachycardia increases myocardial oxygen

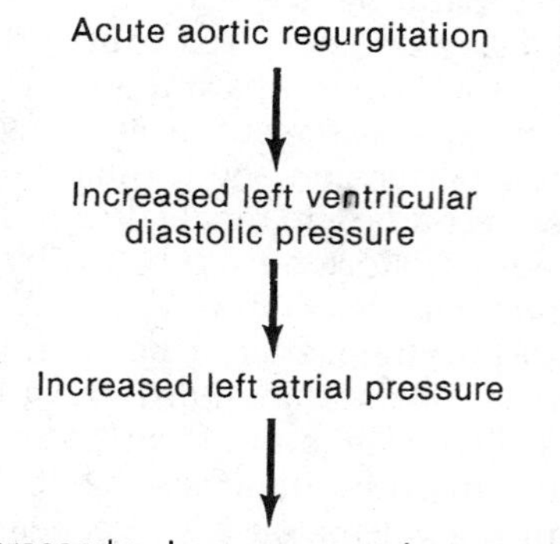

FIGURE 23–15. Pathophysiology of acute aortic regurgitation. (Adapted from Schakenbach, L. H., Physiologic dynamics of acquired valvular heart disease, *Journal of Cardiovascular Nursing, 1*(13), 1–17, with permission of Aspen Publishers, Inc., © 1987.)

demand. Vasodilation decreases diastolic pressure, and tachycardia decreases the time of diastole, thereby decreasing coronary perfusion. Myocardial ischemia may be caused by this mechanism.

Eventually, the left ventricle cannot maintain forward blood flow from the left atrium to the systemic circulation. The high ventricular end-diastolic volumes close the mitral valve prematurely. Blood volume increases in the left atrium, increasing left atrial pressure. In chronic aortic regurgitation there may be dilation; in acute regurgitation there is not. Pulmonary venous volume and pressures rise, followed by pulmonary capillary, pulmonary artery, right ventricular, and right atrial pressures.

Physical Assessment

Patients with chronic aortic regurgitation are often asymptomatic. Some patients perceive palpitations in the head or neck from the forceful ventricular contractions or pulsations due to the elevated systolic pressure. Others are aware of their heart beating, especially while lying down, a sign that is related to the ventricular hypertrophy. Once left ventricular failure occurs with acute or chronic aortic regurgitation, the most common presenting symptom is dyspnea. Other symptoms of left ventricular failure are fatigue, cough, orthopnea, paroxysmal nocturnal dyspnea, pulmonary edema, and syncope. Myocardial ischemia may precipitate other symptoms such as angina, dysrhythmias, and MI. An unexplained symptom is profuse sweating, perhaps related to increased skin perfusion secondary to decreased peripheral resistance and increased sympathetic tone.

Inspection of the patient with severe aortic regurgitation may reveal a head bob with each systole. Carotid or temporal pulsations may be clearly seen, the uvula may pulsate, and when a glass slide is pressed against the patient's lip or a light is pressed to the fingertip, capillary pulsations of the lip or nailbed may be observed. The point of maximal impulse may be observed laterally and caudally. Pulsations of the left chest may be noted if left ventricular hypertrophy exists. If the aorta is dilated, pulsations may be visible in the second and third intercostal spaces. Patients with acute aortic regurgitation may have pale or acrocyanotic extremities and jugular venous distention.

Palpation of the carotid pulse demonstrates a distinctive rapid upstroke and downstroke. It has been called the waterhammer or Corrigan pulse. The point of maximal impulse is larger than normal and may actually be diffuse if left ventricular hypertrophy is present. Pulsations of the digital arteries may be palpable, and the hands may be warm and sweaty. Patients with acute or late chronic aortic regurgitation are tachycardic. There may be a carotid thrill if regurgitation is severe. In acute cases, pulsus alternans characteristic of left ventricular failure may be noted, especially in the femoral arteries.

Auscultation of patients with aortic regurgitation can be difficult. The systolic blood pressure may be normal but is often increased. The diastolic blood pressure is low until the left ventricle fails, then it rises. Korotkoff sounds often continue to 0 mm Hg; in these cases the reading should be taken when the sound changes intensity or muffles. The pulse pressure is widened until the left ventricle fails. Auscultation of the femoral artery may reveal brisk sounds called pistol-shot sounds or double beats of Traube sign.

As chronic aortic regurgitation progresses and also in patients with acute disease, the first heart sound becomes softer from early closure of the mitral valve. The aortic component of the second heart sound becomes softer if the leaflets become immobile. The third heart sound may be heard and more rarely the fourth heart sound. When the aorta is dilated, an ejection click may be heard.

The murmur of chronic aortic regurgitation is a high-pitched, blowing, decrescendo diastolic sound. The murmur is usually best heard in the second right intercostal space while the patient is sitting, leaning forward, and exhaling; alternatively, the murmur may only be heard along the left sternal border at the fourth or fifth intercostal space or in the second or third intercostal space. The duration of the murmur correlates with the severity of the regurgitation. A systolic ejection murmur radiating to the carotids may be heard if the valve is distorted or the aorta dilated. The murmur may be increased by vasopressors, squatting, and isometric exercise and decreased by vasodilators, amyl nitrite, and the Valsalva maneuver. A coarse vibrating sound is usually detected if there is a tear in a cusp or along the annulus.

A second diastolic murmur may be heard at the apex. It is a low-pitched, rumbling sound that is middiastolic, holodiastolic, or presystolic. This sound is called the Austin Flint murmur. It is thought to be caused by the regurgitant flow contacting the anterior mitral leaflet and pushing it up into the flow of blood from the left atrium. Another hypothesis is that the regurgitation murmur is referred to the apex through the thorax. The murmur of acute regurgitation is a midpitched, short diastolic sound. An Austin Flint murmur is usually heard in middiastole. The third heart sound is common. Peripheral arterial sounds are seldom heard.

Laboratory Findings

There are no changes in blood sample values until left ventricular failure affects the pulmonary vasculature (see Table 23–1). Transudates and pulmonary edema will ultimately result in decreased oxygen saturation. The decreased cardiac output leads to acidosis and fluid retention.

Diagnostic Procedures

Chest x-rays may demonstrate the left ventricular hypertrophy characteristic of chronic aortic regurgitation. Dilation of the ascending aorta may be detected. Chronic aortic regurgitation eventually causes left atrial enlargement, which may be evident. Acute and chronic conditions with left ventricular failure will demonstrate pulmonary congestion.

The ECG usually has a left axis deviation and often tall R waves in $V_{4\text{-}6}$ with chronic aortic regurgitation. First-degree AV block is common. Left or right bundle branch blocks and third-degree AV block are also seen. In acute aortic regurgitation nonspecific ST-T wave changes may be seen, and sinus tachycardia is nearly universal.

Echocardiography is used to track the severity of aortic regurgitation (see Table 23–2). In chronic conditions the dilated aorta may be documented. Aortic valve leaflet movement, thickness, and vegetations may be visualized. Left ventricular diameter, wall thickness, and motion can be determined. Tracking the left ventricular end-systolic diameter is often used to determine the best time for surgical intervention. Echocardiography may demonstrate fluttering of the anterior or posterior mitral valve leaflet or the ventricular septum during diastole, caused by the regurgitant blood flow. The size, shape, direction, and velocity of the regurgitant jet may be determined by color Doppler. The size of the left atrium can be determined. Patients with acute aortic regurgitation often demonstrate a delayed slow opening of the mitral valve, diastolic anterior mitral valve leaflet or ventricular septal fluttering, and early mitral valve closure. Indications that the aorta has dissected may also be obtained by echocardiography.

Phonocardiography may be most useful for detecting acute aortic regurgitation when tachycardia alters the sounds and shortens diastole. Recorded simultaneously with the ECG, it can identify both components of the first and second heart sounds. The third heart sound may be depicted. The murmur of aortic regurgitation may be recorded immediately after the aortic component of the second heart sound. In chronic aortic regurgitation, the Austin Flint murmur may also be recorded.

Graded exercise studies may be utilized to document a patient's activity tolerance. Radionuclide studies may be utilized independently or in combination with graded exercise studies. The extent of the regurgitation may be quantified by blood pool imaging, and ejection fractions can be determined.

Cardiac catheterization is employed when surgical intervention is contemplated. The aorta is visualized for dilation and lesions and to determine the degree of regurgitation. Left ventricular pressures, cardiac output, ejection fraction, and regurgitant fraction can be measured and quantified. Left ventricular wall motion is also recorded. The coronary arteries are usually visualized, and CAD may be evaluated. Right heart catheterization is used to determine pulmonary, right heart, and venous pressures.

Clinical Management

The comprehensive health care plan should consider all four elements listed in Table 23–4. The signs and symptoms determine the priority of treatment for aortic regurgitation. Antibiotic prophylaxis (see Table 23–3) for endocarditis should be prescribed for all patients undergoing dental and surgical procedures. Amoxicillin is used, and gentamicin or vancomycin may be added to the regimen. Vigorous sports and heavy exertion should be avoided. Systemic hypertension is treated with hydralazine or nifedipine; propranolol is avoided because left ventricular function may be compromised. Left ventricular failure treatment may include digitalis, diuretics (hydralazine, furosemide), vasodilators (nitrates, sodium nitroprusside, ace inhibitors), and a salt-restricted diet. Once symptoms of ventricular failure present, surgery is the treatment of choice. Dysrhythmias should be treated with antidysrhythmics. Isometric exercises and the use of an intraaortic balloon pump are to be avoided because both increase diastolic pressures and accentuate the regurgitation.

Acute aortic regurgitation usually requires aortic valve surgery at an early stage. Chronic aortic regurgitation may not require valve surgery for many years. The ultimate treatment for both types of aortic regurgitation is usually surgical valve replacement (see Chap. 24). The best time for surgery is before the occurrence of significant left ventricular failure. Valvuloplasty may be attempted in a few cases. Torn leaflets or those torn from the annulus may be surgically repaired. The annulus may be narrowed with a stent or by excising a section of the dilated aorta that is dilating the annulus. The majority of surgical procedures consist of total valve replacements. Considerations relating to prostheses are as follows:

1. Mechanical valves (ball-cage or disc) require the patient to take anticoagulants to prevent thrombus formation as long as the valve is in place.
2. Tissue valves (allografts, xenografts, heterografts, autografts) do not require prolonged anticoagulation, but the leaflets become stiff and sometimes calcify or leak after being exposed to the high-pressure blood flow in the aortic position.
3. The annulus of all valve prostheses and some of the components will create some degree of aortic stenosis (Fig. 23–7). (Refer to the section on mitral regurgitation for criteria for prosthesis selection.)

The aortic valve presents a unique problem compared to the other cardiac valves because of the proximity of the coronary artery ostia and the frequent association with aortic root dilation. Postoperatively, patients will continue to require antibiotic prophylaxis for endocarditis and may require antidysrhythmics or anticoagulation (warfarin).

AORTIC STENOSIS

Pathophysiology

Aortic stenosis may be caused by idiopathic fibrosis and calcification as an individual ages (Fig. 23–16).

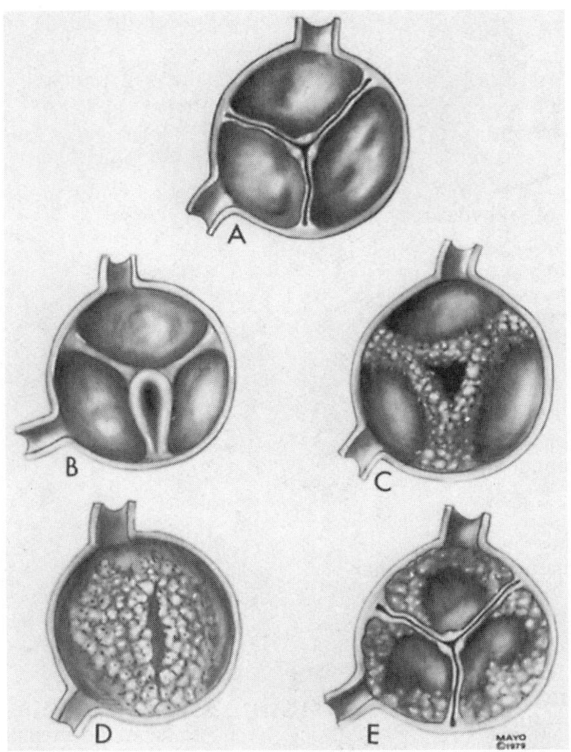

FIGURE 23–16. Types of aortic valve stenosis. *A*, Normal aortic valve. *B*, Congenital aortic stenosis. *C*, Rheumatic aortic stenosis. *D*, Calcific bicuspid aortic stenosis. *E*, Calcific senile aortic stenosis. (By permission of Mayo Foundation.)

The calcification of the leaflets usually begins along the edge of the annulus and slowly moves toward the commissures. Eventually, the leaflet's endothelial layer is injured and becomes fibrous, scarred, and thickened. The aortic valve cusps become less mobile, and the commissures may fuse, narrowing the orifice. Microthrombi may develop on the cusps during and after this process.

Atherosclerotic changes of the aorta or valve may also immobilize the cusps or cause fusion of the commissures. The aortic valve may be immobilized by lipid deposits on the cusps in patients with hyperlipidemia, vegetations of active infection or calcified vegetations due to endocarditis, or accumulation of metabolic products from ochronosis or Fabry disease. Stenosis may be caused by a prosthetic valve that has a narrower orifice because of the mechanical annulus. Prosthetic valves also develop calcifications and stiffening and may develop thrombus, vegetations, or pannus.

Rheumatic endocarditis affects the aortic valve and may cause stenosis (Fig. 23–16). The cusps and annulus thicken, stiffen, and calcify. The commissures fuse and calcify. These changes may be a direct result of the inflammatory process or may predispose the valve to the fibrous, calcific process. In this case, the calcifications begin on the free edges of the leaflets.

Stenosis of the ascending aorta or narrowing of the subvalvular outflow tract by fibroelastic membranes (discrete subaortic stenosis) or muscular tissue (asymmetric septal hypertrophy/IHSS, papillary muscle mass) may mimic aortic valve stenosis. Congenital lesions are a more common cause of aortic stenosis (Fig. 23–16). The lesions are commonly unicuspid and bicuspid valves or malformed tricuspid valves, and calcification precipitates the symptoms. In many cases, the etiology of aortic stenosis is unknown.

Whatever the etiology, the stenotic aortic valve is typically calcified, decreasing both its mobility and its orifice size. Because the process is gradual, the left ventricle compensates for the increased systolic pressures needed by hypertrophy (Fig. 23–17). The hypertrophied ventricle generates high enough pressures to maintain normal stroke volume and cardiac output for a period of time. Left ventricular hypertrophy eventually elevates left ventricular end-diastolic pressures, increasing the work of the left atrium. The left atrium also hypertrophies. The atrial kick component is maintained (Starling's law). As stenosis continues, the left ventricle begins to fail and dilates. Stroke volume decreases, further increasing left ventricular volume and pressure. Strain on the left atrium develops, resulting in backward failure. The left atrial volume and pressures rise, followed by rises in pulmonary venous, capillary, and arterial pressures and then by right ventricular, atrial, and systemic venous pressures.

The rising left ventricular diastolic pressures inhibit coronary artery perfusion. Ventricular oxygen demand is often increased because of hypertrophy, tachycardia, and the need to work against the increased afterload of stenosis, which prolongs isovolumetric contraction. The degree of stenosis may limit stroke volume, which cannot be compensated by increased heart rate, so cardiac output falls.

Physical Assessment

Presenting symptoms of aortic stenosis may be dyspnea, angina, or syncope. Usually the patient is asymptomatic for many years. Dyspnea is usually noted on exertion and is an indication of left ventricular failure, either progressive or as a result of atrial fibrillation. Angina (described in the pathology section) may also be related to calcific emboli or concurrent CAD. Syncope is usually related to exertion and may also be a sign of left ventricular failure or dysrhythmia. Stroke, endocarditis, palpitations, sudden death, and vision disturbances may also be presenting symptoms.

Inspection usually reveals no abnormal findings. If congestive heart failure is present, jugular vein distention, peripheral edema, and respiratory distress may be noted. Palpation may reveal the slowly rising, sustained anacrotic pulse, especially at the carotid and brachial arteries (carotid sinus sensitivity should be considered before palpating the carotid). The carotid may also reveal systolic vibrations called the carotid shudder and, with left ventricular failure, pulsus alternans. The point of maximal impulse is of longer duration than normal and, as the left ventricle dilates, is displaced laterally and caudally. A systolic thrill may be palpable at the second intercostal space on either

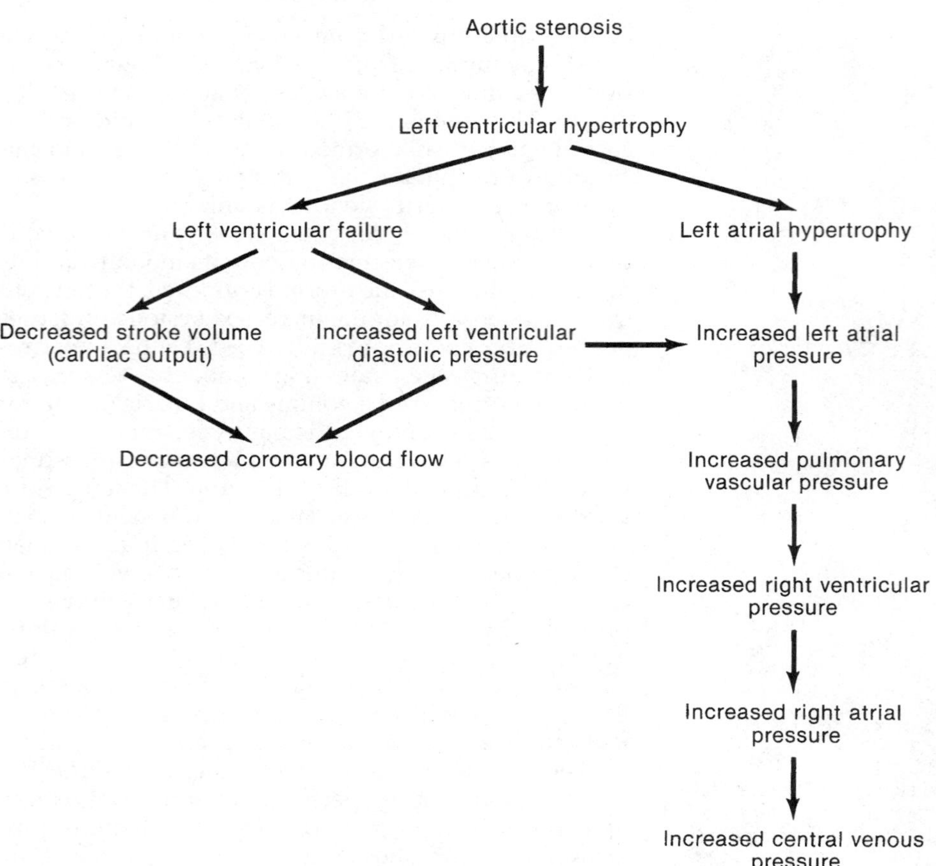

FIGURE 23–17. Pathophysiology of aortic stenosis. (Adapted from Schakenbach, L. H., Physiologic dynamics of acquired valvular heart disease, *Journal of Cardiovascular Nursing, 1*(3), 1–17, with permission of Aspen Publishers, Inc., © 1987.)

side of the sternum, especially during exhalation with the patient sitting and leaning forward. If right heart failure has been prolonged, the liver may be palpable.

Auscultation usually reveals a soft first heart sound as the mitral valve closes early. The second heart sound is variable. While the cusps are mobile, the aortic component may be accentuated, but once they are immobile, the aortic component may be absent. The second heart sound is often single or, with left ventricular failure or left bundle branch block, paradoxical. The third and fourth heart sounds are often heard. An aortic ejection click, a high-pitched sound heard best along the left sternal border, may be heard immediately after the first heart sound if the cusps are mobile. The murmur is a harsh, high-pitched, systolic murmur that is crescendo-decrescendo in nature. The murmur is heard best at the right sternal border at the second intercostal space and may radiate to the neck or apex. The murmur will increase with amyl nitrate, squatting, or lying flat. The murmur will decrease with vasopressors, isometric exercise, the Valsalva maneuver, and standing. Other auscultatory findings may be pulmonary crackles with left ventricular failure and changes in blood pressure. The blood pressure usually demonstrates a low systolic combined with a normal diastolic pressure and, therefore, a narrowed pulse pressure. When the aorta is calcified, the systolic pressure may be elevated.

The ECG usually reveals normal sinus rhythm. First-degree AV block, left bundle branch block, and atrial fibrillation may also be evident. Hemodynamic monitoring may reveal high readings and prominent *a, c,* and *v* waves in the central venous pressure because of right ventricular failure. The PAWP is usually the first to demonstrate backward failure. PAWP may be elevated and may demonstrate prominent *a* waves from left ventricular failure. Pulmonary artery systolic pressure rises; diastolic pressure rises later. Pulmonary vascular resistance may also be elevated. The arterial line waveform may reveal the slow, flat, systolic waveform.

Laboratory Findings

The turbulent blood flow across the stenotic valve may damage red blood cells. Hemolytic anemia is demonstrated by a decreased red blood cell count. The red cell indices will demonstrate normocytic, normochromic red cells. Once left ventricular failure occurs, a decreased arterial oxygen saturation may be found (see Table 23–1).

Diagnostic Procedures

Chest x-rays may be normal with early aortic stenosis. As the left ventricle fails, left ventricular dilation, left atrial dilation, and pulmonary congestion or edema may be seen. The calcified valve or a dilated aorta, caused by the ejection jet of ventricular systole, may be seen on the x-ray.

The ECG may reveal left ventricular strain with large S waves in V_{1-2} and large R waves in V_{4-6} with depressed ST segments and inverted T waves. Left axis deviation may be noted, as well as left anterior hemiblock and right or left bundle branch block. Left atrial hypertrophy may be reflected by the P wave ending negatively in V_1.

Phonocardiograms can be helpful, especially in identifying the fourth heart sound, first heart sound, and ejection click. The second heart sound components can be demonstrated. The ECG and phonocardiogram used together can help to determine the degree of aortic stenosis.

Echocardiography is useful in diagnosing and monitoring the progression of aortic stenosis (see Table 23–2). The M-mode echocardiogram may demonstrate aortic cusp thickness and movement as well as left ventricular diameter and wall thickness. Two-dimensional echocardiography may demonstrate the number, thickness, shape, movement, and calcification of the aortic cusps. Left ventricular function can be documented. Doppler echocardiography may be used to determine the pressure gradient between the left ventricle and the aorta.

Radionuclide studies may be used to document ventricular function, myocardial perfusion, and left ventricular ejection fraction. Graded exercise studies are seldom attempted because of the risk of peripheral vasodilation, decreasing preload, and increasing heart rate. The resultant decrease in cardiac output and coronary perfusion may result in severe left ventricular failure.

Cardiac catheterization is used for definitive diagnosis of aortic stenosis. A catheter is used to measure left ventricular and aortic pressures. The gradient, systolic blood flow, and valve orifice area can be determined. Ventricular and atrial dimensions, wall thickness, and movement can be observed. The number and shape of the aortic cusps may be demonstrated. The functioning of the coronary arteries, aorta, and other valves can be evaluated as well.

Clinical Management

The comprehensive health care plan should consider all four elements in Table 23–4. The primary management of patients with aortic stenosis consists of prophylaxis for endocarditis (see Table 23–3). Amoxicillin is prescribed for all dental and surgical procedures. Gentamicin or ampicillin may be added to the regimen.

Once left ventricular failure develops, digoxin, diuretics (furosemide, hydrochlorothiazide), and low-salt diets may be prescribed to minimize the effects of ventricular failure until surgical repair can be provided. PACs are prophylactically treated with quinidine or disopyramide. Atrial fibrillation is treated with digoxin or quinidine. Electrical cardioversion is used, especially when loss of the atrial kick decreases the cardiac output. Unresolved atrial fibrillation is also an indication for anticoagulant therapy (warfarin, heparin).

When the patient develops left ventricular failure, angina, or syncope or when echocardiography or cardiac catheterization demonstrates significant aortic stenosis, surgical valve replacement is the treatment of choice (see Chapt. 24). Factors requiring consideration in regard to prosthetic valves were discussed in the Clinical Management of Aortic Regurgitation section.

One- and two-balloon percutaneous valvuloplasty, as well as open valvuloplasty procedures, are also options. Unfortunately, the disease process continues, the long-term results have been disappointing, and the procedures may result in aortic regurgitation.

Postoperatively, anticoagulation (warfarin and possibly also dipyridamole) is prescribed for all patients for 6 weeks; it is then discontinued if the valve replacement was a tissue valve. Supraventricular dysrhythmias are treated with digoxin. Ventricular dysrhythmias are treated with lidocaine or procainamide (Pronestyl). If dysrhythmias continue beyond 3 postoperative days, procainamide is continued for 6 weeks. The prophylactic antibiotic regimen should continue as described in Table 23–3.

Subvalvular fibrous membrane and supravalvular aortic stenoses are usually surgically corrected. Subvalvular muscular stenosis is usually treated with propranolol. Surgical intervention is attempted if symptoms persist despite propranolol therapy, but surgical mortality is high.

TRICUSPID REGURGITATION

Pathophysiology

Tricuspid regurgitation is rarely an isolated lesion. Most often, it is a sequela of rheumatic endocarditis (Fig. 23–18) and is highly correlated with mitral stenosis. It is also frequently the result of infectious endocarditis. Tricuspid valve endocarditis most often results from drug abuse but is also a complication of alcoholism, burns, immunodepression, rheumatic disease, untreated infections, and pulmonary artery catheters. The inflammatory reaction may result in thickened, shortened leaflets or fused, shortened chordae tendineae. Patients with infectious endocarditis may also develop vegetations that prevent apposition of the leaflets or that perforate the leaflets or chordae. The tricuspid valve annulus may be distorted by right ventricular dilation (Fig. 23–18). Some causes of right ventricular dilation are right ventricular failure, pulmonary hypertension, and left ventricular failure. Endomyocardial fibrosis and the carcinoid syndrome result in fibrous tissue development on the ventricular aspects of the leaflets. The fibrous tissue eventually causes adhesions between the leaflets and the right ventricular endocardium, preventing leaflet closure.

The tricuspid valve's papillary muscles may be

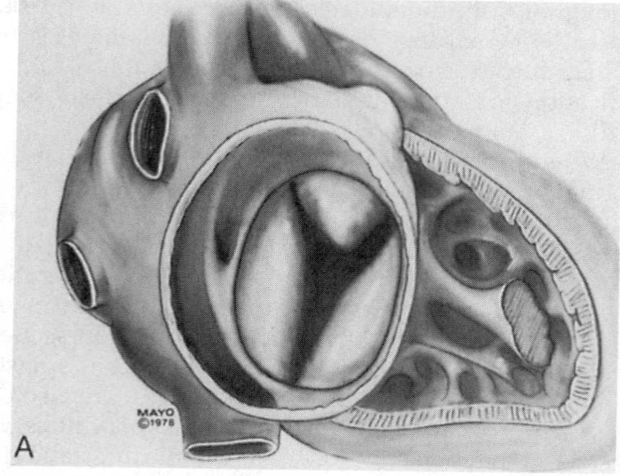

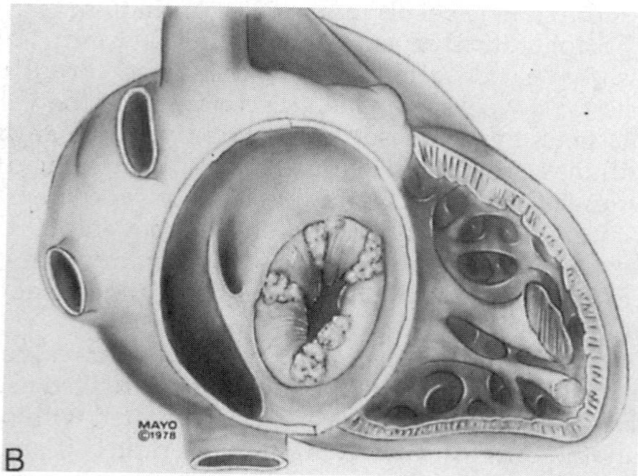

FIGURE 23–18. Types of tricuspid regurgitation. *A*, Functional tricuspid regurgitation secondary to dilation of the right ventricle. *B*, Organic rheumatic tricuspid regurgitation. (By permission of Mayo Foundation.)

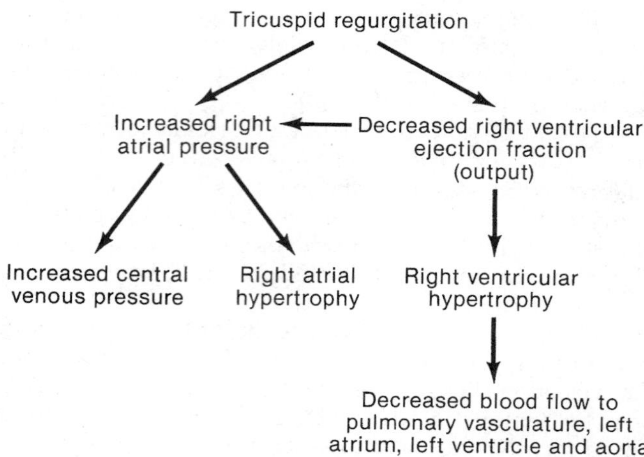

FIGURE 23–19. Pathophysiology of tricuspid regurgitation. (Adapted from Schakenbach, L. H., Physiologic dynamics of acquired valvular heart disease, *Journal of Cardiovascular Nursing, 1*(3), 1–17, with permission of Aspen Publishers, Inc., © 1987.)

ischemic, infarcted, or ruptured as a result of CAD and trauma. The trauma may be blunt (with no symptoms for a number of years) or may result from injury by pacer wires or right heart catheters. The tricuspid valve may develop myxomatous changes in the leaflets, annulus, or chordae tendineae. The central layer of the leaflets, the spongiosa, has an overabundance of myxomatous cells. These cells spread into the supporting layer of the leaflet, the fibrosa, interrupting its continuity. The weakened valve stretches and develops interchordeal hooding and prolapse. The surfaces of the leaflets that contact each other fibrose and thicken over time. The thinned, hooded areas develop collagenous fibrous tissue on the ventricular aspect, thickening the leaflet. The weakening and fibrous processes may also occur in the annulus and chordae. The annulus may become distorted or inflexible. The chordae may stretch or shorten. Myxomatous changes typically result in tricuspid regurgitation secondary to prolapse, usually of the posterior leaflet; the leaflets may also be drawn toward the ventricle and be unable to approximate.

Right atrial tumors may produce friction on a leaflet, stretching or perforating it. Ebstein anomaly is a congenital cause of tricuspid regurgitation. The posterior and septal leaflets develop abnormally. Some patients' leaflets are attached to the ventricular wall; others originate from the ventricular wall distal to the normal position. The anterior leaflet is usually large and fibrotic. The leaflets may be fused. The chordae and papillary muscles may be shortened or attached to the leaflets abnormally. Other congenital causes typically involve deformed leaflets.

In tricuspid regurgitation blood flows from the right ventricle to the right atrium during systole (Fig. 23–19). The increased right atrial volume increases right atrial pressure. The right atrium hypertrophies and dilates. Central venous volume and pressure increase. Peripheral edema and fluid weight gain progress to hepatomegaly and may cause ascites, intestinal vein distention, and splenomegaly. The dilated atrium typically fibrillates. Tricuspid regurgitation decreases right ventricular output through the pulmonary system and decreases left ventricular output. The right ventricle dilates to accommodate large diastolic volumes and hypertrophies in an attempt to increase output to the pulmonary system. The dilated ventricle may displace chordae or papillary muscles and actually increase the regurgitation.

Physical Assessment

Tricuspid regurgitation is asymptomatic in many patients, especially if it is an isolated lesion. Once the right ventricle fails to maintain its cardiac output, signs and symptoms increase. The initial symptoms of right heart failure are increased venous pressure, peripheral edema, fluid retention and, therefore, weight gain. Some patients can feel the systolic pulsations of the jugular vein. Eventually, hepatomegaly, ascites, and splenomegaly develop. Hepatomegaly may cause abdominal pain. Ascites and venous engorgement may cause anorexia and weight loss. The decreased cardiac output may limit activity tolerance. Low cardiac output or perfusion may cause fatigue and peripheral cyanosis due to desaturated hemoglobin. When tricuspid regurgitation develops as a result of severe left ventricular failure, the pulmonary symptoms of left ventricular failure may decrease or resolve. The patient will have decreased dyspnea, will regain the ability to lie supine, and will have fewer crackles. Tricuspid regurgitation is seldom an isolated lesion, and symptoms of other conditions are often more prominent.

Inspection may reveal jugular neck vein distention. In normal sinus rhythm the *a* wave has little or no *x* descent, and the *c* and *v* waves merge and are prominent. The *c-v* wave, also called an *s* wave, is followed by a brisk *y* descent. If atrial fibrillation is the rhythm, no *a* waves are noted, but the *c-v* wave and *y* descent remain. There is a positive hepatojugular reflux, and liver pulsations may be noted in the right flank. Eventually, congestion causes cirrhosis of the liver, and pulsations may cease. Anorexia will cause weight loss. The patient may be jaundiced or may demonstrate ascites as right ventricular failure progresses. Water weight gain may then become evident. Peripheral edema is common, and the veins in the extremities may also pulsate. The lips, tongue, face, and nailbeds are the first to develop cyanosis. The lower sternum and lower left sternal border may pulsate as a result of right ventricular hypertrophy, and the lower right sternal border may pulsate as a result of right atrial hypertrophy.

Palpation of the chest often reveals a lower sternal lift. The liver is palpable, and pulsations may be palpable. While the liver is engorged, it is tender, but once it becomes cirrhotic, it is firm and nontender. The pulse is often tachycardiac and will be regular in sinus rhythm and irregular in atrial fibrillation. Palpation will assist in determining the severity of peripheral edema and in diagnosing ascites. The spleen may be palpated.

On auscultation a normal blood pressure is usually present until cardiac output becomes severely impaired. The first heart sound may be normal if the mitral component is normal and the patient in normal sinus rhythm, or soft, as with atrial fibrillation or an abnormal mitral valve. The second heart sound may be normal or, if pulmonary hypertension is present, the pulmonary component may be louder. When right bundle branch block coexists, the physiologic splitting of the second heart sound will be widened. A third heart sound is often present, originating from the right ventricle; it is heard best along the lower left sternal border. The third heart sound is louder during inspiration. The murmur is a blowing, high-pitched, systolic sound heard best at the lower left sternal border or xiphoid area. The murmur may be enhanced by inspiration, lying down, exercise, and amyl nitrate. It is decreased by standing and the Valsalva maneuver. The murmur is often difficult to identify because right heart pressures are so low.

Hemodynamic monitoring will demonstrate the central venous pressure waveforms that correspond with the jugular vein pulsations noted during inspection. The *a* wave may not be present because of atrial fibrillation. In normal sinus rhythm the *x* descent is small or absent. The *c* and *v* waves merge and are large, and the *y* descent is steep. Pressures are elevated. The cardiac index may be low. ECG monitoring may demonstrate normal sinus rhythm, sinus tachycardia or, most commonly, atrial fibrillation. Incomplete or complete right bundle branch block, PACs, and large, notched P waves may be present.

Laboratory Findings

Chronic liver congestion may be evidenced by hypoalbuminemia. In more advanced cases, coagulopathies may be noted. Low cardiac output conditions may cause venous oxygen saturations to fall below 70%. Blood cultures may be positive if an infectious process is active (see Table 23–1).

Diagnostic Procedures

Chest x-rays may demonstrate right atrial, right ventricular, or superior vena cava enlargement. The azygos vein may be distended, and the resulting pleural effusions may be evident. If ascites has developed, the diaphragm will be displaced cephalically.

Fluoroscopy may be used to identify systolic pulsations of the right atrium and superior vena cava.

Electrocardiograms will provide additional information. The axis can be determined and is usually deviated to the right but may be vertical. Right ventricular hypertrophy may be confirmed by voltage criteria. Right atrial enlargement may be confirmed by Q waves in V_1. Atrial fibrillation is very common.

Phonocardiograms may be helpful because right heart sounds are soft, and tricuspid regurgitation may be overshadowed by other cardiac valve lesions. The components of the first heart sound and murmur can be recorded. The second and, if present, the third heart sounds may be documented.

Echocardiography may be of assistance in diagnosing tricuspid regurgitation (see Table 23–2). M-mode echocardiography can be used to document right atrial and ventricular size, septal movement, vegetations and, especially in systole, leaflet movement. Two-dimensional echocardiography is used to identify vegetations and, in combination with an intravenous contrast agent, will demonstrate blood flow back and forth across the valve. Doppler and transesophageal echocardiography may also be used.

Right heart cardiac catheterization may be useful. Pressure and waveform recordings can be obtained. Contrast material can be injected into the ventricle, but regurgitation may be created or exaggerated by the catheter crossing the tricuspid valve. Indicator–dilution curves have been more useful. An indicator is injected into the right ventricle, and samples are taken from the right atrium and the femoral artery. The indicator appears in atrial samples more quickly or in higher concentrations than in arterial samples and is an indication of tricuspid regurgitation.

Clinical Management

Management of tricuspid regurgitation varies with the symptoms and etiology. The comprehensive health care plan should consider all four elements listed in Table 23–4. Treatment of isolated tricuspid regurgitation is geared to the etiology. Antibiotic treatment and prophylaxis (Table 23–3) for rheumatic disease and for endocarditis during dental and surgical procedures is achieved with amoxicillin. Gentamicin and ampicillin may be added to the regimen. Right ventricular failure is treated with digoxin, diuretics (furosemide, hydrochlorothiazide), vasodilators (nitroglycerin, nitroprusside), low-salt diets, fluid restriction, and activity restriction. Atrial fibrillation is treated with digoxin, quinidine, or electrical cardioversion as well as with anticoagulation (warfarin). Tricuspid regurgitation related to left heart or pulmonary pathology is treated by treating the original cause. Patients with tricuspid endocarditis secondary to substance abuse require treatment for their dependent behavior and personality as well as for the endocarditis.

Surgical intervention is rarely required unless pulmonary artery hypertension is chronic or the leaflets are deformed. Most surgical interventions are associated with mitral valve surgery (see Chap. 24). Two types of valvuloplasty may be performed, plication of the posterior leaflet or narrowing of the annulus. Surgery on the annulus may be comprised by a purse-string suture or a ring/stent. Total valve replacement (see Fig. 23–7) may be done with either mechanical (ball-cage, disc) or tissue (porcine, bovine, human) prostheses; the latter are preferred. Tissue valve stiffening and calcification do not occur with the low right heart pressures characteristic of tricuspid regurgitation; however, most surgeons use anticoagulation (warfarin, dipyridamole) for all patients because of the slow blood flow in the right heart. Endocarditis prophylaxis is prescribed for life. Digoxin and diuretics may be required for a few months after surgery.

TRICUSPID STENOSIS

Pathophysiology

Tricuspid stenosis is most commonly the result of rheumatic disease. It is usually associated with left heart valve involvement. The inflammatory process results in fibrosing of the leaflets, commissures, and chordae. Most commonly, the commissures fuse (usually the anteroseptal commissure), narrowing the orifice. The chordae thicken, shorten, and fuse. Infectious endocarditis may result in the same changes but is rare in the right heart except among intravenous drug users. In addition, vegetations may occlude part or all of the lumen.

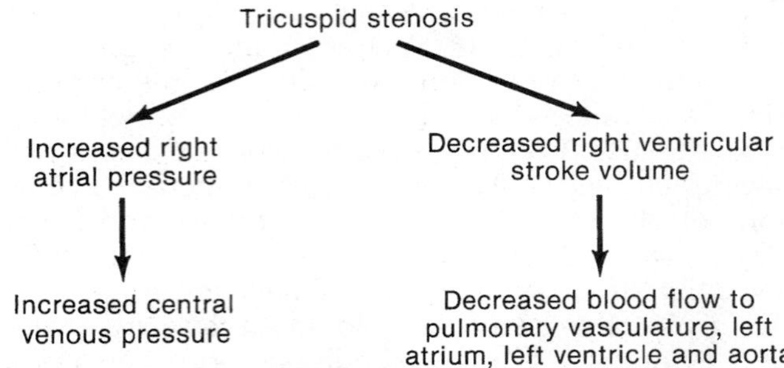

FIGURE 23–20. Pathophysiology of tricuspid stenosis. (Adapted from Schakenbach, L. H., Physiologic dynamics of acquired valvular heart disease, *Journal of Cardiovascular Nursing, 1*(3), 1–17, with permission of Aspen Publishers, Inc., © 1987.)

Atrial myxomas or thrombi may occlude the right ventricular inflow channel. Endocardial fibroelastosis and the carcinoid syndrome result in fibrous tissue development on the leaflets, which may fuse the commissures or stiffen the leaflets, decreasing their movement. A form of Ebstein anomaly with fused leaflets may also cause stenosis.

Tricuspid stenosis results in accumulation of blood in the right atrium and in less blood reaching the right ventricle (Fig. 23–20). The increased volume and pressure dilate and hypertrophy the right atrium. The veins entering the atria dilate as the volume of blood backs into the system. Pressures in the venous organs, such as the liver and spleen, rise, and the organs become engorged; peripheral edema is seen. Eventually, the liver fibroses. Decreased right ventricular filling volumes result in decreased cardiac output throughout the pulmonary and systemic circulations.

Physical Assessment

Dyspnea and fatigue are the most common symptoms of tricuspid stenosis. Patients cannot increase their cardiac output with exertion. Dyspnea and fatigue may also be the result of mitral stenosis, which is nearly always present with tricuspid stenosis. The pulmonary symptoms of mitral stenosis often decrease as tricuspid stenosis progresses. Other symptoms reported by patients result from venous distention, pulsations of the neck (jugular vein), and abdominal fullness or discomfort (hepatic vein).

Inspection demonstrates jugular vein distention with a slow *y* descent and, in normal sinus rhythm, a prominent *a* wave and slow *x* descent. There is a positive hepatojugular reflux. Peripheral, generalized, or central edema may be observed. The right flank may demonstrate diastolic hepatic pulsations. In advanced stages, cyanosis resulting from low cardiac output and jaundice due to hepatomegaly may cause the skin to have a greenish cast.

Palpation may reveal pulsations at the lower right sternal border due to right atrial hypertrophy. A diastolic thrill may also be felt at the lower left sternal border during inspiration.

Auscultation may demonstrate an accentuated first heart sound because the tricuspid valve closure may be intensified. The second heart sound may not demonstrate normal respiratory splitting because right ventricular filling is fixed. The murmur is a rumbling, low-pitched, decrescendo diastolic sound. It is best appreciated at the left sternal border in the fourth intercostal space or lower. The murmur may be increased during inspiration, while lying on the left side or squatting, during isotonic or isometric exercise, while raising the legs, and with amyl nitrate. The murmur is diminished by exhalation and the Valsalva maneuver. Auscultation at the left sternal border at the fourth intercostal space may also demonstrate an opening snap.

Hemodynamic monitoring demonstrates central venous waveforms corresponding with the jugular vein pulsations noted during inspection. Pressures are elevated. The cardiac index may be low, and passing a catheter through the stenotic valve may not be possible. ECG monitoring usually demonstrates atrial fibrillation if the cause is rheumatic disease, but normal sinus rhythm may be present if the cause is right sided.

Laboratory Findings

Chronic liver congestion may be evidenced by hypoalbuminemia. In later stages, coagulopathies may be evident. Low cardiac output conditions may cause venous oxygen saturations to fall below 70%. Blood cultures may be positive if an infectious process is active (see Table 23–1).

Diagnostic Procedures

Chest x-rays may demonstrate right atrial or superior vena cava enlargement. ECGs may demonstrate the increased P wave amplitude and depressed PR interval (atrial repolarization) characteristic of right atrial hypertrophy. The P wave may be deformed. Atrial fibrillation is the most common cardiac rhythm. Phonocardiograms are often very useful for recording the components of the first and second heart sounds as well as the opening snap. The murmur may be better appreciated, especially when other valve lesions are also present.

Echocardiograms may be used to identify the movement and thickness of the leaflets (see Table 23–2). M-mode may be able to demonstrate atrial thrombus, leaflet vegetations, calcification, and atrial and ventricular size. Two-dimensional or transesophageal echocardiography may also document the size of the tricuspid valve orifice.

Cardiac catheterization may be used to record pressures simultaneously in the right atrium and ventricle to confirm a gradient. Contrast medium may be injected into the right atrium to visualize the contour of the blood flow tract. Right atrial wall thickness as well as leaflet mobility and thickening may also be visualized. Right atrial pressures and waveforms may be documented.

Clinical Management

Antibiotic treatment and prophylactic therapy with amoxicillin (see Table 23–3) are prescribed for endocarditis. Gentamicin and ampicillin may be added to the regimen. Symptoms of venous congestion may be treated with low-sodium diet, fluid restriction, diuretics (furosemide, hydrochlorothiazide), and digoxin. Quinidine may be added if atrial fibrillation exists. The comprehensive health care plan should consider all four elements listed in Table 23–4.

Surgical correction of tricuspid stenosis is indicated if the stenosis is severe (see Chap. 24). One- and two-balloon percutaneous valvuloplasty has been used, but may be complicated by tricuspid regurgitation or right bundle branch block. Finger valvulotomies have had limited success and have been complicated by tricuspid regurgitation. Open commissurotomies of either septal leaflet commissure have been successful. Commissurotomy of the anterior-posterior leaflet commissure has been complicated by tricuspid regurgitation. Valve replacement with mechanical (ball-cage, disc) or tissue (porcine, bovine, human) prostheses has been successful (Fig. 23–7). Low blood flow on the right side is an indication for anticoagulation (warfarin, dipyridamole) regardless of what kind of prosthesis is used, although tissue valves are preferred due to lower thrombogenetics. Tissue valves do not stiffen or calcify in the low-flow, low-pressure environment of the right heart. Endocarditis prophylaxis is continued, and digoxin and diuretics may be continued for a few months after surgery.

PULMONIC REGURGITATION

Pathophysiology

Pulmonic regurgitation is often the result of pulmonary hypertension. The annulus stretches, and the leaflets cannot approximate. The same mechanism of dilation may result from a syphilitic aneurysm or an idiopathic or connective tissue abnormality of the pulmonary artery. Regurgitation may be the result of a valvulotomy for pulmonic stenosis. Infective and rheumatic endocarditis and the carcinoid syndrome all result in fibrous plaque formation on the leaflets. The plaques cause contractures of the leaflets, preventing apposition. Pulmonic regurgitation may also be the result of congenitally absent or malformed leaflets.

Pulmonic regurgitation results in blood flowing from the pulmonary artery into the right ventricle dur-

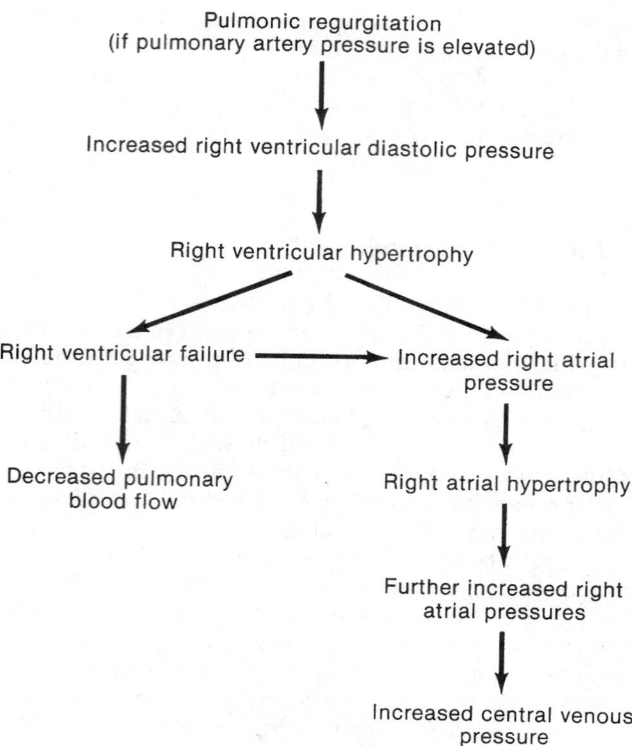

FIGURE 23–21. Pathophysiology of pulmonic regurgitation. (Adapted from Schakenbach, L. H., Physiologic dynamics of acquired valvular heart disease, *Journal of Cardiovascular Nursing, 1*(3), 1–17, with permission of Aspen Publishers, Inc., © 1987.)

ing diastole (Fig. 23–21). Right ventricular volume and pressure will increase if pulmonary artery pressures are high. Increased volume and pressure cause the right ventricle to hypertrophy. Right atrial volume and pressure may increase, causing right atrial hypertrophy and increased central venous pressure. If pulmonary artery pressure remains high, the hypertrophied right ventricle may eventually fail. Pulmonic regurgitation with normal or low pulmonary artery pressure seldom produces pathophysiologic changes.

Physical Assessment

Pulmonic regurgitation without pulmonary hypertension is usually asymptomatic and is well tolerated. There are no visible or palpable signs of the condition. The murmur is a blowing, medium-pitched, crescendo-decrescendo diastolic sound. It is accentuated by inspiration and amyl nitrate. It is heard best at the third or fourth intercostal space at the left sternal border. It follows a short pause after the second heart sound. The second heart sound may be normal, may be more widely split, or may not have a pulmonic component.

Pulmonic regurgitation with pulmonary hypertension may present with signs of right heart failure (weight gain, edema, fatigue, dyspnea) but typically presents with signs and symptoms characteristic of the cause of the pulmonary hypertension. Inspection may rarely reveal distended jugular veins. Palpation of the lower left sternal border may reveal a pulsation characteristic of right ventricular hypertrophy. Palpation of the second intercostal space at the left sternal border may reveal systolic pulsations or the systolic or diastolic thrill of an enlarged pulmonary artery. Auscultation usually reveals a loud second heart sound that is widely split. Third and fourth heart sounds may be found at the fourth intercostal space at the left sternal border. A pulmonary artery ejection click may precede the blowing, high-pitched, decrescendo, diastolic murmur. The murmur is heard best at the left midsternal border and increases with inspiration or amyl nitrate.

Laboratory Findings

There are no specific laboratory findings for pulmonic regurgitation (see Table 23–1).

Diagnostic Procedures

Chest x-rays of pulmonic regurgitation without pulmonary hypertension may reveal an enlarged pulmonary artery and, more rarely, an enlarged right ventricle. The ECG may reveal right ventricular diastolic overload with an rSr′ or rsR′ in leads V_1 and V_2.

Chest x-rays of patients with pulmonic regurgitation and pulmonary hypertension usually demonstrate enlargement of the pulmonary artery, right atrium, and right ventricle. The ECG may reveal right ventricular hypertrophy or right bundle branch block.

Pulmonic regurgitation with and without pulmonary hypertension may be evaluated by other techniques. Phonocardiograms are often useful for differentiating the heart sounds and murmurs. M-mode, transesophageal, and two-dimensional echocardiography may demonstrate leaflet movement, vegetations, and ventricular enlargement or hypertrophy. Pulsed and color Doppler echocardiography may identify the regurgitant flow (see Table 23–2). Cardiac catheterization may be used to measure pressure gradients or record regurgitation of a contrast material from the pulmonary artery into the right ventricle. Some regurgitation will occur because the catheter traverses the pulmonary valve.

Clinical Management

The comprehensive health care plan should consider all four elements listed in Table 23–4. The primary treatment of pulmonic regurgitation is prophylaxis for endocarditis (see Table 23–3) with amoxicillin. Gentamicin and ampicillin may be added to the regimen. If right ventricular failure occurs, it is treated with digoxin. Surgical intervention is rarely required for pulmonic regurgitation but may be utilized for individuals with severe right ventricular failure (see Chap. 24). Tissue prostheses (bovine, porcine, human) are preferred to mechanical (ball-cage, disc) prostheses because less thrombus formation (see Fig. 23–7) is associated with their use. Anticoagulants (warfarin, dipyridamole) are then prescribed because the low blood flow of the right heart predisposes all prostheses to thrombus. The low pressures of the right heart do not stiffen or calcify tissue prostheses as in the left heart. Endocarditis prophylaxis is continued, and digoxin may also need to be continued.

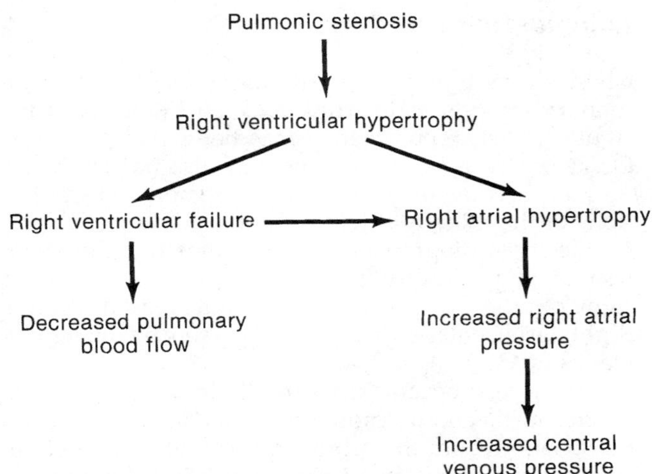

FIGURE 23–22. Pathophysiology of pulmonic stenosis. (Adapted from Schakenbach, L. H., Physiologic dynamics of acquired valvular heart disease, *Journal of Cardiovascular Nursing, 1*(3), 1–17, with permission of Aspen Publishers, Inc., © 1987.)

PULMONIC STENOSIS

Pathophysiology

Pulmonic stenosis is most commonly a congenital lesion and is frequently associated with atrial or ventricular septal defects and tetralogy of Fallot. The congenital malformation is often leaflets fused at the annulus, leaving a small opening at the center and giving a dome shape to the valve. Another configuration is dysplasia, three shortened, thickened, and immobilized leaflets, the result of an overgrowth of myxomatous tissue.

The rare acquired pulmonic stenosis may result from thickened leaflets and commissural fusion resulting from rheumatic endocarditis or the carcinoid syndrome. Calcific pericarditis may immobilize the leaflets or annulus. Pulmonic calcification also occurs as a sequela to pulmonary hypertension or cardiac or pulmonary tumors, or thrombi may occlude blood flow and mimic pulmonic stenosis.

Pulmonic stenosis causes obstruction to right ventricular systolic ejection (Fig. 23–22). Right ventricular volume and pressure increases; right ventricular stroke volume decreases. The right ventricle hypertrophies and may dilate. The stiff, hypertrophied right ventricle and elevated diastolic pressures increase the work of the right atrium. Right atrial volume and pressure rises. The right atrium hypertrophies, and venous volume and pressure rises. Right ventricular failure may occur.

Physical Assessment

Many individuals have no symptoms and very few signs of pulmonic stenosis. The presenting symptom may be pulsations of the neck, exertional dyspnea or fatigue, dizziness, and syncope. Late symptoms are peripheral edema, ascites, weight gain, cyanosis, and hepatomegaly due to right ventricular failure and angina.

Inspection may identify a round or triangular face, cyanosis, distended neck veins or large jugular vein *a* waves, and a left parasternal lift. More rarely, clubbing or flushed fingers or toes may be evident. Palpation may identify a left parasternal or subxiphoid pulsation from right ventricular hypertrophy. A thrill is often found at the second intercostal space at the left sternal border. In the late stages, hepatomegaly, hepatojugular reflux, peripheral edema, and ascites may be found.

Auscultation often identifies the only sign of pulmonic stenosis. The second heart sound eventually softens as the pulmonic component decreases in intensity. The second sound may split on exhalation and widen further during inspiration or may not be audible because of the murmur. An ejection click may be audible at the second intercostal space at the left sternal border as the stenotic valve snaps open. The murmur is often the first sign of pulmonic stenosis. The murmur is a harsh, crescendo-decrescendo, systolic sound heard best at the second intercostal space at the left sternal border. The murmur may radiate along the left sternal border and the neck.

The ECG monitor usually reveals normal sinus rhythm but may demonstrate supraventricular or ventricular tachycardias and AV blocks. Hemodynamic monitoring may reveal elevated central venous or right atrial pressures. Swan-Ganz catheters may be difficult to place, but the waveform often demonstrates a slow upstroke.

Laboratory Findings

There are no laboratory findings specific to pulmonic stenosis (see Table 23–1).

Diagnostic Procedures

Chest x-rays typically reveal enlargement of the pulmonary artery's main trunk and left branches. If the right ventricle is enlarged, it may be seen on the x-ray. Occasionally, a calcified valve may also be visualized.

Fluoroscopy may be used to demonstrate pulsations of the main and left pulmonary arteries.

Electrocardiograms usually demonstrate right ventricular hypertrophy with incomplete or complete right bundle branch block and right axis deviation. Right atrial enlargement may be seen by upright P waves in V_1.

Phonocardiograms are often helpful to differentiate the aortic and pulmonic components of the second heart sound from the murmur. It can also graph both components of the first heart sound and differentiate the ejection click. The changes in timing and intensity of each sound during inhalation and exhalation can be graphed.

Echocardiograms are not able to demonstrate the pulmonic valve definitively (see Table 23–2). M-mode echocardiography cannot visualize the anterior leaflet but can demonstrate atrial contractions and ventricular size and wall motion, which can support the diagnosis. Two-dimensional and transesophageal echocardiography may demonstrate the shape, thickness, and movement of the pulmonic valve leaflets. Vegetations and stenosis may be identified. Ventricular size and wall motion can be determined. Pulsed and color Doppler echocardiograms are utilized to identify flow dynamics.

Cardiac catheterization of the right heart may be used to demonstrate the severity and location of pulmonic stenosis. Central venous, right atrial, and right ventricular pressures may be recorded. Pulmonary pressures may be recorded if the catheter can be maneuvered across the valve and the pressure gradient between the right ventricle and pulmonary artery calculated.

Clinical Management

The comprehensive health care plan should consider all four elements listed in Table 23–4. The primary treatment of pulmonic stenosis is prophylaxis for endocarditis (see Table 23–3) with amoxicillin. Gentamicin and ampicillin may be added to the regimen. Ventricular or pulmonary thromboses are indications for anticoagulation. Right ventricular failure is an indication for surgical correction (see Chap. 24). Valvuloplasty, valvulotomy, commissurotomy for fused commissures, or excision of leaflets may be performed. Pulmonic regurgitation may result and is often tolerated. Pulmonic valve replacement is rare. Tissue prostheses (bovine, porcine, human) are preferred to mechanical prostheses (ball-cage, disc) because there is less thrombus formation (see Fig. 23–7). Anticoagulants (warfarin, dipyridamole) must be prescribed because the low blood flow increases the risk of thrombus formation. The low flow does not stiffen or calcify tissue prostheses as in the left heart. Endocarditis prophylaxis must continue after any surgical intervention.

SUMMARY

This chapter has reviewed some of the specific characteristics of regurgitation and stenosis of each cardiac valve. The primary pathophysiology for each valvular disorder has been discussed in detail; predominant causes are connective tissue disorders, coronary artery disease, and endocarditis. Signs and symptoms develop because the valves cannot maintain unidirectional blood flow. Physical assessment of the patient, including the timing and characteristics of the murmur unique to each valvular condition, was presented. Laboratory analysis was discussed, although it does not usually provide more than supporting data in the diagnosis and tracking of valvular heart disease. Echocardiography was reviewed as the most reliable method of diagnosing and monitoring the progression of cardiac valve disorders. Treatment is prescribed according to symptoms. Surgical intervention is usually late in the course of the disease process. Patients with valvular heart disorders need to be able to manage their chronic disease, and nurses should be prepared to collaborate in the process.

REFERENCES

Arora, R., et al. (1993). Immediate and long-term results of balloon and surgical closed mitral valvotomy: A randomized comparative study. *American Heart Journal, 125,* 1091–1094.

Barlow, J. B. (Ed.). (1987). *Perspective on the mitral valve.* Philadelphia: F. A. Davis.

Baue, A. E., et al. (1991). *Glenn's thoracic and cardiovascular surgery* (5th ed.). Norwalk, Conn.: Appleton & Lange.

Berne, R. M., & Levy, M. N. (1992). *Cardiovascular physiology* (6th ed.). St. Louis: C. V. Mosby.

Bojar, R. M. (1992). *Adult cardiac surgery.* Boston: Blackwell Scientific Publications.

Braunwald, E. (Ed.). (1992). *Heart disease* (4th ed.). Philadelphia: W. B. Saunders.

Cheitlin, M. D., Sokolow, M., & McIlroy, M. B. (1993). *Clinical cardiology* (6th ed.). Norwalk, CT: Appleton & Lange.

Dajani, A. S., et al. (1990). Prevention of bacterial endocarditis: Recommendations by the American Heart Association. *Journal of the American Medical Association, 264,* 2919–2922.

David, T. E., Bos, J., & Rakowski, H. (1991). Mitral valve repair by replacement of chordae tendineae with polytetrafluoroethylene sutures. *Journal of Thoracic and Cardiovascular Surgery, 101,* 495–501.

Davis, E. A., et al. (1993). Valvular disease in the elderly: Influence on surgical results. *Annals of Thoracic Surgery, 55,* 333–337.

Dubin, D. (1989). *Rapid interpretation of EKGs* (4th ed.). Tampa, FL: Cover Publishing Company.

Feigenbaum, H. (1994). *Echocardiography* (5th ed.). Philadelphia: Lea & Febiger.

Frankl, W. S., & Brest, A. N. (Eds.). (1993). *Valvular heart disease: Comprehensive evaluation and treatment.* Philadelphia: F. A. Davis.

Gillum, R. F. (1993). Nonrheumatic valvular heart disease in the United States. *American Heart Journal, 125,* 915–918.

Gregory, F., et al. (1988). A new technique for repair of mitral insufficiency caused by ruptured chordae of the anterior leaflet. *Journal of Thoracic and Cardiovascular Surgery, 96,* 765–768.

Hunt, A. H. (1985). Mitral valve prolapse: Physical assessment, complications and management. *Nurse Practitioner, 10*(4), 15–21.

Katz, A. M. (1992). *Physiology of the heart* (2nd ed.). New York: Raven.

Kaul, U. A., et al. (1993). Long-term results after balloon pulmonary valvuloplasty in adults. *American Heart Journal, 126,* 1152–1155.

Kirklin, J. W., & Barratt-Boyes, B. G. (1993). *Cardiac surgery* (2nd ed.). New York: Churchill Livingstone.

Markowitz, M., & Kaplan, E. L. (1989). Reappearance of rheumatic fever. *Advances in Pediatrics, 36,* 39–65.

Marriott, H. J. L. (1993). *Practical electrocardiology* (8th ed.). Baltimore: Williams & Wilkins.

National Heart, Lung, and Blood Institute Balloon Valvuloplasty Registry. (1992). Multicenter experience with balloon mitral commissurotomy. NHLBI Balloon Valvuloplasty Registry Report on immediate and 30-day follow-up results. *Circulation, 85,* 448–461.

Schakenbach, L. H. (1987). Physiologic dynamics of acquired valvular heart disease. *Journal of Cardiovascular Nursing, 1*(3), 1–17.

Schamroth, L. (1989). *The 12 lead electrocardiogram.* Oxford: Blackwell Scientific Publications.

Schlant, R. C., & Alexander, R. W. (1994). *Hurst's the heart: Arteries and veins* (8th ed.). New York: McGraw-Hill.

Vahanian, A., et al. (1989). Results of percutaneous mitral commissurotomy in 200 patients. *American Journal of Cardiology, 63,* 847–852.

CHAPTER

24 Patients Undergoing Cardiothoracic Surgery and Transplants

Stacey Gross, Bernice Coleman, Carol Flavell, and Johanna Salamandra

Cardiac surgical intervention remains unparalleled as an effective therapeutic approach to coronary heart disease (CHD). As this decade ascends, rapid fluxes on the clinical and fiscal fronts give rise to further challenge for nurses caring for these patients. Heart and lung transplantation procedures have also increased throughout the country as an alternative modality for end-stage cardiopulmonary disease. This chapter on cardiac surgical interventions reviews coronary revascularization, cardiopulmonary bypass conduct, myocardial preservation, surgical conduct, and postoperative physiologic sequelae and common problems. An overview of current modalities in surgical transplants provides a comprehensive perspective on all viable modalities and interventions.

The content is presented with a focus on the current data in these areas. It is hoped that these data will provide critical care nurses with the needed facts to plan better for the "whys" of practice. Likewise, as advances in various areas occur, critical care nurses can appreciate how these innovations can affect the way patients present during the postoperative period, and devise the plan of care accordingly.

CORONARY ARTERY BYPASS GRAFT SURGERY

Cardiovascular disease accounts for 43% of all deaths in the United States (American Heart Association, 1993). The prevalence of CHD is alarming, afflicting an estimated 6.2 million Americans. CHD represents the number one cause of death, claiming approximately 489,171 lives each year. Researchers estimate that in 1995 as many as 1.5 million people will suffer an acute myocardial infarction (MI), and more than one-third will die. More than 156,000 deaths occur before the age of 65 years; women represent more than 50% of all cardiovascular deaths. Consequently, intensive research efforts have focused not only on identification of the causes and contributing factors of CHD but on the best methods of combatting this disease in terms of both prevention and treatment.

During the last decade, a rapid upsurge in technologic and scientific investigations has produced a vast array of treatment options for patients with coronary atherosclerosis. Coronary revascularization procedures include two perspectives, reflecting both the interventional and surgical approach. The limitations associated with percutaneous transluminal coronary angioplasty (PTCA) have led to the emergence of new strategies such as directional/rotational atherectomy, laser angioplasty, and intracoronary stenting. New device development such as the Rotablator (Heart Technology, Inc., Bellevue, WA), Simpson Atherocath (DVI, Inc., Redwood City, CA), excimer laser, holmium laser, Gianturco-Roubin Stent (Cook, Inc., Bloomington, IN), and Palmaz-Schatz Stent (Johnson & Johnson, New Brunswick, NJ) have added increased versatility and improved results in combination with PTCA. Restenosis, however, remains problematic. Thus, the focus of research has shifted in an attempt to secure a method of altering or modulating the hyperproliferative response associated with restenosis. As operator experience is acquired and patient selection criteria are better defined, the challenge at hand remains to determine which procedure or approach will render the greatest benefit in terms of survival, relief of symptoms, and quality of life.

Surgical revascularization in the form of coronary artery bypass grafting (CABG) remains in the forefront of treatment of CHD. Approximately 369,000 CABG operations are performed annually in the United States (American Heart Association, 1993). Within the last three decades, more than 1 million patients have had bypass procedures. Emerging trends reveal a changing demographic profile of patients undergoing cardiac surgery. Current studies demonstrate advancing age, increasing severity and extent of disease (inclusive of increased incidence of prior MI and multivessel and left main stenoses), and reduced ejection fractions commonly depict today's cohort of patients. Elective operations have been less frequent, with a significant rise in the number of emergent or urgent cases (correlating with increased in-hospital mortality) (Disch et al., 1994; Haraphongse et al., 1994). Men were the recipients of 76% of all operations, approximately 270,000 procedures compared with 83,000 procedures performed on women. Fifty percent of the patients were younger than the age of 65 years. Cost expenditure estimates reveal that approximately 6 to 7 billion dollars are spent annually in the treatment of heart disease measured just in direct care services alone (nurse–physician services).

The rationale for performing surgical revascularization or aortocoronary bypass grafting is to restore adequate blood flow or blood supply and to provide nutritional support to the myocardial tissue. A harvested vessel (conduit) is anastomosed between the aortic root and a point distal to the obstructing coronary lesion or stenosis. The restoration of myocardial perfusion aids in preventing further ischemia and in salvaging viable muscle mass and ventricular function.

Historically, the first surgical approach to indirect myocardial revascularization was developed by Vineberg in 1946 (Vineberg, 1946). This technique involved implantation of the internal thoracic artery into the myocardial wall in an attempt to facilitate coronary flow through growth of a vascular network. Limited technology affected the ability to evaluate the results of the initial surgical trials. The advent of extracorporeal circulation and selective coronary arteriography in the 1950s and 1960s ignited renewed interest and investigation into the feasibility of performing direct revascularization procedures (Sones & Shirey, 1962). Reports of varied surgical revascularization attempts emerged during the next decade. In 1968, surgical teams led by Dr. Johnson (Milwaukee) and by Drs. Favalaro and Effler (Cleveland) performed the first successful aortocoronary bypass graft procedures using a reversed saphenous vein as the graft material (Favalaro, 1969; Johnson et al., 1969). By 1972, improvements in extracorporeal circulation and cardioplegic techniques made aortocoronary saphenous bypass graft procedures a common method of revascularization.

TABLE 24–1. **Indications for Coronary Artery Bypass Grafting**

Chronic stable angina refractory to medical therapy
Significant left main coronary occlusion (>50%)

Triple-vessel coronary artery disease
  Left ventricular dysfunction
  Proximal left anterior descending disease (as part of two-vessel disease)

Unstable angina pectoris

Acute myocardial infarction
  Emergent
  Delayed

Intractable ventricular irritability

Left ventricular failure
  Congestive heart failure
  Cardiogenic shock

Percutaneous transluminal coronary angioplasty failure

Indications for Myocardial Revascularization

During the last decade, a number of multicenter clinical investigations have focused attention on patient selection criteria for surgical myocardial revascularization (Table 24–1). Due to the immense cost and large number of CABGs performed each year, this operation has become the most studied surgical procedure. In 1980 a task force was established to examine management strategies used for patients with cardiovascular disease. In March of 1991, as a result of a joint effort of the American College of Cardiology and the American Heart Association, guidelines were released illustrating the recommended indications for CABG (Kirklin et al., 1991). These guidelines represent a framework around which to establish standards for practice and on which to base treatment decisions. The guidelines address which patient populations would obtain the most benefit in terms of relief of angina, survival, and quality of life after CABG. Patients were classified according to severity of disease and, in particular, the most appropriate therapy. With more research emerging regarding revascularization techniques, the question now becomes which mode (interventional vs. surgical) will afford the most positive cost–benefit ratio.

Consequently, several prospective, randomized investigations have compared PTCA to CABG for select patients with multivessel coronary artery disease (CAD) (Table 24–2). In a study of more than 1,000 patients, the Randomised Intervention Treatment of Angina (RITA) trial demonstrated no significant differences among treatment groups in the incidence of death or myocardial infarction. Patients undergoing

TABLE 24–2. **Major Randomized Comparative Trials: PTCA and CABG**

ERACI	Argentine Randomized Trial of Coronary Angioplasty vs. Bypass Surgery in Multiple Vessel Disease
BARI	Bypass Angioplasty Revascularization Investigation
EAST	Emory Angioplasty Surgery Trial
GABI	German Angioplasty vs. Bypass Investigation
CABRI	Italian Coronary Angioplasty vs. Bypass Revascularization Investigation
RITA	Randomized Intervention Treatment of Angina

Abbreviations: CABG, coronary artery bypass grafting; PTCA, percutaneous transluminal coronary angioplasty.

TABLE 24–3. **Results of Prospective Randomized Trials Comparing PTCA and CABG**

	GABI Trial (*n* = 337)		RITA Trial (*n* = 1011)		EAST Trial (*n* = 392)	
	PTCA	*CABG*	*PTCA*	*CABG*	*PTCA*	*CABG*
Sample size	182	177	510	501	198	194
Complication rate						
Death	1.1%	2.5%	3.1% (at 2.5 years)	3.6% (at 2.5 years)	7.1% (at 3 years)	6.2% (at 3 years)
Crossover to CABG						
1 Year	21%		—	—	—	—
3 Years	—	—	15%	—	22%	1%
Freedom from angina	71%	74% (at 12 months)	69% (at 2.5 years)	88% (at 2.5 years)	80%	88%
Repeat procedures	44%	4%	38%	11%	41%	13%
Antianginal medication use	88%	78%	61%	34%		

Abbreviations: CABG, coronary artery bypass grafting; PTCA, percutaneous transluminal coronary angioplasty. See Table 24–2 for full names of trials.

PTCA, however, experienced an increased incidence of recurrent angina, required continued use of antianginal medications, and underwent an increased number of repeat revascularization procedures (repeat angioplasty or surgery). At 2.5 years, the crossover rate to CABG approximated 15%. The Argentine ERACI trial (Randomized Trial of Coronary Angioplasty vs. Bypass Surgery in Multiple Vessel Disease) reported similar findings, noting a 3-year crossover to CABG rate of 25%. Other randomized trials have shown similar outcomes (Table 24–3). The EAST (Emory Angioplasty Surgery Trial) trial found no difference in terms of activity level or employment status/return to work at 3 years between the PTCA and CABG group (King et al., 1994). Recruitment issues arose for many of the trial coordinators due to the vast population with multivessel disease not suitable for PTCA. The GABI (German Angioplasty vs. Bypass Investigation) trial recruited a total sample of 359 patients (4%) from a population of 8,981; the EAST trial ended with 8% enrollment from 5,118 patients. The subset of patients with diffuse, multivessel, or left main CAD were considered poor candidates for angioplasty, thus reinforcing the view that surgical revascularization continues to be the preferred approach for many patients. Further results are expected in 1995 from the BARI trial (with an enrollment of 1,829 patients), spanning a 5-year follow-up period. Thus far, the interim data suggest: (1) no difference in mortality and morbidity between PTCA and surgery; (2) angioplasty still represents a reasonable approach for coronary disease, but is associated with a risk of repeat procedures; and (3) the final decision to undergo either procedure should be determined after a thorough discussion between the patient and clinician, with strong consideration given to individual preference. As the final results of these and other trials become available, more conclusive recommendations can be made regarding patient selection and therapeutic choices. Until these data become available, the decision to perform either procedure is based on clinical findings and patient preference.

At present, chronic angina, left main coronary disease, and acute MI (AMI) are the prime indications for surgical intervention. An increasing number of patients also are referred after failed PTCA. The most significant clinical benefit is derived from relief of symptoms. Conclusive findings reported by several authors demonstrate the effectiveness of CABG in reducing the frequency and severity of anginal pain in 75% to 90% of patients (Yusuf et al., 1994). Improved survival and longevity have been observed with surgical therapy in patients with left main coronary disease, triple vessel disease, and left ventricular dysfunction (Yusuf et al., 1994). Compared with medical therapy alone, surgery has been found to prolong survival in patients with the greatest risk inclusive of poor ventricular function (Killip et al., 1985; Rahimtoola, 1985; Yusuf et al., 1994). Eight-year survival rates approximate 79% in patients with three-vessel disease, compared to 82% in patients with two-vessel disease.

The decision to perform CABG is based on several factors, foremost among them being the alleviation of symptoms and improved survival. An extensive evaluation of the patient's condition is conducted based on the history, symptomatology, and results of coronary arteriography. Some centers also include echocardiography and exercise tolerance testing as components in the diagnostic process. Current controversy over the prognostic value and reliability of exercise testing in women has resulted in limited application of this component in potential surgical candidates. The clinical conditions warranting surgical intervention are reviewed here based on current recommendations.

CHRONIC STABLE ANGINA PECTORIS. Chronic angina pectoris that is unresponsive to medical therapy represents the most widely accepted indication for myocardial revascularization. Stable angina is usually characterized as angina occurring with minimal change in frequency, duration, or severity of symptoms. Stable angina categorized as class I to class II occurs in symptomatic patients who have a varying degree or extent of coronary involvement and ventricular dysfunction. Class III to class IV angina is found in patients who are symptomatic and have one or more severe proximal stenoses, and clearly demonstrate a poor response to medical therapy. Patients in the latter functional category warrant definitive revascularization. Factors such as disability resulting from anginal symptoms, adverse side effects from medications, and noncompliance with medical treatment justify consideration of surgical intervention in this population of patients.

Initial treatment aimed at controlling anginal pain is achieved through the use of long-acting nitrates, aspirin, beta-adrenergic blocking agents, or calcium channel blockers (Willerson, 1992). Failure to alleviate ischemic symptoms after a course of maximum medical therapy warrants surgical consideration. Optimal timing of surgery in patients who have been initially treated medically requires scrupulous evaluation and examination of the nature of the disease process. Evidence from several sources illustrates dramatic relief of pain after surgical intervention. Operative mortality in patients with stable angina ranges from 1% to 3% (Rahimtoola, 1993).

SIGNIFICANT LEFT MAIN CORONARY ARTERY OCCLUSION. Surgical treatment is indicated in patients with severe stenosis of the left main coronary artery. Often, stenosis located within the left main coronary is referred to as the *widow-maker* lesion. Patients with this condition receiving medical treatment alone have demonstrated a diminished prognosis and increased risk of mortality (European Coronary Surgery Study Group [ECSSG], 1982; Yusef, 1994).

A narrowing of greater than 50% of the luminal diameter is considered a significant stenosis (Hurst et al., 1986). Sixty percent of left main coronary artery lesions are associated with significant disease elsewhere in the coronary vasculature (Chaitman et al., 1981). Commonly, patients exhibit triple-vessel disease during angiographic studies. Significant left main stenosis (or stenosis of the proximal left anterior descending artery [LAD]) jeopardizes a large portion of the myocardium because the vascular distribution of these vessels supplies the apex, part of the lateral wall, anterior wall, and two-thirds of the septum. Thus, these patients are at increased risk for acute anterior wall infarction and sudden death (Loop, 1983a, 1983b; Willerson, 1992). Prompt surgical intervention in patients with left main disease has been shown to increase their 3-year survival rates to 85% to 90% compared with medical therapy (65% to 69%) (Rahimtoola, 1985; Coronary Artery Surgery Study [CASS] Investigators, 1983).

TRIPLE-VESSEL CORONARY ARTERY DISEASE. CABG is indicated in patients with high-grade pathoanatomic lesions involving two or more vessels (ECSSG, 1982; Rahimtoola, 1993). Severe coronary artery stenosis, exceeding 70% of the luminal diameter, is classified as significant. Vessels containing *type B* and *type C lesions,* (characterized as diffuse, eccentric, calcified, distal, or thrombus) yield lower success and carry increased procedural risk when treated with PTCA. For surgical consideration, recipient graft vessels must demonstrate adequate perfusion distal to the obstruction, indicating a patent peripheral coronary bed. Poor distal flow in vessels with a luminal diameter of less than 1.0 to 1.5 mm increases the risk of early thrombosis and limits the feasibility of revascularization to the vessel. In patients with single-vessel disease or multivessel CAD, not involving the proximal LAD, with normal left ventricular function, no difference in survival has been observed between medical and surgical treatment. However, patients with impaired ventricular function and three-vessel disease (or multivessel disease with LAD involvement) experience a significant survival benefit and a reduction in mortality with surgical revascularization (Killip et al., 1985; Myers et al., 1989; Yusef, 1994).

UNSTABLE ANGINA PECTORIS. Patients with unstable angina pectoris represent another subgroup of candidates for CABG surgery. The term "unstable angina" has been used to describe a number of clinical conditions such as preinfarction angina, crescendo angina, rest angina, and postinfarction angina. Manifestations of anginal pain that escalates in intensity, frequency, or duration and is unrelieved by rest or pharmacologic therapy typically characterize this syndrome. Unstable angina has been associated with a high risk of subsequent ischemic events. Among patients managed medically, approximately 21% of those with new-onset unstable angina experience a myocardial infarction within 8 months. An associated 41% mortality rate has been observed in this group (Kaiser et al., 1989).

Increasing frequency and severity of chest pain, angina occurring at night or at rest, and ST-T segment changes on electrocardiography (ECG) during anginal episodes correlate with an increased risk (CASS Investigators, 1984). The rationale for surgical intervention in this population is related to the high incidence of MI and death. Significant benefit is obtained in patients with prior subendocardial damage, who frequently have a propensity toward development of transmural infarctions (Kaiser et al., 1985). The CASS investigation focused on coronary care patients who experienced atypical angina that was unresponsive to pharmacologic therapy. Most patients required CABG. The incidence of MI in this group (occurring 6 hours to 30 days before surgery) was 50%, and approximately 75% of patients were found to have extensive three-vessel disease and some degree of left ventricular dysfunction (Rankin et al., 1984). The operative mortality was 4%, approximately twice that of patients with stable angina (Kaiser et al., 1985). Increased age, left ventricular impairment, left main coronary lesions, and female gender represent the variables having a significant impact on operative mortality (Kaiser et al., 1989).

ACUTE MYOCARDIAL INFARCTION. The role of CABG in patients with AMI remains a controversial issue and requires extensive examination of the cost–benefit factors. Multiple therapeutic options exist and provide versatility in the management and support of the patient experiencing an acute event (see Chapter 20). Use of pharmacologic agents (such as propranolol, nitrates, and sodium nitroprusside), thrombolytic agents, and cardiac assist devices such as intraaortic balloon counterpulsation (IABC) represent the various alternative treatment modalities available for patients with AMI. Use of tissue-type plasminogen activator (t-PA), streptokinase (SK), and acylated plasminogen–SK activator complex in the early phases of myocardial injury have been shown to be effective in restoring coronary perfusion to the area in jeopardy (Geltman, 1987; Rentrop, 1985). The efficacy of t-PA administration in reestablishing coronary flow has been recorded as 75% to 85%; efficacy associated with SK ranges from 55% to 65% (Braunwald, 1988; Chesebro et al., 1987; Neuhaus et al., 1992; Tanswell et al., 1992; TIMI Study Group, 1989; Wall et al., 1992). The incidence of restenosis after these therapies is approximately 17% with both t-PA and SK. Close follow-up is vital to detect recurrent angina or ischemic symptoms warranting further intervention with PTCA or CABG.

Therapy in patients with AMI focuses on interrupting the progressive ischemia and myocardial necrosis. The zone of ischemic tissue (the "twilight zone" surrounding the infarcted region) remains viable for 3 to 6 hours. Theoretically, timely performance of CABG aids in restoration of myocardial perfusion to the jeopardized region and potential salvation of viable muscle mass. Readily accessible and expedient treatment options such as thrombolytic therapy or coronary angioplasty often preclude the performance of immediate surgical revascularization. Thus, CABG is not routinely considered the first therapy of choice in AMI.

The question of when to intervene surgically after AMI remains debatable. Statistics during the last 5 years reveal an increasing trend toward surgery performed early after AMI (Fremes et al., 1991; Kennedy et al., 1989). This trend has been attributed to the expanding application of invasive interventional cardiovascular techniques as well as to recognition of the potential risks associated with AMI. In patients who survive an AMI, the 1-year mortality rates are 10% to 15%; approximately 20% incur significant left ventricular damage (left ventricular ejection fraction [LVEF] < 30%) leading to increased risk of death. Recurrent angina after AMI represents a significant predictor for reinfarction, extension, or death. Mortality rates range from 17% to 50% (Curtis et al., 1991). Noninvasive testing and angiographic studies are conducted to evaluate the extent of coronary disease, ventricular performance, or any resultant structural anomalies. Recommendations for PTCA or CABG are established based on test findings and the clinical patient profile. Current guidelines advocate delaying surgery, preferably 1 week after an AMI (Kennedy et al., 1989). The incidence of operative mortality is the same whether surgery is performed 8 days or 30 days after an infarction (Kennedy et al., 1989). In patients who remain free from angina or experience mild angina after an MI, no significant differences exist in 5-year mortality figures comparing surgical with medical treatment (CASS Investigators, 1984).

INTRACTABLE VENTRICULAR IRRITABILITY. Recurrent ventricular irritability due to complications resulting from AMI represents another indication for myocardial revascularization. Left ventricular aneurysm formation after an acute infarction may be the site of electrical instability, which induces reentrant pathways for ventricular dysrhythmias. Symptomatic, persistent dysrhythmias refractory to pharmacologic therapy may increase the risk of sudden cardiac death.

Surgical intervention focuses on interrupting reentrant pathways through myocardial revascularization, myocardial resection of localized infarcted tissue, or excision of a left ventricular aneurysm. The results of such surgical procedures in treating recurrent ventricular dysrhythmias have been variable and inconsistent, with many patients continuing to demonstrate a need for either pharmacologic management with antidysrhythmic agents or placement of an automatic implantable cardioverter–defibrillator.

LEFT VENTRICULAR FAILURE. The efficacy of CABG in the management of left ventricular failure has not been clearly substantiated. In patients with advanced congestive heart failure (CHF), the results of myocardial revascularization have been inconsistent and conflicting with regard to improvement in symptoms or survival benefits. Recent clinical studies have illustrated a positive correlation between heart failure and operative risk (Wechsler & Junod, 1989). In patients with depressed left ventricular performance, further insult from cardiopulmonary bypass (CPB), inadequate myocardial protection, perioperative infarction, or incomplete revascularization may precipitate cardiac decompensation (Wechsler & Junod, 1989). Most evidence indicates that CABG is of limited value in reversing myocardial damage or ventricular function after extensive loss of muscle mass due to an AMI. Patients with CHF who experience severe angina pectoris are considered candidates for surgery after evaluation of the coronary vasculature, left ventricular wall motion, and cardiac performance. Mechanical assist devices are frequently used in the early postoperative period to provide temporary hemodynamic support (Wechsler & Junod, 1989).

Manifestations of CHF may be seen as a complication of AMI. CHF may be precipitated by an acquired ventricular septal defect, acute mitral regurgitation, or ventricular aneurysm (Moore, 1986). Rupture of the intraventricular septum occurs in 1% to 2% of patients with AMI, and survival is about 20% at 2 months after AMI without surgical repair (Moore, 1986). Development of a systolic murmur, CHF, and severe left ventricular failure warrants immediate evaluation to detect the presence of a ventricular septal defect. Interim stabilization with IABC may be required. Pharmacologic agents such as diuretics or vasodilators may be used to unload left ventricular volume. Urgent surgical repair is indicated to close the defect, and concomitant bypass grafting may be necessary to achieve regional perfusion of infarct-related arteries (Nishimura, 1986).

CARDIOGENIC SHOCK. When damage from AMI encompasses more than 40% of the left ventricular muscle mass, marked left ventricular failure and cardiogenic shock ensue (Caulfield et al., 1976). Mortality rates range from 85% to 95% with medical therapy alone (Caulfield et al., 1976). Institution of thrombolytic therapy or PTCA to reperfuse an occluded vessel, within 2 hours of the onset of symptoms, may reverse the spiral of cardiogenic shock (Lee et al., 1988). Aggressive regimens using inotropic agents or mechanical assist devices may provide early means of augmenting systolic performance during an acute insult. Results of CABG on survival in patients suffering from cardiogenic shock vary. Critical determinants of operative mortality depend on the extent of left ventricular dysfunction, myocardial damage, and remaining cardiac reserve. The availability of expert, seasoned medical and surgical teams combined with appropriate mechanical support, timely diagnosis, and surgical technique has had a significant impact on decreasing the incidence of mortality.

PERCUTANEOUS TRANSLUMINAL CORONARY ANGIOPLASTY FAILURE. PTCA has emerged as a viable alternative treatment for selected patients with CAD (see Chapter 19). The increasing number of procedures performed and their growing complexity require continuous surgical support and operative backup. Complications such as coronary artery dissection (most common), complete coronary occlusion, dysrhythmias, and unstable angina resulting in acute ischemia occur in 5% of cases, necessitating emergent surgical intervention (Talley et al., 1989). Careful patient selection, refinements in technique, and the use of reperfusion or "bailout" catheters has aided in limiting myocardial damage and reducing mortality (Hinohara et al., 1988). Advancement of reperfusion catheters through the angioplasty sheath beyond the site of occlusion promotes blood flow distal to the stenosis and maintains supply to the ischemic region. Use of intracoronary stenting in situations of abrupt closure has also assisted in improved outcome. Further support using IABC, femoral bypass, and pharmacologic agents such as intracoronary nitroglycerin has been effective in enhancing hemodynamic stability and cardiovascular function (Murphy et al., 1982).

Emergent CABG (defined in most clinical series as operative intervention within 24 hours after PTCA) carries an obvious increased risk of operative death (7%–11%) and perioperative infarction (29%–50%) compared to planned elective surgical revascularization (Talley et al., 1989). Initial PTCA trials involved patients with single-vessel disease and normal left ventricular function. Emergent CABG undertaken in this patient population revealed little or no added increased operative mortality; the incidence of complications approached 5% in this group. Today, the selection criteria have expanded to include patients with depressed left ventricular function, increased age, left main coronary stenosis, and multivessel disease (Daily, 1989). The presence of one or more of these factors significantly influences the operative outcome, and these factors have been identified as predictors of mortality used to analyze the associated risk of emergent CABG. Complication rates in this patient population approach 28%, prolonging the length of hospital stay (Greene et al., 1991).

Restenosis rates associated with PTCA for single-vessel disease are approximately 20% to 30%; restenosis typically presents within the first 6 months after the initial procedure (Hurst et al., 1986). In patients with multiple lesions, the restenosis rate is higher. Repeat procedures often produce successful results in 70% to 80% of patients (Daily, 1989). Patients with lesions located in the LAD, right coronary artery (RCA), or left circumflex artery; a post-PTCA translesional gradient of greater than 15 mm Hg; a residual stenosis greater than 30%; and unstable angina are at a higher risk for restenosis at the time of initial angioplasty and at repeat PTCA. Various new techniques using laser balloon angioplasty, intracoronary stents, and atherectomy devices hold promise for preventing restenosis. Yet continued patency and complete revascularization in patients with extensive three-vessel disease remain problematic. Consequently, these patients eventually require surgical intervention to correct coronary hypoperfusion. Current statistics indicate that within 1 year of angioplasty, 85% to 90% of patients maintain freedom from the need to cross over to CABG. Subsequently, 81% of patients are free at 3 years, and 75% to 86% are free at 5 years (O'Keefe et al., 1990).

Relative Contraindications

Comprehensive patient assessment is crucial to the identification and elucidation of factors influencing the feasibility of surgical revascularization. Technical constraints imposed by anatomic anomalies create considerable problems for the surgeon. Small, narrowed, atheromatous coronary vessels (<1.0–1.5 mm in diameter) accompanied by diffuse distal disease and poor collateralization may prohibit bypass grafting. An open artery greater than 1 mm in diameter beyond the stenotic lesion must exist. Furthermore, viable myocardial tissue in the area supplied by the recipient vessel must be documented. Lack of a conduit or suitable graft material in patients with severe systemic vascular disease may inhibit revascularization attempts. Aortic root anomalies or severe aortic sclerosis can complicate proximal anastomosis construction, precipitating unsatisfactory results.

Alterations in physiologic and functional states have been used as indicators to determine the relative risk associated with surgery. Left ventricular function has been identified as a significant prognostic indicator of survival and surgical outcome (Gersh et al., 1989).

Left ventricular dysfunction (LVEF < 20%) accompanied by cardiomegaly or elevated left ventricular end-diastolic volume incurs an increased risk of associated surgical mortality (Parsonnet et al., 1989). Preexisting pulmonary disease, renal insufficiency, and carotid disease represent incremental risk factors predisposing the patient to *potential* postoperative complications (Rich et al., 1988). Age as an isolated factor in itself has not been identified as a significant prognostic indicator (Rich et al., 1988), but a consensus exists that patients older than 70 years of age carry a higher risk (Parsonnet et al., 1989). Several reports from septuagenarian and octagenarian studies cite factors such as low body weight, prolonged bypass time, and need for repeated operations as contributing to an increased risk of perioperative complications (Rich et al., 1988).

Selection of Conduits

The saphenous vein and the internal thoracic artery (ITA) are the most commonly used conduits today for myocardial revascularization. Both vessels have been used successfully, alone or in combination, when multiple bypasses are needed.

The greater saphenous vein, located anterior to the medial malleolus, travels upward to join the common femoral vein at the groin. Exposure of the vessel is accomplished through a continuous incision starting at the ankle. Use of the saphenous vein segment below the knee is preferred because of its closer approximation in size (4–5 mm in diameter) to that of the coronary arteries. Usually, 15- to 20-cm vein segments are harvested for each graft. Once the vein has been excised, the tributaries are ligated. Injection of a heparinized plasmolytic or saline solution gently distends the graft segment to detect the presence of any leaks in the vessel. Extreme care is exercised in handling the vein graft material. Excessive manipulation may result in vasospasm or intimal damage, activating a potential thrombotic process that has been implicated in early graft closure (Baumann, 1981). Before aortic anastomosis, vein graft material is placed in a reverse direction to prevent venous valves from impeding the flow of coronary blood. The leg incision is irrigated with antibiotic solution and closed with running nylon or subcuticular sutures (Fig. 24–1).

The patency rate for saphenous vein grafts at 1 year is 98%, but at 10 years falls to 81% (Loop et al., 1986). Use of the saphenous vein graft offers several advantages, such as technical ease and flexibility and less time required to dissect and harvest the vessel, both of which aid in decreasing bypass and operative time. Satisfactory flow rates have been demonstrated with the saphenous vein graft due to the lower resistance and large diameter characteristic of venous vessels. Because the saphenous vein is an accessory vein, circulation in the lower extremity is not usually interrupted because of its removal. In patients with preexisting deep venous obstructions, impaired circulation resulting in edema has been found to occur.

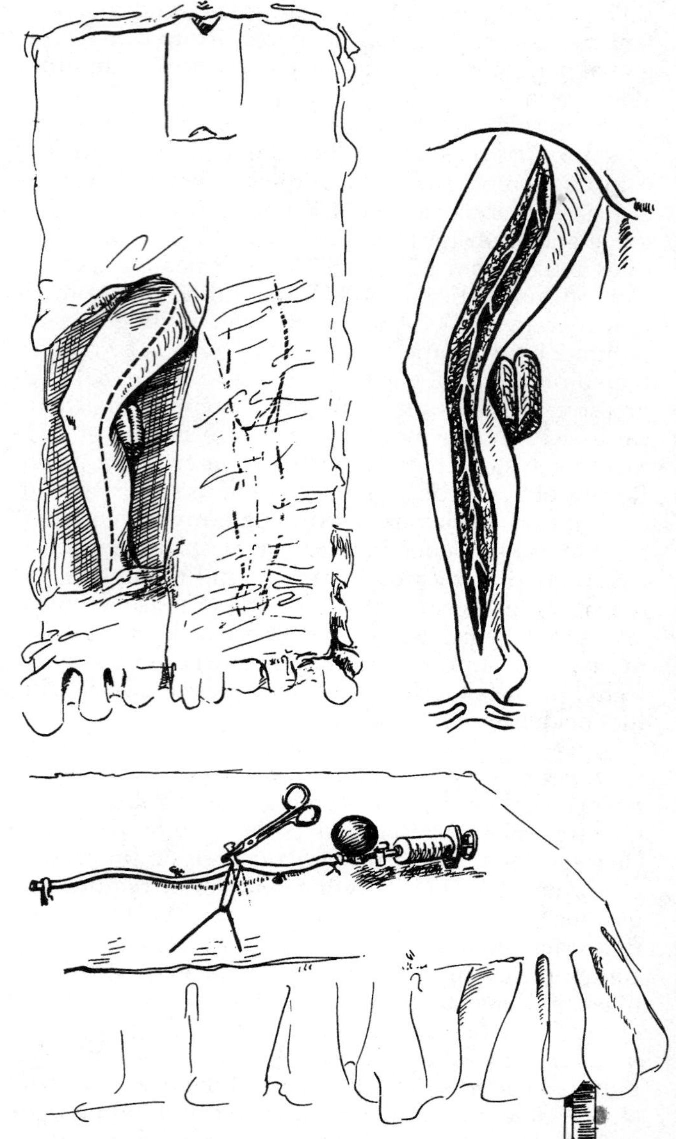

FIGURE 24–1. Harvesting the saphenous vein. (From Dillard, D. H., & Miller, D. W. [1983]. *Atlas of cardiac surgery* [Plate XXXI, p. 81]. New York: Simon and Schuster.)

The ITA has emerged as the conduit of choice for bypass of the LAD (Loop et al., 1986). The ITA arises from the subclavian artery as the second branch. Located 1 to 2 cm lateral to the sternal border, it descends inferiorly through the diaphragm to become the superior epigastric artery. The ITA, used as a pedicle bypass graft, is left attached proximally to the subclavian artery and is transsected distally for anastomosis to the recipient coronary artery. Due to its diminished diameter below the sixth intercostal space, use of the ITA is limited to bypass of anterior coronary vessels such as the proximal LAD, proximal diagonal, or marginal vessels. The longer length and diameter of the left ITA compared to the right ITA provide increased versatility for bypassing obstructed coronary vessels (Fig. 24–2).

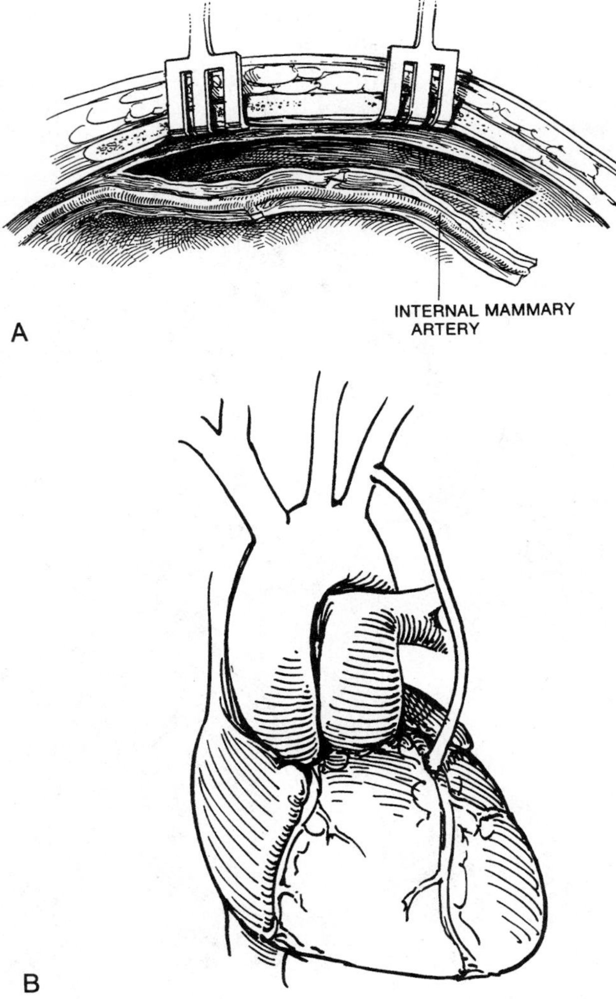

FIGURE 24–2. *A,* Dissection of the left internal thoracic artery from left sternal wall and surrounding tissue. Use of retractors facilitates optimum vizualization. *B,* Aortocoronary bypass of left internal thoracic artery to left anterior descending artery. (From Waldhausen, J. A., & Pierce, W. S. [1985]. *Surgery of the chest* [5th ed., p. 481]. Chicago: Year Book Medical Publishers.)

Applications of the ITA have expanded to include use as a free graft. Some authors report increased technical difficulty, inconsistent flow rates, and a propensity for vasospasm as problems associated with use of the ITA as a free graft (Green, 1989). More recent experiences with free grafts have led to improved results and lower attrition rates (Green, 1989). Bilateral grafting offers additional options for patients with poor-quality lower extremity vessels or calcific lesions. Use of both ITAs in younger patients enhances revascularization results, increasing graft longevity and survival (Green, 1989). However, a slight increase in risk of mediastinitis has been documented with the use of bilateral ITAs (Grover et al., 1994). In women, use of the ITA is particularly advantageous due to the prevalence of small primary vessels (Loop et al., 1989). Some controversy accompanies the use of the ITA in elderly women. However, limited availability of conduits may make the ITA the best choice.

The ITA has demonstrated excellent long-term patency rates approaching 96% at 10 years (Loop et al., 1986). Efforts to explain the increased longevity and durability of the ITA graft have focused on increased prostacyclin synthesis and vasoactive properties inherent within the arterial lumen wall (Chaikhouni et al., 1986). Progression of atherosclerotic disease and subintimal changes appears to be inhibited. The absence of valves minimizes luminal turbulence, reducing the risk of thrombosis and occlusion. Angiographic evaluation has documented the ability of the ITA to enlarge in response to increased demand. Flow rates of ITA grafts have been demonstrated to be equivalent to its vein graft counterpart (Green, 1989).

Some of the limitations associated with ITA grafts include the increased operative time needed for retrosternal dissection, bleeding, postoperative chest wall discomfort, and technical difficulties (Jansen & McFadden, 1986). The incidence of postoperative bleeding can be minimized with careful inspection before chest closure. Grover and colleagues (1994), in a large-scale Veterans Administration study, failed to demonstrate an increase in operative mortality associated with ITA use. Circumstances precluding use of the ITA may include patients with a prior mastectomy, a history of chest wall radiation, brachiocephalic disease, or emergent revascularization for myocardial instability (Loop et al., 1989).

ALTERNATIVE VENOUS AND ARTERIAL CONDUITS. In some patients, the number of available grafts may be limited due to prior vein-stripping procedures, varicosities, or other circumstances previously mentioned that hinder use of the ITA. Upper arm veins, namely, the cephalic vein and basilic vein, have been investigated as alternative venous conduits. Location, accessibility, and length of vessels were noted advantages. Compared to the saphenous vein, the internal diameter of the cephalic and basilic veins is less than 3.5 cm, slightly less than optimal for implantation. The major disadvantage of the upper arm veins is their structural composition. The thin walls of these vessels make anastomotic construction and suturing extremely difficult. Studies have demonstrated poor patency rates. Occlusions were evident in 42% to 47% of patients at 2 years. Basilic and cephalic veins appear to develop significant intimal changes by the second or third postoperative year. Other findings indicate a high rate of aneurysm formation within these vessels. Thus, the use of upper extremity veins has not proved to be a reliable alternative.

The internal thoracic vein (ITV) represents another potential venous conduit. Clinical experience to date is limited, but French surgeons report that ITV characteristics are similar to those of the saphenous vein in terms of resiliency and size. Initial reports indicate that the ITV appears to be suitable as a venous conduit (Stephan et al., 1990). The ITV is dissected and prepared similarly to the saphenous vein graft.

Reports of use of the radial artery as an arterial conduit for CABG emerged in the early 1970s (Foster &

Kranc, 1989). On initial evaluation, properties similar to those of the internal thoracic were apparent. Luminal size equivalent to that of the coronary vessels, long length, superficial position, and ease of removal represented qualities inherent in a good conduit. However, initial trials using free radial artery grafts revealed significant graft occlusion within 1 year (Foster & Kranc, 1989). Most of the grafts were found to be completely occluded and stenosed on repeat angiography. Subsequent studies demonstrated disappointing results, rendering use of the radial artery unsuitable for CABG procedures.

While some researchers examined use of the radial artery, other investigators focused on the feasibility of the splenic artery for myocardial revascularization procedures. The splenic artery as a pedicled artery graft was thought to possess physiologic features similar to those of the ITA. Initial experiences yielded satisfactory results in terms of graft patency. However, preparation and harvesting of this vessel imposed great difficulty, requiring rerouting of the splenic artery from the abdomen through the diaphragm (Foster & Kranc, 1989). A splenectomy was performed concomitantly. Problems with kinking, size, and atherosclerotic lesions precluded continued use of the splenic artery.

Recent attention has focused on use of the right gastroepiploic artery (RGEA) in CABG (Lytle et al., 1987a; Mills & Everson, 1989; Suma et al., 1989). The RGEA has been used both as a pedicle graft and as a free graft (Lytle et al., 1987a). The RGEA, originating from the anterior superior pancreaticoduodenal artery (Fig. 24–3), is routed upward through the diaphragm to the recipient coronary artery. Initial investigations have yielded mixed results. Because the RGEA is part of an arterial system, researchers have suggested that it may possess physiologic characteristics of increased longevity and patency similar to those of the ITA. The RGEA has been used in patients undergoing reoperation where conduit availability is problematic. Further circumstances in which RGEA use is considered are in patients with poor-quality or absent saphenous veins, diabetes mellitus, or aortic stenosis (Mills & Everson, 1989). Use of the RGEA is associated with increased operative time and increased complexity of the procedure due to the need for entrance into the abdominal cavity. This may pose significant problems if future abdominal surgery is necessary. Because of the lack of experience with RGEA grafts, information about flow rates and long-term patency is lacking. Some controversy still exists regarding competitive flow and gastric perfusion after meals and digestion. Initial data at 3 months reveal 93% patency rates compared to 95% patency rates with ITA grafts (Suma et al., 1989). Further research continues, and other investigators have pursued use of the inferior epigastric artery (IEA) as a potential arterial conduit (Puig et al., 1990). The IEA, originating from the external iliac artery, possesses histologic features similar to those of the ITA. Results with IEA grafts are limited but display promise as clinicians explore other sources of viable conduits.

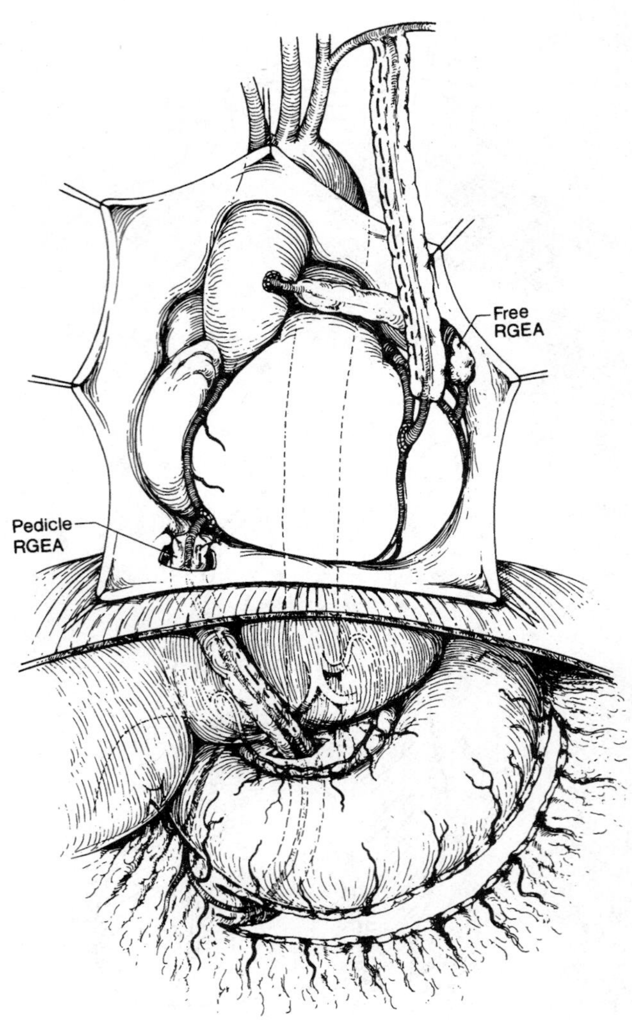

FIGURE 24–3. Right gastroepiploic artery (RGEA) graft to right coronary artery. The RGEA is passed behind the stomach, over the liver, and through the pericardium. (Reprinted with permission from The Society of Thoracic Surgeons. *The Annals of Thoracic Surgery*, Vol. 47, 1989, p. 710.)

There have been a few reports regarding the use of synthetic graft material for myocardial revascularization. Polytetrafluoroethylene (Gore-Tex) has been used in most investigations as the graft material. Graft occlusion represents a significant limitation. Two-year patency rates approach only 32% (Foster & Kranc, 1989). Despite the limited experience and exposure, poor results have precluded the clinical application of synthetic grafts.

Results

The results of CABG have been subject to scrutiny by the general public and health care professionals alike. Controversy fuels the debate over the "need" for the vast number of surgical procedures currently being performed. Questions posed address the efficacy of CABG surgery on survival, relief of symptoms, and quality of life. Current research efforts have refocused on the comparative outcomes of medical and surgical therapy and on risk factor stratification. Results from several large-scale observational investigations have illustrated the relatively low mortality rates, increased survival, longevity, and improved quality of life associated with CABG (Califf et al., 1989).

OPERATIVE MORTALITY. Wide variation exists in reports of operative mortality for patients undergoing CABG. Overall, mortality rates equal 2.1% (Rahimtoola, 1993). This figure has actually declined compared to past statistics in the early era of cardiac surgery. Earlier cohorts of patients demonstrated younger age, shorter long-term survival, and higher operative mortality rates (Rahimtoola, 1993). Despite the increasing severity in patient condition and the complexity of the procedure, this current trend in operative mortality figures reflects improvements in surgical technique, perioperative management, myocardial protection, and CPB.

Multiple factors influence the surgical outcome. The most significant prognostic indicator of operative mortality in patients with chronic stable angina is left ventricular function (Gersh et al., 1989). Risk of operative mortality has been found to be inversely proportional to left ventricular function. Patients with mild left ventricular dysfunction (LVEF > 50%), moderate left ventricular dysfunction (LVEF > 30%–50%), and severe left ventricular dysfunction (LVEF < 30%) incur a risk of operative mortality approximating 1.5%, 3.8%, and 6.1%, respectively (Gersh et al., 1989). Operative mortality rates double in patients with unstable angina compared to those with stable angina. Figures range from 1.2% to 8.5% (Kaiser et al., 1989). Recent data have suggested that duration of CPB is a significant predictor of perioperative MI and mortality in patients with unstable angina. A 16-fold increase in mortality was noted in patients with CPB times longer than 100 minutes. CPB duration also correlated with increased incidence (7.7%) of perioperative MI (Iyer et al., 1993).

Patients undergoing CABG for treatment of recent MI incur an increased risk for operative death. The time interval between the acute event and surgery is a significant factor. Patients operated on within 1 week of the event have been found to have the highest mortality (Kennedy et al., 1989). Advanced age, female gender, presence of left main coronary artery disease, and need for emergent operation have been identified as preoperative factors contributing to an increased risk of operative mortality (Kennedy et al., 1989).

LATE SURVIVAL. Increased longevity and survival is one of the most significant benefits derived from CABG surgery (Califf et al., 1989). Approximately 88% of patients are alive 5 years after surgery; 10-year and 15-year survival rates equal 73% and 55%, respectively (Rahimtoola, 1993). Comparatively, statistics for patients treated medically reveal an 80% 5-year and a 65% 10-year survival rate (Califf et al., 1989).

Impressive findings from several large-scale studies have helped to provide concrete evidence about the survival benefits of CABG. Many studies focus on survival statistics in certain patient subsets. Previous research has documented improved survival after surgery in patients with left main coronary artery disease and three-vessel disease with impaired left ventricular function (Killip et al., 1985). Ten- and 15-year survival rates approximate 66% and 47%, respectively, in patients with reduced left ventricular function. Patients with normal left ventricular function experience 10- and 15-year survival rates of 82% and 64%, respectively (Rahimtoola, 1993). Duke University investigators reported that this survival benefit extends even to patients considered high risk. In particular, older patients with poor left ventricular function or severe angina were found to exhibit the greatest improvement in survival benefits (Califf et al., 1989). The degree of survival benefit correlated proportionally with the severity of symptoms and the presence of a greater number of adverse prognostic indicators. Overall mortality was reduced in patients who were at highest risk for sudden death. Other studies have also noted improved survival benefits in some patients with normal left ventricular function and those with two proximal coronary artery stenoses (Myers et al., 1989).

Consistent findings indicate that the year in which the operation was performed affects survival (Califf et al., 1989; Teoh et al., 1987). Progressive improvements in surgical results are related to advances in CPB procedures, surgical techniques, and perioperative management. Consequently, increased survival benefits have been extended to patients with more complex underlying pathologies.

Incomplete revascularization influences late survival. The number of ungrafted diseased vessels increases the risk for development of future ischemic events. Complete revascularization of all major areas with significant stenoses affords the greatest relief of symptoms and improved survival.

RELIEF OF ANGINA. Relief of angina pectoris gained after CABG clearly represents the outcome of greatest magnitude for patients. In both patient subsets of chronic stable angina and unstable angina, dramatic improvement in chest pain has been noted both subjectively and from graded exercise testing (Kaiser et al., 1989; Kirklin et al., 1989). Nearly 80% to 90% of CABG patients experience complete relief of symptoms (Kaiser et al., 1989; Kirklin et al., 1989). Differences among gender have been noted, with a greater relief of symptoms observed in men than in women. At follow-up, Rahimtoola (1993) reported 81% of men were angina free, versus 74% of women. Relief of symptoms consequently affects the patient's quality of life and return to work. Freedom from disabling anginal symptoms affords patients the opportunity to engage in a more productive lifestyle. As time progresses, the beneficial effects of CABG surgery diminish. A lack of consensus is evident among reports of recurrence of symptoms. Seventy to 80% of patients remain pain free or experience minimal symptoms 7 to 10 years after CABG (Kaiser et al., 1989). Some patients remain asymptomatic despite angiographic evidence denoting severe reocclusion of both native and grafted vessels. Researchers have attributed this phenomenon to the placebo effect of surgery as well as to the possibility of psychological denial or silent ischemia.

REOPERATION. A vast increase in the number of reoperations has been observed during the last several years. Reoperation accounts for approximately 15% to 20% of coronary bypass procedures performed (Lytle et al., 1987b). Most reoperations are performed for recurrent angina unresponsive to medical therapy or in situations where accelerated native and graft disease is rendered unamenable to angioplasty or stenting procedures. Early reintervention within the first year often results from technical problems or conduit viability (Gersh et al., 1989). Young age, nonuse of the ITA, atherosclerotic disease progression, and recurrence of symptoms comprise the most common indicators for late reoperation (Gersh et al., 1989).

Operative mortality figures associated with reoperation are two to three times higher than those of the first operation. Consequences of aging on multiple organ systems influence the surgical outcome. Patients undergoing cardiac reoperation are older, present with increased severity of symptoms, have a higher incidence of left ventricular dysfunction, left main coronary artery disease, and fewer bypass grafts (Lytle, 1993). Increased technical difficulties often prolong the operative time. Perioperative MI, respiratory complications, neurologic injury, and bleeding are common postoperative sequelae associated with reoperation (Gersh et al., 1989). Efforts to minimize complications associated with reoperation have focused on cardioplegia delivery. Use of retrograde cardioplegia in high-risk patients has demonstrated impressive reductions in postoperative myocardial dysfunction in the reoperation subset (Rosengart et al., 1993).

Reoperation enhances survival in patients with late vein graft disease. A significant survival benefit is seen with reoperation compared to medical therapy in patients with saphenous vein graft stenosis to the LAD (Lytle, 1994). Four-year survival rates approximate 74%, compared to 53% with medical therapy. Redevelopment of angina is more common after reoperation and is often contingent on degree or completeness of revascularization. Reports of third-time reoperation appear to indicate acceptable morbidity and mortality rates. Merrill and colleagues (1993) noted the prime indication for third-time reoperation was refractory angina. Smoking and hypercholesterolemia were factors correlating with need for reoperation. Results demonstrated a 7.7% in-hospital mortality and an average 31-month pain-free interval. Overall survival after reoperation, however, is difficult to predict and must be viewed in the light of preoperative risk factors and susceptibility.

GRAFT PATENCY. Graft patency is the pivotal factor that determines the degree of success and the results after CABG surgery. A direct correlation has been established between graft patency and the recurrence of angina, ischemic symptoms, survival, and quality of life (Loop, 1983a, 1983b; Loop et al., 1989).

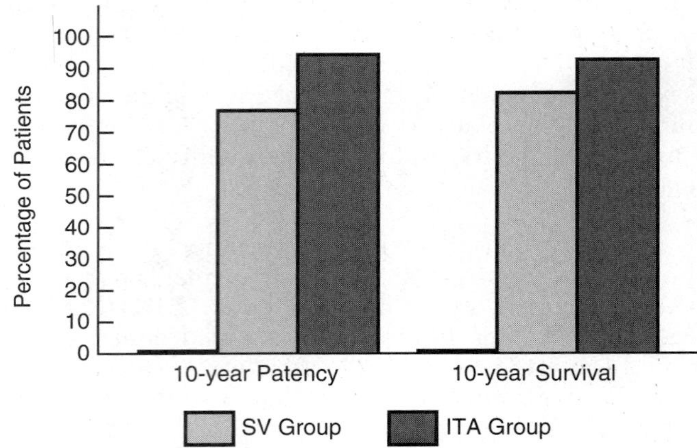

FIGURE 24–4. Comparison of internal thoracic artery (ITA) and saphenous vein (SV) grafts.

Excellent long-term patency rates associated with use of the ITA have led to improved 10-year survival rates (Fig. 24–4) approaching 90% (Loop et al., 1989). Survival statistics in patients with normal left ventricular function indicate significant differences between those who received an ITA graft and those who received saphenous vein grafts. Eighty-seven percent of ITA patients survived 10 years compared to 78% of patients with saphenous vein grafts (Loop et al., 1986, 1989). The most dramatic survival difference emerged in patients with impaired left ventricular function. The ITA group experienced a 16% greater 10-year survival compared to the saphenous vein group (Loop et al., 1986, 1989) (Fig. 24–5). Significantly fewer MIs, fewer reoperations, and longer event-free survivals have been observed in patients with ITA grafts (Loop et al., 1986, 1989). Several reports demonstrate that patients who receive an ITA graft to the LAD exhibit a reduction in risk of mortality by 62% to 65% (Loop et al., 1989).

Ten-year patency rates for ITA grafts approach 96%, compared with 81% for saphenous vein grafts (Zeff et al., 1988). Saphenous vein grafts are associated with a dramatic attrition rate with time. Approximately 8% to 12% of grafts occlude in the early postoperative period (Fitzgibbon et al., 1986; Grondin et al., 1989). Surgical technique, recipient vessel size, and graft flow rates are factors influencing early vein patency. Angiographic studies performed at 1 year revealed that significant morphologic changes affected 12% to 20% of the vein grafts (Grondin et al., 1989). At 5 years, 20% to 30% of grafts were found to display impressive narrowing and luminal changes, compromising flow. This rate doubled to approximately 50% at 10 years (Fitzgibbon et al., 1986; Grondin et al., 1989).

Histologic changes occurring within vein grafts are

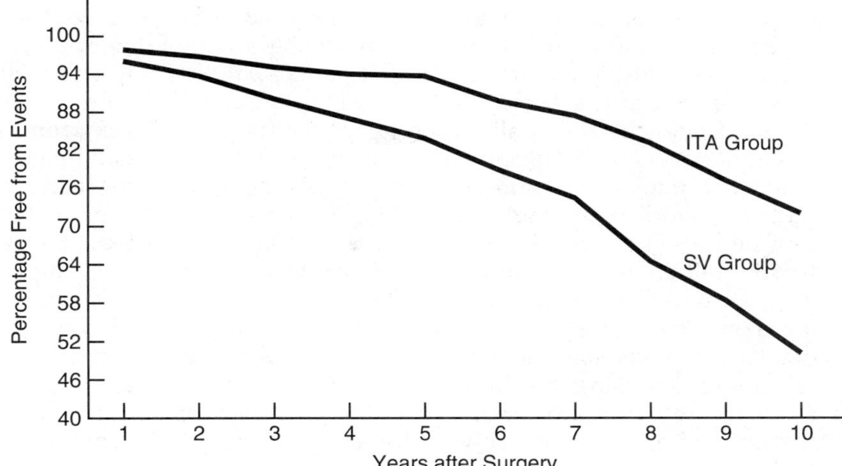

FIGURE 24–5. Occurrence of cardiac events with internal thoracic artery (ITA) and saphenous vein (SV) grafts.

responsible for failure and occlusion. Intimal proliferation and migration of smooth muscle cells precipitate a thickening of the endothelial layer. Platelet deposition and release of thromboxane (a potent vasoconstrictor) further contribute to the development of vein graft atherosclerosis (Goldman et al., 1988). Measures to retard the rapidity and acceleration of atherosclerotic disease have focused on the use of aspirin and dipyridamole. Dipyridamole acts to inhibit platelet aggregation, mural thrombus formation, and thromboxane release (Goldman et al., 1988). Some centers administer dipyridamole 24 to 48 hours before surgery. Institution of antiplatelet therapy before and after surgery has been found to improve early graft patency (Goldman et al., 1988). Emphasis on serum cholesterol and diet warrants continued investigation. Evidence suggests that cholesterol-lowering agents have an important role in potentially limiting both systemic and coronary vein graft atherosclerosis (Grondin et al., 1989).

PREVENTION OF CARDIAC EVENTS. The role of CABG surgery in preventing further myocardial injury is difficult to quantify. Patients who have undergone surgery demonstrate greater freedom from cardiac events compared to patients treated medically. The incidence of MI approaches 1.1% per year in surgical patients. This figure doubles to 2.6% in medically treated patients. Approximately 77% of CABG patients remain free from ischemic or myocardial injury during the first 5 years, and almost 50% report event-free survival at 10 years (Kirklin et al., 1989). Surgical patients demonstrate a 26% reduction in cardiac-related hospital admissions (Kirklin et al., 1989). This result has a significant impact not only on health care costs but on the patient's ability to maintain an uninterrupted quality of life, free from hospital admissions.

QUALITY OF LIFE. Improved quality of life represents one of the most important benefits derived from CABG surgery. From the patient's perspective, the crucial determinant of operative success hinges on the ability to resume an active and productive lifestyle. In patients with unstable angina, CABG has been found to produce superior results compared to medical therapy alone (Booth et al., 1991). The Veterans Administration Cooperative Study demonstrated that surgery enhanced quality of life, as quantified by improved treadmill performance, decreased need for antianginal medications, reduced chest pain, and noted subjective improvement (Booth et al., 1991). Several investigations have focused on patient expectations with regard to postoperative outcome. Patients' expectations represent key determinants of recovery. Most patients achieved the expected benefits of prolongation of life, prevention of infarct, and improved quality of life at 6 months after surgery (Gortner et al., 1989). Typically, however, during the first postoperative month patients report symptoms of decreased appetite, insomnia, weakness, fatigue, and reduced activity tolerance. As time progresses, improved exercise tolerance most often leads to increased participation in daily activities. Increased coronary blood flow is demonstrated on postoperative exercise tolerance testing (Kirklin et al., 1989). Improved left ventricular wall motion and performance after surgery facilitate increased myocardial work capacity. Patients enjoy greater freedom to participate in physical activity and sexual activity, and have fewer and less severe associated symptoms (Gortner et al., 1989). Decreased requirements for medications and reliance on nitrates allows patients greater independence, both physically and psychologically (Gortner et al., 1989).

Patients are encouraged to return to work after successful surgery. The goal of recovery focuses on return to gainful employment. Wide variations exist in figures depicting patients who return to work after surgery. It is estimated that 38% to 81% (average 62%) of patients are employed after surgery (Allen, 1990). Preoperative work status is the major predictor of postoperative employment. However, considerable controversy surrounds the use of return to work as an index or measure of quality of life. There has been some attempt to use return to work figures to examine and justify the economic impact of cardiac surgery.

Caution must be used, however, in outcome analysis of the efficacy of surgical intervention for CAD with regard to quality of life. Many variables affect patient decisions to return to work. Factors such as age, gender, and financial status all play a role. Reports indicate that participation in some form of structured cardiac rehabilitation program increases the likelihood of return to work (Gutmann et al., 1982). Patients who returned to work experienced greater degrees of self-worth, self-confidence, and lifestyle satisfaction. In general, psychosocial factors have been found to be more predictive of return to work and gainful employment than physiologic factors. More researchers are carefully reassessing the clinical utility of work status as an accurate indicator of quality of life, and placing it within a contextual framework for each individual patient.

GENDER. Until recently, data about results and outcomes associated with CABG procedures were derived primarily from studies composed of men. Limited information was available about recovery in women. Thus, a number of recent investigations have focused on examining the impact of gender on recovery from surgical revascularization.

Mortality figures are higher for women undergoing CABG surgery than for men. Women incur an operative mortality rate of approximately 4.6% with first CABG, compared to 2.6% in men. Reasons explaining an almost 50% higher mortality rate have centered on differences in age and functional class. Women are older, being referred for surgery later in the course of disease, which contributes to a higher preoperative functional class before surgery. Other reports have indicated that the predictive accuracy of diagnostic testing (such as exercise testing) has led to a misinterpretation of disease severity. Tobin (1987) noted that when exercise results were abnormal in women with anginal symptoms, recommendations for angiographic study were less likely to occur. Wenger (1990) showed that women displayed significantly greater preoperative symptoms of dypsnea and hypercholesterolemia and had longer postoperative intensive care unit stays and mortality rates than men. Factors such as hypertension, diabetes, family history, and smoking were equitable between the sexes.

Long-term survival rates are similar in men and women. However, women demonstrate lowered rates of graft patency. Consequently, more women have an increased incidence of anginal symptoms, shortness of breath, and MIs. Differences also exist in psychosocial outcomes, denoting a correlation between physiologic status and psychological functioning. Women report decreased levels of postoperative activity compared to men. At 12 to 21 months after surgery, men participate in some form of moderate activity twice as often as women (Stanton et al., 1984). Employment status is closely related to the patient's personal, social, and economic status. Most investigations reveal that fewer women are employed outside the home after surgery. Several reports have shown that women display less postoperative anxiety, anger, and depression than men (Wenger, 1990). Figure 24–6 depicts the differences noted between women and men after cardiac surgery. For nurses caring for these patients, knowledge of postoperative differences will assist in planning interventions and providing support to facilitate optimal postoperative recovery and adaptation.

ELDERLY. The elderly comprise an ever-increasing number of patients undergoing cardiac surgery. There has been more than a fivefold increase in the elderly cohort (age > 70 years as defined in most series). In-hospital mortality figures range from 3.7% to 7.6% (He

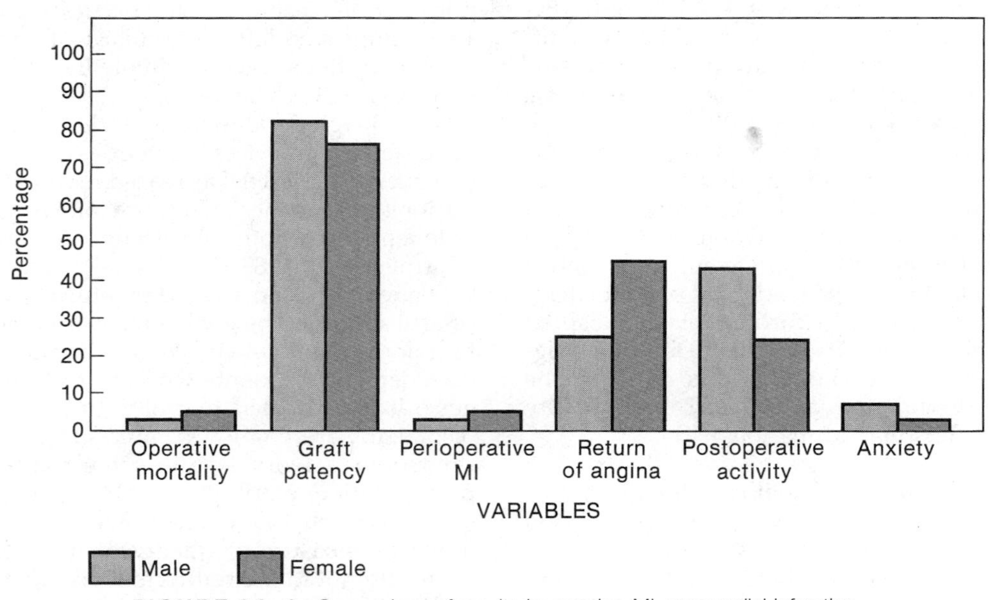

FIGURE 24–6. Comparison of results by gender. MI, myocardial infarction.

et al., 1994). The most common cause of death was cardiac failure. Late mortality has been attributed to noncardiac or organ failure. Probability of 3-year survival approaches 86%. Profiles of elderly patients reflect an increased incidence of CHF and renal disease, with hypertension being more prevalent in the female population. There have been no gender differences noted in complication rates. However, women typically displayed an increased incidence of CHF. Age was positively correlated to length of stay (King et al., 1992). He and colleagues (1994) identified seven risk factors for operative mortality according to a regression analysis. They include right ITA grafting, reoperation, history of MI, age, left main disease, smoking history, and postoperative complications. The role of right ITA grafting will continue to require further study in this population.

In an attempt to study this population further, the Health Care Financing Administration has initiated a demonstration project, Medicare Participating Heart Bypass Center Demonstration. This project exemplifies a multicenter effort to examine creative ways of bundling costs and developing a data base to evaluate the outcomes of bypass surgery over a 5-year period for the Medicare population.

PREOPERATIVE CARE

Initial Assessment

Comprehensive systematic assessment elicits vital information in the preliminary stages to prepare the patient for cardiovascular surgery. The initial assessment of the patient and family, focusing on physiologic, psychological, psychosocial, and spiritual factors and concerns, will enable the critical care nurse to compile an extensive and informative data base. On completion, identification of actual and potential problems will assist the nurse in delineating factors that may affect the surgical outcome and in formulating an individualized plan of care. Sharing the plan and any other vital information among caregivers assists in maximizing continuity of care. Reducing fragmentation of care resulting from the shortened lengths of stay in acute care areas represents a continuous challenge to the health team. Use of case managers has gained increased attention in an attempt to facilitate the coordination of care. Institution of critical pathways and care maps has aided in charting the course of illness for each patient and monitoring progress through shorter hospital stays. As capitation becomes more prevalent, same-day admission for cardiac surgery presents additional challenges for hospitals to implement creative programs for this complex patient population.

Diagnostic Studies

Preoperative laboratory studies are used in the assessment of physiologic function. Many centers have dramatically reduced the number of studies acquired in the preoperative phase. Anecdotal reports have failed to demonstrate negative outcomes with less testing. Modifications should be made, however, on an individual basis, using discretion to determine the need for extensive testing in an attempt to promote cost efficiency.

Routine complete blood count, electrolytes, blood urea nitrogen, creatinine, prothrombin time (PT), and partial thromboplastin time are evaluated. Some centers have stopped testing routine bleeding times; with a large percentage of cases being "urgent" priority, prolonged times have not affected timing of surgery. Chest radiographs and ECGs are done to establish baseline information. Urinalysis may be done to rule out urinary tract infection. In patients about to undergo concomitant valvular surgery, dental consultations are obtained to confirm the absence of any periodontal infection. These measures are enacted to reduce the risk of postoperative endocarditis.

Pulmonary function tests may be obtained to identify patients at high risk for respiratory complications or respiratory failure in the postoperative period. However, there is conflicting evidence about the relationship between preoperative pulmonary status and postoperative outcome. Some reports indicate that vital capacity and flow greater than 80% represents a low risk, and that results that are less than 50% of the predicted value signify a high risk for postoperative pulmonary complications (Braunwald, 1988). Ingersoll and Grippi (1991), however, demonstrated no correlation between diminished pulmonary function and the need for prolonged mechanical ventilation. Thus, the need for preoperative pulmonary function measurements remains questionable.

Cardiovascular performance and valvular function are evaluated through findings from the ECG, echocardiogram, cardiac catheterization, and magnetic resonance imaging. The echocardiogram provides valuable baseline data regarding chamber dimensions, wall excursion, valvular motion, thickening, calcification, and prolapse. Coronary angiography reveals details of the location, severity, and shape of coronary lesions. Close study of the coronary anatomy assists the surgeon in devising and formulating an appropriate plan for revascularization. Valvular function is assessed through calculation of transvalvular pressure gradients and estimation of valve area. Ventriculography determines the LVEF and the degree of mitral regurgitation, and aortography aids in evaluating regurgitant flow in patients with aortic regurgitation. Magnetic resonance imaging is gaining closer attention for use in patients with poor ventricular function or valvular disease to determine the presence of thrombus and the need for prophylactic intervention.

The presence of carotid atherosclerotic disease is significant for the patient about to undergo CABG. The use of angiography or duplex scanning is the most reliable method of detecting carotid disease. Studies have shown a significantly higher neurologic complication rate after CABG in patients with greater than 50%

narrowing of carotid vessels. When indicated, carotid endarterectomy is often performed concomitantly with CABG to reduce the risk of ischemic induced neurologic injury (Hurst et al., 1986). Thus, preoperative carotid screening serves as a valuable tool in identifying patients at risk for stroke after CABG (Faggioli et al., 1990).

Additional attention must be paid to conduit availability. History of prior vein ligation or stripping, extensive varicosities, or severe arterial insufficiency may preclude use of the greater saphenous vein. These situations warrant evaluation with duplex scanning to map venous geography and flow to determine viable options and length of potential conduit material.

Close examination of the coagulation profile is of paramount importance. Consumption of aspirin products, nonsteroidal antiinflammatory agents, or warfarin alters bleeding time, predisposing the patient to an increased risk for coagulopathy as a postoperative complication, potentially requiring transfusion. Type and cross-match, autologous blood donations, and direct donor donations are used to ensure the presence of an adequate blood reserve before surgery.

Autologous blood donation is encouraged in many centers for patients undergoing elective surgery. It is estimated that only 5% of all eligible patients participate in the program, indicating a significant underutilization of this service (Toy et al., 1987). Predonation has been considered safe for patients with cardiovascular disease. Eligibility criteria include patients with chronic angina but preclude those with preinfarction angina. Use of autologous blood programs has helped to reduce the need for homologous transfusions as well as the transmission of blood-borne diseases. Some centers have reported a 50% decrease in the need for homologous blood transfusion after surgery. Approximately 73% to 75% of patients who predonated blood avoided homologous transfusions, compared to 18% to 20% who did not donate (Britton et al., 1989). Most patients donate an average of one unit of blood per week, according to pre-established guidelines from the American Association of Blood Banks. Factors affecting donation are progression of angina, anemia, and development of new symptoms. Current investigations focus on the use of synthetic growth hormones such as erythropoietin to stimulate red blood cell production, increasing the ability of patients to donate. In addition to red cell autologous transfusion, interest has also increased in the readministration of plasma and platelets during CPB to reduce bleeding risk and augment hemostasis (Boldt et al., 1990).

Medications

The value of obtaining a complete medication history cannot be overemphasized. Before surgery, the modification of certain medications is warranted to avert the development of perioperative complications. First and foremost, all aspirin and nonsteroidal antiinflammatory products must be discontinued at least 7 to 10 days before surgery. Aspirin acts to inhibit thromboxane synthesis, thereby inhibiting platelet aggregation and vasoconstriction. This effect persists 5 to 7 days or for the life of the platelet. This action, in combination with the effects of CPB on platelet membranes, has been associated with an increased perioperative blood loss (Ferraris et al., 1988). Resultant bleeding increases the risk of cardiac tamponade, reoperation, and transfusion requirement. Other agents known to interfere with platelet function are ampicillin, carbenicillin, diphenhydramine, furosemide, gentamicin, ibuprofen, indomethacin, nitrofurantoin, papaverine, penicillin, phenothiazines, propranolol, sulfinpyrazone, and tricyclic amines (Bick, 1984). Recent reports have linked the intake of large amounts of omega-3 fatty acids to increased risk of prolonged bleeding times, especially in patients taking coumadin (warfarin) or aspirin (Leaf & Weber, 1988). Patients on warfarin are advised to refrain from consumption of omega-3 fatty acids 5 days before surgery. Knowledge of the impact of these agents on hemostasis assists the nurse in identifying high-risk patients. Postoperative bleeding remains a risk in some cases when PTs have returned to normal. Administration of vitamin K may be considered to ensure adequate reversal and hemostasis. Patients receiving continuous anticoagulation therapy can remain on heparin until line placement or according to anesthetic protocols.

All antianginal agents such as beta-adrenergic blocking agents, calcium channel blockers, and nitrates are continued. With the increased emotional and physiologic stress experienced by patients before surgery, continued administration of antianginal agents is warranted to prevent exacerbation of ischemic symptoms or myocardial damage. Propranolol has been found to be effective for controlling increased adrenergic stimulation, assisting in anesthetic induction, and reducing the incidence of perioperative ventricular dysrhythmias (Hurst et al., 1986). The use of propranolol has not been found to depress postoperative myocardial performance (Hurst et al., 1986).

Recent attention has focused on the use of clonidine, an alpha$_2$-adrenergic agonist. Some of the proposed benefits include blunting of sympathetic discharge and suppression of plasma catecholemines, potentially decreasing risk of perioperative ischemia and reducing the incidence of postoperative tachydysrhythmias. Transdermal administration 12 hours before surgery has been noted to improve hemodynamics, reduce blood pressure lability, and decrease ischemia in the prebypass and intraoperative periods (Dorman et al., 1993). Further benefits include reduction in analgesic use and decreased shivering.

Digoxin is usually withheld 1 to 2 days before surgery except in patients with atrial fibrillation with a poorly controlled ventricular response (Hurst et al., 1986). It has been found that serum digoxin levels tend to rise in these patients, a phenomenon that is poorly understood but is thought to be linked to the effects of CPB.

Additional medications administered include

prophylactic antibiotics, most commonly a broad-spectrum cephalosporin. Many centers recently have added dipyridamole (100 mg three times a day) to the preoperative regimen. Antiplatelet therapy started early has been shown to be effective in reducing the incidence of thrombosis and early vein graft occlusion (Goldman et al., 1988). Some centers also have focused on the administration of preoperative allopurinol. Allopurinol acts to inhibit the formation of cytotoxic free radicals during myocardial ischemia and reperfusion. Johnson and colleagues (1991) found that allopurinol improved postoperative cardiac performance, demonstrated by a reduced need for inotropic support or mechanical support. The recommended dose is 200 mg to 400 mg (depending on patient weight) administered once on the evening before the operation and once 4 hours before surgery.

INTRAOPERATIVE MANAGEMENT

Cardiopulmonary Bypass

The first successful use of extracorporeal CPB in humans was undertaken by Gibbson in 1954 (Gibbson, 1954). CPB is a method by which venous blood is diverted from the arrested heart's right atrium to pass through either a membrane or a bubble oxygenator. In the oxygenator, through the process of diffusion, carbon dioxide is given off and oxygen is bound to hemoglobin. Once arterialized, the blood is returned to the body through the aorta for systemic distribution (Blanche et al., 1990; Edmunds & Stephenson, 1983; Moores & Willford, 1989). The diversion of blood provides the surgeon with a bloodless, immobilized heart muscle on which to work. Improvements in the delivery of hypothermia, myocardial protection, anesthesia, blood conservation, and surgical techniques all have contributed to the ever-decreasing mortality associated with various types of cardiac operations.

Although CPB clearly has contributed greatly to the art and science of cardiac surgery, it is not without consequences. Nurses caring for these patients in the perioperative phase need to understand the operative events that affect common postoperative clinical problems. This section reviews the components of the CPB machine, myocardial preservation, the systemic pathophysiologic responses associated with the conduct of CPB, common nursing problems, and the management of cardiac surgical patients.

Components of CPB

HEMODILUTION. The CPB machine is usually primed with a crystalloid solution. A volume of 1,800 to 2,000 mL of fluid, or the equivalent of 20 mL/kg, is used, resulting in dilution of the serum hematocrit to the range of 20% to 25% (Blanche et al., 1990; Edmunds & Stephenson, 1983; Milam, 1983). Because of loss of pulsatile pressure while on CPB and hemodilution, some of the perfusate becomes translocated into the interstitial space (Milam, 1983). Albumin may be used in the priming solution to balance the changed oncotic pressures and maintain volume in the intravascular space. However, Marelli and associates (1989) conducted a randomized study on the effect of the use of albumin in the priming solution on clinical outcomes. These investigators found no significant difference in the group in which albumin was used.

HEPARINIZATION. After the chest is opened and before cannulation of the great vessels and cardiac chambers, heparin at 3 mg/kg is administered to prevent spontaneous clot formation as blood comes in contact with the approximately 40 feet of polyvinyl chloride tubing associated with the CPB system (Blanche et al., 1990; Milam, 1983). A baseline activated clotting time is measured before the first injection of heparin, which inhibits clotting factors V, IX, XI, XIIa, and thrombin (Blanche et al., 1990; Edmunds & Stephenson, 1983). While on CPB, the ACT is measured every 30 to 60 minutes and should be maintained between 350 and 500 seconds during both normothermic and hypothermic states with supplemental heparin (Gravlee et al., 1990a).

At completion of the cardiac operation, protamine sulfate is given in a dose of approximately 1.3 mg to each 1-mg dose of heparin given, including any used in the priming solution to reverse the clotting inhibition (Blanche et al., 1990; Edmunds & Stephenson, 1983; Milam, 1983). Protamine administration at the completion of CPB has been demonstrated to cause significant hemodynamic effects due to systemic vasodilation, hypotension, and myocardial dysfunction (Levy et al., 1989; Michaels & Barash, 1983). Right ventricular dysfunction caused by pulmonary vasoconstriction due to protamine has also been demonstrated (Lewenstein et al., 1983). Patients with a history of insulin-dependent diabetes using protamine zinc insulin or with allergies to seafood may also be at risk for development of anaphylaxis with protamine administration. Another population at risk is male patients who have had a vasectomy. In this group, it is reported that 1 year after the vasectomy, antibodies to human protamine produced by sperm develop in up to 55% of patients (Samuel, 1977). Because protamine is derived from salmon gonadal tissue, vasectomized patients are at risk for having a potential anaphylactoid reaction because of previous development of sensitivity to the drug (Levy et al., 1989). When a reaction is anticipated, pretreatment using steroids, diphenhydramine hydrochloride (Benadryl; Parke-Davis, Morris Plains, NJ), and ranitidine (Zantac; Glaxo, Research Triangle Park, NC) is recommended. Blanche and associates (1990) recommend that protamine be administered after removal of the venous catheters but before removal of the arterial catheter, because CPB may need to be reinitiated emergently.

CARDIOTOMY SUCTION SYSTEM. Blood conserved from the operative field is removed and returned to

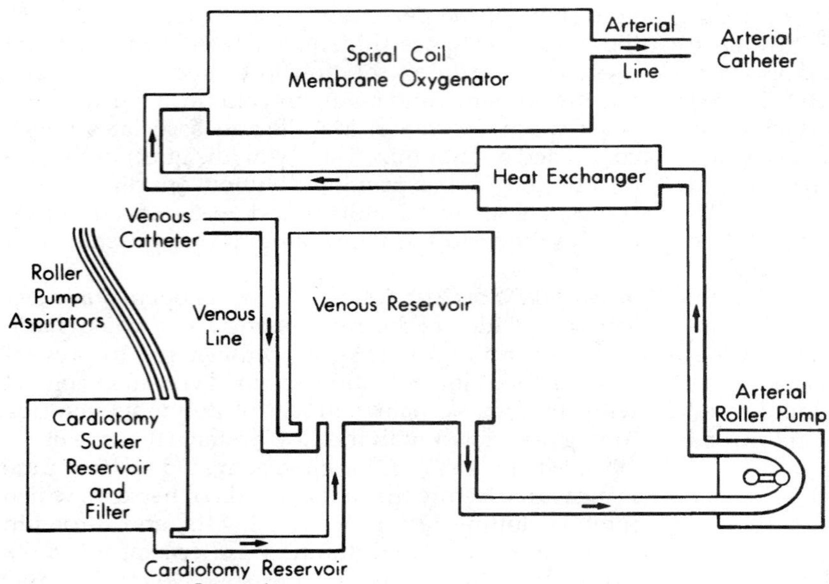

FIGURE 24–7. Diagram of a typical set-up for cardiopulmonary bypass using a spiral coil-type membrane oxygenator. (From Edmunds, H., & Stephenson, L. [1983]. Cardiopulmonary bypass for open heart surgery. In Geha, A., et al. [Eds.], *Thoracic and cardiovascular surgery* [4th ed., p. 1092]. E. Norwalk, CT: Appleton-Century-Crofts.)

the extracorporeal perfusion system by way of the cardiotomy suction system (Edmunds & Stephenson, 1983). This aspirate contains calcium, bits of sutures, fat or fibrin, and foreign materials that are filtered through the CPB system to prevent systemic embolization. Delong and associates (1980) demonstrated that the intense blood–air contact during suctioning has a major effect on blood cell hemolysis in conjunction with use of the CPB oxygenator. Although blood conservation is the objective, some hemolysis does occur.

VENOUS RESERVOIRS. A venous reservoir is a conduit for deoxygenated blood, and is a part of the CPB machine. It is usually positioned 30 cm below the right atrium to facilitate passive venous drainage before blood enters the oxygenator. In the bubble oxygenator system, venous blood enters the oxygenator directly and is arterialized (Blanche et al., 1990; Edmunds & Stephenson, 1983) (Figs. 24–7 and 24–8). These conduits also receive filtered blood from the operative field from the cardiotomy system.

BUBBLE OXYGENATOR. The bubble oxygenator is the most commonly used oxygenator because it is thought to have little hemolytic effect on the red blood cells (Milam, 1983). Oxygenation occurs when venous blood comes in contact with oxygenated bubbles. During this interface, oxygen diffuses from the bubbles and is absorbed by the red blood cells of the venous blood while CO_2 diffuses in the opposite direction. Bubbles in the arterialized blood are removed by passing the blood over a large mesh or sponge surface area that is treated with an antifoam agent. The arterialized blood then enters a large settling chamber or reservoir in which heat exchange occurs (Blanche et al., 1990; Edmunds & Stephenson, 1983). Arterialized blood is then pumped into a chamber, where it is filtered again for potential gaseous emboli before being returned to the aorta for systemic distribution.

MEMBRANE OXYGENATOR. Venous blood passes through a separate heat exchanger before entering the membrane oxygenator. Once inside the oxygenator, blood never comes in direct contact with oxygen, but instead covers a large, semipermeable, capillary-type membrane. Arterialization of the venous blood occurs by diffusion when CO_2 is given off by the red blood cells and oxygen diffuses across the membrane from the oxygenator. A filter is not needed in this system because the arterialized blood is then returned directly to the patient after oxygenation.

The bubble oxygenator causes less damage to blood cells on CPB runs of 3 hours or less (Clark et al., 1979). When CPB runs are anticipated to be longer than 3 hours, the membrane oxygenator causes less damage to blood cells (Boonstra et al., 1986). In clinical use, the bubble oxygenator has the advantages of being easy to prime and assemble, simple to use, and relatively inexpensive.

PUMPS. Both the roller pump and the centrifugal pump are used to conduct cardiac operations. Originally designed by DeBakey in 1934, the roller pump used today is virtually unchanged (DeBakey, 1934) (Fig. 24–9). It is simple to use, reliable, produces low blood trauma, and delivers accurate perfusion rates. Flow through the roller pump is delivered by the degree of partial occlusion applied to the CPB tubing by the roller. Pump output is proportional to the speed of rotation and the internal diameter of the compressible tubing (Edmunds & Stephenson, 1983). Flow rates of 1.6 to 2.2 liters / m^2 per minute in conjunction with hypothermia are thought to deliver adequate blood volume during CPB without causing cerebral dysfunction

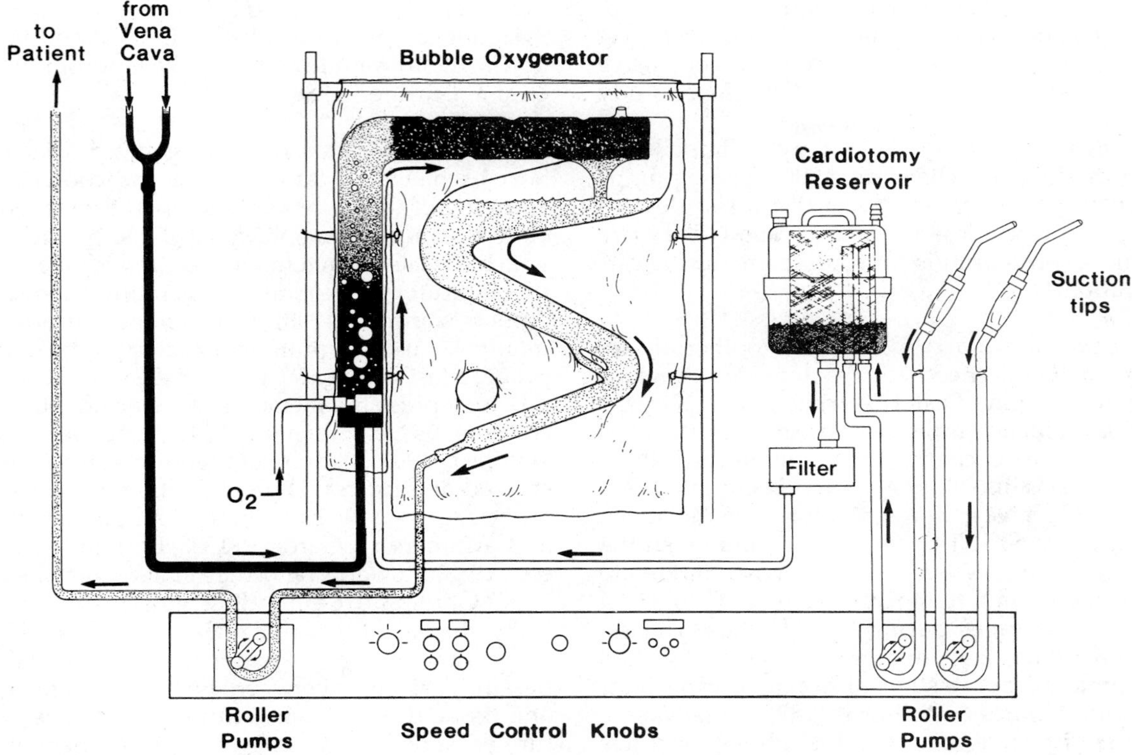

FIGURE 24–8. Composite illustration of a cardiopulmonary bypass system using a bubble oxygenator system. (From Milam, J. [1983]. Blood transfusion in heart surgery. *Surgical Clinics of North America, 63,* 1127–1146.)

(Edmunds & Stephenson, 1983). The roller pump delivers continuous, nonpulsatile blood flow to the tissues. Although adequate for CPB, this flow state contributes to the pathophysiologic systemic changes seen in the postoperative period.

Use of a pump that delivers pulsatile flows during CPB has been thought to be more physiologic. Very little clinical use of this pump has been documented (Moores et al., 1977; Niemmen et al., 1980; Reis et al., 1987; Singh et al., 1980). However, pulsatile flow is thought to produce less metabolic acidosis, lower peripheral arterial resistance, improved cerebral perfusion, less hepatocellular injury, improved myocardial perfusion to the subendocardium, and expedient cooling and warming of body tissues (Reis et al., 1987). Study of the effects of pulsatile flows on the cooling

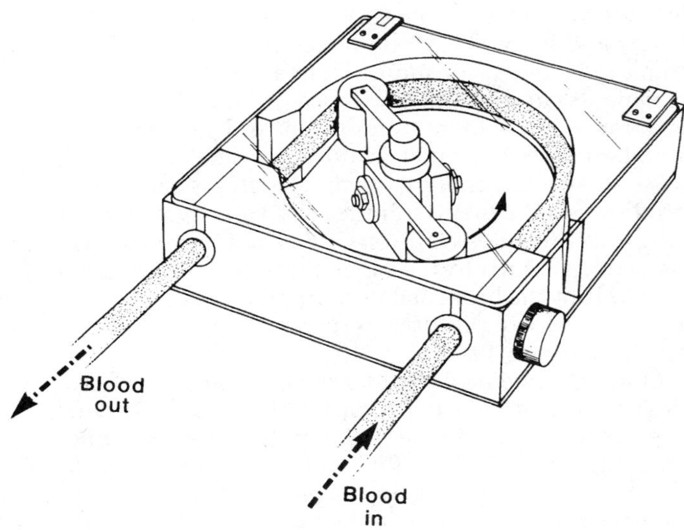

FIGURE 24–9. Diagram of a roller pump used in both the membrane and bubble oxygenator systems. (From Milam, J. [1983]. Blood transfusion in heart surgery. *Surgical Clinics of North America, 63,* 1127–1147.)

and rewarming of tissues has not proved this approach to be beneficial (Niemmen et al., 1983; Singh et al., 1980). Clinical study has not provided conclusive data to support the use of pulsatile CPB; more study is needed on the use of such pumps.

Centrifugal pumps move blood by an impeller or vortexing motion (Blanche et al., 1990). These pumps have been used for long-term cardiac assist devices and appear to cause less trauma to blood. They are gaining more consideration for routine use during cardiac operation.

HYPOTHERMIA AND BLOOD FLOWS. Hypothermia reduces the metabolic need for oxygen and provides an important margin of safety during cardiac surgery (Reitz, 1982). Biochemical reactions are described as a function of a 10°C change in temperature (Milam, 1983; Moores & Willford, 1989). It has been stated that for every 10°C increase in temperature, the metabolic rate increases by 50%. The converse occurs when the temperature decreases by 10°C. Likewise, moderate systemic hypothermia (temperatures of 25°C to 32°C) has several advantages during CPB: lower perfusion flow requirements, less myocardial rewarming, less blood trauma, and protection of organs during brief hypothermia (Moores & Willford, 1989). Initially, surface-induced hypothermia was thought to be safer than core cooling through CPB (Haneda et al., 1982). However, use of the surface method prolonged cooling and was abandoned because of the need for prolonged rewarming time and increased metabolic acidosis. Also, its use was prohibitive in hemodynamically unstable patients (Cameron & Gardner, 1988).

During the hypothermic state, a left shift in the oxyhemoglobin dissociation curve occurs. This results in less unloading of oxygen from the hemoglobin molecule. However, as long as the tissue metabolic need for oxygen is decreased, a balance of oxygen supply and demand is maintained.

While on CPB, perfusion flow rates take the place of the cardiac index and may range from 1.8 to 2.4 liters/minute/m^2 during systemic hypothermia of 25°C (Blanche et al., 1990; Cameron & Gardner, 1988). Hickey and Hoor (1983) conducted a clinical trial that monitored oxygen consumption in a small population of patients undergoing coronary revascularization. Flow rates of 1.2 liters/minute/m^2 did not produce formation of detrimental acidosis or deleterious decreases in mixed venous oxygen saturations compared with flows of 2.2 liters/minute/m^2. The advantage of using low flow rates while on CPB is that they produce less venous return to the heart through noncoronary collaterals of the bronchial and pulmonary vessels because less blood perfuses through the body (Cameron & Gardner, 1988).

Optimal systemic hypothermia and perfusion flow rates are individualized. Patients with few or no collaterals benefit least from deeper hypothermia. Systemic temperatures of 28°C to 30°C with flow rates of 2.2 to 2.4 liters/minute/m^2 are appropriate. In patients with extensive collateralization, anticipated complex procedures, or a compromised heart, the converse is true. Systemic temperatures of 20°C to 25°C and flow rates of 1.6 liters/minute/m^2 may be appropriate (Cameron & Gardner, 1988).

HEAT EXCHANGER. Both oxygenator systems have heat exchangers that allow for the cooling and rewarming of the body. Body temperature is monitored closely using a nasopharyngeal temperature probe, which reflects brain temperature and is the most sensitive indicator of systemic temperature changes (Cameron & Gardner, 1988). Core temperature is usually monitored using a pulmonary artery catheter or rectal probe. Most cardiac surgeons use systemic hypothermia to depress the metabolic cellular rate, thereby decreasing tissue vulnerability to ischemia (Moores & Willford, 1989). Adult temperatures are usually decreased at a rate of 0.7°C to 1.5°C/minute to achieve moderate systemic hypothermia ranging from 25°C to 32°C (Cameron & Gardner, 1988; Edmunds & Stephenson, 1983). Rewarming occurs at a slower rate of 0.2°C to 0.5°C/minute (Edmunds & Stephenson, 1983). Clinically, the rate of systemic rewarming is limited by perfusion flow rates in the extracorporeal circuit and temperature gradients between the heat exchanger, blood, and tissue (Cameron & Gardner, 1988). The temperature of blood generated by the heat exchanger should not exceed 40°C to 42°C during rewarming because a risk of protein denaturation and hemolysis to blood cells occurs at 44°C (Blanche et al., 1990; Cameron & Gardner, 1988; Edmunds & Stephenson, 1983). Close monitoring of temperature gradient differences between the perfusate temperature and the nasopharyngeal temperature is maintained to ensure that the gradient remains between 6°C and 8°C. Such a gradient is maintained during systemic cooling and rewarming because gases may be liberated from solution when cool blood perfuses warmed tissue or when cool blood is rewarmed (Blanche et al., 1990).

Myocardial Protection

This review of the technical aspects of the conduct of CPB is most helpful for nurses caring for cardiac surgical patients. The advent of the use of CPB has allowed surgeons to perform delicate cardiac operations while supporting the patient's systemic metabolic function. However, one of the most crucial aspects of the operation is myocardial preservation. This section gives nurses an understanding of the basic approaches to myocardial preservation as it affects ventricular functioning in the postoperative period. Such information, in conjunction with a knowledge of the conduct of CPB, provides a foundation for anticipating nursing care for these patients.

Optimal subendocardial preservation during cardiac operations has a major impact on morbidity and mortality during the perioperative period. The initial techniques used to protect the subendocardium and provide the surgeon with a bloodless, arrested heart were hypothermic intermittent ischemic arrest with aortic cross-clamping (Olinger, 1988) and the induction of ventricular fibrillation (Buckberg, 1975). These techniques were attempts to decrease the oxygen debt during the period of myocardial anoxia. However, the former approach accentuated changes in anaerobic metabolism, causing increased intracellular acidosis, and altered cellular enzymatic functions (Kirklin & Barratt-Boyes, 1986). Further, the latter approach depleted adenosine triphosphate (ATP) and high-energy phosphate stores within the myocardial cells (Buckberg, 1983; Cameron & Gardner, 1988). Both approaches were associated with subendocardial injury and support the current use of a high-potassium cardioplegic solution to precipitate global myocardial arrest.

The key considerations in preventing subendocardial damage depend on decreasing myocardial energy demands during the ischemic period while salvaging enough energy stores to meet these demands. Care is also taken to prevent both iatrogenic injury due to excessive cold, excessive retraction on the organ, trauma, or potassium-induced fibrosis and damage caused by the reperfusion process (Silverman et al., 1988). Therefore, the goals of myocardial protection are prevention of cardiac muscle injury through induction of rapid electromechanical arrest, adequate hypothermia, buffering of the myocardial and systemic acidotic state, and prevention of intracellular edema (Silverman et al., 1988).

Cardinal to subendocardial protection is the provision of continuous, even myocardial hypothermia. Maintenance of hypothermic myocardial temperatures during aortic cross-clamping depends on maintaining the balance between heat escaping and heat entering the tissues (Rosenfeldt, 1988). Rosenfeldt and colleagues (1988) studied the effects of noncoronary blood flow of pulmonary venous return to the left heart and inadequate systemic venous drainage to the CPB system on rewarming the hypothermic heart. These investigators demonstrated that bronchial venous return increased septal temperatures. Systemic and pulmonary venous return entering the cardiac chambers was found to be a significant heat source that precipitated early rewarming and ischemic injury to the myocardium. These data support the notion that such venous return may also cause injury to the conduction system through early rewarming.

To prevent these injuries from warmed venous blood entering the cardiac chambers, cold cardioplegia and topical cooling techniques are used. Typically, concern about the evenness of cooling the dense ventricular mass, specifically in the hypertrophied left ventricle, warrants the common practice of using adjunctive topical cooling with a cold cardioplegia infusion (Blanche et al., 1990; Rosenfeldt & Watson, 1979). Various methods of topical cooling have been used. For example, recirculating solutions have been used in both open techniques, such as cold saline ice solution poured into the operative field (Edmunds & Stephenson, 1983; McKnight et al., 1985; Silverman et al., 1988), and closed techniques, such as cooling jackets (Bonchek & Olinger, 1981). Although the use of the cooling jacket theoretically has advantages, it has proved to be inadequate in maintaining uniform myocardial temperatures and interferes with surgical logistics (Rosenfeldt & Arnold, 1982). Whichever method is used, myocardial hypothermic temperatures between 12°C and 20°C have been demonstrated to provide adequate protection in both hypertrophic and normal ventricular myocardium (Blanche et al., 1990; Rosenfeldt, 1988). Protection of the subendocardium (i.e., swift induction and maintenance of diastolic arrest), global myocardial hypothermia, and use of cardioplegia are attempts to minimize cell injury.

Investigation into the determinants of adequate myocardial protection has focused on ventricular preservation and recovery. However, an early study has demonstrated that inadequate interatrial temperatures of 25°C to 30°C result from the use of hypothermic antegrade cardioplegic techniques (Smith et al., 1983). Atrial activity secondary to early rewarming of the atrial septum has been suggested as an explanation for the high incidence of postoperative tachydysrhythmias (Ferguson et al., 1986; Tchervenkov et al., 1983) and conduction defects (Ferguson et al., 1987; Williams, 1988). Preliminary data on using warm blood cardioplegia via the retrograde method (Salerno et al., 1991) and the use of the right atrial method of cardioplegia delivery seem to indicate resulting decreased supraventricular dysrhythmias.

On aortic cross-clamping, an intracellular ischemic period occurs just before the onset of rapid diastolic arrest. During this period, endogenous catecholamines are secreted that deplete intracellular high-energy stores while myocardial cells undergo a hyperfunctional and hypermetabolic state. In efforts to reduce these cellular demands quickly, high-potassium crystalloid or blood cardioplegia is widely used in conjunction with systemic hypothermic cooling measures to minimize cellular ischemic injury.

Adequate delivery of cardioplegic solution is cardinal to the prevention of myocardial injury. Although most surgeons use the antegrade or aortic root method, either retrograde or cardioplegic administration via the coronary sinus (Chitwood, 1988) or the right atrial delivery method (Fabiani et al., 1986) is beginning to demonstrate promise. Although popular, antegrade delivery of cardioplegic solutions does have the disadvantages of uneven distribution of the solution past the stenotic native coronaries (Lust, 1988) and a potential for right ventricular intraoperative injury secondary to its thin-walled muscled mass and anatomic position (Morris & Whechler, 1988). The retrograde method has been documented to promote better distribution of the cardioplegic solution (Fabiani et al., 1987; Gates et al., 1993). Exploration of the microvascular distribution of retrograde cardioplegia has demonstrated complete dissemination to all regions of the ventricles and the intraventricular septum. These researchers demonstrated that two-thirds of the cardioplegic solution shunts through the thebesian veins. An

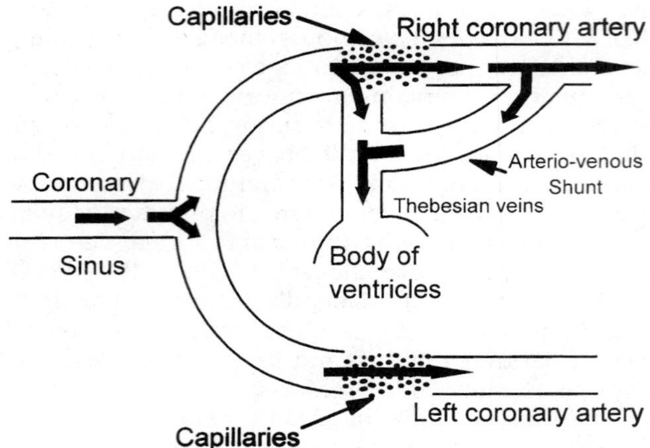

FIGURE 24–10. Basic and complex theoretical pathways of retrograde cardioplegia flow. (From Gates, R., et al. [1993]. Grogs and microvascular distribution of retrograde cardioplegia in explanted human hearts. *Annals of Thoracic Surgery, 56,* 410–417.)

additional one-third traverses the capillaries of the left coronary artery, with less than 5% traveling through the RCA (Fig. 24–10). This research supports the efficacy of this method in providing adequate myocardial protection (Gates et al., 1993). Use of the right atrial method has provided data supporting a lowered incidence of postoperative tachydysrhythmias through the maintenance of even atrial hypothermia and diastolic arrest. Its use may increase as research involving atrial preservation continues.

Cold high-potassium crystalloid solution is the most common cardioplegic solution used to produce global cardiac hypothermic arrest. Cardiac arrest is achieved through perfusion of the high-potassium solution through the native coronary vessels, which ultimately perfuse the myocardial cells. This causes an elevation in the extracellular potassium level, which decreases the resting membrane potential and inactivates the sodium channels. As a result, the cardiac cell is inactive and remains in diastolic arrest (Guyton, 1988; Silverman et al., 1988). Optimal temperature range for the delivery of cold crystalloid cardioplegia is between 10°C and 15°C (Blanche et al., 1990; Buckberg, 1988; Rosenfeldt, 1988). Both the delivery of cardioplegic solution and the continuous maintenance of adequate temperatures may be impeded by perfusion gradients in diseased vessels, ventricular position, and muscle mass differences.

As long as the extracellular potassium level remains high, diastolic arrest will prevail. However, noncoronary flow can lower extracellular potassium and precipitate electrical mechanical activity, causing ischemic damage created by an oxygen debt. Intermittent reinfusion of hyperkalemic cardioplegia every 20 to 30 minutes, through either an antegrade or a retrograde approach, is a common practice used to prevent this washout (Silverman et al., 1988).

The superiority of blood cardioplegia over crystalloid cardioplegia remains controversial. Sanguineous cold cardioplegia has the major advantages of oxygen-carrying capacity (Blanche et al., 1990; Cameron & Gardner, 1988; Edmunds & Stephenson, 1983), excellent buffering capacity supporting a normal pH (Bodenhamer et al., 1983), and oncotic properties (Kresh et al., 1987). However, cold blood cardioplegia demonstrates a leftward shift of the oxyhemoglobin dissociation curve when used in conjunction with hypothermia. This impedes unloading of oxygen to the tissues (Cameron & Gardner, 1988; Cusmano et al., 1988). These effects are counterbalanced by a decrease in cellular oxygen demand. Clinical studies show that optimal temperatures for the delivery of cold blood cardioplegia are 15°C to 20°C (Fermes et al., 1984; Salerno et al., 1991; Singh et al., 1981).

WARM HEART SURGERY. An emerging practice in maintaining myocardial protection is the use of normothermia in conjunction with high-potassium, warm-blood cardioplegia delivered retrograde through the coronary sinus. Avoidance of hypothermia has the advantages of not interfering with biochemical cellular functions, maintaining the normal oxyhemoglobin dissociation curve, and avoiding the clinical problems associated with reperfusion (Salerno et al., 1991). Further, normothermia and the continuous circulation of warm whole blood has the advantages of providing oxygen and needed substrates to the myocardial cells during diastolic arrest. Through using the retrograde method via the coronary sinus, warm-blood cardioplegia is evenly distributed to both the right and left ventricles and the interventricular septum (Drinkwater et al., 1990; Salerno et al., 1991).

Although controversial, there are principles that support the safe initiation of warm cardiac surgery. Under normothermic conditions, the oxygen requirement of the normal pumping left ventricle, assuming 100% saturation and 60% extraction, is 9 to 10 mL of oxygen per 100 g per minute. Only a small amount, 1 mL of oxygen per 100 g per minute, in the beating heart is required for electrical activity. An additional 1 mL per 100 g per minute of oxygen is required for intracellular work and the maintenance of ionic balances. Of interest, this requirement is independent of variables such as end-diastolic stretch, circulating catecholamines, available calcium, and, to a lesser extent, temperature (Litchenstein & Abel, 1992). Thus, the greatest oxygen consumption occurs during the pumping activity of the heart. Inducing heart arrest through the use of hyperkalemic solution and introduction of hypothermia at 20°C results in an additional 20% oxygen consumption (Braunwald, 1979). Myocardial intracellular ability to make energy via the ATP pathways is further inhibited under hypothermic conditions of 10°C or lower (Cameron & Gardner, 1988). Therefore, hypothermic conditions do decrease oxygen consumption. However, in anoxic states, once the cell has used up available oxygen, an oxygen debt is created. Further, cellular capability to produce or utilize oxygen efficiently, especially during reperfusion, is diminished. If electrical mechanical arrest can be carried out using high-potassium solution and ischemia can be minimized through the use of warm or normothermic blood cardioplegia, then hypothermia may not be required for myocardial protection, and in some cases may not be desired (Brown et al., 1993; Litchtenstein & Abel, 1992). Use of blood cardioplegia is thought to have the following advantages: (1) it allows ischemic time to be independent of the cross-clamp time, (2) it provides the endogenous oxygen radical scavengers normally found in blood, (3) it supports continuous intracellular production of ATP, and (4) it reduces the need for countershock at the completion of surgery to promote the return of normal sinus rhythm (Litchtenstein & Abel, 1992). Data regarding its impact on the incidence of perioperative MI, mortality, and phrenic nerve injury await the results of randomized trials.

Salerno and associates (1991) reported the first clinical use of these methods in 113 consecutive patients who underwent both coronary bypass and valve surgery. In this series, 6% of patients experienced perioperative MI, 7% required the use of inotropic support, and 96% spontaneously converted to normal sinus rhythm without the need for intraoperative defibrillation. Although still inconclusive, these data appear to be encouraging and may well change the recovery pattern for cardiac surgical patients.

Another emerging trend that seems to accompany the conduct of warm surgery is the use of systemic normothermia or tepid cooling. These methods have been used to curtail the systemic effects of profound hypothermia. A recent randomized trial comparing normothermia and hypothermia demonstrated a significant decrease in 30-day mortality in the hypothermic group (2.4%) and in the normothermic group (1.4%). No difference was found in incidence of stroke, reoperation for bleeding, tamponade, or infection between groups (The Warm Heart Investigators, 1994).

Operative Procedure

Initial entry into the chest wall is most commonly achieved through a median sternotomy. This approach provides optimal exposure and visualization of the myocardium and related structures. In addition, use of a median sternotomy incision affords less interruption in respiratory mechanics and reduced postoperative chest wall discomfort, which facilitate earlier mobilization and recovery.

The incision extends longitudinally between the suprasternal notch and the xiphoid process. After the spread of soft tissue, a sternal saw is used to open the sternum. Lateral placement of retractors facilitates stabilization and separation of the chest wall. The pericardium is incised and tacked to obtain an unobstructed view of the epicardial surface (Fig. 24–11).

Dissection and mobilization of the ITA from the chest wall is performed while the saphenous vein is harvested from the lower extremities and prepared for implantation. Once the aorta has been cross-clamped, injection of cold, hyperkalemic cardioplegic solution into the aortic root or coronary ostia induces electromechanical diastolic arrest.

The sequencing of anastomotic construction is dictated by the urgency of the situation, the degree of disease, and the preference of the surgical team. Emergent situations resulting from acute coronary closure or occlusion induced during cardiac catheterization or angioplasty procedures require prompt restoration of flow. To expedite the revascularization process, the saphenous vein may be used as the primary conduit. The relative ease in preparation and large graft flow add to the appeal of use of the saphenous vessel in the face of hemodynamic instability or evolving ischemia.

In general, the distal anastomoses to the posterior vasculature (circumflex and right coronary systems) can be performed first. Vessels to be bypassed on the anterior surface of the heart are exposed and incised. Selection of an anastomosis site requires a minimum size of 1 mm in diameter and a disease-free lumen. A vein graft end-to-side anastomosis is constructed to the most distal diagonal branch, and side-to-side anastomoses are made to bypass more proximal obstructions (Fig. 24–12). Finally, the ITA graft is attached to the LAD using an end-to-side technique. Every 20 to 30 minutes, or after each distal anastomosis, infusion of cardioplegic solution distends the vein graft to enhance cardioplegic delivery and distribution to the myocardium in that region, contributing to tissue protection.

Sequential grafting, most commonly used by surgeons, involves attachment of a single conduit to a coronary artery in one or more sites (Fig. 24–13). This technique facilitates the ease and speed of performing multiple-bypass grafts, reducing the number of aortic manipulations. *Simple grafts* bypass a single lesion, usually beginning at the ascending aorta, with the distal attachment below the obstruction. A *skip graft* is used to bypass a coronary vessel that has both proximal and distal lesions, such as is commonly seen in the LAD. *Y grafts* may be used when a conduit shaped like a "Y" is used to bypass two adjacent vessels (Fig. 24–14).

Construction of anastomoses may be performed with either continuous or interrupted sutures. Some evidence suggests that interrupted sutures provide a better anastomosis. Excellent results have been achieved, however, with both techniques. Optical magnification affords the surgeon excellent visualization of the coronary vasculature and minimizes the risk of technical error.

After completion of the distal anastomosis, the cross-clamp is removed. Rewarming is performed gradually, initiated at a rate of 1°C/minute. At this time the vein grafts are directed up to the ascending aorta. Each vein is distended with cold cardioplegic solution each time it is fitted between anastomotic sites, and finally again before aortic attachment. This helps to determine adequate graft length and tension. Evaluation and adjustment of each graft must be performed to ensure proper symmetry and angulation to

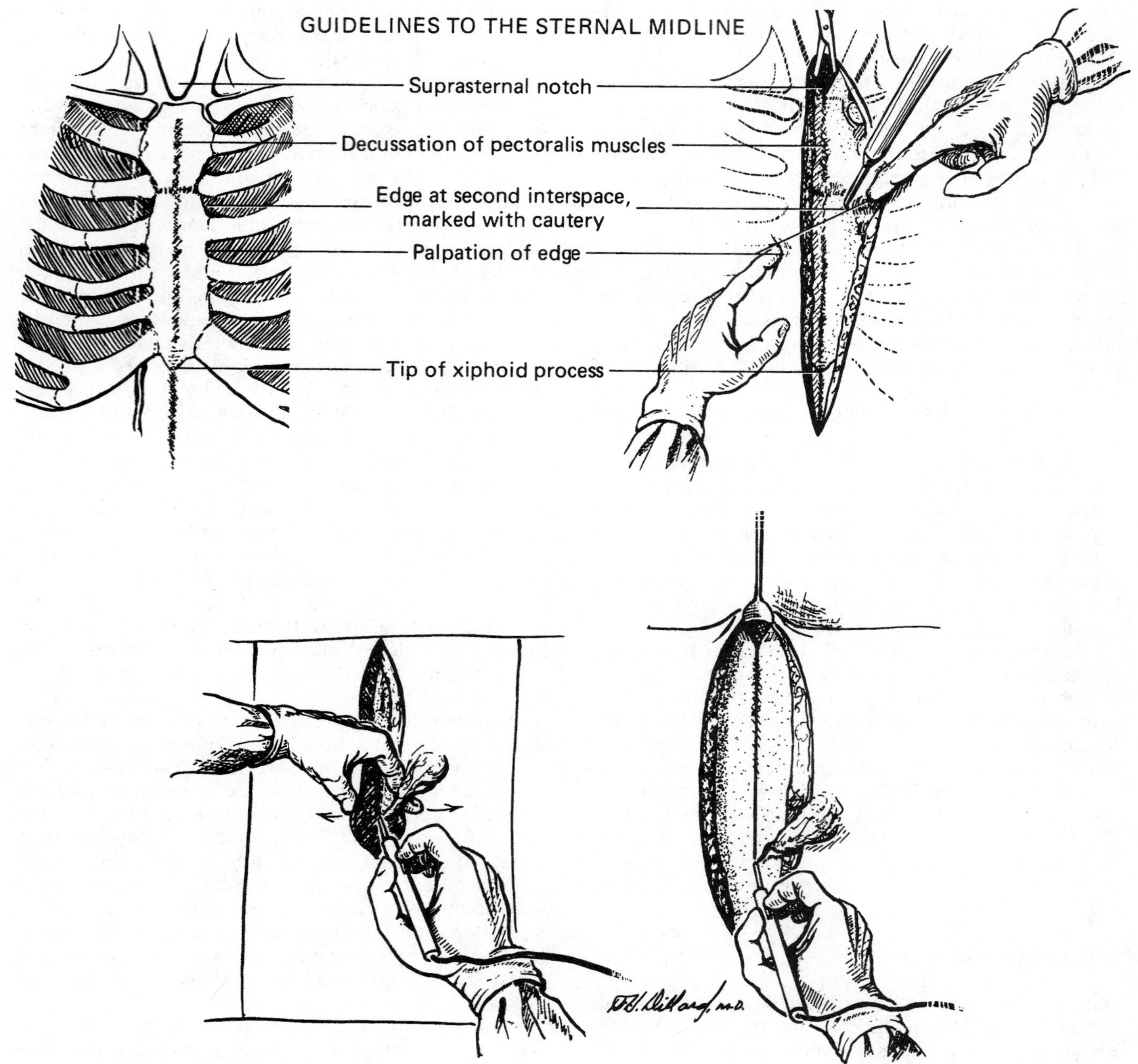

FIGURE 24–11. Median sternotomy incision. (From Dillard, D. H., & Miller, D. W. [1983]. *Atlas of cardiac surgery* [p. 21]. New York: Simon and Schuster.)

prevent kinking or early graft closure. A special device (Goosen aortic punch) is used to punch out circular pieces of aorta for construction of each proximal graft.

Before separation from CPB, basal flow rates are measured within the coronary system. Target flow rates range from 40 to 80 mL/minute, depending on the size of the recipient coronary artery and the particular conduit used. The use of transesophageal two-dimensional Doppler echocardiography (TEE) is gaining increasing popularity. Placement of an esophageal transducer provides continuous, real-time color flow imaging. The information obtained allows rapid assessment of ventricular function and visualization of coronary graft flow. Clinical reports validate the efficacy of TEE in precise detection of undiagnosed lesions and prevention of postoperative myocardial ischemia due to poor graft construction or procedural defects (Currie, 1989). Kato and colleagues (1993) found that TEE was more sensitive in defining and detecting episodes of ischemia in the postbypass period compared to patients receiving conventional monitoring. TEE has proven useful to allow for correction of

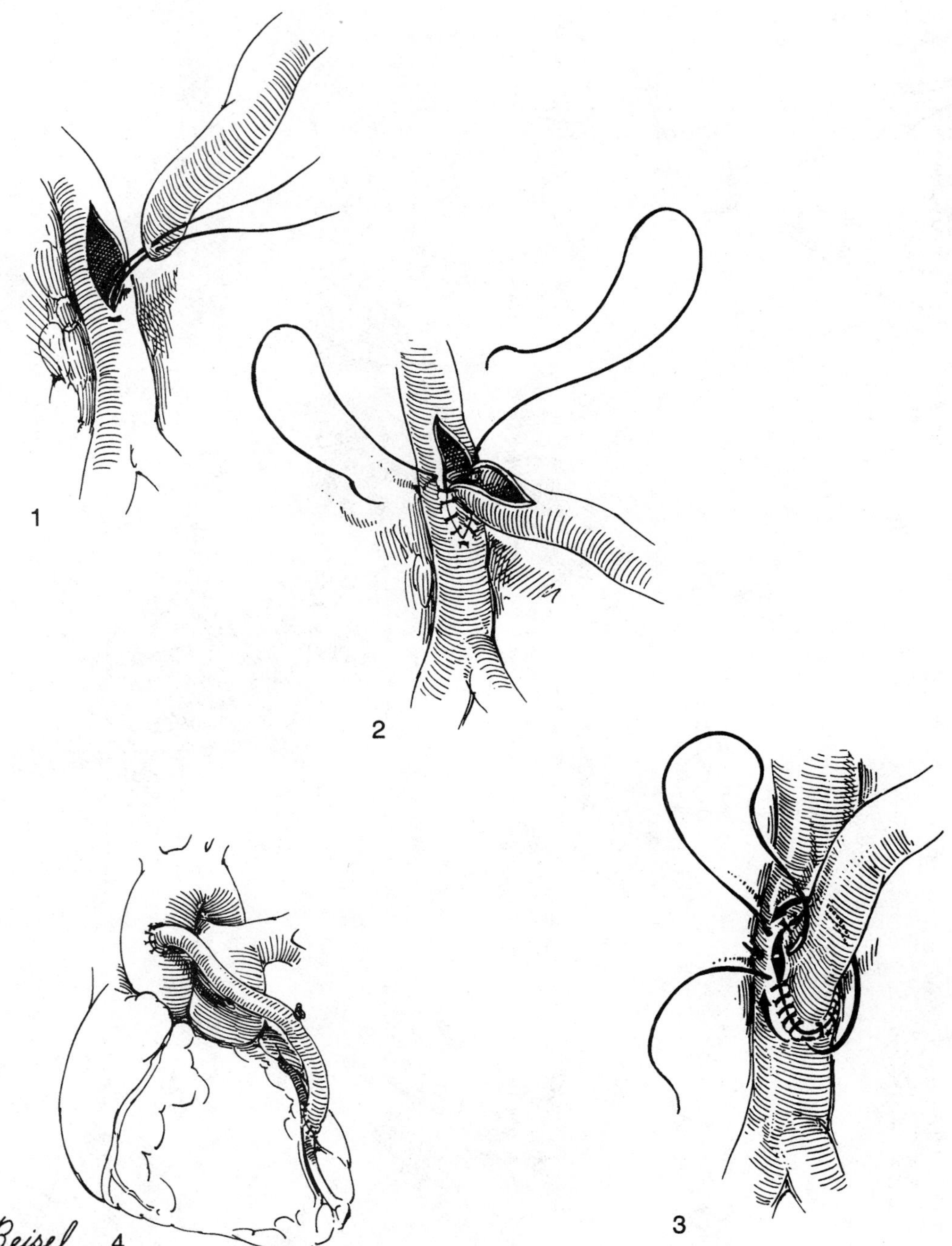

FIGURE 24–12. Saphenous vein anastomosis. Anastomotic construction starts distally (*1*) using Prolene sutures and continues along both edges of arteriotomy (*2*). Cold cardioplegia de-airs graft before completion of suture line (*3*). Completed aortocoronary saphenous vein graft is shown (*4*). (From Waldhausen, J. A., & Pierce, W. S. [1985]. *Surgery of the chest* [5th ed., p. 467]. Chicago: Year Book Medical Publishers.)

intraoperative problems such as inadequate myocardial protection or graft abnormalities to reduce adverse outcome.

Weaning from CPB is accomplished after evacuation of air from the grafts and chambers. The cannulas are removed after satisfactory recovery of cardiovascular and hemodynamic function. Atrial and ventricular pacing wires are implanted on the epicardial surface of the right ventricle and brought out to the skin through the chest wall. Pleural and mediastinal tubes are inserted to evacuate blood and drainage and prevent cardiac tamponade. Administration of protamine sulfate and desmopressin aids in reversing the effects of heparin to minimize postoperative bleeding. The

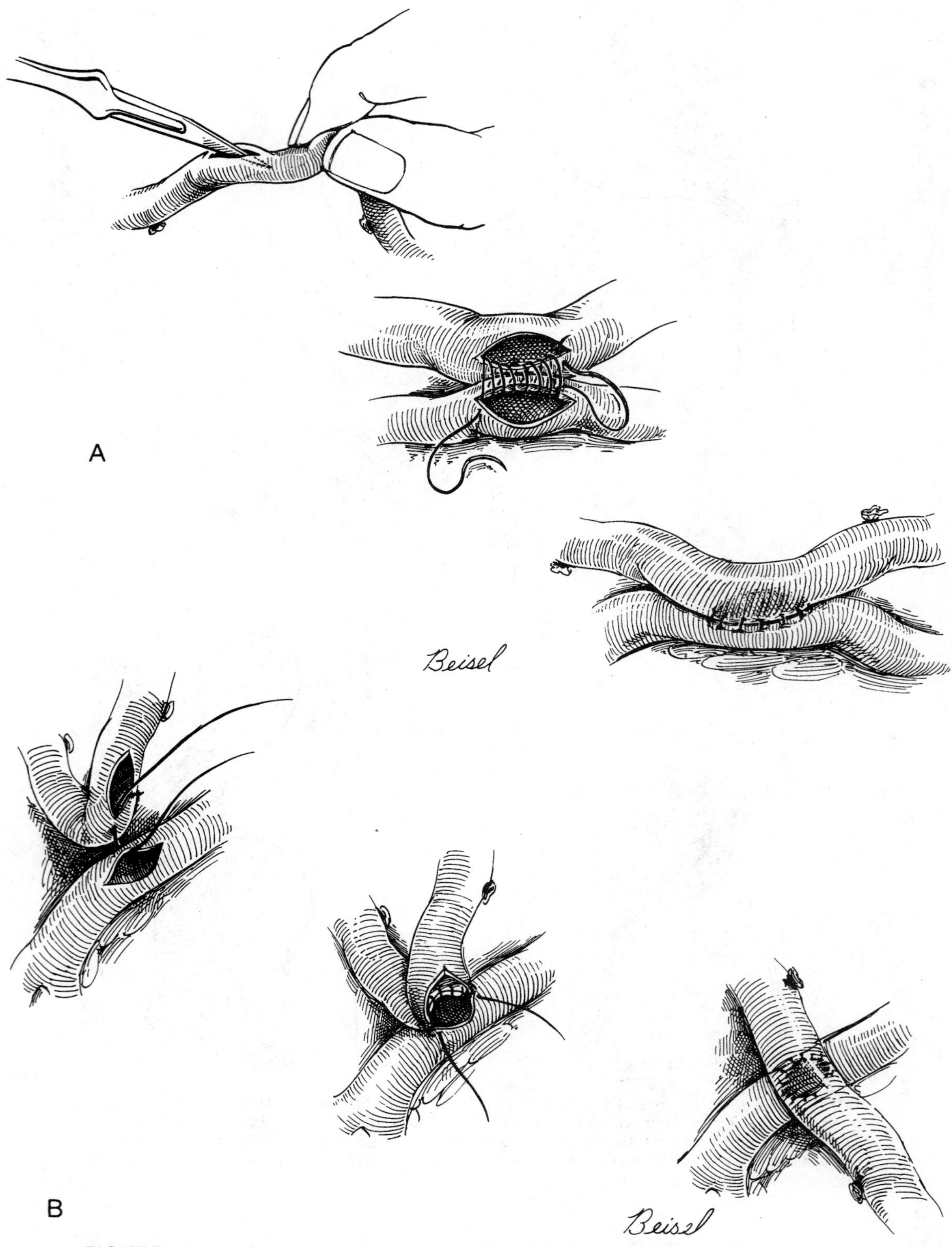

FIGURE 24–13. Sequential graft construction. *A,* Construction of parallel sequential anastomosis is frequently used to revascularize left anterior descending diagonal coronary artery. *B,* Perpendicular anastomosis is used when venotomy lies perpendicular to long axis of coronary artery. (From Waldhausen, J. A., & Pierce, W. S. [1985]. *Surgery of the chest* [5th ed., p. 471]. Chicago: Year Book Medical Publishers.)

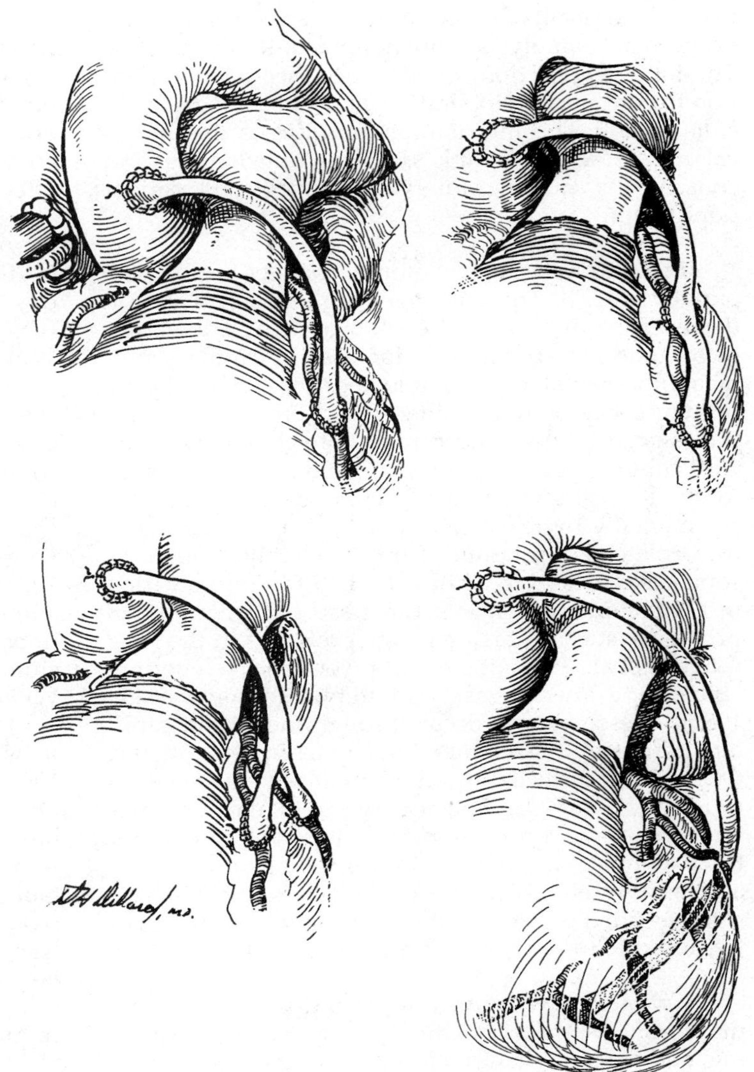

FIGURE 24–14. Types of bypass grafts. (From Dillard, D. H., & Miller, D. W. [1983]. *Atlas of cardiac surgery* [Plate XXIX, p. 77]. New York: Simon and Schuster.)

pericardium may be left open or partially closed and resutured; the sternum is then wired for closure. The skin is approximated with sutures or staples.

After satisfactory hemodynamic recovery, the surgical team prepares the patient for transport to the surgical intensive care unit. Portable monitoring devices are applied to ensure maximum safety during transport. On arrival in the intensive care unit, the patient is carefully assessed and evaluated collaboratively by intensive care nursing and medical staff. After admission and stabilization, a report of intraoperative events is communicated among nursing and medical staff. Information exchanged at this time allows the nurse an opportunity to plan the patient's care and to anticipate the pathophysiologic response during the immediate postoperative period.

An emerging trend is the practice of early extubation. Traditionally, patients remain tracheally intubated for 12 to 24 hours after surgery. Previous standards of care emphasizing use of long-acting narcotic anesthesics lent themselves to prolonged intubation and mechanical ventilation. Use of newer agents such as propofol and short-acting narcotics has allowed clinicians to extubate patients within 4 hours after surgery. Chong and coworkers (1993) described the use of a recovery area for postoperative patients after early extubation. No increase in morbidity or mortality was observed. Goals of such programs focus on "fast-tracking" patients in an effort to decrease length of stay and promote earlier ambulation and earlier discharge. Impact on patient satisfaction and psychological recovery has been positive (Gross, 1995). Yet, this practice will need further investigation as the patient population facing cardiac surgery continues to grow more complex.

Systemic Pathophysiologic Changes Characteristic of Cardiopulmonary Bypass

Although the mortality with cardiac surgery is low, there are many pathophysiologic systemic responses to CPB as a result of hemodilution, heparinization, hypothermia, hemolysis, and nonpulsatile blood flow. The following section reviews these sequelae in relation to common postoperative clinical problems as results of CPB. This information provides cardiac surgical nurses with valuable data for anticipating and constructing nursing interventions for this patient population.

FLUID. Intravascular volume changes occur secondary to CPB. These changes are associated with a decreased serum protein level, producing a lowering of osmotic pressure and an increase in capillary permeability mediated by complement activation. Plasma protein concentration is altered by hemodilution and trauma caused by blood coming into contact with the CPB tubing system. Increased capillary permeability to small proteins and water has been demonstrated experimentally to be caused by the release of serotonin from platelets, histamine from mast cells, and lysosomal enzymes from white cells. In addition, elevation in C3 complement levels can pose particular organ problems, such as gas exchange problems in the lung (Lavelle et al., 1984), increased myocardial cell permeability, and altered gastric motility (McKnight et al., 1985). These changes occur through increasing capillary permeability and interstitial water in these organs. Overall extravascular fluid volume may increase as much as 150 mL/kg. This increase in total body water appears to be proportional to the length of CPB (McKnight et al., 1985) and to increases in aldosterone and antidiuretic hormone (Roth et al., 1981). These changes often precipitate the clinical problem of hypotension due to decreased intravascular volume.

CARDIAC CHANGES. As a result of disruption of normal coronary perfusion, cardioplegia, uneven rewarming, and surgical manipulation, varying degrees of intracellular myocardial edema occur. These changes can contribute to potential injury of the conduction system, which may precipitate dysrhythmias, ventricular dysfunction, and perioperative ischemia or infarction. In addition, alterations in hemodynamics caused by hypotension or hypertension are commonly observed.

During CPB, some degree of cardiac cellular edema occurs (Guyton, 1988; Williams, 1988). These changes may be caused by ischemia, changes in serum oncotic pressures, high cardioplegic perfusion pressures, or ventricular distention (Kirklin & Barratt-Boyes, 1986; Silverman et al., 1988). Restoration of coronary blood flow after global arrest often accentuates cardiac edema produced by ischemia. Changes in cell membrane functions and serum oncotic pressures promote an increase in cell water volume on reperfusion. Damage to the cell membrane has been attributed to cytotoxic hydroxyl (OH) radicals (Silverman et al., 1988). The addition of mannitol to cardioplegic solutions has proved beneficial for reducing reperfusion injury because of its hyperosmolarity effects (Lucus et al., 1980). Experimental data seem to support the notion that mannitol may also have a scavenger effect that eliminates the OH radical, thereby improving postischemic reperfusion injury and coronary blood flow (Magovern et al., 1984). Clinical studies conducted by Johnson and colleagues (1991) demonstrate promising outcomes using preoperative allopurinol to decrease the effects of OH free radicals.

DYSRHYTHMIAS. Commonly, patients who undergo CABG or valvular surgery are observed to have tachydysrhythmias, premature ventricular contractions (PVCs), and bradydysrhythmias (Cox, 1993; Moore & Wilkoff, 1991). These dysrhythmias may range in severity from benign to life-threatening, and are among the most common complications encountered after cardiac operations. Many operative factors can contribute to the development of these dysrhythmias, including premature myocardial rewarming, electromechanical atrial activity during anoxic states (Cox, 1993; Fergusen et al., 1983; Magillian et al., 1985; Smith et al., 1983), hypoxemia, hypotension, increased sympathetic stimulation, fluid shifts (Estanfanous, 1981), metabolic imbalances (commonly due to digitalis and potassium), and irritation due to prosthetic valves (Moore & Wilkoff, 1991).

The incidence of supraventricular tachydysrhythmias is reported to be 48% in CABG patients (Cox, 1993). The most common dysrhythmia after cardiac operation is atrial fibrillation and atrial flutter, which has a reported incidence of 25% to 50% (Cox, 1993). Atrial fibrillation can result in hypotension, congestive failure, pneumonia or stroke. Dysrhythmias most commonly occur on the second to third postoperative day. Age represents the strongest factor correlating to the development of atrial fibrillation (Cox, 1993). An approximate 5% of patients undergoing any surgical procedure, including cardiac surgery, will develop atrial fibrillation. Thirty percent of patients do experience atrial fibrillation. Intra-atrial conduction delay has been correlated with postoperative atrial fibrillation. Identification of this group in the preoperative phase could prevent complications in the postoperative period (Frost et al., 1992; Rubin et al., 1987; Yousif et al., 1990). Vast variability in patient response is supported by the electrophysiologic investigations of Cox (1993).

The notion that vulnerability is variable in select groups of patients who demonstrate dispersion of refractoriness in atrial repolarization patterns is the operating hypothesis (Cox, 1993). Dispersion of refractoriness is the concept related to variability of atrial myocardial repolarization. Typically, once the atrium is depolarized, the relative refractory period follows. This period is thought in global terms. However, Sato and coworkers (1992) have determined through the placement of as many as 256 electrodes on the atrium that there is a local refractory period relative to the atrium. Further, in some individuals, the local refractory period is not uniform, resulting in variability or dispersion of refractoriness in the atrium, leading to increased vulnerability of reentrant atrial fibrillation.

In the cardiac surgery patient, the use of high-potassium cardioplegia and uneven atrial myocardial warming states has been associated with the incidence of atrial fibrillation. Early work by Smith and colleagues (1983) demonstrated that the atria cool quickly after introduction of cardioplegia and their temperature is correlated with the systemic temperature. Therefore, electrical activity may well be occurring in the anoxic state.

Although this new knowledge is helpful in understanding the mechanism of atrial fibrillation, it is still beyond the reach of the clinician to offer direction in screening potential patients for prophylactic intervention. Thus, the controversy surrounding protocols for the treatment of atrial fibrillation continues.

Onset of dysrhythmias usually occurs on the second to third postoperative day, with deleterious consequences stemming from their hemodynamic effects. The increased time spent in systole increases myocardial oxygen demand. However, the diastolic time is decreased, leading to reduced coronary flow, ventricular filling, and cardiac index. These imbalances set the stage for ischemia, ventricular dysfunction, or infarction.

Treatment, which may vary by institution and clinician, is aimed toward control of the ventricular response relative to the individual patient. Once hypoxemia and metabolic derangements are ruled out, the most common pharmacologic medications used are diltiazem, which remains controversial, verapamil, and low-dose beta blockers. Class I antidysrhythmics such as procainamide or quinidine can be used to convert atrial fibrillation or atrial flutter to normal sinus rhythm. These drugs are helpful only after the ventricular rate is controlled in the absence of atrial enlargement (Moore & Wilkoff, 1991). Commonly, atrial overdrive pacing is effective in restoring atrial flutter to normal sinus rhythm (Figs. 24–15 and 24–16).

Ventricular dysrhythmias, ranging from isolated PVCs to nonsustained ventricular tachycardias requiring treatment, occur in 36% of postoperative patients (Moore & Wilkhoff, 1991). Their occurrence is particularly high in the operating room during anesthesia, induction, cardiac cannulation for CPB, rewarming, and weaning from CPB. The most powerful predictor is age greater than 62 years (Ferraris et al., 1991). These investigators did not demonstrate an increase in mortality in the group of patients in whom ventricular dysrhythmia developed. The hemodynamic consequences are related to the frequency and duration of the dysrhythmia as it relates to adequate perfusion pressures.

Once physiologic deficits are ruled out as the cause, lidocaine or bretylium may be used as common first-line medications. In the case of polymorphic ventricular tachycardia, usually a result of drug toxicity, magnesium sulfate is the drug of choice (Gray & Mandel, 1991). The presence of ventricular fibrillation is life-threatening and is treated with defibrillation and cardiopulmonary resuscitation, as recommended by the American Heart Association (1994).

Bradydysrhythmias caused by injury to the conduction system during CABG or valve surgery are common. In CABG patients, 45% are reported to manifest a new bundle branch block (BBB), with a complete atrioventricular block developing in 4%. However, resolution of the new BBB before discharge has been reported to occur in 54% (Moore & Wilkoff, 1991). Development of new conduction defects after aortic valve replacement is reported to occur in 29% (Thompson et al., 1980).

These defects are commonly precipitated by operative events associated with hypothermia, potassium concentration of cardioplegia, number of coronary arteries bypassed, aortic cross-clamp time, and time on CPB (Gray & Mandel, 1991; Moore & Wilkoff, 1991). The clinical significance of these defects depends on their hemodynamic outcome. The most common treatment is the use of temporary atrial or ventricular pacing until the normal intrinsic conduction pathways resume. In rhythm patterns in which loss of the atrial contribution to the cardiac output occurs, temporary atrioventricular sequential or DDD (Cox, 1993) pacing is used.

VENTRICULAR DYSFUNCTION. Transient biventricular dysfunction to a varying degree occurs after CPB. Common contributors to this phenomenon are preexisting ventricular dysfunction, microemboli to the subendocardium, inadequate cardioplegic protection, premature or uneven rewarming, elevation in systemic and pulmonary vascular resistance, or ischemic ventricular injury. These causes are commonly thought to be associated with left ventricular dysfunction after CPB. However, increasing attention is being directed toward factors that specifically put the right ventricle at risk for dysfunction. In addition to the causes previously stated, right ventricular dysfunction is caused by cold potassium cardioplegia (Christakis et al., 1985), RCA air embolism, elevated pulmonary vascular resistance, and left ventricular dysfunction (Coleman, 1989; Hines & Barash, 1985). Likewise, biventricular dysfunction can be caused by independent injury to the right or left ventricle, cardiac cellular edema, or loss of high-energy phosphates due to initiation of global arrest. Recovery of left ventricular function may take up to 8 days (Pennington et al., 1985), whereas right ventricular recovery may be reversed in 3 to 5 days depending on the severity of injury and the absence of pulmonary hypertension (Hines & Barash, 1985). Although multifactorial, any or all of these factors can contribute to the development of low cardiac output states observed after surgery. These patients often need fluid administration, mechanical assist devices, or inotropic support to maintain an acceptable cardiac index, urine output, and mentation level.

CARDIAC TAMPONADE. Careful assessment for signs and symptoms of cardiac tamponade must not be overlooked as a cause of ventricular dysfunction. Cardiac tamponade results from accumulation of blood or fluid in the pericardial space, impairing ventricular diastolic filling, which eventually causes the equalization of all cardiac chamber pressures. A major factor

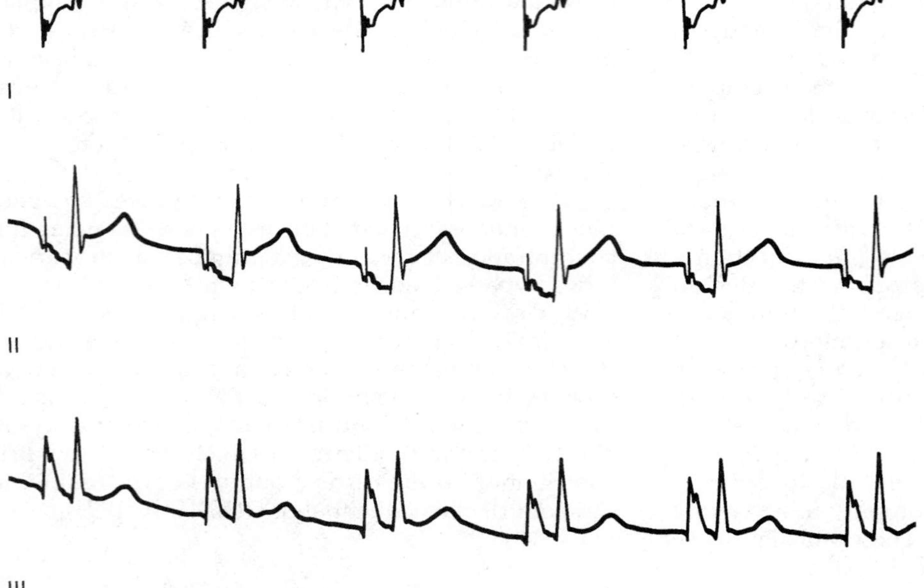

FIGURE 24–15. Atrial electrogram; the rhythm is normal sinus rhythm. The lead I recording is bipolar; note the very small ventricular complex. Leads II and III are unipolar; both the atrial and the ventricular complexes are easily seen. The atrial complex in lead III is significantly larger than that seen in lead II. This signifies that the atrial pacing wire attached to the left arm lead is farthest away from the ventricle and would be the best pacing wire to use for rapid atrial pacing.

in the development of tamponade is the rapidity with which fluid accumulates in the pericardial space. However, slow, subtle bleeding into the mediastinum also can cause tamponade. Occluded mediastinal chest tubes secondary to clot formation in the anterior mediastinum may induce a precipitous fall in drainage output. Manifestations of hypotension, elevation and equalization of diastolic filling pressures, low cardiac output, a decrease in chest tube drainage, and a widening mediastinum on x-ray are the clinical sequelae of cardiac tamponade. TEE is an excellent imagined modality to determine the actual location of a pericardial effusion. Immediate recognition of this situation is imperative to ensure expeditious intervention, which most often requires reexploration.

PERIOPERATIVE MYOCARDIAL INFARCTION. The incidence of perioperative MI in patients after coronary

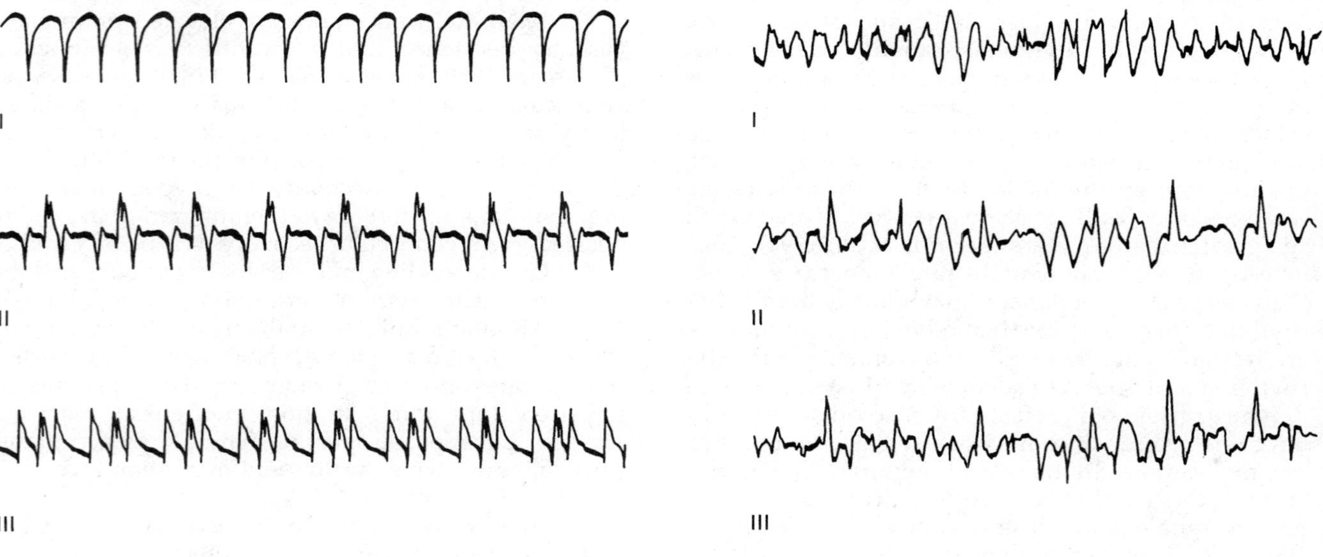

FIGURE 24–16. *A,* Atrial electrograms recorded during atrial flutter. Atrial rate is approximately 290 beats per minute (bpm); ventricular rate is 145 bpm. Lead I is bipolar; only the atrial activity is visible. Leads II and III are unipolar; both atrial and ventricular activity are seen. *B,* Atrial electrograms recorded during atrial fibrillation. Note the chaotic atrial activity seen in both the bipolar (lead I) and the unipolar (leads II and III) atrial electrograms.

revascularization is approximately 5% to 15%, depending on diagnostic criteria (Chaitman et al., 1983; Force et al., 1990; Guiteras Val. et al., 1988; Seitelberger et al., 1991; Van Lente et al., 1989). To date, there is no consensus on the criteria used to determine the presence of perioperative MI. However, the presence of a new Q wave on the ECG (Force et al., 1990) and the presence of a prolonged peak elevation in creatine kinase MB isoenzyme 12 to 15 hours after surgery are criteria often used (Guiteras Val. et al., 1983; Van Lente et al., 1989). Both of these primary criteria have been documented to provide false-negative and false-positive results. A new marker, cardiac troponin T, has been found to demonstrate high sensitivity and specificity for diagnosis of minor perioperative myocardial tissue damage and small infarctions (Mair et al., 1993). Given an index of clinical suspicion for the presence of a perioperative MI, the above criteria, taken in conjunction with myocardial scanning techniques or ventricular contractility assessment, provide additional data that help to determine the presence of a perioperative MI, as well as its functional implications for the patient.

The CASS study demonstrated in a sample of 939 patients that the single most important factor that has decreased the incidence of perioperative MI is the use of potassium cardioplegia (Berger et al., 1981). In a large series of more than 12,000 first-time cardiac surgical patients who underwent CABG over a 12-year period, Iyer and colleagues (1993) found that the type of cardioplegia used was not predictive of perioperative MI. However, the investigators did find that the presence of unstable angina doubled the rate of perioperative MI, from 0.86% to 1.9%. In addition, if the bypass time was less than 94 minutes, the rate was 0.56%, which increased impressively to 7.7% when the bypass time was longer than 100 minutes. Although Iyer and colleagues did not find recent MI a predictor of perioperative MI, Tuman and coworkers (1989) confirmed this variable, using 6 weeks as the criterion. In addition, Tuman and colleagues found that aortic cross-clamp time, presence of life-threatening dysrhythmias, and congestive heart failure further defined this high-risk group.

Conditions in which adequate myocardial preservation might not be achieved promote high-risk states. Patients at risk are those with a left main stenotic lesion greater than 50% with accompanying stenosis of the RCA, prolonged aortic cross-clamp and CPB time, multivessel bypass, or a concomitant valve replacement (Guiteras Val. et al., 1983). In addition to these operative risks, patients who undergo surgery emergently, have cardiomegaly, have unstable angina, or are women are also at risk.

Postoperative consequences associated with a suspected perioperative MI are significant ventricular irritability, low cardiac output, and poor hemodynamic response. The intraaortic balloon pump and pharmacologic inotropic support are common treatment modalities used to support the failing ventricle(s) until recovery. Seitelberger and colleagues (1991) conducted a randomized study on the use of nifedipine in reducing the incidence of MI. These investigators demonstrated a reduction in MI and necrosis with the use of this calcium channel antagonist. Although these results are encouraging, larger clinical trials are needed.

HYPERTENSION. Hypertension is most commonly seen in the immediate postoperative period as a result of peripheral arterial constriction and hypothermia (Leslie, 1993). The incidence varies from 33% to 75%, and is most prevalent in the first 2 to 6 postoperative hours (Chitwood et al., 1992; Halpern et al., 1992). The primary etiology for hypertension is elevation in systemic vascular resistance secondary to increased endogenous catecholamines. Hypertension is rapidly alleviated after administration of sedatives, analgesics, and vasodilators and initiation of the rewarming process. Efforts to control hypertension and reduce arterial blood pressure help to decrease left ventricular workload and wall tension while lessening myocardial oxygen demand. Intravenous nitroglycerin and sodium nitroprusside are effective vasodilating agents used to lower systemic vascular resistance through preload and afterload reduction. Delivery of antihypertensives such as nipride through a closed-loop device has recently been found to control hypertension more consistently, decreasing bleeding and transfusion requirements compared to manual delivery and titration (Chitwood et al., 1992).

Reduced arterial pressure allows more complete left ventricular emptying and ejection, facilitating a rise in stroke volume and a redistribution of coronary blood flow. Maintenance of systolic blood pressure at less than 120 to 140 mm Hg is advocated to prevent adverse effects on the vein graft and suture lines (Gray, 1990; Wheatley, 1986). Excessive pressure exerted on suture lines and anastomosis sites may precipitate serious consequences such as leakage or rupture.

HYPOTENSION. Hypotension may be precipitated by hemorrhage, vasodilation, intravascular volume depletion, or catecholamine depletion. Early recognition and volume reexpansion prevent complications resulting from prolonged episodes of hypotension such as tissue hypoperfusion, organ ischemia, or cardiovascular collapse. Severe volume deficits may induce early vein graft closure and myocardial ischemia and injury (Behrendt & Austen, 1981). Typically, volume replacement of colloidal fluids is the treatment of choice (rather than the use of crystalloid) to improve hypotension. In a two-group, randomized trial, Ley and colleagues (1990) demonstrated reduced fluid replacement needs, improved hemodynamics, and shortened intensive care unit stays in the patient group given replacement volume with colloid compared with the crystalloid group.

CORONARY ARTERY SPASM. Coronary artery vasospasm has been postulated as a cause of postoperative morbidity and mortality after CABG (Tanimoto et al., 1984). It occurs early in the postoperative period in approximately 0.8% of cases (Gurley et al., 1990; Maleki & Manley, 1989). Common manifestations have been identified as ST segment elevations, hypotension, atrioventricular block, ventricular tachycardia, and cardiovascular collapse. Many centers routinely use intravenous nitroglycerin and nifedipine prophylactically in the postoperative period to promote vasodilation and counteract the potential for perioperative MI or ischemia caused by spasm (Maleki & Manley, 1989).

Coronary artery spasm has been found to affect both normal coronaries, endarterectomized vessels, recipient bypassed vessels, and conduits such as the ITA or saphenous vein. The etiology of this syndrome is unknown; researchers propose that calcium infusion, increased catecholamine levels, or myocardial ischemia may be factors linked to the development of coronary artery vasospasm (Behrendt & Austen, 1981). Recognition is extremely difficult. However, many centers now routinely use ST segment monitoring in the postoperative period. Treatment of coronary artery spasm with calcium channel blockers or intracoronary vasodilators has proved effective (Fischell et al., 1989).

HEMATOLOGIC CHANGES. At the time of sternotomy, bone marrow emboli are liberated into the blood and are thought to be the mediators of subclinical disseminated intravascular coagulation associated with a decrease in platelet count seen before initiation of CPB (Milam, 1983; Heyman, 1985). Once on CPB, exposure of blood to nonendothelial surfaces and high shear forces associated with the circuit is associated with hematologic changes (Copeland et al., 1989). Blood is subject to turbulence, causing hemolysis; pressure, producing trauma to the cells; low-flow states, precipitating clumping of cells; and denaturing of blood cells as a result of contact with CPB tubing. Further damage to blood cells results from the direct interface of blood and oxygen in the bubble oxygenator or suctioning of the surgical field (Heyman, 1985; Milam, 1983). Other factors that contribute to alterations in hematologic function are low fibrinogen, primary fibrinogenolysis, and changes in fibrin polymerization (Czer et al., 1987; Holloway et al., 1988). In addition, blood coagulability is further hindered by heparinization, hemodilution, and hypothermia. Although overall clotting factors are reduced by one half, such reduction has been demonstrated to be adequate to establish hemostasis (Kucuk et al., 1986).

One of the most important contributions to the development of postoperative bleeding is platelet dysfunction. The definitive mechanism of injury to platelets as they travel through the oxygenator is unclear. However, there is evidence to support the development of platelet cell membrane receptor injury (Harker, 1986) and impaired platelet binding to fibrinogen (Musial et al., 1985) in conjunction with low levels of factor V or von Willebrand factor (Czer et al., 1985; Salzman et al., 1986). During CPB, the process of platelet activation induces thrombocytopenia. Platelet adherence to the nonepithelial surface results in the formation of aggregates that are removed by filtration mechanisms. Another contributor to thrombocytopenia in the presence of thrombosis is heparin administration. In sensitized patients, the use of prostacyclin has been found to preserve platelet function and prevent thrombosis (Addonozio et al., 1987).

At the completion of bypass, a far less homogeneous population of platelets remains circulating, contributing to platelet dysfunction until the damaged platelets are replaced. In addition, the use of aspirin and antiplatelet medications contributes to the development of this dysfunction (Sethi et al., 1990). Although the outcomes with the use of desmopressin have been conflicting (D'Alauro & Johns, 1988; LoCicero, 1990), its efficacy in patients taking aspirin at the time of operation has been demonstrated (Chard et al., 1990). Administration within 60 to 90 minutes after CPB has demonstrated optimal results (Van Oeveren et al., 1990). Other common alterations in blood indices observed after CPB are slight thrombocytopenia, elevation in fibrin degradation products, increases in factors VII and IX, and a decrease in factor V (Edmunds & Stephenson, 1983; Heyman, 1985; Milam, 1993). Decreased fibrinogen values while on CPB have also been documented; these values elevate immediately after surgery and remain high for 24 to 48 hours (Moores & Willford, 1989). Thorough assessment of clotting factor activity, bleeding time, and platelet function provides an appropriate treatment plan. Interventions commonly used are autologous platelet transfusions (Giordano et al., 1988), desmopressin (Salzman et al., 1986), and cryoprecipitate (Harker, 1986). Treatment should be directed toward repletion of the specific clotting factor(s) needed (Bracey & Radovancevic, 1994). The use of a protease inhibitor, aprotinin, to reduce homologous blood product transfusion has been supported by a multicenter, randomized, double-blind study (Lemmer et al., 1994). However, controversy regarding early graft closure (Lemmer et al., 1994; Royston, 1994), renal dysfunction, particularly in the elderly (Sundt et al., 1993), and cost warrants cautious consideration for the use of this medication.

Postoperative mediastinal bleeding usually stems from a coagulation disturbance or vascular interruption. Care is taken during surgery to avoid unnecessary dissection, although persistent bleeding may result despite precautions taken to achieve intraoperative hemostasis. Identification of the causative factors determines the appropriate therapy. Coagulation abnormalities can result from incomplete heparin reversal, heparin rebound effect, thrombocytopenia, platelet dysfunction, depletion of clotting factors, or disseminated intravascular coagulation (Bojar, 1989).

In the absence of a hemostatic defect, bleeding most likely results from an anastomotic site, warranting return to the operating room for urgent surgical reexploration. Anastomotic bleeding usually occurs in the presence of diseased vessels. When grafts are sutured to thin-walled, poor-quality recipient vessels, excessive intraluminal pressure may cause rupture or tearing. Increased pressure may be a product of vasoconstriction or hypertension. Repair of the anastomosis may induce further compromise or damage to the vessel. Bleeding may also occur from side branches of the vein graft sites, areas of intracardiac cannulation, or acute disruption of sutures at the valve site. All such conditions require emergent reoperation.

ENDOCRINE CHANGES. Controlled trauma of CPB, hypothermia, diversion of circulation from the heart and lung, hemodilution, and the loss of autonomic innervation contribute to changes in the endocrine system (Edmunds & Stephenson, 1983; Philbin, 1985; Reyes, 1985). As a result of these factors, epinephrine may be elevated to nine times normal and norepinephrine to two times normal in response to an empty heart (Reyes, 1985), and changes in glucose regulation have been demonstrated. Reyes found an elevation in endogenous catecholamines when CPB began and during weaning (Reyes, 1985). These elevations have been documented to persist up to 8 hours after surgery (Estanfanous, 1981; Landymore et al., 1979). Such impressive elevations in these potent vasoconstrictors, in combination with hypovolemia and hypothermia, mediate the common problem of hypertension.

Elevations in vasopressin levels have been demonstrated to be 20 times normal after CPB (Edmunds & Stephenson, 1983; Philbin, 1985). These extremely high circulating levels not only cause water retention and result in hyponatremia but exert a potent vasoconstricting effect on the vascular beds (Reyes, 1985). In conjunction with elevations in serum vasopressin levels, renin and angiotensin levels have been found to be elevated, contributing to a 35% to 45% incidence of postoperative hypertension (Estanfanous, 1981; Philbin, 1985). However, a prospective trial conducted by Weinstein and colleagues (1987) found no difference in renin, angiotensin II, or aldosterone levels in subjects who underwent coronary artery bypass as compared to normal subjects. Changes in angiotensin-converting enzyme are also associated with CPB. During the time the lungs are perfused but not ventilated while on CPB, angiotensin-converting levels were found to decrease and return to normal 24 hours after surgery (Gorin & Liebler, 1986). These findings call into question the contributory role of angiotension II in the development of early postoperative hypertension. Treatment focuses on maintaining adequate intravascular volume, slow rewarming, and vasodilation therapy.

Temporary increases in serum glucose patterns can be observed in all patients during CPB, even when exogenous glucose is not used in the priming solution (Kuntschen et al., 1985). During hypothermia, inhibition of both insulin secretion and hepatic glucose production occurs. Under normothermic ischemic conditions in an animal model, elevated serum glucose potentiates anaerobic glycolysis, resulting in increased lactic acid and decreased cellular pH (Ibayashi et al., 1986). The role of hyperglycemia and hypothermia during CPB is unclear; however, it is speculated that hypothermia inhibits these cellular metabolic changes. Hypothermic patients have been found to have no insulin secretion or elevation in serum glucose response during CPB (Kuntschen et al., 1985). However, after CPB and after rewarming occurs, hyperglycemia and hyperinsulinemia (Kuntschen et al., 1985, 1986) with some insulin resistance have been observed in both diabetic and nondiabetic patients (Kuntschen et al., 1986). These data are helpful because hyperglycemia is commonly observed in all patients after CPB and typically does not require treatment. However, diabetic patients may require insulin drips to gain control of the serum glucose.

Crystalloid prime solutions often contain metabolically active substrates that have been thought to modulate the hormonal and metabolite responses to CPB. McKnight and associates (1985) conducted a randomized, controlled trial on the effects of four different crystalloid prime solutions. Patients were randomzied to four groups and received prime solutions containing either glucose, lactate, glucose and lactate, or neither glucose nor lactate. Four hours after surgery, no significant changes in endocrine or metabolic responses were found between the groups. However, in groups in which glucose or lactate were used in the prime, serum glucose and lactate levels were found to be elevated. These findings support the use of nonglucose or lactate additives to the prime solution (McKnight et al., 1985). Whatever solution is used, an increase in total body water results at completion of CPB.

Hypothermic CPB decreases thyroid function, causing low serum levels of thyroxine and triiodothyronine (Robuschi et al., 1986). Triiodothyronine given as a replacement to patients after CPB has demonstrated a positive inotropic effect in a select group of patients with ejection fractions greater than 40% (Novitsky et al., 1989). The inotropic mechanism is mediated through increasing intracellular Ca^{2+}, thereby stimulating pyruvate dehydrogenase and movement of ATP into the cytosol to increase contractility (Novitsky et al., 1989).

PULMONARY CHANGES. The lungs remain deflated and underperfused during CPB. During this process there is a decrease in chest wall compliance with a resultant decrease in functional vital and residual capacity, leading to the collapse of peripheral alveoli (Ingwersen et al., 1993; Weiman et al., 1993). General anesthesia and muscle paralysis cause cephalad movement of the dependent portion of the diaphragm, which decreases static and dynamic spontaneous lung volume. These mechanical factors, in addition to an ineffective cough, contribute to the postoperative development of pulmonary problems (Bevelaqua et al., 1990; Weiman et al., 1993).

Once on CPB, activation of the complement cascade occurs through both the alternative pathway (Howard et al., 1988) and, most recently described, through the classic pathway (Wachtfogel et al., 1989). Both systems were found to be activated by factor XII located on the surface of the bypass circuits (Wachtfogel et al., 1986). Fragments of complement activation, namely C5a, have demonstrated binding to neutrophils, leading to activation and pulmonary sequestration (Tennenberg et al., 1990). The use of heparin-bonded circuits has been shown in an animal model to reduce complement activation and its sequelae in the lung (Nilson et al., 1989). Likewise, Bando and colleagues (1990) found that depleting the level of circulating leukocytes decreased lung injury in an animal model. Although the use of heparin-bonded circuits and leukocyte filters during the conduct of cardiac surgery in humans is evolving, the results of large studies will determine their efficacy.

After CPB, an increase in the alveolar–arterial oxygen difference with a resultant increase in intrapulmonary shunting occurs (Chulay et al., 1982; Edmunds & Stephenson, 1983; Svennevig et al., 1984). Further changes in the pneumocytes as a result of CPB lead to a loss of surfactant (Chulay et al., 1982), increased alveolar permeability secondary to the anaphylatoxins C3a, C4a, and C5a, which are complement fragments, swelling of endothelial cells, sequestering of leukocytes with release of lysosomal enzymes (Downey & Edmunds, 1992; Edmunds & Stephenson, 1983), and development of atelectasis secondary to intraoperative ventilation at high oxygen levels, which dilutes normal alveolar nitrogen and impairs clearance of secretions (Asada & Yamaguchi, 1981).

Left lower lobe atelectasis is the most common sequela of CPB, with a reported incidence of 68% to 88% (Chulay et al., 1982; Wilcox et al., 1988) in cardiac surgical patients. Factors proposed to explain this phenomenon include the operative factors previously stated, the supine position in combination with an enlarged heart, which may interfere with left lower lobe expansion (Sheland et al., 1983), the presence of an endotracheal tube (Freedman & Goodman, 1982), phrenic nerve damage (Benjamine et al., 1982; Curtis et al., 1989; Wilcox et al., 1990), and preexisting lung disease (Bevelaqua et al., 1990). Of interest, patients at high risk for pulmonary complications are those who have restrictive disease or undergo valve surgery (Bevelaqua et al., 1990). Recovery is usually accompanied by return of normal diaphragmatic function. Other reports indicate that exposure to hypothermia interferes with surfactant production (Rousou et al., 1985). Interruption of lung surfactant may produce transient alveolar collapse, potentiating atelectasis. In the population of patients who undergo cauterization of the ITA, development of an ipsilateral pleural effusion further prevents alveolar expansion and predisposes patients to the development of atelectasis (Jansen & McFadden, 1986; Wilcox et al., 1990).

Diaphragmatic dysfunction secondary to phrenic nerve injury, particularly that involving the left hemidiaphragm, has been seen to persist for up to 48 to 72 hours or for up to 2 years after surgery (Asada & Yamaguchi, 1981; Curtis et al., 1989; Lewis, 1980; Luce, 1984). This reported variable recovery pattern is attributed to the severity (i.e., unilateral or bilateral) of involvement and the mechanism of injury to the phrenic nerve (Weiman et al., 1993). Injury to the phrenic nerve may also result from the use of ice slush for myocardial cooling (Curtis et al., 1989), take-down of the ITA for CABG, and electrocautery (Abd et al., 1989). Whatever the cause, these patients are prone to development of atelectasis, may require prolonged mechanical ventilation, and are at risk for respiratory infection. Treatment focuses on managing the airway, strengthening the ventilatory muscles, promoting adequate patient communication, and managing anxiety.

Preoperative variables that predispose patients to postoperative lung problems include chronic obstructive lung disease, poor lung compliance, decreased activity tolerance, advanced age, malnutrition, and a prior long hospitalization with pulmonary complications (Rich et al., 1988). Prevention and management of atelectasis is a primary nursing concern. Interventions such as early turning (Chulay et al., 1982), progressive increases in activity, and the use of incentive spirometry (Lewis, 1980) should be initiated in the intensive care unit and continued throughout the patient's hospital stay.

RENAL AND SERUM ELECTROLYTE CHANGES. CPB decreases overall blood flow distribution to the kidney, impairing autoregulation as a result of hemodilution and hypothermia (Utley et al., 1981). In addition, hypotension, microemboli, and nonpulsatile CPB flow states contribute to development of a drop in glomerular filtration rate (GFR) to 50% to 60% of normal while the patient is on CPB, which usually normalizes by the second postoperative day (Kristensen, 1990). The reported incidence of renal dysfunction is 1.5% to 5% in the cardiac surgical patient population.

Acute tubular necrosis as a result of these factors is not an uncommon clinical problem after cardiac surgery (Davis et al., 1982; Myers & Moran, 1986). Episodes of hypotension or the use of potent vasoconstrictor medications in the perioperative period may precipitate a sudden decrease in renal perfusion and output (Utley et al., 1981). This may be compounded by hypothermia, which contributes to a potential decrease in renal blood flow by increasing renal vascular resistance, resulting in a decrease in free water clearance, urine osmolarity, and a subsequent decrease in urine output (Davis et al., 1982; Edmunds & Stephenson, 1983). Hemolysis of red cells is a common problem of CPB and requires the kidney to clear the degraded byproducts such as hemoglobin. Free hemoglobin binds to plasma albumin, producing methemalbumin, which is secreted in the kidney (Kristensen, 1990). As long as urine output is adequate, free hemoglobin will be excreted and will be of no consequence to the renal tubules. To differentiate between hemoglobinuria and hematuria by observation, hemoglobinuria does not precipitate and usually clears with adequate urine output within the first 1 to 2 hours after CPB (Edmunds & Stephenson, 1983).

With the need to reduce exposure to homologous

blood products, the use of aprotinin has proven very efficacious for both first-time and repeat cardiac surgical patients (Lemmer et al., 1994). However, this medication has negative effects on renal function. Aprotinin inhibits the fibrinolytic system, with resultant preservation of platelet function (Royston, 1992). The definitive mechanism of action in renal dysfunction is unclear. However, aprotinin concentrates in the kidney and is 90% bound to the brush borders of the renal proximal tubules. Its metabolism in the normothermic state typically occurs in 12 to 14 hours (Emerson, 1989). Perhaps a combination of age, decreased GFR, and hypothermia leads to increased risk in the elderly. Sundt and coworkers (1993) demonstrated that over two-thirds of their patients (65%) who received aprotinin developed renal dysfunction, compared to 5% of the age-matched controls who did not receive aprotinin. Further, patients who were older than the age of 65 years were the only ones in whom renal dysfunction developed. There was also a trend, although not statistically significant, toward increases in MI, stroke, and mortality in this study. These findings are not supported in the study by Lemmer and coworkers (1994). However, definitive mortality and morbidity statistics associated with the use of this drug await larger trials.

As a result of these renal perfusion changes and the use of electrolyte-based cardioplegic solutions and diuretics, common changes in serum electrolytes observed after CPB include hypokalemia, hyponatremia, and hypomagnesemia. These serum electrolytes should be monitored closely in conjunction with renal function indices and urine output, and altered as needed.

CENTRAL NERVOUS SYSTEM. Central nervous system problems resulting from CPB are most commonly caused by macroemboli or microemboli or ischemia (Blauth et al., 1992; Santillan et al., 1985). Perfusion pressures below 50 mm Hg, prolonged CPB runs, and advanced age can contribute to postoperative cerebral manifestations (Brewer et al., 1983; Rebeyka et al., 1987; Slogoff et al., 1990). CPB does not cause changes in cerebral blood flow unless perfusion pressures drop below 50 mm Hg (Brewer et al., 1983; Slogoff et al., 1990). If the perfusion pressure decreases to less than 40 mm Hg (Brewer et al., 1983; Johnson et al., 1987), or there is a temperature-corrected carbon dioxide level greater than 40 mm Hg (Prough et al., 1990), cerebral autoregulation is decreased, changing cerebral blood flow and precipitating an ischemic event.

CEREBROVASCULAR ACCIDENTS. Microemboli from the CPB machine, cardiotomy suction system, ischemia, or release of plaque from artery walls can cause stroke (Rankin et al., 1994). Usually, neurologic sequelae due to air embolization elicit transient symptoms that resolve completely. However, neurovascular injury secondary to particulate matter results in less predictable recovery and prognosis. The incidence of this iatrogenic event is increasing, a finding that may be related to whether the methodology of the study in question is retrospective (where findings are typically lower) or prospective (Kuroda et al., 1993; Rankin et al., 1994). The cause is attributed to the advanced age of patients, the presence of calcified aorta (Blauth et al., 1992), or carotid stenosis at the time of bypass. Data from the CASS Study registry of greater than 10,000 subjects revealed an incidence of 1.9% in the aggregate subject pool. The most powerful predictors of stroke are age, use of alpha-adrenergic medications after CPB, and length of time on CPB. Rankin and colleagues (1994) also found in a similar population that age was a strong predictor. Those who were younger than 70 years of age demonstrated a 1.2% incidence, and the over–70-year-old group yielded an increased incidence of 2.6%. Tuman and coworkers (1992) also demonstrated a higher incidence, 8.9% in the over–75-year-old group. Given the current trend in managed care, patients with a preoperative history of hypertension and who have had a previous cerebral vascular event remain at risk for stroke up to 1 year after CPB (Frye et al., 1992). These findings provide nurses with important information for patient teaching and preventive health care.

The mechanism of injury that produces stroke remains unclear. It is thought to be related to the duration of CPB, changes related to altered metabolism, presence of aortic arch disease, sudden blood pressure changes during the postoperative period, and border zone infarction. Infarction results from insult to major vascular distribution or between the branches of the middle cerebral artery, leading to hypoperfusion and ischemia (Brenner et al., 1987; Faggioli et al., 1990; Krul et al., 1989; Rankin et al., 1994; Turnipseed et al., 1980). Reports of permanent deficits range from 2% to 10% (Brewer et al., 1983; Faggioli et al., 1990; Hornick et al., 1994). Usually, the period of improvement in function after reversible injury in edematous, metabolically depressed tissue is 3 to 18 months (Ricotta et al., 1995). Emerging treatments are focusing on rehabilitative restoration of the affected muscles with active therapy to the flaccid extremity based on new hypotheses of neuroplasticity explored in animal models (Dobkins, 1991). These hypotheses suggest that the forced-use notion of exercising the affected limb serves to support reorganization of cortical representation of movement, increasing the function of residual pathways and alternate efferent pathways (Dobkins, 1991).

Cognitive or neuropsychological changes such as short-term memory loss, impaired visual motor ability, difficulty in problem-solving, and lack of ability to concentrate have been found to exist in the absence of stroke (Raymond et al., 1985; Townes et al., 1989; Mattlar et al., 1991). The incidence ranges from 16% to 100%, depending on study methodology. Typically, in patients who are older than the age of 70 years, the incidence approaches 85% (Newman et al., 1994). Risk factors for these changes are age, length on CPB, preexisting cerebral vascular accident, and aortic atherosclerosis (Blauth et al., 1992). These deficits may persist up to 6 months after CPB (Townes et al., 1989). Such changes have implications for nurses in developing teaching strategies for patients, particularly those older than 70 years, in whom the pattern of resolution may not be predictable.

Prevention is an area of emerging efforts. There is evidence that hyperglycemia potentiates cerebral ischemia (Woo et al., 1988). Therefore, treatment of elevated serum glucose during cardiac surgery, which is simple, can improve outcomes. A promising pharmacologic agent in the calcium channel blocker family is nimodipine, which acts as a potent cerebral vasodilator (Gelmers et al., 1988); it moves easily across the blood–brain barrier. It is not approved for use in cardiac surgery. Although promising, it has a negative inotropic effect that requires consideration in this population.

PERIPHERAL NERVE INJURY. Neuralgia and numbness are common symptoms in patients with saphenous vein grafts (Nair et al., 1988). Some patients experience sensory deficits around the ankle and leg, such as pain and paresthesias. Injury to the saphenous nerve at the time of operation may result from surgical handling, trauma, or postoperative compression. Patients experience the most numbness during the first 48 hours. Numbness is attributed to a combination of surgical trauma and tissue inflammation.

Different methods of repairing the leg incision have been proposed to alleviate the problem. A single-layer technique of suture closure may result in improved protection of cutaneous sensation compared to subcuticular sutures (Angelini et al., 1984). The optimum technique of closure is directed toward minimizing pressure on the saphenous nerve as healing progresses (Angelini et al., 1984).

Upper extremity nerve injury has been reported in approximately 10% to 15% of patients undergoing CABG (Green, 1989). The etiology of this syndrome remains unclear. Hickey and colleagues (1993) used somatosensory-evoked potentials (SEPs) to monitor ulnar and median nerve function during surgery. A transient change in SEP was observed during central venous cannulation in 13% of patients. Use of the sternal retractors was correlated with a SEP change in 70% of patients. The majority of patients (eighty-five percent) did not develop permanent neurologic deficit and experienced complete resolution of symptoms.

IMMUNE SYSTEM. Recognition of the systemic inflammatory response associated with CPB has become an emerging area of research. Germane to this response is the activation and adhesion of neutrophils in conjunction with a synergistic cytokine network. Neutrophil adhesion to endothelial surfaces is the first step in promoting chemotaxis to the site of inflammation or injury. Once activated, these cells make cytokines, which further recruit other immune cells to the site. Hill and colleagues (1994) have demonstrated a blunting effect on neutrophil adhesion to endothelial surfaces with the use of steroids given just before CPB initiation, compared to patients not receiving steroids. Such findings hold promise for the control the systemic inflammatory responses commonly observed after CPB.

Cytokines are endogenous polypeptides that serve as communication signals between cells involved in immune function and the inflammatory response. Steinberg and associates (1993) have demonstrated an elevation in plasma levels of cytokines, namely, interleukin (IL)-1B, IL-2, IL-6, and complement mediators as a result of CPB. Repeated measures of these components demonstrated no difference in cytokine elevation from pre-CPB measures except for IL-6, which peaked 3 hours after CPB. IL-6 is the hepatocyte-stimulating factor that mediates the acute-phase proteins. Such a response is associated with fever, leukocytosis, thrombocytosis, and release of prostaglandins, leukotrienes, and vasoactive substances (Kushner, 1982). Complement was elevated during CPB. No improvement was demonstrated with the use of heparin-bonded circuits in preventing the activation of these two systems as a result of translocation of endotoxin into the serum.

Complement activation via the alternative pathway (which liberates C3a and C5a) takes place in response to elevations in serum endotoxin (Casey, 1993) liberated from blood coming in contact with CPB tubing (Hammerschmidt et al., 1981; Nilsson et al., 1988). With the administration of protamine for heparin reversal, complement is further activated via the classic pathway, mediating the formation of C4a (Cavarocchi et al., 1985). In addition to complement activation, other systems such as the coagulation, cytokine network, fibrinolytic, and kallikrein systems work synergistically to produce the systemic inflammatory response associated with CPB (Butler et al., 1993; Steinberg et al., 1993).

Complement activation causes release of polymorphonuclear leukocytes (PMNs) from bone marrow. However, overall PMN levels and lymphocytes are decreased during this hypothermic state because of pulmonary leukosequestration (Quiroga et al., 1985), platelet adherence to the surface of the CPB tubing (Colman, 1990), and the tendency of neutrophils, complement anaphylatoxins (Butler et al., 1993) and platelets (Colman, 1990) to aggregate in small vessels within the lung, leading to pulmonary dysfunction (Howard et al., 1988; Lavelle et al., 1984; Nilsson et al., 1988; Quiroga et al., 1985).

A major source of endotoxemia generated during initiation of CPB is gastrointestinal ischemia (Martinez-Pellus et al., 1993) and blood–air interface associated with suction in the operative field. Recent investigations have focused on alleviation of the gastrointestinal contribution. A significant decrease in IL-6 and endotoxin was demonstrated in patients who underwent digestive decontamination before CPB.

Also observed at the beginning of CPB is an overall increase in the white blood cell count, which continues until rewarming is complete. On rewarming, the serum PMN count is elevated, with further uptake of these white cells in the lung (Quiroga et al., 1985). Significant elevation in the PMN count causes the development of perivascular edema in the endothelial cells of the pneumocytes, impairing gas exchange and increasing pulmonary arterial–alveolar gradients (Edmunds & Stephenson, 1983; Howard et al., 1988; Lavalle et al., 1984; Quiroga et al., 1985).

Lymphocytes are depressed after CPB and return to normal after 7 days. Phenotypically, a reversal of the CD4+/CD8+ ratio was found with a redistribution of CD4+ cells in bone marrow (Ryhanen et al., 1987). Interestingly, no change in B lymphocytes has been demonstrated. A decrease in natural killer cell number and cytotoxicity has been found after CPB (Nguyen et al., 1992). Hisatomi and colleagues (1989) have demonstrated that the T-cell–dependent lymphocyte response was significantly diminished after cardiac operation for the first postoperative week. These findings suggest two major potential areas of vulnerability. First, with the diminished CD4+ cell function, patients are vulnerable to viral infections, such as human immunodeficiency virus (HIV), because CD4+ cells remove intracellular organisms. Second, a decrease in CD4+ lymphocytes, in addition to changing natural killer cell function, suggests potential changes in the cytokine feedback mechanism that mediates competent cellular immune function. These findings suggest a vulnerable period during the first postoperative week in which patients may be susceptible to bacterial and viral infections.

Recent research has demonstrated promising outcomes in attempts to modulate the immune dysregulatory response mediated by IL-1, IL-6, and tumor necrosis factor. Markewitz and colleagues (1993) demonstrated a decrease in IL-6 response after CPB in a group of subjects who received indomethacin (which blocks the synthesis of prostaglandin through cyclooxygenase inhibition) and thymopentin (which acts similarly to the thymic hormone thymopoietin to promote T-cell activation and recruitment). Although these data were not further correlated with clinical outcomes, it is postulated that if immune modulation of T-cell function could be regulated, this could have a significant effect on postoperative infection.

INFECTION. Sternal wound infections infrequently complicate the postoperative period. Approximately 1% to 5% of patients have major wound infections involving the chest wall and mediastinum (Grossi et al., 1985; Jeevanandam et al., 1990; Ko et al., 1992). These patients are at extremely high risk, with potentially fatal consequences. The common practice of shaving patients before surgery was explored by one group to determine whether a manual versus an electric approach affected the incidence of suppurative mediastinitis. In addition, the use of topical povidone–iodine or normal saline was investigated. These researchers found a higher incidence of infection in the manually shaved patients. No benefit was demonstrated in the use of topical skin-cleansing agents (Grossi, 1985).

Signs and symptoms of infection are usually manifested by the second postoperative week but can occur anywhere from 6 to 21 days after surgery. Diagnosis and confirmation of sternal wound infection is made after comprehensive examination and testing. Development of fever, leukocytosis, incisional pain, sternal instability, and wound drainage commonly describe the clinical picture. *Staphylococcus aureus* and *Staphylococcus epidermidis* are the common causative organisms (Grossi et al., 1985).

Bacterial invasion of the myocardium and surrounding structures due to mediastinitis can jeopardize the integrity of the coronary grafts and suture lines. Erosion caused by release of endotoxin may precipitate anastomotic instability and potential rupture. The risk of graft occlusion in these patients arises from the potential formation of septic thrombi.

Factors related to the development of mediastinitis are advanced age (older than 80 years), early chest reexploration, and prolonged low cardiac output (Behrendt & Austen, 1981). Recent data suggest that use of a single ITA graft carries a 1% chance of sternal wound infection. Use of bilateral ITA grafts has been associated with a slightly increased incidence of infection (Culliford et al., 1976; Grover et al., 1994). Multivariate analysis, however, indicates that factors such as age and diabetes have a greater impact than use of the ITA in determining the risk of infection (Cosgrove et al., 1988). Subsequent reports have failed to support a relationship between use of the ITA and mediastinitis (Cosgrove et al., 1988).

Leg wound infections occur in less than 1% of patients (DeLaria et al., 1981). Necrosis or sloughing of wound edges may result from postoperative low cardiac output or poor skin perfusion. The primary goal of saphenectomy care lies in the reduction of extravascular fluid to reduce suture line tension and encourage wound edge approximation. In patients with large hematomas, accumulation of serous fluid acts as a suitable medium for bacterial proliferation. It is recommended that infected hematomas be evacuated and drained to promote granulation. Some data suggest the avoidance of povidine–iodine preparations secondary to toxicity to epithelial cells and decreased subdermal healing. Careful attention must be given to those patients with peripheral vascular disease or diabetes, or who are steroid users or smokers. Proper nutritional intake and iron stores are necessary to deliver adequate substrate and tissue oxygenation. Supplementation with vitamin C and zinc has been proposed to facilitate wound healing and granulation in the immunocompromised patient. Certain wound closure techniques have also been associated with infection. Some authors note that use of subcuticular sutures facilitates improved wound healing compared to metal staples (Angelini et al., 1984).

Management of Cardiac Surgical Patients

Nursing and medical staff collaborate on the management of the patient throughout the postoperative recovery phase. During the acute postoperative phase, patients are monitored continuously as systemic recovery from anesthesia occurs and body temperatures return to normal. The primary goals of management are to ensure the adequacy of the cardiac index and tissue perfusion and to monitor neurologic recovery. Systemic responses to the operative procedure and the cardiopulmonary pump run are monitored. Nursing and medical management of these patients is accomplished through monitoring of direct and derived hemodynamic parameters, clinical assessment, and laboratory tests.

The focus of management for these patients is continuous assessment and prompt intervention to maintain an adequate cardiac index to meet metabolic needs. Concurrently, the critical care nurse assists the family in coping with the situational crisis of the illness, receiving communications about the patient's progress, and verbalizing their feelings. Operative correlations of the clinical problem, nursing interventions, and rationale for treatment are listed in the Coronary Artery Bypass Graft Surgery Multidisciplinary Care Guide.

THORACIC TRANSPLANTS

Thoracic transplantation is rapidly becoming a common option for patients with end-stage cardiac disease not amenable to medical management. Likewise, with the current success of lung transplantation, end-stage lung disease is also treated with various surgical approaches. One of the mainstays of either transplantation surgical procedure is the use of CPB. Inherent in its use are all the clinical problems associated with CPB, most of which have not been studied in the thoracic transplant patient. However, the following section provides an overview of thoracic transplantation focusing on background, evaluation, patient selection, preoperative waiting period, donor management, postoperative care, and common complications.

Cardiac Transplantation

BACKGROUND

The first attempts at heart transplantation, led by Dr. Christiaan Barnard in 1967 (Macdonald, 1990), generated considerable publicity and enthusiasm. Unfortunately, the success of the surgical procedure was not equaled by postoperative medical management, and most patients quickly succumbed to infection, rejection, or both. A better understanding of the immune response, more accurate diagnosis of rejection, development of immunosuppressive agents with greater specificity, and a more balanced approach to immunosuppression have dramatically changed outcomes in heart transplantation.

By 1994, more than 26,700 heart transplants had been performed worldwide. Current 1-year survival posttransplant is 79% to 85%, 5-year survival is 60% to 85%, and 10-year survival is approximately 45% (Hosenpud et al., 1994; Mudge et al., 1993; O'Connell et al., 1993). Heart failure is the principal indication for transplantation in 95% of all recipients (Stevenson, 1994a). The etiology of disease is CAD in 47% and cardiomyopathy in 43%. Valvular disease, congenital abnormalities, retransplantation, and miscellaneous causes account for a few percent each (Hosenpud et al., 1994). According to data from the United Network for Organ Sharing (UNOS), approximately 84% of those listed for transplant are male, and 69% are between the ages of 44 and 64 years (McManus et al., 1993).

The increased success of the procedure has, ironically, led to a crisis in heart transplantation. More than 11,000 patients are placed on the waiting list for donor hearts each year, but the donor supply remains fixed at about 3,000 hearts per year in the United States (Stevenson, 1994a). Waiting time for a heart varies by blood type, geographic region, recipient size, recipient clinical status, and the presence of high levels of circulating antibodies that necessitate a prospective crossmatch with a potential donor. Average waiting time is now 8 months and is continuing to increase (Stevenson et al., 1993). Donor organs are prioritized to the sickest patients, and more than half of all transplants are now performed on patients who are hospitalized while waiting. It has been predicted that in 4 years "there will be virtually no hearts available for outpatient candidates" (Stevenson, 1991). The shortage of donor organs has forced transplant centers to carefully evaluate both the candidacy of potential recipients and the timing of listing for transplantation.

PATIENT EVALUATION AND SELECTION

Inclusion and exclusion criteria are determined individually by each transplant center. The current trend is toward standardization as well as more restrictive criteria (Kubo et al., 1993; Mudge et al., 1993). The evaluation process is aimed at determining three factors: (1) the severity of heart disease; (2) the presence of any other medical condition that would unfavorably affect the outcome of transplantation; and (3) elimination of the possibility of any other medical or surgical therapy as an alternative to transplantation (see Table 24–4).

Cardiac testing during evaluation includes an echocardiogram to evaluate heart size, valve competency, wall motion abnormalities, and ejection fraction. Although ejection fraction is a good assessment of myocardial failure, a low ejection fraction is not in itself a good indicator of the need for heart transplant (Mudge et al., 1993). Functional capacity and cardiac reserve are determined by a bicycle exercise test measuring oxygen uptake (peak V_{O_2}). Peak V_{O_2} of less than 14 mL/kg/minute and patient report of significant limitations in daily activities are indicative of a probable need for transplantation. Peak V_{O_2} less than 10 mL/kg/minute is associated with the worst survival and is a strong indicator for transplantation (Mudge et al., 1993). Cardiac catheterization is performed to evaluate CAD and assess hemodynamics. Elevated pulmonary pressures, particularly pulmonary vascular resistance and resistance index, that do not respond to oxygen or intravenous vasodilator therapy continue to be strong exclusionary criteria for orthotopic heart transplantation. This is because of the high risk of immediate right heart failure in the transplanted donor heart, which is unable to adapt to the high pressures of the recipient's pulmonary vasculature. Patients with elevated pulmonary pressures may be considered for heterotopic ("piggy-back") transplantation, now rare, or, more commonly, for combined heart–lung transplantation. Sudden death accounts for 30% of deaths among patients awaiting transplant (McManus et al., 1993). Dysrhythmia evaluation by Holter monitor or electrophysiologic studies is also an important component of the cardiac evaluation.

During the evaluation process, virtually every organ system is also assessed by laboratory testing, radiographically, or by functional status. Immunosuppressive medications, which must be taken for life, take a heavy toll on both liver and kidneys, and adequate function pretransplant is essential to posttransplant survival. Psychosocial assessment is probably the most important evaluation component after the cardiac evaluation. Psychological stability, good social supports, and the ability to comply with complex medical regimens are crucial to successful transplantation.

The evaluation period is extremely stressful for potential recipients. In addition to dealing with the reality of a terminal disease, patients feel they are literally "on trial for life." The associated tension and anxiety can worsen cardiac problems and often impede the patient–caregiver relationship. Assurance that it is the appropriate therapy that is being evaluated, rather than the patient, often "defuses" the situation and facilitates communication. Patients and their families need to be able to ask questions about the ongoing testing and results, as well as about transplantation, to make an informed choice about the procedure. Meeting another patient who has had a heart transplant is often very helpful in stimulating questions from potential recipients and in providing reassurance about quality of life and the ability to handle a complex medical regimen posttransplant (see Table 24–5).

TABLE 24–4. **Exclusion Criteria for Heart Transplantation**

Older age

Systemic illness with poor prognosis
- Renal dysfunction with serum creatinine >2 mg/dL on creatinine clearance <50 mL/minute
- Liver dysfunction
- Severe cerebral or peripheral vascular disease
- Recent malignancy
- Active infection
- Insulin-dependent diabetes with end-organ damage
- Active gastrointestinal disease
- Pulmonary hypertension with high and irreversible pulmonary vascular resistance (PVR >480 dynes/sec^2 or >240 dynes/sec^2 after therapy
- Pulmonary parenchymal disease
- Recent pulmonary embolus or infarct
- Severe obesity
- Severe osteoporosis

Psychosocial instability or substance abuse

Adapted from Mudge, G. H., et al. (1993). Task force 3: Recipient guidelines/prioritization. *Journal of the American College of Cardiology, 22,* 21–30.

TABLE 24–5. **Current Indications for Heart Transplantation**

Accepted Indications

1. Peak V_{O_2} < 10 mL/kg/minute
2. Severe ischemia limiting daily activities and not treatable by other medical or surgical treatments
3. Recurrent symptomatic dysrhythmias that are refractory to all therapy

Possible Indications

1. Peak V_{O_2} < 14mL/kg/minute
2. Unstable ischemia not treatable by other medical or surgical therapy
3. Unstable fluid balance or renal function in patients who are compliant with sodium and fluid restriction and diuretics

Adapted from Mudge, G. H., et al. (1993). Task force 3: Recipient guidelines/prioritization. *Journal of the American College of Cardiology, 22,* 21–30.

PREOPERATIVE CARE AND WAITING PERIOD

Once all the testing data have been reviewed by the cardiac transplant team, a decision is made about the patient's candidacy and the timing of listing for transplant. Steimle and colleagues (1994) demonstrated that a minority of patients with dilated cardiomyopathy referred for transplant evaluation and who had symptoms for less than 6 months, subsequently had a marked improvement in left ventricular function that permitted deferral of listing for transplant. Patients with symptom duration longer than 3 months, more severe hemodynamic compromise, and low serum sodium levels showed little subsequent improvement. Early listing may be appropriate for this population.

When the patient and the timing are deemed appropriate, the potential candidate is prioritized on a waiting list by blood type, body size, clinical status, and date. Patients are listed with an organ procurement organization (OPO), determined by the transplanting center, within a specific geographic region of the country, and are also listed on a national waiting list maintained by UNOS. Because of the current donor shortage, donor hearts are almost always used within the procuring region and are rarely offered nationally unless a rare blood type or body size makes an in-region match impossible. Throughout the waiting period the patient's medical management and listing status are continually re-evaluated and priority status on the waiting list adjusted for both improvement and worsening of the patient's condition.

Universally, patients describe the uncertainty of

the waiting period as the most difficult time physically, psychosocially, and often financially (Cardin & Clarke, 1985). The analogy most often used is "like living on death row" (Porter et al., 1994). As more patients are hospitalized before transplant, nurses and other caregivers have become an increasingly important part of the pretransplant support system, and often share this stress (Riether & Boudreau, 1988). Anger and depression related to physical and psychological losses, anticipatory grief for the potential donor, and survivor guilt are common issues. The most frequently identified coping strategies to deal with these issues are (1) thinking positively, (2) using humor, and (3) trying to keep life as normal as possible (Porter et al., 1994).

Despite careful medical management, some patients continue to deteriorate and intensive care unit admission may be necessary. Often, patients can be stabilized on intravenous vasoactives such as dobutamine, dopamine, amrinone, or milrinone, but if medication fails, mechanical support may be required. Intubation has been identified as an independent risk for increased mortality after transplantation (Bourge et al., 1993), and should be avoided if at all possible. Counterpulsation with IABC is the usual first-line mechanical support used as a bridge to transplant in low cardiac output states. There are a number of advantages to this device, including (1) general availability, (2) relatively simple and quick insertion, and (3) lower cost than other mechanical assist devices. However, there are also disadvantages and limitations to IABC therapy, such as (1) a limited increase in cardiac output, (2) thromboembolic complications, (3) infection, and (4) vascular damage (Naucke, 1990). When IABC therapy fails or is contraindicated, other forms of mechanical assistance must be considered. Short-term univentricular and biventricular devices have been used in cardiogenic shock and for cardiac surgical patients who cannot be weaned from CPB, but have few applications in the area of bridging to transplant, which usually requires long-term therapy. Several devices are currently under investigation for use in long-term support, and one has recently been approved by the Food and Drug Administration (FDA).

The only biventricular device proposed is the pneumatically driven "total artificial heart," which may be reintroduced for clinical use in the future. Two pulsatile left ventricular devices are currently being evaluated in multicenter trials. Both the Novacor (Baxter Healthcare Corp., Oakland, CA) and the Heartmate TCI (Thermocardiosystems, Inc., Woburn, MA) devices have an implantable left ventricular pump that receives blood from the left ventricular apex and pumps outflow into the ascending aorta via cannula. Both pumps require an external power console and drive line, which is electrical in the case of the Novacor device and pneumatic in the TCI. Early data for both devices indicate approximately 60% of patients underwent subsequent transplantation, and more than 85% of those transplanted survived to discharge. Both devices present some risk of thromboembolism and infection, and are currently very costly. However, the disadvantages are offset by their significant improvement in patient rehabilitation before transplant and their successful long-term use of more than 460 days (Costanzo-Nardin et al., 1993). The use of xenografts (organs or tissues transplanted from one animal species to another) remains experimental and controversial. However, with long waiting times and more patients dying while waiting, bridge to transplant instead of transplant, may assume increasing importance.

HEART DONOR PROCUREMENT AND ORTHOTOPIC TRANSPLANTATION

Organ donors are usually victims of head trauma or patients who have had a primary cerebral event, such as subarachnoid hemorrhage. To be identified as a potential donor, the patient must meet two clinical brain death criteria: (1) there must be a complete loss of brain function, including cortex and brain stem; and (2) the loss of function must be irreversible (Baldwin et al., 1993). The exact procedure for declaration of brain death varies by state, and strict adherence to the guidelines are both legally and ethically imperative. Once brain death has been established, consent for organ donation should be discussed with the next of kin. Both the patient's wishes (if known) and the family's wishes are crucial. Often, it is the nurse who has been caring for the patient who is in the best position to help the families recognize organ donation as a positive outcome from an otherwise tragic loss.

After consent is obtained, the potential donor is screened. A procurement coordinator from the OPO obtains information about donor age and size, blood type, hepatitis and HIV status, cause of death, and other clinical information. If there are no contraindications to transplant, a cardiac surgeon or cardiologist reviews data on the extent of injuries, hemodynamics, need for cardiopulmonary resuscitation or vasoactive medications, chest x-ray, ECG, echocardiogram, and arterial blood gases. Because of the shortage of donor organs, there is increasing interest in carefully evaluating so-called "marginal donors" who might have been declined in the past, due to concerns such as age, ventricular hypertrophy, or low ejection fraction on echocardiogram. Further evaluation, including cardiac catheterization of the donor to assess for CAD, has resulted in the use of healthy hearts that might otherwise have been rejected. The final screening is determined by the cardiac surgeon, who inspects the heart at the time of explanation (Baldwin et al., 1993). Case reports of heart transplant patients using hearts with known coronary disease have shown highly variable early results. As yet, no long-term outcomes have been reported, and this approach remains controversial (Laks et al., 1993).

Most heart donors are multiorgan donors, and the donor cardiectomy often requires coordination with several other transplant teams. A median sternotomy is performed and, after transection of the superior and inferior vena cavae, pulmonary artery and veins, and the aorta, the heart is removed. The heart is cooled topically with saline, and crystalloid cardioplegia is used to arrest and preserve the heart (Madonald, 1990). Current data show increased mortality with ischemic times greater than 4 hours, so every effort is made to keep transit and reimplantation times as short as possible (Bourge et al., 1993). Surgery often begins on the recipient before the donor heart has arrived at the transplant center. After opening the chest with a median sternotomy, the aorta and superior and inferior vena cavae are cannulated and the patient is placed on CPB. Implantation of the donor heart is performed using one of two techniques. The first, described by Shumway and associates in 1966, is referred to as the atrial technique (Shumway et al., 1966). The recipient's pulmonary artery and aorta are transected and the atria are resected, leaving a cuff of atria intact above the atrioventricular groove. The donor heart is trimmed to approximate the recipient atria, and the atria, septal pulmonary artery, and aorta are anastomosed (Fig. 24–17).

The composite atria from the donor transplanted heart and the recipient's right atrium cause both ECG and functional changes. Because the recipient's native sinoatrial node is left intact, an impulse may be generated that travels to, but not across, the atrial suture line and is recorded on ECG as an autonomically responsive, nonconducted P wave. The sinoatrial node of the donor heart generates a conducted impulse that results in contraction, and there may be two P waves visible on ECG. Functionally, the composite atria result in atrial dysynergy and a reduction in the atrial contribution to ventricular filling. (An RBBB is also a common ECG finding posttransplant.)

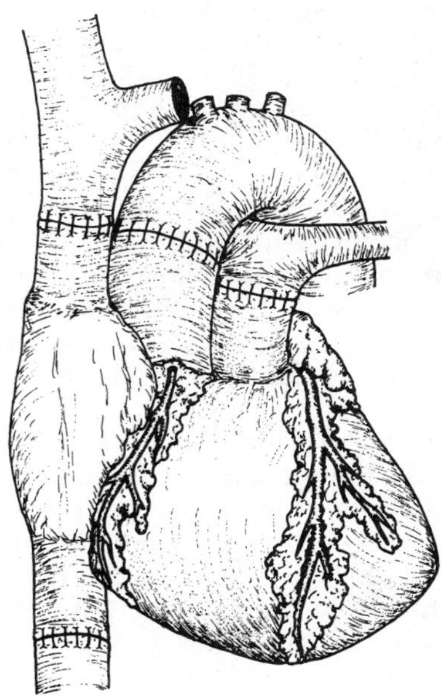

FIGURE 24–17. Reconstructed aorta and pulmonary artery, completed implantation of the donor heart. (From Blanche, C., et al. [1994]. Orthotopic heart transplantation with bicaval and pulmonary venous anastomoses. *Annals of Thoracic Surgery, 58,* 1505–1509.)

All air is evacuated from the heart and the patient is gradually weaned from CPB. If spontaneous defibrillation of the heart does not occur, electrical defibrillation is used to restore rhythm. Monitoring lines, pacing wires, and chest tubes are placed, as in any other cardiac surgical patient.

The transplanted heart, although working better than its predecessor, never functions completely as a normal heart would. The new heart has no autonomic innervation. Immediately after surgery, slow heart rates are common in the cold, ischemic, transplanted heart, and isoproterenol (a beta-adrenergic stimulator) may be required for both inotropic and chronotropic support. Once recovered from the operative insult, the resting heart rate is typically 90 to 110 beats per minute, without the slowing effects of the parasympathetic nerves. Parasympathetic blocking medications like atropine or vagal maneuvers have no effect on heart rate. Without sympathetic innervation, the transplanted heart must rely on circulating catecholamines and increased venous return to increase heart rate and contractility. These mechanisms are effective, but much slower than autonomic responses, and patients must learn to increase activity and exercise slowly. Orthostatic hypotension is also common early in the posttransplant period, due to venous pooling, reduced preload, and absence of a compensatory tachycardia. Without innervation, transplant patients do not usually experience anginal chest pain with coronary disease. Cardiac catheterization remains the only way to evaluate coronary disease, except in the few patients who have developed reinnervation late after transplant (Young et al., 1993).

A new surgical technique (Fig. 24–18) for orthotopic heart transplantation confers some benefits to preserve the physiologic integrity of the conduction system and mechanical function of the right atrium (Blanche et al., 1994). This bicaval approach involves complete excision of the recipient atria and transection of the superior vena cava. The inferior vena cava is divided, leaving a cuff of right atrium. Following completion of the left atrial anastomosis, the superior and inferior vena cavae are then anastomosed in an end-to-end fashion. This technique has yielded less distortion of the right atrium and has led to less tricuspid regurgitation and improved hemodynamic function. The technique takes slightly longer and there is a small risk of caval stenosis and possible anastomic perforation with endomyocardial biopsy.

POSTOPERATIVE MANAGEMENT AND CARE

HEMODYNAMICS. Myocardial dysfunction is a common problem in the immediate postoperative period and is caused by global ischemia, preexisting high pulmonary pressures, right ventricular overload, donor–recipient size mismatch, inadequate organ preservation, and early restrictive myocardial physiology (Young et al., 1993). Vasopressor support, judicious volume management, and chronotropic support with

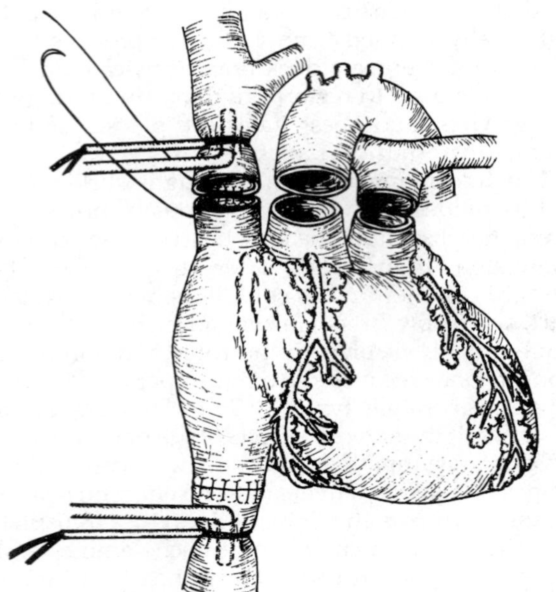

FIGURE 24–18. The superior and inferior venae cavae are anastomosed in an end-to-end fashion. (From Blanche, C., et al. [1994]. Orthotopic heart transplantation with bicaval and pulmonary venous anastomoses. *Annals of Thoracic Surgery, 58,* 1505–1509.)

medication or pacing are routine interventions early posttransplant. In addition to the hemodynamic changes specific to transplant, the patient may experience any of the problems and complications that commonly occur with cardiac surgery such as bleeding, MI, or thromboembolic events.

REJECTION. Once hemodynamic stability is ensured, the focus shifts to protecting the transplanted heart from the immune response of the recipient. Rejection after organ transplantation is believed to be primarily a cell-mediated process in which recipient T lymphocytes recognize donor tissue as foreign, become activated, proliferate, and ultimately destroy the donor organ. Humoral or antibody-mediated rejection also plays a role in graft destruction and is characterized histologically by immunoglobulin and fibrin deposition in the walls of small vessels. Hyperacute rejection is a rare form of humoral rejection in which preformed recipient antibodies cause immediate graft dysfunction (Stevenson, 1994). The greatest risk for rejection occurs early after transplant and diminishes significantly by 6 months. Immunosuppressive medication doses are highest early after transplant and then are gradually tapered based on rejection history, severity, and episodes (Keogh et al., 1992). Most centers use triple-drug therapy, including cyclosporine, prednisone, and azathioprine, to suppress the immune system through multiple mechanisms and to minimize the side effects of any one drug (Miller et al., 1993). Because there are no reliable noninvasive indicators of asymptomatic rejection, patients undergo endomyocardial biopsy frequently during the first year to obtain tissue samples Table 24–6). Therapeutic decisions are based on the severity of rejection according to histologic grade and the presence of clinical or hemodynamic changes. Most rejection episodes are asymptomatic, but the presence of fever, fatigue, malaise, hypotension, decreased ejection fraction, dysrhythmias, and symptoms of congestive heart failure always requires more careful evaluation. Mild rejection episodes in patients without clinical signs of rejection often are not treated but monitored carefully and rebiopsied earlier than usual (Yeoh et al., 1992). There are data to suggest that mild rejection in conjunction with clinical allograft dysfunction can progress to moderate rejection on subsequent biopsy 30% of the time (Yeoh et al., 1992). Moderate rejection with or without clinical symptoms is usually treated either with an intravenous bolus or an oral pulse of high-dose corticosteroid (Billingham et al., 1990). In the case of severe or repeated rejection episodes, monoclonal or polyclonal antilymphocyte antibodies may be used in addition to steroids. Monoclonal or polyclonal antibody therapy is also used in some centers as induction therapy immediately after surgery to delay cyclosporine use in patients with renal dysfunction, to decrease steroid use, or to minimize allograft sensitization (Hook, 1990). This therapy has been shown to delay the time to first rejection, but has not decreased rejection frequency (Miller et al., 1993). Antilymphocyte therapy has also been associated with an increased frequency of infection (Miller et al., 1994).

INFECTION. The severity of infection and the number of types of infections have decreased with the use of more selective immunosuppressives, but infection continues to be a significant cause of morbidity and mortality. Bacteria are the most common cause of infection within the first month after transplant, with *Staphylococcus* and gram-negative species being the most common causes. Most of these infections are catheter- or line-related. Although some transplant centers use maximal to full isolation precautions, there is no evidence that there is any difference in infection or survival rates based on infection control practices (Lange et al., 1992). Strict handwashing and adherence to line-change guidelines appear to be the most important precautions in the early posttransplant phase.

During the second to fifth month, opportunistic infections are the most common, and include cytomegalovirus (CMV), *Pneumocystis carinii* (PCP), and fungal infections. Most centers use trimethoprim–sulfamethoxazole as prophylaxis for PCP, and mycostatin liquid or troches for *Candida* prophylaxis. Some centers are also using ganciclovir for CMV prophylaxis in seronegative recipients receiving a seropositive donor, or to prevent reactivation in seropositive recipients. CMV infection continues to be a significant cause of morbidity and mortality, despite attempts at prevention (Miller et al., 1993).

TABLE 24–6. **Standardized Cardiac Biopsy Grading**

Grade	"New" Nomenclature	"Old" Nomenclature
0	No rejection	No rejection
1	A = Focal (perivascular or interstitial) infiltrate without necrosis B = Diffuse but sparse infiltrate without necrosis	Mild rejection
2	One focus only with aggressive infiltration and/or focal myocyte damage	"Focal" moderate rejection
3	A = Multifocal aggressive infiltrates and/or myocyte damage B = Diffuse inflammatory process with necrosis	"Low" moderate rejection "Borderline/severe"
4	Diffuse aggressive polymorphous ± infiltrate ± edema, ± hemorrhage, ± vasculitis, with necrosis	"Severe acute" rejection

"Resolving" rejection denoted by a lesser grade.

"Resolved" rejection denoted by grade 0.

From Billingham, M. E., et al. (1990). A working formulation for the standardization of nomenclature in the diagnosis of heart and lung rejection: Heart Rejection Study Group. *Journal of Heart Transplantation, 9,* 587–593.

COMPLICATIONS

Accelerated graft atherosclerosis is now the major limitation to posttransplant survival. A diffuse disease characterized by intimal thickening of the coronary arteries with a loss of tertiary vessels and no development of collateral vessels, it is detectable by angiography in 30% to 50% of patients by 5 years and has rarely occurred as early as 6 months after transplant (Miller et al., 1993). The disease is believed to be an immune-mediated process and has been reported in other transplanted organs as well. Medical therapies used for conventional CAD are not effective and the only definitive treatment is retransplantation. However, the 2-year survival rate with retransplant may be as low as 40%, and the issue of retransplant has raised ethical questions about the use of scarce donor organs (Mullins et al., 1991).

Malignancies resulting from immunosuppression usually occur late after transplant. However, lymphoproliferative diseases that appear related to Epstein-Barr virus have been reported as early as a few months posttransplant. The use of enhanced immunosuppression or antilymphocyte globulins is associated with an increased incidence of malignancy. Decreasing immunosuppressive therapy and the use of chemotherapy and radiation may be effective in treatment (Miller et al., 1993).

Immunosuppressive medications alone or in combination induce a number of serious and common complications. Cyclosporine nephrotoxicity is a well recognized problem and the decline in renal function occurs primarily within the first 6 months of transplant. Prevention of renal failure by close monitoring of cyclosporine levels and avoidance of other drugs that may worsen cyclosporine nephrotoxicity is vital. Hypertension, induced by cyclosporine, has been reported to occur in 50% to 90% of patients posttransplant. No one agent has been shown to be effective, and often several medications in combination are required for adequate blood pressure control. Hyperlipidemia is also common and may be seen as early as 3 weeks after transplantation. Early withdrawal of steroids and diet and exercise modifications should be tried before medications are added. Obesity is a significant problem, and most patients who gain weight do so in the first year. Osteoporosis from steroid therapy, older age, postmenopausal status, and lower bone mass pretransplant can result in chronic pain and significant disability from compression fractures and avascular necrosis. Aggressive treatment with calcium, calcitonin, vitamin D, and hormone therapy has been helpful (Miller et al., 1993).

DISCHARGE AND LONG-TERM CARE

The transition to wellness begins immediately after surgery, and both patients and families report significant problems in role adjustment (Hook et al., 1990). Teaching is focused on progressive self-care and may require significant involvement of family members because most patients experience a decreased attention span, impaired thought processes, and emotional lability (Cifani & Vargo, 1990). Providing small amounts of information with frequent repetition is most effective. Most patients can return to the level of activity and employment they experienced before their cardiac disability, and are not significantly limited physically (Stevenson, 1994).

Lung Transplantation

BACKGROUND

Human lung transplantation was first attempted in 1963 (Hardy et al., 1963). Although unsuccessful, technical feasibility of the procedure was demonstrated. Subsequent endeavors over the following two decades suffered dismal results largely due to infection, rejection, and disruption of the bronchial anastomosis. During this period, however, advances in critical care management and thoracic surgery, refinement of immunosuppressive therapy, and success in heart and heart–lung transplantation occurred. Consequently, the first long-term success in single-lung transplantation (SLT) occurred in 1983 in Toronto. Success with en bloc double-lung transplantation was reported in 1986 (Patterson et al., 1988). This procedure was later modified to a bilateral sequential lung transplant (BLT), essentially requiring two SLTs performed consecutively through a common incision (Pasque et al., 1990). The number of lung transplant programs, procedures, and candidates has increased tremendously in the ensuing years as these techniques have been applied successfully to an ever-widening range of indications. Lung donor procurement has been the single most limiting factor in the growth of lung transplantation worldwide. Neurogenic pulmonary edema, contamination and sepsis from aspiration and prolonged intubation, or direct trauma, all common conditions in the donor population, make suitable lung donor grafts the most difficult of all solid organs to procure. In response to this problem, living-related and lobar transplantation has recently emerged as a possible option for critically ill and pediatric patients for whom finding suitable donor organs is unlikely (Starnes et al., 1994).

INDICATIONS

Lung transplantation is reserved for patients with end-stage pulmonary disease that is progressively disabling despite conventional treatment. Patients are usually accepted for transplantation when life expectancy is estimated at less than 18 to 24 months. However, because no reliable tool for measurement of life expectancy in these patients exists and the waiting period for a suitable donor organ depends on unpredictable variables, timing for intervention is not definitive.

Inclusion and exclusion criteria may be center-specific and depend on patient population, experience, and availability of resources. Guidelines and contraindications are listed in Table 24–7.

TABLE 24–7. **Guidelines and Contraindications for Lung Transplantation**

Age:
- Younger than 60–65 years for single lung transplant
- Younger than 55–60 years for bilateral sequential transplant

Reliable psychosocial support

Demonstrated compliance with medical regimens

Pulmonary impairment that interferes with activities of daily living

Absolute and relative contraindications may include any or all of the following:
- Severe systemic disease
- Severe coronary artery disease or left ventricular dysfunction (heart–lung transplant may be an option)
- Malignancy
- Sepsis
- High-dose steroid dependency
- Severe psychiatric disorders
- Current history of substance abuse, including smoking, alcoholism, drug abuse
- Severe malnutrition or morbid obesity

Within the above guidelines, restrictive, obstructive, and pulmonary vascular disorders are amenable to treatment with either SLT or BLT. Choice of operation is designed to limit the surgical risk for the patient while optimizing the donor pool and providing the best chance for survival.

Single-lung transplantation is best suited for patients with restrictive and obstructive disorders, such as pulmonary fibrosis or emphysema. If, however, the disease involves chronic infection, such as cystic fibrosis or bronchiectasis, both lungs must be replaced and BLT becomes the appropriate option. Pulmonary vascular diseases for which SLT is appropriate include Eisenmenger's syndrome (with surgically correctable congenital lesions) and primary pulmonary hypertension (PPH). Previously, heart–lung transplantation was thought to be the procedure of choice for these disorders, which involve severe right ventricular dysfunction secondary to markedly elevated pulmonary artery pressures. In the late 1980s, SLT was successfully used after clinical experience (Daily et al., 1987) demonstrated that severe right ventricular dysfunction was reversible if right ventricular afterload could be significantly reduced by replacing the diseased pulmonary circulation with a normal one (as in single or bilateral transplantation).

PATIENT EVALUATION AND SELECTION

To establish candidacy for lung transplantation, patients must undergo an extensive screening process. Studies are designed to the patient's particular needs and diagnosis. A description of some common screening studies and consults is presented in Table 24–8.

PREOPERATIVE CARE

Formulation of a preoperative plan of care is important for transplant candidates to optimize the patient's condition before the transplant. Patients usually remain under the care of their referring physician until the time of transplant, but are seen at regular intervals by the transplant team to ensure that no change in their condition or candidacy has occurred.

Etiology-based management is most appropriate for these patients. Patients with pulmonary fibrosis and emphysema often have muscle deconditioning secondary to steroids and disability, and should participate in some type of pulmonary rehabilitation. Chronic steroids should be weaned or maintained at low levels when possible to prevent problems of post-operative healing. PPH patients should be monitored for signs of worsening right heart failure and pulmonary hypertension. Drug-resistant infections and malnutrition may require intervention in bronchiectasis and cystic fibrosis patients.

LUNG DONOR PROCUREMENT

As stated previously, lung donors are more scarce than other solid organ donors. Careful screening and management of potential donors is paramount to ensure the survival of lung transplant candidates. Currently, unlike heart and liver transplant patients, there is no ranking of patients according to medical urgency on lung transplant waiting lists, and therefore priority is based only on accrued time on list.

Donor–recipient matching is done by blood type and size. Size is determined by height, weight, and chest x-ray measurements. Cross-match is usually not necessary before the transplant unless the recipient has demonstrated a high percentage of reactive antibodies on histocompatibility testing. Matching by tissue typing is not done. If the donor–recipient match is appropriate, donors are accepted based on criteria listed in Table 24–9.

Before the procurement of the lung graft, critical care management must be aggressive and meticulous. Viability of organ function is monitored by frequent arterial blood gases and chest x-rays. Key to donor maintenance are judicial fluid replacement (maintaining central venous pressure < 10 mm Hg) and good pulmonary toilet. Fluid management should include prompt treatment of diabetes insipidus with vasopressin. Nasogastric tube drainage should be used to prevent aspiration. Ventilator settings are maintained with 0.4 FIO_2 and 5 cm positive end-expiratory pressure. Downward trending of PaO_2 on these settings should raise suspicion as to organ acceptability.

A bronchoscopy is performed and all chest x-rays are reviewed by the procurement surgeon before the removal of the lung bloc. The start of the recipient surgery is contingent on normal radiographic, bronchoscopic, and surgical findings. After dissection, the lung is prepared for transport by first injecting prostaglandin E_1 into the pulmonary artery and then flushing and immersing the organ in a cold electrolyte solution. A single donor bloc consists of the donor lung and its pulmonary artery, bronchus (distal to the carina), and a cuff of the left atrium containing the ipsilateral pulmonary veins (Calhoun & Trinkle, 1993). Ideal ischemic times are less than 4 to 6 hours, but good posttransplant lung function has been established with ischemic times greater than 9 hours.

TABLE 24–8. **Common Screening Tests and Consults for Lung Transplantation**

Pulmonary Assessment

Pulmonary function tests
Arterial blood gases
Pulmonary exercise tests

Chest Imaging and Procedures

Chest x-ray
  Obtain measurements for donor matching
High-resolution computed tomography
  Rule out bronchiectasis
Quantitative ventilation–perfusion lung scan
  Rule out pulmonary emboli
  Assess percentage of blood flow to each lung
Bronchoscopy
  Evaluate cell population, cultures, and anatomy

Cardiac Assessment

Echocardiogram, electrocardiogram
Right and left heart catheterization
  Age over 45 and/or risk for coronary artery disease
  Eisenmenger's syndrome: visualize defect
Resting wall motion study (select cases)
  Differentiate right and left ventricular dysfunction

Consults and Team Members

Cardiothoracic surgeon
Pulmonologist
Cardiologist
Psychiatrist
Transplant coordinator
Nurse
Social worker
Infectious disease (select cases)

Laboratory Tests

Hematology
Chemistries
Serology
Blood bank
Histocompatibility

TABLE 24–9. **Cadaveric Lung Donor Criteria**

Brain death
Age ≤ 55 years (center-specific)
Normal chest x-rays
Arterial blood gases: $PaO_2 \geq 350$ with 1.0 FIO_2 and 5 cm positive end-expiratory pressure
No significant history of smoking or previous lung disease
No pulmonary sepsis
No bilateral chest trauma

RECIPIENT SURGICAL PROCEDURES

SINGLE-LUNG TRANSPLANT. A standard posterolateral thoracotomy approach is used when CPB is not anticipated due to normal pulmonary artery pressures. For those patients with high pulmonary artery pressures in which CPB is required, a median sternotomy is an option. However, cannulation can also be initiated via posterolateral thoracotomy, allowing continued access to the posterior mediastinum. Technique for SLT requires anastomoses of donor–recipient bronchus, pulmonary artery, and a left atrial (pulmonary venous) connection. A telescopine technique for the healing anastomosis of the bronchus reduces the incidence of bronchial problems (Calhoun et al., 1991; Judson, 1993) (Fig. 24–19). The donor left atrial cuff containing the insertion of the pulmonary veins is joined to the left atrium of the recipient. In this fashion, risk of thrombus formation is reduced and unconstrained flow from the pulmonary veins occurs.

At completion of all anastomoses, a bronchoscopy is performed to examine the integrity of the bronchial anastomosis and to remove blood and debris from the

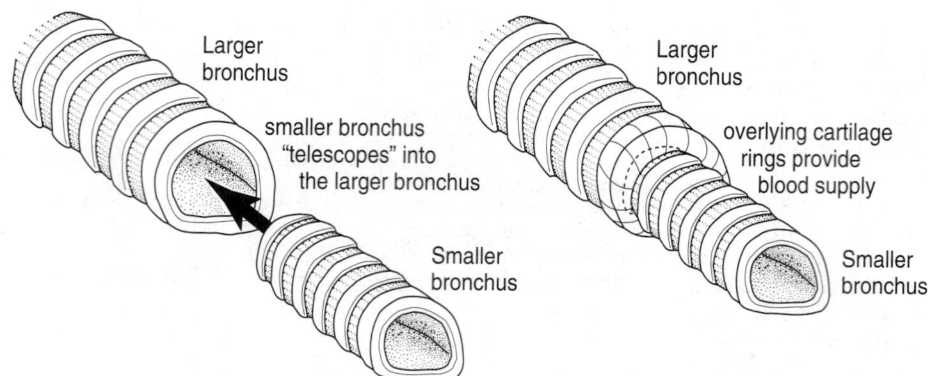

FIGURE 24-19. Telescoping anastomosis. (From Judson, M. A. [1993]. Clinical aspects of lung transplantation. *Clinics in Chest Medicine, 14*(2), 337.)

airway. Chest tubes are inserted for pleural drainage and lung reexpansion.

BILATERAL SEQUENTIAL LUNG TRANSPLANT. Surgical approach is obtained via a bilateral transsternal anterior thoracotomy, which provides wide exposure of both lung fields. BLT has replaced en bloc double-lung transplant for the replacement of both lungs because it does not always require the use of standard CPB, with its inherent risks. In BLT, it is possible for the recipient to be ventilated via the contralateral native lung while the first donor lung is transplanted and then, alternately, on the newly placed donor lung while the second lung is transplanted. When CPB is required, it can usually be instituted after the excision of the recipient's first lung, thereby decreasing the risk of hemorrhage substantially. As in SLT, bronchoscopy and chest tube insertion are performed at the completion of the procedure.

PHYSIOLOGY OF THE TRANSPLANTED LUNG. The preserved, denervated lung with interrupted lymphatic drainage is an environment in which changes can occur rapidly and with devastating effects. Posttransplant pulmonary physiology involves denervation of the organ, altered patterns of ventilation and perfusion, impaired lymphatic drainage, altered rate and rhythm of respirations, impaired mucociliary clearance, and increased lung edema and atelectasis. In addition, there is loss of bronchial artery blood supply and deep cough reflex in the donor segment of the bronchus (Coleman & Salamandra, 1991).

Lung innervation, which is lost, affects the airways, blood vessels, glandular secretions, and ciliary movement (Guyton, 1986; Murray, 1986). The net result is a decline in the ability to clear secretions from the allograft. The phrenic nerves and diaphragm and the chemoreceptors are preserved and help to carry on the work of breathing. The bronchial artery is sacrificed when the donor lung is procured, leaving the subsequent donor segment of the bronchial anastomosis with limited flow from the low-pressure pulmonary artery circulation.

There is a tendency toward fluid overload, which may be caused by interruption of pulmonary lymphatic drainage during recipient pneumonectomy and an increase in extravascular lung water during reimplantation (Kaiser & Cooper, 1992). Lymphatic drainage is achieved via the pleural lymphatics until normal drainage routes are reestablished in 21 to 60 days (LeKander, 1988).

Changes in perfusion and ventilation are affected most by the underlying disease, the degree of intrapulmonary shunting, and the amount of interstitial lung water. In SLT, preferential blood flow should exist in the "normal" transplanted lung. This distinction is much more pronounced in the patient with severe pulmonary hypertension in the native lung. In patients with severe obstructive disorders, overinflation and mediastinal shift may occur in the native lung from overventilation. During episodes of rejection, perfusion may be shunted away from the transplanted organ (Shumway, 1993).

POSTOPERATIVE MANAGEMENT AND CARE

All postoperative lung transplant patients return to the intensive care setting in critical condition and require optimal vigilance and care. They are intubated and sedated and must be monitored frequently for hemodynamic and ventilatory compromise. After initial hemodynamic stability is established and throughout the hospital course, the focus is primarily pulmonary in nature. It is essential to the survival of the patient that optimal pulmonary function and care are promoted and maintained.

HEMODYNAMICS. Lung transplant patients must be monitored carefully for signs of right ventricular dysfunction and fluid overload. The goal of fluid balance should be euvolemia. Low-dose pressors for blood pressure support and renal perfusion are used once adequate filling pressures are established. Right ventricular afterload reduction and vigorous diuresis may be necessary in the early postoperative period, especially in patients with a history of pulmonary hypertension and those requiring CPB. Because patients with severe pulmonary hypertension retain high pressures in the native lung with SLT, they are at greater risk for noncardiogenic pulmonary edema and reperfusion injury when most of the cardiac output is shunted through the transplanted lung. These patients must be kept intubated and sedated until diuresis can occur and the pulmonary artery pressures can be maintained at normal levels.

OXYGENATION AND VENTILATION. The primary sign of allograft dysfunction in critical care is oxygen desaturation. Therefore, continuous pulse oximetry is vital. Arterial blood gases and chest x-rays should be monitored carefully. Positioning the transplanted side up is recommended to improve lung expansion, facilitate drainage of lung water, and promote perfusion of the transplanted lung. Weaning to extubation proceeds as soon as the patient is stable, awake, and easily responsive. Bronchoscopy should be performed before extubation to observe the integrity of the bronchial anastomosis and obtain cultures. The patient is placed on 40% high-humidity mask until activity increases without desaturation, secretion production diminishes, and the patient is able to participate in chest physiotherapy exercises. Often, nasal cannulation is the only method of oxygen delivery needed once the patient is able to eat and ambulate. Oxygen usually can be completely withdrawn before discharge.

Aggressive chest physiotherapy is the cornerstone to proper management for these patients and should continue until discharge. Percussion and postural drainage (especially with transplanted side up), breathing treatments with bronchodilators, endotracheal–nasotracheal suctioning as needed, and coughing and deep breathing exercises should be done around the clock.

IMMUNOSUPPRESSION. Protocols vary from center to center, but lung transplant recipients frequently receive cyclosporine or azathioprine before surgery. Intraoperative methylprednisolone is given at reperfusion. Triple-drug therapy, which includes cyclosporine, azathioprine, and prednisone or a cytolytic agent, is initiated after surgery. Careful monitoring of the serum creatinine and daily cyclosporine trough levels is necessary, especially in those patients who have required CPB. Azathioprine is started at 2 mg/kg and white blood cell counts are monitored. Cytolytic preparations may cause severe initial reactions and therefore require premedication to limit these effects. Patients, especially lung transplant recipients who are already at risk, must be monitored closely for signs of pulmonary edema after the initial administration and before administration of diuretics.

INFECTION CONTROL. Protocols for isolation of transplant patients are diverse and center-specific. Typically, it is not necessary to isolate lung transplant patients more than other transplant patients. Protective isolation and strict handwashing should be observed by all people entering the room. Traffic in and out of the room should be kept to a minimum, especially when the patient is intubated and on high-dose immunosuppression.

Cultures from the donor graft and native lung are monitored. Prophylactic antibiotics are appropriate for the first postoperative week. Inhaled amphotericin, fluconazole, or itraconazole may be used to reduce the incidence of *Aspergillus* and *Candida* infection. Low-dose trimethropin–sulfamethoxazole is used for long-term prophylaxis against PCP infection (Paradis & Williams, 1993). Thrush associated with high-dose steroids can be effectively treated with oral antifungal agents.

Prophylaxis includes coverage against CMV in any recipient who is seropositive and those seronegative recipients who receive seropositive donor organs. The drug of choice is usually ganciclovir, which, at this writing, must be administered intravenously, with length of duration a center-specific decision.

POTENTIAL COMPLICATIONS

BLEEDING. Lung transplantation usually does not necessitate massive transfusions. However, all surgical procedures involving the anastomosis of major blood vessels demand vigilance against the risk of hemorrhage. Previous adhesions and use of CPB may increase this risk significantly. Frequent observations of all hemodynamics, drainage and dressings, and spun hematocrits are essential.

REJECTION. Lung rejection typically occurs between postoperative day 5 and 10. Patients may become hypoxic, short of breath, and manifest temperature elevation, malaise, and leukocytosis. There may or may not be a corresponding change on chest x-ray, with the appearance of fluffy hilar infiltrates. Any trend toward desaturation raises the suspicion for rejection. Spirometry, if done, may show diminished peak flow rates. Lung rejection may be difficult to differentiate from infection and reperfusion injury. A bronchoscopy is performed to rule out infection and obtain transbronchial biopsy for histologic examination. Diagnosis often is confirmed after treatment with a pulse of methylprednisolone (500–1,000 mg). If symptoms and findings begin to resolve within 6 to 12 hours of steroid pulse, the diagnosis is confirmed and the dose is repeated for the next 2 days.

INFECTION. Infection is the leading cause of mortality and morbidity after lung transplantation (Paradis & Williams, 1993). In the early postoperative course, infections are often donor-transmitted and bacterial in nature. Fungal infections are an ever-present danger in light of the need for high-dose steroids and prophylactic antibiotics. At 1 to 2 months after transplant, viral infections begin to arise. CMV pneumonitis is a serious and all-too-prevalent problem for lung transplant patients and has been linked to an increased risk for obliterative bronchiolitis (OB) (Shumway, 1993). Aggressive treatment with ganciclovir is essential. All infections in the immunosuppressed transplant population require prompt attention. Treatment includes pan cultures, appropriate antimicrobials (previously discussed), monitoring of temperatures, white blood cell counts, cultures, and secretions. Patients with cystic fibrosis and bronchiectasis may need broadened coverage for chronically colonizing organisms, such as *Pseudomonas* species.

AIRWAY COMPLICATIONS. As stated previously, the blood flow to the bronchial anastomosis is provided retrograde by flow to the donor segment of the bronchus by the pulmonary artery system only. Rejection, infection, poor graft preservation, and other conditions that compromise pulmonary circulation may cause ischemia at the bronchial anastomosis and lead to stricture or dehiscence. In the past, prednisone was withheld in the first 1–2 postoperative weeks to allow healing of the airway (Goldberg et al., 1983). More recent studies have revealed no increase in airway complications when postoperative steroids are used in patients with telescoped anastomoses (Patterson, 1993).

Signs of airway problems are massive or new air leaks, subcutaneous or mediastinal emphysema, and stridor or wheezing. Any of these symptoms require immediate attention and investigation. Diagnosis is usually made by bronchoscopy. Early dehiscence may respond to surgical repair without subsequent stricture. If the dehiscence occurs beyond the first few days, however, it must be left to heal by granulation, and the risk of stricture, malacia, or worsening dehiscence increases. Stricture can be treated by stent placement or dilatation (Patterson, 1993).

OBLITERATIVE BRONCHIOLITIS. OB occurs in up to 30% of surviving lung and heart–lung transplant recipients, and usually is not encountered before 3 months after transplant. It is characterized by a progressive decline in pulmonary function tests accompanied by shortness of breath. There are no radiologic findings. OB may progress rapidly from diagnosis. The patient often has chronic infections. Attempts at arresting the progress of the disease by using high-dose steroids, FK506, or cytolytic agents have been made with little success. At present, OB in the lung transplant recipient cannot be reversed, and patients may require retransplantation. Chronic rejection may be the causative agent, but patients who have suffered infection from CMV and other viruses seem to be at higher risk (Shumway, 1993).

DISCHARGE AND LONG-TERM CARE

The patient is transferred out of critical care when he or she can be weaned to nasal cannulation and can ambulate in the room. Once the patient is able to participate in his or her care, instructions with regard to medications, aftercare, and pulmonary rehabilitation are begun. On discharge, the patient is seen in the transplant clinic twice a week, where spirometry, laboratory tests, and chest x-rays are monitored by the pulmonologist, surgeon, and transplant coordinator. Patients are expected to keep a record of medications and vital signs. As the patient improves, clinic visits and laboratory tests are scheduled less frequently, and immunosuppression is gradually reduced to maintenance doses.

SUMMARY

During the past decade, innovations in cardiac surgery have produced exciting and provocative information for the scientific community caring for these patients. Coronary artery bypass operations have increased during the last decade by almost 50%. Simultaneously, the interventional arena has also experienced tremendous growth. As continued advances are made in device development, the number of interventional procedures is expected to supercede the number of CABG operations.

What are the implications for the future? What trends can be expected in the twenty-first century? With $7.7 billion currently being spent on PTCA and CABG procedures, the inherent socioeconomic ramifications are evident. Researchers are now focusing on risk factor stratification in an attempt to evaluate the outcomes associated with various modes of therapy. What factors can be derived to indicate or predict operative outcomes of CABG surgery?

As angioplasty and valvuloplasty techniques become more sophisticated, the patient population selected for these procedures will change. Consequently, the patient profile undergoing surgical revascularization is now characterized by advanced age and multiple preexisting pathologic disease states compared to the population observed during the last decade.

The area of thoracic transplantation, including heart and lung transplantation, has undergone a revolution in terms of improvements in operative technique and advancements in immunologic regimens. Yet, as the demand for organ donors grows, the number of patients awaiting transplant represents the greatest management challenge. As we enter the next century, innovations in technology and new strategies for care of cardiac surgical and thoracic transplant patients will be of paramount importance.

REFERENCES

Abd, A., Braun, N., Baskin, M., et al. (1989). Diaphragmatic dysfunction after open heart surgery: Treatment with a rocking bed. *Annals of Internal Medicine, 111,* 881–886.

Addonozio, V., Fisher, C., & Jeffery, A. (1987). Prevention of heparin induced thrombocytopenia during open heart surgery with iloprost (Zk36374). *Surgery, 102,* 796–807.

American Heart Association. (1987). *Textbook of advanced cardiac life support.* Dallas: Author.

American Heart Association. (1993). *1993 heart and stroke facts.* Dallas: Author.

Angelini, G. D., Butchart, E. G., Armistead, S. H., et al. (1984). Comparative study of leg wound skin closure in coronary artery bypass graft operations. *Thorax, 39,* 924–925.

Asada, S., & Yamaguchi, F. (1981). Fine structural changes in the lung following cardiopulmonary bypass: Its relationship to early postoperative course. *Chest, 50,* 478–486.

Baldwin, J. C., Anderson, J. L., Boucek, M. M., et al. (1993). Task force 2: Donor guidelines. *Journal of the American College of Cardiology, 22,* 15–20.

Bando, I., Pilla, R., Cameron, D., et al. (1990). Leukocyte depletion ameliorates free radicals mediated lung injury after cardiopulmonary bypass. *Journal of Thoracic and Cardiovascular Surgery, 99,* 873–877.

Baumann, F. G. (1981). Vein contraction and smooth muscle extensions as causes of endothelial damage during graft preparation. *Annals of Surgery, 194,* 199–210.

Behrendt, D., & Austen, G. (1981). *Patient care in cardiac surgery* (3rd ed.). Boston: Little, Brown.

Benjamine, J., Cascade, P., Rubenfire, N., et al. (1982). Left lower lobe atelectasis and consolidation following cardiac surgery: The effects of topical cooling on phrenic nerve. *Radiology, 142,* 11–14.

Berger, R., Davis, K., Kaiser, G., et al. (1981). Preservation of the myocardium during coronary artery bypass surgery. *Journal of Thoracic and Cardiovascular Surgery, 64,* 66–72.

Bevelaqua, F., Garritan, P., Haas, F., et al. (1990). Complications after cardiac operation in patients with severe pulmonary impairment. *Annals of Thoracic Surgery, 50,* 602–616.

Bick, R. L. (1984). Alterations of hemostasis associated with surgery, cardiopulmonary bypass, and prosthetic devices. In O. D. Ratnoff & C. D. Forbes (Eds.), *Disorders of hemostasis.* New York: Grune & Stratton.

Billingham, M., Cary, N., Hammond, E., et al. (1990). A working formulation for the standardization of nomenclature in the diagnosis of heart and lung rejection: Heart Rejection Study Group. *Journal of Heart Transplantation, 9,* 587–593.

Blanche, C., Matloff, J., & Mackay, D. (1990). Technical aspects of cardio-pulmonary bypass. In R. Gary & J. Matloff (Eds.), *Medical management of the cardiac surgical patient* (p. 55). Baltimore: Williams & Wilkins.

Blanche, C., Valenza, M., Czer, L., et al. (1994). Orthotopic heart transplantation with bicaval and pulmonary venous anastamoses. *Annals of Thoracic Surgery, 58,* 1505–1509.

Blanche, C., Valenza, M., Aleksic, I., et al. (1994). Technical considerations of a new technique for orthotopic heart transplantation. Total excision of recipient's atria with bicaval and pulmonary venous anastomoses. *Journal of Cardiovascular Surgery, 35*(4), 283–287.

Blauth, C., Cosgrove, D., & Webb, B. (1992). Atheroembolism from the ascending aorta: An emerging problem in cardiac surgery. *Journal of Thoracic and Cardiovascular Surgery, 103,* 1104–1111.

Bodenhammer, R., DeBor, L., Geffin, G., et al. (1983). Enhanced myocardial protection during ischemic arrest. *Journal of Thoracic and Cardiovascular Surgery, 86*(5), 769–780.

Bojar, R. M. (1989). *Manual of perioperative care in cardiac and thoracic surgery.* Boston: Blackwell Scientific Publications.

Boldt, J., Kling, D., Zickmann, B., et al. (1990). Acute preoperative plasmapheresis and established blood conservation techniques. *Annals of Thoracic Surgery, 50,* 62–68.

Bonchek, L., & Olinger, G. (1981). An improved method of topical hypothermia. *Journal of Thoracic and Cardiovascular Surgery, 82,* 878–882.

Boonstra, P., Vermenlen, F., Levsink, J., et al. (1986). Hematologic advantages of a membrane oxygenater over a bubble oxygenater in long perfusions. *Annals of Thoracic Surgery, 41,* 297–300.

Booth, D. C., Deupree, R. H., et al. (1991). Quality of life after bypass surgery for unstable angina. *Circulation, 83,* 87–95.

Bourge, R. C., Naftel, D. C., Costanzo-Nordiin, M., et al., and the Transplant Cardiologists Research Database Group. (1993). Pretransplantation risk factors for death after heart transplantation: A multiinstitutional study. *Journal of Heart and Lung Transplantation, 12,* 549–560.

Bracey, A., & Radovancevic, R. (1994). The hematologic effects of cardiopulmonary bypass and the use of hemotherapy in coronary artery bypass grafting. *Archives of Pathology and Laboratory Medicine, 118,* 411–416.

Braunwald, E. (1979). The determinants of myocardial oxygen consumption. *Physiologist, 12,* 65–93.

Braunwald, E. (Ed.). (1988). *Heart disease: A textbook of cardiovascular medicine* (3rd ed). Philadelphia: W. B. Saunders.

Brenner, B., Brief, D., Alpet, J., et al. (1987). The risk of stroke in patients with asymptomatic carotid stenosis undergoing cardiac surgery: A followup study. *Journal of Vascular Surgery, 5,* 269–279.

Brewer, A., Furlan, A., & Hansen, E. (1983). Central nervous system complications of coronary artery bypass graft surgery: Prospective analysis of 421 patients. *Stroke, 45,* 682–687.

Britton, L. W., Eastlund, D. T., & Dziuban, S. W. (1989). Predonated autologous blood use in elective surgery. *Annals of Thoracic Surgery, 47,* 529–532.

Brown, W., Jay, J., Gott, J., et al. (1993). Warm blood cardioplegia: Superior protection after acute myocardial ischemia. *Annals of Thoracic Surgery, 55,* 32–41.

Buckberg, G. (1975). Ventricular fibrillation: Its effects on myocardial flow, distribution, and performance. *Annals of Thoracic Surgery, 20,* 76–81.

Butler, J., Rocker, G., & Westby, S. (1993). Inflammatory response to cardiopulmonary bypass. *Annals of Thoracic Surgery, 55,* 552–559.

Calhoun, J. H., Grover, F. L., Gibbons, W. J., et al. (1991). Single lung transplantation: Alternative indications and technique. *Journal of Thoracic and Cardiovascular Surgery, 101,* 816–825.

Calhoun, J. H., & Trinkle, J. H. (1993). Donor selection and management. *Chest Surgery Clinics of North America, 3,* 19–28.

Califf, R. M., Harrell, F. E., Lee, K. L., et al. (1989). The evolution of medical and surgical therapy for coronary artery disease. *Journal of the American Medical Association, 261,* 2077–2086.

Cameron, D., & Gardner, T. (1988). Principles of clinical hypothermia. *Cardiac Surgery: State of the Art Reviews, 2,* 13–25.

Cardin, S., & Clarke, S. (1985). A nursing diagnoses approach to the patient awaiting cardiac transplantation. *Heart and Lung, 14,* 499–504.

Casey, L. (1993). Role of cytokines in the pathogenesis of cardiopulmonary-induced multisystem failure. *Annals of Thoracic Surgery, 56,* S92–S96.

Caulfield, J. B., Leinbach, R. C., & Gold, H. K. (1976). The relationship of myocardial infarct size and prognosis. *Circulation, 53*(Suppl 1), 141–145.

Cavarocchi, N., Schaff, H., Orszlak, T., et al. (1985). Evidence for complement activation by protamine–heparin interaction after cardiopulmonary bypass. *Surgery, 98,* 525–530.

Chaikhouni, A., Crawford, F. A., Kochel, P. J., et al. (1986). Human internal mammary artery produces more prostacyclin than saphenous vein. *Journal of Thoracic and Cardiovascular Surgery, 92,* 88–91.

Chaitman, B. R., Alderman, E. L., Sheffield, L. T., et al. (1983). Use of survival analysis to determine clinical significance of new Q waves after coronary artery bypass surgery. *Circulation, 67,* 302–310.

Chaitman, B. R., Fisher, L. D., Bourassa, M. G., et al. (1981). Effect of coronary bypass surgery on survival patterns in subsets of patients with left main coronary artery disease: (CASS). *American Journal of Cardiology, 48,* 765–777.

Chard, R., Kann, C., Nunn, G., (1990). Use of desmopressin in the management of aspirin-related and intractable haemorrage after cardiopulmonary bypass. *Australian and New Zealand Journal of Surgery, 60,* 125–128.

Chesebro, J. H., Knatterud, G., Roberts, R., et al. (1987). Thrombolysis in Myocardial Infarction (TIMI) Trial, phase I: A comparison between intravenous tissue plasminogen activator and intravenous streptokinase. *Circulation, 76,* 142–154.

Chitwood, W. (1988). Myocardial protection by retrograde cardioplegia: Coronary sinus and right atrial methods. *Cardiac Surgery: State of the Art Reviews, 2,* 197–218.

Chitwood, W., Cosgrove, D., Lust, R., et al. (1992). Multicenter trial of automated nitroprusside infusion for postoperative hypertension. *Annals of Thoracic Surgery, 54,* 517–522.

Chong, J. L., Grenbenik, C., Sinclair, M., et al. (1993). The effect of a cardiac surgical recovery area on the timing of extubation. *Journal of Cardiothoracic and Vascular Anesthesia, 7,* 137–141.

Christakis, G., Fremes, S., Weiser, R., et al. (1985). Right ventricular dysfunction following cold potassium cardioplegia. *Journal of Thoracic and Cardiovascular Surgery, 90,* 243–250.

Chulay, M., Brown, J., & Summer, W. (1982). Effect of postoperative immobilization after coronary artery bypass surgery. *Clinical Care Medicine, 10,* 176–182.

Cifani, L., & Vargo, R. (1990). Teaching strategies for the transplant recipient: a review and future directions [Review]. *Focus on Critical Care, 17*(6), 476–479.

Clark, R., Beauchamp, R., & McGrath, R. (1979). Comparison of bubble and membrane oxygenators in short and long perfusions. *Journal of Thoracic and Cardiovascular Surgery, 78,* 655–666.

Coleman, B. (1989). Nursing implications for pulmonary artery balloon counterpulsation: A treatment for right ventricular dysfunction after cardiac surgery. *Critical Care Nursing Clinics of North America, 55,* 373–379.

Coleman, B., & Salamandra, J. (1991). Lung transplantation. In B. A. Williams, K. L. Grady, & D. M. Sandiford-Guttenbiel (Eds.), *Organ transplantation: A manual for nurses* (pp. 165–185). New York: Springer Publishing Company.

Colman, R. (1990). Platelets and neutrophils activation in cardiopulmonary bypass. *Annals of Thoracic Surgery, 49,* 32–34.

Cooper, J. D., Pohl, M. S., & Patterson, G. A. (1993). An update on the current status of lung transplantation: report of the St. Louis International Lung Transplant Registry. *Clinical Transplants,* 95–100.

Copeland, J., Harker, L., & Joist, J. (1989). Bleeding and anticoagulation. *Annals of Thoracic Surgery, 47,* 88–95.

Coronary Artery Surgery Study (CASS) Principal Investigators. (1984). Myocardial infarction and mortality in the Coronary Artery Surgery Study (CASS) randomized trial. *New England Journal of Medicine, 310,* 750–758.

Coronary Artery Surgery (CASS) Principal Investigators and Associates. (1983). A randomized trial of coronary artery bypass surgery: Survival data. *Circulation, 68,* 939–950.

Cosgrove, D. M., Lytle, B. W., Loop, F. D., et al. (1988). Does bilateral internal mammary artery grafting increase surgical risk? *Journal of Thoracic and Cardiovascular Surgery, 95,* 850–856.

Costanzo-Nordin, M, R., Cooper, D. K., Jessup, M., et al. (1993). 24th Bethesda conference: Cardiac transplantation. Task Force 6: Future developments. *Journal of the American College of Cardiology, 22*(1), 54–64.

Cox, J. L. (1993). A perspective of postoperative atrial fibrillation in cardiac operations [editorial; comment]. *Annals of Thoracic Surgery, 56*(3), 405–409.

Culliford, A. T., Cunningham, J. N., & Zeff, R. H. (1976). Sternal and costochondral infections following open heart surgery. *Journal of Thoracic and Cardiovascular Surgery, 52,* 714–726.

Currie, P. J. (1989). Transesophageal echocardiography. *Circulation, 80,* 215–217.

Curtis, J., Nawaraawong, W., Walls, J., et al. (1989). Elevated hemidiaphragm after cardiac operation: Incidence, prognosis, and relationship to the use of topical ice slush. *Annals of Thoracic Surgery, 47,* 64–68.

Curtis, J. J., Walls, J. T., Salam, N. H., et al. (1991). Impact of unstable angina on operative mortality with coronary revascularization. *Journal of Thoracic and Cardiovascular Surgery, 102,* 867–873.

Cusmano, R., Ashe, K., Salerno, P., et al. (1988). Oxygenated solutions in myocardial preservation. *Cardiac Surgery: State of the Art Reviews, 2,* 167–180.

Czer, L., Bateman, T., Gray, R., et al. (1985). Prospective trial of DDAVP in treatment of severe platelet dysfunction and hemorrhage after cardiopulmonary bypass. *Circulation, 72*(Suppl 3), 111–130.

Czer, L., Bateman, T., Gray, R., et al. (1987). Treatment of severe platelet dysfunction and hemorrhage after cardiopulmonary bypass: Reduction in blood product usage with desmopressin. *Journal of the American College of Cardiology, 9,* 1139–1147.

Daily, P. O. (1989). Early and five year results for coronary artery bypass grafting. *Journal of Thoracic and Cardiovascular Surgery, 97,* 67–77.

Daily, P. O., Dembitsky, W. P., Peterson, K. L., et al. (1987). Modifications of techniques and early results of pulmonary thromboendarterectomy for chronic pulmonary embolism. *Journal of Thoracic and Cardiovascular Surgery, 93,* 221–233.

D'Alauro, E., & Johns, R. (1988). Hypotension related to desmopressin administration following cardiopulmonary bypass. *Anesthesiology, 69,* 962–963.

Davis, R., Lappas, D., & Kirklin, J. (1982). Acute oliguria after cardiopulmonary bypass: Renal functional improvement with low-dose dopamine infusion. *Critical Care Medicine, 10,* 852–856.

DeBakey, M. (1934). A single continuous blood flow transfusion instrument. *New Orleans Medical Surgical Journal, 87*(1), 386–394.

DeLaria, G. A., Hunter, J. A., & Goldin, M. D. (1981). Leg wound complications associated with coronary revascularization. *Journal of Thoracic and Cardiovascular Surgery, 81,* 403–407.

Delong, J., Ten-Ovis, H., Sibinga, C., et al. (1980). Hematologic aspects of cardiotomy suction in cardiac operations. *Journal of Cardiovascular Surgery, 79,* 227–236.

Disch, D. L., O'Connor, G. T., Birkmeyer, J. D., et al. (1994). Changes in patients undergoing coronary artery bypass grafting: 1987–1990. *Annals of Thoracic Surgery, 57,* 416–423.

Dobkins, B., (1991). Neuroplasticity, key to recovery after central nervous system injury. *Western Journal of Medicine, 159,* 56–60.

Dorman, B. H., Zucker, J. R., Verrier, E. D., et al. (1993). Clonidine improves perioperative myocardial ischemia, reduces anesthetic requirement, and alters hemodynamic parameters in patients undergoing coronary artery bypass surgery. *Journal of Cardiothoracic and Vascular Anesthesia, 7,* 386–395.

Downey, S., & Edmunds, S. (1992). Release of vasoactive substances during cardiopulmonary bypass. *Annals of Thoracic Surgery, 54,* 1236–1243.

Drinkwater, D. K., Laks, H., & Buckberg, G. (1990). A new simplified method of optimizing cardioplegia delivery without right heart isolation. *Journal of Thoracic and Cardiovascular Surgery, 77,* 56–64.

Edmunds, H., & Stephenson, L. (1983). Cardiopulmonary bypass for open heart surgery. In A. Getta, W. Glen, G. Hammond, et al. (Eds.), *Thoracic and cardiovascular surgery* (4th ed., p. 1091). Norwalk, CT: Appleton-Century-Crofts.

Emerson, T. (1989). Pharmacology of aprotinin and efficacy during cardiopulmonary bypass. *Cardiovascular Drug Review, 7,* 127–140.

Estanfanous, F. (1981). Hypertensive episodes during and after open heart surgery. *Cleveland Clinic Quarterly, 48,* 139–141.

European Coronary Surgery Study Group. (1982). Long-term results of prospective randomized study of coronary artery bypass surgery in stable angina pectoris. *Lancet, 2,* 1173–1181.

Fabiani, J., Deloche, A., Swansen, J., et al. (1986). Retrograde cardioplegia through the right atrium. *Annals of Thoracic Surgery, 41,* 101–102.

Fabiani, J., Swansen, J., & Deloche, A. (1987). Right atrial cardioplegia. In A. Roberts (Ed.), *Myocardial protection in cardiac surgery* (p. 505). New York: Marcel Dekker.

Faggioli, G. L., Curl. G. R., & Ricotta, J. J. (1990). The role of carotid screening before coronary artery bypass. *Journal of Vascular Surgery, 12*(6), 724–730.

Favalaro, R. G. (1969). Saphenous vein graft in the surgical treatment of coronary artery disease: Operative technique. *Journal of Thoracic and Cardiovascular Surgery, 58,* 178–185.

Ferguson, T., Smith, P., & Buhrman, W. (1983). Studies of the physiology of the conduction system during hyperkalemic hypothermic cardioplegic arrest. *Surgery Forum, 34,* 302–318.

Ferguson, T., Smith, P., Damiano, R., et al. (1987). Electrical activity on the heart during hyperkalemic hypothermic cardioplegic arrest: Site of origin and relationship to specialized conduction tissue. *Annals of Thoracic Surgery, 43,* 373–379.

Ferguson, T., Smith, P., Lofland, G., et al. (1986),. The effects of cardioplegic potassium concentration on myocardial temperature on electrical activity in the heart during elective cardioplegic arrest. *Journal of Thoracic and Cardiovascular Surgery, 92,* 755–765.

Ferraris, V. A., Ferraris, S. P., Gilliam, H. S., et al. (1991). Predictors of postoperative ventricular dysrhythmias: A multivariate study. *Journal of Cardiovascular Surgery, 32*(1), 12–20.

Ferraris, V. A., Ferraris, S. P., Lough, F. C., et al. (1988). Preoperative aspirin ingestion increases operative blood loss after coronary artery bypass grafting. *Annals of Thoracic Surgery, 45,* 71–74.

Fischell, T. T., McDonald, T., Grattan, M., et al. (1989). Occlusive coronary artery spasm as a cause of acute myocardial infarction after coronary artery bypass grafting. *New England Journal of Medicine, 320,* 400–401.

Fitzgibbon, G. M., Leach, A. J., Keon, W. J., et al. (1986). Coronary bypass conduit fate after operation. *Journal of Thoracic and Cardiovascular Surgery, 91,* 773–778.

Force, T., Hibberd, P., Weeks, G., et al. (1990). Perioperative myocardial infarction after coronary artery bypass surgery. *Circulation, 82,* 903–912.

Foster, E. D., & Kranc, M. (1989). Alternative conduits for aortocoronary bypass grafting. *Circulation, 79*(Suppl 1), 34–40.

Freedman, A., & Goodman, L. (1982). Suctioning the left bronchial tree in the intubated adult. *Critical Care Medicine, 10,* 43–45.

Fremes, S., Christakis, G., Weiser, R., et al. (1984). A clinical trial of blood and crystalloid cardioplegia. *Journal of Thoracic and Cardiovascular Surgery, 104,* 726–741.

Fremes, S. E., Goldman, B. S., Weisel, R. D., et al. (1991). Recent preoperative myocardial infarction increases the risk of surgery for unstable angina. *Journal of Cardiac Surgery, 6*(1), 2–12.

Frost, L., Molgaard, H., Christiansen, E. H., et al. (1992). Atrial fibrillation and flutter after coronary artery bypass surgery: epidemiology, risk factors and preventive trials [Review]. *International Journal of Cardiology, 36*(3), 253–261.

Frye, R. L., Kronmal, R., Schaff, H. V., et al. (1992). Stroke in coronary artery bypass graft surgery: An analysis of the CASS experience. The participants in the Coronary Artery Surgery Study. *International Journal of Cardiology, 36*(2), 213–221.

Gates, R., Laks, H., Drinkwater, D., et al. (1993). Gross and microvascular distribution of retrograde cardioplegia in explanted human hearts. *Annals of Thoracic Surgery, 56,* 410–417.

Gelmers, H., Gorter, K., de Weerdt, C., et al. (1988). A controlled trial of nimodipine in acute ischemic stroke. *New England Journal of Medicine, 318,* 203–207.

Geltman, E. M. (1987). Coronary thrombolysis with intravenous streptokinase. *Cardiology Clinics, 5,* 91–99.

Gersh, B. J., Califf, R. M., Loop, F. D., et al. (1989). Coronary bypass surgery in chronic stable angina. *Circulation, 79*(Suppl 1), 46–59.

Gibbson, J. (1954). Application of a mechanical heart and lung apparatus to cardiac surgery. *Minnesota Medicine, 37,* 171–178.

Giordano, G. F., Rivers, S. L., Chung, G. K., et al. (1988). Autologous platelet-rich plasma in cardiac surgery: Effect on intraoperative and postoperative transfusion requirements. *Annals of Thoracic Surgery, 46*(4), 416–419.

Goldberg, M., Lima, O., Morgan, E., et al. (1983). A comparison between cyclosporin A and methylprednisolone plus azathioprine on bronchial healing following canine lung autotransplantation. *Journal of Thoracic and Cardiovascular Surgery, 85*(6), 821–826.

Goldman, S., Copeland, J., Moritz, T., et al. (1988). Improvement in early saphenous vein graft patency after coronary artery bypass surgery with antiplatelet therapy: Results of a Veterans Administration Cooperative Study. *Circulation, 77,* 1324–1332.

Gorin, A., & Liebler, J. (1986). Changes in serum angiotensin converting enzyme during cardiopulmonary bypass in humans. *American Review of Respiratory Disease, 134,* 79–84.

Gortner, S. R., Gillis, C. L., Paul, S. M., et al. (1989). Expected and realized benefits from cardiac surgery: An update. *Cardiovascular Nursing, 25*(4), 18–24.

Gravlee, G., Haddon, S., Rothberger, H., et al. (1990). Heparin dosing and monitoring for cardiopulmonary bypass. *Journal of Thoracic and Cardiovascular Surgery, 99,* 518–527.

Gray, R. (1990). Postoperative hypertension. In R. Gray & J. Matloff (Eds.). *Medical management of the cardiac surgical patient.* Baltimore: Williams & Wilkins.

Gray, R., & Mandel, W. (1991). Management of common postoperative arrhythmias. In R. Gray & J. Matloff (Eds.), *Medical management of the cardiac surgical patient* (p. 208). Baltimore: Williams & Wilkins.

Green, G. E. (1989). Use of internal thoracic artery for coronary artery grafting. *Circulation, 79*(Suppl 1), 1-30–1-33.

Greene, A., Gray, L. A., Slater, A. D., et al. (1991). Emergency aortocoronary bypass after failed angioplasty. *Annals of Thoracic Surgery, 51,* 194–199.

Grondin, C. M., Campeau, L., Thornton, J. C., et al. (1989). Coronary artery bypass grafting with saphenous vein. *Circulation, 79*(Suppl 1), 24–29.

Gross, S. (1995). Early extubation: Preliminary experience in the cardiothoracic patient population. *American Journal of Critical Care, 4*(4), 262–266.

Grossi, E. A., Culliford, A. T., & Krieger, K. H. (1985). A survey of 77 major infectious complications of median sternotomy: A review of 7949 consecutive operative procedures. *Annals of Thoracic Surgery, 126,* 214–221.

Grover, F. L., Johnson, R. R., Marshall, G., & Hammermeister, K. E. (1994). Impact of mammary grafts on coronary bypass operative mortality and morbidity. *Annals of Thoracic Surgery, 57,* 559–568.

Guiteras Val., P., Pelletier, C., Hernandez, M., et al. (1983). Diagnostic criteria and prognosis of perioperative myocardial infarction following coronary bypass. *Journal of Thoracic and Cardiovascular Surgery, 88,* 878–886.

Gurley, J., Booth, D., & DeMaria, A. (1990). Circulatory collapse following coronary bypass surgery: Multivessel and graft spasm reversed in the catheterization laboratory by intracoronary papaverine. *American Heart Journal, 119,* 1194–1195.

Gutmann, M. C., Knapp, D. N., & Pollack, M. L. (1982). Coronary bypass patients and work status. *Circulation, 66,* 33–38.

Guyton, A. (1986). Respiration. In A. Guyton (Ed.), *Textbook of medical physiology* (7th ed., pp. 466–479). Philadelphia, W. B. Saunders.

Halpern, N., Goldberg, M., Neely, C., et al. (1992). Postoperative hypertension: A multicenter prospective randomized comparison between intravenous nicardipone and sodium nitroprusside. *Critical Care Medicine, 20,* 1637, 1643.

Hammerschmidt, D., Stroncek, D., Bowers, T., et al. (1981). Complement activation and neutropenia occurring during cardiopulmonary bypass. *Journal of Thoracic and Cardiovascular Surgery, 81,* 370–377.

Haneda, K., Thomas, R., & Breasale, D. (1982). Whole body temperature gradients under surface perfusion and combined surface perfusion hypothermia. *Cryobiology, 19,* 119–128.

Haraphongse, M., Na-Ayudhya, R. K., Teo, K. K., et al. (1994). The changing profile of coronary artery bypass graft patients, 1970–1989. *Canadian Journal of Cardiology, 10,* 71–76.

Hardy, J. D., Webb, W., Dalton, M., & Walker, G. (1963). Lung transplantation in man. *Journal of the American Medical Association, 186,* 1065–1070.

Harker, L. (1986). Bleeding after cardiopulmonary bypass. *New England Journal of Medicine, 314,* 446–448.

He, G., Acuff, T. E., Ryan, W. H., & Mack, M. J. (1994). Risk factors for operative mortality in elderly patients undergoing internal mammary artery grafting. *Annals of Thoracic Surgery, 57,* 1453–1461.

Heyman, S. (1985). Effects of cardiopulmonary bypass on coagulation. *Dimensions of Critical Care Nursing, 4*(2), 70–78.

Hickey, C., Gugino, L. D., Aglio, L. S., et al. (1993). Intraoperative somatosensory evoked potential monitoring predicts peripheral nerve injury during cardiac surgery. *Anesthesiology, 78*(1), 29–35.

Hickey, R., & Hoor, P. (1983). Whole body oxygen consumption during low flow hypothermic cardiopulmonary bypass. *Journal of Thoracic and Cardiovascular Surgery, 86,* 903–906.

Hill, G., Alonso, A., Thiele, G., et al. (1994). Glucocorticoids blunt neutrophil CDIIb surface glycoprotein upregulation during cardiopulmonary bypass in humans. *Anesthesia and Analgesia, 79,* 23–27.

Hines, R., & Barash, P. (1985). Right ventricular function in the perioperative period. *Mount Sinai Journal of Medicine, 52,* 529–537.

Hinohara, T., Simpson, J. B., Phillips, H. R., et al. (1988). Transluminal intracoronary reperfusion catheter: A device to maintain coronary perfusion between failed coronary angioplasty and emergency coronary bypass surgery. *Journal of the American College of Cardiology, 11,* 977–982.

Hisatomi, K., Isomura, T., Kawara, T., et al. (1989). Changes in lymphocyte subsets, mitogen responsiveness and interleukin-2 production after cardiac operations. *Journal of Thoracic and Cardiovascular Surgery, 94,* 580–591.

Hoie, J., & ForFang, K. (1980). Arrhythmias and conduction disturbances following aortic valve replacement. *Scandinavian Journal of Thoracic and Cardiovascular Surgery, 14,* 177–183.

Holloway, D., Summaria, L., Sandresara, J., et al. (1988). Decreased platelet number and function and increased fibrinolysis contribute to postoperative bleeding in cardiopulmonary bypass patients. *Thrombosis and Haemostasis, 59,* 62–67.

Hook, M. A. (1990). Immunosuppressive agents in transplantation. In S. Smith (Ed.), *Tissue and organ transplantation: Implications for professional nursing practice* (pp. 48–76). St. Louis: C. V. Mosby.

Hornick, P., Smith, P. L., Taylor, K. M. (1994). Cerebral complications after coronary bypass grafting (Review). *Current Opinion in Cardiology, 9*(6), 670–679.

Hosenpud, J. D., Novick, R. J., Breen, T. J., & Daily, O. P. (1994). The registry of the International Society for Heart and Lung Transplantation: Eleventh official report—1994. *Journal of Heart and Lung Transplantation, 13,* 561–570.

Howard, R., Crain, C., Franzini, D., et al. (1988). Effects of cardiopulmonary bypass on pulmonary leukostasis and complement activation. *Archives of Surgery, 123,* 1496–1501.

Hurst, J. W., King, S. B., & Friesinger, G. C. (1986). *The heart.* New York: McGraw-Hill.

Ibayashi, S., Fujishima, M., Sadoshima, S., et al. (1986). Cerebral blood flow and tissue metabolism in experimental cerebral ischemia of spontaneous hypertensive rats with hyper-, normo-, and hypoglycemia. *Stroke, 17,* 261–266.

Ingersoll, G. L., & Grippi, M. A. (1991). Preoperative pulmonary status and postoperative extubation outcome of patients undergoing elective cardiac surgery. *Heart and Lung, 20,* 137–143.

Ingwersen, U., Larsen, K., & Bertelden, T. (1993). Theree different mask physiotherapy regimens for prevention of postoperative pulmonary complication after heart and pulmonary surgery. *Intensive Care Medicine, 19,* 294–298.

Iyer, V. S., Russell, W.J., Leppard, P., & Craddock, D. (1993). Mortality and myocardial infarction after coronary artery surgery: A review of 12,003 patients. *Medical Journal of Australia, 159*(3), 166–170.

Jansen, K. J., & McFadden, P. M. (1986). Postoperative nursing management in patients undergoing myocardial revascularization with the internal mammary artery bypass. *Heart and Lung, 15,* 48–54.

Jeevanandam, V., Smith, C., Rose, E., et al. (1990). Single stage management of sternal wound infections. *Journal of Thoracic and Cardiovascular Surgery, 99,* 256–263.

Johnson, P., Messter, K., Ryding, E., et al. (1987). Cerebral blood flow and autoregulation during hypothermic cardiopulmonary bypass. *Annals of Thoracic Surgery, 43,* 386–390.

Johnson, W., Flemma, R. J., & Lepley, D. (1969). Extended treatment of severe coronary artery disease: A surgical approach. *Annals of Surgery, 170,* 460–467.

Johnson, W. D., Kayser, K. L., Brenowitz, J. B., et al. (1991). A randomized controlled trial of allopurinol in coronary bypass surgery. *American Heart Journal, 121,* 20–23.

Judson, M. A. (1993). Clinical aspects of lung transplantation. *Clinics in Chest Medicine, 14*(2), 335–357.

Kaiser, G. C., Davis, K. B., Fisher, L. D., et al. (1985). Survival following coronary artery bypass with severe angina pectoris (CASS): An observational study. *Journal of Thoracic and Cardiovascular Surgery, 89,* 513–522.

Kaiser, G. C., Schaff, H. V., & Killip, T. (1989). Myocardial revascularization for unstable angina. *Circulation, 79*(Suppl 1), 60–67.

Kaiser, L. R., & Cooper, J. D. (1992). The current status of lung transplantation. *Advances in Surgery, 25,* 259–307.

Kato, M., Nakashima, Y., Levine, J., et al. (1993). Does transesophageal echocardiography improve postoperative outcome in patients undergoing coronary bypass surgery? *Journal of Cardiothoracic and Vascular Anesthesia, 7,* 285–289.

Kennedy, J. W., Ivey, T. D., Misbach, G., et al. (1989). Coronary artery bypass graft surgery early after acute myocardial infarction. *Circulation, 79*(Suppl 1), 68–72.

Keogh, A., MacDonald, P., Mundy, J., et al. (1992). Five year follow-up of a randomized double-drug versus triple drug therapy immunosuppressive trial after heart transplantation. *Journal of Heart and Lung Transplantation, 11,* 550–556.

Killip, T., Passamani, E., & Davis, K. (1985). Coronary artery surgery study (CASS): A randomized trial of coronary bypass surgery: Eight years follow-up and survival in patients with reduced ejection fraction. *Circulation, 72*(Suppl 5), 102–109.

King, K. B., Clark, P. C., Norsen, L. H., & Hicks, G. L. (1992). Coronary artery bypass graft surgery in older women and men. *American Journal of Critical Care, 1,* 28–35.

King, S. B., Lembo, N. J., Weintraub, W. S., et al. (1994). A randomized trial comparing coronary angioplasty with coronary bypass surgery: EAST trial. *New England Journal of Medicine, 333,* 1044–1050.

Kirklin, J. W., Akins, C. W., Blackstone, E. H., et al. (1991). Guidelines and indications for coronary artery bypass graft surgery. *Journal of the American College of Cardiology, 17,* 543–589.

Kirklin, J. W., & Barratt-Boyes, B. G. (Eds.). *Cardiac surgery.* New York: John Wiley & Sons.

Kirklin, J. W., Naftel, D. C., Blackstone, E. H., et al. (1989). Summary of a consensus concerning death and ischemic events after coronary artery bypass grafting. *Circulation, 170,* 81–91.

Ko, W., Lazenby, W., Zelano, J., et al. (1992). Effects of shaving methods and intraoperative irrigation on suppurative mediastinitis after bypass operation. *Annals of Thoracic Surgery, 53,* 301–305.

Kresh, J., Nastala, C., & Bianchi, P. (1987). The relative buffering power of blood cardioplegic solution. *Journal of Thoracic and Cardiovascular Surgery, 93,* 309–311.

Kristensen, C. (1990). Renal failure. In R. Gray & J. Matloff (Eds.), *Management of cardiac surgical patients.* Baltimore: Williams & Wilkins.

Krul, J., van Gijn, J., & Ackerstaff, A. (1989). Site and pathogenesis of infarcts associated with carotid endarterectomy. *Stroke, 20,* 324–328.

Kubo, S. H., Ornwaza, S. M., Francis, G. S., et al. (1993). Trends in patient selection for heart transplantation. *Journal of the American College of Cardiology, 21,* 975–981.

Kucuk, O., Kwaan, H., Frederickson, J., et al. (1986). Increased fibrinolytic activity in patients undergoing cardiopulmonary bypass operation. *American Journal of Hematology, 23,* 223–229.

Kuntschen, F., Galletti, P., & Hahn, C. (1986). Glucose–insulin interactions during cardiopulmonary bypass: Hypothermia versus normothermia. *Journal of Thoracic and Cardiovascular Surgery, 91,* 451–459.

Kuntschen, F., Galletti, P., Hahn, C., et al. (1985). Alteration in insulin and glucose metabolism during cardiopulmonary bypass under normothermia. *Journal of Thoracic and Cardiovascular Surgery, 89,* 97–106.

Kuroda, Y., Uchimoto, R., Shinjura, R., et al. (1993). Central nervous system complication after cardiac surgery: A comparison between coronary bypass graft and valve surgery. *Anesthesia and Analgesia, 76,* 222–227.

Kushner, I. (1982). The phenomenon of the acute phase response. *Annals of the New York Academy of Science, 389,* 39–48.

Laks, H., Gates, R., Ardhali, A., et al. (1993). Orthotopic heart transplant and concurrent coronary artery bypass. *Journal of Heart Transplantation, 12,* 810–815.

Landymore, R., Murphy, D., & Kinley, C. (1979). Does pulsatile flow influence the incidence of postoperative hypertension? *Annals of Thoracic Surgery, 28,* 261–272.

Lange, S. S., Prevost, S., Lewis, P., & Fadol, A. (1992). Infection control practices in cardiac transplant recipients. *Heart and Lung, 21,* 101–105.

Lavelle, J., Duigan, J., & Neligan, A. (1984). The effects of cardiopulmonary bypass on immune mechanisms of man. *Irish Journal of Medical Science, 153,* 431–436.

Leaf, A., & Weber, P. C. (1988). Cardiovascular effects of Ω-3 fatty acids. *New England Journal of Medicine, 181,* 549–557.

Lee, C., Goh, B., & Chin, L. (1990). The role of protamine dose assay on reversal of heparin following extracorporeal circulation for open heart surgery. *Annals of Academy of Medicine, Singapore, 19,* 41–44.

Lee, L., Bates, E. R., Pitt, B., et al. (1988). Percutaneous angioplasty improves survival in acute myocardial infarction complicated by cardiogenic shock. *Circulation, 78,* 1345–1350.

LeKander, B. (1988). Preventing complications for the heart and lung transplant recipient. *Dimensions of Critical Care Nursing, 7,* 18–27.

Lemmer, J., Stanford, W., Bonney, S., et al. (1994). Aprotinin for coronary bypass operations: Efficacy, safety, and influence on early saphenous vein graft patency. A multicenter, randomized, double-blind, placebo controlled study. *Journal of Thoracic and Cardiovascular Surgery, 107,* 543–551.

Leslie, J. (1993). Incidence and aetiology of perioperative hypertension. *Acta Anaesthesiologica Scandinavica. Supplementum, 99,* 5–10.

Levy, J., Schwieger, I., Zaidan, J., et al. (1989). Evaluation of patients at risk for protamine reactions. *Journal of Thoracic and Cardiovascular Surgery, 948,* 200–204.

Lewis, R. (1980). Management of atelectasis and pneumonia. *Surgical Clinics of North America, 60,* 1391–1401.

Ley, J., Miller, K., Skov, P., et al. (1990). Crystalloid versus colloid fluid therapy after cardiac surgery. *Heart and Lung, 19,* 31–40.

Lichtenstein, S., & Abel, J. (1992). Warm heart surgery: Theory and current practice. *Advances in Cardiac Surgery, 3,* 135–153.

LoCicero, J. (1990). Any value for desmopressin acetate (DDAVP) in cardiopulmonary bypass? (Letter). *Journal of Cardiothoracic Surgery, 99,* 945.

Loop, F. D. (1983a). Progress in surgical treatment of coronary atherosclerosis: Part 1. *Chest, 84,* 611.

Loop, F. D. (1983b). Progress in surgical treatment of coronary atherosclerosis: Part 2. *Chest, 84,* 740.

Loop, F. D., Lytle, B. W., & Cosgrove, D. M. (1989). New arteries for old. *Circulation, 79*(Suppl 1), 40–45.

Loop, F. D., Lytle, B. W., Cosgrove, D. M., et al. (1986). Influence of the internal mammary-artery-graft on 10 year survival and other cardiac events. *New England Journal of Medicine, 314,* 1–6.

Lowenstein, E., Johnston, W. E., Lappas, D. G., et al. (1983). Catastrophic pulmonary vasoconstriction associated with protamine reversal of heparin. *Anesthesiology, 59*(5), 470–473.

Luce, J. (1984). Clinical risk for postoperative pulmonary complications. *Respiratory Care, 29,* 484–495.

Lucus, S., Gardner, F., Flatherty, J., et al. (1980). Beneficial effects of mannitol administration during reperfusion after ischemic arrest. *Circulation, 62,* 1–34.

Lust, R. (1988). Physiologic influences of alterations in coronary anatomy on cardioplegia and reperfusion. *Cardiac Surgery: State of the Art Reviews, 2,* 351–382.

Lytle, B. W., Cosgrove, D. M., Stewart, R. W., et al. (1987a). Right gastroepiploic artery: Alternative coronary bypass conduit. *Circulation, 76,* 351.

Lytle, B. W., Loop, F. D., Cosgrove, D. M., et al. (1987b). Fifteen hundred coronary reoperations: Results and determinants of early and late survival. *Journal of Thoracic and Cardiovascular Surgery, 205,* 847–859.

Lytle, B. W., Loop, F. D., Taylor, P. C., et al. (1993). The effect of coronary reoperation on the survival of patients with stenoses in saphenous vein bypass grafts to coronary arteries. *Journal of Thoracic and Cardiovascular Surgery, 105*(4), 605–612.

Lytle, B. W., McElroy, D., McCarthy, P., et al. (1994). Influence of arterial coronary bypass grafts on the mortality in coronary reoperations. *Journal of Thoracic and Cardiovascular Surgery, 107*(3), 675–682.

Macdonald, S. N. (1990). Heart transplantation: Part I. In S. Smith (Ed.), *Tissue and organ transplantation: Implications for professional nursing practice* (pp. 210–231). St. Louis: C. V. Mosby.

Magilligan, D., Vij, D., Peper, W., et al. (1985). Failure of standard cardioplegic techniques to protect the conduction system. *Annals of Thoracic Surgery, 39,* 403–408.

Magovern, G., Bolling, S., Casale, A., et al. (1982). Failure of blood cardioplegia to protect myocardium at lower temperatures. *Circulation, 62*(Suppl 1), 160–176.

Mair, P., Mair, J., Seibt, I., et al. (1993). Cardiac troponin T: A new marker of myocardial tissue damage in bypass surgery. *Journal of Cardiothoracic and Vascular Anesthesia, 7,* 674–678.

Maleki, M., & Manley, J. (1989). Venospastic phenomena of saphenous vein bypass grafts. *British Heart Journal, 62,* 57–60.

Marelli, R., Paul, A., Samson, R., et al. (1989). Does the addition of albumin to the prime solution in cardiopulmonary bypass affect clinical outcome? *Journal of Thoracic and Cardiovascular Surgery, 98,* 757–766.

Markewitz, A., Faist, E., Lang, S., et al. (1993). Regulation of acute phase response after cardiopulmonary bypass by immunomodulation. *Annals of Thoracic Surgery, 55,* 389–394.

Martinez-Pellus, A., Merino, P., Bru, M., et al. (1993). Can selective digestive decontamination avoid the endotoxemia and cytokine activation promoted by cardiopulmonary bypass? *Critical Care Medicine, 21,* 1684–1691.

Mattlar, C. E., Engblom, E., Vesala, P., et al. (1991). The proportion of patients with cognitive impairment after coronary artery bypass surgery: An 8-month follow-up study. *Psychotherapy and Psychosomatics, 55*(2–4), 145–150.

McManus, R. P., O'Hair, D. P., Beitzinger, J. M., et al. (1993). Patients who die awaiting heart transplantation. *Journal of Heart and Lung Transplantation, 12,* 159–171.

McKnight, E., Elhot, M., Pearson, D., et al. (1985). The effects of four different crystalloid bypass pump priming fluids upon the metabolic response to cardiac operation. *Journal of Thoracic and Cardiovascular Surgery, 90,* 90–97.

Merrill, W. H., Elkins, C. C., Stewart, J. R., et al. (1993). Third-time coronary artery bypass grafting: Midterm results. *Annals of Thoracic Surgery, 55,* 582–585.

Michaels, I., & Barash, P. (1983). Hemodynamic changes during protamine administration. *Anesthesia and Analgesia, 60,* 33–36.

Milam, J. (1983). Blood transfusions in heart surgery. *Surgical Clinics of North America, 63,* 1127–1147.

Miller, L., Naftel, D., Bourge, R., et al. (1994). Infection after heart transplant: A multiinstitutional study. *Journal of Heart and Lung Transplantation, 13,* 381–393.

Miller, L. W., Schlant, R. C., Kobashigawa, J., Kubo, S., & Renlund, D. G. (1993). Task force 5: complications. *Journal of the American College of Cardiology, 22*(1), 41–54.

Mills, N. L., & Everson, C. T. (1989). Right Gastroepiploic Artery: A third arterial conduit for coronary artery bypass. *Annals of Thoracic Surgery, 47,* 706–711.

Moore, C. A., Nygaard, T. W., Kaiser, D. L., et al. (1986). Posinfarction ventricular septal rupture. *Circulation, 74,* 45–50.

Moore, S., & Wilkoff, B. (1991). Rhythm disturbances after cardiac surgery. *Seminars in Thoracic and Cardiovascular Surgery, 3,* 24–28.

Moores, W. Y., Hannon, J. P., Crum, J., et al. (1977). Coronary flow distribution and dynamics during continuous and pulsatile extracorporeal circulation in the pig. *Annals of Thoracic Surgery, 24*(6), 582–590.

Moores, W., & Willford, D. (1989). Modification of cardiopulmonary bypass to optimize myocardial protection. *Cardiac Surgery: State of the Art Reviews, 2*(2), 331–350.

Morris, J., & Wechsler, A. (1988). Right ventricular performance and protection. *Cardiac Surgery: State of the Art Reviews, 2*(2), 303–329.

Mudge, G. H., et al. (1993). Task force 3: Recipient guidelines / prioritization. *Journal of the American College of Cardiology, 22,* 21–30.

Murphy, D. A., Craver, J. M., Jones, E. L., et al. (1982). Surgical revascularization following unsuccessful percutaneous transluminal coronary angioplasty. *Journal of Thoracic and Cardiovascular Surgery, 84,* 342–348.

Murray, J. (1986). Lymphatic and nervous system. In J. Murray (Ed.), *The normal lung* (pp. 61–82). Philadelphia: W. B. Saunders.

Musial, J., Neiwiarowski, S., Hershock, D., et al. (1985). Loss of fibrinogen receptors from the platelet surface during simulated extracorporeal circulation. *Journal of Laboratory and Clinical Medicine, 105,* 514–522.

Myers, B., & Moran, S. (1986). Hemodynamically mediated acute renal failure. *New England Journal of Medicine, 314,* 97–105.

Myers, W. O., Schaff, H. V., Gersh, B. J., et al. (1989). Improved survival of surgically treated patients with triple vessel coronary artery disease and severe angina pectoris (CASS). *Journal of Thoracic and Cardiovascular Surgery, 97,* 487–495.

Nair, U. R., Griffiths, G., & Lawson, R. A. (1988). Postoperative neuralgia in the leg after saphenous vein coronary artery bypass graft. *Thorax, 43,* 41–43.

Naucke, N. A. (1990). Heart transplantation: Part II. In S. Smith (Ed.), *Tissue and organ transplantation: Implications for professional nursing practice* (pp. 231–243). St. Louis: C. V. Mosby.

Neuhaus, K. L., VonEssen, R., Tebbiè, U., et al. (1992). Improved thrombolysis in acute myocardial infarction with front-loaded administration of TPA. *Journal of the American College of Cardiology, 19,* 885–891.

Newman, M. F., Croughwell, N. D., Blumenthal, J. A., et al. (1994). Effect of aging on cerebral autoregulation during cardiopulmonary bypass. Association with postoperative cognitive dysfunction. *Circulation, 90*(5 Pt 2), II243–II249.

Nguyen, D., Mulder, D., & Shennib, H. (1992). The effects of cardiopulmonary bypass on circulating lymphocyte function. *Annals of Surgery, 53,* 611–616.

Niemmen, M., Philbin, D., Roscow, C., et al. (1983). Gradients and rewarming time during hypothermic cardiopulmonary bypass with and without pulsatile flow. *Annals of Thoracic Surgery, 35,* 488–493.

Nieminen, M. T., Rosow, C. E., Triantafillou, A., et al. (1983). Temperature gradients in cardiac surgical patients—a comparison of halothane and fentanyl. *Anesthesia and Analgesia, 62*(11), 1002–1005.

Nilsson, L., Brunnkvist, S., Nilsson, U., et al. (1988). Activation of inflammatory systems during cardiopulmonary bypass. *Scandinavian Journal of Thoracic and Cardiovascular Surgery, 22,* 51–53.

Nilsson, L., Storm, K., Thelin, S., et al. (1989). Heparin-coated equipment reduces complement activation during cardiopulmonary bypass in the pig. *Artificial Organs, 14,* 46–48.

Nishimura, R. A. (1986). Early repair of mechanical complications after acute myocardial infarction. *Journal of the American Medical Association, 356,* 47–54.

Norris, S. O. (1989). Managing postoperative mediastinitis. *Journal of Cardiovascular Nursing, 3,* 52–65.

Novitsky, D., Cooper, D., & Swanepoel, A. (1989). Triiodothyronine as an inotropic agent after open heart surgery. *Journal of Thoracic and Cardiovascular Surgery, 98,* 972–978.

O'Connell, J. B., Gunman, R. M., Evans, R. W., et al. (1993). Task force 1: Organization of heart transplantation in the U.S. *Journal of the American College of Cardiology, 22,* 8–14.

O'Keefe, J. H., Hartzler, G. O., McConahay, D. R., et al. (1990). Procedural risk and long term effectiveness of multi-vessel coronary angioplasty 1980–1989. *Journal of the American College of Cardiology, 15,* 205.

Olinger, G. (1988). Hypothermic intermittent ischemic arrest. *Cardiac Surgery: State of the Art Reviews, 2,* 155–165.

Paradis, I. L., & Williams, P. (1993). Infection after lung transplantation. *Seminars in Respiratory Infections, 8,* 207–215.

Parsonnet, V., Dean, D., & Bernstein, A. D. (1989). A method of uniform stratification of risk for evaluating the results of surgery in acquired adult heart disease. *Circulation, 79*(Suppl 1), 3–12.

Pasque, M. K., Cooper, J. D., Kaiser, L. R., et al. (1990). Improved technique for bilateral lung transplantation: Rationale and initial clinical experience. *Annals of Thoracic Surgery, 49,* 785–791.

Patterson, G. A. (1993). Airway complications. *Chest Surgery Clinics of North America, 3,* 157–173.

Patterson, G. A., Cooper, J. D., Goldman, B., et al. (1988). Technique of successful clinical double-lung transplantation. *Annals of Thoracic Surgery, 4,* 626–633.

Pennington, G., Merjavy, J., & Swartz, M. (1985). Important biventricular failure in patients with postoperative cardiogenic shock. *Annals of Thoracic Surgery, 39,* 16–28.

Philbin, D. (1985). Endocrine response to cardiopulmonary bypass. *Mount Sinai Journal of Medicine, 52,* 508–510.

Porter, R. R., Krout, L., Parks, V., et al. (1994). Perceived stress and coping strategies among candidates for heart transplantation during the organ waiting period. *Journal of Heart and Lung Transplantation, 13*(1 Pt 1), 102–107.

Prough, D. S., Rogers, A. T., Stump, D. A., et al. (1990). Hypercarbia depresses cerebral oxygen consumption during cardiopulmonary bypass. *Stroke, 21*(8), 1162–1166.

Puig, R. B., Ciongolli, W., Cividanes, G. V. L., et al. (1990). Inferior epigastric artery as a free graft for myocardial revascularization. *Journal of Thoracic and Cardiovascular Surgery, 99,* 251–255.

Quiroga, M., Miyagishima, R., Haendschen, L., et al. (1985). The effects of body temperature on leukocyte kinetics during cardiopulmonary bypass. *Journal of Thoracic and Cardiovascular Surgery, 90,* 91–96.

Rahimtoola, S. H. (1985). A perspective on the three large multicenter randomized clinical trials of CABG for chronic stable angina. *Circulation, 72*(Suppl V), 123–135.

Rahimtoola, S. H., Fessler, C. L., Grunkemeier, G. L., et al. (1993). Survival 15 to 20 years after coronary bypass surgery for angina. *Journal of the American College of Cardiology, 21*(1), 151–157.

Rankin, J., Silbert, P., Yadava, O., et al. (1994). Mechanism of stroke complicating cardiopulmonary bypass surgery. *Australian and New Zealand Medical Journal, 24,* 154–160.

Rankin, J. S., Newton, J. R., Jr., Califf, R. M., et al. (1984). Clinical characeristics and current management of medically refractory unstable angina. *Annals of Surgery, 200,* 457–464.

Raymond, M., Conklin, C., Schaeffer, J., et al. (1985). Coping with transient intellectual dysfunction after coronary bypass surgery. *Heart and Lung, 13,* 531–539.

Rebeyka, M., Coles, J., Wilson, G., et al. (1987). The effects of low flow cardiopulmonary bypass on cerebral function: An experimental and clinical study. *Annals of Thoracic Surgery, 43,* 391–396.

Reis, C., Evora, P., Ribeiro, P., et al. (1987). A simple mechanical system for pulsatile cardiopulmonary bypass. *Journal of Cardiovascular Surgery, 28,* 143–144.

Reitz, B. A. (1982). Uses of hypothermia in cardiovascular surgery. In A. K. Ream (Ed.), *Acute cardiovascular management: Anesthesia and intensive care.* Philadelphia: J. B. Lippincott.

Rentrop, K. P. (1985). Thrombolytic therapy in patients with acute myocardial infarction. *Circulation, 71,* 627–631.

Reyes, J. (1985). Adrenergic response to cardiopulmonary bypass. *Mount Sinai Journal of Medicine, 52,* 511–515.

Rich, M. W., Keller, A. J., Schechtman, K. B., et al. (1988). Morbidity and mortality of coronary bypass surgery in patients 75 years of age or older. *Annals of Thoracic Surgery, 46,* 638–644.

Ricotta, J. J., Faggioli, G. L., Castilone, A., et al. (1995). Risk factors for stroke after cardiac surgery: Buffalo Cardiac-Cerebral Study Group. *Journal of Vascular Surgery, 21*(2), 359–363.

Riether, A. M., & Boudreau, M. Z. (1988). Heart transplant. Impact on CCU nurses. *American Journal of Nursing, 88*(11), 1521–1524.

Robuschi, G., Medici, D., Fesani, F., et al. (1986). Cardiopulmonary bypass: a low T4 and T3 syndrome with blunted thyrotropin (TSH) response to thyrotropin-releasing hormone (TRH). *Hormone Research, 23*(3), 151–158.

Rosenfeldt, F. (1988). The theory and practice of cardiac cooling. *Cardiac Surgery: State of the Art Reviews, 2,* 219–240.

Rosenfeldt, F., & Arnold, M. (1982). Topical cooling by recirculation: Comparison of a closed system using a cooling pad with an open system using topical spray. *Annals of Thoracic Surgery, 34,* 138–145.

Rosenfeldt, F., & Watson, D. (1979). Interference with local myocardial cooling by heart gain during aortic cross clamping. *Annals of Thoracic Surgery, 27,* 13–16.

Rosengart, T. K., Kreiger, K., Lang, S. J., et al. (1993). Reoperative coronary artery bypass surgery: Improved preservation of myocardial function with retrograde cardioplegia. *Circulation, 88,* 1330–1335.

Roth, J., Golub, S., Cukingnan, R., et al. (1981). Cell mediated immunity is depressed following cardiopulmonary bypass. *Annals of Thoracic Surgery, 31,* 350–356.

Rousou, J. A., Parker, T., Engelman, R. M., et al. (1985). Phrenic nerve paresis associated with use of iced slush and the cooling jacket for topical hypothermia. *Journal of Thoracic and Cardiovascular Surgery, 89,* 921–925.

Royston, D. (1992). High-dose aprotinin therapy: A review of the first five years' experience. *Journal of Cardiothoracic and Vascular Anesthesia, 6,* 76–100.

Royston, D. (1994). Intraoperative coronary thrombosis: Can aprotinin be incriminated? *Journal of Cardiothoracic and Cardiovascular Surgery, 8,* 137–141.

Rubin, D., Niemanske, K., Reed, G., et al. (1987). Predictors, prevention, and long-term prognosis of atrial fibrillation after coronary artery bypass surgery. *Journal of Cardiothoracic and Vascular Anesthesia, 94,* 331–335.

Ryhanen, P., Llonwn, J., Helja-Marja, R., et al. (1987). Characterization of in vivo activation of lymphocytes found in the peripheral blood of patients undergoing cardiac operation. *Journal of Thoracic and Cardiovascular Surgery, 93,* 109–114.

Salerno, T., Houch, J., Barrozo, C., et al. (1991). Retrograde continuous warm blood cardioplegia. *Annals of Thoracic Surgery, 51,* 245–247.

Salzman, E., Weinstein, M., Weintraub, R., et al. (1986). Treatment with desmopressin acetate to reduce blood loss after cardiac surgery. *New England Journal of Medicine, 314,* 1402–1411.

Samuel, T. (1977). Antibodies reacting with salmon and human protamines in sera from infertile men and from vasectomized men and monkeys. *Clinical and Experimental Immunology, 30*(2), 181–187.

Santillan, G., Chemnitius, M., & Bing, P. (1985). The effects of cardiopulmonary bypass on cerebral blood flow. *Brain Research, 280,* 1–9.

Sato, S., Yamaucho, S., & Schuessler, R. (1992). The effects of augmented atrial hypothermia on atrial refractory period, conduction, and atrial flutter/fibrillation. *International Journal of Cardiology, 36,* 253–261.

Seitelberger, R., Zwolfer, W., Huber, S., et al. (1991). Nifedipine reduces the incidence of myocardial and transient ischemia in patients undergoing coronary bypass grafting. *Circulation, 83,* 460–468.

Sethi, G., Copeland, J., Goldman, S., et al. (1990). Implications of preoperative administration of aspirin in patients undergoing coronary artery bypass grafting: Department of Veteran Affairs Cooperative Study on Antiplatelet Therapy. *Journal of the American College of Cardiology, 15,* 15–20.

Sharples, L. D., Caine, N., Mullins, P., et al. (1991). Risk factor analysis for the major hazards following heart transplantation—rejection, infection, and coronary occlusive disease. *Transplantation, 52*(2), 244–252.

Sheland, J., Hirleman, M., & Hoang, A. (1983). Lobar collapse in the surgical intensive care unit. *British Journal of Radiology, 247,* 531–534.

Shumway, S. J. (1993). Rejection and immunosuppression in lung transplantation. *Chest Surgery Clinics of North America, 3,* 145–156.

Shumway, S., Lower, R., & Stofer, R. (1966). Transplantation of the heart. *Advances in Surgery, 2,* 265–284.

Silverman, N., Del Nadio, P., Kruken-Kamp, I., et al. (1988). Biological rationale for antegrade cardioplegic solution. *Cardiac Surgery: State of the Art Reviews, 2,* 181–195.

Singh, A., Farrugia, R., Teplitiz, C., et al. (1981). Electrolytes versus blood cardioplegia: Randomized clinical and myocardial intrastructural study. *Annals of Thoracic Surgery, 33,* 218–227.

Singh, R., Barratt-Boyes, B., & Morris, E. (1980). Does pulsatile flow improve perfusion during hypothermic cardiopulmonary bypass? *Journal of Thoracic and Cardiovascular Surgery, 79,* 827–832.

Slogoff, S., Reul, G., Keats, A., et al. (1990). Role of perfusion pressures and flow in major organ dysfunction after cardiopulmonary bypass. *Annals of Thoracic Surgery, 50,* 911–918.

Smith, P. K., Buhrman, W., Levett, J., et al. (1983). Supraventricular conduction abnormalities following cardiac operation. *Journal of Thoracic and Cardiovascular Surgery, 85,* 105–115.

Sones, F. M., & Shirey, E. K. (1962). Cine coronary arteriography. *Modern Concepts in Cardiovascular Diseases, 31,* 735–745.

Stanton, B. A., Jenkins, C. D., Savageau, J. A., et al. (1984). Perceived adequacy of patient education and fears and adjustments after cardiac surgery. *Heart and Lung, 13*(5), 525–531.

Starnes, V. A., Barr, M. L., & Cohen, R. G. (1994). Lobar transplantation: Indications, technique, and outcome. *Journal of Thoracic and Cardiovascular Surgery, 108,* 403–410.

Steinberg, J., Kaplanski, D., Olsen, J., et al. (1993). Cytokine and complement levels in patients undergoing cardiopulmonary bypass. *Journal of Thoracic and Cardiovascular Surgery, 106,* 1008–1016.

Stephan, Y., Jebara, V. A., Fabiani, J., et al. (1990). The internal mammary vein: A new conduit of coronary artery bypass. (Editorial). *Journal of Thoracic and Cardiovascular Surgery, 99,* 178.

Stevenson, L. W. (1994a). Selection and management of patients for cardiac transplantation. *Current Opinion in Cardiology, 9,* 315–325.

Stevenson, L. W. (1994b). Cardiac transplantation. In J. Stein (Ed.), *Internal Medicine* (4th ed., pp. 329–338). St. Louis: C. V. Mosby.

Stevenson, L. W., Hamilton, M. A., Tillisch, I. H., et al. (1991). Decreasing survival benefit from cardiac transplantation for outpatients as the waiting list lengthens. *Journal of the American College of Cardiology, 18*(4), 919–925.

Stevenson, L. W., Warner, S. L., Steimle, A. E., et al. (1993). The impending crises awaiting cardiac transplantation. *Circulation, 89,* 451–457.

Suma, H., Takeuchi, A., & Hirota, Y. (1989). Myocardial revascularization with combined arterial grafts utilizing the internal mammary and the gastroepiploic arteries. *Annals of Thoracic Surgery, 47,* 712–715.

Sundt, T., Kouchoukos, N., Saffitz, J., et al. (1993). Renal dysfunction and intravascular coagulation with aprotinin and hypothermic circulatory arrest. *Annals of Thoracic Surgery, 55,* 1418–1424.

Svennevig, L., Linberg, H., Geiran, O., et al. (1984). Should the lungs be ventilated during cardiopulmonary bypass? Clinical, hemodynamic, and metabolic changes in patients undergoing elective coronary artery surgery. *Annals of Thoracic Surgery, 37,* 295–300.

Talley, J. D., Jones, E. L., Weintraub, W. S., et al. (1989). Coronary artery bypass surgery after failed elective percutaneous transluminal coronary angioplasty. *Circulation, 79*(Suppl 1), 126–131.

Tanimoto, Y., Matuda, Y., & Kobayaski, Y. (1984). Coronary spasm as a cause of perioperative myocardial infarction. *Japanese Heart Journal, 25,* 275–281.

Tanswell, P., Tebbe, U., Neuhaus, K. L., et al. (1992). Pharmacokinetics and fibrin specificity of alteplase during accelerated infusions in acute myocardial infarction. *Journal of the American College of Cardiology, 19,* 1071–1075.

Tchervenkov, C., Wynands, J., & Symes, J. (1983). Persistent atrial activity during cardioplegic arrest: A possible factor in the etiology of postoperative supraventricular tachyarrhythmias. *Annals of Thoracic Surgery, 36,* 453–459.

Teoh, K. H., Christakis, G. T., Weisel, R. D., et al. (1987). Increased risk of urgent revascularization. *Journal of Thoracic and Cardiovascular Surgery, 93,* 291–299.

Tennenberg, S. D., Clardy, C. W., Bailey, W. W., et al. (1990). Complement activation and lung permeability during cardiopulmonary bypass. *Annals of Thoracic Surgery, 50*(4), 597–601.

Thompson, R., Mitchell, A., Ahmed, M., et al. (1980). Conduction defects in aortic valve disease. *American Heart Journal, 94*(8), 3–10.

TIMI Study Group. (1989). Comparison of invasive and conservative strategies after treatment with intravenous tissue plasminogen activator in acute myocardial infarction: TIMI trial. Phase II. *New England Journal of Medicine, 320,* 618–627.

Tobin, J. N., Wassertheil-Smoller, S., Wexler, J. P., et al. (1987). Sex bias in considering coronary bypass surgery. *Annals of Internal Medicine, 107,* 19–25.

Townes, B., Bashein, G., Hornbein, T., et al. (1989). Neurobehavioral outcomes in cardiac operations: A prospective controlled study. *Journal of Thoracic and Cardiovascular Surgery, 98,* 774–782.

Toy, P., Strauss, R. G., & Stehling, L. C. (1987). Predeposited autologous blood for elective surgery. *New England Journal of Medicine, 316,* 517–520.

Tuman, J., McCarthy, R., & Najafi, H. (1992). Differential effects of advanced age on neurologic and cardiac risks of coronary artery operations. *Journal of Thoracic and Cardiovascular Surgery, 104,* 1510–1517.

Turnipseed, W., Berkoff, H., & Belzer, F. (1980). Postoperative stroke in cardiovascular and peripheral vascular disease. *Annals of Surgery, 192,* 365–368.

Utley, J., Wachtel, C., & Cain, R. (1981). Effects of hypothermia, hemodilution, and pump oxygenation on organ water content, blood flow and oxygen delivery, and renal function. *Annals of Thoracic Surgery, 31,* 121–133.

Van Lente, F., Martin, A., Ratliff, N., et al. (1989). The predictive value of serum enzymes for perioperative myocardial infarction after cardiac operation. *Journal of Thoracic and Cardiovascular Surgery, 98,* 704–710.

VanOeveren, W., Harder, M., Roozendaal, K., et al. (1990). Aprotinin protects against the initial effects of cardiopulmonary bypass. *Journal of Thoracic and Cardiovascular Surgery, 99,* 788–797

Vecht, R., Nicolaides, E., & Ireuke, J. (1986). Incidence and prevention of supraventricular tachydysrhythmias after coronary bypass surgery. *International Journal of Cardiology, 13,* 125–134.

Vineberg, A. M. (1946). Development of an anastamosis between coronary vessels and transplanted internal mammary artery. *Canadian Medical Association Journal, 55,* 117.

Wachtfogel, Y. T., Harpel, P. C., Edmunds, L. H., Jr., et al. (1989). Formation of C1s-C1-inhibitor, kallikrein-C1-inhibitor, and plasmin-alpha 2-plasmin-inhibitor complexes during cardiopulmonary bypass. *Blood, 73*(2), 468–471.

Wachtfogel, Y. T., Kucich, U., Greenplate, J., et al. (1987). Human neutrophil degranulation during extracorporeal circulation. *Blood, 69*(1), 324–330.

Wachtfogel, Y. T., Pixley, R. A., Kucich, U., et al. (1986). Purified plasma factor XIIa aggregates human neutrophils and causes degranulation. *Blood, 67*(6), 1731–1737.

Waldhausen, J. A., & Pierce, W. S. (Eds.). (1985). *Johnson's surgery of the chest* (5th ed., pp. 433–460). Chicago: Year Book.

Wall, T. C., Califf, R. M., George, B. S., et al., for the TAMI-7 Study Group. (1992). Accelerated Plasminogen Activator Dose Regimens for Coronary Thrombolysis. *Journal of the American College of Cardiology, 19,* 428–429.

Warm Heart Investigators, The. (1994). Randomized trial of normothermic versus hypothermic coronary artery bypass surgery. *Lancet, 343,* 559–563.

Wechsler, A. S., & Junod, F. L. (1989). Coronary bypass grafting in patients with chronic congestive heart failure. *Circulation, 79,* 92–96.

Weiman, D., Ferdinand, F., Bolton, J., et al. (1993). Perioperative management in cardiac surgery. *Clinics in Chest Medicine, 14,* 283–292.

Weinstein, G., Zabetarkis, P., Clavel, A., et al. (1987). The renin–angiotensin system is not responsible for hypertension following coronary artery bypass surgery. *Annals of Thoracic Surgery, 43,* 74–77.

Wenger, N. (1990). Gender coronary artery disease and coronary bypass surgery. *Annals of Internal Medicine, 112,* 557–558.

Wheatley, D. J. (1986). *Surgery of coronary artery disease.* St. Louis: C. V. Mosby.

Wilcox, P., Baile, E., Hards, J., et al. (1988). Phrenic nerve function and its relationship to atelectasis after coronary artery bypass surgery. *Chest, 93,* 693–698.

Wilcox, P., Pare, P., & Pardy, R. (1990). Recovery after unilateral phrenic nerve injury associated with coronary artery revascularization. *Chest, 98,* 661–666.

Willerson, J. T. (1992). *Treatment of heart disease.* New York: Gower Medical Publishing.

Williams, J. (1988). Effects of cardioplegia on arrhythmias and conduction. *Cardiac Surgery: State of the Art Reviews, 2,* 259–269.

Woo, E., Ma, J. Robinson, J., Yu, Y., et al. (1988). Admission glucose levels in relation to mortality. *Stroke, 19,* 1359–1364.

Yeoh, T., Frist, W., Eastburn, T., et al. (1992). Clinical significance of mild rejection of the cardiac allograft. *Circulation, 86*(Suppl II), II-267–II-271.

Young, J. B., Winters, W. L., Bourge, R., & Uretsky, B. F. (1993). Task force 4: Function of the heart transplant recipient. *Journal of the American College of Cardiology, 22,* 31–41.

Yousif, H., Davies, G., & Oakley, C. (1990). Perioperative supraventricular arrhythmias in coronary bypass surgery. *International Journal of Cardiology, 26,* 313–318.

Yusuf, S., Zucker, D., Pedruzzi, P., et al. (1994). Effect of coronary artery bypass graft surgery on survival: Overview of 10 year results from randomised trials by the Coronary Artery Bypass Graft Surgery Trialists Collaboration. *Lancet, 344,* 563–570.

Zeff, R. H., Kongtahworn, C., Iannone, L. A., et al. (1988). IMA vs. SVG to the left anterior descending coronary artery: Prospective randomized study with 10 year follow-up. *Annals of Thoracic Surgery, 45,* 533–536.

CARDIAC SURGERY: CORONARY ARTERY BYPASS GRAFT SURGERY MULTIDISCIPLINARY CARE GUIDE

COORDINATION OF CARE

Diagnosis/Stabilization Phase		Acute Management Phase		Recovery Phase	
Outcome	***Intervention***	***Outcome***	***Intervention***	***Outcome***	***Intervention***
All appropriate team members and disciplines will be involved in plan of care.	Develop plan of care with patient/family, primary nurse(s), primary physicians, cardiovascular surgeon, cardiologist, perfusionist, pulmonologist, hematologist, anesthesiologist, respiratory therapist, social services, chaplain, and clinical nurse specialist/case manager.	All appropriate team members and disciplines will be involved in plan of care.	Update plan of care with patient/family, other team members, physical therapist, cardiac rehabilitation, discharge planner, and dietician. Assess support systems at home. Initiate planning for anticipated discharge and call home health as indicated. Begin teaching patient/family about care at home. Assess ability to manage at home vs. extended care.	Patient will understand how to maintain optimal health at home.	Provide written guidelines concerning care at home and any follow-up visits. Provide patient/family with phone number of resources available to answer questions.

FLUID BALANCE

Diagnosis/Stabilization Phase		Acute Management Phase		Recovery Phase	
Outcome	***Intervention***	***Outcome***	***Intervention***	***Outcome***	***Intervention***
Patient will achieve optimal hemodynamic status as evidenced by: • MAP >70 mm Hg • Hemodynamic parameters WNL • Urine output >0.5 mL/kg/hr • Return to normal thermic state • Free from abnormal ECG changes Patient will remain free from bleeding.	Monitor and treat cardiac parameters: • HR • BP • PA pressures • PCWP • CO • CI • SV • $S\bar{v}O_2$ • SvR/PVR • ST segment • I & O • Level of consciousness • Peripheral pulses • Evidence of tissue perfusion • Dysrhythmias	Patient will maintain optimal hemodynamic status and remain free from dysrhythmias.	Monitor and treat cardiac variables. Assist with chest tube and indwelling line removal and monitor patient afterwards. Monitor and treat dysrhythmias. Consider need for dysrhythmia prophylaxis. Begin patient/family teaching on cardiovascular system, current treatment, and expected clinical course. Monitor lab values: Hgb and Hct, platelets, SMA-6. Monitor daily weight and I & O. Assess need for diuretics and/or K^+ repletion.	Patient will maintain optimal hemodynamic status.	Same as acute management phase. Continue cardiac teaching. Assess for understanding. Reinforce as needed. Assist with pacing wire removal and monitor patient after pacing wires removed.

Care Guide continued on following page

CARDIAC SURGERY MULTIDISCIPLINARY CARE GUIDE *continued*

FLUID BALANCE *continued*

Diagnosis/Stabilization Phase		Acute Management Phase		Recovery Phase	
Outcome	*Intervention*	*Outcome*	*Intervention*	*Outcome*	*Intervention*
	Rewarm slowly and monitor temperature and signs of shivering. Methods of rewarming include head covering, radiant light, warming blankets, and/or vasodilators. Anticipate need for epicardial pacing and/or pharmacologic agents. Monitor lab values: K^+, Mg^{++}, Hgb, Hct, PT, PTT, ACT if available, platelets, total CK, CK-MB, glucose, BUN, and creatinine. Assess for sudden increase or decrease in chest tube drainage, equalization of filling pressures, widening mediastinum, decrease in blood pressure, and pulsus paradoxus.				

NUTRITION

Diagnosis/Stabilization Phase		Acute Management Phase		Recovery Phase	
Outcome	*Intervention*	*Outcome*	*Intervention*	*Outcome*	*Intervention*
Patient will be adequately nourished.	Maintain patient NPO until extubation. If extubation is delayed, assess need for alternative nutritional therapy. Monitor response to clear liquids. Remove NG tube (if utilized), once extubated. Monitor protein and albumin lab values. Administer antiemetics, H_2 blockers, and/or antacids as needed.	Patient will be adequately nourished, remain free from nausea, and demonstrate return of appetite.	Advance to heart healthy (low-fat, low-cholesterol) diet as tolerated. Monitor response to diet. Monitor daily weight. Assess bowel sounds. Administer laxatives/stool softeners as needed.	Patient will be adequately nourished.	Teach patient/family about heart healthy diet: • Total fat <30% of daily intake • Total saturated fat <10% of daily intake • Total daily cholesterol intake <300 mg • Caloric reduction if indicated • Low-sodium diet if indicated Continue laxatives/stool softeners as needed. Assess need for multivitamin.

MOBILITY

Diagnosis/Stabilization Phase		Acute Management Phase		Recovery Phase	
Outcome	**Intervention**	**Outcome**	**Intervention**	**Outcome**	**Intervention**
Patient will maintain normal ROM and muscle strength.	Bed rest until extubation. Begin passive/active-assist range of motion exercises. Turn and position every two hours. Dangle after extubation.	Patient will achieve optimal mobility.	Progress exercise as tolerated: dangle, bathroom privileges, out of bed for meals, and walking 50 feet. Monitor response to increased activity. Decrease if adverse events occur (tachycardia, chest discomfort, dyspnea, ectopy). Provide support as necessary. Begin patient/family teaching on principles of a gradual exercise program.	Patient will achieve optimal mobility.	Walk at least 200 to 300 feet tid to qid. Walk up and down one flight of stairs. Teach patient/family about home exercise program.

OXYGENATION/VENTILATION

Diagnosis/Stabilization Phase		Acute Management Phase		Recovery Phase	
Outcome	**Intervention**	**Outcome**	**Intervention**	**Outcome**	**Intervention**
Patient will have adequate gas exchange as evidenced by: • $Sa_{O_2} > 90\%$/ $Sp_{O_2} > 92\%$ • Arterial blood gases (ABGs) • Clear breath sounds • Respiratory rate, depth, and rhythm WNL • Chest x-ray normal	Monitor ventilator settings and wakefulness and determine readiness to wean. Monitor hemodynamic variables before, during, and after weaning. Wean ventilator and monitor patient response: • Wean F_{IO_2} to keep $Sp_{O_2} > 92$ • Monitor effects of anesthesia and wean ventilator accordingly • After extubation, apply supplemental oxygen Assess respiratory functioning, including lung sounds, respiratory muscle strength, respiratory rate and depth, coughing ability, and chest x-ray. Monitor pulse oximetry. Reinforce use of incentive spirometry (with inspiratory hold) when extubated.	Patient will have adequate gas exchange.	Monitor and treat oxygenation/ventilatory status per ABGs, Sp_{O_2}, chest assessment, and chest x-ray. Monitor closely for hypoxemia or SOB related to atelectasis and/or pleural effusion. Evaluate need for thoracentesis. Assess chest tube for drainage/presence of air leak. Support patient with oxygen therapy as indicated. Reinforce use of incentive spirometry. Provide chest splint pillow and instruct on proper use.	Patient will have adequate gas exchange.	Obtain chest x-ray before discharge. Teach patient/family about incentive spirometry and the use of the chest splint pillow at home.

Care Guide continued on following page

CARDIAC SURGERY MULTIDISCIPLINARY CARE GUIDE *continued*

COMFORT

Diagnosis/Stabilization Phase		Acute Management Phase		Recovery Phase	
Outcome	*Intervention*	*Outcome*	*Intervention*	*Outcome*	*Intervention*
Patient will be as comfortable and painfree as possible as evidenced by: • No objective indicators of discomfort • No complaints of discomfort	Anticipate need for analgesia and provide as needed. Use a pain scale or visual analog tool. Assess response to all analgesics and effects on ability to wean from ventilator when indicated. (Use newer NSAID that have fewer sedative effects) Establish effective communication technique with intubated patient with which he/she can communicate discomfort and need for analgesics.	Patient will be relaxed and as comfortable as possible.	Anticipate need for analgesics and provide as needed; assess response. Provide chest splint pillow and instruct on proper use. Provide uninterrupted periods of rest. Assist patient with relaxation techniques. Use back massage, humor, music therapy, and imagery to promote relaxation. Provide analgesics as needed before chest tube removal, ambulation, and any other procedures.	Patient will be relaxed and as comfortable as possible.	Progress analgesics to oral medications as needed; assess response. Teach patient/family regarding analgesic administration and potential side effects for post discharge. Continue alternative methods to promote relaxation as listed above. Teach patient/family alternative methods to promote relaxation at home. Provide uninterrupted periods of rest.

SKIN INTEGRITY

Diagnosis/Stabilization Phase		Acute Management Phase		Recovery Phase	
Outcome	*Intervention*	*Outcome*	*Intervention*	*Outcome*	*Intervention*
Patient will have intact skin without abrasions or pressure ulcers. Patient will return to normothermia.	Rewarm slowly; monitor temperature and signs of shivering. Assess all bony prominences at least q4h and treat if needed. Maintain integrity of all dressings. Consider mattress overlay.	Patient will have intact skin without abrasions, pressure ulcers, or wound infections.	Assess all bony prominences at least q4h and treat if needed. Use preventive pressure-reducing devices if patient is at high risk for development of pressure ulcers. Treat pressure ulcers according to hospital protocol. Use TED hose and elevate legs to minimize edema. Assess sternotomy incision and leg incisions for drainage, erythema, and induration. Teach patient/family proper skin care at home: incision care, TED hose, signs and symptoms of infection, and how to minimize edema.	Patient will have intact skin without abrasions, pressure ulcers, or infections.	Assess all wounds/incisions for signs/symptoms of infection. Culture if necessary. Reinforce importance of proper hygiene and wound care postop. Continue patient/family teaching on skin care at home. Assess understanding and reinforce as needed.

PROTECTION/SAFETY

Diagnosis/Stabilization Phase		Acute Management Phase		Recovery Phase	
Outcome	*Intervention*	*Outcome*	*Intervention*	*Outcome*	*Intervention*
Patient will be protected from possible harm.	Assess need for wrist restraints while patient is intubated, has a decreased level of consciousness, or is agitated and restless. Explain need for restraints to patient/family. Assess response to restraints and check q1–2h for skin integrity and impairment to circulation. Remove restraints as soon as patient is awake from anesthesia and able to follow instructions. Follow hospital protocol according to use of restraints. Provide sedatives/anxiolytic agents as needed. Isolate pacing wires.	Patient will be protected from possible harm.	Provide support when dangling or getting out of bed; monitor response. Isolate pacing wires.	Patient will be protected from possible harm.	Provide support with ambulation and climbing stairs. Teach patient/family about physical limitations such as no lifting/pulling objects over 10–15 lb, for 2–3 months post discharge. Review signs and symptoms to report to physician. Isolate pacing wires until removed.

PSYCHOSOCIAL/SELF-DETERMINATION

Diagnosis/Stabilization Phase		Acute Management Phase		Recovery Phase	
Outcome	*Intervention*	*Outcome*	*Intervention*	*Outcome*	*Intervention*
Patient will achieve psychophysiologic stability. Patient will demonstrate a decrease in anxiety as evidenced by: • Vital signs WNL • Level of consciousness WNL • Subjective reports	Assess physiologic effects of critical care and/or open heart recovery environment on patient (hemodynamic variables, psychological status, signs of increased sympathetic response). Provide sedatives as indicated. Take measures to reduce sensory overload. Develop effective interventions to communicate with patient while intubated. Use calm, caring, competent, and reassuring approach with patient and family. Allow flexible visiting to meet patient and family needs. Determine emotional impact and coping ability of patient and take appropriate measures to meet needs. Conduct a family needs assessment and employ measures to meet identified concerns.	Patient will achieve psychophysiologic stability. Patient will demonstrate a decrease in anxiety.	Take measures to decrease sensory overload. Provide adequate rest periods. Provide sedatives as needed. Continue to include family in aspects of care. Continue to assess coping ability of patient/family and take measures as indicated. Involve patient/family in health care decisions.	Patient will achieve psychophysiologic stability. Patient will demonstrate a decrease in anxiety.	Provide adequate periods of rest. Continue to assess coping ability of patient and family. Provide information on coping mechanisms for use after discharge. Refer to outside services or agencies as appropriate (chaplain, social services, or home health). Include patient/family in decisions concerning care.

Care Guide continued on following page

CARDIAC SURGERY MULTIDISCIPLINARY CARE GUIDE *continued*

DIAGNOSTICS

Diagnosis/Stabilization Phase		Acute Management Phase		Recovery Phase	
Outcome	***Intervention***	***Outcome***	***Intervention***	***Outcome***	***Intervention***
Patient will understand any tests or procedures that must be completed (vital signs, I & O cardiac output, hemodynamic monitoring, hyperthermia unit, chest x-ray, lab work, chest tube, invasive devices, EKG, suctioning).	Explain all procedures and tests to patient/family. Be sensitive to individualized needs of patient/family for information. Establish effective communication technique with patient while intubated.	Patient will understand any tests or procedures that must be completed (removal of indwelling lines, removal of chest tubes, removal of indwelling urinary catheter, lab work, chest x-ray, incentive spirometry, coughing and deep breathing, increase in activity, TED hose).	Explain procedures and tests needed to assess recovery from surgery. Be sensitive to individualized needs of patient/family for information.	Patient will understand meaning of diagnostic tests in relation to continued health (lab tests, increase in activity, coughing and deep breathing, incentive spirometry).	Review with patient before discharge the results of lab tests, chest x-ray, and surgery. Discuss any abnormal values and appropriate measures patient can take to help return to normal. Provide patient with written guidelines concerning follow-up care. Provide instruction on care at home after discharge (i.e., when to call the doctor, care of incision, activity limitations, medications, diet).

REFERENCE

DeAngellis, R. (1991). The cardiovascular system. In J. G. Alsphach, Ed. *Core Curriculum for critical care nursing* (4th ed., pp. 132–314). Philadelphia: W. B. Saunders.

Patients With Hypertension

Rita M. Barden

Hypertension is a major health problem in the United States, afflicting over 50 million Americans of every age (Joint National Committee on the Detection, Evaluation and Treatment of High Blood Pressure [JNC], 1993). Hypertension is defined as a diastolic pressure (DBP) of greater or equal to 90 mm Hg, or a systolic blood pressure greater than or equal to 140 mm Hg (JNC, 1993), or both. Hypertension is the major contributing factor in the development of cerebral vascular accidents, renal failure, and congestive heart failure. It is a significant risk factor associated with cardiovascular heart disease (Frohlich, 1989). Although in most cases the cause is unknown, the disease is easily detected and treated.

Largely through the efforts of the JNC and other national education programs, detection and treatment of high blood pressure have been successful. Aggressive treatment has resulted in a 57% reduction in deaths from strokes, a 50% reduction in deaths from myocardial infarction, and an overall reduction in mortality from cardiovascular disease (JNC, 1993). Research efforts are currently aimed at finding the cause or causes of primary hypertension and refining treatment regimens.

The JNC (1993) recommends that an individual's blood pressure be obtained at every exposure to the health care system. Mass public screenings for detection of high blood pressure are needed for populations at high risk, especially for cardiovascular disease or lack of access to the health care setting. The emphasis of the JNC is on the development of a national standard for treatment of hypertensive persons in an effort to mitigate untoward vascular events and target organ damage. The critical care nurse is in a pivotal position to administer treatment and evaluate the hypertensive patient's clinical response to medical treatment. Nursing's emphasis on prevention of disease and education of patients makes the profession particularly well suited to address this major health issue.

This chapter addresses the definition, prevalence, and classification of hypertension. A review of the homeostatic mechanisms that maintain normal blood pressure, the pathophysiology of the development of primary (essential) and secondary hypertension, and the clinical treatment of this disease process are discussed. Hypertensive crisis and the intensive nursing care required to manage this emergency effectively are highlighted.

REGULATION OF ARTERIAL BLOOD PRESSURE

Blood pressure is determined by cardiac output (blood flow) and the resistance to flow or total peripheral resistance. Simply put, arterial pressure equals cardiac output times total peripheral resistance (Guyton, 1991). Total peripheral resistance is the sum of resistance in all vascular beds. Direct determinants of arterial pressure include cardiac output, aortic impedence, and vascular resistance. Figure 25–1 diagrams those factors affecting blood pressure regulation. Indirect determinants that maintain control of arterial pressure are the autonomic nervous system, hormonal regulation, the renin–angiotensin pressor system, and the volume of extracellular fluid (Dustan, 1986). Guyton (1991) divides these indirect determinants into rapid-acting systems and long-term control mechanisms. Rapid-acting systems are effective in seconds, whereas long-term control mechanisms may take minutes to hours to manifest their effects on arterial pressure.

Autonomic Nervous System

The autonomic nervous system's mechanisms for control of arterial pressure include the baroreceptor reflex, the chemoreceptor reflex, and the central nervous system ischemic mechanism. Baroreceptors are located in the walls of the large systemic arteries, most notably the internal carotid artery and the aortic arch. When these receptors are stimulated by stretching, they send signals to the medullary area of the brain stem. These signals inhibit the vasoconstrictor center of the medulla and innervate the vagal center, causing vasodilation of the peripheral vascular circuit. Stimulation of the vagus nerve also results in a decrease in heart rate and a decrease in the strength of contractions (Guyton, 1991). Arterial pressure declines secondary to a decrease in peripheral resistance and cardiac output. When arterial pressure is too low, the baroreceptor re-

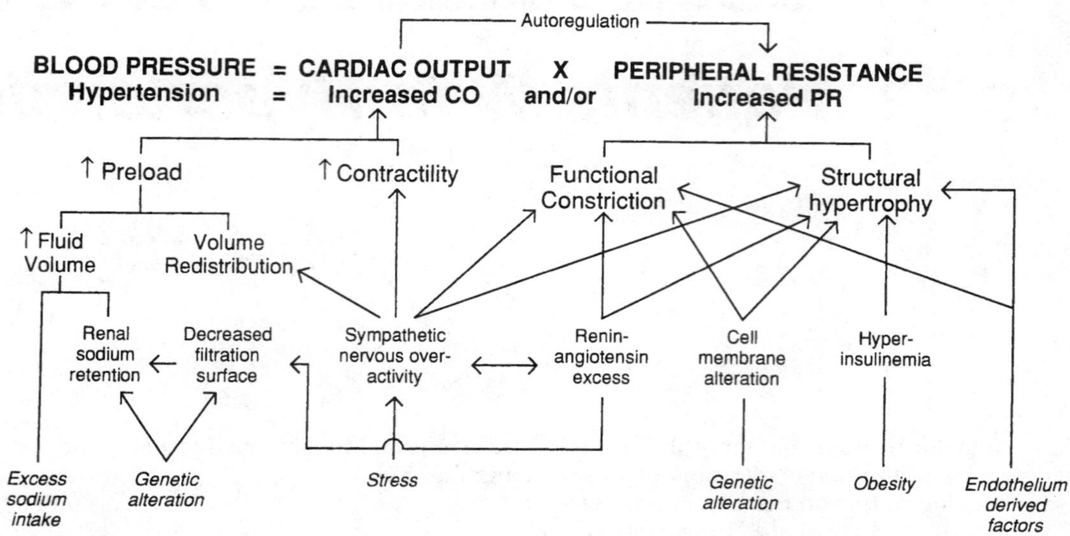

FIGURE 25–1. Some of the factors involved in the control of blood pressure that affect the basic equation: Blood pressure = cardiac output × peripheral resistance. (From Kaplan, N. [1994]. *Clinical hypertension.* Baltimore: Williams & Wilkins).

flex system creates the opposite effect, resulting in a rise in blood pressure. The baroreceptor system reacts immediately to variations in arterial pressure, making it an effective mechanism for short-term control of blood pressure. However, this system adapts to the pressure it is exposed to within 1 to 2 days, making it an ineffective system for long-term arterial pressure control.

Changes in arterial pressure also stimulate chemoreceptors located in small bodies in the carotid artery and the aorta. These bodies are in close contact with the arterial pressure system via an artery that flows through the chemoreceptors. As arterial pressure declines, the chemoreceptors are stimulated because of a decrease in oxygen and the build-up of carbon dioxide and hydrogen. The chemoreceptors stimulate the vasomotor center, which creates a rise in arterial pressure (Guyton, 1991). These receptors respond to low arterial pressures only, not to normal arterial pressures.

Other reflexes located in the atria are stimulated by excess fluid volume. These stretch receptors, when stimulated, cause reflex dilation in afferent arterioles, most notably in the kidneys. As dilation occurs, the glomerular capillary pressure rises, causing increased deposition of fluid into the tubules. As the atria stretch, they also stimulate the hypothalamus to decrease the excretion of antidiuretic hormone (ADH). This results in increased excretion of fluid into the urine. Loss of blood volume results in a decline in arterial pressure (Guyton, 1991).

As atrial pressure increases, the stretching of the sinoatrial node stimulates a 15% increase in heart rate. As the atria are stretched, the receptors of the Bainbridge reflex are also stimulated, resulting in an additional 40% to 60% increase in heart rate. This significant increase in heart rate is the result of stimulation of the vagal and sympathetic nerves. This mechanism increases arterial pressure but does not serve to maintain arterial pressure within the normal range, and may actually be detrimental to blood pressure control for brief periods (Guyton, 1991).

The central nervous system (CNS) ischemic response exerts powerful control over arterial pressure. As arterial pressure declines to below 60 mm Hg, the build-up of carbon dioxide and lactic acid stimulates the vasomotor center, resulting in innervation of the sympathetic nervous system. The sympathetic discharge results in an increase in heart rate and contractile force, causing arterial pressure to rise. The CNS ischemic response is activated in lethal situations of low arterial pressure (Guyton, 1991).

Stimulation of the sympathetic nervous system also results in venous constriction. This constriction decreases capacity in the veins, forcing blood into the heart. As the heart receives an increased blood volume, both the heart rate and the strength of contractions are increased. Venous constriction results in an increase in cardiac output, causing an increase in arterial pressure.

Hormonal Regulation

In addition to neural responses, the body also regulates arterial pressure using certain hormones. Rapid hormonal responses include the release of epinephrine and norepinephrine into the circulation through stimulation of the sympathetic nervous system. These catecholamines increase heart rate and the force of contractions and exert a vasoconstrictive effect on both arteries and veins.

Another hormone involved in the regulation of arterial pressure is ADH, also known as vasopressin. This hormone causes profound vasoconstriction and elevates blood pressure by increasing total peripheral resistance and vascular filling pressure (Guyton, 1991). The principal action of ADH is the reabsorption of water in the renal tubules. With the increase in vascular volume, the arterial pressure rises (Gifford, 1994).

Renin–Angiotensin System

Both vasopressin and the renin–angiotensin system are rapid-acting as well as long-term control mechanisms in the maintenance of arterial pressure. When the blood pressure is inadequate to maintain sufficient blood flow through the kidneys, the juxtaglomerular cells of the kidneys secrete renin. Renin secretion is also increased with sympathetic nervous system stimulation and oliguria (Dustan, 1986). Renin is converted in the bloodstream to angiotensin I, which is converted in the lungs to angiotensin II. Romero and Textor (1991) write that "angiotensin II is about 40 times more potent as a vasoconstrictor than epinephrine." Angiotensin II affects arterial pressure in several ways. It acts as a powerful vasoconstrictor of the arterial system and has a mild vasoconstrictive effect on the venous circulation as well. Angiotensin II inhibits the excretion of salt and water as regulated by the kidneys, and stimulates the production of aldosterone, which further reduces the excretion of salt and water. This results in an increase in blood volume, creating an increase in arterial pressure (Kaplan, 1994). Aldosterone is not a pressor agent in itself; rather, it causes retention of sodium by the kidneys, which results in an excess accumulation of water. Figure 25–2 outlines the renin–angiotensin–aldosterone mechanism. The renin–angiotensin system and the regulation of aldosterone are part of a feedback loop that can either increase or decrease blood volume in an effort to maintain normal arterial pressure.

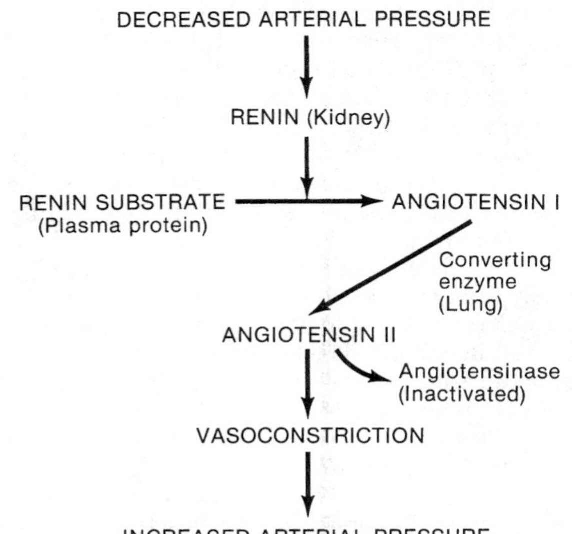

FIGURE 25–2. The renin–angiotensin vasoconstrictor mechanism for arterial pressure control. (From Guyton, A. C. [1991]. *Textbook of medical physiology* [8th ed., p. 212]. Philadelphia: W. B. Saunders).

Extracellular Fluid Volume

The kidneys' ability to regulate the volume of extracellular fluid plays a major role in the maintenance of long-term arterial pressure control. With a rise in arterial pressure, the kidneys are stimulated to excrete water and salt into the urine. This is called pressure diuresis and pressure natriuresis (Dustan, 1986; Guyton, 1991). This decrease in fluid volume causes a decline in the pumping action of the heart and diminishes cardiac output, resulting in a decline in arterial pressure. With a decline in arterial pressure the kidneys reabsorb water and sodium, thereby increasing extracellular fluid volume and blood volume. With an increase in blood volume, the cardiac output increases, and arterial pressure rises. This system is involved in the long-term regulation of blood pressure.

Ingestion of large quantities of water rarely results in a dramatic and sustained elevation in arterial pressure; rather, the ingestion of salt results in an increase in vascular volume. As the amount of salt increases in the body, the osmolality in the plasma volume increases, stimulating the thirst center in the brain, resulting in increased consumption of water. This excess salt intake also stimulates secretion of antidiuretic hormone, which results in reabsorption of more water by the kidneys, all of which increase extracellular fluid volume. Fluid overload results in vasoconstriction resulting in turn in increased peripheral resistance, which, if chronically elevated, quickly leads to abnormal thickening of the vascular wall. This is believed to be one of the mechanisms associated with the development of hypertension.

The inherent ability of the vascular beds to increase or decrease blood flow depending on the metabolic needs of the tissues is called autoregulation. As blood flow in the vascular bed increases beyond demand, vasoconstriction occurs, decreasing the volume of blood in the vascular bed. When blood flow is diminished, the vessels dilate to increase the volume of blood required to meet the metabolic needs of the tissues. As the vascular bed constricts and dilates, it influences resistance to flow, creating a fluctuation in arterial pressure (Guyton, 1991; Kaplan, 1994).

DEFINITION AND PREVALENCE OF HYPERTENSION

Hypertension is defined according to the criteria of the JNC (1993). Hypertension is defined as multiple averaged blood pressure readings in people 18 years of age or older that are greater than or equal to 140/90 mm Hg. The JNC further defines the stage of hypertension depending on the degree of elevation of either the systolic or diastolic reading. In previous years, DBP elevation was the hallmark of hypertension. The JNC (1993), based on new studies, has concluded that in certain populations isolated systolic blood pressure can result in cardiovascular events. For this reason the new guidelines include stages for systolic elevation as well.

The prevalence of hypertension has increased with the growth in our population. There has been a dramatic increase in the last decade of Americans who have been informed they have high blood pressure or are receiving antihypertensive therapy (JNC, 1993). Advancing age correlates with increasing numbers of individuals with hypertension. Recent surveys indicate that hypertension affects 60% of whites, 61% of Mexican-Americans, and 71% of African-Americans older than the age of 60 years (JNC, 1993). Isolated systolic hypertension, defined as a DBP less than 90 mm Hg with a systolic blood pressure (SBP) greater than 160 mm Hg, is common in the elderly and is associated with an increased risk of cardiovascular events (SHEP Cooperative Research Group, 1991). African-Americans continue to sustain increased morbidity and mortality from hypertension, most commonly renal and cerebrovascular disease. Men suffer more cardiovascular morbidity and mortality than women with every degree of severity of hypertension (Vokonas et al., 1988).

CLASSIFICATION OF HYPERTENSION

Classification of hypertension is based on cause and severity. Primary (also known as essential or idiopathic) hypertension accounts for 90% to 95% of all hypertension. The causes of primary hypertension are still unknown. Secondary hypertension has a distinct cause and accounts for 5% to 10% of all hypertension (Dustan, 1986; JNC, 1993; Kaplan, 1994). There are numerous causes of secondary hypertension (Table 25–1). A third classification is hypertensive crisis, which is manifested by a marked elevation in DBP, usually greater than 130 mm Hg, and evidence of target organ damage (Kaplan, 1994; Ram, 1991). Although this phenomenon is rare, it is life threatening and must be promptly and aggressively treated.

TABLE 25–1. **Types and Causes of Hypertension**

- Systolic and diastolic hypertension
  - Primary, essential, or idiopathic
  - Secondary
    - Renal
      - Renal parenchymal disease
        - Acute glomerulonephritis
        - Chronic nephritis
        - Polycystic disease
        - Diabetic nephropathy
        - Hydronephrosis
      - Renovascular disease
        - Renal artery stenosis
        - Intrarenal vasculitis
      - Renin-producing tumors
      - Renoprival
      - Primary sodium retention (Liddle syndrome, Gordon syndrome)
    - Endocrine
      - Acromegaly
      - Hypothyroidism
      - Hyperthyroidism
      - Hypercalcemia (hyperparathyroidism)
      - Adrenal disorders
        - Cortical disorders
          - Cushing syndrome
          - Primary aldosteronism
          - Congenital adrenal hyperplasia
        - Medullary tumors (pheochromocytoma)
      - Extraadrenal chromaffin tumors
      - Carcinoids
      - Exogenous hormones
        - Estrogen
        - Glucocorticoids
        - Mineralocorticoids
        - Sympathomimetics
        - Foods containing tyramine and monamine oxidase inhibitors
    - Coarctation of the aorta
    - Pregnancy
    - Neurologic disorders
      - Increased intracranial pressure
        - Brain tumor
        - Encephalitis
        - Respiratory acidosis
      - Sleep apnea
      - Quadriplegia
      - Acute porphyria
      - Familial dysautonomia
      - Lead poisoning
      - Guillain-Barré syndrome
    - Acute stress (including surgery)
      - Psychogenic hyperventilation
      - Hypoglycemia
      - Burns
      - Pancreatitis
      - Alcohol withdrawal
      - Sickle cell crisis
      - After resuscitation
      - After surgery
    - Increased intravascular volume
      - Alcohol and drug use
- Systolic hypertension
  - Increased cardiac output
    - Aortic valvular insufficiency
    - Arteriovenous fistula, patent ductus
    - Thyrotoxicosis
    - Paget's disease of bone
    - Beriberi
    - Hyperkinetic circulation
  - Rigidity of aorta

From Kaplan, N. (1994). *Clinical hypertension.* Baltimore: Williams & Wilkins.

Classification of hypertension according to severity is based on systolic and diastolic pressure. The JNC (1993) has classified hypertension by stages, as outlined in Table 25–2.

The risk for cardiovascular, renal, and neurologic morbidity and mortality increasing with the severity of hypertension is well documented (Hypertension Detection and Follow-up Program Cooperative Group, 1979; Multiple Risk Factor Intervention Trial Research Group, 1982; Parati et al., 1987; Veterans Administration Cooperative Study Group on Antihypertensive Agents, 1967, 1970).

Structural and Functional Disturbances in Hypertension

The structural and vascular changes of hypertension are the same, regardless of whether the cause of hypertension is known. Hypertension is a disease of resistance resulting in increased arterial wall rigidity. The changes in the arteries and arterioles are similar to the changes undergone by the vascular system with aging, but are far more severe. As the tension in the arterial wall increases due to elevated arterial pressure, damage occurs to the vessel wall, including medionecrosis, atherosclerosis, and development of aneurysms, rupture, and hemorrhages (Kaplan, 1994). The chronic increase in arterial pressure results in more forceful pulsatile flow, which causes endothelial wall damage. This damage causes an increase in smooth muscle contraction and enhances the development of fibrosis and atherosclerosis. Areas of damage to the endothelial lining result in enhanced cell replication. Atherosclerosis is directly related to the rate and number of cell replications (Kaplan, 1994).

Specific arterial lesions associated with chronic elevation of arterial pressure have been identified. These lesions, which are more commonly found in hypertensives, include hyperplastic atherosclerosis, hyaline atherosclerosis, and miliary aneurysms. Hyperplastic atherosclerosis, or increased cell replication, results from vessel damage. This damage is manifested by deposition of fibroblasts, elastin fibers, and other damag-

TABLE 25–2. **Classification of Blood Pressure for Adults Aged 18 Years and Older***

Category	Systolic, mm Hg	Diastolic, mm Hg
Normal†	<130	<85
High normal	130–139	85–89
Hypertension‡		
Stage 1 (mild)	140–159	90–99
Stage 2 (moderate)	160–179	100–109
Stage 3 (severe)	180–209	110–119
Stage 4 (very severe)	≥210	≥120

*Not taking antihypertensive drugs and not acutely ill. When systolic and diastolic pressures fall into different categories, the higher category should be selected to classify the individual's blood pressure status. For instance, 160/92 mm Hg should be classified as stage 2, and 180/120 mm Hg should be classified as stage 4. Isolated systolic hypertension is defined as a systolic blood pressure of 140 mm Hg or more and a diastolic blood pressure of less than 90 mm Hg and staged appropriately (e.g., 170/85 mm Hg is defined as stage 2 isolated systolic hypertension).

In addition to classifying stages of hypertension on the basis of average blood pressure levels, the clinician should specify presence or absence of target-organ disease and additional risk factors. For example, a patient with diabetes and a blood pressure of 142/94 mm Hg, plus left ventricular hypertrophy should be classified as having "stage 1 hypertension with target-organ disease (left ventricular hypertrophy) and with another major risk factor (diabetes)." This specificity is important for risk classification and management.

†Optimal blood pressure with respect to cardiovascular risk is less than 120 mm Hg systolic and less than 80 mm Hg diastolic. However, unusually low readings should be evaluated for clinical significance.

‡Based on the average of two or more readings taken at each of two or more visits after an initial screening.

From Joint National Committee on Detection, Evaluation and Treatment of High Blood Pressure (1993). The fifth report of the Joint National Committee on Detection, Evaluation and Treatment of High Blood Pressure. *Archives of Internal Medicine,* 153, 154–183.

ing substances in the intima. The other layers of the vessel wall are affected; the adventitia becomes fibrotic, and the media is hypertrophied in hyperplastic atherosclerosis (Kaplan, 1994). The abnormal deposition of hyaline and the thickening of the basement membrane of the intima and media are the types of damage associated with hyaline atherosclerosis. Both forms of atherosclerosis result in a significant reduction in lumen size and elasticity of the vessel (Kaplan, 1994). Miliary aneurysms are usually found in the cerebral arterioles. Dilation of the arteriole occurs just past an area of thickening or stenosis in the vessel wall. Miliary aneurysms are closely related to the increased incidence of cerebral vascular accidents found in hypertensive individuals (Kaplan, 1994).

The ischemia and infarction of target organs (kidneys, heart, and brain) probably result from thrombus formation over these arterial lesions. Medial layer damage in the aorta due to chronic arterial pressure elevation may result in development of aortic aneurysms and dissections, which are found more commonly in hypertensive individuals (Kaplan, 1994).

PRIMARY (ESSENTIAL) HYPERTENSION

Several hypotheses have been postulated to explain primary hypertension. The factors that regulate normal arterial pressure, as previously discussed, have all been implicated in the development of hypertension. Dysfunction in these interrelated factors contributes to sustained elevated arterial pressure, indicating the multifactorial aspect of primary hypertension. There are several hypotheses postulated to explain primary hypertension. They are the autoregulatory, the renal volume retention, and the sodium transport theories. There is much debate among clinicians about which theory most likely explains the development of primary hypertension. Kaplan (1994) believes that blood pressure is the result of several complex mechanisms in the body, namely, cardiac output, vessel diameter and resistance, and fluid volume. All of these factors are interrelated in the maintenance of arterial pressure control. All have been implicated in the development of chronic arterial pressure elevation.

The autoregulatory hypothesis explains the increase in arterial pressure as a direct result of an increase in cardiac output, presumably caused by an increase in extracellular volume or increased stimulation of the sympathetic nervous system. This increase in cardiac output causes an elevation in arterial pressure. With this oversupply of blood and nutrients, the autoregulatory mechanism of the arterial vessels will begin vasoconstriction to bring supply and demand into balance. This chronic constriction leads to structural thickening of the vessel wall and the sequence of events discussed in the following section on vascular changes associated with hypertension. Even though cardiac output may fall to normal or low, the vessels remain structurally damaged, resulting in a chronic increase in peripheral resistance (Guyton, 1991).

The renal volume retention hypothesis claims that, with normal elevation in arterial pressure, renal blood flow is increased. This increase in flow increases the glomerular filtration rate, enhancing the excretion of sodium and water into the urine, thus returning blood pressure to normal. This mechanism is called pressure natriuresis–diuresis. In hypertension, there appears to be an increase in renal efferent arteriolar constriction, possibly as a result of overstimulation of catecholamines or increased sensitivity to these catecholamines. This arteriolar constriction results in an increased filtration fraction and peritubular oncotic pressure, which increases reabsorption of sodium and water. The kidneys become accustomed to higher arterial pressures, requiring markedly increased arterial pressures to begin excreting sodium and water. This is labeled the resetting of the pressure–natriuresis curve (Guyton, 1991; Kaplan, 1994).

Alterations in sodium transport recently have been postulated as an explanation for primary hypertension. Because of a genetic defect, the kidneys are unable to excrete sodium in sufficient quantities, resulting in an increase in extracellular fluid. A natriuretic hormone secreted in response to this elevated volume decreases the activity of the intracellular sodium pump. The sodium–potassium ATPase pump is located on receptor sites of the semipermeable membrane and functions to maintain homeostatic balance

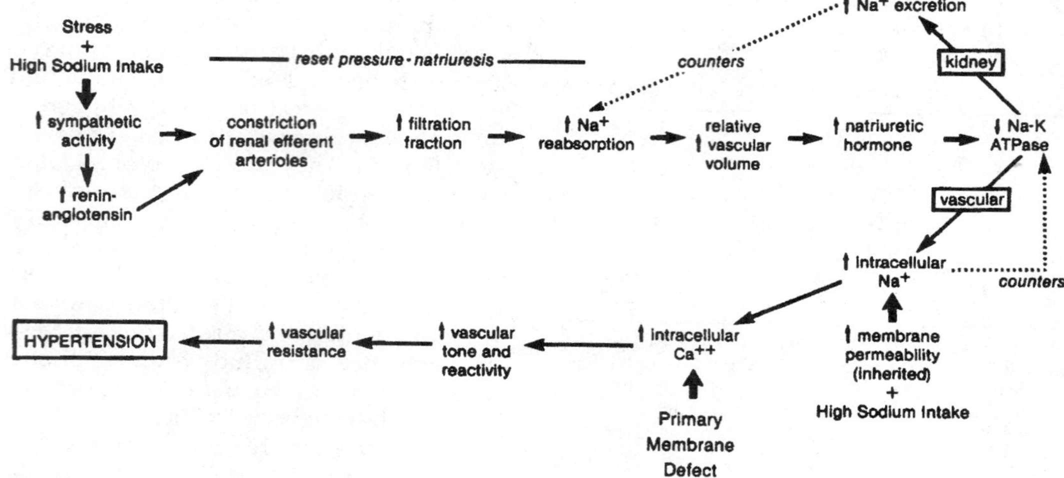

FIGURE 25–3. Hypothesis for the pathogenesis of primary (essential) hypertension, starting from one of three points, shown as *heavy arrows.* The first, starting on the *top left,* is the combination of stress and high sodium intake, which induces an increase in natriuretic hormone and thereby inhibits sodium transport. The second, at the *bottom right,* invokes an inherited defect in sodium transport to induce an increase in intracellular sodium. The third, at the *bottom middle,* suggests a primary membrane defect that directly leads to increased free intracellular calcium. (From Kaplan, N. [1988]. Systemic hypertension: Mechanisms and diagnosis. In Braunwald, E. [Ed.], *Heart disease* [pp. 817–851]. Philadelphia: W. B. Saunders.)

between intracellular and extracellular sodium, potassium, and calcium. This system malfunctions (presumably due to an inherited defect), increasing the amount of intracellular sodium. Sodium heightens contraction of the vascular tissues. Studies also indicate an increase in intracellular calcium, which results in increased vascular tone and reactivity. This increase in intracellular sodium and calcium leads to sustained peripheral resistance, the hallmark of hypertension (Kaplan, 1994).

Figure 25–3 demonstrates the interaction of the various hypotheses suggested for the development of hypertension. These various hypotheses explain the chemical and structural changes found in people with hypertension, but factors such as heredity, obesity, cigarette smoking, diabetes, alcohol, ingestion of excess sodium, and a decrease in potassium intake in American diets, as well as other factors, have been associated with the development of hypertension. Discussion of these factors follows.

Heredity

The role of heredity in the development of hypertension is accepted among scientists and practitioners. Hypertension aggregates in families, and individuals with immediate family members (two or more) with hypertension before the age of 55 years stand a 3.8 times greater risk for development of hypertension (Williams et al., 1991). What is not clearly understood is the exact contribution of heredity and the method of genetic transmission necessary for the development of hypertension. Without a clearer understanding of the causes of primary hypertension, the exact weight of heredity in hypertension may never be known.

The mode of inheritance of hypertension is also a mystery. It is postulated that hypertension may be caused by a genetic defect in cellular transport of sodium, a defect in renal excretion of sodium, or an exaggerated sympathetic response to stress. Hypertension may be the result of one or all of these genetic abnormalities (Kaplan, 1994).

Factors Affecting Hypertension

A variety of factors have been implicated in the acute or chronic elevation of blood pressure. These factors include cigarette smoking, caffeine, alcohol, obesity, diabetes, diet, and stress.

SMOKING. With acute inhalation of nicotine, there is a rise in both systolic pressure and DBP, probably because of the release of norepinephrine. The effects of catecholamines on the vascular system last 15 to 30 minutes. Mann and colleagues (1991), in a study of hypertensives, using ambulatory blood pressure measurements, found a significant increase in blood pressure in smokers. Smoking has been found to increase the development of other cardiovascular diseases and has been linked to an increased death rate in hypertensives. Smoking cessation should be encouraged (Kaplan, 1994).

CAFFEINE. Caffeine does not appear to affect hypertension, although ingestion of this substance in individuals who do not normally ingest it has been found to elevate arterial blood pressure and renin and catecholamine levels. Chronic ingestion results in development of a tolerance, which results in normal secretion of renin and catecholamines as well as a return to a normal blood pressure (Kaplan, 1994).

ALCOHOL. Alcohol has been associated with a rise in arterial pressure in persons consuming more than 2 to 3 ounces daily. Alcohol increases vascular tone, which results in vasoconstriction. Increasing amounts of alcohol appear to correlate with higher blood pressure levels. Therefore, a person who consumes 6 to 7 ounces daily is likely to have higher blood pressure than a person who consumes 4 to 5 ounces daily. A reduction in blood pressure and coronary mortality has been associated with modest (0.5 to 2 ounces daily) consumption of alcohol (Klatsky et al., 1992).

OBESITY. There is a strong correlation between obesity and hypertension. There is a relationship between weight gain and the development of hypertension, especially in young adults and children. The association between obesity and the worsening of atherogenesis was noted in the Framingham Study (Kannel, 1976). Obesity creates an increase in blood volume, resulting in an increase in cardiac output.

DIABETES. Diabetes and hypertension commonly coexist. Recent studies have indicated a link between insulin resistance, hyperinsulinemia, and hypertension (DeFronzo & Ferrannini, 1991; Ferrannini et al., 1987; Kaplan, 1992a). Many hypertensive individuals are insulin resistant, with concommitant hyperinsulinemia. This relationship is not clearly understood, and debate continues on whether hypertension creates or is the result of insulin abnormalities (Kaplan, 1994). It is known that insulin activates the sympathetic system, resulting in vasoconstriction. Insulin is also a vasodilator that serves to maintain normal blood pressure in nonhypertensive people. In obese and hypertensive individuals, insulin enhances and potentiates the sympathetic response, which diminishes the vasodilatory effect, resulting in elevated blood pressure. Kaplan (1992a) notes that much research supports a relationship between hypertension, obesity, diabetes, and hyperlipidemia, but the extent of this relationship needs further study. Hypertension when combined with diabetes results in a significant increase in cardiovascular morbidity and mortality (Assmann & Schulte, 1989).

DIET. Over the past 100 years, food processing has changed the average American diet. Food storage adds sodium and depletes potassium from the food substances (Kaplan, 1994). The correlation between sodium ingestion and blood pressure elevation has been well documented (Cutler et al., 1991; Law et al., 1991). Recent studies have focused on low ingestion of potassium and have found a correlation between decreased potassium levels and hypertension (Tobian, 1988; Veterans Administration Cooperative Study Group on Antihypertensive Agents, 1987). Kaplan (1994) suggests there is a relationship between high sodium and low potassium ingestion that plays a role in hypertension.

STRESS. Stress stimulates the sympathetic nervous system, resulting in increased cardiac output, vasoconstriction, and enhanced excretion of renin. Hyperactivity of the sympathetic nervous system has been demonstrated in response to mental stress, physical activity, exposure to cold, and postural changes in individuals with hypertension (Kaplan, 1994). Whether stress itself or the hypertensive individual's response to stress results in hypertension is unknown. Studies have shown a greater degree of hostility and anger and suppression of these emotions in hypertensive people (Schneider et al., 1986).

SECONDARY HYPERTENSION

Although primary hypertension accounts for the majority of individuals with hypertension, approximately 5% to 10% of all hypertensives have secondary hypertension, or hypertension with a known cause. After identifying the cause, the treatment may be tailored to eradicate the hypertension. An extensive list of possible causes is found in Table 25–1.

Oral Contraceptives

Oral contraceptives containing estrogen are the most common cause of secondary hypertension in women (Kaplan, 1992c). Progestogen, contained in oral contraceptive preparations, has also been shown to increase blood pressure. The hypertensive effects of both estrogen and progestogen are dose dependent. With increasing amounts of each hormone, blood pressure levels elevate (Meade, 1988). The severity of hypertension is usually mild, but does increase over time with oral contraceptive use. Hypertension is one of the major contributors to the increased incidence of cardiovascular mortality seen in women using oral contraceptives. Concomitant use of cigarettes and alcohol in excess of 10 ounces/week increases a woman's risk of cardiovascular mortality. Hypertension is probably caused by stimulation of the renin-angiotensin-aldosterone mechanism, creating volume expansion in oral contraceptive users (Kaplan, 1992c). The structural and functional changes associated with contraceptive use include enhanced blood clot formation, increased coronary artery vascular tone, increased fibroblast deposition, and enhanced cellular replication in vessel walls (Royal College of Practitioners Oral Contraception Study, 1981; Stadel, 1981).

Renal Parenchymal Disease

Renal parenchymal disease resulting in hypertension is associated with chronic glomerulonephritis and acute oliguric renal failure. Both of these entities, if untreated, result in renal damage that alters the renal pressor system and/or inappropriately stimulates the renin–angiotensin mechanisms (Laragh & Pickering, 1991). Acquired infections or polycystic kidney disease can alter renal function as well. Renal parenchymal disease may account for 2% to 5% of the hypertensive population (Kaplan, 1992a).

Renovascular Disease

Another common cause of secondary hypertension is renovascular disease. Estimates indicate that about 3% of the hypertensive population has renovascular disease causing hypertension (Hall et al., 1994). This increase in systemic vascular resistance is the result of stenosis caused by fibrous dysplasia or atherosclerosis of one or more of the renal arteries. This decrease in renal flow results in an overproduction and release of renin–angiotension. Production of renin is also stimulated by the sympathetic nervous system, predominantly through catecholamine release. Hypokalemia is a common finding of renovascular hypertension and is a result of the stimulation of aldosterone by angiotensin II. Aldosterone further elevates peripheral resistance by decreasing absorption of sodium, causing an increase in extracellular fluid (Laragh & Pickering, 1991).

Primary Aldosteronism

Primary aldosteronism is caused by an adenoma on the adrenal gland or an adenomatous hyperplasia of the adrenal gland, resulting in overproduction of aldosterone. This creates an excess of salt and water, which is the mechanism behind the development of hypertension with this disease. The percentage of hypertensives with this disease is estimated at less than 1%. This is the most common of the steroid-induced hypertensions. Other disease entities that alter steroid production and result in hypertension include Cushing syndrome, adrenogenital syndrome, and 17-hydroxylase and 11-hydroxylase deficiencies (Dustan, 1986).

Pheochromocytoma

Pheochromocytoma, a tumor located in the adrenal glands, is a rare cause of hypertension. This tumor oversecretes catecholamine, causing an increase in peripheral resistance through vasoconstriction. This disease may cause fluctuations in blood pressure or may result in sustained hypertension that is often difficult to control. In addition to hypertension, the practitioner will see headache, sweating, palpitations, anxiety, and weight loss. Pheochromocytomas have a strong familiar link. Stroke and myocardial infarction have been associated with rapid, significant elevations in blood pressure in this disease process (Dustan, 1986; Kaplan, 1992a).

Coarctation of the Thoracic Aorta

This localized lesion develops in the thoracic portion of the aorta just below the ligamentum arteriosum. This constriction reduces the lumen of the aorta significantly or may result in complete obliteration (Dustan, 1986; Kaplan, 1992a). The hallmark presentation of coarctation is an elevated arterial pressure in the upper extremities and low or absent pressures in the lower extremities. The mechanisms of hypertension are vasoconstriction and an increase in fluid volume secondary to alterations in renal function (Kaplan, 1992a).

Pregnancy-Induced Hypertension

Pregnancy-induced hypertension (PIH) is an important cause of maternal morbidity and mortality and fetal mortality (Assche et al., 1989). PIH is the term used to include preeclampsia, toxemia, and chronic hypertension exacerbated by pregnancy. It may occur in previously normotensive women or may intensify in chronic hypertensive subjects (Koniak-Griffin & Dodgson, 1987). The definition of hypertension in PIH is a blood pressure greater than 140/90 mm Hg, or a systolic increase of 30 mm Hg or a diastolic increase greater than 15 mm Hg from baseline readings. These measurements need to be obtained on two separate occasions at least 6 hours apart (Cunningham et al., 1993).

Signs of preeclampsia are hypertension, edema, and proteinuria after the twentieth week of gestation. Eclampsia is a severe manifestation of PIH and includes significant alterations in cerebral function that result in grand mal seizures (Cunningham et al., 1993). See Chapter 69 for further discussion.

Another severe manifestation of PIH is the HELLP syndrome. This acronym stands for hemolysis, elevated liver function tests, and low platelets (Weinstein, 1982). Symptoms associated with this syndrome are malaise, nausea with or without emesis, epigastric pain, right upper quadrant tenderness on examination, and edema. Frequently these patients present with blood pressures greater than 160/110 mm Hg. Clinical signs include elevated levels of serum aspartate aminotransferase, formerly called SGOT, serum alanine aminotransferase, also called SGPT, bilirubin, blood urea nitrogen (BUN), creatinine, and more than 2+ proteinuria. Disturbances in the hematologic profile include decreases in the hematocrit and platelet count and an abnormal peripheral blood smear (Weinstein, 1982). HELLP syndrome may be superimposed on preeclampsia or eclampsia. Without rapid and aggressive treatment, infant and maternal mortality is high.

Hypertensive Crisis

Although hypertensive crisis is rare, its recognition and treatment must be rapid and aggressive. Most hypertensive crises occur in patients with preexisting hypertension, primary or secondary. Disease entities commonly associated with hypertensive crisis are essential hypertension, chronic renal disease, toxemia of pregnancy, renovascular hypertension, pheochromocytoma, acute glomerulonephritis, and certain medications (Kaplan, 1994). The determinants of crisis are an elevated DBP (usually 130–140 mm Hg), the rapidity with which the blood pressure rises (often within hours), and evidence of acute target organ damage. Ram (1991) categorized hypertensive crisis into emergencies and urgencies. Emergencies are defined as hypertension causing target organ damage such that prognosis will be poor unless the blood pressure is decreased within 1 to 3 hours. Treatment requires the use of parenteral agents. Urgencies are acute hypertensive episodes that pose a less immediate life threat but if sustained, will result in serious complications. Reduction of blood pressure should occur within 3 to 24 hours, often with the use of oral agents. Table 25–3 provides a list of clinical problems that, combined with hypertension, require an immediate reduction in blood pressure. Hypertensive crisis classified as an urgency may rapidly develop into an emergency (Gonzales & Ram, 1988).

TABLE 25–3. **Circumstances Requiring Rapid Treatment of Hypertension**

Hypertensive Emergencies

Cerebrovascular
- Hypertensive encephalopathy
- Intracerebral hemorrhage
- Subarachnoid hemorrhage

Cardiac
- Acute aortic dissection
- Acute left ventricular failure
- Acute or impending myocardial infarction
- After coronary bypass surgery

Excessive circulating catecholamines
- Pheochromocytoma crisis
- Food or drug interactions with monoamine oxidase inhibitors
- Sympathomimetic drug abuse (cocaine)

Eclampsia
Head injury
Postoperative bleeding from vascular suture lines
Severe epistaxis

Hypertensive Urgencies

Accelerated–malignant hypertension
Atherothrombotic brain infarction with severe hypertension
Rebound hypertension after sudden cessation of antihypertensive drugs
Surgical
- Severe hypertension in patients requiring immediate surgery
- Postoperative hypertension
- Severe hypertension after kidney transplantation

Severe body burns

From Kaplan, N. (1994). *Clinical hypertension* (p. 282). Baltimore: Williams & Wilkins.

TABLE 25–4. **Keith-Wagener Scale for Funduscopic Examination**

KW1 = Minimal arteriolar narrowing and irregularity.

KW2 = More marked narrowing and arteriovenous nicking. Implies arteriosclerotic as well as hypertensive changes.

KW3 = Flame-shaped or circular hemorrhages and fluffy "cotton wool" exudates.

KW4 = Any of the above plus papilledema (i.e., elevation of the optic disk, obliteration of the physiologic cup, or blurring of the disk margins). By definition, malignant hypertension is always associated with papilledema.

From Sokolow, M. (1985). In Krup, M., Chalton, M., & Werdegan, D. (Eds.), *Current medical diagnosis and treatment*. Los Altos, CA: Lange Medical Publications.

Accelerated hypertension is defined as significantly elevated blood pressure (DBP greater than 130 mm Hg) with hemorrhages and exudate (grade 3 on the Keith-Wagener scale; Table 25–4) on funduscopic examination (Ram, 1991; Kaplan, 1992a). Malignant hypertension is defined as a marked elevation in blood pressure (DBP greater than 140 mm Hg) with a grade 4 Keith-Wagener funduscopic examination, which includes the findings of grade 3 and papilledema (see Table 25–4). Kaplan (1994) notes that because the clinical symptoms and prognosis are similar in both, the term used should be accelerated–malignant hypertension. Although the incidence of accelerated–malignant hypertension is declining, the syndrome is more common in young, poor, black, or Hispanic individuals. There is some correlation with smoking and preexisting hypertension and the development of this syndrome (Kaplan, 1994).

PATHOPHYSIOLOGY. It is likely that significant and rapid elevations in blood pressure or involvement of other factors set off a cascade of events resulting in the physiologic changes considered the hallmark of accelerated–malignant hypertension (Kaplan, 1994; Ram, 1991). Figure 25–4 outlines the structural and functional changes that occur in hypertensive crisis. The effects of elevated arterial pressure result in endothelial damage and platelet deposition. With this abnormality, myointimal proliferation occurs, with fibrinoid necrosis found most notably in the interlobular arteries of the kidneys. This vascular damage may occur throughout the arterial system. Sections of the arterioles are constricted and dilated, creating a "sausage"-like pattern that likely enhances platelet deposition and the development of microangiopathic hemolytic anemia. There is an increase in secretion of renin, aldosterone, catecholamines, and vasopressin that sustains and potentially elevates the blood pressure, creating further vascular damage and tissue ischemia (Kaplan, 1994; Ram, 1991).

CLINICAL MANIFESTATIONS. The clinical presentation of accelerated–malignant hypertension is a markedly

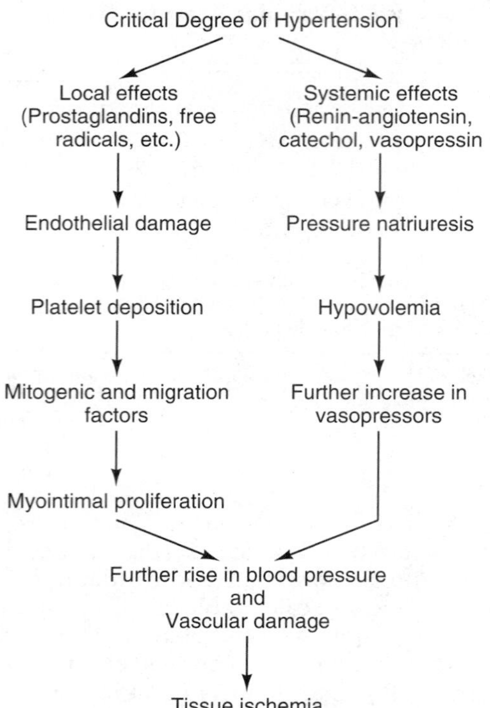

FIGURE 25–4. Scheme for initiation and progression of accelerated–malignant hypertension. (From Kaplan, N. [1994]. *Clinical hypertension.* Baltimore: Williams & Wilkins.)

elevated DBP, usually 130 to 140 mm Hg, with recent onset or progressive end-organ damage (JNC, 1993). Neurologic symptoms may include headache (a frequent presenting symptom), confusion, lethargy, stupor, hemiparesis, seizures, and coma. Visual impairment to include vision loss and diplopia may be present, especially if the funduscopic examination reveals papilledema (Kaplan, 1994; Rubenstein & Escalante, 1989). Renal manifestations include oliguria and azotemia. Urinalysis reveals gross or microscopic blood and is positive for protein and hyaline or red cell casts. Cardiac presentation may include cardiac enlargement, prominent apical pulse, and congestive heart failure. Anemia is especially common in patients with renal insufficiency, as is an elevated BUN and creatinine. Hypokalemia is usually present due to hyperaldosteronism (Kaplan, 1994; Kaplan, 1992b; McKinney, 1992).

Hypertensive Encephalopathy

Because of aggressive detection and treatment of elevated arterial pressure, the occurrence of hypertensive encephalopathy is uncommon. Although any cause of a rapid elevation in blood pressure may precipitate this syndrome, it is more common as a complication of glomerulonephritis, eclampsia, and accelerated–malignant hypertension (Ram, 1991). Encephalopathy may result despite no evidence of other vascular abnormalities seen in accelerated–malignant hypertension. As in eclampsia, the blood pressure need not be markedly elevated to produce the signs and symptoms of encephalopathy. An abrupt rise in a normotensive person may cause hypertensive encephalopathy, whereas a chronically hypertensive individual may require markedly elevated pressures for this syndrome to develop (Kaplan, 1992).

Normally, as arterial blood pressure rises, the cerebral vessels constrict, and as blood pressure falls, vessels vasodilate. Cerebral blood flow is maintained through this mechanism, called autoregulation. As arterial pressure rises significantly, the autoregulatory mechanism is disrupted, and vasodilation results. This causes fluid to be forced into the perivascular space, resulting in cerebral edema. Cerebral ischemia may be a result of vasospasm of the arterioles (Rubenstein & Escalante, 1989). Both of these physiologic abnormalities result in cerebral edema (Ram, 1991).

As cerebral edema worsens, the patient experiences persistent headache and visual impairment ranging from blurred vision to transient blindness. Altered mental status is common and can present anywhere on the continuum from slight disorientation to coma. Seizures are more common in children, but can occur in adults with encephalopathy. Nausea and vomiting may result as intracranial pressure increases.

EVALUATION AND DIAGNOSIS OF HYPERTENSIVE EMERGENCIES

A diagnosis of hypertensive crisis is not made on the basis of one reading; several readings demonstrating markedly abnormal elevations in blood pressure combined with evidence of target organ damage need to be validated to make the diagnosis. A detailed history and physical examination need to be rapidly obtained. The work-up should address the issue of primary versus secondary hypertension, involvement of target organs, and determination of other cardiovascular risk factors (Hall et al., 1994; JNC, 1993; Kaplan, 1994).

A history should include previous medical conditions such as hypertension, coronary artery disease, renal disease, peripheral vascular disease, diabetes, and retinopathy (Rubenstein & Escalante, 1989). Assessment of additional cardiovascular risk factors is important. A thorough history should determine the occurrence of angina, previous myocardial infarction, transient ischemic attacks, stroke, and claudication, and family history needs to be assessed. Other cardiac risk factors need to be assessed such as obesity, cigarette smoking, and hyperlipidemia. A medication history to include prescribed, over-the-counter, and illegal drug use is important (Kaplan, 1992b). Drugs that have been implicated in the development of hypertensive emergencies include steroids, oral contraceptive pills, cyclosporin, monoamine oxidase (MAO) inhibitors, nonsteroidal antiinflammatory agents, tricyclic antidepressants, cocaine, amphetamines, nasal decongestants and other cold remedies, and appetite suppressants (JNC, 1993). Abrupt withdrawal of medications such as clonidine or beta blockers may precipitate a crisis. Dietary information of importance includes ingestion of fat and sodium, and alcohol use.

Stress stimulates the sympathetic nervous system and may create episodic hypertension. Determining relevant socioeconomic factors, including employment, financial status, and compliance may assist in determining causative factors and interventions needed after blood pressure is controlled.

Physical examination, laboratory tests, and diagnostic procedures are performed to determine the extent of target organ damage and to search for clues that might yield a cause for hypertension. A thorough physical assessment is important, but should not delay treatment of this life-threatening condition. The target organs most affected by hypertension are the heart, kidneys, and brain. Each of these systems is reviewed to highlight the sequelae of uncontrolled hypertension.

Cardiovascular System

The Framingham Study found that hypertension was the leading cause of heart failure (Kannel, 1976). Cardiac damage caused by hypertension is manifested as either coronary artery disease or left ventricular hypertrophy (Fig. 25–5).

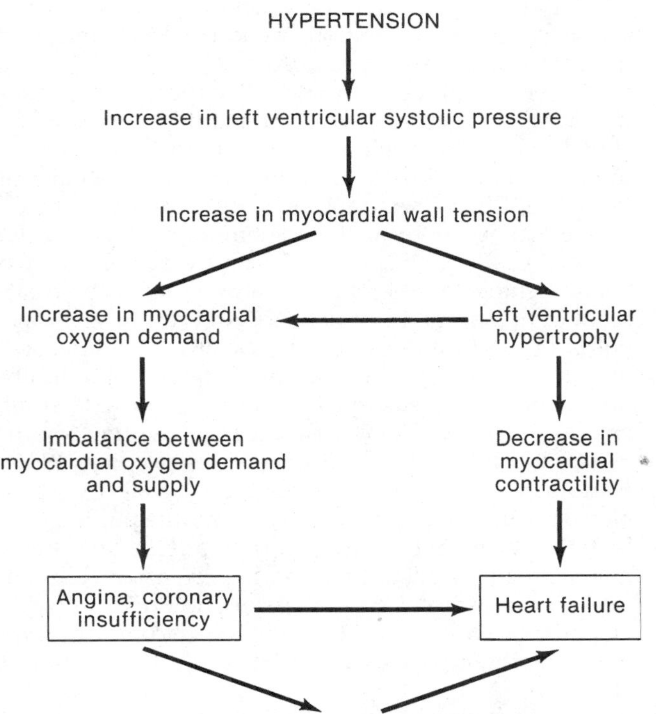

FIGURE 25–5. Effects of hypertension on myocardial function. (From Hollander, W. [1976]. Role of hypertension in atherosclerosis and cardiovascular disease. *American Journal of Cardiology, 38,* 786.)

Clinical signs, including rales, jugular venous distention, ventricular gallop, edema, and an apical impulse diameter greater than 3 cm in the left lateral position indicate left ventricular hypertrophy. A cardiothoracic ratio greater than 0.5 on chest x-ray supports this diagnosis. An electrocardiogram (ECG) is valuable in determining evidence of left ventricular strain as well as for providing a baseline cardiac assessment. Although the chest x-ray and ECG can be of assistance, a more sensitive detector of early left ventricular hypertrophy is the echocardiogram (Savage et al., 1979). Left ventricular mass index, interventricular septal thickness, posterior wall thickness, and mean muscle mass can be determined from the echocardiogram and can provide the practitioner with valuable information about the effects of hypertension on the left ventricle (Kaplan, 1994).

Angina and myocardial infarction are twice as prevalent in hypertensive as in normotensive individuals. Angina may be related to a lack of adequate microcirculation for the increased muscle mass of left ventricular hypertrophy (Kaplan, 1994). Hypertension enhances the development of atherosclerosis. Myocardial infarction, recognized and unrecognized, is twice as common in individuals with hypertension. Frequently after a myocardial infarction the blood pressure normalizes, and hypertension may elude detection. Kannel (1976) suggests performing frequent ECGs in hypertensive patients to assist in earlier detection and prevention of myocardial damage. Arterial blood gases may be warranted if the person displays signs and symptoms of respiratory distress. If cardiac symptoms are present or dysfunction is suspected, serial creatine phosphokinase and lactic dehydrogenase levels with isoenzymes are obtained every 8 hours for 2 days to determine myocardial damage.

Renal System

Uncontrolled hypertension may result in renal failure. It is the second most common cause of end-stage renal disease just after diabetes (Kaplan, 1994). Renal effects include arteriosclerotic lesions, especially in the afferent and efferent tubules and glomerular capillary tufts (Kaplan, 1994). Signs of renal impairment are usually nocturia and albuminuria. Elevated uric acid is a common finding and is probably caused by nephrosclerosis. In most hypertensives, renal impairment is slow and does not affect daily living, but in hypertensive individuals in whom accelerated–malignant hypertension develops, renal damage may progress rapidly and may result in death (Kaplan, 1994). Uncontrolled hypertension leads to progressive renal impairment, causing azotemia, uremia, and death. A complete chemistry panel is important in determining the extent of renal involvement and potential reversible causes of the hypertensive emergency. Glucose levels may be elevated as in diabetes, Cushing syndrome, or pheochromocytoma, which are predisposing conditions for hypertensive crisis.

Cerebral System

Hypertensive hemorrhage, hypertensive encephalopathy, and lacunar infarction almost always occur in the presence of hypertension. Chronic arterial pressure elevation causes damage to the vessel wall, resulting in leakage of plasma into the wall and creating microaneurysms (Kaplan, 1994). This destruction occurs predominantly in the small-resistance vessels in the brain. Occlusion of the larger vessels in the brain is the result of atherosclerosis and thrombosis. Serial neurologic examinations and computed tomography are needed to determine the extent of damage to the brain.

TREATMENT OF HYPERTENSIVE EMERGENCIES

The goal of treatment is to limit damage to target organs and inflict few, if any, treatment-related adverse effects (JNC, 1993). Treatment depends on the degree of severity of hypertension.

For hypertensive emergencies, a fast-acting, potent vasodilator is needed to prevent death or major target organ damage. These patients are admitted to the intensive care unit and arterial lines are inserted. In the event of hypertensive urgency, patients can be managed in an environment where quick administration of rapid-acting oral agents and careful observation can be obtained.

Table 25–5 lists medications commonly used in the treatment of hypertensive crisis. Mean arterial pressure should be lowered 20% to 25% over 2 to 3 hours, because too rapid a decline may result in worsening of target organ damage, especially cerebral (Kaplan, 1994; McKinney, 1992). The parenteral drug selected depends on the patient's clinical condition, fluid status, existing medical problems, target organ impairment, and pharmacodynamics of the medication.

The four most commonly used direct vasodilators are sodium nitroprusside (nipride), nitroglycerin, diazoxide, and apresoline. In hypertensive emergencies, the most common and effective medication used is nipride (Prisant et al., 1993). Onset of action is within seconds and lasts 1 to 5 minutes. The wide range of drug levels allows for the patient's clinical response to quide administration. It is usually not used in patients with ongoing myocardial ischemia. The drug is metabolized to thiocyanate and cyanide in the liver and excreted via the kidneys; therefore, caution should be used in patients with renal impairment. Cyanide toxicity is rare in doses less than 2 μg/kg/minute (Prisant et al., 1993). Nipride has been implicated in coronary steal phenomena, which may decrease blood supply to the heart. Coronary steal phenomena may occur when potent vasodilators shift blood supply from atherosclerotic areas to portions of the coronary arteries that are clean. The myocardium most in need of blood receives a decreased supply, which may result in angina, infarction, or dysrhythmias. Profound hypotension resulting in target organ ischemia can also be a side effect of this drug. Other adverse effects include a tendency toward increased intracranial pressure (Kaplan, 1992a).

Depending on the condition that has caused or complicated the hypertensive emergency, other drugs may be preferred. Nitroglycerin is the antihypertensive of choice in patients who are experiencing myocardial ischemia, because of its cardiac-protective action. A pulmonary artery catheter may be inserted if heart failure is evident or cardiac involvement is hindering control of blood pressure. Nitroglycerin increases intracranial pressure and is contraindicated in hypertensive encephalopathy (Prisant et al., 1993). Side effects include headache, flushing, and reflex tachycardia. Tolerance to the drug has been noted after 24 to 48 hours (Prisant et al., 1993).

Diazoxide, another potent vasodilator, is administered in bolus form. This drug may be useful because it decreases the episodes of uncontrolled drops in blood pressure that may be detrimental in some patients (Prisant et al., 1993). The side effects of this medication include salt and water retention, reflex tachycardia, hyperglycemia, hyperuricemia, and reduced renal blood flow.

Another antihypertensive commonly used in the obstetric patient is hydralazine, because it maintains and increases uterine blood flow. The medication is administered in bolus doses. It is contraindicated in coronary, carotid, and intracranial atherosclerosis (Prisant et al., 1993). Side effects include reflex tachycardia, salt and water retention, myocardial ischemia, and increased intracranial pressure.

Other agents used in specific hypertensive crises include phentolamine, which is helpful in excess catecholamine states, such as pheochromoctoma and the interaction of an MAO inhibitor and a food containing tyramine. Effects are transient and there are reported side effects of myocardial ischemia and tachycardia (Prisant et al., 1993). Labetalol and esmolol are two beta-blocking agents that are being used in the treatment of hypertensive crisis. Labetalol can be given via bolus or continuous infusion, usually at a rate of 2 mg/minute. It is an alpha and beta receptor inhibitor; it decreases vasospasm and may provide some cranial protection. Onset of action is within 5 minutes, and effects last for 3 to 6 hours (Kaplan, 1994). Esmolol is a very short acting, cardioselective beta blocker with effects lasting for 30 minutes. It is given in bolus form and is frequently used in anesthesia management of postintubation hypertension (Kaplan, 1994). Both esmolol and labetalol should be avoided in patients with ventricular failure, chronic obstructive pulmonary disease, and heart blocks (Prisant et al., 1993).

Diuretics may be indicated if the patient is in heart failure or has fluid overload. As blood pressure declines, renal sodium reabsorption occurs and may necessitate the use of diuretics, to maintain desired blood pressure levels. In hypovolemia associated with hy-

TABLE–25–5. **Management of Hypertensive Crisis: Emergencies and Urgencies***

Drug	Dose	Onset	Cautions
Parenteral Vasodilators			
Sodium nitroprusside	0.25–10 μg/kg per min as IV infusion; maximal dose for 10 min only	Instantaneous	Nausea, vomiting, muscle twitching; with prolonged use may cause thiocyanate intoxication, methemoglobinemia acidosis, cyanide poisoning; bags, bottles, and delivery sets must be light resistant
Nitroglycerin	5–100 μg as IV infusion	2–5 min	Headache, tachycardia, vomiting, flushing, methemoglobinemia; requires special delivery system due to drug binding to PVC tubing
Diazoxide	50–150 mg as IV bolus, repeated, or 15–30 mg/min by IV infusion	1–2 min	Hypotension, tachycardia, aggravation of angina pectoris, nausea and vomiting, hyperglycemia with repeated injections
Hydralazine	10–20 mg as IV volus 10–40 mg IM	10 min 20–30 min	Tachycardia, headache, vomiting, aggravation of angina pectoris
Enalapril	0.625–1.25 mg every 6 hours IV	15–60 min	Renal failure in patients with bilateral renal artery stenosis, hypotension
Parenteral Adrenergic Inhibitors			
Phentolamine	5–15 mg as IV bolus	1–2 min	Tachycardia, orthostatic hypotension
Trimethaphan camsylate	1–4 mg/min as IV infusion	1–5 min	Paresis of bowel and bladder, orthostatic hypotension, blurred vision, dry mouth
Labetalol	20–80 mg as IV bolus every 10 min; 2 mg/min as IV infusion	5–10 min	Bronchoconstriction, heart block, orthostatic hypotension
Methyldopate	250–500 mg as IV infusion every 6 hours	30–60 min	Drowsiness
Oral Agents			
Nifedipine (not extended release)	10–20 mg PO, repeat after 30 min	15–30 min	Rapid, uncontrolled reduction in blood pressure may precipitate circulatory collapse in patients with aortic stenosis
Captopril	25 mg PO, repeat as required	15–30 min	Hypotension, renal failure in bilateral renal artery stenosis
Clonidine	0.1–0.2 mg PO, repeated every hour as required to a total dose of 0.6 mg	30–60 min	Hypotension, drowsiness, dry mouth
Labetalol	200–400 mg PO, repeat every 2–3 hours	30 min–2 hours	Bronchoconstriction, heart block, orthostatic hypotension

*It is sometimes appropriate to administer a diuretic agent with any of these drugs.

Abbreviations: IV, intravenous; IM, intramuscular; PO, orally; PVC, polyvinyl chloride.

From Joint National Committee on Detection, Evaluation and Treatment of High Blood Pressure. (1993). The fifth report of the Joint National Committee on Detection, Evaluation and Treatment of High Blood Pressure. *Archives of Internal Medicine, 153,* 154–183.

pertensive crisis, fluid resuscitation with isotonic agents may be indicated (Kaplan, 1994).

Once blood pressure is stabilized, patients require oral agents, which are started before discontinuing the parenteral infusion. Blood pressure is then gradually decreased over several days to prevent unnecessary side effects. Kaplan (1994) notes that patients after hypertensive crisis are most likely to require a multiple-drug regime effectively to control arterial pressure. The search for secondary causes of the crisis should continue once the patient is out of danger (Kaplan, 1994). The next section provides a brief review of the management of secondary hypertension, which is often a precipitator of hypertensive crisis.

MANAGEMENT OF SECONDARY HYPERTENSION

If the blood pressure remains elevated despite pharmacologic treatment of hypertension with a combination of medications, the search for secondary causes may prove fruitful. Medical and surgical interventions are discussed for each of the identified causes.

Oral Contraceptives

Decreasing the dose of estrogen and progestogen found in oral contraceptives may be effective in reducing blood pressure. Discontinuation of oral contraceptives may be necessary; results indicate a return of blood pressure to normal within 3 to 6 months (Kaplan, 1994). Recent studies indicate that oral contraceptives with low-dose estrogen can be prescribed in healthy, nonsmoking, premenopausal women between the ages of 35 and 44 years (Mishell, 1988). Women older than 35 years of age with hypertension or cardiovascular risk factors (obesity, cigarette smoking, or family history) should be encouraged to use alternative means of birth control (Mishell, 1988). If this is not possible, antihypertensives can be effective in controlling hypertension. Close monitoring of blood pressure is necessary in this group of patients.

Renal Parenchymal Disease

Chronic renal disease is one of the most common causes of hypertension. Glomerulonephritis, pyelonephritis, polycystic disease, and diabetic nephropathy damage the kidneys, creating insufficiency and ultimately failure. Glomerulonephritis and pyelonephritis are becoming less common causes; early diagnosis and treatment are preventing their chronic occurrence. Hemodialysis or renal transplantation is the treatment for renal failure. Hypertension may or may not accompany renal failure. If hypertension is present, antihypertensive medications are indicated to control blood pressure (Smith & Dunn, 1991). On occasion, severe refractory hypertension may necessitate a nephrectomy. The advent of potent agents such as minoxidil has decreased the need for surgical removal of the kidney or kidneys.

Renovascular Hypertension

Atherosclerosis, fibromuscular disease, and renal artery aneurysms are common causes of renovascular hypertension. Although medical management can control blood pressure, surgical procedures produce excellent long-term relief of hypertension and preservation of renal function in most patients (Lawrie et al., 1989). Common surgical procedures include Dacron grafting, endarterectomy, and angioplasty. Recurrence of hypertension requires reoperation or medical management. Fibromuscular disease appears to respond favorably to angioplasty, whereas atherosclerotic lesions respond well to grafting and endarterectomy. Angioplasty can be performed only on accessible vessels, and thus its use is limited. There is an approximate reocclusion rate of 20%, necessitating another angioplasty procedure. Lawrie and colleagues (1989), in a retrospective review of 916 patients with renovascular lesions, found that age significantly affected long-term prognosis. Diffuse atherosclerosis in the elderly may have affected their prognosis in that myocardial infarction was the most common cause of death in the age group older than 62 years. These physicians recommend conservative medical management of the elderly unless hypertension is refractory or renal impairment occurs.

Primary Aldosteronism

In those patients with bilateral hyperplasia, those who are unable or unwilling to undergo surgery, and those who remain hypertensive after surgery, medical management is indicated (Kaplan, 1994). Spironolactone and amiloride are the agents of choice. Large doses of spironolactone, 300 to 400 mg daily, are used to initiate treatment. After adequate blood pressure control has been achieved, daily doses may be as low as 50 mg. Low-dose thiazides may be added to maintain adequate blood pressure control and to decrease the dose of spironolactone, thereby mitigating the side effects of both medications.

In patients with solitary adenomas, surgical intervention is indicated. Preoperative management includes administration of spironolactone to assist in determining the hypertensive response postsurgery and to correct fluid and electrolyte deficits. Removal of the adenoma usually results in a return to normal of the fluids and electrolytes within 6 months. Hypertension may persist and can be medically managed. If bilateral hyperplasia is found during surgical exploration, surgical removal of the left adrenal is preferred. There are significant complications from bilateral adrenalectomies. The removal of only one adrenal gland may be a judicious course (Kaplan, 1994; Wells & Santen, 1986).

Pheochromocytoma

Pheochromocytoma results in excessive secretion of catecholamines. These tumors arise from chromaffin cells that may be found anywhere along the sympathetic system, but are most commonly located in the adrenal gland. If missed, a pheochromocytoma may result in fatal hypertensive crisis during anesthesia, childbirth, or other stress (Kaplan, 1994).

Medical management is indicated if the patient is unable to have surgery or is in hypertensive crisis. Alpha-blocking agents such as dibenzyline or prazosin are effective in reducing the blood pressure. Beta blockers may be added only after adequate alpha blockade has been achieved. These agents blunt the tachycardia and dysrhythmias seen with excessive catecholamine excretion. Intravenous administration of phentolamine (an alpha-blocking agent) in 2- to 5-mg boluses every 5 minutes is effective in treatment of hypertensive crisis to achieve rapid control of the arterial pressure (Kaplan, 1994).

Surgical intervention is the preferred treatment for pheochromocytomas. There is a high mortality if blood pressure is not adequately controlled at the time of surgery. Preoperative treatment requires medication to control blood pressure and restore diminished blood volumes. Minimal mortality rates are associated with adequate preoperative treatment and vigorous intraoperative blood volume restoration.

Coarctation of the Thoracic Artery

Surgical correction of this damaged artery is the preferred treatment. The hypertension associated with coarctation can be treated with antihypertensive medications. Balloon angioplasty has been tried in limited numbers and appears to be effective, but requires long-term follow-up to determine its efficacy (Driscoll, 1992).

Pregnancy-Induced Hypertension

The most effective treatment is delivery of the fetus if maturity of the infant allows. Magnesium sulfate is administered to alleviate seizures, and an antihypertensive agent is given intravenously to control DBP greater than 110 mm Hg (Cunningham et al., 1993; Shannon, 1987). When the fetus is immature, the mother is placed on bedrest. If diastolic blood pressure remains greater than 105 mm Hg, antihypertensive medications are indicated. Hydralazine is the most common medication used, but nifedipine and labetalol have been tried with success.

CLINICAL MANAGEMENT

Critical care nurses monitor and provide intervention to numerous patients with all degrees of severity of hypertension. The initial responsibility of the critical care nurse is to assist with line insertion and stabilization of the patient's blood pressure. Continuous ECG and blood pressure monitoring is necessary. The collaborative efforts of the nurse and physician work to optimize patient health and to minimize target organ damage. The JNC (1993) cautions health care providers accurately to assess patients' blood pressure to provide safe and effective treatment. Administering the vasoactive medication of choice and monitoring the patient for response to the drug is essential. Keeping the physician informed of the patient's clinical response and making recommendations for changes in medication or dosages are integral nursing responsibilities.

As a pivotal member of the health care team, the nurse's initial and ongoing assessment of the patient's clinical status is essential to proper management of hypertension. Nurses also play a vital role in identifying hypertension in patients in whom it was previously undiagnosed. Physical examination includes assessment of heart sounds for an S3 or S4, which are present in heart failure, and determination of the width and location of the point of maximal impulse, which, if widened and displaced, indicates cardiac enlargement. Examination of the jugular veins for distention and evidence of peripheral and sacral edema further confirms the diagnosis of heart failure. Auscultation of the lungs every 4 hours to determine the absence or presence of rales is necessary to confirm heart failure and monitor therapy. A review of the patient's 12-lead ECG for signs of left ventricular strain assists the nurse and physician in providing the care needed.

A neurologic assessment is obtained every 4 hours and prn changes in mental status, development of motor disturbance, and rapid, marked elevations in arterial pressure are noted. Close monitoring of the patient for signs and symptoms of cerebral encephalopathy is needed. Scrupulous attention to fluid status with notations of intake and output and daily weights are important in managing hypertension owing to the frequency of renal impairment and fluid retention seen with the vasodilators used to control arterial pressure.

Examination of the abdomen may reveal a bruit over the flank area indicating renal artery stenosis. Weak femoral and popliteal pulses combined with hypertension in the upper extremities may be indicative of coarctation of the thoracic aorta.

Patients in hypertensive crisis are often anxious, and those with cerebral involvement may be agitated. This emotional state worsens the patient's blood pressure. The nurse's calm and caring manner helps to decrease anxiety. Keeping patients and significant others informed of procedures, results, and clinical condition, as well as encouraging verbalization of fears, assists in decreasing anxiety. A quiet, calm environment for the patient may be beneficial.

The nurse's relationship with the patient and family plays a vital role in assessing the patient's response to therapy and his or her understanding of the disease process, health beliefs, degree of compliance, and other psychological and social factors affecting adequate arterial pressure control. These data assist the nurse in developing a plan to address the educational needs of the patient and significant others.

SUMMARY

The physical examination, history, laboratory findings, and radiologic procedures such as echocardiography, aortography, renal artery arteriography, and renal ultrasound provide the nurse and physician with sufficient data to develop and implement a plan of care to meet the needs of patients in hypertensive crisis. The critical care nurse's understanding of the disease process and clinical manifestations, and his or her rapid implementation of care as well as close monitoring of the patient's responses, are necessary for safe and effective treatment of this emergency.

REFERENCES

Assche, F., Spitz, B., & Vansteelant, L. (1989). Severe systemic hypertension during pregnancy. *American Journal of Cardiology, 63,* 22C–25C.

Assmann, G., & Schulte, H. (1989). Diabetes and hypertension in the elderly: Concomitant hyperlipidemia and coronary heart disease risk. *American Journal of Cardiology, 63,* 33H–37H.

Cunningham, F. MacDonald, P., Gant, N., Leveno, K., & Gilstrap, L. (1993). Hypertensive disorders of pregnancy. In F. Cunningham et al. (Eds.), *William obstetrics* (19th ed., pp. 763–817). Norwalk, CT: Appleton and Lange.

Cutler J., Follmann, D., Elliot, P., & Suh, I. (1991). An overview of randomized trials of sodium reduction and blood pressure. *Hypertension, 17*(Suppl I), I27–I33.

DeFronzo, R., & Ferrannini, E. (1991). Insulin resistance: A multifaceted syndrome responsible for NIDDM, obesity, hypertension, dyslipidemia and atherosclerotic cardiovascular disease. *Diabetes Care, 14,* 173–194.

Driscoll, D. (1992). Coarctation of the aorta. In J. Cooke & E. Frohlich (Eds.), *Current management of hypertensive and vascular diseases* (pp. 180–186). St Louis: B. C. Decker.

Dustan, H. (1986). Systemic arterial hypertension. In J. Hurst, R. Logue, C. Rackley, et al. (Eds.), *The heart* (6th ed., pp. 1038–1048). New York: McGraw-Hill.

Ferrannini, E., Buzzigoli, G., Bonadonna, R., et al. (1987). Insulin resistance in essential hypertension. *New England Journal of Medicine, 317,* 350–378.

Gifford, R. W. (1994). Treatment of patients with systemic arterial hypertension. In R. C. Schlant & R. W. Alexander (Eds.), *Hurst's the heart* (8th ed., pp. 1427–1448). New York: McGraw-Hill.

Gonzales, D., & Ram, V. (1988). New approaches for the treatment of hypertensive urgencies and emergencies. *Chest, 93,* 193–195.

Guyton, A. (1991). Arterial pressure regulation: Parts 1 and 2. In A. Guyton (Ed.), *Textbook of medical physiology* (8th ed., pp. 149–157, 185–218). Philadelphia: W. B. Saunders.

Hall, W., Wollam, G., & Tuttle, E. (1994). Diagnostic evaluation of the patient with systemic hypertension. In R. C. Schlant & R. W. Alexander (Eds.), *Hurst's the heart* (8th ed., pp. 1403–1425). New York: McGraw-Hill.

Hypertension Detection and Follow-up Program Cooperative Group. (1979). Reduction in mortality of persons with high blood pressure, including mild hypertension. *Journal of the American Medical Association, 242,* 2562–2573.

Joint National Committee on Detection, Evaluation and Treatment of High Blood Pressure (1993). The fifth report of the Joint National Committee on Detection, Evaluation and Treatment of High Blood Pressure. *Archives of Internal Medicine, 153,* 154–183.

Kannel, W. (1976). Some lessons in cardiovascular epidemiology from Framingham. *American Journal of Cardiology, 37,* 269–282.

Kaplan, N. (1994). *Clinical hypertension* (6th ed.). Baltimore: Williams & Wilkins.

Kaplan, N. (1992a) Treatment of hypertensive emergencies and urgencies. *Heart Disease and Stroke, 1,* 373–378.

Kaplan, N. (1992b). Systemic hypertension: Mechanisms and diagnosis. In E. Braunwald (Ed.), *Heart disease: A textbook of cardiovascular medicine* (4th ed., pp. 817–851). Philadelphia: W. B. Saunders.

Kaplan, N. (1992c). Systemic hypertension: Therapy. In E. Braunwald (Ed.), *Heart disease: A textbook of cardiovascular medicine* (4th ed., pp. 852–874). Philadelphia: W. B. Saunders.

Klatsky, A., Armstrong, M., & Friedman, G. (1992). Alcohol and mortality. *Annals of Internal Medicine, 117,* 646–654.

Koniak-Griffin, D., & Dodgson, J. (1987). Severe pregnancy induced hypertension: Postpartum care of the critically ill patient. *Heart and Lung, 16,* 661–669.

Laragh, J., & Pickering, T. (1991). Essential hypertension. In B. Brenner & F. Rector (Eds.), *The kidney* (pp. 1909–1939). Philadelphia: W. B. Saunders.

Law, M., Frost, C., & Wald, N. (1991). By how much does dietary salt reduction lower blood pressure?: Analysis of observational data among populations. *British Medical Journal, 302,* 811–815.

Lawrie, G. M., Morris, G. C., Glaser, D. H., et al. (1989). Renovascular reconstruction: Factors affecting long term prognosis in 919 patients followed up to 31 years. *American Journal of Cardiology, 63,* 1085–1092.

Mann, S., James G., Wong, R., & Pickering, T. (1991). Elevation of ambulatory systolic blood pressure in hypertensive smokers: A case control study. *Journal of the American Medical Association, 265,* 2226–2228.

McKinney, T. (1992). Management of hypertensive crisis. *Hospital Practice,* 27(3), 133–151.

Meade, T. (1988). Risks and mechanisms of cardiovascular events in users of oral contraceptive. *American Journal of Obstetrics and Gynecology, 158,* 1646–1652.

Mishell, D. (1988). Use of oral contraceptives in women of older reproductive age. *American Journal of Obstetrics and Gynecology, 158,* 1652–1657.

Multiple Risk Factor Intervention Trial Research Group. (1982). Multiple Risk Factor Intervention Trial: Risk factor changes and mortality results. *Journal of the American Medical Association, 248,* 1465–1477.

Parati, G., Pomidossi, G., Albini, F., Malaspina, D., & Mancia, G. (1987). Relationship of 24-hour blood pressure mean and variability to severity of target-organ damage in hypertension. *Journal of Hypertension, 5,* 93–98.

Prisant, L., Carr, A., & Hawkins, D. (1993). Treating hypertensive emergencies. *Postgraduate Medicine, 93*(2), 92–110.

Rahn, K. (1989). How should we treat a hypertensive emergency? *American Journal of Cardiology, 63*(Suppl), 48C–50C.

Ram, C. (1991). Management of hypertensive emergencies: Changing therapeutic options. *American Heart Journal, 122,* 356–363.

Royal College of Practitioners Oral Contraception Study. (1981). Further analyses of mortality in oral contraceptive users. *Lancet, 1,* 541.

Rubenstein, E., & Escalante, C. (1989). Hypertensive crisis. *Critical Care Clinics, 5,* 477–495.

Savage, D., Drayer, J., Henry, W., et al. (1979). Echocardiographic assessment of cardiac anatomy and function in hypertensive subjects. *Circulation, 59,* 623–632.

Schneider R., Egan, B., Johnson, E., Drobny, H., & Julius, S. (1986). Anger and anxiety in borderline hypertension. *Psychosomatic Medicine, 48,* 242–248.

Shannon, D. (1987). HELLP syndrome: A severe consequence of pregnancy induced hypertension. *Journal of Obstetric, Gynecologic, and Neonatal Nursing, 16*(6), 395–402.

SHEP Cooperative Research Group. (1991). Prevention of stroke by antihypertensive drug treatment in older persons with isolated systolic hypertension. *Journal of the American Medical Association 265,* 3255–3264.

Smith, M., & Dunn, M. (1991). Hypertension due to renal parenchymal disease. In B. Brenner & F. Rector (Eds.), *The kidney* (pp. 1968–1996). Philadelphia: W. B. Saunders.

Stadel, B. (1981). Oral contraceptives and cardiovascular disease. *New England Journal of Medicine, 305,* 672.

Tobian, L. (1988). Potassium and salt in hypertension. *Journal of Hypertension, 6*(Suppl 4), S12–S24.

Veterans Administration Cooperative Study Group on Antihypertensive Agents. (1967). Effects of treatment on morbidity in hypertension: Results in patients with diastolic blood pressure averaging 115 through 129 mm Hg. *Journal of the American Medical Association, 202,* 116–127.

Veterans Administration Cooperative Study Group on Antihypertensive Agents. (1970). Effects of treatment on morbidity in hypertension: Results in patients with diastolic blood pressure averaging 90 through 114 mm Hg. *Journal of the American Medical Association, 213,* 1143–1152.

Veterans Administration Cooperative Study Group on Antihypertensive Agents. (1987). Urinary and serum electrolytes in untreated black and white hypertensives. *Journal of Chronic Disease, 40,* 839–847.

Vokonas, P., Kannel, W., & Cupples, L. (1988). Epidemiology and risk of hypertension in the elderly: The Framingham Study. *Journal of Hypertension, 6*(Suppl 1), S3–S9.

Weinstein, L. (1982). Syndrome of hemolysis, elevated liver enzymes, and low platelet count: A severe consequence of hypertension in pregnancy. *American Journal of Obstetrics and Gynecology, 142,* 154–159.

Wells, S. A., Jr., & Santen, R. J. (1986). The pituitary and adrenal glands. In D. Sabiston (Ed.), *Textbook of surgery: The biological basis of modern surgical practice* (13th ed., pp. 639–696). Philadelphia: W. B. Saunders.

Williams, R., Hunt, S., Hasstedt, J., et al. (1991). Are there interactions and relations between genetic and environmental factors predisposing to high blood pressure? *Hypertension, 18*(Suppl I), I29–I37.

Vascular Emergencies

Jane Parthum

Vascular emergencies encompass a wide range of arterial and venous problems, some of which may result in risk to an extremity, vital organ, or loss of life. Vascular emergencies, whether from trauma or secondary to peripheral vascular disease, offer major challenges to the critical care nurse.

Significant advances have been made in caring for patients with vascular emergencies. Delivery of optimal nursing care requires a thorough understanding of vascular anatomy, specific clinical manifestations, pathophysiology, current methods of diagnosis and treatment, and a high index of clinical suspicion for vascular abnormalities.

This chapter addresses selective vascular emergencies, current methods of diagnosis and treatment, and related nursing care in the critical care setting. The topics chosen are limited to conditions that are limb- or life-threatening and that require immediate or emergent attention.

AORTIC ANEURYSM

An aneurysm is an irreversible dilation of an artery secondary to a localized weakness of the arterial wall that may predispose the artery to thrombosis, distal embolization, or rupture (Haimovici, 1989a).

Aneurysms are described and categorized by a variety of criteria, including shape, location, and etiology. There are two types of true aneurysms: fusiform and saccular. A fusiform aneurysm is the most common type of aortic aneurysm and involves dilation and bulging of the entire circumference of the aorta. A saccular aneurysm is an outpouching from the aorta that results from localized thinning and stretching (Dalsing & Sawchuk, 1994; Haimovici, 1989a). In both cases, the arterial wall remains as a barrier (Figure 26–1).

A pseudoaneurysm occurs when the entire aortic wall is disrupted, resulting in communication of blood with the surrounding tissues, producing a pulsatile hematoma. Pseudoaneurysms may be classified as traumatic, anastomotic, degenerative, or mycotic (Ochsner, 1982).

Aortic aneurysms may involve the ascending aorta, the aortic arch, descending aorta, thoracoabdominal aorta, abdominal aorta, or a combination of these. Abdominal aortic aneurysms (AAA) are the most common type; they usually arise just below the renal arteries (infrarenal AAA), and frequently involve the iliac arteries at the bifurcation.

Etiology

Most AAAs are presumed to be caused by atherosclerosis. Factors associated with the development of ath-

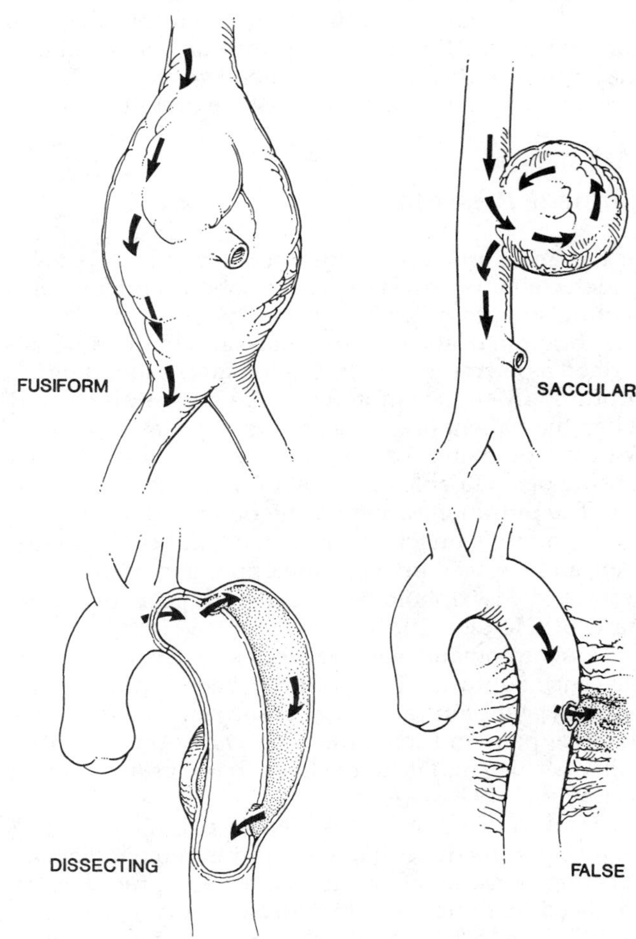

FIGURE 26–1. Types of basic aneurysms. (From Dalsing, M., & Sawchuk, A. [1994]. Surgery of the aorta. In V. Fahey [Ed.], *Vascular nursing* [2nd ed., p. 253]. Philadelphia: W. B. Saunders.)

erosclerosis include hypertension, diabetes, cigarette smoking, hyperlipidemia, and heredity. Other causes of aneurysms may include infections, poststenotic dilation, syphilis, arteritis, congenital abnormalities, and trauma (DeBakey & McCollum, 1991; Haimovici, 1989a; Hertzer, 1989).

Pathophysiology

The infrarenal abdominal aorta is particularly prone to the formation of aneurysms and atherosclerotic occlusive disease. Atherosclerosis causes a weakening of the aortic wall due to destruction of the media, the middle layer containing elastic fibers. The gradual weakening of the media in combination with hemodynamic forces may cause thickening and compression of the vasa vasorum, which supplies nutrition to the aortic wall. The muscle fibers then become damaged and may be replaced with fibrous tissue and calcium deposits (Goldstone, 1991; Hertzer, 1989). As the aneurysm increases in diameter, wall tension increases also, allowing further enlargement.

As dilation occurs, changes in laminar blood flow allow the formation of an intraluminal thrombus. In some cases, the thrombus may become dislodged and may produce distal thromboembolism, causing acute ischemia of vital organs or a distal extremity.

Clinical Presentation

In thoracic aortic aneurysm, the aneurysm is usually undetectable on physical examination, and the presenting symptom is usually chest pain.

Abdominal aortic aneurysms are frequently described as asymptomatic, symptomatic/expanding, or ruptured. Many asymptomatic AAAs are discovered when the patient has presented for unrelated reasons. An asymptomatic AAA is usually discovered by the finding of a palpable mass just proximal to the umbilicus. The pulsations are typically described as pushing the examiner's fingers apart. If the hand of the examiner can be placed between the upper end of the aneurysm and the xiphoid, the aneurysm probably is infrarenal (Hertzer, 1979).

A symptomatic AAA indicates expansion or impending rupture. Excruciating back pain is the cardinal symptom and may be accompanied by abdominal pain and tenderness on palpation. The back pain may also radiate to the lower back, groin, or flank (Haimovici, 1989a).

Frank rupture of an AAA is a medical emergency requiring immediate diagnosis and treatment. Factors affecting outcome after surgery for a ruptured AAA are listed in Table 26–1. Ruptured aneurysms are frequently fatal, with an overall perioperative mortality approaching 80% (Hertzer, 1989; Wakefield, 1991). Diagnosis of rupture is based on the presence of a pulsatile mass or retroperitoneal hematoma accompanied by excruciating abdominal or back pain. Evidence of hemorrhage may include hypotension, tachycardia, diaphoresis, pallor, oliguria, mottling of the abdomen and extremities, and diminished pulses (Haimovici, 1989a).

Diagnostic Findings

X-RAYS. Anteroposterior and lateral abdominal x-rays may suggest the presence of an aortic aneurysm because of mural calcification. Sufficient calcification to permit even an estimate of size is present in only 60% to 70% of cases; therefore, other imaging techniques are routinely employed.

ULTRASOUND. Ultrasound is a simple and safe technique for the diagnosis and measurement of AAA. Ultrasound is not influenced by either thrombus or mural calcification and is more accurate than plain x-ray. It is a good way to follow the size of an abdominal aneurysm in patients who are being treated conservatively. Ultrasound has correlated well with measurements taken at the time of surgery and is considered a reliable diagnostic tool.

COMPUTED TOMOGRAPHY. Computed tomography (CT) scan provides information similar to that of ultrasound. It is more expensive than ultrasound, and its primary superiority in diagnosis is in the suprarenal and thoracoabdominal aneurysms.

MAGNETIC RESONANCE IMAGING SCAN. Magnetic resonance imaging is a powerful diagnostic tool for evaluating both thoracic and abdominal aneurysms. Contrast material is not needed as in a CT scan, so it is a better choice for patients who may have renal compro-

TABLE 26–1. **Factors Affecting Outcome After Surgery for a Ruptured Abdominal Aortic Aneurysm**

Patient	Surgical Procedure
Advanced age Female sex Ischemic heart disease Hypertension Renal failure Chronic obstructive lung disease Large size of aneurysm Suprarenal extension	Long operation time Hypotension Inadvertent venous injury Extensive loss of blood Less experienced surgeon
Rupture	**Postoperative Factors**
Intraabdominal rupture Preoperative hypotension/shock Extensive preoperative loss of blood Preoperative cardiac arrest	Renal failure Myocardial infarction Heart failure Impaired hemostasis Ischemic colitis

From Greenhalgh, M. A., & Hollier, L. H. (Eds.). (1992). *Emergency vascular surgery* (p. 175). Philadelphia: W. B. Saunders.

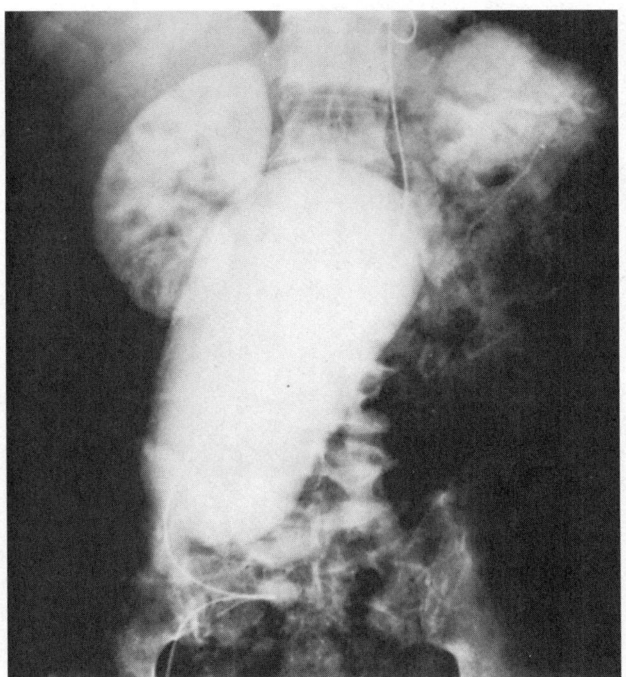

FIGURE 26–2. Angiographic demonstration of an abdominal aortic aneurysm. (Compliments of Larry-Stuart Deutsch, M.D., Chief Cardiac/Vascular/Interventional Radiology, University of California Irvine Medical Center.)

mise. The need for the patient to lie quietly during the test and the expense are two drawbacks to this choice (Hertzer, 1989).

AORTOGRAM. Aortography is not performed routinely for the purpose of diagnosing AAA. Aortography demonstates only the blood flow in the lumen, which may be occupied by thrombus, and cannot estimate the total diameter of the aneurysm (Fig. 26–2). Except with aneurysm rupture, aortography is useful for evaluating the number and location of the renal arteries; for determining the presence of renal, inferior mesenteric, iliac, and distal artery disease or aneurysm; for confirming a suspicion of a thoracoabdominal aneurysm; and for determining whether the AAA extends above the level of the renal arteries.

Management

Generally, the patient with an AAA should undergo surgery. The risk of aneurysmal rupture balanced against the risk of elective operation supports resection. The mortality rate is usually less than 4% provided that the patient is a good operative risk. Untreated aortic aneurysms put the patient at high risk for potential rupture, infection, or embolization of thrombotic debris (Goldstone, 1991; Hertzer, 1989; Hollier & Marino, 1991).

The most important predictor of aneurysmal rupture is the size of the aneurysm. Rupture occurs when the aortic wall can no longer sustain the shear stress. It is known that larger aneurysms rupture more often than smaller aneurysms, and patients with hypertension are at greater risk for rupture. An aneurysm of 4 cm has less than a 15% chance of rupture within 5 years, whereas an aneurysm of 8 cm has a 75% chance of rupture. The risk of rupture is more significant than the risk of operation when an aneurysm reaches 5 cm in diameter; therefore, surgery is recommended for aortic aneurysms greater than 5 cm. The risk of rupture for aneurysms less than 5 cm is small; however, an average growth rate of 0.4 cm / year determined by ultrasound is an indication for surgery (Hertzer, 1989; McIntyre & Bernhard, 1987).

Elective operation for repair of an AAA requires optimal preoperative evaluation of the cardiac, pulmonary, renal, and endocrine systems. A cardiology consultation should be obtained for all patients except in extreme emergencies. Pulmonary function studies may be indicated for patients with emphysema or a long smoking history. Patients with renal disease may have an elevated creatinine level after the aortogram and should be well hydrated before surgery. Diabetes should be well controlled.

Prophylactic antibiotics are usually given the night before or 1 to 2 hours before surgery. A mechanical bowel preparation is usually recommended. Electrocardiographic (ECG) monitoring, arterial pressure, pulmonary artery pressure, urinary catheter, and a nasogastric tube are used to ensure optimal fluid management during surgery.

OPERATIVE TECHNIQUE

Minimal dissection is desired to expose the aneurysm. After proximal and distal control has been obtained, the aneurysmal sac is opened, the intraluminal thrombus is removed, and bleeding lumbar arteries are oversewn. The aortic clamp can be placed below the renal arteries in 90% to 95% of cases. Clamping above the renal arteries (less than 60 minutes) is usually tolerated by the kidneys. If distal perfusion is necessary, partial aortic occlusion for placement of an end-to-side proximal anastomosis or the use of a shunt may allow adequate distal perfusion. The graft limbs are flushed with arterial blood to clear atherosclerotic debris and thrombus to prevent distal embolization. A preclotted, woven Dacron graft is sutured in place, and the remaining aneurysm wall is wrapped around the graft. If the iliac arteries are free from disease, a straight tube graft is used. In the presence of aneurysmal or aortoiliac occlusive disease, a bifurcated graft is placed to the segment with adequate open vessels (Fig. 26–3) (Dalsing & Sawchuk, 1994).

When rupture is impending, the chest may be opened to obtain proximal control of the aorta before resection of the aneurysm.

Ruptured aneurysms require emergent surgery. X-rays, CT scans, and blood tests are avoided to expedite treatment. The site of aneurysmal rupture depends on the location of the aneurysm, but aneurysms most

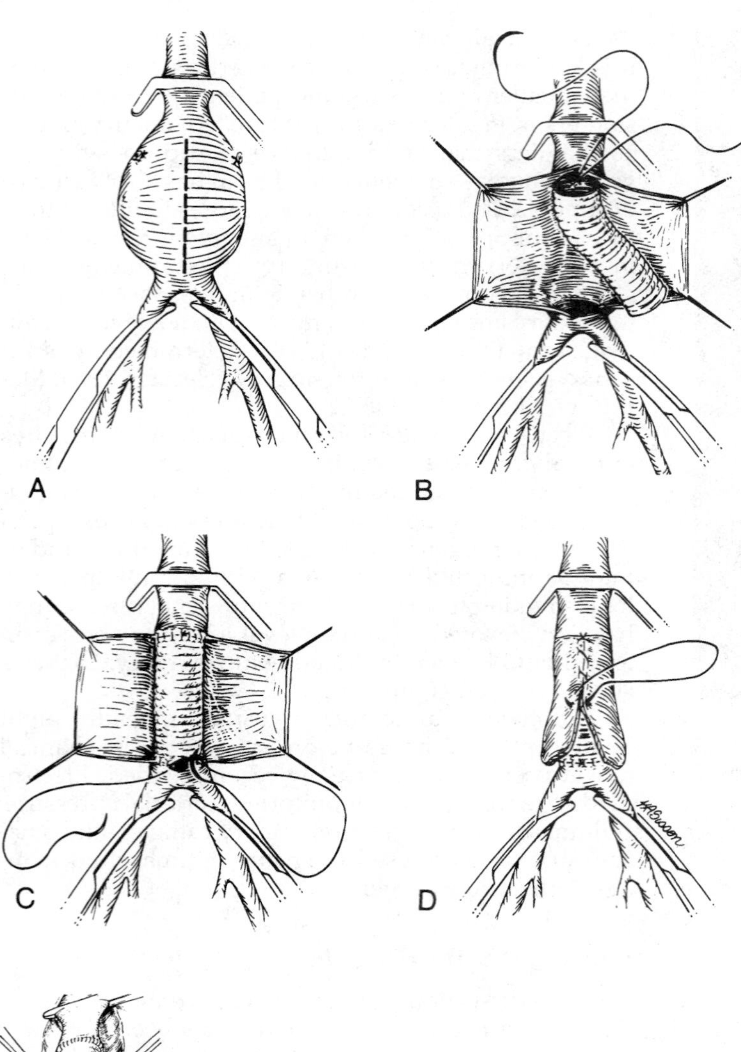

FIGURE 26–3. Repair of abdominal aortic aneurysm not involving the iliac arteries. *A*, Vascular control using clamps. *B*, Aneurysm is opened, and tube graft is inserted. *C*, Proximal and distal anastomosis. *D*, Posterior wall of aneurysm is wrapped around new graft. *E*, Repair of abdominal aortic aneurysm involving iliac arteries. (*A* through *D* from Yao, J., Flinn, W. R., & Bergan, J. [1984]. Technique for repairing infrarenal abdominal aortic aneurysms. In L. M. Nyhus & R. J. Baker [Eds.], *Mastery of surgery* [pp. 1361–1365]. Boston: Little, Brown; *E* from Haimovici, H. [1984]. *Vascular surgery: Principles and techniques* [2nd ed., p. 702]. Englewood Cliffs, NJ: Appleton & Lange.)

commonly rupture into the retroperitoneum. The abdomen is opened and bleeding controlled by compressing the aorta against the vertebrae. Once the aorta has been cross-clamped, the aneurysm is opened, and the preclotted Dacron graft is flushed, sutured in place, and wrapped by the remaining posterior aneurysm wall (Coselli & Crawford, 1989).

POSTOPERATIVE COMPLICATIONS

ACUTE RENAL FAILURE. Renal failure is a relatively rare occurrence in elective AAA repair. It may result from prolonged ischemia, inadequate hydration, or emboli. The incidence of acute renal failure increases in patients with severe shock, prolonged cross-clamping, and massive transfusions. When the aorta is clamped above the renal arteries for longer than 60 minutes, the incidence of renal failure is approximately 8% (Crawford et al., 1989). To reduce the risk of renal failure it may be wise to wait for the patient to be rehydrated after aortography, before surgery. In addition, some surgeons administer mannitol to patients considered at increased risk for renal failure before surgery (Hollier & Rutherford, 1989).

COLON ISCHEMIA. A severe potential complication of AAA surgery is ischemia of the descending and retrosigmoid colon. A major cause of this may be ligation of the inferior mesenteric artery. However, occlusion of the mesenteric artery by mural thrombus as a consequence of the atherosclerotic process may also result in colon ischemia (Hollier & Rutherford, 1989). Manifestations include cyanotic discoloration of the colon, melena, diarrhea, abdominal pain, and leukocytosis.

THROMBOEMBOLISM. Manipulation of the aneurysm during surgery can result in mobilization of intraluminal thrombus and distal embolization. Distal embolization can be prevented by initial distal clamping of the iliac arteries with minimal manipulation of the aneurysm. Distal embolization may result in renal failure or acute tissue ischemia of the lower extremities characterized by areas of discoloration or petechia-like lesions on the toes or bottom of the foot (blue toe syndrome or trash foot).

SPINAL CORD ISCHEMIA. Spinal cord ischemia associated with resection of the infrarenal aortic aneurysm is rare, but may result from interruption of the spinal cord's arterial supply. The incidence of spinal cord ischemia leading to paraplegia or paraparesis may be as great as 6% in aneurysms of the descending thoracic aorta (Goldstone, 1991).

MYOCARDIAL INFARCTION. The coexistence of coronary artery disease (CAD) with AAA has been well documented (Goldstone, 1991; Hollier & Rutherford, 1989). Indeed, CAD is the cause of 50% to 60% of deaths after abdominal aortic surgery. Preoperative evaluation of elective patients can suggest those who might benefit from coronary artery bypass grafting before AAA repair.

INFECTION. Infection may occur in 1% to 2% of aortic procedures, but carries a high mortality when a prosthetic graft is in place. Fevers, prolonged ileus, and leukocytosis may indicate a smoldering infection. A white blood cell scan can indicate a site of infection.

PROGNOSIS

Untreated AAA has a 40% to 50% mortality in 1 year, 75% to 80% at 5 years, and 100% at 10 years. Current operative mortality is 3% to 4%, and overall late survival is approximately 70% to 80% at 5 years and 40% to 50% at 10 years (Dalsing & Sawchuk, 1994; Hollier & Rutherford, 1989).

PREOPERATIVE MANAGEMENT

Preoperative evaluation of the patient for elective aneurysm repair requires a thorough history and physical examination. Baseline data, including risk factors, vital signs, peripheral pulses, breath sounds, and heart sounds should be documented.

Preparation for surgery involves a variety of tasks, including completion of diagnostic tests and laboratory work and carrying out specific preoperative protocols. Four to eight units of blood should be available in the blood bank.

The high-risk patient may be admitted to the intensive care unit before surgery for insertion of a Swan-Ganz catheter for continuous monitoring of the pulmonary artery wedge pressure and cardiac output. Arterial line placement is also done to monitor blood pressure and to secure easy access for blood samples.

Most patients and families have a high level of anxiety about the impending surgery, and lack of knowledge about the surgery and hospital routine. Preoperative education for the patient and family should include explanations of the equipment, routines, procedures, visiting hours, and postoperative pain control plans. When possible, a tour of the intensive care unit (ICU) may help allay anxiety. Specific fears and concerns of the patient and family should be addressed.

POSTOPERATIVE MANAGEMENT

A main goal of postoperative care is prevention of complications. Patients with aortic rupture are at much higher risk for complications than those with elective surgery.

The patient is transferred to the ICU for continuous monitoring of cardiopulmonary, renal, and neurologic systems. Fluid management is one parameter of ICU care, with the goal to optimize cardiac output and maximize renal function.

Aggressive management of the pulmonary system is directly associated with reduced complications. Mechanical ventilation is used only as long as necessary. Early extubation, early activity, and judicious use of suctioning, incentive spirometry, and coughing and deep breathing are important aspects of management.

Tissue perfusion should be evaluated hourly by assessing the extremities for pulses, pain, paresthesia, pallor, and temperature. Capillary refill time should be assessed and documented in seconds. Doppler signals may be helpful in assessing flow to extremities. The femoral pulses should be easily palpable; absence of these pulses may indicate graft failure.

The incidence of postoperative hemorrhage is approximately 1% to 4%, and may result from the extensive retroperitoneal dissection and vascular anastamoses. Intraabdominal bleeding may be suspected with increasing abdominal girth, decreasing urine output, hemodynamic instability, and inability to maintain adequate preload. Significant, uncontrolled hemorrhage necessitates a return to the operating room.

The patient should be routinely assessed for signs and symptoms associated with the previously mentioned potential complications of AAA repair. Renal failure, colon ischemia, thromboembolism, spinal cord ischemia, myocardial infarction, and infection are well known potential complications, and early detection and intervention can reduce the morbidity associated with these problems.

ACUTE AORTIC DISSECTION

Acute aortic dissection is a catastrophic event that is characterized by an intimal tear and separation of the medial layers by a column of blood creating a false lumen. Pulsatile flow in the false lumen may cause proximal or distal extension of the dissection, resulting in compression of the true lumen, occlusion of arterial branches, or rupture through the adventitia, resulting in hemorrhage (Baird & Almond, 1991; Scarris & Miller, 1989).

The term "dissecting aneurysm" was first used in 1761 by Morgagni, who described a hematoma separating the medial layer (Anagnostopoulos, 1975). Although the term is widely applied in the literature, the pathogenesis of acute aortic dissection differs from that of a true aneurysm.

Histology

The aorta consists of three basic layers. The inner layer, or intima, is composed primarily of endothelium and connective tissue. The media is the thick middle layer and is composed of elastin, collagen, and smooth muscle cells. The outer layer, the adventitia, is thin and is composed of connective tissue. This layer serves to anchor the vessel to the surrounding structures, providing strength and stability to the aorta. The blood supply to the media flows through the vasa vasorum, a network of capillaries embedded in the adventitia.

Etiology

CYSTIC MEDIAL NECROSIS. Medial degeneration, specifically cystic medial necrosis, has been considered the primary basis for acute aortic dissection. In medial degeneration, the middle layer of the aorta, which is normally elastic, is replaced by a fibrotic band of collagen. It is not well understood, but may be a final pathway from a variety of conditions that alter the collagen, elastin, and mucopolysaccharides in the arterial wall.

MARFAN SYNDROME. Marfan syndrome is a genetic disorder characterized by premature degeneration of vascular elastic tissue that leads to aortic dissection and aortic root dilation. This leads to aortic valve insufficiency, which will eventually cause heart failure and death.

HYPERTENSION. Approximately 70% of patients with aortic dissection have hypertension, which is thought to contribute to aortic injury.

PREGNANCY. During pregnancy, the body produces hormones to relax smooth muscle and connective tissue for normal uterine expansion. A combination of these hormonal changes, increased blood volume, and hypertension may increase the risk of aortic dissection (Roberts, 1981; Wahlers et al., 1994).

AORTIC COARCTATION. Approximately 10% of untreated patients with aortic coarctation die from aortic dissection and hemopericardium. The dissection usually occurs in the proximal aorta and is thought to be associated with hypertension and a high frequency of congenital bicuspid aortic valve disease (Burchell, 1955; Roberts, 1981).

TRAUMA. Blunt trauma due to deceleration accidents is a well recognized cause of aortic tears and dissection. Most of these are thoracic in origin and occur just distal to the left subclavian artery at the aortic isthmus. Here the mobile aortic arch joins a relatively fixed thoracic aorta and is vulnerable to injury. The abdominal aorta may also be prone to tears and dissection. The mechanism of injury includes motor vehicular crashes both with and without seatbelts, abdominal blows, and crush injuries (Brathwaite & Rodriguez, 1992).

Pathology

Aortic dissection begins with a tear in the intima that allows blood to enter the vessel wall and create a false channel by splitting through the media. In 62% of patients the initial intimal tear is in the ascending aorta, in 26% it is in the descending aorta, 9% in the arch, and 3% in the abdominal aorta. Extension is usually distal, but most patients have some amount of extension proximally. Proximal extension can lead to complications involving aortic insufficiency or coronary artery occlusion. Distal extension can include branch vessel occlusion that can cause cerebrovascular accident (CVA) or ischemia to the viscera or extremities (Coselli & Crawford, 1989).

Classification

Depending on the source, aortic dissection may be classified in many ways. However, the distinguishing feature is the presence or absence of ascending aorta involvement. Dissections including the ascending aorta are classified as type A (Stanford Classification), proximal (MGH Classification), ascending (University of Alabama Classification), and type I (De Bakey Classification.) If the ascending aorta is not involved, it is classified as type B, distal, descending, or type II (Baird & Almond, 1991; Sarris & Miller, 1989, 1993).

Clinical Presentation

The diagnosis of acute aortic dissection should be suspected in any patient who has severe back pain, anterior chest pain, epigastric pain, abrupt onset of a pulseless extremity, acute aortic valve insufficiency without known heart disease, and a history of hypertension or Marfan syndrome (Burruss, 1993; Sarris & Miller, 1989). Despite major advances in diagnostic tools, the correct diagnosis is made in less than half of the cases (Spittell et al., 1993). Acute onset of severe chest pain is the most common initial complaint. Less commonly, patients exhibit heart failure, syncope, CVA, shock, or paraplegia.

Diagnostic

Laboratory findings, ECG, and chest radiographs are not specific enough in their results either to rule in or rule out aortic dissection.

CAT SCAN. Computed tomography is a quick means of making the diagnosis of aortic dissection. When contrast medium is used, the CT scan is highly accurate and can clearly delineate the intimal tear and false channel within the aorta.

MAGNETIC RESONANCE IMAGING SCAN. Magnetic resonance imaging (MRI) is 95% sensitive and 90% specific for detecting aortic dissections. MRI is also highly effective in identifying extension into the branch vessels or the aortic root (Link, 1992). A disadvantage of MRI is that patients with vascular clips, pacemakers, or metal equipment cannot be scanned because of the magnetic forces involved.

TRANSESOPHAGEAL ECHOCARDIOGRAPHY. Much is currently being researched on the role of transesophageal echocardiography (TEE) in the evaluation of aortic dissection. TEE is used before emergency surgery in pending rupture and has a role in the health care team's ability to act quickly in dire situations (Erbel, 1993).

AORTOGRAPHY. Although aortography is an invasive technique that puts the patient at risk for renal compromise, it is still considered by many vascular surgeons the optimal diagnostic tool. Abnormal findings may include demonstration of a false lumen, splitting of the contrast column, evidence of intraluminal thrombus, increased thickness of the aortic wall, narrowing or occlusion of aortic branches, and alterations in flow patterns (Fig. 26–4) (Nienaber, 1992; Peyasnick, 1991).

Management

Immediate therapy for acute aortic dissection requires interventions to prevent extension of the dissection or aortic rupture, and involves control of hypertension, pain relief, and reduction of environmental and emotional stressors. Nitroprusside is begun at 0.5 μg/kg/minute and is titrated to maintain systolic blood pressure at 90 to 110 mm Hg. The increased adrenergic activity of nitroprusside may be counteracted by administration of a beta blocker. All hemodynamic parameters and urine output should be monitored frequently to ensure adequate peripheral tissue perfusion during the acute phase.

Pain control is maintained with morphine sulfate. Any increase or recurrence of the pain may indicate progression of the dissection and should be reported to the surgeon immediately.

A feeling of impending doom is often reported by patients with acute dissection, and this, compounded

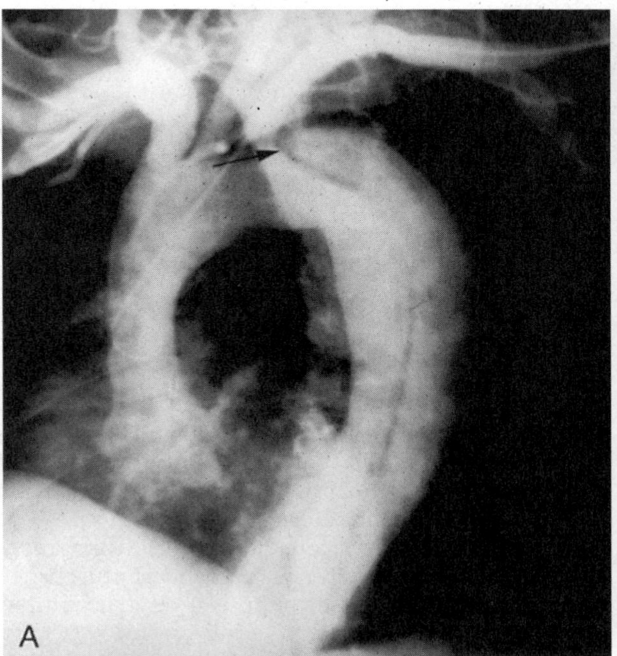

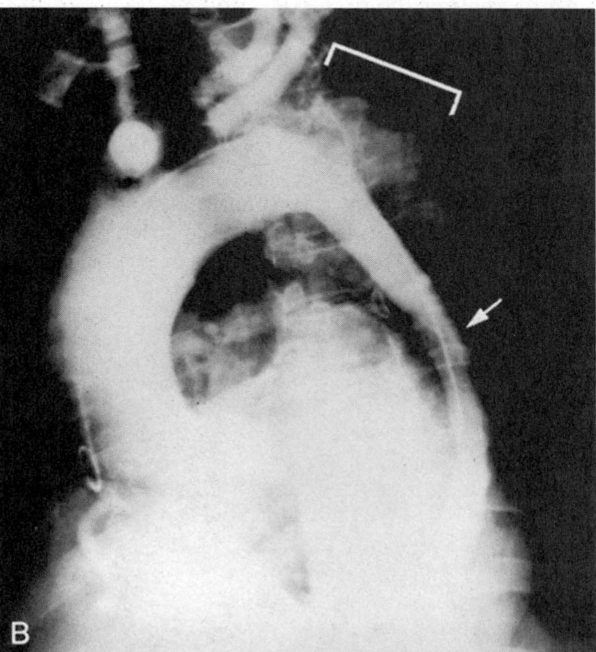

FIGURE 26–4. *A* and *B*, Angiographic demonstration of acute aortic dissection. Note narrowed tube lumen (*arrow in A*) and evidence of double lumen (*arrow in B*) in descending aorta. There is evidence of clotted false lumen (*bracket in B*) just distal to the left subclavian artery. (Compliments of Larry-Stuart Deutsch, M.D., Chief Cardiac/Vascular/Interventional Radiology, University of California Irvine Medical Center.)

by the fear of hospitalization in the patient, can be overwhelming. Such anxieties will increase blood pressure and can worsen the patient's condition; therefore, it is imperative to reduce these stressors when possible. A calm approach to the situation, using relaxation techniques when appropriate, can be an effective strategy. The patient and family should be kept informed of planned diagnostic testing and results, and interventions and their effects. Appropriate resources should be used to assist the patient and family in identifying effective coping skills and supports.

Surgical Treatment

The decision to follow acute medical treatment with surgery rests on the effect of the emergent therapy, the long-term prognosis with medical therapy, and the patient's associated risk factors. In general, patients without associated complications who have descending dissection may be tentatively managed medically. Those with ascending dissection or descending dissection complicated by myocardial infarction, CVA, renal failure, or arterial occlusion require surgical intervention (Masuda et al., 1991).

ASCENDING DISSECTION. Indications for surgical management include aortic valve insufficiency, impending rupture, progression of the dissection, symptoms of cerebral or coronary ischemia, pericardial tamponade, and failure to control the blood pressure with drug therapy (Neya et al., 1992). Surgical treatment for ascending dissection is aimed at preventing aortic rupture and correcting the dissection and related complications. The repair consists of resection of the site of the tear and the false lumen with placement of a prosthetic graft, repair or replacement of the aortic valve if indicated, and restoration of blood flow to the major branches of the aorta (Fig. 26–5) (Sarris & Miller, 1989).

DESCENDING DISSECTION. Indications for surgical intervention in descending dissection include progression of the dissection, hypertension or pain despite adequate drug therapy, evidence of compromise or occlusion of major aortic branches such as the renal or mesenteric artery, impending rupture, and cardiac tamponade (Burruss, 1993).

Operative repair consists of resection of the dissection, obliteration of the false lumen, and graft replacement. A femorofemoral, atriofemoral, or ventriculofemoral bypass or shunt is used to maintain blood supply distally (Fig. 26–6) (DeBakey et al., 1982).

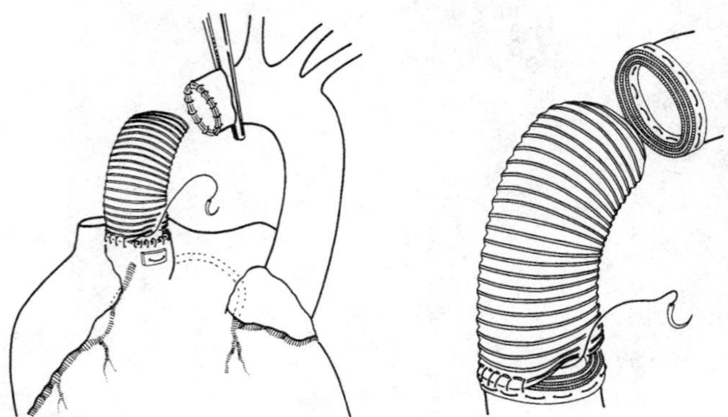

FIGURE 26–5. Repair of ascending dissection. (From Symbas, P. N. [1979]. Treatment of aortic diseases. In J. Lindsay & J. W. Hurst [Eds.], *The aorta* [p. 380]. New York: Grune & Stratton.)

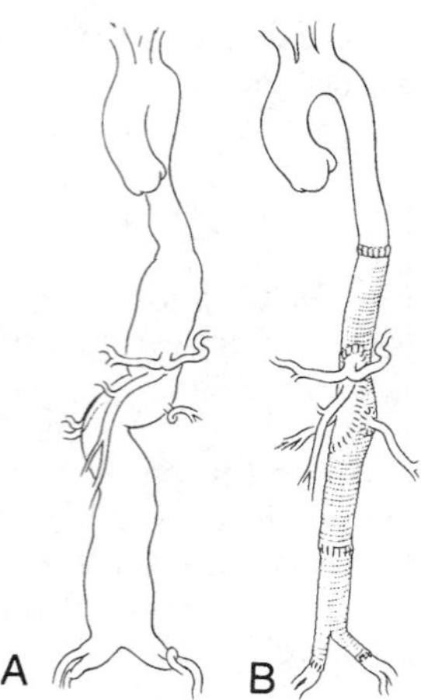

FIGURE 26–6. Illustrations of a degenerative aneurysm that involves the distal half of descending thoracic aorta and the entire abdominal aorta. *A*, Drawing showing the location and extent of disease. *B*, Drawing showing graft in place and functioning. (Courtesy of Baylor College of Medicine, 1987.)

Complications

Major complications of acute aortic dissection are directly related to the extent of the dissection. Complications that carry the greatest threat to the patient include rupture of the aorta, shock, myocardial infarction, CVA, aortic regurgitation leading to heart failure, renal failure, mesenteric infarction, and peripheral arterial occlusion (Masuda, 1991).

Postoperative Care

Postoperative care requires continued control of blood pressure by continuous infusion of nitroprusside and beta blockers. Hemodynamic monitoring via an oximetric pulmonary artery catheter and arterial line is required. The potential for redissection and postoperative bleeding requires constant monitoring of the vital signs, hemodynamic trends, peripheral pulses, neurologic status, and level of pain. Aggressive pulmonary management is required to reduce pulmonary complications. Close monitoring of blood pressure is necessary during suctioning to avoid hypertension.

The patient and family need to be counseled about risk factor reduction such as control of hypertension. An interdisciplinary approach will ensure that areas such as sodium restriction, weight control, appropriate exercise, and adherence to prescribed medication regimens will be addressed.

ACUTE ARTERIAL OCCLUSION

Acute arterial occlusion was first recognized in 1628 by William Harvey, and the first successful embolectomy was performed by Labey more than a century later. In the early 1940s, heparin was discovered, and anticoagulation became the focus of treatment. In 1963, the introduction of the Fogarty embolectomy balloon catheter made it possible to extract emboli and thrombi directly from arteries (Fogarty et al., 1963). Significant tissue ischemia can result from acute arterial occlusion. Prompt diagnosis and treatment are critical to avoid limb loss, tissue or organ ischemia, or death.

Etiology

Acute arterial occlusions are either embolic or thrombotic in origin. Determining the cause will determine appropriate treatment (Fig. 26–7) (Butler & Fahey, 1993; O'Donnell, 1993).

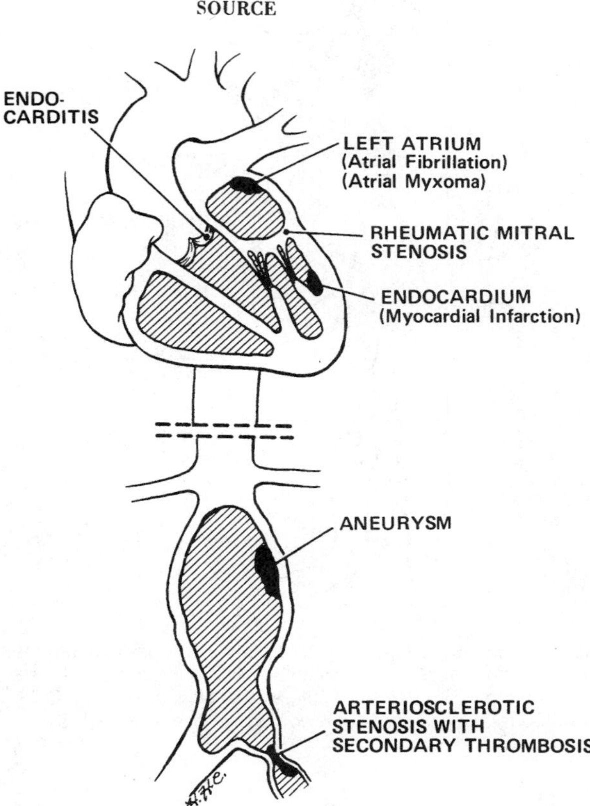

FIGURE 26–7. Emboli may originate from cardiac, aneurysmal, or atherosclerotic disease. (From Zimmerman, J. J., & Fogarty, T. J. [1986]. Acute arterial occlusion. In W. S. Moore [Ed.], *Vascular surgery: A comprehensive review* [p. 694]. New York: Grune & Stratton.)

Emboli can be either cardiac or noncardiac in origin. Major cardiac sources of emboli are rheumatic mitral stenosis, atrial fibrillation, and acute myocardial infarction.

Both mitral stenosis and atrial fibrillation predispose the patient to atrial stasis and thrombus formation. These atrial thrombi can embolize at any time, although classically this is seen in non-anticoagulated atrial fibrillation patients who convert to sinus rhythm. Myocardial infarction with subsequent mural thrombus formation is a precursor to cardiogenic emboli. Ventricular aneurysm, dilated cardiomyopathy, and myocarditis are also sources of emboli. Other cardiac sources include prosthetic heart valves, endocarditis, and cardiac tumors.

Noncardiac emboli may originate from proximal lesions such as atherosclerotic plaque and aneurysms. Iatrogenic embolization is an unfortunate complication of invasive vascular procedures. Embolization of catheter tips, guidewires, and dislodged atherosclerotic debris can result in acute arterial occlusion (Finkelmeier & Finkelmeier, 1991).

More than half of all acute arterial occlusions are caused by arterial occlusive disease with subsequent thrombosis. Spontaneous thrombosis usually occurs in patients in whom a low-flow state exists due to a narrowed atherosclerotic artery. Systemic conditions predisposing to arterial thrombosis include dehydration, congestive heart failure, fever, infection thrombocytosis, disseminated intravascular coagulation, and polycythemia (Brewster, 1991).

Blunt or penetrating trauma may cause arterial injury and thrombosis. Blunt trauma can cause damage to the intima or dislodge preexisting plaque, resulting in embolus. Penetrating trauma may lead to thrombosis, intimal dissection, hematoma, or spasm (Perry, 1991). Closed fractures in the extremities put the patient at risk for compartment syndrome due to bleeding or soft tissue swelling, leading to acute arterial occlusion.

Pathophysiology

Emboli of cardiac origin tend to obstruct large arteries at their bifurcations where the luminal diameter is decreased. Atheroemboli tend to occlude smaller vessels. The size of the obstructed vessel may help to determine the origin of the emboli. For example, an embolus that obstructed the common femoral artery is usually of cardiac origin; an embolus that causes local ischemia of a toe (blue toe syndrome) usually arises from the descending aorta or common iliac artery. Cardiac embolization accounts for most upper extremity, cerebral, and visceral ischemia (Mills & Porter, 1991; Smith et al., 1987).

Most peripheral emboli lodge in the lower extremities (Fig. 26–8). Sudden occlusion of a severely stenotic vessel may produce only mild intermittent claudication because the preexisting atherosclerotic disease has

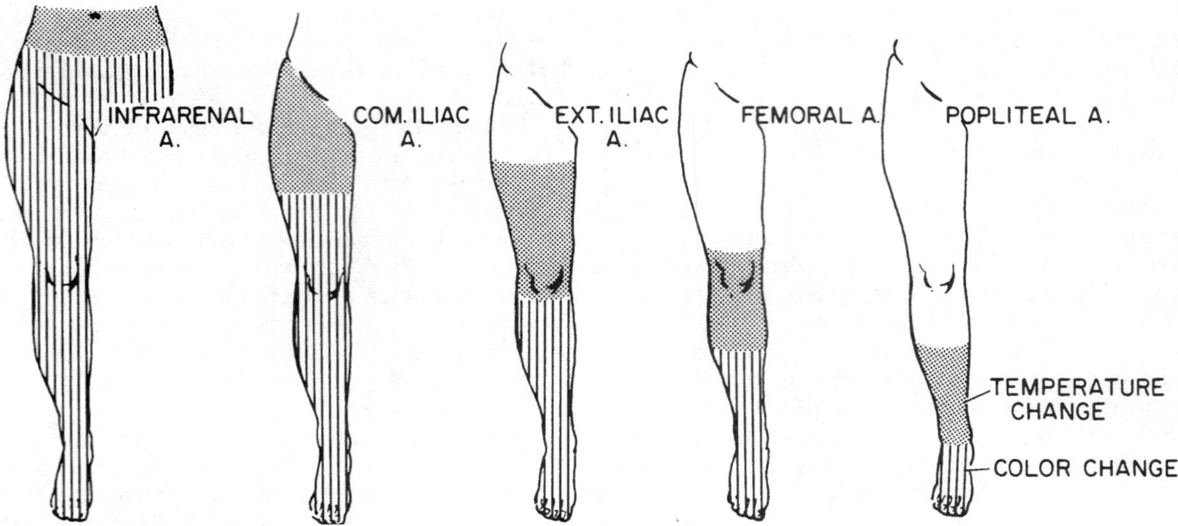

FIGURE 26–8. Level of temperature and color change with occlusion of different arteries. (From Smith, J., Holcroft, J., & Blaisdell, W. [1987]. Acute arterial insufficiency. In S. Wilson, F. Veith, R. Hobson, & R. Williams [Eds.], *Vascular surgery: Principles and practices* [p. 327]. New York: McGraw-Hill.)

prompted the formation of a well developed collateral circulation. Conversely, severe acute ischemia may result from an embolic event in a patient with marginal vascular status in whom the involved artery and collateral circulation are affected with chronic occlusive disease. Severe ischemia may also result from occlusion of a normal artery in the absence of collateral channels (Fig. 26–9) (Chin et al., 1986; Green, 1991).

Once an embolus or thrombus occludes an artery, the vasculature distal to the obstruction goes into spasm for up to 8 hours. The clot propagates distally and proximally from the obstruction, blocking branch vessels and collaterals and worsening the ischemia.

The extent of ischemic damage depends on the adequacy of the collateral circulation, blood viscosity, the oxygen-carrying capacity of the hemoglobin, the patient's underlying cardiovascular status, the extent of the clot propagation, and the promptness of diagnosis and treatment. Skeletal muscle and peripheral nerves can endure acute ischemia for 6 to 8 hours without permanent damage; skin can withstand severe ischemia for up to 24 hours (Blaisdell et al., 1978; Fiorani et al., 1992; Zimmerman & Fogarty, 1983).

Once muscle damage occurs, the muscle becomes paralyzed and acquires a firm, doughy consistency. Peripheral nerve damage results in loss of motor and sensory function. The skin appears blotchy, cold, cyanotic, or pale.

Reperfusion of the extremity poses a risk to the systemic circulation and vital organs. Anaerobic metabolism produces unbuffered acid, injured cells release potassium and myoglobin, microemboli form in areas of stasis and acidosis, and platelet aggregation is enhanced (Fiorani et al., 1992; Karmody & Leather, 1984). When these toxins are released into the circulation, pulmonary, cardiac, renal, and neurologic embarrassment can result. The degree of insult depends on

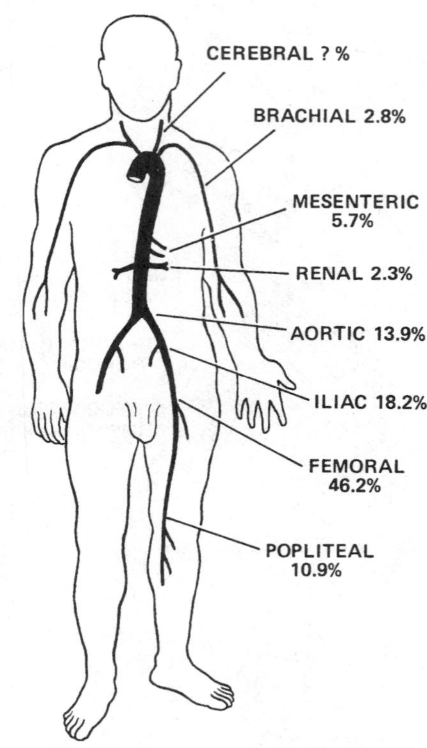

FIGURE 26–9. Emboli may obstruct various arteries but most frequently compromise flow to the extremities. (From Zimmerman, J. J., & Fogarty, T. J. [1986]. Acute arterial occlusion. In W. S. Moore [Ed.], *Vascular surgery: A comprehensive review* [p. 864]. New York: Grune & Stratton.)

the degree of ischemia and necrosis, the length of the revascularization procedure, and the previous condition of the organs (Blaisdell et al., 1978; Fiorani et al., 1992).

Clinical Presentation

A thorough history should include the type of symptoms and their duration. A history of prior cardiac disease, dysrhythmias, vascular disease, claudication, and smoking may help to differentiate between embolic and thrombotic occlusions. If there is no history of peripheral vascular disease, the acute ischemia is most likely to be of cardiac origin. A recent history of chest pain, myocardial infarction, atrial fibrillation, or murmurs is suggestive of cardiac embolus. Pain, paresthesia, pallor, pulselessness, paralysis, and poikilothermia (cold) are the classic signs and symptoms of acute arterial occlusion.

Acute pain is present in most patients. The pain usually worsens with movement of the extremity. Muscle tenderness and rigidity are seen as tissue swelling worsens.

Paresthesia is an early sign of ischemia. It is important to distinguish the perception of light touch from that of pressure, pain, and temperature. The small nerve fibers responsible for soft touch are more sensitive to hypoxemia than the nerve fibers serving the latter functions. The patient may be able to detect a pinprick yet not perceive the touch from a cotton swab.

Pallor results from decreased arterial blood flow and is an ominous sign of arterial occlusion when accompanied by pulselessness and paresthesia. Capillary refill is sluggish or absent. As ischemia worsens, pallor may be replaced by cyanosis or mottling.

Absence of peripheral pulses may be acute or chronic. The pulses are absent distal to the arterial occlusion. Pulses may be bounding proximal to the area of occlusion. Doppler arm and ankle pressures should be done to estimate the extent of ischemia.

Paralysis is a late symptom. It indicates significant neural and skeletal muscle ischemia and is frequently irreversible. Patients presenting with paralysis require immediate revascularization and frequently associated fasciotomy.

Temperature should be compared in both extremities using the back of the hand. An abrupt temperature change distal to the level of the obstruction is common.

Diagnostic Studies

Doppler pressures provide an accurate assessment of the area of acute aortic occlusion. Ankle–brachial indices can provide the baseline by which to measure postoperative results.

Laboratory tests, including coagulation tests and hematologies such as prothrombin time, partial thromboplastin time, antithrombin III, platelet count, and hematocrit need to be evaluated. The presence of myoglobin and creatine phosphokinase indicate muscle damage.

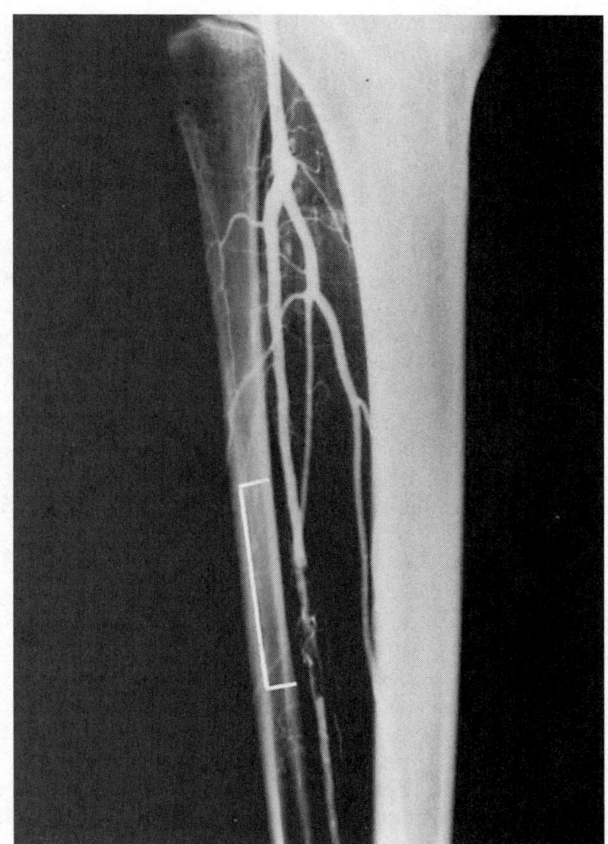

FIGURE 26–10. Angiographic demonstration of distal emboli to anterior tibial artery. Note intraluminal clot (*brackets*). (Compliments of Larry-Stuart Deutsch, M.D., Chief Cardiac/Vascular/Interventional Radiology, University of California Irvine Medical Center.)

An *ECG* can identify the presence of dysrhythmias or a myocardial infarction and can help in judging the overall status of the heart.

Echocardiography can be used to identify heart chamber size and condition of the valves, to estimate ejection fraction, and to identify intracardiac thrombus.

Ultrasound of the abdominal aorta may demonstrate the presence of an aneurysm or intraluminal clot.

Arteriography is frequently performed before embolectomy. A sharp cutoff of the normal artery indicates the presence of an embolus (Fig. 26–10).

Management

All patients with limb-threatening acute arterial occlusion should be given anticoagulation with heparin to prevent propagation of the clot. A bolus of 5,000 to 10,000 units, followed by continuous infusion of 1,000 units/hour should be started immediately. The guidelines of heparin administration are 100 to 200 units/

kg per bolus, followed by 15 to 30 units/kg per minute in a constant infusion (Smith et al., 1987). Heparin should be administered regardless of whether surgical intervention is planned because it can easily be reversed wtih protamine sulfate in the operating room (Fairbairn et al., 1980).

Once anticoagulation has been established, treatment of cardiac disorders should be initiated as soon as possible. Adequate hydration may help to restore perfusion. Appropriate pain management should be provided as necessary.

Continuous emotional support of the patient and family must not be overlooked. Appropriate hospital resources such as clinical nurse specialists, social workers, and chaplains should be used as needed. Effective communication and mutual goal setting will enhance optimal patient care and decrease the sense of powerlessness and anxiety often experienced by the patient.

Fluid status can be optimized by monitoring the pulmonary artery and wedge pressures and cardiac output. The patient should be adequately hydrated to maintain a urine output of 100 mL/hour.

Ischemic pain is excruciating, and the only true relief comes with revascularization and the return of blood flow to the area. Intravenous morphine sulfate is used to reduce pain in some cases.

The ischemic limb should be protected. The extremity should not be elevated because this serves only to diminish capillary perfusion and worsen the ischemia and pain. Ischemia and parasthesia put the extremity at risk for injury. Avoid application of heat, cold, or chemical agents that could burn the skin. Protect the extremity from trauma with an egg crate, airflow mattress, lamb's wool, sheepskin, or bed cradle. No venipunctures or injections should be initiated into the ischemic extremity.

Hourly neurovascular checks should be done and any changes reported immediately.

Hemorrhage is the major complication of anticoagulation or fibrinolytic therapy. Close observation of vital signs, intravenous or injection sites, and operative incisions is necessary.

The management of acute arterial occlusion remains a challenge to the medical and nursing staffs. Early diagnosis and treatment are crucial for limb salvage. The critical care nurse who maintains excellent assessment skills and familiarity with proper treatment measures can greatly increase the success rate in treating acute arterial occlusion.

FIBRINOLYTIC THERAPY

Fibrinolytic therapy is useful in the management of patients with acute arterial occlusion because the fibrinolytic agents lyse the emboli and allow reperfusion of the previously occluded vessel. Streptokinase, urokinase, and tissue plasminogen activator have been used with 80% to 90% improvement in blood flow in some cases (Fiorani et al., 1992; Silver & Cikrit, 1989). Heparin administration usually follows treatment with a fibrinolytic agent. Long-term anticoagulation, angioplasty, or revascularization are used to prevent reocclusion of the artery.

Complications of fibrinolytic therapy can include intracranial hemorrhage, local hematoma, distal embolization, retroperitoneal hemorrhage, and allergic reaction (Comerota, 1991; Smith et al., 1987).

SURGICAL PROCEDURE

The type of surgical procedure used to correct acute arterial occlusion varies with the location and underlying cause of the occlusion. When atherosclerotic occlusive disease or aneurysmal disease is suspected, a reconstructive procedure is indicated. The level of bypass grafting is chosen according to the location of the disease and thrombosis. When arterial occlusion of the graft occurs, thrombectomy of the graft or a new bypass procedure may be necessary.

When acute ischemia is caused by an embolus, balloon embolectomy is the definitive surgical treatment. A Fogarty balloon catheter is inserted through an arteriotomy and is passed through the clot or embolus, the balloon is inflated slowly, and the catheter is withdrawn, dragging out the embolic material (Haimovici, 1989b; Müller-Wiefel & Langkav, 1992). Embolectomy can be done under local anesthesia (Fig. 26–11). Complications of balloon embolectomy include arterial rupture, perforation, intimal injury, arterial dissection, and embolization. These complications can be readily visualized by obtaining an arteriogram after the embolus extraction.

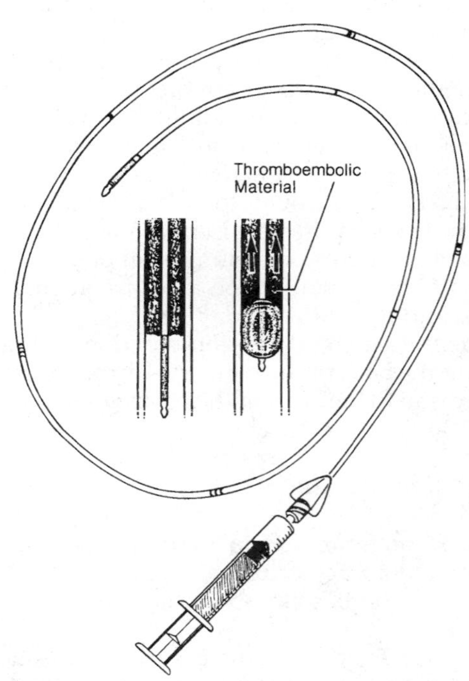

FIGURE 26–11. Demonstration of balloon embolectomy. (Balloon Embolectomy Catheter [Figure 3] from page 45 of *Critical Care Quarterly*, Vol. 8, No. 2 © September 1985.)

Fasciotomy is often required after revascularization in patients with severe ischemia and edema lasting 6 to 8 hours. The fasciotomy is done to release pressure within the muscle compartments and preserve distal circulation. Subcutaneous vertical incisions are made in the involved compartments, releasing the pressure. The major complication of fasciotomy is infection (Ernst et al., 1989; Fiorani et al., 1992).

VASCULAR TRAUMA

More than 50 million injuries occur each year, and more than 100,000 victims die as a result of those injuries, making trauma the fourth leading cause of death in the United States. Many of these patients present with multiple trauma, but injuries to the major vessels are often the cause or major contributing factor in deaths. Patients who survive may suffer from residual disability, impaired function, or amputation. Successful management of vascular injuries depends on prompt evaluation, accurate diagnosis, and skillful management. Major advances in rapid transportation, including helicopter retrieval, and the use of highly trained paramedic and nursing personnel have resulted in the survival of many trauma victims (see Chapter 62).

Etiology

Penetrating trauma from knives and bullets is the most common cause of vascular injuries in urban areas (Jacobs & Jacobs, 1991; Viese-Berry & Beachley, 1994). Other causes include multiple trauma from motor vehicle and motorcycle accidents, farm accidents, fractures, dislocations, lacerations, falls from great heights, crushing injuries, sports-related injuries, and iatrogenic injuries.

Mechanism of Injury

Most penetrating injuries are caused by stab or low-velocity bullet wounds, and damage is usually confined to the wound tract. High-velocity bullet wounds have a cavitation effect that may directly injure vessels, nerves, tissue, and bone. Vascular injuries may occur directly or secondarily to bone fractures. Such injuries may not be appreciated on initial inspection of the surface wound (Perry, 1985; Weigelt & Klein, 1994).

Motor vehicle accidents are also a cause of trauma and vascular injury. More than 1.6 million people have died on the nation's highways in the last century. Motor vehicle crashes caused 46,300 deaths in 1990 (18.6 per 100,000 population), a 2% decrease from 1988 (Viese-Berry & Beachley, 1994). Although seatbelts have proved to save lives, vascular injuries such as contusions, lacerations, and thrombosis of the abdominal aorta and the mesenteric, hepatic, subclavian, and carotid vessels have been reported (States et al., 1987).

Iatrogenic complications are not always avoidable, but many can be prevented. Intravenous infusions of hypertonic solutions may result in thrombophlebitis. Accidental intraarterial infusions may cause arteriospasm and arteritis. Flushing air bubbles through an arterial line can result in necrosis and loss of the distal extremity and digits. Arterial puncture or cannulation for diagnostic studies or therapeutic procedures may cause local hematoma, thrombosis, dissections, and false aneurysms.

Pathophysiology

The usual pathogenesis of blunt trauma is intimal tear or contusion with associated thrombosis. Compression injuries are commonly seen in the femoral, popliteal, brachial, carotid, and renal arteries. Shearing and deceleration injuries may involve the thoracic, innominate, carotid, and subclavian arteries and may result in transection, dissection, thrombosis, aneurysm, or rupture. Penetrating arterial injury may result in hematoma, tamponade, dissection, transection, pseudoaneurysm formation, and arteriovenous fistula formation (Bastnagel Mason, 1994; Mattox, 1989).

Arterial insufficiency and organ ischemia may be a devastating result of arterial injury. Significant cerebral ischemia may result in permanent brain damage within 4 minutes; irreversible renal damage can occur within 1 hour; and skeletal muscle necrosis may occur within 6 hours or more. Compartment syndrome may result after revascularization of tissue that has been ischemic for 3 to 6 hours. This problem is commonly seen as a result of popliteal injury and crushing injuries to the lower leg. The compartments can be relieved by performing a fasciotomy (Mattox, 1989; Strange & Kelly, 1994).

Clinical Manifestations

Injuries of large vessels are usually readily identified because of obvious hemorrhage, but deeper, less extensive wounds may not be as evident. Hemorrhage, hematoma, and pulse deficits are the cardinal signs of vascular injury. Specific presentations are discussed under specific vascular injuries.

DIAGNOSTIC STUDIES

Doppler signals and measurement of distal arterial blood pressure are helpful in detecting vascular injury, but the specificity of these tests depends on the hemodynamics and the presence of preexisting vascular disease. Extensive hemorrhage may be accompanied by a decrease in hemoglobin and hematocrit, especially with hemodilution from fluid resuscitation.

Routine x-rays may reveal retained bullets, bone fragments and fractures, and soft tissue damage.

The CT scan is effective in identifying injuries to

the abdominal organs, hematomas, and displacement of other structures.

Magnetic resonance imaging provides a clear delineation of structures and can detect minor injuries. However, the use of MRI is contraindicated in circumstances where the patient could be suspected of having any embedded metal fragments, such as in shotgun wound.

The use of arteriography in the diagnosis of vascular injury remains controversial. In a stable patient, preoperative arteriography may be quite valuable in identifying vascular injury. Abnormalities may include an abrupt cutoff of a vessel, extravasation of contrast media, and evidence of an intraluminal clot. If the patient is unstable, or when firm indications for operation are present, arteriograms may not be necessary, and further evaluation is best performed in the operating room.

Management

Management of trauma patients is a frequent event in a major emergency department. Priority measures are establishing and maintaining an airway, controlling obvious hemorrhage, stabilizing the cervical spine, and providing fluid resuscitation and pain control.

Patients who arrive in severe hemorrhagic shock and are too unstable to be transferred to the operating room may require surgical control of hemorrhage in the emergency department. An emergency thoracotomy may be necessary to treat the unstable patient with an injury to the aorta or major abdominal vascular structure. The patient should be taken to the operating room for more definitive repair as soon as possible.

Patients who have major hemorrhage but are in less distress should be resuscitated in the emergency department while preparations are being made for surgery. Fluid resuscitation via large-bore catheters, either central or peripheral, should be begun as soon as possible. The choice of colloid or crystalloid fluid is controversial. Crystalloids tend to be eliminated rapidly from the vascular space by the kidneys. Colloids may leak through unstable capillary walls and promote interstitial edema. Blood is replaced as indicated. Regardless of the choice of fluid, it is of the utmost importance to keep central venous pressure (CVP) high enough to provide an adequate preload.

AORTA AND GREAT VESSEL INJURY. Injury to the aorta and great vessels may be the result of penetrating or blunt trauma. Massive hemorrhage resulting in hypovolemia, shock, and death often occurs. The physical examination usually reveals marked hypotension. Cardiac tamponade is a possibility with aortic injury and may be recognized by elevated CVP, tachycardia, paradoxical pulses, and narrow pulse pressure. Abdominal distension due to hemorrhage may be seen, although retroperitoneal bleeding may go undetected.

Radiographic signs of aortic injury include widened mediastinum, loss of the aortic knob, loss of sharpness of the aortic outline, deviation of the trachea and nasogastric tube to the right, depression of the left mainstem bronchus, and hematoma in the left apex. Foreign objects such as bullets may also be seen (Peyton & Wolfe, 1988; Weigelt & Klein, 1994).

If the patient's condition is not deteriorating, a CT scan or aortogram may be useful in identifying injury to the vessels as well as to organs and surrounding structures. Characteristics of an abnormal aortogram include extravasation of contrast medium, interruption of the aorta, intimal tears visualized as filling defects, and medial dissection (Bastnagel Mason, 1994; Peyton & Wolfe, 1988).

Hemodynamically unstable patients should be taken directly to the operating room. The nature of the vascular reconstruction depends on the nature of the injury. Small lacerations may be repaired by simple suturing. More extensive wounds may require extensive vessel repair, cardiopulmonary bypass, bypass grafting, as well as repair of surrounding tissues and organs.

CAROTID INJURY. Approximately 75% of carotid artery trauma is related to penetrating gunshot wounds, and 25% is caused by stab wounds. The mechanism of injury and direction of penetration may be helpful in locating the site of carotid injury. Gunshot wounds frequently cause complete transection of the artery with significant tissue loss. Stab wounds may result in lacerations or perforations (Perry, 1985, 1992). Injuries associated with blunt trauma may present with no external evidence of injury. These injuries may remain undetected until neurologic symptoms develop resulting from thrombus formation.

Physical examination may reveal evidence of local trauma, frank bleeding, tracheal or esophageal trauma, crepitus, stridor, pulse deficits, neurologic deficits, hematoma, thrills, and bruits (Kelly, 1984; Perry, 1992).

Neck x-rays may reveal cervical spine injuries, soft tissue injuries, tracheal deviation, or foreign bodies. Chest x-rays are useful in detecting hemopneumothorax. Noninvasive oculopneumoplethysmography and Doppler scanning are helpful in documenting carotid occlusion.

The carotid arteriogram provides direct assessment of the location and extent of the arterial disruption as well as intraluminal thrombus. Patients who are unstable and hemorrhaging should be taken immediately to the operating room for exploration and repair.

Initial therapy is directed at controlling the bleeding and maintaining cerebral perfusion. Maintenance of blood pressure and adequate oxygenation can help prevent cerebral infarction. An expanding hematoma may cause tracheal compression and respiratory compromise. Penetrating wounds that are not bleeding should not be probed in the emergency room because this may dislodge a thrombus or activate hemorrhage (McCann & Makhoul, 1988; Perry, 1992).

Carotid repair must be done using precise suture

and graft techniques to avoid thromboembolic complications. Isolation and control of the artery both proximal and distal to the injury is obtained. The artery is flushed, any clot is removed, and the artery is then repaired. The various methods of carotid repair include lateral arteriorrhaphy with or without vein patch, end-to-end anastomosis, interposition vein graft, prosthetic graft, and ligation (McCann & Makhoul, 1988; Perry, 1992). Complications include embolus, stroke, bleeding, and death. Maintenance of adequate blood pressure and blood volume is extremely important before and after surgery to preserve cerebral perfusion.

Patients should be closely monitored in the ICU for bleeding and neurologic problems. When occlusion from a thrombus or technical error occurs, rapid restoration of flow is often successful in preventing permanent neurologic deficits (Perry, 1986).

INJURIES TO ARTERIES OF THE EXTREMITIES. Vascular injuries to the upper extremity result primarily from gunshot wounds or stab wounds. Iatrogenic injuries may result from such procedures as venous access, percutaneous angiography, or cardiac catheterization. Although blunt trauma is an infrequent cause of upper extremity vascular injury, fractures and dislocations can potentially lacerate or compress adjacent vessels.

Femoral arteries are among the most frequently injured vessels. Large veins and vital nerves are located near the femoral arteries, and associated injuries are common. Most femoral injuries result from penetrating trauma from stab wounds and gunshot wounds, but they may be associated with femoral fractures (Perry, 1986).

Popliteal artery injuries are frequently associated with lower extremity injury. Although penetrating trauma may be more severe, blunt trauma may cause intimal disruption and thrombosis with no visible external injury. Blunt trauma is frequently seen in hyperextension or posterior dislocations of the knee (Perry, 1986). Failure to diagnose popliteal injury can lead to severe tissue ischemia and limb loss.

The most important factors associated with successful management of vascular wounds of the extremities are the ischemic time and the extent of the associated injuries to bones, muscles, joints, and nerves (McCann & Makhoul, 1988). Most experts agree that muscle can tolerate approximately 6 to 12 hours of ischemia before necrosis and permanent nerve damage occur.

The recognition of vascular injury in the extremity is often difficult in the presence of multiple trauma and hypovolemia. Doppler assessment of the distal circulation may be helpful when pulses are difficult to palpate. A difference of 10 mm Hg between extremities is considered significant.

Arteriography is helpful in identifying the location and extent of the vascular injury. However, if arterial injury is obvious or if the patient is unstable, arteriography can be performed in the operating room (McCann & Makhoul, 1988).

TABLE 26–2. **General Indications for Fasciotomy**

Vascular trauma
Prolonged arterial ischemia
Massive venous stasis
Combined venous–arterial injury
Popliteal arterial or venous injuries
Arterial ligation or failed reconstruction
Prolonged shock
Massive tissue swelling
Distal soft tissue injury
"Crush syndrome"
Massive soft tissue injury
External limb compression (drug overdose, constricting bandages)
Major extremity fractures
Limb reimplantation
Circumferential extremity burns
Stress-induced compartment syndromes (anterior compartment syndrome)
Wringer injuries
High-pressure tissue injections
Snake bite or other envenomation
Bleeding dyscrasia
Phlegmasia cerula dolens

Reprinted from T. F. Sweeney and M. D. Kerstein, Antibiotics in surgery for vascular trauma, in M. Kerstein (Ed.), *Management for Vascular Trauma* (Table 10.1, p. 137). Gaithersburg, MD: Aspen Publishers. Copyright © 1985 Aspen Publishers, Inc.

The type of vascular repair depends on the location and extent of the injury. The opposite extremity should be prepared in case a saphenous vein graft is required. Proximal and distal control is achieved before the hematoma is explored. Damaged tissue is resected, and an end-to-end anastomosis is completed. Once the necessary vascular repairs have been done, stabilization of fractures and other orthopedic repairs can be done.

Complications can include graft thrombosis, thromboembolism, bleeding, infection, and limb loss (Ernst et al., 1989).

Fasciotomy should always be considered when the arterial supply has been disrupted for 3 hours or more and is recommended when ischemic time is greater than 6 hours. Other indications for fasciotomy include crush injuries, closed distal extremity fractures, and swelling and tenseness of the extremity (Table 26–2) (Strange & Kelly, 1994).

Signs and symptoms diagnostic of compartment syndrome are swelling and tenderness of the compartment; pain greater than anticipated for the clinical situation, pain not relieved by analgesics, pain on passive stretch of the compartment, and decreased motor and sensory function (Bess, 1984).

After surgery the patient should be monitored in the ICU. Hourly neurovascular checks should be done by assessing the pulses, color, temperature, sensory and motor function, and level of pain. If there is any question about the patency of the graft or the distal circulation, the surgeon should be notified immediately.

SUMMARY

Remarkable advancements in the diagnosis and treatment of vascular disease and emergencies have been made. Major advances in rapid transportation, including helicopter retrieval and the use of specially trained paramedic personnel, have resulted in successful management of many vascular emergencies. Effective management depends on a high index of clinical suspicion for certain injuries as well as a solid knowledge base of the vascular anatomy and physiology.

Nurses play a vital role in the initial assessment and management of vascular emergencies. Although vascular surgery is an emerging subspecialty of medical practice, the nursing profession as a whole has not recognized the requirements for nursing vascular problems in nursing curricula, continuing education programs, nursing research, or nursing literature.

Recognition of the unique needs of vascular patients and the need for education, research, and publications on vascular disease continue to be a challenge to the nursing profession. Vascular nurses throughout the country are dedicated to the advancement of peripheral vascular nursing and high-quality patient care by supporting basic and advanced education in vascular nursing, providing local and national education programs, developing standards of care for vascular problems, and encouraging clinical research.

Although this chapter has not been all-inclusive, it is hoped that the topics will enhance the reader's understanding of vascular emergencies and the exciting challenges of caring for the patient with peripheral vascular problems.

REFERENCES

Anagnostopoulos, C. E. (1975). *Acute aortic dissections.* Baltimore: University Park Press.

Baird, R. J., & Almond, D. G. (1991). Medical management of the acute thoracic aortic dissection. In C. B. Ernst & J. C. Stanley (Eds.), *Current therapy in vascular surgery* (2nd ed.). Philadelphia: B. C. Decker.

Bastnagel Mason, P. J. (1994). Abdominal injuries. In V. D. Cardona, P. D. Hurn, P. J. Bastnagel, et al. (Eds.), *Trauma nursing from resuscitation through rehabilitation.* Philadelphia: W. B. Saunders.

Blaisdell, F. W., Steele, M., & Allen, R. E. (1978). Management of acute lower extremity arterial ischemia due to embolism and thrombosis. *Surgery, 84,* 822–834.

Brathwaite, C. E., & Rodrigues, A. (1992). Injuries of the abdominal aorta from blunt trauma. *American Surgeon, 58,* 350–352.

Brewster, D. C. (1991). Acute peripheral arterial occlusion. *Cardiology Clinics, 9,* 497–513.

Burchell. H. (1955). Aortic dissection. *Circulation, 12,* 1068–1079.

Burruss, N. (1993). Aortic dissection: Diagnosis and acute care management. *Cardiovascular Nursing, 29*(6), 41–51.

Butler, L., & Fahey, V. (1993). Acute arterial occlusion of the lower extremity. *Journal of Vascular Nursing, 11*(1), 19–22.

Chin, A., Zimmerman, J., & Fogarty, T. (1986). Acute arterial occlusion. In W. Moore (Ed.), *Vascular surgery: A comprehensive approach* (2nd ed., pp. 861–880). Orlando: Grune & Stratton.

Comerota, A. J. (1991). Fibrinolytic therapy for acutely thrombosed lower extremity arteries and grafts. In C. B. Ernst & J. C. Stanley (Eds.), *Current therapy in vascular surgery* (2nd ed.). Philadelphia: B. C. Decker.

Coselli, J. S., & Crawford, E. S. (1989). Thoracic aortic aneurysms. In H. Haimovici (Ed.), *Haimovici's vascular surgery: Principles and techniques* (pp. 591–611). Norwalk, CT: Appleton and Lange.

Crawford, E. S, Coselli, J. S., & Safi, H. J. (1989). Thoracoabdominal aortic aneurysms. In R. B. Rutherford (Ed.), *Vascular surgery* (3rd ed., pp. 927–942). Philadelphia: W. B. Saunders.

Dalsing, M., & Sawchuk, A. (1994). Surgery of the aorta: In V. Fahey (Ed.), *Vascular nursing* (pp. 251–290). Philadelphia: W. B. Saunders.

DeBakey, M., Cooley, D., & Creech, O., Jr. (1995). Surgical considerations of dissecting aneurysms of the aorta. *Annals of Surgery, 142,* 586–610.

DeBakey, M. E., & MeCullum, C. H. (1991). Surgical treatment of nonruptured infrarenal and juxtarenal aortic aneurysms. In C. B. Ernst & J. C. Stanley (Eds.), *Current therapy in vascular surgery* (2nd ed.). Philadelphia: B. C. Decker.

Erbel, R., Oilert, H., Meyer, J., et al. (1993). Effect of medical and surgical therapy on aortic dissection evaluated by transesophageal echocardiography: Implications for prognosis and therapy. The European Cooperative Study Group on Echocardiography. *Circulation, 87,* 1604–1615.

Ernst, C. B., Brennaman, B. H., & Haimovici, H. (1989). Fasciotomy. In H. Haimovici (Ed.), *Haimovici's vascular surgery: Principles and techniques* (pp. 995–1004). Norwalk, CT: Appleton and Lange.

Finkelmeier, B. A., & Finkelmeier, W. R. (1991). Iatrogenic arterial injuries resulting from invasive procedures. *Journal of Vascular Nursing, 3*(9), 12–17.

Fiorani, P., Taurino, M., Novelli, G., et al. (1992). Acute occlusion of the lower limbs. In R. M. Greenhalgh & L. H. Hollier (Eds.), *Emergency vascular surgery.* Philadelphia: W. B. Saunders.

Fogarty, T. J., Cranley, J. J., Krause, R. J., et al. (1963). A method of extraction of arterial emboli and thrombi. *Surgical Gynecology and Obstetrics, 116,* 241–244.

Goldstone, J. (1991). Aneurysms of the aorta and iliac arteries. In W. S. Moore (Ed.), *Vascular surgery: A comprehensive view* (pp. 304–324). Philadelphia: W. B. Saunders.

Green, R. (1991). Balloon catheter embolectomy for macroembolism in the extremities. In C. B. Ernst & J. C. Stanley (Eds.), *Current therapy in vascular surgery* (2nd ed.). Philadelphia: B. C. Decker.

Haimovici, H. (1989). Abdominal aortic and iliac aneurysms. In H. Haimovici (Ed.), *Vascular emergencies* (pp. 622–649). Norwalk, CT: Appleton and Lange.

Haimovici, H. (1989). Arterial embolism of the lower extremity and technique of embolectomy. In H. Haimovici (Ed.), *Vascular emergencies* (pp. 330–353). Norwalk, CT: Appleton and Lange.

Hertzer, N. R. (1989). Abdominal aortic and iliac aneurysms. In H. Haimovici (Ed.), *Haimovici's vascular surgery: Principles and techniques* (pp. 622–649). Norwalk, CT: Appleton and Lange.

Hollier, L. H., & Marino, R. J. (1991). Thoracoabdominal aortic aneurysms. In W. S. Moore (Ed.), *Vascular surgery: A comprehensive view* (pp. 304–324). Philadelphia: W. B. Saunders.

Hollier, L. H., & Rutherford, R. B. (1989). Infrarenal aortic aneurysms. In R. B. Rutherford (Ed.), *Vascular surgery* (pp. 909–927). Philadelphia: W. B. Saunders.

Jacobs, B. B., & Jacobs, L. M. (1991). Injury epidemiology. In E. Moore, K. L. Mattox, & D. V. Feliciano (Eds.), *Trauma* (2nd ed., pp. 15–36). Norwalk, CT: Appleton and Lange.

Link, K. M. (1992). Great vessels. In D. D. Stark & W. G. Bradley (Eds.), *Magnetic resonance imaging* (pp. 1490–1529). St. Louis: C. V. Mosby.

Masuda, Y., Yamada, Z., Morooka, N., Watanabe, S., & Inagaki, Y. (1991). Prognosis of patients with medically treated aortic dissections. *Circulation, 84*(5 Suppl), III7–13.

McIntyre, K., & Bernhard, V. (1987). Aortic aneurysms: Complications of aneurysms of the abdominal aorta and iliac arteries. In S. Wilson, F. Veith, R. Hobson, et al. (Eds.) *Vascular surgery: Principles and practice* (pp. 481–486). New York: McGraw-Hill.

Mills, J. R., & Porter, J. M. (1991). Nonoperative therapy for arterial macroembolism in the extremities. In C. B. Ernst & J. C. Stanley (Eds.), *Current therapy in vascular surgery* (2nd ed.). Philadelphia: B. C. Decker.

Modrall, J. G., Weaver, F. A., Yellin, A. E. (1993). Vascular considerations in extremity trauma. *Orthopedic Clinics of North America 24*(3), 557–563.

Muller-Wiefel, H., & Langkam, G. (1992). Acute occlusion of the upper limb arteries. In R. M. Greenlalgh & L. H. Hollier (Eds.), *Emergency vascular surgery.* Philadelphia: W. B. Saunders.

Neiman, H. L. (1989). Principles of arteriography. In H. Haimovici (Ed.), *Haimovici's vascular surgery: Principles and techniques* (pp. 76–93). Norwalk, CT: Appleton and Lange.

Neya, K., Omoto, R., Kyo, S., et al. (1992). Outcome of Stanford type B acute aortic dissection. *Circulation, 86*(5 Suppl), II1–7.

Nienaber, C. A., Spielman, R. P., von Kodolitsch, Y., et al. (1992). Diagnosis of thoracic aortic dissection: Magnetic resonance imaging versus transesophageal echocardiography. *Circulation, 85,* 434–447.

Nunnelee, J. D. (1994). Medications used in vascular patients. In V. Fahey (Ed.), *Vascular nursing* (pp. 219–234). Philadelphia: W. B. Saunders.

Ochsner, J. (1982). Management of femoral pseudoaneurysms. *Surgical Clinics of North America, 62,* 431–444.

O'Donnell, T. F., Jr. (1993). Arterial diagnosis and management of acute thrombosis of the lower extremity. *Canadian Journal of Surgery, 36,* 349–353.

Perry, M. O. (1991). Vascular trauma. In W. S. Moore (Ed.), *Vascular surgery: A comprehensive view* (pp. 560–577). Philadelphia: W. B. Saunders.

Perry, M. O. (1992). Penetrating carotid injury. In R. M. Greenhalgh & L. H. Hollier (Eds.), *Emergency vascular surgery.* Philadelphia: W. B. Saunders.

Roberts, W. (1981). Aortic dissection: Analogy, consequences and causes. *American Heart Journal, 101,* 195–215.

Sarris, G. E., & Miller, D. C. (1989). Peripheral vascular manifestations of acute aortic dissection. In R. B. Rutherford (Ed.), *Vascular surgery* (pp. 942–951). Philadelphia: W. B. Saunders.

Sarris, G. E., & Miller, D. C. (1993). Long-term results of surgical treatment. In J. Yao & W. Pearce (Eds.), *Long-term results in vascular surgery.* Norwalk, CT: Appleton and Lange.

Silver, D., & Cikrit, D. F. (1989). Thrombogenesis and thrombolysis. In H. Haimovici (Ed.), *Haimovici's vascular surgery: Principles and techniques* (pp. 188–194). Norwalk, CT: Appleton and Lange.

Smith, J., Holcroft, J., & Blaisdell, W. (1987). Acute arterial insufficiency. In S. Wilson, F. Veith, R. Hobson, et al. (Eds.), *Vascular surgery: Principles and practice* (pp. 325–343). New York: McGraw-Hill.

Smith, C. M., Yellin, A. E., Weaver, F. A., et al. (1994). Thrombolytic therapy for arterial occlusion: A mixed blessing. *American Surgeon, 60,* 371–375.

Spittell, P. C., Spittell, J. A. Jr., Joyce, J. W., et al. (1993). Clinical features and differential diagnosis of aortic dissection: Experience with 236 cases (1980–1990). *Mayo Clinic Proceedings, 68,* 642–651.

Strange, J. M., & Kelly, P. M. (1994). Musculoskeletal injuries. In V. D. Cardona, P. D. Hurn, P. J. Bastnagel, et al. (Eds.), *Trauma nursing from resuscitation through rehabilitation.* Philadelphia: W. B. Saunders.

Veise-Berry, S. W., & Beachley, M. (1994). Evolution of the trauma cycle. In V. D. Cardona, P. D. Hurn, P. J. Bastnagel, et al. (Eds.), *Trauma nursing from resuscitation through rehabilitation.* Philadelphia: W. B. Saunders.

Wahlers, R., Laas, J., Alken, A., & Borst, H. G. (1994). Repair of acute type A aortic dissection after cesarean section in the thirty-ninth week of pregnancy. *Journal of Thoracic and Cardiovascular Surgery, 107,* 314–315.

Wakefield, T. W. (1991). Surgical treatment of ruptured infrarenal abdominal aortic aneurysm. In C. B. Ernst & J. C. Stanley (Eds.), *Current therapy in vascular surgery* (2nd ed.). Philadelphia: B. C. Decker.

Weigelt, J. A., & Klein, J. D. (1994). Mechanism of injury. In V. D. Cardona, P. D. Hurn, P. J. Bastnagel, et al. (Eds.), *Trauma nursing from resuscitation through rehabilitation.* Philadelphia: W. B. Saunders.

Zimmerman, J. J., & Fogarty, J. J. (1983). Acute arterial occlusion. In W. S. Moore (Ed.), *Vascular surgery: A comprehensive review.* New York: Grune & Stratton.

VASCULAR EMERGENCIES MULTIDISCIPLINARY CARE GUIDE

COORDINATION OF CARE

Diagnosis/Stabilization Phase		Acute Management Phase		Recovery Phase	
Outcome	*Intervention*	*Outcome*	*Intervention*	*Outcome*	*Intervention*
All appropriate team members and disciplines will be involved in the plan of care.	Develop the plan of care with the patient/family, primary nurse(s), primary physician(s), vascular surgeon, cardiologist, family practitioner, perfusionist (if used), other specialists as needed, respiratory therapist, chaplain, and clinical nurse specialist, social worker.	All appropriate team members and disciplines will be involved in the plan of care.	Initiate planning for anticipated discharge and call home health as indicated. Begin teaching patient/family about care at home. Initiate vascular rehabilitation program if available.	Patient will understand how to maintain optimal health at home.	Provide written guidelines concerning care at home and any follow-up visits. Provide patient/family with phone numbers of resources available to answer questions.

FLUID BALANCE

Diagnosis/Stabilization Phase		Acute Management Phase		Recovery Phase	
Outcome	*Intervention*	*Outcome*	*Intervention*	*Outcome*	*Intervention*
Patient will achieve optimal hemodynamic status as evidenced by: • MAP >70 mm Hg • Hemodynamic parameters WNL • Urine output >0.5 mL/kg/hour • Absence of dysrhythmias • Adequate level of consciousness • Clear lung sounds • Absence of jugular venous distension	Monitor and treat cardiac parameters: • Dysrhythmias • BP • PA pressures • PCWP • CO/CI • SVR/PVR • Stroke volume • $S\dot{v}O_2$ • I & O • Level of consciousness • Evidence of tissue perfusion Monitor lab values: electrolytes, Mg^{++}, Hgb, Hct, PT, PTT, ACT if available, platelets, total creatine kinase (CK), and CK-MB. Assess for fluid overload or deficit and treat accordingly.	Patient will maintain optimal hemodynamic status.	Assess neurologic status q2–4h and PRN. If used, assess intracranial pressure q2–4h and PRN. Continue to assess for complications associated with vascular emergencies. Daily weight.	Same as acute management phase.	Same as acute management phase. Begin teaching patient signs and symptoms of inadequate tissue perfusion and when to seek medical attention.

	Anticipate need for vasopressor agents and assess response and titrate accordingly. Assess neurologic status q1h and PRN. If used, assess intracranial pressure q1h and PRN. Observe for signs of bleeding and administer blood products as needed; assess response. Monitor for signs of complications that can occur with vascular emergencies: hypovolemic shock, aneurysm dissection, aortic dissection, embolism, thrombus formation, cerebral hemorrhage, GI complications, stroke, acute renal failure, colon ischemia, spinal cord ischemia, MI, infection, hypertension, and so forth. Assess heart and bowel sounds q4h and PRN. Assess evidence of tissue perfusion.				

NUTRITION

Diagnosis/Stabilization Phase		Acute Management Phase		Recovery Phase	
Outcome	*Intervention*	*Outcome*	*Intervention*	*Outcome*	*Intervention*
Patient will be adequately nourished.	NPO until extubation, if applicable. Assess bowel sounds, abdominal distension, abdominal pain and tenderness q4h and PRN. Initiate clear liquids and monitor response.	Patient will be adequately nourished.	Assess bowel sounds, abdominal distension, abdominal pain, and tenderness q4h and PRN. Advance to diet as tolerated and monitor response. Monitor protein and albumin lab values. Assess patient risk of hypercholesterolemia and hyperlipidemia and begin assessment of patient's usual diet. For abdominal vascular surgery only—nasogastric tube to low intermittent suction until bowel sounds are present.	Patient will be adequately nourished.	Teach patient/family about heart healthy diet: • Total fat <30% of daily intake • Total saturated fat <10% of daily intake • Total daily cholesterol intake <300 mg • Caloric reduction if indicated • Sodium restriction if indicated Involve dietitian as necessary: • If eating less than half of tray • For unanticipated weight loss • For albumin <3

Care Guide continued on following page

VASCULAR EMERGENCIES MULTIDISCIPLINARY CARE GUIDE *continued*

MOBILITY

Diagnosis/Stabilization Phase		Acute Management Phase		Recovery Phase	
Outcome	*Intervention*	*Outcome*	*Intervention*	*Outcome*	*Intervention*
Patient will achieve optimal mobility.	Turn at least q2h if hemodynamically stable and monitor response. Begin passive/active-assist range-of-motion exercises.	Patient will achieve optimal mobility.	Progress exercise as tolerated: dangle, out of bed tid to qid, and walking 50 feet. Monitor response to increased activity and decrease if adverse events occur (tachycardia, dysrhythmias, syncope, hypotension/hypertension, dyspnea). Provide support as necessary.	Patient will achieve optimal mobility.	Continue to progress exercise as tolerated and monitor response. Walk at least 200–300 feet tid to qid. Assess ability to negotiate stairs if part of home environment. Teach patient/family about home exercise program. Decrease activity if tachycardia, chest discomfort, hypotension, or dyspnea occur.

OXYGENATION/VENTILATION

Diagnosis/Stabilization Phase		Acute Management Phase		Recovery Phase	
Outcome	*Intervention*	*Outcome*	*Intervention*	*Outcome*	*Intervention*
Patient will have adequate gas exchange as evidenced by: • $Sa_{O_2} > 90\%$ $Sp_{O_2} > 92\%$ • ABGs WNL • Clear breath sounds • Respiratory rate, depth, and rhythm WNL • Chest x-ray normal • Absence of dyspnea, cyanosis, and secretions • Hemoglobin and hematocrit WNL	Monitor ventilator settings and hemodynamic variables before, during, and after weaning. Wean ventilator and monitor patient response: • Wean F_{IO_2} to keep $Sp_{O_2} > 92\%$ • Monitor effects of anesthesia and wean ventilator accordingly. Assess respiratory functioning, including lung sounds, respiratory muscle strength, respiratory rate and depth, coughing ability, and chest x-ray. If not intubated, apply supplemental oxygen. Monitor with pulse oximetry. Reinforce use of incentive spirometry when extubated. Assess evidence of tissue perfusion. Monitor lab values: Hemoglobin, ABGs.	Patient will have adequate gas exchange.	Monitor and treat oxygenation/ventilation disturbances. Wean oxygen therapy and/or mechanical ventilation as tolerated. Reinforce the use of incentive spirometry. Use chest splint pillow or abdominal splint pillow if indicated. Have patient demonstrate proper use. Observe effect of increased activity on respiratory status. Observe for complications of vascular emergencies that may impair oxygenation/ventilation: aortic dissection, thrombus formation, embolus, tamponade, shock. If applicable, begin discussion on smoking cessation.	Patient will have adequate gas exchange.	Same as acute management phase. Chest x-ray before discharge. Provide instruction to patient/family on incentive spirometry and the use of chest/abdominal splint pillow at home. Continue discussions on smoking cessation. Refer to Smokers Anonymous or other available support groups.

COMFORT

Diagnosis/Stabilization Phase		Acute Management Phase		Recovery Phase	
Outcome	*Intervention*	*Outcome*	*Intervention*	*Outcome*	*Intervention*
Patient will be as comfortable and pain-free as possible, as evidenced by: • No objective indicators of discomfort • No complaints of discomfort	Assess quantity and quality of pain using pain scale. Administer narcotics and monitor response. Anticipate need for analgesia and provide as needed. If patient is intubated, establish effective communication technique with which patient can communicate discomfort and need for analgesics. Provide a quiet environment to potentiate analgesia. Provide reassurance in a calm, caring, competent manner.	Patient will be relaxed and pain free.	Same as stabilization phase. Provide chest or abdominal splint pillow, if indicated, and instruct on proper use. Have patient demonstrate proper use. Provide uninterrupted periods of rest. Teach patient relaxation techniques. Use back massage, humor, music therapy, and imagery to promote relaxation. Involve family in strategies. Provide analgesics as needed before chest tube removal (if indicated), ambulation, and any other procedures. Use sedatives as indicated. Observe for complications of vascular emergencies that may cause discomfort, as listed earlier.	Patient will be relaxed and pain-free.	Progress analgesics to oral medications as needed; assess response. Use sedatives as indicated and assess response. Continue alternative methods to promote relaxation as listed above. Teach patient/family alternative methods to promote relaxation as home. Teach self-medication for after discharge.

SKIN INTEGRITY

Diagnosis/Stabilization Phase		Acute Management Phase		Recovery Phase	
Outcome	*Intervention*	*Outcome*	*Intervention*	*Outcome*	*Intervention*
Patient will have intact skin without abrasions or pressure ulcers. Patient will be afebrile and without objective signs of infection.	Preoperative shower/scrub with antibacterial agent. Temperature q4h or as indicated. Begin passive/active-assist range-of-motion exercises. Assess all bony prominences at least q4h and treat if needed. Use preventive pressure-reducing devices if patient is at high risk for development of pressure ulcers. Treat pressure ulcers according to hospital protocol.	Patient will have intact skin without abrasions or pressure ulcers. Patient will be afebrile and without objective signs fo infection.	Same as stabilization phase. Temperature q4h unless elevated, then more frequently as indicated. Keep surgical site covered for 24 hours, then open to air unless actively draining. Assess incision sites for signs and symptoms of infection q4h and PRN. Wash incisions daily proximally to distally with sterile soap and water. Assess all bony prominences at least q4h and treat if needed. Assess skin adjacent to surgical wounds for symptoms of tape burns, allergies.	Patient will have intact skin without abrasions or pressure ulcers. Patient will be afebrile and without objective signs of infection.	Assess all bony prominences at least q4h and treat if needed. Assess and cleanse incisions as above. Teach patient/family proper skin care for at home: • Foot care • Care of incision • Appropriately fitting shoes and garments • Diet • Avoidance of tape and restricting garments Provide information concerning wound infection as needed.

Care Guide continued on following page

VASCULAR EMERGENCIES MULTIDISCIPLINARY CARE GUIDE *continued*

PROTECTION/SAFETY

Diagnosis/Stabilization Phase		Acute Management Phase		Recovery Phase	
Outcome	*Intervention*	*Outcome*	*Intervention*	*Outcome*	*Intervention*
Patient will be protected from possible harm.	Assess need for wrist restraints if patient is intubated, has a decreased level of consciousness, or is agitated and restless. Explain need for restraints to patient/family. Assess response to restraints, if used, and check q1–2h for skin integrity and impairment to circulation. Remove restraints as soon as patient is able to follow instructions. Provide sedatives as needed. Follow hospital protocol according to use of restraints.	Patient will be protected from possible harm.	If need still exists for restraints, check q1–2h for skin integrity and impairment to circulation. Provide support when dangling, getting out of bed, and ambulating; monitor response. Use gait belt as indicated for ambulation. Physical therapy consult as indicated.	Patient will be protected from possible harm.	Teach patient/family about any physical limitations in activity after discharge.

PSYCHOSOCIAL/SELF-DETERMINATION

Diagnosis/Stabilization Phase		Acute Management Phase		Recovery Phase	
Outcome	*Intervention*	*Outcome*	*Intervention*	*Outcome*	*Intervention*
Patient will achieve psychophysiologic stability. Patient will demonstrate a decrease in anxiety as evidenced by: • Vital signs WNL • Subjective report of decreased anxiety • Objective signs of decreased anxiety	Assess physiologic effects of critical care environment on patient (hemodynamic variables, psychological status, signs of increased sympathetic response). Provide sedatives as indicated. Take measures to reduce sensory overload. If patient is intubated, develop effective interventions to communicate with patient. Use calm, caring, competent, and reassuring approach with patient and family.	Patient will achieve psychophysiologic stability. Patient will demonstrate a decrease in anxiety.	Same as stabilization phase. Provide adequate rest periods. Continue to include family in all aspects of care. Continue to assess coping ability of patient/family and take measures as indicated. Maintain quiet environment.	Patient will achieve psychophysiologic stability. Patient will demonstrate a decrease in anxiety.	Provide instruction on coping mechanisms after discharge. Refer to outside services or agencies as appropriate (chaplain, social services, home health).

Arrange for flexible visiting to meet patient/family needs.
Determine coping ability of patient/family and take appropriate measures to meet their needs (i.e., explain condition, explain equipment, provide frequent condition reports, use easy-to-understand terminology, repeat information as needed, allow family to visit, answer all questions).

DIAGNOSTICS

Diagnosis/Stabilization Phase		Acute Management Phase		Recovery Phase	
Outcome	***Intervention***	***Outcome***	***Intervention***	***Outcome***	***Intervention***
Patient will understand any tests or procedures that need to be completed (vital signs, intake and output, hemodynamic monitoring, cardiac output, angiography, chest x-ray, echocardiography, Doppler studies, lab work, suctioning, ultrasound, CT scan, x-rays, ECG, MRI).	Explain all procedures and tests to patient/family. Be sensitive to individualized needs of patient/family for information. Establish effective communication technique with patient if he or she is intubated.	Patient will understand any tests or procedures that need to be completed [removal of indwelling lines, removal of chest tubes (if indicated), removal of ET tube (if indicated), lab work, chest x-ray, incentive spirometry, coughing and deep breathing, increase in activity, pulse oximetry].	Explain procedures and tests needed to assess recovery from surgery. Be sensitive to individualized needs of patient/family for information. Anticipate need for further diagnostic tests such as ultrasound or angiography and any intervention that may result from this.	Patient will understand meaning of diagnostic tests in relation to continued health (lab tests, increase in activity, coughing and deep breathing, incentive spirometry).	Review with patient before discharge the results of lab tests, chest x-ray, Doppler studies, angiography, and surgery. Discuss any abnormal values and appropriate measures patient can take to help return to normal. Provide patient with written guidelines concerning follow-up care. Provide instruction on care at home after discharge (i.e., when to call the doctor, care of incision, activity limitations, medications, diet).

REFERENCE

DeAngellis, R. (1991). The cardiovascular system. In J. G. Alspach (Ed.), *Core curriculum for critical care nursing* (4th ed., pp. 132–314). Philadelphia: W. B. Saunders.

UNIT 5

PULMONARY SYSTEM

Respiratory Physiology*

Kathleen S. Stone

Respiration can be defined as two separate processes: *external respiration,* the process of gas exchange within the lungs, which includes the absorption of oxygen (O_2) and the elimination of carbon dioxide (CO_2), and *internal respiration,* the utilization of oxygen at the cellular level in the mitochondria in oxidative phosphorylation and the production of adenosine triphosphate (ATP) and carbon dioxide.

The primary functions of the respiratory system are threefold: (1) regulation of the partial pressure of oxygen, (2) maintenance of the partial pressure of carbon dioxide at a constant, and (3) maintenance of the plasma hydrogen (H) ion concentration.

The components of the respiratory process include (1) pulmonary ventilation, which is the exchange of air between the external atmosphere and the alveoli, (2) the diffusion of oxygen and carbon dioxide between the alveoli and the blood, (3) transport of oxygen and carbon dioxide in the blood to and from the cells, and (4) control of ventilation. This chapter focuses on the anatomy of the respiratory tract and the four components of the respiratory process.

ANATOMY OF THE RESPIRATORY TRACT

The respiratory tract is composed of upper and lower passageways whose primary function is to conduct air in and out of the respiratory system. In contrast, the respiratory gas exchange portion of the respiratory system is the site where oxygen is exchanged from the alveolus into the blood and carbon dioxide from the blood into the alveolus.

Upper Respiratory Tract

Air can enter the respiratory system through either the nose or mouth, the nose serving as the normal route. The nasal cavity is irregularly shaped. It extends from the bony palate on the floor of the mouth upward to the base of the cranial cavity, which comprises the roof. The nose is divided into right and left nasal cavities by the nasal septum. The nostrils have a wide opening called the vestibule, which is lined with coarse hairs in the external nares that trap foreign substances such as dust. The roof of the nasal cavity contains the olfactory receptors for the sense of smell. The sense of smell is diminished by smoking or upper respiratory infections and is enhanced with hunger.

The nasal cavity contains three bony projections called the superior, middle, and inferior conchae. Under each conchae is an air space called a meatus. Air swirls around and under the conchae as it enters the nose, where it is warmed and humidified by the blood vessels in the surface epithelium covering the conchae.

The sinuses (frontal, paranasal, and sphenoidal), located in the face, are large air pockets lined with mucous membrane. Mucus from the sinuses drains into the nasal cavity. The sinuses add resonance to the voice and decrease the weight of the skull.

The posterior nasal opening is called the internal nares. Distal to the internal nares is the nasal pharynx, which contains the pharyngeal tonsils, or adenoids, composed of lymphoid tissue that is responsible for trapping bacteria and foreign particles. The oropharynx, surrounded by the palatine tonsils, serves as the common passageway for food and air. Distal to the oropharynx is the larynx (Fig. 27–1).

The larynx is the air passageway between the pharynx and the lungs. The epiglottis, a thin, leaf-shaped structure located immediately posterior to the root of the tongue, covers the entrance to the larynx. The larynx acts as a sphincter to prevent solids and liquids from passing into the bronchi and the lungs. Contained within the larynx are the vocal cords, which are composed of the true and false cords. The vocal cords are open with inspiration and closed during swallowing. During swallowing, the vocal cords assist in preventing the aspiration of food into the lungs. The vocal cords vibrate during the expiration of air, resulting in the production of sound. The vocal cords are innervated by the recurrent laryngeal nerve, which is a branch of the vagus nerve (cranial nerve X). Stimulation of the vocal cords during endotracheal intubation can cause stimulation of the vagus nerve, resulting in a decline in heart rate.

The major functions of the upper respiratory tract include (1) filtration of dust, dirt, foreign materials, and bacteria larger than 5 to 10 μm, and (2) humidifi-

Please refer to the glossary on page 630.

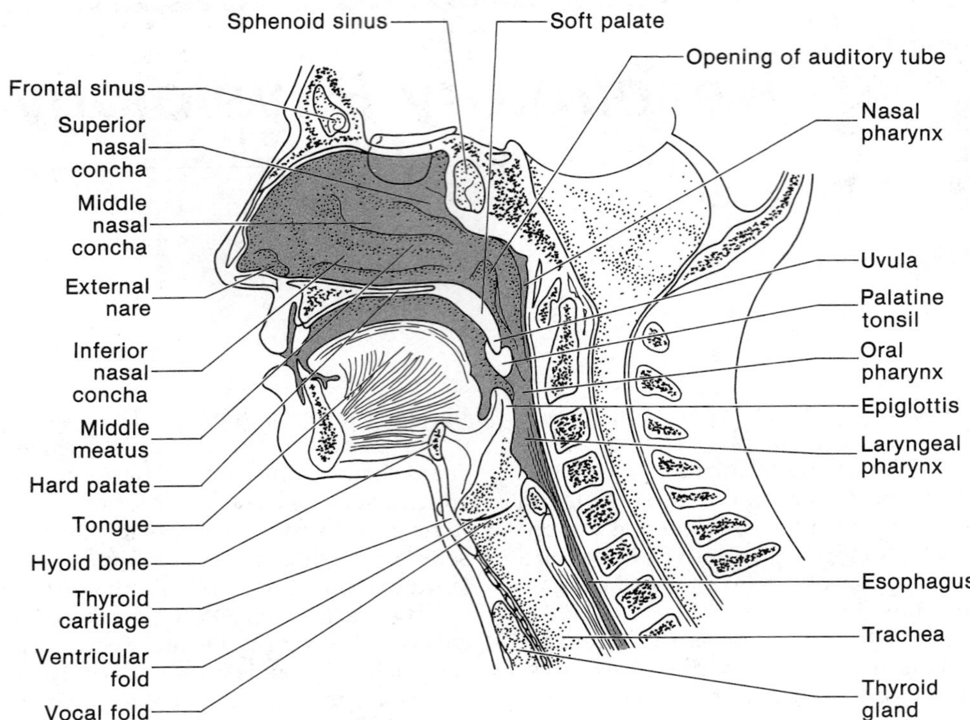

FIGURE 27–1. Sagittal section of the human head, showing the right nasal cavity; superior, middle, and inferior conchae; sinuses, frontal and sphenoidal; and the pharyngeal and laryngeal portions of the respiratory system.

cation and warming of the air. Alteration of these functions is an important consideration when the upper respiratory tract is bypassed with an endotracheal tube or a tracheostomy.

Irritation of the nasal passageways initiates afferent impulses traveling via the fifth cranial nerve, the trigeminal, to the medulla of the brain, where the sneeze reflex is triggered. The sneeze reflex results in the inspiration of atmospheric air, followed by closure of the epiglottis and tightening of the vocal cords, producing air trapping in the respiratory tract. This process is followed by contraction of the abdominal muscles and the expiratory muscles of respiration, resulting in the rapid expulsion of the trapped air and the foreign material that stimulated the reflex. During the sneeze reflex the uvula in the oropharynx becomes depressed to allow large amounts of air to pass rapidly through the nose to clear the nasal passageways.

Lower Respiratory Tract

The lower respiratory tract begins at the level of the trachea. The trachea in an adult is approximately 5 inches long and 1 inch in diameter. The trachea is continuous with the larynx above and terminates at the carina, the point of bifurcation into the right and left mainstem bronchi in the thoracic cavity. The trachea is composed of 16 to 20 regularly placed, horseshoe-shaped cartilaginous rings. The cartilaginous rings are incomplete posteriorly and have a musculomembranous sheath that lies anterior to the esophagus.

The paired lungs occupy most of the space in the thoracic cavity. The right lung is composed of three lobes and the left lung of two lobes. Each lung receives a branch from the right and left mainstem bronchus, respectively. The right bronchus is shorter and wider and has a more vertical position. This anatomic structure increases the risk of aspiration of food and foreign objects as well as the introduction of endotracheal tubes and suction catheters into the right bronchus. The right and left bronchi branch distally into numerous hollow tubes. Bronchi are differentiated into two categories. Bronchi not surrounded by lung tissue are called *extrapulmonary bronchi,* as opposed to bronchi that are surrounded by lung tissue, which are called *intrapulmonary bronchi.* Smooth muscle and irregularly shaped (ovals or crescents) cartilage plates maintain the patency of the intrapulmonary bronchi during lung inflation. With very distant branching, the cartilage becomes less complete. The secondary bronchi give rise to innumerable smaller branches called bronchioli.

The bronchioli are distinguished from the bronchi by a lack of cartilage and a single layer of epithelium. The bronchioli give rise to between 50 and 80 terminal bronchioli in each lobule. The terminal bronchioli are the last purely conducting portion of the bronchial tree where no gas exchange occurs (Fig. 27–2).

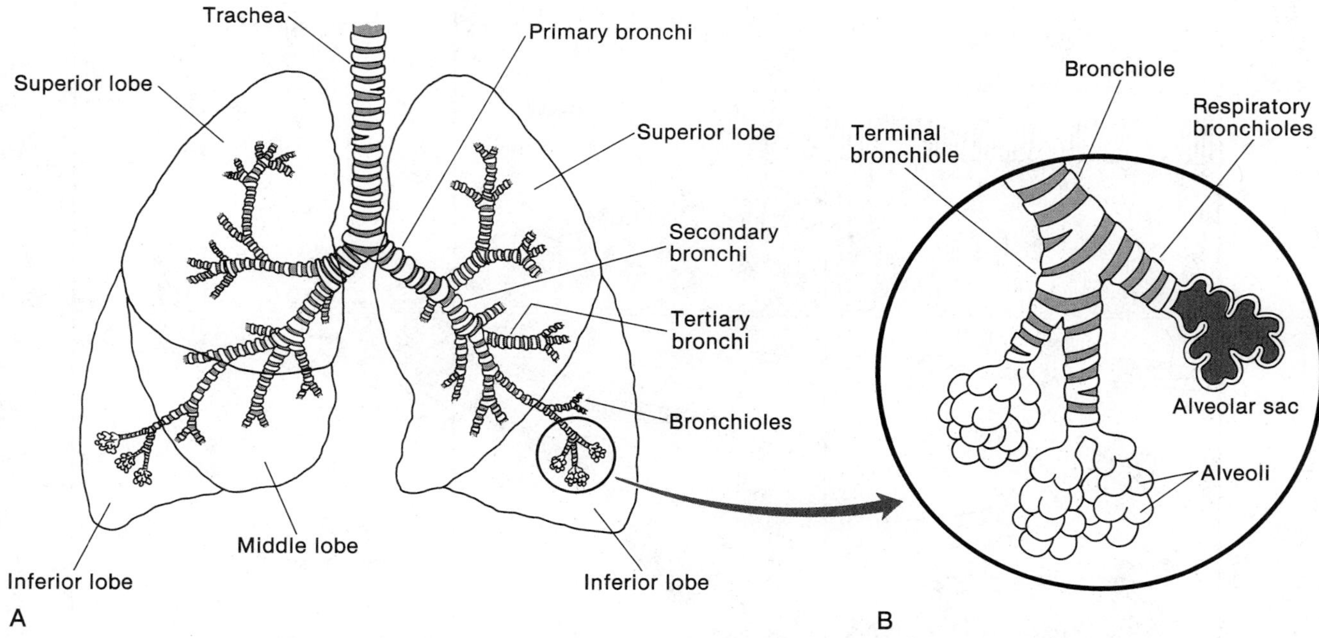

FIGURE 27–2. Gross anatomy of the lower respiratory tract, including the right lung composed of three lobes and the left lung of two lobes; the right and left mainstem bronchus; the extrapulmonary bronchi, intrapulmonary bronchi, bronchioli, and terminal bronchioli.

Histology of the Conduction Portion of the Respiratory Tract

The innermost layer of the respiratory tract is composed of pseudostratified columnar ciliated epithelium. The cells are rectangular-shaped columns that are anchored in a basement membrane. The cells give the appearance of being stratified in layers but are not, because each cell is individually anchored in the basement membrane. Projecting out of each columnar cell are 15 to 200 cilia, which measure 7 μm in height. The name "pseudostratified columnar ciliated epithelium" is reflective of the visual appearance of this layer. Interspersed between the columnar cells are goblet cells, which produce mucus. Mucus is a protective material that traps particulate matter such as dust, foreign material, and bacteria. Mucus is composed of a double (sol–gel) layer on the surface of the epithelium. The innermost layer is the periciliary liquid or sol layer in which the cilia beat. The outermost layer is the viscous gel layer. The viscous layer is nonabsorbent to water and serves to protect the sol phase from desiccation. The tips of the cilia just strike the innermost portion of the gel covering them, thus facilitating the proximal movement of material. The mucus is constantly propelled by the swaying cilia, which move at a rate of 16 times/second, to the pharynx, where it is either expectorated or swallowed and eliminated by the gastrointestinal tract.

The mucus together with the cilia comprise the mucociliary escalator. The escalator is an important protective mechanism to maintain airway clearance. The composition and physical properties of the mucous layer can change dramatically in bronchopulmonary and cardiac disease. Allergic reactions, asthma, cystic fibrosis, circulatory failure, and respiratory tract neoplasms increase the volume and the character of the mucus. Decreased hydration can increase mucus viscosity, thereby decreasing mucociliary clearance. Ciliary movement can be inhibited by many noxious agents, particularly cigarette smoke. The mucociliary escalator is disrupted by endotracheal intubation and by the denuding of the epithelial layer with repeated endotracheal catheter insertions and withdrawal, and the application of vacuum as with endotracheal suctioning. A reduction in mucociliary activity can result in lung infections and airway obstruction by stationary mucus.

The pseudostratified columnar ciliated epithelium lines the entire conducting respiratory passageway. The terminal bronchioli do not have mucus-secreting goblet cells or cilia on the columnar cells. In the terminal bronchioli, the epithelial cells are cuboidal in shape and flattened (Fig. 27–3).

Immediately below the basement membrane is the membrane propria. The membrane propria has a different appearance depending on its location in the upper or lower respiratory tract. In the trachea, the membrane propria is composed of loose elastic fibers, whereas in the bronchi there are strong strips of elastic tissue. The membrane propria contains macrophages—phagocytic cells that engulf bacteria. In addition, the membrane propria is very vascular and assists in warming the inhaled atmospheric air.

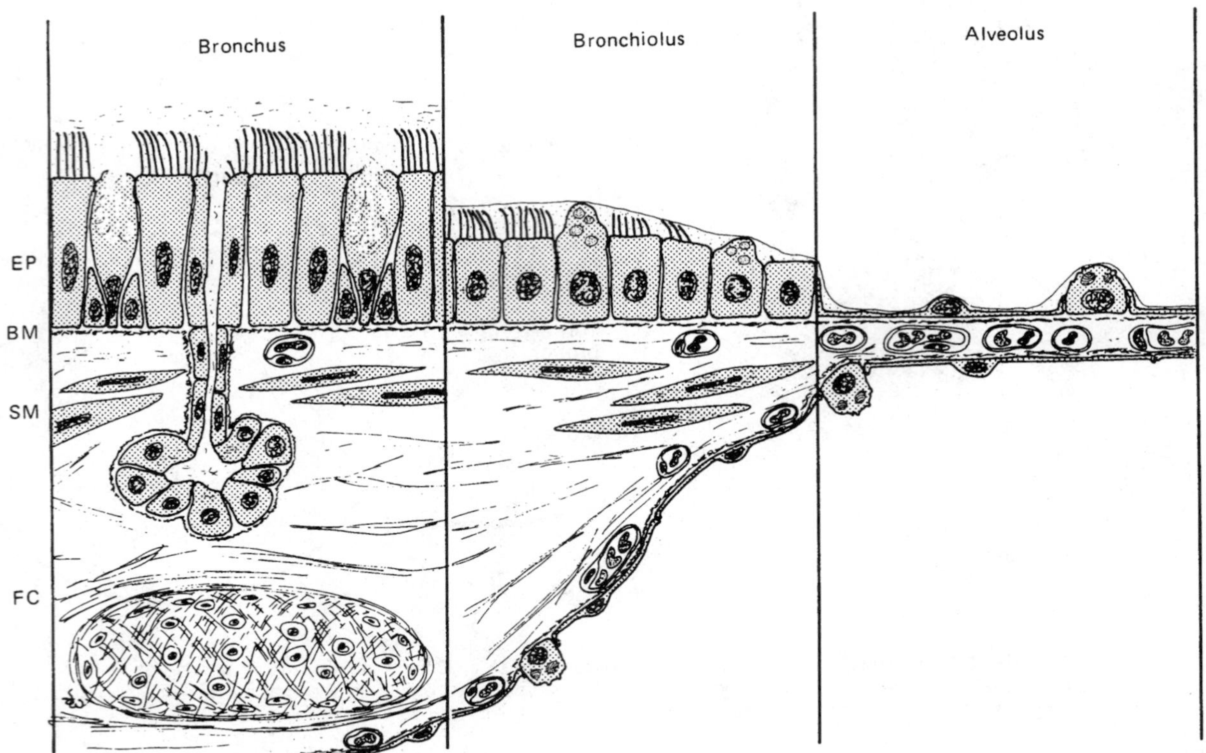

FIGURE 27–3. Change of airway wall structure at the three principal levels. The epithelial layer (*EP*) gradually becomes reduced from pseudostratified to cuboidal and then to squamous but retains its organization as a mosaic of lining and secretory cells. The smooth muscle layer (*SM*) disappears in the alveoli. The fibrous coat (*FC*) contains cartilage only in bronchi and gradually becomes thinner as the alveolus is approached. BM, basement membrane. (From Weibel, E. R., & Burri, P. H. [1973]. *Funktionelle aspekte der lungenmorphologie.* In W. A. Fuchs & E. Voegeli [Eds.], *Aktuelle probleme der roentgendiagnostik* [Vol. 2, pp. 1–17]. Berne: Huber Publishers.)

Smooth muscle is located immediately under the membrane propria in portions of the upper and lower respiratory tracts. Smooth muscle is located in the posterior portion of the trachea and in the extrapulmonary bronchi. In the intrapulmonary bronchi, the smooth muscle constitutes a layer that completely encircles the lumen of the bronchi. There are two sets of spirally arranged smooth muscle fibers, one clockwise, the other counterclockwise. The state of muscle contraction of this smooth muscle layer can significantly affect the size of the bronchial lumen. Contraction and relaxation of the smooth muscle, especially in the bronchioli, can alter resistance to air flow. The smooth muscle fibers are innervated by the autonomic nervous system. Parasympathetic influence through vagal innervation results in bronchial constriction and mucus secretion. Sympathetic innervation as well as stimulation of $beta_2$-adrenergic receptors due to increased circulating epinephrine levels cause bronchial relaxation. Mast cells situated beneath the epithelium near the blood vessels and smooth muscle release histamine in antigen–antibody reactions, causing bronchoconstriction.

The level of carbon dioxide in the respiratory gas in the bronchi influences the degree of muscular contraction. Increased levels of carbon dioxide cause bronchodilation, thus enhancing exhalation of the gas, whereas decreased levels of carbon dioxide cause bronchoconstriction and enhanced carbon dioxide retention. Cooling of the airways due to inhaled cold atmospheric air, as during exercise, can trigger bronchoconstriction. There is a circadian rhythm in bronchial tone, with maximal constriction occurring commonly in the early morning hours and maximal dilation occurring commonly in the early evening hours. As a result, asthma attacks are more severe in the late night and early morning hours.

The inner lining of the trachea and bronchi is very sensitive to light touch, excessive amounts of foreign matter, pollutants, cigarette smoke, or other causes of irritation. The larynx and carina, the point where the trachea divides into the right and left bronchi, are especially sensitive. Stimulation of the inner lining initiates afferent impulses through the vagus nerve to the medulla, causing a cough reflex. The cough reflex initiates the inspiration of approximately 2.5 liters of air. The events of the cough reflex are similar to those of the sneeze reflex except that the pressures generated in the lungs may rise to as high as 100 mm Hg and expel air at velocities as high as 75 to 100 miles per hour, assisting in the removal of foreign material. Endotracheal intubation reduces the effectiveness of the cough reflex because closure of the epiglottis and vocal cords is prohibited.

ANATOMY OF THE RESPIRATORY GAS EXCHANGE UNIT

The functional unit of the lung in which gas exchange occurs (external respiration) is called the primary globule or the acinar. An acinar gas exchange unit is composed of (1) respiratory bronchioli, (2) alveolar ducts, (3) alveolar sacs, and (4) alveoli (Fig. 27–4).

Bronchioli

The respiratory bronchioli are short, tubular structures that have an internal diameter of approximately 0.5 mm. The respiratory bronchioli are continuous with the terminal bronchioli. The epithelial cells in the respiratory bronchioli are cuboidal in shape and lack cilia and interspersed goblet cells. The walls of the respiratory bronchioli consist of collagenous connective tissue, smooth muscle bundles, and sparse elastic fibers. Alveoli appear in the walls of the bronchioli, hence the name *respiratory bronchioli.*

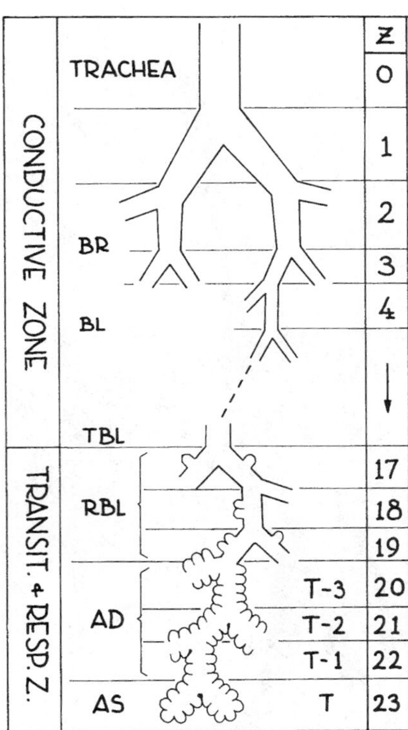

FIGURE 27–4. Airway branching in human lung by regularized dichotomy from trachea (generation z-0) to alveolar ducts and sacs (generations 20 to 23). The first 16 generations are purely conducting: transitional airways lead into the respiratory zone made of alveoli. (From Weibel, E. R. [1963]. *Morphometry of the human lung.* Heidelberg: Springer-Verlag.)

Alveoli

The alveolar ducts are thin-walled, tubular structures that give off numerous branches. The alveolar sacs contain two or more individual alveoli. The alveoli are thin-walled, polyhedral sacs. The walls of the alveoli are really spaces in a huge mesh of sponge-like elastic tissue fibers lined with a layer of epithelium, which is a single cell in thickness. Surrounding the walls of the alveoli are capillary networks for gas exchange between the respiratory system and the blood. In the normal adult there are approximately 300 million alveoli, thereby creating a tremendously large surface area for gas exchange (Fig. 27–5).

The alveolar capillary membranes have four layers.

1. Alveolar squamous epithelium
2. Basement membrane of elastic fibers and collagen
3. Basement membrane of the pulmonary capillary
4. Capillary endothelium

These four layers, which are 0.5 μm thick, form the morphologic interface between the alveoli and the capillary blood for the diffusion of oxygen from the alveoli and carbon dioxide from the blood. In the adult the total surface area of alveoli in contact with the capillaries is 70 m^2 (Fig. 27–6).

The alveoli are lined by two types of epithelial cells. Type I cells are flat cells and are the primary lining cells. Type II cells, or granular pneumocytes, are highly active metabolically and produce surfactant. Alveolar macrophages are present in the alveoli and are responsible for phagocytizing foreign particles and bacteria.

PULMONARY CIRCULATION

The pulmonary artery arises from the right ventricle and branches almost immediately into the right and left pulmonary arteries to join the bronchi in the mediastinum at the hilus of the lung. The pulmonary arterial vessels transport deoxygenated venous blood to the lungs. The pulmonary circulation delivers the cardiac output from the right ventricle and distributes it as a very thin film of blood in the pulmonary capillaries to enhance gas exchange between the alveoli and the capillaries. The pulmonary vascular system is a network of highly distensible vessels with thin, incomplete smooth muscle in the tunica media layer, resulting in a low resistance system. In a normal person the average systolic and diastolic pressures in the pulmonary artery are approximately 25 and 10 mm Hg, respectively, with a mean pressure of 15 mm Hg. These pressures are much lower than those in the aorta, which reflects the lower pressures produced in the right ventricle during systole and the low resistance network. The mean diastolic pressure in the left

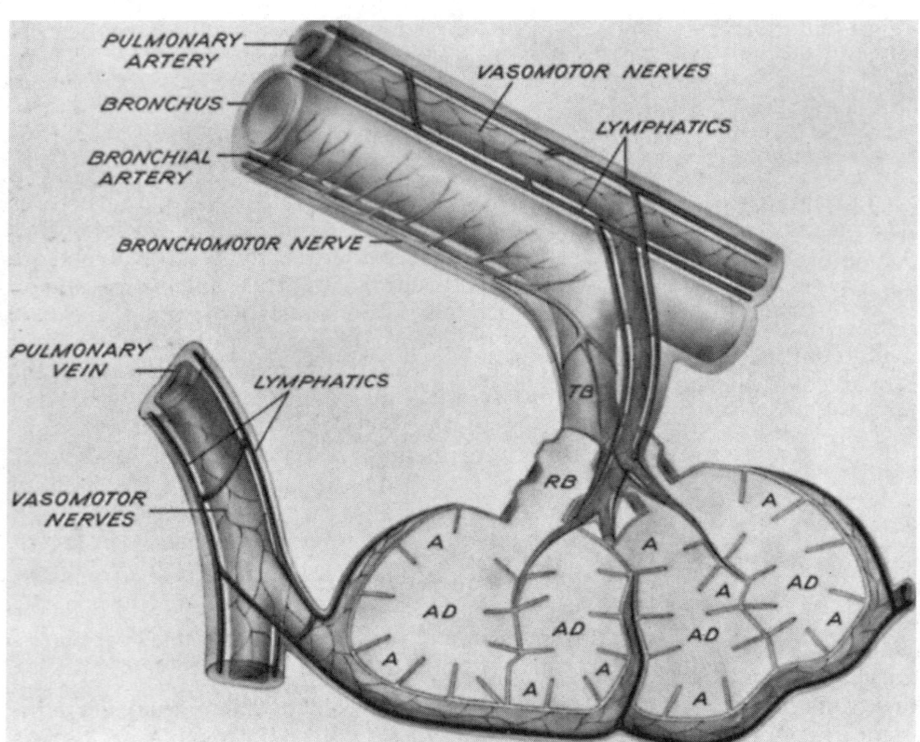

FIGURE 27–5. Structure of the lung. *Abbreviations:* A, anatomic alveolus; AD, alveolar duct; RB, respiratory bronchiole; TB, terminal bronchiole. (From Staub, N. C. [1970]. The pathophysiology of pulmonary edema. *Human Pathology, 1,* 419.)

atrium is 5 to 8 mm Hg, so the total pulmonary arteriovenous pressure gradient is approximately 10 mm Hg, compared to about 90 mm Hg in the systemic circulation. The pressure fall from the pulmonary artery to the pulmonary capillaries is negligible, resulting in a mean hydrostatic pressure in the pulmonary capillaries of approximately 10 mm Hg. The oncotic pressure in the pulmonary capillaries is 25 mm Hg, resulting in an inward-directed pressure gradient of 15 mm Hg, which keeps the alveoli free of fluid. When pulmonary capillary pressure is increased above 25 mm Hg, as in left ventricular failure or mitral valvular disease, pulmonary congestion and edema result. Pulmonary edema is the accumulation of fluid in the interstitial spaces of the lung or in the air spaces. As pulmonary capillary pressure rises, fluid moves out of the capillaries into the interstitial space. The interstitial fluid of the lungs can increase only 100 mL before fluid begins to rupture the alveolar epithelial membranes and enter into the alveoli. If the edema becomes severe enough, death can occur because of suffocation resulting from the decreased diffusion of oxygen from the alveoli to the pulmonary capillaries (see Chapter 32). The lymphatic channels, which end near the terminal bronchioli, drain fluid from the interstitial space and propel the fluid by active contraction of the smooth muscle in the wall of the lymphatics to the hilus of the lung (Fig. 27–7). Lymph flow from the lung is normally about 20 mL/minute and greatly increases in pulmonary edema. The four pulmonary veins that transport oxygenated blood course independent of the bronchial tree and are collected at the hilus to return the blood to the left atrium for distribution through the system circulation.

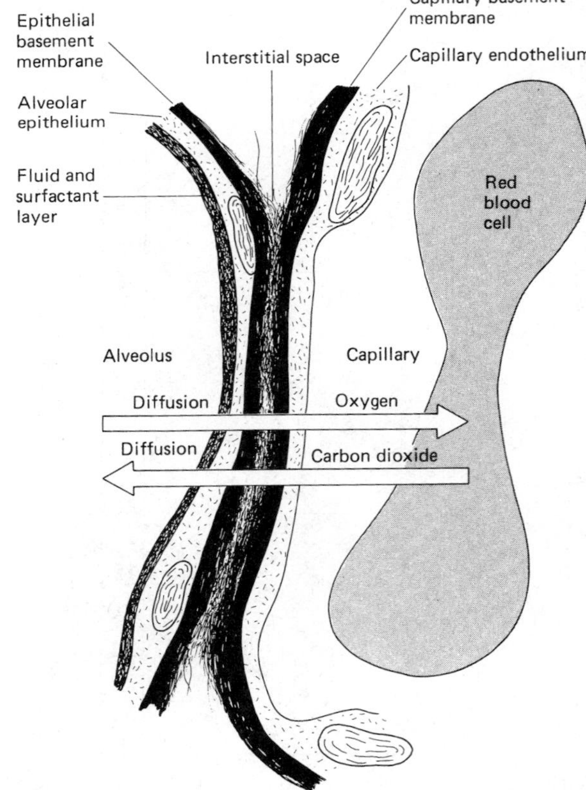

FIGURE 27–6. Ultrastructure of the respiratory membrane as shown in cross section. (From Guyton, A. C. [1991]. *Textbook of medical physiology* [8th ed., p. 429]. Philadelphia: W. B. Saunders.)

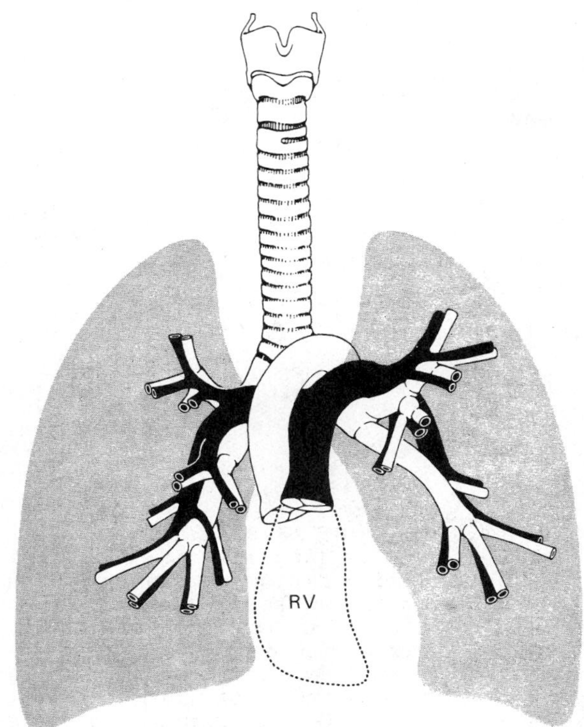

FIGURE 27–7. Schematic diagram of distribution of lymph nodes and main lymphatic channels along bronchial tree. (Reproduced with permission from Fishman, A. P. [1980]. *Assessment of Pulmonary Function* [p. 50]. New York: McGraw-Hill. Reproduced with permission of The McGraw-Hill Companies.)

The pulmonary blood vessels are innervated by the sparse sympathetic vasoconstrictor fibers and by the parasympathetic dilator fibers. The fetal pulmonary circulation responds to both parasympathetic and sympathetic stimulation. The pulmonary arterioles are constricted by such substances as norepinephrine, epinephrine, angiotensin II, thromboxanes, and prostaglandin $F_{2\alpha}$. They are dilated by isoproterenol, acetylcholine, prostaglandin I_2, and nitric oxide. In the body, both constrictor and dilator substances may be released simultaneously, resulting in a mixed response. The pulmonary venula are constricted by serotonin, histamine, and *Escherichia coli* endotoxin. Despite this innervation and the reactivity to vasoactive agents, the overall regulation of pulmonary blood flow is passive, and local adjustments to ventilation and perfusion are determined by the local concentration of oxygen and H^+ ion. This local control will be addressed later in the chapter under Ventilation–Perfusion Ratio.

Because the pulmonary circulation receives all of the venous blood of the body before it is recycled, the lungs play an important metabolic role in regulating the level of vasoactive substances in the circulation. The surface area of the pulmonary capillary endothelium is large, and the cells have many projections and indentations that contain many enzyme-rich sites. Prostaglandins E and F types, serotonin, norepinephrine, and histamine are removed from the blood while passing through the lungs. Angiotensin I is converted to the powerful vasoconstrictor angiotensin II during passage through the lung.

The bronchi and lung tissue receive blood through the bronchial vessels that originate from the midthoracic aorta or from branches of the intercostal, internal mammary, or subclavian arteries. Two or three arteries accompany the bronchi to form a peribronchial plexus. Venous blood drains into the azygous and hemizygous systems. Venous blood from the small bronchi enters the pulmonary veins, thus adding deoxygenated blood to the overall oxygenated blood leaving the lungs.

MECHANICS OF PULMONARY VENTILATION

Relationship of the Lungs to the Thoracic Cage

The lungs are located in a closed compartment called the thoracic cage. The thoracic cage is composed of the sternum anteriorly, the 12 pairs of ribs, and the spine posteriorly. The intercostal muscles, both internal and external, are located between the ribs. The large, dome-shaped muscular diaphragm composed of skeletal muscle, forms the floor of the thoracic cage (Fig. 27–8).

The space inside the thoracic cage is called the thoracic cavity. In addition to the lungs, the thoracic cavity houses the heart, great vessels, esophagus, and mediastinum. The lung is maintained in a stable position within the thoracic cavity by the root or hilus. The hilus is a depression in the lung where the airways and blood vessels enter the lung from the mediastinum. The pulmonary ligament, a long, narrow band of attachment between the visceral and mediastinal pleura, also serves to stabilize the lung. When the lung retracts during a pneumothorax, it remains attached to the mediastinal wall of the thoracic cavity because of these attachments. When the lungs are expanded they fill the entire chest cavity to a total lung capacity of 5 to 6 liters.

Although the lungs are stable within the thoracic cavity, they are very mobile to allow for expansion during inspiration and retraction during expiration. The mobility of the lung is the result of morphologic development from the mesoderm of a serosal space. The interior surface of the thoracic cavity is lined by a delicate sheet of squamous epithelial cells (serosal or mesothelial cells) called the parietal pleura. The surface of the lung tissue is covered by an identical serosal layer called the visceral pleura. The parietal and visceral pleura are so closely apposed that there is only a potential space between the two surfaces called the intrapleural space. The intrapleural space is filled with a thin film of fluid produced by the serosal cells that serves as a lubricant between the two layers. The relationship between the parietal pleura lining the thoracic cavity and the visceral pleura covering the lung tissue can be compared to two glass slides with a drop of water between them. The two pleural surfaces are as closely apposed as the glass slides, which slide easily

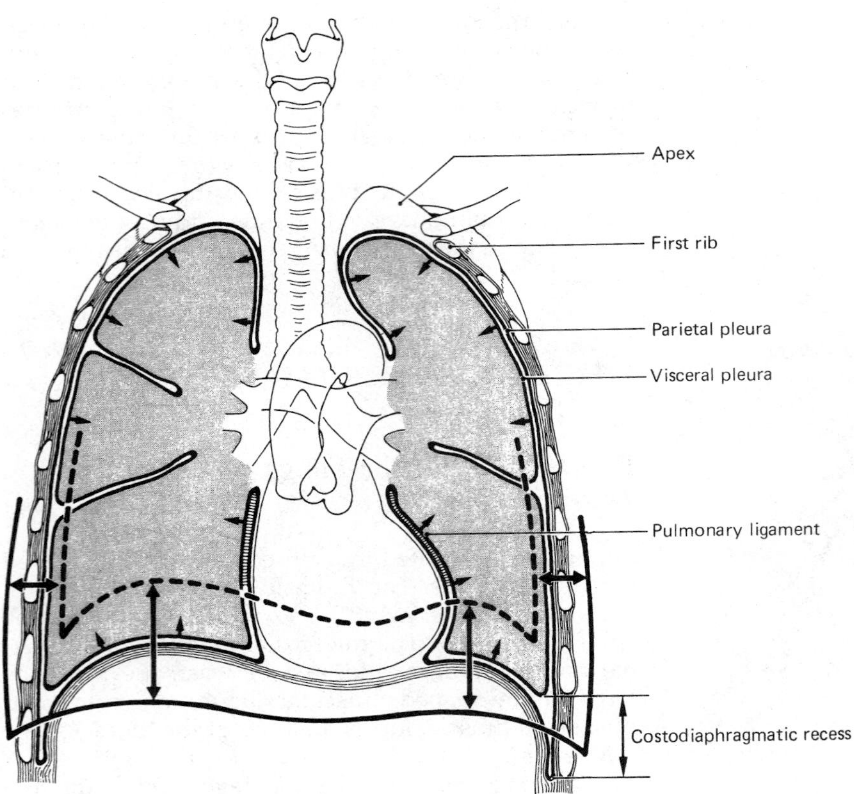

FIGURE 27–8. Frontal section of the chest and lung, depicting the thoracic cage and the structures contained within the thoracic cavity. The single arrows indicate retractive force; the double arrows show the excursion of the lung bases and the periphery between deep inspiration and expiration. (Reproduced with permission from Fishman, A. P. [1980]. *Assessment of pulmonary function* [p. 19]. New York: McGraw-Hill. Reproduced with permission of The McGraw-Hill Companies.)

along one another but are also adherent to one another. This intimate relationship between the two pleural surfaces is important for breathing, as described in the next section.

Inspiration and Expiration

The process of inspiration followed by expiration is called the respiratory cycle, and is the result of pressure gradients. To understand the process of ventilation, it is important to understand the pressures that exist on the thorax and within the lungs at rest and during the respiratory cycle. The external pressure exerted on the thorax is atmospheric pressure, which is equal to 760 mm Hg. The alveoli, which are in direct communication with the atmosphere through the nose or mouth, are also at atmospheric pressure equal to 760 mm Hg. The pressure within the alveoli is termed "intraalveolar."

The pressure between the chest wall and the lungs is called intrapleural pressure and is −2.5 mm Hg subatmospheric, or 757.5 mm Hg. The intrapleural subatmospheric pressure results from the two opposing forces of deflation and inflation (Fig. 27–9).

The forces tending toward deflation in the lung are caused by the elastic recoil of the lung tissue and the surface tension at the liquid–air interface. The lungs have a continual tendency to recoil or collapse because they are composed of elastic fibers that when stretched by inflation attempt to shorten. This process is similar to an elastic band, which, when stretched, will recoil upon the release of tension.

The second and most important force tending toward deflation of the lung is the surface tension of the fluid lining the alveoli. The surface tension is the result of the intermolecular attraction between the water molecules at the surface of the liquid–air interface in the alveoli. The water molecules at the surface are pulled downward toward the water molecules below the surface because of the attraction of unlike charges on the water molecules. This intermolecular attraction results in a sheet of fluid lining the alveolar surface that is continually trying to collapse inward. About one-third of the elastic recoil of the lung and two-thirds of the surface tension account for the forces acting toward deflation in the lung (Fig. 27–10).

Surfactant, a lipoprotein substance secreted by the type II pneumocytes in the alveoli, is important in lowering the surface tension at the air–liquid interface, thereby decreasing the tendency of the alveoli to collapse. Surfactant is composed of dipalmitoylphosphatidylcholine (DPPC). The DPPC molecule has a hydrophilic (water-loving) "head" and two parallel hydrophobic (water-fearing) fatty acid "tails." The surfactant molecules are oriented parallel at the air–liquid interface in the alveoli. The heads of the molecule are oriented toward the water in the alveoli, whereas the tails are oriented toward the air. The orientation of the surfactant molecule disrupts the inter-

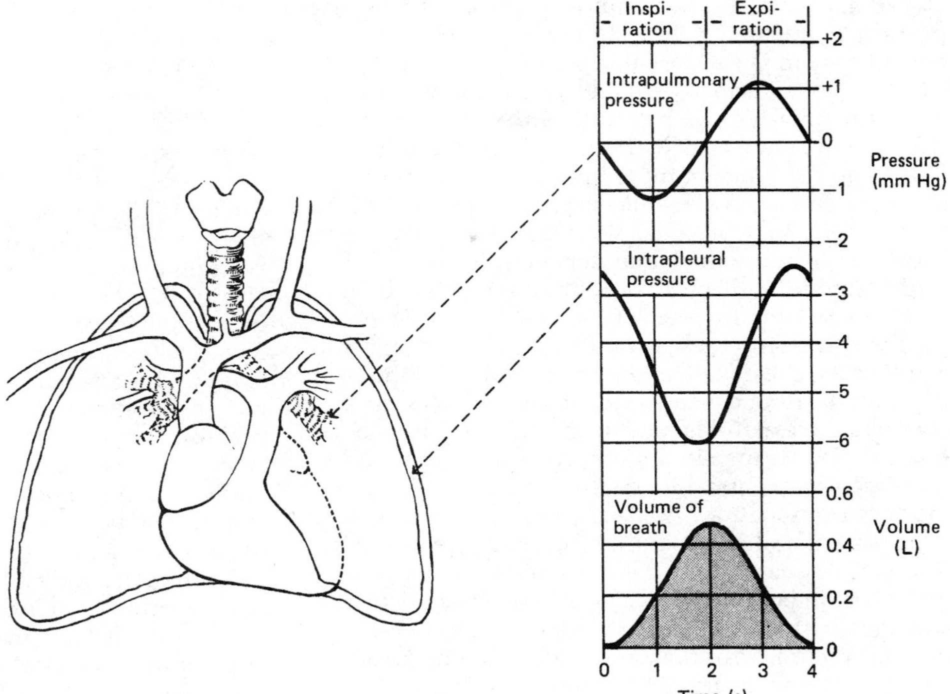

FIGURE 27–9. Changes in intrapleural (intrathoracic) and intrapulmonary pressure relative to atmospheric pressure during inspiration and expiration. (From Ganong, W. F. [1989]. *Review of medical physiology* [14th ed.]. Norwalk, CT: Appleton & Lange.)

molecular interaction between the surface water molecules, thereby decreasing the surface tension. The surfactant molecules are spread apart during inspiration as the alveolar size increases, but move together during expiration, thus adjusting surface tension during breathing.

Surfactant is produced and replaced on a regular basis by type II cells. The importance of surfactant in reducing surface tension in the alveoli is exemplified by commonly seen derangements. Cigarette smoking decreases the amount of surfactant at the air–liquid interface in the alveoli. Fresh-water drowning victims lose their surfactant, resulting in increased alveolar tension that necessitates high pressures to ventilate the individual. Patients who have been on a pump-oxygenator during cardiac surgery have a surfactant deficiency, resulting in patchy atelectasis in the immediate postoperative period.

Surfactant is important at birth, when the infant expands the lungs for the first time. Surfactant prevents the lungs from collapsing. Normally, near term, both maternal and fetal glucocorticoid hormone levels are

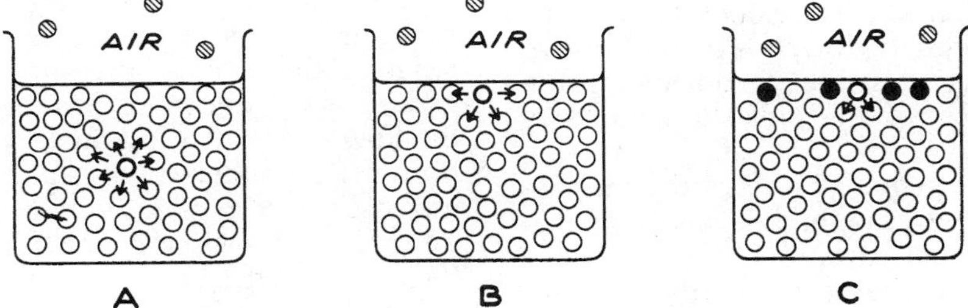

FIGURE 27–10. Surface tension. "In a liquid such as water at rest, the intermolecular forces acting on the molecule in *A* are equal in all directions; molecular forces pull it downward, to the left, to the right, and upward. However, the water molecule in *B*, at the water–air surface, does not experience equal attracting forces in all directions. *B* is attracted by water molecules directly beneath it, but there are relatively few molecules in the gas above it to exert an upward force. Therefore, more molecules pull it down than pull it up, and typical of surface molecules, it tends to dive downward. As a result of this imbalance of intermolecular forces, the surface shrinks to the smallest possible area. The resulting force in the surface is referred to as surface tension" (description from Comroe, 1965). In *C*, surface tension lowering substances (e.g., surfactant), denoted by the black circles, decrease the attraction between the surface water molecules and therefore lower the surface tension at the liquid–air interface. *Abbreviations:* Open circles, molecules of water; shaded circles, molecules of air; black circles, surface-active molecules. (From Comroe, J. H. [1965]. *Physiology of respiration* [p. 106]. Chicago: Year Book Medical Publishers.)

elevated, facilitating the maturation of type II cells that produce surfactant. If the infant is born before the surfactant system is functional, a serious pulmonary disease develops, formerly called hyaline membrane disease and now termed respiratory distress syndrome (RDS) in the newborn. Without surfactant, the surface tension in the lungs of these infants is high, and there are many collapsed alveoli, resulting in atelectasis. The type II cells that produce surfactant have also been shown to increase in size under the influence of thyroid hormone, and hence RDS is more severe in infants with low plasma thyroid levels.

The force acting toward inflation in the lung is the result of the chest wall tending to expand, pulling outward on the lung tissue. The continual tendency of the chest wall to expand is held in check by the intercostal muscles. When the circumference of the chest wall is measured before and after death, it is larger upon postmortem examination. At death, when the chest wall is no longer under the restraining influence of the intercostal muscles, it naturally expands. The opposing forces of deflation in the lungs and inflation of the chest wall create a vacuum between the visceral and parietal pleura, resulting in an intrapleural pressure that is subatmospheric (757.5 mm Hg).

Inspiration

Inspiration is an active process that requires energy for the contraction of the inspiratory muscles to expand the thoracic cavity. The diaphragm is the most important muscle of inspiration. Neural innervation of the diaphragm occurs through the phrenic nerve, which exits from the spinal cord between the third and fourth cervical vertebrae. At rest, the diaphragm is bowed upward into the thoracic cavity to the level of the fourth intercostal space. With neural stimulation, the diaphragm contracts, moving downward and pushing on the abdominal contents while raising the rib margins upward and outward, thus increasing the transverse diameter of the thoracic cavity. The external intercostal muscles, which run obliquely downward and forward from rib to rib, contract to raise the ribs during inspiration and increase the anteroposterior (AP) diameter of the thoracic cavity.

In otherwise healthy people, the accessory muscles of inspiration assist only during high levels of ventilation by enlarging the upper part of the thoracic cavity. The scalene muscles in the neck elevate the first two ribs. The sternocleidomastoid elevates the sternum and enlarges slightly the AP diameter of the chest.

As the thoracic cavity expands, the parietal pleura that lines the thoracic cavity pulls outward on the visceral pleura that surrounds the lung tissue, causing the intrapleural pressure to become more subatmospheric (−6 mm Hg). There is a pressure gradient difference between the intraalveolar air pressure and the intrapleural pressure that causes air to flow from the atmosphere into the alveoli. Air enters the lungs by bulk flow to the region of the terminal bronchioli and by gaseous diffusion to the alveolar spaces. The volume of air entering the lungs during a normal breath at rest is approximately 500 mL or 0.5 L (see Fig. 27–9).

Expiration

Expiration is normally a passive process in the sense that no muscles contract. During expiration the diaphragm relaxes, the external intercostals relax, and the size of the thoracic cage decreases. The elastic tissue of the lungs recoil, pulling the chest back to the expiratory position, where the recoil pressure of the lungs and the chest wall balance. As the stretched lung tissue recoils, the alveolar air is compressed; the intraalveolar pressure exceeds atmospheric pressure, and air flows from the alveoli to the atmosphere by bulk flow. Normally, passive expiration takes one-third longer than inspiration because of the increase in airway resistance during expiration.

Although normally passive, expiration can become active during high levels of ventilation or when resistance to air flow is increased. The accessory muscles of expiration include the internal intercostals and the abdominal muscles. With contraction, the internal intercostals, which run upward and backward between the ribs, cause the ribs to move inward, thus decreasing the anteroposterior diameter of the thoracic cage. The abdominal muscles compress the abdominal contents and raise the intraabdominal pressure.

Relationships Between Pressure Gradients, Airway Resistance, and Compliance

The volume of air that flows in or out of the alveoli during breathing is directly proportional to the pressure gradient. During deep breathing, the accessory muscles of inspiration and expiration are called into play, resulting in greater negative pressure gradients during inspiration and greater positive pressure gradients during expiration. Air moves into and out of the lungs as the alveolar pressure (P_{alv}) is less than and greater than atmospheric pressure (P_{atm}). In addition, the flow of air into and out of the alveoli is inversely proportional to airway resistance. As airway resistance increases, as in patients with asthma, chronic obstructive pulmonary disease, or a tumor, the flow of air into the lungs decreases.

$$\text{Flow} = \frac{\text{Pressure gradient } (P_{atm} - P_{alv})}{\text{Resistance}}$$

A number of factors determine airway resistance, including (1) the number of interactions between the flowing gas molecules, (2) the length of the airway, and (3) the airway radius. The airway radius is extremely important because resistance to air flow is inversely proportional to the fourth power of the airway radius.

$$\text{Resistance} = \frac{1}{r^4}$$

Airway resistance may be altered by physical, nervous, or chemical factors. During normal inspiration, simple expansion of the lungs acts as a physical factor that pulls on the airways and widens them, thereby decreasing airway resistance. Conversely, during expiration, when airway pressures are above atmospheric, airway resistance is increased, and expiration takes one-third longer than inspiration. As discussed earlier, nervous regulation of the bronchiolar smooth muscle through the autonomic nervous system can decrease (sympathetic) or increase (parasympathetic) airway resistance. The bronchiolar smooth muscle is also sensitive to chemicals, such as histamine, and low carbon dioxide levels, causing bronchoconstriction, whereas high levels of carbon dioxide cause bronchodilation. The radius of the airways can become severely decreased with certain disease processes. Asthma is characterized by severe bronchiolar smooth muscle constriction and plugging of the airways by secretions. Airway resistance may become great enough to impede air flow completely despite large pressure gradients. Because of physical factors, asthmatics have much less difficulty with inhaling than with exhaling, resulting in air trapping in the lungs.

Compliance refers to the stretchability, distensibility, or elasticity of the lungs and the thoracic structures. The lungs and thorax have elastic properties—that is, they return to their resting shape after deformation by an external force. When pressure changes are applied to these structures, the resulting volume changes are proportional to the applied force (pressure) within limits. As intrapleural pressure decreases or intraalveolar pressure increases, lung volume increases proportionally according to the following formula:

$$\frac{\Delta V}{\Delta P}$$

in which V equals lung volume and P equals pressure. The compliance of the normal lungs and the thorax combined is 0.1 liters/centimeter of water pressure. That is, every time the alveolar pressure is increased by 1 cm H_2O, the lung volume increases by 100 mL:

$$\frac{1}{\text{Total compliance}} = \frac{1}{C_L} = \frac{1}{C_T} = 0.1\ \text{L/cm}\ H_2O$$

in which C equals compliance, L equals lungs, and T equals thorax.

The compliance of the lungs alone, when removed from the thoracic cage, is 0.2 L/cm H_2O. This highlights the fact that the lungs are twice as distensible as the thorax and that the muscles of inspiration must expend energy to expand the lungs and the thoracic cage. Lung compliance can be determined indirectly in humans by measuring the pressure developed in an intraesophageal balloon during respiration with the glottis open. The pressure changes in the intraesophageal balloon reflect the intrapleural pressure changes. The pressure is recorded at the end of expiration and again while holding the breath after inspiring a known volume of air in increments of 50 to 100 mL.

Lung compliance provides an indication of the elastic recoil of the lung tissue and the surface tension of the lung. Normally, lung compliance decreases with age. Lung compliance also decreases in disease processes such as pulmonary fibrosis and pulmonary edema. Decreased lung compliance is a hallmark sign in adult respiratory distress syndrome (ARDS) and RDS in the newborn and in oxygen toxicity. Deformities of the thoracic cage such as kyphosis, scoliosis, and muscular dystrophy can significantly reduce thoracic compliance. Thoracic compliance can also be reduced with obesity, trauma, and postoperative surgical splinting.

Work of Breathing

The work of inspiration can be divided into three components: (1) work required to expand the elastic forces of the lung, called compliance work; (2) work required to overcome the viscosity of the lung and thoracic cage, called tissue resistance work; and (3) work required to overcome the resistance to the flow of air into and out of the lungs, called airway resistance. During normal quiet breathing, most of the work is expended to overcome compliance, with tissue resistance and airway resistance requiring only a small percentage of the total work of breathing. In pulmonary disease, any or all of the components of the work of breathing may be increased. Expiration is normally passive due to elastic recoil of the lungs and the thoracic cage, thus requiring no work. In rapid breathing or when tissue resistance or airway resistance is increased, expiratory work becomes greater than inspiratory work. To perform work, the respiratory muscles require oxygen. Oxygen consumption by the respiratory muscles is an indirect measure of the work of breathing. The oxygen cost of breathing is assessed by determining the total oxygen consumption of the body at rest and at an increased level of ventilation. The oxygen cost of normal breathing is approximately 1 mL/liter of ventilation and comprises less than 3% to 5% of total body consumption. During rapid respiration, the oxygen requirement may increase 25-fold. In pulmonary disease, respiratory oxygen consumption increases markedly, resulting in respiratory muscle fatigue and overall skeletal muscle fatigue, which limits severely the amount of energy that can be exerted for other daily activities.

PULMONARY FUNCTION MEASUREMENTS

Spirometry is a simple method of measuring pulmonary function by recording the volume of air move-

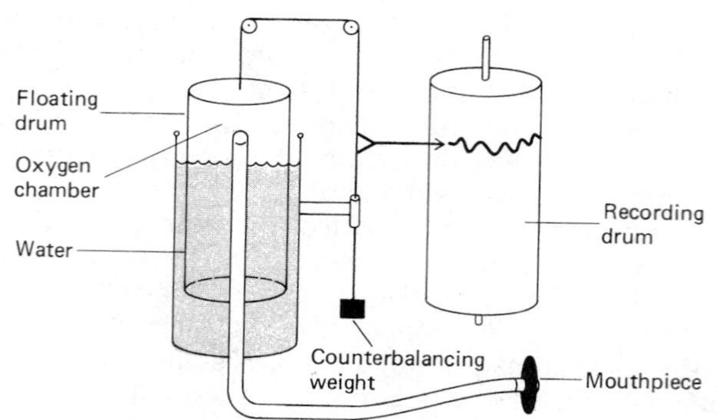

FIGURE 27–11. A spirometer. (From Guyton, A. C. [1991]. *Textbook of medical physiology* [8th ed., p. 407]. Philadelphia: W. B. Saunders.)

ment into and out of the lungs (Fig. 27–11). A spirometer consists of a drum inverted over a chamber of water, with the drum counterbalanced by a weight. The inverted drum is filled with air or oxygen, and a tube connects the mouth of the subject with the gas-filled drum. The water in the chamber prevents the gas mixture from escaping from the inverted drum. When the subject breathes through the tubing, the inverted drum rises and falls with expiration and inspiration, respectively, while a recording (spirogram) is made simultaneously on a moving sheet of paper. Figure 27–12 illustrates a spirogram during different breathing conditions. The values have been divided into four volumes and four capacities. The values reported below are "average" values for a 70-kg man. The values depend on height, weight, sex, and age. The volumes and capacities are 20% to 25% lower in women. With increasing age, all of the values are lower.

Pulmonary Volumes

1. *Tidal volume* (V_T) is the volume of air entering or leaving the lungs during a single breath in the resting state (500 mL)
2. *Inspiratory reserve volume* is the amount of air that can be inspired over and above resting tidal volume (3,100 mL)
3. *Expiratory reserve volume* is the air remaining in the lungs at the end of a normal expiration that can be exhaled by active contraction of expiratory muscles (1,200 mL)
4. *Residual volume* is the amount of air remaining in the lungs after maximum expiration (1,200 mL)

Pulmonary Capacities

1. *Vital capacity* is the sum of normal tidal volume, inspiratory reserve volume, and expiratory reserve volume (4,800 mL)

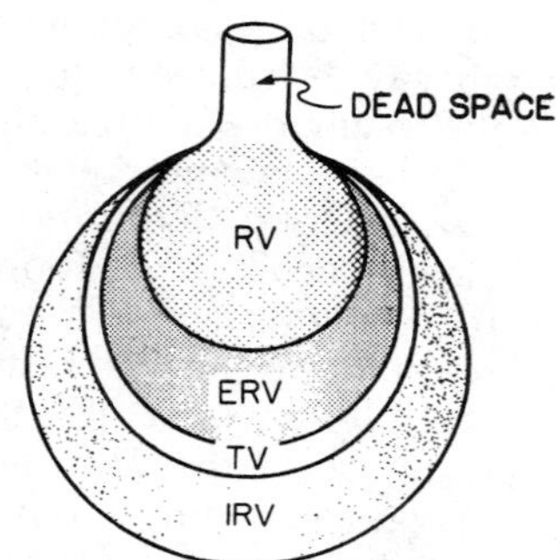

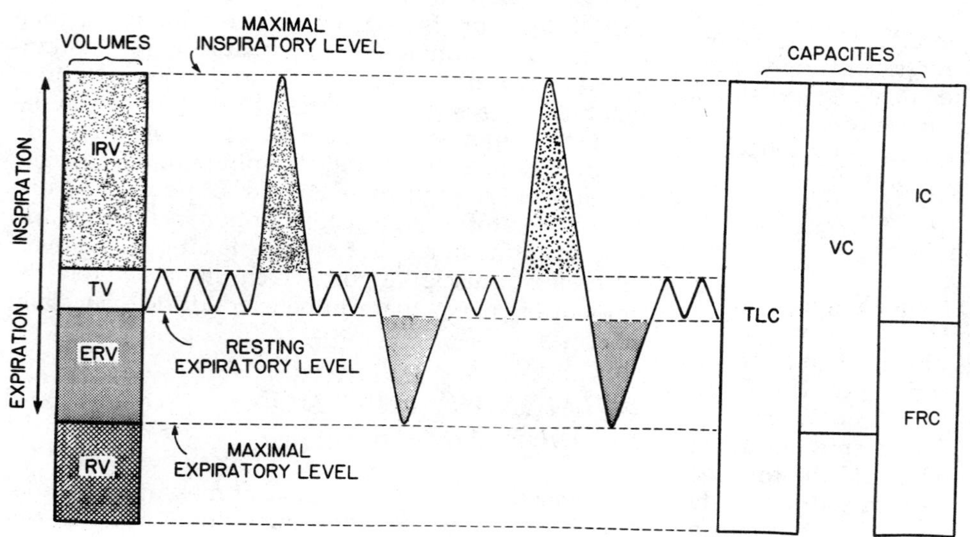

FIGURE 27–12. The lung volumes and capacities. The upper diagram illustrates the four principal lung volumes: RV, residual volume; ERV, expiratory reserve volume; TV, tidal volume; IRV, inspiratory reserve volume. The same shading is used in the lower part of the figure to indicate the same volumes. The four lung capacities are shown to the right of the figure. TLC, total lung capacity; VC, vital capacity; IC, inspiratory capacity; FRC, functional residual capacity. (From Jensen, D. [1980]. *The principles of physiology* [2nd ed., p. 668]. New York: Appleton-Century-Crofts.)

2. *Inspiratory capacity* is the sum of inspiratory reserve volume and tidal volume (3,600 mL)
3. *Functional capacity* is the sum of the expiratory reserve volume and the residual volume (2,400 mL)
4. *Total lung capacity* is the amount of air in the lungs after a maximum inspiration (6,000 mL, the sum of all volumes)

Alterations in body position can affect pulmonary volumes and capacities. When a subject lies down, the values decrease because the abdominal contents exert pressure on the diaphragm and increased pulmonary blood volume decreases available space for pulmonary air. This becomes important in patients with cardiac and pulmonary dysfunction.

Minute Ventilation and Maximum Voluntary Ventilation

Minute ventilation or volume is the volume of air moved in or out of the respiratory tract per minute in the resting state. This volume is equivalent to the product of tidal volume and respiratory rate. Therefore, if the tidal volume is 500 mL during the resting state and respiratory rate is 12 breaths/minute, the minute respiratory volume is 500 mL times 12 breaths/minute = 6,000 mL/minute (or 6 L/minute). During strenuous breathing, the tidal volume can equal vital capacity and the respiratory rate may reach as high as 50/minute, thereby markedly increasing minute ventilation. At extremely rapid respiratory rates, maintenance of tidal volume at much above one-half of vital capacity is limited by the work of breathing.

Maximum voluntary ventilation is the total volume of air that can be moved into and out of the respiratory tract while breathing as rapidly and as deeply as possible for 12 seconds. This volume can be as high as 170 L/minute for short intervals. Because the respiratory system has an enormous reserve, respiratory volume can increase up to 20- to 25-fold for short intervals.

Anatomic and Physiologic Dead Space

Air that enters the purely conducting portions of the respiratory tract, including the nose, mouth, pharynx, larynx, trachea, bronchi, and bronchioli to the respiratory zone where gas exchange does not occur is called the anatomic dead space. The volume is difficult to determine, but rough estimates based on age, sex, and tidal volumes indicate that in the adult anatomic dead space is equal to "ideal weight" in milliliters, or approximately 150 mL in a 70-kg man.

Alveolar dead space is a less well defined volume that consists of a variable number of alveoli whose perfusion is reduced or absent because of gravitational shifts in pulmonary blood flow in the normal person and to impaired blood flow in the diseased person.

Physiologic dead space is the sum of the anatomic and alveolar dead spaces; it is the functional dead space ventilation. In otherwise healthy people, the anatomic dead space is equivalent to the physiologic dead space.

Dead space ventilation (V_{DS}) is the amount of air that ventilates the physiologic dead space per minute, whereas alveolar ventilation (V_A) is the volume per minute that ventilates all perfused alveoli and is the difference between minute ventilation and dead space ventilation.

During a normal breath at rest, the tidal volume is equal to 500 mL. Approximately 150 mL of the total mL ventilates the anatomic dead space, which is composed of the purely conducting portion of the respiratory tract. The alveolar ventilation is 350 mL of the total 500 mL. The relationship between the tidal volume, dead space ventilation, and alveolar ventilation is expressed in the following formula.

$$V_T = V_{DS} + V_A$$
$$500 \text{ mL} \quad 150 \text{ mL} \quad 350 \text{ mL}$$

Single-Breath Nitrogen Analysis

One test to assess pulmonary function is the modified single-breath nitrogen analysis (Fig. 27–13). The anatomic dead space can be measured by this technique. Starting from midinspiration, the subject takes as deep a breath of pure oxygen as possible and exhales steadily while the nitrogen content of the expired gas is continuously measured. When the subject inhales pure oxygen, it fills the conducting portion of the respiratory tract, or the anatomic dead space. Consequently, the initial gas that is exhaled (phase I) contains no nitrogen. The exhaled gas that follows is first a mixture of dead space and alveolar gas (phase II) and then the alveolar gas (phase III) alone. The dead space volume is the volume of gas expired from peak inspiration to the midportion of phase II. Phase III of the single-breath nitrogen curve, the alveolar plateau, terminates at the closing volume, where there is an abrupt in-

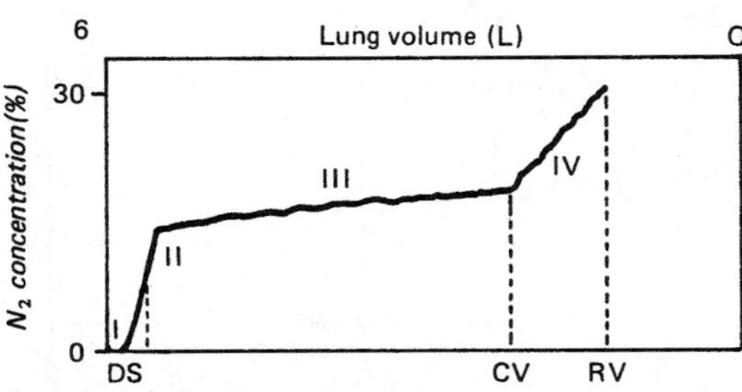

FIGURE 27–13. Single-breath nitrogen curve. From midinspiration, the subject takes a deep breath of pure oxygen, then exhales steadily. The changes in the nitrogen concentration of expired gas during expiration are shown, with the various phases of the curve indicated by roman numerals. *Abbreviations:* DS, dead space; CV, closing volume; RV, residual volume. (Reprinted, by permission, from the *New England Journal of Medicine, 293*, 438, 1975.)

crease in slope of phase IV to residual volume. The closing volume is the lung volume above residual volume where the airways begin to close off because of increasing positive transmural pressure during expiration. The modified single-breath nitrogen test is currently being used in longitudinal studies of healthy subjects and individuals with lung disease. The alveolar plateau increases with age, and the closing volume increases in subjects exposed to pollutants and cigarette smoke. The closing volume is increased in subjects with premature airway closure as with emphysema.

Forced Expiratory Vital Capacity

Forced expiratory vital capacity is measured using a spirometer or a pneumotachograph. The subject inhales to total lung capacity and then exhales in a rapid, forceful maximal expiration. Figure 27–14 illustrates a graph of volume versus time. Several measurements are commonly obtained from the volume–time presentation of the forced vital capacity, including the volume exhaled in one second (FEV_1) and the volume exhaled in 3 seconds (FEV_3). These values can be expressed as a ratio of total forced vital capacity.

$$\frac{FEV_1}{\text{Forced vital capacity}}$$

Patients with airway obstruction show drastic changes in the appearance of the forced vital capacity tracing. There is a flattening of the slope of the curve at any given volume, indicating a reduced rate of air flow on

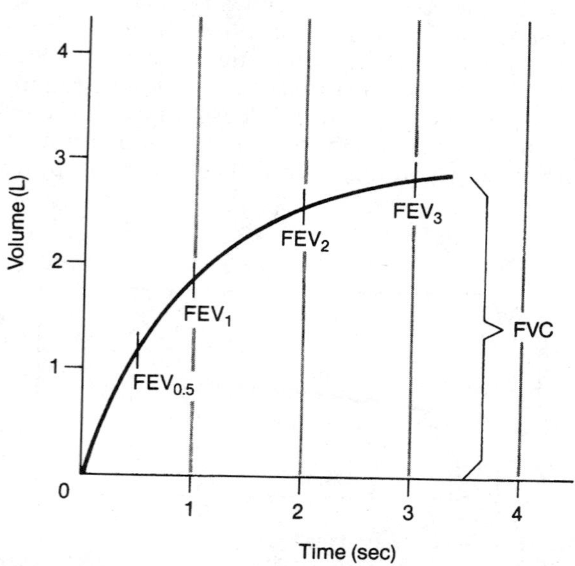

FIGURE 27–14. A spirogram of a forced vital capacity (FVC) maneuver with forced expiratory volume (FEV) labeled at various time intervals. The FEV at 1 second (FEV_1) is the most important measurement. (From Kersten, L. D. [1989]. *Comprehensive respiratory nursing* [p. 375]. Philadelphia: W. B. Saunders.)

expiration. In addition, the duration of the forced expiratory maneuver is prolonged, and the cessation of air flow is delayed as indicated by a plateau at the top of the curve. The smaller the ratio of FEV_1 to forced vital capacity, the more difficult it is to exhale. Pre-expiratory and postexpiratory forced vital capacity tests are used to determine the effectiveness of bronchodilating drugs on patients with airway obstructive disease.

DIFFUSION OF RESPIRATORY GASES

The diffusion of oxygen from the alveoli to the pulmonary capillary blood and the diffusion of carbon dioxide from the blood to the alveolus is the result of the partial pressure gradients of the gases. The partial pressure of a gas is the desire of the gas to escape from the liquid state into the gaseous state. This phenomenon can be exemplified by a carbonated soft drink in an enclosed glass container. With the cap on, the gas is contained within the liquid state. When the cap is removed, the gas in the liquid begins to escape, as visualized by the bubbles escaping into the atmosphere from an area of higher partial pressure in the container to an area of lower partial pressure in the atmosphere. The respiratory gases are carried in the liquid portion of the plasma of the blood and on the hemoglobin molecule and exert a partial pressure. This partial pressure is the result of the individual gas molecules bombarding the walls of the blood vessels. The magnitude of the pressure depends on the concentration of the gas and the temperature. At higher gas concentrations there will be a greater number of molecules colliding with the vessel wall. At higher temperatures the speed of the moving molecules will be greater and the number of collisions with the vessel wall will be greater. The exchange of oxygen from the alveoli and carbon dioxide from the blood is the result of partial pressure gradients. To understand the diffusion of respiratory gases from areas of higher concentration to areas of lower concentration, the composition of atmospheric air must be considered.

Composition of Air

Atmospheric air is composed of the following gases in different percentages:

Nitrogen	78.6%
Oxygen	20.9%
Carbon dioxide	0.04%
Inert gases	0.92%
Water vapor	Variable

The total pressure of a mixture of gases is simply the sum of the individual pressures according to the Dalton law of partial pressures. With the atmospheric pressure at sea equal to 760 mm Hg, the individual partial pressures of the gases can be calculated by taking the percentage of each of the respiratory gases comprising the total pressure. The partial pressures (P) of the inspired atmospheric air are stated in the following formula.

Partial pressure atmospheric	=	PO_2	+	PCO_2	+	PN_2	+	PH_2O
760 mm Hg		158		0.3		597		5

The partial pressure of water vapor depends on the temperature of the atmospheric air. At low temperatures, atmospheric air has very little water in vapor form. At high temperatures, as in the summer months, atmospheric air will have more water in vapor form, as indicated by the increased "humidity" of the air.

Oxygen is consumed by the body at the cellular level for the production of ATP in the process of oxidative phosphorylation, and carbon dioxide is produced as a byproduct. Therefore, oxygen and carbon dioxide are considered essential respiratory gases. Nitrogen is in high concentration in the atmospheric air, and although it is inert (devoid of active properties), it does serve a useful purpose. Nitrogen serves to dilute the concentration of oxygen, thereby protecting the alveolar cells from the effects of oxygen toxicity. In addition, nitrogen is not as soluble as oxygen and therefore does not diffuse as readily from the alveoli into the blood. Nitrogen stays in the alveoli, keeping them inflated and thereby reducing their tendency to collapse.

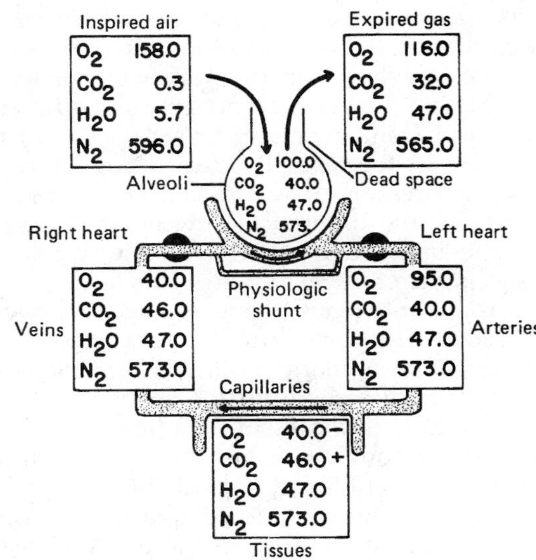

FIGURE 27–15. Partial pressures of gases (mm Hg) in the respiratory and cardiovascular system. (From Ganong, W. F. [1989]. *Review of medical physiology* [14th ed.]. Norwalk, CT: Appleton & Lange.)

Factors Affecting Diffusion

The movement of gas molecules occurs by physical diffusion from a region of higher partial pressure to one of lower partial pressure. The rate of diffusion depends on the following factors:

1. The difference in partial pressure between the two sides
2. The surface area for diffusion
3. The thickness of the tissue separating the two sides
4. The diffusibility of the gas

In the respiratory system, the difference in partial pressures lies in the partial pressure of oxygen and carbon dioxide in the alveoli versus the partial pressure in the blood. The total surface area available for diffusion is 70 m^2 because of the large number of alveoli and pulmonary capillaries surrounding the alveoli. The total surface area available for diffusion in the lungs is the size of a badminton court. In health, the alveolar capillary membrane thickness is 0.5 μm. The diffusibility of a gas is directly proportional to the solubility of the gas in the liquid and inversely proportional to the square root of the molecular weight, and is expressed in the following formula:

$$\text{Diffusibility} \propto \frac{\text{Solubility of the gas}}{\sqrt{\text{Molecular weight of the gas}}}$$

As a result of this relationship, carbon dioxide is 20 times more diffusible than oxygen. The reason for this difference in the two gases is that carbon dioxide is 24 times more soluble than oxygen. Using the formula, carbon dioxide is 24 times more soluble than oxygen, but its molecular weight is greater, resulting in carbon dioxide being 20 times more diffusible than oxygen. Carbon dioxide moves 20 times as fast across the alveolar capillary membrane as oxygen. For this reason, the elimination of carbon dioxide is almost never limited by alterations in the diffusion component of the respiratory process. However, the diffusion of gases between the alveoli and the capillaries can be impaired in a number of disease processes. In emphysema, which is frequently related to cigarette smoking, alveolar capillary walls are broken down, resulting in fewer but larger alveoli and a reduction in the total surface area available for diffusion. Alveolar capillary membrane thickening, as in ARDS or RDS and pulmonary edema, increases the distance needed for the diffusion of gas molecules. The alveolar capillary walls may become denser and less permeable with inhaled substances such a beryllium.

The diffusion of oxygen from the alveoli and carbon dioxide from the pulmonary capillaries is depicted in Figure 27–15. As discussed earlier, the partial pressure of oxygen in the atmospheric air is 158 mm Hg and the partial pressure of carbon dioxide is 0.3 mm Hg. During inspiration, as atmospheric air is inhaled it becomes mixed with the air in the anatomic dead space and the gases contained in the alveoli. As a result, in the alveoli the partial pressure of oxygen is 100 mm Hg, and the partial pressure of carbon dioxide is 40 mm Hg. In addition, the partial pressure of the water vapor is increased because the temperature of the body is higher at 98°F than the atmosphere at 70°F.

As discussed earlier, the pulmonary arteries (right and left) are transporting deoxygenated blood from the right ventricle to the lungs. At the level of the pulmonary capillaries that surround the individual alveoli, the partial pressure of oxygen in the venous blood is 40 mm Hg and the partial pressure of carbon dioxide is 46 mm Hg. Because of pressure gradient differences, oxygen moves from an area of higher partial pressure (100 mm Hg in the alveoli) into the capillaries at a lower partial pressure of 40 mm Hg. The partial pressure gradient (the difference between the two pressures) in the diffusion of oxygen from the alveoli to the capillaries is therefore 60 mm Hg. This large pressure gradient is advantageous to ensure adequate oxygenation of blood. The partial pressure of carbon dioxide in the pulmonary capillaries is 46 mm Hg, whereas the partial pressure of carbon dioxide in the alveoli is 40 mm Hg, resulting in a pressure gradient of 6 mm Hg that "drives" carbon dioxide into the alveoli. Although the pressure gradient for carbon dioxide is only 6 mm Hg, it is sufficient to provide adequate diffusion because carbon dioxide is 20 times more diffusible than oxygen.

The four pulmonary veins return oxygenated arterialized blood to the left atrium and left ventricle to be distributed to the cells of the body through the arterial system. At the tissue level, the partial pressure of oxygen is 40 mm Hg and the partial pressure of carbon dioxide is 46 mm Hg because of the utilization of oxygen and the production of carbon dioxide by the cells in oxidative phosphorylation. The pressure gradient for the diffusion of oxygen to the cells is 60 mm Hg, whereas the diffusion gradient for the movement of carbon dioxide from the cells to the capillaries is 6 mm Hg. The diffusion process results in a partial pressure of 40 mm Hg for oxygen and 46 mm Hg for carbon dioxide in the returning venous blood.

Venous blood returns from the lower portions of the body through the inferior vena cava and from the upper portions through the superior vena cava to the right atrium and right ventricle, exiting into the two pulmonary arteries, which carry the deoxygenated blood to the lung to reinitiate the entire process. Under normal circumstances the diffusion process is immediate and blood flow through the pulmonary capillaries is slow enough (a single red cell remains in the pulmonary capillary approximately 0.75 second) that equilibrium is easily achieved. With strenuous exercise, an increase in cardiac output results in a decrease in the time available for diffusion to 0.3 second, thereby challenging the respiratory system. High altitudes, where the atmospheric pressure is reduced, pose a respiratory challenge. At high altitudes, the partial pressure of atmospheric oxygen is less, thereby reducing the normal "driving" pressure gradients and compromising the diffusion process. As a result, physical activity is limited by the partial pressure of oxygen in the arterial blood.

Ventilation–Perfusion Ratio

Diffusion of the respiratory gases is optimal when both ventilation and blood flow are evenly matched. However, even this ideal situation does not exist in the normal lung. At rest, pulmonary ventilation averages 5.1 L/minute. Cardiac output averages 6.0 L/minute, resulting in a ventilation-to-perfusion ratio (V_A/Q) of 0.85. The discrepancy between ventilation and perfusion is caused by the difference in the distribution of pulmonary gases and pulmonary circulation due to gravity. In an upright subject at rest between breaths, the alveoli in the apex of the lung will be filled with air because of the fact that air rises. During inspiration, more ventilation will be distributed to the base of the lung than to the apex. Similarly, perfusion of the lung is lowest in the apex and greatest in the base due to gravity. However, in the apex of the lung, ventilation is three times greater than perfusion. At the base of the lung, alveolar ventilation is less than pulmonary capillary blood flow, and the V_A/Q is 0.6. This results in an overall V_A/Q of 0.85. The range of V_A/Q throughout the normal lung is relatively narrow, so that differences in arterial blood gases in different regions of the lung are small.

However, in pulmonary diseases in which airway resistance is increased, pulmonary compliance is decreased, and blood vessel caliber is altered, ventilation–perfusion mismatches can occur, resulting in a decreased capacity for gas exchange. Normally, physiologic mechanisms attempt to reduce the degree of ventilation–perfusion mismatch. As discussed earlier, high carbon dioxide concentrations result in bronchodilation, whereas low concentrations result in bronchoconstriction, altering pulmonary ventilation. Pulmonary arteriolar smooth muscle is very sensitive to the partial pressure of oxygen in the alveoli. Increased alveolar oxygen results in vasodilation, whereas decreased alveolar oxygen results in vasoconstriction. This local control permits perfusion of well ventilated alveoli and the "shunting" of blood away from poorly ventilated alveoli. Systemic hypoxia also causes the pulmonary arterioles to constrict, resulting in an increase in pulmonary arterial pressure and pulmonary hypertension. The pulmonary arteriolar smooth muscle is also sensitive to the concentration of H^+ ion, which is indirectly related to the concentration of carbon dioxide. When carbon dioxide combines with water, carbonic acid forms and rapidly breaks down into H^+ and HCO_3^-. An increased concentration of H^+ results in pulmonary vasoconstriction and the "shunting" of blood away from poorly ventilated alveoli with high alveolar carbon dioxide levels to better-ventilated alveoli.

TRANSPORT OF RESPIRATORY GASES

The oxygen delivery system and the carbon dioxide elimination system in the body are composed of the lungs, heart and blood vessels, and the blood. The adequacy of the system depends on the processes of ventilation, diffusion, perfusion, and the capacity of blood to carry the respiratory gases.

Oxygen Transport

Oxygen is transported in the blood in two forms: (1) physically dissolved in the liquid or plasma portion of the blood, and (2) chemically bound to hemoglobin. The amount of oxygen that is physically dissolved in blood is directly proportional to the partial arterial pressure of oxygen (Pa_{O_2}). However, as discussed earlier, oxygen is relatively insoluble in water, and thus only 0.30 mL of oxygen can be dissolved in 100 mL of blood. If the oxygen requirement of the body were to be met simply by the dissolved oxygen in the plasma, then the P_{O_2} would have to be 2,000 mm Hg. The largest amount (98%) of oxygen is transported by hemoglobin, the bright red pigmented protein found in red blood cells. Oxygen binds rapidly (0.01 second) and reversibly with hemoglobin to form oxyhemoglobin (HbO_2). Hemoglobin that is not combined with oxygen is called reduced hemoglobin (Hb).

Hemoglobin is a protein made up of four subunits, each containing a heme moiety attached to a polypeptide chain. The four polypeptide chains comprise the globin portion of the hemoglobin molecule. Two of the subunits, alpha chains, have 140 amino acid residues, whereas the other two subunits, beta chains, have 146 amino acid residues. Individuals who have equal quantities of alpha and beta chains in their hemoglobin are said to have hemoglobin A. The heme moiety is a complex made up of porphyrin and one atom of iron (Fe^{2+}). Each of the four iron atoms can bind reversibly with one O_2 molecule according to the following formulas:

$$
\begin{aligned}
Hb_4 &+ O_2 \rightleftharpoons Hb_4O_2 \text{ (25\% saturated)}\\
Hb_4O_2 &+ O_2 \rightleftharpoons Hb_4O_4 \text{ (50\% saturated)}\\
Hb_4O_4 &+ O_2 \rightleftharpoons Hb_4O_6 \text{ (75\% saturated)}\\
Hb_4O_6 &+ O_2 \rightleftharpoons Hb_4O_8 \text{ (100\% saturated)}
\end{aligned}
$$

The reactions of oxygen with heme are called oxygenation, not oxidation, because the iron remains in the ferrous (Fe^{2+}) state. Frequently, the reactions of oxygen with hemoglobin are abbreviated to $Hb + O_2 \rightleftharpoons HbO_2$, when in reality each molecule of hemoglobin can bind four molecules of O_2. Because there are approximately 280 million hemoglobin molecules per red blood cell, each red blood cell can carry over a billion molecules of oxygen.

The structure of the hemoglobin molecule determines its affinity for oxygen by shifting the position of its four component polypeptide chains, fostering either O_2 uptake or O_2 delivery. The movement of the polypeptide chains results in a change in position of the heme moieties, which assume an R state (relaxed state), favoring O_2 binding, or a T state (tense state), decreasing O_2 binding. The transition from the R state to the T state is the result of the breaking or forming of salt bridges between the polypeptide chains. When hemoglobin binds to oxygen, the two beta chains move close together, and when oxygen is given up they move farther apart. The oxygen–hemoglobin dissocia-

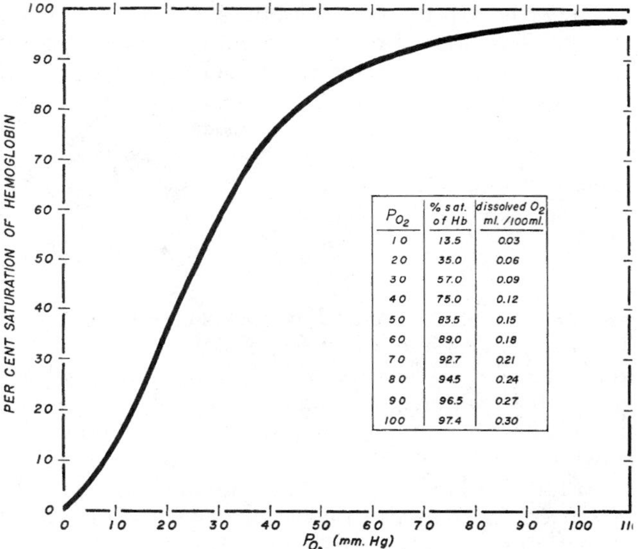

P_{O_2}	% sat. of Hb	dissolved O_2 ml./100ml.
10	13.5	0.03
20	35.0	0.06
30	57.0	0.09
40	75.0	0.12
50	83.5	0.15
60	89.0	0.18
70	92.7	0.21
80	94.5	0.24
90	96.5	0.27
100	97.4	0.30

FIGURE 27–16. Oxyhemoglobin dissociation curve at temperature 38°C, pH 7.40.

tion curve (Fig. 27–16), relating the percentage of oxygen saturation of hemoglobin to the P_{O_2} is characteristically sigmoid-shaped because of the movement of the polypeptide chains of the hemoglobin molecule. The combination of O_2 with the first heme increases the affinity of the second heme for O_2, which in turn increases the affinity of the third, and so on. Similarly, the release of O_2 by each of the four iron atoms enhances the release of O_2 molecules from the remaining iron atoms.

One gram of hemoglobin is capable of combining with 1.34 mL of oxygen, and this is called the oxygen capacity. At a normal hemoglobin concentration of 15 g/100 mL of blood, the blood is capable of carrying approximately 20 mL O_2/100 mL, or 20 volume percent.

$$\frac{15 \text{ g Hb}}{100 \text{ mL blood}} \times \frac{1.34 \text{ mL } O_2}{1 \text{ g Hb}} = 20.1 \text{ mL } O_2/100 \text{ mL blood}$$

Oxygen-carrying capacity of the blood depends on the amount of hemoglobin in the blood. If the hemoglobin concentration falls below normal, as with anemia, the oxygen concentration of the blood is reduced. In contrast, the hemoglobin concentration can be increased above normal, as seen in polycythemia vera, when the red blood cell count is increased in response to high altitudes or hypoxemia. The production of hemoglobin and red blood cells in the bone marrow is controlled by the hormone called erythropoietin, which is synthesized and released by the kidneys. When the delivery of oxygen to the kidney is reduced due to high altitudes or pulmonary or cardiovascular disease, the hormone increases red blood cell production to enhance the oxygen-carrying capacity of the blood. The actual amount of O_2 in combination with hemoglobin is normally less than the capacity. The actual amount of O_2 carried on the hemoglobin is called the oxygen content. The ratio of the O_2 content to the O_2 capacity is expressed as a percentage and is called the oxygen saturation (SaO_2).

$$\frac{\text{How much oxygen carried by hemoglobin (content)}}{\text{How much oxygen hemoglobin is capable of carrying (capacity)}}$$

$$SaO_2 = 100 \times \frac{\text{Content}}{\text{Capacity}}$$

The oxygen content and oxygen saturation of blood increase progressively with increasing PO_2 as depicted in Figure 27–16. The upper flat region of the oxyhemoglobin dissociation curve indicates that the oxygen saturation and hence hemoglobin affinity are relatively constant (92.7%–97.5%) over an approximate range of 70 to 110 mm Hg PO_2. Therefore, small changes in PO_2 produced by changes in alveolar ventilation ordinarily have little effect on oxygen saturation. However, changes in oxygen saturation are more pronounced in the lower PO_2 ranges, below 55 mm Hg. Because of the steep slope of the oxyhemoglobin dissociation curve below 55 mm Hg PO_2, large quantities of O_2 can be unloaded from the blood to the tissues with a relatively small decrease in blood PO_2.

The amount of oxygen bound to hemoglobin is affected not only by the oxygen tension (PO_2) but by the partial pressure of carbon dioxide (PCO_2), the pH, the temperature of the blood, and the concentration of 2,3-diphosphoglycerate (2,3-DPG). The HbO_2 dissociation curve is shifted to the right by an increase in carbon dioxide, a decrease in pH, an increase in temperature, or an increase in the concentration of 2,3-DPG (Fig. 27–17). Therefore, at any given partial pressure of O_2, hemoglobin is less saturated, and the delivery of oxygen from the blood to the tissues is enhanced. Increased tissue metabolism, as occurs with an increase in body temperature, results in increased CO_2 production and a local decrease in pH. The shift in the oxyhemoglobin dissociation curve to the right with increased CO_2, decreased pH, and increased temperature facilitates the unloading of O_2 from the hemoglobin to the blood to meet the increased metabolic needs of the cell.

2,3-Diphosphoglycerate is very plentiful in red cells. It is formed in the erythrocyte by anaerobic glycolysis and has a half-life of 6 hours. It is a highly charged anion that binds to the beta chains of deoxygenated hemoglobin but not to those of oxyhemoglobin, thereby causing the release of oxygen.

$$HbO_2 + 2,3\text{-DPG} \rightleftharpoons Hb\text{-}2,3\text{-DPG} + O_2$$

2,3-DPG concentration in the red blood cells is decreased in patients with acidosis because of red blood cell glycolysis. Thyroid hormone, growth hormone, androgens, exercise in the untrained athlete, high altitude, and chronic anemia increase the concentration of 2,3-DPG, thereby enhancing oxygen delivery to the tissues. In stored bank blood, 2,3-DPG levels fall, reducing the ability of the transfused blood to release O_2 to the tissues.

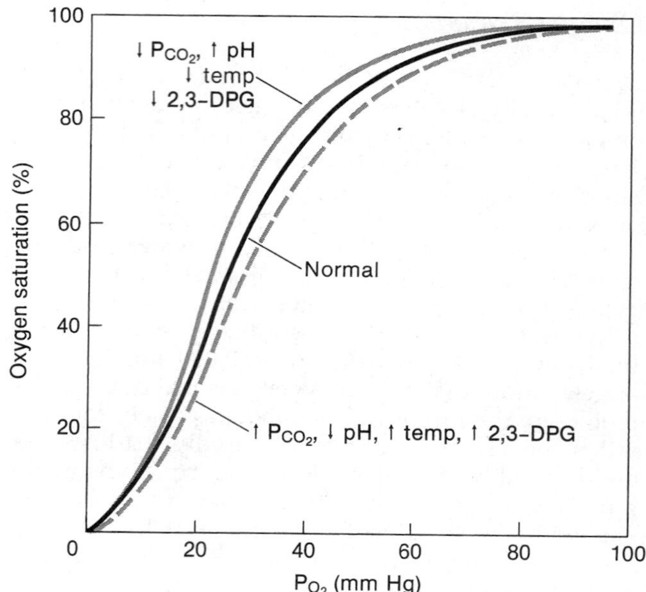

FIGURE 27–17. The effects of changes in PCO_2, pH, temperature, and 2,3-diphosphoglycerate (2,3-DPG) on oxygen binding to hemoglobin. An increase in partial pressure of CO_2, decrease in pH, increase in temperature, or increase in 2,3-DPG produce a shift to the right of the hemoglobin oxygen dissociation curve. The hemoglobin–oxygen dissociation curve is shifted to the left by a fall in carbon dioxide, increase in pH, decrease in temperature, or decrease in concentration of 2,3-DPG. (Modified from Berne, R. M., & Levy, M. N. [1988]. *Physiology* [2nd ed., p. 610]. St. Louis: C. V. Mosby.)

In contrast, the HbO_2 dissociation curve is shifted to the left with decreased carbon dioxide levels, increased pH, decreased temperature, or decreased 2,3-DPG, enhancing the affinity of hemoglobin for oxygen and improving oxygen saturation at lower PO_2 levels. However, the enhancement of hemoglobin's affinity for oxygen decreases the unloading of oxygen at the tissue level. This phenomenon should be kept in mind when caring for patients with hypothermia, which reduces cellular metabolism while simultaneously decreasing the availability of oxygen at the tissue level.

Carbon Dioxide Transport

Carbon dioxide is transported to the lungs in the plasma of blood and in the erythrocyte in three forms: (1) dissolved in the plasma or liquid portion of the erythrocyte, (2) as a carbamino compound combined with blood proteins and plasma proteins, and (3) as bicarbonate (HCO_3^-) ion. The volume of carbon dioxide dissolved in the blood depends on the partial pressure of CO_2, as with oxygen. Because carbon dioxide is 24 times more soluble than oxygen, more is transported in the dissolved form. A small fraction, about 20% of the total CO_2, is carried to the lungs in the blood as carbamino compounds formed by the reaction between CO_2 and the amino groups (NH_2 groups) of the

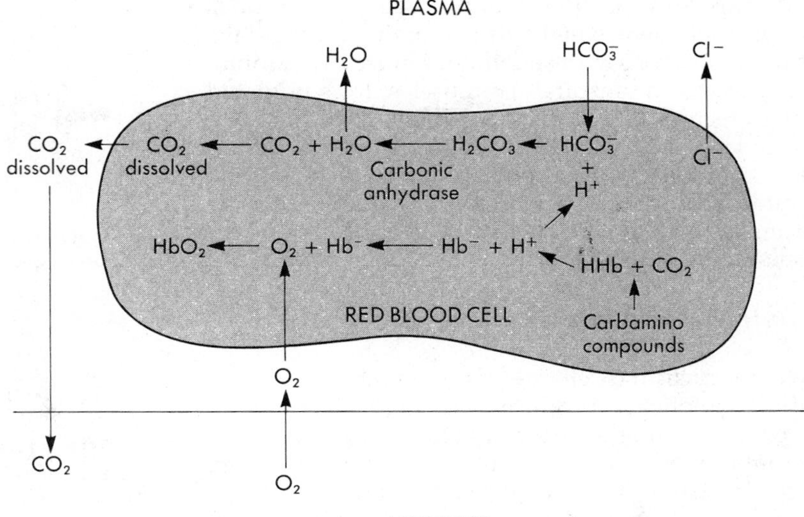

FIGURE 27–18. Carbon dioxide transport in blood. (From Berne, R. M., & Levy, M. N. [1988]. *Physiology* [2nd ed.]. St. Louis: C. V. Mosby.)

proteins in both plasma and erythrocytes. The amino groups of hemoglobin, for example, react with carbon dioxide in the following manner:

$$Hb - NH_2 + CO_2 \rightleftharpoons Hb - NHCOO^- + H^+$$

As oxygen is given up to the tissues from Hb, CO_2 combines very rapidly with Hb. Deoxyhemoglobin is able to form carbamino compounds more readily than oxyhemoglobin, and consequently CO_2 transport in venous blood is achieved more readily than in arterial blood.

The carbon dioxide that diffuses into the plasma and the erythrocytes combines rapidly with water (hydration reaction) in the presence of the enzymatic catalyst carbonic anhydrase to form carbonic acid (H_2CO_3). The H_2CO_3 dissociates rapidly to H^+ and HCO_3^- according to the formula depicted in Figure 27–18. The hydration reaction takes approximately 200 seconds and is rapidly reversed in the lungs to permit the diffusion of carbon dioxide into the alveoli. The H^- ion formed in the hydration reaction is buffered by deoxygenated hemoglobin, and the HCO_3^- enters the plasma. Because the HCO_3^- content rises 70% in the plasma as the blood passes through the tissue capillaries, electrochemical neutrality is maintained by Cl^- entering the red cells in exchange for HCO_3^-; this is called the chloride shift. The hydration reaction allows large amounts of carbon dioxide to be carried to the lungs in the form of HCO_3^- (Fig. 27–18).

Arterial blood gases provide important information about the concentration of the respiratory gases in the arterial blood and about the effectiveness of ventilation, perfusion, and diffusion. The normal arterial blood gas values are as follows:

Pao_2	95–100 mm Hg	Oxygenation status
Sao_2	97%	
pH	7.35–7.45	Acid-base status
$Paco_2$	38–42 mm Hg	
HCO_3^-	23–25 milliequivalents/L	

PaO_2 and the Sao_2 provide information about the oxygenation status of the individual, whereas the pH, $Paco_2$, and HCO_3^- reveal information about acid–base status. For the body to function optimally, these values must remain within these narrow ranges. A complete discussion of acid–base balance is provided in Chapter 28.

CONTROL OF RESPIRATION

The respiratory system has fine controls to adjust the rate of alveolar ventilation to meet the demands of the body exactly and to maintain the partial pressures of oxygen and carbon dioxide and the pH of the blood at normal levels. Control of the respiratory system is achieved through both neural and chemical control.

Neural Control

The nervous system provides both voluntary control through the cerebral cortex via the corticospinal tracts to the respiratory muscles, and automatic control through the medulla and pons of the brain stem. Normal resting respiration requires cyclical respiratory muscle excitation from the brain through the phrenic nerves to the diaphragm and from the spinal nerves to the external intercostals, resulting in active contraction of the inspiratory muscles, thereby producing expansion of the thoracic cage and inspiration. The accessory muscles of inspiration, including the scalene and sternocleidomastoid muscles, are activated in stimulated respiration. Passive relaxation of the inspiratory muscles cause the thoracic cage and the lungs through their own weight to resume a resting state. The motor neurons to the expiratory muscles are inhibited, whereas the inspiratory muscles are stimulated through reciprocal innervation. When expiration must be facilitated, stimulation through the spinal nerves causes contraction of the internal intercostals and the abdominal muscles. A person can voluntarily alter the rate and depth and pattern of breathing through mechanisms in the cerebral cortex.

Medullary and Pontine Neural Control

Rhythmic cyclical discharge of neurons located in the medulla oblongata produces automatic respiration. The precise anatomic and physiologic function of the respiratory medullary neurons is under investigation. Current research indicates that there are two groups of respiratory neurons in the medulla. The dorsal group of neurons is in or near the nucleus of the tractus solitarius and is the source of rhythmic drive to the contralateral phrenic motor neurons. The neurons in the dorsal group project to and drive the ventral group. The ventral group has two divisions: the cranial division is composed of neurons in the nucleus ambiguous that innervate the accessory muscles of respiration on the same side, and the caudal division is composed of neurons in the nucleus retroambigualis that provide inspiratory and expiratory input to the intercostal muscles (Fig. 27–19).

Although the rhythmic discharge of the neurons in the medullary respiratory center is spontaneous, research to date has failed to demonstrate actual pacemaker cells similar to those in the sinoatrial node in the heart, which drive respiration. Research has shown that the rhythmic discharge of the medullary neurons is modified by centers in the pons and by afferent information via the vagus nerve from stretch receptors (mechanoreceptors) in the lungs. Research studies examining the role of the pneumotaxic and apneustic

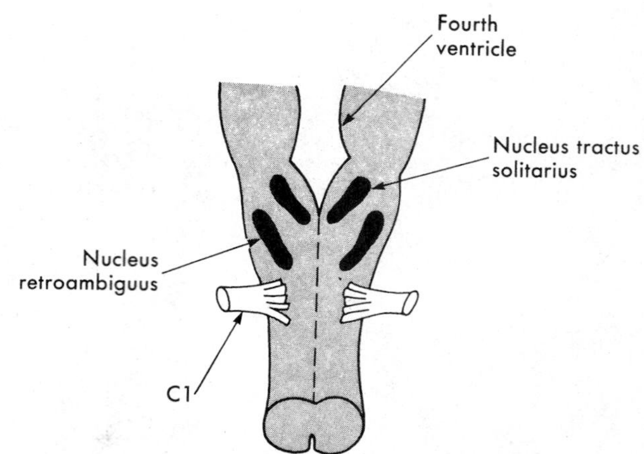

FIGURE 27–19. Neuronal group in the brainstem that controls respiration. (From Berne, R. M., & Levy, M. N. [1988]. *Physiology* [2nd ed., p. 625]. St. Louis: C. V. Mosby.)

centers in the pons have been performed in anesthetized animal models in which the brain stem was transected above the pons. When the brain stem is transected at this point, normal regular breathing occurs (point A in Fig. 27–20). When the pneumotaxic center is intact and the vagus nerve is cut, the depth of respiration is increased, indicating that the vagus nerve sends information from stretch receptors in the lung and provide information about the stretch of the lungs during inspiration. With the vagus intact, stretching of the lungs during inspiration reflexly inhibits the inspiratory drive, reinforcing the function of the pneumotaxic center in producing intermittent inspiratory neuron discharge. The pneumotaxic center causes stimulation of the expiratory neurons and simultaneously inhibits the inspiratory center, thus promoting regular cyclical respirations. Transection of the brain stem in the inferior portion of the pons (point B in Fig. 27–20) results in continuous inspiratory discharge

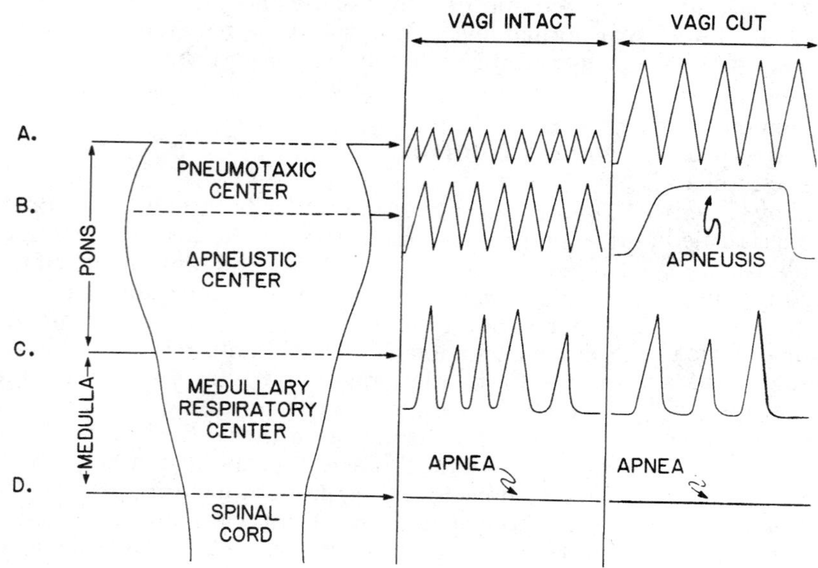

FIGURE 27–20. Respiratory patterns after complete transection of the brain stem at four levels: A, B, C, and D. (From Jensen, D. [1980]. *The principles of physiology* [2nd ed., p. 674]. New York: Appleton-Century-Crofts.)

with the vagus intact. When the vagi are cut, respiration in inspiration is arrested (called apneusis, hence the name apneustic center). When all pontine tissue is separated from the medulla (point C in Fig. 27–20), respirations are irregular and gasping, indicating that the medullary respiratory neurons may be capable of spontaneous rhythmic discharge. Complete transection on the brain stem below the medulla (point D in Fig. 27–20) stops all respirations.

Chemical Control

Central chemoreceptors are located in the medulla and account for 70% to 80% of the increase in ventilation when carbon dioxide levels are elevated. The peripheral chemoreceptors, located in the carotid and aortic bodies, are responsible for 20% to 30%. The exact location of the central chemoreceptors is unknown, but it is hypothesized to be near the ventrolateral surface of the medulla. The medullary chemoreceptors monitor the H^+ ion concentration of the cerebrospinal fluid (CSF) and the brain stem interstitial fluid. Unfortunately, H^+ ion and HCO_3^- ions are unable to cross the blood–brain barrier and the blood–CSF barrier easily. On the other hand, carbon dioxide readily penetrates these barriers and immediately after hydration forms H_2CO_3, which dissociates into H^+ ion and HCO_3^-. The H^+ ion concentration in brain interstitial fluid parallels the arterial P_{CO_2} and acts as the stimulus for increases in respiration. There is a linear relationship between the respiratory minute volume and the alveolar P_{CO_2} to an upper limit of 100 mm Hg Pa_{CO_2}. Accumulation of CO_2 in the body (called hypercapnia) depresses the central nervous system and the respiratory center and produces headache, confusion, and eventually coma.

The peripheral chemoreceptors include the carotid body near the bifurcation of the internal and external carotid arteries and the aortic bodies near the arch of the aorta (Fig. 27–21). The carotid and aortic bodies are composed of islands of type I and type II cells surrounded by capillaries with large openings or fenestration. The carotid bodies receive a tremendous blood supply (0.04 mL/minute or 2,000 mL/100 g of tissue per minute). The type I cells are surrounded by nerve endings from the glossopharyngeal nerve to the carotid bodies and from the vagi to the aortic bodies. Type I cells are sensitive to the concentration of the partial pressure of oxygen dissolved in the liquid plasma of the blood. Afferent nerve fibers from the carotid and aortic bodies ascend to the medulla and cause an increase in ventilation when the Pa_{O_2} falls below 60 mm Hg, which is the point at which hemoglobin saturation declines. Because the receptors are sensitive to Pa_{O_2} dissolved in the plasma, they do not respond in patients with such conditions as anemia or carbon monoxide poisoning, which affect the concentration of hemoglobin or the content of oxygen on the hemoglobin molecule. The carotid and aortic bodies are primarily stimulated by an elevated Pa_{CO_2} or an increased H^+ ion concentration and secondarily by a marked decrease in Pa_{O_2}. Chronic sustained hypoxia appears to depress the carotid and aortic chemoreceptor response to low Pa_{O_2}, and peripheral control depends on the levels of Pa_{CO_2} and H^+ ion to increase ventilation.

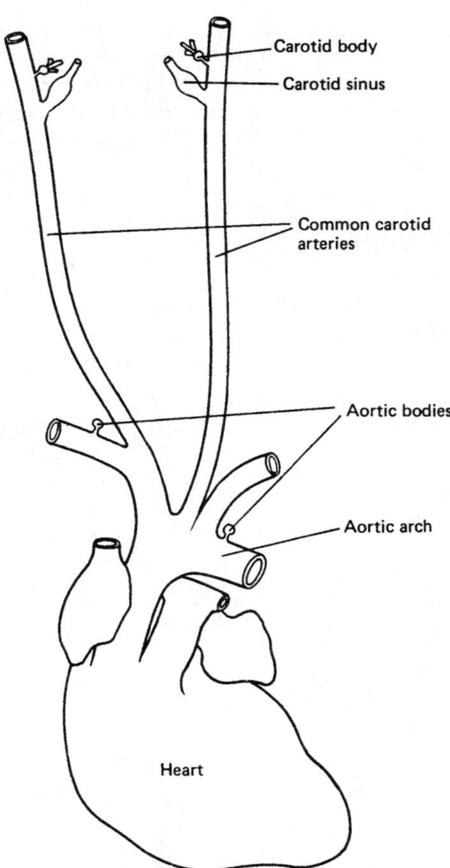

FIGURE 27–21. Location of the carotid and aortic bodies. (From Ganong, W. F. [1983]. *Review of medical physiology* [11th ed.]. Los Altos, CA: Lange Medical Publications.)

SUMMARY

The relationship of the neural and chemical control of the respiratory system is summarized in Figure 27–22.

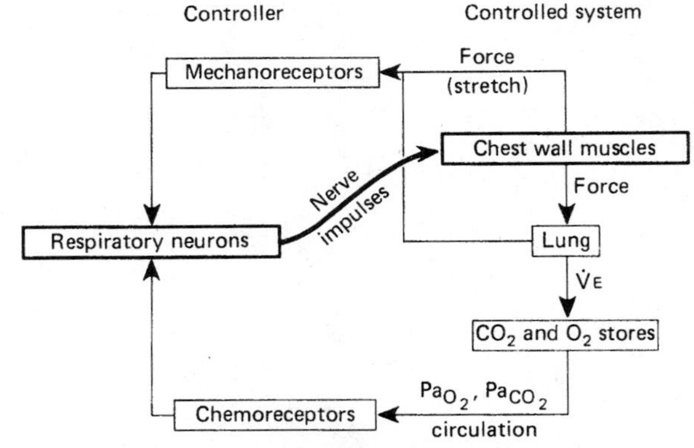

FIGURE 27–22. Control of the respiratory system. (Reproduced with permission from Fishman, A. P. [1980]. *Assessment of pulmonary function.* New York: McGraw-Hill. Reproduced with permission of The McGraw-Hill Companies.)

Control of respiration is an intricate interplay between neural and chemical factors that serve to maintain the levels of PaO_2, $PaCO_2$, and pH at a constant level to promote the optimal functioning of the cells of the body.

REFERENCES

Berne, R. M., & Levy, M. N. (1993). *Physiology* (3rd ed.) St. Louis: C. V. Mosby.

Comroe, J. H., Jr. (1965). *Physiology of respiration*. Chicago: Year Book Medical Publishers.

Fishman, A. P. (1980). *Assessment of pulmonary function*. New York: McGraw-Hill.

Fox, S. I. (1993). *Human physiology* (4th ed.). Dubuque, IA: Wm. C. Brown.

Guyton, A. C. (1991). *Textbook of medical physiology* (8th ed.). Philadelphia: W. B. Saunders.

Kersten, L. D. (1989). *Comprehensive respiratory nursing*. Philadelphia: W. B. Saunders.

Moffett, D. F., Moffett, S. B., & Schauf, C. L. (1993). *Human physiology: Foundations and frontiers* (2nd ed.). St. Louis: C. V. Mosby.

Vander, A. J., Sherman, J. H., & Luciano, D. S. (1990). *Human physiology* (5th ed.). New York: McGraw-Hill.

Acid–Base Physiology

Carol F. Baker

Humans produce acids by means of carbohydrate, fat, and glucose metabolism. The hydrogen ion concentration (H^+) of body fluids is represented by the symbol pH. For human life, the pH of extracellular fluids is normally maintained within a fairly narrow range (7.35–7.45), whereas other fluids of the body such as urine undergo wide fluctuations in pH. The body cells and organs, especially the brain and heart, are very susceptible to changes in pH and tolerate them poorly. The range of blood pH compatible with life is 6.8 to 8.0. Immediately on detecting a change from normal, feedback mechanisms are initiated to compensate for the altered state and usually return the blood pH to the normal range. This regulation of H^+ concentration is one of the most important aspects of homeostasis necessary to maintain health (Guyton, 1991).

The body tolerates acidosis better than alkalosis. Compensatory mechanisms are designed primarily to remove acid and restore base through the lungs or kidneys. Carbon dioxide (CO_2) is normally the most potent stimulus of the respiratory center. Increases in the partial pressure of CO_2 stimulate the respiratory center, causing increased ventilation. CO_2 in water forms carbonic acid (H_2CO_3): $CO_2 + H_2O \rightarrow H_2CO_3$. As CO_2 is lost, H_2CO_3 is reduced and the pH is increased. A primary function of the kidney is to retain base and neutralize or excrete unwanted organic and inorganic acids. Although mechanisms exist to correct alkalosis, they are less powerful and take longer. The body tolerates alkalosis poorly, although it is less severe or life threatening.

KEY DEFINITIONS

To understand the regulation of acid–base balance, appropriate principles and terms need to be defined (Guyton, 1991; Porth, 1990; Preuss, 1993; Rutherford et al., 1992).

1. An *acid* is an ion that releases H^+ in solution. Carbonic acid ionizes in water to form $H^+ + HCO_3^-$, and hydrochloric acid ionizes to $H^+ + Cl^-$. An acid can be a simple or complex ion. Some other acids in the body are acetic, uric, and lactic acids.

2. *Acidosis* is the state of excess addition of H^+ or a loss of basic ions to solutions.

3. A *base* is an ion that combines with H^+ and removes them from solution. Some examples of base in the body are bicarbonate, phosphate, proteins, and hemoglobin.

4. *Alkalosis* is the excess removal of H^+ or the addition of basic ions to solutions. An alkali is the combination of one of the alkaline metals (sodium or potassium, for example) with a highly basic ion such as the hydroxyl ion (OH^-).

5. *Strong versus weak reaction:* A strong acid readily gives up H^+ into solution, such as hydrochloric acid (HCl). A weak acid releases H^+ more slowly, such as H_2CO_3. A strong base readily accepts H^+ and removes them rapidly from solution, such as the hydroxyl ion (OH^-). The bicarbonate ion (HCO_3^-) is a weak base but is the primary buffering system of the body.

6. *pH* is the symbol used to express the concentration of H^+ in solutions. The actual H^+ concentration in extracellular fluid (ECF) is normally regulated at a constant value of approximately 4×10^{-8} mEq/L. A logarithmic figure (pH) was derived for ease of expression. pH is related to actual H^+ concentration by the following formula:

$$pH = 6.1 + \log HCO_3^- / H_2CO_3 + CO_2$$

A low pH (6.7–7.35 in ECF) corresponds to a high H^+ concentration, acidosis. A high pH (7.45–7.9 in ECF) corresponds to alkalosis.

7. *Compensatory mechanisms* are the responses of the buffers, the respiratory or the renal systems, to alterations in the opposite system; that is, respiratory acidosis is compensated by the kidney's reabsorption of bicarbonate, a metabolic process.

An *uncompensated* state is a single or complex acid–base disorder resulting in an abnormal pH and abnormal respiratory or renal signs.

A *compensated* state occurs when the pH returns to normal after an acid–base imbalance, but respiratory or renal signs may remain abnormal until the imbalance is corrected.

8. Measured *anions* are ions with a negative valence, such as HCO_3^- and chloride (Cl^-).

9. Measured *cations* are ions with a positive valence, such as sodium (Na^+), potassium (K^+), calcium (Ca^{2+}). The sum of measured cations is greater than the sum of

measured anions due to the presence of unmeasured anions.

10. An *anion gap* is the difference between the sum of measured anions (HCO_3^- and Cl^-) subtracted from the sum of measured cations (e.g., Na^+, K^+) and is 12 to 16 mmol per liter normally. The unmeasured anions are proteins, phosphates, sulfates, and organic acids.

11. *Base deficit or excess* measures the level of all buffer systems of the blood. Base deficit is the amount of base that must be added to one liter of whole, arterial blood to achieve a pH of 7.4 with normal values of $Pa{O_2}$, $Pa{CO_2}$, and temperature. It indicates metabolic acidosis. Base excess measures the amount of fixed acid that must be added to achieve a pH of 7.4 and indicates metabolic alkalosis. The normal range is ±3.0 mEq/L.

SOURCES OF ACIDS AND BASES IN THE BODY

Through normal diet intake, large amounts of acids are continuously formed from the metabolism of carbohydrates, proteins, and fats. Carbon dioxide is produced and combines with water to form H_2CO_3 ($CO_2 + H_2O \overset{CA}{\leftrightharpoons} H_2CO_3$) in the presence of the enzyme, carbonic anhydrase (CA). The majority of the gas is eliminated through the lungs and is regulated by the rate and depth of pulmonary ventilation. *Fixed acids* consist of all other acids in the body, sulfuric, lactic, acetoacetic, and so on. Most are formed as a result of protein metabolism. Hydrogen ions produced from the dissociation of fixed acids are excreted by the kidneys.

Aerobic Glucose Metabolism

The metabolism of glucose results eventually in the formation of CO_2 and water. Complete oxidation of one mole of glucose releases 686,000 calories of energy to form a total of 38 moles of adenosine triphosphate (ATP) (Guyton, 1991). There are several steps in the oxidation of glucose for energy:

1. Glycolysis is the splitting of glucose to form pyruvic acid, ATP, and hydrogen. The efficiency of energy in the formation of ATP is 43%, whereas 57% of the energy is lost as heat.
2. Pyruvic acid is converted into acetyl coenzyme A (acetyl Co-A), CO_2, and hydrogen.
3. In the citric acid cycle (Krebs cycle), the acetyl portion of acetyl Co-A is degraded to CO_2, hydrogen, and coenzyme A. Two molecules of ATP are formed for each molecule of glucose metabolized.
4. Oxidative phosphorylation is the process by which 95% of ATP is formed. Tremendous quantities of energy are released to form ATP. The overall efficiency of energy transfer into ATP is 66%, whereas the remaining 34% becomes heat. End products of metabolism are CO_2 and water.

Anaerobic Glucose Metabolism

When oxygen becomes unavailable or is insufficient, anaerobic glycolysis occurs. When the build-up of pyruvic acid and H^+ becomes excessive, lactic acid is formed. Lactic acid allows the conversion of ATP to continue and glycolysis to proceed without oxygen. Lactic acid is released in large quantities from skeletal muscles during heavy exercise or with severe tissue hypoxia, such as from a myocardial infarction. This causes metabolic acidosis. When oxygen becomes available, lactic and pyruvic acids are used in the liver to reconvert glucose. Heart muscle is especially capable of converting lactic to pyruvic acid and using it for energy, especially during heavy exercise (Guyton, 1991).

Protein Metabolism

Protein metabolism results in the production of strong organic acids such as sulfuric and phosphoric acids. There is a limit to the amount of protein that can be used in cells. Once that limit is reached, additional amino acids will be degraded in the liver and used for energy or stored as fat. The process of deamination of protein is the removal of amino groups from amino acids. Amino acids can be transferred to another substance, and released in the form of ammonia. Ammonia is converted in the liver into urea, which is excreted by the kidney. A second method of deamination is oxidation of amino acids into pyruvic acid and glucose or into keto (fatty) acids.

Fat Metabolism

Fat metabolism occurs with the oxidation of fatty acids in the cell, resulting in the production of acetyl Co-A. Acetyl Co-A enters the citric acid cycle and is converted into CO_2 and H^+ in the liver. Excess accumulation of acetyl Co-A produces acetoacetic acid, which is converted into beta-hydroxybutyric acid and acetone. During abnormal states such as starvation, diabetes mellitus, or a high-fat diet, ketosis occurs. Ketosis is the production of ketone bodies, which are also converted into beta-hydroxybutyric acid and acetone.

Diet and Medication

Dietary intake of acids occurs from ingesting fruits (citric, acetic, tannic, or ascorbic acids), fat, and especially protein. Heavy meat eaters tend to have an increased production of acid. The major source of alkaline production is from the catabolism of fruits and vegetables into organic anions such as lactate and citrate. Other alkaline sources in the diet include milk products, which contain calcium. Vegetarians tend to have a net production of alkali (Guyton, 1987, 1991). Medications

TABLE 28–1. **pH of Normal Body Fluids**

Extracellular fluid	7.35–7.45
Cerebrospinal fluid	7.35–7.45
Intracellular fluid	6.9–7.2
Bile–gallbladder	5.0–6.0
Pancreatic	7.6–8.2
Urine	4.0–8.0
Gastric	1.0–2.0
Intestine	6.5–7.6
Bile–liver	7.4

such as ammonium chloride and aspirin are sources of acid. Antacids are a source of base.

pH OF NORMAL BODY FLUIDS

Although the range of pH in the ECF, which is compatible with life is narrow, the relative acid or alkaline characteristics of other body fluids vary considerably and depend on the particular organ's function. For instance, gastric fluid is highly acid, reflecting the large concentration of hydrochloric acid in the stomach. On the other hand, fluids containing pancreatic enzymes are alkaline. Urine has the widest range in pH, varying from highly acidic to highly basic, depending on the pH of plasma. Normal values of pH of body fluids are shown in Table 28–1.

DEFENSE AGAINST CHANGES IN ACID–BASE BALANCE

To maintain a homeostatic balance and a normal pH, the body first buffers acids produced by metabolism and then removes excess H^+ through excretion. Three regulatory systems are sequentially available to readjust for constant fluctations in acid–base balance. The chemical buffer system response is both intracellular and extracellular and occurs within seconds. This mechanism is temporary until the other mechanisms go into effect. The respiratory system compensation occurs in a few minutes to hours, and is primarily concerned with the excretion of CO_2. The renal system compensation occurs over a matter of days and is the slowest but most powerful response. It removes excess acid or base from the body and restores or retains the bicarbonate buffer base.

The Buffer System

A chemical buffer is a substance that prevents rapid or great change in the pH of a solution when an acid or a base is added. A buffer system usually consists of a pair of compounds: a weak acid and its conjugate base. For example, when hydrochloric acid is added to water, the strong acid dissociates completely, releasing many H^+ into solution and markedly lowering the pH of the solution. When sodium bicarbonate is added as a weak base, it dissociates in water. The H^+ combine with bicarbonate, forming H_2CO_3, a weak acid, and a salt, sodium chloride:

$$H^+ + Cl^- + Na^+\ HCO_3^- \rightarrow H_2CO_3 + NaCl$$

The strong acid is replaced with a weak acid that dissociates only slightly. If a strong base such as sodium hydroxide were added to the system, H_2CO_3 would dissociate to release H^+, forming a weak base and water:

$$NaOH + H_2CO_3 = Na\ HCO_3 + H_2O$$

A buffer system works most efficiently when the concentrations of the weak acid and conjugate base are equal (McCance & Heuther, 1994; Porth, 1990). There are several major buffer systems in the body. Extracellular buffers include bicarbonate, plasma, proteins, hemoglobin, and bone. The most important buffer of the ECF, especially the interstitial fluid, is the bicarbonate–H_2CO_3 system. However, bicarbonate cannot buffer H_2CO_3 because it would simply regenerate itself ($H_2CO_3 = H^+ + HCO_3^-$). The intracellular compartment may provide up to 50% of the total body buffering response by intracellular proteins, hemoglobin, phosphates, and other organic buffers (Appel & Chase, 1986).

BICARBONATE–H_2CO_3 BUFFER SYSTEM

The bicarbonate buffer system is a mixture of H_2CO_3 and sodium bicarbonate in solution, as seen in the formula above. The concentrations of H_2CO_3 and dissolved CO_2 form the total "H_2CO_3 pool" available for buffer action. Because the amount of H_2CO_3 in body fluids is small, the strength of the buffer pool is determined by the amount of dissolved CO_2 or the partial pressure of CO_2, P_{CO_2}.

Maximal buffering occurs when the ratio of available base (bicarbonate concentration) to the H_2CO_3 pool is 20 to 1. This ratio is measured in terms of the pH of the acid-containing solution. Different acids have various buffering capacities depending on their pK (the pH at which half the acid is undissociated, a constant of 6.1). This ratio is called the Henderson-Hasselbach equation and is expressed as:

$$pH = 6.1 + \log \frac{BHCO_3}{H_2CO_3}$$

where B equals any cation. The buffer pair loses buffering capacity if either the base or H_2CO_3 is totally consumed. Even though considerable amount of base is required to buffer the acid, the strength of the system lies in the fact that each member is capable of being regulated independently by either the kidneys or the lungs.

PHOSPHATE BUFFER SYSTEM

The phosphate buffer system is important in red blood cells and especially in the cells of kidney tubules, where it enables the kidneys to excrete H^+. The buffer system is composed primarily of a weak acid, sodium dihydrogen phosphate ($NaH_2PO_4 = Na^+ + H^+ + HPO_4^{2-}$) and its conjugate base, sodium monohydrogen phosphate (Na_2HPO_4). In the kidneys' intracellular fluid, high concentrations of Na_2HPO_4 are available to combine with H^+, which are secreted into the urine and eliminated along with NaCl. On the other hand, if a strong base is introduced into the body, the NaH_2PO_4 can combine with it, forming a weak base and water (Goldberger, 1986).

PROTEIN BUFFER SYSTEM

The protein buffer system consists of a weak acid (H^+-protein) and a weak base (Na^+-protein) and is found in proteins in cells and in plasma. Carbon dioxide diffuses readily through the cell membranes, followed more slowly by bicarbonate and H^+. This diffusion causes the intracellular pH to change in proportion to changes in the ECF. However, the change occurs over several hours; it cannot respond to rapid changes in the ECF. Fixed acids produced inside the cells, such as sulfuric acid, are also initially buffered by proteins and phosphate before they enter the ECF. Proteins act as anions, carrying many negative charges in the alkaline pH of body fluids (Goldberger, 1986; McCance & Heuther, 1994).

HEMOGLOBIN BUFFER SYSTEM

Hemoglobin of the red blood cells is a protein buffer that is very important in buffering CO_2 while it is being transported to the lungs for elimination. Carbon dioxide enters the blood as a byproduct of tissue metabolism. Some (5%) is immediately transformed into H_2CO_3 and carried in solution by the plasma. This process occurs slowly, and the remainder of the CO_2 diffuses into red blood cells. Twenty percent of it reacts to form a carbamino compound with hemoglobin.

The enzyme carbonic anhydrase is a catalyst for the formation of H_2CO_3 from the remaining 75% of the CO_2:

$$CO_2 + H_2O \rightarrow CA \rightarrow H_2CO_3$$

This compound dissociates into $H^+ + HCO_3^-$ ions, the H^+ ion reacts with reduced deoxygenated hemoglobin ($H^+ + Hb^- \rightarrow HHb$), and the bicarbonate reacts with potassium in the red blood cells to form $KHCO_3$. Bicarbonate later diffuses into the plasma. To maintain electrical neutrality, chloride ions diffuse inside the red blood cells (the *chloride shift*) to form KCl. In the lungs, the opposite reaction occurs. The reduced hemoglobin is oxygenated ($HHbO_2$). Hydrogen ions are released from the hemoglobin and react with bicarbonate salts to form H_2CO_3, which is converted to CO_2 by carbonic

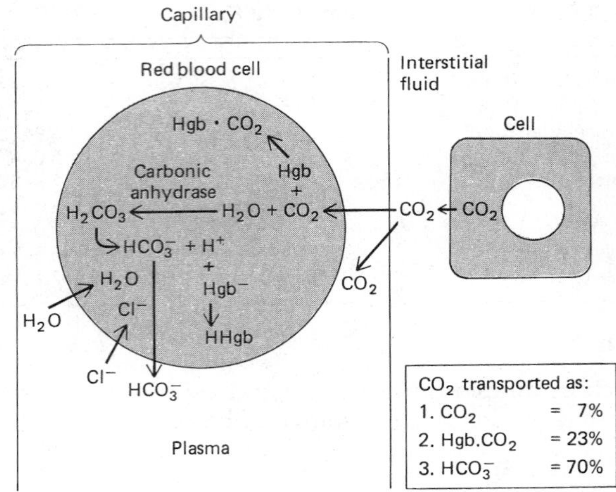

FIGURE 28–1. Mechanisms of carbon dioxide transport. (From Guyton, A. C. [1991]. *Textbook of medical physiology.* Philadelphia: W. B. Saunders.)

anhydrase (Fig. 28–1) (Goldberger, 1986). Chloride diffuses back into the plasma, and potassium reacts with bicarbonate:

$$HHbO_2 + KHCO_3 \rightarrow H_2CO_3 + KHbO_2$$

BONE BUFFER SYSTEM

Carbonate in the bone can act as a cellular buffer when acid is present in the ECF. Hydrogen ions are absorbed into the crystal lattice of bone, and sodium is released into the ECF. This exchange provides a vast buffering capacity in patients with chronic conditions of H^+ retention such as chronic renal failure (Chambers, 1987). Calcium is also released in exchange for the uptake of phosphorus by the bone. When alkaline substances are being buffered, more carbonate is deposited. In acid–base abnormalities, a large proportion of the buffering is carried out in bone: in respiratory alkalosis, 99%; in respiratory acidosis, 97%; in metabolic acidosis, 57%; and in metabolic alkalosis, 32% (Goldberger, 1986).

Respiratory Regulation of Acid–Base Balance

Because the ultimate goal of respiration is to maintain normal levels of carbon dioxide, hydrogen ions, and oxygen, changes in their concentrations are integral to respiratory regulation.

RESPIRATORY CENTER

Excess CO_2 and H^+ have excitatory effects on the respiratory center, causing increased strength of both inspiratory and expiratory signals to the respiratory muscles. This respiratory compensation increases the elimination of CO_2 and H_2CO_3 from the plasma. It is thought that a chemosensitive area, receptive to changes in CO_2 and H^+ concentrations, is located directly beneath the surface of the medulla near the entry of the glossopharyngeal and vagal nerves. The chemosensitive area then excites other portions of the respiratory center, especially the inspiratory center. Although it is believed that H^+ are the only direct stimulus for this area, they are slow to cross the blood–brain barrier. Because CO_2 readily diffuses across all cell membranes, changes in this concentration have the most powerful effect on control of respiration, although the effect is indirect. Carbon dioxide reacts with water of the tissues to form H_2CO_3. This then dissociates into bicarbonate ions and H^+, which have a potent direct stimulatory effect (Guyton, 1991; Shapiro et al., 1982).

STIMULI FOR VENTILATION

CARBON DIOXIDE CONCENTRATION. Changes in metabolism affect the amount of CO_2 produced, whereas changes in pulmonary ventilation affect the rate of excretion of CO_2, creating a cyclical feedback mechanism. Because the CO_2 concentration is directly related to the pH of tissue fluids, tissue fluid P_{CO_2} must be regulated exactly by the respiratory system. Its ability to stimulate ventilation is especially great in the *normal* P_{CO_2} and pH ranges: P_{CO_2} between 30 and 50 mm Hg and pH between 7.5 and 7.3. When venous blood reaches the pulmonary capillaries, the P_{CO_2} is approximately 46 mm Hg. The P_{CO_2} in the alveoli is normally 40 mm Hg. This difference in partial pressure facilitates the diffusion of CO_2 from the plasma into the alveoli for elimination. Increasing the CO_2 concentration can result in an increase in ventilation up to 11-fold. This concentration is the primary chemical regulator of normal respiration. If the P_{CO_2} rises above 65 mm Hg, CO_2 acts as a depressant, and other stimulants to respiration must intervene.

HYDROGEN ION CONCENTRATION. Ventilatory rate also affects H^+ concentration; an increase in ventilation causes the excretion of excess H_2CO_3 with a net increase in pH. On the other hand, H^+ concentration also controls alveolar ventilatory rate by acting directly on the chemosensitive area of the respiratory center (Fig. 28–2). Because of the blood–brain barrier, respiratory regulation is slower when it is dependent on a change in pH. Up to a fourfold increase in hyperventilation occurs when the pH drops to 7.2; however, hyperventilation stops when the pH reaches 7.0.

OXYGEN CONCENTRATION. The respiratory center is affected in varying degrees by the partial pressure of oxygen in the alveolar air. Normally, the respiratory system maintains an alveolar P_{O_2} that is much higher than that needed to saturate the hemoglobin. Ventilation can decrease to as low as one-half normal and the hemoglobin will still remain essentially saturated. Chemoreceptors, located outside the central nervous system in the carotid and aortic bodies of the carotid arteries and aorta, respectively, are sensitive to

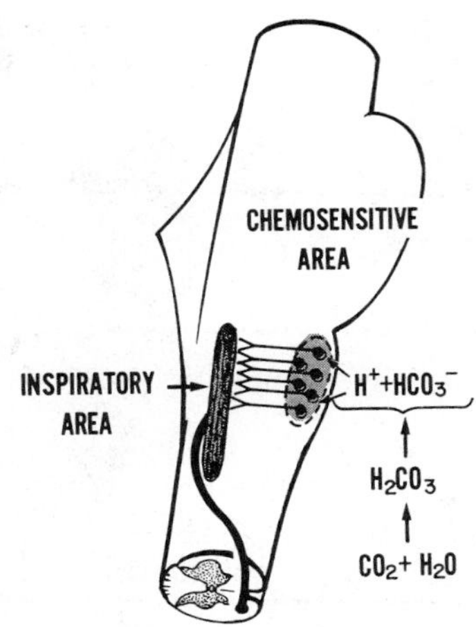

FIGURE 28–2. Stimulus of the respiratory center. (From Guyton, A. C. [1991]. *Textbook of medical physiology.* Philadelphia: W. B. Saunders.)

changes in oxygen concentration. Low blood P_{O_2} will not increase alveolar ventilation appreciably until the P_{O_2} is one-half normal. Hypoxia, a P_{O_2} between 60 and 30 mm Hg, will increase ventilation by 1.5 to 1.7 times, a much weaker effect than occurs with increased CO_2 and H^+ concentrations. A reduced P_{O_2} becomes the primary stimulus to respiration only in conditions of acute or chronic pulmonary disease, when CO_2 and H^+ cannot be excreted and their concentrations remain elevated.

Renal Regulation of Acid–Base Balance

Metabolic control and restoration of acid–base balance are regulated by the kidneys. The kidneys control H^+ concentration primarily by increasing or decreasing the bicarbonate concentration of the body fluids and secreting fixed acids. Although it may take 1 to 3 days for the kidney to restore acid–base balance, the mechanism provides for complete removal of excess acid or base unless an abnormality persists. The pH of the urine can vary from 4.4 to 8.0, depending on the need to conserve or excrete acid. Dietary intake has a major influence on urinary pH; a heavy protein intake will acidify the urine, whereas a vegetarian intake creates an alkaline urine. The usual urinary pH is 6.0, more acidic than the 7.4 pH of blood because 50 to 80 mmol more acid than alkali is produced each day and excreted (Guyton, 1991).

BICARBONATE REABSORPTION AND HYDROGEN ION SECRETION

There are three major processes by which the kidneys excrete acid and retain bicarbonate: bicarbonate-carbonic acid system, phosphate buffers, and ammonia excretion.

THE BICARBONATE–CARBONIC ACID SYSTEM. Sodium bicarbonate is filtered, and then Na^+ is reabsorbed into

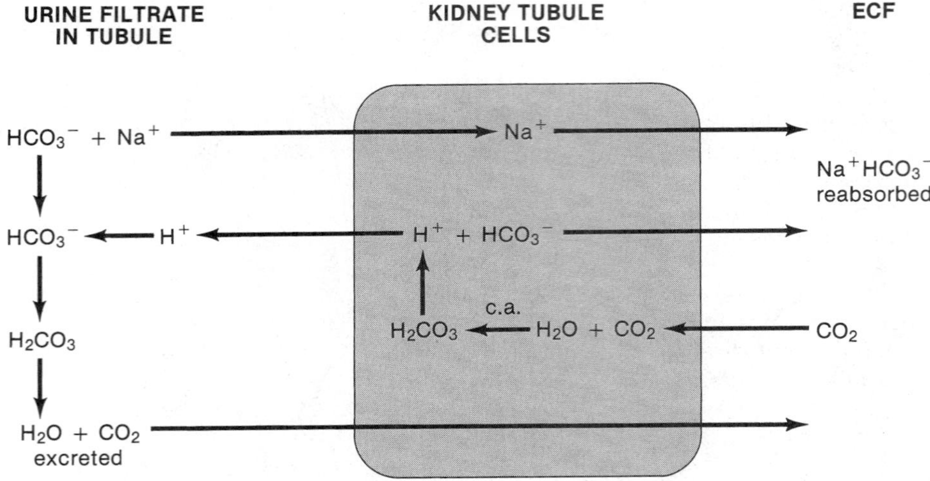

FIGURE 28–3. Renal regulation of hydrogen and bicarbonate ion concentration. *Abbreviations:* ECF, extracellular fluid; c.a., carbonic anhydrase.

the proximal tubule. Carbon dioxide in the tubular cells combines with water, under the catalytic action of CA, to form H_2CO_3. This dissociates, and H^+ are exchanged for Na^+ in the tubular fluid in a process called countertransport. A carrier protein combines with sodium and moves it along a concentration gradient to the interior of the cell. At the same time, hydrogen attaches to the same protein and is moved actively against a concentration gradient into the tubular lumen. As sodium crosses into the ECF, the lumen is electronegative, and H^+ secretion occurs (Fig. 28–3). In this way, hydrogen can be excreted even though acid already exists in the tubular fluid (Puschett & Piraino, 1985). About 84% of all H^+ secretion occurs in the proximal tubules. The gradient is only three to four times the tubular concentration, compared with a gradient of 900 times greater in the collecting ducts.

Under normal conditions, the amount of H^+ secreted from the tubular cells is approximately the same as the amount of bicarbonate filtered through the glomerulus. The H^+ and bicarbonate combine to form CO_2 and water, thereby neutralizing each other. Usually there is an excess of acid to be excreted. However, if an alkalotic condition exists, increased bicarbonate would be filtered and fewer H^+ secreted into the tubules, with a net loss of bicarbonate and a return of the pH toward normal.

The normal process of restoring bicarbonate to the ECF occurs inside the tubular cell. When H_2CO_3 dissociates, it releases bicarbonate as well as H^+. These bicarbonate ions diffuse into the ECF and combine with sodium ions that were reabsorbed from the tubular fluid to form sodium bicarbonate.

PHOSPHATE BUFFERS. The second mechanism facilitates the removal of H^+ through the kidney. In the tubular filtrate, the phosphate buffers become more concentrated. Once filtered, they are relatively impermeable to reabsorption. Although weak in the plasma, they are powerful buffers in the filtrate in transporting a major portion of H^+ into the urine. As excess H^+ are secreted into the filtrate in the distal tubule, they combine with Na_2HPO_4 to form NaH_2PO_4. The remaining sodium ions are reabsorbed into the ECF along with bicarbonate ions (Fig. 28–4). This allows excretion of a titratable acid with a pH of 4.5 (Guyton, 1991; McCance & Heuther, 1994).

AMMONIA BUFFERS. The third potent buffer in the tubular filtrate is ammonia (NH_3) and the ammonium ion (NH_4^+). The epithelial cells of most of the tubule continually synthesize ammonia, which diffuses into the lumen. This combines with hydrogen to form NH_4^+. The tubular cells are less permeable to NH_4^+, helping to excrete the hydrogen. The major anion of the filtrate is chloride. Much of it combines with NH_4^+ to form ammonium chloride, a weak acid that gives urine its characteristic odor. This process facilitates the removal of hydrogen, ammonium, and chloride ions, avoiding the formation of a strong acid, hydrochloric acid, and keeps the pH of the urine within acceptable limits. At the same time, a bicarbonate ion is reabsorbed into the ECF as a substitute for the chloride ion. The ammonia buffer system allows the tubules to secrete many times the number of H^+ that would otherwise be possible and facilitates the retention of bicarbonate, thus enhancing the ability of the kidney to correct acidotic states (Fig. 28–5) (Guyton, 1991; Porth, 1990).

Potassium Exchange

Another process exists at the cellular level to compensate for an acidotic state. It is estimated that 57% of total buffering for metabolic acidosis is intracellular (Preuss, 1993). Normally, extracellular sodium is exchanged for intracellular potassium by means of the sodium pump. If other cations such as excess H^+ or ammonium ions are present, these will compete with potassium. Hydrogen ions can be transported intracellularly in exchange for potassium. To maintain a fairly

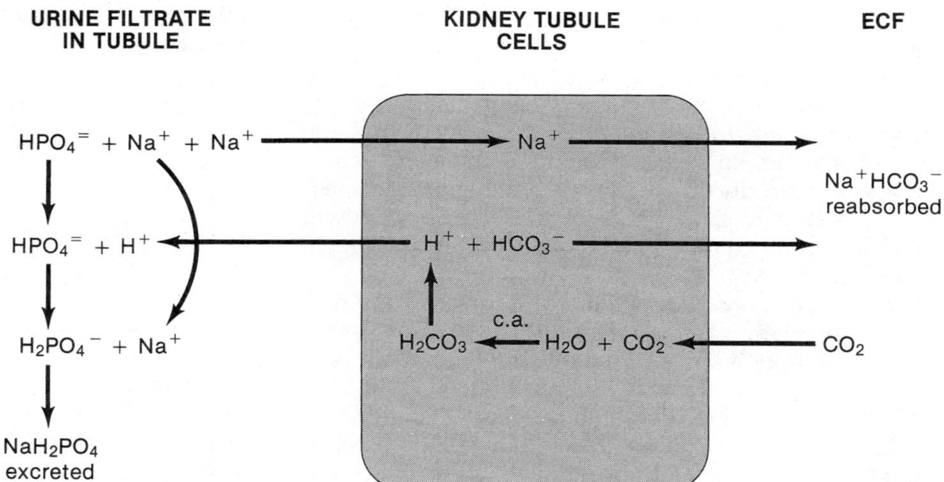

FIGURE 28–4. Renal regulation of the phosphate buffer system.

narrow range of extracellular potassium levels, excess amounts of the ion are excreted in the urine. This mechanism is another means by which the blood pH maintains its delicate balance (Appel & Chase, 1986).

The urine pH is not an indication of the total amount of acid excreted by the kidney. If the concentration of buffer is high, the amount of acid excreted will also be great, but the pH will be maintained above 4.5. Disruption of any of the cell transport mechanisms, NH_3 production, or aldosterone deficiency in the distal tubule will decrease maximal acid production (Appel & Chase, 1986).

Compensation

The relationship of bicarbonate (indicated by HCO_3^-, renal regulation) and carbonic acid (indicated by P_{CO_2}, respiratory regulation) is expressed as a ratio. When the pH is 7.4, the ratio is 20 base:1 acid. The clinical significance of this ratio is that values for HCO_3^- and P_{CO_2} can increase or decrease proportionately, but the 20:1 ratio remains stable. The ability of the unaffected system to adjust to an increase or decrease in the other system and return the pH to normal is the process of *compensation.* A 20:1 ratio is achieved though the actual values of bicarbonate or carbonic acid may remain abnormal (McCance & Heuther, 1994).

When a single disorder of acid or base imbalance occurs, concentration of that ion is either excessive or deficient. *Alkalosis* occurs from excess base, with a ratio of 30:1, or an acid deficit, a ratio of 20:0.5, with an increase in pH. The normal or unaffected system adjusts for the imbalance by either excreting base from the kidneys, or slowing ventilation and retaining CO_2, returning the pH toward normal. *Acidosis* occurs from excess acid (20:2) or a base deficit (10:1), with a decrease in pH. The unaffected system adjusts by excreting acid and retaining bicarbonate from the kidneys, or increasing ventilation to excrete CO_2, returning the pH toward normal. Complete respiratory compensation may take 12 to 24 hours; the kidneys require sev-

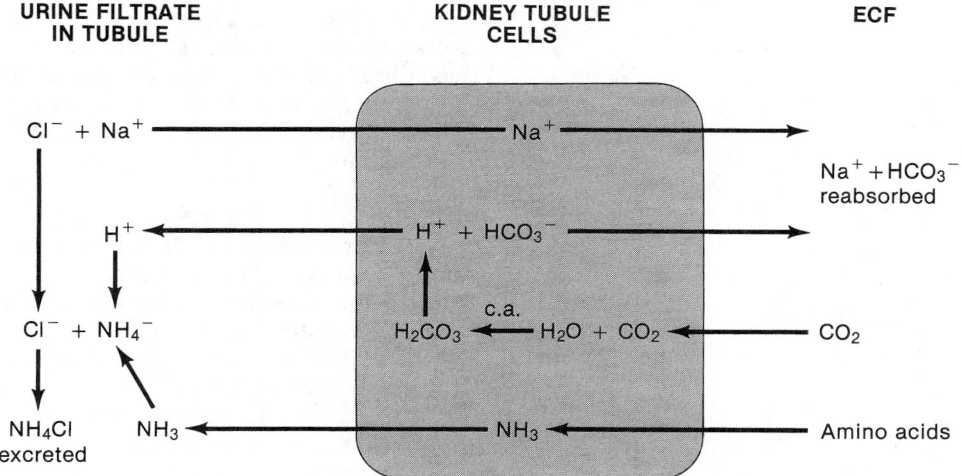

FIGURE 28–5. Renal regulation of ammonia secretion.

eral days for a full compensatory response (Goldberger, 1986; Preuss, 1993).

If there is a shift in the ratio, an imbalance occurs. An excess of base (30:1) or a deficit of acid (20:0.5) produces an alkalotic state and an increase in pH. On the other hand, an excess of acid (20:2) or a deficit of base (10:1) produces an acidotic state and a decrease in pH. A change in the bicarbonate buffer system will be reflected by changes in the other buffer systems in solution.

A *correction* occurs when the pH is returned to normal by alleviating the problem of the primary system; that is, the P_{CO_2} is lowered by putting the patient on a mechanical ventilator and eliminating excess CO_2. All parameters return to normal in a corrected state. *Overcompensation* occurs when one parameter (i.e., metabolic) continues to be abnormal after the primary imbalance has been corrected. If the primary abnormality in acid–base balance persists, the other system will not be able to adjust fully or compensate, and an *uncompensated* state will exist (Guyton, 1991).

ASSESSMENT OF ACID–BASE BALANCE AND IMBALANCE

Laboratory Assessment

NOMOGRAM. To understand the patient's state of acid–base balance, determine the parameters of serum pH and bicarbonate concentration from venous blood. Serum H_2CO_3 can then be calculated from a chart called a nomogram (Fig. 28–6) (McLean, 1938). Bicarbonate concentration and pH are plotted on the chart,

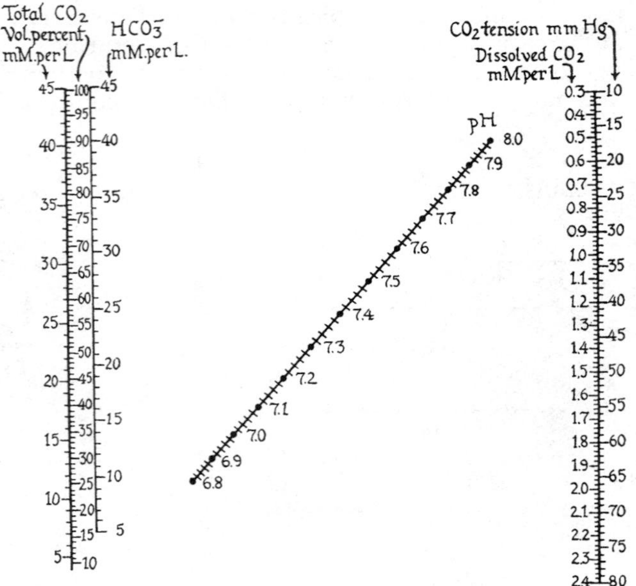

FIGURE 28–6. Nomogram to determine P_{CO_2} from pH and CO_2 content. (From McLean, F. C. [1938]. Application of the law of chemical equilibrium (Law of Mass Action) to biological problems. *Physiological Review, 18,* 495.)

TABLE 28–2. **Normal Blood Gas Values of Acid–Base Balance**

Parameter	Arterial Blood	Mixed Venous Blood
pH	7.35–7.45 (7.4)	7.33–7.43 (7.38)
P_{CO_2}	35–45 mm Hg	41–51 mm Hg
HCO_3^-	22–26 mEq/liter	24–28 mEq/liter
Base excess or plasma anion gap	−3 to +3.0 10–15 mEq/liter	0 to +4

and a line is drawn between them. The point of intersection with the right column represents the H_2CO_3 concentration. This method is useful in patients in whom arterial vascular access is lacking. Normal values for mixed venous blood are variable and represent the extremity from which the blood was drawn. There is less variation from arterial samples if the extremity is warmed and free-flowing blood is drawn without pumping the hand (Preuss, 1993).

ARTERIAL BLOOD GASES. More commonly, four parameters of acid–base balance are measured directly from ABGs: P_{CO_2}, pH, HCO_3^-, and base excess/deficit. Normal values for blood gases are listed in Table 28–2 (Halperin & Goldstein, 1988; Hudak et al., 1986; Romanski, 1986). Respiratory parameters of oxygenation, the partial pressure of oxygen (P_{O_2}) and oxygen saturation (O_2 Sat), are included in blood gas analysis, but their values do not directly affect blood pH. The usual sample for blood gas analysis is obtained from an artery and not exposed to air.

The P_{CO_2} is a measure of the tension exerted by dissolved CO_2 in the blood. It is proportional to the P_{CO_2} in alveolar air. To maintain a normal P_{CO_2}, the rate and depth of ventilation vary with changes in metabolism (Metheny, 1987).

There is a direct relationship between the degree of ventilation and the P_{CO_2} in the blood. If the P_{CO_2} is too high, it is a result of inadequate ventilation and removal of CO_2. This is called "hypoventilation." Increased concentrations of H_2CO_3 accumulate. If the condition persists, respiratory acidosis will develop. A P_{CO_2} that is lower than normal due to excessive ventilation (hyperventilation) causes a depletion of H_2CO_3. Prolonging this condition causes the development of respiratory alkalosis.

Blood pH is the negative log of H^+ concentration. pH is a measure of chemical balance and is a ratio of acids to bases. Low pH numbers (<7.36) represent an acid state, whereas higher pH numbers (>7.44) indicate an alkaline state in the ECF.

Metabolic parameters of acid–base balance include direct or indirect measures of bicarbonate concentration. Base excess and base deficit measure the level of all buffer systems of the blood: bicarbonate, hemoglobin, protein, and phosphate. The total quantity of buffer anions is normally 45 to 50 mEq/L, or twice that of bicarbonate. This gives a more complete picture of the metabolic causes of acid–base imbalances. A deficit of buffer base reflects metabolic acidosis, and a base excess reflects an excess of buffer base or a loss of metabolic acid, metabolic alkalosis (Corbett, 1987). Base deficit has been tested and found to be an accurate estimate of oxygen debt from lactic acidosis in trauma patients. A significant number of patients who were at high risk as defined by base deficit remained normotensive (hypotension is a late sign of inadequate perfusion). Base deficit was a significant predictor of mortality; those with a base deficit of ≤15 mmol/L had a 69.7% mortality (Rutherford et al., 1992).

VENOUS BLOOD PARAMETERS. If ABGs are not available, the concentration of bicarbonate can be determined by using an indirect measure, *CO_2 content*. The approximate bicarbonate ion concentration can be determined by subtracting 1 mEq/L from the CO_2 content, or using the formula:

$$\text{bicarbonate} = CO_2 \text{ content} - (0.03 \times P_{CO_2})$$

The normal values are 24 to 30 mEq/L (Goldberger, 1986; Metheny, 1987). Carbon dioxide content is normally 95% bicarbonate and 5% H_2CO_3. The CO_2 content will rise with a respiratory acidosis and a metabolic alkalosis owing to increased production of bicarbonate. It will drop with a metabolic acidosis or respiratory alkalosis because of depletion of bicarbonate.

ANION GAP. The anion gap is the difference between the total unmeasured anions in serum: phosphate, sulfates, ketones, and lactic acid. Normally these anions are less than 16 mEq/L of the total anion production. The anion gap can be determined by subtracting the sum of the measured anions (HCO_3^- and Cl^-) from the cation concentration (represented by Na^+ and K^+) (Metheny, 1987):

$$\text{Anion gap} = Na^+ + K^+ - [Cl^- + HCO_3^-] = 10\text{–}15 \text{ mEq/L}$$

Plasma proteins usually constitute most of the anion gap. When the gap exceeds the normal range, it is an important diagnostic tool. Figure 28–7 depicts the normal anion gap on the left, with the first bar representing cations and the second bar, anions. An increase in the gap (ratio of 1.0) occurs in metabolic acidosis with an increase in organic acids (starvation, dehydration, ketoacidosis, or lactic acidosis) because bicarbonate is decreased and replaced by an unmeasured anion. This is depicted in the middle set of bars. In metabolic acidosis from bicarbonate or chloride loss, the anion gap changes little, and has a ratio of less than 0.8, depicted in the set of bars on the right. A ratio much greater than 1.0 may indicate a superimposed metabolic alkalosis (Preuss, 1993).

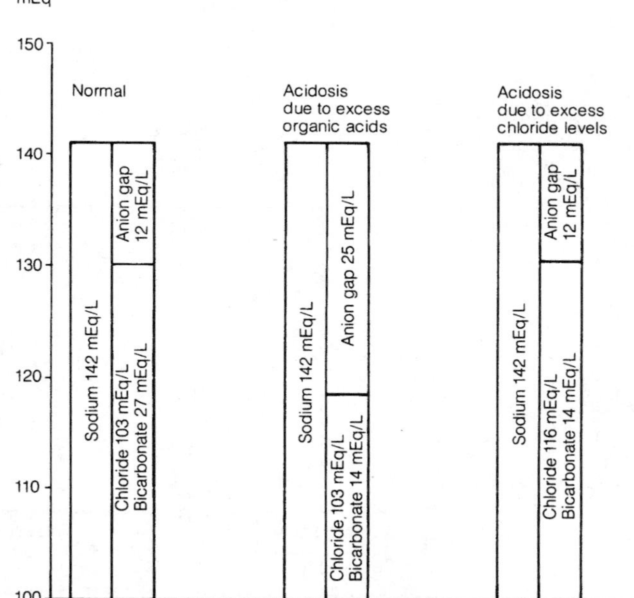

FIGURE 28–7. Comparisons of the anion gap in metabolic acidosis. (From Porth, C. M. [1990]. *Pathophysiology.* Philadelphia: J. B. Lippincott.)

ELECTROLYTE IMBALANCES

SODIUM. Hyponatremia, if associated with hypochloremia, may also be associated with *alkalosis* and a decreased potassium. Bicarbonate is reabsorbed with sodium instead of with chloride, and potassium is lost in exchange for sodium, which is conserved (Holloway, 1984).

POTASSIUM. Hyperkalemia is associated with *acidosis.* This can be precipitated by clinical situations such as hypotension, hemolysis, multiple transfusions, or ketoacidosis (Vaska, 1992). Because an elevated potassium concentration can quickly be fatal owing to its effect on cardiac muscle, an intracellular mechanism exists whereby potassium ions in the ECF can be exchanged for H^+ in the intracellular fluid. The inverse is also true. The kidneys exchange H^+ instead of potassium to retain sodium, resulting in increased potassium. Alkalosis is related to hypokalemia. For example, aggressive ventilation can cause respiratory alkalosis and hyperchloremic alkalosis, creating hypokalemia (Vaska, 1992).

CALCIUM. The ionization of calcium in the ECF increases with acidosis and decreases with alkalosis. Acidosis can mask the muscular signs of true hypocalcemia. With overcorrection of the acidosis, symptoms of tetany, carpopedal spasms, paresthesias, or convulsions may occur.

CHLORIDE. Chloride is primarily an extracellular ion. The concentration varies inversely with that of bicarbonate. A chloride shift occurs across the cellular membrane in exchange for bicarbonate during buffering. The renal reabsorption of chloride varies inversely with bicarbonate, and therefore a decreased chloride level is related to metabolic alkalosis and an

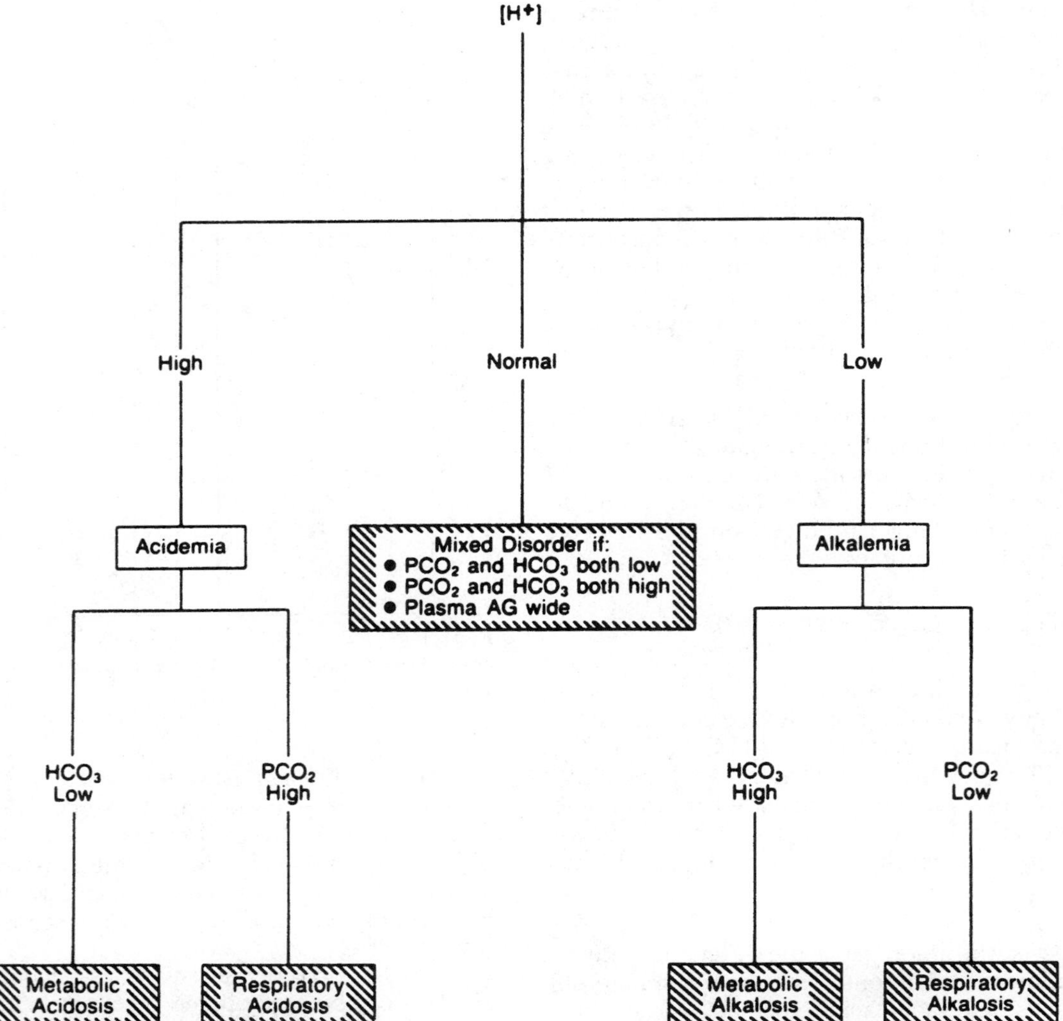

FIGURE 28–8. Systematic assessment of acid–base disorders. AG, anion gap. (From Halperin, M. L., & Goldstein, M. B. [1988]. *Fluid, electrolyte, and acid–base emergencies.* Philadelphia: W. B. Saunders.)

increased chloride concentration to metabolic acidosis. If a patient has lost considerable amounts of sodium and chloride, such as from gastrointestinal drainage or a low-salt diet without chloride replacement, metabolic alkalosis can develop.

Systematic Method of Assessing Acid–Base Balance and Imbalance

To assess acid–base disorders accurately, a systematic method needs to be used to evaluate laboratory values and clinical signs in the specific context of a clinical situation. Although the four basic alterations, respiratory and metabolic acidosis and respiratory and metabolic alkalosis, can occur independently, more frequently a combination of two or more can be observed. The disturbances may be antagonistic to or synergistic of each other. When attempting to interpret laboratory values, the following steps are helpful (Fig. 28–8):

1. First observe the arterial pH to determine whether an acidotic or an alkalotic state exists.
2. Look for the cause, which may be respiratory, metabolic, or both.
3. Look for the expected compensatory response.

Depending on the cause, selected laboratory values will be changed as shown in Table 28–3.

Factors to be considered in the clinical assessment of acid–base disorders include the following (Holloway, 1984):

1. Conditions in the patient's history predisposing to acid–base imbalance
   a. Respiratory: pneumonia, chronic obstructive pulmonary disease, use of a ventilator, extreme anxiety
   b. Renal/metabolic: diabetes mellitus, kidney disease, starvation states (NPO), loss of gastrointestinal fluids, liver disease, hypoxic states, heart disease

TABLE 28–3. **Changes in P_{CO_2}, pH, and Bicarbonate With Different Acid–Base Imbalances**

Acid–Base Imbalance	P_{CO_2}	pH	HCO_3^-/Base Excess
Respiratory acidosis	↑	↓	No change or ↑
Respiratory alkalosis	↓	↑	No change or ↓
Metabolic acidosis	No change or ↓	↓	↓
Metabolic alkalosis	No change or ↑	↑	↑

From Hurray, J., & Saver, C. (1992). Arterial blood gas interpretation: Improving perioperative skills. *Association of Operating Room Nurses Journal, 55,* 180–185.

2. Clinical signs and symptoms of acid–base imbalance
   a. Changes in cerebral status: confusion, coma (acidosis), dizziness, giddiness (alkalosis). Cerebral changes occur sooner with respiratory disorders than with metabolic states because CO_2 crosses the blood–brain barrier faster
   b. Changes in respiratory status (changes are more rapid if acute): hypoventilation or hyperventilation (rate and depth of pattern), restlessness or cyanosis (hypoxia), changes in pattern of respiration
   c. Changes in cardiovascular status: hypoxia or electrolyte imbalances (can lead to arrhythmias, angina, or shock); acute myocardial infarction (results in altered perfusion and lactic acidosis); acid–base imbalances (cause changes in the oxygen dissociation curve: alkalosis causes a shift to the left with decreased dissociation of oxygen from hemoglobin and hypoxia; acidosis causes a shift to the right, allowing oxygen to be released more readily from hemoglobin. Acidosis also results in a decreased response to catecholamines, decreased myocardial contractility, and decreased peripheral vasoconstriction)
   d. Changes in renal status: electrolytes, urine characteristics (color or ammonia odor), urine output

CLINICAL ALTERATIONS IN ACID–BASE BALANCE

Respiratory Acidosis

Respiratory acidosis is an accumulation of CO_2 and H_2CO_3 in the body as a result of hypoventilation, an increase in P_{CO_2} above 46 mm Hg, and a lowering of the pH below 7.34. Respiratory acidosis can result from breathing air with an abnormally high CO_2 content, as is done experimentally or during anesthesia administration. Respiratory acidosis more commonly occurs as a result of pulmonary, abdominal, or central nervous system alterations that interfere with respiration and the elimination of CO_2 (Kersten, 1989).

Respiratory acidosis may occur acutely or may develop chronically over a period of time. For a given increase in P_{CO_2}, there is a greater change in pH with an acute condition. In a chronic condition, a compensatory mechanism exists to increase retention of bicarbonate and enhance secretion of H^+ and chloride ions by the kidneys. For each 10 mm Hg increase in P_{CO_2}, there is a rise in bicarbonate by 35 mEq/L. However, this mechanism takes several days to compensate. Often, hypoxia occurs simultaneously with hypercapnia as a result of hypoventilation. The effect of hypoxia is much more life threatening than that of hypercapnia. The limit to life from hypercarbia is not known.

The pathophysiology of respiratory acidosis is a result of alveolar hypoventilation. This may occur if the tidal volume or respiratory rate is decreased (rapid, shallow breathing to compensate for metabolic alkalosis or central nervous system depression) or if there is obstruction of the diffusion or ventilation of CO_2 (Guyton, 1991).

Because retention of CO_2 interferes with the normal respiratory response to hypercapnia, the following compensatory mechanisms develop (Fig. 28–9): (1) the blood buffers react with H_2CO_3 to form more basic salts; (2) the kidneys increase the secretion and excretion of H^+, ammonium ions are formed and excreted, bicarbonate ions (along with sodium) are retained in exchange for chloride ions, and phosphate ions combine with hydrogen and are excreted; and (3) there is a shift in electrolytes: H^+ and sodium ions move intracellularly, raising the blood pH, in exchange for which potassium enters the ECF, causing a tendency toward hyperkalemia. With these compensatory changes, the bicarbonate concentration and pH rise toward normal, producing a partially compensated respiratory acidosis.

Many patients may actually *overcompensate.* The pH may rise over 7.46 as serum bicarbonate increases, a positive base excess is achieved, and total body potassium decreases as it is excreted in urine. As the P_{CO_2} returns to normal, the lost chloride ions must be replaced before bicarbonate can return to normal. Until this occurs, a metabolic alkalosis exists. Excessive loss of potassium ions due to use of diuretics will also potentiate alkalosis (Goldberger, 1986).

The causes and signs of respiratory acidosis are listed in Table 28–4 according to acute or chronic conditions. Acute conditions are often the result of a temporary and sudden problem occurring in a previously normal respiratory system. Chronic conditions usually result from prolonged disease states in which there is a gradual build-up in the CO_2 concentration. Pulmonary disorders include those in which gas exchange is limited by an abnormal alveolar–capillary membrane, airway obstruction, or inadequate lung tissue, such as pulmonary edema, bronchial obstruction, or emphysema. Neurologic disorders include problems with innervation of the lung (Guillain-Barré syndrome), or central nervous system depression (head injuries). Drugs that reduce respiratory drive, such as sedatives, analgesics, anesthesia, or alcohol, produce hypoventi-

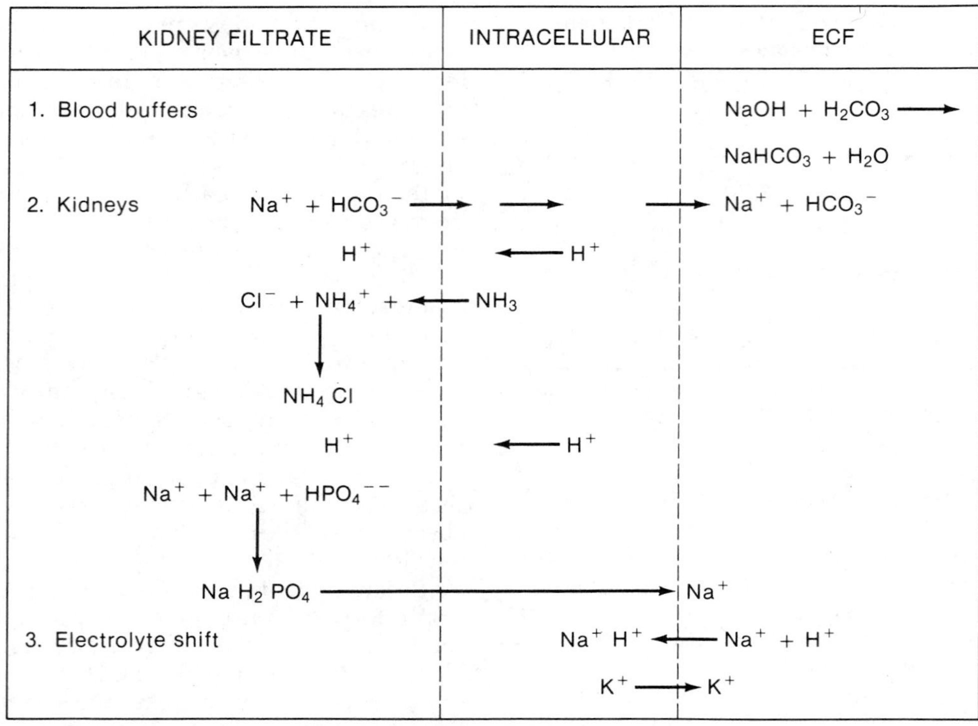

FIGURE 28–9. Compensatory mechanisms in respiratory acidosis.

lation. Abdominal distention may interfere with lung expansion and reduce ventilation, as in pregnancy, obesity, or ascites (Flomenbaum, 1984; Hudak, 1986; Metheny, 1987).

CLINICAL MANAGEMENT

Nursing diagnoses often associated with respiratory acidosis include the following:

1. Alteration in respiratory function: ineffective airway clearance and impaired gas exchange
2. Alteration in acid/base and electrolyte balance
3. Alteration in sensory-perceptual awareness

Implications for interventions revolve around improving ventilation, allowing for rest and comfort, and correcting fluid and electrolyte imbalances.

Improving Ventilation

1. Increase cough and deep breathing by use of unassisted blow bottles or incentive spirometry, postural drainage, or bronchodilators.
2. Humidify secretions mechanically and by encouraging fluid intake.
3. Treat documented infection with antibiotics.
4. Use mechanical ventilation if the patient is in respiratory failure.
5. Adjust nutritional therapy to minimize CO_2 production by giving calculated amounts of calories or carbohydrates according to energy expenditure (Ireton-Jones et al., 1993).

Providing Rest and Comfort

1. Plan activities to allow for rest periods between treatment or care.
2. Provide a position of comfort and support with a backrest, overbed table, or pillows. The use of a chair with arm supports instead of reclining in bed allows the patient to bend his or her legs for better support and chest expansion.
3. Help alleviate anxiety of patient by teaching slow breathing exercises when condition is stable. Use comfort touch measures and relaxation tapes or music.
4. Maintain a cool, low-humidity environment to promote ease of breathing; adjust humidity level to comfort of patient.

Correcting Fluid and Electrolyte Imbalances

1. Diuretics are often necessary to treat edema.
2. If the acidosis and hyperkalemia are corrected, potassium chloride may be given to replace these electrolytes in both the intracellular and extracellular fluids, respectively.
3. If a metabolic alkalosis persists after the respiratory acidosis has been corrected (e.g., as with mechani-

TABLE 28–4. **Respiratory Acidosis**

Cause	Signs	Laboratory Findings
Acute Respiratory Acidosis		
Congestive heart failure and pulmonary edema Massive pulmonary embolism Severe pulmonary infections Bronchial obstruction, atelectasis Aspiration Pneumothorax, open chest wound Hypoventilation with mechanical ventilation Severe abdominal distention Trendelenburg positions Neuromuscular: Guillain-Barré syndrome CNS depression: Head trauma, oversedation, anesthesia, high cord injury	Palpitations Warm, flushed skin Ventricular fibrillation may be first sign in anesthetized patient Fullness in head Mental cloudiness, dizziness Muscular twitching Convulsions Decreased LOC May be respiratory signs: rales, wheezing	pH = 7.4–7.0 P_{CO_2} = 45–120 mm Hg CO_2 content = upper normal or above HCO_3^- = normal or slightly elevated Base excess = upper normal Elevated serum K^+
Chronic Respiratory Acidosis		
Bronchiectasis Emphysema Pulmonary fibrosis Cystic fibrosis Pickwickian syndrome (obesity) Poliomyelitis Amyotrophic lateral sclerosis Myasthenia gravis Multiple sclerosis (advanced)	Hyperpnea (maybe), productive cough, thick-colored sputum Weakness Headache Stupor Irritability, poor judgment and coordination Symptoms of underlying disease: Dependent edema Weight gain Orthopnea Use of accessory muscles Pursed lip breathing	Changes in pH and CO_2 content are similar to above HCO_3^- > 26 mEq/liter pH rises to or near normal Decreased Cl^-, increased Na^+ and K^+

Abbreviations: CNS, central nervous system; LOC, level of consciousness.

cal ventilation), administration of calcium gluconate may be indicated to prevent tetany.

4. Acidosis *may* be treated occasionally with bicarbonate administration (York, 1987).

Respiratory Alkalosis

Respiratory alkalosis results from stimulation of the respiratory center with a resulting decrease of P_{CO_2} in the alveolar air due to hyperventilation. There is an increase in tidal volume or depth of respiration and increased alveolar ventilation; however, respiratory rate may or may not be increased. When this situation occurs, a large amount of CO_2 is eliminated from the body, increasing the acid–base ratio and the pH.

Compensatory processes can occur to restore the pH to within normal limits. The kidney excretes less acid in the urine by suppressing H^+ formation, ammonia production, and chloride excretion, and it conserves less bicarbonate. Potassium moves into the intracellular space in exchange for H^+ and sodium ions, which move extracellularly.

Respiratory alkalosis is the least common type of acid–base disturbance. Some of the *causes* are psychogenic in origin, such as pain or anxiety. Other causes are central nervous system stimulation due to head injury or lesions, early salicylate poisoning, alcohol intoxication, hepatic coma, paraldehyde ingestion, thyrotoxicosis, or fever. Cardiac or pulmonary causes often indicate an attempt to increase oxygenation during conditions of hypoxia, such as congestive heart failure or pulmonary embolism. Patients receiving excessive mechanical ventilation or those with respiratory acidosis who have been treated with a tracheostomy experience a sudden increase in alveolar ventilation. Exercise and change to a higher altitude may precipitate temporary hyperventilation.

The most characteristic *signs* of respiratory alkalosis occur in the "hyperventilation syndrome" associated with anxiety. The patient may complain of lightheadedness or dizziness; circumoral paresthesias; numbness of fingers and toes; sweating, sometimes profusely; palpitations, dyspnea, and a feeling of panic; and muscle cramps or tetany, such as carpopedal spasm. Other sensations in the chest or abdomen may be present. The condition is usually temporary and self-limited.

Laboratory findings are a low P_{CO_2}, an elevated blood pH, and a normal or low bicarbonate concentration. The base excess may be negative in a chronic state. It may be difficult to diagnose a primary respiratory alkalosis; however, tetany does not occur with the compensatory hyperventilation associated with a primary metabolic acidosis. The causes, signs and laboratory findings of a respiratory alkalosis are listed in Table 28–5.

CLINICAL MANAGEMENT

Nursing diagnoses often associated with respiratory alkalosis include the following:

1. Anxiety related to known or unknown factors
2. Alteration in respiratory function: ineffective breathing patterns
3. Alteration in fluid and electrolytes

Implications for nursing interventions revolve around relieving anxiety, correcting hypoxia, and increasing the partial pressure of carbon dioxide.

TABLE 28–5. **Respiratory Alkalosis**

Cause	Signs	Laboratory Findings
Hyperventilation, extreme anxiety Hypoxemia Excessive mechanical ventilation Hypermetabolic states: high fever, thyrotoxicosis Toxic stimulation of resp. center: central nervous system lesions, drug intoxication (early salicylate) Pregnancy Gram-negative septicemia	Dizziness Lightheadedness Numbness of fingers Tinnitus Palpitations Sweating Feeling of panic Muscle cramps Tetany Tightness of chest Dry mouth Blurred vision	pH > 7.45 P_{CO_2} < 35 mm Hg Low CO_2 content, normal or low HCO_3^- Base excess normal in acute and low in chronic Decreasing Ca^{2+} and K^+

Relieving Anxiety

1. Measures to relieve anxiety depend partly on the clinical state of the patient and the underlying psychological mechanisms of each person. A soothing but firm touch on the shoulders and a calm voice, or asking the person to concentrate on when to breathe may greatly facilitate a decrease in ventilatory excursion.

2. If the cause of the hyperventilation is primarily anxiety, use of psychotherapeutic interventions or minor tranquilizers may be indicated.

Correcting Hypoxia

If the patient has an underlying disease of cardiac or pulmonary origin and has some degree of hypoxia, increasing the partial pressure of oxygen should relieve the hyperventilation and respiratory alkalosis. Oxygen therapy, diuretics, cardiotonic drugs, antibiotics, pulmonary hygiene, or mechanical ventilation may be indicated.

Increasing Partial Pressure of Carbon Dioxide

1. Teaching an anxious patient to breathe into a paper bag held closely around the nose and mouth or using rebreathing oxygen masks acts to retain CO_2 momentarily, which the patient then inhales.

2. Adjusting the settings on a mechanical ventilator to decrease tidal volume or rate and perhaps adjusting the pulmonary end-expiratory pressure will help restore a normal P_{CO_2}.

Metabolic Acidosis

Metabolic acidosis results either from an excess of inorganic or organic acids not being freely excreted by the kidney or from a loss of base from the body. As a result, the normal bicarbonate–H_2CO_3 ratio decreases, and the pH falls to less than 7.35. The decreased pH stimulates the respiratory center, and an increased depth and rate of respirations occur in an attempt to lower the H_2CO_3 concentration and restore the pH to a normal range.

As in respiratory acidosis, there is a shift of electrolytes, with H^+ and sodium ions moving intracellularly in exchange for potassium. This creates a tendency toward hyperkalemia. Compensation by the pulmonary system is usually not complete. The renal mechanism involving sodium bicarbonate retention and acid excretion may occur depending on the cause and duration of the metabolic acidosis. The compensatory hyperventilation may persist after the acidotic state has been corrected, especially if sodium bicarbonate or lactate has been used.

Metabolic acidosis can result from a variety of conditions. An acid excess or an increase in the absolute amount of acid in the blood may occur with metabolic conditions that interfere with the normal catabolism of nutrients or with excess tissue breakdown. Accumulation of acid due to abnormal protein and fat metabolism occurs in diabetic acidosis and starvation. The unavailability of glucose for metabolism as a result of either lack of insulin or limited intake results in the mobilization of fats and protein to supply energy. Large amounts of nitrogenous wastes and ketones then accumulate in the blood, causing a metabolic acidosis. The body may be depleted of large amounts of sodium and potassium from a diuresis associated with hyperosmotic plasma.

Increased metabolic demands during surgical anesthesia, fever and infectious disease, and hyperthyroidism cause increased catabolism of all nutrients and acid accumulation. Anaerobic metabolism resulting from violent exercise, shock, acute myocardial infarction, sepsis, pancreatitis, acute leukemia, liver metastasis, and other conditions cause the accumulation of lactic and pyruvic acids. These conditions often occur acutely compared with diabetic or other metabolic conditions, which usually occur on a more chronic basis.

An excess of acids due to retention of those produced under normal conditions of metabolism occurs in renal disease and renal failure. The acidosis is related to several disturbances in renal function. Decreased glomerular filtration causes the retention of urea, creatinine, uric acid, and other nitrogenous products and organic acids. These react with serum bicarbonate, which is excreted as CO_2. Because the kidneys have a limited ability to reabsorb bicarbonate, the acid–base ratio falls, decreasing the pH. The tubules lose part of their ability to conserve water and secrete ammonia and sulfuric, phosphoric, and other inorganic acids. The net effect is a retention of metabolic acids and a decrease in base excess. Due to the chronic nature of renal disease, respiratory compensation usually does not occur until the bicarbonate concentration falls below 10 mEq/liter.

An acute metabolic acidosis can result from *excessive intake* of oral or parenteral acids, such as administration of intravenous fluids containing chloride ions such as hypertonic saline, when given in excessive amounts. The sodium is converted to sodium bicarbonate, and chloride is retained with H^+. Medications such as ammonium chloride, calcium chloride, or CA inhibitors can result in metabolic acidosis, and their administration needs careful monitoring.

The more common cause is a drug overdose: salicylic acid, methanol, or ethylene glycol (antifreeze) poisoning. Methanol breaks down into formic acid; ethylene glycol breaks down into oxalic acid, which crystallizes in the kidney and causes acute renal failure. Salicylic acid poisoning causes two types of acid–base disturbance: a primary respiratory alkalosis and, within 8 hours, a primary metabolic acidosis. Salicylate disturbs carbohydrate metabolism and causes a depletion of liver glycogen, resulting in an accumulation of ketone bodies and lactic and pyruvic acids. When respiratory alkalosis develops, the renal compensatory mechanism causes an excretion of bicarbonate, producing a compensatory metabolic acidosis.

Metabolic acidosis can also result from excessive loss of alkaline body fluids such as intestinal secretions, as with severe diarrhea or a small bowel or biliary fistula. When diarrhea occurs, large amounts of bicarbonate are secreted into the intestinal tract and excreted, lowering the acid–base ratio and the pH. An excess accumulation of H^+ in the serum also contributes to metabolic acidosis.

Two types of metabolic acidosis can occur: (1) an excess fixed acid accumulation or an increased unmeasured anion gap; or (2) a normal anion gap with a net loss of bicarbonate and its replacement in the ECF by chloride (hyperchloremic metabolic acidosis). Table 28–6 lists conditions causing each type of metabolic acidosis.

TABLE 28–6. **Classification of Metabolic Acidosis According to Type**

Elevated Anion Gap

Chronic renal failure
Lactic acidosis
Diabetic ketoacidosis
Starvation
Ingestions and intoxications (methanol, late salicylate poisoning, ethylene glycol)
Alcoholic ketolactic acidosis

Hyperchloremic Metabolic Acidosis

Excessive gain of chloride (large quantities of normal saline, ammonium chloride, hyperalimentation)
Renal tubular acidosis
Administration of carbonic anhydrase inhibitors (Diamox)
Gastrointestinal bicarbonate loss: diarrhea, ureterosigmoidostomy, or fistulas
Hypoaldosteronism and Addison's disease
Renal tubulointestinal diseases: obstruction, infection, sickle cell disease

Data from Metheny, N. M. (1987). *Fluid and electrolyte balance.* Philadelphia: J. B. Lippincott; Preuss, H. (1993). Fundamentals of clinical acid–base evaluation. *Clinics in Laboratory Medicine, 13,* 103–116; Puschett, J. B., & Piraino, B. (1985). Disorders of acid–base balance. In J. B. Puschett & A. Greenberg (Eds.), *Disorders of fluid and electrolyte balance.* New York: Churchill-Livingstone.

TABLE 28–7. **Metabolic Acidosis**

Cause	Signs	Laboratory Findings
Increase in acid retention or production: renal failure, ketoacidosis, acute myocardial infarction, starvation, salicylate intoxication, anaerobic metabolism	Headache Confusion Kussmaul respirations Weakness Nausea Stupor	pH < 7.35 $HCO_3^- < 22$ mEq/liter $P_{CO_2} < 35$ mm Hg Negative base excess Increased K^+
Hyperchloremia: prolonged diarrhea, intestinal fistulas, ureterosigmoidostomy, renal tubular acidosis	Delirium Arrhythmias Warm, flushed skin	Decreased Ca^{2+} in some

Signs of metabolic acidosis may not become readily apparent until the acidosis becomes more advanced. A history of one of the precipitating conditions suggests a diagnosis of metabolic acidosis. When the CO_2 content falls to 18 mEq/liter, the patient may complain of weakness, malaise, dull headache, nausea, vomiting, and abdominal pain. Kussmaul respirations, especially very deep respirations as opposed to a rapid rate, usually develop when the pH is 7.2 or lower. Vasodilation with a flushed face and a bounding pulse may be seen. Other signs depend on the underlying clinical process. Patients with diabetes and renal disease develop a fruity odor on the breath and may show signs of severe water and sodium loss due to diuresis.

The diagnosis is made with laboratory evaluation of pH, HCO_3^-, and P_{CO_2}. If the condition is uncompensated, the pH is low and the P_{CO_2} is normal. The bicarbonate is low, and there is a base deficit. When compensation occurs, because this is a simple disturbance, a compensatory decrease in P_{CO_2} would occur, with the pH rising slightly (see Table 28–2). The second step in the diagnosis is to determine whether an excess anionic gap exists (see Fig. 28–7). The serum bicarbonate level will vary depending on the underlying condition, but usually it remains low. Chloride and potassium levels are often elevated, the potassium producing electrocardiographic changes of a spiked T wave and prolonged QRS complex. A normal or low potassium value is a sign of total body fluid and potassium depletion. The causes and signs of metabolic acidosis are listed in Table 28–7 (Alexander, 1986; Metheny, 1987; Preuss, 1993; Thomas & Dodhia, 1991).

CLINICAL MANAGEMENT

Nursing diagnoses associated with metabolic acidosis are often related to the cause of the disorder or to clinical or laboratory signs. They may include the following:

1. Alteration in nutrition: more or less than body requirements

2. Alteration in electrolytes: potassium excess, sodium deficit
3. Alteration in acid–base: H^+ excess or base deficit
4. Fluid volume excess or deficit: altered elimination
5. Alteration in cardiac output: decreased
6. Potential for injury related to alterations in sensory-perceptual awareness

Implications for nursing interventions revolve around stopping the metabolic disturbance, restoring the electrolytes that have been lost, preventing any further catabolism, and supporting respiration.

Stopping the Metabolic Process and Restoring Electrolytes

1. If the metabolic acidosis results from chloride excess, the chloride salt should be stopped immediately; the kidneys usually can eliminate the excess.

2. If the problem is diabetes, treating the patient with insulin and replacing the sodium, potassium, and water lost in diuresis should reverse the diabetic acidosis. Long-term treatment must be aimed at controlling the diabetes with a balanced dietary, medication, and activity program (Butts, 1987).

3. In patients with chronic renal failure, the acidosis cannot be reversed without dialysis. However, before they need dialysis, patients are often dehydrated. Replacing lost sodium and water will facilitate any remaining renal function. In patients with acute renal failure, water, sodium, and potassium need to be restricted until kidney function returns. Elevations of potassium need immediate treatment because they may be life threatening (Chambers, 1987).

4. In salicylate poisoning, the patient may be supported by dialysis. Sodium bicarbonate may be given; however, it is dangerous because it may cause a metabolic alkalosis with a sodium overload.

5. Lactic acidosis can be treated with adequate oxygenation, optimal volume loading, appropriate monitoring of catecholamine therapy, and limiting the use of sodium bicarbonate for the treatment of hyperkalemia (Grillo & Gonzales, 1993; Nimmo et al., 1991).

Preventing Catabolism

Preventing further catabolism is also necessary. Any additional stress such as invasive lines or wounds that would contribute to tissue trauma or breakdown should be avoided. Preventing the occurrence of or treating existing infection is a major factor in reducing metabolic need. Adequate intake of essential nutrients either orally or by means of total parenteral nutrition will facilitate maintenance of a positive nitrogen balance, reduce excess acid production, and help in building new tissue.

Supporting Respiration

Support respiration by maintaining a patent airway, using positioning to facilitate breathing, and giving oxygen or using mechanical ventilation as necessary. Because hyperventilation is the primary respiratory compensation, this mechanism should be supported while treatment is aimed at correcting the underlying problem. Replacement of fluids and electrolytes will help to rehydrate the patient and loosen respiratory secretions. Mechanical ventilation may be used when the blood pH is very low or when the patient is in respiratory failure.

Metabolic Alkalosis

Metabolic alkalosis results from an accumulation of excess base (bicarbonate) or a loss of H^+ from the body. When H^+ are lost, the bicarbonate–H_2CO_3 ratio increases, and the serum pH rises above 7.46. The kidneys try to compensate by excreting excess bicarbonate and retaining H^+. However, this process seldom fully corrects the serum pH because it is antagonistic to the normal regulatory mechanisms. It is often secondary to volume or chloride ion depletion from diuretic therapy (Preuss, 1993).

Metabolic alkalosis can occur in the following types of conditions: oral or parenteral intake of excessive base, such as sodium bicarbonate; loss of acid from the body through the gastrointestinal tract or in the urine; and electrolyte abnormalities, such as loss of potassium, chloride, or calcium. The expected respiratory compensation of hypoventilation to retain CO_2 and elevate pH is not very efficient in correcting alkalosis. The P_{CO_2} will not exceed 60 mm Hg in patients with metabolic alkalosis, who are breathing room air, because a decreased oxygen saturation and hypoxia would result. The kidneys attempt to compensate by excreting large amounts of bicarbonate in the urine. In prolonged metabolic alkalosis, this renal compensatory mechanism often is impaired due to enhanced bicarbonate reabsorption, decreased filtration if the person is in renal failure, or a low serum potassium.

The pathophysiologic state of metabolic alkalosis is a result of excess concentrations of bicarbonate in the ECF. For instance, when *excessive amounts of base,* such as milk or absorbable alkali salts, are ingested, they combine with the hydrochloric acid of the gastric juice, the H^+ are neutralized, and CO_2 is formed and eliminated, leaving excessive concentrations of bicarbonate and an elevated pH.

When *H^+ are lost* from the gastrointestinal tract, as in vomiting, the base that has been absorbed cannot be neutralized, causing an alteration in the acid–base ratio and an increase in pH. Acids can also be lost through excessive use of diuretics. The ability of the distal tubules to reabsorb sodium and especially chloride ions is reduced with the use of diuretics. Along with the loss of these ions, potassium and ammonium ions are excreted. The excretion of each ammonium ion is associated with the loss of an H^+. When large amounts of salt and water are excreted as a result of diuretic use, the ECF becomes more concentrated around a constant amount of bicarbonate, resulting in a contraction alkalosis.

The reduction of potassium ions with gastrointestinal or renal fluid losses aggravates a metabolic alkalotic state. Potassium loss causes a metabolic alkalosis and vice versa. When potassium is lost from the intracellular fluid, sodium ions and H^+ move into the cells, causing a decreased concentration of hydrogen in the ECF. A similar loss of potassium occurs in the renal tubular cells. Potassium is not available to combine with H^+, and they are lost in the urine, causing an increase in pH (Metheny, 1987).

In addition to losses through the kidneys with diuretics or renal tubular acidosis, many other conditions of metabolic alkalosis are associated with the loss of potassium. Loss of potassium occurs through the gastrointestinal tract from vomiting, gastric suction, intestinal fistulas, or diarrhea. Gastric secretions contain approximately 10 times the amount of potassium in the serum and twice the amount in the intestine. Cirrhosis of the liver and non–insulin-secreting tumors of the pancreas are associated with loss of potassium ions and metabolic alkalosis. Potassium is lost in malnourished or semistarved patients due to a very low intake despite continued urinary excretion. Hypersecretion of adrenal cortical hormones, as in Cushing syndrome or hyperaldosteronism, results in retention of sodium and the secretion of potassium. Certain antibiotics, such as sodium penicillin and amphotericin B, cause potassium loss through the kidneys (Adinaro, 1987).

Signs of metabolic alkalosis may be difficult to differentiate from the signs of the associated disease processes. After ingestion of large amounts of absorbable antacid medication over a long time, symptoms of anorexia, nausea, and painless vomiting may occur. Confusion and mental "unreliability" may develop, followed by drowsiness and coma. Another symptom is tetany. In alkalosis, more calcium is bound to protein, producing a low serum calcium concentration. Tetany does not occur in an acidotic state or with hypokalemia. Electrocardiographic changes can occur in alkalosis and hypokalemia. Sinus tachycardia may be apparent, with a prolonged Q–T interval and the T wave approaching or merging with the P wave. The causes and signs of metabolic alkalosis are listed in Table 28–8.

TABLE 28–8. **Metabolic Alkalosis**

Cause	Signs	Laboratory Findings
Acute loss of H^+: vomiting, nasogastric suction Potassium or chloride loss: diuretics, corticosteroids, liver disease Addition of base: excess use of bicarbonate, lactate administration in dialysis	Tingling of fingers and toes Dizziness Nausea Vomiting Lethargy Coma Paralytic ileus Disorientation Convulsions Weakness Muscle cramps Tetany Depressed respirations Electrocardiographic changes	pH > 7.45 HCO_3^- > 0.26 mEq/liter Positive base excess P_{CO_2} normal or high K^+ normal or low, Ca^{2+} low Urinary Cl^- low with vomiting, higher with K^+ loss

CLINICAL MANAGEMENT

Nursing diagnoses often associated with metabolic alkalosis include the following:

1. Fluid volume deficit: gastrointestinal or renal
2. Alteration in electrolyte balance: potassium, calcium, chloride
3. Alteration in acid–base balance
4. Alteration in thought processes
5. Potential for injury related to neuromuscular irritability

Implications for nursing interventions revolve around restoring fluid and electrolyte balance and limiting alkaline intake.

Restoring Fluid and Electrolyte Balance

1. Restore fluid volume and electrolyte balance either orally or parenterally to correct the cause of the alkalosis. Observe for vomiting, diarrhea, or excess use of diuretics. Electrolytes such as chloride and potassium need to be replaced if diuretics are used or gastrointestinal fluid losses have occurred. Records of intake and output and laboratory results should be noted frequently.

2. Tetany can be corrected either by lowering the pH or raising the serum calcium. A low potassium should be treated only if a low serum calcium is increased at the same time. Correcting the alkalosis will allow the serum calcium to return to normal.

Limiting Alkaline Intake

1. Alkaline antacids should be administered cautiously to patients who have gastric ulcers or a metabolic acidosis.

2. Occasionally, acidifying agents, such as CA inhibitors (Diamox; Lederle Laboratories, Pearl River, NY), are used to treat alkalosis such as that produced from prolonged diuretic use. They should be used with caution.

Mixed Acid–Base Disorders

Frequently, patients have more than one acid–base imbalance due to multiple system disease, normal compensatory mechanisms, or various therapies. A mixed disorder can make the patient's condition better or worse. For instance, the following combinations create a more *abnormal serum pH:* (1) respiratory and metabolic acidosis (e.g., acute pulmonary edema and cardiopulmonary arrest); (2) both increased anionic gap and hyperchloremic metabolic acidosis (e.g., diabetic ketoacidosis and excessive intake of chloride from IV fluid); or (3) both metabolic and respiratory alkalosis (e.g., a patient with cirrhosis who is volume- and chloride-depleted from diuretics.

On the other hand, the following combinations result in an *improved serum pH:* (1) metabolic alkalosis and respiratory acidosis (e.g., a patient with chronic obstructive pulmonary disease who is volume-depleted from diuretics; (2) metabolic acidosis and respiratory alkalosis (e.g., a patient with end-stage renal disease [ESRD] who is on a ventilator); or (3) metabolic acidosis and metabolic alkalosis (e.g., a patient with ESRD with excessive vomiting).

Any of the following conditions would make one suspect that *two or more acid–base disturbances* are present: (1) the compensatory response is less or greater than expected by a nomogram or titration table; (2) the serum pH is normal but abnormal values of HCO_3^- or P_{CO_2} are present; (3) all acid–base parameters are normal but there is an excessive anionic gap; or (4) the compensatory response (increased HCO_3^-) for an event (respiratory acidosis) is greater than 3 to 4 mmol/L beyond expected (Preuss, 1993).

SUMMARY

Maintaining a serum pH within the normal range is essential to life. Critically ill patients often have multiple conditions predisposing them to one or more acid–base imbalances. The critical care nurse can discover changes early through careful history taking and accurate interpretation of clinical assessment findings and laboratory acid–base parameters. Only ABGs will specifically indicate serum pH and respiratory retention of CO_2. ABGs will also yield bicarbonate levels and base excess or deficit. Venous blood samples will indicate renal excretion of bicarbonate and electrolytes for anion gap assessment. Once a respiratory or metabolic disturbance is detected, one can assess if the compensatory responses are expected and whether a single or mixed disorder exists. The presence of an excess anion gap or elevated potassium or chloride ions may be a clue to the cause of the acid–base imbalance. Early detection is essential if appropriate preventive interventions are to be initiated.

REFERENCES

Adinaro, D. (1987). Liver failure and pancreatitis: Fluid and electrolyte concerns. *Nursing Clinics of North America, 22,* 843–851.

Alexander, E. (1986). Metabolic acidosis: Recognition and etiologic diagnosis. *Hospital Practice, 21*(1), 100E–100R.

Appel, G. B., & Chase, H. S. (1986). Diagnosis and treatment of acid–base disorders. In J. Askanazi, P. M. Starker, & C. Weissman (Eds.), *Fluid and electrolyte management in critical care.* Boston: Butterworth.

Butts, D. (1987). Fluid and electrolyte disorders associated with diabetic ketoacidosis and hyperglycemic hyperosmolar nonketotic coma. *Nursing Clinics of North America, 22,* 827–836.

Chambers, J. K. (1987). Fluid and electrolyte problems in renal and urologic disorders. *Nursing Clinics of North America, 22,* 815–825.

Corbett, J. V. (1987). *Laboratory tests and diagnostic procedures with nursing diagnoses* (2nd ed.). Norwalk, CT: Appleton & Lange.

Flomenbaum, N. (1984). Acid–base disturbances. *Emergency Medicine, 16,* 59–89.

Goldberger, E. (1986). *A primer of water, electrolyte and acid–base syndromes* (7th ed.). Philadelphia: Lea & Febiger.

Grillo, J., & Gonzales, E. (1993). Changes in the pharmacotherapy of CPR. *Heart and Lung, 22,* 548–553.

Guyton, A. C. (1987). *Human physiology and mechanisms of disease* (4th ed.). Philadelphia: W. B. Saunders.

Guyton, A. C. (1991). *Textbook of medical physiology* (8th ed.). Philadelphia: W. B. Saunders.

Halperin, M. L., & Goldstein, M. B. (1988). *Fluid, electrolyte, and acid–base emergencies.* Philadelphia: W. B. Saunders.

Holloway, N. M. (1984). *Nursing the critically ill adult* (2nd ed.). Menlo Park, CA: Addison-Wesley.

Hudak, C. M., Gallo, B. M., & Lohr, T. (1986). *Critical care nursing* (4th ed.). Philadelphia: J. B. Lippincott.

Ireton-Jones, C., Borman, K., & Turner, W. (1993). Nutrition considerations in the management of ventilator-dependent patients. *Nutrition in Clinical Practice, 8*(2), 60–64.

Kersten, L. D. (1989). *Comprehensive respiratory nursing: A decision-making approach.* Philadelphia: W. B. Saunders.

McCance, K., & Heuther, S. (1994). The biologic basis for disease in adults and children. *Pathophysiology* (2nd ed.). St. Louis: C. V. Mosby.

McLean, F. C. (1938). Application of the law of chemical equilibrium (Law of Mass Action) to biological problems. *Physiological Review, 18,* 495–523.

Metheny, N. M. (1987). *Fluid and electrolyte balance.* Philadelphia: J. B. Lippincott.

Nimmo, C., Grant, J., & Mackenzie, S. (1991). Lactate and acid base changes in the critically ill. *Postgraduate Medicine Journal, 67*(Suppl 1), 556–561.

Porth, C. M. (1990). *Pathophysiology* (3rd ed.). Philadelphia: J. B. Lippincott.

Preuss, H. (1993). Fundamentals of clinical acid–base evaluation. *Clinics in Laboratory Medicine, 13,* 103–116.

Puschett, J. B., & Piraino, B. (1985). Disorders of acid–base balance. In J. B. Puschett & A. Greenberg (Eds.), *Disorders of fluid and electrolyte balance.* New York: Churchill-Livingstone.

Romanski, S. D. (1986). Interpreting ABG's in four easy steps. *Nursing 86, 16*(9), 27–32.

Rutherford, E., Morris, J., Reed, G., & Hall, K. (1992). Base deficit stratifies mortality and determines therapy. *Journal of Trauma, 33,* 417–423.

Shapiro, B. A., Harrison, R. A., & Walton, J. R. (1982). *Clinical application of blood gases* (3rd ed.). Chicago: Year Book.

Thomas, C., & Dodhia, N. (1991). Common emergencies in cancer medicine: Metabolic syndromes. *Journal of the American Medical Association, 83,* 809–818.

Vaska, P. (1992). Fluid and electrolyte imbalances after cardiac surgery. *AACN Clinical Issues in Critical Care, 3,* 664–671.

York, K. (1987). The lung and fluid–electrolyte and acid–base imbalances. *Nursing Clinics of North America, 22,* 805–814.

Patients With Chronic Obstructive Pulmonary Diseases

Frederick J. Tasota

Although several other terms are often used synonymously with *chronic obstructive pulmonary disease* (COPD), including chronic airflow obstruction and chronic obstructive lung disease. However, COPD remains the most frequently used clinical terminology to describe chronic diseases associated with limitation to airflow within the lungs. This disease alters the anatomy and physiology in varying degrees in three different areas of the lung: the large airways, peripheral airways, and lung parenchyma.

The term COPD initially referred to a group of chronic diseases characterized by diffuse obstruction of airflow. At that time, subcategories of the disease were delineated and included chronic bronchitis, emphysema, and asthma. COPD is now used to describe a process characterized by the presence of either chronic bronchitis, emphysema, or both that leads to the development of airflow obstruction. However, that obstruction need not be present at all times, and it may be potentially reversible in part (Snider, 1989). This more current definition excludes asthmatic patients with airflow obstruction that is completely reversible in nature, but includes those with overlapping components of the various disease entities (Fig. 29–1). In this chapter, COPD (chronic bronchitis and emphysema) is discussed separately from asthma. Cystic fibrosis and bronchiectasis are also categorized as obstructive diseases, but are seen more frequently in the younger age group and will not be discussed in this chapter.

The usual clinical findings indicative of chronic obstructive diseases include:

1. Significant and progressive reduction in expiratory airflow as measured by the forced expiratory volume in 1 second (FEV_1) (Fig. 29–2)
2. Exertional dyspnea
3. Chronic cough and sputum production

Although clinical findings are similar, the consequences and severity of COPD vary over time. "The bottom line becomes the degree of air flow obstruction (or limitation) as measured by FEV_1, the age of the patient when the abnormality is found, the degree of reversibility, and the rate of change of the FEV_1 over time" (Hodgkin & Petty, 1987, p. 5).

EPIDEMIOLOGY

It is estimated that 14.6 million Americans are afflicted with some degree of COPD, 41% more people than a decade ago. Emphysema sufferers number approximately 2 million, whereas chronic bronchitis affects 12.6 million (American Lung Association, 1993). Deaths attributed to this ailment have risen to 90,650 (1991), making it the fourth leading cause of death in the United States, up from fifth in previous years. The death rate for COPD per 100,000 individuals is five times greater today than in 1950 (National Center for Health Statistics, 1993b).

Chronic bronchitis is more frequently found in women, whereas emphysema is more likely to occur in the male population. Morbidity and mortality are related to socioeconomic status, with blue collar workers and those with fewer years of formal education having higher rates. COPD is also seen more frequently in offspring of affected parents as well as in siblings. Several studies indicate correlations between COPD and both genetics and the environment.

Morbidity and mortality statistics portray only a portion of the total picture. Approximately 45% of all people with COPD have some restrictions on their activity level (Weaver & Narsavage, 1992). Disability due to COPD is second only to heart disease in people older than the age of 40 years (MacDonnell et al., 1987). Total costs to the nation amounted to greater than $12 billion in 1988—$5.5 billion in direct health care costs and an additional $6.5 billion in indirect costs (American Lung Association, 1993). The numbers of people diagnosed, treated, and dying from COPD challenge health care providers to deliver high-quality care in the most cost-efficient fashion. As such, critical care

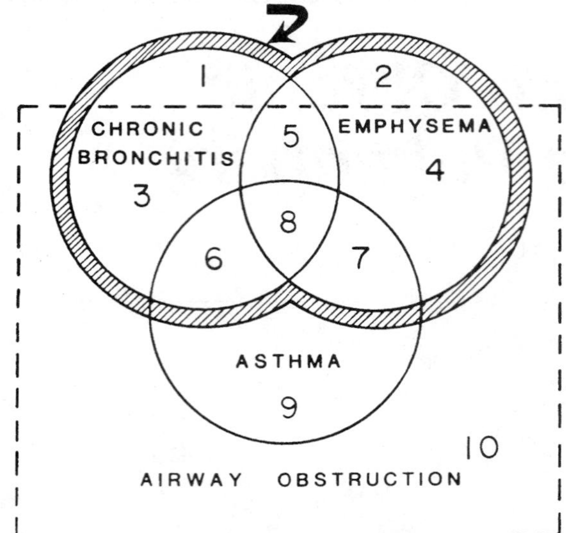

FIGURE 29–1. Scheme of chronic obstructive pulmonary disease. A nonproportional Venn diagram shows subsets of patients with chronic bronchitis, emphysema, and asthma in three overlapping circles. Subsets of patients lying within the rectangle have airways obstruction. Patients with asthma, Subset 9, are defined as having completely reversible airways obstruction and lie entirely within the rectangle. Patients in Subsets 6, 7, and 8 have reversible airways obstruction with chronic productive cough or emphysema; it may be difficult to be certain whether patients in these subsets have underlying asthma or whether they have bronchial hyperreactivity as a complication of chronic bronchitis or emphysema. Patients in Subset 3 have chronic bronchitis with airways obstruction but no emphysema. Patients with emphysema alone fall into Subset 4. Most patients who require medical care for their disease fall into Subsets 5 and 8. Patients in Subsets 1 and 2 do not have airways obstruction as determined by the FEV_1, but have clinical or radiographic features of chronic bronchitis or emphysema, respectively. Patient Subsets 1 to 8 are included within the area outlined by the shaded band that denotes COPD. (Reprinted from Snider, G. L. [1988]. Chronic bronchitis and emphysema. In J. F. Murray & J. A. Nadel [Eds.], Textbook of respiratory medicine [Chapter 44]. Philadelphia: W. B. Saunders.)

nurses will play an ever-increasing role in the coordination and delivery of care for this group of patients.

ETIOLOGY

Approximately 90% of COPD is attributable to cigarette smoke. However, it remains unanswered as to how cigarette smoke actually causes COPD. Although cigarette smoking as a cause of COPD is well established, not all smokers suffer the same effects with regard to frequency or severity of illness. Cigarettes affect the pattern of COPD development depending on differences in cigarette composition, tar and nicotine contents, filters, number of cigarettes smoked, and length of time the person smoked. It is also important to note that clinically significant COPD develops in only 15% of smokers (Snider, 1989).

Fortunately, it appears clear that cessation of smoking is beneficial for the person with COPD. Smoking cessation results in a decrease in symptoms that include chronic cough, sputum production, dyspnea, and wheezing. It also has an impact on the frequency of pulmonary infections, potential improvement in objective measures of pulmonary function, possible arresting of the processes that lead to COPD, and an improvement in the risk of mortality related to the disease process. If permanent lung damage and overt symptoms of COPD are evident, lost function is less likely to return after smoking cessation. Long-term outcomes for the person are influenced by the age at which the person stopped smoking, the amount he or she smoked, and the stage of the disease at the time of smoking cessation (Fiore et al., 1993).

Although it is quite evident that there is a direct link between cigarette smoking and the development of COPD, there are unanswered questions about symptoms resulting from involuntary exposure to smoking or "secondhand smoke." With increasing amounts of information indicating that cigarette smoke not only affects the person smoking, but those exposed to the smoke in the environment, restrictions on smoking are becoming increasingly prevalent. However, a direct link between the development of COPD from exposure to "secondhand" cigarette smoke is not yet confirmed.

Episodes of severe air pollution have been associated with sudden increases in morbidity and mortality, especially among people with heart or lung disease. Yet, Pope and Kanner (1993) and other investigators have concluded that there are, for the most part, only transient, small, negative effects on pulmonary function from exposure to particulate air pollution. Although healthy individuals are affected by exposure to inhaled irritants such as sulfur dioxide

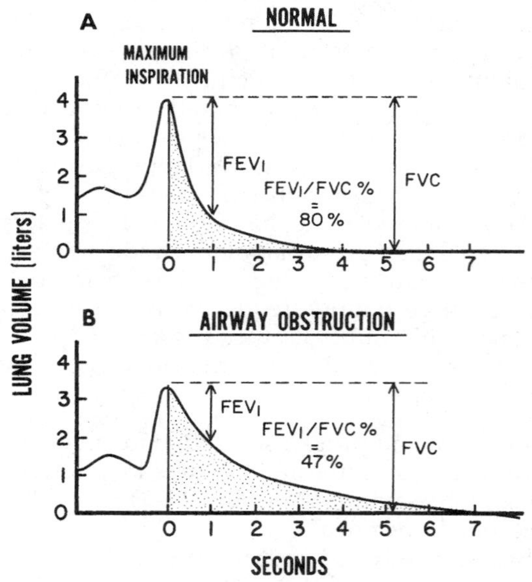

FIGURE 29–2. Recordings during a forced vital capacity maneuver. *A,* In the normal person. *B,* In the person with airway obstruction. *Abbreviations:* FEV_1, forced expiratory volume in 1 second; FVC, forced vital capacity. (From Guyton, A. C. [1986]. *Textbook of medical physiology* [7th ed., p. 477]. Philadelphia: W. B. Saunders.)

and ozone, those with chronic respiratory disease are affected the most. Indoor pollution may be a factor in the development of respiratory problems in some people, but appears to aggravate rather than cause COPD.

Certain occupations place people at higher risk for the development of COPD. People exposed to coal dust, potash, metal molds, stone, glass, clay products, cotton or grain dust, and asbestos are included. Firefighters are also at increased risk (Owens, 1993).

Genetic influences linked to the development of COPD are evident in two distinct areas. One involves a familial predisposition due to bronchial hyperreactivity or hypersensitivity, while the other is related to a specific enzyme-deficiency.

The role of infection as an etiologic factor in the development of COPD (particularly chronic bronchitis) is unproven and controversial despite extensive study in this area. Viral upper respiratory infections in children may precipitate COPD in adult life. Potential contributors to the clinical progression of the disease include chronic colonization/infection and recurrent infectious exacerbations that accelerate airway injury (Murphy & Sethi, 1992).

In 1955, Dornhorst coined the phrases "blue bloater" to characterize chronic bronchitics and "pink puffer" to typify the person with emphysema. Few present in one of these classic fashions because most people with COPD are a combination of the two. However, the differentiation provides the basis for a clinical diagnosis and management. Robin and O'Neill (1963) called the bronchitic patient the "quitter" and the patient with emphysema the "fighter." This distinction emphasizes that the bronchitic patient usually maintains low minute volumes and manifests arterial hypoxemia and hypercapnia, whereas the emphysema patient "fights," thus maintaining a higher minute ventilation and normal arterial blood gases. Table 29–1 highlights these differences between the two.

The remainder of this chapter covers the specific diseases of chronic bronchitis and emphysema. Asthma, with its increased potential for reversibility, is covered separately. Although these diseases are covered separately, they remain closely linked in most patients, and it is not uncommon for patients to exhibit varying degrees of symptomatology related to all of them.

TABLE 29–1. **Clinical Distinctions Between Emphysema and Chronic Bronchitis Pathophysiology**

Feature	Type A	Type B
Commonly used name	Pink puffer	Blue bloater
Disease association	Predominant emphysema	Predominant bronchitis
Major symptom	Dyspnea	Cough and sputum
Appearance	Thin, wasted, not cyanotic	Obese, cyanotic
P_{O_2}	↓	↓↓
P_{CO_2}	Normal or ↓	Normal or ↑
Elastic recoil of lung	↓	Normal
Diffusing capacity	↓	Normal
Hematocrit	Normal	Often ↑
Cor pulmonale	Infrequent	Common

From Weinberger, S. (1992). *Principles of pulmonary medicine* (2nd ed.). Philadelphia: W. B. Saunders.

CHRONIC BRONCHITIS

The commonly accepted definition for chronic bronchitis describes airway changes which result in the symptoms of chronic cough and sputum production. A specific criterion is that a productive cough is present for at least 3 consecutive months in 2 successive years in the absence of other potential causes of a chronic productive cough (i.e., tuberculosis, lung tumor, and congestive heart failure).

Etiology

Cigarette smoking is undeniably the single most important etiologic factor. There is a strong correlation among severity of the illness with the amount of cigarettes smoked and the duration of smoking. The prevalence of chronic bronchitis rises as the lifetime consumption of cigarettes increases beyond approximately 8 pack years of exposure (calculated by the number of packs/day times the number of years smoked) (Tisi, 1983).

The cigarette smoking male has typified the individual with chronic bronchitis. However, as the population of women that have smoked for a number of years has increased, so has the incidence of chronic bronchitis among this group. In 1992, U.S. Department of Health and Human Services statistics show an incidence of chronic bronchitis that is considerably greater for women than men, particularly in the 45- to 64-year-old age category (71.9 per 1,000 vs. 43.6 per 1,000).

Because chronic bronchitis rarely develops in nonsmokers, other factors implicated in the development of COPD (e.g., air pollution, occupational exposure, infection, and genetics) play a relatively unimportant role in the initial development of the disease. Yet, these same factors may be relevant in the overall decline of the person's clinical condition. Of particular importance is the significant role that infection plays in the exacerbation of symptoms, progression of pathology, and mortality.

Pathophysiology

Significant changes in the airways develop as a result of the repeated irritation from cigarette smoke. Bronchial mucous glands hypertrophy and mucus-secreting goblet cells in the airways increase in number and secrete excessive amounts of mucus. Mucus-transporting cilia are destroyed. In addition, bronchial and bronchiolar walls become inflamed and narrowed.

This combination of excess mucus production, diminished ability for mucus transport, and narrowing of the airways leads to mucus plugging, stagnation of secretions, and increased susceptibility to infection. In later stages of the disease, changes associated with emphysema can be seen.

Although the patient with chronic bronchitis may have only minimal changes in airway resistance initially, these tend to become more pronounced over time. This increased resistance results in inspiratory and expiratory obstruction in the airways, overinflation of the alveoli, and abnormal distribution of ventilation. These changes create ventilation–perfusion mismatching with resultant hypoxemia and hypercapnia. The pulmonary vasculature constricts in response to this hypoxemia, increasing the resistance to blood flow throughout the lungs. As a result, there is an increase in the workload placed on the right side of the heart, and it eventually begins to dilate. Over time, the right heart is unable to effectively pump blood through the pulmonary vasculature, resulting in right ventricular hypertrophy and cor pulmonale (Jess, 1992; Wilkins & Dexter, 1993) (Fig. 29–3).

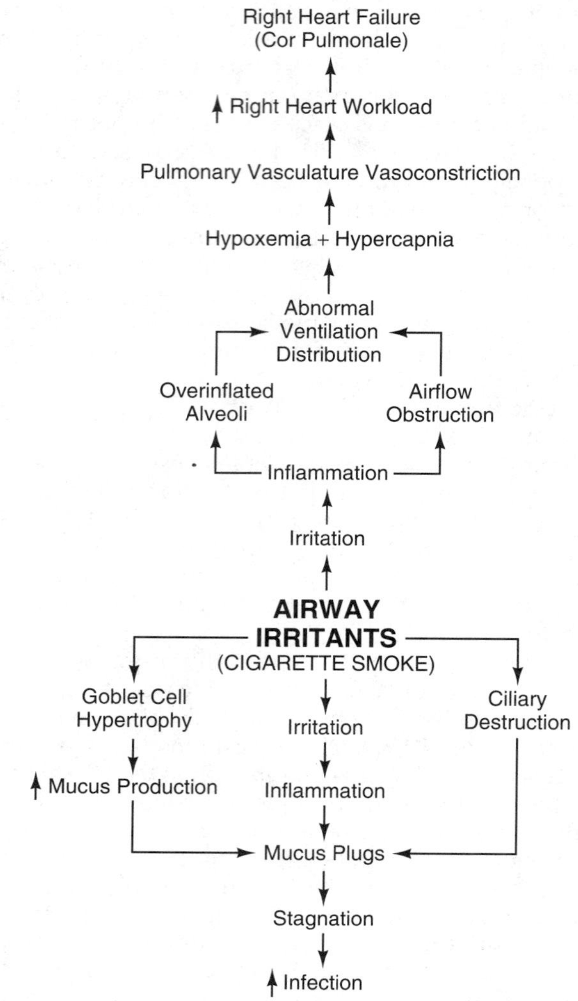

FIGURE 29–3. Proposed pathogenesis of chronic bronchitis.

Clinical Manifestations

The signs and symptoms of chronic bronchitis are variable. For many, the cough and sputum production have been present so long that the person denies any symptoms. Also, the symptoms depend on the severity of the disease and the presence or absence of exacerbation.

The patient whose only changes have been cough and sputum production for a number of years may have simple (or uncomplicated) chronic bronchitis. These individuals, with no evidence of decrease in airflow or other serious complications, have a good prognosis. In contrast, individuals with measurable airflow reduction have increased morbidity and mortality. Prognosis is related less to the symptoms than to the degree of airflow obstruction, as measured by decrease in FEV_1, and the age of the person when the decrease in airflow was first identified. The rate at which this decrease occurs is also significant. Individuals losing function rapidly die sooner than those with a slower rate of decline. Most become symptomatic in their 40s and 50s and become disabled from the disease in their late 50s and early 60s. Mortality related to chronic bronchitis rises dramatically after the age of 65 years and peaks between 75 and 84 years of age (National Center for Health Statistics, 1993a).

Symptoms are usually insidious, with infections precipitating exacerbations. Although people will often adjust their lifestyles to avoid dyspnea, the disease continues to progress so that less exertion or activity causes dyspnea to occur. Eventually, those in whom severe airway disease develops may be dyspneic at rest. At this point, ventilation–perfusion abnormalities and abnormal arterial blood gases are evident. These patients with pulmonary hypertension and cor pulmonale are termed end stage.

During a history and physical examination, the bronchitic individual with mild, stable disease may present with no significant findings. With progressive disease or during periods of acute exacerbation, numerous findings may become apparent. This patient usually gives a history of smoking for years, experiencing chronic smoker's hack for as long as he or she can remember, with multiple episodes of exacerbation and remission. A good history will also uncover a pattern of decreasing activity. Inspection may reveal the use of the accessory muscles of respiration and prolonged expiration. During an exacerbation, fever may be present with change in the amount and color of the sputum. Auscultation may reveal crackles, rhonchi, and wheezing. Pathologic cardiac changes related to right-sided heart failure occur as the disease progresses. These may result in jugular venous distention and pedal edema on inspection, a loud P_2 on auscultation, and hepatomegaly on palpation (Wilkins & Dexter, 1993).

Routine Testing Data

LABORATORY TESTS. Urinalysis and chemistry panel results are routinely normal in the patient with chronic bronchitis. Polycythemia is evident on a complete blood count (CBC) if the client is chronically hypoxemic. In addition, the CBC may exhibit an elevated white blood cell count if there is any type of infectious process present.

Arterial blood gases (ABGs) are quite useful in this population to assess acid–base and oxygenation abnormalities. Individuals with mild chronic bronchitis routinely have normal ABGs. In those with more advanced disease and those experiencing exacerbations requiring hospitalization, hypoxemia and respiratory acidosis (increased $Paco_2$ and decreased pH) are often found. Patients with chronic respiratory acidosis may have a near-normal or even normalized pH along with an elevated serum bicarbonate secondary to compensation for the consistently elevated $Paco_2$.

PULMONARY FUNCTION TESTS. Pulmonary function tests (PFTs) serve a dual purpose in the assessment of the chronic bronchitic by quantifying severity of the disease and documenting the response to treatment. In the early stages PFTs are usually negative. With more severe disease, findings include decreases in vital capacity and increases in residual volume consistent with the degree of hyperinflation present. At the same time, reductions in FEV_1 become more pronounced, even though there may be measurable improvement with bronchodilators.

RADIOGRAPHIC STUDIES. Radiographs are usually normal in uncomplicated chronic bronchitis. As the severity of the disease progresses, however, the chest x-ray becomes increasingly abnormal. Hyperinflation and increased lung markings become more pronounced (Fig. 29–4). An enlarged right heart is seen with cor pulmonale. Evidence of pneumonia may be seen during exacerbations.

ELECTROCARDIOGRAPHIC FINDINGS. Although the electrocardiogram (ECG) is normal in uncomplicated cases, some typical changes are seen in more severe stages of both chronic bronchitis and emphysema. Once pulmonary hypertension, hypoxemia, and airflow obstruction are present, the ECG often reveals specific changes related to the COPD. These include:

1. Right shift of the P and QRS axes due to hyperinflation and flattening of the diaphragm
2. Reduced size of the complexes in the limb leads secondary to hyperinflation
3. P pulmonale (tall, peaked P waves indicative of

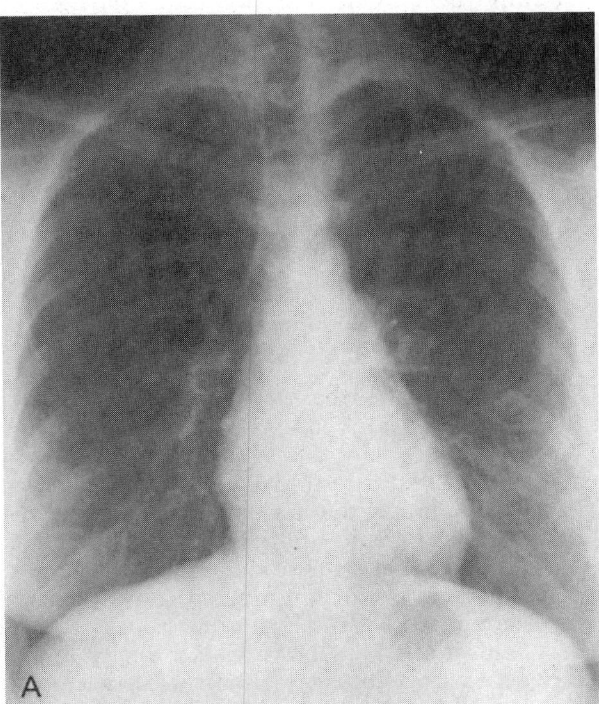

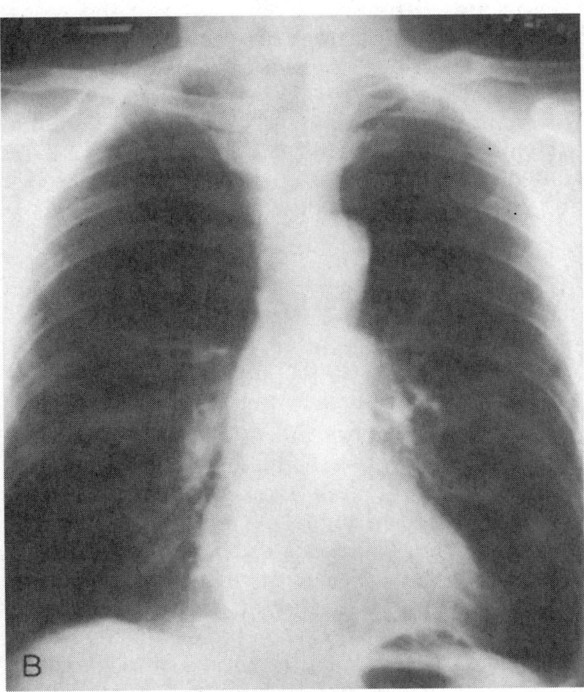

FIGURE 29–4. *A,* Normal chest roentgenogram. Posteroanterior view. *B,* Chest radiograph of a patient with severe chronic obstructive lung disease, showing the arterial deficiency pattern of emphysema. The lungs are hyperinflated, the diaphragms are low and flat, and there is a paucity of vascular markings. (From Weinberger, S. [1992]. *Principles of pulmonary medicine* [2nd ed., pp. 35, 102]. Philadelphia: W. B. Saunders.)

right atrial enlargement), particularly in leads II, III, and aVF
4. Signs of right ventricular hypertrophy
5. Atrial and ventricular dysrhythmias, often managed by treating the underlying respiratory failure, acid–base imbalance, hypoxemia, and potassium or magnesium abnormality (Wilkins & Dexter, 1993). Multifocal atrial tachycardia is a specific atrial dysrhythmia found in a high proportion of COPD patients with respiratory failure and potentially confused with other supraventricular arrhythmias.

Course and Prognosis

Most patients with chronic bronchitis experience years of sputum production and chronic cough, but have limited disability and often live out a normal life span. However, those in whom increased airway obstruction develops and who have progressive loss of pulmonary function and suffer frequent infections will reach a stage of respiratory insufficiency or failure that establishes a much less favorable prognosis. Cessation of smoking in conjunction with appropriate medical and nursing management are essential for the prolongation of life and enhancement of the quality of that life.

EMPHYSEMA

"A blowing into," the Greek derivation of the word "emphysema," appropriately describes the anatomic changes that develop in these individuals. Abnormal expansion of the acinus (the air space distal to the terminal bronchioles), accompanied by destruction of the alveolar walls, creates a pattern of permanent air space enlargement that disrupts the orderly nature of the lung and promotes physiologic impairment.

Etiology

Two primary etiologic factors specifically linked to the development of this form of COPD are a genetic predisposition and cigarette smoking. Both of these factors are implicated secondary to their relationship to elastin (a protein found in the connective tissue of alveolar walls) and proteases (enzymes capable of destroying elastin). Experimental production of emphysema in animal models indicates that the activity of these enzymes leads to the development of the disease, and that the greater the elastolytic activity of the enzyme, the more pronounced the changes in the lung.

These protease enzymes, the most important of which is elastase, are normally kept in balance by an inhibitor of their activity that is also found in the lung. The genetic factor related to the development of emphysema involves a deficiency in this inhibitor, $alpha_1$-protease inhibitor (formerly called $alpha_1$-antitrypsin), a glycoprotein that is manufactured in the liver and

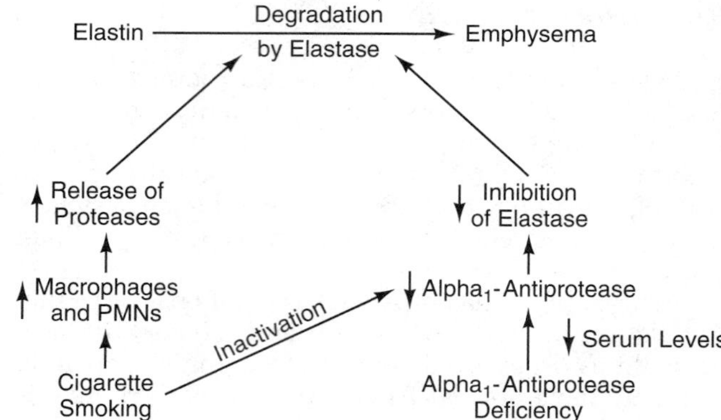

FIGURE 29–5. Schematic diagram of the hypothesized relationship between elastase and $alpha_1$-antiprotease indicating how smoking and $alpha_1$-antiprotease alter the balance, leading to degradation of elastin. *Abbreviation:* PMNs, polymorphonuclear leukocytes. (Adapted from Weinberger, S. [1992]. *Principles of pulmonary medicine* [2nd ed.]. Philadelphia: W. B. Saunders.)

normally circulates in the blood. People with a decreased serum level of this antiprotease or antielastase are strongly predisposed to the premature development of emphysema, as early as in the third or fourth decade of life, particularly if they smoke. Approximately 10% of the cases of emphysema are caused by this problem.

There are also reasons to believe that the balance between elastase and antielastase is disturbed by cigarette smoking and that this promotes the development of emphysema. One reason is that smokers have an increased number of alveolar macrophages and polymorphonuclear leukocytes, both sources of elastase. These cells are found in the lung as part of an inflammatory response secondary to irritation. The increased amount of elastase produced in the lungs of the cigarette smoker and the inactivation of antiprotease are believed to lead to increased destruction of elastin and the development of emphysema (Owens, 1993) (Fig. 29–5).

Pathology

The degradation of the elastic connective tissue in the distal portions of the lung is characterized by destruction of the alveolar walls and enlargement of the air spaces distal to the terminal bronchioles. The terminal bronchioles are purely air-conducting structures, but distal to these are the approximately 300 million alveoli, the functional units of the lung.

In patients with emphysema, flow rates during inspiration are relatively normal unless obstructive bronchitis is also present. However, during expiration, airway narrowing and increased resistance result in airway collapse. In addition, there is decreased elastic recoil. Intrathoracic pressure changes during expiration also predispose to narrowing, collapse, and premature airway closure in the emphysematous patient.

Alteration of the normal alveolar capillary membrane creates a decrease in the surface area available

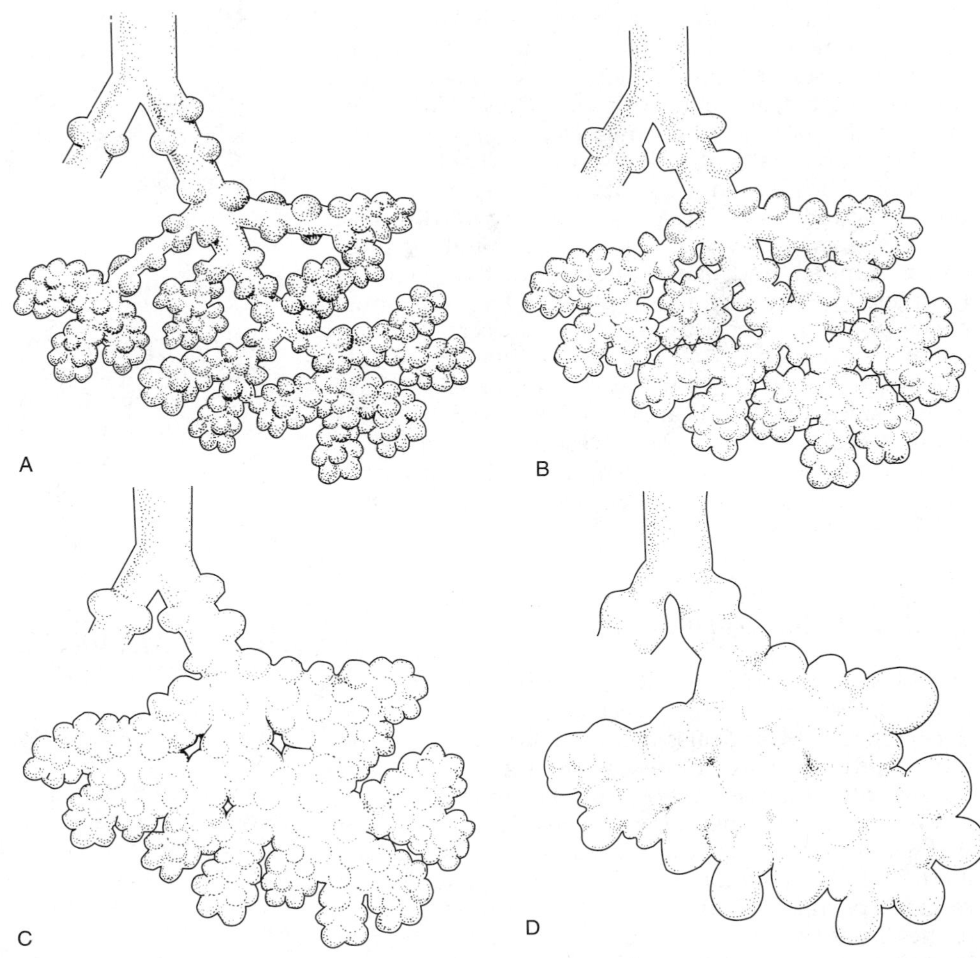

FIGURE 29–6. Comparison of the differences in the distal airways in (*A*) the normal patient, (*B*) simple hyperinflation, (*C*) centriacinar emphysema, and (*D*) panacinar emphysema.

for gas exchange. This causes alterations in oxygen-diffusing capacities and produces ventilation–perfusion abnormalities. These abnormalities contribute to an increase in the work of breathing and lead to the hypoxemia seen in emphysema.

Types of emphysema are often divided according to the site of pulmonary involvement (Fig. 29–6). In centrilobular (centriacinar) emphysema, the pathology is located in the central portion of the acinus and not in its periphery. This form of the disease most often involves the upper zones of the lung and is almost always associated with chronic bronchitis. It is also the most common form of the disease, and is rarely seen in nonsmokers. In the less common panlobular (or panacinar) form of the disease, the entire acinus is involved. The normal architecture of the alveoli is lost as the walls separating distinct alveoli are destroyed, air spaces become grossly enlarged, and there is loss of lung parenchyma. Although this form can occur anywhere in the lung, it is usually seen in the lower and more anterior areas. There is little association between it and chronic bronchitis. It can occur in nonsmokers and is the type usually seen in those with alpha$_1$-protease inhibitor deficiency. Some pathologists believe that the centrilobular type progresses into the panlobular.

Clinical Manifestations

Dyspnea, the chief complaint of the person suffering from the effects of emphysema, initially occurs only during exertion. It gradually increases in intensity as the disease progresses, and most severely limits activity. The rapidity of progression of the shortness of breath varies among individuals. However, all those affected adjust their activity level to minimize the dyspnea. As the disease advances, they find symptoms occurring with less and less activity until they are dyspneic at rest. The fact that some patients' dyspnea does not seem to correlate with the degree of pathology has led some nurse researchers to focus on the association between dyspnea and respiratory muscle function rather than pulmonary function. Based on this research, potential treatment strategies have been investigated (Breslin et al., 1992).

Like chronic bronchitis, the course of emphysema varies, with periods of exacerbations that are most often associated with infections, but may also be related to environmental irritants and bouts of congestive heart failure. Inspection classically demonstrates the frail, debilitated, and elderly "pink puffer." Characteristically, this person is a tachypneic, acyanotic, barrel-chested individual with a thin physique due to muscle wasting. The person may appear dyspneic, using pursed-lipped breathing and leaning forward to best use accessory muscles of respiration. Cough, if present, is minimal and usually nonproductive. Signs of right heart failure may also be evident. Palpation often elicits decreased vocal fremitus and a decrease in respiratory excursion due to hyperinflation. On percussion, hyperresonance is heard due to increased lung volumes. Breath sounds are diminished and often difficult to hear because of the increased anteroposterior diameter of the chest (heart sounds are distant for the same reason). Expiratory wheezes may be evident (Wilkins & Dexter, 1993).

Routine Laboratory Data

In patients with pure emphysema, especially younger patients, the alpha$_1$-antiprotease phenotype should be determined. ABGs are also helpful. ABGs in the person with emphysema are not necessarily representative of the severity of the disease, but can be clinically useful in determining the need for and response to oxygen therapy. In addition, they provide a baseline assessment for future comparison. Moderate hypoxemia and respiratory alkalosis are common with milder forms of the disease, whereas severe hypoxemia and respiratory acidosis are present with end-stage disease, infections, and other complications.

ELECTROCARDIOGRAPHIC FINDINGS. As with chronic bronchitis, assessment of the ECG is not specifically diagnostic for emphysema. ECG changes relate more to the severity of the disease.

RADIOGRAPHIC STUDIES. Classic findings seen in the later stages of the disease include flattening of the diaphragm, hyperlucency, decreased vascular markings, widening of the rib spaces, and increased anteroposterior diameter. Careful interpretation is necessary to rule out other reasons for the hyperinflation, because the most common cause of hyperlucent lung fields is an overexposed film on a thin, elderly patient (Tisi, 1983). Bullous lesions are unequivocal indications of emphysema.

PULMONARY FUNCTION TESTS. Common findings include:

1. Increased functional residual capacity (volume of air remaining in the lungs at the end of expiration) secondary to hyperinflation.
2. Decreased forced vital capacity (FVC), FEV_1, and FEV_1/FVC due to air flow obstruction.
3. Decreased diffusion capacity as a result of loss of surface area for gas exchange.

Although PFTs are not routinely done during exacerbations, they can be useful parameters in evaluating severity and progression of the disease and response to bronchodilators.

Course and Prognosis

Although progression of the disease varies, most patients will experience a fairly predictable decline in pulmonary function, with an average time between onset of disease and severe disability being 20 to 25 years. The correlation between severity of airflow obstruction (as measured by FEV_1) and mortality is good. Few patients survive more than 5 years with an FEV_1 less than 750 mL (Farzan, 1985).

ACUTE MANAGEMENT OF THE PATIENT WITH COPD

Clinical Presentation

Admission of the COPD patient to the intensive care unit (ICU) presents special problems for care providers. Nursing and medical management are truly a challenge, whether the patient is admitted in respiratory failure with acute exacerbation secondary to infection (most common), acute bronchospasm, congestive heart failure, gastrointestinal bleeding, metabolic abnormalities, or after surgery for an unrelated problem.

Acute respiratory failure is the end result of an imbalance between respiratory muscle strength and stamina available and the amount of energy needed to do the work of breathing (see Chapter 31). In the COPD patient, it manifests itself as dyspnea, changes in cough and sputum production, mental changes (irritability or lethargy), and fatigue. Physical examination may reveal tachycardia, tachypnea, use of accessory muscles, paradoxical breathing, along with the presence of abnormal breath sounds and signs of cor pulmonale (Donahoe & Rogers, 1993; Hagedorn, 1992). Physically stressed postoperative COPD patients may not be admitted in this state, but are at high risk for its development.

Laboratory Assessment Data

On the patient's admission to the ICU, it is important to obtain ABGs, sputum for analysis, a chest x-ray, blood for CBC and electrolyte evaluation, and an ECG. This information should serve as a baseline for comparison to past and future data and assist in determining the cause and specific management of acute respiratory failure.

TABLE 29–2. **Priorities for Clinical Management of the COPD Patient**

Acute Stage

Maintaining an effective airway
Improving gas exchange
Decreasing dyspnea and work of breathing
Managing intubation and mechanical ventilation
Hemodynamic monitoring
Maintaining adequate nutrition
Managing drug therapy
Preventing infection
Enhancing psychosocial support for both patient and the family

Recovery Stage

Slowing disease progression
Controlling symptoms
Minimizing exacerbations
Assisting in ability to perform activities of daily living
Smoking cessation
Pulmonary rehabilitation
Meeting educational needs of both patient and the family

Clinical Management

The primary goal of therapy for any patient admitted to the ICU in respiratory failure is to maintain adequate cellular respiration. To achieve this, identifying and reversing the precipitating cause of the failure is critical. Parameters used to identify respiratory failure in non-COPD patients ($Pa{O_2} < 60$ mm Hg; $Pa{CO_2} > 50$ mm Hg) are frequently "normal" values for the COPD patient. Therefore, the key to differentiating life-threatening acute respiratory failure from longstanding but nonthreatening chronic failure often found in these patients is an acidotic pH (< 7.25) in conjunction with an elevated $Pa{CO_2}$ and a decreased $Pa{O_2}$.

Priorities for supporting the patient during the most acute stages of the illness are targeted towards improving oxygen delivery and consumption and include varied interventions. Later, priorities change somewhat, but they continue to need to be holistic and focused on individual patient needs (Table 29–2).

MAINTAINING AN EFFECTIVE AIRWAY (PULMONARY HYGIENE)

Inability to maintain adequate pulmonary hygiene results in retained secretions, an excellent medium for bacterial growth. Patients with thick or copious secretions and those with an ineffective cough are most susceptible to problems. Interventions aimed at managing these symptoms address the mobilization and removal of secretions from the airways. Although some physicians order expectorants, more commonly hydration and humidification of inspired oxygen will be used to thin secretions. However, cardiac and renal contraindications to hydration must be considered. Percussion, vibration, and postural drainage techniques may be quite effective to open occluded airways and mobilize secretions for patients with copious secretions or lobar atelectasis. However, caution must be taken with these procedures because they may be physiologically taxing for the patient and may initiate desaturation and bronchospasm. In most patients, positioning, ambulation, administration of bronchodilators, encouraging deep breathing, and use of proper coughing techniques are appropriate measures to facilitate the removal of secretions. Depending on the person's overall condition, however, oropharyngeal or tracheal suctioning may be indicated (American Thoracic Society, 1989; Wilson & Thompson, 1990).

For a significant number of patients in ARF, with difficulty in clearing their secretions, suctioning is a necessity. However, suctioning is by no means a benign procedure. To realize benefits and avoid complications such as dysrhythmias, hemodynamic instability, hypoxemia, and mucosal damage, appropriate suction techniques must be used. Although a thorough commentary is beyond the scope of this chapter, a brief review is in order because of the importance of the subject.

Many excellent nursing studies have been done to promote optimal suctioning methods. The most accepted recommendations for suctioning include the following:

1. Suction only when needed.
2. Maintain the negative pressure used to suction no higher than 150 mm Hg.
3. Use catheters no larger than one-half the internal diameter of the airway.
4. Monitor vital signs and patient response before, during, and after the procedure.
5. Hyperoxygenate with 100% oxygen.
   - Use caution with manual resuscitation bags because of the interruption of mechanical ventilation and positive end-expiratory pressure (PEEP), inability to maintain consistent volumes, increases in mean arterial pressure, and potential airway contamination
   - Closed suction systems help to maintain PEEP and PaO_2
   - Preoxygenation with the ventilator requires a washout time to achieve 100% oxygen
6. Minimize the number of suction passes.
7. Continuous application of negative pressure during suctioning is not detrimental.
8. The installation of normal saline remains controversial; although it may be helpful to initiate a cough, it could increase the risk of bacteria entering the lungs. A good guideline is to monitor the patient's response to suctioning and individualize the procedure to meet the patient's need.

IMPROVING GAS EXCHANGE

Supplemental oxygen is considered the mainstay of therapy to correct hypoxemia and, at the same time, minimize oxygen-induced hypercapnia (Donahoe & Rogers, 1993). An adequate $Pa{O_2}$, in conjunction with an acceptable hemoglobin level, improves oxygen delivery to body tissues. Supplemental oxygen may reverse the pulmonary hypertension resulting from hypoxemia and in turn improve cardiac output necessary for optimal oxygen delivery by reducing right-sided cardiac afterload.

In acute as well as long-term management, it is the only intervention that has increased longevity with COPD. Oxygen is a necessity for the acute patient and currently is recommended for medically stable patients with a $Pa{O_2}$ below 55 mm Hg (Owens, 1993). The goal of therapy is to maintain the $Pa{O_2}$ between 55 and 65 mm Hg and the $Sa{O_2}$ at or above 90%.

Although pulse oximetry is not accurate 100% of the time and must be used with caution in the COPD patient, it offers an economically sound and clinically practical alternative to frequent ABG evaluations. However, hypercapnia may go undetected when pulse oximetry is used as the sole tool to monitor gas exchange. Venous measurements of CO_2 can be helpful and, again, will minimize the need for ABGs. Capnography is not recommended in this setting (see Chapter 15).

Maintaining oxygenation in the appropriate range provides adequate saturation of hemoglobin while avoiding oxygen-induced hypercapnia. It has previously been proposed that many COPD patients with an increased CO_2 had a reduced hypercapnic and prominent hypoxic drive to breathe. As such, it was believed that supplemental oxygen could potentially suppress the hypoxic drive, decrease minute ventilation, and promote hypercapnia. However, recent studies have demonstrated that despite an increase in $Pa{CO_2}$, ventilation is maintained in these patients while they are receiving supplemental oxygen. Increases in $Pa{CO_2}$ occurring during the administration of supplemental oxygen may be explained instead by changes in ventilation–perfusion relationships that are induced by the oxygen (Donahoe & Rogers, 1993). Therefore, it is important to slowly increase oxygen and closely monitor its effects.

ENDOTRACHEAL INTUBATION AND VENTILATORY MANAGEMENT

The decision to intervene with intubation and mechanical ventilation must be made in light of expected outcomes and quality of life for the patient. These are often difficult decisions, ideally discussed among patient, family, and primary physician before intubation is imminent. Documentation in the form of living wills and durable power of attorney for health care may be helpful to ensure patients' wishes are carried out, in the event they are unable to speak for themselves (see Chapter 3).

Intubation and mechanical ventilation do not remedy the cause of the respiratory failure, but allow the patient to "rest" the muscles of respiration, facilitate suctioning, and improve gas exchange. However, specific management of these patients is difficult, and potential complications are numerous (see Chapter 16). Particular caution must be used to prevent problems due to barotrauma secondary to high positive airway pressures, the use of PEEP, and increased respiratory rates that lead to air trapping. This is particularly true for patients with emphysematous changes.

The most significant problem associated with the use of mechanical ventilation in patients with COPD is the frequent difficulty encountered in weaning. Chronic ventilator dependency is a physical, psychological, and financial stressor for both patients and families. It also presents unique challenges to health care providers (see Chapter 33).

Recently, a potential alternative to intubation has been investigated in controlled studies. The results suggest that mechanical ventilation with a nasal mask can successfully manage acute respiratory failure in some groups of patients in whom intubation is controversial or not immediately necessary (Benhamou et al., 1992; Bott et al., 1993; Hill, 1993).

DECREASING DYSPNEA AND THE WORK OF BREATHING

Inability to manage comfortable breathing results in problems such as increased anxiety, nutritional deficits, and inability to cope with the disease. In the acutely ill ICU patient, it may inhibit ventilator weaning. Interventions aimed at managing dyspnea and decreasing the work of breathing include the use of techniques such as pursed-lip breathing to prolong exhalation and prevent bronchiolar collapse, and diaphragmatic breathing to maximize gas exchange. Other proven methods include optimal positioning to facilitate the use of accessory muscles, relaxation techniques, diversional activities, and optimal scheduling of rest and activity periods. Quantification of dyspnea, using a scale of 1 to 10, may be helpful to assess the patient's subjective sense of shortness of breath, plan appropriate interventions, and evaluate improvement (Nield et al., 1989).

HEMODYNAMIC MONITORING

Hemodynamic monitoring principles are similar for all critically ill patients (see Chapter 13). However, there are differences, depending on the extent of disease present. Secondary to increased pulmonary vascular resistance, pulmonary artery pressures (systolic and diastolic) may be above normal and pulmonary artery diastolic pressures may be 5 to 20 mm Hg above the pulmonary capillary wedge pressure (normally 1–2 mm Hg above the wedge pressure). In addition, changes in compliance of the lungs may affect readings.

The actual measurement technique used is another consideration in the pulmonary patient. It has been demonstrated in multiple studies that patients need not be placed flat in bed to obtain readings. In addition, the potentially restless, uncomfortable, dyspneic COPD patient may change position frequently, necessitating adjustment of the reference point to ensure accurate measurements. Accuracy may also be affected by difficulty in interpreting measurements secondary to an inability to determine end expiration (when airway and intrathoracic pressures are stable) if the patient is being mechanically ventilated. There remains debate concerning whether the patient should be removed from the ventilator for readings particularly when PEEP is being used. Removing patients from the ventilator to obtain readings may result in hypoxemia and sudden increases in venous return to the heart. It is usually recommended that the measurements be made while the patient remains on the ventilator. Finally, consistency in the method of determining measurements is essential.

NUTRITIONAL SUPPORT

Nutrition is particularly important for the person with COPD due to the debilitating nature of the disease. Although more research is needed, relationships between maintenance of normal body weight (with a positive nitrogen balance) and adequate diaphragm muscle mass, susceptibility to respiratory infection, and mortality are evident (Rose, 1992).

Many of these patients show evidence of malnutrition before admission to the ICU. These critically ill patients require adequate calories to meet increased metabolic demand from increased work of breathing and other factors such as fever. Unless definitive measures to provide adequate caloric intake are initiated and maintained, these patients become increasingly difficult to manage, particularly with regard to weaning from mechanical ventilation. Yet, caution must be exercised as to how the calories are provided. Excess carbohydrates in the diet are converted into fats, resulting in increased production of CO_2 and increased respiratory work. Therefore, minimizing carbohydrate load and increasing the amount of fats to provide calories is recommended (Rose, 1992). In addition, electrolyte abnormalities, including hypokalemia, hypophosphatemia, hypocalcemia, and hypomagnesemia, must be corrected via supplementation because they adversely affect respiratory muscle strength (see Chapter 47).

DRUG THERAPY

The appropriate use of medications is invaluable in the management of COPD. Bronchodilators (especially for those with a reversible component to their disease), steroids (in the acute setting), antibiotics (with the presence of infection), and other agents are used as indicated.

BRONCHODILATOR THERAPY. Bronchodilators can significantly reduce airway resistance in the critically ill COPD patient. Due to their efficacy, rapid onset of action, and low toxicity, inhaled beta$_2$ agonists and ipratropium bromide (Atrovent; Boehringer Ingelheim, Ridgefield, CT) are the drugs of choice for early and continued management; the latter appears to be a more potent bronchodilator in COPD (Owens, 1993). Even if pulmonary function tests indicate only a small degree of reversibility of airflow obstruction in the chronic patient (a 15% improvement over baseline is considered significant), treatment with bronchodilators may be able to prevent accelerated loss of lung function, improve PFTs (particularly in chronic bronchitics), and help to minimize signs and symptoms of the disease.

The use of theophylline preparations remains controversial. Although the bronchodilator effects of these agents are not impressive, there is increased discussion about their enhanced effect on mucociliary clearance and impact on diaphragmatic contractility. When theophylline is used, serum levels must be monitored closely because smokers tend to metabolize the drug faster than nonsmokers, and patients with hepatic or cardiac disease and those receiving erythromycin metabolize it more slowly. Therefore, dosages must be individualized. Serum levels should be maintained at 12 μg/mL or less (Owens, 1993). Bronchodilators are discussed further in the Asthma section of this chapter.

STEROIDS. The use of steroids is well documented in the presence of asthma and is discussed later in that section. Long-term steroid use in the acute management of COPD remains controversial. It appears a short course of steroids started early and tapered quickly is a safe and effective therapy, as long as the patient is monitored closely for hyperglycemia.

ANTIBIOTICS. Because infections are a common precipitating cause of respiratory failure in patients with COPD, antibiotics are frequently ordered. Initial choice of the drug used is commonly based on Gram stain of the sputum. It is changed if blood and sputum cultures and sensitivities suggest a more appropriate choice.

ANTIPYRETICS. Treating an elevated temperature in the patient with an already compromised respiratory system is essential. It is estimated that CO_2 production and O_2 consumption increase by as much as 10% for each degree Fahrenheit rise in temperature above normal (Chin & Pesce, 1983). This increase puts additional strain on the respiratory system.

OTHER AGENTS. A multitude of other drugs may be used depending on concomitant problems. The key to appropriate management of the COPD patient is using a holistic approach to optimally maintain all body systems. This includes using diuretics (if congestive heart failure is evident) and mood-altering agents (with caution in depressed patients).

PREVENTING INFECTION

Prevention of this complication is extremely important. Adequate hydration, removal of secretions, proper nutrition, avoidance of sudden changes in climate, and adherence to prescribed antibiotics and physical therapy regimens are crucial. Annual prophylaxis vaccination against influenza and *Streptococcus pneumoniae* are recommended (Owens, 1993). Prevention of infection in the ICU is particularly relevant because of the debilitated state in which these patients often present, and the invasive nature of critical care. Judicious use of invasive procedures, consistent hand washing, and careful monitoring for infection are extremely important.

DISCHARGE PLANNING

Priorities change after the patient leaves the ICU and no longer requires acute care in the hospital setting. Referrals for appropriate follow-up should be made at this time. Two areas that can have a significant impact on the patient's well-being are smoking cessation and pulmonary rehabilitation.

SMOKING CESSATION. Effective management of these diseases includes smoking cessation as the single most important intervention to alter the progression of airflow obstruction. Care providers must address this fact in a realistic, practical manner. Avoidance of further insult to the lung is advantageous to the person's future well-being, as demonstrated in multiple longitudinal studies reporting improvement in symptoms, decreased respiratory infections, improved pulmonary function, and decline in mortality (Fiore et al., 1993).

Multiple techniques to facilitate continued cessation after discharge are available. These include behavior modification, support groups, and the use of nicotine-containing patches that may help combat the addictiveness of nicotine. Nicotine-containing patches may also be used while the patient is acutely ill.

PULMONARY REHABILITATION. Patient compliance and changes in lifestyle often depend on understanding of the illness and treatment regime. Proper education of patients and families is critical to the overall management of COPD. Multidisciplinary pulmonary rehabilitation programs, tailored to the individual, offer advantages. These programs generally include instruction on reconditioning, breathing retraining, energy conservation techniques, smoking cessation, and vocational and sexual counseling. Although they have not proven to increase life expectancy, it is clear that these programs favorably affect the quality of life for the patient with COPD (Table 29–3).

TABLE 29–3. **Demonstrated Benefits of Pulmonary Rehabilitation**

Reduction in respiratory symptoms
Reversal of anxiety and depression and improved ego strength
Enhanced ability to carry out activities of daily living
Increased exercise ability
Better quality of life
Reduction in hospital days required
Prolongation of life in selected patients (i.e., use of continuous oxygen in patients with severe hypoxemia)

From Hodgkin, J., & Petty, T. (1987). *Chronic obstructive pulmonary disease.* Philadelphia: W. B. Saunders.

ASTHMA

Prevalence, mortality, and monetary expenditures related to asthma are on the rise (Aberman, 1991; American Lung Association, 1993; Barnes, 1993). The prevalence of this disease increased 71% between 1970 and 1990. There was a 56% increase in the relative death rate from asthma between 1979 and 1989. Annual direct and indirect costs to the nation continue to rise, reaching $6.2 billion dollars in 1993. This has occurred despite the fact that scientific progress is increasing our understanding of the disease and improving the treatment. This apparent contradiction, the "asthma paradox," only validates the challenge health professionals currently face (Page, 1993).

Asthma, the seventh most prevalent chronic condition in the United States, affects 10.3 million people and remains a common cause of admission to emergency rooms and hospitals (American Lung Association, 1993). Despite maximal drug therapy, some people are incapacitated by the disease and others die because of it (5,106 in 1991 alone) (National Center for Health Statistics, 1993a). There is a growing racial disproportion between blacks and whites in both prevalence and mortality. In 1990, the prevalence among blacks was 13.8% greater than among whites (American Lung Association, 1993). Mortality rates were found to be two times greater in 1992. Women are affected more than men. City dwellers are more likely to have the disease than suburban or rural residents (National Center for Health Statistics, 1993b).

Asthma can begin at any age, although half the cases begin before the age of 10 years, and 3.7 million asthma sufferers are younger than 18 years of age. Approximately half of the children in whom asthma develops will "outgrow" the problem, but the remainder will endure the condition for their lifetime. There appears to be a genetic predisposition in some and definite links with smokers in the family for others (American Lung Association, 1993).

Traditionally, asthma has been characterized as a disease of episodic bronchoconstriction and bronchial hyperreactivity (abnormal, exaggerated airway narrowing in response to a variety of stimuli), manifested by widespread but highly reversible narrowing of the airways. Recently, however, it has been discovered that a cardinal feature of asthma is chronic inflammation of the airways. Bronchial constriction and hyperreactivity depend on the degree of inflammation present (Hillman & Bishop, 1993).

Etiology (Precipitating Stimuli)

The episodic nature of the disease, with asymptomatic periods interspersed with occasions of acute symptomatology, has demonstrated clear patterns of precipitating event and response. When an attack is associated with a specific external source (allergen), the asthma is often referred to as *extrinsic* in nature. This type typically begins in childhood. When specific causative agents cannot be identified, but attacks may be precipitated by a variety of situations, the asthma is referred to as *intrinsic*. This type usually starts in adulthood (Wilson & Thompson, 1990).

Although it is not always possible, identifying and avoiding triggers of the disease is a first step in its management. Some of the stimuli that can precipitate an attack of asthma include the following.

ALLERGENS. Inhaled allergens, although probably the most significant, are but one of the etiologic factors responsible for maintaining symptoms. Dust mites, found throughout the home, but particularly in mattresses, are a common agent responsible for perennial symptoms. Depending on the type of exposure, pets in the household may cause intermittent symptoms. Seasonal forms of the disease are most likely related to exposure to pollens or molds in the air. It is not uncommon for children with severe asthma to have a strong history of allergic conditions such as hay fever or eczema, more strongly positive skin tests, and higher levels of immunoglobulin E than those with milder asthma (Barnes, 1993).

INFECTION. Viral upper respiratory tract infections are common precipitants of asthma attacks and are also the most common cause of severe exacerbations. Bacterial infections, on the other hand, are not implicated as a causative agent and, therefore, antibiotics are of no value during exacerbations (Barnes, 1993).

EXERCISE. Asthma attacks related to exercise are common in children and young adults. When they occur with sudden bursts of exercise they are thought to be due to the sudden cooling of the airways. Normally inspired air is humidified and temperature regulated (37°C). This process occurs by heat exchange and evaporation of water from the airway mucus. Heat loss is proportional to minute ventilation, which, in vigorous exercise, is markedly increased. Heavy exercise in cold, dry air (e.g., ice skating) is much more likely to cause an attack than exercise in warm, humid air (e.g., indoor swimming).

In a similar fashion, simply breathing cold, dry air without exercising may produce symptoms in some people, whereas others may have symptoms triggered by laughing or crying with subsequent airway cooling.

EMOTIONS. There is no evidence indicating a psychological basis for asthma, but sudden emotional reactions or stress reportedly reduce airway caliber in asthmatics. Tachypnea resulting in hypocapnia may increase airway resistance by constricting the smooth muscles of the airways.

TABLE 29–4. **Occupational Irritants Implicated in Asthma**

Tobacco smoke
Ozone
Nickel
Platinum
Pigeon droppings (bird breeder's lung)
Moldy bark exposure (maple bark stripper's lung)
Moldy vegetable compost (farmer's lung/bagassosis)
Contaminated air conditioning systems
Polyurethane fumes
Sulfur dioxide
Formaldehyde
Cotton fiber (byssinosis)

NASAL POLYPS, MEDICATIONS, AND OTHER FACTORS. Recurrent nasal polyps, asthma, and aspirin sensitivity is a well recognized triad. Other nonsteroidal anti-inflammatory agents, including ibuprofen, should be avoided. Acetaminophen is usually safe as an analgesic. All beta blockers should be avoided due to antagonism of $beta_2$ receptors in the airways. Certain foods (dairy products), food additives such as monosodium glutamate, and alcoholic beverage additives (e.g., metabisulfite) are specifically implicated as precipitating agents. Premenstrual worsening occurs in many women with asthma, probably because of a decrease in progesterone levels. Chronic occupational exposure to inhaled irritants can cause fixed airway obstruction in some individuals (Barnes, 1993); some of those implicated are listed in Table 29–4.

Mechanisms Producing Asthma

In the past, sensitized mast cells in the lungs were believed to be a mechanism central to the understanding of the development of bronchoconstriction in asthma. It is now apparent that numerous types of inflammatory cells and multiple chemical mediators are responsible for the multiple pathologic changes evident with asthma (Busse et al., 1993).

Biochemical agents regulate these mediators. Increased levels of cyclic adenosine monophosphate (cAMP) inhibit their secretion, whereas decreased levels facilitate release of mediators. This mechanism of action is the basis for many of the drugs used in the treatment of asthma. $Beta_2$-adrenergics, specific to the airways, increase levels of cAMP by stimulating the conversion of adenosine triphosphate to cAMP. Methylxanthines such as theophylline inhibit phosphodiesterase, the enzyme that breaks down cAMP (Barnes, 1993).

Pathophysiology

In response to precipitating stimuli that act as triggers, different cells within the airways become abnormally active and inflamed. These inflamed cells then release

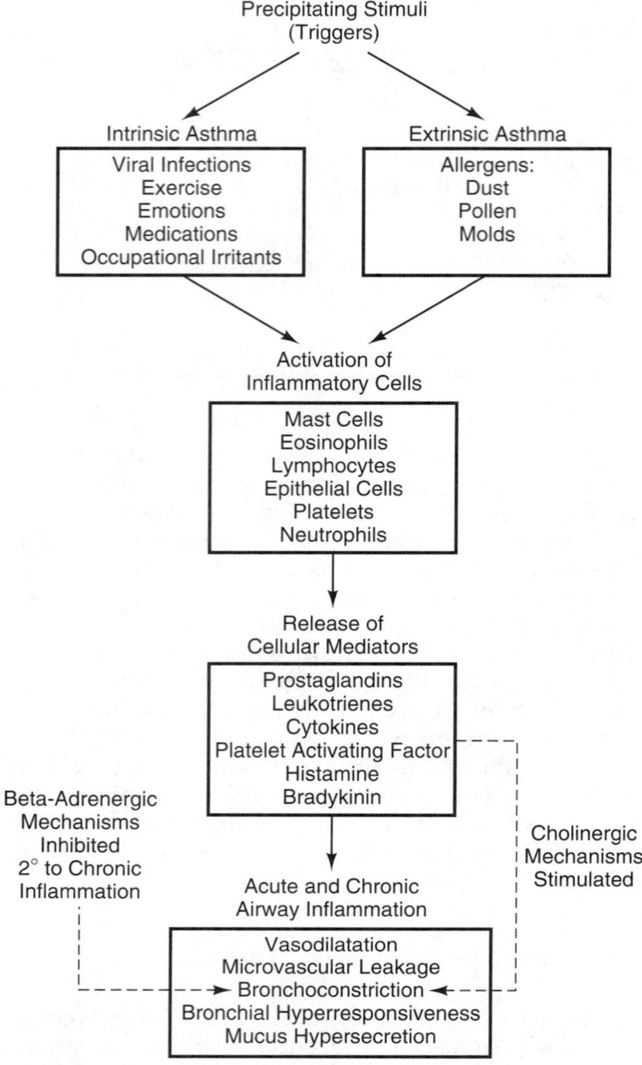

FIGURE 29–7. Proposed pathogenesis of asthma.

inflammatory mediators directly responsible for the pathophysiologic changes of asthma. Vasodilation and microvascular leakage produce edema and plasma exudate. Irritated and inflamed airways hypersecrete mucus that further clogs the airways. This inflammatory process leads to bronchial hyperreactivity and bronchoconstriction. Bronchoconstriction is recurrent and possibly progressive in nature, with thickening and contraction of the smooth muscle of both central and peripheral airway walls, resulting in narrowing (Kaliner et al., 1992). Due to the absence of cartilage in the peripheral airways, they are particularly susceptible to narrowing and collapse.

Collectively, the characteristic pathologic changes seen in asthma are the result of the release of inflammatory mediators that cause significant narrowing of the airways. This narrowing results in obstruction to flow, hyperinflation, ventilation–perfusion abnormalities, and changes in ABGs. Impairment of cardiac function also occurs during severe attacks (Wilkins & Dexter, 1993) (Fig. 29–7).

As a result of narrowing, inspiratory and expiratory flow rates are reduced. Objective measurements of FEV_1 and peak expiratory flow rate (PEFR) are below those predicted and indicate the presence of obstructive disease.

Initially, the response to allergens and irritants causes symptoms to appear quickly and subside after approximately 1 hour. This *early-phase reaction*, as it is known, is followed by a *delayed* or *late-phase reaction* in about half of all asthma patients. This phenomena, producing the same symptoms, occurs 4 to 8 hours after the initial episode and may last for hours to days (Reinke & Hoffman, 1992).

Because the narrowing of peripheral airways is not uniform, there is uneven distribution of ventilation throughout the lungs. Quite early in an asthmatic attack, functional residual capacity (the air remaining in the lungs at the end of expiration) increases as alveoli become overdistended to maintain vital capacity. These hyperinflated areas have excess ventilation and therefore increase dead space. However, other areas are underventilated due to narrowing, increased secretions, and edema. In these areas, perfusion of the pulmonary capillaries exceeds ventilation and a low ventilation-to-perfusion ratio is produced. Initially, hypoxemia may not be a problem, but as the attack continues and worsens, ventilation to affected areas may be minimal, producing a right-to-left shunt and worsening oxygenation (Hillman & Bishop, 1993).

ABGs are a valuable means to evaluate the severity and duration of an acute asthma attack (Dellinger, 1991). If untreated, oxygenation progressively worsens from initially normal Pa_{O_2} levels to severe hypoxemia. Initially, ventilatory drive is normal or increased (anxiety and response to hypoxemia) and produces a hypocapnic state. As work of breathing increases and the patient tires, however, Pa_{CO_2} increases and the patient becomes hypercapnic and at high risk for morbidity and mortality.

With hypoxemic vasoconstriction and overdistention of alveoli, pulmonary artery pressures increase. This subsequently impairs right ventricular function. Pulmonary edema may also occur, due either to left ventricular dysfunction or, more likely, to the highly negative intrathoracic pressures generated on inspiration (Hillman & Bishop, 1993).

Clinical Manifestations

People with asthma are not a homogenous group. Variable signs and symptoms are seen among different patients and in the same patient over time. Astute assessment of various clinical findings and laboratory data assist the practitioner to select appropriate therapies based on the severity of the disease at the time. Chronic mild and moderate asthma are routinely managed outside the hospital. Discussion here is limited to acute, severe manifestations of the disease (status asthmaticus and exacerbation in the critically ill patient), which require close monitoring, numerous treatments, and multiple assessments of pulmonary function.

VITAL SIGNS. A respiratory rate above 30 in an adult indicates an impaired ability to adequately oxygenate and increased use of energy reserves to ventilate. If not associated with changes in activity or other physiologic requirements, increasing respiratory rates may be early indicators of impending problems.

Tachycardia above 120 is associated with increased work of breathing secondary to a decreased PaO_2, increased $PaCO_2$, or both. It is important to discern whether the increased rate is due to the pulmonary pathology, requiring more aggressive therapy, or is a result of the bronchodilator therapy. In addition, tachycardia may be augmented by the patient's anxiety as an asthma attack progresses.

Temperature elevations may indicate infection, necessitating identification of the cause and proper treatment. The use of rectal or tympanic thermometers may be necessary because of the patient's respiratory distress and the inability to perform oral monitoring accurately.

Systemic blood pressure can also be affected during severe attacks. As air trapping occurs secondary to obstruction of flow, hyperinflation develops and pleural pressures become increasingly negative on inspiration. These large intrathoracic pressure shifts can create a reduced cardiac output and subsequent decrease in blood pressure during inspiration. If systolic pressure drops more than 10 mm Hg on inspiration, pulsus paradoxus is present.

PATIENT PRESENTATION. During severe, potentially life-threatening exacerbations, history and symptom assessment can be invaluable. However, it must also be remembered that there is not a strong correlation among the symptoms and the severity of the disease or the response to treatment. Nevertheless, complaints of progressive muscle fatigue with a history of profound exhaustion, lack of sleep, and repeated coughing on mild effort correlate with a more severe attack. Dyspnea, the subjective response to an increase in the work of breathing, and complaints of chest tightness are frequently described by the patient in fragmented speech, between breaths. In addition to being very short of breath, the patient is often diaphoretic, sitting upright (unable to lie supine), or leaning forward, using accessory muscles of respiration. Mentation and personality may be affected as well. Changes in the movement of gas in the airways produce distinctive symptoms evident on chest examination. Wheezing, however, routinely associated with increased bronchoconstriction in asthma, is an unreliable indicator of the degree of air flow obstruction. Decreased wheezing heard on auscultation may indicate an improvement in airflow, but it may just as well indicate that there is increased obstruction and patient deterioration (Aberman, 1991). The presence of complications (e.g., pneumonia, pneumothorax, atelectasis) or any other major organ abnormality (e.g., dysrhythmias or heart failure) may affect the patient's appearance and further worsen the situation.

It is particularly important to appreciate the impact of circadian rhythms on asthma. Many patients may be well during the day and symptomatic at night due to a diurnal rhythm reflecting a decrease in function during the night (lowest at 3 A.M.) and improvement during the day (peak function at 3 P.M.). To avoid exacerbation of symptoms, providing 24-hour therapeutic management is a necessity (Martin, 1993).

Factors that may indicate an impending asthma attack or deterioration in a stable patient are:

1. Increasing dyspnea (although a subjective symptom, patients may be able to quantify their discomfort similarly to the way a pain scale is used)
2. Increased sleep disturbances with increased bronchodilator use at night
3. Early morning chest tightness with progressively less relief from medication
4. Increased frequency and severity of cough
5. Increased allergic state (atopy) with a "runny nose" and early morning sneezing bouts

Laboratory Data

PULMONARY FUNCTION TESTS. Although PFT values vary among patients and in the same patient at different times, they are essential in diagnosis and vital for ongoing assessment of the severity of the disease. These objective measures should be obtained initially to provide a baseline, and periodically thereafter to monitor progression of an attack and response to treatment. PFTs provide the following useful information:

1. Peak expiratory flow rate (PEFR)—maximum flow rate generated during a forced expiration that is measured in liters per second (this simple procedure can be used by the asthmatic in the home for monitoring)
2. Forced vital capacity (FVC)—fully and forcefully exhaling after as deep an aspiration as possible
3. Forced expiratory volume one second (FEV_1)—volume of air exhaled in 1 second after a maximal inspiration
4. FEV_1/FVC ratio—comparison of the two values (used as an excellent means of assessing the degree of obstruction)
5. Functional residual capacity—volume of air remaining in the lungs at the end of expiration (indicates the degree of hyperinflation present).

Between attacks, although some may have normal or near-normal PFTs, most asthmatics show evidence of small airway obstruction. During an acute attack, common findings indicative of increases in this obstruction include marked decreases in exhaled flow, FVC, and FEV_1/FVC ratio and increases in functional residual capacity. These findings are similar to those noted in emphysema, but usually improve to a greater extent after treatment with bronchodilators.

RADIOGRAPHIC STUDIES. The findings on chest x-ray during an asthmatic attack are often normal except for the hyperinflation due to increased lung volumes. However, it is important to obtain the film as a means to rule out other lung pathology.

SPUTUM EXAMINATION. Changes in color, thickness, and amount of sputum, together with microscopic evaluation, provide information regarding the presence of infection and the increased number of eosinophils frequently present during an attack.

ARTERIAL BLOOD GASES. Although they are not always indicated immediately, ABGs may be important adjuncts in management decision-making. Although previously discussed, it should be reemphasized that normal oxygenation or mild hypoxemia and hypocapnia are seen initially. Progressive severity and duration of an attack lead to moderate hypoxemia, with normalization of the $PaCO_2$. Eventually, increasingly severe hypoxemia, hypercapnia, and respiratory acidosis occur. The asthmatic who reaches this point of ventilatory failure may require intubation and mechanical ventilation.

PULSE OXIMETRY. Due to the importance of monitoring oxygenation, pulse oximetry is an invaluable tool for the management of acute asthma. With knowledge of the hemoglobin level and direct or indirect estimation of cardiac output, the practitioner can evaluate oxygen transport to body tissues (see Chapter 15).

CAPNOGRAPHY. Noninvasive monitoring of ventilation can be accomplished by measuring end-tidal carbon dioxide levels (see Chapter 15). However, it is not supported as a means of assessing $PaCO_2$ in the acute asthmatic patient. Assessment of the carbon dioxide content component of an electrolyte panel can provide some information related to the presence of acidosis or alkalosis, but direct measurement of $PaCO_2$ via ABGs remains an important clinical tool for optimal evaluation.

Management of Asthma

Whether the patient presents in the emergency room as an outpatient, is already in the hospital for asthma management, or is an inpatient for an unrelated problem, acute, severe attacks require organization, cooperation, and appropriate management.

Treatment goals include:

1. Rapid reversal of airflow obstruction with the repetitive administration of inhaled beta$_2$ agonists and early addition of systemic corticosteroids to relieve respiratory distress
2. Correction of significant hypoxemia with the administration of oxygen
3. Reduction of the rate of future severe attacks by intensifying medication regimens (National Asthma Education Program, 1991) and improving guided self-management or comanagement (the collaboration among patients, families, and health care providers) with effective teaching (Reinke & Hoffman, 1992).

DRUG THERAPY

The fact that multiple drugs are used in the treatment of asthma highlights the difficulty of adequate management. Because the various agents are used differently depending on the severity of airflow obstruction and presence of symptoms a comprehensive discussion of the use of the drugs is beyond the scope of this chapter. Emphasis therefore is placed on their use in acute, severe exacerbation of asthma and in patients with COPD (Table 29–5).

SYMPATHOMIMETICS. The routine use of inhaled beta$_2$ agonists is being increasingly discouraged, because there is increasing belief that they may mask airway inflammation, enhance airway hyperreactivity, and actually accelerate the disease process (Kaliner, 1993). However, these drugs are the backbone of immediate treatment for severe attacks. As beta$_2$ agonists, they have a direct effect on smooth muscle in the airways, producing bronchodilation. They may also inhibit release of inflammatory mediators from mast cells, and may have beneficial effects on mucociliary transport (National Asthma Education Program, 1991).

Inhaled aerosol delivery directly into the lungs allows a reduced dosage and rapid onset with minimal side effects of tachycardia, tremor, nausea, and vomiting. Delivery by nebulizer is preferable. Although metered-dose inhalers with spacers are equally effective, acutely ill patients may not be able to manage them. Intermittent positive pressure breathing devices may be indicated for select patients, but often offer no advantage and may be potentially hazardous.

Because individual patients vary in their response, dose and frequency must be based on maximally stimulating receptors without inducing side effects. Although the duration of activity is 4 to 8 hours, repeat doses at 20- to 30-minute intervals are recommended to produce more consistent bronchodilation. Continuous nebulization is also possible. Maintenance doses every 4 to 6 hours are appropriate after the acute period (Hillman & Bishop, 1993).

The subcutaneous, intravenous, and inhaled administration of epinephrine with both alpha and beta effects may be useful in certain emergency situations. However, its routine use is not substantiated.

CORTICOSTEROIDS. The prophylactic use of steroids is increasingly being emphasized in the long-term management of asthma. This is due to the fact that chronic inflammation is pivotal to the pathogenesis of asthma and steroids are currently the most effective agent available to counteract this. Although their exact mechanism of action remains unknown (they may in-

TABLE 29–5. **Drug Therapy of Asthma**

Drug	Examples	Possible Routes of Administration	Mechanism of Action
Bronchodilators			
Sympathomimetics	Epinephrine Isoproterenol Isoetharine Metaproterenol Terbutaline Albuterol Bitolterol	Inhaled, oral, parenteral (depending on particular drug)	↑ cAMP via stimulation of adenyl cyclase
Xanthines	Theophylline Aminophylline	Oral Oral, parenteral	? ↑ cAMP via inhibition of phosphodiesterase
Anticholinergics	Ipratropium	Inhaled	Blockade of cholinergic (bronchoconstrictor) effect on airways
Mast cell stabilizers			
Cromolyn		Inhaled	Inhibition of mediator release from mast cells; ? additional mechanisms
Antiinflammatory drugs			
Corticosteroids		Oral, parenteral, inhaled	Decreased inflammatory response in airways; ? additional mechanisms

Abbreviation: cAMP, cyclic adenosine monophosphate.
From Weinberger, S. (1992). *Principles of pulmonary medicine* (2nd ed.). Philadelphia: W. B. Saunders.

terfere with various inflammatory mediators), they significantly reduce inflammation and may potentiate the effects of bronchodilators (National Asthma Education Program, 1991).

Intravenous steroids hasten the resolution of severe attacks and for this reason should routinely be administered to these patients without delay. Side effects, including hyperglycemia and hypokalemia, can be minimized with proper monitoring, reduction of dosage, and converting to oral prednisone after a severe, acute attack subsides. Aerosolized, inhaled steroids, now a mainstay for the management of chronic asthma, are not helpful during acute, severe exacerbations (Hillman & Bishop, 1993).

METHYLXANTHINES (THEOPHYLLINE). Although aminophylline and other, similar agents have been used for almost 60 years and are commonly prescribed for asthma today, their exact mechanism of action remains elusive, and their very use is debatable. This is particularly true in relationship to the management of acute, severe asthma (Dellinger, 1991).

Rarely, if ever, should theophylline be used as a first-line drug, because its bronchodilatory effects are minimal. Other theoretical advantages (enhanced contractility of the diaphragm, accelerated mucus transport, and positive inotropic and diuretic effects) have limited relevance in acute, severe asthma. In addition, there is a higher incidence of side effects (headache, nausea, tachyarrhythmias, seizures) than with beta$_2$ agonists, and levels must be monitored due to significant variability in clearance (increased and decreased) with multiple drugs, age, and concomitant conditions. When used for patients with chronic, severe asthma, it helps to sustain bronchodilator effects throughout the night for those with nocturnal exacerbations. Maintaining levels of 5 to 15 μg/mL provides optimal bronchodilation with low incidence of side effects (Hillman & Bishop, 1993).

ANTICHOLINERGICS. Ipratropium bromide inhibits vagal tone and promotes bronchodilation, but is far less effective than beta$_2$ agonists in chronic asthma. Inhaled anticholinergics, used in conjunction with beta$_2$ agonists, may be most useful in severely ill patients with airway obstruction that is unresponsive to beta$_2$ agonists or slowly resolving. Their onset is much slower than the sympathomimetics (15 vs. 1–2 minutes). Side effects are rare due to poor systemic absorption (National Asthma Education Program, 1991).

CROMOLYN SODIUM. Used most frequently in children, cromolyn sodium is helpful as a prophylactic agent but has no role in acute, severe asthma. Cromolyn's effect lies in its ability to stabilize mast cells and inhibit the release of inflammatory mediators. In adults, it may take 1 to 2 months to determine its effectiveness. Because of this potential delay, inhaled steroids are recommended for adults.

OTHER DRUG THERAPY. The use of sedation in the nonintubated patient is potentially dangerous and should be avoided. There is no evidence that mucolytic agents are beneficial in the treatment of acute, severe asthma. Antibiotics, although frequently abused in asthma management, are not indicated unless there is bacterial infection. Magnesium sulfate has demonstrated potential to improve airflow in patients with acute, severe asthma. Last, in dangerously refractory asthma, the use of anesthetic agents in conjunction with mechanical ventilation may be necessary to promote relaxation of the airways and facilitate oxygenation and ventilation (Hillman & Bishop, 1993).

OTHER CLINICAL MANAGEMENT

Although the mainstay of the treatment of acute, severe asthma is pharmaceutical, additional therapeutic interventions are often critical to complement drug therapy and minimize complications. Specific patient problems frequently observed in the critical care setting are related to ineffective breathing patterns resulting in fatigue, ineffective airway clearance, and anxiety. Knowledge deficits are also observed (Wilson & Thompson, 1990).

The asthmatic patient requires interventions to promote optimal gas exchange and prevent fatigue. Patients often present with complaints of dyspnea, possible changes in behavior and level of consciousness, use of accessory muscles, wheezing, tachypnea, and tachycardia related to an ineffective breathing pattern. Along with maintaining oxygen uptake and monitoring vital signs, ABGs, and response to medications, nursing measures such as proper positioning, use of therapeutic breathing techniques, rest periods, and comfort measures are important to maximize oxygen utilization and minimize fatigue.

Inability to adequately clear secretions is a further impediment to optimal gas exchange. Assessing breath sounds and sputum production helps to identify problems, whereas positioning, assisting with therapeutic coughing, and suctioning as needed, facilitate removal of secretions. Dehydration, due to insensible losses with breathing and inability to take in adequate fluids, requires correction to decrease sputum viscosity. Instillation of saline with suctioning may worsen bronchospasm and should be done with caution, if at all. Percussion, vibration, and postural drainage are contraindicated during the acute phase of management because they have not shown effectiveness and may be detrimental. Later, they may be helpful for specific patients (Hillman & Bishop, 1993).

Anxiety related to the fear of suffocation or memories of previous episodes is a common feature of the attack. Simple, yet effective management strategies include identifying and encouraging use of coping mechanisms, allowing the patient to verbalize, staying with the patient, and using comfort and relaxation techniques. Visitors may be particularly helpful, but their presence may also be detrimental. Therefore, astute observation of patient–visitor interactions and appropriate interventions are important.

Methods to decrease knowledge deficits are vital measures throughout the acute phase. This includes the use of simple, yet specific instruction related to treatments and responses. After the acute phase, nurses can be instrumental in providing teaching to promote increased awareness of triggering stimuli, adequate comanagement of the disease, and minimization of future severe exacerbations.

MECHANICAL VENTILATION

Because of the risks involved in using positive pressure ventilation for patients refractory to other forms of treatment, this should be avoided if at all possible. Yet, the continuation of inadequate ventilation as evidenced by increasing fatigue, refractory hypoxemia, hypercapnia, and respiratory acidosis clearly indicates patient deterioration and the need for intubation and mechanical ventilation. The primary goal therefore is to provide optimal gas exchange while minimizing complications. Complications are directly related to the following:

1. Positive intrathoracic pressure—barotrauma (e.g., pneumothorax) and diminished venous return causing a decreased cardiac output
2. Length of time of mechanical ventilation—atelectasis, pneumonia, tracheal damage, inability to wean, and many others (Hillman & Bishop, 1993) (see Chapter 16).

In selected patients, the use of noninvasive positive pressure ventilation may be indicated. This method of management avoids endotracheal intubation and its complications, is tolerated by patients, and improves gas exchange in appropriately selected patients experiencing acute respiratory failure. Its overall effectiveness and role in patient management remain undetermined (Hill, 1993).

Course and Prognosis

Approximately half of all those with childhood asthma recover spontaneously. Beyond childhood, the incidence of spontaneous recovery decreases. When the onset of asthma occurs later in life, most will continue to suffer with its effects for the remainder of their lives. Chronic management can be difficult. For that reason, many will have progressively more frequent attacks. Pathologic changes due to chronic inflammation and obstruction may predispose the person to changes similar to those with COPD.

SUMMARY

The pulmonary patient with chronic compromise to airflow presents multiple opportunities for the clinical management team. More than ever before, with vigilant assessment, appropriate diagnosis, and knowledgeable, research-based care, the team can compassionately assist the patient to optimally manage the disease itself, as well as the individual response to the disease, in a cost-effective fashion. Although this chapter was directed toward the management of these patients in the critical care setting, it must be recognized that even greater management demands exist outside the hospital. Management of these patients presents the team with multiple opportunities and challenges. Fulfillment of these opportunities can be realized by coordinating and refining care to meet the patients' needs as they change, regardless of the location.

REFERENCES

Aberman, A. (1991). A battle plan for acute asthma. *Emergency Medicine, 23*(13), 67–70.

American Lung Association. (1993). *Lung disease data 1993.* New York: American Lung Association.

American Thoracic Society. (1991). Standards of nursing care for adult patients with pulmonary dysfunction. *Review of Respiratory Disease, 144*(1), 231–236.

Barnes, P. J. (1993). Asthma. In R. C. Bone et al. (Eds.), *Pulmonary and critical care medicine* (Vol. 1). St. Louis: C. V. Mosby.

Benhamou, D., et al. (1992). Nasal mask ventilation in acute respiratory failure: Experience in elderly patients. *Chest, 102,* 912–917.

Bott, J., et al. (1993). Randomized controlled trial of nasal ventilation in acute ventilatory failure due to chronic obstructive airways disease. *Lancet, 341,* 1555–1557.

Breslin, E. H., Roy, C., Robinson, C. R. (1992). Physiological nursing research in dyspnea: A paradigm shift and a metaparadigm exemplar. *Scholarly Inquiry for Nursing Practice: An International Journal, 6*(2), 81–103.

Busse, W. W., Calhoun, W. F., & Sedgwick, J. D. (1993). Mechanism of airway inflammation in asthma. *American Review of Respiratory Disease, 147,* S20–S24.

Chin, R., & Pesce, R. (1983). Practical aspects in management of respiratory failure in chronic obstructive pulmonary disease. *Critical Care Quarterly, 6*(2), 1–21.

Dellinger, R. P. (1991). Acute life-threatening asthma. *Postgraduate Medicine, 90*(3), 63–77.

Donahoe, M., & Rogers, R. M. (1995). Acute respiratory failure in chronic obstructive pulmonary disease. In Shoemaker, W. C., et al. (Eds.), *Textbook of critical care* (pp. 836–847). Philadelphia: W. B. Saunders.

Dornhorst, A. C. (1955). Respiratory insufficiency. *Lancet, 1,* 1185.

Farzan, S. (1985). *A concise handbook of respiratory diseases.* Reston, VA: Reston Publishing Co.

Fiore, M. C., Baker, L. J., & Deeren, S. M. (1993). Cigarette smoking: The leading preventable cause of pulmonary diseases. In R. C. Bone, et al. (Eds.), *Pulmonary and critical care medicine* (Vol. 1). St. Louis: C. V. Mosby.

Hagedorn, S. D. (1992). Acute exacerbations of COPD: How to evaluate severity and treat the underlying cause. *Postgraduate Medicine, 91*(1), 105–112.

Hill, N. S. (1993). Noninvasive ventilation: Does it work, for whom, and how. *American Review of Respiratory Disease, 147,* 1050–1055.

Hillman, K., & Bishop, G. (1993). Acute severe asthma. In R. C. Bone et al. (Eds.), *Pulmonary and critical care medicine* (Vol. 1). St. Louis: C. V. Mosby.

Hodgkin, J., & Petty, T. (1987). *Chronic obstructive pulmonary disease: Current concepts.* Philadelphia: W. B. Saunders.

Jess, L. W. (1992). Chronic bronchitis and emphysema: Airing the differences. *Nursing92, 22*(3), 34–41.

Kaliner, M. A. (1993). Evolution of asthma treatments. *Annals of Allergy, 71,* 300–305.

Kaliner, M. A., et al. (1992). Asthma therapy: Into the 1990s. *Patient Care, 26*(1), 69–100.

MacDonnell, K., Fahey, P., & Segal, M. (1987). *Respiratory intensive care.* Boston: Little, Brown & Co.

Martin, R. J. (1993). Nocturnal asthma: Circadian rhythms and therapeutic interventions. *American Review of Respiratory Disease, 147,* S25–S28.

Murphy, T. F., & Sethi, S. (1992). Bacterial infection in chronic obstructive pulmonary disease. *American Review of Respiratory Disease, 146,* 1067–1083.

National Asthma Education Program. (1991). *Executive summary: Guidelines for the diagnosis and management of asthma.* National Institutes of Health Publication No. 91-3042A. Bethesda, MD: U.S. Department of Health and Human Services.

National Center for Health Statistics. (1993b). *Vital and health statistics: Current estimates from the National Health Interview Survey 1992.* DHHS Publication No. (PHS) 94-1517. Hyattsville, MD: U.S. Department of Health and Human Services.

National Center for Health Statistics. (1993a). *Monthly vital statistics report: Advance report of final mortality statistics, 1991* (Vol. 42, No. 2). Hyattsville, MD: Public Health Service.

Nield, M., Kim, M. J., & Patel, M. (1989). Use of magnitude estimation for estimating the parameters of dyspnea. *Nursing Research, 38,* 77–80.

Owens, G. R. (1993). Chronic obstructive pulmonary disease. In R. C. Bone et al. (Eds.), *Pulmonary and critical care medicine* (Vol. 1). St. Louis: C. V. Mosby.

Page, C. P. (1993). An explanation of the asthma paradox. *American Review of Respiratory Disease, 147,* S29–S32.

Pope, C. A., & Kanner, R. E. (1993). Acute effects of pm_{10} pollution on pulmonary function of smokers with mild to moderate chronic obstructive pulmonary disease. *American Review of Respiratory Disease, 147,* 1336–1340.

Reinke, L. F., & Hoffman, L. A. (1992). Breathing space: How to teach asthma co-management. *American Journal of Nursing, 92*(10), 40–51.

Robin, E. D., & O'Neill, R. P. (1963). The fighter versus the nonfighter. *Archives of Environmental Health, 7,* 125.

Rose, W. (1992). Total parenteral nutrition and the patient with chronic obstructive pulmonary disease. *Journal of Intravenous Nursing, 15*(1), 18–23.

Snider, G. L. (1989). Chronic obstructive pulmonary disease: A definition and implications of structural determinants of airflow obstruction for epidemiology. *American Review of Respiratory Disease, 140,* S3–S8.

Tisi, G. (1983). *Pulmonary physiology in clinical medicine* (2nd ed.). Baltimore: Williams & Wilkins.

Weaver, T. E., & Narsavage, G. L. (1992). Physiological and psychological variables related to functional status in chronic obstructive pulmonary disease. *Nursing Research, 41*(5), 286–291.

Wilkins, R. L., & Dexter, J. R. (1993). *Respiratory disease: Principles of patient care.* Philadelphia: F. A. Davis.

Wilson, S. F., & Thompson, J. M. (1990). *Respiratory disorders (Mosby's Clinical Nursing Series).* St. Louis: Mosby–Year Book.

Pulmonary Infections

Catherine J. Ryan

A complex system of body defense mechanisms keep the respiratory tree free of infection. These mechanisms include the cough reflex, ciliary activity, secretion of mucus lysosome, lactoferrin and immunoglobulins, phagocytic cells, and the lung parenchyma containing the lymphatic system. Intensive care unit (ICU) patients, however, quickly become colonized with potentially pathologic microorganisms. In these patients, invasion of the lower airway by a virulent organism combined with failure of one or more of the components of the pulmonary defense system results in a pulmonary infection.

Six possible mechanisms of infection for the lung have been identified: aspiration, colonization, inhalation, inoculation, direct spread from contiguous sites, and hematogenous spread. Factors that predispose persons to the development of serious cases of pneumonia include advanced age, dehydration, coma, weakness, sedation, malnutrition, chronic lung disease, immunosuppression, drugs that impair mucociliary clearance, and bypass of the upper airway with endotracheal intubation and tracheostomy (Stenberg, 1993; Wisinger, 1993). One or more of these factors is present in virtually all critically ill patients.

INCIDENCE

Pneumonia is the sixth leading cause of death in the United States and the number one cause of death from infectious disease (American Thoracic Society, 1993). During the past decade dramatic changes have occurred in the types of patients with pulmonary infections that require intensive care as well as changes in the infecting organisms. The significance of these phenomena is demonstrated in the changing population seen in hospitals today. Persons with health problems not encountered in the past, such as AIDS, organ transplantation, complex cardiovascular procedures, and cancer with immunosuppressive therapy are now patients in our ICUs. Additionally, the elderly population, who are more susceptible to complicated pneumonia (McCue, 1993), is growing at a dramatic rate.

Pathophysiology

Pneumonia is an inflammation of the lung parenchyma caused by any one of a large number of infectious agents. It is common among older patients and those with coexisting illnesses, including chronic obstructive pulmonary disease (COPD), diabetes, renal insufficiency, congestive heart failure (CHF), and chronic liver disease (American Thoracic Society, 1993). Each of the pneumonias has characteristic clinical findings.

In the literature, pneumonias have been categorized in various ways. Clinically, the presentation of pneumonia can be divided into two categories: bacterial pneumonias and atypical pneumonias. This classification is important for selection of the appropriate method of treatment and for prediction of outcome.

Pneumonia has been defined as a foci of consolidation with intense polymorphonuclear leukocyte accumulations in the bronchioles and adjacent alveoli scattered through several lung sections (Meduri, 1990). Generally, pneumonia produces areas of low ventilation with normal perfusion because alveoli fill with exudate. This process produces tracheobronchial edema with increased production of secretions.

COMMON BACTERIAL PNEUMONIAS

Bacteria cause half of the cases of adult pneumonia. Table 30–1 summarizes causative organisms for various types of bacterial pneumonia. It is most commonly seen in the elderly population or in other adults with impaired immunity (Rello et al., 1992). Bacterial pneumonia may be caused by a number of different organisms. Any anatomic or physiologic alteration in the tracheobronchial tree or in the defenses of the host increases the risk of the infecting organism entering the lungs. Many of the organisms capable of invading the lungs are components of the oropharyngeal or nasopharyngeal flora in states of health and disease. A common cause of pneumonia, especially in the elderly and debilitated population, is aspiration of oropharyngeal or gastric secretions, including their flora, into the lower respiratory tract (McCue, 1993).

Streptococcus pneumoniae

Streptococcus pneumoniae (commonly referred to as pneumococcal pneumonia) is a major cause of community-acquired bacterial pneumonia (Ostergaard & Anderson, 1993). It is spread via inhalation of droplets or airborne nuclei, or it may enter the pharynx from the skin through direct contact. Aspirated bacteria bind

TABLE 30–1. **Etiology of Bacterial Pneumonias**

Gram-Positive Cocci	Gram-Positive Rods
Streptococcus pneumoniae	*Nocardia* species
Staphylococcus aureus	*Actinomyces* species
Streptococcus pyogenes	*Bacillus anthracis*
Anaerobes: *Peptococcus, Peptostreptococcus*	
Gram-Negative Cocci	**Gram-Negative Rods**
Neisseria meningitidis	*Haemophilus influenzae*
	Klebsiella pneumoniae
	Pseudomonas aeruginosa
	Escherichia coli
	Acinetobacter species
	Serratia species
	Proteus species
	Enterobacter species
	Legionella species
	Anaerobes: *Bacteroides* species, *Fusobacterium nucleatum*

to the respiratory epithelial cells and produce local edema with transudation into the alveoli. The transudation produces pulmonary congestion as well as an environment where pneumococci may multiply. Adjacent capillaries become congested, and red cells along with polymorphonuclear leukocytes appear in the alveoli (red hepatization). Later, polymorphonuclear leukocytes ingest the pneumococci and fibrin precipitates in the alveoli (gray hepatization). Finally in many cases there is resolution with complete healing as macrophages clear particulate debris, fibrin, and remaining bacteria. Mortality from this type of bacterial pneumonia is 10% to 25% overall and 50% in the debilitated population (Pachon et al., 1990).

Staphylococcal Pneumonia

Staphylococcal pneumonia occurs most often as a secondary infection occurring with or following influenza. It is frequently seen in infants and children under age 3 and in persons who are chronically ill. *Staphylococcus* usually enters the respiratory tract via inhalation of contaminated air or after aspiration of carrier staphylococci from the nasopharynx (Kaye et al., 1990). It may also enter the lungs as a secondary infection after bacteremia from a septic focus elsewhere in the body (Tsao et al., 1992). There are two types of staphylococcal pneumonia, acute hemorrhagic and subacute.

Acute hemorrhagic staphylococcal pneumonia is most frequently seen in association with influenza. In this type, bronchi and bronchioles are stripped of their mucosa and their walls are infiltrated with polymorphonuclear leukocytes, histiocytes, and fibrin. Abscesses may form and rupture into the pleural space to form a fistula or pneumothorax. Empyemas are not an uncommon complication (Kaye et al., 1990).

Subacute staphylococcal pneumonia causes the lungs to become heavy and engorged. A moderate amount of thin fluid may be present in the pleural cavity. The trachea and bronchi become filled with plugs of yellow-gray tenacious exudate. Abscesses that communicate with the bronchi and bronchioles may be a complication (Kaye et al., 1990).

Gram-negative Pneumonia

Gram-negative pneumonia, with mortality reported to be as high as 50% (Potgieter & Hammond, 1992), is frequent in the elderly as well as the chronically ill populations (Meijer et al., 1990). It is most often attributed to microaspiration of oropharyngeal contents (Rello et al., 1991). Colonization of the upper airway and lungs may occur as a result of the use of broad-spectrum antibiotics in patients with endotracheal tubes. The patient with gram-negative pneumonia may follow a chronic course of disease with a slow response to treatment. The healing process often results in fibrosis of lung tissue and loss of functional lung volume.

Nosocomial Pneumonia

Nosocomial pneumonia is an infection of the lower respiratory tract involving the pulmonary parenchyma that develops in hospitalized patients (Rello et al., 1991). Recent studies reveal that the incidence of nosocomial pneumonia in ICU patients ranges from 10% to 65% and mortality may be as high as 55% (Heyland & Mandell, 1992; Kollef, 1993). It is the second most frequent cause of hospital-acquired infection and the leading cause of mortality directly related to nosocomial infection (Montecalvo et al., 1992). Although nosocomial pneumonias may be caused by any bacterial, viral, or fungal organism, most clinical studies show that enterobacteria, Pseudomonas, and other gram-negative organisms are the main causes (Rello et al., 1992; Potgieter & Hammond, 1992; Kollef, 1993; Stenberg, 1993).

Critically ill patients are most likely to acquire nosocomial pneumonia because of their debilitated state, which is often related to age, severity of illness, and altered immune defenses. Other factors in the critical care environment contributing to the development of nosocomial pneumonia include prolonged tracheal or gastric intubation, repeated tracheal intubation, depressed level of consciousness allowing for aspiration of oropharyngeal secretions that often contain gram-negative bacilli, underlying chronic lung disease, thoracic or upper abdominal surgery, prior episode of large volume aspiration, gastric colonization by gram-negative bacilli, poor oral hygiene, supine positioning, and inhibition of the normal cough (Torres et al., 1990, 1993; Kollef, 1993; Ephgrave et al., 1993; Stenberg, 1993). Endotracheal intubation is the most commonly named risk factor for nosocomial pneumonia (Meduri, 1990; Torres et al., 1990, 1993; Montecalvo et al., 1992; Rello et al., 1992; Kollef, 1993) because the endotracheal tube bypasses the upper airway and the host defense mechanisms of nasopharyngeal filtration and mucociliary clearance. Endotracheal tubes and related respiratory procedures such as suctioning may also create mechanical irritation or injury to the mucosa, predisposing the lungs to inoculation and colonization with bacteria (Meijer et al., 1990; Stenberg, 1993). Respiratory therapy equipment and the persons who care for the equipment may also contaminate the respiratory tract.

A number of studies (Torres et al., 1990; Meijer et al., 1990; Heyland & Mandell, 1992; Apte et al., 1992) have shown that elevation of the gastric pH with antacids and H_2 antagonists may increase the risk of developing nosocomial pneumonia in critically ill patients receiving mechanical ventilation. Elevation of the gastric pH provides an environment for gastric colonization with gram-negative bacilli (Maijer et al., 1990). A number of interventions to eliminate this risk factor are under investigation, including: (1) avoidance of agents that would elevate gastric pH, and (2) gastric and oropharyngeal decontamination via administration of nonabsorbable topical antibiotics.

Widespread and often inappropriate use of antibiotics has also been implicated as a predisposing factor to the development of nosocomial pneumonia (Meduri, 1990). Antibiotics cause suppression of normal upper airway flora, which may permit colonization with drug-resistant organisms.

Atypical Pneumonias

There are numerous causes of atypical pneumonia (see Table 30–2). The most common types seen in critical care will be discussed here.

Viral Pneumonia

Viruses are a common cause of community-acquired pneumonia but may also cause pneumonia in patients who are already hospitalized. Paramyxoviruses are most common in younger populations. Influenza A or B virus is more common in adults and the elderly (McCue, 1993). Transmission occurs by inhalation of aerosolized virus. The virus enters the respiratory tract, attaches to columnar epithelial cells, and replicates with a cycle of 4 to 6 hours. Particles of the replicated viruses are shed, causing illness to occur in 18 to 72 hours after exposure to the virus. The severity of the illness correlates with the quantity of the virus shed and the amount of ciliated columnar epithelial cells damaged (denuded airway) as a result of viral replication. Severe forms of viral pneumonia are more common in pregnant women and persons with cardiovascular disease. Severe viral pneumonia has been shown to carry a mortality rate as high as 50% because it may rapidly progress to a clinical picture of adult respiratory distress syndrome (American Thoracic Society, 1993).

The denuded airway tissue is also more susceptible to colonization and infection by bacteria. The phenomena of secondary bacterial infection in viral pneumonia is more commonly noted in patients with underlying chronic pulmonary disease and the elderly population (McCue, 1993). *Pneumococcus* (*Streptococcus*) and *Staphylococcus aureus* are the secondary bacterial organisms most frequently isolated.

TABLE 30–2. **Etiology of Atypical Pneumonias**

Viruses	Mycoplasma
Paramyxovirus	*Mycoplasma pneumoniae*
Respiratory syncytial virus	
Parainfluenza virus types 1, 2, 3, and 4	**Protozoa**
Influenza viruses A and B	*Pneumocystis carinii*
Adenovirus	*Toxoplasma gondii*
Rhinovirus	
Varicella-zoster virus	**Other**
Herpes simplex virus	*Strongyloides* species
Measles virus	
Coxsackie viruses A and B	
Echovirus	
Cytomegalovirus	

Pneumocystis carinii

Pneumocystis carinii pneumonia is an opportunistic infection whose infecting organism may be a protozoan or a fungus (Henry & Holzemer, 1992; Timby, 1992). The infection was noted to occur primarily in severely immunosuppressed persons who were undergoing chemotherapy until the discovery of AIDS in 1981. Since that time it has become possibly the most well known and most commonly recognized opportunistic pulmonary infection in patients with AIDS (Henry & Holzemer, 1992; Janson-Bjerklie et al., 1992).

P. carinii pneumonia is primarily an alveolar process in which the alveoli are filled with a proteinaceous material that contains cysts and trophozoites (Henry & Holzemer, 1992). Studies show that the risk of *P. carinii* pneumonia is greatly increased once the level of $CD4^+$ lymphocytes falls to 200 / mm^3 (Weinberger, 1993a). Persons with AIDS possess complex immunologic abnormalities that encompass all arms of the immune system. Research suggests that the human immunodeficiency virus (HIV) locks onto alveolar macrophages and monocytes, are antigen presenting cells required for optimal immune responses to invading pathogens, in patients with AIDS, producing an immune deficit (Timby, 1992) that allows the lungs to be infected with *P. carinii.*

Clinical Presentation

The classic symptoms of pneumonia—fever, cough, leukocytosis, and appearance of a new or progressive pulmonary infiltrate—may present with an acute or chronic onset. The clinical presentation of the patient with pneumonia is varied because unique properties of the interaction between the host and the organism determine the presentation (Wisinger, 1993).

Accurate diagnosis of pneumonia generally requires a combination of clinical observations, micro-

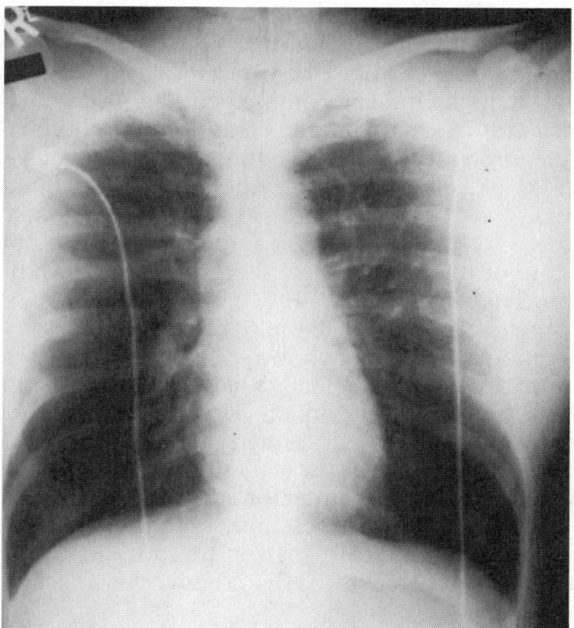

FIGURE 30–1. Chest x-ray of a female patient with bacterial pneumonia. There is a prominent infiltrate in the right base and atelectasis in the upper left lobe.

biological findings, and radiographic findings (Figs. 30–1 and 30–2). Signs and symptoms of infection may be absent in the immunocompromised or elderly patient (McCue, 1993; Stanley, 1992; Stenberg, 1993). The classic symptoms of pneumonia may be unreliable in patients receiving mechanical ventilation because these patients commonly develop other clinical conditions that may also present with fever, pulmonary infiltrates, or production of purulent secretions (Meduri, 1990; Meduri et al., 1992; Stenberg, 1993).

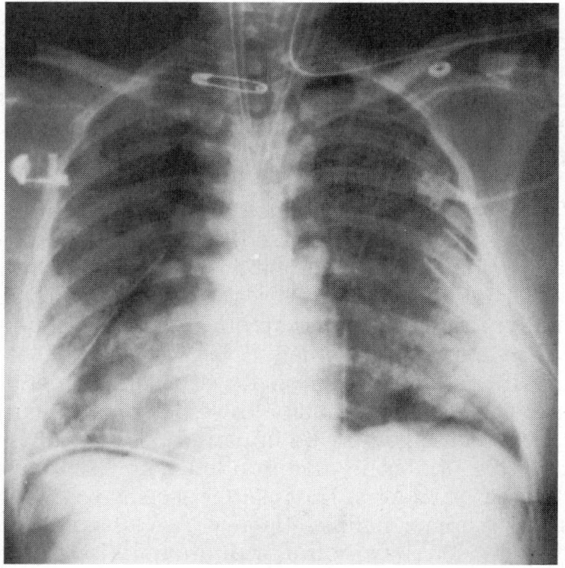

FIGURE 30–2. Chest x-ray of a female patient with viral pneumonia showing diffuse interstitial infiltrates bilaterally.

BACTERIAL PNEUMONIAS

The patient with pneumococcal pneumonia presents with a sudden onset of illness that includes shaking chills, fever of 102° to 105°F (38.8° to 40.5°C), a cough that is initially dry but becomes productive of rusty sputum early and yellow-green sputum later (Wisinger, 1993). Rusty sputum is caused by a mixture of red blood cells (RBCs) and inflammatory cells in infected alveoli. The patient may be dyspneic, tachypneic, diaphoretic, tachycardiac, and cyanotic, and have pleuritic chest pain that is worse on inspiration and with coughing. Accompanying symptoms include malaise, weakness, headache, myalgia, and possibly cyanosis depending on the degree of respiratory compromise. The elderly patient may also present with altered mental state and dehydration.

Complications involve dissemination of the bacteria into a site other than the lungs, causing meningitis, endocarditis, empyema, disseminated intravascular coagulation, lung abscess, or nephritis. Haemophilus influenzae may mimic pneumococcal pneumonia.

Chest examination in the patient with pneumococcal pneumonia will reveal consolidation manifest by dullness to percussion; increased tactile fremitus (palpable vibrations transmitted through the bronchopulmonary system to the chest wall when the patient speaks); bronchophony (voice sounds louder and clearer than usual because the higher pitched components are better transmitted through airless lung tissue); course inspiratory crackles; egophony ("ee" to "ay" change because of altered filtration of sound); and whispered pectoriloquy (whispered sounds louder and more clearly heard than normal because of enhanced transmission through airless lung tissue) indicating that air is being replaced with exudate, and crepitant rales. A pleural friction rub may be present. Pneumococcal pneumonia takes some time to resolve, with consolidation in the lungs taking up to 6 weeks to clear completely.

Staphylococcal pneumonia has an insidious onset in chronically ill and elderly patients and an acute onset in infants. High fever with chills may last up to 1 week in severe cases despite the use of antibiotics. Early in the course of the disease, tachypnea with cyanosis and cough with production of blood-streaked sputum occur; the airways are stripped of mucosa and ulcerated. Lung abscesses and cavitation are not uncommon with this type of pneumonia (Kaye et al., 1990).

The patient with gram-negative bacterial pneumonia has a highly variable clinical presentation dependent on the patient's underlying condition and the infecting organism. It may progress slowly or rapidly over a few days. Patients will have fever with cough that is productive of purulent sputum and pleuritic chest pain as with other bacterial pneumonias. Mortality is most often related to concomitant host disease rather than to the type of gram-negative infection.

ATYPICAL PNEUMONIAS

In contrast to bacterial pneumonia, only 50% of patients with viral pneumonia will have clinical manifestations. Those that do will present with a gradual onset of symptoms and a milder course of illness. The symptoms include rhinorrhea, a dry cough, low grade fever without chills, pharyngitis, and muscle pain (Johnson & Cunha, 1993). Myalgias are the hallmark of influenza A. If sputum is present, it will be scanty and nonpurulent. The chest examination of the patient with viral pneumonia will reveal crackles and rhonchi. In fulminating cases of viral pneumonia, however, the alveoli are filled with fibrin, fluid, RBCs, and macrophages, which causes profound hypoxemia that may respond poorly to oxygen administration.

Pneumocystis carinii pneumonia presents with nonspecific chronic respiratory symptoms that have a more gradual onset. The symptoms include a nonproductive cough, fever, dyspnea, and pulmonary infiltrates (Henry & Holzemer, 1992; Timby, 1992). The patient with *P. carinii* pneumonia may have inspiratory crackles but frequently has normal breath sounds. The patient may be tachypneic.

Laboratory Findings/Diagnostic Procedures

Sputum evaluation is a critical part of the evaluation of the patient with pneumonia. Care must be taken when collecting the sputum culture to avoid the collection of saliva because it can be colonized with many of the organisms that cause pneumonia and be misleading. In addition, previous antibiotic treatment may affect the bacterial culture and inhibit identification of the organism (Meduri, 1990; Meduri et al., 1992). Early morning specimens are preferred because secretions that have pooled during the night can be mobilized. A sputum sample with >25 polymorphonuclear leukocytes and <10 squamous epithelial cells per 100× field is considered to be from the lower respiratory tract and diagnostic of pneumonia (Meduri, 1990; McCue, 1993). If it is impossible to collect an acceptable specimen using traditional methods (cough or endotracheal or nastotracheal tube suction) the physician may elect to obtain a specimen by more invasive means, such as transtracheal aspiration, fiberoptic bronchoscopy with bronchoalveolar lavage or brushed specimens, or open lung biopsy (Meduri, 1990). Serologic studies may reveal a diagnosis when positive microbiologic diagnosis cannot be made.

BACTERIAL PNEUMONIAS

The Gram stain of the sputum helps to determine initial therapy of the patient with bacterial pneumonia. Later verification is required by culture and sensitivity testing. Arterial blood gases (ABGs) may be normal or show significant desaturation depending on the extent of the pneumonia and the presence of other pulmonary pathology. Other laboratory tests helpful in diagnosis may include a complete blood count (CBC), blood cultures, and antigen assays of body fluids. The white blood cell (WBC) count is usually elevated (12,000–30,000/mL) but may be normal in debilitated persons. If a significant pleural effusion is seen on chest x-ray, thoracentesis may be indicated to obtain culture of the pleural fluid (Pachon et al., 1990; Bates et al., 1992; Weinberger, 1993).

The chest x-ray of the patient with pneumococcal pneumonia classically shows a dense infiltrate of one or more lobes or the "patchy" pattern of bronchopneumonia with no consolidation. This pattern may not be seen in the patient with underlying COPD.

The chest x-ray of the patient with gram-negative pneumonia will show interstitial infiltrates early in the course of the disease.These may be unilateral or bilateral and will rapidly progress to consolidation that may be confused with CHF and atelectasis.

ATYPICAL PNEUMONIAS

Traditional laboratory tests will not reveal a diagnosis in viral pneumonia. The total leukocyte count may rise with a neutrophilia and relative lymphopenia with the first 48 hours but will quickly return to normal. Therefore, if the WBC count is performed early in the course of the disease, it will not be significantly elevated. ABGs usually show no arterial desaturation. Although viral pneumonia may be suspected clinically, the diagnosis can only be confirmed with serologic studies, which may take several days to complete. The chest x-ray of the patient with viral pneumonia will show scattered and diffuse interstitial infiltrates involving one or more lobes. Infiltrates are most common in the lower lobes and represent inflammation of pulmonary interstitial areas.

Respiratory complications are among the most common clinical problems in the patient with AIDS. More than one organism is frequently involved in the pulmonary pathology, and thus the diagnosis of *P. carinii* may not be classic. Evaluation of a sputum specimen is the first procedure to be done and may be diagnostic in as many as 50% to 80% of the cases (Weinberger, 1993b). The yield is higher when immunofluorescence stains are used. The typical chest x-ray pattern of *P. carinii* pneumonia is diffuse interstitial or alveolar infiltrates. However, a variety of atypical presentations are not uncommonly seen (Weinberger, 1993b; Henry & Holzemer, 1993; Timby, 1992), especially in patients treated with aerosolized pentamidine. $Pa{O_2}$ may be normal or low when breathing room air. Gas exchange may be impaired because air is unevenly distributed in alveoli filled with *P. carinii* and inflammatory debris. The result is seen as ventilation/perfusion abnormalities (Henry & Holzemer, 1992; Timby, 1992). The amount of pulmonary involvement by *P. carinii* is best evaluated through pulmonary function studies, which will show changes consistent with diffuse alveolar disease. Inflammation decreases pulmonary compliance (Henry & Holzemer, 1992), resulting in decreased total lung capacity, vital capacity, and single breath diffusing capacity for carbon monoxide and increase in expiratory flow rates (Henry & Holzemer, 1992). Other laboratory findings include $CD4^+$ cell count $\leq 200/mm^3$, elevated lactate dehydrogenase (LDH), and elevated erythrocyte sedimentation rate.

Clinical Management

PREVENTION MEASURES

The previous discussion has demonstrated that nearly all patients admitted to the critical care unit who do not already have a pulmonary infection have a potential to develop pneumonia. With this in mind, patient management must first be aimed at prevention of pneumonia. The clinical management team must be aware of the risk factors previously described that lead to the development of pneumonia and which patients are susceptible. Whan caring for susceptible patients, careful attention to aseptic technique, including handwashing and handling of respiratory equipment, must be taken to prevent spread and cross contamination among patients (Meijer et al., 1990). In addition, the pulmonary hygiene measures of frequent turning, coughing and deep breathing exercises, as well as early mobilization of patients on bed rest, must be facilitated. Lateral rotational therapy beds may be indicated for patients who cannot be mobilized or turned.

Assessment of the airway protective mechanisms (cough, gag, and swallowing reflexes) is essential to identify the patient at risk for aspiration of oral secretions and gastric contents. Special attention to oral care may prevent colonization of the oral cavity with gram-negative organisms. Positioning with the head of the bed elevated will decrease gastric reflux and facilitate swallowing. The supine position should be avoided (Kollef, 1993).

Careful and frequent assessment of the temperature, pulse, respiratory rate, chest sounds, and chest x-ray, along with observation of the sputum that is produced, will assist in prompt identification of the development of a pulmonary infection.

TREATMENT MEASURES

When the diagnosis of pneumonia has been made, the focus of care will change to provision of appropriate therapy, maintenance of adequate oxygenation, and prevention of complications. Management of the patient with pneumonia is specific to the needs of the individual patient.

Antibiotic therapy is the basis of medical therapy, but use of empiric broad-spectrum antibiotics in patients at high risk for infection but without infection facilitates colonization and superinfection with more virulent organisms (Meduri, 1990; Meduri et al., 1992). Identification of appropriate antibiotic therapy, prompt administration, and monitoring of the patient response to this therapy must occur in concert with treatment of concomitant medical disorders.

Provision of respiratory support is essential in the care of the patient with a pulmonary infection. Pulmonary treatment begins with providing humidified oxygen. Supplemental oxygen assists to reverse hypoxemia and improves tissue oxygenation; humidification liquefies secretions and assists the patient in secretion mobilization. ABGs must be evaluated and monitored. Continued arterial desaturation with $Po_2 < 60$ mm Hg and a rising Pco_2 indicate that the patient may need to be intubated and mechanically ventilated (see Chapter 31).

AIRWAY PATENCY

The additional pulmonary secretions produced have a potential to compromise the patency of the airway. Airway management techniques include assessment of the effectiveness of the cough, chest percussion and drainage for improved sputum clearance, and possibly nasotracheal or endotracheal suctioning for the patient who is unable to clear secretions. Bronchodilators may be prescribed to promote patency of the airways, but cough suppressants should be avoided unless the cough interferes with rest. The patient should also be placed in a comfortable position for breathing, preferably with the head of the bed elevated. Assessment techniques to evaluate the effectiveness of these measures include observation of the respiratory rate, depth, and use of accessory muscles for breathing; color; and circulation as well as evaluation of the ABGs.

FLUID BALANCE

The patient with a pulmonary infection may also have a poor oral intake and intravascular volume depletion related to increased insensible loss from fever and possible mouth breathing. Assessment of the patient's total volume status and provision of additional fluids is essential. Adequate hydration is critical to maintain intravascular volume. It will also enhance secretion removal because secretions will be thinned and liquefied. Intravenous fluid therapy is necessary for the patient who is unable to ingest adequate amounts of oral fluids. Nutritional assessment must also be done (see Chapter 33 and Chapter 47). If the patient is unable to ingest adequate nutrition orally, enteral or parenteral nutrition must be considered.

Pharmacologic Treatment

Table 30–3 summarizes the pharmacologic treatments commonly recommended for pneumonia. A vaccine is available for pneumococcal pneumonia. It is recommended prophylactically in high-risk groups, including the elderly, those with chronic lung disease, CHF, renal failure, alcoholism, cirrhosis, splenic dysfunction

TABLE 30–3. **Commonly Prescribed Pharmacologic Treatment Specific to Causative Organism**

Organism	Antibiotic
Streptococcus pneumoniae (Pneumococcus)	Penicillin Alternatives: erythromycin, cephalosporin
Staphylococcus aureus	Nafcillin Alternatives: vancomycin, cephalosporin
Haemophilus influenzae	Ampicillin or cefamandole Alternative: trimethoprim-sulfamethoxazole
Escherichia coli	Gentamicin Alternatives: ampicillin, cephalosporin
Klebsiella pneumoniae	Gentamicin with cephalosporin Alternative: chloramphenicol
Pseudomonas aeruginosa	Gentamicin and penicillin Alternatives: gentamicin with cephalosporin
Pneumocystis carinii	Trimethoprim-sulfamothaxazide with or without pentamidine
Virus	Amantadine
Mycobacterium tuberculosis	Isoniazid and rifampin Alternatives: streptomycin, ethambutol, pyrazinamide, ethionamide, cycloserine, *p*-aminosalicylic acid, kanamycin, or capreomycin

From American Thoracic Society, 1993; Henry & Holzemer, 1992; Johnson & Cunha, 1993; Kent, 1993; McCue, 1993; Pachon et al., 1990; Wisinger, 1993.

or splenectomy, Hodgkin's disease, myeloma, and other immunocompromised states. The vaccine should only be given once to adults to avoid significant adverse reactions. Influenza vaccines are also available.

Because *P. carinii* pneumonia occurs primarily in patients with decreased $CD4^+$ counts, the Public Health Service task force recommends prophylaxis against *P. carinii* for HIV-infected persons who have had an episode of *P. carinii* pneumonia or those with $CD4^+$ levels $\leq 200/mm^3$ (Weinberger, 1993). Steroid therapy for HIV-infected patients with respiratory failure remains controversial (Henry & Holzemer, 1992; Weinberger, 1993).

TUBERCULOSIS

Pathophysiology

Tuberculosis (TB) is a serious pulmonary infection whose increasing incidence is causing great concern among health care providers. Before the mid-1980s it was seen most frequently in large cities in areas of poverty and overcrowding. Since 1985, primary infection with TB has increased dramatically (Centers for Disease Control and Prevention, 1993a) in populations at risk, including patients with AIDS, the homeless, the elderly (especially those in nursing homes), minorities, immigrants, and prisoners (Ellner et al., 1993; Weinberger, 1993b). Another recent development is the emergence of multidrug-resistant TB in high-risk populations (Ellner et al., 1993; Jacobs & Starke, 1993).

Mycobacterium tuberculosis is a slow-growing, acid-fast, non–spore-forming bacillus (Marks, 1993). Tuberculosis differs from the other bacterial pulmonary infections because it is a chronic condition that may also affect other organs.

Tuberculosis is an infiltrative disease caused by the tubercle bacillus (*Mycobacterium tuberculosis*). It is spread by droplets from persons infected with cavitary tuberculosis being transmitted through the air and inhaled into the alveoli. In the alveoli, the tubercle bacilli eventually cause a cellular immune response with dilation of the capillaries and moderate swelling of epithelial cells and an increase in fibrin, macrophages, and polymorphonuclear lymphoctyes. The organism grows slowly, spreads to the regional lymph nodes, and within several weeks disseminates via the bloodstream (Dunlap & Briles, 1993). In most instances, cell-mediated immunity to the organism develops and halts further bacterial replication. This prevents clinical development of the disease at that time even though live tubercle bacilli remain in the body. The remaining bacilli may proliferate and cause clinical disease when cell-mediated immunity is weakened long after the initial infection. When cell-mediated immunity does not halt bacterial replication, the organism will infiltrate the alveolar structure. A process of necrosis termed caseation, which is characteristic of tuberculosis, may occur. Infiltration usually occurs in the upper zones of the lung tissues (Weinberger, 1993b) and creates inflammation. The tubercular lesion in the lung may persist as a granuloma, may progress through caseation (necrosis of the center of the lesion), or may heal as a scar. Often the hilar lymph nodes are involved in the infection.

Clinical Presentation

In early stages, the patient may be asymptomatic. As the disease progresses, malaise, fatigue, weight loss, night sweats, cough, and hemoptysis develop (Ellner et al., 1993). In fulminant cases, alveolar and reticular infiltrates and cavitation are seen (Ellner et al., 1993).

Laboratory Findings/Diagnostic Procedures

The chest x-ray is variable but classically will demonstrate cavitary upper lobe infiltrates (Weinberger, 1993a). Diagnosis requires demonstration of the organism in sputum or other body fluid culture. Because the bacterium is very slow growing, it may take several weeks to identify the organism by culture (Ellner et al., 1993). A presumptive diagnosis is made when acid-fast bacilli can be demonstrated with special stains of sputum or other body fluids. Newer tests that show promise for more rapid identification include nucleic acid probes, restriction fragment length polymorphism (RFLP), and polymerase chain reaction (PCR) (Marks, 1993; Ellner et al., 1993). A tuberculin skin test will be positive within 6 weeks of infection in most cases and is therefore of little use in diagnosis of active infection.

Clinical Management

Patient management is primarily aimed at prevention and identification of asymptomatic individuals. Most persons with positive skin reactions to standard tuberculin tests have been infected but may not have clinical symptoms (Miller, 1993; Dunlap & Briles, 1993). Because curative or preventive therapy for TB involves treatment for ≥6 months, compliance to prescribed drug therapy may be a significant problem (Ellner et al., 1993). Nurses can be instrumental in facilitating care, including adherence to the prolonged medication regimen (Pozsik, 1993) and compliance with follow-up chest x-rays (Etkind, 1993).

In 1993 the Occupational Health and Safety Administration mandated a strict method for hospital TB control. The guidelines include immediate development of specialized isolation rooms that have negative pressure and use of high efficiency particulate air filter masks for patients with known or suspected TB infections (Occupational Safety and Health Administration, 1993; Centers for Disease Control and Prevention, 1993b; US Dept of Health & Human Services, 1991).

Special pulmonary treatments are usually not necessary for patients with TB. If, however, the patient develops respiratory compromise, medical management is the same as it would be for pneumonia.

Pharmacologic Treatments

Active TB is treated with combination therapy antitubercular drugs. Isoniazid and rifampin (Brausch & Bass, 1993; Peloquin, 1993) are the most potent agents used to treat tuberculosis, but streptomycin, ethambutol, pyrazinamide, ethionamide, cycloserine, *p*-aminosalicylic acid, kanamycin, or capreomycin may be chosen (Peloquin, 1993; Brausch & Bass, 1993; Ellner et al., 1993). Treament is continued for several months because the organism is slow growing and has long periods of inactivity.

Drug-resistant TB organisms are a major concern in the urban poor and in developing countries. Drug-resistant TB is defined as resistance to one or more first-line antitubercular medications in persons not known to have had previous treatment with antitubercular drugs (Kent, 1993). Drug resistance, caused by random chromosomal mutations, is thought to be due to erratic or incomplete treatment of TB, which creates an environment that favors the growth of drug-resistant bacilli over drug-sensitive bacilli (Kent, 1993). Drug-resistant strains are transmitted in the same manner as drug-sensitive strains. For this reason, all TB isolates must be evaluated for drug sensitivity.

ASPIRATION PNEUMONITIS

Pathophysiology

Pneumonitis is defined as an inflammatory response in the lungs caused by physical or chemical irritation. Aspiration pneumonitis occurs in three different forms: acute chemical aspiration pneumonitis, which is also known as septic pneumonitis or Mendelson syndrome; chronic aspiration pneumonia; and lipoid pneumonia.

Acute chemical aspiration pneumonitis is caused by inhalation of large amounts of gastric contents, primarily hydrochloric acid, into the lungs, resulting in a severe, almost instantaneous, inflammatory response. The pneumonitis is characterized by degeneration of the bronchial epithelium, pulmonary edema, hemorrhage, isolated areas of atelectasis, and necrosis of type I alveolar cells. In 24 to 36 hours, alveolar consolidation is seen and the airways may begin mucosal sloughing. Hyaline membrane appears after 48 hours. By 72 hours, resolution has begun with regeneration of bronchial epithelium.

Chronic aspiration pneumonia leads to localized consolidation of dependent portions of the lungs or bilaterally of the midzones from repeated aspiration of small quantities of infected pharyngeal secretions. It is common in alcoholics, drug abusers, and obtunded patients. Lung abscess is a common outcome.

Lipoid aspiration pneumonia is a result of aspiration of milk- or oil-based substances such as oily nosedrops. Oily substances can be easily aspirated because the material may pass through the vocal cords without exciting the protective cough reflex. Lipoid aspiration pneumonia often occurs in elderly persons with swallowing defects.

Clinical Presentation

Gastric acid aspiration causes aspiration pneumonitis with a rapid onset of dyspnea, bronchospasm, wheezing, fever, leukocytosis, and production of frothy nonpurulent sputum. This will usually occur within 2 to 5 hours of aspiration (Khawaja et al., 1992). The pH of the aspirate appears to be the single most important factor in producing disease. In acute gastric acid aspiration, the patient may become severely hypoxic with a low Pa_{O_2}. The patient may have a normal or low Pa_{CO_2}. Hypoxemia is thought to be caused by a reflex airway closure in response to aspiration of fluid. The chest x-ray will show infiltrates in the dependent lung segments. The endotracheal secretions will be profuse and have an acid pH. Localized consolidation of dependent portions of the lungs is characteristic of chronic aspiration pneumonitis. If aspiration is allowed to continue, necrosis and abscess formation are common.

In lipoid aspiration the chest x-ray shows chronic consolidation that resembles carcinoma. These patients may not appear acutely ill and often have a clinical presentation very similar to that of the patient with a mild case of bacterial pneumonia.

Clinical Management

Because aspiration pneumonitis carries a high mortality, management is primarily aimed at prevention. The ability of each patient to swallow and manage secretion must be carefully evaluated in patients at risk. High-risk groups include patients with a decreased level of consciousness, patients receiving tube feedings, and patients with neuromuscular disorders. Prophylactic endotracheal intubation may be suggested for these high-risk groups. Appropriate positioning during feeding and procedures is essential. Elevation of the head of the bed will decrease gastropharyngeal reflux. Parenteral nutrition via gastrostomy or jejunostomy tubes should be considered for patients who aspirate tube feedings despite appropriate positioning. If gastrostomy or jejunostomy feeding is not possible, use of the smallest-bore feeding tube possible is recommended.

As soon as possible after aspiration, the airway must be suctioned to remove any aspirated material and stimulate coughing. ABGs and shunt studies assess the degree of respiratory embarrassment. If the patient is alert, ventilation with continuous positive airway pressure via mask may be attempted to restore adequate Po_2. Intubation with a cuffed endotracheal tube is recommended to restore adequate oxygenation and to protect the airway from further aspiration in the patient who is not able to manage secretions. Mechanical positive pressure ventilation may be necessary to reverse arterial hypoxemia (see Chapter 33). Fluid therapy is necessary to replace intravascular volume lost to pulmonary edema.

Pharmacologic Treatments

Bronchodilators are used for patients who develop bronchospasms as a result of aspiration. Patients with aspiration do not always develop an infectious pneumonia that can be treated with antibiotics and therefore antibiotics are held until a specific organism can be identified.

SUMMARY

Pulmonary infections remain a significant problem in the critical care environment despite recent advances in pharmacologic treatments and newer therapeutic interventions. In fact, advances in treatment, including ventilatory support equipment, immunosuppressive therapy, and widespread use of antibiotics, have created new populations at risk for the development of pulmonary infections. Nurses can make a significant contribution to patient care and cost containment through early identification of persons at risk, prevention, and aggressive management of persons with pulmonary infections.

REFERENCES

American Thoracic Society. (1993). Guidelines for the initial management of adults with community-acquired pneumonia: Diagnosis, assessment of severity, and initial antimicrobial therapy. *American Review of Respiratory Diseases, 148,* 1418–1426.

Apte, N. M., Karnad, D. R., Medhekar, T. P., Tilve, G. H., Morye, S., & Bhave, G. G. (1992). Gastric colonization and pneumonia in intubated critically ill patients receiving stress ulcer prophylaxis: A randomized, controlled trial. *Critical Care Medicine, 20*(5), 590–593.

Bates, J. H., Campbell, G. D., Barron, A. L., McCracken, G. A., Morgan, P. N., Moses, E. B., & Davis, C. M. (1992). Microbial etiology of acute pneumonia in hospitalized patients. *Chest, 101*(4), 1005–1012.

Brausch, L. M., & Bass, J. B. (1993). The treatment of tuberculosis. *Medical Clinics of North America, 77*(6), 1277–1288.

Centers for Disease Control and Prevention. (1993a). Tuberculosis morbidity—United States—1992. *JAMA, 270*(13), 1525.

Centers for Disease Control and Prevention. (1993b). Draft guidelines for preventing the transmission of tuberculosis in health care facilities (2nd ed.). Notice of comment period. *Federal Register, 58,* 52810–52854.

Dunlap, N. E., & Briles, D. E. (1993). Immunology of tuberculosis. *Medical Clinics of North America, 77*(6), 1235–1252.

Ellner, J. J., Hinman, A. R., Dooley, S. W., Fischl, M. A., Sepkowitz, K. A., Goldberger, M. J., Shinnick, T. M., Iseman, M. D., & Jacobs, W. R. (1993). Tuberculosis Symposium: Emerging problems and promise. *Journal of Infectious Diseases, 168*(3), 537–551.

Ephgrave, K. S., Kleiman-Wexler, U., Pfaller, M., Booth, B., Werkmeister, L., & Young, S. (1993). Postoperative pneumonia: A prospective study of risk factors and morbidity. *Surgery, 114*(4), 815–821.

Etkind, S. C. (1993). The role of public health department in tuberculosis. *Medical Clinics of North America, 77*(6), 1303–1314.

Henry, S. B., & Holzemer, W. L. (1992). Critical care management of the patient with HIV infection who has *Pneumocystis carinii* pneumonia. *Heart & Lung, 21*(3), 243–249.

Heyland, D., & Mandell, L. A. (1992). Gastric colonization by gram-negative bacilli and nosocomial pneumonia in the intensive care unit patient. *Chest, 101*(1), 187–193.

Jacobs, R. F., & Starke, J. R. (1993). Tuberculosis in children. *Medical Clinics of North America, 77*(6), 1335–1352.

Janson-Bjerklie, S., Holzemer, W., & Henry, S. B. (1992). Patients' perceptions of pulmonary problems and nursing interventions during hospitalization for *Pneumocystis carinii* pneumonia. *American Journal of Critical Care, 1*(1), 114–121.

Johnson, D. H., & Cunha, B. A. (1993). Atypical pneumonias: Clinical and extrapulmonary features of chlamydia, mycoplasma, and legionella infections. *Postgraduate Medicine, 93*(7), 69–82.

Kaye, M. G., Fox, M. J., Bartlett, J. G., Braman, S. S., & Glassroth, J. (1990). The clinical spectrum of *Staphylococcus aureus* pulmonary infection. *Chest, 97*(4), 788–792.

Kent, J. H. (1993). The epidemiology of multidrug-resistant tuberculosis in the United States. *Medical Clinics of North America, 77*(6), 1391–1409.

Khawaja, I. T., Buffa, S. D., & Brandstetter, R. D. (1992). Aspiration pneumonia: A threat when deglutition is compromised. *Postgraduate Medicine, 92*(1), 165–177.

Kollef, M. H. (1993). Ventilator-associated pneumonia: A multivariate analysis. *JAMA, 270*(16), 1965–1970.

Marks, G. L. (1993). Genetics of tuberculosis. *Medical Clinics of North America, 77*(6), 1219–1234.

McCue, J. (1993). Pneumonia in the elderly: Special considerations in a special population. *Postgraduate Medicine, 94*(5), 39–51.

Meduri, G. U. (1990). Ventilator-associated pneumonia in patients with respiratory failure: A diagnostic approach. *Chest, 97*(5), 1208–1219.

Meduri, G. U., Wunderink, R. G., Leeper, K. V., & Beals, D. H. (1992). Management of bacterial pneumonia in ventilated patients: Protected bronchoalveolar lavage as a diagnostic tool. *Chest, 101*(2), 500–508.

Meijer, K., van Saene, H. K. F., & Hill, J. C. (1990). Infection control in patients undergoing mechanical ventilation: Traditional approach versus a new development—selective decontamination of the digestive tract. *Heart & Lung, 19*(1), 11–20.

Miller, B. (1993). Preventive therapy for tuberculosis. *Medical Clinics of North America, 77*(6), 1263–1276.

Montecalvo, M. A., Steger, K. A., Farber, H. W., Smith, B. F., Dennis, R. C., Fitzpatrick, G. F., Pollack, S. D., Korsberg, T. Z., Birkett, D. H., Hirsch, E. F., & Craven, D. E. (1992). Nutritional outcome and pneumonia in critical care patients randomized to gastric versus jejunal tube feedings. *Critical Care Medicine, 20*(10), 1377–1387.

Occupational Safety and Health Administration. (1993). *Enforcement policy and procedure for occupational exposure to tuberculosis.* Supplement A & B, 1–9.

Ostergaard, L., & Anderson, P. L. (1993). Etiology of community-acquired pneumonia: Evaluation of transtracheal aspiration, blood culture, or serology. *Chest, 104*(5), 1400–1407.

Pachon, J., Prados, M. D., Capote, F., Cuello, J. A., Garnacho, J., & Verano, A. (1990). Severe community-acquired pneumonia: Etiology, prognosis and treatment. *American Review of Respiratory Diseases, 142,* 369–373.

Peloquin, C. A. (1993). Pharmacology of the antimycobacterial drugs. *Medical Clinics of North America, 77*(6), 1253–1262.

Potgieter, P. D., & Hammond, M. J. (1992). Etiology and diagnosis of pneumonia requiring ICU admission. *Chest, 101*(1), 199–203.

Pozsik, C. J. (1993). Compliance with tuberculosis therapy. *Medical Clinics of North America, 77*(6), 1289–1302.

Rello, J., Quintana, E., Ausina, V., Castella, J., Laquin, M., Net, A., & Prats, G. (1991). Incidence, etiology, and outcome of nosocomial pneumonia in mechanically ventilated patients. *Chest, 100*(2), 439–444.

Rello, J., Ricart, M., Ausina, V., Net, A., & Prats, G. (1992). *Chest, 102*(5), 1562–1565.

Stanley, M. (1992). Elderly patients in critical care: An overview. *AACN Clinical Issues in Critical Care Nursing, 3*(1), 120–125.

Stenberg, M. J. (1993). Postoperative pneumonia. *Today's OR Nurse, 15*(5), 19–22.

Timby, B. K. (1992). *Pneumocystis* in patients with acquired immunodeficiency syndrome. *Critical Care Nurse, 12*(7), 64–73.

Torres, A., Aznar, R., Gatell, J. M., Jimenez, P., Gonzalez, J., Ferrer, A., Celis, R., & Rodriguez-Roisin, R. (1990). Incidence, risk and prognosis factors of nosocomial pneumonia in mechanically ventilated patients. *American Review of Respiratory Diseases, 142,* 523–528.

Torres, A., El-Ebiary, M., Gonzales, J., Ferrer, M., De La Bellacasa, J. P., Gene, A., Martos, A., & Rodriguez-Roisin, R. (1993). Gastric and pharyngeal flora in nosocomial pneumonia acquired during mechanical ventilation. *American Review of Respiratory Diseases, 148*(2), 352–357.

Tsao, T. C., Tsai, Y., Lan, R., Shieh, W., & Lee, C. (1992). Pulmonary manifestations of *Staphylococcus aureus* septicemia. *Chest, 101*(2), 574–576.

US Department of Health & Human Services / Public Health Service. (1991). *Core curriculum on tuberculosis* (2nd ed.). Atlanta: Centers for Disease Control and Prevention.

Weinberger, S. E. (1993a). Recent advances in pulmonary medicine: Part 1. *New England Journal of Medicine, 328*(19), 1389–1397.

Weinberger, S. E. (1993b). Recent advances in pulmonary medicine: Part 2. *New England Journal of Medicine, 328*(20), 1462–1470.

Wisinger, D. (1993). Bacterial pneumonia. *Postgraduate Medicine, 93*(7), 43–52.

Patients With Acute Respiratory Failure

Elizabeth A. Henneman

GLOSSARY	
PAO_2	Partial pressure of alveolar oxygen
PaO_2	Partial pressure of arterial oxygen
$P\bar{v}O_2$	Partial pressure of mixed venous oxygen
$PACO_2$	Partial pressure of alveolar carbon dioxide
$PaCO_2$	Partial pressure of arterial carbon dioxide
FIO_2	Fraction of inspired oxygen
PIO_2	Partial pressure of inspired oxygen
$\dot{V}DS$	Volume of dead space
$\dot{V}E$	Minute ventilation
$\dot{V}A$	Alveolar ventilation
$\dot{V}/\dot{Q}$	Ventilation-perfusion ratio
A-a gradient	Alveolar-arterial gradient
a/A ratio	Arterial/alveolar ratio
$\dot{Q}T$	Cardiac output
$\dot{Q}S/\dot{Q}T$	Shunt fraction
CaO_2	Oxygen content of arterial blood
CcO_2	Oxygen content of end capillary blood
$C\bar{v}O_2$	Oxygen content of mixed venous blood
$C(a\text{-}v)O_2$	Arterial-venous oxygen content difference
$\dot{D}O_2$	Oxygen delivery
$\dot{V}O_2$	Oxygen consumption
$\dot{V}CO_2$	Carbon dioxide production
SaO_2	Oxygen saturation of arterial blood
$S\bar{v}O_2$	Oxygen saturation of mixed venous blood
$ETCO_2$	End-tidal carbon dioxide
DO_2 crit	Critical oxygen delivery

Acute respiratory failure (ARF) is a medical emergency frequently encountered in the critical care setting. Critical care nurses must be able to identify patients at risk for developing ARF, recognize its signs and symptoms, and be able to provide appropriate lifesaving intervention.

Respiratory failure occurs when the body is unable to meet its need for tissue oxygenation or carbon dioxide (CO_2) removal. Events leading to the development of ARF are varied and include primary lung dysfunction as well as extrinsic problems such as circulatory insufficiency (Luce, 1988). The diagnosis of ARF is made on the basis of arterial blood gas (ABG) results. A sudden deterioration in PaO_2 to less than 50 mm Hg or in $PaCO_2$ to greater than 50 mm Hg constitutes ARF. ABGs should serve only as a guide and must be used in conjunction with other data derived from the clinical assessment. Factors such as age and altitude affect ABGs even in healthy people. Patients with chronic obstructive pulmonary disease (COPD) often have ABGs outside the normal range. In these instances, changes from baseline and not absolute values should be considered.

An assessment of a patient's respiratory status depends on more than an evaluation of ABGs. Arterial blood gases reflect only the adequacy of ventilation and the efficiency with which gas is exchanged across the pulmonary capillary membrane. Ultimately, the purpose of respiration is to provide the tissues with oxygenated blood so that normal cellular processes may occur. This cannot happen unless well-oxygenated blood can be delivered to and used by the tissues. Oxygen delivery and consumption are dependent not only on pulmonary function but also on nonpulmonary factors such as cardiac output and hemoglobin levels. This chapter will review the pathophysiology, clinical assessment, and management of patients with ARF.

PATHOPHYSIOLOGY

The process of respiration involves four steps: (1) ventilation, (2) diffusion of gases across the pulmonary-capillary membrane (i.e., arterial oxygenation and CO_2

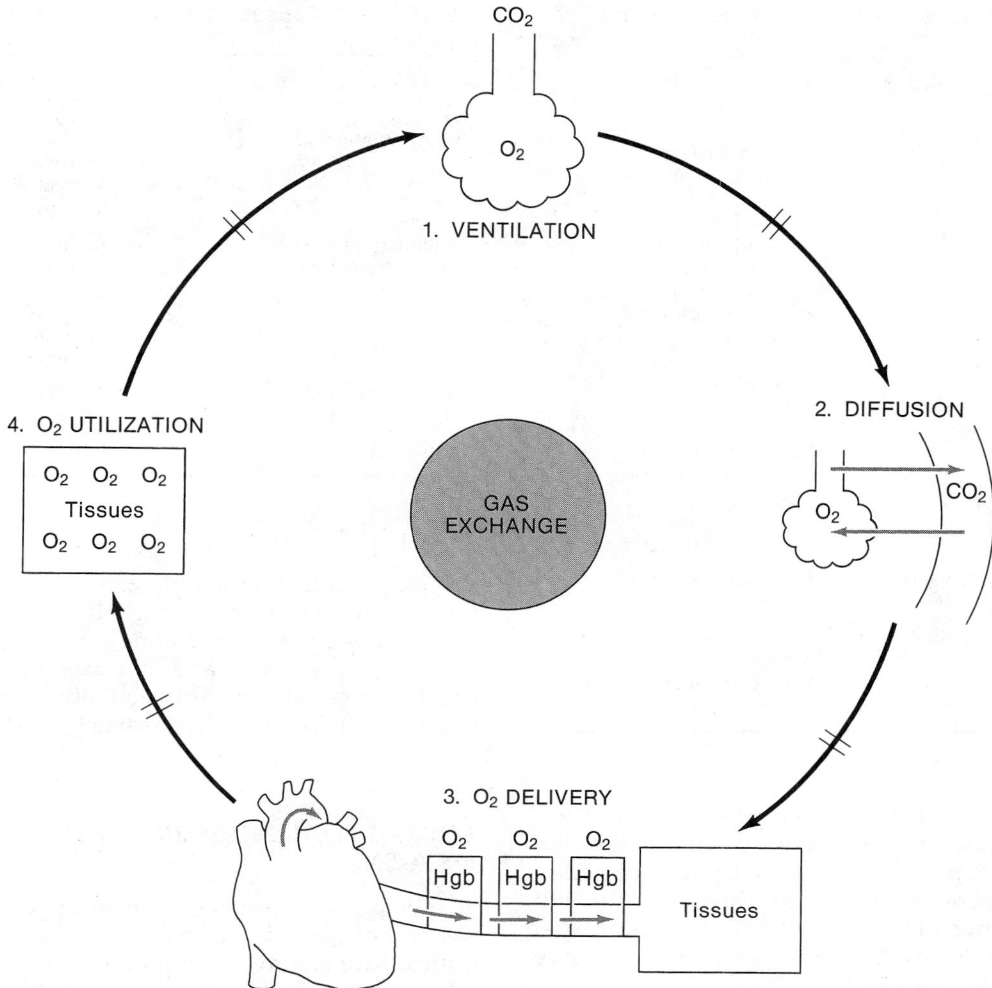

FIGURE 31–1. Process of gas exchange leading to tissue oxygenation. An interruption at any point in the cycle will lead to acute respiratory failure.

elimination), (3) oxygen delivery, and (4) oxygen consumption. A sudden impairment in one or more of these processes will result in acute respiratory failure (Fig. 31–1).

Acute Ventilatory Failure

Acute ventilatory failure (AVF) is a common cause of ARF in trauma patients, drug overdose victims, and patients with neurologic disorders. The result of acute ventilatory failure is alveolar ventilation ($\dot{V}_A$) inadequate for removing the CO_2 produced by the body ($\dot{V}CO_2$). Elevated CO_2 levels result from an inability to eliminate CO_2 or an increase in physiologic dead space ($\dot{V}_{DS}$), or secondary to increased production of CO_2 (Table 31–1). An inability to maintain an adequate minute ventilation ($\dot{V}_E$) to eliminate CO_2 is the most common cause of AVF. As minute ventilation falls, effective ventilation (i.e., alveolar ventilation) also falls, resulting in an increased $PaCO_2$.

$$PaCO_2 = \frac{\dot{V}CO_2}{\dot{V}_A} \frac{(CO_2 \text{ produced})}{(\text{Alveolar ventilation})}$$

Decreased minute ventilation may occur secondary to mechanical obstruction, aspiration, decreased ventilatory drive (head trauma, drug overdose), or restrictive processes (muscle weakness).

Increased dead space, or wasted ventilation, will also contribute to ventilatory failure (Fig. 31–2). This occurs when areas of the lung are ventilated but not perfused. Poor perfusion inhibits the transfer of CO_2 from the pulmonary capillary into the alveoli, resulting in an increased $PaCO_2$. Increased dead space is seen with pulmonary embolism and other disorders that compromise the pulmonary vasculature, such as the adult respiratory distress syndrome (ARDS). In most cases, however, although CO_2 transfer is impaired, the measured $PaCO_2$ will be normal or low because the patient has been stimulated to compensate by hyperventilating (Luce, 1988).

TABLE 31–1. **Causes of Acute Ventilatory Failure**

Decreased minute ventilation ($\dot{V}E$)	Mechanical obstruction Upper airway Edema Hemorrhage Aspiration of solid object Lower airway Asthma Emphysema Chronic bronchitis Pulmonary edema Restrictive disorders Obesity Kyphoscoliosis Muscle weakness Neuromuscular defects Pneumonia Decreased ventilatory drive Drug poisonings Sedatives Head trauma Postoperative complications
Increased dead space ventilation ($\dot{V}D$)	Pulmonary embolus ARDS
Increased CO_2 production ($\dot{V}CO_2$)	Fever Seizures High carbohydrate loads Exercise

Although an increase in CO_2 production is rarely the primary cause of AVF, it may complicate the clinical course of a patient with underlying pulmonary dysfunction. Increases in CO_2 production occur with the administration of high carbohydrate loads or when metabolic activity is increased (e.g., with fever, exercise, seizures, or agitation).

Acute ventilatory failure may occur with or without a concomitant decrease in oxygenation. Ventilatory failure without hypoxemia occurs when the patient's $\dot{V}E$ is affected but gas exchange in the lung is otherwise normal (e.g., after head trauma).

Failure of Arterial Oxygenation

Primary failure of arterial oxygenation is a common cause of ARF in critically ill patients (e.g., those with ARDS, pneumonia, or pulmonary edema). When the level of arterial oxygenation falls below normal, hypoxemia is present. Five conditions lead to impaired arterial oxygenation and hypoxemia: low inspired O_2, hypoventilation, diffusion abnormalities, ventilation–perfusion ($\dot{V}/\dot{Q}$) mismatch, and shunt (Table 31–2).

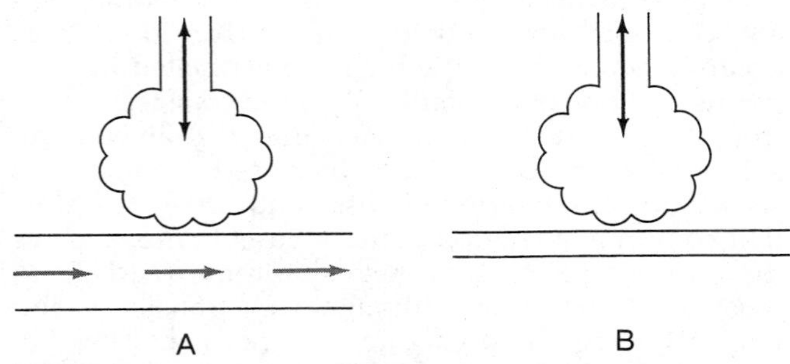

FIGURE 31–2. Relationship between ventilation and perfusion in normal (*A*) and dead space (*B*) units that are underperfused.

TABLE 31–2. **Causes of Impaired Arterial Oxygenation**

Low PIO_2	High altitude Administration of low FIO_2
Hypoventilation	Mechanical obstruction Restrictive disorders Decreased ventilatory drive Increased dead space ($\dot{V}D$)
Ventilation–perfusion ($\dot{V}/\dot{Q}$) mismatch	Asthma COPD Atelectasis Congestive heart failure Pulmonary embolism Pulmonary edema
Intrapulmonary shunt ($\dot{Q}S/\dot{Q}T$)	ARDS (as above but more severe)
Diffusion defects	Pulmonary fibrosis

LOW PARTIAL PRESSURE OF INSPIRED OXYGEN

A low partial pressure of inspired oxygen (PIO_2) is rarely a cause of impaired arterial oxygenation in the critical care setting. At high altitudes (as in Denver), where atmospheric pressure is less than at sea level, the PIO_2 will be lower despite equal concentrations of inspired oxygen (FIO_2).

$$PIO_2 = FIO_2 \times (\text{atmospheric pressure} - 47)^*$$

Decreases in the PIO_2 also occur during a fire, when combustion diminishes the availability of O_2 (Tyler, 1986). Purposeful or inadvertent discontinuation of delivered oxygen (FIO_2) can also decrease the PIO_2, leading to hypoxemia.

HYPOVENTILATION

Hypoventilation results in an increased $PaCO_2$ and therefore decreased PAO_2, as evidenced by the following equation:

$$PAO_2 = FIO_2 \times (PB - 47) - \frac{PaCO_2}{0.8}$$

Only severe hypoventilation accompanied by significant increases in $PaCO_2$ will have an impact on the

*47 = *Vapor pressure of water at 37°C.*

P_{AO_2}. Hypoventilation is a singular problem, therefore, rarely produces hypoxemia.

DIFFUSION ABNORMALITIES

Another rare but potential cause of impaired oxygenation in the critically ill patient is diffusion defects. Optimal diffusion of gases into and out of the alveoli is dependent on the characteristics of the alveolar capillary membrane. Equilibrium between the alveoli and capillaries occurs so rapidly and efficiently that even severe diffusion defects rarely result in hypoxemia. Diffusion abnormalities occur in such conditions as interstitial fibrosis, sarcoidosis, asbestosis, and primary alveolar disease (Albert, 1988).

VENTILATION–PERFUSION ABNORMALITIES

The mismatching of ventilation to perfusion is the primary cause of impaired oxygenation and hypoxemia in the critically ill patient. Hypoxemia results when alveoli are underventilated relative to the amount of perfusion (i.e., blood flow) they receive (i.e., low $\dot{V}/\dot{Q}$) (Fig. 31–3). Unoxygenated blood passing by underventilated alveoli mixes with oxygenated blood and lowers the Pa_{O_2} (Kersten, 1989).

Decreased ventilation relative to perfusion is the mechanism of hypoxemia in such conditions as asthma, COPD, and pulmonary edema. Bronchospasm, mucus plugging, and atelectasis can also reduce ventilation of well-perfused alveoli, resulting in impaired arterial oxygenation.

SHUNT

The most severe form of low ventilation–perfusion mismatch is intrapulmonary shunt. Shunting occurs when alveoli are completely collapsed from atelectasis or are filled with fluid or mucus (Fig. 31–3). Shunted blood returns to the systemic arteries without ever having come in contact with gas-exchanging areas of the lung.

Normal physiologic shunting comprises 3% to 5% of the cardiac output (5 mL/dL) and results from bronchial and thebesian veins emptying into the left side of the heart (Neagley, 1991). The equation for determining the ratio of shunted blood ($\dot{Q}_S$) to cardiac output ($\dot{Q}_T$) is:

$$\frac{\dot{Q}_S}{\dot{Q}_T} = \frac{Cc_{O_2} - Ca_{O_2}}{Cc_{O_2} - C\bar{v}_{O_2}}$$

where Cc_{O_2} = oxygen content of end capillary blood, Ca_{O_2} = oxygen content of arterial blood, and Cv_{O_2} = oxygen content of mixed venous blood.

Because the equation for calculating the shunt fraction is somewhat cumbersome, it can be estimated as follows: when breathing 100% oxygen, each 20 mm Hg reduction in Pa_{O_2} (below 700 mm Hg) is equal to a 1% shunt. This rule holds true until the Pa_{O_2} falls below 150 mm Hg (severe shunt) (Zagelbaum & Pare, 1982).

Example: Pa_{O_2} = 300 mm Hg on 100% oxygen

Shunt = Approximately 20%

Shunting can occur with atelectasis, pneumonia, pulmonary edema, or ARDS and can be differentiated from low ventilation–perfusion abnormalities by administering 100% oxygen to the patient. Hypoxemia due to shunting will not respond to high FI_{O_2}, whereas hypoxemia due to a low ventilation–perfusion ratio will (Demling & Knox, 1993).

Failure of Oxygen Delivery

Patients with normal ventilation and oxygenation may still develop ARF if they are unable to deliver the well-oxygenated blood to the tissues where it is needed. Oxygen delivery is dependent on two variables, oxygen content (Ca_{O_2}) and cardiac output ($\dot{Q}_T$) (Fig. 31–4).

$$O_2 \text{ delivery} = Ca_{O_2} \times \dot{Q}_T$$

OXYGEN CONTENT. The majority of oxygen in the blood is bound to hemoglobin (97%); the rest is dissolved in the plasma. The oxygen content of the arterial blood is calculated by adding the amount of O_2 carried on hemoglobin to the amount of dissolved O_2:

$$Ca_{O_2} = O_2 \text{ saturation} \times \text{hemoglobin} \times 1.34 + (Pa_{O_2} \times 0.0031)$$

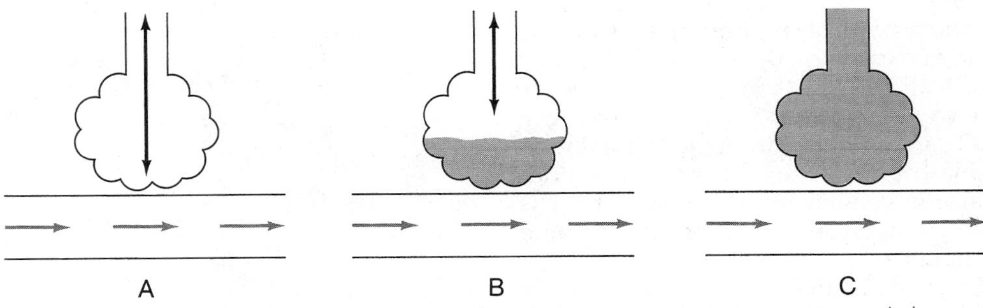

FIGURE 31–3. *A*, Normal ventilation/perfusion. *B*, Low ventilation, normal perfusion (low $\dot{V}/\dot{Q}$). *C*, No ventilation/perfusion (shunt).

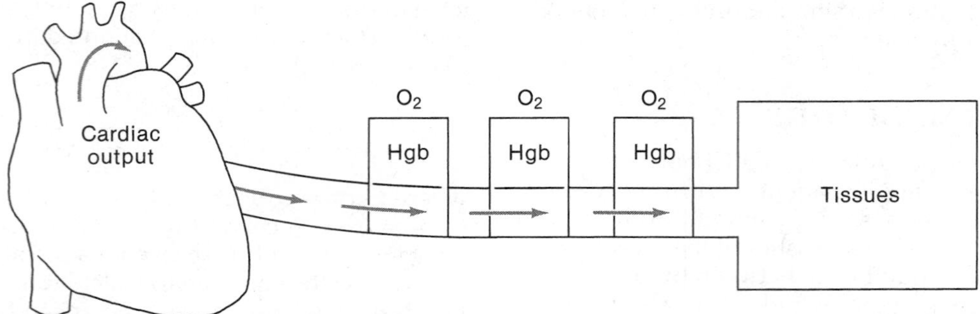

FIGURE 31–4. Components of oxygen delivery: cardiac output, hemoglobin (Hgb), and oxygen saturation.

where 1.34 = the maximal amount of oxygen that can combine with 1 gram of hemoglobin. Oxygen saturation has a significant impact on the O_2 content of the arterial blood. Factors that influence the affinity of hemoglobin for O_2, such as temperature and metabolic factors, will influence O_2 saturation and enhance or impede O_2 delivery. Conditions that shift the oxyhemoglobin-dissociation curve to the right (e.g., acidosis, increased $Paco_2$, fever, increased 2,3-diphosphoglycerate [2,3-DPG]) facilitate the dissociation of O_2 from hemoglobin and decrease the O_2 content of the arterial blood. Alkalosis, hypothermia, decreased $Paco_2$, and decreased 2,3-DPG have the opposite effect, resulting in a greater affinity of hemoglobin for O_2 and higher O_2 saturations (shift to the left).

The amount of hemoglobin available to carry O_2 will also influence the O_2 content of the arterial blood. Anemia resulting either from blood loss, impaired red blood cell production, or increased red blood cell destruction will decrease the oxygen-carrying capacity of the blood.

CARDIAC OUTPUT. The cardiac output ($\dot{Q}T$) also influences the amount of O_2 delivered to the tissues. An inadequate cardiac output results from disturbances in heart rate or stroke volume. Although cardiac output normally increases to compensate for a low oxygen content, this mechanism is often compromised in severely ill patients (Marini, 1988) (Table 31–3).

Failure of Oxygen Consumption

The final step in the process of respiration is the uptake and consumption of oxygen by the tissues. If this final step is impaired, ARF will result. When the tissues are unable to utilize oxygen, aerobic processes in the cell come to a halt. The result is a dramatic reduction in energy (adenosine triphosphate)-producing reactions and a compromise in cellular metabolic activity. The cells become dependent on anaerobic metabolism, and lactic acid accumulates.

The amount of O_2 consumed by the tissues is not related (under normal conditions) to the amount of O_2 delivered to them. Rather, the amount of O_2 consumed determines how much O_2 will be delivered. This process involves local autoregulatory mechanisms, which allow increased blood flow when O_2 requirements are high (Clemmer et al., 1988). However, studies suggest that when O_2 content reaches critically low levels, O_2 consumption becomes dependent on O_2 supply (called the critical Do_2 [Do_2 crit]) (Danek et al., 1980; Abraham et al., 1984).

The relationship between O_2 consumption and delivery is expressed by the Fick principle. Oxygen consumption is calculated by multiplying the cardiac output by the amount of O_2 extracted by the tissues (i.e., the arterial–venous O_2 content difference):

$$\dot{V}o_2 = \dot{Q}T \times C(a\text{-}v)o_2$$

where $\dot{V}o_2$ = oxygen consumption, $\dot{Q}T$ = cardiac output, and $C(a\text{-}v)o_2$ = arterial–venous oxygen content difference.

A primary failure of O_2 consumption occurs in septic shock and cyanide poisoning. Patients in septic shock commonly exhibit signs of tissue hypoxia yet do not consume available O_2, as evidenced by high mixed

TABLE 31–3. **Factors Leading to Failure of O_2 Delivery and Consumption**

O_2 Delivery ($\dot{D}o_2$)

Decreased cardiac output	Decreased O_2 content of arterial blood (Cao_2)
Heart rate	Decreased hemoglobin
Stroke volume	Decreased O_2 saturation
Arrhythmias	
Hypovolemia	
High systemic vascular resistance	
Myocardial infarction	
Cardiac tamponade	
Congestive heart failure	

O_2 Consumption ($\dot{V}o_2$)

Anemia
Fever
Acidosis
Sepsis
Cyanide poisoning

venous O_2 levels (i.e., oxygenation of the blood returning to the right side of the heart). It is presently unclear what mechanism is responsible for this impairment in O_2 uptake, although peripheral tissue damage plays a role (Danek et al., 1980). Cyanide poisoning also results in a failure of O_2 consumption. When cyanide ions react with the enzyme cytochrome oxidase, a complex is formed that interferes with intracellular respiration. The result is a decreased consumption of oxygen, an increased amount of oxygenated blood returning to the heart (partial pressure of venous oxygen [$P\bar{v}O_2$]), and a narrowing arterial–venous oxygen content difference.

TABLE 31–4. **Clinical Manifestations of ARF**

Low PaO_2	Increased $PaCO_2$
Hypoxemia	Hypercapnia
Restlessness	Headache
Confusion	Altered level of consciousness
Poor judgment	Coma
Coma	Cardiovascular collapse
Tachycardia	Arrhythmias
Hypertension (early)	Hypotension
Hypotension (late)	Poor peripheral perfusion
Cyanosis	
Dyspnea	
Tachypnea	

CLINICAL ASSESSMENT

A comprehensive clinical evaluation of the patient with ARF includes a history, physical examination, laboratory studies, and diagnostic testing. Because ARF frequently presents as an emergency situation requiring immediate intervention, the clinical assessment is often limited. It is not uncommon to collect the majority of data after therapy has been initiated.

History

The patient history can be very useful in determining the etiology of ARF. If the patient is unable to provide information, data can be collected from family or other medical personnel. As much information as possible should be obtained about the details of the precipitating event (e.g., trauma, drug ingestion, flu, allergen exposure). The patient's past medical, family, occupational, and travel history may all provide useful data in reaching a diagnosis.

The chief complaint (e.g., cough, chest pain, dyspnea) may also be helpful in making a diagnosis and determining a plan of care. Unfortunately, because the signs and symptoms of ARF are nonspecific, laboratory and diagnostic testing are usually necessary to confirm a diagnosis.

Symptoms and Physical Signs

The presence of cough, sputum production, chest pain, dyspnea, and mental status changes, alone or in combination, may be suggestive of respiratory failure. A cough productive of large amounts of sputum suggests chronic bronchitis or bronchiectasis. Purulent sputum points to an infectious process, and foul-smelling sputum indicates an anaerobic organism. Pink, frothy sputum is seen with pulmonary edema, whereas grossly bloody sputum occurs with pulmonary infarction or malignancy.

If the patient complains of chest pain, attempts must be made to ascertain if the discomfort is of pulmonary or cardiac origin. Pleuritic chest pain is acute, localized, and intermittent and is aggravated by breathing. This type of pain is associated with conditions such as pneumonia, pleurisy, and pulmonary infarction. Cardiac chest pain is more constant than pleuritic pain and is unaffected by respirations.

Dyspnea is a useful diagnostic finding when it is considered together with other clinical signs and symptoms. For example, dyspnea associated with cough and a history of allergen exposure is suggestive of asthma. Paroxysmal nocturnal dyspnea and orthopnea occur with left-sided heart failure. Dyspnea associated with stridor is consistent with upper airway obstruction. Transient episodes of dyspnea at rest may indicate a pulmonary embolism (Zagelbaum & Pare, 1982).

Complaints by the patient or family about mental status changes deserve particular attention. Alterations in level of consciousness (LOC) or mentation may be early signs of respiratory insufficiency.

The clinical manifestations of ARF include those of the underlying disease as well as the signs and symptoms of hypoxemia or hypercapnia (Table 31–4). Respiratory failure may present in a dramatic fashion (e.g., tension, pneumothorax, asthma, massive pulmonary embolism, aspiration) or so subtly that it goes unnoticed and is appreciated only by laboratory testing. Because the brain and heart have high O_2 requirements, they are particularly vulnerable to O_2 deprivation. As a result, the neurologic and cardiovascular systems deserve particular attention during the physical examination of a patient with ARF.

NEUROLOGIC SYSTEM

Headache, restlessness, and confusion are among the most common signs of ARF. Neurologic disturbances arise from both hypoxemia and hypercapnia. Altered LOC can range from a mild inability to concentrate to profound coma. The critically ill patient who experiences an acute change in LOC should be rapidly assessed for impairments in oxygenation or ventilation.

Central nervous system disorders may also be the precipitating event in ARF. Respiratory center depression and hypoventilation result from a number of neurologic insults, including head injury and sedative overdosage. Altered LOC may also precipitate ARF by predisposing the patient to aspiration.

CARDIOVASCULAR SYSTEM

Early cardiovascular changes associated with ARF represent the body's attempt to compensate for hypoxemia. These findings include tachycardia, mild hypertension, peripheral vasoconstriction, and increased cardiac output. However, if left to progress, ARF will result in cardiovascular collapse and inadequate perfusion, manifested by arrhythmias, ischemic pain, and hypotension.

PULMONARY SYSTEM

An in-depth evaluation of the pulmonary system is indicated for all patients with suspected or proved ARF. This comprehensive examination includes observation, palpation, percussion, and auscultation.

Skillful observation may provide useful diagnostic information about the presence and severity of ARF, although not in all cases. For example, patients who are hypercapnic may appear somnolent and not in any acute distress when in fact their Pa_{CO_2} levels are dangerously high. On the other hand, respiratory distress may be suspected in other groups of patients simply by noting their facial expressions (e.g., apprehension or fear in patients with asthma).

Careful attention must be paid during the physical examination to observation of the respiratory rate, pattern, and depth. Irregular or labored respirations may provide early clues to respiratory failure. Patients who are hypoxemic frequently present with tachypnea, whereas hypercapnic patients may have depressed respirations.

Observation of chest and abdominal movements may be useful in assessing ventilatory status. The use of accessory muscles (e.g., sternocleidomastoid) suggests air hunger, whereas the development of inward abdominal retraction indicates diaphragm fatigue, usually an ominous sign.

Palpating the trachea and chest wall is also a useful diagnostic tool in patients with ARF. Tracheal deviation and asymmetric chest wall movements occur in such conditions as pneumothorax and hydrothorax. Areas of abnormal density can be discovered by percussing the chest wall. Pneumothoraces are characterized by hyperresonance, whereas pneumonia and pleural effusions are associated with dullness.

Auscultation is used to identify the presence or absence of breath sounds and to identify obstruction or fluid in the airways or lungs. Breath sounds are diminished or absent when the alveoli are collapsed or underventilated, as in atelectasis or pneumothorax. Upper airway obstruction usually results in inspiratory wheezes (heard best over the trachea), and lower airway obstruction results in expiratory wheezes. When severe, these findings are audible without the aid of a stethoscope. Other adventitious breath sounds such as crackles occur when fluid is present in the airway or alveoli or when collapsed alveoli are opened during inspiration (e.g., in pulmonary edema). Crackles that are gravity dependent are commonly associated with a cardiac cause, such as congestive heart failure, whereas crackles secondary to a pulmonary cause tend not to be related to patient position (i.e., nongravity-dependent). Rhonchi are indicative of large airway obstruction due either to mucus accumulation or stricture. A pleural friction rub—a harsh, grating sound—is suggestive of an inflammation of the pleura or a loss of pleural fluid (as with pulmonary emboli, infarction, or fractured ribs) (Neagley, 1991). See Table 31–5 for specific findings associated with pulmonary embolism.

PSYCHOSOCIAL ASSESSMENT

Acute respiratory failure is a potentially life-threatening problem. The interventions employed in the management of ARF are often invasive (e.g., intubation) and may cause significant discomfort (e.g., suctioning). Patients and their families must be assessed for their response to ARF and its treatment.

The clinician must be alert to signs and symptoms of anxiety. They may herald impending or worsening ARF or be a result of the treatment of the respiratory failure. Anxiety generally presents as a cluster of findings that include restlessness, confusion, tachypnea, tachycardia, and hypertension. The critically ill patient who is anxious may attempt to pull out invasive devices, such as IV lines and endotracheal tubes. Anxiety may be exacerbated in ARF when the patient is unable to communicate secondary to dyspnea or invasive devices (endotracheal or tracheostomy tubes).

Extra effort must be taken to assess for anxiety in patients receiving medications that mask many of the signs of anxiety. Neuromuscular blocking agents, for example, prohibit the patient from exhibiting the restlessness, confusion, and tachypnea that are classic markers of anxiety. In this instance, other indicators of anxiety such as tachycardia and hypertension should be used as assessment parameters. In addition, the neuromuscular blocking agent should be stopped once a day to allow the patient's anxiety level to be assessed appropriately.

The family of the patient with ARF must also be assessed for their response to the patient's condition. Signs of effective family coping include asking appropriate questions, communicating with the patient using words or touch, and seeking out and using resources.

DIAGNOSTIC TESTS

Arterial Blood Gas Monitoring

Critically ill patients with ARF require monitoring of the adequacy of ventilation (Pa_{CO_2}), oxygenation of arterial blood (Pa_{O_2}), oxygen delivery (oxygen satura-

TABLE 31–5. **Pulmonary Embolism**

Predisposing Factors

History of deep vein thrombosis
Immobilization (e.g., bed rest)
Postoperative patients
Right atrial thrombi (e.g., associated with atrial fibrillation)
Hypercoagulability
Trauma
Estrogen therapy
Pregnancy
Obesity

Pathophysiology

Clot lodges in pulmonary vasculature resulting in: (1) increased dead space ventilation ($\uparrow \dot{V}/\dot{Q}$) + pulmonary hypertension → ↑ $\dot{V}_E$ (minute ventilation); (2) platelet aggregation, serotonin, and thromboxane → bronchoconstriction → ↑ alveolar hypoventilation → atelectasis → ↓ $\dot{V}/\dot{Q}$ → hypoxemia

Clinical Presentation

Tachypnea
Tachycardia
Dyspnea
Apprehension
Pleuritic chest pain
Cough
Crackles
Fever
Wheezing
Hemoptysis
Pleural friction rub/pleural effusions

Diagnostic Tests

Laboratory tests
- ABGs: Pa_{O_2} < 80 mm Hg; Pa_{CO_2} < 35 mm Hg; pH > 7.45
- A-a gradient: increased
- Mild leukocytosis
- Elevated fibrin degradation products

Electrocardiographic
- Sinus tachycardia
- Right axis deviation
- Nonspecific T wave changes
- Right bundle branch block

Chest x-ray (rarely diagnostic)
- Elevated hemidiaphragm
- Atelectasis
- Pulmonary infiltrates
- Wedge-shaped density in periphery
- Pleural effusions
- Enlarged hilar pulmonary arteries

Deep vein thrombosis evaluation (impedence plethysmography or ultrasound)
Ventilation–perfusion scans—see multiple segmental or lobar perfusion defects with normal ventilation
Angiography will show "cut off" of blood flow or filling defect

Medical Therapy

Goal: To stabilize cardiopulmonary function (i.e., maintain adequate oxygen delivery), prevent reembolization, and avoid pulmonary damage

1. Stabilize cardiopulmonary function (particularly for patients with hemodynamic compromise; i.e., in shock)
   a. Basic and advanced life support
   b. Ventilatory support/supplemental O_2
   c. Maintenance of cardiac output
      (1) Vasopressors
      (2) Fluids
2. Prevent reembolization with anticoagulation therapy to prevent new clots
   a. Heparin
      (1) Initial dose = 140–200 units/kg IV
      (2) Maintenance dose = 25 units/kg/hr IV to keep PTT at 1.5 to 2.5 times control
   b. Sodium warfarin (Coumadin) = 5–10 mg/day to keep PT at 2.0 to 2.5 times control (long-term up to 12 months)
3. Avoid further pulmonary damage with thrombolytic therapy to dissolve embolus
   a. Indicated for patients with significant hemodynamic disturbances
   b. Streptokinase
      (1) Initial dose = 250,000 IU IV (over 30 min)
      (2) Maintenance dose = 100,000 IU/hr IV for 24–72 hr
   c. Urokinase
      (1) Initial dose = 4400 IU/kg IV (over 30 min)
      (2) Maintenance dose = 4400 IU/kg/hr IV for 12 hr
4. Surgical management—indicated for patients in whom medical management is contraindicated and for patients with recurrent pulmonary embolism despite adequate anticoagulation
   a. Femoral vein ligation
   b. Inferior vena cava ligation
   c. Intraluminal umbrella
   d. Pulmonary embolectomy (rare)

From Arabian, A. A. (1986). In S. V. Spagnolo & A. Medinger (Eds.), *Handbook of pulmonary emergencies* (pp. 193–204). New York: Plenum Publishing Corp.; and Stein, P. D., Hull, R. D., Saltzman, H. R., & Pineo, G. (1993). Strategy for diagnosis of patients with suspected acute pulmonary embolism. *Chest, 103,* 1553–1559.

tion, cardiac output, and hemoglobin), and oxygen consumption. Adequacy of ventilation can be monitored intermittently through ABG analysis of Pa_{CO_2}. The Pa_{CO_2} varies directly with alveolar ventilation and therefore can be used as an indicator of whether or not the patient is ventilating enough to meet metabolic needs. A Pa_{CO_2} less than 35 mm Hg (hypocapnia) occurs in ARF either secondary to pain or anxiety or as a compensatory response to a metabolic acidosis or in an attempt to improve oxygenation. Hypercapnia (Pa_{CO_2} greater than 45 mm Hg) suggests that the patient is unable to ventilate adequately to meet metabolic needs. Hypoventilation and resultant hypercapnia are dangerous in that they will lead to respiratory acidosis if left untreated.

The adequacy of ventilation can also be measured continuously with end-tidal CO_2 ($ETCO_2$) monitoring. This noninvasive technique utilizes mass spectrometry or infrared spectroscopy to detect variations in expired CO_2. It may be used to trend CO_2 levels, particularly if continuous monitoring is indicated such as during weaning from mechanical ventilation.

Arterial blood gas monitoring also allows for intermittent evaluation of Pao_2 and oxygen saturation (Sao_2). A Pao_2 of less than 50 to 60 mm Hg or an Sao_2 of less than 90% on room air (at sea level) is indicative of hypoxemia. A comprehensive evaluation of the cause and extent of hypoxemia requires the use of formulas such as the alveolar-arterial (A-a) gradient and a/A ratio. Calculation of the A-a gradient is useful in determining whether the hypoxemia is caused by a problem with gas exchange in the lung or is secondary to an extrapulmonary event. A normal A-a gradient is 10 mm Hg on room air and 100 mm Hg on an FIO_2 of 1.0. If the A-a gradient is widened (greater than normal), the hypoxemia is caused by a primary lung problem (e.g., diffusion defect, ventilation–perfusion mismatch, shunt); normal A-a gradients are seen with such extrapulmonary causes of hypoxemia as hypoventilation and low PIO_2. Use of the A-a gradient is of limited use in trending changes in oxygenation because the gradient will change when the FIO_2 varies.

$$\text{A-a gradient} = PAO_2 - Pao_2$$

$$PAO_2 = FIO_2 \times (PB - 47) - \frac{Paco_2}{0.8}$$

The arterial to alveolar ratio (a/A ratio) is also useful in evaluating the patient's oxygenation status. Many clinicians prefer the a/A ratio over the A-a gradient because it allows for trending changes in oxygenation despite changes in the FIO_2.

Noninvasive oxygen monitoring that permits continuous evaluation of Sao_2 is available. Although these oximeters (pulse or ear) can assess arterial oxygenation, they may be of limited value in certain situations (e.g., in patients who have hypothermia or vasoconstriction or are agitated).

Monitoring of oxygen delivery and consumption requires a pulmonary artery catheter to determine cardiac output and obtain mixed venous blood gas samples. The newest hemodynamic monitoring technology uses reflectance spectrophotometry to monitor continuously the saturation of mixed venous oxygen ($S\bar{v}o_2$), which is an indicator of the balance between O_2 delivery and consumption. The newest technology allows for the continuous monitoring of both $S\bar{v}o_2$ and cardiac output (Baxter Health Care Corp.; Abbott Critical Care Systems).

Laboratory Tests

As previously mentioned, ABG analysis is critical in diagnosing ARF. In addition to ABGs, a complete blood count and electrolyte levels should be routinely ordered for all patients with ARF, paying particular attention to hemoglobin, potassium, magnesium, phosphorus, and calcium levels. Patients in whom an infectious pulmonary process is suspected (e.g., a patient with COPD who is admitted with an acute exacerbation of the illness) should have a sputum specimen taken and sent for culture and sensitivity. More specific tests such as toxicology screens or thyroid function studies should be ordered if indicated by the patient's history or other clinical findings.

Chest X-ray

An evaluation of the anteroposterior and lateral chest x-ray is valuable in substantiating the findings from the physical examination and determining the etiology of ARF. Possible chest x-ray findings include areas of consolidation (e.g., pneumonia), hyperinflation (e.g., emphysema), pulmonary venous congestion, cardiomegaly (e.g., left heart failure), pleural effusion, collapsed lung (e.g., pneumothorax), fractured ribs, or flail chest.

Pulmonary Function Tests

Measurement of pulmonary function tests are useful in diagnosing obstructive airway disease and in evaluating the effectiveness of bronchodilator therapy. Patients with COPD typically have a reduction in expiratory volume during the first second of a forced exhalation (FEV_1) and a reduction in the ratio of FEV_1 to forced vital capacity (FEV_1/FVC). Asthmatics also have diminished flow rates but experience improvement after bronchodilator therapy. This difference in response of FEV_1 to bronchodilator therapy is used to distinguish reversible (e.g., asthma) from nonreversible (e.g., COPD) airway disease (Zagelbaum & Pare, 1982). Pulmonary function studies require an alert, cooperative patient and are often difficult to perform during a critical illness.

Miscellaneous Tests

A variety of other diagnostic tests are available to assist in the differential diagnosis of ARF, including bronchoscopy, ventilation–perfusion ($\dot{V}/\dot{Q}$) scans, and angiography. Bronchoscopy permits direct visualization of the tracheobronchial tree using a flexible fiberoptic scope. The bronchoscope can also be used to obtain specimens, either by suction or biopsy, to confirm or provide a diagnosis.

Pulmonary $\dot{V}/\dot{Q}$ scans and angiography are used

in the evaluation of pulmonary embolism. Although $\dot{V}/\dot{Q}$ scans are among the major diagnostic tests for pulmonary embolism, they lack specificity and can only suggest a low intermediate, or high probability of pulmonary embolism. Pulmonary angiography is considered the "gold standard" diagnostic tool for pulmonary embolism but is associated with some risk (see Table 31–5).

MANAGEMENT OF ACUTE RESPIRATORY FAILURE

Effective management of ARF requires the combined efforts of a skilled multidisciplinary team. Although each member of the team (nurse, physician, respiratory therapist) has specific functions, the goals of therapy are similar. The critical care nurse's role in management of ARF includes assessing and monitoring the patient, developing a plan of care, administering therapy, and evaluating the effectiveness of the plan. Interventions employed by the nurse include those prescribed by the physician as well as other independent therapies.

A primary goal in the management of ARF is treatment of the underlying condition that precipitated the acute event while supporting respiratory function. The specifics of patient management for the multitude of possible causes of ARF are beyond the scope of this chapter. (See Chapters 29, 30, and 32 for management of COPD, pulmonary infection, and ARDS.) The essentials of management of pulmonary embolism are addressed in Table 31–5 to serve as an example.

Regardless of the underlying cause, the principles of providing airway management, ventilatory support, and supplemental oxygenation are the same. The approach used ultimately depends on the mechanism of respiratory failure present in a particular patient (i.e., ventilatory failure, oxygenation failure, failure of O_2 delivery, or failure of O_2 consumption).

Managing Acute Ventilatory Failure

A patient with AVF requires immediate assessment and stabilization of the airway (basic cardiac life support). If the airway is obstructed, steps must be taken to ensure its patency. This may require repositioning the patient (chin-tilt) or removing foreign material (e.g., Heimlich maneuver, suctioning). Opening the patient's airway may be the only step necessary for treating AVF (American Heart Association, 1994).

If the patient's $\dot{V}_E$ is inadequate, experienced personnel should intubate the patient, allowing for artificial ventilation as well as airway protection. Types of artificial airways are listed in Table 31–6. (See Chapter 33 for a discussion of mechanical ventilators.) Once ventilatory support has been established, the priority of management is treatment of the underlying condition and interventions aimed at preventing complications.

IMPROVING ARTERIAL OXYGENATION

A failure of arterial oxygenation may occur alone or in combination with AVF. As soon as the patient's airway and ventilation are supported, efforts are directed toward maximizing alveolar oxygenation. Hypoxemia is managed by improving ventilation, increasing the F_{IO_2}, decreasing ventilation–perfusion mismatch, and diminishing shunt.

IMPROVING VENTILATION

Any attempt to influence oxygenation will be futile if the patient does not have an adequate airway or effective alveolar ventilation (see previous section on management of AVF). In some patients (e.g., those with COPD or asthma) both ventilation and oxygenation can be optimized by relieving air flow obstruction through such interventions as bronchial hygiene or bronchodilators. In other instances, the need for artificial support may be averted through performing vigorous interventions aimed at improving airway patency (e.g., bronchodilators, bronchial hygiene).

INCREASING F_{IO_2}

Increasing the F_{IO_2} will improve the Pa_{O_2} when a low P_{IO_2}, hypoventilation, diffusion impairment, or ventilation–perfusion mismatch is the cause of hypoxemia. Only intrapulmonary shunting will not respond significantly to increased O_2 administration.

There are a variety of methods available for administration of O_2 therapy (Table 31–7). Because O_2 is a drug, it should be administered cautiously, with an awareness of the dosage being given and potential side effects. Serious complications of O_2 therapy include suppression of hypoxic drive in patients with COPD, absorption atelectasis, and parenchymal damage. Prolonged periods of high Pa_{CO_2} with acidosis in patients with COPD reduce the sensitivity of the medulla to changes in cerebrospinal pH. The result is that hypoxia instead of hypercapnia becomes the stimulus to breathe. If high levels of O_2 are administered without ventilatory support, CNS depression, hypoventilation, and acidosis may occur (Mecca, 1986).

Alveoli are normally filled with a combination of gases, including CO_2, O_2, and nitrogen (N_2). Because N_2 is not absorbed into the pulmonary capillaries, it keeps the alveoli open. However, when 100% oxygen is delivered, N_2 is replaced by O_2, and the alveoli collapse when all their oxygen is absorbed before the next breath (i.e., absorption atelectasis).

Oxygen toxicity may also result in damage to the lung parenchyma itself. If high levels of O_2 are administered for prolonged periods, pulmonary capillary damage can also occur, resulting in an ARDS-like picture of pulmonary edema (Mecca, 1986; Demling, 1992). The actual incidence of oxygen toxicity is difficult to deter-

TABLE 31–6. **Artificial Airways**

Airway	Indications	Precautions	Potential Complications	Miscellaneous
Nasopharyngeal	Pharyngeal obstruction Secretion removal Mouth to nose ventilation		Trauma from insertion (bleeding)	Useful with facial or jaw fractures or when oral airways are inappropriate May be used in conscious or unconscious patients Humidification is necessary to maintain airway patency
Oropharyngeal	Pharyngeal obstruction Secretion removal Hold tongue anteriorly Mouth to mouth ventilation	Will cause gagging in conscious patients	Trauma from insertion Vomiting Aspiration	Improper insertion technique could push tongue back and occlude airway
Endotracheal	Establish airway when nasopharyngeal or oropharyngeal airways are inadequate Allow for mechanical ventilation Secretion removal	Requires skilled personnel to insert	Improper placement (esophageal intubation) Mucosal damage Laryngeal or tracheal edema Vocal cord damage Tracheal stenosis (rare) Obstruction of tube Kinking of tube Cuff herniation Tracheoesophageal fistula Sinusitis	Has cuff to prevent aspiration Cuffs should be maintained below capillary filling pressure of trachea (20 mm Hg) to avoid damage
Tracheostomy	Long-term airway management Allow for mechanical ventilation Secretion removal Upper airway obstruction Assist in prevention of aspiration		Complications associated with insertion (e.g., bleeding, infection, pneumothorax) Obstruction of tube Cuff herniation Tracheoesophageal fistula Dislodged tube Hemorrhage	Requires surgery
Cricothyrotomy	An immediate airway in extreme emergencies	Requires skilled personnel	Bleeding	Only a temporary measure to be used until a more stable airway is secure

mine because it occurs in the context of other lung injuries associated with the same histologic changes.

DECREASING $\dot{V}/\dot{Q}$ MISMATCH

Efforts directed toward improving the ratio of alveolar ventilation to perfusion may also improve hypoxemia. Low $\dot{V}/\dot{Q}$ is managed by decreasing airway obstruction (secretions, bronchospasm) or lung fluid (pneumonia, pulmonary edema). Bronchial hygiene and pharmacologic interventions (bronchodilators, diuretics) are also used in the treatment of patients with low $\dot{V}/\dot{Q}$ ratios.

Bronchial Hygiene

Vigorous bronchial hygiene is frequently the mainstay of therapy for ventilation–perfusion abnormalities. Methods include chest physiotherapy, effective coughing, and suctioning. Chest physiotherapy is used to facilitate the transfer of mucus from the lower to the upper airways, where it can be removed by suctioning or coughing. Theoretically, chest physiotherapy prevents the accumulation of secretions and aids in their removal, thereby improving oxygenation. However, there is little evidence that as a singular modality it improves Pa_{O_2}. Studies do suggest that chest physiotherapy improves mucus clearance and air flow in patients with copious secretions (e.g., cystic fibrosis, chronic bronchitis) (Feldman et al., 1979; May & Munt, 1979). Chest physiotherapy techniques (postural drainage, percussion, vibration) have been described in detail elsewhere (Dean, 1987; Starr, 1992). Typically, a combination of methods is used to optimize removal of secretions.

A variety of conditions are typically considered contraindications to chest physiotherapy, such as cardiovascular instability, coagulopathies, thoracic trauma (e.g., rib fractures), bronchospasm, degenerative bone disease, and elevated intracranial pressure (ICP). The major concern in these situations is the potential for complications associated with vigorous percussion. The clinician must be conscientious in weighing the benefits of any bronchial hygiene program with the potential risks of chest physiotherapy. For example, a patient with a head injury who also has copious amounts of secretions may benefit from the improved oxygenation derived from gentle vibration, but should not be placed in a head-down position.

It is important that the clinician document the

TABLE 31–7. **O_2 Delivery Systems**

System	Amount of O_2 Delivered	Advantages	Disadvantages	Miscellaneous
Nasal cannula	0.5–5 L/min (20%–40%)	Easy to apply Comfortable Patient able to eat	Variable amounts of O_2 delivered depending on patient's $\dot{V}_E$, O_2 flow rate, and the way patient breathes (mouth or nose) Causes mucosal drying at high flow rates (>4L/min)	Requires humidification at flow rates > 4 L/min
Simple face mask	40%–60%	Easy to apply	Variable amounts of O_2 delivered depending on patient's $\dot{V}_E$, O_2 flow rates, and mask fit Must be removed to eat May cause skin irritation if applied too tightly Uncomfortable	May be used with a nebulizer to humidify inspired gas
Partial rebreathing mask	35%–60%	Allows for delivery of higher concentrations of O_2 than a simple mask Humidification of inspired gas is unnecessary	Increases in CO_2 may occur if O_2 reserve bag collapses, allowing the rebreathing of expired gases Uncomfortable	High flow rates are necessary to prevent the reserve bag from collapsing
Nonrebreathing mask	60%–100%	One-way valve prevents rebreathing of expired gases and allows for delivery of higher F_{IO_2} than with partial rebreathing masks	Skin irritation Uncomfortable	Loose masks allow room air to enter during inspiration Requires high flow rates to prevent collapse of reservoir bag
Venturi mask	24%–50%	Maintains F_{IO_2} within a narrow range Allows for minimal rebreathing of CO_2 Humidification not necessary	Uncomfortable	Used in patients with COPD (or other patients with specific O_2 needs) to avoid depression of hypoxic drive
T-piece tracheal mask	21%–100%	Delivers variable amounts of humidified O_2 to intubated patients		May be used with oral or nasal endotracheal tubes or tracheostomy tubes Requires heated nebulizer and large-bore tubing Requires high flow rates to prevent CO_2 accumulation in T-tube reservoir
Mechanical ventilation	21%–100%	Allows for high concentrations of O_2 in patients with concomitant ventilatory failure or in patients requiring constant high F_{IO_2}	Requires skilled personnel to operate	O_2 must be warmed and humidified High F_{IO_2} may be offset with PEEP

Abbreviations: COPD, chronic obstructive pulmonary disease; PEEP, positive end-expiratory pressure.

efficacy of chest physiotherapy as well as the patient's tolerance of the procedure. This documentation should include: the impact on airway clearance (breath sounds), heart rate/rhythm, blood pressure, Sa_{O_2}, and any additional adverse outcomes, such as increased ICP or bleeding (e.g., petechiae).

Postural drainage uses gravity to assist in the drainage of secretions from localized areas of the lung. This technique is commonly used in conjunction with other methods to enhance their effectiveness. Percussion and vibration are used to loosen and dislodge mucus and assist in the movement of secretions into the bronchi and trachea.

Coughing and deep breathing may be employed singly or in combination with the techniques mentioned earlier as part of a bronchial hygiene regimen. It has been suggested that coughing is the most effective method of mobilizing and removing secretions (DeBoeck, 1984; Bateman et al., 1981).

Suctioning the trachea and mainstem bronchi is necessary when patients are unable to cough effectively and clear their secretions or when they are intubated and normal clearance of secretions is impaired. This situation is typically seen in patients with decreased LOC and in those with weak muscular strength. Various techniques have been suggested to improve the efficacy of suctioning. One such technique is the instillation of normal saline into the endotracheal tube before suctioning. This method is believed to improve Pa_{O_2} by loosening secretions and opening the airway. Several studies have been conducted to examine the usefulness of this practice. In one study, investigators instilled technetium-tagged saline solution into tracheal tubes and found that all of the normal saline remained in the trachea or mainstem bronchi even after hyperinflation (Hanley et al., 1978). Instillation of normal saline has also been reported to be of questionable value in facilitating removal of secretions, to be ineffective in improving PaO_2 (Bostick & Wendelgrass, 1987) and has been shown to have an adverse effect on SaO_2 (Ackerman, 1993). Some clinicians theorize that the major benefit of saline is its propensity to elicit a cough. Hyperventilation can also be used to elicit a cough without the deleterious effects of saline instillation on oxygenation.

Despite the fact that suctioning is a mainstay of critical care interventions, most of our practice continues to be ritualistic in nature (e.g., instilling normal saline to loosen secretions). Until recently, suctioning was typically performed on a routine basis (q 2 hr) regardless of whether or not the patient needed to be suctioned. Suctioning practices have changed significantly in the past decade, presenting both the potential for improved patient care as well as more questions for critical care clinicians and researchers.

In-line suction catheters are now commonplace. These sheath-covered catheters allow for instant suctioning availability without the cumbersome task of donning sterile gloves and assembling catheter equipment. In addition, they allow the patient to be suctioned without interrupting the delivery of ventilator tidal volumes or positive end-expiratory pressure (PEEP). Despite these benefits, research suggests that patients may still desaturate if not hyperoxygenated before they are suctioned using the catheter (Harshbarger et al., 1992). The efficacy of these catheters in successfully removing secretions and their cost/benefit ratio relative to traditional methods requires further study.

Routine hyperventilation with a manual resuscitator before suctioning is now considered of questionable benefit, especially in patients who are dependent on significant levels of PEEP to maintain adequate oxygenation (DeCampo & Civetta, 1979). This technique has largely been replaced with the use of in-line suction port adapters or in-line suction catheters, which allow patients to be suctioned without disconnecting the ventilator.

Hyperoxygenation (with or without hyperventilation) before suctioning has been demonstrated to be an important adjunct to the suctioning process in critically ill patients (Kelly et al., 1987; Chulay, 1988; Lookinland & Appel, 1991). The practice of pre-oxygenating with 100% oxygen is based on concerns that suctioning removes vital amounts of oxygen as well as secretions from the patient's tracheobronchial tree. These concerns seem justified in that significant decreases in oxygenation during suctioning have been reported, particularly in patients with decreased PaO_2. Recently, however, research (Rogge et al., 1989) has demonstrated that oxygen support of 20% higher than maintenance is as effective as 100% in maintaining O_2 level in patients with COPD. The use of oxygen insufflation catheters has been suggested as an effective alternative to traditional methods of hyperoxygenation (Dam et al., 1994). This technique uses a dual-lumen catheter that allows for both oxygen insufflation and suctioning. The widespread use of continuous pulse oximetry in critical care has also affected the time-honored use of preoxygenation. Because the clinician has continuous data regarding the patient's SaO_2, the clinician may feel more comfortable assessing the impact of suctioning on the patient and hence does not feel compelled to routinely preoxygenate all patients. This is clearly an area of nursing practice deserving further investigation.

Many questions remain about the best techniques and protocols for suctioning. Research-based algorithms that guide suctioning practice help clinicians make sound decisions about suctioning their patients (Mancinelli–Van Atta & Beck, 1992). There is, in fact, little evidence suggesting that any one method is best for all patients. The optimal approach to suctioning would include the deletion of all ritualistic procedures (e.g., q 2 hr suctioning, instillation of saline) and the adoption of a policy that promotes the individualization of a suctioning plan based on the patient's needs; for example, the use of only soft, red rubber catheters for patients with bleeding dyscrasias. This necessitates removing them from the ventilator and using the manual resuscitator. Although this is not a common "typical" practice, it appears to be the best approach for this group of patients.

Pharmacologic Agents

Bronchospasm, either alone or in combination with increased secretions, can impair ventilation. A variety of bronchodilators are now available, including sympathomimetics and corticosteroids (Table 31–8). The advent of $beta_2$-selective agents has minimized the adverse side effects (e.g., tachycardias) once common with bronchodilator therapy.

Diuretics are indicated in the treatment of low ventilation–perfusion abnormalities secondary to pulmonary edema of cardiac or noncardiac origin (i.e., ARDS). Cardiogenic pulmonary edema is treated by improving left ventricular function (by optimizing preload, afterload, and contractility). Noncardiogenic pulmonary edema is not related to heart function and therefore will not respond to similar interventions. In both instances, however, diuresis may be useful in reducing intravascular hydrostatic pressure and excessive filtration of fluid into the alveoli (Albert, 1988).

Decreasing Shunt

Intrapulmonary shunting is the most extreme form of low $\dot{V}/\dot{Q}$ mismatching. As a result, many of the techniques described in the previous section will also improve shunt. Administration of high FIO_2, however, will be futile in the patient with shunt.

TABLE 31–8. **Pharmacologic Agents Commonly Used in Acute Respiratory Failure**

Drug	Indications	Mechanism of Action	Dosage	Adverse Effects	Miscellaneous
Albuterol (Proventil/Ventolin)	Bronchospasm	Beta adrenergic	2 puffs (90 μg/puff) via metered-dose inhaler q 4–6 hr 0.5 mL of a 0.5% solution via nebulizer q 6–8 hr	Tachycardia Palpitations	
Epinephrine	Bronchospasm	Alpha and beta agonist	0.3–0.5 mL of a 1/1000 solution SC q 20–30 min (may be repeated 3 times)	Cardiac stimulation: Palpitations Arrhythmias Hypertension	Avoid use in patients with ischemic heart disease
Isoproterenol (Isuprel)	Bronchospasm	Nonselective beta agonist	1–2 puffs (131 μg/puff) via metered-dose inhaler based on individual need and response	As above	
Isoetharine (Bronkosol)	Bronchospasm	Selective $beta_2$ agonist	1–2 puffs (0.34 mg/puff) q 4 hr	As above (less severe)	
Metaproterenol (Alupent/Metaprel)	Bronchospasm	Selective $beta_2$ agonist	2–3 puffs (0.65 mg/puff) q 3–4 hr	As above	Longer duration of action than isoproterenol or isoetharine
Racemic epinephrine (Vaponephrin)	Laryngeal edema	Alpha and beta stimulation	0.25–0.5 mL of a 2.25% solution via nebulizer q 2 hr prn	Cardiac stimulation	
Ipratropium bromide (Atrovent)	Bronchospasm Increased secretions	Antimuscarinic	2 puffs (18 μg/puff) via metered-dose inhaler q 6 hr		May cause prolonged pupillary dilation if inadvertently sprayed in the eye
Corticosteroids	Bronchospasm	Anti-inflammatory	Dose dependent on type of corticosteroid administered	Gastric disturbances Hypokalemia Metabolic alkalosis	
Furosemide (Lasix)	Heart failure Pulmonary edema	Loop diuretic Decreases intravascular volume Increases venous capacitance	20–80 mg IV/PO	Volume depletion Hypokalemia Hyponatremia Hypochloremic metabolic alkalosis Ototoxicity	
Antibiotics	Pulmonary infection		Varies	Hypersensitivity reactions Superinfections	Antibiotic therapy should be based on results of culture and sensitivity tests
Heparin	Pulmonary embolism Proved or suspected deep venous thrombosis	Inactivates clotting factors	Loading dose (IV): 140–200 units/kg Maintenance dose (continuous infusion): 20 units/kg/hr	Bleeding	Heparin dosages should be adjusted to maintain PTT at 1.5 to 2.5 times control
Streptokinase	Pulmonary embolism resulting in unstable cardiopulmonary status	Antithrombolytic	Initial dose (IV): 250,000 IU over 30 min Maintenance dose (IV): 100,000 IU/hr for 24–72 hr	Hemorrhage Allergic reactions Fever Hypotension Arrhythmias	Monitor thrombin time to maintain 2.5 times normal
Urokinase	Same as for streptokinase	Same as above	Initial dose (IV): 4400 IU/kg over 30 min Maintenance dose (IV): 4400 IU/kg/hr for 12 hr	Same as above	Same as above

Data from Brenner & Yanos, 1985; Witek & Schachter, 1994; Zagelbaum & Pare, 1982.

Positive end-expiratory pressure in the ventilated patient, or continuous positive airway pressure (CPAP) in the spontaneously breathing patient, is used in the treatment of severe shunt (i.e., hypoxemia refractory to the administration of greater than 60% oxygen for at least 30 minutes) (Demers & Irwin, 1983). PEEP opens collapsed alveoli, increases the lung's functional residual capacity, and improves compliance. When pulmonary edema is present, the application of PEEP converts areas of shunt to areas of low $\dot{V}/\dot{Q}$ by opening alveoli and allowing the edema to spread over a greater surface area. The result is improved transport of gases across the pulmonary capillary membrane, an increased responsiveness to O_2 therapy, and an improvement in Pa_{O_2}.

Potential complications of PEEP include pulmonary barotrauma and a reduction in cardiac output. Barotrauma, the presence of extraalveolar air resulting from positive pressure ventilation, occurs in up to 25% of patients receiving PEEP. Barotrauma may be manifest as subcutaneous emphysema, pneumothorax, tension pneumothorax, pneumopericardium, pneumoperitoneum, interstitial emphysema and, rarely, air embolism.

PEEP reduces cardiac output by impeding venous return and possibly by impairing ventricular distensibility (Dorinsky & Whitcomb, 1983). Of note is that PEEP adversely affects patients with normal, compliant lungs more than those with abnormal lungs (e.g., those with ARDS) because PEEP is dissipated across the stiff lungs more than normal lungs. As a result, patients on PEEP with noncompliant lungs experience less change in intrathoracic pressure, and therefore there is less impact on venous return than in patients with normal lungs.

PEEP is generally applied in small increments (3 to 5 cm H_2O) while ABGs and hemodynamic parameters are being monitored. The goal is to determine the "optimal PEEP"; i.e., the amount of PEEP that allows optimal oxygenation without compromising cardiac output. Monitoring O_2 delivery allows the best evaluation of PEEP therapy because it includes the beneficial effect on oxygen content as well as the detrimental effect on cardiac output. The level of PEEP at which O_2 delivery is maximized is the optimal PEEP.

Improving O_2 Delivery

Optimizing O_2 delivery requires interventions aimed at maximizing O_2 saturation, cardiac output, and hemoglobin. Oxygen saturation can be improved by optimizing Pa_{O_2} and by stabilizing blood pH and temperature so that shifts in the oxyhemoglobin-dissociation curve (i.e., in hemoglobin's affinity for O_2) do not occur.

Anemia also has an impact on O_2 delivery. Fortunately, the body will compensate for a fall in hemoglobin by increasing cardiac output. However, this ability to increase cardiac output in compensation for anemia is often compromised in critical illness. Treatment of anemia is essential to optimize O_2 delivery and may require blood transfusions. Iron replacement may also be used as an adjunctive therapy.

Without an adequate cardiac output, oxygenated blood is unable to reach the tissues. Optimizing cardiac output may necessitate altering heart rate or stroke volume. Abnormal heart rates or rhythms can impede ventricular filling and cardiac function. Treatment of arrhythmias requires normalizing oxygenation and electrolytes and possibly administering antiarrhythmics. Stroke volume can be improved by optimizing preload (left ventricular end-diastolic volume), contractility, and afterload (systemic impedance to ventricular ejection). Preload is optimized by administering fluid or diuretic therapy and noting its effect on the pulmonary capillary wedge pressure and other variables (blood pressure, cardiac output, urine output).

Correction of acid–base and electrolyte imbalances is useful in ensuring optimal cardiac contractility. When necessary, inotropic agents (e.g., digitalis, catecholamines) may be used to improve ventricular performance.

Afterload reduction may be necessary when systemic vascular resistance is impeding ventricular ejection. Nitroprusside is often the drug of choice, although other agents (e.g., hydralazine) may also be effective. The combination of an afterload reducer and a selective inotrope (e.g., dobutamine) may be beneficial in optimizing O_2 delivery.

Optimizing O_2 Consumption

Impaired consumption of O_2 is perhaps the least understood of all the mechanisms of ARF and as a result is difficult to manage. In certain situations, however, it has been shown that improving oxygen delivery also improves oxygen consumption. The current recommendation in patients with septic shock is to increase O_2 delivery until O_2 consumption no longer increases (i.e., supply independent) (Abraham et al., 1984; Danek et al., 1980; Gutierrez et al., 1991).

Patients with cyanide poisoning also suffer from a primary failure of O_2 consumption but are more easily treated. Administration of sodium nitrate and sodium thiosulfate allows cyanide to convert to thiocyanate, a relatively nontoxic, excretable substance (Clemmer et al., 1988).

MANAGING COMPLICATIONS OF ACUTE RESPIRATORY FAILURE

Complications of ARF will arise if hypoxemia and hypercapnia are left untreated. Hypoxemia affects all bodily functions but particularly the central nervous and cardiovascular systems. Hypercapnia associated with respiratory acidosis also affects the central nervous system and may lead to cardiovascular collapse.

Although remedial steps may be helpful in managing the complications of ARF, the underlying condition must ultimately be resolved.

In addition to the complications of hypoxemia that have previously been addressed, acid-base disorders pose particular problems for the patient in respiratory failure. Not only do acid-base disorders interfere with normal cellular processes, but they also aggravate other complications.

Acute respiratory acidosis occurs when the $PaCO_2$ is allowed to rise suddenly without intervention. Treatment of respiratory acidosis involves facilitating the removal of CO_2 by improving alveolar ventilation.

Respiratory alkalosis results from hyperventilation, which may be a compensatory response to hypoxemia or may be iatrogenically induced through mechanical ventilation. Therapy is directed at treating the cause of the hyperventilation; it is seldom necessary to treat the alkalosis itself.

WEANING FROM MECHANICAL VENTILATION

One of the great challenges facing the critical care team is successfully weaning the patient recovering from ARF off the ventilator. The process of weaning can range from simple to complex, depending on the underlying process that necessitated ventilator support as well as the presence of other variables (e.g., history of COPD) (Tobin & Alex, 1994). Regardless of the patient's underlying problem or the methods used to wean, successful weaning is always dependent on the collaborative efforts of the ICU team.

Management of the weaning patient can be divided into the following processes: (1) assessment of weaning readiness, (2) implementation of the weaning trial, (3) evaluation of the weaning process, and (4) documentation.

Assessment of Weaning Readiness

The ability to maintain adequate spontaneous ventilation after an episode of ARF is dependent on a variety of factors. An accurate evaluation of the factors that help in determining readiness to wean is critical in ensuring that a premature and hence unsuccessful weaning attempt is not initiated. An assessment of weaning readiness involves an evaluation of both respiratory and nonrespiratory factors.

The most significant factor influencing weaning readiness is whether or not the underlying problem that resulted in the need for mechanical ventilation has resolved significantly. It should be noted that the etiology of ARF may have been pulmonary (e.g., pneumonia) or nonpulmonary (e.g., neurologic injury). Hence, readiness may depend on a nonpulmonary process being adequately controlled before the consideration of weaning.

Numerous respiratory parameters have been suggested as helpful in determining weaning readiness, although there is little empirical support to suggest their value as predictors of weaning success. Traditional weaning parameters include the measurement of ventilation-related factors such as $PaCO_2$, respiratory rate, tidal volume, vital capacity, inspiratory force, and work of breathing. In addition, an assessment is made of oxygenation status, using variables such as the PaO_2, SaO_2, A-a gradient, and shunt fraction ($\dot{Q}S/\dot{Q}T$).

Some evidence supports using combinations of these factors to assess a patient's weaning readiness (Morganroth et al., 1984; Yang & Tobin, 1991). An example is using the ratio of respiratory frequency to tidal volume during 1 minute of spontaneous breathing (Yang & Robin, 1991). Patients who have high respiratory rates relative to their tidal volume (rapid/shallow breathing) generally are poor weaning candidates.

Many nonrespiratory factors can directly affect the weaning process. A comprehensive assessment of weaning readiness includes an evaluation of the following factors: mental status, oxygen transport capacity, metabolic status, fluid and electrolyte status, nutrition, and psychological readiness (Henneman, 1991).

The Weaning Trial

Several techniques are currently used in weaning, and combination methods are not uncommon. They include synchronized intermittent mandatory ventilation (SIMV), T-piece, (CPAP), and pressure support. The ongoing debate over the superiority of any one weaning method continues despite the lack of support for any one technique. It has been suggested that it is not the technique, but the manner in which the technique is implemented, that influences how well a patient weans (Tobin, 1994).

The SIMV mode is typically used in the postoperative patient who is regaining spontaneous ventilation after the administration of anesthesia. The process of weaning with SIMV is relatively straightforward. The number of preset breaths the patient receives is gradually decreased while the adequacy of ventilation is assessed ($PaCO_2$). One advantage of SIMV is that the clinician has the benefit of the ventilator alarm system if the patient becomes apneic.

T-piece weaning is the process of intermittently replacing ventilator support with a T-piece assembly of corrugated tubing that delivers humidified oxygen. Patients are typically placed on the T-piece for short periods of time initially (10 minutes), then allowed to rest between trials. The amount of time off the ventilator is gradually increased and the rest periods decreased.

The technique of "zero" CPAP is similar to the T-piece method except that the patient does not need to be disconnected from the ventilator, yet like with the T-piece, the patient is totally responsible for meeting ventilation demands. CPAP has the same advantage of SIMV in that the alarm system of the ventilator remains intact. A disadvantage of CPAP relative to the T-piece is the greater resistance to breathing imposed by the inhalation values and circuitry of the ventilator.

The newest method of weaning is pressure support ventilation. It may be used alone, or in combination with the SIMV mode. Pressure support augments the patient's inspiratory effort by providing a predetermined amount of pressure "assist." Weaning by pressure support alone requires supplying a level of pressure support that produces the desired tidal volume, then decreasing the pressure in a stepwise fashion. It should be noted that the pressure support mode requires that the patient have adequate ventilatory drive, because it provides no back-up rate. Pressure support weaning continues to be used as an important adjunct for decreasing work of breathing associated with weaning (Kanek et al., 1985) and improving patient comfort (Burns, 1990) during this sometimes stressful process. When pressure support and SIMV are used in combination, the SIMV rate is gradually decreased, but spontaneous breaths have the advantage of the pressure support (see Chapter 16).

Regardless of the method chosen for weaning, certain steps that promote weaning success must be taken before weaning. This involves preparing the patient both physically and psychologically. Physical preparation includes ensuring a patent airway (e.g., chest physiotherapy, suctioning) and placing the patient in a comfortable position. Although sitting upright allows for maximal diaphragmatic excursion, it is not always the most comfortable for the patient and therefore is not always the optimal position for weaning.

Psychological preparation is especially critical if the patient is awake and alert. The process of breathing on one's own, especially after a prolonged period, can be very frightening. The clinician must provide the patient with an explanation of the weaning process, including what the patient should expect, and when he or she should expect it. As much as possible, the patient should be involved in determining the weaning plan (e.g., what time in the morning the weaning trial will start) in order to give the patient a sense of control.

Evaluation of the Weaning Process

The patient's response to weaning requires an evaluation of the neurologic and cardiovascular systems as well as the respiratory system. Changes in neurologic status frequently occur when weaning is unsuccessful, including restlessness and agitation or lethargy and somnolence, associated with hypoxemia and hypercapnia, or both.

Cardiovascular indices that require monitoring include heart rate and rhythm and blood pressure. Significant increases in heart rate or blood pressure suggest the patient is being overly stressed by the weaning trial.

An evaluation of the respiratory system requires an assessment of both subjective and objective criteria. A common complaint of patients who are weaning is a feeling of being short of breath. Clinicians must be alert to this finding, because it may be an indicator of impending weaning failure. However, patients who have not been alerted to the potential for feelings of increased work that accompany breathing on their own may interpret this effort as "shortness of breath." Differentiation by the clinician of these two responses is critical to decision making concerning whether the weaning trial should be continued. Generally, dyspnea is accompanied by other indices indicative of impaired ventilation or oxygenation, such as tachypnea and tachycardia. The use of a visual analog scale to track the patient's experience of dyspnea during weaning may be helpful in tracking progress (Bouley et al., 1992).

Other criteria that require monitoring include respiratory rate and rhythm and ABGs. When possible, noninvasive monitoring, such as pulse oximetry and $ETCO_2$ monitoring should be used. Researchers suggest that combined use of the two techniques can decrease the use of ABGs without compromising patient outcome (Niehoff et al., 1988).

Documentation

As previously noted, the key to successful weaning is coordination between members of the team, including nurses, respiratory therapists, and physicians. All parties should be involved in the planning and evaluation of this process. Key to this multidisciplinary endeavor is a system of documentation that supports the effort and allows the clinicians to note changes over time. Although critical care practitioners are typically excellent at charting over a 24-hour period, the tracking of day-to-day or week-to-week progress is essentially nonexistent in critical care settings. This becomes a problem for patients recovering from ARF, who typically do not wean in 1 day.

The best documentation system for weaning would be multidisciplinary in nature and allow for documentation of the following: (1) ventilatory mechanics before weaning, (2) type of weaning method used, (3) length of time of weaning trial, (4) why trial was stopped (planned vs. complication), and (5) comments and suggestions to assist in the next weaning trial (e.g., patient does better with family at bedside).

PROVIDING PSYCHOSOCIAL SUPPORT TO THE PATIENT AND FAMILY

Meeting the psychosocial needs of the ARF patient and the family is critical to achieving successful outcomes. Interventions aimed at meeting these needs include providing information and increasing patient/family control over the environment.

Both patients and families need to receive clear, concise information in a manner they can understand.

The stressful nature of the situation demands that information may need to be repeated several times before it is understood. The emergency nature of ARF often requires information to be given almost simultaneously with interventions (e.g., during an emergency intubation). Although this situation is often unavoidable, every attempt should be made to anticipate upcoming procedures and events so that the patient and family can be adequately prepared.

The loss of control that accompanies ARF may be devastating to the patient and family. This loss can be minimized by increasing the amount of control the patient and family have over the environment. Flexible visiting policies allow the patient and family to be together during this stressful period. Family members can provide invaluable support to staff by helping to orient and reassure the patient.

The use of restraints may be necessary to prevent the patients from extubating themselves or pulling out other invasive devices. Sedatives and analgesics should also be used as needed to minimize patient anxiety and discomfort. Neither, however, serves as a replacement for focused interventions that provide psychosocial support.

SUMMARY

Successful management of the patient with acute respiratory failure requires the combined efforts of a skilled multidisciplinary team. The critical care nurse is responsible for the ongoing assessment and treatment of patients with this potentially life-threatening problem. An understanding of the pathophysiology of ARF and current monitoring and treatment modalities provides the nurse with the knowledge base necessary for effective management of these patients.

REFERENCES

Abraham, E., Bland, R. D., Cobo, J. C., et al. (1984). Sequential cardiorespiratory pattern associated with outcome in septic shock. *Chest, 85,* 75–80.

Ackerman, M. H. (1993). The effect of saline lavage prior to suctioning. *American Journal of Critical Care, 2,* 326–330.

Albert, R. K. (1988). Physiology and management of failure of arterial oxygenation. In R. J. Fallot (Ed.), *Cardiopulmonary critical care management* (pp. 37–59). New York: Churchill-Livingstone.

American Heart Association. (1994). *Advanced Cardiac Life Support* (pp. 1–17). Dallas: American Heart Association.

Bateman, J., Newman, S. D., Daunt, K., et al. (1981). Is cough as effective as chest physiotherapy in the removal of excessive tracheobronchial secretions? *Thorax, 36,* 683–687.

Baxter Health Care Corp. Edwards Critical Care Division. Irvine, CA.

Bostick, J., & Wendelgrass, S. T. (1987). Normal saline instillation as part of the suctioning procedure. Effects on Pa_{O_2} and amount of secretions. *Heart & Lung, 16,* 532–537.

Bouley, G. H., Froman, R., & Shah, H. (1992). The experience of dyspnea during weaning. *Heart and Lung, 21,* 471–476.

Brenner, B. E., & Yanos, J. (1985). Asthma. In B. E. Brenner (Ed.), *Comprehensive management of respiratory emergencies* (pp. 315–339). Rockville, MD: Aspen.

Burns, S. M. (1990). Advances in ventilator therapy. *Focus on Critical Care, 17,* 227–237.

Chulay, M. (1988). Arterial blood gas changes with a hyperinflation and hyperoxygenation suctioning intervention in critically ill patients. *Heart and Lung, 17,* 654–661.

Clemmer, A. B., Orme, J. F., & Thomas, F. O. (1988). Physiology and management of failure of oxygen transport and utilization. In R. J. Fallot (Ed.), *Cardiopulmonary critical care management* (pp. 61–87). New York: Churchill-Livingstone.

Dam, V., Wild, C., & Baun, M. M. (1994). Effect of oxygen insufflation during endotracheal suctioning on arterial pressure and oxygenation in coronary artery bypass graft patients. *American Journal of Critical Care, 3,* 191–197.

Danek, S. J., Lynch, J. P., Wey, J. G., et al. (1980). The dependence of oxygen uptake on oxygen delivery in the adult respiratory distress syndrome. *American Review of Respiratory Disease, 122,* 387–395.

Dean, E. (1987). The ICU: Principles and practice of physical therapy. In D. L. Frownfelter (Ed.), *Chest physical therapy and pulmonary rehabilitation* (2nd ed., pp. 377–442). Chicago: Year Book.

DeBoeck, C. (1984). Cough versus chest physiotherapy—a comparison of the acute effects on pulmonary function in patients with cystic fibrosis. *American Review of Respiratory Disease, 129,* 182–184.

DeCampo, T., & Civetta, J. (1979). The effect of short term discontinuation of high level PEEP in patients with acute respiratory failure. *Critical Care Medicine, 7,* 47–49.

Demers, R. R., & Irwin, R. S. (1983). Positive end-expiratory pressure. In J. M. Rippe (Ed.), *Manual of intensive care medicine* (pp. 142–145). Boston: Little, Brown.

Demling, R. H. (1992). Role of oxygen radicals in acute lung injury. In A. Artigas, F. Lemaire, P. M. Suter, & W. M. Zapol (Eds.), *Adult respiratory distress syndrome* (pp. 121–140). London: Churchill Livingston.

Demling, R. H., & Knox, J. B. (1993). Basic concepts of lung function and dysfunction: Oxygenation, ventilation, and mechanics. *New Horizons, 1,* 362–370.

Dorinsky, P. M., & Whitcomb, M. E. (1983). The effect of PEEP on cardiac output. *Chest, 82,* 210–216.

Feldman, J., Traver, G. A., & Taussig, L. M. (1979). Maximal expiratory flows after postural drainage. *American Review of Respiratory Disease, 119,* 239–245.

Fell, T., & Cheney, F. W. (1971). Prevention of hypoxia during endotracheal suctioning. *Annals of Surgery, 174,* 24–28.

Hanley, M., Rudd, T., & Butler, J. (1978). What happens to intratracheal saline instillations? (Abstract). *American Review of Respiratory Disease, 117,* 124.

Harshbarger, S. A., Hoffman, L. A., Zullo, T. G., & Pinsky, M. R. (1992). Effects of a closed tracheal suction system on ventilatory and cardiovascular parameters. *American Journal of Critical Care, 1,* 57–61.

Henneman, E. A. (1991). The art and science of weaning from mechanical ventilation. *Focus on Critical Care, 18,* 490–501.

Kanek, R., Fahey, P. J., & Vanderwarf, C. (1985). Oxygen costs of breathing, changes dependent upon mode of mechanical ventilation, *Chest, 88,* 403–408.

Kelly, R., Yao, F., & Artusio, J. (1987). Prevention of suction induced hypoxemia by simultaneous oxygen insufflation. *Critical Care Medicine, 15,* 874–875.

Kersten, L. O. (1989). *Comprehensive respiratory nursing* (pp. 68–69). Philadelphia: W. B. Saunders.

Lookinland, S., & Appel, P. L. (1991). Hemodynamic and oxygen transport changes following endotracheal suctioning in trauma patients. *Nursing Research, 40,* 133–138.

Luce, J. M. (1988). Pathophysiology and management of ventilatory failure. In R. J. Fallot (Ed.), *Cardiopulmonary critical care management* (pp. 11–35). New York: Churchill-Livingstone.

Mancinelli-Van Atta, J., & Beck, S. L. (1992). Preventing hypoxemia and hemodynamic compromise related to endotracheal suctioning. *American Journal of Critical Care, 1,* 62–79.

Marini, J. J. (1988). Hemodynamic assessment and management of patients with respiratory failure. In R. J. Fallot (Ed.), *Cardiopulmonary critical care management* (pp. 179–214). New York: Churchill-Livingstone.

May, D. B., & Munt, P. W. (1979). Physiologic effects of chest percussion and postural drainage in patients with stable chronic bronchitis. *Chest, 75,* 29–32.

Mecca, R. S. (1986). Complications of therapy. In R. Kirby & R. W. Taylor (eds.), *Respiratory failure* (pp. 583–601). Chicago: Year Book.

Morganroth, M. L., Morganroth, J. L., Nett, L. M., & Petty, T. L. (1984). Criteria for weaning from mechanical ventilation. *Archives of Internal Medicine, 144,* 1012–1016.

Naigow, D., & Powaser, M. M. (1977). The effect of different endotracheal suctioning procedures on arterial blood gases in a controlled experimental model. *Heart & Lung, 6,* 808–816.

Neagley, S. (1991). Pulmonary system. In J. Grif-Alspach (Ed.), *AACN core curriculum for critical care nurses* (4th ed., pp. 1–131). Philadelphia: W. B. Saunders.

Niehoff, J., DelGuercio, C., Lamorte, W., et al. (1988). Efficacy of pulse oximetry and capnography in postoperative ventilatory weaning. *Critical Care Medicine, 16,* 701–705.

Rogge, J., Bunde, L., & Baun, M. (1989). Effectiveness of oxygen concentrations of less than 100% before and after endotracheal suction in patients with chronic obstructive pulmonary disease. *Heart & Lung, 18,* 64–71.

Starr, J. A. (1992). Manual techniques of chest physiotherapy and airway clearance. In C. C. Zadari (Ed.), *Clinics of Physical Therapy* (pp. 99–133). New York: Churchill Livingstone.

Tobin, M. J. (1994). Mechanical ventilation. *New England Journal of Medicine, 330,* 1056–1061.

Tobin, M. J., & Alex, C. G. (1994). Discontinuation of mechanical ventilation. In M. J. Tobin (Ed.), *Principles and practices of mechanical ventilation* (pp. 1177–1206). New York: McGraw-Hill.

Tyler, M. L. (1986). Acute respiratory failure. In M. L. Patrick, S. L. Woods, R. F. Clover, et al. (Eds.), *Medical-surgical nursing* (pp. 449–457). Philadelphia: J. B. Lippincott.

Witek, T. J., & Schachter, E. N. (1994). *Pharmacology and therapeutics in respiratory care* (pp. 137–182). Philadelphia: W. B. Saunders.

Yang, K. L., & Tobin, M. J. (1991). A prospective study of indices predicting the outcome of trials of weaning from mechanical ventilation. *New England Journal of Medicine, 324,* 1445–1450.

Zagelbaum, G. L., & Pare, J. A. (1982). *Manual of acute respiratory care* (pp. 19–50). Boston: Little, Brown.

ACUTE RESPIRATORY FAILURE MULTIDISCIPLINARY CARE GUIDE

COORDINATION OF CARE

Diagnosis/Stabilization Phase		Acute Management Phase		Recovery Phase	
Outcome	*Intervention*	*Outcome*	*Intervention*	*Outcome*	*Intervention*
All appropriate team members and disciplines will be involved in the plan of care.	Develop the plan of care with the patient/family, primary nurse(s), primary physician(s), pulmonologist, intensivist, respiratory therapist, physical or occupational therapist, dietician, pulmonary care specialist, and social services.	All appropriate team members and disciplines will be involved in the plan of care.	Update plan of care with other team members, pulmonary care practitioners, and discharge planners. Begin home care teaching to patient and family. Consult pulmonary rehabilitation if indicated.	Patient will understand how to maintain optimal health at home.	Teach patient/family about need for follow-up health care visits. Coordinate home care with continuing care agency. Involve home care company for home equipment if needed. Provide written guidelines concerning continuing care to patient/family. Provide patient/family with phone number of resources available to answer questions.

FLUID BALANCE

Diagnosis/Stabilization Phase		Acute Management Phase		Recovery Phase	
Outcome	*Intervention*	*Outcome*	*Intervention*	*Outcome*	*Intervention*
Patient will achieve optimal hemodynamic status as evidenced by: • MAP >70 mm Hg • Normal hemodynamic parameters • Free from dysrhythmias • Optimal hydration	Monitor and treat hemodynamic parameters: • BP • CO/CI • SV • SVR/PVR • PA pressures • PCWP • CVP • $S\dot{v}O_2$ • O_2 delivery • O_2 consumption Monitor lab values: electrolytes, ABG, CBC. Monitor and treat dysrhythmias. Assess weight changes from daily weights. Determine hydration needs based on hemodynamics, intake and output, viscosity of pulmonary secretions, vital signs, SaO_2, chest x-ray, and electrolytes.	Patient will maintain optimal hemodynamic status.	Continue as in first phase. Maintain optimal hydration based on continued assessment.	Patient will maintain optimal hemodynamic status.	Teach patient/family: • Patient's optimal fluid balance and how to maintain it • Review signs and symptoms of fluid overload and dehydration • Importance of daily weights • Importance of reporting any changes to physician • Home medications

Care Guide continued on following page

ACUTE RESPIRATORY FAILURE MULTIDISCIPLINARY CARE GUIDE *continued*

NUTRITION

Diagnosis/Stabilization Phase		Acute Management Phase		Recovery Phase	
Outcome	*Intervention*	*Outcome*	*Intervention*	*Outcome*	*Intervention*
Patient will be adequately nourished.	Assess nutritional status. Monitor albumin, prealbumin, total protein, cholesterol, triglycerides, and lymphocyte count.	Patient will be adequately nourished.	Dietary consult if needed. Determine patient's resting energy expenditure. Estimate caloric need and type of intake required. Monitor response to diet. Avoid high carbohydrate load in patients who retain CO_2.	Patient will be adequately nourished.	Assess effectiveness of patient/family teaching that began in acute management phase; reinforce information as needed.
		Patient will be free of bowel and elimination problems.	Treat diarrhea, constipation, or ileus as needed. Teach patient/family on: • Food pyramid and suggested servings per day • Daily caloric requirements • Safe weight-reduction or weight-gaining techniques if needed		

MOBILITY

Diagnosis/Stabilization Phase		Acute Management Phase		Recovery Phase	
Outcome	*Intervention*	*Outcome*	*Intervention*	*Outcome*	*Intervention*
Patient will achieve optimal mobility.	Assess muscle mobility, flexibility, strength, and tone.	Patient will achieve optimal mobility.	Assess physical limitations of mobility. Consult PT and/or OT for specific mobility limitations. Develop progressive activity program. Monitor response to activity and decrease if tachycardia, dyspnea, ectopy, syncope, or hypotension occur.	Patient will achieve optimal mobility.	Continue PT/OT in home if needed. Assist patient in developing realistic goals for home exercise plan. Determine a gradual increasing program of aerobic activity such as walking, swimming, water aerobics, treadmill, or exercise bicycle. Refer to outpatient pulmonary rehabilitation program if indicated.

OXYGENATION/VENTILATION

Diagnosis/Stabilization Phase		Acute Management Phase		Recovery Phase	
Outcome	***Intervention***	***Outcome***	***Intervention***	***Outcome***	***Intervention***
Patient will have a patent airway and optimal ventilation as evidenced by: • Normal chest x-ray • Respiratory rate, depth, rhythm WNL • Clear breath sounds bilaterally • SaO_2 >90%/ SpO_2 >92% • ABGs, vital signs, mental status, and pulmonary function tests WNL for the patient • Demonstrated ability to cough and clear secretions	Constantly monitor breath sounds, respiratory pattern, SpO_2. Be prepared for intubation and mechanical ventilation. Monitor quantity, color, and consistency of secretions. Monitor for signs and symptoms of respiratory distress: • Weak ineffective cough • Shortness of breath, dyspnea • Use of accessory muscles • Adventitious breath sounds • Alterations in LOC • PCO_2 >50 mm Hg or > normal for patient • SaO_2 <90% or SpO_2 <92 Monitor patients at high risk of inadequate ventilation (postoperative, on narcotics or sedation, anxious or in pain, CNS or metabolic disorders). Assist with placement and maintenance of artificial airway if needed. Maintain adequate humidification. Assist with monitoring or adjusting of ventilator settings to obtain appropriate level of assistance and minute ventilation. Assist in correction of underlying disorder. Chest physiotherapy as needed. Administer bronchodilators as indicated.	Patient will have a patent airway and optimal ventilation.	Continue as in first phase. As patient improves, change aminophylline to oral agent and monitor response. Assess readiness to wean. Measure respiratory mechanics: minute ventilation, negative inspiratory force, RR, tidal volume, vital capacity. Assess hemodynamic stability and factors that increase metabolic demand (fever, increased WBCs, bacteremia, sepsis, systemic inflammatory syndrome, hypo- or hyperthyroidism). Monitor electrolytes (including calcium, magnesium, and phosphorus) Assess for improvement in breath sounds, thin white secretions, and adequate cough reflexes. Monitor ventilatory status and hemodynamic variables prior to, during, and after weaning from mechanical ventilation. Assist with extubation. Teach patient effective cough techniques such as cascade coughing.	Patient will have optimal ventilation and gas exchange.	Teach patient about home medications and home treatments; include proper way to use metered-dose inhaler and spacer. Teach patient/family signs and symptoms of respiratory infection and when to report symptoms. Refer to outpatient pulmonary rehabilitation program if indicated.

Care Guide continued on following page

ACUTE RESPIRATORY FAILURE MULTIDISCIPLINARY CARE GUIDE *continued*

OXYGENATION/VENTILATION *continued*

Diagnosis/Stabilization Phase		Acute Management Phase		Recovery Phase	
Outcome	***Intervention***	***Outcome***	***Intervention***	***Outcome***	***Intervention***
Patient will exhibit optimal gas exchange and tissue perfusion as evidenced by: • ABGs, vital signs, and mental status WNL for patient • Normal hemoglobin • Normal intrapulmonary shunting • Urine output >.5 cc/kg • Normal liver enzymes	Monitor patient for signs/symptoms of altered gas exchange: • Dyspnea • Restlessness • Confusion • Headache • Central cyanosis (not peripheral) • $Pa{O_2}$ <50 mm Hg on room air • $Pa{O_2}/PA{O_2}$ ratio <.60 • $Pc{O_2}$ >50 mm Hg • $Sa{O_2}$ <90% • $Sp{O_2}$ <92% • Use of accessory muscles • Dysrhythmias • Hypotension Administer oxygen therapy as needed. Assess intrapulmonary shunt by one of the following: • Classic shunt equation • $Pa{O_2}/PA{O_2}$ ratio • $Pa{O_2}/FI{O_2}$ ratio • a-A gradient Improve $\dot{V}/\dot{Q}$ mismatch and shunt by: • Determining optimal PEEP and monitoring response to PEEP • Suctioning as needed • Chest physiotherapy Optimize oxygen delivery by monitoring and treating cardiac output, blood pressure, heart rate, $Sa{O_2}$, $Sv{O_2}$, Hgb, $Pa{O_2}$ Assess for evidence of adequate tissue perfusion in all organ systems (normal blood pressure, LOC, urine output, liver enzymes). Monitor and treat complications (hypoxemia, hypercapnia, acid/base disturbances, headache, restlessness, tachycardia, and hypertension).	Patient will exhibit optimal gas exchange and normal tissue perfusion.	Continue as in stabilization phase. Wean oxygen therapy as gas exchange improves. Begin patient/family teaching on the pulmonary system, current pulmonary problems, current treatment, and expected clinical course.		

COMFORT

Diagnosis/Stabilization Phase		Acute Management Phase		Recovery Phase	
Outcome	**Intervention**	**Outcome**	**Intervention**	**Outcome**	**Intervention**
Patient will be as comfortable and pain free as possible as evidenced by: • No objective indicators of discomfort • No complaints of discomfort	Plan interventions to provide optimal rest periods. Assess quantity and quality of discomfort. Administer analgesics when indicated. Provide reassurance in a calm, caring, and competent manner. Keep lights dim and a quiet environment to minimize catecholamine response. Keep head of bed elevated to enhance breathing comfort. If intubated, establish effective communication methods. Observe for complications of ARF that can cause discomfort (dyspnea, shortness of breath, bronchospasm).	Patient will be as comfortable and painfree as possible.	Instruct patient on relaxation techniques. Use complementary therapies such as guided imagery, music, humor, or body massage to enhance patient comfort.	Patient will be as comfortable and painfree as possible.	Patient will demonstrate relaxation techniques.

SKIN INTEGRITY

Diagnosis/Stabilization Phase		Acute Management Phase		Recovery Phase	
Outcome	**Intervention**	**Outcome**	**Intervention**	**Outcome**	**Intervention**
Patient will have intact skin without abrasions or pressure ulcers.	Assess all bony prominences q4h. Use preventive pressure-reducing devices when patient is at high risk for development of pressure ulcers. Treat pressure ulcers according to hospital protocol.	Patient will have intact skin without abrasions or pressure ulcers.	Continue as in first phase.	Patient will have intact skin without abrasions or pressure ulcers.	Instruct patient/family on proper skin care interventions to be continued at home.

Care Guide continued on following page

ACUTE RESPIRATORY FAILURE MULTIDISCIPLINARY CARE GUIDE *continued*

PROTECTION/SAFETY

Diagnosis/Stabilization Phase		Acute Management Phase		Recovery Phase	
Outcome	*Intervention*	*Outcome*	*Intervention*	*Outcome*	*Intervention*
Patient will be protected from possible harm.	Assess need for wrist restraints if patient is intubated. Balance the need to protect patient from dislodgement of endotracheal tube with additional fear and anxiety that might be caused by restraints. Use sedatives as indicated (preferably short acting and/or those that have the least effect on respiratory drive).	Patient will be protected from possible harm.	Give appropriate physical support as patient increases mobility to prevent falls or injury.	Patient will be protected from possible harm.	Review with patient/family any physical limitations in activity before discharge home. Consult physical and/or occupational therapy for home follow-up if limitations are present.

PSYCHOSOCIAL/SELF-DETERMINATION

Diagnosis/Stabilization Phase		Acute Management Phase		Recovery Phase	
Outcome	*Intervention*	*Outcome*	*Intervention*	*Outcome*	*Intervention*
Patient will achieve psychophysiologic stability.	Assess physiologic effect of environment on patient. Assess patient for appropriate level of stress. Assess personal responses (affective, feelings) of patient regarding critical illness. Observe the patient's patterns of thinking and communicating.	Patient will achieve psychophysiologic stability. Patient will demonstrate a decreased level of anxiety as evidenced by: • Vital signs WNL • Mental status WNL • Patient reports feeling less anxious	Include patient/family in all health care decisions. Same as Diagnostic/Stabilization Phase.	Patient will achieve psychophysiologic stability. Patient will demonstrate a decreased level of anxiety as evidenced by: • Vital signs WNL • Mental status WNL • Patient reports feeling less anxious	Same as Diagnostic/Stabilization Phase.

Outcome	Intervention
Patient will demonstrate a decreased level of anxiety as evidenced by: • Vital signs WNL • Mental status WNL • Patient reports feeling less anxious	Use calm, competent, reassuring approach to all interventions. Take measures to reduce sensory overload such as providing uninterrupted periods of rest. Allow flexible visiting patterns to meet the psychosocial needs of the patient and family.

DIAGNOSTICS

Diagnosis/Stabilization Phase		Acute Management Phase		Recovery Phase	
Outcome	*Intervention*	*Outcome*	*Intervention*	*Outcome*	*Intervention*
Patient will understand tests and procedures that are needed.	Explain all procedures and tests to patient. Be sensitive to patient's individual needs for information.	Patient will understand tests and procedures that are needed.	Explain procedures and tests needed to assess respiratory ability such as respiratory mechanics and pulmonary function tests.	Patient will understand tests and procedures that are needed.	Review with patient/family before discharge the results of significant tests and how the patient's baseline values compare to normal (ABGs, PFTs). Make sure patient has a copy of tests that may be significant to continuing home care.

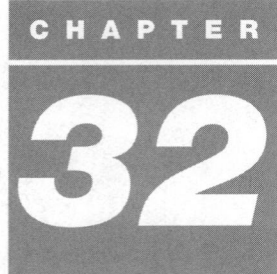

Patients With Adult Respiratory Distress Syndrome

Elaine L. Enger

Adult respiratory distress syndrome (ARDS) is a severe form of acute respiratory failure that can occur in individuals with or without preexisting pulmonary disease as a consequence of acute lung injury. To date, there is no universally accepted definition of this syndrome. In its broadest usage, ARDS refers to the acute onset of pulmonary edema that is not due to cardiogenic factors but to increased permeability factors. Hence, the term noncardiogenic pulmonary edema has been used interchangeably with ARDS. More specifically, ARDS is a term used to encompass the pathophysiologic, clinical, and pathologic alterations that occur when there is a fundamental loss in alveolar-capillary (a-c) membrane integrity. Development of increased permeability resulting from damage to the microvascular endothelial barrier or the alveolar epithelium is common to all cases of acute lung injury. Therefore, the patient will present with pulmonary edema with a high protein content. This, however, represents only the first pathologic response on a continuum of complex responses found in ARDS. Damage to the endothelial capillary membrane will result in an increased permeability interstitial edema. Damage to the alveolar barrier will result in alveolar flooding as well as a series of other gas exchange and metabolic derangements not necessarily encompassed by the term noncardiogenic pulmonary edema. Therefore, the terms are not necessarily synonymous.

In 1967, Ashbaugh and co-workers published a report describing the clinical characteristics of 12 patients who developed acute respiratory failure. These patients, admitted for such conditions as major trauma, pancreatitis, drug overdose, and viral pneumonia, all consequently developed respiratory failure during the course of their hospitalization. The authors noted that the clinical and physiologic characteristics of these patients' respiratory impairment were remarkably similar to those of neonates exhibiting infant respiratory distress syndrome. Therefore, the term adult respiratory distress syndrome was used to describe this respiratory impairment. The recognition that acute respiratory failure could occur as a consequence of nonpulmonary conditions was not new in 1967. Since World War II, the occurrence of severe pulmonary dysfunction had been noted in soldiers suffering from nonthoracic trauma. The terms wet lung, shock lung, and DaNang lung have been applied to the pulmonary edema associated with severe combat injury (Putterman, 1988). The contribution made by Ashbaugh and associates (1967) was grouping the acute respiratory failures that occurred in patients afflicted with a variety of underlying diseases into a single entity. In addition, the authors suggested that there might be a single pathogenic mechanism common to all of these cases despite the diversity of underlying disorders.

Since this report, the term ARDS has become firmly entrenched in medical terminology. There is general agreement that it is characterized by (1) a history compatible with the development of the syndrome, (2) bilateral diffuse infiltrates on the chest roentgenogram, (3) tachypnea, and (4) progressive hypoxemia despite increasing levels of inspired oxygen (Dalnogare, 1989). Although the precise incidence of ARDS is unknown, it is estimated to exceed 150,000 cases annually in the United States alone, making it one of the most common diagnoses in the critical care setting (Murray, 1977).

STRUCTURE OF THE ALVEOLAR-CAPILLARY MEMBRANE

Integral to the understanding of the pathogenesis of ARDS is the comprehension of normal alveolar-capillary membrane structure as well as fluid dynamics in the lung (Fig. 32–1).

The Microvascular Barrier: Capillary Endothelial Layer

The capillaries of the lung comprise the microvascular barrier and consist of primarily endothelial cells. The

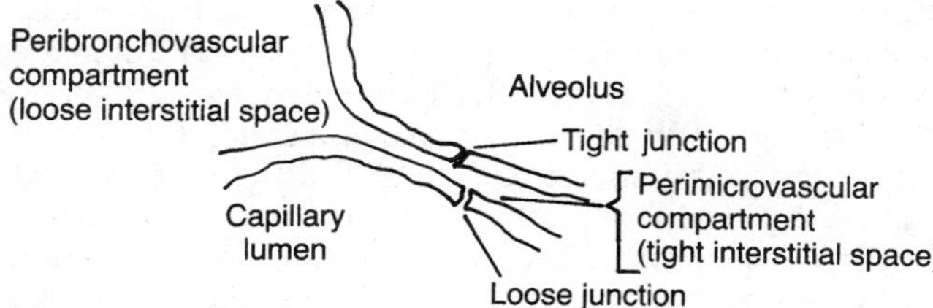

FIGURE 32–1. Schematic representation of the ultrastructure of the alveolar-capillary membrane (see text). (Adapted from Ingram, R. H., & Braunwald, E. [1988]. Pulmonary edema: Cardiogenic and noncardiogenic. In E. Braunwald [Ed.], *Heart disease* [3rd ed., p. 544]. Philadelphia: W. B. Saunders.)

thin cytoplasmic projections of these cells overlap to form a continuous tube, facilitating maximal gas exchange with minimal tissue mass. At each of the areas of overlap are clefts that serve as communication channels between the pulmonary capillaries and the interstitial space. These clefts have been referred to as "loose junctions" because their width can be enhanced as a result of increases in vascular pressures or by toxic damage. It is across these junctions that water, lipid-insoluble molecules, and macromolecules may pass (Simionescu & Simionescu, 1984).

Interstitium and Lung Lymphatics

The interstitium is organized into two interconnecting compartments (Taylor & Parker, 1985), the perimicrovascular compartment, which comprises the alveolar wall interstitium, and the peribronchovascular compartment, which consists of the loose connective tissue spaces around the bronchi and blood vessels. The peribronchovascular interstitium is wider and more compliant than the perimicrovascular interstitium. This makes it more susceptible to liquid accumulation if the capacity of the lymph channels is exceeded. In addition, there is a pressure gradient from the alveolar interstitium (which is exposed to alveolar pressure) to the peribronchovascular interstitium (which possesses a more negative pressure approximating pleural pressure). This pressure gradient encourages fluid drainage from areas of high to low pressure into the peribronchovascular interstitium in an effort to prevent fluid accumulation near the air–blood interface (Havill & Gee, 1984).

Lymphatic channels are not present in the perimicrovascular interstitium (Staub, 1974). They originate in the connective tissue of the peribronchovascular compartment. Under normal conditions, fluid and protein filtered into the interstitium are directed along lymphatic ducts and are pumped via thoracic ducts into the superior vena cava as rapidly as they accumulate. Therefore, the lymph channels serve as an indispensable means of draining extravasated fluid and proteins from the interstitium. Although no method for measuring lymph flow in humans exists, it has been estimated by Staub (1974, 1980) to average 20 mL/hr in the resting 70-kg individual. Drainage away from the alveolar wall also occurs by the filling of loose connective tissue spaces of the peribronchovascular compartment called cuffs. The capacity of these cuffs to fill with fluid increases as the lungs are inflated and the cuff pressures fall (Havill & Gee, 1984). These cuffs are then drained slowly into the surrounding blood vessels or down the prevailing pressure gradient to the openings of lymph channels in the mediastinum.

The Alveolar Barrier: Alveolar Epithelial Layer

The alveolar barrier consists of two types of epithelial cells. The type I cells are thin, flat cells that cover 95% of the surface area. They are extremely vulnerable to injury and possess limited regenerative capabilities. The remaining surface area of the alveolar barrier is covered by the more compact type II cells, which secrete surfactant, a regulatory product that decreases alveolar surface tension. These cells appear to be far less susceptible to injury and possess remarkable reparative abilities (Connors et al., 1981). Like the cells of the capillary endothelium, the alveolar epithelial cells abut and overlap. However, because the areas of overlap in the capillary endothelium are loose junctions, the alveolar epithelium must serve as the principal protector against alveolar fluid accumulation. To achieve this, alveolar epithelial cell clefts are obliterated by complete fusion of the membranes of the adjacent cells. The alveolar barrier, therefore, has a very low permeability, and much greater distending forces are required before any disruption or transport can occur. Therefore, these junctions have been referred to as "tight junctions." In addition, the interstitial pressure gradient favors the movement of fluid away from the alveolar wall so that it may be drained by the lymphatics. This explains why interstitial edema precedes alveolar edema. Even though fluid leaks into the interstitial tissues, it will not accumulate and lead to gas exchange abnormalities because it is efficiently removed by the lymphatics. Therefore, the alveoli will flood only if the rate of fluid filtration increases beyond the capacity of the lymphatics to drain it away and of the peribronchovascular cuffs to sequester it from the alveolar walls (Staub, 1983).

PHYSIOLOGIC BASIS OF FLUID MOVEMENT

The Microvascular Barrier: Capillary–Interstitial Exchange

The lung is not a dry organ. In fact, it has one of the highest water contents of any organ. There is normally a continuous exchange of liquid, colloid, and solutes between the vascular bed and the interstitium due to the loose endothelial capillary junctions as well as to

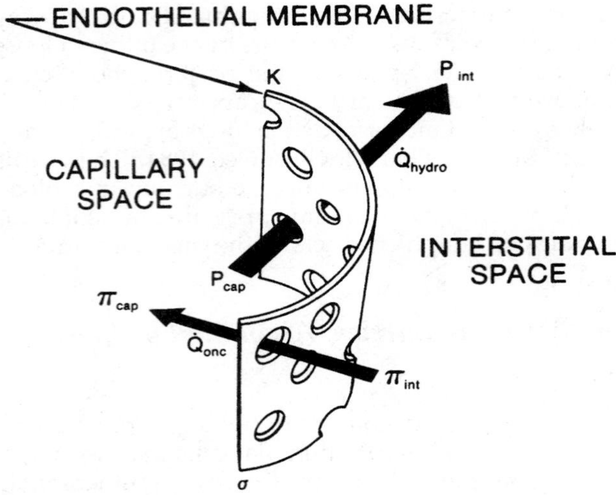

THE STARLING EQUATION

$$\dot{Q}_f = K(P_{cap} - P_{int}) - K\sigma(\pi_{cap} - \pi_{int})$$

FIGURE 32–2. Fluid filtration across the endothelial membrane into the interstitial space is the sum of the fluid filtration generated by the hydrostatic pressure gradient, which tends to push fluid into the interstitial space, and the filtration generated by the oncotic pressure gradient, which tends to pull fluid into the capillary. The final factor influencing fluid filtration is the inherent permeability of the membrane. The relationship of these factors is mathematically expressed by the Starling equation. (Adapted from Connors, A. F., McCaffrie, D. R., & Rogers, R. M. [1981]. The adult respiratory distress syndrome. *Disease-a-Month, 27,* 1–75.)

the balance of the driving filtration forces (Taylor, 1981). These driving forces, including both hydrostatic and osmotic pressures, have been referred to collectively as Starling forces because Ernest Starling first recognized that fluid flow out of a vessel was determined by a balance of these forces acting across a semipermeable membrane. A pathologic state will exist only when there is an increase in the net flux of liquids and colloids from the vascular into the interstitial space. The dynamic equilibrium between the capillary and interstitial forces that determines net transvascular fluid flux is mathematically described by the Starling equation (Staub, 1978). The equation is generally expressed as the balance between hydrostatic and osmotic forces (Connors et al., 1981) (Fig. 32–2).

Although the Starling equation appears quite complex, it can be simplified by summarizing that three major factors influence net transvascular fluid flux across the pulmonary capillary endothelium: hydrostatic pressure, colloidal osmotic pressure, and the integrity of the capillary endothelial membrane (Staub, 1978).

HYDROSTATIC PRESSURE

Transvascular hydrostatic pressure, or the difference between the microvascular and interstitial hydrostatic pressure, will influence the outward movement of fluid from the vasculature. In other words, hydrostatic pressure is considered a "push" pressure, and it is the primary force regulating fluid flux. If hydrostatic pressure is higher in the microvascular space (the capillary) than in the interstitial space, fluid will be pushed out of the capillary. Conversely, if interstitial hydrostatic pressure exceeds capillary hydrostatic pressure, fluid will be pushed out of the interstitial space. An indirect estimate of microvascular hydrostatic pressure or pulmonary capillary pressure can be easily obtained from the pulmonary artery wedge pressure (PAWP) or left atrial pressure measurements. Interstitial hydrostatic pressure is very difficult to measure. It is assumed to be closely related to pleural pressure and thus is estimated to be subatmospheric (Staub, 1974). Consequently, under normal conditions hydrostatic pressure is higher in the intravascular space, and thus the net fluid flux as influenced by this pressure is from capillary to interstitium. In addition, because pulmonary blood flow is gravity dependent and is greater in the basilar regions, filtration of fluid into the interstitium will also be highest in the lung bases.

COLLOIDAL OSMOTIC PRESSURE

Transvascular colloidal osmotic pressure, or the difference between microvascular and interstitial osmotic forces, opposes transvascular hydrostatic pressure at fluid exchange sites. Because molecules smaller than plasma proteins pass unhindered across the microvascular barrier, colloidal osmotic forces are generated primarily by the plasma proteins and macromolecules. Colloidal osmotic (oncotic) pressure is considered a "pull" pressure. Fluid will be pulled or drawn toward the compartment where protein concentration is greatest. Plasma osmotic pressure is generally about 1.3 mOsm or 24 mm Hg (Nitta et al., 1981). Interstitial osmotic pressure is generated by extravasated proteins in the interstitial fluid. Although this pressure has not been measured directly, it has been calculated to be approximately 0.8 mOsm or 14.5 mm Hg (Erdmann et al., 1975). Consequently, under normal conditions the net fluid flux as influenced by colloidal osmotic pressure is from interstitium into capillary (Staub, 1974, 1980).

MICROVASCULAR BARRIER PERMEABILITY

The last factor influencing fluid flux is the inherent permeability of the microvascular barrier. This permeability is expressed in the Starling equation by two descriptors, the Kf and the σf. The Kf is a measure of how easily fluid crosses the barrier per unit of barrier filtering area. It therefore is the primary measure of permeability and is determined by the structure and function of the endothelial cells forming the barrier. Although it cannot be measured directly, it is believed that the Kf is normally quite low because fluid filtration is quite low relative to the large surface area of the lung (Staub, 1980). The σf is a measure of how effectively the barrier hinders the passage of solutes and thus also reflects capillary membrane permeability. It is an intrinsic property of the barrier. The σf of the microvascular barrier appears to be quite high, so the barrier is quite proficient at hindering the passage of solutes (Staub, 1980).

BALANCE OF FORCES: CAPILLARY–INTERSTITIAL FLUID EXCHANGE

In summary, three factors determine the flux of fluid across the microvascular barrier: hydrostatic pressure, colloidal osmotic pressure, and the inherent permeability or integrity of the capillary endothelial membrane. Under normal conditions, both hydrostatic pressure and osmotic pressure are higher in the intravascular space than in the interstitial space. Consequently, there is a relative balance of forces pushing fluid out of and pulling fluid into the capillary across a semipermeable membrane, the net flux being in an outward direction. This fluid flux, which constitutes approximately 20 mL/hr, can easily be drained by the lymphatics. A pathologic state will exist only when there is an increase in the net flux of extravasated fluid.

The Alveolar Barrier: Interstitial–Alveolar Exchange

As previously indicated, fluid and protein do not normally cross into the alveoli because the alveolar barrier possesses a low permeability. In addition, fluid is continuously drained away from the alveolar walls through the interstitium and removed by the lymphatics (Crandell, 1983).

GENERAL PATHOGENESIS OF PULMONARY EDEMA

Pathogenic Mechanisms

From the foregoing discussion of the a-c membrane structure and the regulatory factors of fluid movement, three potential predisposing mechanisms of pulmonary edema can be identified (Bernard & Brigham, 1986). The first of these mechanisms is an imbalance of the Starling forces leading to an increase in fluid filtration into the interstitium that exceeds lymphatic capacity. This situation is generally referred to as an increased pressure edema. Increased microvascular hydrostatic pressure (PAWP) constitutes the most common alteration in Starling forces. Congestive heart failure resulting in increased pulmonary venous pressure is the most frequent clinical cause. For this reason, increased pressure edema is sometimes called cardiogenic pulmonary edema regardless of the fact that other Starling forces besides microvascular hydrostatic pressure may be contributing to the increased extravascular fluid flux.

The second mechanism is a primary lymphatic insufficiency that limits the rate of removal of extravascular fluid. This mechanism is probably responsible for the edema that develops when lymphatics are disrupted following lung transplantation.

The third mechanism is fundamental damage to the a-c membrane that increases the microvascular barrier's permeability to fluid and protein. This renders the normal Starling forces that limit fluid extravasation inoperative. This situation is referred to as increased permeability pulmonary edema, and it is the mechanism responsible for the development of pulmonary edema in ARDS. Normally, the capillary endothelial barrier deters most protein filtration. When this membrane is damaged, permeability to protein is greatly enhanced. On examination of the Starling equation, it is evident that with the loss of barrier integrity, the major determinant of fluid flux will be hydrostatic pressure. Because capillary hydrostatic pressure normally far exceeds interstitial hydrostatic pressure, capillary endothelial damage will result in increased water conductance into the interstitium. Lymphatic capability to pump excess filtrate away will be enhanced even at low capillary hydrostatic driving pressures (PAWP). The increased permeability pulmonary edema witnessed in ARDS, therefore, is identified by a concomitant increase in pulmonary lymph flow and lymph protein content (Sibbald et al., 1983).

Process and Sequence of Fluid Accumulation

Regardless of the specific mechanism involved, the sequence of fluid exchange and accumulation can be described in three separate stages, the last of which consists of two almost simultaneous substages (Fishman, 1980; Staub et al., 1967) (Fig. 32–3).

STAGE I. During this stage, an increase in mass transfer of fluid and colloid from the capillaries occurs across the microvascular barrier to the interstitium. The capillary endothelial junctions may have been widened by an increase in filtrative forces or by toxic damage. However, no measurable increase in interstitial volume is seen because lymphatic outflow also increases. In addition, fluid and protein are pumped down the prevailing pressure gradient away from the alveolar walls into the loose perivascular tissue. As a result, development of pulmonary edema is limited.

STAGE II. Stage II occurs when the amount of fluid filtered out of the capillary approaches and exceeds lymphatic drainage capacity. If the integrity of the microvascular barrier is maintained and there is no alteration in its permeability, the filtered fluid will be relatively free of protein. This will result in a dilution of interstitial protein, a decrease in the osmotic forces pulling fluid into the interstitium, and a maintenance of blood protein osmotic pull. All of these factors will help to deter further progression of edema. If, how-

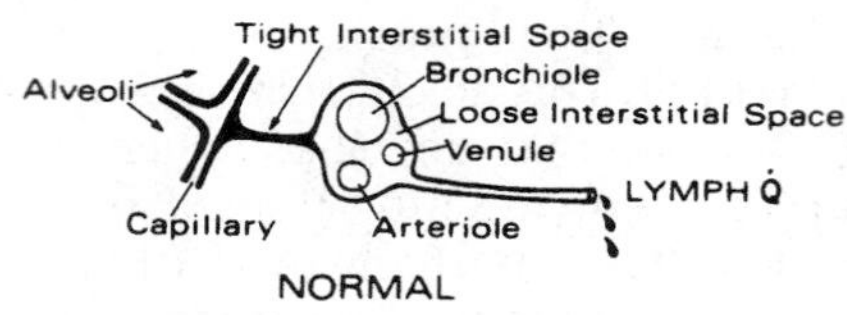

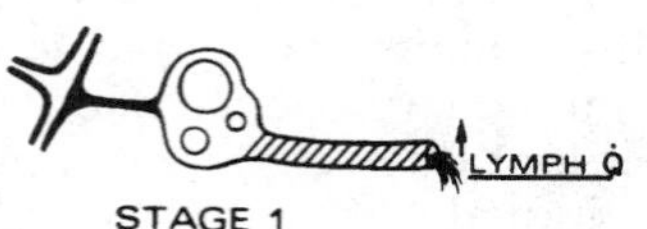

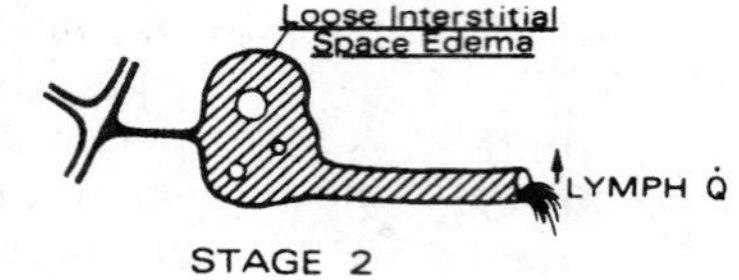

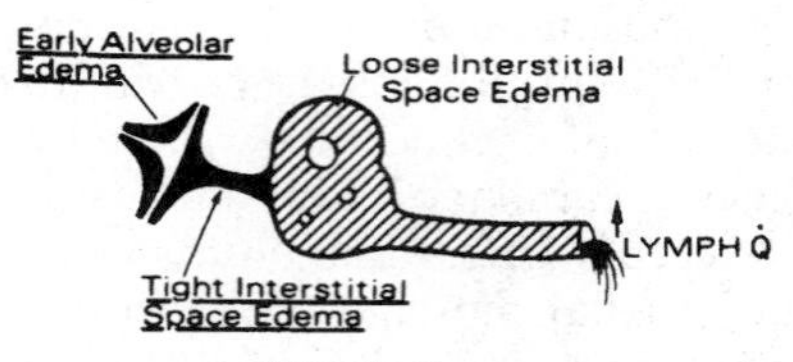

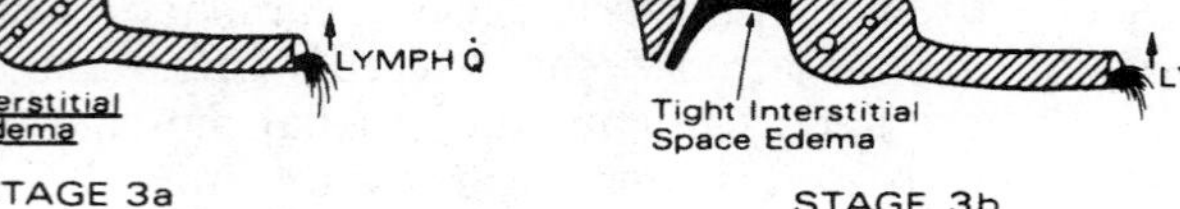

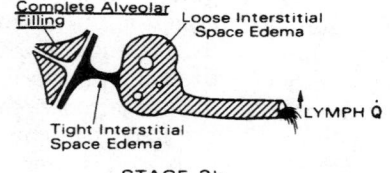

FIGURE 32–3. Schematic representation of the a-c membrane, loose interstitial space, and lymphatic system at the several stages of pulmonary edema. The new feature at each stage from normal to fully developed alveolar edema is underlined. (From Ingram, R. H., & Braunwald, E. [1988]. Pulmonary edema: Cardiogenic and noncardiogenic. In E. Braunwald [Ed.], *Heart disease* [3rd ed., p. 547]. Philadelphia: W. B. Saunders.)

ever, this safety mechanism does not sufficiently protect the interstitium or if the barrier is injured, liquid and colloid will begin to accumulate in the peribronchovascular interstitium. Increases in interstitial volume, however, will result in only small elevations of interstitial pressure until the interstitial volume is quite large. This mechanism serves as an attempt to keep the hydrostatic driving pressure across the alveolar barrier suitably low.

STAGE III. In this stage, the volume limits of the loose interstitium have been exceeded. Therefore, fluid will begin to distend the less compliant perimicrovascular (alveolar wall) interstitium. As fluid fills the alveolar interstitium, several mechanisms come into play in an attempt to protect the alveoli from edema. The first protective mechanism is the alveolar epithelial membrane. The junctions of this membrane are quite tight and thus serve as excellent barriers to fluid flux. In addition, surfactant plays a role in keeping the alveoli dry by reducing surface tension at the air–liquid interface. If, however, the pressure developing in the alveolar wall interstitium is sufficient to disrupt the tight junctions of the alveolar epithelium, alveolar edema occurs in two substages. In the normal adult, the interstitial space can accommodate 200 to 300 mL of fluid before alveolar edema occurs (Staub et al., 1967).

Initially, fluid accumulates in the corners of the alveoli. This small fluid accumulation will, however, eventually alter the surface tension of the alveoli. As a result, alveolar size will be diminished, gas volume will be replaced by edema fluid, and alveolar flooding will ensue. During alveolar flooding, the alveoli are filled individually in an "all or none" fashion (Staub et al., 1967). The exact process by which alveolar flooding occurs remains unclear. However, it is believed that this flooding occurs when alveoli reach a critical configuration, at which point inflation pressures can no longer maintain the existing structure.

PREDISPOSING FACTORS FOR ARDS

Diffuse a-c membrane injury, the hallmark of ARDS, can result from a variety of direct mechanisms such as inhaled or blood-borne toxins as well as from indirect mechanisms such as the release of various intervening mediators or neurohumoral factors. Therefore, a large number of clinical predispositions have been described (Beale & Grover, 1993; Maunder, 1986; Messent & Griffiths, 1992). These can be divided into two groups: those that involve direct damage to the lung and those in which a remote disease process indirectly affects the lung, presumably through the action of humoral inflammatory mediators. The most commonly cited conditions associated with ARDS are listed in Table 32–1. Recent epidemiologic studies suggest that

TABLE 32–1. **Predisposing Factors for ARDS**

Direct Injury	Indirect Injury
Aspiration of gastric contents	Septicemia or septic syndrome
Direct pulmonary trauma	Shock syndrome
Pneumonia	Multiple trauma
Oxygen toxicity	Drug overdose
Inhalation (smoke/noxious gases)	Multiple transfusions
Near-drowning	Disseminated intravascular coagulation
	Fat, amniotic fluid, thrombotic or air embolism
	Acute hemorrhagic pancreatitis
	Cardiopulmonary bypass
	Eclampsia

the incidence of ARDS differs greatly among these predisposed groups.

The highest incidence appears to occur in patients with septic syndrome. This is described as a combination of leukocytosis or leukopenia, a known source of infection, fever or hypothermia, and hypotension regardless of whether blood cultures are positive for a gram-negative bacterial pathogen. More than one-third of these patients develop ARDS (Fowler et al., 1983; Pepe et al., 1982).

The second most common predisposition appears to be aspiration of gastric contents, which has an incidence of associated ARDS of approximately 30%. It has been suggested that aspiration of gastric contents with a pH of less than 2.5 is particularly likely to lead to lung injury (Fowler et al., 1983; Pepe et al., 1982).

All types of shock have been associated with lung injury. Historically, shock was felt to be such an important predisposition for ARDS that the syndrome was termed "shock lung" by many investigators (Ayres, 1982; Shoemaker & Hauser, 1979). The relative importance of the various types of shock as a single risk factor is difficult to ascertain. Only 2% to 7% of patients presenting with hemorrhagic shock alone are reported to develop ARDS (Fowler et al., 1983). Because many of these patients have sustained trauma and have received multiple blood transfusions, it is difficult to implicate hemorrhagic shock as an isolated risk factor. Cardiogenic shock has also been described as a predisposing factor (Keren et al., 1980). However, it is difficult to differentiate increased pressure from increased permeability pulmonary edema in these cases.

The patient who has sustained multiple trauma is at high risk for ARDS. Fulton and Jones (1975) reported post-traumatic pulmonary insufficiency in 22% of patients with multiple trauma associated with pulmonary involvement and in 14% of patients with multiple trauma without primary chest involvement. ARDS has also been associated with head trauma as well as near-drowning.

Many drugs, when taken in excess, have been classified as predispositions to ARDS. These include narcotics, especially heroin, and barbiturates as well as aspirin, colchicine, and thiazides (Taylor & Duncan, 1983).

One of the mainstays in treatment of ARDS is also a potent lung toxin. High concentrations of oxygen may cause significant lung injury by facilitating the production of oxygen-free radicals (Jenkinson, 1982). Other inhalants such as smoke and nitrogen dioxide have also been linked with ARDS (Taylor & Duncan, 1983).

It is most important to note that the risk of developing ARDS has been reported to increase dramatically if more than one predisposing factor exists—25% with one risk factor, 42% with two risk factors, 85% with three risk factors (Beale & Grover, 1993). In addition, it has been shown that the onset of ARDS usually occurs within 48 hours of the occurrence of a risk factor. Thus, patients who survive for 2 days after a risk factor event will usually not develop ARDS (Fowler et al., 1983; Pepe et al., 1982).

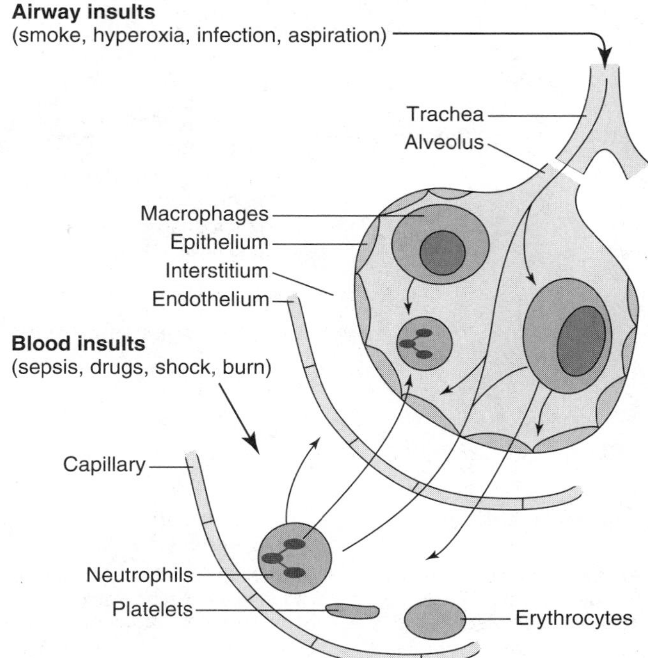

FIGURE 32–4. Progression to ARDS. Interaction between cell types and predisposing factors. (Adapted from Repine, J. E. [1992]. Scientific perspectives on adult respiratory distress syndrome. *Lancet, 339*:446–469.)

MECHANISMS AND MEDIATORS OF ACUTE LUNG INJURY: THE ROLE OF POLYMORPHONUCLEAR LEUKOCYTES

There are many potential mechanisms and mediators of lung injury in ARDS (Boxer et al., 1990). Which mediators are involved and their cells of origin remain unclear. Because information from humans is difficult to obtain and interpret, most of our knowledge about the mechanisms of acute lung injury comes from experimental animal models. From these models it has been learned that many cells and cell interactions are likely to be involved in the pathogenesis of ARDS. These cells include alveolar macrophages, neutrophils, platelets, and endothelial cells. The interaction of these cells as well as how both the direct and indirect factors predisposing ARDS might lead to the progression of acute lung injury is depicted in Figure 32–4 (Repine, 1992). Activation of these cells results in the development of an acute inflammatory response with the release of several critical mediators that can potentiate the physiologic derangements witnessed in ARDS (Fig. 32–5) (Boxer et al., 1990). Most research to date has focused on the role of the neutrophil or polymorphonuclear leukocyte (PMN) because these cells are capable of being activated by and producing most of the potential inflammatory and toxic products that have been linked to acute lung injury. It has been hypothesized that various events known to incite ARDS cause an abnormal accumulation of adherent neutrophils in the vasculature of the lung and that tissue in-

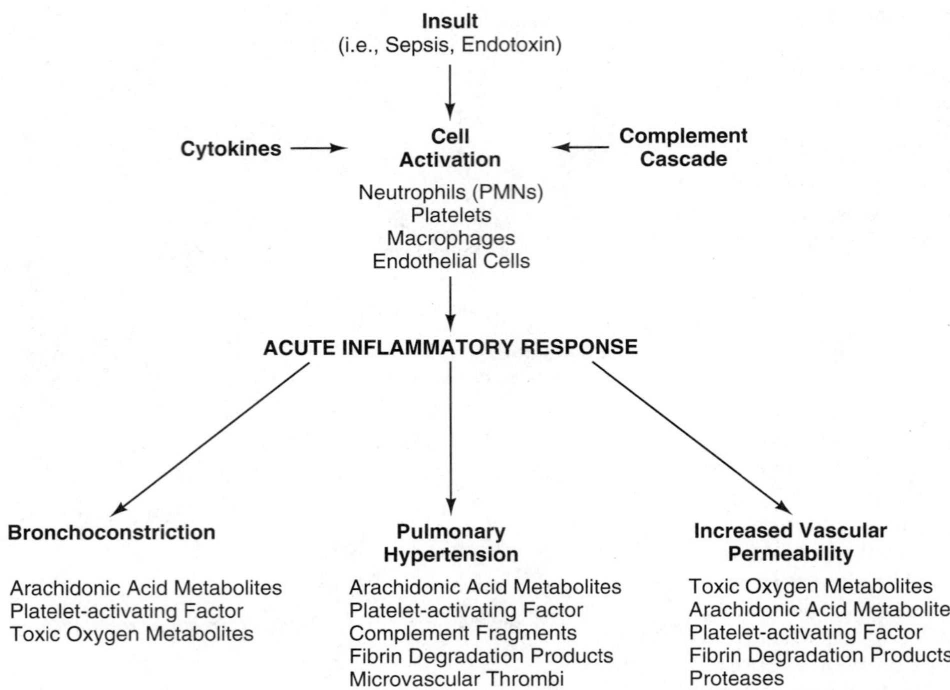

FIGURE 32–5. Potential mediators of the acute inflammatory response and the physiologic derangements in ARDS.

jury resulting from neutrophil stimulation is central to the development of ARDS. Therefore, rather than attempt to describe all the cells and mediators that have been implicated in the pathogenesis of ARDS, this review concentrates on the role of the PMN. The reader should be aware, however, that PMN-independent pathways undoubtedly exist (Rinaldo & Rogers, 1986).

Overview

Normally, the pulmonary circulation contains a large pool of marginated or inactive PMNs (Cooper et al., 1985). The premise is that a catastrophic clinical insult leads to the activation of these PMNs. This activation results in increased PMN adherence and entrapment in the lungs. In this aggregated, trapped state, PMNs generate and secrete toxic substances and degradative enzymes that promote the physiologic derangements in ARDS. Many of these factors can directly injure the microvascular and alveolar barriers, promoting the development of pulmonary edema. They can also disrupt normal pulmonary blood flow and coagulation, thus leading to the onset of pulmonary hypertension. They can amplify the inflammatory response by attracting more neutrophils. Consequently, activated PMNs create a vicious self-perpetuating cycle that inevitably leads to severe lung injury (Putterman, 1988) (Fig. 32–6).

Considerable experimental evidence suggests that PMNs play a critical role in ARDS (Repine & Beehler, 1991). If PMNs are instrumental, it would be expected that activation of leukocytes would be abnormal in patients with ARDS and that their number would be at least transiently diminished in the peripheral blood and increased in bronchoalveolar lavage samples as a consequence of lung sequestration. Indeed, these findings have been reported. Neutrophils obtained from pulmonary artery blood from critically ill patients with ARDS appear to be in a functionally and metabolically activated state compared to those from patients without ARDS (Zimmerman et al., 1983). Increased numbers of neutrophils have been found by several investigators in the bronchoalveolar lavage of patients with

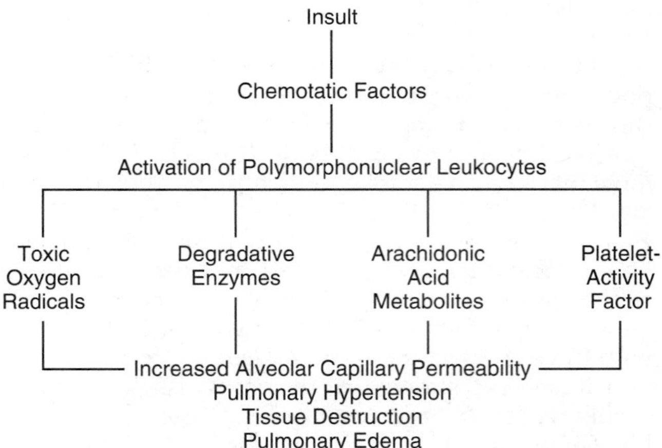

FIGURE 32–6. Flow chart showing the proposed mechanism of PMN activation promoting the physiologic derangements in ARDS.

ARDS. In healthy lungs, neutrophils constitute approximately 1% to 3% of the recovered cells. These studies, however, have reported that within 24 hours of the onset of ARDS, 68% to 82% of the lavaged cells were neutrophils; increased numbers of neutrophils were not present in the bronchoalveolar lavage obtained from intubated patients with non-ARDS respiratory failure (Christner et al., 1985; Parson et al., 1985; Weiland et al., 1986). In a prospective study of 40 patients at risk of developing ARDS, blood leukocyte counts were measured serially (Thommasen et al., 1984). Of the 10 patients who developed ARDS, 8 demonstrated peripheral blood leukocyte counts that fell to extremely low levels. Only 4 of the remaining 30 patients without ARDS demonstrated a similar fall in number of circulating leukocytes. Thommasen and colleagues (1984) found a predictable relation between an acute fall in circulating neutrophils and the onset of ARDS in septic patients. In another study aimed at identifying the reason for this decrease in circulating leukocytes, patients who were injected with indium-labeled autologous neutrophils demonstrated an increased amount of radioactivity accumulating in the lung (Powe et al., 1982). It was inferred, therefore, that the decreased number of reported circulating leukocytes may well be a mark of the sequestration of leukocytes in the lungs.

Mechanism of PMN Activation

If PMN activation is critical to the onset of ARDS, what mediators are responsible for this activation? At least three inflammatory mediators have been postulated: complement, endotoxin, and tumor necrosis factor (TNF).

Several observations support the hypothesis that stimulation of the complement system, which in turn activates PMNs, is essential to the development of lung injury in ARDS (Tate & Repine, 1983). Complement activation during hemodialysis causes hypoxemia and concurrent neutrophil sequestration in the human lung. In addition, several of the predispositions to ARDS, such as trauma, pancreatitis, and sepsis, are associated with complement cascade activation. The premise is that activation of the complement system results in the production of chemotaxins, especially C5a, which induce PMN activation (Goldstein, 1988). A prospective study of 61 patients at risk for ARDS reported an increase in C5a levels before ARDS onset in 31 of 33 patients developing ARDS; only 5 of the 28 patients not developing ARDS had similar elevations of C5a (Hammerschmidt et al., 1980).

Infusion of endotoxin or lipopolysaccharide, a component of the gram-negative bacterial cell wall, produces clinical signs identical to ARDS (Ghosh et al., 1993). The hydrophobic lipid A moiety of lipopolysaccharide possesses a number of proinflammatory direct effects. PMNs exposed to lipopolysaccharide have been reported to develop increased adhesiveness (Pohlman et al., 1986) and to release large amounts of toxins (Strieter et al., 1989). Again, because sepsis frequently precedes ARDS, these direct lipopolysaccharide effects may be important in initiating pulmonary injury.

Cytokines may play a pivotal role in PMN activation in ARDS. Cytokines are communication proteins essential for cell-to-cell signalling. At low levels, these cytokines appear to perform critical homeostatic actions that regulate immunologic and physiologic events. However, at high concentrations, cytokines can exert harmful biological effects, which range from target organ dysfunction to life-threatening systemic inflammatory reactions (Christman, 1992). The primary cytokines implicated in ARDS, which are released from macrophages and monocytes, are TNF and interleukin-1 (IL-1). These cytokines appear to stimulate the elaboration of other cytokines, producing a cascade effect that promotes an uncontrolled inflammatory response and the clinical picture of ARDS (Shapiro & Gelfand, 1993). TNF has been termed a proximal mediator in that it possesses numerous effects at the cellular level which may initiate or amplify the action of other mediators and effector cells that promote ARDS. TNF is known to stimulate not only the release of several other cytokines, but also the production of endothelial adhesion molecules that promote PMN–endothelial cell adherence. TNF primes PMNs for activation and potentiates the release of their toxic enzymes (Klebanoff et al., 1986), which cause injury to endothelial cells, promoting an increase in permeability (Stephens et al., 1987). TNF may also affect tissue procoagulant activity and thus contribute to thrombosis as well as small vessel clotting (Repine, 1992). The infusion of recombinant human TNF into experimental animals causes PMNs to sequester and adhere to lung capillaries, leading to a pattern of lung edema and hemorrhage indistinguishable from ARDS (Tracey et al., 1988). The strongest evidence supporting the role of TNF in the pathogenesis of ARDS, especially related to septic shock, has been gleened from studies that employ anti-TNF antibodies. Specifically, a significant reduction in mortality has been observed in both mice (Beutler et al., 1985) and rabbits (Mathison et al., 1988) that have been passively immunized against TNF with monoclonal antibodies and then subsequently given endotoxin. The polypeptide cytokine IL-1 has likewise been linked to ARDS. IL-1 is a potent inflammatory stimulant with biologic effects that include endothelial cell and PMN activation, fever, hypotension, and increased vascular permeability. IL-1 also promotes the release of other cytokines and acts synergistically with TNF in the production of many of its effects. Raised concentrations of both TNF and IL-1 have been found in blood samples and bronchoalveolar lavage fluid taken from ARDS patients (Hyers et al., 1991; Jacobs et al., 1989). The relative contributions of the direct toxic effects of cytokines and those caused indirectly by the products of activated PMNs and their secondary mediators is unclear. However, in the final fibroproliferative phases of ARDS, locally produced cytokines are thought to regulate the growth, chemotaxis, and metabolic activity of lung fibroblasts, influencing the ultimate balance between fibrosis and remodeling of normal lung tissue (Messent & Griffiths, 1992).

Consequences of PMN Activation

Once activated, PMNs can damage the lung through several mechanisms: (1) release of toxic oxygen metabolites, (2) release of degradative enzymes, (3) release of arachidonic acid metabolites, and (4) release of platelet-activating factor (PAF).

RELEASE OF TOXIC OXYGEN METABOLITES

Reactive, toxic oxygen metabolites represent a group of molecules generated through the reduction of oxygen (Klebanoff, 1980). Activated PMNs possess an enzyme that catalyzes the reduction of oxygen by facilitating the addition of an electron to the oxygen molecule. When oxygen picks up this electron, it becomes a superoxide anion, a free radical (Babior et al., 1973). Oxygen-derived free radicals can participate in a variety of reactions with other molecules as well as with themselves. They can be further reduced to several toxic metabolites, including hydrogen peroxide and the hydroxyl ion, or can react with arachidonic acid to produce chemotactic factors that attract more PMNs to the site of injury. In general, the various molecules formed from superoxide are very reactive. The cell interior is protected by antioxidant enzymes that scavenge toxic oxygen metabolites. Thus, if the release of these metabolites is minimal, the host will maintain organ function through reparative and cellular proliferative mechanisms (McCord, 1993). However, because normal extracellular defenses against oxygen-derived free radicals are not very potent, these compounds are not readily converted to nontoxic products outside cells. As such, when the amount of toxic oxygen metabolites released surpasses the host's ability to counterbalance their injurious effects through antioxidant defense mechanisms, direct endothelial (Varani et al., 1985) and lung parenclymal (Martin et al., 1981) cell damage will ensue. Indeed, experimental administration of agents that generate reactive oxygen species has been reported to cause pathologic changes resembling ARDS (Messent & Griffiths, 1992). Studies of bronchoalveolar lavage fluid in patients with ARDS have produced evidence of increased oxidant activity (Cochrane et al., 1983).

RELEASE OF DEGRADATIVE ENZYMES

When PMNs are activated, granules in their cytoplasm are stimulated to release a variety of degradative enzymes (Ayars et al., 1984). The proteases that degrade elastin, collagen, and basement membranes have been studied the most intensively (Dalnogare, 1989). These proteases have been implicated as major factors contributing to the production of experimental acute lung injury and have been found in the bronchoalveolar lavage fluid from patients with ARDS (Lee et al., 1981). Intravenous administration of elastase has been shown to increase pulmonary vascular resistance, induce pulmonary leukocytosis and microembolization, and increase the venous admixture of oxygen (Stokke et al., 1986).

RELEASE OF ARACHIDONIC ACID METABOLITES

Arachidonic acid is a fatty acid precursor present in all cell membranes that can be released whenever a cell membrane is hormonally, neurally, or mechanically activated. Released arachidonic acid is then metabolized via two major pathways. The cyclooxygenase pathway produces several eicosanoids, sometimes generically termed prostaglandins, including prostaglandins D_2, E_2, $F_{2\alpha}$, thromboxane, and prostacyclin (Lefer, 1987). The lipooxygenase pathway produces leukotrienes. The biologic effects of these arachidonic acid metabolites on vascular and airway smooth muscle as well as on formed blood elements such as platelets have made them attractive candidates for initiating or modulating some of the abnormalities witnessed in ARDS. The role of these metabolites has, therefore, been studied in various models (Brigham, 1985).

The prostaglandins have been shown to have potent effects on lung vascular function in sheep (Ogletree, 1982). Thromboxane, a potent vasoconstrictor and platelet aggregator, has been shown to be elevated in the blood and lungs of sheep with endotoxin-induced ARDS (Brigham & Ogletree, 1981). In addition, it has been reported that the administration of cyclooxygenase inhibitors blunted the early increase in pulmonary artery pressure and lung lymph flow witnessed after infusion of endotoxins into various animals (Brigham & Ogletree, 1981). Thromboxane has also been reported to increase the adhesiveness of PMNs in vitro (Spagnuolo et al., 1980), whereas the vasodilating prostaglandins (prostacyclin and PGE_2) have been shown to increase PMN influx into inflammatory sites (Issekutz & Movat, 1982).

Little information is known about the role of leukotrienes in ARDS. Certain leukotrienes cause longlasting, intense bronchoconstriction in peripheral airways (Lewis & Austen, 1984). Morganroth and coworkers (1984) reported that a variety of inhibitors of leukotriene synthesis or action were found to inhibit hypoxic pulmonary vasoconstriction. Edema fluid concentrations of leukotrienes also were found to be higher in patients with ARDS than in patients with increased pressure pulmonary edema (Matthay et al., 1984).

PLATELET ACTIVATING FACTOR

Disturbed coagulation is common in ARDS (Hasegawa et al., 1994) and is hypothesized to be potentiated by the release of platelet activating factor (PAF) (Braquet & Hosford, 1989). PAF is a glycerophospholipid formed like arachidonic acid from the action of phospholipase A_2 on the membranes of PMNs, platelets, and all of the essential inflammatory cells (Koltai et al., 1993). It has been referred to as a master lipid mediator because of its ability to interact with macrophages that release TNF and to amplify the release of other toxic products from the PMN. Administration of PAF experimentally causes activation of platelets, reactivation of neutrophils and reproduces many of the features of ARDS in vivo, including pulmonary hypertension, pulmonary edema, decreased compliance, and bronchoconstriction (Pinkard, 1988). Two-thirds of patients with ARDS have evidence of thrombocytopenia and increased platelet turnover rates with platelet deposition in the lungs (Schneider et al., 1980). Factor VIII antigen (which participates in platelet adherence to vessel walls) and fibrinogen degradation products (specifically D antigen) are increased in patients with ARDS (Boggis & Greene, 1983). Frank disseminated intravascular coagulation was found in 23% of patients in one study (Bone et al., 1976). Histologically, platelet aggregates and fibrin-rich microthrombi are frequently observed (Stevens & Raffin, 1984). Angiographic examination of the pulmonary vasculature in patients with ARDS frequently demonstrates fibrin thrombi (Boggis & Greene, 1983). Pathophysiologically, platelet and fibrin thrombi may mechanically obstruct the vascular bed, release vasoactive substances, and promote increased permeability pulmonary edema (Stevens & Raffin, 1984). There has also been a recent emphasis on the possible role of fibronectin deficiency in ARDS. There appears to be a reticuloendothelial system suppression in most patients with ARDS due to decreased levels of fibronectin (Saba & Jaffe, 1980). Because the reticuloendothelial system plays a major role in the clearance of particulate debris from the circulation, its depression in ARDS patients may allow this debris to accumulate for long periods and amplify its injurious effects on the pulmonary membranes.

Summary

Although this review has emphasized that the PMN is fully capable of producing ARDS, a fundamental question that remains unanswered is whether pulmonary sequestration of PMNs is both necessary and sufficient for the development of ARDS. Further research on the role of PMN-dependent and -independent pathways in the pathogenesis of ARDS is required.

THE CLINICAL AND PATHOLOGIC PHASES OF ARDS

ARDS can be divided into four major clinical phases. The first three phases parallel the stages of edema formation described earlier, whereas the fourth phase specifically represents a structural response to the alteration in a-c membrane integrity (Modig, 1986; Putterman, 1988).

Latent Phase

During this phase, the primary disorder responsible for the development of ARDS dominates the clinical picture. Unless the underlying disorder is pulmonary in nature, no respiratory distress is apparent and the lungs are clear to auscultation. In fact, little evidence of dysfunction exists except for an increased lymphatic flow. However, it is during this period that the ultrastructural changes in the a-c membrane begin to occur. This phase may last from several hours to a few days.

Acute Interstitial Edema Phase

During this period, pathologic evidence of pulmonary capillary damage and the development of widened endothelial pores exists. The endothelial barrier thus offers less resistance to flow, and hydrostatic pressure is unopposed by osmotic pressure. As a consequence, protein-rich edema fluid rapidly leaks into the lung interstitium, swelling its gel and reducing its compressibility. Alveolar distensibility is reduced, vital capacity is impaired, and mild ventilation–perfusion ($\dot{V}/\dot{Q}$) mismatch is present. However, regardless of the diminished lung distensibility or compliance, the amount of air remaining in the lungs at the end of a normal expiration is not greatly affected. This volume, referred to as functional residual capacity, is normal because alveolar collapse is prevented by normal surfactant activity and airway closure mechanisms. Pulmonary vascular resistance may increase due to morphologic changes of the microvascular endothelium (Wang et al., 1985).

Clinically, the patient is often apprehensive and restless and may complain of dyspnea. Tachypnea is present as a result of excitation of sensory nerve endings called J receptors in the alveolar wall by the interstitial fluid. Therefore, minute ventilation is substantially increased. Capillary hydrostatic driving pressure, measured by PAWP, is generally low to normal unless cardiovascular disease coexists. However, an increase in pulmonary artery pressures with a widening of the pulmonary artery end-diastolic and wedge pressure gradient often exists, reflecting the increase in pulmonary vascular resistance. Chest auscultation reveals few, if any, abnormalities. The chest x-ray may be normal or demonstrate increased interstitial markings if at least a 20% to 30% increase in extravascular lung water is present (Staub, 1981). These interstitial findings might include patchy peripheral clouding as well as poor definition of the vascular markings. Edema of the interlobular septa, which produces radiographic linear densities referred to as Kerley lines, is generally not present in increased permeability edema states. In addition, many of the other findings of increased pressure edema such as peribronchial cuffing, pleural effusions, and an enlarged vascular pedicle are often not seen (Staub, 1985). Arterial blood gas values reveal an acute respiratory alkalosis secondary to hyperventilation as well as moderate arterial hypoxemia. Another method of evaluating pulmonary gas exchange is through the alveolar–arterial oxygen tension gradient (PAO_2-PaO_2), which measures the ability of oxygen to cross the a-c membrane. Normally the gradient is less than 15 to 20 mm Hg on room air, but it will be widened in these patients as a result of $\dot{V}/\dot{Q}$ mismatch.

Acute Intra-alveolar Edema Phase

During this phase, alveolar flooding occurs and thus many alveoli are completely filled with high-protein fluid. There is morphologic evidence that both type I and type II alveolar epithelial cells may be injured or their function altered (Barrett et al., 1979). Type I cells, comprising most of the alveolar surface, appear to be more seriously damaged. Injury to these cells diminishes the geometric stability of the alveoli, lung compliance, the efficacy of gas exchange, and the ability of the alveolar barrier to protect against fluid accumulation. Although type II cells, responsible for surfactant production, appear to be less susceptible to injury, evidence exists that the surface-active material recovered from the lungs of patients with ARDS is abnormal (Hallman et al., 1982). This implies that although surfactant is produced, what is available is functionally abnormal. Mechanisms of surfactant alteration may include: (1) a change in surfactant phospholipid composition, (2) inhibition of surfactant function by plasma proteins in edema, (3) inhibition of surfactant by inflammatory mediators, and (4) inactivation of surfactant by compression at low lung volumes (Massaro et al., 1980; Seeger et al., 1993; Wirtz & Schmidt, 1992). As a consequence, high surface tension promotes alveolar collapse, leading to severe decreases in lung compliance. Functional residual capacity is now markedly diminished, and the work of breathing is tremendously increased. Gas exchange is severely compromised owing to the development of absolute intrapulmonary shunting as perfusion continues to flooded, airless alveoli. However, perfusion is also compromised due to hypoxemic-induced enhancement of pulmonary vascular resistance. This compensatory response is viewed as beneficial in that an attempt is made to reduce perfusion to airless alveoli. This may better preserve ventilation–perfusion matching and minimize the severity of intrapulmonary shunting. Unfortunately, vasoconstriction in gas exchange units that remain aerated will result in wasted or dead space ventilation and further intensify the $\dot{V}/\dot{Q}$ inequality and hypoxemia (Dantzker et al., 1979).

Clinically, the patient is often agitated and markedly short of breath. Tachypnea persists now as a consequence of profound hypoxemia, and changes in mental acuity reflect the severity of respiratory distress. The patient may use the accessory muscles of inspiration to optimize ventilation in noncompliant lungs; thus, intercostal retractions are seen. Excessive work of breathing leads to respiratory muscle fatigue, and the associated increase in oxygen consumption is far too costly in the face of progressing hypoxemia. Even if the patient is being mechanically ventilated, peak inspiratory pressures required to deliver a given tidal volume progressively increase. Increases in pulmonary artery pressures associated with enhanced pulmonary vascular resistance persist, and these may precipitate the development of right heart failure, decreased left ventricular filling volumes, and a deleterious reduction in cardiac output. Auscultation of the chest generally reveals fine, diffuse crackles, but the distinctive fluid-derived crackles of increased pressure pulmonary edema are often notably absent. Breath sounds, however, are diminished, reflecting altered air movement and atelectasis. The chest x-ray demonstrates a diffuse, bilateral, fluffy alveolar filling pattern referred to as white lung (Staub, 1985). Arterial blood gas values generally reveal acute respiratory alkalosis, severe arterial hypoxemia unresponsive to supplemental oxygen even at increased fraction of inspired oxygen (FIO_2) levels, and a markedly widened PAO_2-PaO_2. Because some gas exchange units will have adequate ventilation but limited perfusion whereas others will have adequate perfusion but no ventilation, a rise in physiologic dead space ($\dot{V}D/\dot{V}T$) and an increase in shunt fraction ($\dot{Q}S/\dot{Q}T$), respectively, are also characteristic (Dantzker et al., 1979). $\dot{V}D/\dot{V}T$ reflects underperfused alveoli and thus wasted ventilation. $\dot{Q}S/\dot{Q}T$ reflects the percentage of blood flowing from the right to left heart that does not perfectly exchange with alveolar gas; as such, this is a particularly useful parameter to measure in these patients. Calculated shunts of between 20% and 30% reflect an intrapulmonary abnormality that requires intervention. Any calculated shunt that exceeds the 30% value is considered life-threatening because it is incompatible with maintaining oxygenation (Dalnogare, 1989). Several studies have identified an abnormal relationship between oxygen delivery (DO_2) and oxygen consumption ($\dot{V}O_2$) in patients with ARDS. In normal individuals, the energy requirements of the body determine $\dot{V}O_2$. In addition, generally a reserve of DO_2 in excess of what is required to meet these metabolic demands exists. Under these circumstances, if DO_2 falls, $\dot{V}O_2$ will be maintained by increased oxygen extraction. This relationship is referred to as supply-independent $\dot{V}O_2$. At a critical threshold, the ability of the enhanced oxygen extraction compensatory mechanism will be exceeded as the blood oxygen reserve is depleted, and $\dot{V}O_2$ will fall in proportion to the reduction in DO_2. This relationship is referred to as supply-dependent $\dot{V}O_2$. Unfortunately, in ARDS patients, $\dot{V}O_2$ becomes delivery-dependent above the typical threshold. These patients appear to demonstrate an inability to increase oxygen extraction in response to a primary reduction in DO_2. Consequently, in ARDS, a primary reduction or augmentation of DO_2 will be met with a similar change in $\dot{V}O_2$ over a wide range of DO_2. This linkage has been labeled pathologic supply dependency because $\dot{V}O_2$ is totally dependent on DO_2 rather than metabolic need. The mechanisms underlying this observation are poorly understood, but it has been interpreted as evidence of occult tissue hypoxia and has been associated with a high mortality. An increased plasma lactate concentration, which may reflect an imbalance between metabolic requirements and Do_2, may be a useful marker of pathologic supply dependency (Dantzker, 1993).

Subacute–Chronic Phase

If recovery or death does not occur, a subacute stage results after the development of interstitial and alveolar edema. Pathologic evidence shows that with the natural progression of acute lung injury, alveolar damage appears to be more severe than damage to the capillary endothelium (Barrett et al., 1979). Type I pneumocytes are destroyed, leaving a denuded basement membrane. Condensed aggregates of plasma protein, cellular debris, fibrin strands, and remnants of surfactant adhere to the denuded alveolar surface, forming characteristic hyaline membranes. Over the course of the next few days, fluid is reabsorbed from the air spaces. The alveolar septum thickens markedly and is infiltrated by proliferating fibroblasts, plasma cells, and leukocytes. Hyaline membranes begin to organize, and microatelectasis is seen. These membranes can be a formidable barrier to gas diffusion. In addition, as a result of the limited regenerative properties of type I pneumocytes, proliferation of type II cells occurs. Fibrogenesis may begin at this point. Alveoli may be obliterated, alveolar walls coalesced, and functional lung units lost, leading to end-stage pulmonary fibrosis within a matter of weeks (Bachofen & Weibel, 1982). However, even these very severe changes may be reversible with slow recovery toward normal lung function. Recovery is probably related to the severity of the initial damage to the architecture of the lungs and to the intensity of the fibrotic response. Death can result either from a complicating event or from unrelenting, progressive pulmonary failure.

Clinically, peak ventilator pressures increase progressively, and the chest x-ray shows evidence of interstitial fibrosis. As carbon dioxide normally diffuses with ease across the a-c membrane, an increase in $Paco_2$ represents a grave prognostic sign, suggesting severe membrane damage. Elevated $Paco_2$ levels may also represent increased work of breathing, an increase in wasted ventilation, or muscle respiratory fatigue in patients not supported by mechanical ventilation (Estenne & Yernault, 1984).

TABLE 32–2. **Differentiation of Cardiogenic and Increased Permeability Pulmonary Edema**

	Cardiogenic Pulmonary Edema	Increased Permeability Pulmonary Edema
History	Acute cardiac event	Predisposing condition for ARDS
Clinical examination	S_3/cardiomegaly Jugular venous distention Crackles (wet)	No gallop No jugular venous distention Crackles (dry)
Diagnostic data	Chest x-ray: Perihilar distribution PAWP $\geq$ 18 mm Hg PADP − PAWP gradient $\leq$ 5 mm Hg Intrapulmonary shunt: Small increase Edema fluid/serum protein ratio $<$ 0.6	Chest x-ray: Peripheral distribution PAWP $<$ 18 mm Hg PADP − PAWP gradient $>$ 5 mm Hg Intrapulmonary shunt: Large increase Edema fluid/serum protein ratio $>$ 0.7

Abbreviations: PAD = pulmonary artery diastolic pressure, PAWP = pulmonary artery wedge pressure.

THE CLINICAL DIAGNOSIS OF ARDS

Identifying ARDS in its early stage, increased permeability interstitial edema, is very difficult. Because its onset may be sudden or insidious, any patient presenting with a predisposing condition associated with ARDS should be viewed with a high index of suspicion. This is by far one of the most powerful diagnostic tools. Additional features that are reasonably reliable during this stage include (Dalnogare, 1989; Putterman, 1988):

1. Fio_2 of 0.35 or higher required to maintain a Pao_2 greater than 60 mm Hg
2. Chest x-ray compatible with increased permeability interstitial edema and without pneumonia infiltrates or atelectasis
3. An elevated minute ventilation (greater than 20 L/min) associated with an acute respiratory alkalosis
4. Absence of COPD and increased pressure cardiogenic edema.

The major differential diagnosis is increased pressure cardiogenic pulmonary edema (Sibbald et al., 1983) (Table 32–2). Pulmonary artery and wedge pressure measurements can facilitate this differentiation. In ARDS, the PAWP is generally normal, mild to moderate pulmonary hypertension is often present, and the pulmonary artery diastolic pressure (PADP)–PAWP gradient is often increased to greater than 5 mm Hg. Conversely, in cardiogenic pulmonary edema, the PAWP is increased, and pulmonary hypertension, when present, is secondary to pulmonary venous congestion. Therefore, no significant PADP–PAWP gradient exists. It is, however, important to note that pressures obtained from pulmonary artery catheterization may be misleading in patients who are on mechanical ventilators, in particular those receiving positive end-expiratory pressure (PEEP), because alveolar pressure may exceed capillary hydrostatic pressure in different regions of the lung (Lozman et al., 1974; Rajacich et al., 1989). If the pulmonary artery catheter is located in a vessel where alveolar pressure is greater than capillary hydrostatic pressure, capillary narrowing or collapse can occur, disrupting the continuous column of blood from the catheter tip to the left heart and jeopardizing

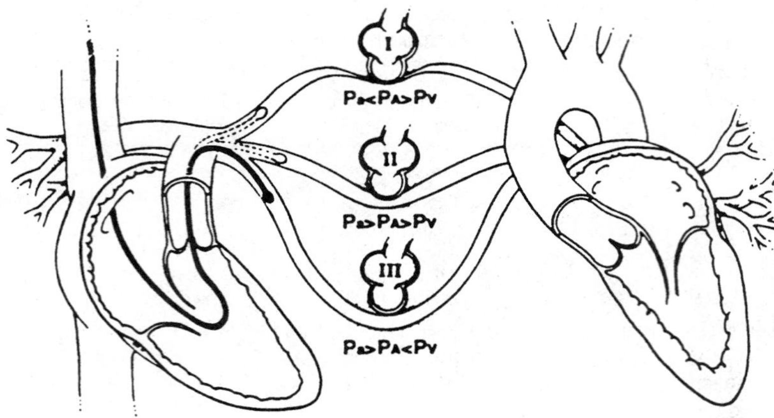

FIGURE 32–7. West lung zones. In lung zone III pulmonary arterial and venous pressures exceed alveolar pressure. PAWP reflects left atrial pressure only under lung zone III conditions, which allow for a continuous column of blood to exist from the tip of the pulmonary artery catheter to the left atrium. (From Enger, E. L. [1989]. Pulmonary artery wedge pressure: When it's valid, when it's not. *Critical Care Nursing Clinics of North America, 1*, 603–618.)

the validity of the PAWP measurement (Enger, 1989) (Fig. 32–7). Confirmation of the position of the catheter tip in a vessel below the level of the left atrium (West lung zone III) by lateral x-ray will minimize this discrepancy because hydrostatic pressure should exceed alveolar pressure in this zone, and therefore PAWP should be reflective of the left atrial pressure (Enger, 1989).

Once the alveolar edema, gas exchange abnormalities, and metabolic derangements of ARDS ensue, the syndrome is more easily identified by the following parameters (Dalnogare, 1989; Putterman, 1988):

1. Refractory hypoxemia (Pa_{O_2} less than 60 mm Hg at an F_{IO_2} of 0.5 or higher)
2. A markedly diminished static lung compliance (less than 50 mg/cm H_2O on mechanical ventilatory assistance)
3. A chest x-ray with diffuse bilateral parenchymal infiltrates
4. An increased shunt fraction ($\dot{Q}_S/\dot{Q}_T$).

An additional diagnostic technique that has been advocated for distinguishing between increased pressure and increased permeability alveolar edema is the edema fluid-plasma protein ratio (Fein et al., 1979). Calculation of this ratio requires the measurement of protein content in edema and plasma collected simultaneously from endotracheal suctioning and blood sampling. Because the microvascular barrier is functionally intact in increased pressure alveolar edema, plasma proteins will remain confined to the intravascular space, and edema fluid protein content will be low relative to plasma protein content, with a ratio generally of less than 0.6. Conversely, with increased permeability alveolar edema, as the barrier is injured, the edema-plasma protein content ratio will be greater than 0.7 (Crandell, 1983; Fein et al., 1979).

MEDICAL TREATMENT

The medical treatment of ARDS is divided into three major areas of concentration: (1) reversing the underlying associated disorder, (2) blocking the specific mechanism of a-c membrane injury, and (3) minimizing the pathologic consequences of acute lung injury through supportive measures. The first two areas address preventing the development of ARDS, whereas the last area focuses on attempting to minimize the morbidity and mortality of ARDS once it occurs. Therapy aimed at reversing the underlying disorder will vary according to the specific precipitating cause. The common disorders associated with ARDS have been discussed earlier, and their therapy can be found in other areas of this text. Therefore, measures addressing only the second two areas of treatment priority will be highlighted here.

Blocking the Specific Mechanism of a-c Membrane Injury

Several agents have been investigated in both human and animal models to determine their efficacy in blocking cell damage and subsequent pulmonary dysfunction. Animal studies, however, cannot totally duplicate the physiologic conditions of human ARDS. In addition, it is difficult to design human studies in which the lung injury is physiologically well defined, in which the time from insult to intervention can be established, and in which endpoints are clearly defined. Therefore, data from these studies are often inconclusive. Until the mechanisms and mediators of acute lung injury in ARDS have been clearly elucidated, all aspects of specific therapy will remain controversial. However, based on the previous discussion, it seems logical that pharmacologic therapy be directed at (1) stabilizing PMNs through the neutralization of those mediators that are responsible for their activation, including complement, endotoxin, and cytokines, and (2) inactivating the toxic products released from aggregating PMNs, including oxygen-derived free radicals, degradative proteases, arachidonic acid metabolites, and PAF (Raffin, 1987; Roberts, 1990).

CORTICOSTEROIDS

Several beneficial effects have been postulated for the use of corticosteroids in ARDS. These include the ability of corticosteroids to inhibit the production of arachidonic acid metabolites, impair PMN adherence, stabilize lysosomal membranes, prevent superoxide damage, and decrease complement activation (Roberts, 1990). Sibbald and colleagues (1981) have demonstrated reduced passage of radiolabeled albumin from serum to pulmonary edema fluid in patients with ARDS after methylprednisolone administration. However, Bernard and associates (1987) conducted a prospective, randomized, double-blind, placebo-controlled trial of high-dose methylprednisolone therapy in 99 ARDS patients with various underlying diseases and observed no statistical difference between groups in pulmonary shunting, oxygenation variables, chest x-ray severity, compliance, pulmonary artery pressures, infectious complications, or mortality. In addition, Bone and co-workers (1987) evaluated whether early methylprednisolone treatment would decrease the incidence or severity of ARDS in 304 patients with septic syndromes. They concluded that early corticosteroid therapy did not prevent the development of ARDS but actually impeded the reversal of ARDS and increased the mortality rate. Based on these and other trials, corticosteroid therapy for patients with ARDS cannot currently be recommended unless they present with shock secondary to or associated with adrenal insufficiency.

NEUTRALIZATION OF ENDOTOXIN EFFECTS

Two large trials have been published recently describing the effects of monoclonal antibodies to endotoxin in the human sepsis syndrome (Greenman et al., 1991; Ziegler et al., 1991). Both showed advantages in terms of survival and resolution of system failures only in subgroups of patients. E5, a murine immunoglobulin M (IgM) antibody, significantly decreased mortality in patients with gram-negative sepsis with no evidence of circulatory shock. In this group, 28% of the total, ARDS resolved in 4 of 10 patients who received E5 compared with 2 of 9 patients given placebo. By contrast, HA-1A, a human monoclonal IgM antibody, was found to be effective regardless of shock, but only in patients with proven gram-negative bacteremia. Data specific to ARDS were not given. However, in the group that responded, all major morbidities including ARDS resolved within 7 days in 38 of 61 patients given HA-1A compared with 26 of 62 patients given placebo. There were no significant side effects attributable to either antibody. Problems, however, that may preclude the more widespread application of these novel treatments include their high cost and difficulties in identifying those patients with gram-negative bacteremia rapidly enough to maximize the therapeutic potential.

MODULATION OF CYTOKINE RESPONSE

It is theoretically possible to block the damaging effects of cytokines at several levels, though most of these potential treatments are as yet untried in vivo (St. John & Dorinsky, 1993). Animal studies have shown that when administered prophylactically, neutralizing antibodies for TNF protect against lethal endotoxemia, although only one study has shown benefit when such antibodies were given after injury (Hinshaw et al., 1989). A Phase I study of a murine immunoglobulin G (IgG) monoclonal antibody to recombinant human TNF in patients with septic shock revealed no serious side effects (Exley et al., 1990). Results of a larger study examining therapeutic efficacy are awaited. Pentoxifylline is a methylxanthine derivative that reduces the production of both TNF and IL-1 as well as decreases the response of PMNs to these cytokines (Sullivan et al., 1988). It also improves red cell deformability and decreases platelet aggregation. The hemodynamic changes associated with sepsis are ameliorated, as are indices of lung injury, when pentoxifylline is used either before or soon after pulmonary insult. Oxygen delivery is maintained in models of hemodynamic shock, possibly by preventing white cell adherence in the pulmonary and systemic microcirculation (Coccia et al., 1989). These data suggest a potential role for pentoxifylline in ARDS.

PROTECTION FROM REACTIVE TOXIC OXYGEN METABOLITES

Scavengers of oxygen-free radicals appear promising as protective agents. In patients with early ARDS and in those at high risk, protection against reactive oxygen species-mediated injury by the use of N-acetylcysteine has been shown to reduce injury (Bernard et al., 1984). Other scavengers, including superoxide dismutase (Parker et al., 1983) and catalase (Milligan et al., 1985), have been reported to attenuate increased microvascular permeability in sheep with endotoxin-induced ARDS. The use of specific antioxidants in ARDS is complicated, however, by the pro-oxidant effect of many of these compounds. Lower concentrations of the antioxidant vitamin E have been found in patients who develop ARDS than in those who do not, but high concentrations of both vitamin E and vitamin C have been shown to promote lipid peroxidation, suggesting they produce damage mediated by free radicals (Bast et al., 1991; Richard et al., 1991).

INHIBITION OF THROMBOXANE ACTIONS

Because the arachidonic acid metabolite thromboxane has been mechanistically implicated in ARDS, agents that inhibit its production have been examined. In animal models, ibuprofen and indomethacin have been shown to alter the course of acute lung injury (Begley et al., 1984). In the early phases, pulmonary hypertension was reduced, arterial hypoxemia diminished, and neutrophilic adherence and activation decreased. The incidence of pulmonary edema was also lower in treated subjects. However, to date, there is no evidence from any large clinical trial to support the use of nonsteroidal antiinflammatory drugs despite encouraging experimental data (Metz & Sibbald, 1991). Thromboxane synthase inhibitors have likewise been examined (Said & Foda, 1989). Although dazoxiben did not appear to be beneficial in the treatment of established ARDS (Leeman et al., 1985), a randomized prospective study in patients at risk for the development of ARDS showed a reduced incidence when prophylactic treatment with ketoconazole was applied (Slotman et al., 1988). Two additional arachidonic acid metabolites with protective actions opposing thromboxane, prostacyclin (Perlman et al., 1986) and PGE_1 (Shoemaker & Appel, 1986), have been shown to inhibit hypoxic vasoconstriction and to stabilize PMN membranes.

ADDITIONAL PHARMACOLOGIC STRATEGIES

Alpha-1 antitrypsin has been shown to combat the degradative effects of several proteases (Vered et al., 1985). Because pulmonary fibrosis is a major sequela of ARDS, the potential beneficial effects of antithrombotic therapy have been investigated. For example, urokinase has been reported to suppress the development of lung fibrosis in ARDS animal models (Shigematsu et al., 1980).

Nitric oxide selectively dilates pulmonary vessels in ventilated areas of the lung when given by inhalation. Unlike other pulmonary vasodilators, which cannot be delivered to ventilated areas of lung alone, nitric oxide appears to successfully reduce pulmonary shunting. Moreover, because nitric oxide is rapidly inactivated by hemoglobin, it has no systemic effects. In a series of 10 patients with ARDS, Rossaint and colleagues (1993) reported that short-term administration of nitric oxide reduced pulmonary artery pressure, decreased intrapulmonary shunting, and improved oxygenation without any systemic hemodynamic effects.

Currently, there is considerable interest in the use of exogenous surfactant to supplement surfactant that may be abnormal in ARDS. It may be that surfactant replacement, which has become an accepted treatment for respiratory distress associated with premature birth, will improve pulmonary compliance in any patient, whether adult or child, with ARDS. Phase III trials are in progress (Lewis & Jobe, 1993).

Although preliminary communications on all of these investigational therapies have been promising, controlled human studies will determine which, if any, of these agents is effective. Until success is achieved, supportive intensive care will remain the focal point of therapy for ARDS.

Minimizing the Pathologic Consequences: Supportive Measures

Supportive measures are divided into three major objectives:

1. Minimizing edema formation
2. Maintaining tissue oxygenation while reducing exacerbating factors
3. Preventing and recognizing complications.

MINIMIZING EDEMA FORMATION

With increased permeability pulmonary edema, the urgent problem is not that the driving pressure for edema formation is abnormally elevated but that the edema will form in great quantities even at low driving pressures (Fig. 32–8). Because of this, microvascular hydrostatic pressure (PAWP) is generally kept as low as possible to minimize fluid flux. Diuretics are often administered to achieve this outcome. However, diuresis often does not decrease lung water considerably. In fact, efforts to minimize fluid exudation may result in microvascular pressures inadequate to maintain effective blood flow to the tissues. It should be clear that the maintenance of cardiac output is of paramount importance because impairment of flow will have a profound effect on oxygen delivery to the tissues. Hence, fluid therapy may be required to maintain adequate cardiac performance even in the presence of wet lungs. This careful balancing of cardiopulmonary performance may be facilitated by invasive hemodynamic monitoring (Snider, 1990).

The choice of fluid to maintain vascular volume has received a great deal of attention. In patients with a low PAWP as well as a low hematocrit, packed red blood cells are effective not only in expanding intravascular volume, but also in increasing the oxygen-carrying capacity of the blood. However, increased blood viscosity may intensify the workload of the right heart, which is already enhanced as a consequence of pulmonary hypertension. In patients with a normal hematocrit, both colloids and crystalloids have been advocated. Those favoring the use of colloid solutions argue that they are more effective for intravascular volume expansion than equal volumes of crystalloid solutions (Hauser et al., 1980). It is further argued that much of the crystalloid solution ends up in the pulmonary interstitium and alveoli, thus worsening gas exchange (Shoemaker et al., 1981). Large volume crys-

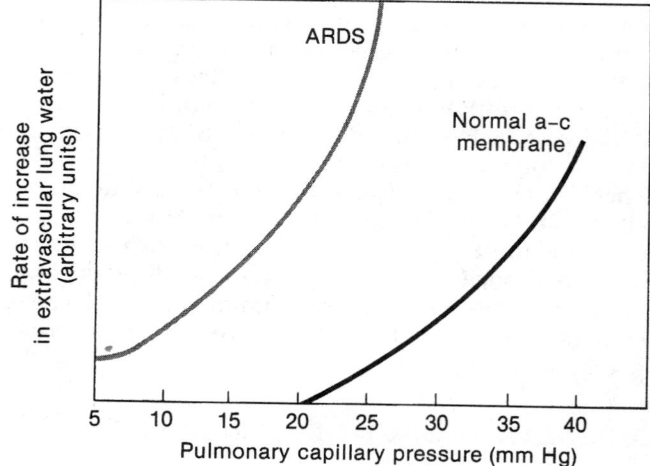

FIGURE 32–8. Schematic representation of the deleterious effects of essentially normal PAWP in combination with the loss of a-c membrane integrity in ARDS.

talloid infusion also lowers colloidal osmotic pressure (Haupt & Rackow, 1982). Proponents of crystalloid therapy suggest that since the barriers restricting colloid movement from the vascular space into the lungs do not function normally when the lungs have been injured, osmotic pressure differences favoring fluid movement into the vascular space cannot be established. Indeed, data from animal studies support the theory that albumin readily crosses into the interstitium (Moss et al., 1981). This would mitigate against using albumin. Therefore, there appears to be no advantage to fluid resuscitation with expensive colloid solutions. In fact, they may even compound edema formation.

The goal of therapy is to maintain the lowest possible PAWP that is consistent with adequate cardiac output and perfusion to vital organs. If cardiac output is adequate, no wedge pressure is considered too low (Putterman, 1988). Vasodilator therapy may be beneficial because it will lower systemic afterload, which may improve cardiac output yet maintain low pulmonary vascular pressures. Blood pressure can then be supported as appropriate with inotropic agents. Vasodilators must be used cautiously, however, because they may increase intrapulmonary shunt in the later stages of ARDS by interfering with hypoxic vasoconstriction, which attempts to preserve ventilation–perfusion matching by decreasing perfusion to airless alveoli (Wood & Prewitt, 1981).

MAINTAINING TISSUE OXYGENATION

Tissue oxygen delivery (transport) is the product of arterial blood oxygen content (primarily determined by hemoglobin concentration and oxygen saturation of that hemoglobin) and cardiac output. Oxygen uptake (consumption) by the tissues is reflected by the product of the difference in oxygen content in arterial and venous blood and cardiac output. Oxygen uptake is determined by the metabolic requirements of the tissues until oxygen delivery falls below these requirements, at which time oxygen uptake becomes dependent on and varies directly with oxygen delivery. Normal oxygen delivery (1000 mL/min) is greater than oxygen consumption (250 mL/min). Therefore, the human body can experience a large fall in oxygen content, cardiac output, or both yet still supply sufficient oxygen to meet metabolic requirements (Snyder, 1987). However, some evidence exists that in ARDS, oxygen uptake is dependent on oxygen delivery over a much greater range and, therefore, that oxygen uptake is extremely delivery dependent. As a result, maintaining oxygen delivery is of paramount importance in establishing adequate tissue oxygenation in ARDS patients (Dantzker, 1990; Karima & Burns, 1985). In addition, oxygen delivery must be maintained with a minimum F_{IO_2} because the lungs are already damaged, making them especially sensitive to the effects of alveolar hyperoxia and consequent oxygen-free radical production, as previously discussed. Fortunately, during the interstitial edema stage of ARDS, if adequate fluid balance and cardiovascular support have been achieved, the patient should be sufficiently oxygenated with F_{IO_2} concentrations below 0.50. In fact, the inability to achieve a Pa_{O_2} of greater than 60 mm Hg with a maximum F_{IO_2} of 0.45 should be considered a warning signal of patient deterioration and the development of intraalveolar edema. The appropriateness and timeliness of therapy directed at the early stage of ARDS will greatly determine whether the patient will progress into later, more severe stages. Hypotension, volume overload, and oxygen toxicity must be strictly avoided (Keogh et al., 1989).

CONVENTIONAL MECHANICAL VENTILATION. Patients with fully developed ARDS invariably require mechanical ventilation to minimize the work of breathing associated with their stiff, noncompliant lungs. When mechanical ventilation is initiated, tidal volumes of 10 to 15 mg/kg of body weight are generally employed to minimize atelectasis. Controversy persists with regard to which mode of ventilation is best suited for these patients. Advocates of the assist-control mode believe that it will better decrease the work of breathing. Advocates of the intermittent mandatory ventilation mode believe that it will diminish respiratory alkalemia, sparing the patient from difficulties in oxygen unloading at the tissues owing to increased pH-induced alterations in oxygen hemoglobin affinity (Keogh et al., 1989).

POSITIVE END-EXPIRATORY PRESSURE. Although conventional mechanical ventilation can eliminate the high work of breathing in this disorder, it does not address the critical problem of impaired oxygen exchange. Keep in mind that no amount of oxygen administration can correct hypoxemia if this oxygen never reaches the alveoli because they are fluid filled. Therefore, the use of positive-pressure ventilation with PEEP has a well-documented role in the management of refractory hypoxemia secondary to intrapulmonary shunting in ARDS (Dalnogare, 1989). PEEP is the artificial maintenance of positive (superatmospheric) pressure after passive exhalation is complete. This technique is termed continuous positive-pressure ventilation (CPPV) when PEEP is added to intermittent positive-pressure ventilation provided by a ventilator, whereas it is called continuous positive airway pressure (CPAP) when PEEP is applied to patients without ventilator assistance. Regardless of the technique used, the effect of PEEP on the lungs is an increase in functional residual capacity, which recruits or maintains open alveoli that are otherwise collapsed. This increase in lung volume, in return, improves pulmonary compliance, minimizes intrapulmonary shunting, and reduces the alveolar–arterial oxygen tension difference (Shapiro et al., 1984). Accordingly, the beneficial use of PEEP generally improves oxygen delivery and allows reduction of the inspired oxygen concentration to levels less likely to produce oxygen toxicity and free radical production. Several additional effects of PEEP have been explored. It has been hypothesized that PEEP may alter surface tension by a yet unproven interaction with surfactant and thus reduce atelectasis. It has also been hypothesized that a relationship exists between PEEP and actual lung water (Shapiro et al., 1984). Despite initial reports, PEEP does not reliably decrease lung water. In fact, in some settings, it has been reported to increase it, possibly by increased filtration through extraalveolar vessels (Permutt, 1979). The question of whether PEEP may reduce the extent of acute lung injury and therefore may be prophylactic if introduced early in patients at risk of developing ARDS has also arisen. Despite early encouraging data that this might be true, most controlled studies have not supported the prophylactic value of PEEP (Pepe et al., 1984).

Considerable controversy exists about how best to establish the optimal level of PEEP. Criteria that have been advocated to determine this optimal level include adjusting the PEEP to attain:

1. A Po_2 of approximately 60 mm Hg with an Fio_2 of 0.5 or less (Weisman et al., 1982)
2. The lowest intrapulmonary shunt percentage (Gallagher et al., 1978)
3. The greatest oxygen delivery (transport) (Suter et al., 1975)
4. The greatest measured lung compliance (Suter et al., 1975)
5. The point where mixed venous oxygen tension and/or saturation falls (Hurewitz & Bergofsky, 1981).

Despite differing emphasis in these approaches to establishing a PEEP level, there is no clear evidence that any one method has a distinct advantage in reducing morbidity or mortality. To better understand how to adjust this modality, its potential deleterious effects must be appreciated, the most significant of which are barotrauma (Balk & Bone, 1983) and a reduction in cardiac output (Weisman et al., 1982). Barotrauma involves the development of pneumomediastinum, pneumothorax, or subcutaneous emphysema. Decreased cardiac output results from a reduction in venous return as well as an increase in pulmonary vascular resistance. As right heart afterload increases, right ventricular emptying is impeded, shifting the intraventricular septum to the left, thus reducing left ventricular internal dimension and compliance (Weisman et al., 1982). Recall that arterial oxygen delivery is the product of arterial blood oxygen content and cardiac output. Any increase in oxygen content that results from the use of PEEP will not beneficially improve oxygen delivery if it is associated with a counterbalancing fall in cardiac output. Therefore, to determine the optimal level of PEEP, it is necessary to determine the level that provides combined optimal respiratory and cardiac function. This level should establish optimal tissue oxygenation (Putterman, 1988). Generally, PEEP is instituted in 3- to 5-cm H_2O increments until a predetermined measure of optimal tissue oxygenation is achieved. The efficacy of levels of PEEP in the range of 1 to 20 cm H_2O has been fairly thoroughly documented. Levels of PEEP in excess of 20 cm H_2O have also been studied, but efficacy remains to be shown (Brandstetter, 1986; Dalnogare, 1989). It has been suggested that excessive PEEP levels may compress alveolar vessels adjacent to well-ventilated alveoli, thus diverting more blood flow to poorly ventilated areas and increasing the shunting phenomenon (Shapiro et al., 1984).

NEW STRATEGIES IN RESPIRATORY SUPPORT. Several nontraditional ventilatory modes have been evaluated in the management of ARDS (Hinson & Marini, 1992; Keogh et al., 1990; MacNaughton & Evans, 1992; Swami & Keogh, 1992; Toben & Lewandowski, 1988). These new approaches aim to maintain a mean airway pressure high enough to recruit unstable alveoli and improve gas exchange while avoiding high peak inflation pressures.

Inverse ratio ventilation (IRV) is a variation on conventional ventilatory treatment in which the inspiratory-expiratory (I:E) ratio is lengthened by prolonging inspiratory time to more than half of the respiratory cycle. Volume-controlled IRV (VC-IRV) delivers a preset tidal volume irrespective of peak inspiratory pressure and, therefore, allows a predictable clearance of carbon dioxide. Although mean airway pressure is increased and oxygenation is improved, substantial air trapping may occur, with a rise in lung volume, high peak airway pressure, and a profound reduction in cardiac output. Pressure-controlled IRV (PC-IRV) delivers a constant preset inspiratory pressure for the desired inspiratory time and so avoids these risks. An early trial of PC-IRV showed improved oxygenation when conventional ventilation failed, while reducing peak airway pressure and without impairing cardiac function (Tharratt et al., 1988). Although reduction in mortality has not been demonstrated, PC-IRV is probably the best existing method of maintaining gas exchange.

Another mode, airway pressure release ventilation, maintains lung volume and oxygenation by CPAP. Carbon dioxide clearance with this mode is achieved by the transient release of circuit pressure, allowing gas to exit and lung volume to fall. Continuous positive pressure is then reestablished, allowing fresh gas to enter the system. The patient may breathe spontaneously throughout the respiratory cycle, and the need for conventional positive-pressure breaths is eliminated. This system is attractive in that it retains the favorable characteristics of spontaneous respiration, enhances carbon dioxide clearance, and should decrease respiratory work in patients with poor respiratory compliance (Downs & Stock, 1987). Although this technique has been used successfully in patients with ARDS, its effects on outcome remain uncertain.

Pressure-limited, low tidal volume, synchronized intermittent mandatory ventilation with permitted hypercapnia has also recently been advocated on the basis of the results of a 5-year retrospective study of 50 patients with severe acute lung injury in whom peak inspiratory pressure was limited to 30 cm H_2O, often necessitating the use of tidal volumes as low as 5 mL/kg. Pa_{CO_2} was allowed to rise and PEEP was manipulated as necessary to achieve adequate oxygenation with inspired F_{IO_2} of less than 0.6. The survival rate for this group was remarkably 84% (Hickling et al., 1990). Although this was a retrospective, uncontrolled study, the results are compelling.

High-frequency jet ventilation uses high-pressure pulses of gas delivered at supranormal frequencies (60–600/min) for a preset percentage of each inspiratory cycle. The use of this technique was most aggressively applied in acute lung injury in the early 1980s. A prospective, randomized trial of high-frequency jet ventilation versus conventional ventilation in acute lung injury reported by Carlo and colleagues (1983) showed high-frequency ventilation to be effective, but not to have any significant benefit over conventional techniques. Interest in high-frequency techniques, therefore, has now been directed to the use of frequency at or near the resonant frequency of the lung (about 5 Hz). This technique is termed ultrahigh-frequency ventilation. Potential advantages of this approach include enhanced alveolar gas kinetics and minimal barotrauma while recruitment and maintenance of alveolar volume are achieved. An important advantage of this approach is that mean airway pressure is maintained to recruit and stabilize alveoli. A multicenter feasibility study using a prototype ultrahigh-frequency ventilation ventilator in patients with acute lung injury deemed refractory to conventional treatment is currently in progress. A preliminary report from this trial confirmed that survival is substantially improved in patients with severe acute lung injury who are identified and switched to ultrahigh-frequency ventilation within 48 hours of the start of mechanical ventilation (Swami & Keogh, 1992).

Finally, the use of the prone position in ventilated patients has been shown to be effective in improving gas exchange in acute lung injury. Langer and colleagues (1988) have used computed tomography to observe redistribution of atelectasis and edema after patients with moderate to severe acute lung injury have been put in the prone position. Eight of thirteen patients in this study responded with improved oxygenation that persisted after reversion to the supine position. These data suggest that the prone position should always be considered in the absence of contraindications and that it should be particularly beneficial in combination with a ventilatory technique capable of alveolar recruitment and maintenance, such as PC-IRV or ultrahigh-frequency ventilation.

The clinical efficacy of all of these respiratory strategies and their ability to improve outcome in patients with ARDS remains to be established. As such, the use of tidal volume preset ventilation, PEEP, and an I:E ratio of less than 1:1 remains the mainstay of respiratory support in patients with ARDS.

EXTRACORPOREAL AND INTRAVASCULAR GAS EXCHANGE. Several attempts to improve gas exchange by the use of extracorporeal membrane lungs have been made in patients with severe ARDS. Extracorporeal membrane oxygenation (ECMO) was first used in patients with ARDS in 1972 (Hill et al., 1972). With this technique, blood is usually taken from the inferior vena cava via the femoral vein, passed through a membrane oxygenator at high flow rates where it undergoes gas exchange, and then is returned to the circulation through the femoral artery. Results of a national multicenter collaborative study (Zapol et al., 1979) as well as several subsequent studies have not shown a significant decrease in mortality with the use of ECMO (Keogh et al., 1990). However, all patients in these studies have been severely ill prior to entry. More recently, a modified form of extracorporeal gas exchange termed extracorporeal carbon dioxide removal has been demonstrated to improve survival in patients with ARDS (Pesenti et al., 1988). With this technique, the lungs are still used for oxygenation and supplied with low-frequency positive-pressure ventilation. However, carbon dioxide is removed through the membrane. This technique has several advantages. Because the removal of carbon dioxide requires a lower rate of blood flow through the extracorporeal circuit than that needed to achieve full oxygenation, it is possible to perform this procedure via a simple venovenous cannulation. In addition, barotrauma is minimized and lung movement reduced, thus providing better conditions for lung repair (Keogh et al., 1990).

Mortensen (1987) has pioneered the construction of an intravenous capillary membrane lung, the IVOX, which is designed to be placed percutaneously into the inferior vena cava. Gas exchange occurs by passive diffusion sufficient to supply 90% of the basal oxygen requirements of a resting adult. This device may prove to be substantially beneficial in decreasing the ventilatory requirements of ARDS patients (Swami & Keogh, 1992).

The future role of these devices in the supportive treatment of patients with ARDS remains to be determined.

NUTRITIONAL SUPPORT. Patients with ARDS are at risk for developing protein–calorie malnutrition, which will further compromise the respiratory system and tissue oxygenation (Rochester & Esau, 1984). In undernourished patients, pulmonary defense mechanisms become impaired (Moriguchi et al., 1983), and an altered ventilatory response to hypoxemia is common (Weissmann et al., 1983). Surfactant function is also abnormal in the malnourished patient (Sahebjami et al., 1978), structural parenchymal changes have been documented (Sahebjami et al., 1978), and diaphragmatic mass may be dramatically decreased (Arora & Rochester, 1977). These responses can lead to markedly altered lung mechanics. Therefore, some form of nutritional therapy that maintains a positive protein balance is imperative. Nutritional supplementation is not, however, without risk. If the carbohydrate load exceeds energy needs, lipogenesis and a greater production of carbon dioxide relative to oxygen consump-

TABLE 32–3. **Medical Complications of ARDS**

Pulmonary	**Infection**
Pulmonary emboli	Sepsis
Pulmonary fibrosis	Nosocomial pneumonia
Oxygen toxicity	
Barotrauma	**Hematologic**
Renal	Anemia
	Thrombocytopenia
Renal failure	Disseminated intravascular coagulation
Fluid retention	
Cardiac	**Other**
Arrhythmia	Hepatic
Hypotension	Endocrine
Low cardiac output	Neurologic
	Psychiatric
Gastrointestinal	Malnutrition
Hemorrhage	
Ileus	
Gastric distention	
Pneumoperitoneum	

tion can predispose to hypercapnia. Therefore, judicious nutritional support must be provided (Majors, 1988).

PREVENTING AND RECOGNIZING COMPLICATIONS

The complications of ARDS can be divided into two broad categories, mechanical and medical complications (Pingleton, 1982). Because the majority of ARDS patients will be receiving mechanical ventilatory assistance, which entails control of the airway either by endotracheal intubation or tracheotomy, all of the mechanical complications associated with these procedures may be experienced. In addition, because virtually every organ system can be involved with ARDS, whether from underlying disease processes, concomitant disease processes, or as a result of therapeutic interventions, a number of medical complications may occur as well (Table 32–3).

PRIMARY OUTCOME PATHWAY: ADEQUACY OF OXYGENATION/ VENTILATION

Throughout this chapter, it has been emphasized that maintenance of a sufficient, balanced amount of oxygen diffusion across the a-c membrane (ventilation) and intrinsic blood flow (perfusion) is essential to tissue oxygenation in ARDS patients. Therefore, a multidisciplinary approach must be targeted at addressing alterations in the pulmonary gas exchange process and at establishing methods to improve oxygenation and ventilation.

Causes and Manifestations of Impaired Gas Exchange

Several factors may potentially impair pulmonary gas exchange in ARDS patients (Roberts, 1990). Adequate ventilation may be threatened by bronchoconstriction, interstitial edema, decreased pulmonary compliance, intraalveolar edema, and atelectasis. Manifestations that signal inadequate ventilation include tachypnea, decreased tidal volume, dyspnea, restlessness, tachycardia, and diminished or adventitious breath sounds. Optimal perfusion may be compromised by hypoxia-induced vasoconstriction, pulmonary microemboli, continuous positive pressure ventilation, and inadequate circulating blood volume secondary to diuresis. Warning signs of insufficient perfusion include tachycardia, arrhythmias, hypotension, decreased urine output, and a decreased level of consciousness.

Desired Outcomes

Collaborative interventions should be directed at attaining the following outcomes consistent with the goal of optimizing pulmonary gas exchange and thus tissue oxygenation (Dalnogare, 1989; Putterman, 1988; Roberts, 1990; Shapiro et al., 1984; Wood & Prewitt, 1981):

1. The lowest PAWP that will minimize the hydrostatic gradient for edema formation yet not compromise the adequacy of left ventricular filling and cardiac output
2. The lowest F_{IO_2} that will minimize toxic lung injury by oxygen-derived free radicals yet not compromise alveolar ventilation or arterial blood oxygen content
3. The lowest PEEP value that will minimize pressure-related barotrauma and cardiac output reduction yet not compromise alveolar expansion, FRC, and $\dot{V}/\dot{Q}$ matching
4. The lowest intrapulmonary shunt percentage that will minimize refractory hypoxemia
5. The highest pulmonary compliance that will minimize the work of breathing
6. The highest arterial oxygen delivery that will optimize tissue oxygen utilization.

Interventions

DECREASE METABOLIC REQUIREMENTS FOR OXYGEN

Anxiety, pain, and dyspnea notoriously increase basal metabolic rate, thus increasing inspired oxygen requirements (Snyder, 1987). Even in patients with good respiratory support, these factors often prevail. Consequently, implementing strategies to control these factors is ultimately beneficial. It is important to ensure that the ventilator's circuit is properly set up and functioning. Sedation can also be used to control the discomfort of the endotracheal tube or other sources of pain as well as to calm the patient.

Fever is another factor that increases the demand for oxygen (Snyder, 1987). However, temperature must be regulated judiciously with cooling blankets and antipyretics because shivering, which increases oxygen consumption and masks sepsis, can be equally detrimental.

MAINTAIN CONTINUOUS PEEP

In patients with ARDS supported by continuous positive-pressure ventilation, removing the ventilator and PEEP for short times has been reported to decrease rapidly arterial oxygen tension as well as functional residual capacity (Enger, 1989; Weisman et al., 1982). An ideal tracheal suctioning or tubing change procedure, therefore, uses principles of preoxygenation, minimal suctioning time, postsuctioning hyperinflation to reverse atelectasis, and uninterrupted PEEP facilitated by an adaptor valve or a closed airway suctioning system (Roberts, 1990; Schumann & Parsons, 1985). Discontinuation of PEEP during measurements of PAWP has also been advocated because PEEP can introduce uncertainty in the validity of the values by inducing changes in left ventricular compliance and intrathoracic pressure. Alveolar pressure in patients on PEEP will equal the PEEP value, and, thus, in less dependent regions of the lung, it will be greater than capillary hydrostatic pressure. In these cases, the alveolar pressure will collapse the pulmonary capillary and the PAWP will reflect the alveolar pressure instead of left heart filling pressures (Enger, 1989). However, because removing PEEP can induce serious gas exchange abnormalities as well as artificial hemodynamic changes, it is recommended that PAWP measurements be done with the patient on PEEP. PAWP is not generally affected by low levels of PEEP (less than 10 cm H_2O) (Lozman et al., 1974). As previously discussed, ensuring that the pulmonary artery catheter is positioned properly below the level of the left atrium will also maximize the accuracy of the values. At higher levels of PEEP, a mathematical adjustment of PAWP has been advocated (Enger, 1989; O'Quin & Marini, 1983).

IDENTIFY HEMOGLOBIN-RELATED ALTERATIONS IN OXYGEN DELIVERY

An important yet often overlooked threat to oxygen delivery and subsequent tissue oxygenation is anemia. In addition, those factors that make it more difficult for hemoglobin to unload oxygen at the tissue level due to an increase in oxygen hemoglobin affinity should be detected and corrected. Conditions predisposing to this state (a leftward shift in the oxyhemoglobin-dissociation curve) include hypophosphatemia, alkalemia, decreased $Paco_2$, and decreased levels of 2,3-DPG that result from administration of banked blood.

ASSESS INTRAPULMONARY SHUNTING ($\dot{Q}s/\dot{Q}T$)

Intrapulmonary shunting refers to blood flowing from the right side of the heart to the left side of the heart that does not perfectly exchange with alveolar gas. Shunting has three potential components: (1) anatomic, (2) capillary, and (3) venous admixture. The first two are absolute shunting mechanisms in that blood reaches the left ventricle without having been exposed to the air–alveolar interface. Absolute shunt mechanisms are, therefore, refractory to oxygen therapy. No matter how much oxygen is available, blood volume that bypasses does not participate in oxygen exchange. Anatomic shunting includes blood flow leaving the right ventricle without passing through the pulmonary capillaries. Normally, this comprises 2% to 5% of the cardiac output. Pathologic anatomic shunting can result from intrapulmonary arteriovenous fistulas and right-to-left intracardiac shunts. Capillary shunting is a result of pulmonary capillary blood passing totally collapsed or airless alveoli. The third type of shunt mechanism is venous admixture, also referred to as the shunt effect. It is the result of perfusion in excess of ventilation, yet some ventilation still exists. This mechanism is responsive to oxygen therapy. In the later stages of ARDS, intrapulmonary shunting is primarily secondary to the absolute capillary mechanism. The percentage of intrapulmonary shunting can be quantified by calculating $\dot{Q}s/\dot{Q}T$ in which $\dot{Q}s$ is the shunted perfusion and $\dot{Q}T$ is the total perfusion. Because pathologic anatomic shunting can easily be ruled out, $\dot{Q}s/\dot{Q}T$ generally reflects the percentage of capillary and venous admixture shunting. If the parameter is abnormal or greater than 10% when measured on an FIO_2 of at least 0.5, it reflects primarily absolute capillary shunting (Reischman, 1988). It then is a very valuable parameter to use to assess the severity of gas exchange abnormalities witnessed in ARDS.

Calculation of $\dot{Q}s/\dot{Q}T$ requires simultaneously drawn arterial and mixed venous (pulmonary artery) blood samples. $\dot{Q}s$ is determined by subtracting the arterial blood oxygen content (Cao_2), which represents the amount of oxygen content in pulmonary capillary blood immediately after it has passed the average alveolus, from the ideal end-pulmonary capillary oxygen content (Cco_2). As such, any difference between ideal pulmonary capillary oxygen content and the actual oxygen content reflected by the systemic arterial sample is attributed to pulmonary shunting. $\dot{Q}T$ is determined by subtracting mixed venous blood oxygen content ($C\bar{v}o_2$) from Cco_2. Dividing $\dot{Q}s$ by $\dot{Q}T$ will yield the shunt fraction, which may be multiplied by 100 to arrive at the percent shunt.

$$\frac{\dot{Q}s}{\dot{Q}T} = \frac{Cco_2 - Cao_2}{Cco_2 - C\bar{v}o_2}$$

Cao_2 is calculated by the following equation:

$$(Hgb \times 1.38 \times Sao_2) + (Pao_2 \times 0.003)$$

$C\bar{v}O_2$ is calculated by the following equation:

$$(Hgb \times 1.38 \times S\bar{v}O_2) + (P\bar{v}O_2 \times 0.003)$$

The calculation of CcO_2 requires some explanation of underlying assumptions. The alveolar gas equation is used to calculate end-pulmonary capillary oxygen tension because ideally they should be the same. The patient's FIO_2, barometric pressure (PB usually equals 760 mm Hg), and water vapor pressure (PH_2O = 47 mm Hg) need to be known to determine the oxygen tension of inspired air. In addition, the patient's $PaCO_2$ needs to be measured. These values are then inserted into the alveolar gas equation. The oxygen saturation of end capillary blood should be 100%. However, to eliminate any source of error induced by carboxyhemoglobin or other mechanisms, it is generally assumed to be 98%. CcO_2 is then calculated by the following equation:

$$(Hgb \times 1.38 \times 0.98) + (PAO_2 \times 0.003)$$

where

$$PAO_2 = FIO_2(PB - PH_2O) - (PaCO_2)\ (1.25)$$

A shunt of less than 10% is considered normal. A shunt of 10% to 20% implies a noncritical pulmonary abnormality. A shunt of 20% to 30% is considered very serious. A shunt of 30% or greater may be life-threatening. It should be clear that calculating and trending this parameter can assist the practitioner in evaluating the efficacy of various interventions in improving gas exchange and $\dot{V}/\dot{Q}$ equality in ARDS patients (Reischman, 1988).

MONITOR OXYGEN DELIVERY

In patients with ARDS, a simple cardiac output determination to evaluate whether the value falls within normal limits is not sufficient. Remember that high cardiac output values do not necessarily benefit the patient if, to attain them, PEEP values must be kept very low or PAWP values representing left ventricular filling pressures must be very high. Low PEEP values can compromise gas exchange by allowing alveolar units to recollapse. High PAWP values can increase the pressure gradient for edema development. Either situation will lead to a compromise in arterial blood oxygen content, and good perfusion to the tissues is wasted if the blood is not well oxygenated. Therefore, the clinician does not need to determine the normality of cardiac output but rather its adequacy in ensuring adequate oxygen delivery to the tissues (Snyder, 1987).

To calculate oxygen delivery, also referred to as transport, arterial blood oxygen content and cardiac output need to be determined. Cardiac output is measured using a pulmonary artery catheter via the thermodilution technique. Arterial blood oxygen content is measured by collecting an arterial sample for blood gas and hemoglobin determination.

$$\text{Oxygen delivery} = CaO_2 \times CO \times 10$$

Recall that CaO_2 is calculated by the following equation:

$$(Hgb \times 1.38 \times SaO_2) + (PaO_2 \times 0.003)$$

An oxygen delivery of 1000 mL/min is considered normal. Although achieving normal may be an unrealistic goal, calculating this parameter following different interventions will assist the practitioner in determining the adequacy of cardiac output as well as which combination of therapies best facilitates tissue oxygenation.

MEASURE STATIC PULMONARY COMPLIANCE

Compliance is an expression of the elastic properties of the lung. It is the change in volume accomplished by a change in pressure. As such, it reflects the distensibility of the lung. When compliance is low, the lung is stiff, work of breathing is increased, and ineffective breathing patterns ensue (McCauley & Von Rueden, 1988). The calculation for measuring static compliance (CST) for patients on ventilatory assistance is:

$$C_{ST} = \frac{\text{Tidal volume } (V_T)}{\text{Plateau pressure} - \text{PEEP}}$$

All of these values are readily available in the ventilatory-assisted patient. A static compliance of greater than 50 mL/cm H_2O is generally considered acceptable. However, calculating CST at different tidal volume and PEEP levels can assist the practitioner in determining at what level compliance is optimum, work of breathing is reduced, and breathing patterns are most effective (McCauley & Von Rueden, 1988).

PROGNOSIS

The prognosis of ARDS is determined by the underlying cause, the extent of injury, the patient's response to therapy, and the development of multisystem organ failure, a dreaded and deadly complication of ARDS (Putterman, 1988). Mortality rates are reported to range from 50% to 90% (Fowler et al., 1983; Montgomery et al., 1985; Pepe et al., 1982; Seidenfeld et al., 1986). However, it is difficult to interpret these mortality rates because no definition of ARDS is uniformly accepted and applied as well as because milder forms of this syndrome probably go unrecognized.

ARDS is often a complication that occurs late in the natural course of other diseases. Although prognostic indicators have not been extensively studied, mortality directly correlates with the number and severity of the underlying disease or diseases (Fowler et al., 1983; Pepe et al., 1982). In addition, severe pulmonary hypertension and multisystem organ failure as a consequence of sepsis are apparently more predominant in

TABLE 32–4. **Outcome in Survivors of ARDS**

Outcome Variable	Number of Patients	Normal (%)	Comments
Clinical status	84	83.3	7.1% mild DOE, 2.4% moderate DOE
Chest x-ray	81	80.2	7.4% hyperinflation, 11.1% interstitial changes
Lung volumes	122	72.1	5.7% hyperinflation, 22.1% restrictive (no improvement after 1 year in the few patients studied serially)
Expiratory flow	122	83.6	5.7% had reversible obstruction; the others had irreversible obstruction
Airway resistance	26	88.5	
Resting Pa_{O_2}	91	73.6	
Exercise Pa_{O_2}	65	52.3	3.1% developed increased Pa_{O_2} with exercise
$\dot{Q}s/\dot{Q}_T$	38	89.5	
DLCO	74	5.14	Those with abnormal values tended to return toward normal over time

Abbreviations: DOE, dyspnea on exertion; $\dot{Q}s/\dot{Q}_T$, shunt fraction; DLCO, diffusing capacity for carbon monoxide, either single breath or steady state.
Adapted from Alberts, W., Michael, M. D., Priest, G. R., et al. (1983). The outlook for survivors of ARDS. *Chest, 84,* 272–274.

nonsurvivors (Bell et al., 1983). Deaths as a result of respiratory failure are less common (Dalnogare, 1989). Patients with self-limited causes of ARDS, such as those with air emboli, isolated trauma, or massive blood transfusions, as well as those with milder degrees of edema also have a greater chance of survival (Lamy et al., 1976).

The outlook for patients who survive diffuse lung injury, even if severe, is favorable. Most recover completely or possess a residual reduction in diffusing capacity. Histologic abnormalities may also gradually regress. Alberts and colleagues (1983) summarized the findings in 21 publications providing prognostic information. The authors included only those publications that they agreed described ARDS based on its association with widely accepted etiologic and clinical descriptors. Their data are summarized in Table 32–4. As is evident, the outlook for those who do survive the acute event appears optimistic. On the other hand, the mortality rates for patients with severe ARDS are unlikely to improve until more is known specifically about how the lungs are injured and repaired. Therapy directed at these mechanisms as opposed to supportive therapy still needs to be identified so that it may be administered prophylactically or very shortly after the lung insult.

REFERENCES

Alberts, W. M., Priest, G. R., & Moser, K. M. (1983). The outlook for survivors of ARDS. *Chest, 84,* 272–274.

Arora, N. S., & Rochester, D. F. (1977). Effect of general nutritional and muscular states on the human diaphragm. *American Review of Respiratory Disease, 115,* 84–87.

Ashbaugh, D. G., Bigelow, D. B., Pelty, T. L., et al. (1967). Acute respiratory distress in adults. *Lancet, 2,* 319–323.

Ayars, G. H., Altman, L. C., Rosen, H., et al. (1984). The injurious effects of neutrophils on pneumocytes in vitro. *American Review of Respiratory Disease, 130,* 964–973.

Ayres, S. M. (1982). Mechanisms and consequences of pulmonary edema: Cardiac lung, shock lung, and principles of ventilatory therapy in adult respiratory distress syndrome. *American Heart Journal, 103,* 97–102.

Babior, B. M., Kipnes, R. S., & Curnutte, J. T. (1973). Biological defense mechanisms: The production of leukocytes of superoxide, a potential bactericidal agent. *Journal of Clinical Investigation, 52,* 741–744.

Bachofen, M., & Weibel, E. R. (1982). Structural alterations of lung parenchyma in the adult respiratory distress syndrome. *Clinical Chest Medicine, 3,* 35–56.

Balk, R., & Bone, R. C. (1983). The adult respiratory distress syndrome. *Medical Clinics of North America, 67,* 685–699.

Barrett, C. R., Bell, A. L. L., & Ryan, S. F. (1979). Alveolar epithelial injury causing respiratory distress in dogs: Physiologic and electron-microscopic correlations. *Chest, 75,* 705–711.

Bast, A., Haenen, G. R. M., & Doeleman, C. J. A. (1991). Oxidants and antioxidants: State of the art. *American Journal of Medicine,* Suppl 3C, 2S–13S.

Beale, R., & Grover, E. R. (1993). Acute respiratory distress syndrome (ARDS): No more than a severe acute lung injury? *British Medical Journal, 307,* 1335–1339.

Begley, C. J., Ogletree, M. L., Meyrick, B. O., et al. (1984). Modification of pulmonary responses to endotoxemia in awake sheep by steroid and nonsteroidal anti-inflammatory agents. *American Review of Respiratory Disease, 130,* 1140–1146.

Bell, R. C., Coalson, J., Smith, J., et al. (1983). Multiple organ system failure and infection in adult respiratory distress syndrome. *Annals of Internal Medicine, 99,* 293–298.

Bernard, G. R., & Brigham, K. L. (1986). Pulmonary edema: Pathophysiologic mechanisms and new approaches to therapy. *Chest, 89,* 594–600.

Bernard, G. R., Luce, J., Sprung, C., et al. (1987). High-dose corticosteroids in patients with the adult respiratory distress syndrome. *New England Journal of Medicine, 317,* 1565–1570.

Bernard, G. R., Lucht, W. D., Niedermeyer, M. E., et al. (1984). Effect of *N*-acetylcysteine on the pulmonary response to endotoxin in the awake sheep and upon in vitro granulocyte function. *Journal of Clinical Investigation, 73,* 1772–1784.

Beutler, B., Milsark, I. W., & Cerami, A. C. (1985). Passive immunization against cachectin/tumor necrosis factor protects mice from the lethal effect of endotoxin. *Science, 299,* 869–871.

Boggis, C. R. M., & Greene, R. (1983). ARDS. *British Journal of Hospital Medicine, 29,* 167–174.

Bone, R. C., Fisher, C., Clemmer, T., et al. (1987). The Methylprednisolone Severe Sepsis Study Group: Early methylprednisolone treatment for septic syndrome and the adult respiratory distress syndrome. *Chest, 92,* 1032–1036.

Bone, R. C., Francis, P. G., & Pierce, A. K. (1976). Intravascular coagulation associated with the adult respiratory distress syndrome. *American Journal of Medicine, 61,* 585–589.

Boxer, L. A., Axtell, R., & Suchard, S. (1990). The role of the neutrophil in inflammatory diseases of the lung. *Blood Cells, 16,* 25–42.

Brandstetter, R. D. (1986). The adult respiratory distress syndrome—1986. *Heart & Lung, 15,* 155–164.

Braquet, P., & Hosford, D. (1989). The potential role of platelet-activating factor (PAF) in shock, sepsis and adult respiratory distress syndrome (ARDS). *Progress in Clinical and Biological Research, 308,* 425–439.

Brigham, K. L. (1985). Metabolites of arachidonic acid in experimental lung vascular injury. *Federation Proceedings, 44,* 43–45.

Brigham, K. L., & Ogletree, M. L. (1981). Effects of prostaglandins and related compounds on lung vascular permeability. *Bulletin of European Physiology, 17,* 703–722.

Carlon, G. C., Howland, S. W., Ray, C., Miodownik, S., & Griffin, J. P. (1983). High frequency jet ventilation: A prospective randomised evaluation. *Chest, 84,* 551–559.

Christman, J. W. (1992). Potential treatment of sepsis syndrome with cytokine-specific agents. *Chest, 102,* 613–617.

Christner, P., Fein, A., Goldberg, S., et al. (1985). Collagenase in the lower respiratory tract of patients with adult respiratory distress syndrome. *American Review of Respiratory Disease, 131,* 690–695.

Coccia, M. T., Waxman, K., & Soliman, M. H. (1989). Pentoxifylline improves survival following hemorrhagic shock. *Critical Care Medicine, 17,* 36–41.

Cochrane, G. C., Spragg, R. C., & Revak, S. D. (1983). Studies on the pathogenesis of ARDS: Evidence of oxidant activity in bronchoalveolar lavage fluid. *Journal of Clinical Investigation, 71,* 754–761.

Connors, A. F., McCaffree, D. R., & Rogers, R. M. (1981). The adult respiratory distress syndrome. *Disease-a-Month, 27,* 1–75.

Cooper, J. A., Bizios, R., & Malik, A. B. (1985). Pulmonary neutrophil kinetics in sheep: Effects of altered hemodynamics. *Journal of Applied Physiology, 59,* 1796–1801.

Crandell, E. D. (Ed.) (1983). Fluid balance across the alveolar epithelium. *American Review of Respiratory Disease, 127*(5), S1–S65.

Dalnogare, A. R. (1989). Southwestern Internal Medicine Conference: Adult respiratory distress syndrome. *American Journal of Medical Science, 298,* 413–430.

Dantzker, D. R. (1990). The role of oxygen supply dependence in the adult respiratory distress syndrome. *Critical Care Report, 1,* 260–265.

Dantzker, D. R. (1993). Adequacy of tissue oxygenation. *Critical Care Medicine, 21,* S40–S43.

Dantzker, D. R., Brook, C. J., Dehart, P., et al. (1979). Ventilation–perfusion distributions in the adult respiratory distress syndrome. *American Review of Respiratory Disease, 120,* 1039–1052.

Downs, J. B., & Stock, M. C. (1987). Airway pressure release ventilation: A new concept in ventilatory support. *Critical Care Medicine, 15,* 459–461.

Enger, E. L. (1989). Pulmonary artery wedge pressure: When it's valid, when it's not. *Critical Care Nursing Clinics of North America, 1,* 603–618.

Erdmann, A. F., Vaughan, T. R., Brigham, K. L., et al. (1975). Effect of increased vascular pressure on lung fluid balance in unanesthetized sheep. *Circulation Research, 37,* 271–284.

Estenne, M., & Yernault, J. C. (1984). The mechanism of CO_2 retention in cardiac pulmonary edema. *Chest, 86,* 936–938.

Exley, A. R., Cohen, J., Buurman, W., Owen, R., Hanson, G., & Lumley, J. (1990). Monoclonal antibody to TNF in severe septic shock. *Lancet, 335,* 1275–1276.

Fein, A., Grossman, R. F., Jones, J. G., et al. (1979). The value of edema fluid protein measurements in patients with pulmonary edema. *American Journal of Medicine, 67,* 32–38.

Fishman, A. P. (1980). Pulmonary edema. In A. P. Fishman (Ed.), *Pulmonary diseases and disorders* (p. 733). New York: McGraw-Hill.

Fowler, A. A., Hamman, R., Good, J., et al. (1983). Adult respiratory distress syndrome: Risk with common predispositions. *Annals of Internal Medicine, 98,* 593–597.

Fulton, R. L., & Jones, C. E. (1975). The cause of post-traumatic pulmonary insufficiency in man. *Surgery, Gynecology and Obstetrics, 140,* 179–184.

Gallagher, T. J., Civetta, J. M., & Kirby, R. R. (1978). Terminology update: Optimum PEEP. *Critical Care Medicine, 6,* 323–326.

Ghosh, S., Latimer, R. D., Gray, B. M., Harwood, R. J., & Oduro, A. (1993). Endotoxin-induced organ injury. *Critical Care Medicine, 21,* S19–S24.

Goldstein, I. M. (1988). Complement: Biologically active products. In J. I. Gallin, I. M. Goldstein, & R. Snyderman (Eds.), *Inflammation* (pp. 55–74). New York: Raven Press.

Greenman, R. L., Schein, R. M. H., Martin, M. A., Wenzel, R. P., MacIntyre, N. R., & Emmanuel, G. (1991). A controlled clinical trial of E5 murine monoclonal IgM antibody to endotoxin in the treatment of Gram negative sepsis. *Journal of the American Medical Association, 266,* 1097–1102.

Hallman, M., Spragg, R., & Harrell, J. H. (1982). Evidence of lung surfactant abnormality in respiratory failure: Study of bronchoalveolar lavage phospholipids, surface activity, phospholipase activity and plasma myoinositol. *Journal of Clinical Investigation, 70,* 673–683.

Hammerschmidt, D. E., Weaver, J., Hudson, L., et al. (1980). Association of complement activation and elevated plasma C_{5A} with adult respiratory distress syndrome. *Lancet, 1,* 947–949.

Hasegawa, N., Husari, A. W., Hart, W. T., Kandra, T. G., & Raffin, T. A. (1994). Role of the coagulation system in ARDS. *Chest, 105,* 268–277.

Haupt, M. T., & Rackow, E. R. (1982). Colloid osmotic pressure and fluid resuscitation with hetastarch, albumin and saline solution. *Critical Care Medicine, 10,* 159–165.

Hauser, C. J., Shoemaker, W. C., & Turpin, I. (1980). Oxygen transport responses to colloid and crystalloid in critically ill surgical patients. *Surgery, Gynecology and Obstetrics, 150,* 811–816.

Havill, A. M., & Gee, M. H. (1984). Role of interstitium in clearance of alveolar fluid in normal and injured lungs. *Journal of Applied Physiology, 57,* 1–6.

Hickling, K. G., Henderson, S. J., & Jackson, R. (1990). Low mortality associated with low volume pressure limited ventilation with permissive hypercapnia in severe adult respiratory distress syndrome. *Intensive Care Medicine, 16,* 372–377.

Hill, J. D., O'Brien, T. G., & Muray, J. T. (1972). Prolonged extracorporeal oxygenation for acute post traumatic respiratory failure (shock lung syndrome). *New England Journal of Medicine, 286,* 629–634.

Hinshaw, L., Olson, P., & Kuo, G. (1989). Efficacy of posttreatment with anti-TNF monoclonal antibody in preventing the pathophysiology and lethality of sepsis in the baboon. *Circulatory Shock, 27,* 362–364.

Hinson, J. R., & Marini, J. J. (1992). Principles of mechanical ventilatory use in respiratory failure. *Annual Review of Medicine, 43,* 341–361.

Hurewitz, A., & Bergofsky, E. H. (1981). Adult respiratory distress syndrome. *Medical Clinics of North America, 65,* 33–51.

Hyers, T. M., Tricomi, S. M., Dettenmeier, P. A., & Fowler, A. A. (1991). TNF levels in serum and bronchoalveolar lavage fluid of patients with the adult respiratory distress syndrome. *American Review of Respiratory Disease, 144,* 268–271.

Issekutz, A. C., & Movat, H. Z. (1982). The effect of vasodilator prostaglandins on polymorphonuclear leukocyte infiltration and vascular injury. *American Journal of Pathology, 107,* 300–309.

Jacobs, R. F., Tabor, D. R., Burks, A. W., & Campbell, G. D. (1989). Elevated IL-1 release by human alveolar macrophages during ARDS. *American Review of Respiratory Disease, 140,* 1686–1692.

Jenkinson, S. G. (1982). Pulmonary oxygen toxicity. *Clinical Chest Medicine, 3,* 109–120.

Karima, N. K., & Burns, S. (1985). Regulation of tissue oxygen extraction is disturbed in adult respiratory distress syndrome. *American Review of Respiratory Disease, 132,* 109–114.

Keogh, B. F., Hunter, D. N., Morgan, C. J., et al. (1989). The management of adult respiratory distress syndrome (Part I). *British Journal of Hospital Medicine, 42,* 468–474.

Keogh, B. F., Hunter, D. N., Morgan, C. J., et al. (1990). The management of adult respiratory distress syndrome (Part II). *British Journal of Hospital Medicine, 43,* 26–30.

Keren, A., Klein, J., & Stern, S. (1980). Adult respiratory distress syndrome in the course of acute myocardial infarction. *Chest, 77,* 161–166.

Klebanoff, S. J. (1980). Oxygen metabolism and the toxic properties of phagocytes. *Annals of Internal Medicine, 93,* 480–489.

Klebanoff, S. J., Vadas, M., Harlan, J., et al. (1986). Stimulation of neutrophils by tumor necrotic factor. *Journal of Immunology, 136,* 4220–4225.

Koltai, M., Hosford, D., & Braquet, P. G. (1993). Platelet-activating factor in septic shock. *New Horizons, 1,* 87–95.

Lamy, M., Fallat, R., Koeniger, E., et al. (1976). Pathologic features and mechanisms of hypoxemia in adult respiratory distress syndrome. *American Review of Respiratory Disease, 114,* 267–284.

Langer, M., Mascheroni, D., Marcolin, R., et al. (1988). The prone position in ARDS patients. *Chest, 94,* 103–107.

Lee, C. T., Fein, A. M., Lippmann, M., et al. (1981). Elastolytic activity in pulmonary lavage fluid from patients with adult respiratory distress syndrome. *New England Journal of Medicine, 304,* 192–196.

Leeman, M., Beoynaems, J. M., & Degaute, J. P. (1985). Administration of dazoxiben, a selective thromboxane synthase inhibitor, in the adult respiratory distress syndrome. *Chest, 87,* 726–730.

Lefer, A. M. (1987). Physiologic and pathophysiologic role of cyclooxygenase metabolites of arachidonic acid in circulatory disease states. *Cardiovascular Clinics, 18,* 85–99.

Lewis, J. F., & Jobe, A. H. (1993). Surfactant and the adult respiratory distress syndrome. *American Review of Respiratory Disease, 147,* 218–233.

Lewis, K. A., & Austen, K. F. (1984). The biologically active leukotrienes: Biosynthesis, metabolism, receptors, functions, and pharmacology. *Journal of Clinical Investigation, 73,* 889–897.

Lozman, J., Powers, S. R., Older, T., et al. (1974). Correlation of the pulmonary wedge and left atrial pressures: A study in the patient receiving positive end-expiratory pressure ventilation. *Archives of Surgery, 109,* 270–277.

Macnaughton, P. D., & Evans, T. W. (1992). Management of adult respiratory distress syndrome. *Lancet, 339,* 469–472.

Majors, M. (1988). Nutritional support of the mechanically ventilated patient. *Critical Care Nursing Quarterly, 11,* 50–61.

Martin, W. J., Gadek, J. E., Hunninghake, G. W., et al. (1981). Oxidant injury of lung parenchymal cells. *Journal of Clinical Investigation, 68,* 1277–1288.

Massaro, D., Thet, L. A., Massaro, G. D., et al. (1980). A hypothesis relating breathing pattern to some forms of the "adult respiratory distress syndrome." *American Journal of Medicine, 69,* 113–115.

Matthay, M. A., Eschenbacher, W. L., & Goetzl, E. J. (1984). Elevated concentrations of leukotriene D_4 in pulmonary edema fluid of patients with the adult respiratory distress syndrome. *Journal of Clinical Immunology, 4,* 479–483.

Mathison, J. C., Wolfson, E., & Ulevitch, R. J. (1988). Participation of tumor necrosis factor in the mediation of Gram negative bacterial lipopolysaccharide-induced injury in rabbits. *Journal of Clinical Investigation, 81,* 1925–1937.

Maunder, R. J. (1986). Clinical predictors of the ARDS. *Clinical Chest Medicine, 6,* 413–426.

McCauley, M., & Von Rueden, K. (1988). Noninvasive monitoring of the mechanically ventilated patient. *Critical Care Nursing Quarterly, 11,* 36–49.

McCord, J. M. (1993). Oxygen-derived free radicals. *New Horizons, 1,* 70–76.

Messent, M., & Griffiths, M. J. (1992). The pulmonary physician and critical care: Pharmacotherapy in lung injury. *Thorax, 47,* 651–656.

Metz, C., & Sibbald, W. J. (1991). Anti-inflammatory therapy for acute lung injury. A review of animal and clinical studies. *Chest, 100,* 1110–1119.

Milligan, S. A., Hoeffel, J. M., & Flick, M. R. (1985). Endotoxin induced acute lung injury in unanesthetized sheep is prevented by catalase. *American Review of Respiratory Disease, 131,* A422.

Modig, J. (1986). ARDS: Pathogenesis and treatment. *Acta Chirurgica Scandinavica, 152,* 241–249.

Montgomery, A. B., Stager, M. A., Carrico, C. J., et al. (1985). Causes of mortality in patients with the adult respiratory distress syndrome. *American Review of Respiratory Disease, 132,* 485–489.

Morganroth, M. L., Reeves, J. T., Murphy, K. C., et al. (1984). Leukotriene synthesis and receptor blockers block hypoxic pulmonary vasoconstriction. *Journal of Applied Physiology, 56,* 1340–1346.

Moriguchi, S., Sone, S., & Kishino, Y. (1983). Changes of alveolar macrophages in protein-deficient rats. *Journal of Nutrition, 113,* 40–46.

Mortenson, J. D. (1987). An intravenacaval blood gas exchange device: A preliminary report. *Transactions of the American Society of Artificial Internal Organs, 33,* 570–572.

Moss, G. S., Lowe, R. J., & Jilek, J. (1981). Colloid or crystalloid in the resuscitation of hemorrhagic shock: A controlled clinical trial. *Surgery, 89,* 434–440.

Murray, G. F. (1977). Mechanisms of acute respiratory failure. *American Review of Respiratory Disease, 115,* 1071–1078.

Nitta, S., Ohnuki, T., Ohkuda, K., et al. (1981). The corrected protein equation to estimate plasma colloid osmotic pressure and its development on a nomogram. *Tohoku Journal of Experimental Medicine, 135,* 43–49.

Ogletree, M. L. (1982). Pharmacology of prostaglandins in the pulmonary microcirculation. *Annals of the New York Academy of Science, 384,* 191–205.

O'Quin, R., & Marini, J. J. (1983). Pulmonary artery occlusion pressure: Clinical physiology, measurement and interpretation. *American Review of Respiratory Disease, 128,* 319–326.

Parker, J. C., Martin, D. J., Rutili, G., et al. (1983). Prevention of free radical-mediated vascular permeability increase in lung using superoxide dismutase. *Chest, 83,* S52–S53.

Parson, P. E., Fowler, A., Hyers, T., et al. (1985). Chemotatic activity in bronchoalveolar lavage fluid from patients with adult respiratory distress syndrome. *American Review of Respiratory Disease, 132,* 490–493.

Pepe, P. E., Hudson, L. D., & Carrico, C. J. (1984). Early application of PEEP in patients at risk for the adult respiratory distress syndrome. *New England Journal of Medicine, 311,* 281–288.

Pepe, P. E., Potkin, R., Holtman-Reus, D., et al. (1982). Clinical predictors of the adult respiratory distress syndrome. *American Journal of Surgery, 144,* 124–128.

Perlman, M. B., Lo, S. K., & Malik, A. B. (1986). Effect of prostacyclin on pulmonary vascular response to thrombin in awake sheep. *Journal of Applied Physiology, 60,* 546–553.

Permutt, S. (1979). Mechanical influences on water accumulation in the lungs. In A. P. Fishman & E. M. Renkin (Eds.), *Pulmonary edema* (p. 175). Bethesda, MD: American Physiological Society.

Pesenti, A., Gattinoni, L., & Kolobow, T. (1988). Extracorporeal circulation in adult respiratory failure. *Transactions of the American Society of Artificial Internal Organs, 34,* 43–47.

Pingleton, S. K. (1982). Complications associated with the adult respiratory distress syndrome. *Clinical Chest Medicine, 5,* 143–151.

Pinkard, R. N., Ludwig, J. C., & McManus, L. M. (1988). Platelet activating factors. In J. J. Gallin, I. M. Goldstein, & R. Syderman (Eds.), *Inflammation: Basic principals and clinical correlates* (pp. 139–167). New York: Raven Press.

Pohlman, T. H., Stanness, K., Beatty, P., et al. (1986). An endothelial cell surface factor induced in vitro by lipopolysaccharide, interleukin 1 and tumor necrosis factor-alpha increases neutrophil adherence by a CDW18-dependent mechanism. *Journal of Immunology, 136,* 4548–4553.

Powe, J. E., Short, A., & Sibbald, W. J. (1982). Pulmonary accumulation of polymorphonuclear leukocytes in the adult respiratory distress syndrome. *Critical Care Medicine, 10,* 712–718.

Putterman, C. (1988). Acute respiratory distress syndrome: Current concepts. *Resuscitation, 16,* 91–105.

Raffin, T. (1987). ARDS: Mechanisms and management. *Hospital Practice, 22,* 65–76; 78–80.

Rajacich, N., Burchard, K. W., & Hasan, F. M. (1989). Central venous pressure and pulmonary capillary wedge pressure as estimates of left atrial pressure: Effects of PEEP and catheter tip malposition. *Critical Care Medicine, 17,* 7–11.

Reischman, R. R. (1988). Impaired gas exchange related to intrapulmonary shunting. *Critical Care Nurse, 8,* 35–49.

Repine, J. E. (1992). Scientific perspectives on adult respiratory distress syndrome. *Lancet, 339,* 466–469.

Repine, J. E., & Beehler, C. J. (1991). Neutrophils and adult respiratory distress syndrome: Two interlocking perspectives in 1991. *American Review of Respiratory Disease, 144,* 251–252.

Richard, C., Lemonnier, F., & Thibault, M. (1991). Vitamin E deficiency and lipoperoxidation during adult respiratory distress syndrome. *Critical Care Medicine, 18,* 4–9.

Rinaldo, J. E., & Rogers, R. M. (1986). Acute respiratory distress syndrome. *New England Journal of Medicine, 315,* 578–580.

Roberts, S. L. (1990). High-permeability pulmonary edema: Nursing assessment, diagnosis and intervention. *Heart & Lung, 19,* 287–300.

Rochester, D. F., & Esau, S. A. (1984). Malnutrition and the respiratory system. *Chest, 85,* 411–416.

Rossaint, R., Falke, K. J., Lopez, F., Slama, K., Pison, U., & Zapol,

W. M. (1993). Inhaled nitric oxide for the adult respiratory distress syndrome. *New England Journal of Medicine, 328,* 399–405.

Saba, T. M., & Jaffe, E. (1980). Plasma fibrinectin: Its synthesis by vascular endothelial cells and role in cardiopulmonary integrity after trauma as related to reticuloendothelial function. *American Journal of Medicine, 68,* 577–594.

Sahebjami, H., Vassallo, C. L., & Wirman, J. A. (1978). Lung mechanics and ultrastructure in prolonged starvation. *American Review of Respiratory Disease, 117,* 77–82.

Said, S. I., & Foda, H. D. (1989). Pharmacologic modulation of lung injury. *American Review of Respiratory Disease, 139,* 1553–1564.

Schneider, R. C., Zapol, W. N., & Corvalb, A. H. (1980). Platelet consumption and sequestration in severe acute respiratory failure. *American Review of Respiratory Disease, 122,* 455–461.

Schumann, L., & Parsons, G. (1985). Tracheal suctioning and ventilator tubing changes in adult respiratory distress syndrome: Use of a positive-end expiratory pressure value. *Heart & Lung, 14,* 362–367.

Seeger, W., Gunther, A., Walmrath, H. D., Grimminger, F., & Lasch, H. G. (1993). Alveolar surfactant and adult respiratory distress syndrome: Pathogenic role and therapeutic prospects. *Clinical Investigator, 71,* 177–190.

Seidenfeld, J. J., Pohl, D. F., Bell, R. C., et al. (1986). Incidence, site and outcome of infections in patients with the adult respiratory distress syndrome. *American Review of Respiratory Disease, 134,* 12–16.

Shapiro, B. A., Cane, R. D., & Harrison, R. A. (1984). Positive end-expiratory pressure in adults with special reference to acute lung injury: A review of the literature and suggested clinical correlations. *Critical Care Medicine, 12,* 124–141.

Shapiro, L., & Gelfand, J. A. (1993). Cytokines and sepsis: Pathophysiology and therapy. *New Horizons, 1,* 13–22.

Shigematsu, N., Matsuba, K., & Shirakusa, T. (1980). The preventive effect of urokinase on experimental bleomycin-induced interstitial pneumonia. *American Review of Respiratory Disease, 121,* 188.

Shoemaker, W. C., & Appel, P. L. (1986). Effect of prostaglandin E_1 in ARDS. *Surgery, 99,* 275–282.

Shoemaker, W. C., & Hauser, C. J. (1979). Critique of crystalloids versus colloid therapy in shock and shock lung. *Critical Care Medicine, 7,* 117–124.

Shoemaker, W. C., Schluchter, M., & Hopkins, J. A. (1981). Comparison of the relative effectiveness of colloids and crystalloids in emergency resuscitation. *American Journal of Surgery, 142,* 73–75.

Sibbald, W. J., Anderson, R. R., & Reid, B. (1981). Alveolocapillary permeability in human septic ARDS: Effect of high-dose corticosteroid therapy. *Chest, 79,* 133–138.

Sibbald, W. J., Cunningham, D. R., & Chin, D. N. (1983). Noncardiac or cardiac pulmonary edema? A practical approach to clinical differentiation in critically ill patients. *Chest, 84,* 453–462.

Simionescu, M., & Simionescu, N. (1984). Ultrastructure of the microvascular wall: Functional correlations. In E. M. Renkin & C. C. Michel (Eds.), *Handbook of physiology* (Section 2), *the cardiovascular system* (Part 2), *microcirculation* (pp. 41–101). Bethesda, MD: American Physiological Society.

Slotman, G. J., D'Arezzo, A., & Gann, D. S. (1988). Ketoconazole prevents acute respiratory failure in critically ill surgical patients. *Journal of Trauma, 28,* 648–654.

Snider, M. T. (1990). Adult respiratory distress syndrome in the trauma patient. *Critical Care Clinics, 6,* 103–110.

Snyder, J. V. (1987). Patterns of hemodynamic response. In J. V. Snyder & M. R. Pinsky (Eds.), *Oxygen transport in the critically ill* (pp. 46–66). Chicago: Year Book.

Spagnuolo, P. J., Ellner, J. J., Hassid, A., et al. (1980). Thromboxane A_2 mediated augmented polymorphonuclear adhesiveness. *Journal of Clinical Investigation, 66,* 406–414.

Staub, N. C. (1974). Pulmonary edema. *Physiological Reviews, 54,* 678–811.

Staub, N. C. (1978). Lung fluid and solute exchange. In N. C. Staub (Ed.), *Lung water and solute exchange* (pp. 3–16). New York: Marcel Dekker.

Staub, N. C. (1980). The pathogenesis of pulmonary edema. *Progress in Cardiovascular Disease, 23,* 53–80.

Staub, N. C. (1981). Clinical measurement of lung water content. *Chest, 79,* 3–18.

Staub, N. C. (1983). Alveolar flooding and clearance. *American Review of Respiratory Disease, 127*(5), S44–S51.

Staub, N. C. (1985). Only the shadow knows. *American Journal of Roentgenology, 144,* 1086–1087.

Staub, N. C., Nagano, H., & Pearce, M. L. (1967). Pulmonary edema in dogs, especially the sequence of fluid accumulation in lungs. *Journal of Applied Physiology, 22,* 227–240.

Stephens, K. E., Ishizaka, A., Larrick, J., et al. (1987). Tumor necrosis factor causes increased pulmonary permeability and edema. *American Review of Respiratory Disease, 137,* 1364–1370.

Stevens, J. V., & Raffin, T. A. (1984). ARDS: Etiology and mechanisms. *Postgraduate Medical Journal, 60,* 505–513.

St. John, R. C., & Dorinsky, P. M. (1993). Immunologic therapy for ARDS, septic shock and multiple organ failure. *Chest, 103,* 932–943.

Stokke, T., Burchardi, H., Hensel, A., Kostering, H., Kartner, T., & Rahlf, G. (1986). Continuous intravenous infusion of elastase in normal agranulocytic minipigs: Effects on the lungs and the blood coagulation system. *Resuscitation, 14,* 61–79.

Strieter, R. M., Kunkel, S., Showell, H., et al. (1989). Endothelial cell gene expression of a neutrophil chemotactic factor by TNF-alpha, LPS and IL-1 beta. *Science, 243,* 1467–1469.

Sullivan, G. W., Carpenter, H. T., Novick, W. J., & Mandell, G. L. (1988). Inhibition of the inflammatory action of interleukin-1 and tumour necrosis factor (alpha) on neutrophil function by pentoxifylline. *Infectious Immunology, 56,* 1722–1729.

Suter, P. M., Failey, H. B., & Isenberg, M. D. (1975). Optimum end-expiratory pressure in patients with acute pulmonary failure. *New England Journal of Medicine, 292,* 284–289.

Swami, A., & Keogh, B. F. (1992). The injured lung: Conventional and novel respiratory therapy. *Thorax, 47,* 555–562.

Tate, R. M., & Repine, J. (1983). Neutrophils and the adult respiratory distress syndrome. *American Review of Respiratory Disease, 128,* 552.

Taylor, A. E. (1981). Capillary fluid filtration: Starling forces and lymph flow. *Circulation Research, 49,* 557–575.

Taylor, A. E., & Parker, J. C. (1985). Pulmonary interstitial spaces and lymphatics. In A. P. Fishman & A. B. Fisher (Eds.), *Handbook of physiology* (Section 3), *The respiratory system* (Vol. 1), *Circulation and nonrespiratory function* (pp. 167–230). Bethesda, MD: American Physiological Society.

Taylor, R. W., & Duncan, C. A. (1983). The adult respiratory distress syndrome. *Res Medica, 1,* 17–40.

Tharratt, R. S., Allen, R. P., & Albertson, T. E. (1988). Pressure controlled inverse ratio ventilation in severe adult respiratory failure. *Chest, 94,* 755–762.

Thommasen, H. V., Russell, J. A., & Boyko, W. J. (1984). Transient leukopenia associated with adult respiratory distress syndrome. *Lancet, 1,* 809–812.

Toben, B., & Lewandowski, V. (1988). Nontraditional and new ventilatory techniques. *Critical Care Nursing Quarterly, 11,* 12–28.

Tracey, K. J., Lowry, S. F., & Cerami, A. (1988). Cachectin/TNF-α in septic shock and septic adult respiratory distress syndrome. *American Review of Respiratory Disease, 138,* 1377–1379.

Varani, J., Fligiel, S. E. G., Till, G. O., et al. (1985). Pulmonary endothelial cell killing by human neutrophils: Possible involvement of hydroxyl radical. *Laboratory Investigation, 53,* 656–663.

Vered, M., Dearing, R., & Janoff, A. (1985). A new elastase inhibitor from *Streptococcus pneumoniae* protects against acute lung injury induced by neutrophil granules. *American Review of Respiratory Disease, 131,* 131–133.

Wang, C. G., Hakim, T. S., Michel, R. P., et al. (1985). Segmental pulmonary vascular resistance in progressive hydrostatic and permeability edema. *Journal of Applied Physiology, 59,* 242–247.

Weiland, J. E., Davis, W., Holter, J., et al. (1986). Lung neutrophils in the adult respiratory distress syndrome. *American Review of Respiratory Disease, 133,* 218–225.

Weisman, I. M., Rinaldo, J. E., & Rogers, R. M. (1982). Positive end-expiratory pressure in adult respiratory failure. *New England Journal of Medicine, 307,* 1381–1384.

Weissmann, C., Askanazi, J., & Rosenbaum, S. (1983). Amino acids and respiration. *Annals of Internal Medicine, 48,* 41–46.

Wirtz, H., & Schmidt, M. (1992). Ventilation and secretion of pulmonary surfactant. *Clinical Investigator, 70,* 3–13.

Wood, L. D. H., & Prewitt, R. M. (1981). Cardiovascular management in acute hypoxemic respiratory failure. *American Journal of Cardiology, 47,* 963–972.

Zapol, W. M., Snider, M. T., Hill, J. D., et al. (1979). Extracorporeal membrane oxygenation in severe acute respiratory failure: A randomized prospective trial. *Journal of the American Medical Association, 242,* 2193–2196.

Zieler, E. J., Fisher, C. J., Sprung, C. L., Straube, R. C., Sadoff, J. C., & Foulke, G. E. (1991). Treatment of Gram negative bacteraemia with HA-1A human monoclonal antibody against endotoxin. *New England Journal of Medicine, 324,* 429–436.

Zimmerman, G., Renzetti, A., & Hill, A. (1983). Functional and metabolic activity of granulocytes from patients with ARDS: Evidence of activated neutrophils in the pulmonary circulation. *American Review of Respiratory Disease, 127,* 290–300.

ADULT RESPIRATORY DISTRESS SYNDROME MULTIDISCIPLINARY CARE GUIDE

COORDINATION OF CARE

Diagnosis/Stabilization Phase		Acute Management Phase		Recovery Phase	
Outcome	*Intervention*	*Outcome*	*Intervention*	*Outcome*	*Intervention*
All appropriate team members and disciplines will be involved in plan of care.	Develop the plan of care with patient/family, primary nurse(s), primary physician(s), pulmonologist, intensivist, other specialists as needed, clinical nurse specialist, respiratory therapist, and chaplain.	All appropriate team members and disciplines will be involved.	Update the plan of care with patient/family, dietician, social services, discharge planner, home health agency, and physical therapist. Initiate planning for anticipated discharge.	Patient/family will understand how to maintain optimal health at home.	Provide written guidelines concerning follow-up care to patient and family. Provide patient/family with phone numbers of resources available to answer questions.

FLUID BALANCE

Diagnosis/Stabilization Phase		Acute Management Phase		Recovery Phase	
Outcome	*Intervention*	*Outcome*	*Intervention*	*Outcome*	*Intervention*
Patient will achieve optimal hemodynamic status as evidenced by: • MAP >70 mm Hg • Normal hemodynamic parameters • Free from dysrhythmias • Optimal hydration • Adequate perfusion to vital organs	Monitor and treat hemodynamic parameters: • BP • CO/CI • PA pressures • PCWP • CVP • SVR/PVR • $S\dot{v}O_2$ Note especially increases in pulmonary vascular resistance, widening of the PA diastolic and PCWP gradient, and changes in $S\bar{v}O_2$ (may be normal to elevated in sepsis, low in oxygen transport disturbances). Monitor lab values: electrolytes, ABG, CBC with differential, platelets, factor VIII, antithrombin III and DIC profile (PT, PTT, thrombin time, fibrinogen level, FDP). Monitor and treat dysrhythmias.	Patient will maintain optimal hemodynamic status.	Same as stabilization phase. Monitor and treat hemodynamic values. Maintain optimal fluid therapy based on cardiopulmonary assessment.	Patient will maintain optimal hemodynamic status.	Same as in other phases. Teach patient/family home medication regimen, signs/symptoms of fluid overload, and what to report to physician.

	Intervention				
	Monitor and treat predisposing clinical conditions commonly associated with and/or complications of ARDS: sepsis, systemic inflammatory response syndrome [SIRS], shock, trauma, drug overdose, pneumonias, multiple blood transfusions, anemia, thrombocytopenia, DIC, embolism (fat, amniotic fluid, thrombotic, or air), hemorrhagic pancreatitis, cardiopulmonary bypass, burns/smoke inhalation, or toxemia in pregnancy. Monitor and treat complications of ARDS such as right-sided heart failure occurring from excessive PA pressures, resulting in decreased left ventricular filling, CO, and BP. Administer fluid therapy to maintain adequate cardiac performance (i.e., lowest possible PCWP consistent with adequate CO and perfusion to vital organs). Other complications of ARDS include renal failure, fluid retention, gastrointestinal bleeding, ileus, liver failure, and neurologic/endocrine disorders. Administer vasodilators and inotropic agents as indicated and monitor response. Assess weight changes from baseline and weigh daily.				

NUTRITION

Diagnosis/Stabilization Phase		Acute Management Phase		Recovery Phase	
Outcome	*Intervention*	*Outcome*	*Intervention*	*Outcome*	*Intervention*
Patient will be adequately nourished.	Assess nutritional status. Monitor albumin, prealbumin, total protein, and lymphocyte count. Involve dietician to determine protein/calorie needs. Anticipate increased protein/calorie needs without excessive carbohydrates. (In undernourished patients, pulmonary defense mechanisms become impaired, including an altered ventilatory response to hypoxemia). Initiate diet as tolerated and monitor response (NPO, enteral feedings, or parenteral nutrition).	Patient will be adequately nourished.	Same as other phases. Continue diet as tolerated and monitor response.	Patient will be adequately nourished.	Same as other phases. Teach patient/family: • Food pyramid and suggested servings per day • Daily caloric intake needed • Safe weight reduction or weight gaining techniques as indicated

Care Guide continued on following page

ADULT RESPIRATORY DISTRESS SYNDROME MULTIDISCIPLINARY CARE GUIDE *continued*

MOBILITY

Diagnosis/Stabilization Phase		Acute Management Phase		Recovery Phase	
Outcome	***Intervention***	***Outcome***	***Intervention***	***Outcome***	***Intervention***
Patient will achieve optimal mobility.	Assess degree of mobility, flexibility, strength, and tone of muscles. Begin passive/active-assist range of motion exercises.	Patient will achieve optimal mobility.	Same as in stabilization phase. Involve physical therapy as indicated. Monitor response to increased activity; decrease activity if adverse events occur (tachycardia, discomfort, dyspnea, or hypotension). Provide support as necessary. Space activities to allow adequate rest periods. Allow patient to assist in activities of daily living as tolerated.	Patient will achieve optimal mobility.	Same as in other phases. Teach patient/family home exercise program.

OXYGENATION/VENTILATION

Diagnosis/Stabilization Phase		Acute Management Phase		Recovery Phase	
Outcome	***Intervention***	***Outcome***	***Intervention***	***Outcome***	***Intervention***
Patient will have adequate ventilation, gas exchange, and adequate tissue perfusion as evidenced by: • ABGs, pulse oximetry, vital signs WNL for the patient • Respiratory rate, depth, and rhythm WNL for the patient • Normal intrapulmonary shunting • Urine output >0.5 mL/kg/hr • Normal liver enzymes • Mental status normal	Constantly monitor respiratory rate, depth, pattern, pulse oximetry, ABGs, lung sounds, and chest x-ray. Be prepared for intubation and mechanical ventilation. Assist with monitoring and adjusting of ventilator settings to maintain appropriate level of assistance and minute ventilation. Monitor peak airway pressures and pulmonary compliance to assess patient's progress. Monitor patient for signs/symptoms of altered gas exchange: dyspnea, increased work of breathing, restlessness, confusion, tachypnea, apprehension, headache, central cyanosis (not peripheral), refractory hypoxemia (Pa_{O_2} <60 mm Hg with an F_{IO_2} >.50), Pa_{O_2}/PA_{O_2} ratio <.40 $\dot{Q}s/\dot{Q}_T$ >20%, P_{CO_2} >50 mm Hg, Sa_{O_2} <.90, use of accessory muscles, dysrhythmias, or hypotension.	Patient will have adequate ventilation, gas exchange, and tissue perfusion.	Same as in stabilization phase. Continue to monitor patient's response to mechanical ventilation. Assess readiness to wean: 1. Measure respiratory mechanics: • Minute ventilation ($\dot{V}_E$) • Negative inspiratory force • Respiratory rate • Tidal volume (V_T) • Vital capacity (VC) 2. Assess hemodynamic stability and factors that increase metabolic demand: • Fever • Increased white blood cell count • Bacteremia • Sepsis or SIRS • Thyroid dysfunction 3. Monitor electrolytes (including Ca^{++}, Mg^{++}, PO_4^{3-}) 4. Assess for improvement in breath sounds.	Patient will have adequate ventilation, gas exchange, and tissue perfusion.	Same as in other phases. Continue patient/family teaching as in acute management phase; assess understanding and reinforce as needed. Teach patient home medications, signs and symptoms of respiratory distress, when to contact physician, and how to avoid respiratory infections. Refer to outpatient pulmonary rehabilitation program when indicated.

Assess intrapulmonary shunting by one of the following:

- Classical shunt equation
- Pa_{O_2}/PA_{O_2} ratio
- Pa_{O_2}/FI_{O_2} ratio

Administer oxygen therapy as ordered when intrapulmonary shunt present. Utilize lowest FI_{O_2} to attain adequate arterial blood oxygen content level. Assist in determining optimal level of PEEP and monitor response (improve $\dot{V}/\dot{Q}$ matching yet not compromise alveolar expansion and/or CO). Assess hemodynamic parameters with any change in PEEP therapy.

Consider use of continuous lateral rotational therapy if severe intrapulmonary shunt present ($\dot{Q}s/\dot{Q}T$ >30% and/or Pa_{O_2}/PA_{O_2} ratio <.25).

Optimize O_2 delivery by monitoring and treating CO, BP, heart rate, Sa_{O_2}, $S\bar{v}_{O_2}$, hemoglobin, Pa_{O_2}, D_{O_2}, $\dot{V}_{O_2}$, and O_2 extraction ratio.

Assess for adequate tissue perfusion in all organ systems (normal BP, LOC, urine output, liver enzymes).

Monitor and treat complications of ARDS that can affect oxygenation/ventilation: bronchoconstriction, interstitial edema, decreased pulmonary compliance, atelectasis, dysrhythmias, pulmonary microemboli, barotrauma (pneumomediastinum, pneumothorax, subcutaneous emphysema), decreased CO, increased PVR, oxygen toxicity, or pulmonary fibrosis.

Monitor chest x-ray closely (diffuse bilateral interstitial and alveolar infiltrates seen early and later fibrotic changes seen).

Administer medications as ordered: antibiotics, nonsteroidal antiinflammatory agents (inhibit thromboxane production), prostacyclin or PGE_1 (oppose thromboxane action).

Monitor ventilatory/oxygenation status and hemodynamic variables before, during, and after weaning patient from mechanical ventilation.

Assist with extubating patient from mechanical ventilation.

Wean O_2 therapy as gas exchange improves.

Consider positioning of patient to enhance gas exchange (i.e., good lung dependent if unilateral lung disease or prone position if bilateral lung involvement).

Begin teaching on the pulmonary system, current pulmonary problems, current treatment, and expected clinical course.

Care Guide continued on following page

ADULT RESPIRATORY DISTRESS SYNDROME MULTIDISCIPLINARY CARE GUIDE *continued*

COMFORT

Diagnosis/Stabilization Phase		Acute Management Phase		Recovery Phase	
Outcome	*Intervention*	*Outcome*	*Intervention*	*Outcome*	*Intervention*
Patient will be as relaxed and pain free as possible as evidenced by: • No objective indicators of discomfort • No complaints of discomfort	Plan interventions to provide optimal rest periods. Assess quantity and quality of discomfort. Provide reassurance in a calm, caring, and competent manner. Keep lights dim and maintain a quiet environment to minimize catecholamine responses. While patient is intubated, establish effective communication technique so patient can communicate. Observe for complications of ARDS that can cause discomfort (dyspnea, breathlessness, bronchospasm). Implement nursing measures to decrease pain, anxiety, and shivering related to fever.	Patient will be as comfortable as possible.	Teach patient relaxation techniques. Use complementary therapies such as guided imagery, music, humor or body massage to enhance patient's comfort. Involve family in strategies.	Patient will be as comfortable as possible.	Patient will demonstrate relaxation techniques to use at home.

SKIN INTEGRITY

Diagnosis/Stabilization Phase		Acute Management Phase		Recovery Phase	
Outcome	*Intervention*	*Outcome*	*Intervention*	*Outcome*	*Intervention*
Patient will have intact skin without abrasions or pressure ulcers.	Assess all bony prominences q4h. Use preventive pressure-reducing devices when patients are at high risk for development of pressure ulcers (based on scoring tool such as Gosnell). Treat pressure ulcers according to hospital protocol.	Patient will have intact skin without abrasions or pressure ulcers.	Same as Stabilization Phase.	Patient will have intact skin without abrasions or pressure ulcers.	Teach patient/family proper skin care after discharge.

PROTECTION/SAFETY

Diagnosis/Stabilization Phase		Acute Management Phase		Recovery Phase	
Outcome	*Intervention*	*Outcome*	*Intervention*	*Outcome*	*Intervention*
Patient will be protected from possible harm.	Assess need for assistance with activities. Provide physical support as needed. Assess need for restraints if patient is untubated, has a decreased LOC, or is agitated and restless. Explain need for restraints to patient/family. Assess response to restraints when used and check q1h for skin integrity and impairment to circulation. Follow hospital protocol for use of restraints. Provide sedatives as needed and monitor response, especially to respiratory system. Monitor pulmonary effects of PEEP and high FIO_2 therapy closely to minimize further pulmonary insults. Monitor peak airway pressures and make ventilatory adjustments to minimize risk of barotrauma.	Patient will be protected from possible harm.	If need still exists for restraints, check q1–2h for skin integrity and impairment to circulation. Provide support when activity increases. Monitor response to activity.	Patient will be protected from possible harm.	Review with patient/family any physical limitations in activity before discharge home. Consult physical therapist or occupational therapist for home follow-up if limitations present.

PSYCHOSOCIAL/SELF-DETERMINATION

Diagnosis/Stabilization Phase		Acute Management Phase		Recovery Phase	
Outcome	*Intervention*	*Outcome*	*Intervention*	*Outcome*	*Intervention*
Patient will achieve psychophysiologic stability. Patient will demonstrate a decrease in anxiety as evidenced by: • Vital signs WNL for the patient • Subjective report of decreased anxiety • Objective report of decreased anxiety	Assess physiologic effects of critical care environment on patient (i.e., hemodynamic variables, psychological status, signs of increased sympathetic response). Assess patient for appropriate level of stress. Assess personal responses (affective and/or feelings) of patient/family regarding critical illness. Take measures to reduce sensory overload. When patient is intubated, develop effective communication techniques. If unresponsive, use tactile and verbal stimuli. Use calm, caring, competent, and reassuring approach with patient/family.	Patient will achieve psychophysiologic stability. Patient will demonstrate a decrease in anxiety as evidenced by: • Vital signs WNL for the patient • Subjective report of decreased anxiety • Objective report of decreased anxiety	Same as stabilization phase.	Patient will achieve psychophysiologic stability. Patient will demonstrate a decrease in anxiety as evidenced by: • Vital signs WNL for the patient • Subjective report of decreased anxiety • Objective report of decreased anxiety	Same as stabilization phase.

Care Guide continued on following page

ADULT RESPIRATORY DISTRESS SYNDROME MULTIDISCIPLINARY CARE GUIDE *continued*

PSYCHOSOCIAL/SELF-DETERMINATION *continued*

Diagnosis/Stabilization Phase		Acute Management Phase		Recovery Phase	
Outcome	*Intervention*	*Outcome*	*Intervention*	*Outcome*	*Intervention*
	Allow flexible visiting to meet the needs of the patient and family. Administer anxiolytics if indicated and monitor response. Involve patient/family care partner in health care decisions. Determine coping ability of patient/family and take measures to help patient cope (allow verbalization of concerns and fears, provide frequent explanations, hold family conferences, consult support services, etc.).				

DIAGNOSTICS

Diagnosis/Stabilization Phase		Acute Management Phase		Recovery Phase	
Outcome	*Intervention*	*Outcome*	*Intervention*	*Outcome*	*Intervention*
Patient/family will understand any tests or procedures that need to be completed (vital signs, intake and output, hemodynamic monitoring, x-rays, lab work, ABGs, electrocardiogram, cardiac monitoring, mechanical ventilation, PEEP therapy, pulse oximetry).	Explain all procedures and tests to patient/family. Be sensitive to individualized needs of patient/family for information.	Patient/family will understand any tests or procedures that must be completed.	Explain procedures and tests necessary to assess progress and recovery of ARDS to patient/family. Anticipate need for further procedures such as ECMO, extracorporeal carbon dioxide removal, IVOX.	Patient/family will understand meaning of diagnostic tests in relation to continued health.	Review with patient and family results of tests prior to discharge (such as ABGs, pulmonary function). Discuss any abnormal findings and appropriate measures patient/family can take to return to normal, if possible. Provide patient/family with written guidelines concerning follow-up care and/or home care (i.e., when to call the physician, physical restrictions, skin care, medications).

REFERENCE

Burns, S. M., Burns, J. E., & Truwit, J. D. (1994). Comparison of five clinical weaning indices. *American Journal of Critical Care, 3*, 342–352.

Care of the Chronic Mechanically Ventilated Patient

Donna J. Wilson

The management of critically ill patients requiring mechanical ventilation for prolonged periods creates many challenges for nurses and other health care providers. Such challenges are related to the repeated weaning trials and common respiratory complications associated with prolonged mechanical ventilation. This chapter focuses on the care of the chronically ventilated patient and includes a review of the causes of respiratory decompensation, approaches to weaning, assessment criteria for weaning, weaning methods, causes of weaning failure, and airway management.

RESPIRATORY DECOMPENSATION

Clinical Signs and Symptoms

It is vital that the critical care nurse, when caring for patients with ventilator failure, is able to recognize early signs of change in respiratory status. Patient assessment and review of physiologic data should be performed throughout the shift. Abnormal findings or significant changes must be evaluated for cause and treated accordingly. There are times when early and often subtle changes in the patient's physical status are recognized and successfully managed, thus preventing a serious complication.

Simple assessment of the patient's breath sounds and breathing pattern can provide the nurse with important information. Discoordinated breathing patterns, including excessive use of the accessory muscles with an increased respiratory rate and a decrease in tidal volume, are indicative of excessive ventilatory workload. This increased workload may be due to many factors, including diaphragmatic fatigue. The following examples illustrate common presentations. In a patient with a lobar pneumonia, the consolidated lung is dull to percussion, breath sounds are decreased or bronchial in nature, and crackles are heard on inspiration. In the asthmatic patient, the hyperinflated lung produces a hyperresonant note with percussion, wheezes are audible, chest wall excursion decreases, and use of accessory muscles is increased. A patient presenting with a tension pneumothorax would exhibit absent breath sounds and hyperresonant sound on percussion over the affected hemithorax, with the potential for trachea shift. Implications of these findings are discussed in the following sections.

Etiology

VENTILATOR MALFUNCTION

Mechanical ventilators are complex machines. Patients are dependent on ventilators to ensure adequate oxygenation and ventilation. Small changes in the delivered tidal volume, respiratory rate, or flow rate can cause major physiologic changes in patients. Ventilator malfunction can be a cause of significant morbidity in any ventilator-assisted patient (Abramson et al., 1980; Feeley & Bancroft, 1982). Malfunctions result from both equipment failure and human error.

Feeley and Bancroft (1982) reviewed 280 incident reports involving equipment problems. The majority were due to disconnection or leaks in the breathing circuits, dysfunction of the exhalation valves, electrical problems, or failure of different components of the ventilator. Failures commonly occur in the ventilator's compressor, control switch, or alarm system. Abramson and colleagues (1980) reviewed incident reports involving 57 patients treated in an intensive care unit (ICU). In these patient incidents, 34 were directly related to equipment problems and 23 were due to human error. The human error–related ventilator malfunctions were inappropriate assembly of the patient's breathing circuit, respiratory parameters not set correctly, deactivated alarms, and failure to restore power after a procedure such as suctioning. Although dependable equipment with excellent alarm systems is available, this does not replace careful monitoring by the nurse or respiratory therapist. Standardization procedures and education of the health care team concerning equipment function should minimize human error.

PNEUMOTHORAX

Patients receiving positive-pressure ventilation are at risk for pneumothorax. Gas accumulates in the pleural space from a communication between the pleural space and the atmosphere or between the pleural space and the lung. In the latter circumstance, the lung may be partially or completely collapsed as pressure exceeds atmospheric pressure. This situation frequently results in acute cardiopulmonary decompensation.

The incidence of pneumothorax in patients receiving positive-pressure ventilation had been reported as 2% to 15% (Gammon et al., 1992; Petersen & Baier, 1983; Pierson et al., 1986). Pneumothorax is caused by chest trauma, placement of a central venous catheter; thoracentesis, chest tube placement, adult respiratory distress syndrome (ARDS), status asthmaticus, and aspiration pneumonia. In a study of 1700 ventilator patients by Pierson and colleagues (1986), only 39 (2%) had a significant bronchopleural air leak. This occurred most frequently in patients who had experienced chest trauma. The other identified causes did not directly result from mechanical ventilation. In a retrospective review of 139 medical ICU patients, Gammon and colleagues (1992) reported an incidence of pneumothorax in 14% of patients. The incidence of ARDS was 60%. Patients with diagnoses such as neurologic disease and congestive heart failure did not experience this complication.

Patients exposed to high peak airway pressure (PAP) (40 to 50 cm H_2O) and high levels of positive end-expiratory pressure (PEEP) appear to be at increased risk for alveolar rupture. In patients with PAP exceeding 70 cm H_2O, the incidence of pneumothorax was 40% (Haake et al., 1987). Other factors that influence the risk of barotrauma are maximal distending pressures, mean airway pressure, the "mechanical stress of hyperventilation," tissue fragility, secretion retention, surfactant depletion, shear forces, and the duration of mechanical ventilation (Marcy, 1993). Utilization of lower airway pressure, tidal volume, and flow rates may help to keep the incidence of this problem at minimum. Pressure-targeted ventilation (permissive hypercapnia), pressure-controlled ventilation, and extended inspiratory time ventilatory modes may be used to limit barotrauma.

PERSISTENT BRONCHOPLEURAL AIR LEAK

Persistent bronchopleural air leak with positive-pressure ventilation can cause loss of the delivered tidal volume and loss of PEEP through the chest tube. In some cases the goal is to minimize the air leak by changing the ventilator setting and maintaining gas exchange. The ventilator pattern can be changed by using smaller tidal volumes and higher respiratory rates to maintain the same minute ventilation. PEEP should be reduced to the lowest possible level, and expiratory retard should not be used. Pressure support ventilation may be used to provide a lower airway pressure throughout the inspiratory phase. If the patient's spontaneous respiratory pattern interferes with this goal, sedation should be used. These changes are made to try to lower the intrathoracic pressures and decrease the air leak. Other approaches to treatment reported in the literature include use of high-frequency ventilation, independent lung ventilation using two mechanical ventilators through a double-lumen endotracheal tube, application of PEEP through the chest tube, and surgical repair (Downs & Chapman, 1976; Rafferty et al., 1980; Sjostrand, 1980). However, none of these methods have proven to be consistently successful.

BRONCHOSPASM

If respiratory distress caused by bronchospasm is suspected, treatment with bronchodilators is generally used. However, if no relief is observed (decrease in respiratory rate, decrease in inspiratory work of breathing), other causes of airway obstruction must be considered. The presence of secretions, airway collapse from poorly supported airways, a foreign body in the airway, or other airway pathology are possible sources.

PATIENT OR VENTILATOR ASYNCHRONY

Another cause of respiratory distress is the patient breathing out of synchrony with the ventilator. When out of phase with the ventilator, the patient is often exhaling while the machine is delivering a breath. This causes an increase in the peak inspiratory pressure, which often exceeds the pressure limit set on the machine. This triggers the pressure alarm. Increasing the delivered minute ventilation by increasing the tidal volume and/or the respiratory rate may gain control of the patient's respirations. If the patient's respiratory status does not change after tracheal suctioning and/or a bronchodilator nebulizer treatment, sedation may be indicated.

Asynchronous movement of the thorax and abdomen during weaning from mechanical ventilation is an indicator of distress and reflects an increased respiratory load (Tobin et al., 1987). This breathing pattern is commonly observed in a patient being weaned from mechanical ventilation. If this pattern continues for a prolonged period, respiratory muscle fatigue may occur, the clinical signs of which are dyspnea, tachypnea, decreased tidal volume, oscillation in blood pressure and tachycardia, agitation, diaphoresis, and ultimately, an elevated Pa_{CO_2} arterial carbon dioxide level (Burns, 1991). Other causes that may potentiate respiratory muscle fatigue are hypoxemia, anemia, poor nutritional status, hypophosphatemia, and reduced cardiac output.

If these causes for respiratory decompensation have been ruled out, systemic abnormalities should be

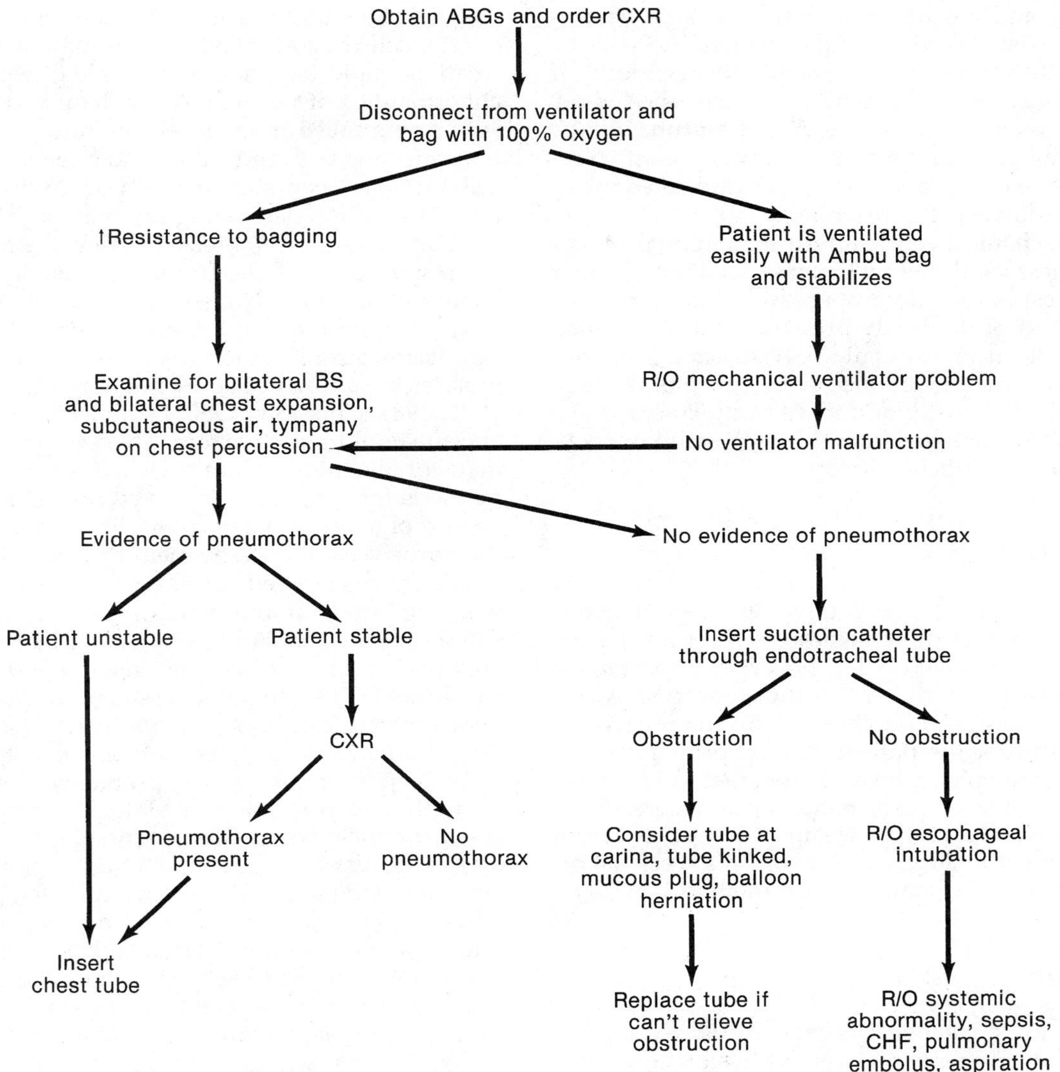

FIGURE 33–1. Approach to the patient who decompensates on a mechanical ventilator. ABGs, arterial blood gases; CXR, chest x-ray; BS, breath sounds; R/O, rule out; CHF, congestive heart failure. (From Hotchkiss, R. S., & Wilson, R. S. [1983]. *Surgical Clinics of North America, 63,* 417–438.)

suspected. These possibilities include sepsis, congestive heart failure, pulmonary embolus, and aspiration.

If respiratory difficulty is suspected, the patient should be disconnected from the ventilator and manually ventilated with 100% oxygen. Troubleshooting the cause of the respiratory difficulty can then be accomplished (Fig. 33–1). If the patient can be manually ventilated with ease, a mechanical ventilator problem should be suspected. An air leak in the system is suspected if the peak airway pressures are noted to be lower than prior recorded values. Other causes of respiratory distress include difficulty in triggering the machine on inspiration, insufficient or excessive volume, or an inspiratory phase that is either too long or too short. The mechanical ventilator should be checked so that the sensitivity will not register a negative pressure of greater than 2.0 cm H_2O just before the beginning of inspiration. If the inspiratory phase is too long or too short, the flow rates should be checked and adjusted (flow rate is decreased if inspiration is too short; flow rate is increased if too long). If the patient complains of difficulty exhaling, the inspiratory/expiratory (I/E) ratio should be evaluated and modified accordingly. To increase the expiratory time, the flow rate should be increased. Once the problem has been corrected, the patient can be safely placed back on the ventilator.

If increased resistance to manual ventilation is noted, the chest should be examined for bilateral breath sounds and chest expansion. If either is abnormal, a pneumothorax should be suspected. Other signs of a pneumothorax include tachypnea, tachycardia, chest pain (side of pneumothorax), tympanic sounds on percussion, tracheal deviation (away from the affected side), and subcutaneous emphysema. If a pneumothorax exists, cardiovascular instability will be present with hypoxemia and respiratory acidosis. If any of these signs are present, a portable chest x-ray should be obtained immediately. A chest tube will be required if a significant pneumothorax is present. Needle or catheter decompression is often indicated if dictated by cardiovascular instability.

If the mechanical ventilator is functioning properly and the chest x-ray shows no pneumothorax, other causes of respiratory decompensation that can cause an increase in peak airway pressure should be ruled out. The artificial airway could be obstructed from mucus plugging or malpositioned with the tip of the tube obstructed by the posterior tracheal wall. Tracheal suctioning is performed to eliminate any possibility of obstruction of the artificial airway.

WEANING

Weaning from mechanical ventilation to spontaneous breathing is often a difficult process for both the patient and staff (Knebel et al., 1994). It is important to realize that weaning is often a complex process, which is time-consuming and psychologically and physiologically stressful for the patient, family, primary nurse, respiratory therapist, physical therapist, and physician. Consistency of care, patience, and persistence will make a difference. The weaning of a patient from chronic ventilator support is usually a very labor-intensive process no matter which method is used.

Evaluation

The ability to be weaned is governed by several factors, including the patient's overall physical condition, respiratory assessment, and psychological state (Burns et al., 1994; Morganroth et al., 1984; Nett et al., 1987). The evaluation process should be performed systematically. No single parameter successfully predicts the patient's ability to wean. During the preweaning phase, information is collected. Weaning is considered when the following conditions are optimized.

The initial pulmonary pathology that necessitated intubation and mechanical ventilation should be resolving (Kersten, 1989). Cardiovascular function should be stable, with a regular heart rate and rhythm and minimal need for vasopressors. Fluid balance is especially important when weaning patients with limited cardiac function; thus, daily weights and strict intake and output should be monitored.

An increased metabolic demand secondary to fever, burns, shivering, pain, agitation, trauma, sepsis, and overfeeding will increase oxygen (O_2) consumption, carbon dioxide (CO_2) production, and the patient's minute ventilation (Marini, 1986). As the patient increases his demand for ventilation, there will be an increased workload on the respiratory muscles; therefore, the weaning process should be temporarily on hold and re-evaluated daily.

The patient's nutritional state should not be overlooked (Majors, 1988). When malnutrition exists, weaning could be hindered because of weakness and abnormalities of pulmonary mechanics. Malnutrition is a leading cause of impaired respiratory muscle function, affecting both endurance and strength (Rochester, 1984). It has been shown that poor nutrition causes muscle wasting, decreasing the mass and strength of the diaphragm and thereby limiting the capability of the respiratory muscle. If muscle wasting exists with abnormalities in nitrogen balance, albumin, phosphate, magnesium, and calcium levels, there will be significant atrophy and weakness of the respiratory muscles, resulting in poor ventilatory effort (Askanazi et al., 1981; Chernow, 1982; Dougherty, 1988). The dietician should be actively involved to provide an estimate of the patient's caloric needs and to suggest methods for achieving improved nutritional support.

A tool to assist the nurse in the weaning process is the Burns Weaning Assessment Program (Burns et al., 1994). This useful bedside checklist helps evaluate the weaning potential and assess if the weaning process should begin. The 26 physiologic variables in the list are divided into two sections, general and respiratory assessment. The general assessment evaluates the patient's overall condition, such as cardiovascular function, fluid and electrolytes, nutritional state, pain control, sleep patterns, bowel problems, general body strength, and psychological state. The respiratory assessment includes evaluation of gas flow, work of breathing, airway clearance, strength, endurance, and arterial blood gases (ABGs). Overall, each physiologic variable is assessed as a "yes," meeting the criteria; "no," not meeting the criteria; and as "not assessed." The number of "yes" answers is divided by the total number of factors ($n = 26$) for the final score. Burns has reported that a score of 65% may indicate that the patient is not ready to wean from mechanical ventilation (Burns et al., 1994). This tool is an excellent way to follow the overall status of the patient and directs the care plan to improve the variables limiting the weaning progress.

Respiratory Parameters

A variety of respiratory parameters and pulmonary tests are available to assess the patient's ability to wean from mechanical ventilation. These parameters should be used as an assessment or guide in the weaning process. None of these parameters have been predictive indicators of successful weaning from mechanical ventilation (Burns et al., 1995). Therefore, it is suggested that these parameters be measured throughout the weaning process and be used as a guide in conjunction with the patient's overall clinical status. This assessment can be divided into three categories: oxygenation, ventilation, and mechanical function (Fitzgerald & Huber, 1976; Sahn & Lakshminarayan, 1973). The arterial oxygen tension during mechanical ventilation should usually be greater than 70 mm Hg with a fraction of inspired oxygen (FIO_2) of 40% and the alveolar-arterial difference in partial pressure of oxygen ($P_{AO_2} - P_{aO_2}$) less than 300 mm Hg. The above condition should exist with a level of PEEP less than 10 cm H_2O. When PEEP is greater than 10 cm H_2O, weaning is usually contraindicated.

The next aspect to be assessed is the patient's ventilation requirement. The necessary level of minute ventilation (tidal volume × respiratory rate) is determined by both CO_2 production and dead space ventilation. The dead space to tidal volume ratio ($\dot{V}_D/\dot{V}_T$) defines that percentage of the tidal volume that does not participate in CO_2 elimination and can be considered wasted ventilation. This dead space ratio is increased in diseases that affect the lung parenchyma and the distribution of gas flow (i.e., ARDS, pulmonary embolism, chronic obstructive pulmonary disease [COPD], and hypovolemia) (Marini, 1986). If the $\dot{V}_D/\dot{V}_T$ is above 0.60 (i.e., 60% of tidal volume), the minute volume required to maintain adequate CO_2 elimination is frequently too great to permit total weaning (Skillman et al., 1971). Thus it is not surprising that a useful estimate of weaning ability is the resting minute ventilation required during mechanical ventilation. Sahn and Lakshminarayan (1973) have shown that a minute ventilation of 10 L/min or less during mechanical ventilation usually indicates that a patient can be safely weaned.

An important relationship exists between $\dot{V}_D/\dot{V}_T$, minute ventilation, and CO_2 production. An increased $\dot{V}_D/\dot{V}_T$ and/or increased CO_2 production will require increased minute ventilation. The CO_2 is elevated with fever, shivering, pain, and sepsis, and with overfeeding or a high-carbohydrate diet. Under such circumstances, weaning may be difficult to accomplish because of the potential need for unusually high respiratory rate and large tidal volumes.

The patient's mechanical function may be assessed by vital capacity, inspiratory force, and the spontaneous respiratory rate. The vital capacity is the maximum volume of gas that can be exhaled after maximal inspiration and serves as an index of ventilatory reserve. The vital capacity should usually be 10 to 15 mL/kg of actual body weight to institute weaning. Inspiratory force (the amount of negative pressure generated against an occluded airway) is used as a measurement of muscle strength. Weaning can be instituted when the inspiratory force is −20 cm H_2O. This measurement has an advantage in that it does not require patient cooperation and can be used in the unresponsive and uncooperative patient. The minute ventilation, vital capacity, and inspiratory force are the easiest bedside parameters to monitor and are important indicators of weaning ability and progress. The respiratory rate generally should not exceed 35 breaths/min because rates greater than this commonly result in fatigue, CO_2 retention, and respiratory acidosis (Morganroth et al., 1984).

Psychological Readiness

The patient must be psychologically prepared to wean. Patient anxiety can stem from fear of ventilator malfunction or of suffocation, and from loss of control (powerlessness). To reduce the patient's fear of ventilator failure, the nurse should explain the safety mechanisms of the ventilator such as alarms, keep the manual resuscitator in the patient's view, and give verbal reassurance that the ventilator is functioning properly. The respiratory therapist should announce to the patient when the ventilator is being checked and explain what changes are being made.

The fear of suffocation and breathlessness is often real. This is frequently related to the weaning process. Monitoring oxygen saturation will provide assurance to the patient that oxygen levels stay within a "safe" range.

The chronic ventilator-dependent patient feels a loss of control. This patient has to rely on others for most care because of his decreased strength and lack of energy. Providing opportunities for the patient to make decisions and keeping the patient informed about his condition may result in a decreased anxiety level. Loss of control over basic activities may cause the patient to develop powerlessness, which may progress to hopelessness (Truesdell, 1992).

Several aspects of treatment on a mechanical ventilator are anxiety-provoking and frustrating for the patient. One major component of this is the patient's impaired ability to communicate. Several communication modalities are available for the mechanically ventilated patient. These include eye signals, lip reading, palm writing, pen and paper, magic slate, alphabet board, flash cards, deflating tracheostomy cuff, talking tracheostomy tubes, Passy-Muir speaking valves, and the use of computers. Encourage the patient to use the least frustrating mode. Remember that whereas weaning is recognized as a sign of improvement for some ventilated patients, for others with chronic respiratory disease it signals a return to ever-increasing respiratory work.

An important aspect in successful weaning is the patient's trust in the staff responsible for his care. The staff should have a consistent approach throughout the weaning process. If there is disagreement among the medical and nursing team and inconsistent information is presented to the patient, the patient becomes distrustful. Repeated explanations help minimize the occurrence of misinterpretation.

Methods of Weaning

Currently, the methods of weaning from mechanical ventilation are the T piece, continuous positive airway pressure (CPAP), synchronized intermittent mandatory ventilation (SIMV), and pressure support ventilation (PSV) (Bendixen et al., 1965; Downs et al., 1973; Sporn & Morganroth, 1988). Each of these techniques can be used alone or in combination with one another.

T PIECE AND CONTINUOUS POSITIVE AIRWAY PRESSURE

The T-piece technique is an accepted and time-honored method that is often modified by application of

CPAP. The patient is placed on a T piece or CPAP system for a specific time and is allowed to breathe spontaneously. CPAP may be used to improve the functional residual capacity and thus improve arterial oxygenation and lung volume. Initially, the weaning begins with short intervals, such as 10 minutes every 1 to 2 hours. As the weaning time increases to 1-hour intervals or longer, the patient often requires a rest period on SIMV for 1 or more hours. Increasing the length of each period of weaning time allows increased respiratory muscle strength and endurance to maintain spontaneous respiration. Thus, monitoring of the patient's vital signs, respiratory pattern of breathing, and pulse oximetry are of utmost value. The first sign of respiratory muscle fatigue is a respiratory rate of 35 breaths/min. The patient's spontaneous tidal volume, vital capacity, minute ventilation, and inspiratory force are measured and recorded. Weaning should not be attempted during the night until the patient can maintain spontaneous ventilation throughout most of the day.

SYNCHRONIZED INTERMITTENT MANDATORY VENTILATION WEANING

Synchronized intermittent mandatory ventilation is a technique by which patients can breathe spontaneously and in addition receive mechanically ventilated breaths at specific, preselected rates (Downs et al., 1973; Feeley & Hedley-Whyte, 1975). This weaning process is achieved by decreasing the number of mechanically delivered breaths. The patient assumes a greater proportion of the total minute ventilation. Ventilators are equipped with a control sensitive enough to regulate the respiratory rate of the mechanical ventilator over a wide range of breaths, ranging from 12 breaths/min to a minimum of 1 breath every 2 to 3 minutes. Weaning is accomplished by instituting a gradual decrease in the frequency of ventilator breaths to rates as low as 1 breath/min or 1 breath every 2 minutes.

The SIMV method is popular for several reasons: (1) maintenance of respiratory muscle tone to decrease muscle atrophy, (2) reduction in the need for sedatives and narcotics, (3) possibly improved distribution of ventilation with the combination of spontaneous and mechanical breaths, (4) initiation of weaning earlier in the course of the disease, (5) less cardiovascular disturbance, and (6) less time needed for direct observation by nurse, therapist, or physician (Luce et al., 1981). The SIMV method is valid when patients are receiving four SIMV breaths or greater, but at the lower SIMV rate, four or less per minute, the patient requires close observation of vital signs and respiratory pattern. This is when the patient assumes most of his total minute volume; at these lower SIMV rates patients fail because of fatigue, increased work of breathing, or other factors, including fever, atelectasis, or poor nutritional state. These problems often are evident when the patient is performing the bulk of total minute ventilation. As this weaning process proceeds with continued reduction in the number of mechanical breaths, ABGs and spontaneous respiratory parameters (tidal volume, vital capacity, inspiratory force) should be measured and recorded every 4 hours. Any significant or adverse trend in vital signs should be noted. If no difficulty is observed, the SIMV rate is decreased until the patient can support his total minute ventilation. Most patients who require short-term mechanical ventilation after major surgery and anesthesia are suitable for SIMV techniques.

PRESSURE SUPPORT VENTILATION

Pressure support ventilation or inspiratory assist is a ventilatory assist technique applied during patient-initiated, ventilator-supported breaths (Kacmarek, 1989). As the patient activates the ventilator demand system, a selected amount of positive airway pressure augments the spontaneous ventilatory effort. The inspiratory phase is terminated when inspiratory flow falls below a predetermined level. This technique allows patients to control their respiratory rate, tidal volume, and inspiratory time. Pressure support can be applied during the spontaneous breaths with the SIMV and CPAP modes.

Pressure support appears to counteract the work of breathing imposed by artificial airways, the ventilator circuit, and the demand system. It has been shown to decrease the inspiratory work of breathing, thereby reducing respiratory muscle fatigue. In the chronic ventilator-dependent patient, pressure support is indicated to decrease the imposed work of breathing. Selecting the appropriate level of pressure support depends on the size of the artificial airway, the ventilator system, and the resistance to ventilation. Some have used the level of ventilatory muscle activity as an indicator of optimal support. In general, clinical observation of the patient's respiratory rate, pulse, and level of accessory muscle activity can provide an estimate of pressure support that reduces work of breathing (Brochard et al., 1989). For most patients, pressure support levels of 5 to 20 cm H_2O appear optimal. Low levels of pressure support ventilation (5 to 10 cm H_2O) with SIMV are provided to reduce the high airway resistance of the endotracheal tube (smaller than 8.0 mm I.D.) and decrease the resistance of the demand valve system. Higher levels of pressure support are used to provide a desired tidal volume, minute ventilation, and a decrease in the patient's peak airway pressure. Once a desired pressure support level is achieved with adequate gas exchange, the patient's respiratory rate, tidal volume, and minute ventilation are monitored. When the patient's respiratory rate is less than 25 breaths/min with a normal breathing pattern, the tidal volume is approximately 3 cc or greater per pound of ideal body weight, and the minute ventilation less than 10 L/min, the pressure support can be reduced. If the respiratory rate increases to greater than 30 breaths/min, tidal volume decreases, and/or the minute ventilation increases, the patient is at risk for respiratory muscle fatigue. Other signs of respiratory muscle fatigue are increased use of accessory muscles and asynchronous chest and abdominal movements. Pressure support levels are commonly weaned down slowly at a rate of 2 to 3 cm H_2O at a time.

Patients who have received long-term mechanical ventilation for acute lung disease or an exacerbation of COPD, are often difficult to wean. Several factors contributing to this include poor nutritional state, muscle weakness and atrophy, and patient fear. If the patient's primary problem for failure to wean is respiratory muscle dysfunction, individualize a weaning approach by using concepts from the T-piece, SIMV, and pressure support ventilation weaning techniques. This method is designed like a training program to improve strength and then endurance of respiratory muscle function. The resting SIMV rate should arbitrarily provide 80% of the patient's minute ventilation and the pressure support set to provide a spontaneous tidal volume of 400 to 500 mL. Incorporating the concept from the T-piece wean, the weaning is done four times a day for 30 minutes to 1 hour on an SIMV rate one-half of the resting SIMV rate and maintaining the same pressure support. At the end of each day, the patient is evaluated; if the spontaneous parameters are normal for that patient and not decreased illustrating respiratory muscle fatigue, the next day the weaning SIMV rate is decreased and the pressure support is maintained. Once the patient progresses to CPAP and pressure support ventilation, increase the four 1-hour intervals. The rest of the wean is accomplished in a fashion similar to a T-piece/CPAP wean. If the weaning process is not successful for a particular patient, individualize your approach and use a combination of weaning modes. Remember, there is no rigid approach to weaning.

Assessment During the Weaning Process

Regardless of the weaning technique employed, the health care team should use sound clinical judgment and pay close attention to detail. First, ensure proper position for the optimal conditions. The patient should ideally be in high Fowler's position whenever possible. Weaning should not be undertaken in the supine position except under certain circumstances such as individuals in the Stryker frame. The obese patient should be out of bed if at all possible. If in bed, a reverse Trendelenburg position helps to allow maximum chest expansion. Attention to airway secretions is vital. The patient should be suctioned, if necessary, before and during weaning.

As weaning begins, pulse, blood pressure, respiratory rate, and spontaneous ventilatory parameters (tidal volume, vital capacity, and inspiratory force) should be measured and recorded. During the period of weaning it may be helpful for the nurse to place a hand on the patient's lateral chest wall and provide verbal instruction to inspire and expire at an appropriate rhythm. For the average patient, an inspiratory to expiratory ratio of 1:2 is desirable. For the patient with COPD, a ratio of 1:4 is often more efficient. This instruction will help to facilitate a slow, regular breathing pattern.

Supervision during the weaning process is most important to alleviate the patient's fear and provide emotional support. At the termination of the weaning period, the vital signs, ABGs, and spontaneous parameters should again be measured and recorded. All of these parameters are useful to predict the length of time the patient can spontaneously breathe before stress, fatigue, hypoxemia, hypercapnia, or a major change in vital signs occur. It is mandatory to stop weaning if the patient appears stressed, demonstrated by a respiratory rate greater than 35 breaths/min, a significant increase in heart rate (i.e., increased by 20 beats/min from the resting heart rate), a dramatic increase in the blood pressure (i.e., systolic pressure increased 20% from resting level), diaphoresis, complaint of air hunger, excessive use of accessory muscles, or a discoordinated breathing pattern. When a patient exhibits such stress, manually ventilate with a self-inflating resuscitator bag for several minutes and do not check spontaneous parameters, because this will stress him too much. After the weaning period mechanical ventilation is instituted at a rate and volume to provide adequate rest. At the next scheduled weaning interval, the patient should be reevaluated.

Causes of Failure to Wean

Failure to wean from mechanical ventilation often has multiple causes: intrinsic pulmonary disease, poor nutritional state, respiratory muscle dysfunction or fatigue, cardiac disease, or sepsis (Norton & Neureuter, 1989).

The major causes of failure to wean because of pulmonary disease are extensive atelectasis, consolidation, edema, fibrosis, and bronchospasm from decreased recruitable airspace and increased airway resistance. Therapy consists of PEEP, bronchodilators, and chest physiotherapy. The nurse should auscultate breath sounds; determine rate, rhythm, and depth of respiration; suction; and monitor ABGs with each ventilator change or change in the patient's clinical status (Carroll, 1986; Daly & Allen, 1987).

POOR NUTRITIONAL STATUS

As previously stated, a very important aspect of weaning is the patient's nutritional status. Nutrition should be considered during the acute phase of illness. It is well-documented that starvation and protein loss causes breakdown of muscle mass for gluconeogenesis (Barrocas et al., 1983; Hyman et al., 1982). This results in a decrease in respiratory muscle (intercostal, diaphragm, and abdominal) function, thus decreasing vital capacity and inspiratory force, contributing to the failure to wean. Studies have indicated that 30% to 40% of adults with COPD are undernourished based on body weight, anthropometrics, and estimates of body fat and muscle mass (Wilson, 1985). The inability to maintain adequate nutritional status has been associated with compromises in pulmonary defense mechanisms, structure, and function (Rochester, 1984).

If patients require central intravenous hyperalimentation for nutritional support, one must appreciate problems that can exist with high-glucose diets (Sheldon & Baker, 1980). Askanazi and others (1981) have documented that high glucose load results in glucose being used for lipogenesis rather than as an energy source. Lipogenesis resulting from excess glucose will result in increased CO_2 production. This is demonstrated by measuring the respiratory quotient (RQ; CO_2 production/O_2 consumption). The normal value is 0.8. When glucose is burned alone, the RQ is 1 or greater. When excess glucose is given, it is converted to fat; thus, CO_2 is produced in excess of O_2 consumed. The excess CO_2 produced must be excreted by the lungs at an energy cost for additional respiratory work, increasing tidal volume, and minute ventilation. Thus, in the patient with compromised pulmonary function and marginal reserve, this can be a cause of inability to wean. Therefore, there should be a balance between dietary intake of fats and carbohydrates. When the patient is able to switch to enteral intake, parenteral nutrition should be withdrawn slowly while enteral nutrition is gradually advanced. Small feeding tubes are generally well-tolerated for enteral diets. These liquid diets are lactose-free and contain a balance of fat and carbohydrate calories. Most standard enteral feedings contain 30% fat and 50% carbohydrates.

Patients' tolerance of tube feedings is essential for the provision of adequate nutritional intake. The effects of intolerance to tube feedings can compound any existing deficiencies and defeat the effort to nourish the patient adequately. Complications that are both critical and frequent in ventilator-dependent patients are aspiration pneumonia, gastric retention, diarrhea, abdominal distension, nausea, vomiting, hypophosphatemia, hypokalemia, and hypomagnesemia (Openbrier, 1985). These complications of tube feedings can contribute to patients' failure to wean. The incorporation of fiber into the diet has been documented to help maintain normal bowel function and decrease the incidence of diarrhea and constipation caused by intolerance to low-residue feedings (Kelsay, 1978). Nursing interventions include auscultation of bowel sounds every 4 hours, monitoring calorie count, and assessment of muscle mass, skin integrity, and wound healing.

RESPIRATORY MUSCLE WEAKNESS

The goal of mechanical ventilation should be to preserve and/or increase the functional capacity of the respiratory muscles. However, respiratory muscle weakness or fatigue is often a major cause of failure to wean (Kim, 1984). Weakness and fatigue are often secondary to poor nutrition, asynchronous breathing pattern, abdominal distension, chest trauma, or phrenic palsy. When one or more of these problems are present, spontaneous respiration is not performed in a coordinated pattern. Discoordination of respiratory muscle activity can develop as a result of prolonged mechanical ventilation. A discoordinated breathing pattern may be a sign of respiratory muscle dysfunction. This results in a lack of synchronized function between the intercostal, diaphragm, and abdominal muscles during spontaneous respiration. The chest wall and abdomen appear to move in a rocking motion. On inspiration the lower chest is pulled inward and the upper chest expands; on expiration the inward movement of the abdomen is interrupted by a bounce as the outward flow of air is suddenly expelled. This may vary in severity. These patients appear to be working much harder, moving less air, and are less able to meet the demands for respiratory work than the average weaning patient. The cause is unknown and there is no known effective treatment. It has been shown that as the ability to breathe spontaneously improves, so does coordination of the breathing pattern. If a discoordinated breathing pattern is observed during weaning, patients generally tire easily because of high respiratory rates and small tidal volumes. Ventilation of the lower lobes will be compromised. Thus, during weaning, it is helpful to institute diaphragmatic and lateral basal expansion breathing exercises with manual resistance to the chest wall and abdomen. These exercises emphasize the synchronized motion of respiratory muscles to increase chest wall expansion, thus requiring less work to maintain ventilation. Frequently respiratory muscle power will be slow to improve. Therefore, by evaluating the patient's mechanical breathing function, the nurse will be able to see changes in the strength and endurance of the respiratory muscles. No one element will determine when the patient needs a rest; this is governed by the overall picture.

CARDIAC FAILURE

Cardiac failure is another reason for failure to wean. Positive-pressure ventilation increases intrathoracic pressure, which can be beneficial to a failing ventricle by decreasing the preload. In the weaning process, as the mean intrathoracic and airway pressure are reduced, the central intravascular volume is increased, causing an increase in preload. This may lead to cardiac ischemia and/or congestive heart failure (Clochesy et al., 1995; Hotchkiss & Wilson, 1983; Mathru et al., 1982). During the weaning process one should monitor the clinical indicators (central venous pressure, pulmonary arterial diastolic and wedge pressures, blood pressure) of preload and afterload. If parameters become grossly abnormal, terminate weaning and return the patient to positive-pressure ventilation. Reevaluation of the weaning process is indicated with consideration for specific therapy with diuretics, nitrates, or inotropic support.

Weaning Centers

Around the United States many units are being organized with a multidisciplinary approach to manage the chronic ventilator patient. These units are being organized because of the long length of stay and high cost in ICUs. There are many different names for this type of unit: chronic ventilator-dependent unit, prolonged respiratory care unit, noninvasive respiratory care unit, and the regional weaning center. These units have all reported successful weaning in the majority of cases (Scheinhorn et al., 1994). The number of days on mechanical ventilation before transfer to a weaning unit ranged from 13 to 55 days. The success rate was reflected in the high percentage of patients who weaned from mechanical ventilation. These units have been cost-effective because of the decreased need for nursing care as compared to ICUs. Most importantly, these units are organized with personnel experienced in the management of the chronic ventilator patient, who provide a complete assessment that often reveals the factor limiting the weaning process.

AIRWAY MANAGEMENT

Airway management is an essential part of nursing care of the ventilator-dependent patient. The artificial airway is either an oral or nasal endotracheal tube or a tracheostomy tube. A discussion on the advantages and disadvantages of each airway and the design of standard and specialized airway appliances follows.

Endotracheal intubation or tracheostomy is performed to provide (1) positive-pressure ventilation, (2) protection of the airway from aspiration, (3) removal of tracheobronchial secretions, and (4) relief of airway obstruction. The three approaches that must be considered are oral endotracheal and nasal endotracheal intubation and tracheostomy. The advantages and disadvantages of each approach are summarized in Table 33–1 (Wilson, 1988). The type of tube selected is based on patient assessment, the need for a long-term artificial airway and mechanical ventilation, patient tolerance, and the related advantages and disadvantages of each situation.

Endotracheal Tubes

Oral endotracheal tubes are generally placed in an emergency situation because of the speed and ease of insertion. Patients tolerate oral endotracheal tubes poorly because it stimulates the gag reflex, increases the production of saliva, and increases the difficulty of swallowing compared to nasal endotracheal tubes. Oral hygiene is often difficult to perform because of the taping necessary to hold the tube in place and the use of bite blocks or oral airways to prevent the patient from biting the tube and causing airway obstruction. Maintaining both the proper position of the endotra-

TABLE 33–1. **Advantages and Disadvantages of Various Airway Appliances**

Type	Advantages	Disadvantages
Oral endotracheal tube	Easy to insert Large bore; work of breathing less Shorter length; easier to suction Less acute angle; less likely to kink	Requires laryngoscopy Easily dislodged Poorly tolerated by some patients Patients require more sedation Occluded by patient biting tube Oral hygiene difficult Patient has difficulty swallowing Unable to communicate Lip laceration Difficult to stabilize Inadvertent extubation common Laryngeal pathology
Nasal endotracheal tube	Easily secured Tolerated better by patient Insert blindly when neck motion or visualization is limited Allow for oral hygiene Able to swallow Requires less sedation Communication; mouthing of words	Skilled personnel for placement Nasal passageway limits size of tube Tube kinking due to curvature Inability to drain sinuses; sinusitis Obstruction of eustachian tube; otitis media Nasal soft tissue injury Laryngeal pathology
Tracheostomy tube	Most comfortable Easiest to suction Communication; mouthing words, talking or fenestrated tracheostomy tubes Ability to swallow Reinsertion of trach tube relatively easy with mature stoma *No* laryngeal injury	Surgical procedure Complications postsurgery Bleeding Pneumothorax Subcutaneous emphysema Infection Posterior tracheal wall rupture during insertion False passage in subcutaneous tissue Stenosis, stoma; cuff Granulation tissue formation Innominate artery erosion

From Wilson, D. J. (1988). Airway appliances and management. In R. M. Kacmarek and J. K. Stoller (Eds.), *Current respiratory care.* Toronto: B. C. Decker. By permission of Mosby–Year Book, Inc.

TABLE 33–2. **Tracheostomy Tube Size Chart**

Size	Portex Standard Length	Portex Extra Length	Shiley Single Cannula Length	Shiley Double Cannula Length	Jackson* Stainless Steel Length
6.0 mm ID	67 mm	—	67	—	69
7.0 mm ID (#6)	73 mm	84 mm	80	78	69
8.0 mm ID	78 mm	95 mm	89	—	69
8.5 mm ID (#8)	—	—	—	84	69
9.0 mm ID	84 mm	106 mm	99	—	69
10.0 mm ID (#10)	84 mm	—	105	84	69

*Jackson #7 extra long = 85 mm.

cheal tube and skin integrity is the responsibility of the nurse.

Nasal endotracheal tubes are better tolerated for extended periods of intubation and are far more comfortable for the conscious patient. Patients can swallow more easily and can communicate with lip motion. Nurses can perform mouth care more effectively. Stabilization of the nasal tube is easier; thus, self-extubation and migration of the tube into the mainstem bronchus are less likely. The disadvantages of a nasal endotracheal tube include size limitation of the nasal passageway, tube kinking from the acute curvature of the nasal route, and poor drainage of sinuses causing sinusitis. If a patient complains of an earache or drainage is observed from the nose, otitis media or sinusitis should be suspected. At this time either the nasal endotracheal tube should be removed and replaced with an oral endotracheal tube or a tracheostomy should be considered.

In the patient on long-term mechanical ventilation, a tracheostomy tube is preferred. Although there are no firm guidelines, it is common practice to place a tracheostomy tube 10 to 14 days after oral or nasal endotracheal intubation if an airway appliance is deemed necessary for the foreseeable future (Whited, 1984; Heffner et al., 1986). The decision for tracheostomy must be individualized in any given situation.

Types of Tracheostomy Tubes

Tracheostomy tubes are available in a variety of designs. The design characteristics—composition, neck flange, sizes, length, and cuff design—differ according to the manufacturer. The most common material used is polyvinylchloride. The tube size is printed on the neck flange. These tubes are sized according to the inner and outer diameter of the tube. The most common tube sizes are a number 7.0 mm and 8.0 mm inner diameter (I.D.), a number 6 Shiley equals a number 7.0 mm I.D. tube. The length of tracheostomy tubes differs depending on design and the manufacturer (Table 33–2). There is a relationship between the size and the length of tubes; the smaller the inner diameter of the tube, the shorter the tube. There are extra-long tubes for the obese patient with a classic short "bull" neck. The need for an extra-long tube is determined at the time of surgery or when there is difficulty sealing a tube because of anatomic variation. The Portex extra-length tracheostomy tube has an increased distance from the flange to the bend and then drops fairly vertically. This tube is a single-lumen cannula available in sizes 7.0 mm I.D. to 9.0 mm I.D. The adjustable hyperflex tracheostomy kits by Bivona Medical Technologies, Inc. (Gary, Indiana) have an adjustable flange to vary the length (Fig. 33–2). This tube can accommodate most airways; for example, in a number 7.0 mm I.D. tube the usable length is up to 120 mm, and for the number 8.0 mm I.D. tube the length is increased to 130 mm. The tube shaft style is a hyperflex wire-reinforced silicone that is kink-resistant. This is a single-lumen tube available in adult sizes 6.0 mm I.D. to 9.0 mm I.D. These extra-length tubes are available in two different cuff designs, the aire-cuf mid-range and the tight to shaft. For the patient with an unusual airway problem, Bivona Medical Technologies provides a customized tracheostomy tube service for the pediatric and adult populations.

Tracheostomy tube cuffs are designed to provide high-volume, low-pressure characteristics. Cuffs are

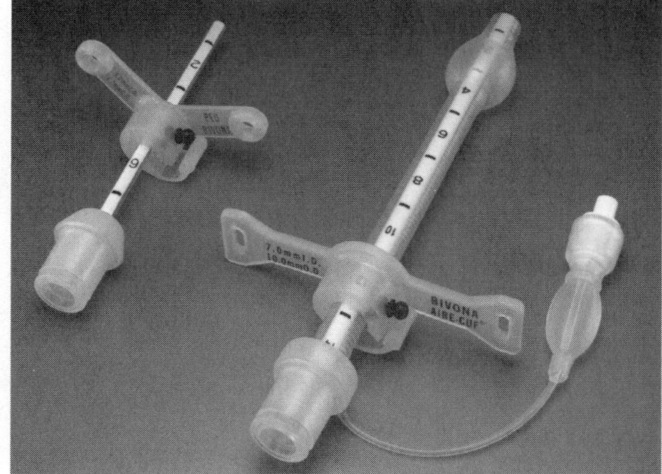

FIGURE 33–2. Adjustable Hyperflex Tracheostomy Tube by Bivona Medical Technologies, Inc.

soft, thin-walled, and compliant to prevent tracheal injury. The large-volume diameter cuff conforms to the shape of the trachea, creating a seal with low lateral tracheal wall pressure.

The two most common cuff inflation techniques are the minimal leak and the minimal occlusive technique (Crabtree-Goodnough, 1988). With the minimal leak technique, the cuff is inflated to adjust for a small air leak audible only at the end of the inspiratory phase with a positive-pressure breath. This technique is recommended to avoid excessive cuff pressures against the trachea while maintaining an adequate seal for positive-pressure ventilation and airway protection. In the minimal occlusive technique, the cuff is inflated so there is no air leak on inspiration. Patients who cannot protect the airway should use the minimal occlusive technique. After reinflation of the cuff, the pressure in the cuff should be measured. The cuff pressure should be maintained at a maximum level of 20 to 30 mm Hg to minimize adverse effects of cuff pressure on blood flow to the tracheal mucosa. The perfusion pressure of tracheal tissue in a normotensive patient has been estimated at approximately 30 mm Hg. Ischemia results whenever the cuff tracheal pressure exceeds the perfusion pressure. The cuff should never be maintained at a volume in excess of that necessary to just prevent a leak from occurring. Maintaining a cuff volume larger than this renders the patient vulnerable to tracheal damage. The lowest possible cuff pressure and cuff volume should be maintained to prevent tracheal injury.

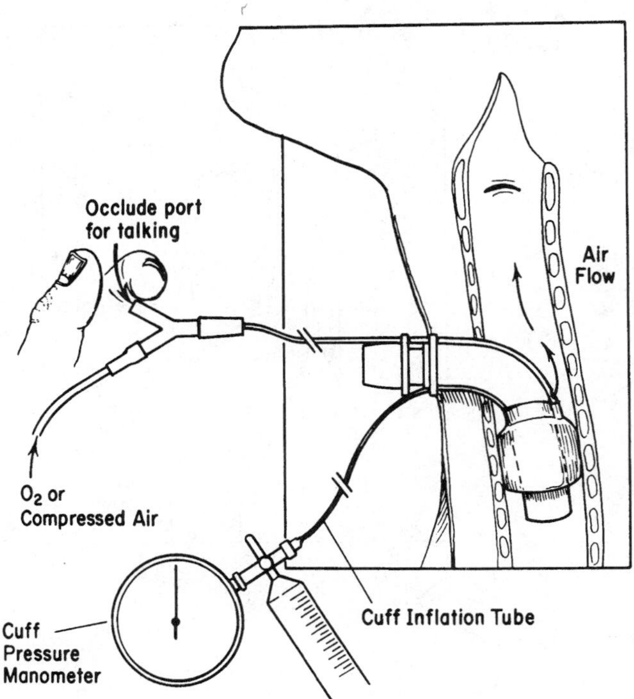

FIGURE 33–3. Talking tracheostomy tube.

Specialized Airway Appliances

The inability to speak with an artificial airway is frustrating for the patient and for the family and health care team. It is often the most stressful problem for the patient (Menzel, 1994). Reports in the literature state that anger, anxiety, fear, insecurity, and the inability to sleep are associated with the inability to speak (Bergbom-Engberg & Haljamae, 1989; Johnson & Sexton, 1990). Patients and nurses are often troubled as a result of the difficulties with lip reading. A variety of appliances are available to promote communication. The talking tracheostomy tubes, fenestrated tracheostomy tubes, and cuffless tracheostomy tubes require that a patient has functioning vocal cords to allow speech.

Several manufacturers supply talking tracheostomy tubes, which allow speech with the cuff inflated, thus providing airway protection and the use of positive-pressure ventilation (Safar & Grenvik, 1985) (Fig. 33–3). The tube is a single-lumen cannula with two external ports: a cuff inflation line and talking port. The talking port is a small tube set into the curvature of the tube that terminates just above the cuff. A flow of gas (compressed air or oxygen) is attached to the two-way connector of the external talking port. The open end of the two-way connector allows for air flow to be regulated via a thumb-controlled valve. The flow of gas exits above the cuff and forces gas through the vocal cords, allowing vocalization. The flow of gas connected to the talking port ranges from 4 to 8 L/min. Some patients have a clearly audible voice at 5 L of flow, whereas others can only whisper even with a higher flow. One reason for poor voice quality is partial obstruction of the talking port with mucus. This can be cleaned by instilling a solution of 50% acetylcysteme (Mucomyst) and 50% saline, then applying suction to the talking port. The patient using this tube must have intact oral motor function and be alert.

Another device used for speaking by the mechanically ventilated patient is the artificial larynx. This is placed against the mandibular triangle; the vibration results in audible speech. This device does not require a patient to have functioning vocal cords to allow speech.

The cuffed fenestrated tracheostomy tube is used in the patient population that is actively weaning and can maintain spontaneous respiration for at least 2-hour intervals and provides airway protection from aspiration with the tracheostomy tube cuff deflated. This type of tube allows preservation of the tracheal air flow and normal glottic function. Before this tube is placed, the patient's ability to swallow must be evaluated.

Swallowing function can be evaluated using a blue dye test and a modified barium swallow. The nurse can perform the blue dye test at the bedside. The nurse performs deep tracheal suctioning, deflates the cuff, and gives the patient 1 ounce (30 ml) of water or ice chips stained with blue food coloring. When the patient has swallowed it completely, the nurse inflates the cuff and performs deep tracheal suctioning again.

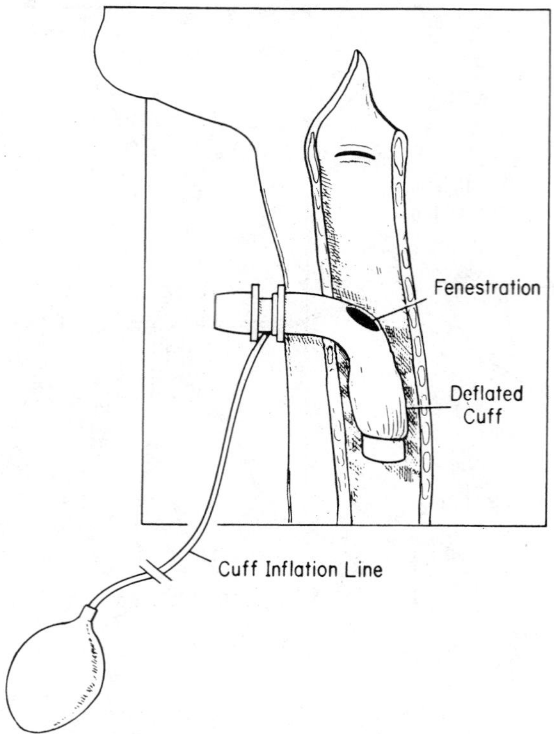

FIGURE 33–4. Proper positioning of a cuffed fenestrated tracheostomy tube in the trachea. The tube is plugged with the fenestration open and the cuff deflated to allow the patient to breathe and speak normally.

The sputum returns are evaluated for color. The test is considered negative if no dye appears in the aspirate, and positive if dye appears in the aspirate. If the test is positive or if a more accurate observation of the swallowing function is preferred, a modified barium swallow is done. The test is often performed by speech pathology and radiology departments.

A fenestrated tracheostomy tube allows patients to breathe, speak, and cough normally, using the upper airway and vocal cord function. The two manufacturers that provide fenestrated tracheostomy tubes are Portex and Shiley. This tube is designed with a standard cuff, precut fenestration, inner cannula, and plug. The fenestration is a hole in the outer cannula of the tube that will direct flow through the vocal cords for speaking (Fig. 33–4). A fenestrated tube must be positioned correctly within the lumen of the trachea. This position is determined with bedside measurement or with a lateral neck x-ray. The bedside measurement is done with sterile pipe cleaners determining the distance between anterior and posterior tracheal wall and skin (Fig. 33–5). The pipe cleaners are placed onto the tracheostomy tube to determine if the fenestration will be positioned correctly in the lumen of the trachea (Wilson, 1988). If the measured distance is larger than the precut tubes, a tube must be custom-designed for proper fit. If the fenestration is not in proper position, there is a potential for the growth of granulation tissue with resultant occlusion of the fenestration, thus causing bleeding with each insertion and removal of the inner cannula. If proper placement is in question, a flexible fiber-optic laryngoscope or bronchoscope can be used for inspection (Snyder, 1983). Nurses should check placement of the fenestration on a routine basis by removing the inner cannula and examining by direct vision, using a flashlight. When in the proper position the fenestration should look like a black hole. If tissue is observed in the fenestration, the physician should be notified and the tube should be repositioned or a new tube inserted to prevent further complications of tracheal injury.

When a cuffed fenestrated tube is in proper position, the patient can breathe, speak, and cough using normal glottic function. To allow use of the upper airway to breathe, the inner cannula must be removed, the cuff deflated, and the tube plugged. Mechanical ventilation and airway protection are provided when the plug is removed, the cuff inflated, and the inner cannula placed to occlude the fenestration.

If a patient cannot tolerate the fenestrated tube being plugged, a one-way speaking valve may be useful. This can be used for patients with vocal cord or tracheal pathology, neuromuscular disease, or COPD (Passy, 1986). The valve, referred to as a Passy-Muir Trach Valve, fits on any tracheostomy tube with a 15-mm adapter. This valve is used for patients who are spontaneously breathing. On inspiration the valve opens to allow air entry through the tube; on expiration it closes, directing the air into the trachea and the upper airway to allow vocalization (Fig. 33–6 and Fig. 33–7).

A method of communication for the ventilator-dependent patient is the Passy-Muir Vent Valve. This valve is designed to be connected directly to disposable flexible ventilator tubing. The goal is to maintain mechanical ventilation and have the patient speak using normal glottic function. The cuff is deflated to

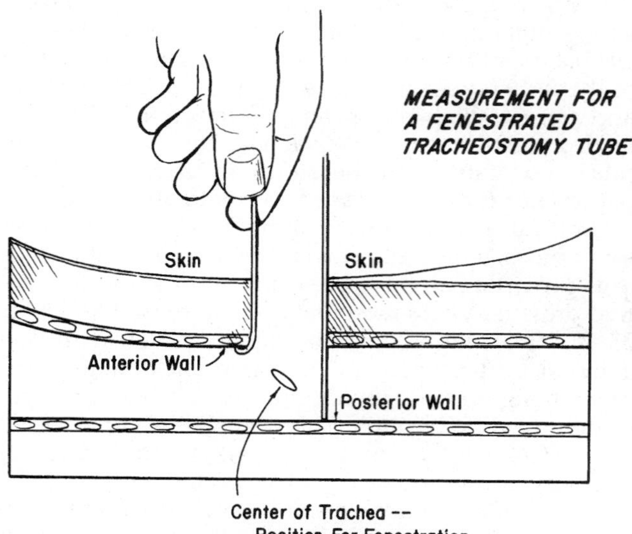

FIGURE 33–5. Bedside technique in measuring for fenestration.

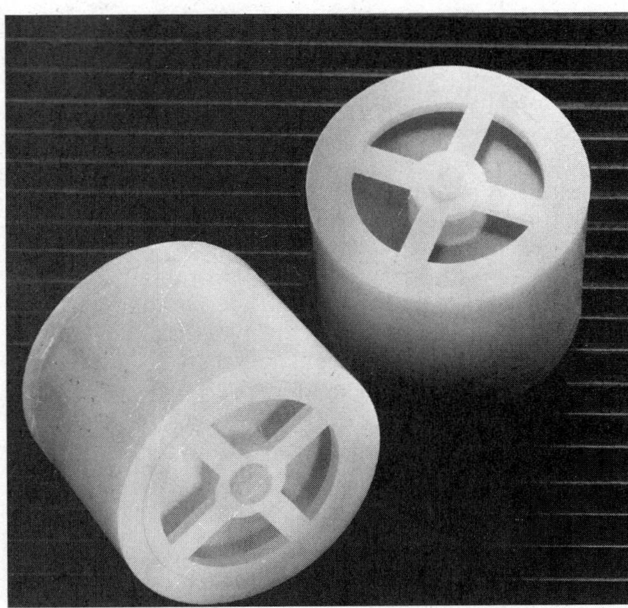

FIGURE 33–6. Passy-Muir speaking valve.

allow exhaled air to pass around the tracheal tube toward the glottis; to compensate for the air leak, the tidal volume is increased until the prior maximum inspiratory pressure is obtained. The Passy-Muir Vent Valve is placed between the tracheostomy tube and the mechanical ventilator tubing. The pressure alarm should be set to detect obstruction, but the expired volume alarm has to be disconnected. Patients are able to speak in full sentences; therefore, the patient's frustration and anxiety are decreased. During the use of the speaking valve, it is necessary to monitor the patient's tidal volume, peak inspiratory pressure, chest expansion, secretion elimination, and air flow through the nose and mouth. Patients with reduced lung compliance and poor oral and laryngeal muscular function, or vocal cord dysfunction will not be able to use the Passy-Muir Vent Valve (Manzano et al., 1993).

Common Problems

The most common problem with artificial airways is a cuff leak. This is evidenced by an audible leak from the patient's mouth or tracheostomy stoma with each positive-pressure breath. The leak is caused by tube position, a crack or slow leak in the housing of the one-way inflation line valve, or cuff rupture. Evaluation of a cuff leak is performed before changing the tube. The tube is examined first. Any pull or torque on the tube should be eliminated. The tracheostomy tube flange should be examined to ensure that it is flush with the patient's neck. The cuff pressure should be measured and the cuff deflated to compare with the known values. The cuff should be reinflated, using minimal leak technique. When an air leak is present, inspect the plastic housing of the one-way valve for cracks. Air leaks can be detected by placing the inflation line under water and observing any air bubbles with each positive-pressure breath. If air bubbles are present, a hemostat is placed on the pilot balloon tubing. The tube should be changed as soon as feasible. If the hemostat is placed on the small-bore tubing of the inflation line, it will collapse the small tubing and will create difficulty in deflating the cuff before a tube change. This procedure will not be helpful for a ruptured cuff. In this situation the tube must be changed immediately.

TRACHEAL STENOSIS

Tracheal stenosis generally develops in one of three regions of the airway: subglottic, cuff site, and stoma site. Subglottic stenosis is rare, but may develop if the tracheostomy is performed too high at the time of surgery, thereby causing damage to the cricoid cartilage (Heffner et al., 1986). Tracheal damage leading to stenosis at the cuff still occurs despite high-volume, low-pressure cuffs. The cuff design does not ensure that low pressure is maintained if the cuff is overinflated. Cuff volumes and pressures higher than necessary can cause this stenosis-related tube pressure necrosis (Grillo et al., 1971). The tracheal mucosa becomes inflamed, ulcerated, and necrotic, resulting in fragmentation of cartilaginous rings when the cuff to tracheal wall pressure exceeds capillary perfusion pressure. Excessive pressure destroys the tracheal architecture, causing scarring and narrowing of the tracheal lumen at the cuff site.

Tracheostomy can produce tracheal damage at the stoma site, resulting in stenosis. Factors that cause this process are the initial dimensions of the tracheal incision, use of an oversized tracheostomy tube, excessive movement of the tracheostomy tube within the stoma, and persistent stomal infection (Collice, 1987). Prevention of stomal injury begins at the time of surgery. Chronic inflammation and infection at the stoma site may lead to the formation of granulation tissue. Granulomas commonly form above and below the anterior tracheal stoma site. Stomal infection and inflammation should be prevented with local care and antibiotics, if necessary. A bacterial culture of the stoma area should be obtained if purulent drainage is present. If the area around the stoma is a large open wound with continuous purulent drainage, and routine care with the application of antibiotic ointment has been done with no results, the area may be swabbed with half-strength povidone-iodine (Betadine) every 4 hours until drainage has ceased. The skin around the stoma area should be examined closely for any irritation from the Betadine. If the area around the stoma is not infected, but irritation and redness is present, place an occlusive dressing (stoma adhesive or Tegaderm) on the area to protect the skin.

TRACHEOMALACIA

Tracheomalacia may develop at the cuff site, stoma site, and the area between the cuff and stoma site. It is

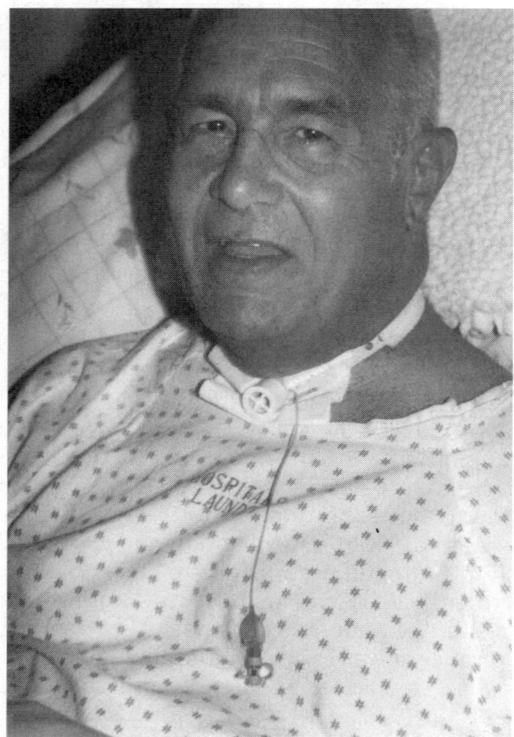

FIGURE 33–7. Patient with muscular dystrophy and COPD finds it easy to speak with the Passy-Muir speaking valve. The valve opens on inspiration and closes as the patient exhales, and the air is directed to the upper airway to allow clear speech.

thought to be due to the thinning of the tracheal wall, secondary to pressure necrosis or infection (Dane & King, 1975). Tracheomalacia should be suspected if the cuff volume required to create a seal progressively increases. Examine the tracheostomy tube and cuff on the chest x-ray. If the cuff diameter is 1.5 times the tracheal diameter, tracheomalacia can be suspected. As a result, a larger or longer tube may be required to change the position of the cuff in the airway.

The complications related to long-term placement of a tracheostomy tube still exist. In a study of 81 patients with the mean duration of a tracheostomy tube of 4.9 months, airway lesions such as granulomas, tracheomalacia, tracheostenosis, and vocal cord and laryngeal dysfunction were observed (Law et al., 1993). In 60% of the patients a tracheal granuloma was found proximal to the stoma, and tracheomalacia was found in 29% of the patients. When the patient is weaned from mechanical ventilation and tracheostenosis or tracheomalacia is suspected, an ENT or thoracic surgery consult is suggested. Consultation should evaluate the need for surgical repair or stinting of the airway with a cuffless tracheostomy tube or T tube. Decannulation of patients with a long-term tracheostomy tube can present problems; thus, bronchoscopy examination is suggested for safe tracheostomy tube removal.

Suctioning

Nurses are required to suction the intubated patient to remove secretions, which potentially interfere with oxygenation and ventilation. The indications for tracheal suctioning include coarse rhonchi and / or crackles on auscultation and an inability to raise secretions. Suctioning should not be done on a routine schedule, but as needed.

Although suctioning is a frequently performed procedure, it should not be considered benign. There are many documented complications, many of which are life-threatening. Recognized complications include hypoxia, arrhythmias, patient discomfort, bronchospasm, and trauma. Nurses must take adequate precautions in patients with cardiovascular instability such as arrhythmias, recent myocardial infarction, and severe hypoxemia with respiratory failure. In these situations, discuss the procedure with the clinical nurse specialist or physician familiar with the case. Remember, suctioning should be done only as often as necessary, not on a preprescribed basis.

Hypoxemia is a hazard of tracheal suctioning, because not only are secretions removed, but large amounts of gas are also evacuated during the suctioning procedure. The patient should be observed for signs of hypoxemia: tachypnea, tachycardia, hypertension, diaphoresis, and restlessness. The patient is also at risk for cardiac arrhythmias from systemic hypoxia. Suctioning may stimulate a vagal response, thus causing bradycardia and other life-threatening arrhythmias. Trauma can occur from the repetition, the vigor, duration, and amount of negative pressure applied while the nurse is suctioning the airway. Trauma is observed by blood aspirated into the catheter. When you note the blood, stop the suctioning procedure and assess the situation.

Another complication is bronchospasm from excessive coughing or stimulation of the airway by a foreign body (catheter). The recommended techniques to reduce the incidence of such complications include the administration of 100% oxygen before and after suctioning, limiting duration of suctioning time to 15 seconds or less, and limiting the amount of negative (suction) pressure applied (Demers & Saklad, 1975; Fell & Cheney, 1971; Rindfleish & Tyler, 1983). Specially designed airway adapters are available to permit suctioning without disconnection from positive-pressure ventilation. These have been shown to decrease the incidence of hypoxemia in postoperative, open-heart, and trauma patients (Brown et al., 1983; Skelley et al., 1980). Similar recommendations have been made by other researchers (Jung & Newman, 1982). This suggests that a closed airway system decreases complications of hypoxia during suctioning. Many studies have demonstrated stable oxygen saturation during the suctioning procedure using a closed suction catheter system (Carlon et al., 1987; Harshbarger et al., 1992).

A study comparing the conventional suctioning technique and a closed suction catheter system reported no significant difference in the effectiveness of secretion clearance (Witmer et al., 1990). The closed system suction catheter is designed for multiple use without need to disconnect the patient from positive-pressure ventilation throughout the procedure. The closed suction catheter system is an aesthetically acceptable technique, being a closed system. It is not uncommon for a patient with a forceful cough to propel saline and secretions out of the tracheostomy tube and thus be a source of contamination to personnel. A study that presented critical care nurses' review of the closed suction catheter system (SteriCath; Concord/ Portex) reported that this system was desirable and safe for the patient and staff (Crimlisk et al., 1994). This method requires further study to determine whether it decreases nursing time for suctioning, constituting a potential decreased cost-benefit ratio. As indicated previously, the complications associated with tracheal suctioning can be fatal. Thus, techniques must be instituted to minimize complications that have been identified with tracheal suctioning.

SUCTIONING PROCEDURE

Suctioning is a frightening experience for the patient; therefore, a nurse should fully explain the procedure and give verbal instruction to the patient throughout the procedure. Once the patient is assessed, the nurse can ready the equipment and begin the procedure, maintaining principles of asepsis. Equipment gathered includes a 100% manual resuscitator bag, oxygen wall outlet, suction regulator connected to the wall suction outlet and pharyngeal suction bottle, sterile suction catheter, sterile gloves, mask, eye protection, and sterile water. The suction regulator is turned on, maintaining −100 to −200 mm Hg. High negative pressure may cause mucosal trauma. The oxygen flowmeter should be set at 15 L for the 100% manual resuscitator bag. The sterile water to be used for clearing suction tubing, sterile gloves, and catheter are opened. The patient is disconnected from the ventilator and preoxygenated with five hyperinflated breaths of 100% oxygen, using the manual resuscitator bag (Chulay & Graeber, 1988). The nurse dons eye protector, mask, and sterile gloves; removes the catheter from the package; and connects it to the suction tubing. If a cough is desired or secretions are very thick, saline may be instilled down the artificial airway, although it is not recommended for routine use, because a decrease in oxygen saturation has been reported when saline was used before tracheal suctioning (Ackerman, 1993). The catheter is gently inserted via the artificial airway as far as it will go, then withdrawn 1 to 2 cm, and suction is applied intermittently for a maximum of 15 seconds, rotating the catheter between the thumb and index finger as the catheter is removed. The patient is postoxygenated with five hyperinflated breaths. The procedure can be repeated or the patient can be returned to the mechanical ventilator or oxygen source system.

SUMMARY

Every step during management of the chronic ventilator patient must be directed toward relieving the patient of his dependency on the mechanical ventilator. The transition from artificial to spontaneous ventilation should be attempted when subjective clinical judgment and objective data indicate that lung function is adequate to permit this changeover. Need for careful monitoring of blood gas exchange, spontaneous parameters, and patient's overall general status during the weaning process cannot be overemphasized. Regardless of the technique used, the responsible nurse needs to organize an individualized plan of care and approach weaning as a priority. The nurse is responsible for coordinating all other services involved in the patient's weaning process, and should proceed with ambulation, muscle training, communication, proper nutrition, and emotional support. Care of the chronic ventilator patient is complex and demanding both in the hospital and home, but with a successful outcome it can be very rewarding.

REFERENCES

Abramson, N. S., Wald, K. S., & Grenvik, A. N. A. (1980). Adverse occurrences in intensive care units. *Journal of American Medical Association, 244,* 1582–1584.

Ackerman, M. H. (1993). The effect of saline lavage prior to suctioning. *American Journal of Critical Care, 2,* 326–330.

Askanazi, J., Carpentier, Y. A., & Elwyn, D. H. (1980). Influence of total parenteral nutrition on utilization in injury and sepsis. *Annals of Surgery, 191,* 40–46.

Askanazi, J., Nordenstrom, J., & Rosenbaum, S. H. (1981). Nutrition for the patient with respiratory failure: Glucose vs. fat. *Anesthesiology, 54,* 373–377.

Barrocas, A., Tretola, R., & Alonso, A. (1983). Nutrition and the critically ill pulmonary patient. *Respiratory Care, 28,* 50–61.

Bendixen, H. H., Egbert, L. D., & Hedley-Whyte, J. (1965). *Respiratory care.* St. Louis: C. V. Mosby.

Bergbom-Engberg, I., & Haljamae, H. (1989). Assessment of the patient's experience of discomforts during respiratory therapy. *Critical Care Medicine, 17,* 1068–1072.

Brochard, L., Harf, A., Lorino, H., & Lemaire, F. (1989). Inspiratory pressure support prevents diaphragmatic fatigue during weaning from mechanical ventilation. *American Review of Respiratory Disease, 139,* 513–521.

Brown, S. F., Merrill, E. J., & Light, R. W. (1983). Prevention of suctioning-related arterial oxygen desaturation. Comparison of off-ventilator and on-ventilator suctioning. *Chest, 4,* 621–627.

Burns, S. M. (1991). Preventing diaphragm fatigue in the ventilated patient. *Dimensions of Critical Care Nursing, 10,* 13–20.

Burns, S. M., Burns, J. E., & Truwit, J. D. (1994). Comparison of five clinical weaning indices. *American Journal of Critical Care, 3,* 342–352.

Burns, S. M., Clochesy, J. M., Hanneman, S. K. G., Ingersoll, G. E., Knebel, A. R., & Shekleton, M. E. (1995). Weaning from long-term mechanical ventilation. *American Journal of Critical Care, 4,* 4–22.

Carlon, G. C., Fox, S. J., & Ackerman, N. J. (1987). Evaluation of a closed-tracheal suction system. *Critical Care Medicine, 15,* 522–525.

Carroll, P. F. (1986). Caring for ventilator patients. *Nursing86, 16,* 34–40.

Chernow, B. (1982). Hypomagnesemia: Implications for the critical care specialist. *Critical Care Medicine, 10,* 193–196.

Chulay, M., & Graeber, G. (1988). Effectiveness of hyperinflation and hyperoxygenation for suctioning interventions. *Heart and Lung, 17,* 15–22.

Clochesy, J. M., Daly, B. J., & Montenegro, H. D. (1995). Weaning chronically critically ill adults from mechanical ventilation: A descriptive study. *American Journal of Critical Care, 4,* 93–95.

Collice, G. L. (1987). Prolonged intubation verse tracheostomy in the adult. *Journal of Intensive Care Medicine, 2,* 85–107.

Crabtree-Goodnough, S. K. (1988). Reducing tracheal injury and aspiration. *Dimensions of Critical Care Nursing, 7,* 324–331.

Crimlisk, J. T., Paris, R., McGonagle, E. G., Calcutt, J. A., & Farber, H. W. (1994). The closed tracheal suction system: Implications for critical care nursing. *Dimensions of Critical Care Nursing, 13,* 292–300.

Daly, B. J., & Allen, M. L. (1987). Nursing care of the mechanically ventilated patient. In: M. L. Nochomovitz & H. D. Montenegro (Eds.), *Ventilatory support in respiratory failure.* Mt. Kisco, N.Y.: Futura Publishing.

Dane, T. E. B., & King, E. G. (1975). A prospective study of complications after tracheostomy for assisted ventilation. *Chest, 67,* 398–404.

Demers, R. R., & Saklad, M. (1975). Mechanical aspiration: A reappraisal of its hazards. *Respiratory Care, 20,* 661–666.

Dougherty, S. (1988). The malnourished respiratory patient. *Critical Care Nurse, 8,* 13–22.

Downs, J. B., & Chapman, R. L. (1976). Treatment of bronchopleural fistula during continuous positive-pressure ventilation. *Chest, 69,* 363–366.

Downs, J. B., Klein, E. P., Desautels, D., Madell, J. H., & Kirby, R. R. (1973). Intermittent mandatory ventilation: A new approach to weaning patients from ventilation. *Chest, 64,* 331–335.

Feeley, T. W., & Bancroft, M. L. (1982). Problems with mechanical ventilators. *International Anesthesiology Clinics, 20,* 83–93.

Feeley, T. W., & Hedley-Whyte, J. (1975). Weaning from controlled ventilation and supplemental oxygen: Weaning from intermittent positive-pressure ventilation. *New England Journal of Medicine, 292,* 903–906.

Fell, T., & Cheney, F. W. (1971). Prevention of hypoxia during endotracheal suction. *Annals of Surgery, 174,* 24–28.

Fitzgerald, L. M., & Huber, G. L. (1976). Weaning the patient from mechanical ventilation. *Heart and Lung, 5,* 228–234.

Gammon, R. B., Shin, M. S., & Buchalter, S. E. (1992). Pulmonary barotrauma in mechanical ventilation. *Chest, 102,* 568–572.

Grillo, H. C., Cooper, J. D., Geffin, B., & Pontoppidan, H. (1971). A low-pressure cuff for tracheostomy tube to minimize tracheal injury: A comparative clinical trial. *Journal of Thoracic and Cardiovascular Surgery, 62,* 898–907.

Haake, R., Schlichtig, R., Ulstad, D. R., & Henschen, R. R. (1987). Barotrauma. Pathophysiology, risk factors, and prevention. *Chest, 91,* 608–613.

Harshbarger, S. A., Hoffman, L. A., Zullo, T. G., & Pinsky, M. R. (1992). Effects of a closed tracheal suction system on ventilatory and cardiovascular parameters. *American Journal of Critical Care, 3,* 57–61.

Heffner, J. E., Miller, K. S., & Sahn, S. A. (1986). Tracheostomy in the intensive care unit. (Part 2: Complications). *Chest, 90,* 430–436.

Hotchkiss, R. S., & Wilson, R. S. (1983). Mechanical ventilatory support. *Surgical Clinics of North America, 63,* 417–438.

Hyman, A. L., Rodriquez, J., & Weissman, C. (1982). Nutritional support of the critically ill patient. *Seminars in Anesthesia, 1,* 354–361.

Johnson, M., & Sexton, D. (1990). Distress during mechanical ventilation: Patient perceptions. *Critical Care Nurse, 10,* 48–57.

Jung, R. C., & Newman, J. (1982). Minimizing hypoxia during endotracheal airway care. *Heart and Lung, 11,* 208–212.

Kacmarek, R. M. (1989). Inspiratory pressure support: Does it make a clinical difference? *Intensive Care Medicine, 15,* 337–339.

Kelsay, J. L. (1978). A review of research on effects of fiber intake on man. *American Journal of Clinical Nutrition, 3,* 142–159.

Kersten, L. D. (1989). *Comprehensive respiratory nursing.* Philadelphia: W. B. Saunders.

Kim, M. J. (1984). Respiratory muscle training: Implications for patient care. *Heart and Lung, 13,* 333–340.

Knebel, A. R., Shekleton, M. E., Burns, S. M., Clochesy, J. M., Hanneman, S. K. G., & Ingersoll, G. L. (1994). Weaning from mechanical ventilation: Concept development. *American Journal of Critical Care, 3,* 416–420.

Landis, K., & Smith, S. (1983). The mechanically ventilated patient. A comprehensive nursing care plan. *Critical Care Quarterly, 6,* 43–52.

Law, J. H., Barnhart, K., Rowlett, W., de la Rocha, O., & Lowenbery, S. (1993). Increased frequency of obstructive airway abnormalities with long-term tracheostomy. *Chest, 104,* 136–138.

Luce, J., Pierson, D., & Hudson, L. (1981). Intermittent mandatory ventilation. *Chest, 79,* 678–685.

Majors, M. (1988). Nutritional support of the mechanically ventilated patient. *Critical Care Nursing Quarterly, 11,* 50–61.

Manzano, J. L., Lubillo, S., Henriquez, D., Martin, J. C., Perez, M. C., & Wilson, D. J. (1993). Verbal communication of ventilator-dependent patients. *Critical Care Medicine, 21,* 512–517.

Marcy, T. W. (1993). Barotrauma: Detection, recognition, and management. *Chest, 104,* 578–584.

Marini, J. J. (1986). The physiologic determinants of ventilator dependence. *Respiratory Care, 31,* 271–282.

Mathru, M., Rao, T. L. K., & Venus, B. (1982). Hemodynamic response to changes in ventilatory patterns in patients with normal and poor left ventricular reserve. *Critical Care Medicine, 10,* 426–432.

Menzel, L. (1994). Need for communication-related research in mechanically ventilated patients. *American Journal of Critical Care, 3,* 165–167.

Morganroth, M. L., Morganroth, J. L., Nett, L. M., & Petty, T. L. (1984). Criteria for weaning from prolonged mechanical ventilation. *Archives Internal Medicine, 144,* 1012–1016.

Nett, L. M., Morganroth, M. L., & Petty, T. L. (1987). Weaning protocols that work: Weaning in specific clinical situations: Weaning the unweanable. *American Journal of Nursing, 87,* 1174–1184.

Norton, L. C., & Neureuter, A. (1989). Weaning the long-term ventilator-dependent patient: Common problems and management. *Critical Care Nurse, 9,* 42–52.

Openbrier, D. (1985). A delicate balance: Strategies for feeding ventilated patients. *American Journal of Nursing, 3,* 247–280.

Passy, V. (1986). Passy-Muir tracheostomy speaking valve. *Otolaryngology, 95,* 247–248.

Petersen, G. W., & Baier, H. (1983). Incidence of pulmonary barotrauma in medical ICU. *Critical Care Medicine, 11,* 67–69.

Pierson, D. J., Horton, C. A., & Bates, P. W. (1986). Persistent bronchopleural air leak during mechanical ventilation. A review of 39 cases. *Chest, 90,* 321–323.

Rafferty, T. D., Palma, J., Motoyama, E. K., Schachter, W., & Ciarcia, M. (1980). Management of a bronchopleural fistula with differential lung ventilation and positive end-expiratory pressure. *Respiratory Care, 25,* 654–657.

Rindfleish, S. H., & Tyler, M. L. (1983). Duration of suctioning: An important variable. *Respiratory Care, 28,* 457–459.

Rochester, D. F. (1984). Malnutrition and the respiratory system. *Chest, 85,* 411–415.

Safar, P., & Grenvik, A. (1975). Speaking cuffed tracheostomy tube. *Critical Care Medicine, 3,* 23–26.

Sahn, S. A., & Lakshminarayan, S. (1973). Bedside criteria for discontinuation of mechanical ventilation. *Chest, 63,* 1002–1005.

Scheinhorn, D. J., Artinian, B. M., & Catlin, J. L. (1994). Weaning from prolonged mechanical ventilation. The experience at a regional weaning center. *Chest, 105,* 534–539.

Sheldon, G. F., & Baker, C. (1980). Complications of nutritional support. *Critical Care Medicine, 9,* 35–37.

Sjostrand, U. (1980). High-frequency positive-pressure ventilation (HFPPV): A review. *Critical Care Medicine, 8,* 345–364.

Skelley, B. F. H., Deeren, S. M., & Powaser, M. M. (1980). The effectiveness of two preoxygenation methods to prevent endotracheal suction-induced hypoxemia. *Heart and Lung, 9,* 316–323.

Skillman, J. J., Malhotra, I., Pallotta, J. A., & Bushnell, L. S. (1971). Determinants of weaning from controlled ventilation. *Surgical Forum, 22,* 198–200.

Snyder, G. M. (1983). Individualized placement of tracheostomy tube fenestration and in-situ examination with the fiberoptic laryngoscope. *Respiratory Care, 28,* 1294–1298.

Sporn, P. H. S., & Morganroth, M. L. (1988). Discontinuation of mechanical ventilation. *Clinics in Chest Medicine, 9,* 113–126.

Tobin, M. J., Guenther, S., Perez, W., et al. (1987). Mead analysis ribcage-abdominal motion during successful and unsuccessful trials of weaning from mechanical ventilation. *American Review of Respiratory Disease, 135,* 1320–1328.
Truesdell, S. K. (1992). Powerlessness in chronically ventilator-dependent patients. *Perspectives in Respiratory Nursing, 3,* 1–5.
Whited, R. E. (1984). A prospective study of laryngotracheal sequela in long-term intubation. *Laryngoscope, 94,* 367–377.
Wilson, D. J. (1988). Airway appliances and management. In: R. M. Kacmarek & J. Stoller (Eds.), *Current respiratory care* (pp. 80–89). Philadelphia: B. C. Decker.
Wilson, D. O. (1985). State of the art: Nutrition and chronic lung disease. *American Review of Respiratory Disease, 124,* 376–381.
Witmer, M. T., Hess, D., & Simmons, M. (1990). An evaluation of the effectiveness of secretion removal with a closed-circuit suction catheter. *Respiratory Care, 35,* 1117–1118.

CHRONIC VENTILATOR DEPENDENT PATIENTS MULTIDISCIPLINARY CARE GUIDE

COORDINATION OF CARE

Diagnosis/Stabilization Phase		Acute Management Phase		Recovery Phase	
Outcome	*Intervention*	*Outcome*	*Intervention*	*Outcome*	*Intervention*
All appropriate team members and disciplines will be involved in the plan of care.	Develop the plan of care with patient/family, primary nurse(s), primary physician(s), pulmonologist, thoracic surgery (for tracheostomy), and other specialists as needed, (clinical nurse specialist, respiratory therapist, physical therapist (PT), occupational therapist (OT), speech therapist, recreational therapist, chaplain, social service).	All appropriate team members and disciplines will be involved in the plan of care.	Update the plan of care with the patient/family, other team members, dietician, discharge planner, and home health agency. Initiate planning for anticipated discharge. Begin teaching patient/family about home care (medications, ventilator care and maintenance, care of tracheostomy tube, diet, skin care).	Patient/family will understand how to maintain optimal health at home.	Provide written guidelines concerning home care for patient/family. Provide patient/family with phone numbers of resources available to answer questions.

FLUID BALANCE

Diagnosis/Stabilization Phase		Acute Management Phase		Recovery Phase	
Outcome	*Intervention*	*Outcome*	*Intervention*	*Outcome*	*Intervention*
Patient will achieve and maintain optimal hemodynamic status as evidenced by: • MAP >70 mm Hg • Hemodynamic parameters WNL for the patient • Urine output >0.5 mL/kg/hr • Free from dysrhythmias • Vital signs WNL for the patient	Monitor and treat evidence of abnormal hemodynamic status such as tachycardia, hypertension, hypotension, increased respiratory distress, increased crackles or wheezes in lungs, murmers, or presence of S_3/S_4 heart sound. Monitor lab values: electrolytes, ABGs, Spo_2, BUN and CBC with differential. Monitor and treat dysrhythmias. Assess and monitor fluid balance. Assess weight changes from baseline and weigh daily. Determine hydration needs based on hemodynamics, I & O, cardiopulmonary assessment, viscosity of pulmonary secretions, V.S., and electrolytes. Monitor and treat complications of chronic ventilator dependence, such as cor pulmonale resulting in right-sided heart failure from prolonged hypoxemia, causing decreased left ventricular filling, CO and BP; CHF or hyper-/hypovolemia. Administer vasodilators and inotropic agents as indicated and monitor response.	Patient will maintain optimal hemodynamic status.	Same as stabilization phase. Maintain optimal hydration based on cardiopulmonary assessment.	Patient will maintain optimal hemodynamic status.	Same as acute management phase. Teach patient/family about the following: • Patient's optimal fluid balance and how to maintain it. Review signs and symptoms of fluid overload and dehydration. Remind patient to weigh daily and report sudden changes to physician. • Antidysrhythmic agents and/or other cardiac medications that will be taken at home.

NUTRITION

Diagnosis/Stabilization Phase		Acute Management Phase		Recovery Phase	
Outcome	*Intervention*	*Outcome*	*Intervention*	*Outcome*	*Intervention*
Patient will be adequately nourished and/or regain nutritional balance.	Assess nutritional status. Monitor albumin, prealbumin, total protein, nitrogen balance, phosphate, magnesium, calcium, and lymphocyte count. Assess skin turgor and inspect oral mucous membranes.	Patient will be adequately nourished. Patient will be absent of bowel or elimination problems.	Involve dietician in plan of care. Determine resting energy expenditure so accurate estimation of caloric need and type can be made. In undernourished patients, response to hypoxemia/hypercapnea is impaired. Avoid high carbohydrate load, which may result in increased CO_2 production. Initiate diet as tolerated and monitor response (enteral feedings, parenteral nutrition, oral foods as able). If patient is eating, deflate cuff of tracheostomy tube to facilitate swallowing function when patient is off positive-pressure ventilation. Treat diarrhea, constipation, or ileus as indicated. Weigh every other day and report changes of ±3 lb.	Patient will be adequately nourished.	Teach patient/family about: • Food pyramid and recommended daily allowances • Daily caloric intake needed • Safe weight reduction or weight gaining techniques as indicated • Dietary supplements for cachectic patients

MOBILITY

Diagnosis/Stabilization Phase		Acute Management Phase		Recovery Phase	
Outcome	*Intervention*	*Outcome*	*Intervention*	*Outcome*	*Intervention*
Patient will achieve optimal mobility.	Assess muscle mobility, flexibility, strength, and tone. Include assessment of respiratory muscle function.	Patient will achieve optimal mobility.	Assess physical limitations of mobility. Involve PT or OT for specific mobility limitations. Nursing/PT to perform range of motion (ROM) at least BID. Develop progressive activity program (sitting on side of bed, transferring from bed to chair, gradual increase in walking, and gradual increase in active ROM/stretching exercises). Monitor response to activity and decrease if adverse events occur (tachycardia, dyspnea, ectopy, syncope, or hypotension).	Patient will maintain optimal mobility. Patient will develop home exercise plan.	Continue PT/OT therapy in home if indicated. Assist patient in developing realistic goals for home exercise plan. Determine a gradually increasing program of aerobic activity such as walking. Refer to outpatient pulmonary rehabilitation program if indicated.

Care Guide continued on following page

OXYGENATION/VENTILATION

Diagnosis/Stabilization Phase		Acute Management Phase		Recovery Phase	
Outcome	*Intervention*	*Outcome*	*Intervention*	*Outcome*	*Intervention*
Patient will have a patent airway and optimal ventilation as evidenced by: • Respiratory rate, depth, and rhythm WNL for the patient • Chest x-ray WNL • Clear airways • ABGs, vital signs, mental status, and pulmonary function tests WNL for the patient • Demonstrated ability to cough and clear secretions • Optimal oxygenation/ventilation on positive-pressure ventilation	Monitor and treat abnormal breath sounds, respiratory pattern (rate, depth, rhythm and work of breathing), and chest x-ray. Monitor and treat signs/symptoms of respiratory distress: • Weak ineffective cough • Shortness of breath, dyspnea • Use of accessory muscles/respiratory alternans • Presence of adventitious breath sounds • Alterations in level of consciousness • P_{CO_2} > 50 mm Hg and/or above normal for patient • Ventilator malfunction Monitor quantity, color, and consistency of pulmonary secretions. Maintain artificial airway. Provide humidification (aerosols), monitor cuff inflation pressure every shift, and monitor for complications of artificial airways such as tracheal stenosis, tracheomalacia, or granulomas causing obstruction. Suction only as often as necessary. Beware of complications of suctioning such as hypoxemia, dysrhythmias, discomfort, vagal stimulation causing bradycardia, bronchospasm, and airway trauma. Avoid routine use of saline installation when suctioning because it has been associated with many adverse effects. Assist with monitoring and adjusting of ventilator settings to maintain appropriate level of assistance and minute ventilation. Administer chest physiotherapy q4h when indicated.	Patient will have a patent airway, optimal ventilation, gas exchange, and adequate tissue perfusion.	As in stabilization phase. Continue to monitor patient's response to mechanical ventilation. Assess readiness to wean per Burns Weaning Assessment Program (Burns, 1994). *General Assessment:* • Free from factors that increase or decrease metabolic rate (seizures, temperature, sepsis, bacteremia, hypo-/hyperthyroid)? • Hematocrit > 25% (or baseline)? • Electrolytes WNL? (Including Ca^{++}, Mg^{++}, PO_4^{3-}) • Chest x-ray improving? *Respiratory Assessment:* • Eupnic respiratory rate and pattern • Absence of adventitious breath sounds (Assess for improvement in breath sounds.) • Secretions thin and minimal? • Absence of neuromuscular disease/deformity • Absence of abdominal distension/obesity/ascites • Oral endotracheal tube >7.5 or trachea >7.0? • Cough and swallowing reflexes adequate? • Negative inspiratory pressure at least −20 mm Hg • Positive expiratory pressure >+30 mm Hg • Spontaneous tidal volume >5 cc/kg? • Vital capacity >10–15 mL/kg? • pH 7.30–7.45 • Pa_{CO_2} approximately 40 mm Hg (or baseline) with minute ventilation <10 L/min • Pa_{O_2} >60 mm Hg on F_{IO_2} <40%	Patient will have adequate ventilation and gas exchange and adequate tissue perfusion.	As in stabilization phase. Teach patient/family on the following if partial or full mechanical ventilatory support will be used at home: • Portable home ventilator care, funtion, and maintenance • How to troubleshoot three most common alarms: high pressure, low pressure, and low exhaled volume • How to perform clean tracheal suction technique • How to perform tracheostomy tube care • How to maintain minimal occlusive pressure in tracheostomy tube cuff • How to breathe with manual resuscitator bag • How to reinsert tracheostomy tube if it becomes displaced • When to call physician • How to use back-up battery power in cases of power failure Organize weekly multidisciplinary discharge rounds to coordinate patient's discharge. Determine which company will supply equipment, be responsible for follow-up care, and contact utility companies, fire department, and police department regarding use of home mechanical ventilator. Teach patient about home medications and signs and symptoms of respiratory distress. Refer to outpatient pulmonary rehabilitation program when indicated.

Diagnosis/Stabilization Phase		Acute Management Phase		Recovery Phase	
Outcome	Intervention	Outcome	Intervention	Outcome	Intervention
	Administer bronchodilators as indicated. Monitor and treat complications that can occur in chronic ventilator-dependent patients such as acute acid-base disturbances, headache, restlessness, hypertension, bronchopleural air leak, or patient/ventilator asynchrony.		Monitor ventilatory/oxygenation status and hemodynamic variables during the weaning process. Use consistent, calm approach to weaning strategy. Provide psychological support and encouragement to allay fears, avoiding increased inspiratory work of breathing.		
Patient will exhibit optimal gas exchange and tissue perfusion as evidenced by: • ABGs, vital signs, and mental status WNL for the patient • Sao_2 >90%/Spo_2 > 92% or WNL for the patient • Normal hemoglobin • Urine output >0.5 mL/kg/hr	Monitor and treat patient for signs and symptoms of altered gas exchange: dyspnea, restlessness, tachycardia, tachypnea, confusion, headache, central cyanosis (not peripheral), Pao_2 <50 mm Hg on room air, Pao_2/PAo_2 ratio <0.50, Sao_2 <90%, use of accessory muscles, dysrhythmias, hypotension. Change Fio_2 or PEEP as indicated and monitor response. Observe for potential complications such as barotrauma or decreased cardiac output. Optimize O_2 delivery by monitoring and treating cardiac output, BP, heart rate, Sao_2, hemoglobin, and Pao_2. Assess for evidence of adequate tissue perfusion in all organ systems (normal BP, LOC, urine output, liver enzyme levels).		Wean Fio_2/PEEP as oxygenation improves. Consider positioning of patient to enhance gas exchange (i.e., good lung dependent if unilateral lung disease or prone position if bilateral lung involvement). Encourage patient to sit up to ease chest expansion. Begin patient/family teaching on pulmonary system, current pulmonary problems, current treatment, and expected clinical course.		

COMFORT

Diagnosis/Stabilization Phase		Acute Management Phase		Recovery Phase	
Outcome	**Intervention**	**Outcome**	**Intervention**	**Outcome**	**Intervention**
Patient will be as comfortable and pain free as possible as evidenced by: • No objective indicators of discomfort • No complaints of discomfort	Plan interventions to provide optimal uninterrupted rest periods. Assess patient's perspective of adequacy of rest. Assess quantity and quality of discomfort or pain and treat as indicated. Provide reassurance in a calm, caring, and competent manner. Keep lights dim and a quiet environment to minimize catecholamine responses.	Patient will be as comfortable as possible.	Teach patient about relaxation techniques. Use complementary therapies such as guided imagery, music, humor, or body massage to enhance patient's comfort. Involve family in strategies. Use diversional therapies such as pet therapy, reading, and listening to book tapes, especially during weaning trials.	Patient will be as comfortable as possible.	Patient will demonstrate relaxation techniques to use at home.

Care Guide continued on following page

CHRONIC VENTILATOR DEPENDENT PATIENTS MULTIDISCIPLINARY CARE GUIDE *continued*

COMFORT *continued*

Diagnosis/Stabilization Phase		Acute Management Phase		Recovery Phase	
Outcome	***Intervention***	***Outcome***	***Intervention***	***Outcome***	***Intervention***
	While patient is intubated, establish effective communication technique so patient can communicate. Encourage patient to write messages or use a Magic Slate, alphabet board, flash cards, or computer to express needs and feelings. Use a Passy-Muir speaking valve, talking tracheostomy tube or cuffed fenestrated tracheostomy tube when patient is able. Value of voicing is very significant to recovery. Observe for complications of prolonged ventilator dependence that can cause discomfort (dyspnea, breathlessness, bronchospasm).				

SKIN INTEGRITY

Diagnosis/Stabilization Phase		Acute Management Phase		Recovery Phase	
Outcome	***Intervention***	***Outcome***	***Intervention***	***Outcome***	***Intervention***
Patient will have intact skin without abrasions or pressure ulcers.	Assess all bony prominences q4h. Use preventive pressure-reducing devices when patient is at high risk for development of pressure ulcers. Treat pressure ulcers according to hospital protocol.	Patient will have intact skin without abrasions or pressure ulcers.	Same as stabilization phase.	Patient will have intact skin without abrasions or pressure ulcers.	Teach patient/family interventions to be continued at home for proper skin care.

PROTECTION/SAFETY

Diagnosis/Stabilization Phase		Acute Management Phase		Recovery Phase	
Outcome	*Intervention*	*Outcome*	*Intervention*	*Outcome*	*Intervention*
Patient will be protected from possible harm.	Monitor cuff pressures to prevent trauma to airway and keep pressure lower than 25 cm H_2O. Monitor peak inspiratory pressures. If peak airway pressure is excessive, may need to adjust ventilatory settings. Evaluate breath sounds, ABGs, and chest x-ray. Secure tracheostomy tube securely to avoid trauma/inflammation at the stoma. Deflate cuff of tracheostomy tube if patient is to eat and is off positive-pressure ventilation. Assess for adequate swallowing function. Have patient perform oral motor exercises if swallowing is impaired. Change tracheostomy tube every 4 to 6 weeks. Assess need for restraints while patient is intubated, has a decreased LOC, or is agitated and restless. Explain need for restraints to patient/family. Assess response to restraints and check q1–2h for skin integrity and impairment to circulation. Follow hospital protocol for use of restraints. Provide sedatives/anxiolytics as needed.	Patient will be protected from possible harm.	Provide support when dangling, getting out of bed, and with increasing activity, and monitor response.	Patient will be protected from possible harm.	Provide support as needed with ambulation. Teach patient/family about any physical limitations the patient might have.

Care Guide continued on following page

CHRONIC VENTILATOR DEPENDENT PATIENTS MULTIDISCIPLINARY CARE GUIDE *continued*

PSYCHOSOCIAL/SELF-DETERMINATION

Diagnosis/Stabilization Phase		Acute Management Phase		Recovery Phase	
Outcome	***Intervention***	***Outcome***	***Intervention***	***Outcome***	***Intervention***
Patient will achieve psychophysiologic stability. Patient will demonstrate a decrease in anxiety as evidenced by: • Vital signs WNL • Subjective report of decreased anxiety • Objective signs of decreased anxiety	Assess physiologic effects of critical care environment on patient (hemodynamic variables, psychological status, signs of increased sympathetic response). Use calm, caring, competent, and reassuring approach with patient and family. Assess for appropriate level of anxiety and nervousness. Allow flexible visiting to meet the needs of the patient and family. Help patient/family to identify and verbalize fears such as dying, being dependent on ventilator, losing control, being dependent on family, or being alone. Plan strategies to help alleviate and/or to help patient process their fears. Determine coping ability of patient/family and take appropriate measures to begin acceptance of long-term ventilator dependence. Provide frequent explanations to patient/family, allow patient to verbalize concerns, consult support services, and hold family conferences. Administer sedatives and anxiolytics and monitor response.	Patient will achieve psychophysiologic stability. Patient will be as relaxed as possible.	Same as stabilization phase.	Patient will achieve psychophysiologic stability. Patient will be as relaxed as possible.	Provide instruction on coping mechanisms after discharge. Refer patient/family to counseling/stress management programs when indicated. Provide support to patient/family in the case of unsuccessful treatment outcomes in reaching difficult decisions and accepting inevitable outcomes.

Common emotional/psychological responses of ventilator-dependent patients include hopelessness, powerlessness, and loss of control. Incorporate the following strategies and others as appropriate into the patient's daily care to minimize these responses:

- Provide daily progress reports for patient/family
- Provide opportunities for patient to participate in care and decisions regarding health
- Keep patient informed of condition, treatment, and results of tests

DIAGNOSTICS

Diagnosis/Stabilization Phase		Acute Management Phase		Recovery Phase	
Outcome	*Intervention*	*Outcome*	*Intervention*	*Outcome*	*Intervention*
Patient/family will understand any tests or procedures that must be completed (vital signs, I & O, cardiac monitoring, x-rays, lab work, ECG, ABGs, Sp_{O_2}, IV lines, PFTs, $\dot{V}_D/\dot{V}_T$ ratio, end-tidal CO_2 levels, bronchoscopy, or swallowing studies).	Explain all tests and procedures to patient/family. Be sensitive to individual's need for information.	Patient/family will understand any tests or procedures that must be completed.	Same as stabilization phase.	Patient/family will understand meaning of diagnostic steps in relation to continued health.	Review with patient/family results of tests before discharge. Discuss abnormal findings and appropriate measures patient/family can take to return to prehospital condition if possible. Provide written guidelines concerning follow-up care and care at home for patient/family.

REFERENCE

Burns, S. M., Burns, J. E., & Truwit, J. D. (1994). Comparison of five clinical weaning indices. *American Journal of Critical Care, 3,* 342–352.

UNIT 6

NERVOUS SYSTEM

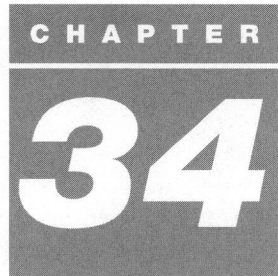

Neurophysiology

Victor G. Campbell and John M. Clochesy

The human nervous system is composed of two constituent cells: neurons and neuroglia. The neurons are the basic structural and functional units for conduction in the nervous system, and the neuroglia cells serve in a supportive capacity for the neurons.

NEUROGLIA CELLS

About 40% of the microscopic structures of the brain and spinal cord are composed of neuroglia cells (Fig. 34–1). The purpose of these cells is to protect, support, and nourish the neuron. There are four different types of neuroglia cells: (1) ependyma, (2) astrocyte, (3) oligodendroglia, and (4) microglia.

EPENDYMA. Ependymal cells are found throughout the epithelial lining of the cerebral ventricles, the choroid plexuses, and the central canal of the spinal cord. Ependymal cells assist in the production of cerebrospinal fluid (CSF).

ASTROCYTE. Astrocytes, or astroglia, are starlike in appearance because of the many processes that extend out from the cell body. The functions of the astrocytes include (1) maintenance of the chemical environment for the conduction of impulses; (2) information storage; (3) maintenance of the blood–brain barrier; (4) maintenance of the nutritional needs of the neuron; and (5) structural support for the neuronal cells.

OLIGODENDROGLIA. Oligodendroglia are cells that synthesize a lipid–protein complex that forms the myelin sheaths around the axons of neurons in the central nervous system (CNS). The functions of the myelin sheath include (1) insulation along the processes of the nerve; (2) holding the nerve fibers together; (3) promotion of ionic flow across the cell membrane of the nerves; and (4) transmission of nerve impulses (this type of transmission is termed saltatory conduction). Although considered homologous to the Schwann cells of the peripheral nervous system, oligodendrogliocytes lack the neurilemma membrane. Therefore, when structures are damaged, they are replaced with astrocytes, which eventually form scar tissue that can disrupt the surrounding tissue and impair neuronal transmission.

MICROGLIA. The microglial cells are formed from the embryonic mesodermal cells that migrated along branches of blood vessels into the CNS (Jensen, 1980). Microglia are found throughout the CNS, primarily in the white matter. The main function of the normally stationary microglia cells is phagocytosis. During this process, the microglia become mobile in order to ingest and digest tissue debris.

THE NEURON

The neuron (Fig. 34–2) is the principal structural cell of the nervous system whose function is transmission of specific nervous stimuli. Neurons have the specialized properties of excitation and electrical–chemical conductivity.

The neuron is composed of a cell body, or perikaryon; an axon, or axis cylinder; and a number of short receptive fibers called dendrites. The axons carry information away from the nerve body and thus are termed *efferent* fibers. The dendrites carry information to the neuron and are therefore called *afferent* fibers.

Neurons are classified according to their structure as unipolar, bipolar, or multipolar (Fig. 34–3). *Unipolar* neurons have one process or pole that divides close to the body of the cell. One branch of this division, termed the *peripheral process,* carries afferent (sensory) impulses from the periphery to the cell body. Another branch, called the *central process,* carries efferent (motor) impulses away from the cell body to the spinal cord and brain stem. *Bipolar* neurons have two processes consisting of one axon and one dendrite. Bipolar neurons are found only in spinal ganglia, the olfactory mucous membrane, and rod and cone cells of the retina. *Multipolar* neurons are found throughout the CNS, including all association (internuncial) and motor neurons. These neurons consist of a cell body, one long projection called the axon, and one or more shorter branches (dendrites).

Functionally, neurons are classified as afferent or efferent. Afferent neurons conduct sensory impulses from the peripheral nerve endings toward the cell

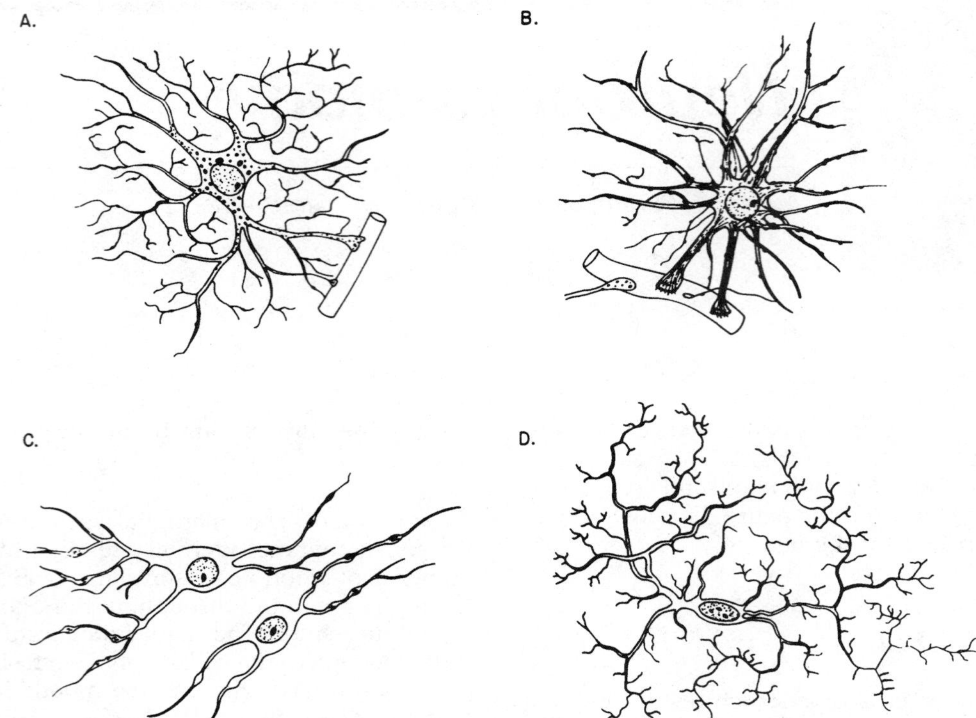

FIGURE 34–1. Neuroglia (interstitial) cells found in the central nervous system. Protoplasmic (*A*) and fibrous (*B*) astrocytes with end feet terminating on capillaries. Oligodendroglia (*C*) and (*D*) are shown. (From Jensen, D. [1980]. *The principles of physiology* [2nd ed.]. New York: Appleton-Century-Crofts.)

body in the CNS. *Efferent* neurons transmit motor impulses away from the cell body via the axon to effector organs and tissues.

Cytologic Features

The neuron is composed of a cell body, or perikaryon, projections called dendrites, and an axon (Fig. 34–4). In the cell body, which is located in the gray matter of the CNS, there is a centrally located *nucleus.* The nucleus is a large structure with a double membrane and contains DNA. Within the nucleus is a single prominent *nucleolus,* which contains RNA. RNA is crucial for protein synthesis and serves as the messenger from the genes of the nucleus.

Surrounding the nucleus is the cellular cytoplasm, which contains numerous organelles including the Nissl bodies, mitochondria, the Golgi complex, neurofilaments, and microtubules. *Nissl bodies* are ordered masses of granular endoplasmic reticulum with ribosomes that function as the protein-synthesizing machinery of the cell. The *mitochondria* are rod-shaped structures that regulate the respiratory metabolism of the cell. Structurally, the mitochondria consist of outer and inner lipid bilayer-protein membranes. The *outer membrane* is smooth. The *inner membrane* forms a number of narrow folds that provide sites of attachment for oxidative enzymes. Between the narrow folds is an inner cavity called the mitochondrion *central cavity.* This cavity is filled with the dense *matrix granules,* which contain large numbers of dissolved enzymes that facilitate energy extraction from nutrients (Guyton, 1991). Mitochondria primarily function as the "powerhouse" of the cell. Specifically, the oxidative enzymes and the enzymes contained in the matrix granules act in a specific sequence to cause oxidation of nutrients. As a result of this oxidative process, water and carbon dioxide are formed, and the liberated energy is used to synthesize the high-energy compound adenosine triphosphate (ATP) from adenosine diphosphate and inorganic phosphate. ATP then is transported from the cell to provide energy where it is needed for cellular functions (Guyton, 1991).

The *Golgi complex* is located in the cytoplasm and condenses and stores substances necessary for transmission of impulses. Throughout the cytoplasm as well as the processes of the axon and dendrites are the dense neurofilaments. Individual *neurofilaments* consist of structures called neurotubules or microtubules. Together, the neurotubules and microtubules make up the *neurofibril.* The neurofibril is involved in intracellular axoplasmic transport.

Neuronal Processes

Neuronal processes consist of the axon and the dendrites. The *axon,* or axis cylinder, is a long smooth projection that extends from the cell body. Generally, the

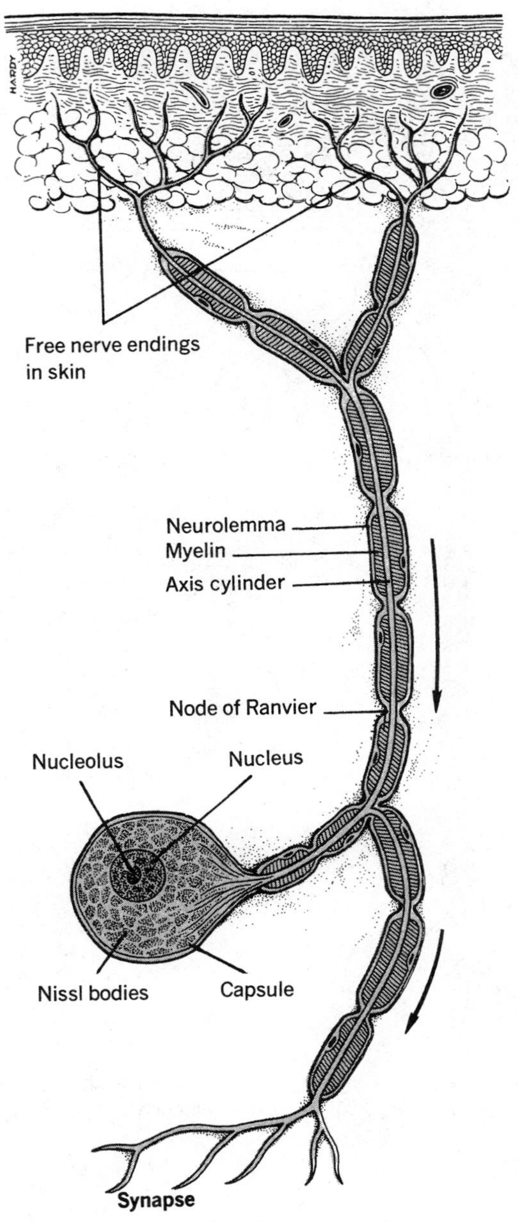

FIGURE 34–2. Typical afferent (sensory) neuron. (From Chaffee, E. E., & Greisheimer, E. M. [1974]. *Basic physiology and anatomy* [3rd ed., p. 164]. Philadelphia, J. B. Lippincott.)

axon originates from the cell body at a point called the *axon hillock.* The axon carries efferent impulses away from the cell body and forms the white matter (myelinated) of the CNS. Surrounding the axon is the myelin, which protects and insulates the axonal structure. The terminal branches of the axon are called *terminal filaments,* or axon telodendria. Short receptive processes called the *dendrites* extend from the cell body to the immediate surrounding areas. The dendrites are unmyelinated and lie in the gray matter of the CNS. The dendritic branches increase the surface area from which neuronal impulses may be picked up. The dendrites transmit afferent impulses to the cell body. Terminal endings of the dendrite, or dendritic spines, provide increased surface area for synaptic transmission of nerve impulses.

THE NERVE

The primary function of the neuron in the peripheral nervous system is the conduction of impulses to and from the CNS. This function of the neuron is accomplished by chainlike groupings of neuronal cell fibers into nerves.

The nerve component responsible for impulse conduction is the axon. Surrounding the axon is the discontinuous layer of the myelin sheath, which protects, insulates, and nourishes the axon (see Fig. 31–4). Periodic interruptions of the myelin sheath in the peripheral nervous system are called *nodes of Ranvier.* These nodes increase the speed of impulse conduction by allowing the nerve impulse to skip from node to node.

All the peripheral nerves are enveloped in a thin cytoplasmic membrane called the neurilemma. The *neurilemma* is formed by the Schwann cells and wraps segmentally around the myelin sheaths of myelinated nerves or the axons of unmyelinated nerves in the peripheral nervous system. The neurilemma protects and supports the vital nerve processes.

Surrounding the nerve are three layers of connective tissue (Fig. 34–5). The innermost *endoneurium* ensheathes the neurilemma cells. Next to the endoneurium is the *perineurium,* which surrounds bundles of nerve fibers (fascicles) with connective tissue. The outermost covering is the *epineurium,* which binds the groups of fascicles together.

As with the neuron, nerve fibers in the peripheral nervous system are classified according to their function. Afferent nerves receive sensory input. *Internuncial,* or association, nerves convey incoming stimuli to the various centers in the CNS. Efferent nerves transmit motor impulses to effector organs.

Impulse Conduction

Like other cells in the body, nerve fibers are charged, or polarized, in their resting state. In this state, the inside of the cell is charged negatively in relation to the outside. This difference in electrical polarity is the result of a high concentration of sodium outside the cell and a high concentration of potassium in the cell, causing unequal electrical charges across the cell membrane. The difference in electrical polarity is caused by the impermeability of the cell membrane to sodium and is maintained by the sodium–potassium pump. The *sodium–potassium pump* is the mechanism by which sodium is pumped continuously out of the cell while potassium is being pumped into the cell.

When a chemical, mechanical, or electrical stimulus of threshold intensity (the amount of stimulus required to elicit tissue response) is applied, there is a rapid, marked change in the permeability of the cell membrane. This change in membrane permeability

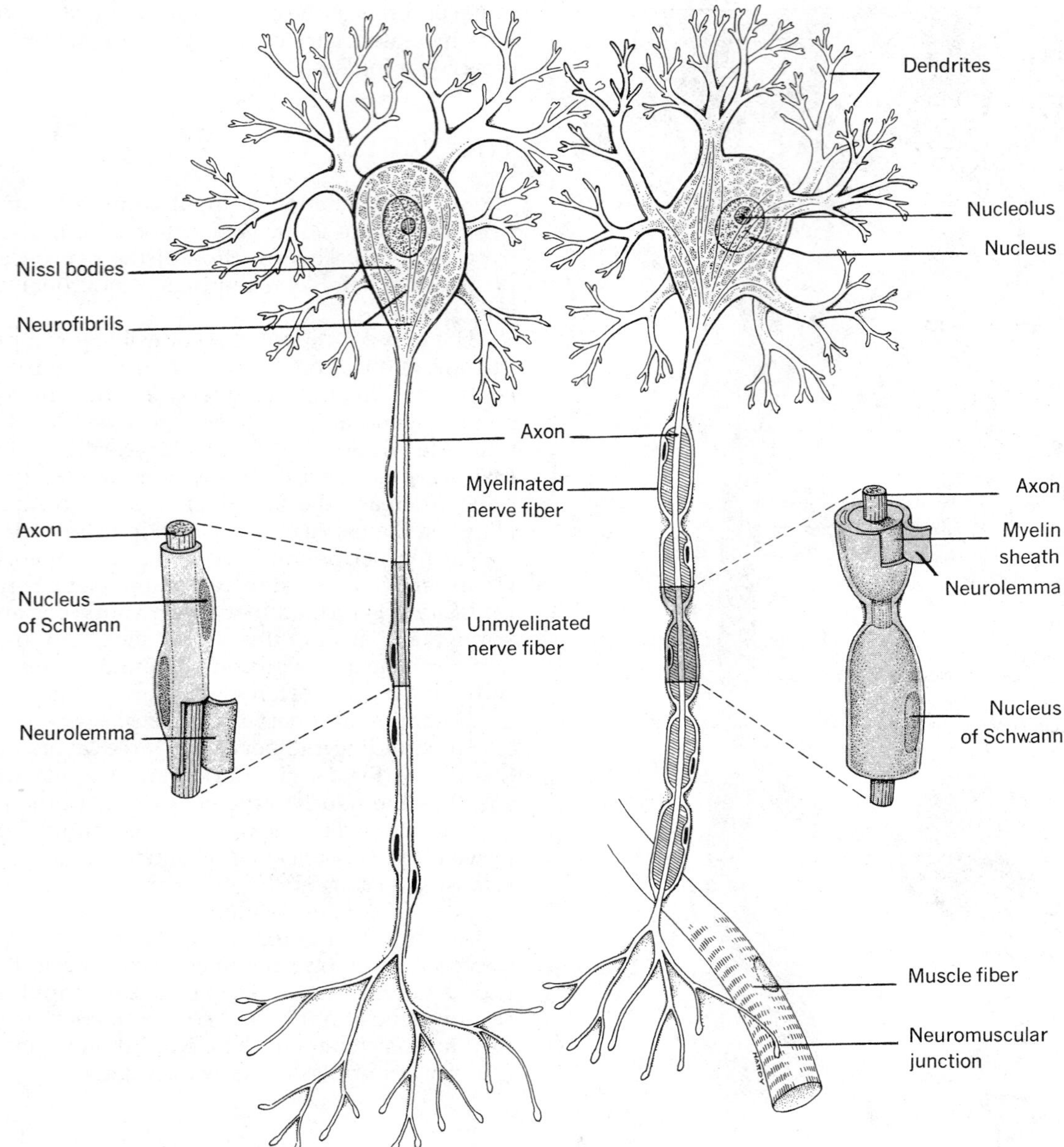

FIGURE 34–3. Typical efferent (motor) neuron. (From Chaffee, E. E., & Greisheimer, E. M. [1974]. *Basic physiology and anatomy* [3rd ed., p. 165]. Philadelphia, J. B. Lippincott.)

causes a rapid influx of sodium and a loss of intracellular potassium via diffusion. As the sodium rushes into the cell, the plasma membrane becomes charged positively in relation to the interstitial space, and an action potential (*depolarization*) results. The depolarization stimulus excites one local area of the cell membrane, which then excites adjacent areas of the cell membrane (conduction), until the whole membrane is stimulated at the same intensity. Consequently, the wave of depolarization is self-propagated along the entire length of the nerve process. Following depolarization, there is a reversal of ionic flow across the cell membrane. Specifically, sodium is pumped out as potassium is pumped back into the cell. This reversal in ionic flow (*repolarization*) restores the membrane polarization, and the membrane returns to its resting potential. To prevent repeated excitation, the neuron cannot be restimulated with another action potential during the entire phase of depolarization and during about one-third of the repolarization phase. This time interval is termed the *absolute refractory period.* Following the absolute refractory period is the *relative refractory period.* During this time interval, which lasts about one-quarter to one-half as long as the absolute refractory period, a stronger than normal stimulus can excite the nerve fiber. The relative refractory period is caused by

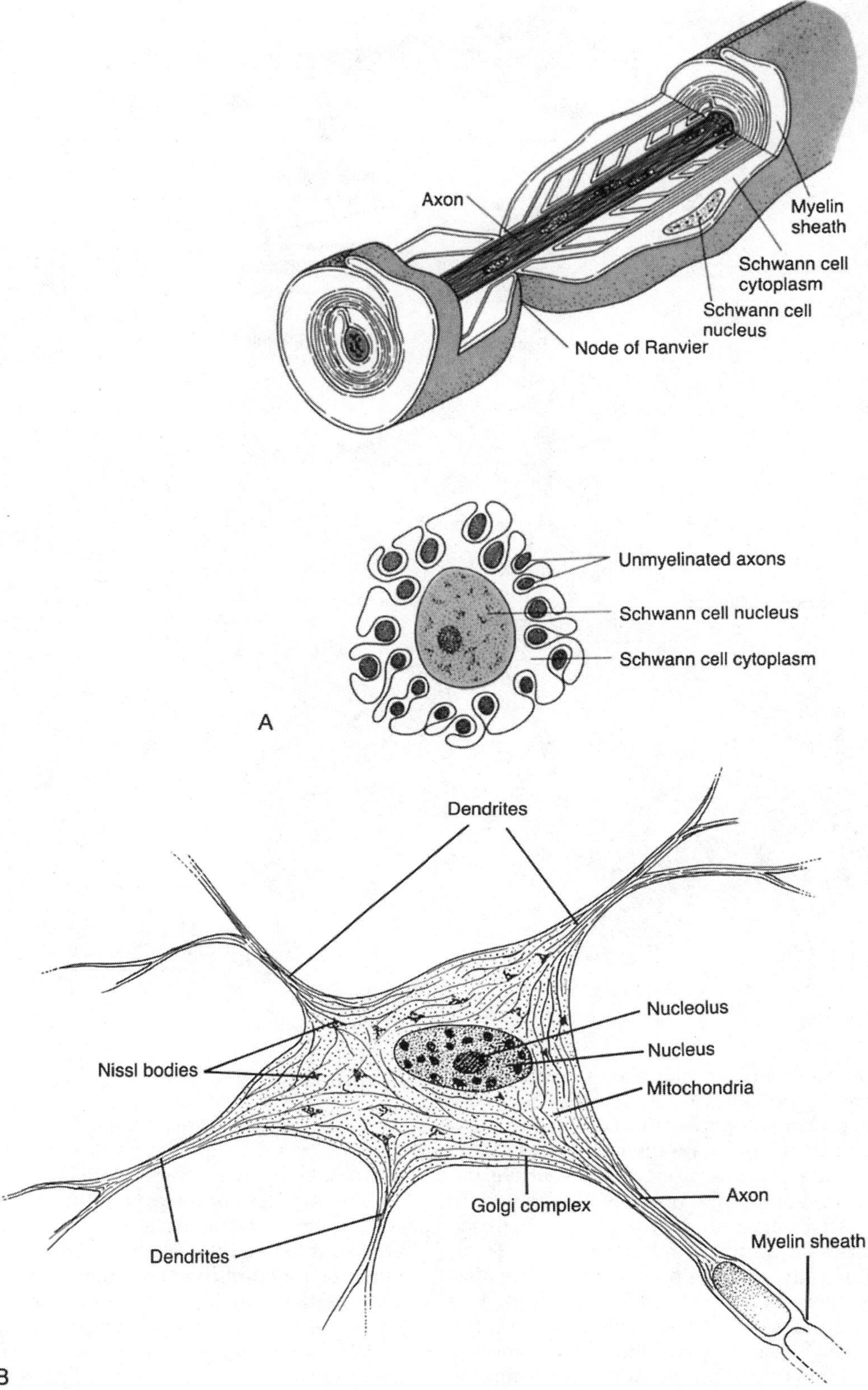

FIGURE 34–4. *A,* Cross-section of a myelinated neuron. *B,* Cell body of multipolar neuron. (*A* modified from Leeson, C. R., & Leeson, T. S. [1979]. *Atlas of histology.* Philadelphia: W. B. Saunders; *In* Guyton, A. C. [1991]. *Basic neuroscience.* [2nd ed., p. 78]. Philadelphia: W. B. Saunders. *B* reproduced by permission from: Conway, B. L. *Pediatric neurologic nursing.* St. Louis, 1977, The C. V. Mosby Co.)

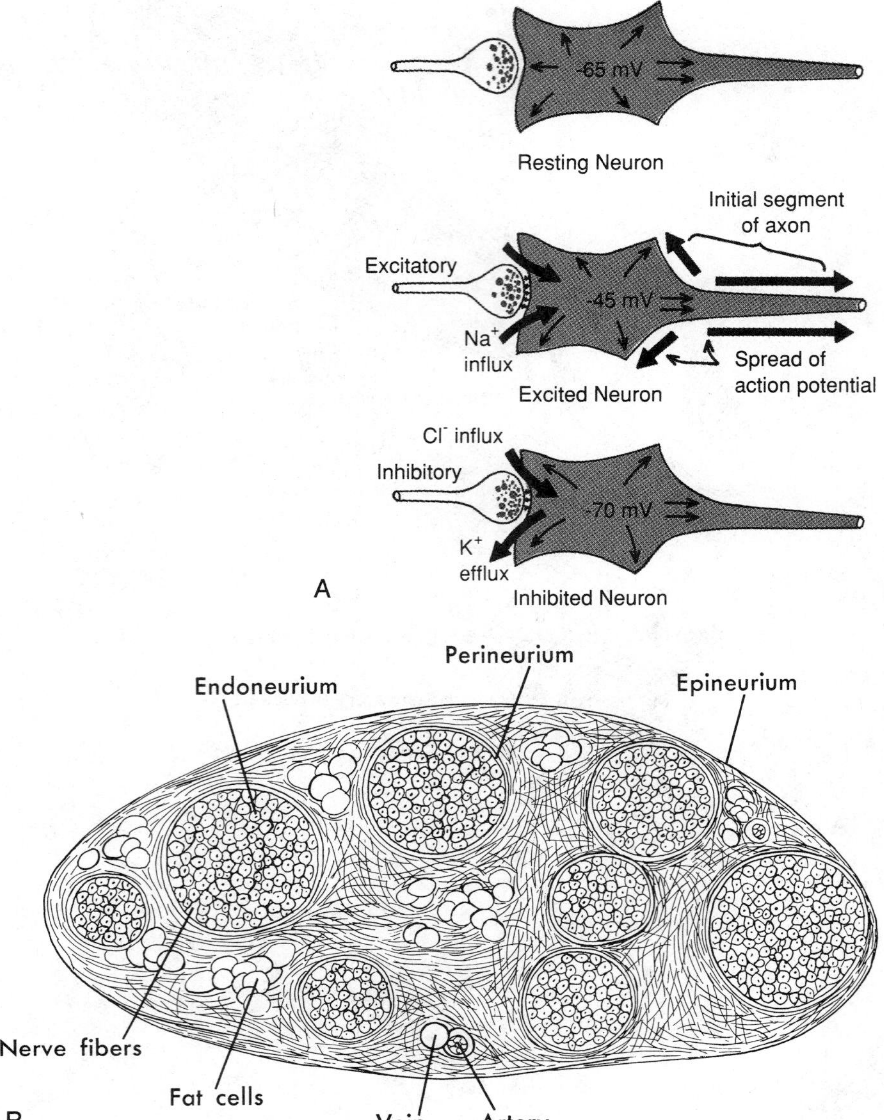

FIGURE 34–5. *A*, Examples of excitatory and inhibitory transmission. *B*, Transverse section of peripheral nerve trunk. (*A* from Guyton, A. C. [1991]. *Basic neuroscience* [2nd ed., p. 95]. Philadelphia: W. B. Saunders; *B* reproduced by permission from: Conway, B. L. *Pediatric neurologic* nursing. St. Louis, 1977, The C. V. Mosby Co.)

(1) sodium channels that have not been reversed from inactivation, and (2) potassium channels that generally are wide open, producing hyperpolarization and making it more difficult to stimulate the nerve fiber (Guyton, 1991). The rate of transmission of the nerve impulse depends on whether the nerve is myelinated. In heavily myelinated nerve fibers, the axon is exposed only at the nodes of Ranvier; therefore, influx of sodium is possible only at these points. When depolarization occurs, there is a rapid influx of sodium ions (termed the sodium sink) at the node. The impulse then "skips" in a discontinuous manner to another node of Ranvier. This node-to-node transmission (termed *saltatory transmission*) results in a more rapid conduction of the action potential, increasing the velocity of impulse transmission and decreasing energy demands. In unmyelinated nerves, the action potential must travel the entire length of the nerve fiber.

Synapse

Because neurons are physically distinct, impulses must travel via "signal transmission" from one neuron to another by way of gap junctions called synapses. Unlike impulse conduction, which is an electrical process, synaptic transmission is a chemical process that is accomplished by substances called *neurotransmitters.* Synaptic junctions between neurons are located in the gray matter. Anatomic structures of the synapse include the (1) presynaptic terminals, (2) synaptic cleft, and (3) postsynaptic membrane. *Presynaptic terminals,* also referred to as presynaptic knobs, store excitatory or inhibitory neurotransmitters in the synaptic vesicles. When the presynaptic terminals are stimulated by an impulse, a specific type of neurotransmitter is released into the synaptic cleft. The synaptic cleft is a microscopic space between the terminals and receptor membranes. The release of the neurotransmitter stimulates specific receptor sites on the postsynaptic membrane (dendrite cell body area) of the next neuron in the pathway. Following synaptic transmission, the neurotransmitter is inactivated chemically or removed by reabsorption to prevent overstimulation of the postsynaptic membrane.

Neurotransmitters

Neurotransmitters (see Fig. 34–5) are chemical substances that conduct impulses from nerve cells to target cells (Hickey, 1992). At least 30 neurotransmitters have now been identified. Each of these synaptic transmitters has a characteristic excitatory (facilitating) or inhibitory effect on the target nerve, muscle, or gland cell. *Excitatory* neurotransmitters stimulate the receptor sites on the postsynaptic membrane to enhance permeability to sodium, chloride, and potassium ions. The influx of the sodium ion lowers the cell membrane potential (depolarization) and forms an excitatory postsynaptic potential. The principal excitatory neurotransmitter of the voluntary nervous system and the parasympathetic division of the autonomic nervous system is *acetylcholine.* In addition to acetylcholine, other central excitatory neurotransmitters include *dopamine, serotonin, norepinephrine, L-asparate,* and *glutamic acid.* Inhibitory neurotransmitters decrease the permeability of the postsynaptic receptor sites to sodium and increase their permeability to potassium and chloride ions. The postsynaptic cell is hyperpolarized (membrane potential is raised) and forms an inhibitory postsynaptic potential (IPSP). Formation of an IPSP is called *direct inhibition.*

Another type of inhibitory action is caused by the stimulation of the excitatory presynaptic terminals by an inhibitory neuron. With presynaptic inhibition, there is a partial depolarization of the terminal fibrils and the excitatory presynaptic terminals, causing less excitatory neurotransmitters to be released from these endings. Consequently, the velocity of the action potential is reduced, and end-excitation of the neuron is decreased. Inhibitory neurotransmitters include *gamma-aminobutyric acid* (presynaptic) and *glycine* (postsynaptic).

CENTRAL NERVOUS SYSTEM

Skull

The *skull* (Fig. 34–6) encloses and protects the vulnerable brain tissue. The two major anatomic divisions of the skull are the cranium and the facial bones. The cranial portion consists of eight irregularly shaped bones that are joined together by fixed joints or sutures. Internally, the cranial cavity is divided into three major areas—the anterior, middle, and posterior fossae. The *anterior fossa* contains the frontal lobes of the brain. The *middle fossa* contains the temporal, parietal, and occipital lobes. The *posterior fossa* contains the brain stem and the cerebellum. The opening at the base of the skull is called the *foramen magnum* and is the area in which the brain and spinal cord join.

The 14 facial bones are fused together as a unit to support the facial structures. The facial skull encloses the eye sockets, a portion of the nasal cavity, and the oral cavity.

Meninges

The brain is covered by three layers of connective tissue referred to collectively as the *cranial meninges* (Fig. 34–7). Each of the three meningeal layers is a continuous sheet of connective tissue that protects the vulnerable brain.

The outermost meningeal layer is the *dura mater* or "hard mother." The dura mater is a double-layered sheath that encloses the brain and separates the skull into various compartments by its folds and processes. The *falx cerebri* process is formed by a vertical fold at the midsagittal line and divides the two cerebral hemispheres. The *tentorium cerebelli* is a horizontal fold that separates the cerebral hemispheres from the brain stem and the cerebellum. Anatomically, structures that lie above the tentorium cerebelli are called *supratentorial,* whereas structures below this fold are termed *infratentorial.* The *falx cerebelli* is a dural process that divides the two cerebellar hemispheres.

The second meningeal layer is the *arachnoid.* The arachnoid has two thin layers of delicate and elastic membranes that create the cobweblike subarachnoid space. Located within the subarachnoid space are a number of cerebral vessels, and it is in this space that CSF circulates around the brain. The CSF is formed from three primary sources: the *choroid plexus,* located in portions of the lateral, third, and fourth cerebral ventricles; the *ependymal cells* that line the ventricles and meningeal blood vessels; and *cerebral* and *spinal blood vessels.*

The third and innermost meningeal layer is the meshlike *pia mater.* This vascular membrane is supplied with blood from the internal carotid and vertebral arteries and provides a large volume of blood to the brain.

Cerebral Circulation

The primary sources of the cerebral blood supply are the two pairs of internal carotid and vertebral arteries (Fig. 34–8). The pair of *internal carotid arteries* provide the brain with approximately 80% of the needed blood supply. These vessels originate from the right and left *common carotid arteries,* respectively, at about the level of the thyroid cartilage. The internal carotid artery enters the skull at the foramen lacerum. At approximately the level of the optic chiasm, the internal carotids give rise to the anterior and middle cerebral arteries. The *anterior cerebral artery* passes medially

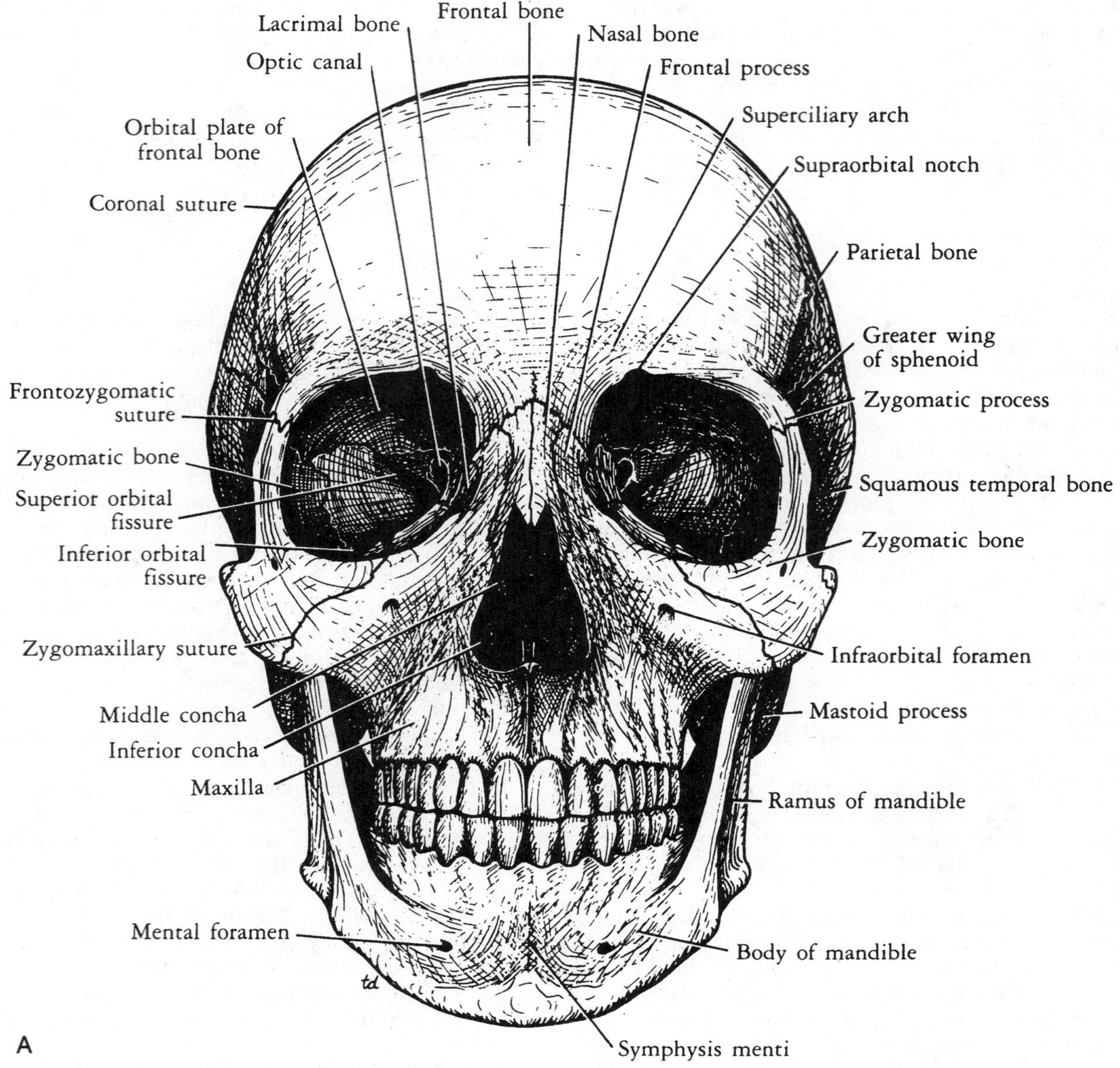

FIGURE 34–6. *A,* Anterior view of the skull. (From *Textbook of Neurological Nursing,* Pallet, P. J., & O'Brien, M. T., © 1985. Reprinted by permission of Scott, Foresman and Company.)

along the base of the brain anterior to the optic chiasm and then runs along the longitudinal fissure between the frontal lobes. The anterior cerebral artery primarily supplies the corpus callosum, medial portions of the frontal and parietal lobes, portions of the internal capsule, and the nuclei of the basal ganglia. The *middle cerebral artery* is the largest branch of the internal carotid artery and supplies the lateral surfaces of the frontal, temporal, and parietal lobes. The middle cerebral artery is the primary source of blood to the precentral (motor) and postcentral (sensory) gyri (wrinkles or convolutions).

The remaining 20% of cerebral blood supply is delivered by the pair of vertebral arteries that originates from the right and left subclavian arteries and enters the skull through the foramen magnum in front of the spinal cord. The arteries run along the anterior surface of the medulla oblongata and unite at the level of the pons to form the *basilar artery.* The basilar artery lies in the median groove of the pons. Branches of the vertebral and basilar arteries provide blood to the brain stem and cerebellum. Within the midbrain, the basilar artery bifurcates into the two *posterior cerebral arteries* that supply inferior and medial portions of the temporal and occipital lobes, the vestibular organs, and the cochlear apparatus.

CIRCLE OF WILLIS. Located at the base of the brain is a small circle of arteries that surround the pituitary stalk and the optic chiasm. This ring of blood vessels,

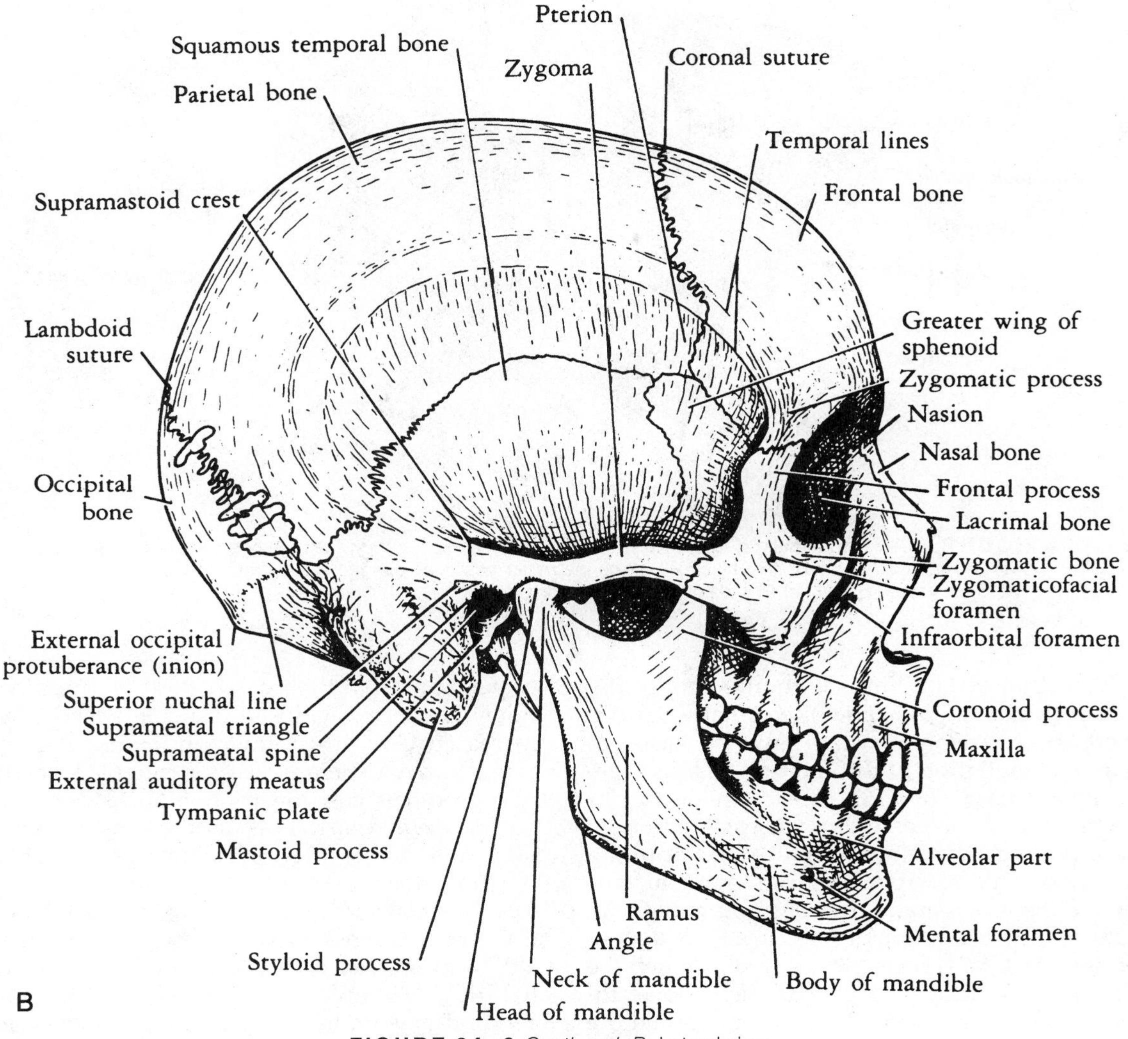

FIGURE 34–6 *Continued. B,* Lateral view.

called the *circle of Willis,* is formed by communicating branches of the posterior and anterior cerebral arteries (Fig. 34–9). Specifically, the posterior and middle cerebral arteries are joined together by the two *posterior communicating arteries.* The two anterior arteries are connected by one *anterior communicating artery.* The circle of Willis is thought to be a protective mechanism by which cerebral circulation is maintained if blood flow from one of the four primary vessels is occluded or interrupted.

VENOUS DRAINAGE. Cerebral venous drainage is accomplished by venous sinuses that are created by two layers of the dura mater. The major venous sinuses include the superior sagittal sinus, the inferior sagittal sinus, the straight sinus, the transverse sinuses, and the cavernous sinuses. The *superior sagittal sinus* arises at the frontal lobe and traverses the top of the falx cerebri. This sinus drains the CSF and the superior cortical veins. The *inferior sagittal sinus* passes along the lower edge of the falx cerebri and drains the medial surface of the brain. The *straight sinus* runs between the superior and inferior sinuses and drains the vein of Galen. The *transverse sinuses* are continuations of the superior sagittal sinus and are found on each side of the skull. The transverse sinuses drain blood from the superior sagittal and straight sinuses into the internal jugular vein. The *cavernous sinuses* run along the sphenoid bone and drain the inferior surfaces of the brain.

Cerebral Blood Flow Regulation

Normal cerebral blood flow (CBF) is approximately 750 mL / min and is maintained by a cerebral perfusion pressure (CPP) of approximately 85 mm Hg (Simon & Sayre, 1987). The cerebral vasculature, and thus CBF, is regulated by a number of mechanisms to maintain sufficient blood flow to meet cerebral metabolic needs. These mechanisms include autoregulation, chemical control, and metabolic regulation.

Autoregulation is a mechanism that permits varia-

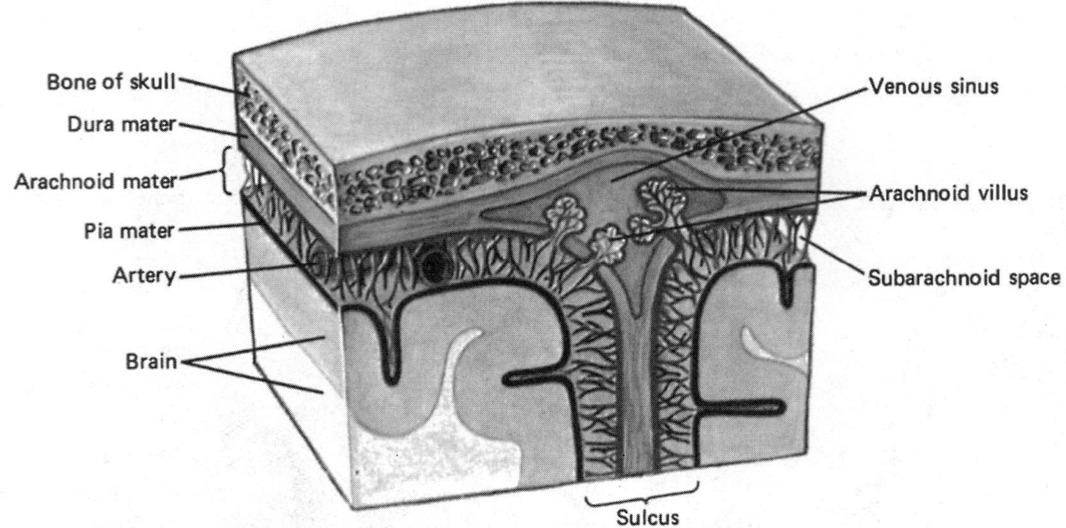

FIGURE 34–7. Schematic diagram illustrating the relationships among the meninges, their spaces, and the ventricles of the brain. Thickness of the pia mater has been exaggerated. (From Guyton, A. C. [1987]. *Basic neuroscience.* Philadelphia: W. B. Saunders.)

tion in CPP within certain limits without significantly altering CBF (Lindsay et al., 1986). Normally, CBF is maintained at a relatively constant level by vasoconstriction and vasodilation of the cerebral vessels. Specifically, an increase in CPP causes the vascular smooth muscles and the vessels to constrict. Similarly, a decrease in CPP produces a myogenic effect resulting in vasodilation. The autoregulatory mechanism fails when the CPP is less than 50 mm Hg or greater than 160 mm Hg. At these extreme pressures, CBF is dependent passively on CPP (Lindsay et al., 1986). When the CPP falls below 50 mm Hg, an extremely powerful sympathetic reflex is initiated. This reflex is called the *Cushing response,* and when stimulated, it produces a rapid elevation in systemic blood pressure.

The Cushing response is an ischemic reflex that occurs when there is an increase in pressure within the cranial vault. Such an increase in pressure occurs when CSF pressure equals arterial pressures, thereby compressing cerebral vessels and cutting off the blood supply to the brain (Guyton, 1991). The purpose of this response is to maintain medullary perfusion, and it is mediated through the vagus nerve and the sympathetic system. When initiated, the Cushing response produces three significant changes in cardiorespiratory physiology. First, there is an increase in arterial pulse pressure that results from a rise in systolic blood pressure. With the increase in arterial pressure above that of the CSF, blood flow is reestablished to the ischemic area. Second, there is a decrease in heart rate. Third, there is a decrease in the respiratory rate (Simon & Sayre, 1987). The main goal in treating the Cushing response is to make a direct attempt to widen the CPP (Simon & Sayre, 1987).

Chemical control of CBF is achieved through alterations in the carbon dioxide, hydrogen, and oxygen concentrations. Increased levels of carbon dioxide (i.e., hypercapnia) and increased hydrogen ion concentrations (i.e., lactic acidosis) result in vasodilatation and increased CBF. In contrast, an increased oxygen concentration or decreased carbon dioxide level (hypocapnia) produces vasoconstriction and lowers the CBF.

Metabolic regulation is another mechanism that significantly affects arteriolar diameter and CBF. During ischemia, large amounts of *adenosine* are released, producing a powerful vasodilating effect. Adenosine levels have been shown to increase in response to falling CPP and increased cerebral metabolic rate of oxygen ($CMRO_2$) (Simon & Sayre, 1987). $CMRO_2$ is the rate of cerebral oxygen utilization during metabolism.

A number of clinical factors can alter CBF significantly. The factors that can produce a decrease in CBF include hypocapnia, hypothermia, and barbiturates. Clinical factors that increase CBF include seizures, fever, narcotics, hypoxia, and anesthetic agents such as halothane (Simon & Sayre, 1987).

Blood–Brain Barrier

The brain tissue is very sensitive to any changes in the concentration of ions. For the CNS to function normally, the brain's internal environment must be delicately balanced. This stable environment is accomplished by the blood–brain and blood–CSF barriers. These barriers are physiologic mechanisms that protect the homeostatic balance of the brain tissue by selective capillary permeability. The *blood–brain barrier* consists of a dense network of astroglial membranes and capillary endothelial cells that form tight junctions around the cerebral capillaries (Hickey, 1992). These tight junctions affect capillary permeability, thus providing selective permeability of substances that cross the neuronal membrane. The *blood–cerebrospinal fluid*

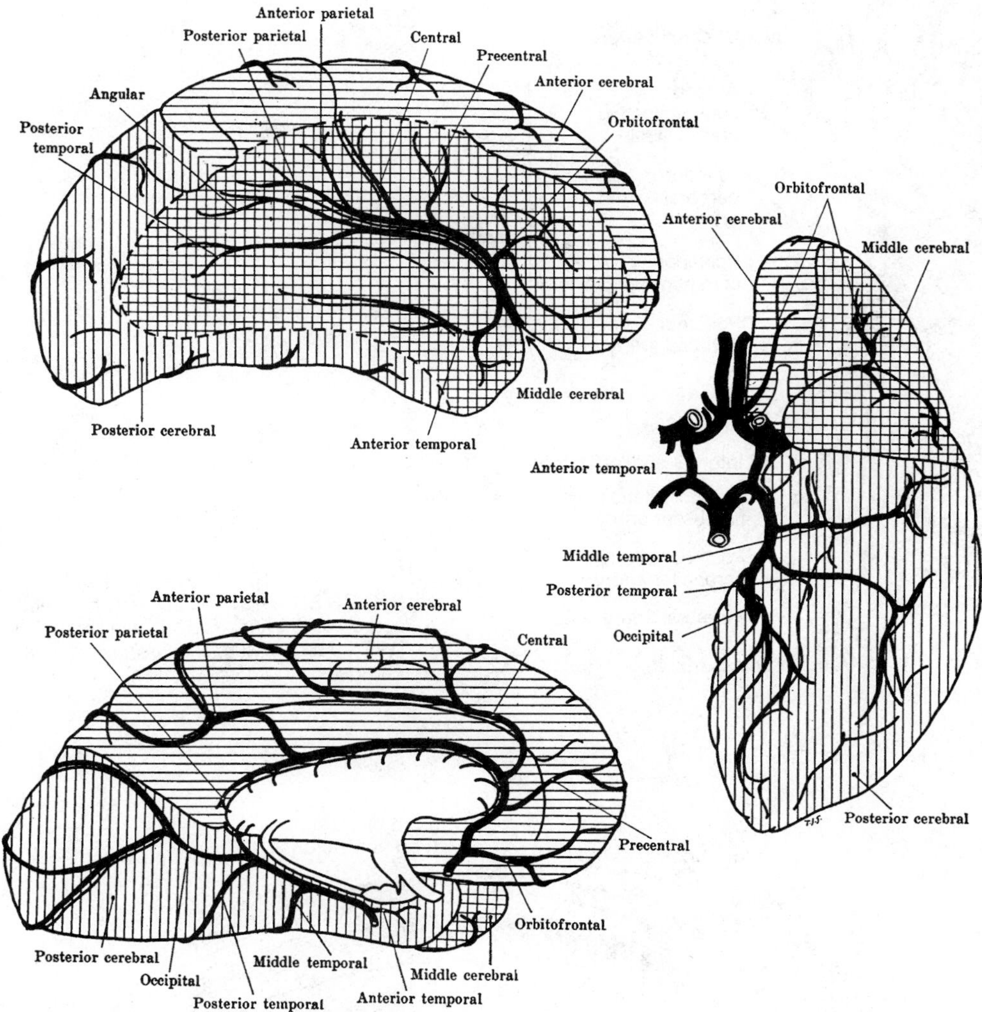

FIGURE 34–8. Diagram of areas of distribution of anterior, middle, and posterior cerebral arteries. (Reproduced by permission from: Mettler, F. A. *Neuroanatomy* [2nd ed.]. St. Louis, 1948, The C. V. Mosby Co.)

barrier is found in the choroid plexuses and also provides selective permeability of substances that gain entrance to the neuron (Hickey, 1992). Both the blood–brain and the blood–CSF barriers are permeable to oxygen, carbon dioxide, water, and glucose. These barriers are somewhat permeable to circulating electrolytes such as Na^+, Cl^-, and K^+, but are impermeable to many drugs, fixed acids, and bases.

Cerebrospinal Fluid

Cerebrospinal fluid is normally a clear, odorless, and colorless fluid that contains oxygen, carbon dioxide, glucose, electrolytes, small quantities of protein, and a few leukocytes. The purpose of the CSF is to protect and cushion the brain and spinal cord by acting as a shock absorber. In addition, the CSF participates in the nutrition and removal of metabolic wastes for the CNS.

CSF FORMATION. CSF is formed from three different sources. The primary source of CSF is the *choroid plexus,* which is a dense network of capillaries located in the lateral, third, and fourth ventricles (Fig. 34–10). The choroid plexus secretes approximately 500 to 750 mL of CSF daily; however, only 125 to 150 mL are present in the cerebral ventricular system at any given time. A smaller amount of CSF is formed by the *ependymal cells* that line the ventricles and meningeal blood vessels. The third source of CSF is the *blood vessels* of the brain and spinal cord (Hickey, 1992).

CSF FLOW. After the CSF is secreted, it passes through the two foramina of Monro to the third ventricle. From the third ventricle, the CSF flows slowly through the aqueduct of Sylvius to the fourth ventricle. The CSF then passes through the medial foramen of Magendie and the paired lateral foramina of Luschke to the cisternal magnum. It then enters the subarach-

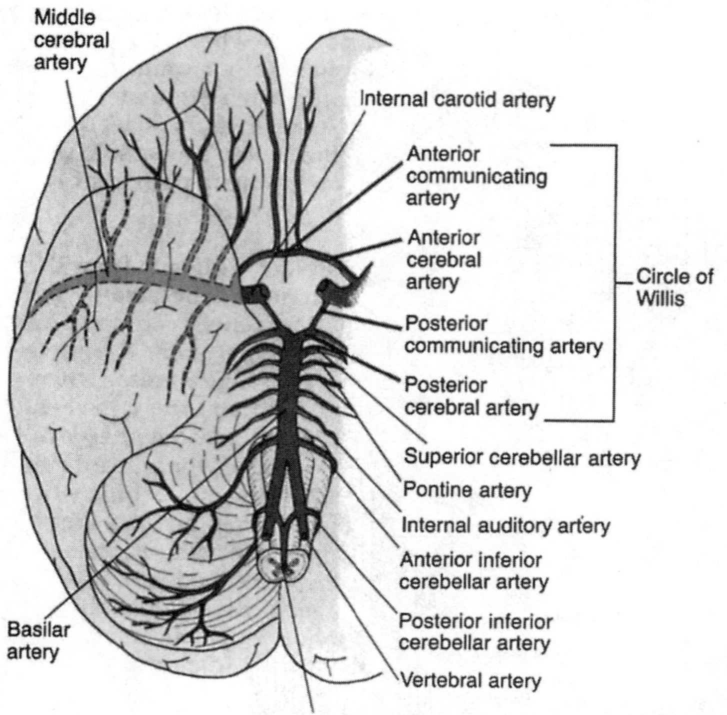

FIGURE 34–9. Diagram of principal cerebral arteries and circle of Willis. (From Ignatavicius, D. D., & Bayne, M. V. [1991]. *Medical-surgical nursing: A nursing process approach.* Philadelphia: W. B. Saunders.)

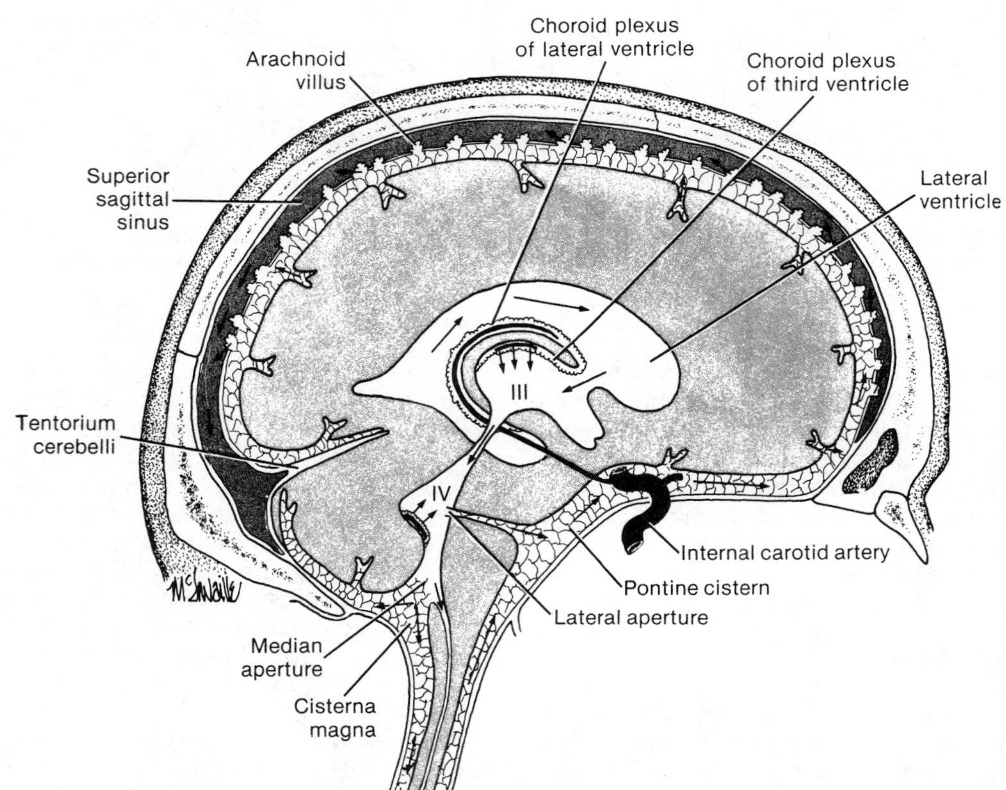

FIGURE 34–10. Path of circulation of cerebrospinal fluid from its formation in the ventricles to its absorption into the superior sagittal sinus. (Reproduced by permission from: Nolte, J. *The human brain* [2nd ed.]. St. Louis, 1988, The C. V. Mosby Co. Redrawn from Hamilton, W. J., ed.: *Textbook of human anatomy* [2nd ed.]. St. Louis, 1976, The C. V. Mosby Co. By permission of Macmillan Press, London and Basingstoke.)

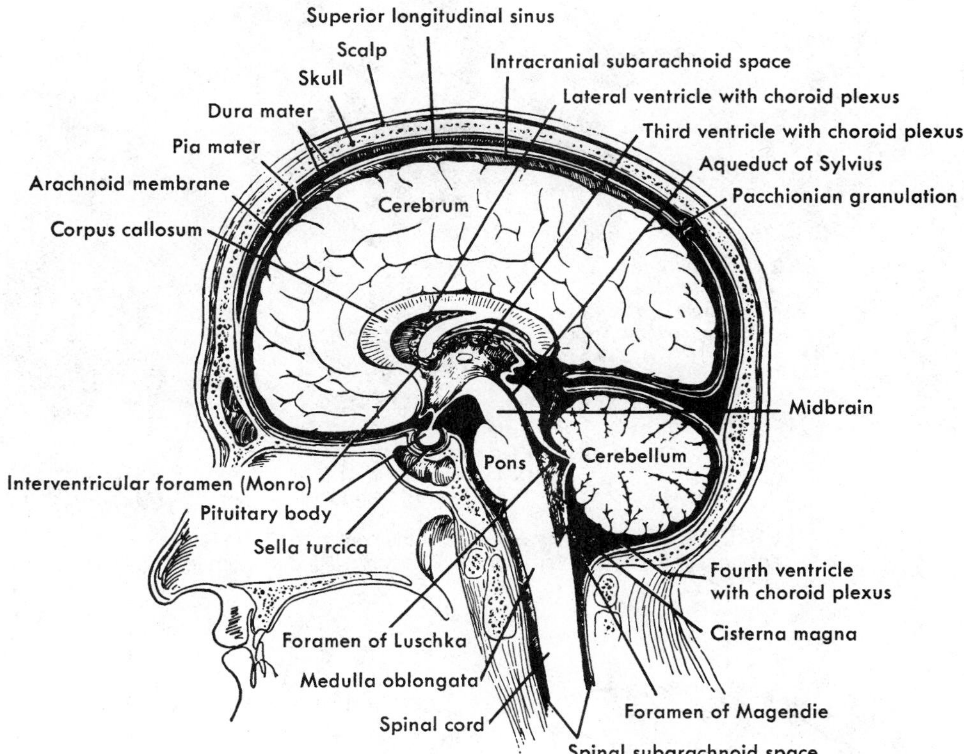

FIGURE 34–11. Sagittal section of the cerebrum. (Reproduced by permission from: Conway-Rutkowski, Barbara Lang: Carini and Owens' *Neurological and neurosurgical nursing*, ed. 8, St. Louis, 1982, The C. V. Mosby Co.)

noid space, where it slowly diffuses upward over the brain and fills the spinal cisterns.

CSF ABSORPTION. Most of the CSF is reabsorbed slowly from the subarachnoid space by the arachnoid villi. The *arachnoid villi* are clusterlike projections from the subarachnoid space into the venous sinuses. The CSF flows through the arachnoid villi into the venous sinuses and is reabsorbed into the venous system.

Cerebral Structures

BRAIN. The brain (Fig. 34–11) constitutes approximately 2% of body weight, receives approximately 20% of the cardiac output, and requires about 20% of the body's oxygen utilization. The brain (encephalon) can be divided into the three anatomic areas—cerebrum, brain stem, and cerebellum.

CEREBRUM. The cerebrum is the largest portion of the brain and consists of two cerebral hemispheres that are divided partially by the *great longitudinal fissure* (Fig. 34–12). The cerebral hemispheres are joined at the bottom of the great longitudinal fissure by a large tract of white commissural fibers, the *corpus callosum.* On the outside of the cerebrum are multiple layers of gray cells called the *cerebral cortex.* Internally, the cerebrum consists of a large number of myelinated nerve fibers and neuroglial cells collectively called the white matter. The major sulci (grooves) and fissures (deep grooves) of the cerebral cortex divide each hemisphere into four pairs of lobes that are named after the overlying cranial bones: frontal, parietal, temporal, and occipital (Fig. 34–12).

Certain areas of the cerebral cortex have been identified as having specific functions. In 1909, Brodmann developed a cytoarchitectural map of 47 primary and association function areas of the human cerebral cortex (Fig. 34–13). Primary function areas include those in which movement or perception of movement occurs. Association function areas surround the primary function areas and provide a higher level of integration for sensory experiences.

FRONTAL LOBES. The frontal lobes are located in the anterior fossa, extending from the front of each cerebral hemisphere to the fissure of Rolando. The function of the frontal lobe is related primarily to motor activity, psychic activity, and higher intellectual activities. Along with the thalamus and hypothalamus, the frontal lobes also control autonomic functions such as respiration, blood pressure, and gastrointestinal activity. Located at the inferior frontal gyrus is Broca's area. *Broca's area* is an association area (areas 44 and 45) that is involved in the formulation of words. When this area is damaged or destroyed, the individual can no longer speak in sentences (expressive aphasia).

PARIETAL LOBES. The parietal lobes lie in the middle fossa in the area between the fissure of Rolando and the parietooccipital fissure. The function of the parietal lobes is the processing of input to the primary sensory cortex. The primary sensory cortex is concerned with

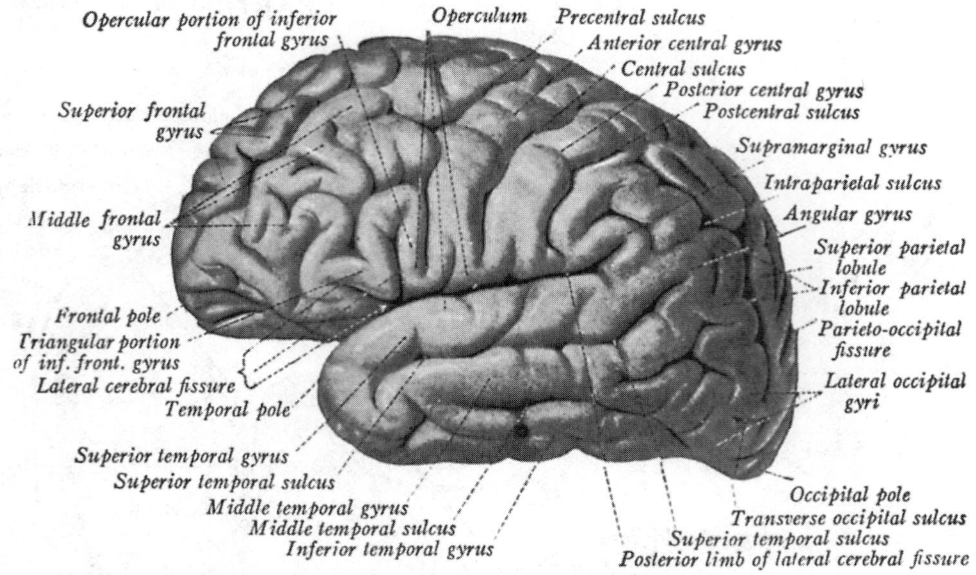

FIGURE 34–12. Lateral surface of the cerebrum. (From Ranson, S. W., & Clark, S. L. [1966]. *The anatomy of the nervous system: Its development and function* [p. 55]. Philadelphia: W. B. Saunders.)

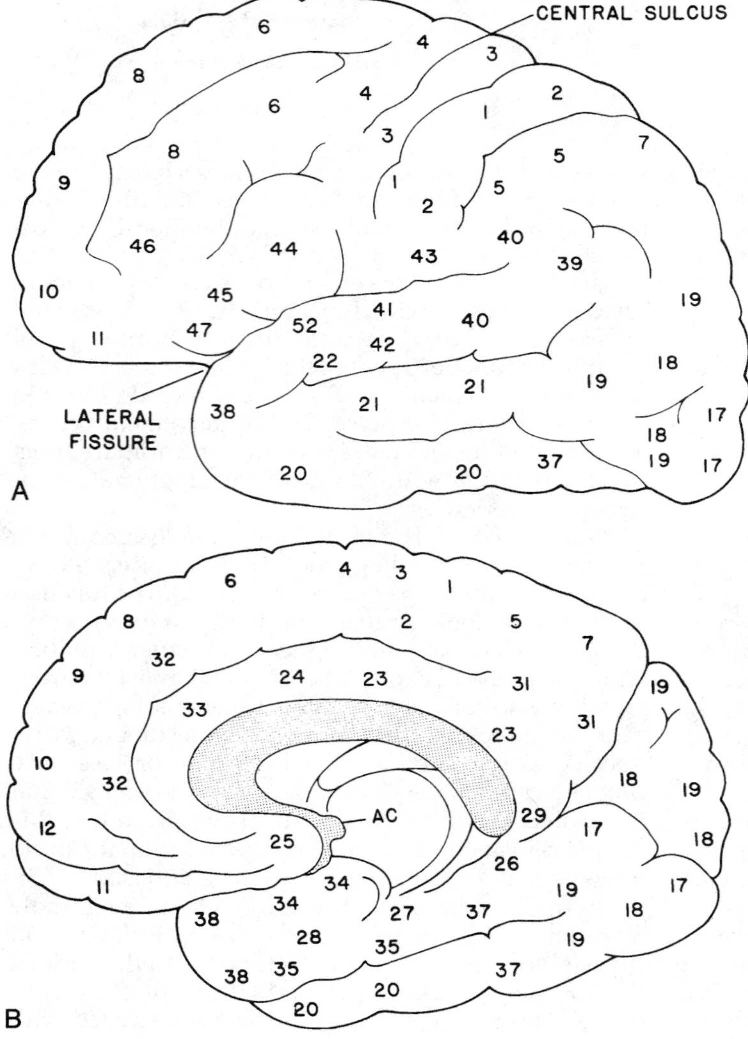

FIGURE 34–13. *A,* Lateral aspect of left cerebral hemisphere showing the cortical areas according to Brodmann. Area 8 = frontal eye movement, pupillary change area. Area 6 = premotor area (portion of extrapyramidal system). Area 4 (precentral gyrus) = primary motor area. Areas 3, 2, 1 (postcentral gyrus) = primary sensory areas. Areas 5, 6, 7 = secondary sensory association areas. Areas 39, 40 = association areas. Areas 18, 19 = visual association areas. Area 17 = primary visual cortex. Area 41 = primary auditory cortex. Area 42 = associative auditory cortex. Area 44 = motor speech area of Broca. *B,* Medical aspect of left cerebral hemisphere showing the cortical areas according to Brodmann. Functions of specific areas are given in the legend to part *A.* AC = anterior commissure. Shaded area indicates the corpus callosum. (From Jensen, D. [1980]. *The principles of physiology* [2nd ed., pp. 229–230]. New York: Appleton-Century-Crofts.)

the gross aspects of sensation and sends input of its interpretation to the thalamus and other cortical structures (Hickey, 1992). The association areas of the parietal lobes are specific to shape, texture, size, and consistency of objects; comprehension of written words; and the ability to discriminate between two simultaneous skin contacts (Rudy, 1984).

TEMPORAL LOBES. The temporal lobes are located in the middle fossa. They lie inferior to the fissure of Sylvius and extend back to the parietooccipital fissure. Primary functions of the temporal lobes are memory storage and hearing. Located in the temporal lobe is an auditory association area called *Wernicke's area.* If Wernicke's area is damaged or destroyed, the individual is unable to understand the meaning of spoken words (receptive aphasia).

OCCIPITAL LOBES. The occipital lobes lie in the middle fossa, just above the cerebellum and posterior to the parietooccipital fissure. The occipital lobes contain the primary vision cortex and the visual association areas. Damage or destruction of the visual association areas will result in an ability to see objects clearly but an inability to recognize or identify those objects (visual agnosia).

LIMBIC LOBES. Anatomically, the limbic lobes are part of the temporal lobes; however, they do have a separate function. The limbic lobes are concerned with visceral activities, self-preservation, moods, and emotions. The limbic lobes also are referred to as the *rhinencephalon.*

BASAL GANGLIA. The basal ganglia are a group of gray nuclei that lie deep within each cerebral hemisphere. The basal ganglia provide a vital subcortical link between the cerebral cortex and the motor cortex (Schmidt, 1985). Paired structures of the basal ganglia include the caudate nucleus, the lenticular nucleus, the amygdaloid body, and the claustrum. Functions of the basal ganglia include the initiation and execution of fine motor movements.

COMMISSURAL FIBERS. Commissural, or interhemispheric, fibers connect the cerebral hemispheres with each other and maintain higher sensory and motor functions of the cortex (Rudy, 1984). Commissural fibers consist of the *corpus callosum, commissure of the fornix, anterior commissure,* and the *habenular commissure.* The largest of these connective pathways is the corpus callosum, which connects every area of one cerebral hemisphere with the corresponding area in the other hemisphere. The connection of the two sides of the brain by the corpus callosum prevents interference between the two hemispheres and ensures coordinated and complementary motor responses and thoughts (Guyton, 1991).

HEMISPHERIC DOMINANCE. The term *hemispheric dominance* refers to the fact that the interpretative functions of the angular gyrus and the temporal lobe are developed more highly in one or the other of the cerebral hemispheres. At birth, both of these regions have almost the same capacity for development. However, Wernicke's area in the left hemisphere is as much as 50% larger in more than half of newborn babies. Because the left side is larger, the temporal lobe in this hemisphere begins to be used to a greater extent than the right (Guyton, 1991). Since the rate of learning occurs much faster in the better developed hemisphere, there is a tendency to continue to direct attention to that hemisphere, resulting in hemispheric dominance. In approximately 90% to 95% of the population, the temporal lobe and the angular gyrus of the left cerebral hemisphere become dominant. In the remaining 10%, there is dual dominance, or, in rare cases, the right side becomes the dominant hemisphere (Guyton, 1991).

DIENCEPHALON. The oval-shaped diencephalon (Fig. 34–14) is a major division of the cerebrum and consists of the epithalamus, thalamus, hypothalamus, and subthalamus. The internal capsule and pituitary gland (hypophysis) also are located in the area of the diencephalon.

EPITHALAMUS. The epithalamus is located in the most dorsal area of the diencephalon and consists of the pineal body, habenula, habenular commissure, posterior commissure, and striae medullares. The most important structure in the epithalamus is the *pineal body,* which is believed to have a role in growth and sexual development. The epithalamus also is believed to have a role in the primitive reflex of getting food (Hickey, 1992).

THALAMUS. The thalamus also is located in the dorsal portion of the diencephalon and is composed of two connected ovoid masses of gray matter located deep within each cerebral hemisphere. The thalamus essentially is the "main entrance" for all sensory input (except that from the olfactory system) to the cerebral cortex (Guyton, 1991). As such, the thalamus is in-

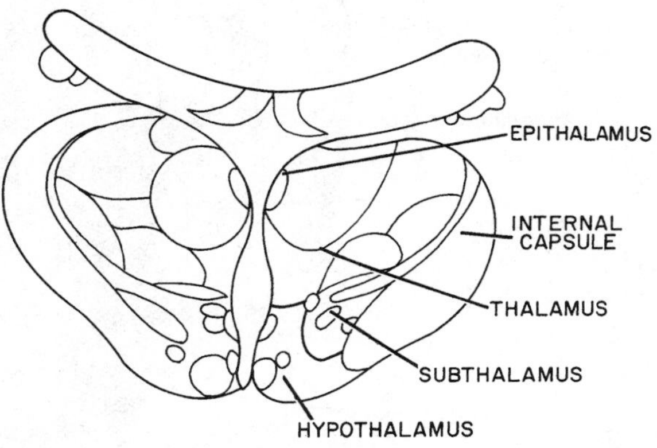

FIGURE 34–14. Diencephalon. Cross-section of the brain stem at the diencephalic level. (From B. Curtis, et al.: *An introduction to the neurosciences.* Philadelphia: Lea & Febiger, 1977. Reprinted with permission.)

volved intricately in several important functions including direction of attention to specific areas of one's mental environment, the sleep-wake cycle, and influence on voluntary movements and motor responses.

HYPOTHALAMUS. The hypothalamus is located under the thalamus, forming the floor and parts of the walls of the third cerebral ventricle. The hypothalamus functionally is the most important efferent pathway by which the limbic system controls many of the essential functions of the body (Guyton, 1991). These functions include:

1. Regulation of body temperature
2. Regulation of body water by controlling water excretion into the urine and creation of the thirst sensation
3. Control of appetite
4. Control of secretions of the pituitary gland such as corticotropin, thyrotropin, luteinizing hormone, and follicle-stimulating hormone
5. Regulation of uterine contractility and expelling of breast milk
6. Cardiovascular regulation including increased or decreased blood pressure, and increased or decreased heart rate
7. Subcortical regulation of somatic and visual activities of the autonomic nervous system
8. Influence on the sleep-wake cycle, motivation, learning, and sexual behavior

SUBTHALAMUS. The subthalamus is located between the tegmentum of the midbrain and the dorsal part of the thalamus. The functions of the subthalamus are related closely to those of the basal ganglia.

PITUITARY GLAND. The pituitary gland (or hypophysis) lies in the sella turcica at the base of the brain and is directly above the sphenoid air sinus and slightly anterior to the optic chiasm. The pituitary gland is connected to the hypothalamus by the *hypophyseal stalk.* Structurally, the gland is divided into two major lobes, the *anterior pituitary lobe* and the *posterior pituitary lobe.* The anterior lobe secretes seven major hormones: (1) growth hormone, (2) prolactin, (3) adrenocorticotropin, (4) thyroid-stimulating hormone, (5) follicle-stimulating hormone, (6) luteinizing hormone, and (7) melanin-stimulating hormone. The posterior pituitary lobe stores oxytocin and antidiuretic hormone.

INTERNAL CAPSULE. Located deep in the region of the thalamus and hypothalamus is a dense mass of white matter called the internal capsule. This area is called

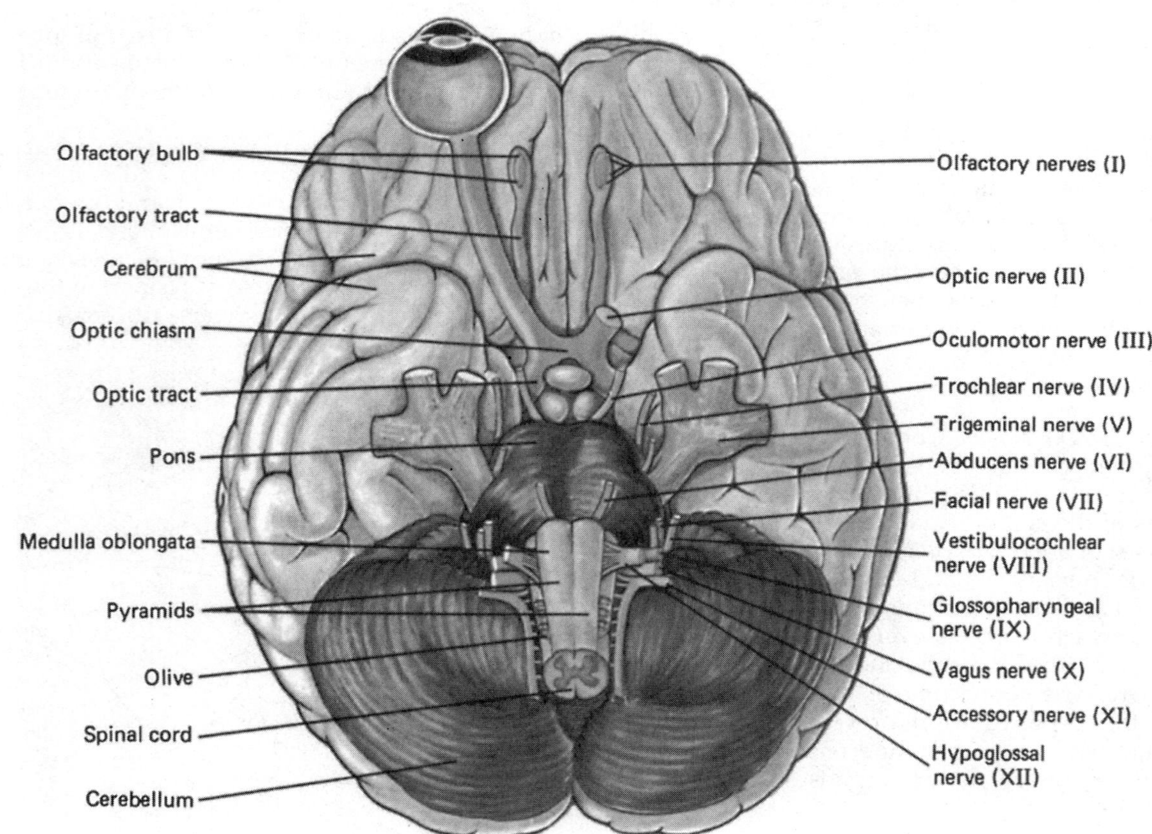

FIGURE 34–15. Anterior brain stem showing the cranial nerves. (From Guyton, A. C. [1987]. *Basic neuroscience.* Philadelphia: W. B. Saunders.)

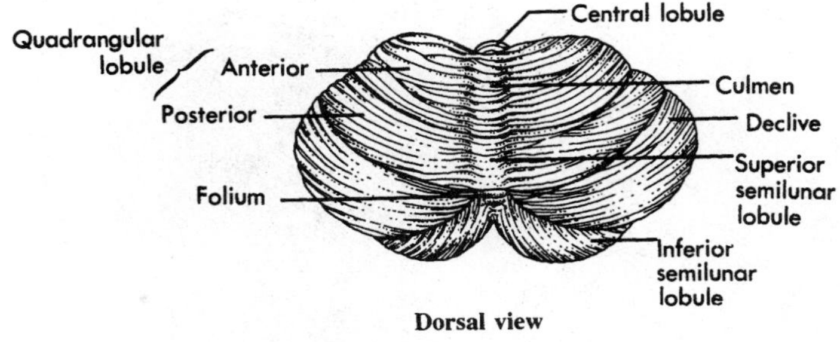

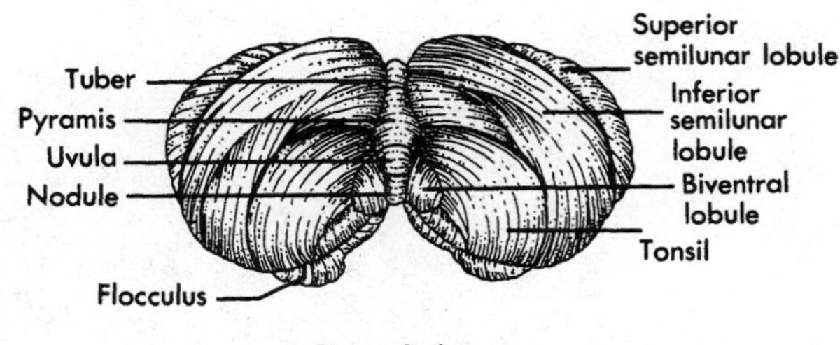

FIGURE 34–16. Cerebellum. (Reproduced by permission from: *Mosby's medical and nursing dictionary,* ed. 2, St. Louis, 1986, The C. V. Mosby Co.)

a capsule because of the way the pyramidal and other tracts essentially encapsulate the thalamus as they pass between it and the basal ganglia (Schmidt, 1985). Damage to the structures of the internal capsule may result in the stroke syndrome due to the blockage of conduction in motor pathways.

Brain Stem

The brain stem (Fig. 34–15) consists of the midbrain, pons, and medulla oblongata. Overall, the purpose of the brain stem is control of involuntary reflexes necessary for maintaining vital functions.

MIDBRAIN. The midbrain, or mesencephalon, lies between the diencephalon and the pons. The top of the midbrain is made up of four rounded elevations called the *corpora quadrigeminal.* The superior pair of colliculi control eye tracking, whereas the posterior pair of colliculi have a role in the auditory system. Cranial nerves III (oculomotor) and IV (trochlear) emanate from the midbrain. The lower surface of the midbrain consists of two fiber bundles called the *crura cerebri.* These bundles are composed of the corticospinal, corticopontine, and corticobulbar tracts of the voluntary nervous system. The primary functions of the midbrain are the relay of stimuli between the cerebrum and the lower brain, and central control of auditory and visual reflexes.

PONS. The pons (metencephalon) lies between the midbrain and the medulla. The pons contains cranial nerve V (trigeminal), and three other cranial nerves (VI, abducens; VII, facial; and VIII, acoustic) originate at the pons–medulla junction. The white matter of the pons is made up of the corticobulbar and corticospinal tracts.

MEDULLA OBLONGATA. The medulla, or myelencephalon, is located directly under the pons and is continuous with the spinal cord at the foramen magnum. The medulla contains cranial nerves IX (glossopharyn-

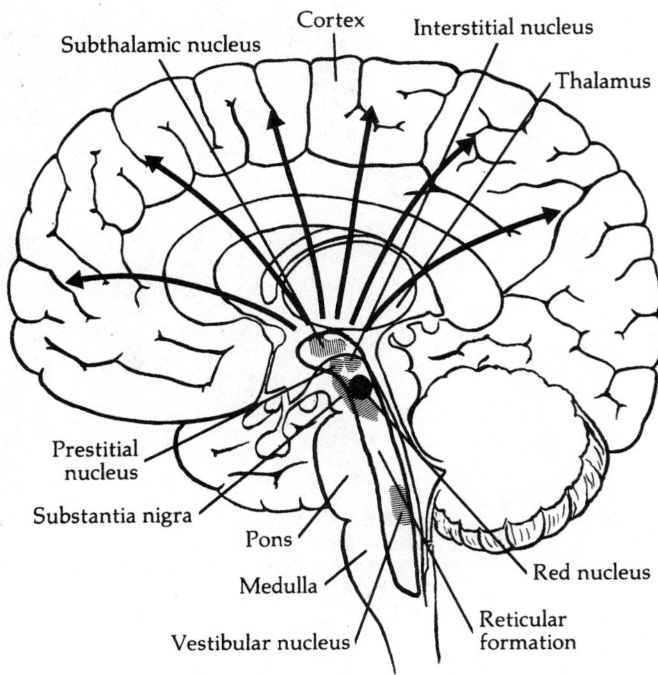

FIGURE 34–17. Reticular activating system. (Reproduced by permission from: Thompson, J. M., et al. *Mosby's manual of clinical nursing,* ed. 2, St. Louis, 1989, The C. V. Mosby Co.)

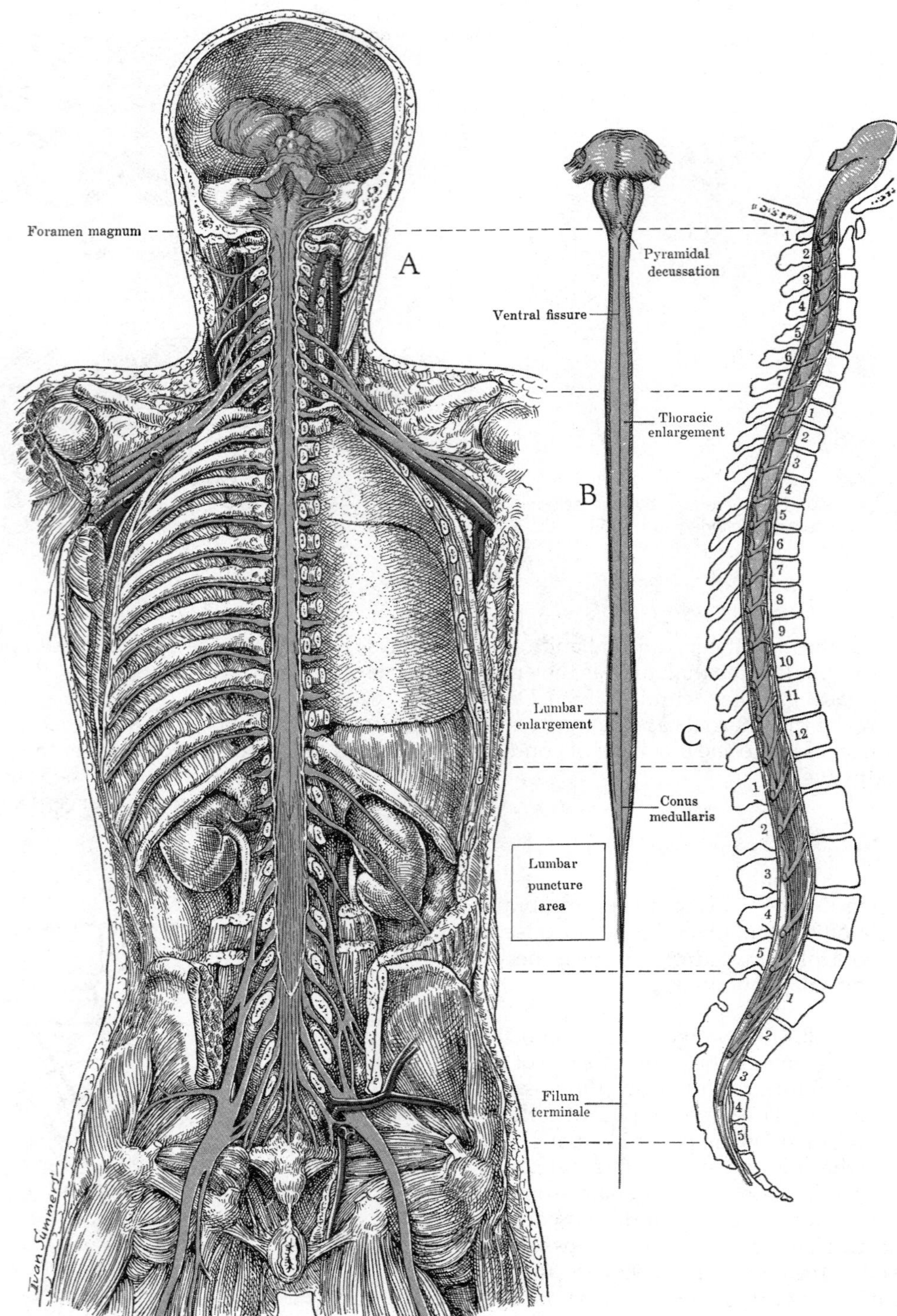

FIGURE 34–18. *A,* Posterior view of brain stem and spinal cord in situ with spinal nerves and plexuses. *B,* Anterior view of brain stem and spinal cord. *C,* Lateral view, showing relationship of spinal cord to vertebrae. (Reproduced by permission from: Mettler, F. A. *Neuroanatomy* [2nd ed.]. St. Louis, 1948, The C. V. Mosby Co.)

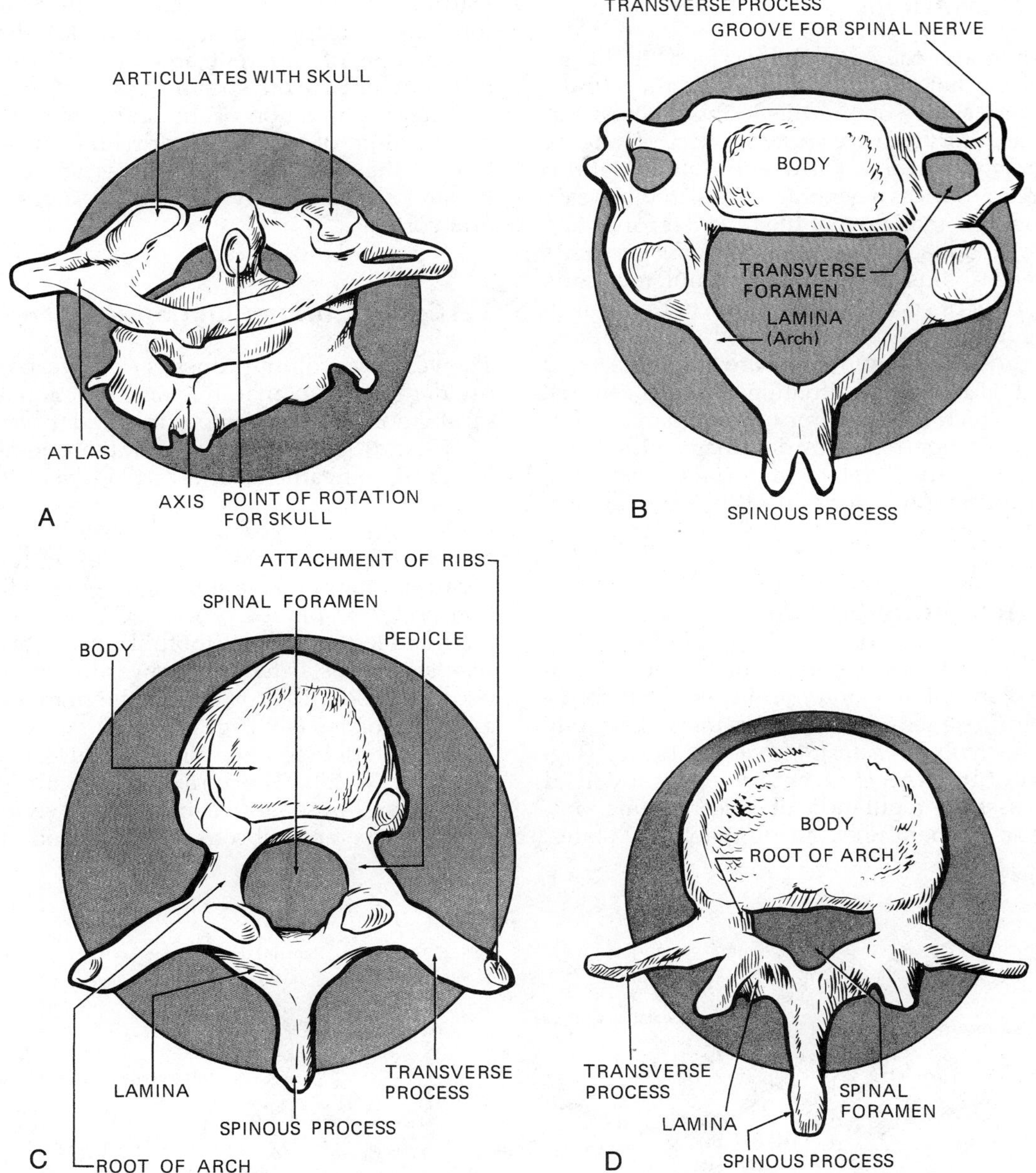

FIGURE 34–19. Types of vertebrae. *A,* Cervical vertebrae. *B,* Atlas and axis. *C,* Thoracic vertebrae. *D,* Lumbar vertebra. (From Snyder, M., & Jackle, M. [1981]. *Neurologic problems: A critical care nursing focus.* Bowie, MD: Robert J. Brady.)

geal), X (vagus), XI (spinal accessory), and XII (hypoglossal). The decussation (crossover) of the pyramidal tract forms a ridge on either side of the median fissure in the medulla. Functionally, the medulla contains important involuntary reflex centers for breathing, sneezing, coughing, swallowing, salivating, vomiting, and vasoconstriction.

Cerebellum

The *cerebellum* (Fig. 34–16) is separated from the cerebrum by the tentorium cerebelli and is connected to the midbrain, medulla, and pons by three pairs of *cerebellar peduncles.* It consists of two lateral hemispheres and a middle section called the *vermis.* The outer covering is composed of a cortex of gray matter, and the inner medulla consists of white matter. Deep within the white matter are four pairs of cerebellar nuclei: *dentate, emboliform, globose,* and *fastigial.* These nuclei receive input from the cerebellar cortex and all sensory afferent tracts to the cerebellum. The major function of the cerebellum is the monitoring and corrective adjustment of motor activities elicited by other parts of the brain (Guyton, 1991).

Reticular Formation

Located throughout the entire brain stem are diffuse areas of neurons that collectively are called the *reticular formation.* The majority of neurons in the reticular formation are excitatory and are known collectively as the *bulboreticular facilatory area.* Diffuse stimulation of this facilatory area produces a general or localized increase in muscle tone. A small area of the reticular formation in the lower medulla, the *bulboreticular inhibitory area,* decreases general muscle tone when stimulated (Guyton, 1991). Under normal circumstances, both the facilitory and inhibitory areas are activated, and therefore the spinal cord's motor functions are neither excited nor inhibited. However, in situations such as cerebral infarction, in which the inhibitory area is damaged or destroyed, facilitation becomes dominant with resultant muscle spasticity. Another important function of the reticular formation is support of the body against gravity.

Reticular Activating System

Extending from the lower portion of the brain stem through the diencephalon and into the cerebral cortex are multiple diffuse sensory pathways that collectively are called the *reticular activating system* (RAS) (Fig. 34–17). Most of the RAS is excitatory and is involved in the processes of regulation of visceral functions; consciousness; temperature control; emotional states; learning; regulation of skeletal muscle activity and tone; and perception of sensory stimuli (Jensen, 1980). Stimulation of different areas of the RAS produces different effects on specific parts of the brain. For example, stimulation of the brain stem (mesencephalic) portion of the RAS provides intrinsic activation of the whole brain, whereas stimulation of the thalamic portion activates specific areas of the cerebral cortex.

Vertebral Column and Spinal Cord

The vertebral column consists of 33 vertebrae that are divided into five anatomic and functional areas: cervical, thoracic, lumbar, sacral, and coccygeal (Figs. 34–18 and 34–19). The vertebrae are joined together by multiple ligaments and cartilage pads called intervertebral discs.

The first two cervical vertebrae differ from the other cervical vertebrae. C1 is referred to as the *atlas* because it supports the skull and does not have a vertebral body or spinous process. C2, or the *axis,* also is modified in that it has a toothlike projection called the *odontoid process,* extending upward from the vertebral body. The odontoid process is the point on which the atlas articulates (see Fig. 34–19).

Most vertebrae have similar anatomic characteristics (Fig. 34–20). The *vertebral body* supports weight bearing and is separated from other vertebral bodies by cartilage and fibrous tissue called *intervertebral*

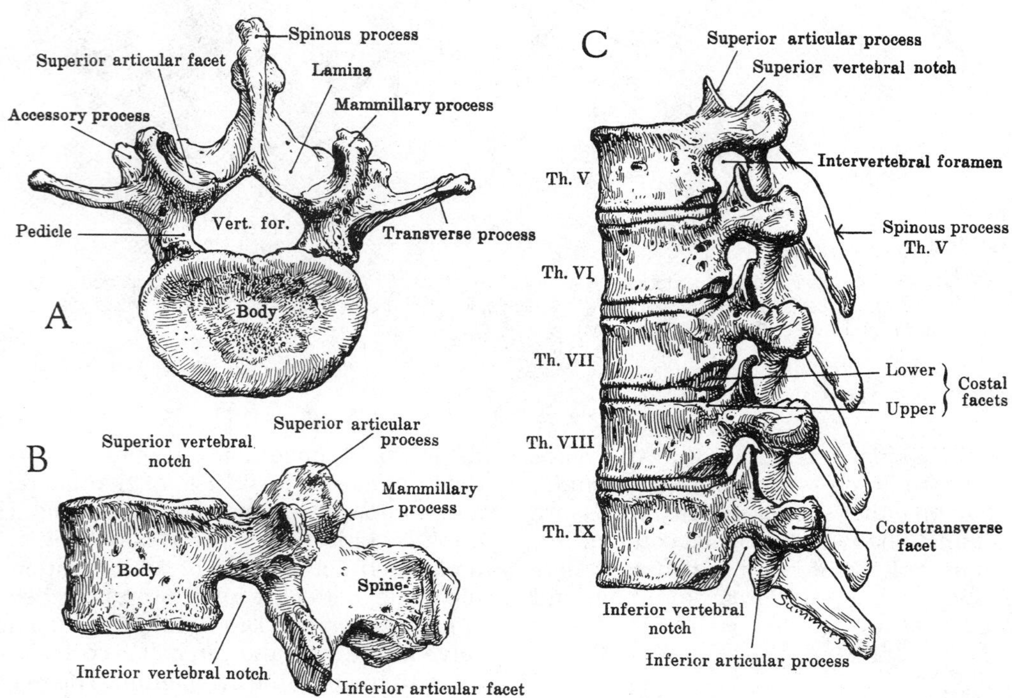

FIGURE 34–20. Vertebral anatomy. *A,* Fourth lumbar vertebra from above. *B,* Fourth lumbar vertebra from side. *C,* Fifth to ninth thoracic vertebrae showing relationships of various parts. (Reproduced by permission from Mettler, Fred A.: *Neuroanatomy* [2nd ed.] St. Louis, 1948, The C. V. Mosby Co.)

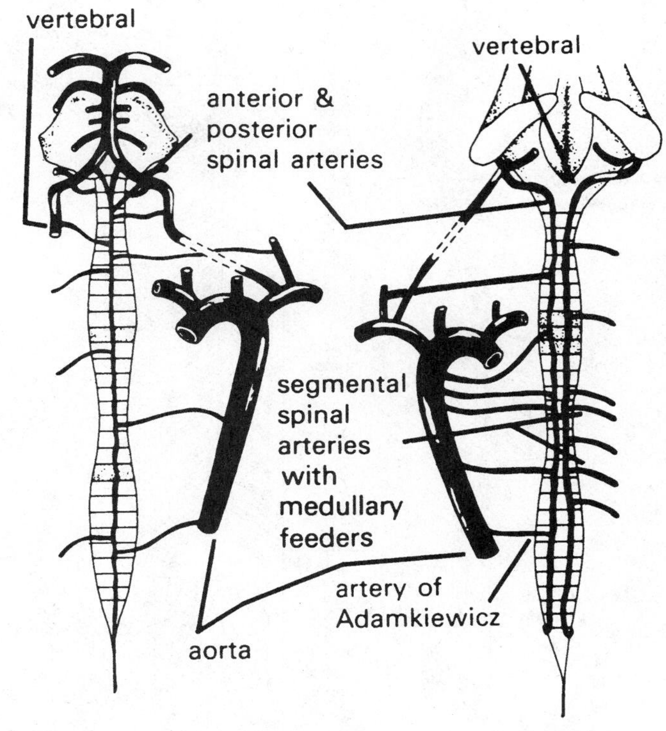

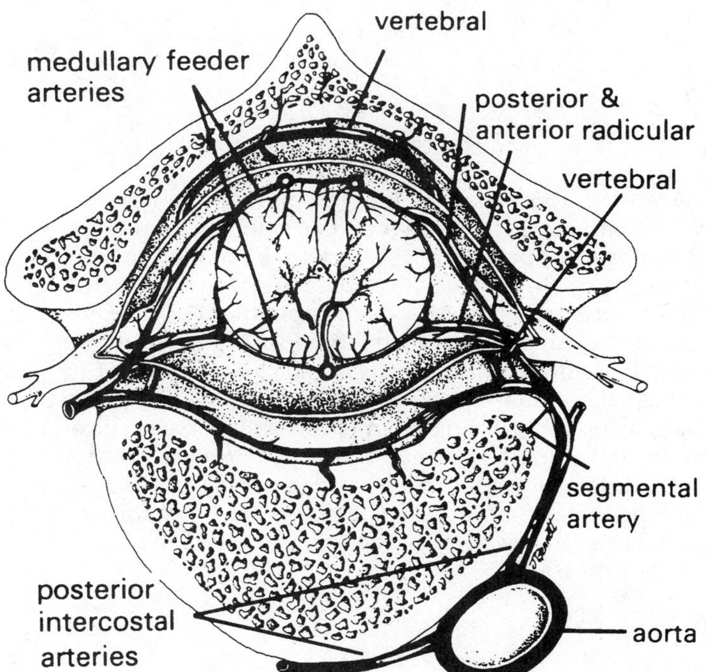

FIGURE 34–21. Vascular supply of the spinal cord. (From Romero-Sierra, C. [1986]. *Neuroanatomy: A conceptual approach.* New York: Churchill Livingstone.)

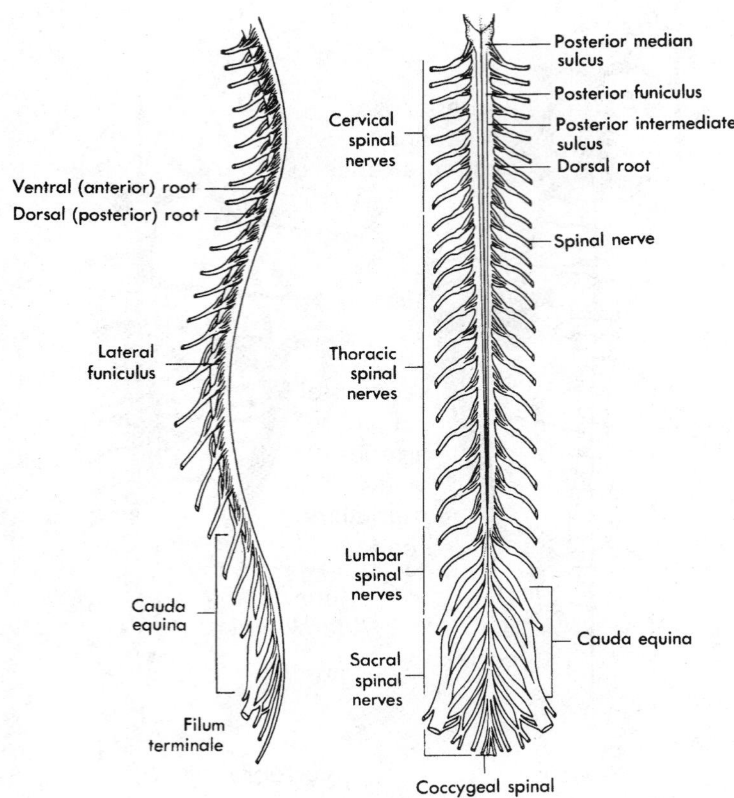

FIGURE 34–22. Two views of gross anatomy of the spinal cord. (Reproduced by permission from: *Mosby's medical and nursing dictionary*, ed. 2, St. Louis, 1986, The C. V. Mosby Co.)

discs. The dorsal part of the vertebrae is the *vertebral arch* that is formed by two pedicles and two laminae. The posterior portion of the vertebrae is called the *spinous process.* In the middle of the vertebrae is the *vertebral foramen.* This foramen is the opening that contains the spinal cord and spinal meninges. A portion of the vertebral foramen, the *vertebral notch,* is the point at which the spinal nerves and blood vessels leave the spinal cord. Extending from either side of each vertebrae are the *transverse processes,* which provide sites for articulation of adjacent vertebrae and for attachment of ligaments and muscles. The *pedicle* is a bony connection between the body of the vertebrae and the transverse process.

SPINAL MENINGES. Like the brain, the spinal cord is surrounded by three meningeal coverings: dura mater, arachnoid, and pia mater. The spinal *dura mater* extends from the cranial dura to the second sacral vertebra, where it fuses with the filum terminale. The dura also covers the roots of the spinal nerves. The second spinal meningeal layer, the *arachnoid,* extends from the foramen magnum to the lower surfaces of the cauda equina and the filum terminale. The spinal arachnoid also covers the spinal nerve roots to the point where they exit the vertebral canal. Between the arachnoid and innermost meningeal layer is the *subarachnoid space,* which contains a delicate network of cells and CSF. The third meningeal layer is the *pia mater.* The

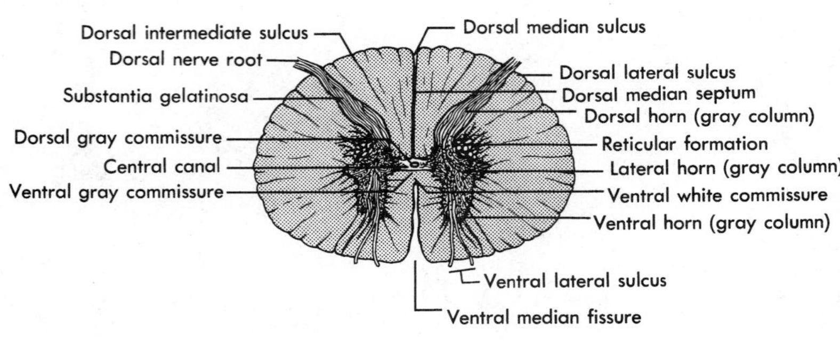

FIGURE 34–23. Cross-section of the spinal cord. (Reproduced by permission from: *Mosby's medical and nursing dictionary*, St. Louis, 1983, The C. V. Mosby Co.)

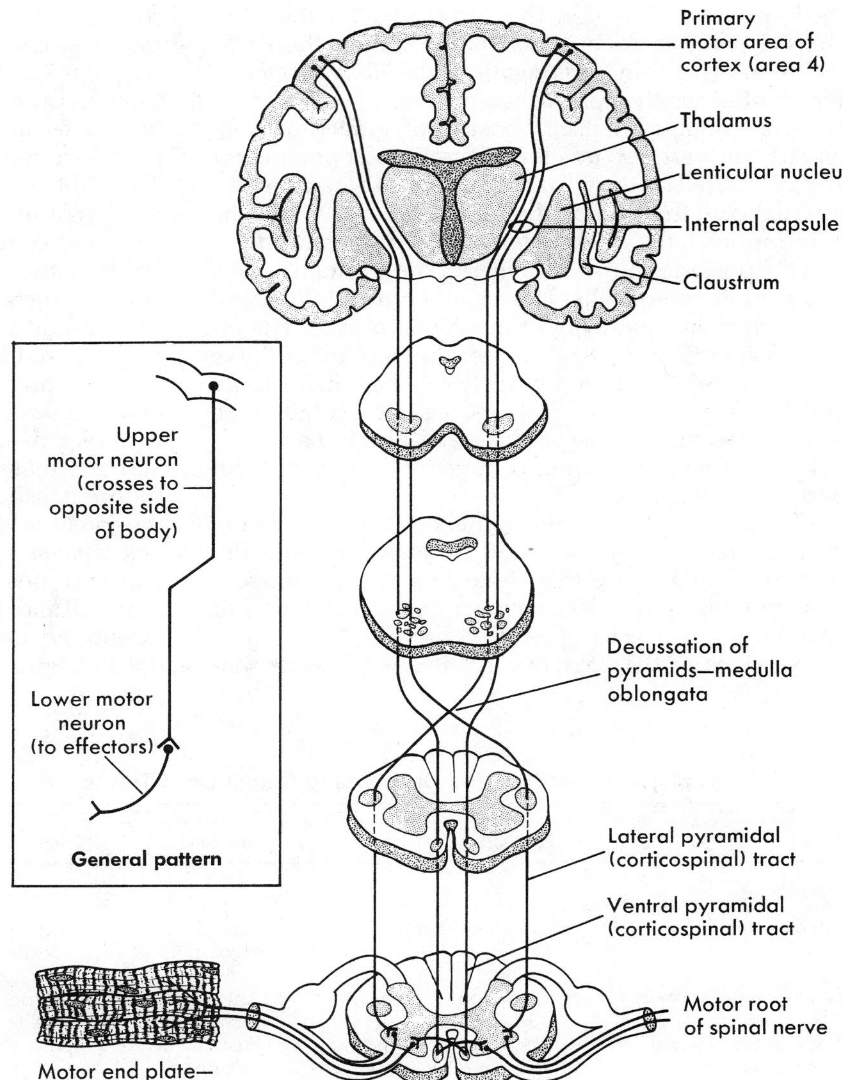

FIGURE 34–24. Pyramidal tracts. Upper motor neurons cross to muscles on opposite side of body. Lateral pyramidal tracts cross high at decussation in medulla oblongata. Ventral tracts cross low. (Reproduced by permission from: Conway-Rutkowski, B. L. *Neurological and neurosurgical nursing* [8th ed.]. St. Louis, 1982, The C. V. Mosby Co.)

fibrous pia mater extends to the filum terminale, where it is attached by denticulate ligaments to the dura mater between the spinal nerve roots.

SPINAL VASCULAR SUPPLY. The primary supply of blood to the spinal cord is provided by the *vertebral artery* and small *spinal arteries* (Fig. 34–21). The spinal arteries enter the intervertebral foramina at successive vertebral levels and divide into a number of *anterior* and *posterior radicular arteries.*

Three longitudinal arteries, the *anterior* and two *posterior spinal arteries,* supply the entire spinal cord. The anterior spinal artery is formed by the fusion of two branches of the vertebral artery at the level of the foramen magnum. Small branches of the anterior spinal artery enter the gray and white matter of the spinal cord and join together in the anterior median fissure to form the anterior central artery. The two posterior spinal arteries have many tiny branches that enter the spinal cord and help to form the posterior central artery (Rudy, 1984).

There are a number of venous plexuses extending along the entire inside and outside of the vertebral canal. Outside the vertebral column, venous plexuses receive blood from the spinous processes, vertebral bodies, facets, laminae, and surrounding muscles. Inside the canal, venous plexuses located between the dura and vertebral surfaces receive blood from the spinal matter and nearby bony structures. A series of venous rings are formed from these venous plexuses at each vertebral level. Blood from the internal and external plexuses drains into the intervertebral veins that exit the canal through the intervertebral foramina.

Intradural veins of the spinal cord follow the general distribution pattern of the spinal arteries and form the *anterior* and *posterior radicular veins.* Blood from the radicular veins and the two venous plexuses at each vertebral level drain into the *intervertebral vein.*

SPINAL CORD. The spinal cord (Fig. 34–22), which originates at the foramen magnum, is essentially a downward continuation of the medulla oblongata. In the lower thoracic region, the cord tapers into the cone-shaped *conus medullaris.* Extending below the *conus medullaris* is a thin prolongation, the *filum terminale,* which attaches the cord to the coccyx.

The spinal cord itself consists of gray (unmyelinated) and white (myelinated) microscopic matter (Fig. 34–23). The gray matter is concentrated into an internal core that can be divided functionally into the anterior horn, the intermediate zone and lateral horn, and the posterior horn. The *anterior horn* contains alpha and gamma motor cells. These cells constitute the final common motor pathway of the spinal nerves. The *intermediate zone* and *lateral horn* of the gray matter give rise to the preganglionic *sympathetic* fibers in T1 to L2 and L3. At the level of S2 to S4, cell bodies give rise to the preganglionic *parasympathetic* fibers. The *posterior horn* of the gray matter contains sensory cells from peripheral neurons.

The white matter of the spinal cord surrounds the gray matter, and is composed of ascending and descending spinal tracts that serve as pathways for sensory and motor impulses between the spinal cord and brain.

Neurons of the *ascending* pathways transmit sensory impulses from peripheral receptors (i.e., skin, muscles, and tendons) to the spinal cord and brain (Fig. 34–24). The sensory pathway is made up of a three-neuron chain. The cell body of the first neuron originates in the spinal ganglion and conducts impulses from the peripheral receptors to the spinal cord. The cell body of the second neuron occurs at different levels within the gray matter of the brain and spinal cord and conducts impulses to the thalamus. The cell body of the third neuron is located in the thalamus and conducts sensory impulses from the thalamus to the cerebral cortex. The major ascending pathways are summarized in Table 34–1.

Descending pathways consist of two primary types of neurons: upper motor neurons and lower motor neurons (Fig. 34–25). *Upper motor neurons,* which originate and terminate within the CNS, transmit impulses from the brain to the motor neurons in the anterior horn cell of the spinal cord and motor neurons in the cranial nerves. *Lower motor neurons* constitute the final common pathway and consist of motor neurons in the anterior spinal horn cell and motor nuclei of the cranial nerves. The major subdivisions of the descending tracts are the pyramidal and extrapyramidal pathways (Table 34–1).

TABLE 34–1. **Major Ascending and Descending Spinal Cord Tracts**

Name	Function	Location	Origin*	Termination†
Ascending				
Lateral spinothalamic	Pain, temperature and crude touch opposite side	Lateral white columns	Posterior gray column opposite side	Thalamus
Ventral spinothalamic	Crude touch, pain, and temperature	Anterior white columns	Posterior gray column opposite side	Thalamus
Fasciculi gracilis and cuneatus	Discriminating touch and pressure sensations, including vibration, stereognosis, and two-point discrimination; also conscious kinesthesia	Posterior white columns	Spinal ganglia same side	Medulla
Spinocerebellar	Unconscious kinesthesia	Lateral white columns	Posterior gray column	Cerebellum
Descending				
Lateral corticospinal (or crossed pyramidal)	Voluntary movement, contraction of individual or small groups of muscles, particularly those moving hands, fingers, feet, and toes of opposite side	Lateral white columns	Motor areas of cerebral cortex (mainly areas 4 and 6) opposite side from tract location in cord	Intermediate or anterior gray columns
Ventral corticospinal (direct pyramidal)	Same as lateral corticospinal except mainly muscles of same side	Lateral white columns	Motor cortex but on same side as tract location in cord	Intermediate or anterior gray columns
Lateral reticulospinal	Mainly facilitory influence on motor neurons to skeletal muscles	Lateral white columns	Reticular formation, midbrain, pons, and medulla	Intermediate or anterior gray columns
Medial reticulospinal	Mainly inhibitory influence on motor neurons to skeletal muscles	Anterior white columns	Reticular formation, medulla mainly	Intermediate or anterior gray columns

*Location of cell bodies of neurons from which axons of tract arise.

†Structure in which axons of tracts terminate.

Reproduced by permission from Anthony, C. P., & Thibodeau, G. M. *Textbook of anatomy and physiology* (12th ed.). St. Louis, 1987, The C. V. Mosby Co.

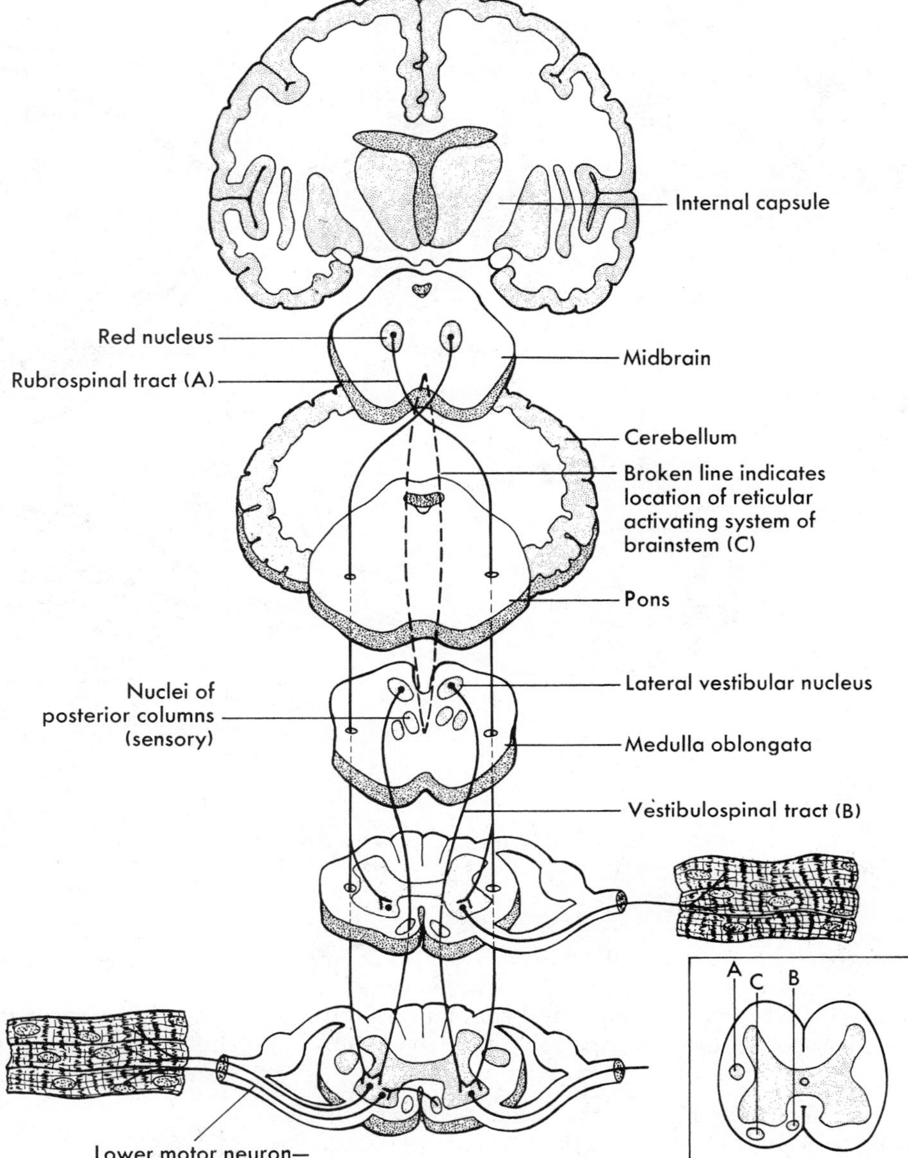

FIGURE 34–25. Extrapyramidal descending tracts. Upper motor neurons originate below level of cortex and converge on lower motor neurons (final common pathway) along with upper motor neurons of pyramidal tracts. *A,* Rubrospinal tract originates in the red nucleus of the midbrain, crosses immediately, and descends contralaterally in opposite cord. *B,* Vestibulospinal tract originates in vestibular nucleus of medulla oblongata and descends ipsilaterally. *C,* Reticulospinal tracts (medial and lateral) originate from reticular activating system of brain stem and descend in general area of *C.* (These are not so well organized as others are.) Interconnections between basal nuclei, midbrain, diencephalon, and cerebellum are extensive. (Reproduced by permission from: Conway-Rutkowski, B. L. *Neurological and neurosurgical nursing* [8th ed.]. St. Louis, 1982, The C. V. Mosby Co.)

REFLEXES. The reflex arc (Fig. 34–26) is the basic unit that maintains the body's integrity by the automatic conduction of impulses from afferent (sensory) receptors to efferent (motor) neurons. The reflex arc consists of the stimulation of a sensory nerve ending that conducts an impulse via sensory (afferent) neurons to the nuclei in the gray matter of the spinal cord. In the gray matter, the sensory neuron may synapse directly with lower motor neurons, or it may synapse with one or more association neurons, which transfer the impulse to the lower motor neuron. The impulse then is carried by the lower motor neurons, via the anterior spinal roots, to the neuroeffector junction. Stimulation of the neuroeffector junction elicits a response in the effector organ such as muscle contraction or glandular secretion (Campbell, 1993).

Peripheral Nervous System

SPINAL NERVES. The 31 pairs of spinal nerves arising from different spinal cord segments are categorized as follows: 8 cervical; 12 thoracic; 5 lumbar; 5 sacral; and 1 coccygeal. Each spinal nerve is composed of an anterior (ventral) and a posterior (dorsal) root in the spinal cord. The *anterior root* lies within the gray matter of the spinal cord and carries motor (efferent) impulses from the cord to the muscles and glands. The *posterior root* is made up of sensory (afferent) fibers that conduct impulses from the body's sensory receptors to the spinal cord. As the anterior and posterior fibers exit the spinal cord, they pass side by side and exit the vertebral column through the intervertebral foramina. Once outside the vertebral column, the two sets of nerve fibers

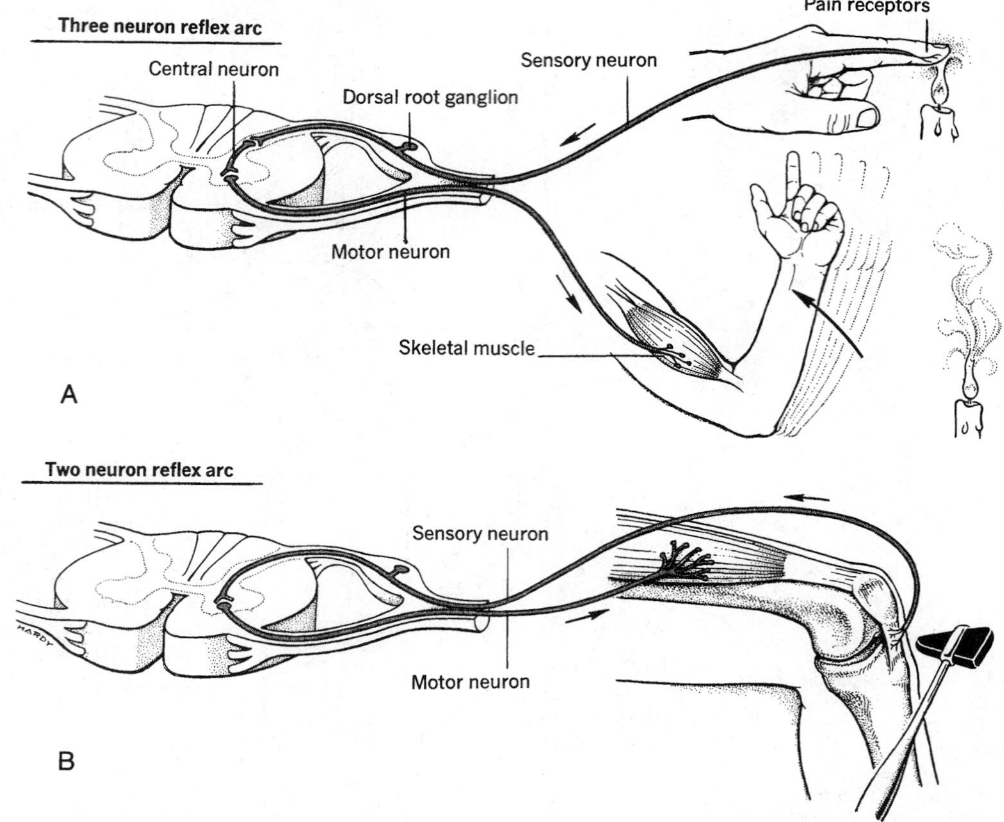

FIGURE 34–26. Diagram of (*A*) flexor reflex and (*B*) stretch reflex. (From Chaffee, E. E., & Lytle, I. M. [1980]. *Basic physiology and anatomy.* Philadelphia, J. B. Lippincott.)

join together and form the *spinal nerve.* Some spinal nerves join together and form dense networks of nerve fibers called *plexuses.* Table 34–2 summarizes the spinal nerves, plexuses, and peripheral innervation.

DERMATOMES. Each of the spinal nerves is distributed to a specific area of the body to receive superficial or cutaneous sensations. The specific body areas supplied by the spinal nerves are known as *dermatomes.* The many sensory fibers of the spinal nerves distributed to each of the dermatome regions provide many types of sensory reception including touch, kinesthetic sensation, vibration, heat and cold, and pain. Figures 34–27*A* and *B* illustrate the anterior and posterior distribution of dermatomes for cutaneous sensation.

CRANIAL NERVES. There are 12 pairs of cranial nerves (Table 34–3). The first two pairs of cranial nerves are not true peripheral nerves but are actually tracts of the CNS. The cranial nerves transmit impulses for sensation, voluntary control of muscles, and autonomic functions in the head and are involved in transmitting impulses for the special senses of vision, hearing, smell, and taste. Table 34–3 summarizes the origin and functions of each of the cranial nerves.

Autonomic Nervous System

The autonomic nervous system (ANS) is considered to be a part of the peripheral nervous system because it is outside of the CNS. However, the function of the ANS is substantially different from that of the rest of the peripheral nervous system. More specifically, the ANS regulates the body's organs and internal environment in close conjunction with the endocrine system. The ANS has two major subdivisions: the sympathetic and parasympathetic systems. These subdivisions differ in (1) type of neurotransmitter released, (2) nerve fiber distribution, and (3) effector organ response (Campbell, 1993) (Fig. 34–28).

The *sympathetic* system, also referred to as the thoracolumbar division of the ANS, is involved in maintaining the body's survival. Therefore, it is activated in situations that produce internal and external stress. Sympathetic stimulation results in a phenomenon called the flight-or-fight response that enables the body to respond to stressful situations. This response affects some of the body systems as follows:

1. Cardiovascular system—increased blood pressure and heart rate; peripheral vasoconstriction
2. Gastrointestinal system—decreased motility, con-

TABLE 34–2. **Spinal Nerves, Plexuses, and Peripheral Innervation**

Spinal Nerves	Plexuses Formed from Anterior Rami	Spinal Nerve Branches from Plexuses	Parts Supplied
Cervical 1 2 3 4	Cervical plexus	Lesser occipital Great auricular Cutaneous nerve of neck Anterior supraclavicular Middle supraclavicular Posterior supraclavicular Branches to numerous neck muscles	Sensory to back of head, front of neck, and upper part of shoulder, motor to numerous neck muscles
		Phrenic nerve	Diaphragm
		Suprascapular and dorsoscapular	Superficial muscles of scapula
		Thoracic nerves, medial and lateral anterior	Pectoralis major and minor
		Long thoracic nerve	Serratus anterior
		Thoracodorsal	Latissimus dorsi
		Subscapular	Subscapular and teres major muscles
		Axillary (circumflex)	Deltoid and teres minor muscles and skin over deltoid
Cervical 5 6 7 8 **Thoracic (or Dorsal)** 1	Brachial plexus	Musculocutaneous	Muscle of front of arm (biceps brachii, coracobrachialis, and brachialis) and skin on outer side of forearm
		Ulnar	Flexor carpi ulnaris and part of flexor digitorum profundus; some of muscles of hand; sensory to medial side of hand, little finger, and medial half of fourth finger
2 3 4 5 6 7 8 9 10 11 12	No plexus formed; branches run directly to intercostal muscles and skin of thorax	Median	Rest of muscles of front of forearm and hand; sensory to skin of palmar surface of thumb, index, and middle fingers
		Radial	Triceps muscle and muscles of back of forearm; sensory to skin of back of forearm and hand
		Medial cutaneous	Sensory to inner surface of arm and forearm
		Phrenic (branches from cervical nerves before formation of plexus; most of its fibers from fourth cervical nerve)	Diaphragm
		Iliohypogastric } Sometimes fused	Sensory to anterior abdominal wall
		Ilioinguinal } Sometimes fused	Sensory to anterior abdominal wall and external genitalia; motor to muscles of abdominal wall
		Genitofemoral	Sensory to skin of external genitalia and inguinal region
Lumbar 1 2 3 4 5 **Sacral** 1 2 3 4 5 **Coccygeal** 1	Lumbosacral plexus	Lateral cutaneous of thigh	Sensory to outer side of thigh
		Femoral	Motor to quadriceps, sartorius, and iliacus muscles; sensory to front of thigh and to medial side of lower leg (saphenous nerve)
		Obturator	Motor to adductor muscles of thigh
		Tibial* (medial popliteal)	Motor to muscles of calf of leg; sensory to skin of calf of leg and sole of foot
		Common peroneal (lateral popliteal)	Motor to evertors and dorsiflexors of foot; sensory to lateral surface of leg and dorsal surface of foot
			Motor to muscles of back of thigh
		Nerves to hamstring muscles Gluteal nerves, superior and inferior	Motor to buttock muscles and tensor fasciae latae
		Posterior cutaneous nerve	Sensory to skin of buttocks, posterior surface of thigh, and leg
		Pudendal nerve	Motor to perineal muscles; sensory to skin of perineum

*Sensory fibers from the tibial and peroneal nerves unite to form the *medial cutaneous* (or *sural*) *nerve* that supplies the calf of the leg and the lateral surface of the foot. In the thigh, the tibial and common peroneal nerves are usually enclosed in a single sheath to form the *sciatic nerve*, the largest nerve in the body with its width of approximately ¾″. About two-thirds of the way down the posterior part of the thigh, it divides into its component parts. Branches of the sciatic nerve extend into the hamstring muscles.

Reproduced by permission from Anthony, C. P., & Thibodeau, G. M. *Textbook of anatomy and physiology* (12th ed.). St. Louis, 1987, The C. V. Mosby Co.

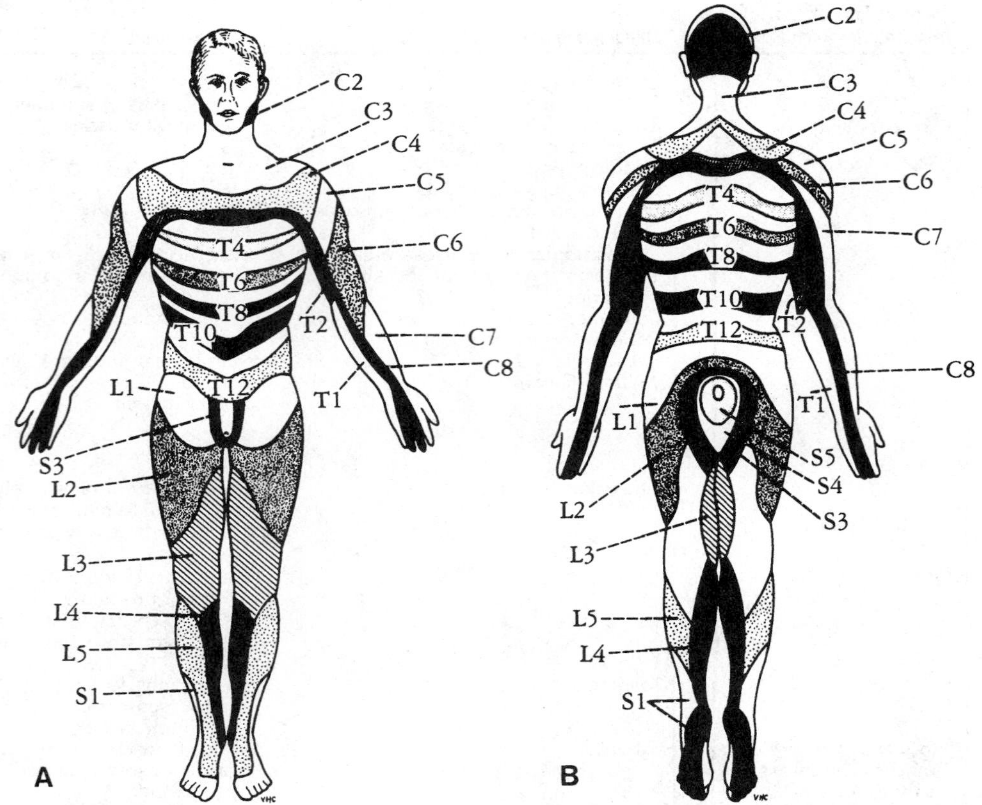

FIGURE 34–27. Dermatomes. *A*, Anterior view. *B*, Posterior view. (From Snell, R. S. [1980]. *Clinical neuroanatomy for medical students.* Boston: Little, Brown.)

traction, and secretions; increased rectal sphincter tone; loss of appetite

3. Genitourinary system—relaxation of bladder muscles and contraction of the urinary sphincter
4. Eyes—pupillary dilation and slight elevation of the upper eyelid

The primary neurotransmitter of the sympathetic nervous system is norepinephrine, thus making the system an adrenergic one. Norepinephrine, or noradrenaline, is secreted by the postganglionic nerve terminals.

Structurally, the preganglionic neurons of the sympathetic system are found in the intermediolateral columns of all the thoracic and the upper two lumbar segments of the spinal cord. After exiting the spinal nerves, the preganglionic sympathetic axons enter, via a connection called the *white ramus,* a chain of ganglia that extends from the upper portion of the neck to the coccyx. This chain of ganglia is called the *sympathetic trunk, ganglionated cord,* or *sympathetic chain.*

Most of the sympathetic fibers synapse with preganglionic neurons in the sympathetic trunk or pass up and down the trunk and synapse with postganglionic neurons in other ganglia of the chain. Some axons pass through the sympathetic trunk and synapse with a peripheral ganglion closer to the organ of innervation. Finally, some axons pass through the sympathetic trunk to the adrenal medulla and act as a preganglionic fiber along the entire path to the innervated organ, gland, or tissue.

Functionally, the *adrenal medulla* is an extension of the sympathetic nervous system. Sympathetic stimulation of the adrenal medulla results in the release of large amounts of epinephrine and norepinephrine. The discharge of adrenal sympathetic hormones produces almost the same response as direct sympathetic stimulation of the afferent organs; however, the effect lasts much longer. Generally, the organs or body tissues are stimulated simultaneously by the sympathetic fibers (direct stimulation) and by the adrenal medulla (indirect stimulation).

The *parasympathetic* division of the autonomic nervous system is involved primarily with vegetative activities that conserve and restore an individual's energy reserves. Such activities include decreased blood pressure, slower respiratory rate, decreased heart rate, and stimulation of the digestive system. The parasympathetic nervous system also is referred to as the *craniosacral system* because the preganglionic neurons exit from the brain stem through the cranial nerves and leave the spinal cord through the second, third, and fourth sacral spinal nerves. Parasympathetic fibers in the cranial and sacral spinal nerves synapse only with terminal ganglia in the effector organ; therefore, preganglionic fibers are long and postganglionic fibers are

TABLE 34–3. **The Cranial Nerves**

Number	Name	Nerve Fiber Type(s)*	Origin; Primary Cell Body	Peripheral Termination(s)	Principal Function(s)
I	Olfactory	SVA	Rhinencephalon; olfactory epithelium	Olfactory epithelium	Olfaction
II	Optic	SSA	Diencephalon; retina, ganglionic layer	Bipolar retinal cells to rods and cones	Vision
III	Oculomotor	GSA, GSE, *GVE*	Superior collicular level; oculomotor nucleus, Edinger-Westphal nucleus	Superior, inferior, medial rectus, and levator palpebrae muscles; pupillary constrictors and ciliary muscles of eyeball	Proprioceptive impulses, eye movements, accommodation reflex
IV	Trochlear	GSA, GSE	Superior cerebellar peduncle; trochlear nucleus	Superior oblique muscle	Proprioceptive impulses, eye movements
V	Trigeminal	GSA, SVE	Pons; masticator nucleus, semilunar ganglion, mesencephalic nucleus	Face, nose, mouth, jaw	Muscles of mastication; sensory to face, nose, mouth; proprioceptive to tooth sockets and jaw muscles
VI	Abducens	GSA, GSE	Pons; abducens nucleus	Lateral rectus	Eye movements
VII	Facial	GVA, SVA, SVE, *GVE*	Pons; facial nucleus, superior salivatory nucleus, geniculate ganglion	Glands of nose, lacrimal glands, palate; sublingual and submaxillary glands; anterior taste buds	Motor and sensory components to facial region, tongue
VIII	Vestibulocochlear:				
	Cochlear division	SSA	Pons; spiral ganglion	Organ of Corti	Audition (hearing)
	Vestibular division	SSA	Pons; vestibular ganglion	Cristae of semicircular canals, maculae of saccule and utricle	Equilibrium
IX	Glossopharyngeal	SVA, GVA, SVE, *GVE*	Medulla; ambiguous nucleus, inferior salivatory nucleus, petrosal ganglion, superior ganglion	Superior constrictor, stylopharyngeus muscles; parotid glands, taste buds (vallate papillae), eustachian tube	Motor to pharyngeal region; gustation (taste); motor to parotids; pain, tactile, thermal sensations from posterior tongue, tonsils, and eustachian tubes; regulates blood pressure
X	Vagus	GSA, GVA, SVA, *GVE*, SVE	Medulla; ambiguous nucleus, dorsal motor nucleus; nodose ganglion; jugular ganglion	Muscles of pharynx and larynx, viscera of thorax and abdomen; pinna of ear	Sensory and motor to thoracic and abdominal viscera, certain skeletal muscles of pharyngeal, laryngeal regions
XI	Spinal accessory	GSA, *GVE*, SVE	Medulla; accessory nucleus	Sternocleidomastoid and trapezius muscles; portions of laryngeal, pharyngeal muscles; heart (?)	Sensory and motor to muscles of larynx and pharynx; may form components of cardiac branches of vagus
XII	Hypoglossal	GSA, GSE	Medulla; hypoglossal nucleus	Tongue muscles	Sensory and motor to tongue muscles

*Special afferent fibers are found only in the cranial nerves. SVA, special visceral afferent (sensory) fibers related only to nerves that subserve olfaction (I) and gustation (VII, IX, X). SSA, special somatic afferent (sensory) fibers that transmit impulses from the special sense organs, i.e., eye (II) and ear (VIII). SVE, special visceral efferent (motor) fibers of cranial nerves that innervate particular skeletal muscles derived embryologically from visceral (branchial) arch mesoderm. Some authors prefer the term "branchial motor fibers" to SVE when referring to the nerves that innervate the muscles derived from visceral arch mesoderm (e.g., the palatine, pharyngeal, laryngeal, and masticatory muscles as well as those of facial expression innervated by branches of cranial nerves V, VII, IX, X, and XI). GSA, general somatic afferent; GSE, general somatic afferent; GVA, general visceral afferent, *GVE*, general visceral efferent; GVE components of cranial nerves III, VII, IX, and X are in italics.

From Jensen, D. (1980). *The Principles of Physiology* (2nd ed.). New York: Appleton-Century-Crofts.

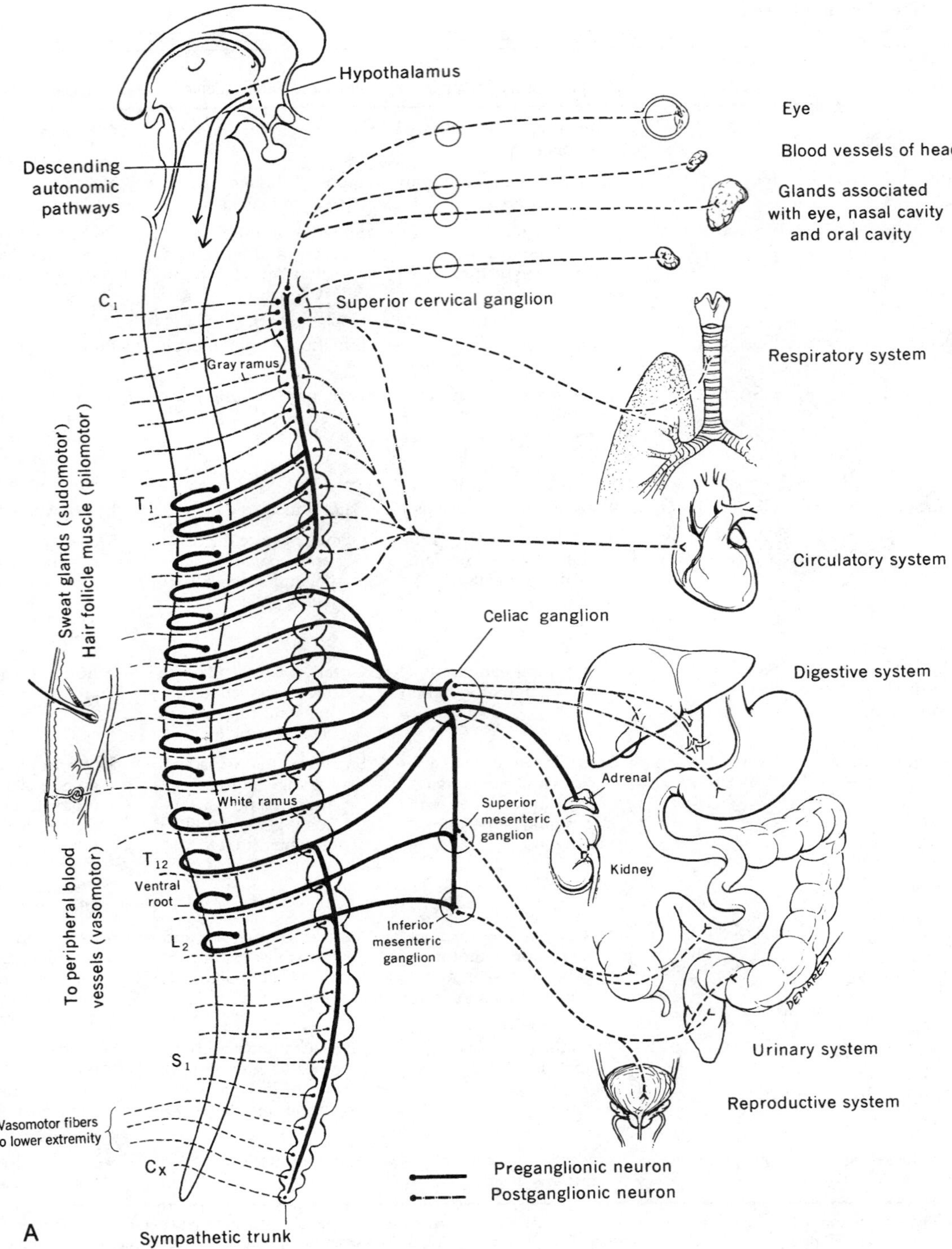

FIGURE 34–28. *A,* Sympathetic nervous system.

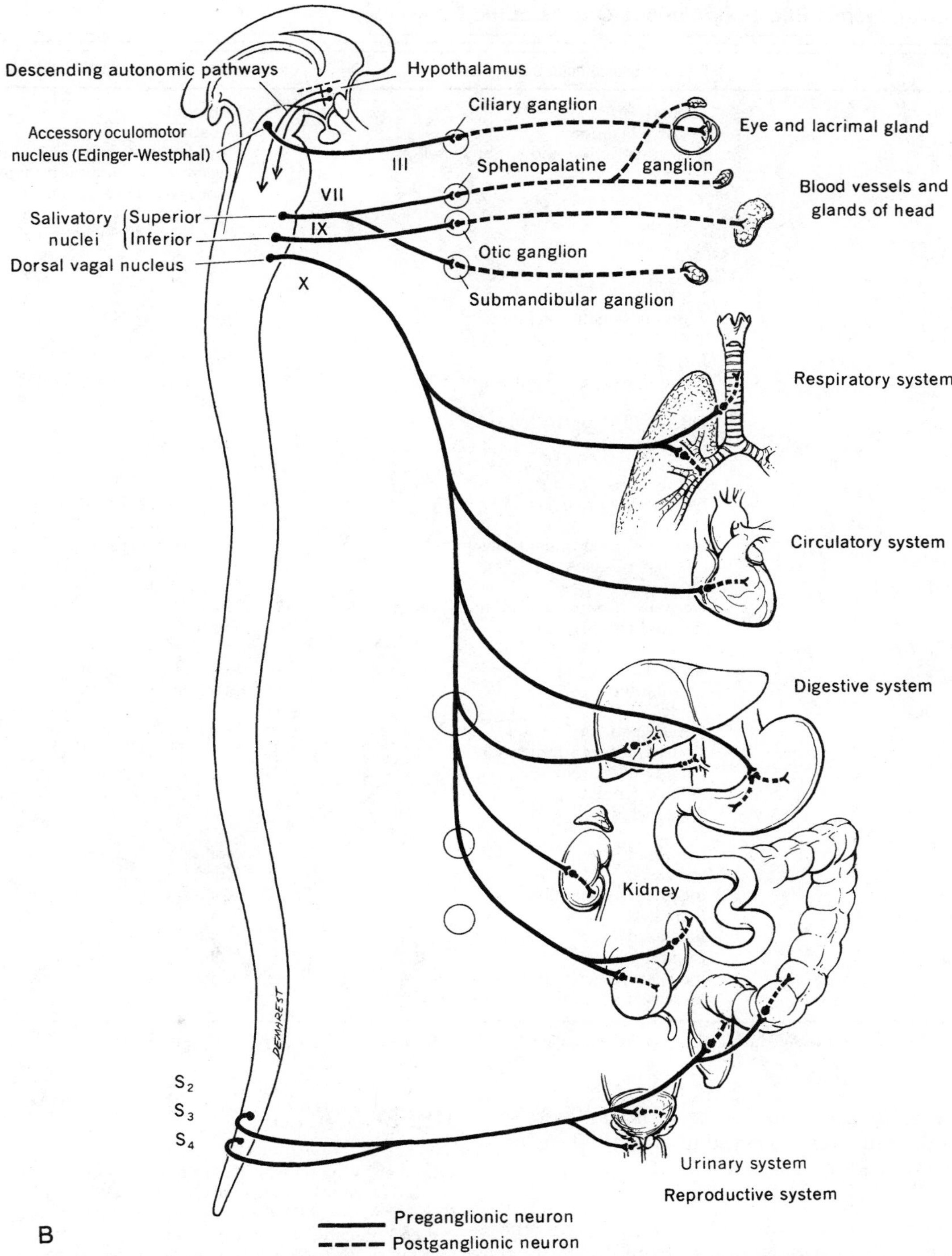

FIGURE 34–28 *Continued. B,* Parasympathetic nervous system. (From Adams, R. D., & Victor, M. [1977]. *Principles of neurology.* New York: McGraw-Hill. Reproduced with permission of McGraw-Hill, Inc.)

TABLE 34–4. **Autonomic Effects on Various Organs of the Body**

Organ	Effect of Sympathetic Stimulation	Effect of Parasympathetic Stimulation
Eye:		
Pupil	Dilated	Constricted
Ciliary muscle	Slight relaxation	Constricted
Glands: Nasal Lacrimal Parotid Submandibular Gastric Pancreatic	Vasoconstriction and slight secretion	Stimulation of copious (except pancreas) secretion (containing many enzymes for enzyme-secreting glands)
Sweat glands	Copious sweating (cholinergic)	None
Apocrine glands	Thick; odoriferous secretion	None
Heart:		
Muscle	Increased rate Increased force of contraction	Slowed rate Decreased force of contraction (especially of atrium)
Coronaries	Dilated (β_2): constricted (α)	Dilated
Lungs:		
Bronchi	Dilated	Constricted
Blood vessels	Mildly constricted	? Dilated
Gut:		
Lumen	Decreased peristalsis and tone	Increased peristalsis and tone
Sphincter	Increased tone (most times)	Relaxed (most times)
Liver	Glucose release	Slight glycogen synthesis
Gallbladder and bile ducts	Relaxed	Contracted
Kidney	Decreased output and renin secretion	None
Bladder:		
Detrusor	Relaxed (slight)	Excited
Trigone	Excited	Relaxed
Penis	Ejaculation	Erection
Systemic arterioles:		
Abdominal	Constricted	None
Muscle	Constricted (α-adrenergic) Dilated (β_2-adrenergic) Dilated (cholinergic)	None
Skin	Constricted	None
Blood:		
Coagulation	Increased	None
Glucose	Increased	None
Basal metabolism	Increased up to 100%	None
Adrenal medullary secretion	Increased	None
Mental activity	Increased	None
Piloerector muscles	Excited	None
Skeletal muscle	Increased glycogenolysis Increased strength	None

From Guyton, A. C. (1986). *Textbook of Medical Physiology* (7th ed.). Philadelphia: W. B. Saunders.

short. Both preganglionic and postganglionic fibers of the parasympathetic nervous system are called *cholinergic* because they secrete *acetylcholine.*

AUTONOMIC EFFECTS. Table 34–4 summarizes the autonomic effects on various organs. From this table, it is evident that both sympathetic and parasympathetic stimulation produce excitatory effects in some body organs and inhibitory effects in others. Also, as can be noted from the table, when sympathetic stimulation excites a specific organ, parasympathetic stimulation usually inhibits that organ. However, most organs are dominated by one or the other system, so that the sympathetic and parasympathetic nervous systems do not oppose one another actively (Guyton, 1991).

REFERENCES

Campbell, V. G. (1993). Neurologic system. In J. Thompson et al. (Eds.), *Mosby's clinical nursing* (3rd ed.). St. Louis: Mosby.

Guyton, A. C. (1991). *Basic neuroscience: Anatomy and physiology* (2nd ed.). Philadelphia: W. B. Saunders.

Hickey, J. (1992). *The clinical practice of neurological and neurosurgical nursing* (3rd ed.). Philadelphia: J. B. Lippincott.

Jensen, D. (1980). *The principles of physiology* (2nd ed.). New York: Appleton-Century-Crofts.

Lindsay, K. W., Bone, I., & Callander, R. (1986). *Neurology and neurosurgery illustrated.* London: Churchill Livingstone.

Rudy, E. B. (1984). *Advanced neurological and neurosurgical nursing.* St. Louis: C. V. Mosby.

Schmidt, R. F. (Ed.) (1985). *Fundamentals of neurophysiology.* New York: Springer-Verlag.

Simon, R. H., & Sayre, J. T. (1987). *Strategy in head injury management.* E. Norwalk, CT: Appleton & Lange.

Patients With Head Injury and Brain Dysfunction

Connie (Walleck) Jastremski

The brain is a very sensitive organ and can be injured in many ways. When the brain is injured, physiologic, behavioral, cognitive, and psychological changes may occur. This chapter reviews some major causes of brain injury, such as traumatic head injury, ischemic injury, metabolic disorders, and the effects of seizure on brain function. The pathophysiology of these events differs, but the medical and nursing interventions have the same goal: to protect the brain throughout the recovery process in order to restore the patient to his or her optimum level of functioning.

TRAUMATIC BRAIN INJURY

Over the years there has been a steady increase in the number of people who sustain traumatic head injuries. Each year approximately 5% of the population sustain a head injury serious enough to result in lost time from normal daily activities (Hickey, 1986; Rimel, 1982). Head injury is the leading cause of all trauma-related deaths (i.e., 70% of all fatal injuries involve the head) (Rimel & Lundgren, 1986). Mortality from head injury alone is approximately 50%, with most of these deaths occurring before hospitalization. Studies in both the United States and Australia have shown that in urban areas almost two-thirds of head injury deaths occur before hospitalization (Marshall et al., 1990).

The incidence of head injury is higher in men than in women (3:1), and highest in people 15 to 24 years of age. Most head-injured people are single and have a low median family income (Krause, 1987; Krause et al., 1984; Rimel and Lundgren, 1986).

The economic consequences of head injury are staggering. According to the National Head and Spinal Cord Survey (based on today's dollar), direct costs for diagnosis, treatment, and rehabilitation and the indirect costs to society from lost productivity total more than 5 billion dollars (Kalsbeck et al., 1981). This figure does not include such psychosocial and emotional issues as pain, suffering, effects on family and significant others, or the symbolic aspects of disability. Therefore, the total costs are probably enormous (Spielman, 1988).

Major causes of head injury are motor vehicle accidents, falls, and assaults. Vehicular accidents account for 48% of head-injured patients and occur most frequently in the 15- to 24-year-old age group (Rimel & Lundgren, 1986). Falls generally occur in the elderly and the under–15-year-old age group. The most significant contributing factor in all accidents is the use of alcohol (Hickey, 1992; Rimel & Lundgren, 1986; Spielman, 1988).

Many preventive programs have been developed to ameliorate the death and disability associated with head injury. Failure to use safety restraint systems increases the risk of head injury in motor vehicle accidents. Most states have mandatory seat belt laws, but there is commonly a lack of compliance with the law. Advocates for passive restraints (e.g., air bags) feel that because compliance with seat belt usage will never be complete, mandatory passive restraints will ensure protection of people involved in motor vehicle accidents.

Motorcycle accidents account for many trauma victims. Laws mandating the use of helmets when riding a motorcycle have met with resistance from motorcyclists. The motorcyclists' lobby in most states has been effective in repealing or preventing the adoption of such laws.

Preventive programs designed to protect the trauma victim provide the means to decrease mortality and morbidity from head injury. Health care professionals involved in the care of trauma patients must become active in designing, implementing, and researching the effectiveness of preventive programs. These professionals then need to be active in sponsoring, supporting, and lobbying for legislation for mandatory safety equipment and more stringent safety requirements.

Types of Injury

"Head injury" is a generic term that refers to any injury of the scalp, skull (either the facial or cranial section), or brain. In this chapter, head injury is divided into injuries of the head and injuries of the brain tissue.

Injuries of the head include scalp lacerations and skull fractures. Traumatic brain injuries are those in which tissue disruption and injury occur. Tissue injuries include concussion, contusion, and laceration.

SCALP LACERATIONS

Scalp lacerations are among the most common head injuries (Nikas & Tolley, 1982). Because of the extensive vascularity of the scalp and poor contractility of these blood vessels, scalp injuries can result in significant blood loss, occasionally resulting in hypovolemia. Diagnosis of scalp injury is made by inspection. Skull radiographs, computed tomography (CT) scans, magnetic resonance imaging (MRI), and other diagnostic procedures may be ordered to rule out concurrent injury.

The bleeding of scalp lacerations is controlled by direct pressure, although sutures may be required for hemostasis in severe injuries. Careful inspection of the wound is important. Digital examination of the wound is conducted after infiltration with lidocaine and 1:1,000 epinephrine for anesthesia and vasoconstriction (Hickey, 1986). Copious irrigation of the wound with normal saline cleanses the wound of dirt and debris. Severe lacerations require debridement of devitalized tissue.

SKULL FRACTURES

Skull fractures are categorized as linear, depressed, or basilar but may also be described as simple, comminuted, and compound. The type of fracture depends on the velocity, direction, and momentum of the object causing the injury (Hickey, 1986, 1992).

Linear skull fractures comprise about 80% of all skull fractures, half of which involve the temporoparietal area (Hickey, 1992; Jennett & Teasdale, 1981). Usually, linear fractures are not displaced and require no treatment. If the fracture extends into the orbit or paranasal sinuses or crosses a major vascular channel (such as the sagittal sinus or middle meningeal artery), the patient should be admitted to the hospital for observation. Surgery may be necessary to correct these secondary injuries (Weiner & Eisenberg, 1985).

A depressed skull fracture is characterized by an inward depression of the outer table of the skull below the inner table of the adjacent bone (Jennett & Teasdale, 1981) (Fig. 35–1). Depressed skull fractures are classified as open, or compound, in the presence of a communicating scalp laceration. Most patients with depressed fractures caused by nonpenetrating injuries have symptoms associated with focal brain damage, and therefore never, or briefly, lose consciousness. Half of the patients with compound fractures have a torn dura, which is associated with a higher incidence of prolonged posttraumatic amnesia and focal signs (Jennett & Teasdale, 1981).

When depressed skull fractures are open, surgical asepsis is used to care for the scalp laceration because of the obvious potential for infection. Surgery to elevate the depressed bone is accomplished within 24 hours with open fractures (Nikas, 1987).

Because of the risk of infection, fracture fragments are removed from grossly contaminated wounds. If these fragments cannot be replaced in the wound, a plate cranioplasty (with a plate made of acrylic or metal) may be needed. The cranioplasty may be delayed to prevent local infection. A course of antibiotics is recommended if removal of fragments is not possible or if more than 24 hours elapses before debridement (Nikas, 1987).

A basilar skull fracture involves the base of the skull, including the anterior, middle, or posterior fossa. Because these fractures are difficult to confirm with radiographs, diagnosis may be based on the clinical presentation of the patient.

The clinical signs of an anterior fossa basilar skull fracture include cerebrospinal fluid (CSF) rhinorrhea (Fig. 35–2) and bilateral periorbital ecchymosis (referred to as "raccoon's eyes"). CSF rhinorrhea occurs in 25% of patients with anterior basilar fractures, and in more than half of these the leak lasts for only 2 or 3 days, until the dura seals itself (Jennett & Teasdale, 1981). Anterior fossa fractures may be associated with other facial injuries.

Middle fossa basilar skull fracture results in ecchymosis over the mastoid bone, called Battle sign, and CSF otorrhea. The leaking fluid from the ear demonstrates a dural tear and a ruptured tympanic membrane. If the tympanic membrane remains intact, blood and CSF may be evident behind the membrane on otoscopic examination. CSF otorrhea is rare, but when it occurs, CSF flow is profuse (Jennett & Teasdale, 1981).

CONCUSSION

Concussion is a clinical diagnosis that involves transient neurogenic dysfunction caused by rapid acceleration–deceleration or by a sudden blow to the head. It is suspected that temporary alteration in function results from transient ischemia or neural depolarization after a sudden release of acetylcholine (Mitchell, 1994; Spielman, 1988).

Mild concussion is the most common brain injury. It is considered a minor injury, generally not requiring hospitalization. Symptoms include confusion, disorientation, and sometimes retrograde amnesia or posttraumatic amnesia. Symptoms usually last only a few minutes and are not related to permanent deficits. Preservation of consciousness is the distinguishing feature of mild concussion as opposed to classic concussion (Gennarelli, 1987). Classic concussion involves temporary loss of consciousness, retrograde amnesia, posttraumatic amnesia, and occasionally mild neurologic impairment. Unconsciousness usually lasts less than 5 minutes and no longer than 6 hours. The duration of posttraumatic amnesia is often a predictor of the severity of the injury (Mitchell, 1984; Spielman, 1988).

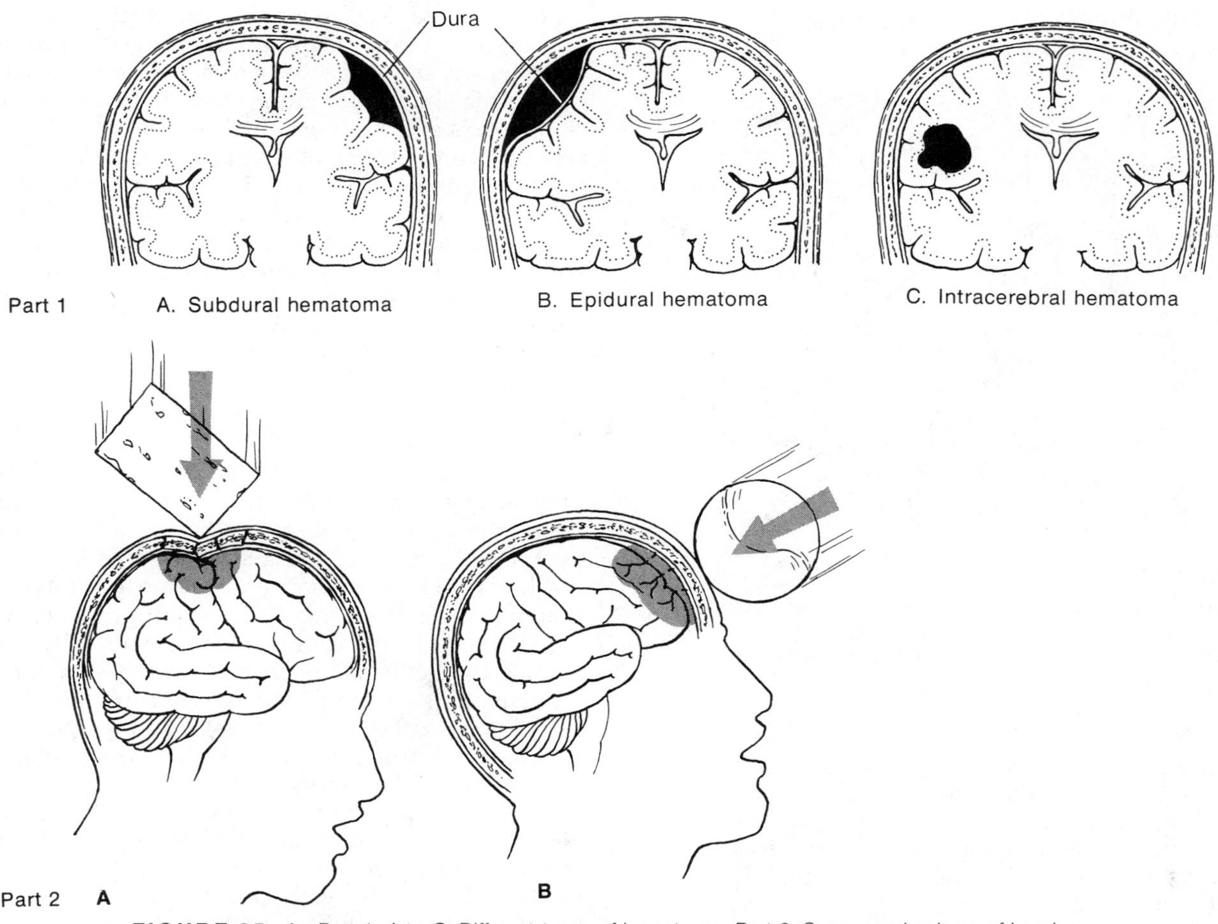

FIGURE 35–1. *Part 1, A* to *C,* Different types of hematoma. *Part 2,* Some mechanisms of head injury. Head injury results from penetration or impact. *A,* A direct injury (blow to the skull) may fracture the skull. Contusion and laceration of the brain may result from fractures. Depressed portions of the skull may compress or penetrate brain tissue. *B,* In the presence of skull fracture, a blow to the skull may cause the brain to move enough to tear some of the veins going through the cortical surface of the dura. Subsequently, subdural hematoma may develop. Note areas of cerebral contusion (*shaded*). In addition to the injuries depicted, secondary phenomena may result from the injury and cause additional brain dysfunction or damage. For example, ischemia, especially cerebral edema, may occur, elevating intracranial pressure. (From Luckmann, J., & Sorensen, K. C. [1987]. *Medical–surgical nursing: A psychophysiologic approach* [3rd ed.]. Philadelphia: W. B. Saunders.)

CONTUSION AND LACERATION

Contusions involve cortical bruising and laceration of vessels and brain tissues with subsequent tissue infarction and necrosis. These injuries usually involve cortical and white matter petechial hemorrhages. The size and severity of the contusion and laceration vary depending on the area of contact between the striking object and the skull. The distinction between contusion and laceration is based on the degree of trauma, a laceration being more serious than a contusion.

The major sites of contusions and lacerations are the frontal and temporal lobes at the frontal poles, the orbital areas, the frontotemporal junction around the sylvian fissure, and the inferior and lateral surfaces of the temporal lobes (the temporal tips) (Hickey, 1986; Mitchell, 1994). The distribution of contusions in these particular areas is explained by the movement of the brain within the cranium, and the bony ridges on the inner plate of the cranium in these areas.

Assessment of the severity of contusion depends on the site and extent of brain injury. Isolated contusions do not usually produce immediate loss of consciousness but may subsequently if there is associated ischemia. Coma is usually the result of diffuse injury. Frontal injuries result in personality, behavior, motor, and speech deficits. Temporal lobe contusions are closely monitored because of their proximity to the tentorium and midbrain, increasing the potential for herniation (Mitchell, 1994; Spielman, 1988).

PENETRATING INJURIES

Penetrating injury may be caused by missile injuries or impalement. Direct injury to the brain can result from

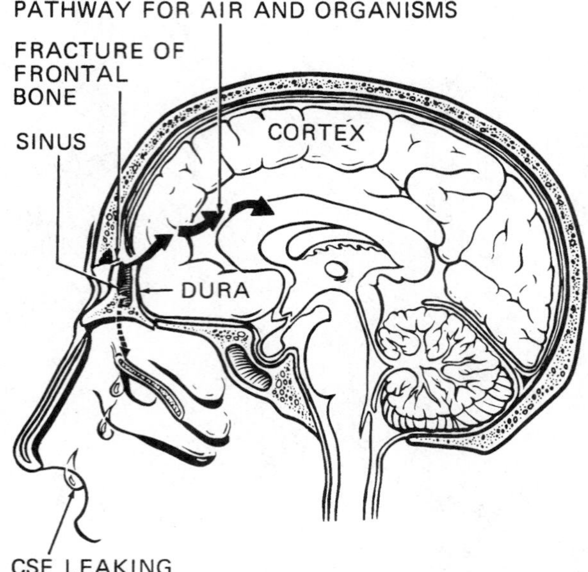

FIGURE 35–2. Frontal bone fracture with cerebrospinal fluid (CSF) leakage. (From Snyder, M., & Jackle, M. [1981]. *Neurologic problems: A critical care focus.* Bowie, MD: Robert J. Brady.)

penetration of the cranium. The wound created by a bullet depends on the size (caliber), shape, velocity, direction, and action within the intracranial space.

Wounds from missiles have been described as (1) tangential, when the missile produces a depressed skull fracture; (2) penetrating, when the missile enters but does not exit, resulting in metal, bone, hair, and skin fragments within the brain; and (3) through-and-through injuries, when the missile enters the cranium, traverses the cranial contents, and passes through an exit wound (Purvis, 1966).

The major effects of missile injuries are focal damage and generalized destruction of the brain from concussion, contusions, and lacerations of the brain. Necrosis of tissue and hemorrhage can occur. The amount of injury depends on the structures involved. The amount of injury depends on the structures involved. There is an 80% mortality rate associated with through-and-through wounds (Hickey, 1986). Patients who are in deep coma on admission seldom survive. Forty-five percent of the patients with missile injuries become epileptic within 5 years (Jennett & Teasdale, 1981).

Impalement injuries include piercing of the scalp, skull, or brain. A foreign body that is protruding from the head should be left in place to control bleeding until it is removed during surgery (Gudeman et al., 1989).

Pathophysiology of Brain Injury

COUP–CONTRECOUP INJURIES

The brain has some movement within the skull, and this results in mass movement of the intracranial contents when the head incurs trauma (Fig. 35–3). An injury directly below the point of trauma can produce a coup injury, caused by the slapping effect of the brain hitting the skull. The contrecoup contusion, or laceration, occurs at the opposite pole of impact as the brain rebounds and strikes other parts of the skull. Whenever the impact occurs on the head, the resulting lesions are usually bilateral and symmetric. These lesions are most marked at the interfaces between tissues that have different physical properties (i.e., compliance or elasticity), such as between white and gray matter or brain and blood vessels (Jennett & Teasdale, 1981).

DIFFUSE AXONAL INJURY

Diffuse axonal injury (DAI) is the most severe form of brain injury and differs from concussion in degree rather than in kind of brain pathophysiology. This injury has also been called a shearing injury. The hallmark of DAI is immediate and prolonged coma (more than 6 hours). The coma is the result of severe, widespread damage to the white matter, essentially disconnecting the hemispheres from the brain stem's reticular activating system (RAS) by stretching and tearing the RAS fibers (Spielman, 1988). There is widespread neurologic dysfunction, diffuse white matter degeneration, and global cerebral edema.

Diffuse axonal injury is classified as mild, moderate, or severe. Gennarelli and colleagues (1982) described mild injury as that restricted to the parasagittal white matter of the cerebral hemispheres; a moderate injury adds to focal injury in the corpus callosum; and a severe injury involves a large degree of axonal abnormality of the white matter of the cerebellum and upper brain stem. Because DAI involves microscopic changes, the severity of injury is not identified through radiographs but by the severity of symptoms and the duration of coma (Spielman, 1988).

The clinical findings of DAI include deep and prolonged coma, initial decortication (flexion) or decerebration (extension), increased intracranial pressure (ICP), hypertension, and an elevated temperature. The clinical course and outcome depend on the severity of axonal injury. The patient may be comatose for up to 3 months and may never regain full consciousness. Major sequelae of severe DAI are deficits in cognition, memory, speech, motor function, and personality (Spielman, 1988). Mortality in severe DAI is around 51%, and only 15% of the survivors have a good outcome (Gennarelli et al., 1982).

Complications of Brain Injury

POSTCONCUSSION SYNDROME

Concussion is considered a mild brain injury, but postinjury sequelae, called postconcussion syndrome, may be devastating for the patient. Major complaints with this syndrome include headache, dizziness, ner-

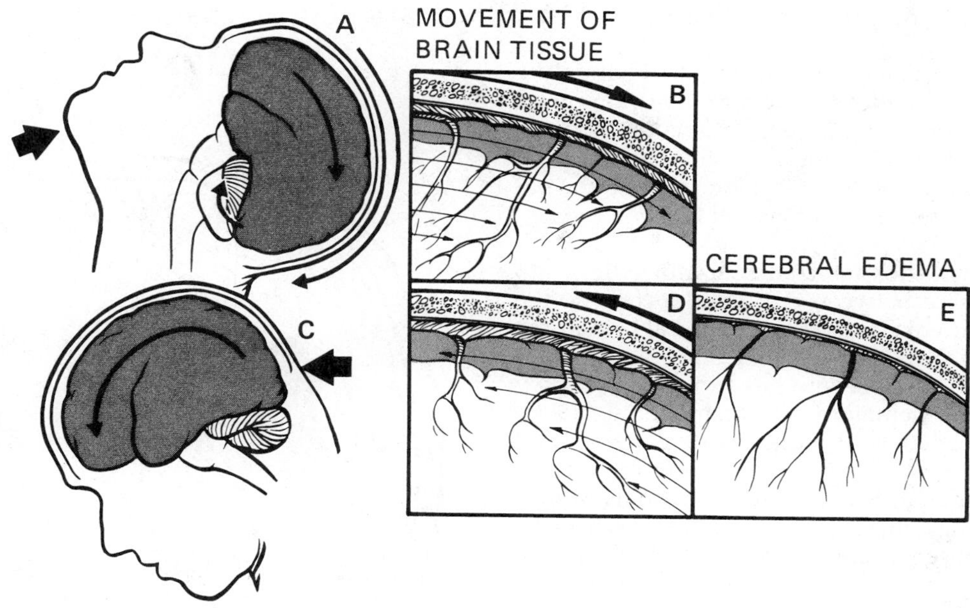

A, C Forceful extension and flexion of the neck

B, D Movement of the brain within the skull

E Cerebral edema

FIGURE 35–3. Acceleration–deceleration injury. *A* and *C*, Forceful extension and flexion of the neck. *B* and *D*, Movement of the brain within the skull. *E*, Cerebral edema. (From Snyder, M., & Jackle, M. [1981]. *Neurologic problems: A critical care focus.* Bowie, MD: Robert J. Brady.)

vousness, irritability, fatigability, insomnia, poor concentration, poor memory, and changes in intelligence. Symptoms may be delayed several weeks to 2 years after the injury. Recognition of this syndrome has led to changes in follow-up for concussion patients. Patients whose symptoms persist have apparently sustained some organic injury and will have difficulty regaining their previous lifestyle and level of function. Referral to a neuropsychologist for follow-up aids in early identification of the syndrome, facilitating the patient in adjusting to any disabilities.

HEMATOMA FORMATION

SUBDURAL HEMATOMA. A subdural hematoma (SDH; see Fig. 35–1) refers to bleeding between the dura mater and the arachnoid layer of the meninges. This bleeding creates pressure on the brain. Bleeding into the subdural space is believed to result from tearing of the bridging veins between the brain and the dura, bleeding from contused or lacerated brain tissue, or extension from an intracerebral hematoma. SDH develops in 10% to 15% of head-injured patients.

Subdural hematomas have a poor prognosis because they are frequently not diagnosed rapidly enough after the injury. Mortality varies from 60% to 80% (Mitchell, 1994). Diagnosis is confirmed by CT scan, which demonstrates the typical half-moon–shaped area of increased density on the surface of the brain (Jennett & Teasdale, 1981).

Acute SDH occurs within 24 to 48 hours of injury and is associated with major cerebral trauma with contusion and laceration. Patients usually present with progressive and marked depression of consciousness, headache, drowsiness, agitation, and confusion. Pupillary and motor changes are present in many of these patients. Treatment consists of craniotomy with evacuation of the hematoma and coagulation of actively bleeding vessels. Patients are monitored in a critical care unit postoperatively.

Subacute SDH can develop 2 to 14 days after injury. Subacute SDH is strongly indicated by a failure to regain consciousness (Hickey, 1986). The prognosis is substantially better in subacute SDH (Marshall et al., 1990).

Chronic SDH can occur up to several months after the initial injury. The pathogenesis of chronic SDH is not known. The hematoma tends to develop slowly, indicated by the same signs as a space-occupying lesion. Symptoms commonly include an increasingly severe headache, confusion, slow cerebration, and drowsiness. Papilledema and ipsilateral pupil dilation may be noted. Chronic SDH is more common in alcoholics or in older people with cerebral atrophy (Nikas, 1987).

Treatment of subacute or chronic SDH involves burr holes and evacuation. Some authors recommend craniectomy for recurrent accumulations of subdural fluid (Tyson et al., 1980). Mortality with chronic SDH has been reported as 5% to 10%, depending on the patient population studied (Marshall et al., 1990).

EPIDURAL (EXTRADURAL) HEMATOMA. Bleeding into the potential space between the inner surface of the skull and the dura mater forms an epidural hematoma (EDH) (see Fig. 35–1). Incidence of EDH is low, comprising only 10% of all severe head injuries and only 20% to 30% of all hematomas (Marshall et al., 1990). EDHs are associated with temporal or parietal skull fractures with involvement of a branch of the meningeal artery (Hirsh, 1980; Jennett & Teasdale, 1981). Fractures crossing a major venous channel, such as the sagittal or transverse sinus, led to EDH of venous origin.

One-third of patients with EDH have the classic triad of symptoms—immediate loss of consciousness at the time of injury, a lucid interval lasting a few minutes to a few hours, then a lapse into unconsciousness again. Other symptoms include increasingly severe headache, seizures, vomiting, hemiparesis, and a fixed and dilated ipsilateral pupil (Hickey, 1992). Emergency surgery to evacuate the hematoma is done to prevent cerebral herniation (Fig. 35–4). Prognosis is good in patients with EDH who undergo surgical evacuation before the onset of neurologic decompensation (Langfitt, 1978). Eighty percent of these patients show a rapid recovery with little neurologic deficit. Mortality rates of 16% to 32% are reported when surgery is done rapidly (Gudeman et al., 1989).

INTRACEREBRAL HEMATOMA. An intracerebral hematom (ICH) is a well defined blood clot within the brain tissue (see Fig. 35–1). Similar to contusion, the most frequent sites for ICH are the frontal and temporal lobes (Jameson & Yelland, 1972). ICH is uncommon, representing only 1.5% to 21% of intracranial mass lesions (Bowers & Marshall, 1980; Miller et al., 1981). Small, deep hematomas within the periventricular, medial, or paracentral area follow shear forces and indicate diffuse axonal injury (Genarelli & Thibault, 1982). Intracerebral bleeding is found with lacerations after closed head injury but may also be found in patients with open or penetrating injury.

Signs and symptoms of ICH are similar to those of contusions, the course and outcome depending on the size and location of the hematoma. ICH is complicated by progressive focal edema and mass effect, which result in neurologic deterioration. Deterioration may be immediate or may follow the injury by 7 to 10 days (Spielman, 1988).

Delayed hemorrhage after ICH is known as delayed traumatic intracerebral hemorrhage (DTICH). DTICH occurs in areas that were injured at the time of impact but appeared normal on the initial CT scan.

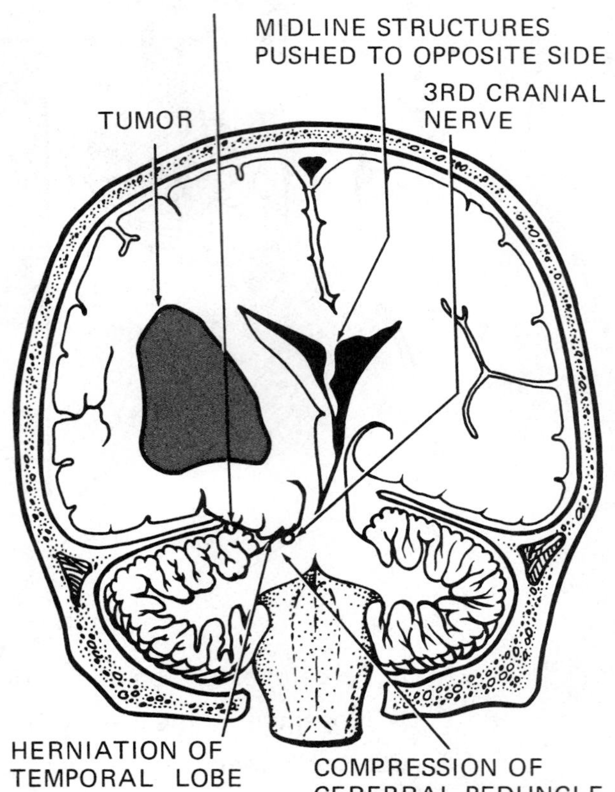

FIGURE 35–4. Cerebral herniation. Lesions or edema in the supratentorial compartment tend to push the uncus of the temporal lobe through the tentorial notch. This is called uncal or tentorial herniation. The downward pressure of the uncus compresses the oculomotor nerve and the posterior cerebral artery. With increasing pressure, the midbrain is compressed against the opposite side of the tentorium. (From Snyder, M., & Jackle, M. [1981]. *Neurologic problems: A critical care focus.* Bowie, MD: Robert J. Brady.)

Clot formation and deterioration occur within a few days of the original trauma (Cooper, 1985). DTICH is associated with a poor outcome and a high incidence of intracranial hypertension. Patients with disseminated intravascular coagulopathy, hypoxia, hypotension, or alcohol abuse have an increased incidence of DTICH (Cooper, 1985; Spielman, 1988).

CEREBRAL EDEMA AND INCREASED INTRACRANIAL PRESSURE

Cerebral edema is a common complication of head injury that affects cerebral function, increases ICP, and may interfere with neural function in edematous brain tissues (Cooper, 1985). Klatzo (1967) was the first to classify brain edema into cytotoxic and vasogenic types. Cytotoxic edema results in cellular metabolism abnormalities that allow the accumulation of fluid that is rich in electrolytes but low in proteins (Klatzo, 1967). The relevance of cytotoxic edema for head injury is unclear (Cooper, 1985).

There appears to be a relationship between the type

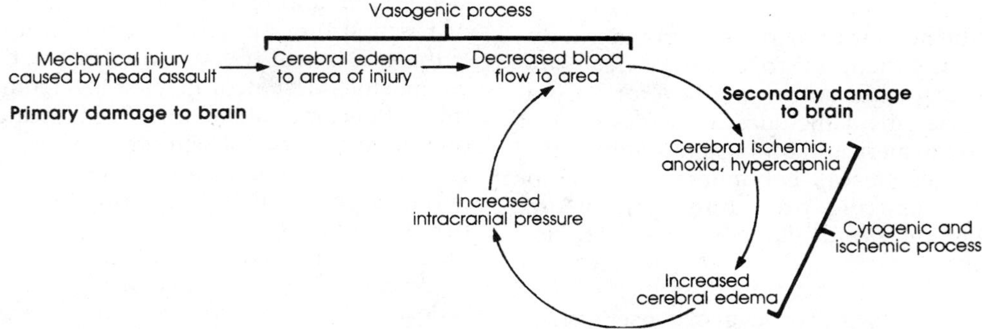

FIGURE 35–5. Mechanisms in cerebral edema from head trauma. (Reproduced by permission from: Rudy E. [1984]. *Advanced neurological and neurosurgical nursing.* St. Louis: C. V. Mosby Company.)

of cerebral injury and vasogenic edema (Fig. 35–5). Vasogenic edema results from a defect in cerebral capillaries that allows extravasation of plasma proteins and electrolytes into the extracellular cerebral tissues (Cooper, 1985). Edema spreads from the site of capillary injury into the white matter, diffusing into areas where capillaries remain intact.

Cerebral edema may be localized or diffuse. Diffuse cerebral edema of one or both hemispheres is common in traumatic brain injury. Cerebral edema exaggerates the amount and severity of any neurologic deficit that is present. The severity and extent of edema are related to the severity of the head injury. As the brain's compensatory mechanisms to accommodate additional brain mass fail, increases in ICP begin.

Intracranial hypertension is a major complication of head trauma and is the most frequent cause of death in head-injured patients (Walleck, 1990). The effects of cerebral edema and increased ICP on cerebral tissues depend on their severity and duration. Compression of blood vessels results in ischemia and infarction of brain tissue.

Normal ICP reflects the intracranial volume within the rigid skull. Intracranial volume is composed of brain tissue (80%), CSF (10%), and blood within blood vessels (10%). Increased ICP results from an increase in the volume of one of these three constituents without a compensatory decrease in one of the other two. The chief compensatory mechanism is a reduction of CSF by increased resorption, displacement into the subarachnoid space, or decreased production of CSF. Vasoconstriction with reduced blood volume or shifts of brain tissue may also occur, but these are of time-limited assistance.

The concept of compliance also contributes to an understanding of increased ICP. Compliance is an index of the volume–pressure relationship within the skull. When compensatory mechanisms fail, compliance is minimal, and a small increase in volume causes a large increase in pressure (Fig. 35–6).

Autoregulation is the automatic change in the caliber of the cerebral blood vessels over a broad range of mean arterial blood pressures to ensure normal perfusion pressure. The brain regulates its blood flow by autoregulation, which is influenced by systemic changes in blood pressure, and metabolic factors. Primary control of ICP occurs through autoregulatory mechanisms. Head trauma interferes with maximum functioning of autoregulation. Most nursing and medical interventions to control increased ICP support these compensatory mechanisms.

Posttraumatic epilepsy is the most common sequela of brain trauma, occurring in 5% of patients with closed head injury and 50% of patients with open head injuries (Hickey, 1986). The interval between trauma and the onset of seizures varies greatly. Fifty percent of patients have seizures within 1 to 6 months of injury; by the end of 2 years, 80% of the patients at risk will have had a seizure. Focal or tonic-clonic seizures are most common. Most seizures are amenable to anticonvulsant therapy. Because seizures tend to decrease in frequency over a period of years, it is estimated that 10% to 30% of these patients will eventually be seizure-free (Hickey, 1986).

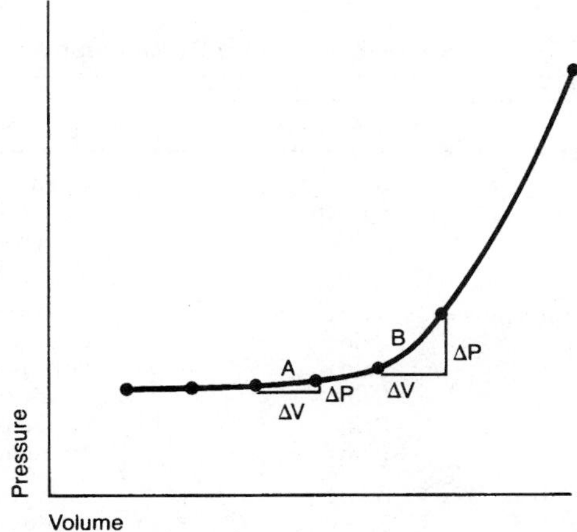

FIGURE 35–6. Pressure–volume curve. *A,* A change in volume (ΔV) causes only a small change in pressure (ΔP), and so elastance ($\Delta P/\Delta V$) is small. *B,* The elastance is high, and the same ΔV causes a much greater ΔP. (Reproduced from Bruce, D. A. [1978]. *The pathophysiology of increased intracranial pressure* [p. 19]. Kalamazoo, MI: The Upjohn Company, with permission from the publisher.)

Clinical Presentation

Assessment of the head trauma patient provides a dynamic overview of patient improvement or deterioration and guides diagnostic or therapeutic efforts. Complete physical assessment includes an assessment of the level of consciousness and brain stem reflexes (primarily pupillary responses). Laboratory data, radiologic procedures, imaging procedures, and neural monitoring techniques aid diagnosis and provide prognostic information.

LEVEL OF CONSCIOUSNESS. The level of consciousness is the most sensitive indicator of neurologic function. The Glasgow Coma Scale (GCS) is an internationally recognized tool for evaluating level of consciousness, both arousal and awareness (Table 35–1 and Fig. 35–7). The arousal component of consciousness depends on the function of the RAS in the brainstem. Awareness is a measure of cortical activity. The three functions assessed with the GCS are eye opening, verbal response, and motor response. The scale ranges from 3 to 15, with a score of 13 to 15 indicating mild head injury; 9 to 12 signifying moderate head injury; and a score of 8 or less indicating severe head injury or coma. This scale aids clinicians in making meaningful comparisons between patients and in predicting head injury outcomes and mortality (Spielman, 1988). The lower the GCS score, the deeper the coma and the higher the mortality and morbidity.

Another useful head injury assessment scale is the Rancho Los Amigos Scale (Table 35–2). This scale was designed by Chris Hagen, a speech and language pathologist (Hagen et al., 1979). The scale is based on standard evaluation criteria that provide a numerical reference for levels ranging from nonresponsiveness (level I) to purposeful and appropriate response (level VIII). This scale generalizes behavior from brain stem reflexes through high cortical activity and is useful in all phases of head injury care.

PUPILLARY RESPONSE. Pupils are normally equal in size, round, and react briskly to light. Changes in size or reaction time should be reported to the physician. If there is lateral transtentorial herniation from brain edema, mass lesion, or EDH or SDH, the ipsilateral pupil will become dilated and fixed because of pressure of brain matter on the oculomotor nerve (cranial nerve III). An oval-shaped pupil occurs with increased ICP and is associated with a poor prognosis (Marshall, Barber, & Toole, 1983a).

Other brain stem reflexes that can be assessed include corneal, gag, oculocephalic, and oculovestibular reflexes. The corneal reflex (cranial nerves V and VII), gag reflex (cranial nerves IX and X), and oculocephalic test, or doll's eye maneuver (cranial nerve VIII), are easily assessed at the bedside. The oculovestibular test involves instillation of ice water into the auditory canal and provides information on the function of cranial nerves III, VI, and VIII. Tests of these reflexes serve to assess the function of the brain stem. Absent brain stem reflexes indicate a poor prognosis.

VITAL SIGNS. Vital signs are routinely monitored on all neurotrauma patients. Blood pressure and heart rate are assessed to ensure adequate perfusion of brain tissues. Cerebral blood flow depends on the cerebral perfusion pressure (CPP) and the diameter of the cerebrovascular bed. CPP is the difference between the mean arterial pressure and the ICP. Normal CPP is 60 to 80 mm Hg (Miller, 1985). Alterations in CPP occur because of changes in the mean arterial pressure, which reflect changes in blood pressure, or changes in ICP. CPP falls when there is arterial hypotension or increased ICP. As ICP rises and cerebral blood flow falls, the systemic arterial blood pressure rises to maintain adequate cerebral perfusion. This is part of the Cushing reflex (i.e., increased systolic blood pressure, widened pulse pressure, and bradycardia). When autoregulation is lost after severe head injury, a rise in arterial pressure may be accompanied by a rise in

TABLE 35–1. **The Glasgow Coma Scale Response Chart**

	Stimulus/Measure	Patient's Response	Score
Eye opening	Spontaneous	Opens eyes independently	4
	Speech	Opens eyes in response to loud command	3
	Pain	Opens eyes with painful stimulus	2
	Pain	Does not open eyes even with painful stimulus	1
Best motor response	Verbal command	Follows simple commands	6
	Pain	Pushes away the source of painful stimulus	5
	Pain	Pulls body part away from painful stimulus	4
	Pain	Flexes body inappropriately in response to pain	3
	Pain	Body becomes rigid in extended position in response to pain stimulus	2
	Pain	No motor response to deep pain (pressure on nailbeds or orbital arch)	1
Verbal response	Speech	Converses appropriately and is oriented to person, place, and time	5
	Speech	Confused or disoriented	4
	Speech	Speech is understandable but nonsensical	3
	Speech	Unintelligible speech	2
	Speech	Makes no sound	1

Adapted from Rimel, R. (1978). Emergency management of the patient with central nervous system trauma. *Journal of Neurosurgical Nursing, 10*(4), 185–188.

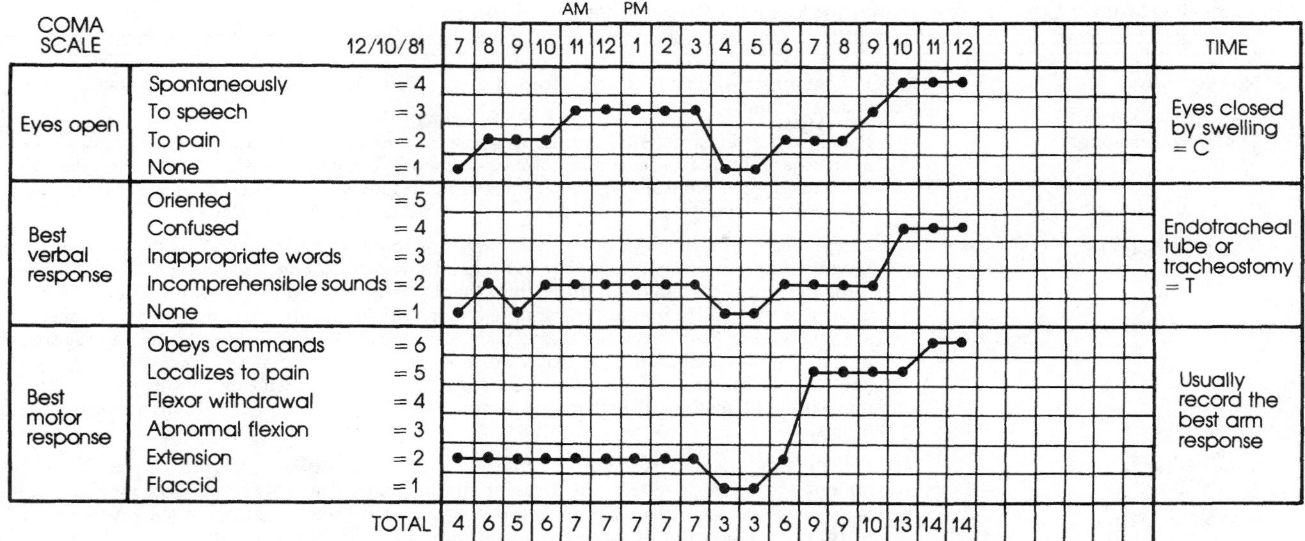

FIGURE 35–7. Glasgow coma scale for recording assessment of consciousness. (Reproduced by permission from Rudy, E. [1984]. *Advanced neurological and neurosurgical nursing.* St. Louis: C. V. Mosby Company.)

ICP, leading to reduced CPP (Miller, 1985). A change in the blood pressure and heart rate without an accompanying change in the level of consciousness indicates nonneurologic pathology. Classic Cushing reflex occurs late in the clinical course in patients whose condition is deteriorating.

Cardiac rate, rhythm, and conduction changes occur with a variety of intracranial injuries and may be neurogenic in origin. Dysrhythmias vary with the initial neurologic pathology. Progressive bradycardia, junctional escape rhythms, and idioventricular rhythms occur with cerebral hemorrhage and increased ICP. Atrial fibrillation and bundle branch blocks are more frequently seen with cerebral contusion. Acute subdural hematoma is associated with atrial and ventricular ectopy and conduction defects (Clifton et al., 1983; Staller, 1987).

ST- and T-wave changes follow cerebral ischemia resulting from severe head injury and increased ICP. Neurogenic T waves (inverted T waves with increased amplitude and duration) are associated with a variety of neurologic pathologies (Conner, 1969; Staller, 1987). The frequent, although inconsistent, electrocardiographic changes associated with intracranial pathology require continuous cardiac monitoring of these patients in the critical care unit (Nikas, 1987).

Changes in respiratory pattern are associated with the level of intracranial injury or the degree of pressure exerted on the brain stem. Centers controlling the regulation of respirations are scattered throughout the cerebral hemispheres and brain stem, and each center is responsible for a unique respiratory pattern (Spielman, 1988). Changes in respiration assist in identifying the area of injury and indicate neurologic deterioration. The earliest and most common respiratory alteration is Cheyne-Stokes respirations, which result from hemispheric compression (Spielman, 1988). Although it is not essential that the nurse know the name of each respiratory pattern, it is vital to identify changes, recognize the potential neurologic origin of the changes, and be prepared to provide neurologic and ventilatory support (Plum & Posner, 1982).

Temperature monitoring is essential after head injury. Hyperthermia increases metabolic demand in already compromised cerebral tissues and may contribute to increased ICP. Fever indicates either infection or hypothalamic dysfunction. Body temperature fluctuations from hypothermia to hyperthermia occur frequently with these patients, requiring continuous temperature monitoring.

Intracranial Pressure Monitoring

Monitoring ICP allows aggressive management of patients with potential or actual increased ICP. Lundberg (1960) introduced ICP monitoring in 1960, using direct cannulation of a ventricle with a catheter. Since Lundberg's work, several other monitoring methods have been introduced, including subdural, epidural, and intraparenchymal monitoring (see Chapter 13 for more information on ICP monitoring).

Overall, ICP monitoring allows early identification and rapid treatment of intracranial hypertension, a complication of head injury. Any head-injured patient with a GCS score of 8 or less is a candidate for ICP monitoring. Ability to monitor ICP allows critical evaluation of treatments used to prevent or control increased ICP. Because nursing activities have been implicated in elevating ICP, use of ICP monitoring allows

TABLE 35–2. **Rancho Los Amigos Hospital: Levels of Cognitive Functioning**

I. No response	Patient appears to be in a deep sleep and is completely unresponsive to any stimuli presented to him.
II. Generalized response	Patient reacts inconsistently and nonpurposefully to stimuli in a nonspecific manner. Responses are limited in nature and are often the same regardless of stimulus presented. Responses may be physiologic changes, gross body movements, and/or vocalizations. Often the earliest response is to deep pain. Responses are likely to be delayed.
III. Localized response	Patient reacts specifically but inconsistently to stimuli. Responses are directly related to the type of stimulus presented as in turning head toward a sound, focusing on an object presented. The patient may withdraw an extremity and/or vocalize when presented with a painful stimulus. He may follow simple commands in an inconsistent, delayed manner, such as closing his eyes, squeezing or extending an extremity. Once external stimuli are removed, he may lie quietly. He may also show a a vague awareness of self and body by responding to discomfort by pulling at nasogastric tube or catheter or resisting restraints. He may show a bias toward responding to some persons (especially family, friends) but not to others.
IV. Confused-agitated	Patient is in a heightened state of activity with severely decreased ability to process information. He is detached from the present and responds primarily to his own internal confusion. Behavior is frequently bizarre and nonpurposeful relative to his immediate environment. He may cry out or scream out of proportion to stimuli even after removal, may show aggressive behavior, attempt to remove restraints or tubes, or crawl out of bed in a purposeful manner. He does not, however, discriminate among persons or objects and is unable to cooperate directly with treatment efforts. Verbalization is frequently incoherent and/or inappropriate to the environment. Confabulation may be present; he may be euphoric or hostile. Thus gross attention to environment is very short, and selective attention is often nonexistent. Being unaware of present events, patient lacks short-term recall and may be reacting to past events. He is unable to perform self-care (feeding, dressing) without maximum assistance. If not disabled physically, he may perform motor activities as sitting, reaching, and ambulating, but as part of his agitated state and not as a purposeful act or on request necessarily.
V. Confused-inappropriate-nonagitated	Patient appears alert and is able to respond to simple commands fairly consistently. However, with increased complexity of commands or lack of any external structure, responses are nonpurposeful, random, or at best, fragmented toward any desired goal. He may show agitated behavior, but not on an internal basis (as in level IV), but rather as a result of external stimuli, and usually out of proportion to the stimulus. He has gross attention to the environment but is highly distractible and lacks ability to focus attention to a specific task without frequent redirection back to it. With structure, he may be able to converse on a social-automatic level for short periods of time. Verbalization is often inappropriate; confabulation may be triggered by present events. His memory is severely impaired, with confusion of past and present in his reaction to ongoing activity. Patient lacks initiation of functional tasks and often shows inappropriate use of objects without external direction. He may be able to perform previously learned tasks when structured for him, but is unable to learn new information. He responds best to self, body, comfort, and often family members. The patient can usually perform self-care activities with assistance and may accomplish feeding with maximum supervision. Management on the ward is often a problem if the patient is physically mobile, as he may wander off either randomly or with vague intention of "going home."
VI. Confused-appropriate	Patient shows goal-directed behavior but is dependent on external input for direction. Response to discomfort is appropriate, and he is able to tolerate unpleasant stimuli (as NG tube) when need is explained. He follows simple directions consistently and shows carry-over for tasks he has relearned (as self-care). He is at least supervised with old learning; maximally assisted for new learning with little or no carry-overs. Responses may be incorrect due to memory problems, but they are appropriate to the situation. They may be delayed to immediate situation and he shows decreased ability to process information with little or no anticipation or prediction of events. Past memories show more depth and detail than recent memory. The patient may show beginning immediate awareness of situation by realizing he does not know an answer. He no longer wanders and is inconsistently oriented to time and place. Selective attention to tasks may be impaired, especially with difficult tasks and in unstructured settings, but is now functional for common daily activities (30 minutes with structure). He may show a vague recognition of some staff, has increased awareness of self, family, and basic needs (as food), again in an appropriate manner as in contrast to level V.

TABLE 35–2. **Rancho Los Amigos Hospital: Levels of Cognitive Functioning** *Continued*

VII. Automatic-appropriate	Patient appears appropriate and oriented within hospital and home settings, goes through daily routine automatically, but frequently robotlike, with minimal to absent confusion, but has shallow recall of what he has been doing. He shows increased awareness of self, body, family, foods, people, and interaction in the environment. He has superficial awareness of, but lacks insight into his condition, decreased judgment and problem-solving, and lacks realistic planning for his future. He shows carry-over for new learning but at a decreased rate. He requires at least minimal supervision for learning and for safety purposes. He is independent in self-care skills for safety. With structure he is able to initiate tasks such as social or recreational activities in which he now has interest. His judgment remains impaired, such that he is unable to drive a car. Prevocational or avocational evaluation and counseling may be indicated.
VIII. Purposeful-appropriate	Patient is alert and oriented, is able to recall and integrate past and recent events, and is aware of and responsive to his culture. He shows carry-over for new learning if acceptable to him and his life role, and needs no supervision once activities are learned. Within his physical capabilities, he is independent in home and community skills, including driving. Vocational rehabilition, to determine ability to return as a contributor to society (perhaps in a new capacity), is indicated. He may continue to show a decreased ability, relative to premorbid abilities, in abstract reasoning, tolerance for stress, judgment in emergencies or unusual circumstances. His social, emotional, and intellectual capacities may continue to be at a decreased level for him, but functional in society.

From Hagen, C., Malkmus, D., Durham, P., et al. (1979). Rancho Los Amigos Hospital, Levels of Cognitive Functioning. Head Trauma Service, Rancho Los Amigos Medical Center, Downey, CA.

assessment while performing these activities and facilitates nursing research into the best methods to use in caring for these patients.

Laboratory Studies

Initial laboratory data provide a baseline for comparison with future laboratory studies. Baseline data also indicate the patient's overall physiologic status.

Because hypoxemia and hypercarbia aggravate brain injury, arterial blood gases (ABGs) should be monitored every 6 hours during intensive care. The $PaCO_2$ should be maintained 27 to 33 mm Hg (Marshall et al., 1990). A normal hemoglobin and hematocrit aid in ensuring adequate oxygen transport to the brain.

White blood cell counts with differential should be done daily to monitor for infection. Daily coagulation profiles assess for disseminated intravascular coagulation, which can be a complication of neurologic injury. Early diagnosis of coagulopathy allows early treatment, reducing mortality and morbidity from this complication.

It is important to monitor serum sodium, potassium, glucose, and chloride levels. Because of their role in nervous system function, changes in sodium and glucose levels may complicate the clinical course of patients with head injury. Iatrogenic fluid and electrolyte imbalance must be monitored for when dehydration or diuresis therapies are used. The serum osmolality should be closely monitored in these patients because diuretics and fluid restriction can cause dangerously high osmolality levels (>310 mOsm). Complications of diabetes insipidus (DI) and syndrome of inappropriate secretion of antidiuretic hormone (SIADH) can lead to hypoosmolar and hyperosmolar states. Blood serum osmolality, urine osmolality, urine specific gravity, and urine electrolytes (Na, K, and Cl) should be monitored as indices of fluid balance.

Diagnostic Procedures

SKULL FILMS. The skull x-ray is used to diagnose skull fractures in the emergency department. This is the most common neuroradiologic procedure used. These films also demonstrate facial fractures, especially orbital rim injuries.

COMPUTED TOMOGRAPHY. CT scanning has revolutionized the care of patients with head injury. CT scanning clearly identifies space-occupying lesions, contusions, and hemorrhagic or edematous areas in the brain. An accurate diagnosis can be made within minutes, allowing rapid initiation of therapy. CT scans have significantly reduced mortality and morbidity from EDH, SDH, and ICH.

MAGNETIC RESONANCE IMAGING. MRI promises to be an improvement over CT scanning. MRI is based on the interaction of protons, moved by radio waves, in a static magnetic field and provides excellent composites of the brain anatomy. No ionizing radiation or x-rays are associated with MRI. MRI surpasses CT scan in differentiating between gray and white matter and in detecting small hemorrhages in DAI (Spielman, 1988).

Because of technical problems, it is extremely difficult to use MRI in critically ill patients who are being mechanically ventilated with a ventilator that is not MRI-compatible, or in patients undergoing ICP monitoring. These problems include the longer time needed for MRI versus CT scanning; the magnetic field of MRI will not function with ferrous-containing compounds in the imaging room; and the radio frequency generator disrupt function of hemodynamic monitoring devices, including ICP monitors. Efforts are underway to correct these problems to allow use of MRI in critically ill patients.

EVOKED POTENTIAL STUDIES. Evoked potential studies have become valuable in locating lesions and in clarifying prognoses in head-injured patients. Evoked potential studies reflect the brain's response to specific sensory stimulation (visual, auditory, or somatosensory). They can be performed at the bedside and are valuable in assessing and monitoring patients who would be considered untestable or in a comatose state because of the influence of central nervous system depressants or barbiturate-induced coma.

CONTINUOUS CEREBRAL BLOOD FLOW STUDIES. A new technology introduced in the care of head-injured patients involves the continuous monitoring of cerebral circulation. Cerebral blood flow studies have been used in the past to define no-flow states in brain death. This technology involves the use of radiologically tagged xenon gas delivered by a computerized ventilator that monitors xenon uptake as a reflection of cerebral blood flow.

Although this technology is at present in limited use, it promises to be very helpful in determining the effect of brain injury on blood flow and monitoring the effects of treatment to improve blood flow in ischemic areas. Monitoring of cerebral blood flow may eventually replace ICP monitoring.

POSITRON EMISSION TOMOGRAPHY. Positron emission tomography (PET) is a major neurodiagnostic tool that has the potential capacity of providing simultaneous measurements of regional cerebral blood flow, metabolism, and biochemistry (Marshall et al., 1990). PET has been available since the late 1970s, but despite its ability to influence clinical care, it has not become widely used. Its complexity and cost (between $3,000 and $5,000 per session in 1990 dollars) plus the need for a cyclotron on site have made its use in most centers impractical (Marshall et al., 1990).

SINGLE PHOTON EMISSION COMPUTED TOMOGRAPHY. Single photon emission computed tomography (SPECT) was developed because of the limitations of PET scanning. The SPECT uses conventional nuclear medicine cameras to image regional cerebral blood flow and regional metabolic activity. Although not as precise as PET, SPECT is commonly used today to study perfusion.

DOPPLER ULTRASOUND. A bedside technique called Doppler ultrasound imaging offers the possibility of noninvasive screening for vascular problems. Transcranial Doppler is used to measure blood flow velocity, which can assist in determining the effect of the cerebral blood volume on the ICP.

OXYGEN SATURATION. The ability to monitor cerebral oxygen saturation is currently available and will be useful in monitoring the oxygen delivery to the brain. Measuring SjO_2 (jugular oxygen saturation) provides the most accurate picture of cerebral oxygenation (Langfitt, 1982; Marshall et al., 1990). If the SjO_2 is between 50% and 55%, one should suspect cerebral hypoxemia. Both of these bedside monitoring techniques are useful in guiding medical and nursing therapeutics.

Assessment of the patient with brain injury involves the use of a variety of techniques to provide a comprehensive picture of the patient's neurologic status. Comparison of current and past assessment data identifies subtle changes in neurologic status, allowing appropriate intervention in the patient's care.

Medical Management

The goals of medical management of patients with closed head injury include creating a brain tissue environment conducive to recovery; avoiding hypoxia, hypercapnia, hypotension; and preventing complications. Use of standard treatment protocols and early institution of therapy appropriate to the underlying pathology improve the potential for favorable outcomes.

OXYGENATION

Severely head-injured patients are intubated and ventilated to maintain their airways and prevent hypoxia and hypercapnia. High levels of supplemental oxygen should be provided to ensure adequate cerebral oxygenation (Nikas & Tolley, 1982). The goal of therapy is to acheive a PaO_2 of 80 to 100 mm Hg.

Ability to maintain adequate oxygenation may be compromised by pulmonary pathology (e.g., pulmonary contusion, atelectasis, pneumonia). Ventilation–perfusion abnormalities are found in many severely head-injured patients (Walleck, 1987). Meticulous pulmonary toilet is essential, including positioning, suctioning, and chest physiotherapy while attempts are made to maintain acceptable levels of ICP. Positive end-expiratory pressure (PEEP) may also be needed. PEEP prevents collapse of the alveoli at the end of expiration, improving gas exchange. In patients with normal pulmonary compliance, PEEP increases intrathoracic pressure, which may also increase ICP (Cepuzzo et al., 1977; Frost & Gildenberg, 1977). With pulmonary pathology, intrathoracic compliance is reduced, decreasing the impact on ICP (Frost & Gildenberg, 1977). Elevation of the head of the bed to 30° reduces the effect of PEEP on ICP (Cepuzzo et al., 1977).

HYPERVENTILATION

Hyperventilation has been part of most head injury protocols for the last two decades. Hyperventilation decreases the $PaCO_2$ and therefore constricts cerebral blood vessels, decreasing cerebral blood volume, which in turn decreases ICP. Each millimeter of mercury decrease in $PaCO_2$ results in a cerebral blood flow decrease of 2 to 3 mL/100 g of tissue per minute. This compromised blood flow can cause ischemia in injured brain tissues. $Paco_2$ of below 25 mm Hg should be avoided (Cooper, 1989). Because of this potential for ischemia, many institutions are no longer using hyperventilation on a routine basis. In patients with severe head injury, the vasoreactivity of cerebral vessels may be reduced, which also limits the therapeutic effectiveness of hyperventilation. Although hyperventilation produces respiratory alkalosis, which combats brain tissue acidosis, this may also lower the seizure threshold (Bruce et al., 1978; Shapiro, 1975; Spielman, 1988). Monitoring Pao_2 is essential to ensure that it remains within 27 to 33 mm Hg.

GLUCOCORTICOSTEROIDS

Glucorticosteroids had been used extensively to treat cerebral edema in patients with head injury. Most frequently used are dexamethasone and methylprednisolone. The usefulness of steroids in severe head injury is questionable—some researchers report positive effects, whereas others find no effect. Researchers who disclaim the effectiveness of steroids also believe that they may do harm by lowering resistance to infection and increasing the risk of gastrointestinal hemorrhage. Proponents of steroids believe that they reduce mortality from head injury as effectively as other therapeutic modalities.

It is speculated that steroids exert a stabilizing effect on the cell membrane. They may also improve neuronal function by improving cerebral blood flow and restoring autoregulation. Large doses and prolonged therapy are associated with complications, including carbohydrate intolerance and hyperglycemia, immunosuppression, decreased resistance to infection, gastric ulceration, and sodium and water retention (Spielman, 1988). New studies are being conducted on the use of high-dose steroids in head injury management.

DIURETIC THERAPY

Osmotically active agents have been used for over 50 years to treat cerebral edema. Hypertonic solutions remove cerebral tissue fluid via the vascular osmotic pressure gradient, reducing brain volume and lowering ICP. To be effective, the agent must remain within the intravascular compartment. If the blood–brain barrier is disupted, the therapy becomes more harmful than beneficial because the hypertonic solution could pass into the already edematous brain, increasing the edema in a rebound phenomenon.

Osmotherapeutic agents include mannitol, glycerol, and urea. Mannitol is most frequently used and has been found to be more effective than glycerol or pentobarbital in reducing ICP (Levin et al., 1979). Twenty percent mannitol is given as an intravenous bolus or continuous infusion in dosages ranging from 0.5 to 2.0 g/kg of body weight. Optimal effect is acquired with rapid administration. Its rapid onset of action makes this the preferred drug for elevated ICP. Hyperosmolality and acute renal failure are complications of hyperosmotic therapy. Monitoring fluids, electrolytes, and serum osmolality is essential to avoid severe dehydration.

Recent research has demonstrated the potential usefulness of nonosmotic diuretics (furosemide and ethacrynic acid) in reducing ICP. Furosemide is a potent loop diuretic that is thought to reduce ICP by decreasing sodium transport within the brain, reducing systemic fluid volume and inhibiting CSF production (up to 70%) (Spielman, 1988; Walleck, 1990). Loop diuretics minimize the potential for electrolyte and osmolality disturbances (Bakay & Wood, 1985).

Fluid dehydration has also been advocated to control ICP. The patient with isolated head injury is not usually hypovolemic and thus does not require large-volume fluid replacment. Fluid replacement should be based on indicators of fluid and electrolyte balance and on serum osmolality. Osmolality in the head-injured person should be between 305 and 310 mOsm/liter (normal, 275–296 mOsm/liter). Osmolality greater than 310 mOsm/liter can be dangerous and indicates a need to reduce or eliminate diuretic therapy (Spielman, 1988).

CONTROLLING METABOLIC ACTIVITY OF THE BRAIN

The pharmacologic control of cerebal metabolism is well established as a means of preventing cerebral dysfunction and controlling ICP. High doses of barbiturates (pentobarbital or thiopental) have been successful in reducing elevated ICP and protecting against cerebral hypoxia and ischemia. High doses of barbiturates stabilize cell membranes and produce superimposed coma, which reduces cerebral metabolism and cerebral blood flow (Marshall et al., 1979; Platt & Schiff, 1984).

Barbiturate therapy requires close monitoring of the patient. Because the ability to assess the neurologic status is lost, it is vital to monitor ICP and cerebral perfusion pressures in these patients. Because large doses of barbiturates may cause hypotension, endangering cerebral blood flow, mean arterial pressure monitoring is mandatory. Vasopressors may be required to maintain an adequate cerebral perfusion pressure. Although barbiturates effectively reduce ICP, they have not been demonstrated to decrease mortality (Marshall et al., 1979, 1990; Spielman, 1988).

Narcotic sedation has been used as an alternative to barbiturate therapy to control agitation and ICP. Fentanyl, a short-acting narcotic, can be administered intravenously in doses of 50 to 250 μg. This agent may be used to blunt the effect of turning or suctioning. The advantage of narcotic therapy is the ability to reverse the effect with naloxone, allowing neurologic assessment. Morphine should be avoided because it dilates cerebral blood vessels and may raise the ICP.

Many agents are being investigated for use in head-injured patients and ICP management, including alfaxalone, dimethyl sulfoxide, lidocaine, and phenytoin. These agents should be used only as part of approved clinical research protocols.

Alfaxalone is an intravenous steroid anesthetic that has properties similar to those of barbiturates. This agent combines the advantages of pentobarbital with the capability for rapid reversal and no systemic hypotension (Spielman, 1988; Versari et al., 1980).

Dimethyl sulfoxide (DMSO) has been used in experiments to treat cerebral stroke, acute brain injury, and spinal cord injury. DMSO is suspected to cause vasodilation, osmotic diuresis, decreased ICP, and decreased cellular oxygen consumption. A side effect, severe hypernatremia, has made this agent unacceptable for current use (Marshall et al., 1984).

Lidocaine is an anesthetic agent that suppresses neuronal activity and cerebral metabolism. This agent has been used to suppress the cough reflex and prevent arterial hypertension with endotracheal intubation. Lidocaine has been used before suctioning in doses of 50 to 100 mg given 2 minutes before the procedure to reduce sudden increases in ICP. This agent has not been shown to be effective in all subjects studied (Donegan & Bedford, 1980), making further study of its efficacy necessary.

Phenytoin is a widely used anticonvulsant, similar to barbiturates, that is known to decrease cerebral oxygen consumption. Clinical studies of this agent are required to test its effectiveness in the head-injured patient (Walleck, 1987).

A new protocol under investigation is known as hypothermic–hypokalemic coma. This therapy should be instituted within a few hours of injury as prophylaxis against secondary injury response. The patient is placed between cooling blankets and the head is surrounded by ice packets. The goal is to lower the body temperature to 30°C (86°F). In addition to cooling the patient, a pentobarbital drip is started and after a loading dose of 10 mg/kg, the drip is maintained at 0.25 mg/kg/hour. Nondepolarizing muscle relaxants and phenothiazines are used to control shivering. The hypothermia and suppressive drug regimen produces a hypometabolism. This protocol requires new management guidelines for the patient in the ICU, including being tolerant of a slight hypotension (a systolic pressure of 90 mm Hg), a lowered urine output, and a reduced metabolism for most drugs (Vise, 1994). This is currently an experimental protocol, with considerable research still needed to determine its efficacy.

FUTURE DRUG THERAPIES

As research continues to unravel the complexities of traumatic brain injury, the management of these patients may change dramatically in the next few years. The focus of the new interventions will be the treatment of the secondary events that follow the primary injury. Those secondary events include loss of calcium homeostasis and the enhanced production of free radicals. The results of the calcium release are the activation of lipolytic enzymes, proteolytic enzymes, and protein kinases, which jeopardizes cellular survival. The production of free radicals causes a pathogenic acidosis that is very difficult to normalize (Siesjo, 1993).

Future drug therapies include agents to compete with or block the receptors for excitatory amino acids that open the calcium channels. Antagonists such as ketamine, dizocilipine (MK-801), and phenylcyclidine block the calcium in channels. There is also evidence that these agents have a beneficial effect on cerebral blood flow (Meyer, 1993).

Calcium antagonists may also be beneficial in decreasing the influx of calcium into the mitochondria. Nimodipine has been demonstrated to decrease the incidence of ischemic deficits after subarachnoid hemorrhage (Meyer, 1993). Perhaps this agent may be useful in the treatment of traumatic brain injury.

The treatment of oxygen-free radicals, which produce a profound acidosis, has been difficult. Free radical scavengers such as polyethylene glycol-conjugated superoxide dismutase and catalase have been demonstrated to decrease infarct size in ischemic injury (Meyer, 1993). Clinical trials with head-injured patients are being conducted. Another group of free acid scavengers has already undergone trial in stroke patients, and is being studied in head injury. These agents are 21-amino steroids (lazaroids). These steroids have no glucocorticoid activity, but have the same properties as glucocorticosteroids, including maintaining the cellular membrane (White & Krause, 1993).

Tris-hydroxy-methyl aminomethane (THAM) is a buffering agent that penetrates the central nervous system, and therefore is theoretically superior to sodium bicarbonate for the treatment of central nervous system acidosis (Narayan, 1993). The agent has been shown to lower ICP.

SURGICAL MANAGEMENT

Recognition and rapid treatment of mass lesions are vital to improving outcomes in head-injured patients. A primary cause of death in patients who "talked and died" was delay in surgical intervention (Marshall, Toole, & Bowers, 1983b; Rose et al., 1977). Causes of delay include failure to identify the rate and significance of neurologic deterioration and inappropriately relating deterioration to alcohol intoxication or other neurologic pathology. CT scanning has significantly reduced the misdiagnosis of mass lesions. Determination of the need for surgery is facilitated by assessment and CT scan findings.

Clinical Management

Nursing care of patients with traumatic head injury is guided by the severity of the injury and the medical plan of care. Nursing diagnoses involve actual and potential problems and focus on preventing secondary brain injury due to hypoxemia, hypercarbia, increased cerebral metabolism, and increased ICP, to maximize functional outcome.

ALTERATION IN CEREBRAL TISSUE PERFUSION

Cerebral injury results in disrupted local blood supply and cerebral edema.

EXPECTED OUTCOMES. Neurologic status improves or remains stable, ICP of the resting patient is less than 15 mg Hg, and cerebral perfusion pressure is more than 50 mm Hg.

Neurologic assessements focus on level of consciousness (using the GCS), pupillary reflexes, and motor function. Careful documentation of findings allows identification of subtle changes of deterioration over time.

Intracranial pressure monitoring is essential in patients with severe head injury. Accuracy of the system is important to ensure that interventions can be accomplished when indicated. ICP monitoring also reflects the impact of nursing care activities and therapy on ICP.

The head of the bed should be elevated 30 to 45 degrees to facilitate venous drainage of the head and decrease ICP. Some recent research has suggested that patients with severe intracranial hypertension should be nursed in the flat position (Feldman et al., 1992; Rosner & Coley, 1992). These researchers state that raising the head of the bed decreases the cerebral perfusion pressure, which increases the ICP. More study is needed in this area. Head and body alignment should also be maintained.

POTENTIAL FOR INJURY DUE TO DECREASED INTRACRANIAL ADAPTIVE CAPACITY

EXPECTED OUTCOMES. ICP remains at less than 15 mm Hg during nursing care activities or returns to baseline immediately, and cerebral perfusion pressure remains above 50 mm Hg.

Because routine care activities may increase ICP, patients with decreased adaptive capacity the nurse should use interventions for positioning, suctioning, and hygiene that are based on research in this area.

Because activities have a cumulative effect on ICP, care activities should be spaced to allow intervals of inactivity that permit the ICP to return to baseline. The patient's baseline should be assessed before any intervention. If ICP is monitored, the cerebral perfusion pressure should be calculated during all activities using the following formula:

$$MAP - ICP = CPP$$

where MAP = mean arterial pressure, and CPP = cerebral perfusion pressure. Nursing care procedures may safely be performed as long as the cerebral perfusion pressure remains at or above 50 mm Hg.

Hyperoxygenation and hyperventilation before, during, and after suctioning blunt the effect of suctioning on ICP. Limiting suctioning to no more than 10 seconds at a time also limits elevation of ICP.

Controlling the cerebral metabolic rate (CMR) increases the adaptive capacity of the brain. A quiet environment with meaningful stimuli should be basic to the care of these patients. Barbiturate coma decreases the CMR for oxygen ($CMRO_2$) and protects the neuroglial cells, but may also cause cardiovascular depression, requiring continuous monitoring and appropriate interventions for hypotension. Narcotic sedation appears to be more beneficial in controlling or decreasing cerebral metabolism.

POTENTIAL ALTERED BODY TEMPERATURE DUE TO LOSS OF THERMOREGULATION OR INFECTION

EXPECTED OUTCOMES. Patient remains normothermic, or temperature elevations are rapidly identified and interventions begun before complications occur.

A rectal temperature probe allows continuous monitoring and identification of rapid temperature changes. Because of increased cerebral metabolism, temperature elevations should be avoided. Interventions to reduce temperature elevations need to be implemented quickly, including use of acetaminophen, tepid water baths, ice packs, or cooling blankets. Rapid cooling and prolonged use of hypothermia blankets should be avoided because of the potential for shivering, which increases cerebral metabolism and ICP. Shivering is avoided by reducing the temperature slowly and discontinuing use of hypothermia when the temperature reaches 38°C (100°F). Sometimes sedation with thorazine is required to control shivering (Spielman, 1988).

POTENTIAL FLUID VOLUME DEFICIT

Fluid volume deficits may be due to therapeutic osmotic diuresis or fluid restriction, or to complications of DI or SIADH.

EXPECTED OUTCOME. Fluid and electrolyte balance is maintained.

Intake and output should be monitored hourly. Taking weights daily or biweekly assists in identifying the presence of fluid retention. Signs of DI that require notification of the physician include thirst, dehydration, diluted urine, diuresis, low specific gravity, decreased urine osmolality, elevated serum osmolality, and elevated serum sodium level. Patients with an altered level of consciousness are often unable to report their thirst and require astute observation by the nurse to recognize symptoms of DI. Therapy for DI involves replacement of free water and administration of aqueous vasopressin or vasopressin tannate in oil.

Syndrome of inappropriate antidiuretic hormone secretion results in continuous resorption of water from the renal tubule, causing a serum osmolality of less than 280 mOsm/kg of water and hyponatremia (>125 mmol/liter). SIADH leads to water intoxication and cerebral edema. Indicators that require notification of the physician include weight gain without obvious edema, neurologic deterioration, and increased urinary sodium. Treatment depends on severity but includes fluid restriction, furosemide, and, possibly, judicious use of hypertonic saline (3% sodium chloride).

Excess fluid loss may also result from "neurogenic sweats," during which 500 to 1,000 mL of fluid may be lost. Calculation of fluid loss should include comment on the number of diaphoretic episodes.

POTENTIAL FOR INJURY DUE TO INCREASED CEREBRAL METABOLISM AND INTRACRANIAL PRESSURE DURING SEIZURES

EXPECTED OUTCOME. Seizures do not occur, or, if they do, no injury results from the seizures.

Anticonvulsants are used to prevent and control seizures. Seizure precautions should be used with all patients with head injury, including keeping the bed in a low position, keeping side rails up and padded (as necessary), and keeping an airway at the bedside.

If a seizure occurs, the onset, characteristics, and duration of abnormal activity should be carefully documented. A patent airway should be maintained and supplemental oxygen provided. Objects that may injure the patient should be removed. Restraint of the patient during the seizure may result in injury, and should be avoided.

INEFFECTIVE FAMILY COPING

Family coping may be impeded by the overwhelming aspects of head injury to a family member.

EXPECTED OUTCOME. Patient and family are able to cope effectively with the situation as shown by their positive adaptations to limitations.

Family members may experience fear, helplessness, and a loss of control. The family can be assisted in identifying tasks they can perform (exercises, repositioning) that aid the patient's recovery. When the patient responds, encourage the family to listen to the patient's concerns and identify problem areas in which the staff can intervene. Encourage the family to talk about current events and reminisce about the patient's past to facilitate communication with the semicomatose or comatose patient. Incorporate the family's efforts into the care of the patient to the extent with which they are comfortable.

Extensive support services are available through the National Head Injury Foundation, Inc. This organization was established by the family of a severely head-injured child and has grown rapidly to become a national organization that emphasizes support for head-injured patients and their families as well as support for research in this area. For local chapters and support group information, families and patients may be referred to the National Head Injury Foundation, 1776 Massachusetts Ave., NW, Suite 100, Washington, DC 20036; telephone (800) 444-6443. (See also Chapter 7, Psychosocial Needs of Families.)

ALTERED THOUGHT PROCESSES DUE TO THE EFFECT OF BRAIN INJURY ON COGNITIVE PROCESSES

EXPECTED OUTCOME. Patient will attain maximal cognitive function, and independent functioning will be encouraged.

Assessment of cognitive function aids in determining level of consciousness. The Rancho Los Amigos scale of cognitive function aids in this assessment (see Table 35–2) (Hagen et al., 1979). When scale scores of level I, II, or III are noted, the patient should receive low-level stimulation of all senses. Most touch stimulation of the patient is the natural outcome of nursing care (e.g., from turning and bathing). Soft, conversational speech or music provides auditory stimuli. Taste is stimulated through oral hygiene or popsicles. Pleasant-smelling substances close to the patient stimulate the olfactory senses. To prevent confusion, stimulation of one sense at a time should be attempted (Spielman, 1988).

Additional nursing diagnoses for these patients may include Self-Care Deficit, Impaired Verbal Communication, and Alteration in Nutrition: Less Than Body Requirements. Holistic patient care will prevent secondary injury to the brain and avoid the many complications to which these patients are prone.

Clinical management of the traumatic head-injured patient has changed dramatically in the past decade. Improved emergency medical care, improved CT scanning in diagnosis, and more aggressive treatment have combined to produce better patient outcomes.

ISCHEMIC BRAIN INJURY

Brain ischemia has many causes, and may be focal or generalized. Focal ischemia may result from traumatic brain injury, cerebral vasospasm, or stroke, whereas generalized ischemia may be caused by asphyxiation, severe hypovolemia, or cardiorespiratory arrest. This section focuses on global ischemia as the cause of brain injury.

Pathophysiology of Ischemic Injury

METABOLIC CONSEQUENCES

Cessation of brain circulation results in depletion of oxygen and a loss of consciousness within about 10 seconds, and in the depletion of glucose and adenosine triphosphate (ATP) within about 5 minutes (Safar, 1983). Without ATP, the cellular sodium–potassium pump fails, leading to cerebral edema (cytotoxic edema). If ischemia continues, the blood–brain barrier is damaged, allowing vasogenic edema to increase the injury (Jordan, 1983). After 4 to 7 minutes of total ischemia, calcium enters the cell and mitochondria (Jordan, 1983; Safar, 1983). The occipital cortex, basal ganglia, and diencephalon are more susceptible to ischemic–anoxic damage than the frontal and temporal cortices (Nemoto, 1978).

REPERFUSION

Once cerebral perfusion is restored, reperfusion occurs nonhomogeneously throughout the brain. The nonuniformity of reperfusion probably results from varied degrees of vasospasm, increased local tissue pressures, capillary compression, and intravascular coagulation (Nemoto, 1978). Reperfusion may provoke secondary changes that evolve into microscopic infarctions (Safar, 1983). These microinfarctions probably result from transient vasoparalysis, hypoperfusion from blood cell sludging, catecholamine-stimulated hypermetabolism, tissue acidosis, free chemical radicals that damage cell membranes, or varying degrees of intracellular or extracellular edema. These secondary changes may be exacerbated by noncerebral organ system failures.

NO-REFLOW PHENOMENON

In 1968, Ames and colleagues described a no-reflow phenomenon as causing continuing neuronal injury despite reestablished circulation (Jordan, 1983). They speculated that lack of perfusion resulted from increased blood viscosity in low- and no-flow states because of red blood cell aggregation, and theorized that during stasis of global ischemia, red blood cells aggregate in dependent areas, increasing blood viscosity. When circulation is reestablished, the vessels are unable to be reperfused, resulting in patchy areas of no flow (Fischer, 1974).

Clinical Presentation

After global ischemia, the patient is usually comatose, with a GCS score of less than 8. Duration of coma after resuscitation from global ischemia is the most reliable indicator of patient outcome (Epstein & Hamilton, 1983).

NEUROLOGIC ASSESSMENT

Neurologic assessment of the patient with ischemic brain injury is performed in the same way as that for traumatic brain injury. The following discussion focuses on predictors of outcomes that are based on assessment data.

LEVEL OF CONSCIOUSNESS

The coma after global ischemic injury implies bilateral diffuse dysfunction of the cerebral hemispheres or, less commonly, damage to the upper brain stem (Koehler & Michael, 1985). Although presentation in coma does not necessarily indicate a poor prognosis, coma lasting more than 2 days is associated with a poor neurologic outcome (Koehler & Michael, 1984; Safar, 1983). Motor unresponsiveness or flaccidity, assessed through the GCS, carries a poor prognosis (Snyder et al., 1977). Flexion and extension posturing are serious indicators, but are not effective as predictors.

PUPIL CHANGES AND OTHER BRAIN STEM REFLEXES

Absence of pupillary light response and oculocephalic (doll's eyes) and oculovestibular (caloric) reflexes at 6 and 12 hours after ischemic insult signifies a poor but not hopeless prognosis (Snyder et al., 1977). Pupil size and spontaneous eye movements are unreliable indicators of prognosis. Synder and colleagues (1981) reported 100% mortality in patients with three or more reflex abnormalities or those without corneal or pupillary light reflexes 3 hours after global ischemic–anoxic injury from cardiac arrest.

VITAL SIGNS

Studies of the predictive powers of vital signs have been inconclusive. The presence or absence of spontaneous breathing shows promise as a predictor, but further study is needed.

INTRACRANIAL PRESSURE MONITORING

Although sudden ischemia results in a fluid shift, causing cerebral edema, this may not raise ICP unless the insult is prolonged and severe (Safar, 1983). Monitoring ICP is not common after an ischemic insult, but most physicians assume that cerebral edema occurs and intervene to prevent elevated ICP.

LABORATORY FINDINGS

Examination of CSF provides important information about the degree of cellular injury. Concentrations of ATP and phosphocreatinine return to normal after brain injury even without functional recovery. Elevations of amino acids persist after injury, and the level of alanine increases in proportion to the duration of global ischemia (Debard, 1983).

The CSF creatinine kinase level appears to be related to the amount of cellular injury and may eventually provide a means of assessing the potential for recovery. Measures of serum and CSF creatinine kinase-BB fraction (CKBB) at 6 hours after cardiac arrest are related to neurologic outcome and survival (Longstreth et al., 1981). CSF CKBB levels of less than 2 units/liter are associated with a good recovery, whereas levels greater than 10 units/liter are associated with a poor outcome or death.

Diagnostic Procedures

A variety of procedures is used to diagnose ischemic injuries. Many of these diagnostic tests were discussed in greater detail in the previous section of this chapter on closed head injury. Only the specific use of these procedures for ischemic injuries is described here.

After 72 hours, CT scans will identify cerebral edema and areas of infarction. CT scans also rule out other causes of coma, such as mass lesions.

Because MRI clearly demonstrates edema, it shows promise as a diagnostic tool in patients with ischemic injuries. MRI also demonstrates small areas of infarction earlier than CT scans. More experience with this tool is necessary to evaluate its effectiveness. The major problem with using MRI to follow global ischemia is that the patient often requires ventilatory support, and no metal can be used in the area of the MRI because the imaging machine creates a strong magnetic field.

Evoked potential studies test neuronal pathway integrity and detect marginally functional neurons missed in neurologic assessment. Relationships between evoked potentials and patient prognosis have been identified (DeBard, 1983).

Electroencephalography (EEG) is most effective as a negative predictor (i.e., for identifying nonsurvivors). It is not effective in predicting survivors or disability (DeBard, 1983).

Monitoring of cerebral blood flow can determine areas of hyperemia and poor reperfusion after ischemic injury. With further research, this procedure may be shown to be effective in guiding treatment to maximize blood flow to ischemic areas.

Medical Management

Neurologic deficit may be intensified after a global ischemic insult by extracranial complications of hypoxemia, hypotension, hypercarbia, hyperthermia, or sepsis. Preventing these complications may ameliorate the neurologic deficit. Safar (1981) outlined the therapeutic goals that should be set after ischemic insult:

1. Control the mean arterial pressure at between 90 and 100 mm Hg, maintaining systolic blood pressure at 100 mm Hg or higher.
2. Maintain Pa_{CO_2} at 100 mm Hg or more.
3. Keep arterial pH within a range of 7.3 to 7.6.
4. Decrease the $CMRO_2$ by immobilizing the patient with sedatives and paralytic agents.
5. Maintain the following blood value limits:
   a. Hematocrit, 30% to 40%
   b. Electrolytes, within normal limits
   c. Plasma colloidal osmotic pressure, 15 mm Hg or higher
   d. Albumin, 3 g/100 mL or above
   e. Serum osmolality, 280 to 315 mOsm/liter
   f. Glucose, 100 to 300 mg/100 mL
6. Maintain normothermia or mild hypothermia for a short interval.
7. Monitor central nervous system status closely using the GCS, EEG, and CT scanning.

These are the immediate goals of therapy, and these procedures are maintained throughout the period of unresponsiveness (usually 2–7 days) (Safar, 1983).

OXYGENATION

The uninjured brain uses 20% of all consumed oxygen (3.5 mL/100 g tissue per minute). Mild hyperoxygenation ($Pa_{O_2} \geq 100$ mm Hg) should be provided immediately after an ischemic insult. Controlled ventilation with an Fi_{O_2} of 1.0 ensures an adequate Pa_{O_2}, Pa_{CO_2}, and pH. Neuromuscular blockade may be needed to ensure controlled ventilation.

HYPERVENTILATION

Hyperventilation decreases Pa_{CO_2} and produces a constriction of the cerebral blood vessels. Careful monitoring of the hyperventilation and Pa_{CO_2} is important because a Pa_{CO_2} of less than 25 mm Hg may result in excessive vasoconstriction in reactive brain areas while also decreasing cardiac output (Jagger & Bobovsky, 1983).

GLUCOCORTICOSTEROIDS

Use of corticosteroids after an ischemic insult with coma is controversial (Safar, 1983). There are no studies of the use of steroids after global ischemic injury. After ischemic brain injury, the use of steroids would be an adjunctive measure as part of a combination of brain resuscitation measures (Safar, 1983).

DIURETIC THERAPY

Short-term, low-dose osmotherapy and mannitol may be used to control increased ICP. Although this therapy may be initially helpful with large doses of osmotic agents, rebound edema may occur, limiting its usefulness (Safar, 1983).

The use of DMSO has been investigated to control ICP. DMSO is a water-soluble, organic industrial solvent. Low concentrations of DMSO have been used in clinical trials in patients with cerebral stroke, spinal cord injury, and acute brain injury. DMSO is suspected to cause cerebral vasodilation, osmotic diuresis, changes in prostaglandin actions, stabilization of mitochondria from tissue injury, decreased cellular oxygen consumption during anoxia, and decreased ICP. In humans this agent also acts as a potent diuretic.

The main side effects of DMSO are nausea, headache, ventricular toxicity demonstrated by dysrhythmias with prolonged use, respiratory stimulation, and hemolysis (Martin, 1983). Hemolysis appears to be related to use of high concentrations of DMSO. More research is needed on the use of this agent in global ischemic injury.

CEREBRAL METABOLIC CONTROL

Barbiturate coma reduces cerebral metabolism and suppresses seizure activity. Barbiturates may also block noxious stimuli through their anesthetic effects; scavenge free chemical radicals resulting from ischemia; alter metabolic pathways; and suppress catecholamine hypermetabolism (Safar, 1983). Clinical trials show promising results with thiopental and pentobarbital. A recently published study reports research done in nine countries using thiopental (30 mg/kg) as the barbiturate. This report noted that barbiturates do not exert a marked improvement on neurologic recovery after global ischemia. Because of the frequent cardiorespiratory side effects, the researchers did not recommend routine use of barbiturates after cardiac arrest (Abramson et al., 1985).

Phenytoin is being investigated for its action in controlling the CMR by decreasing $CMRO_2$. Phenytoin promotes sodium efflux from neurons, stabilizing and protecting the neuron from hyperexcitability. Phenytoin may also enhance cerebral blood flow by promoting vasodilation after ischemia, and may increase brain energy reserves (Martin, 1983). The dosage schedules for brain resuscitation have not been established. Administration of phenytoin should not exceed 50 mg/minute because of the associated potential for cardiac dysrhythmia, hypotension, or arrest.

MAINTAINING HOMEOSTASIS

Facilitating the patient's rapid return to homeostasis is assumed to be beneficial after ischemic injury. Initial therapy involves the ABCs of emergency care (airway, breathing, and circulation). Opening the airway and providing supplemental oxygen will reduce hypoxia and minimize further brain injury. Tracheal intubation and controlled ventilation are usually necessary.

Avoidance of hypotension or severe hypertension is essential; the usual goal is a normotension (mean arterial pressure = 100 mm Hg). Safar (1983) has advocated the benefits of mild sustained hypertension (mean arterial pressure ≥ 150 mm Hg) after the restoration of cerebral circulation. Severe hypertension increases cerebral blood volume and ICP, which may cause cerebral edema or hemorrhage and exacerbate the postischemic neurologic deficit.

Plain dextrose and water solutions should not be used for fluid replacement because they contribute to cerebral edema. Infusions of 5% to 10% dextrose in 0.25 to 0.5 normal saline solutions are preferred (Safar, 1983).

Normothermia or mild hypothermia should be maintained. Hypothermia reduces cerebral metabolism, but the actual mechanism of action after ischemic brain injury has yet to be documented. Complications of hypothermia include cardiac dysrhythmias, increased blood viscosity and reduced tissue blood flow, and increased potential for infection and stress ulcers (Safar, 1983). A study of the risks and benefits of hypothermia is needed to document the efficacy of this therapy.

OTHER INVESTIGATIONAL DRUGS

CALCIUM CHANNEL BLOCKERS. Safar (1983) described the postischemic reperfusion phenomenon as a result of cerebral vasospasm, blood cell sludging, and clotting. Calcium and sodium ions that accumulate within neurons may also contribute to destructive metabolic activity after cerebral ischemia. Calcium channel blockers may deter the increased blood viscosity and decrease vasospasm. For example, nifedipine counters elevated ionized calcium in cytosol and mitochondria, and flunarizine interferes with calcium ion entry into the plasma membrane (Raffsen & Davis, 1989). The future role of calcium channel blockers in patients undergoing brain resuscitation is uncertain (Martin, 1983).

LIDOCAINE. Lidocaine's role in controlling increased ICP was discussed earlier. Lidocaine may also play a role as a calcium channel blocker, so that intravenous or endotracheal administration of lidocaine may eventually be used to treat ischemic injuries.

Other agents currently being studied are prostaglandin-blocking agents, opiate blockers (naloxone), and brain-buffering agents (THAM). These agents may be useful in preventing or correcting the metabolic effects of global ischemia.

Clinical Management

Nursing care of survivors of global ischemic injury is challenging, as is the care of any comatose patient with an unknown prognosis. Recovery from global ischemic injury is determined not only by the course of the pathologic state but by the intensity of the nursing care provided for the patient. In addition to the following nursing diagnoses, those discussed under Traumatic Brain Injury are also applicable.

TOTAL SELF-CARE DEFICIT DUE TO UNCONSCIOUSNESS

EXPECTED OUTCOME. The patient's basic care needs will be met until the patient is able to participate in self-care.

All basic care activities are provided based on the patient's tolerance. Care activities should be done at intervals to prevent the cumulative effects of these activities on ICP.

IMPAIRED VERBAL COMMUNICATION DUE TO COMA, INTUBATION, OR VARYING DEGREES OF UNCONSCIOUSNESS

EXPECTED OUTCOME. Patient maintains optimal communication level for his or her physiologic state. Family members actively communicate with the patient.

An inability to communicate contributes to the overwhelming fear and frustration experienced by patients and families. The nurse needs to use a creative approach to help these patients communicate their needs. Letter and picture boards may be used for selected patients. Although use of communication boards is tedious and time consuming, they may be the only means of communication by the patient with others. It is important to spend time with the patient and family to teach them how to use the communication method adequately. The nurse should acknowledge the patient's frustration about the slowness of communication, while encouraging patience. The family needs to be encouraged to continue to communicate with the patient, reminiscing about past experiences and discussing current events. If the patient has awareness, this will provide sensory stimulation while also allowing the family to feel capable of contributing to the care of the patient.

ALTERATION IN NUTRITION: LESS THAN BODY REQUIREMENTS

Malnutrition may be due to immobility, decreased gastrointestinal mobility, dysphagia, anorexia, or depression.

EXPECTED OUTCOME. Patient maintains ideal body weight. Enteric or parenteral nutrition is necessary with comatose patients to accommodate the increased metabolism due to the stress of the injury. Patients who are receiving tube feedings should be assessed for excessive gastric residual (>50 mL in 2 hours for those on continuous feedings and >100 mL for those on every-4-hour feedings). Metoclopramide hydrochloride may be ordered to facilitate gastric emptying. Most institutions have established regimens for patients receiving total parenteral nutrition to ensure adequate hydration and nutrition while avoiding any iatrogenic influences of the therapy. Weights taken daily or every other day allow monitoring of nutritional status. Serum albumen and total lymphocyte counts also aid in determining the patient's nutritional status.

INEFFECTIVE FAMILY COPING: COMPROMISED OR DISABLING

Family coping abilities may be ineffective due to the overwhelming aspects of the patient's illness.

EXPECTED OUTCOME. Patient, when appropriate, and family are able to cope effectively with the situation as shown by the absence of abnormal reactions.

Family members may experience fear, helplessness, and a loss of control. The family can be helped to identify tasks that they can perform (range-of-motion exercises, sensory stimulation, repositioning) that aid the patient's recovery. Encourage the family to talk about current events and reminisce about the patient's past to distract the patient from the reality of the current situation and foster a sense of hope. The family should be allowed to participate in the care of the patient to the extent that they are comfortable.

METABOLIC DISORDERS

Because the brain is sensitive to changes in homeostasis, disturbances in other body systems often affect brain function. Changes in consciousness are early indicators of most acute and subacute metabolic encephalopathies. Primary metabolic encephalopathies include Creutzfeldt-Jakob disease, Alzheimer syndrome, Huntington chorea, and Pick disease. Secondary encephalopathies, which are related to dysfunction of other organ systems, include pancreatic, liver, or kidney disease; toxic reactions to drugs or heavy metals; and hypoxia. This section focuses on secondary metabolic encephalopathies related to liver failure, hypoglycemia, renal failure, and toxic reactions.

Hepatic Encephalopathy

Severe liver disease eventually involves the central nervous system, usually with progressive mental, cerebellar, or extrapyramidal deterioration (Plum & Posner, 1983). The actual pathogenesis depends on the underlying hepatic disease. Although many toxic agents or deficiencies have been proposed as potential causes of hepatic coma, none has been clearly linked to this process.

Hypoglycemia

Hypoglycemia is a common cause of metabolic coma and is associated with great variation in the presenting findings (Plum & Posner, 1983). The major pathology of hypoglycemia involves the cerebral hemispheres, and the resulting encephalopathy presents in one of the following ways (Plum & Posner, 1982):

1. Delirium with mental changes varying from sleepy confusion to wild mania
2. Coma with signs of multifocal brain stem dysfunction, including central neurogenic hyperventilation, decerebation, and hypothermia with pupillary reaction preserved
3. Stroke-like findings with focal neurologic signs with or without coma and shifting neurologic deficits
4. Single or multiple generalized convulsions and postictal coma

Toxic Reactions

Ingestion of large amounts of alcohol, barbiturates, sedatives, other drugs, poisons, and some heavy metals may result in encephalopathy. Toxic reactions may also follow absorption through the skin or inhalation.

The mechanism of toxic reactions on the nervous system is unclear. With some drugs and alcohol there is a depression of central nervous system function, including the brain stem. Suggested mechanisms of action include interference with neurotransmitter synthesis or release, focal demyelination, axonal edema, or disruption of cellular biochemistry (Hickey, 1986).

Pathophysiology

The normal brain consumes 3.5 mL of oxygen/100 g tissue per minute; this is known as the $CMRO_2$, and represents 15% to 20% of the systemic oxygen consumed. $CMRO_2$ levels of 2.5 mL/100 g per minute are associated with changes in level of consciousness, and coma follows a $CMRO_2$ of 2.0 mL/100 g per minute. Normal cerebral blood flow is 50 to 60 mL/100 g per minute (Plum & Posner, 1982), and interferences in the rate of flow result in changes in consciousness.

Glucose is the main source of energy for the brain, but the brain is unable to store much glucose (only about 2 g). Each 100 g of brain tissue requires 5.5 mg of glucose/minute. Lacking adequate glucose, the brain begins anaerobic metabolism, which results in lactic acidosis.

The severity of symptoms is related to the amount and areas of the brain affected. Symptoms usually are aggravated by the compensatory mechanisms of hyperpnea, hypoventilation, metabolic acidosis or alkalosis, or fluid shifts.

Clinical Presentation

Presenting signs are related to the etiology, depth of coma, complications associated with the primary illness, and treatment of the primary illness. Differential diagnosis of metabolic coma is difficult but is assisted by careful assessment of the level of consciousness, respirations, pupillary response, extraocular movements, motor function, and EEG evaluations.

Level of consciousness varies from mild drowsiness to total unresponsiveness. The pupillary response aids in distinguishing metabolic from structural disease. A preserved pupillary response to light in the presence of decerebrate rigidity or muscle flaccidity and respiratory depression suggests metabolic coma (Plum & Posner, 1982). The eyes in patients with metabolic coma usually rove randomly.

Motor changes may be either nonspecific in strength, tone, and reflexes accompanied by seizures, or they may involve adventitious movement with weakness, loss of tone, grasp reflexes, and prehensile sucking. Tremors may be present in patients with metabolic coma, but are usually absent at rest. Asterixis is associated with metabolic coma and is characterized by sudden palmar or plantar flapping (liver flap), which can occur at rest or in response to dorsiflexion. Some patients manifest multifocal myoclonus, which is a sudden, nonrhythmic, nonpatterned gross twitching of all muscle groups.

Respiratory changes may include hyperventilation, hypoventilation, or Cheyne-Stokes respirations. Hypoventilation may indicate respiratory compensation characteristic of metabolic alkalosis or severe respiratory depression and acidosis.

Electroencephalographic changes aid in diagnosing metabolic coma. These changes usually involve diffuse slowing with no focal change.

A complete history is vital because a past history of diabetes, liver disease, or renal pathology provides clues to changes in the level of consciousness. However, a history is often unobtainable, and neurologic assessment is difficult due to coma. Because hypoglycemia is the most frequent cause of metabolic coma, most patients are given a trial of 25 to 50 g of intravenous glucose in the emergency department.

Laboratory Findings

Laboratory findings are helpful in determining the primary cause of metabolic encephalopathy. Increases in serum ammonia aid in the diagnosis of hepatic encephalopathy. The CSF may also demonstrate bilirubin (Plum & Posner, 1982). In patients with hypoglycemia, serum and CSF glucose levels (normally two-thirds of the serum glucose level) may be useful. Blood urea nitrogen and electrolyte levels do not reflect the presence of uremic encephalopathy. However, it is important to rule out water intoxication (serum osmolality < 260 mOsm/liter and serum sodium $<$ 120 mEq/liter). A toxicology screen is helpful in assessing the presence of toxic etiologies of metabolic coma. Drug, alcohol, and heavy metal levels should be determined as indicated.

Diagnostic Procedures

LUMBAR PUNCTURE. CSF determinations aid in diagnosing the causes of coma. In addition to the changes in CSF mentioned earlier (see discussion under Ischemic Brain Injury), uremia may cause an aseptic meningitis with increased lymphocytes and polymorphonuclear leukocytes in the CSF and increased CSF pressure (160–180 mm H_2O).

ELECTROENCEPHALOGRAPHY. EEG shows generalized diffuse slowing in patients with metabolic coma as opposed to focal changes in structural disease. Seizures often accompany metabolic coma, and EEG can help in diagnosing the seizure type.

COMPUTED TOMOGRAPHY. CT scanning can differentiate between structural and metabolic etiologies, but it cannot determine the cause of metabolic encephalopathy.

Medical Management

Medical management begins with treatment of the primary cause of the metabolic encephalopathy, while providing supportive care of the comatose patient. Most patients require intubation and ventilation for hypoventilation or hyperventilation. ABGs are assessed frequently to evaluate acid–base balance and oxygenation. Brain resuscitation measures (discussed earlier in the section on Ischemic Brain Injury) should be initiated. Because cerebral edema may result from metabolic encephalopathy, management of increased ICP is critical (see discussion in the section on Traumatic Brain Injury).

Prognosis of these patients is good once the primary etiology has been treated. Hypoglycemia and uremic encephalopathy are usually reversed quickly through administration of glucose or dialysis.

Clinical Management

Care of patients with metabolic coma is complex, and the nurse must be aware of the underlying medical illness as well as the neurologic dysfunction. Nursing goals involve preventing further injury while the primary medical condition is being treated. The nursing diagnoses discussed for the patient with traumatic brain injury are also appropriate for the care of these patients.

TABLE 35–3. **International Classification of Epileptic Seizures**

I. Partial seizures (seizures beginning locally)
   A. Partial seizures with elementary symptomatology (generally without impairment of consciousness)
      1. With motor symptoms (includes Jacksonian seizures)
      2. With special sensory or somatosensory symptoms
      3. With automatic symptoms
      4. Compound forms
   B. Partial seizures with complex symptomatology (generally with impairment of consciousness) (temporal lobe or psychomotor seizures)
      1. With impairment of consciousness only
      2. With cognitive symptomatology
      3. With affective symptomatology
      4. With "psychosensory" symptomatology
      5. With "psychomotor" symptomatology (automatisms)
      6. Compound forms
   C. Partial seizures secondarily generalized

II. Generalized seizures (bilaterally symmetrical and without local onset)
   A. Absences (petit mal)
   B. Bilateral massive epileptic myoclonus
   C. Infantile spasms
   D. Clonic seizures
   E. Tonic seizures
   F. Tonic-clonic seizures
   G. Atonic seizures
   H. Akinetic seizures

III. Unilateral seizures (or predominantly)

IV. Unclassified epileptic seizures (due to incomplete data)

From Gastaut, H. (1970). Clinical and electroencephalographical classification of epileptic seizures. *Epilepsia, 11,* 102–113.

SEIZURES

"Epilepsy" is a Greek word meaning "to be seized by a force from without." Epilepsy is a chronic seizure disorder of the cerebral tissues characterized by recurrent paroxysmal episodes of disturbed skeletal motor function, sensation, autonomic visceral function, behavior, or consciousness (Hickey, 1986).

Seizures are a symptom of central nervous system irritability characterized by abnormal neuronal discharge. Epilepsy is a syndrome rather than a disease because seizures are often manifestation of a disease.

Classification of Seizures

Attempts to classify seizures began with Hippocrates, and since then, classification schemes have been based on symptomatology, electrophysiology, anatomic origin, etiology, or response to therapy (Hickey, 1986). Two currently used classifications are partial (focal) and generalized (unlocalized) seizures.

Partial seizures affect certain areas of the brain, the signs and symptoms depending on the area involved. Consciousness is usually present as long as the seizure involves only one hemisphere. If midline structures such as the thalamus, hypothalamus, or midbrain are involved, unconsciousness results.

Both cerebral hemispheres and connections with subcortical nuclei are involved in generalized seizures, and consciousness is always impaired. Some generalized seizures begin as focal or parietal seizure and progress to the generalized form.

Since 1969, the International Classification of Epileptic Seizures by Gastaut has been used (Table 35–3). This classification system is based on the nature of the onset of seizures.

Most seizures are thought to be caused by a few abnormally hyperactive or hypersensitive neurons, which form an epileptogenic focus. These neurons are physiologically and chemically abnormal and are always hyperactive compared to normal neurons (Hickey, 1986). The epileptogenic focus is autonomous and emits an excessive number of paroxysmal discharges.

It is unclear what cellular mechanism initiates a seizure, but it has been postulated that an autonomous discharge may be enhanced or minimized by neurotransmitter substances on the postsynaptic membrane. After neuronal stimulation, depolarization occurs, followed by a period of hyperpolarization that probably results from an inhibitory postsynaptic potential. Hyperpolarization is replaced by depolarization, which then increases in amplitude, causing the cell to "fire" (depolarize) repeatedly, allowing sustained depolarization and seizure activity.

Cessation of seizure activity is associated with membrane hyperpolarization, thought to be the result of an electrical potential generated by the sodium pump. On an EEG this result is evidenced by high-voltage spikes and waves that gradually decrease in size and frequency. Focal cells cease firing, suppressing in turn the abnormal firing of the surface cells.

The period after a seizure is called the postictal period; it is characterized by confusion, headache, lethargy, or a deep sleep. There also may be temporary paresis, aphasia, or hemianopsia (Hickey, 1986).

Cerebral blood flow during a seizure is increased dramatically to approximately 250% of normal to meet the metabolic demands; cerebral oxygen consumption is also increased. Increased cerebral blood flow meets demand as long as hypoxemia, hypoglycemia, and cardiac irregularities do not occur. In these situations the brain may require more energy than it can produce with the limited oxygen or glucose available. Cellular exhaustion and destruction occur in these situations.

Clinical Presentation

Because seizures are associated with numerous primary diseases, it is important to rule out any underlying causes. Diagnosis is based on the history and on the physical and neurologic assessments. Questions about seizure activity should include those relating to age at onset, progression of the seizure, loss of consciousness, subjective and objective details, frequency and length of the seizure, any associated prodome or aura, and resulting injuries (Hickey, 1986). The status of the patient in the postictal phase should also be documented.

Diagnostic Data

Baseline laboratory data should include complete blood count, urinalysis, serum chemistries (especially glucose, urea, sodium, and potassium), and liver enzymes. If indicated, a toxicology screen may be helpful.

The most useful diagnostic tool is the EEG. EEGs not only aid in diagnosing the type of seizure, but may isolate the epileptogenic focus through its abnormal neuronal activity. Certain EEG waveform abnormalities are associated with specific seizure disorders. Absence (petit mal) seizures classically have a 3-second spike wave complex seen on all leads. High-voltage spikes are seen with tonic-clonic seizures. Temporal lobe, psychomotor, or complex partial seizures are illustrated by spike complexes over the involved temporal lobe; these complexes may be square-topped and occur at a rate of four to six per second. Other waves include theta and delta waves. Theta waves may be normal, whereas delta waves are associated with necrotic brain tissue resulting from infarction, tumor, or abscess. Because EEG is frequently normal between seizure events, video EEGs and 24-hour EEGs are more commonly used.

Lumbar puncture may reveal CSF with an increased cell count, indicating infection as the source of the seizures. CSF pressure exceeding 180 mm H_2O may indicate a tumor or other source of elevated ICP as the cause of the seizure.

Computed tomography is frequently used to rule out sources of seizures such as tumor, aneurysm, stroke, and cerebral edema. Normal CT scans rule out these potential causes of the seizure. MRI is becoming the diagnostic tool of choice over CT.

Medical Management

The first principle of therapy is to treat the underlying cause of the seizure when an underlying cause can be identified. When no primary cause is known, the goal of therapy is to control the seizures.

Seventy-five percent of patients with seizures are controlled with medication (Hickey, 1986). It is important to remember that drugs control but do not cure the seizures. Some drugs are more effective than others for specific seizures. Once the seizure type has been identified, the drug of choice is prescribed and dosage regulated until a therapeutic level is achieved. If control is not achieved, then the initial drug is tapered as the alternative drugs are instituted. Some patients require combination therapy (e.g., phenytoin and phenobarbital). Sometimes a second drug is used to decrease the dosage of the initial drug to avoid toxicity. Of the many anticonvulsant drugs available, some appear to be better at controlling specific seizures than others (Table 35–4). Patients on long-term drug therapy should be closely monitored for toxicity. Serum levels should be periodically assessed to ensure that adequate therapeutic levels are maintained.

Surgical Intervention

Patients who fail to respond to drug therapy may be candidates for surgical ablation of the epileptogenic focus. Only 5% of epileptic patients fit this category (Hickey, 1986). Patients with loss of quality of life and a unilateral focus in an area that will not result in major neurologic deficit after surgery are considered for operative intervention (Norman, 1981). The procedure is done under local anesthesia to allow interaction with the patient and to permit EEG and cortical stimulation during the procedure. Once the epileptogenic focus has been identified and removed and the EEG no longer demonstrates abnormal activity, the patient is completely anesthetized to allow closure of the incision. The patient is managed in the same way as any postcraniotomy patient. After postoperative recovery, anticonvulsants are slowly tapered as long as no seizure activity is encountered. Periodic EEG is done to monitor for recurrence. Drug tapering is done slowly

TABLE 35–4. **Drugs Used for Management of Seizures**

Medication	Seizure Type
Phenytoin (Dilantin) Phenobarbital (Luminal) Primidone (Mysoline) Mephenytoin (Mesantoin)	Tonic-clonic (generalized) and focal sensory
Phenytoin (Dilantin) Phenobarbital (Luminal) Primidone (Mysoline) Carbamezepine (Tegretol) Mephenytoin (Mesantoin) Phenacemide (Phenurone) Felbamate (Felbatol)	Partial seizures with complex symptomatology (temporal lobe or psychomotor seizures)
Ethosuximide (Zarontin) Trimehadione (Tridione) Methsuximide (Celontin) Valproic acid (Depakane) Paramethadione (Paradione) Phensuximide (Milontin)	Generalized—absences (petit mal seizures)
Nitrazepam (Mogadon)	Generalized—myoclonus, akinetic seizures
Prednisone Corticotropin (ACTH)	Generalized—infantile spasms
Diazepam (Valium) Paraldehyde Thiopental Lorazepam	Status epilepticus

over a period of 2 years; if no seizure activity occurs, the drug is discontinued.

Status Epilepticus

Status epilepticus is a medical emergency defined as recurrent, generalized seizures that occur at a frequency that does not allow the patient to regain consciousness between tonic-clonic activity. Metabolic exhaustion eventually occurs because of lack of sufficient oxygen and glucose to meet the metabolic demands of the brain. About 10% of all epileptics develop this condition (Borchert & Labar, 1993). Concurrent impaired respirations compound the problem because they contriubte to hypoxemia.

The goals of therapy are to control the seizures and restore normal cerebral metabolism. Establishing and maintaining an airway while providing supplemental oxygen are essential for these patients. An intravenous line should be used to replace fluids and provide medications. Diazepam and lorazepam are the drugs of choice; other drugs that may be used to include phenobarbital, amobarbital, and phenytoin. As long as the seizure continues, a search should be made for a primary cause to allow treatment of the initiating etiology. Brain damage or death may result from status epilepticus, so control of the seizure activity is mandatory.

Clinical Management

Management of patients with seizures focuses on preventing the complications of seizures and avoiding injury during seizures. Teaching the patient and family about seizures and anticonvulsant therapy begins in the intensive care unit.

SUMMARY

Brain injury has serious consequences for the patient. Whether the injury is traumatic, ischemic, or metabolic, these patients require vigilant and continuous nursing care. Accurate and knowledgeable assessment is important to identify the neurologic status and the subtle changes that may occur. Nursing care is aimed at meeting the physical, cognitive, and personal needs of these patients, and can be a challenge for the nurse. This chapter has provided an overview of the major causes of brain injury and the current methods of medical and nursing care. This knowledge will aid the nurse in accepting the challenges of caring for these patients.

REFERENCES

Abramson, N. S., Safar, P., Detre, K., et al. (1985). Randomized clinical study of thiopental loading in comatose survivors of cardiac arrest. *New England Journal of Medicine, 314,* 1982–1983.

Ames, A., Wright, R. L., Kowanda, M., et al. (1968). Cerebral ischemia: II. The no reflow phenomenon. *American Journal of Pathology, 52,* 437.

Bakay, R. A. E., & Wood, J. H. (1985). Pathophysiology of cerebrospinal fluid. In D. P. Becker & J. T. Povlishock (Eds.), *Central nervous system trauma status report 1985* (pp. 89–137). Bethesda, MD: National Institutes of Health/National Institutes of Neurological Disorders and Stroke.

Borchert, L. D., & Labar, D. R. (1993). An organized approach to managing status epilepticus. *Journal of Critical Illness, 8,* 965–972.

Bowers, S. A., & Marshall, L. F. (1980). Outcome in 200 consecutive cases of severe head injury treated in San Diego County: A prospective study. *Neurosurgery, 6,* 237–242.

Bruce, D., Gennarelli, T., & Langfitt, T. (1978). Resuscitation from coma due to head injury. *Critical Care Medicine, 6,* 254–266.

Cepuzzo, M. L. J., Weiss, M. G., & Petersons, V. (1977). Effect of positive end-expiratory pressure ventilation on intracranial pressure in man. *Journal of Neurosurgery, 46,* 227–238.

Clifton, G. I., Robertson, G. S., & Kyper, K. (1983). Cardiovascular responses to severe head injury. *Journal of Neurosurgery, 59,* 447–454.

Conner, R. (1969). Myocardial damage secondary to brain lesions. *American Heart Journal, 78,* 145–148.

Cooper, P. R. (1985). Delayed brain injury: Secondary insults. In D. P. Becker & J. T. Povlishock (Eds.), *Central nervous system trauma status report 1985* (pp. 217–228). Bethesda, MD: National Institutes of Health/National Institutes of Neurological Disorders and Stroke.

Cooper, K. R. (1989). Respiratory complications in patients with serious head injury. In D. P. Becker & S. K. Gudeman (Eds.), *Textbook of head injury* (pp. 255–264). Philadelphia: W. B. Saunders.

DeBard, M. L. (1983). Predictors in brain resuscitation. *Critical Care Quarterly, 5*(4), 91–98.

Donegan, M., & Bedford, R. (1980). Intravenously administered lidocaine prevents intracranial hypertension during endotracheal suctioning. *Anesthesiology, 52,* 516–518.

Epstein, F., & Hamilton, G. (1983). Initial approach to the brain injured patient. *Critical Care Quarterly, 5*(4), 13–29.

Feldman, Z., Kanter, M. J., Robertson, C. S., et al. (1992). Effect of head elevation on intracranial pressure, cerebral perfusion pressure, and cerebral biopatients. *Journal of Neurosurgery, 76,* 207.

Fischer, E. G. (1974). Impaired perfusion following cerebrovascular stasis. *Archives of Neurology, 33,* 91–92.

Frost, E. A. M., & Gildenberg, P. L. (1977). Effect of postive end-expiratory pressure on intracranial pressure and compliance in brain injured patients. *Journal of Neurosurgery, 46,* 227–238.

Gennarelli, T. A. (1987). Cerebral concussion and diffuse brain injuries. In P. Cooper (Ed.), *Head injury* (2nd ed., pp. 108–123). Baltimore: Williams & Wilkins.

Gennarelli, T. A., Spielman, G. M., & Langfitt, T. W. (1982). Influence of the type of intracranial lesion on outcome from severe head injury: A multicenter study using a new classification system. *Journal of Neurosurgery, 56,* 26–32.

Gennarelli, T. A., & Thibault, L. (1982). Biomechanics of acute subdural hematoma. *Journal of Trauma, 22,* 680–685.

Gudeman, S. K., Young, H. F., Miller, J. D., et al. (1989). Indications for operative treatment and operative technique in closed head injury. In D. P. Becker & S. K. Gudeman (Eds.), *Textbook of head injury* (pp. 138–181). Philadelphia: W. B. Saunders.

Hagen, C., Milkmus, D., & Dunham, P. (1979). *Comprehensive physical management* (pp. 87–88). Downey, CA: Professional Staff Association of Rancho Los Amigos Hospital.

Hickey, J. V. (1986). *The clinical practice of neurological and neurosurgical nursing* (2nd ed.). Philadelphia: J. B. Lippincott.

Hickey, J. V. (1992). *The clinical practice of neurological and neurosurgical nursing* (3rd ed.). Philadelphia: J. B. Lippincott.

Hirsh, L. F. (1980). Chronic epidural hematomas. *Neurosurgery, 6,* 508–512.

Jagger, J. A., & Bobovsky, J. (1983). Nonpharmacologic therapeutic modalities. *Critical Care Quarterly, 5*(4), 31–41.

Jameson, K. G., & Yelland, J. D. N. (1972). Traumatic intracranial hematoma: Report of 63 surgically treated cases. *Journal of Neurosurgery, 37,* 528–532.

Jennett, B., & Teasdale, G. (1981). *Management of head injuries.* Philadelphia: F. A. Davis.

Jordan, R. C. (1983). Pathophysiology of brain injury. *Critical Care Quarterly, 5*(4), 1–11.

Kalsbeck, W. D., McLaurin, R. L., & Harris, B. S. H., III (1981). The national head and spinal cord injury survey: Major findings. *Journal of Neurosurgery, 53,* 19–31.

Klatzo, I. (1967). Neuropathological aspects of brain edema. *Journal of Neuropathophysiology and Experimental Neurology, 20*(1), 1–14.

Koehler, R. C., & Michael, J. R. (1985). Cardiopulmonary resuscitation, brain blood flow and neurologic recovery. *Critical Care Clinics, 1*(2), 195–204.

Krause, J. F. (1987). Epidemiology of head injury. In P. Cooper (Ed.), *Head injury* (2nd ed., pp. 1–19). Baltimore: Williams & Wilkins.

Krause, J. F., Black, M. A., & Hessol, N. (1984). The incidence of acute brain injury and serious impairment in a defined population. *American Journal of Epidemiology, 119,* 186–201.

Langfitt, T. W. (1978). Measuring the outcome from head injury. *Journal of Neurosurgery, 48,* 673–678.

Langfitt, T. W. (1982). Increased intracranial pressure and cerebral circulation. In J. R. Youmans (Ed.), *Neurological surgery* (Vol. 2, 2nd ed., pp. 30–46). Philadelphia: W. B. Saunders.

Levin, A., Duff, T., & Javid, M. (1979). Treatment of increased intracranial pressure: A comparison of different hyperosmotic agents and the use of thiopental. *Neurosurgery, 5,* 570–575.

Longstreth, W. T., Jr., Clayson, K. J., & Sume, S. M. (1981). Cerebrospinal fluid and serum creatine kinase BB activity after out-of-hospital cardiac arrest. *Neurology, 31,* 455–458.

Lundberg, N. (1960). Continuous recording and control of the ventricular-fluid pressure in neurosurgical practice. *Acta Psychiatrica Scandinavica, 36*(Suppl 149), 581–590.

Marshall, L. F., Barbar, D., & Toole, B. M. (1983). The oval pupil: Clinical significance and relationship to intracranial hypertension. *Journal of Neurosurgery, 58,* 566–568.

Marshall, L. F., Camp, P., & Bowers, S. (1984). Dimethylsulfoxide for the treatment of intracranial hypertension: A preliminary trial. *Neurosurgery, 14,* 659–663.

Marshall, L. F., Smith, R. W., & Shapero, H. M. (1979). The outcome with aggressive treatment in severe head injuries: I. The significance of intracranial pressure monitoring. *Journal of Neurosurgery, 50,* 20–25.

Marshall, L. F., Toole, B. M., & Bowers, S. A. (1983). The national traumatic coma databank: II. Patients who talk and deteriorate: Implications for treatment. *Journal of Neurosurgery, 59,* 285–288.

Marshall, S. B., Marshall, L. F., Vos, H. R., & Chestnut, R. M. (1990). *Neuroscience critical care: Pathophysiology and patient management.* Philadelphia: W. B. Saunders.

Martin, M. L. (1983). Pharmacologic therapeutic modalities: Phenytoin, dimethyl sulfoxide, and caclium channel blockers. *Critical Care Quarterly, 5*(4), 72–81.

McQuillan, K. A. (1986). *The effects of the Trendelenburg position for postural drainage on cerebrovascular status in head injured patients.* Unpublished Master's thesis. Baltimore: University of Maryland, School of Nursing.

Meyer, F. N. (1993). The intensive care management of cerebral ischemia. In B. T. Andrews (Ed.), *Neurosurgical intensive care* (pp. 329–342). New York: McGraw-Hill.

Miller, J. D. (1985). Head injury and brain ischemia: Implications for therapy. *British Journal of Anesthesiology, 57,* 120–129.

Miller, J. D., Butterworth, J. F., Gudeman, S. K., et al. (1981). Further experience in the management of severe head injury. *Journal of Neurosurgery, 54,* 289–299.

Mitchell, P. H. (1994). Central nervous system: I. Closed head injuries. In V. D. Cardona, P. D. Hurn, P. J. Bastnagel Mason, et al. (Eds.), *Trauma nursing: From resuscitation through rehabilitation* (2nd ed., pp. 383–434). Philadelphia: W. B. Saunders.

Narayan, R. K. (1993). Emergency room management of the head-injured patient. In B. T. Andrews (Ed.), *Neurosurgical intensive care.* New York: McGraw-Hill.

Nemoto, E. M. (1978). Pathogenesis of cerebral ischemia–anoxia. *Critical Care Medicine, 6,* 203–214.

Nikas, D. L. (1987). Critical aspects of head trauma. *Critical Care Nursing Quarterly, 10*(1), 19–44.

Nikas, D. L., & Tolley, M. (1982). Acute head injury. In D. L. Nikas (Ed.), *The critically ill neurosurgical patient* (pp. 89–106). New York: Churchill-Livingstone.

Norman, S. E. (1981). Surgical treatment of epilepsy. *American Journal of Nursing, 81,* 994–997.

Platt, J. H., & Schiff, S. J. (1984). High dose barbiturate therapy in neurosurgery and intensive care. *Neurosurgery, 15,* 427–444.

Plum, F., & Posner, J. B. (1982). *The diagnosis of stupor and coma* (3rd ed.). Philadelphia: F. A. Davis.

Purvis, J. (1966). Craniocerebral injuries due to missile and fragments. In W. Caveness & A. E. Walker (Eds.), *Head injury* (pp. 133–141). Philadelphia: J. B. Lippincott.

Raffsen, M. L., & Davis, W. R. (1989). Cerebral function and preservation during cardiac arrest. *Critical Care Medicine, 17,* 283–292.

Rimel, R. W. (1982). Head injury: A challenging future for neurological nursing. *Journal of Neurosurgical Nursing, 14,* 207–209.

Rimel, R., & Lundgren, J. (1986). The head injured patient. In J. Lundgren (Ed.), *Acute neuroscience nursing: Concepts and care* (pp. 130–146). Boston: Jones and Bartlett.

Rosner, M. I., & Coley, I. (1992). Cerebral perfusion pressure, the ICP and head elevation. *Journal of Neurosurgery, 54,* 596.

Safar, P. (1981). Dynamics of brain resuscitation after ischemic anoxia. *Hospital Practice, 4*(2), 67–72.

Safar, P. (1983). Brain resuscitation. In G. Tinker & M. Rapin (Eds.), *Care of the critically ill patient* (pp. 751–763). Philadelphia: F. A. Davis.

Shapiro, H. M. (1975). Intracranial hypertension: Therapeutic and anesthetic considerations. *Anesthesiology, 43,* 445–467.

Siesjo, B. K. (1993). Basic mechanism of traumatic brain injury. *Annals of Emergency Medicine, 22,* 959.

Snyder, B. D., Gumnit, R. J., & Leppik, I. E. (1981). Neurologic prognosis after cardiopulmonary arrest: IV. Brainstem reflexes. *Neurology, 31,* 1092–1097.

Snyder, B. D., Ramirez-Lassepas, M., & Lippert, D. M. (1977). Neurologic status and prognosis after cardiopulmonary arrest: I. A retrospective study. *Neurology, 27,* 807–811.

Spielman, G. M. (1988). Central nervous system: I. Head injuries. In V. D. Cardona, P. D. Hurn, P. J. B. Mason, et al. (Eds.), *Trauma nursing: From resuscitation through rehabilitation* (pp. 365–418). Philadelphia: W. B. Saunders.

Staller, A. G. (1987). Systemic effects of severe head trauma. *Critical Care Quarterly, 10*(1), 58–68.

Tyson, G., Strachan, W. E., & Newman, P. (1980). The role of craniectomy in the treatment of chronic subdural hematomas. *Journal of Neurosurgery, 52,* 776–781.

Versari, P., Vecci, C., & Arosio, M. (1980). Effects of althesin on intracranial hypertension in patients with severe head injury. In R. Shulman, A. Marmarrou, & J. Miller (Eds.), *Intracranial pressure* (pp. 610–613). New York: Springer-Verlag.

Vise. W. M. (1994). A metabolic approach to the management of neurological trauma. Presented at the University Hospital, SUNY Health Science Center at Syracuse, NY.

Walleck, C. A. (1987). Intracranial hypertension: Interventions and outcomes. *Critical Care Nursing Quarterly, 10*(1), 45–57.

Walleck, C. A. (1990). Acute head injury. In K. VonRueden & C. A. Walleck (Ed.), *Critical care case studies.* Rockville, MD: Aspen.

Weiner, R. L., & Eisenberg, H. M. (1985). Radiologic evaluation of head injury: Key concepts. *Trauma Quarterly, 2*(1), 26–39.

White, B. C., & Krause, G. S. (1993). Brain injury and repair mechanisms: The potential for pharmacologic therapy in closed head trauma. *Annals of Emergency Medicine, 22,* 970.

ACUTE HEAD INJURY MULTIDISCIPLINARY CARE GUIDE

COORDINATION OF CARE

Diagnosis/Stabilization Phase		Acute Management Phase		Recovery Phase	
Outcome	*Intervention*	*Outcome*	*Intervention*	*Outcome*	*Intervention*
All appropriate team members and disciplines will be involved in the plan of care.	Develop the plan of care with patient/family, primary nurse(s), primary physician(s), neurologist, neurosurgeon, family practitioner, and other specialists as needed, including respiratory therapist, chaplain, social services, clinical nurse specialist.	All appropriate team members and disciplines will be involved in the plan of care.	Update plan of care with patient, family/other team members, dietician, discharge planner, home health agency, physical therapist, recreational therapist, occupational therapist, speech and language pathologist. Initiate planning for anticipated discharge. Begin teaching patient/family about care at home if discharge to home is anticipated.	Patient/family will understand how to maintain optimal health at home, extended care facility, or physical rehabilitation facility.	Provide written guidelines concerning follow-up care to patient/family. Provide patient/family with phone number of resources available to answer questions. Provide patient/family with written guidelines concerning follow-up care. Continue to involve physical therapy and physical rehabilitation consults. Prepare for discharge to extended care facility, physical rehabilitation facility, or home. If discharged to home, provide instruction on care at home (i.e., when to call the doctor, physical restrictions, exercise, diet, medications).

Care Guide continued on following page

ACUTE HEAD INJURY MULTIDISCIPLINARY CARE GUIDE *continued*

FLUID BALANCE

Diagnosis/Stabilization Phase		Acute Management Phase		Recovery Phase	
Outcome	*Intervention*	*Outcome*	*Intervention*	*Outcome*	*Intervention*
Patient will achieve optimal hemodynamic status as evidenced by: • Vital signs WNL • Intracranial pressure WNL • Hemodynamic parameters WNL • Adequate level of consciousness • Clear lung sounds • Normothermia Patient will maintain optimal neurologic status, as evidenced by cerebral perfusion pressure >50 mm Hg.	Monitor and treat direct and derived hemodynamic parameters (Svo_2, blood pressure, intracranial pressure, intake and output, level of consciousness, evidence of tissue perfusion). Monitor lab values: electrolytes, SMA-18, total creatine kinase (CK), CK-BB. Assess for fluid overload or deficit and treat accordingly. Anticipate need for vasopressor agents and assess response and titrate accordingly. Assess neurologic status q1h and PRN. If used, assess intracranial pressure q1h and PRN. Anticipate need for diuretics. Monitor for signs of increased intracranial pressure and treat accordingly. Monitor temperature and watch for signs of shivering. Use hypothermia/hyperthermia unit if necessary. Avoid rapid cooling. Raise head of bed 30–45°. If intracranial pressure changes with activity, space activities. Determine baseline intracranial pressure before any activity.	Patient will maintain optimal hemodynamic status. Patient will maintain optimal neurologic status. Patient will remain normothermic.	Same as stabilization phase. Include diaphoretic episodes in estimation of intake and output. Assess neurologic status q2–4h and PRN. If used, assess intracranial pressure q2–4h and PRN. Assess temperature and signs of shivering. Maintain normal temperature with hypothermia/hyperthermia unit or other measures. Avoid rapid cooling. Monitor for complications associated with head injury and treat accordingly: pneumonia, muscle atrophy, infection, embolus, thrombus formation, renal failure, diabetes insipidus, hematoma formation, increased intracranial pressure, hypoglycemia, leukocytosis, hyperglycemia, uremic encephalopathy, hepatic encephalopathy. Monitor urine specific gravity and osmolality. Monitor blood osmolality.	Same outcomes and same interventions as in acute management phase. Assess neurologic status q4–8h and PRN.	

NUTRITION

Diagnosis/Stabilization Phase		Acute Management Phase		Recovery Phase	
Outcome	*Intervention*	*Outcome*	*Intervention*	*Outcome*	*Intervention*
Patient will be adequately nourished. Weight will remain within 10 pounds of normal.	Initiate total parenteral or enteral nutrition as soon as possible and monitor response. Assess bowel sounds, abdominal distention, abdominal pain and tenderness q4h and PRN.	Patient will be adequately nourished.	Same as in stabilization phase. If able, advance to diet as tolerated and monitor response. Assess gag and swallowing reflexes. Monitor protein and albumen lab values.	Patient will be adequately nourished.	Teach patient/family about diet. Involve dietician in plan of care.

MOBILITY

Diagnosis/Stabilization Phase		Acute Management Phase		Recovery Phase	
Outcome	*Intervention*	*Outcome*	*Intervention*	*Outcome*	*Intervention*
Patient will achieve optimal mobility. Patient will be free of joint contractures.	Assess degree of mobility. Keep head of bed elevated 30°. Begin passive/active-assist range-of-motion exercises as tolerated.	Patient will achieve optimal mobility. Patient will be free of joint contractures.	Same as stabilization phase. Continue passive/active-assist range of motion exercises. Obtain physical therapy/rehabilitation consult. Monitor response to increased activity. Decrease if adverse events occur (dyspnea, increased intracranial pressure, syncope, tachycardia, hypotension, hypertension). Provide support as necessary. Take measures to prevent joint contractures. Begin discussion with patient/family about potential physical limitations and required resources post-discharge.	Patient will achieve optimal mobility. Patient will be free of joint contractures.	Prepare for transfer to extended care facility, home, or physical rehabilitation facility. Include family in all plans of continuing care. Teach patient/family about exercise program.

OXYGENATION/VENTILATION

Diagnosis/Stabilization Phase		Acute Management Phase		Recovery Phase	
Outcome	*Intervention*	*Outcome*	*Intervention*	*Outcome*	*Intervention*
Patient will have adequate gas exchange as evidenced by: • O_2 saturation >90% • Arterial blood gases (ABGs) WNL or possibly $Paco_2$ at 27–33 mm Hg • Clear breath sounds • Respiratory rate, depth, and rhythm WNL • Chest x-ray WNL • Absence of dyspnea • Absence of cyanosis • Absence of secretions	Monitor ventilator settings and hemodynamic variables before, during, and after weaning (if applicable). Anticipate need for hyperventilation and hyperoxygenation, particularly before suctioning. Wean ventilator when appropriate and monitor patient response: • Wean Fio_2 to keep Spo_2 >92% • Use humidification to keep secretions thin Assess respiratory functioning including lung sounds, respiratory muscle strength, respiratory rate and depth, coughing ability, ABGs, and chest x-ray. If not intubated, apply supplemental oxygen. Monitor with pulse oximetry. Assess evidence of tissue perfusion. Monitor lab values: ABGs, CO_2, hemoglobin.	Patient will have adequate gas exchange.	Monitor and treat oxygenation/ventilation disturbances as per ABGs, Sao_2, chest assessment, adventitious breath sounds, and chest x-ray. Wean oxygen therapy or mechanical ventilation as tolerated. Begin teaching patient/family mechanical ventilation if home care is expected. Assess effects of increased activity on respiratory status. Observe for complications of head injury that may impair oxygenation/ventilation: embolus, increased intracranial pressure, thrombus formation, seizures, fever, neurogenic shock. Assess need for long-term mechanical ventilation. If indicated, initiate plans to place in extended care facility, physical rehabilitation facility, or in the home. If going home, involve home health agency and home oxygen supply company.	Patient will have adequate gas exchange.	Assess respiratory functioning and intervene as indicated. Provide instruction to patient/family on mechanical ventilation if needed. Continue to assess for complications of head injury that may impair oxygenation/ventilation (i.e., pneumonia, infection, embolus, thrombus formation). Assess patient/family understanding of home care needs. Reinforce knowledge and skills as needed.

Care Guide continued on following page

ACUTE HEAD INJURY MULTIDISCIPLINARY CARE GUIDE *continued*

COMFORT

Diagnosis/Stabilization Phase		Acute Management Phase		Recovery Phase	
Outcome	***Intervention***	***Outcome***	***Intervention***	***Outcome***	***Intervention***
Patient will be as comfortable and pain free as possible, as evidenced by: • No objective indicators of discomfort • No complaints of discomfort	Assess absence of, or quantity and quality of pain. Administer analgesics and monitor response. Administer sedatives cautiously. Monitor response on level of consciousness. Assess response to all analgesics and effects on ability to wean from ventilator if applicable. If patient is intubated, establish effective communication technique with which patient can communicate discomfort. Provide reassurance in a calm, caring, and competent manner.	Patient will be relaxed and comfortable.	Same as stabilization phase. Provide uninterrupted rest periods in a quiet environment. Teach patient relaxation techniques. Use massage, humor, music therapy, and imagery to promote relaxation. Involve family in strategies. Observe for complications of head injury that may cause discomfort.	Patient will be relaxed and comfortable.	Same as other phases. Progress analgesics to oral medications as needed; assess response. Teach patient/family alternative methods to promote relaxation after discharge.

SKIN INTEGRITY

Diagnosis/Stabilization Phase		Acute Management Phase		Recovery Phase	
Outcome	***Intervention***	***Outcome***	***Intervention***	***Outcome***	***Intervention***
Patient will have intact skin without abrasions or pressure ulcers.	Assess all bony prominences at least q4h and treat if needed. Use preventive pressure-reducing devices if patient is at high risk for development of pressure ulcers. Treat pressure ulcers according to hospital protocol.	Patient will have intact skin without abrasions or pressure ulcers.	Same as Stabilization Phase.	Patient will have intact skin without abrasions or pressure ulcers.	Teach patient/family proper skin care for after discharge.

PROTECTION/SAFETY

Diagnosis/Stabilization Phase		Acute Management Phase		Recovery Phase	
Outcome	*Intervention*	*Outcome*	*Intervention*	*Outcome*	*Intervention*
Patient will be protected from possible harm.	Seizure precautions. Assess need for restraints. If indicated, assess response to restraints. Check q1–2h for skin integrity and impairment to circulation. Explain need for restraints to patient/family. Remove restraints when patient is able to follow instructions. Administer sedatives and anxiolytics cautiously and monitor neurologic effect. Follow hospital protocol according to use of restraints.	Patient will be protected from possible harm.	Same as stabilization phase. When activity is increased, provide any necessary support.	Patient will be protected from possible harm.	Same as other phases. Teach patient/family about any physical limitations in activity after discharge.

PSYCHOSOCIAL/SELF-DETERMINATION

Diagnosis/Stabilization Phase		Acute Management Phase		Recovery Phase	
Outcome	*Intervention*	*Outcome*	*Intervention*	*Outcome*	*Intervention*
Patient will achieve psychophysiologic stability. Patient will demonstrate a decrease in anxiety as evidenced by: • Vital signs WNL • Subjective report of anxiety level • Objective signs of anxiety level Patient will begin acceptance process for head injury and possible effects.	Assess physiologic effects of critical care environment on patient (hemodynamic variables, psychological status, signs of increased sympathetic response). If patient is intubated, develop effective interventions to communicate with patient. If patient is unresponsive, maintain verbal and tactile contact with patient. Use calm, caring, competent, and reassuring approach with patient and family. Arrange for flexible visiting to meet patient and family needs. Determine coping ability of patient/family and take appropriate measures to meet their needs (i.e., explain condition, explain equipment, provide frequent condition reports, use easy-to-understand terminology, repeat information as needed, allow family to visit, answer all questions).	Patient will achieve psychophysiologic stability. Patient will demonstrate a decrease in anxiety. Patient will continue acceptance process of head injury and any possible effects.	Same as acute management phase. Provide adequate rest periods. Continue to assess coping ability of patient/family and take measures as indicated (i.e., verbalize feelings, initiate family conferences, use support services). Initiate discharge planning—extended care facility, physical rehabilitation facility, or home. Include patient/family in decisions concerning care.	Patient will achieve psychophysiologic stability. Patient will demonstrate a decrease in anxiety as evidenced by: • Vital signs WNL • Subjective report of anxiety level • Objective signs of anxiety level Patient will begin acceptance process for head injury and possible effects.	Same as acute management phase. Provide patient and family information about support groups.

Care Guide continued on following page

ACUTE HEAD INJURY MULTIDISCIPLINARY CARE GUIDE *continued*

DIAGNOSTICS

Diagnosis/Stabilization Phase		Acute Management Phase		Recovery Phase	
Outcome	***Intervention***	***Outcome***	***Intervention***	***Outcome***	***Intervention***
Patient/family will describe any tests or procedures that need to be completed (vital signs, intake and output, hemodynamic monitoring, intracranial pressure monitoring, x-rays, computed tomography (CT) scan, magnetic resonance imaging [MRI], angiography, lab work, electrocardiogram, lumbar puncture).	Explain all procedures and tests to patient/family. Be sensitive to individualized needs of patient/family for information. Assess patient's ability to understand procedures. If patient is unresponsive, use tactile and verbal methods to communicate. Establish effective communication technique with patient if patient is intubated.	Patient/family will describe any tests or procedures that need to be completed (vital signs, hemodynamic monitoring, intracranial pressure monitoring, lab tests, radiology, CT scan, MRI, chest x-ray, tests to determine physical functioning, EEG).	Explain procedures and tests to assess recovery from head injury to patient/family. Assess individualized needs of patient/family for information. Anticipate need for further diagnostic tests such as EMG, EEG, CT scan, and any intervention that may result from this.	Patient/family will describe or discuss the meaning of diagnostic tests in relation to continued health (MRI, CT scan, EMG, further testing to assess potential for healing/mobility).	Review with patient/family before discharge results of all tests. Discuss abnormal findings and appropriate measures patient/family can take to return to normal or to regain as much physical and mental functioning as possible.

REFERENCE

Nikas, D. L. (1991). The neurologic system. In J. G. Alspach (Ed.), *Core curriculum for critical care nursing* (4th ed., pp. 315–471). Philadelphia: W. B. Saunders.

CHAPTER

36 Patients With Cerebral Vascular Disorders

John M. Clochesy

Cerebrovascular disease, or stroke, is a general term referring to an interruption in blood flow to or hemorrhage in an area of the brain, as shown by transient or permanent neurologic deficit. Since 1900 there have been significant advances in the understanding of the risk factors, etiology, and pathophysiology of stroke. Knowledge of cerebral structure and vascular anatomy, refinements in microneurosurgery, new and more accurate imaging techniques, and improved understanding of pharmacotherapy have enhanced our ability to treat stroke patients successfully. However, stroke continues to be a major cause of disability and is the third leading cause of death in the United States. In 1992, health care costs for stroke were estimated at $12.9 billion, including costs of health care providers, hospital and extended care use, medications, and loss of productivity (American Heart Association, 1992).

Stroke devastates the family and patient. Nearly half of the patients admitted for an acute neurologic condition have had a stroke. Nurses play a critical role in the care of these patients, making it imperative for them to understand thoroughly the etiology, risk factors, medical and surgical therapies, and nursing management of cerebrovascular disease. In addition to the preceding topics, this chapter provides a brief overview of the cerebrovascular system.

CEREBROVASCULAR SYSTEM

The cerebrovascular system is composed of extracranial and intracranial arteriovenous components. The extracranial arterial supply stems from the external carotid artery (ECA) and its main branches, the superficial temporal, posterior auricular, and occipital arteries. The occipital artery supplies the scalp and facial and neck muscles, whereas its terminal branches, through the cranial foramina, supply the meninges of the posterior fossa and dura mater. The supraorbital and supratrochlear branches of the ophthalmic artery, which arises from the internal carotid artery (ICA), supply the skin, muscles, and pericranium of the forehead (Sheldon, 1981).

The central nervous system receives 15% to 20% of the total cardiac output via the ICAs and vertebral arteries (Millikan et al., 1987). The ICA enters the skull through the foramen lacerum. The anterior and middle cerebral arteries and the terminal branches of the ICA and their subdivisions supply the cerebral hemispheres. Vertebral arteries, entering the skull through the foramen magnum, join to form the basilar artery, which branches terminally into the posterior cerebral artery. The vertebrobasilar system supplies the brain stem, cerebellum, and rostral portion of the midbrain.

Both superficial and internal cerebral venous systems drain through the dural sinuses, large collecting channels, which eventually empty into the internal jugular vein.

Collateral Circulation

The collateral vessel circulation may compensate for lost blood supply from an occluded primary vessel. Collateral circulation develops when there is a gradual decrease in cerebral blood flow (CBF) through one of the primary arteries, provided that there has not been a prior occlusion of the collateral vessel. The three major collateral circulations are the extracranial, extracranial–intracranial, and intracranial anastomoses. The ECA is the main source of the extracranial collateral supply. The extracranial–intracranial anastomosis of the ECA and ICA occurs in the orbit. Also, cervical arteries may interconnect with the vertebral arteries (Millikan et al., 1987). The most important intracranial collateral channel is the circle of Willis (Fig. 36–1). The circle of Willis connects the anterior (carotid system) and posterior (vertebrobasilar system) circulations at the base of the brain. The anterior communicating artery allows collateral flow between the ICAs, and the posterior communicating artery connects the anterior and posterior circulations. There are many idiosyncratic variations of the circle of Willis that may affect the amount of collateral circulation provided. The leptomeningeal arteries, formed from the terminal branches of the anterior, middle, and posterior cerebral arteries, may provide intracranial collateral blood flow over the surface of the brain (Millikan et al., 1987).

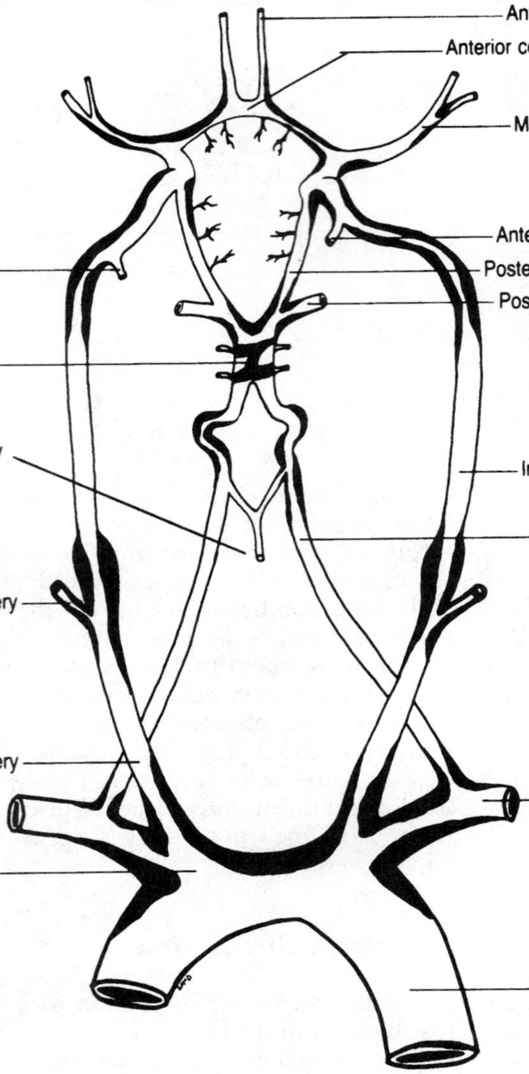

FIGURE 36–1. Diagram showing the carotid and vertebral arteries, their major branches, and the circle of Willis. The diagram also shows the common sites of atherosclerosis in extracranial and intracranial cerebral arteries, which are darkened. (From Millikan, C. H., McDowell, F., & Easton, J. D. [1987]. *Stroke* [p. 41]. Philadelphia: Lea & Febiger.)

Cerebral Blood Flow

Cerebral blood flow is the blood flow (in milliliters) to a given amount of brain (100 g) per minute (Millikan et al., 1987). In a healthy adult the average CBF is 50 to 55 mL/100 g brain per minute. Blood flow to various areas of the brain is related to the activity of the area (Lassen et al., 1978), but cerebral autoregulation ensures constant CBF. The exact mechanism of cerebral autoregulation is incompletely understood (Strandgaard & Paulson, 1984), but by regulating the diameter of arterioles, CBF remains constant despite fluctuations in systemic blood pressure. Therefore, hypertension results in cerebral vasoconstriction, decreasing blood flow, whereas hypotension causes vasodilation and increased CBF. When autoregulation fails, CBF is dependent on changes in systemic blood pressure. Situations associated with these changes are summarized in Table 36–1 (Millikan et al., 1987). The caliber of the resistance vessels is maximal at 40 mm Hg, so that autoregulation fails because no further decrease of resistance is possible, and blood flow becomes a function of pressure. Above 160 mm Hg the converse is true. Additional factors that alter CBF are listed in Table 36–2.

NONHEMORRHAGIC STROKE

Pathophysiology

Nonhemorrhagic, or ischemic, stroke results from significant reduction or obstruction of arterial or venous

TABLE 36–1. **Potential Causes of Failure of Cerebral Autoregulation**

Acute cerebral lesion, either focal or global
Low perfusion pressure (below 40–60 mm Hg)
High perfusion pressure (greater than 160 mm Hg)

TABLE 36–2. **Factors Influencing Cerebral Blood Flow (CBF)**

Increase in CBF (Vasodilation)	Decrease in CBF (Vasoconstriction)
Increased arterial P_{CO_2}	Decreased arterial P_{CO_2}
Decreased arterial P_{O_2}	Increased arterial P_{O_2}
Decreased blood viscosity	Increased blood viscosity
Hyperthermia	Hypothermia
Increased cerebral metabolism	Increased intracranial pressure
	Drugs
	Anesthetics
	Barbiturates

blood flow to or from an area of the brain. The size of the infarct is related to the vessel(s) involved, the length of time of critical reduction in CBF, and the availability of collateral circulation. Central nervous system (CNS) function is affected when CBF is 20 mL/100 g brain per minute for 15 to 30 minutes (Millikan et al., 1987). With this rate of CBF, the amplitude of electrocortical activity on the electroencephalogram (EEG) as well as the amplitude of the evoked cortical responses decreases (Millikan et al., 1987). Changes in intracellular water and electrolyte concentration occur because the sodium–potassium pump is disrupted when the CBF is less than 10 to 15 mL/100 g brain per minute. Below this threshold, cytotoxic (intracellular) edema immediately occurs (Schuier & Hossman, 1980). Cytotoxic edema results from an accumulation of extracellular potassium and intracellular sodium and calcium. A CBF of below 10 mL/100 g brain per minute results in irreversible cellular damage (Millikan et al., 1987). Also, lack of oxygen stimulates anaerobic glycolysis, leading to high lactic acid levels that contribute to permanent cellular damage (Raichle, 1983).

Collateral circulation may maintain CBF at 10 to 20 mL/100 g brain per minute, allowing normal cellular metabolism, avoiding permanent damage, and permitting partial or complete functional recovery. Without adequate perfusion, vasogenic (extracellular) edema resulting from cellular destruction and disruption of the blood–brain barrier occurs. Vasogenic edema occurs within hours of the original insult and peaks within 2 to 4 days (Schuier & Hossman, 1980). Extensive edema may result in shifts of portions of the brain, sometimes leading to transtentorial herniation and death.

Cerebral infarction occurs when an area of brain is deprived of oxygen and nutrients, especially glucose, long enough to produce cellular death (Fig. 36–2). This may result from thrombotic, embolic, or inflammatory processes.

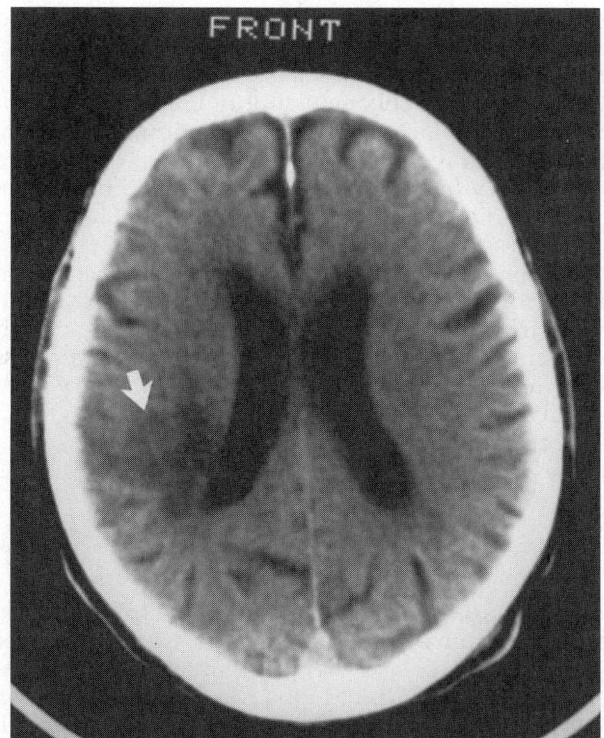

FIGURE 36–2. Axial computed tomography scan of the head demonstrating a hypodense wedge-shaped area (*arrow*) in the right posterior hemisphere consistent with an ischemic infarct.

Thrombosis

Thrombosis is a local obstruction of one or more vessels and is the most common cause of cerebral infarction. Thrombotic stroke most often results from atherosclerosis. In the Framingham study, 60% of all strokes were secondary to atherothrombotic brain infarction (Wolf et al., 1983). Factors that stimulate atheromatous plaque formation are poorly understood. From birth, the intima of the arterial wall begins to thicken. Smooth muscle cells, collagen, elastic fibers (elastin), and glycosaminoglycans contribute to this thickening (Garcia & Geer, 1985). These components may act to trap elements of the plasma, including lipids, that form the core of the atheromatous plaque. Lipids, especially cholesterol, are released into the extracellular spaces, prompting an inflammatory response. Lipids are surrounded by collagen, smooth muscle cells, and fibrous tissue, all of which make up the plaque. Plaques vary in size, involving part or the entire circumference of the arterial wall. Over time, fibrous plaques may thicken, resulting in stenosis of the arterial lumen and restriction in CBF (Millikan et al., 1987). Extension of fibrous plaque is often related to mural thrombus formation. Also, hemorrhage into plaque, connective tissue synthesis, and lipid accumulation are thought to promote plaque enlargement (Garcia & Geer, 1985).

Atherosclerotic changes predominate in large arteries at points of bifurcation (Baker & Ionnone, 1961). The process tends to begin in the aorta and then involve the coronary arteries; by the third decade of life there is evidence of atherosclerotic changes in the cerebral vessels (Moosey, 1959). Common loci of atherosclerosis in intracranial and extracranial vascular systems are shown in Figure 36–1. Location, degree, rate of occlusion, and collateral supply influence the clinical response to a vascular lesion. Gradual narrowing of the arterial lumen allows development of collateral circulation, which may then become the primary blood supply of the area formerly supplied by the thrombosed vessel.

Cerebral venous thrombosis, although uncommon, may also cause ischemic brain disease. Most commonly involved are the dural sinuses and their tributary veins. Meningitis, local infection (e.g., sinusitis, otitis media, peritonsillar abscess), head injury, Behçet's disease, oral contraceptive use, and pregnancy may precipitate venous thrombosis, but the cause may also be idiopathic (Bousser et al., 1985).

Embolism

Ischemic stroke from embolism results from material formed proximally in the vascular tree that travels through the vascular system, lodging in a cerebral vessel and occluding distal blood flow. Although emboli may occur in any vessel, they are most commonly found in the distribution of the middle cerebral artery (Lhermitte et al., 1970). Onset of symptoms is usually sudden, with maximal deficit at the onset, but a fluctuating course does not rule out the possibility of an embolus. Nineteen percent of the Michael Reese Stroke Registry patients with embolic stroke presented with fluctuating, stepwise, or steady progression of a neurologic deficit (Caplan et al., 1983b). Neurologic deficit may quickly resolve after break-up of an embolus or lysis of an associated thrombus (Furlan, 1985). Cardiac disease is the most common source of embolic stroke. Chronic atrial fibrillation, with or without valvular disease, is the most common cause of cardioembolic stroke (Furlan, 1985; Hart et al., 1983; Sage & Van Uitert, 1983; Wolf et al., 1978). Young, healthy adults (<45 years) with no other explanation of their cerebrovascular symptoms should be investigated for mitral valve prolapse as a possible cause of cerebroembolism (Jackson et al., 1984). The risk of emboli after myocardial infarction is greatest in the first 2 to 4 weeks (Komrad et al., 1984; Millikan et al., 1987). Cardiac conditions associated with embolic stroke are listed in Table 36–3.

Other sources of embolic stroke include fat emboli after trauma or long bone fracture, tumor emboli, and atherosclerotic emboli (Sandok et al., 1980; Soloway & Aronson, 1964; Thomas & Ayyer, 1972).

TABLE 36–3. **Cardiac Sources of Cerebral Embolism**

Atrial fibrillation
Rheumatic heart disease
Mitral valve prolapse
Myocardial infarction
Infectious endocarditis
Nonbacterial thrombotic endocarditis
Atrial myxoma
Mitral annulus calcification
Cardiomyopathy
Coronary artery disease
Prosthetic heart valve

Thromboembolism

Sometimes it is difficult to determine clinically whether a cerebral infarct results from emboli, thrombus, or a combination of the two. Thrombus of a vessel can lead to embolism of distal arteries. Nonatherosclerotic thromboembolic disease may result from hematologic disorders, migraine, use of illicit drugs, fibromuscular dysplasia, or moyamoya disease.

HEMATOLOGIC DISORDERS. CBF is reduced when blood viscosity and platelet aggregability are increased. Decreased CBF may lead to ischemic stroke. Elevated hematocrit and fibrinogen indicate increased blood viscosity (Grotta et al., 1982). This occurs in disorders such as polycythemia, thrombocytosis, and sickle cell anemia. Less commonly, ischemic stroke has also been associated with serum lupus anticoagulant and disseminated intravascular coagulation (Levine & Welch, 1988; Reagan & Okazaki, 1974). Oral contraceptives may also cause hypercoagulability that results in thromboembolic stroke (Stadel, 1981).

MIGRAINE. Strokes secondary to migraine, although rare, have been reported (Bogousslavsky et al., 1988; Broderick & Swanson, 1987). At greatest risk are patients with migraines associated with hemianopsia, ophthalmoplegia, or hemiparesis (migraine with aura) (Bogousslavsky et al., 1988; Broderick & Swanson, 1987; Featherstone, 1986). Migraine patients without aura appear to have the same risk of stroke as people without migraine (Featherstone, 1986). The pathogenesis of migraine and its role in stroke are poorly understood, although the clinical picture of stroke in migraine reflects a thromboembolic process (Featherstone, 1986).

DRUG ABUSE. Neurologic sequelae of drug abuse are difficult to study because multiple substances are often used and the subjects are unreliable (Caplan et al., 1982). Reviews of the literature in this area report cerebral infarction related to the intravenous use of heroin, Talwin (Winthrop Pharmaceuticals, New York, NY), and pyribenzamine (Ts and blues); methylphenidate (Ritalin; Ciba Pharmaceutical Co., Summit, NJ); intranasal, intramuscular, or inhaled cocaine and crack; or oral ingestion of lysergic acid diethylamide (LSD) (Caplan et al., 1982; Levine & Welch, 1988). The mechanism of infarction is probably multifactorial, including embolism from endocarditis, injection of foreign matter, or an immune-mediated response altering the cerebral vessels (Caplan et al., 1982).

FIBROMUSCULAR DYSPLASIAS. This idiopathic, nonatheromatous vascular process affects the systemic arteries, especially renal, carotid, and intracerebral vessels. Cerebral ischemia may result from either stenosis or emboli (Paulson et al., 1978).

MOYAMOYA. This rare, idiopathic cerebrovascular abnormality is characterized by acquired stenosis of the carotid arteries resulting in the development of extensive collateral circulation at the base of the brain (Millikan et al., 1987). Focal cerebral ischemia is a common manifestation of moyamoya.

Inflammation

Vasculitis, inflammation, and necrosis of blood vessels may result in ischemic cerebrovascular disease. Rarely, CNS vasculitis presents as an intracranial hemorrhage (Biller et al., 1987). CNS vasculitis occurs in isolation, with peripheral vasculitides, or secondary to infection, toxins, neoplasia, or collagen vascular disease (Moore & Cupps, 1983). Isolated cerebral angiitis may involve any size of artery or vein, but small vessel disease is always present. Untreated, this disease is fatal, usually as a result of recurrent cerebral infarctions. Cerebral vessel involvement may be associated with polyarteritis nodosa, Wegener granulomatosis, Behçet disease, systemic lupus erythematosus, lymphomatoid granulomatosis, hypersensitivity vasculitis, and giant cell arteritis (temporal arteritis and Takayasu arteritis) (Moore & Cupps, 1983). Secondary causes of cerebral vasculitis include bacterial, syphilitic, tubercular, herpetic, and fungal meningitis and drug abuse, especially with amphetamines and phenylpropanolamine (an amphetamine analog found in many over-the-counter nasal decongestants, diet pills, and stimulants) (Caplan & Stein, 1986; Fallis & Fisher, 1985; Stafford et al., 1975). Sarcoidosis also produces cerebral vasculitis, most often affecting the veins, manifested by ophthalmologic, cranial nerve, cortical, and cerebellar involvement (Caplan & Stein, 1986; Caplan et al., 1983a).

Epidemiology

The incidences of stroke and stroke mortality have decreased for both sexes, blacks, whites, and all age groups, although the phenomenon is more pronounced in the elderly (Garraway et al., 1979; Gillum, 1988; Whisnant, 1974). These improvements may reflect better understanding and control of risk factors, especially hypertension.

Age, gender, race, and family history influence the incidence of stroke, but these factors cannot be altered. The incidence of stroke dramatically increases over the age of 55 years, with a twofold increase each decade (Robins & Baum, 1981). Blacks have a greater incidence of stroke and stroke mortality than whites, with black women having the highest rate (Gillum, 1988; Gross et al., 1984). Men have a higher incidence than women (Garraway et al., 1979; Robins & Baum, 1981). There is evidence that family history plays a role in the development of cerebrovascular disease (Gifford, 1966; Heyden et al., 1969). This can partially be attributed to known familial occurrence of several stroke risk factors, such as hypertension and diabetes mellitus.

Risk Factors

HYPERTENSION. Hypertension ($\geq$160/95 mm Hg) is the greatest risk factor for ischemic stroke. The degree of risk is directly related to the magnitude of blood pressure (Kannel et al., 1970). The Framingham study indicated that isolated systolic hypertension (systolic $\geq$ 160 mm Hg, diastolic $<$ 95 mm HG) is significantly related to the risk of stroke, especially in the elderly (Kannel et al., 1981). Diastolic pressures were not demonstrated to be a better indicator of risk for stroke. Labile hypertension was found to be significantly related to stroke and should not be ignored. It was recommended that the diagnosis of hypertension be based on the *average* of serial blood pressure readings taken on different days (Kannel et al., 1980).

CARDIAC DISEASE. People with cardiac disease, regardless of blood pressure, have more than twice the risk of stroke found in people with normal cardiac function (Wolf et al., 1983). Cardiac disease is also associated with increased morbidity among stroke survivors (Sacco et al., 1982). People who have had a transient ischemic attack are at high risk for mortality from myocardial infarction (Toole et al., 1978).

TRANSIENT ISCHEMIC ATTACKS (TIAS). A recent TIA increases the risk of stroke. In the Rochester, Minnesota population study, 21% of the patients had a stroke within a month of suffering a TIA, and 51% within a year (Whisnant, 1974). Although TIAs are a significant risk factor, only 10% to 25% of strokes are preceded by a TIA (Mohr et al., 1978; Whisnant, 1974).

PREVIOUS STROKE. Cumulative recurrence rates vary among studies, but a previous stroke increases the risk of subsequent strokes (Meissner et al., 1988; Sacco et al., 1982). In the Framingham study, concomitant hypertension and cardiac disease increased the potential for recurrent stroke (Sacco et al., 1982). However, the Rochester study showed that management of hypertension after stroke did not decrease the recurrence rate (Meissner et al., 1988).

DIABETES. Adult diabetics, women more so than men, have an increased risk of atherothrombotic brain infarcts (Wolf et al., 1983). However, no evidence suggests that tighter control of serum glucose either decreases the incidence or improves the outcome of strokes (Helgason, 1988). There is some evidence that hyperglycemia at the time of ischemia increases the risk of infarction, and that this is associated with poorer outcomes (Helgason, 1988).

HYPERLIPIDEMIA. Although elevated serum lipids (total and low-density lipoprotein–cholesterol) have been closely associated with coronary artery disease, the same relationship has not been consistently found with cerebrovascular atherosclerosis (Tell et al., 1988; Wolf et al., 1983). The Framingham study demonstrated a significant association between elevated serum cholesterol and atherosclerotic brain infarction only in men younger than the age of 55 years (Kannel et al., 1974).

BLOOD VISCOSITY. Blood viscosity is largely determined by serum fibrinogen concentration and hematocrit. An increase in either component leads to increased blood viscosity, resulting in decreased CBF (Grotta et al., 1982). CBF is significantly lower when the hematocrit is in the upper limits of normal (47% to 53%). Hematocrit in the upper limits of normal has also been associated with an increased incidence of cerebral infarction (Tohgi et al., 1978). Thomas and colleagues (1977) demonstrated that reducing the hematocrit by phlebotomy increased the CBF by 50%.

ASYMPTOMATIC CAROTID BRUIT. Carotid bruits often indicate advanced atherosclerosis and are associated with increased stroke risk. In the asymptomatic individual, however, a carotid bruit is a nonlocalizing sign. Data from the Framingham study showed that less than half of the strokes in people with an asymptomatic carotid bruit occurred in the distribution of the corresponding carotid artery (Wolf et al., 1981).

ORAL CONTRACEPTIVES. Oral contraceptives stimulate platelet aggregability and increase prothrombin-converting factor (factor III) activity (Stadel, 1981). It is believed that these characteristics lead to an increased risk of stroke (thromboembolic and hemorrhagic) and myocardial infarction among users of oral contraceptives. The risk of stroke among oral contraceptive users is greatest in women who also smoke cigarettes, are older than 35 years of age, and have other risk factors, particularly hypertension. With the introduction of a low-estrogen and progesterone pill, the risk of stroke has decreased (Stadel, 1981).

There are many factors that by themselves may not increase the risk of atherothrombotic infarction, but, when combined with other factors, may become significant. Some of these factors include obesity, cigarette smoking, and use of alcohol. Outcomes of the Framingham study delineate five characteristics that, when found together, identify 10% of the population that will have at least a third of all strokes. The profile characteristics include systolic hypertension, left ventricular hypertrophy on electrocardiography, hyperlipidemia (cholesterol), cigarette smoking, and glucose intolerance (Wolf et al., 1983).

Clinical Manifestations

TRANSIENT ISCHEMIC ATTACKS. TIAs are vascular events that result in temporary, focal neurologic dysfunction. Characteristic TIAs are of rapid onset, reaching maximal dysfunction within 5 minutes (often in less than 1 minute), with resolution occurring within 2 to 15 minutes (Millikan et al., 1987). Symptoms rarely persist for 24 hours, but if they do and there is resolution within 21 days, the event is referred to as a reversible ischemic neurologic deficit (RIND) (Millikan et al., 1987). In either case, the patient is without permanent neurologic deficit.

TABLE 36–4. **Common Symptoms of Transient Ischemic Attacks (TIAs)**

Carotid System	Vertebrobasilar System
Amaurosis fugax	Vertigo
Homonymous hemianopsia	Bilateral homonymous hemianopsia; diplopia
Unilateral weakness of one or both limbs	Weakness that may be bilateral or may alternate during subsequent TIAs
Unilateral numbness or paresthesias	Numbness or paresthesias of any or all limbs
Aphasia or dysarthria	Dysarthria Dysphagia Ataxia Perioral numbness

Transient ischemic attacks result from a variety of conditions. Arterial obstruction from thrombus or embolus, arterial inflammation, and hematologic or coagulation abnormalities may reduce CBF to a point that allows transient focal ischemia. Cardiac or atherosclerotic plaque emboli are considered the most common source of TIAs (Barnett, 1979; Millikan et al., 1987). Lysis of emboli from intravascular enzymes or emboli that are small enough to pass through the affected vessel may account for the transient nature of focal abnormalities (Millikan et al., 1987).

The significance of hypotension induced by positional change, cerebral arteriography, or medications in chronically hypertensive patients as a mechanism for producing TIAs has been debated. Ruff and associates (1981) found that rapid lowering of blood pressure in hypertensive patients with hemodynamically significant carotid artery stenosis (greater than 85%) put the patient at risk for a TIA. Others have found no relationship (Kendall & Marshall, 1963). Nevertheless, nurses must be particularly attuned to monitoring postural blood pressure changes and assessing these patients for any transient focal neurologic signs.

Most TIAs are not witnessed by health care workers, making a careful history essential for diagnosis. TIA symptoms may be classified by localization to areas supplied by the carotid or vertebrobasilar systems; however, at times the distinction can be difficult. Common signs and symptoms of TIAs in both distributions are listed in Table 36–4. The most common symptoms associated with the carotid system are contralateral weakness and ipsilateral amaurosis fugax (painless, unilateral blindness). Amaurosis fugax indicates retinal ischemia and is usually the result of atherosclerotic plaque emboli from the ipsilateral ICA. Many patients describe this transient blindness as if a "shade were pulled down over the eye." Others describe a central scotoma that spreads to involve part or all of the visual field within seconds. Each episode is usually brief (<10 minutes), and often normal vision returns, but usually more slowly than the visual defect began (Marshall & Meadows, 1968).

Vertigo and binocular visual complaints are most frequently associated with vertebrobasilar TIAs. Nausea and vomiting may accompany these findings. Less commonly, drop attacks and transient global amnesia (TGA) occur. A drop attack is an unprecipitated loss of strength in both legs, causing the patient to fall. The attack is so sudden that the patient is unable to break the fall. The patient remains conscious, and, usually by the time he or she lands on the ground, his or her strength has returned (Brust et al., 1979; Kubala & Millikan, 1964). TGA is an episode of memory loss that persists minutes to hours. The patient is oriented to self but confused about the environment, has retrograde amnesia, and conversation is vague. The episode gradually resolves with the patient returning to normal except for amnesia for the event. TGA, unless associated with risk factors or other symptoms of cerebral ischemia, is unlikely to recur or lead to stroke (Jensen & de-Fine-Olivarius, 1981; Shuping et al., 1980).

It is important to note that TIAs within the carotid system produce contralateral motor or sensory symptoms, whereas those of the vertebrobasilar system result in alternating or bilateral motor or sensory deficits. TIAs usually present as a constellation of symptoms, as opposed to an isolated abnormality. For example, recurrent vertigo in the absence of other symptoms is probably not secondary to ischemia (Barnett, 1979; Millikan et al., 1987). The nurse should be aware that a TIA signals impaired cerebral circulation. Episodes that increase in frequency over a short period of time, "crescendo" TIAs, indicate the need for immediate medical intervention.

PROGRESSING STROKE. Progression of stroke is a temporal phenomenon defined as the continued worsening of a neurologic deficit or the progressive development of new neurologic signs. Stroke may evolve steadily or in a stuttering fashion over minutes to days. Britton and Roden (1985) found that 43% of the patients admitted for stroke experienced an extension of their neurologic deficits, half of which occurred in the first 24 hours. Progression can result from cerebral edema, recurrent emboli, or failure of collateral blood supply. Complications such as pulmonary embolus, hypotension, and systemic infection may also contribute to a worsening neurologic status.

It is frequently the nurse who first notes deterioration of the patient's neurologic status, especially changes in the level of consciousness. Because this is a critical finding, it should be reported immediately. Repeated neurologic and cardiac assessments, comparing the findings to those of previous examinations, are essential. This information aids the physician in isolating the cause, allowing selection of appropriate diagnostic procedures and rapid institution of medical and surgical interventions to attempt to prevent further progression. Ischemia within the carotid artery distribution is unlikely to progress after 18 to 24 hours of *stable* neurologic status. However, progression of ischemia within the vertebrobasilar system may occur up to after 72 hours of neurologic stability.

COMPLETED STROKE. A completed stroke is defined as a prolonged neurologic deficit, lasting more than 21 days, and is basically stable (Millikan et al., 1987). A completed stroke indicates infarction as opposed to ischemia. However, a completed stroke does not preclude the potential for gradual improvement. The term "completed stroke" does not reflect the cause or degree of associated neurologic dysfunction. Prognosis depends on the size and location of the infarct and the availability of collateral circulation.

Lacunar infarcts are small, deep "holes" that often result from occlusion of small arteries in the basal ganglia, thalamus, internal capsule, or brain stem (Mohr, 1982). Small vessel disease secondary to hypertension is the most likely cause. Lacunar infarcts may result in "pure sensory" or "pure motor" strokes, or dysarthria–clumsy hand syndrome (Fisher, 1982; Fisher and Curry, 1965). Prognosis is generally good for these patients.

Diagnosis

Diagnosis begins with a detailed history, including a family history. Activity and time of onset, first noticed symptom, and progression or resolution of symptoms are essential information. Some patients present with seizures or status epilepticus. Most commonly, focal motor seizures with or without generalization are noted (Cocito et al., 1982; Lesser et al., 1985). Risk factors should be identified, including history of hypertension, cardiac disease, diabetes mellitus, and TIAs. Questions should be very specific, such as, "Have you ever lost vision in one eye which lasted only a few minutes?" (Millikan et al., 1987). When the patient is dysarthric, aphasic, or confused, the history should be taken from family or friends.

Physical assessment focuses on vital signs, cardiac status, and assessment of skin. Hypertension, hypotension, atrial fibrillation, evidence of congestive heart failure, and coagulopathy (petechiae, ecchymosis) should be noted (Millikan et al., 1987). Laboratory studies should include a complete blood count, erythrocyte sedimentation rate, and platelet count; serum electrolytes, glucose, and calcium; coagulation studies; VDRL test; and urinalysis. Serum and urinary toxicology screens should be done for suspected substance abuse. Chest radiographs are also done. Electrocardiography and echocardiography are obtained on all patients with suspected embolic stroke or known cardiac abnormalities.

Neurologic assessment emphasizes the level of consciousness, mental status, cranial nerve function, and motor and sensory function. Frequent neurologic assessments should be carefully documented on a flow sheet. Funduscopic examination and auscultation for subclavian, carotid, and orbital bruits are also useful. Specialized testing procedures used in assessing ischemia and infarction are discussed in the following.

COMPUTED AXIAL TOMOGRAPHY SCAN. Computed tomography (CT) scan of the head is appropriate for most patients with transient or progressive neurologic symptoms. Intracerebral or subarachnoid blood appears as a hyperdensity compared to normal brain. In contrast, a nonhemorrhagic (bland) infarct and cerebral edema are hypodense. Often a bland infarct will not be evident on CT for several days after the insult. CT is also valuable in uncovering previously unsuspected pathology, such as a structural lesion (tumor, abscess) or subdural hematoma, rather than stroke as an explanation for the patient's condition. In an emergency situation, a contrast-enhanced study is not always necessary. Contrast agents should be avoided in patients with renal disease, congestive heart failure, or a known allergy to the contrast medium, although the latter is quite rare.

CEREBRAL ANGIOGRAPHY. Angiography is performed by the direct intraarterial injection of a radiopaque contrast medium into either the carotid or vertebral artery (or both), thus providing visualization of the vascular tree. The catheter is usually inserted through the femoral artery, passed to the aortic arch, and then passed to the carotid or vertebral artery. Angiography is done to delineate extracranial or intracranial occlusive vascular disease (such as that from atherosclerosis or vasculitis) and to guide subsequent treatment, medical or surgical. The major complication, although rare, of angiography is the onset of or progression of neurologic deficit. There is also a very small potential for allergic reaction to the contrast agent.

MAGNETIC RESONANCE IMAGING. Magnetic resonance imaging (MRI) is more sensitive in detecting early changes in cellular water content, allowing new infarcts to be identified within hours (Brant-Zawadzki, 1988). MRI also enhances visualization of the cerebellum and brain stem, permitting better identification of vertebrobasilar infarcts. With multiple infarcts, it is not possible to distinguish the age of infarcts without previous comparison scans (Brant-Zawadzki, 1988). MRI is contraindicated for patients with cardiac pacemakers or intracranial aneurysm clips because of the high magnetic fields generated (Brant-Zawadzki, 1988).

DIGITAL SUBTRACTION ANGIOGRAPHY. Digital subtraction angiography (DSA) may be done intravenously (IV) or, preferably, intraarterially (IA). IV-DSA is accomplished by means of systemic venous injection of contrast media. IA-DSA is done in the same way as cerebral angiography, but it requires less contrast medium, allows electronic subtraction of the overlying bony structures, and takes less time (Millikan et al., 1987).

MAGNETIC RESONANCE ANGIOGRAPHY. Magnetic resonance angiography (MRA) is a new, rapid, noninvasive procedure that promises to define ECA disease as well as invasive IA-DSA (Masaryk et al., 1989). This procedure, with a short increase in examination time, can also image the brain parenchyma. The disadvantages of MRA are its sensitivity to patient movement and positioning (Masaryk et al., 1989).

ULTRASONOGRAPHY. Ultrasound noninvasively detects stenosis of the ECAs through Doppler or B-mode scanners. The Doppler provides a static image, whereas B-mode produces real-time images of the pulsating artery. A duplex scanner combines both of these techniques into a single instrument. The quality of the image is very dependent on the technician and on patient cooperation. This device is unable to distinguish between severe stenosis and complete occlusion (Millikan et al., 1987). Ultrasound results should be confirmed by angiography before considering surgical correction.

LUMBAR PUNCTURE. Since the advent of CT scanning and MRI, the lumbar puncture (LP) has become less crucial in diagnosing ischemic stroke patients. However, patients with unexplained ischemic infarction may require LP for examination of the cerebrospinal fluid (CSF) for evidence of meningitis or vasculitis. LP is always contraindicated with clinical evidence of increased intracranial pressure.

Clinical Management

The goals of treatment of patients with acute cerebral ischemic events are to prevent associated complications and further neurologic insult. Interventions are initiated in an attempt to restore normal perfusion to the injured area and prevent increased intracranial pressure secondary to cerebral edema, cautiously manage blood pressure, and identify and correct contributing systemic processes (e.g., cardiac disease, pneumonia, and pulmonary embolism). Besides transtentorial herniation, the most common causes of death in the initial 35 days after stroke are pneumonia, cardiac disease, and pulmonary embolism (Bounds et al., 1981). Therefore, identification and treatment of these conditions are imperative.

MEDICAL TREATMENT

Platelet antiaggregants, anticoagulation, calcium channel blockers, hemodilution, and thrombolytic therapy are used to treat ischemic stroke. Inflammatory cerebrovascular disease is treated with corticosteroids and cyclophosphamide.

PLATELET ANTIAGGREGANTS. Agents that inhibit platelet aggregability, or adhesiveness, include dipyridamole (Persantine; Boehringer Ingelheim, Ridgefield, CT), sulfinpyrazone (Anturane; Ciba Pharmaceutical Co., Summit, NJ), acetylsalicylcic acid (ASA), and ticlopidine. ASA is more effective for men than women in reducing the incidence of stroke after TIA or atherothrombotic stroke. Side effects of this therapy include gastrointestinal upset or bleeding. Although the optimum dosage has not been determined, as little as 40 mg (1/2 a baby aspirin) daily will inhibit platelet aggregation in vitro. Dipyridamole and sulfinpyrazone, by themselves or with ASA, are no better than ASA alone in preventing cerebral infarction (American–Canadian Study Group, 1985; Bousser et al., 1983; Weksler et al., 1985). Platelet antiaggregants are associated with less severe or disabling strokes (Grotta et al., 1985). Results of a large multicenter trial of ticlopidine, a newer platelet antiaggregant, in the prevention of nonfatal stroke in patients with a history of TIA, RIND, or minor stroke demonstrated that ticlopidine was somewhat more effective in men and women than ASA. The risk of side effects from ticlopidine (diarrhea, skin rash, severe neutropenia), however, was greater than that from ASA (Hass et al., 1989).

ANTICOAGULATION. Anticoagulants are used to prevent recurrent emboli and further formation of thrombus. Use of anticoagulation in an acute ischemic event is controversial. Anticoagulation is considered a treatment option in the treatment of "crescendo" or multiple TIAs and in progressive, acute partial or cardioembolic stroke (Miller & Hart, 1988). This therapy is not indicated in a patient with a completed infarction.

Before beginning anticoagulation, CT or MRI is done to rule out hemorrhagic stroke and allow careful consideration of the risks and benefits for the patient. Lumbar puncture done within an hour of the advent of anticoagulation therapy increases the risk of a spinal hematoma (Ruff & Dougherty, 1981). Contraindications for anticoagulant therapy include hemorrhagic lesions (e.g., gastric ulcer), poorly controlled hypertension, high risk for falls (e.g., ataxia, vertigo), and an inability to adhere to specific instructions (e.g., cognitive impairment or dementia).

Therapy usually begins with a bolus of intravenous heparin (5,000 to 10,000 units) followed by a continuous infusion of heparinized solution. Dose adjustments are made to maintain the activated partial thromboplastin time (APTT) within 1.5 to 2.5 times the control (normal, 35–40 seconds; therapeutic, 60–100 seconds) (Miller & Hart, 1988). A potential risk of anticoagulation is the transformation of an ischemic lesion into a hemorrhagic infarct or an intracerebral bleed. Hypertension and excessive anticoagulation are significantly associated with an increased risk of a fatal intracerebral bleed (Ruff & Dougherty, 1981). Anecdotal reports indicate a need to delay heparinization for 5 to 7 days and avoid bolus administration in patients with large embolic infarcts (Cerebral Embolism Study Group, 1984).

Patients on long-term anticoagulation will be converted to the oral medication warfarin (Coumadin; Du Pont, Wilmington, DE). Dosage is adjusted to maintain a prothrombin time (PT) of 1.5 times normal. Heparin is continued until the PT is within the therapeutic range; hence, there is an overlap of treatment of about 4 days.

Patients beginning anticoagulation therapy need careful neurologic monitoring for intracerebral hemorrhage. Increasing neurologic deficit should be rapidly reported to the physician. Laboratory values, APTT, and PT should be monitored to ensure that therapeutic levels are met and not exceeded.

Patients and family members should be instructed in the rationale for anticoagulation therapy and taught the need to report evidence of petechiae, epistaxis, ecchymosis, hematuria, melena, hematemesis, hemoptysis, bleeding gums, or wounds that continue to bleed.

Coadministration of drugs known to alter the effect of anticoagulation therapy should be avoided, including salicylates, intravenous nitroglycerin, carbamazepine, and phenytoin. The reader is referred to *Drug Interaction Facts* or a similar handbook for a complete listing of potential interactions.

CALCIUM CHANNEL BLOCKERS. Cerebral ischemia results in an influx of calcium into the cell that may contribute to cellular death. Administration of nimodipine, a calcium channel blocker that crosses the blood–brain barrier, may modify this process. Nimodipine has improved outcomes and reduced mortality in patients with acute completed atherothrombotic infarcts, especially men, and those with moderate to severe neurologic deficits at onset of symptoms (Gelmers et al., 1988).

HEMODILUTION. A relationship between increased blood viscosity and decreased CBF has been identified. Hemodilution is used to decrease the hematocrit and increase CBF to ischemic but potentially viable tissue surrounding the infarct, called the ischemic penumbra. If the ischemic area is reperfused, the completed infarct may be smaller, improving patient outcome. Hemodilution is accomplished through phlebotomy and volume replacement (isovolemic hemodilution), administration of a plasma volume expander such as low–molecular-weight dextran (hypervolemic hemodilution), or a combination of both methods (Grotta, 1987). Strand and colleagues (1984) demonstrated that hemodilution through phlebotomy and dextran in the acute phase of ischemic stroke improved patient outcome, whereas others have found no beneficial effect (Scandinavian Stroke Study Group, 1987). This treatment should not be considered for patients with impaired cardiac function, low hematocrit on admission, or evidence of cerebral edema. Further studies are needed to determine the effectiveness of hemodilution and, if found to be effective, to develop a protocol to ensure safe implementation.

THROMBOLYTIC THERAPY. Thrombolytic therapy may be useful in the treatment of cerebral vessels occluded by thrombus or emboli (Del Zoppo et al., 1986). In the past, unacceptable complications such as hemorrhagic transformation of the infarct have precluded clinical use of this therapy. However, development of intravenous tissue plasminogen activator, which has less effect on systemic fibrinogen and clotting factors and tends to have a more specific action against fibrin of fresh thrombi, has renewed interest in this therapy (Sherry, 1985). Bleeding complications, however, are still evident, and controlled studies are needed to document the safety and efficacy of this therapy.

HYPERTENSION. CBF remains constant as long as the autoregulation mechanism is intact. Cerebral edema or ischemia may impair autoregulation, and CBF then becomes dependent on systemic blood pressure. Therefore, lowering the blood pressure in these circumstances may significantly reduce CBF, resulting in clinical deterioration. Most stroke patients are hypertensive on admission, but spontaneous reduction in blood pressure occurs gradually during the next 10 days (Wallace & Levy, 1981). Antihypertensive therapy is discouraged during this period except when there is hypertensive encephalopathy, a diastolic pressure of 130 mm Hg or more, or compromised vital organs (e.g., heart or kidney) (Lavin, 1986; Strandgaard, 1983). Hypertensive therapy should be done cautiously, using short-acting agents that can be precisely adjusted and promptly withdrawn.

CNS VASCULITIS. Cyclophosphamide and prednisone are the agents of choice for isolated CNS vasculitis (Moore, 1989). If cerebral angiitis is due to an infectious process such as bacterial meningitis or neurosyphilis, specific antibiotic therapy is needed.

SURGICAL TREATMENT

Some patients with extracranial vascular disease are candidates for surgery. The goals of surgery are to prevent recurrent TIAs or stroke.

CAROTID ENDARTERECTOMY. Carotid endarterectomy is the most common surgical procedure used for extracranial artery disease. Atherosclerotic occlusive disease usually occurs at the carotid bifurcation, an area easily accessible for surgical intervention (Fig. 36–3). During endarterectomy, the vessels are temporarily clamped and opened, and the atheroma and associated thrombus are excised, leaving a smoother luminal surface. Intraoperative EEG is frequently done to ensure adequate intraoperative perfusion and assess the need for surgical shunting. There is controversy, however, about when and for whom endarterectomy is indicated. The potential surgical mortality and morbidity must be carefully weighed against the risk of stroke.

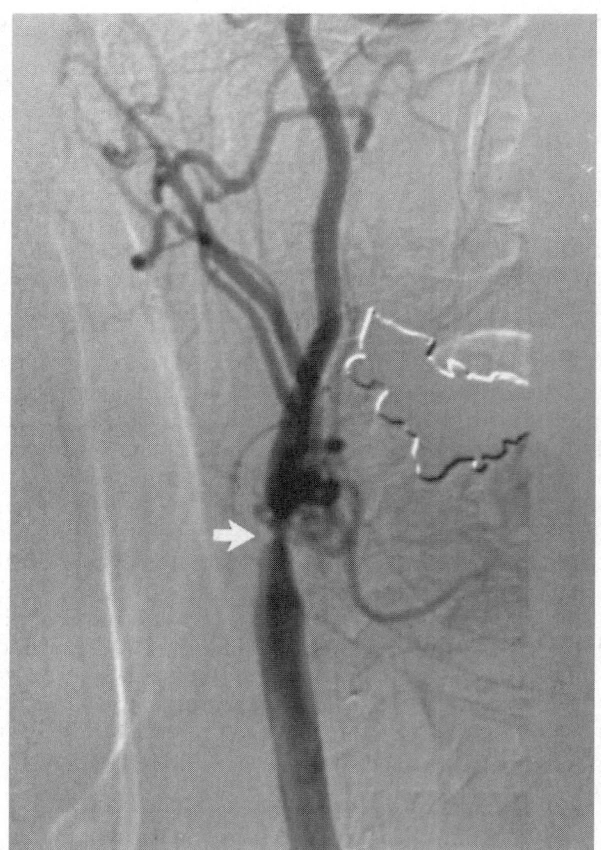

FIGURE 36–3. Intraarterial digital subtraction angiogram demonstrating stenosis (*arrow*) of the right carotid artery at the bifurcation.

The potential for surgical complications increases in patients with major medical, neurologic, or angiographically defined risk factors (Sundt et al., 1987b). Medical risk factors include cardiopulmonary disease, severe hypertension, obesity, advanced peripheral vascular occlusive disease, and age older than 70 years. Neurologic risk factors include crescendo TIAs, progressive neurologic deficit, deficit resolving within 24 hours of surgery, cerebral infarct less than 7 days old, and generalized cerebral ischemia. Occlusion of the contralateral ICA, a large plaque in the operative vessel, or a large plaque protruding from an ulcerative lesion are some angiographically defined risk factors (Sundt et al., 1987b).

Potential neurologic complications of surgery are stroke, TIAs, or cranial nerve injury. Ischemic stroke may result from perioperative embolization, postoperative ICA occlusion, or hyperperfusion syndromes due to significantly increased CBF during surgery. Intracerebral hemorrhage is an uncommon but devastating complication and may result from hyperperfusion. Cranial nerve injury, particularly to the hypoglossal, recurrent, or superior laryngeal branches of the vagus, and facial nerves may occur (Sundt et al., 1987a) (Fig. 36–4). Postoperative assessments should include evaluation of tongue movement, quality and tone of voice, ability to swallow, and facial symmetry. Nonneuro-

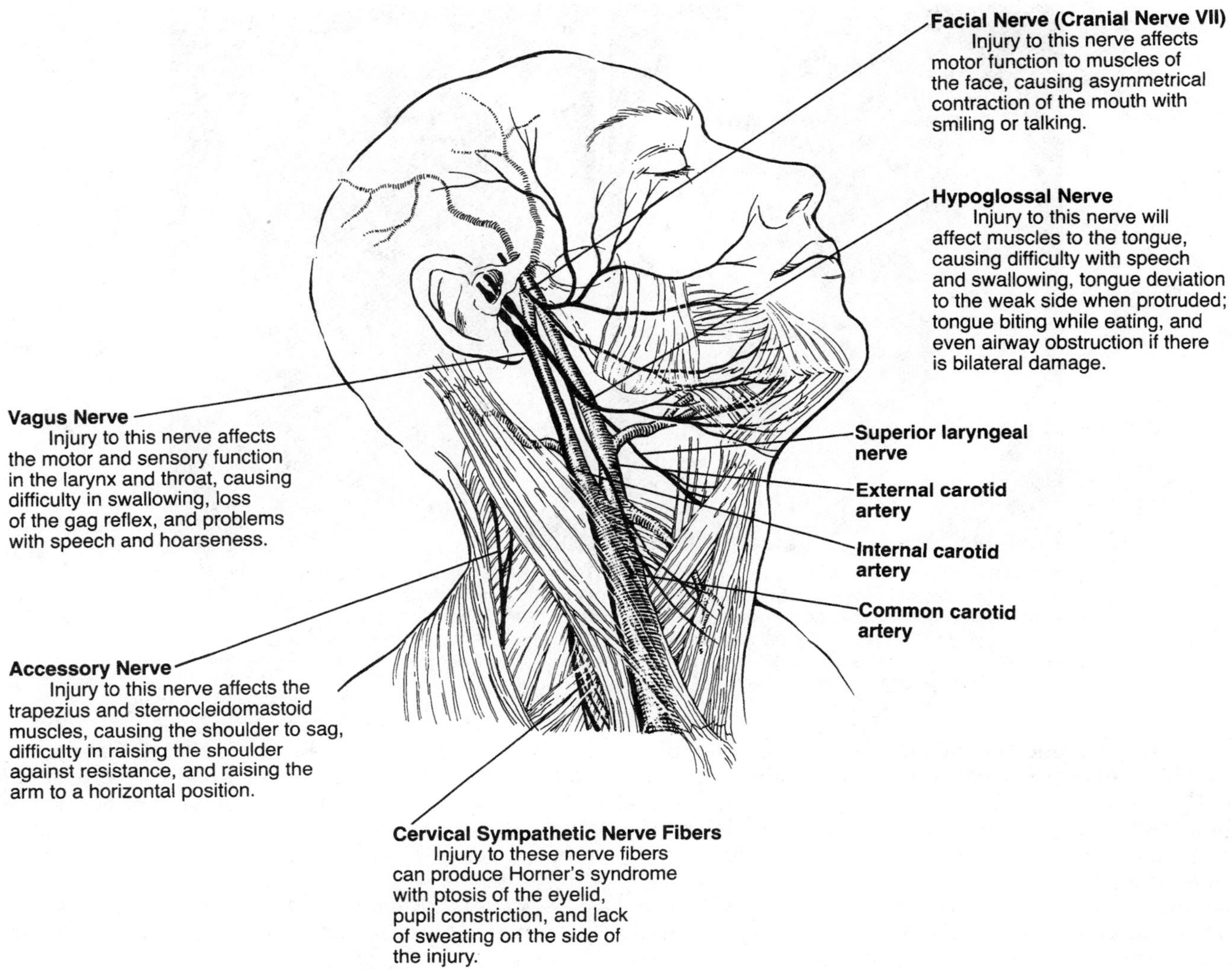
Facial Nerve (Cranial Nerve VII)
Injury to this nerve affects motor function to muscles of the face, causing asymmetrical contraction of the mouth with smiling or talking.
Hypoglossal Nerve
Injury to this nerve will affect muscles to the tongue, causing difficulty with speech and swallowing, tongue deviation to the weak side when protruded; tongue biting while eating, and even airway obstruction if there is bilateral damage.
Vagus Nerve
Injury to this nerve affects the motor and sensory function in the larynx and throat, causing difficulty in swallowing, loss of the gag reflex, and problems with speech and hoarseness.
Superior laryngeal nerve
External carotid artery
Internal carotid artery
Common carotid artery
Accessory Nerve
Injury to this nerve affects the trapezius and sternocleidomastoid muscles, causing the shoulder to sag, difficulty in raising the shoulder against resistance, and raising the arm to a horizontal position.
Cervical Sympathetic Nerve Fibers
Injury to these nerve fibers can produce Horner's syndrome with ptosis of the eyelid, pupil constriction, and lack of sweating on the side of the injury.

FIGURE 36–4. Cranial nerves exposed to trauma during carotid endarterectomy.

logic complications include wound infection, hematoma, carotid artery hemorrhage, and fluctuations in blood pressure. Transient dysfunction of carotid sinus baroreceptors is the suspected cause of postoperative hypotension and hypertension. Hypotension is managed with volume replacement and Trendelenburg positioning because the patient usually fails to respond to vasopressors. Hypertension is dealt with by intravenous nitroglycerin or nitroprusside (Sundt et al., 1987a).

Overall, mortality from carotid endarterectomy is approximately 1.3% (Sundt et al., 1987a). Obviously, the more medically and neurologically unstable a patient is, the greater the risk of surgery. The expertise and experience of the surgical team are critical factors in ensuring a favorable outcome.

EXTRACRANIAL–INTRACRANIAL (EC-IC) ARTERIAL BYPASS. An international randomized study investigated the benefit of EC-IC arterial bypass in patients with symptomatic atherosclerotic disease. Bypass of the superficial temporal or occipital artery to the middle cerebral artery failed to decrease stroke recurrence and stroke mortality (EC/IC Bypass Stroke Group, 1985). Therefore, this procedure does not appear to be warranted for these patients.

HEMORRHAGIC STROKE

Hemorrhagic stroke results from bleeding into the subarachnoid space or brain parenchyma and accounts for approximately 14% of all cerebral infarctions (Wolf et al., 1983).

Subarachnoid Hemorrhage

Subarachnoid hemorrhage (SAH) results from a cerebral vessel that has "leaked" or "ruptured," allowing

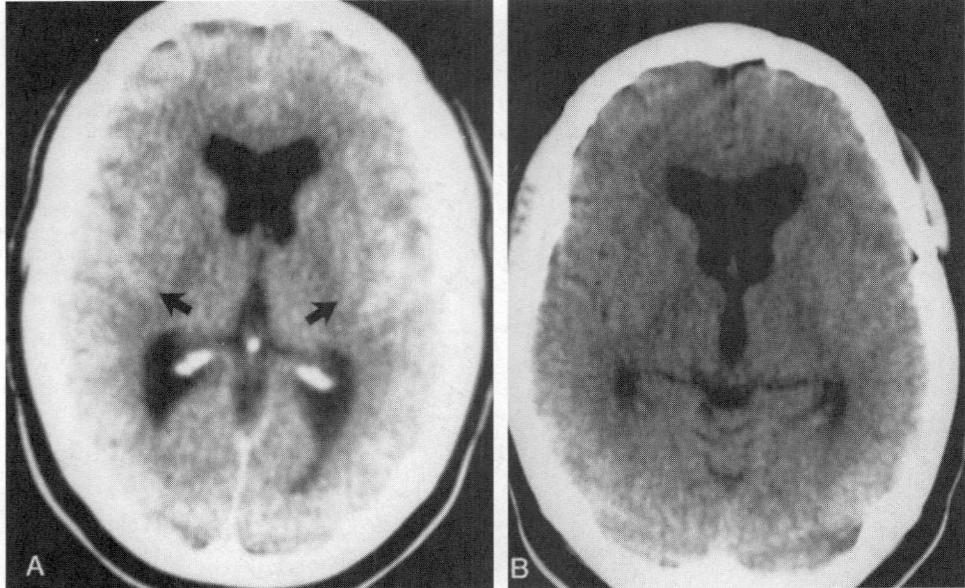

FIGURE 36–5. *A*, Axial computed tomography (CT) scan of the head demonstrating hyperdensity around the cortical convexity, particularly in the area of the sylvian fissures (*arrows*) secondary to recent subarachnoid hemorrhage. Hyperdense areas in the posterior horns of the lateral ventricles and the third ventricle represent normal calcification of choroid plexus. *B*, Axial CT scan of the same patient as in *A* 3½ months later. Note resolution of the subarachnoid blood. (The cut is lower than that in *A*, explaining the absence of calcification.)

blood to flow into the subarachnoid space (Fig. 36–5). This provokes several responses that alter regional CBF. Loss of cerebral autoregulation, decreased cerebral perfusion pressure, increased intracranial pressure, and arterial vasospasm combine to reduce CBF. Consequently, cerebral ischemia and infarction are frequent and devastating complications of SAH. The most common cause of SAH is a ruptured cerebral aneurysm. Less commonly, arteriovenous malformations, head injury, or blood dyscrasias result in SAH.

ANEURYSMS

Aneurysms are formed from a weakness in the arterial wall and result in an outpouching or ballooning appearance. Aneurysms are classified according to their configuration as saccular, fusiform, or dissecting.

SACCULAR ANEURYSMS. Saccular, or berry, aneurysms are most common and usually form at places of arterial bifurcation, especially in the anterior cerebral circulation of the circle of Willis. Saccular aneurysms often have a narrow neck that extends from the parent vessel and expands into a broader portion or dome, giving them a sac-like or berry-like appearance (Fig. 36–6). Size of the neck and dome varies. Although either portion may rupture, the dome is the more common site of hemorrhage.

Saccular aneurysms are thought to originate from a congenital defect of the muscularis of the artery, degenerative changes in the internal elastic lamina, or a combination of both processes that gradually weakens the arterial wall (Mohr et al., 1986a). Rarely, aneurysms form from infectious emboli (mycotic aneurysm), trauma, or neoplastic emboli. Mycotic aneurysms are usually found in the distal branches of major cerebral vessels.

FUSIFORM ANEURYSMS. Fusiform aneurysms are characterized by a spindle-shaped dilatation of an ar-

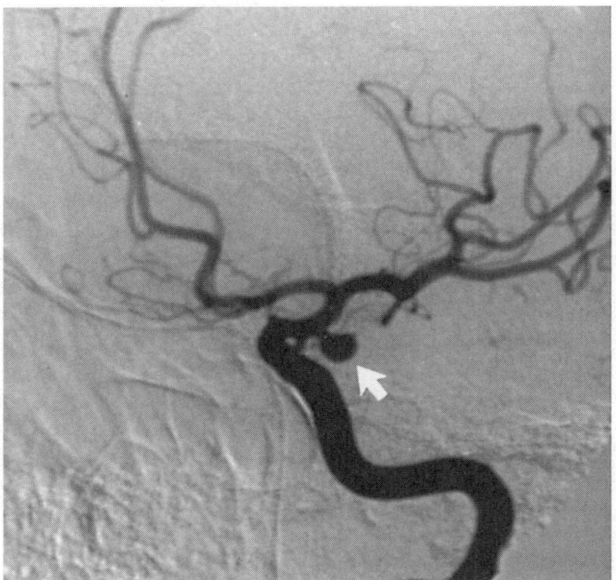

FIGURE 36–6. Cerebral arteriogram demonstrating a saccular aneurysm (*arrow*) of the left internal carotid artery at the origin of the posterior communicating artery.

tery, with tapering at either end. Weir (1987a) described fusiform aneurysms as "shaped like deformed cigars." These are more commonly found in the vertebrobasilar artery and cause symptoms of cranial nerve compression, cerebral ischemia, or impaired CSF circulation (Weir, 1987a).

DISSECTING ANEURYSMS. Dissecting aneurysms, often the result of trauma, form from a tear in the endothelium that creates a false channel. These rarely cause SAH because they usually occur extracranially.

Clinical Manifestations

Aneurysms rupture when the stress on the arterial wall exceeds the wall's strength. This may occur when there is an increase in intraaneurysmal pressure, increased aneurysmal radius, or decreased arterial wall thickness (Ferguson, 1972). This could explain why aneurysms are more likely to rupture during hypertensive episodes, strenuous activity, straining to defecate (Valsalva maneuver), heavy lifting, or sexual intercourse. Spontaneous rupture, however, may occur at any time, even during nonstrenuous activity or sleep. Mortality rates after the initial hemorrhage are 27% to 43% at 1 week and 50% at 1 month (Weir, 1987a). Many patients die before reaching the hospital.

Characteristic symptoms of an SAH include sudden explosive headache, with or without loss of consciousness, and subsequent nuchal rigidity. The headache peaks in severity within seconds. The pain may initially be localized in the area of the bleed, but soon becomes holocephalic. Nausea, vomiting, neck pain, and stiffness are commonly associated with the headache. Frequently, there is loss of consciousness lasting minutes to hours; some patients never regain consciousness. Others may manifest only altered consciousness (e.g., lethargy) and altered mentation, including confusion or disorientation. Additional symptoms may include partial or generalized seizures, photophobia, diplopia, and vertigo. Seizure is most likely to occur at the onset of hemorrhage or with a rebleed (Hart et al., 1981). With extension of the hemorrhage intracerebrally or compression of adjacent brain by hematoma, the patient may exhibit focal neurologic signs such as hemiparesis or aphasia.

Before rupture, many patients (48%) have a warning leak (sentinel hemorrhage) or evidence of aneurysmal enlargement (Okawara, 1973). A warning leak may be enough to cause a headache with nausea, vomiting, and neck pain. Patients usually describe the headache as different from their typical headache. However, many times these symptoms do not prompt the patient to seek health care, or they are misdiagnosed. Cranial nerve palsies, particularly of the oculomotor and abducens nerves, visual field defects, and pain in, behind, or around the eye may indicate aneurysmal enlargement (Mohr et al., 1986b). The striking morbidity and mortality associated with SAH may be reduced through early recognition of these warning signs and rapid institution of definitive therapy before severe SAH occurs.

DELAYED NEUROLOGIC COMPLICATIONS

Major causes of delayed morbidity and mortality after SAH are symptomatic cerebral vasospasm, rebleeding, and delayed hydrocephalus. The onset of these complications is heralded by a change in the findings of the neurologic examination. The importance of consistent and frequent assessment and documentation of the patient's neurologic status by nurses and physicians cannot be overemphasized.

VASOSPASM. Symptomatic cerebral vasospasm (abnormal narrowing of an artery) occurs in about 30% of patients with SAH after rupture of a saccular aneurysm. The incidence in patients with arteriovenous malformation (AVM) is less because AVMs occur less frequently and rarely rupture into large basal cisterns.

Onset of cerebral vasospasm averages 4 to 14 days (range 3–21 days) after the initial hemorrhage (Mohr et al., 1986b). The size and location of SAH can be correlated with the occurrence, severity, and location of vasospasm (Kistler et al., 1983).

Cerebral artery vasospasm can lead to ischemia or infarction, the clinical findings varying with the specific arteries involved. Many patients with vasospasm exhibit altered mental status or consciousness. Signs of severe vasospasm of the anterior cerebral area include urinary incontinence, whispered voice, speaking with eyes closed, pursing lips, grasp reflex, and abulia (impaired ability to initiate spontaneous action) (Kistler et al., 1983). Ischemia of the middle cerebral artery's distribution may produce monoparesis, hemiparesis, facial weakness, anosognosia (nondominant hemispheric lesion), and dysphasia (dominant hemispheric lesion) (Kistler et al., 1983). Homonymous hemianopsia is often seen with posterior cerebral artery ischemia.

REHEMORRHAGE. Aneurysms are most likely to rebleed within the first 2 weeks after the initial hemorrhage, especially in the first 24 hours (Kassell & Torner, 1983). This fact significantly affects decisions about the timing of surgical interventions.

HYDROCEPHALUS. Interruption or impairment of CSF flow due to blood in the subarachnoid space or intraventricular spaces can lead to hydrocephalus. Hydrocephalus is caused by impaired reabsorption of CSF. Communicating hydrocephalus usually occurs 4 to 20 days after aneurysmal rupture, although it may occur at any time. Patients may be completely asymptomatic, requiring no intervention, or they may exhibit marked deterioration of level of consciousness over a few hours, requiring emergency drainage of CSF (Mohr et al., 1986b).

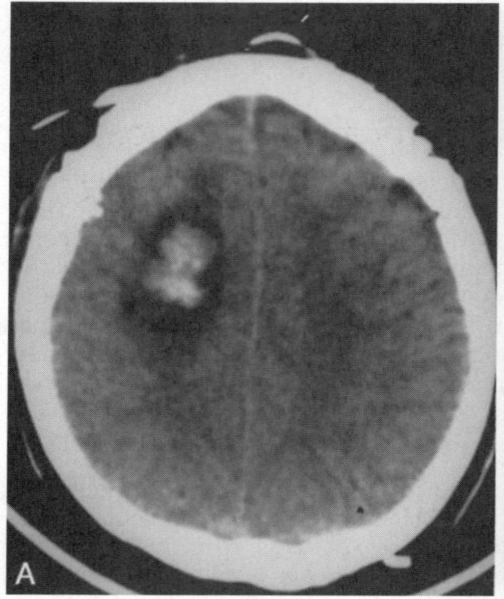

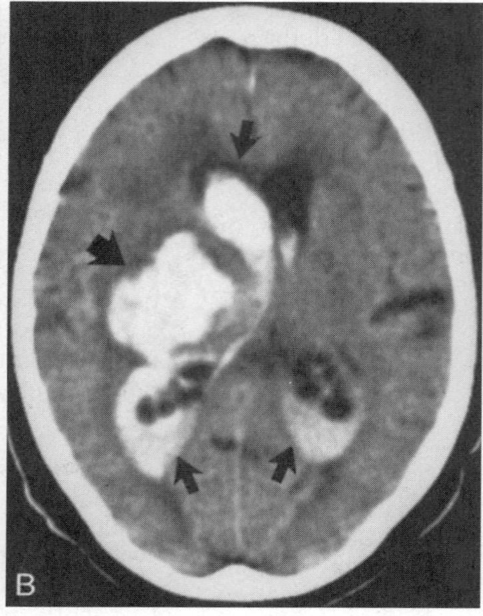

FIGURE 36–7. *A,* Axial computed tomography (CT) scan of the head demonstrating a hyperdense lesion surrounded by a hypodense area in the right hemisphere. This is an intracerebral hematoma with surrounding edema. *B,* Axial CT scan of the head demonstrating a right hemispheric basal ganglian intracerebral hematoma (*wide arrow*) with intraventricular extension (*narrow arrows*).

Intracerebral Hemorrhage

Intracerebral hemorrhage (ICH) results from bleeding into the brain parenchyma (Fig. 36–7). Although the most common source is small penetrating arterioles or capillaries, AVM and aneurysms may also cause ICH. ICH usually develops gradually, over minutes to hours, due to the low pressure of arterioles and capillaries. By comparison, SAH causes a rapid (within seconds) increase in intracranial pressure secondary to rupture of an aneurysm under systemic arterial pressure.

Most ICHs occur in the cerebral hemispheres, particularly within the putamen, thalamus, and lobar regions. A smaller percentage occur in the cerebellum and pons (Kase & Mohr, 1986). Hypertension is the usual cause, with vascular malformations the most common nonhypertensive cause. Oral anticoagulant therapy, cerebral amyloid angiopathy, and intracranial tumors may also result in ICH. Drug abuse may lead to both SAH and ICH.

HYPERTENSIVE HEMORRHAGE

Chronic hypertension causes degenerative changes in cerebral vessels and the formation of microaneurysms (Charcot-Bouchard aneurysms). Blood pressure does not need to be in a critical range for this to occur; moderate hypertension for many years or a few years of severe hypertension produce the same changes (Furlan et al., 1979). ICH occurs when one or more affected vessels rupture. Many ICH patients are hypertensive on admission, the hypertension being either an acute process secondary to increased intracranial pressure or a chronic process, which is the primary cause of ICH. Therefore, a blood pressure history should be obtained for all patients admitted for ICH.

VASCULAR MALFORMATIONS

There are a number of cerebral vascular malformations besides aneurysms. McCormick's (1966) classification of vascular malformations includes venous angiomas, cavernous angiomas, capillary telangiectasis, varix, and AVMs.

VENOUS ANGIOMAS. Venous angiomas are formed by a group of anomalous veins, usually located deep within the white matter. These angiomas may serve to drain areas lacking normal venous drainage (Mohr et al., 1986b; Senegor et al., 1983). These rarely hemorrhage, but may be associated with seizures and headaches (Mohr et al., 1986b).

CAVERNOUS ANGIOMAS. Cavernous angiomas are space-occupying lesions composed of large, vascular, cavernous channels most commonly found in the cerebral hemispheres. A large part of the malformation may be thrombosed. Unlike tumors, cavernous angiomas replace, instead of displace, normal brain and therefore do not create a significant mass-like effect. These lesions are associated with headache, seizures, and occasionally hemorrhage (Mohr et al., 1986b; McCormick, 1966).

CAPILLARY TELANGIECTASIS. This is a small group of thin-walled capillaries often found in the brain stem, cerebellum, or diencephalon. These rarely hemorrhage (Mohr et al., 1986b; McCormick, 1966).

VARIX. A varix is a large, dilated vein or veins, usually found in the parenchyma or leptomeninges. Occasionally multiple veins are involved. These malformations have been associated with hemorrhage (McCormick, 1966).

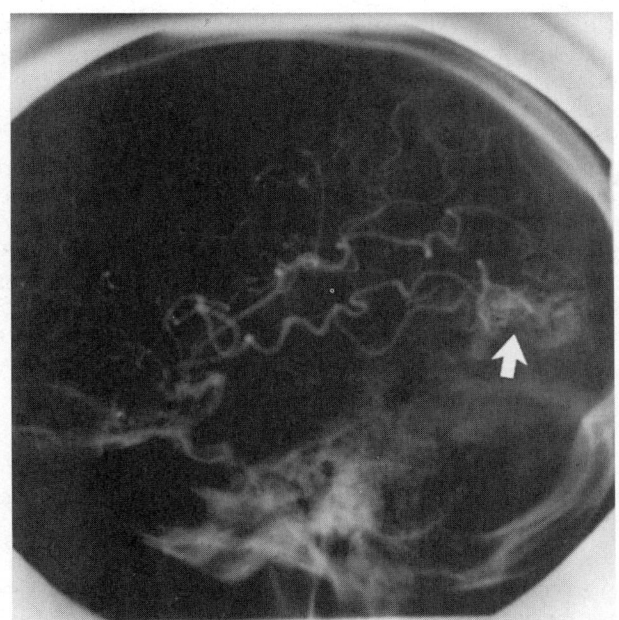

FIGURE 36–8. Cerebral arteriogram demonstrating left posterior temporal and occipital arteriovenous malformation (*arrow*) supplied by branches of the middle cerebral artery.

ARTERIOVENOUS MALFORMATION. AVM, the most common nonaneurysmal vascular anomaly, is composed of a tangle of abnormal arteries and veins larger than capillaries (Fig. 36–8). These are congenital or, less commonly, familial lesions. The normal capillary bed is absent, and blood flow, following the path of least resistance, creates an arteriovenous (A-V) fistula. Vessels supplying the lesion, feeding vessels, may be one or more of the major cerebral arteries and their branches. Venous drainage occurs through superficial and deep veins. Because of absent arteriolar and capillary resistance, blood flow increases and leads to increased venous pressure. Over time, as blood supply demand increases, arterial and venous dilation occurs. These veins transport oxygenated blood (i.e., little oxygen is extracted in the A-V fistula) called nonnutritive flow. In addition, blood shunted through the fistula may cause hypoperfusion of the surrounding brain, called cerebral steal. Cerebral vessels dilate in response to chronic hypoperfusion, and when maximal dilation is reached, autoregulation may be lost. As a result, chronic hypoperfusion can lead to ischemic changes in the surrounding brain and possible focal neurologic deficits (Mohr et al., 1986b).

CLINICAL MANIFESTATIONS

Arteriovenous malformations range in size from very small, cryptic lesions to lesions involving more than one lobe. AVMs enlarge with age and may not become symptomatic until the second or third decade of life. Early manifestations are usually hemorrhage or seizure (Fults & Kelly, 1984). Other findings include headache, progressive neurologic deficit, and, occasionally, bruits.

HEMORRHAGE. Approximately 50% of patients with AVM present with hemorrhage (Fults & Kelly, 1984). AVMs are most likely to cause ICH, but the hemorrhage can extend into the subarachnoid or intraventricular space. Although it is usually the smaller AVM that bleeds, larger lesions may also hemorrhage.

About 10% to 15% of AVMs show evidence of previous hemorrhage when they are operated on (Mohr et al., 1986b). These hemorrhages often were asymptomatic or produced only minor symptoms. Unlike aneurysms, AVMs tend not to rebleed within a short time. The rate of rebleeding after the initial hemorrhage is difficult to determine with certainty. Fults and Kelly (1984) reported rebleeding rates of 17.9% during the first year, 3% per year after 5 years, and 2% per year after 10 years. However, Graf and colleagues (1983) estimated rebleeding at 6% during the first year and 2% per year thereafter.

SEIZURES. Before small hemorrhages, chronic ischemia due to cerebral steal, cerebral cortex hemorrhage, and scarring all contribute to seizures (Berger et al., 1988). Seizures are often focal and correspond to the site of hematoma, but may secondarily generalize or may be primarily generalized. Patients who present with a seizure unassociated with hemorrhage have a more favorable prognosis than those presenting with seizures with hemorrhage (Fults & Kelly, 1984).

HEADACHE. Although headaches are very common in the general population, recurrent headaches may be a premonitory sign of AVM. Sentinel headaches may resemble atypical migraine. Headaches at the onset of ICH are often associated with vomiting (Gorelick et al., 1986).

PROGRESSIVE NEUROLOGIC DEFICIT. The size and location of the hemorrhage determine the extent of the neurologic deficit. Ischemia or direct compression of adjacent brain may result in focal neurologic deficits in the absence of any episode of bleeding.

BRUIT. Depending on the size and location of the AVM, a bruit may be heard over the eyes or skull. The patient may describe hearing a murmur within his or her head.

ANTICOAGULANT THERAPY

Bleeding associated with anticoagulation occurs infrequently, but people who take oral anticoagulants, often to prevent stroke, have a 10-fold risk of ICH (Wintzen et al., 1984). Hemorrhages may occur without systemic bleeding, tend to be larger than those due to hypertension, and are associated with a higher mortality rate (62%) (Kase et al., 1985). Onset of focal neurologic deficit is often insidious, developing over hours to days. Increased risk of ICH is associated with excessively prolonged PT (>1.5 times normal). Other risk factors include hypertension, age, and duration of therapy (Kase et al., 1985).

CEREBRAL AMYLOID ANGIOPATHY

Cerebral amyloid angiopathy is associated with amyloid deposits in the walls of small vessels in the cerebral cortex but not with systemic amyloidosis. Amyloid plaques may be found in patients with Alzheimer disease, senile dementia of the Alzheimer type, and Down syndrome (Vinters, 1987). Cerebral amyloid angiopathy usually presents in normotensive people older than 65 years of age with multiple or recurrent intracerebral hemorrhages, possibly due to vessel wall weakening. Most commonly, lobar hemorrhages occur, occasionally extending into the subarachnoid space. Hemorrhage in the basal ganglia, brain stem, or cerebellum is rare (Gilles et al., 1984; Vinters, 1987).

INTRACRANIAL TUMORS

An uncommon cause of ICH is bleeding into an intracranial tumor. Malignant tumors such as glioblastoma multiforme and metastatic lesions are most likely to hemorrhage because of their rich vasculature and neoplastic characteristics. In addition, some tumors invade and disrupt the vessel walls (Kase & Mohr, 1986).

DRUG ABUSE

Cocaine, amphetamine, pseudoephedrine, and ephedrine abuse have been temporally associated with ICH and SAH (Delaney & Estes, 1980; Loizou et al., 1982; Wojak & Flamm, 1987; Wooten et al., 1983). Bleeding from aneurysms and vascular malformations has been documented shortly after use of cocaine. Cocaine use has been shown to result in transient blood pressure increases that may precipitate the hemorrhage (Wojak & Flamm, 1987; Levine & Welch, 1988). Phenylpropanolamine, even used within dosage guidelines, has been associated with ICH (Fallis & Fisher, 1985; Glick et al., 1987; Kase et al., 1987). Even though ICH after drug abuse is uncommon, it is prudent to obtain a drug history, including use of illicit and over-the-counter medications, especially from young and otherwise healthy patients who present with ICH.

Epidemiology

A population study in Rochester, Minnesota, done between 1945 and 1974, showed decreasing rates of ICH, but not as striking as the decrease in ischemic stroke. No clear trend for SAH was identified (Garraway et al., 1979). The average age at onset for ICH increased from 65 to 71 years (Furlan et al., 1979), perhaps reflecting better control of hypertension, a major risk factor for ICH.

Prevalence of ruptured aneurysm increases with age, peaking in the fifth to sixth decades, after which the frequency declines. Aneurysms rarely are found in children (Weir, 1987a). Intracranial aneurysms are slightly more common in women after the sixth decade, possibly reflecting the longer life span of women (Weir, 1987a). Aneurysms are found in all races, but there are some geographic variations that are difficult to interpret because they may represent varied levels of health care rather than prevalence (Weir, 1987a).

The rate of primary ICH increases with age. Men have a higher rate of spontaneous ICH in all age groups (Furlan et al., 1979). The increased incidence among blacks may reflect a higher incidence of hypertension in this population (Brott et al., 1986; Gross et al., 1984).

Risk Factors

A variety of factors have been associated with hemorrhagic cerebrovascular disease. The most common are described in the following.

HYPERTENSION. As in ischemic cerebrovascular disease, hypertension is considered a major risk factor for both ICH and SAH (Brott et al., 1986; Longstreth et al., 1985; Stemmerman et al., 1984). Conditions transiently elevating blood pressure produce an additive effect, such as cigarette smoking, alcohol consumption, and use of stimulants.

ORAL CONTRACEPTIVES. Current or past use of oral contraceptives increases a woman's risk of SAH, especially if the current oral contraceptive user is older than 35 years of age and smokes cigarettes (Donaldson, 1986; Longstreth et al., 1985; Petitti et al., 1979). This increased risk associated with oral contraceptives may result from hormones that act directly on the arterial wall, weakening it and promoting formation or rupture of cerebral aneurysms (Petitti et al., 1979).

PREGNANCY. Pregnancy increases the risk of both ischemic and hemorrhagic stroke. Although ischemic strokes related to pregnancy are rarely fatal, 5% to 10% of all maternal deaths result from ruptured aneurysms or AVMs (Donaldson, 1986). Aneurysms are most likely to bleed in the third trimester, whereas AVMs are more likely to bleed in the second trimester or during labor. Rebleeding from an aneurysm may occur during childbirth or in the postpartum period. AVMs rarely rebleed postpartum (Donaldson, 1986). Development of pregnancy-related hypertension is another complicating factor.

CIGARETTE SMOKING. Cigarette smoking is a risk factor for hemorrhagic stroke (Petitti et al., 1979). Women who smoke more than a pack a day have twice the risk of hemorrhagic stroke as nonsmokers (Collaborative Group for the Study of Stroke in Young Women, 1975). Increased risk has also been identified for men (Abbott et al., 1986). The risk of hemorrhagic stroke is significantly reduced with cessation of smoking.

Diagnosis

The history, neurologic examination, and baseline laboratory work are similar to those described for ischemic cerebrovascular disease. Clinical presentation is often very suggestive of ICH. Due to the high morbidity and mortality associated with ICH, rapid and accurate diagnosis is important to allow appropriate medical and nursing management. CT scans, MRI, cerebral angiography, transcranial Doppler examination, and LP are used for diagnosis.

COMPUTED TOMOGRAPHY. Noncontrast CT scans done on suspicion of hemorrhage are excellent in detecting and determining the extent of acute bleeds (Mohr et al., 1986a). Although a very small-volume SAH may be missed, most will be detected. CT scans may also identify hydrocephalus, if present. Contrast CT scans may locate and determine the size of an aneurysm or AVM, but this is not a definitive procedure for this condition; it must be confirmed with angiography.

MAGNETIC RESONANCE IMAGING. The appearance of blood on MRI and CT scans changes with time. In the first 24 hours after an SAH, MRI detects an abnormal signal but cannot specify that it is blood, making the CT scan the preferred method during the first 24 hours (Brant-Zawadzki, 1988). The MRI is preferred in the subacute phase because hemorrhage may appear isodense on CT scan. Intracerebral hemorrhage and its relationship to the surrounding brain are readily visualized on MRI. MRI is more effective in identifying small ("cryptic") vascular lesions. MRI angiography may become the best noninvasive method of detection of intracranial AVMs and aneurysms in the future (Ross, 1988).

CEREBRAL ANGIOGRAPHY. Depiction of the vascular anatomy and location of AVMs, aneurysms, and the degree of vasospasm is possible with cerebral angiography. Thrombosed vessels, vessels obliterated by hemorrhage, or very small malformations may not be visualized. Angiography is definitive for AVMs and aneurysms and is required before surgery.

TRANSCRANIAL DOPPLER. Transcranial Doppler is a noninvasive ultrasound procedure used to diagnose and monitor vasospasm in the middle and anterior cerebral arteries. Vasospasm in other cerebral arteries is difficult to detect with this method (DeWitt & Wechsler, 1988). Transcranial Doppler can detect increased blood velocity secondary to a narrowed vessel lumen that may precede symptomatic vasospasm by hours to days (DeWitt & Wechsler, 1988).

LUMBAR PUNCTURE. LP should be done to aid diagnosis if the CT scan is negative for SAH, intraventricular hemorrhage, mass, or obstructive hydrocephalus. The CSF in SAH either contains frank blood that does not clear as the fluid is collected or fluid that is xanthochromic (deep yellow) due to the presence of blood breakdown products. Further examination of the CSF will reveal increased opening pressure, elevated protein, normal glucose, and a pleocytosis (Caplan & Stein, 1986).

Medical Management of the Patient With Acute Intracranial Hemorrhage

Treatment of acute intracerebral hemorrhage is aimed at preventing further hemorrhage, maintaining adequate cerebral perfusion pressure, and preventing neurologic sequelae. These goals are usually accomplished using combined medical and surgical interventions.

MEDICAL TREATMENT

Many of the signs and symptoms of ICH are due to increased intracranial pressure.

To reduce the risk of rebleeding, patients are placed in a quiet, dimly lit room on complete bed rest. If tolerated, the head of the bed is elevated 30 degrees to aid venous drainage. Stool softeners are given to reduce straining during bowel movements. Mild, short-acting sedatives may be used with caution to aid restlessness and anxiety. Sedatives may mask subtle changes in the level of consciousness, thus interfering with accurate neurologic assessment. Platelet antiaggregants, such as ASA, are contraindicated. Anticonvulsants may be prescribed if the patient has had a seizure or as prophylaxis. Corticosteroids have not been shown to be useful in reducing cerebral edema associated with hemorrhage (Mohr et al., 1986a; Poungvarin et al., 1987).

As in ischemic stroke, it is essential to obtain careful control of hypertension. Palliative measures for pain and anxiety may reduce blood pressure. If needed, short-acting antihypertensive medications may be used. It is essential to monitor the neurologic status and blood pressure closely. Mild hypotension may result in clinical deterioration.

Medical treatment of these patients is geared toward preventing rebleeding or treating symptomatic cerebral vasospasm. Several treatment modalities are discussed in more detail.

ANTIFIBRINOLYTICS. The antifibrinolytic agents, aminocaproic acid (Amicar; Lederle Laboratories, Pearl River, NY) or tranexamic acid, may be used to try to prevent rebleeding from a ruptured intracranial aneurysm. These drugs prevent the lysis of thrombus within and on the surface of an aneurysm. This thrombus may support the wall of the aneurysm, reducing the potential for rebleeding (Adams, 1987). The suggested dosage of aminocaproic acid is 5 g given in an IV bolus followed by a continuous infusion of 24 to 36 g/day for 10 to 14 days, unless surgery is attempted. Antifibrinolytic agents considerably reduce the 14-day rebleeding rate but do not significantly alter the overall mortality rate (Kassell et al., 1984) because these agents are associated with a greater incidence of hydrocephalus and ischemic complications (Kassell et al., 1984). Therefore, use of these drugs in patients with SAH is controversial (Adams, 1987; Weir, 1987b).

CALCIUM CHANNEL BLOCKERS. The mechanism for vasospasm is thought to be related to the presence of blood and blood products within the CSF, which stimulate arterial narrowing. Calcium channel blockers, which inhibit vascular smooth muscle contraction by blocking the influx of extracellular calcium, are thought to prevent or reverse vasospasm (Greenberg, 1987). Two agents currently under investigation for this use are nimodipine and nicardipine. Both of these agents have been associated with reduced severity of cerebral vasospasm and improved patient outcomes (Aver, 1984; Flamm et al., 1988; Petruk et al., 1988). Hypotension, a serious potential complication of calcium channel blockers, usually responds to increased intravascular fluid and rarely necessitates discontinuation of the drug (Flamm et al., 1988; Petruk et al., 1988).

INTRAVASCULAR VOLUME EXPANSION. The most common treatment for symptomatic cerebral vasospasm is to increase cerebral perfusion pressure through plasma volume expansion. Vasopressors may be used to increase mean arterial pressure after surgery on an aneurysm. Because autoregulation is lost during vasospasm, an increase in systemic arterial pressure increases CBF. To be effective, this therapy must restore adequate CBF before infarction occurs.

Intravascular volume expansion is accomplished by administering fluid to create a positive fluid balance. The central venous pressure is maintained at 10 to 12 mm Hg, and the pulmonary artery wedge pressure is kept at 15 to 20 mm Hg (Awad et al., 1987; Kassell et al., 1982). Kassell and associates (1982) used albumin or plasma fractionate along with packed cells or whole blood to maintain a hematocrit of 40%. Others advocate hypervolemic hemodilution, reducing the hematocrit to 33% to 38% (Awad et al., 1987). Crystalloid solutions are used to maintain normal serum electrolytes.

Blood pressure is kept at the minimum level necessary to maintain neurologic function. For patients awaiting surgery, the maximum systolic pressure is 160 mm Hg. When the aneurysm has been obliterated, the maximum systolic pressure is 240 mm Hg (Kassell et al., 1982). When necessary, a vasopressor (such as dopamine) may be administered to maintain optimum blood pressure.

Risks associated with intravascular volume expansion include aneurysmal rebleeding, pulmonary edema, myocardial infarction, dilutional hyponatremia, hemothorax, and coagulopathy (Kassell et al., 1982). Intensive monitoring of central venous pressure, pulmonary artery wedge pressure, cardiac function, arterial blood gases, and serum and urinary electrolytes is mandatory.

SURGICAL TREATMENT

Operative treatment of saccular aneurysms involves placing a metal clip across the base of the lesion where it rises from the parent vessel. Definitive treatment of AVM is complete excision, when possible. Optimal timing for surgery (early versus delayed) is controversial. Prognosis and treatment decisions are often based on the size and location of the lesion as well as the clinical status of the patient on admission.

Surgery during the first 48 hours (early) eliminates the risk of aneurysmal rebleeding and may reduce vasospasm by removing the subarachnoid clot. Surgery performed 10 to 14 days after the initial hemorrhage allows resolution of cerebral edema and reduces postoperative vasospasm (Mohr et al., 1986b). The Hunt and Hess (1968) classification of intracranial aneurysms is frequently used to aid these decisions (Table 36–5). The current trend is to operate on grade I and II lesions as soon as diagnostic studies are complete.

The decision to intervene surgically to remove an AVM that has hemorrhaged is based on similar criteria. An unruptured AVM that presents with a seizure or headache may be managed appropriately without surgery. Because of their size or location, some AVMs are not amenable to surgical intervention. Embolization, Bragg-Peak proton beam therapy, or stereotactic radiosurgery may be used in these situations.

EMBOLIZATION. Embolization obliterates inoperable vascular malformations, including some aneurysms. This procedure may precede surgical intervention in an attempt to reduce the size of the lesion. Superselective catheterization and angiography are used to deliver the embolizing material (e.g., particles [radiopaque Silastic spheres], detachable balloons, or liquid adhesive). Best results have been obtained with balloons or adhesive. Transient or permanent neurologic deficits may follow embolization. Some complications are specific to the technique, such as gluing the balloon in place, rupture of the balloon in a small feeder artery, or occlusion of normal arteries (Vinuela & Fox, 1986).

TABLE 36–5. **Classification of Patients With Intracranial Aneurysms According to Surgical Risk**

Category*	Criteria
Grade I	Asymptomatic, or minimal headache and slight nuchal rigidity
Grade II	Moderate to severe headache, nuchal rigidity, no neurologic deficit other than cranial nerve palsy
Grade III	Drowsiness, confusion, or mild focal deficit
Grade IV	Stupor, moderate to severe hemiparesis, possibly early decerebrate rigidity and vegetative disturbances
Grade V	Deep coma, decerebrate rigidity, moribund appearance

*From Hunt, W. E., & Hess, R. M. (1968). Surgical risk as related to time of intervention in the repair of intracranial aneurysms. *Journal of Neurosurgery, 28,* 14.

BRAGG-PEAK PROTON BEAM THERAPY. In this procedure, stereotactic neurosurgery is used to guide proton beam radiation to the AVM. Within 1 to 2 years of treatment, the walls of small vessels thicken and reduce the lumen, causing associated arteries and veins to return gradually to near-normal size. Although this is a low-risk procedure, it is not widely available because of the elaborate equipment needed (Kjellberg et al., 1983).

STEREOTACTIC RADIOSURGERY. In this procedure, gamma radiation is focused stereotactically on an intracranial target. Although individual beams deliver very small doses of gamma radiation, the intersecting focus of all beams receives a large dose of energy that is capable of obliterating a vascular malformation. This procedure is most effective for smaller AVMs of which the entire nidus can be irradiated. The mechanism of occlusion is uncertain, but proliferation of endothelial lining and thrombosis are thought to contribute (Steiner, 1986).

The major drawback to radiosurgery is the length of time that elapses before results are seen. Hemodynamic changes, such as decreased flow rate, may be noted within 3 months, but complete obliteration may take from 6 to 22 months (Steiner, 1986). Angiographic evidence of obliteration has been identified in 85% of the patients who have undergone radiosurgery. Potential complications include delayed radiation necrosis or rebleeding, but the risk of rebleeding is the same as that noted in the natural history of an AVM (Steiner, 1986).

NURSING CARE OF THE PATIENT WITH AN ACUTE CEREBROVASCULAR EVENT

Optimal care of the patient with a stroke is provided through an interdisciplinary approach that includes the primary nurse, physician, social worker, dietitian, and physical, occupational, and speech therapists. Nursing care of the patient with a stroke should focus on stabilization in the acute phase, prevention of complications, psychological needs, rehabilitation, and discharge planning (Hickey, 1986). The quality of the care given during the earlier stages has a significant impact on the overall outcome and rehabilitation potential. Monitoring the neurologic, hemodynamic, and respiratory status throughout the patient's care is essential. Specific nursing care is guided by the patient's actual neurologic deficit. Monitoring activities, selective nursing diagnoses, and interventions are outlined in the following.

Monitoring Activities

NEUROLOGIC STATUS. The patient's neurologic condition can change rapidly and subtly. Hourly assessments of the level of consciousness, mental status, cranial nerves, and general motor and sensory function should be carefully documented until the patient is stable. Decreased level of consciousness is often the first indicator of progression of the stroke. Any deterioration must be promptly reported to the physician.

HEMODYNAMIC STATUS. Cardiovascular monitoring for arrhythmias (particularly atrial fibrillation), congestive heart failure, and variations in blood pressure is important. Blood pressure should be assessed before and after administration of antihypertensive agents. If there is a significant change from previous blood pressure readings or in the patient's condition, the nurse should notify the physician before giving the medication. A precipitous drop or rise in blood pressure may be associated with clinical decline. Fluid balance (intake and output), serum and urinary electrolytes, and osmolality should be closely monitored.

PULMONARY STATUS. Recovery may be impeded by respiratory problems, such as pneumonia, aspiration, or pulmonary embolism. To prevent or promptly treat these conditions, the respiratory status should be frequently monitored. Auscultation of breath sounds, observation of respiratory rate and pattern, and monitoring reports of arterial blood gases and chest x-rays should be included in the nurse's assessment.

Vigorous coughing, suctioning, and chest physiotherapy must be avoided in patients with intracranial hemorrhage or signs of increased intracranial pressure. Repositioning of the patient every 1 to 2 hours will also facilitate mobilization of secretions.

Patients with dysphagia should be carefully assessed before beginning oral feedings. It is important to note that the gag reflex is *not* a reliable indicator of the patient's swallowing ability (Horner et al., 1988). Nurses must assess palatal function and the swallowing reflex. A small amount of water or soft food is given and the swallowing process observed. Speech therapists can be consulted for a formal swallowing evaluation. Dysphonia is present more often in patients who aspirate (Horner et al., 1988), and should prompt the nurse to assess carefully the patient's ability to swallow.

REFERENCES

Abbott, R. D., Yin, Y., Reed, D. M., et al. (1986). Risk of stroke in male cigarette smokers. *New England Journal of Medicine, 315,* 717–720.

Adams, H. P. (1987). Antifibrinolytics in aneurysmal subarachnoid hemorrhage: Do they have a role? Maybe. *Archives of Neurology, 44,* 114–115.

American Heart Association. (1992). *Facts about stroke.* Dallas: Author.

American–Canadian Co-Operative Study Group. (1985). Persantine aspirin trial in cerebral ischemia. Part II: Endpoint results. *Stroke, 16,* 406–415.

Aver, L. M. (1984). Acute operation and preventive nimodipine improve outcome in patients with ruptured cerebral aneurysms. *Neurosurgery, 15,* 57–66.

Awad, I. A., Carter, P., Spetzler, R. F., et al. (1987). Clinical vasospasm after subarachnoid hemorrhage: Response to hypervolemic hemodilution and arterial hypertension. *Stroke, 18,* 365–372.

Baker, A. B., & Ionnone, A. (1961). Cerebrovascular disease: VII. A study of etiologic mechanisms. *Neurology, 11,* 23–31.

Barnett, H. J. M. (1979). The pathophysiology of transient cerebral ischemic attacks therapy with platelet antiaggregants. *Medical Clinics of North America, 63,* 649–679.

Barnett, H. J. M., Jones, M. W., Boughner, D. R., et al. (1976). Cerebral ischemic events associated with prolapsing mitral valve. *Archives of Neurology, 33,* 777–782.

Beck, D. W., Adams, H. P., Flamm, E. S., et al. (1988). Combination of aminocaproic acid and nicardipine in treatment of aneurysmal subarachnoid hemorrhage. *Stroke, 19,* 63–67.

Berger, A. R., Lipton, R. B., Lesser, M. L., et al. (1988). Early seizures following intracerebral hemorrhage: Implications for therapy. *Neurology, 38,* 1363–1365.

Biller, J., Loftus, C. M., Moore, S. A., et al. (1987). Isolated central nervous system angiitis first presenting as spontaneous intracranial hemorrhage. *Neurosurgery, 20,* 310–315.

Bogousslavsky, J., Regli, F., Van Melle, G., et al. (1988). Migraine stroke. *Neurology, 38,* 223–227.

Bounds, J. V., Wiebers, D. O., Whisnant, J. P., et al. (1981). Mechanisms and timing of deaths from cerebral infarction. *Stroke, 12,* 474–477.

Bousser, M., Chiras, J., Bories, J., et al. (1985). Cerebral venous thrombosis—a review of 38 cases. *Stroke, 16,* 199–213.

Bousser, M. G., Eschwege, E., Haguenau, M., et al. (1983). "AICLA" controlled trial of aspirin and dipyridamole in the secondary prevention of athero-thrombotic cerebral ischemia. *Stroke, 14,* 5–14.

Brant-Zawadzki, N. (1988). MR imaging of the brain. *Radiology, 166,* 1–10.

Britton, M., & Roden, A. (1985). Progression of stroke after arrival at hospital. *Stroke, 16,* 629–632.

Broderick, J. P., & Swanson, J. W. (1987). Migraine-related strokes. *Archives of Neurology, 44,* 868–871.

Brott, T. G., Gelfand, M. J., Williams, C. C., et al. (1986). Frequency and patterns of abnormality detected by iodine-123 amine emission CT after cerebral infarction. *Radiology, 158,* 729–734.

Brott, T., Thalinger, K., & Hertzberg, V. (1986). Hypertension as a risk factor for spontaneous intracerebral hemorrhage. *Stroke, 17,* 1078–1083.

Brust, J. C., Plank, C. R., Healton, E. B., et al. (1979). The pathology of drop attacks: A case report. *Neurology, 29,* 786–790.

Canadian Cooperative Study Group. (1978). A randomized trial of aspirin and sulfinpyrazone in threatened stroke. *New England Journal of Medicine, 299,* 53–59.

Caplan, L., Corbett, J., Goodwin, J., et al. (1983a). Neuro-ophthalmologic signs in the angiitic form of neurosarcoidosis. *Neurology, 33,* 1130–1135.

Caplan, L. R., Hier, D. B., & Banks, G. (1982). Current concepts of cerebrovascular disease–stroke: Stroke and drug abuse. *Stroke, 13,* 869–872.

Caplan, L. R., Hier, D. B., & D'Cruz, I. (1983b). Cerebral embolism in the Michael Reese Stroke Registry. *Stroke, 14,* 530–536.

Caplan, L. R., & Stein, R. W. (1986). *Stroke: A clinical approach.* Boston: Butterworths.

Cerebral Embolism Study Group. (1984). Immediate anticoagulation of embolic stroke: Brain hemorrhage and management options. *Stroke, 15,* 779–789.

Cocito, L., Favale, E., & Reni, L. (1982). Epileptic seizures in cerebral arterial occlusive disease. *Stroke, 13,* 189–195.

Collaborative Group for the Study of Stroke in Young Women. (1975). Oral contraceptive and stroke in young women: Associated risk factors. *Journal of the American Medical Association, 231,* 718–722.

Delaney, P., & Estes, M. (1980). Intracranial hemorrhage with amphetamine abuse. *Neurology, 30,* 1125–1128.

Del Zoppo, G. J., Zeumer, H., & Harker, L. A. (1986). Thrombolytic therapy in stroke: Possibilities and hazards. *Stroke, 17,* 595–607.

DeWitt, L. D., & Wechsler, L. R. (1988). Transcranial Doppler. *Stroke, 19,* 915–921.

Donaldson, J. O. (1986). Cerebrovascular disease: Pregnancy, puerperium, and the Pill. *Neurology and Neurosurgery Update Series, 6,* 2–8.

EC/IC Bypass Study Group. (1985). Failure of extracranial–intracranial arterial bypass to reduce the risk of ischemic stroke. *New England Journal of Medicine, 313,* 1191–1200.

Edmunds, L. H. (1982). Thromboembolic complications of current cardiac valvular prostheses. *Annals of Thoracic Surgery, 34,* 96–106.

Fallis, R. J., & Fisher, M. (1985). Cerebral vasculitis and hemorrhage associated with phenylpropanolamine. *Neurology, 35,* 405–407.

Featherstone, H. J. (1986). Clinical features of stroke in migraine: A review. *Headache, 26,* 128–133.

Ferguson, G. G. (1972). Physical factors in the initiation, growth, and rupture of human intracranial saccular aneurysms. *Journal of Neurosurgery, 37,* 666–677.

Fisher, C. M. (1982). Pure sensory stroke and allied conditions. *Stroke, 13,* 434–447.

Fisher, C. M., & Curry, H. B. (1965). Pure motor hemiplegia of vascular origin. *Archives of Neurology, 13,* 30–44.

Flamm, E. S., Adams, H. P., Beck, D. W., et al. (1988). Dose-escalation study of intravenous nicardipine in patients with aneurysmal subarachnoid hemorrhage. *Journal of Neurosurgery, 68,* 393–400.

Fults, D., & Kelly, D. L. (1984). Natural history of arteriovenous malformations of the brain: A clinical study. *Neurosurgery, 15,* 658–662.

Furlan, A. J. (1985). Cardiac disease and stroke. In F. McDowell & L. R. Caplan (Eds.), *Cerebrovascular survey report for the National Institute of Neurological and Communicative Disorders and Stroke* (pp. 97–107). Bethesda: National Institute of Health.

Furlan, A. J., Whisnant, J. P., & Elveback, L. R. (1979). The decreasing incidence of primary intracerebral hemorrhage: A population study. *Annals of Neurology, 5,* 367–373.

Garcia, J. H., & Geer, J. C. (1985). Carotid artery atherosclerotic disease pathology and detection. In F. McDowell & L. R. Caplan (Eds.), *Cerebrovascular survey report for the National Institute of Neurological and Communicative Disorders and Stroke* (pp. 35–45). Bethesda: National Institutes of Health.

Garraway, W. M., Whisnant, J. M., Furlan, A. J., et al. (1979). The declining incidence of stroke. *New England Journal of Medicine, 300,* 449–452.

Gelmers, H. J., Gorter, K., de Weerdt, C. J., et al. (1988). A controlled trial of nimodipine in acute ischemic stroke. *New England Journal of Medicine, 318,* 203–207.

Gent, M., Blakely, J. A., Easton, J. D., et al. (1988). The Canadian–American ticlopidine study (CATS) in thromboembolic stroke. Design, organization, and baseline results. *Stroke, 19,* 1203–1210.

Gifford, A. J. (1966). An epidemiological study of cerebrovascular disease. *American Journal of Public Health, 56,* 452–461.

Gilles, C., Brucher, J. M., Khoubesserian, P., et al. (1984). Cerebral amyloid angiopathy as a cause of multiple intracerebral hemorrhages. *Neurology, 34,* 730–735.

Gillum, R. F. (1988). Stroke in blacks. *Stroke, 19,* 1–9.

Glick, R., Hoying, J., Cerullo, L., et al. (1987). Phenylpropanolamine: An over-the-counter drug causing central nervous system vasculitis and intracerebral hemorrhage. *Neurosurgery, 20,* 969–974.

Gorelick, P. B., Hier, D. B., Caplan, L. R., et al. (1986). Headache in acute cerebrovascular disease. *Neurology, 36,* 1445–1450.

Graf, C. J., Perret, G. E., & Torner, J. C. (1983). Bleeding from cerebral arteriovenous malformations as part of their natural history. *Journal of Neurosurgery, 58,* 331–337.

Greenberg, D. A. (1987). Calcium channels and calcium channel antagonists. *Annals of Neurology, 21,* 317–330.

Greenlee, J. E., & Mandell, G. L. (1973). Neurological manifestations of infective endocarditis: A review. *Stroke, 4,* 958–963.

Gross, C. R., Kase, C. S., Mohr, J. P., et al. (1984). Stroke in south Alabama: Incidence and diagnostic features—a population based study. *Stroke, 15,* 249–255.

Grotta, J. C. (1987). Current status of hemodilution in acute cerebral ischemia (editorial). *Stroke, 18,* 689–690.

Grotta, J., Ackerman, R., Correia, J., et al. (1982). Whole blood parameters and cerebral blood flow. *Stroke, 13,* 296–301.

Grotta, J. C., Lemak, N. A., Gary, H., et al. (1985). Does platelet antiaggregant therapy lessen the severity of stroke? *Neurology, 35,* 632–636.

Hart, R. G., Byer, H. A., Slaughter, J. R., et al. (1981). Occurrence and implications of seizures in subarachnoid hemorrhage due to ruptured intracranial aneurysms. *Neurosurgery, 8,* 417–421.

Hart, R. G., Coull, B. M., & Hart, D. (1983). Early recurrent embolism associated with nonvalvular atrial fibrillation: A retrospective study. *Stroke, 14,* 688–693.

Hass, W. K., Easton, J. D., Adams, H. P., et al., for the Ticlopidine Aspirin Stroke Study Group. (1989). A randomized trial comparing ticlopidine hydrochloride with aspirin for the prevention of stroke in high-risk patients. *New England Journal of Medicine, 321,* 501–507.

Helgason, C. M. (1988). Blood glucose and stroke. *Stroke, 19,* 937–941.

Heyden, S., Heyman, A., & Camplong, L. (1969). Mortality patterns among parents of patients with atherosclerotic cerebrovascular disease. *Journal of Chronic Disease, 22,* 105–110.

Hickey, J. V. (1986). *The clinical practice of neurological and neurosurgical nursing* (2nd ed.). Philadelphia: J. B. Lippincott.

Horner, J., Massey, E. W., Riski, J. E., et al. (1988). Aspiration following stroke: Clinical correlates and outcome. *Neurology, 38,* 1359–1362.

Hunt, W. E., & Hess, R. M. (1968). Surgical risk as related to time of intervention in the repair of intracranial aneurysms. *Journal of Neurosurgery, 28,* 14–20.

Jackson, A. C., Boughner, B. R., & Barnett, H. J. M. (1984). Mitral valve prolapse and cerebral ischemic events in young patients. *Neurology, 34,* 784–787.

Jensen, T. S., & de-Fine-Olivarius, B. (1981). Transient global amnesia—its clinical and pathophysiological basis and prognosis. *Acta Neurologica Scandinavica, 63,* 220–230.

Kannel, W. B., Gordon, T., & Dawber, T. R. (1974). Role of lipids in the development of brain infarction: The Framingham study. *Stroke, 5,* 679–685.

Kannel, W. B., Sorlie, P., & Gordon, T. (1980). Labile hypertension: A faulty concept? The Framingham study. *Circulation, 61,* 1183–1187.

Kannel, W. B., Wolf, P. A., McGee, D. L., et al. (1981). Systolic blood pressure, arterial rigidity, and risk of stroke: The Framingham study. *Journal of the American Medical Association, 245,* 1225–1229.

Kannel, W. B., Wolf, P. A., & Verter, J. (1983). Manifestations of coronary disease predisposing to stroke: The Framingham study. *Journal of the American Medical Association, 250,* 2942–2946.

Kannel, W. B., Wolf, P. A., Verter, J., et al. (1970). Epidemiologic assessment of the role of blood pressure in stroke: The Framingham study. *Journal of the American Medical Association, 214,* 301–310.

Kase, C. S., Foster, T. E., Reed, J. E., et al. (1987). Intracerebral hemorrhage and phenylpropanolamine use. *Neurology, 37,* 399–404.

Kase, C. S., & Mohr, J. P. (1986). General features of intracerebral hemorrhage. In H. J. M. Barnett, J. P. Hohr, B. M. Stein, et al. (Eds.), *Stroke: pathophysiology, diagnosis, and management* (Vol. 1, pp. 497–523). New York: Churchill-Livingstone.

Kase, C. S., Robinson, K., Stein, R. W., et al. (1985). Anticoagulant-related intracerebral hemorrhage. *Neurology, 35,* 943–948.

Kassell, N. F., Peerless, S. J., Durward, O. J., et al. (1982). Treatment of ischemic deficits from vasospasm with intravascular volume expansion and induced arterial hypertension. *Neurosurgery, 11,* 337–343.

Kassell, N. F., & Torner, J. C. (1983). Aneurysmal rebleeding: A preliminary report from the Cooperative Aneurysm Study. *Neurosurgery, 13,* 479–481.

Kassell, N. F., Torner, J. C., & Adams, H. P. (1984). Antifibrinolytic therapy in the acute period following aneurysmal subarachnoid hemorrhage: Preliminary observations from the Cooperative Aneurysm Study. *Journal of Neurosurgery, 61,* 225–230.

Kendall, R. E., & Marshall, J. (1963). Role of hypotension in the genesis of transient focal cerebral ischemic attacks. *British Medical Journal, 2,* 344–348.

Kistler, J. P., Crowell, R. M., Davis, K. R., et al. (1983). The relation of cerebral vasospasm to the extent and location of subarachnoid blood visualized by CT scan: A prospective study. *Neurology, 33,* 424–436.

Kjellberg, R. N., Hanamura, T., Davis, K. R., et al. (1983). Bragg-Peak proton-beam therapy for arteriovenous malformations of the brain. *New England Journal of Medicine, 309,* 269–274.

Komrad, M. S., Coffey, C. E., Coffey, K. S., et al. (1984). Myocardial infarction and stroke. *Neurology, 34,* 1403–1409.

Kubala, M. J., & Millikan, C. H. (1964). Diagnosis, pathogenesis, and treatment of "drop attacks." *Archives of Neurology, 11,* 107–113.

Lassen, N. A., Ingvar, D. H., & Skinhoj, E. (1978). Brain function and blood flow. *Scientific American, 239,* 62–71.

Lavin, P. (1986). Management of hypertension in patients with acute stroke. *Archives of Internal Medicine, 146,* 66–68.

Lesser, R. P., Luders, H., Dinner, D. S., et al. (1985). Epileptic seizures due to thrombotic and embolic cerebrovascular disease in older patients. *Epilepsia, 26,* 622–630.

Levine, S. R., & Welch, K. M. A. (1987). Cerebrovascular ischemia associated with lupus anticoagulant. *Stroke, 18,* 257–263.

Levine, S. R., & Welch, K. M. A. (1988). Cocaine and stroke. *Stroke, 19,* 779–783.

Lhermitte, F., Gautier, J., & Derouesné, C. (1970). Nature of occlusions of the middle cerebral artery. *Neurology, 20,* 82–88.

Loizou, L. A., Hamilton, J. G., & Tsementzis, S. A. (1982). Intracranial hemorrhage in association with pseudoephedrine overdose (letter to the editor). *Journal of Neurology, Neurosurgery, and Psychiatry, 45,* 471–475.

Longstreth, W. T., Koepsell, T. D., Yerby, M. S., et al. (1985). Risk factors for subarachnoid hemorrhage. *Stroke, 16,* 377–385.

Marshall, J., and Meadows, S. (1968). The natural history of amaurosis fugax. *Brain, 91,* 419–434.

Masaryk, T. J., Modic, M. T., Ruggieri, P., et al. (1989). Three dimensional (volume) gradient echo imaging of the carotid bifurcation: Preliminary clinical experience. *Radiology, 171,* 801–806.

McCormick, W. F. (1966). The pathology of vascular ("arteriovenous") malformations. *Journal of Neurosurgery, 24,* 807–816.

Meissner, I., Whisnant, J. P., & Garraway, W. M. (1988). Hypertension management and stroke recurrence in a community (Rochester, Minnesota, 1950–1979). *Stroke, 19,* 459–463.

Miller, V. T., & Hart, R. G. (1988). Heparin anticoagulation in acute brain ischemia. *Stroke, 19,* 403–406.

Millikan, C. H., McDowell, F., & Easton, J. D. (1987). *Stroke.* Philadelphia: Lea & Febiger.

Mohr, J. P. (1982). Asymptomatic carotid artery disease (editorial). *Stroke, 13,* 431–433.

Mohr, J. P., Caplan, J. W., Melski, J. W., et al. (1978). The Harvard Cooperative Stroke Registry: A prospective registry. *Neurology, 28,* 754–762.

Mohr, J. P., Kistler, J. P., Zambramski, J. M., et al. (1986a). Intracranial aneurysms. In H. J. M. Barnett, J. P. Mohr, B. M. Stein, et al. (Eds.), *Stroke pathophysiology, diagnosis, and management* (Vol. 1, pp. 643–677). New York: Churchill-Livingstone.

Mohr, J. P., Tatemichi, T. K., Nichols, F. C., et al. (1986b). Vascular malformations of the brain: Clinical considerations. In H. J. M. Barnett, J. P. Mohr, B. M. Stein, et al. (Eds.), *Stroke pathophysiology, diagnosis, and management* (Vol. 1, pp. 679–705). New York: Churchill-Livingstone.

Moore, P. M. (1989). Diagnosis and management of isolated angiitis of the central nervous system. *Neurology, 39,* 167–173.

Moore, P. M., & Cupps, T. R. (1983). Neurological complications of vasculitis. *Annals of Neurology, 14,* 155–167.

Moosey, J. (1959). Development of cerebral atherosclerosis in various age groups. *Neurology, 9,* 569–574.

Okawara, S. (1973). Warning signs prior to rupture of an intracranial aneurysm. *Journal of Neurosurgery, 38,* 475–580.

Paulson, G. W., Boesel, C. P., & Evans, W. E. (1978). Fibromuscular dysplasia. *Archives of Neurology, 35,* 287–290.

Petitti, D. B., Wingerd, J., Pellegrin, F., et al. (1979). Risk of vascular disease in women smoking, oral contraceptives, noncontraceptive estrogens, and other factors. *Journal of the American Medical Association, 242,* 1150–1154.

Petruk, K. C., West, M., Mohr, G., et al. (1988). Nimodipine treatment in poor-grade aneurysm patients. *Journal of Neurosurgery, 68,* 505–517.

Poungvarin, N., Bhoopat, W., Viriyavejakul, A., et al. (1987). Effects of dexamethasone in primary supratentorial intracerebral hemorrhage. *New England Journal of Medicine, 316,* 1229–1233.

Powers, W. J., & Raichle, M. E. (1985). Positron emission tomography and its application to the study of cerebrovascular disease in man. *Stroke, 16,* 361–376.

Raichle, M. E. (1983). The pathophysiology of brain ischemia. *Annals of Neurology, 13,* 2–10.

Reagan, T. J., & Okazaki, H. (1974). The thrombotic syndrome associated with carcinoma. *Archives of Neurology, 31,* 390–395.

Robins, M., & Baum, H. M. (1981). Incidence. *Stroke, 12*(Suppl 1), I-45–I-55.

Ross, J. S. (1988). MR angiography furnishes detailed vascular images. *Diagnostic Imaging, 10,* 96–103.

Ruff, R. L., & Dougherty, J. H. (1981). Evaluation of acute cerebral ischemia for anticoagulant therapy: Computed tomography or lumbar puncture. *Neurology, 31,* 736–740.

Ruff, R. L., Talman, W. T., & Petito, F. (1981). Transient ischemic attacks associated with hypotension in hypertensive patients with carotid artery stenosis. *Stroke, 12,* 353–355.

Sacco, R. L., Wolf, P. A., Kannel, W. B., et al. (1982). Survival and recurrence following stroke: The Framingham study. *Stroke, 13,* 290–295.

Sage, J. I., & Van Uitert, R. L. (1983). Risk of recurrent stroke in patients with atrial fibrillation and non-valvular heart disease. *Stroke, 14,* 537–540.

Sandok, B. A., von Estorff, I., & Guiliani, E. R. (1980). CNS embolism due to atrial myxoma. *Archives of Neurology, 37,* 485–488.

Scandinavian Stroke Study Group. (1987). Multicenter trial of hemodilution in acute ischemic stroke: I. Results in the total patient population. *Stroke, 18,* 691–699.

Schuier, F. J., & Hossman, K. A. (1980). Experimental brain infarcts in cats: II. Ischemic brain edema. *Stroke, 11,* 593–601.

Senegor, M., Dohrmann, G. J., & Wollmann, R. L. (1983). Venous angiomas of the posterior fossa should be considered as anomalous venous drainage. *Surgical Neurology, 19,* 26–32.

Sheldon, J. J. (1981). Blood vessels of the scalp and brain. *Clinical Symposia, 33,* 3–36.

Sherry, S. (1985). Tissue plasminogen activator (t-PA): Will it fulfill its promise? *New England Journal of Medicine, 313,* 1014–1017.

Shuping, J. R., Rollinson, R. D., & Toole, J. F. (1980). Transient global amnesia. *Annals of Neurology, 7,* 281–285.

Soloway, H. B., & Aronson, S. M. (1964). Atheromatous emboli to central nervous system. *Archives of Neurology, 11,* 657–667.

Stadel, B. V. (1981). Oral contraceptives and cardiovascular disease (Pt. 2). *New England Journal of Medicine, 305,* 672–677.

Stafford, C. R., Bogdanoff, B. M., Green, L., et al. (1975). Mononeuropathy multiplex as a complication of amphetamine angiitis. *Neurology, 25,* 570–572.

Steiner, L. (1986). Radiosurgery in cerebral arteriovenous malformations. In E. Flamm & J. Fein (Eds.), *Textbook of cerebrovascular surgery* (pp. 1161–1215). New York: Springer-Verlag.

Stemmermann, G. N., Hayashi, T., Resch, J. A., et al. (1984). Risk factors related to ischemic and hemorrhagic cerebrovascular disease at autopsy: The Honolulu heart study. *Stroke, 15,* 23–28.

Strand, T., Aspuland, K., Eriksson, S., et al. (1984). A randomized controlled trial of hemodilution therapy in acute ischemic stroke. *Stroke, 15,* 980–989.

Strandgaard, S. (1983). Cerebral blood flow in hypertension. *Acta Medica Scandinavica Supplements, 678,* 11–25.

Strandgaard, S., and Paulson, O. B. (1984). Cerebral autoregulation. *Stroke, 15,* 413–416.

Sundt, T. M., Piepgras, D. G., Ebersold, M. J., et al. (1987a). Postoperative evaluation and management of complications with illustrative cases. In T. M. Sundt (Ed.), *Occlusive cerebrovascular disease: Diagnosis and surgical management* (pp. 243–260). Philadelphia: W. B. Saunders.

Sundt, T. M., Piepgras, D. G., Ebersold, M. J., et al. (1987b). Risk factors and operative results. In T. M. Sundt (Ed.), *Occlusive cerebrovascular disease: Diagnosis and surgical management* (pp. 226–231). Philadelphia: W. B. Saunders.

Szekely, P. (1964). Systemic embolism and anticoagulant prophylaxis in rheumatic heart disease. *British Medical Journal, 1,* 1209–1212.

Tell, G. S., Crouse, J. R., & Furberg, C. D. (1988). Relation between blood lipids, lipoproteins, and cerebrovascular atherosclerosis: A review. *Stroke, 19,* 423–430.

Thomas, D. J., du Boulay, G. H., Marshall, J., et al. (1977). Effect of haematocrit on cerebral blood-flow in man. *Lancet, 2,* 941–943.

Thomas, J. E., & Ayyer, D. R. (1972). Systemic fat embolism. *Archives of Neurology, 26,* 517–523.

Toole, J. F., Yuson, C. P., Janeway, R., et al. (1978). Transient ischemic attacks: A prospective study of 225 patients. *Neurology, 28,* 746–753.

Tohgi, H., Yamanouchi, H., Murakami, M., et al. (1978). Importance of the hematocrit as a risk factor in cerebral infarction. *Stroke, 9,* 369–374.

Vinters, H. V. (1987). Cerebral amyloid angiopathy: A critical review. *Stroke, 18,* 311–324.

Vinuela, F., & Fox, A. J. (1986). Interventional neuroradiology. In H. J. M. Barnett, J. P. Mohr, B. M. Stein, et al. (Eds.), *Stroke pathophysiology, diagnosis, and management* (Vol. 1, pp. 1173–1189). New York: Churchill-Livingstone.

Wallace, J. D., & Levy, L. L. (1981). Blood pressure after stroke. *Journal of the American Medical Association, 246,* 2177–2180.

Weir, B. (1987a). *Aneurysms affecting the nervous system.* Baltimore: Williams & Wilkins.

Weir, B. (1987b). Antifibrinolytics in subarachnoid hemorrhage: Do they have a role? No. *Archives of Neurology, 44,* 116–118.

Weksler, B. B., Kent, J. L., Rudolph, D., et al. (1985). Effects of low dose aspirin on platelet function in patients with recent cerebral ischemia. *Stroke, 16,* 5–9.

Whisnant, J. P. (1974). Epidemiology of stroke: Emphasis on transient cerebral ischemic attacks and hypertension. *Stroke, 5,* 68–70.

Wintzen, A. R., de Jonge, H., Loeliger, E. A., et al. (1984). The risk of intracerebral hemorrhage during oral anticoagulant treatment: A population study. *Annals of Neurology, 16,* 553–558.

Wojak, J. C., and Flamm, E. S. (1987). Intracranial hemorrhage and cocaine use. *Stroke, 18,* 712–715.

Wolf, P. A., Dawber, T. R., Thomas, H. E., et al. (1978). Epidemiologic assessment of chronic atrial fibrillation and risk of stroke: The Framingham study. *Neurology, 28,* 973–977.

Wolf, P. A., Kannel, W. B., Sorlie, P., et al. (1981). Asymptomatic carotid bruit and risk of stroke: The Framingham study. *Journal of the American Medical Association, 245,* 1442–1445.

Wolf, P. A., Kannel, W. B., & Verter, J. (1983). Current status of risk factors for stroke. *Neurologic Clinics, 1,* 317–343.

Wooten, M. R., Khangure, M. S., & Murphy, M. J. (1983). Intracerebral hemorrhage and vasculitis related to ephedrine abuse. *Annals of Neurology, 13,* 337–340.

CHAPTER

37 Brain Death

Ellen B. Rudy

To most people the term "death" is a clear-cut pronouncement. Death occurs when a person stops breathing and the heart stops beating. These criteria, cessation of function of the heart and lungs, continue to be synonymous with death. Biomedical advances, however, have provided us with the means to ventilate the lungs mechanically and ways to restart the heart and maintain circulation. Such advances in medical technology, coupled with pharmacologic support that can maintain physiologic function in patients well beyond any potential for recovery, created the need to reexamine the definition of death.

Along with recognition of the inadequacy of the common law definition of death have come improvements in the area of organ transplantation. Early activities in the transplantation of solid organs, including the kidney, heart, liver, and pancreas, were limited due to surgical techniques, inadequate understanding of the immune system, and subsequent rejection by organ recipients. This picture changed dramatically in the 1960s with perfection of transplant surgery and major advances in the field of immunology. An even greater boost to organ transplantation occurred with the discovery of cyclosporin and its antirejection properties. These advances and subsequently more effective antirejection drugs have led to organ transplantation as an accepted treatment modality, not just an experimental procedure. The need for healthy, viable organs can be met only by cadaveric sources, focusing attention on the necessity to declare a person dead as soon as irreversible brain damage can be established. The object, of course, is to hasten the process of recognizing death early enough to allow transplantable organs to be adequately perfused and kept healthy to increase the potential for successful transplantation.

Biomedical advances that allowed irreversibly brain damaged individuals to maintain cardiopulmonary function coupled with an increasing need for viable organs for transplantation resulted in recognition of the concept of brain death. *Brain death is the irreversible loss of all brain function.* This means loss of the higher centers of the cerebral hemispheres, which are involved in cognitive functioning, and loss of the lower centers of the brain stem, which control many involuntary functions, including respiratory and circulatory activities.

It should be clearly understood that brain death does not introduce a second type of death or a second means of determining death. Death is viewed as a single phenomenon that can be accurately demonstrated either by the traditional means of irreversible cessation of function of the heart and lungs or by irreversible loss of all functions of the entire brain (President's Commission, 1983). The President's Commission for the Study of Ethical Problems in Medicine and Biomedical and Behavioral Research, in its report *Defining Death* (President's Commission, 1981), took special note of the confusion that the term "brain death" has created in the literature by means of public discussions and legislative activity. The Commission advised that terminology such as "brain-based standard of death" be used rather than brain death. Their point was that the term brain death can refer either to "cessation of brain function" or to "the death of a person based on cessation of brain function." Such usage may indeed be confusing, particularly to the lay public. Brain death, however, has become a part of accepted medical and legal terminology. It seems unlikely that the term will be changed, and efforts will continue to be made to inform the public that brain death is not a second type of death apart from cardiac and respiratory death.

The three most common causes of brain death are (1) direct head trauma, such as occurs with motor vehicle accidents and gunshot wounds; (2) massive, spontaneous hemorrhage into the brain; and (3) lack of blood flow to the brain secondary to cardiac arrest or severe systemic hypotension (Cranford & Smith, 1979). In each of these cases, brain death occurs when the brain has inadequate cerebral perfusion to maintain cell integrity. This interruption of blood flow may be the result of inadequate systemic blood pressure (such as occurs with cardiac arrest) or the consequence of increased intracranial pressure that exceeds the cerebral perfusion pressure necessary to deliver blood to the brain cells. When the cerebral circulation is interrupted, all brain functions will cease within a matter of minutes to hours. The relationship between cerebral circulation and brain functioning is essential to the understanding of the clinical tests used to determine brain death and to an appreciation of the certainty of the prognosis in these cases.

Two developments have occurred that directly affect clinical practice and the application of brain death in critical care. First is the development of the legal, or statutory, criteria, to determine brain death, and the second is the development of clinical criteria to determine brain death.

STATUTORY RECOGNITION OF BRAIN DEATH

A variety of lawsuits concerning the determination of death for organ procurement and transplantation and for inheritance and criminal purposes first prompted the medical community to seek legal recognition of brain death. Such recognition has occurred through enactment of state statutes that include brain death along with general death. Not surprisingly, such laws, beginning in 1970 with the Kansas state law, were not uniform in wording or application.

Work began in the later 1970s by the American Medical Association, the American Bar Association, and the National Conference of Commissioners on Uniform State Laws to develop a uniform definition to be used in state statutes. The President's Commission for the Study of Ethical Problems in Medicine and Biomedical and Behavioral Research worked with those organizations and eventually endorsed the Uniform Determination of Death Act to replace earlier proposals. The definition in this act reads:

An individual who has sustained either (1) irreversible cessation of circulatory and respiratory functions, or (2) irreversible cessation of all functions of the entire brain, including the brain stem, is dead. A determination of death shall be made in accordance with accepted medical standards.

The President's Commission recommended adoption of this statute in all jurisdictions in the United States. By the end of 1991, most states gave legal recognition to brain death. As an aid to the implementation of the proposed statute, the President's Commission published *Guidelines for the Determination of Death* (Table 37–1). These guidelines were developed by a group of more than 50 medical and scientific consultants representing a wide range of medical specialties (President's Commission, 1983).

As noted in the statute on brain death, determination of brain death, or cessation of all brain functions, must be made "in accordance with accepted medical standards." Such a phrase allows for altering of clinical criteria to determine brain function as medical technology improves and measurements become more precise. Recognizing the continuing advancements being made in biomedical technology, such leeway only makes sense to members of the health care profession. The lack, however, of any *one* test for brain death leaves questions in the mind of the public as to the validity of the tests used, and again leads people to ask, "Is a person who is brain dead really dead?"

TABLE 37–1. **Guidelines for the Determination of Death**

A. An individual with irreversible cessation of circulatory and respiratory functions is dead.
   1. Cessation is recognized by an appropriate clinical examination.
   2. Irreversibility is recognized by persistent cessation of functions during an appropriate period of observation and/or trial of therapy.

B. An individual with irreversible cessation of the entire brain, including the brain stem, is dead.
   1. Cessation is recognized when evaluation discloses finding of both:
      Absence of cerebral functions, and
      Absence of brain stem functions.
   2. Irreversibility is recognized when evaluation discloses *all* of the following:
      The cause of coma is established and is sufficient to account for the loss of brain functions; and
      The possibility of recovery of any brain functions is excluded.

From Medical Consultants on the Diagnosis of Death to the President's Commission for the Study of Ethical Problems in Medicine and Biomedical and Behavioral Research (1981). Report: Guidelines for the determination of death. *Journal of the American Medical Association, 246,* 2184–2186. Copyright 1981 American Medical Association.

CRITERIA FOR DETERMINING BRAIN DEATH

Many different combinations of clinical criteria have been proposed for determining brain death. The earliest and most frequently cited are those developed by an Ad Hoc Committee of the Harvard Medical School of 1968 (Beecher, 1968), referred to as the "Harvard criteria." However, these criteria have been reported to be unnecessarily restrictive (Walker, 1983), and, as the lay and medical communities have become more confident in the use of brain death as a terminal diagnosis, the original criteria have been modified.

The criteria used to determine death based on irreversible cessation of all brain function provided by the President's Commission (see Table 37–1) require documentation of three items:

1. Cerebral and brain stem functions are absent.
2. The condition of the patient is irreversible. This necessitates that the condition has a known cause and that the possibility of recovery has been excluded.
3. Cessation of all brain functions has persisted for an appropriate period of observation or trial of therapy.

Absence of Cerebral and Brain Stem Functions

Assessment of the function of the entire brain requires testing the functions of both the cerebral cortex and the brain stem. When possible, laboratory tests are used to confirm the clinical diagnosis. At one time, the electroencephalogram (EEG) was considered important in the diagnosis of brain death. However, because an isoelectric EEG only measures the electrical activity of the cerebral hemispheres and not the physiologic function of the brain stem, it does not confirm the diagnosis of brain death. Furthermore, physical, electrical, and ventilator artifacts and variability in reading the EEG contribute to difficulties with interpretation. In a multicenter study funded by the National Institutes of Neurological Diseases and Stroke, investigators found that all functions of the brain considered essential could be lost irreversibly while very small (2-microvolt) electrical potentials could be observed on EEG. For these reasons, an isoelectric EEG is not considered mandatory for the diagnosis of brain death. The most widely used laboratory tests include cerebral blood flow studies by radioisotope cerebral angiography or computed tomography (CT) scanning with contrast media.

Laboratory tests used to confirm brain function usually include only the most commonly available and clinically accepted tests. Laboratory testing is the most likely area of change as advances in medical technology allow more precise information. One example is the positron emission tomography (PET) scanner, which already has the capacity to measure not only cerebral circulation but cerebral metabolism. Some writers believe that cerebral metabolism is the ultimate test of cerebral function. Results of a PET scan would certainly be a more definitive test of cerebral function than that currently used. However, the cost and limited availability of a PET scan prohibited its consideration as a "standard" medical practice for the establishment of brain death.

To establish the absence of cerebral and brain stem functions, tests of cerebral cortex function and tests of brain stem function are used, as described in the following sections.

TESTS OF CEREBRAL CORTEX FUNCTIONING

Cerebral or cognitive functioning is determined by responses to stimuli, such as light, sound, motion, or pain. Absence of cortical functioning is determined by a lack of verbal response, lack of spontaneous or coordinated eye movements, and absence of muscle flexion or extension (decorticate and decerebrate activity) in response to any of the foregoing stimuli. Complex spinal cord reflexes may be preserved in brain-dead people and must be differentiated from true decerebrate and decorticate posturing (Powner & Grenvik, 1979).

Documentation of the absence of cerebral circulation through four-vessel (carotid and vertebral vessels) intracranial angiography in the normothermic patient is considered a definitive test of cerebral death. This test, however, involves considerable practical difficulties and some risks to the patient. For these reasons, tests assessing only the cerebral hemisphere circulation are usually employed. Tests of cerebral blood flow include radioisotope angiography, echo cerebrovascular pulsations, CT scans with contrast media, and regional cerebral blood flow studies.

TESTS OF BRAIN STEM FUNCTION

Brain stem function is determined by testing the cranial nerves whose nuclei are within the brain stem and the presence or absence of spontaneous respirations. The usual tests of brain stem function are as follows (Rudy, 1984):

PUPILLARY LIGHT REFLEX. With an intact optic nerve (cranial nerve II) and oculomotor nerve (cranial nerve III), a light will stimulate the parasympathetic fibers to the iris, causing pupillary constriction. Absence of pupillary response to light indicates nonfunction of cranial nerves II and III. Pupils need not be equal or necessarily dilated, but must be nonreactive to light to meet the criteria.

Pupillary response will be absent after administration of scopolamine, atropine, opiates, neuromuscular blocking agents, or glutamine. It may also be absent after eye trauma or eye disease. In the presence of either medication that interferes with pupillary response, or eye trauma or disease, tests of the pupillary reflex will be omitted. Testing this reflex is not considered mandatory to the determination of brain death.

OCULOVESTIBULAR REFLEX. The patient is positioned with the head elevated 30 degrees, and the ear is inspected with an ophthalmoscope to ensure that the tympanic membrane is intact. Ice water is slowly introduced through a 30-mL syringe into the patient's ear canal. In the person with an intact brain stem, stimulation conducted from the vestibular portion of the acoustic nerve (cranial nerve VIII) via the pons and the abducens nerve (cranial nerve VI) to the midbrain and the oculomotor nerve (cranial nerve III) will result in a horizontal nystagmus, slow movement toward the irrigated ear and rapid movement away. In the absence of brain stem function, ice water will produce no eye movement.

VAGUS NERVE FUNCTION. The tenth cranial nerve, the vagus nerve, with its parasympathetic fibers, acts to slow the heart. Thus, atropine, a parasympathetic inhibitor, given intravenously, inhibits the action of the vagus nerve, causing an increase in pulse rate when the vagus nerve is functioning and the cardiac muscle is capable of responding. Vagus nerve function is tested by administering 0.1 mg of atropine intravenously. The pulse rate is expected to increase by 5 beats per minute if the vagus nerve is functioning.

BRAIN STEM AUDITORY EVOKED RESPONSE. Some physicians believe that one of the last portions of the brain stem to remain intact is the acoustic nerve (cranial nerve VIII). This nerve is tested by using the brain stem auditory evoked response (BAER) technique. An electrode is placed deep within the ear canal, and surface electrodes on the mastoid bone record the electrical evoked responses. After administration of stimuli, evoked responses appear as electrical sequelae on a computer-averaged EEG. The presence of a response reflects activation of the eighth cranial nerve and auditory regions of the brain stem and cerebral cortex by sound stimuli. Absence of a BAER indicates severe, widespread central nervous system dysfunction consistent with brain death. Although the BAER is not widely used at present, there is evidence that the use of such electrophysiologic measurements may soon become more widespread.

OTHER CRANIAL NERVE FUNCTIONS. Although the functions of other cranial nerves are often checked in determining brain stem responses in comatose patients, these are less often used to determine brain death. The *corneal reflex* is elicited by brushing the cornea of the eye lightly with a wisp of cotton. The normal response is an involuntary blink of the eye, indicating intact trigeminal (V) and facial (VII) cranial nerves. The corneal reflex may be absent due to facial muscle weakness or paralysis, and these possibilities should be ruled out before considering this reflex a reliable clinical test. The *gag reflex* may be elicited by touching the back of the throat or tongue, indicating intact glossopharyngeal (cranial nerve IX) and vagus (cranial nerve X) nerves. Assessment of this reflex is not practical in a patient who is intubated or has a tracheostomy tube in place.

Irreversible Condition of the Person

In essence, this criterion requires the physician to establish as nearly as possible the cause of the comatose state and rule out any conditions that may be treated and reversible. Although much attention has been focused on the pros and cons of the clinical tests used, most difficulties with determining brain death have occurred because inadequate attention has been paid to reversible complicating conditions.

When the cause of the patient's condition is well established and loss of brain function is not unexpected, there is little problem. Difficulties may occur when the cause of the comatose state is not known or is complicated by drugs, metabolic abnormalities, hypothermia, or shock. To document adequately the irreversibility of the loss of brain function, the possibility of complicating conditions must be investigated and treated.

DRUG OR METABOLIC INTOXICATION

When the cause of the coma is unknown or when drugs are suspected, comprehensive drug toxicology screening is required. A variety of sedative and anesthetic drugs produce clinical symptoms that mimic brain death, including electrocerebral silence or an isoelectric EEG. Drugs most commonly producing brain dysfunction at toxic levels include barbiturates, benzodiazepines, meprobamate, methaqualone, and trichloroethylene. When toxic serum levels of a drug are present, death may not be declared until the drug is metabolized or until testing demonstrates absent cerebral circulation.

Another category of drugs that may cause complete muscle paralysis and areflexia is the neuromuscular blocking agents such as succinylcholine, pancuronium, or similar agents. Because these drugs can also cause death-like symptoms, patients with prolonged paralysis with these drugs need to be tested for pseudocholinesterase deficiency by low-dose atropine stimulation, electromyography, or peripheral nerve stimulation. If there is any question about the possibility of a drug-induced coma, additional testing or extended observation is required (Medical Consultants, 1981).

Illnesses that cause severe metabolic abnormalities can produce prolonged deep coma, including hepatic coma with encephalopathy, hyperosmolar coma, and severe uremia. It seems unlikely that these metabolic abnormalities would go untreated, but efforts should be made to correct them before brain function is tested. Again, absence of cerebral circulation would be a definitive test.

HYPOTHERMIA

People are considered hypothermic when their core body temperature is below the physiologically normal limits (less than 35.6°C) (Elder, 1989). However, for purposes of establishing brain death, the core body temperature must be above 32.2°C (90°F) for the criteria to apply. Hypothermic victims may appear dead by all clinical signs, but successful resuscitation has been reported after a core body temperature of 28°C and below (DeRouboix, 1980; Pickering et al., 1977)—hence the dictum, "No one is dead until he is warm and dead" (Reuler, 1978). With increased experience and success in treating severely hypothermic patients, brain death is usually not considered until rewarming procedures have been initiated. Hypothermia coupled with drug or alcohol intoxication can produce cerebral dysfunction that mimics brain death at temperature levels above the proposed 32.2°C, making careful diagnosis and toxicology screening essential prerequisites for the diagnosis of brain death.

SHOCK

A state of shock with its accompanying low levels of blood pressure can reduce cerebral circulation to the point where clinical tests can be inaccurate, making a determination of brain death unreliable. This is particularly true in patients with shock with coexisting multiple injuries. Early evidence of the combined effects of multiple injuries with shock came from battlefield determinations of death in soldiers later shown to be in a state of severe shock closely resembling death. In a clinical setting, patients should be treated appropriately for shock before any examination for brain death takes place.

Cessation of All Brain Functions Persisting for an Appropriate Period of Observation or Trial of Therapy

Once the cessation of all brain functions has been established by clinical criteria, the length of time required for observation or for further trials of therapy varies, and is a matter of clinical judgment by the physician. Thus the term "appropriate" will depend on the clinical situation. The report to the President's Commission suggests the following observation guidelines (Medical Consultants, 1981).

SIX HOURS. Once clinical criteria for brain death have been documented and confirmed by appropriate clinical testing and the patient has no complicating conditions (e.g., drug intoxication, hypothermia, young age, shock), an observation period of 6 hours with no change in brain function is considered adequate for determination of brain death.

TWELVE HOURS. In the absence of confirmatory tests (e.g., electrocardiogram, cerebral blood flow) but when an irreversible condition is well established, a period of at least 12 hours of observation is recommended.

TWENTY-FOUR HOURS. In cases of anoxic brain damage, when the extent of damage may be more difficult to ascertain, 24 hours of observation with no evidence of brain function is suggested. This period of observation may be reduced if cerebral blood flow studies or an EEG support the loss of brain function.

MANAGEMENT OF PATIENTS WHO MEET BRAIN DEATH CRITERIA

There is evidence from clinical reports that in patients who are supported on mechanical ventilation, cardiac arrest usually occurs within 72 hours of brain death (Ibe, 1971; Jorgensen, 1973; Kimura et al., 1968; Korein, 1978). However, in a recent reported case, a pregnant woman who was declared brain dead after a craniotomy was kept on mechanical ventilation 53 days until her baby could be delivered by Caesarean section (*Akron Becon Journal,* 1986). Another publication reported a patient with documented brain death after a cardiorespiratory arrest who was kept on mechanical ventilatory support for 68 days before removal from ventilatory support and electrocardiac silence occurred (Parisi et al., 1982). Because of the long duration of external support and attendant circumstances, these two cases are unusual. For the most part, once brain death has been determined, there are few circumstances when intensive care therapy is still indicated. Exceptions include cases in which the brain-dead patient is a pregnant woman with a viable fetus, or when the family (or patient) has agreed to organ donation and organ retrieval is scheduled.

PREGNANT WOMAN. In the case of a brain-dead woman who is pregnant with a viable fetus, there is already evidence that a live birth may occur if the fetus can be maintained through ventilatory and circulatory support to the mother (Dillon et al., 1982). Such circumstances are rare, and the birth can be successful only if the fetus is at least in the second trimester of development at the time of maternal death.

ORGAN DONOR. With improved surgical technology and a more complete understanding of the immune system and improved antirejection drugs, organ transplantation has progressed from an experimental procedure to a recognized therapeutic modality. Publicity and increased long-term survival have resulted in a need for solid organs and tissues (cornea, skin, bones) that has far outstripped the supply. The only source of solid organs such as the pancreas, liver, or heart is brain-dead patients. In many states, statutes have been passed requiring the family of every patient who dies in an acute care setting and meets eligibility criteria for organ donation to be offered the opportunity to donate the patient's organs. If the family agrees to organ donation, the brain-dead patient must be kept on life-support therapy until organ procurement takes place. This is obviously necessary to keep the organ perfused and viable for subsequent transplantation.

FAMILY WISHES. If one believes legally, morally, and ethically that brain death is no different from death that occurs when the heart and lungs stop functioning, there is little reason to maintain patients on intensive therapy after a determination of brain death has been made. In fact, termination of further medical intervention is ethically justifiable when that treatment is no longer deemed useful (Lucas et al., 1987). That is, there is no moral obligation to perform useless or futile therapy, and in the presence of a declaration of brain death, further therapy would be useless. The reality of clinical circumstances, however, sometimes dictates otherwise. In a survey of neurologists and neurosurgeons on the subject of brain death, they were asked what they would do if a patient met the brain death criteria but the family wanted the life support to be continued. A total of 76% said they would continue ventilatory support. There was variability in exactly what that meant, and responses ranged from declaring the patient dead but continuing support, not declaring the patient dead and continuing support, and declaring the patient dead and stopping support regardless of the family's wishes (Black & Zervas, 1984). Many respondents spoke of working with the family to help them accept the patient's death. This type of situation is mentioned to emphasize that family members may require additional time and help to understand that a beating heart and moving lungs are possible even when a person is dead.

PROBLEMS IN DETERMINING BRAIN DEATH

The established criteria for determining brain death and accepted clinical tests have been presented. There remain, however, practical problems in the performance and interpretation of test results.

Motor Response to Stimuli

Decerebrate or decorticate muscle activity is inconsistent with brain death criteria. Spinal reflexes, however, can occasionally produce complex integrated movement of muscle groups, and such movement may be difficult to ascribe to spinal reflexes on clinical evidence alone. If there is any doubt about the origin of muscle activity, cerebral blood flow studies should be done to confirm the absence of perfusion to the brain.

Electroencephalogram

In some places an isoelectric EEG may be required as part of brain death testing. Spontaneous muscle fasciculations may produce EEG tracing artifacts, making interpretation difficult. In such cases, drugs may be used to produce neuromuscular paralysis during the EEG recording. Clinical examination for cerebral and brain stem responses cannot be performed until the drug effects have worn off or a neuromuscular stimulator counteracts the initial drug effect. As mentioned earlier in the chapter, most physicians no longer require an EEG to determine brain death.

Spontaneous Respirations

Testing for the absence of spontaneous respirations is difficult because of the potential for producing further deterioration in the patient's status while he or she is apneic. The first problem is hypoxia, which can occur while the patient is disconnected from the ventilator. This problem is usually handled by preoxygenating the patient with 100% oxygen for several breaths before disconnecting ventilatory support, or providing passive oxygen through a catheter down the endotracheal tube during the disconnect time. Some patients require a hypoxic stimulus to initiate spontaneous breathing, so they must be allowed to become hypoxic to rule out spontaneous respirations. Blood gas determinations are required to validate the P_{CO_2} level.

For most patients, increased carbon dioxide is considered the strongest stimulus for spontaneous respirations. Because many ventilator-dependent patients, particularly head-injured patients, are maintained in a hypocarbic state, the respiratory rate should be decreased before testing, and P_{CO_2} levels should be allowed to rise to near normal values (40–50 mm Hg) before testing for spontaneous respirations is performed. This test is not considered valid unless the P_{CO_2} is at least 45 mm Hg, providing an adequate stimulus for spontaneous respiratory effort. In patients with increased intracranial pressure, increases in P_{CO_2} result in cerebral vasodilatation and subsequent increases in intracranial pressure. This sequence of events obviously has the potential to compromise brain function further. Therefore, tests of spontaneous respirations in patients with increased intracranial pressure should be reserved until all other criteria have been met.

Cerebral Blood Flow

Cerebral blood flow is the test that is probably considered the most definitive test for brain death. However, cerebral blood flow angiography requires visualization of all four vessels supplying the brain. The test is invasive, requires complicated radiologic techniques, and is often impractical for routine use in critically ill patients.

Indirect methods to determine cerebral blood flow include radioisotopic techniques, echoencephalography to demonstrate loss of the midline intracranial pulsations, and cerebral Doppler echoencephalography (Korein et al., 1975; Schwartz et al., 1983). Although not as definitive as four-vessel contrast cerebral angiography, these tests support other clinical determinations of brain death and are useful when clinical criteria are inconclusive or impractical.

Controversy Surrounding Whole-Brain Definition of Death

Brain death has been discussed extensively for more than 25 years. Most nurses and physicians believe that the concept of requiring loss of function of the entire brain (higher brain and brain stem) as the criterion for brain death and the use of standard (but evolving) clinical tests to document loss of whole-brain function have produced a satisfactory resolution to most of the issues surrounding the determination of death. There continues, however, to be a vocal group of writers who challenge the need for the "whole-brain" definition of death.

It is beyond the scope of this chapter to present an in-depth discussion of the ethical and philosophical debate between using the whole-brain criterion for determining death versus the higher-brain criterion, but recognition that such a debate exists and the major points presented seem important.

The general theme of people who challenge the use of the whole-brain definition of death is essentially twofold. First, the legal definition that states "irreversible cessation of *all functions* of the brain, including brain stem" cannot be absolutely determined. That is, some individuals who meet all of the standard clinical tests for brain death may still have certain cellular-level functions, preserved brain stem evoked responses, or even microvolt-level electrical activity on EEG testing (Barelli et al., 1990; Ferbert et al., 1986). These facts, they say, cast doubt on the entire concept and call for an expanded or alternative definition of brain death. Second, the whole-brain definition relates to functioning that is independent of consciousness, and because this is what is essential to human beings, death should be defined as *the irreversible cessation of conscious functioning*. This definition of death is referred to as the "higher-brain criterion" (Halevy & Brody, 1993; Veatch, 1993; Youngner & Bartlett, 1983). The primary premise of this argument equates death to the loss of consciousness and the ability to interact, to reason, and so on.

Although a handful of writers would have you believe that this move to an alternative higher-brain definition of death is just around the corner, the criticisms are many. First, a clear definition of consciousness has not been proposed, let alone the clinical testing required to validate this state. Second, the clear implication in this definition is that vegetative patients who breathe on their own are, in fact, dead and would need to be buried or cremated. Even Youngner and Bartlett (1983) acknowledge the problems with this scenario. Finally, because all of us must at some time face death, the fear that the definition of death can be expanded causes anxieties and a fear that there may be no stopping the expansion of brain functions that are not considered essential for life. This is the so-called slippery slope argument (Bernat, 1992).

Although the constant questioning and challenges of the current definition and clinical judgment of brain death are important, there is little empirical evidence that a higher-brain definition of death is gaining momentum and will be anything more than an academic debate for some time.

One special case currently challenging the whole-brain definition of brain death is that of anencephalic infants. These infants are born with a major portion of the brain, skull case, and overlapping scalp absent. Only the brain stem and spinal cord of the central nervous system remain. Without the cerebral hemispheres, there is no cognition or intellect, and no measurable electroencephalographic activity or cerebral circulation. What does remain is brain stem activity, including conjugate gaze, pupillary light response, voluntary respirations, sucking, smiling, and even crying (Diaz, 1993).

The prognosis for these congenitally afflicted infants is very poor, with the vast majority dying within the first week of life. This time-line may be somewhat misleading because many anencephalic infants are given comfort care only (fluids, nutrition, and warmth) in anticipation of death, and without any intent to provide life-supportive measures. However, even with intensive care, most of these infants die within 2 weeks (Mavroudis et al., 1989). The cost of keeping these infants alive and the need for neonatal organs, particularly hearts for brain-normal infants born with hypoplastic left heart syndrome, have focused attention on the need to reexamine brain death criteria for these special cases.

The controversy over anencephalic infants is fairly straightforward. A child born without a cerebral cortex has no upper brain function but cannot legally be declared brain dead with an intact brain stem. Transplant surgeons who are in critical need of infant heart donors feel that in waiting for brain stem functions to cease—to meet fully brain death criteria—most transplantable organs become unsuitable for living donor transplantation. This push to have viable organs in infants who will ultimately die has led some authors to assert that the anencephalic fetus has never been alive and should be considered brain dead from birth (Holzgreve et al., 1987; Holzgreve & Beller, 1987). Others recommended that the anencephalic infant be considered "brain-absent" and thus excludable from the state Uniform Determination of Death Acts. Although anencephalic births are uncommon and are admittedly a special case, they do highlight the "upper brain" versus "whole-brain" controversy surrounding the definition of brain death.

Non–Heart-Beating Donors

Recognizing the impact that organ transplantation has had on the acceptance of brain death within both the medical and lay public, the move back to organ procurement from patients pronounced dead by cardiopulmonary criteria, *not* brain death criteria, deserves mention. At one time, the only organs available for transplantation were from living donors (as in paired organs such as kidneys) or cadaveric sources. Because of prolonged ischemic time in the case of cardiopulmonary death, the viability of organs for transplantation was very poor. This led, as described earlier, to the development and acceptance of neurologic or brain death criteria to identify people whose hearts were still beating even while they were pronounced dead—"heart-beating cadavers." Because the demand for organs has continued to grow well beyond the supply available from brain-dead donors, there has recently been a move to reconsider and improve organ donation from individuals who are declared dead by the traditional cardiopulmonary criteria—irreversible cessation of circulatory and respiratory functions. These donors are called "non–heart-beating cadavers" (DeVita et al., 1993).

The current practice of obtaining viable organs from non–heart-beating cadavers is discussed in more detail in Chapter 56, but the point that needs to be made here is that although the terminology is confusing, brain death criteria are applicable only for heart-beating donors.

BRAIN DEATH IN CHILDREN

Little information is available on the application of brain death criteria in pediatric patients. The President's Commission warns physicians to "be particularly cautious in applying neurological criteria to determine death in children younger than 5 years" (Medical Consultants, 1981). This warning, however, offers little in the way of explicit information about which clinical tests are to be used or which applications are to be changed in determining brain death. Some authors claim that the brains of infants and children have increased resistance to hypoxic damage and may recover substantial function even after exhibiting unresponsiveness on neurologic examination for long periods of time compared to adults (Green & Lauber, 1972; Pasternak & Volpe, 1979; Rowland et al., 1984). Keeping in mind the potential immaturity of the nervous system in children, the use of cerebral blood flow studies is recommended as a more accurate assessment of irreversible neurologic loss in these patients (Ashwal & Schneider, 1979; Schwartz et al., 1983). The recommended observation periods during which time EEGs are repeated and cerebral blood flow studies can be done depend on the age of the infant and the tests to be used. Some specific time frames are provided by the Task Force for the Determination of Brain Death in Children (1987), but the major point to remember is that the younger the infant, the more difficult it is to confirm brain death. Newborns and premature infants present the most difficulty and require the longest observation times before the extent and reversibility of the brain injury can be determined.

Two additional factors are noteworthy with comatose children. First, many of these children may be hypothermic at the time of testing. Hypothermia occurs commonly in the critically ill child and may mimic brain death in the slowing of responses; it should be assessed and corrected before brain death criteria are examined. Second, barbiturates and muscle relaxants are frequently used to treat increased intracranial pressure in children. These medications make neurological testing suspect, and therefore a serum barbiturate level is recommended before testing for brain death.

SUMMARY

The recognition and diagnosis of death by brain function criteria is an inevitable step in the evolution of twentieth century medical care. The increasing capacity to maintain human physiologic functions through mechanical and medical means makes the concept of brain death increasingly necessary.

Ability to transplant human organs with increased success highlights the demand for viable organs from cadaveric sources. The statutes and the Uniform Determination of Death Act have paved the way for acceptance of brain death within the health care professions. The clinical criteria used to establish brain death require clear evidence of irreversible loss of both cortical and brain stem activity.

REFERENCES

Akron Beacon Journal. (1986, July). Baby girl born to woman legally dead seven and one-half weeks.

Ashwal, S., & Schneider, S., (1979). Failure of electroencephalography to diagnose brain death in comatose children. *Annals of Neurology, 6,* 512–517.

Barelli, A., Della Corte, F., Calimici, R., et al. (1990). Do brainstem auditory evoked potentials detect the actual cessation of cerebral functions in brain dead patients? *Critical Care Medicine, 18,* 322–323.

Beecher, H. K. A. (1968). Definition of irreversible coma. Report of the Ad Hoc Committee of the Harvard Medical School to examine the definition of brain death. *Journal of the American Medical Association, 205,* 337–340.

Bernat, J. L. (1992). How much of the brain must die in brain death? *Journal of Clinical Ethics, 3*(1), 21–26.

Black, P. L., & Zervas, N. T. (1984). Declaration of brain death in neurosurgical neurological practice. *Journal of Neurosurgery, 15,* 170–174.

Cranford, R. E., & Smith, H. L. (1979). Some critical distinctions between brain death and the persistent vegetative state. *Ethics in Science and Medicine, 6,* 199–209.

DeRouboix, J. A. M. (1980). Successful resuscitation in severe accidental hypothermia—a case report. *South Africa Medical Journal, 57,* 375–376.

DeVita, M. A., Snyder, J. V., & Grenvik, A. (1993). History of organ donation by patients with cardiac death. *Kennedy Institute of Ethics, 3*(2), 113–129.

Diaz, J. H. (1993). The anencephalic organ donor: A challenge to existing moral and statutory laws. *Critical Care Medicine, 21,* 1781–1786.

Dillon, W. P., Lee, R. V., Tronolone, M. J., et al. (1982). Life support and maternal death during pregnancy. *Journal of the American Medical Association, 248,* 1089–1091.

Elder, D. T. (1989). Accidental hypothermia. In W. C. Shoemaker, W. L. Thompson, & P. R. Holbrook (Eds.), *Textbook of critical care* (2nd ed., pp. 85–93). Philadelphia: W. B. Saunders.

Ferbert, A., Buchner, H., Ringelstein, E. B., & Hacke, W. (1986). Isolated brain-stem death. *Electroencephalography and Clinical Neurophysiology, 65,* 157–160.

Green, J. B., & Lauber, A. (1972). Return of EEG activity after electrocerebral silence: Two case reports. *Journal of Neurosurgery and Psychiatry, 35,* 103–107.

Halevy, A., & Brody, B. (1993). Braindeath: Reconciling definitions, criteria, and tests. *Annals of Internal Medicine, 119,* 519–525.

Holzgreve, W., & Beller, F. K. (1987). Kidney transplantation from anencephalic donors. *New England Journal of Medicine, 317,* 961.

Holzgreve, W., Beller, F. K., Buchalz, B., et al. (1987). Kidney transplantation from anencephalic donors. *New England Journal of Medicine, 316,* 1069–1070.

Ibe, K. (1971). Clinical and pathophysiological aspects of the intravital brain death. *Electroencephalography and Clinical Neurophysiology, 30,* 272.

Jorgensen, E. O. (1973). Spinal man after brain death. *Acta Neurochirurgica, 28,* 259–273.

Kimura, J., Gerber, H. W., & McCormick, W. F. (1968). The isolectric electroencephalogram. *Archives of Internal Medicine, 121,* 511–517.

Korein, J. (1978). The problem of brain death: Development and history. *Annals of New York Academy of Science, 315,* 1–5.

Korein, J., Braunstein, D., Kricheff, I., et al. (1975). Radioisotopic bolus technique as a test to detect circulatory deficit associated with cerebral death. *Circulation, 51,* 924–939.

Lucas, B. A., Clark, D. B., Belak, A., Jr., et al. (1987). Brain death in a murder victim: A medicolegal dilemma. *Hospital Practice,* April 15, 251–276.

Mavroudis, C., Willis, R. W., & Malais, M. (1989). Orthotopic cardiac transplantation for the neonate: The dilemma of the anencephalic donor. *Journal of Thoracic and Cardiovascular Surgery, 97,* 389–391.

Medical Consultants on the Diagnosis of Death to the President's Commission for the Study of Ethical Problems in Medicine and Biomedical and Behavioral Research. (1981). Report: Guidelines for the determination of death. *Journal of the American Medical Association, 246,* 2184–2186.

Parisi, J. E., Kim, R. C., Collins, G. H., et al (1982). Brain death with prolonged somatic survival. *New England Journal of Medicine, 306,* 14–20.

Pasternak, J. F., & Volpe, J. J. (1979). Full recovery from prolonged brainstem failure following intraventricular hemorrhage. *Journal of Pediatrics, 95,* 1046–1049.

Pickering, B. G., Bristow, G. K., & Craig, D. B. (1977). Case history number 97: Case rewarming by peritoneal irrigation in accidental hypothermia with cardiac arrest. *Anesthesia and Analgesia, 56,* 574–577.

Powner, D. J., & Grenvik, A. (1979). Triage in patient care: From expected recovery to brain death. *Heart and Lung, 8,* 1103–1108.

President's Commission for the Study of Ethical Problems in Medical and Biomedical and Behavioral Research. (1981). *Defining death.* Washington, D. C.: U.S. Government Printing Office.

President's Commission for the Study of Ethical Problems in Medicine and Biomedical and Behavioral Research. (1983). *Summing up.* Washington, D. C.: U.S. Government Printing Office.

Reuler, J. B. (1978). Hypothermia. Pathophysiology, clinical settings and management. *Annals of Internal Medicine, 89,* 519–527.

Rowland, T., Donnelly, J. H., Jackson, A. H., et al. (1984). Brain death criteria. In Reply to Letters to the Editor. *American Journal of Diseases in Children, 138,* 102.

Rudy, E. B. (1984). *Advanced neurologic and neurosurgical nursing* (pp. 255–261). St. Louis: C. V. Mosby.

Schwartz, J. A., Baxter, J., Brill, D., et al. (1983). Radionuclide cerebral imaging confirming brain death. *Journal of the American Medical Association, 249,* 246–247.

Task Force for the Determination of Brain Death in Children: (1987). Guidelines for the determination of brain death in children. *Pediatric Nursing,* 3(4), 242–243.

Veatch, R. M. (1993). The impending collapse of the whole-brain definition of death. *Hasting's Center Report,* 23(24), 18–24.

Walker, E. A. (1983). Current concepts of brain death. *Journal of Neurosurgical Nursing, 15,* 261–264.

Youngner, S. J., & Bartlett, E. T. (1983). Human death and high technology: The failure of the whole-brain formulations. *Annals of Internal Medicine, 99,* 252–258.

Patients With Spinal Cord Injury

Connie (Walleck) Jastremski

Anyone is at risk for a spinal cord injury (SCI). SCI with loss of motor and sensory function is one of the most catastrophic medical conditions possible (Krause, 1985). These injuries not only change the lifestyle of the victim but affect family, friends, the community, and society. SCI can result in permanent paralysis and total loss of sensation below the level of the injury. The ability to breathe may be diminished or destroyed. Bowel, bladder, and sexual function may also be affected. Significant psychological, social, and economic ramifications are associated with SCI.

Care of SCI patients is complex and demanding. The critical care nurse must have a thorough understanding of the effects of SCI to be able to provide comprehensive care of the patient and avoid the associated complications.

EPIDEMIOLOGY

Spinal cord injury occurs most frequently in younger people, with 80% of patients younger than the age of 40 years and 50% between 15 and 25 years. The "typical" SCI victim is a young man (82% men versus 18% women) injured in a motor vehicle accident. Most SCI patients (57%) possess a high school education and were either working or full-time students when they were injured (Young & Northrup, 1981).

A recent report from the National Spinal Cord Injury Statistical Center (1990) has shown a decrease in the number of SCIs in this country from 40.1 per 1 million in 1985 to 32.1 per million, or approximately 8,000 per year, in 1990. About 40% of patients with SCI die before reaching the hospital or during the initial hospitalization. SCI remains a costly disability, with the average hospital charges for a quadriplegic being approximately $80,200 and for paraplegics $72,000 (in 1987 dollars) (Hickey, 1992; National Spinal Cord Injury Statistical Center, 1990).

Motor vehicle accidents account for 45% of cases of SCI, followed by falls (21.5%), acts of violence (15.5%), and sports injuries (13%) (Hickey, 1992; National Spinal Cord Injury Statistical Center, 1990). Penetrating wounds are responsible for 12% of all SCIs, most of these occurring in children (Leader, 1976).

Mortality and morbidity of SCI patients have dramatically changed during the past 50 years. During World War I, the life expectancy for an SCI victim was 6 to 12 months. During the past decade, improvements in acute care and treatment of complications have allowed these patients a near-normal life expectancy. Factors affecting survival include the level at which the injury occurred, the extent of paralysis, associated injuries, age when injured, and survival for the first 3 months after injury. Ten percent of those who survive the initial resuscitation die within 3 months from cardiopulmonary complications.

"Prevention" refers to programs aimed at lowering the incidence of SCI. Because most SCI victims are young (15–25 years old), prevention programs are focused toward the middle and high school populations. In these groups there is a sense of invulnerability and peer pressure for risk-taking behaviors, especially among boys. Boys are also encouraged to be more exploratory during the preteenage and early teenage years. Public education about the consequences of drug and alcohol abuse when driving or during other high-risk activities can be effective in reducing SCIs. Prevention programs should include information about law enforcement of driving within the speed limits, drinking and driving, and use of passenger restraints. An aggressive public education program in Florida focuses on preventing SCI from diving accidents. The program, *Feet First, First Time,* focuses on preventing young people from diving head first into shallow water. In the first year after the initiation of the program there was a 50% decrease in SCI in Florida (Green et al., 1985).

Today's challenge is to motivate the general public to use safety measures and minimize high-risk situations. Public education and media support are essential to disseminate the information needed to avoid this type of preventable trauma.

TABLE 38–1. **Levels of Injury and Expected Functional Ability**

Level	Normal Activity	Functional Expectation
C4	Head control Mouth control Shoulder/scapular elevation Diaphragm movement	Use of a mouthstick for turning pages, typing or writing Control of electric wheelchair ADL dependent
C5	Shoulder flexion Elbow flexion Increased scapular function	Feeds self with special adaptive devices Able to move wheelchair for short distances, does better with electric wheelchair Assists a little in self-care
C6	Good elbow flexion Wrist extension Shoulder rotation and abduction	Independent in feeding and some grooming with adaptive devices Weak hand grasp Can roll over in bed Use regular wheelchair Can drive a car with hand controls Can assist in transfer
C7	Elbow extension Strong wrist extension Good shoulder movement	Transfers independently to chair Independent in most ADLs Excellent bed mobility
T1	Normal hand strength Normal upper extremity strength	Bed and wheelchair independent Performs self-catheterization Wheelchair independent

ADL, activities of daily living.

TYPES OF SPINAL CORD INJURY

Spinal cord injury is classified by level, degree (complete or incomplete), and mechanism of injury. Vertebral injuries are also defined according to their contribution to SCI.

Spinal levels include cervical, thoracic, and lumbar. Cervical and lumbar injuries occur most commonly because these areas have the greatest flexibility and movement. A cervical injury may result in paralysis of all four extremities, called quadriplegia, or, less frequently, tetraplegia. Injuries of the thoracic and lumbar areas leave the patient paraplegic. Table 38–1 provides a list of some levels of injury and the expected functional ability after rehabilitation.

Degree of involvement may be complete or incomplete (partial). Complete SCI results in initial flaccid paralysis and total loss of motor and sensory function below the level of the injury. Losses result from irreversible spinal cord damage. Incomplete cord injury (partial transection) results in a mixed loss of motor and sensory function because some spinal cord tracts remain intact. The degree of loss depends on the level of injury and the specific nerve tract damaged.

Central cord syndrome is an example of partial transection. This syndrome usually follows a hyperextension injury in a peson with cervical spondylosis (degeneration or ankylosis of the spine from osteoarthritis) or stenosis (narrowing of the spinal canal) (Chilton & Dagi, 1985). Central cord syndrome is characterized by microscopic hemorrhage and edema in the central gray matter of the cord (Fig. 38–1). Motor weakness of the extremities occurs, but it is greater in the upper extremities. There is varying sensory and bladder dysfunction. Recovery depends on the number of undamaged spinal cord tracts and on resolution of the edema (Walleck, 1987).

Another partial injury is anterior cord injury, which is characterized by acute compression of the anterior portion of the spinal cord. Compression may impair blood flow through the anterior spinal artery, which supplies the anterior two-thirds to three-quarters of the spinal cord (Ducker et al., 1971). This syndrome may follow flexion injury but is also associated with a herniated intervertebral disc or thrombosis of the anterior spinal artery. Signs of this injury include immediate motor loss, hypesthesia (decreased sensation), or loss of sensation for pain and temperature below the level of injury. Because posterior cord function is preserved, the sensations of touch, position (proprioception), and vibration remain intact. If the syndrome is caused by compression of the anterior cord from bony fragments, surgical decompression is necessary.

Brown-Sequard syndrome, or hemisection of the cord (see Fig. 38–1), results in ipsilateral motor loss and contralateral loss of pain and temperature sensation due to spinothalamic tract involvement. Penetrating injuries may cause pure Brown-Sequard syndrome, whereas blunt trauma may result in a more asymmetric loss (Chilton & Dagi, 1985). The sensorimotor dysfunction seen in this syndrome can be understood by knowing that the corticospinal tracts and posterior columns decussate (cross) in the medulla, but the spinothalamic fibers cross the spinal cord within one or two spinal segments before ascending to the thalamus.

Other incomplete injuries cause varying degrees of

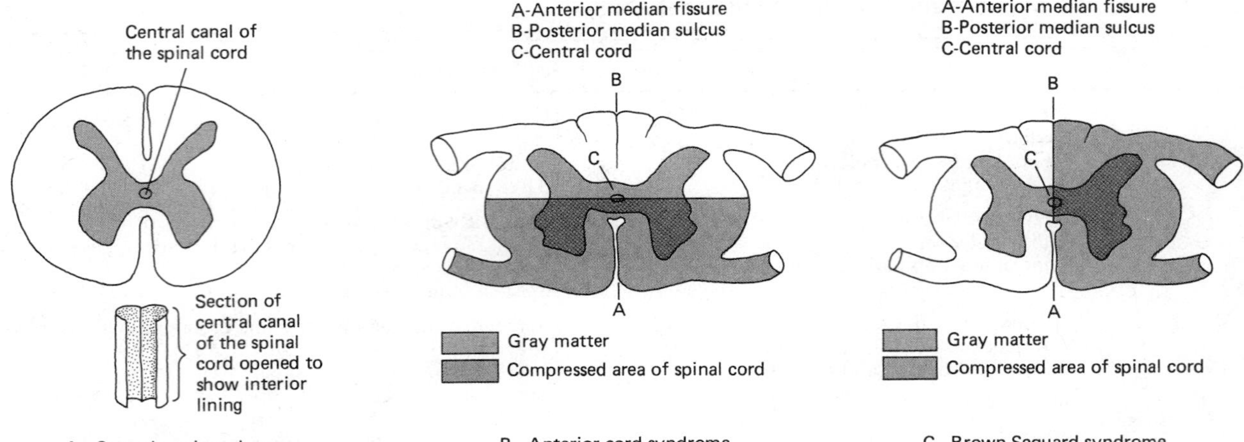

FIGURE 38–1. Three syndromes associated with incomplete cord lesions. (Reproduced by permission from: Lewis, S. M., & Collier, I. C. [Eds.]. *Medical surgical nursing: Assessment and management of clinical problems* [p. 1602]. New York: 1982, McGraw-Hill Book Co.; copyrighted by The C. V. Mosby Co., St. Louis.)

sensorimotor dysfunction, sometimes sparing specific functions.

Spinal cord injury results from compression, contusion, or transection of the spinal cord. The major mechanisms of injury are flexion, flexion–rotation, hyperextension, and compression (axial loading) (Figs. 38–2 and 38–3). Flexion injury with tearing of the posterior ligaments and dislocation is the most unstable injury. This injury is often associated with severe neurologic deficits. Hyperextension injury is the most common mechanism of cord injury.

Vertebral injuries can be classified as simple, compression, and comminuted, or as teardrop fracture, dislocation, subluxation (partial dislocation), and fracture–dislocation (Hickey, 1992; Riggins & Kraus, 1983). Simple fractures usually involve the spinous or transverse processes and are seldom associated with neurologic deficits.

In a wedge or compression fracture the vertebral body is compressed due to hyperflexion injury. Neural compression may or may not occur. This fracture is common in elderly women with osteoporosis. Severe successive fractured vertebral bodies may produce the clinical picture known as "dowager's back," in which the woman's spine is hunched forward.

The burst fracture, or comminuted fracture, results in a shattering of the vertebral body. This fracture is associated with a compression injury and often results in serious SCI.

Dislocation is defined as one vertebra overriding another with unilateral or bilateral facet joint dislocation. The dislocation results from torn or stretched ligaments that allow excessive vertebral movement. Subluxation is a partial or incomplete dislocation. Ligamentous injury and SCI may also be present after subluxation.

Fractures may be stable or unstable. Stability is maintained if all the anterior ligaments and posterior ligaments, plus one additional structure (such as the lamina or spinous process), remain intact (Carol & Ducker, 1987). Even though an injury may be described as acutely unstable, delayed stability can occur after fracture healing. If severe ligamentous damage has occurred, fractures may remain chronically unstable unless they are internally fixed with spinal fusion or internal fixation devices.

PATHOPHYSIOLOGY OF SPINAL CORD INJURY

Spinal cord injury is multiphasic, involving morphologic damage to the spinal cord, hemorrhage, vascular damage, structural changes in the gray and white matter, and subsequent biochemical responses to trauma (Gilbert, 1987).

The hemodynamic changes that occur after SCI are a major factor in the resulting damage to the spinal cord. Autoregulation is lost during the acute phase of injury, profoundly decreasing blood flow and causing ischemic injury to the cord. Concomitant with changes in blood flow are changes in the tissue oxygen tension that ultimately affect metabolic function. As blood flow is compromised, free radicals are released from ischemic areas, increasing the damage in the area of the original injury by means of increased ischemia, vasospasm, and hypoxia. The optimum time for intervention to limit or reverse these destructive processes is within 4 hours of injury, and preferably within 50 to 90 minutes (Senter & Venes, 1979).

In addition to morphologic and histologic changes, the injured spinal cord may also suffer concussion or contusion. Concussion, due to severe shaking of the cord, may cause temporary loss of function lasting 24 to 48 hours. No identifiable neuropathologic changes are usually present (Hickey, 1986). Contusion of the spinal cord is a bruising that includes bleeding, subse-

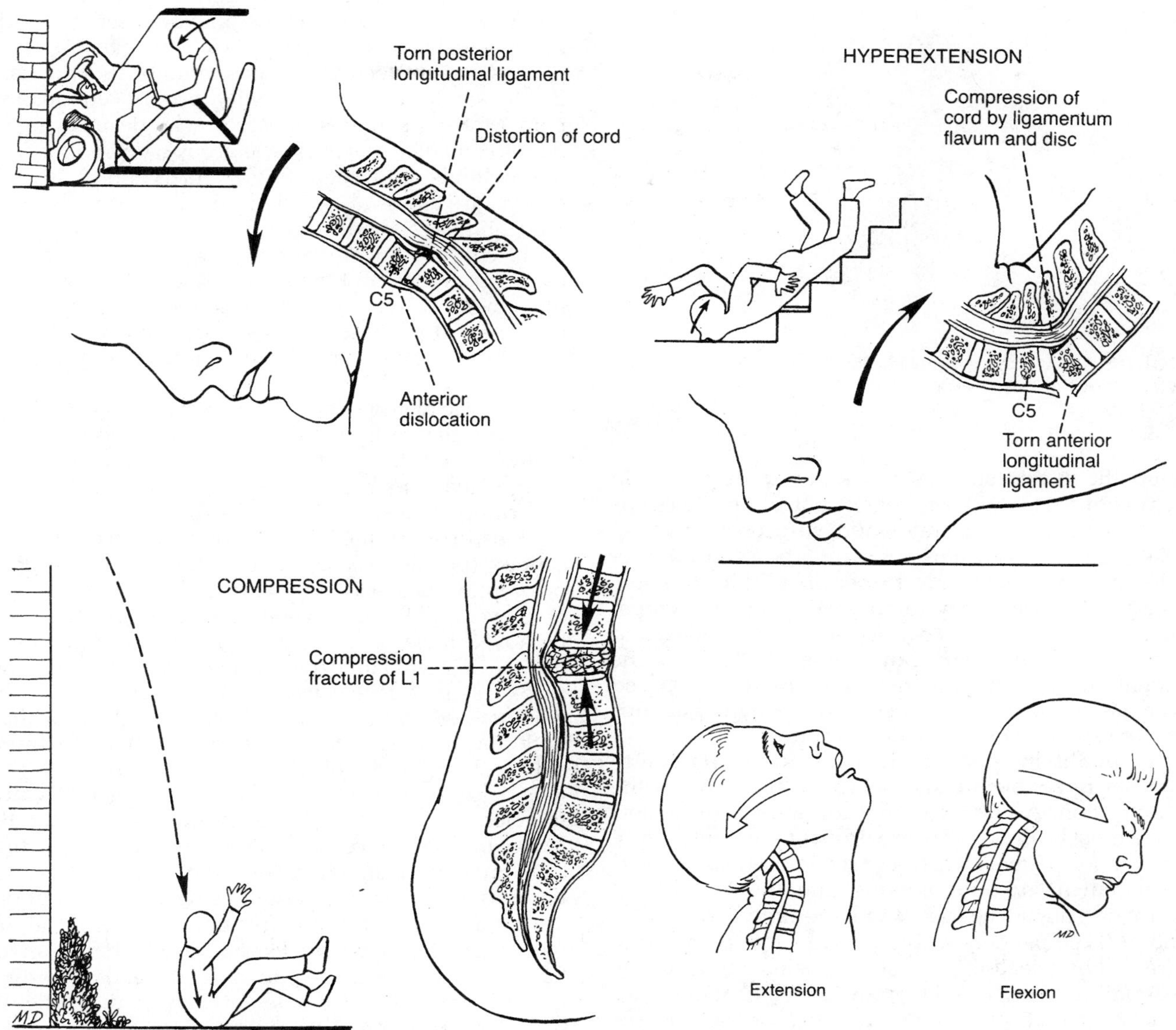

FIGURE 38–2. Closed spinal injury mechanisms. Many situations produce these consequences; this figure shows examples only. (From Luckmann, J., & Sorensen, K. C. [1987]. *Medical–surgical nursing: A psychophysiologic approach* [3rd ed., pp. 417–428]. Philadelphia: W. B. Saunders.)

quent edema, and possible necrosis from the edematous compression. The neurologic involvement depends on the severity of the contusion and necrosis (Hickey, 1986).

SPINAL SHOCK

Bony compression of the spinal cord can result in spinal shock, a temporary suspension of function and reflexes below the level of injury. After acute injury, input from higher brain centers is abruptly lost. Symptoms of spinal shock occur below the level of injury and include flaccid paralysis of all skeletal muscles; loss of all spinal reflexes; loss of pain, proprioception, and other sensations; bowel and bladder dysfunction; and loss of thermoregulation and the ability to perspire.

Spinal shock may last days, weeks, or months. Usually, it subsides within 7 to 10 days. It may be prolonged by infection or other complications (Guttman, 1976). A return of reflexes indicates the end of spinal shock. As spinal shock dissipates, spasticity of involved muscles begins (Nikas, 1988).

Neurogenic Shock

Neurogenic shock occurs after cervical and upper thoracic cord injury. This form of shock is the result of the loss of brain stem and higher center control of the

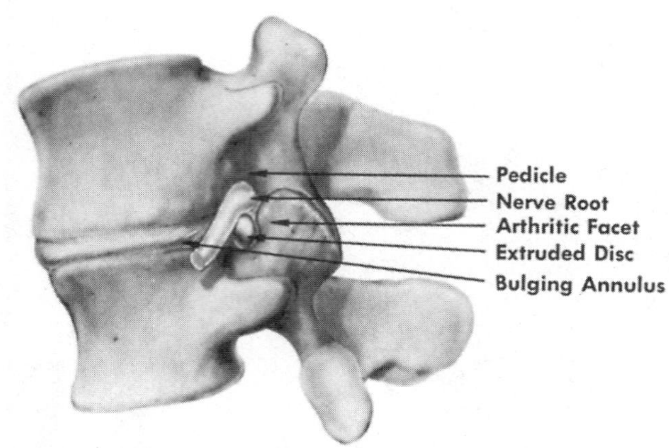

FIGURE 38–3. Normal vertebra. Note the comparatively protected position of the spinal cord relative to the transverse and spinous processes. (From Rothman, R. H., & Simeone, F. A. [Eds.]. [1975]. *The spine: Volume II* [p. 450]. Philadelphia: W. B. Saunders.)

sympathetic nervous system. Input from the brain stem contributes to basic reflex control of vital signs through cardiac accelerator and vasoconstrictive reflexes (Tyson, 1979). Loss of sympathetic outflow results in hypotension due to peripheral vasodilation, bradycardia (secondary to an overriding parasympathetic influence), loss of cardiac accelerator reflex, and loss of ability to sweat below the level of injury. The patient may be hypothermic because of disrupted transmission of impulses between the hypothalamus and the sympathetic nervous system.

In identifying neurogenic shock, it is important to rule out hypovolemic shock, which may worsen the hypotension. An active search for sources of hemorrhage must be done to ensure proper treatment. Hypotension in patients with neurogenic shock reflects displacement of fluid volume into the vasodilated periphery, not a true lack of fluid volume. Overhydration of these patients will not correct low blood pressure and may lead to pulmonary edema or congestive heart failure. The goal of therapy is to combat the cause of lost circulatory volume. The use of vasopressor agents is discussed later under Medical Management.

CLINICAL PRESENTATION

Most patients with acute SCI are in spinal shock. They have lost all sensorimotor and reflex function below the level of injury. Even when transection is incomplete, the patient may appear to have a complete transection. Once spinal cord shock resolves, upper motor neuron (UMN) signs appear. UMN signs include increased muscle tone, flexor spasms in the lower extremities, spasticity of trunk muscles, bowel and bladder incontinence, and increased reflexes. Recovery of voluntary motor function is not temporally associated with spinal shock resolution (Geisler, 1988).

Neurologic Assessment

Assessment of patients with SCI begins at the scene of the accident. It is critical to note the actual time of onset of loss of sensorimotor function. Because treatment within 60 to 90 minutes is thought to limit or reverse neurologic deficits, noting the time of onset can guide the aggressiveness of therapy (Geisler, 1988).

Assessment focuses on sensorimotor function and includes voluntary motor ability, proprioception, and pain. Motor function is assessed by requesting the patient to move all major muscle groups, beginning with the deltoids and biceps (C5 innervation). Muscle groups are assessed by asking the patient to flex, extend, abduct, and adduct each extremity. If the patient is able to move against gravity, resistance is applied by the examiner, and the patient is asked to repeat the movement. A five-point motor scoring system is used to grade muscle function: 5 = normal movement, 3 = movement against gravity, 0 = total paralysis (Fig. 38–4).

Superficial and deep reflexes are also assessed. Although reflex testing does not provide specific information about motor function ability, it aids in identifying spinal shock and differentiates between partial and complete lesions (Nikas, 1988).

Sensory assessment includes evaluation of proprioception (position sense), temperature, and pain. Proprioception is assessed by asking the patient to close both eyes and identify whether the thumb or great toe is moved toward or away from the head (i.e., up or down). Spinothalamic tracts convey pain and temperature sensations. Pain sensation is tested with a pin. The patient closes both eyes, and the face is lightly touched with the pin to determine the patient's ability to differentiate sharp from dull. The pin is then touched to various places on the patient's body, progressing distally, to determine if and where sensation has been lost. Bilateral testing is necessary to rule out sensory sparing. Care must be taken not to break the skin while testing. Light touch is similarly tested using a wisp of cotton.

Initially, sensorimotor function is assessed along with the vital signs to determine whether changes have occurred. Once the patient is stable, daily testing is sufficient. Careful documentation in the patient's record is important to detect neurologic deterioration.

Monitoring of vital signs, including cardiac rhythm, is important during the critical care phase. With the loss of sympathetic outflow, hypotension and bradycardia can occur. An arterial line, pulmonary artery catheter, and electrocardiographic monitoring aid is the assessment of these patients during the spinal and neurologic shock phases (Carol & Ducker, 1987; Dunham & Cowley, 1986). Monitoring temperature carefully is important because hypothermia can result from peripheral vasodilation and loss of thermoregulation.

In addition to hypotension from decreased systemic vascular resistance (SVR), the cardiac preload is decreased. Cardiac output (CO) drops, and tissue perfusion decreases. A pulmonary artery catheter monitors SVR, CO, and pulmonary capillary occlusion pressure.

Heart rate is closely monitored for bradycardia. Atropine should be available at the bedside in case the pulse drops below 40 beats/minute. Left ventricular function can also be depressed. Beta-endorphins re-

UNIVERSITY OF MARYLAND
MIEMSS — UMMS
SPINAL CORD INJURY FLOW SHEET

Muscle Strength

5 Normal
4 Active movement through range of motion against resistance
3 Active movement through range of motion against gravity
2 Active movement through range of motion with gravity eliminated
1 Palpable or visible contraction
0 Total paralysis
U Unable to test strength of extremity

Rectal Tone, Proprioception, Diaphragm

P-Present A-Absent U-Untestable

Medication

Sedation-S
Paralytic-PL
Tranquilizer-T
Pain-P

Sensation

N-Normal
ABN-Abnormal
A-Absent
U-Untestable

Level of bony/ ligamentous injury																
Anatomical Classification					MOTOR LEVEL			***Circled entry means to refer to nurse's note***								
Date																
Time																
Medications																
*Diaphragm (P/A)	C_4															
Deltoid (raise arms) (R/L)	C_5															
*Biceps (elbow flexion) (R/L)	$C_{5.6}$															
Wrist Extensors (R/L)	C_6															
*Triceps (elbow extension) (R/L)	C_7															
*Flexor Digitorum Profundus (finger flexion) (R/L)	C_8															
Hand Intrinsics (finger abduction) (R/L)	T_1															
*Iliopsoas (hip flexion) (R/L)	L_2															
Quadriceps (knee flexion) (R/L)	L_3															
Tibialis Anterior (dorsiflex foot) (R/L)	L_4															
Extensor Hallucis Longus (great toe extenstion) (R/L)	L_5															
*Gastrocnemius (ankle plantar flexion) (R/L)	S_1															
Function	Level															
Proprioception (finger) (R/L)																
Proprioception (toe) (R/L)																
Rectal Tone (P/A)																
INITIALS																
INITIALS/SIGNATURE																

A

FIGURE 38–4. *A* and *B*, Spinal cord injury flow sheet. (*Tested each time.) (Reproduced with permission from University of Maryland; MIEMSS–UMMS.)

SENSATION

DATE														
TIME														
C_2 (R/L)														
C_3 (R/L)														
C_4 (R/L)														
*C_5 (R/L)														
C_6 (thumb and forefinger) (R/L)														
C_7 (middle finger) (R/L)														
C_8 (ring and little finger) (R/L)														
T_1 (R/L)														
T_2 (R/L)														
T_3 (R/L)														
*T_4 (nipple) (R/L)														
T_5 (R/L)														
T_6 (R/L)														
T_7 (R/L)														
T_8 (R/L)														
T_9 (R/L)														
*T_{10} (umbilicus) (R/L)														
T_{11} (R/L)														
T_{12} (R/L)														
L_1 (R/L)														
L_2 (R/L)														
L_3 (R/L)														
L_4 (R/L)														
L_5 (R/L)														
S_1														
S_2														
$S_{3,4,5}$ (sacral sparing)														
Sensory Function														
INITIALS														

B

FIGURE 38–4 *Continued*

leased as a result of SCI have been implicated in exacerbating poor ventricular performance. Left ventricular dysfunction can lead to cardiac dysrhythmias.

Respiratory insufficiency is a serious threat after SCI. Some degree of respiratory insufficiency should be suspected in all quadriplegics and most paraplegics until this is disproved (Carter, 1979). Insufficiency may result from airway obstruction, intercostal or diaphragmatic muscle paralysis, or associated thoracic or tracheal trauma or aspiration.

Respiratory assessment is critical because respiratory failure is the leading cause of death for quadriplegics. Arterial blood gases, chest assessment, vital capacity, and chest radiographs are used to determine the patient's respirtory status. It may be normal for long-term quadriplegics to have a chronically low $Pa{O_2}$ (60–70 mm Hg) and an abnormally high $Pa{CO_2}$ (45–60 mm Hg), but during the immediate postinjury phase a much higher $Pa{O_2}$ of at least 80 mm Hg coupled with normalization of the $Pa{CO_2}$ is recommended.

Assessment of respiratory rate and pattern should be done hourly. Measurements of tidal volume, minute ventilation, and vital capacity should be included in the respiratory assessment.

Laboratory Findings

Laboratory studies include baseline blood studies (serum electrolytes, glucose, hemoglobin, hematocrit, blood gases, and enzymes), urinalysis, and other studies as indicated, including a toxicology screen. This laboratory work provides a baseline for future blood work. If a pulmonary artery catheter is in place, mixed venous blood gases should be monitored.

Diagnostic Procedure

A cervical spine radiograph is obtained right after admission to the hospital. Thoracic and lumbar x-rays should also be taken. These x-rays add to information obtained from subsequent neuroradiologic tests (myelogram, tomograms, computed tomography [CT] scans, and magnetic resonance imaging [MRI]) and facilitate therapeutic decisions.

The x-ray process must be accomplished with the patient in neutral position to prevent further SCI. Immobilization of the spinal column is important to prevent additional trauma. All seven cervical vertebrae must be seen to the top of T1 on anteroposterior and lateral films. It may be necessary to depress the shoulders to visualize C7. A swimmer's view (one arm up and the other at the patient's side, with the x-ray taken through the axilla) may facilitate visualization. Views of the odontoid process (the dens of C2) may require films taken through the open mouth (Fig. 38–5).

If a major neurologic deficit is noted, a myelogram is done to determine any potential sources of pressure on the spinal cord. After reduction, a puncture at the C1–C2 level is made, and radiopaque dye (iophendylate, metrizamide, or iohexal) is instilled with the patient in the supine position (Carol et al., 1980). A CT scan may also be performed with the myelogram.

Computed tomography scans define and delineate bony injury and cord compression. The CT image is extremely helpful in visualizing spinal areas not seen on plain x-ray. Indications for CT scan with myelography include (Dunham & Cowley, 1986):

1. Neurologic deficit in the presence of normal x-rays at the level of the deficit
2. Thoracic spine injury with deficit to allow differentiation of injury of the conus medullaris from cauda equina injury
3. After reduction of the spinal column in patients with a neurologic deficit to ensure adequate bony reduction and cord decompression
4. In preoperative patients if bone is suspected within the spinal canal

Magnetic resonance imaging is a new diagnostic procedure used to determine the extent of SCI. It is difficult to perform MRI on critically ill patients because no metal can contact the patient during the scan. However, newer MRI-compatible devices are being developed. MRI is useful for detecting soft tissue involvement (i.e., spinal cord contusion and edema).

Another diagnostic tool used in SCI is the somatosensory evoked potential (SEP). Evoked responses may establish a prognosis because they reflect neural pathway function. Although SEPs reflect only sensory function, findings in patients with acute cord injury show a high but incomplete correlation with motor function as well (Grundy & Friedman, 1987). In SEP, a peripheral nerve in an arm or leg below the level of injury is stimulated, and the responses of the cord and cerebral cortex are recorded with electrodes. In patients with complete injury, SEPs are absent because no transmissions can pass the site of injury. In patients with an incomplete injury, an altered response is noted. Early persistence and progressive normalization of evoked potentials usually precede clinical improvement (Green et al., 1985).

MEDICAL MANAGEMENT

The medical management of a patient with SCI begins at the scene of the accident. All trauma patients should be treated as if they had SCI until proven otherwise. A thorough assessment at the scene uses the priorities of airway, breathing, and circulation. The goals of treatment are immobilization of the spinal column, stabilization of all systems, ventilatory support, oxygen supplementation, and rapid transportation for emergency care.

Traditionally, fluid replacement is begun in the field using two large-bore (14- to 16-gauge) intravenous lines to treat hypovolemic shock. Dextrose 5% and lactated Ringer's solution is the usual fluid of choice for the initial resuscitation. However, this form of fluid replacement is inappropriate for patients with

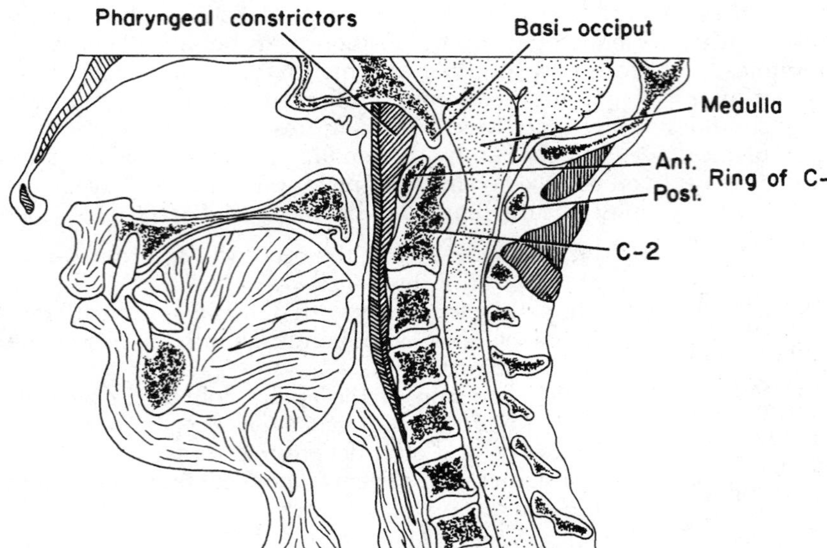

FIGURE 38–5. Sagittal section through the base of the skull and upper cervical spine. Note the ring of CI surrounding the dens of C2; also note the close relationship of the medulla to the basiocciput and upper cervical vertebrae. (From Rothman, R. H., & Simeone, F. A. [Eds.]. [1975]. *The spine: Volume I* (p. 103). Philadelphia: W. B. Saunders.)

SCI because their hypotension arises from systemic vasodilation after neurogenic shock. Cautious fluid management is necessary until hemorrhagic shock is ruled out.

On admission to the emergency department, a report of prehospital management and a history of the injury are rapidly obtained. Immobilization with a spinal board is maintained until spinal x-rays are completed and cleared. The priorities of care are to prevent further injury and reestablish physiologic homeostasis—that is, normalize vital signs and blood gases and establish spinal alignment (Green et al., 1987).

Skeletal cervical traction is useful in patients with upper-level SCI to realign the spinal column and relieve the pressure on the spinal cord from the displaced, bony fragments. Biomechanical knowledge and experience are necessary for optimal application of the traction and to prevent complications (Geisler, 1988).

Patients must be evaluated individually for the amount of instability and damage they have sustained to determine the amount of traction needed. A variety of devices may be used for skeletal traction of cervical vertebrae (Fig. 38–6). At least 10 pounds of traction is initially applied. Weight is applied based on the 5-pound-per-interspace formula (for example, a C5–C6 injury would require between 25 and 30 pounds of traction). Serial x-rays are taken to determine the effect of the traction. Traction weights may be increased to as high as twice the initial weight (Green et al., 1987). If this amount of traction is unable to reduce bony fragment displacement and neurologic deficit persists, muscle relaxants or paralytic agents may aid in reduction. If these agents are used, the patient will be intubated and placed on a ventilator. Open reduction, with or without internal fixation, may be needed. Aggressive reestablishment of spinal alignment is essential for physiologic homeostasis.

The decision to operate on patients with SCI depends on the type of injury and the patient's overall hemodynamic status. Once emergency department stabilization has been accomplished, decisions about immediate or delayed surgery or conservative therapy can be made.

In SCI patients with a flexion or flexion–compression cervical fracture, closed cervical reduction is usually successful. If there are no associated fractures (i.e., unilateral or bilateral locked facet joints), traction is maintained until posterior cervical wire fixation or bony fusion can be performed in the operating room.

Patients with severe ligamentous injuries, compression unrelieved by traction, or a burst fracture require rapid surgical intervention. An anterior corpectomy (removal of the vertebral body) and fusion are performed. Progressive neurologic deficit from edema or intrathecal hemorrhage may require emergency decompression laminectomy (Fig. 38–7). Early surgery may preserve, improve, or restore spinal cord function (Hickey, 1986).

Thoracic and upper lumbar injuries may require surgical intervention using a variety of methods to stabilize the injury. Autograft or allograft bone may be used to perform spinal fusion. A variety of internal fixation devices may be used to stabilize the spine, including Harrington or Luque rods, Dwyer instrumentation, methylmethacrylate, and surgical wire (Fig. 38–8).

Once the airway, breathing, and circulation are stable, the patient should be started on a high dose of methylprednisolone. A bolus of 30 mg/kg is administered over 1 hour, followed by a 23-hour infusion of 5.4 mg/kg per hour. This treatment must be started within 8 hours of the injury to be effective (Brackman et al., 1990). The patient with a neurologic deficit is usually transferred to the critical care unit. The hemodynamic and pulmonary status of the patient is of

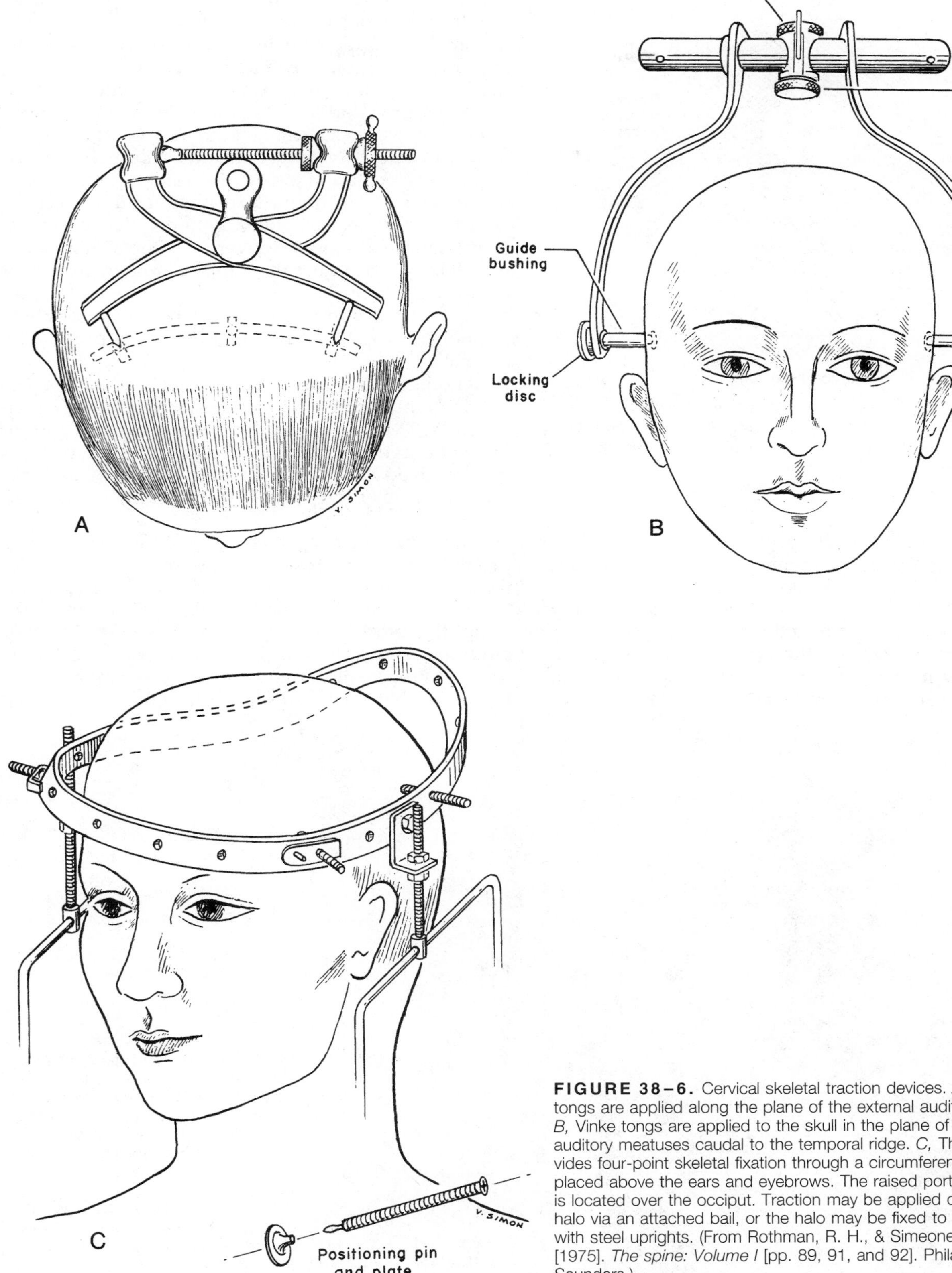

FIGURE 38–6. Cervical skeletal traction devices. *A,* Crutchfield tongs are applied along the plane of the external auditory meatuses. *B,* Vinke tongs are applied to the skull in the plane of the external auditory meatuses caudal to the temporal ridge. *C,* The halo provides four-point skeletal fixation through a circumferential steel ring placed above the ears and eyebrows. The raised portion of the ring is located over the occiput. Traction may be applied directly to the halo via an attached bail, or the halo may be fixed to a body jacket with steel uprights. (From Rothman, R. H., & Simeone, F. A. [Eds.]. [1975]. *The spine: Volume I* [pp. 89, 91, and 92]. Philadelphia: W. B. Saunders.)

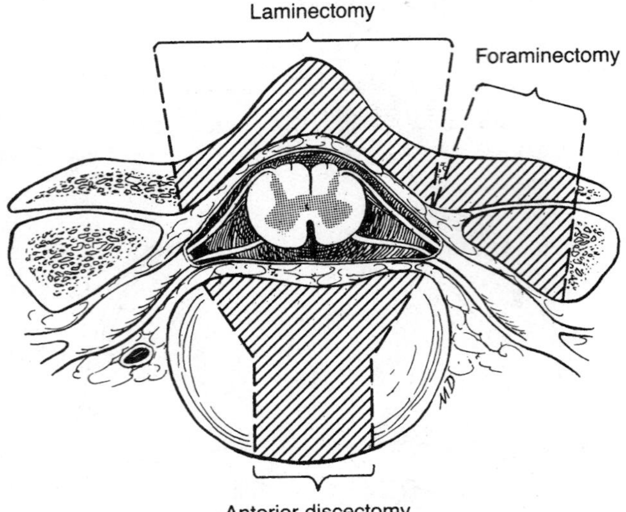

FIGURE 38–7. Operative approaches to the spinal cord. (From Luckmann, J., & Sorensen, K. C. [1987]. *Medical–surgical nursing: A psychophysiologic approach* [3rd ed., p. 537]. Philadelphia: W. B. Saunders.)

major concern. The goal of care is to prevent life-threatening complications while maximizing function of all body systems. A holistic approach to care throughout the acute phase is needed because every system of the body is affected by SCI.

The intensive care of these patients has changed dramatically in the last decade due to the realization that hypotension and bradycardia are the result of neurogenic shock. Hypotension is not the result of circulatory volume deficit but is secondary to vasodilation from lack of sympathetic outflow. The use of inotropic drugs rather than fluid resuscitation is the treatment of choice. Dopamine hydrochloride (3–5 mg/kg per minute) may be supplemented with dobutamine hydrochloride in low doses to maintain mean arterial blood pressures of 80 to 90 mm Hg with an increased cardiac output (1–1.5 times normal) (Geisler, 1988). Augmentation of cardiovascular dynamics is maintained for 72 hours to counteract the effects of neurogenic shock and enhance spinal cord perfusion to promote neurologic recovery. Gilbert (1987) states that dobutamine rather than dopamine is preferred for hemodynamic push because it does not increase pulmonary vascular resistance, which could contribute to pulmonary capillary extravasation and pulmonary edema.

Another study done by Geisler and colleagues (1991) demonstrated that monosialotetrahexoxylganglioside (GM-1), a protein that causes axonal sprouting, enhanced the functional recovery of the patients who received the drug. More study is needed to determine the true efficacy of GM-1 in treating spinal cord injury.

The future of drug therapy holds a great deal of promise in SCI treatment. Lazaroids, 21-aminosteroids, have been used in experimental studies and have shown positive results (Hall, 1988; Tator, 1992). Drugs that block glutamate receptors, such as MK-801, have been shown to reduce the damage caused by the release of this toxic amino acid (Faden & Simon, 1988). It is clear that further research into the exact mecha-

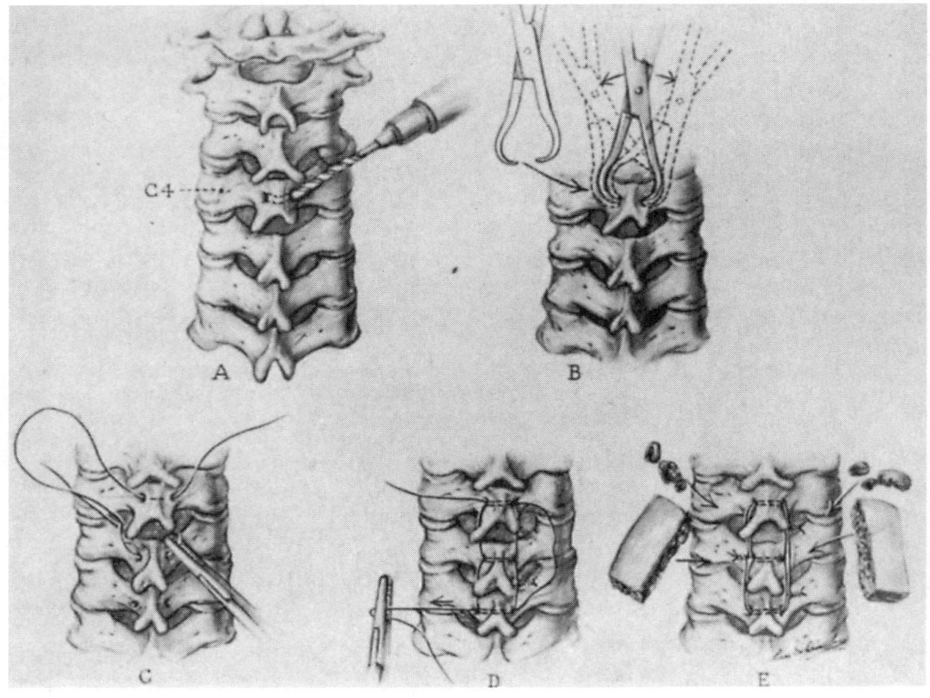

FIGURE 38–8. Posterior interspinous fusion. *A,* Holes are drilled in the outer cortex of the spinous process adjacent to the lamina. *B,* The drill holes are connected with a towel clip. *C,* Wires are passed through the holes and adjacent vertebrae and are twisted in place. *D,* One additional wire is passed, to surround all of the vertebrae involved in the area of intended fusion. *E,* Corticocancellous strips of bone graft are laid down about the posterior elements in the area of intended fusion. (From Rothman, R. H., & Simone, F. A. [Eds.]. [1975]. *The spine: Volume I* [p. 128]. Philadelphia: W. B. Saunders.)

nisms that cause the SCI will lead to further developments in the pharmacologic treatments available.

Cardiovascular System

Bradycardia in patients with SCI complicates increased vascular capacitance and decreased circulatory volumes (Nikas, 1988). Pulse rate may be as low as 40 beats/minute. Slow heart rates are usually tolerated by patients with adequate volume replacement and an adequate cardiac index. Atropine sulfate may be used when hemodynamic changes accompany the low heart rate. Suctioning or turning that causes a vasovagal response with a heart rate below 40 beats/minute should be treated with atropine sulfate.

Although not directly related to cardiovascular function, the sympathectomy resulting from SCI may result in loss of thermoregulation. Hypothermia and poikilothermia are frequently seen in patients with spinal shock. Poikilothermia occurs when the patient's temperature rises and falls in response to the environmental temperature (Nikas, 1982). Normothermia should be maintained. If the patient is hypothermic, warming intravenous fluids and the use of warming lamps and blankets can elevate the patient's temperature. Hyperthermia may result in serious metabolic strain. Cooling may be encouraged by removing excess clothing, altering the environmental temperature, or judicious use of a cooling blanket.

The peripheral vascular system is also affected in patients with SCI. Decreased blood flow increases the risk of venous thrombosis in the legs and pelvis. Venous stasis, intimal damage, and hypercoagulability are reported to exist in all patients with SCI (McCagg, 1986). Prevention of deep vein thrombosis (DVT) is a goal throughout hospitalization. Diagnosis of DVT is difficult because the usual associated signs and symptoms are unreliable. Daily calf and thigh measurements are recommended. Definitive diagnostic studies are indicated if an increase of 2 cm or more in circumference occurs (McCagg, 1986).

There is no agreement on the most effective way to prevent DVT. Elastic hose, pneumatic calf compression devices, elevation, and kinetic therapy have all been used (Becker et al., 1987; Green et al., 1983). Prophylactic anticoagulation has been advocated as a form of definitive therapy (Hull et al., 1982). Anticoagulation may be avoided because of its potential for complications involving hemorrhage, especially in multiple-trauma patients or preoperative or postoperative patients. Low-dose heparin (5,000–7,000 units every 12 hours) is recommended in high-risk patients (e.g., those with long bone fractures, the elderly, or the obese) (Nikas, 1986).

Respiratory System

Altered respiratory function is a major problem for patients with high thoracic or cervical SCI. Injuries at or above C4 result in ventilator dependency because of the inability to breathe spontaneously due to lost phrenic nerve function and paralysis of intercostal muscles. Edema or hemorrhage can result in compression of the spinal cord in patients with injuries below C4, thus interfering with respiration. Prophylactic intubation (nasoendotracheal) is used in quadriplegics (Geisler & Salcman, 1987; Green et al., 1985). Paralysis of the abdominal and intercostal muscles aggravates the respiratory insufficiency, leading to ineffective cough and retention of secretions. Respiratory management of these patients must be aggressive, routinely using chest physiotherapy every 4 hours. Ventilatory support is used to maintain normal blood gases.

Aspiration and pneumonia are common complications in patients with SCI. Aspiration may occur at the time of injury in water or diving accidents, or vomitus may be aspirated in motor vehicle accidents. Pneumonia usually occurs within the first few weeks of hospitalization resulting from hypostasis of secretions due to immobility. Pulmonary edema may follow aspiration or pneumonia but is most commonly caused by fluid overload during resuscitation. Pulmonary emboli occur in about 13% of these patients and are seen in the first few weeks after injury (Gilbert, 1987).

Physical assessment of the chest, including observation, inspection, palpation, percussion, and auscultation, should be done with the vital signs for the initial 72 hours. Chest expansion and abdominal movement should be observed to determine whether accessory muscles are being used for respirations. Bedside pulmonary function studies can determine respiratory function and the need for ventilatory support. Tidal volume, inspiratory and expiratory reserve volume, residual volume, total lung capacity, functional residual capacity, and vital capacity are assessed. Serial blood gas analysis aids in determining the need for ventilatory support. Pulse oximetry may also be used for continuous monitoring of Sa_{O_2}. Daily chest radiographs rule out the presence of pulmonary complications or allow early treatment of complications.

As mentioned earlier, all body systems are affected by SCI. Identification of cardiovascular and pulmonary complications is a high priority in critical care of these patients because they may be life threatening. However, care of patients with SCI also includes identifying and managing complications of the gastrointestinal, urinary, musculoskeletal, and integumentary systems.

Gastrointestinal System

Gastrointestinal complications after SCI include gastric dilation, paralytic ileus, and stress ulcers. A nasogastric, or sump, tube is placed while the patient is in the emergency department to decompress the stomach. Patients are usually started on intravenous hyperalimentation within 24 to 48 hours. When peristalsis returns, nasogastric feedings are begun, emphasizing calories, protein, and high fiber.

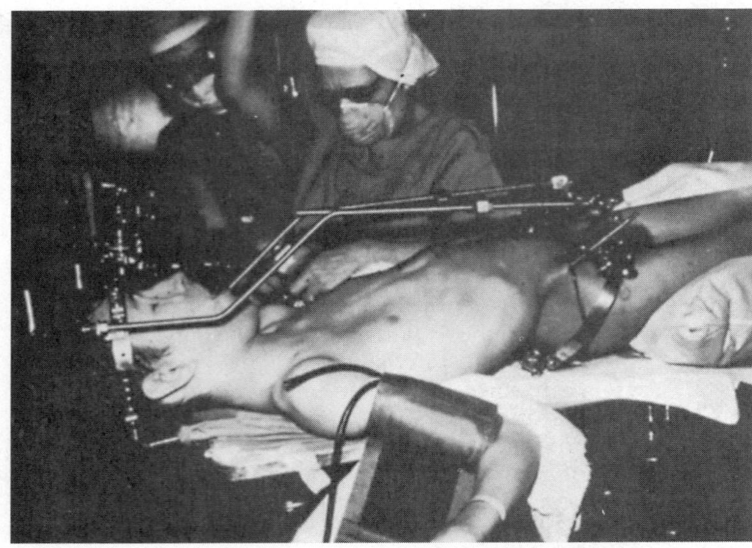

FIGURE 38–9. Halopelvic external fixator. (From Rothman, R. H., & Simeone, F. A. [Eds.]. [1975]. *The spine: Volume I* [p. 304]. Philadelphia: W. B. Saunders.)

Stress ulcers occur in 10% to 20% of patients with SCI (Nikas, 1988). These are thought to be related to vagal stimulation of gastric acid release during spinal shock. Frequent testing of gastric Ph and intravenous H_2 receptor blocking agents (ranitidine, cimetidine, fomotidine) or antacids are used to prevent gastrointestinal hemorrhage. Monitoring for melena and hematochezia is done for all patients with SCI, including hematests of all stools.

Urinary System

Areflexia caused by spinal shock leads to urinary retention. An indwelling catheter is placed on admission. The catheter is maintained until the hemodynamic push is stopped. Once hemodynamic stability is attained, scheduled intermittent catheterizations should be initiated (McCagg, 1986).

Musculoskeletal System

Management of musculoskeletal problems in the intensive care period is a priority. Primary concerns include ensuring stability of the spine and managing the consequences of immobility. Maintaining the mobility of the paralyzed joints while maintaining spinal stability is the key to care of these patients. A variety of devices may be used to maintain spinal stability besides traction and surgery. These include halopelvic external fixators (Fig. 38–9), hyperextension body casts, Minerva jacket casts, and many forms of orthoses.

Integumentary System

Prevention of skin breakdown is another important consideration in the intensive care unit, as it is throughout the patient's lifetime. Pressure necrosis can prolong spinal shock, complicate spasticity, delay rehabilitation, and lead to life-threatening systemic infection (Nikas, 1988). Frequent turning and use of Stryker frames, rotational therapy, and other specialty beds, such as low–air-loss types, can be useful in preventing pressure necrosis and skin breakdown.

Other Experimental Therapies

Hypothermia of the injured cord has also been studied. A small pad through which cooled saline solution is circulated is positioned surgically on the epidural level of the newly injured spinal cord for 3 to 4 hours, or fluid may be directly perfused through a C1–C2 stick and a lumbar drain. The temperature of the coolant is 6°C in most research protocols. The purpose of the procedure is to produce local vasoconstriction, decrease edema formation, and reduce intrinsic destructive processes (Hickey, 1986). Hypothermia in humans with SCI has improved neurologic function in some patients (Hansebout et al., 1984). This therapy requires further study to demonstrate its efficacy. One major problem with this therapy is the potential for infection from prolonged exposure of the spinal cord.

Hyperbaric oxygen therapy is a medical treatment in which the entire body is placed in a chamber under increased atmospheric pressure, and the patient breathes pure oxygen (Hickey, 1986). This treatment has been tried in patients with SCI in the belief that it may reduce ischemia and subsequent cord destruction by improving oxygen diffusion. Studies show conflicting results with this therapy (DeJesus-Greenberg, 1980; Gamache et al., 1981). Further study is needed to document the benefit of this therapy.

NURSING MANAGEMENT

The care of patients with acute SCI is complex because of the effect of this injury on all body systems. During the critical care phase the priorities of nursing care focus on the appearance of changes in major organ systems. The goals of nursing care are to prevent complications and prepare the patient for rehabilitation.

Altered Tissue Perfusion: Spinal Cord

Spinal cord tissue perfusion is altered due to inflammatory responses after injury, sympathetic blockade, and changes in intrathecal oxygen tension.

EXPECTED OUTCOME. Blood pressure and Pa_{O_2} remain within normal limits for these patients; high cardiac output is maintained (1–1.5 times normal); urinary output exceeds 0.5 mL/kg/hour.

Careful monitoring of all hemodynamic parameters is essential. Titration of vasopressor agents to maintain optimal hemodynamic status is often accomplished by the critical care nurse. Special attention should be paid to fluid and electrolyte balance, and careful monitoring of intake and output is essential. Fluid replacement should be judiciously accomplished to maintain adequate blood volume without risking pulmonary edema.

The patient's mental status should be closely monitored as a reflection of cerebral perfusion. Supplemental oxygen therapy should be provided during the first 24 hours and as indicated thereafter. Maintenance of normothermia during neurogenic shock prevents increased metabolic demand from hyperthermia. Vital signs should be monitored every 4 hours or more often as needed.

Ineffective Breathing Pattern

Breathing patterns may be altered due to upper level SCI (C4 and above) and because of possible loss of innervation of the intercostals and diaphragm. In patients with lesions above T1, the diaphragm is the only muscle of respiration. Gastric dilation and paralytic ileus may also limit respiratory excursion. When only the diaphragm is active, fatigue may also contribute to ineffective breathing patterns.

EXPECTED OUTCOME. Ventilation will be adequate as demonstrated by normal arterial blood gases, absence of respiratory distress, absence of pulmonary complications, absence of fever, and lungs that are clear to auscultation.

Physical assessment of the chest, including observation, inspection, palpation, percussion, and auscultation, should be done along with the vital signs during the first 72 hours after injury. Any changes from baseline respiratory function should be noted and reported, particularly the depth and pattern of respirations. As the injured spinal cord becomes edematous, respiratory arrest due to impaired innervation can occur in any patient with a cervical fracture. Serial vital capacity measurements are the most accurate method of predicting mechanical pulmonary failure. When serial vital capacity measurements demonstrate progressive decline, elective intubation and mechanical ventilation are required. Arterial blood gases or pulse oximetry are carefully monitored to detect impaired oxygenation and to guide the type of ventilatory support used. Initially the Pa_{O_2} should be maintained at or above 80 mm Hg because systemic hypoxemia may exacerbate the SCI. Supplemental oxygen should be provided for the first 24 hours and as needed. The Pa_{CO_2} must be monitored carefully because quadriplegic patients retain CO_2 when they hypoventilate. Daily chest x-rays are done to rule out pulmonary complications and to allow early treatment of complications.

Assessment of the abdomen is important because abdominal distention interferes with respiratory excursion. An abdominal binder may be helpful in providing external support.

Ineffective Airway Clearance

Airway clearance may be impaired due to flaccid paralysis of the abdominal and intercostal muscles, which reduces the strength of the patient's cough (Richmond, 1985).

EXPECTED OUTCOME. Patients will participate in assisted cough and will not show indications of retained secretions—that is, they are afebrile, the Pa_{CO_2} is within normal limits, and the sputum is clear and is present in normal amounts.

The "quad-assist" cough augments the abdominal muscles during the expiratory phase of a cough. As in the Heimlich maneuver, the nurse places a fist or heel of the hand between the umbilicus and the xiphoid process and presses downward and upward when the patient coughs. The patient is instructed to take a deep, slow breath and repeat it three times; then, instead of exhaling, the patient coughs on the last breath as the nurse assists. Performing this intervention hourly effectively assists patients in clearing respiratory secretions. Standard nursing interventions of turning and ensuring adequate hydration aid in mobilizing and liquefying respiratory secretions. Patients and family members need to be instructed in the need for frequent pulmonary hygiene, fluid intake, and turning to mobilize secretions.

Aggressive chest physiotherapy is needed to mobilize and clear secretions to prevent atelectasis. Care must be taken when the patient is in the head-down position for chest physiotherapy because of the risk of severe bradycardia resulting from vagal stimulation. Close monitoring of vital signs during and after therapy is necessary. Patients who are able to do so should be encouraged to use incentive spirometry hourly.

If the patient has an endotracheal tube or tracheostomy, suctioning will clear secretions. Care is needed when suctioning because of the vasovagal response, which may result in severe bradycardia.

Impaired Physical Mobility

Mobility is altered due to total loss of motor function below the level of injury during spinal shock. Flaccid paralysis progresses to spastic paralysis following spinal shock. If the patient is not paralyzed, immobility may be necessary to prevent SCI.

EXPECTED OUTCOME. Further injury of the spinal cord does not occur, and range of motion of all joints is maintained.

Continuing assessment of motor function is critical during the acute phase. In-depth muscle testing should be performed every 4 hours. All major muscle groups should be graded for strength on a five-point scale (i.e., 0 equals no movement and 5 equals movement against full resistance). Decreased motor function may accompany swelling at the injury site, loss of vertebral alignment, or intrathecal hematoma formation. Consistent documentation is important to identify trends of dysfunction. Significant changes should be promptly reported to the physician.

Immobilization can be maintained with tongs (see Fig. 38–6). As with other bony injuries, observing the principles of traction is essential, including providing the ordered amount of weight and ensuring that the weights hang free. Maintenance of spinal stability is facilitated with mechanical beds. Two commonly used beds are Stryker frames (see Fig. 38–10), which turn from supine to prone, and kinetic therapy beds (Fig. 38–11), which constantly rotate in a 60- to 60-degree arc. Turning or rotation in these beds should not begin until bony alignment is documented by x-ray and the issue is discussed with the physician.

The halopelvic external fixator (see Fig. 38–9) may be used to maintain vertebral stability. This fixator is a static traction device that permits increased patient mobility. A metal halo ring is secured to the outer table of the skull. Metal struts attach the halo to a metal pelvic ring, which is secured to the bony pelvis with Steinmann pins. Depending on the stability of the fracture, the halo may eventually be attached to a body cast or sheepskin-lined plastic vest for cervical immobilization.

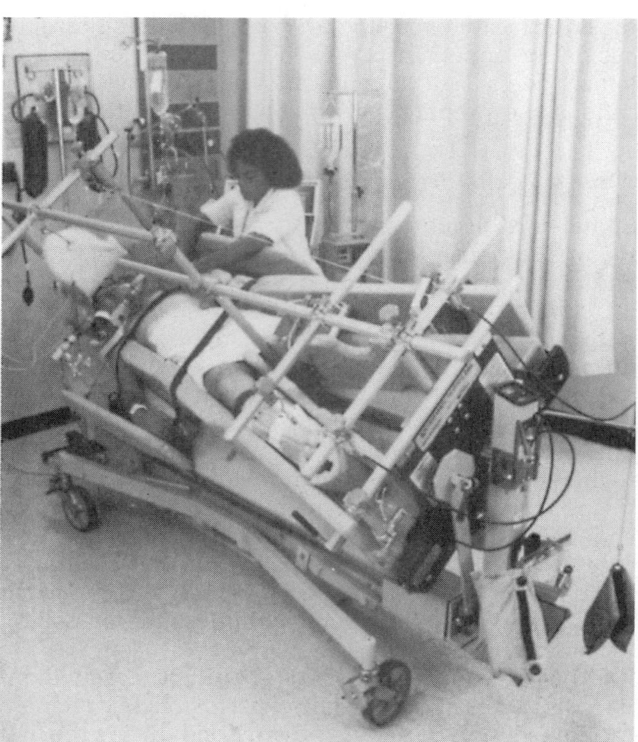

FIGURE 38–11. Kinetic therapy treatment table. (Reproduced by permission from Lewis, S. M., and Collier, I. C. [Eds.]. *Medical surgical nursing: Assessment and management of clinical problems* [p. 1607]. New York, 1987, McGraw-Hill Book Co.; copyrighted by the C. V. Mosby Co., St. Louis.)

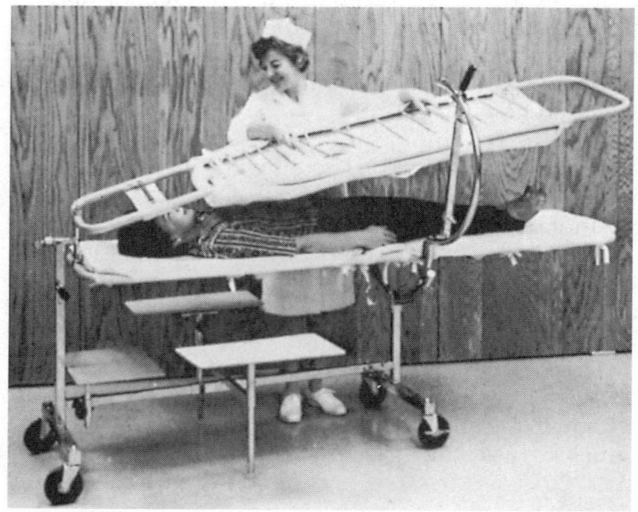

FIGURE 38–10. Stryker frame. (Reproduced with permission from: Lewis, S. M., & Collier, I. C. [Eds.]. *Medical surgical nursing: Assessment and management of clinical problems.* New York, 1987, McGraw-Hill Book Co.; copyrighted by the C. V. Mosby Company, St. Louis.)

Passive range-of-motion exercises should be done every 4 hours to prevent contractures. Poor positioning contributes to contracture formation. Joints should be positioned in the neutral position whenever possible. Adjunctive devices, antirotation boots, antidrop foot splints, trochanter rolls, high-top tennis shoes, and wrist splints are useful in maintaining the correct position. Joints with partial or complete function should also be placed through range of motion. Instructing the patient and family about the need for range-of-motion exercises increases the potential for prevention of contractures of nonparalyzed areas.

Potential for Injury: Deep Vein Thrombosis Due to Venostasis

EXPECTED OUTCOME. Lower extremity circumference will be monitored daily, and increases of more than 2 cm will be promptly reported; antithrombus regimen will be maintained.

Circumference of the lower extremities should be checked daily. Standard measurement sites are ensured by marking the positions on the legs with permanent markers. Measures should be made at midcalf and midthigh on each leg.

Promoting venous return is facilitated by range-of-motion exercises, which should be done every 4 hours. Antiembolism hose or alternating pneumatic pressure devices on the legs aid venous return. Elevating the entire lower extremity 10 to 15 degrees prevents venostasis. Kinetic treatment beds, which rotate the patient for up to 20 hours a day, also promote circulation in the patient with SCI (Green et al., 1983). Mobilization from bed to chair is still the best mechanism for decreasing the cardiovascular sequelae of immobility.

Potential Alteration in Skin Integrity Due to Paralysis and Immobility

EXPECTED OUTCOME. Skin will remain dry, intact, and nonerythemic. Patient and family will verbalize understanding of the need for frequent repositioning.

Thorough assessment of the skin should be accomplished each time the patient is turned and positioned. A turning and positioning schedule should be established and posted at the bedside to ensure that all personnel maintain the same turning routine. Turning should be done every 2 hours unless it is contraindicated.

Encouraging self-care within the patient's abilities will decrease feelings of complete dependence. When possible, incorporating the patient and family in goal setting and decision making increases the patient's sense of autonomy.

The patient should be informed by the physician about the degree of injury, the diagnosis, and the prognosis as soon as possible after the injury. The family or significant others should be part of these discussions. This information will not ease the patient's fears but does allow him or her to begin to grasp the reality of the situation and thus begin to deal with fear (Green et al., 1985).

Patients who are able to talk should be encouraged to verbalize their fears. The nurse should be a receptive listener, making time for the patient to verbalize concerns. The patient's self-worth should be reinforced by making time to spend talking with the patient.

Ineffective Thermoregulation

Thermoregulation may be altered due to loss of hypothalamic control of the sympathetic nervous system in patients with SCI above the level of T6.

EXPECTED OUTCOME. Patients with poikilothermia will receive careful monitoring, and normothermia will be maintained.

Rectal or tympanic membrane temperature should be monitored every 4 hours during the first 72 hours after injury. Palpation of skin surfaces to note areas of warmth, coolness, and moisture augments temperature monitoring.

The nurse should be alert to environmental temperatures, adding blankets when it is cool and removing bedclothes when it is warm. Drafts should be eliminated when possible. Tepid baths should be used first in trying to reduce a fever. Care must be exercised with hypothermia blankets because these may result in a precipitous drop in the patient's temperature.

Constipation Due to Changes in Neural Function and Immobility After SCI

EXPECTED OUTCOMES. The patient will maintain normal bowel habits or pass a formed stool every other day without straining.

The location and degree of SCI determine the degree of alteration in bowel elimination. Bowel sounds generally return within 2 days of injury, but elimination may not return. Patients with cervical or thoracic SCI lose the ability to feel the urge to defecate, but reflex defecation activity may remain intact in patients with nonsacral injuries. Sacral cord injuries may destroy the defecation reflex and anal sphincter tone, resulting in fecal retention and oozing of stool through a flaccid anal sphincter.

A bowel regimen is begun when peristalsis returns. The patient is given a psyllium hydrophilic mucilloid and stool softener daily. Every other day at the same time of day, the patient is given a cup of warm fluid to drink to stimulate the gastrocolic or duodenocolic reflex. If this is unsuccessful, a glycerine suppository is inserted, and digital stimulation of the internal anal sphincter provided. If this is unsuccessful, a laxative or bisacodyl suppository may be required. Use of the bowel regimen makes it possible to establish bowel continence. Avoid the use of enemas, which will dilate the rectum and sigmoid colon. Digital disimpaction may occasionally be necessary. Caution should be exercised when the anus is stimulated because it may create autonomic dysreflexia.

Alterations in Urinary Elimination

Urinary elimination may be altered by disruption of normal neurologic bladder innervation by the SCI. Areflexia resulting from spinal cord shock causes urinary retention. Sacral reflexes normally causing bladder contraction and detrusor muscle opening are lost (McCagg, 1986).

EXPECTED OUTCOME. Urinary output will be maintained at 0.5 mL/kg/hour when an indwelling catheter is in place; there are no findings of urinary tract infection on assessment.

When the patient with SCI is on vasopressor therapy, an indwelling catheter is used. This catheter is removed as soon as possible because it contributes to bladder atonicity, making later reflex emptying more difficult.

Intermittent catheterization should be started as quickly as possible. Criteria for such a program include negative urine culture; patient tolerance of fluid restriction to 1,800 to 2,200 mL/24 hours; and no use of diuretics. The goal of the program is to stimulate reflex emptying of the full bladder. The need for catheterization is based on the amount of urine obtained from each catheterization, usually done every 4 hours initially. Frequency of catheterization decreases as the bladder gains automaticity. After resolution of spinal cord shock, the patient may void spontaneously between catheterizations.

Potential for Injury

Autonomic dysreflexia may occur due to an uninhibited response of the sympathetic nervous system resulting from lack of higher-level control in paraplegic and quadriplegic patients with upper level injury (above T6) (Fig. 38–12).

EXPECTED OUTCOME. Signs of autonomic dysreflexia are rapidly identified and treated before complications occur.

Autonomic dysreflexia may result from a variety of stimuli, including an overdistended bladder, infection, skin stimulation, pressure necrosis, pain, sudden changes in environmental temperature, and, most commonly, a full rectum (Mason, 1981). Symptoms of autonomic dysreflexia include a sudden onset of severe headache, hypertension, bradycardia, tachycardia, diaphoresis and flushing above the level of injury, pallor and coolness below the level of injury, nasal stuffiness, and unusual apprehension. Hypertension may be so severe that it results in cerebral hemorrhage or myocardial infarction (Hickey, 1986). This is most likely to occur in the first year after injury, but it can occur anytime after spinal shock subsides. Patients and families need to be taught that this problem can occur, how to identify it, and the need for rapid intervention.

Once identified, these patients should have the head elevated to a sitting position and the blood pressure and pulse closely monitored. The physician should be promptly notified. If possible, the source should be identified and removed (i.e., check for distended bladder and perform intermittent catheterization; check the indwelling catheter for kinks or plugs). Ganglionic blocking agents may be required to disrupt the hyperreflexic state. Hydralazine hydrochloride, 20 mg, may be ordered and should be given slowly to avoid abrupt hypotension. Diazoxide may also be used. If this situation occurs during a bowel movement, a local anesthetic should be applied to the anal canal to reduce further stimuli (Zejdlik, 1983).

Self-Care Deficit: Partial Due to Partial Loss of Motor Function

EXPECTED OUTCOME. Patient will participate maximally in self-care, the degree of participation being based on his or her physiologic capabilities. The patient will demonstrate feelings of self-worth and exercise some degree of control over his or her care.

Patients with SCI experience a temporary but total loss of physical ability to perform some activities of daily living. The patient is initially dependent on others for most self-care. This dependence decreases self-worth, interferes with role performance, and increases feelings of helplessness, powerlessness, and humiliation (Walleck, 1988). Giving the patient as much con-

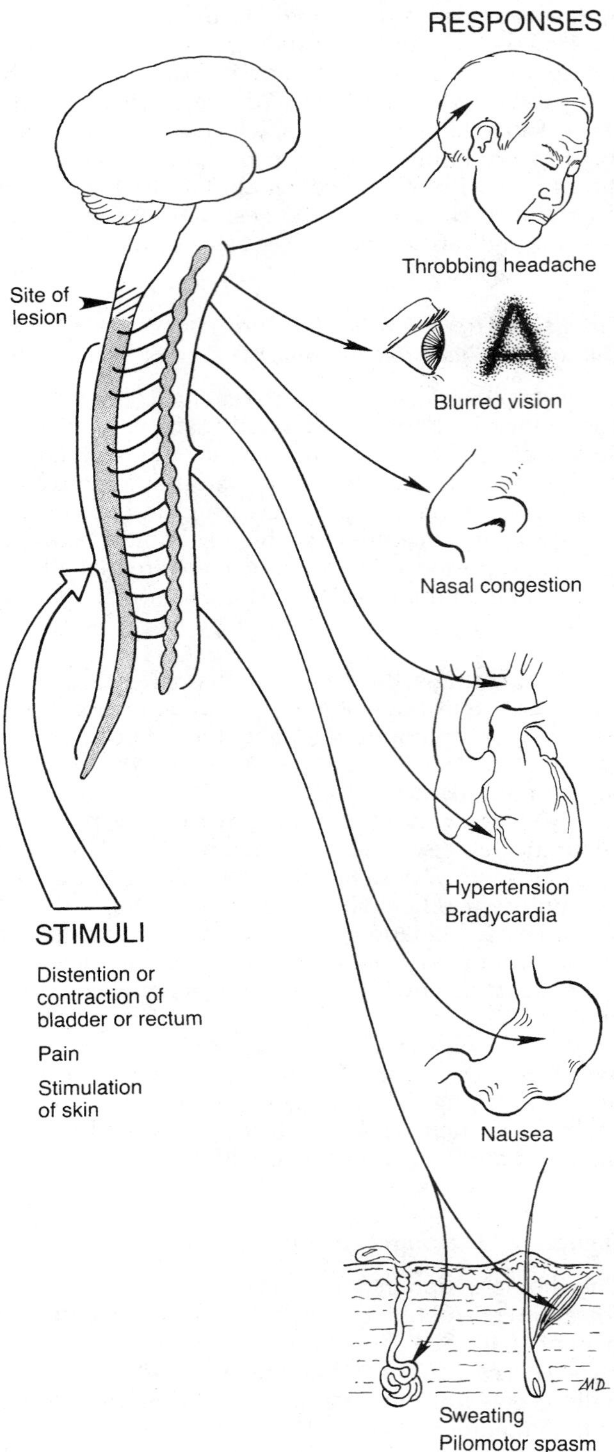

FIGURE 38–12. Causes of hyperreflexia and assessment findings. (From Luckmann, J., & Sorensen, K. C. [1987]. *Medical–surgical nursing: A psychophysiologic approach* [3rd ed., p. 434]. Philadelphia: W. B. Saunders.)

trol as possible over his or her life is essential. Include the patient in planning of care and goal setting; provide instruction that will allow the patient to make knowledgeable decisions. Contracting with the patient and establishing behavior modification programs may be useful in setting limits for some patients.

These patients are often depressed because of their forced dependency. Be honest and consistent about describing the patient's condition, and share realistic goals for the patient's future. Individualize the patient's care to meet the patient's needs. Beginning to teach patients to manage their disability in the intensive care unit (ICU) aids adaptation.

Sexual Dysfunction Due to Disruption of Normal Sexuality

EXPECTED OUTCOME. Patient verbalizes understanding of potential for sexual functioning and demonstrates satisfactory adjustment.

Although sexuality may not be a high-priority issue in the care of ICU patients, it may be of great concern to the patient. Sexuality is a complex physical and emotional response. During the critical care phase, the nurse should be aware that the patient may be worried about sexual function. Sexual counseling is usually delayed until the intermediate phase of care. Create a climate of openness; answer any questions honestly. The degree of sexual function varies with the level of injury and the sex of the patient. Although the capability for orgasm is frequently lost, the ability to bear children remains for most women. For men, orgasm is lost and the ability to reproduce is severely limited, but the capability to engage in sexual intercourse may remain. Reassure the patient that sexual counseling will be available later.

SUMMARY

Care of the patient with SCI has changed dramatically during the past decade. ICU care is complex, and these patients demand aggressive medical and nursing management. These patients represent a unique challenge to the critical care nurse. Every body system is affected by the injury and must be addressed in planning care. Continued research is aimed at reversing the pathophysiology seen at injury in the hope of improving the quality of life for these patients. The care provided by the critical care nurse will allow survivors of SCI to achieve maximal return to functional well-being.

REFERENCES

Becker, D. M., Gonzalez, M., & Gentilli, A. (1987). Prevention of deep vein thrombosis in patients with acute spinal cord injuries: Use of rotating treatment tables. *Neurosurgery, 20,* 675–677.

Brackman, M. B., Shepard, M. J., Collins, W. F., et al. (1990). A randomized controlled trial of methylprednisolone or nalaxone in the treatment of acute spinal cord injury. *New England Journal of Medicine, 322,* 1405–1411.

Carol, M. P., & Ducker, T. B. (1987). Spinal cord injury and spinal shock syndrome. In J. H. Siegel (Ed.), *Trauma emergency surgery and critical care* (pp. 947–981). New York: Churchill-Livingstone.

Carol, M. P., Ducker, T. B., & Byrnes, D. P. (1980). Minimyelogram in spinal cord trauma. *Neurosurgery, 1,* 218–222.

Carter, E. R. (1979). Medical management of pulmonary complications of spinal cord injury. *Advances in Neurology, 22,* 267–268.

Chilton, J., & Dagi, T. F. (1985). Acute cervical spinal cord injury. *American Journal of Emergency Medicine, 3,* 340–351.

DeJesus-Greenberg, D. A. (1980). Acute spinal cord injury—hyperbaric oxygen therapy: A new adjunct in management. *Journal of Neurosurgical Nursing, 12,* 155–160.

Ducker, T. B., & Kindt, G. W. (1971). The effect of trauma on the vasomotor control of spinal cord blood flow. *Current Topics in Surgical Research, 3*(1), 163–181.

Durham, C. M., & Cowley, R. A. (1986). *Shock trauma/critical care handbook.* Rockville, MD: Aspen.

Faden, A. I., & Simon, R. P. (1988). A potential role for excitotoxin in the pathophysiology of spinal cord injury. *Annals of Neurology, 23,* 623–626.

Gamache, F. W., Myers, R. A. M., Ducker, T. B., & Cowley, R. A. (1981). The clinical application of hyperbaric oxygen therapy in spinal cord injury: A preliminary report. *Surgical Neurology, 15,* 85–87.

Geisler, F. H. (1988). Acute management of cervical spinal cord injury. *Trauma Quarterly, 4*(3), 1–22.

Geisler, F. H., & Salcman, M. (1987). Respiratory system: Physiology, pathophysiology and management. In F. P. Wirth & P. A. Ratcheson (Eds.), *Neurological critical care* (pp. 1–50). Baltimore: Williams & Wilkins.

Geisler, F. H., Dorsey, F. C., & Coleman, W. P. (1991). Recovery of motor function after spinal cord injury: A randomized placebo-controlled trial with GM-1. *New England Journal of Medicine, 324,* 1829–1839.

Gilbert, J. (1987). Critical care management of the patient with acute spinal cord injury. *Critical Care Clinics, 3,* 549–567.

Green, B. A., Eismont, F. J., & O'Heir, J. T. (1987). Spinal cord injury—a systems approach: Prevention, emergency medical services, and emergency room management. *Critical Care Clinics,* 471–293.

Green, B. A., Green, K. L., & Klose, K. J. (1983). Kinetic therapy for spinal cord injury. *Spine, 8,* 772–778.

Green, B. A., Klose, K. J., & Goldberg, M. I. (1985). Clinical and research considerations in spinal cord injury. In D. P. Becker & J. Povlishock (Eds.), *Central nervous system trauma status report 1985* (pp. 341–368). Bethesda, MD: National Institute of Neurologic and Communicative Disorders and Stroke/National Institutes of Health.

Grundy, B. L., & Friedman, W. (1987). Electrophysiological evaluation of the patient with acute spinal cord injury. *Critical Care Clinics, 3,* 519–548.

Guttman, L. (1976). *Spinal cord injuries: Comprehensive management and research.* Oxford, England: Blackwell.

Hall, E. D. (1988). Effects of the 21-aminosteroid u74006F on post-traumatic spinal cord ischemia in cats. *Journal of Neurosurgery, 68,* 462–465.

Hansebout, R. R., Tanner, J. A., & Romero-Sierra, C. (1984). Current status of spinal cord cooling in the treatment of acute spinal cord injury. *Spine, 9,* 508–511.

Hickey, J. V. (1986). *The clinical practice of neurological and neurosurgical nursing* (2nd ed.). Philadelphia: J. B. Lippincott.

Hickey, J. V. (1992). *The clinical practice of neurological and neurosurgical nursing* (3rd ed.). Philadelphia: J. B. Lippincott.

Hull, R., Hirsh, J., & Jay, R. (1982). Different intensities of oral anticoagulant therapy in the treatment of proximal vein thrombosis. *New England Journal of Medicine, 307,* 1076–1081.

Krause, J. F. (1985). Epidemiological aspects of acute spinal cord injury: A review of incidence, prevalence, causes and outcomes. In D. P. Becker & J. Povlishock (Eds.), *Central nervous system trauma status report 1985* (pp. 313–322). Bethesda, MD: National Institute of Neurologic and Communicative Disorders and Stroke/National Institutes of Health.

Leader, W. (1976). *Statistical reports for traumatic spinal cord injury*

(1975–1976). Tallahassee, FL: Florida Central Registry for Severely Disabled.

McCagg, C. (1986). Postoperative management and acute rehabilitation of patients with spinal cord injuries. *Orthopedic Clinics of North America, 17,* 171–182.

Mason, R. (1981). Autonomic dysreflexia: A nursing challenge. *Rehabilitation Nursing, 5*(2), 11–15.

National Spinal Cord Injury Statistical Center, University of Alabama at Birmingham. (1990). *Spinal cord injury fact sheet.* Birmingham, AL: National Spinal Cord Injury Statistical Center.

Nikas, D. L. (1982). Acute spinal cord injuries: Care and complications. In D. L. Nikas (Ed.), *The critically ill neurosurgical patient* (pp. 107–124). New York: Churchill-Livingstone.

Nikas, D. L. (1988). Pathophysiology and nursing interventions in acute spinal cord injury. *Trauma Quarterly, 4*(3), 23–44.

Richmond, T. (1985). The patient with a cervical cord injury. *Focus on Critical Care, 12*(2), 23–33.

Riggins, R., & Kraus, J. (1983). The risk of neurological damage with fractures of the vertebrae. *Trauma, 23,* 459–465.

Senter, H. J., & Venes, J. L. (1979). Loss of autoregulation and post-traumatic ischemia following experimental spinal cord trauma. *Journal of Neurosurgery, 50,* 198–206.

Tator, C. H. (1992). Regeneration research: Hope for the future. In C. P. Zejdlik, *Management of spinal cord injury* (2nd ed., pp. 129–135). Boston: Jones and Bartlett.

Tyson, G. W., (1979). Acute care of the spinal cord injured patient. *Critical Care Quarterly, 2,* 45–60.

Walleck, C. A. (1987). Nursing role in management of peripheral nerve and spinal cord problems. In S. M. Lewis & I. C. Collier (Eds.), *Medical–surgical nursing: Assessment and management of clinical problems* (pp. 1591–1621). New York: McGraw-Hill.

Walleck, C. A. (1988). Central nervous system: II. Spinal cord injury. In V. D. Cardona, P. D. Hurn, P. J. Mason, et al., (Eds.), *Trauma nursing: From resuscitation through rehabilitation* (pp. 419–448). Philadelphia: W. B. Saunders.

Young, J. S., & Northrup, N. E. (1981). *Statistical information pertaining to some of the most commonly asked questions about spinal cord injury.* Phoenix, AZ: National Spinal Cord Injury Data Center.

Zejdlik, C. P. (1983). *Management of spinal cord injury.* Monterey, CA: Wadsworth Health Sciences Division.

Patients With Guillain-Barré Syndrome

Kathryn Sabo Thompson

The disorder known as Guillain-Barré syndrome (GBS) is a rare peripheral nervous system disease that is a challenge for the patient, family, and the team caring for the patient. GBS is characterized by an acute, ascending, symmetric weakness that can progress to total paralysis of the extremities, trunk, respiratory musculature, and face. The incidence ranges from 0.75 to 2/100,000 population per year (Ropper, 1992). The syndrome occurs in all seasons and throughout the world; it affects both sexes and all age groups. GBS gained notoriety during the 1976 Swine flu immunization program when an increased incidence was noted and linked to an immune response to the vaccine (Retailiau et al., 1980). This syndrome was first described in 1859 by Jean Landry and again in 1916 by George Guillain, Jean Barré, and Andry Strohl (Guillain et al., 1916; Landry, 1859).

ETIOLOGY

The cause of GBS is unknown, but it has been classified as an acute, demyelinating, inflammatory polyradiculopathy. The myelin sheath that surrounds the axon of the neuron is segmentally destroyed, making nerve impulse conduction impossible. Focal segmental demyelination is associated with infiltration of the endoneurial and perivascular areas by lymphocytes and monocytes (Honovar et al., 1991). Lesions may appear on cranial nerves, spinal nerve roots, and peripheral nerves. At first, the myelin sheath breaks down and the axon remains intact (Figs. 39–1 and 39–2). As lymphocytes and monocytes invade the neuron, the axon may become damaged, resulting in muscle denervation and atrophy. Regeneration and recovery of the axon and myelin sheath depend on the amount of destruction incurred. Complete clinical recovery may take years, and permanent neurologic damage may result when there is extensive demyelination and axonal destruction.

Triggering Events

Although the etiology of GBS is unknown, a variety of preceding or triggering events are associated with its pathophysiology. Triggering events usually occur within 30 days of the onset of symptoms, and the pathophysiology is suspected to involve a delayed hypersensitivity reaction to the trigger. Some evidence suggests that GBS is caused by an immunologically mediated peripheral nerve injury (Korn-Lubetzki & Abramsky, 1986). It has also been suggested that im-

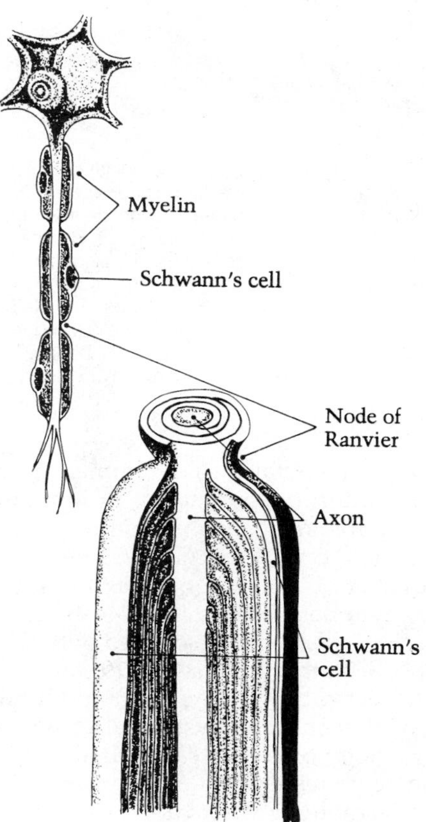

FIGURE 39–1. Microscopic enlargement of the anatomic components of the normal peripheral nerve. (From *Critical Care Nursing: Body-mind-spirit* by Cornelia Vanderstaay Kenner, Cathie E. Guzzetta, and Barbara Montgomery Dossey. Copyright © 1985 by Cornelia Vanderstaay Kenner, Cathie E. Guzzetta, and Barbara Montgomery Dossey. Reprinted by permission of Scott, Foresman and Company.)

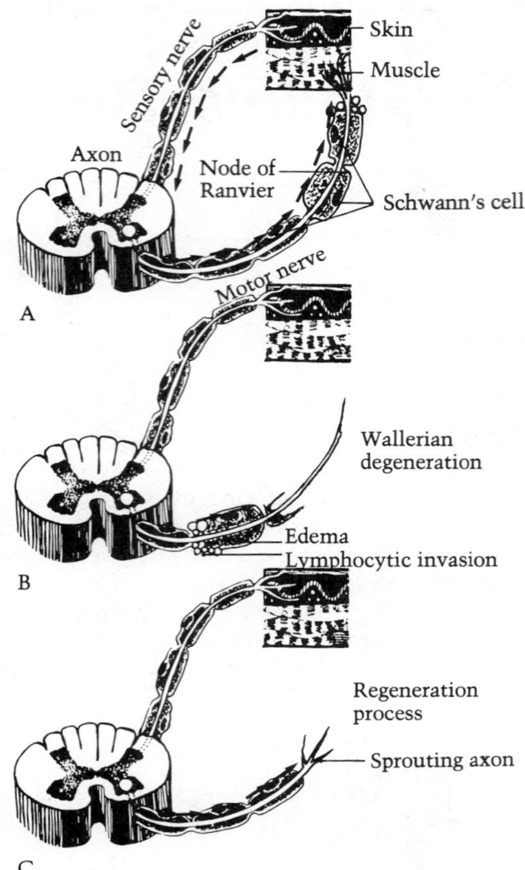

FIGURE 39–2. Cross-section of the spinal cord illustrating the pathologic changes with Guillain-Barré syndrome. *A*, Anatomy of a motor and sensory peripheral nerve; the innervation of a muscle fiber with the sensory receptors is displayed. *B*, Response of a neuron to injury, with wallerian degeneration. *C*, Regeneration with the sprouting axon. (From *Critical Care Nursing: Body-mind-spirit* by Cornelia Vanderstaay Kenner, Cathie E. Guzzetta, and Barbara Montgomery Dossey. Copyright © 1985 by Cornelia Vanderstaay Kenner, Cathie E. Guzzetta, and Barbara Montgomery Dossey. Reprinted by permission of Scott, Foresman and Company.)

munosuppressive states (i.e., human immunodeficiency virus infection, pregnancy, or immunosuppressive therapy for malignant neoplasms or after organ transplantation) can trigger GBS (Cameron et al., 1958; Cornblath et al., 1987; Klingon, 1965). Viral infections, especially cytomegalovirus, Epstein-Barr, and swine influenza, have also been associated with GBS (Kaplan et al., 1983; Schonberger et al., 1979).

It is suspected that both cellular and humoral components of the immune system are involved in the pathophysiology of GBS because there is frequently a preceding acute respiratory or gastrointestinal illness. The illness is thought to activate the cell-mediated immune system by sensitizing T lymphocytes to the person's own myelin sheath, initiating its destruction. Research has also suggested that B lymphocytes may respond to some antigens (the trigger) by producing a demyelinating antibody that activates myelin destruction.

Course of the Disease

Once the destruction of the myelin sheath has begun, the patient begins to experience muscle weakness, which may progress to flaccid paralysis. The disease course is variable but can be divided into three distinct phases: progression, plateau, and recovery. During the *progression phase,* muscle weakness and paralysis increase in severity; this phase may last from a few hours to 4 weeks. The *plateau phase* occurs when the patient does not develop further weakness or paralysis. The *recovery phase* usually begins 2 to 4 weeks after the plateau and is characterized by a slow return of muscular strength. Prognosis for complete recovery is generally excellent (Rantala et al., 1991). The rate and degree of an individual's recovery cannot be predicted. The slow recovery, which may be as long as 6 months to 2 years, can be very frustrating for the patient, family, and caregivers. Most patients recover with no or minor side effects such as distal numbness or foot drop. However, a small percentage of patients suffer from sensory loss, weakness, and imbalance resulting in major changes in activity level and lifestyle (Winer et al., 1988).

CLINICAL PRESENTATION

Although variable, the onset of symptoms is usually sudden, involving pain, muscle weakness, and autonomic dysfunction.

Pain

Pain is a major finding on assessment and varies from mild to extremely severe. Painful sensations can be categorized into paresthesias, muscular aches and cramps, and hyperesthesias. Paresthesias can include numb, prickly, tingling, and burning sensations, especially in the stocking and glove dermatomes. Perception of joint position (proprioception) and vibratory and temperature sensations may diminish. Hyperesthesia may cause the light touch of a hand or bed sheet to be perceived as severe pain. Ropper and Shahani (1984) reported that the patient's pain is usually worse at night and occurs most frequently in the buttocks, quadriceps, and hamstrings and less frequently in the calves, shins, shoulders, and lower back. It is unclear what causes the pain associated with GBS, but it is thought to result from spontaneous discharges in demyelinated nerves (Ropper, 1992).

Muscular Weakness

Progressive muscular weakness usually develops rapidly. Muscle weakness begins distally and progresses in an ascending manner with relatively symmetric muscle involvement. Severity of muscle involvement varies from weakness of the legs to total paralysis of all extremities, the trunk, face, and areas innervated by the bulbar (cranial) nerves. Bulbar nerve involvement can result in weakness or paralysis of the respiratory musculature, necessitating admission to the intensive care unit and ventilatory support.

Cranial nerve involvement can result in facial muscle weakness, dysphagia, and inability to talk or blink. The patient may be paralyzed but remains fully conscious and able to hear. Once the disease process begins to subside, pain and muscle weakness decrease, descending from head to toes.

Autonomic Dysfunction

Autonomic dysfunction is critically important in caring for the GBS patient. GBS may impair autonomic function due to lesions on the afferent limb of the baroreflex arc, interrupting homeostatic reflexes. Lesions may also involve the postganglionic sympathetic fibers of the spinal nerves. Autonomic disturbances are commonly seen in GBS patients with severe muscle involvement and respiratory muscle paralysis (Calleja, 1990). The heralding sign of autonomic dysfunction in GBS is an unexplained sinus tachycardia. The most dangerous autonomic dysfunctions include orthostatic hypotension, hypertension, abnormal vagal responses (bradycardia, heart block, asystole), and the syndrome of inappropriate antidiuretic hormone secretion (SIADH). Other autonomic dysfunctions include bowel and bladder dysfunction, facial flushing, and diaphoresis. The severity of autonomic disturbances varies and is a major cause of mortality (Traux, 1982); there is a 5% mortality rate associated with all of the complications of GBS. The literature describing the duration of autonomic dysfunction is inadequate, making it difficult to determine the length of time necessary for these patients to remain monitored in an intensive care unit.

Clinical Variants

Guillain-Barré syndrome has several regional and functional variations reflecting the area of peripheral nerve demyelination (Ropper, 1986).

ASCENDING GBS. GBS most commonly presents with muscular weakness and pain in the legs, which progresses upward to the trunk, arms, or cranial nerves. In severe cases the patient presents with flaccid quadriplegia involving both spinal and cranial nerves. Deep tendon reflexes are diminished or absent. Life-threatening events associated with ascending GBS include respiratory muscle paralysis and autonomic dysfunction.

PURE MOTOR GBS. This variant is similar to ascending GBS except that the patient retains normal sensory function. Quadriparesis may occur but without muscular pain.

DESCENDING GBS. A less common variation of GBS involves weakness beginning with the cranial nerves and progressing downward to the respiratory muscles, trunk, and extremities. Normal reflexes are present. This type of disease may involve the facial, glossopharyngeal, and vagus nerves as manifested by facial paralysis, ophthalmoplegia, dysphagia, and cardiac dysrhythmias.

MILLER-FISHER SYNDROME (FISHER VARIANT). This variation of GBS is extremely rare and may also be called encephalomyeloradiculopathy. Prominent features include ophthalmoplegia, ataxia, and areflexia. This form is distinguished from descending GBS by the weakness of eye movement, limb and gait ataxia, minimum or no muscular weakness, and normal sensory function.

CHRONIC IDIOPATHIC POLYNEURITIS (CHRONIC OR RELAPSING GBS). This rare process shares features with GBS. Chronic idiopathic polyneuritis is similar in the presentation of peripheral nerve demyelination, areflexia, muscular weakness, and pain. Unlike GBS, weakness in patients with chronic idiopathic polyneuritis develops slowly over 6 to 12 months, and muscular strength may take 2 years or longer to return. In some cases, there are cyclical episodes of progressive weakness and return of muscle strength. Evidence suggests that cell-mediated immunity plays a significant role in the pathogenesis of chronic idiopathic polyneuritis, thus linking it to GBS (Korn-Lubetzki & Abramsky, 1986).

Diagnostic Considerations

Diagnostic criteria for GBS were established in 1978 by the National Institute of Neurological and Communicative Disorders and Stroke (1978). Criteria include clinical assessments and laboratory and electrodiagnostic data. Illnesses such as spinal cord compression, acute intermittent porphyria, poliomyelitis, botulism, and diphtheria must be ruled out before GBS can be definitively diagnosed. Serial lumbar punctures are performed to exclude other illnesses and to identify elevations in cerebrospinal fluid (CSF) protein, which occur during the first week of symptoms. There is usually no increase in mononuclear leukocytes within the CSF. In most cases, electromyographic studies are abnormal, ruling out muscle disease as a cause of the patient's symptoms (Table 39–1).

CLINICAL MANAGEMENT

Recovery from GBS is determined not only by the course of the disease but by the intensity of the care required by the patient. The plan of care frequently

TABLE 39–1. **Diagnostic Requirements for Guillain-Barré Syndrome**

Required for Diagnosis
Progressive motor weakness of more than one limb
Definite hyporeflexia or areflexia
Strongly Supports Diagnosis
Cerebrospinal fluid protein elevated after 1 week of symptoms
Progression of motor weakness develops rapidly over days to 4 weeks
Motor weakness plateaus within 2 to 4 weeks
Relative symmetry of motor weakness
Mild sensory symptoms
Cranial nerve involvement
Recovery begins 2 to 4 weeks after plateau is reached
Autonomic dysfunction
Absence of fever
Abnormal electrodiagnostics (usually)
Possible Variants
Fever at onset
Severe sensory loss with pain
Progression beyond 4 weeks
Major permanent residual deficits
Transient bladder paralysis
Central nervous system involvement
Required to Rule Out Diagnosis
No evidence of:
Porphyria
Lead intoxication
Polio
Botulism
No history of hexacarbon abuse
Symptoms not purely sensory
Organophosphates
Tick paralysis
Diphtheria infection
Toxic neuropathy

Adapted from National Institute of Neurologic and Communicative Disorders and Stroke. (1978). Criteria for diagnosis of Guillain-Barré syndrome. *Annals of Neurology, 3,* 565–566.

changes, given the unpredictable nature of the disease, and requires a high degree of resourcefulness by the clinical management team. Initial management for GBS includes diagnosis, symptom management, and interventions to prevent major complications (such as infection and deep vein thrombosis). Therapeutic plasmapheresis (TP) has been used within 2 weeks of the onset of symptoms and has been associated with decreased length of stay and reduced need for mechanical ventilation (Consensus Conference, 1986). TP removes antibodies and other immunologically active substances that have been implicated in GBS (Fig. 39–3). The most common side effects associated with TP in patients with Guillain-Barré syndrome are hypotension, bradycardia, fever, chills, and skin rash, whereas the reported incidence of adverse events varies from 11% to 82% of patients treated (Bouqet et al., 1993).

Treatment with intravenous immunoglobulin (IVIG) has been attempted with conflicting results, requiring further study of this therapy. It has been suggested that IVIG downregulates antibody production by introducing anti-idiotypic antibodies, making it a potentially useful treatment for GBS (Bleck, 1993). Treatments for respiratory support and autonomic monitoring are collaborative efforts between physicians, nurses, and other team members. The nurse's role in this collaborative care is to monitor the patient for progressive symptoms while also assessing the person's response to therapy.

During the progressive phase, careful evaluation of muscular strength is done every 8 hours to determine further deterioration of clinical status. The Medical Research Council scale provides a consistent, quantitative method for evaluating muscle group function (Griswold et al., 1984) (Table 39–2).

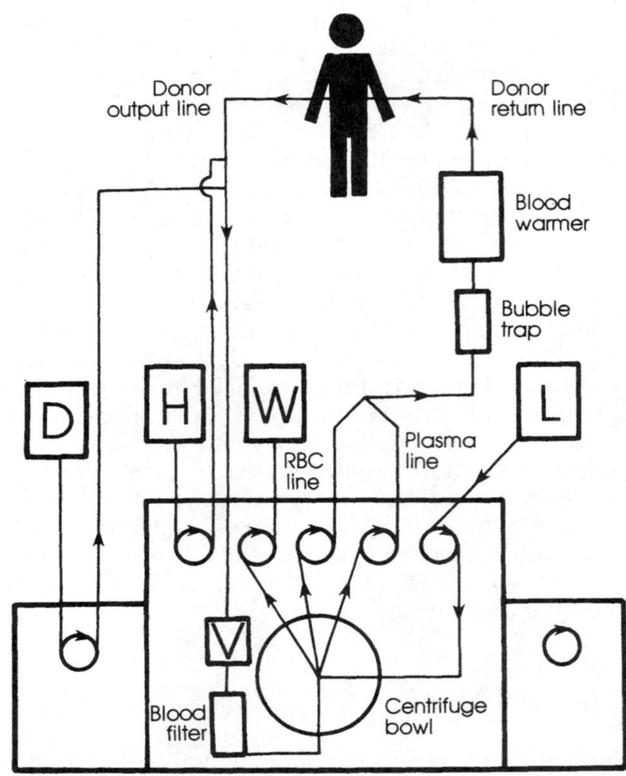

FIGURE 39–3. Plasmapheresis. Diagrammatic representation of leukapheresis procedure using a continuous-flow cell separator. (Reproduced by permission from: Rudy, E. B. [1984]. *Advanced neurological and neurosurgical nursing* [p. 311]. St. Louis: C. V. Mosby.)

TABLE 39–2. **Medical Research Council Scale**

0 = No contraction
1 = Flicker or trace contraction
2 = Active movement with gravity eliminated
3 = Active movement against gravity
4 = Active movement against gravity and resistance
5 = Normal power

Adapted from Griswold, K., McKenna, M., & Ropper, A. (1984). An approach to care of patients with Guillain-Barré syndrome. *Heart and Lung, 13,* 69.

Respiratory Muscle Dysfunction Management

During the progressive phase, the patient is monitored in an intensive care unit for potentially fatal respiratory muscle paralysis and autonomic dysfunction. It is critical to assess the trends of muscle weakness to anticipate acute respiratory dysfunction. It is useful to assess maximum inspiratory pressure and vital capacity every 2 to 4 hours. Testing the gag, cough, and swallow reflexes is mandatory to monitor pharyngeal function.

The danger of atelectasis, aspiration, and hypostatic pneumonia is great for patients with respiratory and pharyngeal muscle weakness. Pleuritic-type chest pain and dyspnea are insidious signs of respiratory tract infection in these patients. It is important to institute meticulous pulmonary toilet every 2 hours to mobilize secretions.

Intubation and mechanical ventilation are recommended when the following clinical signs are noted:

1. Vital capacity is 1 liter or less or 30% or less of predicted value for the patient.
2. Negative inspiratory force is 20 cm H_2O or less.
3. Pharyngeal paralysis and inability to clear oral secretions are present.

Tracheostomy is indicated when the duration of intubation exceeds 10 days, unless there is rapid improvement and the potential for unassisted ventilation (Ropper & Kehne, 1985).

Weaning from mechanical ventilation begins once respiratory muscle strength returns, as evidenced by a vital capacity exceeding 30% of the predicted value for that patient and a negative inspiratory force of 20 cm H_2O or greater. Successful weaning of a patient with respiratory muscle weakness involves training of the respiratory muscles. It is not helpful to push these patients to fatigue during weaning trials (see Chapter 33).

Several methods of weaning have been successful in patients with GBS. The eventual success of weaning involves not only the physical and mental readiness of the patient but the skill of the caregiver. The four methods most commonly used for weaning from mechanical ventilation include T-piece, continuous positive airway pressure (CPAP) mode with pressure support, synchronized intermittent mandatory ventilation (SIMV), and pressure support ventilation (PSV) (see Chapter 16). Researchers have demonstrated no difference in weaning success between SIMV and assist or controlled ventilation (Schacter et al., 1981) and SIMV versus T-piece (Tomlinson et al., 1989). There have been no controlled studies comparing the use of pressure support and other modes of weaning in GBS patients.

Management of Autonomic Dysfunction

Cardiac monitoring is mandatory for GBS patients with respiratory muscle dysfunction and severe motor weakness because of the high incidence of autonomic dysfunction in these patients. Treatment of autonomic dysfunction is preventive and symptomatic.

Orthostatic hypotension may be avoided by maintaining positive pressure ventilation and slowly elevating the head while closely monitoring the blood pressure. Elevation of the head of the bed 30 degrees at night enhances renin secretion, resulting in sodium retention and increased blood volume, which may reduce orthostatic hypotension (Widgiks et al., 1990). Severe or sustained hypertension should be treated with carefully titrated or short-acting antihypertensive agents such as nitroprusside or esmolol. Vagal episodes are avoided by limiting the length of time of tracheal suctioning. Pacemakers may be necessary in patients with severe vagal episodes.

Bladder dysfunction is usually seen in patients with respiratory muscle failure and severe motor weakness. Urinary retention is treated with intermittent catheterization. Continuous catheterization is indicated for patients with severe, prolonged muscle weakness. Catheters are discontinued when the patient regains motor function of the trunk muscles. Often, intermittent catheterization is required for several days after continuous catheterization until the patient regains bladder tone.

Another autonomic dysfunction that occurs with GBS patients is hyponatremia and SIADH. It is important to monitor serum sodium and osmolality in these patients. Treatment of SIADH involves crystalloid fluid restriction (see also Chapter 52).

Management of Potential for Aspiration Due to Dysphagia

The threat of respiratory muscle failure and aspiration is of immediate concern in the progressive phase of GBS and requires intense monitoring, usually in a critical care unit. Inability to clear secretions because of paresis and an ineffective cough due to diaphragmatic paralysis are indications for intubation.

It is crucial that physical assessment include hourly monitoring of the patient's ability to gag, cough effectively, and clear secretions. An increase in oral secretions may signify that the patient is experiencing dysphagia.

Maintaining the head of the bed at 60 to 90 degrees if the patient is not hypotensive may facilitate a patent airway. The patient should be coached to cough forcefully every 2 hours.

Evidence of aspiration includes agitation, abnormal breath sounds, dyspnea, tachycardia, tachypnea, and abnormal arterial blood gases. Elective intubation should be done at the first sign of dysphagia with or without respiratory distress to prevent aspiration and its complications.

It should be explained to the patient and family why the patient's cough and swallow are being evaluated so frequently. The patient should be instructed to notify the nurse if he or she is experiencing increased difficulty in swallowing and coughing.

Management of Pain Due to Paresthesia, Hypesthesia, and Muscle Cramps

Pain is one of the most difficult and frustrating symptoms to treat in GBS patients. The patient with uncontrolled pain may demonstrate varying degrees of anxiety, depression, hopelessness, hostility, and anger. Uncontrolled pain may be interpreted by the patient as a progression of disease, preventing him or her from participating in rehabilitation.

It is important on physical assessment to ask the patient to describe thoroughly the location, quality, and intensity of the pain. Information should also be elicited about what increases or relieves the pain. Sometimes it is possible to reduce the patient's pain by repositioning an extremity, removing a bed sheet, or using a foot cradle. Pain may be so severe that it requires narcotic analgesics. Recording the assessment of pain and the treatment given on a flow sheet helps to track and communicate treatment success.

Pain can overwhelm the patient. Developing rapport with the patient allows the patient to relate his or her fears and demonstrates belief in the patient's pain. Interventions to manage pain can include passive range-of-motion exercises, massage, distraction, ice, heat, cutaneous stimulation, oil of wintergreen, and transcutaneous electrical nerve stimulation. Analgesics used for these patients range from the nonsteroidal antiinflammatory drugs to narcotic analgesics. Pain control needs to be individualized, considering the patient's response to pain and the phase of illness. For instance, if the patient is being weaned from the ventilator or is not intubated, an attempt should be made to use the least amount of narcotic analgesic possible because these drugs depress respirations. In the progressive phase, when the patient is intubated, narcotic analgesics may be very appropriate.

Management of Impaired Verbal Communication Due to Intubation or Progressive Paralysis

An inability to communicate contributes to the overwhelming fear and frustration experienced by the GBS patient and the family. Development of communication tools for these patients has been unsatisfactory to date. Imagination needs to be used to help these patients communicate their needs (see Chapter 7). One successful method, if the patient has little or no facial muscle weakness, is lip reading. It is important to encourage the patient to exaggerate lip movements, articulate key words, and go slowly. This is a skill requiring patience on the part of both nurse and patient. When successful, patients express enormous relief and appreciation when communication is established by means of lip reading.

If the patient has facial paralysis, lip reading is difficult or impossible. Letter and picture boards may be used. Diplopia may occur due to eye muscle involvement, making it difficult for the patient to see the communication board clearly. An eye patch covering one eye may help. Although use of the communication boards is tedious and time consuming, it may be the patient's only means of communicating with others.

A "talk trach" may be useful for patients who have a tracheostomy but do not have vocal cord paralysis. The talk trach has air vents below the vocal cords. When the air port of the talk trach is connected to 4 to 6 liters of air flow, it is possible for the patient to speak. Problems with the talk trach include plugging of the air vents with secretions and gastric distention due to air leaking into the esophagus.

Other communication methods include the electronic artificial larynx and Morse code. Whichever method is used, it is important to spend time with the patient and family teaching them how to use the method adequately. The patient's frustration about the slowness of communication should be acknowledged while encouraging patience. The patient and family should be reminded that verbal communication will return when the patient is extubated. Humor is frequently useful in promoting a positive attitude while using a variety of communication methods.

Because of the inability to communicate verbally, some means of allowing the patient to signal for help must be established. Sometimes patients who cannot call out can still "click" with their tongue to gain attention. Clicking is useful when the nurse is in close proximity to the patient. Some very anxious patients may seem to click excessively. The nurse should investigate whether the patient has an actual physical need or is expressing anxiety indirectly and should deal with the situation accordingly.

There are pressure-sensitive call devices that require minimal pressure to be activated. These may be placed near the part of the patient that has the greatest remaining strength (e.g., the hand or the head). A "Sip-n-Puff" call system works well if the patient cannot use a pressure-sensitive plate. The ability to use a call device allows the patient to retain a sense of some control over the situation. Just one episode of being unable to summon help may cause severe anxiety or mistrust or even result in death if the ventilator-dependent patient becomes dislodged from the ventilator. There has been no documented research describing successful interventions for facilitating communication with intubated, paralyzed patients (see Chapter 7).

Management of Skin Integrity

Because these patients may become completely paralyzed, they are especially prone to pressure necrosis. As long as possible in the progressive and recovery phases, the patient should be encouraged to change position frequently. Family members should be taught the importance of moving the patient and how to avoid shear forces when moving so that they can help the person move appropriately. A turning schedule should be established and posted at the bedside to ensure that turning patterns are followed uniformly. Inspection and massage of, and application of lotion to all bony prominences should be accomplished each time the patient is turned and positioned. Skin should be kept free of excess moisture but not allowed to become dry and scaly; bath oil is preferred to soap for bed baths. Avoid use of plastic incontinent pads in direct contact with the patient's skin because these trap moisture and heat and may macerate the skin (see Chapter 61).

Adjunctive devices cannot replace basic nursing interventions in the prevention of skin breakdown. Air mattresses and mechanical beds (kinetic tables, air fluidized mattresses, Stryker frames) may be useful depending on the patient's condition. Judicious use of heel and elbow pads may also be helpful. When helping the patient into a chair, a gel pad such as the air flotation cushion may decrease excessive pressure.

Management of Potential for Injury from Joint Contractures Due to Muscle Weakness or Paralysis

During the progressive and recovery phases the patient and family should be instructed in the need for and how to perform range-of-motion exercises for paralyzed and weakened extremities. An exercise program should be established that places all joints through their full range of motion each 8 hours. Ideally, the exercise schedule is posted at the bedside to encourage patient and family participation.

Proper positioning is vital to maintain optimal joint function. The ideal joint position is neutral. Splints, orthoses, and adjunctive aids (antirotation boots) may be indicated to prevent or correct joint contracture.

Isometric and isotonic exercises of uninvolved or partially involved muscle groups should accompany range-of-motion exercises. Too frequent or vigorous exercise should be avoided because it may contribute to the demyelination process (Ross et al., 1979). Traction weight systems may be set up on the bed to allow the patient to perform isotonic exercises when confined to bed. Exercise goals set mutually with the patient and family should be posted at the bedside. Attained goals should be celebrated with effusive positive reinforcement and reward.

Management of Activity Intolerance Due to Orthostatic Hypotension from Associated Autonomic Dysfunction

The judgment of when to get the patient out of bed to a chair varies with each individual. Autonomic nervous system stability and trunk muscle strength should be considered. Patients with unstable autonomic nervous system function should have their blood pressure taken and cardiac monitoring performed whenever the patient's head is elevated. If the patient has little or no upper body strength, it is difficult and painful for him or her to sit in a chair. Patients transferred into a cardiac chair should have adequate torso strength to maintain their position in the chair.

Elastic support stockings and elastic wraps applied to the upper legs may provide adequate compression to decrease venous pooling and decrease orthostasis. Slowly elevating the head of the bed over a period of several hours may aid in overcoming orthostasis in the patient who has been on prolonged bed rest. Tilt tables may also be necessary for some patients (see Chapter 61).

Management of Nutrition

Malnutrition may be the result of immobility, decreased gastrointestinal mobility, dysphagia, anorexia, or depression.

Because the threat of aspiration can complicate the patient's ability to maintain adequate nutrition, careful assessment of pharyngeal function is mandatory as a baseline in nutritional interventions. In patients with mild dysphagia, it may be possible to provide semisolid to solid foods while the patient sits upright. Liquids tend to be more easily aspirated. Enteric or parenteral nutrition is necessary with patients who have moderate to severe dysphagia. Careful evaluation of gastrointestinal symptoms may indicate intolerance of the feeding formula or medications bolused through the feeding tube, or may indicate infection by *Clostridium difficile* (Estoup, 1994). Patients on tube feedings should be assessed for excessive gastric residual (>50 mL in 2 hours for continuous feedings and >100 mL for every 4 hour feedings), diarrhea, and constipation. Metoclopramide hydrochloride may be ordered to facilitate gastric emptying. When the patient is again able to begin solid foods, calorie counts may be periodically used to ensure adequate caloric intake. If necessary, the patient should be aided in choosing foods that are nutritious. Encouraging the family to bring in home-cooked foods may be useful for some patients. Weights taken daily or every other day allow monitoring of nutritional status. Serum albumin and total lymphocyte counts also aid in determining nutritional status (see Chapter 47).

Management of Fear Through Patient/Family Education

Fear may be due to lack of understanding of the disease process and prognosis, pain, inability to communicate, loss of control, and thoughts of dying.

Fear is experienced by most if not all GBS patients. The experience of GBS may seem like a nightmare. Fearful feelings may be exacerbated by caregivers' inability to provide a precise estimate of the rate and degree of recovery. It is imperative that the critical care nurse keep the patient and family informed. Information provided varies from details about intensive care unit routines to supplemental information about the disease and its therapy. Whenever possible, sensory information, from the patient's perspective, should be provided, especially for painful or uncomfortable procedures. It is important to spend time with the patient and family to identify misconceptions or distorted perceptions. Identifying a small group of primary caregivers facilitates providing patients and families with reassurance and consistent information.

Fear may be exacerbated by a lack of sleep. ICU psychosis has also been associated with a lack of sleep. This syndrome is described as a gradual loss of ability to perceive reality in response to restraints, sensory overload, sensory monotony, and sleep deprivation. Patients with GBS are prone to ICU psychosis because of changes in their ability to perceive the environment, chronic pain, sleep deprivation, and a feeling of being trapped within their own body. It is important to combat this complication because it can prolong hospitalization.

The patient's sleep routine should be monitored and hypnotics administered, if necessary, to promote rest. A day–night routine should be established and maintained for the patient. Allow the patient optimal control in establishing the daily schedule. A posted schedule of activities aids staff and family in maintaining the schedule for the patient.

The GBS Society has published a booklet for patients and families that provides information about the disease and resources for financial, rehabilitative, and social support (Steinberg, 1994). (The booklet is available from The Guillain-Barré Syndrome Support Group, P.O. Box 262, Wynnewood, PA 19096.) It is sometimes helpful to direct families to the nearest GBS support group to share feelings, hope, and practical information on coping strategies. (The National GBS Support Group Office [telephone 610-667-0131] can direct patients and families to the nearest chapter.)

Visits of former patients with GBS are helpful because they allow the patient to gain insight into the situation. They also provide a role model of the recovered patient and visible evidence of recovery for the patient. The timing of such a visit is crucial and may be best arranged during the plateau or recovery phase after the patient has experienced the illness and gained a sense of ownership of it.

Management of Ineffective Family Coping

Family members may also experience fear, helplessness, and a loss of control. Aid the family in identifying tasks that they can perform (exercises, repositioning) that aid the patient's recovery. Encourage the family to listen to the patient's concerns and to identify problem areas in which the staff can intervene. Encourage the family to talk about current events and reminisce about the patient's past to distract the patient from the reality of the current situation and foster a sense of hope. Incorporate the family as much as possible in the care of the patient to the extent that they feel comfortable (see also Chapter 6).

Discharge Planning

Recovery from the sequelae of GBS can take weeks to months. Approximately 65% have persistent problems, such as foot drop or distal numbness, that do not impede activities of daily living, whereas permanent disabling effects of GBS occur in 5% to 10%, involving imbalance, weakness, and sensory loss (Ropper, 1992). Once the patient no longer requires intensive care (airway management and cardiac monitoring), the patient should be evaluated for a rehabilitation program. Acceptance into a rehabilitation facility usually requires that a patient is able to tolerate at least 3 hours/day of physical therapy. The family should be encouraged to visit the facilities considered for rehabilitation. The patient and family should meet with a social worker to discuss concerns related to insurance coverage and possible loss of income related to the disability. The social worker can discuss options related to community resources.

SUMMARY

Guillain-Barré syndrome is a debilitating neuromuscular disorder characterized by sensory, motor, and autonomic dysfunction. Nursing care is directed toward supportive care of these patients as they progress through the progressive, plateau, and recovery phases of the illness. Successful recovery of these patients is highly dependent on the nurse's ability to prevent complications and support recovery.

REFERENCES

Bleck, T. (1993). Treatment strategies for patients with Guillain-Barré syndrome. *Critical Care Medicine, 21,* 641–643.

Bouget, J., Chevret, S., Chastang, C., & Raphael, J. (1993). Plasma exchange morbidity in Guillain-Barré syndrome: Results from the French prospective, double-blind, randomized, multicenter study. *Critical Care Medicine, 21,* 651–658.

Calléja, M. (1990). Autonomic dysfunction and Guillain-Barré syndrome. *Anaesthesia, 27,* S13–S15.

Cameron, D., Howel, D., & Hutchinson, J. (1958). Acute peripheral neuropathy in Hodgkin's disease: Report of fatal case with histiologic features of allergic neuritis. *Neurology, 8,* 575–577.

Consensus Conference. (1986). The utility of therapeutic plasmapheresis for neurological disorders. *Journal of the American Medical Association, 256,* 1333–1336.

Cornblath, D. R., McArthur, J. C., Kennedy, P. G., et al. (1987). Inflammatory demyelinating peripheral neuropathes associated with human T-cell lymphotropic virus Type III infection. *Annals of Neurology, 21,* 32–40.

Dracup, K. (1993). Helping patients and families cope. *Critical Care Nurse,* (Aug. Suppl), 4–9.

Estoup, M. (1994). Approaches and limitations of medication delivery in patients with enteral feeding tubes. *Critical Care Nurse, 14*(1), 68–79.

Griswold, K., McKenna, M., & Ropper, A. (1984). An approach to care of patients with Guillain-Barré syndrome. *Heart and Lung, 13,* 66–72.

Guillain, G., Barré, J., & Strohl, A. (1916). Sur un syndrome de radiculonervite avec hyperalbuminose du liquide encephalorachidien sans reaction cellaire. *Bull Soc Med Hop, 40,* 1462.

Honovar, M., Tharakan, K., Hughes, R., Liebowitz, S., & Winer, J. (1991). A clinicopathological study of Guillain-Barré syndrome. *Brain, 114,* 1245–1269.

Kaplan, J., Greenspan, J., Bomgaars, M., et al. (1983). Simultaneous outbreaks of Guillain-Barré syndrome and Bell's palsy in Hawaii in 1981. *Journal of the American Medical Association, 250,* 2635–2640.

Klingon, G. (1965). The Guillain-Barré syndrome associated with cancer. *Cancer, 18,* 157–163.

Korn-Lubetzki, I., & Abramsky, O. (1986). Acute and chronic demyelinating inflammatory polyradiculoneuropathy: Association with autoimmune diseases and lymphocyte response to human neuritogenic protein. *Archives of Neurology, 43,* 604–608.

Landry, O. (1859). Note sur la paralysic ascendante aigul. *Gaz Rebd Med Chir, 6,* 472–486.

National Institute of Neurologic and Communicative Disorders and Stroke. (1978). Criteria for diagnosis of Guillain-Barré syndrome. *Annals of Neurology, 3,* 565–566.

Rantala, H., Uhari, M., Niemala, M. (1991). Occurrence, clinical manifestations, and prognosis of Guillain-Barré syndrome. *Archives of Disease in Childhood, 66,* 706–708.

Ratailiau, H., Curtis, A., Storre, G., et al. (1980). Illness after influenza vaccination reported through a nationwide surveillance system, 1976–1977. *American Journal of Epidemiology, 111,* 270–278.

Ropper, A. (1992). The Guillain-Barré syndrome. *New England Journal of Medicine, 326,* 1130–1136.

Ropper, A. (1986). Unusual clinical variants and signs in Guillain-Barré syndrome. *Archives of Neurology, 43,* 1150–1152.

Ropper, A., & Shahani, B. (1984). Pain in Guillain-Barré. *Archives of Neurology, 41,* 511–514.

Ropper, A., & Kehne, S. (1985). Guillain-Barré syndrome: Management of respiratory failure. *Archives of Neurology, 43,* 1150–1152.

Ross, A. J., Herr, B. E., Norwood, M. L., et al. (1979). Neuromuscular diagnostic procedures. *Nursing Clinics of North America, 14,* 107–156.

Slutsky, A. (1993). Mechanical ventilation. *Chest, 104,* 1833–1859.

Schacter, E., Tucker, D., & Beck, G. (1981). Does intermittent ventilation accelerate weaning? *Journal of the American Medical Association, 246,* 1210–1214.

Schonberger, L., Bregman, D., Sullivan-Bolyai, J., et al. (1979). Guillain-Barré syndrome following vaccination in the national influenza immunization program, United States, 1976–1977. *American Journal of Epidemiology, 118,* 105–123.

Steinberg, J. (1994). *Guillain-Barré syndrome: An overview for the lay person.* Wynnewood, PA: Guillain-Barré Support Group.

Tomlinson, J., Miller, K., Lorch, D., et al. (1989). A prospective comparison of IMV and T-piece weaning from mechanical ventilation. *Chest, 96,* 348–352.

Traux, B. (1982). Autonomic disturbances in the Guillain-Barré syndrome. *Seminars in Neurology, 4,* 462–468.

Widgiks, E., Ropper, A., & Nathansjon, J. (1990). Atrial natriuretic factor and blood pressure fluctuations in Guillain-Barré syndrome. *Annals of Neurology, 27,* 337–338.

Winer, J. B., Hughes, R. C., Osmond, C. (1988). A prospective study of acute idiopathic neuropathies: Clinical features and their prognostic value. *Journal of Neurology, Neurosurgery and Psychiatry, 51,* 605–612.

GUILLAIN-BARRÉ SYNDROME MULTIDISCIPLINARY CARE GUIDE

COORDINATION OF CARE

Diagnosis/Stabilization Phase		Acute Management Phase		Recovery Phase	
Outcome	*Intervention*	*Outcome*	*Intervention*	*Outcome*	*Intervention*
All appropriate disciplines will be consulted.	Consult the following as needed: neurologist, internist/family practice, other specialists as needed, respiratory therapist, chaplain, social services, clinical nurse specialist.	All appropriate disciplines and team members will be involved in the plan of care.	Develop plan of care with patient/family, primary nurse(s), primary physician(s), dietician, discharge planner, home health agency, home oxygen supply company, physical therapist, recreational therapist. Initiate planning for anticipated discharge. Begin teaching patient/family about care at home if discharge to home is anticipated.	Patient/family will understand how to maintain optimal health at home, extended care facility, or physical rehabilitation facility.	Provide written guidelines concerning follow-up care to patient/family. Provide patient/family with phone number of resources available to answer questions.

FLUID BALANCE

Diagnosis/Stabilization Phase		Acute Management Phase		Recovery Phase	
Outcome	*Intervention*	*Outcome*	*Intervention*	*Outcome*	*Intervention*
Patient will achieve optimal hemodynamic status as evidenced by: • MAP >70 mm Hg • Hemodynamic parameters within normal limits (WNL) • Adequate level of consciousness • Adequate respiratory functioning • Neurologic status WNL	Monitor and treat hemodynamic parameters: • BP • I & O • LOC • Svo_2 • Evidence of tissue perfusion • Glasgow Coma Scale Constantly monitor level of muscle functioning, paralysis, and paresthesia. Constantly monitor respiratory functioning and anticipate respiratory complications. Be prepared for intubation and mechanical ventilation. Anticipate need for vasopressor agents; assess response and titrate accordingly.	Patient will maintain optimal hemodynamic status.	Same as stabilization phase. Monitor and treat hemodynamic parameters. Continue to monitor for possible complications as listed for stabilization phase and treat accordingly. Daily weight.	Patient will maintain optimal hemodynamic status.	Same as acute management phase.

Assess neurologic status q1h and PRN.
Monitor for possible complications associated with Guillain-Barré syndrome and treat accordingly: respiratory deterioration, autonomic dysfunction, pharyngeal paralysis, dysphagia, aspiration, muscle cramps, hyperesthesia, orthostatic hypotension, respiratory infection, pneumonia, and contractures.

NUTRITION

Diagnosis/Stabilization Phase		Acute Management Phase		Recovery Phase	
Outcome	*Intervention*	*Outcome*	*Intervention*	*Outcome*	*Intervention*
Patient will be adequately nourished.	Assess swallowing and gag reflexes. If present, initiate diet as tolerated. Monitor response to diet. If swallowing and gag reflexes are not present, initiate enteral or parenteral feeding. Assess bowel sounds, abdominal distension, abdominal pain and tenderness q4h and PRN. Begin oral motor exercises if indicated.	Patient will be adequately norished.	Same as stabilization phase. Daily weight. Monitor protein and albumen lab values. Involve dietician in plan of care as necessary. Teach patient/family oral motor exercises. Monitor for signs of aspiration.	Patient will be adequately nourished.	Monitor response to nutrition given. Instruct patient/family on diet.

MOBILITY

Diagnosis/Stabilization Phase		Acute Management Phase		Recovery Phase	
Outcome	*Intervention*	*Outcome*	*Intervention*	*Outcome*	*Intervention*
Patient will achieve optimal mobility. Patient will be free of joint contractures.	Assess degree of mobility, muscle strength, paresthesia, and paralysis. Institute other types of bed therapy as indicated (e.g., kinetic bed). Begin passive/active-assist range-of-motion exercises.	Patient will achieve optimal mobility. Patient will be free of joint contractures.	Same as stabilization phase. Obtain physical therapy/rehabilitation consult. Monitor response to increased activity; decrease activity if adverse events occur. Provide support as necessary. Begin discussing with family potential residual physical limitations and required home resources.	Patient will achieve optimal mobility. Patient will be free of joint contractures.	Same as other phases. Prepare for transfer to extended care facility, home, or physical rehabilitation facility. Include family in all transfer plans. Teach patient/family about progressive exercise program.

Care Guide continued on following page

GUILLAIN-BARRÉ SYNDROME MULTIDISCIPLINARY CARE GUIDE *continued*

OXYGENATION/VENTILATION

Diagnosis/Stabilization Phase		Acute Management Phase		Recovery Phase	
Outcome	***Intervention***	***Outcome***	***Intervention***	***Outcome***	***Intervention***
Patient will have adequate gas exchange as evidenced by: • Sa_{O_2} saturation >90% • Arterial blood gases (ABGs) WNL • Clear breath sounds • Respiratory rate, depth, and rhythm WNL • Chest x-ray WNL • Absence of dyspnea, cyanosis, and secretions • Effective cough	Constantly monitor respiratory status—functioning, respiratory muscle strength, pulse oximetry, rate, rhythm, depth of respirations, lung sounds, coughing ability, ABGs, and chest x-ray. Be prepared for intubation and mechanical ventilation. Encourage coughing and deep breathing at least q2h. If patient is on ventilator, monitor settings and hemodynamic variables before, during, and after weaning. Wean ventilator when appropriate and monitor patient response: • Wean F_{IO_2} to keep $Sa_{O_2} > 90\%$ • Use humidification to keep secretions thin If patient is not intubated, apply supplemental oxygen. Monitor with pulse oximetry. Assess evidence of tissue perfusion. Monitor lab values: ABGs, hemoglobin.	Patient will have adequate gas exchange.	Monitor and treat oxygenation status per ABGs and/or Sa_{O_2}. Monitor and treat ventilation status per chest assessment, ABGs, adventitious breath sounds, and chest x-ray. Support patient with oxygen therapy and/or mechanical ventilation as indicated. Use humidification to keep secretions thin. Monitor lab values: ABGs, hemoglobin. Assess effects of increased activity on respiratory status. Observe for complications of Guillain-Barré syndrome that may impair oxygenation/ventilation: respiratory arrest, pneumonia, infection, thrombus, embolus. If necessary, prepare patient/family for long-term mechanical ventilation and need for tracheostomy. If so, monitor ventilator settings as above. Wean as above. If long-term mechanical ventilation is indicated, initiate plans to place in extended care facility, physical rehabilitation facility, or in the home. If going home, involve home health agency and home oxygen supply company.	Patient will have adequate gas exchange.	Obtain chest x-ray before discharge. Encourage coughing and deep breathing at least q2h. Begin to teach patient/family on mechanical ventilation and/or tracheostomy care if needed. Continue to assess for complications of Guillain-Barré syndrome that may impair oxygenation/ventilation. Teach patient/family potential complications to watch for. Assess patient/family understanding of home care. Reinforce knowledge and skills as needed.

DIAGNOSIS/STABILIZATION

Diagnosis/Stabilization Phase		Acute Management Phase		Recovery Phase	
Outcome	*Intervention*	*Outcome*	*Intervention*	*Outcome*	*Intervention*
Patient will be as comfortable and pain free as possible as evidenced by: • No objective indicators of discomfort • No complaints of discomfort • Absence of dyspnea	Assess absence of, or quantity and quality of pain. Administer analgesics and monitor response, particularly of respiratory system. Administer sedatives cautiously and monitor effects on respiratory status. Reposition extremities. If patient is intubated, establish effective communication technique with which patient can communicate discomfort. Provide reassurance in a calm, caring, and competent manner.	Patient will be relaxed and comfortable.	Same as stabilization phase. Provide uninterrupted rest periods in a quiet environment. Instruct patient on relaxation techniques. Use massage, humor, music therapy, and imagery to promote relaxation. Involve family in strategies. Consider alternative methods to control pain (i.e., cutaneous stimulation of transcutaneous electrical nerve stimulation). Observe for complications of Guillain-Barré syndrome that may cause discomfort: contractures, pulmonary embolus, infection.	Patient will be relaxed and comfortable.	Same as acute management phase. Progress analgesics to oral medications if patient is able to swallow; assess effect on respiratory system. Continue alternative methods to promote relaxation. Teach patient/family alternative methods to promote relaxation after discharge.

SKIN INTEGRITY

Diagnosis/Stabilization Phase		Acute Management Phase		Recovery Phase	
Outcome	*Intervention*	*Outcome*	*Intervention*	*Outcome*	*Intervention*
Patient will have intact skin without abrasions or pressure ulcers.	Assess muscle strength, movement, paresthesia, and paralysis. Assess all bony prominences at least q4h and treat if needed. Use preventive pressure-reducing devices if patient is at high risk for development of pressure ulcers. Treat pressure ulcers according to hospital protocol.	Patient will have intact skin without abrasions or pressure ulcers.	Same as stabilization phase.	Patient will have intact skin without abrasions or pressure ulcers.	Begin plans for transfer to extended care facility, physical rehabilitation facility, or home. Teach patient/family about proper skin care after discharge.

Care Guide continued on following page

GUILLAIN-BARRÉ SYNDROME MULTIDISCIPLINARY CARE GUIDE *continued*

PROTECTION/SAFETY

Diagnosis/Stabilization Phase		Acute Management Phase		Recovery Phase	
Outcome	*Intervention*	*Outcome*	*Intervention*	*Outcome*	*Intervention*
Patient will be protected from possible harm.	Assess need for assistance with activities. Provide physical support as needed.	Patient will be protected from possible harm.	Assess need for assistance with activities. Provide physical support as needed. Teach patient/family about range-of-motion exercises. Have patient/family demonstrate these exercises. Position joints in neutral position if possible. When patient is getting out of bed, consider possibility of orthostatic hypotension and/or autonomic dysreflexia. Monitor all vital signs with any activity and decrease activity if adverse events occur. Elevate head of bed slowly or use tilt table or Stryker frame. Consider TED hose. If used, remove at least q8h and inspect skin.	Patient will be protected from possible harm.	Teach patient/family about any physical limitations in activity after discharge/transfer.

PSYCHOSOCIAL/SELF-DETERMINATION

Diagnosis/Stabilization Phase		Acute Management Phase		Recovery Phase	
Outcome	*Intervention*	*Outcome*	*Intervention*	*Outcome*	*Intervention*
Patient will achieve psychophysiologic stability. Patient will demonstrate a decrease in anxiety as evidenced by: • Vital signs WNL • Subjective report of decreased anxiety • Objective signs of decreased anxiety Patient will demonstrate a decrease in fear.	Assess physiologic effects of critical care environment on patient (hemodynamic variables, psychological status, signs of increased sympathetic response). Administer sedatives cautiously and monitor respiratory effects. Take measures to reduce sensory overload. If patient is intubated, develop effective interventions to communicate with patient. If patient is unresponsive, maintain verbal and tactile contact with patient. Use calm, caring, competent, and reassuring approach with patient and family.	Patient will achieve psychophysiologic stability. Patient will demonstrate a decrease in anxiety. Patient will demonstrate a decrease in fear.	Same as stabilization phase. Provide adequate rest periods. Allow patient to verbalize/communicate feelings of anxiety and fear. Continue to include family in all aspects of care. Continue to assess coping ability of patient/family and take measures as indicated. Initiate discharge planning—extended care facility, physical rehabilitation facility, or home. Include patient/family in decisions concerning care. Continue explanation of process of Guillain-Barré syndrome and required treatment.	Patient will achieve psychophysiologic stability. Patient will demonstrate a decrease in anxiety. Patient will demonstrate a decrease in fear.	Same as acute management phase. Continue to assess coping ability of patient/family and take measures as appropriate (psychological consult, social services, home health agency, chaplain). Explain process of Guillain-Barré syndrome and any anticipated future effects of illness.

	Arrange for flexible visiting to meet patient/family needs. Determine coping ability of patient/family and take appropriate measures to meet their needs (i.e., explain condition, explain equipment, provide frequent condition reports, use easy to understand terminology, repeat information as needed, answer all questions, allow verbalization of fears/concerns). Begin explanation of process of Guillain-Barré syndrome and required treatment to patient and family.				

DIAGNOSTICS

Diagnosis/Stabilization Phase		Acute Management Phase		Recovery Phase	
Outcome	***Intervention***	***Outcome***	***Intervention***	***Outcome***	***Intervention***
Patient/family will understand any tests or procedures that need to be completed (vital signs, intake and output, hemodynamic monitoring, x-rays, CT scan, MRI, lab work, EKG, EEG, lumbar puncture) to rule out other pathology.	Explain all procedures and tests to patient/family. Be sensitive to individualized needs of patient/family for information. Establish effective communication technique with patient if intubated.	Patient/family will understand any tests or procedures that need to be completed (vital signs, hemodynamic monitoring, lab tests, radiology, CT scan, MRI, x-rays, EEG, tests to determine physical functioning).	Explain procedures and tests to assess progress and recovery from Guillain-Barré syndrome to patient/family. Assess individualized needs of patient/family for information. Anticipate need for further diagnostic tests such as EMG, EEG, CT scan, and any intervention that may result from this.	Patient/family will understand meaning of diagnostic tests in relation to continued health (MRI, CT scan, pulmonary function, EMG, further testing to assess potential for healing/mobility).	Review with patient/family before discharge results of all tests. Discuss abnormal findings and appropriate measures patient/family can take to return to normal or to regain as much physical functioning as possible. Provide patient/family with written guidelines concerning follow-up care. Prepare for discharge to extended care facility, physical rehabilitation facility, or home. Continue to involve physical therapy and physical rehabilitation consults. If discharged to home, provide instruction on care at home (i.e., when to call the doctor, physical restrictions, exercise, care of mechanical ventilator [if necessary], diet, medications).

REFERENCE

Nikas, D. L. (1991). The neurologic system. In J. G. Alspach (Ed.), *Core curriculum for critical care nursing* (4th ed., pp. 315–471). Philadelphia: W. B. Saunders.

Craniotomy

Julie Tackenberg and John M. Clochesy

Craniotomy is a surgical approach used for management of a wide variety of cerebral lesions. Aneurysms, abscess, hemorrhage, hematomas, and neoplastic disease are a few of the more common pathologies that justify surgical intervention with craniotomy as well as epilepsy and pain disorders. The extent and location of the craniotomy, as well as that of the surgical intervention, guide nursing care that promotes the recovery of the patient through the intensive care phase to discharge. This chapter focuses on the pathologies of cerebral neoplastic disease and the epilepsies as an indication for craniotomy and reviews the procedure of craniotomy and principles of neuroanesthesia.

INTRACRANIAL TUMORS

At some point in the course of their disease, most patients with oncologic disease are admitted emergently to the intensive care unit (ICU) for various complications of treatment or of the disease. Schulier and Markiewicz (1991) collected data that demonstrated oncology patients are admitted to the ICU for medical emergencies and for administration and monitoring of treatment. Those with intracranial tumors are frequently admitted for management of increasing intracranial pressure (ICP) or status epilepticus. Others are admitted for management of the postoperative period.

Tumor Etiology/Incidence

A tumor is a swelling or a mass of tissue that can be considered benign or malignant depending on its characteristics. The term *tumor* is not to be equated with the term *cancer*. The term *cancer*, however, can be used synonymously with *malignant neoplasm*, which can be defined as uncontrolled new growth capable of metastasis and invasion of the host tissue (Groenwald et al., 1993). Evidence suggests that central nervous system (CNS) tumors occur more frequently in individuals exposed to occupational chemicals such as vinyl chloride, plutonium, and petroleum (Jones, 1986).

Tumors can be identified by histologic, biologic, and cytologic characteristics, which differentiate benign forms from malignant growth. The properties of invasiveness and ability to metastasize are the most important prognostic tumor characteristics.

Tumor growth retains the characteristics of tissue from which it is derived, thus providing identifying histologic properties. The suffix added to the histologic root word designates the benign or malignant nature of the growth. If it is benign, the suffix *-oma* is used. A malignant tumor is indicated by the ending *-sarcoma* or *-carcinoma*. If the tumor is derived from connective tissue, *sarcoma* is attached to the tissue name. Carcinoma is a term used to indicated growth from epithelial cells.

Clinical staging or grading the growth process classifies malignancy by extent of spread or by neurologic signs and symptoms as well as diagnostic results. Pathologic staging is based on histologic evidence. Classification and grading are done to assist treatment planning and prognostic determinations. The most common classification system is the TNM system, which describes the anatomic extent of disease using characteristics of tumor invasiveness (T), lymph node involvement (N), and distant metastasis (M). (See Table 40–1.) Grading of a malignant neoplasm is done descriptively (well-differentiated to poorly differentiated, or numerically on a scale of 1 to 4 with 3 and 4 being the least differentiated). Brain tumors are not suited to the TNM system because they have no associated lymph nodes. According to Beahrs and colleagues (1988), histopathology is the most important feature of CNS tumor classification. Magnetic resonance imaging may be helpful to confirm a diagnosis in cases of disparity between clinical and neuropathologic findings (Dean et al., 1990; Judnick et al., 1992). The nurse also needs to know that despite cell type and invasive characteristics, if a tumor is inaccessible for surgical intervention, it is usually considered malignant.

Intracranial tumors can arise from any structure of the brain, including cranial nerves and meninges. Primary intracranial tumors develop from neuroepithelial (glial) cells. This is due to the capability of glial cells to divide. Gliomas can spread, or metastasize, to other parts of the CNS. A primary tumor reflects the histologic cells of its origin. A metastatic tumor also retains the cells of its origin but often becomes anaplastic beyond recognition.

In the adult population, brain tumors are the second leading cause of death from neurologic disease

TABLE 40–1. **TNM Classification System for Describing the Anatomic Extent of Disease**

TNM Definitions

(T) Primary tumor

TX	Primary tumor cannot be assessed
TO	No evidence of primary tumor
Tis	Carcinoma in situ
T1, T2, T3, T4	Increasing size and/or local extent of the primary tumor

(N) Regional lymph nodes

NX	Regional lymph nodes cannot be assessed
NO	No regional lymph node metastasis
N1, N2, N3	Increasing involvement of regional lymph nodes

(M) Distant metastasis

MX	Presence of distant metastasis cannot be assessed
MO	No distant metastasis
M1	Distant metastasis

TNM Classifications

cTNM or TNM	*Clinical Classification:* Based on information obtained from the physical examination, laboratory and imaging studies, endoscopy, biopsy, and surgical exploration. Clinical staging uses all information available before the initiation of definitive treatment.
pTNM	*Pathologic Classification:* Based on information acquired before treatment, supplemented or modified by information from surgery and the pathologic examination of a resected specimen. This includes resected tumor (pT), lymph nodes (pN), and distant metastasis (pM).
rTNM	*Retreatment Classification:* Based on all information available after a disease-free interval or at the time of a second-look surgery. The extent or absence of disease recurrence is documented before retreatment planning is begun.
aTNM	*Autopsy Classification:* Based on all information available at the time of a postmortem examination. It is helpful in answering questions about the tumor's response to treatment, recurrence patterns, and the extent of disease at the time of death.

Adapted from Beahrs, OH, Henson, DE, Hutter, RVP, et al. (1992). *American Joint Committee on Cancer: Manual for staging of cancer* (4th ed., pp. 6–7). Philadelphia: J. B. Lippincott.

(Bilsky & Posner, 1993). The incidence may be as high as 15% as the population continues to age. Most intracranial tumors are supratentorial.

Types of Brain Tumors

GLIOMAS

GLIOBLASTOMA MULTIFORME. The most common primary adult brain tumor (25% of all intracranial tumors), glioblastoma is found twice as often in men as in women. Diagnosis is usually made during middle age, between the fourth and sixth decades of life. They can occur anywhere in the cerebral hemispheres, but glioblastomas are usually found in the frontal lobe. Spread from one hemisphere to the other is often through the corpus callosum. This is a fast-growing, rapidly invasive neoplasm. Typically a Grade IV astrocytoma, the glioblastoma causes cellular changes such as necrosis, pseudopalisading, fistulous vessels, vascular endothelium proliferation, and areas of hemorrhage, thrombosis, and fibroplastic proliferation (Zulch, 1980).

Early findings include diffuse cerebral edema and generalized seizures. Symptoms become localized as the disease process continues. Focal symptoms reflect the area affected by the presence of the neoplasm. Prognosis for the patient with glioblastoma multiforme is poor, with less than 20% surviving the first year after diagnosis. Chemotherapy has proven to be of little value; radiotherapy may extend the mean survival to 12 to 14 months.

ASTROCYTOMA. A relatively common primary tumor of the brain (third most common in adults) (Kornblith et al., 1987), astrocytomas are infiltrative histologically and tend to be solid tumors that form large cavities; they may also present as cysts in the cerebral tissue. Although found throughout the CNS, the most common sites for this tumor are the cerebral white matter, cerebellum, hypothalamus, optic nerve, optic chiasm, and pons. This tumor type comprises 10% of primary brain tumors. Age of incidence is between the second and sixth decades, with peak incidence between the fifth and sixth decades. Seizures are the most common presenting symptoms.

Histologic changes of astrocytomas range from well-differentiated astrocytes (Grade I) to Grades III and IV, which may demonstrate multiple sites of origin. A Grade IV astrocytoma can also be classified as a glioblastoma multiforme. Astrocytomas are generally considered highly malignant due to their infiltrative nature. Because they are not encapsulated, sloughing of tumor cells around the necrotic focus is often seen with these tumors (del Regato et al., 1985).

Oligodendroglioma

Oligodendroglioma is another form of glioma that arises from the oligodendrocytes, which produce the myelin of the brain. Peak incidence of this tumor is in the fifth and sixth decades. A relatively uncommon tumor type, the oligodendroglioma represents 5% to 7% of intracranial tumors. This tumor is usually found in the frontal lobes and characteristically is a well-marginated, spongy vascular mass often with mixed cell types. Calcification is a frequent concurrent finding as well as multinucleated cells of the Langhans type.

Oligodendrogliomas are slow-growing tumors. Commonly a period of 2 to 3 years exists between the first symptom and surgical intervention. Seizures are the most common symptoms that bring the patient to the physician. Oligodendrogliomas have been found to be sensitive to procarbazine, lomustine (CCNU), and vincristine. Surgical excision has resulted in a survival length of approximately 5 years.

MENINGIOMAS

Meningiomas are usually well-encapsulated, smooth tumors that arise from the meninges. This tumor type comprises 15% to 20% of all primary intracranial tumors. Histologically, meningiomas are well-differentiated tumors that have hyalinized calcified centers known as psammoma bodies (visible on computed tomography [CT] scan). Biologically, these are the most benign of intracranial tumors because they are slow-growing and noninvasive of other tissue, although they can cause cranial deformities. Meningiomas have been found on the parasagittal surface of the frontal and parietal lobes, the lesser wings of the sphenoid, olfactory grooves, tuberculum sellae turcicae, the cerebellum, parasylvian region, intraventricular area, and the spinal canal (Stewardt-Amidei, 1991).

Seizures are a common presenting symptom of meningiomas. Other symptoms are related to the location of the tumor. Radiation therapy of the cranium or scalp has proven to be a significant antecedent to tumor occurrence (Stewardt-Amidei, 1991). Mortality rates associated with meningiomas are low. Incidence of meningiomas is two times greater in women than men, with the occurrence diagnosed during the third and sixth decades. Incidence is higher in women with a history of breast cancer. Malignant meningiomas, which are inoperable by location, have been found with a greater ratio of 3:2 in men vs. women. Malignant, invasive meningiomas are usually treated with radiation after surgical resection. Easily accessible tumors respond to surgical excision.

PITUITARY TUMORS

Pituitary tumors represent 8% to 10% of all primary intracranial tumors. Tumor incidence increases with each decade. Adenomas, the most common neoplasm of the pituitary, may arise from the basophil, eosinophil, or chromophobe cells of this gland. Adenomas are characterized according to clinical characteristics: (1) a space-occupying lesion without endocrine involvement or (2) a space-occupying lesion with endocrine hyperactivity.

Growth of pituitary tumors is predictable and progresses through four phases: (1) stretching of the diaphragma sella with resultant bitemporal headaches, (2) increasing pressure on the pituitary gland with its eventual destruction and development of panhypopituitary syndrome, (3) bitemporal visual field deficits secondary to pressure on the medial fibers of the optic chiasm, and (4) development of hydrocephalus as the tumor invades the third ventricle, obstructing flow of cerebrospinal fluid (CSF). Concurrent symptoms usually include headache, altered mentation, and motor and sensory dysfunction. Without treatment, the patient experiences altered sleep patterns and coma.

A major portion of pituitary neoplasms secrete hormones such as prolactin, growth hormone and, infrequently, arginine vasopressin, resulting in amenorrhea-galactorrhea syndrome or acromegaly. Amenorrhea-galactorrhea syndrome is characterized by periods of amenorrhea, increased serum prolactin, and galactorrhea. Impotence is noted in men with prolactin-secreting tumors. Acromegaly results in the presence of excessive production of growth hormone, resulting in enlarged hands and feet as well as thickening and broadening of facial features.

PRIMARY MALIGNANT LYMPHOMAS

Although relatively rare in the past, primary CNS lymphomas are increasing due to the number of immunosuppressed patients. Those at greatest risk are solid organ transplant recipients, AIDS patients, and those with congenital immunodeficiencies. A slightly higher incidence is found in men than in women. Approximately 3% of all AIDS patients develop CNS lymphomas. Mainly of B-cell origin, these tumors are often seen in the cerebrum, cerebellum, or brain stem. Most common presenting symptoms are hemiparesis, aphasia, seizures, cranial nerve palsies, and headache.

METASTATIC TUMORS

Intracranial metastases occur in 10% to 20% of individuals with systemic cancer. Metastatic tumors are commonly found in the skull and dura, the cortex itself, and the meninges. Meningeal carcinoma is rare. The skull and dura are the secondary sites for metastasis originating from the breast or prostate. Hematogenous spread has been found to be the process of seeding tumors of the cortex via the cerebral arterial pathway. Approximately one-third of cortex metastases have been found to originate from the lungs. Clinical presentation is varied depending on the extent of destruction of cerebral structures and cerebral edema. Seizures are a frequent concurrent symptom.

Signs and Symptoms of Intracranial Tumors

In the ICU, the most common signs and symptoms of an intracranial lesion are secondary to increased ICP. These clinical manifestations are related to the mechanisms of compression, obstruction, and invasion of surrounding tissue by the space-occupying lesion. Location and extent of the tumor determines the focal clinical signs and symptoms that must be monitored. As the tumor continues to cause obstruction and compression, the mass effects become more global, influencing bilateral hemispheric function and the patient's level of consciousness. Seizure activity can occur secondary to the tumor in any location.

FRONTAL LOBE SIGNS

Pressure on the frontal lobe can cause subtle alterations in personality and cognition that may only be recognized by family members. Affective changes include increased irritability, impulsivity or loss of inhibition, and socially inappropriate behaviors. The patient often lacks insight into the unacceptability of the behaviors. Abstract thinking may be compromised as well as initiative and judgment.

Motor deficits ranging from mild weakness to paralysis can be present if the motor cortex becomes affected. Spasticity or flaccidity can develop. Such deficits occur on the contralateral side of the lesion. Motor performance of speech can be affected by a tumor that encroaches on Broca's center of the language-dominant hemisphere. Aphasia will vary depending on the extent of neoplastic invasion or effects of increased ICP.

PARIETAL LOBE SIGNS

Tumors in the parietal lobe affect sensory processing. Contralateral abnormalities such as numbness, tingling, and burning are often noted as well as astereognosis and loss of stimuli localization. If the speech-dominant hemisphere is involved, Broca's center may be involved. Difficulties of spoken and written language can be found.

TEMPORAL LOBE SIGNS

Seizure activity in the presence of temporal lobe lesions are characteristically complex partial behaviors with automatisms such as chewing or swallowing movements. If the hippocampal areas are compromised, psychic abnormalities may be present. These behaviors could include visual hallucinations, feelings of déjà vu, or feelings of jamais vu. Auditory disturbances such as tinnitus and sound distortion are often reported in the presence of temporal lobe lesions.

OCCIPITAL LOBE SIGNS

Visual deficits are the predominant findings with lesions of the occipital lobe. Hemianopsia and diplopia are the most common visual changes. The patient often reports small, seemingly insignificant accidents due to change in depth perception and peripheral field alterations.

CEREBELLAR SIGNS

Lesions of the cerebellum are manifest by incoordination, ataxia, inability to maintain posture, and tremor. Generally ipsilateral involvement is seen. Reflex function is disturbed, and tendon reflexes are slow and prolonged. Nystagmus occurs as well as slurred speech, halting articulation, and explosive articulation. Vestibular involvement with tumors of the vermis produce incoordination of the head and trunk, difficulty maintaining the head midline and upright, as well as retropulsion and propulsion. Subjectively, the patient reports easy fatigability and muscle weakness due to poor muscle contraction and hypotonia.

EPILEPSIES

The term *epilepsy* is generally recognized as the tendency to "experience recurrent seizures of major or minor intensity and varying characteristics" (Wyllie & Lunders, 1993). A seizure is the result of an abnormal electrical discharge by a neuron or neuronal network. This abnormal discharge can result from electrical stimulation, changes in the metabolic environment, neurotransmitter substances, or excitatory drugs. Seizures generally noted in the ICU are related to underlying reversible pathologies such as metabolic acidosis, renal compromise, or hepatotoxicity. Idiopathic epilepsy is the occurrence of abnormal cellular discharge in the absence of such discernible pathology. Postnatal or acquired cerebral insults such as brain injury, CNS infection, cerebrovascular disease, brain tumors, degenerative CNS diseases, and developmental deficits have been noted to greatly increase the incidence of epilepsy. Certain regions of the brain, such as the temporal lobe, motor cortex, and limbic structures, have been found to be sensitive to disturbances in the cellular environment, especially vascular compression and biochemical disturbances related to hypoxia (Dichter, 1989). Surgical resection of epileptogenic focus via craniotomy has gained acceptance with the improvement of diagnostic capabilities such as the positron emission tomography scan and video electroencephalogram (EEG) monitoring. Although these patients are generally young and otherwise healthy, they present a nursing challenge because of the wide scope of seizure behaviors they may present to the ICU nurse familiar only with generalized tonic-clonic seizures.

A classification system currently exists to communicate clinical and EEG characteristics of the seizure behaviors. As with any classification system, the present categories are unable to describe every event or epilepsy syndrome and continue to be revised.

Partial Seizures

In partial seizures, the first clinical and EEG changes are characteristically confined to one cerebral hemisphere. The status of the individual's consciousness during these episodes is an important differentiating characteristic within this classification. If consciousness is not impaired, the event is considered a simple partial seizure. An impairment of consciousness identifies the episode as a complex partial seizure. Partial seizures of either type may produce motor, sensory, autonomic, or psychic symptomatology. Disturbances of higher cerebral functions/psychic symptomatology (e.g., illusions, hallucinations, affective alterations) usually occur with complex partial seizures (Wyllie & Lunders, 1993). Simple partial seizures generally maintain a unilateral spread; complex partial seizures, however, frequently have a secondary bilateral hemispheric spread. Automatisms typically occur in complex partial seizures.

The term *aura* is frequently used to describe the first indications of an impending seizure. The aura is that portion of the seizure experience recalled by the person after the event. It may be a simple partial seizure in its entirety, or that portion of a complex partial seizure that becomes secondarily generalized with its accompanying impairment of consciousness.

Generalized Seizures

Generalized seizures have bihemispheric clinical and EEG changes. Bilateral involvement may occur at the onset of the episode or may represent secondary transmission of the electrical discharge. Within this classification are several distinct seizure types. Nonconvulsive generalized seizures include absence seizures, atonic seizures, and myoclonic seizures.

TONIC-CLONIC SEIZURES

These are the most common form of generalized seizures, characterized by a sharp tonic contraction of muscles. Respiratory muscles may also be involved, producing a stridor or outcry and possible color change if air exchange is inadequate. Loss of consciousness occurs without warning at the onset. This phase progresses to the clonic portion of the seizure, which is associated with convulsive movements. At the conclusion of the convulsions, muscle relaxation occurs, allowing respiration to return to normal. Consciousness may remain impaired for a variable length of time after the event.

ABSENCE SEIZURES

Absence seizures are generalized seizures characterized by sudden onset, arrest of activity and speech, and a blank stare. Additional characteristics include mild clonic, atonic, and tonic components, as well as automatisms.

CRANIOTOMY

Craniotomy is the surgical opening of the skull to provide access to the brain for surgical resection, removal, or repair of lesions. A supratentorial craniotomy is used to access the parietal, frontal, and occipital lobes of the cerebral cortex. The infratentorial approach provides access to the brain stem and cerebellum. The suboccipital or posterior fossa approach are the common infratentorial procedures. Anatomic location of the lesion and craniotomy greatly influence the nursing care in the ICU. Based on knowledge of the function of the structures involved in each approach, the nurse is able to individualize patient care.

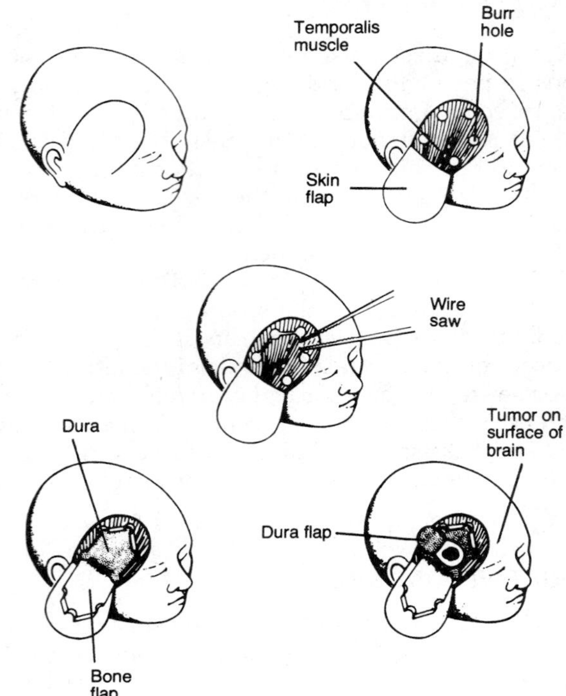

FIGURE 40–1. Stages of craniotomy. (From Hickey, J. [1993]. Care of the patient undergoing cranial surgery. In *The clinical practice of neurological and neurosurgical nursing* [3rd ed., p. 304]. Philadelphia: J. B. Lippincott Co.)

Advanced technology has allowed electronic monitoring to be an integral part of intraoperative management of the patient undergoing craniocerebral surgery. Intraoperative monitoring for CNS function now includes cerebral blood flow (CBF) monitoring, brain electrical activity, somatosensory evoked potentials, ICP monitoring, and Doppler evaluation. These adjunct studies are used for deeper surgical resections as well as to guide surgical resection in superficial eloquent areas of the cortex.

Procedure

Typically, a craniotomy consists of the following steps (Figure 40–1). First, an incision is made through the scalp and underlying muscle. This tissue is dissected from the underlying skull to form a soft tissue flap. Surgical clips are placed along the edges of the excised area to obtain hemostasis. Once this exposure has been achieved, the procedural options will vary in the following manner depending on the purpose and extent of the surgery.

Burr holes are made into the cranium with a drill. Single or small burr holes are used for superficial repairs, such as evacuation of hematomas or cerebral biopsy. Bone from these burr holes may or may not be replaced. The smaller the burr hole (<2 cm), the

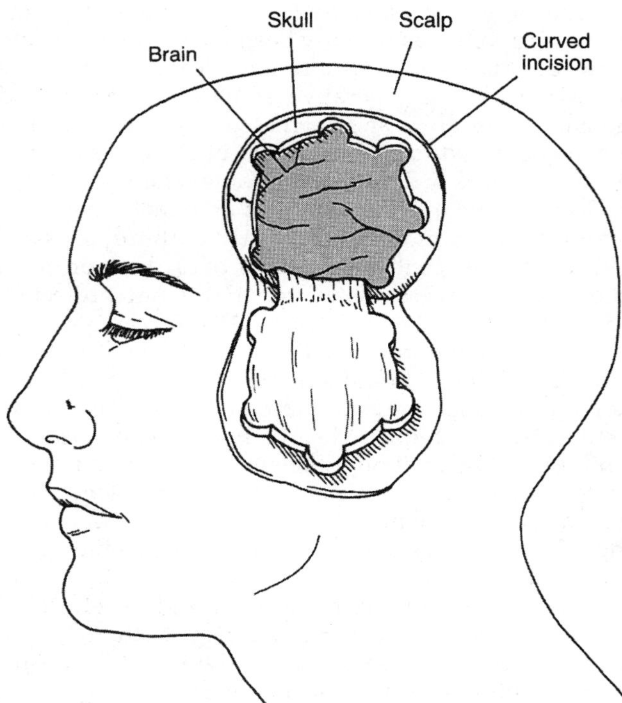

FIGURE 40–2. Craniotomy with osteoplastic bone flap. (From Black, J. M., & Matassarin-Jacobs, E. [1993]. *Luckmann and Sorensen's medical-surgical nursing* [4th ed., p. 734]. Philadelphia: W. B. Saunders.)

greater the tendency not to replace the cranial bone. Bone from larger burr holes (>2 cm) is held within the immediate surgical field with wire or heavy silk sutures until it is replaced at the end of the procedure. Burr holes are enlarged with a rongeur to expose enough brain surface to perform the procedure.

More extensive craniotomies are created by surgically connecting the burr holes with a saw or wire (Gilgi blade). This larger piece of bone may be left attached to the periosteum and muscle to create a hinge that allows retention of a vascular supply (osteoplastic bone flap; see Fig. 40–2). Once the bone flap is turned over and the brain exposed, the dura mater is incised and retracted, exposing the cerebral tissue.

Alternatively, a free-form flap may be created, in which the section of cranium is removed from its attachments and temporarily removed. If the section is permanently removed, a protective prosthesis of methyl methacrylate may be inserted at a later date.

On completion of the surgery, the process of closing the craniotomy reverses the previous steps: suture of the dura, replacement and stabilization of the bone flap, and suturing of the periosteum and muscle. Skin closure is achieved with sutures or staples. Open or closed drainage systems may be left in place depending on the type and extent of surgery.

Pituitary Surgery

Currently two surgical approaches are used for resection of pituitary tumors. Recent advances have made the transsphenoidal hypophysectomy approach the technique of choice for removal of pituitary neoplasms. Technically, this is not cranial surgery. Recent studies have demonstrated a high success rate when this approach is coupled with gamma knife treatment. A second surgical option, the transcranial technique (Figure 40–2), is recommended only in rare circumstances of extremely large tumors due to the high morbidity rate associated with the deep manipulation of the frontal lobes required for adequate exposure of the pituitary.

Stereotactic Assistance

Stereotaxis is the precise localization of a specific tissue target using three-dimensional coordinates. The coordinates are calculated using a special stereotactic frame and other related instruments. This type of precise location is needed for tumors and lesions too deep for traditional resection (Arbor, 1993). After placement of the head frame, the point of intersection of the three coordinates (x = anteroposterior, y = superoinferior, z = left/right) in relation to the stereotactic frame identify the lesion location. A CT scan can also be used concurrently to determine the exact target point. Stereotaxis offers much in terms of surgical precision, but it is not without its complications. Intraoperatively, obstruction of the endotracheal tube can occur despite head fixation. In a study by Korn and colleagues (1993), obstruction occurred due to torso movement rather than the usual flexion of the head.

Placement of the frame usually occurs the day before surgery. Food and fluids are withheld before placement. Sedatives are administered before the patient is taken to radiology for measurement and application. Mild analgesics are ordered for headache and neck pain. Pin sites should be assessed for swelling and loosening.

Many different types of frames are available and continue to be refined. Stereotactic frames are used in conjunction with radiotherapy and laser surgery.

LASERS

Based on the principles of light and electromagnetic radiation, lasers concentrate a single wavelength of light into a beam of light energy that can be focused on specific tissue. As the tissue absorbs the beam of monochromatic light energy, the beam is transformed into heat energy, producing surgical dissection (through vaporization) and coagulation of cerebral blood vessels. The laser beam is directly applied to the tissue or indirectly to heat probes, which in turn are placed on the specified tissue. The advantage of this device in surgery is the decrease in trauma to surrounding tissue seen with traditional surgical techniques. Three types of surgical lasers are currently available, each using a different light energy, allowing for varied degrees of control and application of the energy beam.

Appropriate patient selection is important to clinical application of this technology. Acoustic neuromas, craniopharyngiomas, some brain stem gliomas, ventricular tumors, and meningiomas have all been successfully resected with laser surgery. Tumors extrinsic to the brain but adjacent to delicate cerebral tissue are also amenable to laser surgery.

Neuroanesthesia

When caring for the patient who has undergone a craniotomy, it is important to be familiar with the various anesthetic agents used and the principles of cerebral protection in neurosurgery. The following summary will provide the ICU nurse with the basic information necessary to manage the neurosurgical patient.

Anesthesia, in general, is intended to provide analgesia, sedation, and muscle relaxation. Choice of agents depends on the needs of the patient and the surgeon. The needs of the surgeon include adequate room to work within the cranium and control of bleeding.

General anesthesia provides a controlled and reversible state of unconsciousness, analgesia, appropriate muscle relaxation, and adequate control of the autonomic nervous system. This state is accompanied by a partial or complete loss of protective reflexes such as swallow, gag, and eye blink reflexes. Intravenous drugs or inhalation agents are used to produce this state. Induction of the anesthetized state is accomplished with a barbiturate such as sodium thiopental and maintained with nitrous oxide (N_2O), oxygen O_2, and narcotics or inhalants. Muscle relaxants can be added as needed. Selection of the appropriate anesthetic also considers characteristics of the agent, such as its nonflammability (cautery is often used in neurosurgery), effect on blood pressure, and nonirritability (to avoid coughing and retching).

Many anesthetics are available for neurosurgical procedures, but an ideal agent does not exist. All have side effects that may be detrimental to any one patient. Consideration must be given to the principles of cerebral protection when selecting anesthesia and when providing perioperative management for the craniotomy patient.

PROTECTIVE NEUROANESTHETIC AGENTS

Although the anesthesiologist may select from an array of agents (Table 40–2), isoflurane is currently the most widely used agent for intracranial procedures, especially if brain retraction is necessary. It has proven successful in the presence of ischemia, hypotension, and hypocapnia and with cerebrovascular procedures. Isoflurane is frequently used in combination with N_2O oxide and a narcotic. Ornstein and colleagues (1993) found that desflurane is similar to isoflurane in terms of effects on absolute CBF, response to increasing doses, and preservation of carbon dioxide CO_2 reactivity.

Used only occasionally for neurosurgical procedures, propofol has recently been proven to have several advantages over isoflurane. Propofol produces more reliable intraoperative somatosensory evoked potential recordings and decreased retraction pressure when compared to an isoflurane/N_2O/fentanyl combination (Moss & Price, 1990; Taniguche et al., 1992; Todd et al., 1993). Etomidate is an imidazole anesthetic that has proven more effective than barbiturates as an intraoperative agent. Relative lack of cardiodepression and rapid recovery make this a cerebral protective agent (Lee et al., 1990; Olympia, 1994).

A prospective study by Todd and colleagues (1993) indicated minor differences between propofol/fentanyl, isoflurane/N_2O, and fentanyl/N_2O. This study demonstrated higher heart rates with use of isoflurane/N_2O, although mean arterial pressure was lower during the maintenance phase. Emergence time was more rapid with the fentanyl/N_2O patients, although no relationship existed between emergence time and ICP.

A few recent studies have addressed the effects of anesthetic agents in epilepsy surgery. Although propofol did not increase seizure activity, it was postulated to interfere with recording of EEG spikes, which may be used to direct resection of the epileptogenic tissue. Fentanyl, however, has been found to induce seizure activity in patients with complex partial seizures. Newer opioids, such as sufentanil and alfentanil, when used for awake craniotomy (for epilepsy surgery), have not proven more beneficial than fentanyl (Ganz, 1993).

INTRAOPERATIVE CEREBRAL PROTECTION

Cerebral protection implies that brain function can be maintained and injury can be avoided (Andrews & Bringas, 1993). Patients undergoing a cranial neurosurgical procedure are at risk for compromised physiologic autoregulation due to pathology or the procedure itself. Manipulation of the ICP and all the factors of influence (metabolism, homeostasis, and circulation) during the surgical procedure constitute the practices of cerebral protection.

Patients with lesions from hemorrhage, aneurysm, or tumor are at risk of developing increased ICP. Studies indicate that in 8% of postcraniotomy patients, increased ICP was a significant problem due to cerebral edema, ventricular enlargement, or location of the fluid in the tumor bed (Steen, 1991). Intraoperative management of increased ICP can be achieved by reduction of CSF via a ventricular tap. This technique is also used to provide more operative space. Direct needle tap of the ventricles is used for suprasellar and posterior fossa masses associated with hydrocephalus. More commonly, intrathecal lumbar drainage is initiated once the durae are opened. Mild, transient reduction of CSF volume may also be achieved intraoperatively with acetazolamide or furosemide. Intraoperative use of brain-stem auditory evoked poten-

TABLE 40–2. **Commonly Used Neurosurgical Anesthetic Agents**

Drug	Side Effects/Adverse Reactions	Comments
Halothane (volatile liquid)	Slight cerebral vasodilation and subsequent increase in intracranial pressure (ICP), especially at the time of induction Hypotension Postoperative shivering Decreased cerebral metabolic oxygen requirement ($CMRO_2$)	Begin induction with other drugs using the IV route; hyperventilate the patient Has a hypotensive effect when given with curare and ganglionic blockers Useful in inducing hypothermia Cleared quickly from the body when administration is discontinued
Enflurane (volatile liquid)	Increased ICP Decreased $CMRO_2$ Possible renal failure Hepatotoxicity Slight hypotension	Rapid onset Rapid excretion from the lungs of 85% to 90% of the drug Used in combination with small amounts of skeletal muscle relaxants
Nitrous oxide (inhalant gas)	No effect on ICP Increased cerebral metabolic rate	Increases the risk of air emboli Always used in a mixture with oxygen
Ketamine hydrochloride (dissociation agent)	Elevated blood pressure (tachycardia) Increased ICP Increased $CMRO_2$ Cerebrovasoconstriction Possible tonic-clonic movements	Rapid-acting anesthetic agent Produces analgesia while maintaining normal skeletal muscle tone Associated with a slow recovery from anesthesia with possible vivid dreams or hallucinations Barbiturates or narcotics may increase recovery time
Innovar (a combination of fentanyl and droperidol; a dissociation agent)	Decreased $CMRO_2$ and ICP (fentanyl decreases $CMRO_2$, whereas droperidol has no effect on it) Hypotension Bradycardia Muscle rigidity Respiratory depression	Neuroleptanalgesic agent that produces analgesia, reduces motor activity, and alters consciousness Slow onset and prolonged duration Used in combination with other drugs
Nondepolarizing muscle relaxants—gallamine triethiodide (Flaxedil); pancuronium bromide (Pavulon); tubocurarine (Metubine)	Tachycardia Muscle weakness Salivation (an anticholinergic is administered to reduce this side effect) Dizziness Hypertension Respiratory depression Decreased ICP	Adjunct to anesthetic agents during surgery; produces skeletal muscle relaxation Assists patients on mechanical ventilators Competitive antagonist of acetylcholine at the neuromuscular junction or receptor site Almost immediate onset of effect that lasts 20 to 60 minutes Excreted through urine
Depolarizing muscle relaxant—succinylcholine (Anectine)	Bradycardia or tachycardia Hypotension or hypertension Muscle twitching Respiratory depression Malignant hyperthermia Postoperative muscle pain and stiffness Excessive salivation	Adjunct to anesthetic agents during surgery; produces skeletal muscle relaxation Facilitates intubation Produces initial muscle fasciculations, which are quickly followed by flaccid paralysis Almost immediate onset of effect that lasts 2 to 4 minutes Can be given by IV drip for prolonged muscle relaxation Should not be used with nondepolarizing blockers because this prolongs the effect Excreted through urine Use with great caution in paraplegics because they tend to become severely hyperkalemic
Barbiturates (short acting)—thiopental sodium and pentobarbital	Decreased $CMRO_2$ Cerebrovasoconstriction Decreased ICP	Administered intravenously to decrease the effects on ICP from halothane and intubation

tials in posterior fossa surgery will guide the surgeon in the effects of increased ICP in this area.

Corticosteroids are routinely used as an adjunct to tumor surgery. These agents restore the blood–brain barrier, promoting electrolyte transport and water excretion. If cerebral edema, as commonly found with mass lesions, is present at the time of anesthesia induction, significant elevation of ICP can occur. Based on the preoperative CT scan, studies demonstrate that steroids initiated perioperatively and tapered postoperatively act to minimize the development of increased ICP (Hoff, 1986).

Hyperventilating the patient perioperatively is another measure to control ICP. Hypocapnia, or $Paco_2$ of 25 to 30 mm Hg, provides the maximum beneficial effect, although other parameters may be established in the ICU. This technique reduces cerebral blood volume, resulting in decreased cerebral bulk and ICP immediately. Decrease in cerebral bulk allows the neurosurgeon more work space within the head. Because ischemia and hypoxia may result if the $Paco_2$ falls below 20 mm Hg, hyperventilation must be managed judiciously by the anesthesiologist.

Balanced isotonic solutions, such as mannitol, are used to reduce the brain's water content and achieve brain relaxation during surgery. Mannitol begins to influence ICP within 10 to 15 minutes by causing cerebral water to enter the intravascular compartment. Renal excretion begins 40 minutes after administration. Mannitol alters blood viscosity, improving CBF and reducing blood volume and ICP. The neurosurgeon and anesthesiologist must monitor the dose and rate of administration of mannitol very carefully. Vasodilatation, and therefore an increase in ICP, can occur with large, rapid doses of 25% mannitol. Mannitol is not recommended in the presence of vascular lesions, because further shrinkage of the brain may promote expansion of the hematoma. In the geriatric patient, sudden decrease in brain size may lead to tearing of the parasagittal veins, resulting in a subdural hematoma. Glycerol in a 10% solution can also be used to manage ICP perioperatively as well as loop diuretics. Furosemide in combination with mannitol has a greater effect on increased ICP than either agent alone.

Position of the patient during surgery depends on the region of the craniotomy. This may require the patient to be prone or seated in a barber's chair for surgical accessibility. When selecting the position, the surgeon must be aware of the potential for obstruction of cerebral venous blood flow. It is desirable to keep the head higher than the heart in any selected position. This general principle also allows gravity to facilitate brain exposure, reducing the amount of retraction required for visualization. However, head elevation also produces negative pressure in the dural venous sinuses, placing the patient at risk for a venous air embolism, reduced cerebral perfusion pressure, and right-to-left shunting. Other activities that may obstruct venous return are positive end-expiratory pressure (PEEP), sedation, and sharp flexion of the neck.

Intraoperative use of the Doppler sensor and transesophageal echocardiography are needed to determine the presence of an air embolism in the heart. Entry site of the air must be located, the field flooded with saline, all bleeding points coagulated, and exposed bone sealed with wax. Breathing air is changed to 100% oxygen to decrease expansion of the embolism by N_2O. Vasopressors are given to maintain the blood pressure. Aspiration of the air embolism from the pulmonary artery or the right arterial line is done by the anesthesiologist. Complications of an air embolism include pulmonary infarction and ischemic stroke.

Maintaining adequate CBF for metabolic needs is another goal of cerebral protection during craniotomy. This may be accomplished by raising the systemic blood pressure according to the state of the brain's autoregulation. If autoregulation is intact, the blood pressure must exceed the brain's upper limits of autoregulation before CBF is increased. If cerebral arterial pressure is elevated after cell injury, the blood–brain barrier is compromised and autoregulation is subsequently lost. Measuring CBF with arterial-venous oxygen difference ($avDo_2$) measurements is the most accurate way of determining the optimal blood pressure.

The patient may come to surgery with increased ICP; the practice of brain retraction, necessary for visualization and access of the surgical site, also increases ICP by producing decreased CBF and ischemia. Brain retraction, although often necessary, does place the patient at risk of increasing ICP. Fuchamachi and colleagues (1985) found that 8% to 22% of postoperative clinically significant neurologic deficits are related to retraction-induced injuries. Brain retraction injury is induced by the focal pressure of the retractor blade (especially the tip) on the brain tissue, resulting in a local deformity (Andrews & Bringas, 1993). This deformity results in a reduction of local perfusion. Brain retraction is accomplished by (1) constant pressure retraction or (2) constant exposure. Constant pressure retraction entails periodic readjustment of the blade to maintain a constant pressure. Constant exposure involves placement of the retractor blade once during the procedure. This method requires the brain to adjust to the presence of the blade. Both have their disadvantages: Constant exposure can obviously cause ischemia. Reperfusion injuries occur between the repeated retraction events of constant pressure retraction as well. Current literature recommends that brain retraction be limited to 15 minutes at pressures lower than 40 mm Hg. Recovery periods of 5 minutes should be expended between retraction episodes as well. Use of multiple narrow blades rather than a single wide blade is also suggested. It is imperative that the ICU nurse be cognizant of these intraoperative events because the area of injury will not be evident on CT scan for several days postoperatively although clinical symptoms have been seen as early as 6 hours after surgery (Andrews & Bringas, 1993). The patient with epilepsy undergoing craniotomy for temporal lobectomy generally experiences an uncomplicated recovery due to a relatively brief duration of retraction. Comparatively, the patient undergoing deep tumor resection or aneurysm repair is prone to complications related to deeper and more extensive periods of retraction.

Other measures that may be used perioperatively to protect the brain include administration of calcium channel blockers, hypothermia, hypervolemia, and metabolic depression through administration of anesthetic barbiturates. Barbiturates given before or within 30 minutes of a permanent occlusion as indicated by clinical signs or Doppler have been proven to reduce the size of the infarct. Recently, etomidate has been proven more effective than barbiturates as a cerebral metabolic depressant with minimal cardiotoxic effects (Batjer et al., 1988).

SPECIFIC SURGERIES

Epilepsy Surgery

Craniotomy for management of intractable epilepsy is used diagnostically and for treatment. If scalp EEG is unable to localize the epilepsy focus adequately, burr holes or craniotomy may be used for placement of invasive EEG electrodes. Surgical management follows and may be a focal resection, a corpus callosotomy, or hemispherectomy depending on the location and multiplicity of the foci.

CORPUS CALLOSOTOMY. The corpus callosum is considered to have an important role in the propagation and mediation of bilateral epileptic discharge. Interruption of the discharge by surgical resection is a treatment for generalized seizures. Sectioning of the corpus callosum to disrupt this propagation is achieved in two separate stages. The first procedure resects one-half to two-thirds of the anterior or posterior callosum, depending on the location of the EEG abnormalities. If adequate control is not achieved, further resection can be performed after the initial surgery. This surgical management is appropriate for adults and children when seizures remain medically intractable.

HEMISPHERECTOMY. Hemispherectomy is surgical excision of an involved cerebral hemisphere of children with severe, debilitating generalized seizures. The plasticity of the immature brain allows this procedure to be done in youngsters until ages 10 to 12. This multilobar excision is reserved for children with an atrophic hemisphere and infantile hemiplegia. Children with Sturge-Weber syndrome are also candidates for this elective surgery. A subtotal hemispherectomy, sparing the frontal or occipital lobe, is performed to avoid the complications of hemorrhage, obstructive hydrocephalus, superficial siderosis, and intracranial hematomas seen with complete hemispherectomy.

GENERAL CLINICAL CARE AFTER CRANIOTOMY

After craniotomy, postoperative management entails many general principles of postsurgical care. Among these are the maintenance of a patent airway with good gas exchange, management of pain and discomfort, evaluation of fluid and electrolyte balance, monitoring of intake and output, promotion of adequate nutrition, and prevention of complications secondary to immobility.

During a craniotomy, the patient is positioned for the best cerebral exposure and prevention of complications. The various positions include supine, prone, lateral, and sitting. Pressure sores and peripheral nerve damage may result from prolonged surgery or improper positioning. Postoperative care should include assessment of the skin, peroneal, and brachial plexus, and function of the eyes and eyelids. Cardiac or pulmonary distress may be anticipated if the sitting position was assumed for posterior fossa surgery.

The head dressing should be assessed frequently for comfort and degree of saturation. Inspect the dressing for evidence of bleeding or CSF drainage. The dressing will not be constrictive if you can comfortably place two fingers beneath it. Nurses can reinforce the dressing or replace it to the level of the suture covering, depending on the orders of the neurosurgeon.

Specific clinical interventions related to the patient's baseline status and the neurosurgical procedure can be developed based on knowledge of the concepts of ICP, the anatomy and function of the surgical site, and the effects of the surgical process. Astute assessment and initiation of appropriate interventions by the nurse are critical to the prevention of life-threatening complications of neuropathology and the craniotomy procedure. Collaborative consultation during the acute phase may include neurology for seizure management, dietary for nutritive support of the patient receiving chemotherapy, pastoral services for someone with a terminal prognosis, and physical therapy when balance or truncal weakness problems exist.

Specific Assessment for Postoperative Deficits

Once the patient has arrived in the ICU and initial physical assessment has been done as well as a baseline neurologic evaluation and trending of ICP, a more extensive functional neurologic assessment can be done by the nurse. Postoperative deficits will vary from patient to patient depending on presurgical status, the operative procedure undertaken, and the amount of cerebral edema present. Many deficits will resolve spontaneously within the first few days to months after surgery. Others may do so only with rehabilitation. Collaborative consultation may be helpful to patient adjustment for intermittent deficits as well as those requiring formal rehabilitative therapy.

COMMUNICATION DEFICITS. An understanding of the patient's baseline communication skills is necessary to the determination of any postoperative changes. If the temporal lobe and associated language areas (Broca's,

Wernicke's) are involved in the surgical procedure, verbal output or comprehensive language may be impaired. If the deficits are related to cerebral edema, improvement correlates with resolution of the cerebral edema. Surgery in the language areas may require therapy to minimize permanent deficits.

Assessment of communication is possible only if the patient is alert enough to respond. It is first necessary to determine the areas of language deficits, if any. Ask the patient simple questions and assess expressive speech for spontaneity, appropriateness of content, and fluency. Be aware that rote phrases that are overlearned, such as greetings and profanity, do not represent the full language ability of the individual. Present the patient with written words and pictures to evaluate naming and abstract language. The patient may be fluent in verbal speech but demonstrate a deficit in written and pictorial/abstract language. If the patient is able to execute verbal commands (i.e., touch your nose, tell me your name), comprehension of verbal input is accurate.

Based on the findings of this assessment, an alternative means of communication should be developed if needed and placed in the care plan. Some patients may require only that the nurse speak slowly, use single concepts of instruction, or simply allow the patient more response time. If these adjustments are made by all staff, much frustration for the patient and staff can be avoided.

MOTOR AND SENSORY ALTERATIONS. Motor and sensory deficits can be the result of postoperative cerebral edema or represent permanent deficit. The level of improvement is related to involvement of the motor and sensory regions (temporal/parietal lobes) in the surgical procedure and the presence of a preoperative deficit.

Assessment of motor function should move distal to proximal and include evaluation for muscle tone, movement against gravity, and movement against resistance. Assessment of sensory function should include recognition of hot/cold stimuli, as well as light touch and pressure. An awareness of the patient's capabilities allows development of individualized care, support of the physical therapy program, and prevention of injuries due to patient unawareness of body position or thermal injuries.

For the child who has undergone a hemispherectomy, hemiparesis that existed before surgery should be unchanged. This patient may require frequent scheduled range of motion exercises to maintain preoperative status.

VISUAL DISTURBANCES. Visual disturbances are common after cerebral neurosurgery due to increased ICP or cerebral edema. The changes may be transient for up to 3 months postoperatively or permanent. Gross visual assessment can be accomplished by having the patient focus straight ahead and indicating when an object is brought into the peripheral field. Extraocular movements can be evaluated by asking the patient to focus on an object and to follow it through various movements. Loss of an area of vision after neurosurgery is common. Ask the patient to report changes in vision such as decreased acuity, dimness of vision, or diplopia.

TABLE 40–3. **Cranial Nerve Assessment Following Craniotomy**

Optic nerve (II)	Assess visual disturbances and homonymous hemianopsia
Oculomotor (III)	Ptosis
Oculomotor (III), trochlear (IV), abducens (VI)	Deficits in extraocular movements
Facial (VII)	Absent corneal reflex, ipsilateral paralysis of facial muscles
Acoustic (VIII)	Dizziness, nystagmus, decreased hearing
Glossopharyngeal (IX)	Diminished gag/swallow reflex, orthostatic hypotension
Vagus (X)	Hypotension

CRANIAL NERVE ASSESSMENT. Location of the surgical site and potential cranial nerve involvement dictates the extent of cranial nerve assessment needed. Table 40-3 lists the assessment that should be done for specific neurologic functions of the cranial nerves.

CALLOSAL DISCONNECTION SYNDROME. The individual who has undergone a corpus callosotomy may demonstrate a cluster of symptoms that have been described as the callosal disconnection syndrome. This syndrome, characterized by right-left confusion and denial, is manifested by (1) an inability to identify an object held in one hand when it is transferred to the other hand, (2) an inability to match identical objects seen in different visual fields, and (3) an inability to carry out commands correctly with the left hand (Geschwind, 1965).

A speech deficit characterized by mutism or a decrease in the ability to initiate spontaneous speech is actually a buccofacial apraxia that may also be seen after corpus callosotomy. Residual deficits in any of these areas are unpredictable and must be considered in the global results of the desired seizure control.

CLINICAL MANAGEMENT

Patients undergoing cerebral neurosurgical procedures have several special care needs. Common to both the supratentorial and infratentorial craniotomy are the following interventions: monitoring of the head dressing for blood and CSF drainage, elevation of the head of the bed up to 30 degrees, assessment of incision/skin flap for infection, maintenance of a neutral head position, positioning of the patient off the operative site, avoidance of extreme flexion of the legs and hips, administration of analgesia, and avoidance of clustering of nursing care, which may increase ICP.

After infratentorial surgery, a few exceptions may be noted. The head of the bed may be kept flat without elevation, the patient should not be positioned on his back, a soft collar may be used to maintain a neutral neck position, the patient should have longer periods of bed rest due to orthostatic hypotension, NPO should be maintained for a minimum of 24 hours to ascertain status of cranial nerves, and nausea and vomiting are more frequent, requiring longer administration of IV fluids. If a bone flap was removed for brain decompression, position the patient only to the nonoperative side to facilitate brain expansion.

HYPERTHERMIA. Although some elevation in temperature is expected postoperatively, surgical manipulation in the area of the hypothalamus will bring higher temperatures for periods longer than normal. Elevations above 98.6°F (37°C) indicate irritation or infection of the hypothalamus; petechial hemorrhage or traction on the hypothalamus can produce temperatures of 105°F (40°C) (Arbor, 1993; Kajs-Wyllie et al., 1993). Surgery in the area of the third or fourth ventricles can cause similar temperature increases due to their close proximity to the hypothalamus.

Assessment of body temperature should be more frequent in those patients undergoing surgical manipulation in regions of the hypothalamus. Rectal temperatures should be taken in order to obtain a more accurate body core reading. Because elevations in temperature can contribute to increases in ICP, hyperthermia must be controlled. Antipyretic drugs, hypothermia blankets, and environmental manipulation can be used concurrently to achieve gradual decrease of major elevations of temperature. Shivering also increases ICP and can be avoided with the administration of chlorpromazine (Thorazine).

FATIGUE. Fatigue is a very nebulous and individual symptom. However, following a craniotomy a number of factors may affect the patient's perception of energy level and expected rate of recovery. Neuroanesthetic agents are absorbed and excreted at different rates depending on the agent and site of metabolism and excretion. Lipid-soluble agents are slower to be metabolized, resulting in longer periods of anesthetic effects.

Another factor is the somnolence syndrome that follows chemotherapy. If the patient has completed chemotherapy within the last 6 to 8 weeks before the craniotomy, lethargy and apathy can be related to this treatment as well as to the surgery (Allan et al., 1988). Incorporating this information into the plan of care with frequent rest periods will conserve patient energy and promote realistic expectations of recovery.

Presurgical level of activity can also influence the degree of fatigue experienced by the postcraniotomy patient. Individuals with chronic illness such as intractable epilepsy do not typically engage in sustained aerobic activity for fear of personal injury. An aggressive physical therapy program without an adequate baseline of tolerance may overexert the unconditioned patient.

Possible Complications After Craniotomy

Seizures are common in the postoperative period after cerebral neurosurgery secondary to existing increased ICP, the insult of extensive surgery, and metabolic abnormalities due to tumor treatment. Seizures during the immediate postoperative period are commonly generalized tonic-clonic episodes. Recurrent seizures are noted in 17% of patients undergoing supratentorial craniotomy, although that rate is reduced in individuals who have received prophylactic phenytoin (North et al., 1983). Approximately 2% of patients undergoing posterior fossa surgery will have seizures within the first 2 weeks of the postoperative period (North et al., 1980). At-risk patients may be treated prophylactically with antiepileptic medications. Studies have indicated there is no significant difference in seizure frequency between management with carbamazepine and phenytoin. Selection of antibiotics for the intraoperative and postoperative periods can also be a factor in the occurrence of seizures during the acute surgical recovery period. Early seizures have been noted in patients receiving penicillin during supratentorial craniotomy (Moss & Price, 1990). Maintaining a patent airway and preventing aspiration is a primary concern during the seizure. Astute recognition of seizure behaviors to prevent status epilepticus is also a primary concern.

HEMORRHAGE

Intracranial hemorrhage is a serious occult postoperative complication. Manifesting itself as increasing ICP, the bleeding can occur in the subdural, epidural, or intraventricular spaces. Intracerebral hemorrhage can also occur. At-risk patients for development of hematoma at the surgical site are those with evidence of alcohol intake and preoperative administration of mannitol. Approximately 69% of these hematomas developed in the extradural space, indicating that the potential space underlying the craniotomy bone flap may be a predisposing factor for postcraniotomy hematoma. Diagnosed by CT scan, intracranial hemorrhage often presents as a rapid deterioration in neurologic status as well as signs of shock, such as tachycardia, thready pulse, decreased blood pressure, pallor, and cold, clammy skin. The nurse must monitor the neurologic status of the patient as well as the hematocrit to determine trends and response to treatment.

INFECTION

Occurrence of infection in clean cases is less than 5% in cranial procedures. If debriding is necessary due to open cranial injuries secondary to vehicular accidents or penetrating injuries, the predisposition increases.

Observe the incision for drainage, erythema, and edema. Assess the patient for clinical signs of meningitis or fever. Protect the incision, catheter, or drain by placing a Telfa dressing over the site. Clean as ordered. Soften the dry scalp with baby oil or glycerin, then wash with soap and water once the dressing is removed. Avoid tension on the suture line. Document condition of the scalp and suture line.

HYPOVOLEMIC SHOCK

If the patient experiences general fluid loss during a craniotomy, hypovolemic shock may result. Blood loss occurs from the scalp and bone and the tumor resection as well as fluid loss secondary to the use of osmotic diuretics during the craniotomy. Many patients with recurrent brain tumors experience thrombocytopenia from chemotherapy. Preoperative platelet count should be greater than 100,000/μl and prothrombin time and partial thromboplastin time should be in a normal range to avoid bleeding diathesis. Preoperative preparation should include normalization of coagulation to prevent significant bleeding. Lack of adequate circulating volume results in decreased venous pressure and an increase in peripheral resistance. Signs and symptoms of hypovolemic shock include decreasing blood pressure, tachycardia, rapid respiration, pallor, decreased urine output, and restlessness or coma. With normal coagulation parameters, excessive intraoperative blood loss is unusual. If the coagulation abnormalities are diagnosed, the nurse must manage administration of vitamin K and fresh frozen plasma to reverse the bleeding. Fluid replacement treatments such as volume expanders (dextran, lactated Ringer's solution) and vasopressor drugs (dopamine) can also be implemented.

CEREBRAL EDEMA

Because of the pathology and cerebral surgery, the craniotomy patient experiences brain edema. Management of postoperative cerebral edema can be managed by elevation of the head, maintenance of a slightly dehydrated state through measurement of intake and output, and administration of corticosteroids, as well as management of fever and pain. Clinical findings are confirmed by CT scan.

CARDIAC ARRHYTHMIAS

Blood within the CSF often precipitates cardiac arrhythmias. They are often noted after posterior fossa surgeries as well. During the acute ICU period, the patient should be placed on a cardiac monitor for the first 48 hours. Frequent assessment should be done to identify any abnormalities that may develop. Treatment will be symptomatic of the type of arrhythmia.

RESPIRATORY COMPLICATIONS

Many patients undergoing craniotomy have compromised cranial nerve function and an altered level of awareness, which may precipitate respiratory complications. Airway obstruction can occur from improper positioning or accumulation of secretions. Elevating the head of the bed 30 degrees with the jaw forward and down will relieve the obstruction. If the brain stem or surrounding area is edematous, cranial nerve dysfunction can occur, diminishing protective reflexes such as cough, gag, and swallow. Place the patient in a side-lying position and withhold oral fluids until reflexes are adequate. During the interim, suction secretions as needed.

The nurse also needs to be aware of the potential for adult respiratory distress syndrome and neurogenic pulmonary edema. Symptoms of neurogenic pulmonary edema are thought to be triggered by an acute increase of ICP as seen with head trauma or massive subarachnoid hemorrhage. Symptoms of neurogenic pulmonary edema include dyspnea; restlessness; tachycardia; rapid, wet respirations; cold, clammy skin; and expectoration of mucus or possibly blood.

Related to any surgery are the respiratory complications of atelectasis, pneumonia, and pulmonary emboli. All respiratory complications warrant prophylactic care such as turning, deep breathing, and suctioning. Suctioning should be done with attention to the caution that saline installations before and after suctioning decrease oxygen exchange.

GASTRIC HEMORRHAGE

Cushing's ulcer accompanied by gastrointestinal hemorrhage is a frequent attendant of neurologic pathology. Although the relationship is controversial, these ulcers are seen in patients with tumors around the anterior hypothalamus, acute and chronic disease of the CNS, and craniocerebral trauma. Neurologic procedures as well as medication treatment (dexamethasone [Decadron]) contribute to gastric irritation.

Gastric bleeding may be acute or gradual, necessitating evaluation of the hematocrit, blood pressure, and daily stools by the nurse. Prophylactic administration of Maalox or cimetidine is common precaution. Active bleeding is managed by instillation of iced saline, nasogastric suction, fluid and blood replacement, and administration of sucralfate.

TENSION PNEUMOCEPHALUS

Pneumocephalus is the entrapment of air in the extradural, subdural, subarachnoid, or intraventricular compartments of the brain. This complication is often associated with transsphenoidal and posterior fossa craniotomy due to the sitting position required postoperatively. Air may enter the subarachnoid space through the posterior or pituitary fossa. CSF rhinorrhea can also allow entry of additional air into the intracranial space. The trapped air expands when warmed. Under normal circumstances, the air is absorbed. However, an air pocket of sufficient volume can act as a space-occupying lesion, producing neurologic deficits. Pneumocephalus usually develops within the first 24 hours after surgery, or as late as 1 week postoperatively. Clinical signs of decreased level of consciousness and focal deficits provide the first indicators of the diagnosis, which is confirmed by CT scan (Olympia, 1994).

CSF LEAK

A CSF leak is often seen in conjunction with basal skull fractures and transsphenoidal hypophysectomy. Caused by an opening in the subarachnoid space, a CSF leak will generally seal over spontaneously. A lumbar drain or serial lumbar punctures may be done to assist repair of the torn dura by reducing CSF pressure. This complication places the patient at risk for meningitis. Antibiotics are administered prophylactically. Nurses need to be alert for the drainage on the head dressing and to differentiate CSF drainage from normal serosanguinous drainage. CSF drainage will produce a halo sign—a clear or yellow ring around the outside of the drainage area. Fresh drainage will test glucose-positive if CSF is present.

DIABETES INSIPIDUS

Central diabetes insipidus can occur as a temporary disturbance after supratentorial surgery, especially if resection is in the area of the posterior pituitary gland, hypothalamus, or supraopticohypophysial tract. Because of manipulation and focal edema, the posterior pituitary gland may not produce sufficient amounts of ADH. As a result the patient eliminates large amounts of dilute urine demonstrated by a low specific gravity. Postsurgical diabetes insipidus can be expected within the first 2 weeks after neurosurgery. If left uncorrected, the patient will experience fluid and electrolyte imbalance. Because it is usually a transient problem, treatment is focused on maintenance of fluid and electrolyte balance with intravenous therapy. Vasopressin (Pitressin) subcutaneously or desmopressin acetate (DDVAP) intranasally can be used for severe transient or permanent central diabetes insipidus.

SYNDROME OF INAPPROPRIATE ADH

Syndrome of inappropriate ADH secretion (SIADH) is a common metabolic problem seen in neurosurgical patients who have experienced rupture of an aneurysm or head trauma. If the patient has a craniotomy for surgical repair or resection, you may expect the following clinical signs: serum sodium > 130 mEq/L, spot urine sodium > 20 mEq/L, serum osmolality < 270 mOsm/kg, urine osmolality > serum osmolality. A basic feature of this syndrome is hypervolemia and hyponatremia with natriuresis. Hayward and Smith (1963) postulated that SIADH may be related to a disruption of the limbic-midbrain-supraoptic circuit, which regulates ADH secretion. Fluid restriction is the treatment for SIADH. Vingerhoets and de Tribolet (1988) indicated that it is a common response when clinical symptoms occur within the acute, or first 3 days, following the insult and suggest that a delayed occurrence of hyponatremia and natriuresis may be another phenomenon.

CEREBRAL SALT WASTING SYNDROME

Cerebral salt wasting (CSW) is a condition also marked by hyponatremia and natriuresis. The distinguishing feature is that these patients are hypovolemic. Studies indicate that CSW may be attributed to the peptide atrial natriuretic factor although this remains controversial (Diringer et al., 1988, 1989). Widjicks and colleagues (1991) demonstrated that the natriuresis noted after subarachnoid hemorrhage was associated with decreased plasma level of vasopressin. Others have shown elevated level of atrial natriuretic factor early (within the first few hours of rupture) in the course of subarachnoid hemorrhage and a second, delayed increase greater than the first. The fluid restriction usually ordered if SIADH is suspected can be detrimental to the patient already experiencing undetected hypovolemia resulting from CSW. Determination of intravascular volume can be critical to the patient with subarachnoid hemorrhage when early volume expansion has proven to reduce the risk of vasospasm following subarachnoid hemorrhage (Finn et al., 1986; Solomon et al., 1984, 1988). In patients prone to cerebral vasospasm and subsequent infarct, management of hyponatremia and natriuresis should be evaluated in light of intravascular volume. If the patient is hypovolemic, intravenous fluids and volume expanders should be implemented rather than fluid restriction (Winn & Mayberg, 1992).

Many of the complications after craniotomy require the nurse to have a working knowledge of laboratory studies and values. The more common studies used to determine the effectiveness of treatment as well as development of complications include hemoglobin, hematocrit, blood urea nitrogen, potassium, calcium, sodium, fasting blood glucose, creatinine, serum osmolality, and arterial blood gases.

Collaboration in Management of Care

In the current environment of managed health care and vertical services, the need for individualized care is a priority for the patient and the service institution. Delayed or unnecessary services cannot be tolerated. Collaboration among all professionals involved in the care of the patient is now necessary to meet the dual needs of the patient and the industry. Open, honest, and respectful communication is expected and granted by every member of the health team for collaboration to be present. Although a craniotomy is a conventional procedure, the pathology and need for further treatment for optimal recovery requires the nurse to have a broad perspective on the health care system, its available resources, and the collaborative expertise to activate and direct these resources. Each patient and family will have different resources and needs to be considered.

Because of the delivery of personal care, the nurse at the bedside is in a position to assess these needs first. Studies indicate that nurses in the ICU setting assess and meet the needs of the family with varying degrees of success, which impacts the collaboration and use of resources. Murphy and colleagues (1992) indicated that higher levels of empathy enable the nurse to gauge more accurately some of the needs of the family of a critical care patient. Interestingly, this study indicated a negative correlation between the nurse's length of experience and the ability to accurately estimate the needs of family members. Careful listening, appropriate questioning, and observation and interpretation of body language are other skills that have been identified as promoting accurate assessment of family needs and therefore collaboration for support services (Murphy et al., 1992).

In face of increased acuity and shortened hospital stay, critical care staff now find it necessary to shift the perspective of patient management from illness to wellness and long-term goals without compromising quality of care. Kajs-Wyllie and colleagues (1993) have demonstrated the success of this refocusing and incorporation of collaborative services through implementation of neurologic rehabilitation rounds in a critical care unit. With implementation of this protocol, these authors were able to decrease the length of stay of their neurologically impaired patients, transfer of the patient to appropriate units was expedited, and families were less anxious and better informed regarding status of their family member (Kajs-Wyllie et al., 1993). These changes were possible through early recognition of complications and collaboration of services to best serve the patient in a timely manner. Planning of patient care includes collaboration with the physician and other health professionals, such as respiratory therapists, physical therapists, occupational therapists, dieticians, social workers, and pastoral care, to determine in concrete terms the achievable short- and long-term goals and identification of services required to meet these goals.

Case management of high-risk patients along the continuum of care is another mechanism that helps ensure timely and appropriate health services. This advocacy and utilization of appropriate resources can now be seen in both the institutional and community settings (Bergen, 1992; Rheaume et al., 1994).

Patient and Family Education

Involving the patient and designated others in the plan of care is an important part of the patient's adjustment and recovery. Determination of the "designated others" is an important part of the nursing assessment because many nontraditional family members may not be recognized by the legal system but are nevertheless imperative to the patient's adjustment or recovery. A family conference is one means to clarify issues not only for the patient and family, but also for the primary nurses and physicians involved with them (Bokinskie, 1992).

Education is a collaborative undertaking as the health team moves with the patient through treatment and recovery. Each member of the team must be apprised of the patient plan of care, condition, and procedures in order to accurately respond to questions regarding treatment and condition. Information must be shared with the patient and family in a timely and caring manner. Preoperative information will help everyone adjust to the postoperative condition of the patient as well as provide a baseline of recovery by which to plan short-term future arrangements such as child care, time off from work, and financial coverage. Presentation of information must consider not only the diagnosis and emotional state of the patient, but also the integrity of brain function given that a craniotomy is for treatment of a cerebral pathology. Postoperative appraisal provides opportunity for reevaluation of alternatives of recovery direction and support.

SUMMARY

Craniotomy is a surgical technique that has many applications. Surgical interventions as superficial as cerebral biopsy and as extensive as tumor resection all require craniotomy. An extensive knowledge of cerebral anatomy and function is necessary to care for the acute needs of the patient undergoing this procedure. Astute assessment by the ICU nurse can result in early recognition and intervention of life-threatening complications and facilitate optimal recovery in the community.

REFERENCES

Allan, M. J., et al. (1988). Atrial natriuretic peptide inhibits osmolarity-induced arginine vasopressin release in man. *Clinical Science, 75,* 33–39.

Andrews, R. J., & Bringas, B. S. (1993). A review of brain retraction and recommendations for minimizing intraoperative brain injury. *Neurosurgery, 33*(6), 1052–1063.

Arbor, R. B. (1993). Stereotactic localization and resection of intracranial tumors. *Journal of Neuroscience Nursing, 25*(1), 14–21.

Batjer, H. H., et al. (1988). Use of etomidate, temporary arterial occlusion, and intraoperative angiography in neurosurgical treatment of large and giant cerebral aneurysms. *Journal of Neurosurgery, 68,* 234–240.

Beahrs, O. H., et al. (1988). *Manual for staging of cancer.* Philadelphia: J. B. Lippincott.

Bergen, A. (1992). Case management in community care. *Journal of Advanced Nursing, 17*(9), 1106–1113.

Bilsky, M., & Posner, J. (1993). Intensive and postoperative care of intracranial tumors. In *Neurological and neurosurgical intensive care* (3rd ed., pp. 308–329). New York: Raven Press.

Bokinskie, J. C. (1992). Family conferences: A method to diminish transfer anxiety. *Journal of Neuroscience Nursing, 24*(3), 129–133.

Dean, B. L., et al. (1990). Gliomas: Classification with MRI. *Radiology, 174*(2), 411–415.

del Regato, J., Spjut, H., & Cox, J. D. (1985). *Cancer: Diagnosis, treatment and prognosis* (6th ed., pp. 149–155). St. Louis: C. V. Mosby.

Dichter, M. A. (Ed.). (1986). *Mechanisms of epileptogenesis.* New York: Plenum Press.

Diringer, M., et al. (1988). Plasma atrial natriuretic factor and subarachnoid hemorrhage. *Stroke, 19,* 1119–1123.

Diringer, M., et al. (1989). Sodium and water regulation in a patient with cerebral salt wasting. *Archives of Neurology, 46,* 928–930.

Finn, S. S., et al. (1986). Observations on the perioperative management of aneurysmal subarachnoid hemorrhage. *Journal of Neurosurgery, 65,* 48–62.

Fuchamachi, A., Koizumi, H., & Nukui, P. (1985). Postoperative intracerebral hemorrhages: A survey of computed tomographic findings after 1074 intracranial operations. *Surgery and Neurology, 23,* 575–580.

Ganz, J. (1993). Gamma knife applications in and around the pituitary fossa. In *Gamma knife surgery: A guide for referring physician* (pp. 122–132). New York: Springer-Verlag Wien.

Geschwind, N. (1965). Disconnection syndromes in animals and man. *Brain, 88,* 237–294.

Groenwald, S. L., Goodman, M., Hansen Frogg, M., & Henke Yarbro, C. (Eds.). (1993). *Cancer nursing: Principles and practice* (3rd ed.). Boston: Jones and Bartlett.

Hoff, J. T. (1986). Cerebral protection. *Journal of Neurosurgery, 65,* 579–591.

Jones, R. D. (1986). Epidemiology of brain tumors in man and their relationship with chemical agents. *Ed Chem Toxic, 24,* 99–106.

Judnick, J. W., et al. (1992). Radiotherapy technique integrates MRI into CT. *Radiologic Technology, 64*(2), 82–91.

Kajs-Wyllie, M., et al. (1993). Enhancing recovery via neuro-rehab rounds. *Journal of Neuroscience Nursing, 25*(3), 153–157.

Korn, S., Schubert, A., & Barnett, G. (1993). Endotracheal obstruction during stereotactic craniotomy. *Journal of Neurosurgical Anesthesia, 5*(4), 272–275.

Kornblith, P. L., Walker, M. D., & Cassady, R. R. (1987). *Neurologic oncology.* Philadelphia: J. B. Lippincott.

Lee, S. T., et al. (1990). Early postoperative seizures after posterior fossa surgery. *Journal of Neurosurgery, 73*(4), 541–544.

Moss, E., & Price, D. J. (1990). Effect of propofol on brain retraction pressure and cerebral perfusion pressure. *British Journal of Anaesthesiology, 65,* 823–825.

Murphy, K., et al. (1992). Empathy of intensive care nurses and critical care family needs assessment. *Heart and Lung, 21*(1), 25–30.

North, J. B., et al. (1983). Phenytoin and postoperative epilepsy: A double-blind study. *Journal of Neurosurgery, 58,* 672–677.

North, X., et al. (1980). The prevention of postoperative epilepsy. *Lancet, 1,* 384–386.

Olympia, M. A. (1994). Venous air embolism after craniotomy closure: Tension pneumocephalus implicated. *Journal of Neurosurgical Anesthesia, 6*(1), 35–39.

Ornstein, E., et al. (1993). Desflurane and isoflurane have similar effects on cerebral blood flow in patients with intracranial lesions. *Anesthesiology, 79*(3), 498–502.

Rheaume, A., et al. (1994). Case management and nursing practice. *Journal of Nursing Administration, 24*(3), 30–36.

Schulier, J. P., & Markiewicz, E. (1991). Medical cancer patients and intensive care. *Anticancer Research, 11*(6), 2171–2174.

Solomon, R. A., Post, K. D., & McMurty, J. G., III. (1984). Depression of circulating blood volume in patients after subarachnoid hemorrhage. Implications for management of symptomatic vasospasm. *Neurosurgery, 15,* 354–367.

Solomon, R. A., Fink, M. E., & Lennihan, L. (1988). Early aneurysm surgery and prophylactic hypovolemic hypertensive therapy for the treatment of aneurysmal subarachnoid hemorrhage. *Neurosurgery, 23,* 699–704.

Steen, P. A. (1991). Barbiturates in neuroanesthesia and neurointensive care. *Agressologie, 32*(6-7), 323–325.

Stewardt-Amidei, C. (1991). Meningioma: Nursing care considerations. *Journal of Neuroscience Nursing, 6*(4), 269–278.

Taniguche, M., et al. (1992). Total intravenous anesthesia for improvement of intraoperative monitoring of somatosensory evoked potential during aneurysm surgery. *Neurosurgery, 31,* 891–897.

Todd, M. M., et al. (1993). A prospective, comparative trial of three anesthetics for elective supratentorial craniotomy. Propofol/fentanyl, isoflurane/nitrous oxide, and fentanyl/nitrous oxide. *Anesthesiology, 78*(6), 1005–1020.

Vingerhoets, F., & de Tribolet, N. (1988). Hyponatremia hypo-osmolarity in neurosurgical patients. "Appropriate secretion of ADD" and "cerebral salt wasting syndrome." *Acta Neurochir 91,* 50–54.

Widjicks, E. F., et al. (1991). Atrial natriuretic factor and salt wasting after aneurysmal subarachnoid hemorrhage. *Stroke, 22*(12), 1519–1524.

Winn, H. R., & Mayberg, M. (Eds.). (1992). Stereotactic radiosurgery. In *Neurosurgery Clinics of North America* (pp. 191–205). Philadelphia: W. B. Saunders.

Wyllie, E., & Lunders, H. O. (1993). Classification of seizures. In E. Wyllie & H. O. Lunders (Eds.), *Treatment of epilepsy: Principles and practice* (pp. 359–368). Malvern, PA: Lea & Febiger.

Zulch, K. J. (1980). Principles of the new World Health Organization (WHO) classification of brain tumors. *Neuroradiology, 19,* 59–66.

Infections of the Central Nervous System

Darlene Averell Lovasik

The meninges, brain tissue (parenchyma), and blood vessels of the central nervous system (CNS) may be attacked by a variety of pathogenic microorganisms. Meningitis, encephalitis, and brain abscesses are the most common CNS infectious diseases seen in clinical practice in North America. Frequently, the effect of the inflammatory process may involve more than one structure such as the parenchyma and meninges. Meningoencephalitis describes both meningeal and encephalitic signs.

This chapter will discuss the pathophysiology of CNS infections that may require intensive nursing care, medical therapy, and indications for surgical intervention.

MENINGITIS

Meningitis is an inflammation of the leptomeninges (pia mater and arachnoid), the covering of the brain and spinal cord. This process may result from bacterial or viral infections or meningeal irritation due to encephalitis or a systemic disease. Due to the free flow of cerebrospinal fluid (CSF) through the subarachnoid space around the brain and spinal cord, the organisms may spread throughout the CNS. The causative agent may be bacterial (purulent meningitis) or viral (aseptic meningitis). Bacterial meningitis produces profound and life-threatening symptoms. Viral meningitis is self-limiting, no specific therapy is available, and recovery is usually complete.

Performing a lumbar puncture and obtaining CSF specimens for the presence, type, and antibiotic sensitivities of organisms is essential for the diagnosis of meningitis. However, the lumbar puncture must be done with caution. If an expanding lesion is present in the brain, the change in pressure after the procedure may precipitate transtentorial herniation within 8 hours. If computed tomography (CT) is readily available, the lumbar puncture may be deferred until after it has been established by CT scan that significant mass effect is not present. In addition to Gram stain and culture, analysis of CSF specimens includes cell count and differential and protein and glucose content. Skull, sinus, and chest radiographs may provide additional information in determining the origin of the infection.

General Characteristics

A severe headache is one of the early symptoms of meningitis. The brain tissue itself does not have pain receptors; stimulation of the dura mater and traction on the blood vessels are responsible for the headache. Photophobia, extreme sensitivity to light, is an additional sign of meningeal irritation; however, it may also occur with other neurologic conditions such as vascular headache or subarachnoid hemorrhage. Patients with bacterial meningitis also present with a fever from 38°C to 40°C (101°F to 103°F).

The characteristic stiff neck (nuchal rigidity) associated with meningeal irritation prohibits forward movement of the neck. Flexion of the neck precipitates spasms of the neck extensor muscles and causes severe pain.

The Kernig and Brudzinski signs also indicate meningeal irritation. To evaluate the patient for the Kernig sign, place the patient in a supine position, flex the leg at the knee, then at the hip to a 90-degree angle, and finally extend the knee. In a patient with meningitis, this will trigger pain and spasms of the hamstring muscles due to the inflammation of the meninges and spinal nerve roots. The Brudzinski sign is also elicited with the patient supine, then flexing the head and neck to the chest. The legs will flex at both the hips and knees in response to this maneuver, again secondary to inflammation around the nerve roots.

Bacterial (Purulent) Meningitis

Bacteria may invade the subarachnoid space or meninges through the bloodstream from bacteremia, septic emboli, or metastasis from an infection of the heart or lung. Transmission of microorganisms may occur following a laceration through the dura mater associated with compound fractures of the skull, penetrating trauma, or after neurosurgical procedures. The infection may be spread directly into the cranial cavity as

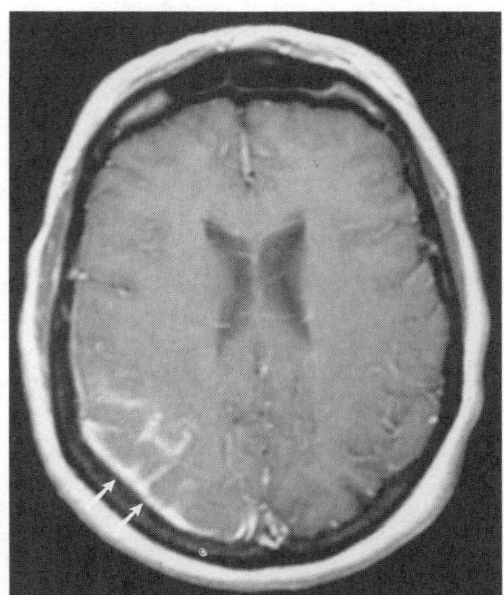

FIGURE 41–1. Contrast-enhanced magnetic resonance image (MRI) of the brain reveals an abnormally thickened meninges *(arrows)* over the right parietal cortex, diagnosed by biopsy to be tuberculous meningitis. (Photographs courtesy of Charles Jungreis, MD, Chief, Division of Neuroradiology and Associate Professor of Radiology and Neurological Surgery, University of Pittsburgh.)

in sinusitis or mastoid infections. The onset of bacterial meningitis may be preceded by an upper respiratory tract infection, otitis media, or pneumonia. The most common pathogenic bacteria identified in recent years include *Haemophilus influenzae, Neisseria meningitidis,* and *Streptococcus pneumoniae. H. influenzae* is responsible for approximately 60% of the cases of bacterial meningitis in children. Infants and immunosuppressed patients may develop meningitis from gram-negative microorganisms such as *Escherichia coli, Enterobacter, Klebsiella,* and *Proteus.*

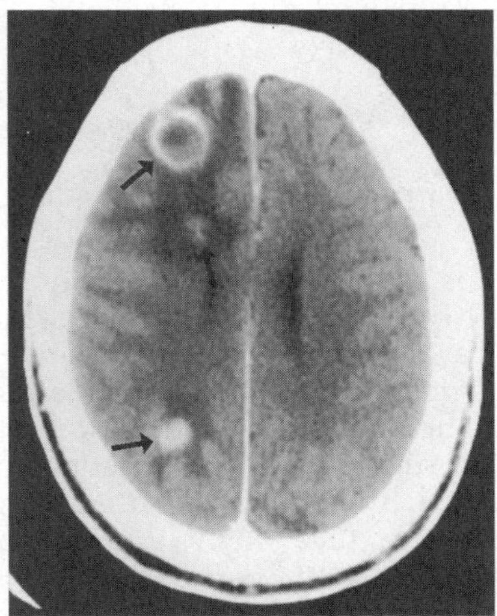

FIGURE 41–2. Contrast-enhanced computed tomography (CT) of the brain demonstrates multiple abnormal enhancing nodules and rings *(arrows)* with surrounding edema identified as pyogenic meningitis. (Photographs courtesy of Charles Jungreis, MD, Chief, Division of Neuroradiology and Associate Professor of Radiology and Neurological Surgery, University of Pittsburgh.)

The symptoms of bacterial meningitis include irritability, chills, fever, headache, stiffness of the neck, and back pain. The "meningeal cry" in children is described as sharp and high-pitched. As the disease progresses, the patient may become lethargic, then decline into a coma. On examination, the patient may be confused and have an elevated temperature, tachycardia, and tachypnea. In acute fulminating cases, the patient may be hypotensive; however, the blood pressure is generally normal. Petechial rashes are common and seizures may also occur, especially in children.

A lumbar puncture is essential for diagnostic purposes. (Table 41–1). The opening pressure is elevated, usually between 200 and 500 mm H_2O. The CSF is cloudy or purulent and contains a large number of cells. The CSF protein content is increased and the glucose content is decreased. The protein is elevated due to the increased protein volume contributed by the bacteria and the white blood cells (WBCs). Glucose is consumed by the bacteria, causing a decrease in the glucose level. Additional laboratory data may reveal the WBC count in the normal range, but generally in the range of 10,000 to 30,000/mm. The combination of purulent material and neutrophils will create an accumulation of exudate over the surface of the brain, which then increases the inflammatory process. This destructive cycle continues and, combined with increasing pressure on the brain tissue and cerebral blood vessels, may result in infarction of areas of the brain. The buildup of exudate will cause the arachnoid villi to become progressively occluded and CSF will accrue, causing hydrocephalus. Over time, this condition may advance to fibrotic changes of the arachnoid and arachnoid villi, causing changes in the flow of CSF and hydrocephalus.

The outcome from bacterial meningitis is dependent on early diagnosis and treatment. If the primary cause of the mengingitis is acute sinusitis, otitis media, or fractures of the skull, further medical and surgical intervention may be necessary.

MENINGOCOCCAL MENINGITIS

Outbreaks of meningococcal meningitis (*N. meningitidis*) may occur in schools, colleges, and other group settings. Such outbreaks require prophylactic treatment of contacts the patient may have had. The entry of the meningococci may be from the nasopharynx or via blood to the meninges, creating a massive inflammatory response. As the infection progresses, the pia-arachnoid becomes dense and may form adhesions. In time, the adhesions may obstruct CSF flow and produce hydrocephalus. Adhesions and fibrous tissue growth may also cause cranial nerve deficits, including damage to the auditory nerve resulting in hearing loss.

Meningococcal meningitis may be complicated by a condition known as Waterhouse-Friderichsen syndrome. In addition to the usual symptoms of meningitis, hemorrhage may also occur in the adrenal glands, causing adrenal insufficiency. This will lead to hypotension, respiratory distress, and circulatory collapse

TABLE 41–1. **Normal and Pathological Characteristics of Cerebrospinal Fluid (CSF)**

CSF Characteristic	Normal	Bacterial Meningitis	Viral Meningitis
Appearance	Clear, colorless	Cloudy, turbid	Clear, occasionally turbid
Opening pressure	80–180 mm H_2O	Elevated (> 180 mm H_2O)	Variable
Cells	0–10 lymphs No polymorphonuclear cells	Increased white blood cells (1000–2000/mm, mostly polymorphonuclear cells)	Increased white blood cells (300/mm, mostly mononuclear cells)
Total Protein	15%–45 mg/dL	Increased (100–500 mg/dL)	Normal or slightly increased
Glucose	60%–80% of blood glucose level	Decreased (<40 mg/dL, or 40% of blood glucose)	Normal
Culture		Bacteria present on Gram stain and culture	No bacteria present; virus demonstration requires special techniques

unless adrenal corticosteroids are administered immediately.

The pharmacologic treatment for meningococcal meningitis is aqueous penicillin G or ampicillin administered intravenously. The treatment regiment should continue for 5 to 7 days after the patient becomes afebrile. Anticonvulsants are prescribed for seizure control. The use of corticosteroids remains controversial; however, they may be prescribed for evidence of cerebral edema or signs of cerebral herniation.

Long term-complications of the disease include deafness, cranial nerve palsies, blindness, changes in mentation, and hydrocephalus.

HEMOPHILUS INFLUENZAE MENINGITIS

H. Influenzae is the most common cause of acute bacterial meningitis (approximately 50%), generally occurring in infancy and childhood. Season patterns are noted, with most cases occurring in the spring and autumn. The signs and symptoms of *H. influenzae* meningitis are similar to those of other forms of bacterial meningitis. Treatment has traditionally been ampicillin; however, ampicillin-resistant strains of *H. influenzae* may require a combination of ampicillin and chloramphenicol or a third-generation cephalosporin.

PNEUMOCOCCAL MENINGITIS

Pneumococcal (*S. pneumoniae*) meningitis occurs more frequently in infants and the elderly. The signs and symptoms are similar to those of other forms of bacterial meningitis. Gram-positive diplococci are found in large numbers in the CSF. The mortality is high when it is associated with pneumonia, bacteremia, and/or endocarditis. Aqueous penicillin is given intravenously for 12 to 15 days. Chloramphenicol is an alternative drug for adults.

OTHER BACTERIAL MENINGITIS

Staphylococci (*S. aureus* and *S. epidermidis*), streptococci, and other bacterial sources of meningitis are less common and must be treated appropriately. Tuberculous meningitis occurs only when there is a primary source for tuberculosis in the body. Significant characteristics of tuberculosis meningitis includes a longer disease course, less pronounced CSF changes, and higher mortality than other bacterial meningitis.

Viral (Aseptic) Meningitis

Viral meningitis is generally a confined illness with symtoms of meningeal irritation such as fever, frontal headache, photophobia, and a stiff neck. It may occur after flulike symptoms of fever, sore throat, or gastrointestinal symptoms. Results of CSF studies in viral meningitis are similar to those in bacterial meningitis, with an increase in opening pressure; however, there is only a moderate elevation in protein, a normal glucose content, and no bacteria identified on culture. "Aseptic" meningitis indicates that no organism was discovered on testing. As with other viral diseases, no specific pharmacologic agent is available. Supportive therapy is provided and patient recovery is usually complete.

ENCEPHALITIS

Encephalitis is the term used for an infection of the parenchymal brain tissue (cortex and white matter), with viruses as the most common causative organism. As a pathologic agent, viral infections are not a common cause of neurologic disease. Most viral infections of the CNS are uncommon complications of systemic illnesses caused by common viruses. However, because viruses reproduce only within the host cell, destruction of healthy brain tissue occurs. Transmission of the virus develops through access through the bloodstream, cranial nerves, or peripheral nerves. Patients who are immunocompromised through chemotherapy, immunodeficiency diseases, or other systemic conditions are particularly susceptible. A generalized inflammation without exudate occurs, followed by widespread edema, hemorrhage, cavitation, and necrosis.

As with other viral diseases, the etiology of viral encephalitis has not clearly been identified. The numerous modes of transmission include mosquito bites (Western and Eastern equine encephalitis) tick-transmitted arboviruses (Colorado tick fever), animal bites (rabies), postvaccination, or following the natural course of measles or mumps.

Clinical manifestations include alterations in the level of consciousness, irritability, behavioral disturbances, seizures, and focal neurologic deficits. The diagnosis is generally based on the clinical findings because most of the diagnostic tests are nonspecific for viral diseases. CSF findings mimic those of viral meningitis with an increase in opening pressure, a moderate elevation in protein content, and a normal glucose content. Brain biopsy and tissue examination may be recommended for diagnostic purposes. There is no adequate pharmaceutical therapy for most viral infections of the CNS.

Health care providers and families are disheartened by the current lack of effective therapy for viral encephalitis, with the exception of herpes simplex encephalitis. Medical care and nursing management is supportive.

Herpes Simplex Encephalitis

Early diagnosis of herpes simplex encephalitis is critical because antiviral treatment is available for this encephalitis. The viral strain is herpes simplex type 1, which is associated with oral herpes lesions (cold sores). It is initially transmitted by respiratory or salivary contact, and 50% of the population has antibody by age 15. It is hypothesized that this encephalitis may arise from an endogenous reactivation of the virus rather than from a primary infection. The chief targets of this virus are the frontal and temporal areas. The early signs and symptoms are fever, headache, changes in mentation or peculiar/bizarre behavior, seizures, or focal neurologic deficits. The cerebral edema and hemorrhage associated with disease progression causes an increase in intracranial pressure (ICP) leading to temporal lobe or brain stem herniation and death.

The electroencephalogram (EEG) is the primary diagnostic tool because it is most likely to reveal early abnormalities such as diffuse slowing over the temporal area. The CSF pressure may be moderately to greatly elevated, and analysis of CSF may reveal increased protein, increased lymphocytes, and a normal or low glucose content. A CT scan may be normal for the first several days of the disease, and so cannot be relied on for early diagnosis. Later in the course of the illness, CT scan reveals hemorrhagic areas with edema in the frontal and temporal regions. The diagnosis is confirmed by brain biopsy with examination of the brain tissue.

Acyclovir sodium is now prescribed for herpes simplex encephalitis and has decreased mortality from 70% to 28% (Hickey, 1992; Rowland, 1989). Corticosteroids may be administered to decrease cerebral edema and anticonvulsants may be prescribed for seizure activity. Patients who survive are generally left with critical neurologic deficits.

BRAIN ABSCESS

Brain abscesses are collections of encapsulated or free pus in the brain tissue. Infections of the middle ear and mastoid produce 40% of brain abscesses (Hickey, 1992). Abscesses may also develop after an infection within the cranium such as the nasal sinuses or osteomyelitis of the skull. Other potential sites of origin are fractures of the skull, neurosurgical or oral surgical procedures, or metastases from infection elsewhere in the body, such as a lung abscess or endocarditis. The most common bacteria identified are *Staphylococcus aureus, Streptococcus* variations, hemolytic streptococcus, Enterobacteriaceae, and gram-negative organisms (Rowland, 1989). Initially, a purulent inflammation of the brain tissue occurs within the white matter deep within the hemispheres. An inflammatory response follows, which mobilizes WBCs, produces edema, then proceeds to necrosis. The area becomes encapsulated by fibrous tissue, and edema surrounds the site. The capsule hampers blood flow and delivery of antibiotics to the region.

Headache is the predominant symptom, followed by nausea, vomiting, and seizure activity. Progressive signs are similar to those of other expanding lesions: change in mentation, hemiparesis or hemiplegia, or other focal neurologic signs. Due to the hazards of lumbar puncture in the presence of an expanding lesion, CT scan is used for diagnosis and is then used to follow progressive changes in the abscess. The lesion is usually ill-defined in the early stages; however, a ring of enhancement soon develops due to the edema surrounding the mass. Small lesions or abscesses from a known cause may be treated by an antibiotic regimen alone for 4 to 6 weeks, usually penicillin G and chloramphenicol given intravenously. Large abscesses or situations that necessitate a differential diagnosis of abscess versus tumor may require a surgical procedure for drainage. Brain abscesses were common before the availability of antibiotic therapy for the underlying disease. With the use of CT scan to monitor response to therapy, the mortality from brain abscess has been reported to be less than 10%.

SUBDURAL EMPYEMA

A subdural empyema is a collection of purulent fluid between the dura and the arachnoid. It may develop from an infection from the nasal sinus (most common), middle ear, or meninges or as a result of a skull fracture. The microorganism responsible for the infection is usually *Streptococcus, Staphylococcus,* or a gram-negative enteric organism.

The symptoms are similar to those of a brain abscess. In addition to local pain and tenderness from the site of origin, symptoms include chills, fever, severe headache, and changes in mentation. Seizures or focal neurologic signs such as hemiplegia or aphasia may also be present. An infection of the nasal sinuses or osteomyelitis of the skull may be noted on skull x-rays. CT scan with contrast will show a crescent-shaped area of hypodensity with enhancement between the empyema and the cortex. In contrast to treatment of brain abscess, immediate neurosurgical evacuation of the empyema is essential followed by treatment with intravenous antibiotics. Delay in therapy may result in fulminant meningitis, multiple intracranial abscesses, and increasing cerebral edema.

INTRACRANIAL EPIDURAL ABSCESS

Epidural abscesses are generally associated with an overlying infection in the cranial bones related to chronic sinusitis, head trauma, or neurosurgical procedures. Severe headache, fever, and malaise are frequently described, although focal neurologic deficits are uncommon. A CT scan revealing an extradural defect will confirm the diagnosis. Neurosurgical intervention to drain the abscess and treatment with intravenous antibiotics is required.

SPINAL EPIDURAL ABSCESS

A spinal epidural abscess is an accumulation of purulent fluid external to the dura in the spinal canal. The presenting symptoms include severe back pain, fever, and weakness of the lower extremities that may progress to paraplegia. The origin of the infection may be through direct extension from decubitus ulcers, bloodstream metastasis from other sites, or from neurosurgical procedures, lumbar puncture, or stab wounds. CT scan with contrast may reveal an abscess; however, a myelogram is generally required for diagnostic purposes. It is essential that the spinal needle not penetrate the abscess and carry the infection into the subarachnoid space. If a partial or complete extradural block is noted, antibiotic therapy is initiated, followed by a laminectomy for surgical drainage. If treatment is delayed, the paralysis is likely to be permanent.

BACTERIAL VENTRICULITIS

Bacterial ventriculitis may be a complication of invasive monitoring of ICP through a ventricular catheter inserted into the lateral ventricle and the use of an external drainage system for CSF. Infection rates varying from 0 to 21.9% have been reported in numerous studies (Schultz, et al., 1993). Contributing factors include the duration of ICP monitoring, patient populations with open head trauma, CSF leaks and/or hemorrhage, drainage of CSF, and manipulation of the system to obtain CSF specimens. Controversy also exists regarding the use of prophylactic antibiotics and care of the insertion site.

Infections also occur after the placement of ventricular shunts, especially ventriculoperitoneal shunts. The most common organism is *Staphylococcus epidermidis* followed by *S. aureus.* It is frequently necessary to remove or externalize the shunt after an infection. Many staphylococci are resistant to multiple agents and will require intrathecal (intraventricular) and intravenous aminoglycosides to achieve therapeutic levels.

CREUTZFELDT-JAKOB DISEASE

Creutzfeldt-Jakob disease is a rare, progressive disease of the cortex, basal ganglia, and spinal cord occurring in middle-aged and elderly adults. The agent responsible for this progressive disease is transmissible spongiform with a long incubation period, a latent period following infection, and a lack of an inflammatory response. The signs of the disease are a gradual onset of dementia, impaired judgment, and unusual behavior, leading to the onset of coma, then death. There are no signs of an infection, and CSF is usually normal. A characteristic EEG pattern of periodic bursts of abnormal activity is noted. In the later stages of the disease, CT scan will reveal enlarged ventricles with cerebral atrophy. The diagnosis is confirmed by brain biopsy with careful pathological tissue examination. There is no known medical treatment, and death occurs in a few months to 1 year from diagnosis.

The method of transmission of Creutzfeldt-Jakob disease is unknown; however, inadvertent human-to-human transmission has been reported following corneal transplantation, use of natural human growth hormone preparation, and the use of a human dura mater graft. Therefore, extreme caution must be emphasized in the operating room and pathology laboratories. In addition, special sterilization and autoclaving procedures are necessary for surgical instruments.

HUMAN IMMUNODEFICIENCY VIRUS

The role of human immunodeficiency virus (HIV) in the CNS continues to be studied; neurologic complications are a frequent cause of morbidity and mortality in HIV-infected patients. There is evidence of HIV and antibodies to HIV in both the brain and CSF of patients with neurologic signs; however, this does not fully explain the progressive and diffuse neurologic symptoms that occur with HIV infections. Primary HIV infections produce HIV encephalitis and atypical aseptic meningitis. Toxoplasmic encephalitis, caused by the parasite *Toxoplasma gondii,* is recognized as the most frequent cause of intracerebral lesions in the patient with HIV (Mocsny, 1992). The fungal agent *Cryptococ-*

cus neoformans, responsible for cryptococcal meningitis, is difficult to cure and may require lifelong therapy (Mocsny, 1992). Secondary viral infections include herpes simplex encephalitis, progressive multifocal leukoencephalopathy, and cytomegalovirus meningoencephalitis. Other fungal and yeast organisms may also cause infections.

AIDS dementia is a syndrome identified in the early stages by impaired memory, confusion, social withdrawal, and apathy. This is the most common neurologic problem in the HIV patient population. Many patients decline over months to severe dementia, incontinence, lower extremity weakness, and occasionally myoclonus. CSF studies are normal or have a slight increase in protein content. EEG may show focal or diffuse slowing. CT scan reveals significant cortical atrophy and enlarged ventricles. There is some evidence that AZT penetrates the blood–brain barrier and may be effective against HIV in the CNS. Nursing care and other therapies are directed toward supportive care.

UNCOMMON VIRAL DISEASES TARGETING THE CNS

*Herpes zoster (shingles), *herpesvirus-varicella zoster*—an extremely painful outbreak of a rash that follows the sensory distribution of a dermatome; caused by a dormant virus of herpes varicella (chickenpox).

*Poliomyelitis, *polioviruses, type 1, 2, or 3*—destruction of the motor cells of the anterior horn cells of the spinal cord; poliovirus transmitted through gastrointestinal tract.

*Rabies, *rhabdovirus*—encephalomyelitis infection that progresses to respiratory and cardiac arrest after several days; relayed to humans through a bite from infected animals.

*Lyme disease, *Borrelia burgdorferi*—systemic disease with potential neurologic manifestations of meningitis, encephalitis, and/or Bell's palsy and arthritic symptoms; spirochete carried by the bite of an infected tick carried on deer and other wild animals.

ISOLATION

Isolation procedures established by the Centers for Disease Control and Prevention and the hospital infection control department will provide guidelines for practices related to specific infections. Although isolation is usually not required for patients with CNS infections, respiratory isolation is recommended for at least 24 hours for patients with acute meningococcal meningitis. This organism can be transmitted through secretions from the nasopharynx and droplets from the respiratory tract; however, the meningococci usually disappear after the patient has received antibiotic therapy for 24 hours.

REFERENCES

Hickey, J. V. (1992). *The clinical practice of neurological and neurosurgical nursing* (3rd ed.). Philadelphia: J. B. Lippincott.

Mocsny, N. (1992). Cryptococcal meningitis in patients with AIDS. *Neuroscience Nurs, 24*(5), 265–268.

Mocsny, N. (1992). Toxoplasmic encephalitis in the AIDS patient. *J Neuroscience Nurs, 24*(1), 30–33.

Rowland, L. P. (1989). *Meritt's textbook of neurology* (8th ed.). Philadelphia: Lea & Febiger.

Schulz, M., Moore, K., & Foote, A. W. (1993). Bacterial ventriculitis and duration of ventriculostomy catheter insertion. *J Neuroscience Nurs, 25*(3), 158–164.

UNIT 7

RENAL SYSTEM

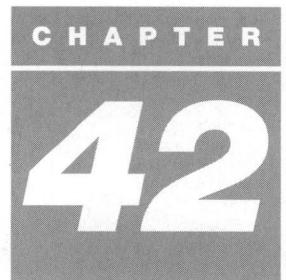

Renal Physiology

Patricia Peschman

The human kidney is a complex organ that performs several major functions essential for survival (Table 42–1). The primary role of the kidney is to maintain the composition and volume of the extracellular fluid, thereby ensuring a constant environment in which normal cellular function can take place. The kidney accomplishes this fine-tuning by removing the waste products of metabolism while conserving substances needed by the body.

The kidney performs several additional functions. It participates in the regulation of blood pressure through the renin-angiotensin-aldosterone system. It contributes to acid-base balance by removing hydrogen ions and conserving bicarbonate. The kidney produces erythropoietin, which promotes red blood cell synthesis. Additionally, the kidney plays a role in the metabolism of vitamin D to its active form.

This chapter addresses the anatomic structures and physiologic principles underlying these functions of the human kidney. A clear understanding of normal renal function is helpful when studying the pathophysiology, symptomatology, and management of renal dysfunction. It will also assist the nurse with problem solving when confronted with concerns about a patient's renal function in the critical care setting.

RENAL ANATOMY

Gross Anatomy

The kidneys are paired, reddish-brown, bean-shaped organs. They are retroperitoneal organs whose posterior surfaces are adjacent to the muscles of the posterior abdominal wall. The kidneys lie on either side of the abdominal aorta, inferior vena cava, and lumbar spine between the twelfth thoracic and third lumbar vertebrae. The right kidney usually sits slightly lower than the left beneath the large right lobe of the liver.

TABLE 42–1. **Functions of the Kidney**

Maintenance of extracellular fluid volume and concentration
Regulation of blood pressure
Regulation of acid-base balance
Production of erythropoietin
Metabolism of vitamin D

Adult kidneys measure 11 to 12 cm in length and 5 to 7.5 cm in width (Tisher & Madsen, 1991). The weight of each kidney ranges between 125 and 170 grams in adult males and 115 and 155 grams in adult females (Tisher & Madsen, 1991). Determination of kidney size by ultrasound may be useful clinically in the differential diagnosis of renal failure. Small kidneys are suggestive of many forms of chronic renal disease. Large kidneys may be indicative of obstruction or polycystic kidney disease. Abdominal palpation is not always helpful in measuring kidney size because the kidneys are usually not palpable.

The kidneys move up and down within the abdominal cavity in association with respiration. This movement is clinically important during the performance of a kidney biopsy. The cooperation of the patient in holding the breath during the biopsy is essential to prevent complications.

The outside of each kidney is protected by a tough white fibrous coat known as the renal capsule. Additional protection is offered by a mass of perinephric fat that surrounds each kidney. An adrenal gland lies above each kidney within the perinephric fat. The renal fascia and surrounding organs help to hold the kidneys in place. On the medial aspect of each kidney there is a central indentation known as the hilum. The renal arteries and nerves enter and the renal veins, lymphatics, and ureters exit the kidney at the hilum.

Internal Structure

When the kidney is cut longitudinally and opened, three distinct sections become apparent: cortex, medulla, and renal sinus (Fig. 42–1). The outer three-quarters of an inch is known as the cortex. The cortex is pale in color and has a granular appearance. Most parts of the nephrons, the primary functional units of the kidney, lie in the cortex.

The middle section, the medulla, is darker in color and has a striated appearance. The medulla is composed of 8 to 18 wedge-shaped structures known as pyramids. Within the pyramids a segment of the nephrons and the collecting ducts descend deep into the

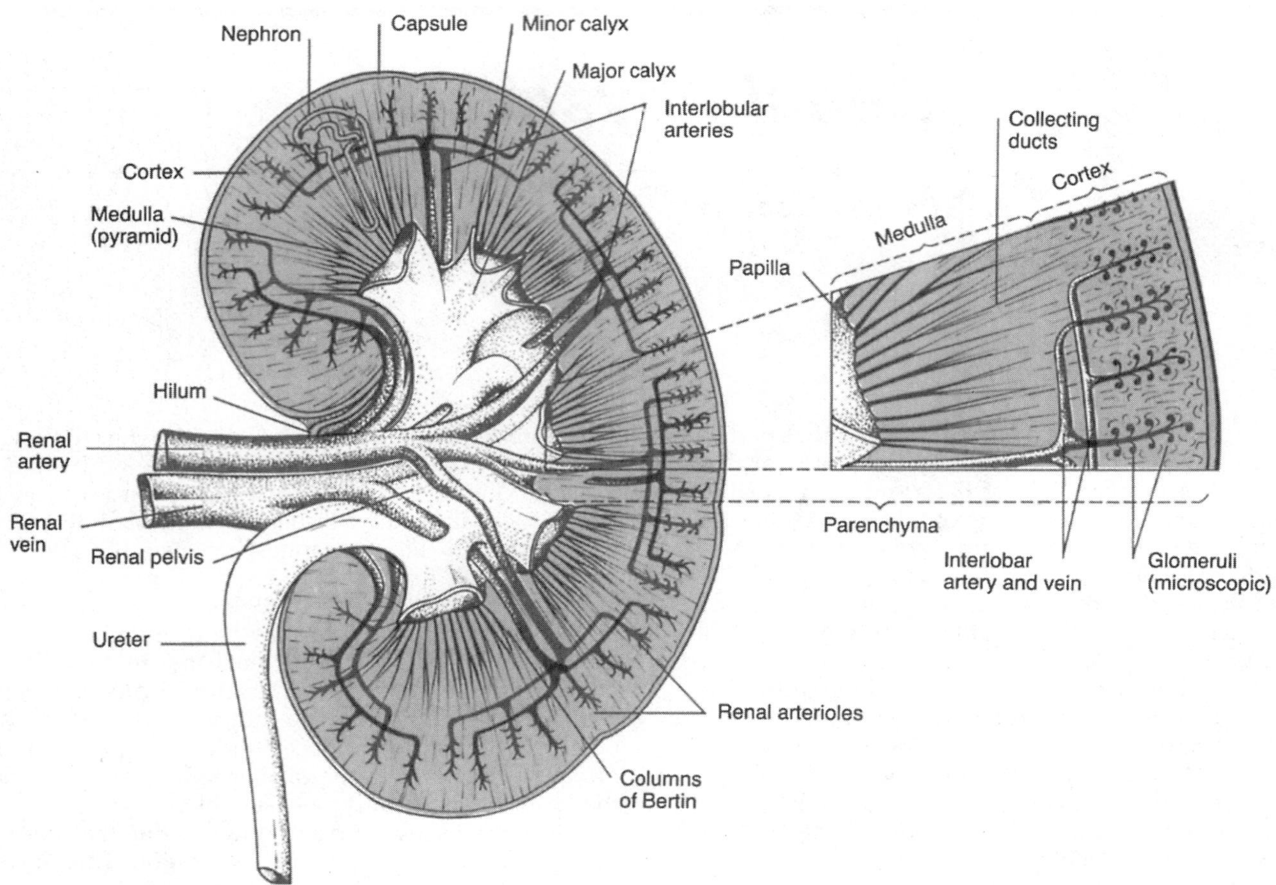

FIGURE 42–1. Major structures of the kidney. (From Ignatavicius, D. D., & Bayne, M. V. [Eds.]. [1991]. *Medical-surgical nursing: A nursing process approach* [p. 1801]. Philadelphia: W. B. Saunders.)

kidney, resulting in the striated appearance. Between the pyramids, blood vessels and nerves run to and from the cortex in areas known as the columns of Bertin. The apex of each pyramid forms a nipplelike projection known as the papilla, as seen in Figure 42–2. The collecting ducts end in the papillae, perforating their surfaces, allowing urine to flow out of the medulla.

The final section of the kidney is the renal sinus, a cavity that is almost completely filled with blood vessels and structures formed by the expanded upper end of the ureter. Before entering the kidney, the ureter dilates to form the renal pelvis. The renal pelvis branches into two or three major divisions known as the major calyces. Each major calyx branches further to form several minor calyces. The upper part of each minor calyx cups itself around one to three papillae, collecting the urine that drains through the papillae from the collecting ducts.

Microscopic Structure

The primary functional unit of the kidney is the nephron, a long, tubular structure composed of several distinct parts. Each kidney contains approximately one million nephrons. Each nephron is capable of performing all the kidney's necessary functions.

The kidney contains two types of nephrons, cortical and juxtamedullary, distinguished by their structure and location in the cortex (Fig. 42–3). Cortical nephrons have glomeruli that lie in the outer region of the cortex. These nephrons have relatively short loops of Henle that end in the cortex or extend only a short distance into the outer medulla. Juxtamedullary nephrons have glomeruli situated in the inner region of the cortex, near the outer zone of the medulla. Juxtamedullary nephrons have long loops of Henle that penetrate deeply into the medulla. The structure of the juxtamedullary nephrons is important to the kidney's ability to concentrate the urine.

Each nephron is composed of three major parts: the renal corpuscle, the renal tubules, and the collecting duct (Fig. 42–4). The renal corpuscle, consisting of the glomerulus and Bowman's capsule, is responsible for the formation of ultrafiltrate from the blood. The renal tubules are responsible for the processes of reabsorption and secretion, which alter the volume and composition of the ultrafiltrate to form the final urine product. The collecting duct, which receives tubular fluid

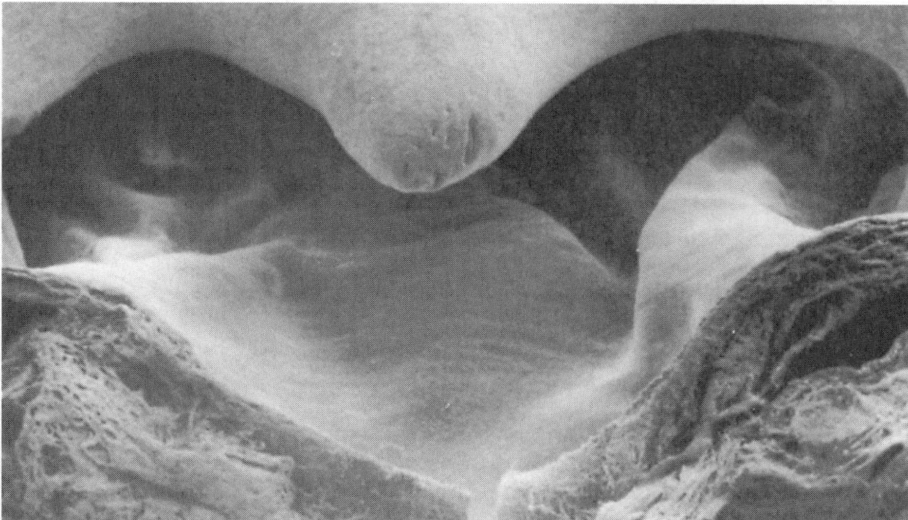

FIGURE 42–2. Scanning electron micrograph of papilla from a rat, illustrating the area cribrosa formed by the slit-like openings where the ducts of Bellini terminate. The renal pelvis surrounds the papilla. (From Tisher, C. C., & Madsen, K. M. [1986]. In B. M. Brenner and F. C. Rector [Eds.]. *The kidney* [3rd ed., p. 5]. Philadelphia: W. B. Saunders.)

from many nephrons, transports the fluid from the cortex to the minor calyx.

RENAL CORPUSCLE. Renal corpuscles are located in the cortex and columns of Bertin between the pyramids and are composed of the glomerulus and Bowman's capsule. The glomerulus is a complex anastomosing tuft of capillaries that branches from the afferent arteriole (Kriz & Kaissling, 1992). Bowman's capsule is the blind initial end of the renal tubules that is invaginated by the glomerular capillaries. Bow-

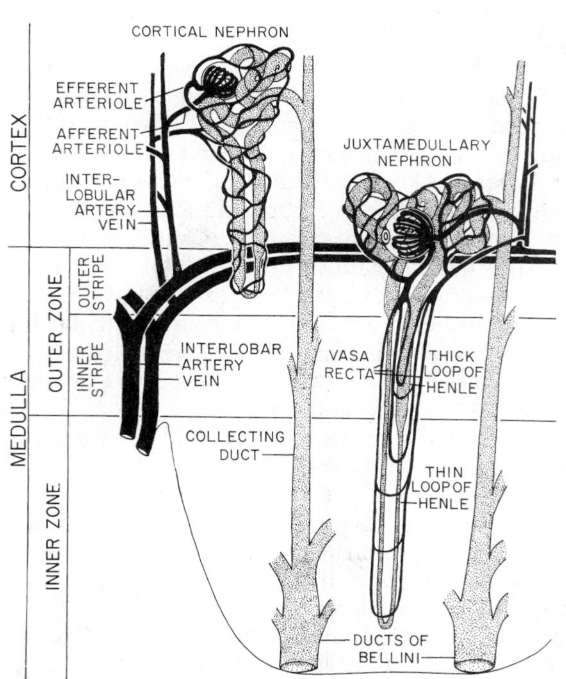

FIGURE 42–3. Differences between a cortical and a juxtamedullary nephron. (From Pitts, R. F. [1974]. *Physiology of the kidney and body fluids* [3rd ed.]. Chicago: Year Book Medical Publishers.)

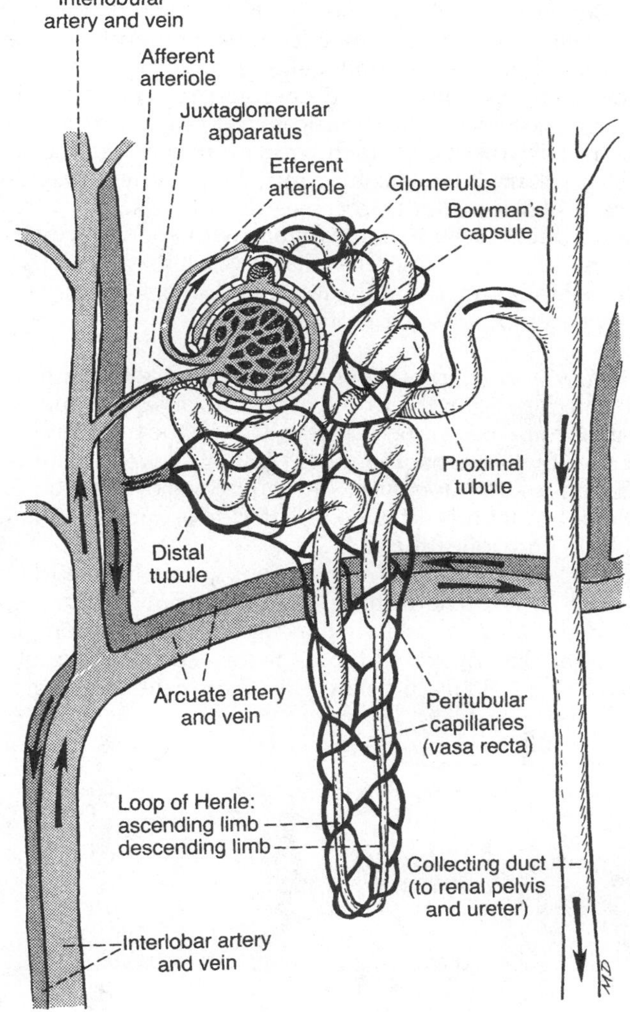

FIGURE 42–4. The nephron. (From Black, J. M., & Matassarin-Jacobs, E. [1993]. *Luckmann and Sorensen's medical-surgical nursing* [4th ed., p. 1407]. Philadelphia: W. B. Saunders.)

man's capsule is composed of an inner (visceral) wall, which covers most sides of the glomerular capillaries, and an outer (parietal) wall. Between the outer and inner walls of Bowman's capsule is an open area, the urinary space, which is continuous with the lumen of the proximal convoluted tubule (Tisher & Madsen, 1991).

GLOMERULAR MEMBRANE. The glomerular capillary membrane is composed of three distinct layers: the capillary endothelium, the basement membrane, and the epithelial cells, or podocytes. The first layer, the endothelium, lines the lumen of the glomerular capillary. The endothelial cells are perforated by regularly spaced pores. The second layer, the glomerular basement membrane, is a filamentous support structure composed of the merged basement membranes of the glomerular endothelium and epithelium. The glomerular basement membrane contains negatively charged sites that influence the filtration of some molecules (Tisher & Madsen, 1991). The third layer of the glomerular membrane is actually the visceral epithelial wall of Bowman's capsule. The tightly interwoven epithelial cells that cover the outside of the glomerular capillaries are known as podocytes. Extending from the body of the podocytes are numerous projections or primary processes. These processes branch further to form foot processes, which wrap around the glomerular capillary loops, contacting the basement membrane. Adjacent foot processes do not arise from the same podocyte but interdigitate with foot processes from other epithelial cells (Tisher & Madsen, 1991). A thin diaphragm, the slit diaphragm, covers the narrow gap between adjacent foot processes.

RENAL TUBULES AND COLLECTING DUCTS. The ultrafiltrate formed in the renal corpuscle leaves Bowman's capsule and begins its journey through the tubular system of the nephron. Figure 42–5 illustrates the distinct anatomic structures of the three sections of the tubule: the proximal tubule, the loop of Henle, and the distal tubule and collecting duct.

PROXIMAL TUBULE. The proximal tubule lies entirely in the cortex. The initial part is convoluted—that is, looped or folded—whereas the later portion is straight. The proximal tubule is formed from a single layer of cuboidal epithelial cells. These cells are characterized by a dense brush border of microvilli on their luminal surface, multiple mitochondria, and relatively open junctions between adjoining cells. These cellular characteristics are responsible for the proximal tubule's ability to rapidly reabsorb and secrete various substances. Approximately 65% of the filtered sodium and water are reabsorbed in the proximal tubule (Vander, 1991).

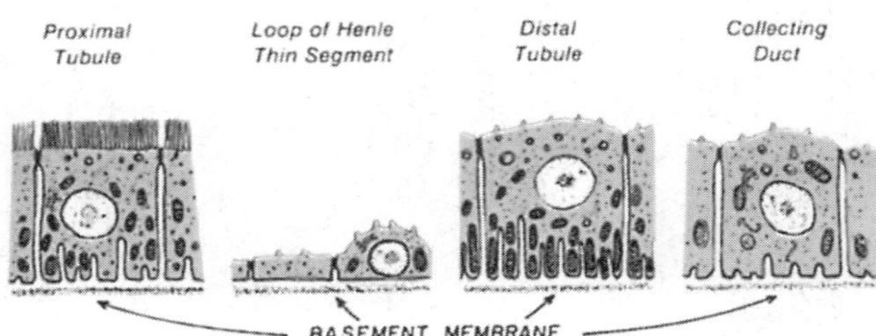

FIGURE 42–5. Characteristics of the epithelial cells in different tubular segments. (From Guyton, A. C. [1991]. *Textbook of medical physiology* [8th ed., p. 402]. Philadelphia: W. B. Saunders.)

LOOP OF HENLE. The straight portion of the proximal tubule turns toward the medulla and tapers to become the thin descending limb of the loop of Henle. At the base of the loop, the tubule makes a hairpin turn, and the ascending limb of the loop of Henle begins. The tubule widens again to form the thick segment of the ascending limb. In juxtamedullary nephrons, the thin segment of the loop of Henle descends deep into the medulla and continues around the turn to form the initial one-third to one-half of the ascending limb. In cortical nephrons the thin segment is shorter and ends shortly before or after the hairpin turn. The result is that all or nearly all of the ascending limb is thick (Tisher & Madsen, 1991). The loop of Henle is made up entirely of cuboidal epithelial cells except for the thin ascending segment of the juxtamedullary nephrons. The thin ascending segment of the juxtamedullary nephrons is composed of squamous epithelial cells.

DISTAL TUBULE. The distal tubule is divided into three distinct sections: the thick ascending limb of the loop of Henle, the macula densa, and the convoluted portion (Tisher & Madsen, 1991). The thick ascending limb of the loop of Henle extends from the outer medulla into the cortex. At one point the distal tubule comes to lie between the afferent and efferent arterioles as they enter and exit the glomerulus. Cells of the distal tubule lying between the afferent and efferent arterioles are known as the macula densa. These cells are distinguished by their taller height and more compact relationship. The macula densa is part of the juxtaglomerular apparatus, which will be discussed later in the chapter. The convoluted portion of the distal tubule extends from the macula densa to the collecting duct. Both the straight and convoluted portions of the distal tubule are made up of cuboidal epithelial cells with sparse microvilli on their luminal surface.

In some nephrons, fluid exiting the distal tubule enters a short, straight connecting tubule before entering a collecting duct. Multiple nephrons eventually connect to a single collecting duct. Small collecting ducts join together to form progressively larger collecting ducts as they progress downward through the medulla. The collecting duct is divided into three sections: the cortical collecting duct, the medullary collecting duct, and the papillary collecting duct or ducts of Bellini. The cells of the collecting duct begin as flat cuboidal epithelium in the cortical section enlarging to taller columnar epithelium in the ducts of Bellini. These cells have few microvilli and mitochondria, indicating that little metabolic activity occurs in this area. The ducts of Bellini finally empty into the minor calyces through the surface of the papillae.

Renal Vascular System

The kidneys are very vascular organs, receiving about 20% of the cardiac output under resting conditions (Divorkin & Brenner, 1991). As shown in Figure 42–1, the renal vascular structure closely follows the pattern of the various parts of the nephrons, an indication of the close link between structure and function.

RENAL ARTERIES, ARTERIOLES, AND CAPILLARY SYSTEM. Arterial blood is supplied to the kidneys by the renal arteries, which branch directly off the abdominal aorta. Most individuals have only one renal artery supplying each kidney. Approximately 30% of individuals have one or more accessory renal arteries that branch off the aorta and supply a portion of the renal parenchyma (Divorkin & Brenner, 1991).

The renal artery divides into an anterior main branch and a posterior main branch before entering the kidney. The anterior main branch further divides into four segmental arteries, which divide the kidney into vascular segments. The segmental arteries give rise to interlobar arteries, which ascend toward the cortex on either side of the pyramid in the renal columns (Divorkin & Brenner, 1991). At the point where the cortex and medulla meet, the interlobar arteries turn at right angles to form the arcuate arteries, which course along the tops of the pyramids. The arcuate arteries have multiple branches known as the interlobular arteries, which ascend at right angles from the arcuate artery into the cortex.

The vascular structure of the kidney has several unique features that distinguish it from vascular beds in other areas of the body (see Fig. 42–3). The afferent arteriole branches off the interlobular artery to supply blood to the glomerular capillaries. Blood leaving the glomerulus does not enter a vein but instead enters a second arteriole, the efferent arteriole. The kidneys are unique in having two separate capillary beds separated from each other by the efferent arteriole. The efferent arterioles leaving the glomeruli of cortical nephrons branch into a network of peritubular capillaries that surround the proximal and distal convoluted tubules. The efferent arterioles from the juxtamedullary nephrons form a very different capillary network known as the vasa recta (Divorkin & Brenner, 1991). The vasa recta is a complex of long, straight capillary loops connected by side branches at various levels that run parallel to the ascending and descending loop of Henle. The vasa recta play an important role in maintaining the concentrated interstitial fluid found within the medulla.

JUXTAGLOMERULAR APPARATUS. The juxtaglomerular apparatus is a specialized anatomic structure made up of the macula densa and the juxtaglomerular granular cells (Fig. 42–6). As discussed previously, the macula densa is the part of the distal tubule that lies in close proximity to the afferent and efferent arterioles as they enter and exit the glomerulus. The arterioles, particularly the afferent arteriole, and the mesangium in this region, contain differentiated smooth muscle cells known as juxtaglomerular granular cells. The enzyme renin is believed to be produced and stored in the juxtaglomerular cells (Tisher & Madsen, 1991). The function of the juxtaglomerular apparatus will be discussed in the section on renal blood flow and blood pressure regulation.

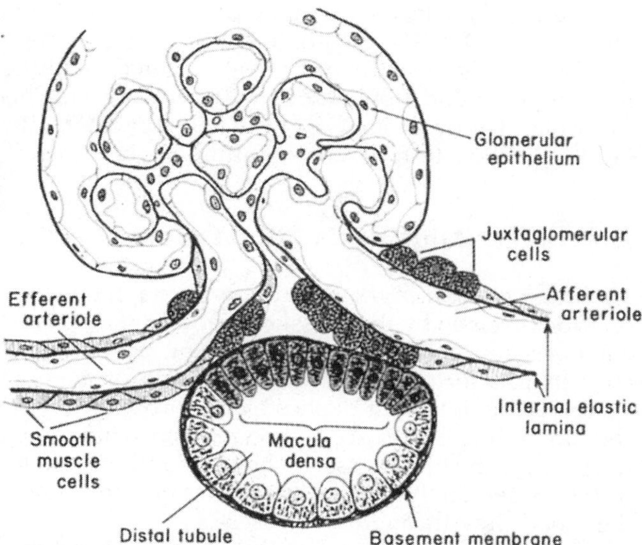

FIGURE 42–6. Structure of the juxtaglomerular apparatus. (From Guyton, A. C. [1991]. *Textbook of medical physiology* [8th ed., p. 411]. Philadelphia: W. B. Saunders.)

RENAL VEINS. Blood drains from the peritubular capillaries and vasa recta into the interlobular veins, beginning the venous system in the kidneys. The veins of the kidney retrace the pattern formed by the renal arteries. Blood flows from the interlobular veins into the arcuate veins and then to the interlobar veins, ultimately forming the renal vein, which empties into the inferior vena cava.

RENAL HEMODYNAMICS

Renal Blood Flow and Distribution

Renal function is largely dependent on maintenance of a normal rate and distribution of renal blood flow (RBF) and normal pressures within the renal vascular circuit. Although the function of the renal vasculature is similar to that of other vasculature in the body, special features and regulatory mechanisms help to maintain normal renal hemodynamics.

The renal fraction—the part of the cardiac output that passes through the kidneys—averages around 20% of cardiac output, or approximately 1000 to 1200 mL/min. Blood flow is not distributed evenly throughout the kidney. About 85% to 90% of RBF is distributed to the cortex under normal circumstances (Divorkin &

Brenner, 1991). The remaining blood circulates through the medulla. Only 1% to 2% of total RBF passes through the vasa recta surrounding the loop of Henle, resulting in sluggish blood flow through the vasa recta. This slow blood flow is an important component of the kidney's ability to form a concentrated urine.

Determinants of Renal Blood Flow

PRESSURE GRADIENTS. Blood flow through any vessel is determined by the pressure gradient and the vascular resistance. The pressure gradient, or the difference in pressure between the two ends of a blood vessel, is the force that pushes blood through the vessel. Blood flow is opposed by the resistance offered by the walls of the blood vessel. The smaller the diameter of the vessel, the higher the resistance and the slower the blood flow through the vessel.

Normally, the diameter of the arterioles is the major determinant of resistance within an organ. This is true in the kidney, where mean arterial pressure (MAP) does not fall significantly until the afferent arteriole is reached.

The MAP inside the arcuate artery averages 100 mm Hg. The mean glomerular capillary pressure is estimated to be 55 to 60 mm Hg. These figures are estimates from animal studies because direct measurements in human kidneys are not available. Glomerular capillary pressure is much higher than in other capillaries throughout the body, where it is believed that mean capillary pressure averages 17 mm Hg (Guyton, 1991). Changes in the diameter of the afferent and efferent arterioles determine resistance to RBF and intraglomerular pressure. The afferent arteriole controls blood flow into the glomerulus, whereas the efferent arteriole offers resistance to blood flow out of the glomerulus. Blood pressure drops significantly across the efferent arteriole, averaging 13 mm Hg in the peritubular capillaries and 8 mm Hg in the renal veins. The low pressure in the peritubular capillaries promotes reabsorption of fluid from the tubules back into the circulatory system (Guyton, 1991).

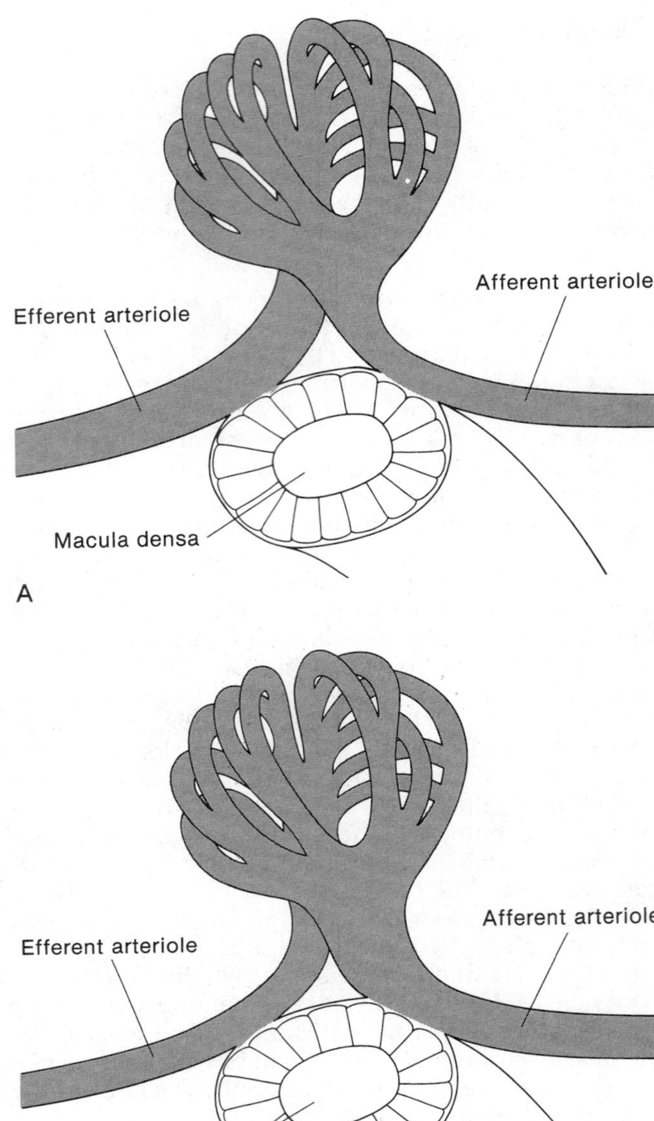

FIGURE 42–7. *A*, Response of afferent arteriole to increased intraglomerular pressure. *B*, Response of afferent and efferent arterioles to decreased intraglomerular pressure.

AUTOREGULATION. Autoregulation refers to the kidney's ability to maintain a relatively constant RBF and intraglomerular pressure despite changes in MAP of between 75 and 160 mm Hg (Guyton, 1991). Autoregulation is extremely important in the fine-tuning of renal regulation of the extracellular fluid. If autoregulation were not present, fluctuations in arterial blood pressure, such as normally occur with changes in activity level, would result in changes in RBF and the intraglomerular pressure. Consequently, the glomerular filtration rate (GFR) would also fluctuate widely. Because even small changes in the GFR can produce significant changes in the volume and content of the urine, the volume and composition of the extracellular fluid would ultimately be altered.

As discussed previously, blood flow through a vessel is determined by the pressure gradient and vascular resistance. It follows that the only way RBF can remain constant despite changes in arterial pressure is through changes in the vascular resistance. In the kidney the predominant location of changes in vascular resistance is the afferent arteriole. The efferent arteriole also participates in autoregulation but to a lesser extent (Divorkin & Brenner, 1991). Increases in the MAP result in constriction of the afferent arteriole, which prevents the increased arterial pressure from raising the intraglomerular pressure (Fig. 42–7*A*). A fall in blood pressure within the range of 75 to 160 mm Hg results in dilatation of the afferent arteriole

(Fig. 42–7*B*). As the diameter of the afferent arteriole increases, more blood is allowed to flow into the glomerulus. The increased glomerular blood flow will increase intraglomerular pressure if efferent arteriolar resistance remains constant. Efferent arteriolar resistance may increase as the arterial blood pressure falls below 100 mm Hg, helping to maintain the intraglomerular pressure (Divorkin & Brenner, 1991).

The exact mechanism by which renal autoregulation occurs is not known. There are two theories of its operation—the myogenic theory and the tubuloglomerular feedback theory (Divorkin & Brenner, 1991). The myogenic theory suggests that changes in the diameter of the arteriole are an intrinsic response to changes in vascular wall tension. A rise in arterial pressure would cause the walls of the afferent arteriole to stretch, triggering a subsequent contraction of the smooth muscle cells of the arteriole. The opposite would occur with a decrease in arterial pressure. Decreased stretch in the afferent arteriolar wall would cause the arteriole to dilate, thereby allowing increased blood flow into the glomerulus and maintaining intraglomerular pressure.

The tubuloglomerular feedback theory is somewhat more complex. Tubuloglomerular feedback is believed to operate in the following way. As arterial pressure increases, intraglomerular pressure also increases, resulting in an increase in the GFR. This increase in the GFR increases the rate of fluid flow through the tubules, preventing them from reabsorbing normal amounts of water and sodium from the filtrate. The cells of the macula densa in the distal tubule sense the increase in fluid flow past them, probably by detecting the increase in the sodium concentration, and respond by releasing a vasoconstrictor substance. The vasoconstrictor substance constricts the afferent arteriole, thereby decreasing the intraglomerular pressure and the GFR. Tubular fluid flow is thereby returned toward normal. A fall in arterial pressure would have the opposite effect, resulting in inhibition of release of the vasoconstrictor substance, thus allowing afferent arteriolar dilation.

A number of other substances are being studied to determine whether they play a role in autoregulation of RBF. These substances, which include prostaglandins, kinins, angiotensin II, and adenosine, are known to affect RBF (Divorkin & Brenner, 1991). Their exact role in the kidney's response to changes in arterial blood pressure remains to be determined.

RENIN-ANGIOTENSIN-ALDOSTERONE SYSTEM. Another important mechanism that affects RBF and the GFR is the renin-angiotensin-aldosterone system, which is illustrated in Figure 42–8. The primary function of the renin-angiotensin-aldosterone system is to maintain an adequate blood pressure and intravascular volume. Activation of this complex system produces a multitude of physiologic effects. Within the kidney these physiologic alterations result simultaneously in a reduction of RBF, maintenance of GFR, and conservation of sodium and water (Ballerman et al., 1991).

A number of stimuli are known to trigger the release of renin by the kidney. These include reduced perfusion pressure in the afferent arteriole, reduced sodium chloride delivery to the macula densa, sympathetic nervous system stimulation, and prostaglandins (Ballerman et al., 1991). The juxtaglomerular cells of the afferent arteriole are believed to act as a baroreceptor. When the pressure against these cells falls, a direct stimulus for renin release results. Changes in tubular sodium chloride concentration, sensed by the macula densa, also result in renin release. Renin release from the juxtaglomerular cells is triggered by a decrease in distal tubular sodium chloride concentration (Guyton, 1991). Additionally, stimulation of renal sympathetic nerves and the presence of prostaglandins have also been shown to be direct stimuli for renin release.

As previously discussed, the juxtaglomerular cells, located primarily in the afferent arteriole, contain many granules that are the site of renin storage. When these cells are stimulated, renin is released into the bloodstream, where it acts on the plasma protein angiotensinogen, splitting off part of the molecule to form angiotensin I. Angiotensin I is then rapidly split to form angiotensin II by a converting enzyme found in vascular endothelial cells throughout the body, particularly in the lung. The formation of angiotensin II then produces a variety of actions, including increased peripheral vascular resistance, altered renal hemodynamics, increased reabsorption of sodium and water by the kidneys, and increased thirst.

The renin-angiotensin-aldosterone system participates in the adjustment of vascular resistance in response to changes in arterial pressure that occur with changes in position and activity level. This system is particularly important in maintaining blood pressure in critically ill patients who experience extracellular fluid volume depletion (Ballerman et al., 1991). Angiotensin II increases blood pressure in several ways. It is a potent vasoconstrictor, directly stimulating contraction of vascular smooth muscle cells. Angiotensin II also directly increases cardiac contractility. Indirectly, angiotensin II increases blood pressure by acting on the central nervous system to stimulate increased sympathetic activity and vasopressin release. Angiotensin II also increases catecholamine release from peripheral nerve endings and from the adrenal medulla.

In the kidney, angiotensin II produces a fall in RBF and GFR. However, researchers have observed that the GFR does not fall as much as would be predicted by the fall in RBF. This observation led to the conclusion that the primary effect of angiotensin II in the nephron is constriction of the efferent arteriole (Guyton, 1991). Constriction of the efferent arteriole raises the intraglomerular pressure. As a result, a greater proportion of the plasma filters across the glomerulus into the tubules, thereby maintaining the GFR.

Other physiologic effects of angiotensin II result in an increased extracellular fluid volume. Angiotensin II stimulates aldosterone release from the adrenal cortex. Aldosterone acts on the collecting duct in the nephron,

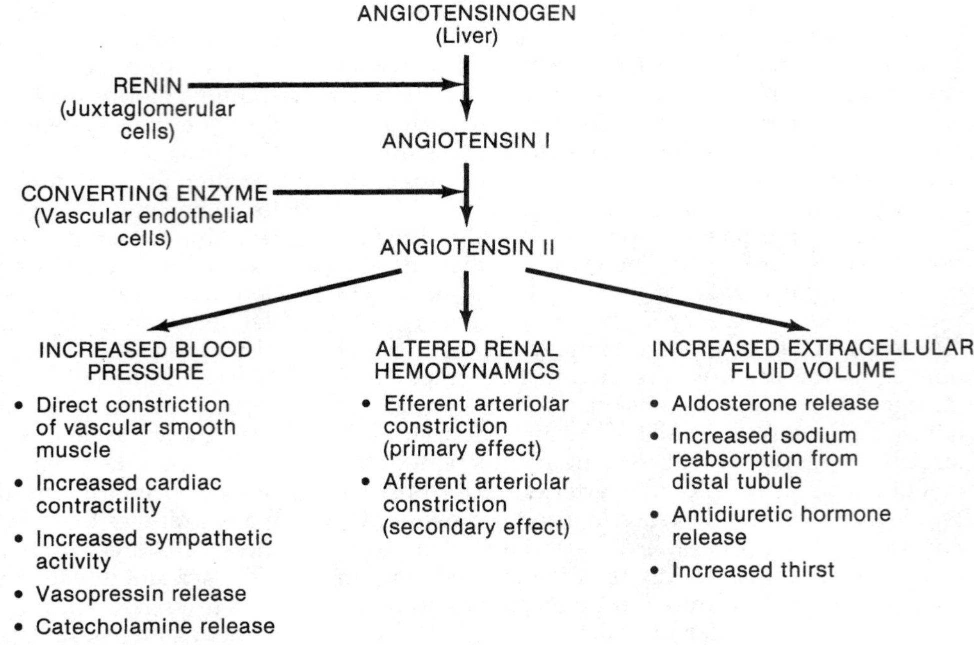

FIGURE 42–8. The renin-angiotensin-aldosterone system.

stimulating increased sodium reabsorption. As sodium is reabsorbed water follows, resulting in increased intravascular volume. Angiotensin II also acts directly to increase sodium reabsorption by the distal tubule (Ballerman et al., 1991). Angiotensin II is also believed to stimulate antidiuretic hormone (ADH) release from the posterior pituitary, though the exact mechanism is not completely understood (Ballerman et al., 1991). As will be discussed later, ADH increases water reabsorption by the distal tubule and collecting duct of the nephron. Finally, angiotensin II increases the sensation of thirst, which should result in increased fluid intake.

SYMPATHETIC NERVOUS SYSTEM. The sympathetic nevous system is the third system that has an effect on RBF. The kidney is richly innervated with sympathetic fibers. Nerve fiber endings have been found in the afferent and efferent arterioles and in all sections of the tubules. Their presence implies that the sympathetic nervous system has a role in alteration of blood flow and reabsorptive processes. Under resting conditions the influence of the sympathetic nervous system on renal function is thought to be minor. At low levels of stimulation, the sympathetic nervous system increases sodium reabsorption within the proximal tubule. At moderate levels of sympathetic nervous system stimulation, both the afferent and efferent arterioles constrict. This results in a decrease in both RBF and GFR, although RBF is more impaired (Navar et al., 1989). With higher levels of sympathetic nervous system stimulation, such as might occur with severe hypotension, afferent arteriolar constriction predominates. RBF may be reduced sufficiently to cause cessation of glomerular filtration. If RBF is reduced for a prolonged period, renal ischemia and acute renal failure may result.

LOCAL HORMONES. Prostaglandin and bradykinin are two hormones produced by the kidney and other tissues. They are considered local hormones because they are synthesized in the same location in which they exert their effect and they are rapidly inactivated. Prostaglandin production is promoted by the presence of angiotensin II, bradykinin, ADH, sympathetic stimulation, and renal ischemia (Mene & Dunn, 1992). Bradykinin release is stimulated by angiotensin II, prostaglandins, and ADH (Mene & Dunn, 1992). Both prostaglandin and bradykinin cause vasodilation in the kidney. They are believed to help modulate the vasoconstricting effects resulting from angiotensin II and sympathetic stimulation, thereby helping to preserve renal blood flow. Nonsteroidal antiinflammatory agents, such as aspirin and ibuprofen, act by inhibiting prostaglandin formation. In individuals with renal insufficiency, these agents may decrease RBF enough to cause severe renal ischemia.

EXTRINSIC VASOACTIVE SUBSTANCES. Renal blood flow may also be altered by a variety of vasoactive drugs administered to patients. Dopamine hydrochloride, epinephrine, and norepinephrine are three common examples of drugs that affect RBF. In low doses of 2 to 5 μg/kg per minute, dopamine acts primarily on the dopaminergic receptors in the renal artery, resulting in dilation of the artery. Low doses of dopamine are frequently used as a means of protecting renal function by improving RBF when blood flow to the kidneys has been impaired. In higher doses greater than 10 μg/kg/min, dopamine may itself impair RBF by causing constriction of the renal artery. Epinephrine and norepinephrine both result in renal artery constriction. Urine output is monitored as an index of RBF during administration of these drugs.

PHYSIOLOGIC FUNCTIONS PERFORMED BY THE KIDNEY

Formation of Urine

The kidney performs its primary function, regulation of the volume and composition of the extracellular fluid, through the processes involved in the formation of urine: glomerular filtration, reabsorption, and secretion. Urine formation begins with glomerular filtration, the movement of fluid across the glomerular membrane as a consequence of pressure gradients. The composition of the resulting filtrate is then altered by the processes of reabsorption and secretion. The process of reabsorption returns filtered substances to the blood. Secretion results in the movement of solutes from the blood into the tubules. The end result of all of these processes is the excretion of waste products and excess water as urine and the selective adjustment of the composition and volume of the extracellular fluid. This section will discuss the specific processes involved in the formation of urine and will introduce the concept of clearance.

GLOMERULAR FILTRATION. Glomerular filtration is similar to filtration of fluid from capillaries in other parts of the body. The rate at which fluid filters out of any capillary is determined by the net filtration pressure and the permeability of the capillary membrane. In nonrenal capillary systems, pressure dynamics result in a net pressure that pushes fluid into the interstitial space at the arterial end of the capillary. The net pressure in the glomerulus moves fluid out of the capillaries into Bowman's capsule. The major difference between the glomerulus and other capillaries is the permeability of the capillary membrane. In comparison to other capillaries, the glomerular membrane is significantly more permeable, allowing a much greater amount of fluid to move out of the capillary for each mm Hg difference in pressure (Vander, 1991).

NET FILTRATION PRESSURE. The net filtration pressure for any capillary is determined by the opposing values of hydrostatic and colloid osmotic pressures across the capillary wall. Hydrostatic pressure refers to the pressure exerted by a fluid—for example, the pressure exerted by the blood in a capillary. Colloid osmotic pressure refers to the pressure that develops across a semipermeable membrane when large molecules, such as protein, are unable to cross the membrane. The net pressure responsible for glomerular filtration is the sum of the hydrostatic and colloid osmotic pressures in the glomerular capillary and Bowman's capsule (Fig. 42–9).

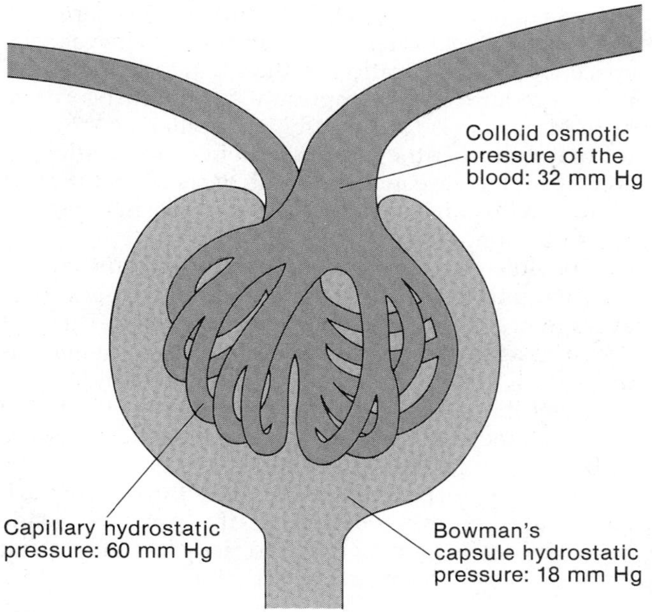

FIGURE 42–9. Average pressures involved in filtration from the glomerular capillaries.

Glomerular capillary hydrostatic pressure and the colloid osmotic pressure of the fluid in Bowman's capsule promote filtration. Under usual circumstances, the glomerular membrane allows only a small amount of protein to filter out of the blood into Bowman's capsule. Therefore, the colloid osmotic pressure of the fluid in Bowman's capsule is too small to have any significant impact on filtration. For this reason, glomerular capillary hydrostatic pressure will be the only force promoting filtration considered in this discussion. Glomerular filtration is opposed by the colloid osmotic pressure of the blood in the glomerular capillary and by the hydrostatic pressure exerted by the fluid inside Bowman's capsule.

The hydrostatic pressure exerted by the blood against the walls of the glomerular capillary has not been measured in humans. It has, however, been calculated to be around 55 to 60 mm Hg (Navar et al., 1989). As discussed previously, many factors have the potential to increase or decrease this pressure. The autoregulatory mechanisms within the kidney normally help to maintain intraglomerular hydrostatic pressure at a relatively constant level.

The normal colloid osmotic pressure of the blood averages 28 mm Hg. As plasma water leaves the glomerular capillary to filter into Bowman's capsule, the concentration of the proteins that are left behind increases. The resulting colloid osmotic pressure is approximately 36 mm Hg. An average colloid osmotic pressure in the glomerular capillaries would then be

32 mm Hg (Guyton, 1991). The osmotic pull exerted by the plasma proteins tends to hold fluid in the vascular space, opposing filtration in the glomerulus. This osmotic pressure is also important for the reabsorption of fluid back into the peritubular capillaries. Any factor that decreases the plasma protein concentration results in an increase in filtration. A decrease in filtration occurs with an elevation in the plasma protein concentration.

The fluid that filters into Bowman's capsule creates a hydrostatic pressure of its own that is believed to average around 18 mm Hg (Guyton, 1991). This is a pressure against which fluid leaving the glomerulus must flow, and thus it opposes filtration. Under normal conditions the hydrostatic pressure of the blood in the glomerulus is much higher than the pressure in Bowman's capsule, and fluid filters easily into the tubules. However, if the flow of urine through the urinary tract becomes obstructed, the pressure inside Bowman's capsule may begin to rise. This may result in a decrease in or even cessation of glomerular filtration.

Calculation of the difference between the forces promoting and the forces opposing filtration results in determination of the net filtration pressure. Using the average pressures that have been discussed, the net filtration pressure in the glomerulus is calculated to be 10 mm Hg.

GLOMERULAR CAPILLARY PERMEABILITY AND COMPOSITION OF THE GLOMERULAR ULTRAFILTRATE. The glomerular capillary membrane is very permeable in comparison to most other capillary membranes (Guyton, 1991). This permeability is the result of the large number of tiny perforations in the various layers of the membrane. Water and solutes of small molecular size filter freely across the glomerular membrane. The size of the perforations in the glomerular membrane, especially in the basement membrane layer, restrict the filtration of large molecules such as protein. As a result, the glomerular ultrafiltrate that enters Bowman's capsule has a composition almost identical to that of plasma except that it is protein free.

FILTRATION FRACTION AND GLOMERULAR FILTRATION RATE. The term renal filtration fraction refers to the portion of the plasma entering the glomerular capillaries that filters out of the capillary into Bowman's capsule. The renal filtration fraction is much higher than the filtration fraction in other capillaries. The filtration fraction in the glomerulus is approximately 20%, compared with 0.5% in most other capillaries (Guyton, 1991). The total amount of plasma flowing through the kidneys is around 650 mL/min. If 20% of this amount were to filter across the glomerular membrane into Bowman's capsule, the GFR would be calculated at 130 mL/min. Actual measurements in man have determined that the average amount of glomerular filtrate formed by both kidneys is 125 mL/min or 180 L/day.

The GFR can be altered by factors that affect the net filtration pressure or the permeability of the glomerular membrane. Disease processes that decrease the permeability of the glomerular membrane, such as acute or chronic glomerulonephritis or diabetes, decrease the amount of fluid that is able to filter across the membrane at a given filtration pressure. In patients with chronic renal disease, the GFR usually decreases slowly over a relatively long period. In most chronic renal diseases the nephrons are not all affected at the same time. Some nephrons cease to function while others remain intact. The nephrons that remain functional increase their GFR to compensate for the filtration capacity lost from diseased nephrons. It is not entirely clear how the intact nephrons are able to increase their GFR, but this mechanism functions so efficiently that little alteration in the composition of the extracellular fluid occurs until 50% to 66% of the nephrons have ceased to function (Guyton, 1991).

TUBULAR REABSORPTION. The process of glomerular filtration results in approximately 180 L of ultrafiltrate entering the renal tubules every day. This huge volume of ultrafiltrate is equal to more than four times the volume of total body water. A carefully controlled process governing the reabsorption of water and solutes is essential to prevent significant alterations in the volume and composition of the extracellular fluid. Ordinarily, the renal tubules reabsorb 99% of the water and sodium from the 180 L that filter into the tubules, resulting in the production of 1 to 2 L of urine each day. Other substances that can be used by the body, such as glucose and amino acids, are also returned to the blood by the process of reabsorption. Some metabolic waste products, such as urea and uric acid, are partially reabsorbed. The majority of these wastes, however, are lost in the urine.

Substances reabsorbed by the nephrons move from the tubular lumen and pass through either the junctions between the tubular cells or the tubular cells themselves to enter the interstitial fluid. From the interstitial fluid, water and solutes readily enter the peritubular capillaries, which are extremely permeable and which together reabsorb about four times as much as all other capillaries in the entire body (Guyton, 1991). The majority of reabsorbed solutes must pass through the tubular cells, crossing both the luminal membrane (separating the tubular lumen from the interior of the cell) and the basolateral membrane (separating the interior of the cell from the interstitial fluid) in the process. A description of diffusion, osmosis, and active transport—the transport mechanisms used in reabsorption—follows.

DIFFUSION. The term diffusion refers to the movement of molecules or ions from an area of higher concentration to an area of lower concentration via the random motion of the molecule or ion (Fig. 42–10*A*). For diffusion to occur, there must be a concentration or electrical gradient across the cell membrane, and the membrane must be permeable to the substance. If the membrane is permeable, net movement of the substance from the area of higher concentration to the area of lower concentration will occur until equilibration is

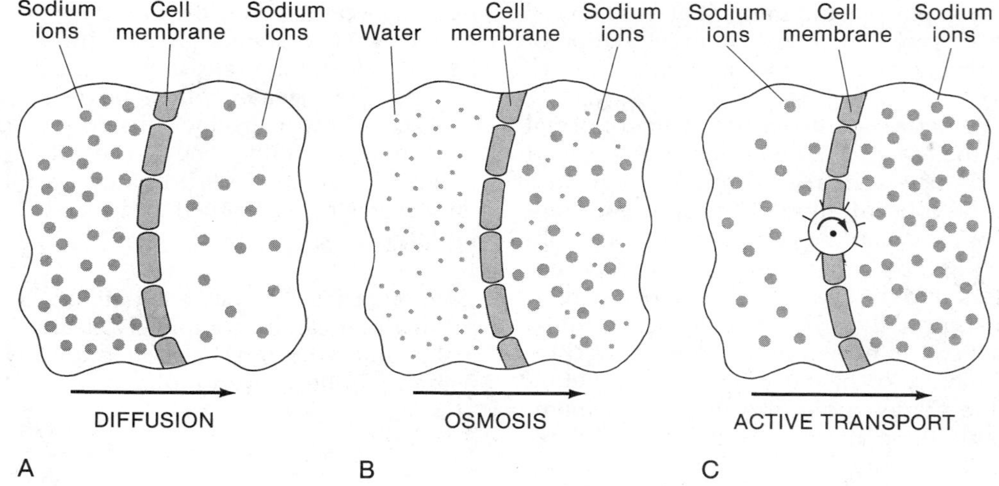

FIGURE 42–10. Movement of molecules across cell membranes. A, movement of sodium ions by diffusion. B, movement of water by osmosis. C, movement of sodium ions by active transport.

achieved. In the nephron, negatively charged ions are most frequently reabsorbed passively due to the electrical gradient created by sodium reabsorption. As sodium and water are transported out of the tubular lumen, the concentration of solutes that are left behind increases. This sets up a concentration gradient and often an electrical gradient for these solutes between the tubular lumen and the interstitial fluid surrounding the tubular cell. If the tubular membrane is permeable to them, solutes will move down their concentration gradient or electrical gradient and will be reabsorbed.

Some solutes that are not lipid soluble are able to cross the tubular membrane only if a specific carrier molecule is available to help them across—a process known as facilitated diffusion. The carrier molecule combines with the solute at the outside surface of the cell membrane, transports the solute across the lipid inside of the membrane, and releases it on the other side. In this type of system, the rate of diffusion is limited by the amount of carrier molecule available and the rate at which the chemical reaction can take place.

OSMOSIS. The movement of water from an area of higher water concentration to an area of lower concentration is referred to as osmosis (Fig. 42–10*B*). In the nephron, osmosis occurs when sodium molecules are transported out of the tubular lumen, decreasing the concentration of solutes in the lumen and increasing the concentration of solutes in the interstitial fluid. Concurrently, the concentration of water in the lumen increases and the concentration of water in the interstitial fluid decreases. If the tubular membrane is permeable, water will move from the lumen to the area of increased solute concentration in the interstitium to equalize the concentrations. Water in the interstitium then rapidly diffuses into the peritubular capillaries due to the movement of sodium and the osmotic pull created by the high concentration of plasma proteins in the blood leaving the glomerulus.

ACTIVE TRANSPORT. The term active transport refers to a cellular transport mechanism that moves a substance against its concentration gradient or electrical gradient, requiring the expenditure of cellular energy (Fig. 42–10*C*). The majority of substances that are reabsorbed leave the tubular lumen through active transport. Sodium is an example of a molecule that is actively transported.

Each actively reabsorbed solute requires a specific carrier system. These systems operate like the mechanism described for facilitated diffusion except that energy is expended in the process. The rate at which reabsorption of the solute can occur is limited by the amount of carrier available and the time it takes for the completion of the chemical reaction between the carrier and the solute. As a result each actively reabsorbed solute has a transport maximum—the maximum rate at which it can be transported across the tubular membrane. If the concentration of the solute in the tubular fluid is greater than the amount of the solute that can be actively reabsorbed, some of the solute in the tubular fluid will not be reabsorbed but will be excreted in the urine. Glucose is a substance that exhibits this property. When the serum glucose is within normal limits, about 125 mg of glucose filters into the tubules each minute and is reabsorbed by its carrier system. As the amount of glucose entering the tubules rises above 200 mg/min, some of the glucose is not reabsorbed and begins to appear in the urine. The point at which it begins to appear in the urine is known as the threshold. The maximum amount of glucose that can be reabsorbed by the tubules is 325 mg/min. The amount of glucose entering the tubules must increase above 400 mg/min before the carrier system will begin to operate at that capacity (Guyton, 1991).

Disease processes within the tubular cell can increase or decrease the transport maximum of various substances. One example is gout, in which an increase in the tubular transport maximum for uric acid contributes to a rise in plasma and interstitial fluid levels. Eventually this elevated level leads to precipitation of uric acid in the joints and other tissues.

FACTORS REGULATING REABSORPTION. Under normal circumstances, the amount of a substance reabsorbed depends on body needs. Its reabsorption is regulated by changes in the concentration of the substance and by body hormones. When the concentration of a substance decreases in the plasma, the amount of that substance that filters into the tubule will also decrease. If the substance is normally reabsorbed by active transport, a fall in its concentration in the tubular fluid results in fewer molecules of the substance competing for the available carrier molecules in the cell membrane. As a result, the percentage of the substance reabsorbed from the tubular fluid will increase with a consequent decrease in the amount lost into the urine. The opposite occurs with an increase in the plasma concentration of a substance. More of the substance is filtered into the tubules, and there are more molecules of the substance competing for the available carrier molecules in the tubular cell membranes. A smaller percentage is reabsorbed and more is excreted in the urine.

Hormones also play a role in regulation of tubular reabsorption. A good example of this is aldosterone. As described previously, aldosterone release is one of the end results of stimulation of the renin-angiotensin-aldosterone system. Aldosterone stimulates the distal convoluted tubule to increase sodium reabsorption, which in turn increases the intravascular volume and RBF. These adjustments of tubular reabsorption occur continuously to maintain a stable composition of the extracellular fluid.

TUBULAR SECRETION. The process of tubular secretion transports substances from blood in the peritubular capillaries into the tubular lumen, adding substances to the urine that either are not filtered or are filtered in small amounts. In general, secreted substances are electrolytes present in excess amounts in the extracellular fluid, metabolic wastes, and chemicals or drugs. Examples of substances secreted by the nephron are hydrogen ion, potassium, creatinine, ammonia, thiamine, histamine, and penicillin. Secretion occurs by diffusion and active transport, though active transport plays a larger role.

The amount of a substance secreted is regulated by body needs and hormones. Tubular handling of potassium illustrates this well. A significant amount of the filtered potassium is reabsorbed in the proximal tubule, leaving a low concentration of potassium in the fluid that enters the distal tubule. As a result, a diffusion gradient is set up between the peritubular capillary blood and the distal tubular fluid, resulting in passive secretion of potassium. The higher the potassium content in the plasma, the wider the gradient and the greater the amount of potassium that is secreted. In addition, potassium is also secreted through a sodium-potassium pump in the cells of the distal tubule. This pump operates under the influence of aldosterone. A high plasma potassium concentration is a direct stimulus for aldosterone release from the adrenal cortex.

The terms net absorption and net secretion are used to discuss how a specific substance is handled by the nephron. Generally, one process takes precedence; however, a molecule or ion may be only reabsorbed, only secreted, reabsorbed and secreted, or it may not undergo either process.

CLEARANCE. Clearance is defined as the volume of plasma that can be completely cleared of a substance in 1 minute. It can be calculated for any substance by using the following formula:

$$\text{Clearance (mL/min)} = \frac{\text{UV} \times \text{UC}}{\text{PC}}$$

where

UV = the volume of urine in mL/min,
UC = the concentration of the substance in the urine, and
PC = the concentration of the substance in the plasma.

Most substances are not completely cleared from the plasma in one pass through the nephron. Instead, a percentage of the substance is actually removed from a given volume of plasma. The concept of clearance is helpful in comparing how much of one particular substance is removed by the kidney relative to another substance.

The clearance of creatinine or inulin may be used as a measure of GFR. These molecules are unique in that they are freely filtered across the glomerulus and are not reabsorbed. Inulin is an exogenous polysaccharide that must be given intravenously to the patient for a clearance to be determined. Inulin is not secreted by the tubules, so the amount of inulin that enters the tubules is the same as the amount excreted in the urine. For this reason, the clearance of inulin is equal to the GFR.

To spare the patient the invasive administration of inulin, most practitioners use creatinine clearance to measure GFR. Creatinine is an endogenous waste product released from muscle tissue. A tiny amount of creatinine is secreted into the tubules from the peritubular capillary blood. The creatinine clearance, therefore, slightly overestimates the GFR. The difference is so slight that in the clinical setting it is considered insignificant.

Transport of Specific Substances Throughout the Nephron

The processes of glomerular filtration, reabsorption, and secretion result in precise regulation of waste removal and conservation of water and other substances required for normal body functioning. Following is a description of how each section of the nephron specifically regulates key substances to accomplish this task.

PROXIMAL TUBULE. The proximal convoluted tubule is structurally designed for reabsorption . Its cells have a large surface area and a large number of mitochondria to supply cellular energy. About two-thirds of the glomerular filtrate is normally reabsorbed in this first section of the tubules. Of particular importance is the reabsorption of electrolytes, water, and substances of nutritional value. Secretion of a few metabolic end-products also occurs in the proximal tubule.

REABSORPTION OF ELECTROLYTES. Approximately 65% of the filtered sodium is actively reabsorbed in the proximal tubule. Figure 42–11 illustrates the processes involved in sodium reabsorption. Sodium moves by facilitated diffusion from the tubular fluid in the lumen of the proximal tubule, across the luminal membrane, and into the cytoplasm of the proximal tubule epithelial cell. Sodium movement occurs as a result of an electrochemical gradient for sodium. The inside of the proximal tubule epithelial cell is negatively charged in relation to the luminal fluid, and the concentration of sodium inside the cell is low. This electrochemical gradient for sodium movement into the cell is maintained by an active transport mechanism or "sodium pump" within the basolateral membrane of the proximal tubule epithelial cell. The sodium pump moves sodium from the interior of the cell into the interstitial fluid. As the concentration of sodium in the interstitial fluid increases, sodium moves by simple diffusion into the blood in the peritubular capillaries.

The reabsorption of several other substances is closely linked to the reabsorption of sodium in the proximal tubule. As large amounts of the positively charged sodium ions leave the tubular lumen, negatively charged ions must also leave to maintain electroneutrality. For example, bicarbonate ions are passively reabsorbed with the sodium ions in the first part of the proximal tubule. Chloride is the preferred ion to accompany diffusion of sodium in the latter portion of the proximal tubule. Sodium is the most abundant ion reabsorbed, and its movement creates a large osmotic gradient, resulting in the reabsorption of water. The reabsorption of other solutes also contributes to the osmotic gradient for water.

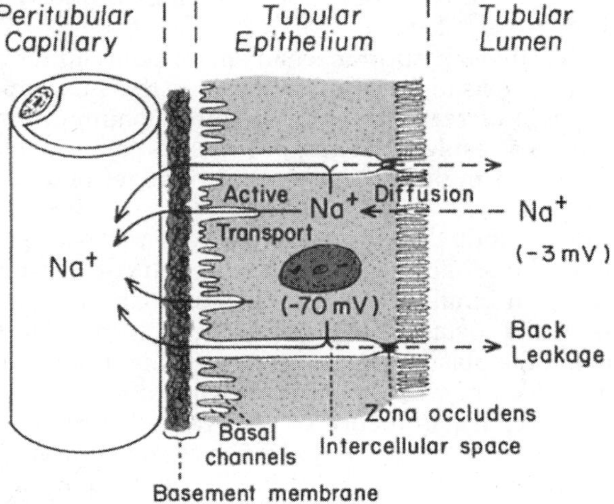

FIGURE 42–11. Mechanism for reabsorption of sodium from the tubular lumen into the peritubular capillary. (From Guyton, A. C. [1991]. *Textbook of medical physiology* [8th ed., p. 400]. Philadelphia: W. B. Saunders.)

Potassium reabsorption in the proximal tubule involves both active transport and diffusion. The concentration of potassium in the lumen of the proximal tubule is around 5 mEq/L. The potassium concentration inside the tubular cells is about 140 mEq/L. This large concentration gradient acts against passive reabsorption. The reabsorption of sodium, however, causes the inside of the tubular cell to become very negative, setting up an electrical gradient for potassium diffusion. In addition, an active transport mechanism is present to assist in moving potassium into the cell against its concentration gradient. Potassium is able to move passively down its concentration gradient from the inside of the cell into the peritubular capillary blood. Ultimately, 65% of the filtered potassium is reabsorbed from the proximal tubule.

Less is known about how the nephron handles calcium and phosphate. A large amount of the filtered calcium is actively reabsorbed from the proximal tubule. Phosphate is also actively reabsorbed under the principles of tubular transport maximum. If the serum phosphate level is low, virtually all filtered phosphate is reabsorbed. As serum phosphorus rises, increasing amounts of phosphate fail to be reabsorbed and are excreted in the urine. The tubular transport maximum for phosphate is under the influence of parathyroid hormone. The presence of this hormone decreases the transport maximum for phosphate, resulting in increased excretion into the urine.

REABSORPTION OF NUTRIENTS. A number of substances are so important for maintenance of nutritional balance in the body that little, if any, of these substances are allowed to leave the proximal tubule. Glucose, amino acids, proteins, vitamins, and acetoacetate ions are all actively reabsorbed (Guyton, 1991). Glucose reabsorption operates by a transport maximum system as previously described. Protein molecules are too large to cross the cell membrane by the usual means and thus are transported into the cell by the process of pinocytosis. First, the protein molecule attaches itself to the cell wall of the tubular epithelial cell. The cell wall then forms a pocket around the protein molecule, which eventually is pinched off into the interior of the cell. Once inside the cell, the protein molecules are broken down into their component amino acids, which are then reabsorbed by diffusion.

REABSORPTION AND SECRETION OF WASTE PRODUCTS. Substances that are considered to be body wastes are either secreted, not reabsorbed, or only partially reabsorbed by the proximal tubule. For example, creatinine is not reabsorbed at all, and only 50% of filtered urea is reabsorbed. Reabsorption of waste substances is regulated by the permeability of the tubular membrane. Hydrogen ion is secreted by the proximal tubule. This process will be discussed in detail later when the kidney's role in maintenance of acid-base balance is addressed.

EFFECT OF DIURETICS ON THE PROXIMAL TUBULE. Osmotic diuretics, such as mannitol, exert their effect primarily in the proximal tubule because that is where most of the water is reabsorbed. Mannitol is a monosaccharide that is freely filtered at the glomerulus and is not reabsorbed by the tubules. The presence of mannitol in the proximal tubule contributes to an osmotic gradient, decreasing the amount of water reabsorbed. The water, held in the tubules by the mannitol, passes into the more distal portions of the tubules and is excreted, thus increasing the urine volume.

LOOP OF HENLE. The loop of Henle also reabsorbs substances from the tubular fluid. Its configuration, cell structures, and management of sodium and water reabsorbtion function to cause a buildup of solutes within the interstitial fluid of the medulla, decreasing the solute concentration of the fluid moving into the distal tubule. This function is essential to the kidney's ability to control the volume and concentration of the urine.

The amount of sodium and water reabsorbed varies greatly from section to section of the loop of Henle. In the descending portion of the thin segment, the membrane is highly permeable to water and moderately permeable to sodium and other ions. Movement of sodium and water in this portion of the loop occurs primarily by diffusion. The cell membrane in the ascending portion of the thin segment is much less permeable to water but remains permeable to solutes. Finally, in the thick portion of the ascending limb sodium is actively transported out of the tubular lumen into the interstitial fluid. The membrane here is almost completely impermeable to water. Because water cannot move along with sodium and other solutes, the fluid leaving the loop is quite diluted.

Potassium is reabsorbed from the loop of Henle. Potassium is actively transported from the thick portion of the ascending limb. Approximately 25% of the filtered potassium is reabsorbed from the loop, allowing only about 10% of the original tubular load of potassium to enter the distal tubule.

Furosemide and bumetanide belong to a class of diuretics known as the "loop diuretics." Their site of action is the thick segment of the ascending limb of the loop of Henle. These diuretics work by blocking sodium reabsorption. As a result, the sodium concentration of the fluid leaving the loop increases. The increased sodium content holds water in the distal tubule and collecting duct, increasing the volume of urine excreted.

DISTAL TUBULE. Fine-tuning of the final urine product occurs in the distal tubule. The concentration of sodium, potassium, calcium, urea, and other substances continues to be altered by reabsorption and secretion. Whereas the fluid leaving the proximal tubule is isotonic at 300 mOsm/L, the fluid leaving the distal tubule may vary between 100 and 300 mOsm/L, depending on the permeability of the tubule to water.

REABSORPTION OF ELECTROLYTES. Sodium is actively reabsorbed throughout the length of the distal tubule. The transport process here is similar to that in the proximal tubule. A major difference is that the transport mechanism for sodium in the distal tubule is under the influence of aldosterone. When aldosterone is present in large amounts, virtually all of the sodium entering the distal tubule is reabsorbed. The final urine normally contains less than 1% of the filtered sodium. If aldosterone is not present, a much smaller amount of sodium will be reabsorbed, resulting in the loss of large amounts into the urine. The exact mechanism by which aldosterone alters the sodium transport process is not known. It is believed that aldosterone either increases the amount of available carrier protein or increases the concentration of a particular enzyme, thus increasing the rate of sodium reabsorption (Guyton, 1991).

Another difference between the proximal tubule and the distal tubule is that sodium reabsorption in the distal tubule is coupled with potassium secretion. Potassium diffuses into the distal tubular cell down an electrical gradient and then diffuses into the tubular lumen down a concentration gradient. Control of potassium secretion is influenced by aldosterone, the plasma potassium concentration, and the amount of sodium that enters the distal tubule. The presence of aldosterone increases potassium secretion by increasing the electrical gradient for potassium diffusion. Potassium secretion is also increased by an elevation of the plasma potassium concentration above normal. The higher plasma potassium concentration creates a wider concentration gradient between the peritubular fluid and the tubular lumen, thus increasing diffusion. Finally, if the amount of sodium entering the distal tubule increases, as occurs after administration of a loop diuretic, sodium reabsorption and potassium secretion also increase.

An active transport mechanism for potassium reabsorption exists in the distal tubule, and this mechanism is capable of reabsorbing all of the remaining potassium. As a result, excretion of excess potassium is dependent on the mechanisms that regulate potassium secretion.

Only about 10% of the filtered calcium reaches the distal tubule. When the plasma calcium concentration is within normal limits, little calcium reabsorption occurs in the distal tubule, and calcium is lost into the urine. If the plasma calcium concentration is low, most of the calcium will be reabsorbed from the distal tubule under the influence of parathyroid hormone. A low plasma calcium concentration is the stimulus for parathyroid hormone release. This hormone stimulates calcium reabsorption from the bone as well as from the distal tubule, leading to correction of the low plasma calcium concentration.

WATER REABSORPTION. Water reabsorption from the distal tubule depends on the presence of ADH. ADH is produced in the supraoptic and paraventricular nuclei of the hypothalamus and is released from the posterior pituitary (Vander, 1991). The two primary stimuli for ADH production and release are a fall in blood pressure that is sensed by the baroreceptors, particularly in the left atrium, and an increase in serum osmolality, sensed by the osmoreceptors located in the hypothalamus and liver. ADH production and release is inhibited by an increase in blood pressure, a decrease in serum osmolality, or the presence of alcohol (Vander, 1991).

When ADH is absent, the distal tubular cell membranes are impermeable to water. Water remains in the distal tubule, so the fluid entering the collecting duct will be dilute. In the presence of ADH, the distal tubular cell membrane becomes more permeable to water. ADH is thought to cause pores within the cell wall to open, allowing water to move with sodium as it is actively reabsorbed. Movement of water equalizes the concentration gradient between the tubular lumen and the peritubular capillary blood.

SECRETION OF WASTE PRODUCTS. Wastes and substances foreign to the body are secreted by the distal tubule and are not reabsorbed from the tubular fluid. As water is reabsorbed from the distal tubule, the concentration of these substances in the tubular fluid increases.

CONNECTING TUBULE AND COLLECTING DUCT. The collecting duct epithelium functions like the distal tubule in the handling of sodium, potassium, water, and wastes. Sodium is actively reabsorbed under the influence of aldosterone. Potassium continues to be secreted, although potassium reabsorption may occur if potassium intake is reduced. It is in the collecting duct that the final volume and concentration of urine are determined. Water reabsorption is dependent on the presence of ADH. As the collecting duct descends through the medulla, the solute concentration of the surrounding interstitial fluid continuously increases. In the presence of ADH, the collecting duct becomes permeable to water. Significant amounts of water may be reabsorbed due to the large concentration gradient. ADH also makes the membrane of the collecting duct more permeable to urea, allowing urea to diffuse into the interstitial fluid of the medulla along with water.

IMPACT OF TUBULAR DAMAGE ON COMPOSITION OF THE EXTRACELLULAR FLUID. Disease processes, such as acute tubular necrosis, damage the tubules of the nephron. Tubular damage may impair the kidney's ability to reabsorb electrolytes, amino acids, and vitamins and to secrete body wastes. As a result, the plasma concentrations of these substances become altered and may eventually impair cellular function in organ systems and tissues.

Regulation of Urine Concentration and Volume

The various mechanisms for controlling urine volumes and concentration have already been described. When fluid intake increases and the extracellular fluid becomes more diluted, the kidney must be able to excrete the excess water without depleting sodium or other solutes. Conversely, when fluid intake is limited, the kidneys must be able to rid the body of waste products while conserving water. Under ordinary circumstances, the kidney manages this by matching urine output closely to fluid intake minus fluid loss from other sources and by varying urine concentration within a range of 70 to 1400 mOsm/L (Guyton, 1991). This section will discuss the integration of the various mechanisms controlling urine volume and concentration. Clinical problems that affect this important renal function will also be addressed.

ANATOMIC AND PHYSIOLOGIC FEATURES CONTRIBUTING TO CONTROL OF URINE CONCENTRATION AND VOLUME. As previously described in the section on renal anatomy, the loops of Henle in the juxtamedullary nephrons are structurally quite different from those in the cortical nephrons. The specialized structure of the juxtamedullary nephrons is critical to the kidney's ability to concentrate the urine. The loops of Henle, distal convoluted tubules, and collecting ducts also play essential roles in the handling of sodium, water, and urea. A summary of water and solute handling is presented in Table 42–2. Table 42–3 outlines the differences between the fluid that filters into the tubules and the fluid that is ultimately excreted as urine.

COUNTERCURRENT MECHANISM. The term countercurrent mechanism refers to the interaction of the specialized anatomic and physiologic features of the loops of Henle in the juxtamedullary nephrons that result in the development of an interstitial fluid that becomes increasingly more concentrated with movement from the outer to the innermost regions of the medulla. An understanding of this mechanism's function in forming a concentrated interstitial fluid is fundamental to understanding how the kidney concentrates urine.

The process begins with entry of fluid from the proximal tubule into the loop of Henle, as seen in Figure 42–12. At this point, the tubular fluid has a concentration of 300 mOsm/L, the same as plasma. On the opposite side, the thick segment of the ascending limb

TABLE 42–2. **Water and Solute Handling by the Nephron**

Loop of Henle	
Descending limb	Very permeable to water and solutes
Thin segment of the ascending limb	Permeable to sodium and chloride Low water permeability
Thick segment of the ascending limb	Active absorption of sodium Impermeable to water and urea
Distal convoluted tubule	Active reabsorbtion of sodium Permeable to water when antidiuretic hormone (ADH) is present Impermeable to urea
Collecting duct	Active reabsorption of sodium Permeable to water and urea when ADH is present

TABLE 42–3. **Relative Concentrations of Substances in the Glomerular Filtrate and in the Urine**

	Glomerular Filtrate (125 mL/min)		Urine (1 mL/min)		Conc. Urine/Conc. Plasma (Plasma clearance/min)
	Quantity/min	*Concentration*	*Quantity/min*	*Concentration*	
Na^+	17.7 mEq	142 mEq/L	0.128 mEq	128 mEq/L	0.9
K^+	0.63	5	0.06	60	12
Ca^{2+}	0.5	4	0.0048	4.8	1.2
Mg^{2+}	0.38	3	0.015	15	5.0
Cl^-	12.9	103	0.134	134	1.3
HCO_3^-	3.5	28	0.014	14	0.5
$H_2PO_4^-$	0.25				
HPO_4^{2-}		2	0.05	50	25
SO_4^{2-}	0.09	0.7	0.033	33	47
Glucose	125 mg	100 mg/dL	0 mg	0 mg/dL	0.0
Urea	33	26	18.2	1820	70
Uric acid	3.8	3	0.42	42	14
Creatinine	1.4	1.1	1.96	196	140
Inulin	—	—	—	—	125
Diodrast	—	—	—	—	560
PAH	—	—	—	—	585

From Guyton, A. C. (1991). *Textbook of medical physiology* (8th ed., p. 407). Philadelphia: W. B. Saunders.

of the loop of Henle actively transports sodium from the tubular lumen into the interstitial fluid. Because the ascending limb is impermeable to water, water cannot follow the sodium into the interstitial fluid.

Consequently, the concentration of the interstitial fluid increases. As a concentration gradient develops between the fluid in the descending limb and the interstitial fluid, water begins to move out of the descending limb and solute diffuses into the descending limb until an equilibrium is reached. As a result, the fluid within the descending limb becomes more concentrated.

Sodium and urea also help to raise the concentration of the interstitial fluid as they are reabsorbed from the collecting duct. The addition of these solutes to the interstitial fluid pulls additional water out of the descending limb, further concentrating the fluid in this part of the tubule. The tubular fluid flows down toward the tip of the loop of Henle, carrying the solutes with it. As the fluid rounds the bend and enters the ascending limb, the transport mechanisms there remove sodium, adding it to the solute accumulating in the interstitial fluid. Solute is constantly being added to the interstitial fluid by the ascending limb and the collecting duct. Therefore, solute becomes concentrated in the interstitial fluid of the medulla. The concentration becomes highest in the deepest regions of the medulla as solute is carried there by the loops of Henle and vasa recta, potentially reaching a concentration of about 1400 mOsm/L.

The tubules of the loop of Henle have the capacity to maintain a concentration difference of up to 200 mOsm/L between the fluid in the ascending and descending limbs. Thus, the distal segment of the ascending limb can reduce the concentration of the tubular fluid to as little as 100 mOsm/L.

EXCRETION OF A DILUTED URINE. When the extracellular fluid becomes hypotonic, secretion of ADH is inhibited. Without ADH, the distal tubules and collecting ducts of the kidney become impermeable to water. Sodium continues to be removed from the tubular fluid and as water cannot follow it, the diluted fluid entering the distal tubule becomes even more diluted as it passes through the collecting duct. The concentration may decrease from 100 mOsm/L at the start of the distal tubule down to 70 mOsm/L in the collecting duct. The end result is the excretion of a large volume of diluted urine.

EXCRETION OF A CONCENTRATED URINE. When body fluids become hypertonic, the normal kidney con-

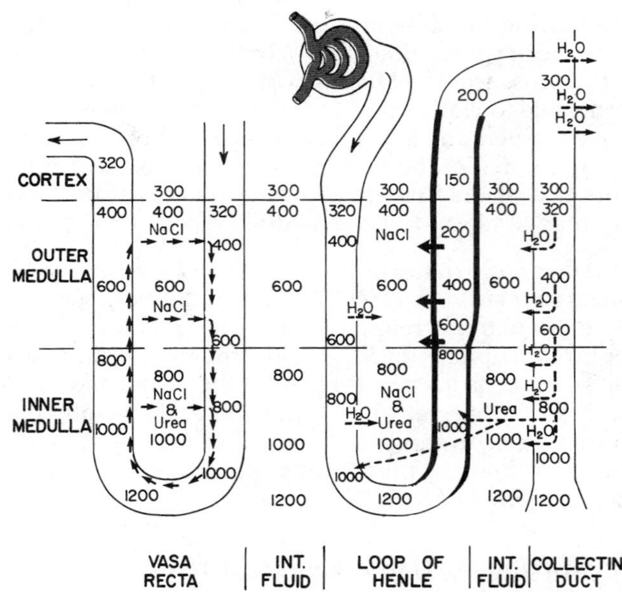

FIGURE 42–12. The countercurrent mechanism for concentrating the urine. (Numerical values are in milliosmoles per liter.) (From Guyton, A. C. [1991]. *Textbook of medical physiology* [8th ed., p. 415]. Philadelphia: W. B. Saunders.)

serves water. At the same time, the kidney must be able to excrete the end-products of metabolism. Increased osmolality of the extracellular fluid stimulates ADH secretion. The presence of ADH increases the permeability of the distal tubule and collecting duct to water. Water can leave the relatively diluted fluid inside the collecting duct to move into the concentrated interstitial fluid of the medulla. If a very large amount of ADH is present, the urine concentration may equilibrate with the concentration of the interstitial fluid, potentially reaching 1400 mOsm/L. The end result is the excretion of a small volume of very concentrated urine.

The amount of ADH secreted determines the permeability of the collecting duct to water, the amount of water reabsorbed from the collecting duct, and therefore the final volume and concentration of the urine. If the urine is maximally concentrated to 1400 mOsm/L, a urine volume of at least 500 mL is required to excrete the waste solutes produced in a 24-hour period (Robertson & Tomas, 1991). If the urine volume is less than 500 mL/24 hr, or if the urine volume is low and the urine cannot be maximally concentrated, waste products will begin to accumulate in the blood.

CLINICAL PROBLEMS AFFECTING URINE CONCENTRATION AND VOLUME. Disease states or drug therapy used to treat illness may alter urine volume and concentration. A common example is diabetes mellitus. As blood glucose levels rise, the amount of glucose being filtered also increases. When the tubular load of glucose exceeds the transport maximum, some glucose fails to be reabsorbed and passes into the urine. The increase in urinary glucose molecules creates an increased osmotic pull, holding water in the tubule and increasing urine output.

Diabetes insipidus can also affect the volume and concentration of the urine. Diabetes insipidus is caused by either the insufficient production of ADH or the kidney's inability to respond to ADH. In either case the distal tubule and collecting duct remain relatively impermeable to water, resulting in significant loss of water as urine. Conversely, when excessive amounts of ADH are present, water is maximally reabsorbed from the distal tubule and collecting duct, and a small volume of concentrated urine is excreted. This may occur in a condition known as the syndrome of inappropriate antidiuretic hormone secretion. Administration of exogenous ADH (vasopressin) for therapeutic reasons may also result in excessive concentration of urine.

Acute or chronic renal failure impairs the kidney's ability to regulate urine volume and concentration. Both forms of renal failure result in a fall in GFR. Many disease processes also damage the tubules, impairing tubular function and the ability to concentrate the urine.

The use of diuretics to treat fluid overload results in a common clinical situation affecting urine volume and concentration. Administration of any of the major categories of diuretics results in an increased excretion of sodium. Table 42–4 describes the mechanisms by which the various categories of diuretics inhibit sodium reabsorption. With a higher sodium concentration in the tubules, water will remain in the tubules, and urine output will increase.

Renal Regulation of Acid-Base Balance

OVERVIEW OF ACID-BASE BALANCE REGULATION. Acid substances are constantly being produced as a consequence of cellular metabolism. These acids must be removed from the body if a stable pH is to be maintained. Two physiologic mechanisms are in place to accomplish this: pulmonary excretion and renal excretion.

Cellular metabolism produces large amounts of carbon dioxide (CO_2). Carbon dioxide leads to the production of acid when it combines with water in the

TABLE 42–4. **Mechanism of Action of the Major Classes of Diuretics**

Class of Diuretic	Representative Drugs	Mechanism of Action
Loop diuretics	Furosemide (Lasix) Bumetanide (Bumex) Ethacrynic acid (Edecrin)	Inhibits sodium reabsorption in the thick segment of the loop of Henle
Thiazide diuretics and thiazidelike diuretics	Hydrochlorothiazide (Hydrodiuril, Esidrix) Metolazone (Diulo, Zaroxolyn)	Inhibit sodium reabsorption in the proximal and early distal tubules
Osmotic diuretics	Mannitol (Osmitrol)	Increase osmolality of the tubular fluid leading to decreased reabsorption of sodium and water
Potassium-sparing diuretics	Spironolactone (Aldactone) Triamterene (Dyazide, Dyrenium, Maxzide)	Aldosterone antagonist Blocks the sodium-potassium exchange mechanism in the distal tubule
Carbonic anhydrase inhibitors	Acetazolamide (Diamox)	Blocks the action of carbonic anhydrase in the proximal tubule, preventing bicarbonate and sodium reabsorption

following reaction:

$$CO_2 + H_2O \rightleftarrows \underset{\text{(carbonic acid)}}{H_2CO_3} \rightleftarrows \underset{\text{(hydrogen ion)}}{H^+} + \underset{\text{(bicarbonate)}}{HCO_3^-}$$

This reaction is reversed as blood passes through the lungs. CO_2 is excreted through the lungs, so normally there is no net gain of H^+.

Cellular metabolism also results in the production of acid substances not amenable to pulmonary excretion known as "nonvolatile acids." Examples of nonvolatile acids are sulfuric, phosphoric, and lactic acids. These substances release a hydrogen ion as they dissociate. Nonvolatile acids can be excreted only by the kidneys (Cogan & Rector, 1991). The kidneys have two functions in regulating acid-base balance. First, hydrogen ions are secreted by the epithelial cells of the kidney tubules and excreted in the urine. Second, the kidneys help to maintain a normal HCO_3^- concentration by reabsorbing filtered bicarbonate ions and forming bicarbonate inside the epithelial cells of the tubules.

Bicarbonate functions as a major buffering mechanism in the body. It combines with H^+ to prevent acidosis through the following reaction:

$$HCO_3^- + H^+ \rightleftarrows H_2CO_3 \rightleftarrows CO_2 + H_2O$$

The CO_2 produced by this reaction is either excreted through the lungs or used to form a bicarbonate ion inside the epithelial cells of the kidney tubules. This latter mechanism will be described later.

REGENERATION OF BICARBONATE BY THE TUBULAR EPITHELIAL CELLS. The processes responsible for renal secretion of H^+ and conservation of HCO_3^- are complex and intertwined. These processes are illustrated in Figure 42–13. Hydrogen ion secretion and regeneration of bicarbonate ion begin with the buildup of CO_2 inside the tubular epithelial cell. Carbon dioxide is either formed by the cell's own metabolic processes or diffuses into the cell from the tubular lumen or peritubular capillary blood. As the CO_2 concentration rises, the rate of H^+ secretion and HCO_3^- formation also increase.

Inside the cell, CO_2 combines with water to form H_2CO_3 under the influence of the enzyme carbonic anhydrase. Carbonic acid then dissociates into H^+ and HCO_3^-. The hydrogen ions are secreted into the tubular lumen. The bicarbonate ions combine with sodium and diffuse out of the cell into the extracellular fluid. In this way, bicarbonate ions, which were used somewhere in the body to buffer hydrogen ions, are reformed and replenished in the extracellular fluid.

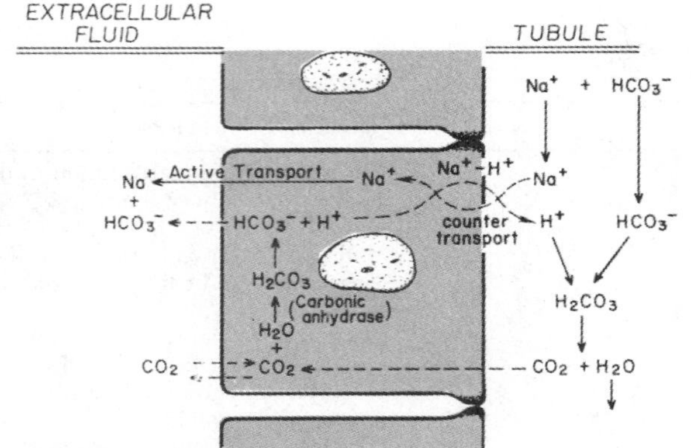

FIGURE 42–13. Chemical reactions for (1) hydrogen ion secretion, (2) sodium ion absorption in exchange for a hydrogen ion, (3) combination of hydrogen ions with bicarbonate ions in the tubules. (From Guyton, A. C., and Hall, J. E. [1996]. *Textbook of medical physiology* [9th ed.]. Philadelphia: W. B. Saunders.)

HYDROGEN ION SECRETION. Secretion of H^+ occurs primarily in the proximal tubule and to a lesser extent in the thick segment of the ascending limb of the loop of Henle, the distal tubule, and the collecting duct. H^+ secretion is linked to the reabsorption of sodium. Sodium combines with a carrier protein in the cell wall and is carried from the lumen of the tubule into the interior of the epithelial cell. Simultaneously, H^+ from the inside of the cell combines with the other side of the carrier protein. As sodium diffuses into the cell, the carrier protein rotates, carrying the hydrogen ion from the inside of the cell and releasing it into the tubular lumen. The energy provided to the carrier protein by sodium diffusion allows the tubules to move hydrogen ion against its concentration gradient. Secretion may continue until the pH reaches approximately 6.8 in the proximal tubule, 6.0 to 6.5 in the ascending limb of the loop of Henle and the distal tubule, and 4.5 in the collecting duct (Guyton, 1991).

REABSORPTION OF FILTERED BICARBONATE. Inside the tubular lumen much of the secreted hydrogen ion again combines with bicarbonate. A small but significant amount of H^+ combines with other tubular buffers. The HCO_3^- in the tubular fluid originates from filtration of sodium bicarbonate from the glomerular capillary blood. As sodium is actively reabsorbed from the tubular fluid, bicarbonate is left behind. If bicarbonate did not combine with hydrogen ion, it would be lost into the urine because the epithelial cells of the tubules are generally not permeable to it. The combination of HCO_3^- and H^+ forms H_2CO_3, which quickly dissociates into carbon dioxide and water under the influence of carbonic anhydrase. The carbon dioxide diffuses rapidly out of the tubule into the epithelial cell. From there, carbon dioxide may diffuse into the blood in the peritubular capillaries to be transported to the lungs. Carbon dioxide may also remain in the epithelial cell to combine with water, ultimately resulting in the reformation of a bicarbonate ion. In essence, this process results in the reabsorption of bicarbonate ions even though they cannot be reabsorbed directly across the tubular membrane. Approximately 80% of the filtered bicarbonate is reabsorbed from the proximal tubule.

TUBULAR BUFFERS. The number of hydrogen ions secreted into the tubular lumen is greater than the number of bicarbonate ions being filtered. This leaves an excess of hydrogen ions in the tubular fluid. Because there are limits on how far the tubular fluid pH may fall, only a small portion of the daily H^+ production would be excreted in the urine if not for the presence of the tubular buffering systems. One method of removing a free hydrogen ion from the tubular fluid is to combine it with a weak acid. The two primary tubular buffers, phosphate and ammonia, combine with free hydrogen ions, allowing excretion of large amounts of H^+ while minimizing the fall in urine pH.

Acid phosphates (H_3PO_4), byproducts of cellular metabolism, are buffered by bicarbonate in the extracellular fluid . . . as illustrated below:

$$(2NaHCO_3) + (H_3PO_4) \rightarrow Na_2HPO_4 + 2CO_2 + 2H_2O$$

This process produces two CO_2 molecules and Na_2HPO_4, which is then filtered. The concentration of Na_2HPO_4 in the tubular fluid increases because the tubular membrane is relatively impermeable to it. It remains in the tubular lumen as water is reabsorbed. Within the tubule Na_2HPO_4 combines with H^+ in the following reaction:

$$Na_2HPO_4 + H^+ \rightarrow NaH_2PO_4 + Na^+$$

In this way, a free hydrogen ion is picked up to be excreted and a sodium ion is returned to the extracellular fluid (Fig. 42–14).

The other major tubular buffer is the ammonia buffer system. Ammonia (NH_3) is formed within the tubular cells of all portions of the tubules except the thin segment of the loop of Henle. It is produced by the metabolism of amino acids, particularly glutamine. Ammonia diffuses easily into the tubular lumen, where it combines with a free hydrogen ion to form ammonium (NH_4^+) (Fig. 42–15). Because the tubular membrane is much less permeable to ammonium than to ammonia, NH_4^+ is trapped within the tubular lumen. Ammonium then combines with chloride or another negative ion and is excreted.

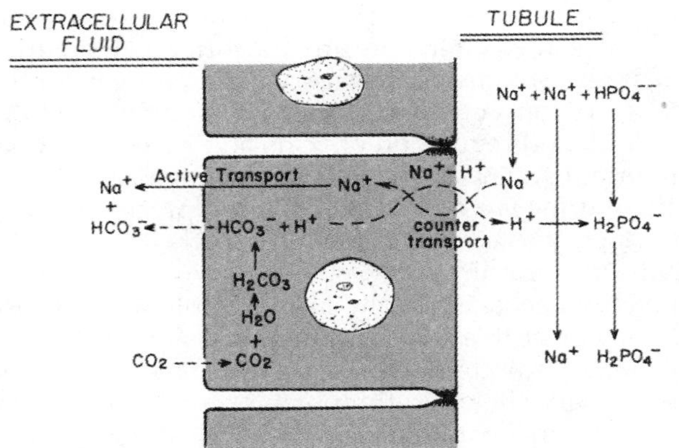

FIGURE 42–14. Chemical reactions in the tubules involving hydrogen ions, bicarbonate ions, sodium ions, and the phosphate buffer system. (From Guyton, A. C. [1991]. *Textbook of medical physiology* [8th ed., p. 446]. Philadelphia: W. B. Saunders.)

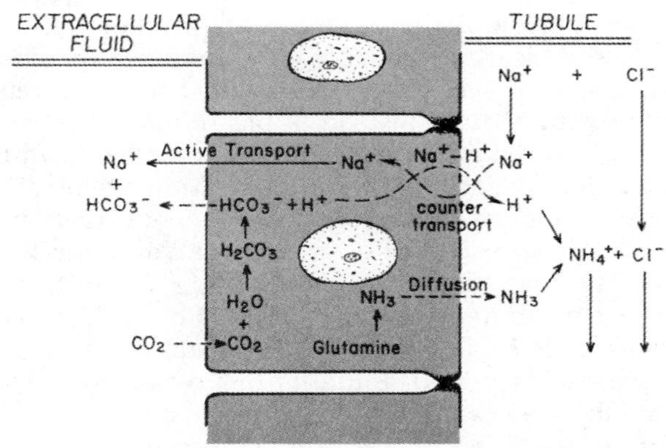

FIGURE 42–15. Secretion of ammonia by the tubular epithelial cells and reaction of the ammonia with hydrogen ions in the tubules. (From Guyton, A. C. [1991]. *Textbook of medical physiology* [8th ed., p. 447]. Philadelphia: W. B. Saunders.)

RENAL RESPONSE TO ACID-BASE IMBALANCE. When acids and bases are in balance in the body, the ratio of the amount of H^+ to the amount of HCO_3^- remains constant. In a state of acidosis H^+ is increased in proportion to HCO_3^-. In response to acidosis, the kidneys increase their secretion of H^+. Increased H^+ secretion by the tubules helps to restore acid-base balance by (1) ensuring reabsorption of all filtered bicarbonate ions, (2) adding large amounts of bicarbonate to the blood via the process of bicarbonate regeneration, and (3) increasing excretion of hydrogen ion.

In a state of alkalosis, the ratio of bicarbonate to hydrogen ion increases. The kidney responds to alkalosis by decreasing H^+ secretion. As a result, insufficient hydrogen ions are available to combine with filtered bicarbonate for reabsorption. Bicarbonate is lost into the urine, and the proportion of bicarbonate to hydrogen ion is brought back into range.

CLINICAL PROBLEMS RESULTING IN ALTERED RENAL HANDLING OF HYDROGEN AND BICARBONATE IONS. The normal renal processes for maintenance of acid-base balance may be impaired by either a defect in the tubular epithelial cells or by some other factor that impairs their ability to conserve bicarbonate and secrete hydrogen ion. Both metabolic acidosis and alkalosis may be the result of alterations in renal handling of hydrogen or bicarbonate ions. Examples of conditions leading to metabolic acidosis include proximal and distal renal tubular acidosis, renal failure, and carbonic anhydrase inhibition. Conditions known to cause metabolic alkalosis include administration of most diuretics and hyperreninemic hyperaldosteronemia.

Proximal renal tubular acidosis is a defect of the epithelial cells that impairs HCO_3^- recovery from the tubular fluid. The problem may be a defect in the carrier protein located on the luminal surface of the epithelial cell that transports Na^+ and H^+. It may also be caused by impaired carbonic anhydrase supply or function. In either case, bicarbonate cannot be reabsorbed and is lost in the urine. Because 80% of HCO_3^-

reabsorption normally occurs in the proximal tubule, this loss of bicarbonate eventually leads to acidosis. In addition, serum chloride levels rise as chloride is reabsorbed with sodium instead of bicarbonate.

In distal renal tubular acidosis the deficit is an inability to move H^+ into the tubular lumen against its concentration gradient. This prevents net excretion of H^+ as well as reabsorption of the small amount of bicarbonate that enters the distal tubule. Both of these factors contribute to the development of acidosis. Hypokalemia is also associated with distal renal tubular acidosis as increased amounts of potassium are secreted by the distal tubule to maintain electroneutrality in the face of decreased H^+ secretion.

Metabolic acidosis is often a component of renal failure. The major defect in renal failure is an inability to produce adequate amounts of ammonia. Without ammonia available as a buffer, the amount of H^+ that can be secreted is significantly reduced. The decreased GFR associated with renal failure also contributes to acidosis because a smaller amount of nonvolatile acids can be filtered and excreted.

The administration of carbonic anhydrase inhibitors may promote the development of metabolic acidosis. Acetazolamide is a commonly used carbonic anhydrase inhibitor. This drug inhibits carbonic anhydrase on the luminal surface of the epithelial cells in the proximal tubule. As a result, carbonic acid formed in the tubular lumen cannot dissociate into carbon dioxide and water, and the indirect mechanism for the reabsorption of filtered bicarbonate cannot occur.

Administration of diuretics may lead to the onset of metabolic alkalosis. Osmotic, thiazide, and loop diuretics all promote increased flow of fluid and decreased sodium reabsorption. Consequently, the sodium load arriving at the distal tubule is greatly increased. As the distal tubule attempts to reabsorb this large amount of positive sodium ions, hydrogen ion is secreted into the tubules in large amounts to maintain electroneutrality. This increase in hydrogen ion loss eventually leads to metabolic alkalosis.

Alkalosis may also result from conditions that cause increased renin secretion, such as renal artery stenosis. Renin initiates a series of reactions that culminate in angiotensin II formation. Angiotensin II then triggers secretion of aldosterone, which directly stimulates the distal tubule and collecting duct to secrete increased amounts of hydrogen ion (Vander, 1991).

Hormonal Function of the Kidney

Though it is not considered an endocrine organ, the kidney does participate in the formation of erythropoietin and in the metabolism of vitamin D, two systemic hormones. Although these functions are not necessary for survival, the kidney is essentially the only place in the body where they occur. Loss of these hormone functions may lead to significant problems for the individual.

Erythropoietin is believed to be produced by the epithelial cells of the proximal tubule and endothelial cells of the peritubular capillaries. Up to 90% of the erythropoietin produced in the body is contributed by the kidney. The stimulus for erythropoietin production and release is tissue hypoxia. Erythropoietin acts on the bone marrow to accelerate the production and release of red blood cells. Maximal erythropoietin production can increase red blood cell production up to 50 times the normal rate (Guyton, 1991). When erythropoietin production is diminished, few red blood cells are formed. Erythropoietin deficiency is one of the principal causes of the anemia seen in renal failure.

The kidney performs an important step in the formation of an active metabolite of vitamin D. It is this active metabolite that acts as a hormone within the body. Under normal circumstances, humans have two sources of inactive vitamin D: vitamin D_3, which is formed by the skin after exposure to ultraviolet light, and vitamin D_2, which is absorbed from ingested food. Both forms have identical biologic activity and are known together as vitamin D. Both forms of the vitamin are stored in the liver, where the initial conversion to 25-hydroxycholecalciferol (25-OHD_3) takes place. This substance is then converted by the mitochondria of the proximal tubular cells to 1,25-dihydroxycholecalciferol (1,25-$(OH)_2D_3$), known as calcitriol. Calcitriol is the active metabolite of vitamin D. Calcitriol stimulates calcium and phosphorus absorption from the gastrointestinal tract and is of critical importance to mineralization of newly formed bone. Individuals whose kidneys are unable to participate in vitamin D metabolism are at risk for hypocalcemia, secondary hyperparathyroidism, and osteomalacia.

SUMMARY

This chapter reviews the anatomic structure and major physiologic functions of the kidney as well as the close relationship between structure and function in this organ. The kidney's primary function is to maintain stability in the composition and volume of the extracellular fluid. This is accomplished through complex processes that culminate in the formation of urine. Each step—glomerular filtration, tubular reabsorption and secretion, concentration and dilution of the tubular fluid, and regulation of acids and bases—plays an important and necessary role in forming urine. The resulting urine is a fluid that eliminates precise amounts of water, waste, and excess electrolytes. Loss of the ability to form urine, which is responsive to changes in bodily needs, is usually incompatible with life. Replacement of this function by dialysis or renal transplantation is necessary for survival. The kidney is also the primary site of erythropoietin production and the final step in vitamin D metabolism. Although these two functions are not necessary for survival, they are required for maintenance of well-being. Integration of these complex functions allows the kidney to play a significant role in maintaining a relatively constant extracellular environment in which cells throughout the body can function normally.

REFERENCES

Ballerman, B. J., Zeidel, M. L., Gunning, M. E., Brenner, B. M. (1991). Vasoactive peptides and the kidney. In B. M. Brenner & F. C. Rector (Eds.), *The kidney* (4th ed., pp. 510–583). Philadelphia: W. B. Saunders.

Cogan, M. G., & Rector, F. C. (1991). Acid-base disorders. In B. M. Brenner & F. C. Rector (Eds.), *The kidney* (4th ed., pp. 737–804). Philadelphia: W. B. Saunders.

Divorkin, L. D., & Brenner, B. M. (1991). The renal circulations. In B. M. Brenner & F. C. Rector (Eds.), *The kidney* (4th ed., pp. 164–204). Philadelphia: W. B. Saunders.

Guyton, A. C. (1991). *Textbook of medical physiology* (8th ed.). Philadelphia: W. B. Saunders.

Kriz, W., & Kaissling, B. (1992). Structural organization of the mammalian kidney. In D. W. Seldin & G. Giebisch (Eds.), *The kidney: physiology and pathophysiology* (2nd ed., pp. 707–777). New York: Raven Press.

Mene, P., & Dunn, M. J. (1992). Vascular, glomerular, and tubular effects of angiotensin II, kinins and prostaglandins. In D. W. Seldin & G. Giebisch (Eds.), *The kidney: physiology and pathophysiology* (2nd ed., pp. 1205–1248). New York: Raven Press.

Navar, L. G., Carmines, P. K., & Paul, R. V. (1989). Renal circulation. In S. G. Massry & R. J. Glassock (Eds.), *Textbook of nephrology* (2nd ed., pp. 43–53). Baltimore: Williams & Wilkins.

Robertson, G. L., & Tomas, B. (1991). Pathophysiology of water metabolism. In B. M. Brenner & F. C. Rector (Eds.), *The kidney* (4th ed., pp. 677–736). Philadelphia: W. B. Saunders.

Tisher, C. C., & Madsen, K. M. (1991). Anatomy of the kidney. In B. M. Brenner & F. C. Rector (Eds.), *The kidney* (4th ed., pp. 3–75). Philadelphia: W. B. Saunders.

Vander, A. J. (1991). *Renal physiology* (4th ed.). New York: McGraw-Hill.

Patients With Fluid and Electrolyte Disturbances

Leanna R. Miller

The kidney provides a myriad of important functions necessary for the maintenance of the body's internal environment. Among these functions is regulation of the physicochemical milieu that supports cellular processes. This chapter deals with problems of fluid volume and composition associated with disease states or trauma frequently seen in the critical care setting. For a detailed discussion of renal regulation of electrolytes, the reader is referred to Chapter 42.

BODY FLUID COMPARTMENTS

Approximately 55% to 60% of the body is composed of water. This solution is crucial to the maintenance of life because essential solutes are dissolved or suspended in this medium. The total body water (TBW) is distributed in several discrete compartments or volumes. The intracellular (IC) fluid volume is the largest compartment, comprising 67% of TBW. IC fluid accounts for approximately 40% of body weight. The extracellular (EC) fluid volume is composed of several small compartments, including interstitial fluid and plasma volume. The vascular volume also contains erythrocytes, which contain a portion of the IC fluid volume. The combined EC fluid makes up approximately 20% of body weight. The smallest compartment is the transcellular volume, which consists of fluid found in the peritoneum and pleural cavities, gastrointestinal tract, joints, and cerebrospinal fluid. The body water compartments and proportional sizes are shown in Table 43–1. Adult males tend to have a TBW of approximately 60% because of a somewhat larger proportion of muscle mass. Adipose tissue contains less water. Thus, the average adult female has a TBW equal to about 50% of body weight, reflecting the gender predisposition to increased body fat. Infants and children up to the age of puberty also have higher values for TBW.

Intracellular water is separated from EC fluid by cell membranes. The plasma volume is confined to the vascular space by capillary membranes. These membranes selectively permit passage of solutes between compartments through a variety of active and passive mechanisms. The cell membranes are freely permeable to water. Thus, body water is distributed in the various anatomic compartments to achieve osmotic equilibrium throughout the total body water.

The cation and anion composition of the respective compartments is shown in Figure 43–1. Sodium salts are the primary osmotically active constituent of the EC fluid. The concentration of sodium in the interstitial subcompartment of EC fluid will be somewhat lower than the plasma concentration due to the effect of the Donnan equilibrium (Guyton, 1991). Because plasma proteins are negatively charged ions, a larger number of positively charged ions are required to achieve electrochemical balance. Concentrations of sodium (Na) and chloride (Cl) may differ in these two subcompartments because of the associated difference in protein concentrations.

The major electrolyte of the IC fluid is potassium (K), which is actively retained within the compartment by energy-consuming sodium–potassium pumps found in the cell walls. These pumps remove sodium from cells in exchange for potassium from the EC fluid. In this way, sodium remains in EC fluid while potassium is confined to IC fluid. Other low-molecular-weight solutes (such as urea and glucose) can be con-

TABLE 43–1. **Body Compartment Volumes**

Plasma volume (liters)	= 4.5% body weight (kg)
Interstitial fluid volume (liters)	= 13% body weight (kg)
Extracellular fluid volume (liters)	= 17.5% body weight (kg)
Intracellular fluid volume (liters)	= 33% body weight (kg)

Total body water (TBW) (liters)
Males, thin females, chronically ill patients—normal hydration:
TBW = 55% to 60% body weight (kg)
Obese patients, normal females—normal hydration:
TBW = 47% to 52% body weight (kg)

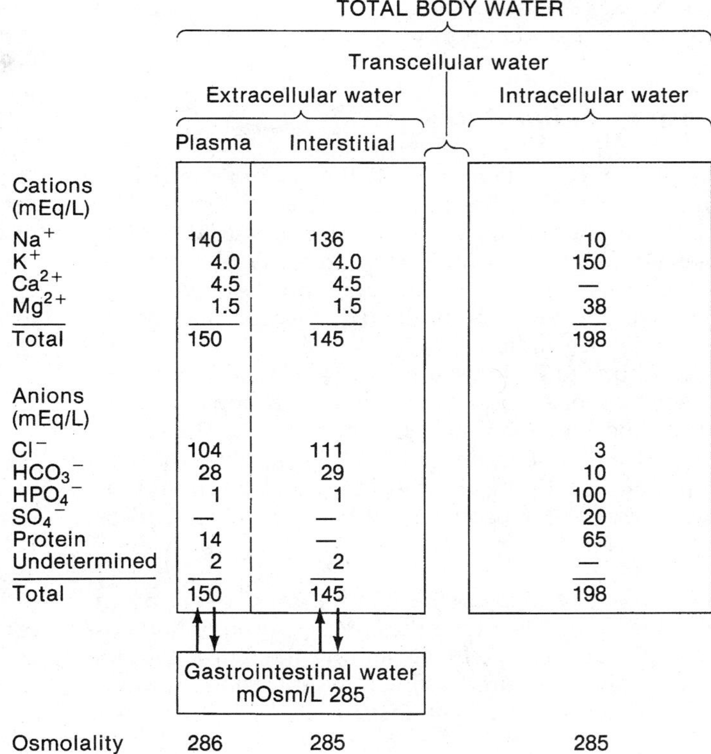

TOTAL BODY WATER
Transcellular water
Extracellular water
Intracellular water
Plasma
Interstitial
Cations (mEq/L)
Na+ 140 136 10
K+ 4.0 4.0 150
Ca2+ 4.5 4.5 —
Mg2+ 1.5 1.5 38
Total 150 145 198
Anions (mEq/L)
Cl− 104 111 3
HCO3− 28 29 10
HPO4− 1 1 100
SO4− — — 20
Protein 14 — 65
Undetermined 2 2 —
Total 150 145 198
Gastrointestinal water mOsm/L 285
Osmolality 286 285 285

FIGURE 43–1. Body water composition.

sidered freely diffusible between IC fluid and EC fluid. Other electrolytes, such as magnesium (Mg), are also osmotically active but exert a much smaller effective osmotic pressure in both the IC and EC compartments.

Exchange of Water Between Plasma and Interstitial Volumes

Water exchange between the plasma and interstitial volumes is dependent on three important pressure relationships. One is the hydraulic or hydrostatic pressure in the capillary. This pressure gradient normally tends to move water out of the capillary into the interstitial space. Opposing that outward flow of water is the capillary oncotic pressure exerted by plasma proteins. About 65% to 70% of this plasma protein oncotic pressure in plasma is due to albumin, with the rest provided by globulins (Guyton, 1991). The third pressure results from a slow albumin leak in the capillary wall, which accounts for a low concentration of protein in the interstitial fluid. The protein in the interstitial fluid exerts an oncotic pressure, which tends to pull water into the interstitial compartment. Under normal conditions of hydration, the net result is that most of the fluid leaving the plasma at the afferent end of the capillary is reabsorbed. However, the net filtration pressure allows a small amount of fluid and solutes to remain in the interstitial fluid. This small volume eventually is returned to the circulation through the lymphatic system.

Effective Arterial Volume

The theoretical concept of effective arterial volume (EAV) associated with circulation and tissue perfusion has important implications for fluid and electrolyte control in health and illness. The EAV is essentially the degree of fullness of the arterial vascular tree relative to its capacity. This volume is a balance between peripheral resistance and cardiac output. Normally, if cardiac output falls, there is a compensatory increase in peripheral resistance. However, there may be situations in which the arterial vascular capacity is abnormally increased such that cardiac output cannot compensate completely. In this situation, EAV will decrease, and there will be renal conservation of sodium and water to augment volume. Major effectors for controlling EAV include the sympathetic nervous system as well as the renin–angiotensin II response.

Sodium regulation is closely associated with maintenance of the EAV. In general, EAV varies as the EC volume varies, and both of these volumes vary with total body sodium. In some instances, EAV may not reflect EC volume or, more specifically, plasma volume. Pathologic sequestration of EC water in the interstitium because of decreased plasma oncotic pressure will produce an expanded interstitial volume but a depleted plasma volume. If cardiac output falls, EAV will be decreased. The kidney will attempt to alleviate this situation by conserving sodium. Water will also be retained but may be sequestered in the already expanded interstitial space. This situation produces a decreased EAV and plasma volume but a greatly expanded interstitial and EC volume.

Cation–Anion Balance

As illustrated in Figure 43–1, the sum of the plasma cations (150 mEq/liter) is balanced by the sum of the plasma anions (150 mEq/liter). Electroneutrality of the plasma is always maintained. Under normal circumstances, any increase or decrease in cation concentration will result in a similar increase or decrease in anion concentration.

Sodium and potassium are the major measured plasma cations, and chloride and bicarbonate are the major measured anions. Bicarbonate is estimated as $CO_2 - 1$ (Goldberger, 1986). Other anions not measured but exhibiting clinical significance in certain disease states are phosphates, sulfates, proteins, and organic acid ions.

ANION GAP. Measurement of the anion gap is a simple method of describing the concentration of unmeasured plasma anions. In calculating the anion gap, the sum of the measured anions is subtracted from the sum of the measured cations:

$$\text{Anion gap} = (\text{Na} + \text{K}) - (\text{HCO}_3 + \text{Cl})$$

The resulting "gap" represents the unmeasured anions present in the plasma. Normally, the anion gap is 8 to 16 mEq/liter.

As described in Table 43–2, the anion gap may be increased or decreased in disease states that alter the unmeasured anions or unmeasured cations. Fluid volume disorders will also affect the anion gap by elevating or lowering plasma sodium. Metabolic acidosis is the most common cause of an increased anion gap in critically ill patients. The most frequent cause of decreased anion gap is hypoalbuminemia.

TABLE 43–2. **Mechanisms Affecting the Anion Gap**

Increased Anion Gap (>16 mEq/liter)	Decreased Anion Gap (<8 mEq/liter)
Increased unmeasured anion	Decreased unmeasured anion
Lactic acidosis	Hypoalbuminemia
Ketoacidosis	
Hyperosmolar coma	
Sodium penicillin	
Phosphate administration	
Sulfate administration	
Decreased unmeasured cation	Increased unmeasured cation
Hypocalcemia	Hypercalcemia
Hypomagnesemia	Hypermagnesemia
	IgG (multiple myeloma)
Water loss	Water excess
Hypernatremia	Hyponatremia
Metabolic alkalosis	

Calculation of the anion gap is clinically useful in differentiating between possible etiologies of metabolic acidosis. For example, the anion gap in patients with diabetic ketoacidosis is frequently greater than 22 mEq/liter. On the other hand, patients with metabolic acidosis resulting from excessive intestinal fluid losses will have a near normal anion gap. Measurement of the anion gap is also helpful in evaluating the efficacy of interventions. If the intervention is decreasing the production of anions, the anion gap will narrow and approach normal. However, if the intervention is ineffective, the anion gap will widen.

FLUID VOLUME AND OSMOLALITY

Distribution of body water follows osmotic pressure relationships within the EC and IC compartments. The terms osmolality and osmolarity often are used interchangeably although they are different. Osmolality is expressed as the number of osmoles per *kilogram* (kg) of *water,* whereas osmolarity refers to the number of osmoles per *liter* of *solution.* With dilute solutions, such as EC or IC fluids, the difference is negligible, and osmolality is the more common term employed. EC volume is determined by the total number of osmoles in the EC compartment. Therefore, EC volume regulation is accomplished through the regulation of EC osmoles. The IC volume generally is not manipulated directly but will change as a consequence of alterations in EC volume and osmolality. Because EC osmolality is equal to IC osmolality, the respective volumes will be dictated by the requirements of osmotic equilibrium. In a state of fluid and solute balance:

$$\text{Osmolality TBW} = \text{osmolality EC fluid} = \text{osmolality IC fluid}$$

Tonicity refers to the osmolality of a solution relative to another. If one solution has a higher osmolality than another, it is described as being hypertonic relative to the second solution. Solutions of the same osmolality are isotonic. A solution with a lower osmolality than a second solution is described as hypotonic.

If sodium is added to EC water, water will flow from the IC to the EC compartment to regain osmotic equilibrium between them. The outcome will be that osmolality will be increased in both compartments, with the EC volume expanded at the cost of a reduced IC volume. On the other hand, if pure water is removed from the EC compartment, the loss will be proportionally distributed between the two compartments. The result will be an increase in osmolality and a decrease in volume in both compartments.

Sodium salts are the primary osmoles in EC water, and therefore regulation of the EC volume involves regulation of Na retention or excretion by the kidney. The principle is that if sodium is retained or excreted, water will follow. Normally, EC volume is controlled through maintenance of the balance of Na intake and renal excretion.

TABLE 43–3. **Regulation of Renal Sodium Excretion**

Mechanism	Action
Afferent	
Baroreceptors Aorta and carotid sinus	Modifies peripheral and renal vascular resistance
Juxtaglomerular apparatus	Produces renin/angiotensin II Direct renal effect Aldosterone Sodium transport in kidney
Low pressure volume receptors	Prostaglandin production Antidiuretic hormone (ADH) secretion
Atrial natriuretic peptide	Vasodilation Natriuresis and diuresis Reduces plasma renin, aldosterone, ADH concentrations
Efferent	
Kidney Proximal tubule Loop of Henle Collecting tubule	Regulates sodium excretion/conservation
Prostaglandins	Renal hemodynamics Sodium excretion/conservation

The afferent and efferent mechanisms of renal Na excretion as well as their respective actions are shown in Table 43–3. No single afferent mechanism dominates this regulatory process. It is worth repeating that the body will protect volume at the expense of osmolality.

Volume Disorders

Volume disorders tend to be classified as either depletion (contraction) or expansion derangements. This refers to both EC and IC compartments, although direct measurement of these states is restricted to the EC compartment, specifically the vascular volume.

VOLUME DEPLETION

Volume depletion is a relatively common disturbance in critically ill patients, occurring when fluid losses exceed intake. The fluid loss must occur acutely and must be of significant magnitude to produce volume depletion. Otherwise, the normal mechanisms for conservation of volume would compensate for the decreased TBW. If left uncorrected, hypovolemia can lead to a variety of serious secondary effects such as shock, myocardial ischemia, acute tubular necrosis, and, depending on the composition of the fluid lost, electrolyte disorders and acid-base disturbances. The severity of symptomatic volume depletion reflects the proportion of volume lost from the EC compartment. An isotonic volume loss of 10% of body weight is considered serious, whereas a loss of 15% may be lethal.

The composition of the fluid lost will have a significant effect on TBW composition after volume depletion. A categorical approach to volume depletion is shown in Table 43–4, and the designation reflects the osmolality of the TBW following acute depletion. The losses come directly from the EC fluid. However, as discussed earlier, compartment volumes are dic-

TABLE 43–4. **Categorization and Laboratory Values in Extracellular Volume Depletion**

	Laboratory Values					
	Urine		*Blood*			
Etiology	*Sodium*	*Osmolality*	*Sodium*	*BUN/Creatinine Ratio*	*Plasma Protein*	*Hematocrit*
Isoosmotic	Decreased	Increased	Unchanged	Increased	Increased	Increased
Solute and water lost in equal proportion Gastrointestinal losses Hemorrhage Third spacing Burns						
Hypoosmotic	Increased	Decreased	Decreased	Increased	Increased	Increased
Solute loss greater than water loss Aldosterone deficiency Diuretic therapy with water replacement Increased insensible loss with water replacement Salt-wasting renal disease Osmotic diuresis						
Hyperosmotic	Increased	Increased	Increased	Increased	Increased	Increased
Water loss greater than solute loss No water or no access to water Increased insensible loss with no replacement Untreated diabetes insipidus						

tated by osmotic equilibrium requirements, so there may well be a secondary effect on IC volume. All disorders will be associated with some depletion of EC volume and thus hypovolemia. However, laboratory and clinical findings associated with each of these volume disturbances will vary. The variability of the composition of these fluids can produce a spectrum of metabolic disturbances when fluid is lost from the body in excessive amounts. Gastrointestinal losses, depending on their origin and composition, may also induce acid-base disturbances. Vomiting and diarrhea will be associated with significant acid loss, with metabolic alkalosis as a possible consequence. Conversely, intestinal, biliary, and pancreatic fluids are alkaline, and large losses of these fluids may be associated with metabolic acidosis. With severe volume depletion, the kidney will conserve sodium bicarbonate even though acid-base status is normal because of the need for sodium and thus volume. As a result, a contraction alkalosis may be present. Chloride and potassium disorders can also occur in conjunction with volume depletion.

The laboratory findings common to EC volume contraction states are shown in Table 43–4. Under the influence of aldosterone, the renal tubule will increase the reabsorption of sodium and water in response to dehydration. This will result in a decreased urine Na level. Urine Na values are often misleading in patients with salt-wasting renal disease, osmotic diuresis, and those who have been treated with diuretics. In renal failure, urinary osmolality (uOsm) may be less than 350 mOsm/kg because of the renal concentrating defect associated with renal disease.

Normal blood urea nitrogen (BUN) and creatinine ratios should be approximately 10:1. This value may be elevated in hypovolemia because of decreased glomerular filtration resulting in elevated BUN values. The ratio is sometimes as high as 40:1 under these circumstances.

Plasma sodium will be variably affected depending on the type of volume depletion. In isoosmotic losses, plasma sodium will probably be unchanged. However, volume depletion will stimulate thirst and antidiuretic hormone (ADH) secretion, so that dilutional hyponatremia may be observed with isotonic contraction. Hypoosmotic contraction, when solute loss exceeds water loss, will generally exhibit a decreased plasma Na level. In hyperosmotic contraction, water is lost in excess of solute, and this may be reflected in hypernatremia.

Potassium may be increased or decreased depending on the etiology of volume loss. Acidosis is associated with increased serum K concentrations due to electroneutrality requirements as hydrogen ion (H^+) moves from the EC into the IC compartment.

Plasma protein and hematocrit values are frequently elevated when hypovolemia is present, reflecting hemoconcentration. These laboratory findings should be evaluated relative to baseline values.

MANAGEMENT OF VOLUME DEPLETION. Both the volume and composition of replacement solutions will depend on the composition and estimated volume deficit. For replacement of a pure water deficit of a hyperosmotic contraction without significant solute loss, fluid replacement can be estimated as follows:

$$\text{Amount of water required (liters)} = \text{weight loss (kg)}$$

Fluid replacement can be given as 5% dextrose in water if only free water is desired, or isotonically if serum sodium is normal (Carroll & Oh, 1989).

For many critically ill patients, both water and sodium are needed to correct volume depletion. For hypoosmotic contraction, isotonic or hypertonic saline solutions are used. The solution chosen depends on the degree of Na deficit and on volume considerations. Normal saline (0.9% sodium chloride) contains approximately 154 mEq/liter of sodium, whereas hypertonic saline contains approximately 513 mEq/liter. The amount of sodium replacement needed can be estimated by the following formula:

$$\begin{aligned}\text{Na required (mEq)} = {} & [(\text{normal PNa} - \text{current PNa}) \\ & \times \text{TBW (liters)}] + [(\text{normal PNa}) \\ & \times \text{weight loss (liters)}]\end{aligned}$$

The amount of water replacement in liters is equal to the weight loss in kilograms.

Depending on the value obtained from this equation, the clinician could prescribe an isotonic solution if renal function is adequate and no significant heart disease is present, or a mix of isotonic and hypertonic solutions. It is also important to consider K stores as well as acid-base status when choosing the appropriate solutions for restoring volume. Common replacement fluids used for critically ill patients and their indications and precautions are shown in Table 43–5.

All patients must receive maintenance fluid. In the critical care setting this usually is accomplished intravenously. This regimen provides for insensible water losses and for water consumed through normal metabolism and tissue maintenance. Maintenance fluid therapy must replace any abnormal ongoing fluid losses such as diarrhea, vomiting, sweating, drainage for open wounds, burns, and abnormally high urine output. The amount of maintenance fluid is estimated by the following formula: 100 mL/kg/24 hr for the first 10 kg of body weight, 50 mL/kg/24 hr for the next 10 kg, and 20 mL/kg/24 hr for each additional kilogram of body weight.

The rate of fluid replacement will be a function of the current or continuing deficit and the type of solution being used. The risk of volume overload from rapid administration of isotonic or hypertonic solutions must be minimized. Rapid addition of sodium to EC fluid can produce a rapid influx of water into the vascular space, overwhelming marginal cardiac function in the critically ill patient.

TABLE 43–5. **Characteristics of Replacement Fluids**

Solution	Composition	pH	Osmolarity	Indications	Precautions
Dextrose in water	5% (5 g dextrose in each 100 mL) 10% (10 g dextrose in each 100 mL)	3.5 to 6.5	5%: 252 mOsm/liter* 10%: 595 mOsm/liter	5%: Hypernatremia as hypotonic replacement fluid Vehicle for many intravenous drug infusions Keep-vein-open solution for sodium-sensitive patients (cardiac, renal) 10%: Hypoglycemia Weaning from total parenteral nutrition	Not appropriate for volume resuscitation Not appropriate as maintenance IV solution Not compatible with blood transfusions (causes hemolysis) Not appropriate for use in patients with increased brain edema
0.2% sodium chloride (1/4-strength saline)	34 mEq Na^+/liter 34 mEq Cl^-/liter 2000 mg NaCl/liter	4.0	67 mOsm/liter	(Usually with dextrose) Treatment of hypernatremia Maintenance IV solution	Not appropriate for rapid volume resuscitation Can lead to hyponatremia
0.45% sodium chloride (1/2-strength saline)	77 mEq Na^+/liter 77 mEq Cl^-/liter 4500 mg NaCl/liter	4.0	150 mOsm/liter	(With or without dextrose) Maintenance IV therapy Hypernatremia	Not appropriate for rapid volume resuscitation Can lead to hyponatremia
0.9% sodium chloride (normal saline)	154 mEq Na^+/liter 154 mEq Cl^-/liter 9000 mg NaCl/liter	5.0	300 mOsm/liter	(Without dextrose) Rapid volume resuscitation Companion solution for blood transfusions Hyponatremia	Not appropriate as maintenance IV solution Can lead to hyperchloremic acidosis
3.0% sodium chloride (hypertonic saline)	513 mEq Na^+/liter 513 mEq Cl^-/liter 30,000 mg NaCl/liter	5.0	1027 mOsm/liter	Correction of severe hyponatremia (sodium < 120 mEq/liter) Hypertonic burn resuscitation Possible benefit in hemorrhagic/septic shock	Do not correct too rapidly (central pontine demyelinolysis) Can lead to hypernatremia Phlebitis
Lactated Ringer's	3 mEq Ca^{2+}/liter 109 mEq Cl^-/liter 28 mEq lactate/liter 4 mEq K^+/liter 130 mEq Na^+/liter	6.5	273 mOsm/liter	Preferred crystalloid resuscitation fluid for rapid intravascular volume expansion May be used as maintenance IV fluid	Not compatible with blood transfusion (causes clotting) Contains potassium, so use with care in renal failure or hyperkalemia Lactate may accumulate in liver failure
Plasmalyte A	3 mEq Mg^{2+}/liter 103 mEq Cl^-/liter 27 mEq acetate/liter 23 mEq gluconate/liter 10 mEq K^+/liter 140 mEq Na^+/liter	7.4	294 mOsm/liter	May be used as maintenance IV fluid Isotonic solution with electrolyte similar to plasma with higher K^+ level Sometimes used to replace intestinal fluid losses	Not compatible with blood transfusion (causes clotting) Contains magnesium, so use with care in renal failure or hypermagnesemia

*Dextrose is rapidly metabolized when administered IV and readily becomes a hypotonic solution.

FLUID VOLUME DEFICIT. Extracellular fluid volume depletion or contraction is frequently seen in critically ill patients. The goals of nursing care are to identify any fluid volume deficit and restore and support the patient's fluid balance.

Clinical manifestations of EC volume depletion may vary depending on the type of volume contraction present. Therefore, it is important for the critical care nurse to carefully assess all aspects of the patient's fluid volume status. Patients with significant volume depletion frequently complain of thirst and dry mouth. Unfortunately, the intubated, elderly, or comatose patient loses this ability, so early volume depletion may go unnoticed. Reduced skin turgor has long been purported to be a hallmark of volume depletion. However, normal skin turgor does not rule out a hypovolemic state. In fact, changes in skin turgor may not appear until late in the volume depletion process. Assessments of the patient's tongue and mucous membranes provide a more reliable indication of the volume status.

Urine output is a sensitive indicator of fluid volume status. Hourly urine volumes are measured, and downward trends are noted and reported. Bedside serial specific gravity measurements may be indicative of the increasing urinary concentration seen in hypovolemia. Accurate daily weights provide the most valuable estimate of TBW loss. Weight loss, as determined by daily weights, is utilized by the physician in calculating fluid replacement.

Hemodynamic parameters provide objective measures of volume depletion. Documentation of hypotension should always be considered relative to baseline blood pressure reference values. Tachycardia is frequently present. Postural hypotension may be observed along with dizziness or syncope on assuming a sitting or erect position.

Central venous pressure (CVP) can be a useful parameter in the assessment of volume status, even without sophisticated monitoring technology. Visual inspection of the external jugular vein just above the clavicle with the patient supine and the neck muscles relaxed can provide useful information. If the external jugular is flat when the patient is supine, the patient is volume depleted. If the fluid wave can be seen in the external jugular vein when the patient is upright, the CVP is approximately 10 cm H_2O. Assessment of the CVP and jugular venous distension is valid in the absence of right or left heart failure. Left ventricular filling pressures, as measured by pulmonary artery wedge pressure, and cardiac output will fall below baseline in patients with hypovolemia.

Although notoriously inaccurate, intake and output records may provide a useful estimate of the balance between fluid lost and fluid gained. The nurse carefully monitors the patient's intake and output for trends indicative of excessive fluid loss or inadequate fluid replacement.

If the patient is at risk of volume depletion, the nurse ensures the availability of intravenous lines. Prescribed infusions are carefully monitored, and the patient's response is closely observed and evaluated.

VOLUME EXPANSION

The kidney normally responds to an increase in Na intake by a compensatory increase in renal Na excretion. This process blunts the change in EC volume that might be associated with the increased Na intake. In some pathophysiologic states, this remarkable balance breaks down, with the immediate consequence of retention of ingested or infused sodium and water. If uncorrected, the increase in vascular volume as well as associated increase in capillary permeability to water leads to accumulation of fluid in the interstitial space and the formation of edema.

The fundamental problem in volume expansion states is that sodium and water are not being excreted. There are two possible reasons why sodium is retained. One is that abnormal kidney function may lead to inappropriately diminished Na excretion in the presence of increased Na intake. The other is that the kidney is responding appropriately to erroneous stimuli indicating that EC volume is contracted. This response is the mechanism that results in the sodium and water retention observed in congestive heart failure (CHF). The classification and clinical features of EC volume expansion are described in Table 43–6.

The interstitial volume is about 75% of that in the EC compartment. As described earlier, movement of fluid into the interstitial space in the capillary bed is influenced by opposing capillary and oncotic pressures. Changes in the hydrostatic pressure before or after the capillary will influence the movement of fluid out of the capillary (Guyton, 1991). Precapillary constriction reduces hydrostatic pressure within the capillary and thus reduces water flux. In contrast, postcapillary vasoconstriction produces increased pressure within the capillary and thus increases water movement into the interstitial space. In hypoalbuminemic states, plasma oncotic pressure is decreased, which also favors movement of fluid out of the capillary. If

TABLE 43–6. **Extracellular Volume Expansion**

Primary Renal Salt Retention	
Cause	Abnormal kidney function
Features	Extracellular and effective arterial volume increased
Associated findings	Hypertension Reduced sympathetic nervous system activity Decreased levels of renin, antidiuretic hormone, aldosterone
Secondary Renal Salt Retention	
Cause	Kidney responds to decreased extracellular volume stimuli
Features	Extracellular volume increased Effective arterial volume decreased
Associated findings	Low blood pressure Increased sympathetic nervous system activity Increased levels of renin, antidiuretic hormone, aldosterone

capillary permeability to plasma protein is increased, migration of these proteins into the interstitium will also encourage water to move (Casley-Smith, 1993; Guyton, 1991).

In normal circumstances, once plasma fluid has entered the interstitial space it eventually returns to the vascular space through the lymphatic system. In clinical conditions in which lymph drainage is obstructed, the normal route of interstitial water return is lost. If lymph obstruction remains uncorrected, edema will result.

Edema may not be evident until interstitial volume is 30% greater than normal (Guyton, 1991). Obviously, if this process is localized, a smaller volume will produce demonstrable edema. Pitting edema is usually not seen until 3 to 4 liters have entered the interstitium from the plasma (Carroll & Oh, 1989). When a significant amount of fluid has left the vascular space, the plasma volume becomes decreased and the kidney begins to conserve sodium and water to restore volume even though the total EC volume is expanded.

In summary, edema occurs through the three primary mechanisms described earlier: (1) increased hydrostatic pressure in the capillary, (2) decreased plasma oncotic pressure, and (3) lymph system obstruction. With the first two mechanisms, the vascular volume decreases and compensatory renal conservation of sodium and water occurs. This renal maneuver attempts to restore the vascular volume to normal despite the accumulation of fluid in the interstitial space, and the EC volume expands. This edema-producing mechanism is seen in disease states such as CHF, cirrhosis, and nephrotic syndrome.

Prostaglandins play a role in Na and water excretion and retention. Prostaglandins are fatty acid compounds whose production by the kidney depends on the availability of arachadonic acids and phospholipase. Prostaglandins are elevated in volume depletion states and decreased in volume expansion conditions, indicating a counterregulatory role in the primary processes of volume regulation. High levels of prostaglandins inhibit Na reabsorption in the kidney and thus counteract the direct effects of the renin–angiotensin II system in volume depletion.

Some drugs commonly used in the critical care environment, including peripheral vasodilators and some calcium channel blockers, also increase Na retention by the kidney. Nonsteroidal antiinflammatory drugs (NSAIDs) may encourage Na retention through their blocking action on prostaglandin synthesis. Estrogens and some synthetic mineralocorticoids also induce primary renal Na retention. The consequence of all these mechanisms of Na and water conservation is an expanded plasma volume and possible edema formation.

Physical findings associated with edema states generally reflect the underlying etiology of the disorder and thus the preferential location of edema formation.

Laboratory findings are not always specific to the underlying pathology. However, all these edema-forming disorders will be reflected in a decreased urine Na concentration, and, in some situations such as nephrotic syndrome, proteinuria may be pronounced. Primary renal Na retention may also produce proteinuria. Elevated BUN and serum creatinine values may be indicative of renal disease. Reduced serum protein values, specifically albumin, are seen in cirrhosis and nephrotic syndrome. Serum Na values are variable depending on the disorder and the degree of plasma volume expansion.

MANAGEMENT OF VOLUME EXPANSION. Pulmonary edema is a life-threatening event and must be treated promptly. Other edematous states require remedial action but are not considered imminently lethal. In fact, in some situations a measured approach to volume correction will avoid secondary complications resulting from treatment.

The goal of treatment should be to resolve the underlying pathology and correct volume status to the degree consistent with adequate tissue perfusion. The objective is to mobilize the expanded interstitial fluid volume without causing a significant reduction in plasma volume, particularly in patients with edema states in which decreased EAV exists. Further reduction in this hemodynamic parameter may potentially decrease cardiac function and tissue perfusion, thereby preventing further volume correction. Diuretics are generally useful in the treatment of edema states. However, volume depletion caused by the overuse of diuretics may induce an increase in renin, aldosterone, and ADH production, all of which will act to conserve sodium and water. An intravenous infusion of low-dose dopamine (<5 μg/kg) is frequently used to increase renal blood flow and enhance Na and water excretion.

Mobilization of interstitial fluid into the vascular volume occurs initially through the mechanism of decreased plasma volume through diuretic action, which decreases capillary hydrostatic pressure. The structure of the interstitial space is such that, normally, the pressure in that compartment is actually below zero. Therefore, there is a point beyond which interstitial fluid will not move, even if the volume is somewhat expanded. Patients with severe generalized edema may experience more rapid mobilization of fluid. Patients with hepatic disease and ascites will tend to have a slower rate of interstitial volume reduction because of the more localized deposition. Forced excretion of water through the use of diuretics may exceed the rate at which ascitic fluid can replace the plasma volume. In this situation, symptoms of volume depletion may be observed. These patients are also more prone to other electrolyte disorders when diuretics are used. To minimize this, an aldosterone-antagonist diuretic is generally used.

Sodium restriction, with or without concurrent administration of diuretics, is often applied successfully in edematous patients because it indirectly diminishes further water retention. In patients with chronic heart failure, the long-term use of diuretics combined with a low-sodium diet may prevent subsequent edema formation.

FLUID VOLUME EXCESS. A number of disease states may cause fluid volume expansion in critically ill patients. Nursing care is directed toward early recognition and prevention of fluid volume excess, monitoring, and evaluation of the patient's response to mobilization of fluid.

Nursing assessment of the patient with fluid volume overload includes identification of edema and the patient's response to changes in TBW. The patient's hemodynamic response to fluid volume overload is carefully monitored. Depending on the underlying cause of volume overload, the patient's blood pressure may be elevated or decreased. If plasma volume is increased, the CVP and pulmonary artery wedge pressure (PAWP) will be elevated. The jugular veins are assessed for distension.

The rate and quality of respirations are assessed. The presence of tachypnea may be indicative of evolving pulmonary edema. The lungs are auscultated for the presence of rales.

In performing a head-to-toe assessment, the nurse observes and documents the presence, location, and severity of peripheral edema. In patients at risk of sequestering fluid in the abdomen, abdominal girth is measured, and the presence or absence of a fluid wave is noted. Skin areas that may be gravitational sites for edema should be evaluated. In patients on bed rest, edema collects along the flanks, lateral chest, lateral abdominal wall, lateral buttocks, and posteromedial thighs. It appears later in the presacral area.

The patient is weighed daily, and changes in body weight are noted and calculated in terms of liters of fluid retained. When fluid restriction is prescribed, the nurse educates the patient and family about the rationale for the restriction. The fluid allotment is appropriately distributed across the 24-hour period to facilitate patient comfort. Fluid administration is individualized to meet the patient's specific needs. Intake and output records assist the nurse to ration fluids appropriately.

The critical care nurse administers the prescribed diuretics and monitors the patient's response. The adequacy of diuresis is assessed. The nurse monitors the patient's serum electrolytes and anticipates the development of hypokalemia following diuretic administration.

IMPAIRED SKIN INTEGRITY. Skin care is an important aspect of nursing care of the volume-overloaded patient. The skin in edematous areas is assessed frequently. Careful attention is paid to relieving pressure areas.

Osmolality Disorders

Plasma osmolality (pOsm) is maintained within narrow limits (280 to 300 mOsm/liter) by body mechanisms that act to conserve or excrete water. This important physiologic parameter is regulated by several integrated neurohormonal–renal mechanisms. The vascular volume is monitored by osmoreceptors and, because it is a subcompartment of the EC volume, is a surrogate for EC osmolality. Changes in the osmolality of the EC compartment have implications for water shifts between the EC and IC compartments.

Thirst is an important mechanism in maintaining plasma osmolality. The thirst mechanism may be brought into play by nonosmotic factors such as hypovolemia (isotonic depletion) or decreased cardiac output. The body will defend volume at the expense of osmolality, which may lead to a situation in which activated drinking occurs in the presence of normal or reduced plasma osmolality. Angiotensin II is thought to be a potent dipsogen, and therefore, clinical events that increase renin production may also increase thirst. To restore plasma osmolality, thirst must be accompanied by the ability of the individual to obtain water. Critically ill patients may lose either their ability to recognize the thirst sensation or their ability to obtain water or both.

Antidiuretic hormone is a second mechanism involved in the regulation of pOsm. Its synthesis and release are stimulated when EC osmolality is increased. This response is marked even when the increase in osmolality is only a 1% to 2% deviation from baseline. In addition to its effect on the renal collecting duct's permeability to water, ADH also plays a role in modulating peripheral vascular resistance and thus blood pressure. When EC fluid volume is lost, ADH and aldosterone secretion is increased regardless of the serum Na concentration. These hormones encourage the conservation of sodium and water. ADH release may also be stimulated by baroreceptor-perceived reduction in plasma volume as well as pain, stress, and drugs such as narcotics, nicotine, and tricyclic antidepressants. Factors stimulating or inhibiting ADH secretion are described in Table 43–7. Thus, as with thirst and drinking, these stimuli and the accompanying change in ADH secretion can cause a change in water excretion that is not indicated by osmolality alone. The action of ADH on the kidney results in the excretion of a small volume of concentrated urine. Enhanced aldosterone secretion results in renal conservation of available sodium. This provides an additional impetus for water conservation and thus volume repletion. Derangements in these important control mechanisms may produce serious perturbations in osmolality.

TABLE 43–7. **Factors Affecting ADH Secretion**

Factor	Effect on ADH Secretion
Hypovolemia	Increased
Low output cardiac failure	Increased
Hyperosmolality/hypernatremia	Increased
Narcotics	Increased
Nicotine	Increased
Tricyclic antidepressants	Increased
Pain	Increased
Stress	Increased
Hypoosmolality/hyponatremia	Decreased
Hypervolemia	Decreased
Excess ADH	Decreased

Osmolality of body water is closely correlated with serum sodium concentration because sodium is the most abundant EC ion. Plasma osmolality can be reasonably estimated by the following formula:

$$\text{Plasma osmolality} = 2(\text{plasma Na}) + \text{BUN}/2.8 + \text{glucose}/18$$

where sodium is measured in mEq/liter, BUN in mg/dL, and glucose in mg/dL. Because sodium is the major osmotically active ion, in the absence of hyperglycemia or renal insufficiency plasma osmolality can be reliably estimated using the following formula:

$$2(\text{plasma Na[mEq/liter]})$$

It is helpful to use the calculated plasma osmolality to explain the effect of various disease states on osmolality. The following examples illustrate the normal calculated pOsm, hyperosmolality caused by hyperglycemia and hypernatremia, and hypoosmolality caused by hyponatremia.

$$\text{Normal: } 2(140) + 12/2.8 + 100/18 = 290 \text{ mOsm/kg}$$

$$\text{Hyponatremia: } 2(130) + 12/2.8 + 100/18 = 270 \text{ mOsm/kg}$$

$$\text{Hyperglycemia: } 2(140) + 12/2.8 + 450/18 = 309 \text{ mOsm/kg}$$

$$\text{Hypernatremia: } 2(152) + 12/2.8 + 100/18 = 314 \text{ mOsm/kg}$$

The normal physiologic range for pOsm is 280 to 300 mOsm/kg H_2O. It should be noted that changes in the serum levels of urea and glucose do have an effect on the calculated pOsm. However, as demonstrated in the examples of calculated pOsm above, small changes in serum Na concentration have the most significant effect on plasma osmolality. Further discussion of osmolality in this chapter will focus on problems with osmolality associated with hyponatremia or hypernatremia.

HYPONATREMIA

Hyponatremia or hypoosmolality results from increased water loading or retention relative to plasma Na levels. The result is a decreased concentration of EC Na ions (<135 mEq/liter). The predominant change occurs in water content, not solute concentration. In this situation, thirst is inactivated, and inhibition of ADH occurs. The outcome of these responses is excretion of a large volume of dilute urine. In situations in which EC volume is severely compromised, the body will override these homeostatic functions to defend volume.

It has been suggested that hyponatremia is the most common electrolyte disorder seen in hospitalized patients. Body fluid losses are usually isotonic or slightly hypotonic. Hyponatremia occurs when the patient drinks or is given hypoosmotic solutions as a replacement for losses. To maintain a hypoosmotic state, there also must be a decreased ability to excrete dilute urine because of diminished reabsorption of sodium or increased reabsorption of water in the kidney. The clinical mechanisms associated with this disorder are shown in Table 43–8. In the critical care setting, hyponatremia is often associated with hypovolemic states in patients with CHF. It frequently results from diuretic therapy.

TABLE 43–8. **Mechanisms Contributing to Hyponatremia**

Mechanism	Effect
Reduced sodium intake	Impairs formation of dilute urine
Excessive free water intake (5% dextrose/water)	
Primary antidiuretic hormone excess (syndrome of inappropriate antidiuretic hormone)	Produces water retention, sodium excretion
Mixed disorders:	
Nonosmotic ADH release	Produces water retention, sodium excretion
Decreased urine sodium excretion	

Factitious hyponatremia and redistribution of water is seen in patients with hyperlipidemia or hyperproteinemia. The concentration is reported as the amount of sodium contained in a certain volume of plasma. When that volume of plasma contains protein or lipids, the amount of water in the sample is decreased. Redistribution of water occurs when a solute that cannot freely penetrate the cellular membrane is added to the EC fluid compartment. This causes an osmotic shift of fluid from the IC fluid compartment to the EC fluid compartment so that a new equilibrium is established. Serum osmolality can help determine whether redistribution of water is the cause of hyponatremia; with the addition of glucose or mannitol to the EC fluid compartment, serum osmolality will be greater than 300 mOsm/kg. Serum osmolality will generally be normal in cases of hyperlipidemia and hyperproteinemia (Sunyecz & Mirtallo, 1993).

Hypertonic hyponatremia, as shown in Figure 43–2, is the result of hyperglycemia or the administration of mannitol. In both situations, the EC compartment tonicity is elevated. In patients with hyperglycemia, glucose does not enter the cells because of the lack of insulin or insulin resistance. Therefore, glucose becomes an osmotically active substance. Mannitol also becomes an effective osmotic agent because it is confined to the EC compartment. Increased EC tonicity leads to a flow of water from the IC compartment to the EC compartment and dilution of plasma sodium. The net result of this osmotic activity is an expanded EC compartment and a contracted IC compartment.

Decreases in total body sodium and water result from nonrenal or renal losses of sodium and fluid. Causes include vomiting, diarrhea, or nasogastric suctioning; excessive loss through the skin due to burns or sweating; and translocation of fluid from vascular

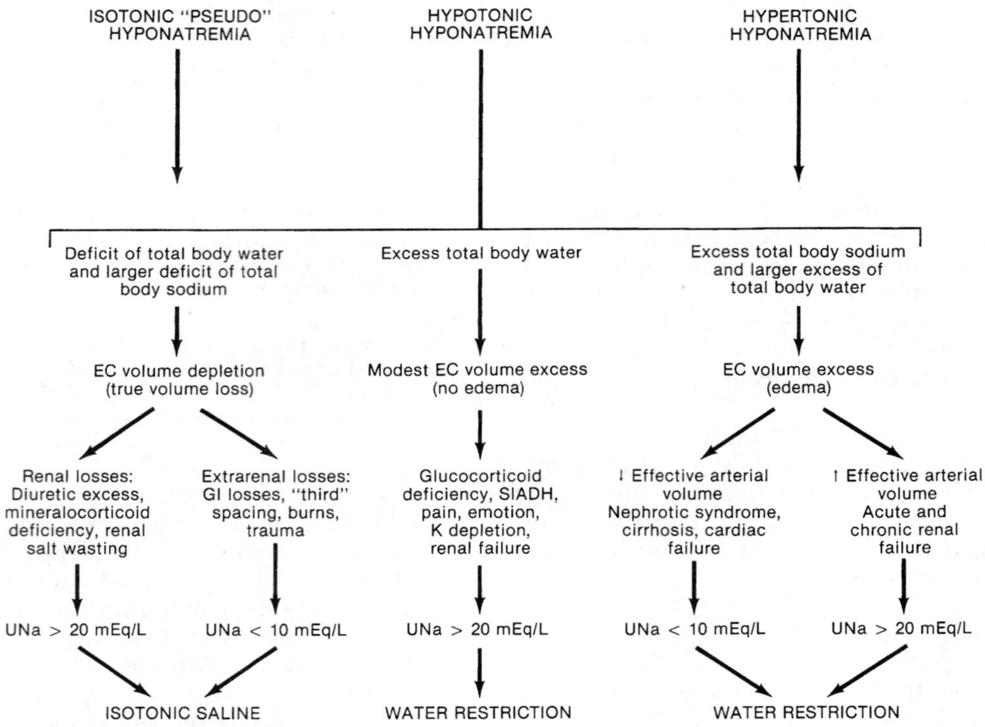

FIGURE 43–2. Clinical approach to patient with hyponatremia. *UNa,* urine sodium.

to interstitial compartments due to burns, pancreatitis, peritonitis, or muscle trauma. Intravascular volume is decreased, and less volume is presented to the kidneys. Causes of renal loss of sodium and fluids include use of diuretics and intrinsic renal disease where water and sodium are wasted. Diuretic use must be monitored closely, especially in elderly patients. Chronic renal disease, especially interstitial disease, can lead to impaired reabsorption of sodium, resulting in sodium wasting and hyponatremia. There is an intravascular fluid deficit due to loss, and the patient may appear dehydrated, exhibiting poor skin turgor, dry mucous membranes, tachycardia, and hypotension. With extrarenal loss leading to hyponatremia, the urine Na concentration generally will be less than 10 mEq/liter because the kidney is retaining sodium and fluid to help correct the intravascular depletion. With diuretic use or impaired kidney function, the urine Na concentration will be variable but in most cases will be greater than 20 mEq/liter.

Another mechanism in the development of hyponatremia occurs with no change in total body sodium with an increase in water. This occurs in the syndrome of inappropriate ADH (SIADH), which results in a large increase of free water reabsorption. The increase in effective arterial volume stimulates salt-excretion mechanisms. The kidneys try to excrete sodium and water, but water is reabsorbed. The urine Na concentration is usually high (>20 mEq/liter) and the urine osmolality is high (>700–800 mOsm/kg), whereas serum Na concentration and serum osmolality are low. Acute water intoxication generally occurs in patients with advanced renal failure due to a decrease in glomerular filtration rate (GFR) that limits the ability to excrete a water load. Occasionally persons with normal GFR can develop this syndrome, psychogenic polydipsia, and consume enough water to overcome the kidney's ability to excrete the water load and become hyponatremic (Sunyecz & Mirtallo, 1993). Causes of SIADH are shown in Table 43–9. The differential diagnosis between hyponatremia caused by

TABLE 43–9. **Causes of Syndrome of Inappropriate Antidiuretic Hormone (SIADH)**

CNS Disorders	**Drugs**
Tumors	Carbamazepine (Tegretol)
Infections	Morphine
Head trauma	Oxytocin
Hemorrhagic events	Thiazide diuretics
	Nicotine
Tumor Production of ADH	Isoproterenol (Isuprel)
Bronchogenic oat cell carcinoma	
Hodgkin's disease	**Miscellaneous**
Cancer of pancreas	Positive-pressure ventilation
Cancer of prostate	Mitral commissurotomy
Pulmonary Conditions (Nonmalignant)	
Tuberculosis	
Chronic obstructive pulmonary disease	
Pneumococcal and viral pneumonia	

SIADH and a modest decrease in serum Na concentration is that in the latter, sodium is conserved so that the urine Na concentration should be less than 10 to 15 mEq/liter. In contrast, in SIADH, the urine Na concentration will be high because of natriuresis.

Decrease in total body sodium with no change in water occurs when sodium is restricted or when there is chronic adrenocorticoid insufficiency. Adrenal insufficiency can lead to Na deficit because aldosterone production is decreased. Without aldosterone, sodium is lost in the urine in exchange for potassium. Adrenal insufficiency must be diagnosed by measuring hormone levels. Increase in total body sodium and water resulting in hyponatremia occurs in CHF, nephrotic syndrome, and cirrhosis. In patients with nephrotic syndrome or cirrhosis, losses of oncotic proteins (albumin) result in a fluid leak from the capillaries into the extravascular space. This results in a decrease in intravascular volume and a decrease in the volume presented to the kidneys. In CHF, the intravascular volume may actually be adequate or increased, but a poor cardiac output decreases the volume presented to the kidneys. The kidney responds as if it is hypoperfused with an increase in the reabsorption of sodium at the proximal tubule, an increase in ADH, and stimulation of the renin-angiotensin-aldosterone pathway. This leads to an increase in the amount of total body sodium and water, with a proportionally greater increase in water content. Diagnosis relies heavily on the clinical examination. Urine Na level will generally be less than 10 mEq/liter; however, the definitive diagnosis should not rely solely on this finding.

The hallmark of hyponatremia is that both pOsm and plasma sodium are reduced. Symptoms associated with this disorder are dependent on the age and sex of the patient as well as the severity and rate of reduction in pOsm and sodium. The primary symptoms are neurologic in origin and reflect the decreased pOsm that leads to IC volume expansion in the brain cells. The relative plasma Na concentrations and associated symptoms are described in Table 43–10. Symptoms related to hyponatremia tend to be more severe in young women (<50 years of age). In some elderly patients, slow salt depletion may occur as a consequence of chronic diuretic therapy and pure water ingestion, leading to a long-term depletion of brain solute. These patients may be less symptomatic until plasma sodium reaches significantly lower levels. Mortality seems to be correlated with symptomatic hyponatremia, which should be considered a medical emergency.

TABLE 43–10. **Clinical Manifestations of Acute Hyponatremia**

Plasma sodium 125 mEq/liter	Nausea, malaise, muscle cramps
Plasma sodium 110–120 mEq/liter	Headache, dizziness, lethargy, obtundation
Plasma sodium < 110 mEq/liter	Seizures, coma, respiratory arrest

MANAGEMENT OF HYPONATREMIA. Treatment of hyponatremia (hypoosmolality) depends on the level of plasma sodium as well as the total body fluid volume and Na status. In edema-forming states, water restriction may be the only therapy required. If hyponatremia is the result of diuretic therapy, the diuretic should be discontinued. Administration of normal amounts of sodium and potassium usually permit a rapid return toward normal osmolality following diuresis.

Symptomatic hypoosmolality must be treated expeditiously to prevent seizures and death. If the plasma Na level is less than 120 mEq/liter and the patient is symptomatic, hypertonic solutions of 3% or 5% saline may be administered intravenously. Hypertonic solutions are given at a rate that allows the serum Na level to increase by approximately 2 mEq/liter/hr.

Hyponatremia can be treated by using a 3% sodium chloride infusion combined with a diuretic to prevent fluid overload. Serum Na concentration should not be corrected by more than 25 mEq/liter in 48 hours, and it should never be increased to hypernatremic levels (Arieff & Ayus, 1991; Sunyecz & Mirtallo, 1993). It is best to correct severe symptomatic hyponatremia rapidly with hypertonic saline, but only partially, to within the range of 120–125 mEq/liter. The remainder of the correction should take place over several days. Central pontine myelinolysis occurs with rapid total correction (or overcorrection) of the serum Na concentration or when correction is associated with insults such as hypoxia/anoxia or hepatic coma (Ayus et al., 1987).

If the EAV is expanded, as in patients with SIADH, the infused sodium will be quickly excreted. To counteract natriuresis, intravenous furosemide may be administered during hypertonic infusion (Carroll & Oh, 1989). This will induce salt and water diuresis. In hyponatremic patients, some or most of the sodium will be retained while excess EC water will be excreted.

Stable, nonsymptomatic patients with SIADH may need only water restriction to restore fluid volume to normal. If water restriction alone is insufficient, an ADH-antagonizing medication, such as demeclocycline, may be administered.

POTENTIAL FOR INJURY. The patient with hyponatremia may experience alterations in central nervous system (CNS) function, including coma and seizures. Early detection of decreased plasma Na level and prevention of patient injury are important nursing goals.

Early hyponatremia is characterized by lethargy and malaise, followed by the development of nausea and vomiting. The nurse carefully assesses the patient's level of consciousness and level of response. The bedside environment is structured to prevent injury to the lethargic or somnolent patient. Suction or other equipment should be available to maintain airway patency in the vomiting patient.

Acute water-loading results in more severe CNS manifestations than a slowly developing hyponatremia. After acute water ingestion, the nurse closely monitors the patient's plasma Na levels. The need for administration of hypertonic saline solutions should be anticipated. Seizure precautions are initiated because the patient is at high risk of convulsions.

HYPERNATREMIA

Hyperosmolality of the EC water is commonly the result of hypernatremia (Na > 145 mEq/liter). The etiology of hypernatremia is either increased water loss in proportion to solute loss or solute gain in excess of water gain. The most common reasons for clinically significant hypernatremia include three pathogenic mechanisms: (1) impaired thirst or decreased access to water, (2) solute or osmotic diuresis, and (3) excessive renal or extrarenal losses of water. Generally, hypernatremia cannot occur in the presence of a normal thirst mechanism and an ability or opportunity to satisfy that sensation. However, the critically ill patient is at risk of developing hypernatremia due to impaired recognition of thirst and an inability to obtain or drink water.

Mortality rate in adults with severe hypernatremia has been reported to be in excess of 75% (Moder & Daniel, 1990). Hypernatremia may occur with volume depletion or expansion or with isovolemia. There have been few cases of survival in adults with severe acute hypernatremia. Factors affecting the survival are the initial serum Na concentration, underlying conditions, the age of the patient, and coexisting infections (Elisaf et al., 1989). The severity of the neurologic dysfunction appears to be related to the rate of the development of the hypernatremia and not the absolute plasma Na concentration. Use of hypotonic dialysis can be used to reverse the hypernatremia. Rapid hydration is associated with worsening of the neurologic status, and seizures often result from cerebral edema. It is suggested that no more than 2 mOsm should be corrected per hour.

The type of volume disorders resulting in hypernatremia are shown in Figure 43–3. These categories reflect the tonicity of fluid lost or gained by the patient relative to EC osmolality. As can be seen, the volume and tonicity changes will affect urine Na losses as well as total body sodium in different ways.

One type of hypernatremia results from no change in total body sodium with a decrease in water from renal or nonrenal losses of free water. Nonrenal losses include evaporation from the respiratory tract or skin in patients with fever or thyrotoxicosis, or in burn patients on air-fluidized beds. Diabetes insipidus, which is the usual cause of renal free-water loss, is due to failure to secrete adequate amounts of ADH (central diabetes insipidus) or failure of the distal tubule to respond appropriately to the hormone (nephrogenic diabetes insipidus). Diabetes insipidus from various causes can lead to severe hypernatremia and permanent brain damage (Vin-Christian & Arieff, 1993).

Causes of central diabetes insipidus include head

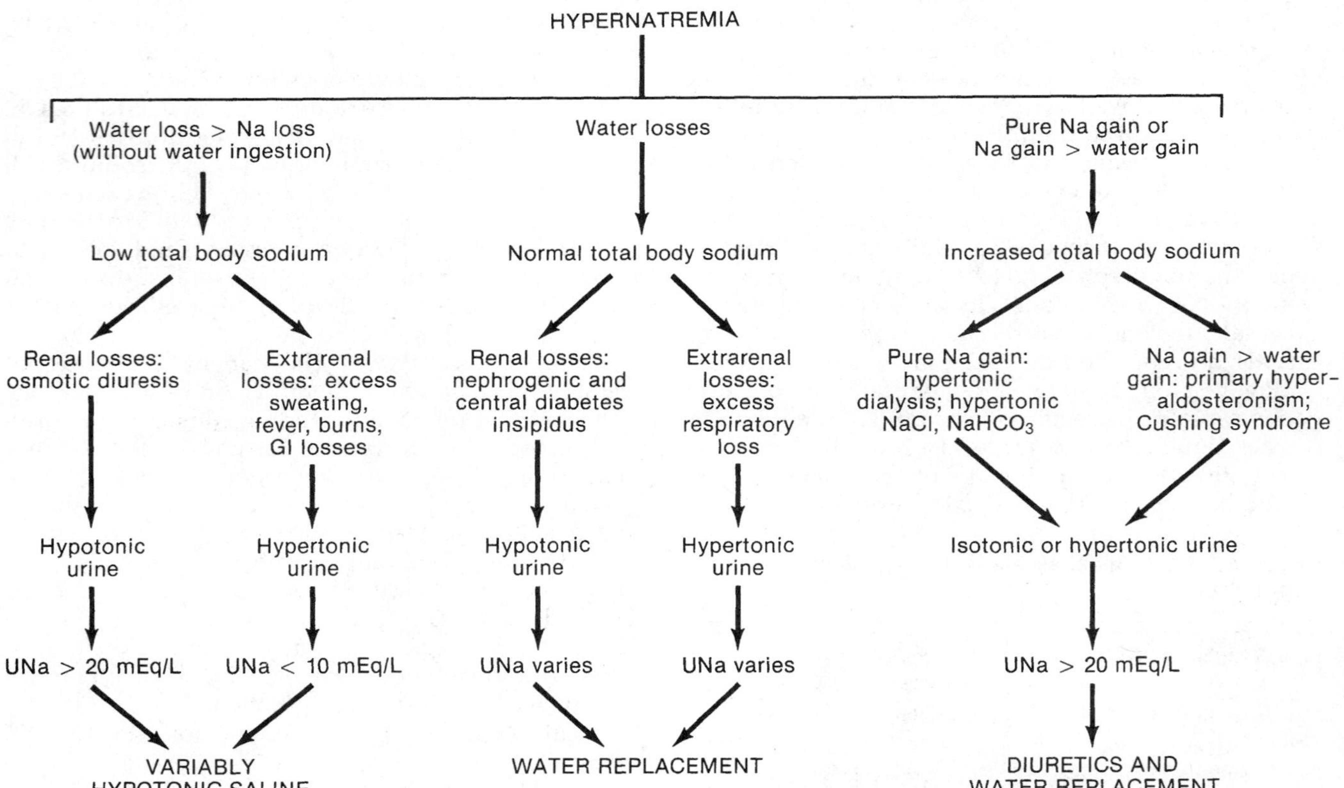

FIGURE 43–3. Clinical approach to patient with hypernatremia. *UNa*, urine sodium.

trauma, tumor, anoxic brain injury, or meningitis. Nephrogenic diabetes insipidus is usually the result of renal disease or drug administration (lithium) but can also be inherited. Loss of free water leads to increased oncotic pressure, which tends to maintain water in the intravascular space. Diagnosis of diabetes insipidus is based on urine output and urine osmolality. Urine output will be high, usually more than 3 liters/day, and can be higher depending on fluid intake. Urine will be dilute, typically less than 300 mOsm/kg. With water deprivation, the urine osmolality of water drinkers will normally become much greater than the serum osmolality; however, this will not occur in patients with diabetes insipidus. Challenge with exogenous vasopressin will differentiate central from nephrogenic diabetes insipidus. Loop diuretics cause a loss of sodium as well as of free water.

A decrease in total body sodium and water results from nonrenal losses through the gastrointestinal tract and skin. Renal losses of hypotonic fluid are due to osmotic diuresis. An osmotic load from urea, glucose, or mannitol can induce not only loss of free water, but also obligatory loss of excess sodium. The serum Na concentration will not be as markedly elevated, typically less than 160 mEq/liter, because there is also loss of sodium. Patients with osmotic diuresis will have hypotension. Continued high urine output will eventually result in increased serum osmolality.

An increase in total body sodium with no change in water occurs with ingestion of salt and is rare and potentially fatal. Salt water as a gargle, saline as an emetic, and pediatric administration when salt was inadvertently used instead of sugar in preparation of a formula have been reported etiologies (Moder & Daniel, 1990).

A final type of hypernatremia occurs with increase in total body sodium and water and results from iatrogenic administration of sodium. The most common etiologies are the use of 3% or 5% sodium chloride to correct hyponatremia, and the use of sodium bicarbonate to correct metabolic acidosis. Patients with this condition and patients with no change in water both have increased EC volume due to the shift of water from the IC space to the EC space in response to an increased solute load. This causes IC cell shrinkage and, if great enough, pulmonary edema. When the patient's kidneys are functioning normally, a brisk diuresis will ensue, with urine Na concentration being much greater than 20 mEq/liter (Sunyecz & Mirtallo, 1993).

Symptoms associated with hypernatremia are related to the rate at which the plasma osmolality increases as well as the degree of increase. The clinical manifestations described in Table 43–11 reflect the CNS intracellular dehydration that occurs with increased pOsm.

TABLE 43–11. **Clinical Manifestations of Hypernatremia**

Early Stage
Thirst/polydipsia
Restlessness/irritability
Confusion/somnolence
Second Stage
Ataxia
Muscle weakness/twitching
Late Stage
Focal or grand mal seizures

MANAGEMENT OF HYPERNATREMIA. Treatment of hypernatremia is designed to address the specific deficits identified. Very rapid correction of hypernatremia can produce cerebral edema, seizures, and death because of rapid IC movement of water. The general approach is to decrease pOsm by 1 to 2 mOsm/kg H_2O per hour. Plasma Na concentrations should be lowered no more than 2 mEq/hr.

When hypernatremia develops quickly, the brain does not have time to adjust to the difference in solute load, so substantial brain cell shrinkage can occur. This can cause meningeal vessels to tear, followed by intracranial hemorrhage. When hypernatremia develops slowly, the brain can manufacture solute to compensate for the increased osmotic load due to sodium and stabilize the osmolar difference so that no brain cell shrinkage occurs. In patients with true free-water loss, replacement of the loss with 5% dextrose injection is generally indicated. Volume replacement is determined by calculating the free-water deficit. In patients who develop acute and symptomatic hypernatremia, half of the calculated replacement volume can be administered rapidly, and the other half can be administered over the next 24 to 48 hours. With chronic hypernatremia, replacement should be done over a longer period (Oh & Carroll, 1992; Moder & Daniel, 1990).

Patients with loss of hypotonic fluids (loss of more total body water than sodium) can develop vascular collapse. Normal saline infusion should be administered until the patient is hemodynamically stable. This fluid is hypotonic to the EC fluid volume and will decrease the serum Na concentration. Once the patient is stable, the fluid can be changed to 5% dextrose and 0.45% sodium chloride (Sunyecz & Mirtallo, 1993).

Patients who have a gain in sodium and those who have a gain in sodium and fluid are managed similarly. Administration of a loop diuretic such as furosemide can cause loss of sodium and fluid. Remember, water is excreted along with sodium, which can worsen the hypernatremia. In patients with isolated Na overload or who have achieved sufficient diuresis, 5% dextrose injection can be added to the loop diuretic to help maintain an adequate fluid volume while eliminating sodium. The serum Na concentration should be monitored at least once a day (Sunyecz & Mirtallo, 1993).

POTENTIAL FOR INJURY. CNS alterations may become manifest from the elevated plasma Na concentration or from cerebral edema resulting from too rapid a reduction in plasma Na level. Nursing care is directed toward ensuring a gradual reduction in plasma Na concentration and protecting the patient from possible injury.

The hypernatremic patient is assessed for signs of CNS irritability. The patient may appear confused and restless. The nurse assesses the patient's level of consciousness frequently and evaluates for change. As plasma Na concentration decreases, the patient's neurologic status should improve. The nurse provides a quiet, calm environment to decrease further stimulation. If the patient is restless and thrashing in bed, protective measures such as placement of bedrail padding are instituted. In patients with significant hypernatremia, seizure precautions are appropriate.

The nurse carefully reviews serial plasma Na measurements and evaluates the patient's response to the hypotonic infusion. The infusion is closely monitored to avoid overhydration and too rapid a reduction in sodium.

Osmolality disorders are frequently the consequence of a number of chronic disease processes. Therefore, the chronically ill patient is at risk for recurring episodes of hyponatremia or hypernatremia. Teaching the patient and family members about the causes and early signs of these osmolality disorders may result in earlier medical attention and may prevent the need for hospitalization.

ELECTROLYTE REGULATION AND BALANCE

Potassium

Potassium is an important electrolyte that serves two major physiologic purposes. One is a regulatory role in cell growth and metabolic processes. In the absence of appropriate K balance, cellular functions are impaired. The second important physiologic role of potassium is in the development of the resting membrane potential in neuromuscular tissue. This resting membrane potential is created by the difference between IC and EC potassium concentrations. The resting membrane potential is important for successful initiation of the action potential in nerve and muscle, including cardiac muscle. If EC potassium is elevated (hyperkalemia), the potential difference between EC and IC is less. The result is a decrease in the resting membrane potential, and the cell becomes more excitable. In the presence of low EC potassium concentration (hypokalemia), the cell membrane is hyperpolarized and is less sensitive to excitation. These pathologic conditions will be discussed in detail in subsequent sections.

The normal plasma concentration of potassium is 3.5 to 5.0 mEq/liter. Potassium homeostasis is achieved through maintaining a balance among (1) K intake; (2) K distribution between the IC and EC compartments; and (3) renal management of filtered potassium. As described previously, potassium is the major IC cation and is preferentially confined to the IC compartment by the energy-consuming Na,K-ATPase pumps located in the cell membrane. The effectiveness of these pumps is demonstrated by the disparity normally maintained between the IC and EC potassium concentrations, as shown in Figure 43–1. Total body K stores in a normal adult are approximately 3000 to 4000 mEq. In normal steady-state conditions, K excretion occurs primarily through the kidney. Some potassium is lost through the gastrointestinal tract and in sweat. Thus, there is an obligatory K excretion regardless of K stores or the plasma concentration. The renal mechanism for EC potassium regulation requires several hours to become effective. Consequently, the more immediate regulation of potassium occurs endogenously through the mechanisms associated with IC and EC potassium distribution.

The mechanisms that influence the distribution of potassium in IC and EC compartments include the presence of Na,K-ATPase, insulin, exercise, and adrenergic nervous activity. In normal circumstances, plasma K concentration is precisely regulated because a small change in plasma concentration could be fatal. The IC concentration acts as a storage or supply depot for the EC compartment depending on the plasma K concentration.

The availability of Na,K-ATPase is an important requirement because the sodium–potassium pump is responsible for the IC and EC distribution of potassium. If the pump is not functioning adequately, the distribution of sodium and potassium will not be maintained in the EC and IC compartments, respectively. Any derangement in pump function has important implications for the fate of potassium added through the diet. Rapid addition of a large amount of potassium into a small EC volume would cause plasma K to rise to potentially lethal levels. Thus, the major body mechanism for handling a dietary load of potassium is rapid incorporation of this electrolyte into cells via the sodium–potassium pump (Carroll & Oh, 1989). This immediate redistribution allows time for the remainder of the K load to be renally excreted. Plasma K concentration may directly affect the Na,K-ATPase pump as well as aldosterone secretion.

Insulin is an important cofactor governing movement of potassium intracellularly, particularly into the liver and skeletal muscle. This explains the useful role played by insulin in conjunction with glucose in the treatment of hyperkalemia. Basal insulin levels also appear to enhance the movement of potassium into cells because suppression of the basal plasma insulin level will lead to an increase in plasma K concentration.

Exercise causes the release of potassium from cells, which, by means of a vasodilatory action, increases blood flow to exercising muscle. This process facilitates nutrient supply and waste removal from the working muscle. Once exercise stops, potassium rapidly moves back into cells. The restoration of potassium to the cellular compartment requires a process that involves the beta-adrenergic system. This mechanism of K distribution can be blunted by beta antagonists such as propranolol. Consequently, severe prolonged exercise in patients taking beta blockers may induce a potentially dangerous hyperkalemia.

Plasma K concentration is itself an influence on K distribution in the body. Plasma K concentration reflects total body stores of potassium, and variations in plasma concentration are correlated with changes in body stores. Exceptions to this clinical observation include significant changes in blood pH, plasma osmolality, and the rate of cell catabolism in the body. Under these circumstances, a change in plasma K concentration may instead reflect a redistribution of potassium between the EC and IC compartments.

Metabolic acidosis leads to an EC shift of potassium. This occurs because the body's attempt to buffer the acid load promotes the movement of hydrogen ion into the IC compartment. This reciprocal shift of K cations into the EC satisfies the requirements of electroneutrality. The effect of alkalosis on K distribution is not as striking, probably because of the decreased magnitude of hydrogen ion movement in patients with this condition. Respiratory acid-base disturbances do not lead to equally significant swings in plasma K concentrations because of the acid source CO_2.

Tissue catabolism will also affect EC potassium concentration. With cell breakdown, potassium will be liberated into the EC compartment. This situation commonly occurs in patients with surgery or trauma. In patients with normal renal function, the effect on plasma K concentration will be minimal. However, in critically ill patients with acute renal dysfunction, plasma K levels may rise rapidly due to tissue catabolism.

Potassium excretion is managed primarily by the kidney, most of it in the distal nephron by means of secretion and reabsorption. Thus, renal excretion is the important mechanism for varying K excretion as a function of K intake.

Aldosterone, synthesized in the zona glomerulosa of the adrenal cortex, plays a powerful role in K homeostasis. When a K load is introduced into the body, aldosterone secretion is stimulated. Aldosterone increases excretion of potassium by the kidney while conserving the other major cation, sodium. Conversely, under appropriate circumstances, decreased aldosterone availability minimizes urinary loss of potassium.

HYPOKALEMIA

A serum K value of less than 3.5 mEq/liter is classified as hypokalemia. The causes of hypokalemia are shown in Table 43–12. Decreased dietary intake is rarely the cause of hypokalemia because urinary losses can be minimized in the presence of a low K intake. Pica involving clay consumption may contribute to hypokalemia because this substance actually binds potassium and iron in the gut.

Increased gastrointestinal losses through the mechanisms of vomiting, nasogastric suction, or diarrhea are common causes of hypokalemia. Because the concentration of potassium in gastrointestinal secretions is relatively low, this loss alone cannot explain the significant degree of hypokalemia seen in these patients. The process by which hypokalemia is induced in this setting is associated with the metabolic alkalosis and volume depletion that accompanies severe vomiting or prolonged gastric drainage. An increase in pH of 0.1 will decrease plasma K concentration by approximately 0.4 mEq/liter (Carroll & Oh, 1989). In the presence of volume and acid-base disturbances, the renal dumping of bicarbonate coupled with high aldosterone levels leads to renal excretion of potassium and preservation of sodium. Metabolic alkalosis favors movement of potassium into the IC compartment. Fecal loss of potassium can be sizable with significant diarrhea and can be responsible for K depletion.

Increased entry of potassium into the IC compartment may result from increased pH, insulin, or beta-adrenergic activity. Any situation in which there is an increase in supply or availability of insulin or catecholamines will promote IC movement of potassium.

Epinephrine in local anesthetic agents does produce hypokalemia and electrocardiographic (ECG) changes. It is well known that epinephrine alone produces hypokalemia and consistent alterations in the ECG as lowering of serum K level progresses: (1) depressed ST segment, typically less than 0.5 mm; (2) a low T wave amplitude; and (3) prominent U waves with amplitude greater than 1 mm. With progressive K depletion, the action potential lengthens as a result

TABLE 43–12. **Etiology and Clinical Manifestations of Hypokalemia**

Etiology	Clinical Findings
Extrarenal	**Neuromuscular**
Decreased potassium intake	Weakness
Increased gastrointestinal losses	Paralysis
Increased potassium entry into cells	**Cardiac**
Increased pH	ST depression
Increased insulin	Decreased amplitude
Increased beta-adrenergic activity	T wave inversion
Dialysis	Increased U wave (>1 mm)
Renal	Prolongation of QT interval
Mineralocorticoid excess	Decreased amplitude of P wave
Hyperaldosteronism	Prolonged PR interval
Cushing's syndrome	Widened QRS complex
Hyperreninemia	**Renal**
Increased sodium delivery to distal nephron	Increased urine potassium (concentration defect)
Diuretics	Sodium retention
Osmotic diuresis	
Bartter syndrome	
Salt-wasting nephropathies	
Nonreabsorbable anions	
Penicillins	
Ketoacids	
HCO_3^- (metabolic alkalosis)	

of phase 3 prolongation. The amplitude of repolarization decreases in systole (depressed T wave) and increased in diastole, resulting in a prominent U wave (Wong et al., 1993). Severe hypokalemia (<2.5 mEq/liter) has been associated with development of serious ventricular tachydysrhythmias, even in the absence of heart disease or digitalis therapy (Kubota et al., 1993).

Epinephrine decreases not only serum potassium, but also magnesium, calcium, and phosphate, and at the same time increases glucose, heart rate, and systolic blood pressure. Pretreatment with mexiletine, a Class I antidysrhythmic, resulted in a still greater fall in serum K concentration than epinephrine alone (Zakowski et al., 1993).

Continuous infusions of epinephrine caused a transient hyperkalemia lasting about 6 to 14 minutes and followed by a prolonged hypokalemia which lasts up to 30 minutes after discontinuation of the infusion. Initial hyperkalemia results from hepatic K release, and the subsequent hypokalemia is due to increased cellular uptake in muscle cells, red blood cells, and eventually liver cells.

Critically ill patients receiving dialysis treatments may become hypokalemic as a result of this therapy. Dialysis utilizing a low potassium bath may produce K depletion because of inappropriate removal of potassium during the treatment. Hypokalemia may be worsened by the correction of metabolic acidosis that occurs during dialysis. This will encourage K movement into cells and a further decrease in serum K concentration.

The more common reasons for hypokalemia involve problems in renal regulation of potassium. As described earlier, the distal nephron plays the major role in regulating K balance. Hypokalemia may occur in the presence of mineralocorticoid excess, an increase in the tubular lumen fluid flow to the distal nephron, or a decrease in the reabsorption of potassium in the presence of a nonreabsorbable anion. If urine K values are 10 mEq/day or more in conjunction with hypokalemia, renal K wasting is probably present.

Hypokalemia is a common sequela of mineralocorticoid excess. This condition causes increased reabsorption of sodium by the kidney and secretion of potassium and hydrogen ion. However, in order for K wasting to occur in the kidney, there must be adequate tubular fluid volume delivered to the distal nephron. Thus, in situations in which effective arterial volume is diminished, serum K values may be relatively normal. Depletion of EC volume stimulates aldosterone secretion but decreases the fluid volume delivered to the distal nephron as a result of the volume restoration effort by the kidney. EC volume expansion produces the opposite effects.

An excess of mineralocorticoid conserves sodium, an effort that, if successful, leads to EC volume expansion and hypertension. As a consequence of the increased volume, the fluid volume delivered to the distal nephron is increased and K wasting may occur. Causes of mineralocorticoid excess include hyperaldosteronism as a consequence of adrenal tumor or hyperplasia. Cushing's disease, in which there is bilateral hyperplasia, produces hypokalemia through glucocorticoid excess. Administration of corticosteroids for treatment of other disease processes may also result in hypokalemia.

Another common mechanism that leads to renal K wasting and hypokalemia is initiated by those states in which there is an increase in the fluid volume delivered to the distal nephron. This disorder is commonly seen in critically ill patients following the administration of diuretics that inhibit proximal Na reabsorption and force water excretion. In this situation, Na reabsorption in the proximal tubule is diminished, resulting in a higher volume of fluid delivered to the distal segment. Consequently, there is an increase in K excretion by the kidney. Chronic use of diuretics can cause EC depletion, which stimulates aldosterone secretion and thus K secretion by the kidney. An osmotic diuresis will also produce hypokalemia in essentially the same way. Hypomagnesemia may produce hypokalemia. This condition will be manifested by elevated aldosterone and renin blood levels but without hypertension.

Hypokalemia has recently been reported in patients with multiple injuries (Vanek et al., 1994). This is contrary to previous investigations. Hypokalemia was significantly more common in trauma patients; however, hyperkalemia was seen in patients exhibiting shock with hypoperfusion and acidosis and was theorized to be caused by an EC shift of potassium. Another factor that often leads to hyperkalemia is soft tissue injury followed by release of potassium from damaged cells. There was no significant difference between patients with and without musculoskeletal injuries, possibly because in this study musculoskeletal injuries were relatively minor and did not involve significant crush injuries (Vanek et al., 1994).

Hypokalemia occurred in 50% to 68% of patients, usually starting within 1 hour and resolving within 24 hours of the trauma. Age, arterial pH, and serum epinephrine were the only significant independent predictors of initial serum K level. The correlation of serum epinephrine and arterial pH with serum potassium are opposite to that predicted by their physiologic effects. However, significantly higher serum K level was seen among patients with cardiac injuries than among other patients.

Intracellular shift of potassium is the probable explanation for hypokalemia seen in the trauma patient. Deficient intake, renal losses, and increased gastrointestinal losses are unlikely to cause an acute onset of hypokalemia. Aldosterone levels are increased in trauma patients; however, the investigators were unable to find any correlation between urine and serum K levels.

The physiologic manifestations of hypokalemia are shown in Table 43–12. The severity of the manifestations tends to be correlated with the degree of hypokalemia, and these signs generally do not appear until serum K values are below 3.0 mEq/liter. A decrease in EC potassium concentration relative to the IC concentration causes hyperpolarization across the cell membrane and reduces the excitability of the cells. The resting membrane potential is below the normal level; thus the cell requires a larger stimulus to reach the threshold value and cause depolarization. The cell then requires a longer time to repolarize to baseline value. These facts have important clinical implications for nerve and muscle function.

One of the important clinical manifestations of hypokalemia is muscle weakness. Progression to muscle paralysis occurs when the plasma K concentration is less than 2.5 mEq/liter (Carroll & Oh, 1989). Muscle dysfunction may first be evident in the lower extremities. With increasing severity, the trunk and upper extremities become involved, and respiratory failure may occur.

Cardiac dysrhythmias induced by hypokalemia are varied and include premature contractions, both atrial and ventricular, tachydysrhythmias, and sinus bradycardia. Serious dysrhythmias are usually not seen until the plasma K level is less than 3 mEq/liter. However, digitalis therapy may make the individual patient susceptible to serious dysrhythmias at a higher plasma K value. The ECG changes commonly seen in hypokalemia are all reversible with K repletion.

Hypokalemia during the first 24 to 48 hours following acute infarction has been advanced as a risk factor for development of ventricular fibrillation. Low plasma K levels exert a variety of electrophysiologic effects (alterations in excitability, conduction velocity, and refractoriness) that may act to promote fibrillation, particularly in infarction, where there are disparities between normal cardiac tissue and the ischemic border zone. Hypokalemia may arise as a result of the profound catecholamine drive that occurs at the onset of infarction. Patients receiving nonselective β-blockers had higher admission plasma K levels than patients on no therapy (Higham et al., 1993).

Incidence of reentry-type dysrhythmias, including ventricular tachycardia and ventricular fibrillation, was found to be inversely related to the levels of serum potassium. Cardiac dysrhythmias are made worse by respiratory alkalosis, digitalis therapy, and myocardial ischemia or infarction in the presence of hypokalemia. The surgical patient should have a preoperative serum K concentration of 3.5 mEq/liter (undigitalized) and 4.0 mEq/liter (digitalized) before receiving anesthesia (Wong, 1993).

Severe muscle dysfunction may also lead to rhabdomyolysis and acute renal failure in patients with severe hypokalemia. This phenomenon appears to be the result of cellular ischemia caused by the lack of available potassium. As described earlier, the release of potassium from IC stores promotes vasodilation in the local area of an exercising muscle. If K depletion exists, this transcellular movement of potassium does not occur. Because there is no increase in blood flow to the area, ischemic necrosis of muscle cells, with release of cellular contents, may occur.

Hypokalemia may have a significant effect on renal function. Polyuria may be associated with low plasma K values. This may be a sequela of impaired urinary concentrating ability associated with K depletion. However, urine osmolality generally stays above 300 mOsm/kg with K depletion. Potassium depletion may lead to renal retention of sodium, resulting in edema formation if Na intake is high.

MANAGEMENT OF HYPOKALEMIA. Treatment of hypokalemia includes identification and correction of the underlying cause as well as the electrolyte disorder. Volume depletion may occur in association with significant extrarenal losses and diuretic usage. Hypovolemia may further cloud the issue with activation of the normal renal response of Na conservation and K secretion. In contrast, primary mineralocorticoid excess is more often associated with volume expansion. The presence of acid-base disturbances may be an important clue to the etiology of the observed hypokalemia. For example, hypokalemia and metabolic alkalosis may indicate excessive diuretic usage or upper gastrointestinal losses.

There is no good correlation between the plasma K concentration and the total K deficit. As noted above, the actual plasma K concentration at which signs and symptoms appear is variable. Symptomatic patients need to be treated promptly. The goal is K repletion to diminish the signs and symptoms of hypokalemia but not necessarily to completely restore body K stores immediately. Rapid administration of K supplements may induce a hyperkalemic state. If the hypokalemia is not acute, oral K supplements may be appropriate. Oral replacement avoids K rebound because there is time for renal regulation to contribute to restoration of K balance. In hypokalemia associated with primary hyperaldosteronism, oral K replacement may not be adequate to replace losses because potassium will continue to be lost through the kidney. Intravenous K supplementation should be administered at an infusion rate of 10 to 20 mEq/hr unless paralysis or potentially fatal dysrhythmias are present. When hypokalemia is severe or when serious ECG abnormalities are evident, intravenous potassium may need to be administered more rapidly, at a rate of up to 80 to 100 mEq/hr. Under these circumstances, the ECG must be monitored closely to prevent *hyper*kalemic changes. Because of the insulin effect on K distribution, glucose solutions, which would stimulate endogenous insulin production, are not usually the solutions of choice for administration of K replacement in patients with severe hypokalemia.

ALTERATION IN CARDIAC OUTPUT. In hypokalemia, the contractility of the cardiac muscle is impaired. The nurse assesses the patient for signs and symptoms of decreased cardiac output and the development of CHF. The effect of digitalis is enhanced in hypokalemia, placing the patient at risk of digitalis toxicity. The critical care nurse monitors the patient's serum K level and confers with the physician regarding withholding or reducing the dosage of digitalis. The ECG is observed for changes indicative of hypokalemia. Particular attention is paid to the patient's ECG during intravenous K repletion. Emergency resuscitation equipment is kept readily available in case cardiac arrest occurs.

POTENTIAL FOR INJURY. The patient with hypokalemia is at risk for injury from several sources. Muscle weakness is a common manifestation of hypokalemia. The patient may not have the strength to perform activities such as transferring himself from bed to chair. The nurse assesses the patient's muscle strength and provides appropriate support and assistance as necessary.

Maintenance of adequate intravenous access is vital in the treatment of K disorders. As with intravenous administration of any drug, K repletion carries some risk to the patient. Rapid repletion of K in a peripheral vein may cause localized pain and irritation of the vein. Therefore, if a peripheral site is used, it may be preferable to infuse lower K concentrations through two sites. Ideally, high K concentrations should be administered through a large-bore central line.

HYPERKALEMIA

Hyperkalemia is defined as a plasma K level of greater than 5.5 mEq/liter, although the level at which hyperkalemic complications occur may vary depending on the steady-state value for a given patient. Adaptation may occur when K intake is gradually increased to very high levels or may be a protective mechanism associated with chronic renal failure. In the case of chronic renal failure, the remaining functioning nephrons are capable of increasing their individual excretion of potassium and avoiding significant hyperkalemia until renal function approaches zero. There can be situations in which serum K level as measured in the blood specimen is erroneously elevated. Hemolysis associated with venipuncture or specimen collection will artificially increase measured serum K values. Spuriously high plasma K values may also be seen in the patient with thrombocytosis or leukocytosis.

Hyperkalemia can be the result of increased oral or intravenous intake of potassium, although this is uncommon in the presence of normal renal function. As discussed earlier, the body first defends against wide swings in EC potassium concentration by rapidly shifting potassium between the body compartments to reestablish appropriate concentrations in each compartment. The secondary regulatory mechanism involving the kidney can then restore true K balance over 6 to 8 hours. Therefore, sustained hyperkalemia is almost always the result of impaired renal K regulation mechanisms. However, there may be instances, either because of the rate of K administration or the size of the patient (infants), in which potentially fatal serum K levels can be reached even with normal renal function.

The most common causes of true hyperkalemia are shown in Table 43–13. These causes are frequently the inverse of those described in the section on hypokalemia. Metabolic acidosis is a frequent cause of hyperkalemia in critically ill patients. With the intracellular

TABLE 43–13. **Etiology and Clinical Manifestations of Hyperkalemia**

Etiology	Clinical Findings
Extrarenal	**Neuromuscular**
Metabolic acidosis	Paresthesias
Decreased insulin availability/hyperglycemia	Paralysis—distal moving to proximal
Beta blockers	
Exercise	**Cardiac**
Tissue catabolism	Peaked T wave
Digitalis overdose	Widened QRS complex
	Widened PR interval
Renal	Disappearance of P wave
Mineralocorticoid deficiency	Appearance of sine wave
Renal failure	
Decreased effective arterial volume	

movement of hydrogen ions, potassium moves out of the cells, thus increasing the EC potassium concentration. Hyperkalemia in patients with diabetic ketoacidosis is partially a consequence of the lack of insulin and thus the inability to move potassium within the cells quickly. Hyperglycemia is also responsible for significant movement of potassium out of cells. The increased EC osmolality accompanying hyperglycemia pulls water out of cells, bringing potassium with it.

Beta blockers may play an indirect role in the production of hyperkalemia by preventing the movement of potassium into cells. This is usually expressed as a modest elevation in serum K concentration. However, when there is a significant addition of potassium to the EC compartment, the normally rapid redistribution of potassium is attenuated. As discussed earlier, this may produce a dangerous situation when vigorous exercise is performed.

Tissue catabolism, either through traumatic injury or surgery, may liberate large amounts of potassium into the EC compartment. This is further exacerbated by renal failure, which often occurs as a sequela to these insults.

Digitalis can also be responsible for the development of hyperkalemia. Large doses of digitalis preparations significantly inhibit the Na,K-ATPase pump, which is instrumental in transporting potassium into cells. Typical therapeutic doses of digitalis may cause an inconsequential increase in serum K values. However, in patients in which the renal regulatory mechanism is compromised or absent, hyperkalemia may be a serious complication of digitalis administration.

Exogenous parathyroid hormone (PTH) impairs extrarenal K disposal. Elevated PTH levels produce a chronic increase in cytosolic Ca levels, and inhibit mitochondrial oxidation and generation of ATP. Low cellular ATP levels inhibit Na,K-ATPase activity, thereby inhibiting K shifts into the IC fluid compartment.

Persistent hyperkalemia may be indicative of an impairment of the mechanisms that regulate K excretion. Mineralocorticoid deficiency may result from either the production of aldosterone or the diminished effect of the hormone on the kidney. Hypoaldosteronism can result from the administration of NSAIDs, potassium-sparing diuretics, or any condition that affects the adrenal synthesis of the hormone.

Renal insufficiency or failure frequently leads to hyperkalemia because of a direct reduction in nephron excretory ability. Hyperkalemia may also result from the secondary problem of decreased flow of water and sodium through the distal tubule. Hyperkalemia occurs more frequently in oliguric acute renal failure than in patients with nonoliguric renal failure.

The development of hyperkalemia should be anticipated when hospitalized hemodialysis patients fast in preparation for surgery or a diagnostic procedure or in protracted nausea and vomiting. A continuous infusion of insulin with dextrose can prevent this complication (add 20 units of regular insulin to a liter of 10% dextrose, and infuse at 50 mL/hr). This prophylactic regimen may produce hypoglycemia in some patients, mandating periodic evaluation of serum glucose concentration (Allon et al., 1993).

Decreased EAV leads to diminished delivery of water and electrolytes to the distal nephron. As described earlier, this will reduce K secretion at this site. Any clinical condition that produces a reduced EAV will encourage K retention by the kidney and the possibility of hyperkalemia. In patients with chronic CHF, the addition of digitalis preparations and the imposition of renal insufficiency may result in significant hyperkalemia.

Clinical manifestations of hyperkalemia are described in Table 43–13. Because of the increase in EC potassium concentration, the cell transmembrane resting potential is reduced (becomes less negative). Thus, the resting potential is closer to the threshold value relative to the normal state. There is a corresponding increase in the velocity of repolarization and a decreased rate of diastolic depolarization (Carroll & Oh, 1989).

The most striking example of this phenomenon is seen in cardiac muscle, where significant conduction abnormalities may be seen in the ECG. Hyperkalemia is manifested by three classic features: (1) peaked, narrow T waves; (2) widened QRS complex; and (3) a shortened QT interval. Peaked, narrow T waves typically are the earliest manifestation of hyperkalemia and are seen in only 20% of patients with hyperkalemia on leads II, III, and V_{2-4}. The peaked T waves result from the increase in the slope of Phase 3. Prolongation of the QRS complex is due to diminished distance between the resting membrane potential and the threshold potential with a reduction in the number of Na channels. Additional changes often seen include a decrease in the amplitude of the R wave, appearance of a prominent S wave, depression of the ST segment, and occasional elevation of the ST segment (Wong et al., 1993). Figure 43–4 illustrates the cardiac effects of hyperkalemia.

The neuromuscular manifestations may be less common but are frequently the initial patient com-

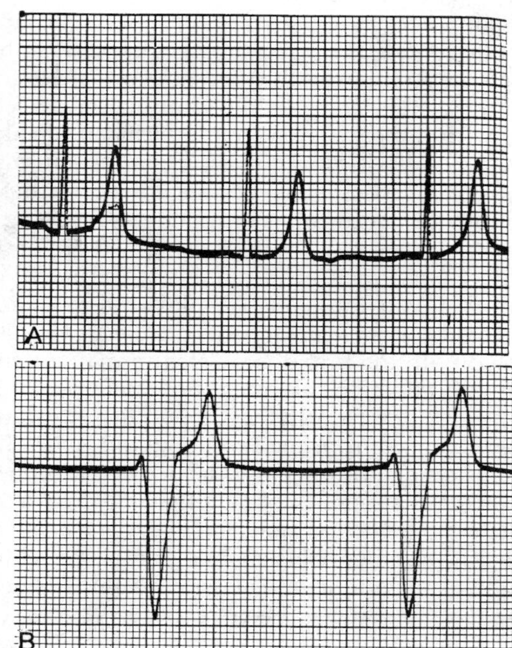

FIGURE 43–4. Characteristic electrocardiographic changes during hyperkalemia.

plaint. Paresthesias of the extremities may be present. Flaccid paralysis of the distal extremities with proximal progression may also be evident. Neuromuscular involvement tends to remain localized to the extremities.

MANAGEMENT OF HYPERKALEMIA. Management of the hyperkalemic patient is directed toward treatment of the underlying etiology as well as the signs and symptoms of hyperkalemia. ECG changes warrant prompt treatment to avoid progression of cardiac toxicity to ventricular fibrillation and cardiac arrest. The absolute value at which treatment must be initiated will vary, and management should be instituted based on ECG and physical findings. Hyperkalemia in the presence of ECG abnormalities or muscular weakness should be treated immediately.

A number of approaches can be used to reduce EC potassium concentration effectively. Treatment is directed toward removal of potassium from the body or effective redistribution of potassium into the IC compartment. The therapeutic techniques most often used are shown in Table 43–14.

TABLE 43–14. **Therapy for Hyperkalemia**

Membrane Antagonism	Removal of Potassium
Calcium	Diuretics
Hypertonic sodium	Exchange resin
	Dialysis
Redistribution of Potassium	
Insulin and glucose	
Bicarbonate	

Calcium acts to antagonize the cell membrane effects of hyperkalemia directly by resetting the interval between the resting and the threshold potential. In cardiac muscle, this reverses the conduction defect observed with hyperkalemia. Acute infusion of calcium increases Na flux through the Na channels in muscle tissue, which also enhances conduction of the impulse. The action of Ca infusion is rapid, the effect being seen in 1 to 3 minutes. The action is sustained for up to 60 minutes. Continuous ECG monitoring must be done during acute Ca infusion. Administration of repeat doses of this agent will depend on the ECG changes produced with the first dose. Calcium may potentiate the digitalis effect. In this situation, calcium should be diluted in 5% dextrose and water and the infusion rate reduced to an appropriate level to avoid toxic effects.

Hypertonic sodium chloride administration in a hyponatremic patient may be effective in correcting the cardiac conduction defect. This agent acts by increasing the number of Na channels in the muscle cells, which helps to conduct the electrical impulse once the threshold potential has been reached. The effectiveness of this technique with normal serum Na values is less obvious.

Rapid redistribution of potassium from the EC to the IC compartment is effective in reducing the toxic effects of hyperkalemia. Insulin in association with a glucose infusion is used for this purpose. Insulin is effective in moving potassium intracellularly, and glucose prevents hypoglycemia resulting from the additional exogenous insulin. This combination is administered over 30 minutes and should be effective for 4 to 6 hours.

The potassium-lowering effect of bicarbonate is quite variable, and may be delayed as long as 4 hours. It therefore is not reliable in the acute management of hyperkalemia. Sodium bicarbonate therapy is still indicated in chronic renal failure patients with severe acidosis ($pH < 7.20$) regardless of the plasma K level. If volume expansion is present, the addition of this Na load may increase the risk of CHF or fluid volume overload.

Administration of $\beta 2$ agonists may have utility in the acute treatment of hyperkalemia. A 0.5-mg intravenous dose of albuterol acutely decreased plasma K concentration by a mean of 1.1 mmol/liter in hyperkalemic patients with acute or chronic renal failure. The effect occurred within 30 minutes and was sustained for up to 6 hours. The albuterol dose required to lower plasma K level was four- to eightfold higher than that used for the treatment of asthma where only a small fraction of inhaled albuterol is absorbed into the systemic circulation, and only that fraction stimulates extrarenal K disposal. The use of albuterol in critically ill patients with acute renal failure or in hemodialysis patients, who are likely to have a high incidence of CAD, has the potential to produce serious adverse effects. The mean increase in heart rate varied between 8 to 20 beats/min, and a modest increase in plasma glucose was also seen. Albuterol therapy is both efficacious and safe for the acute treatment of hyperkalemia in patients with renal failure.

Insulin plus dextrose and nebulized albuterol were equally effective in lowering plasma K concentration. Onset of action of insulin occurred within 15 minutes and of nebulized albuterol, within 30 minutes. The addition of albuterol to insulin therapy not only produces an additive potassium-lowering effect, but also protects against insulin-induced hypoglycemia (Allon, 1991; Allon, 1993).

The maneuvers described above will not reduce total body potassium. They serve as temporary measures that allow the physician and nurse time to consider ways in which potassium can be effectively removed from the body. If kidney function is adequate, diuretics such as furosemide will be useful in delivering increased water and Na flow to the distal tubule, thus enhancing K secretion by the kidney. More frequently, hyperkalemia is associated with renal impairment. In this case, extrarenal removal of potassium may be warranted. Hemodialysis with a zero K dialysate rapidly removes potassium from the body. However, this treatment requires a vascular access device, dialysis equipment, and skilled personnel, all of which may be difficult to obtain in an emergency situation. If time permits, however, this is the most efficient method of reducing serum K level rapidly. Using standard operating parameters, approximately 40 mEq of potassium can be removed in the first hour of dialysis. Peritoneal dialysis can also be used to lower serum K levels, although this therapeutic technique will be much slower than hemodialysis.

Exchange resins, such as Kayexalate, are also effective in removing potassium from the body. The resin exchanges a Na ion for potassium and calcium in the gastrointestinal tract. It can be given either as an oral preparation or by retention enema to accomplish K removal. It is usually given with sorbitol to enhance K loss via the bowel. A 25-g dose will remove approximately 12.5 to 25 mEq of potassium. This method of K removal is slower and requires 1 to 2 hours before onset of action. In general, 50 g of Kayexalate will lower serum K concentration by approximately 0.5 to 1.0 mEq/liter. The additional sodium from the resin, approximately 3 mEq per mEq of potassium exchanged, may be contraindicated in patients with serious cardiac disease.

ALTERATION IN CARDIAC OUTPUT. Nursing care of a patient in hyperkalemic crisis is directed toward supporting and monitoring the patient's cardiac status while administering therapies designed to reduce the plasma K level. Hyperkalemia has no significant effect on cardiac contractility but can cause alterations in cardiac output owing to abnormalities in rhythm and conduction. Careful, ongoing evaluation of ECG monitoring in the hyperkalemic patient before and during treatment is an important nursing responsibility.

The critical care nurse observes the ECG for peaked T waves, shortened QT interval, and prolonged PR interval. After administration of prescribed medications and fluids, serial plasma K measurements are taken and monitored. Response is evaluated by observing the patient for resolution of the ECG changes. If bicarbonate, glucose, and insulin are used, the nurse anticipates the return of hyperkalemia in several hours.

The nurse maintains adequate intravenous access and monitors medication infusions carefully. Several of the drugs used to treat hyperkalemia are incompatible. Calcium and bicarbonate solutions should not be placed in the same intravenous line because Ca salts will precipitate out of solution. At least two intravenous lines should be maintained for emergency drug therapy in the hyperkalemic patient.

Calcium

Calcium, phosphate (P), and magnesium have important roles in bone structure, neuromuscular transmission, and regulation of many enzyme systems. These three electrolytes are maintained in balance by a careful coupling of intestinal absorption and renal excretion. Calcium and magnesium are divalent cations that are also secreted by the intestine in digestive fluids.

Calcium plays an important role in the following body functions: (1) bone structure, (2) neuromuscular transmission, (3) secretions of exocrine and endocrine glands, (4) cardiac action potential, (5) regulation of many enzyme systems, and (6) blood clotting and activation of the complement system.

Calcium is believed to bind with proteins in cellular Na channels, thereby closing the Na channels in the cell membrane after depolarization has occurred. This allows the cell membrane to repolarize and return to its resting membrane potential (Guyton, 1991). When a stimulus of sufficient magnitude occurs, Ca ions are displaced, sodium enters the cell, and depolarization begins. This process is of particular importance in tissues requiring repetitive rhythmic discharge such as the heart. Calcium is an essential participant in cardiac conduction and contractility.

Calcium is also vital to the secretory activity of many endocrine and exocrine glandular cells through the process of stimulus-secretion coupling. Moreover, calcium is a regulator of various enzyme activities within cells. It is essential to many cAMP–mediated responses.

Calcium plays a number of roles in blood coagulation. It is essential in the formation of prothrombin activator. Calcium also interacts with fibrin-stabilizing factor (Factor XIII) to convert the fibrin strands into a stable clot.

Because of its significant contribution to these important functions, Ca concentration is maintained within narrow limits in both the IC and EC compartments. The normal plasma Ca level is 9 to 10.5 mg/dL (4.5 to 5.25 mEq/liter). Calcium exists in the plasma as two separate fractions—40% of plasma calcium is protein bound, primarily to albumin, and 50% exists as an ionized or active fraction. The remainder of total plasma calcium is complexed with other ions such as citrate or phosphate. There is a difference between total serum calcium and the ionized Ca concentration. Direct measurement of the ionized or active fraction of calcium is not routinely performed because of technical difficulties. However, the ionized Ca fraction is an important parameter because this is the free calcium that is physiologically relevant.

If the ionized Ca value is not available it may be necessary to analyze the total calcium in relation to albumin level before a decision to treat the patient is made. The following formula will allow for a more accurate accounting of the Ca level:

$$\text{Correct calcium} = \text{total calcium} + 0.8(4.0 - \text{albumin})$$

The level of plasma proteins also plays a role in determining total serum Ca concentration. Any state associated with increased albumin will increase total calcium. Hypoalbuminemia produces the opposite effect. Protein binding of calcium is reversible and may be affected by blood pH and PTH.

Regulation of calcium is multifactorial. Intestinal absorption of calcium is under the influence of vitamin D-1,25. Renal excretion of calcium is influenced by both PTH and serum Ca levels. Bone deposition and resorption are regulated by vitamin D, PTH, and serum phosphorus levels.

Under normal conditions, constant bone formation and resorption lead to little net change in serum Ca concentration. However, when either the intake or excretion pathways are disturbed, bone acts as a reservoir to stabilize serum Ca levels. PTH in concert with vitamin D-1,25 can change the rate of bone resorption. High levels of PTH increase the liberation of calcium from the skeleton. Alterations in the bioavailability of either PTH or vitamin D-1,25 subsequently affect the utilization of bone as a source of calcium.

Renal regulation of Ca balance is accomplished through reabsorption in the proximal tubule. Final regulation of renal Ca excretion occurs in the distal nephron under the influence of PTH. There is a direct relationship between PTH and Ca reabsorption. As serum PTH levels increase, renal Ca reabsorption increases. It should be noted that clinical disorders that affect Na transport tend to affect Ca transport in a similar direction. Metabolic acidosis promotes Ca excretion by the kidney, whereas alkalosis leads to Ca conservation. Diuretics also influence Ca excretion depending on the site of action. Furosemide, ethacrynic acid, and osmotic diuretics inhibit Na reabsorption and thus force excretion of both sodium and calcium. Thiazide diuretics result in decreased renal excretion of calcium.

HYPOCALCEMIA

Hypocalcemia is defined as a plasma Ca level of less than 9 mg/dL (4.5 mEq/liter). The primary causes of hypocalcemia are shown in Table 43–15. In many of these states, there is a defect in either PTH or vitamin D-1,25. The normal synergistic relationship between PTH and vitamin D cannot compensate for this defect. As described earlier, low serum albumin affects the fraction of calcium bound to protein, thus lowering the total serum Ca level. However, this state may have lit-

TABLE 43–15. **Etiology and Clinical Manifestations of Hypocalcemia**

Etiology	Clinical Findings
Hypoalbuminemia	Neuromuscular
Parathyroid dysfunction	Tetany
Hypoparathyroidism	Seizures
Surgical excision	Muscle cramps
Idiopathic	Weakness
Pseudohypoparathyroidism	Cardiovascular
Hypomagnesemia	Hypotension
Vitamin D abnormalities	Electrocardiographic changes
Malnutrition/malabsorption	Shortened QT interval
Liver disease with decreased production of 25(OH) D	Neurologic or cognitive
Drugs—increased metabolism of 25(OH) D	Cognitive impairment
Nephrotic syndrome—increased loss of 25(OH) D	Affective disorders
Renal failure—decreased production of 1,25-vitamin D	
Excessive removal of calcium	
Hyperphosphatemia	
Acute pancreatitis	
Rapid bone formation	
Massive transfusion of citrated blood	

tle clinical effect if the biologically important ionized fraction is normal.

Hypoparathyroidism is one of the common causes of hypocalcemia. Hypoparathyroidism may be the result of trauma or of surgical removal or injury to the parathyroid gland during neck or thyroid surgery. Idiopathic hypoparathyroidism may occur at any time in life but is most common in childhood or adolescence. True hypoparathyroidism is manifested by low PTH levels. Pseudohypoparathyroidism, in contrast, is characterized by normal circulating PTH levels and an inadequate tissue response to the hormone. In critically ill patients, hypocalcemia is frequently associated with hypomagnesemia. Hypomagnesemia is most often caused by inadequate magnesium content in total parenteral nutrition (TPN), although it can also result from prolonged diarrhea or renal Mg wasting. Hypomagnesemia is generally thought to be responsible for depressing PTH secretion. It may also decrease the responsiveness of bone to PTH action.

As described earlier, vitamin D-1,25 enhances absorption of dietary calcium as well as the effect of PTH on bone. Abnormalities in the chain of vitamin D metabolism and its transformation to the active form can affect these important processes and produce hypocalcemia. Vitamin D abnormalities include inadequate intake of this vitamin. Although this cause is uncommon in the general population, it must be considered in critically ill patients who may be NPO or on clear liquid diets for long periods of time. In addition, clinical states such as partial gastrectomy, pancreatitis, and intestinal resection may be associated with malabsorption, which also contributes to a vitamin D-1,25 deficiency. Also common in critically ill patients are vitamin D abnormalities resulting from disturbances in conversion of the vitamin to its intermediate and active forms. Liver dysfunction may impair conversion of vitamin D to the intermediate form because of a lack of bile salts. Anticonvulsant drugs, such as phenobarbital and phenytoin, may increase metabolism of the intermediate form to inactive metabolites, which then cannot undergo renal conversion to the active form. Nephrotic syndrome may cause increased excretion of the intermediate form. Acute or chronic renal failure renders the kidney incapable of converting the intermediate form to the biologically active vitamin D-1,25. Renal failure is accompanied by metabolic acidosis, which also may adversely affect the metabolism of vitamin D. The consequence of these pathologic states is decreased intestinal absorption of calcium and altered bone deposition and resorption, leading to hypocalcemia.

Abnormalities in P excretion can also result in hypocalcemia. Excessive removal of calcium from the serum may be the consequence of hyperphosphatemia. Mechanisms in this situation may include impaired conversion of vitamin D-1,25, extravascular calcification resulting from the phosphate–calcium complexes, and reduced bone resorption. These mechanisms occur most often in the presence of an acute rise in serum phosphorus. Acute hyperphosphatemia may occur following acute ingestion of phosphate or administration of multiple phosphate enemas. Acute phosphatemia also occurs in rhabdomyolysis, when damaged muscle cells release intracellular phosphate ions into the blood.

Hypocalcemia is seen in conjunction with acute pancreatitis, although the exact mechanism is not known. It is believed that Ca ions combine with fatty acids, released from areas of lipolysis and fat necrosis, to form soaps. Elevated levels of glucagon may also play a role. The reduction in total serum Ca level occurs at the expense of the ionized fraction. Severe hypocalcemia ($<$7 mg/dL) in patients with acute pancreatitis is not common and is associated with a poor prognosis.

Rapid bone formation can also produce hypocalcemia. This condition may appear after correction of hyperparathyroidism, thyrotoxicosis, or nutritional rickets. In these situations, calcium is rapidly restored to the bone to replace that resorbed during the pathologic state.

Binding of calcium by citrate can cause hypocalcemia in critically ill patients who have received massive blood transfusions ($>$6 to 8 units in 24 hours). This is a particular problem in patients with liver dysfunction because liver disease causes decreased metabolism of citrate.

Hypocalcemia may be seen in AIDS related to HIV nephropathy, in renal dysfunction secondary to anti-HIV therapy, or as a consequence of HIV-related malabsorption resulting in the deficiency of vitamin D and calcium (Grinspoon & Bilezikian, 1992). Cytomegalovirus and *Mycobacterium* may directly infect the parathyroid glands, although there has been no clinical evidence of parathyroid dysfunction. Ketoconazole therapy for fungal infections may be associated with hypocalcemia by interfering with the generation of calcitriol by virtue of its inhibitory effects on α_1-hydroxylase activity. Foscarnet, an agent used for cytomegalovirus infection, may decrease serum ionized Ca levels and result in symptomatic hypocalcemia (Ahmed & Jaspan, 1993).

The physiologic manifestations of hypocalcemia are shown in Table 43–15. The most common manifestations are expressed as neuromuscular irritability. Characteristic clinical findings include stiffness, muscle spasms, and cramps. These findings are seen most often in the hand, with carpopedal spasm. More serious complications of laryngeal stridor and respiratory muscle spasm may compromise respiratory effort.

Tetany is described as intermittent tonic spasms. Tetany can occur at variable levels of serum Ca deficiency, depending on coexisting conditions such as alkalosis and hypomagnesemia. However, this neuromuscular manifestation usually occurs when serum Ca level is below 7 to 7.5 mg/dL. Tetany may be elicited by tapping over the facial nerve to produce twitching (Chvostek sign) or by prolonged blood pressure cuff inflation (>3 min) to elicit carpopedal spasm (Trousseau sign). These diagnostic signs may not be present in all hypocalcemic patients. Seizures of any magnitude may be an early sign of disordered serum Ca level. Muscle cramps occur as a consequence of the tetany.

Cardiovascular manifestations of hypocalcemia include hypotension and decreased myocardial contractility. ECG changes include a characteristic increase in the QT interval, which reflects a delay in ventricular repolarization. In contrast to hypokalemia, hypocalcemia usually does not cause ST depression. If hyperkalemia is present, which is frequently the case in critically ill patients with acute renal failure, the T waves may be peaked.

Cognitive and affective disorders may accompany hypocalcemia. Anxiety, lethargy, depression, confusion, and overt psychosis may be seen. These acute changes can be reversed with Ca replacement. Mental retardation may be a sequela of chronic hypocalcemia in children.

MANAGEMENT OF HYPOCALCEMIA. The correction of hypocalcemia includes fluid management as well as administration of calcium-containing medications. A complete evaluation to elicit the underlying cause of the disorder is also required and will help to guide treatment. A history of neck surgery, anticonvulsant therapy, or familial occurrence of hypoparathyroidism is valuable in helping to determine the etiology. In addition, laboratory assessment of serum albumin, Mg, and P levels is useful in the diagnostic process. Each 1 g/dL reduction in serum albumin produces a decrement of approximately 0.7 mg/dL in total serum Ca concentration. Hypomagnesemia (<0.8 mEq/liter) may prove to be the cause of hypocalcemia. Serum P level may provide additional information, although its concentration is dependent on PTH levels in the absence of renal failure.

Severe acute hypocalcemia may present with serious cardiac and neuromuscular complications that require prompt and aggressive therapy with intravenous calcium. Solutions available for use include calcium gluconate and calcium chloride. Calcium gluconate is preferred because calcium chloride is known to produce thrombophlebitis and tissue necrosis should it infiltrate into the extravascular space. It should be noted that standard preparations of calcium chloride contain four times as much calcium as an equal volume of calcium gluconate. The rate of Ca infusion should not exceed 50 mg/min. A total dose of 2 g should not be exceeded without a repeat measurement of the serum Ca level. Continued correction of serum Ca level requires slow Ca infusion and careful monitoring of serum Ca levels.

Magnesium repletion may also be required to treat hypocalcemia. The presence of renal failure is a contraindication to Mg administration unless severe hypomagnesemia exists.

If onset of hypocalcemia is slower, such as that occurring after parathyroid surgery, acute intravenous administration of calcium may still be necessary. However, if the patient is able to take oral medications, further Ca restoration may be accomplished with oral agents in combination with phosphorus restriction. If vitamin D deficiency is the underlying cause of hypocalcemia, vitamin D supplementation may be useful.

POTENTIAL FOR INJURY. Acute symptomatic hypocalcemia is a medical emergency requiring immediate nursing attention. In addition to assisting the physician in monitoring and correcting the serum Ca deficit, nursing care is directed toward preventing patient injury due to seizures or airway obstruction.

Because hypocalcemia increases the irritability of the CNS, the hypocalcemic patient is at risk of developing seizures. The critical care nurse assesses the patient for signs and symptoms of neuromuscular irritability. Specific assessments include patient complaints of numbness or tingling in the digits, muscle cramps, and the presence of the Chvostek or Trousseau signs. In addition, the nurse observes the patient for changes in mentation, mood, and memory. If hypocalcemia is severe or if the patient demonstrates neuromuscular irritability, seizure precautions are instituted.

In addition to the risk of injury from the disease process itself, the hypocalcemic patient is also at risk of injury from therapy with intravenous medications. Ca solutions are not compatible with bicarbonate-containing fluids. When mixed, precipitation of Ca salts will occur. Ca infusions should be accompanied by careful ECG monitoring. During the infusion, the nurse closely monitors the patient for the onset of ventricular irritability or heart block. If either of these cardiac changes occurs, the infusion should be immediately stopped.

IMPAIRED BREATHING PATTERN. Among the life-threatening consequences of severe hypocalcemia are laryngospasm, airway obstruction, and respiratory arrest. The critical care nurse carefully assesses the patient's airway status for evidence of spasm or obstruction. The patient is observed for restlessness, tachypnea, and subtle arterial blood gas changes. These early signs are followed by inspiratory stridor, hoarseness, and decreased air movement. The nurse prepares for the possibility of airway obstruction by assembling emergency airway equipment and preparing for possible intubation.

HYPERCALCEMIA

Hypercalcemia can be classified as mild (<12 mg/dL), moderate (12 to 15 mg/dL), or severe (>15 mg/dL). The causes of hypercalcemia are listed in Table 43–16 and can be categorized as either increased gut absorption or increased bone resorption. The two most common causes of hypercalcemia are malignancy and hyperparathyroidism. The incidence in each category may differ as a function of age, with malignancy a more common cause in the older patient. Bony metastatic lesions are thought to be responsible for most cases of malignancy-related hypercalcemia. The major types of primary malignancy associated with bony metastases and hypercalcemia are breast and lung cancer, multiple myeloma, lymphoma, and renal cell carcinoma (Hall & Burns-Schaiff, 1993). Granulomatous disorders such as sarcoidosis, tuberculosis, histoplasmosis, and coccidioidomycosis can also produce hypercalcemia.

Primary hyperparathyroidism is a major cause of hypercalcemia. The pathogenesis of this disorder remains unknown, although many patients have a past history of head and neck radiation. Primary hyperparathyroidism may also occur in conjunction with a more generalized syndrome of tumors in various endocrine organs. Hypercalcemia may occasionally occur in the presence of endocrine disturbances such as hyperthyroidism, acromegaly, and adrenal insufficiency. Prolonged immobilization, particularly following severe trauma with multiple fractures or spinal cord injury with paralysis, may lead to an increase in bone resorption. This heavy load of calcium exceeds the kidney's regulatory capacity, resulting in hypercalcemia.

Patients with a markedly increased intake of calcium through milk products and antacids for ulcer therapy may exhibit hypercalcemia. Preexisting renal failure is a necessary prerequisite for this mechanism to produce hypercalcemia. The role of alkalosis due to ingested antacids may also be a cofactor because it promotes renal reabsorption of calcium. Vitamin D intoxication will lead to increased intestinal absorption of calcium as well as bone resorption, and hypercalcemia may be a consequence.

Administration of thiazide diuretics may be associated with hypercalcemia. This is usually expressed as a transient elevation in serum Ca concentration, which reflects volume contraction and increased plasma protein as a result of hemoconcentration. If these drugs are used in patients with coexisting disease processes, which tend to increase serum Ca values, significant hypercalcemia may result.

Recovery of renal function via transplantation has been associated with hypercalcemia, probably because the prolonged hypocalcemia that occurs during chronic renal failure often leads to secondary hyperparathyroidism. With successful renal transplantation, it takes a variable period of time for the body to reset PTH secretion.

Hypercalcemia is also seen during the diuretic phase of acute renal failure. The exact mechanism is not known but may be correlated with the extent and severity of muscle damage associated with rhabdomyolysis.

Acute hypercalcemic crisis may produce acute renal failure and a markedly depressed sensorium, a situation that represents a medical emergency. In general, hypercalcemia causes decreased neuromuscular excitability or muscle hypotonicity. The various clinical manifestations associated with hypercalcemia are shown in Table 43–16. The cardiac changes are the most specific indicator of hypercalcemia; both contractility and conduction changes are observed. Shortening of the QT interval is considered the most characteristic sign of hypercalcemia; however, it is not present in all hypercalcemic patients. In hypercalcemic crisis, the S and T waves merge. Other arrhythmias associated with hypercalcemia include varying degrees of heart block and cardiac arrest. Hypercalcemia also increases the patient's susceptibility to digitalis toxicity.

Renal tubular nephropathy is a relatively common occurrence and is related to the degree of serum Ca

TABLE 43–16. **Etiology and Clinical Manifestations of Hypercalcemia**

Etiology	Clinical Findings
Malignancy	Cardiovascular
Breast	Positive inotropic effects
Lung	Increased myocardial contractility
Multiple myeloma	Decreased heart rate
Lymphoma	Shortened systolic time interval
Renal	Shortened ventricular ejection time
Granulomatous disorders	Conduction abnormalities
Endocrine disorders	Shortened QT interval
Primary hyperparathyroidism	Widened T wave
Thyrotoxicosis	Metastatic calcifications in cardiovascular system
Acromegaly	Gastrointestinal
Immobilization	Anorexia
Milk-alkali syndrome	Nausea, vomiting
Excess vitamin D	Constipation
Thiazide diuretic administration	Renal
Renal failure	Acute renal insufficiency
	Nephrolithiasis
	Metastatic calcifications
	Neurologic
	Confusion
	Stupor
	Coma

elevation. Calcification of cellular debris within the renal tubules leads to tubular obstruction and renal failure. This renal damage is frequently reversed when therapy is initiated. Renal calculi formation may occur in patients with chronic hypercalcemic states such as hyperparathyroidism.

Widespread soft tissue calcification can be a serious complication of chronic hypercalcemia. Calcifications are more common in the presence of hyperphosphatemia and chronic renal failure.

MANAGEMENT OF HYPERCALCEMIA. A serum Ca level of greater than 15 mg/dL combined with stupor or coma represents a hypercalcemic crisis and requires prompt treatment. Management efforts are directed toward determining the underlying cause of the hypercalcemia and instituting therapy to lower the serum Ca level. Diagnostic efforts to identify hyperparathyroidism include measurement of immunoreactive PTH levels. The presence of an elevated PTH level tends to support hyperparathyroidism as the cause. A history of neoplastic disease is an important clue to the presence of malignancy-associated hypercalcemia.

In moderate or severe hypercalcemia, prompt reduction of serum Ca concentration is essential. The most important factor in treating hypercalcemia is to ensure adequate hydration (Carroll & Oh, 1989). The polyuria, nausea, and vomiting common with hypercalcemia cause volume depletion, which further decreases the glomerular filtration and excretion of calcium. Administration of 1 to 2 liters of 0.9% sodium chloride is recommended. If symptoms persist after rehydration, a forced saline diuresis can further reduce serum Na level. Furosemide (80–100 mg every 1–2 hours IV) decreases Ca reabsorption in the loop of Henle. Volume and electrolyte replacement (especially potassium and magnesium) must continue throughout this aggressive diuretic therapy. If renal function is good, 6 to 12 liters of intravenous fluid can be administered over 24 hours. Usually 0.9% to 0.45% sodium chloride is infused because this solution promotes excretion of both sodium and calcium. Dextrose 5% may be used if the patient is hypernatremic or has CHF. Intravenous administration of furosemide every 4 to 6 hours will prevent fluid volume overload (Carroll & Oh, 1989).

Reduction of bone resorption can be achieved through administration of pharmaceutical agents. Administration of glucocorticoids has been useful in decreasing bone resorption and may also decrease gut absorption of calcium. Calcitonin is useful when a rapid response to therapy is required. It decreases bone resorption and increases renal excretion of calcium. A dose of 4 IU/kg subcutaneously or intramuscularly achieves a response within a few hours and may be repeated every 12 hours and increased every 1 to 2 days to a maximum of 8 IU/kg every 6 hours. It often loses its effectiveness after 2 to 6 days, possibly due to antibody formation. An allergic reaction could occur, so a test dose is recommended. Nausea and vomiting are potential side effects. Plicamycin (Mithracin) is an antineoplastic antibiotic that inhibits response of osteoclasts to PTH. A dose of 25 μg/kg IV is given every day for 3 to 4 days. It should be given slowly over 4 to 6 hours to decrease the risk of thrombophlebitis. The hypocalcemic effect begins within the first 48 hours and may last for 3 to 15 days. Other side effects include thrombocytopenia, increased bleeding tendency, leukopenia, nausea, and vomiting. Gallium nitrate is absorbed into the bone and provides a direct, dose-dependent resistance to osteoclast activity that produces hypocalcemia primarily by inhibition of bone resorption. The dose is 200 mg/m^2 every day for 5 days as a continuous infusion. Adequate urine output is necessary before gallium nitrate is started and should continue at 2 liters/day during treatment. It should be discontinued if the serum creatinine exceeds 2.5 mg/mL. Etidronate disodium is a biphosphonate that lowers serum Ca level by adsorbing onto the surface of the bone matrix and rendering it more resistant to osteoclastic resorption. This drug has been associated with nephrotoxicity (Healey, 1993).

Intravenous administration of phosphate causes Ca complex formation, which is a rapid method of lowering serum Ca levels. Unfortunately, this method is associated with significant risk. The complex of calcium and phosphate that is formed is usually deposited at extravascular sites and can result in renal failure or sudden death. Oral phosphate is generally considered a safer approach in patients who are not hyperphosphatemic.

Hemodialysis with a dialysate low in calcium is the most efficient way to correct serum Ca concentration, particularly in patients with renal insufficiency. Severe hypercalcemia from hyperparathyroidism can usually be alleviated by surgery.

Mild hypercalcemia may not require major intervention, such as volume expansion with diuretics or agents inhibiting bone resorption. Alleviation of the underlying process may restore serum Ca levels to normal or near-normal values without aggressive intervention.

ALTERED URINARY ELIMINATION AND POTENTIAL FLUID VOLUME EXCESS. Severe hypercalcemia (serum Ca levels of greater than 15 mg/dL accompanied by neurologic or cardiac complications) requires prompt and aggressive treatment. The critical care nurse collaborates in lowering the serum Ca level by administering prescribed fluids and medications. The goals of nursing care include preventing calcium-induced renal insufficiency while maintaining optimal fluid balance.

The primary treatment for severe hypercalcemia is to enhance renal excretion of calcium by administering large volumes of intravenous fluid along with diuretics. The critical care nurse facilitates fluid administration by ensuring that intravenous access is adequate. At least two large-bore intravenous lines are necessary because fluid administration may need to be as high as 500 mL/hr. Urine volumes are assessed hourly, and careful intake and output records are maintained. The BUN and serum creatinine are monitored for elevations indicating renal tubular damage.

While promoting Ca excretion, the critical care nurse must also assess the patient's cardiovascular response to the large fluid load. The patient's hemodynamic parameters, including CVP, PAWP, blood pressure, heart rate, and cardiac output, are monitored frequently for evidence of impending CHF. The jugular veins are observed for distension, and the lungs are auscultated for the development of rales or crackles.

ALTERATION IN CARDIAC OUTPUT. Hypertension is one cardiovascular change that the nurse should anticipate in hypercalcemia. Elevated blood pressure may be partially the result of renal insufficiency; however, it is also seen in patients with normal renal function. It is thought that calcium increases peripheral resistance as well as exerting a positive inotropic effect on the cardiac muscle.

Hypercalcemia is also associated with a number of cardiac dysrhythmias that can adversely affect cardiac output. The critical care nurse carefully monitors the patient's ECG. The PR, QRS, and QT intervals are measured and evaluated for change. If heart block does occur, the nurse evaluates the patient's response by assessing the available hemodynamic parameters as well as the patient's level of consciousness.

Hypercalcemia potentiates the effect of digitalis. The digitalized patient must be carefully observed for signs of digitalis toxicity.

Cardiac standstill may occur at serum Ca levels greater than 17 mg/dL. The nurse anticipates this emergency by keeping resuscitation equipment and medications readily available.

Phosphate

Phosphorus is one of the principal IC anions and in the body is found as organic and inorganic P salts, the latter form occurring in small amounts in EC water and blood. Normal serum P values range from 2.5 to 4.5 mg/dL, whereas the IC concentration may be as much as 300 mg/dL.

Phosphate plays a number of important roles in the body. It is a structural element of bone. In fact, approximately 85% of total body phosphate is found in bone. Phosphate is the major IC anion and plays a role in the metabolism of lipids, carbohydrates, and proteins. As a component of ATP, phosphate is essential to oxidative phosphorylation, the main energy source of muscle tissue. It is also a critical component of 2,3-diphosphoglycerate (2,3-DPG), and is therefore involved in oxygen delivery to peripheral tissues. Phosphate is also a participant in one of the major renal buffering mechanisms controlling acid-base balance in the body.

Phosphate balance is maintained by dietary intake and by urinary and gastrointestinal losses. Protein is a significant source of phosphorus, particularly dairy products. There is little direct regulation of gastrointestinal absorption, so the major influence on body P content is the kidney. Renal excretion of phosphate is influenced by the plasma P concentration and by PTH. Under normal circumstances, as plasma P concentration rises, renal excretion increases. PTH also increases P excretion by the kidney and is accepted as the major factor controlling renal excretion of phosphate. PTH as well as vitamin D-1,25 shifts phosphate from bone to EC water as a consequence of Ca homeostatic mechanisms (Carroll & Oh, 1989). Because the EC concentration is so small, a shift of phosphate across the cell membrane can have a significant effect on EC concentration. Acid-base disturbances also affect the transcellular distribution of phosphate.

HYPOPHOSPHATEMIA

Hypophosphatemia can occur as a consequence of the events described in Table 43–17. Serum P concentrations of less than 1.0 mg/dL are classified as profound hypophosphatemia. Reduced intake alone is rarely the reason for hypophosphatemia of this magnitude because renal excretion can compensate for low intake. Phosphate-binding antacids, such as aluminum hydroxide, bind with phosphate in the gut to decrease absorption and force elimination through the gastrointestinal tract. Vitamin D-1,25 deficiency results in decreased gastrointestinal absorption of phosphate and causes some renal tubular dysfunction, which impairs P reabsorption. In addition, lack of vitamin D retards movement of phosphate from bone to the EC fluid. Malabsorption due to gastrointestinal disease may produce hypophosphatemia. This clinical problem causes a decrease in both vitamin D and Ca absorption and leads to secondary hyperparathyroidism, which in turn leads to increased renal excretion of phosphate.

Increased renal excretion of phosphate can be the consequence of either intrarenal or extrarenal mechanisms. Fanconi syndrome and vitamin D-resistant rickets are intrinsic renal disorders that produce tubu-

TABLE 43–17. **Etiology and Clinical Manifestations of Hypophosphatemia**

Etiology	Clinical Findings
Decreased phosphate intake	Neurologic
Anorexia, starvation	Confusion
Vomiting	Irritability
Decreased gastrointestinal absorption	Obtundation
Phosphate-binding antacids	Seizures
Vitamin D deficiency	Coma
Malabsorption syndromes	Musculoskeletal
Diarrhea	Myopathy
Increased renal phosphate excretion	Weakness
Hyperparathyroidism	Bone pain
Osmotic diuresis (drug-induced or diabetic ketoacidosis)	Bone resorption
Metabolic acidosis	Hematopoietic
Transcellular redistribution	Hemolysis
Acute respiratory alkalosis	Platelet dysfunction
Glucose infusion	Impaired resistance to infection
Insulin administration	
Total parenteral nutrition without phosphate	
Rapid anabolism	

lar transport abnormalities. Extrarenal factors that promote renal wasting of phosphate include hyperparathyroidism, glucosuria, some diuretics, and acute expansion of EC volume. Hyperparathyroidism, either primary or secondary, causes a decrease in renal tubular reabsorption of phosphate. Glucosuria (e.g., in diabetic ketoacidosis) produces an osmotic diuresis that also limits P reabsorption in the kidney. Acute EC volume expansion increases urine flow through the renal tubules, thereby decreasing P reabsorption. Factors that may promote a redistribution of phosphate from the EC to the IC compartment include respiratory alkalosis, glucose infusion, and insulin administration. Hypophosphatemia associated with acute alkalosis is the result of rapid movement of hydrogen ion from the IC space. The cellular response is to increase glycolysis, which results in a shift of phosphate from the EC space into the IC space. Critically ill patients at risk of developing hypophosphatemia from acute alkalosis include those with heatstroke, acute salicylate poisoning, alcohol withdrawal, and thyrotoxicosis.

Administration of intravenous glucose may be the most common cause of hypophosphatemia in hospitalized patients. Administration of glucose, along with endogenous or exogenous insulin, facilitates the transport of both glucose and phosphate into skeletal muscle and liver cells. This response may be particularly severe in the malnourished alcoholic patient. Another common cause of hypophosphatemia in critical care patients is the administration of TPN without an adequate P content.

Phosphate is an ubiquitous electrolyte; a deficiency in serum or body stores is reflected in multisystem abnormalities. The two primary mechanisms through which cellular processes are disturbed by hypophosphatemia are (1) impairment of cellular synthesis of ATP, and (2) decreased amount of red cell 2,3-DPG, which adversely affects oxygen release in the tissues. Thus, energy for cell functions and processes is reduced. The primary manifestations of hypophosphatemia are shown in Table 43–17 and reflect the disordered cellular functions that result from hypophosphatemia. Signs and symptoms are usually not present unless severe hypophosphatemia is present (<1.5 mg/dL). The muscular abnormality associated with ATP depletion may be severe enough to compromise respiratory effort. Myocardial function may also be affected, as manifested by decreased stroke volume and possible development of congestive cardiomyopathy.

A variety of hematologic derangements may occur as a result of hypophosphatemia and may cause significant problems in critically ill patients. Decreased 2,3-DPG levels may result in reduced oxygen delivery to peripheral tissues. Tissue anoxia is manifested by pain and a buildup of lactic acid. Low ATP levels in the erythrocytes lead to red blood cell fragility and hemolytic anemia. Impaired leukocyte function places the patient at increased risk of infection.

Bone resorption and development of bone disease are associated with total body P depletion. With erosion of the skeleton, calcium and magnesium will also be released, resulting in increased Ca and Mg excretion by the kidney.

MANAGEMENT OF HYPOPHOSPHATEMIA. Management of hypophosphatemia includes identification of the etiology and repletion of P stores. If possible, the underlying cause of hypophosphatemia should be identified and corrected. Urine P concentration may be helpful in determining the cause. A high urine P concentration in the presence of low serum P levels indicates an intrinsic renal disturbance or elevated PTH secretion. If urinary losses are in accord with the measured serum P concentration then problems with gastrointestinal absorption or EC distribution are the likely cause. Phosphate administration may not be necessary if the underlying problem is corrected.

The presence of severe neurologic or muscle disturbances necessitates P supplementation. As with hypocalcemia, intravenous administration of phosphate may lead to soft tissue deposition of calcium–phosphate complexes. Oral administration is less likely to lead to untoward effects. However, intravenous administration of phosphate may be the only route available in the critically ill patient. Intravenous phosphate must be diluted and administered slowly. Careful monitoring of the patient as well as serial serum P measurements is necessary. Regardless of the route of administration, P repletion is usually continued only until the serum P level reaches 2.5 to 3.0 mg/dL. Rapid elevation of the serum P level can result in hypocalcemia.

IMPAIRED BREATHING PATTERN. When caring for the hypophosphatemic patient, the critical care nurse must keep in mind that the pathologic manifestations result from decreased levels of ATP and 2,3-DPG. Particular attention must be paid to problems associated with muscle weakness and those related to diminished peripheral tissue oxygenation.

Weakness of the muscles of respiration is a particular nursing concern in the hypophosphatemic patient. The nurse assesses the patient for changes in muscle strength. Hand-grasp strength can be tested to determine general muscle strength. More specifically, changes in the patient's speech may be indicative of muscle weakness. Particular attention is paid to assessment of muscle strength in patients with chronic obstructive pulmonary disease (COPD) who utilize accessory breathing muscles. The nurse should carefully monitor the rate and quality of respirations in these patients. Changes in the patient's sensorium are evaluated in light of the potential for hypoventilation. Arterial blood gases are monitored for a rising $Paco_2$.

The hypophosphatemic patient may lack sufficient respiratory muscle strength to be weaned from mechanical ventilation. Repletion of the serum P concentration and careful evaluation of respiratory muscle function should be done before weaning and extubation.

DECREASED PERIPHERAL TISSUE PERFUSION. The decrease in 2,3-DPG results in peripheral tissue anoxia.

This condition is manifested by muscle weakness, fatigue, and pain. The skin and muscles may be very tender to the touch. The patient may complain of extreme fatigue and muscle pain resulting from such nursing care activities as turning, range of motion exercises, and transferring from bed to chair.

Nursing goals are to reduce the oxygen requirements of peripheral tissues and promote the patient's comfort. The patient's physical activity is reduced to the level of the essential. Adequate rest periods are scheduled. Comfort measures, including patient positioning and analgesics, are administered. These interventions may need to continue for several days following serum P repletion because the clinical manifestations of severe hypophosphatemia do not immediately resolve.

HYPERPHOSPHATEMIA

Hyperphosphatemia (P > 4.5 mg/dL) represents a breakdown in the normal regulatory process, either through an acute increase in EC phosphate concentration or as a consequence of renal dysfunction. The causes of hyperphosphatemia are listed in Table 43–18. Oral intake of phosphate is unlikely to produce elevation of the serum P level because the kidney quickly responds by decreasing P reabsorption. The chronic use of phosphate-containing laxatives or administration of phosphate enemas in a susceptible individual may produce hyperphosphatemia. Severely injured patients may be at risk of hyperphosphatemia. Rhabdomyolysis liberates a large amount of phosphate into the EC fluid, and if renal failure is present, marked serum P elevation may occur. Cytotoxic drugs used to treat leukemia may cause hyperphosphatemia as a result of cell lysis. These clinical situations reflect a shift of phosphate from the IC to the EC compartment rather than an increase in total P load. Acidosis also encourages a transcellular shift of phosphate. Phosphate ions are released from the cell as a result of tissue hypoxia and ATP degradation.

Decreased renal excretion of phosphate is most often the result of hypoparathyroidism. This hormonal disorder is characterized by elevated serum P level, hypocalcemia, and chronic tetany. PTH levels are usually depressed but may be elevated if tissue resistance to the hormone is present. Hypoparathyroidism may occur following neck surgery, most commonly for removal of the parathyroid glands or the thyroid.

TABLE 43–18. **Etiology and Clinical Manifestations of Hyperphosphatemia**

Etiology	Clinical Findings
Increased phosphate load	Neuromuscular
Phosphate enemas	Tetany
Oral phosphate supplementation	Seizures
	Muscle cramps
Rhabdomyolysis	Weakness
Cytotoxic drugs	Cardiovascular
Decreased phosphate excretion	Hypotension
Hypoparathyroidism	Shortened QT interval
Renal insufficiency	Neurologic/cognitive
	Cognitive impairment
	Affective disorders

Renal insufficiency leads to reduced renal excretion of phosphate. In chronic renal failure, hyperphosphatemia tends to occur after 75% of renal function has been lost. Patients with acute renal failure may have more severe episodes of hyperphosphatemia, possibly related to the cause of the acute renal failure (e.g., rhabdomyolysis), in concert with decreased renal excretion. Fortunately, hyperphosphatemia quickly resolves once renal function returns.

The clinical manifestations of hyperphosphatemia are related to the hypocalcemia that frequently accompanies this disorder. Signs and symptoms are more likely to occur when the increase in serum P level occurs rapidly. Soft tissue calcifications occur when the Ca × P product exceeds 70. Calcium–phosphate complex deposition most commonly occurs in the aorta, kidneys, lungs, conjunctiva, and skin. Such deposits may produce other clinical complications such as hypoxia and renal failure.

MANAGEMENT OF HYPERPHOSPHATEMIA. Treatment of hyperphosphatemia is directed toward correction of the underlying pathophysiologic mechanisms and removal of phosphate from the circulation. Phosphate can be removed by dietary restriction of P intake, and the use of phosphate binders to bind intestinal phosphate. In the critically ill patient these methods may not be appropriate. Acute dialysis is often the best method of lowering serum P levels in the critically ill patient.

Careful and judicious monitoring of serum P level during the treatment of *hypo*phosphatemia can help to avoid *hyper*phosphatemia. Maintaining adequate urine volumes through the use of intravenous fluids and diuretics is helpful in preventing hyperphosphatemia in patients at risk.

IMPAIRED TISSUE INTEGRITY. Because serum phosphate and calcium have a reciprocal relationship, hyperphosphatemia is often associated with hypocalcemia. For this reason, the nursing assessments and interventions described for the hypocalcemic patient are also appropriate for the patient with elevated serum P concentration. The critical care nurse is concerned with assessing soft tissue calcification and maintaining tissue integrity.

Pruritus is frequently associated with calcium–phosphate complex deposition in the skin. This may represent a significant problem in the already compromised integument of the critically ill patient. Uncontrolled patient scratching may lead to skin breakdown and infection. The nurse observes for signs of scratching and inspects the skin for areas of breakdown.

A variety of skin care protocols are available to promote patient comfort and protect skin integrity. The patient's fingernails should be clipped short. If pruritus is particularly severe, sedation may be helpful.

Magnesium

Magnesium is an abundant IC cation, although the normal serum concentration is only 1.5 to 2.5 mEq/liter (1.6 to 2.2 mg/dL). Sixty percent of total body magnesium is found in the bone, which serves as a source for exchange with the plasma; 55% to 60% of plasma magnesium is in the ionized form, which is the physiologically active fraction, and 17% is complexed with other compounds such as citrate, phosphate, and bicarbonate. The remaining 25% is protein bound, primarily to albumin. This fraction varies directly with plasma protein concentration.

Magnesium is an important element of bone structure. It also functions as a cofactor in cellular enzyme systems. Magnesium has a direct effect on the neuromuscular junction and therefore plays a role in neuromuscular irritability and muscle contraction.

The exact mechanism of action of magnesium is likely due to its effect on Ca homeostasis. Magnesium is a natural antagonist of calcium, blocking the voltage-sensitive Ca channels and the receptor-operated Ca channels in bronchial and vascular smooth muscle, which then inhibits smooth muscle contraction. Magnesium may also antagonize the action of calcium required for histamine release from basophils, release of mediators from mast cells, and acetylcholine secretion at nerve endings. Serum Mg levels are known to poorly reflect body stores of magnesium because the large majority of magnesium is intracellular (Agus & Morad, 1991; Kuitert & Kletchko, 1991; McNamara et al., 1989).

Magnesium has been reported to successfully reverse bronchospasm in patients refractory to β-agonists (Fesmire et al., 1993). It relaxes bronchial smooth muscle and produces dilation of the airways. Magnesium influences the function of respiratory muscles. Diminished respiratory muscle power has been reported in alcoholics and patients with COPD who have abnormally low serum Mg levels. Increase in Mg concentration may have improved respiratory muscle power and thus improved respiratory function (Skobeloff et al., 1989). Pretreatment with magnesium sulfate decreased airway reactivity to bronchoconstricting agents. This occurs due to inhibition to degranulation of mast cells and by blocking uptake and release of calcium in bronchial smooth muscle (Chande & Skoner, 1992).

Magnesium is found in many foods, vegetables and cereals being the primary dietary source. The major site of gastrointestinal absorption is the small intestine. A number of factors influence intestinal absorption, including availability of sodium and water, lactose, and, most importantly, Mg concentration in the body. There appears to be an inverse relationship between Mg absorption and the amount of magnesium ingested. Magnesium absorption in the gut is at least partially stimulated by vitamin D and PTH (Carroll & Oh, 1989).

Gastrointestinal loss of magnesium cannot be reduced to zero in the face of low intake, nor is there a protective mechanism to decrease gastrointestinal absorption with very large Mg loads. The kidney is responsible for blunting low Mg intake by decreasing renal Mg losses. Despite renal conservation, hypomagnesemia may occur as a result of continued gastrointestinal loss.

The kidney is quite effective in increasing renal excretion of magnesium when the serum Mg level is elevated. Renal excretion of magnesium is primarily regulated by the plasma Mg level. Renal regulation is also partially under the control of PTH, vitamin D, and thyrocalcitonin. The action of these hormones on Mg excretion appears to be a consequence of their role in calcium regulation. Any clinical disorder that increases urine volume results in increased renal excretion of magnesium.

HYPOMAGNESEMIA

A serum Mg concentration of less than 1.6 mg/dL is classified as hypomagnesemia, although the serum level is not always a good indicator of total body magnesium. Significant symptoms usually are apparent at serum Mg levels of less than 1.0 mg/dL.

The primary causes of hypomagnesemia are shown in Table 43–19 and are classified into three categories:

TABLE 43–19. **Etiology and Clinical Manifestations of Hypomagnesemia**

Etiology	Clinical Findings
Decreased intake/reabsorption	Neuromuscular
Protein-calorie malnutrition	Vertigo
Prolonged NPO status	Ataxia
Magnesium-free parenteral nutrition	Nystagmus
Malabsorption	Athetoid and choreiform movements
Diarrhea	Muscle tremors
Increased renal magnesium losses	Weakness
Pharmacologic agents	Hyperreflexia
Alcohol	Tetany with Chvostek sign
Diuretics	Muscle cramps
Digitalis glycosides	Seizures
Aminoglycosides	Cardiac
Cisplatin	Tachycardia
Diuretic phase of acute renal failure	Increased QT interval
Metabolic disturbances	Decreased ST segment
Diabetic ketoacidosis	
Hypercalcemia	
Hyperparathyroidism	
Hyperaldosteronism	
Redistribution to intracellular compartment	
Recovery from severe bone disease	
Acute hemorrhagic pancreatitis	
Recovery from protein-calorie malnutrition	

(1) decreased intake/absorption, (2) increased renal losses, and (3) redistribution into the IC compartment. Diminished intake is a common cause of hypomagnesemia in critically ill patients. Prolonged periods of use of magnesium-poor TPN may lead to Mg depletion. Malabsorptive states including diarrhea can interfere with gastrointestinal absorption of magnesium. Large amounts of gastric or biliary fluid losses postoperatively have been demonstrated to result in hypomagnesemia. Chronic ingestion of large amounts of alcohol also produces hypomagnesemia. Poor nutrition is the major cause of hypomagnesemia in alcoholic patients. Chronic alcohol intake also results in impaired gastrointestinal absorption and increased renal excretion of magnesium.

Increased renal loss of magnesium is a frequent cause of hypomagnesemia. Renal losses of magnesium may be induced by a variety of pharmacologic and pathologic states. Loop or thiazide diuretics inhibit reabsorption of magnesium, and continued use of these agents risks total body Mg depletion. Digitalis preparations also reduce renal Mg reabsorption, placing the patient at risk of hypomagnesemia-related digitalis toxicity. Administration of carbenicillin and gentamicin may lead to hypomagnesemia, although the exact mechanism is unknown.

The mechanism of Mg loss in hyperglycemia and glycosuria is enhanced tissue catabolism, which allows IC magnesium to move into the EC space, and eventually be excreted during the glycosuric osmotic diuresis. Shift of magnesium from the EC to the IC space has been seen during acute administration of insulin, glucose, and amino acids and during alkalemia.

Hormonal disturbances may produce hypomagnesemia. These disorders include hyperaldosteronism and hyperparathyroidism. Hyperparathyroidism is associated with hypercalcemia, which also increases renal Mg losses. Prolonged exercise (marathon running), especially in heat, may be complicated by Mg deficiency. It may persist up to 3 months and increase the release of catecholamines, heighten the possibility of coronary vasospasm, and potentiate the vasoconstrictor effects of catecholamines. Magnesium deficiency may thus be at least partly responsible for the permanent cardiac injury that develops in endurance athletes with normal coronary arteries.

Redistribution of magnesium to the IC compartment is seen with rapid restoration of bone following treatment of hyperparathyroidism. Acute hemorrhagic pancreatitis may lead to Mg deposition in tissue and may produce hypomagnesemia. During the recovery period of protein-calorie malnutrition, hypomagnesemia occurs as a result of rapid incorporation of magnesium into regenerating cells. In critical care, this is commonly seen in the alcoholic patient.

Clinical manifestations of hypomagnesemia are primarily observed in the neuromuscular and cardiac systems. These signs and symptoms are described in Table 43–19. The clinical picture may be complicated by the presence of other abnormalities such as renal potassium-wasting, producing hypokalemia. Hypocalcemia results from the impaired PTH secretion or action present in hypomagnesemia.

MANAGEMENT OF HYPOMAGNESEMIA. The severity of the signs and symptoms will guide the treatment of hypomagnesemia. Treatment will include correction of the underlying disorder as well as Mg repletion. The presence of renal impairment influences management strategies because Mg repletion must be done with great caution in patients with renal insufficiency. Mild hypomagnesemia is treated by oral Mg replacement or by increasing the Mg content of parenteral nutrition infusions. Severe symptomatic hypomagnesemia requires parenteral administration of magnesium. Dosage of intravenous magnesium will depend on the severity of symptoms. In the presence of convulsions, a bolus loading dose of 500 mg is administered. An infusion of up to 3 mEq/kg of body weight is then administered over a 4-hour period. Less severe hypomagnesemia is treated with 0.5 to 1.25 mEq/kg body weight (Carroll & Oh, 1989). These suggested dosages should be administered only to patients with normal renal function. If renal insufficiency exists, the dose must be decreased. The patient's serum Mg concentration must be measured frequently to prevent hypermagnesemia. In hypomagnesemia associated with chronic states such as malabsorption, continued Mg supplementation may be necessary.

Low concentrations of magnesium may be responsible for arrhythmias. A small decrease in serum Mg level occurs with myocardial infarction and is believed to be related to diuretic therapy. It is likely that the benefits of early therapy with intravenous magnesium after infarction (possible reduction in the incidence of ventricular fibrillation) are due more to a pharmacologic action of magnesium than to replacement of a specific physiologic deficit (Higham et al., 1993). Decreased ionized magnesium also enhances atherogenesis by promoting lipid deposition and enhances reactivity of vascular smooth muscle to vasoconstrictor substances, all leading to an increase in cardiac symptoms (Altura et al., 1990; Markell et al., 1993). Magnesium in pharmacologic doses reduces both systemic and pulmonary vascular resistance and potentiates a number of endogenous and exogenous vasodilators. It works as an antihypertensive agent. It inhibits binding of several endogenous pressors to their receptors on vascular smooth muscle and suppresses exercise-induced angina (Matz, 1993).

The clinical manifestations of hypomagnesemia are very similar to those of hypocalcemia. Major problems include irritability of the CNS with possible development of seizures, and the potential for laryngospasm and airway obstruction.

POTENTIAL FOR INJURY. Up to this point, the discussion has centered around administration of parenteral magnesium to hypomagnesemic patients. The critical care nurse may also be called on to care for a critically ill obstetric patient receiving parenteral magnesium as treatment for preeclampsia. For specifics regarding the care of the obstetric patient, the reader is referred to

Chapter 69. Regardless of purpose, the goal of nursing care is to prevent complications during Mg infusion.

Parenteral Mg preparations are available in several concentrations ranging from 10% to 50% solutions. Before administering a loading dose or infusion, the critical care nurse must carefully check the concentration and dosage against the physician's prescription.

Pertinent nursing assessments during Mg infusion include deep tendon reflexes, urine output, blood pressure, respirations, and level of consciousness. Deep tendon reflexes are checked at least hourly during Mg infusion. Patellar reflexes are the most commonly assessed; however, antecubital reflexes can also be used. Reflexes are usually reported on a scale of 1+ to 4+. The nurse observes for a trend toward diminishing reflexes. If deep tendon reflexes are absent, the Mg infusion must be stopped and the physician notified.

Because magnesium is excreted by the kidneys, urine output is an important nursing assessment. Ideally, urine output should remain at or above 0.5 mL/kg body weight per hour. If urine output falls below this level, deep tendon reflexes must be assessed more frequently.

Blood pressure, pulse, respirations, and level of consciousness are checked at least hourly during Mg infusion. A sudden, significant fall in blood pressure or a decrease in respiratory rate is a sign of Mg toxicity.

Any sudden or sustained change in deep tendon reflexes, urine output, or vital signs should alert the nurse to the development of Mg toxicity. The infusion must be stopped, and the nurse should prepare for the possible need for emergency resuscitation.

HYPERMAGNESEMIA

Significant hypermagnesemia (>5 mg/dL) rarely occurs in patients with normal renal function. Even in patients with chronic renal insufficiency, the kidney responds by increasing the efficiency of the remaining nephrons, thereby maintaining serum Mg concentration at normal or near-normal levels. The causes of hypermagnesemia are listed in Table 43–20. Salt depletion, volume contraction, and mineralocorticoid deficiency all lead to increased Mg retention by the kidney despite normal body magnesium. Significant reduction in thyroid function has also been shown to reduce Mg excretion by the kidney.

Magnesium salts that are administered to treat hypomagnesemia or preeclampsia/eclampsia can increase serum Mg levels acutely. Injudicious use of magnesium-containing laxatives and antacids may provide a sizable intake of magnesium; these agents are particularly problematic in patients with diminished renal function. Hypermagnesemia may also result from liberation of magnesium from the muscle cells. Clinical examples of the latter include rhabdomyolysis following crush injuries or soft tissue trauma and severe burns. When renal function is normal, the increase in serum Mg level should be transient. Unfortunately, many of these severely injured patients also develop acute renal failure and are then unable to excrete the high Mg load.

TABLE 43–20. **Etiology and Clinical Manifestations of Hypermagnesemia**

Etiology	Clinical Findings
Decreased renal magnesium excretion	Neuromuscular
Acute/chronic renal failure	Muscle weakness
Salt depletion	Hyporeflexia
Volume depletion	Cardiovascular
Mineralocorticoid deficiency	Increased PR interval
Hypothyroidism	Increased QRS complex
Increased exogenous magnesium load	Increased QT interval
Magnesium salts in diet or parenteral nutrition	Complete heart block
Magnesium-containing antacids or laxatives	Cardiac arrest
Magnesium-containing enemas	Hypotension
High magnesium dialysate	
Increased endogenous magnesium load	
Burns	
Traumatic soft tissue injury	
Rhabdomyolysis	

Significant hypermagnesemia is associated with a variety of signs and symptoms, as listed in Table 43–20. Nonspecific nausea and vomiting may be the earliest symptoms of hypermagnesemia. Muscle weakness is also an early symptom. At serum Mg levels of 3 to 5 mg/dL, peripheral vasodilation occurs. This may result in significant hypotension. Hyporeflexia in deep tendons may be seen when serum Mg concentration approaches 7 mg/dL. Respiratory paralysis occurs when the serum Mg level exceeds 8 mg/dL. Intracardiac conduction defects are varied and will adversely affect cardiac output. Usually the ECG changes of prolonged PR and QRS intervals are not seen until the serum magnesium level is above 15 mEq/liter.

MANAGEMENT OF HYPERMAGNESEMIA. In patients with normal renal function, withdrawal of the exogenous source of magnesium may be sufficient to lower serum Mg concentration to near-normal levels. In patients with renal failure, hemodialysis or peritoneal dialysis is the most effective way to remove excess magnesium from the body.

Patients with severe neuromuscular or cardiac symptoms may require additional support until the serum Mg level is corrected. Intravenous administration of calcium is the emergency treatment for hypermagnesemia in the presence of life-threatening symptoms. A dose of 10 mL of 10% calcium gluconate is administered slowly over a few minutes. Glucose and insulin can also be administered to facilitate the temporary IC movement of magnesium. Forced diuresis with large volumes of intravenous saline solutions can also be used in patients with normal renal function.

DECREASED TISSUE PERFUSION. The critically ill patient with hypermagnesemia is at risk for several life-threatening complications. The goals of nursing care include early recognition and response to the development of neuromuscular complications.

Peripheral vasodilation occurs at Mg levels of more than 3 mg/dL, resulting in hypotension and decreased tissue perfusion. The nurse assesses the blood pressure and heart rate for change. The level of consciousness and urine output are monitored, and these measurements are used to evaluate the patient's response to blood pressure changes. Symptomatic patients may be placed in the head-down position to facilitate blood flow to the core. Volume expansion with intravenous fluids may be helpful in stabilizing the blood pressure.

IMPAIRED BREATHING PATTERN. Paralysis of respiratory muscles followed by respiratory arrest is a life-threatening complication in patients with hypermagnesemia. Pertinent nursing assessments include monitoring muscle strength and respiratory status. Deep tendon reflexes, grasp strength, and head lift are all measures of muscle strength that can be used to assess the extent of neuromuscular depression. Respiratory rate, quality, and depth must be carefully monitored for minute changes. Continuous pulse oximetry monitoring, end-tidal carbon dioxide measurements, and arterial blood gas analysis may all be used to detect diminishing ventilation. In addition to ongoing assessment, the nurse prepares for the possibility of emergency intubation and ventilation.

SUMMARY

Fluid volume and electrolyte disorders are common occurrences in critical illness or injury. The critically ill patient may present with one or several of these alterations in the course of illness. The critical care nurse, in collaboration with the physician, is responsible for monitoring the patient's fluid and electrolyte status. Careful nursing assessment may uncover early manifestations of imbalance. This chapter has presented the etiology, clinical presentations, and management of common fluid and electrolyte disorders. Appropriate nursing diagnoses and nursing interventions have been identified.

REFERENCES

Agus, Z., & Morad, M. (1991). Modulations of cardiac ion channels by magnesium. *Annual Review of Physiology, 53,* 299–307.

Ahmed, B., & Jaspan, J. B. (1993). Case report: Hypercalcemia in a patient with AIDS and *Pneumocystis carinii* pneumonia. *American Journal of the Medical Sciences, 306*(5), 313–336.

Allon, M. (1991). Albuterol and insulin for treatment of hyperkalemia in hemodialysis patients. *Kidney International, 38,* 869–872.

Allon, M. (1993). Treatment and prevention of hyperkalemia in end-stage renal disease. *Kidney International, 43,* 1197–1209.

Allon, M., Takeshian, A., & Shanklin, N. (1993). Effect of insulin-plus-glucose infusion with or without epinephrine on fasting hyperkalemia. *Kidney International, 43,* 212–217.

Altura, B. T., Brust, M., Bloom, S., et al. (1990). Magnesium dietary intake modulates blood lipid levels and atherogenesis. *Proceedings of the National Academy of Sciences of the USA, 87,* 1840–1844.

Arieff, A., & Ayus, J. (1991). Treatment of symptomatic hyponatremia: Neither haste nor waste. *Critical Care Medicine, 19,* 748–751.

Ayus, J. C., Krothapalli, R. K., & Arieff, A. I. (1987). Treatment of symptomatic hyponatremia and its relation to brain damage. *New England Journal of Medicine, 317,* 1190–1195.

Carroll, H. J., & Oh, M. S. (1989). *Water, electrolyte and acid-base metabolism: Diagnosis and management* (2nd ed.). Philadelphia: J. B. Lippincott.

Casley-Smith, J. R. (1993). A model of the factors affecting interstitial volume in edema. Part II: Their effects at various abnormal steady-states. *Biorheology, 30*(1), 9–30.

Chande, V. T., & Skoner, D. P. (1992). A trial of nebulized magnesium sulfate to reverse bronchospasm in asthmatic patients. *Annals of Emergency Medicine, 21*(9), 1111–1115.

Elisaf, M., Litou, H., & Siamopoulos, K. C. (1989). Survival after severe iatrogenic hypernatremia. *American Journal of Kidney Disease, 14,* 230–231.

Fesmire, F. M., Spivey, W. H., Pugh, G., et al. (1993). Intravenous magnesium for acute asthma. *Annals of Emergency Medicine, 22*(3), 616–619.

Goldberger, E. (1986). *A primer of water, electrolytes and acid-base syndromes* (7th ed.). Philadelphia: Lea & Febiger.

Grinspoon, S. K., & Bilezikian, J. P. (1992). HIV disease and the endocrine system. *New England Journal of Medicine, 327,* 1360–1365.

Guyton, A. C. (1991). *Textbook of medical physiology* (8th ed.). Philadelphia: W. B. Saunders.

Hall, T. G., & Burns-Schaiff, R. A. (1993). Update on the medical treatment of hypercalcemia of malignancy. *Clinical Pharmacology, 12,* 117–125.

Healey, P. (1993). The medical treatment of hypercalcemia. *Connecticut Medicine, 57*(9), 619–621.

Higham, P. D., Adams, P. C., Murray, A., et al. (1993). Plasma potassium, serum magnesium and ventricular fibrillation: A prospective study. *Quarterly Journal of Medicine, 86,* 609–617.

Horner, S. M. (1992). Efficacy of intravenous magnesium in acute myocardial infarction in reducing arrhythmias and mortality. *Circulation, 83,* 774–779.

Kamoi, K., Tamura, T., Tanaka, K., et al. (1993). Hyponatremia and osmoregulation of thirst and vasopressin secretion in patients with adrenal insufficiency. *Journal of Clinical Endocrinology and Metabolism, 77*(6), 1584–1588.

Krohn, J. S. (1993). Dilutional hypocalcemia in association with dilutional hyponatremia. *Anesthesiology, 79*(5), 1136–1138.

Kubota, Y., Toyoda, Y., Kubota, H., et al. (1993). Epinephrine in local anesthetics does indeed produce hypokalemia and ECG changes. *Anesthesia and Analgesia, 77,* 864–873.

Kufs, W. M. (1990). Intravenous magnesium sulfate in acute asthma. *Journal of the American Medical Association, 263*(4), 516–517.

Kuitert, L. M., & Kletchko, S. L. (1991). Intravenous magnesium sulfate in acute, life-threatening asthma. *Annals of Emergency Medicine, 10*(11), 1243–1245.

Markell, M. S., Altura, B. T., Sarn, Y., et al. (1993). Deficiency of serum ionized magnesium in patients receiving hemodialysis or peritoneal dialysis. *ASAIO Journal, 39,* M801–M804.

Matz, R. (1993). Magnesium: Deficiencies and therapeutic uses. *Hospital Practice, 30*(28), 79–92.

McNamara, R. M., Spivey, W. H., Skobeloff, E., et al. (1989). Intravenous magnesium sulfate in the management of acute respiratory failure complicating asthma. *Annals of Emergency Medicine, 18*(2), 197–199.

Moder, K., & Daniel, H. (1990). Fatal hypernatremia from exogenous salt intake: Report of a case and review of the literature. *Mayo Clinic Proceedings, 65,* 1587–1594.

Oh, M., & Carroll, J. (1992). Disorders of sodium metabolism: Hypernatremia and hyponatremia. *Critical Care Medicine, 20,* 94–103.

Skobeloff, E. M., Spivey, W. H., McNamara, R. M., et al. (1989). Intravenous magnesium sulfate for the treatment of acute asthma in the emergency department. *Journal of the American Medical Association, 262*(9), 1210–1213.

Sunyecz, L., & Mirtallo, J. M. (1993). Sodium imbalance in a patient receiving total parenteral nutrition. *Clinical Pharmacology, 12,* 138–149.

Vanek, V. W., Seballow, R. M., Chong, D., et al. (1994). Serum potassium concentrations in trauma patients. *Southern Medical Journal, 87*(1), 41–46.

Vin-Christian, K., & Arieff, A. I. (1993). Diabetes insipidus, massive polyuria, and hypernatremia leading to permanent brain damage. *American Journal of Medicine, 94,* 341–342.

Wong, K. C., Schafer, P. G., & Schultz, J. R. (1993). Hypokalemia and anesthetic implications. *Anesthesia and Analgesia, 77,* 1238–1260.

Zakowski, M. I., Ramanathan, S., & Trundorf, H. (1993). Epinephrine in local anesthetics does indeed produce hypokalemia and ECG changes. In response. *Anesthesia and Analgesia, 77,* 867–868.

Patients With Acute Renal Failure

Alice (Ali) Whittaker

Acute renal failure (ARF) is a serious sequela of critical illness and traumatic injury. Despite advances in prevention, diagnosis, and medical treatment, the mortality associated with ARF remains high. Overall mortality rates in patients with acute loss of renal function approach 40% to 50%. In surgical and traumatically injured patients, mortality may be as high as 60% to 86%. (Jacobsen et al., 1990; Jochimsen et al., 1990).

Loss of renal function has a potentially negative impact on all body systems. This chapter will focus on the clinical challenge presented by the critically ill patient with oliguric ARF.

PATHOPHYSIOLOGY

Acute renal failure can be defined as a sudden decrease in renal function manifested by rapid accumulation of waste metabolites in the patient's body. In the majority of cases, the patient becomes oliguric. Oliguria exists when the urine flow is less than the volume required to excrete the body's metabolic waste load. In the adult patient, this obligatory urine volume is approximately 400 mL/24 hr.

Oliguria is considered to be the classic finding in ARF, but the syndrome also manifests in a more benign nonoliguric form. Although patients with nonoliguric renal failure pass normal amounts of urine, they demonstrate the renal pathology and metabolic changes seen in oliguric failure.

Etiology

Acute renal failure is a syndrome of multiple etiologies. The various etiologies can be classified into three major categories: prerenal, postrenal, and renal.

PRERENAL CAUSES. Prerenal causes of ARF are characterized by diminished renal perfusion resulting from a reduction in the volume of blood reaching the kidney. As listed in Table 44–1, the most common causes of renal hypoperfusion are related to an absolute loss of extracellular fluid volume or redistribution of extracellular fluid from the cardiovascular system into other body compartments. Prerenal oliguria may also be caused by a reduction in the effective circulatory volume resulting from impaired cardiac function.

The kidneys react to the prerenal hypoperfusion state by increasing tubular reabsorption of sodium and water and by selective vasoconstriction of the glomerular arterioles. These are normal regulatory mechanisms designed to increase blood volume and improve renal perfusion. The urine volume falls and the patient becomes oliguric.

Renal function remains intact in prerenal states. Oliguria can be reversed if the underlying hypoperfusion disorder is corrected and normal blood flow is restored to the kidneys before ischemic damage occurs.

POSTRENAL CAUSES. Disease states that interrupt or obstruct the outflow of urine from the body cause post-

TABLE 44–1. **Prerenal Causes of Acute Renal Failure**

Cause	Clinical Example
Absolute Extracellular Volume Reduction	
Hemorrhage	Traumatic injury, postoperative bleeding, GI bleeding
GI loss	Diarrhea, vomiting, GI drainage tubes
Urinary loss	Excessive diuretics, diabetes insipidus, diabetic ketoacidosis
Skin loss	Burns, excessive sweating
Extracellular Volume Redistribution	
Third spacing	Bowel obstruction, peritonitis, pancreatitis, soft tissue injury
Vasodilatory states	Sepsis, anaphylaxis, vasodilating medications
Decreased Effective Circulatory Volume	
Decreased cardiac output	Congestive heart failure, cardiomyopathy, pericarditis, cardiac tamponade, pulmonary embolism, cardiogenic shock

TABLE 44–2. **Postrenal Causes of Acute Renal Failure**

Cause	Clinical Example
Obstruction	
Ureteral	Calculi, crystals Retroperitoneal tumor Blood clot
Bladder	Prostatic hypertrophy, carcinoma Tumor Neurogenic, functional Calculi, blood clot
Urethral	Stricture, stenosis
Traumatic Interruption	Severed ureter Bladder tear

renal ARF. Table 44–2 lists the major obstructive and traumatic processes seen in critically ill patients.

Impairment of renal function in postrenal ARF occurs as the intratubular pressure increases proximal to the obstruction. Glomerular filtration ceases as the pressure in Bowman's capsule becomes equal to the hydrostatic pressure in the glomerular capillaries. High intratubular pressure damages the tubular cells, resulting in impaired transport and concentration mechanisms (Finn, 1990). If the postrenal disorder is rapidly corrected, renal function can be preserved. Prolonged postrenal obstruction results in permanent damage to the neprons.

RENAL CAUSES. A variety of diseases and injuries intrinsic to the actual kidney tissue may lead to the development of ARF. As listed in Table 44–3, damage to the renal parenchyma can be related to abnormalities of the glomerulus, tubules, or interstitium. Tubular damage, referred to as acute tubular necrosis (ATN), is the most frequently encountered form of ARF seen in critically ill patients (Racusen, 1992).

TABLE 44–3. **Renal Causes of Acute Renal Failure**

Cause	Clinical Example
Glomerular	
Primary	Poststreptococcal glomerulonephritis
Secondary to systemic disease	Systemic lupus erythematosus, vasculitis, endocarditis Malignant hypertension
Tubulointerstitial	
Ischemic	Uncorrected prerenal hypoperfusion Alpha-adrenergic drug administration Renal artery thrombosis
Nephrotoxic	
Drugs or chemicals	Antibiotics: aminoglycosides, cephalosporins, penicillins, tetracyclines, amphotericin Heavy metals Organic solvents Pesticides, fungicides Cisplatin Radiographic contrast media
Endogenous toxins	Hemoglobinuria Myoglobinuria Hypercalcemia

Both ischemic and toxic insults impair nephron function; however, renal cellular ischemia is the most common cause of ATN. In many patients, renal ischemia is preceded by severe, uncorrected hypoperfusion, as seen in hypovolemia or sepsis. Prolonged administration of alpha-adrenergic drugs, resulting in intense renal vasoconstriction, is another frequent cause of renal ischemia in critically ill patients.

Loss of nephron function may occur after exposure to a number of nephrotoxic chemicals and drugs. Damage to the renal tubules is a frequent sequela to accidental or intentional ingestion of organic solvents, such as carbon tetrachloride or ethylene glycol. Critically ill patients often receive a number of potentially nephrotoxic antibiotics. Approximately 10% to 26% of patients receiving aminoglycoside antibiotics will develop some degree of renal dysfunction. The risk of developing ATN is greatly increased when aminoglycoside antibiotics are administered to patients with fluid volume depletion, sepsis, or fever (Zager, 1992).

Among the endogenous nephrotoxins, hemoglobin and myoglobin are implicated as causes of ATN accompanying critical illness. Hemoglobinuria, resulting from hemolytic transfusion reaction or other hemolytic process, may result in renal tubular injury. Following intravascular hemolysis, hemoglobin is released into the circulating plasma and exerts a toxic effect on the renal tubular epithelium. Myoglobin is a respiratory pigment present in muscle cells. When muscle injury occurs, myoglobin is released into the blood and filtered by the glomeruli, resulting in myoglobinuria. Rhabdomyolysis, with accompanying myoglobinuria, is a frequent cause of ARF in traumatically injured patients (Dayer-Berenson, 1994).

Pathogenesis of Acute Tubular Necrosis

Several theories have been proposed to explain the diminished glomerular filtration rate (GFR) that occurs in patients with ATN. As shown in Figure 44–1, either tubular factors or vascular factors contribute to the reduction in GFR. Different modes of injury may preferentially affect either the tubules or the renal vasculature.

TUBULAR FACTORS. The renal tubular cells maintain very high metabolic demands to fuel their transport and enzymatic activities. For this reason, they are particularly vulnerable to ischemic or toxic injury. When renal ischemia occurs, intracellular adenosine triphosphate (ATP) is rapidly depleted. Cellular energy (ATP) depletion and the accumulation of waste metabolites results in loss of tubular cell polarity and reduced activity of the cells' ionic pump activity (Na^+/K^+-AT-

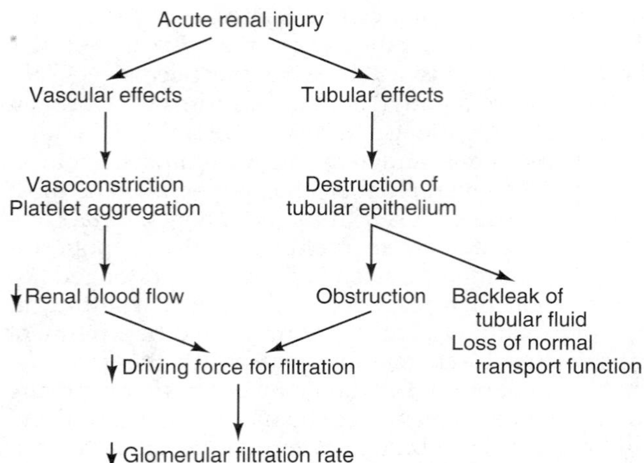

FIGURE 44–1. Schematic representation of the mechanisms theorized to initiate and maintain the reduction in glomerular filtration rate in acute renal failure. (Adapted from Brenner, B. M., and Rector, F. L. [Eds.] [1988]. *Acute renal failure* [2nd ed.]. Philadelphia: W. B. Saunders.)

Pase) (Brezis & Epstein, 1993; Hohenfellner et al., 1992). Impaired Na^+/K^+-ATPase leads to a shift of sodium ions (Na^+) and water into the tubular cell, causing the cell to swell. Calcium ions (Ca^{++}) also enter the hypoxic cell. Increased intracellular Ca^{++} concentration further impairs energy production by preventing generation of ATP. As shown in Figure 44–2, ischemia alters the activity of intracellular enzymes, leading to lysis of the tubular cell wall. Microscopic examination of the renal tubules reveals alteration of the apical brush border with areas of epithelial cell loss along the tubular basement membrane (Racusen, 1992).

Nephrotoxic agents bind to the proximal tubular brush border and enter the cell by endocytosis. After entering the tubular cell, the nephrotoxin can induce alterations in cell membrane and energy production similar to those seen in the ischemic kidney (Humes, 1988; Zager, 1992).

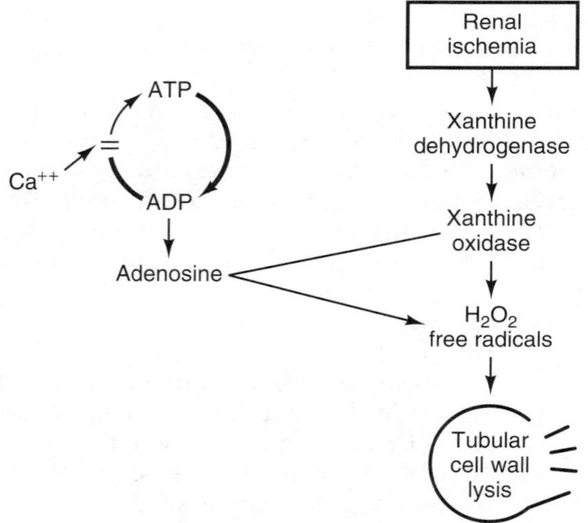

FIGURE 44–2. Schematic representation of how increased intracellular calcium (Ca^{++}) and cellular ischemia interact to produce free oxygen radicals, which cause cell wall lysis (Brezis & Epstein, 1993; Hohenfellner et al., 1992.)

Proximal tubular dilatation and the presence of intraluminal casts and detached tubular cells are common findings in ATN (Racusen, 1992). Desquamated microvilli fill the proximal tubule in the first hours after ischemic injury. Later these cellular debris combine with Tamm-Horsfall protein to form tubular casts, which further obstruct the tubules and the loop of Henle (Bayati et al., 1990a). The tubules remain obstructed until the casts are dissolved by proteolytic enzymes or flushed out by increased glomerular filtrate flow.

Disruption of the integrity of the tubular epithelium permits glomerular filtrate to leak back into the peritubular circulation. This backleak of filtrate is thought to result in interstitial edema and tubular collapse (Racusen, 1992). It is likely that variations in glomerular vasoconstriction and backleak of glomerular ultrafiltrate influence the rise of intratubular pressure in the obstructed nephron.

VASCULAR FACTORS. During the initial phase of ATN, renal blood flow (RBF) decreases by more than 50% (Kasgarian et al., 1976). In addition, there is a significant rise in the renal vascular resistance. The reduction in RBF is preferential. Blood flow to the renal cortex is sharply decreased while perfusion to the medulla is maintained. The mechanisms responsible for these changes in the renal vasculature are not well understood. There is evidence to indicate that damaged endothelial cells swell, reducing the diameter of the renal arterioles. RBF falls as the arteriolar diameter diminishes. Increased peritubular capillary permeability results in a massive extravasation of plasma, leading to an elevated intracapillary hematocrit (Bayati et al., 1990a). Aggregation of red blood cells in the peritubular capillaries of the outer medulla has been shown to cause congestion and possible intravascular coagulation (Mason et al., 1984). Impaired tubular reabsorption of sodium chloride activates the renin–angiotensin system, resulting in afferent arteriole constriction (Shapira et al., 1976). Alterations in intracellular Ca^{++} levels are also thought to play a role in abnormal renal vasoconstriction (Racusen, 1991).

Each of these proposed vascular mechanisms can be demonstrated in the early stages of ARF. However, none can be shown to be totally responsible for maintaining the suppressed GFR beyond the initial phase. Most likely, sustained decreased GFR is a result of both tubular and vascular factors. The relative contribution of each factor varies with the mode of injury and individual patient characteristics.

Metabolic/Biochemical Disturbances

The physiologic disturbances seen in ARF are a result of the kidney's decreased ability to form and excrete urine. As the blood level of metabolic wastes and tox-

TABLE 44–4. **Physiologic Disturbances in Acute Renal Failure**

Protein Metabolism	Fluid/Electrolyte Balance
Increased protein degradation Decreased protein synthesis	Fluid volume overload Hyponatremia Hyperkalemia Hypocalcemic/hyperphosphatemia
Acid-Base Balance	
Metabolic acidosis	
Carbohydrate Metabolism	**Hematologic Function**
Insulin resistance Hyperglycemia Decreased ATP production	Anemia Platelet dysfunction Leukopenia

ins rises, a variety of metabolic and biochemical derangements occur. As shown in Table 44–4, these disturbances range from mild to life-threatening and involve all of the body systems.

CATABOLISM. Two terms are commonly used to describe the physiologic disturbances seen in ARF. The abnormal retention of nitrogenous waste products, such as urea, creatinine, uric acid, and amino acids, is known as *azotemia. Uremia* refers to the symptoms of the clinical illness caused by renal failure.

In ARF, the intensity of azotemia and the uremic syndrome is closely correlated with the patient's rate of catabolism. ARF is characterized by an increased rate of cellular decomposition. The breakdown of cells releases intracellular products and their metabolites into the circulatory system. When renal excretion is suppressed, the blood level of these metabolites rises rapidly and the patient becomes azotemic. In mildly catabolic patients, the blood urea nitrogen (BUN) increases approximately 10 to 20 mg/100 mL/day. When severe catabolism is present, the BUN may rise as much as 40 to 50 mg/100 mL/day (Cameron & Ogg, 1967).

The explanation for the high rate of catabolism in ARF is not well understood. Patients who are stressed by critical illness or traumatic injury demonstrate elevation of circulating catecholamines, cortisol, and glucagon. It is theorized that these hormones play an important role in stimulating catabolism. In addition to protein degradation, protein synthesis is also suppressed in ARF.

ACID-BASE IMBALANCE. Under normal conditions, the kidney regulates acid-base balance by excreting hydrogen ion and selectively reabsorbing bicarbonate. When acute renal damage has occurred, organic and inorganic acids are retained, leading to metabolic acidosis. In catabolism, disintegrated cells release a number of organic acids and sulfate- and phosphate-containing acids into the circulation, thereby greatly increasing acid production. This is evidenced by a rapid fall in plasma bicarbonate levels of 15 to 20 mEq/24 hr.

The presence of uremia intensifies the harmful effects of metabolic acidosis in critically ill patients. Metabolic acidosis further stimulates protein degradation. Carbohydrate metabolism is impaired, and energy production is reduced.

ALTERED CARBOHYDRATE METABOLISM. Patients with ARF are unable to metabolize glucose normally. Hyperglycemia occurs during fasting, and there is a delay in the fall of blood glucose after a glucose challenge (Reaven et al., 1974). Insulin response to high blood glucose levels in acutely uremic patients is greater than in normal patients, indicating that the defect in insulin activity is not impaired secretion. Rather, glucose intolerance is apparently a result of an inappropriate response of target tissue to insulin (Giordano et al., 1987). Peripheral muscle tissue is thought to be the site of insulin resistance in patients with acute uremia.

ELECTROLYTE DISTURBANCES. Acute loss of renal function results in a variety of fluid and electrolyte disturbances.

SODIUM. Hyponatremia is the most common sodium disturbance observed in patients with ARF and is usually attributed to dilution. The serum sodium may become diluted by three mechanisms. First, administration of free water, such as 5% dextrose and water (D_5W) or oral water, may exceed the kidney's ability to excrete it. Second, metabolic water production in patients with ARF may be significantly increased. In catabolic patients, additional water is released as body tissues are destroyed.

Disturbances in ion transport across the cellular membrane also contribute to hyponatremia in ARF. As cellular injury occurs, intracellular potassium is exchanged for sodium. Failure of the sodium–potassium pump results in increased intracellular osmolality and inward movement of water. Cell volume increases and cellular transmembrane potential is depressed.

POTASSIUM. Hyperkalemia is common and is often severe in patients with oliguric ARF. Intracellular potassium concentration is approximately 155 mEq/liter. When cellular injury occurs, potassium is released into the extracellular fluid and the serum potassium rises.

Hyperkalemia is aggravated by hyperglycemia and metabolic acidosis, both of which are commonly present in oliguric patients. It is theorized that the intracellular accumulation of hydrogen ions displaces potassium ions into the extracellular fluid (Knochel, 1985). Lowering of the intracellular pH decreases the rate of glycolysis, leading to reduction of energy needed to run the sodium–potassium pump.

CALCIUM AND PHOSPHATE. Calcium and phosphate derangements are expected in patients with ARF. Because phosphate ions are normally excreted in the urine, serum phosphate levels climb as renal function decreases. In hypercatabolic patients, phosphate levels rise rapidly as phosphate is released from injured tissue. Hyperphosphatemia is aggravated by metabolic acidosis. Acute acidosis interferes with intracellular glycolysis and causes hydrolysis of sugar-phosphates.

The resulting free inorganic phosphate ions are released into the extracellular fluid.

As hyperphosphatemia develops, phosphate ions interact with calcium ions to form calcium-phosphate salts. These salts are deposited in body tissues. Deposition of calcium salts leads to a fall in serum calcium levels (Andreucci, 1984). Synthesis of vitamin D is also suppressed in patients with ARF. Low levels of vitamin D decrease calcium mobilization from bone and have a negative effect on intestinal calcium absorption.

HEMATOLOGIC ABNORMALITIES. Several alterations in hematologic function are commonly seen in ARF.

ANEMIA. Anemia may develop rapidly in patients with ARF. Often these patients have sustained significant blood loss from injury or surgery. The rapid onset of severe azotemia results in hemolysis of red blood cells. Uremic hemolysis is believed to be the major cause of anemia in the early phase of ARF (Steinman & Lazarus, 1988). As the course of acute uremia progresses, anemia is sustained by a decrease in erythropoiesis. Diminished erythropoiesis may be caused by a fall in erythropoietin-stimulating factor or by the action of an erythropoietin inhibitor (Radtke et al., 1979, 1981).

HEMOSTASIS. Thrombocytopenia, platelet dysfunction, and abnormal prothrombin consumption are clotting abnormalities common to acutely uremic patients. Because these abnormalities are associated with other underlying disease processes in critically ill patients, it is difficult to specify the exact role of renal failure in inducing or augmenting them. It is known that the bleeding tendency is well correlated with the degree of renal dysfunction.

LEUKOPENIA. Almost invariably, patients with ARF demonstrate immunologic abnormalities. Leukocytosis of neutrophils, lymphopenia, abnormal chemotaxis, and impaired inflammatory response are common findings. Infection with septicemia is the most common cause of death in acutely uremic patients.

CLINICAL PRESENTATION

Acute oliguria may be attributed to a number of causes, including prerenal, postrenal, and intrinsic renal factors. Because of the critical impact of ARF and the fact that treatment depends on the underlying problem, it is essential that an accurate etiologic diagnosis be made.

Laboratory Analysis

Table 44–5 presents a comparison of the common laboratory findings observed in prerenal and postrenal disease and ATN. Although many of the blood and urine findings appear similar, the correct etiologic diagnosis can usually be made based on laboratory tests, patient history, and physical examination.

Urine from the prerenal kidney shows marked sodium and water reabsorption. Urine volume is low and highly concentrated and contains a minimal amount of sodium. The BUN to serum creatinine ratio is elevated because an increased amount of urea is reabsorbed into the peritubular vascular circulation.

Urine chemistry results in early postrenal oliguria are very similar to those seen in prerenal states. However, after several hours of bilateral obstruction, the concentration of the urine decreases and the excretion of sodium rises. Urine volume may remain high, even

TABLE 44–5. **Comparison of Laboratory Findings in Prerenal, Postrenal, and Intrinsic Renal Acute Oliguric States**

Value	Prerenal	Postrenal	Intrinsic Renal (ATN)
Urine volume	Decreased	May alternate between anuria and polyuria	Anuria <100 mL/24 hr Oliguria 100–400 mL/24 hr Nonoliguria >400 mL/24 hr
Urine osmolality	Increased (>500 mOsm)	Isotonic (≤350 mOsm)	Isotonic (≤350 mOsm)
Urine specific gravity	Increased (>1.020)	Fixed (1.008–1.012)	Fixed (1.008–1.012)
Urine sodium	<20 mEq/liter	>40 mEq/liter	>40 mEq/liter
Fractional excretion of sodium (FE_{Na})*	<1%	>1%	>1%
Renal failure index†	<1%	>1%	>1%
Urine pH	<6.0	>6.0	>6.0
Urine protein	Minimal	Minimal	Increased
Urine sediment	Normal, few casts	Normal, histiocytes and crystals	Granular casts, tubular epithelial cells
Urine creatinine: plasma creatinine ratio	>40	<20	<20
BUN:serum creatinine	>20:1	10–15:1	10–15:1

*Fractional excretion of sodium = U/P sodium ÷ U/P creatinine × 100.

†Renal failure index = U sodium ÷ U/P creatinine.

Adapted from M. Brezis, S. Rosen, & F. H. Epstein (1991). Acute renal failure. In B. M. Brenner and F. C. Rector (Eds.), *The kidney* (4th ed., pp. 993–1061). Philadelphia: W. B. Saunders.

in the presence of severe partial obstruction. The BUN and serum creatinine are both elevated.

Patients with ATN are usually oliguric; however, anuria may also occur. In nephrotoxic ATN, urine volumes may remain relatively normal. Damaged nephrons do not adequately process the glomerular filtrate. The resulting urine is high in sodium with a concentration close to that of the plasma. Serum creatinine levels increase by 1 to 2 mg/dL/day in noncatabolic patients with ATN. The BUN to serum creatinine ratio remains 10 to 15:1, because the BUN and creatinine rise proportionately.

Diagnostic Studies

Occasionally the patient with acute oliguria has inconclusive laboratory and physical findings. In these cases, a number of diagnostic studies may be performed to determine the cause of renal failure.

RADIOLOGIC STUDIES. Intravenous urography (IVU) may provide useful information about renal perfusion and patency of the renal collection system in the patient with ARF. After rapid injection of a radiocontrast agent, serial films (nephrograms) of the renal tubules and collecting system are taken. Normally, the contrast agent enters the tubules by glomerular filtration within a few minutes after injection and is rapidly cleared from the kidneys. Severe reduction in renal perfusion and glomerular filtration, as seen in ATN, produces characteristic changes in the nephrogram. Uptake of the contrast agent is usually delayed, and achievement of normal density may be delayed or prolonged. IVU is most reliably used to rule out urinary tract obstruction. The procedure is not without risk. Injection of an iodinated, hyperosmolar contrast medium may result in hypersensitivity reactions and has been observed to worsen congestive heart failure. Development of nephrotoxic ATN after exposure to radiocontrast agents is well documented and especially problematic in diabetic patients and patients with severe renal hypoperfusion (VanZee et al., 1978; Whalley et al., 1987).

ULTRASONOGRAPHY. Renal ultrasonography is a safe, highly reliable technique used to rule out urinary tract obstruction in the acutely oliguric patient. Dilatation of the renal calyces and collecting ducts can be detected by ultrasonography within the first 24 to 36 hours after acute obstruction. In addition, intrarenal and ureteral calculi can be identified using renal ultrasonography.

RENAL BIOPSY. Biopsy of the renal tissue may be useful in the diagnosis of acute glomerular disease, when cortical necrosis is the cause of ATN, and when ATN is suspected but no known cause can be found for it. Because of the risks involved in tissue biopsy and the usefulness of other diagnostic tests, renal biopsy is not indicated in the majority of patients with acute oliguria.

Physical Findings

The patient with ARF presents with alterations in urine output and increasing azotemia. As ARF progresses, all body and organ systems demonstrate abnormalities. Table 44–6 lists the physical findings commonly observed in patients with acute oliguric failure.

CARDIOVASCULAR. Patients with ARF show several cardiovascular abnormalities. Hypertension is a common finding, resulting from fluid volume overload and increased peripheral resistance. Cardiac output may be elevated as the patient becomes progressively anemic. Fluid volume overload frequently results in congestive heart failure. Impaired contractility, secondary to metabolic acidosis, also decreases cardiac function in the acutely uremic patient. Physical findings include peripheral edema, pulmonary rales, elevated central venous pressure (CVP), and increased jugular venous distention.

Changes in the patient's electrocardiogram (ECG) demonstrate the electrolyte disturbances accompanying ARF. ECG changes are generally noted when the serum potassium level exceeds 5.5 mEq/liter. The typical progression of the ECG abnormalities seen in a patient with ARF with hyperkalemia is presented in Figure 44–3.

Pericarditis is an infrequent complication of acute uremia. The patient with uremic pericarditis usually does not complain of significant chest pain. A pericardial friction rub may be the initial clinical finding.

PULMONARY. Pulmonary edema is a frequent complication of ARF, occurring in patients with congestive heart failure as well as in those with normal cardiac function. Acutely uremic patients demonstrate in-

TABLE 44–6. **Physical Findings in Acute Oliguric Renal Failure**

Cardiovascular	**Gastrointestinal**
Hypertension	Increased gastrointestinal hormones
Congestive heart failure	Increased gastric ammonia
Arrhythmias	Gastritis/pelvic ulcers
Pericarditis	Gastrointestinal hemorrhage
Pulmonary	**Integument**
Pulmonary edema	Edema
Hypoxemia	Pallor
	Hair loss
Neurologic	
Lethargy	
Disorientation	
Seizures	
Coma	

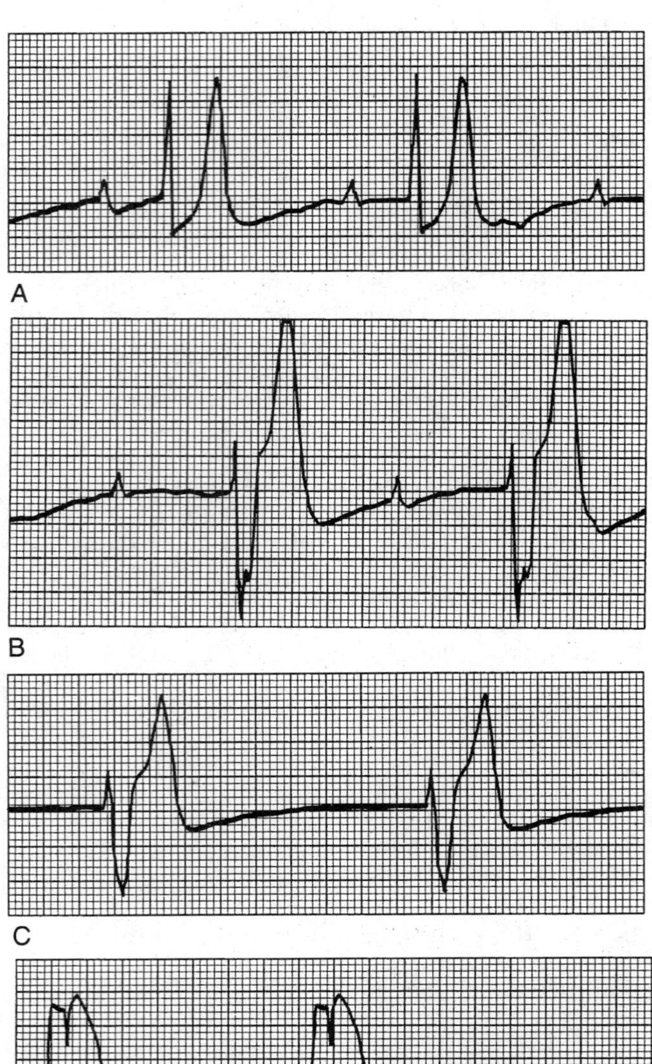

FIGURE 44–3. Electrocardiographic changes in hyperkalemia. *A*, Peaked T waves and AV block are evident at serum potassium levels of 5.5–6.5 mEq/liter. *B*, As the serum potassium concentration reaches 7.0–7.5 mEq/liter, the QRS interval widens and AV nodal conduction is further slowed. *C*, Atrial standstill occurs at serum potassium levels of 8.0–9.0 mEq/liter. *D*, As the serum potassium level exceeds 9.0 mEq/liter, the QRS and T wave merge. Conduction through the His bundle and Purkinje system is further delayed, leading to ventricular fibrillation or asystole.

creased pulmonary capillary permeability, allowing plasma proteins to leak into the alveolae, and resulting in impaired gas diffusion. Arterial blood gas analysis demonstrates hypoxemia. Physical findings include tachypnea and tachycardia. The patient may complain of shortness of breath.

NEUROLOGIC. Neurologic disorders may be caused by the underlying disease process as well as by acute uremia. When the onset of ARF is rapid, neurologic abnormalities are the earliest and most common symptoms. At the onset of acute uremia, the patient complains of fatigue and may appear lethargic or somnolent. As the oliguric phase progresses, the patient may reveal irritability, twitching, disorientation, and possibly psychosis. In advanced uremia, tonic-clonic seizure activity may occur, and the patient will eventually become comatose.

GASTROINTESTINAL. The kidney plays a major role in the inactivation and removal of gastrointestinal (GI) hormones from the blood. When renal function is suppressed, plasma gastrin levels rise. In addition, the gastric ammonia level rises as a result of the increased BUN level. Patients complain of loss of appetite and nausea. Vomiting is a common occurrence. When gastritis or peptic ulcers develop, the patient may complain of abdominal pain. GI hemorrhage is manifested by occult blood in the stool or by frank upper intestinal bleeding.

INTEGUMENT. Generalized subcutaneous edema will be present in the patient with fluid volume overload. As anemia develops, the skin and mucous membranes become pale. Hair loss and abnormal nail growth may also be observed.

Clinical Course of ATN

The clinical course of ATN can be divided into three phases: an oliguric phase, a diuretic phase, and a recovery phase. Patients with nonoliguric ATN progress through a similar course.

The oliguric phase may last a few hours or several months. The average duration of oliguria is 10 to 14 days. In general, a prolonged oliguric phase is associated with a longer and less complete renal recovery. It is during the oliguric phase that the BUN and serum creatinine rise rapidly and the complications of uremia are most severe.

After the onset of the diuretic phase, urine production begins to rise. In most cases, urine output increases incrementally over a period of days or weeks. A small number of patients have a profuse diuresis. The urine produced during the diuretic phase is not well concentrated. It contains less urea and creatinine than is produced by daily metabolic processes. Once urine output has exceeded 1 liter for several days, the BUN and serum creatinine levels will begin to fall. Uremic complications continue to be a threat during the diuretic phase.

The BUN and serum creatinine return to normal levels in the recovery phase. The biochemical and metabolic derangements of acute uremia resolve. Although renal function appears normal, defects in filtration and concentration remain for months to years after the renal injury.

CLINICAL MANAGEMENT

Because there is no cure for ARF once nephron damage occurs, clinical management is focused first on prevention and then on management of the complications arising from the various physiologic alterations accompanying uremia. Table 44–7 summarizes the medical management of the patient with acute oliguric renal failure.

Prevention

Renal injury may be caused by either ischemic insult or nephrotoxic exposure; therefore, it is essential that the physician and nurse assess the patient's clinical status to identify and correct factors that contribute to renal damage. Because the most common cause of ARF in critically ill patients is prolonged renal ischemia, careful attention is paid to signs and symptoms that suggest impending renal hypoperfusion (Davda and Guzman, 1994; Whittaker, 1985). Assessment of extracellular fluid volume loss includes careful consideration of all sources of fluid loss and fluid intake. Intake and output records provide useful information about fluid balance trends. Progressive loss of body weight is a very reliable indicator of fluid volume loss (Baer & Lancaster, 1992). If the patient is experiencing fluid shifts between body compartments (third spacing), body weight may not demonstrate significant change. Assessment focuses on urine output trends and hemodynamic findings. It is crucial that a baseline urine output be obtained and monitored for a downward trend. Periodic specific gravity measurements may be used to detect changes in urine concentration resulting from extracellular fluid volume depletion. Hemodynamic assessment reveals a falling pulmonary artery wedge pressure (PAWP) and CVP. Tachycardia may be present. The blood pressure may show orthostatic changes.

If assessment findings indicate that the patient is at risk of renal hypoperfusion, interventions must be implemented to restore and support circulating volume. The collaborative efforts of medical and nursing management are directed toward maintaining glomerular filtration and urine flow. Preventive management is focused on two areas: fluid challenge and pharmacologic support.

TABLE 44–7. **Clinical Management of Acute Oliguric Renal Failure**

Prevention	Management of Hyperkalemia
Fluid challenge	Potassium restriction
Diuretic challenge	Intravenous insulin/glucose/bicarbonate
Mannitol	Ion exchange resin
Furosemide	Dialysis
Vasoactives	**Nutritional Management**
Dopamine	Minimal carbohydrate requirement 100 g
Calcium channel blockers	Minimal protein requirement 20–30 g
Fluid Management	**Medication Management**
Fluid restriction	Peak/trough serum drug levels
Daily serum sodium monitoring	

FLUID CHALLENGE. A number of clinicians advocate the use of fluid challenge when acute oliguria occurs. If the patient is in a hypovolemic prerenal state, administration of fluid should improve renal perfusion, and the kidney will respond by increasing urine output. Unfortunately, patients with postrenal disease or ATN may also respond to fluid challenge by increasing urine output (Rudnick et al., 1988). In these patients, the additional fluid contributes to worsened hydronephrosis and may result in increased fluid volume overload. For these reasons, many clinicians reserve fluid challenge for patients whose hemodynamic and physical findings strongly suggest hypovolemia.

DIURETIC CHALLENGE. In the oliguric patient with fluid volume overload, administration of a diuretic challenge is preferred to a fluid challenge. Diuretics must be used with caution in the presence of prerenal azotemia, because they may contribute to further fluid volume depletion. In addition to their diagnostic value, diuretics are thought to offer protection against development of ATN. These protective mechanisms include increasing renal blood flow, increasing tubular urine flow, and decreasing nephron cellular energy requirements (Brezis et al., 1984; Davda & Guzman, 1994). Both osmotic and loop diuretics have been used to treat ARF in the clinical setting.

Mannitol, an osmotic diuretic, is theorized to prevent tubular obstruction by increasing tubular urine flow. Increased flow washes out the solutes in the tubules, resulting in decreased tubular cast formation. Mannitol may also decrease endothelial cell swelling, thereby reducing renal vasoconstriction. Administration of mannitol has been shown to reduce the frequency of ATN development in patients receiving nephrotoxic agents (Zager, 1983).

Loop diuretics such as furosemide also have been observed to cause renal vasodilation and to increase tubular urine flow. A number of clinicians have used furosemide to convert oliguric ARF to a nonoliguric state. It is theorized that treatment with loop diuretics reduces the total number of tubules blocked by Tamm-Horsfall casts (Bayati et al., 1990b). Because loop diuretics do not cause shifts of interstitial fluid into the intravascular space, they are safer than mannitol for use in patients with acute volume overload.

VASOACTIVE DRUGS. Because renal vasoconstriction is a consistent finding in ARF, a number of clinicians have advocated the use of vasoactive agents to increase RBF. Infusion of dopamine, a beta-receptor agonist, has been demonstrated to increase RBF in patients with ARF. A number of studies confirm that the combination of dopamine and furosemide is particularly effective in converting oliguric to nonoliguric ARF (Duke & Bersten, 1992; Finn, 1990; Graziani et al., 1984). Other studies suggest that infusion of calcium channel blockers may offer protection against renal ischemia. Administration of calcium channel blockers has been found to attenuate both the vascular and tubular changes that occur in ischemic ARF (Jacobsen et al., 1990; Schrier & Burke, 1991).

HIGH RISK FOR INJURY. Nursing interventions for the patient with impending ARF include assessment of the patient's fluid volume status and evaluation of the patient's response to the prescribed fluid replacement regimen. Significant changes or imbalances are reported to the physician. Changes in fluid therapy are monitored for efficacy. Prescribed diuretics or renal vasoactive infusions are administered and carefully evaluated for their effect on renal function.

Nursing assessment of patient exposure to toxic drugs or chemicals is a valuable aid in the prevention of nephrotoxic injury. A thorough nursing history may reveal evidence of toxin ingestion. In addition, the nurse possesses knowledge of numerous drugs, chemical agents, and endogenous substances known to cause renal damage. Identification of the ingested substance and knowledge of its toxic effects assist the nurse in planning appropriate interventions to prevent or minimize nephrotoxic injury.

The nephrotoxic effects of exogenous and endogenous agents are accentuated by hypovolemia (Zager, 1992). Maintenance of adequate fluid volume status before and during nephrotoxic exposure is essential. Prescribed diuretics may be given on a schedule to increase urine flow during antibiotic administration. Hypokalemia increases the potential for aminoglycoside toxicity. Therefore, serum potassium level must be closely monitored when aminoglycoside antibiotics are administered. The nurse arranges for collection of peak and trough serum drug levels, and monitors for rising trough levels.

Fluid Management

The patient with oliguric ARF will rapidly become fluid volume overloaded unless water intake is restricted. The prescribed fluid restriction will take into account the patient's daily urine output and the daily insensible fluid loss, which is approximately 500 mL. For example, if the patient produces 300 mL of urine in 24 hours, the daily fluid restriction would be 800 mL. Infusion of hypotonic intravenous (IV) fluids is discouraged, because it may lead to hyponatremia. Daily serum sodium measurements will assist in maintaining water and solute balance.

Many critically ill patients sequester fluid in the extravascular compartments. This "third spacing" may significantly increase the patient's fluid volume requirements. Therefore, the clinician must rely on the CVP or the artery PAWP to guide fluid administration. As the patient begins to produce increased amounts of urine, fluid requirements will need to be adjusted to prevent underhydration and hypovolemia.

HIGH RISK FOR FLUID VOLUME EXCESS. The patient with oliguric ARF requires close monitoring for fluid volume overload. Serial daily weights provide a reliable estimate of the patient's fluid status. An increase in weight of 1 kg is approximately equal to a fluid volume increase of 1 liter. Physical findings that provide evidence of volume overload include peripheral edema, pulmonary rales, and increased jugular venous distension. The patient may become hypertensive as a result of increased cardiac output. The CVP and PAWP will increase above baseline.

The patient's daily fluid requirements are prescribed by the physician. Because the daily restriction may frequently be less than 1000 mL, creative nursing strategies will be needed to stretch the allotment over the 24-hour period. Oral and IV fluid allotments must be appropriately divided among shifts. When possible, vasoactive infusions are mixed double strength to increase the amount of discretionary fluid available. Intake and output records can be used to guide the distribution of allowed fluids.

Management of thirst in the conscious patient who is able to take oral fluids is a particular challenge. The nurse explains the reasons for fluid restriction to the patient and family members. The patient may be very uncomfortable, and family members will feel pressured to provide extra fluids. Therefore, frequent explanations and support by the nurse will be necessary. Actions to minimize thirst include providing periodic sips and ice chips. Some patients feel that chewing gum or hard sour candy is helpful. Others may prefer to have a cold wet gauze sponge available to suck on. Frequent, meticulous mouth care is essential to control thirst and maintain the integrity of the oral mucosa.

A large number of critically ill patients will need vasoactive drug infusions and total parenteral nutrition (TPN) in volumes greatly in excess of their calculated daily fluid restriction. These patients will require dialysis therapy to prevent fluid volume overload.

Management of Hyperkalemia

Hyperkalemia is a common complication of oliguric ARF, and is particularly problematic in patients with severe catabolism. The nurse collaborates with the physician and clinical dietician in evaluating sources of potassium intake and facilitating potassium removal from the body. The patient is placed on a low-potassium diet and potassium is removed from IV fluids. Medications containing potassium salts should be discontinued. Restriction of potassium intake may be all that is necessary to control serum potassium elevations of less than 6.0 mEq/liter.

DECREASED CARDIAC OUTPUT RELATED TO DYSRHYTHMIAS. Hyperkalemia is the serious complication of oliguric ARF. Unless treatment is initiated the patient will develop life-threatening cardiac dysrhythmias within a few days after the onset of oliguria. The serum potassium level is monitored at least daily. More frequent measurements will be required if the potassium is rising rapidly. The patient's ECG is monitored for the presence of peaked T waves, widened QRS complexes, and development of heart block or other rhythm disturbances (see Fig. 44–3). Hyperkalemia greater than 6.0 mEq/liter will be actively treated, even in the absence of ECG changes.

Life-threatening dysrhythmias may be emergently treated with IV calcium gluconate. Calcium stabilizes the cardiac cell membrane, but does not actually lower the serum potassium level. IV administration of 4 to 10 units of regular insulin followed by one ampule of 50% dextrose can be used to temporarily lower the extracellular potassium level. Administration of insulin and glucose causes extracellular potassium ions to shift into the intracellular space. Because potassium is not actually removed from the body, hyperkalemia will recur within a few hours as potassium shifts back into the extracellular space (Innerarity, 1992).

Ion exchange resin (Kayexalate) may be effective in controlling serum potassium in noncatabolic patients. Potassium is exchanged across the GI mucosa, and is removed from the body in the feces. Kayexalate can be given rectally or orally. If given as an enema, Kayexalate is effective only if it is retained for at least 30 to 60 minutes. Oral administration is more effective because it allows the resin to remain in contact with the GI mucosa for a longer time. Kayexalate can be very constipating when it is mixed with water. Therefore, it should be mixed with an osmotic agent such as sorbitol. Sorbitol produces an osmotic diarrhea that further increases potassium excretion. Kayexalate is of limited benefit in patients who do not have bowel function; dialysis therapy will be required to control extreme hyperkalemia in such patients.

Nutritional Management

Optimal caloric and protein intake is of critical importance in the treatment of ARF. The goals of nutritional management are to minimize endogenous catabolism and to prevent malnutrition. Adequate caloric intake is essential to prevent protein catabolism. At least 100 g of carbohydrates are necessary to supply energy requirements. Administration of hypertonic glucose solutions, in the form of TPN, is often necessary to supply the required carbohydrates. Fat is an essential nutrient and is useful in providing a concentrated source of calories for the fluid-restricted patient (Mitch & Wilmore, 1988).

Sufficient protein intake is necessary for wound healing to occur. In mildly catabolic patients, 20 to 30 g of protein is usually necessary to maintain neutral nitrogen balance (Mitch & Wilmore, 1988). Administration of additional essential and nonessential amino acids will be required in the more catabolic patient.

ALTERATION IN NUTRITION: LESS THAN BODY REQUIREMENTS. Management of the acutely oliguric patient's nutritional status is a challenge. If the patient is able to eat, the nurse will collaborate with the dietician in obtaining a dietary history. The patient and family will need a thorough explanation of the dietary restrictions. The patient may be anorectic and have periods of nausea and vomiting. Measures to maintain adequate intake include providing small meals or snacks at frequent intervals, and performing mouth care often. If necessary, prescribed antiemetics are administered.

When TPN is used for nutritional management, the nurse carefully monitors the infusion and evaluates the patient's response to the fluid load. The serum glucose is routinely monitored, and an insulin prescription is obtained to correct hyperglycemia.

Prevention of Complications

The kidneys play an important role in many metabolic and hormonal processes in the body. When ARF occurs, these processes are altered and in some cases lost, thereby placing the patient at risk of developing a number of serious complications.

HIGH RISK FOR INJURY: DRUG TOXICITY. A large number of drugs are excreted wholly or partially by the kidneys. In patients with ARF, the dosage of these drugs must be adjusted to prevent toxicity to the kidneys and other organ systems. If the patient is receiving aminoglycoside antibotics, peak and trough serum drug levels are closely monitored. High serum trough levels appear to correlate best with nephrotoxicity and rising serum creatinine (Bernstein & Erk, 1990). Formulas for adjusting drug dosages based on the serum creatinine level may be useful once the serum creatinine reaches a steady state (Bennett, 1986).

HIGH RISK FOR INFECTION. Patients with ARF are at increased risk of infection because of leukopenia and impaired inflammatory response. Nursing actions to prevent infection emphasize careful technique and minimal manipulation of lines and catheters. Frequent pulmonary care will be required to prevent pooling of secretions in the lungs. The patient's body temperature curve is closely monitored, and elevations are reported. Blood, sputum, urine, and wound drainage are cultured. A white blood cell (WBC) count with microscopic differential is monitored for increases in total WBC count and in the number of bands.

HIGH RISK FOR IMPAIRED GAS EXCHANGE. The clotting abnormalities associated with ARF place the patient at increased risk of hemorrhage. In addition, synthesis of new red blood cells is depressed. Loss of red blood cell volume places the patient at risk of anemia, which results in a decrease in the oxygen-carrying capacity of the blood. Because of the high potential for significant blood loss, clinical management is directed toward assessment of bleeding and minimizing blood loss. Hemoglobin and hematocrit levels are monitored for significant downward trends. Observations of the patient include noting the presence of bruising, petechiae, and hematoma formation. The urine, stool, and nasogastric drainage are tested for occult blood. Measures to decrease blood loss incude minimizing the number of times blood samples are drawn and ensuring that only minimal amounts of blood are collected for each specimen. Careful attention is paid to avoiding tissue trauma during tracheal suctioning and insertion of nasogastric tubes.

If the clinical course of renal failure is prolonged, the patient may benefit from administration of recombinant erythropoietin (epoetin). Epoetin can be administered intravenously or subcutaneously. Response to epoetin is usually seen in 2 to 6 weeks (Binkley & Whittaker, 1992). Management of the ARF patient receiving epoetin therapy includes monitoring of the hemoglobin and hematocrit. Because critically ill patients often lack sufficient iron stores to respond to epoetin, the serum ferritin level and transferrin saturation levels will be carefully assessed. The patient's blood pressure must also be closely monitored, because hypertension is a common response to epoetin therapy.

DIALYSIS THERAPY

Dialysis is a process in which waste materials in the blood are filtered through a semipermeable membrane and removed from the body. In ARF, the indications for dialysis therapy include fluid overload, rapidly progressing azotemia, hyperkalemia, and metabolic acidosis. Current clinical practice suggests that dialysis should be initiated early and at frequent intervals (Jameson & Weigmann, 1990). Early, aggressive dialysis minimizes fluctuations in serum chemistries and may decrease uremic complications.

Three dialysis methods are available for use in patients with ARF: hemodialysis, peritoneal dialysis, and continuous renal replacement therapy (CRRT). The advantages and disadvantages of each method are summarized in Table 44–8.

Hemodialysis

Hemodialysis is a highly efficient method of removing water and solutes from the body. The patient's blood is passed across a semipermeable membrane contained in a dialysis hemofilter. Dialysate fluid, containing prescribed concentrations of electrolytes, passes on the outside of the membrane. Water, electrolytes, and nitrogenous waste products diffuse freely across the membrane, both plasma proteins and blood cells are too large to pass through it. The patient's electrolyte balance can be regulated by varying the ion concentration of the dialysate bath. For example, hyperkalemia is treated by using a low potassium concentration in the dialysate.

Water is removed during hemodialysis by means of ultrafiltration. Ultrafiltration depends on the presence of a pressure gradient across the semipermeable membrane. The hydrostatic pressure that produces this transmembrane pressure gradient has both positive and negative components (Peschman, 1992). Positive hydrostatic pressure is applied to the blood compartment and acts to push water from the blood. Negative hydrostatic pressure is applied to the dialysate compartment and creates a vacuum that pulls water from the blood compartment. At any given transmembrane pressure, the amount of fluid removed by ultrafiltration can be predicted. If the patient requires a higher rate of fluid removal, the ultrafiltration rate can be increased by increasing either positive pressure on the blood side or negative pressure on the fluid side.

INDICATIONS FOR HEMODIALYSIS. The greatest advantage offered by hemodialysis to the patient with ARF is efficiency. The patient's fluid and electrolyte abnormalities can be corrected by an average of 4 hours of treatment every other day. Hemodialysis is particularly beneficial for patients with fluid volume overload and rapidly rising BUN and potassium levels (Stark, 1992). In extremely catabolic patients, daily hemodialysis treatments may be required to control azotemia and hyperkalemia.

Although hemodialysis is the dialysis therapy used most frequently in patients with ARF, it is not always well tolerated by critically ill patients. Cardiovascular instability is a common problem in patients undergoing acute hemodialysis. The rapid fluid shifts frequently result in severe hypotension. Other untoward cardiovascular effects include cardiac dysrhythmias, shortness of breath, and chest pain. Hemodialysis may be contraindicated in patients with severe brain injury. The rapid solute removal promotes movement of water across the blood–brain barrier, resulting in increased cerebral edema (Fraser & Arieff, 1988).

CLINICAL MANAGEMENT OF ACUTE HEMODIALYSIS. Although critical care nurses do not routinely perform hemodialysis, the nursing care they provide between treatments is vital to the success of the dialysis regimen. Nursing management of the patient undergoing acute hemodialysis is guided by the nursing diagnoses previously discussed in this chapter. In addition, special nursing consideration is given to maintaining the integrity of the patient's vascular access site. Assessments and interventions are directed toward keeping the access patent and infection-free.

TABLE 44–8. **Comparison of Hemodialysis, Peritoneal Dialysis, and Continuous Renal Replacement Therapy (CRRT)**

	Hemodialysis	Peritoneal Dialysis	CRRT
Effectiveness of therapy	Rapid removal of water and solutes	Slow removal of water and solutes	Rate of removal of water and solutes varies with mode of treatment
Time required for treatment	3–4 hr per treatment; treatments 2–4 times per week	Continuous hourly exchanges or 4–6 exchanges per day with dwell times of 4–8 hr	Continuous hourly therapy
Access requirements	Vascular access—subclavian catheter, femoral catheter, fistula, or shunt—is required	Requires presence of an intact peritoneal membrane and placement of a peritoneal catheter	Arterial and venous access usually required
Technical requirements	Complex equipment; highly specialized dialysis personnel	Manual exchanges easily performed by bedside critical care nurse; peritoneal cycler is moderately complex and requires trained personnel	Moderately complex system; performed by bedside critical care nurse
Anticoagulation requirements	Systemic or regional heparinization required; can be reversed	Minimal heparinization required	Heparinization of hemofilter system required; minimal systemic anticoagulation
Common complications	Bleeding; cardiovascular instability; hypotension, arrhythmias	Peritonitis; protein loss in dialysate, hyperglycemia	Clotting of hemofilter; blood loss in system; potential hypovolemia

Peritoneal Dialysis

Peritoneal dialysis is a renal replacement therapy that uses the peritoneum as the dialyzing semipermeable membrane. Sterile dialysate is instilled into the peritoneal cavity. Water, electrolytes, and metabolic wastes diffuse across the peritoneum from the blood in the peritoneal capillary network. These products are removed from the body when the dialysate is drained out of the peritoneal cavity. Diffusion of electrolytes, such as potassium, can be achieved by instilling dialysate with a concentration lower than that of the plasma. Water removal is enhanced by using a more hypertonic dextrose solution.

Peritoneal dialysis is a slow, continuous dialysis therapy. Initially, hourly exchanges may be required to control fluid and electrolyte abnormalities in the patient with ARF. After the BUN has been controlled, exchanges may be done less frequently. Exchanges of 2000 mL performed every 3 hours achieve approximately the same solute clearance as 3- to 4-hour hemodialysis treatments performed every other day (Maher, 1990).

INDICATIONS FOR PERITONEAL DIALYSIS. Because peritoneal dialysis does not cause rapid shifts in fluid and electrolyte balance, it does not contribute to cardiovascular instability (Ash & Mertz, 1994). Critically ill patients with low mean arterial blood pressures and those with cardiac arrhythmias can be effectively dialyzed. Solutes are removed slowly over a period of hours to days. Because the blood solute level does not fluctuate rapidly, peritoneal dialysis can safely be used in patients with cerebral edema. Anticoagulation is not required, so peritoneal dialysis may be indicated for patients with bleeding tendencies.

One disadvantage of peritoneal dialysis is that solute removal is relatively inefficient. Even hourly exchanges may not be sufficient to control the extreme elevations in BUN and potassium seen in hypercatabolic patients (Kronfol, 1994). In addition, significant amounts of plasma proteins and amino acids may be lost through the peritoneal drainage (Ash & Mertz, 1994). Protein losses of up to 0.5 g/liter further compromise the nutritional status of the catabolic patient. Peritoneal dialysis can only be used in patients with intact peritoneal membranes. The procedure is contraindicated in most patients with abdominal trauma and after surgery that disrupts the peritoneal space.

CLINICAL MANAGEMENT. The critical care nurse is responsible for performing and monitoring the peritoneal dialysis procedure. Careful assessment of the patient's fluid volume status is performed on an ongoing basis. Specific attention is paid to intake and output records and to changes in the patient's body weight. Strict aseptic technique is used while performing exchanges and in performing care of the catheter exit site.

In addition to fluid management and infection control, the nurse observes for potential complications associated with peritoneal dialysis. The most common complications are pain, drainage problems, and the development of peritonitis.

Continuous Renal Replacement Therapy

Continuous renal replacement therapy is an extracorporeal blood treatment used to control both fluid and solute balance in patients with ARF. The therapy does not require the use of hemodialysis machinery but relies instead on the patient's own arterial blood pressure to power the system. As shown in Figure 44–4, the ultrafiltration system is composed of arterial and venous tubing, the hemofilter, and ultrafiltrate collection receptacle.

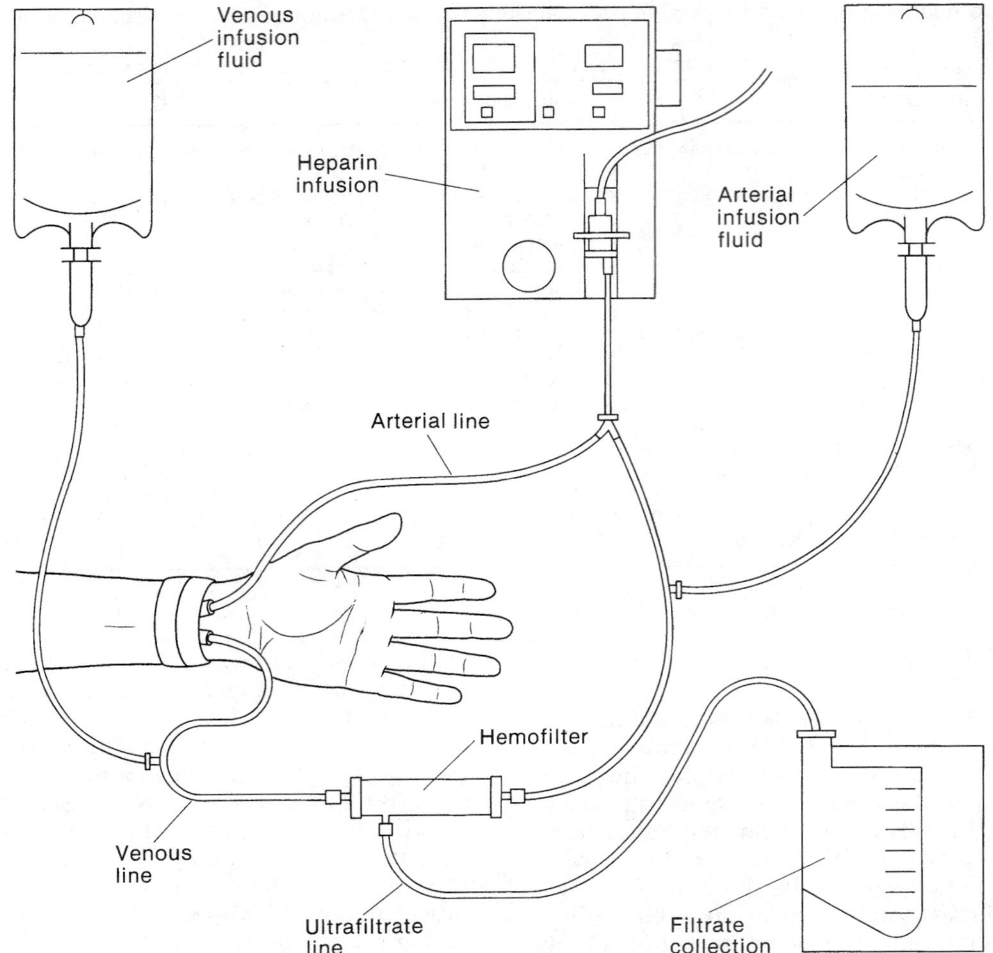

FIGURE 44–4. Continuous renal replacement therapy system.

The success of CRRT depends on maintenance of blood flow through the hemofilter. Both arterial and venous vascular accesses are required. Blood flows of up to 200 mL/min can be obtained using an external arteriovenous shunt or percutaneous femoral catheters. In most patients, a mean arterial blood pressure of 60 mm Hg is required to maintain adequate blood flow.

During CRRT, water, electrolytes, and other solutes are removed as the patient's blood passes over semipermeable membranes contained in a hemofilter. The resulting ultrafiltrate is a protein-free fluid with a solute and electrolyte concentration similar to that of plasma. The plasma proteins and cellular components of the blood remain in the hemofilter circuit and return to the venous circulation. Mass transfer of water and solutes across a semipermeable membrane is a result of convection and diffusion. In CRRT, the convective forces applied across the hemofilter membrane depend primarily on the patient's arterial blood pressure. The higher the blood pressure, the greater the hydrostatic pressure within the hemofilter. Diffusion is a process in which solutes are passively transferred across a membrane. Passive transfer of solutes is dependent on the presence of a concentration gradient across the membrane. In CRRT therapy, a concentration gradient can be established by infusing dialysate fluid into the nonblood side of the hemofilter.

INDICATIONS FOR CRRT. Removal of plasma water and electrolytes by CRRT is a gradual process that closely resembles the kidney's normal function. Because it is a gradual process, rapid fluctuations in fluid and electrolyte status do not occur. Therefore, CRRT is indicated for ARF patients with cardiovascular instability and those with cerebral edema (Nahman & Middendorf, 1990). There are three distinct variations of CRRT in current clinical use. As summarized in Table 44–9, each of these treatment variations is designed to meet the renal replacement needs of a specific group of patients.

SLOW CONTINUOUS ULTRAFILTRATION. Slow continuous ultrafiltration (SCUF) is a therapy in which small amounts of plasma, water, and solutes are slowly removed from the patient. In most patients, fluid removal occurs at rates of 100 to 300 mL/hr. The thera-

TABLE 44–9. **Clinical Application of Continuous Renal Replacement Therapy**

	Slow Continuous Ultrafiltration (SCUF)	Continuous Arteriovenous Hemofiltration (CAVH)	Continuous Arteriovenous Hemofiltration Dialysis (CAVHD)
Therapeutic goal	Prevention of hypervolemia	Control of fluid and solute balance	Control of fluid and solute balance
Indications	Volume overload in CHF; adjunct to hemodialysis	Noncatabolic patients with oliguric ARF	Catabolic or noncatabolic patients with oliguric ARF
Rate of fluid removal	<300 mL/hr	400–800 mL/hr	Approximately 100 mL/hr
Efficiency of solute removal	Minimal solute removed	Solute control achieved dilution with large volume exchanges	Steady-state plasma, urea, and creatinine levels by 24–48 hours
Mechanism of solute removal	Convection resulting from hydrostatic pressure exerted by the arterial blood pressure	Convection	Primary—diffusion of solutes from blood into dialysate; Secondary—convection
Fluid replacement requirements	Fluid requirements usually met by maintenance IV infusions	Up to 20 liters/24 hr of prescribed IV fluids	Fluid requirements usually met by maintenance IV infusions

Abbreviations: ARF, acute renal failure; CHF, congestive heart failure.

peutic goal of SCUF is to control fluid balance and prevent fluid volume overload (Price, 1992). Because only small amounts of solutes are removed, SCUF is unsuitable as the primary dialysis therapy for patients with azotemia or significant electrolyte abnormalities. SCUF is highly effective in controlling fluid volume overload in patients with severe congestive heart failure who do not respond to diuretic therapy. Fluid removal by ultrafiltration can achieve significant preload reduction in these patients. SCUF can also be used as an adjunct to hemodialysis in patients with ARF who require large volumes of maintenance IV fluids. The patient is placed on SCUF between hemodialysis treatments to prevent hypervolemia and decrease the need for additional hemodialysis treatments.

CONTINUOUS ARTERIOVENOUS HEMOFILTRATION. Continuous arteriovenous hemofiltration (CAVH) is a renal replacement therapy in which large amounts of plasma water and solutes are removed on a continuous basis. Fluid removal rates may range from 400 to 800 mL/hr. Because CAVH removes large volumes of plasma water, significant amounts of plasma electrolytes and solutes are also removed. Control of fluid volume and electrolyte balance is achieved through large-volume fluid exchanges. Hourly ultrafiltrate loss is replaced by prescribed amounts of sterile IV electrolyte solution. CAVH provides a mechanism of diluting the patient's plasma by selective replacement of solutes. Therefore, CAVH can be used as the primary dialysis therapy for ARF patients with mild to moderate azotemia and electrolyte disturbances (Olbricht, 1986).

CONTINUOUS ARTERIOVENOUS HEMODIALYSIS. Continuous arteriovenous hemodialysis (CAVHD) combines the convective transport of CAVH with diffusion dialysis. Sterile dialysate fluid is infused into the ultrafiltration compartment of the hemofilter shown in Figure 44–5. The dialysate flows countercurrent to the blood flow, which increases diffusion of solutes from the blood to the ultrafiltrate compartment. Solute removal in CAVHD is much greater than that in CAVH (Stark, 1992). Therefore, CAVHD can be effectively used as the primary dialysis therapy in a wide variety of critically ill patients, including ARF patients with severe azotemia and electrolyte imbalance. Plasma urea and creatinine levels have reached a steady state after 24 to 48 hours of CAVHD treatment (Geronemus, 1986). Electrolyte abnormalities and acid-base disturbances are also well controlled.

CLINICAL MANAGEMENT. The major nursing goal in CRRT is optimization of the patient's fluid volume status (Price, 1992). The large amount of fluid removed by ultrafiltration places the patient at risk of fluid volume depletion. Maintenance of the patency of the ultrafiltration system and prevention of blood loss are additional nursing goals.

DISCHARGE PREPARATION

As discussed previously, the course of ARF varies considerably, with the diuretic and recovery phases lasting up to several months. As hospital length of stay continues to decrease, it is common for the patient with ARF to be discharged home on dialysis therapy. Preparation of the ARF patient for discharge includes teaching the patient about the particular dialysis therapy that he/she is receiving. Content areas that must be considered include care of the vascular access or peritoneal catheter, dietary restrictions, fluid restrictions, medication management, and emphasis on preventive health care. If peritoneal dialysis is being used,

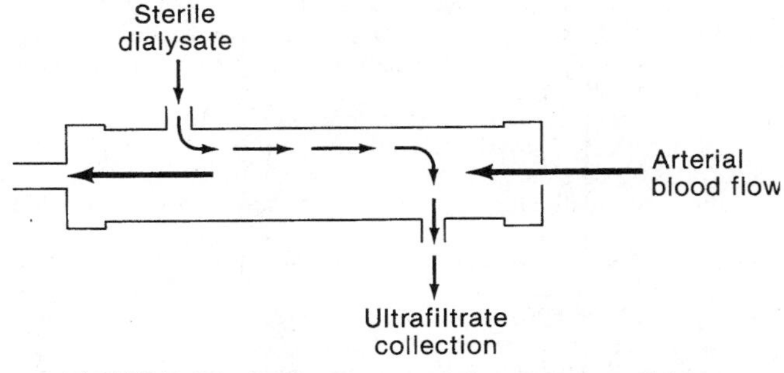

FIGURE 44–5. Continuous arteriovenous hemodialysis.

the patient and/or caretaker must be taught to perform the exchanges using appropriate technique.

SUMMARY

Acute renal failure is a serious complication of critical illness in which renal function is severely compromised. ARF may be caused by renal hypoperfusion, obstruction of the urinary tract, or ATN resulting from renal ischemia or exposure to toxic agents. Oliguria is the most common manifestation, and may persist from days to months. Goals of therapy include control of fluid and solute balance, adequate nutrition, and prevention of infection. Most patients who survive ARF recover near normal renal function, although some deficits in tubular function may remain for months to years after the renal injury.

REFERENCES

Andreucci, V. E. (1984). Myoglobinuria and acute renal failure. In V. E. Andreucci (Ed.), *Acute Renal Failure: Pathophysiology, prevention and treatment* (pp. 250–255). Boston: Martinus Nijhoff.

Ash, S. R., & Mertz, S. L. (1994, January). Peritoneal dialysis for acute renal failure: The safe, effective, and low cost modality. Paper presented at the 14th Conference on Peritoneal Dialysis, Orlando, Florida.

Baer, C. L., & Lancaster, L. E. (1992). Acute renal failure. *Critical Care Nursing Quarterly, 14*(4), 1–21.

Bayati, A., Nygren, K., Kallskog, O., et al. (1990a). The long-term outcome of post-ischaemic acute renal failure II. A histopathological study of the untreated kidney. *Acta Physiologica Scandinavia, 138,* 35–47.

Bayati, A., Nygren, K., Kallskog, O., et al. (1990b). The effect of loop diuretics on the long-term outcome of post-ischaemic acute renal failure in the rat. *Acta Physiologica Scandinavia, 139,* 217–279.

Bennett, W. M. (1986). Update on drugs in renal failure. In J. P. Greenfield, M. H. Maxwell, J. F. Back, et al. (Eds.), *Advances in Nephrology* (Vol. 15, pp. 287–299). Chicago: Year Book.

Bernstein, J. M., & Erk, S. D. (1990). Choice of antibiotics, pharmacokinetics, and dose adjustments in acute renal failure. *Medical Clinics of North America, 74,* 1059–1076.

Binkley, L. S., & Whittaker, A. A. (1992). Erythropoietin use in the critical care setting. *AACN Clinical Issues in Critical Care Nursing, 3*(3), 640–649.

Brezis, M., Rosen, S., Silva, P., et al. (1984). Renal ischemia: A new perspective. *Kidney International, 26,* 375–383.

Brezis, M., & Epstein, F. H. (1993). Cellular mechanisms of acute ischemic injury in the kidney. *Annual Review of Medicine, 44,* 27–37.

Cameron, J. J., & Ogg, C. (1967). Peritoneal dialysis in hypercatabolic acute renal failure. *Lancet, 1,* 1188–1191.

Davda, R. K., & Guzman, N. J. (1994). Acute renal failure: Prompt diagnosis is key to effective management. *Postgraduate Medicine, 96*(5), 89–98.

Dayer-Berenson, L. (1994). Rhabdomyolysis: A comprehensive guide. *ANNA Journal, 21*(1), 15–18.

Duke, G. J., & Bersten, A. D. (1992). Dopamine and renal salvage in the critically ill patient. *Anaesthesiology and Intensive Care, 20*(3), 277–287.

Finn, W. F. (1990). Diagnosis and management of acute tubular necrosis. *Medical Clinics of North America, 74,* 373–380.

Fraser, C. L., & Arieff, A. I. (1988). Nervous system complications in uremia. *Annals of Internal Medicine, 109,* 143–153.

Geronemus, R. (1986). Continuous arteriovenous hemodialysis—Clinical experience. In E. Paginini (Ed.), *Acute continuous renal replacement therapy* (pp. 247–254). Boston: Martinus Nijhoff.

Giordano, C., Castellano, P., Pluvio, M., et al. (1987). Glucose metabolism. In A. Americo, P. Coratelli, R. M. Campese, et al. (Eds.), *Acute renal failure: Clinical and experimental* (pp. 105–111). New York: Plenum.

Graziani, G., Cantaluppi, S., Casati, S., et al. (1984). Dopamine and furosemide in oliguric acute renal failure. *Nephron, 37,* 39–42.

Hohenfellner, M., Thuroff, J. W., & Thurau, K. (1992). Cellular changes in acute renal failure: Functional and therapeutic consequences. *European Urology, 22*(4), 265–270.

Humes, H. D. (1988). Aminoglycoside nephrotoxicity. *Kidney International, 33,* 900–911.

Innerarity, S. A. (1992). Hyperkalemic emergencies. *Critical Care Nursing Quarterly, 14*(4), 32–39.

Jacobsen, W. K., Cole, D. J., Stewart, S. C., et al. (1990). Effect of calcium entry blocker nitrendipine on renal function after renal vascular occlusion. *Critical Care Medicine, 18,* 1403–1407.

Jameson, M. D., & Wiegmann, T. B. (1990). Principles, uses and complications of hemodialysis. *Medical Clinics of North America, 74,* 945–960.

Jochimsen, R., Schafer, J. H., Mauler, A., & Distler, A. (1990). Impairment of renal function in medical intensive care: Predictability of acute renal failure. *Critical Care Medicine, 18*(5), 480–485.

Kashgarian, M., Siegel, J. J., Ries, A. L., et al. (1976). Hemodynamic aspects in development and recovery phases of experimental post-ischemic acute renal failure. *Kidney International, 10,* 160–168.

Knochel, J. P. (1985). Potassium gradients and neuromuscular excitability. In D. N. Seldin & G. Giebisch (Eds.), *The kidney: Physiology and pathology* (pp. 1207–1221). New York: Raven Press.

Kronfol, N. O. (1994). Acute peritoneal dialysis prescription. In J. T. Daugirdas & T. S. Ing (Eds.), *Handbook of dialysis* (2nd ed., pp. 301–309). Boston: Little, Brown & Co.

Maher, J. F. (1990). Physiology of the peritoneum. *Medical Clinics of North America, 74,* 985–996.

Mason, J., Torhorst, J., & Welsh, J. (1984). Role of the medullary perfusion defect in the pathogenesis of ischemic renal failure. *Kidney International, 26,* 283–286.

Mitch, W. E., & Wilmore, D. W. (1988). Nutritional considerations in the treatment of acute renal failure. In B. M. Brenner & J. M. Lazarus (Eds.), *Acute renal failure* (2nd ed., pp. 743–765). New York: Churchill Livingstone.

Nahman, N. S., & Middendorf, D. F. (1990). Continuous arteriovenous hemofiltration. *Medical Clinics of North America, 74,* 975–984.

Olbricht, C. (1986). Continuous arteriovenous hemofiltration—The control of azotemia in acute renal failure. In E. Paginini (Ed.), *Acute continuous renal replacement therapy* (pp. 123–142). Boston: Martinus Nijhoff.

Peschman, P. (1992). Acute hemodialysis: Issues in the critically ill. *AACN Clinical Issues in Critical Care Nursing, 3*(3), 545–557.

Price, C. A. (1992). An update on continuous renal replacement therapies. *AACN Clinical Issues in Critical Care Nursing, 3*(3), 597–604.

Racusen, L. C. (1991). Structural correlates of renal electrolyte alterations in acute renal failure. *Mineral and Electrolyte Metabolism, 17*(2), 72–88.

Racusen, L. C. (1992). Alterations in tubular epithelial cell adhesion and mechanisms of acute renal failure. *Laboratory Investigation, 67*(2), 158–165.

Radtke, H. W., Claussner, A., Erbes, P. M., et al. (1979). Serum erythropoietin concentration in chronic renal failure: Relationship to degree of anemia and excretory function. *Blood, 54,* 877–884.

Radtke, H. W., Rege, A. B., LaMarche, M. B., et al. (1981). Identification of spermine as an inhibitor of erythropoiesis in patients with chronic renal failure. *Journal of Clinical Investigation, 67,* 1623–1629.

Reaven, G. M., Wisinger, J. R., & Swenson, R. S. (1974). Insulin and glucose metabolism in renal insufficiency. *Kidney International, 6,* 63–69.

Rudnick, M. R., Bastl, C. P., Elfinbein, I. B., et al. (1988). The differential diagnosis of acute renal failure. In B. M. Brenner & J. M.

Lazarus (Eds.), *Acute renal failure* (2nd ed., pp. 177–232). New York: Churchill Livingstone.

Schrier, R. W., & Burke, T. J. (1991). Role of calcium channel blockers in preventing acute and chronic renal injury. *Journal of Cardiovascular Pharmacology, 18* (Suppl 6), 38–43.

Shapira, J., Iaina, A., Eliahou, H. E., et al. (1976). High renin activity accompanying angiotensin II inhibition in rats with ischemic renal failure. *Israel Journal of Medical Sciences, 12,* 124–130.

Stark, J. L. (1992). Dialysis options in the critically ill patient. *Critical Care Nursing Quarterly, 14*(4), 40–44.

Steinman, T. I., & Lazarus, J. M. (1988). Organ-system involvement in acute renal failure. In B. M. Brenner & J. M. Lazarus (Eds.), *Acute renal failure* (2nd ed., pp. 705–742). New York: Churchill Livingstone.

VanZee, B. O., Hoy, W. E., Talley, T. E., et al. (1978). Renal injury associated with intravenous pyelography in nondiabetic and diabetic patients. *Annals of Internal Medicine, 89,* 51–54.

Whalley, D. E., Ibels, L. S., Eckstein, R. P., et al. (1987). Acute tubular necrosis complicating bilateral retrograde pyelography. *Australian and New Zealand Journal of Medicine, 17*(5), 536–538.

Whittaker, A. (1985). Acute renal dysfunction: Assessment of patients at risk. *Focus on Critical Care, 12,* 12–17.

Zager, R. A. (1983). Glomerular filtration rate and brush border debris excretion after mercuric chloride and ischemic acute renal failure: Mannitol versus furosemide diuresis. *Nephron, 33,* 196–201.

Zager, R. A. (1992). Endotoxemia, renal hypoperfusion, and fever: Interactive risk factors for aminoglycoside and sepsis-associated acute renal failure. *American Journal of Kidney Disease, 20*(3), 223–230.

ACUTE RENAL FAILURE MULTIDISCIPLINARY CARE GUIDE

COORDINATION OF CARE

Diagnosis/Stabilization Phase		Acute Management Phase		Recovery Phase	
Outcome	*Intervention*	*Outcome*	*Intervention*	*Outcome*	*Intervention*
All appropriate team members and disciplines will be involved in the plan of care.	Develop the plan of care with the patient/family, primary nurse(s), primary physician(s), nephrologist, cardiologist, pulmonologist, hematologist, chaplain, clinical nurse specialist, and dialysis staff.	All appropriate team members and disciplines will be involved in the plan of care.	Update the plan of care with patient/family, other team members, nephrologist, social services, dietician, physical therapist, occupational therapist, and discharge planner. Initiate planning for anticipated discharge. Begin teaching patient/family about home care (i.e., hemodialysis, peritoneal dialysis) if indicated.	All appropriate disciplines will be consulted.	Provide written instructions for dialysis and/or follow-up care. Provide patient/family with phone numbers of resources available.

FLUID BALANCE

Diagnosis/Stabilization Phase		Acute Management Phase		Recovery Phase	
Outcome	*Intervention*	*Outcome*	*Intervention*	*Outcome*	*Intervention*
Patient will achieve optimal renal/fluid and electrolyte status as evidenced by: • Normovolemic state (adequate circulatory volume) • Optimal achievable renal function • Normal electrolytes (including Ca^{++} and phosphorus) • Normal serum glucose • Normal hematologic parameters such as hemoglobin, platelets and WBCs	Monitor renal parameters, including: • Urine output • BUN • Serum creatinine • BUN/serum creatinine ratio • Serum electrolytes • Acid-base status • Urine electrolytes • Urine osmolality • Specific gravity Monitor fluid status, including intake and output (fluid restriction), daily weights, urine output trends, vital signs, CVP, and PCWP. Monitor for signs and symptoms of hypervolemia such as hypertension, tachycardia, pulmonary edema, peripheral edema, distended neck veins, and elevated CVP. Monitor and treat cause of acute renal dysfunction, including: • Hypoperfusion (prerenal) states • Obstructions in the outflow of urine from the body (postrenal) states • Nephrotoxic agents and/or severe renal ischemia	Patient will achieve optimal renal/fluid and electrolyte status.	Same as stabilization phase. Monitor, support, and treat during dialysis treatments. Monitor, support, treat, and assess patient's response to dialysis therapies. Begin teaching patient and family about renal function, current clinical problems, current treatment, and expected clinical course.	Patient will achieve optimal renal/fluid and electrolyte status.	Same as stabilization phase. Prepare and instruct patient on necessary ongoing therapies (peritoneal dialysis vs. hemodialysis). Instruct patient in follow-up care indicated. Teach patient/family signs and symptoms of fluid overload and/or electrolyte disturbances. Teach patient/family about fluid restriction. Teach patient importance of daily weights.

Direct treatment goals aim toward maintaining glomerular filtration and urine flow. Monitor patient closely for response of fluid and/or diuretic challenges. Support and monitor patient closely during the three typical phases of acute renal failure:

- Oliguric phase
- Diuretic phase
- Recovery phase

Monitor and treat for signs of complications that can occur with acute renal failure: hypertension, cardiac dysfunction, pulmonary edema, dysrhythmias, lethargy, decreased LOC, electrolyte disturbances, acid-base disturbances, abnormal glucose metabolism, anemia, thrombocytopenia, leukopenia, nausea, vomiting, and subcutaneous edema.

Monitor, support, and treat patient with dialysis therapies if indicated:

Assess vital signs, fluid status, CVP, PAWP, and patient response to dialysis therapies.

Hemodialysis:

Assure that vascular access to hemodialysis remains patent:

- Palpate the thrill and auscultate buzzing sound over shunt periodically
- Avoid constrictions above access such as tourniquets or BP cuffs
- Assure that access is free from infection

Peritoneal Dialysis:

- Warm dialysate to body temperature and slowly infuse
- Monitor dialysate infusion and drainage closely to evaluate effectiveness of peritoneal dialysis
- Weigh patient daily after the drain cycle is complete
- Monitor for signs and symptoms of fluid overload
- Monitor closely for signs and symptoms of infection. (Report cloudiness or color change in drained fluid.) Culture drainage daily

Care Guide continued on following page

ACUTE RENAL FAILURE MULTIDISCIPLINARY CARE GUIDE *continued*

FLUID BALANCE *continued*

Diagnosis/Stabilization Phase		Acute Management Phase		Recovery Phase	
Outcome	***Intervention***	***Outcome***	***Intervention***	***Outcome***	***Intervention***
	Continuous Ultrafiltration: • Monitor and regulate ultrafiltration rate hourly based on patient's response and fluid status • Assess and trouble-shoot hemofilter and blood tubing hourly • Monitor closely for signs/symptoms of infection				

NUTRITION

Diagnosis/Stabilization Phase		Acute Management Phase		Recovery Phase	
Outcome	***Intervention***	***Outcome***	***Intervention***	***Outcome***	***Intervention***
Patient will be adequately nourished.	Obtain a dietary consult. Monitor caloric intake and percentages of fats, carbohydrates, and proteins closely. • Protein intake should be somewhat restricted (sufficient yet not excessive; usually 20–30 g/day) • Carbohydrates—100 g/day • Assess need for essential and nonessential amino acids Restrict potassium and sodium intake. Restrict fluid intake. Monitor serum protein, albumin, hematocrit, and urea levels and daily weight to assess effectiveness of nutritional therapy.	Patient will be adequately nourished.	Monitor patient's response to dietary restrictions. Consider activity level when assessing caloric need. Teach patient/family rationale for diet restrictions.	Patient will be adequately nourished.	Teach patient/family protein, carbohydrate, and potassium requirements and sodium/fluid restrictions.

MOBILITY

Diagnosis/Stabilization Phase		Acute Management Phase		Recovery Phase	
Outcome	*Intervention*	*Outcome*	*Intervention*	*Outcome*	*Intervention*
Patient will achieve optimal mobility.	Assess muscle strength, flexibility, and mobility. Begin passive/active-assist range of motion exercises.	Patient will achieve optimal mobility.	Progress exercise as tolerated: Dangle, out of bed for meals, and walking 50 feet. Monitor patient's response to activity. Decrease activity if adverse events (tachycardia, dyspnea, ectopy, syncope, hypotension) occur. Provide support as needed. Consult physical or occupational therapist if indicated.	Patient will achieve optimal mobility.	Assist patient/family in developing home exercise program.

OXYGENATION/VENTILATION

Diagnosis/Stabilization Phase		Acute Management Phase		Recovery Phase	
Outcome	*Intervention*	*Outcome*	*Intervention*	*Outcome*	*Intervention*
Patient will have adquate gas exchange as evidenced by: • $Sa_{O_2} > 90\%/Sp_{O_2} > 92\%$ • ABGs WNL for patient (CO_2 decreased to compensate for metabolic acidosis) • Clear breath sounds • Respiratory rate, depth, and rhythm WNL • Normal chest x-ray Patient will have adequate tissue perfusion as evidenced by: • Normovolemic status • Adequate hemoglobin • Optimal urine output depending on phase of ARF • Alert and oriented • Appropriate LOC	Monitor and treat oxygenation status per ABGs and/or Sa_{O_2}. Assess sensorium and LOC q1h. Assess evidence of tissue perfusion. Monitor for signs and symptoms of pulmonary distress from fluid overload. Monitor acid-base status per ABGs. Support patient with O_2 therapy and/or mechanical ventilation as indicated.	Patient will have adequate gas exchange and adequate tissue perfusion.	Monitor and treat oxygenation/ventilation disturbances. Wean oxygen therapy and/or mechanical ventilation as tolerated and monitor response. Observe for complications of acute renal failure that may impair oxygenation/ventilation (i.e., congestive heart failure, pulmonary edema, fatigue, lethargy, somnolence).	Patient will have adequate gas exchange.	Monitor and treat oxygenation/ventilation disturbances. Teach patient/family pulmonary symptoms of fluid overload and what signs and symptoms to report to the physician.

Care Guide continued on following page

ACUTE RENAL FAILURE MULTIDISCIPLINARY CARE GUIDE *continued*

COMFORT

Diagnosis/Stabilization Phase		Acute Management Phase		Recovery Phase	
Outcome	***Intervention***	***Outcome***	***Intervention***	***Outcome***	***Intervention***
Patient will be as comfortable and pain free as possible as evidenced by: • No objective indicators of discomfort • No complaints of discomfort	Monitor and treat breathing status closely for signs and symptoms of respiratory distress related to fluid overload. Keep head of bed elevated and review breathing techniques such as pursed-lip breathing to minimize respiratory distress. Creatively plan fluid restriction over 24 hours, including periodic sip of water and ice chips to minimize thirst. Offer gum, hard candy, mouth swab, and frequent oral care. Assess quantity and quality of discomfort. Provide a quiet environment and reassurance in a calm, competent, caring manner. Observe for complications that may cause discomfort (i.e., infection of vascular access for hemodialysis, peritonitis, or inadequate draining during peritoneal dialysis, nausea, or vomiting. Administer analgesics, antiemetics, sedatives, or anxiolytics as needed and monitor response.	Patient will be as comfortable and pain free as possible.	Same as stabilization phase. Provide adequate rest periods, especially if patient is anemic. Teach patient relaxation techniques, including complementary therapies such as back massage, humor, or music therapy. Involve family in strategies.	Patient will be as comfortable and pain free as possible.	Teach patient/family breathing techniques, relaxation, and complementary therapy techniques. Teach patient/family interventions to alleviate thirst. Teach patient/family creative ways to maintain fluid restriction and alleviate thirst.

SKIN INTEGRITY

Diagnosis/Stabilization Phase		Acute Management Phase		Recovery Phase	
Outcome	***Intervention***	***Outcome***	***Intervention***	***Outcome***	***Intervention***
Patient will have intact skin without abrasions or pressure ulcers.	Assess skin integrity and all bony prominences q4h. Use superfatted or lanolin-based soap for bathing and apply emollients for itching. Use preventive pressure-reducing devices if patient is at high risk for pressure ulcer development. Treat pressure ulcers according to hospital protocol.	Patient will have intact skin without abrasions or pressure ulcers.	Same as stabilization phase.	Patient will have intact skin without abrasions or pressure ulcers.	Avoid tight-fitting shoes or clothing that may create pressure points susceptible to breakdown. Teach patient/family skin care management postdischarge.

PROTECTION/SAFETY

Diagnosis/Stabilization Phase		Acute Management Phase		Recovery Phase	
Outcome	**Intervention**	**Outcome**	**Intervention**	**Outcome**	**Intervention**
Patient will be protected from possible harm.	Assess need for wrist restraints if patient is intubated, has a decreased LOC, is unable to follow commands, or for affected extremity during hemodialysis. Explain need for restraints to patient/family. If restrained, assess response to restraints and check q1–2h for skin integrity and impairment to circulation. Follow hospital protocol for use of restraints. Maintain a patent and infection free vascular access device for hemodialysis or catheter for peritoneal dialysis. Follow seizure precautions.	Patient will be protected from possible harm.	Same as stabilization phase. Provide support when dangling or beginning progressive exercise program, and monitor response.	Patient will be protected from possible harm.	Teach patient/family about physical limitations the patient might have.

PSYCHOSOCIAL/SELF-DETERMINATION

Diagnosis/Stabilization Phase		Acute Management Phase		Recovery Phase	
Outcome	**Intervention**	**Outcome**	**Intervention**	**Outcome**	**Intervention**
Patient will achieve psychophysiologic stability. Patient will demonstrate a decrease in anxiety as evidenced by: • Vital signs WNL • Level of consciousness WNL • Subjective reports of decreased anxiety level • Objective assessment of decreased anxiety level Patient will begin acceptance process of long-term illness.	Assess physiologic effects of critical care environment on patient. If intubated, develop interventions for effective communication. Assess patient for appropriate level of stress. Arrange for flexible visiting to meet patient and family needs. Assess personal responses and coping ability of patient/family and take appropriate measures to meet their needs and reduce their anxiety. (i.e., explain condition and equipment, provide frequent condition reports, use easy-to-understand terminology, repeat information as needed, allow family to visit, and answer all questions). Use sedatives and antidepressants as appropriate.	Patient will achieve psychophysiologic stability. Patient will demonstrate a decrease in anxiety. Patient will continue acceptance process of acute renal failure and extended illness.	Same as stabilization phase. Initiate discharge planning. Include patient/family in decisions concerning care. Provide information on local support groups, kidney centers, and agencies such as the National Kidney Foundation.	Patient will achieve psychophysiologic stability. Patient will demonstrate a decrease in anxiety. Patient will continue acceptance process of acute renal failure and extended illness.	Same as acute management phase.

Care Guide continued on following page

ACUTE RENAL FAILURE MULTIDISCIPLINARY CARE GUIDE *continued*

DIAGNOSTICS

Diagnosis/Stabilization Phase		Acute Management Phase		Recovery Phase	
Outcome	***Intervention***	***Outcome***	***Intervention***	***Outcome***	***Intervention***
Patient will understand any tests or procedures that need to be completed (serum labs, urine electrolytes, urine osmolality, specific gravity, x-rays, ABGs, intravenous urography studies, ultrasound, and renal biopsy).	Explain procedures and tests to patient/family. Be sensitive to patient/family's individual need for information.	Patient will understand any tests or procedures that need to be completed.	Same as stabilization phase.	Patient will understand meaning of diagnostic tests in relation to continuing care.	Review with patient before discharge results of lab tests and renal function. Review with patient/family what to expect in renal function/health.

Patients With End-Stage Renal Disease

Barbara Albee, Nancy J. Beckman, and Hildegarde M. Schell

When the patient with chronic renal failure is admitted to a critical care unit, a critical illness or injury is superimposed on the existing renal pathophysiology. The critical care nurse may care for a number of patients along the continuum of renal failure, including those with mild renal insufficiency, those approaching end stage, and those who are already long-term dialysis patients. An understanding of chronic renal failure is the foundation on which development of nursing diagnoses and appropriate nursing interventions are based. The focus of this chapter is on the patient with end-stage renal disease (ESRD). However, the assessments and interventions presented are applicable to any patient with chronic renal disease.

HISTORICAL PERSPECTIVE ON ESRD AND DIALYSIS

End-stage renal disease was considered a uniformly fatal disease before the development of hemodialysis and transplantation. Before the 1960s, the patient with ESRD could be offered only conservative medical management of diet and fluids. Although hemodialysis and peritoneal dialysis were available, they could be used only in the acute care setting. Chronic hemodialysis first became a reality in 1960 when Scribner and Quinton developed an all-Teflon arteriovenous shunt—the first permanent access to the circulatory system. This shunt heralded the means of obtaining easy, repeated access to the circulation and the start of long-term therapy (McCormick, 1993). Technologic advances have continued over the past three decades and include improved access to the circulation, improved catheters for peritoneal dialysis, sophisticated equipment for dialysis therapies, efficient dialyzers, and advanced immunosuppressive therapy for transplantation. Morbidity and mortality rates have been reduced despite a marked rise in the mean age of patients on dialysis as well as an increased percentage of patients and multiorgan diseases.

In 1972, the End Stage Renal Disease Program was enacted through federal legislation. This provided funding, under Medicare, to cover nearly the entire U.S. population with this catastrophic illness. During the first year of funding in 1973, 10,000 patients enrolled.

By the end of 1992, there were approximately 157,000 patients on dialysis (131,000 on hemodialysis and 26,000 on peritoneal dialysis) (Health Care Finance Administration, 1992). Over 10,000 kidney transplants were performed (Levinsky, 1993). For 1991, the government's financial obligation to the ESRD program was approximately $6.6 billion (Iglehart, 1993). It is estimated that in 1994 there will be about 200,000 U.S. ESRD beneficiaries, at a cost of $10 billion (Burton et al., 1993). According to the United Network for Organ Sharing Research Department (1994), 27,498 patients were on the national waiting list for a kidney transplant at the end of 1994.

PATHOPHYSIOLOGY OF ESRD

A variety of mechanisms are responsible for kidney injury that ultimately progresses to ESRD. These include abnormal immunologic processes, coagulation disorders, vascular disorders, infection, and biochemical and metabolic disturbances. Several of these mechanisms may occur concurrently to cause advancing renal disease.

The typical clinical course of chronic renal failure culminating in ESRD is slow, progressive, and irreversible. The process may take from a few months to many years to become clinically evident. Clinical signs and symptoms may not occur until the glomerular filtration rate (GFR) is decreased by approximately 80%.

Diagnosis of ESRD is based on blood chemistry, 24-hour urine collections for total protein and creatinine clearance, ultrasound of the kidneys to rule out obstruction, and nuclear or computed tomography scans. Kidney biopsy may be done to determine the specific cause of ESRD, if unknown.

Etiology

Determination of the etiology of ESRD is often difficult. There is pathologic and histologic variability in the renal diseases as well as in their rate of progression. However, each results in a similar presentation of chemical and physiologic abnormalities. The hallmark of chronic renal disease is an irreversible, progressive decrease in GFR over a period of months to years. This results in a loss of the kidney's ability to excrete wastes and regulate the body's internal environment. The excretory failure can be treated with dialysis. The loss of biochemical and metabolic regulation leads to disturbances such as anemia and renal osteodystrophy.

The classification of disease states that progress to ESRD is variable and is constantly evolving. Collectively, glomerular disease, polycystic kidney disease, hypertensive nephropathy, and diabetic nephropathy account for approximately 75% of all cases that progress to ESRD. A more extensive review of a particular disease can be found in any text specific to kidney disease.

Progression of Chronic Renal Failure

It is hypothesized that the kidney is able to maintain homeostasis in spite of a significant loss of functional nephrons because of its compensatory mechanisms. Bricker's intact nephron hypothesis suggests that nephrons, which are unaffected by the disease process, are essentially intact and increase their filtration rates (Brenner et al., 1986). This enables them to control solute and water excretion far along the course of the disease. The compensatory hyperfiltration that occurs in the intact nephrons is able to maintain the GFR despite the disease activity until renal deterioration is quite severe. It has been proposed that the elevation in glomerular capillary hydrostatic pressure, which maintains the GFR, is the very mechanism that results in progressive glomerular damage (Fine, 1991).

The progression of chronic renal failure occurs in three stages. Each stage reflects an increasing loss of nephrons, as summarized in Table 45–1 (Richard, 1995). The first stage, diminished renal reserve, reflects a 50% loss of nephron function. During this stage, the patient is asymptomatic with serum creatinine levels within the high normal range. It is important to understand that serum creatinine concentrations above the normal range are highly significant in terms of the magnitude of nephron loss. Serum creatinine concentration doubles with a 50% loss of nephron function. Thus, a rise from 0.6 to 1.2 mg/dL is significant even though this level is still within the normal range.

TABLE 45–1. **Decline of Renal Function With Loss of Nephrons**

Stage	Functional Nephron Loss	Serum Creatinine
Diminished renal reserve	40%	2
Renal insufficiency	75%	4
End-stage renal disease	90%	8

The second stage, renal insufficiency, reflects a nephron loss of 75% to 80%. Due to the decreased GFR and reduced clearance of solutes, the patient exhibits mild azotemia (elevated levels of plasma urea and creatinine), impaired ability to concentrate urine, and anemia. Conservative management with diet, fluid control, and medications may be adequate to control uremic symptoms. Chronic renal insufficiency, once established, tends to progress to the last stage (i.e., ESRD). Progression is influenced by the severity of hypertension, dietary protein intake, infection, nephrotoxic drugs, and other metabolic disturbances.

ESRD represents the final stage in which there is a 90% nephron loss. Homeostasis can no longer be maintained, and all body systems are affected. An accumulation of uremic waste products, fluid and electrolyte abnormalities, and disordered regulatory and hormonal functions are a few of the multiple chemical and physiologic changes that occur.

The patient with ESRD requires renal replacement therapy to maintain life. The options available include conservative management, home- or center-based hemodialysis or peritoneal dialysis, and renal transplantation. Despite the fact that decline of renal function tends to be a gradual process, diagnosis of ESRD may seem to the patient to be a sudden event. Even patients who are aware that their kidneys are failing frequently experience shock and disbelief when confronted with the reality of dialysis.

RENAL REPLACEMENT THERAPY

There is no magic number with regard to creatinine clearance that determines when a patient must begin dialysis or receive a kidney transplant. Initiation of renal replacement therapy depends on the signs and symptoms displayed by the patient. However, as a rough index, considering that ESRD reflects a 90% nephron loss, we can predict that the patient may require dialysis or transplantation when the GFR is 10% of normal or less. For clinical purposes, the creatinine clearance closely approximates the GFR. Serial measurements of GFR show a linear decline with time before initiation of dialysis therapy. GFR may be maintained at varying levels after initiation of dialysis. In most patients who are on dialysis, GFR falls substantially after 6 months to 1 year. The presence of any residual renal function (RRF) is important in determining the optimal pharmacologic management and dialysis prescription. Recent studies show that peritoneal dialysis preserves RRF for extended periods and contributes substantially to weekly creatinine clearance (Lutes et al., 1993). The rate of decline of RRF in hemodialysis patients is twice that of peritoneal dialysis patients (Lysaught et al., 1991).

It is important that patients facing renal replacement therapy be provided with adequate information to make an informed choice. Although this responsibility generally lies with the nephrology team, the critical care nurse may be asked to provide information about the different treatment modalities.

Laboratory findings in patients with ESRD vary. Table 45–2 presents a range of acceptable values for patients on hemodialysis. These values differ somewhat for patients using peritoneal dialysis, with variations for continuous compared to intermittent therapy.

Pharmacologic Management

The effects of renal failure on the absorption, distribution, metabolism, and excretion of drugs present a challenge to both the physician in modifying the dosage and the nurse in monitoring the effects of the medication. The kidney, by means of glomerular filtration and tubular secretion, is responsible for excreting at least part of most drugs. Drugs that are effectively bound to plasma protein are poorly filtered. Conversely, drugs that are not protein bound are cleared from the blood at a rate approximately equal to the creatinine clearance. The most obvious influence of renal failure on the pharmacokinetics of drug activity involves the distribution and excretion of drugs.

Renal failure prolongs the half-life of drugs. There is a gradual increase in half-life until the creatinine clearance falls below 30 mL/minute. As creatinine clearance falls below this level, the half-life of drugs increases rapidly (Baer, 1987). The extent of drug accumulation and the associated risk of toxicity will be more pronounced unless the usual dose or the dosage interval is modified. When dialysis is used, the intermittent or continuous elimination of drugs through the dialyzer or peritoneal membrane must also be taken into consideration. Because some drugs are removed readily by dialysis, the timing of administration in relation to hemodialysis treatments can be important.

Patients with ESRD have other associated medical problems for which a variety of different drugs are routinely prescribed. A review of drugs commonly used by these patients is presented in Table 45–3. The purpose and special considerations for each drug are included.

As a general rule, lipid-soluble compounds are not readily dialyzable. Water-soluble drugs are more readily removed from the body. Drugs that are highly protein bound and those with high molecular weights are not dialyzable because the drug–protein complexes are too large to cross the dialysis membrane effectively. Drugs with large volumes of distribution are not substantially dialyzed because most of the drug remains in tissue storage sites rather than in the blood compartment (Alexander & Gambertoglio, 1985).

Dialysis Therapy

The basic principles and complications of hemodialysis and peritoneal dialysis have been covered previously in Chapter 44. For the patient with ESRD, the goal of maintenance dialysis is to allow the individual to achieve the optimal level of functioning.

Dialysis cannot replace the metabolic and endocrine functions of the kidney. Improvements occur in the function and some organ systems, but reversal of all the adaptive and maladaptive changes does not occur. Successful renal transplantation resolves many of the organ system problems. However, immunosuppression therapy brings with it a new set of systemic consequences.

HEMODIALYSIS

The patient receiving chronic hemodialysis therapy usually requires treatments lasting from 2 to 4 hours three times a week. Residual renal function, urea kinetic modeling, dialyzer capabilities, patient response, and ongoing clinical assessment by the nephrology team are used as parameters in determining the dialysis prescription for the individual patient. It is common for dialysis requirements to change during periods of acute illness or injury. The critically ill patient may require more frequent dialysis treatments due to administration of large amounts of total parenteral nutrition. More frequent dialysis will also be required when catabolism is increased after traumatic injury.

PERITONEAL DIALYSIS

Several treatment options are available to the patient with ESRD selecting chronic peritoneal dialysis. Intermittent peritoneal dialysis requires treatments of 10 to 14 hours each three to four times a week, or 8 to 12 hours nightly. No solution is left to dwell in the peritoneal cavity between dialysis treatments. Continuous cyclic peritoneal dialysis (CCPD) uses a machine to perform four or more overnight cycles, of 2 to 3 hours each. Solution may or may not be left in the peritoneal cavity between treatments. Continuous ambulatory peritoneal dialysis takes place 24 hours a day, 7 days a week, and usually involves four exchanges each day. Solution is left to dwell in the peritoneal cavity from 4 to 6 hours between exchanges during the day, and 8 to 10 hours at night. The method chosen is determined by individual patient desires, physical and medical condition of the patient, and availability of these options for the patient.

Peritoneal dialysis is being used more often than it once was in acute situations. It is very effective in removing excess fluid volume in pulmonary edema and congestive heart failure, and may be less traumatic than hemodialysis in elderly or otherwise unstable patients.

Improved catheters and insertion techniques have reduced the incidence of catheter-related infections and made long-term peritoneal dialysis possible. There are many types of catheters available. Most are made of Silicone rubber and have one or two Dacron felt cuffs to anchor the catheter and prevent infection. Surgical placement of the catheter involves creating a subcutaneous tunnel. The catheter is brought to the surface through a separate exit site, thereby reducing the possibility of infection.

Refinements in peritoneal dialysis delivery systems have resulted in greatly reduced peritonitis rates as well as greater convenience and freedom of movement

TABLE 45–2. **Laboratory Values for ESRD Patients**

	Adult Normal Value	Acceptable Predialysis Range for Dialysis Patients	Usual Causes of Abnormal Values	Important Considerations
Na^+	135–145 mEq/liter	135–145 mEq/liter	High: excessive Na intake; dehydration Low: dilution due to excessive water intake	Indicator of body hydration
K^+	3.5–5.5 mEq/liter	3.0–6.0 mEq/liter	High: excessive K intake; trauma; significant infection; respiratory/metabolic acidosis; rapid transfusion of stored bank blood Low: vomiting, diarrhea; excessive diuretic administration	High levels can cause cardiac dysrhythmias Hyperkalemia must be considered in acute muscle weakness Hypokalemia can potentiate digitalis toxicity
CO_2	25–28 mEq/liter	15–18 mEq/liter	Metabolic acidosis	Dialysate bath to correct acidosis: acetate (39–41 mEq/liter) or Bicarbonate (36–39 mEq/liter)
Ca^{2+}	8.5–10.5 mg/dL (4.5–5.5 mEq/liter)	8.5–10.45 mg/dL	High: secondary hyperparathyroidism; vitamin D metabolite overdose Low: excessive phosphorus intake; noncompliance with phosphate binders	Maintain calcium in upper normal range to minimize PTH stimulation
PO_4	3.0–4.5 mg/dL	3.0–5.0 mg/dL	High: excessive dietary intake; PO_4 in TPN Low: phosphate binder overdose	Calcium–phosphorus product ($Ca \times PO_4$) should be below 50. At 70, soft tissue calcification will occur
Alkaline phosphatase	30–130 IU/liter	30–130 IU/liter	High: bone disease; liver disease	
Mg^+	1.5–2.5 mEq/liter	1.5–2.5 mEq/liter	High: ingestion of exogenous Mg (e.g., antacids, laxatives); Mg in TPN	Hypermagnesemia suppresses neuromuscular transmission
Blood urea nitrogen	10–20 mg/dL	80–100 mg/dL	High: excessive protein ingestion; gastrointestinal bleeding; catabolic state; inadequate dialysis Low: inadequate protein intake	Protein requirements may be increased in critically ill patients
Creatinine	0.6–1.3 mg/dL	6–25 mg/dL	High: inadequate dialysis; increasing muscle mass	Not influenced by diet or metabolic state
Albumin	3.5–5.0 g/dL	2.5–5.0 g/dL	Low: inadequate nutrition	Low plasma oncotic pressure can result in edema formation
Glucose	70–115 mg/dL	70–115 mg/dL	High: diabetes mellitus; persistent uremia Low: excess insulin administration	Uremia is associated with glucose intolerance and insulin resistance
Hematocrit	Male 40%–54% Female 37%–47%	20%–30%	High: dehydration; polycystic disease Low: bleeding; anephric	Recent change in hematocrit is more important than the absolute value Transfuse only if symptomatic

Abbreviations: ESRD, end-stage renal disease; TPN, total parenteral nutrition; PTH, parathyroid hormone.

(Nolph, 1992). Systems with preattached fill and drain bags and disposable tubing offer the continuous ambulatory peritoneal dialysis (CAPD) patient increased safety in performing exchanges. These disconnect systems require air to be purged from the lines, or pneumoperitoneum may ensue. Chest, shoulder, or back pain in a CAPD patient should be evaluated with this phenomenon in mind.

When a chronic peritoneal dialysis patient is admitted to the critical care unit, every possible means should be used to continue the usual dialysis routine. In some cases, as when the patient must undergo major abdominal surgery, peritoneal dialysis may be contraindicated. In these cases, a temporary vascular access is inserted, and the patient is hemodialyzed.

It is common for diabetic patients on CAPD to have

TABLE 45–3. **Medications Commonly Prescribed for ESRD Patients**

Drug	Purpose	Special Considerations
Propranolol Minoxidil Clonidine Terazosin Captopril Verapamil	Beta-adrenergic blocker Vasodilator Antiadrenergic—centrally acting Antiadrenergic—peripherally acting Ace inhibitor Calcium channel blocker	Dose is usually held until after dialysis to prevent hypotension resulting from fluid removal during hemodialysis
Sodium bicarbonate	Treatment of metabolic acidosis	Sodium can enhance fluid retention
Calcium carbonate Calcium acetate	Phosphorus binders	Must be taken with meals in order to bind with dietary phosphorus Can cause constipation Calcium-phosphorus product must be carefully monitored when calcium is used
Digoxin	Management of chronic congestive heart failure	Digitalis toxicity can develop when hypokalemia results from low potassium concentration in the dialysate bath
Furosemide Metolazone	Diuretic	Diuretics may be administered to ESRD patients with some residual renal function Administration schedule may need to be adjusted to avoid hypotension during dialysis
Folic acid	Required for red blood cell synthesis	Water soluble; lost during dialysis
Vitamin B complex Vitamin C	Replacement vitamins	Give after dialysis
Ferrous sulfate Ferrous fumarate	Iron repletion	Do not administer with antacids or when absorption is decreased
Iron dextran	Iron repletion	IV administration generally given during dialysis Test dose is critical to avoid severe allergic response
Activated vitamin D Calcitriol	Management of hypocalcemia May reduce elevated PTH levels Necessary for dietary calcium absorption from gastrointestinal tract	Monitor serum calcium levels during administration Fat-soluble so drug is not lost in dialysis
Epoetin	Increase production of red blood cells	Subcutaneous route preferred; may be given IV at end of hemodialysis
Deferoxamine	Chelates aluminum for removal during dialysis	IV or intraperitoneal administration Iron is also chelated; monitor serum ferritin levels

Abbreviations: ESRD, end-stage renal disease; ACE, angiotensin-converting enzyme; PTH, parathyroid hormone; IV, intravenous.

either subcutaneous or intraperitoneal insulin administered according to the results of blood sugar monitoring. Accurate results are best obtained if samples are scheduled before meals and dialysis exchanges due to the dextrose in the dialysate.

POTENTIAL FOR INFECTION. Care of the peritoneal dialysis catheter varies and may include cleaning daily with soap and water or hydrogen peroxide, followed by application of povidone–iodine ointment. The use of dressings varies, also, but is always indicated if infection is present. Occlusive dressings are not used. The dressing should be changed immediately if it becomes wet from bathing or leakage of dialysate. Leaking around the catheter should be reported. Care should be taken to avoid trauma to the catheter and exit site.

CLINICAL MANAGEMENT

The systemic consequences of renal failure are evident to the nurse caring for the patient with ESRD. Admission of these patients into the critical care unit may involve a number of acute problems such as congestive heart failure, pulmonary edema, hyperkalemia, sepsis, and gastrointestinal bleeding. A review of systems for the patient with ESRD is presented along with a discussion of medical management and specific nursing care. Because most of these patients are maintained by dialysis therapy, specific problems relating to this group are emphasized.

Cardiovascular System

Cardiovascular complications account for approximately 50% of the mortality that occurs in the ESRD population, making it the leading cause of death (Held et al., 1992). In fact, risk factors for cardiovascular disease, including hypertension, lipid abnormalities, left ventricular hypertrophy, and glucose intolerance are present more frequently in patients with chronic renal failure than in the general population, even before starting renal replacement therapy (Ma et al., 1992). For patients on hemodialysis, the mortality rate due to myocardial infarction and cerebrovascular disease is three times that of nonuremic, age-matched controls (Hakim & Lazarus, 1986). This may be due in part to the cardiovascular effects of uremic toxins. Hyperlipidemia has a role in vascular atherosclerosis and occurs in 50% of the dialysis population. In peritoneal dialysis, hyperlipidemia can be aggravated by the continuous transperitoneal glucose absorption that occurs during dialysis exchanges.

HYPERTENSION. Seventy to 90% of patients with severe renal insufficiency are hypertensive. In most of these patients, hypertension can be controlled by a combination of dietary sodium and fluid restriction and sodium and water removal (ultrafiltration) during dialysis. This therapy reflects an expanded extracellular fluid volume.

Many ESRD patients require antihypertensive therapy for optimal blood pressure control. Antihypertensive therapy is commonly instituted before the time of ESRD because there is evidence that reduction of systemic blood pressure slows the progression of renal failure (Baldwin & Neugarten, 1987).

If hypertension persists despite adequate volume control, elevated renin and angiotensin levels may be the cause. Angiotensin-converting enzyme inhibitors, such as captopril, are commonly used to treat this. If there is also a neurogenic cause of the hypertension, agents commonly used include prazosin or methyldopa and clonidine. To enhance the effects of these drugs and to minimize their side effects, a vasodilator may be added.

ALTERATION IN CARDIAC OUTPUT: HYPERTENSION. Normally, hypertension in the patient with ESRD is managed in the outpatient setting with dialysis and antihypertensive medications. In some patients, however, severe hypertension is accompanied by cardiac or central nervous system manifestations (e.g., chest pain, pulmonary edema, syncope, visual disturbances) that require admission to the critical care unit.

Nursing assessment of the hypertensive patient with ESRD includes a careful history of the patient's antihypertensive medication regimen and his or her adherence to that regimen. The physical assessment includes auscultation of heart and lungs, cardiac monitoring for arrythmias, and observation for central nervous system symptomatology. The patient's usual blood pressure values can be obtained from a self-monitoring log or the nephrology team and compared with current readings. Blood pressures are monitored frequently to assess the effect of antihypertensive medications.

The nurse assesses the patient's understanding and compliance with the prescribed medication and the fluid and diet regimen. A dietitian is consulted to provide appropriate diet instruction for the patient and family members. The critical care nurse reviews the patient's antihypertensive medications and teaches the patient the purpose, dosage, and effects of each drug. The patient may need to review proper technique in monitoring blood pressure at home. The pathophysiologic complications of noncompliance are identified, and adherence to the regimen is encouraged.

HYPOTENSION. It is important to recognize hypotension as a less frequent but clinically significant problem for the patient with ESRD. If the blood pressure falls during hemodialysis, fluid removal becomes impossible and congestive and cardiac compromise result.

The etiology of the hypotension seen in ESRD varies. It may be caused by a variety of pharmacologic agents. Anemia and intrinsic heart disease may aggravate hypotension. Pericardial effusion may precipitate hypotension during dialysis. In addition, the incidence of autonomic dysfunction is reported to be as high as 50% in dialysis patients (Henrich, 1986). Altered sympathetic tone in uremia may decrease compensatory responses to hypotension. Acetate, which is commonly used in dialysis baths, has been implicated as a contributor to peripheral vasodilation during dialysis. Patients on peritoneal dialysis may become volume depleted due to excessive use of hypertonic dialysis solution or during periods of acute illness such as influenza.

ALTERATION IN CARDIAC OUTPUT: HYPOTENSION. The critical care nurse monitors the patient's blood pressure between dialysis treatments, noting and reporting significant hypotension. A sitting and standing blood pressure reading will identify orthostatic hypotension. Patients who experience orthostatism may also report dizziness, light-headedness, or syncopal attacks.

It is common to withhold antihypertensive medications for 6 hours before hemodialysis; however, this practice must be individualized for each patient. The critical care nurse should discuss the appropriateness of withholding antihypertensive drugs with the nephrology team. Hypotension in the peritoneal dialysis patient is usually addressed by restoring blood volume with fluids and increased sodium intake, or adjustment of antihypertensive medications.

CONGESTIVE HEART FAILURE. Congestive heart failure secondary to fluid volume overload is often a result of the dialysis patient's noncompliance with dietary restrictions, although it can also be caused by low ejection fraction due to cardiomyopathy. Prevention of heart failure requires sodium and fluid restrictions between dialysis treatments, control of hypertension with adequate fluid removal during dialysis, and adequate antihypertensive drug therapy. The increased cardiac output due to the anemia seen in most patients with ESRD, in addition to large arteriovenous (AV) shunts or grafts, contributes to the development of heart failure. If congestive heart failure persists despite correction of these factors, it may be necessary to digitalize the patient. Digoxin is commonly administered to patients on dialysis in its usual dosage every other day.

FLUID VOLUME EXCESS. Fluid volume excess is a common cause of congestive heart failure in these patients.

Nursing care of the patient with ESRD with volume overload is directed toward returning fluid balance to normal and teaching the patient how to prevent future recurrences (American Nephrology Nurses Association, 1993). The critical care nurse should compare the patient's baseline weight obtained from the physician or dialysis nurse to the current weight to estimate the degree of fluid overload. The peritoneal dialysis patient should be weighed during the first exchange in the morning, after the effluent has been drained but before the new dialysate is instilled. Weight increases are frequently evident before symptoms become apparent. The patient is assessed for evidence of peripheral or dependent edema. Neck veins are observed for distention. The lungs are auscultated for the presence of rales. Patients with ejection fractions of less than 20% may become compromised with relatively small increases in fluid volume.

Pertinent nursing interventions include maintaining the prescribed fluid restrictions. The anuric patient with ESRD is often restricted to 500 to 1,000 mL/day. If the patient requires multiple vasoactive infusions, this restriction will be rapidly exceeded. Mixing the infusion in double or quadruple strength will give the nurse a larger amount of discretionary fluid. Serial daily weights are important in evaluating response to treatment and to guide dialysis requirements.

PERICARDITIS. Pericarditis was once considered the hallmark of ESRD before the availability and early initiation of dialysis. Today it does not often occur after dialysis therapy is begun. The etiology is unknown, although circulating immune complexes have been detected in the blood of dialysis patients with pericarditis. Uremic pericarditis causes a hemorrhagic fibrinous exudate on the pericardial surfaces (Smith, 1993). Myocardial contractions may perpetuate continued trauma to the inflamed pericardial surfaces. Myocarditis can occur with an increased risk of acute and chronic complications.

A major concern is the development of pericardial effusion. Echocardiography is used to monitor and assess the quantity of fluid in the pericardial sac; it can detect small collections of pericardial fluid. When the effusion is large or expands rapidly, the patient must be monitored for signs of impending cardiac tamponade. Chest x-ray will reveal a rapid change in heart size and shape. The treatment of choice if significant effusion occurs is intensification of dialysis. Nonsteroidal antiinflammatory drugs, particularly indomethacin, are frequently used. Corticosteroids may help also (Smith, 1993). Pericardiocentesis may be necessary if the situation does not resolve.

ALTERATION IN CARDIAC OUTPUT: PERICARDITIS. The presenting signs of pericarditis in the patient on dialysis include the triad of low-grade fever, chest pain, and pericardial friction rub. The pulse and blood pressure are monitored for development of pulsus paradoxus of greater than 10 mm Hg. The electrocardiogram may show ST segment elevation with an upward concavity, a depressed PR segment, and low QRS voltage (Lancaster, 1995). After diagnosis of pericarditis, the nurse prepares the patient for intensive dialysis. Equipment for pericardiocentesis is kept available.

DYSRHYTHMIAS. In the ESRD patient, dysrhythmias may be precipitated by multiple factors. These include pericarditis, atherosclerotic heart disease, conduction system calcifications, calcific or congestive cardiomyopathy, acute volume changes, electrolyte disorders, anemia, and congestive heart failure. Premature atrial contractions and premature ventricular contractions are the most frequently noted dysrhythmias. Atrial fibrillation and ventricular tachycardia may also occur.

Dialysis-related dysrhythmias are usually transient and remain unrecognized. During hemodialysis, there may be an increase in myocardial oxygen consumption due to the effects of acetate in the dialysate bath. Limited delivery of oxygen occurs as a result of the anemia and possible hypotension in patients with coronary artery stenosis. Many dysrhythmias are related to these episodes of hypotension during dialysis treatment. Hypotension can often be avoided by administering antihypertensives, tricyclic antidepressants, or tranquilizers after the dialysis treatment.

Dysrhythmias associated with hypokalemia can be a result of intracellular movement of potassium due to glucose administration or to the metabolic alkalosis that may develop from the acetate or bicarbonate buffer used in the dialysis bath. Hypokalemia and hypomagnesemia may precipitate digitalis toxicity with associated dysrhythmias. Thus, it is usual to use a 3-mEq/liter potassium bath in the patient on hemodialysis therapy, who is also taking digoxin, to avoid this occurrence.

Dysrhythmias related to hyperkalemia can be life-threatening. Hyperkalemia usually results from noncompliance with dietary restrictions. Traumatically injured ESRD patients are also at high risk for development of hyperkalemia due to release of intracellular potassium from injured tissue.

ALTERATION IN CARDIAC OUTPUT: HYPERKALEMIA. The goals of nursing care for the hyperkalemic patient with ESRD are to prevent injury, reduce the serum potassium level, and assist the patient to prevent recurrences. Serial serum potassium levels are closely monitored. Serum potassium measurements will be required more frequently if acidosis is also present. The nurse closely monitors the elctrocardiogram for peaked T waves, depressed ST segments, and widened QRS complexes.

The nurse prepares for emergency treatment of hyperkalemia. Intravenous insulin, glucose, and bicarbonate may be given as a temporary measure to reduce serum potassium. If the serum potassium level is not imminently life-threatening, ion exchange resins can be given as a retention enema. Emergency hemodialysis may be necessary to lower life-threatening hyperkalemia.

The nurse assesses the events leading to the hyperkalemic episode. If noncompliance with the dietary regimen is the cause, the nurse assesses the patient's

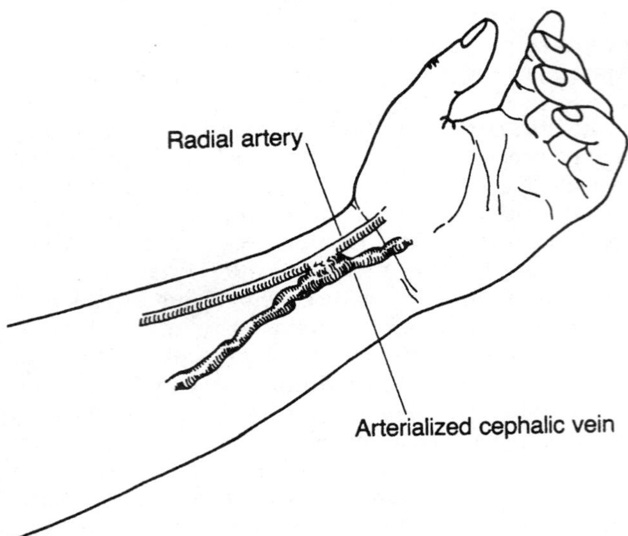

FIGURE 45–1. The native arteriovenous fistula. (Courtesy of Alice A. Whittaker.)

level of understanding, provides the necessary patient instruction, and encourages the patient to adhere to the prescribed diet. Patients with hyperkalemia should be cautioned not to use salt substitutes containing potassium chloride. Hyperkalemia can result from administration of blood transfusions. When possible, blood should be transfused during hemodialysis so that the excess potassium can be removed.

VASCULAR ACCESS. Adequate access to the circulation is the single most important factor in the delivery of adequate hemodialysis therapy. Thrombosis, stenosis, and infections of the vascular access site account for a significant number of hospitalizations for the hemodialysis patient.

An internal AV fistula is the vascular access route usually used in patients with ESRD. These can be composed of either a native vein or a prosthetic graft (e.g., polytetrafluoroethylene). As illustrated in Figure 45–1, the native vein fistula commonly involves the anastomosis of the cephalic vein to the radial artery (Brescia-Cimino fistula). Anastomosis of the basilic vein to the ulnar artery is also used. Approximately 4 to 6 weeks after the anastomosis is created, the venous walls hypertrophy, making repeated venipuncture for dialysis possible (Krupski et al., 1985).

Because patients with ESRD are often diabetic or elderly, and have inadequate or arteriosclerotic vessels, it may be possible to create a native vein fistula. In these patients, placement of a prosthetic graft is necessary. The graft material is implanted subcutaneously to serve as a conduit between an artery and a vein. The superficial implant is made to facilitate easy needle placement. The forearm is the preferred site. Upper arm or thigh grafts can be done, but they increase the chance of high-output failure due to the increased blood flow rates in these larger vessels (Golding, 1986). These large proximal grafts have been implicated in intractable pulmonary edema, which usually occurs in combination with fluid overload and myocardial dysfunction. Other complications of internally created fistulae include thrombosis, stenosis, steal syndrome (numbness or pain in the hand due to diversion of blood), aneurysms, and localized and systemic infections. The two most common causes of fistula loss are thrombosis and infection (Schwab, 1991).

Percutaneous cannulation of the subclavian or femoral vein provides temporary access to the bloodstream for hemodialysis. Percutaneous catheters are used while waiting for a permanent fistula to heal, when acute rejection occurs after renal transplantation, or when hemodialysis is employed as a temporary measure before long-term peritoneal dialysis.

ALTERATION IN PERIPHERAL TISSUE PERFUSION. Maintenance of a patent and infection-free vascular access device is the goal of nursing care. Strict aseptic technique must be used when accessing a fistula, especially one with a prosthetic graft. Prolonged pressure after removal of dialysis needles may cause thrombosis and should be avoided (Schwab, 1991). The nurse monitors the color, temperature, and sensation of the extremity. A cool, pale, or cyanotic extremity may indicate vascular occlusion and should be reported. The patency of the access route is assessed by palpating for the thrill and auscultating for the bruit.

Temporary subclavian or femoral dialysis catheters are not ordinarily used for administration of intravenous fluids or medications. The critical care nurse should consult the dialysis nurse as to how much heparin has been instilled in the catheter after dialysis and whether the catheter should be accessed for nondialysis purposes.

Particular care must be taken to prevent infection in femoral catheters that are left in place after dialysis. Because of their location, femoral catheters are easily contaminated by urine and fecal material. Frequent sterile dressing changes may be required.

Pulmonary System

There is a wide spectrum of pulmonary disease in the patient with renal failure. Abnormalities include asymptomatic changes in pulmonary capillary permeability, pulmonary edema, uremic pneumonitis, pleural effusion, and infectious pulmonary calcifications. Pulmonary edema is the most common problem in the patient with ESRD who is being treated by dialysis. In these patients, pulmonary edema is primarily caused by fluid overload with subsequent left ventricular failure. There may also be increased pulmonary capillary permeability in the uremic patient; this would account for the development of pulmonary edema in the presence of low to normal pulmonary artery pressures (Kaupke & Vaziri, 1991).

Pleural effusions can occur as a result of congestive heart failure and fluid overload. Treatment is first directed at fluid removal through dialysis. If this fails, thoracentesis can be done. Correction of hypoalbuminemia can increase plasma oncotic pressure, which helps to prevent pleural effusion.

Pulmonary infections may occur more frequently in the ESRD patient due to decreased activity of pulmonary macrophages (Lancaster, 1995). The immunocompromised state that exists in patients with renal failure makes them more susceptible to a wide variety of infections. Dialysis patients have an incidence of tuberculosis 10 to 15 times that of the general population (Kaupke & Vaziri, 1991).

As a consequence of calcium and phosphorus imbalances, pulmonary calcifications can lead to impaired pulmonary function. Dyspnea, arterial hypoxemia, and decreased lung volume may result. Partial resolution may occur after good control of calcium and phosphorus concentrations through dietary restrictions, adherence to a phosphate binder regimen, and subtotal parathyroidectomy if appropriate. Pulmonary calcifications also tend to resolve after renal transplantation.

IMPAIRED GAS EXCHANGE. Maintenance of adequate ventilation and prevention of nosocomial pneumonia are major challenges for the nurse caring for the critically ill patient with ESRD. Breath sounds are frequently auscultated for the presence of rales, wheezes, and rubs. The respiratory pattern is assessed for tachypnea and the amount of breathing work required. The patient's subjective complaint of dyspnea is carefully assessed. Baseline data are compared with ongoing assessments to monitor increasing respiratory dysfunction.

Aggressive pulmonary toilet, including coughing, suctioning, percussion/postural drainage, turning, deep breathing, and incentive spirometry, is performed frequently. The patient's sputum is monitored for changes in amount and consistency.

Gastrointestinal System

Gastrointestinal disturbances are often the most disturbing problems experienced by the patient with ESRD before the initiation of renal replacement therapy.

ANOREXIA AND NUTRITIONAL DISORDERS. Anorexia, nausea, and vomiting, especially in the morning, are common complaints associated with uremia. As a consequence, malnutrition may occur if renal replacement therapy is not instituted early enough. Nutritional status may be further compromised if the patient has a catabolic illness. Patients may also experience gastroparesis and nephrotic albumin losses, placing them at higher nutritional risk. In addition, prolonged dietary protein restrictions prescribed to delay the initiation of renal replacement therapy may also result in a suboptimal nutritional status (Maroni, 1994). Even when dialysis therapy is initiated, morbidity and mortality depend on an adequate state of nutrition. Recent studies have focused on the increase in morbidity and mortality that occurs when serum albumin is below 3.0 g/dL (Erroa, 1992; Spiegel et al., 1992).

Albumin should not be lost during hemodialysis treatments. However, it is predicted that 9 to 10 g/day may be lost in patients on CAPD. These losses are increased during episodes of peritonitis.

NUTRITION LESS THAN BODY REQUIREMENTS. The goal of nutritional therapy for the patient with ESRD is provision of a diet adequate for repletion and maintenance of desirable body weight. Acceptable plasma levels of urea, sodium, potassium, magnesium, calcium, phosphorus, and albumin also must be maintained. Nutritional adjustments are necessary throughout the course of renal deterioration. During the stress of a critical illness or injury, further modifications become necessary, depending on individual requirements, rate of catabolism, and any changes made in renal replacement therapy.

For the nonstressed patient on hemodialysis, kinetic modeling is useful for individualizing the dialysis treatment and nutrition plan by determining the patient's protein catabolic rate. The typical recommendation is 1 g of protein per kilogram of ideal body weight, 2 to 3 g of sodium, 40 to 50 mEq of potassium, and 1,200 mg of phosphorus per day. Calcium supplements are given if needed when phosphorus levels are controlled. Water-soluble vitamins are supplemented. Supplemental iron is given if stores are inadequate. Fluid is usually restricted to the sum of the urine output plus 500 to 1,000 mL/day.

Dietary recommendations for the patient on peritoneal dialysis are similar to those for patients receiving hemodialysis. Protein losses are generally greater with peritoneal dialysis. Thus, recommended protein intake is usually 1.2 to 1.5 g/kg per day under normal circumstances. Protein loss is increased in the presence of peritonitis; therefore, dietary protein intake must also be increased. Critically ill patients also have increased protein requirements. It is important for the nurse to encourage the patient to eat a sufficient amount of protein. It may be necessary to use protein supplements, either orally or through enteral feedings.

Potassium restrictions are generally much more liberal for the patient on peritoneal dialysis. Dietary potassium prescriptions range from 75 to 90 mEq/day for patients on intermittent peritoneal dialysis to 3 to 4 g per day for patients on CAPD or CCPD. For patients on CAPD and CCPD, there are usually no fluid restrictions due to the ease of controlling fluid loss through the dialysate glucose concentration (Devine, 1994). If gastroparesis is a problem, it must be addressed to ensure absorption of nutrients. Medications to improve motility in the gastrointestinal tract are frequently prescribed to minimize the need for antiemetics.

If the critically ill patient with ESRD is able to eat, it is important for the nurse to assess the patient's oral mucosa. Stomatitis is a common problem in these patients (Lancaster, 1995). Patients may complain of a dry mouth and an unpleasant taste in the mouth. Frequent mouth care will enhance the patient's ability and desire to eat.

Many critically ill patients with ESRD require total parenteral nutrition (TPN) to meet their nutritional needs. The prescription for TPN will follow the general dietary prescriptions previously described. Potassium and sodium are prescribed according to the patient's serum levels. Phosphate salts are usually not used because of the lack of renal phosphate excretion. Because magnesium excretion is also impaired, magnesium is given in TPN only if serum levels are low.

The patient's fluid balance and ability to handle the TPN fluid load will determine the amount of protein administered in the TPN. In general, if the patient requires fluid restrictions, the amount of amino acids is decreased, and a higher (70%) dextrose concentration is used. The nurse carefully assesses the patient's response to the TPN fluid load, specifically noting the presence of any signs of increasing congestive heart failure or pulmonary edema. The patient's serum glucose concentration is closely monitored and treated with the prescribed insulin dosage.

If the patient is catabolic, a higher TPN protein concentration is required to facilitate tissue or wound healing. These patients are at high risk of fluid volume overload and must be monitored closely. Daily hemodialysis or continuous peritoneal dialysis may be used to prevent fluid volume overload. An alternative method of fluid management is continuous ultrafiltration, described in Chapter 44.

It is now possible to administer amino acids during dialysis. This is referred to as interdialytic parenteral nutrition in hemodialysis, and intraperitoneal nutrition in peritoneal dialysis. Standard peritoneal dialysis solutions that include amino acids are under development (Burrowes et al., 1993).

GASTROINTESTINAL DISORDERS. The most frequent disorders occurring in the patient with ESRD include gastroparesis, gastritis, gastric and duodenal ulcers with bleeding in the upper gastrointestinal tract, diverticulosis, colonic perforation, and obstruction in the lower gastrointestinal tract. Ulcerations can occur at any point in the gastrointestinal tract. It is thought that urea conversion to ammonia influences the pathologic changes seen in the gastrointestinal mucosa.

The increased incidence of gastrointestinal blood loss is probably related to a number of factors. The platelet dysfunction seen in renal failure and the chronic heparinization used for hemodialysis are two contributing factors. It is common for ESRD patients to take histamine-2 antagonist medication to reduce the risk of ulcers.

There is a higher incidence of diverticulosis and colonic perforation in the ESRD population, probably because of the chronic constipation experienced in this group due to ingestion of phosphate binders.

ALTERATION IN BOWEL ELIMINATION: CONSTIPATION. Maintenance of the patient's normal bowel elimination pattern is an important nursing goal for the critically ill patient with ESRD. A detailed history of the patient's bowel patterns and laxative use guides the nursing plan. The patient is assessed for abdominal distention, abdominal discomfort, presence of bowel sounds, and frequency of bowel movements. A prescription for the patient's usual laxative or stool softener should be obtained and administered on a regular basis. When the patient is able to tolerate an oral diet, the nurse encourages high-fiber/high-bulk foods.

Hematopoietic System

Chronic renal failure results in a number of changes in the hematopoietic system, placing the patient at increased risk for tissue hypoxia, bleeding, and infection.

ANEMIA. A common but not universal consequence of chronic renal failure is anemia. Anemia becomes evident when renal function falls below 50% and becomes progressively worse as kidney function deteriorates.

The cause of anemia is primarily related to the decreased secretion of erythropoietin by the kidney. Although the exact secretory site of this substance in the kidney is unknown, it is presumed to be damaged with progression of renal failure. Consequently, erythropoietin levels are inadequate to stimulate the erythroid precursors in the bone marrow to maintain red blood cell (RBC) production (Rosenberg, 1992).

A variety of other factors contribute to the anemia of ESRD. RBC survival rates are decreased due to uremic toxins. External blood losses due to platelet dysfunction as well as those relating to the hemodialysis procedure itself may worsen the anemia. Aluminum has been shown to interfere with iron uptake in the RBC. Aluminum toxicity is evident in some ESRD patients and is associated with ingestion of aluminum hydroxide phosphate binders. Folic acid, a water-soluble vitamin vital to normal RBC production, is lost during dialysis.

Apart from successful renal transplantation, complete reversal of anemia has not been possible. Good control of uremia with dialysis results in some increase in the hematocrit. Present methods of management include minimizing the chronic blood loss related to hemodialysis and laboratory sampling. Routine blood transfusions are discouraged to avoid depression of the individual bone marrow production of RBCs, thereby causing transfusion dependency. The potential for transmission of hepatitis B, non-A, non-B hepatitis, and human immunodeficiency virus is also an important consideration.

An important new development since 1989, recombinant human erythropoietin (Epoietin) is the primary treatment for anemia in ESRD when the hematocrit falls below 30%. Epoietin corrects anemia by stimulating the bone marrow to produce RBCs. Epoietin can be administered subcutaneously, intravenously or intraperitoneally, but studies have shown the subcutaneous route produces a sustained release that more closely resembles endogenous erythropoietin production (York et al., 1991). Side effects are minimal and tend to develop with improvement of the hematocrit level. These include hypertension and embolic incidents (Harnett & Le, 1993). The occurrence of hypertension may require changes in the antihypertensive medication regimen.

Chronic administration of Epoietin depletes iron stores, necessitating supplemental iron administration. Although many oral iron preparations are available, recent studies demonstrate the efficacy of parenteral iron in maintaining transferrin saturation and target hemoglobin levels (Kupferman et al., 1994; Lui et al., 1990). Patients who are able to maintain adequate iron stores generally require smaller doses of erythropoietin.

Many patients self-administer Epoietin similarly to insulin. Monitoring includes testing hemoglobin and hematocrit levels every 2 to 4 weeks, and serum iron, iron-binding capacity, and transferrin saturation monthly. The dose is titrated to the hemoglobin and hematocrit, with 33% to 36% the generally accepted therapeutic range for hematocrit. Epoietin has reduced the need for blood transfusions in anemic ESRD patients, as well as improved the quality of life, increased exercise time, and improved cardiovascular functioning (Alpert et al., 1994; Guthrie et al., 1993; Levin, 1992).

ACTIVITY INTOLERANCE. Nursing care of the patient with ESRD is directed toward minimizing blood loss, thereby maintaining the patient's hematocrit at an adequate level. The patient's hematocrit and hemoglobin are monitored for downward trends. The nurse minimizes the number and amount of blood samples drawn from the patient (Kirlin, 1993). Iron, folate, and Epoietin are administered as prescribed. The blood pressure should be monitored for elevation secondary to improved hematocrit with Epoietin.

PLATELETS. There is a qualitative defect of platelet adhesiveness in the renal failure patient. Platelet factor III, necessary for conversion of the prothrombin to thrombin, is also abnormal. Although there is some improvement with dialysis therapy, these defects do account for some of the increased bleeding tendencies associated with ESRD (Watson & Gimenez, 1991).

POTENTIAL FOR BLEEDING. The critical care nurse anticipates the complication of bleeding in the patient with ESRD. Nursing care is directed toward early detection and prevention of bleeding. Stool, vomitus, and nasogastric aspirate are checked for occult blood. Antacids are administered as prescribed. Manipulation of the nasogastric tube is minimized. Tracheal suctioning is performed carefully to avoid tissue trauma.

Line insertion sites are assessed for bleeding. Manual pressure is applied to the fistula site until hemostasis is achieved after hemodialysis treatment.

LYMPHOCYTES. Infection remains a major cause of morbidity in patients with ESRD. Although the white blood cell (WBC) count is normal, the patient's susceptibility to infection is increased. An immunosuppressed state in which the absolute numbers of T cells and helper T cells are reduced exists in the dialysis patient (Hakim & Lazarus, 1986).

A transient leukocytosis occurs at the beginning of hemodialysis, especially when a Cuprophane or cellulose dialyzer membrane is used. The complement activation induced by these membranes results in neutrophil aggregation and sequestration in the lungs. In the critically ill patient, this process should also be recognized as a possible cause of hypoxemia. More biocompatible membranes, which should eliminate this problem, are now available.

POTENTIAL FOR INFECTION. The critically ill patient with ESRD is at high risk for development of infection. Nursing care is directed toward prevention and early detection of infection processes. Nursing assessment includes monitoring of the patient's temperature curve and WBC count and observing for changes in odor, color, or consistency of drainage and secretions. Meticulous care is taken with line insertion and line maintenance in hemodialysis patients. Peritoneal dialysis patients need catheter exit site care and strict sterile technique during exchanges to prevent peritonitis. Vigorous pulmonary toilet is initiated to minimize pooling of pulmonary secretions. Wounds are carefully inspected for evidence of inflammation and infection.

Neurologic System

The nervous system is one of the earliest systems to show clinical signs and symptoms of advancing renal failure. These signs include impaired mentation, sleep disturbances, lethargy, gait abnormalities, and asterixis. If these are left untreated, the final result will be seizures and coma (Lancaster, 1995). Peripheral neuropathy and electroencephalographic abnormalities improve with dialysis but show even more improvement after renal transplantation.

UREMIC ENCEPHALOPATHY. Metabolic encephalopathy is thought to result from a combination of electrolyte disturbances, acidosis, and an accumulation of middle molecules. The symptoms of metabolic encephalopathy range from mild changes in concentration to deteriorating levels of consciousness, including obtundation, stupor, and coma. The psychological stresses imposed by dealing with some of the early symptoms may result in depression and sometimes even psychotic episodes (Nissenson et al., 1991).

ALTERATIONS IN THOUGHT PROCESSES. The patient with ESRD is at high risk for alterations in mentation, not only as a complication of uremia but due to the many electrolyte and metabolic disturbances that accompany critical illness. It is important that the critical care nurse obtain a baseline assessment of the patient's cognitive functioning on admission. This baseline assessment may be obtained by talking with the patient or from family members if the patient is unable to communicate. Information is obtained about the patient's orientation to person, place, and time, length of attention span, sleep disturbance, fatigue, increasing somnolence, irritability, and signs of depression. The patient's ability to understand requests or instruction is assessed. This information is then used to guide communication with the patient and, when appropriate, to develop a patient education plan. The effects of medication and treatment on the patient's mentation are observed and reported.

SLEEP DISORDERS. Sleep disorders are common in ESRD patients and can significantly detract from quality of life. One study reported that 63% of ESRD patients complain of sleep disturbances. Sleep apnea is thought to result from metabolic acidosis, associated with compensatory lowering of blood P_{CO_2}. The lower P_{CO_2} may be insufficient to stimulate respiration. Other possible causes include autonomic neuropathy, the effects of uremic toxins on airway muscle tone, and instability of respiratory control secondary to central effects of uremia. Diagnosis of sleep apnea is done with polysomnographic sleep studies. Treatment involves surgically correcting anatomic problems, such as deviated nasal septum; weight loss in obese patients; discontinuing sedatives and alcohol; avoiding supine position during sleep; use of continuous positive airway pressure (CPAP) or oxygen at night; and prescribing tricyclic antidepressants to alter sleep patterns (Kimmel, 1991).

Insomnia is another commonly reported sleep disorder in ESRD patients that has a number of causes, including inadequate dialysis, depression, stress, and anxiety. Some patients are helped by mild sedatives, although their effectiveness tends to abate with repeated use.

ALTERATIONS IN SLEEP PATTERNS. The goal of nursing care is to promote restful sleep, which can be difficult to accomplish in the critical care unit. Observation of the patient's breathing patterns during sleep can aid in the diagnosis of sleep apnea. The patient should be taught to avoid ingesting stimulants such as caffeine and to avoid engaging in exercise or other stimulating activity before sleep. Compliance with CPAP therapy should be encouraged, as well as adherence to the dialysis regimen to ensure adequate dialysis. Diabetics tend to sleep better when blood sugars are under control.

PERIPHERAL NEUROPATHY. Uremic neuropathy cannot be distinguished from other types of neuropathy. Decreased motor and sensory nerve conduction is thought to be due to demyelination and axonal degeneration of the large distal nerve fibers. Sensory symptoms usually involve the lower extremities.

The "restless leg syndrome" is a sensory neuropathy that occurs at night and has been associated with inadequate dialysis. It is characterized by numbness, burning, and pain in the feet and lower legs that is often relieved by continuous leg movement. Slowing of motor nerve conduction velocity may result in muscle atrophy with irreversible damage. Treatment of the restless leg syndrome may require changes in the dialysis prescription. Clonazepam at bedtime has provided relief for some patients (Kimmel, 1991).

ALTERATION IN COMFORT. Nursing goals for the patient with ESRD with peripheral neuropathy include ensuring that adequate dialysis is being delivered, providing comfort measures, and encouraging ambulation. Assessment findings may include numbness or burning in the feet, restless leg movements, decreased muscle strength, cramps, paresthesias, and decreased deep tendon reflexes. Nursing measures that promote patient comfort include avoiding unexpected touching of the feet and keeping heavy bed linens off the feet. If there is sensory loss, the nurse teaches the patient how to inspect the feet visually for signs of injury. The nurse encourages and assists the patient with ambulation and collaborates with the physical therapist in developing an exercise program for the patient in the critical care unit.

Skeletal System

The term "renal osteodystrophy" encompasses a broad range of bone diseases that develop in patients with chronic renal failure. The disorders include osteitis fibrosa, vitamin D–deficient osteomalacia, aluminum-induced osteomalacia, osteosclerosis, and combinations of these (Preisig, 1990).

Hyperphosphatemia develops in the patient with ESRD because the kidney is no longer able to excrete phosphate ions. Phosphates are also poorly dialyzable. Because calcium and phosphorus function on a reciprocal basis, when the phosphorus rises, the calcium falls. The failed kidney is no longer able to convert vitamin D to its active form, 1,25-dihydroxyvitamin D_3. This further disrupts calcium homeostasis because the vitamin D–activated metabolite is necessary to facilitate dietary calcium absorption from the gastrointestinal tract. Hypocalcemia triggers excessive secretion of parathyroid hormone in an attempt to maintain normal calcium ion concentration. Secondary hyperparathyroidism often results as part of the tradeoff for calcium and phosphorus balance. Unfortunately, parathyroid hormone causes an increase in the activity of osteoclasts, resulting in bone dissolution to maintain plasma calcium levels. The metabolic acidosis accompanying renal failure further promotes bone demineralization (Preisig, 1990).

Because of the progressive nature of bone disease associated with renal failure, management of serum calcium, phosphorus, and parathyroid hormone levels is critical. Therapy may include a combination of phosphate-binding medications, active vitamin D supplements, calcium supplements, and, if indicated, a subtotal parathyroidectomy.

Treatment of renal osteodystrophy must begin with control of serum phosphorus before instituting calcium and vitamin D therapy. If calcium levels are raised when serum phosphorus levels are elevated, a high calcium–phosphorus product will result, leading to metastatic calcification of soft tissues. Dietary phosphorus restriction and the use of calcium carbonate or acetate to bind the phosphate in the gut are the most common approaches (Wikström et al., 1991). As discussed previously, use of aluminum hydroxide complicates existing bone disorders, although it is still necessary in some cases. Peritoneal dialysis patients now have low calcium dialysate available, which liberalizes the use of calcium-based phosphate binders (Honkanen et al., 1992; Hutchison et al., 1991).

ALTERATION IN COMFORT. Although renal osteodystrophy is considered a chronic problem in patients with ESRD, it is important to direct nursing care in the critical care unit toward preventing immobility and maintaining acceptable calcium and phosphorus levels. The patient is assessed for muscular weakness, gait changes, and the presence of joint pain or deep bone pain. A history of any pathologic fractures is noted. The nurse encourages and assists the patient with ambulation or exercises to maintain mobility.

Baseline serum calcium and phosphorus levels are obtained. The patient is monitored for development of hypocalcemia. Phosphate-binding medications are administered as prescribed. It is important to teach the patient to take these binders with meals for maximum effectiveness.

INTEGUMENT. Pruritus is reported to occur in as many as 86% of patients with renal failure (Mujais et al., 1986). The cause is unknown, but it is thought to be correlated with a variety of factors. Atrophy of the oil-secreting sebaceous glands and the sweat glands contributes to dry skin with resulting pruritus. Also implicated are urochrome deposits in the skin as well as disturbances in calcium and phosphorus metabolism, which may lead to deposition of calcium phosphate crystals in the cutaneous layer. The skin can become excoriated and infected secondary to scratching. If edema is present, the situation worsens. Widespread ecchymosis and purpura are associated with capillary fragility and the clotting abnormalities seen in the uremic state.

The yellow or gray-bronze skin coloration seen in the patient with ESRD is caused by the retained urochromes and pigmented metabolites normally excreted by the kidneys. The underlying pallor is attributed to anemia (Lancaster, 1995).

Wound healing is delayed in the patient with ESRD. This is even further magnified in the patient with chronic renal failure who has malnutrition secondary to uremia. In this situation, protein wasting with associated hypoalbuminemia may be evident by thin, brittle fingernails with pale, paired bands in the nail beds (Muerchke's lines).

IMPAIRED SKIN INTEGRITY. An important goal of nursing care for the critically ill patient with ESRD is maintenance of intact, infection-free skin. The patient's skin is assessed for dryness, signs of infection, inflammation, excoriation, edema, and ecchymosis. Superfatted or lanolin-based soaps are used for bathing. Emollients are applied to relieve itching. The patient is turned frequently to prevent development of pressure areas. If prolonged immobility is expected, therapeutic mattresses or beds should be used to prevent skin breakdown.

Psychosocial Factors

Chronic renal failure and maintenance dialysis impose a number of stressors on the patient and family. The patient may feel that he or she has lost control of his or her life and is now controlled by the weekly schedule of dialysis. The presence of a fistula or peritoneal catheter, along with the outward changes that accompany ESRD, may lead to an alteration in body image. The patient may grieve for the loss of body functions, such as the loss of kidney or urinary function or the decrease in sexual and reproductive function (Finkelstein & Finkelstein, 1986). Critical illness or injury adds additional stress to the patient and family system.

INEFFECTIVE COPING. Nursing care of the critically ill patient with ESRD is directed toward assisting the patient and family to understand and adapt to the changes imposed by the critical illness. The patient and family are assessed for signs of depression, anger, withdrawal, and dependent behaviors. The nurse is alert for evidence of noncompliance or nonparticipation in therapy.

Nursing interventions that facilitate coping by the patient and family include providing an environment that is as quiet and nonstressful as possible. The patient and family are encouraged to express their feelings about the illness and treatment. The nurse assists them to identify their strengths and coping abilities. Information is provided in response to the patient's and family's readiness and ability to learn. The nurse encourages the patient and family to set realistic goals and offers positive reinforcement toward meeting those goals.

As the number of patients choosing dialysis steadily increases, many ethical issues have arisen. Advanced directives have helped health care professionals and patients to define boundaries, but have not eliminated the expected controversy that accompanies any life-preserving treatment (Cohen, 1993; Colvin et al., 1993; Miller, 1993). On occasion, the critically ill patient and family members may decide to withdraw from dialysis treatment. When this occurs, the critical care nurse must recognize and honor the patient's right to choose his own treatment option—including the option of no treatment. In this case the nurse provides emotional support and comfort measures to ease the discomfort of advancing uremia and impending death.

RENAL TRANSPLANTATION

In 1954, the transplantation of a kidney between identical twins was considered a hallmark in the progression of transplantation, although kidney transplantation was proven technically possible in 1902. In 1972, when the End Stage Renal Disease Program was enacted, kidney transplantation became a viable option for thousands of Americans. As of June 1995, there were over 29,000 people waiting for a kidney transplant on the United Network for Organ Sharing (UNOS) national registry (UNOS, 1995b). There are an additional 970 people waiting for a kidney combined with a pancreas transplant, which is a treatment option that has become more widely available to diabetic patients since 1977 (Weber, 1988).

Patients choose transplantation over dialysis for a variety of reasons related to medical and quality-of-life issues. These include the desire not to undergo lifelong dialysis, improved feelings of health, and the ability to be more active and to return to work (Hathaway et al., 1990). When addressing these quality-of-life issues, it is important to base the success of rehabilitation on those positive changes the patient views as important, rather than merely on the number of ways a patient's life does or does not improve (Hauser et al., 1991). In 1993, 10,920 patients received kidney transplants (UNOS, 1994). Although many transplant centers now use living nonrelated donors, in addition to living related and cadaveric donors, the demand for organs continues to exceed the supply.

Medical research continues to develop new drugs with increased specificity and less harmful side effects. Graft survival has increased with the advent of cyclosporine (Sandimmune; Sandoz Pharmaceuticals, East Hanover, NJ) in 1983. For those transplanted in 1992, graft survival at 1 year was 84% for cadaveric organs, and 92% for organs from a living donor. Patient survival rates at 1 year for recipients of cadaveric donors was 93%, and 97% for recipients of living organs (UNOS, 1995a). Meanwhile, research protocols abound in university settings, and patients may be treated with immunosuppressive agents for which little information is available through routine pharmacy channels.

In addition to pharmaceutical research, other frontiers are being explored. Patients who are 65 years of age and older are now being transplanted and have graft survival at 1 year of 78%, and patient survival of 86% (UNOS, 1995a). Immunologic research is abundant and has explored techniques ranging from total lymphoid irradiation (Thomas et al., 1992) to the transfusion of cryopreserved donor-specific bone marrow (Barber et al., 1991). Current medical research is evaluating a "hybrid immune system" in which cells from both the recipient and donor live in a chimeric state (Caldwell, 1992). In theory, this diminishes the risk of rejection, allows for minimal or no immunosuppressive agents, and decreases the risk of infection. Some transplant centers have research protocols that call for low-level preoperative total lymphoid irradiation and a postoperative infusion of donor bone marrow.

Pretransplant Considerations

Patients with ESRD or rapidly approaching ESRD are referred by the nephrologist to the transplant center for a pretreatment evaluation. An extensive medical screening, with a thorough cardiac evaluation, is crucial because the leading cause of morbidity and mortality is cardiovascular in origin (Perryman & Stillerman, 1990). Histocompatibility studies, which include ABO and human leukocyte antigen typing, a psychosocial assessment, and preoperative teaching are part of the initial work-up. Contraindications for kidney transplantation are positive lymphocytotoxic cross-match, active infections, malignant tumors, advanced cardiopulmonary disease, marked obesity, drug abuse, and psychosocial instability.

The preoperative work-up and teaching may take place on the surgical/transplant unit, or may in the future shift to an outpatient focus for recipients of kidneys from living donors. If the patient is to receive a cadaveric kidney, the work-up must be done expediently to minimize preservation injury of the kidney. In addition to routine laboratory tests, a repeat cross-match and cultures of urine and peritoneal dialysate may be ordered. Some immunosuppression protocols call for the patient to receive preoperative immunosuppressive agents.

The Surgical Procedure

The iliac fossa is the position used by most surgeons for placement of the transplanted kidney. It is close to the iliac artery, iliac vein, and the bladder. Placement in this location facilitates assessment by palpation and auscultation, and provides for easier access if a kidney biopsy is required. The right iliac fossa is favored because exposure of the vessels is easier, although the left may be used.

After the patient is anesthetized, a urinary catheter is inserted into the bladder. The bladder is irrigated with an antibiotic solution, which is left in to distend the bladder. After the abdomen is prepped, a curved incision is made that extends from near the symphysis pubis to approximately 1 inch above the iliac crest. The preferred technique for vascular anastomosis is end-to-side, external iliac artery/vein to graft renal artery/vein. (Salvatierra, 1991). A drain may or may not be placed near the kidney hilum. After the anastomoses are completed and blood flow has been established, the kidney changes color from gray to pink, becomes firm, and should begin to produce urine.

There are two common techniques for ureteral anastomosis. The first technique involves incising the dome of the bladder. The ureter is pulled through a small tunnel made between the mucosal and muscular layers of the bladder and anastomosed to the bladder mucosa. The intact muscular layer helps to prevent reflux with each bladder contraction (Whitten & Toledo-Pereyra, 1988). The second technique involves an incision through the muscular layer of the bladder to the mucosa. A small stab wound is made in the mucosa, and the ureter is anastomosed. The muscular layer of the bladder is closed to form a submucosal tunnel to prevent reflux. There is decreased hematuria associated with this technique because there is less disruption to the bladder mucosa (Whitten & Toledo-Pereyra, 1988).

Postoperative Clinical Management

Immediately after surgery, transplant recipients are managed in the intensive care unit or in the postanesthesia care unit and surgical/transplant unit, depending on hospital specific practice. Patients at high risk for complications related to their underlying illness, technical complications, or complications of fluid overload may be admitted to the intensive care unit after surgery for close monitoring. ESRD patients typically have some degree of coronary artery disease and are at risk for cardiac ischemia and infarction with the stress of anesthesia and surgery. Transplant recipients are also admitted to the intensive care unit if they manifest pulmonary edema and hypoxemia, sepsis syndrome, bleeding, or other life-threatening complications. It is important for the critical care nurse to be aware of the normal and abnormal postoperative clinical findings unique to the kidney transplant patient.

FLUID AND ELECTROLYTE MANAGEMENT. Posttransplant kidney function can vary from sufficient clearance of solutes and fluid removal, to decreased clearance with good fluid removal, to both diminished clearance and fluid removal. These variations in kidney function are related to preservation injury.

Most alterations in fluid and electrolyte balances are seen when acute tubular necrosis (ATN) occurs secondary to preservation injury. In ATN, renal tubules are damaged, which results in diminished clearance and fluid removal. A rise in creatinine and blood urea nitrogen (BUN) levels and oliguria or anuria are signs of ATN. Diagnosis of ATN is made by ruling out rejection and technical complications and by biopsy. ATN may last from several days to months; most often, kidney function gradually returns over time. Intermittent hemodialysis treatments are usually necessary during the recovery period.

FLUID VOLUME DEFICIT. Maintaining an adequate fluid balance is a nursing priority in the immediate postoperative period. Ineffective fluid volume status may result from an osmotic diuresis secondary to renal tubular dysfunction that prevents sodium reabsorption, new ability and high clearance of BUN, intraoperative overhydration, and hyperglycemia related to corticosteroids or diabetes mellitus (Haggerty & Sigardson-Poor, 1990). Urine outputs of up to 1 liter per hour may occur, necessitating large volumes of replacement fluids. Prolonged hypovolemia increases the risk of prerenal failure and renal artery thrombosis leading to kidney dysfunction and potential loss of the transplant. Renal-dose dopamine (1–3 μg/kg/minute) infusions cause renal vasodilation and may be used to increase perfusion to the kidney (Flancbaum et al., 1994). Monitoring for high urine outputs, central venous pressures less than 4 to 6 mm Hg, pulmonary artery wedge pressures (PAWP) less than 6 mm Hg, tachycardia, and systolic blood pressures less than 110 mm Hg aid the diagnosis of hypovolemia and guide volume replacement therapy.

FLUID VOLUME EXCESS. Fluid overload results from overhydration or the presence of ATN or decreased urine output. The patient is carefully assessed for signs and symptoms of fluid volume overload. Management includes decreasing intravenous fluid intake, administering diuretics, and possibly plasma ultrafiltration or hemodialysis.

Recognizing and treating abnormal electrolytes helps avoid potentially harmful complications. Diuretics are commonly administered via a continuous infusion or intermittently for decreases in urine output. Furosemide is a potent diuretic that enhances excretion of potassium, magnesium, and hydrogen and blocks reabsorption of sodium. Rapid diuresis may result in hypokalemia, hypomagnesemia, metabolic alkalosis, and hyponatremia. Electrolyte replacement and changing diuretics can correct these electrolyte abnormalities. Metabolic alkalosis may be treated by replacing furosemide with acetazolamide, which produces an alkaline diuresis.

Patients with delayed kidney function or ATN need to be monitored closely for hyperkalemia, hypermagnesemia, hyperphosphatemia, hypocalcemia, and metabolic acidosis. It is important to remember that these electrolyte abnormalities may occur even when there is moderate urine output. Calcium replacement and phosphate binders may be administered until kidney function improves. Hemodialysis is indicated when severe metabolic acidosis is present.

Potassium levels and signs of hyperkalemia should be monitored closely in transplant recipients with ATN. Signs of hyperkalemia typically manifest when levels exceed 6.5 mEq/liter. Emergent temporary treatment for hyperkalemic electrocardiographic changes include hyperventilation to blow off CO_2, intravenous sodium bicarbonate or dextrose and insulin to shift potassium into cells, and intravenous calcium gluconate or calcium chloride to lesson cardiac toxicity. These temporary measures are followed by hemodialysis or polystyrene sulfonate administration.

ALTERED URINARY ELIMINATION. ESRD patients may have deconditioned, neurogenic, or thin-walled, friable bladders. Large urinary catheters are placed during surgery and maintained up to 1 week to decompress the bladder. Continuous drainage of urine prevents stress on suture and anastomosis sites of the bladder.

Abrupt decreases in urine output need to be carefully worked up because they can be related to rejection, ATN, hypovolemia, vascular thromboses, bladder leaks, ureteral stenosis, or obstructions of the ureter, bladder, or urinary catheter. Urine color and consistency ranges from clear pale yellow to hematuria with clots. Patients with obstructed bladder drainage may complain of suprapubic pain and have a distended bladder. Continuous sterile irrigations of the catheter with an antibiotic solution should be attempted before treating the decrease in urine output with fluids or diuretics. The catheter may be replaced if the irrigation fails to relieve an obvious obstruction.

Patients commonly experience painful bladder spasms and require relief with bella and opium suppositories, oxybutynin chloride, or propantheline bromide. These agents should be discontinued at least 24 hours before catheter removal to ensure complete bladder emptying.

Management of Cardiopulmonary Complications

Preoperative anemia, hypertension, atherosclerosis, and coronary artery disease can be exacerbated by the stress of anesthesia and surgery, fluid overload, and electrolyte imbalances. Patients should be monitored for dysrhythmias, hypotension, ischemic electrocardiogram changes, vascular thromboses, and uncontrollable hypertension in the postoperative period.

Hypotension can be the result of overdiuresis, cardiac ischemia, or immunosuppressive agent-induced fever. Hypotension can lead to decreased renal perfusion causing prerenal failure, exacerbation of ATN, or renal artery thrombosis. Patients may lose patency of their AV fistula with hypotensive episodes. The underlying cause of the hypotension should be treated (i.e., volume, vasopressors, inotropic agents, or antipyretics).

The prevalence of posttransplant hypertension is 81% at 1 and 5 years (Ponticelli et al., 1993). Preoperative hypertension, abrupt cessation of antihypertensive medications, and fluid volume overload are associated with postoperative hypertension. Severe hypertension should be managed aggressively because it may disrupt vascular anastomoses, precipitate seizures, or result in a cerebrovascular accident. Agents used are nitrates, calcium channel blockers, and beta blockers.

Pulmonary edema is usually a result of fluid overload, but may also be related to decreased left ventricular function or an adverse reaction to monoclonal or polyclonal antibody immunosuppressive agents. Polyclonal antibody preparations have been associated with noncardiogenic edema leading to adult respiratory distress syndrome (Dean et al., 1987).

Patients are monitored for tachypnea or bradypnea, shallow or labored breaths, crackles, dyspnea, and abnormal sputum production. Pulse oximetry, capnography, and arterial blood gases aid in assessment for adequate oxygenation and ventilation. Pulmonary edema is treated by managing fluid overload and administering oxygen, morphine sulfate, and nitrates. Pulmonary edema resulting in hypoxemia or respiratory failure may require temporary endotracheal intubation and mechanical ventilation. Prevention and treatment for atelectasis include encouraging coughing and deep breathing, incentive spirometry, or adding positive end-expiratory pressure or sigh breaths to ventilator settings.

Management of Gastrointestinal Problems

Transplant patients are at risk for the complications of decreased peristalsis related to anesthesia, narcotics, antacids, and preoperative gastroparesis. Stools are monitored for occult blood because patients are at risk for gastrointestinal irritation and ulcer disorders. Persistent diarrhea requires a thorough infection workup. A low-sodium diet is typically advanced as tolerated. Complaints of anorexia and dysphagia may be early symptoms of a gastrointestinal infection.

Management of Central Nervous System Complications

Patients may experience tingling or numbness near the transplant incision site or in the thigh of the surgical side. This is the result of cutaneous sensory nerve irritation from the retractors used during surgery. Femoral nerve irritation manifests as knee buckling, which may require physical therapy and a temporary knee brace.

Incisional pain is typically treated with opioid analgesics, such as morphine sulfate and fentanyl citrate. Liberal, yet cautious, amounts of analgesics are encouraged to make patients comfortable enough to advance their activity level as soon as possible. Meperidine should be avoided because accumulation of its renally excreted metabolite lowers seizure threshold. Nonsteroidal antiinflammatory agents are also avoided because they inhibit prostaglandin synthesis, which alters renal blood flow.

Management of Hematologic and Immunologic Complications

A goal of transplantation is to create an immunologic state where the graft is not rejected and infections do not occur. See Chapter 57 for immunosuppressive agents used in transplantation. Several new agents are currently in clinical trial. Early detection of hematologic and immunologic abnormalities is a key role of nurses working with transplant patients. Their underlying medical condition, combined with surgery and immunosuppressive agents, puts them at risk for postoperative anemia, thrombocytopenia, bleeding, rejection, and infection.

REJECTION. Rejection is the leading cause of graft loss in kidney transplantation (Rao, 1990). The four types of rejection described are hyperacute, accelerated, acute, and chronic. Rejection is diagnosed by clinical signs and symptoms, a nuclear medicine renal

TABLE 45–4. **Kidney Transplant Rejection**

Type	Time Frame	Clinical Manifestations	Mechanism	Treatment
Hyperacute	Minutes to hours after transplant	Anuria, fever, hypertension, metabolic acidosis, hyperkalemia, potentially disseminated intravascular coagulopathy	Preformed cytotoxic antibodies attack graft cells	Graft removal
Accelerated	Hours to day after transplant	Acutely anuric, similar to hyperacute	Lower antibody levels than in hyperacute, and/or newly formed graft-specific antibodies (Rao, 1990)	Graft removal
Acute	Days to months after transplant	Malaise, fever, oliguria, weight gain, pain over the kidney, rise in serum creatinine	T cells and white blood cells infiltrate graft, causing inflammation and edema	High-dose corticosteroid pulse therapy, or monoclonal or polychlonal antibody therapy, possibly dialysis
Chronic	One year or later after transplant	Slow, irreversible decline in graft function; oliguria, proteinuria, hypertension	Postulated antibodies and T cells involved (Rao, 1990)	Symptom management, resume dialysis, retransplant

scan, and renal biopsy. Acute rejection is the most common, is treated with increased immunosuppression, and is often reversible. Table 45–4 provides a summary of the clinical manifestations and treatment of rejection.

INFECTION. Sixty-five to 80% of kidney recipients have at least one infection during the first year posttransplant, and 40% of deaths result from infectious complications despite antimicrobial prophylaxis (Brayman et al., 1992; Doran & Rubin, 1990). The potential sources of infection are an infected graft, environmental contaminants, wound hematomas, reactivated latent infections, and pretransplant endogenous infections exacerbated by administration of immunosuppressive agents. Figure 45–2 provides an outline of the nosocomial and opportunistic infections and the time at which they typically manifest posttransplant (Rubin & Tolkoff-Rubin, 1991).

Most posttransplant infections are bacterial. Common sites include the urinary tract, wounds, lungs, and invasive catheters (Brayman et al., 1992; Dunn, 1990). Common bacterial pathogens responsible for these infections are *Escherichia coli, Klebsiella, Pseudomonas, Streptococcus,* and *Staphylococcus* (Rubin & Tolkoff-Rubin, 1991). Prompt administration of appropriate antibiotics is important.

Fifty to 75% of patients have viral infections, usually cytomegalovirus (CMV) or herpes simplex virus, even with prophylactic antiviral agents (Payne, 1992). CMV infections manifest as pneumonitis, hepatitis, gastroenteritis, and retinitis. Malaise, constant low-grade fevers, leukopenia, and myalgias are common signs and symptoms of CMV. Herpes simplex virus infection manifests as mucocutaneous lesions or esophagitis. Epstein-Barr virus and varicella-zoster virus are less frequent, but potentially severe viral infections. Reducing therapeutic immunosuppression and providing antiviral therapy are indicated for viral infections.

Common fungal pathogens are *Candida, Torulopsis, Aspergillus,* and *Cryptococcus.* Localized *Candida* infections affect the mouth, esophagus, urinary tract, wounds, and blood. *Aspergillus* typically infects the nasal sinuses and lungs because it is inhaled. Metastasis to the central nervous system is common. Low-grade fevers, nonproductive cough, and radiologic evidence of pulmonary or brain lesions are signs and symptoms of this often fatal infection. Mortality rates for pulmonary and central nervous system aspergillosis in immunosuppressed patients receiving antifungal therapy is 90% to 100% (Demming & Stevens, 1990).

Pneumocystis carinii pneumonia (PCP) is the most common protozoal infection in kidney transplant patients. Signs and symptoms of PCP are fever, dyspnea, nonproductive cough, small infiltrates on x-ray, and severe hypoxemia. The incidence of PCP has decreased tremendously with trimethoprim–sulfamethoxazole prophylaxis.

Prevention of infection in transplant recipients is key. The Centers for Disease Control and Prevention recommends aseptic technique, strict handwashing, and masks for care providers with upper respiratory infections. Studies have not revealed better outcomes for those patients in which extensive isolation techniques were used. Transplant patients may not present with usual signs and symptoms of infection because of their state of immunosuppression. Subtle signs and symptoms such as complaints of vague discomfort, mental status changes, or constant low-grade fevers may be the only manifestation of infection before sepsis syndrome ensues. Nurses are in an optimal position to affect patient and graft survival through assessment and early detection of infection.

Patient Education and Discharge Planning

After the immediate postoperative period, the emphasis of nursing care is on patient education. The success

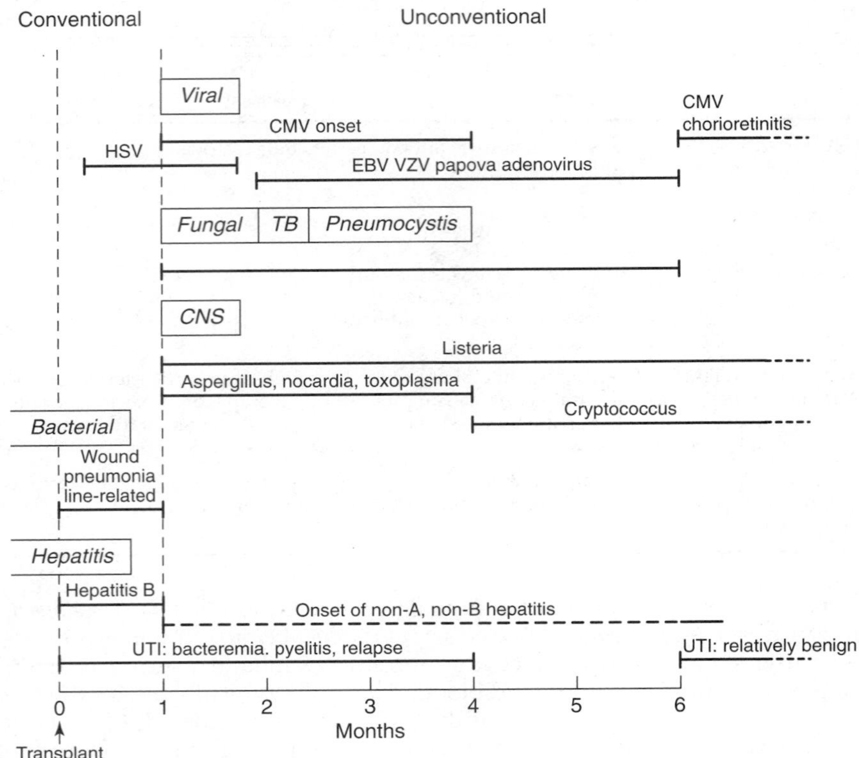

FIGURE 45–2. Timetable for the occurrence of infection in the renal transplant patient. *Abbreviations:* CMV, cytomeglovirus; CNS, central nervous system; EBV, Epstein-Barr virus; HSV, herpes simplex virus; TB, *Mycobacterium tuberculosis;* UTI, urinary tract infection; VZV, varicella-zoster virus. (Reprinted with permission from Rubin, R. H., Wolfson, J. S., Cosimi, A. M., & Tolkoff-Rubin, N. E. [1981]. Infection in the renal transplant patient. *American Journal of Medicine, 70,* 405–410.)

of kidney transplantation lies in more than graft survival alone, and includes an improvement in quality of life and return to activities of daily living (Norris, 1991). These factors, the educational component and promoting self-care, are crucial to the success of kidney transplantation.

Most transplant centers use a systematized educational program that includes: (1) a transplant handbook; (2) patient education classes; (3) a daily log book to record weight, temperature, blood pressure, pertinent laboratory data, and exercise regimen; and (4) a "self-administration of medications" program. With shortening lengths of stay, nursing needs to find creative ways to provide patients with adequate information. This becomes more difficult when patients' readiness to learn is affected by side effects from the corticosteroids, and they are distracted by delayed graft function (Perryman & Stillerman, 1990). Sensory deficits, illiteracy, noncompliance, and the challenge of providing culturally sensitive care are additional obstacles in teaching patients the self-care regimen. The increased use of videotapes, computer-assisted instruction, and patient-oriented pathways (Mosher et al., 1992) are several ways in which patients can independently enhance their learning.

A patient's hospital stay, barring complications, ranges from 1 to 2 weeks. The kidney transplant diagnosis-related group reimbursement is for a 10-day length of stay. Many transplant centers are beginning to use a case management model with accompanying critical pathways to ensure that high-quality care is provided in a timely, cost-effective manner (Cohen, 1991). Historically inpatient needs such as the administration of complex antirejection medication, are shifting to outpatient settings (Campbell & Runner-Heidt, 1993).

Transplant patient groups, providing support and education, are held in both the inpatient and outpatient settings. This is an ideal format for covering topics such as medical follow-up, lifestyle changes, family role changes, sexuality, dietary issues, and reimbursement and work issues.

Medical follow-up may continue at the transplant center, or may be done by the referring nephrologist, with the transplant team acting as consultants. During the first 3 months, clinic visits are frequent, but they decrease as the patient's condition stabilizes. Dental examinations are encouraged every 6 months, with antibiotic prophylaxis. Ophthalmology visits are suggested yearly, although patients should wait 6 months after transplant for lens prescription changes. Women are reminded to perform monthly breast self-examination and to obtain Papanicolaou smears every 6 months. Men receive instruction on testicular self-examination, to be performed monthly. All patients are reminded to wear sun block to decrease the risk of skin cancer.

SUMMARY

Since the early 1970s, the dialysis and renal transplant population has steadily increased. Advances in renal replacement therapy have resulted in longer life expectancy for these patients. The science of dialysis continues to evolve, with emphasis being placed on studies that will demonstrate the superiority of one modality over the other in treating specific types of patients, including diabetics, children, the elderly, or those with increased cardiovascular risk. Attention is focused on improving the quality of life for dialysis patients, as well as the overall quality of the dialysis care itself. And finally, efforts are being directed at finding ways to prevent ESRD or to delay its onset in high-risk populations.

Although chronic renal failure and ESRD are not considered critical illnesses, the pathophysiology of renal disease frequently results in a need for hospitalization in a critical care unit. The medical and nursing management of these patients is complex, involving aspects of both the acute problem and the chronic disease process.

REFERENCES

Alexander, D. P., & Gambertoglio, J. G. (1985). Drug overdose and pharmacologic considerations in dialysis. In M. G. Cogan & M. R. Garovoy (Eds.), *Introduction to dialysis* (pp. 261–292). New York: Churchill-Livingstone.

Baer, C. L. (1987). The pharmacologic aspects of renal failure. In L. E. Lancaster (Ed.), *Core curriculum for Nephrology Nursing* (pp. 157–183). Pitman, NJ: American Nephrology Nurses Association.

Baldwin, D. S., & Neugarten J. (1987). Hypertension and renal diseases. *American Journal of Kidney Diseases, 10,* 186–191.

Barber, W. H., Mankin, J. A., Laskow, D. A., et al. (1991). Long-term results of a controlled prospective study with transfusion of donor-specific bone marrow in 57 cadaveric renal allograft recipients. *Transplantation, 51,* 70–75.

Brayman, K. L., Stephanian, E., Matas, A. J., et al. (1992). Analysis of infectious complications occurring after solid-organ transplantation. *Archives of Surgery, 127,* 38–48.

Brenner, B. M., Dworken, L., & Ichikawa, I. (1986). Glomerular ultrafiltration. In B. M. Brenner & F. C. Rector (Eds.), *The kidney* (3rd ed., pp. 124–144). Philadelphia: W. B. Saunders.

Burrowes, J., Alto, A., & Kaufman, A. (1993). Intradialytic parenteral nutrition: A practical approach. *American Nephrology Nurses Association Journal, 20,* 671–677.

Burrows-Hudson, Sally (Ed.). 1993. *Standards of clinical practice for nephrology nursing.* Pitman, NJ: American Nephrology Nurses Association.

Burton, B., et al. (1993). Can a global payment system work for the ESRD program? *Nephrology News and Issues,* October, 1993, 18–23.

Caldwell, M. (1992). The transplanted self. *Discover, 13*(4), 62–68.

Campbell, P. A., & Runner-Heidt, C. M. (1993). A collaborative approach to home OKT3 therapy. *Journal of Nursing Administration, 23*(11), 63–66.

Cohen, D. (1993). Dialytic care is an unprecedented privilege. *Nephrology News and Issues,* October, 1993, 36–38.

Cohen, E. (1991). Nursing case management: Does it pay? *Journal of Nursing Administration, 21*(4), 20–25.

Colvin, E., et al. (1993). Moving beyond the patient self-determination act: Educating patients to be autonomous. *American Nephrology Nurses Association Journal, 20,* 564–571.

Dean, N. C., Amend, W. C., & Matthay, M. A. (1987). Adult respiratory distress syndrome related to antithymocyte globulin therapy. *Chest, 91,* 619–620.

Demming, D. W., & Stevens, D. A. (1990). Antifungal and surgical treatment of invasive aspergillosis: Review of 2,121 published cases. *Reviews of Infectious Diseases, 12,* 1147–1201.

Devine, W. (1994). Review of nutritional status and diet in dialysis and renal transplant patients. *Dialysis and Transplantation, 23,* 38–48.

Doran, M., & Rubin, N. E. (1990). Infection in the renal transplant patient: New approaches to treatment in a compromised host. *Nephrology Nursing Update, 2*(3), 1–8.

Dunn, D. L. (1990). Problems related to immunosuppression, infection and malignancy occurring after solid organ transplantation. *Critical Care Clinics, 6,* 955–977.

Erroa, M., et al. (1992). Predictor of one-year survival in CAPD (Abstract). *Peritoneal Dialysis International, 12*(1), 88.

Fine, L. (1991). How little kidney tissue is enough? *New England Journal of Medicine, 325,* 1097–1098.

Finkelstein, S. H., & Finkelstein, F. O. (1986). Sexual dysfunction in chronic renal failure. In A. R. Nissenson & R. N. Fine (Eds.), *Dialysis therapy* (pp. 174–177). St. Louis: C. V. Mosby.

Flancbaum, L., Choban, P. S., & Dasta, J. F. (1994). Quantitative effects of low-dose dopamine on urine output in oliguric surgical intensive care unit patients. *Critical Care Medicine, 22,* 61–66.

Golding, A. L. (1986). Complications of vascular access for chronic hemodialysis. In A. R. Nissenson & R. N. Fine (Eds.), *Dialysis therapy* (pp. 9–13). St. Louis: C. V. Mosby.

Guthrie, M., et al. (1993). Effects of erythropoietin on strength and functional status of patients on hemodialysis. *Clinical Nephrology, 39*(2), 97–102.

Haggerty, L. M., & Sigardson-Poor, K. M. (1990). Kidney transplantation. In K. M. Sigardson-Poor & L. M. Haggerty (Eds.), *Nursing care of the transplant recipient* (pp. 343–365). Philadelphia: W. B. Saunders.

Hakim, R. M., & Lazarus, J. M. (1986). Medical aspects of hemodialysis. In B. M. Brenner & F. C. Rector (Eds.), *The kidney* (3rd ed., pp. 1791–1844). Philadelphia: W. B. Saunders.

Harnett, J., & Le, H. (1993). Cardiovascular effects of erythropoietin. *Dialysis and Transplantation, 22,* 536–540.

Hathaway, D., Strong, M., & Ganza, M. (1990). Posttransplant quality of life expectations. *American Nephrology Nurses Association Journal, 17,* 443–449.

Hauser, M. L., Williams, J., Strong, M., Ganza, M., & Hathaway, D. (1991). Predicted and actual quality of life changes following renal transplantation. *American Nephrology Nurses Association Journal, 18,* 295–304.

Health Care Finance Administration. (1992). *ESRD Program highlights.* Baltimore: Bureau of Data Management and Strategy.

Held, P., Levin, N., & Port, F. (1992). Cardiac disease in chronic uremia: An overview. In P. S. Parfrey & J. Harnett (Eds.), *Cardiac dysfunction in chronic uremia.* Boston: Kluwer Academic Publishers.

Henrich, W. L. (1986). Hemodynamic instability during hemodialysis. *Kidney International, 30,* 605–612.

Honkanen, E., et al. (1992). CAPD with low calcium dialysate and calcium carbonate: Results of a 24-week study. *Advances in Peritoneal Dialysis, 8,* 356–361.

Hutchison, A., et al. (1991). Renal osteodystrophy in CAPD. *Advances in Peritoneal Dialysis, 7,* 237–239.

Inglehart, J. (1993). Health policy report—the American healthcare system: The ESRD Program. *New England Journal of Medicine, 328,* 366–371.

Kaupke, C., & Vaziri, N. (1991). Pleural complications in end-stage renal disease. *Seminars in Dialysis, 4,* 189–197.

Kimmel, P. (1991). Sleep apnea in end-stage renal disease. *Seminars in Dialysis, 4,* 52–57.

Kirlin, L. (1993). Case management of the anemic patient: Epoietin Alfa: Focus on iron supplementation. *American Nephrology Nurses Association Journal, 20,* 678–681.

Krupski, W. C., Bruks, M. D., Webb, R. L., & Effency, D. J. (1985). Access for dialysis. In M. G. Cogan & M. R. Garovoy (Eds.), *Introduction to dialysis* (pp. 41–71). New York: Churchill-Livingstone.

Kupferman, J., et al. (1994). Iron dextran therapy in ESRD patients on peritoneal dialysis receiving erythropoietin (Abstract). *Peritoneal Dialysis International, 14,* 68.

Lancaster, L. (1995). Manifestations of renal failure. In L. E. Lancaster (Ed.), *Core curriculum for nephrology nursing* (3rd ed., pp. 73–108). Pitman, NJ: American Nephrology Nurses Association.

Levin, N. (1992). Quality of life and hematocrit level. *American Journal of Kidney Diseases, 20*(Suppl 1), 16–20.

Levinsky, N. (1993). Lessons from the Medicare ESRD Program. *New England Journal of Medicine, 329,* 1395–1399.

Lui, S., et al. (1990). Pharmacokinetics and pharmacodynamics of subcutaneous and intraperitoneal administration of recombinant human erythropoietin in patients on continuous ambulatory peritoneal dialysis. *Clinical Nephrology, 33,* 47–51.

Lutes, R., et al. (1993). Loss of residual renal function (RRF) in patients on peritoneal dialysis. *Advances in Peritoneal Dialysis, 9,* 165–168.

Lysaught, M., Voneh, E., & Farrell, P. (1990). Improved maintenance of residual renal function with CAPD relative to hemodialysis. In K. Nolph (Chair), *10th Annual Peritoneal Dialysis Conference conducted by the University of Missouri, Columbia.* Dallas.

Ma, K., Greene, E., & Ray, L. (1992). Cardiovascular risk factors in chronic renal failure and hemodialysis populations. *American Journal of Kidney Disease, 19,* 505–513.

Maroni, B. (1994). Nutrition in the predialysis patient. *Dialysis and Transplantation, 23,* 76–93.

McCormick, T. (1993). Ethical issues in caring for patients with renal failure. *American Nephrology Nurses Association Journal, 20,* 549–555.

Miller, R. (1993). Dialysis should be withdrawn when the burdens outweigh the benefits. *Nephrology News and Issues,* October, 1993, 33–38.

Mosher, C., Cronk, P., Kidd, A., et al. (1992). Upgrading practice with critical pathways. *American Journal of Nursing, 91*(1), 41–44.

Mujais, S. K., Sabatini, S., & Kurtzman, N. A. (1986). Pathophysiology of the uremic syndrome. In B. M. Brenner & F. C. Rector (Eds.), *The kidney* (3rd ed., pp. 1587–1630). Philadelphia: W. B. Saunders.

Nissenson, A., et al. (1991). Central nervous system dysfunction in dialysis patients: A practical approach. *Seminars in Dialysis, 4,* 115–123.

Nolph, K. (1992). What's new in peritoneal dialysis: An overview. In *12th Annual Peritoneal Dialysis Conference, University of Missouri–Columbia* (pp. 3–7).

Norris, M. K. G. (1991). Applying Orem's theory to the long-term care of adolescent transplant recipients. *American Nephrology Nurses Association Journal, 18,* 45–47.

Payne, J. L. (1992). Immune modification and complications of immunosuppression. *Critical Care Nursing Clinics of North America, 4,* 43–61.

Perryman, J. P., & Stillerman, P. N. (1990). Kidney transplantation. In S. L. Smith (Eds.), *Tissue and organ transplantation: Implications for professional nursing practice* (pp. 176–209). St. Louis: Mosby Year Book.

Ponticelli, C., Montagnino, G., Aroldi, A., et al. (1993). Hypertension after renal transplantation. *American Journal of Kidney Diseases, 21*(5), 73–78.

Preisig, P. (1990). Aluminum-related bone disease. *Nephrology Nursing Update, 2*(1), 1–8.

Rao, K. V. (1990). Mechanism, pathophysiology, diagnosis and management of renal transplant rejection. *Medical Clinics of America, 74,* 1039–1057.

Richard, C. J. (1995). Causes of renal failure. In L. E. Lancaster (Ed.), *Core curriculum for nephrology nursing* (3rd ed., pp. 53–73). Pitman, NJ: American Nephrology Nurses Association.

Rosenberg, M. (1992). Role of transferrin measurement in monitoring iron status during RhEPO therapy. *Dialysis and Transplantation, 21*(2), 81–90.

Rubin, R. H., & Tolkoff-Rubin, N. E. (1991). The impact of infection on the outcome of transplantation. *Transplantation Proceedings, 23,* 2068–2074.

Salvatierra, O. (1991). Renal transplantation. In J. Glenn (Ed.), *Urologic surgery* (4th ed., pp. 243–251). Philadelphia: W. B. Saunders.

Schwab, S. (1991). What can be done to preserve vascular access for dialysis? *Seminars in Dialysis, 4,* 152–153.

Smith, S. (1993). Uremic pericarditis in chronic renal failure: Nursing implications. *American Nephrology Nurses Association Journal, 20,* 432–436.

Spiegel, D., et al. (1992). Serum albumin—a marker for morbidity in peritoneal dialysis patients (Abstract). *Peritoneal Dialysis International, 12,* 266.

Thomas, J., Algaisi, M., Cunningham, P., et al. The development of posttransplant TLI treatment strategy that promotes organ allograft acceptance without chronic immunosuppression. *Transplantation, 53,* 247–258.

United Network for Organ Sharing (1995a). *1994 annual report of the U.S. Scientific Registry for Transplant Recipients and the Organ Procurement and Transplantation Network—transplant data: 1988–1991.* Contract Nos. 240-90-0051 and 240-90-0064. Richmond, VA: Author; Bethesda, MD: Division of Organ Transplantation, Bureau of Health Resources Development, Health Resources and Services Administration, U.S. Department of Health and Human Services.

United Network for Organ Sharing Update. (July 1995b). *11*(7), 26–27.

Watson, A., & Gimenez, L. (1991). The bleeding diathesis of uremia. *Seminars in Dialysis, 4*(2), 86–93.

Weber, M. M. (1988). Pancreas transplantation: Implications for nephrology nursing practice. *American Nephrology Nurses Association Journal, 15,* 289–292.

Whitten, J., & Toledo-Pereyra, L. H. (1988). Surgical techniques. In L. H. Toledo-Pereyra (Ed.), *Kidney transplantation* (pp. 81–103). Philadelphia: F. A. Davis.

Wikström, B., Danielson, B., & Fellstrom, B. (1991). Calcium acetate used as phosphate binding treatment in uremic hyperphosphatemia. *Advances in Peritoneal Dialysis, 7,* 221–224.

York, S., Kinney, R., & Taber, T. (1991). Self-administration of Epoetin Beta by peritoneal dialysis patients. *American Nephrology Nurses Association Journal, 18,* 549–552.

END-STAGE RENAL FAILURE/KIDNEY TRANSPLANTATION MULTIDISCIPLINARY CARE GUIDE

COORDINATION OF CARE

Diagnosis/Stabilization Phase		Acute Management Phase		Recovery Phase	
Outcome	***Intervention***	***Outcome***	***Intervention***	***Outcome***	***Intervention***
All appropriate team members and disciplines will be involved in the plan of care.	Develop a plan of care with the patient/family, primary nurse(s), primary physicians, nephrologist, kidney transplant coordinator, cardiologist, pulmonologist, hematologist, social services, chaplain, clinical nurse specialist, dietitian, and dialysis staff.	All appropriate team members and disciplines will be involved in the plan of care.	Update the plan of care with the patient/family, other team members, physical therapist, occupational therapist, recreational therapist, and discharge planner.	All appropriate team members and disciplines will be involved in the plan of care.	Provide written instructions for continuing care (physician's office visit and/or clinic visit, medication regimen, and signs/symptoms to report to physician). Provide patient/family with phone numbers of resources available.

FLUID BALANCE

Diagnosis/Stabilization Phase		Acute Management Phase		Recovery Phase	
Outcome	***Intervention***	***Outcome***	***Intervention***	***Outcome***	***Intervention***
Patient will achieve and maintain stable fluid and electrolyte status with renal replacement therapy as evidenced by: • Fluid balance remains at or near baseline • Stable hematologic parameters such as hemoglobin, platelets, and WBCs • Optimal cardiopulmonary function • Stable hemodynamic status • Stable hemodialysis regimen	Monitor and treat signs/symptoms of hypervolemia such as hypertension, tachycardia, pulmonary edema, frothy sputum, peripheral edema, distended neck veins, inspiratory crackles, S3, or increased CVP. Monitor renal parameters, including urine output (if any), BUN, serum creatinine, BUN/Scr ratio, serum electrolytes, and acid–base status. Assess effect of prescribed antihypertensive agents on blood pressure and heart rate. Assess patient's understanding and compliance with prescribed medication, fluid, and diet regimen. Determine patient's baseline weight and weigh daily. Maintain patient's fluid and sodium restriction.	Patient will achieve and maintain stable fluid and electrolyte status after kidney transplant.	Monitor kidney function closely per urine output, creatinine clearance, Scr levels, BUN and BUN/Scr ratio. Anticipate possible acute tubular necrosis secondary to preservation injury. Prepare patient for possible temporary intermittent hemodialysis treatments when necessary. Maintain adequate fluid balance. Monitor for signs/symptoms of fluid volume deficit (CVP < 4 mm Hg, PCWP <6 mm Hg, tachycardia, systolic BP <110) which may occur from an osmotic diuresis posttransplant. Monitor for signs and symptoms of fluid overload. Administer diuretics, renal dose dopamine (1–3 μg/kg/minute), and/or antihypertensives as indicated postoperatively.	Patient will maintain stable fluid and electrolyte status after kidney transplant.	Teach patient/family on posttransplant care, including: • Daily log of weight, temperature, blood pressure, pertinent laboratory data, and exercise regimen • Medications, including cardiac medications, antihypertensives, immunosuppressants, and antirejection medications Teach patient/family signs and symptoms of fluid overload and/or electrolyte disturbances.

Care Guide continued on following page

END-STAGE RENAL FAILURE/KIDNEY TRANSPLANTATION MULTIDISCIPLINARY CARE GUIDE *continued*

FLUID BALANCE *continued*

Diagnosis/Stabilization Phase		Acute Management Phase		Recovery Phase	
Outcome	*Intervention*	*Outcome*	*Intervention*	*Outcome*	*Intervention*
Patient will be evaluated for kidney transplantation.	Assess dysfunction in other organ systems caused by impaired renal function such as pericarditis, dysrhythmias, lethargy, decreased LOC, electrolyte disturbances (especially hyperkalemia, hyperphosphatemia, hypocalcemia), acid–base disturbances, anemia, platelet dysfunction, anorexia, nausea, vomiting, bleeding tendencies, and subcutaneous edema. Minimize number of blood samples drawn. Monitor, support and treat patient during dialysis therapy: Assess vital signs, fluid status, and patient response to dialysis. Monitor and treat signs/symptoms of hypovolemia secondary to dialysis. Assess and maintain vascular access device: • Palpate the thrill and auscultate bruit over shunt periodically • Avoid constrictions above access such as tourniquets or cuffs • Ensure that access is free from infection • Monitor perfusion (color, temperature and sensation) of related extremity Assist with pretransplantation screening, including: • Extensive cardiopulmonary evaluation • Psychosocial assessment (rule out psychosis, severe personality disorder, or history of noncompliance) • Histocompatibility studies (ABO and human leukocyte antigen) Administer preoperative immunosuppressive agents if indicated.		If kidney function is delayed posttransplant, monitor and treat abnormal electrolytes such as hyperkalemia, hypermagnesemia, hyperphosphatemia, hypocalcemia, and metabolic acidosis. Administer calcium replacements and phosphate binders when indicated. Monitor and assess dysfunction in other organ systems that can occur posttransplant such as dysrhythmias, hypotension, ECG changes, vascular thromboses, hypertension, pulmonary edema, ARDS, diarrhea, GI bleeding or infection. Administer immunosuppressive agents as ordered and monitor closely for infection, rejection, anemia, thrombocytopenia, or leukopenia. Maintain Foley catheter up to 1 week.		

NUTRITION

Diagnosis/Stabilization Phase		Acute Management Phase		Recovery Phase	
Outcome	*Intervention*	*Outcome*	*Intervention*	*Outcome*	*Intervention*
Patient will be adequately nourished.	Dietary consult. Monitor caloric intake and percentages of fats, carbohydrates, and proteins closely. Dietary recommendations are: • 1 g of protein per kg of ideal body weight • 2–3 g of sodium • 40–50 mEq of potassium (remind patient/family not to use salt substitutes containing potassium chloride) • 1,200 mg of phosphorus per day • Calcium supplements if needed when phosphorus controlled • Vitamin and iron supplements; folate if anemic Restrict fluid intake to 500–1,000 mL/day (+ sum of urine output, if any) and weigh daily. Monitor serum protein, albumin, hematocrit, urea levels, and daily weight to assess effectiveness of nutritional therapy. Keep serum albumin >3.0 g/dL. Medications to improve gastric motility may be necessary to enhance absorption of nutrients and minimize need for antiemetics. Assess oral mucosa and provide frequent oral hygiene. Monitor bowel function and encourage use of laxatives, stool softeners, or high-fiber diet when indicated. Administer H_2 antagonists if ordered.	Patient will be adequately nourished.	Advance diet as tolerated after kidney transplant. Dietitian consult. Monitor bowel function as above. Monitor and treat anorexia and dysphagia. Encourage PO fluid intake to thirst (not restricted). Teach patient/family to avoid simple sugars and limit sodium intake. Encourage patient to eat a high-protein diet up to 4 weeks posttransplant.	Patient will be adequately nourished.	Teach patient/family to follow low-fat diet and limit simple sugars and sodium intake. Teach patient/family to eat less protein after 4 weeks as prednisone is tapered.

Care Guide continued on following page

MOBILITY

Diagnosis/Stabilization Phase		Acute Management Phase		Recovery Phase	
Outcome	**Intervention**	**Outcome**	**Intervention**	**Outcome**	**Intervention**
Patient will achieve optimal mobility.	Monitor patient's tolerance to activity (may be decreased if anemic). Decrease activity if adverse events occur (tachycardia, dyspnea, ectopy, syncope, hypotension). Progress as patient tolerates. Assess for muscle weakness, gait changes, and the presence of joint pain or deep bone pain.	Patient will achieve optimal mobility.	Consult physical or occupational therapist as indicated. Increase activity as tolerated posttransplant. Assess for muscle weakness, joint pain, tingling, or numbness of upper thigh on operative side of transplant.	Patient will achieve optimal mobility.	Instruct patient to avoid lifting or strenuous exercise for 3 months. Continue to progress exercise as tolerated and monitor response. Assist patient/family in developing home exercise program.

OXYGENATION/VENTILATION

Diagnosis/Stabilization Phase		Acute Management Phase		Recovery Phase	
Outcome	**Intervention**	**Outcome**	**Intervention**	**Outcome**	**Intervention**
Patient will have adequate gas exchange as evidenced by: • $Sao_2 > 90\%$/ $Spo_2 > 92\%$ • ABGs WNL • Clear breath sounds • Respiratory rate, depth, and rhythm WNL • Normal chest x-ray • Thin, white pulmonary secretions Patient will have adequate tissue perfusion as evidenced by: • Normovolemic status • Adequate hemoglobin • Alert and oriented • Appropriate level of consciousness	Monitor and treat oxygenation status per ABGs and/or Spo_2. Assess sensorium and level of consciousness frequently. Monitor for signs and symptoms of pulmonary distress from fluid overload. Monitor acid–base status per ABGs. Monitor for signs and symptoms of pulmonary infection/pneumonia. Support patient with O_2 therapy and/or mechanical ventilation as indicated. Monitor for complications of chronic renal failure that may impair oxygenation/ventilation status (congestive heart failure, pulmonary edema, fatigue, lethargy, somnolence).	Patient will have adequate gas exchange after kidney transplantation.	Same as stabilization phase. Anticipate complications related to kidney transplantation that may impair oxygenation/ventilatory status (ARDS, sepsis, pulmonary edema, hypoxemia). Wean oxygen therapy and/or mechanical ventilation as tolerated. Encourage use of incentive spirometer and/or deep breathing with inspiratory hold q2h.	Patient will have adequate gas exchange.	Teach patient/family abnormal respiratory symptoms such as shortness of breath, dyspnea on exertion, wheezing, chest pain, and tachypnea, and importance of reporting these to physician.

COMFORT

Diagnosis/Stabilization Phase		Acute Management Phase		Recovery Phase	
Outcome	*Intervention*	*Outcome*	*Intervention*	*Outcome*	*Intervention*
Patient will be as comfortable and pain free as possible, as evidenced by: • No objective indicators of discomfort • No complaints of discomfort	Monitor and treat breathing status closely for signs and symptoms of respiratory distress related to fluid overload. Keep head of bed elevated and review breathing techniques such as pursed-lip breathing, and coughing techniques to minimize respiratory distress. Creatively plan fluid restriction over 24 hours, including periodic sips of water, ice chips, or popsicles to minimize thirst. Offer gum, hard candy, mouth swab, and frequent oral care. Assess for signs/symptoms of uremic neuropathy or renal osteodystrophy (numbness or burning in feet, restless leg movements, decreased muscle strength, cramps, paresthesias, and decreased tendon reflexes). Avoid unexpected touching of the feet. Keep heavy bed linens off of feet. Ensure that serum calcium and phosphate levels are adequate. Administer phosphate-binding antacids as prescribed. Instruct patient to inspect feet visually for signs of injury. Observe patient for complications of end-stage renal disease that may cause discomfort (dyspnea, joint/bone pain, nausea, lethargy, weakness).	Patient will be as comfortable and pain free as possible.	Teach patient to rate pain on 1–10 scale and administer analgesics as indicated postoperatively. Provide adequate rest periods, especially if patient is anemic. Teach patient relaxation techniques, including complementary therapies such as back massage, humor, or music therapy. Involve family in strategies.	Patient will be as comfortable as possible.	Teach patient/family on comfort measures, including: • Breathing exercises to help control dyspnea • Relaxation techniques • Complementary therapy techniques to decrease dyspnea

Care Guide continued on following page

END-STAGE RENAL FAILURE/KIDNEY TRANSPLANTATION MULTIDISCIPLINARY CARE GUIDE *continued*

SKIN INTEGRITY

Diagnosis/Stabilization Phase		Acute Management Phase		Recovery Phase	
Outcome	*Intervention*	*Outcome*	*Intervention*	*Outcome*	*Intervention*
Patient will have intact skin without abrasions or pressure ulcers.	Assess skin integrity and all bony prominences (including feet) q4h Use superfatted or lanolin-based soap for bathing and apply emollients for itching. Use preventive pressure-reducing devices if patient is at high risk for pressure ulcer development. Treat pressure ulcers according to hospital protocol. Avoid tight-fitting shoes or clothing that may create pressure points susceptible to breakdown if applicable.	Patient will have intact skin without evidence of wound dehiscence.	Evaluate patient's skin integrity. Assess healing of transplant incision.	Patient will have intact skin without evidence of wound dehiscence.	Teach patient/family skin care and incision management postdischarge. Remind patient that sutures/staples may be in for 2–3 weeks due to slower healing rate related to prednisone therapy. Teach patient/family not to lift anything over 10 pounds for 3 months.

PROTECTION/SAFETY

Diagnosis/Stabilization Phase		Acute Management Phase		Recovery Phase	
Outcome	*Intervention*	*Outcome*	*Intervention*	*Outcome*	*Intervention*
Patient will be protected from possible harm. Patient will maintain a patent and infection-free vascular access device before kidney transplant.	Assess need for wrist restraints if patient is intubated, has a decreased level of consciousness, is unable to follow commands, or for affected extremity during hemodialysis. Explain need for restraints to patient/family. Provide support when dangling or beginning progressive exercise program.	Patient will be protected from possible harm.	Provide support as needed as patient increases physical activity posttransplant. Monitor for signs/symptoms of infection (symptoms may be subtle due to immunosuppression). Instruct patient/family to report any vague discomforts, mental status changes, or constant low-grade fevers.	Patient will be protected from possible harm.	Teach patient potential complications of immunosuppressive agents and interventions to alleviate or minimize such complications. Teach patient signs and symptoms of infection. Encourage patient to avoid crowds in first 3 months.

Outcome	Intervention	Outcome	Intervention	Outcome	Intervention
	Monitor the color, temperature, and sensation of extremity with vascular access. Assess for signs and symptoms of infection and maintain strict sterile technique when accessing the device. Assess patency by palpating thrill and auscultating for the bruit. Avoid constriction of affected extremity with BP cuff or tourniquet. Avoid sticks in affected extremity.		Teach patient/family early signs of rejection: fever, pain, tenderness, swelling at graft site, weight gain, decrease in urine output, hypertension, and elevation in serum creatinine. Monitor stools for occult bleeding.		

PSYCHOSOCIAL/SELF-DETERMINATION

Diagnosis/Stabilization Phase		Acute Management Phase		Recovery Phase	
Outcome	***Intervention***	***Outcome***	***Intervention***	***Outcome***	***Intervention***
Patient will achieve psychophysiologic stability. Patient will demonstrate a decrease in anxiety as evidenced by: • Vital signs WNL for the patient • Level of consciousness WNL for the patient • Subjective report of decreased anxiety • Objective assessment of decreased anxiety	Assess physiologic effects of acute care environment on patient. Assess patient for appropriate level of stress. Assess coping mechanisms for chronic illness. Assess personal responses (affective and/or feelings) of patient/family regarding critical care illness and their patterns of thinking/communicating. Assess patient/family for signs of depression, anger, withdrawal, and dependent behaviors. Assist patient/family in decision-making process for transplantation as a treatment alternative. Use calm, competent, reassuring approach to interventions. Observe factors that make patient/family anxious and take measures to reduce their anxiety. (Initiate family conferences, refer support services, and use consistent caregivers). Allow flexible visiting to meet the needs of the patient/family. Use sedatives, antidepressants as appropriate.	Patient will achieve psychophysiologic stability. Patient will demonstrate a decrease in anxiety.	Teach patient/family continuing care. Provide information on local support groups, kidney centers, and agencies such as the National Kidney Foundation.	Patient will achieve psychophysiologic stability. Patient will demonstrate a decrease in anxiety.	Same as acute management phase.

Care Guide continued on following page

END-STAGE RENAL FAILURE/KIDNEY TRANSPLANTATION MULTIDISCIPLINARY CARE GUIDE *continued*

DIAGNOSTICS

Diagnosis/Stabilization Phase		Acute Management Phase		Recovery Phase	
Outcome	*Intervention*	*Outcome*	*Intervention*	*Outcome*	*Intervention*
Patient will understand any tests or procedures that need to be completed to assess renal function (hemodynamic assessments, frequent vital signs, serum labs, calcium and phosphate levels, CBC with differential, platelet count, and renal ultrasound). Patient will understand evaluation and assessment for kidney transplantation potential (echocardiogram, cardiac work-up, pulmonary function studies, histocompatibility studies [human leukocyte antigen test, ABO blood typing, mixed lymphocyte culture, serum blood test to assess for cytoxic antibodies, level of supressor T cells], clotting factors, ABGs, x-rays).	Explain procedures and tests to patient/family. Be sensitive to patient/family's individual need for information.	Patient will understand meaning of diagnostic tests in relation to continuing care.	Review with patient before discharge results of lab tests and renal function posttransplant. Review with patient/family what to expect in renal function/health. Teach patient/family various treatments when rejection is suspected such as ultrasound, renal scan, renal biopsy, and drug regimen.	Patient will understand meaning of diagnostic tests in relation to continuing care.	Same as acute management phase.

REFERENCE

Stark, J. L. (1991). The renal system. In J. G. Alspach (Ed.), *Core curriculum for critical care nursing* (4th ed., pp. 472–608). Philadelphia: W. B. Saunders.

UNIT

8

GASTROINTESTINAL SYSTEM

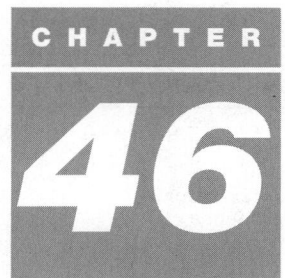

Gastrointestinal Physiology

Una E. Westfall and Margaret Heitkemper

The gastrointestinal (GI) tract is responsible for the digestion and absorption of nutrients. The accomplishment of this task requires appropriate and timely movement of nutrients through the GI tract (motility), the presence of specific enzymes to break down nutrients (digestion), and transport mechanisms to move nutrients from the GI tract lumen to the vascular system (absorption). The term *GI system* denotes the entire system responsible for these functions, whereas *GI tract* refers only to those organs that connect the mouth with the anus (Fig. 46–1). The anatomic parts of the GI tract include the mouth, esophagus, stomach, small intestine, and large intestine. The small intestine is further divided anatomically into duodenum, jejunum, and ileum, the duodenum being closest to the stomach. The large intestine is divided into the cecum, ascending colon, transverse colon, descending colon, sigmoid colon, and rectum. Accessory organs of the GI system include the liver, pancreas, and gallbladder. Each of these organs plays an important role in the digestion of nutrients.

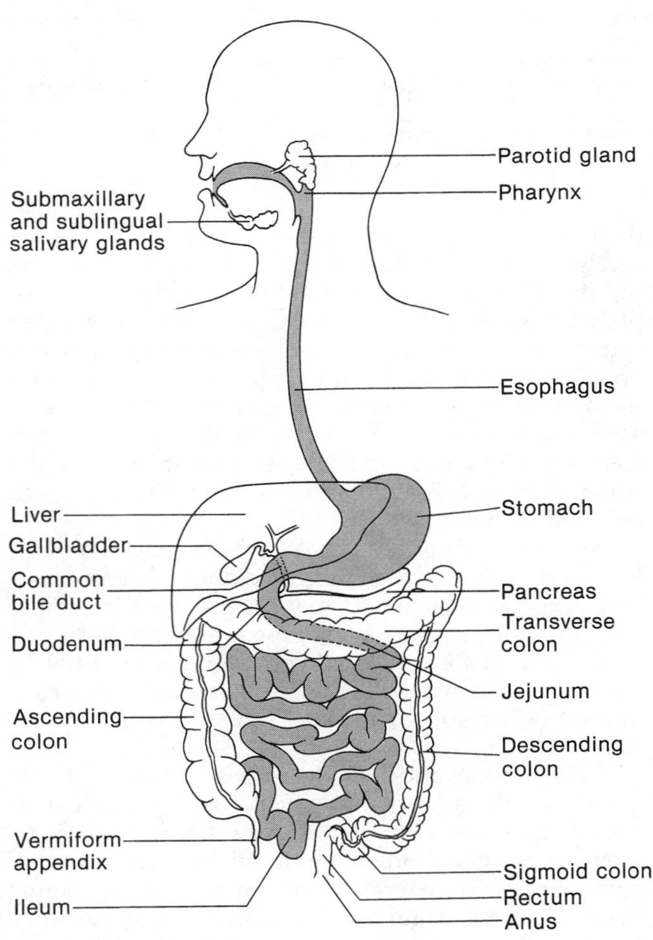

FIGURE 46–1. Digestive tract of the human being.

ANATOMY OF THE GUT WALL

Beginning in the esophagus and extending to the rectum, the GI tract is composed of multiple tissue layers.

MUCOSA. The innermost layer that is exposed to dietary nutrients is the mucosa. The thickness and function of the mucosa vary according to the anatomic segment examined. The mucosal layer is composed of epithelial cells. These epithelial cells are connected by tight junctions, which produce an effective barrier against the entry of large molecular substances and bacteria. In addition, the mucosa contains goblet cells that produce and secrete mucus. In the stomach, the anatomic arrangement of epithelial cells as well as the production of mucus and the relatively rapid regeneration of cells provide what is known as the gastric mucosal barrier. However, some substances, such as salicylates and alcohol, are able to penetrate this barrier and thus are absorbed in the stomach. It is the disruption of this anatomic and physiologic barrier that is thought to play a role in ulcer development.

SUBMUCOSA. Beneath the mucosa is a nerve plexus known as the submucosal plexus. Plexus neurons receive input from and supply innervation to the mucosa and muscle layers. In addition, the plexus neurons communicate with the sympathetic and parasympathetic branches of the autonomic nervous system.

SEROSA. Next is the first of two smooth muscle layers comprising the gut wall. The innermost muscle layer is the circular muscle, and the next is the longitu-

TABLE 46–1. **Responses of Selected Effector Organs to Autonomic Nerve Impulses**

Effector Organs/Adrenergic	Receptor Type	Adrenergic Impulses: Responses†	Cholinergic Impulses: Responses†
Stomach			
Motility and tone	Alpha-1, Alpha-2; beta-2	Decrease (usually)*+	Increase +++
Sphincters	Alpha-1	Contraction (usually)+	Relaxation (usually) +
Secretion		Inhibition (?)	Stimulation +++
Intestine			
Motility and tone	Alpha-1, Alpha-2, beta-1; beta-2	Decrease*+	Increase +++
Sphincters	Alpha-1	Contraction (usually) +	Relaxation (usually) +
Secretion	Alpha-2	Inhibition	Stimulation ++
Gallbladder and Ducts	Beta-2	Relaxation+	Contraction +
Liver	Alpha; beta-2	Glycogenolysis and gluconeogenesis‡+++	
Pancreas			
Acini	Alpha	Decreased secretion+	Secretion++
Islets (beta cells)	Alpha-2,	Decreased secretion+++	—
	beta-2	Increased secretion+	—
Fat Cells	Alpha; beta-1 (beta-3)	Lipolysis‡+++	—
Salivary Glands	Alpha-1	Potassium and water secretion+	Potassium and water secretion+++
	Beta	Amylase secretion+	
Nasopharyngeal Glands		—	Secretion++

*It has been proposed that adrenergic fibers terminate at inhibitory beta receptors on smooth muscle fibers, and at inhibitory alpha receptors on parasympathetic cholinergic (excitatory) ganglion cells of Auerbach's (myenteric) plexus.

†Gives estimated importance of autonomic nervous system control for selected responses by organ.

‡There is significant variation among species in the type of receptor that mediates certain metabolic responses; alpha and beta responses have not been determined in humans. Beta-3 receptor may mediate responses in fat cells in some species.

Adapted from Gilman, A. G., Rall, R. I., et al. (1990). *Goodman and Gilman's the pharmacological basis of therapeutics* (8th ed., pp. 89–90). New York: Macmillan. Reproduced with permission of McGraw-Hill, Inc.

dinal muscle. Both are so named because of their muscle fiber orientation. Combined, these muscle layers form what is called the serosa. Between the two muscle layers is another nerve plexus known as the *myenteric plexus.*

The anatomic arrangement of the gut wall, including the nerve and muscle layers, persists throughout the length of the GI tract. However, in the stomach there is an additional muscle layer known as the muscularis mucosa, which is located between the mucosa and the circular muscle layer.

NEURAL INNERVATION

Extrinsic

Functions of the GI system are influenced by neural as well as hormonal factors.

AUTONOMIC NERVOUS SYSTEM. The autonomic nervous system exerts multiple effects. Table 46–1 summarizes some of the common effects of the ANS on the GI system.

PARASYMPATHETIC NERVOUS SYSTEM. The GI tract is innervated by preganglionic fibers of the parasympathetic nervous system (Fig. 46–2). The upper GI tract receives fibers from the vagus nerve; the distal GI tract receives fibers from the sacral division of the parasympathetic nervous system. As stated earlier, these fibers synapse on the enteric nervous system neurons, which are located between the muscle layers of the gut wall. In addition, these nerve bundles contain afferent (sensory) fibers whose receptors are located within GI tissues. The afferent nerve fibers relay information to the spinal cord and brain about such sensations as pain and distention.

SYMPATHETIC NERVOUS SYSTEM. The GI tract is also innervated by fibers from the sympathetic nervous system. Preganglionic fibers synapse on leaving the spinal cord in ganglia located adjacent to the vertebral column. Long postganglionic fibers then travel to the GI tract organs to synapse on blood vessels and neurons located within the gut wall as well as some secretory cells.

Sympathetic and parasympathetic preganglionic fibers as well as postganglionic parasympathetic neurons release acetylcholine as their neurotransmitter, whereas postganglionic sympathetic fibers release norepinephrine. In general, parasympathetic cholinergic fibers (through vagal efferent fibers) are stimulatory to GI secretion and propulsive activity, in contrast to

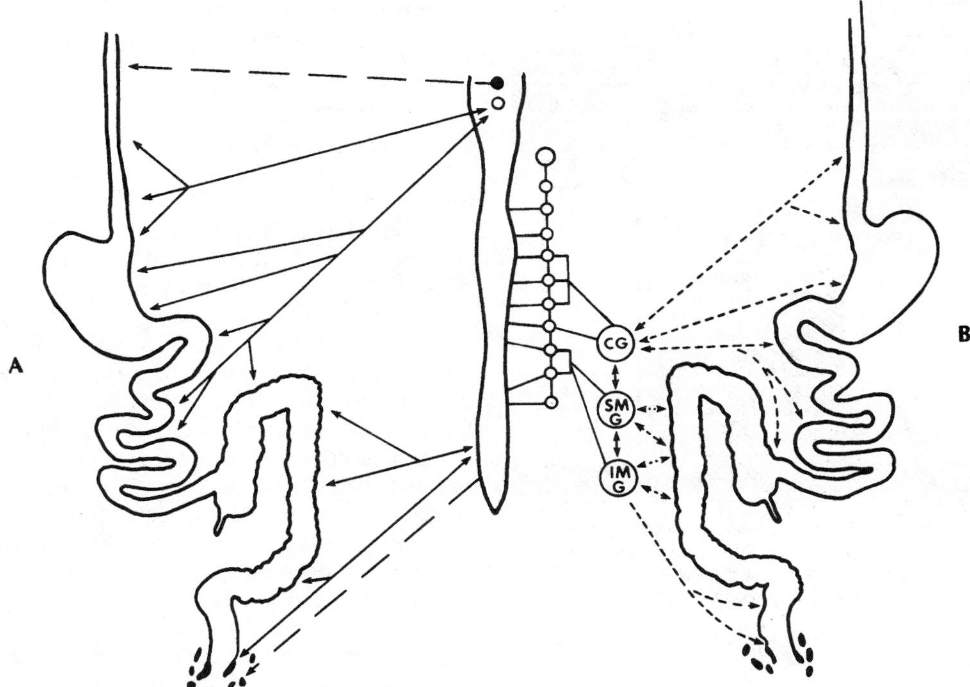

FIGURE 46–2. Extrinsic branches of the autonomic nervous system. *A*, Parasympathetic. Dashed lines indicate the cholinergic innervation of striated muscle in the esophagus and external anal sphincter. Solid lines indicate the afferent and preganglionic efferent innervation of the rest of the gastrointestinal tract. *B*, Sympathetic. Solid lines denote the afferent and preganglionic efferent connections between the spinal cord and the prevertebral ganglia (CG, celiac; SMG, superior mesenteric; IMG, inferior mesenteric). Dashed lines indicate afferent and postganglionic efferent innervation. (Reproduced by permission from: Johnson, L. [1991]. *Gastrointestinal physiology* [4th ed., p. 16]. St. Louis: C. V. Mosby.

sympathetic nervous system input, which inhibits GI motor and secretory activity and produces contraction of GI sphincters and blood vessels. Clinical consequences include gastric stasis, adynamic or paralytic ileus, or colonic ileus. Parasympathetic and sympathetic fibers also innervate the gallbladder and pancreas.

Intrinsic

Extrinsic preganglionic parasympathetic and postganglionic sympathetic fibers synapse on neurons of the myenteric and submucosal plexuses. The submucosal and myenteric nerve networks combined are referred to as the enteric nervous system of the gut. These enteric neurons innervate target cells, including smooth muscle cells, secretory cells, and absorptive cells. In addition, enteric neuron plexuses communicate with each other throughout the length of the gut and contribute to intrinsic coordination. Enteric nerves generate propulsive activities (e.g., peristalsis, segmental contractions) and coordinate activities of the GI sphincters. Disturbances of these enteric neurons in a given segment of GI tract are related to lack of motility or movement. This is seen most dramatically in congenital megacolon (Hirschsprung disease), in which a segment of distal colon lacks enteric neurons. As a result, there is lack of movement of intestinal contents through this region, leading to distention of the region preceding the aganglionic segment.

HORMONAL CONTROL

Hormones that influence GI function include those produced by specialized cells within the GI tract as well as those synthesized by other endocrine organs (Fig. 46–3). In general, the GI tract is considered the largest endocrine organ in the body. Protein and peptide hormones produced by GI tissue are secreted into the portal venous circulation, pass through the liver and heart, and return to the GI tract to modulate activities such as motility, secretion, and absorption. Gastrointestinal hormones (e.g., gastrin) as well as other hormones (e.g., cortisol) may be involved in the normal maturation of GI tissues. There is some overlap in the function of gut hormones in that two or more hormones may produce similar effects in relation to motility, acid secretion, or fluid and electrolyte secretion.

The first hormone "discovered" was secretin in 1902. In 1905 gastrin was described, and in 1928 cholecystokinin (CCK) was named for its ability to cause gallbladder contraction. These three hormones were isolated and characterized in the 1960s. In the late 1960s, gastric inhibitory peptide was isolated and char-

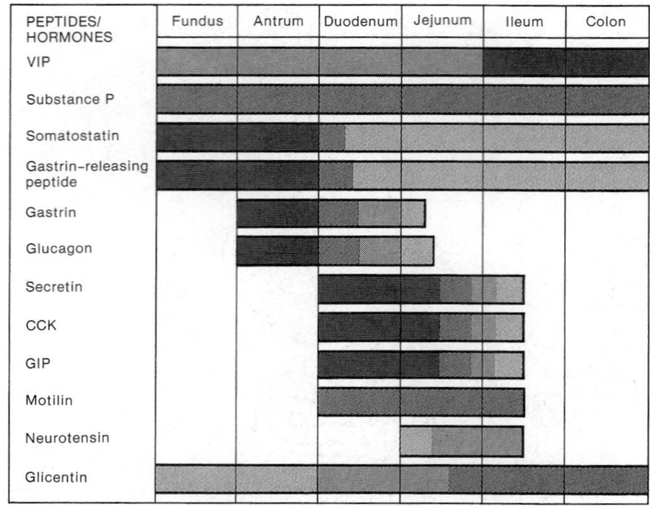

FIGURE 46–3. Distribution of gastrointestinal peptides along the gastrointestinal tract. The shading of each bar is proportionate to the concentration of the peptide in the mucosa. *Abbreviations:* CCK, cholecystokinin; GIP, gastric inhibitory peptide; VIP, vasoactive intestinal polypeptide.

acterized. A variety of other peptide hormones have been found in various segments of the gut; however, their physiologic functions remain to be clarified. These peptides (Table 46–2) include motilin, enteroglucagon, pancreatic polypeptide, vasoactive intestinal polypeptide, gastrin-releasing peptide, and enkephalins.

Table 46–3 lists the better known GI hormones and their actions. Gastrin, which is secreted by cells located in the gastric antrum and duodenum, stimulates release of hydrochloric acid. Serum levels of gastrin can be measured by radioimmunoassay, which may be performed in patients with Zollinger-Ellison syndrome, in which tumor cells produce gastrin. CCK has the widest range of action. CCK is secreted by intestinal cells in response to the presence of fat and protein breakdown products and is a stimulant of pancreatic enzyme secretion and gallbladder smooth muscle contraction. Secretin, which is produced and secreted by the small intestine in response to the presence of acid, is known to stimulate secretion of pancreatic juice with a high bicarbonate content. These hormones also influence GI motility.

BLOOD SUPPLY

Of the various body organ systems, the GI system receives the largest percentage of the cardiac output. Approximately one-third of the cardiac output supplies these tissues. Blood supply to organs within the abdomen is referred to as the splanchnic circulation (Fig. 46–4). The stomach, small and large intestines, pancreas, and gallbladder are supplied by the superior and inferior mesenteric and celiac arteries, whereas the liver receives part of its blood supply from the hepatic artery. Circulation in the GI system is unique in that venous blood draining the GI tract empties into the portal vein, which then perfuses the liver. The portal vein supplies approximately 70% to 75% of blood flow to the liver. Because such a large percentage of cardiac output perfuses the tissues of the GI tract, the GI tract is a major source from which blood flow can be diverted to more vital organs during times of need, such as during exercise or hemorrhage.

At the tissue level, there is an overlap in perfusion that ensures to some degree that occlusion of one artery due to, for example, thrombus or embolus will not completely deny the mucosa its blood supply. However, prolonged occlusion of a major artery supplying the GI tract can produce ischemic changes of the mucosal lining and, ultimately, necrosis. Nonocclusive intestinal ischemia or hemorrhagic necrosis of the gut is an example of potentially fatal damage produced by a prolonged reduction in intestinal blood supply. In the presence of a systemic problem such as congestive heart failure or a peripheral problem such as arteriosclerosis, there could be a reduction in the blood supply to the GI tract. As a result, necrosis of intestinal villi occurs, which can ultimately destroy the GI tract's barrier to harmful toxins and bacteria normally present in the intestinal lumen. These bacteria then enter the blood supply and can produce septic shock and, depending on the severity, death of the patient. This process is referred to as bacterial translocation.

Critically ill patients who do not receive adequate

TABLE 46–2. **Candidate Hormones and Neurocrines**

Peptide	Source	Action	Hormone/Neurocrine
Enkephalin	Gut mucosa and muscle	Increases smooth muscle tone	Neurocrine
Enteroglucagon	Intestinal mucosa	Glycogenolysis	Candidate hormone
Gastrin-releasing peptide or bombesin	Gastric mucosa	Gastrin release	Neurocrine
Motilin	Duodenal mucosa	Increases gastric motility Intestinal motility	Candidate hormone
Pancreatic polypeptide	Pancreas	Decreases pancreatic HCO_3^- Decreases enzyme secretion	Candidate hormone
Vasoactive intestinal polypeptide	Gut mucosa and muscle	Relaxation of gut and circular smooth muscle	Neurocrine

TABLE 46–3. **Gastrointestinal Hormone Actions**

	Hormone			
Action	***Gastrin***	***Cholecystokinin***	***Secretin***	***Gastric Inhibitory Peptide***
Acid secretion	S*	S	I*	I*
Gastric emptying	I	I*	I	I
Pancreatic HCO_3^- secretion	S	S*	S*	0
Pancreatic enzyme secretion	S	S*	S	0
Bile HCO_3^- secretion	S	S	S*	0
Gallbladder contraction	S	S*	S	—
Gastric motility	S	S	I	I
Intestinal motility	S	S	I	S
Insulin release	S	S	S	S*
Mucosal growth	S*	S	I	—
Pancreatic growth	S	S*	S*	—

Abbreviations: S, stimulates; I, inhibits; 0, no effect; —, not yet tested.
*Important physiologic response to endogenous hormone level after normal stimulus.
Reproduced by permission from Johnson, L. (1985). *Gastrointestinal physiology* (3rd ed., p. 8). St. Louis: C. V. Mosby.

oral or enteral feedings are nutritionally supported by total parenteral nutrition (TPN). TPN can result in mucosal atrophy, intestinal bacterial overgrowth, increased intestinal permeability, and deficits in intestinal cellular and hormonal immunity. Together, these changes in gut physiology and immunity lead to bacterial and endotoxin escape from the gut, a process called microbial translocation. Studies in rats demonstrate that 70% to 80% of rats fed TPN or incomplete oral–duodenal elemental diets develop bacterial translocation to their mesenteric lymph nodes as well as a 30% to 40% reduction in intestinal mucosal mass (Go-

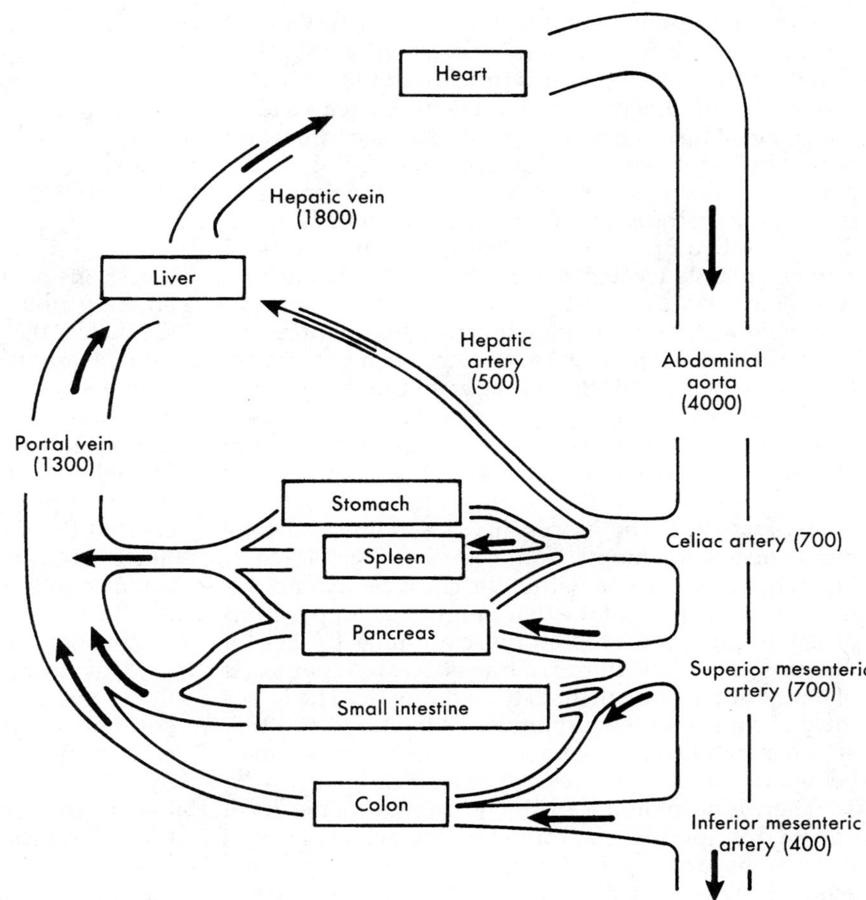

FIGURE 46–4. Blood flows and distributions within the major splanchnic vessels (mL/minute). (Reproduced by permission from: Johnson, L. [1991]. *Gastrointestinal physiology* [4th ed., p. 143]. St. Louis: C. V. Mosby.)

nella et al., 1992; Moore et al., 1992; McGeer et al., 1989). Similarly, in the trauma patient with hemorrhagic shock in whom prolonged hypotension occurs, there is an increased risk for translocation.

MAJOR FUNCTIONS OF THE GI TRACT

Anatomic structures of the GI tract will be discussed as they pertain to the three main functions of the gut: motility, digestion, and absorption. To accomplish these functions, the segments of the GI tract secrete fluids that are important for lubrication, digestion, and absorption. Secretions are presented as they pertain to these functions.

Motility

The term *motility* denotes the timely movement of nutrients through the GI tract. Under normal circumstances, nutrients move through the GI tract at a rate that allows the digestive enzymes to break down nutrients and absorption to occur. Increased motility can result in decreased time for digestion and absorption of nutrients, which can be manifested in the whole-body changes as well as in GI symptoms such as diarrhea.

MOUTH. Normally, food and fluid enter the GI tract through the mouth. Here food is mechanically broken down into smaller pieces in a process known as mastication. During this process, food is mixed with saliva, which facilitates its transit to the back of the throat and down the esophagus. In addition, saliva facilitates exposure of taste receptors located along the tongue to the chemical properties of food. Approximately 1 to 2 liters of saliva are secreted each day. Three pairs of salivary glands located within the oral cavity are responsible for saliva production.

Swallowing is a complex function that requires an intact nervous system. Once food has been voluntarily moved to the back of the throat, it stimulates afferent nerve endings that travel by way of the vagus, glossopharyngeal, and trigeminal nerves to the brain stem to initiate the swallowing response.

ESOPHAGHUS. The esophagus is a cylindrical tube that connects the mouth to the stomach (Fig. 46–5). It lies behind the trachea within the chest cavity and terminates at the level of the diaphragm. The upper third of the esophagus is striated muscle similar to skeletal muscle. The middle third is a transition area composed of a mixture of smooth and striated muscle. The lower third is similar to the remainder of the GI tract—that is, it has two layers of smooth muscle, the inner layer being circular and the next layer longitudinal.

There is no anatomic sphincter separating the distal end of the esophagus from the stomach. However, there is an area of high pressure called the lower esophageal sphincter (LES). This high-pressure zone

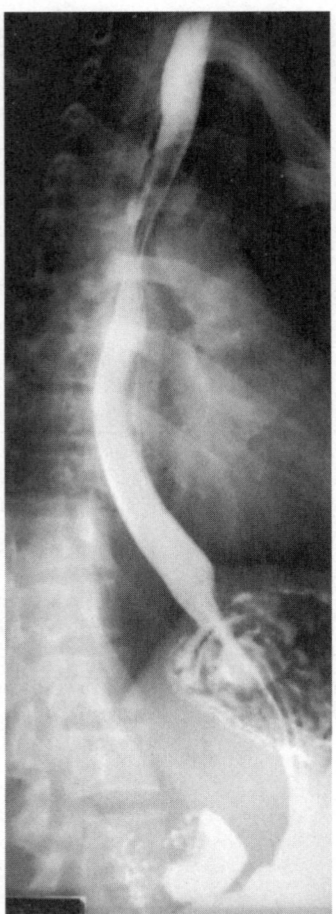

FIGURE 46–5. X-ray film of the entire barium-filled esophagus, showing the course of this organ through the mediastinum from hypopharynx to stomach. Note the three indentations produced by the aorta, left main stem bronchus, and left atrium.

is responsible for preventing the gastric contents from entering the esophagus. Without this physiologic sphincter, the risk of acidic gastric contents moving into the esophagus (regurgitation) when an individual is in a supine position is much greater. A number of clinical conditions can decrease the competency of the LES. Examples include the pathologic states such as a hiatal hernia; pregnancy, with a concomitant elevation in serum progesterone level, which is thought to decrease LES pressure; and cigarette smoking, which reduces LES pressure. In addition, dietary substances can also influence LES pressure. The presence of protein in the stomach elevates the closing pressure; fat diminishes the closing pressure.

Movement of a food bolus from the mouth down the esophagus is promoted by a pressure gradient. In addition, contraction of the esophageal wall (peristalsis) behind the bolus promotes movement. When an individual swallows, the LES relaxes, allowing the bolus to enter the stomach. In the clinical condition known as achalasia, the lower esophagus fails to relax or a spasm of the muscle prevents passage of the bolus into the stomach. Due to distention of the lower portion of the esophagus by the bolus, this condition is frequently painful. Patients often describe a sensation of pain that radiates down both arms. In patients with achalasia, symptoms frequently occur after eating.

STOMACH. Anatomically, the stomach is divided into three parts—the fundus, body, and antrum. The distal portion of the antrum is known as the pylorus. The pylorus is a thick band of muscle that separates the stomach from the upper small intestine and thus acts like a physiologic sphincter. The stomach, like the lower esophagus, has longitudinal and circular muscle layers as well as two nerve layers. When food or liquids are ingested, the stomach acts like a reservoir that empties food into the small intestine at the optimum rate for digestion and absorption. This rate is normally dependent on the characteristics of the diet. That is, foods that have a high osmolarity, such as "rich" foods with a high fat content, tend to empty more slowly than calorically less dense foods. In addition, the volume of liquid or food consumed can also modulate the rate of gastric emptying.

Motility of the stomach serves two purposes: (1) to promote movement of chyme (food mixed with GI secretions) through the pylorus, and (2) to mix and grind food, allowing exposure of food to gastric secretions. Stomach motor activity is controlled in part by extrinsic neural fibers and hormones as well as by intrinsic nerve fibers that respond to distention of the stomach wall. In addition, the rate of gastric emptying is influenced by chyme characteristics such as fat content, acidity, and osmolarity. The caloric concentration, or nutrient density, of a solution is believed to play a major role in gastric emptying. When the calorie count of a fluid rises, the rate of gastric emptying declines (Murray, 1987). Temporal differences in gastric emptying rates have also been reported (Goo et al., 1987). Particularly for solid meals, more rapid emptying occurs with the morning meal rather than the evening one. Figure 46–6 summarizes other common factors influencing gastric emptying.

DELAYED GASTRIC EMPTYING. The motor activity of the stomach is often reduced in response to major body insults such as surgery and trauma. Hypomotility or inertia of the stomach results in delayed gastric emptying. When present, this precludes the use of gastric feedings in some patients immediately after surgery or trauma. The small intestine appears to be less affected, and thus, nasointestinal feedings (minimal enteral feedings) may be used. Such delayed emptying may potentially contribute to aspiration in patients receiving enteral nutrition. Delayed gastric emptying is also associated with diabetic neuropathy, in which neurodegenerative changes result in decreased neural input (Roudebuch, 1994). Patients may report nausea, fullness, loss of appetite, or symptoms of gastric regurgitation. The development of prokinetic drugs such as cisapride, metroclopramide, and erythromycin have proven clinically beneficial in stimulating gastric emptying and decreasing nausea.

VOMITING. Vomiting is the forceful expulsion of gastric or intestinal contents up through the esophagus and out of the mouth. Frequently, vomiting is preceded by a variety of physiologic changes, including increased salivation, sweating, tachycardia, retching, bradycardia, tachypnea, and nausea. The act of vomiting is a complex physiologic function that involves coordination of the GI organs and respiratory system. During vomiting there is relaxation of the upper stomach and esophagus and increased pressure in the duodenum due to contraction of the abdominal wall against these relaxed organs. This promotes the move-

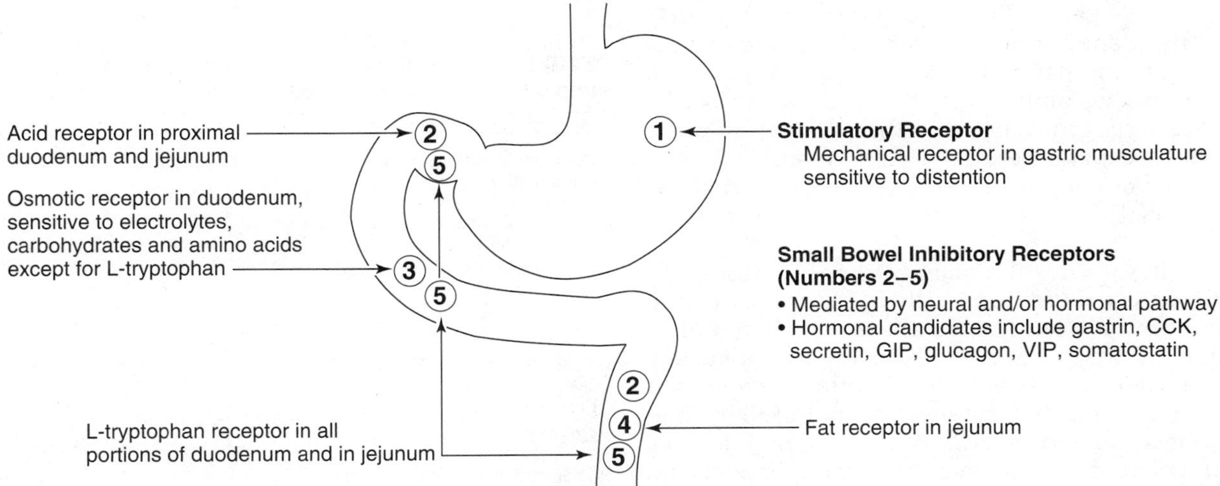

FIGURE 46–6. Physiology of gastric emptying. Various factors that influence gastric emptying are depicted. Location of mechanical and osmotic receptor (*1*and *3*) as determined by human studies. Other receptors localized by studies in dogs. *Abbreviations:* CCK, cholecystokinin; GIP, gastric inhibitory peptide; VIP, vasoactive intestinal polypeptide. (Reprinted with permission from Physiology and pathophysiology of gastric emptying in humans, by H. Minami and R. McCallum. GASTROENTEROLOGY, *86*[6], p. 1594. Copyright 1984 by the American Gastoenterological Association.)

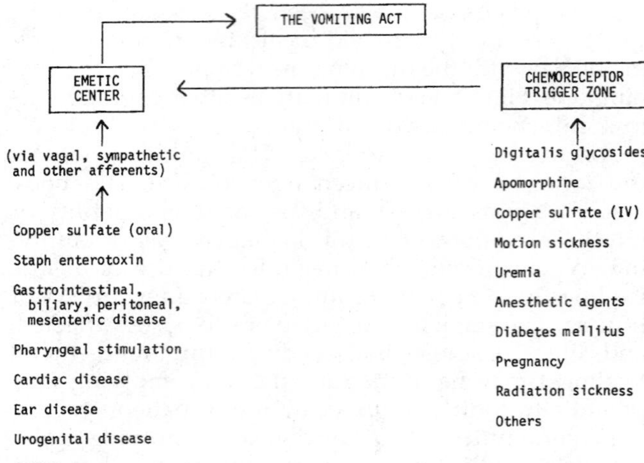

FIGURE 46–7. Diagram of proposed pathways in the act of vomiting. (From Greenberger, N. [1989]. *Gastrointestinal disorders: A pathophysiologic approach* [4th ed., p. 117]. Chicago: Year Book Medical Publishers.)

ment of chyme out of the small intestine and into the stomach. Contractile activity of the antrum then facilitates movement of chyme to the upper stomach and into the esophagus. During vomiting, respiration ceases, and the chyme moves past the pharyngoesophageal sphincter and out of the mouth.

The mechanics of vomiting are controlled by an area in the brain stem frequently referred to as the vomiting or emetic center (Fig. 46–7). Electrical stimulation of this area in animals results in projectile vomiting without retching. This center receives input from its blood supply and from a variety of peripheral organs. Chemicals carried in the blood can activate the chemoreceptor trigger zone of the vomiting center, as can afferent fibers that are activated by noxious stimuli such as severe pain or injury to abdominal structures such as the kidney or bladder. Increases in intracranial pressure or stimulation of the vestibular system can also activate the vomiting center. Vomiting can also be induced psychogenically by the thought of unpleasant or noxious experiences. Conditions associated with nausea or vomiting, or both, in critically ill patients and potential adverse outcomes are shown in Table 46–4.

Drug therapy for the management of nausea and vomiting acts either peripherally to reduce peripheral input or centrally to decrease afferent nerve impulses in brain pathways. Peripherally acting drugs include topical anesthetics and antacids. Centrally acting antiemetics include antihistamines, phenothiazines, and anticholinergics. Drugs such as metoclopramide have a central effect on the chemoreceptor trigger zone and also increase gastric motility, which may decrease gastric distention and thus afferent stimulation.

SMALL INTESTINE. Most digestion and absorption activities occur in the small intestine (i.e., duodenum, jejunum, ileum). Motility of the small intestine is classified as either peristaltic (moving in one direction) or segmental (moving back and forth within an area). The primary purpose of segmentation is to promote the mixing of chyme with digestive enzymes and to allow greater exposure of chyme to the mucosa for digestion and absorption. However, such movement can also propel chyme in a caudal direction. Normal passage of chyme takes 3 to 5 hours from the pylorus to the ileocecal valve. Such movement in the small intestine is enhanced after meals.

Small intestinal motility is controlled by neural and hormonal inputs. Pathologic conditions, such as electrolyte imbalance (particularly hypokalemia) and pharmacologic agents can also influence small intestinal motility. A common condition associated with altered small intestinal motility is paralytic ileus, which is often associated with abdominal surgery. In this condition, manipulation of the intestinal tissue results in release of neurochemicals, which are thought to inhibit contraction of the intestine temporarily. This condition is most persistent in the left colon and is usually self-limiting (lasting until the third to fourth postoperative day); its resolution is evident by the presence of bowel sounds on auscultation.

The distal portion of the small intestine is separated from the large intestine by the ileocecal junction. This is an important anatomic sphincter, which can control the rate of movement from the small intestine to the large intestine and prevents movement of colonic contents back into the small intestine. Flora of the colon include bacteria, which, if allowed to move into the small intestine, can produce malabsorption and diarrhea. At the junction of the ileum and cecum there is a blind tube approximately the size of a little finger known as the vermiform appendix. This structure has no known purpose in humans; however, problems encountered with this structure include inflammation (appendicitis) and rupture.

TABLE 46–4. **Selected Clinical Conditions Leading to and Adverse Consequences of Nausea and Vomiting**

Common Conditions in Critically Ill Patients Associated With Nausea and Vomiting
Cholecystitis
Drug toxicity
Gastrointestinal obstruction
Hepatitis
Infection, including sepsis
Intracranial lesion
Increased intracranial pressure
Myocardial infarction, acute
Pancreatitis
Peritonitis
Selected Adverse Consequences
Acid–base imbalances
Aspiration pneumonia
Electrolyte imbalances
Esophageal rupture
Fluid depletion
Mallory-Weiss syndrome (nonperforating gastric mucosal tear at or near gastroesophageal junction)

LARGE INTESTINE. The colon is similar to the small intestine with regard to motor activity. Segmentation in an adult colon is called haustral formation. Haustral formation allows greater exposure of the colonic mucosa to the luminal contents. Multihaustral formation can propel the contents through the colon.

Expulsion of feces out of the rectal colon is under voluntary control. In the rectum there is an internal and an external sphincter. Under normal conditions, the internal sphincter, which is not voluntarily controlled, is contracted. The external sphincter is composed of striated muscle and is under voluntary control. Distention of the rectum results in an urge to defecate. As the pressure in the rectum increases, the internal and external sphincters relax, allowing the fecal material to pass.

CONSTIPATION. Constipation refers to delayed expulsion of the fecal contents. Because there is wide variation in what constitutes normal bowel function, constipation is usually denoted as a decrease in the individual's usual number of bowel movements or the passage of hard, dry stool or pellets. Constipation, which frequently is accompanied by abdominal discomfort and distention, is common in hospital patients, who experience marked changes in dietary and fluid intake and activity level.

DIARRHEA. Diarrhea refers to the passage of frequent liquid or semiliquid stools. Diarrhea is the result of increased fluid secretion or decreased fluid absorption in the small intestine or colon. Secretagogues such as bacterial endotoxins (e.g., cholera enterotoxin) stimulate colonic fluid and electrolyte secretion through cyclic adenosine monophosphate activation. The ingestion of lactose by lactase-deficient individuals results in an increase in fecal water loss due to increased secretion of fluid in the small intestine and decreased net absorption in the colon.

Diarrhea as a symptom accompanies a number of pathophysiologic conditions. In immunocompromised patients, whose immune systems are impaired as a result of exogenous immunosuppressive therapy or acquired immune deficiency disease, diarrhea may result from the presence of viruses such as cytomegalovirus. This virus is a herpes virus that is widely observed in people across all age ranges from newborns to adults. In healthy people, its presence does not create problems. Like other herpes viruses, it is a lifelong infection that is usually latent (Dieterich, 1987). However, when T-cell–mediated immunity decreases, as in the immunosuppressed patient, this virus is activated. Such a virus creates lesions related to acute and chronic inflammation throughout the length of the GI tract and liver, and the patient may experience symptoms of abdominal pain, diarrhea, hematemesis, distention, and even perforation.

Digestion

As noted earlier, the bulk of digestion and absorption occurs in the small intestine. However, some minor digestive processes occur in the upper GI tract. In the mouth, amylase, which is secreted into salivary secretions, is the only digestive enzyme present. Amylase begins the breakdown of starch. The enzyme is inactivated by the acidity of the stomach and thus does not contribute substantially to carbohydrate digestion. No digestion or absorption occurs in the esophagus. Table 46–5 lists the volume, content, and major regulators of secretions throughout the GI system.

STOMACH. In the stomach there are several secretions that contribute to digestion. Hydrochloric acid (HCl) is secreted by the parietal (oxyntic) cells, which are located primarily in the stomach body and fundus (Fig. 46–8). Under basal conditions, the intragastric pH is acidic (pH 2–4), and the rate of HCl secretion is approximately 2 to 3 mEq/hour. Stimulation of HCl secretion by a number of known stimulants can increase this rate 10-fold. Those factors known to stimulate HCl secretion include vagal stimulation, hormonal stimulation (e.g., gastrin), and chemical properties of the chyme. The antral hormone gastrin and the cholinergic neurotransmitter acetylcholine both directly stimulate the release of HCl by parietal cells. Diagnostic tests used to determine the ability of the stomach to secrete acid under "stimulated" conditions use pentagastrin, a synthetic form of the hormone gastrin. Because acetylcholine also stimulates release of gastrin, acetylcholine both directly and indirectly stimulates HCl secretion. Histamine, which is present throughout the GI tract, is also a stimulant of HCl secretion. Common drug therapies for peptic ulcer disease include histamine (H_2) receptor blockers (e.g., cimetidine, ranitidine) to decrease acid secretion, and omeprazole, a proton pump inhibitor which then blocks the secretion of HCl. There appears to be some age-related decrease in gastric acid secretion; however, this decrease is much greater in patients with chronic atrophic gastritis. When acid secretion is reduced, there is a decrease in iron absorption, often an important element for the trauma or critically ill patient.

The acid environment of the stomach promotes the conversion of pepsinogen, a proteolytic enzyme secreted by gastric chief cells, to pepsin. Pepsin begins the initial breakdown of proteins; however, it does not appear to be essential for normal protein breakdown and absorption.

A necessary protein secreted only by the stomach's parietal cells is intrinsic factor. Intrinsic factor binds to vitamin B_{12} and is essential for transport and absorption of this vitamin in the terminal ileum. Vitamin B_{12} is critical for formation of red blood cells; thus, surgical removal or atrophy of cells that secrete intrinsic factor can result in anemia. Similarly, resection of the terminal ileum, where absorption occurs, can also result in anemia.

In addition to HCl and pepsinogen, the stomach secretes fluid that is rich in electrolytes, including sodium and potassium. Loss of these fluids through vomiting or gastric suction places the individual at risk for fluid and electrolyte imbalances as well as acid–base disturbances.

Although not actively contributing to digestion,

TABLE 46–5. **Gastrointestinal Secretions**

Site	Volume (daily)	Content	Major Regulator
Oral cavity	1–2 liters	Mucus Water Electrolytes and amylase Immunoglobulins	Neural
Esophagus	300–800 mL	Mucus	Neural
Stomach	2 liters	Mucus Hydrochloric acid Water, electrolytes Intrinsic factor Pepsinogen	Neural Hormonal
Liver (bile)	500 mL–1 liter	Bile salts Water, electrolytes Bilirubin	Hormonal
Pancreas	1,200–1,800 mL	Water Electrolytes Enzymes	Hormonal Neural
Small intestine	3–4 liters	Water Electrolytes Mucus Brush border enzymes	Neural
Large intestine	Variable	Mucus	Neural

mucus is secreted by the surface cells located in the body and fundus of the stomach. This mucus coats the organ mucosa and is believed to contribute to the gastric mucosal barrier. This barrier protects the gastric mucosa from autodigestion by gastric secretions, HCl, and pepsin.

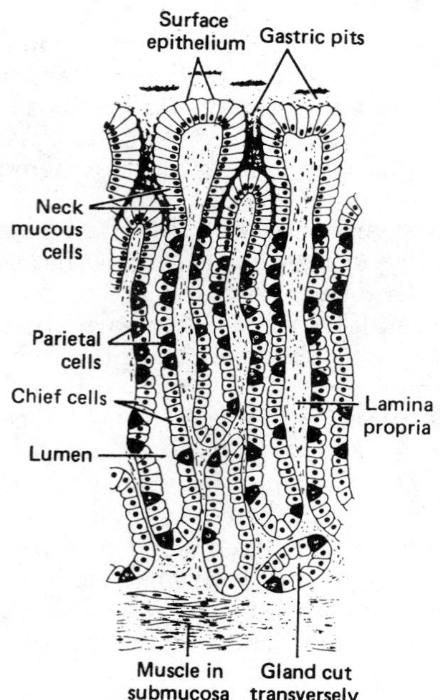

FIGURE 46–8. Diagram of glands in the mucosa of the body of the human stomach. (From Ganong, W. [1987]. *Review of medical physiology* [13th ed., p. 409]. Norwalk, CT: Appleton and Lange; adapted from Bell, G. H., Davidson, N., & Scarborough, G. [1965]. *Textbook of physiology and biochemistry* [6th ed.]. Edinburgh: Churchill-Livingstone.)

In a significant number of people, the bacteria *Helicobacter pylori* lives in the gastric mucus layer. This bacteria induces a chronic inflammatory response (chronic active gastritis) and can result in ulceration and, potentially, gastric neoplasm (Blaser, 1993). It is a commonly found organism. In a study of 404 female and 534 male army recruits (17–26 years of age) in whom serologic testing was performed, 26.3% tested positive (Smoak et al., 1994). Close person-to-person contact in childhood is an important determinant of seroprevalence of *H. pylori* in adulthood, suggesting that infection is transmitted directly (i.e., from person to person), and is commonly acquired in childhood (Webb et al., 1994). Diagnosis of *H. pylori* infection can be done by urease testing, biopsy, culture, and histology. Current medical regimens to eliminate the bacteria include bismuth, antibiotics, and antisecretory agents.

In addition to the parietal, chief, and neck mucous cells, endocrine cells are interspersed among the gastric epithelial cells. The most abundant of these are the gastrin–producing cells in the gastric antrum. Gastrin, a peptide hormone, is produced by specialized cells in the gastric and duodenal mucosa and is released by neural stimulation as well as by chemical properties of the diet and distention of the stomach wall. The stomach also contains enterochromaffin cells, which release serotonin.

SMALL INTESTINE. Digestion of foodstuffs occurs primarily in the small intestine. The anatomic arrangement of the small intestine facilitates the digestive and absorptive processes that occur there. The small intestine is lined with villi and microvilli, which greatly increase the surface area (Fig. 46–9).

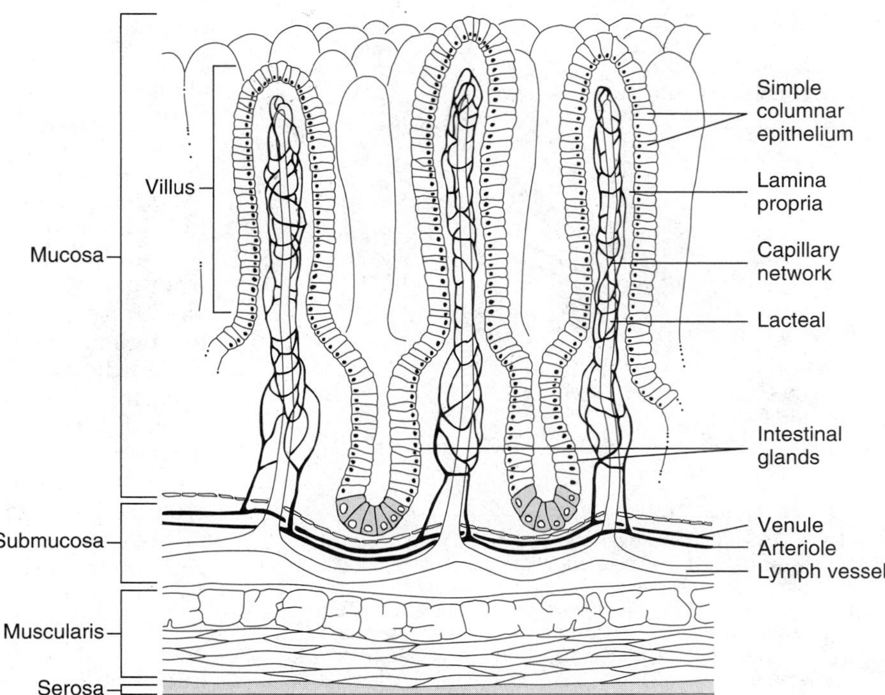

FIGURE 46–9. Small intestine. Enlarged aspect of several villa of the small intestine. (Figure from *Principles of anatomy and physiology* by G. J. Tortora and N. P. Anagnostokos. Copyright © 1981 by G. J. Tortora and N. P. Anagnostokos. Reprinted by permission of Harper & Row, Publishers, Inc.)

The functional unit of the small intestinal mucosal layer is the villus. Villi are composed of an inner core of lymph and capillary vessels surrounded by epithelial cells (i.e., enterocytes) and goblet cells. On each of the epithelial cells there are tiny projections known as microvilli. These tiny projections are referred to as the brush border and contain enzymes that are responsible for final breakdown of disaccharides and peptides. One characteristic of these epithelial cells is their relatively fast turnover rate. Cells migrate up from the crypts during a period of 5 to 7 days to replace cells that are sloughed off during the normal turnover process. This rapid turnover of epithelial cells makes intestinal epithelial cells particularly sensitive to regional radiation or systemic chemotherapy, which interrupts cell division. This feature allows rapid repair of the mucosa after injury.

The mucosa also contains goblet cells, which secrete mucus. The function of this mucus is not precisely known. However, it may play a protective role.

In the small intestine, digestion of proteins, fats, and carbohydrates begins with degradation of these food elements by pancreatic enzymes that are secreted into the duodenum. Additional enzymes located along the mucosal brush border complete the digestive processing of proteins and carbohydrates.

PROTEIN. As stated earlier, protein digestion to a very limited extent begins in the stomach with pepsin. However, most protein digestion occurs after chyme has entered the small intestine. Proteolytic enzymes are synthesized in the pancreas and are secreted in an inactive form into the duodenum through the pancreatic duct. This duct often joins with the common bile duct to empty through the greater duodenal papilla. Once in the small intestine, enterokinase, an enzyme secreted into the small intestinal lumen, cleaves these enzymes to their active forms. This is a protective process that prevents proteolytic and lipolytic enzymes from destroying or autodigesting pancreatic or surrounding tissues outside the GI tract.

Within the small intestinal lumen, pancreatic proteolytic enzymes break down proteins to peptides. Final digestion of peptide fragments to their constituent amino acid components is accomplished by proteolytic enzymes (i.e., peptidases) located on the microvilli brush border.

CARBOHYDRATE. Digestion of carbohydrates is minimally influenced by salivary amylase. Stomach HCl causes some hydrolysis of starches and simple sugars. In the small intestine, carbohydrates are exposed to pancreatic amylase, which breaks down starches to their constituent disaccharides. There is also an enteric amylase. However, this amylase does not contribute significantly to the breakdown of starches. Because carbohydrates are absorbed in the form of monosaccharides, further digestion is required. Along the brush border of the intestinal mucosa there are disaccharidases, which cleave disaccharides to their constituent monosaccharide forms. Problems with carbohydrate maldigestion can result in abdominal discomfort, diarrhea, and possible malabsorption when the disaccharide is ingested. Such problems usually are secondary to lack of or insufficient brush border disaccharidase. Normally, in adults approximately 7 to 8 liters of water are absorbed by the small intestine each day.

FAT. Compared with proteins and carbohydrates, digestion of fats is somewhat more complicated (Fig.

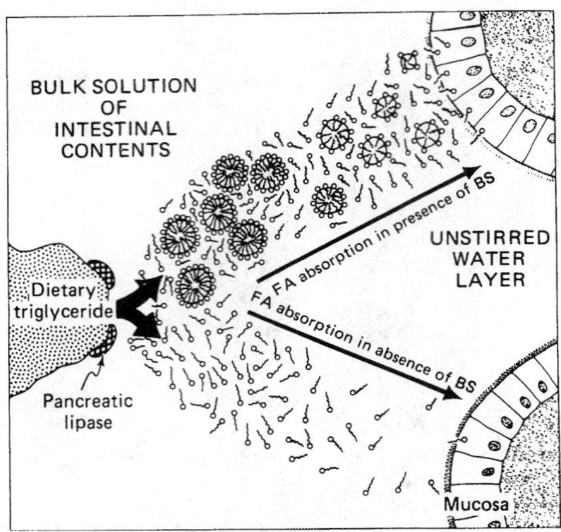

FIGURE 46–10. Lipid digestion and passage to intestinal mucosa. Fatty acids *(FA)* are liberated by the action of pancreatic lipase on dietary triglycerides and, in the presences of bile salts *(BS)*, form micelles (the circular structures), which diffuse through the unstirred water layer to the mucosal surface. (From Ganong, W. [1987]. *Review of medical physiology* [13th ed., p. 396]. Norwalk, CT: Appleton and Lange; Thomson, A. B. R. [1978]. Intestinal absorption of lipids: Influence of the unstirred water layer and bile acid micelle. In J. M. Dietschy, A. M. Gotto, Jr., & J. A. Ontko [Eds.], Disturbances in lipid and lipoprotein metabolism. American Physiological Society.)

46–10). The most common fats in the diet are neutral fats called triglycerides. Triglycerides are composed of glycerol and fatty acids. In the small intestine, dietary fats are emulsified by bile salts. Bile salts are synthesized in the liver, stored in the gallbladder, and secreted into the small intestine as the gallbladder contracts. The bile salts emulsify fat, allowing pancreatic lipase further to break down the fat molecules into monoglycerides and fatty acids. These breakdown products are surrounded by a water-soluble barrier (i.e., micelle) and transported to the absorptive surface. After fat products enter the epithelial cells, bile salts diffuse back into the lumen and either are reused for micelle formation or are reabsorbed in the ileum and returned to the liver.

The processes of digestion are completed within the small intestine. No digestion occurs in the colon.

Absorption

Absorption of dietary constituents occurs primarily in the small intestine. However, absorption of some substances such as ethanol and aspirin can occur in the stomach as well as in the small intestine.

As stated earlier, carbohydrates are absorbed in the form of monosaccharides, and proteins are absorbed in the form of amino acids. Multiple mechanisms, including active and passive transport and facilitated diffusion, contribute to absorption of nutrients. These substances then move into the blood supply. On the other hand, fats that are absorbed in the form of fatty acids and glycerol are reconstituted into triglycerides, cholesterol, and phospholipids to form what are known as chylomicrons. These chylomicrons are absorbed into the lymphatic system, and from there they enter the venous system. Figure 46–11 illustrates the expected absorptive locations for digested nutrients. In addition to nutrients, the small intestine also absorbs fluid and electrolytes arising from the diet or from gastric and intestinal secretions. Refer to Table 46–5 for expected adult daily fluid volumes secreted throughout the GI system.

No dietary absorption occurs in the colon. However, the colon is capable of absorbing certain drugs, as evidenced by the use of rectal suppositories. In addition, the large intestine is involved in the absorption of fluid and electrolytes. Of the 1,500 mL of fluid delivered to the large intestine each day, only 100 to 200 mL is excreted in the feces. However, this fluid and electrolyte absorptive function is not vital to life. Nonetheless, for individuals who have had part or all of the large bowel removed, fluid and electrolyte imbalances are a major concern, particularly during the initial period after surgery and during times of illness when there is reduced intake or increased output of fluids.

PHYSIOLOGIC ADAPTATION TO PATHOLOGY

The body is resourceful in adjusting to changes. Moore-Ede (1986) proposes that the body normally prepares itself for regularly recurring events, such as intermittent food intake, by predictive homeostasis. Body physiology, including such activities as cellular turnover in the gut, sectional motility, and gastric volumes and pH, changes over the course of a 24-hour period (Touitou & Haus, 1992). Knowledge of such intraindividual variations may assist in identifying times of patient vulnerability or resistance, and be one way to enhance care for an already compromised person placed in an alien environment. Surgical resection of parts of the GI tract can result in a number of problems, including diarrhea and malabsorption, leading to the ultimate outcome of malnutrition. The severity and duration of these problems are related to both the location of the tissue removed and the amount of tissue resected. An example of the former is surgical removal of the terminal ileum for a disease such as Crohn's disease (inflammatory bowel disease). Because of tissue loss in this area, which is necessary for bile salt and vitamin B_{12} absorption, the patient may have problems related to fat malabsorption and anemia. Resection or loss of large sections of the intestine decreases the amount of absorptive surface area available for nutrient absorption. However, after resection the tissue remaining usually adapts to compensate for this loss of tissue. Therefore, symptoms of malabsorp-

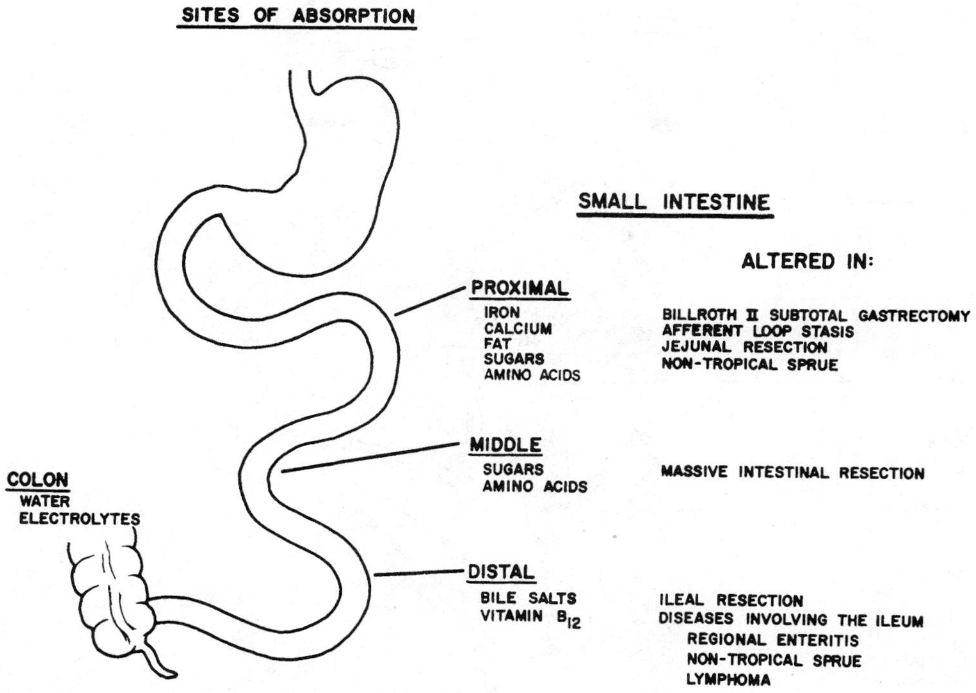

FIGURE 46–11. Sites of absorption of major nutrients across the small intestinal and colonic mucosa. (From Greenberger, N. [1989]. *Gastrointestinal disorders: A pathophysiologic approach* [4th ed., p. 132]. Chicago: Year Book Medical Publishers.)

tion are likely to decrease with time as adaptive changes occur in the remaining tissue.

Nutritional therapies such as total parenteral nutrition and tube feedings have also been associated with structural changes in the gut. Animal studies have demonstrated that colon length is reduced in response to parenteral feeding. Mucosal atrophy has been associated with both prolonged use of liquid diets and total parenteral nutrition. The impact of these structural changes on segmental function such as motility, digestion, and absorption is not known, however.

ACCESSORY GASTROINTESTINAL ORGANS

Liver

The liver is an important and essential organ that performs multiple and complex functions. In an adult the liver weighs approximately 1,500 g, making it the largest organ in the body. It is located primarily in the upper right quadrant of the abdomen and is divided into four lobes. These lobes are further subdivided into lobules. The liver has a rich blood supply that receives blood from both the hepatic artery and the portal vein, which drains the structures of the GI tract. Oxygen saturation of blood from the portal vein approaches 85%. This amount of oxygen is enough to meet about 30% to 35% of the oxygen requirements of the liver. Capillaries surrounding the hepatocytes are known as sinusoids. The sinusoids are lined with phagocytic cells known as Kupffer cells. In addition, the liver contains bile ducts called canaliculi that secret bile salts produced by the hepatocytes.

Multiple functions of the liver include (1) bile formation, (2) drug and hormone metabolism, (3) substrate metabolism, (4) protein synthesis including proteins important in blood coagulation, (5) detoxification of noxious substances, and (6) phagocytosis by means of the liver Kupffer cells. A detailed description of liver functions is found in Chapter 48.

Gallbladder

The gallbladder is a sac-like structure that lies beneath the right lobe of the liver (Fig. 46–12). The gallbladder holds approximately 30 mL of bile. Its primary function is to store and concentrate bile once it has been delivered from the liver. The gallbladder is connected to the duodenum via the common bile duct. Bile salts are delivered into the duodenum when nutrients are ingested. The flow of bile into the duodenum is controlled by contraction of the gallbladder and relaxation of the sphincter of Oddi, which is located at the junction of the common bile duct and the duodenum. The sphincter normally remains closed between meals and during fasting. Contraction of the gallbladder is mediated by hormonal and neural signals initiated by the presence of food.

The most common clinical problem associated with

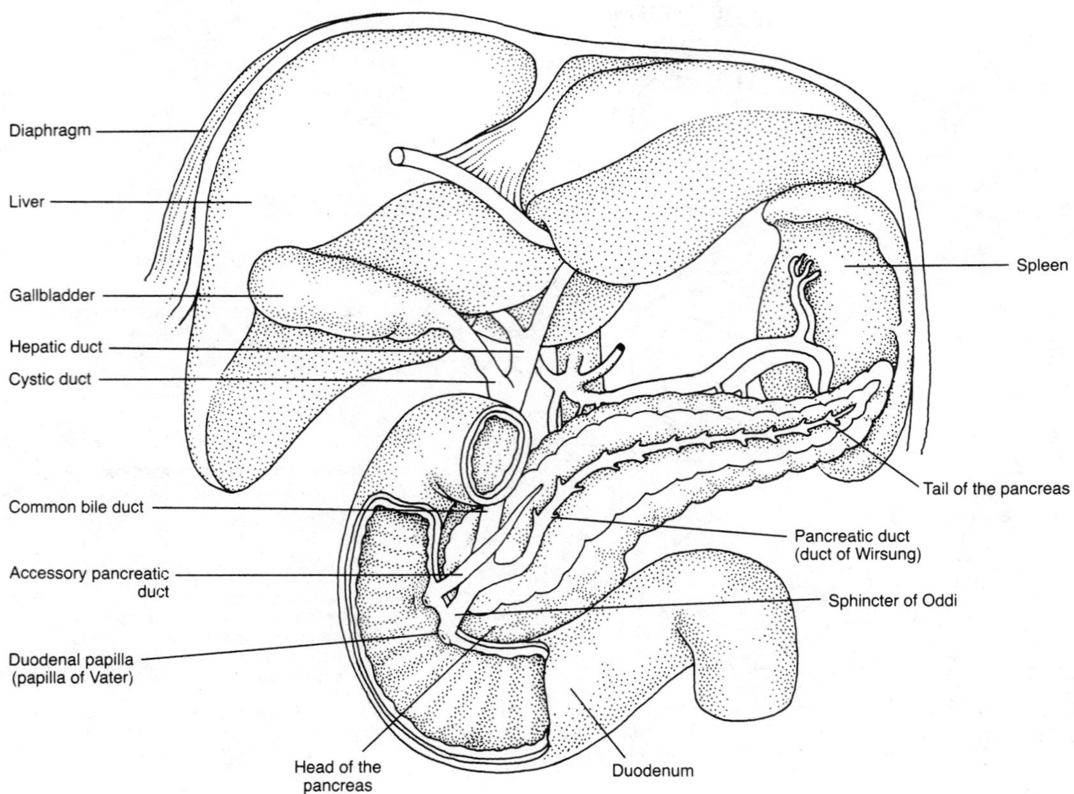

FIGURE 46–12. The gallbladder and its connections to the liver and intestine. (Adapted from Ignatavicius, D. D., & Bayne, M. V. [Eds.]. [1991]. *Medical–surgical nursing: A nursing process approach* [p. 1223]. Philadelphia: W. B. Saunders.)

the gallbladder is cholecystitis (gallbladder inflammation), which is frequently secondary to cholelithiasis (gallstones). Gallbladder stones are frequently composed of cholesterol and occur most commonly in middle-aged women. In addition to cholecystitis, gallstones can occlude the common bile duct and produce posthepatic jaundice or acute pancreatitis. In the patient with major trauma, surgery, or sepsis, cholecystitis can also occur, usually sometime after the initial injury. Although the etiology is unknown, it may be due to ischemia, bacterial invasion of the nonfunctioning gallbladder, or bile stasis.

Pancreas

The pancreas is a long, slender organ located behind the spleen and duodenum. It is anatomically divided into head, body, and tail (see Fig. 46–12). The pancreas has both endocrine and exocrine (e.g., production of digestive enzymes) functions. Hormones are produced in specialized cells (e.g., alpha, beta, and delta cells) located in what is known as the islets of Langerhans. These specialized cells comprise only about 1% of the total pancreatic cells. The beta cells produce insulin, alpha cells glucagon, and delta cells somatostatin (Taborsky, 1989). The hormones are secreted into the rich organ blood supply and influence multiple tissues. Digestive enzymes produced by the clusters of exocrine cells known as acini are secreted into a central duct that runs the length of the pancreas. This duct then often connects to the common bile duct before it enters the duodenum.

The digestive enzymes are secreted in a small volume of fluid. Cells that line the ducts actively secrete bicarbonate into the duct lumen, producing a physiologically basic solution. This secretion of alkaline fluid into the intestine acts to buffer the acidic chyme entering the duodenum. The acinar cells are innervated by the vagus nerve, and thus their activity is also influenced by neural input.

In response to acute illness and hypotension, pancreatic ischemia can occur. This ischemia is thought to contribute to the release of cardiotoxic factors (e.g., myocardial depressant factor), which can lead to further complications of the critical illness. In addition, pancreatic ischemia can result in acute pancreatitis.

REFERENCES

Blaser, M. J. (1993). *Helicobacter pylori:* Microbiology of a "slow" bacterial infection. *Trends in Microbiology, 1,* 255–260.

Dieterich, D. T. (1987). Cytomegalovirus: A new gastrointestinal pathogen in immunocompromised patients. *American Journal of Gastroenterology, 82,* 764–765.

Gonella, P. A., Helton, W. S., Robinson, M. K., & Wilmore, D. W. (1992). O-side chain of *Escherichia coli* endotoxin 0111:B4 is transported across the intestinal epithelium in the rat: Evidence for increased transport during total parenteral nutrition. *European Journal of Cell Biology, 59,* 224–227.

Goo, R. H., Moore, J. G., Greenberg, E., et al. (1987). Circadian variation in gastric emptying of meals in humans. *Gastroenterology, 93,* 515–518.

McGeer, A. J., Detsky, A. S., & O'Rourke, K. (1989). Parenteral nutrition in patients receiving cancer chemotherapy. *Annals of Internal Medicine, 110,* 734–736.

Moore, F. A., Feliciano, D. V., Andrassy, R. J., et al. (1992). Early enteral feeding, compared with parenteral, reduces septic complications. *Annals of Surgery, 216,* 172–183.

Moore-Ede, M. (1986). Physiology of the circadian timing system: Predictive versus reactive homeostasis. *American Journal of Physiology, 250,* R735–R752.

Murray, R. (1987). The effects of consuming carbohydrate–electrolyte beverages on gastric emptying and fluid absorption during and following exercise. *Sports Medicine, 4,* 322–351.

Roudebuch, R. L. (1994). Diabetic gastroparesis: What to do when gastric emptying is delayed. *Postgraduate Medicine, 95,* 195–204.

Smoak, B. L., Kelly, P. W., & Taylor, D. N. (1994). Seroprevalence of *Helicobacter pylori* infection in a cohort of U.S. Army recruits. *American Journal of Epidemiology, 139,* 513–519.

Taborsky, G. (1989). The endocrine pancreas: Control of secretions. In H. Patton, A. Fuchs, B. Hille, et al. (Eds.), *Textbook of physiology* (21st ed. Vol. 2, pp. 1522–1543). Philadelphia: W. B. Saunders.

Touitou, Y., & Haus, E. (Eds.). (1992). *Biologic rhythms in clinical and laboratory medicine.* New York: Springer-Verlag.

Webb, P. M., et al. (1994). Relation between infection with *Helicobacter pylori* and living conditions in childhood: Evidence for person to person transmission in early life. *British Medical Journal, 308,* 750–753.

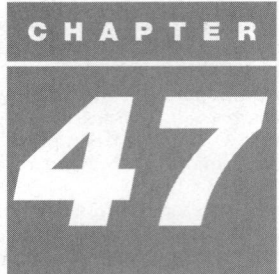

Nutrition in the Critically Ill

Melanie H. Shuster

Malnutrition has been shown to negatively influence patient outcomes. Dempsey and coworkers (1988) observed that the recognition and treatment of malnutrition can positively influence patient outcomes. Moore and colleagues (1989) prospectively studied previously well nourished people and found a reduction in septic complications in patients who were fed within 48 hours after major abdominal trauma. Because of these and other research findings, nutrition in the critical care setting has received increased attention. Nutrition and metabolism in the critically ill must be maximized to prevent organ failure, improve cellular and organ function, and ultimately improve patient outcome.

In the past, assessment of nutritional intervention was primarily subjective. Improvement in objective nutritional assessment parameters was not detectable for weeks to months after the nutritional therapy had been instituted. Clearly, this is not acceptable in the critical care area, where minute-to-minute assessment of the patient's response to therapy is required. Currently, safe and effective nutritional support can be delivered to patients in critical care areas because of advancements in physiologic monitoring and better understanding of how traditional nutritional markers change with critical illness.

Technological advances in enteral and parenteral feeding have also influenced the practice of nutritional support in critical care. Improvements in placement procedures, enteral and parenteral feeding devices, and nutritional products have permitted alimentation in patients who previously would not have been candidates for nutritional support. Critical care nurses must be aware of current nutritional practices to provide nutritional care most effectively to critically ill patients.

NUTRITION AND METABOLISM

The processes of digestion and absorption in the gastrointestinal (GI) tract begin the process of nourishing. The GI tract is responsible for changing food into cellular nutrients. After digestion the nutrients move through the GI mucosa into the venous and lymphatic systems. Nutrients are brought to the liver and then directed into various metabolic pathways. Hepatic energy production or storage or synthesis of proteins (e.g., clotting factors or enzymes) may be performed based on need. Eventually the nutrients are incorporated into cells and are used in various cellular metabolic pathways.

All cells of the body require various amounts of all nutrients to perform their specific functions. The basic nutrients are carbohydrates, fats, proteins, vitamins, minerals, and water. All cells require energy. In general, energy is provided by the macronutrients of carbohydrates and fats. Adipose tissue is the storage form of energy in humans, and may be readily available in critical illness. Protein is usually reserved for protein synthesis, repair, or replacement functions, but can be used for fuel or energy in the absence of carbohydrates or fats. Skeletal muscles and organs are usable sources of proteins in humans, but this process is not without harm.

Vitamins and minerals, including the trace elements, are micronutrients that are required to catalyze or complete various metabolic processes. Water is required to initiate, sustain, or complete metabolic processes. Although oxygen is not a nutrient, it is necessary for metabolic processes to occur without the accumulation of noxious byproducts from anaerobic metabolism. Lack of oxygen, even in the presence of all other nutrients, alters cellular function. Thus, cellular and systemic function is maintained when all nutrients and oxygen are provided in appropriate amounts.

Normal Metabolism

Normal metabolism includes several biochemical reactions in which one or more substances are converted to different products. The fundamental concepts of metabolism include transport, energy, regulation, and two types of reactions: anabolic and catabolic.

TRANSPORT

An intact GI tract is required to change food nutrients into a form that is usable by the cells. Through this process of digestion and transport, ingested nutrients are moved from the external environment to the internal environment. This movement is further facilitated by the cardiovascular and lymphatic systems. Digestion occurs primarily in the small intestine. However, carbohydrate digestion begins in the mouth with salivary amylase and is completed in the small intestine when carbohydrates are broken into their smallest components of glucose, fructose, and galactose. Fats are digested to fatty acids, triglycerides, and glycerol. Proteins are digested to amino acids and dipeptides. The digestion of fat and protein occurs in the presence of bile and pancreatic enzymes. Vitamins, minerals, and trace elements are also absorbed in the small intestine.

Absorption of completely digested nutrients occurs primarily at the brush border of the villi of the small intestine. Various methods of transport across the intestinal mucosa are used for different nutrients, including osmosis, passive diffusion, or active transport, which requires energy. After the absorption of these nutrients into the portal and lymphatic circulation, with subsequent delivery to the liver, other organ and cellular metabolic processes can ensue.

ENERGY

Energy is not created or destroyed. Because of this principle, energy must be transformed from ingested food into cellular energy, which is stored in the chemical bonds of adenosine triphosphate (ATP). ATP is formed from the oxidation of biologic fuels or other energy-yielding reactions of the metabolic pathways. Energy is then used by the body for the performance of work or is lost as heat. Only a small amount of energy is required to maintain body temperature. Energy consumption for the performance of bodily functions ranges from great, as with physical activity, to small, as in the circulation of blood or active transport of nutrients. In adults, when food energy is consumed at the level equal to bodily expenditure, no weight gain or loss occurs. However, if food energy intake exceeds expenditure, energy is stored in the body in the form of adipose tissue. Any form of food—carbohydrate, fat, or protein—in excess is converted by the body to adipose. Storage of glucose or amino acids does not occur. A small amount of glucose is converted to glycogen and stored in the liver and large muscles; the remainder is stored as fat.

REGULATION

Regulation of metabolic processes depends on the availability of enzymes, cofactors, and reactants. Enzymes are synthesized by the body, and, for the most part, vitamins are ingested via food intake. Food energy or the reactants are also ingested, but availability of these substances is influenced by several mechanisms. The digestive process influences the rate of absorption or formation of reactants, hemodynamic status influences the transport of the nutrients throughout the body, and neural and hormonal factors shift various reactants between body compartments. Furthermore, should nutrient intake be inadequate, the body compartments of fat and lean mass can serve as reactant sources.

REACTIONS

Anabolic and catabolic reactions are the two major components of metabolism. Anabolic reactions are those that build or synthesize new products, such as the formation of red and white blood cells or the growth of children. Catabolic reactions are those that break down substances to yield energy, such as the breakdown of fat during starvation. In critical illness, muscle mass is also catabolized to provide energy. Because of this, anabolism and catabolism of both energy and protein must be considered in the critically ill. Calorie or energy anabolism results in the formation of adipose. Calorie or energy catabolism will result in weight loss, and both fat and muscle may be lost. Protein or lean muscle mass loss is referred to as protein catabolism. Protein anabolism in the adult is regulated by insulin, insulin-like growth factor, and growth hormone (Fong & Pisters, 1994).

Catabolic reactions create energy, whereas anabolic processes use energy released from catabolism. Ideally, anabolism and catabolism occur at equal rates, and body compartments of fat, lean muscle mass, and extracellular water are maintained. This is referred to as a state of dynamic equilibrium: change takes place, but mass neither increases nor decreases.

Metabolism Associated With Critical Illness

Disease states and critical illness can influence energy expenditure and protein balance. Metabolic changes of critical illness occur in reaction to the physiologic or neuroendocrine response to stress, and have been described as occurring in two phases, ebb and flow (Table 47–1). The ebb phase usually lasts 12 to 24 hours. Physiologic changes are characterized by alterations in cardiovascular status related to increased autonomic activity and altered fluid status. Restoration of cardiovascular function and oxygen transport are often the goals of therapy during this phase. The flow phase can begin at 24 hours and lasts days to weeks depending on the patient's recovery. This phase is characterized by hypermetabolism and hypercatabolism.

Hypermetabolism is an increase in oxidative metabolism manifested as an increase in cardiac output, oxygen consumption, and metabolic rate due to increased cellular activity and temperature. The increase in energy expenditure increases fuel or energy need.

Hypercatabolism is the degree of muscle wasting measured by increased losses of urinary nitrogen. Additional sources of nitrogen loss in the critically ill include wound drainage, drainage from pleural effusions or ascites, and protein-losing enteropathies or nephropathies. The goals of therapy during this phase

TABLE 47–1. **Metabolic Response to Injury**

Physiologic Response		Ebb Phase	Flow Phase
System	**Physiologic Changes**		
Cardiovascular instability	Cardiac output	Decreased	Increased
Impaired O_2 transport	O_2 consumption	Decreased	Increased
	Lactate level	Increased	Normal
Endocrine response			
Altered circulating blood volume	ACTH released		Cortisol released
	ADH released		Sodium and water retention
	Blood sugar	Increased	Normal or slight increase
	Glucose production	Normal	Increased
	Insulin concentration	Decreased	Normal or increased
	Glucagon	Increased	Increased
Autonomic activity	Catecholamines	Increased	High normal or increased
	Free fatty acids	Increased	Normal or slight increase Flux increased
Temperature	Core temperature	Decreased	Increased

are to minimize the hypermetabolic and hypercatabolic effects of injury and provide nutrients without inducing complications.

Hypermetabolism and hypercatabolism are caused by the physiologic and biochemical alterations of the nervous and endocrine systems. The anterior pituitary releases adrenocorticotropic hormone, which stimulates the release of cortisol from the adrenal cortex, resulting in muscle catabolism. Antidiuretic hormone is released in response to hypovolemia, causing water reabsorption in the kidney, and aldosterone causes renal sodium retention. This increase in volume influences the cardiovascular response to stress. The autonomic nervous system releases catecholamines, which cause mobilization of lipid or fatty acids. Epinephrine and norepinephrine also cause hepatic glycogenolysis, which increases blood glucose. In addition, the pancreas initially decreases insulin production. This causes fatty acids and amino acids to be released from adipose and lean muscle to serve as products for gluconeogenesis, thereby contributing to hyperglycemia. With continued stress, insulin as well as blood glucose levels increase, suggesting insulin resistance. Both hepatic and pancreatic responses to stress result in hyperglycemia. Because of the stress response, alterations in carbohydrate, fat, and protein metabolism occur.

Critically ill patients catabolize lean mass for energy. Amino acids liberated from this catabolism will also be used to manufacture acute-phase reactants, or other critical proteins. However, endogenous proteins are inadequate because the essential amino acids are not available. Essential amino acids can be obtained only from exogenous sources of protein, such as proteins found in food, enteral feeding products, or the amino acids in PN. Rapid depletion of the critically ill patient's protein stores results from increased energy demand and limited protein synthesis attributed to the lack of essential amino acid ingestion. Even with protein administration, accretion of muscle mass does not occur in the critically ill (Schonheyder et al., 1954). Energy intake directly influences protein balance, in that energy prevents the utilization of protein as a fuel source (Paradis et al., 1979). It is also important to note that although weight gain occurs in the critically ill patient, this may not reflect repletion of lean body mass (Hill et al., 1979). This is not to say that benefit is not derived, but that evaluation of nutritional status in the critically ill patient requires different assessment parameters than those traditionally used (Jeejeebhoy, 1994).

Critically ill patients perform many energy-requiring anabolic activities (e.g., synthesis of enzymes). Energy is derived from glucose ingested, the breakdown of glycogen that is stored in liver (glycolysis) and muscles (glycogenolysis), the catabolism of fat stores (lipolysis), or the synthesis of glucose from amino acids (gluconeogenesis). The latter process requires energy before liberating energy, which is an inefficient means of energy production. The stressed, critically ill patient often reverts to this form of metabolism, requiring more energy to make energy—hypermetabolism. Sometimes this process cannot be altered. Calories and protein provided at levels equal to energy expenditure and nitrogen needs may curtail the protein-wasting effects of surgical stress, and may have application to the hypermetabolic effect of critical illness (Almond et al., 1989). Therefore, provision of nutrients may prevent or retard the catabolism of lean mass in the critically ill.

Providing excessive calories will not prevent these metabolic aberrations from occurring. Excessive calories can also result in an increase in body fat mass, an increase in the energy requirement to store unused energy as fat, and have no appreciable influence on the accretion of lean tissue (Almond et al., 1989). Research has shown that provision of adequate calories and protein may slow or prevent further nutritional demise, maintaining cellular stability, even though improvements in visceral proteins or anthropometric measurements are not observed (Jeejeebhoy, 1994). It is not clear if the provision of adequate calories or excessive and specific proteins to critically ill patients results in the restoration of lost muscle mass or improved organ function.

GOALS OF NUTRITIONAL THERAPY

The goals of nutritional therapy for the critically ill patient are to (1) correct obvious deficits, such as hypokalemia, hypophosphatemia, and so forth; (2) maintain energy needs by providing adequate calories and preventing overfeeding or underfeeding; (3) promote nitrogen equilibrium; and (4) prevent nutrition-related complications. All patients admitted to the critical care area require timely nutritional intervention. Critically ill patients are often intubated, which precludes oral nutrition. In patients with functional GI tracts, access must be accomplished. Although informed consent is required for invasive procedures, (e.g., gastrostomy), nasoenteric tube placement usually is within the realm of the general consent to treatment, and the patients' or their representative's consent is considered given. In the current medical–legal–ethical environment, with advance directives and living wills, placement of more invasive nutritional therapy devices (e.g., jejunostomy) may not fall within the delineated guidelines of advance directives. Most important, all therapies must be congruent. Providing vasoactive drugs, ventilatory support, and other forms of invasive therapy without consideration of nutritional therapy is questionable. The oversight of nutritional therapy can be rationalized by contrasting nutritional therapy to vasoactive therapy. Because of the emergent indications for therapy, and the subsequent fatal result if postponed, initiation of vasopressors for hypotension occurs rapidly. Conversely, in the case of nutrition, death does not result in minutes to hours if nutritional therapy is not provided, and delay in provision of nutrients can stretch to days or weeks. Initiation of nutritional therapy is based on the patient's medical condition, the presence of overnutrition or undernutrition, and the severity and anticipated length of illness. Ideally, nutritional therapy is initiated when the patient is stabilized and within 48 to 72 hours of admission to the critical care unit, with the absolute limit of 7 days (American Society for Parenteral and Enteral Nutrition [ASPEN], 1993). Controversy exists regarding this issue, and exactly when to begin invasive nutritional intervention is debatable (DeBiasse & Wilmore, 1994; Koretz, 1994).

Well nourished, critically ill patients who are hypermetabolic and hypercatabolic secondary to the poststress state require endogenous substrates. Moore and colleagues (1989) demonstrated improvements in patients who were fed within 48 hours of injury. In addition, obese patients with an abundance of body fat should not be overlooked and have nutrition withheld for a prolonged period. Malnourished patients require timely nutritional intervention. Although the provision of nutrition will not immediately reverse the malnutrition or replete body stores, the severity of malnutrition should not worsen during the time of hospitalization (Long, 1979). Even with the best efforts, this is not possible. These patients often become the chronic patients in the critical care unit, developing complications and becoming ventilator dependent. In the case of the chronic patient, the nutritional goals include repletion of body stores, in addition to the nutritional goals appropriate for the acute critically ill patient. When the patient is stable, the repletion of body mass can begin. Nitrogen balance studies, visceral proteins (albumin, prealbumin), and weight are nutritional markers for evaluating the effectiveness of nutritional therapy in the chronic patient in critical care.

Nutritional Assessment

Determining the nutritional needs of a patient to prevent, maintain, or improve the nutritional status requires a nutritional assessment. This assessment determines nutritional therapy in the critically ill, and guides modifications of the nutritional treatment plan. A comprehensive nutritional assessment is completed by the registered dietitian. Nurses and physicians, through physical assessment and diagnosis, further contribute to the nutritional assessment.

A nursing nutritional assessment, which includes observations for deficiencies in macronutrients and micronutrients, must be performed and documented. Vitamin deficiencies, especially of vitamins B and C, the water-soluble vitamins, may be present or develop during hospitalization (Table 47–2). Additional components of the nutritional assessment include: (1) evaluation of anthropometric measurements (e.g., weight, height, triceps skinfolds, and arm muscle circumference); (2) evaluation of visceral protein stores (e.g., serum albumin and prealbumin values); (3) total lymphocyte count, which reflects immune competence, although this may not be accurate in the critically ill secondary to increases in the white blood cell count; and (4) calculation of the patient's energy expenditure. Nurses are in an ideal position to monitor the weight, serum albumin or prealbumin, serum electrolytes, complete blood count, and physiologic responses (e.g., respiratory rate, heart rate, and physical strength) to evaluate the effectiveness of the nutritional regimen.

Serum albumin and weight may not be reliable markers of nutritional status. Serum albumin levels fluctuate with volume status. Therefore, a dehydrated patient may appear to have a normal albumin, and an overhydrated patient may appear to be hypoalbuminemic. Vascular permeability allows redistribution of albumin into the extracellular compartment from the intravascular space, decreasing serum values. Furthermore, albumin has an 18-day half-life, and it may not be synthesized in a critical illness because synthesis of other acute proteins (e.g., interleukin-1) takes priority.

TABLE 47–2. **Clinical Signs and Symptoms of Nutritional Deficiencies**

Area of Examination	Water/Fat-Soluble Vitamins	Protein/Calorie	Essential Fatty Acids	Minerals and Trace Elements
Neurologic	Absent vibratory sense in feet Decreased position sense Disorientation Confabulation (B_{12}) Hyporeflexia (thiamine) Weakness Paresthesia of legs (thiamine, pyridoxine, pantothenic acid, B_{12})			Confusion (magnesium, phosphorous) Flaccid paralysis (potassium) Irritability (potassium, calcium, magnesium) Convulsions (calcium) Lethargy (potassium, calcium, iron)
Eyes	Xerosis of conjunctivae Bitot's spots (A) Keratomalacia (riboflavin) Blepharitis (B complex, biotin) "Spectacle eye" (biotin) Pale conjunctivae (B_{12}) Angular palpebritis (riboflavin, niacin)			Pale conjunctivae (iron)
Tongue	Bald (niacin, B_{12}) Glossitis (B_6, riboflavin, folic acid) Magenta (riboflavin)	Edema		Glossitis (iron, zinc)
Lips	Cheilosis (riboflavin, B_6) Angular stomatitis (riboflavin)	Cheilosis		Angular stomatitis (iron)
Mouth	Spongy, bleeding gums (C)			
Hair		Lack of luster Easy pluckability Sparse	Alopecia	Decreased pigmentation (copper) Alopecia (zinc)
Face	Nasolabial seborrhea (riboflavin)			Seborrhea dermatitis (zinc)
Glands	Tachycardia (thiamine, B_{12})	Hepatomegaly Splenomegaly (protein)	Parotid enlargement (protein)	Thyroid enlargement (iodine) Tachycardia (iron)
Skin	Follicular hyperkeratosis (A) Petechiae (C) Purpura (C, K) Pellagrous dermatitis (niacin)	Subcutaneous fat loss	Scaly dermatitis	Dilated superficial veins Pallor superficial (copper)
Extremities	Painful calf muscles Weak thigh muscles (thiamine) Ends of long bones enlarged, with pain (C); without pain (D)	Temporal muscle wasting Intercostal muscle wasting Wasting calf muscles Edema		Weakness (potassium, magnesium)
Nails	Brittle Lined Ridged (Nonspecific)			Thin Brittle Spoon-shaped (iron)

Reprinted with permission from Shuster, M. H., & Mancino, J. M. (1994). Ensuring successful home tube feeding in the geriatric population. *Geriatric Nursing, 15,* 67–82.

For these reasons, albumin is an unreliable nutritional marker in the critically ill.

Prealbumin has a half-life of approximately 2 to 4 days and is responsive to short-term nutritional repletion (Tuten et al., 1985). Therefore, serum measurements of prealbumin can be used to guide nutritional interventions. Increases in weekly measurements of prealbumin imply nutritional improvement. Unfortunately, distribution, synthesis, and loss affect serum levels of prealbumin just as with albumin. Albumin follows prealbumin, and the serum albumin levels begin to increase after several weeks of increases in prealbumin have been noted.

The evaluation of energy expenditure in the criti-

TABLE 47–3. **Harris-Benedict Equation**

Basal energy expenditure (BEE) = Kcal per day

Male: BEE = 66 + (13.7 × weight) + (5 × height) − (6.8 × age)

Female: BEE = 665 + (9.6 × weight) + (1.7 × height) − (4.7 × age)

From Harris, J. A., & Benedict, F. G. (1919). *A biometric study of basal metabolism in man.* Publication 279. Washington, DC: Carnegie Institute of Washington.

cally ill can be accomplished by using indirect calorimetry or predictive equations. Indirect calorimetry, as measured with the metabolic cart, actually predicts the patient's energy requirements in kilocalories per day. The patient is connected to the metabolic cart, and during a steady state for 20 to 30 minutes, oxygen consumption and carbon dioxide production are measured, reflecting the metabolism of substrates. Various calculations are then applied to these values and the energy needed by the patient is reported as kilocalories per day. Repeat measurements validate energy needs.

Predictive equations such as the Harris-Benedict equation (1919) can also be used to estimate energy needs (Table 47–3). This formula uses height, weight, and age to estimate the basal energy needs of patients, and has been shown to closely approximate the measured energy expenditure (Hunter et al., 1988). Weight can greatly influence the energy prediction of the Harris-Benedict equation (McClave & Snider, 1992). Daily weights are a routine nursing measure in the critical care setting, and are very effective in determining volume status. Weights should not be used as a nutritional marker in the critically ill, except perhaps in the chronic, stable, ventilator-dependent patient. Rapid changes related to fluid resuscitation and edema may result in a false weight being used in calculating a patient's energy requirements. Overestimation or underestimation of the patient's energy needs will result. Usual weight or ideal body weight may be used in the equation if the patient is edematous or obese. Ideal body weight can be determined based on height (Table 47–4).

Body mass index normalizes for height and is used to categorize weight status: under, over, or normal:

$$\text{Body mass index} = \frac{\text{Body weight (kg)}}{(\text{height})^2\ (\text{m})}$$

A normal body mass index is 20 to 25. (Determination of body mass index has primarily been used to predict the risk of disease. Although a valid assessment tool in stable patients, body mass index has not been used in the critically ill.) The obese, critically ill patient presents a unique challenge. Energy needs must be met to prevent protein catabolism, but overfeeding must be avoided. Consultation with the registered dietitian is warranted to prevent overfeeding or underfeeding in the critically ill patient.

Blood samples from pulmonary artery and arterial catheters can be used to measure oxygen utilization and also to determine energy expenditure in the critically ill (Williams & Fuenning, 1991). The following equation is used (Schlichtig & Ayres, 1988):

$$\dot{V}O_2\ (\text{mL/min}) = \text{Energy expenditure (kcal/day)}$$

where $\dot{V}O_2$ is oxygen consumption per unit time (mL/min). Circulatory indirect calorimetry has also been shown to correlate with metabolic cart measurements.

Nutritional assessment leads to the diagnosis of malnutrition. Malnutrition in adults can be classified according to type: marasmus (calorie or starvation), protein (hypoalbuminemic or stress related), and mixed. Protein–calorie (mixed) is more commonly observed in hospitalized patients (Table 47–5). Patients should be considered malnourished or at risk for development of malnutrition if intake has been inadequate for more than 7 days or if weight loss greater than 10% of preillness weight has occurred (ASPEN, 1993). The medical treatment plan is influenced by malnutrition, because some diseases increase energy and protein needs, while others do not.

Disease states can influence energy expenditure.

TABLE 47–4. **Calculation of Weight for Height (Hamwi Equation)**

Males: 106 pounds for the first 5 feet and 6 pounds for each inch thereafter ±10%

Example: 5′8″ = 106 + 48 = 154 lbs

Females: 100 pounds for the first 5 feet and 5 pounds for each inch thereafter ±10%

Example: 5′4″ = 100 + 20 = 120 lbs

From Lang, C. E., & Schulte, C. V. (1987). The adult patient in nutritional support. In C. E. Lang (Ed.), *Nutritional support in critical care.* Rockville, MD: Aspen Publishers.

TABLE 47–5. **Characteristics of Malnutrition**

	Types of Malnutrition		
Weight (% UBW)	***Hypoalbuminemic (Stress) >80***	***Marasmus (Starvation) <80***	***Combined <80***
Albumin (mg/dL)	<3.5	>3.5	3 or more of visceral proteins less than normal
Transferrin (mg/dL)	<220	>220	
TLC (cells/mm³)	<1,500	<1,500	
Prealbumin (mg/dL)	<17	>17	

Adapted with permission from McClave, S. A., Mitoray, T. E., Thielmeier, K. A., & Greenburg, R. A. (1992). Differentiating subtypes (hypoalbuminemic vs. marasmic) of protein–calorie malnutrition: Incidence and clinical significance in a university hospital setting. *JPEN. 16,* 337–342.

Hypermetabolism requires additional energy, whereas hypometabolism results in a decreased energy need. Hypercatabolism can occur if energy intake is inadequate (i.e., hypermetabolism without the provision of adequate exogenous energy). During hypercatabolism, the rate of protein breakdown exceeds synthesis, with the end result of a negative nitrogen balance. Body protein is broken down and used for energy when energy intake is not adequate; protein loss can be decreased when adequate calories are provided (Shaw et al., 1987).

Physiologic mechanisms that can result in hypermetabolism include (1) sympathetic nervous system stimulation with release of catecholamines, (2) increases in oxygen transport (delivery and extraction) to peripheral tissue, (3) increase in thyroid hormones, (4) increase in temperature, and (5) increase in activity. Decreases in the preceding would result in hypometabolism. Chronic renal failure, chronic obstructive pulmonary disease, and cancer are some of the medical conditions that influence the energy and protein needs of patients. Critical illness in addition to a chronic condition only heightens the effect.

PROVISION OF NUTRITION

Once the patient's energy and protein needs are established, the method of nutritional therapy can be decided. Artificial invasive nutritional support is often indicated in the critically ill patient. The decision to enterally or parenterally nourish patients is determined by gut function, disease state, and ability to access the GI or vascular system. Decisions regarding the type and volume of nutritional products are governed by the energy needs, estimated from equations or the metabolic cart, protein needs, estimated by weight and nitrogen balance, and concomitant disease conditions. General guidelines for critically ill patients approach 2,000 kcal and 1 g of protein per kilogram per day. However, small or thin adults may need less and larger adults may need more energy. Approximately 100 to 150 g of carbohydrate per day is necessary for basal function (Langkamp-Henken et al., 1992). Protein may also need to be increased to 2 g/kg based on the patient's protein need and tolerance. A 24-hour urine collection to evaluate nitrogen balance can be used to determine protein and energy needs. Increases in calories can increase the retention of protein or nitrogen (Schlichtig & Ayres, 1988). Therefore, periodic reassessment is required to ensure nutritional success.

The recommended distribution of energy for the critically ill patient closely resembles the recommendations of a prudent diet. Therefore, carbohydrates should provide approximately 50% to 60% of the total calories, with less than 30% of the total calories from fat. Protein should provide 10% to 20% of the daily calories (Davis & Sherer, 1994).

Enteral or tube feeding products require digestion, which consumes approximately 10% of the ingested energy. This is referred to as the thermogenic effect of food. In contrast, PN is infused into the venous system and does not require digestion. Therefore, caloric intake via total parenteral nutrition (TPN) equals measured energy expenditure. Ideally, adequate calories are provided in addition to amino acids to prevent the use of protein as an energy source and to provide amino acids for protein synthesis (Shaw et al., 1987). Fifty to 60% of calories in TPN are from carbohydrates and less than 30% are from fat, and 20% are from protein. A minimum of 1,000 fat calories per week is necessary to prevent essential fatty acid deficiency. Excessive fat calories are not recommended because this may lead to increased risk of infection (Seidner et al., 1989).

A nitrogen balance study that requires a 24-hour urine collection may help determine the relationship between calories and protein. Positive nitrogen balance implies that more protein or nitrogen has been taken in compared to what has been excreted or lost. Negative nitrogen balance suggests that more protein or nitrogen has been lost compared to what has been taken in. A positive nitrogen balance of 4 to 6 is desired, but this may not be possible in critically ill patients (Pitkänen et al., 1991). Larsson and coworkers (1990) found that even though positive nitrogen balance might be achieved, the breakdown of lean tissue may not be reversed. This finding suggests that ingested nitrogen is not incorporated into lean body mass.

The type of nutritional support given to a critically ill patient is influenced by the medical diagnosis, treatment, and condition of the patient. The more critical the illness, the greater the metabolic aberrations. Because nutritional regimens improve patient outcomes, it is important that nursing responsibilities include the administration and monitoring of enteral nutritional and PN therapies to ensure nutritional success.

Enteral Nutrition

Enteral nutrition in critical care has become the preferred method of feeding. Oral nutrition is the best option; however, for many critically ill patients this is not possible. Therefore, artificial, invasive enteral nutrition support is considered when the gut is functional and the patient cannot eat adequately. Table 47–6 summarizes indications for enteral feeding in the critically ill. Nasoenteral feeding tubes are most frequently used to access the gut when oral nutrition is not possible; these include nasogastric, nasoduodenal, and nasojejunal tubes. These are usually temporary interventions. More permanent devices include gastrostomy and jejunostomy tubes, which can be placed percutaneously or openly during surgery. Gastrostomy and jejunostomy tubes can be temporary, or they can be permanent, as in the case of a patient with a progressive upper GI obstruction that is not resectable.

SELECTION OF THE ENTERAL FEEDING PRODUCT

Commercial nutritional products are readily available. Enteral formulas are manufactured from various foods

TABLE 47–6. **Indications for Enteral Feeding in the Critically Ill**

Indications

Patients who are or will become malnourished with:
- Functional gastrointestinal tract
- Inability to ingest nutrients safely due to:
  - Altered level of consciousness
  - Endotracheal intubation
  - Neurologic disorders with dysphagia (CVA)
  - Trauma
  - Dysphagia related to mechanical obstruction (e.g., head and neck tumors)
  - Aspiration

Relative Contraindications*

- Pancreatic dysfunction
- Inability to gain access to the GI tract (e.g., tumors of the stomach, liver, and pancreas contributing to gastric outlet obstruction)
- Obstruction of the GI tract (e.g., tumors involving the small and large bowel and the peritoneum)
- Impaired absorption of nutrients, radiation enteritis, ulcerative colitis, and inflammatory bowel disease

*Parenteral nutrition may be indicated in these circumstances.

Abbreviations: CVA, cerebrovascular accident; GI, gastrointestinal.

and chemicals, and have reached a high degree of sophistication to meet the various nutrient needs of specific patient populations. The products vary as to the amounts and types of each nutrient. Selection of the appropriate product for each patient is an essential part of the nutritional care plan. Enteral products must meet the person's nutritional requirements and be well tolerated during initiation and throughout the course of therapy. Nurses are encouraged to consult with the dietitian and the physician to optimize the patient's nutrition while limiting the side effects or complications.

Enteral feeding products can be classified in a variety of ways. Critically ill patients usually tolerate standard "polymeric" formulas. In general, all products (e.g., Isosource, Sandoz Nutrition, Minneapolis, MN; Ensure Plus, Ross Laboratories, Columbus, OH; Isocal HCN, Mead-Johnson, Evansville, IN) contain carbohydrates, fats, proteins, vitamins, minerals (including trace elements), and water, and require digestion. These products are designed to meet average nutritional needs. Complete or polymeric formulas can be delivered through gastric or proximal small bowel feeding tubes. Polymeric formulas are also available in specific caloric densities (1.0, 1.3, 1.5, or 2.0 calories/mL). The primary difference between some of these products lies only in the percentage of water they contain.

Food sources of the essential amino acids are necessary daily for the body's synthesis of proteins. Amino acids are found within the protein of foods or enteral nutrition products. Most enteral products have complete or intact proteins constructed from soy or milk protein sources. Critically ill patients require 0.8 to 1.0 g of protein per kilogram of body weight per day, but may need as much as 2 g/kg/day (Larsson et al., 1990). People who are malnourished may require 1.5 to 2.0 g of protein per kilogram per day. Evidence suggests adequate calories and protein must be delivered together for repletion to take place (Schlichtig & Ayres, 1988). Formulas can be compared as to which delivers the appropriate amount of calories and protein with respect to the patient's needs.

After protein requirements are met and carbohydrate needs are calculated, the remaining calories can be adjusted so that approximately 30% of the total calories are provided from fat. In enteral formulas, fat is most often supplied from long-chain fatty acids, such as corn, safflower, sunflower, or soy oil, which are precursors for linolenic acid, the essential fatty acid. Standard commercial formulas contain approximately 30% of calories from fat, which meets current recommendations for a prudent cardiovascular diet.

Vitamin and mineral content of formulas varies. Most formulas provide 100% of the Recommended Daily Allowance (RDA), but the amount that provides this varies between products. Micronutrient supplements may need to be added if the volume of tube feeding formula does not supply them in adequate amounts. The registered dietitian should make recommendations as to the nutritional adequacy of the prescribed enteral feeding and the need for vitamin and mineral supplementation. The RDA is used as a guide to provide adequate nutrients.

Attention should also be given to the trace elements. Enteral formulas contain trace elements, such as chromium, molybdenum, and selenium, but in varying amounts. Critically ill, tube-fed patients are at risk for trace element deficiency. Unfortunately, there are inadequate data available to make standard recommendations regarding intensive care unit patients and supplementation of trace elements.

Water is one of the essential nutrients, and adequate supply is vital for normal hydration status. Fluid requirements for critically ill patients without cardiac, pulmonary, hepatic, or renal disease are approximately 2,500 to 3,000 mL/day, or 1 mL/Kcal (Davis & Sherer, 1994; Lang & Schulte, 1987).

Most commercial tube feeding products contain approximately 75% water. The amount of additional fluids necessary to meet daily fluid requirements varies with each patient. Water that meets physiologic requirements, in addition to that supplied by the feeding, can include fluid used to flush the feeding tube, water given through the day as water boluses, liquids given with medications, and liquid oral intake. In the critically ill patient, this is further complicated by the infusion of multiple intravenous fluids. Patients may require a more calorically dense formulation to prevent overhydration.

There are numerous specialized enteral products available; these can be reviewed according to modifications in protein, fat, or carbohydrate.

Protein can be altered by the amount or type of amino acid. Patients with increased protein needs can use standard high-protein formulas. Essential and branch-chain amino acid formulas for renal and liver disease are available. These formulas also vary as to whether they are nutritionally complete, and therefore may need specific nutrient supplementation. Patients can also be fed with elemental (predigested) formulas. Patients with feeding tubes placed in the distal small bowel or those who have altered digestive function (pancreatic insufficiency) may benefit from this type of formula.

The type or amount of carbohydrates contained within the product also can be altered. Most products contain polysaccharides from grain sources, and most are lactose free. Another carbohydrate alteration is the inclusion of dietary fiber in enteral formulas. Soluble fiber can help to stabilize blood glucose levels, whereas insoluble fiber aids in bowel function by treating and preventing both diarrhea and constipation. Before using fiber formulas, their influence on bowel function, fluid needs, and interactions with medications should be considered (Kohn & Keithly, 1982; Raymond & Farjood, 1993). The amount and type of fiber optimal for critically ill, tube-fed patients have not been defined. When a fiber product is selected for a patient, it should be added gradually, and it is crucial that adequate fluid be provided. The patient's response to the fiber formula can vary, and adjustment of the formula or fluid regimen may be indicated. Of particular concern in the critically ill is the use of narcotics, presence of electrolyte imbalances, and immobility, all of which have an impact on gut motility. Fiber formulas without adequate fluid could cause further problems.

Many critically ill patients have preexisting diabetes mellitus, or may contract diabetes mellitus secondary to the stress of critical illness. Alteration of their carbohydrate intake for blood glucose control may be indicated. Diabetic patients placed on tube feeding demand more rigorous management (Orr, 1992; Pitts et al., 1993). The goals of therapy are to maintain nutritional status and blood glucose levels within an acceptable range of 150 to 200 mg/dL. These goals are accomplished by manipulation of tube feeding products and insulin. Tube feedings are begun at a low rate of infusion, and blood sugars are monitored every 2 hours, with adjustment of insulin. Peters and Davidson (1992) suggested total carbohydrate is more influential on postprandial blood glucose than the amount of simple carbohydrate (sucrose or corn syrup). Therefore, although formulas without simple carbohydrates may be beneficial, the primary objective is to achieve tube feeding tolerance, maintenance of nutritional status, and blood glucose stability. Standard polymeric formulas may be appropriate to begin tube feeding. Careful monitoring of blood glucose, nutrient intake, and insulin is required to ensure adequate nutrient intake and blood glucose control. Blood glucose control and insulin requirements should be established prior to increasing the rate of tube feeding administration to prevent hyperglycemia. Once this ratio is established, both insulin and tube feeding are advanced appropriately. If hyperglycemia persists, an enteral feeding product that contains soluble fiber or an intermittent administration schedule may be helpful in providing nutrition and gaining control of blood sugars (Phillips, 1987; Vinik & Jenkins, 1988).

In contrast to alterations in type of carbohydrate, there are products with decreased amounts of carbohydrate relative to fat. This mix of nutrients has been suggested to decrease carbon dioxide production (Angelillo et al., 1985), which is assumed to decrease the work of breathing and facilitate the weaning process in ventilation-dependent patients. However, patient intolerance of a higher-fat feeding, with the associated complications of delayed gastric emptying or diarrhea, needs to be considered when using these products.

SELECTION OF THE FEEDING DEVICE

The easiest and most common method of providing nutrients to the GI tract is via nasoenteric feeding tubes. These tubes are usually small bore (8–12 Fr), are made of soft, pliable plastic materials that increase patient comfort, come in various lengths that are capable of reaching the small bowel, and may be weighted, which may or may not facilitate placement into the small bowel or maintain position (Lord et al., 1993; Rees et al., 1988). Table 47–7 summarizes the various feeding devices. Clinicians must be aware of the advantages and disadvantages of the various types of feeding tubes.

NASOENTERIC TUBES. Placement of feeding tubes into the stomach or the small bowel can be done at the bedside or in a special procedures room with fluoroscopic or endoscopic guidance. Verification of placement of the initial feeding tube traditionally has been done radiographically. However, recent nursing research by Metheny and colleagues (1993) has shown that gastric aspirate pH can verify placement. Gastric placement was confirmed with pH readings between 0.0 and 6.0, and intestinal placement was found to provide readings greater than 6.0. Respiratory tract aspirates were found to have a pH greater than 6.0. These preliminary findings suggest that pH readings may be able to distinguish gastric from pulmonary or small bowel intubation. However, administration of acid inhibitors may cause the pH value to rise, causing problems with intestinal tubes because the intestinal pH is expected to be greater than 6.0. Using the color of the aspirate to further verify placement may be useful, because gastric contents are clear to white mucus, and intestinal contents are green and yellow from bile (Table 47–8). Bile can reflux into the stomach, altering the pH as well as the color of the aspirate. Gastric pH and observation of intestinal aspirates can be used to determine if the tube has been malpositioned. Abdominal radiography remains the standard to verify placement and should be used when the position of the feeding tube is questioned.

Small bowel placement can be facilitated by measures such as body positioning, using unweighted feeding tubes, or administering metoclopramide hydrochloride. Small bowel placement using air insuf-

TABLE 47–7. **Enteral Feeding Devices**

Enteral Access	Tube Size, Length	Indications	Advantages	Disadvantages
Nasogastric				
Small-bore feeding tube	8 to 12 Fr 17 to 36 inches	Functional stomach Upper GI tract obstruction Dysphagia to solids Not at risk for aspiration	Placed at the bedside Low morbidity Easily inserted	Patient discomfort Potential for aspiration
Nasoenteric				
Nasoduodenal Nasojejunal	18 to 14 Fr 36 to 45 inches	Gastric atony Risk of aspiration	May decrease the risk for aspiration of tube feeding Continued use of the GI tract	Patient discomfort More difficult placement Easily malpositioned
Combination tubes	18 Fr Gastric port 9 Fr Jejunal feeding port 16 to 30 Fr Gastric port 9 Fr Jejunal feeding port	High risk for pulmonary aspiration of gastric contents Functional small bowel	May decrease the risk for aspiration of tube feeding Continued use of the GI tract	Increased cost for tube and skilled professional needed to place the tube Easily malpositioned
Combination tubes				
Gastric decompression	20 to 28 Fr	Long-term feeding Dysfunctional stomach	Can decompress a dysfunctional stomach and prevent regurgitation of gastric contents while feeding the small intestine	Requires skilled professional to place the tube Expensive process Jejunal feeding
		Functional small bowel		Can be dislodged from original position
		Short term Postoperative care	Use of GI tract Plastic less durable	Placed during surgery
Gastrostomy				
Surgical	14 to 30 Fr	Unable endoscopically to place PEG GI surgery	Permanent gastric access	Difficult removal General anesthesia Invasive procedure
Foley catheter	14 to 30 Fr	Not indicated but frequently used	Easily removed	Tube migration Easily obstructed Local stoma site complications
Percutaneous	14 to 22 Fr	Long-term tube feeding	Traction removal Body image Placement without general anesthesia	Invasive procedure
Gastrostomy replacement tubes	14 to 22 Fr*	Original gastrostomy in need of changing Long-term tube feeding in nonambulatory patients	External bumper to prevent tube migration More durable plastic for longer tube life	Open-end design results in less tube obstruction
Low-profile gastrostomy device	18 to 24 Fr	Long-term tube feeding in ambulatory patients Disoriented patients who pull at the gastrostomy tube	Increased mobility Decreased cost over time due to device longevity Decreased nursing time compared to replacement tube change	Requires skilled professional for placement Increased trauma to patient compared to replacement tube
				Increased cost compared to gastrostomy tube change Requires second procedure after gastrostomy tube placement
			Device placed at the time of initial gastrostomy, no need for second procedure	With weight gain device may impact in abdominal wall
Jejunostomy				
Temporary	11 gauge (5 Fr) Needle Catheter	Short-term enteral nutrition	Continued use of the GI tract	Surgical placement Easily obstructed Costly elemental feeding products
	14 Fr Jejunostomy	Usually ≤2 weeks	Silicone plastic	

TABLE 47–7. **Enteral Feeding Devices** *Continued*

Enteral Access	Tube Size, Length	Indications	Advantages	Disadvantages
Permanent	14 to 18 Fr Witzel	Long-term jejunal feeding	Use of GI tract Easily replaced when fistula tract is formed Larger bore Location is proximal jejunum, therefore does not require elemental products	Requires continuous or slow intermittent tube feeding administration due to location

*Internal balloon size can vary from 5 to 30 mL.

Abbreviations: GI, gastrointestinal; PEG, percutaneous endoscopic gastrostomy.

Adapted with permission from Shuster, M. H., & Mancino, J. M. (1994). Ensuring successful home tube feeding in the geriatric population. *Geriatric Nursing, 15,* 67–82.

flation and auscultating the movement across the abdomen while advancing the tube has been shown to be 85% effective (Ugo et al., 1992). Should an unweighted tube be used, it is recommended that the length be greater than 36 inches (85 cm) to maintain position in the small bowel.

Care of the feeding tube includes maintaining the feeding schedule (see Table 47–9) and the patency of the feeding tube. Patency can best be ensured by flushing the tube with water or fluids before and after medication administration, and whenever tube feeding is interrupted or stopped for any length of time. Feeding tubes do not need to be changed routinely. However, if the tube begins to malfunction, a tube change may be necessary.

GASTRIC TUBES. When enteral feeding is expected to continue for more than 3 months, a permanent feeding tube may be placed. Gastric tubes before the 1970s were placed surgically and often carried a high mortality rate. Gauderer and colleagues (1980) dramatically changed gastrostomy tube placement with the development of the percutaneous endoscopic gastrostomy (PEG) procedure. These tubes can be placed using endoscopy and local anesthesia with conscious sedation, thereby decreasing the associated risks of general anesthesia.

Initial PEG tubes can last several months to years, depending on the material, care of the tube, and the feeding schedule. Many PEG tubes can be removed with traction and do not require endoscopic removal. This decreases cost because a repeat endoscopy is avoided, and also decreases the inherent risk to the patient by eliminating an invasive procedure. However, should a traction-removal PEG tube malfunction and the internal bumper be retained, endoscopic retrieval is suggested to prevent the complications associated with intestinal obstruction (Mutabagani et al., 1994). After removal of PEG tubes, replacement with more patient-convenient and comfortable devices, such as a PEG replacement tube or a low-profile gastrostomy device, may be undertaken (see Table 47–7). This can be performed after a well healed and matured tract has developed, approximately 4 to 6 weeks after PEG placement (Gauderer & Stellato, 1986).

A plethora of gastrostomy feeding devices exists (see Table 47–7). Appropriate tube selection for each patient minimizes postoperative complications. Malecot, de Pezzer, or Foley catheters are usually placed at surgery, and are poor tubes. These tubes are often large, made of latex rubber, lack an external bolster, and cannot be easily and securely stabilized. This contributes to stoma site complications, particularly leaking and development of granulation tissue. These catheters can also migrate into the GI tract, causing gastric outlet obstruction, which can lead to nausea, vomiting, or increased residual volumes (Fig. 47–1). Furthermore, Foley catheters may obstruct more easily than Malecot gastrostomy tubes or gastrostomy replacement tubes because they have side-hole exit ports instead of an open end.

The Janeway is another type of surgical gastrostomy, and may be performed on patients who require long-term tube feeding. This is a continent stoma and does not require a feeding tube or other feeding device to be placed in the fistula tract to maintain patency. The Janeway gastrostomy requires intubation of the os for each feeding, is permanent, and will not close.

TABLE 47–8. **Normal Aspirates of Intestinal Tubes**

Location	pH	Color	Aspirate
Esophagus	6.0–7.0	Clear	Saliva
Stomach	1.0–3.5	Clear	Hydrochloric acid Water
		White	Mucus
Duodenum	7.8–8.3	Green Yellow	Bile
			Pancreatic enzymes Sodium bicarbonate
Jejunum	≥8.0	Green Yellow	Bile
			Pancreatic enzymes Sodium bicarbonate
Lung	>6.0	Clear White	Sputum

Should gastrostomy feedings be discontinued, a surgical procedure is required to close the gastrostomy.

After removal of the initial PEG or surgical gastrostomy, due to dysfunction or accidental removal, a replacement gastrostomy tube may be placed to continue gastrostomy tube feedings in the patient requiring long-term tube feedings. PEG replacement tubes are more costly than Foley-type catheters, which have been used as replacement gastrostomy tubes. In current practice, Foley catheters used as gastrostomy tubes do not have external bumpers (see Fig. 47–1). The external bumper is the major advantage in commercially manufactured replacement PEG tubes. The second advantage is the shorter length of the tube, which prevents movement into the small bowel.

The low-profile gastrostomy device (LPGD) is flush with the skin of the abdomen. Feeding adapters or administration sets are attached when necessary for the administration of medication or tube feeding. Should an LPGD be placed in lieu of a PEG, constant and close daily monitoring to ensure the device is properly positioned is required. Weight gain could cause the tube to impact within the fistulous tract (Fig. 47–2). This can be recognized by the inability of the LPGD to rotate 360 degrees without resistance and by leaking around the device during tube feeding.

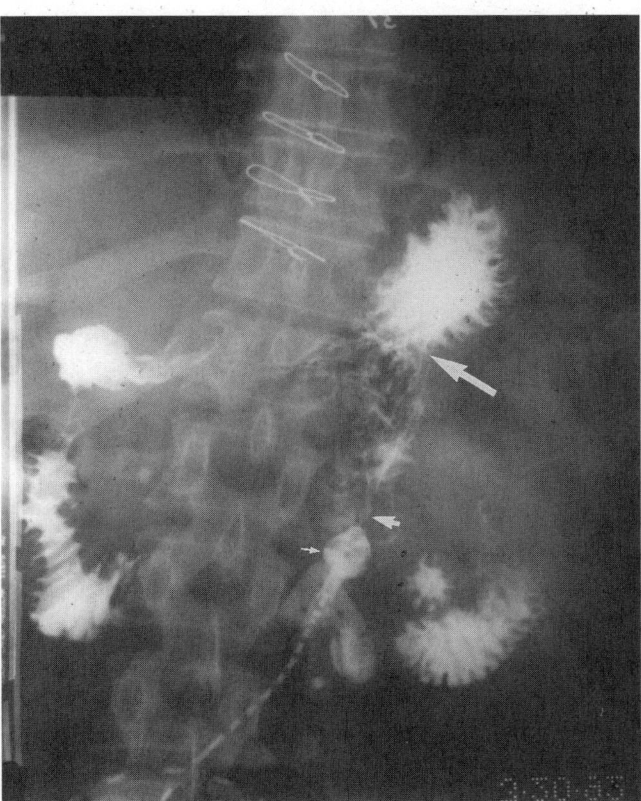

FIGURE 47–2. Low-profile gastrostomy device *(small white arrow)*. The device is impacted within the gastrocutaneous fistulous tract *(medium white arrow)*. The stomach is indicated by the *large white arrow.* Leaking during enteral feeding was noted and inability of the device to rotate was identified.

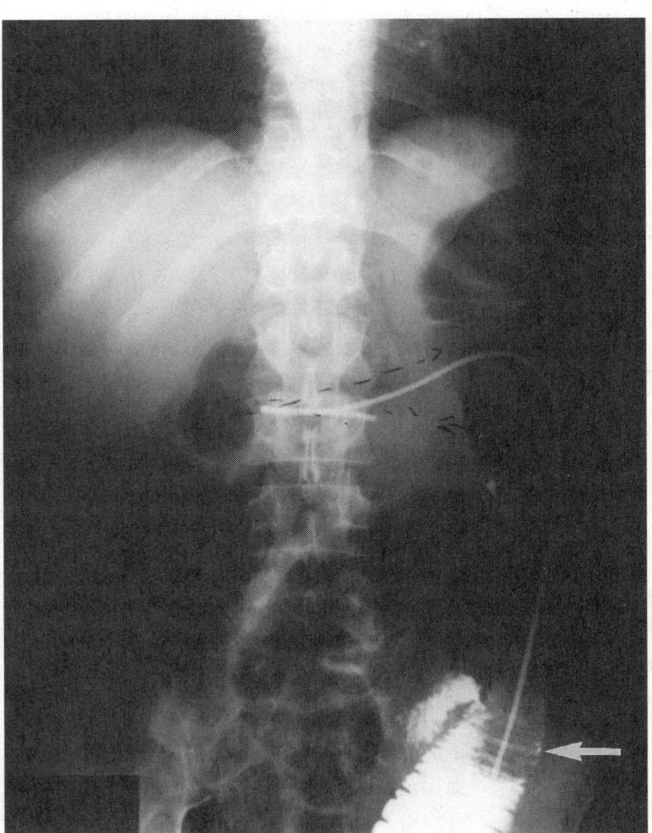

FIGURE 47–1. Foley catheter as gastrostomy tube. The catheter enters stomach *(black arrows)* and passes through duodenum to proximal jejunum. Balloon of the Foley catheter *(white arrow)* is obstructing the intestinal lumen.

COMBINATION TUBES. Combination tubes (i.e., the Moss tube) can be placed during GI surgical procedures when feeding over anastomosis sites is not preferred, and gut function is desired. These tubes are designed for short-term use. The tubes are made of firm plastic that allows gastric decompression and duodenal feeding simultaneously. If not placed correctly, the duodenal port could move into the stomach. Since their initial use in surgical patients, more durable, softer, and longer tubes have been developed to benefit patients with diabetic gastroparesis, multiple sclerosis, or other conditions resulting in gastric atony that require simultaneous gastric decompression and jejunal feeding. In addition to gastric decompression, the gastric port can also serve as a monitoring port. Should tube feeding product delivered via the jejunal port be observed in the gastric secretions, malposition of the feeding tube tip should be suspected. Abdominal radiographs and contrast injected into the tube may be necessary to confirm placement.

Gastrostomies, surgical or PEG, may also be converted to jejunostomies, creating combination tubes. Many enteral nutrition companies now manufacture small (9 Fr) jejunal feeding tubes that can be passed through a gastrostomy tube (20 Fr). Endoscopic or fluoroscopic guidance is used to position the tube in the distal portion of the duodenum or the proximal jejunum. These tubes are referred to as percutaneous endoscopic gastrostomy–jejunostomy (PEG-J) tubes. These combination tubes allow gastric decompression or administration of medications into the stomach while delivering the tube feeding product into the small bowel. This serves two purposes: (1) preventing pulmonary aspiration of gastric contents, or of jejunal contents if refluxed into the stomach; and (2) feeding the small bowel. In addition to decompression, the gastric port allows delivery of gastric-specific medications, such as protectants or antacids, while providing the benefits of maintaining gut function and perhaps preventing the complications associated with gut rest (Langkamp-Henken et al., 1992).

A nasal–jejunal combination tube has recently been introduced. This 18-Fr tube allows gastric decompression and jejunal feeding, which may be of particular benefit in critical care. This tube eliminates the need for placing two nasal tubes. In the past, a separate nasogastric tube for gastric decompression or administration of gastric-specific medications often was needed, while another feeding tube was placed in the opposite nares to feed the small bowel. Dual nasal–intestinal intubation for nasogastric decompression and feeding may interrupt the integrity of the lower esophageal sphincter, contributing to an increased potential for aspiration (Metheny et al., 1986; Mittal et al., 1992).

JEJUNAL TUBES. Patients who have upper GI tract obstruction or those at great risk for aspirating gastric contents may have a jejunostomy feeding tube (JFT) placed. Traditionally, when oral or gastric feedings were not possible due to the surgical procedure, a JFT was placed during the surgical procedure. Recently, interventional radiologists have been successful in placing JFT percutaneously under fluoroscopic guidance (Gray et al., 1987).

The needle catheter jejunostomy (NCJ) is a temporary type of jejunostomy feeding tube commonly seen in clinical practice. This catheter is expected to be used for a period of less than 6 weeks. These are small-diameter tubes placed at the time of surgery, usually distal to the ligament of Trietz, which is distal to the entry of the biliary and pancreatic ducts in the duodenum. Polymeric feeding products have been administered via NCJ without complications (Collier et al., 1994). However, because most enteral feeding products require digestion, administration of these polymeric products (at a point distal to the digestive secretions) may result in maldigestion of some nutrients. To prevent this, predigested or elemental feeding products are used that ensure absorption of nutrients across the gut mucosa without biliary and pancreatic enzymes; due to increased osmolality, however, these products can cause diarrhea. In addition, some enteral feeding products are quite viscous, and modular supplements (i.e., powdered protein and carbohydrates or oils) that can be added to them may obstruct this catheter. The NCJ has been increased in size from 18 gauge (1.25 mm) or 5 Fr to 13 gauge (2.33 mm) or 7 Fr, which has increased the longevity of the tube. Caution should be exercised when administering any tube feeding or modular product through the NCJ. Obstruction of this tube in the immediate postoperative period will most likely require surgical replacement. Recently, endoscopic techniques have been successful in reestablishing a jejunostomy (Pritchard & Bloom, 1994). Should NCJ tubes malfunction, obstruct, or accidentally be removed, manipulation or blind catheterization of the site must not be undertaken by unskilled professionals.

Another jejunal feeding tube that may reduce the risk of aspiration is the surgical jejunostomy or Witzel jejunostomy, which can be more permanent and is usually larger (14 Fr) than the NCJ (7 Fr). This catheter is placed in the proximal jejunum and therefore does not require the use of predigested or elemental feeding products. Should the catheter be obstructed, accidently removed, or malfunction, caution with replacement is suggested. Once a fistulous tract has formed, after about 4 to 6 weeks, catheters can be replaced with ease if done in a timely manner after removal.

A Roux-en-Y jejunostomy has recently been described and offers the benefits of (1) permanent stoma, (2) elimination of a permanent feeding device, (3) no potential for closure of the tract should the feeding tube be displaced, and (4) lessened risk of gastroesophageal reflux and aspiration. This procedure requires general anesthesia and open laparotomy, and is similar to the Janeway gastrostomy, but offers the advantage of jejunal feeding as opposed to gastric feeding. This type of jejunostomy is indicated in severely neurologically impaired patients (DeCou et al., 1993). The major disadvantages of the Roux-en-Y jejunostomy is mucus production, which occurs naturally from the jejunum. An ostomy appliance may be required to protect the skin. Again, the placement of a feeding tube for the delivery of each feeding is required. Finally, because of its anatomic location, the jejunostomy may be mistaken for an ileostomy or colostomy (McGinnis & Matson, 1994).

Percutaneous jejunostomy has also been accomplished in select patients (Gray et al., 1987). This technique offers the advantages of a percutaneous procedure, eliminating general surgical and anesthetic procedures, while providing the advantages of jejunal feeding.

CLINICAL MANAGEMENT OF ENTERAL NUTRITION

Clinical management of enteral feeding includes placing nasoenteric tubes, verifying placement, caring for the skin at exit sites, maintaining tube patency, delivering medications and tube feeding products through the feeding tube or device, preventing complications associated with tube feeding, and monitoring the patient's physiologic response to and tolerance of the tube feeding regimen. In spite of the evolution of feeding devices and nutritional products designed to minimize the complications of enteral nutrition, complications can still occur. Therefore, nursing interventions to prevent the complications associated with enteral nutrition are discussed at length.

SKIN CARE. Skin at the insertion site must be cared for daily. With nasogastric tubes, the nose should be cleaned daily. Because mucus crusting within the nares can be quite uncomfortable, the use of a cotton swab to clean the nares and application of a non–water-soluble lubricant may be necessary to keep mucous membranes clean and moist. Mouth care must be continued, to prevent complications of dry mucous membranes, and to prevent potential bacterial contamination of the pulmonary system should aspiration of the oral secretions occur.

The stoma sites of gastrostomy and jejunostomy tubes must also be cleaned daily. Soap and water is all that is necessary. Leaking gastrostomies or jejunostomies require further evaluation. Gastrostomy tube movement can cause the stoma site to leak and subsequently enlarge. There are a variety of tubes commercially available that are specifically designed to control tube movement and leakage (see Table 47–7). Foley catheters and surgical gastrostomy tubes such as the Malecot type, which lack external bumpers, can migrate into the gastric outlet tract, causing obstruction and leakage of gastric or bilious fluids from the stoma site (see Fig. 47–1). Therefore, Foley catheters and Malecot-type tubes are not acceptable for use as feeding tubes. If encountered in clinical practice, consultation with a qualified professional to change to an appropriate device is recommended.

Unlike gastrostomy tubes, a leaking jejunostomy tube usually indicates a more serious problem, with tube migration into the abdominal wall and possible peritonitis. Immediate cessation of feeding, assessment of vital signs and the site for infection, and physician notification are indicated.

Proper care at the time of insertion is the best prevention against the development of leaking tube sites. Complications occur when excessive manipulation of the tube takes place within 48 hours of placement. This allows mucosa to migrate through the fistula tract instead of permitting epithelium to line the tract, thus creating a leaking stoma site instead of a dry skin site. Actually, the site is not leaking; the mucous membrane is performing its natural function, but in an area that is not appropriate. It is crucial that jejunostomy tubes not be dislodged within 6 weeks of placement. If a fistula tract is not well formed, the patient may require surgical, endoscopic, or radiologic procedures to replace the tube.

ADMINISTRATION TECHNIQUE

Administration of tube feeding products in the critical care unit is the responsibility of the nurse. Various tube feeding administration methods can be used. The location of the feeding tube tip and the patient's tolerance dictate the method of administration (See Table 47–9).

GASTRIC. In general, critically ill patients should not be bolus fed. Bolus feeding is defined as the delivery of a large volume of tube feeding into the stomach (e.g., 500 mL over 30 minutes four times per day). This is not usually tolerated by critically ill patients for a variety of reasons. Therefore, to minimize the complications of rapid delivery and meet the nutritional needs of the patient, a continuous infusion is preferred.

TABLE 47–9. **Methods of Enteral Feeding in the Critically Ill**

Type	Hourly Rate (mL/hour)	Hours/Day	Frequency (times/day)
Continuous	10–125	24	1
Intermittent	50–125	12–16	1
	50–200	3–4	3–4

Intermittent feeding can be a several-hour infusion a few times per day (e.g., 150 mL/hour for 3 hours every 8 hours), or intermittent feeding can be for a longer period (12–16 hours) at an hourly rate (e.g., 100 mL/hour for 16 hours). This allows a fasting period (Table 47–9). The intermittent method of feeding may restore the gastric pH to normal, which may prevent the aspiration pneumonia associated with continuous feeding (Jacobs et al., 1990). Intermittent feedings may also be of greater benefit in the chronically critically ill patient who may have other therapies during the day that require tube feeding to be discontinued.

SMALL BOWEL. Unlike the stomach, the small bowel has no reservoir for food to be stored. Tube feeding administration via duodenal or jejunal feeding tubes needs to be delivered by a feeding pump at a prescribed hourly rate to meet the patient's assessed nutrient needs. The normal role of the stomach in gastric feeding is to liquefy food and deliver chyme slowly to the small intestine. This process is bypassed with small bowel feedings, and bolus feeding to the small intestine can result in dumping syndrome, signs of which include hypoglycemia, diaphoresis, palpitations, nausea, cramping, and diarrhea. An intermittent or continuous schedule is most commonly seen in the critically ill patient to prevent the complications associated with dumping syndrome.

Noctural feedings may be used with both gastric and small bowel feeding tubes. Nocturnal feeding allows other therapies to continue during the day without nutritional compromise. Fluid status and diuretic therapy may need to be adjusted because the fluids are not evenly dispersed throughout the day. Fluid overload could occur when 1,200 to 1,500 mL of tube feeding is administered over 8 to 12 hours. This is particularly true when weaning ventilator-dependent patients. Noctural feeding could contribute to volume overload and ventilatory failure with morning weaning trials.

Nocturnal feeding also permits oral intake in the tracheotomized patient who is ventilator dependent.

The patient who is not capable of eating adequate calories and requires supplemental tube feeding may also benefit from 8 to 12 hours of feeding overnight.

MEDICATION MANAGEMENT. Care must be taken when administering medications through NCJ feeding tubes. Any medication that is site specific must be evaluated closely before administration, because the desired action may not be obtained. In the case of small bowel feeding tubes, the medication would act on the jejunum and not benefit the gastric mucosa (e.g., gastric protectants or antacids). Meticulous care in appropriately administering medications helps to prevent complications. Physical alteration of medications, such as crushing tablets, opening capsules, or dissolving sustained-release or enteric-coated pills, must be done in consultation with the pharmacist because these actions may inactivate the medication in addition to obstructing the tube. In some cases, intravenous (IV) forms of medication may be administered via feeding tubes. However, the bioavailability of these IV drugs given through the GI tract must be evaluated pharmacodynamically, and alterations in dose may be indicated after pharmacokinetics are determined. Phenytoin may not be adequately absorbed in the presence of tube feeding. Subtherapeutic levels may be observed with phenytoin suspension during continuous tube feeding administration. Therefore, it is recommended that enteral feedings be held 1 to 2 hours before and after phenytoin administration. Theophylline absorption has also been noted to be affected by enteral nutrition. Monitoring serum levels is indicated to maintain therapeutic drug levels.

Finally, with regard to small bowel feeding tubes in critical care, should histamine receptor antagonists not be used, passing a nasogastric tube for antacid or protectant therapy may be indicated to protect the stomach.

Prevention of Complications

The complications or side effects of enteral nutrition can be classified according to etiology: infectious, mechanical, functional, and metabolic. Critical care nurses must be alert to all of these potential complications to administer enteral nutritional therapy effectively and safely. The etiology and treatment of the common complications of enteral feeding are summarized in Table 47–10.

INFECTIOUS COMPLICATIONS. Preventable infectious complications include contamination of enteral feeding products and malposition of feeding tubes, which can lead to aspiration. Contamination of enteral feeding products must be avoided. Hand-washing before manipulation of the tube feeding system, closed feeding systems, and avoidance of adding medications, tap water, or modular food products in areas other than the tube feeding preparation area of the diet kitchen can prevent these complications (Fagerman, 1992). Open or reconstituted tube feeding formulas not used within 24 hours should be discarded, and tube feeding administration sets should be discarded every 24 hours. Life-threatening diarrhea can occur in immunocompromised patients (Moe, 1991).

OTITIS MEDIA. Sinusitis and ear infections can occur with any tube that passes through the nasopharyngeal cavity. Critically ill patients may not be able to express the discomfort associated with these infections. Nurses should observe for nasal or ear drainage. Also, in the event the patient appears infected and a source cannot be localized, it should be borne in mind that the presence of a nasoenteric tube can contribute to infection. Radiologic evaluation of the sinuses and otologic examination are indicated. Removal of the feeding tube, antibiotic therapy, and PN therapy may be indicated until the infection has cleared and the feeding tube can be replaced. Placement of a gastrostomy or jejunostomy feeding tube may be indicated if the tube feeding is expected to continue for longer than a few weeks.

ASPIRATION. Preventing the development of an aspiration pneumonia from GI contents or tube feeding product is vital. This can be done in a variety of ways. First, the selection of a feeding tube must be considered. Decompression tubes such as Salem Sump or Levine tubes should not used for enteral feeding (Ibáñez et al., 1992; Metheny, 1993). These tubes are made of polyvinylchloride, a hard and nonpliable plastic. They are large bore (18 Fr) and may interrupt the normally closed position of the lower esophageal sphincter (LES) (Mittal et al., 1992). This, compounded with positive pressure ventilation, increases the potential for airway contamination. The rigidity of these tubes, which increases over time, can erode gastric mucosa. Last, these tubes can be quite uncomfortable for patients, and may contribute to otitis media or sinusitis.

The only exception to use of a decompression tube for feeding may be in the case of oropharyngeal, tracheal, or esophageal surgery, where the decompression tube is precisely placed and perhaps even sutured into position during the surgical procedure. The tube is used for decompression immediately after surgery, and then during the recovery process enteral nutrition is begun via this tube. Because the decompression tube cannot be removed and replaced with an SBFT, tube feeding through the decompression tube is begun within days of surgery and continued until oral nutrition can be resumed. Ideally, SBFT would be placed into the small bowel during surgery to permit feeding while the decompression tube is used for air and fluid removal. In the event oral nutrition does not begin within several days or oral intake is not adequate, and the decompression tube has been removed, placement of an SBFT is indicated. An SBFT may decrease the risk of gastric reflux and pulmonary contamination because the LES can remain competent in the presence of an SBFT (Mittal et al., 1992). SBFT placement is usually performed when anastomosis sites are healed and the decompression tube can be removed safely, usually within 7 days postsurgery.

Another factor that may contribute to aspiration is

TABLE 47–10. **Complications of Enteral Tube Feeding**

Complication and Clinical Findings	Cause	Intervention
Mechanical		
Leaking at site	Tube malpositioned	Gently pull up on tube Slide external bumper against the abdominal wall
	Internal balloon volume decreased	Check volume of balloon If volume less than initial amount, add additional water
Tube migration Site usually appears red and may also have some drainage	Usually occurs shortly after placement Can occur if the *external* abdominal bumper is sutured to the abdominal wall and weight gain occurs; the *internal* bumper could become lodged in the fistulous tract or peritoneum	Stabilize tube after placement Patient may require restraints or loose binder to protect tube Notify physician May need to arrange for abdominal x-ray with gastrograffin injection
Tube obstruction Tube feeding leaking at insertion site	Distal tip of the tube may be obstructed, tube feeding formula may exit the side holes, wick along the catheter, and exit the fistulous tract	Notify physician May need to arrange for abdominal x-ray with gastrograffin injection
Metabolic		
Electrolyte Fluctuations	Related to blood sugar Can occur in individuals who are malnourished, and then nourished serum levels can decrease dramatically secondary to anabolism	Monitor blood sugar; 150–200 mg/dL is desirable Monitor serum electrolytes Replete as needed
Dehydration	Related to blood sugar	Monitor blood sugar
Blood sugar Increased	Usually in a diabetic who has an underlying infection	Assess for infection
Decreased	Abrupt stopping of continuous feedings Related to dumping syndrome with rapid delivery of tube feeding and subsequent diarrhea	Gradually taper tube feeding Slow administration of tube feeding formula
	Administration of insulin and tube feeding product not done concurrently	Short-acting insulin to be delivered until insulin need is determined, then change to long-acting insulin
Infection	Aspiration pneumonia Local at the insertion site	Prevent gastrointestinal complications Clean daily Maintain tube position
Technical		
Usually at the time of insertion if percutaneous procedure	GI tract not accessible Anatomically impossible	Surgical gastrostomy
Gastrointestinal		
Delayed gastric emptying Residual	Gastric dystonia Diabetic gastroparesis GI dysfunction Gastritis Influenza	Monitor blood sugar Change tube feeding formula Increased fat content of formula Medications to increase motility Consider prokinetic agents Monitor vital signs Check gastric aspirate Notify physician if coffee grounds or bleeding noted
Vomiting	Obstruction Tube feeding intolerance Gastritis/ulcers	Monitor vital signs Assess abdomen for distention and rigidity Notify physician Laboratory blood tests may be ordered WBC Electrolytes
Aspiration	Inability to protect the airway Elevated head of the bed Small-bore feeding tubes Small bowel feeding	Prevent delayed emptying Prevent nausea and vomiting Assess swallowing mechanism Perform meticulous mouth care

Table continued on following page

TABLE 47–10. **Complications of Enteral Tube Feeding** *Continued*

Complication and Clinical Findings	Cause	Intervention
Diarrhea	Contamination of tube feeding product or administration sets and equipment Suppression of normal flora by antibiotic therapy Medications that can cause diarrhea	Diagnostic studies may be ordered Stool cultures *Clostridium difficile* toxin Stool for WBC Identify medications Magnesium-containing antacids Stool softeners with laxatives Lactulose Document Amount of stool loss Consistency of stool Occult blood Frequency of bowel movements
Constipation	Narcotics Electrolyte imbalance Lack of fiber in diet	Establish bowel regimen Fiber Water and fluids Laxatives Enemas

Abbreviation: WBC, white blood cell count.

Reprinted with permission from Shuster, M. H., & Mancino, J. M. (1994). Ensuring successful home tube feeding in the geriatric population. *Geriatric Nursing, 15,* 67–82.

tube location. Nurses must verify placement of the feeding tube after initial insertion, and before and during each subsequent feeding. Results of research on the risk of aspiration with more distally placed tubes are controversial. Strong and colleagues (1992) found no statistically significant difference in the rate of aspiration in gastric compared to jejunally fed patients. Montecalvo and coworkers (1992), in a prospective, randomized study, demonstrated no aspiration, higher calorie intake, and greater increases in prealbumin in the jejunally fed group compared to the gastrically fed group. Placement may be confirmed radiographically or with the use of pH (Metheny et al., 1993). Color and consistency of the intestinal aspirate may further contribute to verification of placement (see Table 47–8).

Although aspiration of tube feeding product may be decreased with feeding tubes placed in the small intestine, oropharyngeal aspiration can continue. Bacteria-laden oral secretions can be as noxious as GI contents. Nursing care must include meticulous oral hygiene. The propensity for GI contamination of the pulmonary tract is further increased by the use of histamine antagonists, which alters the acid medium of the stomach, thus decreasing the natural ability of the stomach to destroy bacteria. Use of an intermittent feeding schedule may decrease the incidence of pneumonia, because restoration of the normal gastric pH may occur during the fasting period, exerting an antimicrobial effect (Ruddell et al., 1980). Table 47–9 describes various methods of feeding.

Known gastroesophageal reflux disease (GERD), esophagitis at endoscopy, or the presence of a hiatal hernia can contribute to aspiration pneumonia through regurgitation of stomach contents into the esophagus. These findings, in combination with the inability to protect the airway (as with intubation) and neurologic or neuromuscular impairment, can lead to aspiration of stomach contents. Therefore, the patient's ability to protect his or her airway must be assessed by the nurse, and interventions to protect the lungs must be undertaken. Elevation of the head of the bed and stopping tube feeding before nursing care that requires the patient to be recumbent can minimize the aspiration risk. Torres and colleagues (1992) demonstrated that patients who maintained a semirecumbent position (45 degrees) were less likely to have contaminated endobronchial secretions compared to supine patients. In addition, they observed a direct relationship between length of time spent supine and degree of endobronchial contamination. Ibáñez and colleagues (1992) found no difference in gastroesophageal reflux with positioning.

Gastrostomy tubes do not always prevent aspiration (Mittal et al., 1992). A competent LES with a gastrostomy tube may prevent aspiration of tube feeding. However, if aspiration is secondary to inability to protect the airway, it can still occur from the oropharynx. In this case, an esophagotracheal diversion, a radical surgical procedure that separates the GI and respiratory tracts, may be considered. This will prevent aspiration, but the patient will lose his or her voice. This may be a therapeutic option in selected patients with repeated hospitalizations and intensive care unit admissions for aspiration pneumonia.

Fever, adventitious lung sounds, and an increased white blood cell count with changes in the chest radiograph may be indicative of aspiration pneumonia. Antibiotic therapy may be warranted. If possible, the etiology of aspiration should be determined. Referral to a speech pathologist, who may perform a modified barium swallow, can help in isolating the mechanism of aspiration and prevent future episodes of aspiration by modifying the feeding technique.

MECHANICAL COMPLICATIONS. Mechanical complications include tube displacement, obstruction, and fracture, and pump failure. Mechanical complications can be avoided if meticulous care is given to the feeding tube. As previously discussed, leaking at the gastrostomy or jejunostomy tube sites must always be considered abnormal. Tubes that are unstable can move and cause the stoma to enlarge. Nurses must maintain stability of these tubes with tape or drainage attachment devices to help decrease the problem. PEG replacement tubes with external bumpers also minimize this pivoting action.

Another mechanical complication is tube migration, which occurs when a gastrostomy tube migrates from the stomach into the antrum or gastric outlet of the stomach, or into the small bowel. Leaking occurs, but secretions are usually bilious in color. Gastrostomy tubes can also migrate into the fistula tract. Again, leaking can be the first sign, but patients may complain of pain and tenderness at the tube insertion site. Diatrizoate meglumine and diatrizoate sodium (e.g., Gastrografin [Squibb, Princeton, NJ]) injected through the tube is the definitive diagnostic test to determine tube impaction in the fistulous tract.

Obstruction of feeding tubes can be attributed to several factors, from exit port design to internal diameter. Tubes vary in internal and external diameter; they may have a larger external diameter, but because of the material used to manufacture the tube, the internal diameter may be less than desirable, and may contribute to obstruction. Exit port design can also contribute to obstruction (Silk et al., 1987). The most common cause of obstruction is inadequate flushing (Metheny et al., 1988). Medications and tube feeding products, as well as monitoring for gastric residuals with tube aspirates, can also cause obstruction (Powell et al., 1993). Medications that are not in a liquid form can obstruct the exit holes. Liquid medications not the consistency of water, such as suspensions or syrups, may also obstruct tubes. Liberal flushing (50 mL) with water before and after medication administration, whenever tube feeding is interrupted for any reason, and every 3 to 4 hours during continuous tube feeding, assists in minimizing the potential for tube obstruction (Metheny et al., 1988). Protein contained within tube feeding products is liquid on delivery. However, when protein is heated, it denatures and becomes a solid. This solid protein also obstructs the exit ports of the feeding tube.

Should feeding tubes become obstructed, several methods to relieve the obstruction can be attempted before replacing the tube. Several attempts at irrigation with warm tap water while exerting gentle pressure should clear most obstructed tubes.

Other interventions to relieve obstruction have been recommended. Pancreatic enzymes or meat tenderizer to digest the protein have been tried, as well as carbonated cola beverages, cranberry juice, and water. These three liquids were compared in a research design by Metheny et al. (1988). Water was as effective as cola; cranberry juice was not as good as water or cola. Often the energy, effort, and expense involved may be better expended in replacing the tube. Bommarito and coworkers (1989) have developed a cleaning device to clear obstructed feeding tubes. Blind use of guidewires or stylets to reestablish patency is not recommended because of the possibility of perforation.

Fracture or rupture of feeding tubes usually requires replacement of the tube. Again, in difficult situations interventional radiologists may be of great benefit in replacing these tubes.

Pump failure can range from complete mechanical failure to delivery failures. Pumps can malfunction, delivering less than the amount programmed, or can free-flow, delivering large quantities of tube feeding product. Although the former would compromise the nutrition delivered to the patient, the effect may not be life-threatening. In the event of overdelivery, aspiration secondary to increased volume in the stomach may have graver implications. Dumping syndrome secondary to delivery of a large volume of tube feeding into the small bowel can also occur.

FUNCTIONAL COMPLICATIONS. Functional problems are usually related to GI dysfunction, with diarrhea, constipation, bloating, excessive gas and abdominal distention, cramping, nausea, vomiting, or increased residuals related to delayed gastric emptying being the most common. Leaking, especially of gastrostomy or jejunostomy sites, can be the result of mechanical or functional complications. Gastrostomy or jejunostomy tubes should not leak, and the occurrence of leaking from these sites requires investigation to identify the cause.

Patients in whom nausea, vomiting, or diarrhea develop after having tolerated tube feedings for a period of time may show intolerance to the formula, and changing the formula may be indicated. However, other etiologies for nausea, vomiting, and diarrhea must be investigated. This includes evaluating medications that can induce nausea and vomiting as well as medications that may be prescribed for bowel regimens that can precipitate diarrhea.

Multiple medications can also cause nausea and vomiting, especially if introduced into the stomach without food. The occurrence of gastritis and ulcers as an etiology for nausea and vomiting in the critically ill patient should not be overlooked. Stress gastritis in the critically ill population has been reported to occur in approximately 30% of patients (Martin et al., 1993). This rate may be increased with jejunal feeding because physiologic stimulation of the small intestine causes an increase in gastric secretions. Magnesium-containing antacids used in the critically ill patient to treat ulcers or prevent gastritis can result in diarrhea. Acid inhibitors in preference to antacids or protectants to prevent GI bleeding are widely used in critical care settings, but pH cannot be used to predict when GI bleeding will occur (Moore et al., 1992). Therefore, antacids may need to be used in addition to other therapy.

Diarrhea is thought to be the most common complication of tube feeding. In the critically ill population, a multitude of other reasons can be the cause of diarrhea (Guenter et al., 1991; Kohn & Keithley, 1982). Diarrhea can be classified as secretory, such as with *Clostridium difficile* infection secondary to antibiotic therapy, or can be osmotic, such as that caused by lactulose. Tube feeding products that provide 1 calorie/mL are usually isotonic and do not cause an osmotic diarrhea. In patients in whom diarrhea develops, quantification and characteristics of stool must be noted. Stool specimens for electrolytes, blood, white blood cells, cultures, Sudan stain, and *C. difficile* toxin should be obtained, along with abdominal radiographs. Administration of antidiarrheals without the evaluation of stool for infectious causes is discouraged. Patients treated with antibiotics can contract pseudomembranous colitis secondary to *C. difficile* toxin. Administration of an antidiarrheal without the appropriate antimicrobial therapy directed at the specific microbe could be catastrophic (Kohn & Keithly, 1982). Once stool specimens are obtained and antibiotic therapy is begun, antidiarrheals and tube feeding may be administered. Tube feedings should not be held, nor should parenteral therapy be instituted, unless obstruction or perforation is imminent (Eisenberg, 1993). Another factor that can cause diarrhea is the administration of liquid medications. The vehicle for a variety of liquid medications is sorbitol, a nonabsorbable carbohydrate that causes an osmotic diarrhea. Medications contributing to diarrhea should be discontinued if possible.

Finally, the definition of diarrhea varies among practitioners. If the patient has liquid stool in excess of 250 mL/day, by definition this is diarrhea. However, if this occurs only once per day, the patient may not have diarrhea. The critically ill patient may be incontinent of liquid stool because the rectum is not capable of holding liquids. Quantification and frequency of stools must be recorded by the nurse.

The addition of soluble and insoluble fibers may also change the consistency of the stool. Although the amount of stool production may be the same, the patient may gain the ability to control bowel movements. This would prevent the skin breakdown associated with prolonged diarrhea. The addition of fiber in the form of psyllium powder to tube feeding is not recommended because this may obstruct the feeding tube. A number of tube feeding products contain fiber.

Usually the gut is capable of digesting the nutrients of polymeric formulas. However, the gut may lose its ability to adequately digest the nutrients, as in the case of pancreatitis or prolonged TPN. Nutrients are administered in a predigested or elemental form to prevent maldigestion and malabsorption, which would result in diarrhea. However, by reducing the nutrients to their smallest and most absorbable form, the number of particles per liter increases, and the resulting increased osmolality could cause an osmotic diarrhea.

There are a number of tube feeding products that are hyperosmolar. These products are usually specialty products used for renal or hepatic failure, and may be elemental or calorically dense. Products that are calorically dense (i.e., 1.5 or 2 cal/mL) are hyperosmolar because of the removal of water. These products can be administered to appropriate patients without the side effect of osmotic diarrhea, but the manner in which the tube feeding is delivered requires alteration. Variations in the strength and hourly infusion rates may be required to establish patient tolerance before advancing the formula to the required rate and strength. Beginning at full strength and a high rate may contribute to diarrhea. Consultation with the clinical dietitian or the nutrition support service may prevent these problems.

Dumping syndrome may be mistaken for diarrhea. Dumping syndrome occurs when high concentrations of carbohydrates or large volumes are administered to the GI tract. It occurs most often in patients who have had gastric resections, but can be caused by rapidly bolus feeding the stomach or the small intestine. Dumping syndrome can be observed as loose stools or diarrhea minutes after infusing the formula, and, more important, it is accompanied by the signs and symptoms of hypoglycemia. The presence of food causes pancreatic endocrine stimulation. Hypoglycemia is secondary to the presence of insulin without sugar; sugar was not adequately absorbed from the tube feeding product because increased GI motility triggered by osmoceptors and baroceptors rapidly removed the food from the GI tract. The end result is hypoglycemia. Interventions to decrease the infusion rate, decrease volume of the infusion, or change the tube feeding product (if hyperosmolar or the primary source of calories is from carbohydrate) should not be undertaken indiscriminately. Manipulation of tube feeding has implications as to the quantity of nutrients delivered. Consultation with a nutritionist is warranted before intervening.

Patients who have constipation, cramping, abdominal distention, and bloating need to be evaluated for the cause of their symptoms. Common causes of constipation in the critically ill include the administration of narcotics and other medications, aerophagia secondary to positive pressure ventilation, or electrolyte imbalances. Protectants and aluminum-containing antacids may also contribute to constipation. Medications, especially narcotics and psychotropic medications, may contribute to decreased motility. Often, discontinuation of these medications is not possible, and therefore the development of a bowel regime would be indicated.

Interventions directed at the treatment of constipation include the administration of fiber-containing tube feeding products. Patients may benefit from a change in the tube feeding product (i.e., to a fiber-containing product) if the primary problem is constipation, but this may increase bloating. The addition of simethicone may help to decrease bloating and flatulence. To prevent constipation with fiber products, additional water may be required. If the feeding product contains less than 70% water, or a fluid restriction is imposed, a fiber product can cause constipation.

Careful attention to electrolytes, particularly potassium, and to constipating medications, especially narcotics, may also help maintain gut motility. Any activity that promotes gut motility is also encouraged. Increased blood sugar or enteral feeding products high in fat content can delay gastric emptying and may contribute to the above symptoms. Finally, liquid stool can be passed around an impaction. If liquid stool is noted, a rectal examination is performed, and removal of the impaction and establishment of a bowel regimen to prevent further impaction is indicated.

Delayed gastric emptying may be indicated by persistent large volumes of tube feeding residuals. A nuclear emptying scan may be ordered to confirm gastroparesis. The assumption is that accumulation of any substance in a large volume can contribute to gastric distention, esophageal reflux, and vomiting, placing the patient at risk for aspiration. Therefore, monitoring for residuals is indicated. Unfortunately, there is no consensus as to how often residuals should be obtained or the volume of the residual that should determine when tube feedings be discontinued. Definitions of what constitutes increased residual volumes vary, and range from two times the hourly rate, which could be as little as 20 or 30 mL, to 200 mL (McClave et al., 1992; Silberman, 1989). It is reasonable clinical practice to ascertain the presence of residual volumes several hours after tube feedings are begun, or when the rate of tube feeding is increased. Further research will need to be conducted to give definitive guidance to nursing practice regarding specific volumes and appropriate interventions.

Gastric residuals are measured to determine the patient's ability to tolerate and move the nutrients through the GI tract. When tube feeding is initiated, gastric residuals are checked frequently. The volume aspirated can vary, but increased residuals imply that the GI tract is not moving. The volume of aspirate also increases as the rate of infusion increases. Increased volume and pressure in the stomach or GI tract could cause nausea and vomiting and increase the potential for gastroesphageal reflux and aspiration. Metoclopramide hydrochloride may be of benefit in these patients to increase gut motility.

Several other factors can influence residual volumes. Patient position and tube location can influence the amount of residual obtained. It is recommended that the head of the bed be elevated at 30 to 45 degrees to prevent aspiration. If the feet or knees are also elevated to maintain the patient's position, air may be trapped in the large bowel. Air moves through the intestine more quickly than solids, but when it reaches the large intestine the position of the patient inhibits movement to the sigmoid and rectum, contributing further to bloating and distention. Placing the patient on his or her right side may help evacuate the air and also facilitate movement of fluids from the stomach into the small intestine.

Residual volumes may not be collected from gastrostomy tubes because the tubes are usually placed on the anterior gastric wall. If the patient is supine, pooling of gastric contents or tube feeding product may occur in the posterior stomach. If the tip of the feeding tube is not advanced into the pool, no residual volume will be noted (McClave et al., 1992). Turning the patient, especially onto the right side, can facilitate movement of contents into the small bowel, whereas positioning on the left side may increase residual volumes.

In checking small bowel feeding tubes for residual volumes, motility is assessed as well as tube position. The small bowel is not a distensible organ or reservoir like the stomach. Therefore, the small bowel should not contain a residual volume. Should a small intestinal tube be aspirated, and a residual volume in excess of a few milliliters be noted, tube migration into the stomach should be suspected. Also, the length of the feeding tube exiting the nares should be noted. A greater length exiting the nares may indicate the tube has been pulled out of position. This observation, in addition to residual volumes, pH, and color and consistency of aspirates, may suggest misplacement. Radiographic confirmation is warranted to determine the exact position of the tube. Careful assessment of the abdomen for bowel sounds, distention, and pain and radiographic confirmation of dysmotility and tube location are indicated. Powell and colleagues (1993) also noted an increased rate of tube obstruction with monitoring of residuals. Flushing of feeding tubes after assessing the residual volume is necessary to clear the tube of feeding product and prevent obstruction.

Terminating tube feeding and not replacing the gastric aspirate, or placing the tube to drain by gravity may prevent vomiting. Reinstilling the aspirate but not resuming tube feeding, or initiation of tube feeding after withdrawing and discarding the large residual volume, may be among several options ordered by the physician. However, reinstilling the volume and resuming the tube feeding is not recommended because both of these volumes together may be excessive and lead to aspiration. Furthermore, discarding the aspirate and *not* resuming the tube feeding will not assist in determining whether the problem is related to motility. In any case, whether withholding the tube feeding or trying to feed the patient, careful observation of the patient by the nurse is required to prevent further complications.

METABOLIC COMPLICATIONS. Metabolic alterations related to nutritional intervention include variances in laboratory markers such as electrolytes, minerals, renal and hepatic function tests, glucose, and serum proteins. Patients who may have been malnourished on admission to the intensive care unit may exhibit dramatic changes in electrolytes with administration of nutrition. Awareness of potential metabolic complications allows preventive measures to be incorporated. For the malnourished patient, monitoring and administrating electrolytes in the early stage of feeding is necessary to prevent rapid, potentially life-threatening cardiac dysrhythmias or respiratory arrest (Patrick, 1977). Although monitoring and administering electrolytes is commonplace in critical care areas, magnesium and phosphorus are often overlooked because these are not contained within the standard electrolyte panel. Feeding critically ill patients without adequate repletion of these electrolytes could result in rapid and potentially life-threatening cardiac dysrhythmias or respiratory arrest. This has been referred to as "refeeding syndrome." The reason for this is that with the provision of nutrients, the patient becomes anabolic and incorporates the minerals into cells, thereby depleting the serum levels (Solomon & Kirby, 1990). Constant exogenous repletion in addition to what the enteral product provides is necessary to maintain normal serum levels.

The volume of enteral product given to a patient determines if the RDA of nutrients is met. The RDA is a recommendation for healthy people; standards have not been developed for the critically ill. Also, these products contain the minerals required for the metabolism of the nutrients in the product, but do not contain additional nutrients required by the stressed, critically ill patient. Sustained synthesis or anabolic activity requires additional administration of these nutrients.

Laboratory values must be monitored, and minerals repleted as necessary. Once normal serum levels have been reached, a daily maintenance amount of these minerals must be provided in the nutritional formulation. Depending on the amount of enteral or parenteral product delivered to the patient in a 24-hour period, additional supplementation may also be required. Also, if serum values are life-threatening, parenteral correction is warranted. Oral or tube mineral supplementation can also cause osmotic diarrhea, which contributes to additional electrolyte losses.

Glucose intolerance can also develop in critically ill patients. Patients with diabetes normally controlled by diet or oral agents will often require insulin during their critical illness. Patients with insulin-dependent diabetes may require additional insulin to cover the amount of carbohydrate in the tube feeding product. Patients who contract stress diabetes mellitus also require insulin if blood sugars remain elevated. Blood sugar regulation in the critically ill patient can be challenging.

Hyperglycemia (≥400 mg/dL) has been reported by Orr (1992) to occur in 10% to 30% of patients receiving enteral nutrition. This is related to a number of reasons, including infection, insulin resistance, steroid use, and endocrine response to stress. Regardless of the cause, blood sugars must be controlled within a reasonable range. Hyperglycemia usually responds to an adequate amount of insulin. Hyperglycemia should not prevent or limit the administration of adequate nutrition to patients. Careful monitoring of nutrition and blood sugar, often combined with insulin infusions, allows delivery of required nutrients without the side effects of hyperglycemia.

Enteral feeding products designed to decrease hyperglycemia have been developed. Peters and Davidson (1992) suggest total calories may have a greater influence on blood sugar control in type I diabetics than the type of calories (i.e., carbohydrate versus fat). Should hyperglycemia ensue, additional free water must be given to compensate for the water lost in the natural diuresis of hyperglycemia. If water balance is not addressed in the presence of hyperglycemia, dehydration may result. From the current and usual weight and the serum chemistries, a fluid volume deficit can be calculated and additional water administered to correct the deficit (Paskin, 1989).

Overhydration also frequently occurs in the critically ill patient. This may result from aggressive resuscitation and decreased oncotic pressure, which allows third spacing, and further disturbances in serum chemistries are noted (e.g., hyponatremia or hypernatremia). Because enteral feeding formulations have fixed volumes of water and nutrients, careful bedside evaluation and monitoring of serum chemistries is necessary to prevent these complications (Bowman et al., 1989). Indiscriminate dilution of formulas or use of hyperosmolar formulas may result in severe fluid and electrolyte imbalances, especially in the elderly. Evaluation of renal function with careful recording of intake and output is imperative.

Liver function tests, although more commonly associated with PN, have been noted to be affected with enteral nutrition, and should be monitored at regular intervals during nutritional therapy. Renal function tests (blood urea nitrogen and creatinine) are not direct nutritional markers, but monitoring of these values is indicated because they may be directly affected by the nutritional regimen. The type and the amount of nutrients delivered to patients may need to be adjusted based on organ function. Volume-restricted patients may require more calorically dense formulas, or protein may need to be restricted. Patients with intravascular volume depletion also require additional fluids.

Parenteral Nutrition

Parenteral nutrition is indicated when the GI tract is nonfunctional, inaccessible, or incapable of adequately digesting and absorbing nutrients. Short gut syndrome is an example of the latter. Inflammatory bowel disease may also preclude enteral nutrition, and, finally, enteral feeding in the presence of an obstruction is contraindicated (Table 47–11). Nursing responsibilities with regard to PN include administration and monitoring for complications.

TYPES OF CATHETERS

Parenteral nutrition is a frequent temporary means of nutritional therapy in the critically ill, because critical illness often renders the gut nonfunctional. Long-term PN can also be used to maintain patients' lives when gut failure is permanent.

Parenteral nutrition is delivered via intravenous

TABLE 47–11. **Indications for Total Parenteral Nutrition in the Critically Ill**

Patients who are or will become malnourished who:
- Cannot or should not be orally or enterally fed
- Have no or very limited access to the GI tract
- Have an obstruction of the GI tract
- Cannot tolerate enteral nutrition
- Are severely malnourished with impending abdominal or thoracic surgery

Patients may benefit from partial or peripheral parenteral nutrition, which may be used for up to 2 weeks, when:
- Central access cannot be obtained
- Oral or enteral nutrition is inadequate
- Total parenteral nutrition is not feasible

Abbreviation: GI, gastrointestinal.

catheters, which can include single-, double-, or triple-lumen catheters (TLC). Pulmonary artery catheters that have an additional central venous infusion port have also been used to infuse TPN during critical illness. Other central catheters used to deliver TPN have antimicrobial cuffs or an antimicrobial sheath to reduce the incidence of infection (Kamal et al., 1991; Maki et al., 1988; Norwood et al., 1992).

Intermediate catheters may be indicated in patients in whom central venous catheters must remain in place for several weeks to months, as in the case of acute complicated pancreatitis. These catheters have biodegradable cuffs impregnated with silver ions that exert an antimicrobial effect for 4 to 6 weeks, permitting the catheter to remain in place for the duration of therapy provided it is less than the 4- to 6-week period (Maki et al., 1988; Norwood et al., 1992).

Permanent catheters are usually used in home or long-term TPN patients. These devices may be seen in the intensive care unit, especially in oncologic patients, or in patients with short gut syndrome. These catheters can be used during the intensive care unit admission; however, the primary purpose of the catheter should be maintained (i.e., if the catheter was placed for PN, then TPN should be administered via this catheter).

Peripheral PN usually is not adequate to meet the critically ill patient's nutritional needs. Peripheral PN as an adjunct to enteral therapy may be of benefit, especially if patients are experiencing GI complications that prevent maximal use of the GI tract.

CLINICAL MANAGEMENT OF PARENTERAL NUTRITION

Complications of PN can be grouped in several broad categories. The infectious complication of sepsis is the most feared complication of PN. Mechanical and technical complications may occur. Finally, metabolic complications, including alterations in serum electrolytes, blood sugar, and liver function and injury values, and renal function abnormalities can also occur.

INFECTIOUS COMPLICATIONS. Catheter-related sepsis (CRS) has been described in the literature as a significant risk of PN. This necessitates performance of semiquantitative blood cultures. Semiquantitative cultures require the catheter to be cultured, as well as a peripheral sample. Colony counts are taken and a determination regarding the source of the septicemia is presumed. Positive blood cultures without line cultures preclude identification of the catheter as the source of infection. A line or catheter infection by definition is a positive catheter culture but a negative peripheral blood culture. It is unclear if these infections go on to become sepsis. The Centers for Disease Control and Prevention make specific recommendations regarding the routine changing of central venous catheters. Research has shown conflicting data. Nussbaum and Fischer (1994) report a greater rate of CRS in pulmonary artery catheters used for TPN with routine changes, but Horowitz et al. (1990) found that routine changes of TLC every 3 to 4 days may decrease the risk of infection.

Research regarding the use of single-lumen catheters versus TLC and the location of catheters (subclavian versus femerol) has also noted differences in infection rate. Kemp and colleagues (1994) found a decreased CRS rate with the subclavian approach. The rationale for choosing the subclavian over the jugular or femoral approach is based on the difficulty of maintaining catheter stability and sterility. Clark-Christoff and associates (1992) found a 2.6% CRS rate for single-lumen catheters compared to 13.1% for TLC. The subclavian approach may be superior for administering TPN through multilumen catheters in critically ill patients. Every effort to stabilize these catheters must be attempted. Nurses also must change catheter dressings whenever the dressing is not occlusive.

Markers of infectious complications in patients who are recipients of TPN include increased white blood count, with elevation of bands, and increased temperature. Should these clinical indicators be present, evaluation of blood cultures is indicated. Blood cultures should be drawn from a peripheral site, as well as through the catheter, if the catheter is suspect. The catheter may be changed over a guidewire and sent for semiquantitative cultures to determine CRS. Should the catheter and blood culture be negative, the catheter is not the source of infection. However, should the catheter and blood cultures be positive for the same organism, the catheter is the most likely source, and if the catheter was exchanged over a guidewire, this catheter should be removed and a virgin site be used to place a new catheter for the administration of TPN.

MECHANICAL COMPLICATIONS. Occlusion of a temporary catheter requires changing the catheter. Occlusion often occurs secondary to clot or fibrin sheath formation. Silicone or polyurethane catheters are less thrombogenic. Catheter occlusion not only renders the catheter nonfunctional, but can harbor bacteria. Antimicrobial cuffs and antibiotic and antiseptic agents bonded to catheters have been shown to decrease sepsis rates. Reestablishing patency of an occluded catheter that may be contaminated could shower bacteria from the catheter into the circulation, increasing the potential for septicemia. Unless central venous access is very limited, thrombolytic therapy to reestablish patency of an occluded catheter should not be undertaken.

Another complication of PN is catheter perforation. Central venous catheters can cause vessel erosion, which can result in perforation and pleural effusions. Makau and colleagues (1991) retrospectively studied TPN central venous catheters and found that catheters that originated from the left side and were 14-gauge or larger were more likely to perforate the superior vena cava.

METABOLIC COMPLICATIONS. Refeeding syndrome is a metabolic complication of PN. This phenomenon has been observed in malnourished patients who were subsequently fed. Refeeding is usually associated with TPN, but also is seen with enteral feedings. Specific assessments and interventions were described in the section on Enteral Nutrition. Dramatic decreases in electrolytes—specifically, potassium, magnesium, and phosphorus—are noted with refeeding. Solomon and Kirby (1990) suggest that changes in glucose metabolism, vitamins, and fluid status occur with refeeding. Profound decreases in these minerals can be observed and are thought to be related to the incorporation of minerals into cell structure and utilization in metabolic processes such as the formation of ATP.

Formation of ATP requires phosphorus. Should serum levels of phosphorus become depleted, vital energy-requiring (e.g., breathing) functions will be impaired. Serum phosphorus levels below 1.0 mmol/dL are considered an emergent situation, and must be repleted with IV phosphorus. Usually an IV infusion of 40 to 60 mmol over 4 to 6 hours is indicated. Once the repletion dose is given, a daily maintenance dose of phosphorus must be added to the TPN to maintain normal serum levels. Phosphorus requirements are estimated based on the amount of carbohydrate or protein administered. Usual daily phosphorus requirements in TPN approach 30 mmol.

Calcium and magnesium requirements also need to be addressed. If a deficiency is present, correction is indicated, followed by a daily maintenance dose. One gram of calcium and 2 g of magnesium are the daily requirements. In the critically ill patient, additional magnesium may be administered to prevent cardiac dysfunction.

Potassium is often lost in diuresis or through GI losses. Potassium can be added to TPN based on serum levels. Consultation with the pharmacist may be indicated to prevent precipitation. Calcium, magnesium, and potassium are cations, and in combination with phosphates can precipitate. This may not be observed immediately on mixing the TPN formula, but can occur several hours after the TPN bag has been hanging. A white particulate matter may be seen in the TPN solution. Any change in the appearance of the TPN admixture necessitates discontinuation. Discontinuation of the TPN, administration of dextrose 10% at the same rate as the TPN was ordered, and returning the TPN solution to pharmacy are indicated.

Another metabolic complication commonly seen in the critically ill is hyperglycemia. Hyperglycemia can occur for a number of reasons, as previously discussed. Insulin resistance can occur in critically ill patients. *Central* insulin resistance occurs when the liver continues to produce glucose in the presence of hyperglycemia, whereas *peripheral* insulin resistance occurs when the cells are unable to absorb glucose across the cell membrane even in the presence of insulin. Therefore, an increase in serum glucose as well as insulin levels is present (McMahon & Rizza, 1994). Both of these phenomena may be operational in the critically ill patient. The hyperglycemia must be treated, and nutrition should not be withheld to control glucose. Various methods for determining insulin need have been developed (McMahon & Rizza, 1994). Blood sugars greater than 500 mg/dL may benefit from a continuous insulin infusion. Once blood sugars are controlled with the insulin infusion, insulin may be added to the TPN solution on a daily basis. Should a sliding scale or algorithm be used, the prior day's insulin requirement may be added to the TPN solution. Jovanovic-Peterson and Peterson (1991) have recommended that the addition of one-half to two-thirds of the previous day's insulin requirement be added to the TPN. Only one route of administration for insulin is suggested. In critical care, this usually would be the IV route. Due to edema, immobility, and altered perfusion of subcutaneous tissue, subcutaneous injections may not be effective (Pitts et al., 1993). IV administration ensures delivery. Other means to control blood sugar may include decreasing the amount of carbohydrate in the TPN. Patients should not be overfed because this will contribute to hyperglycemia; this is especially true when patients are fed based on measured energy expenditure, and hyperglycemia continues. Last, in patients with diabetes mellitus who require TPN, Jovanovic-Peterson and Peterson (1991) recommend the addition of insulin to TPN at the ratio of 1 U/10 g of carbohydrate. Pitts and colleagues (1993) recommend 0.3 units of regular insulin per kilogram for mild stress, 0.5 U/kg for moderate stress, and 1.0 U/kg of weight for severe stress or steroid therapy.

Hepatic complications of TPN are seen as elevated liver function tests, including bilirubin, alkaline phosphatase, serum glutamic oxalic transaminase, and serum glutamic pyruvic transaminase (Buchmiller et al., 1992; Klein & Nealon, 1988). Transaminases usually increase within 1 to 2 weeks after therapy is begun, and resolve without intervention. Bilirubin and alkaline phosphatase increase in 2 to 3 weeks after TPN is started. Increases in total and direct bilirubin with the development of jaundice may be noted. This may be attributed to high dextrose concentrations, which may cause a fatty liver due to carbohydrate excess or a diabetic state. The relationship between steatosis, or fat accumulation in the liver, and associated changes in liver function tests is unknown. Intrahepatic cholestasis does not occur until 2 to 3 weeks of TPN have been administered. Treatment includes decreasing the total amount of calories provided because overfeeding may be the cause of these abnormalities. If possible, the TPN should be cycled to allow a fasting period and reversal of the insulin-driven state that continues to promote fat storage. When possible, the GI tract should be used. This may stimulate gallbladder function and relieve the biliary tree of the stasis. However, cholelithiasis and acalculous cholecystitis can present as acute cholecystitis. Imaging studies are required to make the diagnosis. Enteral feeding may not be indicated in this situation, and the patient may require cholecystectomy.

DISEASE-SPECIFIC NUTRITIONAL THERAPY IN THE CRITICALLY ILL

Various disease states may require alterations in the type of nutrition provided. Patients with dysfunction of the cardiac, pulmonary, renal, or hepatic systems have specific nutritional requirements that must be addressed.

Nutrition for Cardiac Dysfunction

In general, cardiac nutrition maintains the basic premises of an oral diet, even though the patient may be receiving enteral nutrition or PN. Sodium restriction, less than 30% of calories from fat, and fluid status need to be addressed. In critical illness, fluid balance can contribute to acute changes in ejection fraction and cardiac performance, and nutrition is affected if volume is restricted. Concentrated tube feeding formulas and TPN solutions can be used. However, as patients recover, additional fluid may be needed. Careful monitoring of intake and output is required. Patient education regarding maintenance of sodium and water balance to prevent readmission is indicated.

Chronic changes of the myocardium can influence cardiac performance (Ansari, 1987; Webb et al., 1986). Decreased muscle mass, changes in myofibrils, edema, and even necrosis can limit the volume the heart can withstand. Nutritional therapy may need to be delivered within volume constraints. In the acute setting, providing the obligatory carbohydrate needs of approximately 150 to 200 g/day and providing protein at maintenance needs is recommended. In chronic conditions, attempting to meet metabolic demands without overfeeding is recommended. Should these patients be in the critical care unit for longer than 7 days, additional calories may need to be provided in an attempt to achieve positive nitrogen balance. If these patients are malnourished, repletion or correction of their underlying malnutrition will not be accomplished during their stay in critical care.

Nutrition for Pulmonary Dysfunction

Hunter and colleagues (1981) and Openbrier and associates (1983) have shown that respiratory dysfunction is associated with malnutrition. Rothkopf and coworkers (1989) demonstrated that pulmonary dysfunction can contribute to malnutrition. Chronic changes with chronic obstructive pulmonary disease (COPD) include decreases in transdiaphragmatic pressure, inspiratory force, tidal volume, and intercostal muscle strength. This can lead to increased infections, further increasing metabolic demands and contributing to malnutrition. Nutritional assessment in these patients reveals decreased weight for height, decreased skinfolds, decreased total lymphocyte count, normal serum albumin, and increased basal energy expenditure.

Goals of therapy in the acute setting include normalization of serum electrolytes, particularly phosphorus, but also magnesium and potassium, and providing adequate carbohydrate and protein. Askanazi and colleagues (1980) observed an increase in oxygen consumption and carbon dioxide production in hypermetabolic patients fed carbohydrates at one to one and one-half times the resting energy expenditure. This increases the stress on both the cardiac and the pulmonary systems. Based on the respiratory quotient alone, which is the ratio of carbon dioxide production to oxygen consumption during substrate utilization, a greater amount of fat calories could be provided to decrease the oxygen consumption and carbon dioxide production, and may assist with ventilatory weaning. This is based on stoichiometry in which the respiratory quotient of fat is 0.7 and that of carbohydrate is 1.0. Talpers and coworkers (1992) demonstrated that the total calories may be more important than the ratio of carbohydrate to fat contained within a product. The minute production of carbon dioxide was greater in patients who were overfed compared to patients fed a greater amount of carbohydrate. Therefore, hypercapnia may result during weaning in patients who are overfed. The key finding in these studies is the fact that patients were overfed. The respiratory quotient of lipogenesis (storage of carbohydrate as fat) is 8.0, which would increase oxygen consumption and carbon dioxide production. The importance of whether to feed increased amounts of fat compared to carbohydrate remains controversial. The efficacy of fat in preventing hypercapnia has not been shown. Should carbohydrate calories be reduced and fat calories increased in an attempt to wean and prevent hypercapnia, it should not be undertaken for long periods of time because fat may contribute to infections (Seidner et al., 1989). Should weaning fail, a return to a more normal caloric distribution is indicated.

Chronic pulmonary patients can become ventilator dependent. Nutrition is important in the ventilator-dependent patient because without nutritional support, weaning is almost impossible (Ireton et al., 1993). However, a host of factors contributes to successful weaning (Burns et al., 1991). Wilson and coworkers (1990) have demonstrated an increase in metabolic demands in COPD patients. However, feeding these patients at levels of approximately 1.7 times their basal energy expenditure may increase their work of breathing (Askanazi et al., 1980). A variety of products for pulmonary nutrition are available that are higher in fat content compared to carbohydrate. It is suggested, however, that more than 110 mg/kg/min of IV lipids may contribute to infection (Seidner et al., 1989).

Nutrition for Renal Dysfunction

Renal and hepatic dysfunction influence protein metabolism and subsequently alter nutritional therapy. Urea is synthesized by the liver from ammonia, and is the end product of protein metabolism. Urea is excreted by the kidney. Because of this, protein can be restricted in both renal and hepatic disease.

For acute renal failure, regardless of the cause (i.e., nephrotoxins or decreased perfusion), a protein restriction of approximately 0.5 g/kg is applied (Andris & Krzywda, 1994). Protein is reduced to preserve kidney function, but as the kidney recovers, protein can be increased. Should recovery not occur, and the patient is dialyzed, protein can be administered at 1.25 g/kg/day or more, depending on the patient's need and renal function.

Chronic renal failure patients maintained with dialysis therapy who become critically ill may require additional protein depending on their protein requirements. Acute renal failure superimposed on chronic renal insufficiency may require protein restriction initially and liberalization of the protein restriction as the patient tolerates. Once patients are committed to dialysis, protein need not be restricted. Should dialysis not be possible secondary to hemodynamic status, volume restriction and use of essential amino acids may be of benefit. The use of continuous arterial venous hemofiltration has allowed clinicians to control fluid volume status while providing maximal nutritional support.

Essential amino acids cannot be synthesized by the body, and daily ingestion is required. With exclusive provision of essential amino acids, the circulating urea pool is used to synthesize the nonessential amino acids (Schlichtig & Ayres, 1988). Essential amino acids provide twice the amount of protein per gram (i.e., 0.5 g of essential amino acids equals 1 g of protein). Essential amino acids are administered at 0.5 g/kg, and can be increased to meet the patient's needs as determined by urea kinetic modeling. This should not cause an increase in blood urea nitrogen; in fact, the blood urea nitrogen should decrease with use of essential amino acids (Schlichtig & Ayres, 1988). More than 2.0 g/kg/day of essential amino acids can induce encephalopathy secondary to an arginine deficiency. Often a mix of essential amino acids and protein is used.

A variety of products for renal failure are available. Complete or elemental products can be administered orally or via feeding tubes. These products also are calorically dense, thus decreasing the amount of free water in the formula. Parenteral products contain only the essential amino acids. Patients with critical illness may require as much as 1.5 to 2.0 g of protein per day in the presence of renal failure. This may be challenging to provide, but various nutritional interventions can assist with providing adequate nutrition during the treatment of renal failure. Nutrition should not be decreased or limited secondary to fluid volume restriction or electrolyte imbalances accompanying renal failure.

Nutrition for Hepatic Dysfunction

The liver is the body's primary metabolic organ. Alterations in the ability of the liver to metabolize various nutrients will readily be apparent. Therefore, special considerations must be given to providing nutrition to critically ill patients with hepatic dysfunction. The most common nutritional intervention for hepatic dysfunction is protein restriction. This is often ordered in liver disease regardless of the presence or absence of encephalopathy, and results in loss of protein mass and decreased protein synthesis. Protein needs to be restricted only in patients who are protein intolerant and who have encephalopathy (Burns et al., 1991).

In times of stress, skeletal muscle can metabolize branched-chain amino acids (BCAA), which theoretically can decrease the workload of the liver. There is some evidence to suggest that use of BCAA improves outcomes of patients with hepatic failure; however, more research is needed in this area.

Patients admitted to the critical care unit in hepatic failure with mental status changes should initially be protein restricted to approximately 0.5 to 0.8 g/kg/day of protein. Should mental status improve, protein may be increased while monitoring mental status and serum ammonia levels. Lactulose may also be added to maintain serum ammonia.

Chronic hepatic failure with protein intolerance evidenced by mental status changes requires protein restriction. Approximately 0.8 g/kg/day of protein is recommended. Protein, regardless of the source (GI bleeding, infection), can cause mental status changes. If patients have no protein intolerance, there is *no need for protein restriction,* and 1.0 to 1.2 g/kg/day of protein may be ingested by the patient. Additional protein may be required based on individual need.

Protein contributes to encephalopathy because the liver is not able to metabolize ammonia and synthesize urea. Monitoring of serum ammonia is often ordered, and arterial measurements are more accurate than venous measurements because of the amount of shunt that occurs in liver disease. It is important to correlate ammonia levels with mental status changes for each individual patient because ammonia levels do not directly correlate with mental status changes. Finally, when administering lactulose and protein, only one variable should be manipulated at a time. Increasing protein intake while maintaining lactulose therapy and noting the ammonia level and mental status is recommended. As ammonia decreases and mental status improves, the daily regimen of lactulose should be maintained and protein gradually added at approximately 10 g/day. If ammonia increases, the protein is maintained and the dose of lactulose is increased. Increasing lactulose and decreasing protein will be confounding. Lactulose therapy should produce four to six soft-formed bowel movements per day, while maintaining a mental status that allows daily functioning.

Several nutritional products are available for liver failure. Parenteral products include BCAA-enriched formulas and formulas which contain only the BCAA. The latter does not contain any other amino acid and is considered inadequate alone. It must be used in combination with other amino acids or essential amino acids.

The use of any specialty product requires close supervision. These products often contain minimal water and high concentrations of protein, lack vitamins and minerals, and can contribute to complications of nutritional support. Specialty products also are not meant for long-term use. As the patient improves, changing to standard enteral and parenteral products is indicated. Specialized nutritional support can increase the expense of enteral nutrition and PN by one- to twofold.

SUMMARY

There is much controversy surrounding all the facets of nutritional therapy, and conflicting data cloud the specifics of critical care nutrition. However, it is important to provide nutrition to the critically ill. Nutritional intervention based on a complete and thorough nutritional assessment that defines the degree of malnutrition and includes the concomitant medical problems is paramount to establishing a sound nutritional plan of care. The role of critical care nursing is to administer the therapeutic nutritional interventions and monitor the patient's response. The goal for all critically ill patients is to provide nutrients that meet protein, energy, and metabolic needs without negative consequence.

Proper nutrition does improve critically ill patient outcomes. Nurses are a critical link in initiating and maintaining nutritional therapy.

REFERENCES

Almond, D. J., King, R. F. G. J., Burkinshaw, L., Laughland, A., & McMahon, M. J. (1989). Influence of energy source upon body composition in patients receiving intravenous nutrition. *JPEN. Journal of Parenteral and Enteral Nutrition, 13,* 471–477.

American Society for Parenteral and Enteral Nutrition (ASPEN). (1993). Guidelines for the use of parenteral and enteral nutrition in adult and pediatric patients. *JPEN. Journal of Parenteral and Enteral Nutrition, 17,* 50SA–51SA.

Andris, D. A., & Krzywda, E. A. (1994). Nutrition support in specific diseases: Back to basics. *Nutrition in Clinical Practice, 9,* 28–32.

Angelillo, V. A., Sukhdarshan, B., Durfee, D., et al. (1985). Effects of low and high carbohydrate feedings in ambulatory patients with chronic obstructive pulmonary disease. *Annals of Internal Medicine, 103,* 883–885.

Ansari, A. (1987). Syndromes of cardiac cachexia and the cachectic heart: Current perspective. *Progress in Cardiovascular Diseases, 30,* 45–60.

Askanazi, J., Carpentier, Y. A., Elwyn, D. H., et al. (1980). Influence of total parenteral nutrition on fuel utilization in injury and sepsis. *Annals of Surgery, 191,* 40–46.

Bommarito, A. A., Heinzelmann, M. J., & Boysen, D. A. (1989). A new approach to the management of obstructed enteral feeding tubes. *Nutrition in Clinical Practice, 4,* 111–114.

Bowman, M., Eisenberg, P., Katz, B., & Metheny, N. (1989). Effect of tube-feeding osmolality on serum sodium levels. *Critical Care Nursing, 9,* 22–28.

Buchmiller, C. E., Kleiman-Wexler, R., Ephgrave, K. S., Booth, B., & Hensley, C. E. (1992). Liver dysfunction and energy source: Results of a randomized clinical trial. *JPEN. Journal of Parenteral and Enteral Nutrition, 17,* 301–306.

Burns, S. M., Fahey, S. A., Barton, D. M., & Slack, D. (1991). Weaning from mechanical ventilation: A method for assessment and planning. *AACN Clinical Issues, 2,* 372–389.

Clark-Christoff, N., Watters, V. A., Sparks, W., Snyder, P., & Grant, J. P. (1992). Use of triple lumen subclavian catheters for administration of total parenteral nutrition. *JPEN. Journal of Parenteral and Enteral Nutrition, 16,* 403–407.

Collier, P., Kudsk, K. A., Glezer, J., & Brown, R. O. (1994). Fiber-containing formula and needle catheter jejunostomies: A clinical evaluation. *Nutrition in Clinical Practice, 9,* 101–103.

Davis, J., & Sherer, K. (1994). *Applied nutrition and diet therapy for nurses.* Philadelphia: W. B. Saunders.

DeBiasse, M. A., & Wilmore, D. W. (1994). What is optimal nutritional support? *New Horizons, 2,* 122–130.

DeCou, J., Shorter, N. A., & Karl, S. R. (1993). Feeding Roux-en-y jejunostomy in the management of severely neurologically impaired children. *Journal of Pediatric Surgery, 28,* 1276–1280.

Dempsey, D. T., Mullen, J. L., & Buzby, G. P. (1988). The link between nutritional status and clinical outcome: Can nutritional intervention modify it? *American Journal of Clinical Nutrition, 47,* 352–356.

Eisenberg, P. (1993). Causes of diarrhea in tube-fed patients: A comprehensive approach to diagnosis and management. *Nutrition in Clinical Practice, 8,* 119–123.

Fagerman, K. E. (1992). Limiting bacterial contamination of enteral nutrient solutions: 6 year history with reduction of contamination at two institutions. *Nutrition in Clinical Practice, 7,* 31–36.

Fong, Y., & Pisters, P. W. T. (1994). Growth factors and the care of the injured patient. In G. P. Zaloga (Ed.), *Nutrition in critical care* (pp. 833–864). St. Louis: Mosby-Year Book.

Gauderer, M. W. L., Ponsky, J. L., & Izant, R. F. Jr. (1980). Gastrostomy without laparotomy: A percutaneous endoscopic technique. *Journal of Pediatric Surgery, 15,* 872–875.

Gauderer, M. W. L., & Stellato, T. A. (1986). Gastrostomies: Evolution, techniques, and complications. *Current Problems in Surgery, 23,* 657–719.

Gray, R. R., Ho, C. S., Yee, A., Montanera, W., & Jones, D. P. (1987). Direct percutaneous jejunostomy. *American Journal of Roentgenology, 149,* 931–932.

Guenter, P. A., Settle, G., Perlmutter, S., et al. (1991). Tube feeding-related diarrhea in the acutely ill patients. *JPEN. Journal of Parenteral and Enteral Nutrition, 15,* 277–280.

Harris, J. A., & Benedict, F. G. (1919). *A biometric study of basal metabolism in man.* Publication 279. Washington, DC: Carnegie Institute of Washington.

Hill, G. L., King, R. F. G. J., Smith, R. C., et al. (1979). Multi-element analysis of the living body by neutron activation analysis: Application to critically ill patients receiving intravenous nutrition. *British Journal of Surgery, 66,* 868–872.

Horowitz, H. W., Dworkin, D. M., Savrno, J. A., et al. (1990). Central catheter-related infections: Comparison of pulmonary artery catheters and triple-lumen catheters for the delivery of hyperalimentation in a critical care setting. *JPEN. Journal of Parenteral and Enteral Nutrition, 14,* 588–592.

Hunter, A. M. B., Carey, M. A., & Larsh, H. W. (1981). The nutritional status of patients with chronic obstructive pulmonary disease. *American Review of Respiratory Diseases, 124,* 376–381.

Hunter, D. C., Jaksic, T., Lewis, D., et al. (1988). Resting energy expenditure in the critically ill: Estimations versus measurement. *British Journal of Surgery, 75,* 875–878.

Ibáñez, J., Peñafiel, A., Raurich, J. M., et al. (1992). Gastroesophageal reflux in intubated patients receiving enteral nutrition: Effect of supine and semirecumbent positions. *JPEN. Journal of Parenteral and Enteral Nutrition, 16,* 419–422.

Ireton Jones, C. S., Borman, K. R., & Turner, W. W. (1993). Nutritional considerations in the management of ventilator-dependent patients. *Nutrition in Clinical Practice, 8,* 60–64.

Jacobs, S., Chang, R. W. S., Lee, B., & Bartlett, F. W. (1990). Continuous enteral feeding: A major cause of pneumonia among ventilated intensive care unit patients. *JPEN. Journal of Parenteral and Enteral Nutrition, 14,* 353–356.

Jeejeebhoy, K. N. (1994). How should we monitor nutritional support: Structure or function? *New Horizons, 2,* 131–135.

Jovanovic-Peterson, L., & Peterson, C. M. (1991, Spring). Prescribing insulin for patients on enteral and parenteral nutrition. *Diabetes Professional,* 15–18.

Kamal, G. D., Pfaller, M. A., Rempe, L. E., & Jebson, P. J. (1991). Reduced intravascular catheter infection by antibiotic bonding. *Journal of the American Medical Association, 266*(18), 2364–2368.

Kemp, L., Burge, J., Choban, P., et al. (1994). The effect of catheter type and site on infections in total parenteral nutrition patients. *JPEN. Journal of Parenteral and Enteral Nutrition, 18,* 71–74.

Klein, S., & Nealon, W. H. (1988). Hepatobiliary abnormalities associated with total parenteral nutrition. *Seminars in Liver Disease, 8,* 237–244.

Kohn, C., & Keithley, J. K. (1982). Techniques for evaluating and managing diarrhea in the tube-fed patient. *Nutrition in Clinical Practice, 2,* 250–257.

Koretz, R. L. (1994). Feeding controversies. In G. P. Zaloga (Ed.), *Nutrition in critical care* (pp. 283–296). St. Louis: Mosby-Year Book.

Lang, C. E., & Schulte, C. V. (1987). The adult patient in nutritional support. In C. E. Lang (Ed.), *Nutritional support in critical care.* Rockville, MD: Aspen Publishers.

Langkamp-Henken, B., Glezer, J. A., & Kudsk, K. A. (1992). Immunologic structure and function of the gastrointestinal tract. *Nutrition in Clinical Practice, 7,* 100–111.

Larsson, J., Lennmarken, C., Mårtensson, J., Sandstedt, S., & Vinnars, E. (1990). Nitrogen requirements in severely injured patients. *British Journal of Surgery, 77,* 413–416.

Long, C. L. (1979). Metabolic response to injury and illness: Estimation of energy and protein needs from indirect calorimetry and nitrogen balance. *JPEN. Journal of Parenteral and Enteral Nutrition, 3,* 452–456.

Makau, L., Talamini, M. A., & Stizmann, J. V. (1991). Risk factors for central venous catheter-related vascular erosions. *JPEN. Journal of Parenteral and Enteral Nutrition, 15,* 513–516.

Maki, D. G., Cobb, L., Garman, J. K., et al. (1988). An attachable silver-impregnated cuff for prevention of infection with central venous catheters: A prospective randomized multicenter trial. *American Journal of Medicine, 85,* 307–313.

Martin, L. F., Booth, F. V. M., Karlstadt, R. G., et al. (1993). Continuous intravenous cimetidine decreases stress-related upper gastrointestinal hemorrhage without promoting pneumonia. *Critical Care Medicine, 21,* 19–30.

McClave, S. A., & Snider, H. L. (1992). Use of indirect calorimetry in clinical nutrition. *Nutrition in Clinical Practice, 7,* 207–221.

McClave, S., Snider, H., & Lowen, C. (1992). Use of residual volume as a marker for enteral feeding intolerance: Prospective blinded comparison with physical examination and radiograph findings. *JPEN. Journal of Parenteral and Enteral Nutrition, 16,* 99–105.

McGinnis, C., & Matson, S. W. (1994). How to manage patients with a Roux-en-y jejunostomy. *American Journal of Nursing, 94,* 43–45.

McMahon, M. M., & Rizza, R. A. (1994). Diabetes mellitus. In G. P. Zaloga (Ed.), *Nutrition in critical care* (pp. 801–813). St. Louis: Mosby-Year Book.

Metheny, N. A., Eisenberg, P., & Spies, M. (1986). Aspiration pneumonia in patients fed through nasoenteral tubes. *Heart and Lung, 15,* 256–260.

Metheny, N. A., Reed, L., Wiersema, L., et al. (1993). Effectiveness of pH measurements in predicting feeding tube placement: An update. *Nursing Research, 42,* 324–331.

Metheny, N. (1993). Minimizing respiratory complications of nasoenteric tube feedings: State of the science. *Heart and Lung, 22,* 213–223.

Metheny, N., Eisenberg, P., & McSweeney, M. (1988). Effect of feeding tube properties and three irrigants on clogging rates. *Nursing Research, 37,* 165–169.

Mittal, R. K., Stewart, W. R., & Schirmer, B. D. (1992). Effect of a catheter in the pharynx on the frequency of transient lower esophageal sphincter relaxations. *Gastroenterology, 103,* 1236–1240.

Moe, G. (1991). Enteral feeding and infection in the immunocompromised patient. *Nutrition in Clinical Practice, 6,* 55–64.

Montecalvo, M. A., Steger, K. A., Farber, H. W., et al., The Critical Care Research Team. (1992). Nutritional outcome and pneumonia in critical care patients randomized to gastric versus jejunal tube feedings. *Critical Care Medicine, 20,* 1377–1387.

Moore, F. A., Moore, E. E., Jones, T. N., McCroskey, B. L., & Peterson, V. M. (1989). TEN versus TPN following major abdominal trauma: Reduced septic morbidity. *Journal of Trauma, 29,* 916–923.

Moore, J. G., Clemmer, T. P., Taylor, S., Bishop, A. L., & Maggio, S. (1992). Twenty-four-hour intragastric pH patterns in ICU patients on ranitidine. *Digestive Diseases and Sciences, 37,* 1802–1809.

Mutabagani, K. H., Townsend, M. C., & Arnold, M. W. (1994). PEG ileus. *Surgical Endoscopy, 8,* 694–697.

Norwood, S., Hajjar, G., & Jenkins, L. (1992). The influence of an attachable subcutaneous cuff for preventing triple lumen catheter infections in critically ill surgical and trauma patients. *Surgery, Gynecology and Obstetrics, 175,* 33–40.

Nussbaum, M. S., & Fischer, J. E. (1994). In G. P. Zaloga (Ed.), *Nutrition in critical care* (pp. 297–305). St. Louis: Mosby–Year Book.

Openbrier, D. R., Irwin, M. M., Rogers, R. M., et al. (1983). Nutritional status and lung function in patients with emphysema and chronic bronchitis. *Chest, 93,* 17–22.

Orr, M. E. (1992). Hyperglycemia during nutrition support. *Critical Care Nurse, 12,* 64–70.

Paradis, C., Spainier, A. H., Shizgal, H. M., et al. (1979). Total parenteral nutrition with lipid. *American Journal of Surgery, 135,* 164–171.

Paskin, D. L. (1989). Fluid, electrolyte and acid base balance. In A. Skipper (Ed.), *Dietitian's handbook of enteral and parenteral nutrition* (p. 21). Gaithersburg, MD: Aspen Publishers.

Patrick, J. (1977). Death during recovery from severe malnutrition and its possible relationship to sodium pump activity in the leukocyte. *British Medical Journal, 1,* 1051–1054.

Peters, A. L., & Davidson, M. B. (1992). Effects of various enteral feeding products on postprandial blood glucose response in patients with type I diabetes. *JPEN. Journal of Parenteral and Enteral Nutrition, 16,* 69–74.

Phillips, M. L. (1987). Enteral nutrition support in diabetes mellitus. *Nutrition in Clinical Practice, 2,* 152–154.

Pitkänen, O., Takala, J., Pöyhönen, M., & Kari, A. (1991). Nitrogen and energy balance in septic and injured intensive care patients: Response to parenteral nutrition. *Clinical Nutrition, 10,* 258–265.

Pitts, D. M., Kilo, K. A., & Pontious, S. L. (1993). Nutritional support for the patient with diabetes. *Critical Care Nursing Clinics of North America, 5*(1), 47–56.

Powell, K. S., Marcuard, S. P., Farrior, E. S., & Gallagher, M. L. (1993). Aspirating gastric residuals causes occlusion of small-bore feeding tubes. *JPEN. Journal of Parenteral and Enteral Nutrition, 17,* 243–246.

Pritchard, T. J., & Bloom, A. D. (1994). A technique of direct percutaneous jejunostomy tube placement. *Journal of the American College of Surgeons, 178,* 173–174.

Raymond, J. L., & Farjood, L. (1993). Adding fiber to enteral formulas: Yes or no? (Letter). *Journal of the American Dietetic Association, 93,* 527.

Rees, R. G. P., Payne-James, J. J., King, C., & Silk, D. B. A. (1988). Spontaneous transpyloric passage and performance of fine bore polyurethane feeding tubes: A controlled clinical trial. *JPEN. Journal of Parenteral and Enteral Nutrition, 12,* 469–472.

Rothkopf, M. M., Stanislaus, G., Haverstick, L., Kvetan, V., & Askanazi, J. (1989). Nutritional support in respiratory failure. *Nutrition in Clinical Practice, 4,* 166–172.

Ruddell, W. S., Axon, A. T., Findlay, J. M., Bartholomew, B. A., & Hill, M. J. (1980). Effect of cimetidine on the gastric bacterial flora. *Lancet, 1,* 672–674.

Schlichtig, R., & Ayres, S. M. (1988). *Nutritional support of the critically ill.* Chicago: Year Book Medical Publishers.

Schonheyder, F., Heilskov, N. C. S., & Oleson, K. (1954). Isotopic studies on the mechanism of negative nitrogen balance produced by immobilization. *Scandinavian Journal of Clinical and Laboratory Investigation, 6,* 178–188.

Seidner, D., Mascioli, E., Istfan, N. W., et al. (1989). Effects of long-chain triglyceride emulsions on reticuloendothelial system function in humans. *JPEN. Journal of Parenteral and Enteral Nutrition, 13,* 614–619.

Shaw, J. H. F., Wildbore, M., & Wolfe, R. R. (1987). Whole body protein kinetics in severely septic patients. *Annals of Surgery, 205,* 288–294.

Silberman, H. (1989). *Parenteral and enteral nutrition* (2nd ed.). Norwalk, CT: Appleton-Lange.

Silk, D. B. A., Rees, R. G., Keohane, P. P., & Attrill, H. (1987). Clinical efficacy and design changes of fine-bore nasogastric feeding tubes: A seven-year experience involving 809 intubations in 403 patients. *JPEN. Journal of Parenteral and Enteral Nutrition, 11,* 378–383.

Solomon, S. M., & Kirby, D. F. (1990). The refeeding syndrome: A review. *JPEN. Journal of Parenteral and Enteral Nutrition, 14,* 90–97.

Strong, R. M., Condon, S. C., Solinger, M. R., et al. (1992). Equal aspiration rates from postpylorus and intragastric-placed small-bore feeding tubes: A randomized, prospective study. *JPEN. Journal of Parenteral and Enteral Nutrition, 16,* 59–63.

Talpers, S. S., Romberger, D. J., Bunce, S. B., & Pingleton, S. K. (1992). Nutritionally associated increased carbon dioxide production. *Chest, 102,* 551–555.

Torres, A., Serra-Batles, J., Ros, E., et al. (1992). Pulmonary aspiration of gastric contents in patients receiving mechanical ventilation: The effect of body position. *Annals of Internal Medicine, 116,* 540–543.

Tuten, M. B., Wogt, S., Dasse, F., & Leider, Z. (1985). Utilization of prealbumin as a nutritional marker. *JPEN. Journal of Parenteral and Enteral Nutrition, 9,* 709–711.

Ugo, P. J., Mohler, P. A., & Wilson, G. L. (1992). Bedside postpyloric placement of weighted feeding tubes. *Nutrition in Clinical Practice, 7,* 284–287.

Vinik, A. I., & Jenkins, D. J. A. (1988). Dietary fiber in the management of diabetes. *Diabetes Care, 11,* 160–173.

Webb, J. G., Kiess, M. C., & Chan-Yan, C. C. (1986). Malnutrition and the heart. *Canadian Medical Association Journal, 135,* 753–758.

Williams, R. R., & Fuenning, C. R. (1991). Circulatory indirect calorimetry in the critically ill. *JPEN. Journal of Parenteral and Enteral Nutrition, 15,* 509–512.

Wilson, D. O., Donahoe, M., Rogers, R. M., & Pennock, B. (1990). Metabolic rate and weight loss in chronic obstructive lung disease. *JPEN. Journal of Parenteral and Enteral Nutrition, 14,* 7–11.

Patients With Gastrointestinal Bleeding

Susan D. Ruppert and DeAnn M. Englert

Throughout most of the gastrointestinal (GI) tract, the lumen of the gut is separated from the capillary blood supply only by a layer of epithelial cells. Any degree of injury to the epithelium may therefore cause bleeding. Blood loss can range in severity from chronic, intermittent, or nearly inconsequential bleeding to sudden-massive hemorrhage that may be life-threatening or fatal.

Acute upper GI bleeding is a common health problem that affects 50 to 150 people/100,000 population and results in 250,000 admissions at an annual cost of almost $1 billion (Henneman, 1992). Despite a number of recent advancements in diagnosis and treatment, the overall mortality rate associated with GI bleeding has remained 10% for the past several decades (Eckhauser et al., 1992). Most patients with moderate to severe upper GI bleeding, regardless of whether they are clinically stable at the time of initial presentation, are admitted to the critical care unit for observation, evaluation, and treatment. Many patients cease bleeding spontaneously. For those who do not, treatment is usually invasive and not always effective. Mortality is often disproportionately high in these individuals. Patients with esophageal varices and peptic ulcer disease must be carefully monitored because they have a propensity for future hemorrhagic episodes. Fortunately, there is a lower mortality rate among patients with lower GI bleeding because of basic and improved diagnostic techniques such as guaiac testing, arteriography, and colonoscopy. In either event, the patient with acute GI hemorrhage represents an urgent and challenging opportunity for the critical care nurse.

PATHOPHYSIOLOGY

General

Because copious blood loss rarely occurs in the midjejunal or ileal segments of the bowel, GI bleeding is usually classified as either upper or lower in origin. Upper GI bleeding, defined as a loss of blood from the GI system at a site above the ligament of Treitz at the duodenojejunal junction, accounts for 85% of all gastrointestinal bleeding episodes (Severance, 1986). Bleeding from a source below the ligament of Treitz is classified as lower GI bleeding.

The patient's presenting clinical signs may differentiate between an upper and a lower source of GI bleeding (Table 48–1). Upper GI bleeding is associated with hematemesis (vomiting of blood) or melena (passage of black, tarry stools), or both, whereas lower GI bleeding results in hematochezia (passage of bright red blood from the rectum). If bleeding is rapid and massive from an upper GI source, both hematemesis and hematochezia will certainly occur. Concomitantly, patients with substantial blood loss will have clinical evidence of hypovolemic hemorrhagic shock.

Blood in the GI tract below the level of the duodenum rarely enters the stomach. Thus, the patient who is vomiting blood or coffee-ground material is usually bleeding from a site in the upper GI tract somewhere above the ligament of Treitz. The nature of the vomited blood can vary from bright red to a coffee-ground color. Red blood, with or without clots, indicates a more recent or ongoing hemorrhage. Coffee-ground material may be present when blood that has accumulated in the stomach for a longer period of time is converted to acid hematin in the presence of gastric hydrochloric acid. Hematemesis may occur when as little as 100 mL of blood has been lost.

In passing through the GI tract, blood becomes progressively darker and eventually black. The change in color depends on the bleeding site, amount, rapidity of bleeding, and intestinal transit time. A transit time

TABLE 48–1. **Clinical Differentiation of Gastrointestinal (GI) Bleeding**

	Upper GI Bleeding	Lower GI Bleeding
Presenting Sign	***Hematemesis or Melena***	***Hematochezia***
Nasogastric aspirate	Positive for blood	Negative for blood
Bowel sounds	Hyperactive	Normal
Blood urea nitrogen	Elevated	Normal

of 8 hours is typically required for melena to appear. The patient will describe the bowel movement as a "black" stool that is somewhat "sticky," with a characteristic foul odor. Melena is usually seen when there is prolonged bleeding from the upper GI tract. As little as 50 to 100 mL of blood injected into the stomach can produce a melanotic stool. However, 400 to 500 mL is the usual amount necessary to produce melena consistently.

After an acute episode of blood loss of 1 liter, melena persists for 1 to 3 days. Although the patient's stools may then return to a normal color, occult blood may be guaiac positive for up to 12 days thereafter. Even when detected only by occult blood in the stool, GI bleeding always represents a potentially serious sign that must be investigated further.

Hemorrhagic Shock

Hemorrhagic or hypovolemic shock occurs when there is an acute loss of 15% to 20% of the circulatory blood volume (Porth, 1994). The clinical findings seen in patients with hypovolemic shock have been correlated with the magnitude of the volume deficit (Table 48–2).

There are four stages of hypovolemic shock as blood loss increases (Porth, 1994). Initially, the circulatory blood volume is decreased, but not enough to cause serious effects. During the second phase, compensatory mechanisms work to maintain blood pressure and tissue perfusion at levels sufficient to prevent cell damage. Unfavorable clinical changes become evident during the third or progressive stage. The blood pressure begins to fall, blood flow to the heart and brain is impaired, capillary permeability is increased, fluid begins to leave the capillaries, blood flow becomes sluggish, and body cells and their enzyme systems are injured. The fourth and final stage is irreversible. In this stage, death is imminent even though blood volume may have been temporarily restored and vital signs stabilized. Although the factors that determine recovery from severe shock have not been clearly identified, it appears that they may be related to blood flow at the level of the microcirculation.

Sudden loss of blood volume (hemorrhage) decreases venous return to the heart and thereby lowers cardiac output. After bleeding begins, the arterial baroreceptors note the decrease in blood pressure and signal a sympathetic response. The compensatory changes in heart rate, cardiac contractility, and vascular tone that develop in shock are mediated through the sympathetic nervous system. During the early stages, vasoconstriction causes a reduction in the size of the vascular compartment and an increase in peripheral vascular resistance. As blood loss increases, release of epinephrine and norepinephrine causes the alpha receptors in the skin, liver, lungs, intestines, and kidneys to constrict and the beta receptors in the striated muscle, heart, and brain to dilate. This reaction, a vascular response to decreased cardiac output and decreased right atrial pressure, shunts blood toward the cerebral and cardiopulmonary system. As vasoconstriction becomes more intense, heart rate and cardiac contractility increase. Decreased blood flow to the kidneys can then result in medullary tube dysfunction or acute tubular necrosis and renal failure. The organs of the GI tract can be equally affected, resulting in ischemia of the gut, liver, and pancreas.

Compensatory mechanisms to replace fluid lost from the vascular compartment also exist. During shock, the decline in capillary pressure causes water to be drawn into the vascular compartment from the interstitial spaces. Maintenance of vascular volume is further enhanced by renal mechanisms that conserve fluid. As renal blood flow decreases during vasoconstriction, there is a decrease in the glomerular filtration rate and an increase in the reabsorption of sodium and water due to activation of the renin–angiotensin–aldosterone mechanism. The decrease in blood volume also stimulates the centers in the hypothalamus that regulate antidiuretic hormone (ADH) release and thirst.

The decreased tissue perfusion associated with vasoconstriction also causes cellular dysfunction. The body cells attempt to extract oxygen from the available blood until this mechanism is no longer adequate. As cellular hypoxia becomes manifest, metabolism of glucose changes from an aerobic to an anaerobic process (Crawford, 1994). Energy production is decreased, and large quantities of lactic acid are produced. The depressed blood flow to the kidneys and liver impairs the ability of these systems to break down lactic acid or remove it from the bloodstream. The patient hyperventilates to exhale the waste products, but pulmonary circulation is also depressed. A profound metabolic acidosis develops as lactic acid accumulates.

TABLE 48–2. **Correlation of Clinical Findings and the Magnitude of Volume Deficit in Hemorrhagic Shock**

Severity of Shock	Clinical Findings	Estimated Blood (Loss mL)
None	None	500*
Mild	Minimal tachycardia (<110 bpm) Slight decrease in blood pressure Cool hands and feet	750–1,250
Moderate	Tachycardia (100–120 bpm) Decrease in pulse pressure Systolic pressure 90–100 mm Hg Restlessness Pallor Diaphoresis Oliguria	1,250–1,750
Severe	Tachycardia (≥120 bpm) Systolic pressure <90 mm Hg Mental stupor Extreme pallor Cold extremities Anuria	2,500

*Based on blood volume of 7% in a 70-kg man of medium build.

Adapted from Weil, M., & Shubin, H. (1967). *Diagnosis and treatment of shock* (p. 118). Baltimore: Williams & Wilkins. Copyright Max H. Weil, MD, PhD.

During hypovolemic shock, the hematopoietic system produces an increase in white blood cells and platelets. As the bone marrow is stimulated, red blood cell production and peripheral reticulocytosis result. Correction of abnormal hemoglobin can then occur naturally over a period of weeks after the hemorrhage.

When blood loss continues, cerebral blood flow becomes compromised. The patient may be confused at first, and these mental changes can progress to a loss of consciousness and brain damage. In patients with severe hypotension, there is decreased coronary perfusion while the shift of body fluids from the extravascular areas into the vascular space continues. Coronary blood flow insufficiency is detected by the presence of flattened T waves and ST-segment depression in the electrocardiogram.

Gastrointestinal hypoxia leads to decreased GI tract motility, venous congestion, edema, and small focal hemorrhages in the gut. Normal bacterial flora begin to release endotoxins in the absence of peristalsis. When circulation is decreased, normal colonic bacteria decompose and release ammonia. Metabolic wastes accumulate, and there is clumping and sludging of red blood cells in the microcirculation. This culminates in widespread microinfarctions, a condition known as disseminated intravascular coagulation (Porth, 1994). In prolonged shock, when all of the patient's clotting factors have been expended, there is a strong tendency for the patient to bleed even more.

CAUSES OF GASTROINTESTINAL HEMORRHAGE

The major causes of GI bleeding in the United States are summarized in Table 48–3 (Henneman, 1992). These various pathophysiologic conditions can be divided into upper GI and lower GI disturbances.

Upper Gastrointestinal Bleeding

Peptic ulcer disease (gastric and duodenal) is responsible for 45% of GI bleeding episodes. Duodenitis has been the cause of bleeding in 6% of patients, and the incidence of hemorrhage from esophageal varices is approximately 10%. Mallory-Weiss tears and esophagitis are seen in 13% of patients with upper GI bleeding (Henneman, 1992).

TABLE 48–3. **Major Causes of Gastrointestinal (GI) Hemorrhage in the United States**

Upper GI	Lower GI
Duodenal ulcer	Carcinoma of left colon
Erosive gastritis	Diverticular disease
Gastric ulcer	Inflammatory bowel disease
Esophageal varices	Polyps
Mallory-Weiss tears	Carcinoma of right colon
Esophagitis	Angiodysplasia of right colon
Duodenitis	

Adapted from Rosen, P. (1988). *Emergency medicine* (Vol. 2, pp. 1423, 1490). St. Louis: C. V. Mosby.

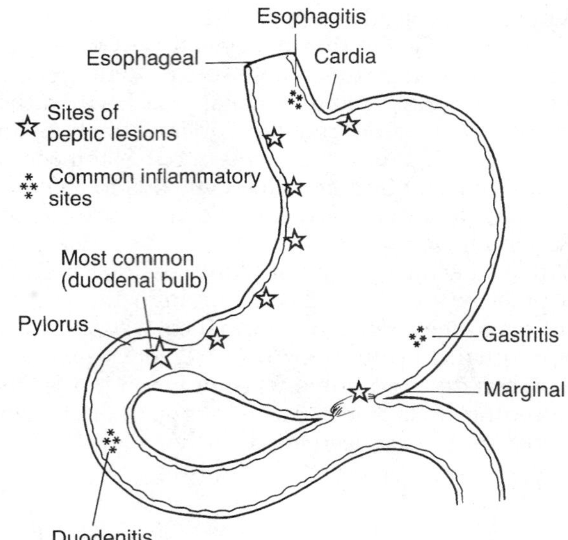

FIGURE 48–1. Upper gastrointestinal tract ulcer and inflammation sites.

PEPTIC ULCER DISEASE. An ulcer is defined as a loss of substance on a mucous surface causing a gradual disintegration and necrosis of the tissues extending below the musculous mucosae into the submucosa or deeper (Crawford, 1994). Peptic ulcers can occur in any area of the GI tract that is exposed to acid–pepsin secretions (Fig. 48–1).

Peptic ulcer disease is a common disorder; 5% to 10% of people will have peptic ulcer in their lifetime (Schiller, 1992). Men are affected three to four times as frequently as women. Duodenal ulcers make up 80% of peptic ulcers (Wilson & Lester, 1992). Duodenal ulcers occur at any age and are frequently seen in young adults, whereas gastric ulcers affect the older age group, with peak incidence occurring in the sixth to seventh decades (Wilson & Lester, 1992). Interestingly, duodenal ulcers seem to have a seasonal trend, with a higher incidence of recurrence in the spring and fall.

In general, it can be said that peptic ulcer formation reflects either an imbalance between acid and pepsin production or an inability of the affected mucosal layer to resist the destructive action of these digestive agents (Porth, 1994). Evidence suggests that hydrochloric acid may be the causative agent in duodenal ulcers, whereas decreased tissue resistance has a greater role in the genesis of gastric ulcers. Patients with gastric ulcers are known to have low hydrochloric acid secretion and a normal gastric emptying time. On the other hand, patients with duodenal ulcers have a high gastric acid secretion, a low pH in the duodenum, and an abnormal gastric emptying time. Patients with duodenal ulcers may have an increased vagal drive or a greater mass of parietal cells than is normally present. More often than not, a number of factors contribute to the development of a peptic ulcer.

Hydrochloric acid is influenced by a number of factors, including neural and hormonal stimulation. The hormone gastrin, which is produced in the antrum of the stomach, is a potent stimulus for the production of hydrochloric acid. Increased levels of gastric acid have also been attributed to (1) increased acid- or pepsin-producing cells in the stomach, (2) increased sensitivity of the parietal cells to food and other stimuli such as alcohol and caffeine, (3) excessive vagal stimulation, and (4) impaired inhibition of gastric secretions as food passes into the intestine. The intractable peptic ulcers associated with Zollinger-Ellison syndrome are caused by a gastrin-secreting tumor of the pancreas.

The defenses of the mucosal surface depend on an adequate blood flow and an intact mucosal barrier. Any disruption of the mucosal barrier therefore reduces these defenses and renders the mucosal surface more susceptible to injury.

It has been suggested that a basic abnormality in people with gastric peptic ulcers is an increased permeability of the epithelial layer of the stomach to hydrogen ions. Bile is known to disrupt the mucosal barrier, and reflux of bile from the intestine into the stomach has been implicated in the pathogenesis of peptic ulcer disease.

The duodenum, acting as a passageway for digestive enzymes and acid-laden chyme, is a common site of peptic ulcers. Brunner's glands, which are located between the pylorus and the site where bile and pancreatic enzymes enter the duodenum, produce copious amounts of viscid mucus, which serves to protect this area. Because the activity of these glands is inhibited by sympathetic stimulation, this may explain why anxiety and stress contribute to the development of duodenal ulcers.

More recent evidence suggests that *Helicobacter pylori*, a bacterium, may contribute to the development of peptic ulcers. Ninety percent of people with duodenal ulcer and 70% of individuals with gastric ulcer have been found to be colonized with this organism (Porth, 1994). This bacterium is thought to destroy the protective mucosal layer, leaving the mucosa susceptible to erosion.

Certain drugs may contribute to the development of GI ulceration, but the exact mechanisms for this are not clearly understood. Table 48–4 identifies some of these offending pharmacologic agents and the proposed action of injury that can lead to GI bleeding. Nonsteroidal antiinflammatory drugs (NSAIDs) such as indomethacin decrease mucosal resistance, are potentially ulcerogenic, and are contraindicated in patients with active or past ulcer disease. Caffeine, commonly contained in coffee, tea, and many soft drinks, stimulates acid production. Phenylbutazone impairs epithelial cell metabolism and makes these cells more susceptible to injury. Antimetabolites and other chemotherapeutic agents damage the nuclei and cytoplasm of both normal and neoplastic cells, inhibiting mitosis and mucosal regeneration. Alcohol stimulates acid production and produces gastric mucosal hemorrhages.

TABLE 48–4. **Pharmacologic Agents Associated With Gastrointestinal Bleeding**

Possible Mechanism of Injury	Drugs
Acid stimulation	Reserpine, caffeine
Decreased mucosal blood flow	Vasopressors
Hydrogen back-diffusion	Aspirin, alcohol, bile salts, cinchopen, indomethacin, phenylbutazone, corticosteroids
Decreased mucus secretion	Corticosteroids, phenylbutazone
Decreased cell renewal	Antineoplastic agents, corticosteroids, phenylbutazone

STRESS ULCERS. "Stress ulcer" is a nonspecific term that has been attached to a variety of gastric lesions and commonly refers to antral and duodenal ulcers. Changes in the mucosa can range from small petechial hemorrhages to deep ulceration with perforation. Endoscopic examinations have demonstrated that gastric erosions develop in up to 100% of critical care patients within a few hours of admission to the unit (Gottlieb et al., 1986).

The development of stress ulcers has been associated with such conditions as sepsis, shock, renal failure, hepatic failure, major trauma, adult respiratory distress syndrome, major operative procedures, and respiratory management using mechanical ventilation. In addition, burns and brain injury have been linked to ulcerative lesions. Curling's ulcers occur in patients who have sustained burns to 35% or more of the total body surface. This type of ulcer is thought to result from local ischemia. Decreased blood flow impairs mucus secretion and tends to make the mucosal surface less resistant to the damaging effects of hydrochloric acid. Cushing's ulcer is a special type of stress ulcer that is associated with severe brain injury, including brain tumors, lesions, and head trauma. It occurs when the vagus nerve is overstimulated by way of the central nervous system. Cushing's ulcers are usually deep and can occur anywhere along the GI tract.

The clinical diagnosis of stress ulcers may be difficult because patients may be asymptomatic. The onset of hemorrhage occurs typically between 2 and 10 days after the original insult. Once stress ulceration has produced significant hemorrhage requiring surgery, mortality usually exceeds 70% (Chamberlain & Peura, 1989).

Although the pathogenesis of stress ulcers is not completely understood, several mechanisms have been implicated. These mechanisms include mucosal

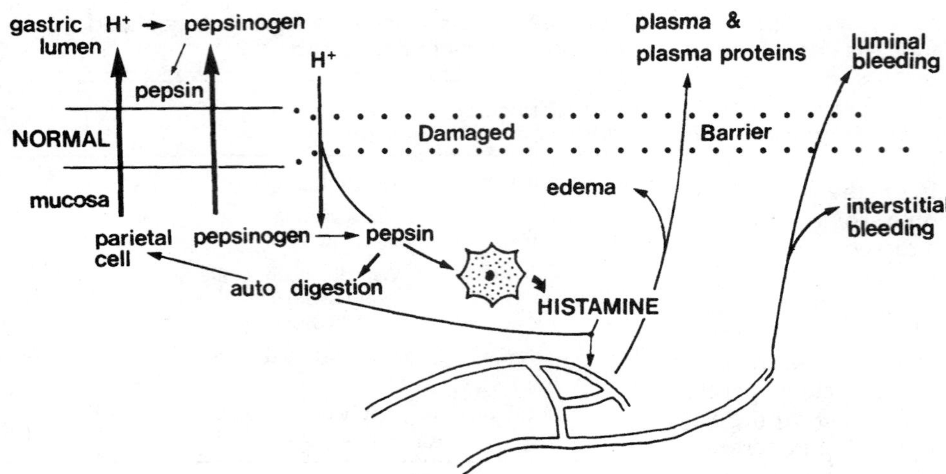

FIGURE 48–2. Pathophysiology of stress ulceration. (From Konopad, E., & Noseworthy, T. [1988]. Stress ulceration: A serious complication in critically ill patients. *Heart and Lung, 17,* 339–346.)

barrier breakdown, lowered intramural pH, decreased mucosal blood flow, increased acid secretion, decreased epithelial regeneration, and alteration in prostaglandin synthesis. The gastric mucosal barrier impedes the back-diffusion of hydrogen ions from the lumen into the interstitium. With barrier disruption, tissue damage results from the increase in permeability of the gastric mucosa to luminal hydrogen ions. Hydrogen ion back-diffusion leads to the formation of edema. The subsequent release of histamine, serotonin, and other vasoactive substances exaggerates the changes in permeability and increases acid secretion. When pepsinogen is activated, mucosal autodigestion occurs. In addition, the mucous–bicarbonate gastric barrier, which normally delays hydrogen ion back-diffusion and acts as a neutralizer, loses its ability to maintain a gradient when hypersecretion lowers the pH (DiPalma, 1992) (Fig. 48–2). Barrier breakers include such substances as bile salts, urea, NSAIDs, salicylates, ethanol, and corticosteroids.

Endocrine hormones such as adrenocorticotropic hormone and cortisone may alter the structure of the mucosa or the production of glycoprotein mucus that overlies the gastric epithelium. In addition, it is theorized that emotional stress may play a significant role in ulcer formation. Sympathetic stimuli cause constriction of blood vessels in the duodenum, thus making it more susceptible to trauma due to gastric acid and pepsin. Activation of the adrenal cortex during the stress state may impair mucous production and stimulate gastric secretion. There is also a reduction in epithelial restoration and cellular proliferation during stress.

Another causative factor implicated in stress ulcer formation is an alteration in the synthesis of prostaglandins E and I (PGE and PGI) in the stomach. A deficiency in these prostaglandins results in a thinner mucous layer. NSAIDs are a causative factor because they block the synthesis of PGE and PGI.

Management of stress ulcers is aimed at prevention by decreasing the underlying risk factors, identifying patients at high risk early, and decreasing the hydrogen ion concentration in the stomach. Treatment of existing stress ulcers is basically the same as that used for other forms of ulcer disease.

GASTRITIS. Acute erosive or hemorrhagic gastritis is a transient irritation of the gastric mucosa that usually appears regional or patchy in nature. Mucosal destruction, however, does not extend beyond the muscularis mucosae. The mucosa may be red and friable, or it may appear normal. Multiple bleeding lesions may be distributed throughout the gastric mucosa or may be localized to the fundus, body, or antrum of the stomach. Pathologic changes may include vascular congestion, edema, acute inflammatory cell infiltration, and degenerative changes in the epithelium. The surface epithelium becomes depleted of mucus, and blood extravasates into the lamina propria (McGuigan, 1994).

The seriousness of acute hemorrhagic gastritis cannot be overemphasized. Its onset may be precipitated by a single mucosal insult, which may be chemical, thermal, mechanical, bacterial, or viral in nature. Spontaneous remission may occur when the offending agent is removed. An acute, fulminating form of gastritis has been reported in patients with acquired immunodeficiency syndrome who have cytomegalovirus or opportunistic infections (Haeney, 1989). Drugs such as alcohol, salicylates, iodine, digitalis, chemotherapeutic agents, and chlortetracycline may cause gastritis. NSAIDs, phenylbutazone, cinchopin, caffeine, ferrous salts, ammonium chloride, and steroids are potentially caustic to the gastric mucosa. Reserpine in large doses stimulates gastric secretion by accentuating the vagal release of gastrin. The *H. pylori* bacterium has also been implicated as a cause of chronic gastritis. Uremia, shock, cirrhosis, severe stress, portal hypertension, and lesions of the central nervous system have been associated with erosive gastritis. Finally, certain foods such as tea, coffee, mustard, paprika, and cloves have the potential to precipitate a bleeding episode when an ulcer is present. Foods high in roughage and those at extreme temperatures may also be irritating to the mucosa.

The signs and symptoms of acute gastritis may vary according to the local irritant. For example, gastritis caused by infectious organisms such as the *Staphylococcus* species usually has an abrupt and violent onset with gastric distress and vomiting about 5 hours after the ingestion of a contaminated food source. Often, patients with aspirin-related gastritis are totally unaware of their condition or may complain only of heartburn. Gastritis associated with excessive alcohol consumption is a different situation. In these patients, transient gastric distress may lead to vomiting and, in more severe cases, to bleeding and hematemesis. Acute gastritis may be a self-limiting disorder, and complete regeneration and healing can occur within several days. It also can lead to major, life-threatening situations.

Chronic gastritis, a separate entity from acute gastritis, is characterized by progressive and irreversible atrophy of the glandular epithelium of the stomach. The pepsin-producing chief cells and the acid-producing parietal cells of the epithelial layer are atrophied in patients with chronic gastritis. There appear to be two forms of chronic gastritis. The more common form, referred to as simple atrophic gastritis, is seen in elderly people and those who drink or smoke heavily. Atrophic gastritis predisposes to gastric ulcer, pernicious anemia, and cancer of the stomach. The second form of the disorder, autoimmune atrophic gastritis, is thought to be caused by autoantibodies that destroy the gastric mucosal cells. Acid and pepsin secretion is thereby impaired. This retention of acid production in a mucosal surface that has impaired defenses predisposes the patient to peptic ulcer formation.

ESOPHAGEAL VARICES. A detailed description of the pathophysiology of bleeding esophageal varices is covered in Chapter 49.

MALLORY-WEISS TEARS. A Mallory-Weiss (MW) tear is defined as a longitudinal laceration in the cardioesophageal region (Peterson & Laine, 1994). This disorder may be related to prolonged retching and vomiting. It is sometimes seen in patients with anorexia nervosa. In other patients, increased abdominal pressure caused by severe coughing, straining, convulsions, trauma, or childbirth has been implicated. Frequently, MW tears occur in alcoholics. They are also associated with a hiatal hernia. About 49% of the tears are located at the gastroesophageal junction, whereas other tears may be found in the gastric mucosa and the esophagus (Spiro, 1993). The condition usually occurs suddenly and requires immediate treatment. MW tears are responsible for 11% to 13% of massive episodes of GI bleeding (Spiro, 1993).

Lower Gastrointestinal Bleeding

Lower GI bleeding results in fewer hospital admissions than upper GI bleeding. The ratio of patients with upper and lower GI bleeding depends on the patient mix at a specific hospital. For example, at Harbor-UCLA Medical Center, which is an urban county hospital, three to four patients with upper GI bleeds are admitted for every patient with lower GI bleeding. Both upper and lower GI bleeding stops spontaneously in 80% of admitted patients (Henneman, 1992).

The causes of lower GI bleeding vary with age. Significant lower GI bleeding is commonly found in elderly patients, usually due to diverticulosis or angiodysplasia. In young adults, massive lower GI bleeding is most commonly caused by ulcerative colitis. In children, significant blood loss from the colon is most often due to Meckel's diverticulum or intussusception (Henneman, 1992).

DIVERTICULOSIS. Diverticulosis occurs in about 49% of patients older than the age of 60 years, but significant hemorrhage develops in only 3% to 5%. The majority (75%) of bleeding from diverticula occurs in the right side of the colon (Henneman, 1992). It is thought that a lack of sufficient fiber content in the diet, a decrease in physical activity, poor bowel habits in which the urge to defecate is neglected, and the effects of aging are contributing factors to development of the disease. Diverticulosis is a condition in which herniation of the mucosal layer of the colon occurs through the muscularis layer (Porth, 1994). Most diverticula occur in the sigmoid colon. In the large intestine, the longitudinal muscle does not form a continuous layer but consists of three separate bands called the taeniae coli. It is between these muscles, in the area where the blood vessels pierce the circular muscle layer to carry blood to the mucosa, that diverticula develop.

An increase in intraluminal pressure provides the force creating these herniations. The greater pressure is thought to be related to the volume of the colonic contents. The more scanty the contents, the more vigorous the contractions, and the greater the pressure. When forceful contractions continue for a period of time, both the circular and longitudinal muscle layers hypertrophy. Sometimes the haustra may become so thick that they are approximated during contractions, causing a marked increase in the pressure within the isolated segment. According to the laws of physics, the pressure within a tube increases as its diameter decreases. The sigmoid colon, which was mentioned earlier as the segment most vulnerable to the development of diverticulosis, is the segment of the colon with the narrowest diameter.

VASCULAR ANOMALIES. Figure 48–3 outlines the normal arterial and venous blood supply to the organs of the alimentary tract. Vascular malformations, known as angiodysplasia, are an important cause of lower GI bleeding. Although they most often produce chronic or recurrent bleeding, these vascular malformations are responsible for up to 11% of cases of massive, recurrent lower GI bleeding (DiPalma, 1992). Angiodysplasias are most commonly found in the cecum and ascending colon, although they may be found in any part of the GI tract from the mouth to the rectum. Arte-

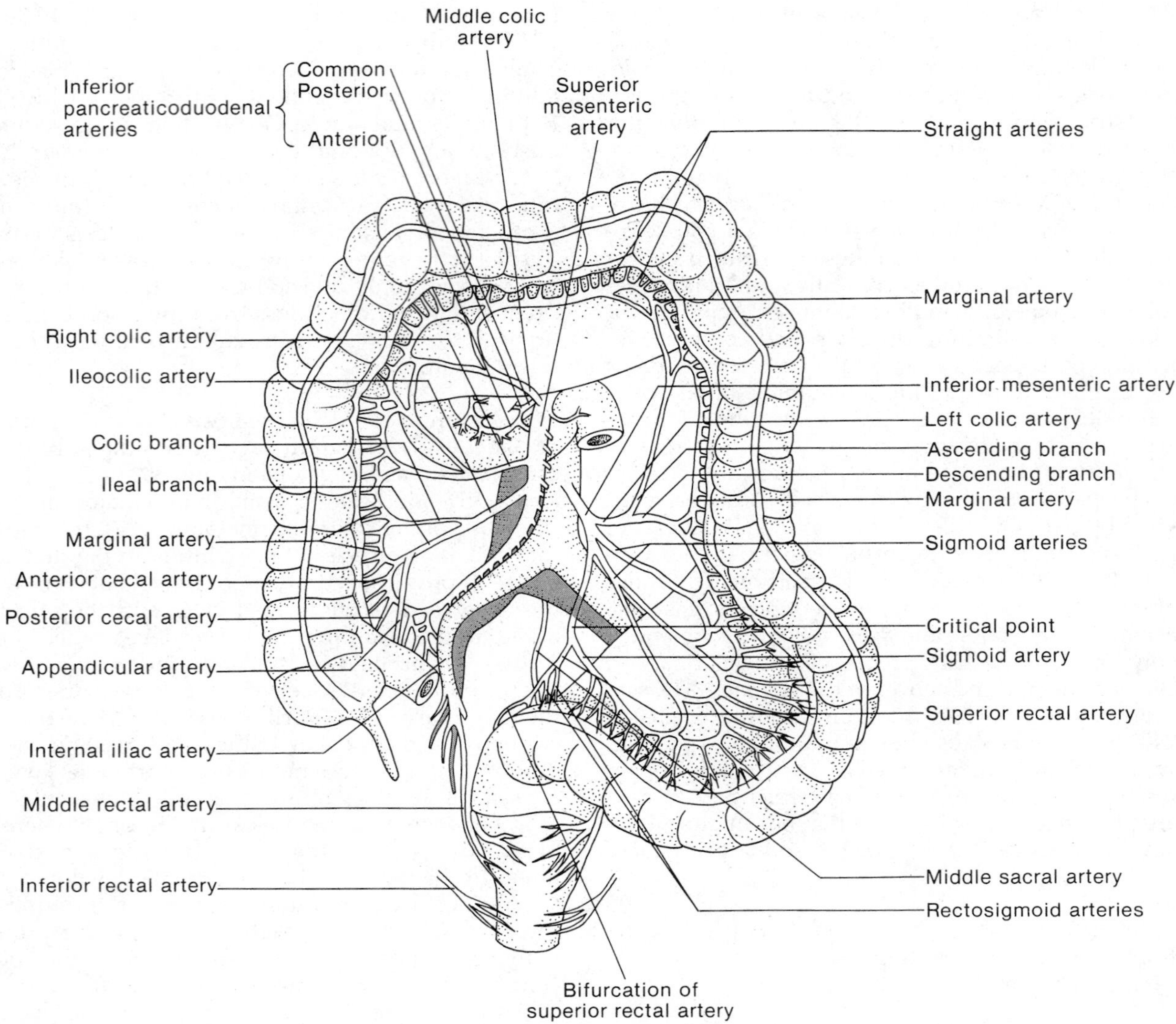

FIGURE 48–3. Arterial and venous blood supplies to primary and accessory organs of the alimentary canal.

riovenous malformations may be found in 25% of patients older than 60 years of age. Many authorities believe that angiodysplasia is at least as common a cause of bleeding as is diverticulosis (Henneman, 1992).

COLORECTAL CANCER. Colorectal cancer is the second most frequent cause of fatal malignancy in the United States today (Kafonek et al., 1988). Almost all cancers of the colon and rectum are carcinomas. Although the cause of cancer of the colon and rectum is unknown, its incidence increases with age, as evidenced by the fact that 95% of people in whom this type of malignancy develops are over age 50 (Porth, 1994). Its incidence is increased in people with a family history of cancer, in people with ulcerative colitis, and in those with familial polyposis of the colon.

Neoplasms do not often produce exsanguinating hemorrhage, but tend to present with chronic, occult bleeding or with intermittent bouts of acute, self-limited bleeding (Peterson & Laine, 1994). Usually cancer of the colon and rectum is present for a long period of time before it produces symptoms. Bleeding is a highly significant early symptom and usually prompts the patient to seek medical attention. Commercially prepared tests for detecting occult blood in the stool and colonoscopy are used to diagnose lower GI bleeding caused by cancer. The only recognized treatment for cancer of the colon and rectum is surgical removal of the tumor mass.

ULCERATIVE COLITIS. Ulcerative colitis is a nonspecific inflammatory condition of the colon affecting primarily the mucosa, although it can extend into the submucosal layer. The disease is relapsing and usually follows a course of remissions and exacerbations. The cause of ulcerative colitis is largely unknown, but certain features of the disease have suggested several areas of importance. These include familial or genetic, infectious, immunologic, and psychological factors (Glickman, 1994).

The inflammatory process tends to be confluent and continuous, causing pinpoint mucosal hemorrhages to appear. These bleeding sites may suppurate and develop into crypt abscesses. Although the ulcerations are usually superficial, they can extend to become large, denuded areas. Bloody diarrhea is always present during the fulminating form of the disease. Major complications of this disease include massive hemorrhage, perforation of the colon, and toxic megacolon (dilation and hypertrophy of the colon).

OTHER LESIONS. Hemorrhoids are probably the most common cause of lower GI bleeds, but with these, usually only small amounts of bright red blood are present on the outside of formed stools (Peterson & Laine, 1994). Anal fissures and hemorrhoids are the most common cause of rectal bleeding in children (most commonly before age 1 year), and adults, respectively. Anal disorders rarely result in significant blood loss (Henneman, 1992).

CLINICAL ASSESSMENT

History

It is often difficult or even impossible to elicit a complete nursing history in critically ill patients with upper GI hemorrhage. When the patient is incapable of providing this important information, the nurse may consult with family members or close friends who have some knowledge of the health history. Not only is the nursing history helpful in ascertaining the origin of the hemorrhage, but it provides a data base with which to monitor the patient's progress, reactions, and complications throughout hospitalization.

An accurate history is important in determining if presenting signs and symptoms are in fact due to GI bleeding. Emesis with red discoloration is often misinterpreted as "bloody" vomiting. Ingestion of beets, iron, charcoal, and bismuth-containing preparations gives the stool a dark red color or tarry appearance that is erroneously thought to be blood. Nosebleeds and hemorrhage secondary to recent oropharyngeal trauma have also been mistaken for GI bleeding.

Demographic data such as age, gender, and ethnic origin can be pertinent in patients with GI bleeds. For example, the incidence of gastric ulcers is twice as common in men as in women until menopause (Crawford, 1994). More than 50% of all bleeding patients are older than 60 years (Quigley, 1989). Ulcerative colitis has a high incidence among the Jewish population (Glickman, 1994).

The presence of pain with GI bleeding is diagnostic and should be thoroughly investigated during the nursing history. Pain is often suggestive of mucosal lesions associated with peptic ulcer, esophagitis, and gastritis. A history of gradually increasing epigastric pain that resolves with the onset of bleeding suggests a duodenal ulcer. Blood in the stomach acts as a buffer for gastric acid, and the pain resolves in much the same way as it does with the ingestion of antacids. Patients with erosive gastritis also may have epigastric distress. On the other hand, MW tears and bleeding from esophageal varices are almost always painless. Whenever possible, the critical care nurse should ask the patient to describe (1) the location of the pain, (2) its radiation or extent, (3) the quality of the discomfort, (4) its quantity or frequency, (5) factors that alleviate or aggravate the distress, (6) its timing and patterns, and (7) the setting in which it occurs.

A careful history of the patient's medications and alcohol intake can be of great value. For instance, there is a high association between erosive gastritis and aspirin or alcohol intake. Besides predisposing to gastritis, alcohol causes an increase in gastric acid production. Alcohol-induced cirrhosis is the most common cause of esophageal varices in the United States. Also, alcohol ingestion is present in 75% of patients with MW tears (Henneman, 1992). A detailed history concerning ingestion of over-the-counter drugs may be beneficial in identifying how much aspirin the patient has actually ingested, because many of these preparations contain aspirin.

A history of vomiting preceding the onset of bleeding is present in at least 50% of patients with MW tears (Henneman, 1992). Chronic weight loss is reported in patients with malignancy and mesenteric vascular insufficiency. A previous history of dysphagia suggests esophageal carcinoma or reflux esophagitis and may indicate a possible bleeding site. Questions should be geared to screen for a history of bleeding disorders and blood dyscrasias. A history of previous GI bleeding is helpful but can also be misleading. Forty percent of hemorrhaging patients who have a known lesion in the upper GI tract, for example, are actually bleeding from a different site (Henneman, 1992).

Physical Examination

An extensive physical examination is not always possible in patients with massive upper GI bleeding, nor should it ever take precedence over the immediate treatment of shock. Clinical manifestations of GI bleeding depend on volume of blood loss, rate of bleeding, associated diseases, and extent of cardiovascular compensation. Unless anemia is present before the onset of bleeding, loss of less than 500 mL of blood is not usually associated with signs or symptoms (Bogoch, 1985).

The vital signs are crucial in evaluating the patient's clinical condition at the time of the initial examination. A body temperature elevation may occur within 24 hours of GI hemorrhage. This temperature elevation may persist for several days to weeks (Porth, 1994). The presence of hypothermia is ominous in patients with GI hemorrhage and suggests severe shock. Pulse and blood pressure are key indices in the evaluation of the patient's hemodynamic status. Following the trend in pulse pressure, which indirectly reflects stroke volume, is one of the simplest ways to predict or diagnose hypovolemia. A narrowing pulse pressure is seen in an advancing shock state. The patient's pulse may be increased from 100 to 120 beats/minute, even when blood pressure remains normal. Of course, the pulse may be an unreliable indicator in certain cases, especially in people accustomed to vigorous sports and in those taking medications, such as digitalis or propranolol, that prevent an increase in heart rate.

Orthostatic changes in blood pressure can be diagnostic in bleeding patients. A systolic blood pressure drop of greater than 20 mm Hg, a diastolic blood pressure drop of greater than 10 mm Hg, and a pulse increase of greater than 20 beats/minute indicate a major blood loss (DiPalma, 1992). The presence of a "normal" blood pressure in a patient with other signs of clinical shock does not necessarily indicate a stable hemodynamic status. The patient may experience tachycardia, a thready peripheral pulse, and an increased respiratory rate in response to lactic acidosis.

The skin should always be examined in patients with upper GI hemorrhage. The skin may be pale, cool, and clammy with or without peripheral cyanosis. These changes, which indicate the presence of shock, represent a sympathetic response to hypovolemia. Petechial and purpuric lesions may signal blood dyscrasias as the cause of bleeding. In patients with cirrhotic liver disease, the nurse may discover ecchymoses, spider angiomas, palmar erythema, and jaundice while inspecting the skin.

An abdominal examination is also relevant in bleeding patients. The size of the liver and spleen is assessed by palpation, even though the spleen cannot be palpated until it is at least two to three times its normal size. Splenomegaly suggests the presence of portal hypertension. Hepatomegaly may be found in patients with malignancy and those with Laennec's cirrhosis or acute hepatitis. The patient with gastritis or peptic ulcer disease may experience epigastric pain during palpation.

Bowel sounds are auscultated during the physical examination. Bowel sounds are typically hyperactive in patients with upper GI bleeding, whereas hypoactive or normal bowel sounds are more commonly heard in patients with lower GI bleeding (Peterson & Laine, 1994). Blood is a potent cathartic that stimulates peristalsis. Decreased or absent bowel sounds in a patient with upper GI bleeding raise the question of whether there is a perforated bowel or intestinal ileus.

Diagnostic Procedures

LABORATORY. A complete blood count is obtained immediately in all patients with acute upper GI hemorrhage, and the hematocrit and hemoglobin are monitored serially to follow the clinical course of the bleeding and the extent of blood loss. In patients with chronic blood losses, the initial values may be low and do not accurately reflect an acute blood loss in the differential diagnosis. This information must be considered to avoid erroneous interpretations during subsequent laboratory studies.

After an acute episode of GI hemorrhage, 24 to 72 hours may elapse before the hematocrit reflects the true extent of the blood loss (Peterson & Laine, 1994). A normal hematocrit in a patient with active GI bleeding does not imply that the blood loss is not extensive. On the contrary, a normal or high hematocrit in the presence of severe hemorrhage suggests that the blood loss has occurred too rapidly to allow for equilibrium of the hematocrit by dilution. A low hematocrit, on the contrary, suggests that the blood loss has occurred at a much slower rate, allowing some equilibrium to occur, or that an acute bleeding episode has been superimposed on a chronic bleeding condition. Blood urea nitrogen (BUN) is frequently elevated in GI bleeding above the level of the colon due to the breakdown of blood by digestive enzymes with resultant nitrogenous end-products. Table 48–5 summarizes the pertinent changes in laboratory values that may occur during GI hemorrhage. The patient's blood values are carefully considered along with the history, physical examination, and other diagnostic findings.

NASOGASTRIC INTUBATION. Passing a nasogastric (NG) tube to obtain gastric aspirate will confirm active bleeding in the upper GI system. NG intubation is indicated in patients with melena or hematochezia and in those reporting bloody emesis. If no blood is present in the aspirated contents, it can be assumed that there is no active bleeding from the distal duodenum. If no blood is present initially, the NG tube is left in place to empty the stomach and aspirate bilious material. Some clinicians do not use NG intubation when esophageal varices are suspected because irritation from the tube may precipitate bleeding episodes.

ENDOSCOPY. Endoscopy is considered the diagnostic test of choice in most patients with persistent bleeding. This study can detect 78% to 95% of bleeding lesions in the upper GI system (Henneman, 1992). For upper GI endoscopy, a flexible tube is passed through the mouth into the stomach and duodenum to allow complete examination of the mucosal lining. Proctosigmoidoscopy allows visualization of the distal sigmoid colon, the rectum, and the anal canal. If a flexible sigmoidoscope is used, the descending colon can also be seen. Colonoscopy is performed to examine the lining of the large intestine, using a flexible endoscope inserted anally. Endoscopic procedures enable the gastroenterologist performing the procedure to remove tissue specimens for microscopic examination or to control localized bleeding.

GUAIAC TESTING. The presence of occult blood should be confirmed in patients without melena or hematochezia whenever GI blood loss is suspected. Because some medications and food products may simulate melena, the stool should always be tested for

TABLE 48–5. **Changes in Laboratory Indices During Gastrointestinal Hemorrhage**

Laboratory Index	Change	Comment
Hematocrit	↑ or ↓	Results can be misleading (see text)
White blood cell count	↑ Up to 40,000 cells/mm^3	Cause of leukocytosis is unknown. White blood cell count usually returns within normal range 24 to 48 hours after bleeding stops
Platelet count	↑ Sometimes within 1 hour after bleeding begins	Thrombocytosis may be absent in patients with bone marrow suppression or cirrhosis
Reticulocyte count	↑	Reticulocytosis is found within 24 hours after bleeding begins and may persist for 14 days after bleeding stops
Mean corpuscular volume	↓ Or within normal limits	Decreased levels suggest chronic bleeding
Hypochromic microcytic red blood cells	↓ Or absent	Presence indicates chronic blood loss
Blood urea nitrogen	↑ As high as 80 mg/dL in patients who otherwise have normal renal function	Usually begins to fall 12 hours after bleeding stops
Sodium	Within normal limits or ↑ in dehydration	Low levels may indicate hemodilution or chronic blood loss

the presence of blood. False-negative results may occur in patients who are taking vitamin C or magnesium-containing antacids. False-positive results may occur after ingestion of iron preparations or red meats, or from methylene blue (Henneman, 1992).

ELECTROCARDIOGRAPHY. An electrocardiogram is necessary in all elderly patients with GI bleeding and those with significant anemia (Henneman, 1992). In shock states, low voltage is usually present because of decreased central vascular volume. Although ischemic changes in the anterolateral precordial leads are common in patients with hypovolemic shock, these usually resolve spontaneously after adequate fluid resuscitation. Persistence of an ischemic state 24 to 36 hours after the bleeding episode suggests myocardial infarction. Of course, patients who have had abnormal electrocardiographic results before the hemorrhage must be carefully evaluated according to their previous history. In general, the incidence of myocardial infarction with upper GI bleeding is 1% to 2% (Palmer, 1992). Most of these myocardial infarctions, which may be subendocardial or transmural, are "silent" and are not manifested in the usual manner by substernal pain.

CHEST AND ABDOMINAL FILMS. Chest radiographs and supine and upright abdominal films may be obtained to rule out perforation, masses, bowel obstruction, and signs of mesenteric vascular ischemia. If a central venous catheter has been placed for fluid replacement, the anteroposterior chest x-ray will enable the physician to confirm placement of the tip of the cannula in a central location. These large-bore catheters are placed in critically ill patients with profound blood loss when the patient's survival may depend on the rapidity of fluid replacement.

ANGIOGRAPHIC THERAPY. When GI bleeding is so brisk that it is impossible to perform endoscopy, selective mesenteric arteriography will localize the site of bleeding and in some instances determine whether the lesion is a diverticulum, vascular anomaly, cancer, or peptic ulcer. Angiographic studies using intraarterial infusion of vasopressin or occlusion of the bleeding artery with embolic agents may be used in patients with bleeding ulcers. Intraarterial vasopressin is successful in 50% or less of cases, whereas embolization has a better chance of success (Peterson & Laine, 1994).

BARIUM RADIOGRAPHS (UPPER GI SERIES AND BARIUM ENEMA). Barium radiographs are not usually the diagnostic procedure of choice, especially in patients with acute active bleeding, due to the patient's vomiting and unstable condition. Double-contrast barium x-rays are more diagnostic than single-contrast x-rays for determining the bleeding site; however, both are less accurate than endoscopy. Furthermore, the ability to visualize the lesion on radiographs does not necessarily confirm that it is bleeding. MW lacerations are not seen well with x-ray (Peterson & Laine, 1994). When barium studies are done, endoscopy has to be postponed temporarily because the presence of barium precludes accurate endoscopic results.

CLINICAL MANAGEMENT OF GASTROINTESTINAL BLEEDING

The goals for immediate treatment of GI bleeding include (1) stabilizing the patient's condition, (2) identifying the source of the bleeding, (3) stopping the bleeding, and (4) initiating treatment to prevent further bleeding. Of patients with acute upper GI bleeding,

70% will stop spontaneously regardless of treatment (DiPalma, 1992). However, 25% will rebleed during the hospitalization, and 10% will die. Accurate assessment and vigorous treatment are required until the patient has been successfully stabilized.

Fluid Replacment

Depending on the magnitude of blood loss, the primary nursing objective is volume replacement. One or more large-bore intravenous devices are started, and crystalloid solutions such as normal saline and Ringer's lactate are infused to replace volume during the initial phase of fluid resuscitation. A central venous pressure cannula or pulmonary artery catheter may be placed to achieve rapid fluid replacement and closer hemodynamic monitoring. Blood samples are obtained for complete blood count, clotting studies, type and cross-match, BUN, serum electrolytes, creatinine, and blood glucose levels. An arterial line may be placed to monitor blood pressure and arterial blood gases.

Blood products may be necessary depending on the estimated amount of blood loss. Estimated losses of 20% or more necessitate replacement with blood to restore oxygen transport. In the hemodynamically unstable patient, saline or lactated Ringer's solution should be infused as rapidly as the cardiopulmonary system will allow to correct the abnormalities in the patient's vital signs. A good rule of thumb is to replace vascular volume as quickly as it was lost. Patients whose bleeding has ceased require predominantly red blood cells. Blood products are used to improve systemic oxygen delivery (with red blood cells) or improve coagulation (with plasma or platelets). Albumin or plasmanate may also be used as volume expanders. Fresh frozen plasma or platelets should be given only if a patient requires more than 10 or more units of blood (Peterson & Laine, 1994). Massive transfusion with 10 or more units necessitates administration of platelets (Peterson & Laine, 1994). Hematocrit and hemoglobin are monitored at least every 2 to 4 hours initially. With hydration, each unit of packed red blood cells increases the hematocrit by approximately 4% and the hemoglobin by 1 g.

The patient must be carefully monitored for complications during massive transfusion therapy (Table 48–6). Hyperkalemia may occur if the aging red blood cells release potassium in the banked blood. Hypocalcemia results when ionized calcium in the banked blood binds to the citrate derivative used as a preservative and anticoagulant. Preservatives in large amounts can also decrease the oxygen-carrying capacity of the blood. Supplemental oxygen is used, and oxygen saturations are monitored until the patient is stabilized. Microaggregate filters may be used for blood administration.

During high-volume fluid replacement therapy, the critcal care nurse observes the patient carefully for signs and symptoms of fluid overload. Hemodynamic indices are monitored as well as physical signs and symptoms such as dyspnea, neck vein distention, and rales. An indwelling urinary catheter is inserted, and hourly urine outputs are measured as an index of volume replacement and renal perfusion.

TABLE 48–6. **Complications of Massive Blood Transfusions**

Complication	Mechanism
Hyperkalemia	Due to release of potassium from breakdown of aging RBCs in stored blood
Hypocalcemia	Due to binding of ionized calcium in stored blood with the preservative citrate–phosphate–dextrose
Hypothermia	Due to rapid administration of large amounts of cold blood
Circulatory overload	Due to infusion of large fluid volumes
Metabolic acidosis	Due to acidity that gradually occurs in stored blood
Decreased tissue oxygenation	Due to a decrease in 2,3-diphosphoglycerate in stored blood, which results in a left shift on the oxyhemoglobin dissociation curve (impaired oxygen transfer at tissue level)
Infections	Due to risk of exposure to hepatitis, AIDS, and other infections despite increased processing precautions
Coagulopathies	Due to a decrease in clotting components because packed RBC infusions do not contain plasma or platelets
Disseminated intravascular coagulation	Due to release of a thromboplastin-like substance from RBCs during hemolysis and the antigen–antibody complex as seen in transfusion reactions
Febrile transfusion reactions	Due to formation of antileukocyte antibodies after previous transfusions
Adult respiratory distress syndrome	Thought to be due to aggregation of microemboli in the pulmonary system from transfusions

Abbreviations: AIDS, acquired immunodeficiency syndrome; RBCs, red blood cells.

NASOGASTRIC INTUBATION OR LAVAGE

A large-bore NG tube is inserted to obtain a gastric specimen for occult blood testing and to clear the stomach for endoscopic examination. After confirmation of upper GI bleeding, the tube remains indwelling to evacuate blood from the stomach. An Ewald tube in which additional side holes have been cut is sometimes used to remove large clots. It is very important to remove as much clot and intragastric material as possible because emptying the stomach allows its walls to collapse, contributing to hemostasis and helping to prevent vomiting and aspiration.

Lavaging the stomach with iced saline has long

been used to stop upper GI bleeding. However, the efficacy of this practice has never been firmly established (Tobin, 1989). Some evidence suggests that iced saline may actually damage the stomach's mucosa and promote bleeding (Dworken, 1989). The use of vasoconstrictors in lavage fluid also has not been proved to be effective. Either room temperature saline or tap water may be used for lavage. Lavage is done to cleanse the stomach for endoscopy and provide an indication of the rapidity of bleeding. Procedurally, 500 to 1,000 mL of fluid is instilled and then removed by gravity drainage or gentle suction. As much as 10 liters may be necessary for optimal results.

The duration of NG intubation varies according to the patient's condition. After the patient's condition is stabilized, the tube can be used for instilling antacids and for obtaining gastric aspirate for pH testing. Newer NG tubes are now available that contain a disposable electrode for continuous and more accurate pH monitoring. When the use of the tube becomes unimportant, it should be removed. Besides being uncomfortable, prolonged NG intubation may predispose the patient to gastroesophageal reflux and esophagitis.

Pharmacologic Therapy

HISTAMINE RECEPTOR ANTAGONISTS. Histamine (H_2) receptor antagonists (cimetidine, ranitidine, famotidine, nizatidine) competitively inhibit the action of histamine on the H_2 receptors of parietal cells, thus reducing gastric acid output and concentration. Some studies indicate that H_2 antagonists may be effective for the treatment of stress ulcers and GI bleeding when hemorrhage is not caused by the erosion of major blood vessels (Quigley, 1989).

Side effects of H_2 receptor antagonists include confusion, lethargy, seizures, hypotension, hepatotoxicity, thrombocytopenia, gynecomastia, and male impotence. Because of its binding with the hepatic cytochrome P-450 enzyme, cimetidine reduces the clearance of drugs such as warfarin, phenytoin, theophylline, propanolol, and the benzodiazepines (Morgan, 1993). This does not occur with other H_2 receptor antagonists. The usual intravenous or oral dose of cimetidine is 300 mg four times daily. Ranitidine can be given at a dosage of 150 mg twice daily to obtain the same effect. For the critically ill patient, a constant infusion of ranitidine has been shown to provide better pH control than bolus infusions (Ballestros et al., 1990). Because antacids may interfere with the oral absorption of ranitidine, administration of the drug and antacids should be separated by 1 hour. Nizatidine can be given at a dosage of 300 mg at bedtime or 150 mg twice daily. Maintenance dosage is 150 mg at bedtime. Famotidine 40 mg orally at bedtime is recommended for use in patients with an active duodenal ulcer or pathologic hypersecretory conditions. During acute situations, the drug can be given at a dosage of 20 mg IV orally every 12 hours.

ANTACIDS. Antacids are the common pharmacologic agents used to treat upper GI bleeding (Table 48–7). Antacids are inorganic salts that dissolve in gastric acid secretions, releasing anions that partially neutralize gastric hydrochloric acid. The clinical use of antacids is based on their ability to increase the pH of gastric acid secretions.

There are four major classifications of antacids. They are, in decreasing order of their ability to neutralize gastric acids, calcium carbonate, sodium bicarbonate, magnesium hydroxide, and aluminum hydroxide. Although aluminum hydroxide antacids usually do not raise the gastric pH above 5, magnesium hydroxide can increase the gastric pH above 9 (Thompson & Mahachai, 1985). Although antacids do not usually neutralize all gastric acids, increasing the gastric pH from 1.3 to 2.3 neutralizes 90%, and raising the pH to 3.3 neutralizes 99%. Consequently, the amount of gastric acid back-diffusing through the gastric mucosa and reaching the duodenum is decreased.

Although generally uncommon, some side effects are associated with the chronic use of antacids. All antacids promote some degree of metabolic alkalosis. Because of its high propensity for this, as well as its high sodium content, sodium bicarbonate is not commonly used for antacid effect. Calcium carbonate is not usually prescribed because it may produce hypercalcemia and impair renal function. Aluminum-containing antacids are known to cause constipation, whereas magnesium-containing antacids may produce diarrhea. To avoid these undesirable colonic effects and to balance the neutralizing effects, many commercially prepared antacids are combinations of aluminum and magnesium compounds. Aluminum-containing antacids may occasionally contribute to phosphate depletion. Magnesium-containing antacids may cause hypermagnesemia, but this is rare and occurs primarily in patients with impaired renal function. Amphogel, composed only of aluminum hydroxide, can be used for patients in renal failure to help control hyperphosphatemia.

In the management of patients with GI bleeding, antacids may be administered to maintain gastric pH around 3.5. A greater increase in pH is unnecessary and can trigger acid rebound (Shlafer, 1994). In some patients, treatment may require the use of both H_2 receptor antagonists and antacids for adequate results. Doses of H_2 antagonists and antacids should be staggered to allow for maximum absorption when both are administered orally.

The use of antacids for critically ill patients is decreasing due to the high volume load and need to monitor gastric pH.

SULCRALFATE. Sucralfate, an ionic, sulfated disaccharide, is an inhibitor of pepsin and an antiulcer agent. The exact mechanism of its pharmacologic action is unclear, but the therapeutic effects of the drug are the results of local rather than systemic activity. It does not appreciably affect gastric acid output or concentration.

TABLE 48–7. **Compositions of Commonly Used Antacids (mg/30 mL)**

Name	Aluminum Hydroxide	Magnesium Hydroxide	Other	Sodium	Acid-Neutralizing Capacity (mEq/30 mL	GI Effects
ALternaGEL*	3,600	—	—	<15	96	Constipation
Amphojel†	1,920	—	—	<13.8	60	Constipation
Gelusil‡	1,200	1,200	Simethicone (150 mg)	4.2	72	Constipation or diarrhea
Maalox§	1,200	1,200	—	8.4	79.8	Constipation or diarrhea
Maalox TC§	3,600	1,800	—	4.8	163.2	Constipation or mild diarrhea
Mylanta*	1,200	1,200	Simethicone (120 mg)	4.1	76.2	Constipation or diarrhea
Mylanta II*	2,400	2,400	Simethicone (180 mg)	7.8	152.4	Constipation or diarrhea
Riopan‖	—	—	Magaldrate (3,240 mg)	0.6	90	Mild constipation or diarrhea
Basaljel†	—	—	Aluminum carbonate (2,400 mg, equivalent to aluminum hydroxide)	17.4	72	Constipation

*Stuart Pharmaceuticals, Wilmington, DE.
†Wyeth Laboratories, Philadelphia, PA.
‡Parke-Davis, Morris Plains, NJ.
§Rorer Consumer Pharmaceuticals, Fort Washington, PA.
‖Ayerst Laboratories, New York, NY.
Abbreviation: GI, gastrointestinal.

The negatively charged sucralfate molecule binds to positively charged molecules such as leukocytes, mucosal debris, and fibrinogen in gastric and duodenal ulcer craters. This provides a protective barrier against hydrogen ions and pepsin. The drug has a greater affinity for the ulcer site than for normal GI mucosa, although binding to normal mucosa does occur. Sucralfate also binds to acute gastric erosions produced by alcohol or other gastric-irritating drugs such as heparin.

The usual dose is 1 g every 6 hours by mouth. The most common side effect is constipation.

Recent studies have advocated the use of sucralfate rather than antacids and H_2 receptor antagonists in mechanically ventilated patients because those agents appear to raise the gastric pH and allow growth of microorganisms (Driks et al., 1987; Tryba, 1987). This is thought to increase the risk of nosocomial pneumonia or bacteremia. More controlled studies are needed before definitive conclusions can be drawn.

PROSTAGLANDINS. Prostaglandin therapy is a relatively new treatment for ulcer disease. The E series of prostaglandins acts by suppressing parietal cell activity and curtailing gastric acid secretion. These agents also are considered cytoprotective in that they potentiate the effects of gastric mucus and bicarbonate. Further studies are needed to substantiate their effectiveness as prophylactic therapy. Side effects are mainly GI in nature and include nausea, vomiting, diarrhea, and abdominal cramping. This therapy is strictly contraindicated in pregnant patients because it can cause spontaneous abortion. Misoprostal, a synthetic PGE_1 analogue, is given at a dosage of 200 μg four times a day by mouth. Because this drug is available only in oral form, it is not used during acute bleeding episodes.

VASOPRESSIN INFUSION. Systemic infusion of vasopressin (Pitressin; Parke-Davis, Morris Plains, NJ) has been shown to be effective in the treatment of massive GI hemorrhage. Vasopressin acts by constricting the arteries and contracting the bowel wall. Thus, mucosal blood flow is reduced, and thrombus formation can occur.

Vasopressin is a polypeptide hormone secreted by the hypothalamus and stored in the posterior pituitary gland of mammals. Exogenous vasopressin elicits all the pharmacologic responses usually produced by endogenous vasopressin (ADH). The primary physiologic role of vasopressin is to maintain serum osmolality within a normal range and to conserve up to 90% of the water that might otherwise be excreted in the urine. In larger doses, the hormone causes vasoconstriction, particularly of capillaries and of small arterioles, resulting in decreased blood flow to the splanchnic, coronary, GI, pancreatic, skin, and muscular systems (DiPalma, 1992). When injected into the celiac or superior mesenteric artery, vasopressin constricts the gastroduodenal, left gastric, superior mesenteric, and splenic arteries. In the intestinal tract, vasopressin increases peristaltic activity, particulary in the large bowel. Vasopressin also causes an increase in GI sphincter pressure and a decrease in gastric secretion, but has no effect on gastric acid concentration.

Vasopressin may be given by regional perfusion using an angiographically placed arterial catheter or

TABLE 48–8. **Selective Vasoactive Infusion Therapy**

Bleeding Source	Vessel Used
Esophageal	Superior mesenteric artery or left gastric artery
Gastric	Left gastric artery
Duodenal	Gastroduodenal artery
Large bowel (right half)	Inferior mesenteric artery
Large bowel (left half)	Superior mesenteric artery

by systemic venous infusion (Table 48–8). The usual dosage is 0.2 to 0.4 units/minute given through an infusion pump. The intravenous route of administration is usually the first choice when bleeding is massive and endoscopy has not yet been performed to identify its source. Most authors believe that intraarterial vasopressin is more effective than intravenous vasopressin. However, some patients who do not respond to the intravenous route may respond positively to an intraarterial infusion. The use of vasopressin in such situations is a temporary measure for controlling bleeding because there is no clinical evidence that its use substantially improves the overall survival rate (Zuckerman et al., 1992).

Because vasopressin can have major cardiovascular complications, its use may be contraindicated in patients with preexisting cardiovascular disease. Vasopressin reduces coronary blood flow, thus leading to such complications as angina, dysrhythmias, hypertension, and myocardial infarction. Other side effects include fluid retention, water intoxication, oliguria, pulmonary edema, confusion, headache, nausea and vomiting, and peripheral or intestinal ischemia. Extravasation of vasopressin can result in subcutaneous tissue sloughing. Nursing assessment of patients on vasopressin therapy should include monitoring of the electrocardiogram, vital signs, lung sounds, level of consciousness, intake and output, and daily weights. Any symptoms of chest pain or abdominal pain should be reported to the physician immediately. Intravenous catheter insertion sites should be inspected frequently for signs of infiltration.

Studies have shown that combining vasodilator therapy (such as nitroprusside or nitroglycerin with vasopressin) reduces the detrimental cardiac effects of vasopressin by reducing cardiac oxygen demand and increasing coronary blood flow (Gelman & Ernst, 1978; Gimson et al., 1986). These agents may actually augment the effect of vasopressin in controlling bleeding from esophageal varices because they reduce portal venous resistance. More clinical studies are needed to establish definitive protocols for the use of vasopressin and vasodilators in combination.

PROTON PUMP INHIBITOR. Omeprazole is the newest pharmacologic agent being used in the treatment of ulcer disease. It has also been shown to be effective in treating Zollinger-Ellison syndrome and may indeed become the medical therapy of choice in these patients. Omeprazole is thought to bond to the proton pump of the parietal cell, acting as a hydrogen–potassium pump inhibitor. This results in inhibition of acid secretion regardless of the source of stimulation (acetylcholine, gastrin, or histamine). This drug is administered in an oral dosage of 20 mg daily after bleeding is controlled. The regime is short-term, for a period of up to 8 weeks. The oral form should be given on an empty stomach. Side effects include dizziness, weakness, headache, fatigue, nausea, diarrhea, numbness of the extremities, and transient elevations of hepatic enzymes.

OTHER. Eradication of *H. pylori* can be difficult due to the development of resistant strains. The most popular treatment consists of a 2-week, triple-drug regime of tetracycline or amoxicillin, metronidazole, and bismuth subsalicylate (Pepto-Bismol; Procter & Gamble, Cincinnati, OH) (McCarthy, 1993).

Technical Interventions

ENDOSCOPIC ELECTROCOAGULATION. In a variety of upper GI lesions, electrocoagulation can be accomplished through the use of a bipolar probe. This form of therapy uses an electric current that flows between two electrodes in close proximity to each other to induce coagulation of bleeding lesions. Coagulation can also be achieved with the use of a heater probe. In this method, direct heat is used to seal the vessel thermally. Both types of therapy can be done using endoscopy. With the portability of this form of therapy and lower cost than laser therapy, endoscopic coagulation is becoming an accepted and popular form of treatment.

TRANSCATHETER EMBOLIZATION. An angiographic modality may be used if vasopressin is unsuccessful in controlling bleeding lesions in patients who are considered to be poor surgical candidates. Once the bleeding artery has been identified through angiography, embolic material is injected through the catheter selectively into the bleeding artery. The material proximally occludes the artery. Substances such as Gelfoam, cyanoacrylate glue, coils autologous clots, and polyvinyl alcohol have been used for embolization. The choice of material depends on the desired length of action of embolization. Complications include tissue ischemia or infarction if collateral circulation is inadequate.

PHOTOCOAGULATION. The use of lasers for coagulation of bleeding sources has gained in popularity as a treatment modality. The neodymium:yttrium–aluminum-garnet laser can be used to treat bleeding esophageal varices, MW tears, ulcers, and gastric erosions. Results are similar to those achieved with endoscopic electrocoagulation. However, it is a more expensive form of therapy and may require endotracheal intubation and general anesthesia.

TABLE 48–9. **Types of Vagotomies**

Name	Effect	Comments
Truncal vagotomy	Denervates stomach, upper abdominal organs, and intestine as far as left flexure of colon	Most widespread method used; used as treatment for duodenal ulcer as well as recurrent ulcers and marginal jejunal ulcers
Selective gastric vagotomy	Denervates stomach only; weakens motility of the antrum	Used for treatment of duodenal ulcer or pyloric/prepyloric ulcer
Proximal gastric vagotomy or	Denervates only proximal acid-producing portion of stomach; innervation and motility of antrum undisturbed	Decreased incidence of "dumping" and diarrhea; used as treatment of duodenal ulcer
Selective proximal vagotomy (also known as highly selective vagotomy and parietal cell vagotomy)		Need for drainage anastomosis eliminated

SCLEROTHERAPY. A detailed description of this form of therapy is covered in Chapter 49.

Surgical Interventions for Upper Gastrointestinal Bleeding

Although most lesions that cause upper GI bleeding are treated primarily medically, there are several indications for surgical treatment (Knauer & Silverman, 1989). Surgery is indicated (1) if healing is not accomplished with medical treatment, (2) if ulcer recurrence is a problem, (3) when malignancy is suspected, or (4) if complications such as perforation, obstructive pyloric stenosis, or intractable hemorrhage occur.

TYPES OF SURGICAL PROCEDURES. A gastric oversew may be indicated as treatment for a subcardial gastric ulcer. This procedure, which is usually considered palliative, involves suture ligation of the bleeding vessel and closure of the ulcer crater. Ulcer excision or gastric resection is preferred to prevent the possibility of rebleeding or the development of malignancy.

To decrease stomach acid production, two surgical approaches are used. The approaches involve (1) severing the nerves that stimulate cellular acid production, and (2) removing the acid-production section of the stomach. A vagotomy to eliminate the stimulus to gastric cells is accomplished by severing the vagus nerve to the stomach. Several types of vagotomy are possible (Table 48–9). Because the vagus nerve also stimulates motility, this procedure necessitates a gastroenterostomy or pyloroplasty to provide for gastric emptying. This is not necessary with the highly selective vagotomy, because motility is preserved.

Surgical treatment for gastric ulcer also includes gastric resection as a means of removing the acid-secreting parietal cells or gastric acid–secreting cells in the antrum of the stomach (Fig. 48–4). Resection is accomplished with either a Billroth I or Billroth II procedure. In the Billroth I procedure, the distal portion of the stomach is removed with an anastomosis of the proximal portion of the duodenum (gastroduodenos-

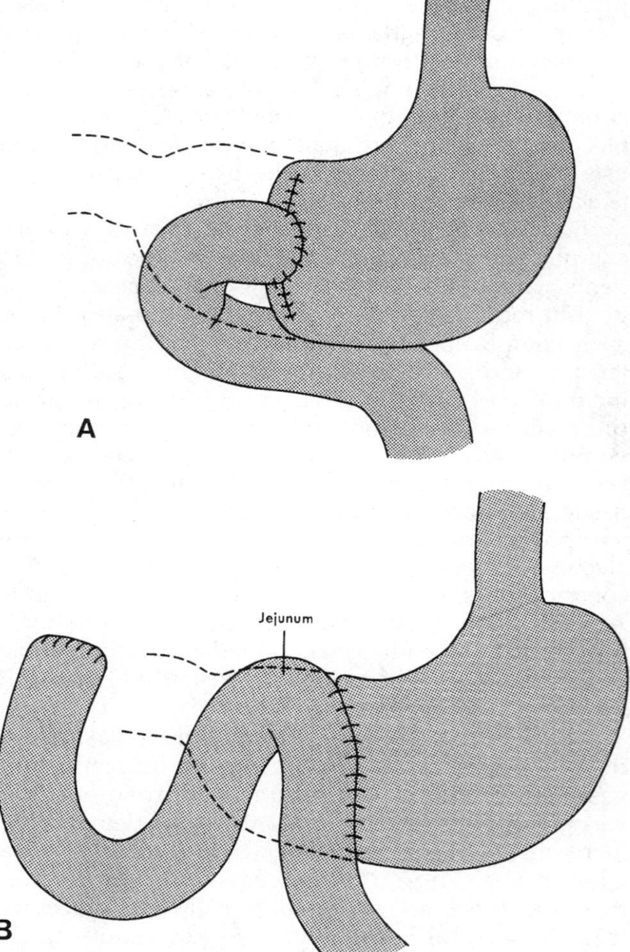

FIGURE 48–4. *A*, Billroth I procedure (gastroduodenostomy). Removal of distal portion of stomach with anastomosis to duodenum. Dotted lines show portion removed. *B*, Billroth II procedure (gastrojejunostomy). Removal of lower portion of stomach with anastomosis to jejunum. Dotted lines show portion removed. A duodenal stump remains and is closed. (From Given, B. A., & Simmons, S. J. [1984]. *Gastroenterology in clinical nursing* [4th ed., pp. 274–275]. St. Louis: C. V. Mosby.)

TABLE 48–10. **Pathologic Sequelae of Gastrojejunostomy**

Dumping syndrome
Diarrhea
Weight loss
Steatorrhea
Iron deficiency
Calcium metabolism disturbances

tomy). The Billroth II procedure involves removal of the lower portion of the stomach with anastomosis of the jejunum (gastrojejunostomy). The duodenal stump is closed. The Billroth II procedure is more frequently performed as a treatment for duodenal ulcer because the incidence of ulcer recurrence is lower than that after the Billroth I. However, postoperative sequelae occur more frequently after the Billroth II (Table 48–10).

A total gastrectomy with anastomosis of the esophagus to the jejunum (esophagojejunostomy) is a radical procedure reserved for intractable ulcer disease such as that seen with Zollinger-Ellison syndrome (Fig. 48–5). Multiple ulcers of the stomach and duodenum occur with this syndrome as a result of hypersecretion of gastric acid caused by a pancreatic non–islet cell gastrinoma. Although the success of medical regimes is improving, the only definitive treatment is removal of all gastric acid-secreting tissue.

IMPLICATIONS FOR CARE. Immediate postoperative nursing care is aimed at providing the routine care needed for an abdominal surgery patient, assessing for immediate postoperative complications, and providing support as the patient adapts to the changes in the gastrointestinal system (Table 48–11).

The patient who undergoes emergency gastric surgery is at risk for development of numerous complications (Table 48–12). Due to the extent of the anastomosis, the potential for postoperative hemorrhage is

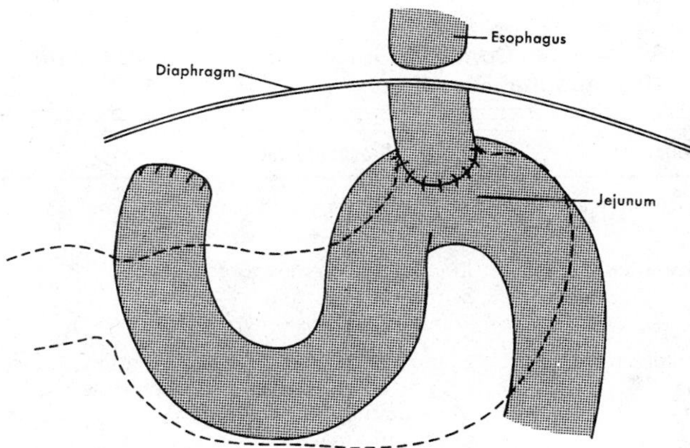

FIGURE 48–5. Total gastrectomy with anastomosis of esophagus to jejunum (esophagojejunostomy). Dotted lines show portion removed. (From Given, B. A., & Simmons, S. J. [1984]. *Gastroenterology in clinical nursing* [4th ed., p. 288]. St. Louis: C. V. Mosby.)

TABLE 48–11. **Primary Nursing Diagnoses for the Patient After Gastric Surgery**

Pain related to	Incision
Impaired Gas Exchange related to	Anesthesia effects Location of incision Aspiration of gastric material
Altered Nutrition: Less Than Body Requirements related to	Loss of intrinsic factor for vitamin B_{12} absorption Reduced absorption of calcium and vitamin D Reduction in pancreatic juices and bile (in Billroth II and gastrectomy) Iron deficiency (in duodenal bypass procedures) Increased metabolic need
Diarrhea related to	Dumping syndrome
High risk for Infection related to	Organism invading wound Hematoma formation Decreased local blood flow Malnutrition
High risk for Fluid Volume Deficit related to	Operative fluid losses Postoperative bleeding Nasogastric losses Diarrhea (dumping syndrome) Inadequate intake
Knowledge Deficit related to	Wound care Dietary needs or restrictions Possible complications or treatments
Anxiety related to	Body function changes Dietary needs or restrictions Lifestyle changes Body image changes

significant. Other causes of hemorrhage may be intraluminal or extraluminal in nature (Table 48–13). The mortality rate for patients with postoperative bleeding is as high as 57% (Haring & Berger, 1988). After surgery, the patient will have an NG tube, which should not be manipulated or irrigated unless specifically ordered. Normally, the patient may lose up to 300 mL of bloody drainage within the first 24 hours (Haring & Berger, 1988). There is less drainage after a total gastrectomy because there is no reservoir to collect the drainage. Excessive drainage or failure of the tube to drain should be reported immediately. A clogged tube may lead to gastric distention and in-

TABLE 48–12. **Postoperative Complications**

Wound infection	Afferent loop syndrome
Dehiscence/evisceration	Stomach wall necrosis
Hemorrhage	Anastomotic loop necrosis
Peritonitis	Postoperative enteritis or necrosis
Pancreatitis	Subphrenic/subhepatic abscesses
Anastomotic leak	Postoperative jaundice
Duodenal stump leak	Gastric retention

TABLE 48–13. **Causes of Hemorrhage After Gastric Surgery**

Extraluminal	Intraluminal
Slipped arterial ligatures	Missed ulcers
Unligated vessels	Stress ulcers/erosions
Liver lacerations	Mucosal injuries
Pancreatic injuries	Loose anastomotic sutures
Coagulation disturbances	Suture dehiscence
	Coagulation disorder

creased pressure at the site of the anastomosis. An anastomotic leak usually occurs between the first and the eighth postoperative days. The result may be peritonitis, cellulitis, or abscess formation. Signs and symptoms include sudden severe pain, high fever, chills, tachycardia, abdominal rigidity, absent bowel sounds, tachypnea, and leukocytosis. Relaparotomy usually is necessary.

Afferent loop syndrome is a complication associated with the Billroth II. In this syndrome, pancreatic secretions and bile fill the afferent loop of the duodenal stump due to obstruction or stenosis of the afferent loop. As the afferent loop becomes distended, there is pressure, pain, and gastric backflow. Typically, the patient experiences vomiting of bilious material after feedings.

After gastric surgery the patient is likely to experience nutritional problems. Removal of the proximal portion or all of the stomach results in loss of intrinsic factor, which is necessary for absorption of vitamin B_{12}. In addition, deficiencies in iron, folic acid, calcium, and vitamin D may occur. Malabsorption of nutrients can occur due to decreased pancreatic secretions and bile. The dumping syndrome is a postprandial problem that often occurs after gastric resection. Rapid passage of a hypertonic bolus of food into the jejunum results in an osmotic shift of fluid into the bowel. Symptoms include abdominal distention, vertigo, palpitations, sweating, and diarrhea. Late manifestations, including sweating, vertigo, hunger, and headache, may occur 1 to 3 hours after eating. The pathogenesis of these systemic symptoms is excessive carbohydrate absorption, which triggers an excessive release of insulin. Patient teaching includes instructing the patient to eat small, frequent meals, avoid high-carbohydrate foods, restrict fluids with meals, and rest after meals.

Surgical Procedures for Lower Gastrointestinal Bleeding

With adequate medical therapy, most lower GI bleeding stops spontaneously. However, surgical treatment is indicated when complications such as uncontrolled hemorrhage, perforation, or obstruction occurs. Extent of surgical resection depends on the source of the problem (Table 48–14).

IMPLICATIONS FOR CARE. Removal of any part of the intestinal tract has an effect on the normal digestive, absorption, and elimination functions. Although operations involving segmental resection with reanastomosis affect these functions only minimally, major resections involving removal of large sections or all of the large intestine with creation of an ostomy produce significant changes for the patient. Removal of the entire colon as treatment for ulcerative colitis necessitates the creation of an ileostomy. Because of the loss of the large bowel for fluid reabsorption, drainage through the ileostomy is very liquid and unformed. With the conventional ileosotomy, an appliance must be worn at all times. Skin protection is important because the drainage contains digestive enzymes that cause extreme excoriation of the skin. The area surrounding the stoma should be kept clean and dry. Protective barriers such as karaya gum and Stomahesive (Squibb, Princeton, NJ) provide skin protection from the corrosive drainage. Appliances must be applied snugly around the stoma.

Two alternative surgical approaches are also used in creating an ileostomy (Fig. 48–6). These approaches give the patient more control over elimination. The continent Kock pouch involves creation of a pouch from the terminal ileum that is sutured to the abdominal wall. A nipple valve is constructed as an outlet. The pouch reservoir retains the feces until the patient drains it with a catheter. This must be done several times a day. No appliance is necessary unless the valve becomes incompetent. The other approach involves construction of an ileal pouch–anal anastomosis. Because the anal sphincter is intact, the patient retains voluntary control of elimination.

Resection of the colon may necessitate the creation of a temporary or permanent colostomy. A temporary colostomy is done if the goal is to divert the fecal flow from an inflamed area to allow healing. Because fluid absorption occurs in the large intestine, the stool eliminated from the colostomy is more formed than that eliminated from an ileostomy. The stool becomes more formed when the colostomy is nearer the terminal por-

TABLE 48–14. **Common Surgical Treatment of Lower Gastrointestinal Bleeding***

Condition	Surgical Procedure Used
Ulcerative colitis	Total colectomy with creation of an ileostomy
Diverticulitis	Ligation and removal of sac(s) Segmental resection Temporary colostomy may be necessary
Colorectal cancer	Colon resection (right hemicolectomy, transverse colon resection, left hemicolectomy, abdominal–perineal resection) Colostomy may be necessary
Hemorrhoids	Hemorrhoidectomy

*Surgical procedures may vary based on patient's condition and physician preference.

tion of the colon. An appliance is not always necessary depending on the location of the colostomy and the preferences of the patient. Some patients are able to control elimination through daily irrigations. Skin protection from drainage is necessary to prevent skin excoriation and breakdown.

Postoperative concerns during the critical care phase include assessment of the stoma for signs of ischemia such as cyanosis or necrosis, abdominal assessment for distention, and observation of patient status for signs and symptoms of fluid and electrolyte imbalances. Function of the ostomy, including the color, amount, and consistency, should be noted. Temperature and white blood cell count should be monitored for signs of infection. As patient recovery progresses, patient and family teaching about the ostomy and its care is necessary. Referral to the nurse enterostomal therapist and local support groups will help the patient deal physically and psychologically with the change in body image and function.

If an abdominal–perineal resection is done, the patient will have a perineal wound in addition to a colostomy and abdominal incision. Frequent dressing changes are necessary because drainage is usually profuse in the first 24 to 48 hours. Wound irrigations and packings are usually done to debride the wound and stimulate granulation. Profuse bleeding or purulent drainage should be reported immediately. The patient should be positioned to avoid pressure on the perineal wound. Postoperative complications include hemorrhage, wound infection, dehiscence, peritonitis, obstruction, and pneumonia.

Although patients with lower GI bleeding are not seen as frequently in critical care units as those with an upper GI bleed, their care provides unique challenges for the critical care nurse. Astute assessment and systemic support can result in stabilization. If surgical intervention becomes necessary, nursing care is aimed at preventing postoperative complications, implementing patient teaching, and providing emotional support in dealing with alterations in body image, body function, and lifestyle (Table 48–15).

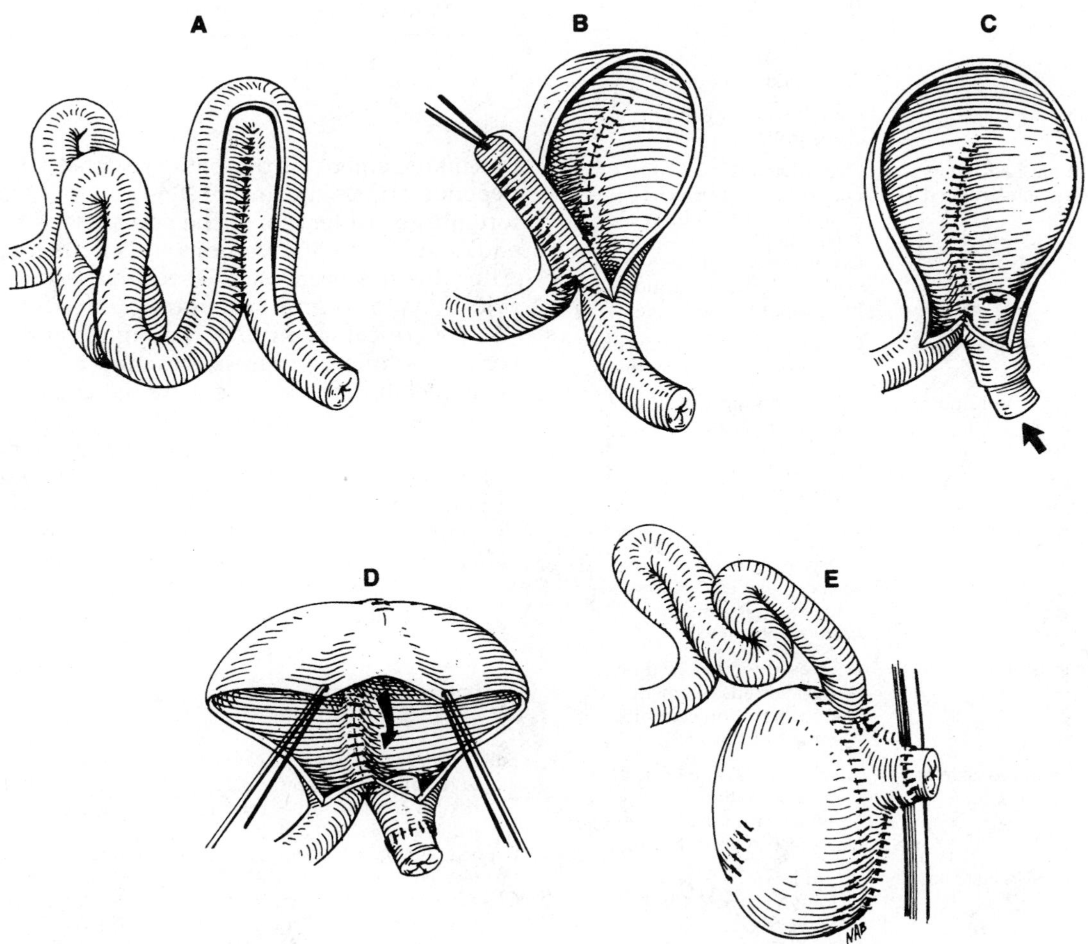

FIGURE 48–6. Continent Kock pouch. *A,* Loop of bowel sewn together. *B,* Removal of anterior portion. *C,* Nipple valve made by pushing bowel back on itself. *D,* Pouch formation. *E,* End brought through stoma. (From Long, B., & Phipps, W. [1989]. *Medical–surgical nursing: A nursing process approach* [p. 1099]. St. Louis: C. V. Mosby.)

DISCHARGE PLANNING

Long-term prevention of GI bleeding includes risk factor identification and lifestyle changes. Patient and family teaching should be incorporated into the discharge plan. Table 48–16 identifies areas that should be addressed within the teaching plan.

SUMMARY

Most patients who require admission to the critical care unit are bleeding from an upper GI source, and 1 of 10 of these will die (Hurst, 1988). GI bleeding is caused by a myriad of primary disease processes. Clinical management of the patient with GI hemorrhage depends on the site, extent, and rate of bleeding. The foremost consideration is the necessity to maintain adequate intravascular volume and circulatory stability. After this has been established, the second treatment priority is to control the source of bleeding.

The critical care nurse can significantly affect the patient's clinical progress. Nursing assessment must be astute and accurate. Because the acuity level of the patient is often labile, it is frequently necessary to update the nursing care plan. Preparing the patient and family for discharge through appropriate education is imperative (see Table 48–16). Prognosis depends on the pathophysiology, but outcome is often positive because most patients cease bleeding spontaneously before medical or surgical intervention is required.

TABLE 48–15. **Primary Nursing Diagnoses for the Patient After Intestinal Surgery**

Pain related to	Incision/wound Surgical manipulation
Impaired Gas Exchange related to	Anesthesia effects Location of incision Postoperative pain
Diarrhea related to	Loss of route for fluid absorption
Altered Nutrition: Less Than Body Requirements related to	Electrolyte losses (Na, K, Ca) Loss of fat and protein digestion (in small intestine resection) Decreased fat-soluble vitamin (A, D, E, K) absorption Increased metabolic need
Body Image Disturbance related to	Change in elimination route (ileostomy or colostomy)
High risk for Fluid Volume Deficit related to	Operative fluid losses Nasogastric losses Diarrhea Decreased fluid absorption Inadequate intake
Anxiety related to	Altered body functions Lifestyle changes Real or perceived alterations in sexual function Loss of control
High risk for Infection related to	Decreased wound healing (poststeroid treatment) Disruption of bowel with spread of flora
High risk for Impaired Skin Integrity related to	Surgical incision or resection Fistula formation Drainage from ostomy Decreased wound healing
Knowledge Deficit related to	Wound care Ostomy care or ostomy products Dietary needs or restrictions Possible complications Need for local support groups (i.e., ostomy, cancer)

TABLE 48–16. **Patient/Family Discharge Teaching**

Assess understanding of cause of present condition (if known). Consult with physician for patient teaching plan concerning etiology.

When patient is ready, institute teaching concerning the purpose, dose, schedule, and side effects of medications (i.e., antacids, H_2 receptor antagonists).

Review the signs and symptoms of recurrent bleeding (i.e., pain, tarry stools, bloody or coffee-ground emesis) for which medical attention should be sought.

Assess risk factors (i.e., smoking, alcohol use) that contribute to delayed healing and gastric irritation. Institute teaching accordingly.

Discuss dietary changes if necessary (i.e., restrictions on coffee, chocolate, hot and spicy foods, high roughage, and milk products, which may contribute to mucosal irritation, acid secretion, or varices irritation).

Discuss lifestyle modifications to reduce stress and instruct the patient about stress management techniques (i.e., deep-breathing exercises, physical exercise, imagery). Refer to counseling groups if warranted.

Discuss the effects of medications such as aspirin and nonsteroidal antiinflammatory drugs on the gastrointestinal system. Educate the patient and family about reading labels on over-the-counter drugs for such ingredients.

REFERENCES

Ballestros, M., Hogan, D., Koss, M., et al. (1990). Bolus or intravenous infusion of ranitidine: Effects on gastric pH and acid secretion: A comparison of relative efficacy and cost. *Annals of Internal Medicine, 112,* 334–339.

Bogoch, A. (1985). Bleeding. In J. E. Berk (Ed.), *Bockus gastroenterology* (4th ed., Vol. 1, pp. 65–110). Philadelphia: W. B. Saunders.

Chamberlain, C., & Peura, D. (1989). Stress ulceration and prevention. In J. DiPalma (Ed.), *Problems in critical care: Gastrointestinal complications* (pp. 371–384). Philadelphia: J. B. Lippincott.

Crawford, J. M. (1994). The gastrointestinal tract. In R. S. Cotran, V. Kumar, & S. L. Robbins (Eds.), *Robbins pathologic basis of disease* (5th ed., pp. 755–830). Philadelphia: W. B. Saunders.

DiPalma, J. (1992). Gastrointestinal bleeding. In J. Covetta, R. Taylor, & R. Kirby (Eds.), *Critical care* (2nd ed., pp. 1537–1545). Philadelphia: J. B. Lippincott.

Driks, M. R., Craven, D. E., Celli, B. R., et al. (1987). Nosocomial pneumonia in intubated patients given sucralfate as compared with antacids or histamine type 2 blockers. *New England Journal of Medicine, 317,* 1376–1382.

Dworken, H. J. (1989). Gastrointestinal hemorrhage. In W. C. Shoemaker, S. Ayers, A. Grenvik, et al. (Eds.), *Textbook of critical care* (2nd ed., pp. 697–703). Philadelphia: W. B. Saunders.

Eckhauser, F., Raper, S., & Knol, J. (1992). Upper gastrointestinal bleeding. In G. Schwartz et al. (Eds.), *Principles and practice of emergency medicine* (3rd ed., pp. 1735–1744). Philadelphia: Lea & Febiger.

Gelman, S., & Ernst, E. (1978). Nitroprusside prevents adverse hemodynamic effects of vasopressin. *Archives of Surgery, 113,* 1465–1471.

Gimson, A, Westaby, D., Hegarty, J., et al. (1986). A randomized trial of vasopressin and vasopressin plus nitroglycerin in the control of acute variceal hemorrhage. *Hepatology, 6,* 406–409.

Glickman, R. M. (1994). Inflammatory bowel disease (Ulcerative colitis and Crohn's disease). In K. J. Isselbacher, E. Braunwald, J. D. Wilson, et al. (Eds.), *Harrison's principles of internal medicine* (13th ed., pp. 1403–1417). New York: McGraw-Hill.

Gottlieb, J., Menaske, P., & Cruz, E. (1986). Gastrointestinal complications in critically ill patients: The intensitivist's overview. *American Journal of Gastroenterology, 81,* 227–238.

Haring, R., & Berger, G. (1988). Postoperative complications and postoperative care. In H. D. Becker, C. Herforth, W. Lierse, et al. (Eds.), *Surgery of the stomach: Indications, methods, complications* (pp. 331–366). New York: Springer-Verlag.

Henneman, P. (1992). Gastrointestinal bleeding. In P. Roseu, R. Barkin, et al. (Eds.), *Emergency medicine: Concepts and clinical practice* (Vol. 2, pp. 1515–1532). St. Louis: C. V. Mosby.

Hurst, J. (1988). Gastrointestinal bleeding. In J. Civetta, R. Taylor, & R. Kirby (Eds.), *Critical care* (pp. 1271–1281). Philadelphia: J. B. Lippincott.

Kafonek, D. R., Herlong, F., Giardiello, F. M., et al. (1988). Gastrointestinal bleeding. In A. M. Harvey, R. J. Johns, V. A. McKusick, et al. (Eds.), *The principles and practices of medicine* (26th ed., pp. 805–812). Norwalk, CT: Appleton & Lange.

Knauer, C. M., & Silverman, S. (1993). Alimentary tract and liver. In S. A. Schroeder, M. A. Krypp, L. M. Tierney, et al. (Eds.), *Current medical diagnosis and treatment* (pp. 343–428). Norwalk, CT: Appleton & Lange.

McCarthy, D. (1993). The stomach and duodenum. *Current Gastroenterology, 13,* 37–63.

McGuigan, J. E. (1994). Peptic ulcer and gastritis. In K. J. Isselbacher, E. Braunwald, J. D. Wilson, et al. (Eds.), *Harrison's principles of internal medicine* (13th ed., pp. 1362–1382). New York: McGraw-Hill.

Morgan, A. (1993). Chronic gastric ulcer. In I. Bouchier, R. Allan, H. Hodgson, & M. Keighley (Eds.), *Gastroenterology: Clinical science and practice* (2nd ed., pp. 254–270). Philadelphia: W. B. Saunders.

Palmer, E. (1992). Gastrointestinal bleeding. In G. Schwartz et al. (Eds.), *Principles and practice of emergency medicine* (3rd ed., pp. 1733–1735). Philadelphia: Lea & Febiger.

Peterson, W. L. & Laine, L. (1994). Gastrointestinal bleeding. In M. H. Sleisenger & J. S. Fordtran (Eds.), *Gastrointestinal disease: Pathophysiology, diagnosis, management* (15th ed., pp. 162–192). Philadelphia: W. B. Saunders.

Porth, C. M. (1994). Alterations in gastrointestinal function. In C. M. Porth (Ed.), *Pathophysiology: Concepts of altered health states* (4th ed., pp. 817–841). Philadelphia: J. B. Lippincott.

Quigley, E. M. (1989). Acute upper gastrointestinal hemorrhage. In L. A. Turnberg (Ed.), *Clinical gastroenterology* (pp. 54–86). Boston: Blackwell Scientific Publications.

Schiller, L. R. (1992). Epidemiology, clinical manifestations, and diagnosis. In J. B. Wyngaarden, L. H. Smith, Jr., & J. C. Bennett (Eds.), *Cecil textbook of medicine* (19th ed., pp. 656–657). Philadelphia: W. B. Saunders.

Severance, S. R. (1986). Gastrointestinal bleeding. In D. A. Zschoche (Ed.), *Mosby's comprehensive review of critical care* (3rd ed., pp. 540–552). St. Louis: C. V. Mosby.

Shlafer, M. (1994). Pharmacologic management of peptic ulcer disease. In M. Shlafer (Ed.), *The nurse, pharmacology and drug therapy: A prototype approach* (2nd ed., pp. 793–815). Redwood City, CA: Addison-Wesley.

Spiro, H. M. (1993). *Clinical gastroenterology* (4th ed., pp. 69–96). New York: McGraw-Hill.

Thompson, A. B., & Mahachai, V. (1985). Medical management of uncomplicated peptic ulcer disease. In J. E. Berk (Ed.), *Bockus gastroenterology* (4th ed., Vol. 2, pp. 1116–1154). Philadelphia: W. B. Saunders.

Tobin, M. J. (1989). *Essentials of critical care medicine* (pp. 409–419). New York: Churchill-Livingstone.

Tryba, M. (1987). Risk of acute stress bleeding and nosocomial pneumonia in ventilated intensive care unit patients: Sucralfate versus antacids. *American Journal of Medicine, 83*(Suppl. 3B), 117–124.

Wilson, L., & Lester, L. (1992). Stomach and duodenum. In S. Price & L. Wilson (Eds.), *Pathophysiology: Clinical concepts of disease processes* (4th ed., pp. 292–306). St. Louis: C. V. Mosby.

Zuckerman, G., Benitez, J., & Cort, D. (1992). Medical therapy of nonvariceal upper gastrointestinal hemorrhage. In M. B. Taylor (Ed.), *Gastrointestinal emergencies* (pp. 117–125). Baltimore: Williams & Wilkins.

GASTROINTESTINAL BLEEDING MULTIDISCIPLINARY CARE GUIDE

COORDINATION OF CARE

Diagnosis/Stabilization Phase		Acute Management Phase		Recovery Phase	
Outcome	*Intervention*	*Outcome*	*Intervention*	*Outcome*	*Intervention*
All appropriate team members and disciplines will be involved in the plan of care.	Develop the plan of care with the patient/family, primary nurse(s), primary physician(s), gastroenterologist, other specialists as needed, clinical nurse specialist, acute care nurse practitioner, respiratory therapist, chaplain, social services.	All appropriate disciplines will be consulted.	Update the plan of care with the patient/family, other team members, dietitian, discharge planner, home health agency, physical therapist (if indicated). Initiate planning for anticipated discharge. Begin teaching patient/family about home care (medications, dietary restrictions, signs/symptoms of bleeding, fluid volume deficit).	Patient/family will understand how to maintain optimal health at home.	Provide written guidelines concerning follow-up care to patient/family. Provide patient/family with phone numbers of resources available to answer questions.

FLUID BALANCE

Diagnosis/Stabilization Phase		Acute Management Phase		Recovery Phase	
Outcome	*Intervention*	*Outcome*	*Intervention*	*Outcome*	*Intervention*
Patient will achieve optimal hemodynamic status as evidenced by: • MAP ≥ 70 mm Hg • Vital signs WNL for the patient • Hemodynamic parameters WNL for the patient • No bleeding • Urine output ≥0.5 mL/kg/hr	Monitor and treat hemodynamic parameters: • BP • CO • CI • Stroke volume • PA pressures • CVP • PCWP • SVR/PVR • Svo_2 Monitor vital signs q1h and prn until stable. Monitor for orthostatic changes in blood pressure and narrowing pulse pressure. Assess intake/output q1h. Measure and record gastric drainage every shift or as indicated during acute bleed. Monitor lab values: CBC, electrolytes, coagulation studies, BUN, creatinine, platelets, reticulocyte count, mean corpuscular volume (MCV), and hypochromic microcytic red blood cells.	Patient will maintain optimal hemodyamic status.	Same as in stabilization phase. Monitor and treat hemodynamic parameters, vital signs, intake and output (I & O), and fluid volume status q2–4h and prn. Monitor lab values (CBC, electrolytes, coagulation studies, platelets, BUN, and creatinine). Begin teaching patient/family about GI system, current problems, treatment, and expected clinical course.	Patient will maintain optimal hemodynamic status.	Same as in stabilization phase. Monitor and treat hemodynamic parameters, vital signs, I & O, and fluid volume status q4h and prn. Teach patient/family risk factors that increase gastric acidity, thus increasing chance of bleeding (smoking, alcohol abuse, antiinflammatory agents, reserpine, caffeine, aspirin, corticosteroids, birth control pills). Instruct patient on purpose, dose, schedule, and side effects of antacids, H_2 receptor antagonists, prostaglandins, and any other antiulcer medications as prescribed. Teach patient/family signs and symptoms of recurrent bleeding and fluid volume deficit (pain, tarry stools, bloody or coffee-ground emesis, dry skin, weight loss).

	If acute upper GI bleeding continues, use room temperature saline and lavage stomach until clear. Monitor patient for abdominal pain and rebound tenderness. Monitor for signs/symptoms of fluid volume deficit (sluggish skin turgor, dry mouth, skin and mucous membranes, sunken eyes, weight loss). Administer crystalloids, colloidal agents, and blood products as ordered. Assess gastric pH and check GI aspirate for blood q1–4h and administer antacids or sucralfate as ordered. Administer H_2 receptor antagonists as ordered. Guiaic all stools. Monitor for complications that can occur from GI bleed (hypovolemic shock, acute tubular necrosis, hepatic failure, metabolic acidosis, loss of consciousness, neurologic insult, dysrhythmias, cardiac ischemia, DIC, sepsis). If massive blood transfusion is necessary, monitor for complications of massive blood therapy (hyperkalemia, hypocalcemia, hypothermia, metabolic acidosis, infections, coagulopathies, DIC, ARDS, hypervolemia, or febrile transfusion reactions). Assist with endoscopic or angiographic procedures to assess and treat bleeding. Prepare patient/family for surgery if indicated.				

NUTRITION

Diagnosis/Stabilization Phase		Acute Management Phase		Recovery Phase	
Outcome	***Intervention***	***Outcome***	***Intervention***	***Outcome***	***Intervention***
Patient will be adequately nourished.	NPO if acutely bleeding in GI tract. Assess total protein, albumin, prealbumin, and lymphocyte count. Begin alternative nutrition such as total parenteral nutrition if bleeding precludes enteral route. Assess bowel sounds q4h (hyperactive in upper GI bleed, hypoactive/normal in lower GI bleed). Daily weight.	Patient will be adequately nourished.	Begin clear liquids and monitor patient's response. Continue to monitor daily weight and nutritional parameters. Involve dietitian for diet counseling.	Patient will be adequately nourished.	Teach patient dietary changes necessary (restrictions on coffee, chocolate, hot and spicy foods, high roughage, and milk products, which may contribute to mucosal irritation, acid secretion, or varices irritation).

Care Guide continued on following page

GASTROINTESTINAL BLEEDING MULTIDISCIPLINARY CARE GUIDE *continued*

MOBILITY

Diagnosis/Stabilization Phase		Acute Management Phase		Recovery Phase	
Outcome	*Intervention*	*Outcome*	*Intervention*	*Outcome*	*Intervention*
Patient will achieve optimal mobility.	Assess degree of mobility and muscle strength. Begin passive/active-assist range-of-motion exercises.	Patient will achieve optimal mobility.	Same as in stabilization phase. Obtain physical therapy consult if indicated. Monitor response to increased activity; decrease activity if adverse events occur (tachycardia, discomfort, dyspnea, or hypotension). Allow patient to assist in activities of daily living as tolerated.	Patient will achieve optimal mobility.	Instruct patient/family about exercise program.

OXYGENATION/VENTILATION

Diagnosis/Stabilization Phase		Acute Management Phase		Recovery Phase	
Outcome	*Intervention*	*Outcome*	*Intervention*	*Outcome*	*Intervention*
Patient will have adequate gas exchange and tissue perfusion as evidenced by: • SaO_2 >90% (SpO_2 >92%) • ABGs WNL for the patient • SvO_2 60%–80% • Urine output ≥0.5 mL/kg/hour • Alert and oriented ×3 • Respiratory rate, depth, and rhythm WNL • Absence of dyspnea, cyanosis, and secretions • Hemodynamic parameters WNL for the patient • Hemoglobin WNL for the patient	Constantly monitor respiratory status—rate, rhythm, and depth of breathing, chest x-ray, ABGs, pulse oximetry, and SvO_2. Be prepared for intubation and mechanical ventilation. If necessary, assist with monitoring or adjusting of ventilator settings to maintain appropriate level of assistance and minute ventilation. Monitor hemoglobin/hematocrit q2–4h until stable. Monitor ABGs or SpO_2/SvO_2 closely. Apply supplemental oxygen if indicated and monitor response. Monitor for signs of adequate tissue perfusion: alert and oriented, BP and pulse WNL for the patient, SvO_2 60%–80%, SpO_2 > 90%, urine output 0.5 mL/kg/hour, normal skin color and temperature. Reduce tissue oxygen demands through bed rest and comfort measures. Reduce fever if present.	Patient will have adequate gas exchange and tissue perfusion.	Same as in stabilization phase. Monitor hemoglobin q12–24h. Monitor and treat oxygenation/ventilation disturbances as per ABGs or SaO_2/SvO_2. Wean oxygen therapy/mechanical ventilation as indicated. Teach patient/family about oxygenation needs and treatments provided. Assess effects of increased activity on oxygenation status.	Patient will have adequate gas exchange and tissue perfusion.	Same as acute management phase. Teach patient/family about home care O_2 needs if applicable.

COMFORT

Diagnosis/Stabilization Phase		Acute Management Phase		Recovery Phase	
Outcome	*Intervention*	*Outcome*	*Intervention*	*Outcome*	*Intervention*
Patient will be as comfortable and pain free as possible as evidenced by: • No objective indicators of pain • No complaints of discomfort	Assess quantity and quality of pain. Administer analgesics and monitor response. Monitor effect on respiratory status and BP. Provide mouth care frequently, especially if patient is NPO to minimize oral discomfort. Avoid the use of lemon and glycerin swabs, which can be drying to the mucosa. Provide reassurance in a calm, caring, and competent manner. Keep lights dimmed and environment as quiet as possible to keep physical and verbal stimulation at a minimum.	Patient will be as comfortable as possible.	Same as stabilization phase. Instruct patient on relaxation techniques. Use complementary therapies such as back massage, music therapy, humor, and imagery to promote relaxation. Involve family members in strategies. Observe for complications of GI bleed that may cause discomfort: bleeding, abdominal distention, infection.	Patient will be as comfortable as possible.	Instruct patient/family on alternative methods to promote relaxation after discharge. Refer to outpatient clinic or stress management program.

SKIN INTEGRITY

Diagnosis/Stabilization Phase		Acute Management Phase		Recovery Phase	
Outcome	*Intervention*	*Outcome*	*Intervention*	*Outcome*	*Intervention*
Patient will have intact skin without abrasions or pressure ulcers.	Assess all bony prominences at least q4h and treat if needed. Turn q2h as hemodynamic status allows. Use preventive pressure-reducing devices if patient is at high risk for development of pressure ulcers. Treat pressure ulcers according to hospital protocol. Use superfatted or lanolin-based soap for bathing and apply emmollients for dry skin.	Patient will have intact skin without abrasions or pressure ulcers.	Same as stabilization phase.	Patient will be as comfortable as possible.	Same as stabilization phase. Teach patient/family proper skin care after discharge.

Care Guide continued on following page

GASTROINTESTINAL BLEEDING MULTIDISCIPLINARY CARE GUIDE *continued*

PROTECTION/SAFETY

Diagnosis/Stabilization Phase		Acute Management Phase		Recovery Phase	
Outcome	***Intervention***	***Outcome***	***Intervention***	***Outcome***	***Intervention***
Patient will be protected from possible harm.	Assess need for restraints and institute if needed. If used, check skin integrity and circulation q1h. Explain need for restraints to patient/family. Follow hospital protocol for use of restraints. Assess need for assistance with activities. Provide physical support as needed. Maintain nasogastric suction at low level to avoid further trauma to gastric mucosa.	Patient will be protected from possible harm.	Same as stabilization phase.	Patient will be protected from possible harm.	Teach patient/family about any physical limitations in activity after discharge.

PSYCHOSOCIAL/SELF-DETERMINATION

Diagnosis/Stabilization Phase		Acute Management Phase		Recovery Phase	
Outcome	***Intervention***	***Outcome***	***Intervention***	***Outcome***	***Intervention***
Patient will achieve psychophysiologic stability. Patient will demonstrate a decrease in anxiety as evidenced by: • Vital signs WNL for the patient • Subjective report of decreased anxiety • Objective signs of decreased anxiety	Assess physiologic effects of critical care environment on patient (hemodynamic variables, psychological status, signs of increased sympathetic response). Administer sedatives and antianxiolytics, and monitor response. Use calm, caring, competent, and reassuring approach with patient/family. Allow flexible visiting to meet patient/family needs. Determine coping ability of patient/family and take appropriate measures (provide frequent explanations, allow patient to verbalize concerns, consult support services, allow family to visit often, and have family conferences).	Patient will achieve psychophysiologic stability. Patient will demonstrate a decrease in anxiety.	Same as stabilization phase.	Patient will achieve psychophysiologic stability. Patient will demonstrate a decrease in anxiety.	Provide support to patient/family in the case of unsuccessful treatment outcomes in reaching difficult decisions and accepting inevitable outcomes. If patient is discharged, refer to outpatient counseling or stress management programs.

DIAGNOSTICS

Diagnosis/Stabilization Phase		Acute Management Phase		Recovery Phase	
Outcome	*Intervention*	*Outcome*	*Intervention*	*Outcome*	*Intervention*
Patient/family will understand any tests or procedures which need to be completed (vital signs, I & O, hemodynamic monitoring, x-rays, CT, MRI, lab work, GI tubes, cardiac monitoring, endoscopy, sclerotherapy, arteriography, barium radiographs, EKG, ABGs, pulse oximetry, IV lines, and blood therapy).	Explain all tests and procedures to patient/family. Be sensitive to individuals' needs for information.	Patient/family will understand any tests or procedures that need to be completed.	Anticipate need for and prepare patient/family for further treatment such as surgery, endoscopy, photocoagulation.	Patient/family will understand meaning of diagnostic tests in relation to continued health.	Review with patient/family results of tests before discharge. Discuss abnormal findings and appropriate measures patient/family can take to return to prehospital condition. Provide written guidelines concerning follow-up care for patient/family. Provide written instructions on care at home (when to call physician, physical restrictions, dietary restrictions, skin care, and medications).

CHAPTER 49

Patients With Liver Dysfunction

Susan L. Smith

ANATOMY OF THE LIVER AND HEPATOBILIARY SYSTEM

The Liver

The liver is the largest solid organ in the body, weighing about 1.5 kg in the adult. It is located mostly in the right upper quadrant (RUQ) but extends across the midline into the left upper quadrant. In the RUQ the superior aspect of the liver lies at about the level of the fifth rib or, more simply stated, at the level of the nipples (Fig. 49–1). The inferior aspect does not extend more than 1 to 2 cm below the right costal margin in normal conditions.

The liver can be anatomically divided into two main lobes, right and left (Fig. 49–2*A*). The imaginary line that separates the two lobes runs from the fossa of the inferior vena cava (IVC) above to the notch of the gallbladder below. The right lobe can be further divided into anterior and posterior segments (Fig. 49–2*B* and *C*), which can be further divided into superior and inferior subsegments. The left lobe can likewise be divided into medial and lateral segments and further subdivided into superior and inferior subsegments.

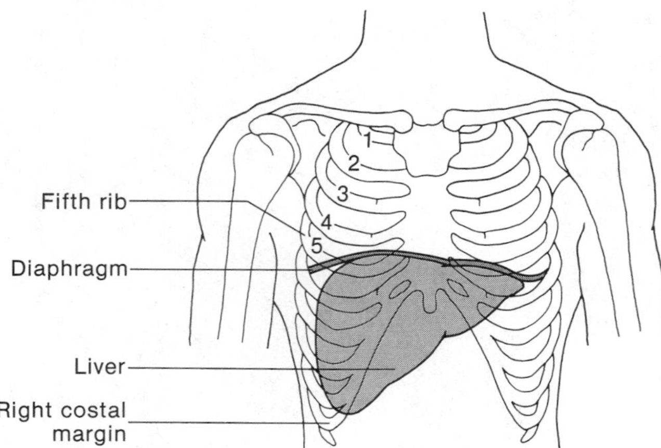

FIGURE 49–1. Anatomic location of the liver. The upper border normally lies at the level of the fourth intercostal space or fifth rib, and the lower border does not normally extend more than 1 to 2 cm below the right costal margin.

Portal Circulation

The liver is a highly vascular organ that holds about 600 mL of blood at any given time. However, the venous capacitance of the liver is much greater, allowing for expansion of its blood volume to approximately 1 liter in conditions such as hypervolemia or right heart failure. Approximately 25% of the cardiac output flows through the liver before it is returned by the IVC to the right atrium.

The liver has an unusual vascular system in that both a vein and an artery supply blood to the liver. The larger portal vein is formed behind the pancreas by the confluence of the superior mesenteric and the splenic veins (Fig. 49–3). The portal vein delivers about two-thirds of the liver's blood supply. The superior mesenteric vein and the portal vein drain the splanchnic circulation; portal venous blood therefore is rich in nutrients and insulin. The smaller hepatic artery branches off the aorta at the celiac axis and divides into the right and left hepatic arteries just before it enters the liver adjacent to the portal vein. It delivers about one-third of the liver's blood supply and is the liver's chief source of oxygen.

Glisson's capsule is an innervated membrane that covers the liver and lies beneath the visceral peritoneum. This capsule converges at and enters the liver at the porta hepatis. Inside the porta hepatis this membrane branches to form the division tracts for the portal vein and the hepatic artery. Within the liver the portal vein and hepatic artery divide and form thousands of branches to the right and left lobes. Portal and arterial inflow vessels unite at the level of the hepatic sinusoids.

Normal hepatic structure consists of functional units called simple hepatic acini or lobules. Lobules are composed of small cords of hepatocytes supported by a reticulin framework and arranged around their afferent (portal venule and hepatic arteriole) and efferent (hepatic venule) blood supply (Fig. 49–4). Small,

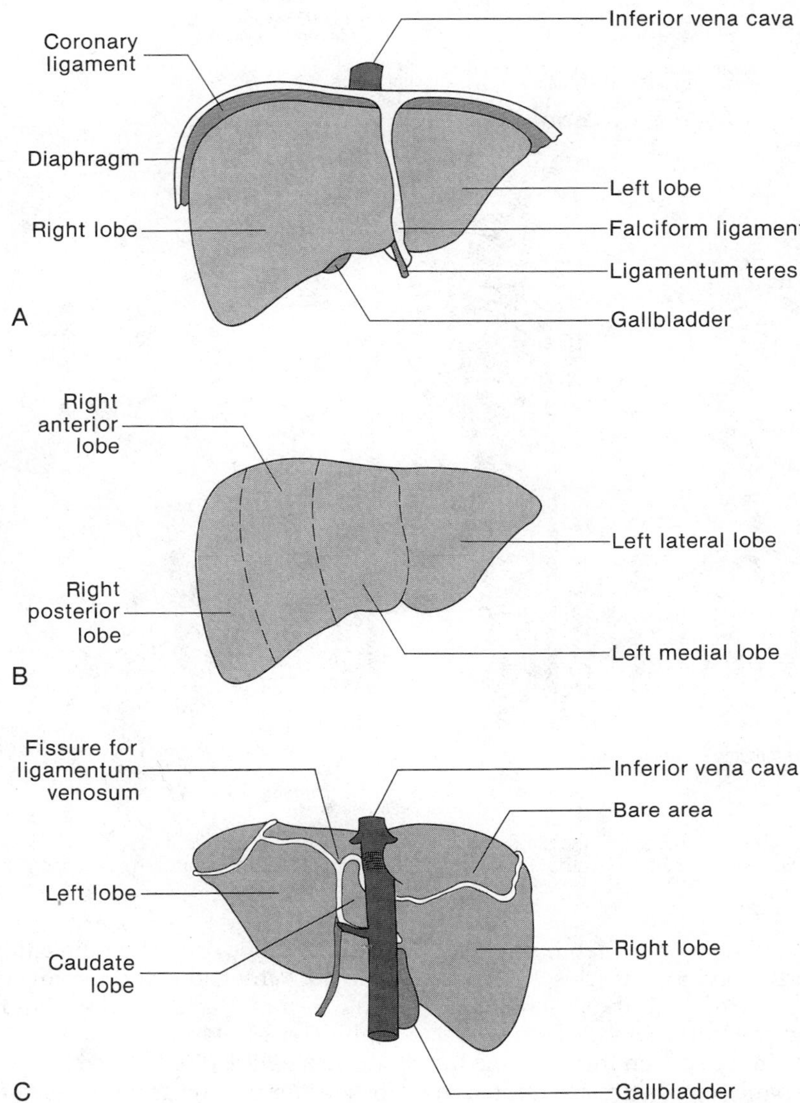

FIGURE 49–2. *A*, Anterior view of the liver. *B*, Segments of the liver, anterior view. *C*, Posterior view of the liver.

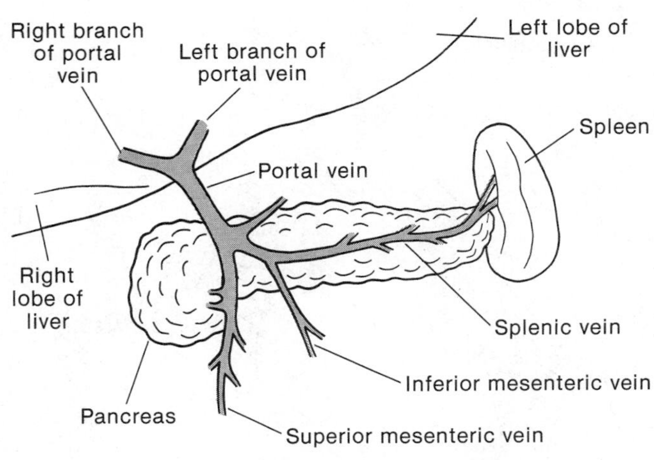

FIGURE 49–3. Portal venous circulation.

parallel branches of the portal vein and hepatic artery, called venules and arterioles, respectively, perfuse the lobules. Blood from these vessels flows through structures called sinusoids before it empties into tributaries of the hepatic veins and is carried from the liver. Sinusoidal blood is a mixture of blood from the portal venous and hepatic arterial systems. Exchange of oxygen, nutrients, and waste between blood and hepatocytes occurs in the sinusoids. Normally, two or three hepatic veins drain blood from the liver into the IVC. Together with small bile ducts that *exit* the lobules, portal venules and hepatic arterioles make up what are referred to as *portal triads*. Portal triads lie at the center of each lobule, and hepatic venules lie at the periphery of each lobule.

The walls of hepatic sinusoids contain highly phagocytic cells called *Kupffer cells*. Kupffer cells are members of the mononuclear phagocytic system. They

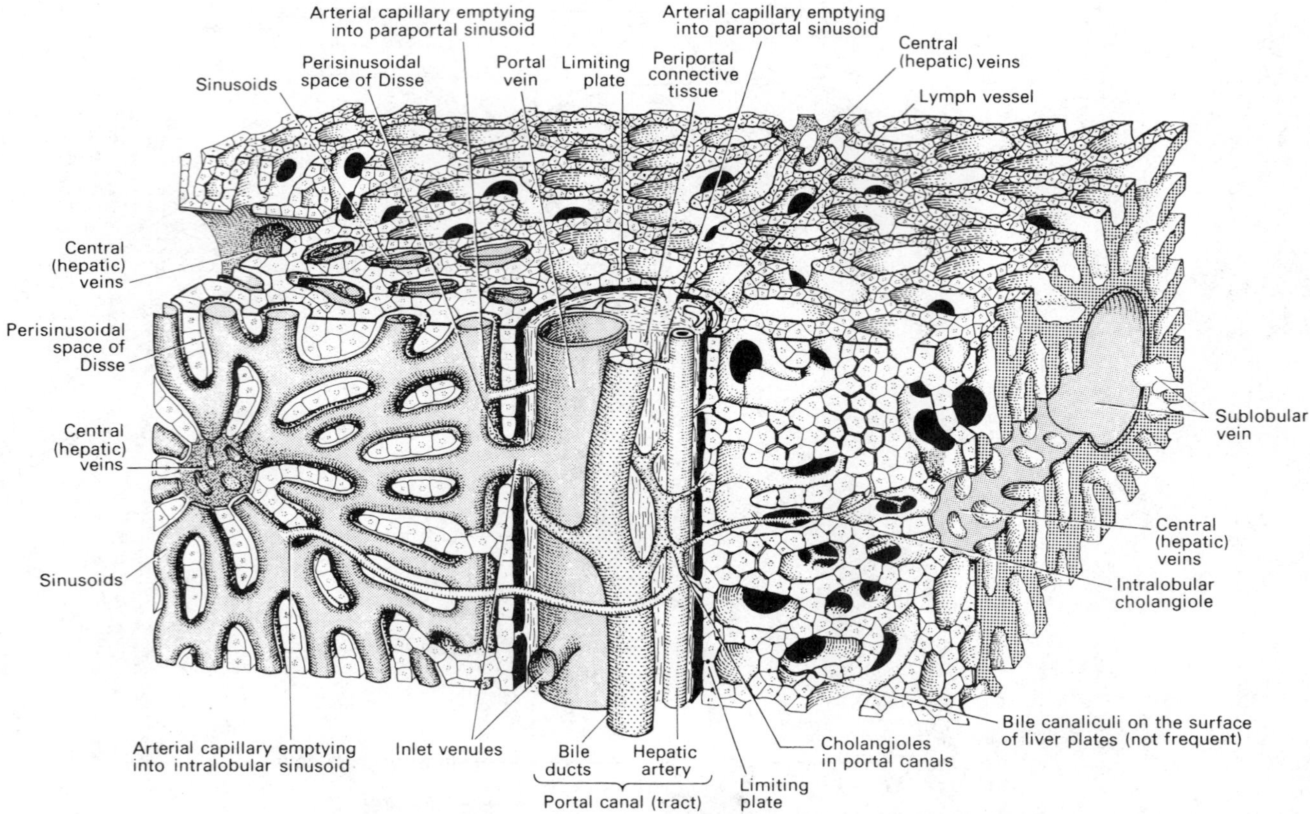

FIGURE 49–4. Synopsis of the structure of the normal human liver. (From Sherlock S. [1985]. *Diseases of the liver and biliary system* [7th ed., p. 7]. London: Blackwell Scientific Publications.)

function to remove particulate matter (denatured protein, lysosomal enzymes, foreign particles, bacteria, yeasts, viruses, and endotoxin) from the vascular system by removing it from the portal blood. The *space of Disse* is a tissue space located between the hepatocytes and sinusoidal cells. Hepatic lymphatics are located in periportal connective tissue and are lined with endothelial cells that allow uptake of hepatic interstitial fluid. When sinusoidal pressure increases, lymph production in the space of Disse increases, contributing to ascites formation when hepatic outflow obstruction occurs. To summarize, blood enters the liver by the portal vein and hepatic artery, is filtered free of foreign matter through hepatic sinusoids, and empties into the central veins. The central veins drain into two or three large hepatic veins that empty into the IVC.

Excretory System of the Liver

A major function of the liver is the production and secretion of bile. The bile excretory system begins as tiny bile canaliculi that emerge from hepatocytes and drain into terminal bile ductules. Terminal ductules branch into larger and larger ducts, until eventually large right and left hepatic ducts are formed (Fig. 49–5). The right and left hepatic bile ducts join to form the common hepatic duct. The common bile duct is then formed by the confluence of the common hepatic duct and the cystic duct from the gallbladder. The common bile duct enters the duodenum at the ampulla of Vater. The terminal end of the common bile duct is the sphincter of Oddi.

The gallbladder is a small, pear-shaped organ that lies under the surface of the right lobe of the liver. The

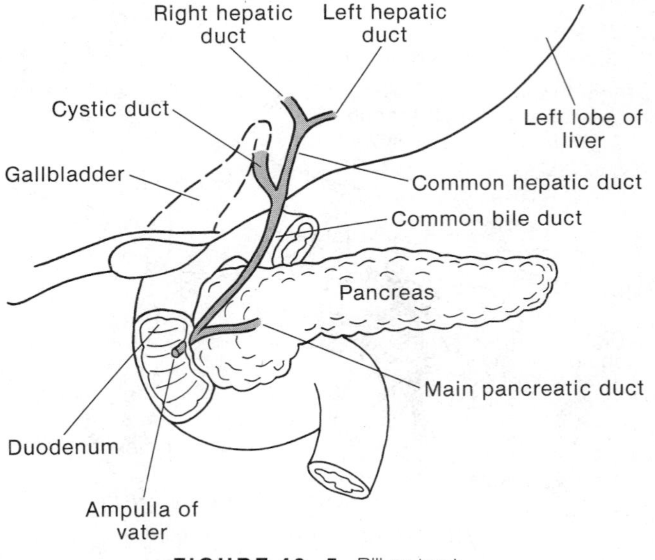

FIGURE 49–5. Biliary tract.

function of the gallbladder is to store and concentrate bile. Although the liver produces about 1 liter of bile/day, the capacity of the gallbladder for bile is only about 50 mL. When chyme enters the duodenum from the stomach, the hormone cholecystokinin is secreted from the duodenum, causing the gallbladder to contract and the sphincter of Oddi to relax so that bile can flow into the intestine to participate in digestion and metabolism of fats.

PHYSIOLOGY OF THE LIVER AND HEPATOBILIARY SYSTEM

Liver Function

The chemical versatility of the liver allows it to perform hundreds of separate functions (Zakim & Boyer, 1990). However, liver function can be summarized to include the synthesis of bile acids and excretion of bilirubin, carbohydrate metabolism, synthesis and release of plasma proteins, amino acid metabolism, conversion of ammonia to a less toxic substance, lipid metabolism, storage of fat-soluble vitamins and iron, detoxification of drugs, inactivation of hormones, control of procoagulants and removal of products of coagulation, and phagocytosis of foreign antigen.

BILE PRODUCTION AND BILIRUBIN METABOLISM

Bile acids, which largely consist of bile salts, are synthesized only by the liver as derivatives of cholesterol synthesis. Bile acids are conjugated in the liver with glycine or taurine to form bile salts. Bile salts are then excreted by active transport mechanisms into bile canaliculi and carried to the small intestine, where they are used to solubilize cholesterol in bile, emulsify and absorb fat, assist the pancreas with lipolysis, and secrete gastrointestinal (GI) hormones. In the ileum bile salts are reabsorbed and are eventually circulated through the liver by portal venous blood, where they are reconjugated and reexcreted. Bile salt deficiency results in cholelithiasis (the formation of gallstones) and the malabsorption of fats.

Cholestasis, the failure of normal amounts of bile to reach the duodenum, can result from inhibition of bile flow anywhere from the conjugating site in the hepatocytes to the duodenum. Cholestasis results in the accumulation of bile in the hepatocytes and bile ducts and is manifested clinically by elevation of serum bile acid levels and differing degrees of jaundice. Prolonged cholestasis leads to biliary cirrhosis. Bilirubin is the chief bile pigment and is the end product of heme released during the metabolism of hemoglobin, myoglobin, and respiratory enzymes. Approximately 80% of bilirubin is formed in the reticuloendothelial cells of the liver, and 20% is formed in the bone marrow. Approximately 6 g of hemoglobin is metabolized to approximately 30 mg of bilirubin each day. Bilirubin formed in the liver and bone marrow is called *unconjugated* bilirubin. Unconjugated bilirubin is lipid soluble and is tightly bound in the plasma to albumin. In this form it is extracted by the liver and *conjugated* to a water-soluble form so that it can be excreted.

Normal serum bilirubin level is 0.2 to 0.9 mg/dL. Serum bilirubin can be measured as *total* bilirubin, *indirect* (unconjugated) bilirubin, or *direct* (conjugated) bilirubin. The normal indirect bilirubin level is 0.1 to 0.5 mg/dL, and the normal direct bilirubin level is 0.1 to 0.4 mg/dL. Therefore, the total bilirubin level is about 0.2 and 0.9 mg/dL. Indirect bilirubin is elevated in conditions such as hepatocellular necrosis and hemolysis, whereas direct bilirubin is elevated during cholestasis.

Jaundice, the most visibly apparent manifestation of altered bilirubin metabolism, can be obstructive, hepatocellular, or hemolytic in etiology. *Obstructive jaundice* occurs most commonly from biliary duct stones but also from cancer of the head of the pancreas, duodenum, or hepatocellular ducts and from metastatic or granulomatous intrahepatic lesions. Obstructive jaundice is associated with an increase in serum levels of enzymes (alkaline phosphatase [ALP] is the most commonly measured one) that are released when the bile duct epithelium is damaged. Intrahepatic biliary duct obstruction (e.g., primary biliary cirrhosis) produces higher elevations in ALP than extrahepatic obstruction (Widmann, 1987). ALP is elevated in growing children and during pregnancy and is therefore not diagnostic in these conditions. In these situations, biliary duct obstruction can be diagnosed by measuring other enzymes such as 5'-nucleotidase, leucine aminopeptidase, and gamma-glutamyl transpeptidase (GGT). In obstructive jaundice the direct bilirubin is also increased, the aspartate aminotransferase (AST) and alanine aminotransferase (ALT) are normal or slightly elevated, and the prothrombin time (PT) is increased due to vitamin K malabsorption. *Hepatocellular jaundice* results from acute destruction of hepatocytes and is associated with such conditions as acute viral hepatitis and acute toxic or ischemic liver injury. The enzymes most commonly associated with hepatocellular jaundice are the aminotransferases. Hepatocellular jaundice is associated with an increase in the AST and ALT. Both indirect and direct bilirubin are elevated, ALP is normal, and PT is normal or slightly elevated. If hepatocellular damage is extensive, the PT will be extremely elevated. *Hemolytic jaundice* occurs when the heme load in the circulation is increased to such a level that the liver cannot metabolize it. Conditions causing hemolytic jaundice are hemolysis of a large volume of red blood cells such as occurs with massive blood transfusion or a hemolytic transfusion reaction (mismatched ABO type). Hemolytic jaundice is associated with an increased indirect bilirubin and normal AST, ALT, ALP, and PT.

METABOLISM OF NUTRIENTS

The liver is the principal site of carbohydrate, protein, and fat metabolism necessary for normal cellular function and growth. Malnutrition is therefore common in patients with end-stage liver disease due to a variety of factors: inadequate nutritional intake (due to nausea, vomiting, anorexia, dietary restrictions, and early satiety), increased energy expenditure, GI hormonal imbalances, intestinal malabsorption, maldigestion (due to decreased intraluminal bile salts, bacterial overgrowth of GI mucosa, and intestinal diseases), increased gluconeogenesis at the expense of muscle protein stores, decreased protein synthesis, increased fat oxidation, medication (diuretics and cathartics) induced losses, and repeated hospitalizations for complications of end-stage liver disease (Palombo et al., 1987; Porayko et al., 1991; Shronts et al., 1987).

Carbohydrate Metabolism

A major function of the liver is to maintain normal serum glucose for energy metabolism. Regulation of circulating levels of blood glucose is necessary because: (1) exogenous carbohydrates circulate through the liver before reaching the systemic circulation, (2) the liver is exposed to high concentrations of insulin, and (3) hepatocytes contain glucokinase and glucose 6-phosphate dehydrogenase. Three mechanisms are responsible: *glycogenesis, glycogenolysis,* and *gluconeogenesis.* Carbohydrates in the diet are converted to simple sugars that can be metabolized by the liver for energy substrate. Excess carbohydrates can be converted to glycogen and stored in the liver for metabolic reserve. This process is called glycogenesis. Approximately 900 kcal are stored in the liver as glycogen in the adult (Keithley, 1985). A much larger reserve of glycogen is stored in skeletal muscle. When glucose is needed but unavailable, the first response by the liver is to convert stored glycogen to glucose. This process is called glycogenolysis. If glycogen reserves are depleted, the liver has the ability to manufacture glucose from noncarbohydrate sources, namely, fat (glycerol and fatty acids) and protein (amino acids). This catabolic process is called gluconeogenesis.

Protein Metabolism

An exclusive role of the liver is the production and secretion of the majority of circulating plasma proteins, particularly albumin, prealbumin, and transferrin. Protein metabolism by the liver involves both the synthesis of plasma proteins from available amino acids and amino acid metabolism. With the exception of gamma globulins and immunoglobulins, all plasma proteins are manufactured by the liver (Donohue et al., 1990). Plasma proteins include albumin, clotting factors, transferrin, haptoglobin, ceruloplasmin, alpha$_1$-antitrypsin, the C_3 component of complement, and alpha-fetoprotein. The most sensitive indices of severity of liver disease are serum albumin and the vitamin K-dependent clotting factors.

Albumin is a low–molecular-weight protein responsible for exerting about 60% to 70% of the serum colloid osmotic pressure. Approximately 10 g of albumin is produced by the normal liver each day; production drops to about 4 g daily in the cirrhotic patient (Galambos, 1979). Because the half-life of serum albumin is approximately 14–20 days, a decreased serum albumin level will not be apparent in patients with acute liver dysfunction unless there is predisposing malnutrition. Serum albumin levels will not normally decrease from liver dysfunction that lasts less than 3 weeks. Prealbumin, a precursor of albumin, has a much shorter half-life than albumin (7–9 days). Decreased plasma protein production is therefore more quickly identified by measuring serum prealbumin levels.

Liver cells synthesize and secrete all proteins necessary for coagulation. Hepatic synthesis of clotting factors II, VII, IX, and X is dependent on hepatocellular function and vitamin K. Vitamin K is lipid soluble and therefore depends on the presence of bile salts in the intestine for absorption. Failure of bile salt secretion leads to inadequate vitamin K absorption and deficiency of vitamin K-dependent clotting factors. Sterilization of the gut with antibiotics also inhibits the synthesis of vitamin K to some degree.

The most commonly used tests of coagulation are the PT and the partial thromboplastin time (PTT). Deficiencies in vitamin K-dependent clotting factors prolong the PT and PTT. The PT and PTT are therefore extremely sensitive indices of liver function. A PT greater than 3 seconds over the control time and a PTT greater than 10 seconds over the control time are significant. Prolongation indicates a deficiency of clotting factors, which may be a sign of acute or chronic liver dysfunction.

Metabolism of amino acids in the diet and from senescent tissue occurs either through the process of deamination (removal of an NH_2) or through the process of conversion of amino acids to ammonia and conversion of ammonia to urea. Deamination must occur before amino acids in the diet can be used for energy, tissue growth, or healing. Ammonia, as a byproduct of protein metabolism, can be formed as a result of deamination, from degradation of protein by gut flora, or from metabolism of blood in the gut secondary to upper GI bleeding. Hepatocellular dysfunction leads to elevated serum ammonia levels, which are associated with hepatic encephalopathy. However, there is evidence that ammonia is not the only toxic compound responsible for this condition (Jacques, 1985).

Lipid Metabolism

The liver is the principal site of lipid synthesis and degradation. Cholesterol, phospholipids, and lipoproteins are formed in the liver, and excess carbohydrates are converted by the liver to triglycerides, which are then stored in adipose tissue. When needed for energy production, triglycerides are metabolized to glycerol and fatty acids. Fatty acids are split into acetyl CoA, which is used in the Krebs cycle in the liver mitochondria for energy production. Phospholipids are necessary for cellular wall integrity and many chemical cellular reactions. Lipoproteins are necessary for lipid transport.

The liver produces about 1,000 mg of cholesterol a day, which is all that is necessary for health. Lipids are unable to circulate freely in the plasma; therefore, to be mobilized, they must be combined with a protein, in this case a lipoprotein. Within the intestine, cholesterol is solubilized into mixed micelles containing fatty acids, triglycerides, lecithin, lysolecithin, and bile acids. The transportation of cholesterol from the intestine to the liver occurs via lipoproteins, called chylomicrons, synthesized in intestinal mucosal cells. Chylomicrons undergo hydrolysis when they come into contact with the enzyme lipoprotein lipase. This results in the release of free fatty acids (FFAs) and the apolipoproteins A and C into the circulation. The residual lipoprotein, called chylomicron remnant, is removed rapidly by the liver. This process constitutes the exogenous pathway of lipoprotein metabolism.

The liver also plays a major role in the endogenous pathway of lipoprotein metabolism. The major lipoprotein synthesized by the liver is very low-density lipoprotein cholesterol (VLDLc). VLDLc interacts with lipoprotein lipase on the surface of capillary and endothelial cells, resulting in hydrolysis and release of FFAs, and a smaller VLDLc remnant. Approximately two-thirds of the VLDLc remnants are removed directly from the circulation by the hepatocytes. Approximately one-third of the VLDLc remnants interact with hepatic lipase and are converted to low-density lipoprotein cholesterol (LDLC). Approximately 75% of LDLc is cleared by the liver via LDLc receptors.

The number of LDLc receptors synthesized by the liver is regulated by the amount of cholesterol in the cell. High levels of intracellular cholesterol lead to suppression of transcription of the gene encoding the LDLc receptor, which leads to a decreased number of LDLc receptors. Reduction of LDLc receptor sites causes delayed clearance of LDLc and VLDLc remnants and results in higher plasma LDLc concentrations. There is, therefore, more free-floating LDLc in the circulation to contribute to atherogenesis.

The liver also acts as a storage depot for fat. There are fat-storing cells in the sinusoidal walls in the space of Disse. These cells store triglycerides and the fat-soluble vitamins A, D, E, and K. The healthy human adult has about a 2 years' supply of vitamin A and about a 6 months' supply of vitamin D stored in the liver.

DRUG AND HORMONE METABOLISM

Another metabolic function of the liver is the metabolism of a wide variety of drugs commonly administered to critically ill patients such as bronchodilators, antibiotics, corticosteroids, and histamine blockers. Hepatic clearance of drugs depends on the presence of drug-metabolizing enzymes, hepatocyte integrity, liver blood flow, and the plasma protein-binding affinity of the particular drug. Chronic ingestion of the same drug initially increases metabolism of that drug and therefore shortens the drug's half-life. However, with time and with hepatocellular damage and hepatic dysfunction, drug metabolism may be significantly impaired. Many drugs, including alcohol, are potentially toxic to the liver. Toxic agents are converted in the endoplasmic reticulum of the hepatocyte to water-soluble substances that can be excreted either in the urine or in the bile.

The adrenal response to stress or alterations in fluid volume status is to secrete glucocorticoids (cortisol) and mineralocorticoids (aldosterone). The liver plays an important role in inactivating these and other hormones when they are no longer needed to maintain homeostasis. Antidiuretic hormone is also cleared by the liver.

VASCULAR CLEARANCE FUNCTION

As mentioned earlier, Kupffer cells within the liver sinusoids function as tissue macrophages for the clearance of potentially pathogenic microorganisms. Patients with cirrhosis have a predisposition to bacterial infections due to shunting and decreased clearance of bacteria by the liver. Procoagulants, or activated clotting factors, and byproducts of coagulation are also cleared by these cells in the liver.

ASSESSMENT OF LIVER FUNCTION

Liver function, liver dysfunction, and effects of liver disease can be assessed or evaluated in various ways. The effects of liver disease on other organ systems can be assessed by laboratory techniques and physical examination. The degree of liver dysfunction is routinely assessed by standard laboratory tests, and true liver function is assessed by using sophisticated quantitative studies.

Physical Assessment

The four components of physical assessment—inspection, auscultation, percussion, and palpation—can be employed to elicit significant physical findings in the patient with suspected or known liver disease. These findings, however, are not evident until the disease is advanced.

INSPECTION. Typical physical findings in the patient with advanced liver disease are described in Table 49–1.

AUSCULTATION. The patient with advanced liver disease has a hyperdynamic cardiovascular system. There are several reasons for this. First, the vascular space increases as a result of extensive collateral vessel development, and vascular volume is not necessarily increased adequately to fill this space. Therefore, cardiac output, as part of the oxygen transport system, accelerates to meet tissue oxygen requirements. Second, anemia due to malnutrition, splenomegaly, and coagulopathy is common in the patient with advanced liver disease. Cardiac output accelerates for the same reason in this condition to increase oxygen transport.

TABLE 49–1. **Physical Assessment Findings in Advanced Liver Disease**

Finding	Rationale
Jaundice	Yellowish discoloration of skin, sclera, and secretions. Due to alteration in bilirubin metabolism. If the problem is "prehepatic" such as hemolysis, the light-skinned patient will manifest mild jaundice and appear mildly yellow. If the problem is "hepatic," such as acute hepatocellular necrosis, the light-skinned patient will appear deep yellow or orange. If the problem is cholestasis, jaundice will become manifest insidiously, and the light-skinned patient will appear greenish.
Spider nevi (Fig. 49–6)	Cutaneous angiomas commonly seen on the anterior thorax, shoulders, neck, and face, and rarely on the posterior thorax. They are part of the arteriovenous (AV) collateral system that develops as a result of portal hypertension. A central arteriole feeds each clump of dilated blood vessels and will blanch when suppressed. The tiny vessels are quickly refilled as pressure is released. This is one feature distinguishing spider nevi from petechial hemorrhages.
Caput medusae	Dilated abdominal veins radiating from the umbilicus. Part of the AV collateral vessel system that develops as a result of portal hypertension.
Striae	"Stretch marks" prominent on inner aspect of arms, lower abdomen, thighs, and buttocks seen in both males and females. Due to increased levels of circulating cortisol.
Palmar erythema	Palmar surfaces of hands appear bright red. Thought to be due to (1) diffuse formation of AV collaterals in hands, and (2) increased levels of circulating estrogen.
Hepatomegaly	Enlarged liver in acute hepatitis, early alcoholic cirrhosis, and early primary biliary cirrhosis.
Splenomegaly	Enlarged spleen as a consequence of portal hypertension.
Clubbing of fingers	Thought to be due to extensive peripheral collateral vessel formation and alteration in hormone metabolism.
Easy bruising	Due to insufficient coagulation factors and thrombocytopenia; seen especially on the legs.
Dry skin and scratch marks	Due to chronic cholestasis and formation of bile crystals in skin. Pruritus is most common skin symptom. It often precedes onset of jaundice and clears as liver insufficiency progresses except in patients with cholestatic liver disease.
Brittle hair, hair loss	Body hair is thinned or lost; nails become white and flat with white striations. Due to increased levels of circulating estrogen and zinc deficiency.
Hypogonadism, feminization in men	Manifested by testicular atrophy, impotence, decreased beard and pubic hair, female escutcheon, and gynecomastia. Exact etiology is unclear, but chronic alcohol abuse is thought to be a significant factor (Van Thiel et al., 1974).
Peripheral edema	Due to hypoalbuminemia.
Xanthomas	Flat, round lesions on eyelids, extensor surfaces of palms, creases of hands, and sometimes on the trunk, face, and extremities. Due to hyperlipidemia and seen commonly in patients with primary biliary cirrhosis.
Cachexia	Appearance of malnutrition due to protein calorie malnutrition with muscle wasting and depletion of subcutaneous fat stores.
Hyperpigmentation	Dark spots on skin, frequently on lower extremities due to chronic cholestasis
Poor oral health status	Loss of dentin on teeth, dental caries, gingivitis, and halitosis due to malnutrition and vitamin deficiencies.

Third, GI peptides responsible for vasodilation are normally cleared from the circulation by the liver. In advanced liver disease they remain in the systemic circulation and cause a compensatory increase in cardiac output. An auscultatory abdominal finding associated with the hyperdynamic circulatory system in advanced liver disease is the *venous hum*. A venous hum is usually heard on auscultation of the abdomen over the upper aspect of the liver. This sound is a murmur that is continuous throughout the cardiac cycle and is associated with rapid flow through collateral portacaval vessels.

PERCUSSION. Although advances in radiographic and angiographic technology are more frequently used, percussion is sometimes useful for determining liver size, splenic enlargement, and the presence of ascites. Liver size can be estimated by percussing from the right clavicle straight down the right midclavicular line (MCL) (Fig. 49–7). Over lung tissue the percussion tone is resonant. At about the level of the fifth intercostal space the percussion tone becomes dull; this marks the upper edge of the liver. The percussion tone over the bowel is normally tympanic. Percussing upward from the level of the umbilicus, again at the MCL, over tympanic bowel until a dull percussion tone is heard locates the lower edge of the liver. The distance between the upper and lower edges of the liver at the midclavicular line, as determined by percussion, is normally about 12 cm (see Fig. 49–7). The liver enlarges in acute inflammatory states such as alcoholic and viral hepatitis. In most advanced forms of disease, the liver atrophies.

The spleen cannot normally be percussed. However, in conditions in which the spleen is grossly enlarged (such as in portal hypertension), it may be percussed at the left MCL, very low in the abdomen. Dull percussion tones are heard over the intercostal spaces and below the left costal margin.

Although ascites may be obvious on inspection,

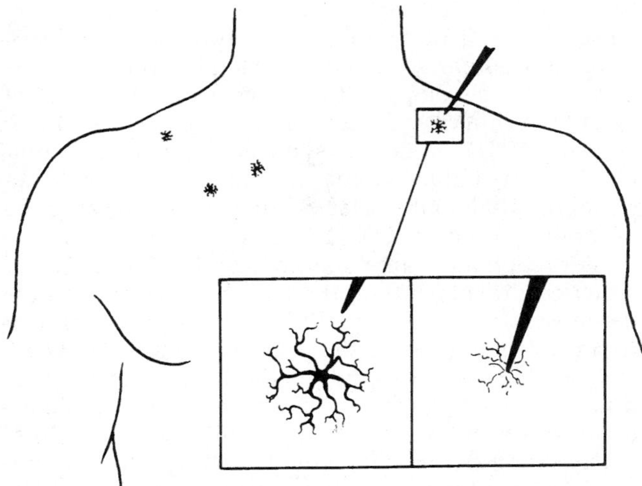

FIGURE 49–6. Cutaneous angiomas, or spider nevi. Notice blanching produced by pressure on central arteriole. (From Prior, J. A., Silberstein, J. S., & Stang, J. M. [1981]. *Physical diagnosis: The history and examination of the patient* [6th ed.]. St. Louis: C. V. Mosby.)

smaller collections of peritoneal fluid that are not visible can sometimes be detected by percussion.

PALPATION. This technique is most useful for assessing liver size. Palpation of the liver is performed at the patient's right side by supporting the right flank area with the left hand and sliding the fingertips of the right hand under the right costal margin using firm pressure. The fingertips are advanced as the patient inhales deeply. The liver edge moves 1 to 3 cm downward during inspiration. Position of the fingertips is held steady as the patient exhales and inhales again. As the patient inhales, exhales, and inhales, the smooth edge of the liver may be felt moving past the fingertips. The liver is more easily palpated in thin individuals. Liver palpation is deep palpation and is therefore slightly uncomfortable in most people if it is done correctly.

Normally, the liver cannot be palpated more than 1 to 2 cm below the right costal margin. However, there is one condition in which the liver may be palpated far below the right costal margin when it is not enlarged. This occurs in the patient with advanced chronic obstructive pulmonary disease when the diaphragm becomes flattened and immobile. The flattened diaphragm pushes the liver farther down into the right abdominal quadrant.

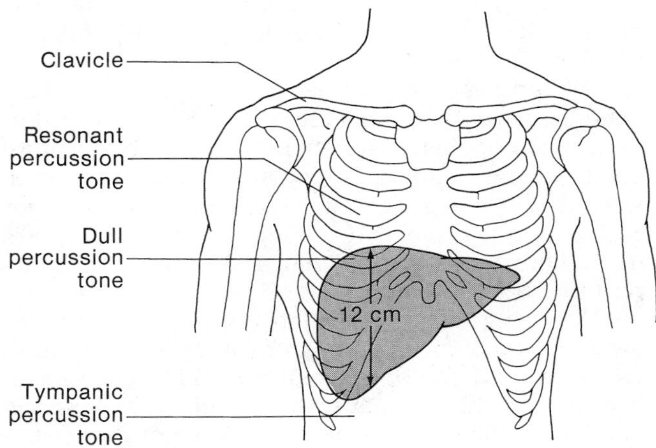

FIGURE 49–7. Percussion to determine liver size.

Standard Laboratory Assessment

Liver function is the capacity of the liver to perform specific tasks or functions. The conventional tests of bilirubin, albumin, PT, and liver enzymes, although referred to as "liver function" tests, do not actually assess liver function. Instead, these tests provide information about liver "dysfunction" and, to some extent, the specific type of liver injury.

The serum bilirubin value indicates the efficiency of the hepatic uptake and excretory system and the rate of production of bilirubin, Serum bilirubin, albumin, and PT were discussed in a previous section.

Liver enzymes are released during cellular injury and stop being released as injured hepatocytes heal. If hepatocellular injury is severe enough to cause massive necrosis, serum enzyme levels will be initially extremely high and then decline because there are no more enzymes to be released. Liver enzymes can be classified into two major types: *aminotransaminases* and *phosphatases.*

Liver aminotransaminases include serum, AST, and ALT. AST is released into the circulation when cells of the heart, skeletal muscle, kidney, or liver are injured. Therefore, an increased AST level is not specific to hepatocellular injury. ALT is released in the same conditions but in much larger quantities from injured liver cells, and is considered a more specific liver cell enzyme. However, in liver disease, elevations in AST and ALT are most often parallel.

The phosphatases include ALP and GGT. Although serum phosphatase levels increase with hepatocellular damage, these increases are more specific to bile duct injury or cholestasis. GGT is more likely to be elevated during biliary obstruction than during hepatocellular damage, and GGT is elevated in alcoholics. Normal serum aminotransferase and phosphatase values are listed in Table 49–2.

Quantitative Liver Function

As previously stated, the traditional laboratory methods for assessing liver function can be grossly misleading. Acute hepatocellular damage can produce significant changes in serum values of bilirubin, liver enzymes, and PT. However, as acute damage resolves, these values can return to normal. Conversely, these values may be practically normal in the patient who has far-advanced liver disease and little functional capacity of the liver. Reliance on the patient's physical appearance and the laboratory evaluation can result in

TABLE 49–2. **Normal Values for Hepatic Function Tests**

Test	Normal Value
Bilirubin (total)	1.0 mg/dL
Indirect	0.5 mg/dL
Direct	0.5 mg/dL
Urobilinogen (urine)	0.2–3.0 mg/24 hours
Urinary bilirubin	0
AST	40.0 units
ALT	45.0 units
ALP	1.5 U/dL (Bodansky)
	4.0–13.0 U/dL (King-Armstrong)
	0.8–2.3 U/mL (Bessey-Lowry)
	15.0–35.0 U/mL (Shinowara-Jones-Rinehart)
GGT	5–55 U/liters
Prothrombin time	Greater than 3 seconds over control
Fibrinogen	200–400 mg/dL
Albumin	3.5–5.0 g/dL
Ammonia	11–35 Umol/liter
Cholesterol	100–250 mg/dL

Abbreviations: AST, aspartate aminotransferase; ALT, alanine aminotransferase; ALP, alkaline phosphatase; GGT, gamma-glutamyl transpeptidase.

errors in diagnosis, prognosis, and treatment for the patient with liver dysfunction and disease.

Liver function can be quantified by assessing the metabolic and clearance functions of the liver, which depend on functional liver cell mass and blood flow. Some of the more useful quantitative tests are the galactose elimination capacity (GEC) and galactose clearance.

The GEC measures the functional hepatocyte mass by calculating the maximal removal rate of galactose, which is exclusively and rapidly converted to glucose in the liver. In this test, a known quantity of galactose is administered intravenously (IV), and several blood samples are taken over a given time span. Assays of these samples are plotted on a semilogarithmic plasma concentration curve over time. The maximal rate of galactose removal is calculated from the slope of this curve. Normal GEC is 500 mg/minute or 33 mg/kg per minute (Henderson & Warren, 1986).

The galactose clearance is used to evaluate hepatocyte function and is an index of "nutritive" liver blood flow. In this test, a 5% solution of galactose is administered IV, and several blood samples are taken over time. Assays of these samples are plotted on a standard plasma concentration versus time curve, and galactose clearance is calculated using a steady-state equation. Normal galactose clearance is between 1,100 and 1,600 mL/minute (Henderson & Warren, 1986).

ACUTE FULMINANT HEPATIC FAILURE

Acute fulminant hepatic failure (AFHF) is a rare clinical syndrome characterized by sudden clinical and biochemical presence of liver disease or severe impairment of liver function due to massive hepatocellular necrosis in someone with previously normal liver function. Liver biopsy reveals massive necrosis, collapse of the reticulin network, and little or no evidence of hepatocellular regeneration. Hepatic encephalopathy usually develops within 8 weeks of the onset of symptoms, but may develop much sooner (Williams & Gimson, 1984). A similar syndrome, subacute fulminant hepatic failure, occurs in which the onset of hepatic encephalopathy is later—up to 6 months after the onset of symptoms (O'Grady et al., 1988).

Although there are many causes of AFHF, in North America viral hepatitis and acetaminophen toxicity are the most common causes. Other causes include mushroom poisoning, acute Budd-Chiari syndrome, acute Wilson's disease, acute fatty liver of pregnancy, infectious organisms such as *Aspergillis,* acute hepatic artery thrombosis, massive blastic infiltration of the liver such as may occur with acute leukemia and lymphoreticular malignancies, Reye syndrome, anesthetic agents, industrial toxins (carbon tetrachloride), pesticides (DDT), and herbicides (paraquat).

The prognosis for the patient with AFHF is poor. With the exception of the patient with acetaminophen toxicity, the outcome is almost always fatal unless liver transplantation is performed in time (Smith & Ciferni, 1993).

Acetaminophen-Induced Acute Fulminant Hepatic Failure

The sudden ingestion of 7.5 g or the chronic ingestion of 3 g/day of acetaminophen in adults can induce AFHF. Alcohol ingestion enhances acetaminophen toxicity. Two metabolic pathways are involved in the detoxification of acetaminophen: conjugation and the cytochrome P450 mixed function oxidase pathway. Approximately 97% of acetaminophen is metabolized through conjugation. During conjugation, a potentially hepatotoxic metabolite combines with hepatic glutathione to form the nontoxic compound mercapturate, which is excreted in the urine. When excessive amounts of acetaminophen are ingested, the conjugation pathway becomes saturated, and increased amounts of the hepatotoxic metabolite accumulate. As hepatic glutathione is depleted, this metabolite combines with hepatocellular proteins and causes hepatocellular necrosis.

The serum acetaminophen level is a good prognostic indicator of the probability of hepatic necrosis, but the acetaminophen level should not be drawn until about 4 hours after ingestion because absorption is slowed with large quantities. The normal range for acetaminophen level is 10–20 mg/L. Hepatotoxicity is likely with levels greater than 200 mg/L at 4 hours postingestion.

The clinical presentation of acetaminophen-induced AFHF is different from AFHF due to other causes. In acetaminophen-induced AFHF, the patient becomes diaphoretic, nauseated, anorexic, and usually vomits within 24 hours of the toxic ingestion. Dehydration may occur. The onset of clinical signs is delayed for 3 to 4 days, when the patient experiences RUQ pain and becomes jaundiced, oliguric, and encephalopathic. Laboratory evidence of elevated serum aminotransferase and phosphatase levels, elevated serum bilirubin, and prolonged PT peaks at approximately 4 days after ingestion.

Non–Acetaminophen-Induced Acute Fulminant Hepatic Failure

The patient with non–acetaminophen-induced AFHF may report vague, flu-like signs and symptoms including nausea, vomiting, malaise, and fatigue. This prodromal period is followed by a variable period of rapidly progressive liver failure and multisystem organ failure. Rapid deterioration of hepatic function is associated with severe systemic alterations: hyperventilation and respiratory alkalosis, coagulopathy and bleeding, hypoglycemia, peripheral edema and ascites, hepatorenal syndrome, sepsis, metabolic acidosis, cardiovascular collapse, and increased intracranial pressure (ICP) with hepatic encephalopathy. Frequently, progression from a fully alert and productive state to encephalopathic coma occurs in a period of only a few days.

Clinical Presentation

Subtle mental status changes are often the first sign of acute liver failure. Cerebral dysfunction is attributed to three factors: (1) decreased synthesis of glucose required by the brain for metabolism; (2) faulty detoxification of nitrogenous byproducts of protein metabolism; and (3) replacement of normal neurotransmitters by "false" neurotransmitters that induce sedation (Galambos, 1979). Increased levels of free ammonia stimulate the respiratory center, causing hyperventilation and respiratory alkalosis. The electroencephalogram (EEG) shows generalized slowing and nonspecific changes consistent with metabolic encephalopathy (Jacques, 1985). Neurologic complications (e.g., cerebral edema, increased ICP, and cerebral herniation) account for most deaths (Daas et al., 1995; Cordoba and Blei, 1995). The signs of progressive hepatic encephalopathy in the patient with AFHF are consistent with the signs of increased ICP: progressive alteration of mental status (deepening coma), brisk deep tendon reflexes, clonus, decortication, decerebration, and dilated pupils. Unfortunately, computed tomography (CT) scans are of little value in detecting cerebral edema in patients with AFHF (Munoz et al., 1991). Therefore, without direct ICP monitoring, the clinical diagnosis of increased ICP is difficult until tentorial herniation occurs. An accurate initial assessment is important to establish a baseline from which to identify subtle changes that may support life-saving treatment decisions. Signs and symptoms of hepatic encephalopathy or coma are outlined in Table 49–3.

On physical examination, the patient's liver is found to be enlarged during the inflammatory phase but becomes progressively smaller with massive necrosis. Rapid reduction in liver size, increasing bilirubin concentration with severe jaundice, severely prolonged PT with hemorrhagic complications, and hypoglycemia are prognostic of impending death. The hemodynamic changes seen in patients with AFHF characterize the hyperdynamic patient and are similar to those associated with septic shock—a decrease in systemic vascular resistance with a compensatory increase in cardiac output (Iwatsuki et al., 1985).

Laboratory findings are remarkable. Serum transaminase levels are markedly elevated early in the course of disease as high as 20,000 U/mL but fall toward the normal range as the liver mass becomes necrotic. Therefore, a decrease in serum transaminase levels is not always a sign of improvement. In addition to signaling that the necrotic process has been arrested, this finding may also indicate that complete necrosis of the liver has occurred. The serum bilirubin is elevated, and coagulation times are significantly prolonged. Serum ammonia levels are elevated, but values do not correlate well with the degree of encephalopathy. The patient may be profoundly hypoglycemic. Serum albumin levels remain normal unless the patient is already malnourished.

As the liver dies, multisystem shock and failure ensue. The clinical syndromes of circulatory collapse secondary to hypovolemia and sepsis, acute respiratory failure, acute renal failure, disseminated coagulopathy, and increased intracranial hypertension become manifest.

Interventions

The goal of initial management of the patient with acetaminophen toxicity is to prevent continued drug absorption. Interventions include evacuating the stomach and adsorbing acetaminophen with activated charcoal. However, charcoal will also absorb another therapeutic drug used to treat acetaminophen overdose, *N*-acetyl-L-cysteine. Treatment with *N*-acetyl-L-cysteine, which is a glutathione precursor, can prevent severe liver damage if it is administered within 8 hours of the acetaminophen overdose (Leoni, 1985). Considerable psychosocial support is necessary for the patient who has taken an intentional overdose, and a psychiatric consultation is indicated.

Survival depends on the capability of hepatocellular regeneration or preservation of organ systems until hepatic regeneration occurs or until definitive treatment such as liver transplantation can be employed. The need for intensive care and multisystem support is obvious. However, in spite of the fact that neurologic complications account for most deaths, prompt and appropriate interventions to decrease cerebral edema are often overlooked.

TABLE 49–3. **Clinical Assessment of Hepatic Encephalopathy**

	Grade I	Grade II	Grade III	Grade IV
Level of consciousness	Awake	Decreased, but opens eyes spontaneously	Patient sleeps, but is arousable to verbal and painful stimuli; does not open eyes spontaneously	Comatose; no response to pain
Orientation	Total orientation with progression to confusion; then disorientation to time and place	Disoriented to time and place; severe confusion	Complete disorientation when aroused	Comatose
Intellectual functions	Mental clouding; slowness in answering questions; impaired handwriting; subtle changes in intellectual function, psychometric test scores decrease	Amnesia for past events; psychometric test scores decrease	Inability to make computations	Comatose
Behavior	Forgetful, restless, irritable, untidy, apathetic, disobedient	Decreased inhibitions, lethargic	Bizarre behavior (rage)	Comatose
Mood	Euphoria, depression, crying	Apathetic, paranoid	Apathy increases	Comatose
Neuromuscular	Muscular incoordination, tremors, yawning, insomnia	Hypoactive reflexes, asterixis, ataxia, slurred speech	Cannot cooperate; nystagmus and Babinski sign; clonus, decortication, decerebration, rigidity, seizures	Seizures; rigidity decreases to flaccidity; dilated pupils
Electroencephalography	Mild to moderate abnormalities	Moderate to severe abnormalities	Severe abnormalities	Severe abnormalities

The patient with AFHF is critically ill. The severity of the situation and the rapidity of deterioration must be recognized early by the health care team, and a protocol for managing this patient population should be in place to avoid unnecessary delays in diagnosis and interventions. Endotracheal intubation should be done before the patient loses consciousness to prevent pulmonary aspiration. A nasogastric (NG) tube is also necessary to allow gastric decompression, administer antacids, and serve as an alert to upper GI bleeding, a common complication of AFHF. Replacement of clotting factors with fresh frozen plasma is necessary to treat coagulopathy. Placement of any invasive catheters or other devices should be done before coagulopathy becomes so severe that these procedures are prohibited. Hemofiltration may be necessary for stabilization of fluid, electrolyte, and acid–base imbalances if acute renal failure and oliguria occur. It is important to avoid overhydration because it can increase cerebral edema.

The goals of treatment of the patient with hepatic encephalopathy are to remove the precipitating factors of encephalopathy, decrease ICP, and preserve cerebral integrity. Prophylactic insertion of an ICP monitoring device is useful for managing intracranial hypertension, but its contribution to increased survival is less clear (Daas et al., 1995). However, neurosurgeons may be reluctant to perform this procedure because of the risks associated with coagulopathy.

Stimuli that increase ICP should be avoided: physical and verbal stimulation should be kept to a minimum, and the lights should be dimmed. Increases in intraabdominal and intrathoracic pressure should be prevented. Cerebral edema can be treated temporarily in the traditional manner with mannitol.

Parenteral amino acids are avoided, and the GI tract should be evacuated to minimize interactions between nitrogenous substances and enteric bacterial flora that produce ammonia. Colonic irrigation with tap water enemas until there is a clear return is one effective method. Lactulose enemas can also be used, and the gut can be sterilized with nonabsorbable antibiotics such as neomycin. Other methods of removing toxins from the body have also been used with varying degrees of success. In general, modalities such as exchange blood transfusions, plasmapheresis, hemodialysis, and charcoal hemoperfusion have not been very successful (O'Grady et al., 1988).

The advances made in liver transplantation have drastically improved the treatment options and outcomes for patients with AFHF (Smith & Ciferni, 1993; Wall & Adams, 1995). Preserving cerebral integrity by early identification and treatment of increased ICP, and early referral for liver transplantation are key factors in patient survival.

The patient in AFHF presents not only physiologic but also intense psychosocial challenges to the critical care nurse. Family members often cannot comprehend how someone can be well one day or week and dying the next. Explaining the link between a failing liver and unconsciousness is difficult at best. Preparing a family for organ transplantation is a process that is optimally done over days or weeks. In this situation, there may not be time to assess important psychosocial factors vital to the long-term success of transplantation or to provide preoperative education. If the patient is not a candidate for liver transplantation, then, in most cases, the critical care team and family will have to cope with the death of the patient.

HEPATITIS

Hepatitis is an important cause of acute and chronic liver disease worldwide. Causes of hepatitis include viral, drug-related, and autoimmune disease processes. There are multiple viruses that may cause hepatitis in humans; they are generally classified as RNA or DNA viruses. The most common RNA viruses that cause hepatitis in the United States are the hepatitis A virus (HAV) and the hepatitis C virus (HCV). In addition, the hepatitis D virus (HDV) and the hepatitis E virus (HEV) are RNA viruses. The most common DNA virus is the hepatitis B virus (HBV). The herpesviruses (cytomegalovirus, Epstein-Barr virus, herpes simplex viruses, varicella zoster virus) are also DNA viruses. This chapter specifically addresses viral hepatitis—HAV, HBV, and HCV.

Hepatitis is defined as an acute inflammation of the entire liver, characterized by centrilobular necrosis and infiltration of the portal tracts by leukocytes (Galambos, 1979). Hepatitis can present as an acute fulminant, acute, or chronic process. Approximately 500,000 new cases of viral hepatitis are diagnosed in the United States each year (Alter et al., 1990b; Mahoney et al., 1993). The incidence in the general public is less than 5%, but the incidence in health care workers is about 30% (Mahoney et al., 1993).

Those at high risk in the general population include those with lepromatous leprosy, homosexuals or heterosexuals with multiple partners, drug abusers, those institutionalized with Down syndrome, hemophiliacs, those of ethnic origin from a country with a high carrier rate, those receiving blood transfusions in underdeveloped countries, and neonates of carrier mothers. Health care personnel who are at high risk are surgeons, hemodialysis personnel, those caring for transplant or oncology patients, those caring for patients with GI bleeding, burn unit personnel, laboratory and pathology personnel, and dentists.

The basic pathophysiology of viral hepatitis is the same. Acute hepatitis can become manifest clinically anywhere along a spectrum ranging from an anicteric, nearly asymptomatic episode to AFHF. Nearly 50% of those contracting acute hepatitis are asymptomatic.

In symptomatic cases of acute nonfulminant hepatitis, an icteric attack occurs that includes a prodromal period of a few days to several weeks. During this time the patient feels "flu-like" with RUQ tenderness, malaise and fatigue, and experiences a lack of desire to smoke cigarettes or drink alcohol. Serum aminotransferase levels are slightly elevated at this time. The urine then becomes dark and the feces colorless; this is followed by jaundice and an elevated serum bilirubin. There is tender enlargement of the liver and an elevated white blood cell count. After a few weeks symptoms begin to decrease and the patient usually recovers without sequelae other than persistent fatigue. A diagnosis of acute viral hepatitis can usually be made from clinical findings; however, only virus-specific tests can identify the virus responsible for a specific infection. The laboratory diagnosis of HAV, HBV, HCV, HDV, or HEV depends on detection of specific antigens or antibodies, viral DNA or RNA, or DNA or RNA polymerase-containing virions. A list of serologic markers used to diagnose hepatitis is shown in Table 49–4.

There are three types of chronic hepatitis: the asymptomatic carrier state, chronic persistent hepatitis, and chronic active hepatitis (CAH). Chronic hepatitis is a chronic inflammation in the liver due to HBV or HCV infection for at least 6 months. A carrier state occurs when the infected individual is unable to clear the antigen from the serum, presumably due to ineffective cellular immunity. Immunosuppressed individuals such as organ transplant recipients, oncology patients, and those with chronic renal failure are at high risk for becoming chronic carriers. When the virus is HBV, HBsAg and HBsAb are found in the serum. The chronic carrier suffers no liver damage but can transmit the virus to others. There are approximately 200 million carriers in the world. In the United States about 5% to 10% of the population and 1% of health care workers are carriers (Mahoney et al., 1993). Chronic persistent hepatitis is characterized by swelling of the portal zones with inflammatory infiltrates, and there is some fibrosis. Piecemeal necrosis is absent. Chronic lobular hepatitis is characterized by intralobular inflammation and necrosis. CAH is characterized by greatly expanded portal zones with extension into the lobules. There is erosion of the limiting plates and piecemeal necrosis.

In CAH liver damage is progressive. Continued viral replication in the liver leads to progressive hepatocellular necrosis. CAH is more likely to occur in the individual who has had a mild or asymptomatic case of acute HBV, HCV, or hepatitis non-A, non-B, non-C infection (Seef & Koff, 1986). The most important sequela of CAH is primary hepatocellular carcinoma (Seef & Koff, 1986). Cirrhosis can develop after a severe case of acute hepatitis, in which case it is called postnecrotic cirrhosis, and it can develop as the end stage of CAH.

Hepatitis A

The HAV is an enterovirus similar to the polio virus. Hepatitis A ("infectious hepatitis") accounts for approximately 20% to 25% of all hepatitis cases world-

TABLE 49–4. **Nomenclature of Serologic Testing for Viral Hepatitis**

Serologic Test	Description and Purpose
Hepatitis A Virus (HAV)	
anti-HAV (total)	Antibody to HAV; detectable at onset of disease before jaundice; presence in serum confers life-long immunity
IgM	Rises early during infection (detectable at 4–6 weeks after exposure and within 1 week after signs and symptoms develop, disappears within 8–12 weeks); indicates acute infection; persists for approximately 6 months
IgG	Rises slowly during infection (detectable at 8–12 weeks after exposure and persists for life)
Hepatitis B Virus (HBV)	
HBsAg	HBV *surface* antigen; most important and commonly used marker for HBV infection; detectable within 30 days of exposure and persists up to 3 months after jaundice unless a carrier state develops, in which case it will persist longer; presence in serum (serpositivity) indicates that disease is infectious
HBcAg	HBV *core* antigen; not detectable in serum, only detectable in hepatocytes
HBeAg	HBV *e* antigen; found only in sera positive for HBsAG; presence in serum (seropositivity) indicates high titer of HBV (extensive vitral replication) and increased infectiousness (ongoing viral replication); detectable 4–6 weeks after exposure
anti-HBs	Antibody to HBsAg; presence in serum (seropositivity) indicates HBV immunity due to HBV infection or vaccination; detectable 4–8 weeks after HBsAg disappears
anti-HBc (total)	Antibody to HBcAg; detectable 6–14 weeks after exposure during what is referred to as the "window phase" (after HBsAg disappears but before HBsAb appears); persists for life; high titers may indicate persistent infection (carrier state)
IgM	Rises early in infection; if persistent, may indicate chronic infection
IgG	Rises slowly during infection; persists for life
HBeAb	Antibody to HBeAg
HBV-DNA	HBV-DNA detected by process of nucleic acid hybridization
PCR for HBV DNA	Polymerase chain reaction (PCR) for HBV DNA; test detects polymerase-containing virions; PCR process amplifies DNA in blood so that it is easily detected; very sensitive test
Hepatitis D Virus (HDV; delta hepatitis virus)	
HDAg (total)	Antigen to HDV; detectable only concurrently with HBV infection
IgM	Rises early in infection; if persistent, may indicate chronic infection
IgG	Rises slowly during infection; persists for life
anti-HDV	Antibody to HDV; detectable only concurrent with HBV infection
HDV-RNA	HDV-RNA detected by process of nucleic acid hybridization
Hepatitis C Virus (HCV)	
anti-HCV	Antibody to HCV; presence (seropositivity) in serum is diagnostic for chronic infection only; absence (seronegativity) does not exclude the diagnosis of HCV infection; may see false positive results
HCV-RNA	HCV-RNA is detected by process of nucleic acid hybridization; presence of HCV-RNA in serum is diagnostic of viremia in acute or chronic HCV hepatitis; the HCV-RNA test is also used to monitor response to interferon-alpha therapy
PCR for HCV-RNA	Polymerase chain reaction for HCV RNA; test detects polymerase-containing virions; PCR process amplifies RNA in blood so that it is easily detected; very sensitive test
bDNA	Quantitative test of HCV-RNA for determining amount of virus; research assay not yet licensed by FDA
Hepatitis E Virus (HEV)	
PCR for HEV-RNA	Polymerase chain reaction (PCR) for HEV RNA; test detects polymerase-containing virions; PCR process amplifies RNA in blood so that it is easily detected; very sensitive test

Serologic Criteria for Diagnosing Acute Hepatitis A Virus Infection

HAVAb-IgM positive

Serologic Criteria for Diagnosing Acute Hepatitis B Virus Infection

HBsAg positive *or*
HBsAb positive *or*
HBcAb-IgM positive *or*
HBV-DNA positive *or*

Serologic Criteria for Diagnosing Acute Hepatitis C Virus Infection

HCVAb positive *or*
Anti-HCV *or*
HCV-RNA positive *or*
Quantitative HCV RNA-bDNA positive

wide (Lettau, 1992). About 20,000 people with hepatitis A are hospitalized in the United States each year.

The mode of transmission is the fecal–oral route. The virus is found in the stool from about 2 weeks before until 1 week after the onset of jaundice. The incubation period is from 2 to 6 weeks. As the stool becomes negative for HAV, serum HAVAb appears and is detectable for years. Therefore, the virus is transmissible before it is apparent that the disease exists. Serum anti-HAV IgM suggests recent infection, and serum anti-HAV IgG confers immunity to HAV.

Hepatitis A is more common in children than adults because of the route of transmission. Those at highest risk for hepatitis A are those of lower socioeconomic status living in crowded conditions, those confined to crowded psychiatric wards, and those living in or traveling to areas with contaminated food and water sources.

Although asymptomatic cases of acute hepatitis can occur, clinical presentation usually involves an acute onset of signs and symptoms including malaise, jaundice, and diarrhea. Often this condition is mistaken for gastroenteritis. Hepatitis A is more severe in adults than in children, but recovery in almost all cases is complete without sequelae. Chronic states do not develop after an acute HAV infection.

Hepatitis B

Hepatitis B infection ("serum hepatitis") is a serious health problem in the United States and worldwide. Hepatitis B is a very different disease in North America and Western Europe, however, than in the Subsahara and the Far East. In North America and Western Europe, the incidence is relatively low, infection occurs mostly during early adulthood, the mode of transmission is most commonly IV drug abuse paraphernalia and sexual intercourse, and the risk of hepatocellular carcinoma is low. By contrast, in the Subsahara and Far East, the incidence is much higher, infection occurs in infants and toddlers, the mode of transmission is perinatal, chronicity is likely, and the risk of hepatocellular carcinoma is high. Approximately 200,000 new cases of hepatitis B are diagnosed in the United States each year (Mahoney et al., 1993).

Carriers are the major source of disease transmission. The major vector is blood and body fluids of infected individuals. The virus is known to be transmitted through whole blood, semen, and saliva. Other body fluids (urine, tears, wound drainage, bile, peritoneal and synovial fluid) of infected individuals contain the HBsAg but not the complete virus, so it is not clear whether these fluids are vectors as well (Hoofnagle & Schafer, 1986; Seef & Koff, 1986).

Hepatitis B disease transmission patterns have changed in the last decade. Previously, male homosexuals were the largest risk group, but currently, IV drug users and heterosexuals with multiple sexual partners are at highest risk (Alter et al., 1990a). Thus, hepatitis B is considered a sexually transmitted disease.

The HBV is a DNA virus, originally referred to as the Dane particle, that belongs to the class of viruses called hepadnaviruses. The HBV has an outer component of surface antigen (HBsAg or "Australia antigen") and an inner component called the HBcAg. HBV is not highly virulent (likely to produce severe illness), but it is highly infective (easily transmissible). It is estimated that 300,000 new cases occur each year, with approximately 18,000 occurring in health care workers (United States Department of Labor, 1987).

The incubation period for HBV is 6 to 26 weeks. In the initial stage of the infection the HBsAg is found in the serum for 4 to 12 weeks. This is the replicating phase when the virus enters the liver cells, replicates, and produces complete virions (Dane particles) and excess surface antigen (HBsAg and HBeAg), which are components of the viral capsid. During this time the infection is very contagious. Then a period of time occurs called the "window" phase between the disappearance of antigen (HBsAg) from the serum and the appearance of antibody (HBsAb). During this time the only serologic marker present is the antibody to HBcAg (HBcAb). This is why it is important that a complete hepatitis serology panel be done in the individual with suspected hepatitis infection. Failure to look for the HBcAb can lead to a false assumption that the patient does not have or has not had HBV infection. The window phase lasts for 2 to 12 weeks. Eventually (after 2 to 10 months), HBsAb appears in the serum.

As stated previously, an acute hepatitis B infection can be entirely asymptomatic. Subclinical disease is frequent, as suggested by the high incidence of HBcAb found in those with no knowledge or history of infection. In symptomatic cases the onset of signs and symptoms is insidious. A prodromal period of flu-like symptoms of fatigue, nausea, taste changes, and anorexia occurs approximately 2 weeks before the onset of jaundice and dark urine. Complete recovery can take as long as several months.

Hepatitis B is associated with serum sickness or immune complex disease. Fever, malaise, liver tenderness, arthralgias, and rashes are common. Less common are arthropathies such as rheumatoid arthritis or polyarteritis, and necrotizing vasculitis. Elevated serum transaminase and bilirubin levels accompany this phase.

Delta Hepatitis

Delta hepatitis is always associated with a coexistent HBV infection. Delta virus and HBV may coinfect, or delta virus hepatitis may be superimposed on the HBV carrier state. The mode of transmission is similar to that of HBV. Diagnosis is made by detection of the delta antigen in the serum or liver, or by detection of the IgM antibody to the delta virus in the serum.

Hepatitis C

The major cause of what was previously referred to as non-A, non-B (NANB) hepatitis has been identified as the HCV (Cuthbert, 1990). HCV is a single-stranded, linear RNA virus similar to flavivirus. Multiple strains of HCV exist.

HCV is the most common cause of posttransfusion-associated and post–liver transplant-associated chronic liver disease (Sherlock, 1993a). Of patients who acquire posttransfusion HCV infection, 50% to 60% develop chronic HCV hepatitis and 20% develop cirrhosis (Sherlock, 1993b). The incidence of posttransplant HCV hepatitis and cirrhosis is currently being studied. HCV has been implicated in autoimmune liver disease, CAH in patients with alcoholic cirrhosis, and hepatocellular carcinoma (Cuthbert, 1990). IV drug users are at higher risk, and others at risk include heterosexuals with multiple sexual partners or an infected partner, health care personnel exposed to blood and blood products, hemophiliacs, and chronic hemodialysis patients (Alter et al., 1990b).

Hepatitis E

Hepatitis E virus is also called enterically transmitted NANB hepatitis, epidemic NANB hepatitis, and fecal–oral NANB hepatitis, but should not be confused with HBV e antigen. The epidemiologic and clinical courses are similar to those of HAV infection, except that the incidence and prevalence are highest in young adult men.

Caring for the Patient With Hepatitis

The patient presenting with suspected or known acute hepatitis should be questioned about specific risk factors and close personal contacts so that follow-up with those who are potentially infected can be done. Treatment of acute hepatitis has very little effect on outcome. The patient needs to rest until symptoms disappear, the liver is no longer tender, and the serum bilirubin has decreased to within normal range. A low-fat, high-carbohydrate diet is most palatable, but does not necessarily play a role in recovery. Corticosteroid therapy does not favorably alter the course of acute hepatitis; in fact, this treatment has been shown to enhance viral replication (Perillo, 1986). Recombinant interferon-alpha offers some hope for patients with early persistent viral hepatitis (Sherlock, 1993a). Interferon-alpha is administered by subcutaneous injection in the dose range of 3 million units, three times per week, for 6 to 12 months. The overall response rate is approximately 25% to 30% (Sherlock, 1993a).

The major implication for nurses caring for the patient with suspected or known acute viral hepatitis is protection of self, coworkers, and other patients from the highly contagious virus. Exposure to blood and possibly other body fluids is the risk, not the patient. Strict observation of universal precautions or maintenance of body substance isolation procedures is crucial.

ALCOHOLIC LIVER DISEASE

Alcoholism is one of the most important public health problems in the United States, directly affecting an estimated 10 to 20 million people, and indirectly affecting hundreds of thousands more. The effects of alcohol abuse and alcoholism are pervasive, with biologic, psychological, and social consequences for the abuser; psychological and social consequences for families; increased risk of injury and death to self, family, and others; and derivative social and economic consequences for society.

Alcoholism is at best difficult to define. Debate over the definition of alcoholism centers around whether it is hereditary or environmentally induced, a psychological or physiologic addiction, a symptom or a disease, the cause or result of mental illness, a sin or a sickness, a moral failing or a disease. The definition by Vaillant is widely accepted. According to Vaillant (1983), alcoholism is a complex disease centering on the loss of voluntary control over alcohol, as it becomes a necessary and sufficient cause for much of an individual's social, psychological, and physical morbidity associated with its use.

Although the association between alcohol and cirrhosis was recognized as early as 1793 (Galambos, 1979), the problem continues to affect the young and old, women and men, and knows no social barriers. Approximately 50% to 80% of all cirrhosis is caused by alcohol abuse. Alcoholic cirrhosis usually, but not always, develops after many years of persistent alcohol consumption. The incidence of serious liver disease begins to rise with an average daily consumption of greater than 40 to 60 g ethanol for men, and as little as 20 g for women (Loft et al., 1987). The type of alcohol consumed is not relevant. The widely held belief that chronic consumption of beer or wine is less harmful (or not harmful at all) than chronic consumption of distilled liquor is a fallacy.

There are two major pathways of ethanol metabolism. The oxidative pathway is the primary pathway. Ethanol oxidation is catalyzed by enzymes in the cytosolic compartment and by enzymes attached to the endoplasmic reticulum of the liver cell. Ninety to 95% of ethanol is oxidized by the liver to acetaldehyde, and then to acetate. The remainder is excreted intact via the lungs, kidneys, and sweat glands. In the nonoxidative pathway, ethanol reacts with long-chain fatty acids to form ethyl esters, which can accumulate in tissues.

Alcohol has a direct toxic effect on liver cells. Ethanol is oxidized in the liver to acetaldehyde, which is oxidized to acetate. Acetaldehyde disrupts cell membranes, resulting in water retention, swelling, hepatomegaly, and eventually permanent hepatocellular damage. Acetate is oxidized to FFAs, which accumulate in the liver (fatty infiltration of the liver).

The amount of fatty acids in the liver depends on the balance between the process of delivery to and removal of fatty acids from the liver. Fatty acids are de novo synthesized in the liver and are constantly released from the adipose tissue to the liver. Normally, fatty acids are oxidized in the liver to triglyceride and resecreted as VLDLc. As synthesis and delivery of triglyceride increases, the secretion of VLDLc increases. The ingestion of excessive amounts of ethanol alters these processes and disrupts the balance. Ethanol increases the synthesis of fatty acids by the liver (increased fat in the liver) and increases the lipolytic rate in adipose tissue (increased release of fatty acids from the adipose tissue), and decreases the ability of the liver to remove triglyceride. Thus, the rate of resecretion cannot keep up with the rate of synthesis and delivery. It is in this setting that fatty liver occurs.

Chronic excessive consumption of alcohol results in a progressive form of liver disease called alcoholic liver disease. The earliest stage of alcoholic liver disease, acute fatty infiltration or hepatic steatosis, is characterized by hepatocellular fat deposition. This lesion is usually reversible if the person stops drinking. The middle stage is alcoholic hepatitis. Alcoholic hepatitis is associated with patchy necrosis, which stimulates phagocytosis. Alcoholic hepatitis is a precirrhotic lesion that progresses to cirrhosis in about 30% of cases (Galambos, 1979). This lesion is also reversible; the prognosis is best in patients who are asymptomatic and stop drinking, but abstinence does not guarantee that cirrhosis will not develop (Zakim & Bouer, 1990). The final stage of alcoholic liver disease is alcoholic cirrhosis. The changes that occur with cirrhosis are described in the following section.

Chronic effects of alcoholism on other body systems must be taken into consideration when caring for the patient with alcoholic liver disease. Cardiovascular effects include hypertension, hyperlipidemia, atherosclerosis, and cardiomyopathy. Patients with alcoholic liver disease may have a significant cigarette smoking history and may have chronic obstructive pulmonary disease. In addition, chronic bronchitis, tuberculosis, and aspiration pneumonia are common. GI effects include peptic ulcer disease, gastritis, reflux esophagitis, and pancreatitis. Malnutrition is associated with hypoalbuminemia, hypomagnesemia, hypocalcemia, hypophosphatemia, and vitamin K deficiency. Megaloblastic anemia secondary to folate deficiency is common. Chronic alcoholism is associated with cerebral degeneration and atrophy.

CIRRHOSIS

Cirrhosis is the ninth leading cause of all adult deaths in the United States, and the seventh leading cause of adult disease-related deaths if trauma and suicide are excluded. Cirrhosis, the end stage of most chronic liver diseases, accounts for more than 26,000 deaths annually in the United States. Cirrhosis is irreversible, but patients may be stable and compensated, allowing for a normal life expectancy in some. On the other hand, if advanced and progressive, cirrhosis becomes refractory to conventional medical or surgical therapy and is a life-threatening condition.

Cirrhosis is a chronic and usually slowly progressive disease involving diffuse formation of connective tissue (fibrosis) and nodular regeneration after hepatic parenchymal necrosis and inflammation. The pathophysiologic mechanism can be greatly simplified into three major events: hepatocellular injury, nodular regeneration, and loss of the original lobular architecture.

Causes of hepatocellular injury and necrosis are many: ischemia, toxemia, and viremia. Persistent necrosis stimulates hepatocellular regeneration, which involves the laying down of increased amounts of connective tissue, particularly collagen, by portal fibroblasts. Regenerating hepatocytes and fibrous connective tissue form nodules that distort the normal hepatic lobular and acinar structure. The septa connecting the hepatocytes become fibrous as well, creating increased resistance to venous flow through the septa and across the liver.

The major consequences of nodular regeneration of the hepatic parenchyma are (1) obstruction of normal portal venous flow and diversion of this blood past functional liver tissue through intrahepatic and perihepatic collateral vesels; (2) formation of basement membranes in the space of Disse; and (3) impedance of metabolic exchange leading to loss of functional capacity of the liver.

Two major physiologic changes occur as a result of advanced cirrhosis; loss of hepatocellular synthetic and metabolic functions, and development of portal hypertension (increased hydrostatic pressure within the portal venous and collateral portacaval vascular systems). The metabolic consequences of cirrhosis are numerous, and include alterations in the synthesis, metabolism, and transport of proteins, carbohydrates, and lipids, which ultimately affect nutritional status. Portal hypertension may lead to recurrent life-threatening variceal hemorrhage, refractory ascites associated with recurrent spontaneous bacterial peritonitis and sepsis, and spontaneous hepatic encephalopathy. It is the combination of these alterations and complications that ultimately leads to death. The most common causes of cirrhosis are listed in Table 49–5.

Portal Hypertension

Portal hypertension is defined as increased hydrostatic pressure within the portal venous system. Specifically, portal hypertension is defined as a portal venous pressure of greater than 5 to 10 mm Hg. There is very little or no pressure drop across the hepatic sinusoid because blood flows from the portal venous system to the hepatic veins. Therefore, if hepatic venous outflow is blocked, 100% of the increase in pressure is transmitted back to the sinusoids and portal venous system. Normal pressures in the sinusoids and hepatic venous system are slightly lower than portal venous pressure, thus creating the pressure gradient necessary for blood flow through the liver and into the IVC.

Portal hypertension can be classified according to the site of obstruction as *presinusoidal, sinusoidal,* and

TABLE 49–5. **Etiology of Chronic Liver Disease**

Postnecrotic Cirrhosis
Cholestatic diseases
Primary biliary cirrhosis
Primary and secondary sclerosing cholangitis
Familial cholestatic syndromes
Hepatocellular diseases
Chronic virus-induced liver disease
Chronic drug-induced liver disease
Alcoholic liver disease
Idiopathic autoimmune liver disease
Vascular diseases
Budd-Chiari syndrome
Venoocclusive liver disease
Metabolic Disease
Alpha$_1$-antitrypsin deficiency
Organic acidurias
Wilson's disease
Homozygous type II hyperlipoproteinemia
Hemochromatosis
Erythropoietic protoporphyria
Fatty liver disease (e.g., postintestinal bypass)

postsinusoidal. Portal hypertension resulting from cirrhosis is considered sinusoidal in nature. In the United States, cirrhosis is the most common cause of portal hypertension. Presinusoidal implies that the site of obstruction is before the sinusoids. Causes of presinusoidal portal hypertension include extrahepatic portal vein thrombosis, tumors, schistosomiasis, congenital hepatic fibrosis, and primary biliary cirrhosis. Postsinusoidal implies that the site of obstruction is beyond the sinusoids. Causes of postsinusoidal portal hypertension include Budd-Chiari syndrome (hepatic vein thrombosis) and other venoocclusive diseases.

Portal venous flow is normally "hepatopedal," or toward the liver. Portal flow can be assessed by visualizing contrast medium in the portal venous branches during the venous phase of superior mesenteric artery arteriography. As cirrhosis develops, resistance to flow increases, resulting in dilation of portal veins proximal to the site of obstruction and increased portal venous pressure. Dilation of the portal veins initially helps to maintain portal blood flow. But eventually portal flow is impeded, and reversal of flow may occur, in which case it is said to be "hepatofugal," or away from the liver. Portal flow is classified according to arteriographic studies from grade I to grade IV, with grade I defined as good hepatopedal flow with contrast medium visible to the periphery of the liver, and grade IV defined as nonvisualization of the portal vein and reversal of flow documented on wedged hepatic venography.

Collateral Vessel Formation

Another consequence of increased resistance to portal venous flow is the development of collateral vessels that bypass the obstruction as a compensatory mechanism to maintain venous return to the right heart. These vessels are called portacaval vessels because they develop between the portal venous system and the caval system (IVC or superior vena cava) (Fig. 49–8).

Portasystemic collateral circulation develops at several sites, particularly within the peritoneal, retroperitoneal, and thoracic cavities. An arteriogram of the patient with severe portal hypertension shows hundreds of collateral vessels that use the abdominal wall, duodenum, stomach, and esophagus as "bridges" between the portal and systemic circulations (Fig. 49–9). Collateral branches can also form in the rectum and may be visible as large hemorrhoidal vessels. For this

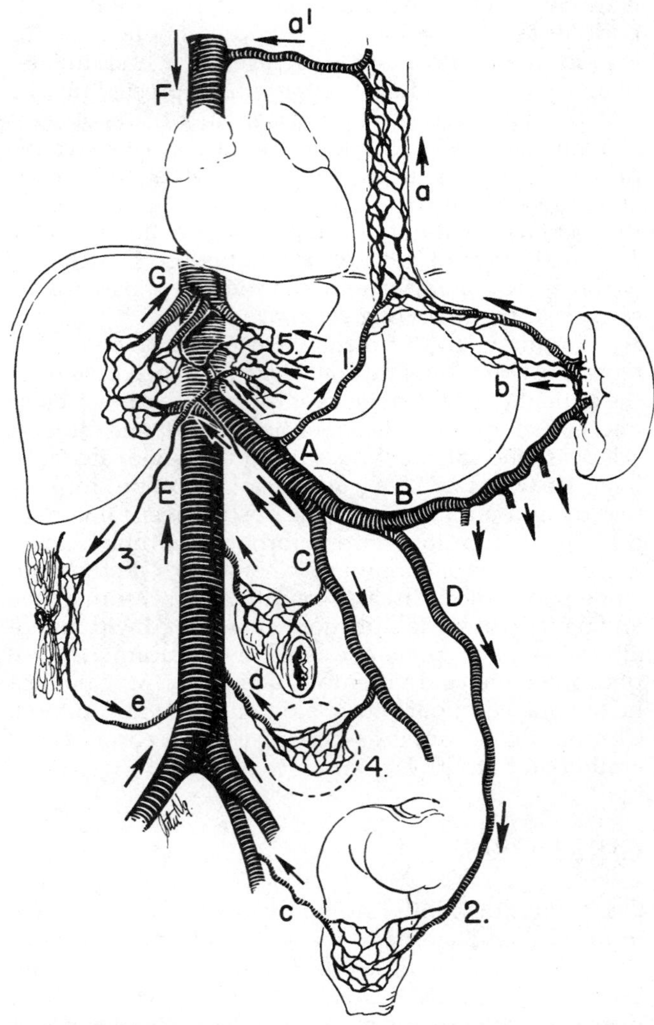

FIGURE 49–8. Collateral circulation. *1,* coronary vein; *2,* superior hemorrhoidal veins; *3,* paraumbilical veins; *4,* veins of Retzius; *5,* veins of Sappey: *A,* portal vein; *B,* splenic vein; *C,* superior mesenteric vein; *D,* inferior mesenteric vein; *E,* inferior vena cava; *F,* superior vena cava; *G,* hepatic veins; *a,* esophageal veins; *a*^{1}*,* azygos system; *b,* vasa brevia; *c,* middle and inferior hemorrhoidal veins; *d,* intestinal; *e,* epigastric veins. (From Schwartz, S. I. [1964]. *Surgical diseases of the liver.* Reproduced with permission of McGraw-Hill, Inc.)

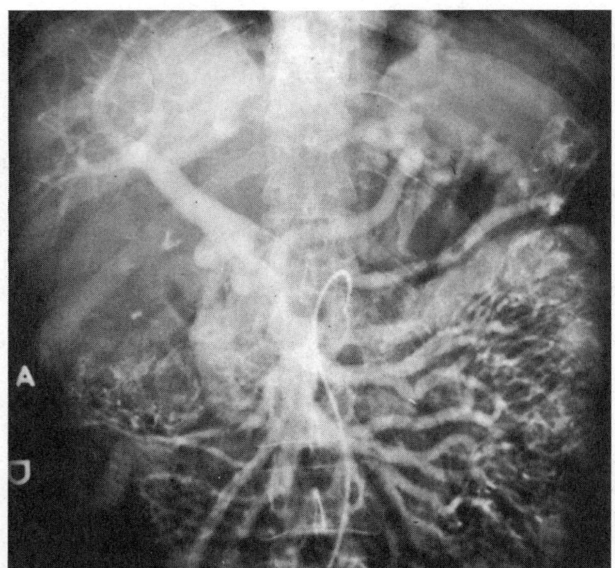

FIGURE 49–9. Venous-phase superior mesenteric artery arteriogram showing extensive collateral vessel formation in a patient with portal hypertension secondary to advanced liver disease.

reason, insertion of anything into the rectum such as a thermometer or rectal drainage tube should be done with great caution.

The collateral vessels of greatest clinical significance are the gastric and esophageal vessels called varices. Varices are fragile, dilated, convoluted veins with very little elastic tissue in their walls. Therefore, they are vulnerable to spontaneous rupture and hemorrhage. The risk of variceal bleeding, however, does not correlate with the degree of portal hypertension (Henderson & Warren, 1988). About 50% of deaths in cirrhotics are due to variceal hemorrhage (Rector, 1986).

A crucial component in the initial management of the patient with upper GI bleeding suspected to be due to gastric or esophageal varices is diagnostic endoscopy. Fifty percent of patients with varices experience upper GI bleeding from other causes such as gastritis, peptic ulcer disease, or Mallory-Weiss tears (Clark et al., 1980). Potentially fatal complications of GI bleeding such as exsanguination, aspiration pneumonia, adult respiratory distress syndrome, hepatic encephalopathy, and acute renal failure can occur (Carrithers & Fairman, 1989). The differential diagnosis is important because the treatment for these conditions varies widely and must be timely for patient survival.

INTERVENTIONS FOR BLEEDING VARICES

ENDOSCOPY. A responsibility of the nurse caring for the patient requiring endoscopy is to reassure the patient and family that the procedure is necessary and safe. Explanations that the procedure will cause some gagging may help the patient to be more cooperative. Gastric lavage with a large-bore (Ewald) tube may be necessary before endoscopy to allow adequate visualization. Approximately 5 minutes before the procedure, the patient is sedated, usually with lorazepam, midazolam, or meperidine. Care is taken not to oversedate the uncooperative patient.

Endoscopy is performed with an instrument called a fiberoptic endoscope or gastroscope. This instrument has a fiberoptic light source that permits an undistorted view of the entire upper GI tract. It is equipped with multiple channels for water, air, and the passage of instruments such as sclerosing needles, biopsy forceps, lasers, and banding devices. The patient is placed in the left lateral recumbent position. After a rubber mouthpiece is inserted to protect the patient's teeth and facilitate passage of the endoscope, the endoscope is gently advanced, first through the cricopharynx into the esophagus, and then down into the stomach and duodenum. Complications of diagnostic endoscopy include aspiration of gastric contents into the lungs, perforation of a viscus, and rupture of stable varices.

ENDOSCOPIC INJECTION SCLEROTHERAPY. Endoscopic injection sclerotherapy, or injection of a "sclerosing" or coagulating substance into varices to stop or decrease the risk of bleeding, was first used in 1939 (Sivak, 1982) in a 16-year-old girl who was hemorrhaging from varices after a splenectomy (Sivak, 1982). Sclerotherapy was abandoned as a treatment for varices with the advent of surgical portacaval shunt procedures (Terblanche et al., 1979). But, because history often repeats itself, sclerotherapy has made a comeback as a first-line treatment option for varices.

Sclerotherapy, in combination with intravenous vasopressin (Pitressin; Parke-Davis, Morris Plains, NJ) is the mainstay of treatment for acute variceal bleeding today and has an 85% to 90% success rate (Henderson & Warren, 1988). Sclerotherapy is usually indicated for the individual who has had at least one variceal hemorrhage, but it is performed prophylactically in some patients. Control of hemorrhage with sclerotherapy is attempted before balloon tamponade.

Several prospective, randomized trials have shown no difference in long-term survival between patients treated with sclerotherapy and those who have distal splenorenal shunts (Alwmark et al., 1982; Cello et al., 1986; Copenhagen Esophageal Varices Sclerotherapy Project, 1984; Korula et al., 1985; Larson et al., 1986; Warren et al., 1986; Westaby et al., 1985). Although the rebleeding rate is significantly lower in the shunt group (Rikkers et al., 1987; Teres et al., 1987; Warren et al., 1986), sclerotherapy with surgical back-up in case of failure of the procedure achieves a better quality of life and long-term survival than distal splenorenal shunt (DSRS) alone (Warren et al., 1986).

Sclerotherapy is performed using a modified fiberoptic endoscope with an injection port through which a flexible cable injector is inserted. The injector is equipped with a needle for injection at one end and a Luer-lok attachment for the syringe filled with the sclerosing agent at the other end. The actual injection technique requires two people who simultaneously visualize the varix, one placing the needle in the varix and the other injecting the sclerosing agent. Injection can be "paravariceal" or "intravariceal." Paravariceal injection is done into the tissue surrounding the varix. This induces formation of fibrous tissue around the varix and obliterates bleeding. Intravariceal injection is done directly into the lumen of the varix, which causes thrombus formation in the vein and obliterates bleeding. The number of injections required depends on the number of varices and the patient's response to sclerotherapy. Usually, regular injection sessions are required every 2 to 3 months to prevent and control bleeding. During each session as many as 10 to 20 injections may be made. The sclerosing agent used most commonly in the United States is a 5% solution of sodium morrhuate.

Sclerotherapy can be performed during acute variceal bleeding or, preferably, when the patient is stable. It may be performed in the patient's hospital room, or general anesthesia may be required to protect the airway and keep the patient still to prevent complications. On the other hand, general anesthesia may be contraindicated in the patient with decompensated liver disease. During the procedure the patient is placed on the left side with the head of the bed elevated 30 degrees to prevent aspiration. The confused or agitated patient who cannot tolerate general anesthesia may require neuromuscular paralysis to facilitate a complication-free procedure. In this situation, of course, mechanical ventilation is necessary. Close monitoring of the patient's respiratory status is necessary during and after sclerotherapy.

The mortality rate related to the procedure is less than 1% (Waye, 1987), but the complication rate is 10% to 15% (Bradford, 1983; Waye, 1987). Complications include esophageal ulceration and mucosal sloughing usually associated with chronic sclerotherapy, perforation of the esophagus, esophageal stenosis after chronic sclerotherapy, variceal bleeding, venous embolism, fever, substernal chest pain due to esophageal spasm, allergic reaction to the sclerosant, and aspiration pneumonia.

The success of sclerotherapy depends on the technical expertise of the sclerotherapists and on whether obliteration of the varices is complete (Cello et al., 1986). In several prospective, randomized trials rebleeding occurred in 23% to 75% of patients (Alwmark et al., 1982; Cello et al., 1986; Copenhagen Esophageal Varices Sclerotherapy Project, 1984; Korula et al., 1985; Larson et al., 1986; Terblanche et al., 1981; Warren et al., 1986; Westaby et al., 1985). Short-term results comparing operative time, number of blood transfusions, and hospital costs favor sclerotherapy over portacaval shunt procedures, although more blood transfusions are required after sclerotherapy and the mortality rates of the two groups do not differ (Cello et al., 1986).

ENDOSCOPIC BAND LIGATION. Endoscopic band ligation or banding is a relatively new intervention for bleeding varices. The indications are the same as for sclerotherapy—temporary control of bleeding or prevention of bleeding from esophageal varices. Banding involves the placement via an endoscope of a small, tight band (O ring) around a varix for the purpose of thrombosing it. Banding is usually performed on several varices at one time. The advantages of banding over sclerotherapy are that the results are similar, but there is no risk of ulcers, strictures, or perforation.

INTRAVENOUS VASOPRESSIN (PITRESSIN). Intravenous Pitressin was first introduced as a treatment for bleeding varices in 1956 (Kehne et al., 1986), but it was not until 1968 that it was applied clinically (Nussbaum et al., 1968). Pitressin is a vasoconstrictor of precapillary arterioles of the gut. It contracts smooth muscle in the arterioles and thus decreases blood flow to the gut. The result is decreased portal flow and pressure.

Pitressin infusion is indicated when sclerotherapy is contraindicated or fails to control an acute bleeding episode. It is indicated before balloon tamponade because it is associated with fewer complications (Rector, 1986). Although Pitressin can be administered intraarterially, the IV route is as effective and is associated with fewer complications. Pitressin is effective in controlling hemorrhage in 50% of cases, but rebleeding is likely to occur (Rector, 1986).

A reasonable protocol for IV administration of Pitressin is a loading dose of 20 U in 100 mL of 5% dextrose given over 20 minutes followed by a maintenance continuous infusion of 0.1 to 0.5 U/minute, titrated to the patient's bleeding status. The safe maximal infusion rate is 0.9 U/minute (Rector, 1986). Discontinuation of the infusion should be done by tapering it slowly over at least 24 hours.

Administration of Pitressin is not a benign treatment. Intravenous Pitressin is associated with several important side effects: coronary vasoconstriction, cardiac arrhythmias, myocardial ischemia, decreased heart rate, decreased cardiac output, systemic hypertension, abdominal cramps, and a hypermotile bowel. Continuous electrocardiographic (ECG) monitoring is necessary to detect ST segment changes associated with myocardial ischemia. IV nitroglycerin may be useful or necessary during Pitressin infusion to prevent myocardial ischemia. The nitroglycerin infusion is started after the Pitressin infusion and is titrated to blood pressure, ST segment on the ECG, and chest pain (if present).

Because Pitressin is a synthetic antidiuretic hormone, another side effect is salt and water retention. Water intoxication and hyponatremia can occur. Pitressin is also a potent vasoconstrictor that causes tissue necrosis and sloughing when it infiltrates into the subcutaneous tissue. Tissue damage due to inadvertent Pitressin infiltration is frequently of such a magnitude that skin grafting is required. For this reason, administration through a central venous access is recommended. Phentolamine mesylate (via subcutaneous injection) is an antidote for Pitressin extravasation (Hill, 1991).

PROPRANOLOL. Propranolol has been used with variable results for the treatment of variceal bleeding.

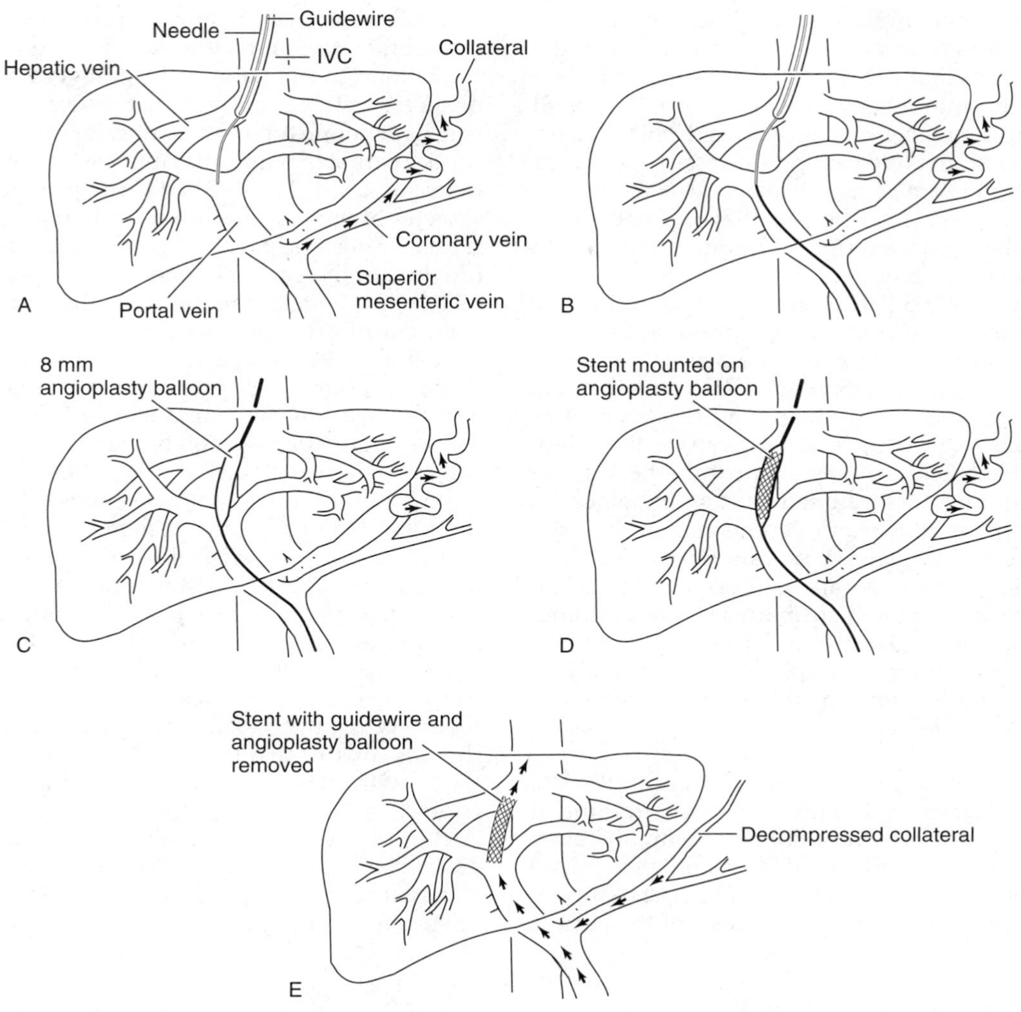

FIGURE 49–10. Transjugular intrahepatic portasystemic shunt. *A,B.* A 10-F introducer sheath is inserted into the right (preferably) jugular vein and a 16-gauge needle is then advanced into a hepatic vein and tunneled through hepatic parenchyma to a portal vein. A guidewire is then advanced through the needle into the superior mesenteric vein. *C,* An 8-mm diameter angioplasty balloon is then advanced over the guidewire and expanded. *D,* A metal stent is then mounted on the angioplasty balloon. *E,* The guidewire and angioplasty balloon are removed, leaving the stent in place. (Adapted from Zemel, G., et al. [1991]. Percutaneous transjugular portosystemic shunt. *Journal of the American Medical Association, 266,* 390–393.)

The proposed benefit of propranolol is that it decreases heart rate, cardiac output, and hepatic venous pressure through beta receptor blockade (Lebrec et al., 1980). Other studies, however, do not support these findings (Colman et al., 1985). The dose response is extremely variable; patients require between 40 and 280 mg/day for results (Fleig et al., 1987).

TRANSJUGULAR INTRAHEPATIC PORTASYSTEMIC SHUNT. Transjugular intrahepatic portasystemic shunt (TIPS) is a relatively new, minimally invasive treatment option for decreasing portal hypertension and variceal bleeding. The TIPS procedure (Fig. 49–10) is performed under fluoroscopy in the radiology department. A nonsurgical shunt is created within the liver, connecting the portal and systemic venous systems and allowing blood to flow from the portal vein directly into the hepatic vein and IVC. The goal of the TIPS is to decrease the portasystemic gradient—the pressure gradient between the hepatic outflow system (hepatic veins) and the hepatic inflow system (portal vein)—to approximately 10 mm Hg.

A 10 F-introducer sheath is inserted into the right (preferably) jugular vein. A 16-gauge needle is then advanced into a hepatic vein and tunneled through hepatic parenchyma to a portal vein, which has been identified with ultrasound, arteriogram, or a wedged hepatic venogram. A guidewire is then advanced through the needle into the superior mesenteric vein. Simultaneous portal and hepatic vein pressures are measured to calculate the portasystemic gradient. Contrast medium is also injected to visualize varices.

An 8-mm diameter angioplasty balloon is then advanced over the guidewire and expanded across the hepatic parenchymal tract. A metal stent is then mounted on the angioplasty balloon to form the actual bridge or shunt between the hepatic and portal veins. Repeat portal and hepatic vein pressures are measured and contrast medium is again injected to determine that varices can no longer be visualized. If necessary, the stent can be expanded up to 12 mm in diameter to reduce the pressure gradient.

Although the TIPS procedure is considered a safe and effective means of portal decompression for treatment of variceal bleeding, there are several potential complications (Adams & Soulen, 1992; Zemel et al., 1991). Bleeding can occur at the puncture site or intrahepatic vessels (e.g., hepatic artery) can be lacerated. Hepatic artery thrombosis can occur if the hepatic artery is injured. Bile duct trauma resulting in hemobilia can occur. Intrahepatic arteriovenous or arterioportal fistulas can develop. The stent can thrombose, and stent migration, although rare, can occur. This is unlikely because the stent will normally become endothelialized within about 10 days. And, as with other types of portasystemic shunts, encephalopathy is likely to occur. Other complications include reaction to the contrast medium and infection.

BALLOON TAMPONADE. From the 1930s until the late 1950s, balloon tamponade was a standard treatment for bleeding varices even though the potentially lethal complications of this mode of therapy were recognized (Conn, 1958; Conn et al., 1981). Today balloon tamponade is reserved for temporary treatment of the patient with bleeding varices refractory to sclerotherapy, Pitressin therapy, and TIPS.

Balloon tamponade of bleeding varices is accomplished most frequently with a device called a Sengstaken-Blakemore tube. This tube is a triple-lumen, red rubber catheter with inflatable gastric esophageal balloons attached (Fig. 49–11*A*). The proximal end of the catheter branches into three clearly marked ports, each representing a separate lumen. One port is used for inflation of the gastric balloon, one is used for inflation of the esophageal balloon, and the third is used for gastric aspiration and suction.

Before insertion, the tube is lubricated, the patient's posterior pharynx is sprayed with a topical anesthetic, and the head of the bed is elevated 30 to 45 degrees. The necessity for insertion of the tube and the insertion procedure are explained to the patient. Patient cooperation is helpful for smooth and uneventful insertion of the tube. Unfortunately, patients requiring this intervention are often in crisis due to upper GI hemorrhage, or they are encephalopathic. The patient is instructed to swallow as the tube is passed through a nostril and into the esophagus. Although the tube has two balloons, gastric balloon tamponade is attempted first; if this is successful, the esophageal balloon remains deflated. When the 50-cm mark on the tube is even with the patient's nostril the gastric balloon is partially inflated with 50 mL of air while the area over the epigastrium is auscultated for the sound of air insufflation. A chest x-ray is then taken to verify placement of the gastric balloon below the gastroesophageal (GE) junction before it is fully inflated. Failure to verify correct balloon placement could result in full inflation of the

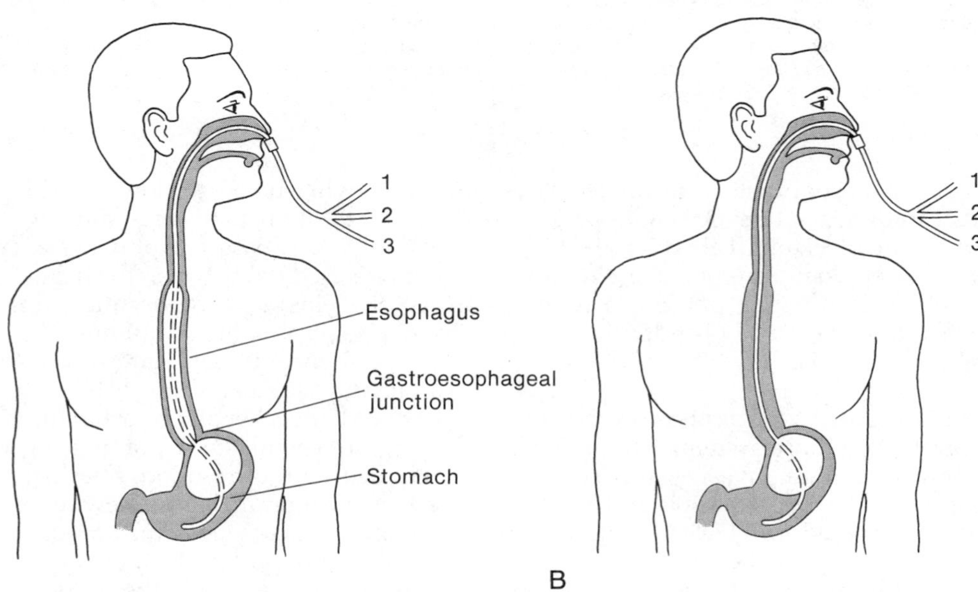

FIGURE 49–11. *A*, Sengstaken-Blakemore tube. *B*, Linton-Nachlas tube.

balloon within the esophagus with resultant esophageal rupture, mediastinitis, and death.

When balloon placement below the GE junction is verified, it is filled with 300 to 500 mL of air, and the gastric balloon port is double-clamped with rubber-shod clamps. The result is a tamponading effect on the bleeding varices located in the proximal gastric and GE junction mucosa. The gastric aspiration port is connected to low, intermittent suction. Initially, the stomach may need to be lavaged until the return fluid is clear to prevent clotting of the gastric aspiration lumen and to monitor control of bleeding.

Secretions can pool in the esophagus above the inflated balloon, increasing the risk of pulmonary aspiration. For this reason, an NG tube is inserted just to the level of the GE junction and connected to low, intermittent suction.

Traditionally, traction has been applied at the proximal end of the tube to ensure that the gastric balloon is placed tight against the cardia of the stomach and the GE junction. Methods used to maintain traction include pulling the tube taut and attaching it to the face bar of a football helmet or baseball catcher's mask, or attaching orthopedic traction to the proximal end of the tube. Regardless of the method used, this intervention is uncomfortable for the patient and family, and the psychosocial implications can be significant. The nursing literature is void of studies comparing outcomes of patients in whom traction is applied with those in whom it is not. However, Teres and colleagues found that this practice is not necessary, that adequate tension of the balloon can be maintained without traction, and that application of traction is associated with more patient discomfort and complications (Teres et al., 1978). In spite of these findings, the use of traction remains a common practice.

If bleeding cannot be controlled using gastric balloon tamponade alone, the esophageal balloon is also inflated to 25 to 40 mm Hg using a mercury manometer, and the esophageal lumen is double-clamped with rubber-shod clamps. Pressure in the esophageal balloon should be checked every 30 to 60 minutes. Continual monitoring of gastric secretions for blood is necessary to determine whether hemostasis is attained. If not, the pressure in the esophageal balloon can be increased to 45 mm Hg, and the gastric balloon can be inflated to hold up to 400 mL of air. However, at these high pressure levels ulceration of the mucosa will occur in only a few hours. Therefore, esophageal balloon pressure should be maintained at the lowest pressure that will control bleeding, and it should be continued only as long as necessary.

Balloon tamponade achieves primary hemostasis in 70% to 80% of cases, but results are rarely permanent (Rector, 1986). Balloon tamponade is not meant to be used as a long-term therapy. Esophageal balloon pressure should not be maintained for longer than 72 hours and should be discontinued in less than 72 hours if possible. When hemostasis is attained, the tube is left in place and the balloons are deflated 12 to 24 hours before removal.

The major complications of balloon tamponade are (1) rupture or deflation of the balloon(s) and subsequent upper airway obstruction, (2) pulmonary aspiration and (3) rupture of the esophagus. Scissors should be kept visible at the bedside at all times to be used in case the balloons migrate proximally and occlude the upper airway. In this life-threatening situation, the lumens are immediately cut to facilitate prompt removal of the tube. Application of suction above the most proximally inflated balloon helps prevent pulmonary aspiration. Esophageal rupture is manifested by a sudden onset of upper abdominal or back pain and a sudden decrease in blood pressure. Necrosis of the affected nare can occur if it is not protected from constant pressure from the tube. Just as after nasotracheal intubation with an endotracheal tube, nasoesophageal intubation can lead to a life-threatening sinusitis. The onset of fever associated with purulent and foul-smelling nasal and nasopharyngeal drainage are signs of sinusitis. One study found that the in-hospital mortality rate was 60% when the Sengstaken-Blakemore tube was used as the only mode of therapy (Sivak, 1982).

Other tubes are commercially available and are used for the same purpose as the Sengstaken-Blakemore tube. The Linton-Nachlas tube (Fig. 49–11*B*) is also a triple-lumen tube, but has only one large gastric balloon. The gastric balloon can be inflated with up to 800 mL of air. The two remaining lumens are for gastric and esophageal aspiration, a distinct advantage over the Sengstaken-Blakemore tube. The Linton-Nachlas tube is used to control bleeding from gastric varices. Because the tube does not have an esophageal balloon, varices in the middle and proximal esophagus cannot be tamponaded with this tube. The Minnesota tube is a quadruple-lumen tube. It has the advantages of both the Sengstaken-Blakemore tube and the Linton-Nachlas tube: gastric and esophageal aspiration capabilities, and both gastric and esophageal balloons.

SUMMARY OF MEDICAL TREATMENT CONSIDERATIONS FOR THE PATIENT WITH BLEEDING VARICES. Medical therapy is employed as a first-line treatment for bleeding varices. Patients who continue to bleed acutely in spite of sclerotherapy or banding are first administered Pitressin. If Pitressin fails to stop the bleeding, angiography is indicated. An emergent TIPS or portacaval shunt may be necessary to control acute variceal bleeding before other forms of medical intervention are tried. The Sengstaken-Blakemore tube may be necessary to maintain hemostasis in the patient who bleeds rapidly and profusely and who does not respond to Pitressin. Emergent portacaval shunts are required more often in this group of patients.

The patient who is bleeding from varices is at risk for hypotension and decreased tissue perfusion. The nurse should routinely assess the patient for end-organ effects of decreased tissue perfusion such as oliguria, signs of myocardial ischemia, altered mentation, adult respiratory distress syndrome and ileus. The goal of treating hemorrhage is prevention of end-organ ischemia and associated complications. The patient's cardiac history is very important. The patient with a compromised cardiac reserve is at high risk for acute myocardial infarction.

Volume resuscitation with packed red blood cells, fresh frozen plasma for clotting factors, and crystalloids is a priority intervention. However, the potential harm in maintaining adequate plasma volume for organ perfusion is the risk of increasing portal pressure and thus the chances of variceal bleeding. Placement of a pulmonary artery catheter is necessary to ensure optimal fluid resuscitation and management. Supplemental oxygen is also indicated.

The patient with upper GI bleeding from varices requires vigorous mouth care for both infection control and aesthetic reasons. This patient will also be passing melanotic stools, which may be frequent enough to cause breakdown of the perianal tissue. Attention to skin and mucous membrane care is important in this high-risk patient.

ASCITES

Ascites is an abnormal accumulation of fluid in the peritoneal cavity. Although there are many causes of ascites (malnutrition, severe congestive heart failure, nephrotic syndrome, pancreatitis, and neoplastic disease, to name a few), the most common cause of ascites in cirrhotics is the cirrhosis itself. Ascitic fluid of cirrhosis is normally clear with a yellow tinge. If the patient is deeply jaundiced the fluid is a deeper shade of yellow. Ascites is a late sign in the continuum of cirrhosis; in other words, its presence indicates advanced disease. The patient in whom ascites develops has only a 40% chance of being alive after 2 years (Sherlock, 1979).

Another form of ascites, "chylous" ascites, is rare in patients with cirrhosis (Schumann, 1983). The most common cause of chylous ascites is malignant disease that results in occlusion and rupture of intestinal lymphatics with leakage of fluid rich in triglycerides into the peritoneal cavity. The triglyceride level of chylous ascites is greater than the plasma level. Chylous ascites also occurs in some patients after DSRS surgery when intestinal lymphatics are transected during the procedure.

There are two theories of ascites formation (Lautt & Greenway, 1987). The first is called the *underfilling theory.* According to this theory, the triad of portal hypertension, decreased colloid osmotic pressure, and increased hepatic lymph transudation results in retention of sodium and water and accumulation of ascites. Because there is no pressure gradient from the sinusoids to the hepatic veins, 100% of the increase in pressure due to blockage of venous outflow is transmitted back to the sinusoids and the portal system, resulting in increased lymph production. Hepatic lymph is returned to the systemic circulation by the large thoracic duct. Normal thoracic duct flow is about 800 to 1,000 mL/day, but this can increase to 20 liters/day in patients with severe portal hypertension (Cattau et al., 1982). Hepatic flow increases by about 60% for every milliliter of mercury increase in intrahepatic venous pressure (Cattau et al., 1982). Fluid weeping from the hepatic vasculature and the splanchnic bed increases thoracic duct flow. Ascites develops when maximal thoracic duct flow is exceeded. There is a net movement of fluid into the peritoneal cavity, resulting in a reduced "effective" plasma volume.

The second theory is called the *overflow theory.* In this theory it is postulated that the diseased liver releases substances that cause renal vasoconstriction and excessive tubular reabsorption of sodium. Expansion of blood volume results in increased hepatic lymph formation. In other words, retained sodium and water are the initiating factors.

Ascites results in plasma volume contraction and stimulation of neuroendocrine compensatory responses of epinephrine, renin–angiotensin, and antidiuretic hormone release. Consequently, renal blood flow is decreased, and urinary sodium is retained.

Several important problems and complications are associated with ascites. From a pathophysiologic perspective, the most important are the predisposition to renal failure and variceal bleeding. The most obvious are the related physical disfigurement and physical dysfunction. Not only are the body and the body image changed, ascites also interferes with erect posture and balance and adds to muscle fatigue in the already malnourished and fatigued individual. Minor complications include incisional, inguinal, and femoral hernias. Premature satiety interferes with nutritional intake at a time when nutrient metabolism is compromised. Reflux esophagitis can exacerbate esophageal varices and predispose the individual to esophageal ulceration.

An elevated diaphragm displaces the heart, causing increased right heart filling pressures and jugular venous distention. Right heart filling pressures may be falsely normal or elevated when the patient is hypovolemic and are almost always falsely elevated in the supine position. An important factor to consider when assessing hemodynamic parameters is the position of the patient. Depending on the extent of accumulation of ascites, the patient may not be able to tolerate the supine position. This is another reason why it is important to measure heart pressures in the upright position that is best tolerated by the patient. The patient's baseline pressures with an elevated diaphragm are established and used for comparison with changing trends. These pressures will of course change if ascitic fluid is drained, necessitating reestablishment of baseline pressures. Other parameters such as urine output may be more useful in assessing volume status and tissue perfusion.

Pleural effusions occur in 5% to 10% of patients with ascites (Carrithers & Fairman, 1989). Fluid transgresses upward through the transdiaphragmatic lymphatics and through tiny ruptures of the diaphragm that occur secondary to increased intraabdominal pressure created by the ascites. End-stage patients may require regular thoracenteses to control reaccumulating pleural effusions. Atelectasis and pleural effusions increase the risk of infection in these already immunocompromised individuals.

Infection of ascitic fluid is common. Peritonitis develops in approximately 8% of cirrhotic patients with ascites (Gregory et al., 1977), and is more common in those with decompensated cirrhosis. Spontaneous bacterial peritonitis is diagnosed when the polymorphonuclear granulocyte count of the ascitic fluid is greater than 250/mm^3 and culture of ascitic fluid is positive. Associated signs and symptoms include localized abdominal pain, fever, leukocytosis, and increased serum bilirubin and creatinine. The development of spontaneous bacterial peritonitis is often the cause of a sudden deterioration in the patient's condition. Frequently, such a patient is admitted to the critical care unit in a "septic" state.

Ascitic fluid in the immunocompetent individual contains humoral substances that are active against gram-negative organisms. Gram-positive organisms are more often the cause of peritonitis than gram-negative organisms (Sherlock, 1985). However, in the cirrhotic patient, both gram-positive and gram-negative organisms cause peritonitis and lead to seeding of infection in other organs, particularly the lungs. Treatment consists of broad-spectrum antibiotics.

Interventions for Ascites

The treatment regimen for ascites in general consists of diuresis and fluid and salt restriction (Perez & Schiff, 1988). Parecentesis may be necessary to prevent pulmonary compromise and immobility.

SODIUM RESTRICTION. Sodium restrictions of from 0.5 to 2.0 g/day may be prescribed. These diets are not generally palatable and can be expensive. Therefore, patient compliance is not likely to be good, especially if the patient is not hospitalized. If the patient is hospitalized, restriction to a low-sodium diet may lead to significant decreases in food intake and further catabolism. Care must also be taken to identify sources of sodium intake such as sodium-rich antacids and antibiotics and drugs that can interfere with renal sodium excretion such as nonsteroidal antiinflammatory agents and beta blockers.

DIURETICS. Diuresis must be accomplished at a safe rate to avoid precipitating hypovolemia, prerenal azotemia, and encephalopathy. According to Sherlock (1985), it may be better to have a patient who is "wet and wise instead of one who is dry and demented." Therefore, replacement of effective plasma volume with plasma should accompany induced diuresis, and the serum creatinine, creatinine clearance, and blood urea nitrogen (BUN) are monitored closely.

The maximal rate of ascites reabsorption is 700 to 900 mL/day (Galambos, 1979). Therefore, diuresis of amounts greater than this results in removal of fluid from spaces other than the peritoneal cavity. This is relatively safe in the patient who also has peripheral edema, but can be very hazardous in the patient who does not, resulting in renal failure.

The aim of diuretic therapy is to inhibit renal sodium conservation mechanisms. Potassium-sparing diuretics such as the aldosterone antagonist spironolactone (Aldactone; Searle Laboratories, Chicago, IL) and triamterene are used for initial control. The onset of action of spironolactone occurs in 2 to 3 days, whereas the effects of triamterene can be seen in a few hours. A side effect of long-term use of spironolactone in men is gynecomastia. Serum potassium levels are monitored regularly in patients taking spironolactone because hyperkalemia is another side effect. Potassium-wasting or loop diuretics (e.g., furosemide) may be necessary. In more severe cases, a combination of IV plasma, furosemide, and mannitol may be employed. Bed rest, up to 18 hours a day, is prescribed by some physicians because this initiates diuresis (Galambos, 1979). Compliance with this prescription is also difficult to control in the nonhospitalized patient.

Hyponatremia can occur after urinary excretion of sodium in the already sodium-restricted patient. Overhydration can also exacerbate this condition, leading to a state of water intoxication. Unless the serum sodium level is less than 130 mEq/liter, it is usually not treated. Treatment may consist of restriction of water intake and osmotic diuresis with mannitol to increase free water clearance. Hypokalemia can also occur after administration of loop diuretics or from secondary hyperaldosteronism, which develops as a compensatory response to decreased effective plasma volume.

PARACENTESIS. Paracentesis may be indicated for removal of ascites when it is interfering with breathing, eating, and activities of daily living. It is also indicated when ascites is resistant (responds to IV therapy but reaccumulates) or refractory (does not respond to other therapies). Repeated paracenteses for the removal of large amounts of fluid are frequently necessary in combination with administration of diuretics and salt-poor albumin. The patient's hemodynamic response to removal of large fluid volumes must be monitored closely. With release of pressure on the IVC, venous return and cardiac output usually improve, resulting in increased diuresis. Also, ventilatory status and appetite improve.

A protocol for sterile insertion of a peritoneal drain and for sterile management of the catheter and drainage system must be developed to prevent peritonitis. Abdominal assessment for peritoneal signs indicative of acute abdomen or peritonitis is an ongoing nursing responsibility.

PERITONEOVENOUS SHUNTING. The LeVeen valve (Fig. 49–12) for peritoneovenous shunting was described as a procedure for "continual reinfusion of ascitic fluid into the circulation via a pressure-activated valve inserted into the peritoneum and connected to a larger interthoracic vein through subcutaneous tub-

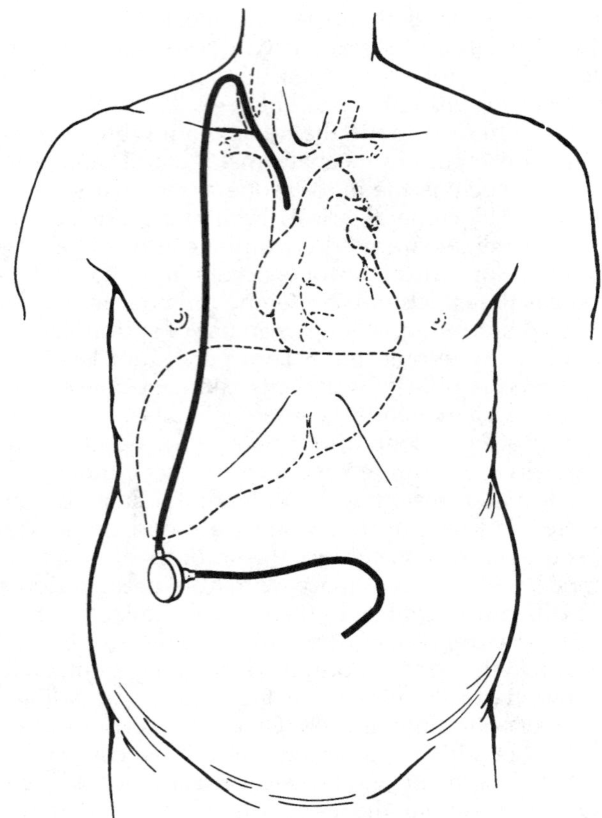

FIGURE 49-12. Placement of the peritoneovenous shunt. The collecting cannula lies within the peritoneal cavity, the valve is positioned extraperitoneally, and the outflow tubing extends from the valve through the subcutaneous tissue on the chest wall to an entrance point in the internal jugular vein. This tip is advanced to the superior vena cava within 1 to 2 cm of the right atrium, or within the right atrium. (From Schumann, D. [1983]. Correction of ascites and arteriovenous shunting; A study of clinical management. *Heart and Lung, 12,* 248–255.)

ing'' (Schumann, 1983). Other similar devices (e.g., the Denver shunt) have been developed more recently. Only the LeVeen valve is discussed.

The LeVeen valve is contraindicated in patients who are encephalopathic, have had recent abdominal surgery, or have congestive heart failure, disseminated intravascular coagulation, or severe decompensated liver disease. One reason for the decrease in the initial popularity of the LeVeen valve is the high associated operative mortality (13%) (Sherlock, 1985). Infection is the major fatal complication. Plugging of the valve with proteinaceous material also occurs, rendering it ineffective and in need of replacement. Less than 50% of LeVeen valves remain patent for 1 year (Sherlock, 1985). For these reasons, the LeVeen valve is a therapeutic option for only a select few patients with intractable ascites.

A functional LeVeen shunt leads to the following changes in the patient's condition: hemodilution, diuresis and urinary loss of potassium, weight loss, decreased abdominal girth, and more comfortable respirations. Mobilization of ascitic fluid into the systemic circulation can lead to acute volume overload, congestive heart failure, and pulmonary edema. Excessive diuresis can trigger the hepatorenal syndrome. Patients receiving LeVeen shunts may require intensive care to provide close observation of and treatment for these problems.

HEPATORENAL SYNDROME

Hepatorenal syndrome is defined as progressive acute renal failure in the patient with advanced liver disease, most commonly alcoholic liver disease, when the etiology of the renal failure cannot be explained by other causes (Carrithers & Fairman, 1989; Clive, 1985). This diagnosis is made on clinical grounds in the patient with manifestations of liver disease, or is based on biopsy findings. Causes other than liver disease of acute renal failure in the patient with liver disease, such as metabolic, toxic, and septic causes, must be ruled out before the diagnosis of hepatorenal syndrome can be made. Hepatorenal syndrome is a ''functional'' disorder of the kidneys characterized by renal hypoperfusion that develops as a result of decreased effective plasma volume. Vasoconstrictive mechanisms such as the release of endotoxins (Hollenberg, 1983), activation of the renin–angiotensin system (Zipser et al., 1983), thromboxanes (Zipser et al., 1979), and prostaglandins (LeVeen et al., 1976) have been implicated as precipitating factors of hepatorenal syndrome. The production of vasoconstrictive substances is increased while production of vasodilatory substances is decreased, favoring renal hypertension. The hepatorenal syndrome can be induced by excessive diuresis or diarrhea, hemorrhage, infection, or administration of nephrotoxic or nonsteroidal antiinflammatory drugs to the patient with a decompensated liver disease.

Sodium-reabsorptive and urinary-concentrating ability of the kidneys remain intact during hepatorenal syndrome. Therefore, the condition is reversible, as demonstrated by the fact that kidneys from patients with hepatorenal syndrome have been successfully transplanted (Finn, 1988).

The differential diagnosis for hepatorenal syndrome includes prerenal azotemia and acute tubular necrosis. Prerenal azotemia can be ruled out by the fluid challenge test. The patient with prerenal azotemia will respond to a fluid challenge by increasing urine output; the patient with hepatorenal syndrome will not. A fluid challenge is not recommended when the patient has pulmonary or venous congestion. If the patient has extreme ascites, rapid volume expansion increases the risk of variceal bleeding. In patients with acute tubular necrosis, urine sodium concentration is greater than 40 mEq/liter, and in those with hepatorenal syndrome it is less than 10mEq/liter (Frakes, 1980).

Hepatorenal syndrome is manifested by progressive oliguria in the presence of normovolemia, azotemia with anorexia, weakness, nausea, vomiting, increased thirst, highly concentrated urine that is free of sodium, and elevated serum creatinine and BUN. Even though the patient's cardiovascular system is hyperdynamic, renal blood flow is diverted away from the renal cortex. Because of this, the patient's ability to excrete free water is decreased. As with any patient in renal failure, the patient with hepatorenal syndrome must be closely monitored for electrolyte imbalances (hyperkalemia, hyponatremia), hypervolemia with pulmonary edema, pleural effusions, and sepsis. In patients with decompensated cirrhosis the serum creatinine is not the most reliable index of renal function. Creatinine clearance is a better index. Therefore, 24-hour urine collections are commonly done on a regular basis to manage this problem.

Patient survival depends on reversing the initiating factors such as restoring effective plasma volume to optimal levels and restoring some degree of liver function. Dialysis may be used as a life-saving measure while initiating factors are being reversed in the patient who has the potential for long-term survival, or as a bridge to transplantation if the patient is a candidate for liver transplantation.

Care of the patient with hepatorenal syndrome is complex because so many other problems coexist. Efforts at multisystem stabilization are ongoing. Finding the right balance between fluid volume deficit and overload can be difficult. The patient in acute renal failure is at high risk of acquiring an infection; the most frequent cause of death resulting from acute renal failure is sepsis (Cascino et al., 1978). Therefore, diligent observation of infection control measures is a vital component of the overall plan of care for this patient. Correction of etiologic factors is a primary goal, with protection of renal perfusion during diuresis and dialysis a secondary goal.

HEPATIC ENCEPHALOPATHY

The brain of the person with advanced liver disease is particularly sensitive to insults that do not affect the brain of the otherwise healthy person. Hepatic encephalopathy is defined as neuropsychiatric dysfunction resulting from liver disease and failure. In general, hepatic encephalopathy is characterized by a deterioration in intellectual function, personal behavior, and level of consciousness. Hepatic encephalopathy may occur spontaneously, or it may be precipitated by several important factors, to be discussed later.

The patient in whom hepatic encephalopathy develops has an altered circulation pathway through which toxic substances in the portal blood enter the systemic circulation and reach the brain without first being metabolized by the liver. This altered pathway consists of intrahepatic and perihepatic collateral vessels that develop because of portal hypertension. The result is that brain cells are poisoned by these toxic substances, which are usually intestinal in nature and which are not metabolized by the liver (Maddrey & Weber, 1975).

Development of spontaneous hepatic encephalopathy indicates that at least 50% of the liver's ability to synthesize urea has been lost (Galambos, 1979). Spontaneous hepatic encephalopathy usually occurs in patients who are deeply jaundiced with ascites and heralds the end stage of advanced liver disease. Not surprisingly, the prognosis for the patient with precipitated encephalopathy is better than that for the patient with spontaneous encephalopathy.

Ammonia is postulated to be the key toxic stimulus to hepatic encephalopathy. Ammonia uptake normally occurs in the brain, liver, and skeletal muscle. Changes in brain, liver, and skeletal muscle metabolism contribute to increased serum ammonia accumulation. Cirrhosis is associated with muscle wasting and portasystemic shunting, both of which interfere with hepatic uptake of ammonia. Decreased hepatic uptake of ammonia increases the uptake of ammonia by the brain. Ammonia concentrations in the cerebrospinal fluid and blood increase in hepatic encephalopathy, and interventions that decrease serum ammonia concentrations improve encephalopathy. However, there is an inconsistent correlation between ammonia levels and the degree of neurologic impairment. For this reason, it is thought that other factors must also be responsible.

The patient in whom hepatic encephalopathy develops is thought to have increased cerebral sensitivity and possibly a deficiency of an essential factor required for normal brain metabolism, resulting in decreased energy utilization by the brain. Mercaptans, which are derived from bacterial metabolism of toxic methionine, are normally removed by the liver. The patient in a state of hepatic encephalopathy, however, excretes mercaptans through pulmonary respiration, which produces the characteristic fruity, odorous breath called fetor hepaticus. The presence of fetor hepaticus is used by some clinicians as a criterion for diagnosing hepatic encephalopathy. Hypovolemia decreases hepatic perfusion and cerebral blood flow and decreases clearance of ammonia. Diuretics that induce a hypokalemic alkalosis with an increased extracellular fluid pH promote diffusion of ammonia from blood into tissues such as the brain.

Failure of deamination functions and altered ammonia metabolism by the diseased liver result in increased levels of aromatic amino acids and decreased levels of branched chain amino acids in the central nervous system (Bouletreau et al., 1979). Aromatic amino acids have an inhibitory effect on normal neurotransmitters, favoring sedation, and branched-chain amino acids have arousal properties, favoring wakefulness. Tryptophan, the most toxic of the aromatic amino acids, is converted to serotonin, which produces sedation.

Accumulated systemic ammonia may impair normal synaptic transmission. Normal neurotransmitter synthesis is controlled by brain concentrations of precursor amino acids. Under normal conditions, phenylalanine is converted by hydroxylation to tyrosine, which is further hydroxylated to dopa for the synthesis of the neurotransmitters dopamine and norepinephrine. In hepatic encephalopathy it is postulated that (1) phenylalanine is hydroxylated to phenyl ethylamine, which is further hydroxylated to phenyl ethanolamine, and (2) tyrosine is hydroxylated to tyramine, which is further hydroxylated to octopamine (Kaplan, 1987). Phenyl ethanolamine and octopamine are "false" neurotransmitters that replace norepinephrine at synaptic junctions, altering cerebral metabolism and favoring sedation.

Common precipitants of hepatic encephalopathy in the cirrhotic patient include hypoxia, infection, electrolyte abnormalities, increased amounts of ammonia in the diet, certain drugs (sedatives, alcohol, anesthetics), GI bleeding, hypovolemia, altered renal function, and surgically created portacaval shunts. It is important not to lose sight of the cause of encephalopathy when caring for a patient with advanced liver disease in whom encephalopathy has been precipitated by iatrogenic measures. Appropriate interventions to correct the underlying problem usually reverse this type of encephalopathy.

The most common precipitant of hepatic encephalopathy in the cirrhotic patient is vigorous diuresis followed by azotemia (Sherlock, 1985). Diuretics can precipitate encephalopathy by increasing ammonia production in either of two ways. First, prerenal azotemia secondary to reduced circulating plasma volume and decreased renal perfusion provides substrate for ammonia production. Renal tubular acidosis impairs hydrogen ion and ammonia transport in the urine, resulting in increased serum ammonia. Second, hypokalemia and metabolic alkalosis that occur as a result of hyperaldosteronism and as a side effect of administration of potassium-wasting diuretics, particularly the thiazides, increase renal production of ammonia. The higher the pH, the more freely ammonia penetrates the blood–brain barrier. Therefore, invasive and noninvasive measurements of plasma volume, as well as serum potassium and ammonia levels, are followed closely in the cirrhotic patient treated with diuretics.

Infection is often found to be the cause of unexplained hepatic encephalopathy. Remember that the patient with advanced liver disease is inherently immunosuppressed and has other risk factors related to the potential for infection such as ascites, malnutrition, and the frequent necessity for hospitalization. Fever increases the metabolic rate of tissues, which in turn increases the rate of amino acid metabolism and ammonia production. Fever can also contribute to decreased extracellular fluid and plasma volume. Detection of septicemia based on hemodynamic assessment of the critically ill patient with advanced liver disease is difficult because the classic signs of septicemia, increased cardiac output, and decreased systemic vascular resistance are normal findings in this patient. Exaggerated changes from the patient's baseline do occur and can be used in this assessment.

Gastrointestinal bleeding places an increased protein load on the GI tract, leading to increased amino acid and ammonia levels. An increased demand for hepatic detoxification occurs at a time when hepatic perfusion is decreased. Hemorrhage that is significant enough to decrease renal perfusion also increases BUN and provides additional substrate for intestinal ammonia production.

An individual with hepatic encephalopathy may be entirely asymptomatic in the very early stages. The clinical manifestations of hepatic encephalopathy may fall anywhere on a continuum from completely asymptomatic to deep coma. Hepatic encephalopathy can be classified clinically into four grades. Table 49–3 outlines the clinical signs and defining characteristics of these stages.

In grade I hepatic encephalopathy, sometimes referred to as the prodromal stage, early signs include decreased intellectual capacity and mild alterations in level of consciousness. Because of the vague nature of these signs, early diagnosis is difficult. Later signs of grade I hepatic encephalopathy include loss of memory, confusion, and insomnia. It is important not to treat the insomnia of the patient with encephalopathy, even in this early stage, with sedatives or hypnotics. To do so would exacerbate the condition. Methods for assessing early encephalopathy include testing the ability of the patient to subtract by ones from 20 and adding or subtracting serial sevens, testing for apraxia by serial comparison of the patient's signature and the patient's attempts to draw a well known object such as a star or house, and the Reitan trailmaking test. In this test the patient is asked to connect successively numbered dots with a line. The time it takes the patient to do this mental exercise is compared to a normal standard. As the degree of encephalopathy increases, the patient's ability to perform these simple tasks deteriorates.

In grade II hepatic encephalopathy, speech becomes slower and slurred, and spontaneous movement decreases. The patient becomes intermittently confused, agitated, and drowsy. Asterixis, the characteristic "flapping" tremor of advanced liver disease, can be elicited in this stage. Asterixis is a condition in which the patient cannot maintain a fixed position or posture. To test for this response, ask the patient to hold his or her arms straight out at right angles to the body for 10 seconds. A loss of posture of the extremities is recovered by a flapping motion. To elicit this response, the patient must be able to cooperate. Asterixis can also be elicited by dorsiflexing the patient's wrist and watching for the characteristic downward flapping motion of the hand. The patient may also have a positive Babinski reflex, seizures, or myoclonic twitching. Myoclonic twitching must be differentiated from status epilepticus to avoid treatment with phenobarbital, which would exacerbate the condition.

In grade III hepatic encephalopathy, severe bilateral forebrain involvement occurs, manifested by somnolence, stupor, decortication, and decerebration. The patient will respond to noxious stimuli. In grade IV hepatic encephalopathy, the patient cannot be awakened and is said to be in a deep coma. Cerebral edema can be diagnosed in about 50% of cases (Sherlock, 1985).

The EEG is useful in diagnosing hepatic encephalopathy and in differentiating metabolic encephalopathy from other conditions that can alter the level of consciousness. The EEG changes of hepatic encephalopathy are those of high-voltage slow waves in the delta range. In the early stages of encephalopathy, changes occur in the frontal lobe. As encephalopathy progresses, the posterior lobes are affected as well, and by grade IV changes are evident in the entire brain. Although most patients who suffer hepatic encephalopathy recover completely, the condition can lead to permanent neurologic damage and even death, especially if it progresses to grade IV.

Laboratory assessment of hepatic encephalopathy is nonspecific. As previously stated, serum ammonia levels do not necessarily correlate with the grade of encephalopathy. Again many precipitating factors may be reflected in analysis of fluid and electrolyte and acid–base status.

Treatment of hepatic encephalopathy involves searching for and treating all possible precipitants. Treatment of the encephalopathy of AFHF, as discussed earlier, is very different from the treatment of encephalopathy that develops with end-stage liver disease. The following discussion relates to interventions for encephalopathy of chronic liver disease.

Dietary protein may be decreased or deleted altogether. Sufficient calories and carbohydrates are important because, according to Galambos (1979), a "low calorie diet in a cirrhotic is a high protein diet" due to catabolism and endogenous protein production. Most patients can tolerate at least small amounts of protein. Excessive amounts of fats, which delay gastric emptying, and glucose, which is hyperosmolar and can exacerbate nausea, are avoided.

Blood in the gut of the cirrhotic can significantly contribute to the ammonia load. Catharsis, or vigorous cleansing of the gut, is one method of removing bacteria that produce ammonia, ammonia itself, and blood. Any ongoing bleeding, of course, must be stopped. Interventions are aimed at interfering with the colonic production and absorption of ammonia. Neomycin and lactulose are the most commonly used pharmacologic agents for this purpose.

Neomycin is a nonabsorbable antibiotic that is effective against ureolytic gram-negative organisms. It also induces regular bowel movements and is gentler in this respect than lactulose. Neomycin is administered in amounts of up to 4 to 6 g/day in divided doses. An important responsibility of the nurse caring for the patient receiving neomycin is monitoring for signs of nephrotoxicity and ototoxicity. Because of these undesirable side effects, neomycin is not intended for long-term use. It is used as a short-term treatment to return patients to a compensated state with regard to dietary intake and ammonia metabolism.

Lactulose is a saline laxative that is converted in the gut to lactic acid and acetic acid. One effect of lactulose is that ammonia in the gut remains in the ionized form and hence cannot cross the gut membranes into the systemic circulation. Another effect is a decrease in fecal pH (5.0), which inhibits growth of ammonia-forming bacteria. Lowering fecal pH creates a gradient of 2.4 between the extracellular fluid pH (7.4) and fecal pH (5.0). This promotes diffusion of ammonia from the systemic circulation into the acidified bowel contents and produces diarrhea. The amount of lactulose administered must be sufficient to decrease the fecal pH to create this gradient. Thirty milliliters of lactulose syrup every 6 to 8 hours of a 20% retention enema solution usually accomplishes this goal. Side effects of lactulose include abdominal cramps and gas. Protection of the perianal area with barrier cream may be necessary depending on the length of treatment and the amount of diarrhea produced. Caution is needed to prevent trauma to hemorrhoidal vessels when inserting rectal tubes for administration of an enema.

Evacuation of blood from the gut of the patient with a GI hemorrhage can also be accomplished with phosphorus or magnesium purgatives or with plain tap water. Although these interventions are time consuming, the results are worth it. Equally important in the hemorrhaging patient, of course, is the replacement of lost circulating volume. Compensatory mechanisms for hypovolemia exacerbate the condition by decreasing hepatic and renal perfusion.

If encephalopathy is precipitated by diuretic therapy, these drugs should be discontinued. Alterations in plasma volume and electrolyte and acid–base balance should be promptly corrected. Potassium supplements are indicated if loop diuretics have been used. In intractable cases of hepatic encephalopathy, colon resection may be indicated to remove the major source of ammonia production.

A primary nursing responsibility in care of the encephalopathic patient is protection of the patient from self-harm to whatever degree is necessary. It is fruitless to try to reason with or expect compliance with normally accepted behavior in an encephalopathic patient. Entering this vicious cycle will only lead to frustration and may further agitate the patient. Family members or friends often need emotional support to cope with observing the sometimes bizarre behavior changes in the encephalopathic patient. Particularly upsetting can be failure of the patient to recognize a significant other.

SPLENOMEGALY

Splenic enlargement occurs as a direct consequence of portal hypertension. In fact, splenic enlargement is the single most important diagnostic sign of portal hypertension (Sherlock, 1993b). However, the exact size of the spleen does not necessarily correlate with the degree of portal hypertension. Unless the spleen is quite enlarged, noninvasive diagnosis of splenic enlargement is difficult. Because the spleen must enlarge to two to three times its normal size (Fig. 49–13) before it can be palpated, the diagnosis of splenic enlargement is usually made radiologically or angiographi-

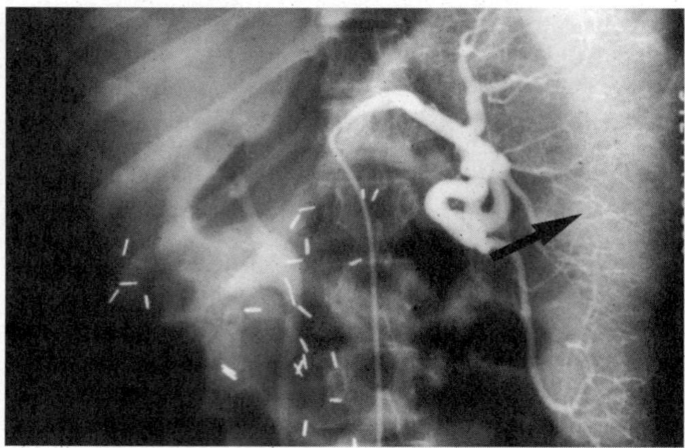

FIGURE 49–13. Greatly enlarged spleen shown *(arrow)* on film of venous-phase superior mesenteric artery arteriogram in patient with portal hypertension and splenomegaly secondary to advanced liver disease.

cally. In contrast to palpation of the liver, the enlarged spleen must be palpated gently to prevent injury and rupture.

The most prominent finding associated with an enlarged spleen is pancytopenia: leukopenia, anemia, and thrombocytopenia. Therefore, frequent laboratory monitoring of these parameters is needed, especially before invasive procedures are performed. Invasive procedures may be precluded until platelets and clotting factors can be replaced. In extreme cases, the patient may complain of left-sided "spleen" pain and may unconsciously physically protect his or her left side.

METABOLIC BONE DISEASE

Bone disease (hepatic osteodystrophy) is a metabolic complication of some types of advanced liver disease, especially chronic cholestasis and alcoholism (Micheson et al., 1988). The primary mechanism of hepatic osteodystrophy is decreased bone formation due to inhibition of osteoblast function, possibly related to toxic effects of systemic substances present in chronic liver disease and cholestasis (bilirubin may inhibit osteoblast activity). Secondary causes include dietary deficiencies, decreased ultraviolet light exposure, and bed rest. Osteoporosis is the primary lesion, but osteomalacia secondary to steatorrhea associated with vitamin D deficiency and altered calcium metabolism can occur.

The mechanism of bone disease associated with cholestatic liver disease is impaired calcium absorption and vitamin D deficiency. Vitamin D_2 (ergocalciferol) is absorbed in the gut, and vitamin D_3 (cholecalciferol) is synthesized in the skin. Both are transported in the serum by a vitamin D-binding globulin that is synthesized in the liver, and both are hydroxylated in the liver. The main defect is a lack of vitamin D substrate, either from lack of exposure to the sun or from malnutrition. Intraluminal (duodenal) bile acids necessary for vitamin D absorption are decreased or absent in patients with cholestatic disease, and because calcium will not be absorbed in the absence of vitamin D absorption, calcium malabsorption occurs. The parathyroid glands stimulate calcium resorption from bones in response to this perceived hypocalcemia. In alcoholic liver disease a defect in this process does contribute to bone disease, but other factors such as malnutrition and hypogonadism are thought to play a role (Stone, 1977). In the acutely ill or chronically debilitated patient, immobility and lack of weight-bearing exacerbate this condition.

The bone diseases that complicate life for these patients are osteomalacia and osteoporosis. Osteomalacia is a condition characterized by inadequate and delayed mineralization of osteoid in mature compact and spongy bone (Kaplan, 1987). Mineral calcification and deposition are inhibited in an otherwise normal bone remodeling cycle (a three-phase process whereby existing bone is resorbed and new bone is laid down to replace it), resulting in normal bone volume that is soft. The most significant factor in development of osteomalacia is vitamin D deficiency. Diffuse skeletal tenderness and pain, muscular weakness, gait disturbances, and fractures occur with osteomalacia. Bone loss is usually not recognized until a fracture occurs. Osteomalacia is specifically associated with primary biliary cirrhosis (Eastell et al., 1991; Herlong et al., 1982). Cholestyramine also induces osteomalacia by decreasing serum 25-hydroxyvitamin D concentration secondary to malabsorption of vitamin D, binding of vitamin D to choleystyramine, and increased urinary secretion of water-soluble vitamin metabolites. The bones are weakened, kyphosis occurs, and pseudofractures are common. Bone pain is a frequent complaint. Dental problems arise as the lamina dura around the teeth disappears and the teeth fall out. The oral cavity can become a source of infection and sepsis, and loss of teeth can contribute to poor dietary intake. A thorough dental or oral surgery consultation is often indicated.

Osteoporosis is a state of decreased bone mass per unit volume (density) of normally mineralized bone (Kaplan, 1987). The bone that remains is histologically and biochemically normal. However, there is not sufficient mass to maintain skeletal integrity or mechanical support. The most prevalent complications are pain; compression fractures of the vertebral bodies, ribs, hip, humerus, and distal radius related to minimal trauma; and deformity. Affected bone is trabecular bone (axial skeleton [vertebrae, ribs, iliac crest], and cortical bone [appendicular skeleton—long bones, metacarpals, radius]). Osteoporosis is specifically associated with sclerosing cholangitis (Hay et al., 1991). Steroid-induced osteoporosis has been described. Mechanisms proposed are (1) decreased bone formation, and (2) increased bone resorption. Decreased bone formation occurs due to direct inhibition of osteoblast function. Increased bone resorption occurs due to direct stimulation of osteoclast function, and the indirect effect of increased parathyroid hormone secretion secondary to decreased intestinal calcium absorption and impaired tubular reabsorption of calcium by kidneys.

The most common symptom is back pain secondary to spontaneous vertebral compression. Pain occurs in the middle to low back (thoracic or high lumbar region) acutely. The pain is constant while the patient is at rest and is exacerbated by activities of daily living. Osteoporosis is more important clinically than osteomalacia because it is not usually diagnosed in this patient population until spontaneous fractures occur.

Although the efficacy of various treatment modalities for metabolic bone disease has not been proved, the most common treatments for this problem include calcium supplementation, vitamin D or vitamin D metabolite supplementation, and estrogen therapy. Regular, weight-bearing exercise is also important in the patient without spinal fractures.

SURGICAL TREATMENT OF PORTAL HYPERTENSION

Patients with portal hypertension sufficient to cause variceal bleeding face a 30% risk of death with each bleeding episode. A variety of medical treatments for control of variceal bleeding have been described, but none has been successful in long-term prevention of recurrent bleeding. Surgical procedures, however, have been perfected that do accomplish this goal.

In 1877, Nickolai Eck demonstrated the feasibility of portacaval anastomosis in a dog, and in 1903 Vidal performed the first portacaval shunt in a human (Henderson & Warren, 1988). This early patient suffered some of the same problems associated with portacaval shunts today, including encephalopathy. This procedure, therefore, fell out of favor with the surgical community for a time, but was repopularized in 1945 by Whipple, who showed that portacaval shunts could be used effectively to treat portal hypertension (Henderson & Warren, 1988).

Evaluation of the Patient With Portal Hypertension

Evaluation of the patient with portal hypertension includes analysis of clinical, hematologic, biochemical, endoscopic, histologic, radiologic, and quantitative liver function data. Many of these parameters have been discussed. *Clinical* data include the patient's presenting symptoms and the presence of cutaneous stigmata suggestive of advanced liver disease. *Hematologic* data include the coagulation status of the patient and evidence of pancytopenia secondary to hypersplenism. *Biochemical* data include the standard laboratory tests associated with liver disease, as well as hepatitis serologies, nutritional status, and fluid and electrolyte status. All patients evaluated for portal hypertension undergo upper GI endoscopic examination either to identify the exact site of bleeding or define the extent of collateral vessel development in the esophagus, stomach, and duodenum.

Percutaneous liver biopsy is performed in some patients to determine the exact nature and extent of disease. The most widely used method is needle biopsy without x-ray visualization using an intercostal transthoracic approach. While the patient is in a supine position under local anesthesia, a small aspiration needle is inserted through the eighth or ninth intercostal space at the midaxillary line. The patient is asked to take a deep breath and hold it. At this time the liver is lower in the abdominal cavity, and the biopsy needle is quickly inserted and withdrawn. This procedure is repeated two or three times to obtain adequate pathologic specimens.

Regardless of the method used, this procedure is not without complications. The major complication is hemorrhage, which can be significant enough to cause shock. A branch of the portal vein or hepatic artery within the liver, or an intercostal artery, can be lacerated. Because branches of the hepatic artery and portal vein lie in juxtaposition to a bile ductule (the portal triad), injury of either vessel through the bile ductule can cause hemobilia, or bleeding into the bile ductule. If the patient has a T-tube, this will be immediately evident as frank bleeding or blood-stained bile in the drainage bag. This is abnormal and should be brought to a physician's attention promptly. Intraperitoneal hemorrhage from a lacerated liver vessel or tumor can occur. Significant hemorrhage will become manifest by a slowly decreasing hematocrit and compensatory cardiovascular signs such as increasing heart rate and decreasing pulse pressure. Other complications include laceration of a diluted bile duct, peritonitis, and pneumothorax.

Nursing responsibilities to the patient who has had a liver biopsy include close monitoring of vital signs and physical assessment parameters for signs of vascular or pulmonary compromise. Postbiopsy protocols vary from institution to institution, but usually the patient is required to be on bed rest, lying on his or her right side for 6 to 8 hours.

Radiologic evaluation of the patient with portal hypertension can be extensive. CT scanning is used to measure liver and spleen size (normally 1,100 to 1,500 cm^3 and 150 to 250 cm^3, respectively) and to detect the presence of lesions within the liver. Hepatoma is associated with some types of advanced liver disease, particularly chronic active hepatitis B. Angiography (portography) is used to visualize portal venous anatomy and sometimes to determine portal pressure. Splenoportography during venous-phase imaging of the superior mesenteric artery and splenic artery allows visualization of the portal vein, splenic vein, and collateral vessels. Retrograde catheterization of the hepatic vein using the balloon occlusion method allows measurement of the wedged and free hepatic vein pressures in much the same way as wedged and free pulmonary artery pressures are measured with a pulmonary artery catheter. The hepatic vein pressure gradient (hepatic vein wedged pressure minus the free hepatic vein pressure) correlates well with and is used to calculate the portal venous pressure. Doppler ultrasound can be used to assess patency and flow velocities of the portal and superior mesenteric veins and the hepatic artery.

Anesthesia and the Patient With Liver Disease

The patient requiring surgery for treatment of portal hypertension is at particular risk. The overall condition of the patient is an important preoperative predictor of outcome. Anesthetic agents decrease hepatic blood flow, so there is a potential for hepatic hypoxia. In this situation, drug delivery to the liver is decreased and drug effects are enhanced, especially drugs with high hepatic extraction ratios such as lidocaine and propranolol. The presence of ascites places the patient at increased anesthetic risk for at least three reasons. First, it is unusual for significant ascites to exist without at least some degree of atelectasis and pleural effusion. Second, the patient with ascites in a supine position is more likely to vomit. Third, ascites increases the distribution and disposition of IV drugs. The onset of drug action is delayed, but the duration of action is prolonged. Actively bleeding varices also pose anesthetic risks, namely, pulmonary aspiration and hypovolemia. A Sengstaken-Blakemore tube left in place may also be vomited into the airway during induction of anesthesia.

The alcoholic patient undergoing surgery for portal hypertension presents special problems. These patients are often systemically debilitated, with poor cardiac and pulmonary status. They frequently go to surgery emergently to stop acute, life-threatening hemorrhage. The amount of anesthesia required may be increased, but again the duration of action will be prolonged, potentially affecting postoperative recovery. Alcoholic patients undergoing surgery, elective or emergent, may have minor withdrawal signs within 6 to 8 hours after anesthetics are metabolized. These signs include tremors, irritability, and insomnia. More severe signs of alcohol withdrawal usually occur after 48 to 72 hours and include disorientation, hallucinations, diaphoresis, hyperpyrexia, tachycardia, hypertension, and seizures. This is truly a medical emergency. Treatment involves prompt sedation, thiamine replacement, and electrolyte balance.

Shunt Surgery

Shunt surgery is one of several treatment options for the patient with bleeding varices, including pharmacotherapy, endoscopic sclerotherapy, TIPS, and liver transplantation. The rationale for choosing one of these therapies is based on the patient's risk for continued bleeding and the risk for acute liver failure (Henderson et al., 1990).

Shunt surgery for decompression of varices falls into two main categories: nonselective and selective. In nonselective shunt surgery all of the portal blood flow can or does enter the systemic circulation without first circulating through the liver. In other words, total portal blood flow is diverted around the liver. In selective shunts, portal venous flow through the liver is preserved. Regardless of the type of shunt performed, it must be remembered that these procedures are not curative but palliative in nature. Shunt surgery for portal hypertension is performed for one reason, and that is to prevent death from variceal bleeding. Eventually the patient will succumb to liver failure. Shunts are not performed prophylactically for variceal bleeding because of the morbidity associated with shunts compared with sclerotherapy or TIPS.

NONSELECTIVE SHUNTS

Nonselective or "total" shunts accomplish total portal decompression. Total shunts fall into two categories: (1) end-to-side shunts, and (2) side-to-side shunts.

END-TO-SIDE PORTACAVAL SHUNT. The end-to-side portacaval shunt (Fig. 49–14*A*) divides the portal vein at its bifurcation before it enters the liver at the porta hepatitis; this access of the portal vein to the liver is then tied off. The proximal segment of the transected portal vein is then anastomosed to the side of the infrahepatic IVC, hence the term "portacaval" shunt (from the portal venous system to the caval system, bypassing or shunting around the liver). Portal venous flow now empties into the IVC instead of the liver, and venous return to the right heart is ensured. Therefore, resistance to flow is decreased, varices are decompressed, and bleeding is prevented. Although the splanchnic bed is decompressed, the liver is not. Pressure can no longer back up through the portal vein and collaterals (varices), and this is the mechanism that prevents variceal bleeding.

SIDE-TO-SIDE PORTACAVAL SHUNTS. There are several versions of side-to-side portacaval shunts, including portacaval, mesocaval, central splenorenal, mesorenal, portorenal, and the Clatworthy cavomesenteric shunt. In the side-to-side portacaval, mesocaval, and mesorenal shunt (Fig. 49–14*B*), the portal vein is left intact and serves as the hepatic outflow tract. Therefore, the liver and splanchnic bed are decompressed. Not only is variceal bleeding prevented, but development of postoperative ascites is inhibited. Long-term patency of side-to-side portacaval shunts is better if the shunt is short and direct. In the longer, curved shunts (mesocaval, mesorenal, and central splenorenal), the risk of thrombosis is greater (Henderson & Warren, 1988). The preferred procedure, should a total shunt be necessary, is the short portacaval H-graft anastomosis (Henderson & Warren, 1988). In this procedure, a short synthetic graft (14- to 18-mm Gore-Tex) is placed between the portal vein and the IVC. This procedure is

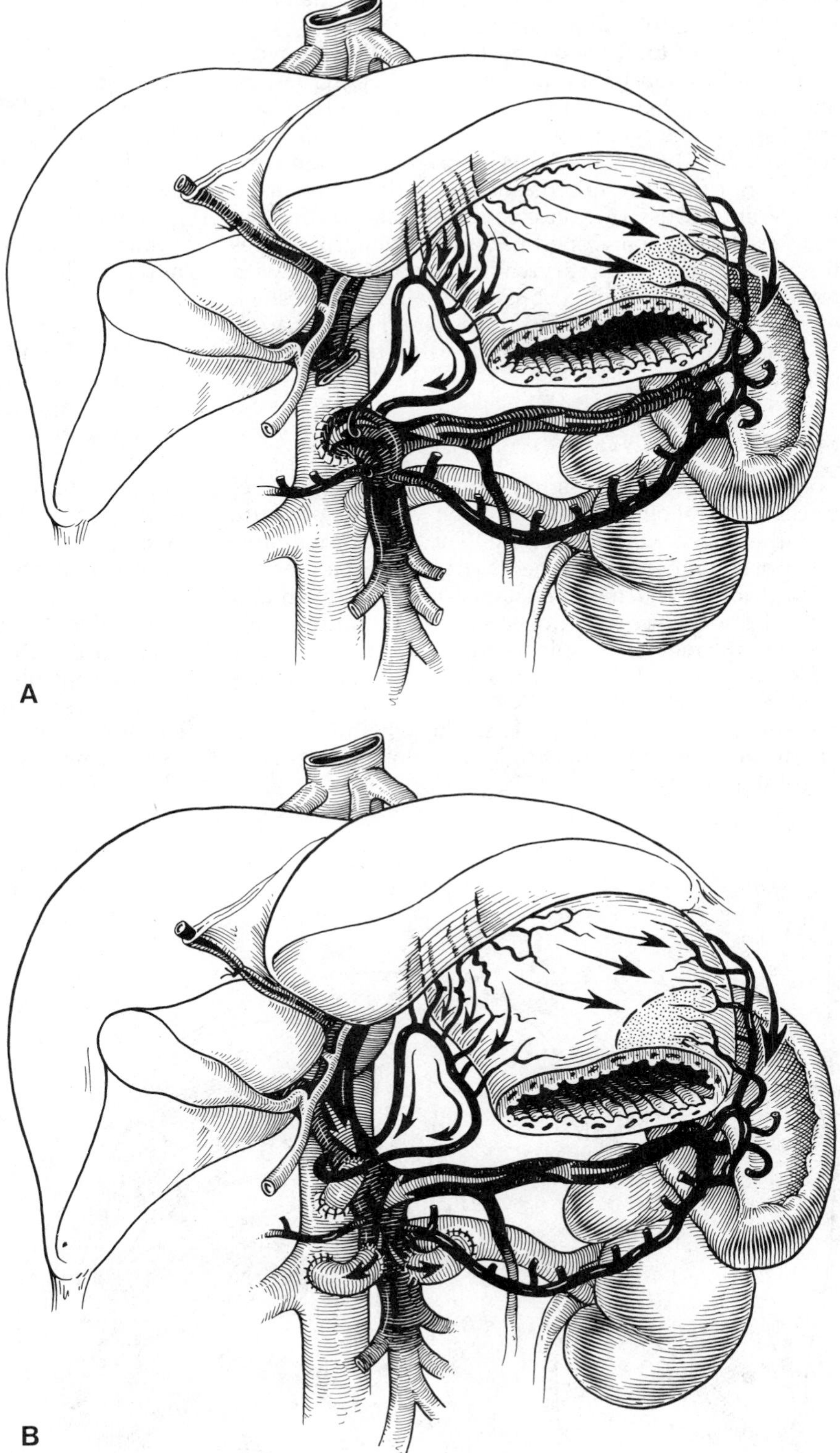

FIGURE 49–14. *A,* Schematic representation of an end-to-side portacaval shunt. Division of the portal vein at its bifurcation irrevocably interrupts portal flow. The splanchnic bed venous hypertension is relieved, but the hepatic sinusoidal hypertension is maintained. *B,* Three examples of side-to-side total portal systemic shunts: portacaval, mesocaval, and mesorenal interposition grafts. The same physiologic effects are achieved with side-to-side portacaval, central splenorenal, and Clatworthy shunts: venous hypertension is lowered in both the liver and the splanchnic bed. The portal vein now serves as a hepatic outflow tract. (From Henderson, J. M., & Warren, W. D. [1988]. Portal hypertension, *Current Problems in Surgery, 25,* 151–223.)

relatively easy to perform and affords the same benefits as the side-to-side portacaval shunt.

The cost of total loss of portal blood flow is eventual deterioration of the patient from hepatic failure and encephalopathy. Although these procedures are still used in emergent situations to control acute variceal bleeding or when sclerotherapy fails in someone who is not for anatomic reasons a candidate for a selective shunt, use of nonselective shunts has for the most part been abandoned because several investigators have found that survival is not prolonged with total portacaval shunts (Millikan et al., 1985; Resnick et al., 1974; Reynolds et al., 1981; Rueff et al., 1976). If possible, a selective shunt is the procedure of choice.

SELECTIVE SHUNTS

The DSRS is a low-pressure, high-flow shunt that reduces esophagogastric and splenic variceal pressure and thereby controls bleeding. The DSRS maintains the portal hypertension necessary to sustain portal flow through the high-resistance cirrhotic liver and provides a low-pressure decompression pathway for varices through the splenorenal anastomosis. The DSRS is reserved for patients who still have hepatopedal or prograde portal flow. There would be no advantage in performing this shunt, which is in general technically more challenging, in someone with retrograde portal flow.

Suitability of a patient for a DSRS also depends on the status of portal and systemic venous anatomy, because anomalies of these structures may make the surgery technically more difficult, and the extent of liver disease. The ideal candidate for a DSRS has stable liver disease with good hepatocellular reserve.

The goals for a DSRS are (1) selective reduction of pressure and volume of flow through gastroesophageal varices, (2) maintenance of portal venous perfusion of the liver, and (3) maintenance of venous hypertension in the splanchnic bed (Warren et al., 1967).

In this procedure (Fig. 49–15), the splenic vein is detached from the portal vein and anastomosed to the left renal vein. Portal flow is not diverted, but varices are decompressed through the short gastric veins, spleen, and splenic vein to the left renal vein, which empties into the IVC. The advantages of the DSRS are prevention of bleeding and preservation of whatever portal flow the patient had before surgery. Ascites after DSRS is common due to the maintenance of portal hypertension, but it is manageable with diuretic therapy and dietary sodium restrictions. Hepatic encephalopathy is not a problem after successful DSRS.

Six controlled, randomized trials have compared the results of DSRS to those achieved with portacaval shunts (Conn, 1958; Fischer et al., 1981; Harley et al., 1986; Langer et al., 1987; Reichle et al., 1979; Rikkers et al., 1978). The DSRS was not found to be superior in

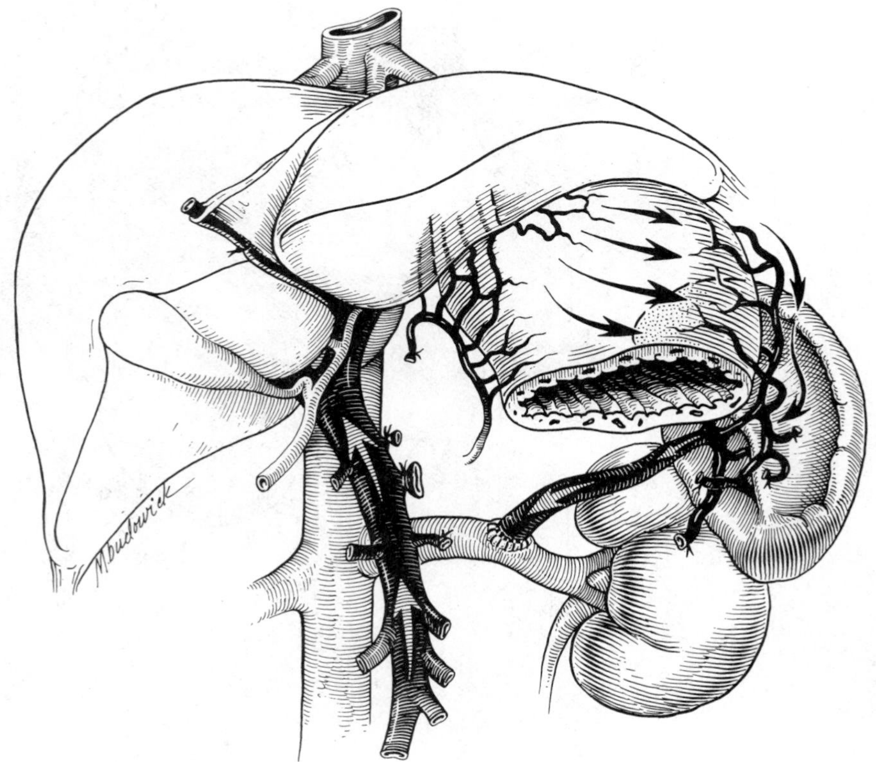

FIGURE 49–15. The distal splenorenal shunt decompresses gastroesophageal varices through the short gastric veins, spleen, and the splenic vein to the left renal vein. Portal hypertension and prograde portal flow are maintained in the superior mesenteric and portal veins. (From Henderson, J. M., & Warren, W. D. [1988]. Portal hypertension. *Current Problems in Surgery, 25,* 151–223.)

improving long-term survival, but, for reasons already stated, the patient's quality of life was better after DSRS.

SPLENOPANCREATIC DISCONNECTION

The survival pattern after DSRS is different between alcoholics and nonalcoholics. Survival after DSRS is better in nonalcoholic patients than in alcoholic patients (Henderson et al., 1983; Van Thiel et al., 1974; Warren et al., 1986; Zeppa et al., 1978). The metabolic response of the nonalcoholic patient after DSRS differs from that of the alcoholic patient after DSRS. In nonalcoholic patients, portal perfusion, liver blood flow, and cardiac output do not change postoperatively. However, in alcoholics, approximately 50% of portal perfusion is lost through a siphon effect created by pancreatic and colonic collaterals. This loss in portal perfusion is compensated for by an increase in cardiac output and hepatic arterial flow, but vital nutrients and insulin are lost from the enterohepatic circulation.

A surgical intervention to prevent this problem and improve portal perfusion is the splenopancreatic disconnection. In this procedure the splenic vein is completely dissected out of (or disconnected from) its normal route of passage through the pancreas. This disconnection prevents siphoning of portal venous flow through the pancreas, and the metabolic response to DSRS is similar in alcoholics and nonalcoholics.

DEVASCULARIZATION PROCEDURES

Occasionally, both selective and nonselective shunts are contraindicated or unsuccessful in the patient with portal hypertension and bleeding varices. In such cases a surgical devascularization procedure to remove collateral bleeding sources may be performed. These procedures include splenectomy, esophageal transection, and gastric and esophageal devascularization. Regardless of the procedure performed, portal hypertension and hepatic perfusion are maintained, but the rebleeding rate approaches 50% (Henderson & Warren, 1988).

CARING FOR THE POSTOPERATIVE SHUNT PATIENT

Shunt surgery for complications of portal hypertension may be done electively or emergently. Certainly the precipitating factors and the condition of the patient just before surgery have an important bearing on postoperative recovery. The sicker the patient before surgery, the greater is the anticipated morbidity and mortality directly related to any surgical procedure. Problems encountered in the immediate postoperative period are related directly to the underlying liver disease. As stated previously, there is nothing curative about shunt surgery for portal hypertension. All of the complications and manifestations, except bleeding varices, of preexisting liver disease will be present in the postoperative period. Taking the patient's past and immediate history into consideration when planning care for this patient is therefore important. In addition, the full impact of intraoperative events, such as severe hemorrhage and hemodynamic instability, is often not realized until the postoperative phase, when the patient is in the intensive care unit.

There is a potential for large interstitial (third space) fluid loss due to the physiologic response to stress and the dissection of abdominal lymphatics. The aldosterone response to stress and interstitial fluid loss is exaggerated in the patient with liver disease. Hemodynamic assessment for adequate circulating plasma volume based on right and left heart pressures, mean arterial pressure, and urine output is routine. Crystalloid replacement is accomplished with 5% dextrose in the DSRS patient. Saline solutions are avoided to help prevent ascites, which usually is not apparent until about 2 weeks after surgery. Fresh frozen plasma may be indicated for replacement of clotting factors and osmotic proteins, depending on the patient's condition. Optimal blood pressure control is necessary to protect the integrity of the graft from hypertension and prevent thrombosis secondary to hypotension. Just as before surgery, the patient's circulation is hyperdynamic. The "normal" cardiac output for this patient is relatively high, in the range of 10 to 15 liters/minute. A functional systolic ejection murmur is a common and normal finding. Commonly, the central venous pressure and pulmonary artery wedge pressure are low due to increased venous capacitance and rapid movement of vascular volume into interstitial spaces.

Gastric decompression with an NG tube is necessary until ileus resolves. Abdominal assessment is important to monitor for (1) gastric and abdominal distention due to failure of the NG tube to decompress the gut, (2) ascites formation, and (3) intraabdominal bleeding. The abdominal incision is a large "rooftop" incision below the right and left costal margins, the apex of the roof being below the xiphoid process. This wound is assessed for progression of healing and evidence of infection.

Because of the likelihood of compromised pulmonary status before surgery, mechanical ventilation is sometimes necessary for as long as several days after surgery. Mechanical ventilation combined with a large abdominal incision increases the potential for atelectasis and pneumonia. Pulmonary hygiene and meticulous attention to aseptic technique are most important in these patients, who have compromised immune defenses.

Finally, assessment for rebleeding and of liver function compared with the patient's baseline indicators are important because shunt thrombosis may occur. Shunt thrombosis is the primary cause of rebleeding after a DSRS (Henderson et al., 1990).

LIVER TRANSPLANTATION

In 1963, Dr. Thomas Starzl performed the first human liver transplant procedure on a young boy for biliary atresia at the University of Colorado. Twenty years later, the National Institutes of Health (NIH) convened worldwide experts in the treatment of liver disease at a Consensus Development Conference on Liver Transplantation. The most important outcome of this historic conference was the acceptance of liver transplantation as a therapeutic option for some patients with liver disease (NIH, 1983). Before this conference, liver transplantation was considered experimental. Access up to this point was limited, not only because of financial constraints, but from geographic constraints. Initially, there was only one center in the United States performing liver transplantation. As of July 1995, there were 117 liver transplantation programs approved by the United Network for Organ Sharing (UNOS) (UNOS, 1995).

Pioneering attempts at liver transplantation met with little success owing to a variety of problems: (1) complexity of the surgical procedures involved in donor hepatectomy (removal of the donor's liver) and recipient grafting (transplanting the donor's liver into the recipient), (2) inefficient donor organ preservation techniques, (3) loosely defined patient selection criteria, and (4) underdeveloped biomedical technology in the field of transplantation immunobiology (Starzl & Demetris, 1990). In spite of numerous attempts from 1963 to 1967, the first successful human liver transplantation was not achieved until 1967, when a 19-month-old girl with cancer of the liver received a transplant. She lived an unprecedented 400 days after the surgery. Before 1980 and the introduction of the drug cyclosporine as an antirejection therapy, 1-year and 5-year patient survival rates after liver transplantation were only 25% and 20%, respectively (Iwatsuki et al., 1988). The Scientific Registry maintained by UNOS began keeping national patient and liver graft survival data in 1988. In an analysis of patients transplanted in 1991–1994 in the United States, 1-year, 2-year, and 3-year patient survival rates were 78%, 72%, and 65%, respectively (UNOS, 1995).

In 1989, it was estimated that approximately 15,000 people in the United States each year could benefit from liver transplantation (Swerdlow, 1989). This estimate, however, excluded patients with alcoholic cirrhosis. Since that time, Medicare reimbursement for liver transplantation, including for alcoholic cirrhosis, has been guaranteed, which has significantly increased the potential pool of liver transplant recipients.

To be eligible for liver transplantation, a person must have end-stage liver disease and must be free of absolute contraindications such as most forms of neoplastic disease or advanced heart disease that would significantly decrease the chance for long-term survival. Evaluating patients for liver transplantation is a complex, multidisciplinary process that usually takes place over at least several weeks. The goals of medical evaluation are to (1) determine the medical indications and appropriate timing for surgery, (2) determine the technical or surgical feasibility, (3) identify extrahepatic or systemic diseases or other conditions that may contraindicate transplantation, and (4) determine overall physiologic, psychological, and psychosocial suitability.

The 1983 NIH Consensus Conference on Liver Transplantation established clear guidelines for absolute and relative contraindications to liver transplantation that became quickly outdated as major advances were made in transplantation technology in the 1980s (NIH, 1983). Absolute and relative contraindications to liver transplantation continue to change as experience and knowledge are gained and further technologic advances are added. For example, because of the highly experimental nature of liver transplantation, it was first indicated and performed only in patients hopelessly ill with carcinoma of the liver. Now, with few exceptions, carcinoma of the liver is an absolute contraindication to liver transplantation because the incidence of tumor recurrence is as high as 100% with some types of tumors (Van Thiel et al., 1989).

Considerable variation in practice has developed nationwide, and controversies over indications for transplantation, patient selection criteria, timing of transplantation, institutional criteria for performing transplantation, and financing of transplantation continue. In 1990, the National Digestive Diseases Advisory Board (NDDAB) sponsored a conference on liver transplantation to develop position statements on these issues. This conference proceeded on the proposition that the clinical conditions that warrant liver transplantation should not be based on etiologic diagnosis of the disease; rather, the decision should be based on the presence of irreversible organ failure and the likelihood that transplantation will significantly improve the health of the potential recipient (NDDAB, 1990).

SOCIAL ASPECTS OF LIVER DISEASE

There is a social stigma attached to "liver" disease. It is true that most liver disease in the United States is alcohol related, and it is this fact that leads the average American to assume that the person with liver disease must be a drinker. A common frustration and complaint of patients with nonalcoholic liver disease is that they have to defend themselves repeatedly, even to those close to them, against this stigma. Another feeling expressed by those with nonalcoholic liver disease is "Why me? I've never even had a drink!"

Ascites creates special problems. Aside from the physical restraints and discomfort associated with ascites, the patient suffers from an alteration in body image due to the changes and disfigurement that occur. Women with ascites are frequently asked by strangers, "When is the baby due?" This is distressing to some, especially young girls or women in their 50s and older. Men with ascites are assumed to have "beer bellies." Regardless of sex, their clothes no longer fit, and there may not be funds to purchase new ones.

The cost of liver disease, like that of any other chronic progressive disease, is high. As advanced liver disease begins to take its toll on bodily functions and robs its host of energy and motivation, gainful employment and providing for oneself or a family may no longer be possible. Roles and family dynamics change. The burden of responsibility on the spouse, child, or parent of the patient with end-stage liver disease is heavy. Even the most productive members of society may be forced to accept financial support from others or apply for disability payments. Too often, insurance coverage is lost after many years of payments, just when it is needed most. Homes and other worldly possessions are sold to provide living and medical expenses. In the final years, patients with chronic liver disease bounce in and out of hospitals for palliative management of ascites, encephalopathy, and infections. The cost of medical treatment during these final years averages $25,000 per year.

SUMMARY

Caring for the critically ill patient with liver dysfunction or liver disease challenges the nurse to understand the complex and vital role the liver plays in health and disease. The patient with AFHF usually demands prompt assessment and appropriate referral to a liver transplant center, because medical treatment is not effective in this life-threatening condition. The patient with cirrhosis may become critically ill for a variety of reasons that are most often related to the end effects of portal hypertension. The prognosis for many patients with cirrhosis has improved with the successes that have been achieved in the field of liver transplantation. Therefore, caring for the patient with end-stage liver disease is no longer a palliative process in most cases, which further emphasizes the need for critical care nurses to understand the nature of the pathophysiologic processes of and interventions for these patients.

REFERENCES

Adams, L. & Soulen, M. C. (1992). TIPS: A new alternative for the variceal bleeder. *American Journal of Critical Care, 2,* 196–201.

Alter, M. J., Hadler, S. C., Margolis, H. S., et al. (1990a). The changing epidemiology of hepatitis B in the United States. *Journal of the American Medical Association, 263,* 1218–1222.

Alter, M. J., Hadler, S. C., Judson, F. N., et al. (1990b). Risk factors for acute non-A, non-B hepatitis in the United States and association with hepatitis C virus infection. *Journal of the American Medical Association, 264,* 2231–2235.

Alwmark, A., Bengmark, S., Borjesson, B., et al. (1982). Emergency and long term transesophageal sclerotherapy of bleeding esophageal varices: A prospective study of 50 consecutive cases. *Scandinavian Journal of Gastroenterology, 17,* 409–412.

Bouletreau, P., Delafosse, B., Auboyer, C., et al. (1979). Role of branched chain amino acids in cirrhotic encephalopathy. In *Postgraduate course: XIth international meeting of anesthesiology and resuscitation* (pp. 239–254). Paris.

Bradford, K. S. (1983). Injection sclerotherapy in the management of bleeding esophageal varices. *Critical Care Nurse, 3*(2), 36–40.

Carrithers, R. L., & Fairman, R. P. (1989). Critical care of patients with severe liver disease. In W. C. Shoemaker, C. Ayers, A. Grenvik, et al. (Eds.), *Textbook of critical care* (2nd ed.). St. Louis: C. V. Mosby.

Cascino, A., Cangiano, C., Calcaterra, V., et al. (1978). Plasma amino acid imbalance in patients with liver disease. *American Journal of Digestive Diseases, 23,* 591–598.

Cate, E. H., & Laudicina, S. S. (1991). *Transplantation white paper.* Northwestern University, Annenberg Washington Program, and Richmond, VA: United Network for Organ Sharing.

Cattau, E. L., Benjamin, S. B., & Knuff, T. E. (1982). The accuracy of the physical exam in the diagnosis of suspected ascites. *Journal of the American Medical Association, 247,* 1164–1169.

Cello, J. P., Grendall, J. H., Crass, R. A., et al. (1986). Endoscopic sclerotherapy versus portacaval shunt in patients with severe cirrhosis and acute variceal hemorrhage. *New England Journal of Medicine, 316,* 11–15.

Clark, A. W., Westaby, D., Silk D. B. A., et al. (1980). Prospective controlled trial of injection sclerotherapy with cirrhosis and recent variceal hemorrhage. *Lancet, 2,* 552–554.

Clive, D. M. (1985). Renal dysfunction in the patient with liver disease. In J. M. Rippe, R. S. Irwin, J. S. Alpert, et al. (Eds.), *Intensive care medicine* (pp. 755–757). Boston: Little, Brown, and Co.

Colman, J., Magnot, P., & Dudley, F. (1985). The effect of acute and chronic propranolol on portal venous pressure (Abstract). *Gastroenterology, 86,* 1315.

Conn, H. O. (1958). Hazards attending the use of esophageal tamponade. *New England Journal of Medicine, 259,* 701–707.

Conn, H. O., Resnick, R. F., Grace, N. D., et al. (1981). Distal splenorenal shunt versus portacaval shunt: Current status of a controlled trial. *Hepatology, 1,* 151–160.

Copenhagen Esophageal Varices Sclerotherapy Project. (1984). Sclerotherapy after first variceal hemorrhage in cirrhosis; A randomized multicenter trial. *New England Journal of Medicine, 311,* 594–600.

Cordoba, J., & Blei, A. T. (1995). Cerebral edema and intracranial pressure monitoring. *Liver Transplantation and Surgery, 1,* 187–194.

Daas, M., Plevak, D. J., Wijdicks, E. F. M., Rakela, J., Weisner, R. H., Piepgras, D. G., Dunn, W. F., & Steers, J. L. (1995). Acute liver failure: Results of a 5-year clinical protocol. *Liver Transplantation and Surgery, 1*(4), 210–219.

Donohue, T. M., Jennett, R. B., Tuma, D. J., & Sorrell, M. F. (1990). Synthesis and secretion of plasma proteins by the liver. In D. Zakim & T. D. Boyer (Eds.), *Hepatology* (pp. 124–137). Philadelphia: W. B. Saunders.

Eastell, R., Dickson, E. R., Hodgson, S. F., et al. (1991). Rates of vertebral bone loss before and after liver transplantation for women with primary biliary cirrhosis. *Hepatology, 2,* 296–300.

Finn, F. (1988). Recovery from acute renal failure. In B. M. Brenner & J. M. Lazarus (Eds.), *Acute renal failure* (2nd ed.). New York: Churchill-Livingstone.

Fischer, J. E., Bower, R. H., Atamian, S., et al. (1981). Comparison of distal and proximal splenorenal shunts: A randomized prospective trial. *Annals of Surgery, 194,* 531–544.

Fleig, W. E., Stange, E. F., Hunecke, R., et al. (1987). Prevention of recurrent rebleeding in cirrhosis with recent variceal hemorrhage: Prospective randomized comparison of propranolol and sclerotherapy. *Hepatology, 7,* 355–361.

Frakes, J. (1980). Physiologic considerations in the medical management of ascites. *Archives of Internal Medicine, 140,* 620–621.

Galambos, J. T. (Ed.). (1979). *Cirrhosis: Major problems in internal medicine* (Vol. 17). Philadelphia: W. B. Saunders.

Gregory, P., Broekelschen, P., Hill, M., et al. (1977). Complications of diuresis in the alcoholic patient with ascites: A controlled trial. *Gastroenterology, 73,* 534–538.

Harley, H. A. J., Morgan, T., Redeker, A. G., et al. (1986). Results of a randomized trial of end-to-side portacaval shunt and distal splenorenal shunt in alcoholic liver disease and variceal bleeding. *Gastroenterology, 91,* 802–809.

Hay, J. E., Lindor, K. D., Wiesner, R. H., et al. (1991). The metabolic bone disease of primary sclerosing cholangitis. *Hepatology, 14,* 257–261.

Henderson, J. M., Millikan, W. J., & Galloway, J. R. (1990). The Em-

ory perspective of the distal splenorenal shunt in 1990. *The American Journal of Surgery, 160,* 54–58.
Henderson, J. M., Millikan, W. J., Wright-Bacon, L., et al. (1983). Hemodynamic difference between alcoholic and nonalcoholic cirrhotics following distal splenorenal shunt: Effect on survival? *Annals of Surgery, 198,* 325–334.
Henderson, J. M., & Warren, W. D. (1986). A method of measuring quantitative hepatic function and hemodynamics in cirrhosis: The changes following distal splenorenal shunt. *Japanese Journal of Surgery, 16,* 158–168.
Henderson, J. M., & Warren, W. D. (1988). Portal hypertension. *Current Problems in Surgery, 25,* 151–223.
Herlong, H. F., Recker, R. R., & Maddrey, W. C. (1982). Bone disease in primary biliary cirrhosis: Histologic features and response to 25-hydroxy vitamin D. *Gastroenterology, 83,* 103–108.
Hill, J. M. (1991). Phentolamine mesylate: The antidote for vasopressor extravasation. *Critical Care Nurse, 11,* 58–62.
Hollenberg, N. K. (1983). Renin, angiotensin and the kidney: Assessment by pharmacological interruption of the renin–angiotensin system. In M. Epstein (Ed.), *The kidney in liver disease* (2nd ed., pp. 395–411). New York: Elsevier.
Hoofnagle, J. H., & Schafer, D. F. (1986). Serologic markers for hepatitis B infection. *Seminars in Liver Disease, 6,* 1–10.
Iwatsuki, S., Esquivel, C. O., Gordon, R., et al. (1985). Liver transplantation for fulminant hepatic failure. *Seminars in Liver Disease, 5,* 325–328.
Iwatsuki, S., Starzl, T. E., Todo, S., et al. (1988). Experience in 1000 liver transplants under cyclosporine–steroid therapy: A survival report. *Transplantation Proceedings, 20,* 498–504.
Jacques, E. A. (1985). Hepatic encephalopathy. In J. M. Rippe, R. S. Irwin, J. S. Alpert, et al. (Eds.), *Intensive care medicine* (pp. 753–757). Boston: Little, Brown, and Co.
Kaplan, F. S. (1987). Osteoporosis: Pathophysiology and prevention. *Clinical Symposia, 39*(1), 1–32.
Kehne, J. H., Hughes, F. A., & Gompertz, M. L. (1956). The use of surgical pituitrin in control of esophageal varix bleeding: Experimental study and report of two cases. *Surgery, 39,* 917–925.
Keithley, K. J. (1985). Nutritional assessment of the patient undergoing surgery. *Heart and Lung, 14,* 449–454.
Korula, J., Balart, L. P., Radvan, G., et al. (1985). A prospective randomized controlled trial of chronic esophageal variceal sclerotherapy. *Hepatology, 5,* 584–589.
Langer, B., Taylor, B. R., Mackenzie, D. R., et al. (1987). Further report of a prospective randomized trial comparing distal splenorenal shunt with end-to-side portacaval shunt. *Gastroenterology, 88,* 424–429.
Larson, A. W., Cohen, H., Zweiban, B., et al. (1986). Acute esophageal variceal sclerotherapy: Results of a prospective, randomized controlled trial. *Journal of the American Medical Association, 225,* 497–500.
Lautt, W. W., & Greenway, C. V. (1987). Conceptual review of the hepatic vascular bed. *Hepatology, 7,* 952–963.
Lettau, L. A. (1992). The A, B, C, D, and E of viral hepatitis: Spelling out the risks for health care workers. *Infection Control and Hospital Epidemiology, 13*(2), 77–81.
LeVeen, H. H., Wapnick, S., Grosberg, S., et al. (1976). Further experience with peritoneo-venous shunt for ascites. *Annals of Surgery, 184,* 574–581.
Lebrec, D., Nouel, O., Corbic, M., et al. (1980). Propranolol, a medical treatment for portal hypertension? *Lancet, 2,* 180–182.
Leoni, M. P. (1985). Management of acetaminophen overdose. *Critical Care Nurse, 5,* 44–47.
Loft, S., Olesen, K. L., & Dossing, M. (1987). Increased susceptibility to liver disease in relation to alcohol consumption in women. *Scandinavian Journal of Gastroenterology, 22,* 1251–1254.
Maddrey, W. C., & Weber, F. J. (1975). Chronic hepatic encephalopathy. *Medical Clinics of North America, 59,* 937–944.
Mahoney, F. J., Burkholder, B. T., & Matson, C. C. (1993). Prevention of hepatitis B virus infection. *American Family Physician, 47,* 865–872.
Micheson, H. C., Malcolm, A. J., Bassendine, M. F., et al. (1988). Metabolic bone disease in primary biliary cirrhosis at presentation. *Gastroenterology, 94,* 463–470.
Millikan, W. J., Warren, W. D., Henderson, J. M., et al. (1985). The Emory prospective randomized trial: Selective versus non-selective shunt to control variceal bleeding; Ten-year followup. *Annals of Surgery, 201,* 712–722.
Munoz, S. J., Robinson, M., Northrup, B., et al. (1991). Elevated intracranial pressure and computed tomography of the brain in fulminant hepatic failure. *Hepatology, 13,* 209–212.
National Digestive Diseases Advisory Board (NDDAB). (1990). *Conference on liver transplantation.* Crystal City, VA, February 11–12.
National Institutes of Health (NIH). (1983). National Institutes of Health development conference statement: Liver transplantation. *Hepatology, 4*(Suppl) 1075–1105.
Nussbaum, M., Baum, S., Kuroda, K., et al. (1968). Control of portal hypertension by selective mesenteric arterial drug infusion. *Archives of Surgery, 97,* 1005–1113.
O'Grady, J. G., Gimson, A. E. S., O'Brien, R. D., et al. (1988). Controlled trials of charcoal hemoperfusion and prognostic factors in fulminant hepatic failure (Part 1). *Gastroenterology, 94,* 1186–1192.
Palombo, J. D., Lopes, S. M., Zeisel, S. H., Jenkins, R. L., et al. (1987). Effectiveness of cholesterol metabolism in patients with end-stage liver disease. *Gastroenterology, 93,* 1170–1171.
Perez, G., & Schiff, E. R. (1988). The hepatorenal syndrome. *Critical Care State of the Art, 9,* 100–123.
Perrillo, R. P. (1986). Corticosteroid therapy for chronic active hepatitis: Is a little too much? *Hepatology, 6,* 1416–1418.
Porayko, M. K., DiCecco, S., & O'Keefe, S. J. D. (1991). Impact of malnutrition and its therapy on liver transplantation. *Seminars in Liver Disease, 11,* 305–311.
Rector, W. G. (1986). Drug therapy for portal hypertension. *Annals of Internal Medicine, 105,* 96–107.
Reichle, F. A., Fahmy, W. E., & Golsorkhi, M. (1979). Prospective comparison clinical trial with distal splenorenal and mesocaval shunts. *American Journal of Surgery, 137,* 13–21.
Resnick, R. H., Iber, F. L., Ishihara, A. M., et al. (1974). A controlled study of the therapeutic portacaval shunt. *Gastroenterology, 67,* 843–857.
Reynolds, T. B., Donovan, A. J., Mikkelsen, W. P., et al. (1981). Results of a 12 year randomized trial of portacaval shunts in patients with alcoholic liver disease and bleeding varices. *Gastroenterology, 80,* 1005–1011.
Rikkers, L. F., Rudman, D., Galambos, J. T., et al. (1978). A randomized controlled trial of the distal splenorenal shunt. *Annals of Surgery, 188,* 271–282.
Rikkers, L. F., Burnett, D. A., Volentine, G. D., et al. (1987). Shunt surgery versus endoscopic sclerotherapy for long term treatment of variceal bleeding: Early results of a randomized trial. *Annals of Surgery, 206,* 261–271.
Rueff B., Degos, R., Prandi, D., et al. (1976). A controlled study of the therapeutic portacaval shunt in alcoholic cirrhosis. *Lancet, 1,* 655–659.
Schumann, D. (1983). Correction of ascites with arteriovenous shunting: A study of clinical management. *Heart and Lung, 12,* 248–256.
Seef, L. B., & Koff, R. S. (1986). Evolving concepts of the clinical and serologic consequences of hepatitis B virus infection. *Seminars in Liver Disease, 6,* 11–22.
Sherlock, S. (1985). *Diseases of the liver and biliary system* (7th ed.). London: Blackwell Scientific Publications.
Sherlock, S. (1993a). Chronic hepatitis C. *Disease-a-Month, 60,* 119–196.
Sherlock, S. (1993b). *Diseases of the liver and biliary system* (8th Ed.). London: Blackwell Scientific Publications.
Shronts, E. P., Teasley, K. M., Thoele, S. L., & Cerra, F. B. (1987). Nutrition support of the adult liver transplant candidate. *Journal of the American Dietetic Association, 87,* 441–447.
Sivak, M. V. (1982). Therapeutic endoscopy of the esophagus. *Surgical Clinics of North America, 62,* 807–820.
Smith, S. L., & Ciferni, M. L. (1993). Liver transplantation for acute hepatic failure: A review of clinical experience and management. *American Journal of Critical Care, 2,* 137–144.
Stone, H. H. (1977). Preoperative and postoperative care. *Surgical Clinics of North America, 57,* 409–419.

Starzl, T. E., & Demetris, A. J. (1990). *Liver transplantation: A 31-year perspective.* Chicago: Yearbook Medical Publishers.

Swerdlow, J. L. (1989). *Matching needs, saving lives.* Chicago: Northwestern University, Annenberg Washington Program.

Terblanche, J., Northover, J. M. A., Bornman, P., et al. (1979). A prospective controlled trial of sclerotherapy in the long-term management of patients after esophageal variceal bleeding. *Surgery, Gynecology and Obstetrics, 148,* 323–333.

Teres, J., Cecelia, A., Bordas, J., et al. (1978). Esophageal tamponade for bleeding varices: Controlled trial between the Sengstaken-Blakemore tube and the Linton-Nachlas tube. *Gastroenterology, 75,* 566–569.

United Network for Organ Sharing. (1995). UNOS Center specific report produced. *UNOS Update, 11*(2), 2–4.

Vaillant, G. E. (1983). *The natural history of alcoholism.* Cambridge, MA: Harvard University Press.

Van Thiel, D. H., Makowka, L., & Starzl. T. E. (1989). Liver transplantation: Where it's been, where it's going. *Gastroenterology Clinics of North America, 17,* 1–18.

Van Thiel, D. H., Lester, R., & Sheras, R. J. (1974). Hypogonadism in alcoholic liver disease: Evidence for a double effect. *Gastroenterology, 67,* 1188–1199.

Wall, W. J., & Adams, P. C. (1995). Liver transplantation for fulminant hepatic failure: North American experience. *Liver Transplantation and Surgery, 1*(3), 178–182.

Warren, W. D., Millikan, W. J., Henderson, J. M., et al. (1986). Splenopancreatic disconnection: Improved selectivity of distal splenorenal shunt. *Annals of Surgery, 204,* 346–355.

Warren, W. D., Zeppa, R., & Foman, J. S. (1967). Selective transplenic decompression of gastroesophageal varices by distal splenorenal shunt. *Annals of Surgery, 166,* 437–442.

Waye, J. D. (1987). Expanding uses of therapeutic endoscopy. *Hospital Practice, 22*(8), 143–148.

Westaby, D., Macdongall, B. R. D., & Millikan, W. J. (1985). Improved survival following injection sclerotherapy for esophageal varices: Final analysis of a controlled trial. *Hepatology, 5,* 827–830.

Widmann, F. K. (Ed.). (1987). *Clinical interpretation of laboratory tests* (9th ed.). Philadelphia: F. A. Davis.

Williams, R., & Gimson, A. E. S. (1984). An assessment of orthotopic liver transplantation in acute liver failure. *Hepatology, 4*(Suppl), 225–245.

Zakim, D., & Bouer, T. D. (1990). *Hepatology* (2nd ed.). Philadelphia: W. B. Saunders.

Zemel, G., Katzen, B. T., Becker, G. J., Benenati, J. F., & Sallee, S. (1991). Percutaneous transjugular portosystemic shunt. *Journal of the American Medical Association, 266,* 390–393.

Zeppa, R., Hensley, G. T., & Levi, J. U. (1978). Factors influencing survival after distal splenorenal shunt. *Annals of Surgery, 187,* 510–542.

Zipser, R. D., Hoefs, J. C., Speckart, P. F., et al. (1979). Prostaglandins: Modulators of renal function and pressor resistance in chronic liver disease. *Journal of Clinical Endocrinology and Metabolism, 48,* 895–890.

Zipser, R. D., Radvan, G. H., Kronberg, K. J., et al. (1983). Urinary thromboxane B_2 and prostaglandin E_2 in the hepatorenal syndrome: Evidence for increased vasoconstrictor and decreased vasodilator factors. *Gastroenterology, 84,* 697–703.

CIRRHOSIS AND PORTAL HYPERTENSION MULTIDISCIPLINARY CARE GUIDE

COORDINATION OF CARE

Diagnosis/Stabilization Phase		Acute Management Phase		Recovery Phase	
Outcome	*Intervention*	*Outcome*	*Intervention*	*Outcome*	*Intervention*
All appropriate team members and disciplines will be involved in the planning of care.	Develop the plan of care with the patient/family, primary nurse(s), primary physician(s), family practice, gastroenterologist, other specialists as needed, clinical nurse specialist, respiratory therapist, chaplain, social services.	All appropriate team members and disciplines will be involved in the planning of care.	Update the plan of care with all team members and dietitian, discharge planning team, home health agency, home equipment supply company, physical therapist. Initiate planning for anticipated discharge. Begin teaching patient/family about home care.	Patient will understand how to maintain optimal health at home.	Teach patient about any follow-up health care visits. Coordinate home care with continuing care agency. Provide written guidelines concerning continuing care to patient/family. Provide patient/family with phone number of resources available to answer questions. Confer as needed with continuing care team members.

FLUID BALANCE

Diagnosis/Stabilization Phase		Acute Management Phase		Recovery Phase	
Outcome	*Intervention*	*Outcome*	*Intervention*	*Outcome*	*Intervention*
Patient will achieve optimal hemodynamic status as evidenced by: • MAP > 70 mm Hg • Hemodynamic parameters WNL • Urine output > 0.5 mL/kg/hr • No bleeding • Free from cardiac dysrhythmias	Monitor and treat: • Hemodynamic parameters • BP • SvO_2 • I & O Monitor LOC. Monitor evidence of tissue perfusion. Monitor lab values: bilirubin, albumin, aspartate aminotransferase, alanine aminotransferase, ABGS, PT, PTT, CBC, ammonia level, creatinine. Monitor and treat cardiac dysrhythmias. Observe for signs of obvious or insidious bleeding and administer blood products as needed and assess response.	Patient will maintain optimal hemodynamic status.	Same as in stabilization phase. Daily weight. Administer diuretics if required. Begin patient/family teaching on liver dysfunction, current treatment, and expected clinical course.	Patient will maintain optimal hemodynamic status.	Same as acute management phase. Teach patient/family signs of fluid overload (peripheral edema, ascites, weight gain). Teach patient/family signs of complications (jaundice, bleeding tendencies, neurologic changes) and when to seek medical attention.

	Intervention (continued)				
	Anticipate the need for vasopressor agents; assess response and titrate accordingly. Assess for peripheral edema and ascites. Monitor for possible complications associated with liver dysfunction and treat accordingly (coagulopathy, pleural effusion, renal insufficiency, upper GI hemorrhage, bacteremia). Assess for ascites; be prepared for paracentesis. Assess need for referral for liver transplantation evaluation.				

NUTRITION

Diagnosis/Stabilization Phase		Acute Management Phase		Recovery Phase	
Outcome	**Intervention**	**Outcome**	**Intervention**	**Outcome**	**Intervention**
Patient will be adequately nourished.	Assess nutritional status. Use dietitian or nutritional support team for treatment of protein/caloric malnutrition. Initiate recommended diet and monitor response. Sodium and protein intake restriction if appropriate. Assess bowel sounds, abdominal distention, and ascites. Monitor albumin, prealbumin, total protein, cholesterol, triglycerides, and lymphocyte count.	Patient will be adequately nourished.	Continue recommended diet and monitor response. Continue utilization of dietitian or nutritional support team. Monitor serum protein and albumin lab values.	Patient will be adequately nourished.	Teach patient/family: • Daily caloric requirements • Low-fat, low-sodium, low-protein diet restrictions as recommended for patient

MOBILITY

Diagnosis/Stabilization Phase		Acute Management Phase		Recovery Phase	
Outcome	**Intervention**	**Outcome**	**Intervention**	**Outcome**	**Intervention**
Patient will achieve optimal mobility.	Assess degree of mobility, muscle strength, and tone. Use physical therapist if immobile. Begin passive/active range-of-motion exercises.	Patient will achieve optimal mobility.	Same as in stabilization phase. Monitor response to increased activity. Provide support with activity as necessary. Space activities to allow for adequate rest periods. Allow patient to assist in activities of daily living as tolerated.	Patient will achieve optimal mobility.	Instruct patient/family about activity limitations. Instruct patient/family about progressive activity program if needed.

Care Guide continued on following page

CIRRHOSIS AND PORTAL HYPERTENSION MULTIDISCIPLINARY CARE GUIDE *continued*

OXYGENATION/VENTILATION

Diagnosis/Stabilization Phase		Acute Management Phase		Recovery Phase	
Outcome	*Intervention*	*Outcome*	*Intervention*	*Outcome*	*Intervention*
Patient will have adequate gas exchange as evidenced by: • Normal chest x-ray • Respiratory rate, depth, rhythm within normal limits • Clear breath sounds bilaterally • Sa_{O_2} >90% • ABGs, vital signs, WNL • Absence of dyspnea, cyanosis, and secretions	Monitor respiratory pattern, Sa_{O_2}, breath sounds, muscle strength, coughing ability, ABGs, hemoglobin and chest x-ray. Be prepared for intubation and mechanical ventilation.	Patient will have adequate gas exchange.	Same as in stabilization phase. Monitor and treat oxygenation disturbances with ABGs and Sa_{O_2}. Observe for complications of liver dysfunction that may impair oxygen/ventilation: ascites, pleural effusion, infection. Monitor and treat ventilation disturbances with chest x-rays, chest assessment, ABGs, breath sounds. Wean from oxygen therapy or mechanical ventilation as indicated. Encourage coughing and deep breathing at least q2h if indicated. Use humidification to thin secretions if indicated. Assess effects of increased activity on respiratory status.	Patient will have optimal ventilation and gas exchange.	Teach patient home medications. Teach patient/family signs and symptoms of respiratory infection and when to report symptoms. Refer to outpatient pulmonary rehabilitation program if indicated.

COMFORT

Diagnosis/Stabilization Phase		Acute Management Phase		Recovery Phase	
Outcome	*Intervention*	*Outcome*	*Intervention*	*Outcome*	*Intervention*
Patient will be as comfortable and pain free as possible as evidenced by: • No objective indicators of discomfort • No complaints of discomfort • Normal vital signs	Assess absence of, or quantity and quality of pain. Administer analgesics when indicated. Monitor effect of analgesics on respiratory status and liver function. Provide reassurance in a calm, caring, and competent manner. If intubated, establish effective communication methods so that patient can communicate discomfort.	Patient will be as comfortable and pain free as possible.	Continue as in stabilization phase. Observe for complications of liver dysfunction which may cause discomfort: ascites, bleeding, pleural effusion. Teach patient relaxation techniques. Use complementary therapies such as guided imagery, music, humor, or body massage to promote relaxation.	Patient will be as comfortable and pain free as possible.	Teach patient/family alternative methods to promote relaxation and comfort after discharge.

SKIN INTEGRITY

Diagnosis/Stabilization Phase		Acute Management Phase		Recovery Phase	
Outcome	Intervention	Outcome	Intervention	Outcome	Intervention
Patient will have intact skin without abrasions or pressure ulcers.	Assess for jaundice, erythema, dry skin. Assess all bony prominences q4h and treat if needed. Use preventive pressure-reducing devices when patients are high risk for development of pressure ulcers.	Patient will have intact skin without abrasions or pressure ulcers.	Same as in stabilization phase.	Patient will have intact skin without abrasions or pressure ulcers.	Same as in stabilization phase. Instruct patient/family about interventions to be continued at home for proper skin care.

PROTECTION/SAFETY

Diagnosis/Stabilization Phase		Acute Management Phase		Recovery Phase	
Outcome	Intervention	Outcome	Intervention	Outcome	Intervention
Patient will be protected from possible harm.	Assess need for assistance with activities and provide physical support as needed. Assess need for wrist restraints if patient is intubated. Explain need for restraints to patient/family. Follow hospital protocol for use of restraints.	Patient will be protected from possible harm.	Give appropriate physical support as patient increases mobility to prevent falls or injury.	Patient will be protected from possible harm.	Review with patient/family any physical limitations in activity before discharge home.

PSYCHOSOCIAL/SELF-DETERMINATION

Diagnosis/Stabilization Phase		Acute Management Phase		Recovery Phase	
Outcome	Intervention	Outcome	Intervention	Outcome	Intervention
Patient will achieve psychophysiologic stability. Patient will demonstrate a decreased level of anxiety as evidenced by: • Normal vital signs • Normal mental status • Patient reports feeling less anxious	Assess physiologic effect of environment on patient (hemodynamic variables, psychological status, signs of increased sympathetic response). Assess patient for appropriate level of stress. Assess personal responses (affective, feelings) of patient regarding critical illness. Determine coping ability of patient/family and take appropriate measures (provide explanations, allow patient to verbalize, consult support services, allow flexible visiting to meet the patient and family needs, have family conferences).	Patient will achieve psychophysiologic stability.	Same as in stabilization phase.	Patient will achieve psychophysiologic stability.	Same as in stabilization phase.

Care Guide continued on following page

CIRRHOSIS AND PORTAL HYPERTENSION MULTIDISCIPLINARY CARE GUIDE *continued*

PSYCHOSOCIAL/SELF-DETERMINATION *continued*

Diagnosis/Stabilization Phase		Acute Management Phase		Recovery Phase	
Outcome	*Intervention*	*Outcome*	*Intervention*	*Outcome*	*Intervention*
	Observe the patient's patterns of thinking and communicating. Use calm, competent, reassuring approach to all interventions. Take measures to reduce sensory overload such as providing uninterrupted periods of rest.				

DIAGNOSTICS

Diagnosis/Stabilization Phase		Acute Management Phase		Recovery Phase	
Outcome	*Intervention*	*Outcome*	*Intervention*	*Outcome*	*Intervention*
Patient will understand tests and procedures that are needed.	Explain all procedures and tests to patient. Be sensitive to patients' individual needs for information.	Patient will understand tests and procedures that are needed.	Explain procedures and tests needed to assess progress and prognosis of liver dysfunction. Anticipate any need for further diagnostic tests and needed interventions.	Patient will understand tests and procedures that are needed in course of disease.	Review with patient/family before discharge the results of significant tests and how the patient's baseline values compare to normal). Discuss any measures patient will need to take to cope with abnormal findings. Provide patient/family with written guidelines concerning follow-up care. Provide instruction on care at home (when to call health care providers, physical restrictions, dietary restrictions, skin care, and medications).

REFERENCE

Briones, T. L. (1991). The gastrointestinal system. In J. G. Alspach (Ed.), *Core curriculum for critical care nursing* (4th ed., pp. 970–1007). Philadelphia: W. B. Saunders.

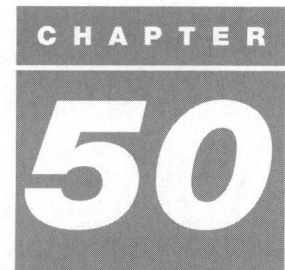

Patients With Acute Pancreatitis

Kathryn Hennessy

Pancreatitis is an inflammation of the pancreas that may be acute or chronic. The intensity of the disease may vary from mild edema to a partial or generalized pancreatic necrosis. The course of acute pancreatitis is largely determined by the presence and extent of the pancreatic necrosis. The manifestations of acute pancreatitis disappear when the causative factors are eliminated. Chronic pancreatitis is a degenerative process that causes pathologic structural and functional changes in the absence of a causative agent. Although most patients presenting with acute pancreatitis recover rapidly, the disease can run a fulminant and fatal course in 10% of all patients (Sabesin, 1987).

PATHOPHYSIOLOGY

Acute pancreatitis is an autodigestive disease resulting from the "premature activation of zymogens to active enzymes within the pancreas" (Soergel, 1983). Zymogen activation may take place in one of three pancreatic tissue compartments: intraductal, interstitial, or intracellular (Figs. 50–1 and 50–2). The events that trigger the sequence of enzyme activation and subsequent autodigestion of the pancreas remain unknown. Acute pancreatitis can be divided into two stages. The mild stage, acute edematous pancreatitis, is characterized by interstitial edema with exudation of small numbers of polymorphonuclear leukocytes. Exocrine, endocrine, and ductular cells are not damaged. Progression of the disease process leads to hemorrhagic or necrotizing pancreatitis, which is characterized by coagulation necrosis of the gland and the surrounding fatty tissue. The factors that promote this disease progression are unknown (Soergel, 1983).

Theories of Pathophysiologic Events of Pancreatic Autodigestion

Six theories have been proposed to explain the process of enzyme activation and autodigestion that overcomes the body's protective mechanisms:

1. One theory is that some agents act as direct cellular toxins or in some way alter the metabolic and secretory processes of the acinar cells (Sabesin, 1987).
2. The bile reflux or common channel theory proposes that a stone may obstruct the flow of bile, allowing it to flow through a common channel into the pancreatic duct (Soergel, 1989).
3. The duodenal reflux theory is that duodenal contents containing activated enzymes enter the pancreatic duct, causing inflammation (Soergel, 1989).
4. Another possibility, called ductal hypertension, is that distal obstruction of the biliary ductal system causes pancreatic outflow obstruction and continued secretion of pancreatic enzymes into the occluded areas. This leads to ductal hypertension, resulting in pancreatitis (Sabesin, 1987).
5. The theory of intracellular protease activation refers to the process of crinophagy, in which lysosomes and zymogen granules are fused, and these, when extruded across the acinar cell wall, lead to the delivery of digestive and lysosomal enzymes to the interstitial and peripancreatic fatty tissue. The lysosome hydrolases include cathepsin B, which can activate trypsinogen, and trypsin will then activate other protease precursors. The normal pancreatic trypsin inhibitor protein is inactive at the acidic pH that exists in lysosomes (Soergel, 1989).
6. The use of alcohol has been implicated in the development of chronic pancreatitis and is said to promote duct obstruction through precipitation of pancreatic secretory proteins (Grendell & Cello, 1989). Whether this mechanism can initiate acute pancreatitis remains unknown (Table 50–1).

Enzyme Activation

The process of enzyme activation, regardless of etiology, is the basis of the disease process (Fig. 50–3). Initial damage to the acinar cells causes a cycle of local inflammation and necrosis as well as systemic complications (Table 50–2).

Trypsinogen, a pancreatic enzyme, may undergo spontaneous activation to trypsin in the presence of an

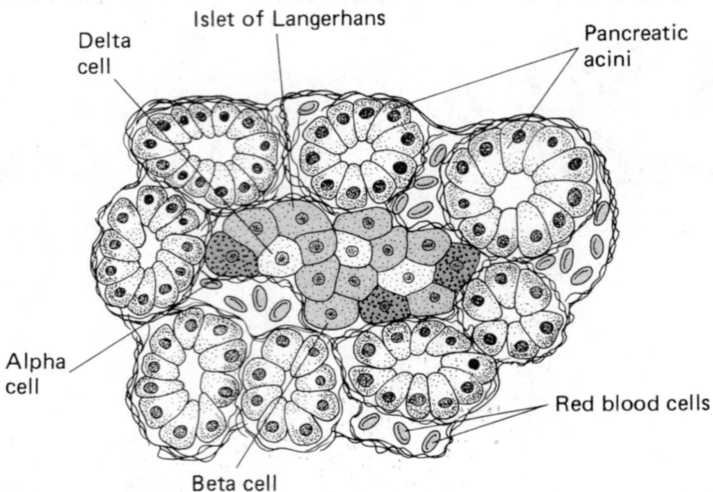

Islet of Langerhans
Delta cell
Pancreatic acini
Alpha cell
Red blood cells
Beta cell

FIGURE 50–1. Physiologic anatomy of the pancreas. (From Guyton, A. C. [1986]. *Textbook of medical physiology* [7th ed., p. 923]. Philadelphia: W. B. Saunders.)

alkaline pH. This release of trypsin can convert kallikrein, a vasoactive substance, to bradykinin, which produces effects on the vascular system such as capillary permeability, vasodilation, and hypotension. The release of these vasoactive substances may be a major pathogenetic mechanism in the production of shock and the cadiovascular complications of acute pancreatitis. Trypsin also produces abnormalities in blood coagulation and thrombotic tendencies. Trypsin can convert prothrombin to thrombin, leading to the formation of clots and the conversion of plasminogen to plasmin, a fibrinolytic enzyme, which leads to clot lysis.

Phospholipase A and elastase, other pancreatic enzymes, have been proposed as the primary enzymes responsible for autodigestion. Phospholipase A, in the presence of bile that has refluxed into the pancreas, causes severe pancreatic parenchymal and adipose tissue necrosis and fluid accumulation. It is believed that this release of phospholipase is instrumental in producing the pulmonary abnormalities characteristic of acute pancreatitis, especially that of adult respiratory distress syndrome (ARDS). Pulmonary surfactant, a phospholipid, may be decreased in the presence of circulating phospholipases. Elastase dissolves the elastic fibers of the blood vessels and is responsible for the hemorrhage seen in patients with necrotizing pancreatitis. Local venous thrombosis, splenic or portal vein thrombosis, and rare instances of disseminated intravascular coagulation result from the activation of elastase.

Fat necrosis in the pancreas occurs as a result of the digestion of lipid by lipase and the precipitation of insoluble calcium and magnesium salts. The formation of calcium soaps causes a sequestration of calcium, thus leading to hypocalcemia.

Precipitating Causes

Acute pancreatitis can have a variety of causes, but the most common are biliary tract stone disease and alcohol abuse. These account for at least 80% of cases (Sabesin, 1987). Other causes are listed in Table 50–3.

CLINICAL PRESENTATION

Abdominal pain can be very severe in patients presenting with acute pancreatitis. The pain is usually located in the epigastric region but may be present in the left upper quadrant radiating to the back. It may

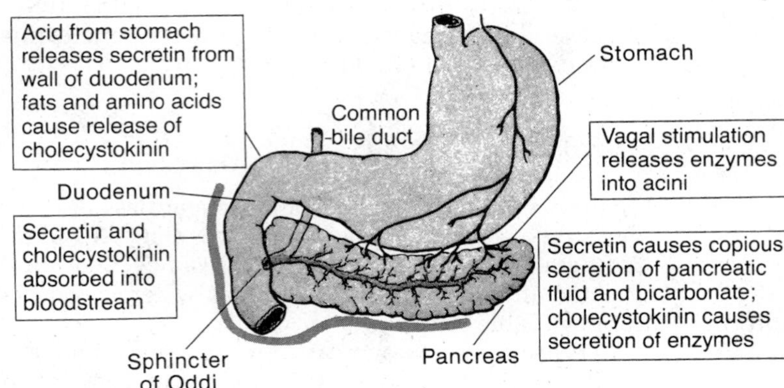

Acid from stomach releases secretin from wall of duodenum; fats and amino acids cause release of cholecystokinin
Common -bile duct
Stomach
Vagal stimulation releases enzymes into acini
Duodenum
Secretin and cholecystokinin absorbed into bloodstream
Secretin causes copious secretion of pancreatic fluid and bicarbonate; cholecystokinin causes secretion of enzymes
Sphincter of Oddi
Pancreas

FIGURE 50–2. Regulation of pancreatic secretions. (From Guyton, A. C. [1986]. *Textbook of medical physiology* [7th ed., p. 781]. Philadelphia: W. B. Saunders.)

TABLE 50–1. **Possible Effects of Alcohol on Pancreas**

Increased secretion of pancreatic enzymes with decreased water and bicarbonate output
Formation of protein plugs in pancreatic ducts that may cause partial outlet obstruction (increased concentration of protein and volume of pancreatic secretions)
Increased tone of sphincter of Oddi with increased pressure in biliary tract and pancreas
Increased reflux of duodenal contents into pancreas (alcohol bile more toxic than pure bile)
Direct toxic effect on acinar cells

Data from Creutzfeldt & Lankisch, 1985.

increase gradually for several hours before reaching maximum intensity, or it may begin suddenly after a large meal. This sudden onset of pain may mimic an acute vascular condition or a gastrointestinal disorder. Once the pain begins, it persists without diminishing for hours and even days. Abdominal pain that fluctuates in intensity or ceases for periods of time is generally not related to pancreatitis but is more often a result of biliary tract disease.

Nausea, vomiting, and retching occur frequently in patients with acute pancreatitis. Abdominal pain persists even after episodes of vomiting and is considered a hallmark sign of acute pancreatitis.

Fever is common in patients with acute pancreatitis but can be a result of other infectious processes. If the temperature is greater than 102° F (31.3°C) it is probably related to peritonitis, cholecystitis, or perhaps an intraabdominal abscess.

Jaundice occurs in 15% to 50% of patients with acute pancreatitis (Sabesin, 1987). Mild elevations in liver enzymes may also be present and reflect pancreatic edema. Hyperbilirubinemia greater than 3 mg/dL may be present (Thompson et al., 1986).

Changes in the circulatory system such as tachycardia, hypovolemia, and hypotension may be present and may progress to circulatory shock and coma in the late stages of the disease.

Patients with severe disease have symptoms that reflect the late stages of pancreatitis. These patients may have pleural effusion and infiltrates, pleuritic

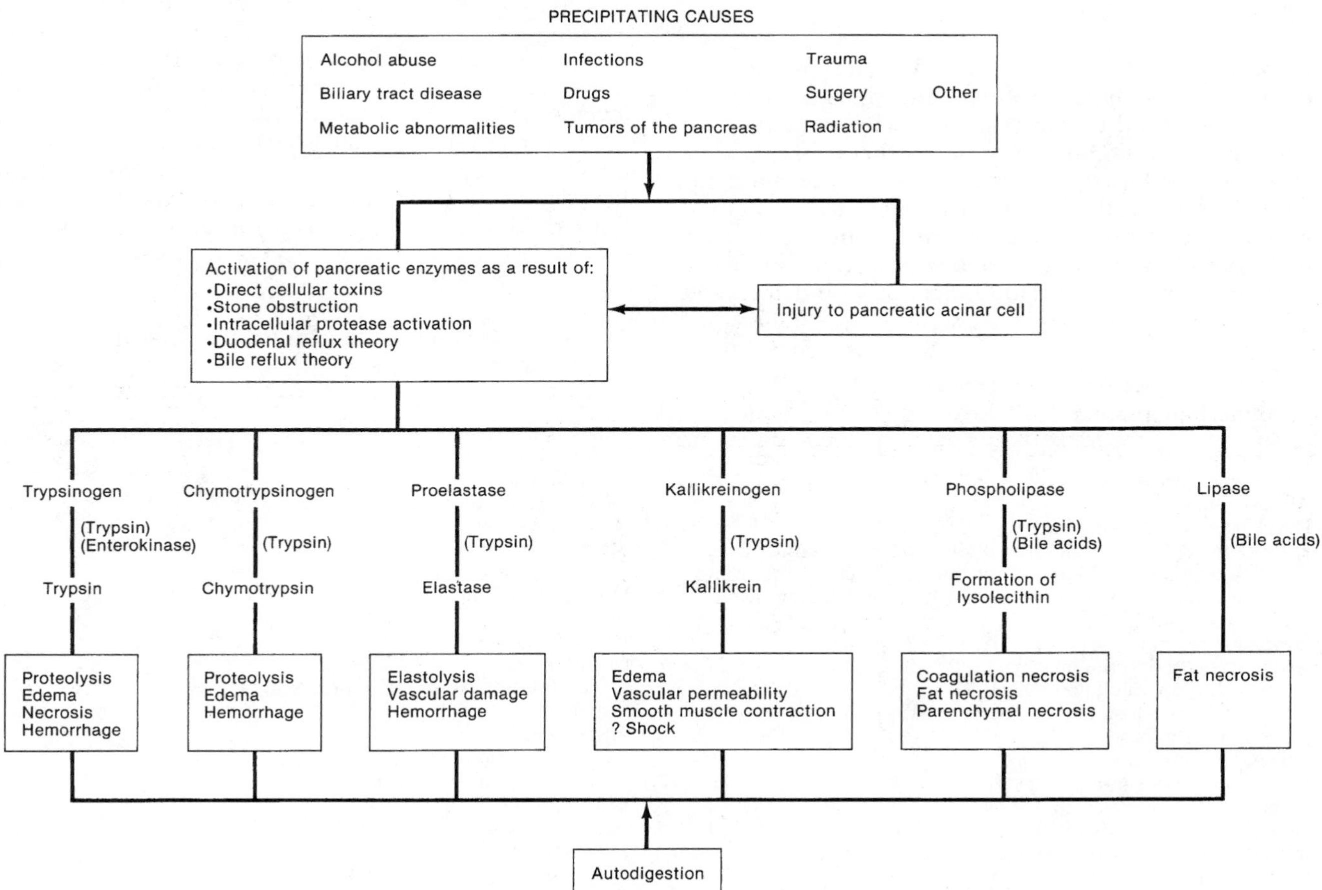

FIGURE 50–3. The activation of pancreatic enzymes in acute pancreatitis. (Adapted from Creutzfeldt, W., & Schmidt, H. [1970]. *Scandinavian Journal of Gastroenterology, 6,* 47, by permission of Scandinavian University Press.)

TABLE 50–2. **Complications of Acute Pancreatitis**

Systemic

Cardiovascular: Hypotension, nonspecific ST-T segment changes, pericardial effusion
Pulmonary: Pleural effusion, adult respiratory distress syndrome, atelectasis
Renal: Acute renal failure
Gastrointestinal: Gastritis, peptic ulcer disease, bacterial translocation
Hematologic: Disseminated intravascular coagulation, involvement of adjacent organs
Metabolic: Hypocalcemia, hyperglycemia, hypertriglyceridemia, acidosis
Central nervous system: Psychosis, mental status changes

Pancreatic

Pseudocyst: Collection of pancreatic juice enclosed by a wall of fibrous or granulation tissue
Abscess: Intraabdominal collection of pus, usually in proximity of pancreas with little or no pancreatic necrosis
Necrosis: Diffuse or focal areas of nonviable pancreatic parenchyma associated with peripancreatic fat necrosis
Ascites
Retinopathy: Purtscher's angiopathic retinopathy

Other

Fat necrosis: Subcutaneous, bone

pain, diaphragmatic irritation with referred shoulder pain, and possibly respiratory compromise and ARDS. Abdominal rigidity, masses, and ascites may be present as a result of fat necrosis, hemorrhage, pseudocyst, or abscess. A bluish-brown discoloration of the flank, Grey Turner sign, signifies the presence of hemorrhagic pancreatitis and the retroperitoneal dissection of blood into that area. Cullen sign is a bluish-brown discoloration in the periumbilical area and indicates blood in that region. Renal function may also be altered as a result of the combined effect of hypovolemia, shock, and mild disseminated intravascular coagulation. Oliguria is usually associated with acute tubular necrosis.

Although the clinical appearance of acute pancreatitis has a wide range of symptoms, most patients present with epigastric pain unrelieved by nausea and vomiting and with guarding of the upper abdominal area. A careful interview should elicit precipitating causes such as alcohol ingestion or biliary tract disease and possibly a history of similar attacks during the preceding years.

TABLE 50–3. **Precipitating Causes of Acute Pancreatitis**

Biliary tract disease
Alcohol abuse
Duodenal disease, peptic ulcer
Drugs—thiazide diuretics, furosemide, estrogens, azathioprine, asparaginase, methyldopa, sulfonamides, pentamide, procainamide, tetracycline, mercaptopurine, excessive vitamin D, dideoxyinosine
Pancreatic tumors
Severe hypertriglyceridemia (type I, IV, V)
Trauma, surgery, radiation injury
ERCP (ionic-hyperosmolar contrast media)
Autoimmune disease, AIDS
Postorgan transplant
Post–Open-heart surgery
Pregnancy/third trimester
Hereditary pancreatitis (pancreas divisium)
Infectious agents (viruses, bacterial, parasites)
Hypercalcemia
Vascular insufficiency
Idiopathic—no cause known (possibly pancreas divisium or occult biliary microlithiasis, and biliary sludge)

DIAGNOSTIC STUDIES

A variety of laboratory and diagnostic tests are ordered in an attempt to confirm the diagnosis of acute pancreatitis.

Laboratory Tests

AMYLASE. Amylase is the digestive enzyme released from the pancreas into the duodenum to assist in the digestion of carbohydrates. The serum amylase level is a widely used, sensitive test for the diagnosis of acute pancreatitis, but it is in no way a specific or exclusive test. Other illnesses can increase the serum amylase level as well (Table 50–4) (Banks, 1985).

Serum amylase is metabolized rapidly and cleared by the kidney, and in the absence of continued inflammation, a transient elevation occurs. In patients with mild pancreatitis, serum amylase may be ele-

TABLE 50–4. **Disease Conditions That Elevate Serum Amylase Levels**

Biliary colic—biliary tract disease
Perforated peptic ulcer
Mesenteric infarct
Salivary gland dysfunction
Renal insufficiency
Macroamylasemia
Tumors of lung and ovary
Diabetic ketoacidosis
Pregnancy
Prostatic disease
Cerebral trauma
Gynecologic disorders—ruptured ectopic pregnancy or ovarian cyst
Pneumonia
Acquired bisalbuminemia
Burns and traumatic shock
Chronic alcoholism
Pancreatic carcinoma, pseudocyst, abscess, ascites
Intestinal obstruction
Aortic aneurysm with dissection
Peritonitis
Acute appendicitis

Data from Banks, 1985; Sabesin, 1987.

vated for 24 to 48 hours and then return to normal levels. The patient may present for treatment after the initial elevation has returned to normal, making a diagnosis of pancreatitis difficult using this laboratory value. A serum amylase level five times the upper limit of normal is a strong indicator of acute pancreatitis. Serum amylase levels remain elevated longer in those conditions previously mentioned (see Table 50–4). Serum amylase may be falsely low in patients with hypertriglyceridemia (Sabesin, 1987).

Serum amylase isoenzymes have been used to improve the diagnostic specificity of increased amylase levels (Banks, 1985). There are two types of serum amylase isoenzymes, pancreatic type (p type) and salivary type (s type). In patients with acute pancreatitis, p-type isoenzymes are elevated, and in those with salivary gland dysfunction and tumors, s-type isoenzymes are increased. Elevations in p-type isoenzymes also occur in patients with other intraabdominal conditions such as perforated ulcer or mesenteric infarction (Banks, 1985).

When serum amylase is elevated, an increased urine amylase level also occurs. In patients with acute pancreatitis the urine amylase rises just before the serum amylase, although this correlation does not always occur. Elevated urine amylase levels may persist for 7 to 10 days after serum amylase levels have returned to normal. There is little practical advantage to using urine amylase over serum levels.

An increase in the amylase–creatinine clearance ratio of greater than or equal to 5% has been proposed as a diagnostic tool in acute pancreatitis (Sabesin, 1987). However, it appears that the serum amylase level must be elevated, and even with this elevation, the clearance ratio can be nonspecific and is affected by other conditions. With the increasing use of isoenzyme measurements, the amylase–creatinine ratio is losing favor as a specific diagnostic test (Sabesin, 1987).

SERUM LIPASE. Serum lipase concentrations are increased in patients with acute pancreatitis and usually remain elevated longer than serum amylase. However, serum lipase, like amylase, can be elevated in patients with other serious abdominal illnesses such as those listed in Table 50–4. Normal serum lipase levels can rule out some nonpancreatic conditions such as macroamylasemia, tumors, pelvic inflammatory disease, and salivary dysfunction. Hyperlipidemia may also interfere with serum lipase results (Banks, 1985).

TRYPSIN. Trypsin is found exclusively in the pancreas. It does not circulate in free form and is measured by radioimmunoassay (RIA), which measures the presence of alpha-1 globulin, a trypsin inhibitor. Trypsin RIA levels tend to parallel the degree and duration of serum amylase levels. There is no correlation between the degree of elevation and the severity, complications, or prognosis of acute pancreatitis. Trypsin RIA levels may also be elevated in patients with pancreatic carcinoma (Bell & Go, 1985).

NONSPECIFIC LABORATORY TESTS. Other nonspecific laboratory tests are used to evaluate the extent of acute pancreatitis (Table 50–5). Although these test results do not identify pancreatitis as the cause of the process, they help to identify the complications of the process.

Procedures

RADIOGRAPHS AND BARIUM STUDIES. Radiographs of the chest and abdomen may be the first diagnostic studies done when the patient presents with acute abdominal pain. These x-rays are taken with the patient in the recumbent and upright positions to exclude the presence of free air in the abdominal cavity, which suggests a perforated hollow viscus. Some findings that point to acute pancreatitis as the cause include regional or localized ileus, sentinel loop (distended small intestinal loop near the pancreas), presence of pancreatic pseudocyst, blurring of the renal outline and left psoas margin, elevation of the diaphragm, pleural effusion, pericardial effusion, atelectasis, and pulmonary edema (Baltaxe, 1985). Pancreatic calculi may also be seen on x-ray.

Contrast studies for patients with acute pancreatitis have been largely replaced by ultrasound and computed tomography (CT) because they provide such limited information. Barium studies are helpful only when the head of the pancreas is inflamed. Contrast studies will demonstrate pancreatic enlargement, widening of the duodenal c-loop, and enlargement of the papilla of Vater. The stomach may also be displaced by a pseudocyst (Baltaxe, 1985).

ENDOSCOPIC RETROGRADE CHOLANGIOGRAPHY (ERCP). This test is not routinely indicated in the evaluation of patients during an attack of acute pancreatitis except in the following situations: (1) preoperative trauma evaluation before abdominal surgery to rule out pancreatic duct disruption, (2) patients with suspected biliary pancreatitis with severe pancreatitis who are not improving, and (3) patients over age 40, with no identifiable cause once the attack is over, to identify the etiology of the disease (Calleja & Barkin, 1993). ERCP is performed to determine the patency of the pancreatic and common bile ducts and to remove bile duct stones if present and / or obstructing the duct.

ULTRASOUND. Ultrasound imaging of the pancreas can be very accurate in the thin person. It shows enlargement or abnormal texture of the pancreas, gallstones, enlargement or distention of the common bile duct, pancreatic mass, pseudocyst, or accumulation of fluid in the abdominal cavity. It can also be used to localize a cyst for percutaneous drainage. Limitations on the use of ultrasound occur in obese patients and in patients with excessive bowel gas because the loops of bowel obscure the imaging process. Because ultrasound is available in most hospitals, this procedure plays an important part in diagnosing acute pancreatitis.

TABLE 50–5. **Nonspecific Laboratory Tests Used to Evaluate Acute Pancreatitis**

Diagnostic Test	Test Result	Cause
White blood count	Moderately elevated	Infectious process
Serum glucose	Transient mild elevation in glucose in initial attacks	Excess glucagon released from alpha cells of islets of Langerhans in pancreas
	Hyperglycemia greater than 200 mg/dL	Widespread pancreatic necrosis, stress response, injury to pancreatic islet cells
Serum calcium	Hypocalcemia 2 to 3 days after onset of disease	Possibly related to hypoalbuminemia; deposition and sequestration of ionized calcium in fat necrosis
	Calcium levels less than 8 mg/dL indicate poor prognosis	Inadequate parathyroid hormone release and end-organ refractoriness to parathyroid hormone
Hematocrit	Elevated on admission	Hemoconcentration is a result of extensive fluid sequestration
	Continuing or declining hematocrit after fluid restoration	Bleeding site, rare in acute pancreatitis
Serum albumin	Hypoalbuminemia	Fluid restoration
PaO_2	Decreased PaO_2	Development of ARDS; pulmonary edema caused by increased permeability of the alveolar-capillary membrane
Serum lipids	Hyperlipidemia—serum triglyceride levels increased (>1000 mg/dL); serum cholesterol normal or moderately elevated	Serum triglycerides elevated in alcohol-induced pancreatitis; lipemic serum is due to the cause of acute pancreatitis (hyperlipidemia I, IV, V)
Serum C-reactive protein	Markedly elevated	Predicts progression of disease to severe, necrotizing pancreatitis (95% accuracy)
Liver enzymes	AST, ALT, alkaline phosphatase elevated	Biliary tract disease
Serum bilirubin	Slight increase	Compression of common bile duct
Serum methemalbumin	Present	Breakdown of hemoglobin in and around pancreas, followed by hematin entering plasma and combining with albumin
Blood urea nitrogen	Elevated	Significant hemoconcentration as a result of fluid sequestration
Serum magnesium	Decreased	Found in patients who abuse alcohol; may contribute to hypocalcemia
Electrocardiography	ST-T segment alteration (depression or elevation), inversion of T waves, extended T-wave negativity, dysrhythmias	May be due to 1. Cardiac damage due to shock 2. Electrolyte imbalance 3. Effect of severe pain on coronary circulation 4. Influence of circulating pancreatic trypsin 5. Vagal influences on cardiac function arising from stimuli from inflamed pancreas

Data from Ammann, 1985; Bell & Go, 1985; Soergel, 1989.

COMPUTED TOMOGRAPHY. CT scanning provides better imaging of the pancreas and abdominal cavity compared with that provided by ultrasound. Unlike ultrasound, the pancreas surrounded by adipose tissue shows up well on CT scans. Although textural changes caused by edema cannot be identified as on ultrasound, enlargement of the gland can be identified. Essentially patients with at least moderate severity will show abnormalities on CT scan. Enlargement of the gland is the most frequent CT finding in patients with acute pancreatitis (Neff & Ferrucci, 1984) (Figs. 50–4, 50–6, and 50–7).* The development of a pancreatic phlegmon, a diffuse inflammation with induration of peripancreatic tissues, is the second most common finding on CT scan in patients with acute pancreatitis (Fig. 50–5). Overall, CT scans can detect at an early stage such complications of pancreatitis as phlegmon, pseudocyst, and abscess and can also monitor the treatment response of these complications and of overall pancreatitis. Contrast-enhanced CT scans can detect pancreatic necrosis, an important marker for assessing severity of pancreatitis.

The author would like to acknowledge the valuable assistance of Michael Powalish, Supervisor of CT Scan, Alexian Brothers Medical Center, Elk Grove Village, IL. Without his enthusiasm and expertise, these CT scan photographs would not have been possible.

Balthazar (1989) developed a severity grading system for CT scans to assist in forming a prognostic assessment. A type A designation denotes a normal pancreas; B, pancreatic enlargement alone; C, inflammation confined to the pancreas and parapancreatic fat; D, one parapancreatic fluid collection, and

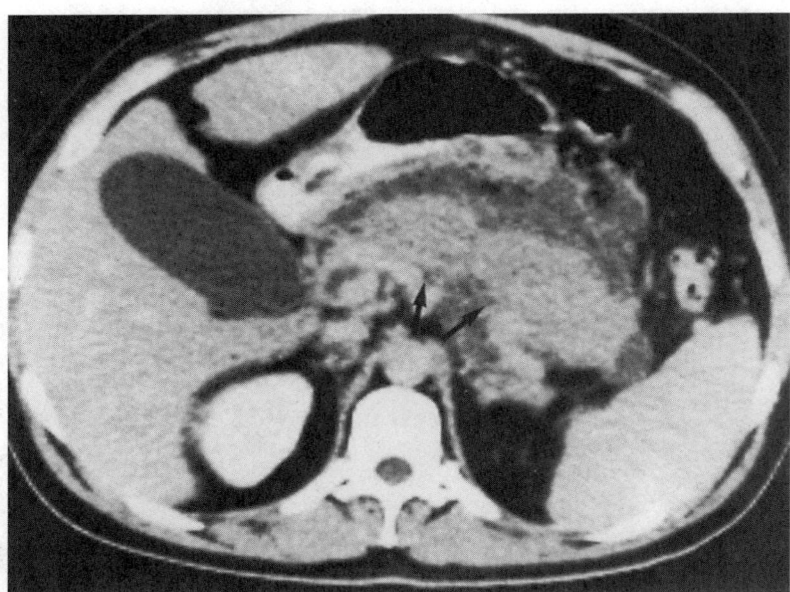

FIGURE 50–4. Computed tomography scan showing marked enlargement of the pancreas with severe peripancreatic inflammatory changes extending into the mesenteric fat anteriorly *(arrows)*.

E, two or more fluid collections. Mild pancreatitis is usually associated with stage A and B and more severe pancreatitis with CT grades C, D, and E. Percutaneous needle aspiration and drainage can be guided with the aid of these imaging procedures. Finally, these noninvasive procedures provide insight into the acute disease process.

MAGNETIC RESONANCE IMAGING. The development of magnetic resonance imaging (MRI) is the most promising diagnostic technique. With the use of contrast media, it may prove useful in the diagnosis of acute pancreatitis. At present, inflamed pancreatic tissue is difficult to differentiate from viable pancreatic tissue, and MRI currently has no advantage over CT scan as the procedure of choice in diagnosing acute pancreatitis.

PROGNOSTIC ASSESSMENT

Patients with acute pancreatitis present with a wide spectrum of clinical conditions. Steady, dull, or boring pain located in the epigastric area is the hallmark of acute pancreatitis. This pain may be accompanied by nausea, vomiting, fever, or jaundice and by cardiovascular, respiratory, or renal complications. The outcome is often unpredictable at the onset of the disease. The overall mortality is 10%, and it exceeds 50% in patients with acute hemorrhagic pancreatitis (Sabesin, 1987). The need to predict outcome at the time of admission is invaluable in determining the type and aggressiveness of treatment and also for providing a comparison between the results of prospective studies. It is for these reasons that researchers have attempted to estab-

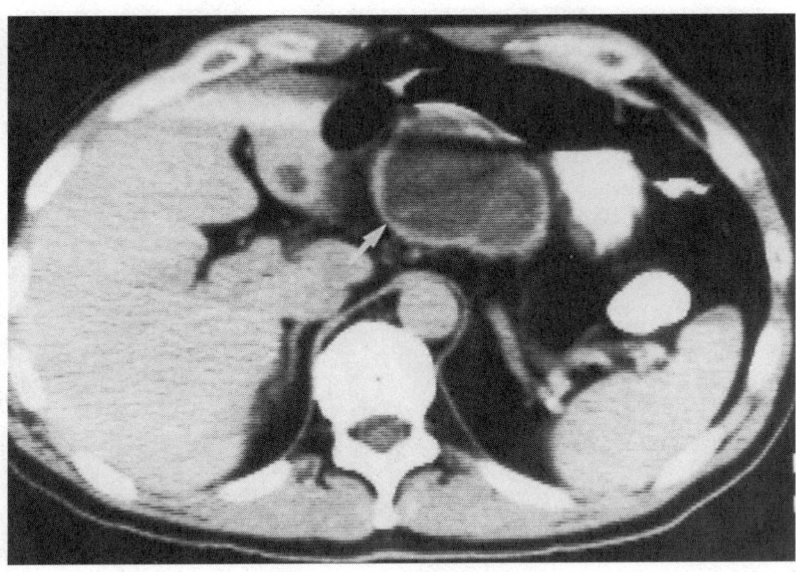

FIGURE 50–5. Computed tomography scan showing an 8 × 6 cm sized well-demarcated space-occupying process in the projection of the body of the pancreas *(arrow)*. This mass appears to be solid in nature.

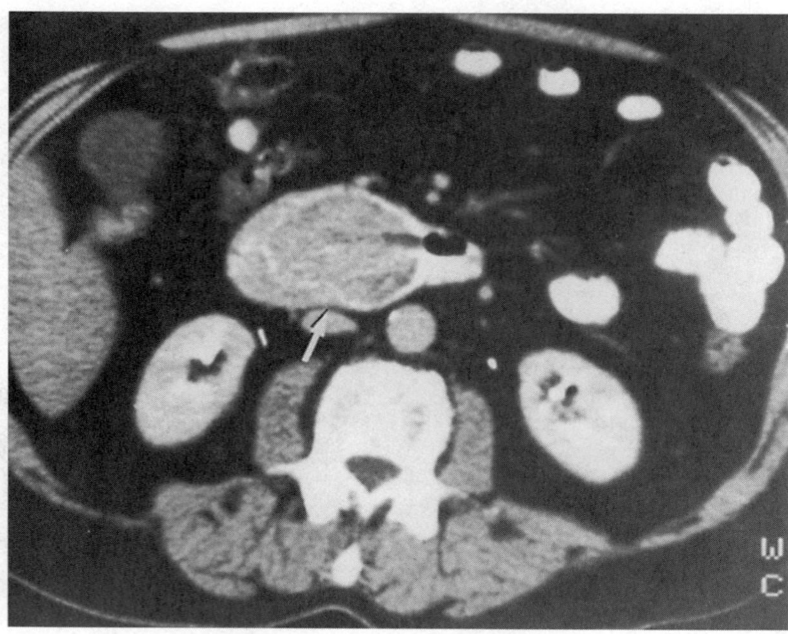

FIGURE 50–6. Computed tomography scan showing a 7 × 5 cm sized well-encapsulated, solid type of mass involving the head of the pancreas, which could be consistent with malignant neoplasm *(arrow)*. Dilatation of the biliary duct and gallbladder is seen. This could be due to obstruction of the distal common duct, where there is a mass.

lish criteria that assess prognosis early in the course of acute pancreatitis.

RANSON'S PROGNOSTIC SIGNS. Of the many protocols that have been developed, the most widely accepted is the list of 11 prognostic signs devised by Ranson, which are determined within the first 48 hours of the hospital stay (Ranson, 1979). This scale has a 96% accuracy rate in predicting severity and outcome in patients with acute pancreatitis (Table 50–6). In Ranson's study, mortality as a result of acute pancreatitis can also be predicted (Table 50–7).

APACHE II (ACUTE PHYSIOLOGY AND CHRONIC HEALTH EVALUATION). The Apache II has also been used to assess acute pancreatitis. It is a complex system that uses 12 routinely available physiologic and laboratory measurements to calculate a severity score within hours of admission. The Apache II also allows for sequential monitoring, which is an advantage over the Ranson criteria.

SINGLE PROGNOSTIC INDICATORS. Other researchers have looked at single prognostic factors to predict disease severity and outcome. Many tests are currently being evaluated to predict pancreatic necrosis (and thus, predict poor patient outcome). Several of those being clinically evaluated are: C-reactive protein, polymorphonuclear neutrophil, elastase, and trypsinogen

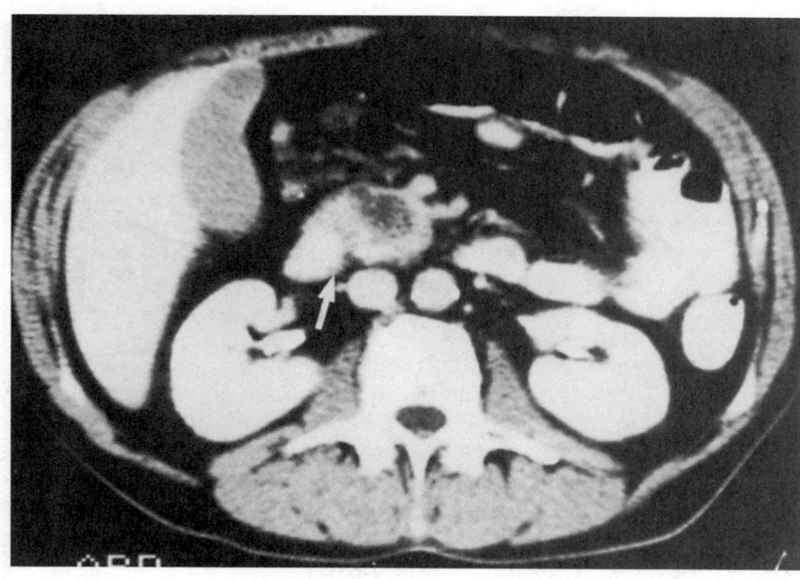

FIGURE 50–7. Computed tomography scan showing a 3.5-cm sized lobulated lucent space-occupying process in the head of the pancreas with suggestion of neoplasm *(arrow)*. Diffuse enlargement of the pancreas is noted. The pancreatic duct and common bile duct are dilated.

TABLE 50–6. **Ranson's Prognostic Signs Used to Predict Severity and Outcome in Patients With Acute Pancreatitis**

On admission to hospital:
- Age greater than 55 years
- Blood glucose greater than 200 mg/dL (no history of diabetes)
- White blood cell greater than 16,000 μl
- Serum aspartate transaminase greater than 250 units/L

During first 48 hours of hospitalization:
- Decrease in hematocrit greater than 10%
- Serum calcium less than 8 mg/dL
- PaO_2 less than 60 mm Hg
- Increase in blood urea nitrogen of greater than 5 mg/dL
- Base deficit of greater than 4 mEq/L
- Fluid sequestration greater than 6 L

From Ranson, J. H. C. (1979). Acute pancreatitis. *Current Problems in Surgery, 16*(11), 1–84.

activation peptide. Further work needs to be conducted to validate these indicators.

CLINICAL MANAGEMENT

In 85% to 90% of patients with acute pancreatitis, the disease is self-limiting and will subside within 3 to 7 days after treatment is initiated (Greenberger et al., 1987). Treatment of the patient with acute pancreatitis is aimed at identifying the cause, stopping the progression of damage to the pancreas, and preventing and treating the local complications. Because specific therapeutic agents for the prevention and treatment of pancreatitis have not been identified, medical interventions are symptomatic and supportive in nature.

Supportive Treatment

In keeping with the overall goals of nursing management, several key areas of treatment have been identified. They include provision of

1. Intravenous fluids and colloids to maintain normal intravascular volume and restore electrolyte balance
2. Nasogastric suction to decrease gastrin release from the stomach and prevent gastric contents from entering the duodenum
3. Elimination of oral intake
4. Analgesics for pain control
5. Respiratory support.

TABLE 50–7. **Using Ranson's Prognostic Signs to Predict Mortality in Patients With Acute Pancreatitis**

Presence of Ranson's Prognostic Signs	Mortality Rates (%)
One to two signs	1
Three to four signs	15
Five to six signs	40
Seven signs or more	100

From Banks, P. A. (1985). Clinical manifestations and treatment of pancreatitis. *Annals of Internal Medicine, 103,* 91–97.

The following sections will address these key areas as they relate to the management of acute pancreatitis.

FLUID REPLACEMENT. In patients with acute pancreatitis large quantities of fluid collect in the retroperitoneal spaces and occasionally within the peritoneal cavity itself. As a result of this third spacing, patients usually experience some degree of dehydration. Fluid replacement is a high priority in preventing systemic hypotension. Hypovolemia and shock are major causes of death early in the disease process. Intravenous fluids, especially high-volume electrolyte and colloid solutions, need to be given to replenish losses. An accurate flow sheet of intake and output should be maintained so that all losses can be replaced with an equal amount of intravenous solution. Patients who are significantly dehydrated should receive isotonic solutions such as Ringer's lactate to replace plasma volume. Leese and colleagues (1987) conducted a study that suggested that fresh frozen plasma be used as a specific therapy for acute pancreatitis because it would replenish the naturally occurring antiprotease system. The results, however, showed no significant difference in terms of clinical outcome between the control group who received colloids and the experimental group. Regardless of the type of fluid used for replacement, fluid restoration helps to prevent the development of acute renal failure as well as to maintain perfusion of the pancreas and possibly diminish the severity of the pancreatitis. An indwelling urinary catheter is inserted to monitor the adequacy of renal perfusion by measuring urine output hourly. Adequate volume resuscitation is indicated when the patient has a stable blood pressure, a stable pulse, and adequate left and right ventricular filling pressures (Crist & Cameron, 1987). Other indications of successful fluid replacement are a urine output of 30 to 50 mL/hr and the presence of warm extremities, indicating an adequate peripheral circulation.

For patients who fail to respond to intravascular fluid replacement, a pulmonary artery catheter needs to be inserted and intravenous fluids administered until the pulmonary artery wedge pressure reaches 15 mm Hg. If hypotension persists, medications to support circulation are administered. The preferred drug is dopamine, which should be started at a dose of 3 to 5 μg/kg per min (Burch, 1988). Adjustments of the dopamine dosage can be made according to hemodynamic parameters and urine output. Patients with severe hemorrhagic pancreatitis may require 6 to 8 L of fluid or more during the initial 24 hours. They may require packed red blood cells or, rarely, whole blood. Albumin has also been shown to be effective in restoring intravascular volume in patients with marked hypoalbuminemia (Cris & Cameron, 1987). Renal failure may occur as a result of hypovolemia and shock and is prerenal in nature.

ELECTROLYTE REPLACEMENT. Along with fluid replacement, electrolyte replacement is extremely important in preventing the complications of acute pancreatitis. The monitoring and replacement of calcium is of particular significance in the early stage of the disease because hypocalcemia reflects a graver prognosis. Hypocalcemia is generally related to a decrease *in* albumin. Calcium replacement is reserved for patients with clinical signs of hypocalcemia such as a positive Chvostek or Trousseau sign or a decreased ionized calcium level. Low calcium levels are related to disease severity, and it is believed that calcium and magnesium are sequestered in the area of pancreatic necrosis (Shearson & Finlayson, 1982).

Hypomagnesemia may be present alone or in combination with a decreased serum calcium level; it requires parenteral administration of magnesium sulfate. Correction of the magnesium level may be necessary before the calcium level can be restored.

Potassium levels must also be monitored carefully because hyperkalemia and acidosis may result from excess tissue destruction. Hypokalemia may result from vomiting, nasogastric (NG) suction, or loss of potassium into an atonic bowel lumen (Burrell & Burrell, 1982).

Another metabolic complication in patients with severe disease is hyperglycemia, which is a result of extensive damage to the pancreas. Regular insulin, on a sliding scale, should be given cautiously because glucagon levels are elevated only transiently in patients with acute pancreatitis. Serum glucose should be monitored frequently.

MINIMIZING PANCREATIC SECRETIONS. Nasogastric suction has been considered part of standard therapy for patients with acute pancreatitis for years (Crist & Cameron, 1987). Theoretically, NG suction should indirectly suppress pancreatic exocrine secretion by preventing acid-induced release of secretin from the duodenum, thereby resting the pancreas (Crist & Cameron, 1987). However, clinical studies have not demonstrated that the use of NG suction alters the course of acute pancreatitis. Therefore, because NG suction has no specific therapeutic effect, it should be reserved for patients with ileus, persistent vomiting, or gastric distension or those with a decreased level of consciousness to prevent pulmonary aspiration.

ORAL INTAKE. Oral intake should be eliminated in patients with acute pancreatitis and should not be resumed until after abdominal pain, tenderness, and ileus have resolved and serum amylase levels have returned to normal or near normal (Banks, 1985). Resumption of oral intake before this time may lead to recurrence of abdominal pain and continued inflammation of the pancreas and may increase the risk of pancreatic abscess formation (Crist & Cameron, 1987). In patients with mild to moderate disease, oral fluids can usually be resumed in 3 to 6 days and a regular diet by day 5 to 7 (Greenberger et al., 1987).

NUTRITIONAL SUPPORT. Intravenous nutritional support is indicated for patients with moderate to severe disease who develop complications or who have pancreatic pseudocyst or abscesses. Levine (1981) proposes that patients who meet four of the criteria established by Ranson are candidates for total parenteral nutrition (TPN). TPN is also beneficial if the patient will require surgery during hospitalization. Central catheter–related sepsis is increased in patients with acute pancreatitis (Kohn et al., 1993), so extreme care must be exercised when managing central lines in these patients. The goal of nutritional support is to provide adequate amounts of calories and protein to meet the patient's increased metabolic demands and to promote anabolism without stimulating the pancreas. Both essential and nonessential amino acids with dextrose can be used to provide the necessary calories and protein. Supplemental vitamins and minerals, especially calcium, are also indicated in patients with acute pancreatitis (Boudeman et al., 1985). Insulin may be necessary if the patient has extensive pancreatic damage. The addition of lipids to the parenteral nutrition regimen is still somewhat controversial due to the etiologic factor of lipid metabolism. Silberman concluded that patients with underlying hyperlipidemia and those with elevations of serum cholesterol and triglycerides without hyperlipidemia should not be given lipids (Rombeau & Caldwell, 1993). Lipids should not be given in patients with marked thrombocytopenia (Kohn et al., 1993). In patients without these abnormalities, lipids can be given safely and effectively. Lipids are usually given two to three times per week to prevent fatty acid deficiency or daily for patients with glucose intolerance. Triglyceride levels should be checked before lipid administration and at least once per week thereafter.

Total parenteral nutrition should be continued until the symptoms abate. Once the acute phase has resolved, patients may be fed orally. Pancreatic enzyme replacement may be needed. In summary, although TPN cannot change the pathophysiology of acute pancreatitis, by promoting bowel rest it can reduce the length of time needed for recovery, decrease complications, and prevent malnutrition.

Elemental enteral diets have been used successfully in patients with acute pancreatitis. These formulas are easily absorbed and fed directly into the jejunum, thereby avoiding stimulation of the pancreas. Jejunostomy tubes are placed during surgery or advanced into the jejunum from the stomach (via gastrostomy or PEG).

DRUG THERAPY. Anticholinergic drugs such as atropine have been used as therapy for patients with acute pancreatitis, their purpose being to decrease the stimulation of the pancreas. However, there have been no controlled trials demonstrating the effectiveness of anticholinergics (Greenberger et al., 1987). Because the use of anticholinergics may decrease urine output and cause bowel hypomotility, tachycardia, increased need for fluid replacement, and signs of toxicity, it is difficult to determine whether the side effects are medication-related or are signs of worsening pancreatitis.

TABLE 50–8. **Pain Rating Scale: McGill-Melzack Present Pain Intensity**

0—No pain
1—Mild pain
2—Discomforting
3—Distressing
4—Horrible
5—Excruciating

Data from Meissner, J. E. (1980). *Nursing80, 10*(1), 50.

The use of histamine (H_2) receptor antagonists such as cimetidine or ranitidine (Zantac) has also not been shown to be effective in reducing pancreatic secretions as an indirect result of the decrease in gastric acid. Although pancreatic secretions are not affected, these drugs may be useful in preventing stress ulcers in the critically ill patient.

PAIN CONTROL. Pain control is essential in the management of the patient with acute pancreatitis. The abdominal pain is constant and severe and can persist for several days; analgesics are needed to control it. However, analgesics that may cause spasm of the sphincter of Oddi, such as morphine, have been routinely avoided; meperidine is administered instead (Banks, 1985). Recent studies have shown that morphine has little effect on the sphincter so morphine may become more widely used for pain control. Because the quantity and quality of the pain are hallmark signs of pancreatitis, assessment should be carefully completed and maintained on an ongoing basis. The use of a pain rating scale can provide qualitative and quantitative assessment (Table 50–8). Frequent administration, at least every 2 to 3 hours, of the analgesic should control acute pain. Patient-controlled analgesia may be more effective in relieving the patient's pain because it allows self-administration of the analgesic as needed. When the pain is severe and is unrelieved by analgesics, sympathetic, splanchnic, or epidural block may be necessary. The benefit of epidural block is that it interrupts the sensory pathways of both visceral and cerebrospinal afferent fibers. Also, an epidural catheter can remain in place for more frequent use (Ammann, 1985). General comfort measures, including knee-chest or fetal positioning, may help to provide additional relief to the patient.

RESPIRATORY SUPPORT. Respiratory complications are well recognized in patients with acute pancreatitis. Pleural effusion, atelectasis, pneumonia, and acute respiratory insufficiency (arterial hypoxemia) have been documented in a significant number of patients (Crist & Cameron, 1987). Ranson (1979) found early arterial hypoxemia in patients with mild to moderate disease in the absence of clinical or radiologic findings. It has been recommended that arterial blood gases be measured every 12 hours for the first 3 to 5 days in all patients with acute pancreatitis (Crist & Cameron, 1987). If arterial hypoxemia is found, oxygen should be administered. In mild to moderate disease the hypoxemia should resolve as the pancreatic inflammation subsides (Crist & Cameron, 1987). Two possible causative agents in the development of acute respiratory insufficiency may be the presence of circulating phospholipase, which may destroy pulmonary surfactant, or the free fatty acids produced by lipolysis of triglycerides in pulmonary capillaries. To date, there is no clinical evidence supporting either of these two theories (Crist & Cameron, 1987).

Treatment of respiratory insufficiency is primarily supportive. Frequent turning and vigorous pulmonary hygiene will reduce the risk of atelectasis. Supplemental oxygen should be used to maintain an adequate $Pa{O_2}$. Careful monitoring of the amounts of intravenous fluid administered is necessary to prevent fluid overload.

Respiratory failure is common in patients with severe pancreatitis and is indistinguishable from ARDS (Burch, 1988). For patients with arterial hypoxemia who have persistent tachypnea and a falling $P{O_2}$, endotracheal intubation and mechanical ventilation may be required. Positive end-expiratory pressure may be helpful in maintaining an adequate $P{O_2}$ in patients who require high fractional inspiratory oxygen concentrations ($FI{O_2}$ greater than 50%). Weaning from mechanical ventilation may begin when patients show improvements in $P{O_2}$, lung compliance, tidal volume, and vital capacity (Burch, 1988).

PERITONEAL LAVAGE. Peritoneal lavage was first suggested as treatment for acute pancreatitis in 1965. Its efficacy is attributed to the removal of toxic substances such as vasoactive kinins, phospholipase A, trypsinogen, and prostaglandinlike histamine that are present in the peritoneal fluid. These substances are thought to cause many of the adverse systemic effects characteristic of pancreatitis, such as decreased blood pressure, increased vascular permeability, and respiratory failure. By removing these substances before they can be absorbed, many of the early systemic complications should be eliminated. Peritoneal lavage for the treatment of severe acute pancreatitis has lost favor since the publications by Mayor and colleagues (1985) and Ihse and colleagues (1986) of studies that concluded no benefit from peritoneal lavage. The first study used 3 days of lavage and the second study, 4 days. However, Ranson and Berman (1990) published results of a small study (29 patients) that compared short peritoneal lavage (2 days) with long lavage (7 days) in severe acute pancreatitis. In the most severely ill patients (five Ranson's signs), long-term peritoneal lavage reduced the frequency and mortality of pancreatic sepsis. Additional studies need to be done to confirm this benefit.

ANTIBIOTICS. Finally, even the use of antibiotics is controversial in the management of patients with acute pancreatitis. There have been no clinical trials that have shown prophylactic antibiotics to be effective in patients with mild to moderate disease

(Greenberger et al., 1987). There is a high incidence of infection in these patients. Additional studies with imipenem, ciprofloxacin, and ofloxacin showed high bacterial activity against most of the bacteria in pancreatic infections. Pederzoli and colleagues (1993) showed the beneficial effects of imipenem-cilastatin in penetrating necrosis and decreasing the incidence of infection. More research needs to be done in this area.

EXPERIMENTAL AGENTS. Steinberg and Schlesselman (1987) reviewed 13 studies of human acute pancreatitis and 25 studies involving experimentally induced pancreatitis in animals. These studies evaluated the use of aprotinin, glucagon, fluorouracil, somatostatin, and peritoneal lavage as possible therapeutic agents in the treatment of acute pancreatitis. Although 81% of the animal studies showed a positive outcome, only 7.7% of the human studies showed a positive outcome on survival. These reviewers concluded that experimentally induced pancreatitis in animals does not compare to the pathophysiology of human pancreatitis and, therefore, animals may not be effective in the testing of therapeutic agents for use in humans. It is their belief that these negative studies have influenced the lack of development of therapeutic agents for acute pancreatitis. Glucagon, fluorouracil, and somatostatin may prove beneficial with the development of studies based on large sample sizes and prolonged therapeutic regimens (Steinberg & Schlesselman, 1987).

Surgical Management

Although patients with acute pancreatitis generally do not require surgery, four categories of conditions necessitate surgical intervention (Martin et al., 1984). They are (1) uncertain diagnosis, (2) deterioration of patient's clinical condition, (3) presence of cholelithiasis, and (4) suspicion of intraabdominal infection or infected pancreatic necrosis. The first three categories are indications for immediate surgery because they usually occur within the first 24 to 48 hours after admission. Late surgical intervention is usually reserved for patients with complications of intraabdominal infection.

When acute pancreatitis cannot be differentiated from other intraabdominal emergencies, exploratory surgery may be necessary. During diagnostic surgery, the pancreas should be inspected for edema, necrosis, and hemorrhage. Peritoneal fluid can be obtained for culture and for amylase and lipase determinations. Cholelithiasis should also be ruled out. It remains controversial whether to drain the pancreas or place lavage catheters. Pancreatic resection or debridement is debatable, and little evidence suggests that pancreatic resection is indicated if there is no secondary infection (Crist & Cameron, 1987).

The most controversial indication for surgical intervention is severe necrotizing pancreatitis in patients who fail to respond to conventional supportive management. Both pancreatic drainage and resection have been proposed for this group of patients. Pancreatic resection has ranged from local debridement of necrotic tissue to total pancreatectomy. However, there is a lack of clinical data supporting these approaches. Crist and Cameron (1987) suggest that patients whose condition continues to deteriorate with supportive care should be managed with nonoperative peritoneal lavage. Operative exploration should then be reserved for these patients and should be limited to local debridement of nonviable tissue and the placement of drainage catheters.

It is generally a well-accepted practice to operate on patients with gallstone pancreatitis to reduce the risk of recurrent attacks. Because there is little evidence to suggest that immediate surgical intervention is required, most surgeons provide initial supportive care followed by biliary surgery during the same hospitalization (Crist & Cameron, 1987). A cholecystectomy and operative cholangiogram are usually performed to remove gallstones in the gallbladder and common bile duct (Shearson & Finlayson, 1982). An alternative approach advocated recently is the use of early ERCP and endoscopic sphincterotomy to remove stones.

The final indication for surgical intervention is the presence of abdominal infection. A pancreatic abscess is a life-threatening complication of acute pancreatitis, and without surgical intervention it has a mortality of 100% (Crist & Cameron, 1987). Pancreatic abscess formation involves the secondary infection of necrotic pancreatic and peripancreatic tissues. The most common causative agents include *Escherichia coli, Klebsiella, Proteus, Enterobacter, Pseudomonas,* and *Enterococcus.* Most abscesses are polymicrobial and may be single or multiple (Crist & Cameron, 1987). They usually form between the first and fourth weeks of hospitalization and present with abdominal pain, distension, tenderness, fever, leukocytosis, tachycardia, and hypotension. A palpable mass may be present (Soergel, 1989). Persistent elevations of amylase, bilirubin, and alkaline phosphatase levels are present in 50% of patients with abscesses. Antibiotics are given before surgical drainage. Surgical debridement is followed by percutaneous catheter drainage and lavage of the infected area. Postoperative complications are common and include chest infections, fistula, upper gastrointestinal bleeding, intestinal obstruction, and perforation (Shearson & Finlayson, 1982). Reoperation is necessary in about 25% of patients as a result of further abscess formation, acute bleeding, and involvement of the adjacent organs (Soergel, 1989).

Pseudocysts are collections of tissue, fluid, debris, enzymes, and blood within the pancreas (Greenberger et al., 1987). They develop over a period of 1 to 4 weeks after the onset of acute pancreatitis. About 30% of patients with pseudocysts present with an abdominal mass (Soergel, 1989). Other signs and symptoms may include abdominal pain, nausea, vomiting, jaundice, and weight loss (Shearson & Finlayson, 1982). Because pseudocysts cause a variety of complications such as bleeding and obstruction, early surgical drainage is indicated if these cysts continue to enlarge or if they persist for greater than 6 to 8 weeks without resolution.

An external pancreatic fistula may develop after drainage of either a pancreatic abscess or a pseudocyst. Fluids, electrolytes, and pancreatic juice are lost through the fistula opening. These losses may lead to dehydration and electrolyte imbalance. The abdominal wall can become infected and irritated from the pancreatic enzymes. Meticulous skin care is necessary to prevent skin breakdown and infection. Pancreatic fistulas usually heal in 6 months with adequate nutritional and electrolyte maintenance.

SUMMARY

The patient with acute pancreatitis presents a challenge to critical care nurses to recognize and initiate supportive and life-saving interventions. The patient's recovery from this devastating disease is due in part to the knowledge and expert clinical skills of the critical care nurse.

REFERENCES

Ammann, R. (1985). Acute pancreatitis: Clinical aspects and medical and surgical management. In J. E. Berk (Ed.), *Bockus gastroenterology* (4th ed., pp. 3993–4008). Philadelphia: W. B. Saunders.

Baltaxe, H. A. (1985). Diagnostic imaging of the pancreas. *Annals of Internal Medicine, 103,* 90–91.

Balthazar, E. J. (1989). CT diagnosis and staging of acute pancreatitis. *Radiology Clinic of North America, 27,* 19–37.

Banks, P. A. (1985). Clinical manifestations and treatment of pancreatitis. *Annals of Internal Medicine, 103,* 91–97.

Batra, S. K. (1987). Pancreatitis. In F. H. Messerk (Ed.), *Current clinical practice* (pp. 428–430). Philadelphia: W. B. Saunders.

Bell, J. S., & Go, U. L. W. (1985). Laboratory diagnosis of pancreatic disease. In J. E. Berk (Ed.), *Bockus gastroenterology* (4th ed., pp. 3877–3892). Philadelphia: W. B. Saunders.

Boudeman, K. A., Cherlock, P. A., & Rowley, S. G. (1985). Pancreatic disease—Special feeding problems. *Nutritional Support Services, 5*(11), 22–27.

Bradley III, E. L. (1993a). A clinically based classification system for acute pancreatitis. *Archives Surgery, 128,* 586–598.

Bradley III, E. L. (1993b). A fifteen year experience with open drainage for infected pancreatic necrosis. *Surgery, Gynecology, and Obstetrics, 177*(3), 215–222.

Browder, W., Patterson, M. D., Thompson, J. L., & Walters, D. N. (1993). Acute pancreatitis of unknown etiology in the elderly. *Annals of Surgery, 217*(5), 469–475.

Browder, W., Sherwood, E., Williams, D., et al. (1986). Protective effect of glucan-enhanced macrophage function in experimental pancreatitis. *American Journal of Surgery, 153,* 25–32.

Burch, J. M. (1988). Acute pancreatitis. In R. E. Rakel (Ed.), *Conn's current therapy* (pp. 438–442). Philadelphia: W. B. Saunders.

Burrell, L. O., & Burrell, Z. L., Jr. (1982). *Critical care* (pp. 319–324). St. Louis: C. V. Mosby.

Calleja, G. A., Barkin, J. S. (1993). Acute pancreatitis. *Medical Clinics of North America, 77*(5), 1037–1056.

Carr, M. R., Dick, S. P., Bordley, J. D., et al. (1987). Gentamicin dosing requirements in patients with acute pancreatitis. *Surgery, 103*(5), 533–537.

Carr-Locke, D. L. (1993). Role of endoscopy in gallstone pancreatitis. *The American Journal of Surgery, 165,* 519–521.

Creutzfeldt, W., & Lankisch, P. G. (1985). Acute pancreatitis: Etiology and pathogenesis. In J. E. Berk (Ed.), *Bockus gastroenterology* (4th ed., pp. 3971–3992). Philadelphia: W. B. Saunders.

Crist, D. W., & Cameron, J. L. (1987). The current management of acute pancreatitis. *Advances in Surgery, 20,* 69–123.

Drewelow, B., Koch, K., Otto, C., Franke, A., & Riethling, A. K. (1993). Penetration of ceftazidime into human pancreas. *Infection, 21*(4), 229–234.

Fan, S.-T., Lai, E. C. S., Mok, F. P. T., et al. (1993). Early treatment of acute biliary pancreatitis by endoscopic papillotomy. *New England Journal of Medicine,* 228–232.

Freeny, P. C., Lewis, G. P., Praverso, L. W., et al. (1988). Infected pancreatic fluid collections: Percutaneous catheter drainage. *Radiology, 167*(2), 435–441.

Greenberger, N. J. (1986). *Gastrointestinal disorders* (3rd ed., p. 250). Chicago: Year Book Medical Publishers.

Greenberger, N. J., Joskes, P. P., & Isselbacher, K. J. (1987). Diseases of the pancreas. In E. Braunwald, K. J. Isselbacker, R. G. Petersdorf, et al. (Eds.), *Harrison's principles of internal medicine* (pp. 1372–1380). New York: McGraw-Hill.

Grendell, J. H., & Cello, J. P. (1989). Chronic pancreatitis. In M. H. Sleisenger & J. S. Fordtran (Eds.), *Gastrointestinal disease: Pathophysiology, diagnosis, management* (4th ed., p. 1844). Philadelphia: W. B. Saunders.

Grönroos, J. M., Hietaranta, A. J., Nevalainen, T. J. (1992). Renal tubular cell injury and serum phospholipase A2 activity in acute pancreatitis. *British Journal of Surgery, 79,* 800–801.

Ihse, I., Evander, A., Holmberg, J. T., Gustafson, I. (1986). Influence of peritoneal lavage on objective prognostic signs in acute pancreatitis. *Annals of Surgery, 204,* 122–127.

Imrie, C. W., Buist, L. J., & Shearer, M. G. (1988). Importance of cause in the outcome of pancreatic pseudocysts. *American Journal of Surgery, 156,* 159–162.

Jain, J. A., & Amato-Vealey, E. (1989). Acute pancreatitis: A gastrointestinal emergency. *Critical Care Nurse, 8*(5), 47–64.

Johanson, B. C., Wells, S. J., Hoffmeister, D., et al. (1988). *Standards for critical care* (pp. 374–378). St. Louis: C. V. Mosby.

Johnson, C. D. (1993). Timing of interventions in acute pancreatitis. *Postgraduate Medical Journal, 69,* 509–515.

Kohn, C. L., Brozenec, S., Foster, P. F. (1993). Nutritional support for the patient with pancreatobiliary disease. *Critical Care Nursing Clinics of North America, 5*(1), 37–45.

Krumberger, J. M. (1993). Acute pancreatitis. *Clinical Care Nursing Clinics of North America, 5*(1), 185–202.

Leach, S. D., Gorelick, F. S., & Modlin, J. M. (1992). New perspectives on acute pancreatitis. *Scandinavian Journal of Gastroenterology Supplement, 27*(192), 29–38.

Leese, J., Holliday, M., Heath, D., et al. (1987). Multicentre clinical trial of low volume fresh frozen plasma therapy in acute pancreatitis. *British Journal of Surgery, 74,* 907–911.

Leibowitz, A. B., O'Sullivan, P., & Iberti, T. J. (1992). Intravenous fat emulsions and the pancreas: A review. *The Mount Sinai Journal of Medicine, 59*(1), 38–42.

Levine, G. M. (1981). Nutritional support in gastrointestinal disease. *Surgical Clinics of North America, 61*(3), 701–708.

Levitt, M. D. (1988). Pancreatitis. In J. B. Wyngaarden & L. H. Smith (Eds.), *Cecil textbook of medicine* (18th ed., pp. 774–780). Philadelphia: W. B. Saunders.

Marshall, J. B. (1993). Acute pancreatitis: A review with an emphasis on new developments. *Archives Internal Medicine, 153,* 1185–1198.

Martin, J. K., Jr., Vanheerden, J. A., & Bess, M. A. (1984). Surgical management of acute pancreatitis. *Mayo Clinic Proceedings, 59,* 259–267.

Mayor, A. D., McMahon, M. J., Corfield, A. P., et al. (1985). Controlled clinical trial of peritoneal lavage for the treatment of severe acute pancreatitis. *New England Journal of Medicine, 312,* 399–404.

Meguid, M. M., & Muscaritoli, M. (1993). Current uses of total parenteral nutrition. *American Family Physician, 47*(2), 383–394.

Meissner, J. E. (1980). McGill-Melzach Pain Questionnaire. *Nursing 90, 10*(1), 50–51.

Neff, C. C., & Ferrucci, J. T. (1984). Pancreatitis. *Surgical Clinics of North America, 64*(1), 23–36.

Pederzoli, P., Bassi, C., Vesentini, S., & Canpedelli, A. (1993). A randomized multicenter clinical trial of antibiotic prophylaxis of septic complications in acute necrotizing pancreatitis with imipenem. *Surgery, Gynecology, and Obstetrics, 176,* 480–483.

Pellegrini, C. A. (1993). Surgery for gallstone pancreatitis. *The American Journal of Surgery, 165,* 515–518.

Pisters, P. W. T., & Ranson, J. H. C. (1992). Nutritional support for acute pancreatitis. *Surgery, Gynecology, and Obstetrics, 175,* 275–284.

Ranson, J. H. C. (1979). Acute pancreatitis. *Current Problems in Surgery, 16*(11), 1–84.

Ranson, J. H. C., & Berman, R. S. (1990). Long peritoneal lavage decreases pancreatic sepsis in acute pancreatitis. *Annals of Surgery, 211,* 708–716.

Rombeau, J. L., & Caldwell, M. D. (1993). *Parenteral nutrition* (pp. 442–461). Philadelphia: W. B. Saunders.

Sabesin, S. (1987). Countering the dangers of acute pancreatitis. *Emergency Medicine, 19*(17), 71–96.

Saunders, C. E., & Gentile, D. A. (1986). Treatment of mild exacerbations of recurrent alcoholic pancreatitis in an emergency department observation unit. *Southern Medical Journal, 81*(3), 317–320.

Sax, H. C., Warner, B. W., Talamini, M. A., et al. (1986). Early total parenteral nutrition in acute pancreatitis: Lack of beneficial effects. *American Journal of Surgery, 153,* 117–124.

Shearson, D. J. C., & Finlayson, N. D. C. (1982). *Diseases of the gastrointestinal tract and liver* (pp. 783–785). Edinburgh: Churchill Livingstone.

Soergel, K. H. (1989). Acute pancreatitis. In M. H. Sleisenger & J. S. Fordtran (Eds.), *Gastrointestinal disease: Pathophysiology, diagnosis, management* (4th ed., pp. 1814–1842). Philadelphia: W. B. Saunders.

Steer, M. L., Meldolesi, J., & Figarella, C. (1984). Pancreatitis: The role of lysosomes. *Digestive Diseases and Sciences, 29*(10), 934–938.

Steinberg, W. M., & Schlesselman, S. E. (1987). Treatment of acute pancreatitis: Comparison of animal and human studies. *Gastroenterology, 93*(6), 1420–1427.

Thompson, J. M., McFarland, G. K., Hirsh, J. E., et al. (1986). *Clinical nursing* (pp. 1261–1265). St. Louis: C. V. Mosby.

UNIT 9 ENDOCRINE SYSTEM

CHAPTER

51

Patients With Disorders of Glucose Metabolism

Diana W. Guthrie

Diabetes mellitus is a group of metabolic disorders characterized by a relative or absolute deficiency in insulin, resulting in a glucose intolerance. The two main types of diabetes are type I, or insulin-dependent diabetes mellitus, and type II, or non–insulin-dependent diabetes mellitus. Diabetic ketoacidosis (DKA), hyperglycemic hyperosmolar nonketotic syndrome (HHNK), and severe hypoglycemia are three of the most common acute complications of diabetes that may necessitate admission to the intensive care unit. These complications have the potential to result in death if not treated appropriately. In addition, critically ill patients with diabetes may develop severe alterations in their glucose balance as a response to the stress of infection, illness, trauma, or surgery.

DIABETIC KETOACIDOSIS

Diabetic ketoacidosis is a metabolic disorder characterized by hyperglycemia with a blood sugar level usually exceeding 300 mg/dL, ketonuria, ketonemia, acidosis with a pH reduced to less than 7.3, and plasma bicarbonate possibly less than 15 mEq/liter (White & Henry, 1992). It occurs primarily in patients with type I diabetes mellitus and has a mortality of 4% (Diabetes Surveillance, 1991). DKA can be precipitated by infection, stress, trauma, or an imbalance between the intake of food and the amount of exogenous insulin received. Sauve and Kessler (1992) note "between 10% and 15% of patients admitted to intensive care units experience complications of acute hyperglycemia."

Pathophysiology

INSULIN AND COUNTERREGULATORY HORMONES

To understand the pathophysiology of DKA, one must first understand the role of insulin in the body. Insulin is an anabolic hormone produced by the pancreatic beta cells in the islets of Langerhans. It permits glucose to be transported into the cells throughout the body, especially in the muscle, fat, and liver, to be used as an energy source. It facilitates the storage of glucose as glycogen in the liver, the storage of amino acids as proteins in the muscles, and the storage of free fatty acids as triglycerides in the fat. The nerve tissue, intestinal mucosa, liver cells, kidney tubules, and formed blood elements are the only cells that do not depend on insulin to transport extracellular glucose across the cell membrane. Hepatic breakdown of glucose is also inhibited in the presence of insulin.

Insufficient levels of circulating insulin result in cellular starvation. This causes a catabolic process in which glycogen from the liver (glycogenolysis), proteins (amino acids to glucose 56%; gluconeogenesis), and fats (10% to glycerol) are broken down in an effort to provide an energy source for the cells. The speed of this catabolic process is determined by the counterregulatory hormones that are stimulated by stressors to the body.

Cortisol, glucagon, growth hormone, and catecholamines (epinephrine and norepinephrine) are the major hormones that oppose the action of insulin. In their presence insulin requirements increase. The breakdown of glycogen to glucose (glycogenolysis) is stimulated by the presence of glucagon or the catecholamines. Growth hormone assists with the breakdown of proteins to amino acids. Cortisol promotes gluconeogenesis (i.e., amino acid conversion to glucose). Epinephrine increases blood glucose by inhibiting glucose uptake by the muscles, decreasing insulin release, and, as noted before, enhancing glycogenolysis. These hormones, in their effort to provide glucose to the cells, compound the problem of hyperglycemia in DKA.

Insulin deficiency is the major endocrine abnormality responsible for the metabolic changes of DKA. This deficiency allows unrestricted production of glucose without peripheral utilization of the glucose by the body. This results in a marked hyperglycemia leading to glycosuria, osmotic diuresis, and ketosis.

HYPERGLYCEMIA

As plasma glucose concentrations rise, the renal threshold for glucose reabsorption by the proximal tubules of the kidneys is exceeded. This causes an osmotic diuresis in which water and glucose are excreted from the body in the urine. Large amounts of water can be lost by the body in this way (polyuria), leading to dehydration and oliguria. The body attempts to compensate for this pathologic condition by stimulating the thirst center in the brain to increase fluid intake (polydipsia). The kidneys are also stimulated to secrete renin, which facilitates the conversion of renin to angiotensin I. Angiotensin I is then converted to angiotensin II, stimulating the adrenal glands to secrete aldosterone. This hormone stimulates the kidneys to reabsorb additional sodium and water in order to reduce fluid loss. Antidiuretic hormone is also secreted from the posterior pituitary gland in an effort to reduce free water loss.

Marked hyperglycemia also causes a change in the osmotic gradient at the cellular level. The presence of excess glucose throughout the extracellular free water results in movement of water from the intracellular to the extracellular compartment. This occurrence may mask the clinical severity of the body's dehydration.

The body is unable to compensate for this ongoing water loss indefinitely. Water loss increases, depending on the severity and the duration of the illness, and may be as great as 150 mL/kg of body weight. Severe dehydration, hypovolemia, and eventually a reduced glomerular filtration rate (GFR) occur. This reduction in GFR limits the body's attempt to excrete glucose, augments hyperglycemia, and exacerbates hypertonicity and cellular dehydration.

Besides dehydration, lack of insulin prevents calories from getting into the cells as glucose or amino acids. This leads to polyphagia (frequent intake of food). As hyperglycemia increases, the stimulation of increased polyuria promotes caloric loss in spite of polyphagia. Weight loss is due to a combined caloric loss and a loss of body fluid. As this imbalance increases, nausea and vomiting, oliguria, and finally anuria occur. Nausea and vomiting, hemoconcentration, hypotension, and vascular collapse may ensue if the patient with DKA is not treated.

KETOSIS/KETOACIDOSIS

Increasing hyperglycemia and cell starvation initially lead to polyphagia. During this period the counterregulatory hormones are activated. Glucagon, produced by the alpha cells in the islets of Langerhans, stimulates glycogenolysis in the liver and muscle cells. When the glycogen stores are exhausted, gluconeogenesis begins. Gluconeogenesis is the process by which fats are converted into glycerol and proteins are converted to glucose.

When glycogen and protein stores are low or depleted or when glucose is unable to get into the cell, the fatty acids in the fat cells are broken down (lipolysis) and transported to the liver in the form of free fatty acids to be formed into ketones (ketogenesis). In the liver, these free fatty acids are converted to "ketone bodies" of acetone, acetoacetic acid, and beta-hydroxybutyric acid. These ketones are transported via the peripheral circulation where they are used by the cells as an alternative source of energy. Accumulation of ketones eventually result in ketonemia and ketonuria. These ketone bodies dissociate to yield hydrogen ions that lower the normal serum pH and produce a metabolic acidosis.

The body attempts to buffer this acidosis with bicarbonate. Bicarbonate reserves in the body, however, are depleted by the osmotic diureses. As the blood pH drops to approximately 7.2, the respiratory center attempts to remove the excess carbonic acid from the body by "blowing off" carbon dioxide (CO_2). This results in an increase in the rate and depth of respirations known as Kussmaul breathing. The acetone formed during the ketogenic process gives the breath a characteristic fruity or sweet odor.

Kussmaul breathing results in hypocapnia, which promotes cerebral vasoconstriction, reduces cerebral blood flow, and breaks down carbonic acid, leading to the release of CO_2 and water. As this respiratory compensatory mechanism fails to maintain the acid–base balance, carbon dioxide passes freely through the blood–brain barrier. The reduced cerebral blood flow and the accumulation of CO_2 lowers the central nervous system (CNS) pH, leading to a decreased level of consciousness.

ELECTROLYTE IMBALANCES

Patients in DKA present with a myriad of electrolyte imbalances resulting from the marked hyperglycemia. Potassium moves from the intracellular to the extracellular compartment with free water during the change in the osmotic gradient. When dehydration is profound, this potassium shift may give the illusion that the patient has a high serum potassium value. If the patient has experienced a significant fluid loss from osmotic diuresis or vomiting, large amounts of potassium can be passively lost, resulting in hypokalemia.

Sodium and phosphate are also transported into the extracellular compartment. An initial low sodium value may be obtained due to a dilution effect in the blood. Aldosterone activity also causes retention of sodium and may produce an abnormally high serum value if large amounts of this hormone have been secreted in an effort to control sodium and water loss. Phosphate is lost passively in the urine. This occurrence may be masked by the shift of the electrolyte to the extracellular space. When treatment for DKA is initiated, the electrolytes will shift back into the intracellular space as the body tissues are rehydrated and the metabolic acidosis corrected.

Clinical Presentation

The patient with DKA presents with a history of lethargy, polyuria, polydipsia, and polyphagia, often accompanied by weight loss. Various signs of dehydration such as loss of skin turgor, sunken eyeballs, flushed dry skin, low blood pressure, and a weak but rapid thready pulse may be observed. The patient may complain of mild to acute abdominal pain, have nausea accompanied by vomiting, and may even report chest pain. Kussmaul respirations (deep, labored breathing) with the accompanying fruity odor to the breath may also be present.

Laboratory tests show an elevated serum glucose and decreased serum bicarbonate and blood pH. Ketonemia, ketonuria, and glycosuria are present. The total white blood cell count may be elevated with a marked shift to the left. This may be due to a predisposing infection or to elevated catecholamine activity. Blood urea nitrogen (BUN), creatinine, hematocrit, and hemoglobin values are usually elevated due to dehydration. Arterial oxygen levels may be lowered if the respiratory status is compromised.

The patient with DKA may present with an altered level of consciousness due to the high serum osmolality. Osmolality can be estimated by the osmolarity calculation:

$$2(\text{Na} + \text{K}) + \text{blood sugar}/18 + \text{BUN}/2.8$$

or, in some texts,

$$2(\text{Na}) + \text{blood sugar}/18 + \text{BUN}/3.0$$

If this number is higher than 350 mOsm/kg, in the presence of blood glucose levels greater than 600/800 mg/dL and little if any presence of ketonuria, HHNK, rather than DKA, should be suspected (Davidson, 1993).

Clinical Management

The three goals of managing DKA are (1) improve the circulatory volume and tissue perfusion, (2) decrease blood glucose levels, and (3) correct electrolyte imbalances. Table 51–1 delineates the clinical management of these patients.

FLUID VOLUME MANAGEMENT

Intravenous fluids are required to improve circulatory blood volume and tissue perfusion. Fluids are given initially as a bolus of an isotonic solution (0.9% sodium chloride or lactated Ringer's). Hyperosmolality is an important consideration for these patients due to the marked hyperglycemia. An isotonic solution will allow a gradual decline in osmolality, which is desirable. Too rapid a decline is thought to contribute to the development of cerebral edema. A hypotonic solution (0.45% sodium chloride) is administered after the initial bolus to compensate for the loss of sodium by the body in the urine. This volume expansion reduces hemoconcentration, improves hemodynamics, improves GFR, and lowers the serum glucose. A 5% dextrose solution is added to the infusate when the blood sugar reaches 200 to 300 mg/dL. A 10% solution may be added when the blood sugar reaches 150 mg/dL to prevent hypoglycemia.

TABLE 51–1. **Clinical Management of Diabetic Ketoacidosis for Adults**

IV Fluids	
First hour	200 to 1000 mL/hr of 0.9% sodium chloride, depending on the degree of dehydration
Second and subsequent hours	200 to 1000 mL/hr of 0.45% sodium chloride, depending on the degree of dehydration
Within the first 12 hours	Add 5% dextrose to the IV fluid when serum glucose reaches 250–300 mg/dL If being maintained on IV fluids, add 10% dextrose to the IV fluid when serum glucose reaches 150 mg/dL or start subcutaneous injections
Insulin	
Initial	IV bolus of 0.1 units/kg of fast-acting insulin
First and subsequent hours	Continuous IV infusion of 0.1 units/kg/hr of fast-acting insulin. When serum glucose falls to 150 mg/dL, start the subcutaneous use of insulin based on 0.5–1.0/kg for adults and 1.0–2.0/kg for children (Guthrie, 1993)
Electrolytes	
First hour	If initial serum K^+ is greater than 3.5 mEq/liter, give 40 mEq/liter in the IV maintenance fluid, one-half as potassium chloride, one-half as potassium phosphate
Second and subsequent hours	If urine output is adequate with serum K^+ of less than 5.5 mEq/liter, give 20 to 30 mEq/liter of IV fluid
Laboratory Tests	
Initial	Serum glucose, pH, bicarbonate, electrolytes, calcium, phosphate, serum osmolality, complete blood count, blood urea nitrogen, creatinine, arterial blood gases, blood culture, urine culture
Subsequent	Hourly monitoring of blood glucose; electrolytes, and bicarbonate every 2–4 hours
Monitoring	Hourly vital signs, neurologic checks, intake and output Central venous pressure monitoring or pulmonary artery pressure may be necessary for patients with a compromised respiratory status Continuous electrocardiographic monitoring needed to evaluate abnormalities with K^+ balance
Ancillary measures	Plasma expanders may be necessary for persistent hypotension Antibiotic and oxygen therapy as needed

FLUID VOLUME DEFICIT RELATED TO OSMOTIC DIURESIS. During fluid replacement therapy the patient must be closely monitored. Vital signs, intake and output, central venous pressure, and pulmonary artery wedge pressure are monitored to prevent unrecognized shock, overhydration, or worsening dehydration. The patient must also be observed for signs and symptoms of cardiovascular overload, pulmonary edema, or inadequate central perfusion during fluid volume restoration. Laboratory values will be assessed to monitor the progression of the patient's hydration status and to guide fluid and electrolyte replacement. Oral hygiene and skin care should be maintained for the patient's comfort and to prevent skin breakdown.

BLOOD GLUCOSE MANAGEMENT

Insulin therapy to lower the blood glucose level is given by continuous low-dose infusion after an initial bolus of fast-acting insulin has been given. This method is simple and effective and results in a lower incidence of hypoglycemia and hypokalemia. It allows a steady cellular metabolic response without fluctuations in the blood sugar that occur from intermittent injections of insulin. This low-dose infusion allows a linear decline in the serum glucose, with an average drop of 75 to 100 mg/dL/hr. A more rapid drop of serum glucose appears to be associated with a higher incidence of cerebral edema. Usually the patient is switched to subcutaneous insulin injections when blood glucose levels reach 150 to 200 mg/dL.

ALTERATION IN NUTRITION: LESS THAN BODY REQUIREMENTS RELATED TO INSULIN DEFICIENCY. Nursing interventions are aimed at providing close observation of the patient's serum glucose level and at maintaining the insulin infusion at a rate that allows for a drop of serum glucose of 75 to 100 mg/dL/hr. Hourly glucose values are needed to assess the status of the hyperglycemia. Bedside glucose monitoring and laboratory tests can provide this information. Intravenous (IV) insulin should be delivered in a separate line to allow for immediate changes in dosage as the patient's condition warrants. Standard solutions of insulin infusions vary from institution to institution. A convenient mix is 20 units of fast-acting insulin in 20 mL of normal saline administered with an infusion pump based on the calculation of 0.1 unit/kg/hr.

An alternative method is putting 100 units of fast-acting insulin in 500 mL of normal saline. This concentration delivers 0.2 units of insulin with every milliliter of fluid. It is thought by many that insulin molecules will adhere to plastic IV tubing, thereby decreasing the amount of drug delivered to the patient. Flushing of the IV line before administration with 50 to 100 mL of the insulin solution limits the amount of insulin absorbed by the IV tubing. Placing insulin in a larger volume of solution will increase the chance of precipitating a greater amount of insulin to the plastic bottle and tubing.

The patient must be monitored for signs of hypoglycemia and hyperglycemia. The physician will need to be notified when serum glucose levels reach between 250 and 300 mg/dL and again at 150 mg/dL to order the necessary dextrose to be added to the hydration line or for orders to start subcutaneous insulin injections.

Once fluids are tolerated by mouth, the replenishment of body nutrients may be instituted at about 30 cal/kg of body weight in adults.

ELECTROLYTE MANAGEMENT

Electrolytes are added to the IV fluids after the initial bolus has been given and when renal function has been assessed as adequate. Potassium supplements are begun early in therapy, and serum levels are monitored frequently. Potassium supplementation should be given as half potassium chloride and half potassium phosphate. This treatment avoids delivery of an excess of chloride to the patient and restores phosphate and calcium balance.

The use of bicarbonate replacement in the treatment of patients with DKA is controversial. Bicarbonate concentrations in the blood are depleted because extracellular bicarbonate is the body's first buffer against metabolic acidosis. Proponents of its use recommend that it be used only in patients with severe acidosis with the blood pH less than 7.1 or CO_2 less than 7 mm Hg. The use of bicarbonate to correct acidosis above a pH of 7.1 may result in a paradoxical CNS acidosis, lead to severe hypokalemia, and may also be a cause of cerebral edema. If bicarbonate is needed, it must be given very slowly. If cerebral edema occurs, treatment includes IV osmotic diuretics such as mannitol and possibly high doses of glucocorticoids such as dexamethasone.

SENSORY PERCEPTUAL ALTERATION RELATED TO INCREASED PLASMA OSMOLALITY AND ELECTROLYTE IMBALANCE. Interventions are directed toward evaluating the patient's neurologic status and monitoring him for physical signs of electrolyte imbalances. The patient's electrocardiogram is observed for changes related to hyperkalemia or hypokalemia. Laboratory values for potassium, chloride, phosphorus, and calcium will be monitored frequently, so that the needed changes in electrolyte supplements can be made. Potassium is usually added once the patient has voided but may be added when the hydrated state of the body and the potassium needs are determined.

MAINTENANCE AND PREVENTION

When the patient's serum glucose is less than 250 mg/dL, the pH is greater than 7.3, the serum bicarbonate is greater than 15 mEq/L, and the patient is able to take food by mouth, conversion to subcutaneous insulin may be initiated. Initially four doses of regular insulin may be used with approximately 35% of the total calculated dose given before breakfast, 22% before lunch, 28% before supper, and 15% between midnight and 1 A.M. (Guthrie, 1992). If four doses are maintained as a management program, the last dose of the day might be changed to an intermediate-acting insulin (Lente or NPH) and given at bedtime. The dosage may also be changed to a three-dose or two-dose schedule. In a two-dose schedule, two-thirds of the previous day's total dose is given as an intermediate-acting insulin, and the remaining one-third is given as a short-acting insulin. The patient receives two-thirds of his total subcutaneous dose before the morning meal and one-third of the total dose before the evening meal. For a three-dose schedule, especially if the fasting blood glucose levels are elevated, the pre-supper dose could be split into regular insulin before supper and intermediate-acting insulin before bedtime. Blood glucose monitoring should continue before meals and at bedtime to assess glycemic control.

KNOWLEDGE DEFICIT RELATED TO THE PRECIPITATING EVENTS, SIGNS AND SYMPTOMS, AND PREVENTION OF DKA. A nursing assessment of the patient's knowledge of the events leading to his hospitalization needs to be made. The patient needs to be able to verbalize the factors of diabetes that predispose to these emergency situations. The patient must be educated about the early signs and symptoms of hyperglycemia, how to manage diabetes when he is ill, and when to call the physician based on blood glucose with or without urine ketone readings. This education can be incorporated into the patient's daily care when his condition has stabilized. Frequent occurrences of DKA indicate a need not only for education, but also for a team approach to meet the patient's psychosocial needs (Henderson, 1991).

HYPERGLYCEMIC HYPEROSMOLAR NONKETOTIC SYNDROME

Hyperglycemic hyperosmolar nonketotic syndrome is a metabolic disorder characterized by hyperglycemia with blood sugar of greater than 800 mg/dL, serum osmolality greater than 350 mOsm/kg, absent or minimal serum ketones, an arterial pH higher than 7.3, serum bicarbonate greater than 20 mEq/liter, and mild to severe mental obtundation. It most commonly occurs in the elderly and people with type II non–insulin-dependent diabetes mellitus. It is differentiated from DKA by the absence of significant ketosis or acidosis.

The most common cause of HHNK is undiagnosed type II diabetes accompanied by a delay in seeking medical treatment after an associated illness. Other predisposing factors include stress, infections, steroid or diuretic usage, dialysis, or hyperalimentation. Mortality has been reported to be as high as 60% to 70% if the condition is not recognized and treated quickly (Kitabachi & Murphy, 1988).

Pathophysiology

Unlike type I diabetes, the patient with type II diabetes has only a "relative" deficiency in insulin production. These patients may control their diabetes with diet management or oral antidiabetic agents.

The patient with HHNK experiences the effects of marked hyperglycemia in the same way as a patient with DKA. Blood glucose levels are considerably higher and result in a more severe osmotic diuresis. This results in increased intracellular and extracellular dehydration and a higher serum osmolality.

The reason for the absence of ketosis in HHNK is not well understood. Several theories have been proposed to explain this occurrence. One prevalent theory is that the patient with HHNK has enough beta cell function to produce the needed insulin to inhibit fatty acid mobilization and the formation of ketones (ketogenesis) but not enough insulin to prevent hyperglycemia. Another theory proposes that the patient with HHNK may lack a substrate for hepatic ketogenesis. The hyperosmolar state may itself inhibit protein breakdown. Hyperosmolarity depresses pancreatic insulin secretion, inhibits adipose tissue lipolysis, and impairs CNS control of growth hormone and cortisol response.

The patient with HHNK presents with electrolyte imbalances similar to those seen in DKA, but usually does not demonstrate a significant decrease in pH or bicarbonate level. Due to the higher serum osmolality, these patients may have an altered sensorium. They may experience grand mal seizures, positive Babinski reflexes, nystagmus, or other neurologic deficits.

Clinical Management

The management for patients with HHNK is very similar to that for patients with DKA (Table 51–2). IV hydration is given more rapidly over the first 8 hours and then as a continuous infusion of 0.45% sodium chloride. This solution is given only if the patient is hypotensive due to the high serum osmolality. Half of the water deficit is given in the first 12 hours as 0.45% sodium chloride. The remainder is given during the next 24 hours as 5% dextrose and 0.45% sodium chloride, or 5% dextrose and 0.9% sodium chloride. Insulin is given as an initial IV bolus of 0.1 unit/kg followed by a continuous infusion of 0.1 unit/kg/hr. The goal of reducing the blood glucose level between 75 and 100 mg/dL/hr is considered a safe guide because most patients in HHNK have some endogenous insulin available and therefore the insulin requirements needed to correct hyperglycemia are usually less than those in DKA. If blood glucose levels are dropping too dramatically (i.e., greater than 100 mg/dL/hr), the insulin infusion should be turned down or off as needed until the blood glucose levels stabilize.

Electrolytes, laboratory studies, and ancillary measures are the same as those used for patients with DKA. Because these patients are usually older and have preexisting illnesses, their response to treatment must be carefully monitored. The patient with type II diabetes who has recovered from HHNK may require small amounts of subcutaneous insulin daily or may be able to control the diabetes with diet or oral medica-

TABLE 51–2. **Clinical Management of HHNK**

IV Fluids	
Hours 1 to 12	0.9% sodium chloride may be used if the serum sodium is less than 130 mEq/liter or if the calculated plasma osmolarity (2(Na + K) + blood sugar/18 + blood urea nitrogen/2.8) is less than 350 mOsm/liter 0.45% sodium chloride is used if serum sodium is above 145 mEq/liter May require 8 to 12 liters of fluid over a 24-hour period; replace half of the water deficit in the first 12 hours When the blood glucose reaches 250 to 300 mg/dL, add 5% dextrose to the infusate to prevent brisk lowering of calculated serum osmolarity
Insulin	
Initial	IV bolus of 0.1 units/kg of fast-acting insulin
Subsequent hours	0.1 units/kg/hr of continuous fast-acting insulin (Guthrie, 1993)
Electrolytes	
Initial	Same as for DKA
Laboratory Tests	Same as for DKA
Monitoring	Same as for DKA
Ancillary Measures	Same as for DKA

tions. Potassium by mouth may be continued for a period of time after the infusion is discontinued.

The nursing diagnoses described for the patient with DKA are also appropriate for the patient with HHNK. It is necessary to educate the family as well as the patient about this disease because the patient may not be able to identify the subtle changes in mental status that often are the early indicators of HHNK.

SEVERE HYPOGLYCEMIA

Hypoglycemia is not usually dealt with in a critical care setting unless a severe insulin reaction (also called insulin shock or insulin coma) has occurred. It is possible for this and milder states of hypoglycemia to be confused with some of the symptoms of hyperglycemia (see Table 51–3). Mild reactions (blood glucose levels of 40 to 60 mg/dL) are often treated by a small snack such as ½ to 1 cup of milk or 2 to 4 crackers and 1 to 2 slices of cheese. Moderate reactions (blood glucose levels of 20 to 40 mg/dL) are more symptom-associated and need to be treated initially with some form of simple sugar (i.e., 2 or 3 glucose tablets or 2 or 3 tsp of glucose gel) followed in 10 to 15 minutes by a small snack if the blood sugar level has climbed to greater than 40 mg/dL. A severe insulin reaction may be treated at home, by emergency medical technicians, or by hospital personnel. In rare instances, severe sequelae such as status epilepticus occur and then the continued treatment and follow-up would occur in the critical care setting.

Glucagon is the treatment of choice for severe hypoglycemia occurring in the home. The recommended adult dosage is 1 mg subcutaneously or intramuscularly for more rapid absorption (Guthrie & Guthrie, 1991). The response time is about 15 to 20 minutes. Nausea is the only side effect. If the blood glucose level is low enough to require glucagon or 50% glucose, nausea is often present. Once the person has regained consciousness simple sugar-containing fluids are administered until any nausea has subsided. Then a snack may be given. If a seizure has accompanied the hypoglycemic episode, a postictal state may last from 6 to 12 hours.

For the hospitalized adult patient, 50% glucose is the drug of choice. Glucagon may also be given in circumstances, under protocol, when the patient does not have an IV access. Although a full 50 mL of 50% glucose is often administered to the teenage patient, it is possible to determine a response (by noting a slower pulse rate in 1½ to 2 minutes) when about 25 mL are administered.

With intensive insulin therapy may come more frequent severe insulin reactions, especially if blood glucose levels are not knowledgeably treated with insulin supplements. The goal is for premeal blood glucose levels to fall between 60 and 120 mg/dL (ideally between 70 and 110 mg/dL) and 2-hour postprandial glucose levels less than 150 mg/dL (ideally less than 120 mg/dL). Although less frequently observed, se-

TABLE 51–3. **Hypoglycemia versus Hyperglycemia**

Hypoglycemia	Hyperglycemia
Differences	
Strong pulse	Weak, thready pulse
Blood pressure high (initially)	Blood pressure low (related to level of hydration)
Face pale	Face flushed
Skin clammy	Skin dry
Pupils dilated	Pupils WNL or constricted
Urination WNL	Polyuria
Thirst WNL	Polydipsia
Similarities	
Adrenalin flush (with circumoral pallor)	Face flushed
Nausea	Nausea
Vomiting	Vomiting
Unconscious	Unconscious
Pulse rapid	Pulse rapid
Staggering gait	Staggering gait
Weak	Weak
Headache	Headache
Irritable	Irritable
Vision impaired (double or blurred)	Vision impaired (blurred)
Seizure	Seizure (very high blood sugar)
Hunger	Hunger

vere insulin reactions also occur in combination therapy (Spollett, 1993). Whatever the methodology used, careful consideration needs to be given when trying to treat "after the fact" with sliding scale insulin administration. Maintaining a baseline level of insulin at all times more closely approximates normal physiology. This baseline insulin is present in both the pattern approach and the algorithm approach. The pattern approach bases insulin changes on previous four times a day comparison blood glucose levels; the algorithm approach maintains baseline insulin with supplements of insulin based on immediate blood glucose levels.

SENSORY PERCEPTUAL DEFICITS RELATED TO GREATER INSULIN LEVELS THAN NEEDED FOR NORMAL FUNCTIONING. When severe hypoglycemia occurs, the individual's level of consciousness may be inadequate, and his memory may possibly be impaired. Adaptive fine motor and gross motor responses may also be delayed. Holmes (1989) reported on the sequelae of acute blood glucose occurrences. Delay of fine and gross motor responses compared to lack of frequency were not noted on a long-term basis. Frequency of severe insulin reactions appear to be more closely associated with permanent changes in cognition (Langan et al., 1991).

The goal is to stabilize the acute situation and to educate the individual and / or family member to prevent further occurrences, to alter medical management as determined by the physician, and to teach other members in the family or a friend, coworker, or teacher how to administer glucagon.

KNOWLEDGE DEFICIT RELATED TO PRECIPITATING EVENTS AND PHYSICAL SYMPTOMS. The individual may have a knowledge deficit related to precipitating events or response to signs as well as symptoms for the prevention of hypoglycemia. A nursing assessment of knowledge of hypoglycemia is essential. Determination of hypoglycemia unawareness (i.e., no symptoms experienced by the patient) must be documented (MacDonald, 1992). The patient is taught to recognize similarities and differences between hyperglycemia and hypoglycemia. Assessment of communication obstacles and levels of knowledge in the hospital or home will facilitate the management of the client's condition. Monitoring of blood glucose levels needs to be more frequent when hypoglycemia unawareness is present. Frequency of blood glucose monitoring should be an inherent part of the program to prevent severe insulin reactions, maintaining intensive insulin therapy, and preventing hypoglycemia in patients with hypoglycemia unawareness (Gaston, 1992).

SURGERY AND TRAUMA

Surgical procedures that require the person with diabetes to be NPO over an extended period of time or the occurrence of nausea and vomiting during the perioperative period will require the use of IV fluids and altered insulin dosages. Surgery or trauma act as a stressor to the body and will raise the blood glucose levels through the action of the counterregulatory hormones. Blood glucose levels must be stabilized and controlled during the procedure and during the time of healing (Terranova, 1991). Maintenance of normal blood glucose levels during the healing time allows the wound to close within the expected time period with fewer complications (Schumann, 1990).

Special consideration should be given to the traumatically injured patient who has a history of poor blood glucose control, renal impairment, parathyroid dysfunction, or chronic alcoholism or who has been treated with antineoplastic agents. These patients frequently have abnormal electrolyte profiles along with their elevated blood glucose levels. Magnesium and phosphorus are usually not included in routine laboratory profiles of standard electrolyte values. Workman (1992) reports that serious tissue damage, including myocardial damage, can occur when these particular electrolytes are not in balance.

ILLNESS

Illness, whether physical or mental, can lead to a hyperglycemic state that, if not controlled, can develop into DKA. To prevent such occurrences, supplemental insulin is usually administered or a specially set protocol is instituted.

Basic guidelines may be similar to those for the treatment of DKA. Blood glucose levels will be checked frequently, and if the blood glucose is >240 mg / dL, ketones should also be monitored. If the person's blood glucose levels have risen beyond 240 mg / dL and ketones are present, insulin 0.1 unit / kg / hr may be administered intramuscularly until the subsequent blood glucose levels are lower than 240 mg / dL.

Oral fluids should be encouraged; if not tolerated, fluids should be given intravenously. As the blood glucose levels fall below 250 to 300 mg / dL, glucose is usually added orally or intravenously.

PANCREAS TRANSPLANTS

Diabetes mellitus predisposes the patient to many serious long-term complications such as diabetic retinopathy, neuropathy, end-stage renal disease, and premature atherosclerosis. Researchers believe that establishing a constant euglycemic state would reduce the risk of these complications (Diabetes Control and Complications Trial Research Group, 1993). For those who have already developed end-stage problems, a pancreas transplant has provided this albeit too late ideal blood glucose state.

Pancreas transplants are usually reserved for those individuals who are receiving a kidney transplant or who for whatever reason are already on immunosuppressive therapy. One-year graft survival rates are nearing 80% when a combined kidney / pancreas transplant is done (Bartucci et al., 1992). Since 1980, many centers have begun transplanting nonuremic, nonkidney transplant patients whose developing diabetes-related complications are more serious than the potential side effects of the antirejection therapy.

The patient who is a candidate for a pancreas transplant must undergo an extensive pretransplant evaluation (Nettles, 1992). Baseline studies to measure serum glucose, insulin, and C-peptide levels as well as pancreatic hormone levels are required. Nerve function studies, an ophthalmic examination, and a renal evaluation are performed. A psychiatric examination is done to ensure that the patient has a thorough understanding of the magnitude of the operation and the potential complications, including lifetime follow-up.

Procedure

Cadaver or living related donors are used for the pancreas transplant procedure. Whole pancreas or segmental grafts are used. Islet cell transplants or beta cell transplants are still in the research phase. The most important technical problem in pancreas transplantation is the need to provide drainage of the exocrine secretions of the transplanted organ.

Postoperative Care

The postoperative care of the patient with a pancreas transplant includes observing the patient for potential complications. The most common complications with this procedure include rejection, infection, venous thrombosis, technical problems with duct anastomoses, and the potential recurrence of diabetes.

The patient's vital signs are monitored closely. Indicators of fluid volume status, such as central venous pressure, intake and output, and nasogastric drainage, are also carefully assessed. A triple-lumen catheter may be used for total parenteral nutrition and for drawing blood samples. Laboratory studies include a complete blood count, electrolyte measurements, and coagulation profiles every 6 hours. Plasma glucose levels are monitored according to protocol. Daily laboratory work includes electrolytes, complete blood count, hemoglobin, and serum and urine amylase measurements. Blood samples for insulin, glucagon, and human C-peptide levels are done three to four times per week. Pancreatic scans and ultrasound examinations are performed on the first day and then once a week until discharge. The patient may require some exogenous insulin for 1 to 2 days postoperatively and will be placed on a program of immunosuppressive agents and antirejection drugs.

DIABETES MONITORING

Bedside blood glucose monitoring has become one of the keystones in the care of the person with diabetes (Walker, 1993). It can assist the nurse in the intensive care setting to monitor a patient's serum glucose level quickly, using only one drop of blood, a reagent strip, and a meter. This technique has replaced urine tests for glucose due to the body's inconstant renal threshold. Any changes in a patient's diabetes control can affect the GFR and tubular glucose reabsorption in the kidneys, thus affecting the blood glucose concentration at which urine glucose excretion normally occurs. Urine tests are still needed to check for ketones, especially when the blood glucose level is greater than 240 mg/dL.

Ketone test strips, for testing of the urine when the blood glucose levels are greater than 240 mg/dL, are sensitive enough to analyze the urine for acetoacetic acid and acetone. Beta-hydroxybuteric acid is found in greater proportion, in comparison to the other acids, when the person is in a more acutely ill state. This may be assayed in the hospital laboratory setting but, as yet, no home testing method is available.

Long-Term Glucose Monitoring

Glycosylated or glycated hemoglobin tests and fructosamine tests aid in determining glucose control over long periods. Fructosamine tests and glycated serum protein tests give values comparative to average blood glucose levels over a 7- to 10-day period. Glycosylated hemoglobin tests give averages over a 2- to 3-month period. One of these, Hgb A1c, is less influenced by more recent elevated or lowered blood glucose levels than Hgb A1. Both of these tests represent the percentage of glucose attached to the protein found in the red blood cells. Because the known life span of a red blood cell is about 120 days, calculated comparisons may be made between the sample and normative values. The fructosamine test measures glycosylated albumin. Glycated serum protein or glycosylated serum protein is measured by assaying the amount of glucose attached to the protein found in the serum of the blood.

The normative values of these various testing methodologies vary in relation to the manufacturer's methodology. For the best interpretation, as in all laboratory tests, the results of the test should be compared against normative values. Comparison of one methodology to another is presently a problem being addressed by the American Diabetes Association.

SUMMARY

Diabetic ketoacidosis, HHNK, and severe hypoglycemia, as emergencies, are a threat to any person with diabetes. Table 51–4 summarizes the expected outcomes for individuals with life-threatening disorders of glucose metabolism.

The chance of these emergencies occurring can be reduced with increased quality and appropriateness of patient education accompanied by the most up-to-date medical management regimen. Landis (1991) recog-

TABLE 51–4. **Expected Outcome of DKA, HHNK, and Severe Hypoglycemia**

Outcome Criteria
Urine output greater than 30 mL/hr
Central venous pressure 7 to 12 cm H_2O
Blood glucose levels greater than 70 mg/dL pre-meal and less than 150 mg/dL post-meal
No ketones in blood or urine
Vital signs within normal range
Moist mucous membranes and good skin turgor
Laboratory data normal:*
Blood urea nitrogen, 10 to 15 mg/dL; pH, 7.4; hematocrit, 35% to 40%+; sodium, 132 to 140 mEq/liter; potassium, 3.5 to 5 mEq/liter; plasma osmolality, 280 to 300 mOsm/liter
Pupils equal and reactive to light
Moves all extremities
Level of consciousness WNL

*Laboratory norms dependent on method of analysis.

nized that any chronic illness and especially diabetes is filled with uncertainties. Such uncertainties are associated with frequency of hospitalizations, poor health due to lack of coping skills, and negative emotional affect resulting, in turn, in more frequent occurrence of DKA, HHNK, and severe hypoglycemia. Adequate education and support by the health care team has the potential to lead to a more stabilized physiologic state. The statistics for risk reduction (Diabetes Control and Complications Trial Research Group, 1993) with normalized, supportive physiologic functioning the majority of the time, are most profound: retinopathy, a 76% risk reduction; nephropathy, a 56% risk reduction; and neuropathy, a 60% risk reduction. The resulting outcome will be well worth the time and quality of care given to the person who has diabetes.

REFERENCES

Bartucci, M. R., Loughman, K. A., & Moir, E. J. (1992). Kidney-pancreas transplantation: A treatment option of ISRD and type I diabetes. *ANNA Journal, 19*(5), 467–474.

Davidson, M. B. (1993). Hyperglycemia. In V. Peragallo-Dittko, K. Godley, & J. Meyer (Eds.), *A core curriculum for diabetes education* (2nd ed., pp. 305–328). Chicago: American Association of Diabetes Educators.

The Diabetes Control and Complications Trial Research Group (1993). The effect of intensive treatment of diabetes on the development and progression of long-term complications in insulin-dependent diabetes mellitus. *New England Journal of Medicine, 329*(14), 977–986.

The Division of Diabetes Translation (1991). *Diabetes surveillance.* Atlanta: U.S. Department of Health and Human Services, Centers for Disease Control.

Gaston, S. F. (1992). Outcomes of hypoglycemia treated by standardized protocol in a community hospital. *Diabetes Educator, 18*(6), 491–494.

Guthrie, D. W., & Guthrie, R. A. (1991). Acute complications. In D. W. Guthrie & R. A. Guthrie (Eds.), *Nursing management of diabetes mellitus* (3rd ed., pp. 187–197). New York: Springer.

Guthrie, R. A. (1992). Intensive insulin therapy for insulin-dependent diabetes. *Internal Medicine, 13*(9), 35–44.

Henderson, G. (1991). The psychosocial treatment of recurrent diabetic ketoacidosis: An interdisciplinary team approach. *Diabetes Educator, 17*(2), 119–123.

Holmes, C. (1989). Neuropsychological sequelae of acute and chronic blood glucose disruptions in adults with insulin-dependent diabetes. In C. S. Holmes (Ed.), *Neuropsychological and behavioral aspects of diabetes* (pp. 122–154). New York: Springer-Verlag.

Kitabachi, A., & Murphy, M. (1988). Diabetic ketoacidosis and hyperosmolar hyperglycemic nonketotic coma. *Medical Clinics of North America, 72*(6), 1545–1563.

Landis, B. J. P. (1991). Uncertainty, spiritual well-being, and psychosocial adjustment to chronic illness. Dissertation. Austin, TX: The University of Texas at Austin.

Langan, S., Deary, I., Hepburn, D., & Frier, B. (1991). Cumulative cognitive impairment following recurrent severe hypoglycemia in adult patients with insulin-treated diabetes mellitus. *Diabetologia, 34,* 337–344.

MacDonald, F. (1992). Asymptomatic hypoglycemia: Overcoming fear. *Beta Release, 16*(1), 21–23.

Nettles, A. T. (1992). Pancreas transplantation: A University of Minnesota perspective. *Diabetes Educator, 18*(3), 232–240.

Sauve, D. O., & Kessler, C. A. (1992). Hyperglycemic emergencies. *AACN Clinical Issues in Critical Care Nursing, 3*(2), 350–360.

Schumann, D. (1990). Postoperative hyperglycemia: Clinical benefits of insulin therapy. *Heart and Lung: Journal of Critical Care, 19*(2), 165–173.

Spollett, G. R. (1993). Intensive insulin therapy in insulin dependent diabetes and combination therapy. *Nurse Practitioner: American Journal of Primary Health Care, 189*(7), 27–38.

Terranova, A. (1991). The effects of diabetes mellitus on wound healing. *Plastic Surgical Nursing, 11*(1), 20–25.

Walker, E. A. (1993). Quality assurance for blood glucose monitoring: The balance of feasibility and standards. *Nursing Clinics of North America, 28*(1), 61–70.

White, N. H., & Henry, D. N. (1992). Special issues in diabetes management. In D. Haire-Joshu (Ed.), *Management of diabetes mellitus* (pp. 249–257). St. Louis: Mosby Year Book.

Workman, M. L. (1992). Magnesium and phosphorus: The neglected electrolytes. *AACN Clinical Issues in Critical Care Nursing, 3*(3), 635–636.

DIABETIC KETOACIDOSIS MULTIDISCIPLINARY CARE GUIDE

COORDINATION OF CARE

Diagnosis/Stabilization Phase		Acute Management Phase		Recovery Phase	
Outcome	*Intervention*	*Outcome*	*Intervention*	*Outcome*	*Intervention*
All appropriate team members and disciplines will be involved in the plan of care.	Develop the plan of care with the patient/family, primary nurse(s), primary physician(s), endocrinologist, other specialists as needed, respiratory therapist, diabetes clinical nurse specialist, social services, and dietician.	All appropriate team members and disciplines will be involved in the plan of care.	Update the plan of care with the patient/family, team members, and dietitian, physical therapist, discharge planner, and home health agency. Initiate planning for anticipated discharge. Begin teaching patient/family about diabetes diet. Begin teaching patient/family about care at home.	Patient/family will understand how to maintain optimal health at home.	Provide written guidelines concerning follow-up care to patient and family. Provide patient/family with phone numbers of resources/diabetes education classes/diabetes clinical nurse specialist available to answer questions.

FLUID BALANCE

Diagnosis/Stabilization Phase		Acute Management Phase		Recovery Phase	
Outcome	*Intervention*	*Outcome*	*Intervention*	*Outcome*	*Intervention*
Patient will achieve optimal hemodynamic status as evidenced by: • MAP > 70 mm Hg • Hemodynamic parameters WNL • Adequate level of consciousness • Adequate respiratory functioning • Neurologic status WNL • Urine output > 0.5 mL/kg/hr • Good skin turgor Patient will achieve normal serum glucose level.	Monitor and treat hemodynamic parameters: • BP • I & O • LOC • Evidence of tissue perfusion • SvO_2 • Serum glucose levels • CVP • JVD • Abnormal heart sounds • Abnormal lung sounds Monitor for signs of dehydration and hypovolemia. Constantly monitor respiratory functioning and anticipate respiratory complications. Be prepared for intubation and mechanical ventilation. Assess neurologic status q1h and PRN. Administer insulin bolus followed by an infusion; monitor response.	Patient will maintain optimal hemodynamic status. Patient will maintain normal serum glucose level.	Same as in stabilization phase. Begin teaching patient/family regarding diabetes, symptoms of hypoglycemia/hyperglycemia, and blood glucose monitoring.	Patient will maintain optimal hemodynamic status. Patient will maintain normal serum glucose level.	Continue diabetes education and tell patient/family when to seek medical attention. Monitor lab values, particularly serum glucose levels.

Outcome	Intervention	Outcome	Intervention	Outcome	Intervention
	Monitor blood glucose levels q30–60 min. Progress to serum glucose and whole blood glucose levels q1–4hr and PRN. Anticipate need for vasopressor agents; assess response and titrate accordingly. Initiate IV therapy with an isotonic solution (normal saline or lactated Ringer's) first, followed with a hypotonic solution (0.45% sodium chloride [½NS]). This may be followed with D_5W or D_5½NS once the serum glucose is < 300 mg/dL. Monitor for possible complications associated with diabetic ketoacidosis (DKA): dysrhythmias, dehydration, renal failure, vascular collapse, decreased LOC, congestive heart failure, pulmonary edema, seizures. Monitor lab values: electrolytes, glucose, ABGs, glomerular filtration rate, bicarbonate, urinalysis for ketonuria and glycosuria, CBC, BUN, creatinine. Monitor for signs of fluid overload or deficit. Anticipate need for potassium replacement therapy.				

NUTRITION

Diagnosis/Stabilization Phase		Acute Management Phase		Recovery Phase	
Outcome	**Intervention**	**Outcome**	**Intervention**	**Outcome**	**Intervention**
Patient will be adequately nourished.	Assess bowel sounds, abdominal distention, and abdominal pain and tenderness q4h and PRN. NPO until extubated, if applicable. Assess ability to take fluids. If not able, maintain enteral or IV feedings as necessary. If able to take fluids, administer clear to full liquids and assess response.	Patient will be adequately nourished.	Same as stabilization phase. Progress diet as tolerated to diabetes diet. Monitor protein, albumin, and glucose levels. Consult dietician as necessary. Begin teaching patient/family about diabetes diet requirements.	Patient will be adequately nourished.	Continue teaching patient/family diabetes diet requirements.

Care Guide continued on following page

DIABETIC KETOACIDOSIS MULTIDISCIPLINARY CARE GUIDE *continued*

MOBILITY

Diagnosis/Stabilization Phase		Acute Management Phase		Recovery Phase	
Outcome	***Intervention***	***Outcome***	***Intervention***	***Outcome***	***Intervention***
Patient will achieve optimal mobility. Patient will be free of joint contractures.	Assess degree of mobility and muscle strength. If comatose, begin passive range of motion (ROM) exercises.	Patient will achieve optimal mobility. Patient will be free of joint contractures.	If able, continue active-assist ROM exercises and progress activity as tolerated. Monitor response to increased activity. Decrease activity should adverse events occur (tachycardia, dysrhythmias, dyspnea, hypotension, etc.) Obtain physical therapy consult if indicated. Provide support as necessary.	Patient will achieve optimal mobility. Patient will be free of joint contractures.	Teach patient/family about recommended exercise program and any activity limitations.

OXYGENATION/VENTILATION

Diagnosis/Stabilization Phase		Acute Management Phase		Recovery Phase	
Outcome	***Intervention***	***Outcome***	***Intervention***	***Outcome***	***Intervention***
Patient will have adequate gas exchange as evidenced by: • $Sao_2 > 90\%$/$Spo_2 > 92\%$ • ABGs WNL • Clear breath sounds • Respiratory rate, depth, and rhythm WNL • Chest x-ray WNL • Absence of dyspnea, cyanosis, secretions, Kussmaul's respirations • Effective cough	Constantly monitor respiratory status—respiratory muscle strength, ABGs, Spo_2, rate, rhythm, and depth of respirations, lung sounds, coughing ability, and chest x-ray. Be prepared for intubation and mechanical ventilation. If on ventilator, monitor settings and hemodynamic variables prior to, during, and after weaning. Wean ventilator when appropriate and monitor patient response: • Wean Fio_2 to keep $Spo_2 > 92\%$ • Use humidification to keep secretions thin If not intubated, apply supplemental oxygen. Monitor with pulse oximetry. Assess evidence of tissue perfusion. Monitor lab values: ABGs, hemoglobin.	Patient will have adequate gas exchange.	Monitor and treat oxygenation disturbances as per ABGs and/or Sao_2. Monitor and treat ventilation disturbances as per ABGs, chest assessment, adventitious breath sounds, and chest x-ray. Wean oxygen therapy/mechanical ventilation as indicated. Assess effects of increased activity on respiratory status. Observe for complications of DKA that may impair oxygenation/ventilation: pneumonia, aspiration, infection, etc.	Patient will have adequate gas exchange.	Obtain chest x-ray before discharge. Encourage coughing and deep breathing at least q2h.

COMFORT

Diagnosis/Stabilization Phase		Acute Management Phase		Recovery Phase	
Outcome	*Intervention*	*Outcome*	*Intervention*	*Outcome*	*Intervention*
Patient will be as comfortable and pain free as possible as evidenced by: • No objective indicators of discomfort • No complaints of discomfort	Assess absence of, or quantity and quality of, pain. Administer sedatives cautiously and monitor effects on respiratory status. If patient is intubated, establish effective communication technique with which patient can communicate discomfort. Assess need for analgesics and administer accordingly. Provide reassurance in a calm, caring, and competent manner.	Patient will be relaxed and comfortable.	Same as stabilization phase. Teach patient relaxation techniques. Use massage, humor, music therapy, and imagery to promote relaxation.	Patient will be relaxed and comfortable.	Teach patient/family alternative methods to promote relaxation after discharge.

SKIN INTEGRITY

Diagnosis/Stabilization Phase		Acute Management Phase		Recovery Phase	
Outcome	*Intervention*	*Outcome*	*Intervention*	*Outcome*	*Intervention*
Patient will have intact skin without abrasions or pressure ulcers.	Assess all bony prominences at least q4h and treat if needed. Use preventive pressure-reducing devices if patient is at high risk for development of pressure ulcers. Treat pressure ulcers according to hospital protocol.	Patient will have intact skin without abrasions or pressure ulcers.	Same as stabilization phase.	Patient will have intact skin without abrasions or pressure ulcers.	Teach patient/family proper skin care, particularly of feet.

PROTECTION/SAFETY

Diagnosis/Stabilization Phase		Acute Management Phase		Recovery Phase	
Outcome	*Intervention*	*Outcome*	*Intervention*	*Outcome*	*Intervention*
Patient will be protected from possible harm.	Assess need for assistance with activities. Provide physical support as needed. Assess skin integrity and circulation q1h. Institute seizure precautions.	Patient will be protected from possible harm.	Same as stabilization phase.	Patient will be protected from possible harm.	Teach patient/family about any physical limitations in activity after discharge.

Care Guide continued on following page

DIABETIC KETOACIDOSIS MULTIDISCIPLINARY CARE GUIDE *continued*

PSYCHOSOCIAL/SELF-DETERMINATION

Diagnosis/Stabilization Phase		Acute Management Phase		Recovery Phase	
Outcome	***Intervention***	***Outcome***	***Intervention***	***Outcome***	***Intervention***
Patient will achieve psychophysiologic stability. Patient will demonstrate a decrease in anxiety as evidenced by: • Vital signs WNL • Subjective report of anxiety • Objective signs of anxiety Patient will demonstrate a decrease in depression as evidenced by: • Subjective report of decreased depression • Objective report of decreased depression	Assess physiologic effects of critical care environment on patient (hemodynamic variables, psychological status, signs of increased sympathetic response). Take measures to reduce sensory overload. If patient is unresponsive, use verbal and tactile stimuli. If intubated, develop effective interventions to commmunicate with patient. Use a calm, caring, competent, and reassuring approach with patient and family. Arrange for flexible visiting to meet patient and family needs. Determine coping ability of patient/family and take measures to help patient cope (allow verbalization of concerns and fears, provide frequent explanations, allow family to visit, use easy-to-understand terminology, support services, etc.). Begin teaching patient and family about DKA.	Patient will achieve psychophysiologic ability. Patient will demonstrate a decrease in anxiety.	Same as in stabilization phase. Initiate discharge planning with instruction to patient/family on activities at home, diabetes diet, proper skin care, foot care, medications, etc. Administer antidepressants/sedatives cautiously if used.	Patient will achieve psychophysiologic ability. Patient will demonstrate a decrease in anxiety.	Same as other phases.

DIAGNOSTICS

Diagnosis/Stabilization Phase		Acute Management Phase		Recovery Phase	
Outcome	*Intervention*	*Outcome*	*Intervention*	*Outcome*	*Intervention*
Patient/family will understand any tests or procedures that must be completed (vital signs, I & O, hemodynamic monitoring, x-rays, glucose, ABGs, bicarbonate, electrolytes, calcium, phosphate, serum osmolality, CBC, BUN, creatinine, ECG, EEG, etc.).	Explain all procedures and tests to patient/family. Be sensitive to individualized needs of patient/family for information.	Patient/family will understand any tests or procedures that must be completed.	Explain procedures and tests to assess progress and recovery from DKA to patient and family. Assess individualized needs of patient/family for information. Anticipate need for further diagnostic tests such as EEG, pancreas transplant workup, and any intervention that may result from this.	Patient/family will understand meaning of diagnostic tests in relation to continued health (serum glucose monitoring at home, etc.).	Review with patient/family before discharge results of all tests. Discuss abnormal findings and appropriate measures patient/family can take to return to normal. Provide patient/family with written guidelines concerning follow-up care. Teach patient technique for home glucose monitoring. Have patient demonstrate procedure several times before discharge. Teach patient administration of insulin if necessary. Have patient demonstrate procedure several times before discharge. Provide teaching on care at home (when to call the doctor, skin care, foot care, diabetes diet, administration of insulin, medication, home glucose monitoring, physical restrictions, signs of hypo-/hyperglycemia, management of diabetes when ill).

REFERENCE

Gotch, P. M. (1991). The endocrine system. In J. G. Alspach (Ed.). *Core curriculum for critical care nursing* (4th ed., pp. 609–674). Philadelphia: W. B. Saunders.

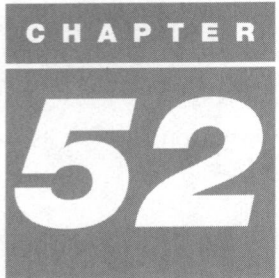

Patients With Disorders of the Neurohypophysis, Thyroid, and Adrenals

Danni Brown

Cellular metabolism largely depends on and is regulated by the nervous system and the endocrine system. Therefore, alterations in hormonal function, regardless of the cause, commonly result in systemic manifestations. This chapter will discuss disorders of the pituitary, thyroid, and adrenal glands. Emphasis will be placed on primary diseases of these endocrine glands rather than on changes in hormonal function as a result of other system failure (i.e., renal failure). Acute alterations that are commonly encountered in the critical care patient population will be highlighted.

PITUITARY GLAND

The pituitary gland, located in the sella turcica, consists of two lobes. The anterior lobe, also known as the adenohypophysis, is under the hormonal control of the hypothalamus. There is blood-borne communication between the hypothalamus and the anterior pituitary via the hypothalamic–pituitary portal system. Six hormones are synthesized and secreted from the anterior pituitary: corticotropin, thyrotropin (thyroid-stimulating hormone; TSH), growth hormone, follicle-stimulating hormone, luteinizing hormone, and prolactin. This lobe of the pituitary will not be discussed further in this chapter.

The posterior pituitary, also known as the neurohypophysis, is derived from different embryonic tissue than the anterior lobe and is connected to the hypothalamus via nervous tissue. The posterior pituitary stores two major hormones, arginine vasopressin (AVP), also known as antidiuretic hormone (ADH), and oxytocin. These hormones are actually synthesized in the hypothalamus and move by axonal transport into the posterior pituitary for storage. They are then secreted from the pituitary into the systemic blood circulation following appropriate stimulation. Oxytocin regulates uterine contractions at parturition and milk release after parturition (Hadley, 1983). Alterations in oxytocin levels will not be discussed in this chapter.

DISORDERS OF THE NEUROHYPOPHYSIS

Diabetes Insipidus

PATHOPHYSIOLOGY

Arginine vasopressin is one of several hormones that regulate the conservation of water to maintain fluid osmolality and systemic blood pressure and volume. It works on receptors in the distal renal tubules. Stimulation of these receptors causes the reabsorption of water and subsequent concentration of urine. Diabetes insipidus (DI) results from the absolute or relative lack of AVP, which causes excessive amounts of dilute urine output. This condition can be either neurogenic or nephrogenic (Blevins & Wand, 1992).

Neurogenic, or central, DI is the result of a defect in either the synthesis or secretion of AVP in the hypothalamus or pituitary, respectively. Some causes of this reduction in hormone include defective osmolreceptors, decreased numbers of secretory cells in the hypothalamus, impaired transport or release of AVP, and production of antibodies to the hormone (Rice, 1983).

The most common cause of an abnormal reduction in circulating AVP is a tumor of the hypothalamus or pituitary (Ingbar, 1987). These tumors may be either primary, such as chromophobe adenomas and craniopharyngiomas, or metastatic, most commonly from breast cancer (Rice, 1983). Some cases of idiopathic DI may result from a tiny lesion localized in the neurohypophyseal system. These lesions are usually nonmalignant (Hoshimaru et al., 1992).

The second most common cause of neurogenic DI is trauma. Trauma can be either accidental or iatrogenic from a surgical procedure. Severe head injury with resultant basilar skull fractures is the most common accidental cause of DI (Smith, 1981). Surgical procedures for tumor removal or aneurysm repair also often result in central DI (Smith, 1981). Traumatic DI is often transient in nature. Determining factors include the area of the lesion and the amount of destruction produced. Lesions of the hypothalamus and of the axonal tract above the median eminence produce permanent DI. However, lesions below the median eminence, even total removal of the pituitary gland, result in only temporary cessation of circulating hormone.

Certain medications also may have a central effect, decreasing the amount of circulating hormone. Some of these drugs are ethanol, reserpine, morphine sulfate, chlorpromazine, and phenytoin (Germon, 1987). Discontinuing the drug usually corrects the condition.

Local ischemia to the hypothalamus or the pituitary can cause neurogenic DI. This ischemia can be the result of decreased blood supply due to hemorrhage, thrombus formation, or severe hypotension.

Other causes of DI include central nervous system infections such as encephalitis, meningitis, tuberculosis, and syphilis. The granulomatous diseases sarcoidosis and eosinophilic granuloma also may cause central DI (Rice, 1983).

Nephrogenic diabetes insipidus results when the kidneys do not respond appropriately to the hormone. The renal tubules are resistant to AVP and therefore do not reabsorb water. Any renal disease in the advanced stages may cause nephrogenic DI; the more common causes include polycystic kidney disease, medullary cystic disease, and pyelonephritis. It may also occur after renal transplantation (Rice, 1983).

Other causes of nephrogenic DI include dietary factors, medications, pregnancy, and electrolyte imbalance. A rare familial form may also be seen; it is an X-linked recessive or autosomal dominant disease that is seen in male infants (Germon, 1987).

Nephrogenic DI is usually less severe than central DI. Fluid loss averages only 3 liters a day. An intact thirst mechanism will allow an individual to maintain an adequate fluid balance.

CLINICAL PRESENTATION

Regardless of the cause, patients with DI have abnormal water loss. Urine output can be as high as 16 to 17 liters/day. The patient with an intact thirst mechanism who is able to obtain enough water will prevent severe dehydration simply by drinking sufficient quantities. The hospitalized patient, however, may not have access to sufficient amounts of water, either because of physical limitations (i.e., too weak or too ill) or environmental limitations (i.e., too little water left at the bedside).

The patient with DI presents with polyuria and polydipsia. Profound weight loss is usually present. If fluid intake is insufficient, dehydration will occur. The patient will be hypotensive and have poor skin turgor and dried mucous membranes. In an attempt to conserve fluid, there will be decreased amounts of saliva and sweat.

Laboratory findings will include a high serum osmolarity (above 300 mOsm/liter) and hypernatremia (above 150 mmol/liter). Urine studies show an osmolarity under 200 mOsm/liter and a specific gravity of less than 1.005.

The diagnosis of DI is based on these laboratory findings and on diagnostic tests, such as the dehydration test and the hypertonic saline infusion test. The dehydration test is used most often. It provides adequate stimulation for AVP release and therefore readily identifies an abnormal state. During the test the patient is fluid restricted. Urine output, osmolality, and specific gravity are recorded. The patient with DI will continue to void dilute urine despite the fluid restriction. The patient should be watched closely due to the risk of severe dehydration resulting from the lack of fluid intake.

Differentiation of neurogenic DI or nephrogenic DI can be made by administering an exogenous form of the hormone, commonly aqueous vasopressin. If the urine osmolality shows a moderate to marked increase (greater than 9%), neurogenic DI is diagnosed. Nephrogenic DI will show little to no response to the exogenous hormone because abnormal endogenous hormone production is not the cause of the disorder.

The hypertonic saline infusion also provides a stimulus for AVP release—a hyperosmolar state. If the infusion of hypertonic saline does not increase the urine concentration, then DI is confirmed. Other laboratory findings include an assay of the serum hormone level both before and after the infusion.

CLINICAL MANAGEMENT

Clinical management of a patient with DI is aimed at adequate fluid replacement, prevention of complications during the acute phase, and providing patient education for long-term control. Medical treatment depends in part on the etiology. Fluid replacement is essential regardless of the cause. Adequate replacement is monitored by following patient weight, intake and output recorded hourly, as well as a cumulative body balance over the acute phase. Fluid intake should be adjusted to match output plus 10% for insensible loss. If the patient is febrile and/or tachypneic, higher fluid replacement may be necessary. Blood pressure and heart rate should be monitored hourly. Both can indicate hydration state.

Neurogenic DI is treated with hormone replacement. Aqueous vasopressin may be administered through either the subcutaneous or the intramuscular route. It is used with patients who have experienced an acute onset of DI, commonly after accidental trauma or surgery. Return of normal neurohypophyseal function can be recognized more easily because of the short duration of aqueous vasopressin. Urine specific gravity should be checked at least every 2 to 4 hours during therapy. This will help prevent fluid overload and water intoxication in patients receiving hormone replacement and intravenous fluids. Other, longer-acting forms of AVP are also available. Several nonhormonal agents are available for patients who have some AVP production. These agents increase AVP release or potentiate its actions on the renal tubules.

Nephrogenic DI is more difficult to treat. The only drugs of clinical value are diuretics. These drugs produce sodium depletion, which leads to a fall in the glomerular filtration rate. This in turn causes an increase in fluid reabsorption from the proximal section of the nephron. Because less sodium reaches the ascending loop of Henle, the ability to dilute the urine is reduced (Ingbar, 1987). The patient with nephrogenic DI must restrict his or her sodium intake.

This disorder may persist for weeks to months, or may be permanent. Therefore patient/family teaching should be started as soon as possible. The disease process and the treatment should be explained to both the patient and family/significant other, as appropriate. The patient/family/significant other must be taught and be able to return demonstrate how to administer the medication as well as how to identify signs of hormonal imbalance, particularly excessive urine output.

Syndrome of Inappropriate Antidiuretic Hormone

PATHOPHYSIOLOGY

The opposite of DI, the syndrome of inappropriate antidiuretic hormone (SIADH), is the result of excessive amounts of circulating AVP. There is a breakdown in the normal negative feedback system regulating the release and inhibition of the hormone. Circulating AVP acts directly on the renal tubules, causing reabsorption of water inconsistent with the body's needs. This leads to water overload and dilutional hyponatremia.

There are multiple causes of SIADH. Tumor tissue, commonly oat cell carcinoma, can produce AVP and release it independent of normal stimuli (Mundy, 1987). Nontumorous lung diseases also can cause SIADH either by independent synthesis and secretion of AVP or by altering left atrial filling pressures, thereby altering the stimulus for AVP release from the pituitary. Disorders of the central nervous system (CNS) can affect the neurohypophysis, thereby increasing AVP release. These disorders include head trauma with skull fractures, cerebrovascular accidents, CNS infections, and Guillain-Barré syndrome (Ingbar, 1987). Certain medications increase the secretion of AVP from the pituitary. These include chlorpropamide, the antineoplastic drugs vincristine and vinblastine, general anesthetics, and tricyclic antidepressants (Ingbar, 1987).

Physiologic SIADH occurs when plasma hypoosmolality and urine hyperosmolality are associated with severe hypovolemia and/or hypotension. This results when a stronger physiologically appropriate stimulus to AVP secretion overrides the osmotic stimulus. This can occur at times of acute severe blood loss, excessive fluid intake together with nausea and vomiting, infections, trauma, surgery, or other stresses (Streeten & Moses, 1993).

CLINICAL PRESENTATION

Patients with SIADH produce a small amount of very concentrated urine. If the symptoms—a result of the increased water retention—are not recognized and treated, they may progress to water intoxication. The symptoms are weight gain, anorexia, weakness, nausea, vomiting, diarrhea, confusion, aberrant respirations, hypothermia, and coma (Johndrow & Thornton, 1985).

Laboratory findings for the client with SIADH are a serum sodium level of less than 130 mmol/liter and a serum osmolality of less than 275 mOsm/liter. Other laboratory values, such as blood urea nitrogen, creatinine, hematocrit, and albumin, may also be decreased. Hypokalemia is rare in SIADH. Urine sodium is usually greater than 20 mmol/liter. The diagnosis of SIADH is suspected in any patient with the above laboratory findings. Care should be taken to exclude other causes of hyponatremia. If SIADH is suspected and no cause can be identified, a malignancy should be strongly considered. SIADH may occur before a lesion can be detected by chest x-ray (Ingbar, 1987).

Also helpful in the diagnosis is a water load test. To prevent any serious side effects from the fluid load, the patient must have a sodium level greater than 125 mmol/liter and must not display any symptoms consistent with hyponatremia before administration of the test. The patient is then given an oral fluid load (usually 20 mL/kg body weight). Urine is collected over the next 5 to 6 hours. Patients with SIADH will excrete less than 40% of the water load in this period of time. Normal individuals will excrete 80%.

Other diagnoses that produce similar signs and symptoms should be excluded before the diagnosis of SIADH is made. These include congestive heart failure, renal failure, and liver failure. Also, adrenal insufficiency and hypothyroidism should be excluded from the differential diagnoses through appropriate laboratory testing (Batcheller, 1992).

CLINICAL MANAGEMENT

Medical management of SIADH is largely dependent on the etiology. Treatment is biphasic, the fluid overload being treated first and the underlying cause afterward. At present there are no drugs that successfully inhibit the secretion of AVP from either the pituitary or a tumor. Treatment therefore consists of restricting fluid intake. If the condition is mild to moderate a fluid restriction of 800 to 1000 mL/24 hr is usually sufficient to increase the serum sodium concentration. If the client has any signs of more severe water intoxication such as mental confusion, seizures, or coma more expedient correction of the hyponatremia must be implemented. The treatment of choice for the acute phase is infusion of 3% hypertonic saline solution and intermittent doses of furosemide. Although this will be only a temporary measure to increase the serum sodium, it will prevent the deleterious effects of severe hyponatremia, and the diuresis from the furosemide will help prevent pulmonary edema that might otherwise occur as a result of the fluid overload.

Achievement and maintenance of a euvolemic state can be monitored by hourly intake and output along with a cumulative total body balance. Vital signs should be taken every 1 to 2 hours, along with auscultation of breath sounds to monitor for edema. Daily assessment of the patient's weight is extremely helpful in following the patient's fluid balance.

Long-term management of SIADH includes strict water restriction. Certain drugs that interfere with the actions of AVP at the nephron can be used to limit the effect of the hormone on water reabsorption and prevent fluid overload and hyponatremia. The most commonly used drug is demeclocycline. Other pharmacologic agents that have been used, but with less success, in the treatment of SIADH are lithium and phenytoin (Streeten & Moses, 1993).

Patient/family/significant other education should be started as soon as possible. They must understand the causes of SIADH, the therapy, and the signs and symptoms of fluid overload that must be reported to the physician.

THYROID GLAND

The thyroid gland is located below the larynx and anterior to the trachea. It consists of two lobes connected by the isthmus. The lobes are situated on either side of the trachea.

The thyroid gland is directly regulated by the anterior pituitary gland and indirectly by the hypothalamus. The hypothalamus secretes thyrotropin-releasing hormone (TRH). This hormone travels through the hypophyseal portal system to the anterior pituitary. In response to TRH, the anterior pituitary secretes TSH. This hormone is secreted into the general circulation and has as its target tissue the thyroid gland. This is called the hypothalamic-pituitary-thyroid axis.

The thyroid gland in response to TSH secretes thyroxine (tetraiodothyronine or T_4) and triiodothyronine (T_3). Synthesis of both hormones within the thyroid gland depends on sufficient quantities of iodine. Both hormones are bound to carrier proteins in the bloodstream. The largest amount of circulating hormone is T_4. This hormone is also relatively physiologically inactive. In the peripheral tissue, however, T_4 is converted to T_3 by the enzymatic removal of an iodine atom from the T_4 outer ring. Unbound T_3 has considerable effect on cellular metabolism. Thyroid hormones affect tissue growth and maturation, energy expenditure, and vitamin and hormone degradation.

Secretion of the thyroid hormones is under negative feedback control. High serum levels of circulating hormones (T_3 and T_4) decrease the pituitary's response to TRH. Thyrotropin-releasing hormone is secreted in response to sleep, cold temperatures, and nonspecific stress.

SICK EUTHYROID SYNDROME

Alteration in hormone levels results in widespread systemic dysfunction. Abnormal levels of thyroid hormones can result from either dysfunction of an organ in the physiologic axis or from other severe illness, physical trauma, or stress; the latter conditions result in a condition referred to as sick euthyroid syndrome (Wartofsky & Burman, 1982).

There are several variants of sick euthyroid syndrome. The concentration of T_4 may be normal with a decreased concentration of T_3. This is a result of a decrease of peripheral conversion of T_4 to T_3. The total T_3 concentration depends on the severity of the illness. This variant can be separated from intrinsic hypothyroidism by the presence of normal T_4 and TSH levels.

A second variant involves a low T_4 concentration and occurs in severely ill individuals. T_3 levels are also low. The low T_4 levels may be a result of hyposecretion of TSH. Low T_4 sick euthyroid syndrome hypothyroidism can be differentiated from pituitary hypothyroidism by rT_3 levels. (rT_3 is produced by removal of an iodine atom from the inner ring of T_4. It is physiologically inactive.) rT_3 concentrations are increased in sick euthyroid syndrome and decreased in pituitary hypothyroidism (Ingbar, 1987).

Sick euthyroid syndrome has been shown to occur in a wide variety of critically ill patients. Surgical patients demonstrate changes in thyroid hormone levels within 6 hours of surgery, but normalize within 1 week. The degree of alteration in hormone levels relates to the severity of the surgical trauma, and few if any adverse effects have been demonstrated (Zaloga et al., 1984).

Patients undergoing open-heart surgery demonstrate changes in hormone levels related to cardiopulmonary bypass. Although sick euthyroid syndrome is adaptive during times of stress, it also has been demonstrated that it contributes to low cardiac output syndrome in open-heart surgery patients (Holland et al., 1991). Replacement therapy remains controversial.

Patients with septic shock have shown marked disturbance of oxygen uptake autoregulation with a causative role related to sick euthyroid syndrome (Palazzo & Suter, 1991). The syndrome has also been studied in patients with AIDS (Raffi et al., 1991) and in hemorrhagic shock (Vitek et al., 1982).

THYROID DISORDERS

Goiters

Patients with nontoxic goiters (thyroid gland enlargement) can also become hypothyroid. Nontoxic goiters are the result of an imbalance between the supply of hormone produced and the demand by the body's needs. To provide for the supply required the thyroid enlarges. Lack of iodine, a necessary element in the production of thyroid hormones, can lead to a goitrous state. In most individuals enlargement of the gland allows the production of sufficient hormone to maintain normal metabolic functioning. Some individuals, however, are unable to meet the body's demands despite the glandular enlargement. They become both goitrous and hypothyroid. The addition of iodine to table salt has effectively decreased the incidence of endemic goiters.

Simple goiters can cause problems solely as a result of their size. The trachea and the esophagus can be compressed and displaced. Obstruction of either structure can occur if the goiter is large enough. Large retrosternal goiters can cause superior mediastinal obstruction.

Treatment of simple goiters is aimed at reducing the size and therefore the obstructing nature of the goiter. Exogenous hormone therapy is used to suppress the secretion of TSH from the pituitary. If the cause of the enlargement can be determined, treatment can be aimed more specifically. If iodine deficiency has resulted in the goitrous state, supplemental iodine should be used to treat the condition rather than hormone therapy.

Sodium L-thyroxine (levothyroxine) is the drug most commonly used to treat simple goiters. The dose usually starts at 100 μg/24 hr and is increased up to 200 μg/24 hr. Adequate suppression can be determined by measuring radioactive iodine uptake. Suppression of the thyroid gland is successful if the uptake of radioactive iodine (^{131}I or ^{123}I) is less than 5%.

Surgical intervention is used to treat simple goiters only if the goiter is causing severe obstruction and other medical means to reduce its size have failed. If a subtotal thyroidectomy is done, levothyroxine should be used (150 μg/24 hr) to prevent recurrence of the goiter from hyperplasia of the remaining tissue.

Hypothyroidism

PATHOPHYSIOLOGY

Hypothyroidism, regardless of the cause, is the condition that results when the levels of circulating T_3 and T_4 are inadequate. A variety of causes, both structural and functional, affect hormonal synthesis. Primary disease of the thyroid itself accounts for approximately 95% of hypothyroid conditions. The remaining 5% of cases arise from secondary (pituitary) and tertiary (hypothalamic) causes.

Failure of the thyroid gland to synthesize and secrete sufficient amounts of hormone (primary disease) can arise from several causes. These include congenital defects, surgical removal of the gland or radioiodine ablation, and dysfunction as a result of radiation for another condition such as lymphoma. Thyroid dysfunction can also be idiopathic.

Primary thyroid failure results in high levels of circulating TSH. Low to absent levels of T_3 and T_4 do not provide the negative feedback that is inhibitory to TSH production. The high levels of TSH stimulate tissue enlargement and the formation of a goiter. In the United States the most common cause of goitrous hypothyroidism is Hashimoto's disease, which results from defective organic binding of iodide and abnormal secretion of iodoproteins (Ingbar, 1987).

Hypothyroidism can be induced in critically ill individuals by other mechanisms. A drug commonly used in critically ill individuals, dopamine, is known to induce hypothyroidism. Dopamine inhibits TSH release from the pituitary gland.

Cretinism is a hypothyroid state seen in infancy. If left untreated it will result in both physical and mental developmental handicaps. Most infants in the United States today are tested for thyroid function before leaving the hospital and between 7 and 10 days of age. Early detection and proper treatment with hormone replacement prevent any disability.

CLINICAL PRESENTATION

Early symptoms of hypothyroidism are nonspecific. They may include lethargy, constipation, and weight gain. Hair and skin may become dry. Obstructive sleep apnea may also occur. The range of symptoms associated with hypothyroidism is found in Table 52–1. If left untreated, severe hypothyroidism may develop.

Severe hypothyroidism in adults can lead to accumulation of mucopolysaccharides in tissue. Lack of thyroid hormones also causes fluid retention and electrolyte imbalance. The excess fluid leaks into the tissue due to increased capillary permeability and the osmotic pull of the mucopolysaccharides. This results in nonpitting edema in the eyelids, periorbital tissue, hands, and feet. This condition is collectively called myxedema. This state can be treated and, more appropriately, prevented by early detection and prompt treatment of hypothyroidism.

CLINICAL MANAGEMENT

The clinical management of the patient with hypothyroidism is aimed at restoring adequate circulating hormone levels, and preventing or limiting the effects of the clinical manifestations of the disorder. It is essential to carefully monitor the patient's response to therapy to meet these outcomes. Hypothyroidism in the critically ill patient is treated with a synthetic thyroid preparation, levothyroxine, because of its uniform potency. The drug may be given orally or intravenously. Maintenance dose varies with individuals, some as low as 50 μg/24 hr to as high as 400 μg (Gilman et al., 1990). Blood tests to monitor thyroid function must be done periodically to assure adequate replacement.

Hormonal replacement therapy increases cellular metabolism. This results in increased cellular demand

TABLE 52–1. **Clinical Manifestations of Hypothyroidism**

Cardiovascular

Cardiomegaly
Pericardial effusions
Decreased beta-adrenergic receptors
Impaired contractility
Decreased intravascular volume
Hypotension
Peripheral edema
Defect in baroreceptor responses
Increased sensitivity to digitalis
ECG: sinus bradycardia; low voltage QRS complexes, prolonged PR and QT intervals, flattening of T waves

Renal

Decreased renal blood flow and glomerular filtration rate
Urine retention

Gastrointestinal

Ascites
Ileus
Atonic bowel
Constipation

Miscellaneous

Cold intolerance
Periorbital edema
Hypothermia
Arthralgias
Joint effusions
Pseudogout
Decreased drug metabolism
Hypercholesterolemia
Hypoglycemia
Hyperuricemia
Hyponatremia
Elevated creatine kinase, lactate dehydrogenase, AST, aldolase
Decreased cortisol response to stress

Respiratory

Hypoventilation
Impaired ventilatory response to hypoxia and hypercapnia
Pleural effusions
Edema and thickening of vocal cords
Airway obstruction (i.e., enlarged tongue)
Muscle discoordination
Decreased diffusing lung capacity for carbon monoxide, vital capacity

Neurologic

Obtundation, coma
Slowed mentation
Dementia
Psychosis
Seizures
Slowed relaxation of deep tendon reflexes
Decreased hearing
Vertigo
Peripheral neuropathy
Abnormal EEG
Elevated CSF protein

Muscular

Myopathy
Aches and pains
Cramps

Hematologic

Anemia
Coagulopathy
Capillary fragility

Skin

Cool, dry skin
Dry, coarse hair; brittle fingernails
Nonpitting edema
Alopecia

From Shoemaker, W. C., Ayres, S. M., Grennik, A., et al. (1989). Society of Critical Care Medicine: *Textbook of critical care* (2nd ed.). Philadelphia: W. B. Saunders.

for oxygen. In critically ill patients the subsequent increase in heart rate and contractility to match supply with demand may result in myocardial ischemia. Also, patients with hypothyroidism commonly have coronary artery disease. Therefore patients should be monitored for heart rate, dysrhythmias, and morphologic changes indicative of ischemia during therapy (McMillan, 1988).

Support of the patient until hormonal replacement has achieved normal physiologic function is essential to prevent or limit the clinical manifestations. Profound hypoventilation and hypercapnia may require intubation and mechanical ventilation. Drugs that suppress respirations should be avoided. Hypothermia should be treated by slowly warming the patient with blankets. Rapid rewarming could lead to vasodilation and cardiovascular collapse. Hypotension and decreased intravascular volume should be treated with volume expansion. The patient response to fluid should be carefully monitored and electrolytes checked to prevent exacerbation of the dilutional hyponatremia common in severe hypothyroidism (Spittle, 1992).

Hyperthyroidism

PATHOPHYSIOLOGY

Multiple etiologies can produce the clinical state of excessive circulating thyroid hormone. All produce essentially the same clinical picture. Treatment, however, varies depending on the cause.

The most common cause of hyperthyroidism is Graves' disease, an autoimmune disorder sometimes referred to as diffuse toxic goiter. The thyroid gland is enlarged and highly vascular. The follicles are both hyperplastic and hypertrophic. Excessive TSH is not the cause of enlargement of the gland. Abnormal immunoglobulins that have TSH-like properties are found in the plasma of individuals with Graves' disease. These immunoglobulins are termed thyroid-stimulating immunoglobulins (TSI). The first immunoglobulin discovered had a much longer physiologic effect than TSH and it was named long-acting thyroid stimulator. TSIs bind to the thyroid membrane, activate adenylate cyclase, increase the accumulation of iodide within the follicle, and induce glandular hyperplasia. The high circulating hormone levels that result inhibit TSH secretion from the pituitary gland.

Much less common than Graves' disease, hyperthyroidism can result from a toxic nodular goiter in a hyperfunctioning state. Adenoma of the thyroid gland may secrete thyroid hormones inappropriate to stimuli and may cause hyperthyroidism. Rare causes include thyroiditis, metastatic thyroid carcinoma, and overtreatment for hypothyroidism.

Secondary causes of hyperthyroidism are related to disorders of the pituitary or hypothalamus. Inappropriate secretion of thyrotropin results in excessive amounts of TSH with respect to the clinical picture. This elevation can result from a TSH-secreting tumor or resistance to thyroid hormone, thereby eliminating the negative feedback component (Faglia et al., 1987).

Thyrotoxic crisis, or thyroid storm, is a complication of hyperthyroidism. Although it is seen rarely, it is associated with a high mortality. The exact etiology is unknown. Several factors are thought to contribute to the development of this complication. They include an abrupt release of thyroid hormones or an increased sensitivity of peripheral receptors to the circulating hormones (Evangelisti & Thorpe, 1983).

TABLE 52–2. **Clinical Features of Hyperthyroidism**

Signs	Symptoms
Thyroid enlargement	Nervousness, anxiety
Thyroid bruit	Diaphoresis
Ophthalmopathy	Emotional lability
Lid retraction	Heat intolerance
Lid lag	Palpitations
Hyperkinesis	Dyspnea
Tremor	Fatigue and weakness
Hyperactive reflexes	Weight loss
Tachycardia	Increased appetite
Atrial fibrillation	Eye complaints (e.g., irritation, pain, diplopia)
Hot and moist skin	Hyperdefecation
Thin and fine hair	Personality change
Onycholysis	Impaired concentration and cognitive function
Hyperpigmentation and/or vitiligo	Insomnia
Impaired renal concentrating ability	Difficulty swallowing
Muscle weakness	
Hoarseness	
Gynecomastia	
Amenorrhea, oligomenorrhea	
Congestive cardiomyopathy	

Laboratory Tests:
Elevated total and free T_4
Elevated total and free T_3
Elevated RT_3U
Elevated (Graves' disease), normal and low (thyroiditis) RAIU
No response of TSH to TRH
Low creatine kinase, cholesterol, and triglycerides

RT_3U, T_3 resin uptake; RAIU, radioiodine uptake; TSH, thyrotropin; TRH, thyrotropin-releasing hormone.

From Shoemaker, W. C., Ayres, S. M., Grennik, A., et al. (1989). Society of Critical Care Medicine: *Textbook of critical care* (2nd ed.), Philadelphia: W. B. Saunders.

CLINICAL PRESENTATION

The clinical presentation of the client with hyperthyroidism is quite variable. The thyroid gland is palpable in approximately 95% of the cases. A bruit can usually be heard over the superior thyroid arteries. Other signs and symptoms include excessive sweating, heat intolerance, tachycardia, tremor, nervousness, and excitability. Wasting of the skeletal muscles often occurs and results in a proximal myopathy. The muscle wasting may be severe even when the client has only mild to moderate hyperthyroidism. The cardiovascular findings—sinus tachycardia, systolic flow murmurs, and atrial fibrillation—develop in severe cases of long duration and are more common in the elderly. Chest pain may occur with myocardial infarction in 4% to 10% of patients with thyrotoxicosis. Patients in thyroid storm present with exaggerated symptoms of hyperthyroidism. There is a rapid rise in temperature, quickly reaching up to and in excess of 41°C (Table 52–2).

Diagnosis of advanced hyperthyroidism typically is not difficult and is based on the clinical findings. However, the insidious onset often delays diagnosis well into the disease course. Thyroid function tests are diagnostic in most cases. If the T_4 and free T_4 index are borderline or normal, plasma T_3 should be measured. In approximately 5% of patients with hyperthyroidism T_3 alone will be elevated.

CLINICAL MANAGEMENT

Clinical management of the critically ill patient with hyperthyroidism involves three strategies. The first is to suppress the thyroid hormones, the second is to inhibit conversion of T_4 to T_3, and the third is to ameliorate the patient's symptoms (Table 52–3). Definitive therapy aimed at decreasing the overproduction of thyroid hormone often involves radioactive iodine or surgery.

Nurses must monitor these patients carefully for signs of thyroid storm. Fever, tachycardia, hypertension, and myocardial ischemia can all be life-threatening. It is important to watch for these symptoms and to the patient's response to drug therapy such as propranolol.

ADRENAL GLANDS

The adrenal glands are small structures located at the apex of each kidney. The adrenals consist of two sec-

TABLE 52–3. **Treatment of Hyperthyroidism**

Antithyroid Therapy

Drugs
  Propylthiouracil 100–400 mg q6h
  Methimazole 20–40 mg q day
  Iodide
  Lithium 300 mg q8h
Radioactive iodine
Thyroidectomy

Agents Inhibiting Peripheral Conversion of T_4 to T_3

Propylthiouracil
Glucocorticoids
Propranolol 40–60 mg q6h
Ipodate (Oragrafin) 1 gqday

Agents Ameliorating Symptoms

Propranolol 40–60 mg q6h
Reserpine 1.0–2.5 mg/day
Guanethidine 50–150 mg/day

From Shoemaker, W. C., Ayres, S. M., Grennik, A., et al. (1989). Society of Critical Care Medicine: *Textbook of critical care* (2nd ed.). Philadelphia: W. B. Saunders.

tions: the medulla and the cortex. The adrenal medulla is a part of the sympathetic nervous system. It synthesizes and secretes epinephrine (80%) and norepinephrine (20%).

The adrenal cortex surrounds the medulla and is divided into three zones. The outermost zone, zona glomerulosa, produces the mineralocorticoids. The most common mineralocorticoid, aldosterone, has an essential role in potassium, sodium, and water balance. Mineralocorticoid secretion is under the control of the renin–angiotensin system.

The middle zone, the zona fasciculata, produces glucocorticoids. The most common glucocorticoid is hydrocortisone. Glucocorticoids have an essential role during stress states. They regulate metabolism (glucose, protein, and fat) and the inflammatory response.

The innermost zone, the zona reticularis, also produces glucocorticoids and in addition androgen sex hormones. The zona fasciculata and the zona reticularis are under the control of the pituitary and hypothalamus. The glucocorticoid steroids are regulated by negative feedback on the hypothalamic-pituitary-adrenal axis.

Adrenal Insufficiency

PATHOPHYSIOLOGY

Adrenal insufficiency is simply the lack of adequate circulating hormone concentration (supply) to meet the needs (demand) of the cells. Primary adrenal insufficiency occurs when the supply of hormone is decreased due to disease/destruction of the adrenal glands. The most common reason for destruction of the glands is autoimmune adrenalitis leading to atrophy of the adrenal tissue. Other causes include tuberculosis of the adrenal glands, adrenal hemorrhage, and fungal infections. Adrenal hemorrhage can occur from infections, such as meningococcal or pseudomonal infections, or from anticoagulant therapy. Both glands must be affected to have any clinical significance. The production of adrenocortical hormones may also be suppressed by exogenous steroid therapy.

Acute adrenal insufficiency is rare but life-threatening if left untreated. It is usually associated with a stress state or abrupt withdrawal of exogenous therapy. During stress states (e.g., infection, trauma, surgery) the demand for glucocorticoids and mineralocorticoids increases. The differences between demand and supply will dictate the severity of the illness.

CLINICAL PRESENTATION

The clinical manifestations of acute adrenal insufficiency are related to the lack of hormones from the adrenal cortex, glucocorticoids and mineralocorticoids. Acute adrenal insufficiency usually leads to profound hypotension and hypovolemic shock. Patients may also complain of generalized weakness, weight loss, confusion, lethargy, and vomiting. The patient's condition may quickly progress to a comatose state if left untreated.

Laboratory data will reveal hypoglycemia, hyponatremia, and hyperkalemia. If the patient has an acute exacerbation of a chronic process, mild eosinophilia may also be present. Hyperpigmentation occurs in patients with chronic adrenal insufficiency (Werbel, 1993).

CLINICAL MANAGEMENT

Acute adrenal insufficiency should be suspected in any critically ill patient for whom a cause of profound hypotension cannot be readily identified. Therapy should be initiated as quickly as possible to prevent death. The clinical management of a patient in acute adrenal crisis is aimed at hormonal replacement, restoration of fluid volume, adequate tissue perfusion, and normalized electrolyte and glucose levels (Bruton-Maree & Maree, 1993). Hormonal replacement is essential. The drug of choice is intravenous hydrocortisone. Other supportive measures should be used as necessary. These may include a rapid infusion of 0.9% sodium chloride and 5% dextrose to prevent vascular collapse and elevate serum glucose. If an infective cause is suspected, appropriate antibiotic therapy should also be used.

The assessment of the patient's status will guide therapy. Hemodynamic parameters such as heart rate and blood pressure, along with invasive hemodynamic measurements in patients with pulmonary artery catheters, should be assessed frequently (Lee & Gumowski, 1992). The patient's temperature should also be monitored.

Fluid balance and tissue perfusion are assessed continuously by meticulous intake and output monitoring and assessment of mentation. Laboratory tests should be obtained every 2 to 4 hours to follow electrolyte levels. A complete blood count and differential should be obtained periodically to monitor for infection. Bedside capillary glucose levels are obtained every 2 hours until normalized, then every 4 to 6 hours until the patient is stabilized on an oral steroid regimen.

Prompt and aggressive therapy is necessary to treat the crisis, but the cause of the deficiency should also be investigated so appropriate long-term therapy may be prescribed. These patients may require long-term steroid replacement.

Once the crisis has passed and the patient is stable, patient education regarding the causes of adrenal crisis, precipitating signs and symptoms, and early treatment is essential. Patients requiring long-term steroid therapy (commonly lifelong therapy) will require extensive education regarding drug therapy. They must understand the increased need for hormonal replacement during times of stress and the extreme dangers of abrupt cessation of drug therapy (Schira, 1987).

SUMMARY

Dysfunction of the endocrine system presents a major challenge to the critical care nurse. Clinical management of the patient with an endocrine crisis includes careful assessment of the patient's clinical status, administration of replacement hormones, and collaborative interventions directed toward prevention of complications.

REFERENCES

Batcheller, J. (1992). Disorders of antidiuretic hormone secretion. *AACN Clinical Issues in Critical Care Nursing, 3*(2), 320–378.

Blevins, L. S., & Wand, G. S. (1992). Diabetes insipidus. *Critical Care Medicine, 20,* 69–79.

Bruton-Maree, N., & Maree, S. M. (1993). Acute adrenal insufficiency: A case report. *CRNA, 4*(3), 128–132.

Evangelisti, J., & Thorpe, J. (1983). Thyroid storm—a nuring crisis. *Heart and Lung, 12*(2), 184–193.

Faglia, G., Beck-Peccoz, P., Piscitelli, G., et al. (1987). Inappropriate secretion of thyrotropin by the pituitary. *Hormone Research, 26,* 79–99.

Germon, K. (1987). Fluid and electrolyte problems associated with diabetes insipidus and syndrome of inappropriate antidiuretic hormone. *Nursing Clinics of North America, 22*(4), 785–796.

Gilman, A. G., Rall, T. W., Nies, A. S., et al. (1990). *The pharmacological basis of therapeutics* (8th ed.). New York: Pergamon Press.

Hadley, M. E. (1983). *Endocrinology.* Englewood Cliffs, NJ: Prentice-Hall.

Holland, F., Brown, P., Weintraub, B., & Clark, R. (1991). Cardiopulmonary bypass and thyroid function: A "euthyroid sick syndrome." *Annals of Thoracic Surgery, 52,* 46–50.

Hoshimaru, M., Hashimoto, N., & Kikuchi, H. (1992). Central diabetes insipidus resulting from nonneoplastic tiny mass localized in the neurohypophyseal system. *Surgical Neurology, 38*(1), 1–6.

Ingbar, S. (1987). Diseases of the thyroid. In E. Braunwald et al. (Eds.), *Harrison's principles of internal medicine* (11th ed., pp. 1732–1752). New York: McGraw-Hill.

Johndrow, P., & Thornton, S. (1985). Syndrome of inappropriate antidiuretic hormone: A growing concern. *Focus on Critical Care, 12*(5), 29–34.

Lee, L., & Gumowski, J. (1992). Adrenocortical insufficiency: A medical emergency. *AACN Clinical Issues in Critical Care Nursing, 3*(2), 319–330.

McMillan, J. (1988). Preventing myxedema coma in the hypothyroid patient. *Dimensions of Critical Care Nursing, 7*(3), 136–144.

Mundy, G. (1987). Ectopic hormonal syndromes in neoplastic disease. *Hospital Practice,* April 15, 179–194.

Palazzo, M., & Suter, P. (1991). Delivery dependent oxygen consumption in patients with septic shock: Daily variations, relationship with outcome and the sick-euthryoid syndrome. *Intensive Care Medicine, 17,* 325–332.

Raffi, F., Brisseau, J., Planchon, B., Remi, J., Barrier, J., & Grolleau, J. (1991). Endocrine function in 98 HIV-infected patients: A prospective study. *AIDS, 5*(6), 729–733.

Rice, V. (1983). Problems of water regulation: Diabetes insipidus and syndromes of inappropriate anti-diuretic hormone. *Critical Care Nurse, 3*(1), 63–82.

Rubin, E., & Farber, J. (1994). Adrenal cortical insufficiency. In E. Rubin & J. L. Farber (Eds.), *Pathology* (2nd ed., pp. 1131–1133). Philadelphia: J. B. Lippincott.

Schira, M. (1987). Steroid-dependent states and adrenal insufficiency. *The Nursing Clinics of North America, 22*(4), 837–841.

Smith, J. (1981). Nursing management of diabetes insipidus. *Journal of Neurosurgical Nursing, 13*(6), 313–317.

Spittle, L. (1992). Diagnoses in opposition: Thyroid storm and myxedema coma. *AACN Clinical Issues in Critical Care Nursing, 3*(2), 300–308.

Streeten, D., & Moses, A. (1993). The syndrome of inappropriate vasopressin secretion. *The Endocrinologist, 3*(5), 353–358.

Vitek, V., Shatney, C., Lang, D., & Cowley, R. (1982). Thyroid hormone responses in hemorrhagic shock: Study in dogs and preliminary findings in humans. *Surgery, 93*(6), 768–777.

Wartofsky, L., & Burman, K. (1982). Alterations in thyroid function in patients with systemic illness: The "euthyroid sick syndrome." *Endocrine Reviews, 3*(2), 164–217.

Werbel, S. (1993). Acute adrenal insufficiency. *Endocrinology and Metabolism Clinics of North America, 22*(2), 303–328.

Zaloga, G., Chernow, B., Smallridge, R., et al. (1985). A longitudinal evaluation of thyroid function in critically ill surgical patients. *Annals of Surgery, 201*(4), 456–464.

PATIENTS WITH ADRENAL CRISIS MULTIDISCIPLINARY CARE GUIDE

COORDINATION OF CARE

Diagnosis/Stabilization Phase		Acute Management Phase		Recovery Phase	
Outcome	*Intervention*	*Outcome*	*Intervention*	*Outcome*	*Intervention*
All appropriate team members and disciplines will be involved in the plan of care.	Develop the plan of care with the patient/family, primary nurse(s), primary physician(s), endocrinologist, intensivist, other specialists as needed, clinical nurse specialist, respiratory therapist, chaplain, and social services.	All appropriate team members and disciplines will be involved in the plan of care.	Update the plan of care with the patient/family, other team members, dietician, discharge planner, and home health.	Patient/family will understand how to maintain optimal health at home.	Provide written guidelines concerning follow-up care to patient/family. Provide patient/family with phone numbers of resources available to answer questions. Consult home health to provide continuity of care.

FLUID BALANCE

Diagnosis/Stabilization Phase		Acute Management Phase		Recovery Phase	
Outcome	*Intervention*	*Outcome*	*Intervention*	*Outcome*	*Intervention*
Patient will achieve and maintain optimal hemodynamic status as evidenced by: • MAP > 70 mm Hg • Hemodynamic parameters WNL for the patient • Urine output > 0.5 mL/kg/hr • Normovolemic state (balanced intake and output) • Adequate LOC • Free of cardiac dysrhythmias • Vital signs WNL for the patient Suspect acute adrenal insufficiency in patients with profound hypotension without identifiable cause.	Assess history for use of corticosteroids (more than 20 mg of hydrocortisone for longer than 7–10 days can suppress hypothalamic-pituitary-adrenal axis). Monitor and treat: • Hemodynamic parameters • BP • HR • I & O • LOC • Evidence of tissue perfusion • PA pressures • CO/CI • CVP • SVR/PVR • Svo_2 • Temperature • Abnormal heart and lung sounds Monitor lab values: electrolytes and bedside glucose checks q2h until stable, then q4–6h. CBC with differential (eosinophilia may be present in acute exacerbation of a chronic process), ABGs, Spo_2 as indicated. Assess plasma corticotropin, plasma aldosterone, and thyrotropin level.	Patient will maintain optimal hemodynamic status.	Same as stabilization phase. Maintain optimal hydration, hemodynamics, and tissue perfusion based on cardiopulmonary assessment and laboratory values. Begin teaching patient/family regarding cause of adrenal crisis, precipitating events, and signs and symptoms of adrenal crisis.	Patient will maintain optimal hemodynamic status.	Same as other phases. Continue teaching patient/family about: • Long-term steroid therapy if indicated. Include instruction on increasing hormonal replacement during stressful times. Emphasize danger of stopping drug therapy abruptly. Remind patient that if they vomit and are unable to take the oral dose of corticosteroids, notify physician immediately or go to emergency department for parenteral hydrocortisone • Precipitating signs/symptoms of adrenal crisis so patient can seek medical therapy early • Optimal fluid balance and how to maintain it. Review signs and symptoms of fluid overload and dehydration. Remind patient to weigh daily and report sudden changes to physician

Care Guide continued on following page

PATIENTS WITH ADRENAL CRISIS MULTIDISCIPLINARY CARE GUIDE *continued*

FLUID BALANCE *continued*

Diagnosis/Stabilization Phase		Acute Management Phase		Recovery Phase	
Outcome	*Intervention*	*Outcome*	*Intervention*	*Outcome*	*Intervention*
	Administer IV hydrocortisone, IV fluids (usually 0.9% sodium chloride and 5% dextrose to increase glucose and vascular volume) and inotropes as indicated. Monitor and treat dysrhythmias. Assess and monitor fluid balance. Assess weight changes from baseline and weigh daily. Determine hydration needs based on hemodynamics, intake/output, cardiopulmonary assessment, vital signs, and electrolytes. Monitor and treat complications of adrenal crisis such as profound hypotension, hypovolemic shock, generalized weakness, weight loss, confusion, lethargy, hypokalemia, vomiting, and severe dehydration.				

NUTRITION

Diagnosis/Stabilization Phase		Acute Management Phase		Recovery Phase	
Outcome	*Intervention*	*Outcome*	*Intervention*	*Outcome*	*Intervention*
Patient will be adequately nourished.	Assess nutritional status. Assess for vomiting, diarrhea, anorexia, nausea, or weight loss. Monitor albumin, cholesterol, prealbumin, total protein, nitrogen balance, phosphate, magnesium, calcium, and lymphocyte count.	Patient will be adequately nourished.	Involve dietician if needed. Initiate diet as tolerated and monitor response (clear liquids, regular meals, enteral feedings or parenteral nutrition).	Patient will be adequately nourished.	Teach patient/family: • Recommended daily allowances • Daily caloric intake needed • Safe weight reduction or weight gaining techniques as indicated

MOBILITY

Diagnosis/Stabilization Phase		Acute Management Phase		Recovery Phase	
Outcome	*Intervention*	*Outcome*	*Intervention*	*Outcome*	*Intervention*
Patient will achieve optimal mobility.	Assess muscle mobility, flexibility, strength, and tone. Begin passive/active-assist range of motion exercises.	Patient will achieve optimal mobility.	Assess physical limitations of mobility. Involve physical or occupational therapist for specific mobility limitations. Develop progressive activity program. Provide support as needed. Monitor response to activity and decrease if adverse events occur (tachycardia, dyspnea, ectopy, syncope, or hypotension).	Patient will maintain optimal mobility. Patient will develop home exercise plan.	Assist patient/family in developing home exercise plan. Determine a gradually increasing program of aerobic activity such as walking, swimming, and jogging.

OXYGENATION/VENTILATION

Diagnosis/Stabilization Phase		Acute Management Phase		Recovery Phase	
Outcome	*Intervention*	*Outcome*	*Intervention*	*Outcome*	*Intervention*

Patient will have adequate gas exchange and adequate tissue perfusion as evidenced by:
• $Sa_{O_2} > 90\%$ ($Sp_{O_2} > 92\%$)
• ABGs WNL
• Clear lung sounds
• Respiratory rate, depth, and rhythm WNL
• Normal chest x-ray
• Normal hemoglobin
• Evidence of tissue perfusion to major organs:
  • Urine output > 0.5 mL/kg/hr
  • Appropriate LOC
  • Skin warm and dry
	Monitor respiratory status closely, including respiratory rate, depth, rhythm, lung sounds, ABGs, Sp_{O_2}, and chest x-ray. Be prepared for intubation and mechanical ventilation.
	If on ventilator, monitor settings and hemodynamic variables before, during, and after weaning.
	Wean ventilator when appropriate and monitor patient response.
	Wean F_{IO_2} to maintain $Sp_{O_2} > 92\%$.
	If not intubated, use supplemental oxygen if indicated.
	Assess for evidence of tissue perfusion.
	Monitor lab values: ABGs and hemoglobin.
		Patient will maintain optimal gas exchange and tissue perfusion.	Same as stabilization phase.
			Monitor and treat oxygenation/ventilation disturbances as per ABGs, pulse oximetry, chest assessment, adventitious breath sounds, and chest x-ray.
			Wean mechanical ventilator/oxygen therapy as indicated.
			Assess effects of increased activity on cardiopulmonary function.
			Observe for complications associated with adrenal insufficiency which may impair oxygenation/ventilation: infection, tuberculosis, hypovolemic shock, or hypotension.
				Patient will maintain optimal gas exchange and tissue perfusion.	Same as other phases.
					Monitor and treat oxygenation/ventilation disturbances.
					Instruct patient/family on signs and symptoms of respiratory distress and when to seek medical care.

Care Guide continued on following page

PATIENTS WITH ADRENAL CRISIS MULTIDISCIPLINARY CARE GUIDE *continued*

COMFORT *continued*

Diagnosis/Stabilization Phase		Acute Management Phase		Recovery Phase	
Outcome	*Intervention*	*Outcome*	*Intervention*	*Outcome*	*Intervention*
Patient will be as comfortable and pain free as possible, as evidenced by: • No objective indicators of discomfort • No complaints of discomfort	Assess absence of, or quantity and quality of pain. Administer sedatives and analgesics as ordered, and monitor response. If patient is intubated, establish effective communication technique with which patient can communicate discomfort. Provide reassurance in a calm, caring, and competent manner.	Patient will be comfortable and pain free.	Same as stabilization phase. Instruct patient on relaxation techniques. Use complementary therapies such as massage, humor, music, and imagery to promote relaxation. Involve family in strategies.	Patient will be comfortable and pain free.	Same as other phases. Teach patient/family complementary methods to promote relaxation once discharged.

SKIN INTEGRITY

Diagnosis/Stabilization Phase		Acute Management Phase		Recovery Phase	
Outcome	*Intervention*	*Outcome*	*Intervention*	*Outcome*	*Intervention*
Patients will have intact skin without abrasions or pressure ulcers.	Assess all bony prominences at least q4h and treat if needed. Use preventive pressure-reducing devices if patient is at high risk for development of pressure ulcers. Treat altered skin integrity according to hospital protocol. Assess skin and mucous membranes for dryness. Assess for thirst and/or decreased skin turgor.	Patients will have intact skin without abrasions or pressure ulcers.	Same as stabilization phase.	Patient will have intact skin without abrasions or pressure ulcers.	Same as acute management phase. Instruct patient/family on skin care management postdischarge.

PROTECTION/SAFETY

Diagnosis/Stabilization Phase		Acute Management Phase		Recovery Phase	
Outcome	*Intervention*	*Outcome*	*Intervention*	*Outcome*	*Intervention*
Patient will be protected from possible harm.	Assess need for wrist restraints if patient is intubated, has a decreased LOC, or is unable to follow commands. Explain need for restraints to patient/family.	Patient will be protected from possible harm.	Same as stabilization phase.	Patient will be protected from possible harm.	Teach patient/family regarding any physical limitations in activity after discharge.

If restrained, assess response to restraints and check q1–2h for skin integrity and impairment to circulation. Follow hospital protocol for use of restraints.
Assess need for assistance with activities and provide physical support as needed.
Institute seizure precautions if severe electrolyte imbalances exist.

PSYCHOSOCIAL/SELF-DETERMINATION

Diagnosis/Stabilization Phase		Acute Management Phase		Recovery Phase	
Outcome	***Intervention***	***Outcome***	***Intervention***	***Outcome***	***Intervention***
Patient will achieve psychophysiologic stability. Patient will demonstrate a decrease in anxiety as evidenced by: • Vital signs WNL for the patient • Subjective reports of decreased anxiety level • Objective reports of decreased anxiety level	Assess physiologic effects of critical care environment on patient (hemodynamic variables, psychological status, signs of increased sympathetic response). Use calm, caring, competent, and reassuring approach with patient and family. Take measures to reduce sensory overload. If patient is unresponsive, use verbal and tactile stimuli. Arrange for flexible visiting to meet the patient and family needs. Determine coping ability of patient/family and take measures to help patient cope (allow verbalization of concerns and fears, provide frequent explanations, encourage family to visit and participate in care, use easy to understand terminology, and utilize support services when indicated). Administer sedatives and anxiolytics as ordered and monitor response. Begin explanation of adrenal insufficiency to patient/family.	Patient will achieve psychophysiologic stability. Patient will demonstrate a decrease in anxiety.	Same as acute management phase. Initial discharge planning. Teach patient/family about: • Home medications; long-term steroid replacement include dose, increase in greater stress periods, and inform of danger in stopping abruptly • Signs and symptoms of adrenal crisis • Refer to outside services as appropriate	Patient will achieve psychophysiologic stability. Patient will demonstrate a decrease in anxiety.	Same as acute management phase.

Care Guide continued on following page

PATIENTS WITH ADRENAL CRISIS MULTIDISCIPLINARY CARE GUIDE *continued*

DIAGNOSTICS

Diagnosis/Stabilization Phase		Acute Management Phase		Recovery Phase	
Outcome	***Intervention***	***Outcome***	***Intervention***	***Outcome***	***Intervention***
Patient will verbalize any tests or procedures that need to be completed (vital signs, hemodynamic measurements, I & O, cardiac monitor, chest x-ray, oxygen therapy, pulse oximetry, lab work including plasma ACTH levels, cortisol levels and aldosterone levels, ACTH stimulation test to confirm presence of adrenal insufficiency).	Explain all tests and procedures to patient/family. Explain what the patient's role in the diagnostic test will be (i.e., lie still when hemodynamics obtained, keep digit with pulse oximeter on it straight and relaxed.) Be sensitive to individualized needs of patient/family for information.	Patient will understand the meaning of diagnostic tests or procedures that need to be completed.	Same as in stabilization phase.	Patient will understand the meaning of diagnostic tests in relation to continued health.	Review with patient and family results of tests before discharge. Discuss abnormal findings and appropriate measures patient/family can take to help correct whatever is abnormal. Review meaning of individual's stress response and necessity to adjust hydrocortisol for high-stress times.

REFERENCE

Gotch, P. M. (1991). The endocrine system. In J. G. Alspach (Ed.), *Core curriculum for critical care nursing* (4th ed., pp. 609–674). Philadelphia: W. B. Saunders.

UNIT

10

HEMATOLOGIC SYSTEM

CHAPTER 53

Hematologic Physiology

Diane K. Dressler

Critical care nurses are confronted daily with clinical problems related to cellular respiration, immunity, and hemostasis. All these functions depend directly on blood. The nursing care of patients with hematologic disorders is challenging. It requires knowledge of the anatomy of the hematologic system (much of which continually moves around), the physiology of the blood elements, the effects of deficiencies of blood elements, and the processes of hemostasis and thrombosis. The purpose of this chapter is to present the anatomy and physiology of the hematologic system with an emphasis on blood coagulation.

THE COMPOSITION OF BLOOD

Blood is a mixture of living cells and plasma. The major functions of blood include the transportation of oxygen and food products, the removal of carbon dioxide and metabolic wastes, the transport of hormones from endocrine glands, and the protection of the body from infection. In addition, the flow of blood plays a role in the regulation of body temperature.

The average adult has 5 to 6 liters of blood in the intravascular compartment. Fifty-five percent of this is in the form of plasma, and 45% is solid suspended cellular components. The solid suspended cellular component is commonly referred to as the hematocrit. Table 53–1 outlines the more specific composition of plasma and cellular components. The red blood cells (RBCs) are by far the most numerous of the cellular components. It is important to note that the RBCs and platelets remain in the intravascular compartment. Most white blood cells (WBCs) are extravascular, and the blood serves mainly as a transport system for these cells (Lancaster, 1992).

TABLE 53–1. **Composition of Blood**

Plasma (55%)	Cellular Components (45%)
Water (92%)	Red blood cells (erythrocytes): 5 million/mm^3
Protein (7%)	White blood cells (leukocytes): 5,000–10,000/mm^3
Albumin	Granulocytes
Other plasma proteins	Neutrophils (60–70%)
Immunoglobulins	Eosinophils (1–3%)
Fibrinogen	Basophils (.05–1%)
Prothrombin	Monocytes (macrophages) (4–8%)
Other (1%)	Lymphocytes (20–40%)
Metabolites	B-cells
Respiratory gases	T-cells
Enzymes	Platelets (thrombocytes): 150,000–400,000/mm^3
Hormones	
Clotting factors	

All blood cells originate from primordial cells in the bone marrow, as shown in Figure 53–1. The marrow is considered to be one of the largest organs in the body. It produces 2.5 billion RBCs, 2.5 billion platelets, and 1 billion WBCs daily (Williams et al., 1990). The bone marrow is stimulated to differentiate cells into RBCs, platelets, and specific types of WBCs according to physiologic requirements. As the cells mature, they proceed through developmental stages before being released from the bone marrow and becoming fully functional. These stages will be described in more detail as the specific cell types are discussed.

Red Blood Cells

Normal RBCs have a unique structure that facilitates the transport of oxygen from the lungs to the tissues. They are shaped like biconcave discs, allowing greater flexibility as they pass through tiny capillaries. Their biconcave structure also increases the surface area for absorption of oxygen.

The production of RBCs is regulated by tissue oxygenation. Under conditions of hemorrhage, hypoxia, and anemia, the bone marrow is stimulated to produce more RBCs. As the cells are formed, they begin to synthesize hemoglobin during the primitive stages. The cytoplasm eventually fills with hemoglobin, the cell nucleus becomes extremely small, and the cells are released into the circulation as reticulocytes. The number of reticulocytes can be measured to assess the rate of erythrocyte production. The reticulocytes mature in a few days into functional erythrocytes.

The process of erythropoiesis, or RBC production, is controlled by a feedback mechanism involving a circulating hormone, erythropoietin. Cellular hypoxia leads to increased production of erythropoietin by the kidney, which produces 95% of this hormone. Erythropoietin then circulates to the bone marrow, where it

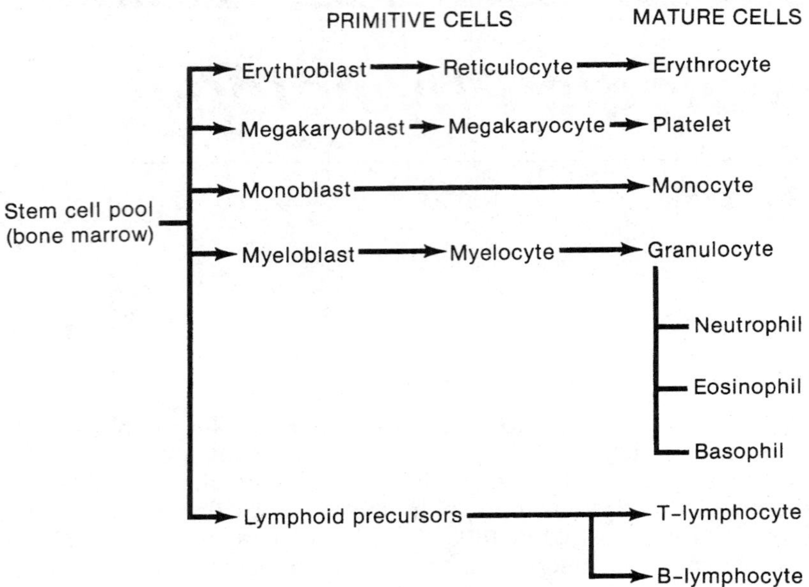

FIGURE 53–1. The production of cellular components.

causes stem cells to differentiate into erythrocytes. In addition, when severe hypoxia is present, more erythropoietin is produced, and the rate of production increases. When the kidneys are nonfunctional, anemia results because the other sites of erythropoietin production (possibly the liver and macrophages) can produce only a fraction of the needed amount (Guyton, 1991). Until recently, transfusion therapy was the only treatment option available for these individuals, but genetically engineered recombinant human erythropoietin is now standard treatment for chronic anemia.

Specific nutrients are necessary for RBC production. Vitamin B_{12} is essential for all tissue growth and is especially important for rapidly proliferating tissues. Lack of vitamin B_{12} inhibits the rate of RBC production and leads to the formation of abnormal RBCs. This maturational failure can be caused by inadequate intake of vitamin B_{12} or failure to absorb it (pernicious anemia). Folic acid, like vitamin B_{12}, is also a necessary nutrient for RBC production. Iron absorbed from the small intestine is formed into a substance called transferrin, which allows the iron to circulate to the parts of the body where it is needed. Excess iron is stored in the liver in the form of ferritin. When the plasma iron level falls, iron is transported to the bone marrow, where transferrin molecules bind with erythroblasts. Transferrin moves into the cells, where mitochondria synthesize heme from iron and porphyrin. The heme molecule then combines with a long polypeptide chain to form hemoglobin. The most important feature of this molecule is its ability to combine with oxygen in a bond that is easily reversible, allowing the oxygen to be readily released into the tissues (Guyton, 1991).

Red blood cells live an average of 120 days. When the cells become old and fragile, they rupture or are taken up by the red pulp of the spleen. The iron from the used cells is transported by macrophages into the blood, where it can be carried as transferrin back to the liver to be stored or to the bone marrow to be used in more hemoglobin production. The porphyrin portion of the hemoglobin molecule is converted by the macrophages into bilirubin, which is eventually secreted by the liver as bile (Guyton, 1991).

White Blood Cells

Six types of WBCs are found in peripheral blood and are known to participate in either nonspecific or specific immune responses. The granulocytes, also called polymorphonuclear leukocytes, are named for their granular appearance and for the fact that mature cells have multiple nuclei. These cells engulf and digest invading organisms through the process of phagocytosis. The three types of granulocytes include neutrophils, eosinophils, and basophils. The monocytes and lymphocytes, which include plasma cells, comprise the nongranulocytic leukocytes. A seventh type of leukocyte found in the bone marrow, the megakaryocyte, produces platelets.

The production of WBCs takes place in the bone marrow. Production of sufficient numbers of WBCs depends on adequate nutrition. Both amino acids and B vitamins are used in production of WBCs. It is thought that specific hormones stimulate immature granulocytes to increase the rate of production. The bone marrow is thought to contain approximately 30 granulocytes for each granulocyte found in the peripheral blood. Because the life span of many of these cells is short, the granulocyte pool can be quickly depleted during an acute infection, especially if the body does not have the resources to increase production (Lee et al., 1993).

White blood cells play a major role in the body's defense against infection. Granulocytes, the most numerous type of WBC, have a relatively short life span.

Neutrophils, the most abundant type of granulocyte, play a major role in the destruction of microorganisms, particularly bacteria. A much smaller number of eosinophils are found in the blood. These cells seem to have less phagocytic activity than neutrophils. Eosinophils are found in high concentrations during parasitic infections and during allergic reactions (Lancaster, 1993). Even fewer basophils are found in peripheral blood. They are associated with the inflammatory response and are known to release both histamine and heparin.

The monocytes are the largest cells found in the peripheral blood and are a unique type of WBC. In both blood and tissues they recognize and phagocytize foreign organisms and particles. After transport through the blood, monocytes can travel to the tissues, where they are transformed into much larger cells called tissue macrophages. Both circulating and fixed macrophages are extremely phagocytic and serve to filter unwanted particles and organisms from the blood and body fluids (Lancaster, 1993).

In addition to the nonspecific inflammatory response initiated by neutrophils and macrophages, a sophisticated, immune response can develop, enabling the body to mount a defense against specific invading organisms, toxins, or cells. This response is carried out by the lymphocytes. The two major types of specific immunity are humoral immunity, which is mediated by B-lymphocytes and involves the production of specific antibodies; and cellular immunity, which is mediated by T-lymphocytes and involves the production of small sensitized lymphocytes that can bind to and destroy invaders. For more detailed information about WBC function and the immune system, see Chapter 57.

Platelets

Platelets are the smallest and most fragile of the cellular components of the blood. They normally circulate as flattened discs (Williams et al., 1990). They originate as small particles that bud from large megakaryocytes. Platelets contain granules that in turn contain substances that directly affect the coagulation process. The granules contain actin and myosin molecules, which can cause platelet aggregation. They also contain enzyme systems capable of forming adenosine triphosphate and adenosine diphosphate (ADP), enzymes that synthesize prostaglandins, and a growth factor that facilitates the repair of damaged vessels. The platelet cell membranes contain glycoproteins that cause the platelets to adhere to damaged cells. The membranes also contain phospholipids, which can activate the intrinsic pathway of blood coagulation (Guyton, 1991).

Platelets play several roles in the hemostatic process. They nurture the vascular endothelium, increasing its structural integrity. Without this nurturing by adequate numbers of platelets, petechiae develop easily. Platelets are able to plug small tears in capillaries physically. When a blood vessel is severed, platelets aggregate and release mediators that cause vascular constriction and initiate clot formation (Kimbrell, 1993).

Platelet production is under the control of a hormone called thrombopoietin. The site of synthesis of this hormone is unknown, but production of the hormone is stimulated by thrombocytopenia. Thrombopoietin increases the number of megakaryocytes formed and appears to speed their maturation and the release of platelets.

After the platelets are released, they circulate as cytoplasmic discs. Approximately 80% of the body's platelets circulate; the rest are stored in the spleen. Normal length of platelet survival is 8 to 10 days, but this is influenced by many factors, including the need for hemostasis.

THE NORMAL HEMOSTATIC MECHANISM

The hemostatic mechanism prevents blood loss from normal vessels and stops bleeding from injured vessels. Normally blood circulates through smooth endothelial-lined vessels without platelet aggregation, coagulation, or hemorrhage (Colman et al., 1991). Injury to the blood vessel is the usual trigger of the hemostatic process. Effective hemostasis is accomplished through the harmonious interplay among three factors: the blood vessel wall, the platelets, and the plasma coagulation factors. The precise mechanisms governing hemostasis are somewhat complex, but it is essential to understand these basic processes to understand coagulopathies.

Physical Events in Blood Clotting

Several mechanisms assist in achieving hemostasis after injury to a blood vessel. As shown in Figure 53–2, these mechanisms include vascular constriction, platelet plugging, clot formation, and fibrinolysis plus wound healing (Atkins, 1993).

VASCULAR CONSTRICTION. When a blood vessel is injured, it constricts to slow the flow of blood. This constriction is thought to result from nervous reflexes in the vessel walls and local myogenic contraction of the vessel. It is also thought that platelets release a powerful vasoconstrictor, thromboxane A_2, at the injury site (Lee et al., 1993). Later, this effect is reversed when the vessel walls, under the influence of the procoagulant thrombin, release a powerful vasodilator called prostacyclin (PGI_2). The greater the trauma, the greater the vascular spasm that occurs. This process can last from minutes to hours while the subsequent processes of platelet plugging and actual clot formation are under way (Guyton, 1991).

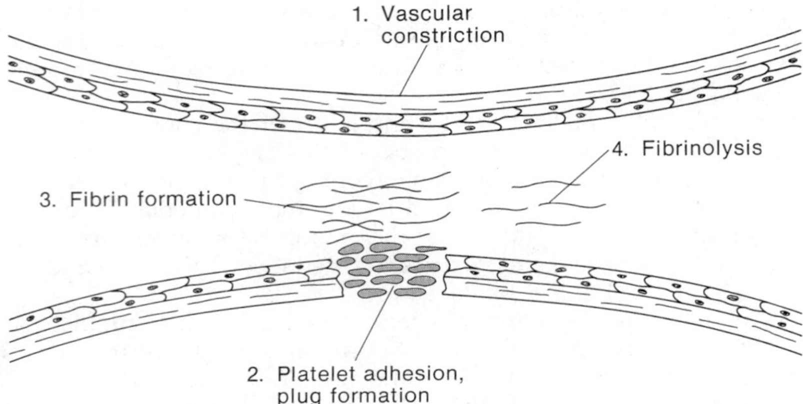

FIGURE 53–2. Physical events in blood clotting.

PLATELET PLUGGING. After an injury, the platelets change their form from discs to spheres (Colman et al., 1991). They become sticky and immediately begin to adhere to the damaged endothelium. They then release ADP and thromboxane A_2. These substances act on nearby platelets to activate them, resulting in their adhesion to the original platelets. The platelet adhesion process requires the presence of von Willebrand factor and normal receptor sites for this substance.

Contact with tissue collagen on the damaged endothelium is the signal that sparks the platelet release reaction. The chemical mediators act quickly to promote platelet aggregation, and an unstable platelet plug may form over the injured site within seconds (Lee et al., 1993). If the tear in the vessel is very small, it may be sealed by a platelet plug. This process is particularly important in sealing ruptured capillaries. The larger vessels damaged in more severe injuries are not sealed with platelet plugging. Here the aggregated platelets provide a surface on which blood coagulation can occur. Once a fibrin clot forms, the platelet plug is strengthened.

BLOOD CLOT FORMATION. A blood clot will begin to form within minutes after a vessel is damaged. The clot develops even faster if the trauma has been severe. Activating substances are released from platelets; others are released from the vessel wall and from plasma proteins. These substances activate the extrinsic and intrinsic blood coagulation pathways to initiate clotting. Fibrin strands appear over the injured site and eventually form a mesh that traps RBCs. The fibrin clot should form within 3 to 6 minutes (the normal bleeding time) unless the opening in the vessel is very large. After about 30 minutes to an hour, serum is expressed from the clot, and it retracts. This further closes the vessel and stabilizes the clot (Guyton, 1991).

FIBRINOLYSIS. Fibrinolysis is the process that eventually dissolves the clot. The fibrin is digested by enzymes from the plasma fibrinolytic system. WBCs also move in to phagocytize the debris by a process known as cellular fibrinolysis. Dissolution of the clot prepares the way for formation of fibrous scar tissue and wound healing.

The Biochemical Steps in Clot Formation

The process of blood clotting occurs as a series of steps that result in the formation of fibrin, the main substance of a clot. The physical events in blood clotting are controlled by biochemical reactions occurring between the procoagulant proteins and enzymes present in blood. There are four essential steps in clot formation:

1. Initiation of the extrinsic or intrinsic pathway
2. Formation of prothrombin activator
3. Conversion of prothrombin to thrombin
4. Conversion of fibrinogen to fibrin

Each of these important steps will be discussed in greater detail subsequently.

THE PLASMA COAGULATION FACTORS. All steps in the coagulation process involve interaction among the plasma coagulation factors. These factors, listed in Table 53–2, play a role in the initiation and completion of the clotting process. The first four factors—fibrino-

TABLE 53–2. **Plasma Coagulation Factors**

Factor I	Fibrinogen
Factor II	Prothrombin
Factor III	Tissue thromboplastin
Factor IV	Calcium
Factor V	Proaccelerin
Factor VII	Proconvertin, serum prothrombin conversion accelerator
Factor VIII	Antihemophilic factor (AHF)
Factor IX	Plasma thromboplastin component (Christmas factor)
Factor X	Stuart-Prower factor
Factor XI	Plasma thromboplastin antecedent
Factor XII	Hageman factor
Factor XIII	Fibrin-stabilizing factor

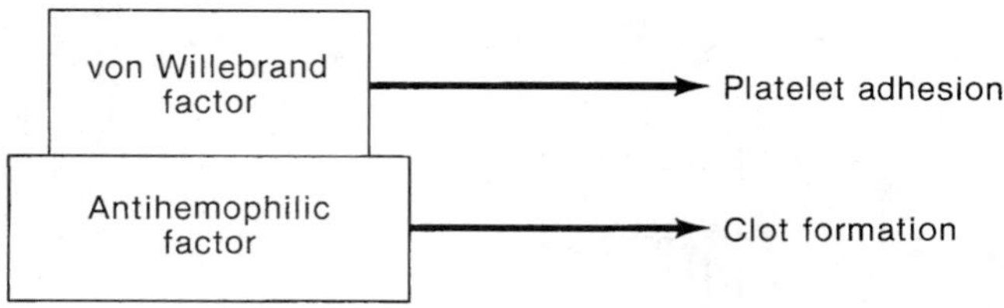

FIGURE 53–3. The factor VIII molecule.

gen, prothrombin, tissue thromboplastin, and calcium—are usually referred to by their common names. The other factors are most frequently referred to by their designated roman numeral. No factor VI is listed because the substance initially designated factor VI was found to be an activated form of factor V.

Most coagulation factors are produced in the liver, many in conjunction with vitamin K. Many of the factors are basically inactive forms of proteolytic enzymes. When activated, these enzymes cause the cascading reactions that result in clotting.

A few factors require a closer look. Factor VIII, the antihemophilic factor, actually has two components. Each component has its own function and genetic control. First, there is the coagulant protein known as antihemophilic factor, which has a role in the intrinsic pathway. People who lack this factor have hemophilia A. The other portion of factor VIII is a large polymeric protein known as von Willebrand factor, as illustrated in Figure 53–3. This component is necessary for normal platelet adhesion to collagen in a damaged vessel wall.

Factor XII is unique in that it functions not only in coagulation, but also in interaction with other related processes that occur during an injury. As seen in Figure 53–4, surface activation of factor XII also activates the kinin system and the fibrinolytic system. In this way, factor XII links the initiation of clotting with the subsequent activation of the inflammatory process and fibrinolysis during the contact phase of coagulation (Secor, 1993).

The clotting process is initiated through two basic mechanisms termed the extrinsic and intrinsic pathways. Both pathways have the same endpoint, the activation of factor X, which becomes what is called prothrombin activator.

THE EXTRINSIC PATHWAY. The extrinsic pathway is associated with trauma to body tissues. When an injury occurs, blood comes in contact with the damaged tissues, which release tissue thromboplastin. As seen in Figure 53–5, this substance, along with factor VII and calcium, forms activated factor X. The activated factor X then interacts with platelet phospholipids and factor V to produce the prothrombin activator complex. This complex is then able to split prothrombin to thrombin within seconds.

The extrinsic pathway is a much faster pathway of coagulation than the intrinsic pathway. The addition of tissue thromboplastin enables clotting to begin without some of the early time-consuming steps involved in the intrinsic system (Colman et al., 1991).

THE INTRINSIC PATHWAY. The intrinsic pathway is thought to be the more important coagulation pathway (Colman et al., 1991). All factors necessary to activate this pathway are already present in the intravascular compartment. The intrinsic pathway is activated when blood comes in contact with a foreign surface, such as a damaged vessel, or when the blood itself is traumatized (Guyton, 1991).

The intrinsic pathway has been called the *coagulation cascade.* It involves a series of reactions through which each inactive precursor is converted in turn into an active enzyme, which then goes on to convert another precursor. When a blood vessel is damaged and the subendothelium is exposed, the "contact" phase of coagulation begins. As shown in Figure 53–5, activated factor XII subsequently activates factor XI. This factor in turn activates factor IX. Factor IX then acts with factor VIII and the phospholipids released from traumatized platelets to activate factor X. A deficiency of any of these factors interferes with this process and prevents adequate initiation of the intrinsic pathway. It should also be noted that calcium ions are necessary for many steps in this process.

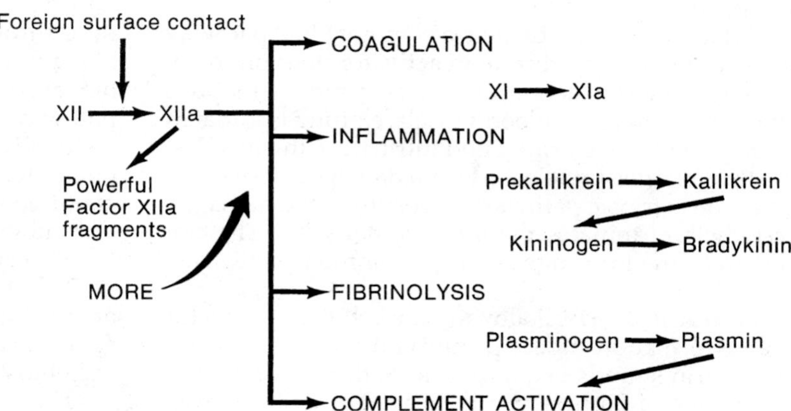

FIGURE 53–4. The activation of factor XII links a number of homeostatic reactions. It promotes blood coagulation through activation of factor XI, inflammation through kinins, fibrinolysis through plasmin, and subsequent complement activation.

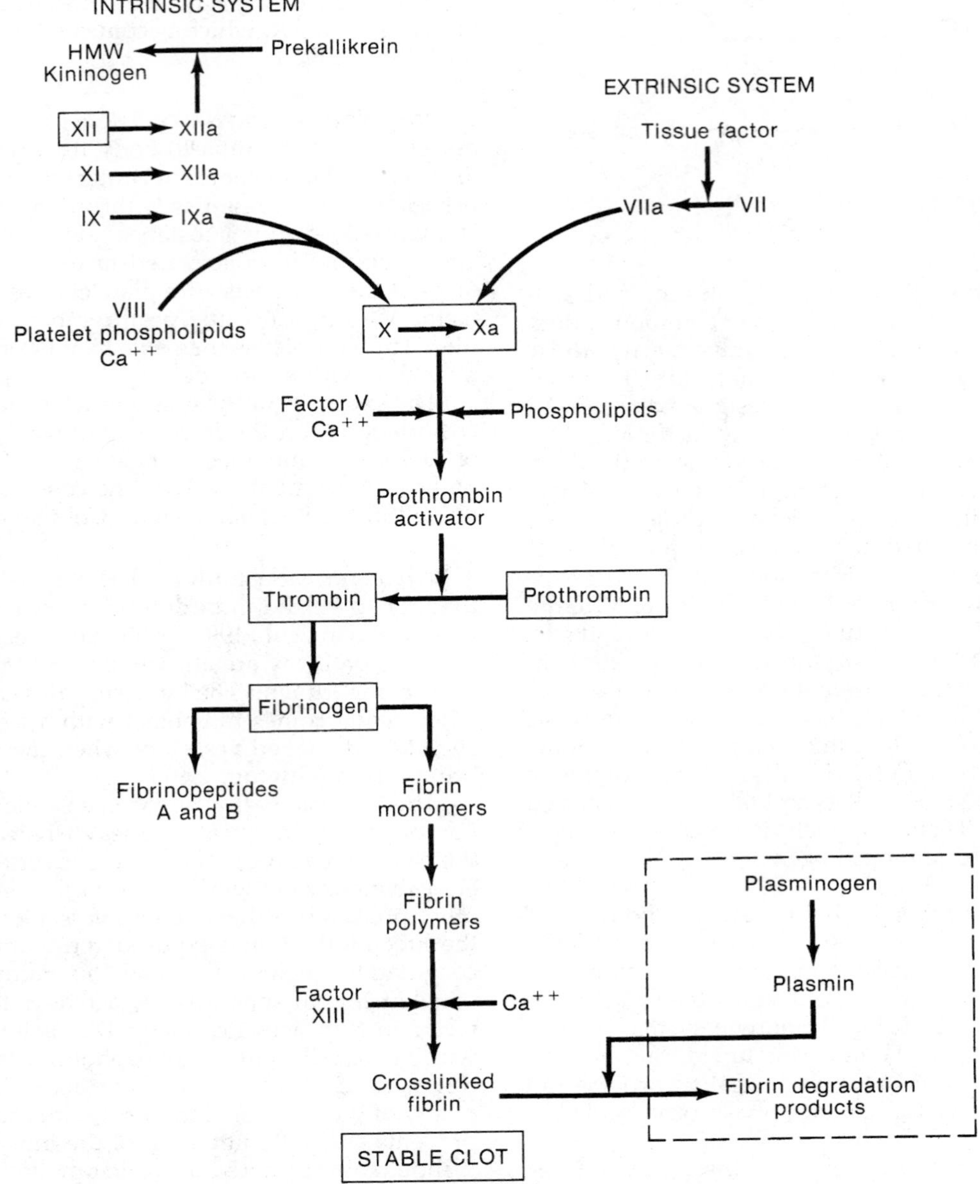

FIGURE 53–5. The coagulation process. HMW, high molecular weight.

After factor X is activated, a common final pathway is used in which prothrombin activator goes on to begin the actual formation of a clot. In most situations involving damage to blood vessels, clotting is initiated through both the extrinsic and intrinsic pathways. Tissue thromboplastin released from damaged tissues initiates the extrinsic pathway. Exposure of the damaged endothelium initiates the intrinsic pathway. The clot is then formed through the final common pathway.

CLOT FORMATION. Following the activation of factor X and formation of the prothrombin activator complex, fibrin strands begin to form within seconds. The production of fibrin depends on a rapid series of reactions through which prothrombin is cleaved to thrombin, a powerful procoagulant. The presence of thrombin accelerates clotting by stimulating the intrinsic pathway. It is thought that the extrinsic pathway may yield only small amounts of thrombin and fibrin. Adequate clot formation depends largely on activation and continued stimulation of the intrinsic pathway. Thrombin stimulates platelets to release ADP and continue to aggregate, and also stimulates the production of PGI_2 and is thus responsible for vessel relaxation after formation of the clot (Colman et al., 1991). Figure 53–6 illustrates the complex role played by thrombin in hemostasis.

The reactions described so far take place on the sur-

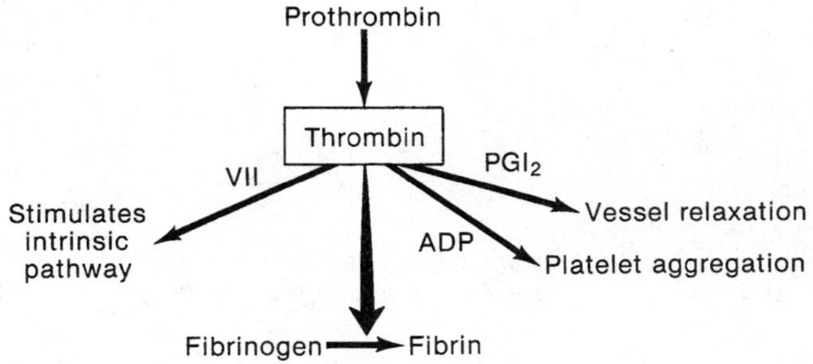

FIGURE 53–6. The role of thrombin in hemostasis. VII, factor VII; PGI_2, prostaglandin I_2; ADP, adenosine diphosphate.

face of platelets and involve platelet phospholipids, as shown in Figure 53–7. Specific glycoproteins in the platelet membrane act as receptors for coagulants such as activated factor X. After the thrombin is formed, it detaches from the platelet surface and goes on to cleave fibrinogen enzymatically into fibrinopeptides and fibrin monomers, an unstable form of fibrin. The fibrin monomers spontaneously become polymers and develop into fibrin threads, which become the basis for the clot. Fibrin-stabilizing factor (factor XIII) is present in the plasma and can also be released from platelets. Fibrin-stabilizing factor converts the fibrin strands by cross-linking them into a strong fibrin mesh. This mesh then traps cellular components of the blood and becomes the stable clot (Guyton, 1991).

The clot retraction that follows is yet another reaction that depends on platelets. Platelets attach to the fibrin threads, where they release fibrin-stabilizing factor and the contractile proteins actin and myosin. These substances cause both the platelets themselves and the clot to retract. Contraction of the edges of the injured vessel further stops the loss of blood.

THE FIBRINOLYTIC SYSTEM. The fibrinolytic system provides the mechanism through which clots are eventually dissolved. This promotes the clearing of clot material from tissues and blood vessels. The fibrinolytic process is particularly important in small peripheral vessels, which can easily become occluded by microclots (Guyton, 1991).

Both plasma fibrinolysis and cellular fibrinolysis are important in accomplishing the process of clot dissolution. The plasma fibronolytic system can physically break apart the fibrin clot, as shown in Figure 53–5. When a clot forms, a certain amount of plasminogen becomes part of the clot along with other plasma proteins. Both tissues and blood contain factors that can activate plasminogen to become plasmin, the substance capable of chemically lysing clots. These factors include a substance released from the vascular endothelium called tissue plasminogen activator (t-PA). Genetically engineered t-PA is used clinically as thrombolytic therapy. Plasmin is also thought to be activated by thrombin, activated factor XII, and lysosomal enzymes from damaged tissues (Colman et al., 1991).

Plasmin is an active proteolytic enzyme that can hydrolyse fibrin and dissolve clots. The lysis of fibrin by plasmin takes place on the surface of the clot because both plasminogen and the activator substances are located there. This reaction results in the formation of fibrin degradation products, also called fibrin split products (Colman et al., 1991). The fibrinolytic system's activity is ultimately limited by an inhibitor, $alpha_2$ antiplasmin. This substance rapidly inactivates plasmin in the circulation, preventing uncontrolled fibrinolysis. If this inhibitor of fibrinolysis is exhausted, as it might be during fibrinolytic therapy, continuous fibrinolysis can occur.

Cellular fibrinolysis has recently been found to make a significant contribution to clot destruction. WBCs release proteolytic enzymes that break down fibrin (Secor, 1993).

Hemostasis ultimately results in the fibrinolytic breakdown of fibrin, relaxation of the blood vessel, and healing. As a result of these processes, the vessel is usually returned to its normal state.

Control of Hemostasis

The hemostatic process is controlled by a number of mechanisms that prevent uncontrolled activity and help to ensure that clots form only where they are needed. The blood contains at least 40 substances that influence clotting. The procoagulant substances promote clotting, whereas the anticoagulant substances

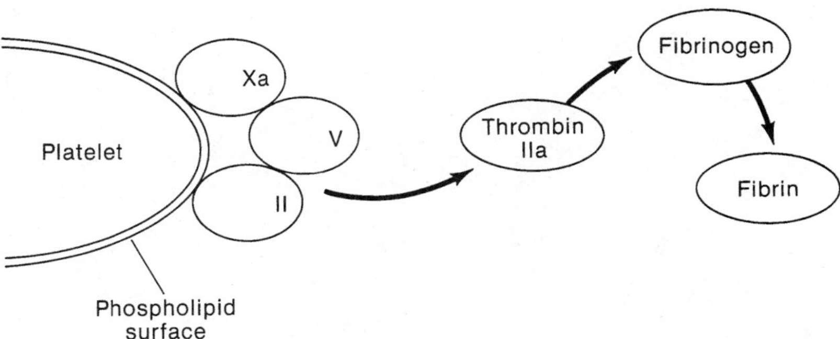

FIGURE 53–7. Coagulation on the platelet surface.

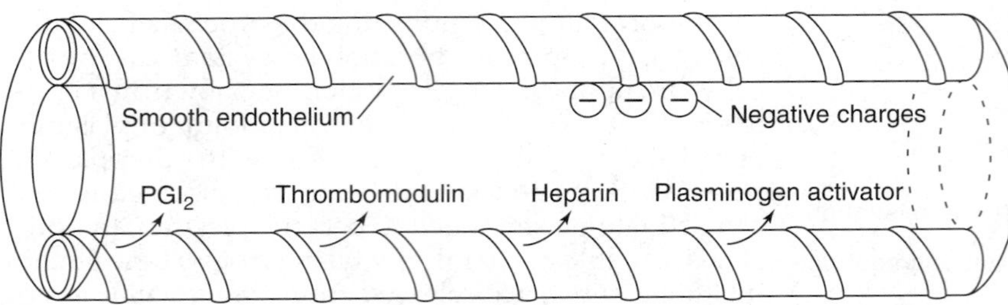

FIGURE 53–8. Anticoagulation characteristics of the vascular endothelium.

inhibit it. In the normal situation, the anticoagulants predominate, and the blood does not clot.

Some properties of the vascular endothelium also discourage clotting in normal blood vessels. As shown in Figure 53–8, endothelial cells are negatively charged and tend to repel the negatively charged platelets. Endothelial cells also synthesize PGI_2, an inhibitor of platelet aggregation, and other substances that inhibit thrombin. Thrombomodulin, a substance released by the vascular endothelium, inhibits clotting. It inactivates thrombin and interacts with another natural anticoagulant, protein C, to inhibit other activated clotting factors (Colman et al., 1991).

Other naturally occurring coagulation inhibitors circulate in the blood. One of the most important is antithrombin III. The role of antithrombin III is removal of the powerful procoagulant thrombin from the circulation. Excess thrombin that is not used in the clotting process is inactivated by antithrombin III so that excessive clotting does not occur (Guyton, 1991).

Heparin is another naturally occurring substance that interferes with blood clotting. It is produced by a number of different cells, particularly the mast cells located near the capillaries. These cells and basophils secrete small amounts of heparin, which is thought to help prevent clots in the capillaries, particularly those of the lungs and liver. Heparin acts by combining with antithrombin III to remove thrombin from the circulation, thereby preventing clot formation (Guyton, 1991).

SUMMARY

The complex system of the checks and balances related to hemostasis enables the body to control bleeding rapidly. Inappropriate clot formation away from the site of injury is prevented, and clots are broken down when they are no longer needed. Alterations in any part of this ongoing process can lead to clinically significant problems involving either hemorrhage or thrombosis.

REFERENCES

Atkins, P. J. (1993). Postoperative coagulopathies. *Critical Care Nursing Clinics of North America, 5*(3), 459–473.

Colman, R. W., Hirsh, J., Marder, V. J., et al. (1991). *Hemostasis and thrombosis: Basic principles and clinical practice* (2nd ed.). Philadelphia: J. B. Lippincott.

Guyton, A. C. (1991). *Human physiology and mechanisms of disease* (8th ed.). Philadelphia: W. B. Saunders.

Kimbrell, J. D. (1993). Acquired coagulopathies. *Critical Care Nursing Clinics of North America, 5*(3), 453–458.

Lancaster, L. E. (1993). Immunogenetic basis of tissue and organ transplantation and rejection. *Critical Care Nursing Clinics of North America, 4*(1), 1–24.

Lee, G. R., Bithell, T. C., Foerster, J., et al. (1993). *Wintrobe's clinical hematology* (9th ed.). Philadelphia: Lea & Febiger.

Secor, V. H. (1993). Mediators of coagulation and inflammation. *Critical Care Nursing Clinics of North America, 5*(3), 411–433.

Williams, W. J., Beutler, E., Erslev, A. J., et al. (1990). *Hematology* (4th ed.). New York: McGraw-Hill.

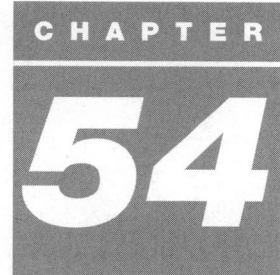

Patients With Coagulopathies

Diane K. Dressler

Few clinical problems are more challenging to the critical care nurse than hemorrhage. With advances in hematologic screening tests, it might be expected that bleeding problems would be predictable and preventable. However, most coagulopathies are difficult to predict. Even exhaustive screening for clotting abnormalities may not correlate with a patient's clinical course.

Nurses play a key role in the recognition and management of patients in a coagulation crisis. Because of this, it is essential for nurses to understand the complexities of both the clinical and laboratory manifestations of coagulation disorders. Acquired coagulation disorders rather than the inherited disorders are seen most commonly in critical care and in general clinical practice. This chapter will present the bleeding disorders associated with disseminated intravascular coagulation (DIC), vitamin K deficiency, liver insufficiency, renal insufficiency, excessive anticoagulation, pathologic fibrinolysis, thrombocytopenia, and postoperative coagulopathy.

DISSEMINATED INTRAVASCULAR COAGULATION

The syndrome of DIC is known by many names—diffuse intravascular coagulation, defibrination syndrome, consumption coagulopathy, and intravascular coagulation–fibrinolysis syndrome (Lee et al., 1993). This syndrome is a unique disorder of coagulation in which both hemorrhage and thrombosis, conditions that are usually diametrically opposed, occur simultaneously. DIC always occurs as a secondary process or a complication of another disease process. The syndrome has both acute and chronic forms. In critical care the acute form is seen most often and is usually considered a medical emergency (Bell, 1993). The chronic form of DIC is associated with certain chronic disease states, particularly oncologic disorders.

Pathophysiology

The pathophysiology of DIC is somewhat complicated and not yet completely understood (Lee et al., 1993). The major pathophysiologic feature is the formation of fibrin in the bloodstream and the deposition of fibrin in the microcirculation. This excessive and inappropriate fibrin formation depletes the blood of essential clotting components, which is why DIC is referred to as a "consumption coagulopathy." As illustrated in Figure 54–1, microclots form where they are not needed. The blood becomes so depleted of coagulation factors that a stable clot cannot form at a site of injury. The ultimate result of this process is determined by the balance between the rate of fibrin formation and the rate of its clearance from the circulation. In general, clotting components are often used up faster than the liver and bone marrow can replace them.

The intravascular clotting of DIC is different from the physiologic clotting that occurs in response to an injury. In DIC clots form within the blood in response to a thrombogenic stimulus that has overwhelmed the normal inhibitors of coagulation. Multiple microclots develop and subsequently embolize into the microcirculation, where they can cause ischemia of organs and tissues (Colman et al., 1991). As shown in Figure 54–2, the process of DIC begins as a thrombotic problem and eventually becomes manifest clinically as a bleeding problem. The vascular occlusion, hemorrhage, and shock that result from this process produce profound alterations in the function of many organ systems.

The bleeding manifestations of DIC are perpetuated by the activation of the fibrinolytic system. In DIC, plasminogen activators are released from the vascular endothelium after fibrin deposition and may also be released from platelets and leukocytes (Lee et al., 1993). The plasminogen activators activate fibrinolysis, the physiologic process that breaks up fibrin clots and eventually reopens blood vessels. In DIC the fibrinolysis is often extensive and results in the release of large amounts of fibrin degradation products (FDPs) or fibrin split products. When FDPs are released, they exert an anticoagulant effect that results in more bleeding (Bick, 1992). The FDPs act like antithrombins, which prevent the formation of normal fibrin and impair platelet function. The presence of large amounts of FDPs in the circulation is thought to be a major factor in the hemorrhagic features of DIC (Lee et al., 1993).

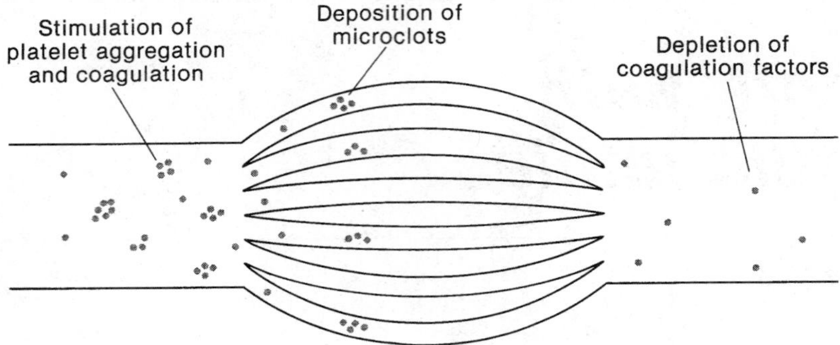

FIGURE 54–1. The process of disseminated intravascular coagulation.

The syndrome of DIC was first described in the 1950s in connection with obstetric disorders. However, it may have been described around 1900 as "temporary hemophilia" (Colman et al., 1991). It was identified as a specific disorder of coagulation in the 1960s. The DIC syndrome is associated with many disease processes and can occur as a complication of a variety of disorders ranging from shock to snake-bite. As shown in Table 54–1, many disorders commonly seen in critical care can be complicated by DIC (Bell, 1993; Bick, 1992). Chronic DIC is associated with disseminated cancer, giant hemangiomas, aneurysms, and intrauterine fetal death. Shock states and sepsis are the most common precipitators of DIC in critically ill patients. It is thought that a clinical situation that includes hypoxia, hypotension, acidosis, and liver dysfunction may predispose the patient to DIC.

There is little information about the incidence of DIC because much of the literature is in the form of case reports. The overall incidence may be as common as 1 in 1000 hospital admissions (Lee et al., 1993). Because DIC is not always manifested clinically, it may remain unrecognized in some patients.

Factors Triggering DIC

To initiate the DIC process, physiologic changes that are capable of altering the normal blood coagulation sequence must be present. So many disease processes are associated with the syndrome that most authors feel that the many types of DIC do not have a common pathogenesis (Bick, 1992). As shown in Figure 54–3, three of the processes associated with the triggering of DIC include tissue factors, factors that produce platelet aggregation, and factors that damage the blood vessel endothelium.

TISSUE FACTORS. The addition of procoagulant tissue factors to the blood can be an initiating factor in DIC. When tissue damage occurs, tissue thromboplastin is released into the circulation, activating factor VII and the extrinsic coagulation pathway. This release of thromboplastic material is associated with massive trauma, obstetric complications, and tissue breakdown due to various neoplasms (Bell, 1993). When DIC is associated with trauma, major surgical procedures, or

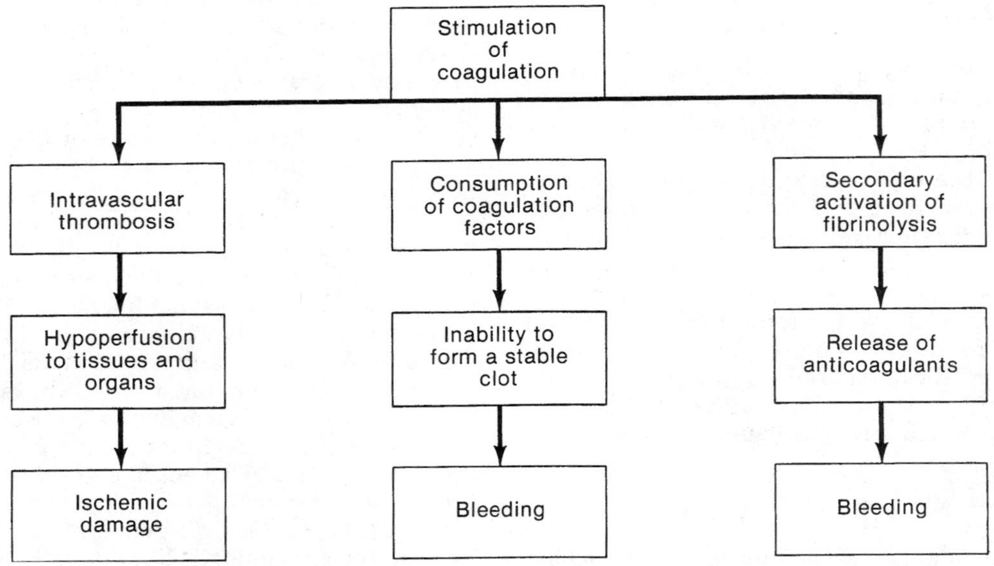

FIGURE 54–2. The pathophysiology of disseminated intravascular coagulation.

TABLE 54–1. **Clinical Conditions Associated With Disseminated Intravascular Coagulation**

Category	Associated Conditions
Septic processes	Bacterial infections (gram-negative most common); viral, rickettsial, protozoal, and mycotic infections
Shock states	Traumatic, septic, hemorrhagic, and cardiogenic shock
Obstetric complications	Abruptio placentae, amniotic fluid embolism, intrauterine fetal death, saline or urea-induced abortion, toxemia
Extensive trauma	Traumatic injury, severe burns, extensive surgical procedures, extracorporeal circulation, head injury
Neoplastic disorders	Acute and chronic leukemia; solid tumors of the prostate, pancreas, breast, lung, ovary, colon, and stomach
Immunologic disorders	Allograft rejection, incompatible blood transfusion, immune complex disease, anaphylactic drug reaction
Intravascular disorders	Dissecting aneurysm, giant hemangioma, vasculitis, pulmonary embolism
Miscellaneous	Venomous snake bite, heat stroke, liver failure, diabetic acidosis

extensive burns, it is thought that thromboplastic substances released from the damaged tissues initiate DIC (Bick, 1992). In patients with obstetric complications such as amniotic fluid embolism, abruptio placentae, or intrauterine fetal death, thromboplastic substances enter the material circulation and activate the coagulation process. In patients with neoplasms, tissue fragments and tumor microemboli may enter the circulation and act like thromboplastins.

PLATELET AGGREGATION. Platelet aggregation is an early and necessary step in physiologic clotting. However, it is thought that extensive stimulation of platelet aggregation may lead to the inappropriate clotting seen in DIC. Septic processes may be associated with platelet aggregation. As endotoxin is released from the infectious organisms, the endothelium of the blood vessel walls and red blood cells may be injured. The injury may stimulate contact activation and platelet aggregation. The eventual result is excessive platelet aggregation and deposition of fibrin in the microcirculation.

The generalized Shwartzman reaction is an important experimental model of DIC. Endotoxin injected into animal models results in fibrin formation in the glomerular capillaries with subsequent renal tubular necrosis. Changes in blood coagulation parameters are similar to those seen in patients with DIC. It is thought that the endotoxin damages the platelets themselves as well as the endothelium, although it is unclear whether platelet injury is the cause or the result of the coagulopathy (Colman et al., 1991).

VASCULAR ENDOTHELIAL INJURY. In addition to the vascular damage done by endotoxins, the vascular endothelium may be injured during shock, acidosis, and hypoxia. This damage may directly activate the intrinsic pathway as collagen is exposed and mediators are released (Colman et al., 1991). Damage to the vascular endothelium initiates a number of interactive processes. Hypoperfusion, acidosis, and hypoxemia are known to initiate hypercoagulability and platelet aggregation. In addition, the inflammatory process is triggered, causing increased capillary permeability and chemotaxis of white blood cells (WBCs). The WBCs may further damage the vascular endothelium as they migrate through the blood vessel walls. Monocytes in particular may play a major role in perpetuating the DIC process (Lee et al., 1993). Hypoxia contributes to this process by causing a rise in chemotactic substances.

Shock is thought to play an important role in the pathophysiologic process. Widespread endothelial damage is known to be extensive in the presence of hypoperfusion. The process of DIC is also enhanced by stasis, which inhibits the inflow of inhibitors of coagulation and impairs clearance of activated factors by the reticuloendothelial system (Colman et al., 1991). Because of this, all forms of shock can both precipitate and perpetuate DIC.

Although the specific initiating processes may vary, the pathophysiologic result is the same. Excessive production of activated coagulation factors overwhelms the normal inhibitors of coagulation, triggering DIC. In addition to the clotting and inflammation characteristic of DIC, the fibrinolytic process is initiated in an attempt to reopen the microcirculation. FDPs then perpetuate the vicious circle by contributing to the bleeding diathesis.

Three physiologic mechanisms aid recovery from this complex and destructive disorder. Reticuloendothelial cells in the liver and other organs phagocytize activated coagulation factors and remove them from the circulation. The fibrin that has been deposited in the microcirculation can be broken down by fibrinolysis, reopening the vessels. Leukocytes also assist in removing microcirculatory deposits of fibrin and fibrin complexes.

Clinical Presentation

The major clinical manifestation of acute DIC is bleeding, often from multiple sites (Colman et al., 1991). The bleeding may begin abruptly and can become a serious problem in a short period of time (Bell, 1993). Blood loss is often followed by shock, and the degree of shock may be out of proportion to the observed blood loss. The clinical signs of DIC are outlined in Table 54–2. There may be oozing of blood from incisions, injury sites, and puncture sites (Williams et al., 1990).

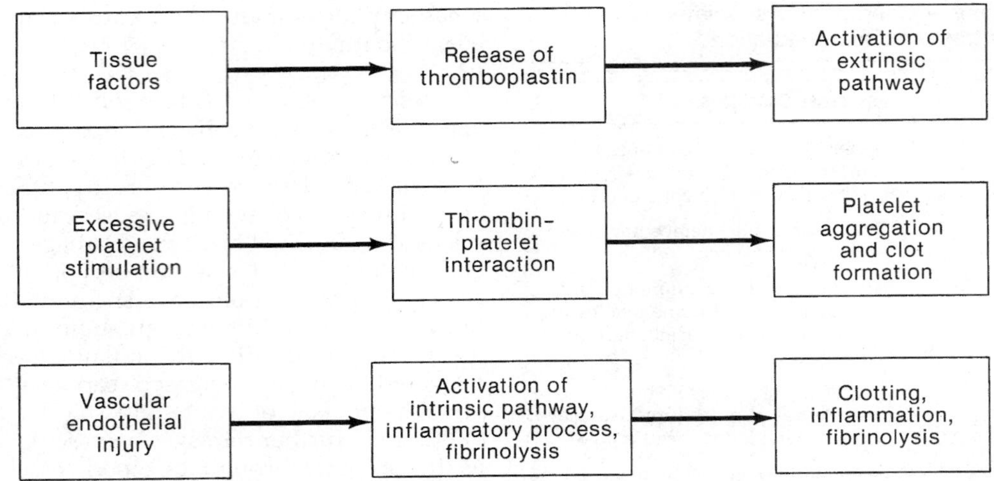

FIGURE 54–3. Triggering factors in disseminated intravascular coagulation.

Sites that were previously observed to be dry and healing may begin to bleed as fibrinolysis begins to dissolve clots. Petechiae or purpura may be observed as well as expanding hematomas. Bleeding from apparently healthy mucous membranes may occur.

In some patients a major hemorrhagic event is the first sign of DIC. Bleeding may begin in the gastrointestinal (GI) tract, genitourinary tract, or central nervous system (CNS). In surgical patients, postoperative hemorrhage may be precipitated.

The deposition of fibrin in the microcirculation can produce hypoperfusion and ischemic damage to tissues and organs. An unusual type of skin discoloration called acral cyanosis may develop on the patient's lips, nose, ears, fingers, and toes (Bell, 1993; Bick, 1992).

TABLE 54–2. **Clinical Features in Disseminated Intravascular Coagulation**

Hemorrhagic	Thrombotic
Obvious cutaneous bleeding	Cutaneous ischemia
Incisions	Acral cyanosis
Mucous membranes	Tissue necrosis
Recent trauma sites	Gastrointestinal tract
Old trauma sites	Diarrhea
Petechiae	Abdominal pain
Purpura	Genitourinary/renal
Hematoma formation	Oliguria
Gastrointestinal tract	Anuria
Active bleeding	Increased blood urea nitrogen and creatinine levels
Genitourinary/renal	Central nervous system
Active bleeding	Convulsions
Hematuria	Coma
Pulmonary	
Interstitial bleeding	
Adult respiratory distress syndrome	
Central nervous system	
Fatal hemorrhage	

This type of cyanosis is characterized by gray to purple discoloration of the skin with sharp irregular lines of demarcation from normal areas. It results from the obstruction of the microcirculation and in some instances can lead to tissue necrosis.

Ischemia of major organs can occur as a result of DIC. Acute tubular necrosis (ATN) is the most common example of this process, as fibrin begins to block the glomerular capillaries (Colman et al., 1991). Respiratory insufficiency may develop as the alveolar capillaries are affected. Diarrhea and abdominal pain may indicate involvement of the GI tract. Confusion and seizure activity may indicate that the CNS is affected. The circulatory and hypovolemic shock that occur in addition to vessel thrombosis further contribute to organ ischemia.

The clinical signs of DIC vary considerably depending on the initiating process, the extent of tissue and organ damage, and the severity of bleeding. In general, signs of DIC result from bleeding and from microcirculatory occlusion. However, in the subacute form of DIC, thrombosis may dominate the clinical picture. Occasionally, patients in whom DIC is suspected may have no obvious signs or symptoms, and DIC is detected only by abnormal laboratory results (Bick, 1992).

Laboratory Findings

Acquired disorders of blood coagulation such as DIC are associated with multiple abnormalities in the clotting scheme. There is no one diagnostic test for DIC. When this disorder is suspected, a complete coagulation panel should be obtained. Key laboratory tests that screen for DIC include the prothrombin time (PT), the activated partial thromboplastin time (APTT), the thrombin time (TT), fibrinogen level, platelet count, and the presence of FDPs (Lee et al., 1993).

TABLE 54–3. **Coagulation Tests for Disseminated Intravascular Coagulation (DIC)**

Test	What Is Measured	Normal Result	Result in DIC
Prothrombin time	Extrinsic and common pathways	12 seconds; INR 1.0	Prolonged
Activated partial thromboplastin time	Intrinsic and common pathways	≤33 seconds	Prolonged
Thrombin time	Rate of conversion of fibrinogen to fibrin	25–45 seconds	Prolonged
Fibrinogen level	Amount of fibrinogen available to form fibrin	150–400 mg/dL	Usually low; fibrinogen consumed
Platelet count	Platelets available for clot formation	150,000–400,000/mm^3	Low; platelets consumed
Fibrin degradation products	Action of plasmin on fibrin or fibrinogen	<10 μg/mL	Often >100 μg/mL
D-dimer	Products of fibrin breakdown	Negative	Positive
Red blood cell (RBC) morphology	Look for abnormal RBCs	Normal RBCs	Schistocytes present
Plasminogen	Amount of plasminogen available to become plasmin	75%–125%	Low due to excessive fibrinolysis
Protamine sulfate test	Presence of normal fibrin strands	Monomers negative	Monomers (unstable fibrin) positive
Antithrombin III assay	Amount available to inactive thrombin	80%–120%	Low

The PT, APTT, and TT are general screening tests of coagulation. As seen in Table 54–3, they test the intrinsic, extrinsic, and common pathways of coagulation and may all be prolonged in a patient with DIC (Williams et al., 1990). The fibrinogen level is usually low in patients with DIC. The level may drop precipitously as fibrinogen is consumed in the formation of fibrin. Thrombocytopenia is an early and consistent indicator of DIC (Colman et al., 1991). The platelet count usually falls to less than 50,000/mm^3 and may be depressed out of proportion to other coagulation abnormalities. It is thought that platelets may be readily consumed as they adhere to damaged surfaces (Lee et al., 1993).

Measurement of the FDPs assesses the rate of fibrinolysis that is occurring. FDPs are frequently elevated to over 100 μg/mL in patients with DIC, indicating excessive fibrinolysis. Other tests for fibrinolysis may be done as well. Studies have shown that the newer test for D-dimers, products of fibrin breakdown, is a better test for fibrinolysis (Bell, 1993; Halfman-Franey & Berg, 1991). The plasminogen level may be assessed; decreased plasminogen indicates that plasminogen has been converted to plasmin, and fibrinolysis is taking place (Colman et al., 1991). The euglobulin clot lysis time may be measured and is shortened when excessive fibrinolysis is taking place.

Other coagulation panel results may indicate DIC. Factors V and VIII may be depleted. The peripheral blood is examined for schistocytes, which are distorted and fragmented red blood cells. The red cells become physically damaged when they try to pass through the fibrin strands that obstruct the microcirculation (Bick, 1992). A test for fibrin monomers, an unstable form of fibrin, such as the protamine sulfate test may be performed. This test is indicative of abnormal fibrin formation, and a positive result is a strong indicator of DIC. Severe depletion of antithrombin III usually occurs in DIC and can be revealed through an antithrombin III assay (Lee et al., 1993).

Some physiologic and pathophysiologic states may change a patient's baseline coagulation panel. In patients with hepatic insufficiency the liver is often unable to synthesize normal levels of prothrombin, fibrinogen, and other factors. Certain stress states such as pregnancy, neoplasms, and infection can increase the levels of fibrinogen and factor VIII (Colman et al., 1991). When coagulation parameters are monitored, serial tests are usually done to detect trends in clotting times and factor levels. Trends are the most important assessment parameters because often the patient's baseline values are unknown.

Even after analysis of multiple coagulation panel results, laboratory diagnosis of DIC can be difficult. At times a definite laboratory diagnosis of DIC cannot be made. A hematologist may be consulted to assist in the interpretation of coagulation parameters and to discuss treatment options.

Clinical Management

The DIC syndrome usually is a complication of a serious underlying disorder, and the original problem must be considered in the treatment plan. Treatment of DIC is challenging because three hematologic abnormalities—thrombosis, hemorrhage, and fibrinolysis—may be occurring simultaneously. The major treatment options for DIC are outlined in Figure 54–4.

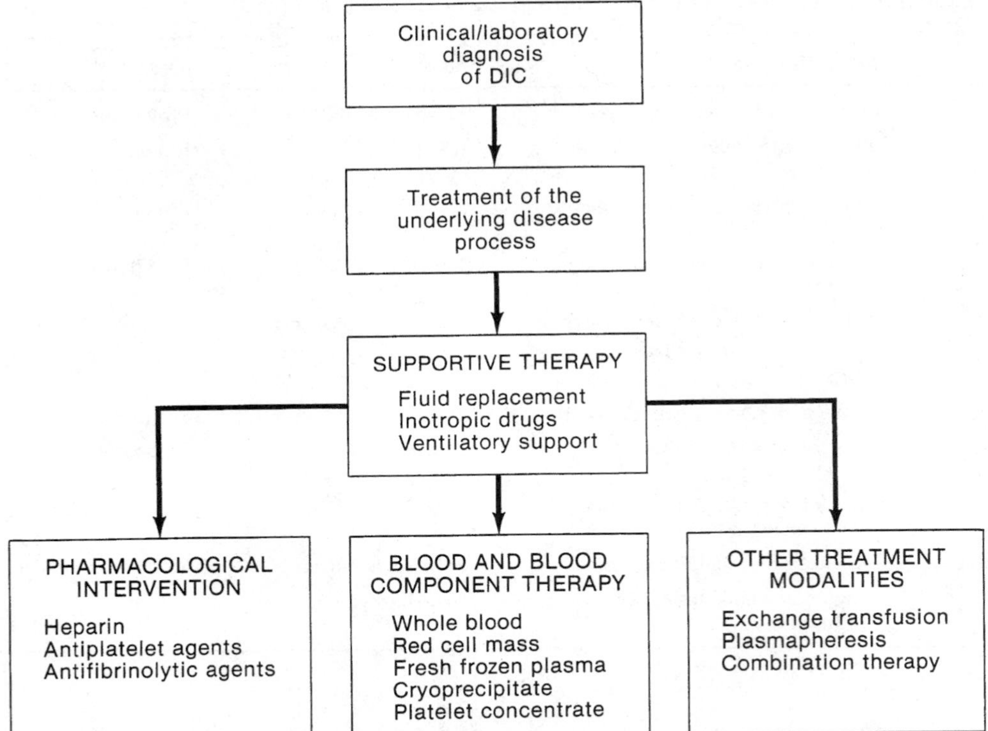

FIGURE 54–4. Medical management of disseminated intravascular coagulation.

Most sources agree that reversal of the DIC syndrome depends first on prompt treatment of the underlying disorder (Bell, 1993; Bick, 1992). For example, if the syndrome was precipitated by gram-negative sepsis, appropriate intravenous antibiotic therapy is begun immediately. Nonspecific supportive therapy is also very important in preventing further deterioration in the patient's condition. Ventilatory assistance may be necessary to ensure adequate oxygenation. Circulatory support with fluid replacement and inotropic drugs are often needed until hemodynamic factors are stabilized. When ATN complicates the situation, hemodialysis may eventually be necessary. The circulatory shock that accompanies the DIC syndrome contributes to the degree of shock and acidosis. Because DIC is perpetuated by these pathophysiologic alterations, every attempt is made to reverse them. Aggressive treatment of the underlying disorder and appropriate supportive treatment will halt the DIC process in some patients.

ANTICOAGULANT THERAPY. Anticoagulant therapy may be used in the treatment of DIC, and although no randomized clinical trials have documented the efficacy, numerous case reports describe the effective use of heparin (Bell, 1993). Heparin therapy is used in patients with acute and chronic DIC. Heparin activates the antithrombin III system and interrupts the intravascular generation of thrombin, preventing further deposition of fibrin in the microcirculation. Although heparin does not alter clots that have already formed, it does slow down the coagulation process enough to allow clotting factor replacement and restore a normal balance (Bell, 1993). When heparin is used, the antithrombin III level may be measured first. Fresh frozen plasma may then be administered to increase the plasma antithrombin III level. Therapeutic or low doses of heparin may be given, and the patient is carefully monitored for response to the drug. Some clinicians prefer subcutaneous to intravenous heparin (Bick, 1992). Laboratory control of heparin therapy is difficult due to the multiple alterations in coagulation parameters already present. Administration of heparin to a patient with actual or potential bleeding seems paradoxical, and this is probably the only time heparin may be given to a bleeding patient (Williams et al., 1990). It may be contraindicated in some patients such as those with CNS or GI tract bleeding or recent surgery.

Other pharmacologic agents may be used in the treatment of DIC. Platelet inhibitors such as dipyridamole and aspirin are being investigated for use in DIC. Antifibrinolytic agents such as aminocaproic acid (Amicar) may be avoided because of the potential complication of fatal thromboembolism associated with their use. When antifibrinolytic agents are used, heparin is administered first (Colman et al., 1991). Investigational protocols using synthetic antithrombin agents and newer antifibrinolytic agents such as tranexamic acid are being studied (Bell, 1993; Bick, 1992).

BLOOD COMPONENT THERAPY. The value of whole blood and blood component therapy in DIC is somewhat controversial. Some sources caution that administration of components may be adding "fuel to the fire" because more fibrinogen and platelets are available for further clotting (Bell, 1993). However, in patients who develop a bleeding diathesis due to DIC, it is usually necessary to replace the losses. In clinical practice, the greater the blood loss, the more blood and blood components will be given to replace lost volume and restore hemostasis and oxygen-carrying capacity. Most commonly, red cell mass, whole blood, fresh frozen plasma, platelet concentrate, and cryoprecipitate are given. Fresh frozen plasma restores factor V, prothrombin, and other essential clotting factors. Fibrinogen and factor VIII can be replaced with cryoprecipitate. Whole blood and blood components do not contain active platelets, so platelet concentrate may be given to replace these (Coffland & Shelton, 1993).

OTHER THERAPEUTIC MEASURES. As in all situations involving hypovolemic shock, intravenous fluid resuscitation is necessary to restore depleted intracellular and extracellular fluid volume. Lactated Ringer's solution, normal saline, and plasma protein fraction (albumin) are titrated to maintain adequate blood pressure, central venous pressure (CVP), pulmonary artery wedge pressure (PAWP), and urine output. Hemodynamic monitoring facilitates appropriate fluid resuscitation. Optimizing ventilation and oxygenation with ventilatory support enhances tissue respiration and assists in maintaining organ viability.

Other therapeutic measures may include exchange transfusions and plasmapheresis. It is thought that exchanging the patient's plasma removes FDPs and supplies fresh clotting components. Often a combination of therapies may be used such as heparin and blood transfusion. Research on these and other therapeutic measures for DIC continues.

Even with prompt and aggressive treatment, it may take hours to days to control the bleeding (Colman et al., 1991). Mortality from DIC is estimated to range from 50% to 80% (Bell, 1993). Mortality increases with the patient's age, the number of clinical manifestations prsent, and the severity of alterations in the coagulation parameters.

OTHER ACQUIRED COAGULATION DISORDERS

In addition to DIC, other acquired coagulation problems are commonly seen in critical care. The basic pathophysiology, clinical features, laboratory features, and medical management of the more common disorders will be described next.

Vitamin K Deficiency

Vitamin K is normally obtained from food, especially green leafy vegetables. It is also synthesized by microbiologic flora in the normal GI tract. As shown in Figure 54–5, vitamin K is absorbed by the GI tract in the presence of bile salts and pancreatic lipases. It is required for the hepatic synthesis of prothrombin (factor II) and factors VII, IX, and X (Kimbrell, 1993). A deficiency of vitamin K is uncommon in healthy people but can result from inadequate intake in critically ill and chronically ill patients. Patients receiving total parenteral nutrition are at risk because this vitamin is not metabolized when it is administered through a central venous line (Colman et al., 1991); it must be administered separately.

Other patients may have inadequate absorption of

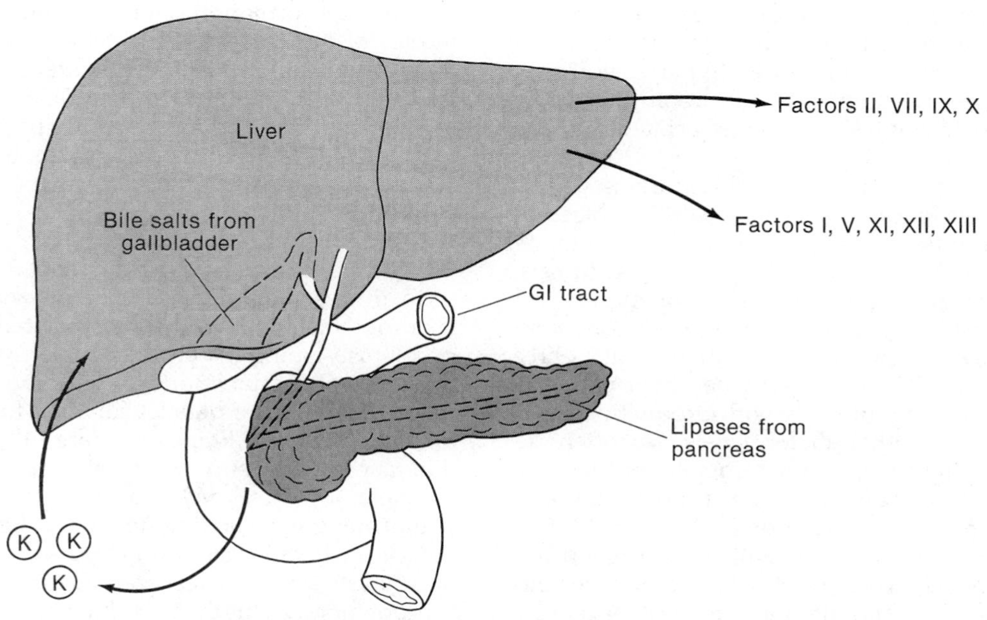

FIGURE 54–5. Production of coagulation factors by the liver.

the vitamin due to fat malabsorption or a lack of bile salts, as might occur in patients with biliary obstruction or pancreatic disease. Antibiotic therapy, especially therapy with broad-spectrum antibiotics, may interfere with the synthesis of vitamin K by intestinal flora. The amount of vitamin K available for production of coagulation factors may be significantly decreased.

Clinical features of vitamin K deficiency include cutaneous ecchymosis, epistaxis, GI bleeding, and the potential for postoperative hemorrhage. There are no specific laboratory tests diagnostic of vitamin K deficiency. In most instances, the PT is prolonged. The patient's history is important in making the diagnosis.

Treatment of vitamin K deficiency generally involves administration of vitamin K preparations. Attempts are also made to correct the cause of the disorder. Transfusion therapy may be appropriate if severe hemorrhage and factor deficiencies develop.

In addition to acquired vitamin K deficiency, the syndrome is commonly present in newborn babies (Lee et al., 1993). During the first few days of life, the liver may be unable to synthesize vitamin K–dependent clotting factors, and intestinal flora are not yet present to synthesize the vitamin. This syndrome, called hemorrhagic disease of the newborn, is generally treated with prophylactic administration of vitamin K at birth.

Liver Disease

Alterations in liver function often result in coagulation abnormalities. As shown in Figure 54–5, the liver synthesizes almost all coagulation factors (except factor VIII), including fibrinogen, factor V, and the vitamin K–dependent factors (Colman et al., 1991). Liver problems such as cirrhosis and hepatic failure limit the production of these coagulation factors, resulting directly in clotting deficiencies. In addition, thrombocytopenia may complicate the situation because patients with chronic liver disease and portal hypertension may have congestive splenomegaly and pooling of platelets. Increased fibrinolysis is also associated with hepatic insufficiency.

Easy bruising is a mild clinical feature associated with these deficiencies. However, serious bleeding may follow trauma or surgery. Local lesions in the GI tract such as esophageal varices or peptic ulcer can also lead to severe bleeding. Portacaval shunt surgery, fulminating hepatitis, and terminal liver disease are associated with severe hemorrhage (Colman et al., 1991).

The PT is usually prolonged when liver problems are severe enough to interfere with production of coagulation factors. Other factor levels are often depressed, including the vitamin K–dependent factors.

Treatment of bleeding due to liver disease involves treatment of the underlying problem. Vitamin K may be administered. Transfusion with whole blood and blood components is often necessary and may be helpful but is only a temporary measure unless there is hope for recovery of hepatic function. Desmopressin (DDAVP) may also be administered to reduce bleeding in patients with liver disease (Schulman, 1991).

Bleeding Due to Anticoagulant Therapy

Clinical indications for the use of anticoagulants include actual or potential thromboembolism. This suppression of the normal coagulation process always carries with it the risk of bleeding, either spontaneous or provoked. Spontaneous bleeding most often occurs in the form of ecchymoses, GI bleeding, hematuria, and retroperitoneal hemorrhage. Bleeding may also be precipitated during trauma from surgery or invasive procedures. Patients at increased risk of bleeding complications from anticoagulant therapy include those who have had recent surgery and those with a history of GI bleeding.

WARFARIN. Warfarin, because of its predictable action and duration of effect, is the oral anticoagulant most commonly used. It inhibits production of vitamin K–dependent factors, including the pivotal factor prothrombin (Dunn & Senerchia, 1993). The PT is monitored in patients receiving warfarin; the usual therapeutic goal is to achieve a PT of 1½ times to 2 times the control value, between 15 and 26 seconds or International Normalized Ratio (INR) of 2.0 to 3.0. Antiplatelet agents may be given concurrently, so that the PT does not need to be prolonged beyond 1½ times the control, decreasing the incidence of bleeding. The effects of warfarin can be reversed by stopping the drug. More rapid reversal can be achieved by administering vitamin K and fresh frozen plasma.

HEPARIN. Heparin, the most commonly used intravenous anticoagulant, acts by combining with antithrombin III to inhibit thrombin and other factors, preventing clot formation (Dunn & Senerchia, 1993). The modes of heparin therapy include full-dose intravenous therapy and low-dose subcutaneous heparin. The APTT is most commonly monitored in patients receiving heparin. Therapeutic levels are usually considered to be 1½ to 2 times the control value. Intravenous protamine sulfate can be given to reverse the effects of heparin.

ANTIPLATELET DRUGS. Antiplatelet drugs such as aspirin are used commonly in patients with cardiovascular problems and have been associated with bleeding problems. Aspirin affects the platelet synthesis of prostaglandin and thus interferes with the platelet release reaction, inhibiting platelet function for the life of the platelet (Halfman-Franey & Berg, 1991). Because of this, aspirin ingestion will have an effect on blood platelets for 4 to 7 days. In most patients, this effect will prolong the bleeding time only slightly. However, defects in hemostasis are magnified in patients who have taken aspirin. Ingestion of a single aspirin tablet can potentially lengthen the bleeding time to 30 min-

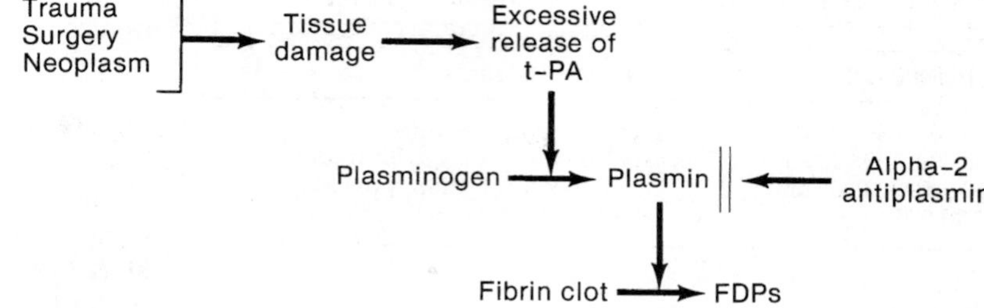

FIGURE 54–6. Primary fibrinolysis. FDP, fibrin degradation products.

utes (from a normal of 5 to 8 minutes) and can induce hemorrhage in patients who are prone to coagulation problems. The drug desmopressin may be used to promote hemostasis in patients who have ingested aspirin (Colman et al., 1991).

Renal Failure

The coagulation derangements that accompany renal failure can result in serious clinical problems. The bleeding tendency in these patients is thought to be caused mainly by a qualitative platelet defect (Colman et al., 1991). The metabolic imbalances that result from uremia have an adverse effect on platelet function.

Treatment of the renal failure itself, such as with dialysis and a low-protein diet, often improves coagulation abnormalities because the problem is proportional to the blood urea nitrogen. Blood and blood component therapy may be used to treat acute anemia. Recombinant erythropoietin is administered to stimulate erythrocyte production (Coffland & Shelton, 1993). Desmopressin has also been used to improve platelet function temporarily in patients with renal failure.

Pathologic Fibrinolysis

Primary pathologic fibrinolysis is an acute and severe bleeding disorder that can resemble DIC. However, it must be distinguished from DIC because the treatment differs. As shown in Figure 54–6, excessive fibrinolysis results when tissue plasminogen activator (t-PA) is suddenly released into the blood (Lee et al., 1993). This syndrome can be induced by cardiothoracic surgery, metastatic cancer of the prostate, injury to the genitourinary tract, or other extensive trauma. Following the release of t-PA, newly formed clots are broken down, and recently injured blood vessels resume bleeding. The disorder is most severe when it occurs in conjunction with hepatic insufficiency because in this condition there is insufficient production of alpha-2 antiplasmin, the naturally occurring substance that inactivates plasmin and controls fibrinolysis. A fibrinolytic state may also be produced intentionally with administration of fibrinolytic agents such as streptokinase, urokinase, and recombinant t-PA. Bleeding resulting from excessive fibrinolysis may be a complication of the drug therapy.

The major clinical feature of pathologic fibrinolysis is posttraumatic or postoperative bleeding. In addition to bleeding from injury sites, internal bleeding from ulcerations in the GI tract may occur.

Coagulation parameters pertinent to fibrinolysis are abnormal. The level of FDPs and D-dimers are elevated, the euglobulin clot lysis time short, and the plasminogen level decreased. Factors such as platelets may not be depleted as they are in DIC. Differential diagnosis can be difficult because fibrinolysis occurs as a secondary process in DIC.

The usual treatment for pathologic fibrinolysis is administration of an inhibitor of fibrinolysis such as aminocaproic acid (Amicar). This agent prevents lysis of microvascular thrombi and the subsequent release of FDPs. After a series of intravenous doses of this drug, bleeding will usually cease (Colman et al., 1991). The drug is usually contraindicated in DIC because of the risk of major thrombosis after administration in these patients (Lee et al., 1993).

Thrombocytopenia

Platelets play a role in many places in the coagulation process, from plugging small tears in capillaries to providing phospholipids for clot formation and retraction. An inadequate number of platelets inhibit the coagulation process and can lead to both minor and major bleeding problems.

Thrombocytopenia can occur as a result of decreased production, increased destruction, or pooling of platelets in the spleen (Coffland & Shelton, 1993). Decreased production of platelets in the bone marrow is associated with leukemia, various anemias, and uremia. This is also a well-recognized side effect of cancer chemotherapy and radiation therapy. Increased destruction of platelets can occur in patients with severe infectious processes, diseases of the liver and spleen, and autoimmune disease. Reduced platelet survival is also associated with cardiopulmonary bypass and the intraaortic balloon pump. Pooling of platelets in the spleen is associated with disorders that produce splenomegaly.

A platelet count of under 150,000/mm^3 is diagnostic of thrombocytopenia. The clinical features of thrombocytopenia may include petechiae, bleeding from mucous membranes, and actual hemorrhage. However, bleeding due to thrombocytopenia is difficult to predict. Some patients with a severely low

TABLE 54–4. **Bleeding from Thrombocytopenia**

Platelet Count	Effect on Hemostasis
150,000–400,000/mm^3	No abnormal bleeding
50,000–150,000/mm^3	Abnormal bleeding with trauma
10,000–50,000/mm^3	Spontaneous bleeding possible
<10,000/mm^3	Severe spontaneous bleeding common

platelet count may not bleed, whereas others with moderately depressed counts may experience major bleeding. As shown in Table 54–4, spontaneous bleeding usually does not occur until the platelet count falls below 50,000/mm^3 (Guyton, 1991). As the platelet count falls, the risk of bleeding increases, and below 10,000/mm^3 there is considerable risk of spontaneous CNS or GI hemorrhage (Halfman-Franey & Berg, 1991).

When possible, thrombocytopenia is treated by treating the underlying cause. For example, if it is thought to be a side effect of a drug, the drug is stopped. Platelet transfusions are indicated in patients at risk of spontaneous or provoked bleeding.

It must also be recognized that there are qualitative disorders of platelet function. The number of platelets present in the blood may not always predict their hemostatic capability, especially in patients who have received platelet-inhibiting drugs. When platelet dysfunction is suspected, platelet concentrate may be administered to provide active platelets. The drug desmopressin may be given to increase the plasma level of von Willebrand factor and improve hemostasis in conditions associated with defective platelet function (Schulman, 1991).

Another type of thrombocytopenia that is not associated with bleeding is seen in conjunction with heparin administration. Heparin can cause two types of thrombocytopenia (Dunn & Senerchia, 1993). There may be a transient fall in the platelet count with an initial loading dose of heparin due to the direct action of heparin on platelets. In addition, a second and more serious reaction can occur, involving a delayed but precipitous fall in the platelet count following the administration of full- or low-dose heparin (Harrington & Hufnagel, 1990). The mechanism is thought to involve the production of antiplatelet antibodies that induce clotting. This syndrome of heparin-induced thrombocytopenia is associated with recurrent venous and arterial thrombosis. Major thrombotic events such as stroke, myocardial infarction, pulmonary emboli, and thrombotic occlusion of major vessels may occur. The documented incidence of this syndrome in patients receiving heparin is as high as 10%. Because of this risk, it is recommended that platelet counts be monitored before and during heparin administration. Laboratory testing for heparin antibodies may also be appropriate in certain patients who have received heparin on numerous occasions. When the syndrome is suspected, heparin must be discontinued, including even small amounts used in hemodynamic monitoring lines.

Postoperative Coagulopathy

Postoperative coagulopathy can occur after many surgical procedures, but is most commonly associated with cardiovascular surgery (Atkins, 1993). The patient undergoing these procedures may be predisposed to bleeding problems due to preoperative anticoagulation or previous surgical procedures and consequent development of adhesions. Excessive bleeding is a serious complication that can lead to hypovolemic shock, decreased oxygen transport, and cardiac tamponade (Halfman-Franey & Berg, 1991).

It is important to distinguish between bleeding due to incomplete surgical hemostasis and coagulopathy. Increased blood loss from chest tubes alone is usually an indicator of surgical bleeding. Patients who develop oozing or bleeding from all surgical sites and invasive monitoring sites, hematuria, petechiae, or purpura may have coagulopathy.

Platelet functional impairment is thought to be the most common cause of postoperative bleeding (Mongan & Hosking, 1992). Mechanical damage to platelets, adhesion to foreign surfaces, and consumption of platelets are known to occur during cardiopulmonary bypass. The degree of platelet dysfunction is proportional to the duration of cardiopulmonary bypass and depth of hypothermia (Halfman-Franey & Berg, 1991). Contact between the blood and the oxygenator results in platelet alteration and activation of both the coagulation and fibrinolytic systems.

In addiiton to the use of cardiopulmonary bypass, the associated heparinization, hypothermia, and hemodilution are intraoperative elements that contribute to the potential for bleeding (Atkins, 1993). Heparin is given to prevent blood clotting within the tubing and oxygenator, and needs to be reversed with adequate amounts of protamine as circulatory support is discontinued. Inadequate reversal of heparin with continuing inability to form clots is a potential problem. Hypothermia decreases metabolic oxygen requirements during surgery, but can adversely affect coagulation by causing vasoconstriction with resultant hypertension that stretches suture lines. Hypothermia can also lead to platelet dysfunction, prolonged coagulation, and increased fibrinolytic activity. Finally, hemodilution reduces the concentration of clotting components.

Treatment of postoperative bleeding is directed by clinical and laboratory evaluation. Reoperation and surgical hemostasis are indicated when excessive surgical bleeding or cardiac tamponade are suspected. Because quantitative and qualitative platelet defects are a common problem, intervention may be directed toward restoring platelet function through platelet infusions or administration of desmopressin. Replacement of blood and blood components containing active coagulation factors is guided by serial coagulation determinations (Atkins, 1993). Antifibrinolytic agents may be given when hyperfibrinolysis is suspected. Aprotinin, a new inhibitor of fibrinolysis, has been shown to improve hemostasis and reduce intraoperative blood loss (Harder et al., 1991). In addition to the antifibrinolytic effect, aprotinin has been shown to be particularly effective when given to patients who have been taking aspirin or who have renal impairment (Halfman-Franey & Berg, 1991).

CLINICAL MANAGEMENT OF THE PATIENT WITH COAGULOPATHY

In addition to medical diagnosis and treatment, specific nursing interventions are necessary to treat existing problems and prevent potential problems during a coagulation crisis. An understanding of the pathophysiology of bleeding disorders plus their clinical recognition and medical management suggests the following priorities of clinical management.

Recognition of Coagulopathy

In patients with coagulopathy, essential clotting components are often depleted, and fibrinolysis may be activated, predisposing the patient to potential hemorrhage and severe volume depletion. The expected outcomes of nursing care include early recognition of overt and covert bleeding and early control of bleeding.

The critical care nurse plays a key role in the recognition of a bleeding problem. Critically ill patients may be unable to report signs and symptoms of coagulopathy. All incisions, puncture sites, and skin lesions are observed for signs of bleeding. Because the mucous membranes bleed easily, it is important to watch for epistaxis and bleeding from the gums after mouth care is given. Expanding hematomas and swollen extremities need to be measured and monitored because bleeding into the muscles and compartments can occur insidiously. Abdominal girth should be assessed at intervals when peritoneal bleeding is suspected.

Exit sites of tubes and catheters are inspected periodically. Surgical drainage containers need to be checked for increased drainage. Tracheal secretions are observed for evidence of pulmonary hemorrhage. It is particularly important to watch for bleeding from more than one source. Bleeding from multiple sites is often a sign of a coagulation problem and must be reported. Early identification of bleeding and initiation of treatment can minimize blood loss.

In critically ill patients, bleeding can lead to shock within a short period. Vital signs are evaluated for evidence of hypotension, labile blood pressure, low CVP or low PAWP, tachycardia, and weak thready pulse. These signs may be indicative of occult bleeding. Extremities are inspected for evidence of poor perfusion such as coldness, delayed capillary refill, weak or absent peripheral pulses, and cyanosis. Urine output is assessed frequently because oliguria may result from hypotension, decreased blood volume, or thrombi in the renal vasculature.

Urine, stools, and nasogastric drainage are tested for occult blood. X-rays are checked for unexpected fluid collection. Changes in the level of consciousness are carefully evaluated because cerebral anoxia can occur as a result of hypovolemia, hypoxemia, and emboli. Patient reports of headache, joint pain, or abdominal pain are carefully assessed.

When a coagulation problem is suspected, laboratory data are monitored for a drop in hemoglobin and hematocrit and for changes in coagulation parameters. A flow sheet or computerized report that displays trends in laboratory data may be helpful in detecting problems, such as a falling platelet count. Changes in the laboratory data may be evident before clinical bleeding occurs, and likewise, improvement in coagulation parameters may be evident before bleeding decreases.

Management of Coagulopathy

In patients with a coagulopathy, a large amount of blood may be lost within a short period. Expected outcomes of nursing care include prevention of acute anemia, acute anoxia, and hypovolemic circulatory failure.

When a bleeding problem is identified, nursing care is directed toward minimizing the loss of blood. The patient is placed on bed rest, and oxygen therapy is adjusted to meet specific needs. The amount and character of the bleeding are reported to the physician. Care is taken not to disturb any clots during dressing changes because patients with coagulopathy may be unable to form new clots. Local measures such as pressure and cold compresses may be used to control bleeding from skin sites. Topical hemostatic agents may be prescribed. Bleeding from the GI tract, genitourinary tract, or respiratory tract may require specific medical intervention.

The patient with a coagulopathy must be continuously monitored for signs and symptoms of hypovolemic shock. Fluid volume replacement is initiated to replace extracellular and intracellular volume and restore adequate blood pressure and cardiac filling pressures.

It is important to be aware of all drug actions and interactions related to coagulation. For example, aspirin or other anticoagulants should not be given unintentionally to a patient with a coagulopathy. When anticoagulant medication such as heparin is ordered for patients with DIC, the patient must be closely monitored for increased bleeding or other untoward effects. Laboratory values such as APTT are checked periodically but are often difficult to interpret due to multiple abnormalities. Because of this, clinical assessment of the patient is particularly important.

When active hemorrhage occurs, whole blood and

TABLE 54–5. **Blood and Blood Components**

Component	Contents	Indication	Shelf Life	Comments
Whole blood cells	Red blood cells (RBCs), plasma, all components	Acute active hemorrhagic, hypovolemic shock	42 days	Restores blood volume and oxygen-carrying capacity
Red cell mass	RBCs, little plasma, white blood cells (WBCs), or platelets	Anemia, hypovolemic shock	Same as whole blood	Same oxygen-carrying capacity as whole blood; less volume, less plasma decreases reactions
Fresh frozen plasma	Plasma with most coagulation factors; no platelets	Many coagulation disorders, factor deficiencies	12 months frozen, 2 hours thawed	Give as soon as thawed
Cryoprecipitate	Factors I and VIII	Disseminated intravascular coagulation, hemophilia, von Willebrand factor deficiency	12 months frozen, 4 hours thawed	Give as soon as thawed
Platelet concentrate	Platelets, few WBCs, and some plasma	Bleeding due to thrombocytopenia	5 days	No refrigeration; multiple units given together. Each unit should raise count by 5000 to 10,000
Albumin, plasma protein fraction	Heat-treated fraction of pooled plasma	Volume or colloid deficiency	3 to 5 years	Use as volume expander while blood is cross-matched

blood components need to be administered by methods which ensure maximum effectiveness. Transfusion therapy aims to restore oxygen-carrying capacity with red cells, and to replace deficient factors needed for hemostasis. Component therapy supplies the specific factors needed, with less risk of fluid overload than whole blood.

Table 54–5 outlines the blood components used most often to treat coagulopathies. Whole blood may be used in patients with acute hemorrhagic shock. It restores blood volume and oxygen-carrying capacity. Red cell mass is used more commonly. Each unit of red cell mass has the same oxygen-carrying capacity as whole blood but less volume and less serum containing the undesirable amounts of potassium, glucose, ammonia, and anticoagulant. After transfusion, the hemoglobin and hematocrit should increase and stabilize. An increase in SaO_2 and $S\bar{v}O_2$ are indicative of increased tissue perfusion (Coffland & Shelton, 1993).

Fresh frozen plasma contains most active coagulation factors except platelets. It is used for patients with specific factor deficiencies, such as a low level of factor V. Fresh frozen plasma may also be administered when the specific deficiency is unknown because it contains so many essential components. This particular component should be infused as soon as it is thawed because some of the coagulation factors become inactive with time.

Cryoprecipitate is also commonly prescribed to treat patients with coagulation disorders such as DIC. It contains fibrinogen and factor VIII. Infusion of multiple units is required to replace depleted factors. Cryoprecipitate should also be infused as soon as possible after thawing.

Platelet concentrate is frequently given for bleeding due to thrombocytopenia or qualitative platelet disorders. Multiple donor units are given to attempt to raise the platelet count above 50,000 / mm^3 and prevent spontaneous bleeding (Coffland & Shelton, 1993).

Patients with a coagulopathy frequently undergo massive blood transfusion. They must be closely monitored for adverse reactions related to the infusion of blood and blood components. Table 54–6 outlines the adverse reactions that may be observed.

During massive transfusion it is particularly important to measure hemodynamic parameters, including CVP and PAWP, before, during, and after the infusion of each unit of blood or blood component. Replacing the patient's blood loss is important to prevent shock, yet volume overload can easily become a complication of transfusion therapy. The appearance of dyspnea, rales, and pulmonary congestion may indicate fluid volume overload.

Hypothermia can result from rapid infusion of cold blood and blood components, leading to chills, decreased body temperature, and ventricular dysrhythmias. These symptoms are especially prevalent when

TABLE 54–6. **Transfusion Reactions**

- Complications of massive transfusion
  - Fluid overload
  - Hypothermia
  - Hyperkalemia
  - Citrate intoxication, hypocalcemia
  - Massive transfusion syndrome
- Febrile reaction
- Hypersensitivity reaction
- Hemolytic reaction
- Bacterial reaction
- Late reactions
  - Hepatitis
  - Cytomegalovirus
  - Human immunodeficiency virus infection

the blood is infused through a central venous line. It may be necessary to use a blood warmer when infusing multiple units.

Hyperkalemia can result from the infusion of multiple units of blood as potassium diffuses from the intracellular space into the extracellular fluid in stored blood, increasing the serum potassium level in the plasma. When large volumes of blood are infused, the electrocardiogram should be continuously monitored for changes indicative of hyperkalemia, such as peaked T waves, widening QRS complexes, and bradycardia.

Citrate intoxication and hypocalcemia may also result from the infusion of large amounts of stored blood. The anticoagulant that prevents blood from clotting in the blood bag is citrate. Citrate acts by precipitating the serum calcium. Because calcium is necessary for blood coagulation, the blood does not clot. Infusion of large amounts of citrate can potentially precipitate the patient's serum calcium. This further decreases the ability of the blood to clot and may result in signs of hypocalcemic tetany. Because of these potential problems, the physician may prescribe intravenous calcium chloride to be administered in patients undergoing multiple blood transfusions.

Massive transfusion syndrome, a severe depletion of coagulation components, can occur as blood is lost and replaced with stored blood. When blood is stored, platelets and coagulation factors are inactivated over hours to days. Following transfusion, the patient's blood becomes diluted and deficient in active coagulation factors (Atkins, 1993). This problem is magnified in patients who are unable to produce new coagulation factors, such as those with liver disease. Because of the potential for this problem in patients undergoing massive transfusion, periodic coagulation panels are analyzed to determine the need for specific component replacement.

In addition to the complications associated with massive transfusion, other reactions to the transfusion of blood and blood components may occur. The most common reaction is a febrile response caused by the reaction to donor platelets, lymphocytes, and granulocytes (Coffland & Shelton, 1993). Fever, chills, and tachycardia may be observed during or following transfusion, and the transfusion may need to be stopped. Patients known to have a history of this type of reaction can be premedicated with an antipyretic such as acetaminophen. Leukocyte-poor blood can be administered to avoid febrile reactions.

Hypersensitivity reactions can occur when a patient is hypersensitive to transfused allergens. These reactions may be mild or serious. Urticaria and wheezing occur most commonly, but an anaphylactic reaction is possible. The transfusion is stopped when a hypersensitivity reaction occurs, and the patient is given an antihistamine. For severe reactions, steroids or vasopressors may be necessary. Allergy-prone patients may be premedicated with an antihistamine such as diphenhydramine hydrochloride.

With current blood banking standards and typing and crossmatching techniques, hemolytic reactions due to incompatible blood are extremely rare. However, it is always necessary to follow policies related to checking patient and blood identification. Patients are observed closely for signs of hemolytic reaction such as chest tightness, chills, low back pain, hemoglobinuria, and shock. Bacterial contamination is also rare. Nevertheless, blood should be examined prior to administration for unusual color, separation, or gas bubbles. Clinical manifestations of diseases transmitted by transfusion such as hepatitis, cytomegalovirus, and other organisms do not appear for many weeks. Patients who have received multiple transfusions of components containing pooled plasma are at greatest risk.

With current attention to transmission of blood-borne disease, blood conservation techniques are used whenever possible. For some bleeding patients, autotransfusion of shed blood may be an option (Johnson & Bowman, 1992). Autotransfusion of mediastinal blood is used in many centers during and after cardiac surgery. The growing availability of autotransfusion systems and the concern about disease transmission from homologous blood have resulted in an increase in the use of autotransfusion. The advantages of autotransfusion include high oxygen-carrying capacity due to high levels of 2,3-diphosphoglycerate, normal pH, and normal temperature. Shed blood contains near-normal clotting factors but a lower hematocrit. It is relatively inexpensive, and there is little risk of disease transmission.

An option for the future may be the use of artificial blood. Currently artificial blood substitutes (perfluorochemicals) can be used on an investigational basis for patients who refuse blood transfusion for religious or other reasons (Marelli, 1994). Fluosol DA can be administered intravenously to support the severely anemic patient. It is an emulsion of water and two perfluorochemicals that has the ability to transport oxygen. This blood substitute can be used to provide temporary support, but will not help the patient who is actively bleeding. Other nonblood options may include folic acid, multiple vitamins containing B_6 and B_{12}, intravenous iron, and erythropoietin.

Prevention of Complications

Because of the patient's potential for bleeding, trauma and hemorrhage can occur with routine critical care procedures. Prevention of vascular and tissue trauma is a crucial expected outcome of nursing care.

Bleeding precautions need to be instituted immediately when a patient develops a coagulopathy. Needle sticks must be avoided to minimize the risk of bleeding and hematoma formation. Indwelling arterial and venous lines are used whenever possible to draw blood and to administer medications. If needle sticks are necessary, a small-gauge needle should be used, and pressure should be applied to the site for 5 to 10 minutes with periodic inspection of the site later.

All staff members must be alerted to the patient's potential for bleeding when invasive procedures are planned. Invasive and surgical procedures may need to be postponed in patients with a coagulopathy until hemostasis is restored. The risk of inserting hemodynamic monitoring lines may be too great during periods of active bleeding.

Other measures can be taken to prevent trauma in these high-risk patients. Patients need to be bathed and turned with enough assistance to prevent trauma. Side rails and sharp objects in the environment need to be padded if the patient is restless. Gentle skin care can be carried out with a mild lotion to minimize skin trauma. Only electric razors should be used for shaving. The teeth should be brushed gently using a foam toothbrush or swab. Frequent mouth care prevents drying and cracking of the oral mucosa, which bleeds easily in patients with coagulation disorders. In patients who are able to take food and fluids orally, liquids and soft foods are tolerated best because there may be irritated or ischemic areas within the oral cavity.

It may be necessary to avoid using a blood pressure cuff because the pressure of the inflated cuff can cause petechiae and ecchymotic skin lesions. Rectal temperature taking and suppositories are also avoided to prevent trauma to the mucous membranes.

If oral or tracheal suctioning is necessary, very low suction is used to prevent trauma to the trachea. Continuous humidity is provided to the respiratory tract to minimize drying and bleeding of mucous membranes.

Pain Management

Painful hematomas can result from bleeding into the tissues. Ischemic tissue pain can result from the deposition of fibrin in the peripheral circulation. Fear and anxiety in patients experiencing hemorrhage or thrombosis can increase the perception of pain and block the effectiveness of usual coping behaviors. Expected outcomes of nursing care include the verbalization of increased comfort and demonstration of a relaxed posture and facial expression.

Patients who are ill with a coagulopathy may be unable to communicate that they are having pain. It may be necessary to observe them for physiologic indicators of discomfort, such as diaphoresis, pallor, tachycardia, and tachypnea. The skin and extremities need to be carefully assessed for the presence of joint or muscle pain, which indicate bleeding into these tissues.

Intervention for pain is difficult because these patients are often hypovolemic and easily become hypotensive after administration of intravenous analgesics. It may be necessary to give small doses of medication and monitor the blood pressure frequently. In addition to analgesic medication, all other comfort measures need to be provided. These patients may benefit from the use of a flotation mattress. Periodic repositioning with pillows or soft bath blankets will also enhance comfort.

Patients with DIC or other coagulopathies can easily become exhausted because of the need for continuous care. This can further increase their degree of stress and discomfort. Allowing rest periods of 30 minutes after activities such as turning, bathing, or x-rays can help to prevent exhaustion.

Isolation from the patient's family tends to increase as the complexity of care increases. Short visits by the family can help to minimize the distress experienced by the bleeding patient and promote relaxation and comfort. Providing reassurance to a patient and family during events as distressing as hemorrhage is always difficult. The situation can be particularly distressing because the coagulopathy is often a complication of another life-threatening disorder such as sepsis, extensive trauma, or malignancy. It may be helpful to list all the measures being used to control the bleeding such as transfusion of blood components and medications. It can also be helpful to point out any signs of improvement that may not be obvious, such as a rising platelet count. Providing honest information and emotional support can help the patient and family set realistic short-term goals and enhance their coping abilities during what is obviously a complex situation.

PREVENTION OF COAGULOPATHIES

Prevention of bleeding problems is a combined medical and nursing responsibility. The following strategies can be helpful in minimizing bleeding problems.

A careful patient history related to bleeding should be obtained before performing invasive procedures or surgery. A history of repeated bleeding problems such as epistaxis, bleeding following dental procedures, and bleeding following labor and delivery can be a reliable predictor of postoperative problems. Patients with a history of chronic renal failure, liver failure, cancer, or inflammatory diseases are predisposed to bleeding (Coffland & Shelton, 1993). A careful history should also include the family history related to spontaneous bleeding or bleeding following trauma.

Each patient's medication history is very important, especially that related to the times anticoagulants were started and stopped. With the increasing number of drugs that affect coagulation in common use, it has become an important role of nurses to assist in the identification of patients at risk of bleeding. Nurses may also be involved in coordinating regimens prescribed by different physicians who are unaware of the patient's cumulative medication profile. For example, in a patient who develops complete heart block and is scheduled for insertion of a permanent pacemaker, the cardiologist may be unaware that warfarin has been prescribed by another physician.

Table 54–7 lists some of the drugs commonly used in critically ill patients that have a known effect on coagulation. Use of aspirin, nonsteroidal antiinflammatory drugs, warfarin, or broad-spectrum antibiotics

TABLE 54–7. **Drugs With Anticoagulant Effects**

Major anticoagulants	Corticosteroids
Heparin	Platelet-inhibiting agents
Warfarin	Dipyridamole
Dicumarol	Sulfinpyrazone
Thrombolytic agents	Clofibrate
Streptokinase	Dextran
Urokinase	Aspirin
Tissue plasminogen activator	Antibiotics
Nonsteroidal antiinflammatory agents	Carbenicillin
Aspirin	Ampicillin
Indomethacin	Penicillin
Naproxen	Chloramphenicol
Ibuprofen	Ethanol
Phenylbutazone	Antidysrhythmic agents
	Fish oil supplements

can increase the risk of bleeding (Atkins, 1993). It should be recognized that many drugs can potentially cause thrombocytopenia. Other drugs may not affect coagulation by themselves but may potentiate the effect of anticoagulants through drug interactions.

During physical examination, patients should be assessed for evidence of hematologic abnormalities. The skin is inspected for petechiae, easy bruising, and jaundice. The abdomen is palpated for hepatosplenomegaly.

Before invasive and surgical procedures, laboratory work is done to assess liver and kidney function. Coagulation parameters are measured when indicated, depending on the patient's history and the nature of the proposed procedure. However, it is recognized that laboratory values may not always accurately predict the potential for bleeding. A new screening test is the Sonoclot or thromboelastograph tracing of whole blood clotting time. This test has been shown to be a sensitive predictor of coagulation problems, including postoperative bleeding (Halfman-Franey & Berg, 1991; Morgan & Hosking, 1992).

Patients themselves can be involved in the prevention of coagulation problems. Teaching patients about the anticoagulant effects of their medications can begin in the critical care unit and continue thoughout the recovery period. Discharge planning for patients receiving anticoagulants should include verbal instructions, clear written information, and facilitation of follow-up care to monitor therapy.

SUMMARY

Few patients challenge the critical care nurse as do those with coagulopathies. Clinical management of the patient with a coagulation disorder includes careful assessment of the patient's clinical status and identification of bleeding risk factors. Individualized interventions are directed toward prevention of bleeding. The nurse collaborates with the physician in treating coagulation problems through the use of pharmacologic agents, blood component therapy, and other appropriate therapeutic interventions.

REFERENCES

Atkins, P. J. (1993). Postoperative coagulopathies. *Critical Care Nursing Clinics of North America, 5*(3), 459–473.

Bell, T. N. (1993). Disseminated intravascular coagulation. *Critical Care Nursing Clinics of North America, 5*(3), 389–410.

Bick, R. L. (1992). Disseminated intravascular coagulation. *Hematology/Oncology Clinics of North America, 6*(6), 1259–1285.

Coffland, F. I., & Shelton, D. M. (1993). Blood component replacement therapy. *Critical Care Nursing Clinics of North America, 5*(3), 543–556.

Colman, R. W., Hirsh, J., Marder, V. J., et al. (1991). Hemostasis and thrombosis: Basic principles and clinical practice (2nd ed.). Philadelphia: J. B. Lippincott.

Dunn, S. M., & Senerchia, C. B. (1993). Bleeding complications in the patient with cardiac disease following thrombolytic and anticoagulant therapies. *Critical Care Nursing Clinics of North America, 5*(3), 511–523.

Halfman-Franey, M., & Berg, D. E. (1991). Recognition and management of bleeding following cardiac surgery. *Critical Care Nursing Clinics of North America, 3*(4), 675–689.

Harder, M. P., Eijsman, L., Roozendaal, K. J., et al. (1991). Aprotinin reduces intraoperative blood loss in membrane oxygenator cardiopulmonary bypass. *Annals of Thoracic Surgery, 51,* 936–941.

Harrington, L., & Hufnagel, J. (1990). Heparin-induced thrombocytopenia and thrombosis syndrome: A case study. *Heart & Lung, 19*(1), 93–98.

Johnson, G. M., & Bowman, R. J. (1992). Autologous blood transfusion—current trends, nursing implications. *Journal of the Association of Operating Room Nurses, 56*(2), 282–291.

Kimbrell, J. D. (1993). Acquired coagulopathies. *Critical Care Nursing Clinics of North America, 5*(3), 453–458.

Lee, G. R., Bithell, T. C., Foerster, J., et al. (1993). Wintrobe's clinical hematology (9th ed). Philadelphia: Lea & Febiger.

Marelli, T. R. (1994). Use of a hemoglobin substitute in the anemic Jehovah's Witness patient. *Critical Care Nurse, 14*(1), 31–38.

Mongan, P. D., & Hosking, M. P. (1992). The role of desmopressin acetate in patients undergoing coronary artery bypass surgery. *Anesthesiology, 77*(1), 38–46.

Secor, V. H. (1993). Mediators of coagulation and inflammation. *Critical Care Clinics of North America, 5*(3), 411–433.

Schulman, S. (1991). DDAVP—the multipotent drug in patients with coagulopathies. *Transfusion Medicine Reviews, 5,* 132–144.

Williams, W. J., Beutler, E., Erslev, A. J., et al. (1990). *Hematology* (4th ed.). New York: McGraw-Hill.

UNIT 11

IMMUNE SYSTEM

Physiologic Response to Infection

M. Linda Workman

Advances in science and technology have led to the development of complex and high-risk therapeutic medical interventions. Interventions such as organ transplantation and ablative cytotoxic chemotherapy directly affect immune function. Patients receiving these aggressive therapies more and more frequently require nursing support in critical care settings. Esperson (1986) suggests that all patients exposed to a critical care enviornment may have lowered immunologic defenses. Thus, a working knowledge of the parts of the immune system and their interaction is essential. Knowing how the immune system works will allow nurses to increase and protect the natural defenses of patients in the critical care setting. This chapter introduces readers to the science of immunology and highlights aspects of immune function most relevant to the critical care setting.

The term *immune* derives from the Latin word *immunis,* which means free from taxes or free from burden. Classically, immunity referred to resistance of the host to reinfection by a given pathogen. A more contemporary definition focuses on the physiologic mechanisms involved in immunity. Immunity enables the body to recognize certain microbes as foreign and to metabolize, neutralize, or eliminate them with or without injury to its own tissues (Abbas et al., 1991). Note that the immune response is a physiologic reaction to the introduction into the body of foreign material, regardless of whether such material is harmful.

BASIC CONCEPTS OF IMMUNOLOGY

Three basic concepts describing the fundamental aspects of immune function are presented before a more complete discussion of immune function. Antigens are the primary stimulants of all immune responses. The major histocompatibility complex provides the basis for discerning foreign substances from our own molecules. Antibody is the key product of immune cell stimulation by antigen. These three concepts lay the foundation for a more complex discussion of the interaction between antigen and antibody in distinguishing self from nonself, which is the hallmark of all immune response (Jackson, 1991).

Antigens and Antigenicity

Antigen is any substance that, when introduced parenterally into an animal, elicits an immune response specifically directed at the inducing substance (Barrett, 1988). Immunogen is a term used to clarify the fact that antigens foster both antibody production and activation of specific immune cell responses. Now the terms antigen and immunogen are used interchangeably. Before describing antigens further, it is necessary to define antibody briefly. Antibodies are proteins produced by specific immune cells. These proteins bind specifically to antigen.

Several characteristics of antigen foster stimulation of an immune response. Both the molecular shape and size of antigen are important. Antigen triggers an immune response only after immune cells recognize the specific shape of parts of the antigen molecule. A better immune response occurs as the molecular weight of a substance increases. The larger the antigen, the stronger the immune response. With bigger antigens, more parts of the molecule (antigenic determinants) stimulate production of specific antibody. Antigenic determinants are important in stimulating the production of many different antibodies during one immune response. Increased complexity of an antigen's molecular structure also enhances the stimulating properties of the antigen. The more "foreign" a substance is considered by the body, the more antigenic the substance is. Solubility and availability of a substance for degradation by cellular mechanisms enhance the antigenic property of that substance (Barrett, 1988). Table 55–1 lists the physical and chemical properties associated with antigenicity.

Mitogens, substances that induce mitosis, mimic antigens. Mitogens, like antigens, induce the activation of immune cells and the production of antibodies (Barrett, 1988). However, the mechanisms by which mitogens and antigens produce an immune response are

TABLE 55–1. **Properties Associated With Antigenicity**

Characteristics	Property That Enhances Response
Size	Large molecule
Complexity	Very complex structures
Stability	Fixed structural configuration
Degradability	Timing of degradation process allows for interaction of antigen and processing cells
Foreignness	Greatest molecular difference from self antigen

different. Both mitogens and antigens are used experimentally to assess the function of the immune system.

The Major Histocompatibility Complex

The ultimate purpose of the cells that compose the immune system is to neutralize, destroy, or eliminate those microorganisms that penetrate or invade the internal environment before the invaders have a chance to multiply and overwhelm body defenses. To accomplish this action, the cells that make up the immune system must be able to recognize "undesirable invaders" from normal, healthy cells. This ability to distinguish "self" from "nonself," necessary so that normal healthy body cells are not neutralized, destroyed, or eliminated along with the invaders, is called *self-tolerance.* Nonself cells include infected or debilitated body cells, self cells that have undergone malignant transformation into cancer cells, and all foreign cells (Gallucci, 1987; Workman, 1993). Recognition and self-tolerance are possible because of the unique ability of immune system cells to examine and interpret the surface proteins present on any cell or organism they contact directly.

All organisms are made up of cells. Each cell is surrounded by a plasma membrane. Protruding through the membranes of all cells are a variety of different protein types. Each protein type differs from all other protein types in its amino acid sequence. Some of the proteins found on the cell membranes of any one person are unique to that person and serve as a cellular fingerprint or a "universal product code" for that person. These universal product codes are as unique as the individual and would be exactly the same only on the surfaces of cells from identical twins and other monozygotic multiple births (Roitt, 1991; Workman, 1993). Because these unique personal proteins can be recognized as foreign by the immune system of another person, these proteins are called *antigens.*

Part of this unique universal product code for each person is composed of the *human leukocyte antigens* (HLA). The term "leukocyte antigen" is not actually correct because these antigens also are present on the surfaces of all cells containing a nucleus, not just on leukocytes. These antigens form the specific "tissue type" of the individual. Other names for these antigens include the human transplantation antigens, human histocompatibility antigens, and class I antigens.

Chromosome 6 has a region that contains the genes that code for a person's HLA (Fig. 55–1). This gene region is called the *major histocompatibility complex* (MHC). The complex contains three different classes of genes that are responsible for at least three different types of activities related to immune function. Class I genes code for the HLAs. Class II genes code for proteins that control or regulate immune function (these proteins are called "Ir" proteins, for "immune regulation"). Class III genes code for proteins that regulate complement synthesis and activity.

Class I antigens are coded for by the HLA genes HLA-A, HLA-B, and HLA-C. At each of the three gene locations on chromosome 6 for HLA, more than one alternative form can exist for each of the genes (these alternative gene forms are called "alleles"). For example, HLA-A has 27 known different possible alleles, and HLA-B has 47 known different possible alleles (Roitt, 1991). Therefore, because all normal humans have a pair of number 6 chromosomes and each chromosome of the pair contains three HLA class I genes, any one person can only have up to six different HLA class I proteins on the surfaces of all their nucleated cells. However, more than 80 different forms of these three genes have been identified among the human

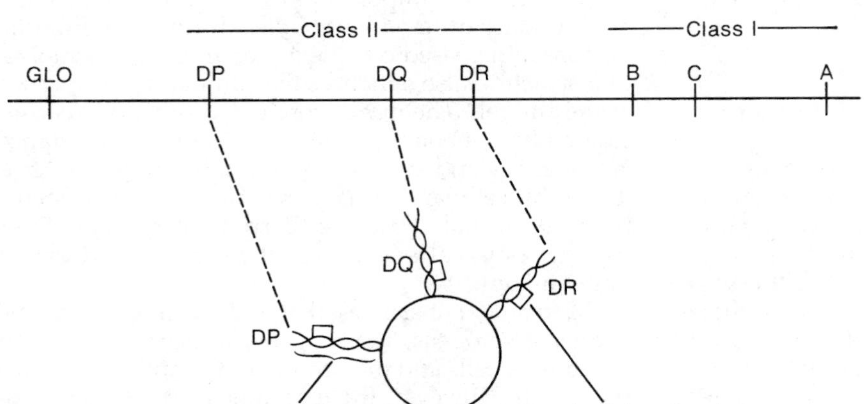

FIGURE 55–1. Schematic representation of major histocompatibility complex located on short arm of chromosome 6. The DP, DQ, and DR loci encode for class II molecules; the A, B, and C loci encode for class I molecules. The products of the MHC, DP, DQ, and DR genes are randomly expressed on cells (e.g., macrophages, B cells, and some activated T cells). These class II molecules express antigenic determinants that are detected by antibodies. (From Lockey, R., & Bukantz, S. [Eds.]. [1987]. *Fundamentals of immunology and allergy* [p. 70]. Philadelphia: W. B. Saunders.)

population (Roitt, 1991). For any one person, three of the HLA genes were inherited from their father (and the father had up to six gene forms to choose from) and three were inherited from their mother (who also had up to six HLA gene forms to choose from). Therefore, the HLA class I proteins present on a person's cells may not be exactly the same as either the father's, the mother's, or the sibling's.

These six class I proteins form the most obvious or major part of a person's universal product code. In addition, it is thought that a number of *minor* antigens also compose part of each person's universal product code. Immunologists speculate that the number of minor antigens may far exceed the number of major antigens, and that these also are genetically determined. It is the major HLAs that must be closely matched between donor and recipient for the best outcome of solid organ transplantation. Currently, matching the minor antigens is not possible, although mismatched minor antigens are likely to be responsible for some degree of rejection among recipients of solid organ transplants.

TABLE 55–2. **Classification of Immunoglobulins**

Class	Mean Survival: Percentage of Total	Mean Survival: Half-life (Days)	Biologic Function
IgG	75	23	Fix complement Cross placenta Active against many blood-borne infectious organisms (e.g., bacteria, viruses, parasites, and some fungi) Primary antibody of the secondary antibody response
IgA	15	6	Secretory antibody Activate complement through alternate properdin pathway
IgM	10	5	Fix complement Primary antibody of the primary antibody response
IgD	1	2.8	Unknown but proposed as lymphocyte surface receptor
IgE	0.002	1.5	Reaginic antibody (allergy) Homocytotropic antibody

Adapted from Bernier, G. M. (1985). In J. A. Bellanti (Ed.), *Immunology III* (p. 91). Philadelphia: W. B. Saunders.

Antibodies

In developing methods of vaccination, Pasteur recognized the protective nature of serum. Antibody was the part of serum thought to confer immunologic protection (Tizard, 1984). Antibodies refer to a vast array of proteins produced by B lymphocytes after stimulation by antigen. The major function of antibody is to bind a specific antigen and remove that antigen from the body (Jackson, 1991; Jeske & Capra, 1984). In a specific response to a specific antigen, a single antibody is produced. Thus, for each antigen there is a matching antibody. There are hundreds of thousands of potential antigens, and there is an equal number of antibodies. Each of these antibodies has slightly different characteristics and specificities.

The many individual types of antibodies are grouped into five different immunoglobulin (Ig) classes: IgG, IgM, IgA, IgE, and IgD. Table 55–2 describes some physical and biologic properties of the five major immunoglobulin classes.

IgG, the most abundant of the immunoglobulins, makes up about 75% of the total concentration of immunoglobulins in the serum. Vascular and extravascular spaces contain high concentrations of IgG. IgG has a relatively long half-life (23 days), can cross the placenta, and can activate complement. This class of immunoglobulin provides immunity against many blood-borne infectious agents such as bacteria, viruses, parasites, and some fungi. Receptors for IgG exist on many immune cells, including monocytes, polymorphonuclear leukocytes, accessory cells in spleen and liver, and some lymphocytes.

IgA provides immunity through the external secretory system. Through this system, IgA moves across mucous membranes within body secretions. Fifteen percent of the total serum concentration of immunoglobulins consists of IgA, making it the second most abundant immunoglobulin. The lympoid tissues lining the gastrointestinal, respiratory, and genitourinary tracts secrete IgA. Saliva and tears contain large amounts of IgA. IgA combines with a protein that confers IgA protection with proteolytic enzymes found in these lymphoid tissues. IgA does not cross the placenta; however, it gives immunity to the newborn by virtue of its high concentration in colostrum. Lymphocytes, polymorphonuclear cells, and monocytes have receptors for IgA.

IgM accounts for 10% of the total serum concentration of immunoglobulins. IgM is the largest immunoglobulin. It is confined almost entirely to the intravascular space because of its large size. IgM molecules have the ability to fix complement and are highly efficient agglutinators of particulate antigens such as red blood cells and bacteria. Both of these properties make IgM an important participant in host defense. IgM antibodies are the first class of antibody synthesized after primary stimulation by antigen. The level of IgM antibodies peaks within days and declines more rapidly than does the level of IgG antibodies.

IgD accounts for only 1% of the total serum concentration of immunoglobulins; its specific biologic role as a humoral antibody is unclear. This immunoglobulin class is found on the surface of lymphocytes much more frequently than in serum. IgD is expressed on neonatal lymphocytes more often than on adult lymphocytes. Both of these findings suggest that IgD serves as a specific surface receptor in the initiation of the immune response. Penicillin hypersensitivity is another instance of IgD participation in the immune response.

IgE is present in only trace amounts in the serum. It has the ability to attach to human skin and to start an allergic reaction. Also called the reaginic antibody, IgE functions to mediate the severe anaphylactic type of hypersensitivities. Like IgA, IgE is produced chiefly in the linings of the respiratory and intestinal tracts. Both IgA and IgE are part of the external secretory system of antibody (Barrett, 1988).

THE BASIC FUNCTIONS OF THE IMMUNE SYSTEM

The basic function of the immune system is to detect and eliminate from the body any substance recognized as foreign or nonself. Typically, each encounter of the body with a foreign substance activates an immune response. When analyzed individually, immunologic responses serve three functions—defense, homeostasis, and surveillance (Bellanti, 1985; Gawlikowski, 1992).

Defense

Response to infection is one defense function commonly attributed to the immune system. The defense action of the immune system has important consequences not only for the invading organism but for normal human tissue. When immune system components or interactions between components are hyperactive, allergy or hypersensitivity may occur (Kirkpatrick, 1987). Conversely, when these elements are hypoactive, increased susceptibility to repeated infections may occur. The immune deficiency disorders are examples of repeated infections in the presence of a hypoactive immune system (Church & Schlegel, 1985).

Homeostasis

By maintaining homeostasis, the immune system preserves the internal environment. Cellular components of the body continually grow, mature, die, and are replaced. In this process of orderly senescence, antigens defining the cells as self become altered. The immune system is thus able to mount a response against normal cells that are no longer functioning competently. Specialized immunocompetent cells serve as scavengers that degrade and remove damaged or dead cells from the body. Other immunocompetent cells serve to control and regulate the homeostatic function of the immune system. The regulation of homeostasis is an important normal immunologic function. Failure of the regulation of homeostatic mechanisms often results in autoimmune disease (Barrett, 1988).

Surveillance

Controversy surrounds the surveillance function of the immune system. The *immune surveillance theory,* first posited by Thomas (1959) and later changed by Burnet (1967), suggests that T lymphocytes of the immune system serve to detect and remove the abnormal cells that constantly arise within the body. These abnormal cells arise through spontaneous neoplastic transformation or induction by certain viruses and chemicals. Failure of this surveillance mechanism is thought to play a causal role in the development of malignant disease. Evidence supporting or refuting this theory is equivocal. Supporting evidence includes (1) the increased incidence of cancer in the elderly, (2) failure of rejection of tumor transplant by genetically thymectomized mice, and (3) a 300-fold increased incidence of cancer in individuals on long-term immunosuppressive therapy (Groenwald et al., 1993). Contradictory evidence suggests that the proposed mechanism of immune surveillance is too simplistic (Mitchell & Bertram, 1985). More recently, non-T lymphocytes (natural killer [NK] cells) have been reported to have the primary role in surveillance rather than T lymphocytes (Herberman & Gorelik, 1989). A further change in the immune surveillance theory suggests that the target of surveillance is the immunogen or stimulus of the immune response (Groenwald et al., 1993).

TISSUES OF THE IMMUNE SYSTEM

Lymphoid or immune tissues are the special tissues that participate in the development of competent immune cells. These tissues, as shown in Figure 55–2, are located throughout the entire body and are subdivided into central and peripheral lymphoid tissues. Differentiation of lymphoid stem cells into lymphocytes that can react with antigen takes place in the central lymphoid tissues. The central lymphoid system has three major subdivisions: (1) the bone marrow, (2) the thymus, and (3) the bursa of Fabricius. The peripheral lymphoid tissues are found in areas in which the lymphocytes can later react with antigen (Barrett, 1988). The peripheral lymphoid system includes lymph nodes, spleen, tonsils, bronchus-associated lymphoid tissue, Peyer patches, and appendix and other gut-associated lymphoid tissue. Many patches of lymphoid tissue are scattered throughout tissues that initially confront antigens from the external environment. Characteristics of primary and secondary lymphoid organs are compared in Table 55–3.

The Central Lymphoid Organs

BONE MARROW. Cells of the immune system originate, mature, and move from the bone marrow into the circulatory system. Erythrocytes, platelets, granulocytes, monocytes, and lymphocytes arise from a primitive, undifferentiated stem cell. Figure 55–3 shows the development of the cells of the bone marrow. The granulocytic, monocytic, and lymphocytic

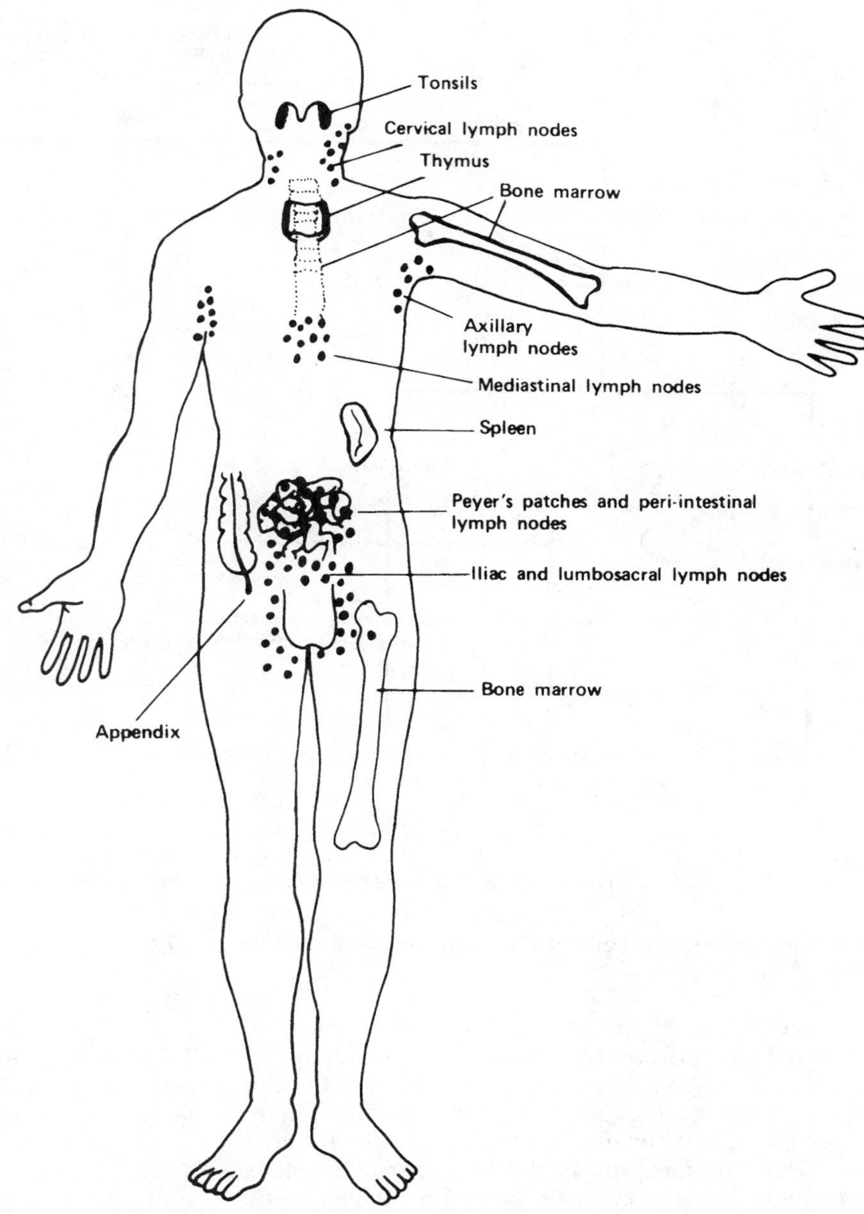

FIGURE 55–2. Diagrammatic representation of the distribution of lymphoid tissues in humans. (Reprinted from Virella, G. J. M., Fudenberg, H., & Patrick, C. [Eds.]. [1986]. *Introduction to medical immunology* [p. 13]. By courtesy of Marcel Dekker, Inc., New York, NY.)

TABLE 55–3. **Comparison of Primary and Secondary Lymphoid Organs**

	Primary Lymphoid Organ	Secondary Lymphoid Organ
Origin	Ectoendodermal junction	Mesoderm
Time of development	Early in embryonic life	Later in fetal life
Persistence	Involutes after puberty	Persists through adult life
Effect of removal	Loss of lymphocytes	No effect or only minor consequences
Response to antigen	Unresponsive	Fully reactive
Examples	Thymus; (bursa)	Spleen; lymph nodes

Table from *Immunology: An Introduction*, by Ian R. Tizard, copyright © 1984 by Holt, Rinehart and Winston, Inc., reproduced by permission of the publisher.

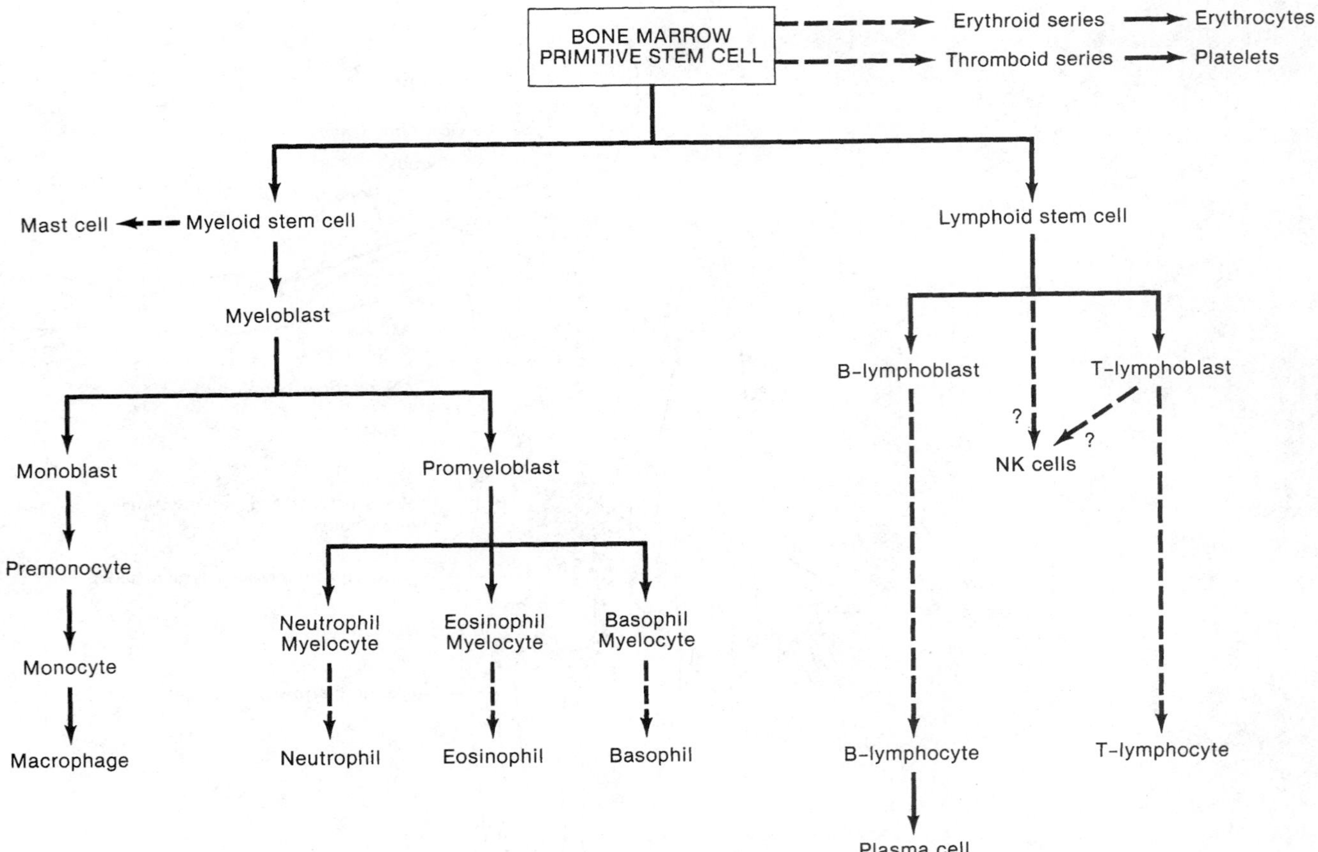

FIGURE 55–3. Differentiation of primitive stem cell in the bone marrow. NK, natural killer.

cell lines are effector cells of the immune system (Barrett, 1988).

THYMUS. The thymus consists of a bilobed sack of epithelial cells surrounding an interior core of lymphocytes. Structurally, each lobe of the thymus divides into an exterior cortex and an interior medulla. Lymphocytes coalesce primarily in the cortex of the thymus. These thymic lymphocytes are morphologically indistinguishable from lymphocytes in other tissues. Thymic lymphocytes are, however, antigenically isolatable by Thy 1, a surface marker antigen, and are called T lymphocytes (Barrett, 1988).

BURSA OF FABRICIUS. The bursa of Fabricius is a lymphoid organ located in the gut of fowl. The bursa serves as the site of B cell maturation in birds. Within the bursa there are three main types of cells: macrophages, B lymphocytes, and plasma cells. Mammals do not have a bursa, but do have B lymphocytes. The major site of B-cell maturation in mammals is the spleen (Abbas et al., 1991). Several other tissue sites also contribute to B-cell maturation.

Another potential tissue is gut-associated lymphoid tissue (GALT). B-lymphocyte activity is impaired with the removal of GALT in the early development of experimental animals (Barrett, 1988).

The Peripheral Lymphoid Organs

The spleen and lymph nodes are the two major peripheral lymphoid organs. Lymphocytes leave the central lymphoid organs, enter the circulatory system and peripheral lymphoid organs, and reenter the thymus. The tonsils, appendix, Peyer patches, and other lymphoid tissues play a lesser role in immune response (Barrett, 1988). Many other lymphoid tissues are scattered throughout the body. All of these tissues are capable of trapping antigen and are sites of immune response.

The spleen is physically divided into two sections—one as a storage site for erythrocytes and the second as the site of immunologic response. The spleen acts as a filter for antigen from the blood. The spleen also sequesters scavenger cells called macrophages and is a site of B-lymphocyte activation in response to antigen stimulation. Lymph nodes trap antigen in the lymph and provide maximal exposure of antigen to antigen-sensitive cells. Antigen-sensitive cells in lymph nodes include lymphocytes, macrophages, and other accessory cells.

CELLS OF THE IMMUNE SYSTEM

One of the most interesting features of the immune system is the great diversity of white blood cells

(WBCs) involved in the events comprising the immune response. Four categories of WBCs involved in the immune response are (1) macrophages and antigen-processing and antigen-presenting cells (accessory cells), (2) granulocytic phagocytes, (3) B lymphocytes, and (4) T lymphocytes. The lymphocytes are primarily participants in the recognition of nonself elements. Other WBCs, including monocytes and granulocytes, help lymphocytes in either the early or late stages of the immune response. In the early stages, accessory cells present antigen in such a way that lymphocytes can recognize the antigen as nonself. In the later stages of an immune response, macrophages and granulocytes ingest and digest nonself elements set for destruction (Barrett, 1988; Roitt et al., 1985).

Each cell type within the immune system has at least one specific function or activity that contributes to host protection. Most immune system cells communicate with each other for activation and regulation. Such communication, resulting in induction and regulation of immunity, is controlled through the selected production and acivity of *cytokines*. Cytokines are small protein hormones synthesized in the various leukocytes. Cytokines synthesized by the mononuclear phagocytes are termed *monokines*, and the cytokines produced by T lymphocytes are termed *lymphokines* (Van Snick, 1990).

Cytokine activity is similar to the action of any other kind of hormone in that one cell produces and secretes a cytokine that then exerts its effects on other cells of the immune system (Guyton, 1991). The cells responding to the cytokine may be right next to the cytokine-secreting cell or quite remote from the cytokine-secreting cell. The cells that change their activity in response to the cytokine are known as "responder" cells. For a responder cell to be able to respond to the presence of a cytokine, the membrane of the target cell must have a specific receptor for the cytokine to bind to and initiate changes in the target cell's activity (Nicola, 1989).

The purpose of cytokines is to induce and regulate a wide variety of inflammatory and immune responses. Most cytokines are produced as they are needed, and are not stored to any great extent (Balkwill & Burke, 1989). The actions of some cytokines are *pleiotropic*, in that the effects are widespread within the immune system, setting into motion a variety of immunomodulating actions. Other cytokines have very specific actions limited to only one type of cell. Table 55–4 summarizes the origins and activities of the currently known cytokines.

Antigen-Presenting and Antigen-Processing Cells

The term *accessory cells* refers collectively to monocytes, macrophages, and many other antigen-presenting and antigen-processing cells. Accessory cells include cells that either participate in the initiation of an immune response or help the lymphocytes with their effector or inflammatory functions. Two broad groups of accessory cells are antigen-presenting cells and granulocytic phagocytes. Mononuclear phagocytes (monocytes and macrophages) and dendritic cells are nonlymphocytic antigen-presenting cells. These cells aid in the presentation of antigen to lymphocytes. A common characteristic of these cells is their ability to participate in the induction of the immune response. Macrophages also are active participants in the elimination of dead or damaged cells through phagocytosis.

MONONUCLEAR PHAGOCYTES. Mononuclear phagocytes arise from a single stem cell in the bone marrow and consist of a series of cells that develop from premonocyte to monocyte to macrophage. In the bone marrow, premonocytes undergo proliferation and move to the blood as monocytes after a period of maturation. After about 1 to 2 days in the blood, monocytes migrate to the main tissue site of their action. Monocytes become fixed in these tissues, where they differentiate into macrophages (Unanue, 1989).

Under normal conditions neither macrophages nor monocytes divide. Proteins secreted by T lymphocytes, fibroblasts, macrophages, and epithelial cells stimulate monocytes to mature. Colony-stimulating factors (CSFs) start the differentiation of the premonocyte to monocyte and monocyte to macrophage. CSFs increase in amount during infection and during strong immune response (Unanue, 1989). Table 55–5 lists the actions of some CSFs involved in mediating the activity of mononuclear phagocytes.

Monocytes represent 3% of the circulating WBCs in the adult, or about 300 cells/mL^3 of blood. Both monocytes and macrophages process and then present antigen to T cells and B cells. Processing of antigen requires internalization of antigens by the monocyte or macrophage. The exact biochemical events that take place within antigen-presenting cells remain unclear. Internalization and biochemical processing result in cell surface expression of antigen fragments (Unanue, 1989).

Most monocytes and macrophages express class II MHC molecules. Chemical mediators influence the amount of MHC protein found on the accessory cell membrane. These chemical mediators include both enhancers (gamma-interferon) and suppressors (prostaglandins) of monocyte/macrophage participation in the immune response. The expression of MHC on monocytes enhances the ability of the monocyte to present antigen fragments to lymphocytes and thus strengthens the lymphocyte response to antigen. Interleukin-1 (IL-1), a lymphokine secreted by monocytes, also enhances antigen presentation by monocytes (Unanue, 1989).

Macrophages are found in all tissues, often surrounding the blood vessels, near the epithelium. At times, macrophages attach to vascular endothelial cells (Unanue, 1989). Macrophages serve at least three distinct functions in host defense: (1) secretion of biologically active molecules, (2) removal of excess antigen,

TABLE 55–4. **Summary of Cytokine Activity**

Cytokine	Cellular Origin	Inducing Event	Cytokine Action
Interleukin-1 (IL-1)	Macrophage	Contact with gram-negative bacterial products Contact with CD4 cell Presence of TNF	Stimulates increased production of prostaglandins Induces fever Increases proliferation of CD4 cells Stimulates growth and differentiation of B lymphocytes Induces further secretion of IL-1 and IL-6
Interleukin-2 (IL-2)	T helper cells (CD4+) CD8+ T cells	T-cell activation by antigens	Increases the growth and differentiation of T lymphocytes Stimulates increased production of IL-2 from activated lymphocytes
Interleukin-3 (multilineage colony-stimulating factor, IL-3)	T helper cells (CD4+)	Infection or invasion	Stimulates production of immature bone marrow stem cells (pluripotent)
Interleukin-4 (B-cell stimulatory factor, IL-4)	T helper cells (CD4+) Activated mast cells	Presence of anti-Ig antibody	Stimulates growth and proliferation of B lymphocytes Stimulates increased production of IgE Induces further secretion of IL-4, IL-5, and IL-6 Acts as a macrophage-activating factor
Interleukin-5 (B-cell growth factor, IL-5)	T helper cells (CD4+) Activated mast cells	Helminth infections	Stimulates growth and differentiation of eosinophils Stimulates mature B lymphocytes to increase the synthesis of immunoglobulins (especially IgA)
Interleukin-6 (IL-6)	Macrophage Vascular endothelial cells Fibroblasts Activated T cells	Infection or inflammation Presence of IL-1 and TNF	Stimulates hepatocytes to make fibrinogen, macroglobulin, and C protein Stimulates the growth of activated B lymphocytes Serves as a cofactor in stimulating production of bone marrow hematopoietic stem cells
Interleukin-7 (IL-7)	Bone marrow stromal cells	Presence of antigen	Stimulates growth and differentiation of committed B-lymphocyte stem cells
Interleukin-8 (monocyte chemotactic factor, IL-8)	Activated T cells, macrophage endothelial cells, platelets, fibroblasts, and epithelial cells	Infection or inflammation Presence of TNF or IL-1	Chemotactic factor for neutrophils, basophils, and eosinophils Neutrophil activation
TNF	LPS-activated macrophage Antigen-stimulated T cells Activated NK cells Activated mast cells	Gram-negative bacterial infection	Increases leukocyte adhesion to endothelial cells Induces fever Stimulates fibroblasts and endothelial cells to secrete colony-stimulating factors Enhances cytolysis of virally infected cells Induces coagulation Stimulates marophages to secrete IL-1 and IL-6 Stimulates metabolic changes that result in cachexia
Granulocyte–macrophage colony-stimulating factor	Activated T cells Macrophages Vascular endothelial cells Fibroblasts	Infection or inflammation	Increases growth and differentiation of committed myeloid stem cells Minor activator of macrophages

TABLE 55–4. **Summary of Cytokine Activity** *Continued*

Cytokine	Cellular Origin	Inducing Event	Cytokine Action
Monocyte–macrophage colony-stimulating factor	Macrophages Vascular endothelial cells Fibroblasts	Infection or inflammation	Enhances proliferation and maturation of the committed progenitor cells for monocytes–macrophages (CFU-M)
Granulocyte colony-stimulating factor	Macrophages Vascular endothelial cells Fibroblasts	Infection or inflammation	Enhances neutrophil maturation and release from bone marrow
Interferon (INF) (α, β, γ)	Macrophages (INF-α) Fibroblasts (INF-β) T-helper cells (INF-γ) CD8+ cells (INF-γ) Natural killer cells	Viral infection	Limits viral infection by: inhibiting viral replication increasing NK-mediated lysis increasing cytolytic T-lymphocyte recognition of virally infected cells Activates macrophages (INF-γ) Promotes differentiation of T and B lymphocytes (INF-γ) Activates neutrophils (INF-γ) Activates NK cells (INF-γ)

Abbreviations: TNF, tumor necrosis factor; Ig, immunoglobulin; LPS, lipopolysaccharide; CFU-M, colony-forming unit—monocyte–macrophage; NK, natural killer.

From Workman, M. L., Ellerhorst-Ryan, J., & Koertge, V. (1993). *Nursing care of the immunocompromised patient* (pp. 53–55). Philadelphia: W. B. Saunders.

and (3) antigen presentation. The secretory products of macrophages include prostaglandin E_2, leukotrienes, IL-1, tumor necrosis factor, interferon, growth factors, complement proteins, and enzymes (Table 55–6). IL-1, tumor necrosis factor (TNF), and alpha- and beta-interferon are particularly important in the promotion of host defense (Unanue, 1989).

Tissue macrophages have specific names according to their anatomic location. Histiocytes are found in connective tissue, Kupffer cells in liver, alveolar macrophages in lung, and microglial cells in the neural system (Werb, 1987). Both free and fixed macrophages reside in the spleen, lymph nodes, and other organs. Blood monocytes have a half-life of only a few hours. However, tissue macrophages have a long lifespan, possibly extending for many months or years. Macrophages participating in inflammatory lesions have short lifespans because they die or fuse with other macrophages.

DENDRITIC CELLS. Dendritic accessory cells reside primarily in the epithelium, lymphatics, spleen, and lymphoid organs. Morphologically distinct from mononuclear phagocytes, dendritic accessory cells express characteristically high levels of class II MHC molecules. Dendritic accessory cells are believed to be

TABLE 55–5. **Colony-Stimulating Factors (CSF) Involved in Differentiation of Monocytes**

Colony-Stimulating Factors	Secreted By	Action
Multi-CSF (interleukin-3)	T lymphocytes	Stimulates growth of granulocytes, mast cells, and lymphocytes
M-CSF	Macrophages	Stimulates differentiation of premonocyte to monocyte to macrophage; increases longevity of mature macrophages
GM-CSF	Granulocytes Macrophages	In vitro administration of GM-CSF increases circulation of neutrophils, eosinophils, and macrophages
G-CSF	Granulocytes	Stimulates differentiation of myeloid precursor cell to granulocytes and monocytes

Compiled from Ihle, J. N., & Weinstein, Y. (1985). Interleukin 3. In J. D. Watson & J. Marbrook (Eds.), *Recognition and regulation in cell-mediated immunity* (pp. 291–324). New York: Marcel Dekker.

Young, D., Lowe, L., & Clark, S. (1990). Comparison of the effects of IL-3, granulocyte-macrophage colony-stimulating factor, and macrophage colony-stimulating factor in supporting monocyte differentiation in culture. *Journal of Immunology, 145*(2), 607–615.

Gillis, S. (1989). T-cell–derived lymphokines. In W. Paul (Ed.), *Fundamental immunology* (2nd ed., pp. 621–638). New York: Raven Press.

Roitt, I. (1991). *Essential immunology* (7th ed.). Boston: Blackwell Scientific Publications.

Guilbent, L. J. (1985). Mononuclear phagocyte progenitors and growth factors. In R. vanFurth (Ed.), *Mononuclear phagocytes: Characteristics, physiology, and function* (pp. 233–241). Boston: Martinus Nijhoff Publishers.

TABLE 55–6. **Some Secretory Products of Macrophages**

Factors synthesized and secreted continuously	Lysozyme Complement components C2, C3, C4, C5 Fibronectin
Factors released during phagocytosis	Plasminogen activators Procoagulants Collagenase Elastase Lysosomal proteases Leukotrienes Thromboxanes Thromboplastin
Regulatory factors released during immune responses	Interferon Interleukin-1 Lymphocyte-activating factors Prostaglandins E_1 and E_2 Cyclic adenosine monophosphate

important in presenting antigens that have been introduced into the body through skin or other epithelial tissues. Details of the exact mechanism of antigen presentation by accessory cells have not yet been clarified (Unanue, 1989).

Of all the accessory cells, the follicular dendritic cells are the least understood. Follicular dendritic accessory cells are found in lymph nodes. These accessory cells participate with B lymphocytes in antigen trapping within the follicles. These follicular dendritic cells have, however, been studied by indirect immunologic techniques only and have not been isolated or cultured. Thus, their exact nature, origin, and role in antigen trapping or in presentation of antigen to lymphocytes are not known.

Granulocytic Phagocytes

Most granulocytes have large, lobular nuclei, leading to the name polymorphonuclear leukocytes. Three varieties of circulating granulocytes exist—neutrophils, basophils, and eosinophils. Of the 5,000 to 10,000 WBCs in each cubic milliliter of blood, about 60% to 70% are neutrophils, 1% to 3% are eosinophils, and only 0.5% to 1% are basophils.

NEUTROPHILS. Neutrophils go through a five-stage maturing process, beginning with the myeloblast, myelocyte, metamyelocyte, and nonfilamented neutrophil and ending with the mature neutrophil. Neutrophils contain large cytoplasmic granules that produce enzymes with bactericidal activity (Patrick et al., 1986). During cell maturation the granules become more concentrated in the center of the cell. This readies the cell edges for movement to the sites of injury. At the metamyelocyte stage, complement and IgG receptors are expressed on the cell surface. These surface antigens are important facilitators of bacterial ingestion and cell motility. Only fully mature neutrophils are able to respond maximally to foreign particles (Densen & Mandell, 1987).

Neutrophils can migrate in response to chemical stimuli. Chemotactic factors also enhance the adhesiveness of neutrophils to endothelial cells, thus providing a mechanical means for motion (Werb, 1987). Chemotactic factors attract neutrophils to areas where antigen is present. Neutrophils engulf and destroy foreign substances such as bacteria and represent an important primary line of defense. Pus forms from neutrophils that die during the inflammatory process and their debris (Patrick et al., 1986).

Neutrophils synthesize and store in granules chemicals that are destructive to bacteria and cause injury in the surrounding tissue. Neutrophil degranulation has been implicated as a source of local tissue injury in adult respiratory distress syndrome and pulmonary emphysema (Densen & Mandell, 1987). Neutrophil secretory products include leukotrienes (slow-reactive substance of anaphylaxis), vasoactive kinins, and toxic oxide metabolites such as hydrogen peroxide and myeloperoxidase (Bellanti & Kadlec, 1985).

EOSINOPHILS. Eosinophils share many features with neutrophils in that both are removed from the body at the tissue site and do not return to the circulation. Like neutrophils, eosinophils contain many granules. Eosinophils concentrate at the mucosal surfaces of the respiratory and gastrointestinal tracts. Eosinophils do engage in phagocytosis; however, they are less efficient in the phagocytic process than neutrophils. Eosinophils concentrate in tissues during allergic reactions and parasitic infections, yet their specific role is unknown. Major roles postulated include destruction of some parasites, ingestion of immune complexes, and limitation of inflammatory reactions (Tizard, 1984).

Eosinophilia occurs in diseases involving increased levels of IgE, such as allergic gastroenteropathy and IgE-mediated anaphylaxis (Goust, 1986). Eosinophils are chemically attracted to sites of IgE concentration. These cells carry certain enzymes that neutralize chemicals responsible for anaphylaxis; however, the overall effect of eosinophilic degranulation is cell destruction. Eosinophils cause inflammation, bronchospasm, and tissue damage by releasing potent chemical mediators.

Some cytotoxic proteins within the eosinophilic granules include major basic protein, eosinophilic peroxidase, eosinophilic cationic proteins, eosinophil-derived neurotoxin, and a variety of enzymes (Gleich & Butterfield, 1987). These cytotoxic proteins not only exert a direct cytolytic effect on the microorganism, but some proteins elicit the support of other cells. For example, eosinophilic peroxidase binds to another granulocyte, the mast cell, and triggers mast cell degranulation and subsequent destruction of the microorganism.

BASOPHILS. Basophils play an important role in cutaneous hypersensitivity reactions but show little phagocytic action. Basophils contain many cytoplasmic granules containing histamine and heparin, two chemical mediators involved in immunologic reactions. Structurally, the basophil is very delicate and is susceptible to easy rupture and release of granule contents into blood and tissues. Both the anticoagulant properties of heparin and the vasoactivity of histamine increase the severity of IgE-dependent allergies (Barrett, 1988).

Basophils contain a variety of vasoactive substances, such as histamine and serotonin. The mediators released from basophils cause a variety of biologic activities, including increased vascular permeability, contraction of smooth muscle, and enhancement of the inflammatory response (Barrett, 1988).

MAST CELLS. Mast cells arise in the bone marrow from a myeloid stem cell. Found at the point of antigen entry into the body, mast cells are called the sentinels of the immune system. Mast cells reside primarily in cutaneous and mucosal surfaces (Austen, 1983). They are the only immunologically active cells that can immediately recognize nonself antigens without presensitization in the blood or lymph systems. Mast cells function as effectors of immediate hypersensitivity or allergic reactions.

Mast cells concentrate most of the body's IgE on their cell membranes. Complexing of antigen and surface-expressed IgE triggers degranulation of the mast cells and alters the cell membrane. Degranulation releases histamines and other mediators into the extracellular environment. Changes in the cell membrane lead to arachidonic acid metabolism and the secretion of prostaglandin D_2 and leukotrienes, potent mediators of immediate hypersensitivity responses (Austen & Fisher, 1987).

Lymphoid Cells

The lymphoid cells of the immune system differ from other cells in their ability to react specifically with antigen and to produce specific cell products. Lymphoid cells include B and T lymphocytes, plasma cells, and large granular lymphocytes. The most well defined population of large granular lymphocytes is NK cells.

Lymphocyte is a morphologic term that describes a population of cells with many different immune functions. About 30% of the total WBC count is lymphocytes. One subset of lymphocytes (T lymphocytes) participates in the primary recognition of antigen. Structurally similar but functionally different, B lymphocytes produce circulating antibody.

Both B and T lymphocytes arise from a single lymphoid stem cell. As shown in Figure 55–4, the process of maturation differentiates B cells from T cells. Morphologic separation of T and B lymphocytes by visual inspection through blood smears is not possible. These lymphocytes can, however, be separated by function and cell surface markers (antigens). Some distinguishing functional and antigenic features of T and B lymphocytes are listed in Table 55–7.

B LYMPHOCYTES. B lymphocytes are those cells that contain completely formed chains of immunoglobulin. These immunoglobulin molecules, expressed only on the cell surface of the B lymphocyte, allow in vitro identification of B cells (Kincade & Gimble, 1989). Immunoglobulin serves as a unique surface marker for B lymphocytes. There are, however, many other proteins expressed on the cell membrane of the B lymphocyte. The function of many of these surface markers remains unknown (Kincade & Gimble, 1989). One functionally important surface marker expressed on B lymphocytes is MHC class II antigens. The MHC binds antigen frag-

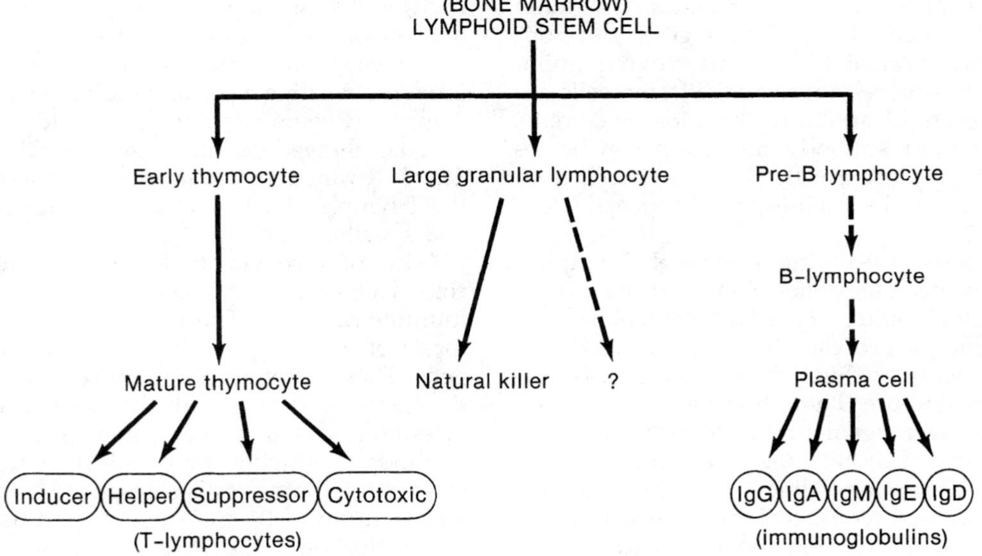

FIGURE 55–4. Maturation process of lymphocytes.

TABLE 55–7. **Relative Comparison of T and B Lymphocytes**

Characteristic	T Lymphocytes	B Lymphocytes
Immune mechanism	Cell-mediated immunity	Humoral immunity
Site of precursor origin	Thymus	Bursal equivalent (fetal liver, bone marrow, gastrointestinal tract)
Distribution in tissue	High in thoracic duct (90%), blood (80%), lymph (75%)	High in bone marrow (>75%), gut-associated lymphoid tissue (70%)
Functions	Protection against most viruses, fungi, and slow-acting bacteria via macrostimulation and complement activation Mediation of cutaneous delayed hypersensitivity reactions Rejection of foreign grafts Regulation of the immune response Immunologic surveillance	Differentiation into plasma cells that secrete antibody Medication of immediate phage hypersensitivity reaction (allergy) Protection against pyogenic infections and toxic reactions
Cell product	Lymphokines	Immunoglobulins
Surface markers	T antigen	Surface immunoglobulin
Immune tolerance	Occurs early and persists	Less sensitive than T cells

ments to the B-cell surface and helps B cells interact with other immune cells (Kincade & Gimble, 1989).

Immunoglobulins are one of the few surface marker proteins made only by B cells. The proteins expressed on the cell surface of B cells change according to the stages of B-cell maturity. A certain number of receptors and glycoproteins are required for proper immune function; however, there can be great diversity in how and when these molecules are acquired (Kantor, 1991; Kincade & Gimble, 1989).

In the resting state, B lymphocytes have not been exposed to antigenic stimuli. On stimulation, many biochemical changes take place in the resting B cell. These changes result in an increase in cell size and in the cellular structures responsible for protein synthesis (Kincade & Gimble, 1989). B lymphocytes undergo a distinct developmental process. Early identifiable pre-B cells, which express incomplete immmunoglobulin molecules, go through intermediate stages of development and activation. Final differentiation of B lymphocytes leads to plasma cell formation. Plasma cells are the major secretors of antibody (Kincade & Gimble, 1989). Thousands of antibody molecules can be released by a single plasma cell. The plasma cell does not usually divide, and has a lifespan of approximately 4 days (Stobo, 1987).

One of the most mystifying aspects of B-lymphocyte function has been the generation of an endless variety of immunoglobulins. Two complementary and antigen-independent processes that create this diversity have been identified. First, the specific genes (variable region genes) in pre-B lymphocytes undergo a series of orderly rearrangements. Each rearrangement creates a new type of B cell clone. The second process is polyclonal proliferation. Almost 1 million clones of B cells, never exposed to antigen and each with a different antigen specificity, bring about the wide variety of antibodies (Cooper, 1987).

Activation of the B lymphocyte requires extensive short-range communication between antigen, B cells, and other immune cells. Communication occurs through a host of cytokines and lymphokines. B cells have receptors for IL, interferon, growth factors, and transferrin. Note that these lymphokines act in concert to enhance and counteract each other. The concentration of these lymphokines varies considerably throughout a specific immune response. Expression of class II molecules is greatly increased when resting B cells are activated, thus enhancing antigen presentation.

T LYMPHOCYTES. From 65% to 80% of all lymphocytes in the blood are of the T-type. These cells, which have a longer lifespan than B cells, are the major recirculating cell in the lymph nodes. The T-cell receptor (TcR) is perhaps the most critical surface marker protein on the cell membrane of the T lymphocyte. The amino acid and DNA sequence of the receptor is known, revealing a pentameric T3–Ti antigen receptor complex (Royer & Reinherz, 1987). Identification of the TcR has allowed definitive isolation of T lymphocytes. The TcR functions as an identity marker and allows the T lymphocyte to interact with antigen, other cells, and specific antibodies.

There are several types of functionally distinct T cells. Helper T lymphocytes aid the triggering of the immune response. These cells help B cells in the synthesis of immunoglobulins to T-cell–dependent antigens. These antigens are more complex than antigens that activate B cells directly. Suppressor T lymphocytes hold back immune responses. These cells restrict antibody production by B cells. Cytotoxic T lymphocytes can kill other cells recognized as nonself, for example, tumor cells and transplanted tissues.

In addition to the three functional groups of T cells just described, T lymphocytes are grouped by distinct proteins expressed on the cell membrane. At least four different taxonomies are used in the literature to identify these T-lymphocyte surface markers (Sprent, 1989). These taxonomic structures include a system developed in mice (Lyt), two human T-lymphocyte models (T_1, T_H), and a universal nomenclature proposed by the World Health Organization (CD). The T-lymphocyte subsets identified by any one taxonomic system correspond only partially with the functional categories of inducer, helper, suppressor, and cytotoxic T lymphocytes.

The monoclonal antibodies specific for CD4+ and CD8+ have identified two T-lymphocyte subsets that are functionally distinct. Mature T cells express CD4+ or CD8+, but rarely both. The ratio of CD4+ to CD8+ varies considerably with disease, but is usually 2:1. The functional role of the CD8+ subset is restricted by class 1 MHC antigens. CD4+ functional activity is restricted by class II MHC antigens. This means that T lymphocytes that are CD4+ bind to class II MHC molecules, and T lymphocytes that are CD8+ bind to class I molecules. Because class I antigens are present on nearly all cells, CD8+ cells interact with virtually every cell in the body. Class II antigens are expressed only on immune cells, and therefore CD4+ cells interact primarily with B cells and macrophages. One must keep in mind that MHC molecules help lymphocytes interact with antigens, thus strengthening the immune response.

After the initial identification of these two T-lymphocyte subsets, CD8+ cells were mistakenly identified as suppressor cells, and CD4+ cells were identified as helper cells. CD4+ cells consist primarily of helper T lymphocytes and to a lesser extent cytotoxic T lymphocytes. CD8+ cells consist of both cytotoxic and suppressor lymphocytes (Royer & Reinherz, 1987).

The major functions of the T lymphocytes include mediation of cytolytic reactions, regulation of delayed hypersensitivity reactions, and overall regulation of immune responses (Fig. 55–5). The regulatory function of T cells can be either positive or negative. The subpopulations of T cells act in a variety of ways to enhance or suppress the immune response. Cytotoxic T lymphocytes provide protection against most viral, fungal, and slow-acting bacterial infections and against some tumor cells. Delayed hypersensitivity is a localized immune reaction to a previously encountered antigen. Activation of T lymphocytes requires the carefully orchestrated interaction of the TcR, the lymphokine IL-2, and the receptor for IL-2 (Royer & Reinherz, 1987).

Activation of T cells is triggered by the interaction of immunogen, the TcR, and MHC antigens and leads to the surface expression of IL-2 receptors. Activated T lymphocytes synthesize and secrete IL-2, which becomes bound to IL-2 receptors on T lymphocytes (Royer & Reinherz, 1987). Once a critical number of IL-2 receptors have been bound, DNA synthesis and T-cell proliferation occur. Activation responses are maximized in the presence of IL-1, a cytokine secreted by

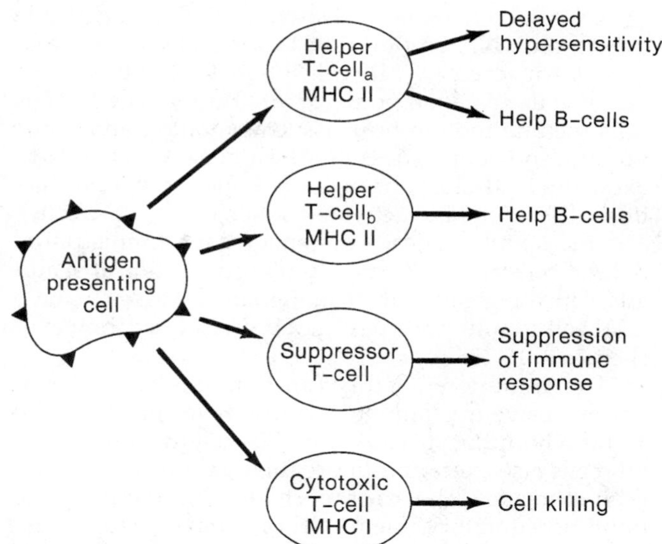

FIGURE 55–5. Major functions of T lymphocytes. MHC, major histocompatibility complex. T-cell$_a$, subclass associated with delayed hypersensitivity; T-cell$_b$, subclass associated with modulation of B-cell response.

macrophages. Activated T cells release soluble lymphokines that influence growth and differentiation of other cells (Lowry, 1993; Sprent, 1989).

These cytokines are not dependent on the specific antigen-inducing activation response or on the MHC antigens expressed by macrophages. The lymphokines produced through lymphocyte activation amplify the immune reaction (Dinarello & Mier, 1987). The same cytokines are also produced by lymphocytes and macrophages. These lymphokines are able to stimulate or inhibit a variety of functions in T and B lymphocytes and macrophages. Table 55–4 lists the functional activities of cytokines involved in lymphocyte activation.

NATURAL KILLER CELLS. Large granular lymphocytes make up almost 3% of the peripheral blood cells. These lymphocytes share some T-lymphocyte, B-lymphocyte, and macrophage surface antigens, but are clearly a distinct subpopulation of lymphocytes (Trincheri & Perussia, 1984). Several different cell lines are included under this term. NK cells are the cells most frequently described (Barrett, 1988).

Natural killer cells participate as effector cells in immune reactions and do not require prior sensitization to exhibit cytotoxicity. NK cells act directly as cytotoxic cells and also produce cytotoxicity by combining with antibody-coated target cells (termed the antibody-dependent cellular cytotoxic reaction). MHC class I or II proteins do not restrict NK cytotoxicity (Bolhuis, 1989). In their resting state, NK cells exhibit maximal killing potential.

The cytotoxic mechanisms of NK cells are not fully understood. The lytic action of agents such as perforins offers one possible mechanism (Anegon et al., 1988). Cytokines also increase the cell-killing ability of NK cells. Cytokines released by NK cells include interferon, TNF, and growth factor. Release of cytokines is triggered by NK cell interaction with IL-2 or target cells (Anegon et al., 1988). Target cells for NK cells include foreign host tissue as in allografts, some viruses, and neoplastic cells (Nakamura, 1989). In vitro exposure to IL-2 has been used to induce the production of lymphokine-activated killer cells (LAK cells). The therapeutic efficacy of concurrent administration of LAK cells and IL-2 is now undergoing clinical evaluation in the treatment of malignant disease. In vivo LAK cell counterparts have not been isolated, however (Lefor et al., 1989).

The immunoregulatory function of NK cells is under extensive exploration. Lymphokines produced by T and B lymphocytes influence NK cell function. Some NK cells also exert immunoregulatory effects on T and B lymphocytes. The exact mechanisms underlying the immunoregulatory role of NK cells have yet to be defined (Kumagai et al., 1989; Tilden & Clement, 1989).

The cells and tissues of the immune system have been reviewed. Some of the interactions between different cell types have been briefly described. In the next sections, the interactions among immune system components are described more fully in the context of how the immune system protects body integrity.

NONSPECIFIC IMMUNITY

Nonspecific immunity (innate immunity) refers to the type of natural resistance each individual characteristically exhibits. Innate immunity varies widely between species and to a lesser extent between individuals (Barrett, 1988). Each exposure to a foreign substance activates nonspecific immune responses. These responses are the body's first line of defense (Roitt et al., 1985). Although selective in differentiating self from nonself, innate immunity is not dependent on specific antigenic recognition.

In comparison, specific immune responses (or acquired immune responses) depend on exposure to a foreign substance and later recognition of and reaction to the substance (memory) (Barrett, 1988). When foreign agents penetrate the innate immune defenses of the body, the acquired immune system specifically recognizes and selectively eliminates them.

Natural Resistance: External Defense System

Nonspecific immunity enables the individual to resist the penetration of foreign substances, fosters the inhibition or destruction of agents invading tissues, and promotes the elimination of toxic wastes (Graziano & Bell, 1985). The first resistive forces met by an invading organism are those outside the physiologic milieu of the body and therefore are categorized as the external defense system (Table 55–8). These forces do not represent a coordinated system and indeed function independently of one another. Nevertheless, they are effective against a variety of potential pathogens.

TABLE 55–8. **External Defense System**

Respiratory System
Mucus
Cilia
Macrophages
Antiviral and antimicrobial secretions
Gastrointestinal System
Acid pH in stomach
Normal flora
Integumentary System
Anatomic barrier
Antimicrobial secretions
Genitourinary System
Flow rate of urine
Acid pH of urine
Lysozyme
Vaginal lactic acid
Eyes
Tears have physical cleansing action
Lysozyme

ANATOMIC BARRIERS. The first line of defense encountered by most potential pathogens is the skin and mucous membranes. These tissues act in nonspecific immunity by providing a physical barrier to invasion. The skin is the more resistant barrier because of its thick outer layer. However, the skin is more than a mere anatomic barrier. The antimicrobial functions of the skin are an important defense mechanism and are discussed more fully in the next section (Adams, 1985). Breaks in skin integrity increase the risk of infection. The skin should be kept relatively dry because in the presence of continuous moisture, skin tends to break down. On the other hand, if the skin is too dry, lubrication should be provided to maintain its integrity. Appropriate skin care of the hospitalized patient will maintain this important defense barrier.

The mucous membranes are structurally more susceptible to penetration than the skin. However, mucosal tissues are protected by several antimicrobial activities. The mucous secretions themselves tend to trap and inactivate organisms. The mucous membranes of the respiratory tract not only act as a trapping mechanism but, together with the action of the ciliated epithelial cells, sweep away foreign microbes (Janson-Bjerklie, 1983). In addition, alveolar macrophages patrol the surface of the mucous membranes. The major function of these cells is the phagocytic destruction of inhaled objects. Tobacco smoke decreases the viability of these macrophages, thus putting smokers at increased risk for respiratory problems (Barrett, 1988).

Lymphoid tissues line the gastrointestinal, respiratory, and genitourinary tracts. IgA and secretory component, found in the secretions from these tissues, increase the protective capacity of lymphoid tissues. IgA also provides antibacterial and antiviral properties to mucosal membranes (Barrett, 1988).

MICROBIAL BARRIERS. There are many microorganisms that colonize the skin and mucosal surfaces. Both internally and externally, a normal flora develops. This flora acts to suppress overgrowth and later infection by pathogenic organisms. The importance of the normal flora of the intestine is often demonstrated in patients receiving long-term antibacterial therapy with a broad-spectrum antibiotic. After about 1 week of therapy, patients may complain of increased flatulence. Stool cultures frequently reveal an increase in number of the yeast *Candida albicans.* This organism is part of the normal intestinal flora and is resistant to antibacterial antibiotics. When antibiotics remove the normal bacterial flora, the yeast thrives and overpopulates the bowel. Continued drug therapy may cause candidiasis of the intestine, in which erosion of the mucous membranes may occur. By this means, the yeast can enter the body and produce a disseminated candidiasis. Normal flora also protect other regions of the body such as the nasopharynx and the vagina.

PHYSIOLOGIC BARRIERS. Secretions of the stomach, skin, and female genitourinary system provide a physiologic barrier against antigens. Hydrogen chloride is secreted in the stomach. Lactic acid and saturated and unsaturated fatty acids are secreted in sweat and on the skin. Lactic acid is secreted in the female genitourinary system. Lysozyme and mucus of the upper respiratory tract and lung are also physiologic barriers (Barrett, 1988).

The gastric juice is an unfavorable environment for many pathogenic orgnisms, which are destroyed in the stomach after ingestion. The lactic acid in sweat and the unsaturated fatty acids in the exogenous secretions from the sebaceous glands are potent antibacterial agents. The saturated fatty acids in these secretions are fungistatic.

Normal urine flow clears bacteria from the urinary tract, preventing infection. Inside the mature female reproductive tract, cells synthesize and store glycogen. As the cells die, the glocygen degrades to lactic acid, creating a bacteriostatic environment in the vagina (Adams, 1985; Bellanti & Kadlec, 1985).

Ciliary action in the respiratory tract is another important physiologic mechanism of resistance. Cilia constantly sweep mucus upward toward the throat. This movement allows organisms trapped in the mucus to be swallowed, exposing them to the potent bactericidal actions of the gastric juices (Adams, 1985; Bellanti & Kadlec, 1985).

The tendency to weep when objects enter the eye is an effective cleansing action and protects the mucosal surfaces of the eye. In the absence of weeping, the action of the enzyme lysozyme is far more important. Lysozyme has the ability to split the bacterial cell wall, causing destruction of the cell. This enzyme is present in high concentration in tears and to a lesser extent in nasal mucus, urine, and plasma and within phagocytic cells. Gram-negative bacteria are highly resistant to lysozyme, but gram-positive microorganisms are not (Adams, 1985; Bellanti & Kadlec, 1985).

Natural Resistance: Internal Defense Systems

PHAGOCYTOSIS. When a foreign substance or antigen enters the body, a chain of events called the phagocytic response is set in motion. The primary role of phagocytosis is to localize an antigen, destroy it or inactivate it, and process it for handling by other parts of the immune system. Phagocytosis is a multiphasic act requiring the following steps: recognition of the material to be ingested, movement toward the object (chemotaxis), attachment, ingestion, and subsequent intracellular digestion by several antimicrobial mechanisms (Fig. 55–6). Very little phagocytosis occurs in the blood because the movement of the blood tends to hold cells apart. Phagocytosis is best accomplished on surfaces and is described as a surface phenomenon (Barrett, 1988).

First, phagocytes are drawn to the area of antigen invasion by a process called chemotaxis. A chemical is released by the antigen itself or by the tissue it has injured. This chemical, the chemotactic factor, stimulates the body's initial efforts to search and destroy. The next step in the sequence is phagocytosis, the process by which a particle is ingested by a phagocytic cell. This process has two steps: the attachment phase and the ingestion phase. During the attachment phase, firm contact occurs between the cell and the particle (Densen & Mandell, 1987). Such contact is largely dependent on the surface properties of the particle. Many bacteria are unencapsulated and are rapidly taken up by phagocytes and destroyed. Encapsulated strains such as the pneumococcus, however, are poorly ingested and hence are not destroyed.

Molecular factors that promote attachment of phagocytes to the objects they will engulf are called opsonins (Densen & Mandell, 1987). Virtually any substance that improves phagocytosis is an opsonin. The best opsonin is antibody against the cell targeted for ingestion. If it is coated with antibody, its surface charge is unable to repel the phagocytic cell. These phagocytic cells tend to carry immunoglobulins of the IgM and IgG class on their surfaces. When an antigen contacts its specific antibody on the phagocytic surface, it is held there by the serologic reaction that takes place. This activity enables phagocytosis to occur. Immunoglobulins are opsonins and share this property with other blood proteins (Barrett, 1988).

The ingestion process is the next step of phagocytosis, and includes engulfment of the particle. The phagocyte extends its cell membrane to form a vacu-

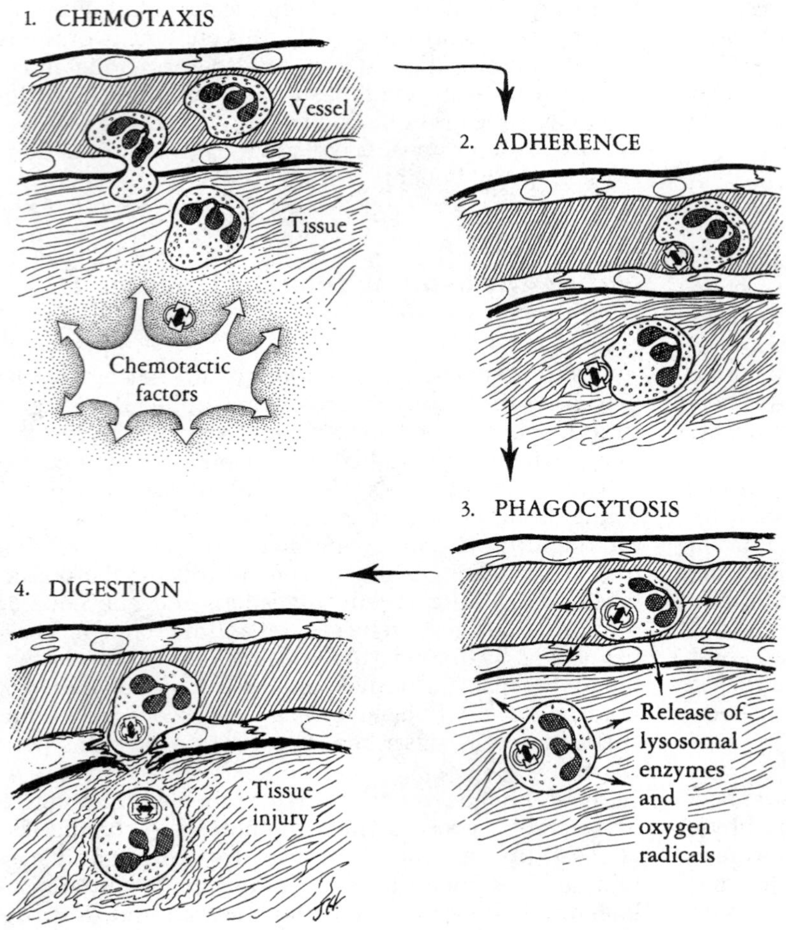

FIGURE 55–6. Sequence of reactions leading to tissue injury associated with neutrophil influx. Note that in addition to chemotaxis, adherence, phagocytosis, and digestion processes that normally result in particle inactivation, there may also be release of neutrophilic granule content (lysosomal enzymes) that results in tissue injury. (From Henson, P. M. [1985]. In J. A. Bellanti [Ed.], *Immunology III* [p. 255]. Philadelphia: W. B. Saunders.)

ole, which surrounds and encloses the antigen. The membrane enclosing the antigen pinches off from the cell surface. Finally, the antigen is internalized and digested by lysosomal enzymes contained within the phagocyte (Densen & Mandell, 1987).

The fate of the ingested antigen depends on its interaction with the phagocyte. Usually antigen is completely destroyed; however, antigen fragments can stay within the phagocyte. Occasionally, both the antigen and the phagocyte die. The necrotic debris that results becomes purulent matter or pus. Another outcome of the interaction between the antigen and the phagocyte is survival of the antigen. If the phagocyte lives, it may spread disease as it travels through the body carrying a live organism. With death of the phagocyte, release of antigen may trigger specific immunologic defense mechanisms.

INFLAMMATION. Inflammation is a complex series of events that occurs when the body is injured (Ward, 1985). There is a tendency to consider the inflammatory response harmful to the body. Inflammation is, however, a protective mechanism in which the body tries either to return to the preinjury condition or to repair itself after injury.

The clinical signs of inflammation are well known. They include swelling, redness, heat, pain, and altered function. The inflammatory response depends on both intact blood vessels and the circulating cells and fluids within these channels. According to histologic criteria, three states of inflammation exist—acute, subacute, and chronic. The acute inflammatory response begins by the dilatation of blood vessels and the outpouring of leukocytes and fluids. Clinically, this results in redness (erythema) due to blood vessel dilation, swelling (edema) due to escape of fluids into soft tissues, and firmness (induration) due to accumulation of fluids and cells. The result of these processes leads to a loss of the normal capacity of blood vessels to keep fluids and cells within the vasculature. The release of certain factors, such as histamine, from tissue mast cells may make the vessel more permeable to plasma fluids. The acute inflammatory response reflects the effects of mediators acting on the blood vessels rather than a nonspecific injury to the vessel. The mediators cause selective release of fluids and cells from the inflamed tissues (Gallin, 1989).

Within 30 to 60 minutes of injury, neutrophils appear, representing the first line of defense against invading microorganisms. As discussed earlier, the prime function of neutrophils is to ingest and destroy pathogens. If the acute inflammatory response progresses, mononuclear cells (including monocytes and lymphocytes) appear within 4 to 5 hours. Monocytes also phagocytose pathogens, whereas lymphocytes respond to foreign agents by specific humoral and cell-mediated phenomena that are discussed later (Ward, 1985).

Although the inflammatory response is protective, if it becomes aberrant, serious consequences may occur. For example, the outpouring of too much fluid from the vasculature into the brain may cause a serious rise in intracranial pressure. Accumulation of fluid due to inflammation in the pleural or pericardial cavities may compromise organ function in these areas. In addition, the arrival of excessive numbers of neutrophils and the subsequent release of their enzymatic contents may result in serious structural damage (e.g., vasculitis, nephritis) (Ward, 1985).

The subacute inflammatory response is a somewhat delayed phase of the acute inflammatory response and is characterized by the accumulation of lymphocytes and monocytes and the formation of granulation tissue. For example, 1 to 3 days after a skin laceration, a dramatic proliferation of endothelial cells and fibroblasts occurs. Within 5 days, a bridge of connective tissue has formed across a previously open and exposed area (Ward, 1985).

If the inflammatory response is not completely successful in restoring the injured tissue to its original state or if repair of tissue is not accomplished, a state of chronic inflammation may ensue. This is characterized by the continued presence of lymphocytes, monocytes, and plasma cells. Persistence of foreign material that mobilizes immunologic reactions may also cause chronic inflammation. For example, in patients with viral hepatitis, replicating virus may persist within the liver (Ward, 1985).

Depending on the severity of the inflammatory response, a variety of systemic effects may occur. Many microorganisms and certain WBCs produce pyrogenic materials, which act on the hypothalamus to increase body temperature (McCarron, 1986; Norwood, 1988). Although there is a tendency to consider fever as harmful to the body, it has several beneficial effects. An elevation in body temperature of only a few degrees results in inhibition or death of a variety of microorganisms. Pneumococci are killed by temperatures as low as 40°C. It has been suggested that one of the reasons why fever may be beneficial during viral infections is that it leads to lysosomal breakdown. Perforation of lysosomes causes autodestruction of the infected cell and prevents viral replication (Cunha, 1985; Cunha et al., 1984). Release of interferons by T cells and fibroblasts during inflammation also inhibits viral replication. Temperature increases of only 2° to 3°F are necessary to increase the production of antiviral interferons. It has frequently been observed that patients who are unable to mount a febrile response or who have subnormal temperatures have a poorer prognosis than those who mount a normal febrile response (Cunha et al., 1984).

Another systemic effect of inflammation may be an increased production of WBCs. A serum WBC level of greater than 10,000/mm^3 is called leukocytosis. Extreme elevations of WBCs may indicate a lymphoproliferative disease such as leukemia. Low-grade WBC elevations can occur with cell injury due to myocardial infarction and bone fracture or with other events such as indigestion, exercise, and increased stress. Total elevation of the WBC count is, therefore, a nonspecific phenomenon (Gurevich, 1985).

The WBC differential count provides more specific information. In this test, white cells in the peripheral blood are classified according to the two major types of leukocytes—granulocytes (neutrophils, eosinophils, and basophils), and nongranulocytes (lymphocytes and monocytes). The percentage of each is also determined. The differential count is the relative number of each type of white cell in the blood. The absolute number of each type of white cell is obtained by multiplying the percentage value of each type by the total WBC count. When the total number of immature neutrophils (blasts, bands, or stabs) is increased in the differential count, it is termed a "shift to the left" because cell maturation is visualized from the left side to the right side, with less mature cells on the left (Gurevich, 1985).

Prolonged bacterial infections tend to cause a shift to the left. In such infections, mature cells are killed by bacterial action and are replaced by immature white cells. In an attempt to replace the mature neutrophils, the bone marrow releases cells prematurely. The release of immature cells results in an increased number of circulating neutrophils, but these immature neutrophils are poor participants in phagocytosis (Gurevich, 1985). Overwhelming infection may result from an imbalance in the proportion of immature to mature neutrophils. Careful attention to the results of WBC differential counts is essential in critically ill patients. A "shift to the right" signifies the presence of mature neutrophils with the more nuclear segments than normal. Commonly, this occurs with hepatic disease and pernicious anemia. A "degenerative shift" indicates an increased number of band cells and a low WBC count, and reflects bone marrow depression. A "regenerative shift" occurs with bone marrow stimulation. Stimulation of the bone marrow causes increased numbers of band cells, metamyelocytes, and myelocytes and a high WBC count. This situation frequently occurs with pneumonia and appendicitis (Gurevich, 1985).

The hallmark of leukopenia is a decreased serum WBC count of less than 4,500 cells/mm^3. Leukopenia commonly occurs in viral infections, typhoid fever, or toxic reactions that depress the bone marrow. Viral and tuberculous infections usually produce an increase in mature lymphocytes (Gurevich, 1985).

An increased erythrocyte sedimentation rate may occur as another systemic effect of inflammation. The technique for determining the sedimentation rate requires the addition of an anticoagulant to blood in a test tube. The red blood cells settle to the bottom more rapidly than normal in patients with an elevated sedimentation rate. An increase in the sedimentation rate occurs during the acute inflammatory stage of infection, coinciding with an increase in the protein fibrinogen, which is essential for the healing process.

It is vital for the nurse to understand the physiologic changes that occur during the inflammatory process. One can then better understand the many defense mechanisms that may be operating during different disease states.

THE COMPLEMENT SYSTEM. One of the most complex and powerful results of antigen–antibody binding is the activation of complement. Discovery of complement within serum occurred in the nineteenth century. The bactericidal activity of fresh serum required not only antibody but also a nonspecific component that enchanced antibody activity (Barrett, 1989). That nonspecific component was later identified as complement.

Recent research has shown a broad role for complement as a participant in inflammation, immune tissue injury, and modulation of the immune response. Elevated levels of activated complement are associated with pulmonary injury in adult respiratory distress syndrome (Langlois et al., 1989). There are at least 20 complement proteins and fragments that circulate in the plasma in an inactive form. Activation of complement proteins results from splitting the inactive protein into two parts. The larger part attaches to target cells and bacteria. The smaller part is released into the fluid around the cell. Most small complement fragments have biologic activity and interact with other proteins in the complement sequence (Frank & Fries, 1989). Table 55–9 describes some of the major complement proteins.

TABLE 55–9. **Some Proteins of the Complement Cascade**

Protein	Concentration in Serum (mg/mL)	Biologic Function
C1 q	80	Binds to Ag-Ab complexes
r	34	Subunit of C1
s	30	Enzymatic activity cleaves C4 and C2
C4	350	C4a anaphylatoxin C4b viral neutralization
C2	15	
C3	1,200	C3a anaphylatoxin, immunoregulatory C3b key component of alternative pathway; major opsonin in serum C3e fragment induces leukocytosis
C5	75	C5a anaphylatoxin; principal chemotactic factor in serum; induces neutrophil attachment to endothelium C5b initiates membrane attack
C6	70	Participates with C5b in formation of membrane attack complex that lyses cells
C7	60	
C8	80	
C9	60	
Factor B	225	Bb causes macrophage spreading on surfaces
Factor D	1	
Properdin	25	Stabilizes alternative pathway convertase

From Lockey, R., & Bukantz S. (1987). *Fundamentals of immunology and allergy* (p. 42). Philadelphia: W. B. Saunders.

The role of biologically active byproducts of complement activation assumes great importance in the immune response. First, the coating of bacteria or other immune complexes with components of complements aids ingestion of the bacteria by phagocytic cells. The cooperation of complement and immune complexes demonstrates the opsonic function of complement. Second, several of the products of complement proteins serve as chemotactic factors that attract phagocytes to the site of the reaction (inflammatory function of complement). When certain complement proteins are activated, other complement fragments are released. Some complement fragments act to release histamine from mast cells and are chemoattractants for polymorphonuclear leukocytes. Histamine increases vascular permeability and enhances smooth muscle contraction. The result is very similar to that seen in the classic anaphylactic reaction. Third, the late-acting proteins of the complement cascade form the complex that attacks and causes the death of target cells. The cytotoxic activity of complement is directed against viruses, bacteria, fungi, parasites, virus-infected cells, and tumor cells (Barrett, 1988).

Several cell types synthesize complement proteins. Two of the most important cell types are the liver hepatocyte and mononuclear phagocytic cells. Activation of complement proteins results in a rapid cascade of protein degradation. Degraded complement protein fragments activate the later steps in the cascade. These proteins are activated by two independent pathways, termed the classic pathway and the alternative pathway (Fig. 55–7).

Activation of the classic complement pathway, C1 through C9, starts with complexing of antigen to antibody. Antibody and complement proteins circulate in the blood and lymph. Antibody undergoes a conformational change on interaction with antigen. This requisite change in antibody structure allows interaction between antibody and complement. It is the antibody conformational change that is the basis for specific activation of the classic complement pathway (Barrett, 1988; Cooper, 1987). Table 55–10 lists the activators of the classic pathway.

Another group of activators of the complement system includes many types of aggregated proteins, bacterial and other microbial membranes, and various cell walls (Table 55–11). These components activate the complement sequence through the alternative pathway (also known as the properdin pathway). This pathway is an alternative to the classic pathway in that this system begins the complement sequence at C3. The alternative pathway does not absolutely require antibody, C1, C4, or C2 for activation (Cooper, 1987).

Parts of bacterial membranes from gram-negative bacteria and the walls of certain gram-positive organisms are some of the most powerful activators of the

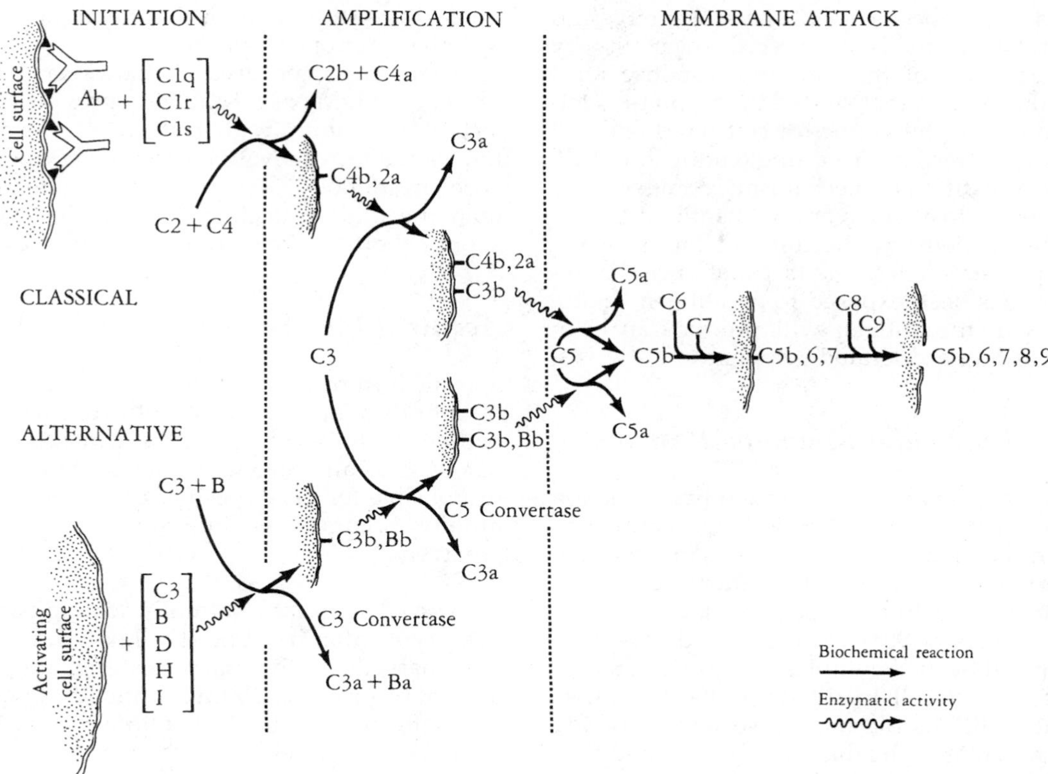

FIGURE 55–7. Schematic representation of the two pathways of complement activation. (From Kimkel, S. L., et al. [1985]. In J. A. Bellanti [Ed.], *Immunology III* [p. 107]. Philadelphia: W. B. Saunders.)

alternative pathway. Consider, for example, an infection with a gram-negative organism. Because we have low levels of antibody to most bacteria, some limited classic pathway activation occurs in response to such an infection. In the presence of large numbers of bacteria, low levels of specific antibody are absorbed from the serum by the antigenic complexes. This allows uncoated bacteria to escape the classic pathway. Before production of specific antibody, the alternative pathway components (C3b, factor B, factor D, and properdin) are spontaneously deposited on the bacteria, thus beginning the alternative complement sequence. Most bacteria, fungi, and viruses activate the alternative pathway to some degree (Barrett, 1988; Cooper, 1987). Hence, activation of this pathway is extremely important during the early phase of infection when specific antibody is limited. After the formation of antibodies, the classic and alternative pathways work in tandem.

SPECIFIC IMMUNITY

There are three general characteristics of the specific immune response that distinguish it from nonspe-

TABLE 55–10. **Activators of the Classic Pathway**

Immunoglobulins
IgG (human subclasses 1, 2, and 3)
IgM
Nonimmunoglobulin Activators
Bacterial lipopolysaccharide (lipid A portion)
C-reactive protein bound to pneumococci
Retroviruses
Heart mitochondrial membranes
Polyanions (e.g., polynucleotides)
Urate crystals

From Kunkel, S. L., et al. (1985). In J. A. Bellanti (Ed.), *Immunology III* (p. 108). Philadelphia: W. B. Saunders.

TABLE 55–11. **Activators of the Alternative Pathway**

Polysaccharides (e.g., inulin)
Yeast cell walls (zymosan)
Bacterial cell wall components (lipopolysaccharide, peptidoglycan)
Influenza and other viruses
Schistosoma and other parasites
Cryptococci and other fungi
Certain tumor cells
Cobra venom factor
Nephritic factor (autoantibody that stabilizes C3b, Bb)
X-ray contrast media
Dialysis membranes

From Kunkel, S. L., et al. (1985). in J. A. Bellanti (Ed.), *Immunology III* (p. 110). Philadelphia: W. B. Saunders.

cific responses: (1) specificity, (2) heterogeneity, and (3) memory. Specificity is the precise selectivity by which the products of the immune response react solely with the antigen that started the response. Heterogeneity refers to the variety of cell types and cell products that can respond to a single antigen but do so through many different mechanisms. Some of these cells also give rise to a wide variety of antibodies (immunoglobulins). Memory, the third hallmark of the immune response, refers to the fact that once the immune system has been exposed to an antigen, future encounters with the antigen will produce an even more vigorous and accelerated response.

Primary and Secondary Immune Response

On initial exposure to an antigen, antibody production and distribution are delayed. Antibody reaches detectable levels in the blood 3 to 4 days after the injection of foreign erythrocytes, 5 to 7 days after exposure to soluble proteins, and 10 to 14 days after exposure to bacterial cells (Barrett, 1988). During these delays, antigen is recognized by the B lymphocyte. Antigen recognition causes the B cell to divide and differentiate into a plasma cell. The plasma cell secretes antibody specific to the antigen. In this primary antibody response, the first antibody class synthesized is usually IgM. Later, IgG antibodies predominate over IgM antibodies. The ratio between IgM and IgG antibodies is a useful index for discriminating between recent and past infections, particularly in viral infections.

Antibody does not reach a high level or persist without a second dose of antigen. The combination of antibody with antigen decreases detectable antibody in the blood. Within 1 to 2 days, a rapid rise in the level of antibody occurs that can be from 10 to 50 times higher than the primary response. The persistent high level of anibody characterizes this secondary response. Antibody levels decline slowly over a period of months. Once an individual has responded to an antigen, the immune system retains a memory of that antigen. It is IgG that carries the memory of exposure. IgG remains in the bloodstream for long periods. Later exposure of IgG to the same antigen stimulates B-lymphocyte memory cells. Even after an interval of months or years, the immune system may mount a secondary response. Such a response is possible because presensitized antibody-secreting cells are mobilized within 1 to 2 days (Barrett, 1988).

A common example of an immunizing antibody response occurs in people with hepatitis A virus infection. It is during the acute phase that specific hepatitis A IgM is detectable. Once IgG titers become elevated, IgM disappears, and the patient enters the recovery phase. Levels of IgG remain detectable for life, a reminder of past infection and immunity. After a second encounter with the hepatitis A virus, IgG titers rise rapidly. The rapid presence of antibody precludes viral takeover and prevents a repeat infection. Vaccinations against the common childhood illnesses produce a similar immune response.

There are some diseases, however, in which the presence of IgM or IgG antibody provides neither protection nor immunity (Barrett, 1988). Herpes virus reinfection and reactivation can occur even in the presence of antibody. Recurrences are often less severe than the initial infection because the rapid IgG response shortens their duration to some extent.

Acquired Immunity

Specific host resistance can be acquired. Acquired immunity develops as a result of exposure to a specific pathogen. Unlike phagocytosis, which is a nonspecific response to an antigen, acquired immune defense is responsible for very specific responses. Acquired immunity occurs after infection with pathogens or passively.

ACTIVE IMMUNITY. Naturally acquired active immunity occurs after overt or subclinical infection. During the illness, the individual receives an antigenic stimulus that begins production of antibody against the specific pathogen involved. On reinfection by the same or an antigenically related pathogen, the antibodies are ready to help defend the body. This naturally acquired defense system lasts for months or years.

Exposure to an antigen (immunogen) by vaccination produces artificially acquired active immunity. Some infections, such as diphtheria, whooping cough, smallpox, and mumps, usually induce a lifetime immunity. Others, such as the common cold, influenza, and pneumococcal pneumonia, induce immunity for a shorter time, sometimes for only a few weeks. The organisms producing these diseases undergo frequent mutations, resulting in a constant supply of new strains. Acquisition of immunity to one strain does not prevent infection by another strain of the same organism. Regardless of the type of infection, active immunity appears only after a specified lapse of time after exposure to the antigen (Barrett, 1988). Like naturally acquired immunity, artificially induced immunity endures for years.

PASSIVE IMMUNITY. Natural and artificial methods are also used to confer passive immunity. In humans, the classic example of naturally acquired passive immunity is the passage of maternal antibody across the placenta during the latter part of pregnancy. IgG alone is transferred from mother to fetus. IgM, IgE, IgD, and IgA do not cross the placental barrier. During breastfeeding, colostrum contains IgA and IgM. Ingestion of colostrum provides passive immunity to infants during the early days postpartum.

Artificially introduced passive immunity develops in one individual after injection of antibodies produced by another individual. Pooled human immunoglobulin (gamma globulin) is a source of antibody used to confer passive immunity. Given during the incubation period of measles infection or infectious hepatitis, pooled human immunoglobulin modifies the intensity of disease symptomatology.

Because passive immunity acquired naturally or artificially involves the transfer of preformed antibodies, its onset of action is immediate. Nonetheless, because there may be no stimulus for continued production, its effect is usually of short duration (Barrett, 1988).

Specific Mechanisms of Immune Response

Specific immunologic defense mechanisms recognize antigens as nonself, as do nonspecific immune mechanisms. They are also capable of more precise immunologic reactions and respond in a manner unique to each antigen's composition. There are two mechanisms that mediate specific immune responses—antibody-mediated (humoral) immunity and cell-mediated immunity. Antibody production by lymphoid tissues is the focal point of antibody-mediated immunity. Cell-mediated immunity focuses on specifically sensitized lymphocytes.

ANTIBODY-MEDIATED IMMUNITY. It is now accepted that the triggering of a humoral (antibody) response to antigens requires the cooperation of B cells, macrophages, and T cells. For participation in an antibody response, B cells require more than one signal before activation. Macrophages and helper T cells aid B-lymphocyte activation. The precise mechanism by which B-cell activation occurs is unknown (Fig. 55–8). Many pieces of the puzzle are, however, emerging. Both specific subsets of cells and cell products called cytokines influence antibody-mediated immunity.

The first step involves antigen processing by the macrophage. During antigen processing, the macrophage releases IL-1, a cytokine that fosters differentiation of inducer T cells. This subset of T cells releases a second cytokine, IL-2. The second cytokine promotes the maturation of helper T lymphocytes.

CELL-MEDIATED IMMUNITY. The primary component of cellular immunity is the T lymphocyte. A basic misconception formerly held about cell-mediated immunity was that T lymphocytes acted independently of antibody. A variety of cell types, antibody, humoral substances, and combinations of these constitute most cell-mediated immune responses.

Like antigen–antibody reactions, cell-mediated immune reactions are divided into primary, secondary, and tertiary stages. After initial processing by the phagocytes, antigens travel to the regional lymph node that drains the area invaded by antigens. The primary stage of the cell-mediated reaction begins when the T lymphocyte binds antigen with an antigen receptor on its surface. During the secondary stage, a variety of morphologic and biochemical changes occur that include DNA, RNA, or protein synthesis. The tertiary stage consists of the generation of helper, suppressor, cytotoxic, and memory T cells. In the tertiary stage, the T cells that release the mediators of cell-mediated immunity emerge.

It is the tertiary stage that is the most complex. Initially, macrophages activate the small number of helper T cells that have receptors for the antigen. In response to contact with the antigen, helper T cells release cytokines. Some of these cytokines activate macrophages and recruit other cytokines and monocytes–macrophages to participate in the reaction. Activated macrophages produce monokines. Monokines are

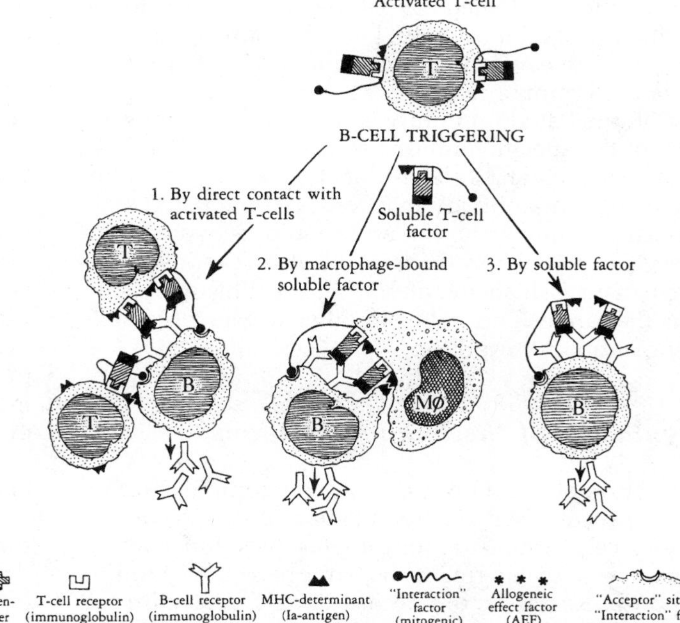

FIGURE 55–8. B cells may be activated and triggered to grow and produce antibody in three ways: (1) by direct contact with antigen-bearing activated T cells; (2) by macrophage-bound soluble factors; or (3) by soluble antigen-specific T-cell factors. (Adapted from Herscowitz, H. B. [1985]. In J. A. Bellanti [Ed.], *Immunology III* [p. 148]. Philadelphia: W. B. Saunders.)

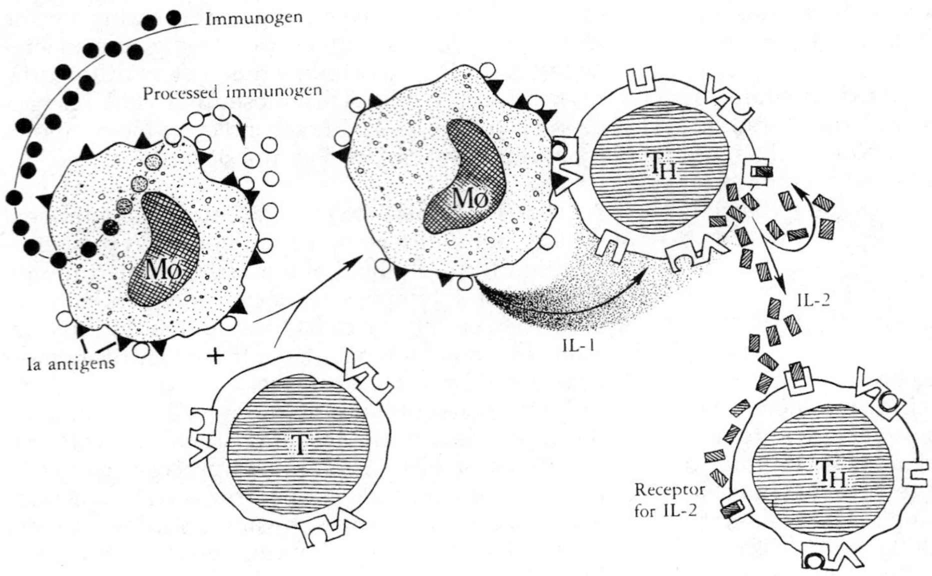

FIGURE 55–9. Schematic representation of the cellular events involved in T-cell activation. Mo, macrophage; T_H, helper T cell. (From Herscowitz, H. B. [1985]. In J. A. Bellanti [Ed.], *Immunology III* [p. 146]. Philadelphia: W. B. Saunders.)

secretory products of monocytes or macrophages. Monokines and cytokines often are the same chemical but are secreted by different cell types.

Some monokines, such as IL-1, are necessary for T-cell activation (Fig. 55–9). The release of IL-1 by macrophages expands the activation of a single T cell by antigen to activation of many T cells. IL-1 is released locally into tissue and into blood and activates all T lymphocytes within its reach. Therefore, a reaction that initially involves a small number of sensitized cells is amplified. Now the immune response includes many T cells that were not directly sensitized by antigen.

Like the antibody-mediated immune response, the cell-mediated immune response results in the formation of long-lived, memory T lymphocytes. Due to the production of memory cells, later exposure to the same antigen will evoke a more rapid and intense cell-mediated immune response.

Cell-mediated immunity includes those manifestations of the specific immune response expressed by a variety of cells and cell products. As opposed to humoral antigen–antibody reactions, cell-mediated reactions have a delayed onset and require activated lymphocytes or their products to elicit a response. This mechanism is instrumental when dealing with antigens that are cell bound or in other ways inaccessible to the antibody response.

Regulation of the Immune Response

Regulation of immune responses is a complex and intricate process. Many different subpopulations of regulatory cells interact among themselves and with effector cells to augment or suppress the immune response. Research to date has largely been directed toward identification and characterization of individual subpopulations of regulatory cells, effector cells, and their secretory products. Understanding how each cell type and mediator interact to provide careful and controlled regulation of each immune response is the true challenge. Figure 55–10 depicts the current understanding of the interplay between immunocompetent cells and immunoregulatory mediators.

IMMUNOCOMPETENCE

The word *immunocompetence* is used by lay persons and many health professionals to describe the effectiveness of the immune system in warding off disease. Although this definition oversimplifies the meaning of immunocompetence, it serves as a common interdisciplinary starting point. The key to the multiple interpretations of this concept is our inherent understanding of the mechanism by which disease can or should be warded off. For example, in medicine immunocompetence describes the ability of humans to respond to a particular infectious or tumorigenic challenge (Wyngaarden & Smith, 1988). In contrast, the lay literature implies that a state of immunocompetence will prevent an individual from succumbing to disease. For example, to the layman, the immunocompetent individual is perceived to be less likely to get a cold than the immunocompromised individual. This view of immune functioning is not supported by empirical evidence.

In nursing, the meaning of immunocompetence has been derived from an exploration of human responses in disorders that suppress immune function. Examples include cancer, acquired immunodeficiency syndrome, genetic immune system defects, and the effects of therapeutic modalities that assault the immune system. Specific pharmacologic agents and radiation ther-

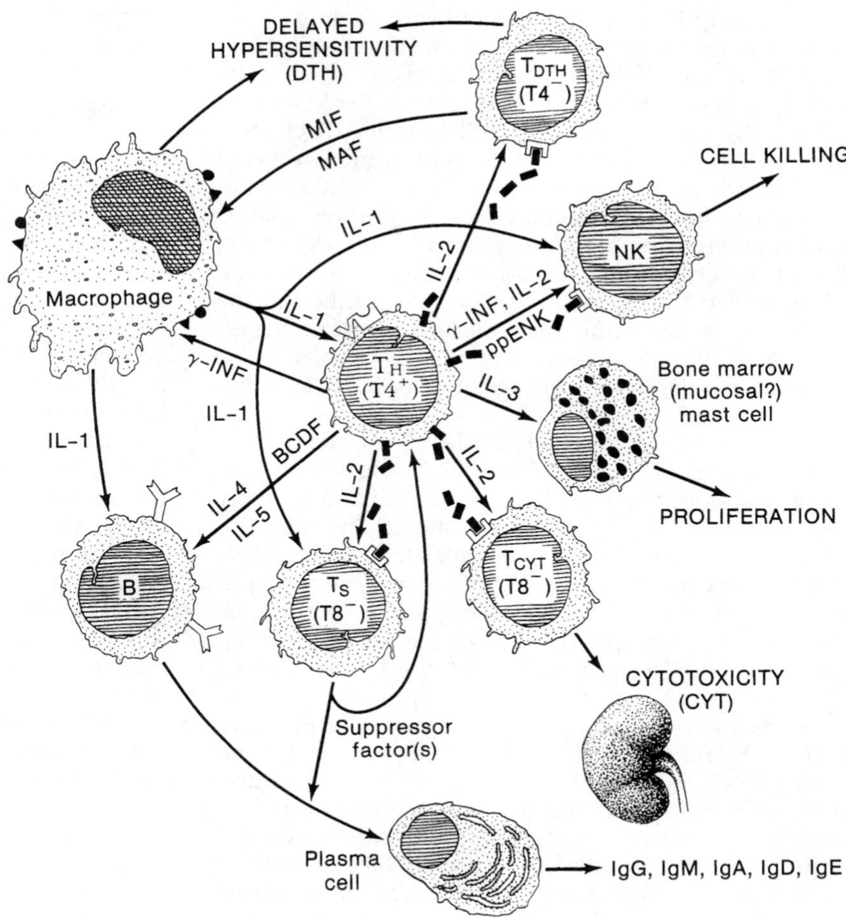

FIGURE 55–10. Cellular events that make up the tertiary stage of cell-mediated immunity in the human, illustrating the central role of the T cell in the immunoregulatory network, γ-INF, interferon-gamma; IL-1, interleukin-1; IL-2, interleukin-2; IL-3, interleukin-3; IL-4, interleukin-4; Il-5, interleukin-5; MIF, migratory inhibitory factor; MAF, macrophage activating factor; CSF, colony stimulating factor; BCDF, B-cell differentiating factor; ppENK, preproenkephalin. (Adapted from Bellanti, J. A., & Rocklin, R. E. [1985]. In J. A. Bellanti [Ed.], *Immunology III* [p. 181]. Philadelphia: W. B. Saunders.)

apy also compromise immune function. Halliburton (1986) describes an immunocompetent person as a host that responds adequately to an antigenic stimulus. An adequate response maintains bodily integrity. She further states that immunocompetence is a human response that is within the nature and scope of nursing practice.

Nurses in critical care settings need to take advantage of what is known about the immune system and the effects of the environment on immunocompetence. We are only beginning to realize that the immune system can be artificially controlled. In vitro enhancement of immune function is a burgeoning area of research. Knowledge of potential threats to immunocompetence will help critical care nurses protect patients from or ameliorate the effects of immunosuppressive agents.

Threats to Immunocompetence

There are many factors that modify immune function. External and internal defense forces do not function at the same level of efficiency in all individuals. Patients requiring intensive medical and surgical treatment are exposed to additional immunosuppressive conditions. Age, hormonal balance, nutrition, surgery, trauma, and psychological distress influence both specific and nonspecific immunity.

AGE. Age influences immunity, and infectious diseases are more severe at the extremes of life. In the very young, immaturity of the immune system leads to poor antigen recognition or antibody production. In the elderly, there is evidence that a hypofunctional state of the immune system occurs (Adler, 1989).

Diminished responsiveness to externally administered antigens and increased responsiveness to internal antigens are the immunologic changes associated with aging (Effros, 1984). Functional changes at the cellular level occur in both T and B lymphocytes (Gillis et al., 1981; Whisler et al., 1985). Immune responses of elderly subjects vary greatly from individual to individual, even in the absence of disease. Responses range from those that are no different from responses in the young adult to responses that are significantly diminished. The most overt change is that of thymic involution (atrophy of the thymus). This change leads to decreased ability of immune cells to discriminate between self and nonself. Thymic involution also causes diminished T-cell proliferation responses to mitogens, self antigens, and conventional antigens. There is conflicting evidence on whether the numbers and proportion of B cells change in old age. There is, however, general agreement that serum immunoglobulin does show age-related changes (Effros, 1984). The defects in humoral immunity associated with old age are related to defective T-cell collaboration, defective monocyte function, and regulation of B-cell responses.

Changes in immune function occur gradually and are not precipitated by achieving a certain chronologic age. A greater proportion of the very old (>85 years) do, however, exhibit diminished immune function compared to younger adults. Therefore, although the aging process does influence immune function, the effects are subtle in nature and appear to be most influential in the extreme age ranges (Whisler et al., 1985).

HORMONES. Changes in the levels of many hormones modulate immune function. These changes occur in response to nonpathogenic stimuli and in many disease states. Insulin deficiency affects the integrity of cell membranes, making diabetics more susceptible to infectious agents. Thus, diabetics are more susceptible to staphylococcal, streptococcal, and several fungal diseases. There is also an increased susceptibility to infection in both hypoadrenal and hypothyroid states.

NUTRITION. Nutrition plays a major role in maintaining the functional capacity of the immune system (Gross & Newberne, 1980; Shronts, 1993). Some clinical studies of cancer and obesity conclude that an imbalance in nutrient intake correlates with decreased immune function (Brookes & Clifford, 1981; Chandra, 1980). Severe, prolonged protein–calorie malnutrition profoundly alters cell-mediated immunity (Chandra, 1980). Severe malnutrition has less effect on humoral immunity and phagocytic function (Stiehm, 1980).

Dietary factors other than protein and calories, such as vitamins and minerals (Lahita et al., 1984), also contribute to these alterations. Insufficient intake of vitamin A, pyridoxine, biotin, folic acid components, zinc, and iron alters immune function (Halliburton, 1986).

Altered cellular immune function occurs in association with gross obesity. Chandra (1981) reported that the altered cellular immunity seen with obesity correlated with subclinical deficiencies of zinc and iron. In addition, high caloric intake, particularly fat-related calorie intake, can affect immune function. Excess cholesterol, saturated fatty acid, and polyunsaturated fatty acid decrease immune function (Beisel, 1981).

SURGERY AND ANESTHESIA. Surgical intervention and anesthesia lead to impaired immune function (Browder & Williams, 1988). A transient, severe lymphopenia occurs in the immediate postoperative period. Complete return of normal immune function may take 10 days to 2 weeks (Lundy & Ford, 1983). The complement system is activated in certain types of operations, particularly abdominal and cardiovascular surgery (Watkins & Salo, 1982). Anesthesia partially inhibits T-cell function and reduces phagocytosis. Length of exposure to anesthetic agents and degree of surgical trauma affect both the quality and the quantity of these immune changes (Halliburton, 1986).

TRAUMA. Burn injury suppresses all aspects of immune function (Moran & Munster, 1987). The exact mechanisms of the pervasive immunosuppressive effect of thermal injury are not well understood. There is a decrease in the regulation of the immune response, with a marked decrease in IL-2 production. Nonspecific immune response is also diminished. Most of these responses are seen in patients about 4 to 5 days after injury (Antonacci, 1986). Because of the many possible contributing factors such as age and infection, it is difficult to discern what causes the persistence of immune dysfunction.

Blunt injury is primarily associated with alterations in nonspecific immune responses. Neutrophil migration to the site of inflammation is impaired. The degree of dysfunction is related to the magnitude of the injury. Immune dysfunction occurs almost immediately after injury and is most intense in the first 24 hours. Although immune dysfunction is of short duration, this time period is associated with a higher rate of infection and septicemia.

THERAPEUTIC AGENTS. A wide variety of drugs used to treat many clinical diseases display immunosuppressive activity (Chang et al., 1993). The most common therapeutic immunosuppressive agents are corticosteroids, azathioprine, cyclophosphamide, actinomycin, mercaptopurine, and antithymocyte globulin. Many of these agents were first developed to treat cancer. These drugs are now used to treat overactive immune responses in autoimmune diseases, including rheumatoid arthritis, multiple sclerosis, and inflammatory bowel disease (Halliburton, 1986; Chang et al., 1993).

The use of corticosteroids is pervasive in the critical care settings. Treatment with corticosteroids reduces the inflammatory response, depresses phagocytosis, alters the functional ability of T lymphocytes, and inhibits immunoglobulin synthesis (Smith, 1986). Corticosteroids thus increase susceptibility to bacterial infection (e.g., staphylococcal infection) as well as to certain viral diseases (e.g., varicella) (Sheagren & Young, 1987).

PSYCHOLOGICAL DISTRESS. Studies of the psychological influence on immune function have explored the relationship of acute stressors to a variety of humoral cellular indicators of immune function. Studies have also measured immune function during events considered by investigators to be distressing. More recently, research has focused on the relationship between emotional distress and immune function in the context of distressing situations (Groer, 1991; Rabin et al., 1989).

Emotionally distressing experiences influence many parameters of immune function, including cellular and humoral responses. Most recent studies have focused on examination of cellular immune function, perhaps due to the relative insulation of this response to transient external stimuli. Transient external stimuli such as engaging in conversation are reported to affect humoral immune function. For example, salivary IgA levels are particularly sensitive to events that represent a change in the environment. Changes in IgA levels do not solely reflect responses to specific distressing situations (Stone et al., 1987). On the other hand, measures of cellular immune function change in response to intense and focused emotional distress.

Suppression of in vitro T- and B-lymphocyte proliferation in response to antigenic and mitogenic stimulation occurs in people experiencing loss. Immunosuppression occurs in bereaved spouses (Bartrop et al., 1977), spouses of people admitted to critical care units with life-threatening diseases (Schleifer et al., 1983), unemployed women (Arnetz et al., 1987), and separated and divorced women (Kiecolt-Glaser et al., 1987a). Immunosuppression has also been reported in students when they take major examinations (Halvorsen & Vassend, 1987; Kiecolt-Glaser et al., 1984, 1986). Research is only beginning in patients with acute medical problems.

Augmentation of Immune Function

Although popular interest in stimuation or boosting of the immune system is high, little research has been done in this arena. Three main avenues of exploration are (1) therapeutic agents, (2) nutrition, and (3) psychological stimulation. To date, most research in these areas has focused on the ability to modulate single cells or mediators of specific immunologic responses reliably. Dietary supplementation with arginine increases in vitro lymphocyte proliferation (Daly et al., 1990). Pavlovian conditioning techniques are used to enhance lymphocyte proliferation in vitro. Importantly, the clinical or in vivo effect of these reported modulators have not been determined, nor have the mechanisms of effect been clearly elucidated. Thus, the area of immune function augmentation is ripe for further research (Rabin et al., 1989).

SUMMARY

The manifestations of the immune response may be viewed as the capacity of the host to recognize and dispose of foreign substances. Once an antigen has been introduced, the body attempts to eliminate it by phagocytosis. During this first encounter, there is no preexisting antibody to facilitate engulfment. Disposal of the antigen is determined by the efficiency of the phagocytic process. If phagocytosis is successful, the organism is eliminated, and disease symptoms are not seen or are minimal. The specific immune response may be induced to stimulate activity of cells capable of either producing antibody or inducing cell-mediated events. Further encounters with the same organism result in a more rapid and intense response. Regulation of the immune system is now recognized to be orchestrated by a host of chemical mediators interacting with many different types of cells.

Immunocompetence depends not only on the state of health of an individual but on biologic and environmental factors. Surgery, trauma, nutrition, and many therapeutic drugs pose a particular threat to the immune function of critically ill patients. Phagocytosis or cellular immune responses may be unsuccessful if the immune system is suppressed by medication or a state of poor health. Impairment of the immune system can lead to active disease or even death.

Competency of both nonspecific and specific immune responses is critical to the body's management of infections. The course of many diseases is determined by the efficiency of the immune response. Antigen must be successfully recognized and removed. This requires not only lymphocyte and macrophage involvement but a granulocytic response. Production of antibody, synthesis and secretion of mediators, and many other chemicals including complement further enhance the effectiveness of the immune response. Effective immune system component responses are not enough to achieve an immunocompetent state; the timing and coordination of individual component responses must be carefully regulated as well.

There is much yet to be learned about the immune system. It is essential that all parts of the system work together to maintain health, including the primitive responses of phagocytosis and inflammation, which can dispose of most foreign substances. In the case of pathogens that escape these responses, the specific immune response leads to release of products that facilitate or enhance these primitive responses. The outcome of this encounter of the host with a pathogen can be either beneficial or harmful, depending on the efficiency of the immune system.

REFERENCES

Abbas, A., Lichtman, A., & Pober, J. (1991). *Cellular and molecular immunology.* Philadelphia: W. B. Saunders.

Adams, A. (1985). External barriers to infection. *Nursing Clinics of North America, 20,* 145–149.

Adler, W. H. (1989). Immune function in the elderly. *Geriatrics, 44*(suppl A), 7–10.

Anegon, I., Cuturi, M., Trinchieri, G., et al. (1988). Interaction of Fc receptor (CD16) with ligands induces transcription of IL-2 receptor (CD25) and lymphokine genes and expression of their products in human natural killer cells. *Journal of Experimental Medicine, 167,* 452–472.

Antonacci, A. C. (1986). Immune dysfunction and immunomodulation following trauma. In J. I. Gallin & A. S. Fauci (Eds)., *Advances in host defense mechanism* (Vol. 6, pp. 81–109). New York: Raven Press.

Arnetz, B., Wasserman, J., Petrini, B., et al. (1987). Immune function in unemployed women. *Psychosomatic Medicine, 49,* 3–12.

Austen, K. F. (1983). Tissue mast cells in immediate hypersensitivity. In F. Dixon & D. Fisher (Eds.), *The biology of immunologic disease* (pp. 223–233). Sunderland, MA: Sinauer Associates.

Austen, K. F., & Fisher, D. (1987). The biology of the mast cell. In R. Lockey & S. Bukantz (Eds.), *Fundamentals of immunology and allergy* (pp. 177–192). Philadelphia: W. B. Saunders.

Balkwill, F., & Burke, F. (1989). The cytokine network. *Immunology Today, 10,* 299.

Barrett, J. (1988). *Textbook of immunology* (5th ed.). St. Louis: C. V. Mosby.

Bartrop, R., Luckhurst, E., Lazarus, L., et al. (1977). Depressed lymphocyte function after bereavement. *Lancet, 1,* 834–836.

Beisel, W. (1981). Impact of infectious disease upon fat metabolism and immune function. *Cancer Research, 41,* 3797–3798.

Bellanti, J. A. (Ed.). (1985). *Immunology III.* Philadelphia: W. B. Saunders.

Bellanti, J. A., Kadlec, J. (1985). Introduction to immunology. In J. A. Bellanti (Ed.), *Immunology III* (pp. 1–15). Philadelphia: W. B. Saunders.

Bolhuis, R. (1989). T-cell responses to cancer. In M. Feldman, J. Lamb, & M. Owen (Eds.), *T cells* (pp. 347–364). New York: John Wiley & Sons.

Brookes, G. B., & Clifford, P. (1981). Nutritional status and general immune competence in patients with head and neck cancer. *Journal of The Royal Society of Medicine, 74*(2), 32–39.

Browder, W., & Williams, D. (1988). Immunosuppression and surgery. *Journal of the National Medical Association, 80,* 531–536.

Burnet, F. M. (1967). Immunologic aspects of malignant disease. *Lancet, 1,* 1171–1174.

Chandra, R. K. (1980). Cell-mediated immunity in nutritional imbalance. *Federation Proceedings, 39,* 3088–3092.

Chandra, R. (1981). Immune response in overnutrition. *Cancer Research, 41,* 3795–3796.

Chang, C., Naiki, M., Halpern, G., & Gerswin, M. (1993). Pharmacological regulation of the immune system. *Journal of Investigational Allergy and Clinical Immunology, 3*(1), 8–18.

Church, J., & Schlegel, R. (1985). Immune deficiency disorders. In J. A. Bellanti (Ed.), *Immunology III* (pp. 471–507). Philadelphia: W. B. Saunders.

Cooper, N. (1987). The complement system. In D. Stites, J. Stobo, & J. V. Wells (Eds.), *Basic and clinical immunology* (6th ed., pp. 114–127). Norwalk, CT: Appleton & Lange.

Cooper, M. (1987). B lymphocytes: Normal development and function. *New England Journal of Medicine, 317,* 1452–1456.

Corman, L. (1985). The relationship between nutrition, infection, and immunity. *Medical Clinics of North America, 69,* 519–529.

Cunha, B. (1985). Significance of fever in the compromised host. *Nursing Clinics of North America, 20,* 163–169.

Cunha, B., Digamon-Beltran, M., & Gobbo, P. (1984). Implications of fever in the critical care setting. *Heart and Lung, 13,* 460–465.

Daly, J., Reynolds, J., Sigal, R., et al. (1990). Effect of dietary protein and amino acids on immune function. *Critical Care Medicine, 18*(Suppl), 86–93.

Densen, P., & Mandell, G. L. (1987). Phagocytosis. In R. Lockey & S. Bukantz (Eds.), *Fundamentals of immunology and allergy* (pp. 51–64). Philadelphia: W. B. Saunders.

Dinarello, C. A., & Mier, J. W. (1987). Lymphokines. *New England Journal of Medicine, 317,* 940–945.

Effros, R. (1984). Aging and immunity. In E. L. Cooper (Ed.), *Stress, immunity, and aging* (pp. 277–290). New York: Marcel Dekker.

Esperson, S. (1986). Nursing support of host defenses. *Critical Care Quarterly, 9,* 51–56.

Frank, M., & Fries, L. (1989). Complement. In W. Paul (Ed.), *Fundamental immunology* (pp. 679–701). New York: Raven Press.

Gallin, J. (1989). Inflammation. In W. Paul (Ed.), *Fundamental immunology* (pp. 721–733). New York: Raven Press.

Gallucci, B. (1987). The immune system and cancer. *Oncology Nursing Forum, 14*(Suppl), 3.

Gawlikowski, J. (1992). White cells at war. *American Journal of Nursing, 92*(3), 44–51.

Gillis, S., Kozak, R., Durante, M., et al. (1981). Immunological studies of aging. *Journal of Clinical Investigation, 67,* 937–942.

Gleich, G., & Butterfield, J. (1987). Eosinophilia. In Lockey, R. & Bukantz, S. (Eds.), *Fundamentals of immunology and allergy* (pp. 217–234). Philadelphia: W. B. Saunders.

Goust, J. (1986). Immediate hypersensitivity. In G. Virella, J. Goust, H. H. Fundenberg, et al. (Eds.), *Introduction to medical immunology* (pp. 317–332). New York: Marcel Dekker.

Graziano, F., & Bell, C. (1985). The normal immune response and what can go wrong. *Medical Clinics of North America, 69,* 439–451.

Groenwald, S. (Ed.) (1993). *Cancer nursing: Principles and practice* (3rd ed.). Boston: Jones and Bartlett.

Groer, M. (1991). Psychoneuroimmunology. *American Journal of Nursing, 91*(8), 33–38.

Gross, R., & Newberne, P. (1980). Role of nutrition in immunologic function. *Physiology Review, 60,* 188–302.

Gurevich, I. (1985). The competent internal immune system. *Nursing Clinics of North America, 20,* 151–161.

Guyton, A. C. (1991). *Textbook of medical physiology* (8th ed.). Philadelphia: W. B. Saunders.

Halliburton, P. (1986). IMpaired immunocompetence. In V. Carrieri, A. Lindsey, & C. West (Eds.), *Pathophysiological phenomena in nursing.* Philadelphia: W. B. Saunders.

Halvorsen, R., & Vassend, O. (1987). Effects of examination stress on some cellular immunity functions. *Journal of Psychosomatic Research, 31,* 693–701.

Herberman, R., & Gorelik, E. (1989). Role of the natural immune system in control of primary tumors and metastasis. In C. Reynolds & R. Wiltrout (Eds.), *Functions of the natural immune system* (pp. 3–37). New York: Plenum Press.

Jackson, R. (1991). The immune system: Basic concepts for understanding transplantation. *Critical Care Nursing Quarterly, 13*(4), 83–88.

Janson-Bjerklie, S. (1983). Defense mechanisms: Protecting the healthy lung. *Heart and Lung, 12,* 643–649.

Jeske, D., & Capra, J. D. (1984). Immunoglobulins: Structure and function. In W. Paul (Ed.), *Fundamental immunology* (pp. 131–166). New York: Raven Press.

Kantor, A. (1991). A new nomenclature for B-cells. *Immunology Today, 12,* 388–393.

Kiecolt-Glaser, J., Garner, W., Speicher, C., et al. (1984). Psychosocial modifiers of immunocompetence in medical students. *Psychosomatic Medicine, 46,* 7–14.

Kiecolt-Glaser, J., Fisher, L., Ogrocki, P., et al. (1987a). Marital quality, marital disruption, and immune function. *Psychosomatic Medicine, 49,* 13–34.

Kiecolt-Glaser, J., Glaser, R., Strain, E., et al. (1986). Modulation of cellular immunity in medical students. *Journal of Behavioral Medicine, 9,* 5–21.

Kincade, P., & Gimble, J. (1989). B Lymphocytes. In W. Paul (Ed.), *Fundamental immunology* (pp. 41–67). New York: Raven Press.

Kirkpatrick, C. H. (1987). Mechanisms of allergic injury. In Lockey, R. & Bukantz, S. (Eds.), *Fundamentals of immunology and allergy* (pp. 153–176). Philadelphia: W. B. Saunders.

Kumagai, K., Suzuki, S., & Suzuki, R. (1989). Role of the natural immune system in the antibody response: Regulatory effects of NK cells. In C. Reynolds & R. Wiltrout (Eds.), *Functions of the natural immune system* (pp. 213–227). New York: Plenum Press.

Lahita, R., Levy, J., Weksler, J., et al. (1984). Effects of sex hormones, nutrition and aging on the immune response. In D. Stites, J. Stobo, H. Fundenberg, et al. (Eds)., *Basic and clinical immunology* (5th ed., pp. 288–311). Los Altos, CA: Lange Medical.

Langlois, P. F., Gawryl, M. S., Zeller, J., et al. (1989). Accentuated complement activation in patient plasma during the adult respiratory distress syndrome: A potential mechanism for pulmonary inflammation. *Heart and Lung, 24*(1), 71–84.

Lefor, A., Mule, J., and Rosenberg, S. (1989). Lymphokine-activated killer cells. Biology and therapeutic efficacy. In C. Reynolds & R. Wiltrout (Eds.), *Functions of the natural immune system* (pp. 39–56). New York: Plenum Press.

Lowry, S. (1993). Cytokine mediation of immunity and inflammation. *Archives of Surgery, 128,* 1235–1241.

Lundy, J., & Ford, C. (1983). Surgery, trauma, and immune suppression: Evolving the mechanism. *Annals of Surgery, 197,* 434–438.

McCarron, K. (1986). Fever—the cardinal vital sign. *Critical Care Quarterly, 9,* 15–18.

Mitchell, M., & Bertram, J. (1985). Immunology and biomodulation of cancer. In P. Calabresi, P. Schein, & S. Rosenberg (Eds.), *Medical oncology.* New York: Macmillan.

Moran, K., & Munster, A. M. (1987). Alterations of the host defense mechanism in burn patients. *Surgical Clinics of North America, 67,* 47–56.

Nakamura, I. (1989). Involvement of natural effector cells in bone marrow transplantation and hybrid resistance. In C. Reynolds &

R. Wiltrout (Eds.), *Functions of the natural immune system* (pp. 321–339). New York: Plenum Press.

Nicola, N. (1989). Hematopoietic cell growth factors and their receptors. *Annual Review of Biochemistry, 58,* 45.

Norwood, S. (1988). An approach to the febrile ICU patient. In J. Civetta, R. Taylor, et al. (Eds.), *Critical care.* Philadelphia: J. B. Lippincott.

Patrick, C., Goust, J., & Virella, G. (1986). Tissues and cells in the immune response. In G. Virella, J. Goust, H. H. Fundenberg, et al. (Eds.), *Introduction to medical immunology* (pp. 7–24). New York: Marcel Dekker.

Rabin, B., Cohen, S., Ganguli, R., et al. (1989). Bidirectional interaction between the central nervous system and the immune system. *Critical Reviews in Immunology, 9,* 279–312.

Roitt, I. (1991). *Essential immunology* (7th ed.). London: Blackwell Scientific Publications.

Roitt, I. M., Brostoff, J., & Male, D. K. (1985). *Immunology.* St. Louis: C. V. Mosby.

Royer, H., & Reinherz, E. (1987). T lymphocytes, ontogeny, function, and relevance to clinical disorders. *New England Journal of Medicine, 317,* 1136–1142.

Schleifer, S., Keller, S., Camerino, M., et al. (1983). Suppression of lymphocyte stimulation following bereavement. *Journal of the American Medical Association, 250,* 374–377.

Sheagren, J., and Young, M. (1987). Glucocorticoids. In J. Parrillo & H. Masur (Eds.), *The critically ill immunosuppressed patient* (pp. 245–263). Rockville, MD: Aspen.

Shronts, E. (1993). Basic concepts of immunity and its application to clinical nutrition. *Nutrition in Clinical Practice, 8*(4), 171–183.

Smith, S. (1986). Immunosuppressive drugs used in clinical practice. *Critical Care Quarterly, 9,* 19–24.

Sprent, J. (1989). T lymphocytes and the thymus. In W. Paul (Ed.), *Fundamental immunology* (pp. 69–93). New York: Raven Press.

Stiehm, E. (1980). Humoral immunity in malnutrition. *Federal Proceedings, 39,* 3093–3097.

Stobo, J. (1987). Lymphocytes: T cells. In D. Stites, J. Stobo, & J. V. Wells (Eds.), *Basic and clinical immunology* (6th ed., pp. 65–72). Norwalk, CT: Appleton & Lange.

Stone, A., Cox, D., Valdimarsdottir, H., et al. (1987). Secretory IgA as a measure of immunocompetence. *Journal of Human Stress, 6,* 136–140.

Thomas, L. (1959). *Cellular and humoral aspects of the hypersensitive states.* New York: Harper & Row.

Tilden, A., & Clement, L. (1989). Role of natural effector cells in the regulation of cell-mediated immune responses. In C. Reynolds & R. Wiltrout (Eds.), *Functions of the natural immune system* (pp. 229–247). New York: Plenum Press.

Tizard, I. (1984). *Immunology: An introduction.* Philadelphia: Saunders College Publishing.

Trinchieri, G., & Perussia, B. (1984). Human natural killer cells: Biologic and pathologic aspects. *Laboratory Investigation, 50,* 489–513.

Unanue, E. (1989). Macrophages, antigen-presenting cells, and the phenomena of antigen handling and presentation. In W. Paul (Ed.), *Fundamental immunology* (2nd ed., pp. 95–115). New York: Raven Press.

Van Snick, J. (1990). Interleukin-6: An overview. *Annual Review of Immunology, 8,* 253.

Ward, P. (1985). Inflammation. In J. A. Bellanti (Ed.), *Immunology III* (pp. 208–217). Philadelphia: W. B. Saunders.

Watkins, J., & Salo, M. (Eds.) (1982). *Trauma, stress, and immunity in anaesthesia and surgery.* Boston: Butterworth Scientific.

Weigle, W. (1983). Immunologic tolerance and immunopathology. In F. Dixon & D. Fisher (Eds.), *The biology of immunologic disease* (pp. 107–116). Sunderland, MA: Sinauer Associates.

Werb, Z. (1987). Phagocytic cells: Chemotaxis and effector functions of macrophages and granulocytes. In D. Stites, J. Stobo, & J. V. Wells (Eds.), *Basic and clinical immunology* (6th ed., pp. 96–113). Norwalk, CT: Appleton & Lange.

Whisler, R., Newhouse, Y., Ennist, D., et al. (1985). Human B-lymphocyte colony responses: Suboptimal colony responsive ness in aged humans associated with defective function of B cells and monocytes. *Cellular Immunology, 94,* 133–146.

Workman, M. (1993). The immune system: Your defensive partner and offensive foe. *AACN Clinical Issues in Critical Care, 4,* 453–470.

Wyngaarden, J. B., & Smith, L. H., Jr. (Eds.). (1988). *Cecil textbook of medicine* (18th ed.). Philadelphia: W. B. Saunders.

CHAPTER 56

Organ Donation

Marilyn Rossman Bartucci

OVERVIEW OF TRANSPLANTATION

The art and science of transplantation have developed a great deal since the first kidney transplant was performed in 1954. The advances made in surgical techniques, tissue typing and matching, understanding the immune system, preventing and treating rejection with powerful and effective immunosuppressive drugs, and improved organ procurement and preservation techniques have brought a dramatic increase in the demand for organs and tissues for transplantation. In 1993, there were 42,369 cornea transplants, 10,928 kidney transplants, 2,298 heart transplants, 3,443 liver transplants, 772 pancreas transplants, 60 heart/lung transplants, and 664 lung transplants performed in the United States (Eye Bank Association of America, 1994; United Network for Organ Sharing [UNOS]. 1994). Approximately 280,000 patients benefitted from bone allografts, 1,200 from heart valves, 668 from arterial and venous allografts, and 5,262 from tendon and cartilage allografts (American Association of Tissue Banks, 1994). Transplantation has offered new life to individuals dying of heart, liver, and lung failure and an improved quality of life for individuals with kidney failure, diabetes, blindness, and bone diseases. Implementation of an efficient national computerized system has made it possible to distribute organs equitably to patients with the greatest need and the greatest chance of a successful outcome. Conservative medical management of patients with end-stage kidney, liver, heart or lung disease is costly. Although transplant procedures are expensive, the current success rates have made transplantation a cost-effective treatment option compared with traditional medical management. For example, a patient undergoing chronic hemodialysis costs the federal government, through Medicare, about $40,000/year. The cost of a kidney transplant is approximately $40,000 for the first year and $5,000/year for follow-up care. If the transplant functions for 5 years (the actual rate approaches 75%), the cost is $60,000, as opposed to $200,000 for 5-year chronic hemodialysis. Likewise, patients with end-stage heart, lung, or liver disease have multiple, extended, and costly intensive care unit admissions for conservative management of the disease before death occurs as the final outcome. Table 56–1 shows the estimated cost of each transplant procedure and the current success rates. Other financial factors that increase the cost effectiveness of transplantation are the potential earning power of the transplant recipient and the discontinuation of disability benefits previously required. In short, transplantation is a therapy that can restore dignity and quality to the lives of patients and families dealing with end-stage organ disease and provide the potential for patients to become productive members of society again.

SHORTAGE OF DONOR ORGANS

During the last 5 years, the number of patients awaiting organs and tissues for transplantation has grown exponentially because the advances made in transplantation have made it possible to transplant both a larger number and a larger variety of organs and tissues. Currently, there are over 36,000 people awaiting vital organs for transplantation (kidney, heart, liver, heart/lung, lung, pancreas) in the United States (UNOS, 1994). It is predicted that by the year 2000, there will be nearly 50,000 people awaiting organ transplantation (Niemcryk et al., 1994). Every day, approximately eight people die because of the large gap that exists between the small available supply and the great demand for organs (UNOS, 1994). The shortage of organs does not result from a lack of suitable donors as documented by the Centers for Disease Control and

TABLE 56–1. **Organ Transplant Success Rates and Average Costs**

	Success Rate (%)	Average Cost ($)
Kidney		
Cadaver	93	40,000
Live donor	97	40,000
Heart	80–85	125,000
Heart/lung	60	155,000
Lung	65–70	155,000
Liver	70–75	100,000
Pancreas	60	41,000
Kidney/pancreas	89	70,000

Success rates are reported by the percentage of functioning grafts after one year since the greatest number of organs fail within the first year from rejection, technical problems, or other complications.

Prevention (CDC). In the early 1980s, the CDC revealed that only 15% of the 20,000 people who die each year meeting donor eligibility criteria actually become organ donors (Kolata, 1983). A recent study revealed that the number of people who die each year meeting donor eligibility criteria is more realistically 10,000 to 12,000, and therefore approximately 40% actually donate (Evans et al., 1992). However, despite extensive public awareness campaigns and the institution of required request laws, efforts to increase the ratio of potential to actual donors have been disappointing. Another study attributed the shortage to a failure to identify suitable donors and obtain consent from the next-of-kin rather than to a lack of suitable donors (Siminoff et al., 1993).

Some of the difficulties in initiating the organ procurement process are related to the definition and declaration of death. In the past, both the medical and lay public agreed that the absence of a heart beat and respirations were acceptable criteria for a declaration of death. However, the advances in life-support technology enabling health care professionals to maintain respiration and circulation in individuals whose brain function is minimal or absent have also created uncertainty about death. Although the Uniform Definition of Death Act adopted by the President's Commission for the Study of Ethical Problems in Medicine and Biomedical and Behavioral Research (1981) includes the cessation of all functions of the entire brain as a criterion for death, many health care professionals continue to feel uncertainty about implementing these criteria. People are strongly conditioned to view a breathing body with a beating heart as alive even when those functions continue only as a result of life-support systems.

ALTERNATIVE ORGAN SOURCES

Because of the disparity between the supply and demand for organs, there is a growing interest in increasing the potential organ donor pool by turning to alternative sources, including reliance on living donors, the use of non–heart-beating cadaver donors, marginal donors, and animals.

Living donors have been used in kidney transplantation since 1954. In the past, donors were blood relatives (i.e., parents, children, siblings). More recently, living unrelated donors have added to the pool of available kidneys. These donors are not blood relatives, but they have an emotional relationship with the recipient (i.e., spouses, step-parents, step-children). The graft survival rates, even with unrelated donors with no human leukocyte antigen match, have surpassed the graft survival rates in cadaver kidney transplants (Sollinger, 1994). Of the 10,928 kidney transplants performed in 1993, 2,760 kidneys came from live donors (UNOS, 1994). In the past 3 years, hearts from recipients needing a heart–lung transplant and segmental portions of liver, pancreas, and lung from live donors have been equally successful, with minimal donor risk (Piper, 1994). Although their numbers are much smaller than live kidney donors, these segmental transplants alleviate some of the need for cadaver donor organs.

Patients who have been declared dead by traditional cardiopulmonary criteria rather than brain-oriented criteria are another potential source of transplantable organs. These patients are non–heart-beating cadaver donors because their hearts are no longer beating at the time of organ procurement. Although before the institution of brain death criteria these donors were the major source of transplantable kidneys, problems with extended warm ischemia time, leading to cell and tissue damage, limited their usefulness. Recently, two different methods of procuring organs from non–heart-beating donors have been designed to circumvent this problem: (1) in situ organ preservation immediately after uncontrolled cardiopulmonary arrest, and (2) procurement from patients who have died after choosing to forego life-sustaining treatment (Youngner & Arnold, 1993).

In situ organ preservation involves the placement of a double- or triple-lumen catheter into the abdominal aorta via the femoral artery and the infusion of cooled preservation solution, after death has been declared according to cardiopulmonary criteria. One problem with this technique is that it must be instituted as soon as possible after asystole. Unfortunately, obtaining family consent for this procedure immediately after the pronouncement of death presents some practical difficulties. In this situation, the likelihood of denied consent is high because the family would not have time to adjust to the death before having to make a decision about organ/tissue donation.

The alternative method, allowing patients and families the option of donating organs after they have decided to forego life-sustaining treatment, has two advantages. First, because the decision for organ donation is made by the patient or family before death, there is time for discussion, reflection, and adequate consent before initiating any invasive procedure. Second, the time and place of death are controlled to minimize warm ischemia time. The patient is taken to the operating room where a waiting surgical team removes organs immediately after the pronouncement of death. Fifteen kidneys and four livers have been recovered from these donors. Of the 12 kidneys transplanted, all were functioning after 6 to 29 months follow-up. Two of the four transplanted livers were functioning after 9 and 30 months' follow-up. These results, at least for kidney transplants, equal those achieved using brain-dead donors. Only anecdotal reports of organs obtained from this source are available. There are no reliable data about the numbers these patients would add to the potential donor pool. Nathan (1992) estimated that, based on current patterns of referrals to Organ Procurement Organizations (OPOs), and the mechanics of organ recovery, the use of severely brain-impaired, but not brain-dead, patients would increase the potential donor pool by 20% to 25%.

Recovering organs from marginal donors, that is, donors who would have been rejected in the past, has increased the organ supply. Organs from older donors, diabetics, and hypertensives with normal renal function have been used with good outcomes (Alexander et al., 1994; Orlowski et al., 1994). A careful evaluation, including histologic assessment of the recovered organs, must be made before transplantation, and careful, long-term follow-up must be maintained to ensure that patient and graft survival rates at least equal those obtained using traditional cadaver donors.

Xenografting, the transplantation of animal organs into humans, has become a very attractive option in clinical transplantation, but the aim must be to get results as good as those achieved with human-to-human transplants. Although significant advances in our understanding of many aspects of xenotransplantation have been achieved since the first endeavors of Jaboulay and Princeteau in 1905 and 1906, they have not been good enough to enable the procedure to become clinically useful (Hammer, 1994). However, it could be as little as 2 years before genetically altered pig organs are available for transplantation into humans. Genes for two essential antigens to protect pig organs from rejection by human recipients have already been injected into pig cells and the animals crossed with normal pigs to produce heterozygous offspring—animals with one copy of each of the protective human genes and one copy of natural pig genes. But it will be 2 years before these animals can be crossed to produce homozygous piglets with two copies of the protective genes. Only organs from these animals could be considered for the first human transplants.

The major obstacle to overcome is hyperacute rejection. Hyperacute rejection occurs when the organ recipient produces xenoreactive antibodies that lodge on the cells lining the blood vessels of the new organ. These antibodies trigger the release of complement, inflammation, swelling, and ultimately blockage of the blood vessels, leading to the death of the organ. Two new drugs currently undergoing human clinical trials have the potential to overcome this antibody-mediated destruction of xenografts (Makowka & Cramer, 1994; White, 1994). Another possible obstacle is the potential risk of transmitting viral diseases from animal to human. Potential advantages of xenografting include a predictable and readily available organ supply, fewer deaths while waiting, lower procurement costs, a more elective surgical procedure, and size matching for donor and recipient. Because successful xenografting is at least 2 years away, this will not be an immediate solution to the organ shortage problem, and may bring new ethical issues to the forefront.

METHODS OF OBTAINING CONSENT

Various methods have been tried in an effort to keep pace with the growing demand for organs and tissues for transplantation. Public education and media coverage of transplant success stories were implemented to raise the consciousness of the general public about the need for donated organs and the success rates achieved through transplantation. In 1968, the Uniform Anatomical Gift Act (UAGA) was passed, legalizing donor cards and the right of next-of-kin to consent to organ/tissue donation. In the past, health care providers relied on *voluntarism,* through which the next-of-kin initiated the offer to donate their loved one's organs or tissues after death. In the United States, voluntarism was ineffective even though it was encouraged by the passage of the UAGA. In Europe, an attempt was made to increase organ/tissue donation by the passage of *presumed consent* laws. These laws gave physicians authority simply to remove needed organs or tissues from cadavers unless the individual carried a card prohibiting such donations or the next-of-kin objected. These laws, however, did not succeed in narrowing the gap between the need for and the availability of organs or tissues for transplantation.

In an attempt to overcome the reluctance of health care professionals to ask grieving families for organ/tissue donation, required request laws were passed in the United States. These laws mandate that all families be given the opportunity to donate the organs or tissues of a loved one who has died if the deceased meets eligibility criteria. The premise of the law is that all families have the right to decide about donation. If this decision-making opportunity is not provided by health care professionals, then these professionals are, in a sense, making the decision for the family *against* donation. A policy of required request can lead hospital personnel to consider the need for transplantable organs or tissues routinely. It can ensure that the burden of decision concerning donation is equitably allocated among all families whose relatives might serve as donors. This policy may standardize the process of routine inquiry about organ/tissue donation in such a way that it lessens the psychological burden on both health care professionals and family members at a time of great stress and emotional upheaval. It removes the chance that a family may not be offered this option to donate while preserving their right to refuse consent, because voluntary choice remains the ethical foundation on which organ/tissue donation rests (Caplan, 1984).

The federal government has required all hospitals to establish organ/tissue procurement protocols to obtain Medicare reimbursement for patient care. Some states have made a similar requirement for Medicaid reimbursement. Government legislation is certainly one mechanism for increasing the likelihood that families of dying patients will be asked for organ/tissue donation, but the chronic shortage of organs and tissues cannot be alleviated solely by the passage of required request laws. Experience with this legislation has shown as much as a 300% increase in the number of tissue donors but no significant increase in the number of organ donors. This result does not necessarily mean that required request laws have been ineffective in increasing the number of organ donors. Changes in other public health policies are in a state of flux and may have clouded the issue. For example, in some states laws about drunk driving have been enacted and strictly enforced. In others, the age for legally purchasing alcohol has been raised. Still other states have enacted mandatory seat belt laws, lowered speed limits, and improved their ability to transport accident victims quickly to tertiary care centers through air transport. The fact that organ donation has remained constant despite the significant decrease in traffic fatalities provides some evidence that the laws have had a small positive impact on the organ supply.

Since required request laws were implemented, some states have reported a greater percentage of families saying "no" to the request. Part of the difficulty in evaluating this claim lies in the incomplete, inconsistent data collected before implementation of the laws compared to the more complete data currently collected. Certificates on every death are now required. These certificates include information about whether the deceased met donor eligibility criteria and the family's response to the request for an anatomic gift. Second, health care professionals formerly relied on voluntarism or carefully evaluated families, making the request only of families they were certain would respond favorably. A careful selection process was used before required request. Now, all potential donor families are offered the opportunity to make an anatomic gift. Another criticism is that there has not been enough preparation of health care professionals on how to identify potential donors and approach grieving families to implement the law effectively. If required request is to have a positive impact on the supply of organs and tissues for transplantation, health care providers must acquire the necessary knowledge to identify potential donors and the skills to enable them to communicate sensitively and effectively with grieving families. In addition, education of the public must continue, emphasizing the need for individuals to discuss their wishes regarding organ/tissue donation with loved ones before a tragedy occurs. The public's attitude toward organ donation and the ability of the medical community to influence that attitude will have a profound effect on the future availability of organs and tissues for transplantation.

Failure to obtain consent is one of the most important causes of donor loss. At least 40% of requests for organ/tissue donation are denied. Why is the refusal rate so high when public surveys suggest that the great majority of Americans strongly approve of organ donation? Unfortunately, very few take advantage of the UAGA to make an advanced directive regarding their wishes to donate organs/tissues on their deaths. Therefore, at the time of death the wishes of the deceased are often unknown. In such cases, under the UAGA, the question of organ donation is left for the family to decide. This can be a very heavy burden for the family to bear. During this time of grief, clear thinking may be impossible. Unfortunately, the need to obtain family approval presents a major barrier to effective organ procurement. One potential solution to this dilemma is mandated choice.

Mandated choice is another proposed system for obtaining consent that is designed to combine the advantages of voluntarism, presumed consent, and required request, while avoiding their problems. Under this system, all adults would be required to decide and record whether they wish to be organ/tissue donors on their deaths. This could be accomplished by asking about donation on driver's license applications or tax returns. To obtain the license or have the tax return accepted, the question would have to be answered. Each person's decision would be legally binding and could not be overridden by the family. A change of mind could be accomplished easily at any time with a written directive. The advantages to this approach are: (1) the system would reach almost all potential adult donors; (2) family consent would neither be required nor requested; (3) the heightened awareness of the great value of and need for organ/tissue donation, which this system fosters, would likely increase participation; (4) mandated choice would be more efficient because it would eliminate the current time-consuming consent process that can jeopardize the quality of organs; and (5) despite the requirement for an answer, the laudable philosophical foundations of our current system of obtaining consent, namely altruism and voluntarism, would be preserved. For mandated choice to have any chance of succeeding, the public must accept the idea of being required to answer the question of organ/tissue donation for themselves and must also be willing to accept advanced directives as ethically and legally binding, unable to be overridden by family members at the time of death. A gallup poll of 1,000 randomly selected U.S. adults regarding this proposal revealed nearly two-thirds of respondents support such a system and three-quarters believe that the family should not be able to override their loved one's wishes (Spital, 1993).

ROLE OF NURSING IN DONATION PROCESS

The most recent nation-wide survey conducted by UNOS and The National Kidney Foundation (1993) showed that 87% of the general public is knowledgeable about transplantation and willing to donate organs/tissues at the time of death. Although many families have discussed their wishes in regard to organ/tissue donation, in an emergency situation the surviving loved one cannot be expected to initiate the idea of donation.

Nurses are frequently the first health care professionals to identify a potential organ donor and make the appropriate referral to the local OPO. Ninety-eight percent of actual organ donors die in a critical care unit. Approximately 20% die within 6 hours of admission, and 50% die within 24 hours (Hawke et al., 1990). Therefore, critical care nurses play a key role in the donation process. The ongoing physical assessment and hemodynamic monitoring provided by critical care nurses help direct care to maintain all transplantable organs and tissues in optimal condition. In addition, they provide both the factual information and the emotional support necessary for the next-of-kin to arrive at a decision about organ/tissue donation. Nurses are in the best position to provide compassionate support because they usually have a close relationship with the family and are well prepared both educationally and through experience to help the family through their crisis. Research by Morton and Leonard (1979) showed that the families' positive attitudes about organ donation and transplantation were strengthened by their donation experience in the hospital. Donor families' attitudes toward the health care team were closely related to the amount of time spent with them. The nursing staff was complimented without exception by all of the families interviewed.

DONOR FAMILY SUPPORT

Dealing With the Family's Reaction to Sudden Illness and Death

In our society, people expect to live until the seventh or eighth decade. The death of a younger family member, which is common in the organ donation situation, in which the mean age of the donor is 26 years, is outside the natural order of life events. When a sudden illness or accident and death occur earlier in an individual's life span, the family is not psychologically prepared for the death. Shock and disbelief interfere with the family's ability to accept the fact of death. Caregivers can help by providing emotional support to families and by gently and sensitively assisting them to recognize the gravity of the loved one's condition.

Providing information to the family about the progress of their loved one consistently, simply, and repeatedly is the way caregivers can gradually assist the family to understand, assimilate, and accept the gravity of the situation. The critical care nurse is in the best position to assess constantly and evaluate the accuracy of the family's perception of the loved one's condition by asking questions like "What did the doctor tell you?" Any misconceptions should be corrected immediately. It may be helpful to convey to the family the recognition that it must be very hard for them to understand all that is happening to their loved one, and to offer to call the physician to return and further clarify information about the clinical condition. It is very effective to provide explanations repeatedly because when anxiety is high, perceptions are narrowed. With narrowed perceptions, family members may hear only a small portion of what they are told in each interaction. In most instances of sudden illness, the family is looking for information that supports the hope that their loved one will survive, and therefore they may listen to information selectively.

Hope is a multidimensional, dynamic life force characterized by a confident yet uncertain expectation of achieving some future good. To the hoping person, the future good is realistically possible and personally significant (Dufault & Martocchio, 1985). Although it is important to be honest and straightforward with the family about the clinical situation, it is important not to destroy hope. The hope that families cling to can be therapeutic because it gives strength and energy at a time when sickness, pain, and fear are threatening to take over. It is important to remember that the family's hope for recovery can evolve into hope for their loved one's release from suffering and hope for meeting the person again in the afterlife.

Anxious family members often seek opinions from many staff members. Because nurses are most accessible to families at all hours, they are often the target of such requests for information. It is therefore critical that a nurse hears what the physician tells the family so that the information can be consistently reinforced during subsequent interactions with other caregivers.

Providing Emotional Support to Family Members

It is helpful if the family is permitted to visit their loved one as often as they wish. This is a good opportunity for the nursing staff to build trust and rapport. These interactions provide the foundation for the initial task of grieving, which is the recognition of the loss by the family when the patient dies. Conveying interest and concern about the patient as a unique individual by asking the family to tell about the patient during these interactions can strengthen the nurse–family relationship. The nurse must understand that the family may need to recount the circumstances leading up to the sudden illness or accident over and over again. It is important that the family be allowed to work through this situation with the help of an empathic listener.

The intensive care unit is a busy place, and extended conversations are not always possible. In such instances, simply personalize the care as much as possible to build rapport. The caregiver can engage the family in talking about the patient while providing care in the room. The family may feel less helpless in this crisis situation if they are able to provide simple comfort measures for their loved one, such as wiping the face, applying skin lotion, combing hair, and shaving.

A family's response to a crisis is variable. It is influenced by the specific circumstances of the illness or accident, the relationship to the loved one, and sociocultural factors. Often rage or anger is expressed initially, particularly if the family feels responsible for the illness. Angry reactions are often directed at staff because there is no other target. Listening attentively and with empathy is the most effective intervention. It is important to remember to avoid becoming defensive because this will only provide fuel for their anger.

Donor Identification and Referral

One of the biggest obstacles to organ donation in the past has been a failure to identify potential donors early in the process. Nurses must be knowledgeable about potential donor eligibility criteria and be able to activate the resources necessary to evaluate the situation. Referral of a potential organ donor does not commit the physician, nurse, or family to donation. Early awareness can prevent the unfortunate circumstance of families being approached unnecessarily or not being approached at all. It is imperative that the local OPO be contacted to determine suitability for organ/tissue donation and to initiate appropriate donor management.

Certain basic information is needed by the OPO to assess the suitability of the potential donor. This includes the potential donor's name, age, sex, race, diagnosis, cause of death, date of admission, availability of next-of-kin, the attending physician's name, and a brief summary of vital signs and pertinent laboratory values (Hawke et al., 1990).

Eligibility criteria are different for organ and tissue donors. Cadaver organ donors (donors of heart, lung, liver, kidney, and pancreas) are previously healthy individuals who have suffered irreversible brain injury of a known cause. The most common causes of injury are cerebral trauma from motor vehicle accidents or gunshot wounds, intracerebral or subarachnoid hemorrhage, and anoxic brain damage resulting from drug overdose or cardiac arrest. The brain-dead donor must have effective cardiovascular function and must be supported on a ventilator to preserve organ viability. The age range of most suitable donors is newborn to 70 years of age. The age of the donor, however, is generally less important than the quality of organ function. The donor must be free of intravenous drug abuse, malignancies, sepsis, and communicable diseases including hepatitis, syphilis, tuberculosis, and human immunodeficiency virus. The organ donor eligibility criteria and necessary laboratory tests are listed in Tables 56–2 and 56–3. The specific criteria used may vary from transplant center to transplant center. Always contact the local OPO for more information. These agencies have health care professionals on 24-hour call to answer questions, evaluate potential donors, make recommendations about proper donor management, and help provide information to potential donor families about the organ donation process.

Unlike organ donors, tissue donors (donors of eyes, bone, skin, heart valves) need not have a beating heart. Death may be pronounced and tissue recovered hours after the heart has stopped beating. Again, it is imperative to determine whether the donor meets eligibility criteria as specified by the local OPO. The general tissue donor eligibility criteria are listed in Table 56–4.

Treatment of the patient changes to management of the donor when brain death is determined, declared, and documented in the medical record and the legal next-of-kin has provided consent for organ donation. The priority of next-of-kin consent is listed in Table 56–5.

Consent may be obtained by phone conversation if witnessed by one other person in person, or by fax. The nurse can help in this situation by asking any family member or friend present at the time of admission the identity of the legal next-of-kin. Health care professionals are protected in obtaining consent by the "good faith" law. This means that the family members actually are who they represent themselves to be and that the professional accepts this in good faith (Caplan, 1988).

TABLE 56–2. **Organ Donor Eligibility Criteria**

	Heart	Heart/Lung	Lung
Age	Term newborn to 55 years	Term newborn to 55 yrs	1–55 years
Cardiac arrest, resuscitated	Center-specific	Center-specific	Possibly OK
Blood type	Yes	Yes	Yes
Laboratory Studies			
Hematology	CBC with differential, platelets, PT/PTT		
Chemistry	Electrolytes, osmolality, arterial blood gases		
	CPK-MB	CPK-MB	N/A
Culture	Blood	Blood Sputum and Gram stain	Blood Sputum and Gram stain
Procedures			
Chest x-ray	Yes, within last 6 hours	Yes, within last 6 hours	Yes, within last 4 hours
12-lead electrocardiogram	Yes, within last 6 hours	Yes, within last 6 hours	Yes
Echocardiogram	Yes	Yes	Yes
Central venous pressure	Yes	Yes	Yes
Arterial line	Yes	Yes	Yes
Miscellaneous	Weight Height	Weight Height	Weight Height
		Chest circumference, left main stem bronchus measurement Tidal volume and lung compliance 100% Oxygen challenge	

Abbreviations: CBC, complete blood count; CPK-MB, creatine phosphokinase, heart; PT, prothrombin time; PTT, partial thromboplastin time.

The Asking Process

A common question that arises in the minds of caregivers about organ/tissue donation is related to religious beliefs. Although the answers vary from denomination to denomination and from individual to individual within each denomination, research by the American Council on Transplantation (1987) found the major religious groups in the United States support donation and transplantation. Many groups, such as Roman Catholics, Amish, Moslems, and Jews, view organ donation as an act of charity, fraternal love, and self-sacrifice. Other religions, such as the Buddhists, Christian Scientists, Hindus, Jehovah's Witnesses, and various Protestant groups, express the belief that donation is a matter of individual conscience. Gypsies are

TABLE 56–3. **Organ Donor Eligibility Criteria**

	Kidney	Liver	Pancreas
Age	2–70 years	Term newborn to 55 years	10 months to 50 years
Cardiac arrest, resuscitated	OK	Possibly OK	Possibly OK
Blood type	Yes	Yes	Yes
Laboratory Studies			
Hematology	Complete blood count with differential, platelets, prothrombin time/partial thromboplastin time		
Chemistry	Electrolytes, arterial blood gases, osmolality		
	Blood urea nitrogen Creatinine Urinalysis	Liver Profile	Amylase Lipase Fasting blood glucose
Culture	Blood Sputum Urine	Blood	Blood
Procedures			
Chest x-ray	Yes	Yes	Yes
12-lead electrocardiogram	Yes	Yes	Yes
Central venous pressure	Yes	Yes	Yes
Arterial line	Yes	Yes	Yes
Miscellaneous		Height Weight Abdominal girth	

the only group opposing donation. Their opposition is associated with the belief that for 1 year after a person dies, the soul retraces its steps. It is believed that all of the body parts must be intact because the soul maintains a physical shape.

Timing is critical to sensitive and effective requests for organ/tissue donation. Only after the physician conveys the hopelessness of the clinical situation and the family has had time to assimilate this information can the donation process be initiated. The success of the request is related primarily to how the caregiver deals with a family during this sensitive period. The family should be approached, not to acquire organs, but to show compassion and offer assistance and support during their bereavement. The request for donation must be handled only as part of the natural support provided to a family at the time of their loved one's death. It is the death that is the most important event, not the organ/tissue donation. Research by Morton and Leonard (1979) showed that some family members were dissatisfied with the manner in which they were approached. Some found the person who approached them blunt and callous, especially if they had not understood the donor's hopeless prognosis until donation was requested. Nevertheless, most families were pleased that they were offered the opportunity to donate their loved one's organs or tissues.

Once the next-of-kin have been informed of their family member's death by the physician, the physician, nurse, procurement coordinator, or hospital designee can offer the family the opportunity to donate organs or tissues. The discussion should take place in a comfortable, private area, conducive to the family's expression of grief. The approach to the family should be planned after they have had time to assimilate the news that their loved one's brain is dead. It is very effective and conveys sensitivity to begin the conversation with an extension of sympathy. Allowing time for the family to express their feelings at this time further conveys the sympathy of the caregivers. It is important then to elicit the family's understanding of the loved one's condition and to re-explain, if necessary, why the patient is considered dead. The caregiver can say something like, "Tell me what you understand about your son's condition." If the family does not understand what has occurred, it may be necessary to bring the physician back to explain the clinical situation. Likewise, if the family needs more time to absorb the idea that their loved one is dead, the interaction is stopped and the caregiver returns after a specified interval. At this point, the caregiver might say, "I can see the news of your son's death is still very overwhelming. I will leave you alone together for awhile . . . . I will return in 20 minutes."

It has been shown that making the request for organ/tissue donation before the family has had time to assimilate the news of their loved one's death results in a high denied consent rate. The process by which there is a clear temporal separation of the explanation of death or the certainty of the family's acceptance of death and the request for organ/tissue donation is called decoupling. Garrison and colleagues (1991) analyzed 155 consecutive medically suitable organ donor referrals for the process and timing of the request for donation. In 143 potential donors, decoupling was documented, and yielded a 60% consent rate and subsequent procurement of transplantable organs/tissues. When the request for donation was coupled with the explanation of brain death, the consent rate was only 18%. There was a statistically significant differ-

TABLE 56–4. **Tissue Donor Eligibility Criteria**

	Bone	Skin	Eye	Heart Valve	Middle Ear	Saphenous Vein
Age	15–65 years	12–75 years	2–75 years	Newborn to 60 years	6–80 years	5–55 years
Cardiac arrest resuscitated	N/A	N/A	N/A	No	N/A	N/A
Malignancy	No	No	Yes	No	N/A	N/A
Culture	Blood	Blood	N/A	Blood	N/A	N/A

TABLE 56–5. **Priority of Next-of-Kin Consent**

Donors Over 18 Years of Age

Spouse
Adult son or daughter
Either parent
Adult brother or sister
Legal guardian
Any person authorized or under obligation to dispose of the body, for example, the coroner in the case of a John Doe

Donors Under 18 Years of Age

Both parents
One parent if both parents not readily available, provided there are no known contrary indications of the absent parent
Custodial parent, if parents are divorced or legally separated
Noncustodial parent, if custodial parent absent and there are no known contrary indications
Legal guardian
Any person authorized or obligated to dispose of the body

Adapted from Caplan, A. L. (1988). Beg, borrow or steal: The ethics of solid organ procurement. In D. Mathieu (Ed.), *Organ substitution technology: Ethical, legal, and public policy issues* (pp. 59–68). Boulder, CO: Westview Press.

ence ($p < 0.05$) between the decoupled and coupled approaches to the request for organ/tissue donation.

Making the Request

If trust and rapport with family members have been established successfully, a conversation about donation can be a major step toward recognition of the loss. The subject can be introduced with a simple question such as, "Did your son ever mention the desire to donate his organs or tissues at the time of death?" The first sentence is the most difficult to get out, but once the subject has been introduced, the caregiver can follow the family's cues. Then pause to allow the family to think about and respond to the question. If the family asks questions, answer and explore any concerns they express.

A decision to donate is personal and voluntary. It is important for families to recognize the request is just another option to consider and a personal decision. It is often the first time families feel in control after the tragic death of a loved one. The caregiver should not feel like a failure as an asker if the family refuses. The refusal can mean many things, ranging from an informed decision to an expression of anger and anguish over the loss, to concern about what body parts are needed in the afterlife. Families have the right to say no. So, how is a negative response handled? Simply, the caregiver can thank the family for considering organ/tissue donation and then close the conversation by saying, "Would you like to see your son one more time?"

If the family seems positive about donation or needs more information or time, continue to discuss their questions. Nurses cannot be expected to be able to answer every question a family asks. They can consult a procurement coordinator. The coordinator will explain the donation procedure to the family in more detail, including the fact that life supports are continued until the organs are removed in the operating room, as well as answering any other questions. In addition, the coordinator may handle communication with the coroner or funeral director about the donor's burial, when appropriate.

Questions frequently asked by the family concern pain experienced by the donor, payment, disfigurement, funeral delays, and confidentiality. A brief explanation of brain death again can allay family fears about their loved one experiencing pain during the organ/tissue procurement surgery. With regard to payment, once an organ or tissue donor has been identified, the procurement agency pays all costs associated with the care of the donor and organ/tissue procurement. These costs include additional laboratory tests, operating room costs, and intravenous fluids and medications required to maintain viable organs or tissues for transplantation. The family is financially responsible, however, for all health care costs before the pronouncement of death. Families are often concerned about whether donation interferes with an open casket funeral. Assurance can be given that the donor will appear normal, and donation does not preclude an open casket. Funeral delays usually do not occur unless procurement teams are coming from various parts of the country. It can take up to 18 hours in some instances, but family members are kept informed of the delays. If delays are causing additional stress for the family, a decision may be made to proceed with the donation of those organs or tissues for which procurement teams are immediately available. After procurement, the body is released to the funeral home. If it is logistically possible, the family should be offered the opportunity to see their loved one after the heart has stopped beating. This can ease the transition from the hospital to the funeral home and again reinforce the family's recognition of the loss. This viewing can take place in the recovery room, the intensive care unit, or the morgue. Most families, however, leave the hospital when the deceased is taken to surgery. Often a telephone call informing them that the procurement has been completed is all the communication the family desires. This can be accomplished by the organ procurement coordinator, who is present in the operating room. Gifts of organs or tissues are confidential. No one who receives a transplant is told the identity of the donor. Likewise, donor families are only told the age and sex of the various recipients and how they are doing after transplantation. The organ procurement agency provides this information in a letter within a few weeks after the donation.

DONOR MANAGEMENT

Before a declaration of brain death, therapeutic modalities are used to maximize neurologic recovery. Ventilation and fluid therapy are altered to reduce intracranial pressure. Systemic blood pressure is supported with vasopressors to maintain adequate cerebral perfusion pressure. When brain death has been declared, therapy changes to optimize organ function. At this point, the management of the donor becomes the responsibility of the organ procurement team.

The goals of donor management are to maintain organ perfusion and organ oxygenation. Organ perfusion is a function of intravascular volume, vascular resistance, and cardiac function. Failure to maintain and balance these three components will result in impaired tissue perfusion, cellular dysfunction, organ deterioration, and organ death. Organ donors usually have conditions such as thoracic injuries, shock, pneumonia, atelectasis, and other clinical problems that may result in diminished oxygenation and ventilation. Delivery of oxygen is essential to the maintenance of viable organ function.

BEREAVEMENT

Teaching family members about what to expect during the grieving process can help prepare them for the next few months. Bereaved families need others for continued comfort and support, such as extended family, friends, and clergy. Grief needs to be shared. It is important to tell families that the mourning process varies from person to person, but for most people healing occurs without complications with time. A variety of thoughts, feelings, behaviors, and physical sensations may be experienced by the family. It is important for family members to understand that these are a normal part of healthy grieving.

Family Reactions to Donation

Health care professionals often fear that asking grieving families for organ/tissue donation will have negative consequences or that it will add to the family's grief. However, studies have shown that the strongest advocates of organ/tissue donation are donor families because they view donation as the highest form of charity, believing that they are giving the ultimate gift, life, to another person (Bartucci, 1987; Bartucci & Seller, 1986; Goldsmith & Montefusco, 1985; Morton & Leonard, 1979; Stocks et al., 1992).

In addition to the gift-giving aspect of donation, families have reported that the grief experienced due to an abrupt and tragic loss of a loved one was lessened when they knew that other people were leading new lives because of donation. The donation of vital organs was reported to be a meaningful part of the normal grief process (Bartucci, 1987; Bartucci & Seller, 1986; Goldsmith & Montefusco, 1985; Morton & Leonard, 1979; Stocks et al., 1992). Furthermore, it was found that families maintain very favorable attitudes over time because they view donation as the one positive aspect of death, seeing it as a chance for their loved one to achieve a type of immortality by living on in another human being through transplantation (Bartucci, 1987; Bartucci & Seller, 1986; Stocks et al., 1992).

In a recent study of families who donated the organs of loved ones, Bartucci (1987) found that 85% identified organ donation as something positive during their time of grief. Ninety-one percent had no regrets about the decision to donate their loved one's organs. The three respondents who regretted the donation identified some problem with the procurement process, but later they reported extremely positive feelings about the recipients of their loved one's organs. One wife stated, "You'll never know how good (for the first time) I felt knowing that a part of my husband was helping a little boy to live a normal life." The two most common reasons cited in the decision to donate were: (1) their loved one would have wanted to help someone, and (2) organ donation seemed to be a way of deriving something positive from the loss.

Most donor families studied had good feelings about their donation experience because they were able to help someone else. It comforted them to know that the death of their loved one was not in vain, and the donation itself gave some meaning to the sudden, untimely death of a previously healthy person. If health care professionals consider the perspective of donor families, they may be less fearful about offering this life-giving, life-sustaining opportunity. Donation can be a vehicle for beginning the resolution of grief and an opportunity for the donor family to turn a tragic death into a heroic gesture. One mother's organ donation experience is described on the facing page.

PSYCHOSOCIAL IMPLICATIONS

There are many sources of stress for caregivers involved in the organ donation/procurement process. One major stressor is the declaration of brain death and the issues surrounding the termination of treatment. There is a great deal of uncertainty and ambivalence about the determination of brain death because there are no absolute rules. A physician makes the diagnosis based on state law, hospital policy, and the criteria currently accepted by experts in the neurosurgical and neurologic professions. The haunting question of whether one can ever be certain there is no potential for recovery remains. Even caregivers who understand and accept the concept of brain death may find it difficult to ignore the signs of life they see. In addition, ambivalent feelings may be exacerbated by interactions with family members who are clinging to the hope for recovery and are less intellectually and emotionally prepared to accept the finality of death despite so much apparent life (Youngner et al., 1985). Caregivers are forced to examine their own concerns about the meaning of a declaration of death made on brain death criteria because they must be able to answer the family's questions and respond to their concerns or misperceptions.

Other stressors include questions of professional competence because of the inability of the health care team to save the life of this previously healthy individual. In addition, there are feelings of conflict and dissonance because the intensive care unit and operating

Jeffrey's Story

Peggy Rickard Bishop

During the Christmas season of 1982, my three-year-old son Jeffrey died of an intracerebral hemorrhage. There had been no indication that anything was wrong with Jeffrey. The day had been a very ordinary day in his life. He played with his two older brothers and exhibited normal three-year-old behavior. Several times that day he went to a corner of the living room, patted the floor, and announced to the family that was where he wanted the Christmas tree.

Because Jeffrey had a long nap and was quite cheerful he stayed up to play with his brothers. At 11:00 P.M., after his prayers and good night kisses, he went to bed with his favorite stuffed animal and a Christmas book. I heard him talking and singing in his bed shortly before I heard a cry I had never heard before. I found Jeffrey holding the left side of his head, rolling back and forth in his crib. I carried him to the living room and as he lay on the couch, he began to vomit.

The rescue squad was called and by the time the paramedics arrived, Jeffrey was unconscious. He was transported to the local community hospital. Within minutes after arrival, he had a respiratory arrest and was placed on a respirator. After three hours, Jeffrey was transferred to a university-affiliated children's hospital where a CAT scan revealed a massive hemorrhage in his brain. At 4:00 A.M., I learned my son was brain dead, that nothing could make him well again. I was stunned and could not believe what was happening. I soon became aware Jeffrey's condition was deteriorating. His body was being artificially warmed, his blood pressure maintained with medications, and his heart beat and respirations dependent upon a machine.

I offered to donate any of Jeffrey's organs for transplant. The physician was very surprised when I brought up the subject of organ donation. A transplant coordinator from the local Organ Procurement Agency arrived at 12:00 noon and began preparations for the removal of Jeffrey's kidneys, eyes, and liver. My only stipulation to the donation was the organs be sent not only as gifts of life, but with the message they were also gifts of love.

During the course of the day, Jeffrey's brothers, grandparents, and a few close friends came to the hospital to spend time with him and give each other much needed support. It was an extremely painful experience to explain to Jay and Michael that their little brother, who had been running around the house hours before, was now being kept alive by a machine. My own pain of trying to cope with the loss was only heightened by experiencing their pain.

The atmosphere in the Intensive Care Unit was one of extreme caring. I was provided with a rocking chair in which I could sit and hold Jeffrey. I was given time to cuddle him, talk to him, and say a very special good-bye to my youngest child. When I requested hand and foot prints, the nurses found ink pads and I got my prints. I was also given a pair of scissors to cut a lock of his hair.

The director of the Intensive Care Unit gave the family much consideration during that day and the following weeks. He spent time explaining what most likely caused Jeffrey's death, what kind of medical care was being provided, and the procedure for donating his organs. He took special time with Jay and Michael, explaining what had happened to Jeffrey and answering their many questions in terms they could understand.

At 4:00 P.M., eighteen hours after Jeffrey became ill, he was taken to surgery for the removal of his kidneys, eyes, and liver. As he left for the operating room, the family prepared to leave for home. I had Jeffrey's hand and foot prints, a lock of his hair, and the belief he had received the best possible care available. I spoke with the Director of the Intensive Care Unit and asked him to take care of Jeffrey for me. I left behind his favorite blue blanket that went everywhere with him and asked the doctor to cover Jeffrey with it following surgery. The doctor assured me he would be cared for as the little boy he was and my wish would be carried out.

Many people have made the comment that the decision to donate Jeffrey's organs must have been difficult. For me, it was a decision bringing comfort, not additional pain. Facing the death of my son was nearly unbearable, but because I had previously thought about organ donation, the decision was much easier. When I was twelve, a friend and I made our own non-legal wills donating our organs to their respective organ banks. It was at this time I first became aware of such medical advances as transplantation. While visiting my parents a few months after Jeffrey's death, I found the copy of the "pretend" will. It was so ironic to relate its contents to the events that had transpired in my life.

Another seed relating to organ donation was planted when I was taking a Medical Terminology class just six months before Jeffrey's death. After a serious class discussion about transplant, I continued to give the idea of organ donation much thought, and expressed the wish to donate my organs by signing the back of my driver's license. Although I decided to donate my organs, I had not allowed myself to consider what I would do if one of my sons was to die. For several weeks after the class the subject of organ donation was in my thoughts. I finally made up my mind, I would donate my child's organs if faced with the decision, so very unaware that within six months I would carry out that decision.

My purpose in sharing this experience is to convey to others that even in this dark tragedy new hope and new life can result. I view Jeffrey as a very precious gift, just as I view Jay and Michael, and through organ donation Jeffrey was again a gift, to five other people and their families.

From Bartucci, M. R., & Bishop, P. R. (1987). The meaning of organ donation to donor families. *ANNA Journal, 14*(7), 369–372, 410.

room suddenly became the places where one life is given to save another through transplantation. The conflict occurs because the donor's welfare no longer provides the rationale for aggressive management, treatment, and surgery. This violation of the general belief that human beings should be treated as ends in themselves, rather than as means to other ends, creates dissonance.

Further conflict arises because these caregivers are also responsible for other critically ill patients in the intensive care unit. Caring for the organ donor requires intense hemodynamic monitoring and careful management to preserve organ viability for transplantation. Legitimate concerns arise about donor management detracting from the care of living patients.

Responsibility for donor management is stressful in itself. A study of intensive care unit nurses' perceptions of cadaver organ procurement revealed that nurses are fearful of making a mistake in the nursing management of a potential donor, thus jeopardizing the donor's ability to donate (Sophie et al., 1983).

Implementing interventions and strategies to help caregivers deal with the psychosocial and stress factors surrounding the care of donors can help to alleviate the stresses or teach caregivers to deal with the stresses in a healthy, constructive manner. The most critical intervention is professional education. A program should be designed to help caregivers evaluate their personal feelings about their own mortality and their beliefs about the benefits of organ donation and transplantation. In addition, there should be discussion about what constitutes brain death, how the determination is made, and what the implications are for making such a declaration. Becoming informed about the documented beliefs of organ donation to donor families can help caregivers view donation in a positive way (Kiberd & Kiberd, 1992). Learning and practicing the words to say when making a request for organ/tissue donation can lessen the fear of approaching a grieving family.

Development of a detailed orientation program for new staff before involving them in organ procurement is critical. The new staff member must be adequately prepared emotionally as well as technically to deal with donor management and supportive care of family members. A preceptorship or buddy system can be beneficial because it provides not only good role models for teaching new staff how to handle their personal feelings but opportunities for practicing appropriate behaviors. Mutual support benefits not only the new staff members but also the more experienced caregiver. It is helpful to use established guidelines and procedures to prepare the new caregiver to function with confidence and to gain the ability to deal with the most common complications that may occur. All caregivers may not be able to participate in organ donation/procurement for a variety of reasons, and should not be required to do so.

Many organ donation/procurement procedures occur in hospitals not involved in transplantation. The process becomes very one-sided because the caregivers involved in donor management do not have the chance to benefit from caring for the recipients and seeing the fruits of their labor. One way to accomplish this is to request and share feedback from the OPO about the recipients of the organs they helped to procure. It is also valuable to provide special recognition for all who participated.

A mechanism for providing support to staff is vital for encouraging positive coping behaviors. It is imperative for staff members to receive the message that emotional upset is legitimate. There must be a forum for discussing these feelings on a regular basis or after each donor experience. If problems occur with the approach to a family or in management of a donor, it is constructive to review what might have been done differently so that all staff can learn what needs to be changed for the next time.

In summary, participation in donor care is emotionally draining because of the support and comfort needed by the grieving family. It is time consuming and requires intense monitoring and expert application of physical and psychosocial assessment skills. In addition, it requires the caregiver to be in touch with his or her personal feelings about death in general, brain death specifically, and beliefs about organ/tissue donation and transplantation.

SURGICAL RETRIEVAL

Organ recovery is undertaken in the operating room of the donor hospital only after an important series of events takes place: timely recognition of a potential donor, notification of an OPO, declaration of brain death, family consent, optimal donor management, and identification of potential recipients for each organ. The operating room at the donor hospital typically has several hours to prepare for organ recovery because of the time involved in identifying the potential recipients and then coordinating the arrival of multiple surgical teams, many times geographically distant. It is during this process that the invaluable role of the organ procurement coordinator is realized.

Multiple organ donor information, including age, weight, and blood type, is entered into a 24-hour computerized network, UNOS, in Richmond, Virginia. A list of potential recipients is generated by a prioritized point system that determines those individuals best suited for the available organs. The preservation time of each organ is always considered when calling a recovery team. There must be enough time to get the organ back and transplanted within the critical time frame.

The surgical teams come prepared with their own specialized equipment, organ preservation solutions, and packaging materials. The assistance of a scrub nurse, circulating nurse, and anesthesia personnel from the donor hospital is needed. No anesthetic agent is required, but a paralyzing agent may be administered initially to inhibit spinal reflexes during the incision. In addition, the anesthesia team helps to monitor vital signs, volume status, and administer intravenous drugs as directed until the aorta is clamped. Diuretics are given for renal cortical dilation and to protect donor renal integrity during the ischemic period. Heparin is given to prevent blood clotting during circulatory arrest.

A multiple organ procurement procedure will last approximately 3–5 hours, depending on which organs are being removed. The operating room nurse prepares the surgical suite the same as for any large abdominal and thoracic case. In addition, there is a need for extra table space with sterile basins for each organ being removed so the organs can be prepared and packaged for transport to the respective transplant centers.

Transport of the donor from the intensive care unit to the operating room is a critical time in the organ recovery process. The donor has multiple intravenous catheters, inotropic drugs infusing, and the need for continuous ventilatory support. Extreme care is taken not to interrupt any of these interventions imperative to maintaining organ viability.

Surgery for multiple organ donation routinely includes the removal of the heart, liver or pancreas (or both), and kidneys. All surgical teams are present and the organs are removed in a coordinated fashion. At no time is collaboration more important in the operating room. The future viability of all recovered organs depends on this cooperative effort.

The heart team makes the initial incision from the sternal notch to the symphysis pubis. The sternum is cracked and retracted for complete visualization. The heart is inspected for any evidence of damage or congenital anomaly. Next, the liver team inspects the liver for color and texture and any sign of injury or anomaly. Dissection begins by removing the adhesions and muscles holding the liver in place. The liver is extremely vascular. All blood vessels must be dissected and tied. The major vessels that supply the liver are left intact until the last minute to prevent ischemic damage. Dissection of the liver can take 2 to 4 hours. If the pancreas is also being removed, it is dissected at the same time as the liver. The kidney team then steps in and dissects the kidneys free.

Once the organs are dissected free, the aorta is clamped and all organs are flushed in situ with a cold electrolyte solution specific for each organ. This initial flush causes immediate cellular standstill, decreasing the risk of damage due to warm ischemia. The heart is the first organ to be physically removed. A limited preservation time of 4 to 6 hours currently forces the recovery team to return immediately to the transplant center to begin transplantation. Lung removal is done in conjunction with removal of the heart. The preservation time for lungs is 6 hours.

The liver is the next organ to be removed. The preservation time for a liver is 8 to 12 hours. The liver team also immediately returns to the transplant center to begin transplantation.

If the pancreas is removed instead of the liver, it would be done after the heart is removed. The preservation time for the pancreas is approximately 12 hours.

If both the liver and the pancreas are to be removed, the portal vein and a patch of aorta with the celiac and superior mesenteric artery are dissected and removed with the pancreas. The hepatic artery and the portal vein above the ligament to the liver are dissected with the liver.

The kidneys are the final solid organs to be removed. They are removed en bloc (i.e., together), attached to the vena cava and aorta. Most often, the kidneys are placed in a serile container, packed in ice, and then refrigerated until transplantation. Infrequently, a pulsatile perfusion machine that pumps a cold plasma solution through the kidneys to control their metabolic activity until transplant is used. The maximum preservation time for both methods is 72 hours, although most surgeons prefer to transplant within 24 to 36 hours. Kidney recipients are not always identified at the time of procurement.

Once the organs are removed, the kidney surgeon closes the abdomen and chest cavity. All care and respect are given to the donor so that there is no disfigurement. If the family has also consented to tissue donation, these procurement teams become involved. Tissue procurement can take approximately 3 hours of operating time.

The eyes are usually the first tissue to be removed. They must be removed within 4 to 6 hours after asystole. In most cases the entire eye is enucleated, although some technicians are trained to remove only the corneas. The technicians bring all the necessary equipment to the donor hospital. If the donor is not an organ donor, the enucleation can be performed at the bedside or in the morgue. The face is sterilely draped, the eyelid retracted, and the muscles surrounding the sclera sterilely incised to free the eyeball. The eye is placed in a sterile container with an antibiotic solution and transported to the local eye bank. The cornea is microscopically removed and examined. It is placed in a preservation medium and transplanted within 2 to 3 days. A plastic prosthesis with a cotton ball is inserted so that the eye cavity retains its natural shape. No external incisions are made.

Bone is recovered within 24 hours after asystole as long as the body has been refrigerated within 12 hours. The bones of the upper and lower extremities, every other rib, every other vertebra, and the iliac crest can be removed. This procedure can be done either in the morgue or sterilely in the operating room. Multiple incisions are made to remove bone. Once the bone is recovered, wooden dowels are used to replace the long bones so the body retains its natural shape. The incisions are then sutured closed. The bone team comes prepared with the necessary equipment and prosthetics. If the procedure is done in the operating room, the team will need the assistance of a circulating nurse. Once the bone is removed, it is packaged and transported to the bone bank. If the bone was removed in the morgue, it is secondarily sterilized before it is frozen. Bone can be preserved for 2 years.

Skin is the last tissue to be removed. It is used in the treatment of burns. The team brings a surgical dermatome to remove the skin either in the operating room or the morgue. Only 8 to 10 one-thousandths of an inch is removed from large body surface areas like the abdomen, back, buttocks, and thighs. No skin is removed from any area that would be seen during an open casket service. The skin is preserved in an antibiotic solution for a period of time and then placed in a −70°C freezer until it is needed. The preservation time is approximately 2 years.

SUMMARY

Tremendous progress has been made in transplantation in the last 10 years, with 1-year graft survivals reaching 90% and 5-year survivals averaging 70%. With the increasing success rates, more and more patients suffering from end-stage organ disease are opting for transplantation. Although more than 14,000 organ transplants are performed annually, the national waiting list continues to grow. There are currently almost 18,000 patients awaiting organs for transplantation. These people and their families are in limbo, walking a tightrope of hope and despair. Many patients will die before an organ becomes available.

The challenge of the 1990s is to prevent the organ supply and demand problem from escalating. The future of organ transplantation rests partially in the hands of critical care nurses. They have the ability to identify and refer potential donors and possess the necessary expert physical assessment and hemodynamic monitoring skills to help direct care toward maintaining organ and tissue viability. Critical care nurses are caring and empathic and have the skills to communicate with families in crisis. They have developed the ability to assess and evaluate the accuracy of the family's perception of a loved one's condition and therefore can identify when a family is ready to hear about the option of donation. They are able to provide both the factual information and emotional support necessary to allow the next-of-kin to arrive at a decision about donation, and they have the support of their colleagues through this often emotionally draining experience.

REFERENCES

Alexander, J. W., Bennett, L. E., & Breen, T. J. (1994). Effect of donor age on outcome of kidney transplantation. *Transplantation, 57,* 871–876.

American Association of Tissue Banks. (1994). *Tissue bank statistics.* Washington, DC: Author.

American Council on Transplantation. (1987). *Religious views of organ/tissue donation.* News Release, National Organ and Tissue Donation Awareness Week Promotional Kit. Alexandria, VA: Author.

Bartucci, M. R. (1987). Organ donation: A study of the donor family perspective. *Journal of Neuroscience Nursing, 19,* 305–309.

Bartucci, M. R., & Seller, M. C. (1986). Donor family responses to kidney recipient letters of thanks. *Transplantation Proceedings, 18,* 401–405.

Caplan, A. L. (1988). Beg, borrow or steal: The ethics of solid organ procurement. In D. Matthieu (Ed.), *Organ substitution technology: Ethical, legal, and public policy issues* (pp. 59–68). Boulder, CO: Westview Press.

Caplan, A. L. (1984). Ethical and policy issues in the procurement of cadaver organs for transplantation. *New England Journal of Medicine, 311,* 981–983.

Dufault, K., & Martocchio, B. (1985). Hope: Its spheres and dimensions. *Nursing Clinics of North America, 20,* 379–391.

Evans, R., Orians, C., & Ascher, N. (1992). The potential supply of organ donors: An assessment of the efficiency of organ procurement efforts in the United States. *Journal of the American Medical Association, 267,* 239–246.

Eye Bank Association of America. (1994). *Eye bank statistics.* Washington, DC: Author.

Garrison, R. N., Bentley, F. R., Raque, G. H., et al. (1991). There is an answer to the shortage of organ donors. *Surgery, Gynecology and Obstetrics, 173,* 391–396.

Goldsmith, J., & Montefusco, C. (1985). Nursing care of the potential organ donor. *Critical Care Nurse, 5*(6), 22–29.

Hammer, C. (1994). Nature's obstacles to xenotransplantation. *Transplantation Reviews, 8*(4), 174–184.

Hawke, D., Kraft, J., & Smith, S. (1990). Tissue and organ donation and recovery. In S. Smith (Ed.), *Tissue and organ transplantation: Implications for professional nursing practice* (pp. 83–102). St. Louis: Mosby Year Book.

Kiberd, M. C., & Kiberd, B. A. (1992). Nursing attitudes towards organ donation, procurement, and transplantation. *Heart and Lung, 21,* 106–111.

Kolata, G. (1983). Organ shortage clouds new transplant era: Organs are used from only one in ten potential donors; some say legislation is needed to make more organs available. *Science, 221,* 32–33.

Makowka, L., & Cramer, D. V. (1994). The pathogenesis of xenograft rejection. *Clinical Transplantation, 8,* 145–154.

Morton, J., & Leonard, D. (1979). Cadaver nephrectomy: An operation on the donor's family. *British Medical Journal, 1,* 239–241.

Nathan, H. (1992). *Would non–heart-beating cadaver donors really increase the organ supply?* Presented at the Conference on Ethical, Psychosocial, and Public Policy Implications of Recovering Organs from NHBCDs, University of Pittsburgh, Pittsburgh, PA.

National Kidney Foundation. (1993). *Controversies in organ donation* (pp. 1–22). New York: Author.

Niemcryk, S., Aronoff, R., Marconi, K., & Bowen, G. (1994). Projections in solid organ transplantation and wait list activity through the year 2000. *Journal of Transplant Coordination, 4,* 23–30.

Orlowski, J. P., Spees, E. K., Aberle, C. L., & Fitting, K. M. (1994). Successful use of kidneys from diabetic cadaver kidney donors: 67 and 44 month graft survival. *Transplantation, 57,* 1133–1134.

Piper, J. (1994). Living donor liver transplants preferable to cadavers. *UNOS Update, 10*(6), 3–5.

President's Commission for the Study of Ethical Problems in Medicine and Biomedical and Behavioral Research. (1981). *Defining death: Medical, legal, and ethical issues in the determination of death.* Washington, DC: U.S. Government Printing Office.

Siminoff, L. A., Arnold, R., Virnig, B., & Caplan, A. (1993). Can we ever solve the shortage problem? American public policy on organ, tissue, and corneal procurement from cadaver sources. *Journal of Transplant Coordination, 3,* 51–59.

Sollinger, H. (1994). LURD kidney transplant survival rates better than cadavers. *UNOS Update, 10*(6), 4.

Sophie, L. R., Salloway, J. C., Sorock, G., et al. (1983). Intensive care nurses' perceptions of cadaver organ procurement. *Heart and Lung, 12,* 261–267.

Spital, A. (1993). Consent for donation: Time for a change. *Clinical Transplantation, 7,* 525–528.

Stocks, L., Cutler, J., Kress, T., & Lewino, D. (1992). Dispelling myths regarding organ donation: The donor family experience. *Journal of Transplant Coordination, 2,* 147–152.

United Network for Organ Sharing (UNOS). (1994). *U.S. scientific registry for organ transplantation.* Richmond, VA: Author.

White, D. (1994). Xenografts no longer unrealistic dream: Animal organs to play important role in future transplants. *UNOS Update, 10*(10), 17.

Youngner, S., & Arnold, R. (1993). Ethical, psychosocial, and public policy implications of procuring organs from non–heart-beating cadaver donors. *Journal of the American Medical Association, 269,* 2769–2774.

Youngner, S., Allen, M., Bartlett, T., et al. (1985). Psychosocial and ethical implications of organ retrieval. *New England Journal of Medicine, 313,* 321–324.

Immunocompromised Patients

Jan L. Hawthorne

In recent years, the treatment of cancer has become progressively more aggressive with the use of immunotherapies and high-dose chemotherapy. Although the success of these treatments is encouraging, the intensity of treatment has created new challenges for nurses caring for these patients. The nurse must be knowledgeable about these therapies to be able to provide the intensive support needed by patients and their families.

Immunotherapy, chemotherapy, and the resultant granulocytopenia can combine with the systemic effects of cancer to compromise the immune system of the patient. The immunocompromised patient has an increased risk of life-threatening infection (Oniboni, 1985; Reheis, 1985; Ristuccia, 1985). It is vital that the immunocompromised patient be protected from sources of infection, and in this area nurses play a significant role.

Leukocytes (white blood cells [WBCs]) act primarily to protect the host from invading foreign bodies. WBCs may be classified as nongranular (or mononuclear) and granular. Nongranular leukocytes include lymphocytes and monocytes. Granulocytes may be subclassified, based on their staining properties, as neutrophils, basophils, or eosinophils. Granulocytes are primarily responsible for combating infection. The total WBC count is usually 4.7 to 11.4 thousand cells/ mm^3. Of this total, 27% to 39% (1,700–3,400) are usually nongranulocytes, and 61% to 73% (3,000–7,000) are usually granulocytes (Corbett, 1987). If the granulocyte count is below 3,000 cells/mm^3, the condition is termed granulocytopenia. Because granulocytes are primarily responsible for combating infection, granulocytopenia significantly increases the patient's risk of acquiring an infection. When neutropenia (less than 1,000 cells/mm^3) occurs, patients should be hospitalized. Neutropenic patients are placed in a protective environment to prevent infection while neutrophil counts return to normal (Smith, 1986a).

Granulocytopenia and neutropenia can be either the direct result of chemotherapy or immunotherapy or the systemic effect of cancer (Table 57–1). Cancer may develop from or metastasize to the bone marrow. Because the hematopoietic tissues of the marrow are responsible for the production of blood cells, bone marrow cancer directly affects the production of WBCs. The altered nutrition and metabolism of cancer patients also have a direct effect on the production of these cells. Chemotherapeutic and immunotherapeutic agents attack rapidly dividing cells, including granulocytes. Therefore, the therapy itself frequently depresses granulocyte counts. Whatever the actual cause, the result of granulocytopenia is an exaggerated risk of infection.

NURSING ASSESSMENT

Granulocytopenia is associated with more frequent and severe infections and increased difficulty in diagnosing the infection (Becker, 1981; Oniboni, 1987; Reheis, 1985; Ristuccia, 1985). In patients with a decreased inflammatory response, infections may develop and spread rapidly. The nurse must be alert for subtle signs of infection (e.g., exudate, edema, erythema, tenderness, localized warmth, fever, regional adenopathy) because these signs will be attenuated due to the inadequate numbers of granulocytes. In patients with granulocytopenia, the only signs of infection may be fever, erythema, and pain (Becker, 1981; Oniboni, 1985; Reheis, 1985).

Fever is the most important indicator of infection in the granulocytopenic patient (McCarron, 1986; Oniboni, 1985). In these patients vital signs should be monitored at least every 4 hours (Becker, 1981). Temperatures above 38°C should be reported to the physician and assessments begun to attempt to identify the source of infection (Reheis, 1985).

The most frequent source of infection is through breaks in the skin (Oniboni, 1985; Reheis, 1985; Smith, 1986a), especially those made by venipuncture and intravenous catheters (Becker, 1981; Reheis, 1985). These sites should be inspected daily for indications of infection; if noted, the physician should be notified (Becker, 1981). Povidone–iodine ointment should be applied to the site, but not until all necessary cultures are obtained. To decrease the potential for infection, meticulous care should be taken with the routine changing of peripheral intravenous catheters every 48 hours and intravenous tubing every 24 hours (Becker, 1981).

TABLE 57–1. **Causes of Neutropenia**

Bacterial—typhoid, paratyphoid

Viral—influenza, measles, infectious hepatitis, infectious mononucleosis, chickenpox, rubella, yellow fever

Rickettsia—rickettsial pox, typhus, Rocky Mountain spotted fever

Protozoal—malaria, kala-azar

Overwhelming Infections (Especially in Debilitated Patients Such as Alcoholics or Malnourished Individuals)

Miliary tuberculosis
Pneumococcal pneumonia
Gram-negative bacteremia

Physical Agents—Chemicals and Drugs

Chemical and physical agents that always produce marrow hypoplasia and aplasia if given in sufficient dose
- Ionizing radiation
- Benzene
- Alkylating agents (nitrogen mustards, busulfan, chlorambucil, cyclophosphamide)
- Urethane
- Antimetabolites (methotrexate, 6-mercaptopurine, 5-fluorocytosine)
- Periwinkle alkaloids (vinblastine, vincristine)
- Antibiotics (daunomycin, Adriamycin)

Chemicals and drugs that occasionally cause neutropenia
- Analgesics (aminopyrine, salicylates)
- Anticonvulsants (Dilantin)
- Antithyroid drugs (propylthiouracil, methimazole)
- Antiinflammatory drugs (phenylbutazone)
- Antimicrobial agents (Chloramphenicol, penicillins, sulfonamides)
- Tranquilizers (meprobamate)
- Phenothiazine (chlorpromazine, promazine)
- Cardiac antiarrhythmic drugs (lidocaine, quinidine, procainamide, phenytoin)

Hematologic and Other Conditions

Those due to decreased or ineffective production
- Anemias (pernicious, aplastic, chronic hyperchromic)
- Leukemia

Those due to increased utilization, destruction, or sequestration
- Cirrhosis of the liver with splenomegaly
- Lupus erythematosus
- Felty's syndrome
- Gaucher's disease
- Hemodialysis

Cachexia and Debilitated States

Alcoholism (folate deficiency)
Vitamin B_{12} deficiency
Copper deficiency

Anaphylactoid Shock and in Early Stages of Reaction to Foreign Protein

Hereditary, Congenital, or Familial and Miscellaneous Disorders

Cyclic neutropenia
Chronic idiopathic neutropenia
Infantile genetic agranulocytosis
Primary splenic neutropenia

From Wintrobe, M. M., et al. (1981). *Clinical hematology* (8th ed.). Philadelphia: Lea & Febiger.

In addition to the obvious invasive sources that interrupt skin integrity, the entire body, including the oral mucosa, should be frequently inspected. Pressure necrosis is a frequent source of infection in immunocompromised patients. Side effects of chemotherapy combined with poor nutrition due to accompanying anorexia leave these patients at risk for breakdown of the oral mucosa. Frequent diarrheal stools, another side effect of chemotherapy, increase the patient's risk of perianal abscess, anal fissures, and excoriation. These areas should be assessed at least daily and more frequently as indicated by the individual's clinical condition (Reheis, 1985). Thorough abdominal assessments should be performed, including a search for distention, listening for bowel sounds in each quadrant, and feeling for abdominal wall firmness. Instruct the patient to report promptly abdominal pain, tenderness, feelings of fullness, nausea, and vomiting.

The respiratory tract is also at risk for infection in patients with granulocytopenia. Complaints of chest pain, discomfort, dyspnea, or shortness of breath require close follow-up. Breath sounds should be auscultated at least every 8 hours. It is possible for a chest radiograph to demonstrate pulmonary infiltrates without clinical findings of decreased or absent breath sounds, rales, or consolidation. In addition to noting patient complaints and performing chest assessment, the nurse should monitor the patient for changes in the amount and quality of sputum, the rate and rhythm of respirations, and fever.

Because of the granulocytopenic patient's increased risk of life-threatening infection, it is vital that the nurse monitor these patients vigilantly and rapidly report untoward findings.

COLLABORATIVE MANAGEMENT

In the granulocytopenic patient, a medical work-up is begun when infection is first suspected in an attempt to identify the source of infection rapidly (Fig. 57–1). This work-up should include cultures of the nasopharynx, urine, blood, sputum, perianal area, and any draining wounds (Oniboni, 1985; Reheis, 1985). The urine should also be examined for bacterial sediment. Chest radiographs should be taken to identify pulmonary infiltrates, pneumonia, and atelectasis.

After cultures are taken, broad-spectrum antibiotic therapy is promptly initiated in granulocytopenic patients to prevent rapid and life-threatening spread of infection (Oniboni, 1985; Reheis, 1985). Untreated infection in these patients has a 48-hour mortality rate of 18% to 40% (Reheis, 1985). Infection-related morbidity increases proportionately with delayed antibiotic therapy.

Granulocyte transfusions have been suggested for patients with infections that do not respond to antibiotic therapy (Oniboni, 1985; Reheis, 1985). However, the expense and risks of these transfusions may outweigh the benefits. Risks of granulocyte transfusion include viral infection, acute hypersensitivity reaction, and sensitization to human leukocyte antigens (HLA) (Oniboni, 1985; Reheis, 1985). One research study has shown that use of granulocyte transfusions was no more effective than appropriate antibiotic therapy (Winston et al., 1982).

The following problems along with the expected outcomes and proposed interventions are those that are most frequently used with the immunocompromised patient.

Potential for Infection

Infection may arise because of the immunocompromised status.

EXPECTED OUTCOMES. No signs or symptoms of infection will be noted, or, if identified, they will receive rapid intervention and not become life-threatening. Patient will verbalize understanding of indicators and symptoms that should be reported to caregivers.

INTERVENTIONS. As already noted, a priority in granulocytopenic patients is monitoring for infection. Vital signs should be routinely monitored every 4 hours, and elevated temperature, the cardinal indicator of infection, should be reported immediately. Decreased blood pressure may precede bacterial sepsis, and tachypnea may indicate pneumonia or atelectasis.

The patient should be encouraged to perform oral hygiene every 4 hours. Supplemental oral hygiene with normal saline or bicarbonate solution and sponge sticks should be initiated in patients with oral lesions. Half-strength hydrogen peroxide solution aids in debriding significant oral lesions.

Similar ulcerations can occur throughout the gastrointestinal tract, and these may be monitored by performing Hematests (Ames Co., Elkhart, IN) on stools. Patients with diarrhea may be afforded some protection of the perianal area through the application of petroleum jelly or A + D ointment (Schering Corp., Kenilworth, NJ) to irritated skin.

Soap with hexachlorophene should be used in the axillary and perineal areas to decrease colonization of these areas. However, excessive use of such soaps may result in dry skin, which is prone to cracking, thus allowing bacterial invasion. Bath oil should be used to bathe the rest of the body when bed baths are necessary.

Careful handwashing is important in any intensive care situation, but it is absolutely mandatory with these patients. Effective handwashing alone has proved effective in reducing infectious episodes (Armstrong, 1984; Garner & Simmons, 1983). The need for careful handwashing by caregivers cannot be overemphasized with the immunocompromised patient.

Granulocytopenic patients should be placed in a protective environment. Inform the patient and family why this is necessary and what it entails. The degree and form of isolation varies from institution to institution. The protective environment can be as simple as a private room, meticulous handwashing, and the omission of plants and flowers from the patient's environment, or as complex as the use of near-sterile environments with laminar flow rooms, high-energy particulate area filtration, and use of a sterile diet (Crane et al., 1980; Daly, 1983; Foon & Gale, 1982; Nauta, 1979) (Figs. 57–2, 57–3, and 57–4). Although protective isolation protects these patients from infection, it may produce negative psychological effects, including depression, anxiety, and, in extreme cases, even psychosis.

Ineffective Individual Coping

Poor coping abilities may result from social and physical separation enforced by protective isolation measures.

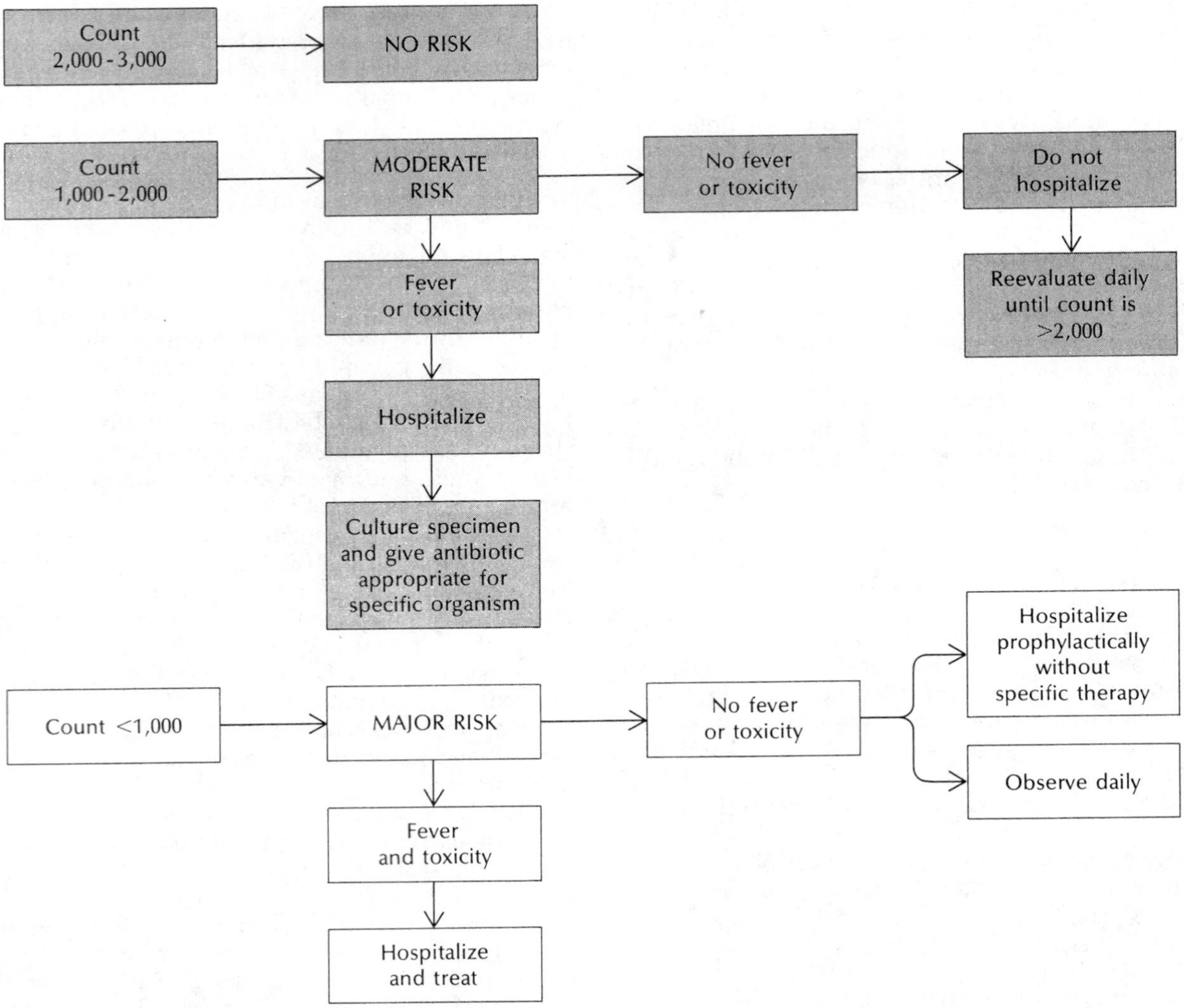

Count 2,000-3,000 → NO RISK

Count 1,000-2,000 → MODERATE RISK
- → No fever or toxicity → Do not hospitalize → Reevaluate daily until count is >2,000
- → Fever or toxicity → Hospitalize → Culture specimen and give antibiotic appropriate for specific organism

Count <1,000 → MAJOR RISK
- → No fever or toxicity → Hospitalize prophylactically without specific therapy / Observe daily
- → Fever and toxicity → Hospitalize and treat

FIGURE 57–1. Managing chemotherapy-induced leukopenia (granulocytopenia): a selective approach. (Reproduced with permission from Lokich, J. J. [1976]. Managing chemotherapy-induced bone marrow suppression in cancer. *Hospital Practice, 11*[8], 61–67.)

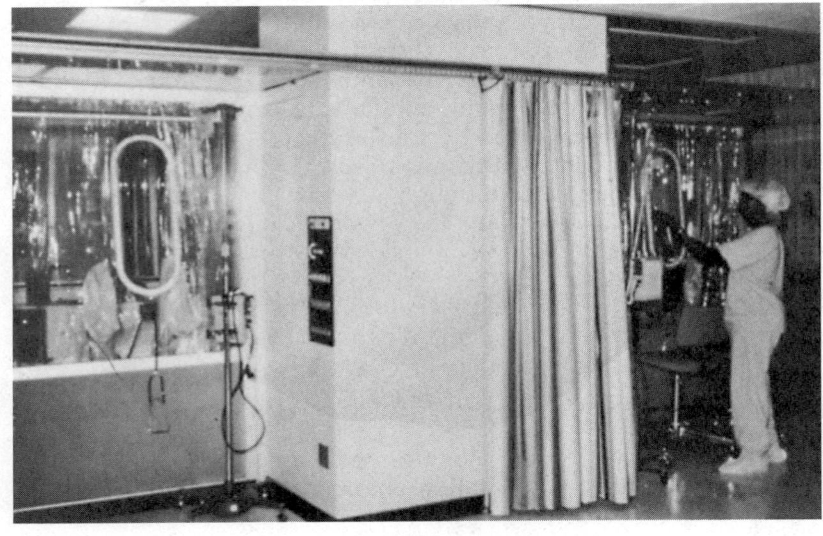

FIGURE 57–2. The Harper Hospital protective environment unit. (From Crane, L. R., Emmer, D. R., & Grguras, A. [1980]. Prevention of infection on the oncology unit. *Nursing Clinics of North America, 15,* 843–856.)

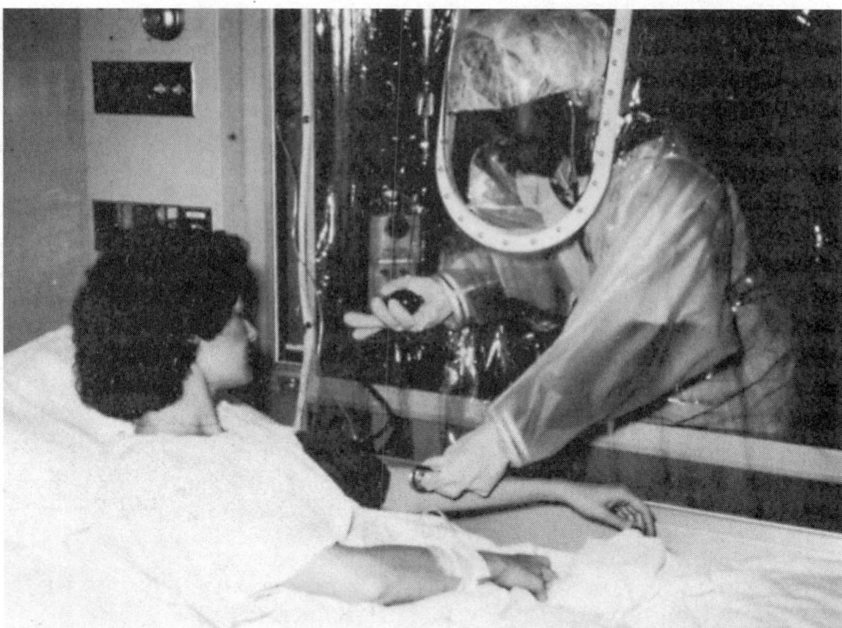

FIGURE 57-3. Clear, sliding plastic barriers allow the nurse to perform many necessary procedures without entering the laminar flow room. (From Crane, L. R., Emmer, D. R., & Grguras, A. [1980]. Prevention of infection on the oncology unit. *Nursing Clinics of North America, 15,* 843–856.)

EXPECTED OUTCOMES. The patient appears to cope with physical and social isolation and does not demonstrate any impaired adjustment.

INTERVENTIONS. The nurse, patient, and family should work together to identify problems related to isolation and alternative activities that the patient can use as distractions during the length of confinement. Sources of distraction include television, computer games, puzzles, music, and similar activities in which the patient has an interest. To decrease isolation, family and friends should be encouraged to spread visits throughout the day. In-person visits should be interspersed with telephone calls from family and friends. Hospital volunteers, social workers, housekeeping staff, and clergy should be encouraged to visit outside the confines of the isolation. When problems in adjustment occur, a psychiatric nurse clinician may be consulted.

Altered Nutrition

The patient may be malnourished due to altered gustatory sense, nausea, vomiting, and excessive diarrhea resulting from chemotherapy.

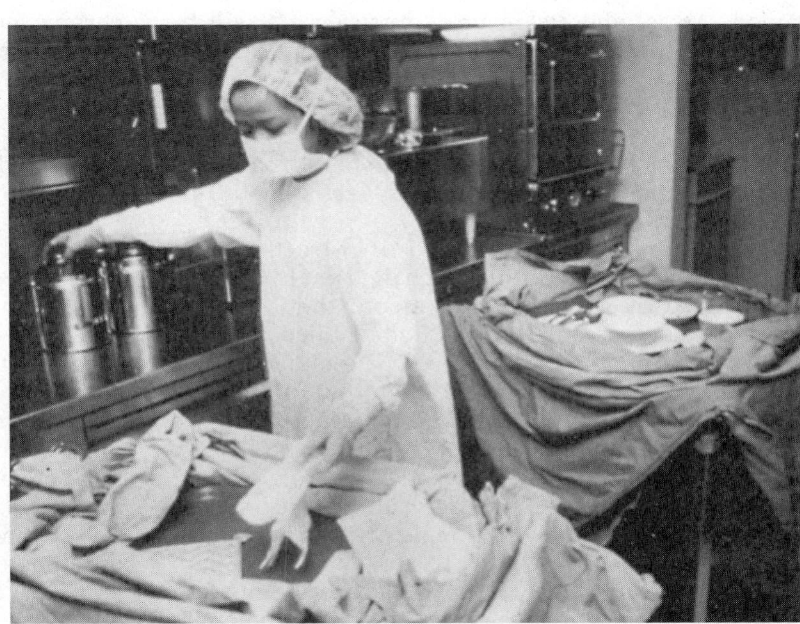

FIGURE 57-4. Bacteria, particularly *Pseudomonas aeruginosa,* can be transmitted by hospital food. (From Crane, L. R., Emmer, D. R., & Grguras, A. [1980]. Prevention of infection on the oncology unit. *Nursing Clinics of North America, 15,* 843–856.)

EXPECTED OUTCOMES. Patient maintains adequate nutrition as demonstrated through maintenance of body weight and total protein and serum albumin levels within normal limits. The patient and family verbalize their understanding of food sources appropriate to the needs of the patient. The patient takes in adequate amounts of calories through meals and between-meal snacks.

INTERVENTIONS. The nurse, patient, and family should identify nutritious foods that the patient enjoys, and these should be provided to the patient whenever possible. Encouraging smaller and more frequent meals (six per day) may avoid bloating, nausea, and diarrhea, which can cause the patient to become discouraged. The availability of a continuous supply of high-protein snacks ensures that the patient always has something to eat when he or she wants it. Warm foods and fluids should be served warm and cold foods and fluids cold, or at the temperature preferred by the patient. Instruct the patient and family about the need for high-protein foods that allow adequate tissue repair after chemotherapy. Instruct the family about sources of high-protein foods, including meats, poultry, fish, eggs, milk, cheese, yogurt, legumes, and nuts.

Monitor the patient's dietary intake closely. Perform daily weights and monitor appropriate laboratory values. Initiate a dietary consultation and calorie counts in patients at risk.

Impaired Skin Integrity

Skin integrity may be impaired due to side effects of chemotherapy, intravenous therapy, and other invasive procedures.

EXPECTED OUTCOMES. Skin integrity will be maintained. Areas where skin breakdown occurs will be promptly reported and therapy initiated immediately.

INTERVENTIONS. Strict surgical asepsis should be used for care of intravenous catheters. Scheduled dressing and luminal cap changes should be maintained. Routine care of invasive catheters should be maintained without fail.

The patient and family should be instructed about the need for frequent positional changes, at least every 2 hours. Areas subjected to pressure should be inspected and massaged and lotion applied every 2 hours. A turning schedule should be established and posted at the bedside to ensure uniformity in turning by all caregivers. Skin should be kept free of excessive moisture but not allowed to become dry and scaly; bath oil is preferred to soap for bed baths. Avoid direct contact of the patient's skin with plastic incontinent pads because these may trap moisture and heat, macerating the skin.

Adjunctive devices cannot replace basic nursing measures to prevent pressure necrosis, but they can help. Air mattresses, heel protectors, elbow pads, sheep skins, and similar devices should be considered for immobile patients.

BONE MARROW TRANSPLANTATION

Bone marrow transplantation is a specialized treatment for certain neoplastic and hematologic diseases that places the patient at particular risk through its disruption of the entire immune system. Transplantation is an aggressive treatment with inherent risks, but the incidence of risks has decreased with refinements in techniques. As a mode of therapy, its increased use makes it highly likely that a nurse may be involved in referring a patient for bone marrow transplantation or caring for a patient who has had a bone marrow transplant.

Types of Bone Marrow Transplantation

Autologous transplantation involves the patient's own tissues (Fig. 57–5). The patient's bone marrow is harvested and frozen and then can be reconstituted for later use. This form of transplantation is used for patients who have had a relapse or have a high potential for relapse on standard therapy. When relapse occurs, patients may receive potentially lethal high-dose chemotherapy alone or in combination with total body irradiation in an attempt to halt the progression of the disease. An autologous transplant rescues patients imperiled by high doses of chemotherapy (Stewart & Thomas, 1985).

Allogeneic bone marrow transplantation involves bone marrow harvested from HLA-compatible or HLA-identical donors. The patient's sibling is frequently used as a donor. This type of transplantation has been most successful in patients with acute or chronic leukemia.

Syngeneic bone marrow transplantation uses bone marrow from a genetically identical twin donor. It reduces the potential for tumor contamination, which can occur with autologous transplantation, or for incompatibility, which can occur with allogeneic transplantation (Table 57–2).

Bone Marrow Harvesting

Patients who undergo bone marrow transplantation require intense medical and nursing care. An interdisciplinary, collaborative effort is necessary to be able to meet the multiple needs of these patients and provide high-quality care.

A bone marrow transplant begins with the harvesting of bone marrow from a donor to obtain viable stem cells. Stem cells are immature hematopoietic cells that differentiate as they mature to form erythrocytes, granulocytes, lymphocytes, and platelets. Bone marrow harvesting is a relatively short procedure (30–45

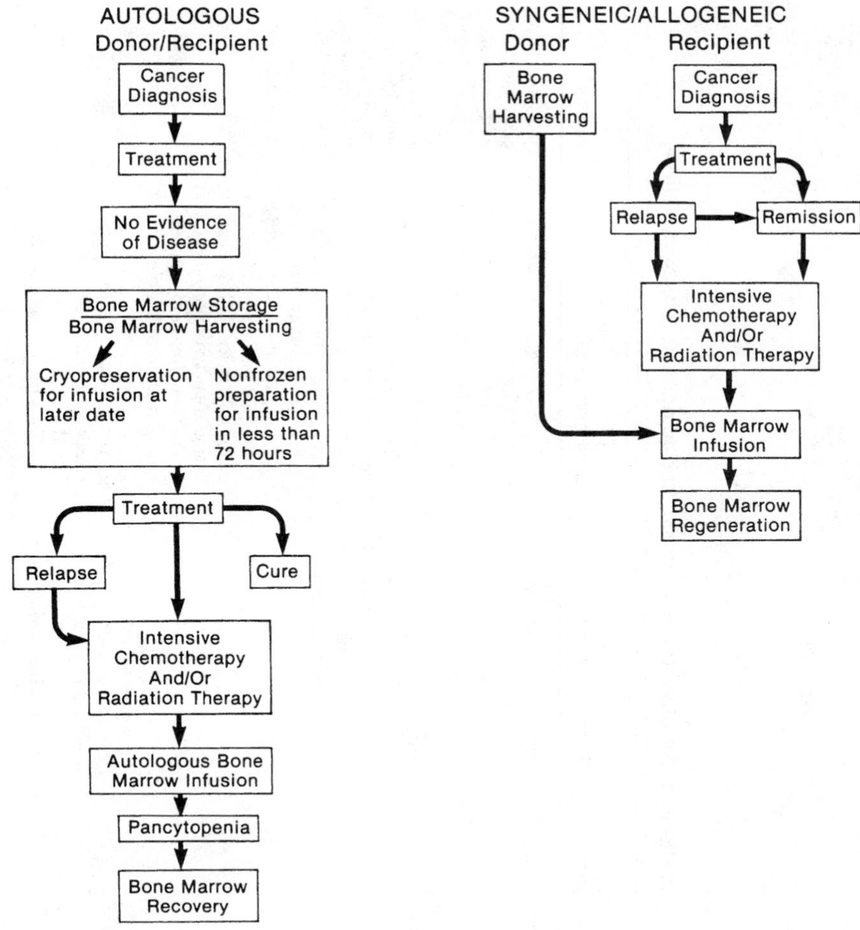

FIGURE 57–5. A comparison of autologous, syngeneic, and allogeneic treatment regimens. (From Cogliano-Shutta, N. A., & Broda, E. J. [1985]. Bone marrow transplantation: An overview and comparison of autologous, syngeneic, and allogeneic treatment modalities. *Nursing Clinics of North America, 20,* 49–66.)

minutes) done under general anesthesia in an operating room. The marrow is obtained by multiple aspirations from the posterior iliac crest. The goal is to extract 10 mL of marrow/kg body weight (i.e., an 80-kg man would donate approximately 800 mL of marrow) (Cogliano-Shutta & Broda, 1985; McGlave, 1985; Stewart & Thomas, 1985). The number of stem cells obtained is more important than the amount of marrow. The number of nucleated marrow cells required for consistent hematopoietic reconstitution is 0.5×10^8 cells/kg.

Processing bone marrow begins in the operating room, where the marrow is immediately mixed with preservative-free heparin in culture media. The marrow is then filtered to remove large particles. Allogeneic and syngeneic transplants are infused within 3 hours. Autologous transplants are treated with a cryoprotective agent, dimethylsulfoxide (DMSO), to prevent lysis of stem cells and stored in liquid nitrogen at −40° to −50°C. When needed, the autologous transplant marrow is reconstituted in sterile isotonic normal saline and warmed to body temperature before being infused intravenously.

After harvesting, pressure dressings are applied to aspiration sites. The donor returns to his or her room after recovery in the postanesthesia recovery room. Hematocrit and hemoglobin levels are monitored carefully for the first 24 hours to assess the need for blood replacement. Dressings are closely monitored for bleeding. This procedure is painful and requires careful management of postoperative pain with narcotic analgesics. New sources of donor marrow that may be used in the future are cadaveric marrow and clones of a patient's healthy peripheral blood stem cells (Gianni et al., 1989; Lucas et al., 1988).

Recipients of marrow transplants require intensive supportive therapy, including antibiotic therapy, parenteral nutrition, multiple blood products, and hydration. Because of the long-term intravenous therapy required for these patients, an indwelling central venous line is usually placed, most commonly a Hickman or Broviac catheter. The catheter is placed when the patient is in the operating room in the external cephalic or internal jugular vein. Placement is done under local or general anesthesia. Fluoroscopy is used to ensure proper positioning of the proximal tip of the catheter. Two small incisions are needed, one to secure the access port of the catheter to the thoracic wall and one to enter the chosen vein (DeVita, 1985). Each device has a Dacron cuff that allows ingrowth of fibroelastic

TABLE 57–2. **Comparison and Contrast of Side Effects and Nursing Interventions in Autologous, Syngeneic, and Allogeneic Transplantation**

Transplantation Procedure	Complication	Pathophysiology	Time of Presentation	Signs and Symptoms	Nursing Intervention	Comments
Autologous, syngeneic, autologous	Discolored urine (red)	Excretion of phenol used in culture media	Time of infusion to 24 hours postinfusion	First void discolored	Note color changes, alleviate possible anxiety	Urine will gradually clear. Seen primarily with autologous
	Fever	Infusion of pyrogenes and TBI	Evening of the bone marrow infusion	Elevated temperature	Frequent vital signs, acetaminophen	
	Venoocclusive disease	Hepatic central vein fibrosis	1 to 3 weeks posttransplant	Hepatomegaly, ascites	Abdominal girth measurements, fluid management	About half of cases are progressive
	Acute GVHD	Donor T cells react to host	5 to 70 days	Skin: erythema, maculopapular eruption, bullae, desquamation	Mild rash: Lubricate skin with oil-based lotions, such as Alpha Keri; antihistamine and steroid creams may be helpful Frank desquamation: Use sterile technique, sterile sheets, debride skin twice daily; cover major areas with normal saline/Betadine-impregnated gauze, and antimicrobial creams	Note: Rash in syngeneic BMT must have GVHD ruled out. Also note temporal change in medications
				Liver: elevations of liver enzymes, bilirubin	Observe for jaundice, bleeding; check liver enzymes, coagulation	
				Gut: diarrhea to greater than 2 L/day	Meticulous intake and output; weights twice daily; good rectal care including sitz baths	
	Chronic GVHD	Primary immunologic	Greater than 100 days postransplant	Increased skin pigmentation/thickening, contractures, conjunctivitis, photosensitivity	Physical therapy, sunscreens, Alpha Keri lotion, sunglasses	
	Infections: bacterial, fungal, viral	Loss of immune function	Primarily during aplasia or GVHD	Fever, chills, malaise, rise in pulse, fall in blood pressure	Prevention: Ensure compliance with oral prophylactic antibiotics, maintain protective isolation. With possible infection: monitor vital signs carefully, fever/sepsis evaluation, anticipate use of broad-spectrum antibiotics with blood level determinations of drug; remember perirectal area as possible site of infection in these patients. Meticulous catheter care is of prime importance.	

	Common preparative regimen toxicities					Note: Increased severity of toxicities is secondary to higher doses
	Cystitis	Cytoxan metabolites in bladder TBI	Shortly after administration; may be delayed	Hematuria, pain	Hydration before, during, and after drug administration; forced voiding every 2 hours for 24 hours after drug is given; careful intake and output	Drug may cause fluid retention, so intake and output is critical
	Anxiety, depression	Isolation, concerns of complications	Any time during and after transplant	Emotional reactions	Encourage verbalization, reinforce reasonable expectations, activity, family involvement	
	Respiratory distress	Transient pulmonary hypertension secondary to infusion of cell particles from cell lysis, volume overload	During bone marrow infusion	Tachycardia, hypertension, anxiety, cyanosis	Monitor vital signs, oxygen, and drugs as ordered; monitor intake and output weights	
	Cardiomyopathy	Associated with high-dose Cytoxam	Shortly after administration	Decreased ECG voltage; decreased cardiac function by any of several laboratory tests; signs/symptoms of congestive heart failure	Baseline ECG with follow-up tracings; observation for clinical evidence of congestive heart failure	
	Mucositis	Multifactorial: radiation, virus, drug	5 days onward	Initially small oral lesions progressing to full oral cavity, perioral involvement	Meticulous oral care with frequent normal saline rinses; antimicrobial rinses may be of use if lesions progress	Emphasis is on prevention; new antiviral drugs are of significant help
	Marrow depression	Direct toxicity of preparative regimen	5 to 7 days after therapy	Depression in all counts of all three cell lines	See failure to engraft	
	"Capillary leak"	Probably direct toxicity of preparative regimen	3 to 5 days	Decreased FVC, decreased P_{O_2}	Weigh twice daily, careful intake and output	
Autologous	Garlic smell, unpleasant taste	Excretion of DMSO by lungs	Time of infusion to 36 hours postinfusion	Decreased appetite, garlic odor	Give patient hard candy, room deodorizer, peppermint oil	
	Transient hemoglobinuria	Release of hemoglobin during lysis after thawing	Within 48 hours after infusion	Positive Hemastix	Hematest all urine, monitor results for 48 hours	

Table continued on following page

TABLE 57–2. **Comparison and Contrast of Side Effects and Nursing Interventions in Autologous, Syngeneic, and Allogeneic Transplantation** *Continued*

Transplantation Procedure	Complication	Pathophysiology	Time of Presentation	Signs and Symptoms	Nursing Intervention	Comments
	Potential for infusion of tumor cells	Related to the harvest of unsuspected tumor cell and subsequent infusion after ablative therapy	After transplant	Tumor recurrence	Plan therapy as feasible	
Primarily allogeneic	Interstitial pneumonitis	Multifactorial including virus (CMV) and pneumocystis	Most commonly in the first 4 months, especially at end of second month	Fall in FVC, fall in Po_2 dyspnea	Monitor for compromise of pulmonary function by daily FVC, careful fluid balance in patients with interstitial pneumonitis	Thirty to 40% of patients develop interstitial pneumonitis; half have no demonstrated etiologic agent, mortality is high
	Graft rejection	Not well understood	Either no engraftment or transient engraftment	No rise in blood counts or rise followed by fall	Continued protection as severely immunocompromised patient; continued colonization surveys and observation for infection; minimize invasive procedures; bleeding precautions; continued irradiated blood product support	
	Chronic GVHD	Primarily immunologic	Greater than 100 days posttransplant	Liver: jaundice coagulopathy Gut: malabsorption, chronic diarrhea Musculoskeletal: arthritis Pulmonary insufficiency; SOB, DOE, cough Immunopathy: opportunistic infection	Enzyme replacement; early recognition Diet manipulation; antidiarrheal medications Encourage increased ROM; physiotherapy Encourage increased activity to preserve function Teach importance of good hygiene and environment protection; observe for signs of any infectious disease—systemic, superficial, or fungal	
Syngeneic	Skin rash	Etiology unclear, question mild GVHD	1 Week	Variable in character and distribution, maculopapular, erythematous, pruritic	Lubricate skin with oil-based lotion; may require antihistamines and steroid creams	

Abbreviations: TBI, total body irradiation; GVHD, graft-versus-host disease; BMT, bone marrow transplantation; DMSO, dimethylsulfoxide; CMV, cytomegalovirus; FVC, forced vital capacity; ROM, range of motion; DOE, dyspnea on exertion; SOB, shortness of breath; ECG, electrocardiography.

From Cogliano-Shutta, N. A., & Broda, E. J. (1985). Bone marrow transplantation: An overview and comparison of autologous, syngeneic, and allogeneic treatment modalities. *Nursing Clinics of North America, 20,* 49–66.

tissue, anchoring the device to the thorax and decreasing potential migration of bacteria along the outer surface of the device. During recovery, the nurse must carefully monitor the patient for hemorrhage (external bleeding or hematoma) from the site of vascular entry.

Autologous Transplantation

To be considered for autologous transplantation, the patient must meet the following criteria (Cogliano-Shutta & Broda, 1985):

1. Bone marrow must be free of detectable tumor.
2. The patient must be able to tolerate anesthesia and bone harvesting.
3. The patient's disease is expected to respond to increased chemotherapy using agents with myelosuppression as the main dose-limiting toxic factor.
4. The patient must be able to tolerate prolonged myelosuppression resulting in a WBC count of less than 1,000 cells/mm^3 and a granulocyte count of less than 500 cells/mm^3 for 2 to 3 weeks.

The bone marrow transplant patient may be asked to choose between low-dose therapy with fewer life-threatening side effects and a low chance of cure, and higher-dose therapy plus bone marrow transplant with more life-threatening complications but a higher rate of cure. Reports in the literature suggest that high-dose chemotherapy and autologous bone marrow transplantation prolong survival in patients with some malignant conditions (Cogliano-Shutta & Broda, 1985). Patients with relapsed solid tumors that are resistant to conventional therapy who received high-dose chemotherapy and bone marrow transplantation had a 30% complete response rate with 16% in remission for at least 15 months after therapy (Deisseroth et al., 1982). Patients with acute leukemia who were treated with autologous bone transplants harvested during remission had response rates equal to those seen in patients who received syngeneic transplants. Autologous transplants were also effective for long-term survival of patients with non-Hodgkin's lymphoma. However, tumor cell contamination may result in recurrence, the rate of recurrence varying with the malignant condition (Cogliano-Shutta & Broda, 1985). The effectiveness of the transplant procedure is predicated on the ability of the preceding chemotherapy to eradicate malignant cells.

POST-TRANSPLANTATION/ENGRAFTMENT PERIOD

The induction phase (i.e., the period before transplantation) varies with the underlying disease and the treatment protocol. Patients typically receive high-dose chemotherapy alone or with radiation therapy. After the treatment regimen is complete, the bone marrow is transfused intravenously, allowing the stem cells to repopulate the recipient's depleted marrow. After transplantation, it takes several weeks for the transplanted marrow to engraft (i.e., to replace the patient's existing marrow as it is slowly destroyed). During this period the patient's blood cell counts drop precipitously, leaving the patient profoundly granulocytopenic.

Many complications may arise and require prompt nursing intervention. Platelet transfusions are required when the platelet count falls below 20,000 cells/mm^3. If the hematocrit falls below 30% and hemoglobin levels below 10 g/100 mL, the patient may require transfusion of packed red cells. Blood products for these patients are usually irradiated to inactivate immunologically competent cells and avoid possible graft-versus-host reactions.

The bone marrow begins to regenerate about 14 days after transplantation. For recipients of autologous transplants, it may take up to 4 weeks for the granulocytes to recover to 500 cells/mm^3. It may take up to 6 weeks for platelets to reach 50,000 cells/mm^3. Autologous bone marrow recovery rates are slower than those with allogeneic and syngeneic transplants because of the myelosuppressive therapy needed before harvesting and the effect of freezing and storage on the bone marrow.

COLLABORATIVE MANAGEMENT

GUSTATORY SENSORY ALTERATIONS. These changes are due to side effects from the preservative DMSO used to freeze the bone marrow for autologous transplantation.

EXPECTED OUTCOMES. Patient states that he or she can tolerate the altered sensation and does not develop nausea or vomiting.

SIDE EFFECTS. Side effects of autologous transplantation include a garlic breath odor and an unpleasant taste that results from the excretion of DMSO by the lungs. The patient should be informed of this side effect before the transplantation procedure to reduce anxiety when it occurs. Patients with sensitivity to taste may become nauseated and vomit. These side effects last up to 36 hours and may be diminished by sucking on hard candy or drinking sweet beverages. Some patients may require antiemetics to control nausea and vomiting.

ALTERED PATTERNS IN URINARY ELIMINATION. Urination is altered due to the presence of phenol dye in the transplant culture media and to lysis of erythrocytes during reconstitution.

EXPECTED OUTCOMES. Patient verbalizes understanding of the reason why urine becomes red after autologous transplantation.

INTERVENTIONS. After autologous transplantation, the patient's urine usually becomes dark red, gradually lightening to an amber color within 24 hours. The patient should be informed about this change before the transplant to reduce anxiety. Clearing of this discoloration is facilitated by forcing fluids. The patient should be instructed about the need for increased fluid intake and his or her fluid preferences determined. The patient's intake and output should be closely monitored to ensure adequate output. Patients should be informed about the need to monitor urinary output.

POTENTIAL FOR ALTERED BODY TEMPERATURE. Temperature is increased due to pyrogens released from WBCs injured during reconstitution.

EXPECTED OUTCOMES. Patient verbalizes understanding of expected temperature elevations; elevations above 38°C will be rapidly identified and reported.

INTERVENTIONS. Patients and families should be informed about the potential for post-transplant fever and told to inform caregivers if the patient feels warm. Vital signs should be monitored every 4 hours for the first day after transplantation. Temperatures exceeding 38°C should be reported to the physician. Acetaminophen may be required as an antipyretic.

FEAR. Fear may be due to the known potential for infusion of malignant cells with the transplanted bone marrow.

EXPECTED OUTCOMES. Patients freely verbalize their concerns and do not demonstrate uncontrolled fear.

INTERVENTIONS. The patient and family should be allowed and encouraged to verbalize their concerns about recurrence of malignancy. The nurse can remind the family that precautions are taken at the time of the harvest to avoid malignancy (e.g., by means of chemotherapy or radiation therapy). Patients and family experiencing uncontrolled fear may require referral to psychiatric nurse clinicians for assistance.

Allogeneic Transplantation

Allogeneic bone marrow transplantation is the treatment of choice for the first remission of acute myelogenous leukemia (AML) and for other hematologic malignancies that are refractory to standard therapy. Data from major transplant centers show the following survival rates with allogeneic transplantation for leukemia (Champlin & Gale, 1983; Stewart & Thomas, 1985): AML, 60%; acute lymphoblastic leukemia, 40%; chronic myelogenous leukemia, 65%; aplastic anemia, 60%.

Although rates varied with the stage of each disease, these results indicate a potential benefit in the use of allogeneic bone marrow transplantation. Variations may have been due to the nature of each disease process or the resistance of the individual patient to the induction therapy.

HLA TYPING. Allogeneic bone marrow transplantation is preceded by HLA typing to determine the compatibility of the donor and recipient. A blood specimen is used to perform HLA typing. There is a one-in-four chance of a sibling being HLA-compatible with the recipient.

Genes encoding the HLA antigens are found on chromosome 6. One set of genes is inherited from each parent. Each set of HLA genes has components labeled A, B, C, DP, DQ, DR, MB, MT, and Te, each of which has numerous subcategories. HLA-A and HLA-B antigens are identified serologically. Because of the large number of combinations of the five major antigens and the subgroups, it is unlikely for a close HLA match to be found outside of the family.

PREPARATION OF THE RECIPIENT. Induction therapy for an allogeneic bone marrow transplant usually includes high-dose chemotherapy and total body irradiation (TBI). The goal of these therapies is to eradicate malignant cells and suppress host immune function to prevent rejection of the allogeneic bone marrow.

High-dose intravenous cyclophosphamide (50 μmol/kg per day) for 2 days followed by a high dose of TBI (1,000 rad) in divided doses or a single dose is an example of an induction therapy (Cogliano-Shutta & Broda, 1985; DeVita, 1985; McGlave, 1985; Stewart & Thomas, 1985). TBI has proved effective because of its immunosuppressive effects and its ability to penetrate tumor growth areas (central nervous system [CNS] and testicles) that are inaccessible to chemotherapy.

COMPLICATIONS OF THERAPY. The first complications encountered are usually related to the induction therapy (e.g., immunosuppression and gastrointestinal side effects). There are also complications unique to allogeneic transplantation (see Table 57–2).

Graft-versus-host disease (GVHD) is unique to allogeneic bone marrow transplantation because of the potential for reaction of the donor's marrow to the recipient. Once infused, the immunologically competent donor T cells may recognize the recipient's tissue as foreign (Cogliano-Shutta & Broda, 1985; McGlave, 1985; Stewart & Thomas, 1985). Organs most commonly affected by this reaction are the skin, liver, and gastrointestinal tract. Clinical findings include erythema and sloughing of skin, elevated liver aminotransferases, jaundice, diarrhea, and fluid and electrolyte imbalances. The severity of GVHD for any one of the target organ systems may be graded on a scale of one to four, with four being most severe.

Graft-versus-host disease has been divided into acute and chronic forms. Acute GVHD occurs within the first 100 days after transplantation (Cogliano-Shutta & Broda, 1985; McGlave, 1985). GVHD persisting after 100 days is labeled chronic GVHD. Chronic GVHD results in changes similar to those seen in collagen vascular diseases, including joint contractures, skin thickening, and dry eyes and mouth. Although not immediately life threatening, chronic GVHD has a high long-term mortality rate if it remains untreated (Cogliano-Shutta & Broda, 1985).

Approximately 60% of all patients with allogenic transplants have some degree of GVHD. Of this group, 30% to 50% will succumb to complications of GVHD. Prevention of GVHD includes use of prophylactic methotrexate or cyclosporine after transplantation. Severe GVHD may be treated with high doses of steroids or antithymocyte globulin (Cogliano-Shutta & Broda, 1985; Doney & Weiden, 1981).

LONG-TERM COMPLICATIONS OF ALLOGENEIC TRANSPLANTATION. Most long-term complications of allogeneic transplantation are the result of high-dose chemotherapy, TBI, or chronic GVHD or are related to the original disease (Table 57–3). As allogeneic transplantation becomes more successful in controlling disease outcomes, the care of these patients becomes more challenging for nurses.

Cataracts that occur after allogeneic transplantation are thought to result from TBI or long-term steroid therapy for GVHD (Corcoran-Buchsel, 1986). Fifty percent of patients who receive single-dose TBI experience cataracts, compared to 20% of those who receive in TBI in divided doses. Age has not been identified as a risk factor for the development of cataracts. The average length of time for cataract formation is 3 years after transplantation (range, 1–5.5 years). Cataract formation is usually bilateral. The treatment of choice is intraocular lens replacement (Corcoran-Buchsel, 1986). The nurse should instruct the patient and family about the potential for this complication and encourage yearly eye examinations.

Because patients with allogeneic transplantation have an immature immune response, they are at risk for numerous opportunistic infections for the first year after transplantation. About half of these patients contract herpes zoster–varicella infections in the first year (Atkinson & Meyers, 1980). Patients with chronic GVHD or mismatched transplants are at greater risk for development of herpes zoster infections because of the profound immunosuppression that occurs after the transplant. Chronic GVHD patients remain at high risk for development of bacterial pneumonia, septicemia, and sinusitis because of their immature immune response (Witherspoon & Storb, 1981).

Most transplant recipients experience some degree of gonadal dysfunction because of the high-dose chemotherapy or TBI. The incidence of gonadal dysfunction and sterility is related to the patient's age at the time of transplantation and the total dose and length of chemotherapy (Ruccione & Fergusson, 1984). When high-dose chemotherapy is used alone, especially cyclophosphamide, patients of either sex who are prepubertal will have normal sexual development. However, the long-term prognosis for postpubertal patients is uncertain. Menses and luteinizing hormone (LH) and follicle-stimulating hormone (FSH) levels in postpubertal women may return to normal, but early menopause and elevations of both LH and FSH have been noted. Outcomes for postpubertal men include the possibility of a return to normal gonadotropin levels and low-to-normal sperm counts, or there may be elevated FSH levels and azoospermia.

The effects of TBI on reproductive function and sexual development are more predictable—that is, sterility usually occurs. Prepubertal girls experience primary ovarian failure, do not achieve menarche, and do not develop secondary sex characteristics (Sanders & Buckner, 1985). Some prepubertal boys develop secondary sex characteristics, but most will have delayed sexual maturity and permanent azoospermia. Postpubertal women experience primary ovarian failure and early menopause, whereas men have primary gonadal failure and azoospermia (Sanders & Buckner, 1985).

The long-term psychological effects of bone marrow transplantation vary with the complications experienced. Patients with recurrent complications report situational depression and anxiety resulting from continued therapy and prolonged restricted activities after transplantation (Gardner & August, 1977). Some patients report residual psychological effects of the primary illness and fears of its recurrence and of dying, especially when chronic complications occur after transplantation. Patients who are able to resume normal activities and return to work have less anxiety about their quality of life and economic stability. Psychological adjustment after transplantation is very dependent on the patient's health status.

DRUGS USED IN TRANSPLANTATION

Cyclosporine

Cyclosporine is an immunosuppressive agent that suppresses allograft rejection and hypersensitivity reactions. This agent selectively inhibits T lymphocytes by interfering with the production of effector T lymphocytes and lymphokines while impairing the cloning of helper T cells (Smith, 1986b). Cyclosporine is more effective when used prophylactically than when treating an acute rejection. Therefore, cyclosporine is begun on the day before or the day of transplantation and is continued indefinitely (Klemm, 1985).

ROUTES OF ADMINISTRATION

ORAL. Cyclosporine is administered orally in an olive oil–based solution, diluted as 1 part cyclosporine to 10 parts of diluent. Although many patients prefer to use chocolate milk, some dilute the drug with regular milk, orange juice, or Ensure. The mixture should be taken at room temperature and mixed in a glass container because cyclosporine will adhere to the walls of other containers. Once the dose has been taken, the container should be rinsed with additional diluent, and this should then be taken by the patient to ensure that the complete dose is ingested. Food interferes with the absorption of this drug, so it should be taken between meals, at least 1 hour before or 2 hours after food is ingested.

INTRAVENOUS. Cyclosporine is supplied in 2-mL ampules in a concentration of 50 mg/mL (41.5 μmol/mL). This amount is further diluted in 20 to 50 mL of 5% dextrose and water or normal saline and administered over 4 to 6 hours. Too-rapid administration has been associated with complaints of burning palms and soles of the feet (Klemm, 1985).

DOSAGE. Dosages are based on body weight and range from 12.5 mg/kg per day (10 μmol/kg per day)

TABLE 57–3. **Possible Late Effects of Bone Marrow Transplantation Caused by High-Dose Chemotherapy and/or Irradiation in Conditioning Regimens**

Late Effect	Incidence Rate	Time Post-BMT	Signs and Symptoms	Nursing Management	Diagnostic Tools	Medical Treatment
Late infectious complications Bacterial, viral fungal infections with or without chronic GVHD	>50%	100–365 days	Fever, wheezing, rales, postnasal drip, signs of infection	Preventive teaching Mask-wearing until 6 months post-BMT Good hand-washing techniques Avoid infectious people (measles, chickenpox, mumps) Avoid school/work until 6 months post-BMT Avoid hot tubs, public swimming pools until 6–9 months post-BMT Limit number of sexual partners Avoid live virus vaccines	Positive blood culture for bacteria, fungus, virus Abnormal chest x-ray studies, PFT Pulmonary infiltrates Open lung biopsy Changes in CBC	Appropriate antibiotic support
Varicella zoster virus without chronic GVHD with chronic GVHD	<50% >75%	100–365 days	Lesions, pain, malaise, tenderness, neurologic manifestation	Relieve pruritus with calamine lotion Cool compresses Prevent secondary infection	Positive HZV cultures	Strict isolation until lesions are crusting IV acyclovir, 10 mg/kg/dose, q8h × 7 days
Pulmonary complications Interstitial pneumonia Cytomegalovirus *Pneumocystis carinii*	70%	100–400 days	Fever, sepsis, hypotension, lethargy, cough	Anticipatory preventive teaching Routine vital signs Chest A&P Monitor PFT, ABG	Chest x-ray studies, CBC, ABG, PFT Positive cultures for bacterial, fungal, and viral microorganisms Bronchoscopy IgA, IgG levels	
Restrictive disease	5%		May be asymptomatic or Cough	Anticipatory teaching of pulmonary toilet Routine vital signs Chest A&P	Total lung capacity, diffusion capacity	Respiratory therapy Bronchodilation
Obstructive disease	11%		Decreased ability to perform daily living activities due to pulmonary insufficiency	Monitor PFT and ABG		

Abbreviations: BMT, bone marrow transplantation; GVHD, graft-versus-host disease; PFT, pulmonary function tests; CBC, complete blood count; HZV, herpes zoster–varicella; A&P, auscultation and percussion; ABG, arterial blood gases; IgA, IgG, immunoglobulins A, G.

From Corcoran-Buchsel, P. (1986). Long-term complications of allogeneic bone marrow transplantation: Nursing implications. *Oncology Nursing Forum, 13*(6), 61–70.

to 25 mg/kg per day (20 μmol/kg per day) (Klemm, 1985). Because this agent has a narrow therapeutic range, peak and trough levels may be determined daily. Daily dosages are adjusted according to the results of these assessments.

SIDE EFFECTS AND PRECAUTIONS. Table 57–4 summarizes the side effects of cyclosporine and the associated nursing interventions.

Colony-Stimulating Factors

Bone marrow transplantation is associated with many serious complications, including infection during the period of profound neutropenia. Recombinant human colony-stimulating factors, such as granulocyte colony-stimulating factor and granulocyte–macrophage colony-stimulating factor, have been used in clinical trials to reduce the period of neutropenia associated with myelosuppressive chemotherapy (Singer, 1992). Colony-stimulating factors have been shown to be beneficial for shortening the neutrophil/recovery time for both autologous and allogeneic bone marrow transplants.

Interleukin-2 Therapy

It is postulated that people with impaired immune response may be at high risk for development of cancer (Jassak & Sticklin, 1986). The evolution of interleukin-2 (IL-2) therapy over the past 10 years has been based on the premise that it could restore or augment immune responses (Dudjak, 1993). Thus, IL-2 is thought to enhance the immune system's ability to destroy cancer cells.

Interleukin-2 is a naturally occurring substance produced by helper T cells in response to specific antigens. It mediates a wide variety of immunoregulatory phenomena (Jassak & Sticklin, 1986). Specific immune responses include enhanced production of T lymphocytes, stimulated responses of B and T cells, augmented cell-killing activity of natural killer cells and cytotoxic T cells, and increased production of lymphokine-activated killer cells.

ADMINISTRATION OF IL-2. IL-2 was approved by the Food and Drug Administration (FDA) in May, 1992 for use in metastatic renal cell carcinoma. Before its approval, no effective treatment regimen was available for renal cell cancer. Other clinical trials have shown that IL-2 has activity in other types of advanced cancer, such as melanoma (Dudjak, 1993).

The regimen on which the FDA based its approval has become known as high-dose IL-2. Current research studies are testing low-dose treatments administered on an outpatient basis. Some researchers are combining IL-2 with other biologic agents or with chemotherapy in an attempt to reduce toxicity while maintaining efficacy (Fisher, 1993).

PRETREATMENT. The care of patients receiving high-dose IL-2 begins with a careful assessment of the patient. Patients who are the best candidates for therapy are those with limited disease and slow-growing tumors. As with other immunologic therapies, IL-2 alters the immune response to the tumor and may require 8 weeks to 1 year to produce a response (Shelton, 1993). Most adverse effects associated with IL-2 therapy are related to the dose administered and the total cumulative dose (Table 57–5).

ALTERED THOUGHT PROCESSES. Mental changes result from CNS toxicity of IL-2 therapy.

EXPECTED OUTCOMES. Toxic reactions and altered thought processes will be rapidly identified and the patient's safety maintained.

INTERVENTIONS. The major CNS effect of IL-2 therapy is severe mental confusion. Disorientation, combativeness, increased anxiety, and psychosis have also been noted (Jassak & Sticklin, 1986). The etiology of this toxicity is unknown. Because of the severe toxicities of high-dose IL-2 regimens, these patients must receive the therapy in an intensive care unit. Lower-dose regimens can be safely administered to nonhospitalized patients (Viele & Moran, 1993). It may be difficult to differentiate the CNS effects of toxicity from those resulting from the stress of being hospitalized in an intensive care unit. Frequent assessment of mental status, orientation, and level of consciousness every 1 to 4 hours is necessary (Shelton, 1993). Documentation of mental status should be carefully made to allow evaluation over time. Administration of medications that affect CNS function should be avoided. CNS side effects may require the interruption or discontinuation of the therapy.

FLUID VOLUME DEFICIT. A volume deficit results from cumulative doses of IL-2, which are associated with increased capillary permeability, extravasation of fluid, and fluid shifts to the extravascular space.

EXPECTED OUTCOMES. Significant deviations from the patient's normal vital signs and indicators of fluid shift will be rapidly identified and reported. The patient will not have complications of fluid volume deficit.

INTERVENTIONS. Weight gains of more than 10% of baseline have been reported with IL-2 therapy (Lotze, 1985; Rosenberg, 1985). Fluid retention is shown by peripheral edema, ascites, and, eventually, pulmonary interstitial edema (Jassak & Sticklin, 1986). Patients with decreased oxygenation, dyspnea, and respiratory distress may require intubation. Blood gas results should be carefully monitored. Daily weights should be begun in prone patients. Lung auscultation, abdominal girth measurements, and assessment for peripheral edema should be performed along with the vital signs. Careful intake and output measurements should be taken and recorded. Inform the patient of appropriate symptoms that should be promptly reported (e.g., dyspnea, dyspnea on exertion, shortness of breath, orthopnea, peripheral edema, and abdominal pain).

TABLE 57–4. **Nursing Actions for the Identification and Management of Cyclosporine Side Effects**

Late Effect	Incidence Rate	Time Post-BMT	Signs and Symptoms	Nursing Management	Diagnostic Tools	Medical Treatment
Cataracts						
Total body irradiation, fractionated	20%	1.5–5 years	Poor vision	Anticipatory teaching of BMT risk factors Ophthalmologist recommendation	Examination with slit lamp microscopy	Intraocular lens replacement
Total body irradiation, single dose	50%	1.5–5 years				
Neurologic complications						
Leukoencephalopathy	7%	1–5 months	Lethargy Somnolence Dementia Seizures Spastic quadriplegia Coma Personality changes	Early intervention Multidisciplinary approach with special education program Routine neurologic assessments	Periodic head computer-assisted tomography and psychometric evaluation	Symptomatic and supportive management
Psychological complications	Unknown	Months to years	Depression, weight change Altered body image Survival syndrome Sibling rivalry	Allow patient/family to verbalize feelings Identify coping mechanisms, personal strengths Refer to mental health resources	Psychological testing	Mental health evaluation and treatment from appropriate source
Impaired growth in children						
Irradiation only	100%	Months to years	Subnormal growth and development	Anticipatory teaching to patients/parents Annual evaluation of growth pattern Serial height/weight	Adrenocortical function Growth hormone Thyroid hormone	Possible appropriate hormone replacement Long-term follow-up

Abbreviations: BMT, bone marrow transplantation.

From Klemm, P. (1985). Cyclosporin A: Use in preventing graft versus host disease. *Oncology Nursing Forum, 12*(5), 25–32.

TABLE 57–5. **Toxicities**

Central Nervous System	Miscellaneous
Confusion Disorientation Combativeness Psychoses Anxiety	Headache Malaise Chills, fever Flu-like syndrome Nasal congestion Glossitis Xerostomia
Gastrointestinal	**Integumentary**
Nausea Vomiting Diarrhea Mucositis ↓ Appetite	Erythematous rash Pruritus Skin desquamation
Renal	**Hematologic**
Oliguria ↑ Creatinine ↑ BUN Proteinuria	Anemia Thrombocytopenia
Pulmonary	**Hepatic**
Pulmonary edema Dyspnea	↑ Bilirubin ↑ AST, ↑ ALT, ↑ LDH
Cardiovascular	
Hypotension Weight gain Edema Ascites Dysrhythmias	

Abbreviations: BUN, blood urea nitrogen; AST, aspartate aminotransferase; ALT, alanine aminotransferase; LDH, lactic dehydrogenase.

From Jassak, P. F., & Sticklin, L. A. (1986). Interleukin-2: An overview. *Oncology Nursing Forum, 13*(6), 17–22.

Hypotension associated with IL-2 is thought to be related to reduced vascular system resistance (Jassak & Sticklin, 1986). Continuous blood pressure monitoring or arterial pressure monitoring is required for these patients. Hypotension may be treated with intravenous colloid solutions (e.g., 5% human serum albumin or 5% plasma protein fraction). Sometimes vasopressors such as dopamine hydrochloride or phenylephrine hydrochloride are needed. Fluid replacement therapy is contraindicated because of the danger of pulmonary edema.

ALTERATIONS IN URINARY ELIMINATION. Changes in urination are due to toxicities resulting from IL-2.

EXPECTED OUTCOMES. The patient's urinary output will be over 30 mL per hour or, if less, it will be rapidly identified and reported to the physician.

INTERVENTIONS. Urinary complications of IL-2 are dose related and include oliguria, proteinuria, elevations of serum creatinine, and increased blood urea nitrogen (BUN). Renal function usually returns to normal within 48 hours of the cessation of IL-2 therapy. Fluid challenges are usually contraindicated (see above), but diuretics may be used if central venous pressure and blood pressure levels are adequate. Intake and output need to be carefully monitored, and each voided specimen should be assessed for proteinuria. Daily serum creatinine and BUN levels should be monitored.

ALTERATIONS IN BOWEL ELIMINATION. Diarrhea results from the toxicity of IL-2.

EXPECTED OUTCOMES. Patient will maintain normal bowel habits with formed stool; if diarrhea develops, it is rapidly identified, and complications are avoided.

INTERVENTIONS. The patient should be instructed about the potential for diarrhea and asked to report any associated symptoms. If diarrhea develops, a record of stools should be maintained. If more than three liquid stools per day are passed, an antidiarrheal medication should be started. The patient should be instructed about the need to take in additional oral fluids to meet fluid losses (2,500–3,000 mL/day); the patient's fluid preferences are determined. The patient is instructed in the appropriate foods to add to the diet (high bulk) and those to avoid (bowel-irritating foods include caffeine, spices, milk products). If diarrhea continues, the need for associated fluid and electrolyte replacement is assessed. The perianal area is carefully cleansed after each stool and white petroleum jelly applied if irritation develops.

ALTERATIONS IN NUTRITION. Intake of less than bodily requirements occurs due to nausea, vomiting, anorexia, and mucositis resulting from side effects of IL-2 therapy.

EXPECTED OUTCOMES. Patient is able to maintain adequate fluid and food intake, weight remains stable, and intake and output are in balance and in adequate amounts.

INTERVENTIONS. The patient should be carefully assessed for indications of nutritional difficulties at each meal. Abdominal assessments should be performed along with the vital signs. Nausea and vomiting may be dealt with by improving the eating environment (removing odors, serving warm foods warm and cold foods cold, and preventing unpleasant sights). Decreasing the size of meals and providing six feedings a day may be helpful (American Cancer Society, 1974). Oral hygiene before meals may remove foul taste. Orally irritating foods (citrus, spices, and mouthwash with alcohol) should be decreased in patients with stomatitis or mucositis. Gargling with a teaspoon of bicarbonate in 8 ounces of water may reduce oral membrane inflammation. Antiemetics may be necessary. The patient is taught about the need to take in adequate amounts of fluids, and goals for fluid intake are set mutually. Parenteral nutrition may be required in severe cases.

POTENTIAL FOR INJURY. Hepatotoxicity may result from toxicity from IL-2.

EXPECTED OUTCOMES. Patients will be carefully assessed for abnormal liver function, and abnormalities will be rapidly identified and therapy initiated.

INTERVENTIONS. Liver function tests (lactic dehydrogenase, serum aspartate aminotransferase, serum alanine aminotransferase, and alkaline phosphatase) levels should be carefully monitored. The skin and sclera should be assessed for icterus. Urine should be assessed for darkening, and stools should be assessed for pasty, clay color. Abdominal assessments should include careful assessment of the position of the liver to note hepatomegaly. Patient complaints of abdominal fullness, nausea, and pain should be carefully evaluated as indicators of hepatomegaly. Abnormalities should be rapidly identified and reported to the physician, who will make the decision about discontinuing this agent.

POTENTIAL FOR INJURY. Anemia and thrombocytopenia may result from toxic reactions to IL-2.

EXPECTED OUTCOMES. Patient will verbalize understanding of the symptoms that should be reported and the precautions that need to be taken. Complete blood count results will be carefully monitored, and abnormal values will be rapidly reported to the physician.

INTERVENTIONS. Patients should be told to report dizziness and abnormal bleeding (epistaxis, bleeding gums, hemoptysis, hematemesis, melena, hematuria, or bleeding from wounds). Monitor laboratory values for hematocrit, hemoglobin, prothrombin time, partial thromboplastin time, fibrinogen, and fibrinogen degradation products (Bindon, 1983; Jassak & Sticklin, 1986). Patients should be discouraged from using safety razors. There is no evidence suggesting that these patients are at risk for disseminated intravascular coagulation (Jassak & Sticklin, 1986).

POTENTIAL IMPAIRED SKIN INTEGRITY. Skin integrity may be impaired due to toxicity of IL-2.

EXPECTED OUTCOMES. Patients verbalize an understanding of the potential skin reactions and the need to report any untoward findings immediately.

INTERVENTIONS. Instruct the patient to report potential skin reactions, including erythema, rash, pruritus, and desquamation. Assess the skin every 8 hours for problem areas. Application of medicated lotions may control most symptoms. Systemic antihistamines may be required for pruritus.

POTENTIAL ALTERATIONS IN TEMPERATURE. Temperature may be elevated due to the side effects of IL-2.

EXPECTED OUTCOMES. The patient's temperature will remain within normal limits or elevations will be rapidly identified and treated.

INTERVENTIONS. Chills and temperature elevations of up to 40.5°C have been reported (Jassak & Sticklin, 1986). The patient should be instructed to report chills or feelings of being too warm. Temperature should be monitored with vital signs every 4 hours. Careful assessments for concurrent infection should be made for each temperature elevation. Forcing fluids, tepid baths, and antipyretics may be necessary.

ALTERATIONS IN FAMILY PROCESSES. Families may be disturbed by having a family member hospitalized for a prolonged period of time.

EXPECTED OUTCOMES. The patient and family members demonstrate an appropriate stress response for the situation and do not demonstrate maladaptive behavior (excessive anger, displacement, inappropriate anxiety).

INTERVENTIONS. Assess the family for causative and contributing factors. Encourage the family to ventilate their feelings about the situation and acknowledge their feelings. Allow maximum family and patient interaction time. Involve the patient and family in the patient's care and in decision making and goal setting. Assist the family in assessing the situation. Aid them in identifying their strengths and previously successful coping mechanisms. Provide health teaching and referrals to a psychiatric nurse clinician if necessary.

POTENTIAL FOR INFECTION. Immunosuppression may increase the potential for respiratory tract infection.

EXPECTED OUTCOMES. Patient will not exhibit indications of respiratory tract infection (e.g., the patient remains afebrile, lungs clear to auscultation, and normal sputum color and amount). Patient will actively participate in pulmonary hygiene.

INTERVENTIONS. A protective environment should be effectively maintained. Patients should be instructed in the need to maintain careful oral and personal hygiene. Instruct the patient about the need to perform pulmonary hygiene exercises (coughing, deep breathing, use of incentive spirometry) every 2 hours. Instruct the patient to report chest discomfort, changes in the color or amount of sputum produced, shortness of breath, and the feeling that he or she may have a fever. Monitor vital signs every 4 hours. Auscultate breath sounds with the vital signs. Increase fluid intake to 2,500 to 3,000 mL/day to aid in liquifying secretions and aiding their mobilization.

BODY IMAGE DISTURBANCE. Changes in body image may occur due to weight loss and alopecia resulting from IL-2.

EXPECTED OUTCOMES. The patient will state his or her acceptance of changes and not demonstrate indicators of maladaptation (excessive anger, dwelling on physical appearance).

INTERVENTIONS. Discuss the changes that can be expected because of therapy (e.g., weight loss and alopecia). Encourage purchase of a wig before the onset of alopecia. When appropriate, encourage use of scarves, cosmetics, hats, or similar devices. Discuss the patient's feelings and allow adequate time for ventilation. If necessary, seek assistance from a psychiatric nurse clinician.

ADDITIONAL CONSIDERATIONS. IL-2 therapy is physically and emotionally taxing, and patients often consider stopping therapy before completing the regimen. It is uncertain whether the nature of the side effects, the compounding neurologic effects, or other factors influence this problem. Patient teaching, combined with empathy, coaching and prompt resolution of adverse effects, can help patients to continue the regimen and thus potentially improve their response rates. Self-care or family assistance in abrogating side effects may also enhance patients' commitment to therapy (Shelton, 1993).

SUMMARY

The treatment of cancer has become increasingly more successful and aggressive in recent years. Nurses are challenged to provide patients and their families intensive and holistic support. The care of immunosuppressed patients receiving bone marrow transplants and IL-2 therapy has been discussed. The nurse must be knowledgeable about these therapies and their effects on patients. Nurses must be prepared to intervene as needed to assist patients and families to complete the therapy successfully, both physically and emotionally.

REFERENCES

American Cancer Society. (1974). *Nutrition for patients receiving chemotherapy and radiation treatment.* Atlanta: Author.

Atkinson, K., & Meyers, J. D. (1980). Varicella-zoster virus infection after marrow transplantation for aplastic anemia or leukemia. *Transplantation, 29,* 47–50.

Armstrong, D. (1984). Protected environments are discomforting and expensive and do not offer meaningful protection. *American Journal of Medicine, 76,* 685–689.

Becker, T. M. (1981). *Cancer chemotherapy: A manual for nurses.* Boston: Little, Brown.

Bindon, C. M. (1983). Clearance rates and systemic effects of intravenously administered interleukin-2 containing preparations in human subjects. *British Journal of Cancer, 47,* 123–133.

Champlin, R. E., & Gale, R. P. (1984). Role of bone marrow transplantation in the treatment of hematologic malignancies and solid tumors: Critical review of syngeneic, autologous, and allogeneic transplants. *Cancer Treatment Reports, 68,* 145–161.

Cogliano-Shutta, N. A., & Broda, E. J. (1985). Bone marrow transplantation: An overview and comparison of autologous, syngeneic, and allogeneic treatment modalities. *Nursing Clinics of North America, 20,* 49–66.

Corbett, J. V. (1987). *Laboratory tests and diagnostic procedures with nursing diagnoses* (2nd ed.). Norwalk CT: Appleton & Lange.

Corcoran-Buchsel, P. (1986). Long-term complications of allogeneic bone marrow transplantation: Nursing implications. *Oncology Nursing Forum, 13*(6), 61–70.

Crane, L. R., Emmer, D. R., & Grguras, A. (1980). Prevention of infection on the oncology unit. *Nursing Clinics of North America, 15,* 843–856.

Daly, P. A. (1983). Supportive care for the patient with myelosuppression and immunosuppression. *Irish Medical Journal, 76,* 466–470.

Deisseroth, A. B., Abrams, R., & Holohan, T. (1982). Blood component replacement, applications of the continuous flow centrifuge, and bone marrow transplantation. In A. S. Levine (Ed.), *Cancer in the young.* New York: Masson.

DeVita, V. T. (1985). *Cancer: Principles and practice of oncology* (2nd ed.). Philadelphia: J. B. Lippincott.

Doney, K. C., & Weiden, P. L. (1981). Treatment of graft versus host disease in human allogeneic marrow graft recipients: A randomized trail comparing ATG and corticosteroids. *American Journal of Hematology, 11,* 1–18.

Dudjak, L. A. (1993). Rationale and therapeutic basis for patients receiving recombinant interleukin-2. *Seminars in Oncology Nursing, 9*(3, Suppl 1), 3–7.

Fisher, R. I. (1993). Introduction: Interleukin-2—Advances in clinical research and treatment. *Seminar in Oncology, 20*(6, Suppl 9), 1–2.

Foon, K. A., & Gale, R. P. (1982). Controversies in the therapy of acute myelogenous leukemia. *American Journal of Medicine, 72,* 963–978.

Gardner, G. G., & August, C. S. (1977). Psychological issues in bone marrow transplantation. *Pediatrics, 60,* 625–630.

Garner, J. S., & Simmons, B. P. (1983). Modification of isolation precautions. *Infection Control, 4,* 324–325.

Gianni, A. M., Bregni, M., Siena, S., et al. (1989). Rapid and complete hemopoietic reconstitution following combined transplantation of autologous blood and bone marrow cells: A changing role for high dose chemo-radiotherapy. *Hematological Oncology, 7,* 139–148.

Jassak, P. F., & Sticklin, L. A. (1986). Interleukin-2: An overview. *Oncology Nursing Forum, 13*(6), 17–22.

Klemm, P. (1985). Cyclosporin A: Use in preventing graft versus host disease. *Oncology Nursing Forum, 12*(5), 25–32.

Lotze, M. T. (1985). In vivo administration of purified human interleukin-2. *Journal of Immunology, 135,* 2685–2875.

Lucas, P. J., Quinones, R. R., Moses, R. D., et al. (1988). Alternative donor sources in HLA-mismatched marrow transplantation: T-cell depletion of surgically resected cadaveric marrow. *Bone Marrow Transplantation, 3,* 211–220.

McCarron, K. (1986). Fever—the cardinal vital sign. *Critical Care Quarterly, 2*(1), 15–18.

McGlave, P. B. (1985). The status of bone marrow transplantation for leukemia. *Hospital Practice, 20*(11), 97–110.

Nauta, E. H. (1979). Infection in the compromised host. In G. Dick (Ed.), *Immunological aspects of infectious disease.* Baltimore: University Park Press.

Oniboni, A. C. (1985). Understanding and preventing infection in the patient with cancer. *Oncology Nursing Forum, 12,* 56–64.

Reheis, C. E. (1985). Neutropenia: Causes, complications, treatment, and resulting nursing care. *Nursing Clinics of North America, 20,* 219–225.

Ristuccia, A. M. (1985). Hematologic effects of cancer chemotherapy. *Nursing Clinics of North America, 20,* 235–239.

Rosenberg, S. A. (1985). Special report observations on the systemic administration of autologous lymphokine–activated killer cells and recombinant interleukin-2 to patients with metastatic cancer. *New England Journal of Medicine, 313,* 1485–1492.

Ruccione, K., & Fergusson, J. (1984). Late effects of childhood cancer and its treatment. *Oncology Nursing Forum, 11*(5), 54–64.

Sanders, J. E., & Buckner, C. D. (1985). Growth and development following marrow transplantation for hematologic malignancy. *Blood, 66*(5, Suppl 1), 253a.

Shelton, B. K. (1993). Clinical pharmacological research with interleukin-2: Implications for nursing. *Seminars in Oncolony Nursing, 9*(3, Suppl 1), 8–13.

Singer, J. W. (1992). Role of colony-stimulating factors in bone marrow transplantation. *Seminars in Oncology, 19*(3, Suppl 7), 27–31.

Smith, S. L. (1986a). Immunosuppressive drugs used in clinical practice. *Critical Care Quarterly, 9*(1), 19–24.

Smith, S. L. (1986b). Physiology of the immune system. *Critical Care Quarterly, 9*(1), 7–13.

Stewart, F. M., & Thomas, R. M. (1985). Bone marrow transplantation: Three treatments for disease. *ACORN Journal, 42,* 196–205.

Viele, C. S., & Moran, T. A. (1993). Nursing management of the nonhospitalized patient receiving recombinant interleukin-2. *Seminars in Oncology Nursing, 9*(3, Suppl 1), 20–24.

Winston, D. J., Winston, G. H., & Gale, R. P. (1982). Therapeutic granulocyte transfusions for documented infections. *Annals of Internal Medicine, 97,* 509–515.

Witherspoon, R. P., & Storb, R. (1981). Recovery of antibody production in human allogeneic marrow graft recipients: Influence of time post-transplantation, the presence or absence of chronic graft-versus-host disease, and antithymocyte globulin treatment. *Blood, 58,* 360–368.

Patients With HIV Disease

Kathleen McMahon Casey

HISTORICAL DEVELOPMENT

In 1981 the established health community became aware of the illness that has since become known as acquired immunodeficiency syndrome (Centers for Disease Control and Prevention [CDC] 1981; Gottlieb et al., 1981). Young, primarily homosexual men who had been previously healthy and had not been treated with immunosuppressive therapies were seeking medical care for opportunistic infections and a malignancy, Kaposi's sarcoma (KS). This heralded the development of an epidemic. In the major metropolitan areas of the east and west coasts of the United States (primarily New York City, Los Angeles, and San Francisco) there were increasingly frequent reports of this new phenomenon, then called GRIDS (gay-related immunodeficiency syndrome), a name that reflected the major risk group and characteristic. Later, when it became clear that other groups were acquiring the disease through other means such as needle-sharing and sexual relations, the name was changed to acquired immunodeficiency syndrome (AIDS). Before the etiologic agent was discovered, it was becoming increasingly evident that an infectious agent was involved. At first, cytomegalovirus (CMV) was thought to be the causative agent, but questions remained about why the syndrome was a recent development. Transmission data cited blood contacts, sexual behaviors, and perinatal acquisition, which framed hepatitis B as a model for this new and still undiscovered agent. In addition, because transmission presumptively occurred between people not obviously ill, a prodromal period of illness or infectivity was probable.

It became clear that the illness was a clinical consequence of infection with a virus. Other co-factors such as recent trends in recreational drug use, use of nitrites as inhalants in sexual pleasure experience, a scientific experiment gone awry, other viral cofactors, and genocidal sabotage were suggested at the time as possible intervening variables. Table 58–1 summarizes the historical development of the illness in the United States.

EPIDEMIOLOGY

Since its clinical emergence, AIDS has claimed the lives of 220,736 adults and children in the United States (CDC, 1994). With 361,164 known cases diagnosed, another 1,000,000 Americans are estimated to be infected with human immunodeficiency virus (HIV). Worldwide, there are approximately 17 million cases of HIV infection, with 6,000 new people infected daily.

In terms of sheer numbers of cases, New York, Los Angeles, and San Francisco continue to be the hardest-hit areas. Data summarizing case rates and reported numbers of cases for the leading metropolitan areas are summarized in Table 58–2. Table 58–3 contrasts the situation in metropolitan and nonmetropolitan areas. The metropolitan areas with the highest numbers of AIDS cases in 1993 were New York, Los Angeles, San Francisco, Miami, Washington, DC, Philadelphia, Houston, Chicago, Boston, and Newark in rank order. But the rate of infection within the population of these metropolitan areas in 1993 demonstrates its impact. In rank order, they are San Francisco, Miami, New York, Jersey City, Newark, San Juan, Fort Lauderdale, Baltimore, Houston, and Los Angeles (CDC, 1994).

AIDS is a leading cause of death for men and women in their late twenties. The data on age and sex distribution of the cases are presented in Table 58–4. Men who have sex with men (MWHSWM) comprise the leading exposure category in adult AIDS cases (54%), with intravenous (IV) drug users (25%) second and MWHSWM who also use IV drugs (7%) third. In children's cases, the highest risk factor is a mother with or at risk for HIV (89%), followed by receipt of a blood transfusion or blood components or tissue (6%). Minorities are unequally represented compared with their representation in the population. Among children younger than 5 years of age, 369 of the 582 HIV cases are in black, non-Hispanics. Among women aged 25 to 29 years, 1,720 of the 2,793 HIV cases are in black women (CDC, 1994). Among young women, HIV was the leading cause of death in nine cities. Among young men, it was the leading cause of death in 64 cities (given a city population of 100,000 or more).

TABLE 58–1. **Historical Development of AIDS: The United States Experience**

1969	A mid-1980s retrospective analysis into the causes of death of a teenage boy in St. Louis, Missouri who died in 1969, shows Kaposi's sarcoma and HIV.
1976–1981	Few but significant changes appear in demographics of Kaposi's sarcoma in New York City cancer registry (i.e., never-married men, unusual sites of presentation of the illness, geographic clustering of cases in New York City's Greenwich Village).
1978–1981	Physicians, community leaders, and others in contact with vast social network of gay men begin to detect unusually high rate of nonspecific illness. Some public health officials are concerned about the rate of venereal disease and hepatitis.
1981	First AIDS-related publication: *Morbidity and Mortality Weekly Report* (CDC) reports clustering of PCP in homosexual men in Los Angeles. CDC forms task force to undertake surveillance and conduct epidemiologic and laboratory investigations. Makes formal request for all state health departments to report all biopsy-proven Kaposi's sarcoma cases in people less than 60 years old if not on immunosuppressive treatment *and* all cases of documented opportunistic infections in patients with no known underlying illness or history of immunosuppressive treatment. Total of 159 cases reported, with 5 to 6 additional cases being reported weekly.
1981–1983	Emergence of cases in other major metropolitan areas; other risk behaviors and groups identified; general acceptance of a prodromal illness and period of infectivity before outright AIDS.
1984	Discovery in France and the United States of a virus as the causative agent.
1985	Blood tests available for detection of HIV in the blood supply.
1986	Name HIV (human immunodeficiency virus) formally endorsed by International Committee on Taxonomy of Viruses (ICTV).
1987	Anti-HIV clinical trials programs started (AIDS Cooperative Trial Group).
1988	A few cases of HIV-2 reported in New Jersey (West African–born patient).
1991	122,905 U.S. deaths reported (cumulative) 191,601 U.S. cases reported (cumulative) 1,000,000 U.S. infected people (estimated) The approximately 44,000 new cases reported in 1991 reflect 25% of *all* cases reported in the previous decade.
1992	Latest definition of AIDS introduced
1993	220,736 U.S. deaths reported (cumulative) 361,164 U.S. cases reported (cumulative) 106,949 U.S. cases reported in 1993

Abbreviations: CDC, Centers for Disease Control and Prevention; PCP, *Pneumocystis carinii* pneumonia.

TABLE 58–2. **AIDS Case Rate per 100,000 Population, by Metropolitan Area With 500,000 Mass Population, Reported in 1992 and 1993; and Cumulative Totals, by Area and Age Group, Through December, 1993, United States**

City	1992 Cases	1993 Cases	1992 Rate	1993 Rate	Cumulative Adults/ Adolescents	Cumulative Children (<13 years of age)	Cumulative Totals
San Francisco	2,115	4,670	130.1	287.5	18,114	28	18,142
Miami	1,216	3,514	60.6	172.9	10,636	283	10,919
New York	7,190	14,716	84.1	171.8	57,556	1,259	58,815
Jersey City, NJ	296	735	53.3	132.0	3,145	72	3,217
Newark, NJ	805	2,109	41.8	109.3	8,027	203	8,230
San Juan, PR	1,045	1,960	55.7	103.4	7,087	188	7,275
Ft. Lauderdale	849	1,274	65.2	96.7	5,405	110	5,515
Baltimore	767	1,780	31.5	72.7	4,907	127	5,034
Houston	1,016	2,569	28.8	70.7	9,451	88	9,539
Los Angeles	3,268	6,040	36.11	66.6	22,652	146	22,798
Washington, DC	1,393	2,788	31.9	63.0	10,023	145	10,168
Atlanta	938	1,912	29.81	59.1	7,224	43	7,267
Philadephia	995	2,656	20.1	53.6	7,860	110	7,970
Boston	735	2,426	13.0	42.6	6,943	123	7,066
Chicago	1,667	2,497	22.0	32.7	9,589	127	9,716

From Centers for Disease Control and Prevention. (1994). *HIV/AIDS Surveillance Report, 5*(4), 6–7.

TABLE 58–3. **Metropolitan Areas by Total Area, by Central Counties, and by Outlying Counties and Nonmetropolitan Areas (by Years, Number of Cases, Case Rates, and Age), 1992–1993, United States**

	1992 Cases	1993 Cases	1992 Rate	1993 Rate	Cumulative Adults/ Adolescents	Cumulative Children (<13 years of age)	Cumulative Totals
Metropolitan areas with 500,000 or more population	39,876	89,407	24.9	55.3	302,570	4,428	306,998
Central counties	39,181	87,742	26.7	59.3	297,407	4,343	301,750
Outlying counties	745	1,665	5.6	12.1	5,163	85	5,248
Metropolitan areas with 50,000 to 500,000 population	4,840	11,128	10.4	23.7	33,758	501	34,259
Central counties	4,583	10,517	11.1	25.0	31,727	458	32,185
Outlying counties	257	611	5.1	11.9	2,031	43	2,074
Nonmetropolitan areas	2,647	5,809	5.0	10.9	18,028	280	18,308
Totals	47,572	106,949	18.4	140.8	355,936	5,228	361,164

From Centers for Disease Control and Prevention. (1994). *HIV/AIDS Surveillance Report, 5*(4), 7.

TABLE 58–4. **AIDS Cases by Sex and Age at Diagnosis, Reported Through December 1993, United States**

	Total*	
Age at Diagnosis (Years)	***No.***	***(%)***
Male		
Under 5	2,142	(1)
5–12	605	(0)
13–19	1,070	(0)
20–24	10,947	(3)
25–29	46,530	(15)
30–34	73,349	(23)
35–39	70,439	(22)
40–44	49,378	(16)
45–49	27,743	(9)
50–54	14,926	(5)
55–59	8,534	(3)
60–64	4,791	(2)
65 or older	3,870	(1)
Male subtotal	314,325	(100)
Female		
Under 5	2,079	(4)
5–12	402	(1)
13–19	484	(1)
20–24	2,943	(6)
25–29	8,063	(17)
30–34	11,208	(24)
35–39	9,490	(20)
40–44	5,493	(12)
45–49	2,536	(5)
50–54	1,454	(3)
55–59	979	(2)
60–64	655	(1)
65 or older	1,051	(2)
Female subtotal	46,838	(100)
Total†	**361,164**	

*Includes 545 males, 86 females, and 1 person of unknown sex whose race/ethnicity is unknown.

†Includes 1 male and 1 female whose age at diagnosis is unknown, and 1 person whose sex is unknown.

From Centers for Disease Control and Prevention. (1994). *HIV/AIDS Surveillance Report, 5*(4), 14.

It is estimated that 60,000 to 70,000 children in New York City will lose at least one parent to AIDS. The high minority representation reflects the impact of culture, economics, power, and health care systems.

INTERNATIONAL STATISTICS

The World Health Organization (WHO) reports 985,119 AIDS cases worldwide, with sub-Saharan Africa and Brazil affected the most (personal communication WHO hotline, Dec., 1994). WHO also estimates the number of HIV infections as 15 million worldwide. Frequent underreporting due to discrimination, scarcity of medical care, lack of public health resources, and other social causes is rampant.

It is postulated that HIV-1 first emerged in central Africa as a new disease, originating from a recent simian-to-human retrovirus transmission (Kanski et al., 1985). The virus was probably transported to the western hemisphere in the 1970s and began infecting Americans around 1978 (Osborn, 1986). HIV-2 is believed to be endemic in West Africa. Several well documented cases of HIV-2 infection have been reported in Europeans and among West Africans residing abroad. By 1991, there were only 18 reported cases of HIV-2 in the United States, and all were associated with immigration from, or travel to, West Africa (O'Brien et al., 1991). Both HIV-1 and HIV-2 are considered to be the causes of AIDS. Differences in the global spread is attributed to differences in transmissibility and duration of infectiousness (De Cock et al., 1993).

Many countries owe acquisition of HIV infection in their population to contact with American blood products that were exported before the 1985 HIV screening procedures, or to sexual transmission (Osborn, 1986).

Worldwide epidemiologic studies indicate that there are three broad but distinct geographic patterns of AIDS transmission. In pattern I, typical of industrialized countries with large numbers of reported cases, most cases occur among homosexual or bisexual men and among urban IV drug users. Only a small percentage of cases is attributed to heterosexual transmission, but this percentage is increasing. Transmission due to exposure to HIV-contaminated blood or blood products occurred between the late 1970s and 1985, but this has since been largely controlled through routine blood screening procedures. The ratio of male-to-female patients ranges from 10:1 to 15:1, and perinatal transmission is relatively rare. The overall population seroprevalence is less than 1%, but this is significantly higher (up to 50% higher) in high-risk behavior groups such as IV drug users and men with multiple male sex partners (CDC, 1988a).

Pattern II is seen in areas of central, eastern, and southern Africa and in some Caribbean countries. Most cases occur among heterosexuals, and the male-to-female ratio is approximately 1:1. Perinatal transmission is relatively more common than in other areas. Transmission through IV drug use and homosexual transmission either does not occur or occurs at a very low rate. The overall population seroprevalence is estimated to be over 1%, and in a few urban areas up to 25% of all sexually active people are infected. Transmission through contaminated blood and blood products remains a significant problem (CDC, 1988a).

Pattern III occurs in areas of eastern Europe, the Middle East, Asia, and most of the Pacific basin. It appears that HIV has been introduced to these areas only since the mid-1980s, and only small numbers of cases have been reported. Generally, cases have occurred among those who have traveled to endemic areas or who have had sexual contact with individuals from endemic areas, such as homosexual men and prostitutes. Only a small number of cases has been reported due to receipt of imported HIV-contaminated blood (CDC, 1988a). The exception to pattern III in eastern Europe is the large-scale nosocomial transmission of HIV in Rumania associated with lack of needle and syringe sterilizations and blood and blood product screening prior to transfusion (Beldescu et al., 1990). This transmission rate is elevated due to the common national medical practice of microtransfusion for newborns. Other developing countries also have a substantial risk of disease transmission owing to the lack of testing and sterilization capabilities and to cultural attitudes toward needles in disease treatment.

HUMAN IMMUNODEFICIENCY VIRUS

Immunopathogenesis

It has become evident that AIDS is the most severe form of a spectrum of clinical consequences resulting from the immunologic reaction to HIV infection. A working knowledge of the virus's life cycle, characteristics, and immune system response assists the clinician in preparing interventions.

HIV-1, discovered in 1983, is a retrovirus belonging to the lentivirus family of viruses. They are generally known to result in neurotropic and lymphotropic viremic disease as a result of an indolent infection process characterized by a long clinical latency period (Libman, 1993). HIV-1 is one of five retroviruses, along with HIV-2 and human T-lymphotropic viruses I, II, and III, associated with human disease. Retroviruses are found in nearly all animal species. Infection can occur through sexual activities, through exposure to blood, and perinatally.

HIV-1 Structure and Genetic Composition

HIV is a piece of RNA surrounded by a lipid envelope that measures slightly over 100 mm in diameter. Electron microscopy reveals a characteristic dense cylindrical nucleoid containing core proteins, genomic RNA, and an enzyme, reverse transcriptase (RT), that classifies it as a retrovirus (Ho et al., 1987). HIV selectively infects the T4 (or CD4+) cell (Bowen et al., 1985; Gallo, 1987; Lawrence, 1985; Margolick et al., 1987; Urba & Longo, 1985), but infects other cell types as well, which may also possess the CD4 receptor molecule. These cell types include monocytes–macrophages, transformed B cells, dendritic cells, microglial cells, endothelial cells, astrocytes and oligodendrocytes, transformed colon cells, neurons, and CD8+ and CD4− cells (Koenig & Fauci, 1988). Very little cell-free virus is found in HIV-infected persons (Ho et al., 1987).

These structural components make up the viral genome and code for essential protein components. These genes are found on the terminal repeat sequences. These genes are called *pol, gag,* and *env.* The second, *gag,* codes for p24, which is also found in the viral core and surrounds the viral RNA. Currently, p24 is measurable in patients' serum, and this test serves as a marker for viral replication (Libman, 1993).

Mechanism of Infection

HIV enters the host and then attaches to a particular surface molecule receptor on the T4 cell membrane (McDougal et al., 1986). T4 cell glycoprotein is essential for HIV binding, but additional factors may be required for penetration (Isobe et al., 1986). One infected T lymphocyte may bind to other CD4+ cells, forming a syncytium with up to 50 cells (Nash & Said, 1992). HIV enters the cell and becomes uncoated. As a retrovirus, HIV has the ability to reverse the usual flow of genetic information with the enzyme RT, using viral RNA as a template for making DNA. Viral RNA is then transcribed into DNA by RT, is circularized, and then becomes integrated into the host T4 genome (Ho et al., 1987). The HIV replication cycle is restricted at this stage until the infected cell is "activated." In vitro, activation takes place through mitogenic, antigenic, or allogenic stimulation. In vivo, potential activators include other pathogens (i.e., hepatitis B virus, CMV, herpes virus) and allogenic exposure to semen, blood, or allografts (Ho et al., 1987). On activation, transcription occurs, and then protein synthesis. Viral proteins, and genomic RNA are then assembled at the cell surface, and mature virions are formed by budding. With HIV replication, the T4 cell is killed (Ho et al., 1987). Other cells that become infected survive. Macrophages and monocytes continue and carry virus in their travels through the lymphoid and blood systems.

Immunologic Abnormalities

HIV has been found in only a few types of cells in infected people. The cell population most profoundly affected is the helper subset of T lymphocytes that express the cell surface (leu 3/T4) molecule. In vitro studies allow the detection of HIV genes in infected cells in tissues of HIV-infected patients at a rate of 1 in 10,000 to 1 in 1,000,000 lymphocytes. Both acute and chronic effects are demonstrated after successful HIV infection (Lane & Fauci, 1985). The most devastating effect, however, is the gradual, progressive depletion of the helper T lymphocytes, which leads to irreversible immunodeficiency.

T-CELL ABNORMALITIES

HIV eventually destroys human T4 lymphocytes, reducing their overall number and function (Bowen et al., 1985; Lane & Fauci, 1985; Lawrence, 1985; Margolick et al., 1987; Seligmann et al., 1987). In vitro, a major mechanism of T-cell death involves cell–cell fusion and the formation of multinucleated giant cells, which die within 24 to 48 hours.

Immunologically normal people have 600 to 1,200 T4 cells/mm^3, whereas people with HIV infection may have only 0 to 500. Decreased T4 cell counts are associated with an increase in clinical problems, especially infection (Lane & Fauci, 1987). The cytotoxic T-cell subpopulation is responsible for attaching virally infected and malignant cell populations and removing them from the body. The overall lymphocyte count is low, and the T4/T8 cell ratio is also decreased (Bowen et al., 1985; Lane & Fauci, 1985; Lawrence, 1985; Margolick, 1987).

Besides having fewer T4 cells, a person with AIDS has absent or depressed T4 cell function. In AIDS there is (1) decreased ability to release lymphokines, (2) decreased cytotoxicity, (3) decreased T-cell to B-cell mediation necessary for antibody production, (4) decreased ability of T cells to proliferate in mixed lymphocyte cultures, and (5) lack of antigen-induced T-cell function (Bowen et al., 1985; Lane & Fauci, 1985; Margolick, 1987).

CD4+ helper T lymphocytes are the regulating cells within the immune system. These cells interact with monocytes, macrophages, cytotoxic T cells, natural killer cells, and B cells (Casey, 1995). Interactions between cells during HIV-1 infection can result in laboratory abnormalities. These abnormalities are summarized in Table 58–5.

TABLE 58–5. **Laboratory Abnormalities in Immune System Testing Related to HIV-1 Infection**

1. Normal or decreased white blood cell count
2. Decreasing lymphocyte values
3. Dramatic changes in CD4+/CD8+ ratio
4. Decreased CD4+ function tests
5. Absent or impaired skin test reactivity (anergy)
6. Increased immunoglobulin levels

From Grady, C., & Vogel, S. (1993). Laboratory methods for diagnosing and monitoring HIV infections. *JANAC, 4*(2), 11–21.

B-CELL ABNORMALITIES

B-cell abnormalities in AIDS patients are due perhaps to the aforementioned T-cell abnormalities; to direct B-cell activation by HIV, CMV, or another virus; or possibly to excessive secretion of B-cell–stimulating lymphokines (Bowen et al., 1985; Lane & Fauci, 1985; Margolick et al., 1987). B cells in patients with AIDS are polyclonal activated, resulting in oversecretion of IgG, IgA, and IgM (hypergammaglobulinemia) and increased levels of circulating immune complexes and autoantibodies (Lane & Fauci, 1985). B cells, however, will not mount an antibody in response to a new antigen. Therefore, a patient with AIDS will not respond to immunization with appropriate antibody production (Lane & Fauci, 1985), and most patients should not be vaccinated with a live virus vaccine (Amman, 1984). An exception is made, however, for HIV-infected children, who are vaccinated for measles, mumps, and rubella (MMR). After reports of severe measles in symptomatic HIV-infected children, and no report of serious or unusual adverse effects of MMR vaccination, the Immunization Practices Advisory Committee recommended MMR vaccination for all HIV-infected children (CDC, 1988b).

MONOCYTE AND MACROPHAGE ABNORMALITIES

Monocyte–macrophage abnormalities may be due to a lack of gamma-interferon and other monocyte-stimulating lymphokines from the T cell as well as to direct infection of monocytes–macrophages with HIV. Frequent infections may result from these monocyte–macrophage abnormalities (Bowen et al., 1985; Margolick et al., 1987). Enhanced release of monokines, such as interleukin-2 (IL-2), tumor necrosis factor, and cachectin may explain the chronic fevers and wasting associated with AIDS. Involvement of alveolar macrophages may explain the high incidence of pulmonary infections in AIDS (Nash & Said, 1992).

In addition, monocytes and macrophages serve as important reservoirs for the persistence of HIV in the host. They are the vehicles that transport HIV across the blood–brain barrier and into the central nervous system (Ho et al., 1987; Libman, 1993).

LYMPHOID ORGANS

There is greater viral activity than had been previously appreciated in the lymphoid tissue during the clini-

TABLE 58–6. **Risks and Benefits of HIV Testing**

Risks	Benefits
Relationship problems	Protection of blood supply
Blaming	Protection of organ recipients
Sexual dysfunction	Support for medical diagnosis
Disrupted ability to make plans as a couple	Avoiding medical mismanagement of asymptomatic patients
Employment problems	Examination of cerebrospinal fluid in asymptomatic persons with syphilis infection of more than 1 year's duration
Insurance problems	Interpretation of a purified protein derivative test as positive if it shows at least 5 cm of induration (and stated prophylaxis with longer duration of treatment)
Spiritual distress	Administration of influenza and pneumovax vaccines and use of inactivated oral polio vaccine
Stigmatization, discrimination	Help women decide about pregnancy, giving birth, and breast-feeding
Self-imposed social withdrawal	Access to clinical trials
Preoccupation with bodily symptoms, fear	Identification of contacts
Desire for revenge, homicidal thoughts	Close medical follow-up; treatment and prophylaxis information on which to make life plans
Psychological impairment	
Anxiety	
Nightmares	
Depression	
Suicidal ideology	

Adapted from McMahon, K. M. (1988). The integration of HIV testing and counseling into nursing practice. *Nursing Clinics of North America, 23,* 814.

cally latent period. Once virus is introduced into the body, it is swiftly disseminated via the bloodstream. The lymphoid organs become heavily seeded with virus (Pantaleo et al., 1993). Although the lymphoid tissue exerts control and contains infection, this protective system wanes over time and the lymphoid microenvironment is destroyed. Replication of the virus has continued within the lymph system, and virus eventually spills out into the bloodstream.

Newer Concepts of Pathogenesis

It has been identified that various HIV strains can be described as either rapid or slow, high or low, or syncytium-inducing or non–syncytium-inducing. This distinction is important because these biologic features can determine tissue tropism (whether the virus goes to the bowel or brain) and the inherent ability to destroy the immune system (Casey, 1995). In addition, Levy (1993) has provided data that suggest that a relatively noncytopathic strain compromises the function of CD4+ cells, producing a gradual, persistent loss of these cells in time by means other than direct cell killing.

Testing for HIV

Testing for HIV is useful for personal health maintenance and for early medical intervention and public health considerations. Table 58–6 shows the risks and benefits of testing. Very serious issues of confidentiality, occupational and public safety, civil liberties and rights, and ethics are involved. Background information on the purposes, possible outcomes, and types of testing are central to handling HIV testing issues well.

The risk that testing may impede a person's ability to function emotionally and socially is one of the components of counseling required during the pretest session. Others include information on the tests, the clinical significance of positive results, potential difficulties (legal, insurance, relational, health care), and review of the benefits. Informed consent is required in most situations, with laws governing practice in some states. Table 58–7 lists the components of the counseling sessions.

HIV ANTIBODY TESTING

Testing serum for antibodies to HIV is currently the most cost-effective and accurate method of screening

TABLE 58–7. **Essential Components of HIV Counseling and Testing Sessions**

Pretest Sessions
Review of meaning and significance of test, positive or negative results; time frames; testing procedures
Identification of client's motive for testing
Elaboration of risk-reduction behaviors; availability of education and supportive counseling
Description of confidentiality and limits
Discussion of possible psychological, emotional, social, legal, spiritual, and medical consequences and benefits
Exploration of coping strengths and support; availability of anonymous test sites
Informed consent
Posttest Sessions
Interpretation of results
Recommendations for medical follow-up
Referral for education and counseling services, such as drug rehabilitation, early intervention program, support group, partner notification program, mental health professional, or clinical trial
Education about transmission and partner or contact notification
Discussion of discrimination, social and psychological crisis needs
Review of immediate posttest counseling session plans for safety and confidentiality
Appointment for medical care

Adapted from McMahon, K. M. (1988). The integration of HIV testing and counseling into nursing practice. *Nursing Clinics of North America, 23,* 814–815.

TABLE 58–8. **HIV-1 Tests**

I. Virus culture techniques
   A. Peripheral blood mononuclear cells coculture for HIV-1
   B. Quantitative cell counts
   C. Quantitative plasma culture
II. HIV antibody tests
   A. Enzyme-linked immunosorbent assay (ELISA)
   B. Western blot
   C. Radioimmunoprecipitation assay (RIPA)
   D. Indirect immunofluorescence assay (IFA)
III. Antigen detection assays
   A. HIV p24 antigen test
   B. Acidified p24 antigen procedure
   C. Polyethylene glycol precipitation
IV. Viral genome amplification tests
   A. Polymerase chain reaction (PCR) techniques
   B. Quantitative PCR

Data from Sang, M. S. (1992). AIDS testing: Now and in the future. In M. A. Sande & P. A. Volberding (Eds.), *The Medical Management of AIDS* (3rd ed., pp. 33–53). Philadelphia: W. B. Saunders.

for infection. Table 58–8 summarizes HIV-1 tests. Since March, 1985, when the first serologic assay became available, many more methods have become commercially available. Others are primarily research tools without clear commercial uses. Enzyme-linked immunosorbent assay (ELISA) and Western blot confirmation continue to be the testing methods most widely used worldwide. A venipuncture specimen of 5 to 7 mL of sterile, whole clotted blood is sufficient for performing repeated tests as well as any needed supplemental tests. Specimens should be refrigerated but can be transported at ambient temperatures. They can be frozen. At-home test kits may be commercially available soon.

ELISA. There are many licensed manufacturers of ELISA tests for antibody to HIV. All have been shown to have a sensitivity and specificity of 98% to 100% (Wilber, 1994). These assays, however, do not detect HIV antibody in the earliest stages of infection. The time interval between HIV infection and appearance of antibody in the blood varies, but is usually less than 6 months. There is also a period late in the course of AIDS when antibody may not be detected because it forms complexes with excess HIV antigen in the patient's serum (Wilber, 1994). ELISA has become a useful screening tool for blood donors and populations at risk for AIDS and helps in diagnosing cases in which AIDS is suspected. When a person is adequately exposed to HIV, an antibody is made that is usually detectable by ELISA within 3 months of exposure. A positive result does not, however, mean that the person has AIDS. It is estimated that approximately 54% of all people who test positive for HIV antibody will develop AIDS within 10 years (Pedersen et al., 1989). The test is widely available through private physicians, health departments, clinics, and other health care providers.

WESTERN BLOT ANALYSIS. Westen blot analysis detects various antibodies made in response to HIV proteins of particular molecular weights. Most HIV antibody-positive sera react with many bands, and the interpretation is not difficult. However, both very early and very late in HIV infection, the patient may not have detectable antibody to some of the viral antigens. It is therefore important to know which reactive bands make a Western blot positive. An indeterminate pattern may represent a nonspecific reaction or a stage in the progression of HIV disease. Repeated testing in 2 weeks is then warranted (Wilber, 1994). A person who tests positive on both ELISA and Western blot analysis is believed to be infected and is considered infectious.

HIV-1/HIV-2 COMBINATION TESTING. In 1992, the Food and Drug Administration (FDA) recommended that blood banks screen for HIV-1 and HIV-2. HIV-2 licensed tests include an ELISA for HIV-2 alone and HIV-1/HIV-2 combination tests. There are also research tests available that have not yet received FDA approval (Wilber, 1994).

HIV Antigen Testing

Commercial tests are available to detect HIV p24 antigen in the serum, plasma, and cerebrospinal fluid of infected individuals as well as in the supernatant media of viral cultures. These assays also have clinical application in evaluating the virologic efficacy of antiretroviral therapy. Tests for p24 antigen can be helpful in diagnosing newborns. Commercial HIV antigen assays are solid-phase antigen capture enzyme immunoassays. A color density identifies p24. The quantity of p24 antigen in the test serum is determined by plotting the value against the reference curve.

HIV Isolation and Quantitation Methods

To define better the virologic aspects of the pathogenesis of HIV disease and to provide objective criteria for the assessment of the efficacy of antiviral therapeutics, much research is focused on developing quantitative assays to gauge better the magnitude of infection and the extent of active viral replication in HIV-infected individuals (Wilber, 1994). A few of these methods are described.

POLYMERASE CHAIN REACTION

By means of a selective DNA amplification technique called the polymerase chain reaction (PCR), HIV proviral sequences can be identified directly in DNA isolated from peripheral blood mononuclear cells of seropositive people (Ou et al., 1988). A single viral DNA molecule can be detected among a million white blood cells. Results are usually available within 3 days. Potential uses of PCR technology include HIV detection in research settings, for early diagnosis, or as a prognostic indicator (Cohen et al., 1990). It has been difficult to quantify accurately the absolute amount of the pathogen in a clincal specimen. Only recently has reproducible and truly quantifiable data on the amount of HIV DNA or RNA been demonstrated (Elbeik & Feinberg, 1994).

QUANTITATIVE COMPETITIVE POLYMERASE CHAIN REACTION

The quantitative competitive (QC) PCR method is of sufficient sensitivity to detect HIV RNA in the plasma of all infected people. Higher levels of HIV RNA correlate with the more advanced clinical stages of disease and lower $CD4^+$ T-cell counts, which is a very important benefit. Currently, the test is expensive and difficult to perform, making it unsuitable for widespread clinical use (Elbeik & Feinberg, 1994).

BRANCHED DNA ASSAY

The branched DNA strategy to measure the amount of HIV RNA in plasma of infected patients has been developed only recently. It involves the use of highly sensitive (so-called branched DNA) probes to detect and quantify RNA sequences. Although it is less sensitive than the QC-PCR assay, it is faster, less expensive, and easier to perform. It may be found to be useful in routine clinical monitoring if its measurements are validated (Elbeik & Feinberg, 1994).

HIV Isolation and Culture Isolation

The first isolate of HIV was derived from in vitro cultures made from a person with lymphadenopathy syndrome. Since then, HIV has been isolated from a wide variety of sources. It has been frequently obtained from human peripheral blood lymphocytes obtained from HIV-seropositive individuals. Rarely, it has been isolated from seronegative individuals with a history of HIV exposure (Mayer et al., 1986). HIV has also been isolated from lymph nodes, serum, brain, saliva, semen, breast milk, urine, tears, cerebrospinal fluid, cervical secretions, pericardial and pleural fluids, and blood (McMahon & Sutterer, 1988).

Cultivation

HIV can be isolated through in vitro cultivation of suspected infected T lymphocytes with the T-cell growth factor, IL-2. Fluid suspected of containing free HIV can be added to cultures of normal T lymphocytes, which will replicate to provide progeny virus. A high ELISA antibody test result correlates best with viral culture isolation. Most results are available in 3 weeks; however, certain body fluids, including tears and cervical secretions, have cultured viruses at 60 days (Wofsky et al., 1986). Cultures cannot be used to quantify the extent of HIV infection because lymph nodes and other structures harbor HIV, reflecting the true status of the disease not present in peripheral blood lymphocytes. Because of cost, laboratory skill, quality assurance, and time factors, viral isolation is not used to analyze large numbers of samples for general clinical use (Cohen et al., 1990; Elbeik & Feinberg, 1994).

Sexual Transmission of HIV

HIV has been isolated from blood, seminal fluid, preejaculate, vaginal secretions, urine, cerebrospinal fluid, saliva, tears, and breast milk of infected individuals. Whether HIV infects spermatozoa is controversial. Recent reports of the removal of infected cells from semen, allowing artificial insemination without seroconversion, supports the idea that spermatozoa are not infected. No cases of HIV infection have been traced to saliva or tears. Virus is found in greater concentration in semen than in vaginal fluids, leading to a hypothesis that male-to-female transmission could occur more easily than female-to-male. Sexual behavior that involves exposure to blood is likely to increase transmission risks. Transmission could also occur through contact with infected bowel epithelial cells in anal intercourse, in addition to access to the bloodstream through breaks in the rectal mucosa. Although all HIV-seropositive people are potentially infectious, there is widespread variation in the seropositivity and seroconversion of their sexual partners. Factors that could explain this variability include differences in sexual practices and numbers of sexual contacts, susceptibility of the partner, differences in viral strains, changing degrees of infectiousness of the HIV-infected person over time, cofactors that enhance or limit transmission, genetic resistance, or a combination of these factors (Osmond & Padian, 1994). Sexually transmitted diseases play a significant role in transmission of HIV in Africa. Azidothymidine (zidovudine; AZT) may play a small role in preventing transmission. Posing the highest risk of infection is anal receptive intercourse, followed by vaginal intercourse. Table 58–9 reviews sexual behaviors with categories of risk.

Risk is reduced through use of the latex condom. For the wearer, condoms provide a mechanical barrier limiting penile exposure to infectious cervical, vaginal, vulvar, or rectal secretions or lesions. For the wearer's partner, proper condom use should prevent semen deposition, contact with urethral discharge, and exposure to lesions on the head or shaft of the penis. Oil-based lubricants may make condoms ineffective, so should not be used. Water-soluble lubricants are considered safe. Natural membrane condoms (made from lamb cecum) contain small pores and do not block HIV passage in laboratory studies (CDC, 1998c). A meta-analysis of several studies of HIV transmission found that condom efficacy was 69% overall (Weller, 1993). Condom failure is greatly reduced by proper use.

Abstinence from sexual intercourse is the sole safe way to prevent transmission. Over a period of time, precautions tend to fail due to breakage of condoms or failure to maintain precautions. Sexual activity in a

TABLE 58–9. **Sexual Practice: Risk Categories for HIV Transmission**

Safe	Moderate to Low	High Risk
Fantasy	French kissing	Unprotected anal receptive intercourse
Hugging	Cunnilingus	Unprotected vaginal intercourse
Massage	Fellatio with ingestion	Unprotected anal insertive intercourse
Social kissing	Fisting (manual-anal intercourse)	Blood contact during sex
Mutual masturbation	Intercourse using a latex condom	
Nonshared sex toys		

mutually monogamous relationship in which neither partner is HIV-infected and no other risk factors are present is considered safe.

Blood Products

It has been estimated that an HIV-infected drop of human blood contains 1 to 100 live virus particles. In comparison, a drop infected with hepatitis B virus has 100 million to 1 billion organisms (Favero, 1987). Even so, blood transmission of HIV does occur, primarily through sharing of contaminated needles among IV drug users and through blood transfusion. Transmission of HIV-1 has occurred after transfusion of the following components: whole blood, packed red blood cells (including washed and buffy coat poor), fresh frozen plasma, cryoprecipitate, platelets, and plasma-derived products, depending on the production process. With the implementation in March 1985 of a donor screening program of the nation's blood supply, blood transfusion is now even safer; the current risk of transmission of AIDS through this route is estimated to be 1 in 225,000. A somewhat higher estimate of 1 in 40,000 to 1 in 60,000 is reported from areas that have a high prevalence of HIV-1 infection. It is possible that before blood screening implementation, more than 12,000 people were infected. A large percentage of hemophiliacs acquired HIV in this manner. Donor screening, HIV testing, and heat treatment of clotting factor have greatly reduced the risks. To decrease further the possibility of HIV transmission through transfusion of blood and blood products, patients scheduled to undergo elective surgery are increasingly advised to make predeposited blood donations for intraoperative autotransfusion.

Current screening tests cannot detect either recently HIV-1–infected people who have not yet developed antibody (the "window period") or HIV antibody-negative patients who have AIDS. Donating procedures include an interview for risk factors and the ability of the potential donor to exclude their blood from being used. Although no transfusion-related cases of HIV-2 infection have been reported in the United States, as of June 1, 1992, all U.S. blood centers test donations for antibodies to both HIV-1 and HIV-2.

Clinicians should recommend HIV-1 antibody testing for all people transfused between January 1978 and March 1985.

Needlesticks and Splashes

Transmission due to occupational exposure of health care workers has occurred in needlestick accidents and blood splashes to the oral mucosa (McMahon & Sutterer, 1988). Needlestick is the most common route. Thousands of health care workers who were so exposed have been studied, and only 32 cases of well documented infection have been reported in the United States. The risk of infection through this route is estimated to be 0.02%, and every effort should be made to decrease the exposure rate. Educational efforts, implementation of engineering controls in needled and sharp-edged medical devices, the use of hard plastic needle disposal units where these devices are most frequently used, and the development of procedural details to avoid blood and body fluid contact would greatly reduce the exposure rate (Jagger et al., 1990). Health care workers must apply universal precautions to all activities to avoid contact with potentially HIV-infected human fluids. Safer medical equipment, particularly needled and sharp-edged devices, must be designed.

Needle-Sharing

Transmission of HIV among IV drug users occurs primarily through contamination of injection paraphernalia with infected blood. Behaviors such as needle-sharing, "booting" the injection with blood, using a shooting gallery, and performing frequent injections increase the risk. Cocaine use (by injection or smoking) is associated with a higher prevelance of HIV infection. This may in part be attributed to the exchange of crack for sex. Sharing of equipment is common due to legal and financial restrictions and cultural norms. Geographically, the rate of infection varies: 80% of New York City addict needle-sharers are infected, as opposed to much lower rates in other metropolitan area clusters. Secondary transmission occurs to women, children, and sexual partners.

Preventative strategies include drug treatment, onsite medical care in a drug treatment program, recruitment of "street" outreach workers for intensive drug and sex "risk reduction" educational campaigns, teaching addicts to sterilize their equipment between use, the free provision or exchange of sterile injection equipment (as allowed by law), distribution of condoms and bleach to clean drug use equipment, or a combination of these interventions.

Maternofetal Transmission

HIV is transmitted to infants by transplacental spread from mother to fetus in utero, during parturition, or through breast feeding after birth (Ziegler et al., 1985). Because infants have underdeveloped natural resistance systems, they are highly susceptible to many infections, including HIV. In vivo transmission is the most common route. Studies of infected mothers reflect a 0% to 65% rate of transmission with a mean about 30%. Both uninfected and infected infants have been born to mothers who have previously borne an infected infant. Recent studies have dramatically demonstrated the beneficial effect of treating pregnant women and newborns with AZT to prevent transmission to the child.

Organ Transplantation

Because these procedures are much less common than other transmission-related activities, there have been very few case reports of HIV acquisition by this route. HIV has been transmitted via the kidneys, liver, heart, pancreas, bone, and, possibly, skin grafts and through artificial insemination (Osborn, 1986). HIV testing is used in these circumstances to rule out infection (CDC, 1988d). Most cases of transmission through transplants of organs, bone, or tissue occurred before HIV screening was available. As with blood transfusions, donors testing antibody seronegative may pass HIV infection on to recipients.

CLASSIFICATION OF HIV INFECTION

The system of classification of HIV infection, developed by the CDC for public health purposes, divides manifestations of the disease into four mutually exclusive groups. The groups are not intended to have prognostic significance, nor do they indicate severity. They are hierarchical, however, in that people classified in one group have met the criteria for the preceding group. Refer to Table 58–10 for the 1993 revised classification system by the CDC.

TABLE 58–10. **1993 Revised Classification System for HIV Infection and Expanded AIDS Surveillance Case Definition for Adolescents and Adults**

	Clinical Categories		
CD4$^+$ T-Cell Categories	*(A) Asymptomatic, Acute (Primary) HIV or PGL*	*(B) Symptomatic, not (A) or (C) Conditions*	*(C) AIDS-Indicator Conditions*
1. ≥500 mm^3	A1	B1	C1
2. 200–499 mm^3	A2	B2	C2
3. <200 mm^3 AIDS-indicator T-cell count	A3	B3	C3

From Casey, K. M. (1995). Pathophysiology of HIV-1, clinical course, and treatment. In J. H. Flaskerud & P. J. Ungvarski (Eds.), *HIV/AIDS: A guide to nursing care* (3rd ed., pp. 64–80, Table 3-6). Philadelphia: W. B. Saunders.

NATURAL HISTORY

Acute HIV Infection

Most patients have signs and symptoms that appear transiently at the time of, or shortly after, the initial acquisition of the virus. Descriptions of illness include a mononucleosis-like ailment lasting several weeks, during which malaise, fever, a maculopapular rash, diarrhea, and lymphadenopathy predominate. Other signs and symptoms include myalgias, headache, encephalitis, neuropathy, and splenomegaly. One study (Pedersen et al., 1989) described a correlation between the length of the "seroconversion" illness and an accelerated progression along the spectrum of HIV infection. Of those with a primary illness of more than 14 days' duration, 78% progressed to symptomatic AIDS within 3 years. Of those with a minor illness, less than 10% progressed as fast. Case reports describe oral and esophageal candidiasis and a profound, transient decrease in the CD4+ lymphocyte count, suggesting that the host is truly immunocompromised at this point. Perhaps most patients experience this acute syndrome, but for most it is unrecognized and passes as an episode of a generalized, benign viral syndrome. Those recently exposed to the virus, including percutaneous or needlestick exposures, should be counseled to seek medical care if this syndrome develops. Almost all patients who acquire the infection will be HIV antibody positive within 6 months.

Asymptomatic HIV Infection

Patients who have no signs or symptoms of HIV infection and have not had previous clinical findings comprise the asymptomatic group. They may be subclassified on the basis of a laboratory evaluation that includes a complete blood count with differential white blood cell count and a platelet count. Immunologic tests, such as the T-lymphocyte helper and suppressor cell counts, are also an important part of the overall evaluation. Patients with test results that are within normal limits and those who have not yet had complete evaluations should be differentiated from patients whose test results are consistent with HIV-associated defects—lymphopenia, thrombocytopenia, and a decreased number of T-helper (T4) lymphocytes. The median duration of this asymptomatic period is 10 years.

Persistent Generalized Lymphadenopathy

Patients may have persistent but painless generalized lymphadenopathy (PGL) but without further disease findings. PGL is defined as palpable lymph node enlargement of 1 cm or greater at two or more extralinguinal sites that persists for more than 3 months in the absence of a concurrent illness or condition other than HIV infection to explain the findings. In some cases, lymphadenopathy actually regresses as HIV disease advances, probably because the architecture of the lymph node is gradually destroyed.

The Middle Stage of Infection

After a period of relative asymptomatic infection, various episodic conditions begin to develop. These may include herpes zoster, thrush, seborrheic dermatitis, skin and nail infections, and bacterial infections such as sinusitis, bronchitis, or pneumonia. Subtle manifestations of neurologic disease may manifest in AIDS dementia complex or peripheral neuropathy. Anergy to skin testing develops. Idiopathic thrombocytopenia purpura may develop.

Patients also may have fevers, involuntary weight loss, and persistent diarrhea. This constellation of symptoms was formerly called AIDS-related complex (ARC).

Other HIV Diseases

NEUROLOGIC DISEASE. Patients may have one or more of the following: dementia, myelopathy, or peripheral neuropathy and an absence of any concurrent illness or condition other than HIV to explain the findings.

SECONDARY INFECTIOUS DISEASES. Patients have been diagnosed with an infectious disease that is either associated with HIV infection or is at least moderately indicative of a defect in cell-mediated immunity. Table 58–11 lists the primary opportunistic infections seen in AIDS.

SECONDARY CANCERS. Patients have been diagnosed with one or more kinds of cancer known to be associated with HIV infection, as listed in the CDC surveillance definition of AIDS, and at least moderately indicative of a defect in cell-mediated immunity: KS, non-Hodgkin's lymphoma (small, noncleaved lymphoma or immunoblastic sarcoma), primary lymphoma of the brain, or cervical cancer. Table 58–11 lists the major cancers seen in AIDS along with the other opportunistic illnesses.

TABLE 58–11. **Opportunistic Diseases Commonly Associated With HIV Infection**

A. Infections
   1. Bacterial
      - Tuberculosis
      - *Mycobacterium avium* complex
      - *Salmonella*
      - *Shigella*
      - *Pseudomonas aeruginosa*
      - *Hemophilus influenzae*
      - *Streptococcus pneumoniae*
      - *Camphylobacter*
      - *Staphylococcus aureus*
      - Listeriosis
      - Bacillary angiomatosis (*Bartonella*)
      - *Rhodococcus equi*
   2. Fungal
      - *Cryptococcus neoformans*
      - *Candida* species
      - *Histoplasma capsulatum*
      - Cuccidioides immitis
      - *Aspergillis* species
      - Blastomycosis
   3. Viral
      - Cytomegalovirus
      - Herpes simplex
      - Varicella zoster
      - Epstein-Barr
      - Progressive multifocal leukoencephalopathy
      - Hepatitis A–E
      - Cervical and anal papilloma
      - Molluscum
   4. Parasitic
      - *Pneumocystis carinii*
      - *Cryptosporidium parvum*
      - *Isospora belli*
      - *Strongyloides stercoralis*
      - *Toxoplasma gondii*
      - *Enterocytozoon bieneusi* (*Microsporidia*)

B. Malignancies
   - Kaposi's sarcoma
   - Non-Hodgkin's lymphoma
   - Primary central nervous system lymphoma
   - Invasive cervical cancer

C. Wasting Syndrome

D. AIDS Dementia Complex (HIV encephalopathy)

E. Idiopathic Thrombocytopenic Purpura

Late-Stage HIV Disease

As the immune system progressively fails, certain illnesses become more prevalent or increase in severity. Central nervous system (CNS) lymphoma, *Mycobacterium avium* complex disease, CMV disease, toxoplasmosis, and cryptococcal meningitis are prevalent as the T-cell count drops below 100.

DEFINITION OF AIDS

The definition of AIDS has undergone several revisions as the clinical syndromes and diseases associated with HIV expanded. The latest definition is given in Table 58–12. It labels AIDS patients as those HIV-infected individuals who have T4 cell counts of 200 or

TABLE 58–12. **The 1993 AIDS Surveillance Case Definition**

Candidiasis of bronchi, trachea, or lungs
Candidiasis, esophageal
Cervical cancer, invasive
CD4+ T-lymphocyte count <200 mm⁴ (<14%)
Coccidiodomycosis, disseminated or extrapulmonary
Cryptococcosis, extrapulmonary
Cryptosporidiosis, chronic intestinal (>1 month in duration)
Cytomegalovirus disease (other than liver, spleen, or nodes)
Cytomegalovirus retinitis (with loss of vision)
Encephalopathy, HIV related
Herpes simplex: chronic ulcer(s) (>1 month in duration) or bronchitis, pneumonitis, or esophagitis
Histoplasmosis, disseminated or extrapulmonary
Isosporiasis, chronic intestinal (>1 month in duration)
Kaposi's sarcoma
Lymphoma, Burkitt's (or equivalent term)
Lymphoma, immunoblastic (or equivalent term)
Lymphoma, primary, of brain
Mycobacterium avium complex or *Mycobacterium kansasii*, disseminated or extrapulmonary
Mycobacterium tuberculosis, any site (pulmonary or extrapulmonary)
Mycobacterium, other species or unidentified species, disseminated or extrapulmonary
Pneumocystis carinii pneumonia
Pneumonia, recurrent
Progressive multifocal leukoencephalopathy
Salmonella septicemia, recurrent
Toxoplasmosis of brain
Wasting syndrome caused by HIV

From Casey, K. M. (1995). Pathophysiology of HIV-1, clinical course, and treatment. In J. H. Flaskerud & P. J. Ungvarski (Eds.), *HIV/AIDS: A guide to nursing care* (3rd ed., pp. 64–80, Table 3–5). Philadelphia: W. B. Saunders.

less. The expanded AIDS surveillance case definition resulted in a 204% increase in the number of AIDS cases reported in the first quarter of 1993, compared with the same period in 1992.

OPPORTUNISTIC ILLNESSES FREQUENTLY ASSOCIATED WITH AIDS

Opportunistic infections are caused by a diverse spectrum of infectious agents that rarely cause disease in people with normal, intact immune systems. They reflect the specific immune defects related to HIV, geographic clustering (i.e., New York City and tuberculosis [TB], south central states and histoplasmosis), age-appropriate illnesses, a relationship to lifestyle, and an impressive consistency in the clinical presentations of certain infections. In many cases, the infections are a reactivation or secondary appearance of a previously acquired pathogen. The opportunistic infections are rarely curable, and at best are controlled during the acute phase and suppressed in the maintenance phase, which usually involves long-term treatment. Many infections become disseminated as the illness advances. Patients usually have concurrent infections that are difficult to treat. The morbidity and mortality of AIDS are chiefly an effect of the major OIs. The most common infections and malignancies are listed in Table 58–11.

Opportunistic Infections—Protozoal

PNEUMOCYSTIS CARINII *PNEUMONIA.* *Pneumocystis carinii* pneumonia (PCP) is the most common opportunistic infection seen in patients with AIDS, occurring in at least 60% and recurring in many (Kovacs & Masur, 1988). Patients generally present with an insidious onset of fever, dyspnea on exertion, and a nonproductive cough. Respiratory rate is slightly increased, PA_{O_2} is decreased, and chest x-ray reveals diffuse interstitial infiltrates (Kovacs and Masur, 1988). A high degree of suspicion for PCP should accompany the clinical evaluation of any HIV-positive patient with fever and cough. Approximately 80% of the general population has detectable antibodies to *P. carinii*, indicating primary infections early in life. Diagnosis is usually made from identification of pneumocysts from induced sputum specimens or from tissue examination after bronchoscopy with bronchial lavage and transbronchial biopsy.

With treatment, 72% of patients with AIDS with *P. carinii* infection survive their first episode. Without treatment, PCP can progress to a fulminant and life-threatening infection. This mortality risk has changed, however, as prevention efforts have improved and clinical treatment expertise has developed. Since 1987, with the advent of prophylaxis in the form of sulfamethoxazole–trimethoprim (Bactrim; Roche Laboratories, Nutley, NJ) or aerosolized pentamidine, incidence has decreased significantly.

Early detection of PCP improves survival and the course of illness dramatically. Zidovudine (ZDV) and prophylaxis with aerosolized pentamidine, Bactrim, or dapsone can greatly reduce the severity and frequency of PCP. Most patients do require initial hospitalization for treatment with sulfamethoxazole–trimethoprim or pentamidine, with continued at-home treatment. Others can be successfully treated at home if the illness is caught early enough. Other agents used to treat PCP are trimethoprim dapsone, clindamycin–primaquine, atovaquone, and trimetrexate glucoronate. Corticosteroids reduce the mortality rate and need for mechanical ventilation (Weinberger, 1993), but may increase the incidence of CMV disease (Nelson et al., 1993).

TOXOPLASMA GONDII. Toxoplasmosis is a common source of CNS disease in patients with AIDS. Presenting symptoms include fever, headache, seizures, lethargy, and focal neurologic findings. Some patients have personality or cognitive changes (Kovacs & Masur, 1988). Diagnosis is usually difficult; however, most patients display multiple space-occupying lesions on brain computed tomography (CT) scan (Kovacs & Masur, 1988). Definitive diagnosis can be made on brain biopsy of an accessible lesion and identification of the *Toxoplasma* trophozoite (Kovacs & Masur, 1988). A presumptive clinical diagnosis is usually made based on signs and symptoms, recent onset of focal neurologic abnormality, brain imaging evidence, and serum antibody to *Toxoplasma* or successful response to therapy for toxoplasmosis. Patients often require adjuvant therapy with phenytoin, folinic acid, and decadron. The mainstay of treatment is sulfadiazine and pyrimethamine, but adverse events are frequent. Clindamycin is used for patients who cannot tolerate sulfa drugs. Most patients respond well to therapy but need to be treated indefinitely.

A standard prophylactic therapy has not been established. The major means of transmission of *Toxoplasma* to humans is through ingestion of meats and vegetables containing oocysts. Patients should cook meat well to avoid contact with *T. gondii* cysts if they have no serologic evidence of prior infection. Reactivation and dissemination of latent toxoplasmosis cannot yet be prevented, but prophylaxis with sulfamethoxazole–trimethoprim, used to prevent PCP, also confers some protection.

CRYPTOSPORIDIUM. Cryptosporidiosis is an intestinal infection manifested by watery diarrhea that occasionally causes severe dehydration and wasting (Kovacs & Masur, 1988). The most common site of infection is the small intestine. Common symptoms include anorexia, malaise, weight loss, and abdominal cramping. Malabsorption is frequently present. No therapy has yet been shown to be consistently effective, and the AIDS patient with *Cryptosporidium* gastroenteritis is at great risk for severe weight loss, fluid and electrolyte imbalance, malnutrition, and debility. Whether cryptosporidiosis is a reactivation of a previous infection or is a newly acquired one has not been determined (Gellin & Soave, 1992).

The disease is highly infectious; it is transmitted from person to person or from animal to person and has an incubation period of 5 to 14 days. In AIDS patients, although cryptosporidiosis is typically associated with a severe, profuse, usually chronic diarrhea, the degree of symptomatology is highly variable. Symptoms of cryptosporidiosis can be exactly mimicked by another parasite, *Isospora belli.*

Diagnosis is established through stool testing, biopsy of the large or small bowel, and serologic techniques. Response to treatment has been very poor. Supportive care, nutritional repletion, and hydration are used to combat the effects of cryptosporidiosis. There is currently no prophylactic therapy, and enteric precautions and infection control measures are the key to controlling nosocomial transmission. Cryptosporidiosis has been known to regress spontaneously as the patient's T cells increase in number. Diarrheal disease can also be caused by other parasites, bacteria, and malabsorption (Kotler, 1989).

Mycobacterial Infections

MYCOBACTERIUM AVIUM *COMPLEX DISEASE*

Infection with *Mycobacterium avium–intracellulare* has developed in 50% of patients with AIDS (Gold & Armstrong, 1989) and is usually a disseminated disease. It is noncommumicable, with little evidence of person-to-person transmission. *M. avium* complex is acquired orally or inhaled. It is usually the result of a primary acquisition of the organism, but can result from a reactivation. It occurs evenly in all risk groups and is a late complication of AIDS. Symptoms include fever, rigor, diarrhea, weight loss, and abdominal cramping. Enlarged lymph nodes and positive blood cultures indicate illness. Medical treatment with four or five drug regimens has been somewhat successful. Recent use of rifabutin as a prophylactic agent has reduced the incidence of this disease.

MYCOBACTERIUM TUBERCULOSIS

One hundred years ago, TB was the leading cause of death from infectious diseases in America. Although evidence of TB has been found in neolithic and pre-Columbian skeletons (Des Prez & Heim, 1990), it was not until the crowded living conditions of the Industrial Revolution that transmission occurred easily among the population. Treatment programs consisting of various pulmonary surgeries, prolonged rest, and fresh air were implemented, and sanitariums to house sick TB patients were developed. With the advent of isoniazid (INH) in 1952, the rate of TB infection declined substantially. It was even anticipated that TB might be eradicated. However, since the mid-1980s there has been a rise in the anticipated number of cases. This infection rate is fueled by poverty, the immigration of people from endemic areas, and underlying HIV infection.

Mycobacterium tuberculosis is an aerobic, obligate parasitic, acid-fast bacillus. Infection is spread by inhalation of droplet nuclei, which are produced when the source patient talks, coughs, or sneezes. A cough can produce 3,000 infectious droplet nuclei, and particles remain suspended in the air for a long time (Des Prez & Heim, 1990). Infection occurs when inhaled particles settle in the peripheral lung and multiply. Chance and the underlying diseases of malnutrition, alcoholism, HIV, and immunologic disorders combined with long-term exposure create a high-risk situation. In HIV-infected patients, most new cases reflect reactivation of a latent infection, and the risk of progression to clinical illness is greater. Secondary spread of infection occurs among social contacts of these patients and others who share their air space.

Because AIDS patients may become anergic, Mantoux testing for TB should be done early in the course of the patient's disease. The clinical presentation of tuberculosis (afternoon fevers, weight loss, cough, fatigue, night sweats) is hard to distinguish from that of other HIV-related ailments. In AIDS patients, extrapulmonary sites of TB can be common; these include lymph nodes, bones, genitourinary tract, miliary sites, and bone marrow. Diagnosis is usually made from the Mantoux test, chest x-ray, and sputum cultures for acid-fast bacillus in a patient with clinically suspect signs. HIV patients with TB need to be treated more aggressively and for a longer period of time than non–HIV-infected patients.

Infection control efforts are challenged by the presence of droplet nuclei in the area (Nardell, 1990) and by the fact that a laboratory may take 6 to 8 weeks to culture the TB organism. Use of disposable particulate respirators, engineering controls in room design, ultraviolet lighting, air ducts, room air flow, and cough suppression or avoidance mechanisms are critical. Case finding in HIV-infected patients with early therapy is very important (Ungvarski, 1990). In addition, interventions that assist patients to comply with the prolonged treatment regimen are necessary. Failure to take medication as prescribed permits development of resistant strains of TB that may be lethal (Division of Tuberculosis Control et al., 1990).

Among the increasing numbers of TB cases reported, there have been large outbreaks of multiple drug-resistant TB (MDR-TB). The principal causes of MDR-TB are thought to be the ingestion of single anti-TB agents for prolonged periods or erratic compliance with therapy (Barnes & Barrows, 1993). Most patients reported with MDR-TB are HIV infected. Many of the outbreaks of MDR-TB have been associated with nosocomial transmission, affecting health care workers as well as patients. Factors contributing to these outbreaks include (1) delayed diagnosis, (2) delayed recognition that the TB was in fact drug resistant, (3) delayed initiation and inadequate duration of isolation, (4) inadequate ventilation in TB isolation rooms, (5) lapses in TB isolation practices, and (6) inadequate precautions for cough-inducing procedures (Barnes & Barrows, 1993; Casey, 1993; Ungvarski & Staats, 1995). Mahmoadi and Iseman (1993) studied the records of 35 MDR-TB patients to identify medical mismanagement practices that deviated from established guidelines and determine the impact of these practices on the development of MDR-TB and adverse medical sequelae. Medical mismanagement was detected in 80% of the cases, with an average of 3.93 errors noted per patient record (Ungvarski & Staats, 1995). Drug-susceptibility tests should be performed on the first isolate of TB and reported to the health department. Care should be planned under the advisement of a physician experienced in the treatment of MDR-TB (Ungvarski & Staats, 1995).

Fungal Infections

CANDIDIASIS

Candida albicans is the most common infection in AIDS patients. The fungus is a commensal organism that in humans exists in the gastrointestinal tract, the female genital tract, the oropharynx, and on diseased skin. Most AIDS patients contract *Candida* infection, although the exact relationship of this organism to T-cell depletion is not understood. Patients manifest a mucocutaneous disease that is rarely systemic. Vulvovaginal candidiasis may be the initial manifestation of AIDS disease in women. It may become chronic and refractory.

Thrush is characterized by creamy, curd-like patches on the tongue and buccal mucosa. Diagnosis is established by inspection and oral scrapings treated with potassium oxide. Clotrimazole troches, nystatin, and ketoconazole are used medically for treatment.

Candidal esophagitis should be suspected in AIDS patients with thrush, odynophagia, and substernal chest pain. It is usually diagnosed presumptively by contrast radiology, and definitively by esophagoscopy. Other infectious agents can cause esophagitis (herpes, CMV). Candidal esophagitis is often difficult to treat. Topical antifungals, troches, and suspensions may fail because swallowing does not allow sufficient time for the antifungal agent to act on the esophageal infection. Oral ketoconazole is often needed. Patients at times require low-dose treatment with amphotericin B.

CRYPTOCOCCOSIS

Cryptococcosus neoformans infection occurs in about 7% of AIDS patients (Kovacs & Masur, 1988), with meningitis being the most common presentation. In the normal host, the initial pulmonary infection is usually asymptomatic. The onset of cryptococcal meningitis in AIDS patients is usually subtle, with nonspecific complaints of fever, headache, nausea, vomiting, and malaise. The headache is usually frontal or temporal, and close associates of the patient notice subtle personality and behavioral changes. Besides its CNS manifestation, cryptococcosis can also be a disseminated disease or a pulmonary disease. These manifestations may coexist. Cryptococcosis is the most common life-threatening fungal infection associated with AIDS (Ungvarski & Staats, 1995).

Diagnosis is established by detection of fungal infection in cerebrospinal fluid, detection of cryptococcal antigen, or fungal culture. Treatment is fluconazole or amphotericin B. Relapse is so common that continued suppressive therapy is warranted.

Viral Infections

HERPES SIMPLEX VIRUS

Most herpes simplex virus (HSV) infections in AIDS patients are reactivations of latent infection. The principal mode of transmission is contact with oral secretions (for HSV-1) or genital secretions (for HSV-2). HSV-1 can occur in the genital or perirectal area by means of oral-sexual contact or by autoinoculation (hands). The same is true of HSV-2 if it occurs orally. Higher rates of HSV-2 infection are seen in patients with higher numbers of sexual partners, in prostitutes, with lack of condom use, in adults of lower socioeconomic class, in people attending sexually transmitted disease clinics, and in homosexual men (Corey & Spear, 1986).

After the initial HSV infection resolves, it becomes dormant within the nerve ganglia. The severity of an acute attack of reactivated infection is related to the patient's degree of immunosuppression. Oral and labial infections may be mild or may involve pain, fever, and cervical lymphadenopathy. Illness in a patient with HIV infection may last for weeks. Genital or perianal lesions also demonstrate a prolonged healing time and carry a risk of dissemination. Intervention in the form of topical, oral, or intravenous acyclovir is initiated when the prodromal symptoms of burning, tingling, and itching begin. Lesions usually occur in the same place as the prior infection. A rare presentation of HSV in AIDS patients is acute encephalitis. Mental status change, fever, headache, and nausea are associated with it. Perianal, anorectal, and esophageal HSV infections also occur. A diagnosis of HSV is made by culture of the lesion. If acyclovir treatment fails, foscarnet is used.

HERPES ZOSTER

The development of herpes zoster (shingles) may signal the progression of HIV illness in an HIV-infected patient. It is the result of a reactivation of a prior primary infection. Herpes zoster produces characteristic painful, red lesions in the skin region of the affected dermatome. Disseminated lesions may appear in the hands and feet. A biopsy to establish the diagnosis is usually not needed, and treatment with intravenous acyclovir is begun. Strict isolation, avoidance of infection, and measures to prevent dissemination and afford pain relief are implemented quickly.

CYTOMEGALOVIRUS

Cytomegalovirus disease, like the herpes family viruses, begins with an initial infection (although it is often unnoticed), and a life-long infection, although usually dormant, results. CMV causes disease by directly destroying organ tissue, impairing immunologic responses, and aiding neoplastic transformation. The initial infection is usually a result of in vitro birth canal or breast milk infection, childhood contact with other children who are infected (via respiratory secretions), or sexual intercourse (vaginal or anal). Alternative routes of CMV transmission include transfusion of blood products. Reexposure to the virus can result in the acquisition of a different strain of CMV. Immunosuppressive drugs such as corticosteroids can permit reactivation of latent disease.

In AIDS patients, CMV is the most common opportunistic pathogen detected at autopsy. It causes over 95% of the chorioretinitis seen in AIDS patients. The patient complains of blurred vision, decreased visual acuity, or floaters. IV ganciclovir is used as a suppressive therapy in patients. Neutropenia is a common dose-limiting toxic reaction. In some cases of CMV retinitis, intravitreal injections are used instead with good results (Heinemann, 1989). In 1991, foscarnet was also made available as a treatment. Foscarnet does not cause neutropenia, but renal toxicity is a common side effect. Concurrent or alternating ganciclovir and foscarnet are also administered. An oral form of ganciclovir was approved in 1995.

Cytomegalovirus also infects and affects all parts of the gastrointestinal tract. CMV colitis is associated with weight loss, anorexia, fever, and diarrhea (Kotler et al., 1991). Kotler and colleagues (1989a) found that IV ganciclovir treatment for CMV colitis repleted body cell mass and body fat, raised the serum albumin level, and allowed patients to gain weight.

Cytomegalovirus pneumonia most frequently occurs concurrently with another pneumonia. Other forms of CMV disease include encephalitis, adrenalitis, esophagitis, cholangitis, and conjunctivitis (Ungvarski & Staats, 1995).

PROGRESSIVE MULTIFOCAL LEUKOENCEPHALOPATHY

Progressive multifocal leukoencephalopathy (PML) is a subacute demyelinating disease of the central nervous system. Multiple lesions develop in the white matter of the cerebrum, brain stem, or cerebellum, resulting in focal neurologic deficits. The disease progresses rapidly to dementia with blindness and paralysis. Death usually occurs within 1 year.

Progressive multifocal leukoencephalopathy is caused by infection with the JC virus, named after the first patient diagnosed with the illness. By adulthood most people are infected. Only 4% of all AIDS patients have been diagnosed with PML; it is considered a reactivation of a latent infection.

Initial symptoms of extremity weakness, gait disturbance, speech disturbance, and visual loss are compounded by altered mentation. A diagnosis is established by a brain biosy, although magnetic resonance imaging, CT scans, electroencephalography, and other studies to rule out CNS lymphoma, toxoplasmosis, and cryptococcal meningitis contribute heavily to the diagnosis. There is no clear treatment. Small trials have demonstrated some benefit from prolonged use of cytosine arabinoside (Ragland, 1993). There have also been isolated reports of spontaneous remissions (Ragland, 1993).

Malignancies

KAPOSI'S SARCOMA

Kaposi's sarcoma is the most common type of malignancy seen in AIDS patients. It occurred in approximately 30% of all AIDS patients diagnosed in 1981, but now occurs in 10% of patients at the time of AIDS diagnosis. Before AIDS was discovered, forms of KS had occurred in various clinical settings. The disease was first described in an 1872 report published by Dr. Moriz Kaposi, entitled "Idiopathic Multiple Pigmented Sarcoma of the Skin" (Friedman-Kien et al., 1989). The original disease described by Kaposi is referred to as classic KS, whereas many other authors have described an indolent disease mainly confined to the lower extremities and frequently occurring in men from the Mediterranean area (Friedman-Kien et al., 1989; Volberding, 1990).

In 1984, Breimer reviewed the original paper and uncovered striking similarities between this "classic" KS and our "epidemic" KS (usually described as being much more aggressive and largely affecting the gastrointestinal tract, skin, and upper extremities). According to Breimer's review, Kaposi described an incurable, rapidly lethal (death within 2 to 3 years), generalized illness composed of lesions affecting the gastrointestinal tract and liver. Before the era of AIDS, KS was considered very rare, and most cases were distinctly clustered among the following groups: elderly men of Mediterranean or eastern European Jewish descent, young black men and children in equatorial Africa, and organ transplant patients who receive immunosuppressive therapy.

Kaposi's sarcoma is believed to originate from the endothelial cell wall. There has been extensive investigation into the possible cofactors (nitrite inhalers, CMV, genetic factors, other infectious agents) that may predispose an HIV-infected person to development of KS. The latest medical thinking is that KS is caused by an as-yet unidentified agent transmitted sexually, perinatally, or through blood; this agent may also be a cofactor (Beral et al., 1990). It is even considered that KS may not be a true malignancy but a stimulated response to HIV in which lymphatic endothelial cells proliferate (Kaplan, 1994a). Although in this country KS is firmly associated with MWHSWM, primarily in California and New York, it also occurs commonly in adults who acquire HIV heterosexually in Puerto Rico, Haiti, Mexico, Central America, and Africa. Women who acquire HIV heterosexually from MWHSWM have a fourfold incidence of KS compared to women who acquire HIV from heterosexual partners (Beral et al., 1990). Friedman-Kien and coworkers (1990) even reported KS in six homosexual men without HIV. Kumar and associates (1989) reported a fatal case of KS in a white heterosexual man without HIV.

Kaposi's sarcoma usually develops in multicentric fashion in asymptomatic nodules, which range in color from red-brown to violet, pink, and dark purple. KS invades other organs besides the skin. New multifocal lesions may appear at any time, and characteristic sites include the tip of the nose, eyelid, hard palate, posterior pharynx, glans penis, thigh, and sole of the foot (Kaplan, 1994a). The most common extracutaneous sites are the gastrointestinal tract, lymph nodes, and lungs. KS causes both structural and functional damage, with internal organ involvement signaled by weight loss, emaciation, hemorrhage, and diarrhea (Safai, 1989). Lymphadema can occur in the face, penis, scrotum, and lower extremities.

When KS is localized to the skin, cryosurgery, laser therapy, and surgical excision have been used, but radiotherapy is the most promising treatment (Myskowski, 1989). Radiotherapy is also useful for palliative or cosmetic purposes. Various chemotherapy regimens and zidovudine with interferon have also been used.

NON-HODGKIN'S LYMPHOMA

The case definition of AIDS was expanded in 1987 to include patients with HIV who have an intermediate or high-grade lymphoma. In patients with AIDS, the lymphoma is usually of B-cell origin. Lymphoma develops in approximately 4% to 10% of all AIDS patients (Gail et al., 1991; Levine, 1988). Non-Hodgkin's lymphoma tends to occur late in the course of HIV infection and is related to progressive immunosuppression (Levine, 1992). The earliest sign is usually a unilateral, painless, enlarged lymph node. As the condition progresses, it spreads through the lymphatic channels to nearby nodes and organ systems, especially the spleen, liver, gastrointestinal tract, skin, lungs, CNS, and bone marrow. Fevers, weight loss, and night sweats commonly occur.

A biopsy of affected tissue clearly makes the diagnosis. Patients with PGL have an 850-fold rate of lymphoma based on incidence rates in America, age adjusted for lymphoma. Because of this, PGL patients should have serial biopsies to monitor for malignant conversion.

Much of the non-Hodgkin's lymphoma that occurs in AIDS patients is confined to the CNS. The most frequent presenting symptoms are hemiparesis, aphasia, seizures, cranial nerve palsies, and headache (Kaplan, 1990). The second most common site is the gastrointestinal tract, with tumors arising in the mouth, esophagus, stomach, duodenum, and other sites. Bone marrow involvement is also commonly seen. Lymph node–based non-Hodgkin's lymphoma is uncommon in AIDS patients; 80% to 90% of the disease is extranodal, involving the CNS, gastrointestinal tract, bone marrow, and liver. Other sites include the gallbladder, rectum, jaw, earlobe, lung, skin, gingiva, and paranasal sinuses, among others (Levine, 1992).

Staging of the illness requires bone marrow aspiration and biopsy bilaterally, lumbar puncture, chest x-ray, CT scans of the chest and abdomen, and assorted blood work. Treatment is initiated with intent to cure. Lymphoma is very responsive to chemotherapy, but if the patient has had a prior opportunistic infection, control or palliation can be the only realized goal. A rapid remission can be achieved, but neutropenia may delay subsequent courses of therapy. Colon-stimulating factors are used to combat this time loss. Successful treatment has been associated with methotrexate, bleomycin, doxorubicin, cytoxan, vincristine, and dexamethasone (M-BACOD modified), but therapy is usually individualized. Responses have been short in duration and have not had any major impact on survival (Kaplan, 1994b).

HIV-RELATED CONDITIONS

Wasting Syndrome

Wasting syndrome in patients with HIV-related disease has a myriad of presentations because there are several mechanisms by which people with HIV disease might become malnourished, including oral lesions that affect food intake, carcinomatosis, disseminated infections, and, possibly, endocrine malfunction. Other factors affect wasting, including neurologic or psychological conditions, finances, lack of facilities to store or prepare food, lack of nutrition knowledge, fatigue, and side effects of medication (Ungvarski & Staats, 1995). Studies have shown that protein–energy malnutrition is a common problem in patients with AIDS (Kotler et al., 1985). Deficiencies in macronutrients and micronutrients have adverse effects on immunologic function, and studies have strongly suggested that the timing of death may be influenced by the extent of tissue depletion (Kotler et al., 1989b). The debilitation caused by starving and malnutrition probably also contributes to hospitalization, diminished quality of life, poor functional living habits, and absence of clear mentation. Nutritional malabsorption is related to injury to the small intestine, and, in some cases, diseases of the digestive organs. Kotler (1992) identified three categories of intestinal disease—primary infection of the enterocytes (e.g., cryptosporidiosis, isosporidiosis), secondary involvement from systemic or disseminated disorders (e.g., CMV or KS), and inflammatory bowel disease (e.g., intestinal infection caused by HIV itself) (Ungvarski & Staats, 1995).

Several studies have documented the ability of malnourished AIDS patients to be repleted (Kotler et al., 1989a; Tierney et al., 1991; Von Roenn et al., 1991). Repletion has been successful using various methods depending on the reason for the malnutrition. Home total parenteral nutrition, home enteral feedings through a percutaneous feeding tube, oral diet change to an elemental diet if the patient is a malabsorber, use of megestrol acetate to stimulate appetite, and aggressive counseling by a dietitian early in the course of illness are among the methods that have been used successfully. A key consideration is that, in the presence of an active opportunistic infection, most forms of nutritional support will not lead to nutritional repletion. If the patient is put into a positive caloric balance, the excess calories are deposited as fat, not protein. The point is that AIDS patients require aggressive evaluation and prompt treatment of opportunistic diseases (Task Force on Nutritional Support in AIDS, 1989). Innovative therapies such as intralesional and oral steroid therapy for CMV esophageal ulcers and thorough examinations to detect the parasite causing enteropathy are necessary. HIV patients should have routine consultations with a dietitian.

Feeding the patient enterally or parenterally may also slow the psychomotor retardation seen in these patients. It is possible that some of the slowing of thought processes thought be related to a patient's dementia or CNS infection may be a profound effect of malnutrition on personality.

Currently, the tools needed to evaluate nutritional status in ill patients are lacking. Weight can be confounded by hydration; caliper skinfold measurements do not have generalized interrater reliability and take time; caloric counts measuring intake do not provide data on a patient's use of the calories to make protein stores. Body cell mass can be estimated by determining body potassium content, nitrogen content, and total body water. However, these calculations are not widely available. Newer equipment such as the electrical impedance analyzers, which can measure fat-free mass and estimate total body water, could provide this clinical information.

Text continued on page 1250

TABLE 58–13. **Major Signs and Symptoms of AIDS Dementia Complex**

Early	Late
Cognitive	Cognitive
Impaired concentration	Global dementia
"Memory loss"	Confusion
Mental slowing	Disorientation
	Disinhibition
Motor	Motor
Unsteady gait	Paralysis
Loss of coordination	Hemiparesis
Tremor	Incontinence
Leg weakness	Psychomotor slowing
Behavioral	Behavioral
Apathy	Mutism
"Depression"	
Withdrawal	
Hallucinations (rare)	

TABLE 58–14. **Staging System for AIDS Dementia Complex**

Stage	Features
0	Normal function
0.5	Equivocal or subclinical
1	Mild Able to work and perform activities of daily living Unequivocal evidence of functional, intellectual, or motor impairment
2	Moderate Able to do basic self-care Unable to work or maintain more demanding activities of daily living Ambulatory
3	Severe Major cognitive and motor incapacity
4	Nearly vegetative

TABLE 58–15. **Drugs Used to Treat HIV Infection and AIDS-Related Conditions (*Under Investigation)**

Generic Name (Trade Name)	Route of Administration	Indications	Side/Adverse Effects
Acyclovir (Zovirax)	PO IV Topical	Herpes simplex virus infection Herpes zoster infection Varicella infection	Parenteral: skin rash, hives, hematuria, lightheadedness, headache, diaphoresis, confusion, tremors, abdominal pain, difficulty in breathing, decreased frequency of urination, nausea, vomiting, unusual thirst, extreme fatigue Oral: changes in menstrual period, skin rash, diarrhea, dizziness, headache, joint pain, nausea, vomiting, acne, anorexia, somnolence Topical: mild pain, burning, itching, skin rash
Adenine arabinoside (Vidarabine) (Vira-A)	IV Ophthalmic	Herpes simplex virus infection Herpes zoster infection Progressive multifocal leukoencephalopathy Varicella infection	Anorexia, nausea, vomiting, diarrhea, tremors, dizziness, confusion, hallucinations, ataxia, psychosis, leukopenia, thrombocytopenia, elevated aspartate aminotransferase and bilirubin levels, anemia
Albendazole (Eskazole) (Zentel)	PO	Microsporidiosis Cryptosporidiosis	Stomach upset, headache, dizziness, rash, fever, elevated liver function tests, alopecia
*All trans retinoic acid	PO	Kaposi's sarcoma	None yet reported
Amikacin (Amikin)	IV IM	*Mycobacterium avium* complex infection	Increase or decrease in frequency of urination or amount of urine, increased thirst, loss of appetite, nausea, vomiting, muscle twitching, numbness, any loss of hearing, ringing or buzzing, clumsiness, dizziness, unsteadiness, difficulty in breathing
Amitriptyline (Elavil)	PO	Peripheral neuropathy Depression	Drowsiness, dizziness, excitation, tremors, weakness, confusion, headache, nervousness, orthostatic hypotension, tachycardia, hypertension, blurred vision, tinnitus, mydriasis, dry mouth, constipation, nausea, vomiting, anorexia, paralytic ileus, urine retention, rash, urticaria, sweating
Amphotericin B (Fungizone)	IV	Candidiasis Coccidioidomycosis Cryptococcosis Histoplasmosis	Fever, chills, hypokalemia (irregular heartbeat, muscle cramps or pain, extreme fatigue), pain at site of infusion, anemia, blurred or double vision, renal failure (increased or decreased urination), paresthesias, impaired hearing, tinnitus, seizures, shortness of breath, skin rash or itching, agranulocytosis or leukopenia, thrombocytopenia
*Amphotericin B colloidal dispersion	IV	Cryptococcosis	*See* Amphotericin B
*Anti-B4-blocked ricin	IV	Lymphoma	Allergic reactions, weight gain, can affect liver
Ampicillin (Omnipen) (Omnipen-N) (Polycillin) (Polycillin-N) (Principen) (Totacillin) (Totacillin-N)	PO IM IV	Salmonellosis	Anaphylaxis, serum sickness, neutropenia, platelet count dysfunction, skin rash, fever, hives, itching, pseudomembranous colitis, seizures, diarrhea, nausea, vomiting, thrush, abdominal pain or cramps
*Atevirdine mesylate	PO	HIV infection	Rash, fever, palpitations
Atovaquone (Mepron) (formerly 566C80)	PO	*Pneumocystis carinii* pneumonia	Rash, nausea, diarrhea, headache, vomiting, fever, insomnia, asthenia, pruritus, thrush, abdominal pain, constipation, dizziness, anemia, neutropenia, elevated liver enzymes
Azithromycin (Zithromax)	PO	Cryptosporidiosis *Mycobacterium avium* complex infection Toxoplasmosis	Diarrhea, nausea, vomiting, abdominal pain, palpitations, chest pain, dyspepsia, flatulence, melena, cholestatic jaundice, *Monilia* infection, vaginitis, nephritis, dizziness, ototoxicity, vertigo, somnolence, fatigue, rash, photophobia, angioedema
*BACI	PO	Cryptosporidiosis	None yet reported

Table continued on following page

TABLE 58–15. **Drugs Used to Treat HIV Infection and AIDS-Related Conditions (*Under Investigation)** *Continued*

Generic Name (Trade Name)	Route of Administration	Indications	Side/Adverse Effects
Bleomycin (Blenoxane)	IV	Kaposi's sarcoma Non-Hodgkin's lymphoma Cervical cancer	Cough, shortness of breath, pneumonitis, fever, chills, stomatitis, confusion, syncope, diaphoresis, changes in skin color and texture, rashes, swelling of fingers, nausea, vomiting and anorexia, weight loss, hair loss
*Brovavir	PO	Herpes simplex virus infection Varicella-zoster virus infection	None yet reported
*CD4, recombinant soluble	IV IM	HIV infection	Local reactions at injection site, fever
Ceftriaxone (Rocephin)	IM IV	Neurosyphilis	Bleeding, bruising, abdominal cramps/pain, diarrhea, melena, fever, bronchospasm, hypotension, Stevens-Johnson syndrome, decreased urine output, skin rash, joint pain, itching, redness, swelling, seizures, thrombophlebitis, pseudolithiasis
Chloramphenicol (Anocol) (Chloromycetin)	PO IM IV	Salmonellosis	Blood dyscrasias, abdominal distention, blue–gray skin color, low body temperature, difficulty in breathing, coma, cardiovascular collapse, skin, rash, fever, confusion, delirium, headache, loss of vision, paresthesias, extremity weakness, diarrhea, nausea, vomiting, pale skin, sore throat, bleeding
Chlorhexidine gluconate Oral Rinse (Peridex)	Oral Rinse	Prophylaxis for thrush	Change in taste, increased tartar, staining of teeth, fillings, and dentures, mouth irritation
Cimetidine (Tagamet)	PO	HIV infection	Diarrhea, headache
Ciprofloxacin (Cipro)	PO	*Mycobacterium avium* complex infection	Restlessness, tremors, seizures, crystalluria, blood in urine, dysuria, low back pain, skin rash, itching, redness, swelling of face or neck, joint pains, stiffness, visual disturbances, photosensitivity, dizziness, headache, abdominal pain, diarrhea, nausea, vomiting, insomnia, unpleasant taste in mouth
Cisplatin (Platinol) (Platinol-AQ)	IV	Cervical cancer	Leukopenia, thrombocytopenia, anemia, nephrotoxicity, ototoxicity
Clarithromycin (Biaxin)	PO	*Mycobacterium avium* complex infection	Nausea, vomiting, headache, rash, hearing loss, hepatotoxicity, abnormal taste, diarrhea, stomach pain or discomfort
Clindamycin (Cleocin)	PO IM IV	Toxoplasmosis Pneumocystosis	Pseudomembranous colitis, skin rash, neutropenia, thrombocytopenia, abdominal pain, nausea and vomiting, diarrhea, fungal growth
Clofazimine (Lamprene)	PO	*Mycobacterium avium* complex infection	Colicky or burning abdominal or stomach pain, nausea, vomiting, pink or red to brownish black discoloration of skin (two suicides have been reported as a result of mental depression secondary to skin discoloration), visual changes, gastrointestinal bleeding, hepatitis or jaundice, dry rough scaly skin, anorexia, dizziness, drowsiness, dryness, burning, itching, or irritation of eyes, skin rash, photosensitivity
Clotrimazole (Mycelex Troches)	PO	Candidiasis (oropharyngeal)	Abdominal or stomach cramping or pain, diarrhea, nausea or vomiting
*CMV Immune globulin	IV	Cytomegalovirus	Flushing, chills, muscle cramps, back pain, fever, nausea and vomiting, wheezing
Colony-stimulating factors (Leukine) (Neupogen)	IV SC	Neutropenia	Hypersensitivity reactions (urticaria, angioedema, bronchoconstriction, anaphylaxis), fever, chills, rigors, bone pain, arthralgias, adult respiratory distress syndrome, rash, pericarditis, local erythema at site of injection, hypoxia

TABLE 58–15. **Drugs Used to Treat HIV Infection and AIDS-Related Conditions (*Under Investigation)** *Continued*

Generic Name (Trade Name)	Route of Administration	Indications	Side/Adverse Effects
Cyclophosphamide (Cytoxan) (Neosar)	PO IM IV	Non-Hodgkin's lymphoma	Missing menstrual cycles, darkening of skin and fingernails, loss of appetite, nausea, vomiting, diarrhea, stomach pain, flushing and redness of face, headache, increased sweating, swollen lips, skin rash, hives, loss of hair
Cycloserine (Seromycin)	PO	*Mycobacterium avium* complex infection *Mycobacterium tuberculosis*	Anxiety, confusion, dizziness, drowsiness, increased irritability, increased restlessness, mental depression, muscle twitching or trembling, nervousness, nightmares, other mood or mental changes, speech problems, skin rash, numbness, tingling, burning pain or weakness in the hands or feet, headache, seizures
Cytarabine (Ara-C) (Cytosine arabinoside) (Cytosar-U)	PO IM IV	Non-Hodgkin's lymphoma Progressive multifocal leukoencephalopathy	Fever, chills, cough, hoarseness, lower back or side pain, difficult urination, diarrhea, sores in mouth or on lips, unusual bleeding or bruising, numbness or tingling in fingers, toes or face, unusual tiredness, swelling of feet or lower legs, pain at injection site, skin rash, reddened eyes, chest pain, shortness of breath, itching of skin, headache
Dapsone (Avlosulfon) (DDS)	PO	Pneumocystosis	Hemolytic anemia, Stevens-Johnson syndrome, agranulocytosis (fever and sore throat), hepatic damage, methoglobinemia (bluish fingernails, lips, or skin, fatigue, dyspnea), mood changes, peripheral neuritis
Dextroamphetamine (Dexedrine)	PO	HIV dementia	Restlessness, tremor, hyperactivity, insomnia, dizziness, headache, chills, dysphoria, tachycardia, palpitations, hypertension, hypotension, nausea, vomiting, cramps, dry mouth, diarrhea, constipation, metallic taste, anorexia, weight loss, urticaria, impotence, altered libido
*Diclazuril	PO	Cryptosporidiosis	Nausea, vomiting, fever, flu-like symptoms
Didanosine (ddl) (Videx)	PO	HIV infection	Diarrhea, abdominal pain, pancreatitis, peripheral neuropathy, seizures, headaches, abnormal bone marrow function, abnormal liver function, electrolyte abnormalities, cardiac arrhythmias, allergic reactions
Doxorubicin hydrochloride (Adriamycin)	IV	Kaposi's sarcoma Non-Hodgkin's lymphoma	Leukopenia or infection (fever, chills, sore throat), stomatitis, esophagitis, flank, stomach, or joint pain, pain at infusion site, peripheral edema, fast or irregular heartbeat, shortness of breath, gastrointestinal bleeding, thrombocytopenia (unusual bleeding or bruising), changes in skin color, diarrhea, nausea, vomiting, skin rash or itching, hair loss, reddish color to urine
Dronabinol (Marinol)	PO	HIV wasting	Irritability, insomnia, restlessness, hot flashes, sweating, rhinnorhea, loose stools, hiccups, anorexia, tachycardia, mood changes, confusion, personality changes, hallucinations, depression, nervousness, anxiety, dry mouth, vision changes, hypotension
Epoetin alpha, recombinant (Epogen) (Eprex) (Procrit)	IV SC	Anemia associated with HIV infection or zidovudine therapy	Chest pain, edema, tachycardia, headache, hypertension, polycythemia, seizures, shortness of breath, skin rash, arthralgias, asthenia, diarrhea, nausea, fatigue, flu-like syndrome after each dose *Note:* Should be temporarily discontinued if the hematocrit reaches or exceeds 36%

Table continued on following page

TABLE 58–15. **Drugs Used to Treat HIV Infection and AIDS-Related Conditions (*Under Investigation)** *Continued*

Generic Name (Trade Name)	Route of Administration	Indications	Side/Adverse Effects
Ethambutol (Myambutol)	PO	*Mycobacterium avium* complex infection *Mycobacterium tuberculosis*	Acute gout, chills, pain and swelling of joints, skin rash, fever, arthralgias, numbness, tingling, burning pain, weakness of hands or feet, blurred vision, eye pain, red–green color blindness, any loss of vision, abdominal pain, anorexia, nausea, vomiting, headache, mental confusion
Ethionamide (Trecator-SC)	PO	*Mycobacterium avium* complex infection *Mycobacterium tuberculosis*	Yellow skin and eyes, tingling, burning, or pain in hands or feet, mental depression, clumsiness or unsteadiness, confusion, mood or mental changes, changes in menstrual periods, coldness, decreased sexual ability, dry puffy skin, weight gain, hyperglycemia, blurred vision or loss of vision, skin rash
Etoposide (VePesid)	IV	Kaposi's sarcoma Non-Hodgkin's lymphoma	Leukopenia, thrombocytopenia, stomatitis, ataxia, paresthesias, tachycardia, shortness of breath or wheezing, pain at site of injection, nausea, vomiting and loss of appetite, diarrhea, fatigue, loss of hair
Fluconazole (Diflucan)	PO IV	Candidiasis Cryptococcosis	Abnormal liver function, Stevens-Johnson syndrome, nausea, headache, skin rash, vomiting, abdominal pain, diarrhea
Flucytosine (Ancobon) (5-Fluorocytosine) (5FC)	PO	Candidiasis Cryptococcosis	Anemia, yellow eyes or skin, skin rash, redness, itching, sore throat, fever, unusual bleeding or bruising, confusion, sensitivity to sunlight, abdominal pain, diarrhea, loss of appetite, nausea, vomiting, dizziness, lightheadedness, drowsiness, headache
Foscarnet sodium (Foscavir)	IV	Cytomegalovirus infection Herpes simplex virus infection HIV infection	Increased thirst, headaches, nausea, anorexia, flank pain, muscle twitching, elevated creatinine, mild proteinuria, renal failure, decrease in calcium, hyperphosphatemia, fatigue, irritability, tremors, seizures, genital ulcers
Ganciclovir (Cytovene) (formerly known as DHPG)	PO IV Intravitreal implants	Cytomegalovirus infection	Granulocytopenia, thrombocytopenia, anemia, mood changes, tremors, nervousness, fever, skin rash, abnormal liver function, phlebitis, abdominal pain, loss of appetite, nausea, vomiting
*Gentamicin liposome injection	IV	*Mycobacterium avium* complex infection	Urinary frequency, increased thirst, anorexia, nausea, vomiting, muscle twitching, paresthesias, seizures, impaired hearing, itching, skin rash, impaired vision
*gp 120 vaccines *gp 160 vaccines	IM	Preventive, therapeutic, and perinatal vaccines	Malaise, myalgia, headache, fever, tenderness and induration at injection site
*Human growth hormone (Humatrope) (Protropin)	SC	Immunomodulation	Sodium and water retention, edema, carpal tunnel syndrome, increased intracranial pressure
*Hypericin	IV	HIV infection	Elevated liver function tests, photosensitivity, paresthesias
Interferon alpha recombinant (Intron-A) (Roferon-A) (Kemron) (Alferon)	IM SC PO	HIV infection Kaposi's sarcoma	Parenteral: flu-like syndrome (fever, myalgias, and malaise), leukopenia, elevation in liver enzymes, weight loss, hair loss, fatigue, proteinuria, reversible congestive cardiomyopathy (weight gain and signs of right- or left-sided congestive heart failure) Oral: no side effects have been reported with low-dose oral interferon alpha

TABLE 58–15. **Drugs Used to Treat HIV Infection and AIDS-Related Conditions (*Under Investigation)** *Continued*

Generic Name (Trade Name)	Route of Administration	Indications	Side/Adverse Effects
*Interleukin-2 recombinant	IV	HIV infection	Fluid retention, hypotension, fever, chills, elevated creatinine, elevated blood urea nitrogen, oliguria, anuria, azotemia, fatigue, weight gain, tachycardia, nausea, vomiting, transient changes in liver function studies, headache, lightheadedness, dizziness, mental changes, pulmonary symptoms, anemia, leukocytosis, skin rash, myalgia, arthralgia
Isoniazid (INH) (Isotamine) Laniazid) (Nydrazid) (Tubizid)	PO IM	*Mycobacterium avium* complex infection *Mycobacterium tuberculosis*	Loss of appetite, nausea, vomiting, diarrhea, unusual tiredness or weakness, dark urine, yellow eyes and skin, clumsiness or unsteadiness, numbness, tingling, burning or pain in hands or feet, fever, sore throat, unusual bleeding or bruising, skin rash, pain at injection site, arthralgia, seizures, depression, psychosis, blurred vision with or without eye pain
Itraconazole (Sporanox)	PO	Maintenance therapy for: Cryptococcosis Histoplasmosis	Nausea, vomiting, headaches, fatigue, abdominal cramps, rash, loss of potassium, edema, diarrhea, anorexia, fever, dizziness, pruritus, hypotension, hypokalemia, elevated liver enzymes, impotence
Kanamycin sulfate (Kantrex)	IV IM PO	Drug-resistant tuberculosis	*See* Amikacin
Ketoconazole (Nizoral)	PO	Candidiasis	Hepatitis, nausea, vomiting, diarrhea, dizziness, drowsiness, gynecomastia, headache, skin rash, itching, impotence, insomnia, photophobia
*Lamivudine	PO	HIV infection	Neutropenia, rash, insomnia, fever, headache, fatigue, diarrhea, vasculitis, photophobia, paresthesias
*Letrazuril	PO	Cryptosporidiosis	Nausea, vomiting, rash
Liposyn III–2%	IV	HIV wasting	Fever, chills, sore throat, dyspnea, hives, anemia, chest pain, cyanosis, diarrhea, flushing, dizziness, nausea, vomiting, thrombocytopenia, jaundice
Leucovorin (Citrovorum) (Folinic acid) (Wellcovorin)	PO IM IV	Prophylaxis and treatment of toxic effects related to: Methotrexate Pyrimethamine Trimethoprim	Skin rash, hives, itching, wheezing
Megestrol acetate (Megace)	PO	HIV wasting	Alteration of menstrual pattern with unpredictable bleeding, pain in chest, visual disturbances, headache, insomnia, pain in abdomen, groin, calf, or leg, loss of coordination, slurred speech, weakness or numbness in extremities, yellow eyes and skin, depression, skin rashes, peripheral edema, brown spots in skin, acne, increased body hair, increased breast tenderness, loss of scalp hair
Methotrexate (Folex) (Folex PFS) (Mexate) (Mexate-AQ)	PO IM IV	Non-Hodgkin's lymphoma	Gastrointestinal ulceration or bleeding, enteritis, intestinal perforation, leukopenia, bacterial infections, septicemia, thrombocytopenia, stomatitis, renal failure, azotemia, hyperuricemia, nephropathy, cutaneous vasculitis, hepatotoxicity, pulmonary fibrosis, pneumonitis, central nervous system toxicity, anorexia, nausea, vomiting, acne, boils, skin rash
Methylphenidate PMS-methylphenidate (Ritalin)	PO	HIV dementia	Tachycardia, hypertension, chest pain, tremors, allergic reactions, anemia, blurred vision, convulsions, leukopenia, agitation, confusion, anorexia, nervousness, insomnia, headache, nausea, vomiting, stomach pain

Table continued on following page

TABLE 58–15. **Drugs Used to Treat HIV Infection and AIDS-Related Conditions (*Under Investigation)** *Continued*

Generic Name (Trade Name)	Route of Administration	Indications	Side/Adverse Effects
Mexiletine (Mexitil)	PO	HIV peripheral neuropathy	Chest pain, rapid or irregular heart beats (premature ventricular contractions), shortness of breath, leukopenia, thrombocytopenia, dizziness, lightheadedness, tremors, ataxia, heartburn, nausea, vomiting, confusion, impaired vision, headache, diarrhea, constipation, tinnitus, rash, insomnia, slurred speech
Miconazole (Micatin) (Monistat Derm) (Monistat IV)	PO IM IV Topical	Candidiasis Coccidioidomycosis Cryptococcosis	Fever, chills, skin rash, itching, redness, swelling at injection site, unusual tiredness, weakness, unusual bleeding or bruising, anorexia, diarrhea, nausea, vomiting
Mitomycin (Mutamycin)	IV	Cervical cancer	Leukopenia, thrombocytopenia, pneumopathy, nephrotoxicity, stomatitis
*Nevirapine	PO	HIV infection	Rash, thrombocytopenia, fever
Nimodipine (Nimotop)	PO	HIV dementia	Decreased blood pressure
Nystatin (Mycostatin) (Nilstat) (Nystex)	PO	Candidiasis (oropharyngeal)	Diarrhea, nausea, vomiting, stomach pain
Octreotide (Sandostatin)	SC	HIV-related diarrhea	Hyperglycemia, hypoglycemia, abdominal pain, diarrhea, nausea, vomiting, pain at injection site, headache, fatigue, dizziness, lightheadedness, edema, flushing of face, hepatic dysfunction
*Oxandrolone	PO	HIV wasting	Anabolic steroid side effects, masculinizing effects in women (facial hair growth, deepened voice), feminizing effects in men (breast development), edema, jaundice, hepatic carcinoma, nausea, vomiting
Paromomycin sulfate (Humatin) (Aminosidine)	PO	Cryptosporidiosis	Nausea, vomiting, diarrhea, renal damage
Pentamidine isethionate (Nebupent, inhalation) (Pentam parenteral)	IM IV Inhalation	Pneumocystosis	Parenteral: blood dyscrasias, rapid and irregular pulse, diabetes mellitus, skin rash, hyperglycemia, hypoglycemia, hypotension, pain or tenderness at site of injection, redness or flushing of face, metallic taste in mouth Inhalation: chest pain, congestion, coughing, dyspnea, pharyngitis, wheezing, skin rash, metallic taste in mouth, pneumothorax
*Peptide T	SC Intranasal	Immunomodulation HIV dementia Neuropathy	None reported yet
*PMEA	IV	HIV infection	None reported yet
Prednisone (Deltasone) (Meticorten) (Orasone) (Prednicen-M) (Sterapred)	PO	HIV myopathy *Pneumocystis carinii* pneumonia (as adjunctive therapy)	Allergic reaction, rectal irritation, bleeding, impaired vision, diabetes mellitus, psychic disturbances, skin problems, muscle cramping, delayed wound healing, infection
Pyrazinamide (PZA)	PO	*Mycobacterium tuberculosis*	Joint pain, loss of appetite, unusual tiredness or weakness, yellow eyes and skin, swelling of joints, itching rash, nausea
Pyrimethamine (Daraprim)	PO	Pneumocytosis Toxoplasmosis	Folic acid deficiency (loss of taste, glossitis, diarrhea, sore throat, dysphagia, ulcerative stomatitis), fever, bleeding, bruising, fatigue, skin rash, trembling, unsteadiness or clumsiness, seizures, anorexia, vomiting
Rifabutin (Ansamycin)	PO	*Mycobacterium avium* complex infection (for prophylaxis and treatment of disease)	Increase in both liver enzymes and creatinine, rash, fever, leukopenia, gastrointestinal distress, hemolysis, arthralgias

TABLE 58–15. **Drugs Used to Treat HIV Infection and AIDS-Related Conditions (*Under Investigation)** *Continued*

Generic Name (Trade Name)	Route of Administration	Indicators	Side/Adverse Effects
Rifampin (Rifadin) (Rifadin IV) (Rimactane)	PO IV	*Mycobacterium avium* complex infection *Mycobacterium tuberculosis*	Chills, difficult breathing, dizziness, fever, headache, muscle and bone pain, shivering, rash, itching, skin redness, sore throat, yellow eyes and skin, unusual bleeding or bruising, loss of appetite, nausea, vomiting, unusual tiredness or weakness, bloody or cloudy urine, stomach cramps, diarrhea, sore mouth or tongue, discoloration of urine, feces, sputum, sweat, or tears
*SP303T	Topical	Herpes simplex virus infection	None yet reported
*Spiramycin	PO IV	Cryptosporidiosis	Parenteral: paresthesias, irritation at injection site, dysesthesia, giddiness, pain, stiffness, burning sensation, hot flashes Oral: nausea, vomiting, diarrhea, fatigue, indigestion, sweating, heaviness in the chest, cool sensation in mouth or pharynx
Stavudine (Zerit) (formerly known as d4T)	PO	HIV infection	Peripheral neuropathy, hepatotoxicity, anemia, headache, nausea
Sulfadoxine and pyrimethamine (Fansidar)	PO	Pneumocystosis	Stevens-Johnson syndrome, toxic epidermal necrolysis, fulminant hepatic necrosis, agranulocytosis, aplastic anemia, photosensitivity, bleeding or bruising, folic acid deficiency (loss of taste, glossitis, diarrhea, sore throat, dysphagia, ulcerative stomatitis), skin rash, fatigue, aching in joints or muscles, hematuria, dysuria, goiter, tremors, seizures, headache, dizziness, nausea, vomiting
Sulfamethoxazole and trimethoprim (Bactrim) (Bethaprim) (Cheragan W/TMP) (Cotrim) (Septra) (Sulfamethoprim) (Sulfaprim) (Sulfatrim) (Sulfoxaprim) (Triazole)) (Uroplus)	PO IV	Isosporiasis Pneumocystosis Salmonellosis Toxoplasmosis	Skin rash, itching, Stevens-Johnson syndrome (myalgia, arthralgia, redness, blistering, peeling or loosening of the skin, extreme fatigue), dysphagia, fever, leukopenia (sore throat), thrombocytopenia (unusual bleeding or bruising), hepatitis (dark urine, pale stools, yellow skin and sclerae), crystalluria, hematuria, diarrhea, dizziness, headache, anorexia, nausea, vomiting
Sulfamethoxazole (Gantanol)	PO	Toxoplasmosis	Fever, itching, skin rash, hepatitis, photosensitivity, blood dyscrasias, difficulty in swallowing, redness, blistering, peeling of skin, hematuria, crystalluria, thyroid dysfunction, dizziness, headache, anorexia, nausea, vomiting, diarrhea
Sulfisoxazole (Gantrisin)	PO	Toxoplasmosis	Fever, itching, skin rash, hepatitis, photosensitivity, blood dyscrasias, difficulty in swallowing, redness, blistering, peeling of skin, hematuria, crystalluria, thyroid dysfunction, dizziness, headache, anorexia, nausea, vomiting, diarrhea
Taxol (Paclitaxel) (Taxol A)	IV	Kaposi's sarcoma	Neutropenia, thrombocytopenia, headache, fatigue, peripheral neuropathy, bradycardia, nausea, vomiting, diarrhea, mucositis, hair loss, arthralgia, fever, taste alterations, urticaria, rashes
Testosterone	PO IM	Depression Muscle wasting	In females: menstrual irregularities, deepened voice, excessive hair growth In males: bladder irritability, breast soreness, frequent or continuing erections

Table continued on following page

TABLE 58–15. **Drugs Used to Treat HIV Infection and AIDS-Related Conditions (*Under Investigation)** *Continued*

Generic Name (Trade Name)	Route of Administration	Indicators	Side/Adverse Effects
			Both sexes: edema, dizziness, headache, fatigue, flushing or redness of skin, bleeding, nausea, vomiting, yellowing of eyes and skin, itching, diarrhea, redness or pain at injection site
*Thalidomide	PO	Immunomodulation	Sedation, severe congenital abnormalities in developing fetuses, neurotoxicity
*Thymic humoral factor	IM	Immunomodulation	Pain on injection, redness, swelling, fatigue, mental fogginess
*Thymopentin	SC	Immunomodulation	Respiratory congestion, pain at injection site, headache, sleep disorders, fatigue, gastrointestinal side effects, pruritus, elevated liver enzymes
*TNP-470	IV	Kaposi's sarcoma	Anorexia, anemia, thrombocytopenia, neutropenia, seizures, ataxia, hemorrhages in lung, brain, and retina, abnormal liver function
Trimethoprim (Proloprim) (Trimpex)	PO	Salmonellosis	Blood dyscrasias (bleeding), headache, methemoglobinemia, skin rash, itching, alteration in taste, sore mouth or tongue, anorexia, diarrhea, nausea, vomiting, abdominal pain, cramping
Trimetrexate glucuronate (Neutrexim)	IV	Pneumocystosis	Decrease in neutrophil and platelet counts, nausea, vomiting, diarrhea, reversible liver function abnormalities, skin rash, fever, mucositis, abdominal pain, kidney damage
Vinblastine (Velban) (Velsar)	IV	Kaposi's sarcoma	Fever, chills, cough, hoarseness, lower back pain, side pain, painful or difficult urination, pain or redness at site of injection, sores in mouth and on lips, rectal bleeding, dizziness, difficulty in walking, double vision, drooping eyelids, headache, jaw pain, mental depression, numbness or tingling in fingers and toes, pain in fingers or toes, pain in testicles, weakness, nausea, vomiting, loss of hair
Vincristine (Oncovin) (Vincasar PES) (Vincrex)	IV	Kaposi's sarcoma Non-Hodgkin's lymphoma Cervical cancer	Constipation, stomach cramps, bed-wetting, decrease or increase in urination, dizziness, lightheadness, dysuria, lack of sweating, joint pain, lower back or flank pain, visual changes, ataxia, drooping eyelids, headache, jaw pain, numbness or tingling in fingers or toes, pain in testicles, weakness, hyponatremia, leukopenia, thrombocytopenia, stomatitis Syndrome of inappropriate antidiuretic hormone evidenced by agitation, confusion, dizziness, hallucinations, anorexia, mental depression, seizures, insomnia, loss of consciousness
*Wobenzym	PO	Immunomodulation	
Zalcitabine (HIVID) (ddC)	PO	HIV infection	Pancreatitis, peripheral neuropathy, oral aphthous ulcers, fever, rash, stomatitis
Zidovudine (Retrovir) (formerly known as AZT)	PO IV	HIV infection	Anemia, leukopenia, neutropenia, platelet count changes (either increased or decreased), anorexia, asthenia, diarrhea, dizziness, fever, headache, nausea, insomnia, malaise, myalgia, pain in abdomen, rash, somnolence, taste alteration

Abbreviations: IM, intramuscular; IV, intravenous; PO, oral; SC, subcutaneous.

Sources: American Foundation for AIDS Research. (1993). Opportunistic infections and related disorders. *AIDS/HIV treatment directory*, 4(4), 1–108; United States Pharmacopeial Convention, Inc. (1994). *USPDI* (Vol. I) (14th ed.). Rockville, MD: The Convention.

Table reproduced from Flaskerud, J. H., Ungvarski, P. J. (1995). Appendix III: Drugs used to treat HIV infection and AIDS-related conditions. In J. H. Flaskerud & P. J. Ungvarski (Eds.), *HIV/AIDS: A guide to nursing care* (3rd ed., pp. 495–511). Philadelphia: W. B. Saunders.

TABLE 58–16. **Primary Prevention: Health History Taking to Identify People at Risk for HIV Disease**

A. Social history
  1. Sexual activities
    a. Absolutely safe behavior: abstinence or mutually monogamous with a noninfected partner
    b. Very safe behavior: noninsertive sexual practices
    c. Probably safe behavior: insertive sexual practices with the use of condoms and spermicide
    d. Risky behavior: everything else
    e. Use of condoms (both male and female), including application, removal, use of lubricants, and difference in condom efficacy
    f. Engaging in sex with multiple partners
    g. Use of mood-affecting drugs before or during sexual activities
    h. Determination of whether HIV disease has been diagnosed in anyone with whom the client has had sex
  2. Use of mood-affecting drugs
    a. Drugs such as alcohol, marijuana, cocaine, crack, LSD, methaqualone (Quaalude), amphetamines, barbiturates, tranquilizers, amyl or butyl nitrate (called "poppers"), and heroin
    b. Route of administration: oral, inhalation (including sniffing, snorting, and smoking), intravenous, or subcutaneous ("skin popping")
    c. Any current or previous treatment for substance abuse
  3. Needle exposure
    a. Use of drugs via intravenous route, and sharing of needles, syringes, and other drug paraphernalia
    b. Other needle-exposure activities such as application of tattoos, acupuncture, treatment by "folk doctors" or other unlicensed individuals, or sharing of prescribed drugs between friends
    c. Determination of whether HIV disease has been diagnosed in anyone with whom client has shared needles
  4. Occupational history
    a. Client's occupation and responsibilities in relation to risk potential for HIV exposure
    b. Any exposure of the client to HIV
    c. The type of health care follow-up that the client has pursued since exposure
    d. The client's knowledge level regarding the signs and symptoms of seroconversion and the need for follow-up
  5. Travel
    a. Within the past 10 years
    b. Sexual activities when traveling in areas where the number of AIDS cases is high, such as New York, California, New Jersey, Texas, or Florida, or countries such as Haiti or Zaire
    c. Treatment of illnesses while traveling
    d. Immigration history and potential exposures in country of origin

B. Medication history: current or previous use of medication that suppresses the immune system, such as steroids; current treatment of chemical dependence if applicable

C. Medical history
  1. Major diseases including (but not limited to) tuberculosis; hepatitis A, B, C, or D; mononucleosis; and hemophilia; receiving treatment with clotting replacements such as factor VIII
  2. Treatment for psychiatric/emotional disorders
  3. Transfusion donor or recipient

D. Surgical history

E. Childhood illnesses, including (but not limited to) varicella; immunization history

F. Sexually transmitted diseases, including (but not limited to) syphilis; gonorrhea; amebiasis; herpes simplex (herpes labialis or herpes genitalis); *Giardia lamblia* enteritis; and *Chlamydia* infection

G. Review of systems
  1. General: a comment from the client concerning a self-appraisal of his or her current state of health should be elicited
  2. Skin: eruptions, lesions, itching, dryness, redness, rashes, lumps, color changes, changes in hair or nails
  3. Head: headaches, lightheadedness, other sensations
  4. Eyes: blurred vision, diplopia, loss of visual fields, "floaters"
  5. Ears: impaired hearing, tinnitus
  6. Nose and sinuses: obstruction, pain, discharges, nosebleed, chronic infections
  7. Mouth and throat: creamy white patches, lesions, bleeding gums, dysphagia, odynophagia, changes in taste, sore throat
  8. Respiratory tract: dyspnea with or without certain activities, coughing, wheezing, chest pain, "cold" or "flulike" symptoms; date and results of last chest x-ray examination and tuberculin test
  9. Cardiovascular system: chest pain, palpitations, edema, known hypertension or hypotension
  10. Gastrointestinal tract: changes in appetite, involuntary weight loss, abdominal pain or cramping, changes in bowel habits, loose stools, diarrhea, blood in stool, rectal and perianal pain and itching
  11. Genitourinary system: dysuria, nocturia, pain, itching, discharges, lesions
  12. Gynecologic concerns: changes in menstruation, dyspareunia, vaginal discharge, breast abnormalities, obstetric history, abortions, chronic infections
  13. Musculoskeletal system: arthralgia, myalgia
  14. Neurologic and emotional concerns: loss of memory, nervousness, personality changes, confusional states, stiff neck, photophobia, tremors, paresthesias, seizures, syncope
  15. Endocrine system: polyuria, polyphagia, polydipsia, fevers, night sweats
  16. Hematopoietic changes: lymphadenopathy, bruising or bleeding, history of anemia

From Ungvarski, P. J., & Schmidt, J. (1995). Nursing management of the adult client. In J. H. Flaskerud & P. J. Ungvarski (Eds.), *HIV/AIDS: A guide to nursing care* (3rd ed., pp. 138–139, Table 5-1). Philadelphia: W. B. Saunders.

TABLE 58–17. **Secondary Prevention: Baseline Physical Examination of the HIV-Infected Client**

A. General: weight, height, temperature, respiratory rate, pulse, blood pressure
B. Neurologic examination
  1. Cerebral functions: impaired cognitive functions, decreased level of consciousness, anger, inattentiveness, depression, denial
  2. Cranial nerve (CN) examination
    a. CN II (optic nerve): papilledema, white retinal spots, yellow-white retinal infiltrates, retinal hemorrhage, visual field deficiencies, blurred vision
    b. CNs III, IV, VI (oculomotor, trochlear, abducens nerves): impaired extraocular movements, unequal pupils, diplopia, ptosis, nystagmus
    c. CN V (trigeminal nerve): photophobia
    d. CN VII (facial nerve): hemiparesis
    e. CN VIII (acoustic nerve): tinnitus, vertigo, impaired hearing
    f. CNs IX, X (glossopharyngeal and vagus nerves): dysphagia, dysarthria
  3. Motor examination: motor weakness, hemiparesis, paraparesis
  4. Sensory examination: dysesthesias, paresthesias, areas of anesthesia
  5. Cerebellar examination: ataxia, dysmetria, tremors
  6. Reflexes: abnormal reflexes, positive Babinski's sign
  7. Meningeal signs: nuchal rigidity, Brudzinski's sign, Kernig's sign
C. Mouth and throat examination: lesions, discoloration, exudates
D. Cardiovascular examination
  1. Heart: disturbances in cardiac rate and rhythm, presence of pericardial friction rub
  2. Peripheral vascular system: edema, decrease in peripheral pulse(s)
E. Respiratory examination: tachypnea, lag of excursion on palpation, dullness to percussion, presence of rales (crackles) or rhonchi (wheezes)
F. Lymphatic examination: lymphadenopathy
G. Abdominal examination: masses, tenderness, hepatomegaly, splenomegaly, hyperactive bowel sounds
H. Breast examination: lesions, masses, discoloration, tenderness, discharges
I. Examination of genitalia (both men and women) and perianal region: lesions, discharges
J. Musculoskeletal examination: pain on range of motion, evidence of muscle wasting
K. Skin examination: lesions or discolorations, dryness, thinning of hair, alopecia

From Ungvarski, P. J., & Schmidt, J. (1995). Nursing management of the adult client. In J. H. Flaskerud & P. J. Ungvarski (Eds.), *HIV/AIDS: A guide to nursing care* (3rd ed., p. 139, Table 5-2). Philadelphia: W. B. Saunders.

A few years ago, AIDS patients were not managed for nutritional impairments as aggressively as they are now. Since protein–calorie malnutrition has been demonstrated to be an independent predictor of death, much has been done to improve nutrition-related services (Kotler et al., 1989b). This development, coupled with more treatment options for opportunistic infections and a growing sophistication about nutritional support for patients with HIV illness (Bradley-Springer, 1991), has wrought substantial change in a few short years.

AIDS Dementia Complex

At least 65% of AIDS patients undergo clinically significant progressive dementia (Navia et al., 1986) and changes consistent with dementia are present in 90% of autopsied patients (de la Monte et al., 1987). AIDS dementia complex is thought to be a direct result of HIV infection of the brain. Although the brain is infected by HIV from the time of the patient's initial seroconversion from HIV negative to HIV positive, patients are asymptomatic until their T4-cell levels drop. AIDS dementia complex may be the first manifestation of AIDS, but usually occurs with other AIDS-defining ailments. It is a progressive disease that waxes and wanes. Table 58–13 lists the major signs and symptoms, and Table 58–14 highlights the functional staging system. A battery of neuropsychiatric tests labels the deficits that are not adequately assessed by the standard minimental status examination. Sensitive neuropsychiatric tests include the timed gait test and the nondominant finger tapping test.

Not all patients have moderate to severe dementia. More recently, the terms "HIV-1–associated cognitive/motor disorder" or "HIV-1–related cognitive impairment" have been applied to HIV-infected individuals with subtle or mild cognitive impairment that has not yet progressed to full-blown AIDS dementia complex (Boccellari et al., 1993). Patients who have clinical symptoms have improved on antiretroviral therapy such as AZT and psychostimulants. Cognitive stimulation therapy should be provided along with medication (Ungvarski & Staats, 1994).

PATIENT CARE PLANNING

The care of HIV-infected patients is complex and multifaceted. Patients exhibit a myriad of diseases and symptoms related to HIV itself and to the multiple infections, cancers, and conditions associated with it. Tables 58–15 through 58–18 provide highlights of selected care considerations.

SUMMARY

This chapter has outlined the historical development of HIV disease, its definition, natural history, testing,

TABLE 58–18. **AIDS-Associated Problems and Nursing Care**

Sensory–Perceptual Alterations

Many symptoms may be associated with this nursing diagnosis. They include impaired memory, "slowed" thinking, impaired concentration, dementia, headache, obtundation, confusion, lethargy, impaired vision, blindness, peripheral neuropathy, social isolation, social withdrawal, forgetfulness, or confusion. Etiologic factors to be considered include opportunistic CNS malignancies and infections, HIV infection of the CNS or peripheral nervous system, site-specific opportunistic infection such as CMV retinitis or herpes zoster, the adverse effects of medications, fluid and electrolyte imbalances, metabolic and vascular disruptions, social ostracism, discrimination, and malnutrition.

Blindness/Decreased Visual Acuity

Probable Cause	Special Features	Nursing Interventions
CMV retinitis	May develop suddenly Antiviral intervention should be started as soon as possible to prevent extension of visual loss	Instruct on symptoms Ensure prompt ophthalmic consult on development of initial symptoms
Rare causes of visual disturbances *Toxoplasma gondii* *Cryptococcus neoformans* Mycobacteria / fungi	Many patients cannot remain on ganciclovir due to neutropenia Many patients dread the development of blindness Full rehabilitation is frequently not a realistic goal. The use of a guide dog or proficiency at Braille may never be achieved Medical treatment is life-long Foscarnet therapy was approved by the FDA in 1991	Provide psychosocial and spiritual support Combat social isolation and withdrawal Focus on anxiety and frustatation management Arrange for outpatient or home care infusion therapy Active referrals as appropriate to blind organizations—assocation for the blind occupational retraining programs, home care agencies, Meals on Wheels, mental health professionals Promote assistive devices Talking clocks, books, newspapers, cane, traveling with a sighted person, tactile identification markers Teach measures enhancing independence and safety Fire prevention and response Hygiene and grooming Meal preparation Communication Transportation Housekeeping and laundry

Dementia

Probable Cause	Special Features	Nursing Interventions
HIV *Other causes in a differential diagnosis* CNS malignancy CNS infection Metabolic complications Cerebrovascular complications Adverse effects of medications Malnutrition	Many patients and care partners dread the development of dementia Diagnosis may be difficult to establish. It involves a thorough assessment The vast majority of AIDS patients have some evidence of early-stage dementia ADC patient's symptoms can wax and wane. Progression ensues at a variable rate	Assist with neuropsychiatric assessment and medical evaluation Provide support, guidance for families/friends. Refer for home care, "buddy" volunteer, day care residential living, or respite care as appropriate Patient may need to move to more structured living arrangements Assess need for medication. Administer and supervise (i.e., Haldol, Ativan) as prescribed. Promote timed drug dosage, pill box alarms, checklists Obtain physical therapy consult for gait, assistive devices Use reminder devices: telephone calls, appointment book, "to do" lists, checklists, maps of food store Advocate antiviral research therapy as appropriate Model interactive techniques. Simplify communications and logistics

Table continued on following page

TABLE 58–18. **AIDS-Associated Problems and Nursing Care** *Continued*

Altered Breathing Patterns

Many symptoms may be associated with this nursing diagnosis. The most common are the constellation of signs and symptoms that patients who are contracting PCP demonstrate. They include a fever with a dry, nonproductive cough; chills; exercise intolerance; and dyspnea.

There are other etiologic agents that cause altered breathing patterns in patients with AIDS. The symptoms include productive coughs, wheezing, and dyspnea. These other underlying concerns include bacterial endocarditis with resulting valvular disease, congestive heart failure, CMV pneumonia, KS lesions in the main lung structures, pleural effusion, pneumothoraxes, recurrent bacterial respiratory infections, or tuberculosis.

Cough

Probable Cause	Special Features	Nursing Interventions
PCP *Other common causes of cough* Bacterial mycobacterial, or CMV pneumonia KS lesions in the lungs Pneumothorax	Those HIV-infected patients, whose T-cell count is below 300, are most at risk for PCP Symptoms may worsen during first days of treatment for PCP Bactrim and aerosolized pentamidine treatments are used to prevent PCP episodes	Instruct patients on initial symptoms and signs of PCP Instruct patient on PCP prophylaxis therapy. Ensure compliance Encourage patient to seek urgent treatment at the initiation of symptoms of PCP Assist in diagnostic work-up (i.e., sputum induction cultures, bronchoscopy) Administer Bactrim, pentamidine, dapsone, Solu-Medrol, or other experimental agent as ordered for PCP

Potential Fluid Volume Deficit: Impaired Tissue Integrity

Many symptoms may be associated with these diagnoses. They include anorexia, nausea, vomiting, candidiasis, oral warts, weight loss, perirectal infections, inability to sustain or gain weight, oral hairy leukoplakia, diarrhea, stomatitis, gingivitis, and marked change in taste. Etiologic factors to be considered include malabsorption, opportunistic cancers or infections, underlying viral infections (CMV, Epstein-Barr, herpes simplex virus), the unrelenting wasting syndrome, and complications due to CNS disease or noncompliance.

Altered Mucous Membranes

Probable Cause	Special Features	Nursing Interventions
Oral candidiasis Vaginal candidiasis *Other common causes of impaired membranes* KS Herpes virus Inadequate mouth care Malnutrition	The development of candidiasis in the asymptomatic, HIV-infected patient signifies progression of illness The development of esophageal candidiasis may be complicated by viral esophageal lesions such as CMV	Normal saline mouth rinses; tub baths. Vitamin A & D ointment to lips. Avoid agents that are drying (i.e., contain alcohol, hydrogen peroxide, Betadine) Use oral irrigation and suction if unable to adequately rinse mouth Administer prescribed oral, vaginal, or systemic antifungal, antiviral, or analgesic medications Oral powder sprays to debride mildly and stimulate circulation if necessary Use rigid oral suction catheter if patient is having difficulty swallowing

Moderate to Severe Diarrhea

Probable Cause	Special Features	Nursing Interventions
Infections, parasitic and viral *Other common causes of diarrhea* Malabsorption KS Other infections, (cryptosporidiosis, *Salmonella, Shigella, Isospora belli*)	Despite aggressive use of antidiarrheals, diarrhea can be unrelenting Extreme diligence in making a diagnosis of a gastrointestinal infection is warranted Nutritional repletion is a vital component of treatment	Assist in aggressive work-up for causative agents Contain diarrhea. Use panty liners, sanitary napkins, adult diapers, ostomy equipment, soft rectal tube, or bed with chamber pot opening ("cholera" bed), depending on severity. Consult with physician before using rectal tube Institute caloric and volume intake and volume output investigation Instruct to clean, rinse, and dry perirectal area after bowel movements Protect perianal skin integrity using Vitamin A & D ointment, Skin Prep, and other skin barriers. Avoid using Stomadhesive-like barriers Reinstruct patient to avoid anal sexual practices Avoid orthostatic hypotension-related syncope Promote hydration

TABLE 58–18. **AIDS-Associated Problems and Nursing Care** *Continued*

Impaired Skin Integrity

Many symptoms may be associated with this diagnosis. They include pruritus, lesions, dryness, rash, skin breakdown with decubitus ulcer formation, wounds, impetigo, psoriasis, xerosis, folliculitis, vasculitis, and dermatitis. Etiologic factors to be considered include contagiosum, *Staphylococcus*, syphilis, herpes simplex virus, and malignancies).

Ulcerative KS Lesions

Probable Cause	Special Features	Nursing Interventions
Terminal-stage illness of AIDS/KS	Lesions are unsightly Healing of wound is not a realistic goal Lymphadenopathy with edema complicates healing process Radiation may assist in palliative and cosmetic improvements	Inform patient to discontinue using make-up to hide KS lesions once they open Clean nondraining, noninfected open lesions. Cover lightly or leave open to air and light Clean open, draining, infected lesions with potassium permanganate soaks followed by normal saline rinse daily. Betadine foam with hydrogen peroxide can be used in place of potassium permanganate If malodorous, use air purifier, air freshener, spirits of peppermint, activated charcoal, vinegar, baking soda, or hospital trash odor control agent, depending on severity Use strips of iodoform Nugauze to pack deep wounds. Use Kerlix to avoid tape contact with skin Maintain wound and skin precautions Simplify dressing technique as much as possible and teach skill to patient or care partner Consult with dermatologist about other measures used Avoid the use of occlusive barrier dressings (e.g., Stomadhesive) which depend on mature neutrophils to clear infection Refer patient to enterostomal therapy nurse's caseload

Pruritus

Probable Cause	Special Features	Nursing Interventions
Infections and underlying systemic, advanced disease	Often, complaints of pruritus have to be solicited	Inform patient that scratching enhances itching. It also leads to escoriated skin with a resultant medium for infection Question patient about the development of pruritus, because it may be a symptom of an underlying infection, drug reaction, or disease Promote hydration, frequent use of emollient creams (i.e., Nivea, Eucerin), tepid water in bathing, and a mild soap (i.e., Dove) Add oil to bath water toward the end of bathing or to moist skin after a shower (i.e., Aveeno) Provide humidified air Use distraction, relaxation, guided imagery, music at night, when pruritus usually worsens Aggressively assist in the treatment of underlying disease to lessen pruritus. Administer antihistamines, antibiotics, or corticosteroids as prescribed

Table continued on following page

TABLE 58–18. **AIDS-Associated Problems and Nursing Care** *Continued*

Body Images Disturbance; Impaired Social Interaction

Many symptoms may be associated with these diagnoses. They may include social isolation, social withdrawal, fearfulness, and body image changes. Etiologic factors to be considered include anxiety; discrimination; stigmatization; generalized weakness; HIV transmission; visible signs of illness; and reaction of family, friends, or society in general.

Body Image Changes

Common Causes	Special Features	Nursing Interventions
KS lesions Premature aging Substantial weight loss	Be sensitive to age of patient May be helpful to compare "before" and "after" photographs to grasp amount of change	Provide psychosocial and spiritual support Discuss the handling of uncomfortable social situations, questions from acquaintances, and stares Facilitate the use of make-up cover for KS lesions if desired Promote the wearing of loosely fitting clothing, turtlenecks, long sleeves, caps, and other camouflaging means if desired Attune yourself to patient's grieving process and feelings of loss

Decreased Socialization

Common Causes	Special Features	Nursing Interventions
Fear of transmission Feelings of uncleanliness Stigmatization Rejection of others Continued substance abuse	Behavior change in these areas is difficult to attain and maintain Group and social network support is advantageous to maintenance of behavior change Education and reinforcement must be ongoing Health care professionals often need professional supervision in these areas due to low knowledge base, cultural insensitivity, and countertransference issues	Reinforce safer sex and drug use teaching Discuss with patient and loved ones specifics of body substance isolation Advocate pregnancy avoidance Refer patient's contacts for HIV testing and counseling Promote the participation in HIV/AIDS support groups. Initiate such a group if needed Encourage maintenance of predisease activities, routine, schedule, network if feasible Confront and guide patient to drug treatment service as needed. Refer to a Twelve-Step anonymous program Familiarize patient with local AIDS advocacy group, governmental departments on discrimination, other community services Form multidisciplinary team to meet patients' and loved ones' needs

Abbreviations: ADC, AIDS dementia complex; CMV, cytomegalovirus; CNS, central nervous system; KS, Kaposi's sarcoma; PCP, *Pneumocystis carinii* pneumonia.

Adapted from McMahon, K. M., & Coyne, N. (1989). Symptom management in patients with AIDS. *Seminars in Oncology Nursing, 5,* 294–298.

many of its clinical manifestations, pharmacologic management, and highlights of nursing care in symptom management. It is an evolving illness, pandemic in nature, requiring tremendous financial, research, care, and social resources. Imposing a relentless assault on the immune system, its attacks become ever stronger if it is given time to ravage—physically, psychologically, financially, and socially—the diseased person and those he or she loves. The human toll cannot be adequately conveyed. However, many patients are living well and living longer. Much of this benefit is due to devoted clinicians and tireless researchers who have prevailed. There remains much pioneering clinical work to be done to put a dent into the needs that are evident. Satisfying intellectual challenge, participation in our century's great human drama, the ability to integrate spiritual, psychological, and biophysical care in alternative practice settings, and an opportunity to contribute on many levels to relieve suffering and help frightened but proud and courageous people with AIDS await these pioneers.

REFERENCES

Amman, A. J. (1984). Immunodeficiency disease. In D. P. Sites, J. D. Stobo, H. H. Fudenberg, et al. (Eds.), *Basic and clinical immunology.* Los Angeles: Lange Medical Publications.

Barnes, P. F., & Barrows, S. A. (1993). Tuberculosis in the 1990s. *Annals of Internal Medicine, 119,* 400–410.

Beldescu, N., Apetrei, R., & Calumfirescu, A. (1990). Nosocomial transmission of HIV in Romania. *Sixth International Conference on AIDS (Abstracts).* TH. C.104, 159.

Beral, V., Peterman, T. A., Berlkelman, R. L., et al. (1990). Kaposi's sarcoma among persons with AIDS: A sexually transmitted infection? *Lancet, 2,* 123–128.

Boccellari, A. A., Dilley, J. W., Chambers, D. B., et al. (1993). Immune function and neuropsychiatric performance in HIV-1-infected homosexual men. *Journal of Acquired Immune Deficiency Syndromes, 6,* 592–601.

Bowen, D., Lane, H., & Fauci, A. (1985). Immunopathogenesis of the acquired immunodeficiency syndrome. *Annals of Internal Medicine, 103,* 704–709.

Bradley-Springer, L. (1991). Nutritional support in HIV infection: A multilevel analysis. *Image, 23*(3), 155–160.

Breimer, L. H. (1984). Did Moriz Kaposi describe AIDS in 1872? *Clio Media, 19*(1–2), 156–158.

Casey, K. M. (1993). Fighting MDR-TB. *RN, 56*(9), 26–30.

Casey, K. M. (1995). Pathophysiology of HIV-1, clinical course and treatment. In J. H. Flaskerud & P. J. Urgvarski (Eds.), *HIV/AIDS: A guide to nursing care* (3rd ed., pp. 64–80). Philadelphia: W. B. Saunders.

Centers for Disease Control and Prevention (CDC). (1981). *Pneumocystis pneumoniae*—Los Angeles. *Morbidity and Mortality Weekly Report, 30,* 250–252.

Centers for Disease Control and Prevention (CDC). (1988a). Quarterly report to the domestic policy council on the prevalence and rate of spread of HIV and AIDS in the United States. *Morbidity and Mortality Weekly Report, 37,* 181–183.

Centers for Disease Control and Prevention (CDC). (1988b). Immunization of children infected with human immunodeficiency virus—supplementary ACIP statement. *Morbidity and Mortality Weekly Report, 37,* 181–183.

Centers for Disease Control and Prevention (CDC). (1988c). Condoms for prevention of sexually transmitted diseases. *Morbidity and Mortality Weekly Report, 37,* 133–137.

Centers for Disease Control and Prevention (CDC). (1988d). Semen banking, organ and tissue transplantation and HIV antibody testing. *Morbidity and Mortality Weekly Report, 37,* 57–58.

Centers for Disease Control and Prevention (CDC). (1994). *HIV/AIDS surveillance report, 5*(4), year-end edition.

Cohen, P. T., Sande, M. A., & Volberding, P. A. (Eds.). (1990). *The AIDS knowledge base.* Waltham, MA: Medical Publishing Group.

Corey, L., & Spear, P. G. (1986). Infection with herpes simplex virus. *New England Journal of Medicine, 314,* 686–691.

De Cock, K. M., Adjorlolo, G., Ekpini, E., et al. (1993). Epidemiology and transmission of HIV-2: Why there is no HIV-2 pandemic. *Journal of the American Medical Association, 270,* 2083–2086.

de la Monte, S. M., Ho, D. D., Schooley, R. T., et al. (1987). Subacute encephalomyelitis of AIDS and its relation to HTLV-III infection. *Neurology, 37,* 562–569.

Des Prez, R. M., & Heim, C. R. (1990). *Mycobacterium tuberculosis.* In G. L. Mandell, R. G. Douglas, Jr., & J. E. Bennett (Eds.), *Principles and practices of infectious disease* (3rd ed., pp. 1877–1906). New York: Churchill-Livingstone.

Division of Tuberculosis Control, Centers for Disease Control and American Thoracic Society. (1990). *National tuberculosis training initiative: Core curriculum on tuberculosis.* New York: American Lung Association.

Elbeik, T., & Feinberg, M. B. (1994). HIV isolation and quantitation methods. In P. T. Cohen, M. A. Sande, & P. A. Volberding (Eds.), *The AIDS knowledge base: A textbook on HIV disease from the University of California, San Francisco, and the San Francisco General Hospital* (2nd ed., pp. 2.4-1–2.4-19). Boston: Little, Brown & Co.

Favero, M. (1987, May). *AIDS.* Paper presented at 18th National Symposium, American Nephrology Nurses Association, New York.

Friedman-Kien, A. E., Ostreich, R., & Saltzman, B. (1989). Clinical manifestations of classical, endemic African, and epidemic AIDS-associated Kaposi's sarcoma. In A. E. Friedman-Kien (Ed.), *Color atlas of AIDS* (pp. 11–48). Philadelphia: W. B. Saunders.

Friedman-Kien, A. E., Saltzman, B. R., Mirabile, M., et al. (1990). Kaposi's sarcoma in HIV-negative homosexual men [letter]. *Lancet, 335,* 168–169.

Gail, M. H., Pluda, J. M., Rabkin, C. S., et al. (1991). Projections of the incidence of non-Hodgkin's lymphoma related to acquired immunodeficiency syndrome. *Journal of the National Cancer Institute, 83,* 695–701.

Gallo, R. C. (1987). The AIDS virus. *Scientific American, 256*(1), 46–56.

Gellin, B., & Soave, R. (1992). Coccidian infections in AIDS: Toxoplasmosis, cryptosporidiosis and isosporiasis. *Medical Clinics of North America, 76,* 205–234.

Gold, J. W. M., & Armstrong, D. (1989). Opportunistic infections in AIDS patients. In P. Ma & D. Armstrong (Eds.), *AIDS and infections of homosexual men* (2nd ed., pp. 325–335). Boston: Butterworths.

Gottlieb, M. S., Schroff, R., Schranker, H. M., et al. (1981). *Pneumocystis carinii* pneumonia and mucosal candidiasis in previously healthy homosexual men. *New England Journal of Medicine, 305,* 1425.

Heinemann, M. H. (1989). Long term intravitreal ganciclovir therapy for cytomegalovirus retinopathy. *Archives of Ophthalmology, 107,* 1767–1772.

Ho, D. D., Pomerantz, R. J., & Kaplan, J. C. (1987). Pathogenesis of infection with human immunodeficiency virus. *New England Journal of Medicine, 317,* 278–286.

Isobe, M., Huebner, K., Madden, P. J., et al. (1986). The gene encoding the T-cell surface protein T4 is located on human chromosome 12. *Proceedings of the National Academy of Science, USA, 83,* 4399–4402.

Jagger, J., Hunt, E. H., & Pearson, R. D. (1990). Sharp object injuries in the hospital: Causes and strategies for prevention. *American Journal of Infection Control, 18,* 227.

Kanski, P. J., Alroy, J., & Essex, M. (1985). Isolation of T-lymphotrophic retrovirus related to HTLV-III/LAV from wild-caught African monkeys. *Science, 230,* 951–954.

Kaplan, L. D. (1994a). Pathogenesis of HIV-associated Kaposi's sarcoma. In P. T. Cohen, M. A. Sande, & P. A. Volberding (Eds.), *The AIDS knowledge base: A textbook on HIV disease from the University of California, San Francisco, and the San Francisco General Hospital* (2nd ed., pp. 7.2-1–7.2-5). Boston: Little, Brown, & Co.

Kaplan, L. D. (1994b). Treatment of HIV-associated non-Hodgkin's lymphoma. In P. T. Cohen, M. A. Sande, & P. A. Volberding (Eds.), *The AIDS knowledge base: A textbook on HIV disease from the University of California, San Francisco, and the San Francisco General Hospital* (2nd ed., pp. 7.6-1–7.6-9). Boston: Little, Brown, & Co.

Kaplan, L. D. (1990). The malignancies associated with AIDS. In M. A. Sande & P. A. Volberding (Eds.), *The medical management of AIDS* (2nd ed., pp. 335–364). Philadelphia: W. B. Saunders.

Koenig, S., & Fauci, A. S. (1988). Immunology of the acquired-immunodeficiency syndrome. *Kansenshgaku Zasshi March, 62*(Suppl), 252–263.

Kotler, D. P., Wang, J., & Pierson, R. N. (1985). Body composition studies in patients with the acquired immunodeficiency syndrome. *American Journal of Clinical Nutrition, 42,* 1255–1265.

Kotler, D. P. (1992). Causes and consequences of malnutrition in HIV/AIDS. In G. Nary (Ed.), *Nutrition and HIV/AIDS* (Vol. 1, pp. 5–8). Chicago: PAAC Publishing.

Kotler, D. P. (1989). Diarrhea in AIDS: Diagnosis and management. *Medical Times, 117*(3), 101–108.

Kotler, D. P., Tierney, A. R., Altilio, D., et al. (1989a). Body mass repletion during ganciclovir therapy of cytomegalovirus infections in patients with acquired immunodeficiency syndrome. *Archives of Internal Medicine, 149,* 901–905.

Kotler, D. P., Tierney, A. R., Ferraro, R., et al. (1991). Enteral alimentation and repletion of body cell mass in malnourished patients with acquired immunodeficiency syndrome. *American Journal of Clinical Nutrition, 53,* 149–154.

Kotler, D. P., Tierney, A. R., Wang, J., et al. (1989b). The magnitude of body cell mass depletion determines the timing of death from wasting in AIDS. *American Journal of Clinical Nutrition, 50,* 444–447.

Kovacs, J. A., & Masur, H. (1988). Opportunistic infections. In V. T. De Vita, S. Hellman, & S. A. Rosenberg (Eds.), *AIDS: Etiology, diagnosis, treatment, and prevention* (2nd ed., pp. 199–225). Philadelphia: J. B. Lippincott.

Kumar, S., Schade, R. R., Peel, R., et al. (1989). Kaposi's sarcoma with visceral involvement in a young heterosexual male without evidence of acquired immune deficiency syndrome. *American Journal of Gastroenterology, 84,* 318–321.

Lane, H. C., & Fauci, A. S. (1985). Immunodeficiency abnormalities in the acquired immunodeficiency virus. *Annual Review of Immunology, 3,* 477–500.

Lawrence, J. (1985). The immune system in AIDS. *Scientific American, 253,* 84–93.

Levine, A. (1992). AIDS-associated malignant lymphoma. *Medical Clinics of North America, 76,* 253–268.

Levine, A. M. (1988). Reactive and neoplastic lymphoproliferative disorders and other miscellaneous cancers associated with HIV infection. In V. T. De Vita, S. Hellman, & S. A. Rosenberg (Eds.), *AIDS: Etiology, diagnosis, treatment, and prevention* (2nd ed., pp. 263–265). Philadelphia: J. B. Lippincott.

Levy, J. A. (1993). HIV pathogenesis and long-term survival. *AIDS, 7,* 1401–1410.

Libman, H. (1993). Pathogenesis, natural history and classification of HIV infection. *Primary Care, 19,* 1–17.

Mahmoadi, A., & Iseman, M. D. (1993). Pitfalls in the care of patients with tuberculosis: Common errors and their association with the acquisition of drug resistance. *Journal of the American Medical Association, 270,* 65–68.

Mayer, K. H., Stoddard, A. M., McCuster, J., et al. (1986). Human T-lymphotropic virus type III in high risk, antibody negative homosexual men. *Annals of Internal Medicine, 104,* 194–196.

McDougal, J. S., Kennedy, M. S., Sligh, J. M., et al. (1986). Binding of HTLV III/LAV to T4 and T-cells by a complex of the L10 K viral protein and the T4 molecule. *Science, 231,* 382–385.

McMahon, K. M., & Sutterer, M. G. (1988). Safety precautions and hospital practices in dealing with seropositive individuals. In V. T. De Vita, S. Hellman, & S. A. Rosenberg (Eds.), *AIDS: Etiology, diagnosis, treatment, and prevention* (2nd ed., pp. 396–420). Philadelphia: J. B. Lippincott.

Margolick, J. B., Volkman, D. J., Folks, T. M., et al. (1987). Amplification of HTLV-III/LAV infection by antigen-induced activation of T cells and direct suppression by virus of lymphocyte blastogenic responses. *Journal of Immunology, 138,* 1719.

Myskowksi, P. (1989). Treatment of Kaposi's sarcoma. In P. Ma & D. Armstrong (Eds.), *AIDS and infections of homosexual men* (2nd ed., pp. 317–327). Boston: Butterworth.

Nardell, E. A. (1990). Dodging droplet nuclei [letter]. *American Review of Respiratory Disease, 142,* 501.

Nash, G., & Said, J. W. (Eds.). (1992). *Pathology of AIDS and HIV infection.* Philadelphia: W. B. Saunders.

Navia, B. A., Jordan, B. D., & Price, R. N. (1986). The AIDS dementia complex I: Clinical features. *Annals of Neurology, 19,* 517–524.

Nelson, M. R., Erskine, D., Hakins, D. A., et al. (1993). Treatment with corticosteroids: A risk for the development of clinical cytomegalovirus disease in AIDS. *AIDS, 7,* 375–378.

O'Brien, T. R., Polm, C., Schable, C. A., et al. (1991). HIV-2 infection in an American. *AIDS, 5,* 85–88.

Osborn, J. E. (1986). AIDS, social sciences, and health education: A personal perspective. *Health Education Quarterly, 13,* 287–299.

Osmond, D. H., & Padian, N. (1994). Sexual transmission of HIV. In P. T. Cohen, M. A. Sande, & P. A. Volberding (Eds.), *The AIDS knowledge base: A textbook on HIV disease from the University of California, San Francisco, and the San Francisco General Hospital* (2nd ed., pp. 1.9-1–1.9-17). Boston: Little, Brown.

Ou, C., Kwok, S., Mitchell, S. M., Mach, D. H., et al. (1988). DNA amplification for direct detection of HIV-1 in DNA of peripheral blood mononuclear cells. *Science, 239,* 295–297.

Pantaleo, G., Graziosi, C., Fauci, A. S., et al. (1993). The immunopathogenesis of human immunodeficiency virus infection. *New England Journal of Medicine, 328,* 327–335.

Pedersen, C., Lindhardt, B. O., Jensen, B. L., et al. (1989). Clinical course of primary HIV infection: Consequences for the subsequent course of the infection. *Abstracts volume: Fifth International AIDS Conference* (Abstracts). No. TAO 30, 60.

Ragland, J. (1993). Progressive multifocal leukoencephalopathy. *AIDS Clinical Care 5,* 17–19.

Safai, B. (1989). Clinical manifestations of Kaposi's sarcoma. In P. Ma, & D. Armstrong (Eds.), *AIDS and infections of homosexual men* (2nd ed.). Boston: Butterworth.

Seligmann, M., Pinching, A. J., Rosen, F. S., et al. (1987). Immunology of human immunodeficiency virus infection and the acquired immunodeficiency syndrome: An update. *Annals of Internal Medicine, 107,* 235–242.

Task Force on Nutritional Support in AIDS. (1989). Guidelines for nutrition support in AIDS. *Nutrition, 5,* 39–46.

Tierney, A. R., Cuff, P., & Kotler, D. P. (1991). The effect of megestrol acetate (Megace) on appetite, nutritional repletion, and quality of life in AIDS cachexia. *Proceedings: Seventh International Conference on AIDS,* MB 2263.

Ungvarski, P. J. (1990). Human immunodeficiency virus (HIV) and *Mycobacterium tuberculosis* (TB). *Journal of the New York State Nurses Association, 21*(4), 7.

Ungvaraski, P. J., & Staats, J. A. (1995). Clinical manifestations of AIDS in adults. In J. H. Flaskerud & P. J. Ungvarski (Eds.), *HIV/AIDS: A guide to nursing care* (3rd ed., pp. 81–133). Philadelphia: W. B. Saunders.

Urba, W. J., & Longo, D. L. (1985). Clinical spectrum of human retroviral-induced diseases. *Cancer Research 45*(a)(Suppl), 4637s–4643s.

Volberding, P. A. (1990). Non-HIV Kaposi's sarcoma: Classic KS and KS associated with immunosuppression. In P. T. Cohen, M. A. Sande, & P. A. Volberding (Eds.), *The AIDS knowledge base* (pp. 712.1–712.2). Waltham, MA: Medical Publishing Group.

Von Roenn, J., Roth, E., Murphy, R., et al. (1991). Controlled trial of megestrol acetate for the treatment of AIDS related anorexia and cachexia. *Proceedings: Seventh International Conference on AIDS,* WB 2392.

Weinberger, S. E. (1993). Recent advances in pulmonary medicine [second of two parts]. *New England Journal of Medicine, 328,* 1462–1470.

Weller, S. C. (1993). A meta-analysis of condom effectiveness in reducing sexually transmitted HIV. *Social Science and Medicine, 36,* 1634–1644.

Wilber, J. C. (1994). HIV-antibody testing: Methodology. In P. T. Cohen, M. A. Sande, & P. A. Volberding (Eds.), *The AIDS knowledge base: A textbook on HIV disease from the University of California, San Francisco, and the San Francisco General Hospital* (2nd ed., pp. 2.2-1–2.2-9). Boston: Little, Brown, & Co.

Wofsky, C. B., Cohen, J. B., Haver, L. B., et al. (1986). Isolation of AIDS-associated retrovirus from genital secretions of women with antibodies to virus. *Lancet, 1,* 527.

Ziegler, J. B., Cooper, D. A., Johnson, R. O., & Gold, J. (1985). Postnatal transmission of AIDS-associated retrovirus from mother to infant. *Lancet, 1,* 896–898.

UNIT 12

INTEGUMENTARY SYSTEM

Wound Healing

Nancy A. Stotts and JoAnne D. Whitney

Healing is a central concept in caring for patients in the critical care unit. Injured tissue is repaired or replaced, and tissue continuity is restored. Disruption in the physiologic function of various systems occurs frequently in the critically ill patient and has potential for disruption of normal wound healing. Impairment in wound healing in critically ill patients has serious consequences, including localized wound infection, delayed healing, dehiscence, and sepsis.

Early identification of the patient at risk for impaired healing, manipulation of factors that place the patient at increased risk of impaired healing, support of therapies to facilitate healing, and mitigation of the effects of impairment are the responsibility of the critical care nurse. Often staff members from many medical subspecialties care for the critically ill patient, each with his or her own focus of concern. The critical care nurse frequently is the person who acts to coordinate the prescribed treatments to maximize therapeutic effects, to suggest medical treatments that have been overlooked, and to initiate nursing interventions to facilitate healing; thus, the critical care nurse's role in supporting healing is central to the patient's welfare. A substantial scientific foundation is essential to enactment of this role and to the care of critically ill patients with wounds.

This chapter addresses the physiology of wound healing; pathophysiology, which results in disrupted healing; clinical representation of normal and disrupted healing; and care of patients with disrupted tissue integrity and impaired healing. Throughout the chapter, the emphasis is on healing of acute injuries in the critically ill; chronic wounds seen in the critically ill are addressed but in less detail.

PHYSIOLOGY OF WOUND HEALING

Classically, wound healing has been divided into three phases and presented as having sequential but overlapping processes (Table 59–1). Although this paradigm is correct for full-thickness injuries, it does not address those wounds that are partial thickness. Advances in the field of wound healing have led investigators to describe wound healing by the type of tissue being formed (e.g., epithelium, collagen) or by the cells involved in the healing process (e.g., fibroblasts, endothelial cells, macrophages). Application of research on the physiology of healing to clinical care might best be approached by using the model of partial-thickness and full-thickness injuries, in which the focus is on the type of tissue involved in healing. This approach allows the clinician to examine the full range of wounds seen in critically ill patients and to examine differences in the healing processes in various types of wounds. Partial-thickness injuries involve the epidermal layer of the skin and may extend to the dermis. They include tape burns, abrasions, and the donor site for a skin graft. Full-thickness injuries involve the epidermis and the dermis and may extend into the subcutaneous fat, muscle, and bone.

Anatomy of the Skin

The skin is composed of an epidermal and a dermal layer separated by the basement membrane (Fig. 59–1). The outer layer of the skin, the epidermis, is composed of the stratum corneum and the stratum germinativum. The stratum corneum provides external protection, whereas the stratum germinativum is important because of its intense mitotic activity during healing. The dermis is composed of elastic fibers, colla-

TABLE 59–1. **Phases of Wound Healing**

Inflammatory Phase: Healing Initiated
Hemostatic responses
Vascular responses
Cellular responses
Proliferative Phase: Major Repair Phase
Collagen synthesis
Angiogenesis
Epithelialization
Remodeling Phase: Repair Process Completed
Changes in collagen

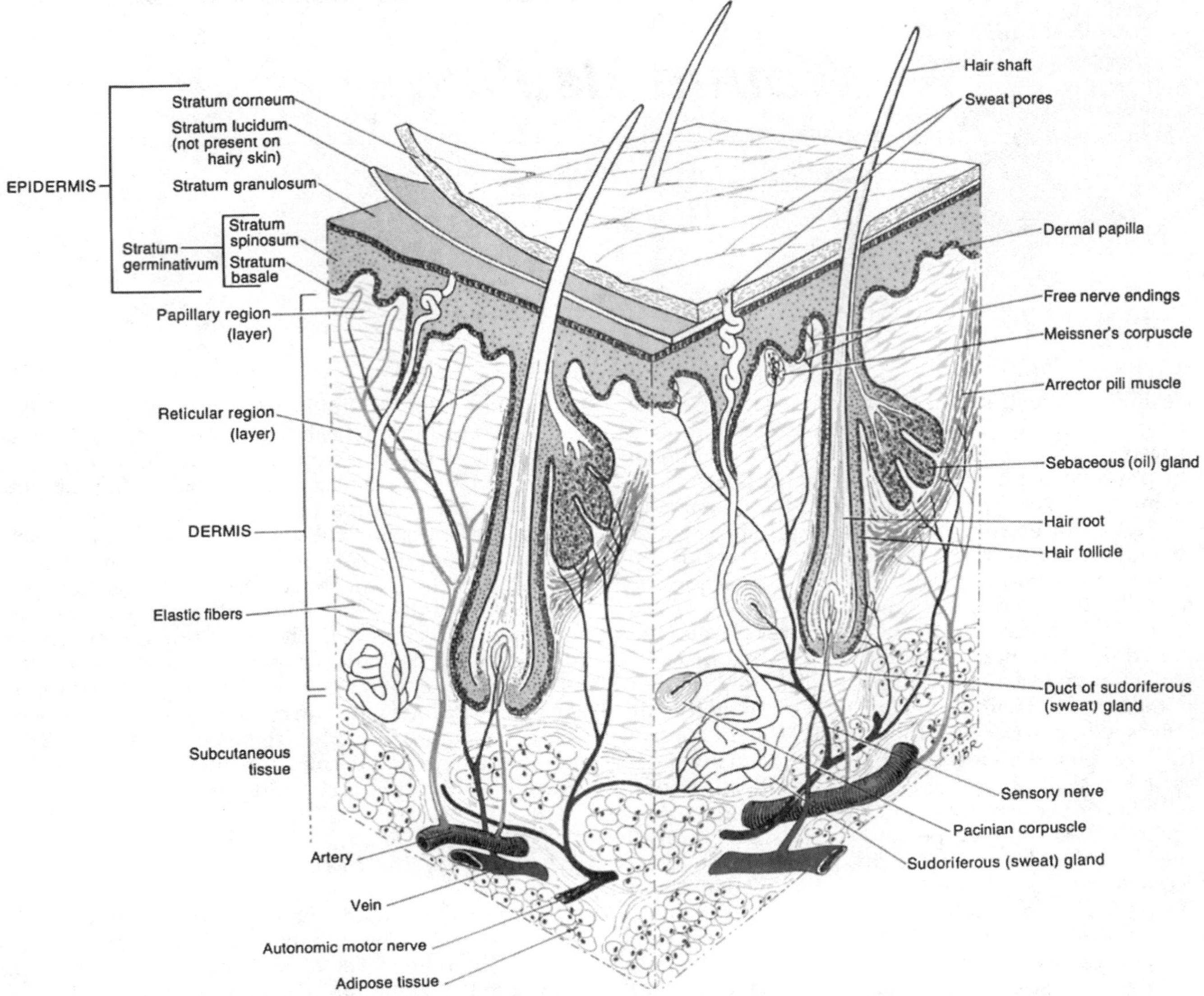

FIGURE 59–1. Structure of the skin and underlying subcutaneous layer. ("The Conduction System," page 311 from *Principles of Human Anatomy*, 4th ed. by Gerard J. Tortora. Copyright © 1986 by Biological Science Textbooks, Inc. Illustrations copyright © 1986 by Leonard Dank. Reprinted by permission of HarperCollins Publishers, Inc.)

gen, fibroblasts, ground substance, blood vessels and adnexal structures, hair follicles, and sebaceous, eccrine, and apocrine glands, all of which are a rich reservoir of keratinocytes to replace damaged epidermis (Jakubovic et al., 1985). The dermis is critical to epidermal function because it provides blood flow and structural support. In addition, the primary cell of the dermis is the fibroblast, which is essential for synthesis of connective tissue.

The skin is a major epithelial structure; however, the epithelia of the tracheobronchial tree, the gastrointestinal (GI) tract, and other tissues and organs respond in the same way to injury and repair as does the skin. Variations in rates of mitosis, migration, and healing are related to the type of epithelial cell involved (Jakubovic et al., 1985).

Repair of Partial-Thickness Injuries

Partial-thickness injuries involve the epidermal layer of the skin and may extend into the dermis. With injury, mitosis of epithelial cells is stimulated. The epithelial cells at the wound edge migrate toward the open wound; mitosis and differentiation into mature epidermal cells then takes place. In a partial-thickness injury, epithelial cells move from the adnexal structures as well as from the wound edges. Migration goes on until epithelial cells reach other epithelial cells and undergo contact inhibition. Epithelial migration continues until the area denuded of epithelial cells is entirely re-covered; then migration ceases and the epithelium is built in layers until it reaches its original thickness. When the injury involves loss of part of the epithelium, plasma is lost onto the surface. When drying of the wound fluid occurs and a scab is formed, epidermal cells must migrate under the scab, and this requires more energy than unimpeded migration.

Epidermal cells migrate, undergo mitosis, and differentiate most efficiently in a moist, well-oxygenated environment (Hinman & Maibach, 1963; Winter & Scales, 1963). Adequate nutrients for cell function must be present in order for cellular activities to take place (Young, 1988).

Repair of Full-Thickness Injuries

Closure of full-thickness injuries occurs by primary, secondary, or tertiary intention (Table 59–2). These three approaches to wound closure all involve the development of a blood supply across the injured tissue, filling of the tissue defect with scar tissue, and covering of the scar tissue with epithelial cells. Differences exist among these three types of healing, but the differences are primarily in the size of the defect requiring repair and the time required for healing.

Healing occurs in a predictable fashion (see Table 59–1). At the time of injury, blood vessels in the area vasoconstrict, the coagulation cascade is initiated, and platelet factors are released, which results in hemostasis at the site. Multiple growth factors have been implicated in healing, including platelet-derived growth factor, transforming growth factor beta, and epidermal growth factor. Platelet activation is thought to be the first step in their release, ultimately resulting in chemotaxis, angiogenesis, and collagen formation (Nemeth et al., 1988). After a few minutes, vasodilatation occurs and vessels proximal to the injury dilate and capillary permeability increases. Fluid and cells leak out of the injured vessels into the interstitium, resulting in edema. The edema is localized by fibroblasts that plug the lymphatics.

Chemotactic substances released at the site of injury attract white blood cells (WBCs) and complement to the area. The WBCs present in the greatest quantity at this time are polymorphonucleocytes (poly), and the neutrophil is the poly that is preponderant. Neutrophils phagocytose foreign material and bacteria and are a major factor in removing debris in the new injury. However, neutrophils have a short half-life (about 24 hours) and are not replaced at the wound site after their death. Monocytes, the preponderant WBCs at the wound site after 24 to 48 hours, are transformed into macrophages and become the most prevalent WBC present in the wound on a long-term basis. Macrophages are essential for phagocytosis, stimulating angiogenesis, replication of fibroblasts, and release of collagen from fibroblasts. Wounds will heal in the absence of neutrophils; however, without macrophages, wounds will not heal. Another important factor in wound cleansing is complement. Complement functions to lyse some bacteria and mark other bacteria for later phagocytosis by WBCs (Clark, 1985; Stotts, 1993).

TABLE 59–2. **Wound Closure Techniques**

Primary intention: Edges of wound well approximated and closed with suture, clips, or tape
Secondary intention: Left open to close by formation of granulation tissue, covered by epithelial tissue, and undergo contraction
Tertiary intention: Left to heal by secondary intention until bacteria count falls and then wound edges approximated

Growth factors are important to angiogenesis and the development of scar tissue. (Hunt et al., 1984; Knighton et al., 1982; Ross, 1987). The stimulus for angiogenesis is not entirely understood but seems to be some combination of the mitogenic factors, lactate, and hypoxia. When these factors are present in the wound space, capillary buds come out from the opposing edges of the wound space and grow until they reach a capillary bed from the opposite wound edge. As the new capillaries stretch out into the hypoxic acidotic wound space, intravascular cells and plasma are pushed into the advancing capillary bed. When the two ends of the capillary meet, flow occurs across the capillary. As the bed of capillaries is built, the amount of plasma and red blood cells traversing the new capillary bed in the wound space increases; over time, the hypoxia abates, the acidotic wound fluid is absorbed into the circulation, and the stimulus for angiogenesis ceases (Clark, 1985; Stotts, 1993).

Collagen formation also is dependent on growth factors. Among the substances recognized as growth factors that stimulate collagen formation are platelet-derived growth factor and macrophage-derived growth factor (Knighton et al., 1982; Ross, 1987). Collagen is synthesized and released by fibroblasts. There is a continual turnover of collagen as the scar tissue matures, and the tensile strength of the wound increases as the biochemical nature of the collagen changes over time. Collagen formation is a complex process; oxygen, vitamin C, zinc, iron, and alphaketoglutarate are critical to this formation (Goodson & Hunt, 1988).

Wounds healing by secondary intention undergo the process of wound contraction, in which wound size decreases. The controls for this process are not entirely understood, but the myofibroblast is thought to be a critical factor in this process.

To close the wound healing by secondary intention, epithelial cells migrate across the base of the wound. Epithelial tissue formation and migration also depend on growth factors to stimulate the epithelial cells to migrate, undergo mitosis, and differentiate as previously described.

DETERMINANTS OF HEALING

Factors in the internal and external environment of the patient affect healing (Fig. 59–2). The internal environ-

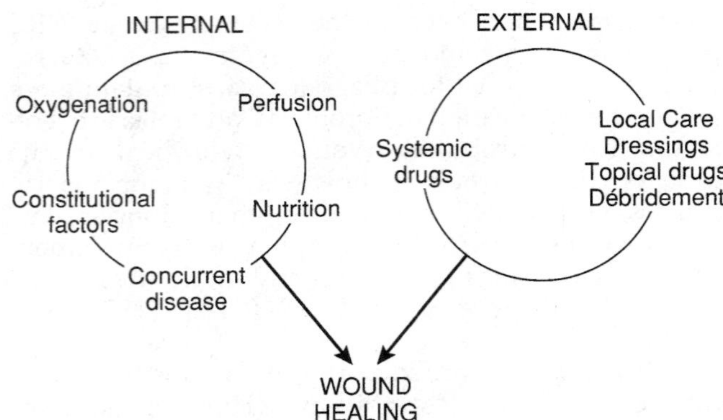

FIGURE 59-2. Environmental factors critical to healing.

ment is within the patient's own body; the external environment is outside the patient. Dimensions of the internal environment important to healing are tissue perfusion, oxygenation, nutrition, concurrent disease, and constitutional factors. Aspects of the external environment that affect healing are local wound treatment and systemic drugs and treatments. Some of these factors can be manipulated to provide an environment favorable to healing. Other factors need to be recognized so that appropriate monitoring can be initiated and realistic goals can be established about the rate and nature of healing.

Internal Environment

TISSUE PERFUSION

Adequate perfusion of tissue is important to bring substances to the injury for healing. Sufficient intravascular volume is needed to carry the substances for healing to the wounded tissue as well as dispose of metabolic wastes. Hypovolemia results in impaired healing, and most patients with hypovolemia show classic signs of increased heart rate, decreased blood pressure, and decreased urine output (Chang et al., 1983; Heughan et al., 1974). Chang and coworkers (1983) found a small proportion of subjects who had impaired wound perfusion and did not show clinical signs of decreased intravascular volume; currently, these patients cannot be identified using standard clinical parameters. Recently it has been shown in patients having GI surgery that fluid replacement that is titrated to tissue oxygen levels in the first 24 postoperative hours increases collagen formation in wounds (Hartmann et al., 1992). Data indicate that support needs to be provided to assist in maintaining the circulating volume in all patients and that frank hypovolemia needs to be aggressively avoided.

In addition to decreased volume, edema increases the space across which substrates must move to get from the vasculature to the tissue, and thus has been accepted as a deterrent to healing (Reed & Clark, 1985). The mechanism by which the edema formation occurs is complicated and not entirely understood at this time (Hargens & Akeson, 1986). Hunt and colleagues (1986) proposed that edema may not always be deleterious to wound healing and therefore may not need to be treated. They suggest that when perfusion is disrupted, it is obvious that edema is deleterious and needs to be treated. On the other hand, they suggest that when edema is the result of fluid replacement, its harmful effects are not as clear cut and it is not known at this time whether attempts should be made to remove edema of this etiology. These investigators acknowledge that additional data are needed to understand this process.

OXYGEN

Oxygen is critical to wound healing. It is an essential component in the transport of collagen from the fibroblast and in the cross-linking of collagen. In the absence of oxygen, the synthesis of collagen is halted but the action of the collagenases is not hindered, such that in a hypoxic environment, collagen lysis exceeds synthesis.

Oxygen also is important for the function of WBCs. WBCs remove debris and bacteria from wounds by phagocytosis and degranulation. When WBCs phagocytose foreign material and bacteria, they have a respiratory burst and use up to 20 times as much oxygen as in their resting state. During the respiratory burst, they use additional oxygen, ingest bacteria, and produce high-energy radicals such as superoxides, hypochlorite, hydroxyl radicals, peroxides, and aldehydes. Radicals are toxic to foreign cells and host cells and are responsible for some of the bactericidal action of the WBCs as well as some local tissue damage; however, enzymes present in healthy tissue quickly inactivate radicals, so that their action in healthy tissue is short lived (Knighton et al., 1984). Once phagocytosis has taken place, bacteria are killed by degranulation when intracellular enzymes are released. In the absence of oxygen, WBCs do not function as efficiently; bacteria may proliferate at a rate greater than phagocytosis, and infection may develop (Knighton et al., 1984).

Anemia also has been linked to impaired healing. Yet when concomitant conditions such as decreased volume are controlled, anemia has not been shown to be implicated in impaired healing except when the hematocrit drops below about 20 mg/dL (Heughan et al., 1974; Jensen et al., 1986; Jonsson et al., 1991). Research is currently in progress to determine which interventions best support oxygenation in the wound. Preliminary data in healthy subjects suggest physical activity may slightly lower tissue oxygen levels, but not to harmful levels (Whitney et al., 1993). Work is underway to further explore the effects of activity in postsurgery patients. Similarly, postoperative rewarming has been studied for its effects on perfusion and oxygenation (West et al., 1993).

Toxins associated with smoking tobacco—nicotine,

hydrogen cyanide, and carbon monoxide—impair healing. Nicotine, a potent vasodilator, and carbon monoxide, which occupies binding sites on hemoglobin, severely limit tissue oxygenation (Jensen et al., 1991). Cigarette smoking decreases tissue oxygenation. Further, nicotine impairs proliferation of erythrocytes, macrophages, and fibroblasts (Asakura et al., 1966; Erikssen et al., 1977). Although the implications of these effects are not fully understood, data indicate that smoking has a negative effect on healing. Until such research data are available, measures used to support systemic oxygenation need to be applied to these patients; these include inspiratory maneuvers, early mobilization and activity, positioning of the patient to support an optimal ventilation–perfusion ratio, secretion clearing techniques, manipulation of ambient oxygen, and/or ventilation as needed.

NUTRITION

Nutrients are critical to all of the processes that take place during healing. Angiogenesis, collagen formation, and epithelialization all require energy, vitamins, and minerals (Goodson & Hunt, 1988; Young, 1988).

Energy substrates include proteins, fats, and carbohydrates. The need for all of them is increased by injury; however, the most significant increase is in protein (Long et al., 1979). Protein is needed to provide the nitrogenous structure for new cell formation. The new cells and biologic factors of importance are those in the wound module itself (macrophages, fibroblasts, endothelial cells) and those that provide immunologic protection (WBCs, complement prostaglandins). Deficiencies of protein result in decreased fibroblast proliferation, proteoglycan and collagen synthesis, angiogenesis, and remodeling (Fitzpatrick & Fisher, 1982; Irvin, 1978; Rhodes et al., 1942; Temple et al., 1975; Williamson & Fromm, 1955).

Carbohydrates are an important source of energy for the body, and in times of stress, the need for energy is increased. Fats provide the substrate from which the intracellular structures and cell walls are made. They also provide an important source of concentrated calories, especially important in situations such as massive trauma when energy needs are great and the patient's ability to manage large volumes of high protein–high carbohydrate fluid is limited. The effects of deficiencies are seen only in prolonged starvation, when fat stores become a primary source of energy for the body.

Vitamins also are important to healing. All of the vitamins play a role in wound healing. Water-soluble vitamins especially important to healing are vitamins B and C. The B vitamins serve as cofactors in the enzyme system. Vitamin B_1 (thiamine) is necessary for the strength of collagen (Alvarez & Gilbreath, 1982). Vitamin B_5 (pantothenic acid) deficiency is associated histologically with decreased fibroblasts and experimentally with decreased tensile strength (Grenier et al., 1982). Vitamin C is critical to collagen formation and angiogenesis. In addition, needs are increased with injury because vitamin C is required for efficient WBC function. When vitamin C intake is depressed, improper sequencing of amino acids occurs, such that collagen formation is disrupted. In addition, because collagenases continue to function even during starvation, lysis of collagen may exceed synthesis. New wounds may not heal well, and old wounds may come apart. Administration of vitamin C rapidly restores this dimension of collagen formation and healing.

Vitamins A, D, E, and K are fat-soluble vitamins. Deficiencies related to healing occur only in prolonged starvation and/or severe injury, because there are reserves of these vitamins in body fat. Vitamin A is important to the inflammatory response and is a cofactor in collagen synthesis and cross-linking as well as in epithelialization (Pollack, 1979). Vitamin A also reverses the stabilizing effect of steroids on lysosomal membranes (Bark et al., 1984; Ehrlich & Hunt, 1968).

Vitamin D is needed for bone repair, because it is an essential component in calcium absorption and excretion. Liver stores of vitamin D are usually adequate in patients with uncomplicated injuries, but patients with multiple long bone fractures may require supplementation (Hey et al., 1982).

Vitamin E is an important component in normal fat metabolism. Scientific data indicate that supplemental vitamin E retards healing and fibrosis (Ehrlich et al., 1973; Kagoma et al., 1985).

Vitamin K is needed for coagulation, one of the first responses to tissue injury. Inadequate levels of vitamin K may result in bleeding into the wound space with hematoma formation and delay of the healing process. However, coagulation is one of the most fundamental body processes and factors needed for coagulation are not decreased unless severe and/or prolonged depletion of vitamin K occurs. Only in prolonged starvation, acute life-threatening hemorrhage, or feeding with total parenteral nutrition does vitamin K supplementation become a consideration.

Minerals also are important to healing; however, very small quantities of them are needed for normal bodily function and deficits related to healing have not often been reported. Zinc, iron, and manganese are important to collagen formation. Zinc is important in nucleic acid formation and protein synthesis. Deficiencies of serum zinc have been documented to impair healing, and impairment has been shown to be reversed by supplemental zinc (Barcia, 1970; Pories et al., 1967; Sandstead et al., 1982). Zinc deficiency is a threat in the elderly, the malnourished, and those with chronic metabolic stress and chronic diarrhea. Zinc is widely distributed in the body and is protein bound; therefore, measurement of serum zinc is not a sensitive measure of decreased intake and deficiencies are not seen until intake has been restricted for a long period.

Iron deficiency has been noted as a factor in impaired healing; however, only in children have deficiencies been related to impaired healing. Theoretically, the elderly may have iron deficiency secondary to changes in absorption of iron, increasing their risk for healing impairment, but clinically this has not been reported. Manganese functions as a cofactor in collagen formation. Deficiencies of this mineral have not been reported, but it must be considered when supplementation is provided.

CONCURRENT CONDITIONS

Patients with diabetes, perfusion problems, fluid and electrolyte disruptions, cancer, malnutrition, immunologic suppression, and infection are all at risk for impaired healing. The mechanism of impairment is different in each case.

Diabetics are a population known to be at risk for impaired healing. They have small vessel disease and experience periods of excessive hyperglycemia with injury (Goodson & Hunt, 1977). Increased glucose levels impair WBC function and often result in wound infection (Bagdale et al., 1974). If glucose levels can be kept to below 200 mg/dL in the first 72 hours after injury, healing will progress with fewer problems (Goodson & Hunt, 1977). Neuropathy that accompanies longstanding disease is important. The neuropathy may play a part in the initial cause of wounds. With decreased peripheral sensation, the patient may not feel pain as damage occurs and therefore the source of injury may not be relieved, leading to more severe injury. The neuropathy may also predispose the patient to iatrogenic injury during his stay in the critical care unit. Excessive pressure or mechanical trauma may lead to tissue damage, and because it is not perceived, pressure-relieving strategies may not be initiated.

Patients in the critical care unit with problems of perfusion also are at risk for impaired healing. Commonly, these patients have cardiac disease with its central pump problems or have vascular disease that results in decreased tissue blood flow. The mechanism by which impaired healing occurs is related directly to impaired delivery of substrates to the injury and wastes not being removed in a timely manner. In many critical care units, patients with actual or potential perfusion problems are the primary population and the potential for impaired wound healing needs to be considered.

Fluid and electrolyte disorders seen in the critically ill may impair healing. Normal sodium and potassium levels are important to cell function. Sodium excess and hyperosmolarity are seen in dehydrated patients and in patients with hemoconcentrations. Potassium loss often occurs with GI fluid losses. In addition, the aldosterone secretion that occurs with stress may result in a period of potassium loss and sodium retention. Phagocytosis is inhibited by high glucose levels and serum osmolarity of greater than 300 mmol/L. Acid-base balance affects healing. Acidosis reduces the inflammatory response to healing, and alkalosis inhibits wound contraction (Schilling, 1976).

Cancer patients are immunologically impaired and at risk for impaired healing. In addition, the radiation therapy and chemotherapy that they often receive disrupt the cell, so that cancer patients have multiple factors that place them at risk for impaired healing.

Other major groups of patients who are at risk for impaired healing are those who have malnutrition and those who are immunosuppressed. In malnutrition, substrates needed for healing are not present in sufficient quantities and the processes of angiogenesis, collagen formation, and epithelialization are slowed. When substrate stores are entirely depleted, healing cannot progress and/or infection develops. Among the patients who are immunosuppressed are transplant patients, those being treated for inflammatory disorders such as arthritis and inflammatory bowel disease, those with AIDS, patients with severe metabolic stress, and patients who have undergone anesthesia. These patients cannot mount a cellular defense to heal tissue and are at risk for infection.

Infection impairs healing because energy substrates needed for healing are used to support the life of the foreign organisms. In the process, complement factors and leukocytes are depleted, energy needed for repair is consumed, and, unless other events intervene, healing is delayed. The byproducts of bacterial action also are toxic and inhibit activities of healthy cells. Immunocompetence is the critical determinant of whether an infection can be controlled and healing returned to its usual rate.

CONSTITUTIONAL FACTORS

The very young and the very old are at risk for impaired healing. In the very young, the immunologic support system is immature and in the presence of heavy bacterial contamination they cannot provide efficient protection against infection. Older patients do not replicate cells as rapidly as younger ones do; the decreased rate of cell formation decreases the ability of these patients to mount an inflammatory response, fight infection, and produce new tissue. The inflammatory response and classic signs of infection may not be as marked as in the younger adult (e.g., redness, warmth, and temperature). This requires that the nurse look for the more subtle changes in the patient's wound status and act on those. Because cell production is slowed in the elderly, the ability to make macrophages and complement is decreased, so these patients are at increased risk of infection. Concomitantly, the rate of epithelialization is delayed; therefore, the wound does not heal from external contamination as rapidly in the elderly.

In the older population, development of connective tissue and scar tissue in wounds healing by primary intention also is delayed and tensile strength builds slowly, increasing the length of time these wounds are at risk for dehiscence. In wounds healing by secondary intention, development of a healthy bed of granulation tissue takes longer in the elderly than in the younger critically ill patient; until this bed of tissue is robust, the wound is at increased risk of infection. Knowledge of this risk is translated into increased efforts to prevent cross-contamination and aggressive local and systemic care that will support healing. The activities involved in the care of the elderly are the same as those with any population, yet they differ because the elderly require greater protection and more prompt and aggressive treatment for less overt signs and symptoms of wound impairment.

External Environment

LOCAL TREATMENT

Local treatment of wounds is an important determinant of healing or a significant deterrent to it. The principles of therapy and available therapies are discussed in detail later in the chapter.

Systemic Drugs and Treatments

Steroids are anti-inflammatory agents that affect healing. Their most potent effects are seen when they are given in the first few days after injury because they inhibit the inflammatory response, which is critical to all phases of healing. Administration of steroids immediately after injury inhibits the migration of the WBCs and the extent of the inflammatory response. The anti-inflammatory effects of steroids also result in suppression of the immunologic response to bacteria. Thus, patients receiving steroids may have only subtle signs of infection when the bacterial load in the wound is very great. The immunosuppression mutes the inflammatory response, and fairly advanced infection may be present before signs and symptoms are overt (e.g., suppuration, increased temperature). Small changes in signs and symptoms of infection in immunosuppressed patients demand attention and exploration to determine whether they are related to the wound. In addition, it should be recognized that steroids impair all phases of healing, interfering with angiogenesis, collagen formation, epithelialization and wound contraction (Ehrlich & Hunt, 1969; Sandberg, 1964).

Vitamin A is used as an inflammatory agent to reverse all of the effects of steroids except wound contraction. It is prescribed in an aqueous form or ointment base and is applied topically for 7 to 10 days to stimulate healing (Ehrlich et al., 1973; Hunt, 1986). Topical use confines the majority of the effects of vitamin A to the local wound and does not disrupt the systemic effects of steroids prescribed for other therapeutic purposes.

Recent animal studies show that corticosteroids reduce the amount of local insulin-like growth factor-I (IGF-I) and that locally administered IGF-I reverses the corticosteroid-induced impairment in healing (Suh et al., 1992). In addition, superior healing was achieved using systemically administered IGF-I and insulin-like growth factor binding protein-3 (Hamon et al., 1993). Work on human subjects is the next step in the research process.

Radiation and chemotherapy slow wound healing. Both interrupt the cell cycle of tumor and healthy cells. In the patient undergoing elective surgery, these therapies may be withheld before the procedure to allow the body to restore cells critical to the cellular response to healing. In patients with recent exposure to these therapies or for whom these therapies are continued, the inflammatory response is depressed. Clinically, this results in delayed healing and also in muting of the signs and symptoms of infection. Thus, the patient receiving chemotherapy or radiation therapy bears a double burden: he is not replicating cells in the wound module, and he also is immunosuppressed.

CLINICAL PRESENTATION OF IMPAIRED TISSUE

Integrity in Partial-Thickness Wounds

Partial-thickness wounds heal primarily by epithelialization. Epithelial cells arise from the adenyl structures of the skin, and closure of these defects usually occurs rapidly. Normal epithelialization is seen in pink tufts of epithelial cells arising around the adenyl structures.

In critical care patients, partial-thickness injuries in themselves are not usually a problem because they rarely become infected. Impairment most commonly becomes manifested when these areas do not close in a timely manner and/or epithelial cells dehydrate and scabs form. They are, however, a serious concern because they are a site for entry of foreign organisms into the body because the skin, the body's first line of defense, is disrupted.

Full-Thickness Wounds

Impairment in healing may manifest itself in several different ways because full-thickness wounds are closed by varying methods. Closure of full-thickness wounds occurs by primary, secondary, or tertiary intention (see Table 59–2).

PRIMARY INTENTION

Immediately after injury, wounds closed by primary intention generally have an initial inflammatory response seen at the wound site as redness, induration, and warmth. Pain and loss of function may be seen, depending on the extent of injury and the body part involved. The incision line normally is well approximated.

Epithelialization begins soon after injury, and in the patient with an uncomplicated injury, the epithelial layer seals the wound from external contamination within 24 to 48 hours. If wound drainage along the incision line is allowed to dry, a scab will form. The scab eventually falls off, revealing pink scar tissue below. Connective tissue needed to bridge the wound

TABLE 59–3. **Abnormal Findings in Wounds Healing by Primary Intention**

Drainage from the incision line 48 or more hours after wound closure
Severely decreased or absent inflammatory response
Inflammatory response lasting more than 5 days
No healing ridge by days 7–9

space is limited in wounds healing by primary intention. A sign that connective tissue repair is proceeding normally is the presence of a healing ridge by days 7 to 9 after injury. The healing ridge is palpable collagen and is an expected finding in all patients except those undergoing cosmetic surgery. Wound closure techniques used in patients having cosmetic surgery minimize scar formation and the associated healing ridge.

Impairment in the wound closed by primary intention is characterized by three alterations: drainage along the incision (in the absence of a drain) that continues after the first 48 hours, lack of a normal inflammatory response, and absence of a healing ridge by days 7 to 9 (Table 59–3). Drainage along the incision line indicates that the wound has not been sealed by epithelialization. Lack of a normal inflammatory response is described as edema and redness 0.5 cm on both sides of the incision line. When the inflammatory response is depressed, WBCs and growth factors are not brought to the area and healing cannot occur at its normal rate. Also, inflammation that lasts more than 5 days signals potential impairment. Absence of a healing ridge by the seventh to ninth day indicates that dehiscence and evisceration may occur.

SECONDARY INTENTION

Assessment and management of wounds healing by secondary intention provide the nurse with a challenge. The size and location of these wounds must be assessed. Size needs to be measured across several dimensions of the wound, and depth of the wound at the deepest area is measured perpendicularly with a sterile swab. Each time size and depth are measured, it is important that the patient be in the same position because shift of tissues with different positions will alter the size and depth of the wound. The wound is examined for the presence of tracts or tunnels that extend into the tissue. The number and location of the tracts are noted, and the size of each tract is measured and recorded. Tracts vary in area, and it is important to obtain an accurate measure so that changes can be appraised over time.

The wound itself then is examined. The granulation tissue is first examined, and then the exudate. Expected findings in wounds that are healing normally include the presence of granulation tissue that initially is pink and progresses to bright red. The change in the color of the tissue reflects the vascularization of the wound. As angiogenesis proceeds, capillary buds connect with similar buds from the opposite side of the wound and RBCs traverse the new capillaries, increasing the red color in the wound. This bright red color has been called "beefy red" because the color is that of a fresh beefsteak. When the tissue color does not progress from pink to red, the nurse needs to be concerned that healing is delayed. Granulation tissue normally is moist, and moisture needs to be maintained so that cells remain hydrated and do not have their cellular processes disrupted. When granulation tissue becomes dry, healing is delayed.

The presence of exudate in the wound then is assessed. Exudate is the byproduct of bacteria. The color and odor of the exudate are related to the specific organism involved. Colors frequently seen are serosanguineous, yellow, brown, and green. Black indicates that the tissue is necrotic. However, color may be deceptive because topical agents affect the color of the exudate; for example, povidone-iodine stains exudate yellow. Also, color becomes darker when it gets drier. Exudate may have no odor or may be musty, sweet, or foul smelling.

The wound edges are surrounded by pink epithelial tissue that normally is continuous around the wound. Over time, it becomes pearly white and extends down into the wound. When healing is abnormal in wounds closing by secondary intention, the epithelial edge may not be present or it may not be continuous around the wound. In addition, over time it may not extend down into the wound. Table 59–4 lists the abnormal findings in wounds healing by secondary intention.

Pressure Ulcers: Additional Evaluation of Wounds Healing by Secondary Intention

Pressure ulcers are a special case of wounds healing by secondary intention. A pressure ulcer is a localized area of tissue necrosis that develops when soft tissue is compressed between a bony prominence and a firm surface. Intrinsic factors that determine susceptibility to pressure ulcers are malnutrition, sensory loss, impaired mobility, altered mental status, incontinence, and old age. Extrinsic factors that contribute to ul-

TABLE 59–4. **Abnormal Findings in Wounds Healing by Secondary Intention**

Granulation tissue
Very pale or not progressing from pink to beefy red
Excessively moist or excessively dry
Wound size
Unchanged or increasing after it is exudate free
Tracts
Unchanged or increasing in size or number
Exudate
Present; thick with or without an odor
Epithelial edge
Not present or continuous around the wound

TABLE 59–5. **Grading of Pressure Ulcers**

Stage I	Nonblanchable erythema of intact skin
Stage II	Partial-thickness skin loss involving epidermis and/or dermis
Stage III	Full-thickness skin loss involving damage that may extend down to, but not through, the fascia
Stage IV	Full-thickness skin loss with intensive destruction, tissue necrosis, or damage to muscle, bone, or supporting structure

cer formation are excessively high or prolonged tissue pressure, shear force, friction, and moisture (Macklebust, 1987). Ulcers are graded, or classified, according to depth, as well as assessed as described previously. Grading of ulcers helps the health care team predict when the ulcer will heal and determine whether the ulcer will heal with conservative medical treatment or whether it will require surgical treatment. Grades III and IV ulcers are the most serious. Grade III ulcers extend into subcutaneous tissue and muscle. Grade IV ulcers involve tissue down to the bone and are the most problematic, often requiring surgical intervention. Table 59–5 lists the grading system used under the Pressure Ulcer Prediction and Prevention in Adults Guidelines from the Agency for Health Care Policy and Research (1992).

Documenting Clinical Status

Although the format each institution uses to organize data may vary, the content important to accurate documentation should be present in any system used, whether organized according to a nursing theory, nursing diagnosis, concepts, or problems. For wounds healing by primary intention, assessment parameters previously discussed are documented. Guidelines for documenting the status of wounds healing by secondary intention are found in Table 59–6. The Wound Healing Society recommends that assessment of the patient with a wound include extent of the wound, a history and physical, the wound severity, and status of the patient (Lazarus et al., 1994).

External Environment: Local Treatment

Wound treatment is planned so that an environment that supports granulation tissue formation and reepithelialization is maintained while contamination and dehydration are kept to a minimum. The characteristics of wounds help to direct treatment.

TABLE 59–6. **Guidelines for Documentation of Wounds Healing by Secondary Intention**

Use a consistent protocol to describe the wound.
Assess the wound rather than its dressing.
Assess granulation tissue, exudate, and epithelialization.
Record wound length, width, and depth at multiple locations.
Use the same terminology as other members of the staff to describe the wound.

TABLE 59–7. **Characteristics of Wound Exudate**

Organism	Color	Consistency	Odor
Streptococcus	Pink	Thin, watery	None
Clostridia	Brown	Thick	Sweet
Staphylococcus aureus	Serosanguineous/creamy	Thin/thick	None
Endogenous bacteria (e.g., *Bacteroides fragilis, Escherichia coli, Bacteroides oralis*)	Purulent	Thick	Foul

Data from Alexander, J. W. (1983). Infection, host resistance, and antimicrobial agents. In American College of Surgeons, *Manual of preoperative and postoperative care* (3rd ed., pp. 106–136). Philadelphia: W. B. Saunders.

The treatment for wounds healing by primary intention requires a protective dressing and in some cases an absorbent dressing as a cover for 2 to 3 days until the wound surface is sealed with a layer of epithelial cells.

Treatment for wounds healing by secondary intention is based on assessment to establish whether the wound is clean, exudative, or necrotic. Clean wounds are usually healthy with a bed of red granulation tissue and an edge of new epithelial tissue. Clean wounds with mature granulation tissue resist infection and generally heal well. Exudative wounds may have patches of granulation tissue but are preponderantly covered with exudate and debris. Characteristics of exudate color, odor, and viscosity vary with the type of organism present in the wound (Table 59–7). The exudate serves to enhance bacterial growth and retard tissue regeneration. Necrotic wounds are covered completely or in part with hard black eschar, which must be removed before healing can proceed.

Local treatment of wounds includes the use of dressings, topical application of antiseptics and drugs, debridement, and experimental treatment with growth factors (Knighton et al., 1988). Within each of these therapies there exist a myriad of treatment choices. Decisions about which therapy to use involve understanding the physiologic events of healing, establishing the state of the wound in the progression of healing, and having knowledge of the therapy and its influence on the physiologic processes of healing.

DRESSINGS

Biosynthetic Dressings

Traditionally, dressings have been used to protect and stabilize the wound; more recently, it has been recognized that dressings help to create an environment that supports healing. Research findings in the 1960s documented the beneficial effects of a moist environment for healing, demonstrating an increased rate of reepi-

TABLE 59–8. **Categories of Biosynthetic Dressings**

Category	Definition
Transparent films	Polyurethane sheets permeable to water vapor, oxygen, and other gases but impermeable to water. Nonabsorbent, maintain moisture
Hydrogels	Polyethylene oxide gel permeable to oxygen and water vapor. Absorbent, cooling, and maintain moist environment
Hydrocolloids	Gelatin, pectin, and hydroactive particles. Impermeable to gas and moisture until moist. Absorbent, maintain moisture, contour to wound
Absorbent dressing	Dextran polymer beads or alginates. Oxygen and water permeable. Absorbent
Foam dressing	Polyurethane. Impermeable to gas and moisture. Maintains contour

thelialization (Hinman & Maibach, 1963; Winter, 1962; Winter & Scales, 1963). Wounds epithelialize twice as fast in a moist environment without the presence of a scab (Winter & Scales, 1963). Epithelial cell migration across a wound is impeded by the presence of dehydrated wound fluid that forms a scab. Recognition of the influence of a moist environment on healing has led to the development of many types of wound dressings, which vary in their permeability to gas or fluids and are generally classified as biosynthetic dressings. Biosynthetic dressings can be further categorized as transparent films, hydrogels, hydrocolloids, absorbent dressings, and foam dressings (Cuzzell, 1990). Definitions of these dressing categories and the properties of the dressings are summarized in Tables 59–8 and 59–9. Indications for the use of these dressings and their advantages are found in Tables 59–10 and 59–11.

GENERAL EFFECTS OF BIOSYNTHETIC DRESSINGS

Dressings support healing through varying mechanisms. They protect the wound's new epithelial edge from injury due to friction, prevent desiccation of tissue and allow epidermal cell migration, promote autolytic digestion of necrotic material by polymorphonuclear leukocytes and macrophages in the wound fluid, and stimulate fibroblasts to synthesize collagen (Witkowski & Parish, 1986).

Relief of pain is associated with all of the biosynthetic dressings, particularly for wounds such as dermabrasions and skin graft donor sites. Hydrogel dressings may provide the most comfort because of their cooling effect. The mechanism for the relief of wound pain with occlusive dressings is not clear. A possible explanation is offered by the fact that some prostaglandins cause pain and these products may be limited by this type of dressing. Specifically, the prostaglandin synthetase system, which participates in the formation of prostaglandin E_2 (PGE_2), is oxygen dependent. Less PGE_2 may result from the reduction in oxygen under the occlusive dressing with less oxygen available for use in synthesizing these prostaglandins (Silver, 1985).

The wound fluid contained under biosynthetic dressings has antibacterial components such as complement, immunoglobulins, and lysozymes as well as growth factors and chemoattractants (Buchan et al., 1981; Hebda & Lee, 1992; May, 1984). Along with the active WBCs in wound fluid, the presence of these factors and an acidic environment created by the dressings may help to explain the infrequent reports of infections associated with these dressings. However, biosynthetic dressings should be used cautiously in the presence of gram-negative bacteria, which thrive in a moist environment and increase after 48 hours (Mertz et al., 1985), and in patients who are immunosuppressed. It also has been shown that although occlusive dressings provide physical barriers to exogenous bacteria, once pathogens are introduced, the local environment will support their growth (Katz et al., 1986). Thus, gauze dressings and hydrogels are more appropriately used in patients whose cultures show gram-negative organisms than more occlusive dressings.

Depending on the patient's general condition, the schedule for changing the dressing will vary. More frequent changes are indicated in critically ill individuals, who are more likely to be colonized with pathogens, and in cases in which gram-negative organisms are present or suspected. Also, heavily exudative wounds require frequent dressing changes.

The higher cost of biosynthetic dressings compared with gauze or other traditional dressings is often raised as a concern. Determination of the cost of wound treatment should include not only the cost of

TABLE 59–9. **Properties of Biosynthetic Dressings**

Category	Permeability		Absorbent	Excludes Bacteria	Damage to New Epidermis
	Gas	Fluid			
Polymers	Yes	No	No	Some	Yes
Hydrogels	Yes	Yes	Yes	No	No
Hydrocolloids	No	No	Yes	Yes	No
Absorbent dressing	?	?	Yes	No	No
Foam dressing	No	No	Yes	Yes	No

TABLE 59–10. **Clinical Indications for Dressings**

Type of Wound	Appropriate Dressing(s)
Partial-Thickness Wounds	
Blisters; dermabrasions; stage I and II ulcers; skin graft donor sites	Transparent films, hydrogels, hydrocolloids, wet-to-wet gauze
Exudative	Hydrogels, hydrocolloids, absorbent dressing, wet-to-damp gauze
Necrotic	Hydrocolloids, wet-to-damp gauze
Full-Thickness Wounds	
Primary intention	Dry gauze
Secondary intention:*	
Healthy, granulating	Wet-to-damp or wet-to-wet fine mesh gauze, hydrocolloid granules
Exudative	Absorbent dressing, damp coarse mesh gauze
Necrotic	Wet-to-dry or wet-to-damp coarse mesh gauze

*Includes stage III and IV ulcers.

the product, but also the time associated with dressing changes. Biosynthetic dressings do not need to be changed as often as gauze dressings and may significantly reduce time required for wound care (Kurzuk-Howard et al., 1985). When these factors are considered, the use of biosynthetic dressings may provide a cost-effective alternative for wound care.

The major categories of dressings are discussed in the following sections.

TRANSPARENT DRESSINGS

Transparent polymer dressings are composed of polyurethane and are marketed as thin, transparent sterile sheets (e.g., Opsite, Tegaderm, Bioclusive, Ensure). They are permeable to gases such as oxygen and carbon dioxide and also transmit moisture vapor. It was thought that a dressing's ability to increase oxygen tension at the wound surface enhances the rate of reepithelialization (Silver, 1972). However, this has not been substantiated in more recent studies that show that even though these dressings are gas permeable, oxygen tensions at the wound surface are very low (Eaglstein, 1985; Varghese et al., 1986).

The transparent dressings are fluid impermeable and have no absorptive properties, so pooling of fluid under the dressing occurs. The dressings adhere to intact epithelium surrounding the wound but not to the denuded wounds. However, as healing progresses and the wound has less exudate, the dressings may adhere to the wound surface and damage new epithelium during their removal (Witkowski & Parish, 1986). Transparent dressings have been used to cover decubitus and stasis ulcers, surgical incisions, and skin graft donor sites (Barnett et al., 1983; Linsky et al., 1981). Donor sites covered with transparent dressings have healed faster than those covered with fine mesh gauze (6.9 days compared with 10.5 days) (Barnett et al., 1983). A reduction in wound pain also has been associated with the transparent dressings (Witkowski & Parish, 1986). The effects of these dressings on surgical incisions in humans when compared with gauze dressings included faster reepithelialization, less eschar formation, less inflammation, and better wound apposition in 70% of 19 cases. In an animal study of incisions closed by primary intention, transparent dressing–treated wounds demonstrated diminished influx of fibroblasts, less collagen synthesis, and a decreased breaking strength when compared with wounds exposed to air (Linsky et al., 1981). Partial-thickness wounds dressed with polyurethane have shown increased collagen synthesis compared with wounds exposed to air and wounds dressed with wet-to-dry gauze. However, the increase in collagen does not ensure that bursting strength is greater (Alvarez et al., 1983). This finding can be understood by remembering that breaking strength is related to maturity of collagen with the cross-linking of fibers. Hence, polyurethane dressings provide moist environments that pro-

TABLE 59–11. **Advantages and Limitations of Dressings**

Dressing	Advantages	Limitations
Wet-to-damp or wet-to-wet gauze	Keeps tissue moist; vehicle for application of solutions; absorbs exudate; inexpensive	Damage to new tissue if removed when dry; may require frequent changing; can macerate new tissue.
Transparent films (e.g., Tegaderm)	Keep tissue moist; preserve wound fluid; relieve pain; easy to apply	Nonabsorbent; can damage new tissue on removal; aspiration may be needed for excessive fluid; does not exclude all bacteria
Hydrogels (e.g., Vigilon)	Keep tissue moist; no damage to new tissue; relieve pain; easy to apply	Require frequent changing; not bacteria resistant; can macerate normal tissue
Hydrocolloids (e.g., Duoderm)	Keep tissue moist; absorb some exudate; relieve pain; easy to apply	Cannot assess wound directly, due to opacity
Absorbent (e.g., Sorbsan)	Highly absorbent; dressing relieves pain; reduces bacteria	May dehydrate tissue excessively
Foam dressing	Insulating; relieves pain	Opaque, so cannot directly assess wound

mote wound comfort and reepithelialization. Their effect on fibroblast activity and ultimate scar strength raises questions about their use for incisions closed primarily. Further research on the effects of these dressings beyond 7 days is needed to answer questions about the long-term effects of polyurethane dressings on wound strength.

HYDROGEL DRESSINGS

Hydrogel dressings (e.g., Vigilon, Spenco Second Skin, Geliperm) are a mixture of 96% water and 4% polyethylene oxide suspended between two sheets of polyethylene, providing a semitransparent dressing. Like transparent dressings, they are permeable to oxygen and water vapor; however, they do not adhere well to either intact or wound tissue and a gauze cover and/or tape is required to secure them. The hydrogel material has absorbent properties and can absorb nearly its own weight in wound exudate (Mandy, 1983). The hydrogel material is placed on the wound after removing one of the encasing polyethylene sheets. If desired, the top sheet also can be removed and a gauze dressing applied so that exudate moves from the wound bed to the outer dressing layers. In addition to their absorptive qualities, hydrogel dressings produce a cooling sensation, a reduction in pain, and rapid reepithelialization, making them an ideal choice for dermabrasion and friction blisters with exudate and fluid production (Wheeland, 1987).

Bacterial proliferation has been shown to occur under hydrogel dressings in an animal model in which wounds were inoculated with *Staphylococcus aureus, Escherichia coli,* or *Pseudomonas aeruginosa* (Leaper et al., 1984). Wounds inoculated with *S. aureus* or *E. coli* did not have delayed wound contraction. In these wounds, the numbers of organisms increased for about a week but were decreasing after 10 days. However, wounds with *Pseudomonas* did have delayed healing and a large increase in organisms after 10 days of occlusion. These results suggest that hydrogel dressings should be changed frequently in order to avoid bacterial growth, especially if *Pseudomonas* is present.

HYDROCOLLOID DRESSINGS

Hydrocolloid dressings (HCDs) such as DuoDerm and Comfeel consist of hydroactive particles, gelatin, pectin, and carboxymethylcellulose in a hydrophobic polymer base. The dressing is applied after removal of the silicone release paper that covers one side of the dressing. It adheres to intact epithelium, but over the wound, fluid interacts with the dressing materials and forms a semisolid gel that expands into the wound cavity (Turner, 1985). Hydrocolloid dressings are opaque, impermeable to gases or fluid, and absorbent to the extent that there is gel available. The wound fluid–gel formation keeps the wound bed moist, supporting epithelial cell migration and also protecting newly formed tissue from injury when the dressing is removed. Angiogenesis has been shown to be significantly greater after 7 days of healing in wounds dressed with hydrocolloid as compared with gauze dressings (Cherry & Ryan, 1985). The HCD wounds had a 29% decrease in size compared with 23% for gauze-covered wounds. This finding is explained by the fact that hydrocolloid dressings are impermeable to oxygen, and the authors hypothesized that a hypoxic stimulus for angiogenesis may be produced by the dressings (Cherry & Ryan, 1985).

Hydrocolloid dressings are appropriate coverings for skin graft donor sites and also may prove to be useful for incisions closed by primary intention. Comparisons of healing time for skin graft donor sites covered with HCDs or saline gauze have been reported (Biltz et al., 1985; Madden et al., 1985). Both reports show that reepithelialization was significantly faster for HCDs, and those patients with HCDs had significantly less pain at the donor site in both reports. HCDs have also been used as an alternative to conventional postoperative dressings for incisions closed by primary intention. Young and Weston-Davies (1985) compared comfort, convenience, incidence of complication (skin sensitivity or infection), and cosmetic appearance of the wound for HCDs and standard postoperative dressings. There were no differences in complications associated with either dressing, and the researchers reported that HCDs were easier to apply and required less changing; they also reported how HCDs affect collagen synthesis and strength in incisions closed by primary intention.

Bacterial proliferation of normal skin flora (micrococci, diphtheroid bacilli, and *S. aureus*) in normal volunteers decreased over a 4-day period of occlusion with an HCD (Lawrence & Lilly, 1985). In another study of venous leg ulcers treated either with an HCD plus compression or a double-layer bandage (inner layer impregnated with zinc oxide paste), *S. aureus* and other pathogenic bacteria decreased as healing progressed with both dressings (Eriksson, 1985).

ABSORBENT DRESSINGS

Debrisan is an absorbent dressing made of hydrophilic dextran polymer porous beads. The beads are used for exudative wounds because of their ability to absorb wound fluid. They are placed into the wound dry or in combination with anhydrous glycerin and then covered with a polymeric transparent dressing. The beads act to draw wound exudate into the interspaces between beads by capillary action; the fluid is then absorbed by the beads. Substances in wound fluid also are absorbed into the beads, depending on molecular weight and size. Larger molecules and bacteria are not absorbed into the beads but become trapped in the interspaces between beads. Beads draw fluid and bacteria away from the surface of the wound and into the upper gel layer that forms as the beads swell. The use of absorptive beads for chronic leg ulcers, pressure sores, surgical sites, and chemical necrosis wounds has been associated with decreased wound inflammation, decreased exudate, and an improved granulation bed in the wound (Jacobsson et al., 1976a, 1976b; Pace, 1978). These effects have been helpful in reducing the time to prepare a wound or ulcer for split-thickness skin grafting (Jacobsson et al., 1976a). Although it is not clear whether the beads expedite the healing process, they have improved healing in patients with wounds resistant to other treatments (Pace, 1978). The beads have also been noted to reduce pain associated with skin graft donor sites (Jacobsson et al., 1976b). In one report, excessive dehydration of several wounds treated with absorptive beads occurred in patients with decreased arterial blood supply, suggesting the need for cautious use in some patients, particularly the elderly (Pace, 1978). The primary action of absorptive beads is to reduce bacterial load on the wound surface and absorb exudate effectively, reducing mediators of inflammation or infection. There is no evidence that they debride wounds, and although the beads draw bacteria away from the wounds, bacteria proliferate within the dressing after 24 hours (Jacobsson et al., 1976b). They seem to be most beneficial for treatment of heavily exudative wounds or those unresponsive to other therapies.

Alginate dressings are another type of absorbent dressing. They are made from the salts of alginic acid, a polymer that is a critical component of the cell wall of brown seaweed. These dressings come as a fiber and display their hydrophilic properties when in contact with the small amount of sodium present in wound exudate. An ion exchange results in the formation of a gel. The gel wicks exudate into the dressing and away from the wound while maintaining an ambient environment that is moist and physiologic. The dressing is removed with saline irrigation, and so dressing change does not interfere with the new granulation tissue that has been formed.

Alginate dressings have been used for a variety of purposes over time,—for example, as a hemostatic agent (Oliver & Blaine, 1950) and in the management of exudating wounds such as pressure ulcers, vascular ulcers, diabetic ulcers, and superficial wounds. They augment the rate of wound closure and reduce pain at the wound site (Gilchrist & Martin, 1983; Odugbesan & Barnett, 1987; Thomas, 1985). Reports also indicate that they have been used in cavity wounds (Dealey, 1989). Dressings initially are changed daily and as exudate abates, as infrequently as every 4 days before another product replaces it.

Foam Dressings

Foam dressings are a two-surfaced dressing with a nonabsorbable polyurethane that faces the wound and a foam that provides the outer layer. Thus foam dressings combine the properties of an absorption control dressing that maintains a moist environment with those of an insulating and protecting dressing (Cuzzell, 1990; Krasner, 1991). The value of the insulation has not been established with empirical studies, but temperature variations among parts of the body have been associated with the rate of healing—that is, warmer areas heal faster.

The foam dressings are designed for use with more superficial types of wounds (Cuzzell, 1990), such as radiation reactions, first- and second-degree burns, pressure ulcers, vascular ulcers, and dermabrasion. Some are self-adhesive, whereas others require sealing with tape. All are opaque, making observation of the wound possible only when the dressing is changed.

Gauze Dressings

Gauze dressings, especially for full-thickness open wounds, provide a moist healing environment when dampened with solutions such as physiologic saline or antimicrobial agents. Selection of the type of gauze (coarse or finer mesh) depends on the characteristics of the wound. The use of coarse gauze is recommended for exudate removal and is based on the principle that exudate and wound fluids will move away from the wound into the interstices of gauze and be absorbed and removed when the dressing is changed (Noe & Kalish, 1976). A finer gauze with smaller interstices is appropriate for wounds that are clean and granulating. When gauze dressings are applied to wounds that are healing by secondary intention, the dressing should first be opened completely and then moistened with normal saline or another solution as prescribed. The gauze is placed into the wound cavity so that a layer of gauze is in contact with all of the wound surface. Other layers of dressings are then added as necessary, care being taken to avoid packing the wound too tightly, which might apply unwanted pressure to the healing tissues.

Gauze "wet to dry" or "wet to damp" or "damp to damp" dressings are inserted into wound cavities; the damp layer keeps the granulating tissue and wound margin moist. The outer layers of these gauze dressings protect the wound from external contamination. Wet-to-damp dressings are removed before the dressing has dried completely and while the inside layer is still damp. This allows the removal of exudate and wound debris without disrupting new tissue. Wet-to-wet dressings are not permitted to dry and therefore require frequent changing. These dressings maintain a moist environment for the wound that appears to promote cleansing and offer a small amount of debridement (Rudolph & Noe, 1983).

Controversy exists as to whether the gauze should be allowed to dry before removal as in wet-to-dry dressings, but current thinking on the subject supports removal of the dressing when it is moist and not stuck to the tissue (Sawyer et al., 1980). Dressings that are removed when still moist, or moistened before removal, will be less likely to disrupt and damage fragile new granulation and epithelial tissue. Bleeding that occurs with the removal of a dressing indicates that capillaries have been injured and will have to undergo repair. Continual damage to new tissue by removal of dressings needs to be avoided.

Another important issue with this type of dressing is the number of bacteria shed when the dressing is changed. Data indicate that removal of gauze liberates significant bacteria into the air and that they are slow to clear when compared with hydrocolloids (Lawrence, 1994). Further work remains to be done to establish whether the liberated organisms are related to delay in healing or to infection, or sepsis.

TOPICAL SOLUTIONS AND OINTMENTS

Topical treatment of wounds often includes the use of antiseptic solutions and antimicrobial ointments employed to limit the growth of microorganisms. Although many of the agents are recognized for their efficacy as antibacterial agents, their effects on wound healing are less clear and thus controversial (Table 59–12).

Antiseptic Solutions

Bacterial contamination of wounds producing infection delays healing. However, the prolonged use of antiseptics on healing wounds has been debated because of their effects on physiologic processes of healing. Antiseptics are toxic to microbes as well as to host cells. Topical antiseptics aid healing only through bacterial control and are probably more detrimental than helpful to processes of cellular repair unless a wound is heavily contaminated or infected (Goodman et al., 1990). They are absorbed irregularly and unpredictably, particularly when the skin is not intact, and can have adverse systemic effects.

Popular antiseptic solutions used in wound care include sodium hypochlorite (0.5%), povidone-iodine (1%), acetic acid (0.25%), and hydrogen peroxide (3%). These solutions have been shown to be toxic to human fibroblasts and to retard epithelialization in animal wounds (Lineaweaver et al., 1985). Hypochlorite solutions are intended for disinfecting contaminated wounds (Goodman et al., 1990). Sodium hypochlorite, a component of Dakin's solution, is a bleaching agent that kills bacteria by the release of free chlorine into the wound. It is recommended that half-strength (0.25%) Dakin's solution be applied using wet-to-wet coarse mesh gauze dressings that are not allowed to dry (Rudolph & Noe, 1983). Studies have shown that hypochlorite solutions have damaging effects on wound healing. One study documented less collagen synthesis and prolonged inflammatory response in animal wounds treated with 1% hypochlorite–containing solutions compared with wounds treated with normal saline (Brennan et al., 1986). A solution of 1% hypochlorite applied directly to granulation tissue was also found to be toxic to the new vessels of granulation tissue (Brennan & Leaper, 1985). These results suggest that chlorine-containing solutions be used with caution and that their use in healthy granulating wounds be avoided.

TABLE 59–12. **Adverse Effects of Antiseptic Solutions**

Solution	Effect on Wound
Sodium hypochlorite (Dakin) (0.5%)	Decreased epithelialization; toxic to fibroblasts, new granulation tissue
Povidone-iodine (1%)	Toxic to fibroblasts; decreased epithelialization; increased susceptibility to infection
Hydrogen peroxide (3%)	Damage to new epithelium
Acetic acid (0.25%)	Toxic to fibroblasts; may delay healing time

Iodine is complexed with polyvinylpyrrolidone to produce povidone-iodine, which liberates free iodine in solution. Its mechanism of killing bacteria and spores is unknown, but it is considered an effective germicide when used on intact skin (Goodman et al., 1990). Its use in wounds healing by secondary intention is controversial and has been described as indiscriminate (Rodeheaver, 1989). Reports on the effects of povidone-iodine on healing are variable. When used on full- and split-thickness wounds in animals or human skin graft donor sites, it has not produced a delay in mean healing time (Gruber et al., 1975). Rodeheaver and associates (1982) reported that wounds exposed to the scrub form of povidone-iodine actually had increased susceptibility to infection, probably due to cytotoxic action of the detergent on WBCs. Furthermore, povidone-iodine antiseptic solution–treated wounds did not differ from saline-treated wounds in terms of bacteria counts. Another study of patients with contaminated pressure ulcers showed povidone-iodine to be the least effective agent in reducing bacterial load when compared with saline and silver sulfadiazine (Kucan et al., 1981). Wounds treated with 1% povidone-iodine also have been reported to be significantly weaker than control wounds when irrigated three times per day for a 4-day period (Lineaweaver et al., 1985). On the other hand, when 1% povidone-iodine was used once as a wound soak for 15 minutes prior to surgical closure, there was no difference in development of wound strength compared with control wounds (Mulliken et al., 1980).

A recent review article focused on in vivo studies of povidone-iodine products. The authors showed that detergent-containing products delay healing but that other povidone-iodine solutions do not delay healing, and that ointments and creams may enhance it (Mayer & Tsapogas, 1993).

The use of povidone-iodine in cases in which large areas of tissue are exposed to the solution merits careful consideration. Iodine can be absorbed from dressings into the systemic circulation. This absorption has been associated with metabolic acidosis and renal failure (Aronoff et al., 1980). Povidone-iodine should be used cautiously not only because of its potentially damaging effects to reparative cells and questionable efficacy for bacterial control, but also because of its documented systemic consequences.

Hydrogen peroxide is an oxidizing agent; contact

with tissues releases oxygen, producing a short period of antimicrobial action (Goodman et al., 1990). It acts as a surface cleanser and is often used in solution with normal saline as a wound irrigant. Wounds treated with a solution of 3% hydrogen peroxide showed shorter healing times in one study; however, the solution produced bullae on skin graft donor sites, suggesting damage to new epithelium (Gruber et al., 1975). Because of this effect, Gruber and colleagues (1975) recommended that hydrogen peroxide not be used on newly epithelialized wounds. In addition, hydrogen peroxide (0.3% and 3% solutions) is toxic to fibroblasts and therefore would have deleterious effects on collagen formation (Lineaweaver et al., 1985).

Acetic acid as an antimicrobial agent is effective against gram-negative organisms, especially *Pseudomonas aeruginosa* (Goodman et al., 1990). In one study, a solution of 0.25% acetic acid had no significant effects on healing time or microscopic findings (Gruber et al., 1975). Conversely, a solution of 0.25% acetic acid has been shown to be toxic to fibroblasts (Lineaweaver et al., 1985).

Antimicrobial Agents

Treatment of wounds with topical antimicrobial agents has not demonstrated as many negative effects on healing as antiseptic solutions; however, reports are limited. Three antimicrobial agents were investigated for their effect on epidermal wound healing (Eaglstein & Mertz, 1981). Neosporin ointment (a mix of neomycin, polymyxin, and bacitracin-zinc) promoted healing by 25% compared with untreated controls. Furacin-soluble dressing (nitrofurazone) slowed healing by 30%, and Silvadene (silver sulfadiazine) produced the fastest healing rate, 28% greater than nontreated control wounds. It is possible that the medium containing the antimicrobial agents plays a role in altering the rate of reepithelialization, since antimicrobial agents of the different ointments alone did not account for the healing differences (Eaglstein & Mertz, 1981).

Summary of Topical Agents

The available data indicate that topical antimicrobial solutions and ointments need to be used with caution, due to documented adverse effects on healing. They are indicated for wounds that are necrotic and/or heavily contaminated and may in fact assist in the debridement and sloughing of necrotic material and debris (Leaper & Simpson, 1986). Once the wound is clean, these agents are no longer necessary, and a change to a moist saline gauze, occlusive, or semiocclusive dressing is preferable.

DEBRIDEMENT

Necrotic tissue that is left undisturbed in a wound acts to encourage infection in the wound and delay the healing process. Infection is promoted by necrotic tissue through its action as a culture medium and through its inhibiting effect on leukocyte phagocytosis and function (Edlich et al., 1979). Removal of devitalized tissue is critical for healing to proceed and can be accomplished through several methods.

Surgical Debridement

Surgical debridement is often the treatment of choice and most quickly rids the wound of the necrotic debris. However, sometimes the patient's condition or the involvement of specialized tissues such as tendons or nerves in the necrotic wound limits the extent to which surgical debridement can be used. Other methods include mechanical debridement using irrigation or gauze dressings; chemical-debridement with topical enzymes; and biologic debridement, described as autolysis occurring with biosynthetic dressings.

Chemical Debridement

Proteolytic enzyme products (e.g., Travase, Elase, Collagenase) are available for use in wound debridement. This type of product is often selected for the treatment of necrotic pressure ulcers and vascular ulcers of the lower extremities. Enzymes are also used as an adjunct to surgical debridement or alone as a wound treatment. They are tissue-specific enzymes that act by digesting denatured and undenatured collagen and by dissolving fibrinous exudates and clots without damaging healthy tissue (Reuler & Cooney, 1981).

Debriding enzymes are applied topically to the wound eschar and are covered with a moist dressing. Because they do not penetrate eschar well, it is recommended that the eschar be crosshatched first to promote their effectiveness (Fowler, 1987). Results are usually obtained within 14 days. Manufacturer recommendations need to be followed closely to obtain the best results; some enzymes are inactivated by acidic environments and should not be used. Wound solutions such as acetic acid may interact with metals and cannot be used with products containing chlorine, iodine, or silver (Alterescu, 1984).

Mechanical Debridement

Wound irrigation, usually in combination with dressings, is used to clean and debride exudative or necrotic wounds mechanically. Debris and necrotic material present in the wound are removed when the irrigation pressure exceeds the adhesive forces of the contaminants (Edlich et al., 1979). High-pressure irrigation, defined as pressure that is 8 or more psi, has been found to be more effective than low-pressure irrigation for wound debridement (Brown et al., 1978; Hamer et al., 1975; Rodeheaver et al., 1975). High-pressure irrigation producing 8 psi can be accomplished using an 18-gauge plastic catheter attached to a 35-mL syringe

(Edlich et al., 1979; Stevenson et al., 1976). Although pulsatile high-pressure irrigation is more effective in cleaning wounds compared with continuous low-pressure irrigation, it damages the wound's resistance to infection (Wheeler et al., 1976). These studies suggest that high-pressure, continuous irrigation using a syringe will provide effective cleaning that does not compromise host resistance.

NURSING OF PATIENTS WITH WOUNDS

Nursing care of patients with wounds is based on data from the patient's history and physical examination and knowledge of the patient's underlying disease and how it is being treated. The history gives the nurse data about risk factors the patient has brought to the critical care unit (e.g., diabetes, age, steroid therapy). The physical examination provides data about the patient's wound status as well as about his general status (e.g., oxygenation, volume, nutrition). These data, together with knowledge of the patient's underlying disease state, allow the nurse to develop a plan of nursing care that addresses local and systemic support for healing in the context of the multitude of other clinical problems that patients in the critical care unit experience.

Systemic support is provided for the patient with wounds. Major concerns include adequate tissue perfusion, normal acid-base status and electrolyte levels, fluid balance, good control of glucose, sufficient oxygenation, and adequate nutrients. To the best of our knowledge, critically ill patients with wounds need care directed at establishing and maintaining normal laboratory values and usual amounts of intravascular volume, oxygen, and nutrients for healing.

Intravascular volume in patients with wounds is maintained most often through intravenous fluids, with the goal being good circulating volume without having the patient develop congestive heart failure or hypovolemia. Strategies used for balancing volume status are consistent with those used for any patient in the critical care unit.

Research has shown that tissue oxygenation is consistently higher than wound oxygen levels (Chang et al., 1983); however, data are not currently available that indicate whether specific nursing activities influence wound oxygenation (e.g., coughing, deep breathing, ambulation, positioning). Until such data are available, activities that support systemic oxygenation as seen in Pa_{O_2} levels and oxygen saturations need to be pursued in patients with wounds.

Similarly, nutritional support based on patients' metabolic needs should be adequate to meet the energy and substrate needs of critically ill patients with wounds. Attention also needs to be given to vitamin and mineral support. Data from recent studies focusing on perioperatve feeding show that enteral feeding immediately after GI surgery is feasible and results in improved healing as measured by hydroxyproline accumulation (Schroeder et al., 1991).

The effect of specific substrates on healing has been examined. Data from a study using a two-group nonrandom design show that chronic ulcers heal faster with a high-protein versus low-protein diet (Breslow et al., 1993). Also, enteral feeding supplemented with arginine, RNA, and omega-3 fatty acid has been shown to improve immunologic, metabolic, and clinical outcomes in patients who underwent major GI surgery (Daly et al., 1992). Similarly, ornithine alpha-ketoglutarate used enterally and parenterally in burn, trauma, and surgical patients has been shown to enhance healing (Cynober, 1991). Further work is needed in this area.

The local and systemic effects of drugs also need to be factored into the care of patients with wounds. Patients receiving steroids are at increased risk for impaired healing because these drugs inhibit all phases of healing. The use of vitamin A to reverse all the effects of the steroids except contraction has been recommended by some investigators but has not been recommended universally. Chemotherapeutic drugs also delay healing. When these medications cannot be stopped, nursing care needs to focus on increased support of aseptic technique to minimize wound contamination and the possibility of infection. In wounds that have been closed by primary intention, additional splinting of the incision line needs to be provided to support the tensile strength of the wound and prevent dehiscence. Anticoagulants are another group of drugs that may impair healing. Their effects are prominent in patients in the early postinjury period, when the coagulation cascade participates most fully in stopping bleeding into the wound. Awareness of the possibility of this complication will allow the nurse to assess wounds for continued bleeding and/or oozing so that early intervention can be undertaken to reverse the effects of anticoagulants, use measures to stop the bleeding (e.g., pressure to the area), and/or provide local evacuation of wound hematomas so that the site does not become a nidus for infection.

Local wound care is based on the appearance of the wound and knowledge of the patient's underlying disease and its treatment. Fundamentally, wounds healing by primary intention need treatment aimed at providing moisture to support epithelialization, preventing external contamination, and mitigating mechanical trauma. For these wounds, a dry sterile dressing is most frequently used. When in contact with the patient's skin, this dressing traps skin moisture and promotes epithelialization. If the wound is in an area where it may be threatened by external contamination (e.g., tracheostomy secretion), a hydrophobic layer such as Vaseline gauze may be used next to the incision to prevent contamination of the wound. Similarly, if the area may be subject to trauma, as is seen in lateral thoracic incisions with turning, extra padding may be needed to prevent mechanical damage to the tissue. Although newer dressings at times have been used on wounds closed by primary intention, they probably cannot be recommended as routine treatment until research establishes their safety, especially for use in the critically ill, who frequently experience multiple confounding factors that increase the risk of impaired healing. For the most part, wounds healing by primary intention seal within 48 hours of closure and risk of impairment in healing is more related to the success of the intraoperative intervention and support of systemic factors than to very sophisticated, unusual, or newer approaches to local wound care.

Wounds healing by secondary intention can be a challenge to the critical care nurse. Many products and approaches have been developed to treat these wounds. A paradigm has been developed to aid the nurse in determining the type of local care required by wounds healing by secondary intention (Stotts, 1990). This approach, called the *three color concept,* provides guidelines for therapy based on the color of the wound. Although untested, this approach uses principles of care established over time in care of patients with all types of wounds. The paradigm is based on knowledge of healthy granulating tissue, the ideal for this type of wound. Optimal tissue appearance is beefy red, and healing is supported when the wound is kept moist. Delay in healing is seen when the wound surface is yellow or black. Yellow and all of its shades from a very pale creamy yellow to the yellows with more green in them indicate that exudate is present and the wound is contaminated. Yellow exudate needs to be removed from the wound by cleansing. A black appearance to a wound indicates that necrotic issue is present. Necrotic tissue is an ideal medium for growth of bacteria and is treated by debridement.

The paradigm indicates that red wounds are kept moist, yellow wounds are cleansed, and black wounds are debrided. These three principles guide care, yet do not dictate the specific product or approach that is to be used (Table 59–13). For example, debridement may be performed with enzymes or moist-to-moist dressings, mechanically (high-pressure irrigation or a whirlpool), surgically (with a scalpel), or by autodebridement (patient's own body cleans area). Similarly, cleansing may be accomplished with hydrophilic beads, with hydrogel polymers, mechanically (high-pressure irrigation), with antibiotic ointment, or with moist-to-moist dressings. Maintaining moisture of the wound can be facilitated by a number of methods; approaches such as transparent dressings, hydrogels, moist-to-moist dressings, and drug-impregnated dressings have been used.

TABLE 59–13. **Three Color Concept**

Color	Goal of Treatment	Examples
Red	Keep moist	Transparent dressing; hydrogel
Yellow	Clean	Irrigation, moist-to-moist dressings
Black	Debride	Enzymes, whirlpool

Data from Stotts, 1990.

To use the three color approach, the critical care nurse must know the products and therapies that are available in her institution, the advantages and limitations of each, and how those therapies fit with the overall goals for the patient. Such an approach will allow the nurse to plan local wound care that is based on current scientific knowledge, maximizes use of available products and therapies (which vary among settings), and provides local care in the context of the overall goals of care for the patient.

Recent nursing research in the care of patients with healing wounds has focused on the effect of the environment on healing. Studies have examined the effects of noise on healing in a rat model (Wysocki, 1986) and the use of guided imagery to reduce stress and enhance wound healing in patients with surgical incisions (Holden-Lund, 1988). Although these studies were not conducted in the critical care unit with critically ill patients, they laid the foundation for research that addresses these concepts with critical care patients. In addition, the concept of pain management during dressing changes of patients with wounds healing by secondary intention has received attention. Music has been used to augment narcotics in pain management during dressing changes of surgical patients with wounds healing by secondary intention (Angus & Faux, 1989). Also, pain control during dressing changes of similar wounds has been shown to be augmented with the use of transcutaneous electrical nerve stimulation (Hargreaves & Lander, 1989). Although additional research is reported that establishes the value of these approaches to pain management and wound healing during dressing changes, such strategies might also be considered for individual patients who present with difficult or complex management problems.

COLLABORATION

Physicians and nurses in critical care units often work together to determine the best treatment for the patient systemically as well as to establish a plan for local care of wounds. With the patient who is admitted to a unit primarily for prevention or treatment of wound healing impairment, the physician often takes the lead in determining the nature of treatment the wound is to receive locally as well as the appropriate supportive care. However, probably more common is the patient who is admitted to a unit for another problem and happens to have a wound. Often in fact, the wound in such a patient is a secondary concern and may be neglected in the more immediate needs of perfusion, oxygenation, and maintenance of organ viability that characterize the critically ill population. In this case, the nurse often takes the initiative to assess the wound and recommend therapy. Probably the third category of patients with wounds seen in critical care units are those who develop iatrogenic wounds such as pressure ulcers, fistulas, or skin tears. These are situations in which the nurse often is the first to diagnose the problem and recommend a plan of care or seek to develop one cooperatively with the physician. In all cases, the institution's standards of care and unit protocol establish routine nursing therapies that are employed independently and those treatments that require prescription by the physician.

REFERENCES

Alterescu, V. (1984). Debriding enzymes. *Journal of Enterostomal Therapy, 11*(3), 122–124.

Alvarez, O. M., & Gilbreath, R. L. (1982). Thiamine influence on collagen during the granulation of skin wounds. *Journal of Surgical Research, 32,* 24–31.

Alvarez, O. M., Mertz, P. M., & Eaglstein, W. H. (1983). The effect of occlusive dressings on collagen synthesis and reepithelialization in superficial wounds. *Journal of Surgery Research, 35,* 142–148.

Angus, J. E., & Faux, S. (1989). The effect of music on adult postoperative patients' pain during a nursing procedure. In S. G. Funk et al. (Eds.), *Key aspects of recovery* (pp. 116–172). New York: Springer-Verlag.

Aronoff, G. R., Friedman, S. J., Doedens, D. F., & LaVelle, K. J. (1980). Increased serum iodide concentration from iodine absorption through wound treated topically with povidone-iodine. *American Journal of Medical Science, 219,* 173–176.

Asakura, R., Sato, Y., & Minikam, S. (1966). Effects of deoxygenation of intracellular hemoglobin on red cell glycolysis. *Journal of Biochemistry, 59,* 525–526.

Bagdale, J. D., Root, R. K., & Bulger, R. J. (1974). Impaired leukocyte function in patients with poorly controlled diabetes. *Diabetes, 23,* 9–15.

Barcia, P. J. (1970). Lack of acceleration of healing with zinc sulfate. *Annals of Surgery, 172,* 1048–1050.

Bark, S., Rettura, G., Goldman, D., et al. (1984). Effect of supplemental vitamin A on the healing of colon anastomosis. *Journal of Surgical Research, 36,* 470–474.

Barnett, A., Bekowitz, R. L., Mills, R., & Vistnes, L. M. (1983). Comparison of synthetic adhesive moisture vapor permeable and fine mesh gauze dressings for split-thickness skin graft donor sites. *American Journal of Surgery, 145,* 379–381.

Biltz H., Kiessling, M., & Kreysel, H. W. (1985). Comparison of hydrocolloid and saline gauze in the treatment of skin graft donor sites. In T. J. Ryan (Ed.), *An environment for healing: The role of occlusion* (pp. 125–128). London: The Royal Society of Medicine.

Brennan, S. S., & Leaper, D. J. (1985). The effect of antiseptics on the healing wound: A study using the rabbit ear chamber. *British Journal of Surgery, 72*(10), 780–782.

Brennan, S. S., Foster, M. E., & Leaper, D. J. (1986). Antiseptic toxicity in wounds healing by secondary intention. *Journal of Hospital Infections, 8*(3), 263–267.

Breslow, R. A., Hallfrisch, J., Guy, D. G., et al. (1993). The importance of dietary protein in healing pressure ulcers. *Journal of the American Geriatrics Society, 41*(4), 357–362.

Brown, L. L., Shelton, H. T., Bornside, G. H., & Cohn, I. (1978). Evaluation of wound irrigation by pulsatile jet and conventional methods. *Annals of Surgery, 187,* 170–173.

Buchan, I. A., Andrews, J. K., & Lang, S. M. (1981). Clinical and laboratory investigation of the composition and properties of human skin wound exudate under semi-permeable dressing. *Burns, 7,* 326–334.

Chang, N., Goodson, W. H. III, Gottrup, F., & Hunt, T. K. (1983). Direct measurement of wound and tissue oxygen tensions in postoperative patients. *Annals of Surgery, 197,* 470–478.

Cherry, G. H., & Ryan, T. J. (1985). The physical properties of a new hydrocolloid dressing. In T. J. Ryan (Ed.), *An environment for healing: The role of occlusion* (pp. 61–68). London: The Royal Society of Medicine.

Clark, R. A. (1985). Cutaneous tissue repair: Basic biological considerations. *Journal of the American Academy of Dermatology, 13*(1), 701–725.

Cuzzell, J. Z. (1990). Choosing a wound dressing: A systematic approach. *AACN Clinical Issues in Critical Care Nursing, 1*(3), 566–577.

Cynober, L. (1991). Ornithine alpha-ketoglutarate in nutritional support. *Nutrition, 7*(5), 313–322.

Daly, J. M., Lieberman, M. D., Goldfine, J., et al. (1992). Enteral nutrition with supplemental arginine, RNA, and omega-3 fatty acids in patients after operation: Immunologic, metabolic and clinical outcome. *Surgery, 112*(1), 56–67.

Dealey, C. (1989). Management of cavity wounds. *Nursing, 3*(39), 25–27.

Eaglstein, W. H. (1985). Experiences with biosynthetic dressings. *Journal of the American Academy of Dermatology, 12*(2), 434–439.

Eaglstein, W. H., & Mertz, P. M. (1981). Effect of topical medicaments on the rate of repair of superficial wounds. In P. Dineen & G. Hildlick-Smith (Eds.), *The surgical wound* (pp. 150–170). Philadelphia: Lea & Febiger.

Edlich, R. F., Rodeheaver, G. T., Thacker, J. G., & Edgerton, M. (1979). Technical factors in wound management. In T. K. Hunt & J. E. Dunphy (Eds.), *Fundamentals of wound management* (pp. 408–413). New York: Appleton-Century-Crofts.

Ehrlich, H. P., & Hunt, T. K. (1968). Effects of cortisone and vitamin A on wound healing. *Annals of Surgery, 167,* 324–341.

Ehrlich, H. P., & Hunt, T. K. (1969). The effects of cortisone and anabolic steroids on the tensile strength of healing wounds. *Annals of Surgery, 170,* 203.

Ehrlich, H. P., Traver, H., & Hunt, T. K. (1973). Effect of vitamin A and glucocorticoids upon inflammation and collagen synthesis. *Annals of Surgery, 177,* 222.

Erikssen, J., Hellem, A., & Stormorken, H. (1977). Chronic effects of smoking on platelet adhesiveness in presumably healthy, middle-aged men. *Thrombosis and Haemostasis, 38,* 606–611.

Eriksson, G. (1985). Comparative study of hydrocolloid dressing and double layer bandage in treatment of venous stasis ulceration. In T. J. Ryan (Ed.), *An environment for healing: The role of occlusion* (pp. 111–113). London: The Royal Society of Medicine.

Fitzpatrick, D. W., & Fisher, H. (1982). Carnosine, histidine and wound healing. *Surgery, 91,* 56–60.

Fowler, E. M. (1987). Equipment and products used in management and treatment of pressure ulcers. *Nursing Clinics of North America, 22*(2), 449–461.

Gilchrist, T., & Martin, A. M. (1983). Wound treatment with Sorbsan: An alginate fibre dressing. *Biomaterials, 4,* 317–320.

Goodman, A. G., Gilman, L. S., Rall, T. W., & Murad, F. (Eds.), (1990). *Pharmacologic basis for therapeutics* (8th ed.). New York: Pergamon Press.

Goodson, W. H., III, & Hunt, T. K. (1977). Studies of wound healing in experimental diabetes mellitus. *Journal of Surgical Research, 22,* 221–227.

Goodson, W. H. III, & Hunt, T. K. (1988). Wound healing. In J. M. Kinney, K. N. Jeejeebhoy, G. L. Hill, & O. E. Owen (Eds.), *Human metabolism and nutrition in patient care* (pp. 635–642). Philadelphia: W. B. Saunders.

Grenier, J. F., Aprahamian, M., Genot, C., & Dentinger, A. (1982). Pantothenic acid (vitamin B_5) efficacy on wound healing. *Acta Vitaminologica et Enzymologica, 4,* 81–85.

Gruber, R. P., Vistnes, L., & Pardoe, R. (1975). The effect of commonly used antiseptics on wound healing. *Plastic Reconstructive Surgery, 55*(4), 472–476.

Hamer, M. I., Robson, M. C., Krizek, T. J., & Southwick, W. O. (1975). Quantitative bacterial analysis of comparative wound irrigations. *Annals of Surgery, 181,* 819–822.

Hamon, G. A., Hunt, T. K., & Spencer, E. M. (1993). In vivo effects of systemic insulin-like growth factors alone and complicated with insulin-like growth factor binding, protein-3 on corticosteroid suppressed wounds. *Growth Regulation, 3*(1), 53–56.

Hargens, A. R., & Akeson, W. H. (1986). Stress effects on tissue nutrition and viability. In A. R. Hargens (Ed.), *Tissue nutrition and viability* (pp. 1–24). New York: Springer-Verlag.

Hargreaves, A., & Lander, J. (1989). Use of transcutaneous electrical nerve stimulation for postoperative pain. *Nursing Research, 38*(3), 159–161.

Hartman, M., Jonsson, K., & Zederfeldt, B. (1992). Effect of tissue perfusion and oxygenation on accumulating of collagen in healing wounds. *European Journal of Surgery, 158*(10), 521–526.

Hebda, P. A., & Lee, C. I. (1992). Occlusive dressing for surgical and other acute wounds. *Wounds, 4*(3), 84–87.

Heughan, C., Chir, B., Grislis, G., & Hunt, T. K. (1974). The effect of anemia on wound healing. *Annals of Surgery, 179,* 163–167.

Hey, H., Lund, B., Sørensen, O. H., & Lund, B. (1982). Delayed fracture healing following jejunoileal bypass surgery for obesity. *Calcified Tissue International,* 34, 13–15.

Hinman, C. D., & Maibach, H. (1963). Effect of air exposure and occlusion on experimental human skin wounds. *Nature (London), 200,* 377–378.

Holden-Lund, C. (1988). Effects of relaxation with guided imagery on surgical stress and wound healing. *Research in Nursing & Health, 11,* 235–244.

Hunt, T. K. (1986). Vitamin A and wound healing. *Journal of the American Academy of Dermatology, 15*(4), 817–821.

Hunt, T. K. (1988). Prospective: A retrospective perspective on the nature of wounds. In A. Barbul, E. Pines, M. Caldwell, & T. K. Hunt (Eds.), *Progress in clinical and biological research. Growth factors and other aspects of wound healing* (Vol. 266, pp. xiii-xx). New York: Alan R. Liss.

Hunt, T. K., Knighton, D. R., Thakral, K. K., et al. (1984). Studies on inflammation and wound healing: Angiogenesis and collagen synthesis stimulated in vivo by resident and activated macrophages. *Surgery, 96,* 48–54.

Hunt, T. K., Rabkin, J., & von Smitten, K. (1986). Effects of edema and anemia on wound healing and infection. *Current Studies in Hematology & Blood Transfusion, 53,* 101–111.

Irvin, T. T. (1978). Effects of malnutrition on wound healing. *Surgery, Gynecology and Obstetrics, 146,* 33–37.

Jacobsson, S., Jonsson, L., Rank, F., & Rothman, U. (1976a). Studies on healing of Debrisan-treated wounds. *Scandinavian Journal of Plastic and Reconstructive Surgery, 10*(2), 97–101.

Jacobsson, S., Rothman, U., Arturson, G., et al. (1976b). A new principle for the cleansing of infected wounds. *Scandinavian Journal of Plastic and Reconstructive Surgery, 10*(1), 65–72.

Jakubovic, H. R., Ackerman, A. B., Pochi, P. E., et al. (1985). Structure and function of the skin. In S. L. Moschella & H. J. Hurley (Eds.), *Dermatology* (pp. 1–103). Philadelphia: W. B. Saunders.

Jensen, J. A., Goodson, W. H. III, Vasconez, L., et al. (1986). Wound healing in anemia: A case study. *Western Journal of Medicine, 144,* 465–467.

Jensen, J. A., Goodson, W. H. III, Hopf, H. W., et al. (1991). Cigarette smoking decreases oxygen. *Archives of Surgery, 126,* 1131–1134.

Jonsson, K. J., Jensen, J. A., Goodson, W. H. III, et al. (1991). Tissue oxygenation, anemia, and perfusion in relation to wound healing in surgical patients. *Annals of Surgery, 214,* 605–613.

Kagoma, P., Burger, S. N., Seifter, E., et al. (1985). The effect of vitamin E on experimentally induced peritoneal adhesions in mice. *Archives of Surgery, 120,* 949–951.

Katz, S., McGinley, K., & Leyden, J. J. (1986). Semipermeable occlusive dressings. *Archives of Dermatology, 22*(1), 58–62.

Knighton, D. R., Doucette, M., Fiegel, V. D., et al. (1988). The use of platelet derived wound healing formula in human clinical trials. In A. Barbul, E. Pines, M. Caldwell, & T. K. Hunt (Eds.), *Progress in clinical and biological research. Growth factors and other aspects of wound healing* (Vol. 266, pp. 313–329). New York: Alan R. Liss.

Knighton, D. R., Halliday, B., & Hunt, T. K. (1984). Oxygen as antibiotic: The effect of inspired oxygen. *Archives of Surgery, 119,* 199–204.

Knighton, D. R., Hunt, T. K., Thakral, K. K., & Goodson, W. H. III (1982). Role of platelets and fibrin in the healing sequence. *Annals of Surgery, 196*(4), 379–388.

Krasner, D. (1991). Resolving the dressing dilemma: Selecting wound dressings by category. *Ostomy/Wound Management, 35,* 62–70.

Kucan, J. O., Robson, M. C., Heggers, J. P., & Ko, F. (1981). Comparisons of silver sulfadiazine and physiologic saline in the treatment of chronic pressure ulcers. *Journal of the American Geriatric Society, 29,* 232–235.

Kurzuk-Howard, G., Simpson, L., & Palmieri, A. (1985). Decubitus ulcer care: A comparative study. *Western Journal of Nursing Research, 7*(1), 58–75.

Lawrence, J. C. (1994). Dressings and wound infection. *American Journal of Surgery, 167,* (I A Suppl.), 215–245.

Lawrence, J. C., & Lilly, H. A. (1985). Bacteriological properties of a new hydrocolloid dressing on intact skin of normal volunteers. In T. J. Ryan (Ed.), *An environment for healing: The role of occlusion* (pp. 51–53). London: The Royal Society of Medicine.

Lazarus, G. S., Cooper, D. M., Knighton, D. R., et al. (1994). Definitions and guidelines for assessment of wounds and evaluation of healing. *Archives of Dermatology, 130,* 489–493.

Leaper, D. J., and Simpson, R. A. (1986). The effect of antiseptics and topical antimicrobials on wound healing. *Journal of Antimicrobial Chemotherapy, 17*(2), 135–136.

Leaper, D. J. Brennan, S. S., Simpson, R. A., & Foster, M. E. (1984). Experimental infection and hydrogel dressings. *Journal of Hospital Infection, 5*(Suppl A), 69–73.

Lineaweaver, W., Howard, R., Soucy, D., et al. (1985). Topical antimicrobial toxicity. *Archives of Surgery, 120*(3), 267–270.

Linsky, C. B., Rovee, D. T., & Dow, T. (1981). Effect of dressing on wound inflammation and scar tissue. In P. Dineen & G. Hildick-Smith (Eds.), *The surgical wound* (pp. 377–378). Philadelphia: Lea and Febiger.

Long, C. L., Schaffel, N., Grieger, J. W., et al. (1979). Metabolic response to injury and illness: Estimation of energy and protein needs from indirect calorimetry and nitrogen balance. *Journal of Parenteral and Enteral Nutrition, 3*(6), 452–456.

Macklebust, J. (1987). Pressure ulcers: Etiology and prevention. *Nursing Clinics of North America 22*(2), 359–377.

Madden, M. R., Finkelstein, J. L., Hefton, J. M., & Yurt, R. (1985). Optimal healing of donor site wounds with hydrocolloid dressings. In T. J. Ryan (Ed.), *An environment for healing: The role of occlusion* (pp. 133–136). London: The Royal Society of Medicine.

Mandy, S. H. (1983). A new primary wound dressing made of polyethylene oxide gel. *Journal of Dermatologic Surgery, 9*(2), 153–155.

May, S. R. (1984). Physiology, immunology and clinical efficacy of an adherent polyurethane wound dressing: Op-site. In D. L. Wise (Ed.), *Burn wound coverings* (Vol. 2, pp. 54–78). Boca Raton, FL: CRC Press.

Mayer, D. A., & Tsapogas, M. J. (1993). Povidone-iodine and wound healing in critical review. *Wounds, 5*(1), 14–23.

Mertz, P. M., Marshall, D. A., & Eaglstein, W. H. (1985). Occlusive wound dressings to prevent bacterial invasion and wound infection. *Journal of the American Academy of Dermatology, 12*(4), 662–668.

Mulliken, J. B., Healey, N. A., & Glowacki, J. (1980) Povidone-iodine and tensile strength of wounds in rats. *Journal of Trauma, 20*(4), 323–324.

Nemeth, G. G., Bolander, M. E., & Martin, G. R. (1988). Growth factors and their role in wound and fracture healing. In A. Barbul, E. Pines, M. Caldwell, & T. K. Hunt (Eds.), *Progress in clinical and biological research. Growth factors and other aspects of wound healing* (Vol. 266, pp. 1–17). New York: Alan R. Liss.

Noe, J. M., & Kalish, S. (1976). The mechanism of capillarity in surgical dressings. *Surgery, Gynecology and Obstetrics, 143,* 454–456.

Odugbesan, O., & Barnett, A. H. (1987). Use of a seaweed-based dressing in management of leg ulcers in diabetics. *Practical Diabetes, 4,* 46–47.

Oliver, L. C., & Blaine, G. (1950). Hemostasis with absorbable alginates in neurological practice. *British Journal of Surgery, 174,* 1.

Pace, W. E. (1978). Beads of a dextran polymer for the local treatment of cutaneous ulcers. *Journal of Dermatology, Surgery, and Oncology, 4*(9), 678–682.

Panel for the Prediction and Prevention of Pressure Ulcers in Adults. *Pressure ulcers in adults: Prediction and prevention.* Clinical Practice Guidelines, Number 3. AHCPR Guideline Publication No. 92–0047. Rockville, MD: Agency for Health Care Policy and Research, Public Health Service, U.S. Dept of Health and Human Services, May 1992.

Pollack, S. V. (1979). Wound healing: A review. *Journal of Dermatology, Surgery, and Oncology, 5*(6), 477–481.

Pories, W. J., Henzel, J. H., Robb, C. G., et al. (1967). Acceleration of wound healing in man with zinc sulphate given by mouth. *Lancet, 1,* 121–124.

Reed, B. R., & Clark, R. A. F. (1985). Cutaneous tissue repair: Practical implications of current knowledge. *Journal of the American Academy of Dermatology, 13,* 919–941.

Reuler, J. B., & Cooney, T. G. (1981). The pressure sore: Pathophysiology and principles of management. *Annals of Internal Medicine, 94,* 661–666.

Rhodes, J. E., Fliegelman, M. T., & Panzer, L. M. (1942). The mechanism of delayed wound healing in the presence of hypoproteinemia. *Journal of the American Medical Association, 118,* 21–25.

Rodeheaver, G. (1989). Controversies in topical wound management. *Wounds, 1,* 19–27.

Rodeheaver, G., Bellamy, W., Kody, M., et al. (1982). Bactericidal activity and toxicity of iodine-containing solutions in wounds. *Archives of Surgery, 117*(2), 181–186.

Rodeheaver, G. T., Pettry, D., Thacker, J. G., et al. (1975). Wound cleansing by high pressure irrigation. *Surgery, Gynecology and Obstetrics, 141,* 357–362.

Ross, R. (1987). Platelet derived growth factor. *Annual Review of Medicine, 38,* 71–79.

Rudolph, R., & Noe, J. M. (1983). *Chronic problem wounds.* Boston: Little, Brown.

Samela, K., & Ahonen, J. (1981). The effect of methylprednisolone and vitamin A on wound healing. I. *Acta Chirurgia Scandinavica, 147,* 307–312.

Sandberg, N. (1964). Time relationship between administration of corticosterone and wound healing in rats. *Acta Chirurgica Scandinavica, 127,* 446.

Sandstead, H. H., Henricksen, L. K., Greger, J. L., et al. (1982). Zinc nutrituse in the elderly in relation to taste acuity, immune response and wound healing. *American Journal of Clinical Nutrition, 36,* 1046–1059.

Sawyer, P. N., Bergan, J., Dagher, F. J., et al. (1980). Treatment alternatives for pressure sores. *Modern Medicine, 48,* 49–56.

Schilling, J. A. (1976). Wound healing. *Surgical Clinics of North America, 56,* 859–874.

Schroeder, D., Gillanders, L., Mahr, K., et al. (1991). Effects of immediate postoperative enteral nutrition on body composition. *Journal of Parenteral and Enteral Nutrition, 15*(4), 376–383.

Silver, I. A. (1972). Oxygen tension and epithelialization. In H. I. Maibach & D. T. Rovee (Eds.), *Epidermal wound healing* (pp. 291–305). Chicago: Year Book Medical Publishers.

Silver, I. A. (1985). Oxygen and tissue repair. In T. J. Ryan (Ed.), *An environment for healing: The role of occlusion* (pp. 15–21). London: The Royal Society of Medicine.

Stevenson, T. R., Thacker, J. G., Rodeheaver, G. T., et al. (1976). Cleansing the traumatic wound by high pressure syringe irrigation. *Journal of the American College of Emergency Physicians, 5,* 17–21.

Stotts, N. A. (1993). Impaired healing. In V. Carrieri-Kohlman, A. M. Lindsay, & C. West (Eds.), *Pathophysiological phenomena in nursing* (2nd ed.). Philadelphia: W. B. Saunders.

Stotts, N. A. (1990). Seeing red . . . and yellow . . . and black: The three-color concept of wound care. *Nursing '90, 20*(2):59–61.

Suh, D. Y., Hunt, T. K., & Spencer, E. M. (1992). Insulin-like growth factor-I reverses the impairment of wound healing induced by corticosteroids in rats. *Endocrinology, 13*(5), 2399–2403.

Temple, W. J., Voitk, A. J., Snelling, C. F. T., & Crispin, J. S. (1975). Effect of nutrition, diet, and suture material on long-term wound healing. *Annals of Surgery, 182,* 93–97.

Thomas, S. (1985). Use of a calcium alginate dressing. *The Pharmaceutical Journal, 235,* 188–190.

Turner, T. D. (1985). Semiocclusive and occlusive dressings. In T. J. Ryan (Ed.), *An environment for healing: The role of occlusion* (pp. 5–14). London: The Royal Society of Medicine.

Varghese, M. C., Balin, A. K., Carter, M., & Caldwell, D. (1986). Local environment of chronic wounds under synthetic dressings. *Archives of Dermatology, 122,* 52–57.

West, J. M., Hopf, H. W., Sessler, D. I., & Hunt, T. K. (1993). The effect of rapid postoperative rewarming on tissue oxygenation (abstract; p. 80). Proceedings of the Joint Meeting of the Wound Healing Society and the European Tissue Repair Society, Amsterdam, Netherlands, August 22–25.

Wheeland, R. G. (1987). The newer surgical dressings and wound healing. *Dermatologic Clinics, 5*(2), 393–407.

Wheeler, C. B., Rodeheaver, G. T., Thacker, J. G., et al. (1976). Side-effects of high pressure irrigation. *Surgery, Gynecology and Obstetrics,* 143, 775–778.

Whitney, J. D., Stotts, N. A., Goodson, W. H. III, et al. (1993). The effect of activity and bed rest on tissue oxygen tension, perfusion, and plasma volume. *Nursing Research, 42,* 349–355.

Williamson, M. B., & Fromm, H. J. (1955). The incorporation of sulfur amino acids into the proteins of regenerating wound tissue. *Journal of Biological Chemistry, 212,* 715–712.

Winter, G. D. (1962). Formation of the scab and the rate of epithelialization of superficial wounds in the skin of the young domestic pig. *Nature (London), 193,* 293–294.

Winter, G. D., & Scales, J. T. (1963). Effect of air drying and dressings on the surface of a wound. *Nature (London), 197,* 91–92.

Witkowski, J. A., & Parish, L. C. (1986). Cutaneous ulcer therapy. *International Journal of Dermatology, 25*(7), 420–426.

Wysocki, A. B. (1986). The effect of intermittent noise exposure on the rate of wound healing in albino rats. Unpublished dissertation, University of Texas at Austin.

Young, M. E. (1988). Malnutrition and wound healing. *Heart & Lung, 7*(1), 60–69.

Young, R. A. L., & Weston-Davies, W. H. (1985). Comparison of a hydrocolloid with a conventional island dressing as a primary surgical wound dressing. In T. J. Ryan (Ed.), *An environment for healing: The role of occlusion* (pp. 153–156). London: The Royal Society of Medicine.

CHAPTER

60 Patients With Burns

Randy M. Caine

Burns are immediately or potentially life-threatening traumatic injuries. In the United States alone, more than 2 million persons suffer burn injuries each year; of those, 500,000 seek medical attention and approximately 70,000 will be hospitalized. Despite the advances in burn treatment and intervention more than 12,000 will die as a result of their burns (American Burn Association, 1990). Prevention as well as emergency care and critical care interventions for burns is necessary.

Burn nursing is both complex and challenging. Nurses involved in the emergent, acute, or rehabilitative aspects of burn care must be knowledgeable about the pathophysiologic and psychosocial changes that occur in the burned patient. These patients are traumatically injured and have multisystem organ involvement, and therefore present with an abundance of difficulties and special challenges. It is for these reasons that the care of the burned patient, as well as the family, cannot be provided by critical care nurses alone but must involve a team effort.

TYPES OF BURN INJURIES

Thermal Injuries

Thermal injuries, or heat-related injuries, account for almost three-quarters of all burn injuries in the United States, and range from hot-water scalds to flame burns to direct contact with a heat source. Because of the diverse mechanisms of injury, treatment must be tailored to the specific etiologic agent.

When we think of thermal injuries, we most often think of house fires. Only 5% of all burn victims, however, are injured as a result of house fires. Smoke inhalation from house fires causes the largest number of burn-related deaths. Hot-water scalds account for approximately 22% of all burns, with most victims under age 4 (Choctaw et al., 1987). Flammable liquids, grease, vehicle fires, and explosions also account for thermal injuries. Despite the cause of injury, all thermal burns are classified according to the depth of injury.

Chemical Injuries

Chemical agents generally do not "burn" in the sense that they destroy tissue through the effect of heat, although some chemicals can act in this manner. Tissue damage and destruction result from the chemical coagulation of protein, precipitation of chemical compounds in the cell, severe cellular dehydration, and protoplasmic poisoning or complete dissolution of tissue proteins (Hersperger & Dahl, 1978; Trofino, 1991). The effects of chemical damage on tissues are determined by the following factors: (1) strength or concentration of the chemical, (2) length of contact with tissue, (3) quantity, (4) extent of tissue penetration, and (5) mode of action of the chemical.

It should be remembered that the skin and the underlying structures will continue to be injured until the chemical source is removed or inactivated by reaction with cellular components. Most chemicals can be washed off the skin with water.

Several types of chemical agents that cause burns include oxidizing agents, reducing agents, corrosive agents, protoplasmic poisons, desiccants, and vesicants. *Oxidizing agents* such as sodium hypochlorite, chromic acid, and potassium permanganate become oxidized on contact with body tissue. *Reducing agents,* including nitric acid and hydrochloric acid, cause tissue damage through a denaturing effect on the cellular proteins. *Corrosive agents* are phenols, white phosphorus, sodium metals, and lyes. *Protoplasmic poisons* such as tannic acid, picric acid, formic acid, oxalic acid, and hydrofloric acid produce tissue damage by forming salts with the cellular cations, resulting in protein coagulation. *Desiccants* such as sulfuric acid and muriatic acid are mineral acids that produce tissue damage through extreme cellular dehydration and generate considerable heat when in contact with tissue fluids. *Vesiccants* include cantharides, dimethyl sulfoxide, and mustard gas. Their burn mechanism of action is not known; however, tissue ischemia and anoxia are the end results of this chemical reaction.

Gasoline burns are due to prolonged contact of gasoline with tissue (without ignition). Unleaded gasoline contains 0.5% to 3% benzene, an absorbable, potentially toxic agent. Gasoline can cause central nervous system depression with the potential for further injury (Edelman, 1987; Trofino, 1991).

Management of chemical injuries depends on the type of agent involved. In general, all chemicals should be flushed with copious amounts of water until definitive therapy can be provided. Regional poison centers maintain specific guidelines and should be contacted immediately. Once tissue damage is complete, standard burn care is instituted.

Electrical Injuries

Approximately 1000 people die each year in the United States as a result of electric shock (Uehara et al., 1986). Electrical injuries occur less frequently than scald injuries but are potentially life-threatening. Tissue damage due to electricity may be caused by either direct contact with the current or the flash caused by electrical arcing. Although actual damage to the body depends on the current passing through it, a number of other factors influence the severity of the injury as well, including (1) amperage, the amount of resistance applied to the voltage; (2) voltage, a measure of force of the flow of current; (3) type of current—alternating (AC) or direct (DC). AC is found in homes and most industries, whereas DC is used in chemical and metallurgic industries and street car systems, and onboard ships; (4) duration of contact—the greater the duration of contact, the more severe the damage; (5) surface area of contact—the larger the surface area, the greater the damage; and (6) tissue resistance, because the body conducts current as a result of its electrolyte content. In declining order, the human tissues may be listed according to the resistance they offer: skin, bone, fat, nerve, muscle, blood and body fluids (Somogyi & Tedeschi, 1977; Trofino, 1991). This means that a given current flowing through bone will generate more heat in the local tissues than will the same current in blood. The resistance of skin also varies with the thickness and moisture content of the skin.

Electric current may cause death directly by ventricular fibrillation, asphyxiation secondary to tetanic contractions of the muscles of respiration, or respiratory arrest. Indirect causes of death are severe thermal injury, nervous system damage, vascular injury, and renal failure (Hersperger & Dahl, 1978). Electric current may also cause long-bone fractures resulting from tetanic contractions as well as associated injuries from falls.

Radiation Burns

Ionizing radiation burns are significantly different from burns caused by flame, steam, chemical agents, or electricity. These burns have long-term biologic effects that result in chronic health care concerns that may be seen years after the initial injury. The critical care nurse will most likely care for these patients as an immediate result of ionizing radiation exposure or a catastrophic nuclear disaster or accident.

The term ionizing radiation includes alpha and beta particles, gamma rays, and roentgen or x-rays. The intracellular destruction of DNA molecules and the resultant loss of genetic information is a significant consequence of radiation injuries. This loss is shown most prominently in the altered replicative ability of the cell (Nicosia & Petro, 1983; Trofino, 1991). For example, mucosal cells of the intestine, which normally reproduce rapidly, demonstrate cellular changes earlier as a result of radiation injury.

Acute radiation injury caused by localized irradiation appears much like the initial stages of thermal injury, with erythema, edema, pain, and tissue ischemia. The potential for acute and chronic infection and necrosis is apparent. Whole-body irradiation, on the other hand, causes systemic symptoms, termed radiation sickness, which are dose dependent. Death may result in as little as hours or days with high radiation doses, whereas lower doses of radiation may cause chronic ulceration, osteoradionecrosis, skin changes, or malignancy. Treatment of whole-body irradiation is primarily supportive in terms of skin care, pain management, infection control, and emotional support.

Tar Injuries

Hot tar burns account for approximately 5% of all burn injuries in adults. When tar is in its liquid form it may be as hot as 500°F (260°C). After coming in contact with the skin, the tar quickly cools, solidifies, and becomes enmeshed in the hair. The cooling process should be expedited by the addition of cool water. The literature states that the tar can be removed with any petroleum-based ointment; however, removal of the tar has been shown to be of lesser concern than the cooling process (Hill et al., 1984). Once the tar has been cooled, the burning process has ended, and the tar can be slowly removed in a matter of days as it is lifted with silver sulfadiazine cream. No increased incidence of bacterial colonization has been shown by leaving the tar in place (Hill et al., 1984). Once the tar has lifted, the burn is treated like any other burn.

PATHOPHYSIOLOGY

Anatomy and Physiology of Skin

The skin comprises the largest organ of the body. It is composed of three layers—the thin, nonvascular outer layer termed the epidermis, the middle tissue layer termed the dermis, or corium, and the subcutaneous fat layer (Fig. 60–1). The epidermis consists of stratified epithelial tissue, whereas the dermis consists of fibrous connective tissue. Subcutaneous tissue is made up of loose areolar and, in some cases, adipose tissue.

The epidermis has five layers, which include the stratum corneum, stratum lucidum, stratum granulosum, stratum spinosum, and stratum germinativum. Two of these layers, the stratum corneum and the stratum germinativum, figure prominently in an understanding of burn wound healing. The stratum corneum is composed of keratin fibers surrounded by a monolipid layer that is water repellent. This layer functions as a vapor barrier that prevents fluid loss. Thus, in extensive burn injuries involving this layer,

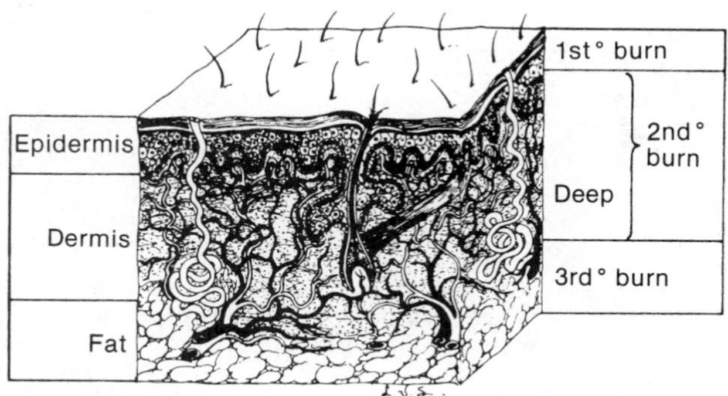

FIGURE 60–1. Cross-section of the skin. (From Demling, R. H. [1989]. In W. C. Shoemaker et al. [Eds.], *The society of critical care medicine textbook of critical care* [2nd ed., p. 1301]. Philadelphia: W. B. Saunders.)

large fluid losses occur. The stratum germinativum is also important because it is constantly producing new cells that move to the surface to replace other epidermal layers that are continually being sloughed off. Melanin may also be found in this layer; it affects the color of the skin.

The dermis, or corium, serves as both a supportive and a nutritional basis for the epidermis. The complex dermis is composed of blood vessels; sensory receptors for touch, pain, and pressure; and the epidermal appendages that include the hair follicles, sebaceous glands, and sweat glands. Collagen fiber is also found in the dermis. Scattered throughout the collagen are connective tissue cells called *mast cells,* which are responsible for secretion, phagocytosis, and repair. Increased amounts of histamine are released by these mast cells in patients with burn injury. When burn injuries destroy the epidermis, epithelial cells from the epidermal appendages begin to form new epithelium.

The subcutaneous fat layer contains the roots of the hair follicles and the sweat glands. Collagen fibers from the dermis extend to this layer to ensure adhesion of the dermis to the subcutaneous tissue. The collagen found here plays a significant role in burn injury because it is collagen that anchors the eschar in place, thus making removal of eschar difficult.

The largest of the skin arteries are found in the subcutaneous tissue just beneath the dermis. Thus, in burn injury, plasma leaking from the arteries may cause edema and blistering.

The skin plays an active role in the prevention of infection as the first line of defense. In addition, it conserves body fluids, regulates body temperature, produces vitamin D when exposed to ultraviolet light, secretes oil to lubricate and soften skin, allows excretion of excess water and waste products, and serves as a sensory organ for touch, pain, and pressure.

Tissue death associated with burn injuries can be described in terms of the histopathologic characteristics related to the concentric zones of the burn injury. The tissues in direct contact with the burn source are in the central zone of protein coagulation and cell death. This is termed the *zone of necrosis.* In full-thickness injury, all dermal elements are destroyed; partial-thickness injury may be characterized by incomplete necrosis. Surrounding the central zone and extending radially are areas of damage called the *zone of stasis* and *zone of hyperemia.* These areas may be characterized by decreased microvascular blood flow and inflammatory response, respectively (Mozingo et al., 1994).

Classification of Burn Depth

In the past, burns were described in terms of degree—first-, second-, third-, and fourth-degree. More recently, first- and second-degree burns have been described as superficial (first-degree) and partial-thickness (second-degree); any burn deeper than the dermis is described as full-thickness (third-degree). Classification of fourth-degree burns includes injuries extending into the subcutaneous fat, muscle, and bone. These injuries are now included in the full-thickness classification (Table 60–1).

SUPERFICIAL BURNS. These burns result either from prolonged exposure to low-intensity heat (e.g., sunburn) or from a short-duration flash exposure to a high-intensity heat source. Erythema of the skin with local edema is the result. Superficial burns do not require treatment other than local pain relief and are not calculated in the amount of body surface area burned when determining the extent of a burn. Comfort measures include aspirin, fluids, local topical pain relief, and frequent application of water-soluble lotion. Superficial burns heal in 3 to 5 days after desquamation and do not cause scarring or require further treatment.

PARTIAL-THICKNESS BURNS. A superficial partial-thickness burn is equal to the classic second-degree burn characterized by fluid-filled blisters appearing immediately after injury and by pain when the blisters are removed and the burn is exposed to air. The blister membrane, in its intact condition, forms a sterile environment that prevents excessive water loss from the burn wound.

Since the dermal layer of the skin is for the most part intact, healing takes place between 10 and 14 days after injury, and scarring is minimal. In some cases, there is a significant loss of melanocytes, which can result in a minor and sometimes permanent color change.

The deep partial-thickness burn consists of a disruption of the epidermis and most of the dermis, sparing the appendages such as hair follicles and sweat glands. This sparing of appendages is what allows the wound potentially to regenerate (thus it is a partial-thickness burn). Blistering of the wound may occur as in the more superficial partial-thickness burn, but this is not an essential component. The wound is more often characterized by eschar formation. Deep partial-thickness burns exhibit massive fluid losses because

TABLE 60–1. **Classification of Burn Injury**

By Depth	First-Degree	Second-Degree		Third-Degree
By skin thickness	Superficial partial thickness	Moderate partial thickness	Deep partial thickness	Full thickness
By anatomic description	Epidermal	Superficial dermal	Deep dermal	Subdermal (fat, muscle, bone)
Appearance/diagnosis of depth	Pink to red; no blisters; skin remains intact when rubbed gently; may appear slightly edematous	Red or mottled red and pink; contains blisters; skin easily rubbed off; moist weeping, edematous; if pulled, hair remains intact; blanches with pressure	Pink to pale ivory; can see a reticulated pattern; wound may appear somewhat dry; contains blisters and bullae; hair removes easily; does not blanch with pressure or return of color is slow	White, cherry red, brown, or black; may or may not contain blisters; may contain thrombosed vessels; appears dry, hard, leathery; and may be depressed
Cause	Radiation (sunburn), flash from low-intensity explosion	Brief contact with hot liquids, steam, or hot objects; high-intensity flash	Longer contact with hot liquids or hot objects; chemicals; and brief contact with flames	Prolonged contact with hot liquids or objects; flames; chemicals; electrical
Pain response	Uncomfortable to touch	Very painful	Pain response variable; hyper- and hypoalgesia	Painless to pinprick; pain is aching in nature
Time to heal	3–5 days	<3 weeks	>3 weeks	Requires grafting

From Marvin, J. (1994). Thermal Injuries. In V. D. Cardona et al. (Eds.), *Trauma nursing: From resuscitation through rehabilitation.* Philadelphia: W. B. Saunders.

the cellular barrier that normally protects against bacterial invasion and wound sepsis is no longer present.

Sensation is usually present in deep partial-thickness burns but may be decreased because of actual destruction of nerve endings in the dermal layer of the skin. Wound healing takes longer at this depth, usually 21 to 28 days, and more scar is formed.

FULL-THICKNESS BURNS. In a full-thickness burn the epidermis, dermis, and all the dermal appendages are destroyed. The burn may extend into the subcutaneous fat, muscle, or bone. A thick, leathery eschar forms that allows copious amounts of fluid loss through the wound and fails to protect against bacterial invasion and wound sepsis. Because dermal appendages have been destroyed by the burn, the wound will heal by contraction and epithelial growth from the edges. If allowed to heal by this means, the scar will be deformed and unstable; therefore, in clinical practice, skin grafts are applied to promote function and stability.

If the full-thickness burn extends into the muscle, myoglobinuria can become a significant problem. This may lead to renal failure in poorly hydrated patients.

Most experienced burn practitioners can determine burn depth correctly by visual inspection only approximately 50% of the time. Visual inspection tends to be very subjective. Objective means for determining burn depth, such as the use of lasers, fluorescein, and magnetic resonance imaging (MRI), have been studied for some time. The laser Doppler technique is another technique used to determine burn depth. In this technique a laser beam is used to look at the flow of blood through burn tissue, providing information about the circulatory physiology of the burn wound. Normal skin has a relatively low basal blood flow, whereas burn tissue increases blood flow remarkably in response to local heating. Full-thickness burn wounds that fail to heal have low blood flow and minimal or no increase of flow in response to local heating. Partial-thickness burns that do heal have elevated blood flow, which may increase even further with local heating (Waxman et al., 1989).

Fluorescein has also been used to attempt to determine the depth of injury. Fluorescein is injected intravenously. If the drug is present in the burn wound, it means that blood flow is adequate to allow the wound to heal. Results of fluorescein injection have been found to be less accurate than those achieved with Doppler study and close to those characteristic of visual inspection.

Magnetic resonance imaging is another tool that may be used to assess the level of injury in patients with electrical burns, in whom there can be significant internal damage. MRI remains in very limited use, however, due to its high cost and the requirement that the patient must be stable to be transported to an MRI center.

Severity of Burn Injury

Both the American Burn Association and the American College of Surgeons rate the severity of burns as minor, moderate, or major (Table 60–2). Both agree that minor burns can be treated on an outpatient basis. Moderate burns can usually be cared for in a general hospital if a burn center is unavailable; however, all

TABLE 60–2. **Criteria of Burn Injury Severity**

	American Burn Association		American College of Surgeons	
	Adults Degree %	*Children Degree %*	*Adults Degree %*	*Children Degree %*
Minor	2nd—<15 3rd—<2	2nd, 3rd } <10	2nd, 3rd } <15	2nd, 3rd } <10
Moderate	2nd—>15–25 3rd—<10	2nd—>10–20 3rd—<10	2nd, 3rd } 15–25	2nd, 3rd } 10–20
Major	2nd—>25 3rd—>10	2nd—>20 3rd—>10	2nd—>25 3rd—>10	2nd—>20 3rd—>10

From Achauer, B. M. (Ed.) 1987. *Management of the burned patient*. Norwalk, CT: Appleton & Lange; Prentice-Hall.

major burns should be cared for in a burn center. In addition, moderate burns of the hands, feet, eyes, ears, face, and perineum should also be cared for in a burn center because of the high risk of either infection or functional disuse in these areas.

CALCULATION OF TOTAL BODY SURFACE AREA BURNED. American Burn Association standards require that the extent of burn injury be calculated on entry to the health care system. Two methods are used for calculating the amount of total body surface area (TBSA) burned. The first is the rule of nines (Fig. 60–2), which is commonly used in the prehospital setting, the primary assessment of the burn patient, and the triage of mass casualties. It is a simple, quick method of estimating the extent of injury. There is a rule of nines for adults and another for children. Because infants and small children have larger heads and smaller legs than adults, the Lund and Browder formula (Fig. 60–3) is commonly used for them. The Lund and Browder chart is also a more specific method of estimating burn extent in the adult.

When estimating TBSA burned, only partial- and full-thickness burns are included. Superficial burns are not part of this calculation nor of the amount of fluid needed for fluid resuscitation, which is based on the concept that superficial burns have intact skin that still functions normally.

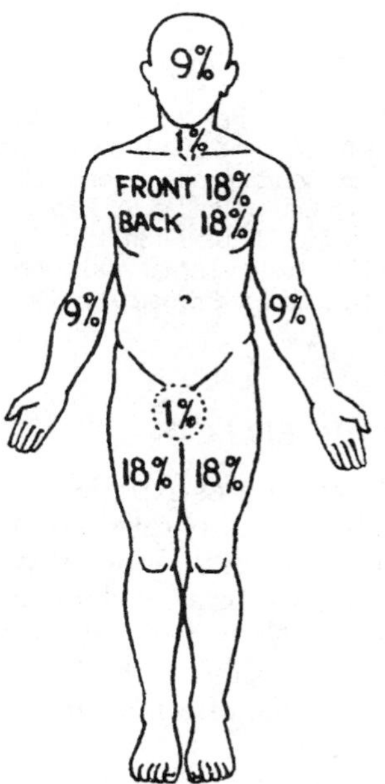

FIGURE 60–2. Rules of nines for calculating the total body surface area burned. (Adapted from Wallace, A. B. [1951]. The exposure treatment of burns. *Lancet, 1*, 501.)

PHASES OF BURN PHYSIOLOGY AND PATIENT CARE MANAGEMENT

When burns cause major destruction in the skin's integrity, numerous physiologic and hemodynamic changes occur throughout each of the body systems. The primary physiologic changes occur in the cardiovascular system in terms of the phases of fluid shifts. Other systemic changes become evident in the period immediately after burn trauma, and, as time from burn injury progresses, these systems undergo additional physiologic alterations. Three general phases in burn physiology and patient care management have been identified; these include the *emergent* or *shock phase*, the *acute* or *fluid remobilization phase*, and the *rehabilitation* or *recovery phase*. For each of these phases, a discussion of the physiology, including the multisystemic effects, and patient care management will be provided.

Emergent (Shock) Phase

PHYSIOLOGY

The emergent phase of burn pathophysiology is characterized primarily by capillary permeability and a shift of fluid from the plasma into the interstitial space as well as loss of plasma through the skin. Along with the shifting fluid goes debris from hemolyzed blood cells, proteins, and electrolytes. In major burns, the fluid loss results in decreased cardiac output and hypovolemic shock. To compensate, vasoconstriction oc-

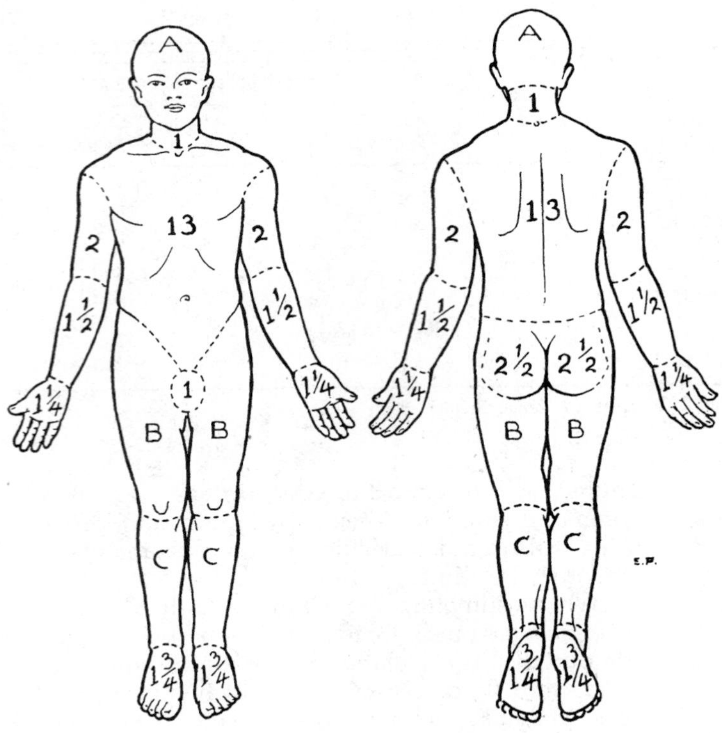

Age	Birth	1	5	10	15	Adult
Area						
Head	19	17	13	11	9	7
Neck	2	2	2	2	2	2
Anterior trunk*	13	13	13	13	13	13
Posterior trunk‡	13	13	13	13	13	13
Buttocks	5	5	5	5	5	5
Genitalia	1	1	1	1	1	1
Upper arms	8	8	8	8	8	8
Forearms	6	6	6	6	6	6
Hands	5	5	5	5	5	5
Thighs	11	13	16	17	18	19
Legs	10	10	11	12	13	14
Feet	7	7	7	7	7	7
Total	100	100	100	100	100	100

*Without neck or genitalia.
‡Without neck or buttocks.

FIGURE 60–3. Lund and Browder chart for estimation of areas of burns. *Abbreviations:* A, one-half of head; B, one-half of thigh; C, one-half of leg (A, B, and C refer to areas affected by growth). (Modified from Lund, C. C., and Browder, N. C. [1944]. The estimation of areas of burns. By permission of *Surgery, Gynecology & Obstetrics, 79,* 353.)

curs. Capillary permeability occurs within 30 minutes of the burn injury, but the most significant changes begin to occur 6 to 8 hours after the burn. This phase generally lasts from 36 to 48 hours after the burn but may last as long as 96 hours depending on the extent of TBSA burned and when fluid resuscitation was initiated. Hypovolemic shock now occurs less frequently in burn patients because of improved early resuscitation efforts.

Every system is affected by the devastating nature of burn injury. The critical care nurse must be aware of the effect of burn injury on each of the primary systems to provide knowledgeable care to the patient.

MULTISYSTEMIC EFFECTS

Patients with burn injuries experience massive physiologic trauma. The mortality rate in patients with extensive burn injuries is high, not only because of the consequences of burn injuries themselves and the resulting sepsis, but also because of the effects of the injury on all major systems of the body. The following describes the systemic effects of burn injuries during the emergent phase.

CARDIOVASCULAR SYSTEM EFFECTS. The most significant cardiovascular response to burn injury is the marked fluid alterations that result from capillary damage. When burn injury occurs, the normal equilibrium maintained among the various fluid compartments is disturbed. To appreciate this phenomenon, an understanding of the normal physiology is necessary. Fluid is normally compartmentalized into intracellular and extracellular areas. In the average adult, 60% of the body is composed of fluid. The intracellular fluid, which consists of the fluids found in all body cells, makes up approximately 40% of that total. The extracellular fluid, comprising plasma and interstitial fluid, constitutes the remaining 20%. Of the extracellular fluid, three-fourths is found in the interstitial spaces and one-fourth in the intravascular space. Equilibrium is maintained between the fluid in the interstitial and intravascular spaces by balancing hydrostatic and osmotic pressures. *Hydrostatic pressure* is the driving force of a liquid pushing against a surface that causes the liquid to move. *Osmotic pressure* is a counterbalancing, pulling force that causes water to move from low to high concentrations of solute particles through a semipermeable membrane. Within the circulatory system, as a result of arterial blood pressure that is higher than the pull of plasma proteins, hydrostatic pressure at the proximal end of the capillaries is normally greater, resulting in fluid being pushed into the interstitial spaces. Capillaries are not normally permeable to plasma proteins. Osmotic pressure, however, is greater at the distal end of the capillaries because blood pressure here is lower than the pull of the plasma proteins. This results in fluid being pulled back into the blood vessels. When capillary integrity is lost in the immediate postburn period, osmotic pressure is negative (Porth, 1994).

Lymph is also responsible for maintaining fluid balance. Lymphatic vessels are particularly numerous in the skin and contain terminating valves that open into the interstitial spaces and absorb excess fluid. Eventually, these vessels empty into the larger venous channels (Minar, 1978; Porth, 1994).

Fluid balance also is maintained between the interstitial and intracellular compartments through the distribution of sodium, potassium, and proteins. Sodium is the chief cation of extracellular fluid and is present in both the intravascular and interstitial spaces in approximately the same amounts. Potassium is the chief cation in intracellular fluid. The relative distribution of sodium and potassium is maintained by a pump mechanism that normally pushes sodium from the cell in exchange for potassium. Protein, found in large quantities within the cell in the form of protoplasm, exerts osmotic pressure to attract and maintain fluid inside the cell. This pull is counterbalanced by the sodium in the extracellular fluid, thus contributing to the balance between the interstitial and intracellular fluid compartments.

In burn injuries, the major physiologic alteration in the fluid compartments involves the extracellular compartment, in which a shift of fluid occurs from the intravascular into the interstitial space as a result of the disruption in balance between the hydrostatic and osmotic pressures. Capillary damage results in increased permeability and decreased selectivity. The increased permeability allows fluid to pass more rapidly and freely from the intravascular into the interstitial space. The decreased selectivity allows the plasma protein to leave the interstitial space. Because these proteins, or *colloids,* are the main solutes responsible for exerting osmotic pressure, there is a resulting decrease in osmotic pressure within the blood vessels and an increased osmotic pressure in the interstitial spaces. Thus, while hydrostatic pressure continues to drive fluid into the interstitial space, osmotic pressure is unable to pull the excess fluid back into the intravascular space. Ultimately, the major loss of fluid from the intravascular compartment results in retention of fluid in the tissues in the form of massive edema. If patients have circumferential burns or if a large body surface area has been burned, the fluid under the overwhelming eschar produces a tourniquet effect on the underlying structures, causing increased interstitial pressure, destruction of nerve endings, and circulatory collapse. To relieve this pressure, escharotomy or fasciotomy may be required.

After a burn, more sodium than water is drawn into the interstitial spaces. The sodium pump becomes less efficient, and more water and sodium enter the intracellular spaces. To attempt to compensate for the loss of water and sodium from the intravascular space, increased secretion of aldosterone and antidiuretic hormone (ADH) occurs, further contributing to the retention of sodium and water. After a major burn, several liters of fluid may be retained.

Fluid losses in patients with burn injuries may also result from water evaporation, blistering, or wound drainage. Approximately 20 times as much fluid is lost through evaporation when the skin is destroyed as when the skin is intact (Busby, 1979; Hayter, 1978; Trofino, 1991). Both sodium and potassium, essential electrolytes, are lost through burned skin as well. Potassium is released from injured tissue and cells and escapes into the extracellular fluid, resulting in a temporary increase in serum potassium levels.

Proteins from the injured cells or from the intravascular fluid freely pass through the injured capillaries into the interstitium. However, this protein is not lost as quickly as electrolytes and water. Therefore, the protein concentration initially increases, in turn increasing the osmotic pressure gradient. This pulls fluid from the interstitial spaces throughout the body to maintain cardiac output and adequate circulating fluid volume. When the interstitial fluid is depleted, the intracellular fluid is used next. If these events are untreated, death of the patient follows.

In addition to massive fluid volume changes, the cardiovascular system is further compromised because of decreased myocardial perfusion. Circulating myocardial depressant factors, liberated as a result of the shock, cause an increase in production of lactic acid and endotoxins.

Serial electrocardiograms (ECG) are indicated in all victims of electrical injuries and in any patient over

TABLE 60–3. **Signs and Symptoms of Smoke Inhalation**

Burned in an enclosed space	Carboxyhemoglobin >10%
Chest, face, or neck burns	Wheezing
Singed nasal hair or eyebrows	Hoarseness of the voice
Carbonaceous material in the mouth	Deep, labored respirations
Carbonaceous sputum	Altered level of consciousness

age 40 with a history of cardiovascular disease. ECGs, although not diagnostic of the burn injury, can be diagnostic of other problems, and a baseline ECG can be invaluable later in the patient's course of treatment.

Lysis and entrapment of red blood cells as well as alterations in coagulation and fibrinolysis, sometimes resulting in disseminated intravascular coagulation (DIC), can occur in patients with burn injuries (Ohura, 1988). These events may cause anemia or, in extreme cases, thrombi may form in the capillaries as a result of stasis or heat from the burn. The ischemia or necrosis of tissue that results is sometimes treated with anticoagulant therapy. More recently, anticoagulant therapy using heparin with antithrombin III is reserved for a severely burned victim unless DIC is documented (Ohura, 1988; Trofino, 1991; Zawacki, 1974).

Anemia in the burn patient may be masked by the initially high hematocrits caused when fluid is lost from the intravascular space. If the patient's hematocrit is within normal values, the critical care nurse should suspect anemia, particularly if the patient has suffered other traumatic injuries. If bleeding from these traumatically injured sites remains undetected or untreated, the anemia may progress.

PULMONARY SYSTEM EFFECTS. After burn injury, pulmonary sequelae such as the loss of respiratory cilia, development of a chemical pneumonitis, destruction of respiratory cell protein, and atelectasis as a result of inhalation injuries are common. Inhalation injuries are caused by a variety of substances toxic to the respiratory passages. Inhalation injuries should be suspected in the patient who has obvious burns to the face, neck, or chest. Patients found burned in an enclosed space should also be assessed for inhalation injury; however, inhalation injuries should not be ruled out in patients burned in open areas.

Inhalation burns may be classified according to the relationship of the burn to the glottis (i.e., supraglottic or subglottic). Burns to the respiratory tract below the glottis are extremely rare; if present, they are usually the result of inhalation of live steam. The trachea is an excellent heat exchanger, effectively cooling hot inspired air. In addition, hot air causes a reflex closure of the vocal cords, further protecting the lower airways from direct heat injury. The usual signs associated with inhalation injury are listed in Table 60–3.

Bronchospasm, alveolar damage, or carbon monoxide poisoning may be responsible for respiratory distress in the burn patient. These pulmonary complications of inhalation injury can be complex and may constitute a major threat to the patient's survival.

Acute airway obstruction can also result from severe facial, oral, or laryngeal edema. Most cases of airway obstruction occur within 24 to 48 hours after burn injury (Wiener & Barrett, 1986). Edema may be a direct result of heat injury in patients with orofacial burn trauma, or it may result from fluid administration.

Smoke is a suspension of small particles in hot air or gas. This particulate matter becomes trapped in the nose, mouth, and throat and during inhalation the gaseous fraction of the particulate matter enters the respiratory passages. Carbon monoxide and hydrogen cyanide, known to be toxic substances, are present in this gaseous fraction of the smoke. Another major concern with smoke inhalation is the possibility of subsequent inhalation of lung-damaging and highly toxic gases that result from the burning of plastic material (e.g., polyvinyl chloride). Polyvinyl chloride alone has been shown to produce 75 toxic gases when burned, the most lethal of which is hydrogen chloride (Desai, 1984; Dyer & Esch, 1976). On entering the lungs, these gases react to form strong acids or alkalis that ultimately destroy the pulmonary epithelium and cilia. Inhaled carbon monoxide binds with hemoglobin, thereby displacing the oxygen-carrying capacity of the hemoglobin and causing a rise in the carboxyhemoglobin (COHb) level to greater than 10% and a shift to the left of the oxygen-dissociation curve. Less oxygen is transported, and cerebral hypoxia results, even though the Pa_{O_2} may be normal. Although patients may be asymptomatic, COHb levels of over 10% are diagnostic of carbon monoxide poisoning, and early intubation may be required (Cioffi & Rue, 1991); COHb levels of less than 10% do not rule out carbon monoxide poisoning because of the short half-life of COHb (Fig. 60–4). It is therefore imperative that COHb levels be monitored judiciously.

Arterial blood pH and gases should be tested periodically because they have the greatest diagnostic clinical value for the majority of patients. When inhalation

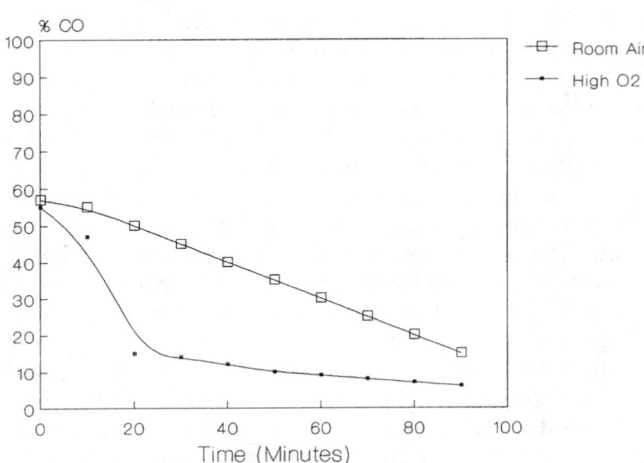

FIGURE 60–4. Half-life of carboxyhemoglobin.

TABLE 60–4. **Symptoms Associated With Pulmonary Injury**

Early Symptoms	Late Symptoms
Laryngeal edema	Parenchymal infection
Stridor	Hypoxemia
Hoarseness	Atelectasis
Bronchospasm	$\dot{V}/\dot{Q}$ mismatch
	Adult respiratory distress syndrome

injury is suspected, fiberoptic bronchoscopy, fiberoptic laryngoscopy, or a xenon-133 (^{133}Xe) ventilation–perfusion lung scan is performed to confirm the diagnosis. Bronchoscopy aids in the diagnosis of smoke inhalation and is indicated whenever there is a question of whether a patient should be intubated. The vocal cords should be visualized along with other structures as the presence of carbonaceous material or edema around the vocal cords is an indication for immediate intubation. If there is no carbonaceous material but slight edema is seen around the vocal cords, the physician may choose to perform serial bronchoscopies every 6 to 8 hours to follow the edema. Carbonaceous sputum at or below the larynx may suggest the need for pulmonary lavage during bronchoscopy. Ventilation–perfusion lung scans involve the intravenous administration of a small bolus dose of ^{133}Xe. Because this isotope is poorly soluble in water, it is almost entirely excreted in the alveoli. If the xenon fails to clear the lung in 90 seconds, the test result is abnormal and strongly indicates inhalation injury in the absence of previous pulmonary pathology. In the patient with inhalation injury, washout of the ^{133}Xe is delayed. Patients with red, swollen vocal cords or supraglottic area should have a nasogastric tube inserted before edema of the hypopharynx and larynx makes intubation difficult (Carrougher, 1993; Wiener & Barrett, 1986).

The consequences of gaseous and thermal injury are typically time dependent, and the immediate effects of burn injury are related to the combination of gases and the temperature involved. Relatively mild inhalation injuries, if left untreated, may progress to adult respiratory distress syndrome. Table 60–4 lists the early and late pulmonary symptoms associated with pulmonary injury.

All of the pulmonary manifestations, when accompanied by an increased percentage of TBSA burned, result in a decreasing functional residual capacity, atelectasis, ventilation–perfusion ($\dot{V}/\dot{Q}$) mismatch, progressive hypoxemia, and eventual death. Chest x-rays are often normal in the early postburn period after inhalation injury and therefore are unreliable early indicators for assessment. X-rays first become abnormal approximately 24 hours after the injury.

Patient care management of pulmonary sequelae involves administration of warm humidified oxygen, use of bronchodilators, postural drainage, percussion, incentive spirometry, intermittent positive-pressure breathing, and use of ultrasonic nebulizers. Hyperbaric oxygenation has been advocated by some for individuals with high COHb levels because of its ability to accelerate the dissociation of COHb from hemoglobin. A decreasing Pa_{O_2} may require nasotracheal intubation and the use of positive end-expiratory pressure (PEEP) in patients with upper airway injuries. Management of lower airway injuries may involve intubation accompanied by humidification, bronchodilation, and aggressive pulmonary hygiene.

Support of ventilation may be achieved through the use of established measures such as volume-cycled mechanical ventilation; however, pressure support, pressure control-inverse ratio ventilation, high-frequency jet ventilation, auto-PEEP, airway pressure release ventilation, negative-pressure ventilation, and differential lung ventilation may be used clinically (Burns, 1990; Cioffi et al., 1991; Kacmarek, 1988; Shelledy et al., 1988a, 1988b; St. John, 1990; White et al., 1990). Clinical trials of high-frequency percussive ventilation in patients with inhalation injury demonstrated significant improvement compared with patients treated with conventional therapy (Cioffi, 1989; Cioffi et al., 1991).

Even in the absence of inhalation injuries, burn patients with circumferential full-thickness injuries to the upper chest and neck also are at risk for respiratory complications. The inelastic eschar formation that results from these injuries impedes adequate respiratory excursion, causing hypoxia, hypoxemia, and respiratory distress. Immediate life-saving escharotomy permits the chest wall to expand and decreases the respiratory distress.

Other respiratory complications can arise from a decreased cough reflex and the patient's inability to expectorate pulmonary secretions. Arterial blood gas changes can be caused by hyperventilation associated with fear or anxiety. In addition, preexisting pulmonary pathology, such as bronchitis, pulmonary emphysema, or asthma, can affect the patient's survival. A compromised respiratory status can ultimately lead to death, and therefore an astute critical care nurse continues to monitor the patient to prevent compromised respiratory status.

IMMUNOLOGIC SYSTEM EFFECTS. The burned patient has an altered host defense response. The granulocytic functions of chemotaxis, phagocytosis, and destruction of ingested bacteria are abnormal, and breakdown of the skin and the mucosal barriers is often responsible for infection in the patient with burns. Infection has long been recognized as potentially the most lethal complication of burn injuries. More recently, however, it has become clear that the increased incidence of fatal sepsis after major burn insult is associated with the immune system (Mozingo et al., 1994; Wardenn, 1987). Of importance is the active cell-mediated suppression of the antigen-specific immune response to burn injury. The cellular events that precipitate this include altered interleukin-2 (IL-2) production. There is a relationship between decreased IL-2 production by lymphocytes and septic complications. Further, immunoglobulin G (IgG) levels are decreased after a burn.

Researchers have demonstrated the involvement of other immunosuppressant factors in the presence of burns, including immunosuppressive polypeptides, complement degradation products, immunoglobulin fragments, prostaglandins, granulocyte chemotaxis, production of oxygen-free radicals, and complement (Mozingo et al., 1994). Suppression of the cell-mediated immune response in thermally injured patients is associated with significantly compromised biologic activity of helper T-lymphocytes. Research studies by Teodorczyk-Injeyan and colleagues showed that IL-2 can promote the synthesis of immunoglobulin M (IgM) by human B-lymphocytes in the presence of functional T-lymphocytes. T-lymphocytes respond to IL-2 by releasing other soluble mediators of the humoral immune response (Teodorczyk-Injeyan et al., 1989). Current research has investigated the roles of human leukocyte surface antigen and neutrophil respiratory burst phenomena, as well as various cytokines such as epidermal growth factor, tumor necrosis factor-α, and basic fibroblast growth factor on burn wounds (Grayson et al., 1993a; Zapata-Sirvent & Hansbrough, 1993a) to accelerate the healing of burns, as well as recipient and donor sites. Steroids increase mortality and infection rates in burn patients and are therefore nearly always contraindicated (Jacobson et al., 1988).

GASTROHEPATIC SYSTEM EFFECTS. The gastrohepatic system is primarily responsible for providing a continual supply of nutrients, fluids, and electrolytes for tissue building and repair. The mouth, pharynx, esophagus, stomach, and small intestines are primarily responsible for ingestion and movement of products through the system, the secretion of essential enzymes and electrolytes to break down the materials ingested, and the absorption of the end-products of digestion into the blood. The liver, an accessory organ, is responsible for the metabolism of proteins, carbohydrates, and fats. During stress, such as that occurring following a burn, these functions are compromised. Increased glucose is released from the pancreas, resulting in an increase in some plasma proteins and in nonesterified fatty acid concentration. Hyperglycemia may also be due to an altered storage of glycogen in the liver, muscle, and brain or to the sympathoadrenal stress response that alters glucose production and breakdown through the effects of the catecholamines on alpha- and beta-adrenergic receptors. A decrease in serum albumin, plasma amino acids, and liver and muscle glycogen also occurs (Jacoby, 1974; Trofino, 1991) in burn injuries. Storage and filtration of blood are other essential activities assumed by the liver. Because a functioning liver is critical to the burn patient's successful recovery, liver function tests are performed routinely. In particular, the critical care nurse should be alert to a prolonged prothrombin time (PT), elevated serum transaminases and serum bilirubin, and retention of sulfobromophthalein as a result of liver reserve functions. It must be noted that in the presence of associated traumatic injuries, these values may also become abnormal. Other factors contributing to abnormal liver function include infectious processes, poor nutrition, blood transfusions, drugs, and anesthesia.

Redistribution of hepatic blood flow was once considered the primary reason for alterations in gastrointestinal and hepatic function in burn patients. Because these alterations continue to occur in the presence of adequate fluid replacement, it is felt that three factors may contribute to gastrohepatic alterations in the burn patient: (1) decreased mucosal mass, (2) decreased rate of DNA synthesis, and (3) enhanced permeability of the small intestine to bacteria (Carter et al., 1988). Further, these factors may predispose the burn patient to bacterial and endotoxin migration across the mucosal barrier and into the systemic circulation, where they may contribute to immunosuppression and end-organ failure (Zapata-Sirvent & Hansbrough, 1993b; Zapata-Sirvent et al., 1994).

The use of narcotic analgesics accompanied by prolonged bedrest or inadequate fluid intake predisposes the patient to constipation, whereas antibiotic therapy or hypertonic enteral tube feedings may cause diarrhea. These bowel problems create a constant challenge for the critical care nurse, requiring diligent assessment and intervention.

GENITOURINARY SYSTEM EFFECTS. The kidney responds immediately to the decreases in circulating blood volume, cardiac output, and blood pressure that occur with burns. With these decreases, renal vasoconstriction also occurs, giving rise to a decrease in the glomerular filtration rate. ADH, secreted by the posterior pituitary, controls water reabsorption through active transport at the distal tubules. Release of ADH causes retention of water as a compensatory mechanism resulting in oliguria. Blood urea nitrogen and creatinine levels become elevated. Glomerular filtration may be reestablished if adequate fluid resuscitation measures are undertaken and monitored. This reaction may occur on a temporary or permanent basis. If decreased glomerular filtration is treated with adequate fluid resuscitation, it will return to normal; however, if the patient has a history of kidney disease, it may not. Tubular damage is a likely possibility if decreased glomerular filtration is untreated; therefore, the critical care nurse must report a urine output of less than 0.5 mL/kg/hr in the adult and less than 1 mL/kg/hr in the child.

Myoglobin is a pigment that is released when muscle tissue is damaged. After massive flame and electrical injuries, myoglobin sludges in the kidney along with hemolyzed red blood cells. The urine in patients with myoglobinuria or hemoglobinuria has a characteristic rust or burgundy color. It is imperative that these substances are flushed from the kidney before acute tubular necrosis occurs. Patients may be diuresed by flushing with fluids or osmotic diuretics such as mannitol (Osmitrol) or urea. During the initial period after burn injury, when edema is most acute, a Foley catheter is essential to monitor fluid resuscitation efforts regardless of the potential infection risk associated with catheterization. Dialysis is not usually necessary if adequate fluid resuscitation is employed.

Glycosuria may occur initially as a result of pseudodiabetes related to the stress of the burn injury. This usually clears spontaneously.

NEUROENDOCRINE SYSTEM EFFECTS. Neurologic effects usually occur as later sequelae to burn injuries. If manifested early, two major effects may be seen. Although rare, direct nerve injury may occur after electrical injury because the low resistance of nerve tissue conducts the electric current. This nerve injury generally resolves, and partial or complete recovery of nerve function occurs. The major goal is to prevent further injury to the nerve (Achauer, 1987). The other immediate effect of burn injury is encephalopathy, which may occur as a result of other systemic alterations such as hypoxemic states.

Loss of skin integrity is accompanied by profound metabolic responses. Catabolic negative nitrogen balance is the primary characteristic associated with the metabolic response to burn injuries. Because of the large urinary nitrogen losses, progressive wasting of skeletal muscle mass and muscle weakness occur, accompanied by loss of skeletal muscle protein.

The neuroendocrine response to stress is activated immediately after a burn injury. The hypothalamic-pituitary system attempts to stabilize the body by activating the target organs. All major burns are accompanied at various times by exaggerated endocrine and metabolic responses. In particular, increases in corticotropin, ADH, cortisol, aldosterone, catecholamines, glucagon, immunoreactive insulin, calcitonin, parathyroid hormone, renin, angiotensin II, 17-ketosteroids, 17-ketogenic steroids, and 17-hydroxycorticosteroids are found. Decreased levels of triiodothyronine, thyroxine, testosterone in males, follicle-stimulating hormone, and progesterone are also found (Dolecek, 1985; Trofino, 1991). Increased corticotropin is produced as a result of anterior pituitary stimulation. The adrenal cortex is then stimulated to produce increased amounts of corticoids, which increase glucose production.

The adrenal medulla, under sympathetic response, secretes the catecholamines epinephrine and norepinephrine, which assist in the "fight or flight" response to stress. The increased epinephrine increases heart rate, constricts the vessels in the skin and kidneys, and may depress pancreatic and insulin production. Cardiac output rises along with blood pressure and a subsequent decrease in peripheral resistance. The bronchi and bronchioles dilate, and the individual becomes hyperpneic. Blood supply is increased to the heart, muscles, and nervous system. These increased circulating catecholamines in the emergent phase of burn physiology cause an increase in circulating white blood cells and a decrease in circulating eosinophils.

Burn injuries, more than any other traumatic injury, cause increased stress on the human body. The burn patient sustains a hypermetabolic state from the time of injury usually until the time of wound closure. The increased metabolic activity leads to loss of weight and a negative nitrogen balance. Energy and protein reserves are quickly used up, depleting the body of necessary resources for tissue repair and building. In an effort to supply the tissues with available energy, the body undergoes gluconeogenesis and ureagenesis. The catabolism that occurs as a result of these activities is related to the extent and severity of burn injury. The caloric needs of burn patients are staggering. Calculations to determine the caloric and protein requirements following massive thermal injury are usually based on body weight in kilograms and TBSA burned. Nomograms to calculate nutritional requirements use age, sex, TBSA burned, and basal metabolic rate to determine caloric and nitrogen requirements.

Decreased nutritional intake, particularly of proteins, increases the patient's risk of poor wound healing because insufficient nutrients will be available for tissue repair. Loss of one-fourth to one-third of the protein mass from the body is predictably fatal in the absence of nutritional support (Kravitz, 1988). The increased nutritional requirements mandate early and aggressive alimentation.

OTHER ASSOCIATED SYSTEMIC CHANGES. Burn-related infection presents an acute risk to the burn patient and a challenge to the entire health care team. Pneumonia, burn wound infection, urinary tract infection, and septicemia caused by fungi, bacteria, or viruses are only a few of the potentially lethal infections that may occur.

Joint function is a major challenge in the rehabilitation of the burn patient. Preservation of joint mobility begins early in the care of the patient to permit a return to functional use. Active participation by physical and occupational therapists begins during the emergent phase of burns.

Corneal abrasions may result after facial burns. Ectropion or exposure keratitis may result from eyelid contractures. Chronic complications of electrical burns may involve cataracts or glaucoma. Ophthalmic examination is necessary in patients with burns to the face. Fluorescein strips can aid in the diagnosis of corneal abrasions or burns.

Burns of the face, hands, feet, and genitalia need special consideration in the emergent phase of burn care. Special care often involves shaving the hair if necessary, preventing pressure on these sites, exposure of the area, elevation (e.g., scrotum), and frequent cleaning and use of topical agents.

PATIENT CARE MANAGEMENT DURING THE EMERGENT PHASE

During the emergent phase, members of the health care team systematically assess various phenomena to classify information about the patient with burns. Major goals during this phase are to maintain adequate pulmonary function, maintain intravascular volume and cardiac output, maintain renal function, preserve joint function and mobility, preserve self-concept, and prevent complications associated with this period after burn injury. Although the patient should be considered an integral member of the collaborative health care team and every attempt made to have the patient participate in decision-making, it is not always possible given the patient's condition. It is at this most critical time in the patient's recovery that the family must be allowed and encouraged to participate in that decision making.

PHYSICAL ASSESSMENT. Assessment of the burn victim begins in much the same way as that of any other trauma victim; in fact, a burn injury is one of the greatest traumas the body can suffer. Airway, breathing, and circulation must first be established. A secondary trauma survey should then be performed because the burn victim may present with concomitant traumatic injuries. Special attention should be paid to respiratory assessment, even though the patient may not be obviously compromised.

A verbal history from the patient should be taken immediately on arrival in the emergency department because the burn victim is generally lucid and able to provide pertinent information about the event and about preexisting health problems. If the history is delayed until a more convenient time, the nurse may find the patient intubated, sedated, or in a state of shock.

In taking a history from the patient who is burned, specific emphasis should be placed on the history of the accident, including the time and location of the incident, how the incident occurred, whether it was indoors or outdoors, and whether drugs or alcohol were involved. The nurse should also obtain a history of preexisting health problems such as allergies, diabetes, or heart or lung disorders that could interfere with fluid resuscitation and wound healing.

The burn victim should be weighed as soon as possible after arrival at the hospital because the preburn weight is of vital importance in providing adequate fluid resuscitation, nutrition, and drug dosages. Table 60–5 is a sample of admission orders used for the burned patient.

Other orders may relate to hemodynamic parameters, nutritional guidelines, respiratory support, consultations, and depth determination studies. Standard orders for admission such as these can shorten the admission process and assist in ensuring that important areas of care are not overlooked.

LABORATORY TESTS. Alterations in laboratory values are carefully monitored during this critical time. The following laboratory tests are usually performed on admission and monitored throughout the patient's recovery:

Arterial blood gases
COHb level
Chemistry panel
Complete blood count (with differential)
Clotting studies (PT and partial thromboplastin time [PTT])
Type and crossmatch
Drug and alcohol screen (if indicated)
Urinalysis
Other tests as indicated, such as HIV titer, 24-hour urine urea nitrogen (UUN)

Metabolic acidosis develops after a major burn injury. This is easily correctable with adequate fluid resuscitation and normalization of the cardiac output. Even in the presence of smoke inhalation, if the patient is adequately oxygenated, blood gases may be abnormal. Elevated carbon monoxide levels should not be depended on to indicate smoke inhalation injuries. Metabolic acidosis also occurs when mafenide acetate (Sulfamylon) is applied topically over a large portion of the body surface area.

Acid-base derangements also occur secondary to shock states, renal failure, and pulmonary failure. The primary causes of the acid-base imbalance should be treated when possible.

Carboxyhemoglobin levels of more than 10% are diagnostic of carbon monoxide poisoning, and early intubation may be required (Cioffi & Rue, 1991). It is important to remember, as stated previously, that the opposite does not hold true, and the absence of an elevated COHb does not rule out an inhalation injury.

Following the burn injury the intracellular sodium concentration increases. This creates an osmotic pressure gradient that pulls water into the cell. In exchange, potassium leaves the cell and concentrates in the serum. This, in addition to the hemolysis of red blood cells, leads to hyperkalemia, which is often seen early, following the burn injury.

Serum electrolyte values are also affected by the fluid status of the patient. Sodium and chloride ions are often increased secondary to the hemoconcentrated state of the patient. The actual number of ions has not changed, but the percentage of solute has decreased.

The patient who has sustained a major burn injury is also unable to regulate the loss of electrolytes through the skin. Sodium is often lost through the skin and requires replacement. Chlorides, on the other hand, are reabsorbed by the kidney.

Alterations in the complete blood count (red blood cells, white blood cells, and platelets) occur in response to burn injury. There is some cellular destruction of red cells (<10%), which occurs as a response of the local heat damage to the burned area. The burn patient initially experiences an increase in hematocrit due to a loss of plasma volume into the interstitial space and hemoconcentration. Hematocrit values are usually obtained every 2 to 4 hours during the first 48 hours after the burn and as needed thereafter to assess fluid status. Anemia often develops during hospitalization due to the progressive hemolysis of red cells.

Leukocytosis occurs early in the postburn period, the white blood cell count often going as high as $30{,}000/mm^3$. This situation generally resolves within

TABLE 60–5. **Sample Admission Orders for the Severely Burned Patient**

1. Diagnosis: _____ % TBSA _____ % full-thickness
2. Condition: Allergies:
3. Vital signs (T, BP, P, R) every _____ min
4. Daily weight
5. Intake and output every 1 hour
6. Foley to gravity drainage
7. IV fluids: Ringer's lactate at _____ mL/hr for _____ hours, then _____ mL/hr for _____ hours. 5% albumisol at _____ mL/hr for _____ hours; then _____ mL/hr for _____ hours
8. Titrate IV fluids to maintain urine output at _____ mL/hr, CVP _____ mm Hg, PAP _____ mm Hg
9. Neurovascular checks of circumferential extremity burns every 1 hour
10. Humidified oxygen by face mask at 6 L/hr or
    Ventilator: Type _____ Mode _____
    PEEP _____ F_{IO_2} _____
    Tidal volume _____ Pressure support _____
    Pulse oximetry: Keep saturation above _____
    Respiratory therapy treatments _____
11. Admission chest x-ray, then daily for _____ days
12. Wound care with _____ dressings q _____
13. Venodyne placement per protocol
14. Physical and occupational therapy consults
15. Medications:
    Morphine sulfate IV continuous drip for pain per protocol _____
    Diphtheria/tetanus 0.5 ml IM _____
    Docusate sodium 250 mg PO/NG bid _____
    Multivitamins 1 tablet/5 ml PO/NG qd _____
    Ascorbic acid 500 mg PO/NG bid _____
    Other _____
16. Hemodynamic parameters: CVP q _____, PAP q _____, PAWP q _____, Cardiac output/index q _____
17. Diet:
    Insert feeding tube/NG tube.
    Obtain post-tube insertion to verify placement.
    Tube feeding type: _____
    Strength: _____
    Rate: _____
    Check gastric pH q 4 hours _____
    Check gastric residual q 4 hours _____
18. Laboratory studies:
    CBC with differential now and q _____
    Electrolyte panel now and q _____
    Clotting studies now and q _____
    Albumin now and q _____
    Urinalysis now and q _____
    Arterial blood gases now and q _____
    Carboxyhemoglobin level now and q _____
    Toxicology and drug screen _____
    Other _____

Abbreviations: TBSA, total body surface area; T, temperature; BP, blood pressure; P, pulse; R, respirations; CVP, central venous pressure; PAP, pulmonary artery pressure; PEEP, positive end-expiratory pressure; F_{IO_2}, fraction of inspired oxygen; NG, nasogastric; PAWP, pulmonary artery wedge pressure; CBC, complete blood count.

24 to 48 hours. Persistent leukocytosis may indicate infection. Leukopenia often occurs as a side effect of topical therapy with silver sulfadiazine but generally resolves within 24 to 48 hours without withdrawal of the therapy or other treatment (Fuller & Engler, 1988).

Thrombocytopenia is often seen during the first 72 hours after the burn. This temporary decrease in platelets may result from the dilutional effects of fluid resuscitation and some degree of microvascular thrombosis or DIC.

Clotting studies are often abnormal in the initial period as well. The PT and PTT are often elevated during the first 72 hours after the burn. As plasma leaks out of the vascular space and into the interstitial space, clotting factors follow. Clotting factors generally return to normal during the first week and need not be treated as long as active bleeding is not observed.

The kidneys perform a major role in regulating the fluid and electrolyte balance and in excreting waste products. Hourly measurements and testing of urine output are required to determine how well the kidney is functioning. During the first 48 hours after a burn, a urine output of 50 to 100 mL/hr indicates adequate renal perfusion. After the first 48 hours, 30 mL/hr is acceptable in the adult. Urine output in children should equal 1 mL/kg/hr during the first 48 hours and 0.5 to 1 mL/kg/hr thereafter.

Specific gravity should be maintained within normal values (1.002 to 1.035). Elevated specific gravity may indicate decreased intravascular fluid volume and dehydration.

A urinalysis that is positive for protein indicates that the body is using protein stores rather than food, an indicator that the patient is in a negative nitrogen balance. Urine that is positive for glucose may indicate that the body is not utilizing ingested glucose, or it may indicate either diabetes or pseudodiabetes, which is often associated with the stress of this major injury. Glucose intolerance is also a sign of sepsis and should be reported and followed. Insulin may be required to assist the body to utilize glucose. Acetone is normally negative on urinalysis. A positive reading may indicate that the body is burning its own fats and proteins and is in a state of starvation.

The urine should normally be yellow or straw-colored. A rust or burgundy appearance indicates myoglobinuria due to the breakdown of muscle tissue secondary to a deep burn injury. Green urine may indicate a *Pseudomonas* infection; a urine culture is indicated.

Urine that tests positive for blood may indicate red blood cell breakdown, which is secondary to hemolysis from the initial injury or from septic shock.

A blood alcohol level may be indicated on admission if the patient has an overwhelming odor of alcohol or if the circumstances surrounding the accident are suspicious. Drug screens are also indicated if the patient is behaving in an inappropriate manner or if the injury is more severe than might be expected. Screening the patient's HIV status continues to be controversial at the present time and may have legal ramifications in some states but can be useful. If there is reason to suspect a positive HIV titer, the reason for the test should be discussed with the patient and his consent obtained if possible. Patients with a positive HIV titer who have major burns usually do not respond to treatment as would be expected because their immune system is compromised, causing infection and nonhealing of wounds. It is important to discuss this subject with the patient early in the course of treatment because it may influence treatment plans and outcomes.

Alterations in laboratory values are carefully monitored during this critical time. Table 60–6 lists the typical laboratory findings found in burn patients in the emergent phase.

TABLE 60–6. **Expected Emergent Phase Laboratory Values**

Serum potassium elevated	Prolonged prothrombin time and partial thromboplastin time
Serum sodium elevated	Metabolic acidosis
Hematocrit elevated	Thrombocytopenia
Serum glucose elevated	Leukocytosis
Bicarbonate deficit	

FLUID RESUSCITATION. In 1952 Evans published the first successful surface area/weight formula for calculating fluid resuscitation in the burn-injured patient. Since that time various other formulas have been developed. In general, patients with a burned area greater than 20% of the TBSA require intravenous fluid resuscitation because of the physiologic fluid shifts. Time is the major factor in determining fluid management of the burned patient. Administration of fluids is calculated from the time of the initial burn injury, not from the time the patient enters the facility or resuscitation is commenced. All fluids must be infused using a large-bore needle or subclavian or subclavicular lines (Dressler et al., 1988). If at all possible, these lines should not be placed through burned tissue to prevent the possibility of infection.

Each patient presents a unique challenge in that fluid requirements must be estimated correctly to ensure adequate cardiac output while preventing shock. The type and amount of fluid to be used in fluid resuscitation remain extremely controversial (Williams & Porvaznik, 1989). Fluid resuscitation therapy for children with burns depends on careful matching of the selected therapy with the patient's tolerance to injury and subsequent treatment (Graves et al., 1988).

Although there is no standard formula for all patients, neither is there a standard for the type of solution chosen for fluid resuscitation or the parameters used to monitor the efficacy of fluid therapy. Most clinicians agree, however, that the burn patient requires electrolyte solutions during the first 24 hours after the burn. Crystalloid solutions chosen most frequently include a balanced salt solution such as lactated Ringer's solution without dextrose or normal saline. Free water, given as a 5% dextrose in water solution, is administered to replace insensible water loss. Additional electrolytes may be added to this solution. Colloids are added anywhere from 6 to 24 hours after injury (Williams & Porvaznik, 1989) when capillary integrity begins to be restored. Some clinicians suggest the use of hypertonic saline (250 mEq sodium/liter of water) as the resuscitation or backup fluid. Advocates of this therapy state that this solution delivers less free water, acts to draw extravascular fluid into the vascular compartment, lessens edema away from the burn site, decreases the need for escharotomy, increases cardiac output, eliminates ileus, and decreases intrapulmonary water in the inhalation-injured patient, but others argue that this solution poses a risk of severe electrolyte disturbances (Williams & Porvaznik, 1989).

The fluid regimens presented in Table 60–7 and the measurements commonly monitored to determine fluid resuscitation efficacy (Table 60–8) are therefore intended as guides and should be geared toward the individual patient's needs and responses. Children with massive burn injuries require a greater volume of fluid relative to body weight and burn size than the average adult (Graves et al., 1988). In children who initially fail to respond to fluid resuscitation, it is often determined that the burn size was underestimated.

The modified Parkland (Baxter) formula is based

TABLE 60–7. **Fluid Resuscitation Formulas**

Formula Name	Electrolyte	Colloid	Water	First 24 Hours*	Second 24 Hours
Artz	Lactated Ringer's: 3.0 mL × kg weight × %TBSA			Half of total given in first 8 hours; balance over remaining 16 hours	
Brigham		5% albumin: 10% body weight	80 mL/hr D_5W	Half of total given during first 8 to 12 hours; balance over following 36 hours	
Brooke	Lactated Ringer's: 1.5 mL × kg weight × %TBSA	0.5 mL × kg weight × %TBSA	2000 mL D_5W	Half of total in first 8 hours; balance over remaining 16 hours	Half of colloids and electrolyte solutions and all water
Burn Budget of F. D. Moore	Lactated Ringer's: 1000 mL titrating to 4000 mL 0.45 normal saline: 1200 mL	7.5% kg weight	1500–5000 mL D_5W	All electrolyte, colloid, and water	All electrolyte, colloid = 2.5% of kg weight, and all water
Evans	Normal saline (0.9%): 1.0 mL × kg weight × %TBSA	1.0 mL × kg weight × %TBSA	2000 mL D_5W	All electrolyte, colloid, and water	Half electrolyte, half colloid
HALFD (hypertonic, albuminated fluid-demand resuscitation)	Hypertonic saline (240 mOsm Na, 120 mOsm Cl, 120 mOsm lactate) to maintain urine output > 40 mL/hr and MAP at 60 mm Hg	1.5 g albumin/liter	0	All electrolytes and colloid	
Hypertonic formula	300 mEq Na, 200 mEq dextrose, 1 liter lactate, 100 mEq Cl to maintain urine output > 30 mL/hr in adults	0	0		One-third to one-half of first day's requirements
Hypertonic saline solution (New Mexico formula)	250 mEq Na/liter: Volume to maintain urine output > 30 mL/hr	0	0	All electrolyte	One-third of sodium solution up to 3500 mL orally
Modified Brooke	Lactated Ringer's: 2.0–3.0 mL × kg weight × %TBSA, titrating to 4 mL/kg per %TBSA	0	0		
Parkland	Lactated Ringer's: 4.0 mL × kg weight × %TBSA	0	0	Half of total in first 8 hours, balance over remaining 16 hours	No formula
Rambam†	Lactated Ringer's: 2000 mL	Plasma: 75.0 mL × kg		All electrolytes and plasma over 36 hours	

*Fluid requirements for the first 24 hours are calculated from time of injury, not entry into the facility.
†Aharoni et al., 1989.

TABLE 60–8. **Monitored Parameters in Thermal Injury**

Level of consciousness
Arterial blood pressure
Pulse rate and rhythm
Central venous pressure
Pulmonary artery and capillary wedge pressures
Cardiac output including cardiac index, stroke index, systemic vascular resistance, left ventricular stroke index, right ventricular stroke index, pulmonary vascular resistance
Arterial blood gases
Hematocrit and hemoglobin
Urine output including specific gravity and urine sodium concentration
Electrolyte values

on the concept that colloid molecules do not remain in the intravascular space during the first 24 hours after a burn; thus, the formula recommends giving only crystalloid solution during the first 24 hours and colloid thereafter. This formula has been adopted by the American College of Surgeons based on its ease of use, the fact that it is readily available, and its reduced cost (Aharoni et al., 1989).

Colloid solutions such as salt-poor albumin or fresh frozen plasma are used infrequently during the first 24 hours after a burn; however, some burn units currently use colloid solutions (Brigham formula) exclusively in the first 24 hours. These solutions are usually costly, and their efficacy compared with crystalloid in the critical first 24 hours has not been proved. After the first 24 hours, other fluid regimens recommend colloid to increase the intravascular oncotic pressure.

A typical burn patient receives large volumes of fluid. Using the Parkland formula, for example, a 70-kg patient with a 40% TBSA would require 11,200 mL (11.2 liters) of fluid during the first 24 hours after the burn. Although the volume of fluid administered seems high, the critical care nurse must remember that unless the patient has cardiovascular compromise because of prior cardiovascular disease, all fluid infused into such a hypovolemic patient will diffuse through the capillary sieve as quickly as it is infused. Regardless of the solution chosen, it must be emphasized that careful titration of the fluid is necessary to prevent shock and maintain the adequacy of urine output, vital signs, acid-base balance, tissue perfusion, and level of consciousness.

Fluid resuscitation in burn patients is not without hazards. Overresuscitation with fluids becomes a priority, as pulmonary morbidity requires vigilance on the part of the critical care nurse to avoid a life-threatening event. Overresuscitation may also cause increased peripheral edema, which can impede wound blood flow, in turn altering healing or converting burn injury from a partial- to a full-thickness injury (Graves et al., 1988).

PAIN MANAGEMENT. Pain control is of major concern during all phases of burn treatment. The pain of a burn injury is more intense and longer lasting than any other acute injury or illness. The pain is often both physical and emotional. No member of the burn team should assume that the patient does not have pain because he or she is not complaining of pain. There continues to be widespread institutional denial of a burned patient's pain assessment and treatment (Acute Pain Management Guideline Panel, 1992). Patients with full-thickness burns do have pain, even though by definition viable nerve endings are not exposed in full-thickness burns and therefore do not hurt. Pure full-thickness burns are rare; more often these burns are mixed with areas of partial-thickness burns.

During the emergent phase of burn care patients with massive burns often suffer pain continuously, and because of the increased metabolic rate, they metabolize drugs very rapidly. Intramuscular injections are usually not given during this phase due to altered capillary permeability and muscular blood flow. Even continuous infusions of opioids may not offer complete relief, possibly due to damage of underlying nerves, yet this remains the accepted standard regimen for pain relief. Lidocaine, administered in a continuous low-dose infusion, has been shown to decrease neuropathic pain and may be a useful adjunct in the treatment of refractory pain (Jonsson et al., 1991). Additional adjuncts include the use of anxiolytics such as lorazepam and midazolam in the treatment of the pain experience (Marvin et al., 1992). Moreover, patients with burn pain may benefit from psychological techniques such as mental imagery, self-talk, reappraisal techniques, relaxation training and reinforcement conditioning, and hypnotherapy (Patterson, 1992).

Environmental temperature plays a role in the pain experience of patients with burns. A temperature maintained between 76°F and 82°F (25°C and 28°C) ensures warmth and comfort of the patient who has lost skin, a source of preserving body heat.

NUTRITIONAL SUPPORT. Major thermal injuries result in a hypermetabolic response that is proportional to the burn injury. Basal metabolic needs may be increased as much as 1 to 2 times above normal in patients with burns (Giel, 1987; Mozingo et al., 1994; Trofino, 1991). Nutritional support for the burned patient can be started as soon as the patient is stabilized in the intensive care unit, usually within 24 hours after the burn. Careful attention is paid to the nutritional needs of the patient, including an estimate of preburn nutritional status. Enteral feedings are always preferred over parenteral feedings because the latter require large amounts of calories that necessitate a central line through which high concentrations of glucose are given, thus increasing the patient's risk of infection. Enteral feedings are usually successful if they are started slowly and increased progressively until the patient's caloric needs are met.

The Curreri formula (Table 60–9) is most commonly used to estimate the caloric needs of adult burn patients, and a similar formula developed by Suth-

TABLE 60–9. **Estimating Caloric Needs**

Curreri formula: 25 kcal × weight (kg) + 40 × TBSA burn
Sutherland formula for children: 60 kcal × kg + 35 × TBSA burn

Abbreviations: TBSA, total body surface area.

erland is used to estimate the caloric needs of children under age 12 (Giel, 1987). Additional calories are sometimes given to compensate for calories not provided during the initial hours of fluid resuscitation and before and after surgical procedures.

The skin is the first line of defense against infection, and loss of this protective defense along with the formation of eschar provides an excellent medium for growth of bacteria. In addition, the patient with a burn has a compromised immune response. Multiple invasive interventions as well as nonadherence to aseptic precautions contribute to the risk of infection to the patient.

The health care provider uses body substance precautions and determines the type of isolation techniques to be used (i.e., gowns, gloves, masks, head coverings per institutional protocol) to keep bacterial counts to a minimum and prevent the spread of infection. All providers of care must use strict sterile technique when changing dressings, and an aseptic environment must be maintained using sterile equipment and supplies. The critical care nurse observes for signs of infection (e.g., malodorous drainage, elevated white blood cell count, elevated temperature) or sepsis. Antibiotics are administered and their effect observed through appropriate laboratory tests and clinical response. Topical antimicrobials and bacteriostatic agents are applied, and their effects on burn wounds are observed. The critical care nurse explains the purpose of hydrotherapy treatment and eschar debridement to the patient and family. Patients must be adequately prepared for numerous grafting procedures, maintaining asepsis and protection of donor and recipient sites. Wound cultures are obtained as ordered, preventing contamination by adjacent skin flora. Skin surfaces should be avoided to prevent autocontamination, and body hair that may harbor bacteria is often shaved or clipped; special site care for face, eyes, ears, or perineum is completed.

Acute (Fluid Remobilization) Phase

The acute phase is characterized by eschar separation and fluid remobilization. This phase lasts until spontaneous healing of the burn wound occurs or until autografts are in place. Primary patient care management involves removal of burn eschar, wound coverage, and prevention of complications. It is during this phase that patients are most likely to develop complications such as septicemia and cardiovascular collapse. This phase may last weeks to months depending on the severity of the burn injury and resultant treatment protocols. Again, as during the emergent phase, multisystemic effects occur during the acute phase of burn injuries.

CARDIOVASCULAR SYSTEM EFFECTS. In this phase, the capillary leak begins to resolve, and the intravascular fluid volume begins to stabilize. There is a decrease in capillary permeability that results in stabilization of the fluid shifts. The large amounts of fluid required for resuscitation in the emergent period are no longer necessary during the acute phase other than for maintenance of hydration and electrolyte balance. In addition, the lymphatic tissue is better able to withstand the fluid load, restoring equilibrium. It is during this phase that the intravascular oncotic pressure must be maintained to preserve physiologic function. This may be achieved through the judicious use of colloids such as salt-poor albumin or fresh frozen plasma. Care must be maintained in this process, particularly in elderly patients and patients with a history of cardiovascular pathology.

Decreased tissue perfusion as a result of edema in the emergent phase causes aggregation of cellular byproducts in the microcirculation during the acute phase. This debris prevents adequate blood flow, which is necessary for healing. Septicemia is also a major concern during this phase. Wound infections as well as other systemic infections such as bacterial infections of the heart may occur; such infections may result from the collection of debris or the administration of steroids.

PULMONARY SYSTEM EFFECTS. If the patient survives the respiratory distress that occurs during the early phases of smoke inhalation, increased cellular permeability in the alveoli results in noncardiogenic interstitial and intraalveolar edema, which interferes progressively with gas exchange. Infusion of large amounts of crystalloid solutions in the fluid resuscitation of the burn patient may further compound the pathogenesis of pulmonary edema. Bronchopneumonia may occur during the acute phase as a result of imposed immobility, increased fluid volume infusions, changes in pulmonary capillary permeability, and pulmonary parenchymal damage. Respiratory failure in this stage is a poor prognostic sign.

Patients may continue to be intubated during the acute phase, and this is associated with the risk of infection. Patients with endotracheal tubes are at risk of nosocomial infections. In addition, nasotracheally intubated patients are at risk for sinus infections.

IMMUNOLOGIC SYSTEM EFFECTS. During the acute phase of burn injury, critical interventions include removal of necrotic or devitalized tissue and coverage of the wound with grafts to prevent infection leading to septicemia. Because the patient continues to be immunosuppressed, infectious organisms are more easily able to invade the body, further compromising the patient's condition.

GASTROHEPATIC SYSTEM EFFECTS. Approximately 90% of burned patients have erythema, punctate hemorrhages, and erosion of the duodenal and gastric membranes. Curling's ulcer, a duodenal ulcer, is a devastating source of gastrointestinal hemorrhage and perforation and can occur during the acute phase of burn injury. Gastric dilatation and paralytic ileus may also occur, caused by fear, anxiety, or sepsis. Paradoxically, these ulcers are not associated with gastric acid secretion but arise from the gastric mucosa, which is altered as a result of back-diffusion of H^+ ions, ischemia, and inadequate mucosal cell proliferation (McAlhany et al., 1979; Trofino, 1991; Wiener & Barrett, 1986). These ulcers can be prevented by providing adequate nutritional support, gastric intubation, and pH monitoring, and by administering H_2 receptor antagonists, antacids, and/or sucralfate.

The presence of blood in the nasogastric aspirate, emesis, or stool should be carefully monitored. Early in the postburn period it may be caused by gastric irritation, whereas later it may be duodenal in origin. Early congestion in the gastric mucosa may be a factor in the development of this phenomenon, which may be caused by hemoconcentration, neurohumoral stimulation, or infection (Trofino, 1991). Colon ulcers may also occur in the presence of hypovolemia, sepsis, or multiple organ failure. These ulcers serve as a source of bacteremia.

Although rare, bacteremia may also cause acalculous cholecystitis. Patients may complain of acute right upper quadrant pain and may present with jaundice. Ultrasonography and radioisotopic scans confirm the diagnosis (Trofino, 1991; Wiener & Barrett, 1986).

GENITOURINARY SYSTEM EFFECTS. Renal failure can occur during any phase of burn injury. During the acute phase, it may be the result of infection, sepsis, or pharmacologic agents. Knowledge of the route of excretion of drugs accompanied by careful monitoring of renal function may prevent further renal damage.

NEUROENDOCRINE EFFECTS. Severe metabolic strain continues in the acute phase of burn injury. Symptoms of adrenal insufficiency are found occasionally in the first week after burn injury and may occur anytime until the burn wound is healed. If adrenal insufficiency occurs, the nurse assesses for hypotension, hyponatremia, hyperkalemia, elevated urine sodium, decreased urine potassium, alterations in temperature, leukopenia, and anorexia.

PATIENT CARE MANAGEMENT DURING THE ACUTE PHASE

Assessment and prevention of complications during this phase cannot be minimized because the patient is always susceptible to them. It is important for the nurse to be vigilant with respect to assessment parameters and laboratory data.

TABLE 60–10. **Expected Initial Acute Phase Laboratory Values**

Serum potassium decreased
Serum sodium decreased
Hematocrit decreased
Bicarbonate decreased

LABORATORY STUDIES. During the acute phase laboratory values are followed periodically for changes from normal. When necessary, daily laboratory studies may be ordered, and when the patient is more stable they may be ordered once or twice a week. Generally, if the patient is undergoing a surgical procedure or is septic, laboratory studies are required more often. Table 60–10 lists the expected laboratory findings in the acute phase.

WOUND CARE. If the skin is broken, it is unable to protect the body against bacterial invasion. The burn may be sterile initially due to the heat causing the burn; however, soon after the injury the normal flora from adjacent areas can invade the burn wound. The burned patient is at risk for wound sepsis until the wound is either healed or has been grafted during the acute or rehabilitative phases of care. To prevent bacterial invasion of the wound until that time, hydrotherapy is performed at least once a day. During hydrotherapy the wound is cleansed either in a whirlpool-type bath or a shower. Cleansing solutions such as povidone-iodine (Betadine), chlorhexidine (Hibiclens), or a 1:240 sodium hypochlorite solution is added to the bath or shower water (Martin, 1989).

Burn wounds are debrided to rid the wound of necrotic tissue and to remove previously applied topical agents. Debridement can be either surgical, mechanical, or enzymatic. Mechanical debridement takes place daily when the patient receives hydrotherapy. This is accomplished using a washcloth with long, firm strokes. At times this procedure must be done with the aid of an anesthetic agent because of the degree of pain it causes.

Surgical debridement is done in the operating room under a general anesthetic. Guarded knives are used to remove burn eschar. Devitalized skin is removed in layers until viable tissue is observed. If the tissue bed is healthy and clean, the patient can be grafted immediately; if an infection is present, the wound is dressed, and grafting takes place at a later date.

Enzymatic debridement to remove eschar has been used effectively in some burn centers. To be effective, the burn eschar must be soft and moist. These enzymatic agents include Elase and Travase. Travase has been known to sting on application to the burn, causing patients increased pain. The enzymatic debridement process usually takes a minimum of a week and will debride only through the layers of the skin. If the burn eschar extends into the subcutaneous fat, this tis-

TABLE 60–11. **Topical Antimicrobial Therapy of Burns**

Topical Preparation	Indication for Use	Advantages	Disadvantages
Mafenide acetate (Sulfamylon)	Deep burns (i.e., electrical, ear burns)	Wide-spectrum antimicrobial coverage	Painful on application and for 20 to 30 minutes afterwards; potent carbonic anhydrase inhibitor, causing decreased renal bicarbonate production; metabolic acidosis is a problem, especially if patient already has respiratory compromise; potassium is also lost in the urine; does not adhere to burn well and requires frequent reapplication
Silver sulfadiazine (Silvadene)	Partial- and full-thickness thermal injuries	Wide-spectrum antimicrobial action; painless on application; eschar remains soft, pliable, easily debridable	Not effective against fungal organisms; may cause leukopenia (self-limiting); resistant organisms can occur with prolonged use
Silver nitrate	Partial- and full-thickness burns	Chemoprophylactic; no reported sensitivities; painless on application	Depth of penetration is only 1 to 2 mm of eschar; hypotonicity of solution will pull Na, Ca, K, and Cl from the burn wound—these effects are seen when larger surface areas are treated; dressings must be kept wet. Dry silver nitrate can injure tissue when allowed to concentrate by evaporation. Range of motion is limited by thick dressings. Silver nitrate stains everything black (clothing, floors, skin, linens)
Acetic acid	Infected partial-thickness burns, after grafting	Sensitive to *Pseudomonas* infection; debridement of grafts by bacterial lysis of eschar; inexpensive	Must be a wet-to-dry dressing; range of motion is limited by thick dressings; removal of dressings may be painful
Sodium hypoclorite (Dakins)	Debridement of grafts	Dries "soupy" wounds; inexpensive	Must be a wet-to-dry dressing; range of motion is limited by thick dressings; removal of dressings may be painful

sue will remain undigested. These agents are generally used after mechanical debridement and rarely after surgical debridement. One disadvantage of these agents is that wound sepsis is difficult to manage because topical enzymatic agents are not antimicrobial. If the patient has signs of wound-related sepsis, enzymatic debridement is discontinued, and appropriate topical antimicrobial therapy is begun.

After debridement a topical antimicrobial agent is applied to the burn. Table 60–11 lists the most commonly used topical agents, their advantages, disadvantages, and method of use.

After debridement down to healthy tissue has been performed, grafting, if necessary, can be performed. Split-thickness skin grafts are most common and can be either meshed or sheet. These can be taken from any donor site but usually are not taken from cosmetic areas such as the arms, upper chest (if possible), or face. Ideal donor sites are the scalp, thighs, and buttocks. Full-thickness skin grafts are also possible. The donor site for these grafts is most commonly the groin, and because this forms a full-thickness deficit from the donor site, it is closed by primary intention. Full-thickness skin grafts are never meshed because this would defeat the purpose of being full thickness.

Grafts may be meshed (expanded) to 1½:1, 3:1, or 6:1 times their original size. Meshing is prepared using a mechanical meshing device. The greater the mesh, the less the initial wound is covered, but within 1 to 2 weeks the graft epithelializes into the interstices of the mesh with new epidermis. The larger the mesh the greater the amount of scarring because as the wound matures there is more wound contracture. For this reason, the smallest amount of meshing possible is used.

Sheet split-thickness skin grafts are used for cosmetic areas such as the hand or face as well as for highly functional areas. Sheet grafts contract less than meshed grafts and therefore are excellent for grafting the hands and neck. Once healed, sheet grafts blend into the normal skin better than meshed grafts.

Full-thickness skin grafts are used for cosmetic areas such as the eyelid. Skin taken from the groin is applied directly to the defect. Once grafted, both the donor site and the recipient area require wound care. Biobrane or Xeroform gauze, among others, is frequently applied to the donor site.

The method of care of the recipient site varies from institution to institution. Graft take should be expected to be 90% to 100%. Burn centers vary with respect to inspection of graft sites. Each burn center has its own dressing protocols.

For burns that do not require grafting or are waiting to be grafted, two types of dressing techniques are used—open and closed. In the open dressing a topical agent is applied to the burn, but no gauze dressings are placed over the topical agent or the burn. Closed dressings consist of layers of gauze dressings over the burn plus topical agents, virtually excluding outside elements from the burn. A semi-open method combines elements of both. Usually one layer of gauze is placed over the burn together with a topical agent. This method permits the burn to "breathe" while providing a means to hold the topical agent in place.

Biologic dressings consist primarily of viable tissues used to cover the burn temporarily as a substitute for conventional dressings or for leaving the burn wound exposed. The benefits of these materials are reduced loss of fluid, electrolytes, and protein; decreased pain; inhibition of bacterial growth; and faster healing of the burn wound. Materials used include allograft (cadaver skin), porcine xenografts (pig skin), and, less frequently, amniotic membrane.

Allograft continues as a popular biologic dressing. Skin harvest should always be considered when organ donation is being considered from a cadaver. Skin banks are able to store harvested skin indefinitely. Cyclosporine has been used in skin allografts to increase the likelihood of adherence. Although allografts are considered a temporary wound covering, permanent coverage has been achieved with the use of cyclosporine (Achauer et al., 1986). Generally, lower doses of cyclosporine are used than in other organ grafts. The risk of sepsis is omnipresent and must be evaluated continuously. Although no permanent synthetic wound covering is currently available, there are several materials that can be advantageous in the treatment of both minor and moderate burns. The first is Biobrane. Biobrane is an ultrathin, polydimethyl-siloxane rubber-like membrane that is bonded to a mixture of hydrophilic collagen peptides. This flexible, nylon-like fabric is used to cover clean partial-thickness burns or to cover temporarily clean, excised full-thickness burns. Biobrane will actually adhere to a partial-thickness burn and acts as an artificial skin until the patient's own skin reepithelializes.

Synthetic dressings such as OpSite or DuoDERM are also used on burn wounds. OpSite is permeable to oxygen and carbon dioxide, but not to water or bacteria. Hydron, another barrier-type dressing, is made into a paste at the time of application and is applied directly over the burn. Hydron allows drainage through the material and may remain in place for up to 7 days.

A synthetic dressing, Sildimac, is a sustained-release drug delivery system composed of polyethylene glycol, poly-2-hydroxyethyl methacrylate, dimethyl sulfoxide, and silver sulfadiazine. When these components are mixed they form an elastic, flexible sheet that is adherent to dry surfaces and conforms closely to body contours. When incorporated into the delivery system, silver sulfadiazine is released in a sustained fashion. Studies have shown that Sildimac dressings on partial-thickness burns can be left in place for 5 to 7 days while bacterial levels are controlled and twice daily dressings with silver sulfadiazine are continued (Deitch et al., 1989; Miller et al., 1990). Treatment of burn wounds with systemic antibiotics has long been a challenge. DepoFoam particles, an encapsulated local drug delivery system, has been shown to reduce colonization at the site of injection and offers a promising method for administering sustained high concentrations of antibiotics to local tissues while at the same time avoiding toxic systemic levels (Grayson et al., 1993b). Inspection of the wound takes place at least daily, looking for signs of infection, odors, and exudate. There is much controversy over what isolation techniques should be required for burn patients. Some burn centers use strict isolation techniques, including hats, masks, caps, shoe covers, and scrub attire. Other centers require only scrub attire and universal isolation precautions. The type of isolation used should be decided in consultation with the epidemiologists at each institution. Culture results should be obtained at least weekly and followed for trends. Although some burn centers have serious cross-contamination and infection problems, others have none.

PAIN MANAGEMENT. Pain management remains a priority during the acute phase of recovery. Without adequate pain relief the patient cannot be expected to participate in his own care or to tolerate necessary procedures and therapies. During this phase the patient usually participates in activities, is more aware of his surroundings, and generally has little to concentrate on other than his burn care. There are many options for managing pain, including those previously discussed. During the early part of the acute phase the patient is generally weaned off the morphine drip and can be placed on patient-controlled analgesia (PCA) if he is free of handsplints and able to understand and use the equipment. PCA sometimes provides the patient with the only independence he experiences. Time-released oral morphine preparations, oral Dilaudid, methadone, and vicodin are among the other drugs that have been shown to work well in patients with burns. Antianxiety medications continue to be an adjunct.

NUTRITIONAL SUPPORT. Nutritional support during this phase is one of the top priorities of care. The patient with massive burns continues to receive enteral feedings, which can be supplemented with oral feedings until the patient is able to take in enough calories orally to meet his needs. Generally, this situation occurs when the patient has only 30% to 40% TBSA left unhealed. Patients are often provided with oral supplements (e.g., Ensure Plus) to assist in attaining adequate caloric intake.

If the patient becomes septic and develops ileus during the acute phase, nutrition continues to remain a high priority. A duodenal tube can be inserted, either through gravity or by gastroscopy, and feedings can continue despite ileus; otherwise, total parenteral nutrition (TPN) must be started through a central venous line. TPN carries an additional risk of intravenous line sepsis, given the large concentrations of glucose that must be administered to meet the patient's high caloric needs.

During the acute phase of recovery periodic urine tests for nitrogen may be done to assess the patient's nitrogen balance. Maintenance of a positive nitrogen balance is important, as is assessment of other nutritional parameters such as serum protein and serum albumin levels.

COLLABORATIVE INTERVENTIONS. There is a substantial degree of overlap in care between the emergent and acute phases of burn injury. The major goals are to maintain intravascular pressure, volume, and cardiac output; maintain electrolyte balance; provide nutritional support; promote continued joint function and mobility; promote continued autonomy and self-concept; and prevent complications associated with the acute phase of burn injury.

Rehabilitation Phase

Rehabilitation actually begins immediately after burn injury. This process is managed by a multidisciplinary network of professionals who contribute to the patient's eventual return, functionally and cosmetically, to his usual roles and responsibilities. The major goals of this phase of burn injury include enabling the patient to adapt emotionally to the burn injury, achieve maximum function of the involved body parts, and achieve rehabilitation within the limits of the disabilities.

PATIENT CARE MANAGEMENT DURING THE REHABILITATIVE PHASE

PAIN MANAGEMENT. Most patients continue to experience pain until the burn is totally healed and for some time thereafter. Pain medications are prescribed during this phase, although they tend to be less potent than the PCA and oral medications prescribed earlier. Tylenol with codeine is often used.

Pruritus is also a major complaint during this phase of recovery but is a normal part of the healing process. Diphenhydramine (Benadryl) and hydroxyzine (Atarax) are often prescribed to help control the symptoms. Lanolin-based skin lotions assist in maintaining lubrication for the healed skin, something that is not always present after a burn injury. Applications of lotion as frequently as every 2 hours may be necessary.

NUTRITIONAL SUPPORT. During this phase of recovery the patient is generally able to take in his caloric needs orally and is weaned from enteral feedings. It is important for the patient to continue to ingest a high-protein, high-calorie diet until the burns are completely healed. After healing has occurred, the patient's caloric intake should revert back to his preburn level.

PSYCHOSOCIAL ASSESSMENT AND SUPPORT. The skin is the defining feature of each person and serves to influence an individual's identity as well as his body image and concept of self. The nurse must be cognizant of the importance of the relationship between the burn patient's appearance and his attitudes and behavior toward care.

It should be noted that increasing numbers of patients are being admitted with burns resulting from abuse or self-inflicted burns. Patients with self-inflicted burns fall into two categories, those with burns suffered without suicidal intent and those who are suicidal (Klasen et al., 1989).

The burn patient and the family are unprepared for the traumatic nature of the devastating injury. They may be unable to manage both internal and external stressors as a result of compromised resources. This inability may continue well into the rehabilitation phase following burn injury, and thus the critical care nurse plays a key role in the assessment and early intervention to aid the patient and family. Most burn-related suicide patients are between ages 20 and 40 and attempt suicide at home (Klasen et al., 1989). This fact points to the need for family intervention for this group in particular.

The most frequent psychological responses encountered after burn trauma include loss, pain, and fear of physical discomfort, disfigurement, mutilation, or death. Disequilibrium caused by inability to manage the stressful event of the burn along with a distorted perception of the event may precipitate a psychological crisis. In addition, patients may demonstrate concerns about abandonment, reliance on life-support equipment, surgical procedures, loss or change of role, and a lengthy convalescence. These concerns may be grounded in reality or unfounded. Resolution in either event may take several weeks to months or years depending on the severity of the burn, the course of recovery, and individual response to treatment (Caine & Bufalino, 1987, 1988, 1991).

Individual patients react differently to the actual and perceived disfigurement associated with burn injuries. The importance of providing support and as-

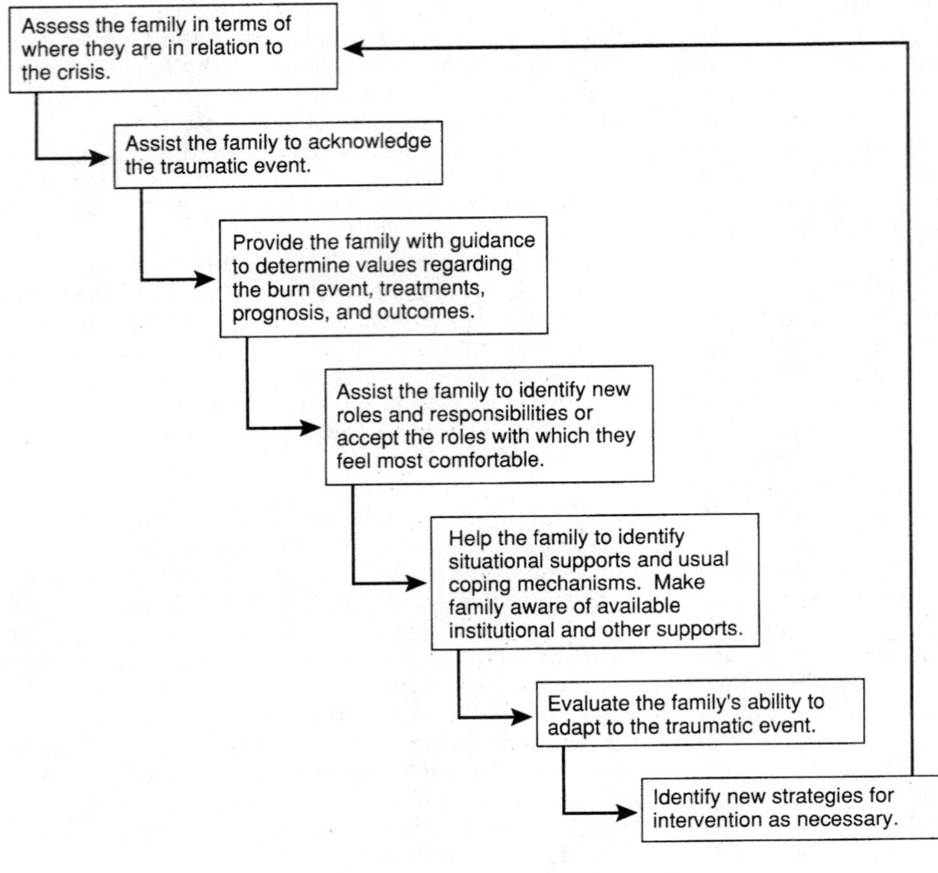

FIGURE 60–5. Framework for care of families of critically ill patients. (Adapted from Caine, R. M. [1989]. Families in crisis: Making the critical difference. *Focus on Critical Care, 16*[3], 188.)

sisting with adaptive coping cannot be minimized. Others who have had similar experiences can provide a valuable resource in the adjustment of both burn patients and families.

The problem of overwhelming helplessness for both the patient and family (Caine & Bufalino, 1988) and dependency in the early stages of postburn psychological processes (Flashman & Shapiro, 1983) needs to be taken seriously by the critical care nurse. The nurse must assess both the patient and family comprehensively to plan for psychological equilibrium. A framework for assessment of the patient and family is given in Figure 60–5 and suggestions for questions that may assist in the family assessment may be found in Table 60–12. Social support is important for the adjustment of burn-injured patients. The presence of caring and knowledgeable individuals rather than the performance of selected activities is important (Cheng & Rogers, 1989). Suggestions for psychosocial interventions are provided in Table 60–13.

OCCUPATIONAL AND PHYSICAL THERAPY. Considerable overlap may exist between occupational and physical therapy, depending on the institution. These two disciplines usually include assisting the patient with positioning, splinting, exercise, ambulation, and activities of daily living and begin within 24 hours of the patient's admission to the burn center. The goal of these therapies is to maintain and regain optimal functioning at the earliest possible time.

Because the rehabilitative process begins at admission, the therapists provide once or twice daily passive and active range of motion (ROM) exercises. Although

TABLE 60–12. **Burn Family Assessment Tool**

1. Who are the significant family members?
2. Who does the family identify as the leader?
3. Who makes health care decisions for the family members?
4. What are the family's spiritual/religious and ethnic orientations? How important are these to the family?
5. What is the developmental level of the patient? The family?
6. What is the educational level of family members?
7. Where does the family live in relationship to the hospital? How far must they travel?
8. What time of the day does the family plan to visit?
9. What information does the family need or want to know?
10. Which significant family members need to be consulted in decision making?
11. Has the family experienced something like this before? How did they cope? What resources did they use?
12. What emotional support do the family members need?
13. What are the family members' expectations regarding the patient's outcome? What are their goals for the patient?

Adapted with permission from Caine, R. M. (1989). Families in crisis: Making the critical difference. *Focus on Critical Care, 16*(3), 186.

TABLE 60–13. **Collaborative Psychosocial Interventions**

Give as much information as patient/family wants to help decrease fear and anxiety.
Encourage to talk about current situation and feelings; provide empathic listening.
Encourage participation and cooperation in care.
Continue to help to express feelings about current status, fears; listen actively; incorporate other health care personnel as appropriate.
Reinforce use of adaptive defenses while patient/family moves through grieving stages.
Plan experiences for the patient to control, manipulate, and succeed in to decrease feelings of powerlessness (e.g., allow to make some decisions regarding own care, schedule).
Refer patient for cosmetic counseling as appropriate, since an enhanced physical appearance may improve patient's body image.
Assess importance and impact of appearance changes; discuss with patient/family.
Provide careful explanation of procedures to dispel fears.
Organize care to prevent undue pain and anxiety.
Inform patient/family of any signs of progress.
Project calm, unhurried attitude while performing procedures.
Demonstrate respect for patient/family.
Allow for privacy when visitors are with patient.
Provide for financial and spiritual counseling as desired.

Adapted with permission from Caine, R. M., and Bufalino, P. (1987). *Nursing care planning guides for adults;* and Caine, R. M., and Bufalino, P. (1988). *Critically ill adults: Nursing care planning guides.* © 1987, 1988, The Williams & Wilkins Co., Baltimore.

both active and passive ROM exercises are difficult during the emergent phase, the patient's recovery is thought to progress faster and with less initial edema if exercises are instituted then.

Hand splints are custom-made to fit each patient and are used in patients with circumferential burns of the wrist and burns of the dorsal surface of the fingers involving the joints. Initially, splints are worn 23 hours a day, but as the burns heal the patient is allowed to wear the splints at night only.

Pain often deters the inexperienced therapist from performing the needed ROM exercises. Careful coordination with the nursing staff is necessary to ensure that the patient is adequately medicated and each form of therapy is allotted a space of uninterrupted time during the day. This therapy may be difficult while the patient's condition is extremely critical, but even 5 minutes at a time is useful.

The occupational therapist is specially trained to assist with the management of scars as the wounds heal. Pressure garments can be fitted for any part of the body and are worn for 6 months to 1 year. They provide pressure on the burn scar, helping to keep it flat and thin. Without the pressure garment, burn scars become raised and thick. Each garment is custom measured and created to fit that one patient.

SPEECH THERAPY. The speech therapist is another member of the burn team. Although most patients do not require this therapy, those who require long-term intubation and tracheostomy will. The speech therapist can assist in helping the patient develop communication techniques, either by means of an alphabet board or other techniques, depending on the needs of the patient. When both hands are splinted, the patient may even have difficulty in pointing.

RELEVANT RESEARCH

During the past two decades tremendous improvements in burn care and survival have occurred, including improved quality of life. Ongoing research has been vital in these improvements. Research ranges from pain management and wound care to immunologic concerns.

A major focus of current research involves the use of cultured human autologous tissue in burn wound closure. Cultured epithelium is not a new idea; however, the ability to perform the procedure in a clinically practical way is new. Cultured epithelium is used in patients with extensive burns when available donor sites are minimal and would not provide the patient with adequate skin coverage (Compton et al., 1989). Dermagraft, a living skin replacement that uses cultured, proliferating human keratinocytes, has been shown to vascularize beneath meshed skin grafts used to close full-thickness wounds and, although limitations exist, may offer a significant advantage in the care of the extensively burned patient (Hansbrough, 1994; Hansbrough et al., 1989, 1993; Zapata-Sirvent & Hansbrough, 1993b).

Hyperbaric oxygenation continues to be a controversial treatment in the care of the burn patient. Administration of hyperbaric oxygen to patients with carbon monoxide poisoning to prevent acute and delayed neurologic symptoms is also an option, but its benefits have yet to be proved.

Cyclosporine has been used for many years with increasing success in the treatment of patients with transplants of various organs. Studies have shown that patients who have undergone cadaver allograft skin transplantation, usually a temporary wound closure procedure, may experience permanent wound closure with the use of cyclosporine (Achauer et al., 1986).

SUMMARY

The consequences of burn injury can be devastating for the patient and his family. Physiologic changes following burn injury are life-threatening if left untreated. The initial phase following burn injury is characterized by a massive fluid shift from the intracellular to the interstitial compartment. This emergent period has a short duration and is followed immediately by a period of fluid remobilization, during which fluid shifts back. It is during these first two phases that the most critical changes occur and the critical care nurse must be most alert. The rehabilitation phase is the final phase after burn injury and can last months to years. The psychological changes that occur after burn injury cannot be minimized, and the astute critical care nurse balances the physiologic care of these traumatically injured patients with the intense psychological care that must also occur.

ACKNOWLEDGMENT. The author wishes to thank Rhonda Martin, RN, MSN, CCRN, and Megan Whalen, RN, MSN, CCRN, for their assistance in the preparation of this chapter.

REFERENCES

Achauer, B. M. (1987). Extremities. In B. M. Achauer (Ed.), *Management of the burned patient* (pp. 121–131). Norwalk, CT: Appleton & Lange.

Achauer, B. M., Black, K. S., Waxman, K. S., et al. (1986). Long-term skin allograft survival after short-term cyclosporine treatment in a patient with massive burns. *Lancet, 1,* 14–15.

Acute Pain Management Guideline Panel (1992). *Acute pain management: Operative or medical procedures and trauma clinical guidelines.* AHCPR Pub. No. 92–0032. Rockville, MD: Agency for Health Care Policy Research. Public Health Service, U.S. Dept. of Health and Human Services.

Aharoni, A., Abramovici, D., Weinberger, M., et al. (1989). Burn resuscitation with a low-volume plasma analysis of mortality. *Burns, 15*(4), 230–232.

American Burn Association (1990). Hospital and prehospital resources for optimal care of patients with burn injury: Guidelines for development and operation of burn centers. *Journal of Burn Care and Rehabilitation, 11,* 98–104.

Burns, S. M. (1990). Advances in ventilation therapy. *Focus on Critical Care, 17*(3), 227–237.

Busby, H. C. (1979). Acute burn patient and nursing management of optimal burn recovery. *The Journal of Continuing Education in Nursing, 10*(4), 16–30.

Caine, R. M., & Bufalino, P. (1987, 1991). *Nursing care planning guides for adults.* Baltimore: Williams & Wilkins.

Caine, R. M., & Bufalino, P. (1988). *Critically ill adults: Nursing care planning guides.* Baltimore: Williams & Wilkins.

Carrougher, G. J. (1993). Inhalation injury. *AACN Clinical Issues in Critical Care, 4*(2), 367–377.

Carter, E., Tompkins, R. G., & Burke, J. F. (1988). Hepatic and intestinal blood flow following thermal injury. *Journal of Burn Care and Rehabilitation, 9*(4), 347–350.

Cheng, S., & Rogers, J. C. (1989). Changes in occupational role performance after a severe burn: A retrospective study. *American Journal of Occupational Therapy, 43*(1), 17–24.

Choctaw, W. T., Eisner, M. E., & Wachtel, T. L. (1987). Causes, prevention, prehospital care, evaluation, emergency treatment, and prognosis. In B. M. Achauer (Ed.), *Management of the burned patient* (pp. 3–19). Norwalk, CT: Appleton & Lange.

Cioffi, W. G., & Rue, L. W. (1991). Diagnosis and treatment of inhalation injuries. *Critical Care Clinics of North America, 3,* 191–198.

Cioffi, W. G., et al. (1989). High-frequency percussive ventilation in patients with inhalation injury. *Journal of Trauma, 29,* 350–354.

Cioffi, W. G., et al. (1991). Prophylactic use of high-frequency percussive ventilation in patients with inhalation injury. *Annals of Surgery, 213,* 575–580.

Compton, C. C., Gill, J. M., Bradford, D. A., et al. (1989). Skin regenerated from cultured epithelial autografts on full-thickness burn wounds from six days to five years after grafting. *Laboratory Investigation, 60*(5), 600–612.

Deitch, E., Sittig, K., Heimbach, D., et al. (1989). Results of a multicenter outpatient burn study on the safety and efficacy of DIMAC-SSD. A new delivery system for silver sulfadiazine. *Journal of Trauma, 29*(4), 430–434.

Desai, M. H. (1984). Inhalation injuries in burn victims. *Critical Care Quarterly, 7*(3), 1–6.

Dolecek, R. (1985). The endocrine response after burns: Its possible correlations with the immunology of burns. *Journal of Burn Care and Rehabilitation, 6*(3), 281–294.

Dressler, D. P., Hozid, J. L., & Nathan, P. (1988). *Thermal injury.* St. Louis: C. V. Mosby.

Dyer, R., & Esch, V. (1976). Polyvinyl chloride toxicity in fires. *Journal of the American Medical Association, 235*(4), 293–297.

Edelman, P. E. (1987). Chemical and electrical burns. In B. M. Achauer (Ed.), *Management of the burned patient* (pp. 183–202). Norwalk, CT: Appleton & Lange.

Flashman, A., & Shapiro, E. (1983). Emotional care of the burned patient. In J. E. Nicosia & J. A. Petro (Eds.), *Manual of burn care.* New York: Raven Press.

Fuller, F. W., & Engler, P. E. (1988). Leukopenia in non-septic burn patients who received topical 1% silver sulfadiazine cream therapy: A survey. *Journal of Burn Care and Rehabilitation, 9*(6), 606–609.

Giel, L. C. (1987). Nutrition. In B. M. Achauer (Ed.), *Management of the burned patient* (pp. 135–148). Norwalk, CT: Appleton & Lange.

Graves, T. A., Cioffi, W. G., McManus, W. F., et al. (1988). Fluid resuscitation of infants and children with massive thermal injury. *Journal of Trauma, 28*(12), 1656–1659.

Grayson, L. S., Hansbrough, J. F., Zapata-Sirvent, R. L., Dore, C. A., Morgan, J. L., & Nicolson, M. A. (1993a). Quantitation of cytokine levels in skin graft donor site wound fluid. *Burns, 19*(5), 401–405.

Grayson, L. S., Hansbrough, J. F., Zapata-Sirvent, R. L., Kim, T., & Kim, S. (1993b). Pharmacokinetics of DepoFoam gentamicin delivery system and effect on soft tissue infection. *Journal of Surgical Research, 55,* 559–564.

Hansbrough, J. F. (1994). The promises of excisional therapy of burn wounds: Have they been achieved? *Journal of Intensive Care Medicine, 9,* 1–3.

Hansbrough, J. F., Boyce, S. T., Cooper, M. L., & Foreman, T. J. (1989). Burn wound closure with cultured autologous keratinocytes and fibroblasts attached to a collagen-glycosaminoglycan substrate. *Journal of the American Medical Association, 262,* 2125–2130.

Hansbrough, J. F., Morgan, J. L., Greenleaf, G. E., & Bartel, R. (1993). Composite grafts of human keratinocytes grown on a polyglactin mesh-cultured fibroblast dermal substitute function as a bilayer skin replacement in full-thickness wounds on athymic mice. *Journal of Burn Care and Rehabilitation, 14,* 485–493.

Hayter, J. (1978). Emergency nursing care of the burn patient. *Nursing Clinics of North America, 13*(2), 223–234.

Hersperger, J. E., & Dahl, L. M. (1978). Electrical and chemical injuries. *Critical Care Quarterly, 1*(3), 43–49.

Hill, M. B., Achauer, B. M., & Martinez, S. (1984). Tar and asphalt burns. *Journal of Burn Care and Rehabilitation, 5*(4), 271–274.

Jacobson, B. K., Cuono, C. B., Kupper, T. S., et al. (1988). Immunologic alterations following excisional wounding and immediate repair with syngeneic or allogeneic skin grafts. *Journal of Burn Care and Rehabilitation, 9*(4), 354–358.

Jacoby, F. G. (1974). *Nursing care of the patient with burns.* (2nd ed.). St. Louis: C. V. Mosby.

Jonsson, A., Cassuto, J., & Hanson, B. (1991). Inhibition of burn pain by intravenous lidocaine infusion. *Lancet, 338,* 151–152.

Kacmarek, R. M. (1988). The role of pressure support ventilation in reducing the work of breathing. *Respiratory Care, 33*(2), 99–120.

Klasen, H. J., van der Tempel, G. L., & Sauer, E. W. (1989). Attempted suicide by means of burns. *Burns, 15*(2), 88–92.

Kravitz, M. (1988). Thermal injuries. In V. D. Cardona, P. Hurn, P. J. B. Mason, et al. (Eds.), *Trauma nursing: From resuscitation through rehabilitation.* Philadelphia: W. B. Saunders.

Martin, L. M. (1989). Nursing implications of today's burn care techniques. *RN, 52*(5), 26–33.

Marvin, J. A., Carrougher, G., Bayley, E., Knighton, J., Rutan, R., & Weber, B. (1992). Burn nursing Delphi study: Pain management. *Journal of Burn Care and Rehabilitation, 13,* 685–694.

McAlhany, J. C., Czaja, A. J., & Rosenthal, A. (1979). Acute gastrointestinal disease after burns. In C. P. Artz, J. A. Moncrief, & B. A. Pruitt (Eds.), *Burns: A team approach* (pp. 512–522). Philadelphia: W. B. Saunders.

Miller, L., Hansbrough, J., Slater, H., Goldfarb, I. W., Kealey, P., Saffle, J., Kravitz, M., & Silverstein, P. (1990). Sildimac: A new delivery system for silver sulfadiazine in the treatment of full-thickness burn injuries. *Journal of Burn Care and Rehabilitation, 11,* 35–41.

Minar, V. (1978). Fluid resuscitation of the burn patient. *Journal of Emergency Nursing, 4,* 39–43.

Mozingo, D. W., Cioffi, W. G., & Pruitt, B. A. (1994). Burns. In F. S. Bongard & D. Y. Sue (Eds.), *Current: Critical care diagnosis and treatment* (pp. 657–685). Norwalk, CT: Appleton & Lange.

Nicosia, J. E., & Petro, J. A. (1983). *Manual of burn care.* New York: Raven Press.

Ohura, T. (1988). The Everett Idris Evans Memorial Lecture—1987: Twenty-five years' experience treating burns. *Journal of Burn Care and Rehabilitation, 9*(1), 106–117.

Patterson, D. R. (1992). Practical applications of psychological techniques in controlling burn pain. *Journal of Burn Care and Rehabilitation, 13,* 13–18.

Porth, C. M. (1994). *Pathophysiology: Concepts of altered health states.* Philadelphia: J. B. Lippincott.

Shelledy, D. C., et al. (1988a). Newer modes of mechanical ventilation: Pressure support part 1. *Respiratory Management, 18*(4), 14.

Shelledy, D. C., et al. (1988b). Newer modes of mechanical ventilation: Pressure support part 2. *Respiratory Management, 18*(4), 21–28.

Somogyi, E., & Tedeschi, C. G. (1977). Injury by electrical force. In C. G. Tedeschi, W. G. Eckert, & L. G. Tedeschi (Eds.), *Forensic medicine.* Philadelphia: W. B. Saunders.

St. John, R. (1990). Alternate modes of mechanical ventilation. *AACN Clinical Issues in Critical Care, 1*(2), 248–259.

Teodorczyk-Injeyan, J. A., Sparkes, B. G., & Peters, W. J. (1989). Regulation of IgM production in thermally injured patients. *Burns, 15*(4), 241–247.

Trofino, R. B. (1991). *Nursing care of the burn-injured patient.* Philadelphia: F. A. Davis.

Uehara, D. T., Baumgartner, E. A., & Eisner, R. F. (1986). Burns. In S. H. Cahill & M. Balkus (Eds.), *Interventions in emergency nursing: The first 60 minutes* (pp. 225–240). Rockville, MD: Aspen Publications.

Wardenn, G. (1987). Immunology. In B. M. Achauer (Ed.), *Management of the burned patient* (pp. 49–63). Norwalk, CT: Appleton & Lange.

Waxman, K., Lefcourt, N., & Achauer, B. (1989). Heated laser Doppler flow measurements to determine depth of burn injury. *American Journal of Surgery, 157*(6), 541–543.

White, C., et al. (1990). High frequency ventilation and extracorporeal membrane oxygenation. *AACN Clinical Issues in Critical Care, 1,* 427–444.

Wiener, S. L., & Barrett, J. (1986). *Trauma management.* Philadelphia: W. B. Saunders.

Williams, R., & Porvaznik, J. (1989). Initial resuscitation of major burn patients. *Journal of Family Practice, 28*(4), 449–456.

Zapata-Sirvent, R. L., & Hansbrough, J. F. (1993a). Temporal analysis of human leukocyte surface antigen expression and neutrophil respiratory burst activity after thermal injury. *Burns, 19*(1), 5–11.

Zapata-Sirvent, R. L., & Hansbrough, J. F. (1993b). Cytotoxicity to human leukocytes by topical antimicrobial agents used for burn care. *Journal of Burn Care and Rehabilitation, 14,* 132–140.

Zapata-Sirvent, R. L., Hansbrough, J. F., Wolf, P., Grayson, L. S., & Nicholson, M. (1993). Epidermal growth factor limits structural alterations in gastrointestinal tissues and decreases bacterial translocation in burned mice. *Surgery, 113*(5), 564–573.

Zapata-Sirvent, R. L., Hansbrough, J. F., Greenleaf, G. E., Grayson, L. S., & Wolf, P. (1994). Reduction of bacterial translocation and intestinal structural alterations by heparin in a murine burn injury model. *Journal of Trauma, 36*(1), 1–5.

Zawacki, B. (1974). Reversal of capillary stasis and prevention of necrosis in burns. *Annals of Surgery, 180*(1), 98–102.

BURNS
MULTIDISCIPLINARY CARE GUIDE

COORDINATION OF CARE

Diagnosis/Stabilization Phase		Acute Management Phase		Recovery Phase	
Outcome	***Intervention***	***Outcome***	***Intervention***	***Outcome***	***Intervention***
All appropriate team members and disciplines will be involved in the plan of care.	Develop a plan of care with the patient/family, primary nurse(s), primary physician(s), surgeon, plastic surgeon, infectious diseases, other specialists as needed, clinical nurse specialist, respiratory therapist, and chaplain.	All appropriate team members and disciplines will be involved in the plan of care.	Update the plan of care with patient/family, other team members and physical therapist, dietician, discharge planner, social worker, recreational therapist, and occupational therapist. Initiate planning for anticipated discharge and call home health and home medical equipment company as needed. Begin teaching patient/family about care at home.	Patient will understand how to maintain optimal health at home.	Provide written guidelines concerning care at home and any follow-up visits. Provide patient/family with phone number of resources/support groups available to answer questions.

FLUID BALANCE

Diagnosis/Stabilization Phase		Acute Management Phase		Recovery Phase	
Outcome	***Intervention***	***Outcome***	***Intervention***	***Outcome***	***Intervention***
Patient will achieve optimal hemodynamic status as evidenced by: • MAP >70 mm Hg • Hemodynamic parameters WNL • Urine output >0.5 mL/kg/hr • Absence of dysrhythmias • Adequate level of consciousness (LOC) • Clear lung sounds • Adequate intake and output • Normothermia • Normal CVP	Assess degree, extent, and severity of burns. Monitor and treat cardiac • dysrhythmias • $S\bar{v}O_2$ • BP • I & O • LOC • evidence of tissue perfusion • jugular venous distention • CVP Monitor lab values: electrolytes, CBC, clotting factors, carboxyhemoglobin, ABGs. Monitor respiratory status and be prepared for mechanical ventilation. Assess lung sounds q1–2h. Assess fluid deficit and treat accordingly. Administer electrolyte solutions the first 24 hours after injury.	Patient will maintain optimal hemodynamic status.	Same as for stabilization phase. Monitor and treat hemodynamic parameters. Assess neurologic status q2–4h and as needed. Measure circumference of burned areas to determine if edema is present. Elevate burned extremities. Stay prepared for mechanical ventilation should respiratory status deteriorate. Anticipate and be prepared for electrolyte replacement therapy. Continue to assess for complications associated with burns. Obtain daily weight.	Same as in acute management phase.	Same as in acute management phase.

	When estimating fluid loss, consider loss through evaporation, blistering, or wound drainage. Anticipate and be prepared for electrolyte replacement therapy. Anticipate need for vasopressor agents; assess response and titrate accordingly. Assess neurologic status q1h and as needed. Monitor and treat dysrhythmias. Weigh patient daily. Obtain 12-lead ECG. Monitor temperature and take measures to return to normal: hypo/hyperthermia unit, warm blankets, antipyretics. Monitor for signs of complications that can occur with burns: inhalation injuries, ARDS, respiratory failure, renal failure, liver failure, infection, sepsis, hypovolemia, DIC, clotting disorders, anemia, atelectasis, bronchospasm, acute airway obstruction, encephalopathy, decreased tissue perfusion, pulmonary edema, ulcers.				

NUTRITION

Diagnosis/Stabilization Phase		Acute Management Phase		Recovery Phase	
Outcome	***Intervention***	***Outcome***	***Intervention***	***Outcome***	***Intervention***
Patient will be adequately nourished.	NPO if intubated or until able to take fluids. Initiate enteral or intravenous feedings as necessary. Provide high-calorie diet. Calculate caloric and protein requirements based on body weight and body surface burned. Monitor response to diet. Assess bowel sounds, abdominal distention, and abdominal pain and tenderness q4h and as needed.	Patient will be adequately nourished.	Same as in stabilization phase. Progress diet as tolerated. Maintain a high-calorie, high-protein diet. Involve dietician in plan of care.	Patient will be adequately nourished.	Monitor response to diet. Instruct patient/family on dietary needs after discharge.

Care Guide continued on following page

BURNS MULTIDISCIPLINARY CARE GUIDE *continued*

MOBILITY

Diagnosis/Stabilization Phase		Acute Management Phase		Recovery Phase	
Outcome	*Intervention*	*Outcome*	*Intervention*	*Outcome*	*Intervention*
Patient will achieve optimal mobility. Patient will be free of joint contractures.	Turn at least q2h if hemodynamically stable and monitor response. Institute alternative bed therapy if indicated, (i.e., kinetic therapy, Stryker frame). Begin passive/active-assist range of motion exercises.	Patient will achieve optimal mobility. Patient will be free of joint contractures.	Increase activity as tolerated. Monitor response to increased activity and decrease if adverse events occur (tachycardia, dyspnea, syncope, dysrhythmias, hypotension). Provide support as necessary. Obtain physical therapy consult. Begin teaching patient/family progressive activity and how to assist patient with program goals.	Patient will achieve optimal mobility.	Continue to progress activity as tolerated and monitor response. Decrease activity if adverse events occur. Continue teaching patient/family about home exercise program.

OXYGENATION/VENTILATION

Diagnosis/Stabilization Phase		Acute Management Phase		Recovery Phase	
Outcome	*Intervention*	*Outcome*	*Intervention*	*Outcome*	*Intervention*
Patient will have adequate gas exchange as evidenced by: • O_2 saturation >90% • ABGs WNL • Clear breath sounds • Chest x-ray normal • Respiratory rate, depth, and rhythm WNL • Absence of dyspnea, cyanosis, and secretions • Effective cough *O_2 saturation must be measured in a blood gas laboratory and not per pulse oximetry because pulse oximetry does not measure carboxyhemoglobin.	Monitor ventilator settings and hemodynamic variables before, during, and after weaning. Avoid prolonged administration of 100% FIO_2. Monitor respiratory status constantly, particularly if inhalation injury has occurred—lung sounds, respiratory muscle strength, respiratory rate and depth, coughing ability, ABGs, and chest x-ray. Anticipate need for hyperventilation and hyperoxygenation, particularly before suctioning. Apply supplemental oxygen if not intubated. Assess evidence of tissue perfusion. Monitor lab values: hemoglobin, ABGs, carboxyhemoglobin.	Patient will have adequate gas exchange.	Monitor and treat oxygenation disturbances as per ABGs and/or SaO_2. Monitor and treat ventilation disturbances as per chest assessment, ABGs, adventitious breath sounds, and chest x-ray. Wean from oxygen therapy/mechanical ventilation as indicated. Administer warm humidified oxygen. Consider use of postural drainage and percussion. Anticipate and prepare for bronchoscopy in the event of pulmonary/inhalation burns. Observe for complications of burns that may impair oxygenation/ventilation: pneumonia, infection, thrombus formation, embolus, ARDS, sepsis, hypovolemia, $\dot{V}/\dot{Q}$ mismatch, atelectasis.	Patient will have adequate gas exchange.	Same as acute management phase. Obtain chest x-ray before discharge. Provide instruction to patient on coughing and deep breathing at home. Have patient give return demonstration. Observe effects of increased activity on respiratory status. Continue to assess for complications of burns that may impair oxygenation/ventilation.

COMFORT

Diagnosis/Stabilization Phase		Acute Management Phase		Recovery Phase	
Outcome	*Intervention*	*Outcome*	*Intervention*	*Outcome*	*Intervention*
Patient will be as comfortable and painfree as possible as evidenced by: • No objective indicators of discomfort • No complaints of discomfort	Assess quantity and quality of pain. Administer IV narcotic analgesics as needed and monitor response. A titrated morphine drip may be used. Establish effective communication technique with which patient can communicate discomfort and need for analgesics if intubated. Provide quiet environment to potentiate analgesia. Provide reassurance in a calm, caring, competent manner.	Patient will be relaxed and as painfree as possible.	Same as stabilization phase. Administer narcotic analgesics before any painful procedures, such as wound debridement or dressing changes. Teach patient relaxation techniques. Use massage, humor, music therapy, and imagery to promote relaxation. Involve family in strategies. Observe for complications of burns that may cause discomfort (embolus, thrombus, infection).	Patient will be relaxed and as painfree as possible.	Progress to oral analgesics and nonnarcotic analgesics when possible. Monitor response. Continue alternative methods to promote relaxation as listed above. Teach patient/family alternative methods to promote relaxation at home.

SKIN INTEGRITY

Diagnosis/Stabilization Phase		Acute Management Phase		Recovery Phase	
Outcome	*Intervention*	*Outcome*	*Intervention*	*Outcome*	*Intervention*
Patient will have intact skin without abrasions or pressure ulcers. Burns will remain free of infection.	Maintain strict aseptic technique. Assess all bony prominences at least q4h and treat if needed. Use preventive pressure-reducing devices/kinetic therapy if patient is at high risk for development of pressure ulcers. Treat pressure ulcers according to hospital protocol.	Same as stabilization phase.	Same as stabilization phase. Begin teaching patient/family on assessment of burn areas/grafted areas, treatment, skin care, and how to evaluate effectiveness of treatment.	Patient will have intact skin without abrasions or pressure ulcers. Burns will be free of infection. Skin grafts will be free of infection.	Continue teaching patient/family care of burn/skin graft wounds at home: • Aseptic technique • Dressing changes • Pressure bandages • Assessment of healing progress • Potential complications (rejection, infection)

PROTECTION/SAFETY

Diagnosis/Stabilization Phase		Acute Management Phase		Recovery Phase	
Outcome	*Intervention*	*Outcome*	*Intervention*	*Outcome*	*Intervention*
Patient will be protected from possible harm. Patient will be protected from infection.	Assess need for restraints if patient is intubated, has a decreased LOC, or is agitated and restless. Explain need for restraints to patient/family. Assess response to restraints, if used, and check q1h for skin integrity and impairment to circulation.	Patient will be protected from possible harm. Patient will be protected from infection.	If need still exists for restraints, check q1–2h for skin integrity and impairment to circulation. Provide support when activity increases. Monitor response to activity.	Patient will be protected from possible harm. Patient will be protected from infection.	Provide support with activity increases and monitor response. Teach patient/family about any physical limitations in activity after discharge. Teach patient/family about the importance of maintaining sterile technique with dressing changes.

Care Guide continued on following page

BURNS MULTIDISCIPLINARY CARE GUIDE *continued*

PROTECTION/SAFETY *continued*

Diagnosis/Stabilization Phase		Acute Management Phase		Recovery Phase	
Outcome	*Intervention*	*Outcome*	*Intervention*	*Outcome*	*Intervention*
	Remove restraints as soon as patient is able to follow instruction. Provide sedatives as needed and monitor response, especially to respiratory system. Follow hospital protocol for use of restraints.				

PSYCHOSOCIAL/SELF-DETERMINATION

Diagnosis/Stabilization Phase		Acute Management Phase		Recovery Phase	
Outcome	*Intervention*	*Outcome*	*Intervention*	*Outcome*	*Intervention*
Patient will achieve psychophysiologic stability. Patient will demonstrate a decrease in anxiety as evidenced by: • Vital signs WNL • Subjective reports of decreased anxiety • Objective signs of decreased anxiety Patient will begin acceptance process of burns.	Assess physiologic effects of critical care environment on patient (hemodynamic variables, psychological status, signs of increased sympathetic response). Provide sedatives as indicated. Take measures to reduce sensory overload. Develop effective interventions to communicate with patient if intubated. Use tactile and verbal stimuli if unresponsive. Use calm, caring, competent, and reassuring approach with patient and family. Arrange for flexible visiting to meet patient and family needs.	Patient will achieve psychophysiologic stability. Patient will demonstrate a decrease in anxiety. Patient will accept burns and long-term effects.	Same as stabilization phase.	Patient will achieve psychophysiologic stability. Patient will demonstrate a decrease in anxiety. Patient will accept burns and long-term effects.	Provide instruction on coping mechanisms after discharge. Refer to outside services or agencies as appropriate (chaplain, social services, support group, home health, medical equipment supplier).

Determine coping ability of patient/family and take appropriate measures to begin acceptance of long-term therapy for burns and long-term results (provide frequent explanations, encourage patient to ask questions, encourage patient to verbalize feelings and concerns).

DIAGNOSTICS

Diagnosis/Stabilization Phase		Acute Management Phase		Recovery Phase	
Outcome	***Intervention***	***Outcome***	***Intervention***	***Outcome***	***Intervention***
Patient will understand any tests or procedures that must be completed (vital signs, I & O, hemodynamic monitoring, C.O., CXR, carboxyhemoglobin level, SMA-18, CBC, clotting studies, type and crossmatch, urinalysis, electrolytes, wound management, bronchoscopy, ABGs).	Explain all procedures and tests to patient/family. Be sensitive to individualized needs of patient/family for information.	Patient will understand any tests or procedures that must be completed to recover from burns (i.e., hydrotherapy, debridement, grafting).	Same as stabilization phase. Anticipate need for further diagnostic tests or procedures such as skin grafting and prepare patient for these.	Patient will understand meaning of diagnostic tests and procedures in relation to continued health (wound care, diet, skin grafting).	Review with patient before discharge the results of lab tests, chest x-ray, and skin grafting. Discuss any abnormal findings and appropriate measures patient can take to help return to normal. Provide patient with written guidelines concerning follow-up care. Provide instruction on care at home after discharge and have patient give return demonstration when appropriate (when to call the doctor, wound care, sterile technique, activity restrictions, exercise program, dietary needs, medications, etc.). Provide patient with phone number of resources available to assist if necessary.

UNIT

13

MULTISYSTEM DISORDERS

Immobility Phenomena in Critically Ill Adults

Nancy L. Szaflarski

Mobility is a fundamental characteristic of humans and is vital to independence. Mobility serves to promote physical fitness, prevent disability, and slow the onset of degenerative processes. Maintenance of optimal health requires a proper balance of rest, sleep, exercise, and time in an upright position. The upright, standing position serves to trigger physiologic responses that counteract gravity effects and maintain a state of homeostasis. Even at rest, the healthy adult normally turns or changes position an average of every 11.6 minutes, emphasizing the important role of mobility in life (Milazzo & Resh, 1981). This standard of movement has been defined as the "minimal physiological mobility requirement."

Bedrest has been traditionally used as a cornerstone, therapeutic measure for critically ill patients. Its benefits result mainly from decreasing oxygen consumption ($\dot{V}O_2$), preventing or reducing trauma to a body part, and allowing energy resources to be directed toward healing. Numerous studies have examined the physiologic and psychological consequences of bedrest. The bulk of these studies were conducted during the 1960s and 1970s for the United States space program because bedrest was used as an analogue of weightlessness. Clinical studies have further defined the pathophysiologic consequences of bedrest, and these have highlighted the use of bedrest as a double-edged sword.

Immobility is a disuse phenomenon that evokes interrelated physiologic, psychological, and psychosocial effects. The stimulus for this akinetic phenomenon in critically ill adults is bedrest. The prevalence of bedrest in this population approaches nearly 100%. An observation of any critical care unit reveals adults confined to bed in supine, Trendelenburg, lateral recumbent, and Fowler positions. Few studies have defined the length and degree of immobility in critically ill patients.

The reasons for immobility in critically ill adults are listed in Table 61–1. The increased use of sophisticated technology has had a major impact on imposing supine immobilization in critically ill adults. The length of immobilization is nearly directly proportional to the length of stay in the intensive care unit (ICU), because many patients are not fully ambulatory on discharge from the ICU.

The high morbidity rate associated with immobility is related to the length of immobilization. Although studies of healthy young adults have demonstrated the presence of significant physiologic changes from bedrest within as few as 3 to 4 days (Greenleaf, 1982; Lamb et al., 1965), the occurrence of pathophysiologic changes is associated with longer immobilization periods. Critically ill patients with long-term disease processes such as multisystem failure, Guillain-Barré syndrome, adult respiratory distress syndrome, and sepsis are at greater risk for morbidity than are elective

TABLE 61–1. **Reasons for Immobility in Critically Ill Adults**

Therapeutic Gain

1. Decrease $\dot{V}O_2$ and carbon dioxide production (refractory hypoxemic–hypercarbic respiratory failure; acute myocardial infarction; congestive heart failure)
2. Attain and maintain cardiopulmonary stability (cardiopulmonary arrest; postarrest states; postcardiopulmonary bypass; shock states; severe burns; intraaortic and pulmonary artery balloon pumping)
3. Promote healing or minimize trauma (intracranial bleeding; disseminated intravascular coagulation; aortic or arterial graft approximations; large wounds with questionable tensile strengths; burns; acute spinal cord injuries; acute stroke)
4. Maintenance of spinal or bone alignment (acute spinal cord injuries, orthopedic fractures)

Safety

1. Altered mental states (coma; confusion; postanesthesia states; sedation or narcotization)
2. Maintenance of intravascular access lines and associated drug or fluid infusions
3. Secure provision for artificial airways and ventilatory modes
4. Provision for accurate invasive monitoring and therapy (hemodynamic and intracranial pressure lines; oximetry or capnography; intraaortic and pulmonary artery balloon pumping; transesophageal echocardiography)
5. Altered motor or sensory function (generalized weakness; stroke; peripheral neuropathies; neuromuscular blockade; paralysis)

TABLE 61–2. **Risk Factors Associated With Complications of Immobility in Critically Ill Adults**

Length and degree of immobility
Past medical history (peripheral vascular disease, DVT, PE, decubitus ulcers, pneumonia)
Altered motor or sensory function
Altered level of consciousness
Incontinence
Poor nutrition
Advancing age
Obesity
Altered skin integrity
Present infection
Extensive surgery
Significant sustained hypotension
Hypoxemia
Altered immunocompetence
Malignancy
Exogenous steroid administration

Abbreviations: DVT, deep venous thrombosis; PE, pulmonary embolism.

postoperative patients who are subjected to a 1- or 2-day recovery period. Consequences of immobility are greatest in the elderly due to concomitant age-related factors (Mobily & Kelley, 1991). Other factors associated with increased risk of morbidity from immobilization in critically ill adults are listed in Table 61–2. The signs and symptoms of complications resulting from immobility may not be fully apparent at the time of discharge from the ICU because many patients remain on bedrest and have not begun the remobilization process.

Major forms of morbidity resulting from immobility include infection, sepsis, muscle atrophy, pressure ulcers, respiratory failure, thromboembolism, pulmonary embolism, and ICU psychosis or delirium. Such morbidity results in increased length of ICU or hospital stay, increased caregiver and equipment costs, and increased duration and extent of suffering for the patient. The critical care nurse can play a major role in preventing these complications by understanding the physiologic, pathophysiologic, and psychological effects of immobility.

PHYSIOLOGIC AND PATHOPHYSIOLOGIC EFFECTS OF IMMOBILITY

Many of the physiologic effects induced by immobility occur immediately as a recumbent position is achieved. Other physiologic and pathophysiologic effects are associated with longer periods of immobility. An appreciation of the time course of the effects is essential to project potential complications.

Cardiovascular Effects

FLUID SHIFTS

When an individual moves from an upright to a supine position, central fluid shifts occur. Eleven percent of total blood volume is shifted from the legs to other parts of the body (Rubin, 1988). Of this shifted volume, 78% is directed to the thorax and 20% to the head and neck (Rubin, 1988). These shifts result in an increased central venous pressure, left ventricular end-diastolic pressure, and stroke volume. A successful adaptation to the supine position activates volume receptors and renal and hormonal mechanisms to produce a diuresis. This diuresis results in a reduction of plasma volume, total blood volume, and end-diastolic filling pressures and volumes, and is independent of total fluid intake. Plasma volume losses occur during short periods of bedrest but then level off and do not regain normal levels. Total blood volume losses parallel plasma volume losses, but are not as great (Winslow, 1985). If bedrest continues, the initial decrease in extracellular volume is restored by an increase in interstitial volume, although plasma volume remains low.

PHYSICAL WORK CAPACITY

Prolonged bedrest results in cardiovascular deconditioning as reflected in a decreased physical work capacity and orthostatic intolerance. Cardiovascular deconditioning effects from bedrest can also be quantified by a measure of physical working capacity known as maximal or peak $\dot{V}O_2$ (oxygen uptake). Peak $\dot{V}O_2$ is the maximal rate at which oxygen can be delivered to the tissues during periods of exhaustive isotonic exercise. It is the product of the maximal cardiac output and the maximal arteriovenous oxygen difference. Maximal $\dot{V}O_2$ is a well recognized measure of cardiopulmonary fitness, maximal aerobic capacity, and deconditioning adaptation of bedridden subjects. Significant decreases of 13% to 46% in maximal $\dot{V}O_2$ after prolonged bedrest were found to occur in men during treadmill testing after 3 to 4 weeks of bedrest (Miller et al., 1965; Saltin et al., 1968).

ORTHOSTATIC CAPACITY

When a healthy adult assumes the erect position from a supine position, approximately 500 mL of blood shifts largely from the intrathoracic cardiovascular compartment to the lower parts of the body. This loss of blood volume from the thorax decreases venous return, stroke volume, cardiac output, and arterial pressure. Neurovascular stretch receptors located in the carotid arteries and aorta and in the walls of the heart are stimulated by a lack of stretch. Their activation results in increased heart rate, increased myocardial contractility, vasoconstriction, and antidiuresis, which maintain arterial pressure and adequate perfusion pressure to the vital organs. Movement of the lower extremities in an erect position causes skeletal muscle contraction, which exerts pressure against the veins and lymph vessels in the legs. Such movement aids in increasing venous return in the presence of competent venous valves.

Orthostatic hypotension occurs in individuals placed on bedrest. Orthostatic intolerance can occur even after as little as 6 hours of bedrest. The sudden development of hypotension, weakness, faintness, or dizziness in a recumbent patient who is placed upright is explained by two contributing factors. Neurovascular reflexes have become dormant during the period of bedrest despite adequate epinephrine output. The peripheral vessels thus fail to constrict appropriately in response to the stress. The general loss of muscle tone that occurs with bedrest also depresses the normal venopressor mechanism, resulting in venous pooling of blood in the dependent lower extremities. The compensatory tachycardia that usually occurs is evoked to sustain cerebral perfusion pressure. Occasionally, individuals have been reported to exhibit a bradycardiac response to the falling blood pressure of orthostasis. The ability of the cardiovascular system to respond appropriately to the upright posture is regained slowly after resumption of activity.

VENOUS FLOW

Due to the decreased use of leg muscles associated with bedrest, the frequency and strength of skeletal muscle contractions are decreased, resulting in unaided venous blood return. Decreased venous flow results in venous blood pooling and stasis in the lower extremities. This phenomenon alone may result in venous thrombosis. Damage to the venous intima also may occur with bedrest when a flaccid leg is subjected to sustained pressure from a supporting surface or another body part (Roberts, 1987). Intimal damage of veins has been a well recognized contributory factor in the development of thrombophlebitis. Hypercoagulability due to associated decreases in plasma volume with immobility also predisposes to thrombophlebitis. These three risk factors—venous stasis, intimal damage, and hypercoagulability—comprise Virchow's triad.

Critically ill patients should be considered as being at high risk for deep vein thrombosis (DVT) based solely on the prevalence and extent of their immobility. Immobility has been defined as a prime risk factor in the development of venous stasis and DVT (Coon et al., 1987; Pingleton, 1985). Plate and associates (1986) reported that prolonged immobility was the most frequent etiologic factor for acute iliofemoral venous thrombosis in 25% of 128 medical–surgical patients. Other factors, identified in Table 61–3, elicit one or more arms of Virchow's triad in predisposing to DVT (Coon et al., 1987; Fahey, 1984; Pingleton, 1985). The frequent synergism of these risk factors in critically ill adults places most such patients at high risk for this complication.

Although the major complication of DVT is pulmonary embolism, it is important to note that DVT may also result in recurrent venous thrombosis and the postphlebitic syndrome. Venous hypertension is present with DVT. As lysis of the clot occurs, subsequent recanalization of the vein may cause destruction of valves in deep and communicating veins. Chronic venous insufficiency may result, causing chronic leg pain, edema, and stasis ulceration. Even when DVT is clinically silent, the postphlebitic syndrome may result (Coon et al., 1987).

TABLE 61–3. **Risk Factors for Deep Venous Thrombosis in Critically Ill Adults**

Immobilization
Major abdominal or orthopedic surgery
Nonsurgical trauma
Advancing age (>40 years)
Obesity
Cardiopulmonary disease
Past medical history (DVT, PE, leg trauma)
Pregnancy or parturition
Malignancy
Altered coagulation (thrombocytosis, polycythemia vera)

Abbreviations: DVT, deep venous thrombosis; PE, pulmonary embolism.

Pulmonary Effects

LUNG VOLUMES

On assuming a recumbent position, all lung volumes decrease except for tidal volume (Fig. 61–1). Residual volume and functional residual capacity (FRC) are decreased due to the increase in intrathoracic blood volume associated with recumbency. Recumbency-induced diaphragmatic elevation secondary to the gravitational redistribution of the abdominal contents also reduces FRC.

The clinical relevance of changing lung volumes and capacities with the supine and lateral recumbent positions depends on the newly altered relationship between the closing volume and FRC. The FRC needs to be greater than the closing volume to keep airways open. If the closing volume is greater than the FRC, some alveoli will be closed, thus creating areas of ventilation–perfusion ($\dot{V}/\dot{Q}$) mismatch in the lung. The sensitivity of closing volumes to changes in posture and overall higher closing volumes have been associated with obese and older adults.

VENTILATION–PERFUSION RELATIONSHIPS

In the upright, normal lung, ventilation and perfusion both increase from the upper to the lower areas of the lung (Fig. 61–2). Perfusion is greater in the bases due to the profound influence of gravitational forces sequestering greater blood flow. Although there is less lung expansion in the bases due to the weight of the lung, ventilation remains greatest in the bases in the upright position because of less negative intrapleural pressures, which are determined by gravitational forces and the weight of the lung. Because increases in perfusion are greater than increases in ventilation down the lung in the upright position, $\dot{V}/\dot{Q}$ ratios decrease from the lung apex to the lung base.

Assumption of the supine, lateral recumbent, or prone position causes a redistribution of ventilation

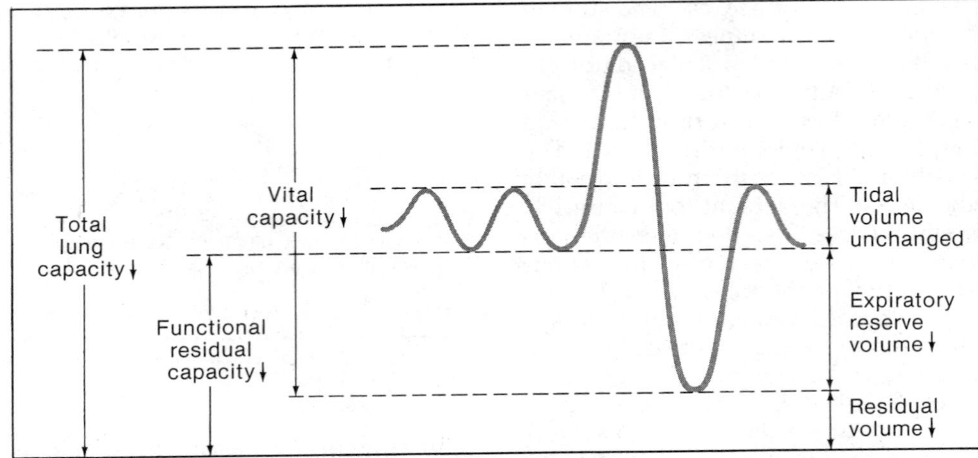

FIGURE 61–1. Effect of supine position on lung volumes and capacities in normal lungs.

and perfusion in the lung. The dependent lung portion in the supine position becomes the dorsal portion of the lung; in a lateral recumbent position it becomes the lung portion that meets the supporting surface; and in a prone position it becomes the anterior lung region. Changes in $\dot{V}/\dot{Q}$ ratios associated with position changes may result in decreases in the partial pressure of oxygen in arterial blood (PaO_2) and increases in the alveolar–arterial oxygen content differences.

Factors impairing ventilation in patients on bedrest may also contribute to altered $\dot{V}/\dot{Q}$ relationships. Restriction of chest excursion and diaphragmatic descent can occur with abdominal distention, abdominal or chest binders, use of pharmacologic agents, and a slumped sitting position, which is a common sight in an ICU. The effects of anesthesia on decreasing diaphragmatic excursion, FRC, and diaphragmatic activity for 24 hours after surgery are also well known factors in impairing ventilation in immobilized patients.

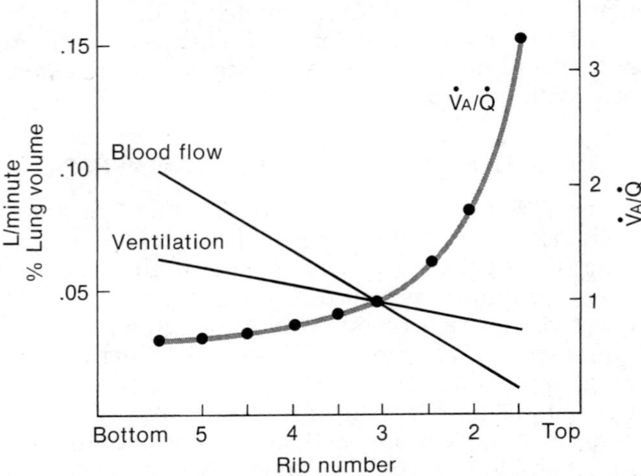

FIGURE 61–2. Ventilation and blood flow distribution in the upright, normal lung. Although ventilation and blood flow both increase down the lung, perfusion increases remain greatest. The ventilation–perfusion ratios ($\dot{V}/\dot{Q}$) thus decrease from apex to base. (Redrawn from West, J. B. [1977]. *Ventilation/blood flow and gas exchange* [3rd ed.]. Oxford: Blackwell.)

ATELECTASIS AND PNEUMONIA

Atelectasis is a known consequence of prolonged bedrest. Due to weakened thoracic muscles, decreased ciliary movement in the tracheobronchial tree, and impaired cough mechanisms, respiratory secretions may easily accumulate in dependent lung areas and block bronchioles. Lung gas distal to these blockages is absorbed, resulting in alveolar collapse. Decreased surfactant production due to decreases in regional blood flow has also been implicated in the development of atelectasis (Memmer & Kozier, 1987). The stasis and pooling of pulmonary secretions can lead to hypostatic pneumonia and may create an excellent medium for bacterial growth. The confounding factors of dehydration and use of anticholinergic drugs in immobile patients may result in secretions that are thick, tenacious, and hard to raise. The clinical consequence of atelectasis and pneumonia is hypoxemia due to low $\dot{V}/\dot{Q}$ units and intrapulmonary shunting.

Pennington (1987) reported a rate of nosocomial pneumonia as high as 20% in patients in a respiratory ICU. Yannelli and Gurevich (1988) have defined the major risk factor of nosocomial pneumonia in critically ill patients as endotracheal intubation because host defenses are bypassed with this therapeutic adjunct. Pennington (1987) found a four times greater incidence of nosocomial pneumonia in intubated patients than in those who were not. Other risk factors for critically ill patients identified by Yannelli and Gurevich (1988) included the presence of nasogastric tubes, assisted ventilation, immunosuppression, impaired mental status, antibiotic use, surgical procedures, and gastric or oropharyngeal aspiration. Hoyt (1990) identified the factors of increased gastric volume/pressure, reduced lower esophageal sphincter tone, decreased gastric pH, and reduced airway protective mechanisms as contributing to aspiration pneumonitis, which may lead to nosocomial pneumonia in critically ill patients. Immobility as a factor in predisposing critically ill adults to nosocomial pneumonia has not been independently defined or controlled for. Because most ICU patients are on bedrest, the factor of immobility remains implied in the identified risk factors.

ASPIRATION

Elpern and colleagues (1987) reported an overall 77% aspiration rate in a study of 31 critically ill intubated adults. A risk factor for aspiration identified in this study was the flat or head-down position, which was a potential cause of retrograde movement of gastroesophageal contents. Subjects placed in these positions were limited in number in this study, limiting the statistical inference of this finding. Elpern and colleagues (1987) also found that the head-up position in these 31 intubated patients did not prove beneficial in protecting against aspiration because the aspiration rate was 27% in this subgroup. The assumption that a Fowler's position protects the airway from aspiration may indeed not be thoroughly true. The major clinical consequences of aspiration are nosocomial pneumonia, chemical pneumonitis, acute lung injury, hypoxemia, and mechanical obstruction. The volume and pH of the aspirate are critical factors in determining the patient's clinical response to aspiration.

PULMONARY EMBOLISM

The release, travel, and lodging of a venous thrombus into a lobar artery or distal arterial branch in the lung can occur in an immobile, critically ill patient without warning. Occasionally associated with no prior symptoms or signs, pulmonary embolism (PE) represents a serious, often fatal, complication. Frequently, DVT and PE are not diagnosed until autopsy. This finding suggests that prophylactic diagnosis and treatment of thromboembolism remain inadequate (Anderson et al., 1991; Moser, 1990). Significant and fatal emboli originate as thrombi in the iliofemoral veins (Matzdorff & Green, 1992).

The clinical consequences of PE depend on the percentage of the pulmonary vascular bed that is occluded. Acute pulmonary hypertension usually results when greater than 50% of the pulmonary vascular bed is occluded (Roberts, 1987). The result of the embolus is a decrease in the cross-sectional area of the lung vasculature, resulting in increases in pulmonary artery pressures, pulmonary vascular resistance, and right ventricular workload. Shock may result from right ventricular failure secondary to the acute increase in afterload to the right ventricle. The stimulation of intrapulmonary receptors in the alveolar–capillary wall may produce dyspnea. Dyspnea also may result from severe arterial hypoxemia, which has been reported in 85% to 90% of critically ill patients experiencing a PE (Roberts, 1987). Hypoxemia occurring during a massive PE is related to overperfusion of the nonembolized lung, resulting in low $\dot{V}/\dot{Q}$ units that cause pulmonary shunting. Increases in dead space ventilation develop due to areas of high $\dot{V}/\dot{Q}$ units created by poor or absent pulmonary perfusion.

Gastrointestinal Effects

CONSTIPATION

Immobility contributes to the development of constipation due to several factors. Overall skeletal muscle weakness can affect the primary muscles of elimination (the diaphragm, abdominals, and levator ani), which may result in a decrease in expulsive power secondary to the loss of ability to increase intraabdominal pressure. Loss of the defecation reflex may occur if patients fail to defecate when the reflexes are excited. If ignored, these reflexes become weaker over time. The use of a bedpan is often refused or is nonproductive of stool due to its uncomfortableness and forced, unnatural position. Patients may repeatedly postpone using the bedpan because of the embarrassment, lack of privacy, and dependence on others (Memmer & Kozier, 1987). Such postponement suppresses the defecation reflex and results in greater water absorption from the stool in the colon. Hardened and dry stool in the colon may lead to fecal impaction, resulting in partial or complete mechanical obstruction of the colon. Colonic contractures may result in excessive intraluminal pressures, whereby liquid stool may be forced around the impaction and expelled as a ribbon of diarrhea or a fecal-colored smear (Memmer & Kozier, 1987). If the impaction is not effectively treated, mechanical bowel obstruction may result in impaired bowel circulation secondary to intraluminal compression of the mesenteric vessels, abdominal distention, impaired fluid and substrate absorption, and venous thrombi formation secondary to large abdominal vein compression resulting from increased abdominal pressure.

In contrast to constipation associated with immobility is the reported incidence of diarrhea in critically ill patients, which has been reported to be as high as 41% (Kelly et al., 1983). Often due to enteral feedings, the enhanced gut motility may serve to prevent impaction or confound a preexisting impaction or obstruction.

Urinary Effects

The human kidney and urinary bladder are anatomically designed to function optimally in an erect position. Erect positions allow most of the urine to flow out of the renal pelvis because the hilus emerges from the medial aspect of the kidney. A minimal amount of urine is left in the dependent calyces. The urethra is the dependent path for urine flow in an erect position.

URINARY STASIS

Supine positions result in the renal pelvis filling with urine before urine can be expressed into the ureter. The result is urinary stasis. Urinary stasis provides a focus for bacterial growth and renal calculus formation. Accumulation of urine in the dependent portion of the urinary bladder in a supine position potentially results in a medium for bacterial growth, urinary retention, and urinary incontinence. Bladder distention may result, inhibiting the urge to void due to chronic stretching of the bladder and loss of bladder tone. Some involuntary urinary incontinence may also occur with considerable distention. The process of voiding in bed is also inhibited by the difficulty of relaxing the perineal muscles and the external sphincter and by ignoring the sensation to void.

URINARY MINERAL EXCRETION

On assuming a supine position, circulatory blood volume is increased, which normally evokes a diuresis and a natriuresis to maintain a normal plasma concentration. Bedrest also affects urinary calcium excretion owing to the hypercalcemia that results from bone disuse. Hwang and associates (1988) reported increases in mean urinary calcium and phosphorus excretion during the first week of bedrest; these increases were sustained throughout 5 weeks of bedrest in healthy subjects. Due to this increased urinary load, calcium deposits may occur in the renal pelvis or bladder, leading to nephrolithiasis and potentially to postrenal failure. Hematuria, dull flank pain, backache, and severe bouts of colic-like pain with nausea and vomiting are classic signs and symptoms of urinary stones. Four factors favor the precipitation of calcium salts in the kidney or bladder: urinary stasis, hypercalciuria, hyperphosphaturia, and alkaline urine. Increased urine alkalinity occurs with immobility due to fewer acid end-products of metabolism. Increases in urine pH cause calcium salts to precipitate. The incidence of nephrolithiasis has been reported to be as high as 15% to 30% in individuals immobilized for extended periods (Mitchell, 1981).

URINARY TRACT INFECTION

Factors favoring the development of urinary tract infections (UTIs) associated with immobility include urinary stasis, bladder distention, increased urinary alkalinization, nephrolithiasis, the presence of an indwelling urinary catheter, and host susceptibility. Stasis and alkaline urine provide a susceptible medium for bacterial growth. Urinary retention with distention along with nephrolithiasis may cause minute tears in the mucosal lining of the urinary tract, providing routes for infection. Bacteriuria has been reported in 50% of patients requiring indwelling urinary catheters for more than 7 to 10 days (Stamm, 1986).

Urinary tract infections are frequent nosocomial infections in critically ill patients. Nosocomial bacteriuria usually represents urinary tract colonization in hospitalized patients (Yannelli & Gurevich, 1988). The most serious complication that can arise from bacteriuria in immobilized patients is urosepsis.

Metabolic Effects

HYPERCALCEMIA AND HYPERCALCIURIA

Immobility results in increased calcium excretion from bones, due to the removal of weight-bearing forces from the long bones rather than to inactivity. Osteoblastic activity decreases in all weight-bearing bones subjected to bedrest, and osteolytic activity increases, resulting in osteoporosis and hypercalcemia (Maynard, 1986). Normally this leads to hypercalciuria and an eventual return to normal serum calcium levels. Hypercalciuria has been associated with prolonged immobility in all age groups.

The incidence of immobilization hypercalcemia has been reported to range from 10.8% to 23.6% in spinal cord–injured patients (Maynard, 1986). Clinically significant hypercalcemia also occurs in patients with fractures of the lower limbs and pelvis (Van Zuiden et al., 1982) and in patients with Guillain-Barré syndrome (Meythaler et al., 1986). Weissman and colleagues (1983) reported a case of hypercalcemia and hypercalciuria in a 50-year-old critically ill patient subjected to prolonged immobility.

GLUCOSE-INSULIN INTOLERANCE

Physical inactivity alters glucose homeostasis in humans. Glucose intolerance results, which requires increasing levels of serum insulin to maintain normal glucose levels. The mechanisms explaining the unresponsiveness of glucose to hyperinsulinemia remain unclear. One theory focuses on the existence of insulin inhibitors altering cellular membrane function.

Musculoskeletal Effects

BONE LOSS

Weight bearing is a critical factor in the normal functioning of osteoblasts and osteoclasts. Loss of longitudinal pressure on the long bones results in decreased osteoblastic activity. Osteoclasts continue to destroy bone matrix even in lieu of increased osteoblastic activity, which results in bone demineralization and decreased bone density. Short-term immobility results in hypercalciuria, which usually does not present significant problems. During continued bedrest, total body calcium losses have been estimated at 0.5% per month (Rubin, 1988). Demineralization continues with bedrest despite the amount of dietary calcium consumed (Memmer & Kozier, 1987). The porous, soft bones characteristic of disuse osteoporosis may result in bone pain, bone fractures, or nephrolithiasis. The bone loss associated with immobility, coupled with the bone loss associated with aging, can easily place the geriatric, critically ill patient at the fracture threshold (Holm & Hedricks, 1989).

MUSCLE ATROPHY

One of the most obvious effects of prolonged immobility is muscle atrophy. Muscle atrophy is the loss of actual muscle mass and results in a decrease of the cross-sectional area of the whole muscle (St. Pierre & Gardiner, 1987). Muscle atrophy resulting from disuse leads to weakness and fatigue. The rate of muscle atrophy is rapid in the early immobilization phase and continues more slowly with long-term immobility (Summers & Hines, 1951). The rate of muscle atrophy has also been found to be faster if the muscle has been denervated rather than just immobilized (Domonkos & Herr, 1965). The muscles of the thigh and calf usually undergo the greatest reduction in circumference during immobility, with the arm muscles being affected least (Greenleaf, 1982).

JOINT CONTRACTURES

Decrease in skeletal muscle activity along with muscle atrophy associated with immobility may limit the normal range of motion (ROM) of a joint. Because flexor muscles are stronger than extensor muscles, joints often remain in a flexed position in bed. If exercise of the joints does not occur, the flexor muscles become permanently shortened, and the joint becomes stiffened in a flexed position. A contracture may result when fibrofatty tissue proliferates within the immobile joint, forming adhesions and maturing as scar tissue. Impairment of the normal gliding motion between collagen fibrils and abnormalities of the mechanical properties of ligaments also contribute to contracture formation (Frank et al., 1984).

Common contracture sites include the hip, knee, and plantar flexor of the ankle. Critically ill patients who are placed and maintained in varying degrees of the Fowler's position with the knees elevated are at risk for development of hip and knee contractures. The reversibility of joint contractures is heavily dependent on their course of development.

PERIPHERAL NERVE INJURY

The immobile patient who is on bedrest is at risk for ulnar nerve injury secondary to compression resulting from improper positioning techniques. Due to the anatomic relationship of the ulnar nerve to structures around the elbow, supination of the forearm in a supine position frees the nerve from external compression at the cubital tunnel (Fig. 61–3*A*). Pronation of the forearm in a supine position, however, traps the ulnar nerve in the cubital tunnel (Fig. 61–3*B*). Flexion of the elbow adds an additional 11 to 24 mm Hg of pressure on the ulnar nerve (Pechan & Julis, 1975).

Chuman (1985) found that ulnar nerve compression occurred in 23% of a patient population composed of orthopedic, neurologic, neurosurgical, and rehabilitative patients who were on bedrest for a minimum of 12 hours per day for 3 consecutive days. Identified risk factors for ulnar nerve compression in this study included diabetes mellitus, bedrest for more than 22 hours per day, injury or pathology of the wrist or elbow, alcoholism, family history of nerve damage, and an age of 50 years or more.

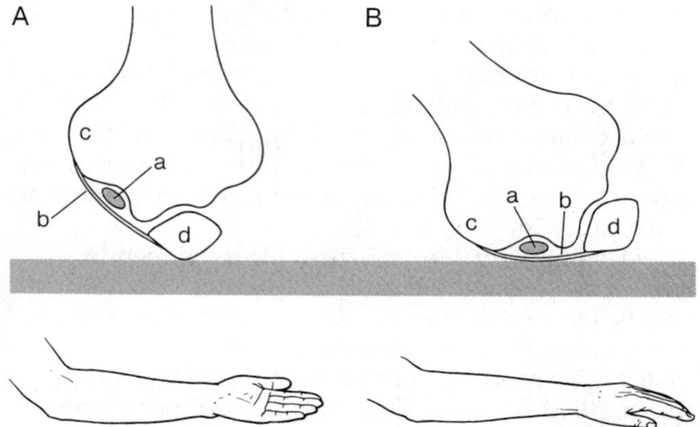

FIGURE 61–3. Relationship of ulnar nerve (*a*), arcuate ligament (*b*), medial epicondyle (*c*), and olecranon process of ulna (*d*). The arcuate ligament normally holds the ulnar nerve within the cubital tunnel. *A*, The supine position with the forearm supinated keeps the cubital tunnel free of external pressure. *B*, The supine position with the forearm pronated creates external pressure at the cubital tunnel that may result in ulnar nerve injury. (Redrawn from Chuman, M. A. [1985]. Risk factors associated with ulnar nerve compression in bedridden patients. *Journal of Neurosurgical Nursing*, *17*, 339.)

Integumentary Effects

PRESSURE ULCERS

Being confined to bed implies that a patient will incur any damage resulting from the pressure of his or her body against the supporting surface and from the friction and shearing effects that occur with confined movement. Integumentary damage resulting from immobility is an iatrogenic complication in the ICU and is often casually accepted as a normal result of prolonged bedrest. Data on the incidence or prevalence of pressure ulcers in the critically ill are scant. One study documented that pressure ulcers developed in 40% of patients while in the ICU (Bergstrom et al., 1987). The term "pressure ulcer" is used to describe integumentary damage on any body surface that is related to immobility and that results from the forces of pressure, friction, shearing, or moisture.

Pressure remains the primary cause of pressure ulcers (Maklebust, 1987). Perpendicular forces exerted by gravity on any skin surface must exceed mean capillary pressures in the skin to produce tissue ischemia and necrosis (Larsen et al., 1979). Normal pressure gradients in the capillary arteriolar limb have been reported as 32 mm Hg, and as 12 mm Hg in the venous capillary limb. Pressures exceeding these levels in the arteriolar capillary limb lead to lymphatic occlusion, increased interstitial fluid pressure, and filtration of fluid from the capillaries, resulting in edema and tissue ischemia (Burn et al., 1987; Glavis & Barbour, 1990). Factors affecting the critical arteriolar closing pressure are skin pressure, systemic hypotension, vascular shunting, and shock.

Development of pressure ulcers depends on a time–pressure relationship (Dinsdale, 1973; Koziak, 1959). The higher the pressure, the less time is needed for necrosis to occur (Brooks and Duncan, 1940). Dinsdale (1974) reported that a constant pressure of 70 mm Hg applied for more than 2 hours produced irreversible tissue damage.

After a skin surface has been compressed, the skin immediately appears blanched due to decreased local blood flow. Reactive hyperemia normally then results as a compensatory measure to enhance blood flow to the compromised area and to decrease the risk of microvascular thrombosis. If the skin remains reddened after the pressure source has been removed, tissue damage can be inferred. The severity of pressure ulcers has been described according to four standard stages (Table 61–4).

Pressure is not equally distributed across the skin surface in any position in bed. Pressure is often concentrated over the bony prominences, where a cone-shaped pressure gradient develops (Fig. 61–4). Generation of this type of gradient results in compression of the soft tissues that lie between the skin and the bony prominence. Although redness may be visible on the skin surface, the damage caused to the underlying tissues from this process may not be clinically evident. Brunner and Suddarth (1986) reported that 75% of all pressure ulcers were located at weight-bearing bony prominences. Most pressure ulcers occur in the lower half of the human body. Common sites prone to pressure ulceration include the sacrum, coccygeal areas, ischial tuberosities, greater trochanters, lateral malleoli, medial and lateral condyles of the tibia, and the heels. Figure 61–5 delineates common pressure sites in a variety of bedrest positions.

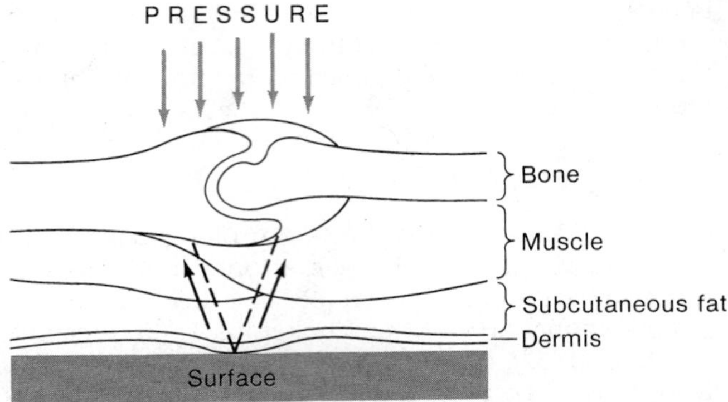

FIGURE 61–4. The creation of a cone-shaped pressure gradient between the skin's surface and the underlying bony prominence. The full extent of soft tissue damage may not appear at the skin surface because the base of the cone resides on the bone surface. (Reproduced, with permission, from Reuler, J. B., & Cooney, T. G. [1981]. The pressure sore: Pathophysiology and principles of management. *Annals of Internal Medicine, 94*, 662.)

TABLE 61–4. **Classification of Severity of Pressure Ulcers**

Stage I	Nonblanchable erythema of intact skin; the heralding lesion of skin ulceration
Stage II	Partial-thickness skin loss involving epidermis and/or dermis; the ulcer is superficial and presents clinically as an abrasion, blister, or shallow crater
Stage III	Full-thickness skin loss involving damage or necrosis of subcutaneous tissue that may extend down to but not through underlying fascia; the ulcer presents clinically as a deep crater with or without undermining adjacent tissue
Stage IV	Full-thickness skin loss with extensive destruction, tissue necrosis or damage to muscle, bone, or supporting structures (e.g., tendon, joint capsules)

Data from the National Pressure Ulcers Advisory Panel. (1989). *Pressure ulcers: Consensus development statement.* West Dundee, IL: S-N Publications.

Friction is the force created when two surfaces in contact with each other move in opposite directions. Skin friction results in the removal of the protective stratum corneum, leading to potential skin breakdown. Pulling rather than lifting patients up in bed remains the classic source of friction frequently experienced by critically ill patients. Continuous, spontaneous skeletal muscle motion due to seizures, agitation, or combativeness may also contribute to friction from bed surfaces or restraining devices in critically ill adults.

Shearing forces are created when the skin is pulled along a surface in the opposing direction of the underlying tissue. Stretching and angulation of blood vessels may occur, resulting in dermal damage. Shearing occurs commonly when a bedridden patient slumps toward the foot of the bed after being placed in a Fowler's position. As the body slides down, pressure is created on the sacral tissues. At the same time, friction is created between the posterior sacral skin and tissues and the bed surface. Shearing forces occur in the sacral area when the head of the bed is raised more than 30 degrees (Maklebust, 1987).

Moisture contributes to skin maceration because it softens the epidermal tissue and decreases its tensile strength. In the critically ill adult on bedrest, moisture accumulation may result from perspiration, fecal or urinary incontinence, or wound drainage. Incontinence is a major predictor of the development of pressure ulcers. Allman and coworkers (1986) also found that fecal soiling was a major risk factor for the development of pressure ulcers in hospitalized patients.

Table 61–5 identifies major risk factors that have been implicated in pressure ulcer development (Allman et al., 1986; Batson et al., 1993; Braden & Bergstrom, 1987; Brunner & Suddarth, 1986; Gosnell, 1987; Macklebust, 1987; Stotts, 1987). Although many of

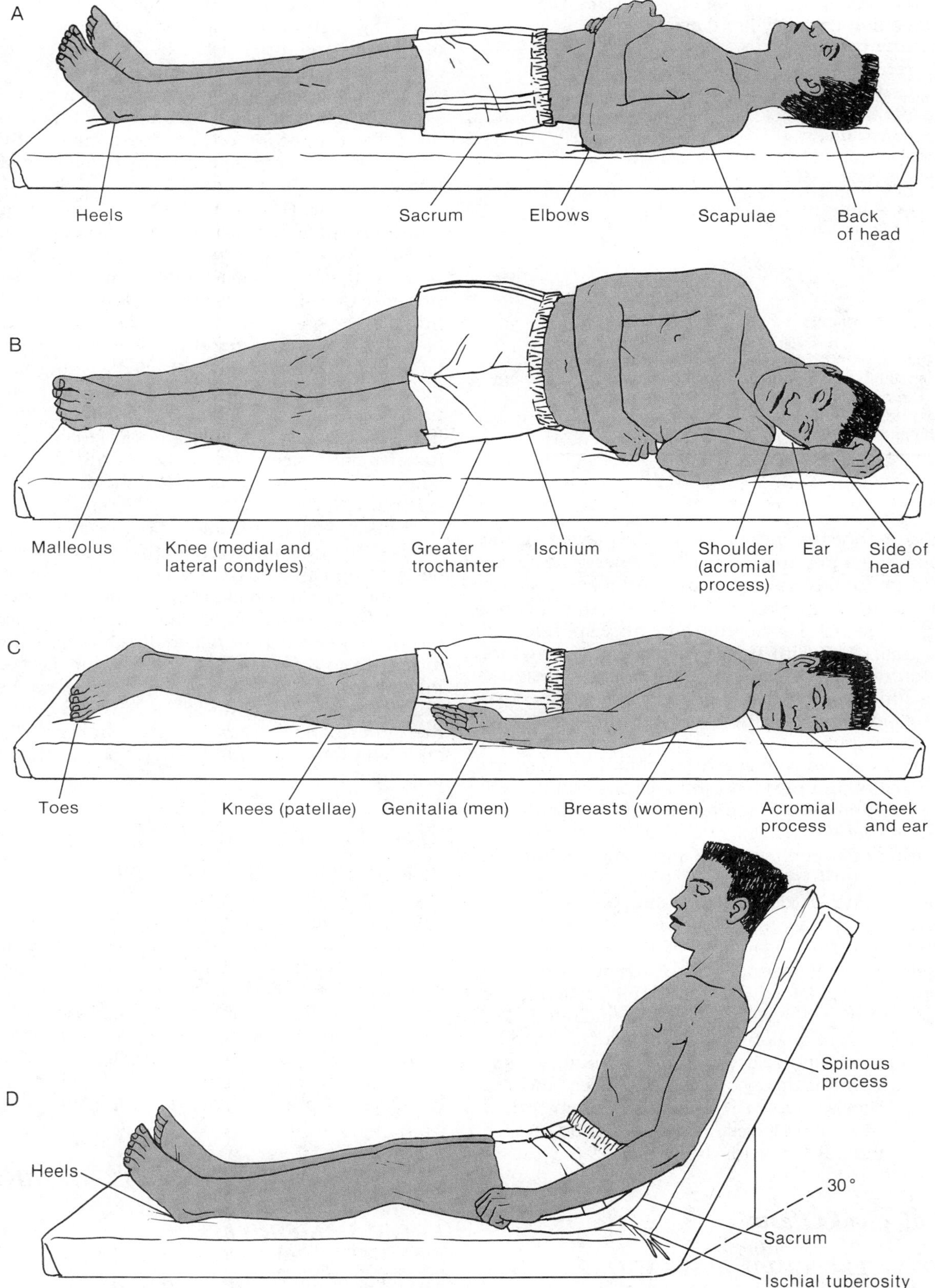

FIGURE 61–5. Body areas susceptible to pressure, friction, and shearing forces. *A,* Supine position. *B,* Lateral position. *C,* Prone position. *D,* Fowler's position. (Redrawn from *Fundamentals of Nursing,* Fourth Edition, by B. Kozier, G. Erb, and R. Olivieri. Copyright © 1991 by Addison-Wesley Publishing Company. Reprinted by permission.)

TABLE 61–5. **Major Risk Factors for Pressure Ulcer Development in Critically Ill Adults**

Immobilization
Altered mental status
Incontinence
Length of hospitalization
Altered motor or sensory function
Advancing age (>40 years)
Altered cardiac output
Orthopedic fractures
Altered nutritional status
Cachexia or obesity
Hypoalbuminemia
Dehydration or edema
Anemia
Exogenous corticosteroids
Diabetes
Administration of intravenous epinephrine or norepinephrine
Technology inhibiting movement (e.g., intraaortic balloon pumping, hemofiltration)
Physiologic instability
Body temperature alterations

these factors operate independently in predicting the development of pressure ulcers, the synergistic action of two or more factors cannot be overlooked because so many of them are present in critically ill patients.

Recent research has begun to identify specific risk factors associated with the development of pressure ulcers in critically ill patients. Batson and colleagues (1993) examined 50 critically ill adults for prospective development of pressure sores. Five factors that were found to be significant were diabetes, "too unstable to turn," restricted movement (e.g., hemofiltration, intraaortic balloon pump), and intravenous administration of epinephrine or norepinephrine. The significant association between intravenous administration of epinephrine or norepinephrine and the development of pressure ulcers was postulated to be due to vasoconstriction leading to decreased tissue perfusion and viability.

Other researchers (Marchette et al., 1991) examined 161 elderly surgical patients in ICUs for pressure ulcer development. Six factors were found that related to the development of pressure ulcers. These included skin condition, surgery, incontinence, state of consciousness, steroid use, and selected serum laboratory tests.

Clinical complications of pressure ulcers include infections, sepsis, and osteomyelitis. Polymicrobial wound infections tend to result that frequently involve obligate anaerobes, particularly *Bacteroides fragilis.*

Psychological Effects

SENSORY–PERCEPTUAL ALTERATIONS

Conscious, critically ill patients who are immobile may experience a state of waiting. Waiting is the perceived process of the passage of time. Waiting may lead to hypervigilance and the overestimation of time. Because of the perceived "dragging of time," the nonoptimal stimulation of the ICU environment, and the lack of patient-structured activities, the patient may become unable to maintain temporal integrity.

The ICU environment is often the stimulus for sensory and perceptual changes in the immobilized patient. The connection of patients to quantitative invasive lines and equipment can create feelings of forced immobility or the sense of being "tied down" in conscious patients (Halm & Alpen, 1993). The underload and overload of auditory, visual, olfactory, kinesthetic, and tactile sensory experiences can lead to aberrant processing of perceived thoughts and sensations. The presence of restraints and side rails along with the ceiling and dependent view that accompanies a recumbent position may restrict the field of vision. Social isolation may occur due to restricted visiting hours and decreased interpersonal contact. Other factors contributing to the development of ICU psychosis resulting from sensory alterations include communication impairments, sleep deprivation, and pharmacologic agents (Geary, 1994; Inaba-Roland & Maricle, 1992; Wilson, 1993).

Sensory–perceptual alterations become manifest as states of confusion, disorientation, restlessness, incoherency, and anxiety or fear along with hallucinations, delusions, and illusions. This symptomatology has frequently been described in the literature by use of the term ICU psychosis or ICU delirium. Estimates of the incidence of ICU psychosis range from 12.5% to 50% in conscious patients admitted to critical care settings (Easton & MacKenzie, 1988). (Chapter 8 contains further information regarding the etiology, diagnosis, and symptoms of sensory alterations in the critically ill patient.)

ALTERED BODY IMAGE

Mobility allows individuals to exercise and maintain control over their environment. Body image is formed from the level of independence that one chooses to maintain. Immobility affects body image because bed confinement gravely alters independence (Baird, 1985; Christian, 1982). Body image disturbances may result in intense feelings of inferiority, anxiety, withdrawal, self-destructive behavior, anger, despair, or noncompliance with medical and nursing regimens. Body image disturbances associated with immobility may also be related to pressure sore development.

CLINICAL MANAGEMENT OF MAJOR COMPLICATIONS RESULTING FROM IMMOBILITY

The focus of care for the immobilized patient is on prevention. Prevention of complications results in significant cost savings to the patient and family, the multidisciplinary team, and the health care system. An astute awareness of, and vigilance for, early symptomatology may also expedite the application of preventive and therapeutic measures.

Deep Vein Thrombosis

Deep vein thrombosis and pulmonary embolism are two major consequences of immobility that have been highlighted as the two easiest consequences to prevent. It should be stressed that physical activity and ambulation should occur at the earliest time possible for critically ill patients to prevent these devastating complications. Acknowledging that 90% of thrombi in the iliofemoral venous system will embolize (Matzdorff & Green, 1992), appropriate management goals should first focus on identifying which patients are at high risk for DVT (see Table 61–3) and then start prophylactic therapy for those patients. Table 61–6 lists the various alternatives for DVT prophylaxis that can be used independently or in combination with each other.

The objective of conventional heparin therapy in DVT prophylaxis is to arrest the thrombotic process by enhancing the inhibitory action of antithrombin III on factor X. Low-dose heparin therapy has been found to be efficacious in preventing DVT in a variety of medical diseases. Cade (1982) reported a reduction in DVT incidence from 30% to 12% with the administration of low-dose heparin therapy in a medical ICU. Low-dose heparin is recommended as prophylaxis for all medical–surgical ICU patients except those at risk for hemorrhage. Such patients include those with bleeding disorders, head injury, general trauma, and severe hypertension. Low-dose heparin prophylaxis has not been found to increase upper gastrointestinal bleeding episodes, but does slightly increase the risk of wound hematoma in surgical patients (Coon et al., 1987). Standard adult doses are 5,000 units administered subcutaneously every 8 to 12 hours. Such doses do not require monitoring of clotting times. Anticoagulants may also be used in an adjusted-dose regimen in high-risk patients in whom fixed low doses are ineffective. Adjusted-dose heparin or warfarin requires frequent monitoring of coagulation times to ensure its efficacy and safety.

Low–molecular-weight heparins (LMWH) for prophylaxis against DVT have recently been introduced.

TABLE 61–6. **Measures for Deep Venous Thrombosis Prophylaxis**

Anticoagulants
Fixed low-dose heparin
Adjusted-dose heparin
Warfarin
Low–molecular-weight heparins
Early mobilization
Intermittent pneumatic compression
Graduated compression elastic stockings
Active or passive leg exercises
Intravenous Dextran

LMWH possess excellent bioavailability after subcutaneous injection and a longer half-life than unfractionated heparin (Hull & Pineo, 1993). LMWH produce their major anticoagulant effect by binding to antithrombin III. The pharmacokinetic properties of LMWH allow for administration of this treatment in fixed doses subcutaneously without laboratory monitoring (Hull & Pineo, 1993). A recent meta-analysis of multiple randomized clinical trials evaluating LMWH for DVT prophylaxis suggested that LMWH was more effective than low-dose heparin and was not associated with increased risk of bleeding (Nurmohamed et al., 1992). Many other studies have documented the efficacy of LMWH (e.g., enoxaprin, lomoparin) in DVT prophylaxis in a variety of populations (Farkas et al., 1993; Leclerc et al., 1991; Turpie et al., 1986).

Compressive forces applied to the lower limbs have been shown to decrease the incidence of DVT by increasing venous blood flow (Hull et al., 1990; Pidala et al., 1992). Graduated compression elastic stockings and intermittent pneumatic compression (IPC) boots represent methods of compression. IPC involves the wearing of plastic leg sleeves that intermittently fill with air and decompress in a sequential manner that enhances blood flow in the calf and thigh. An advantage of IPC is that it is associated with rare complications and can become the best choice of prophylaxis in patients at hemorrhagic risk. IPC remains contraindicated in patients with peripheral vascular disease (Hirsh & Hull, 1987). If patients have been on bedrest or immobilized for longer than 72 hours without any form of prophylaxis, IPC is not recommended because of the chance of dislodging newly formed clots (Merli, 1993). A recent study also revealed that simultaneous use of IPC with graduated compression stockings had a synergistic effect on lowering the incidence of DVT in patients undergoing major general surgery (Scurr et al., 1987). IPC is efficacious only when the compression boots are applied correctly to the critically ill patient. Recent research has revealed that improper use of IPC frequently leads to failure of DVT prophylaxis (Comerota et al., 1992). This study revealed that proper application of IPC is accomplished more frequently in ICUs than in other hospital units.

Dextran may be used to prevent DVT because it decreases blood viscosity and platelet adhesiveness and enhances fibrinolysis (Coon et al., 1987). Disadvantages of this intravenous therapy include the cost of the product, associated fluid volume overloads, and increased tendency to bleed.

Development of DVT may remain clinically silent if the thrombus fails to occlude the inner lumen of the vein or if adequate collateral circulation is present. Signs and symptoms often develop when the thrombus occludes the entire lumen and impedes venous flow or creates an inflammatory process of the vessel wall or perivascular tissue. Swelling of the affected limb occurs, often with an associated increase in circumference distal to the occlusion and increased temperature. Pain and tenderness in the calf or thigh may be present, with fever and malaise. Evidence of Homans' sign should be cautiously weighed because its presence has not been reliable in defining states of DVT.

Clinical signs and symptoms alone have not proved sufficiently reliable to diagnose DVT. Diagnostic tests for DVT include venography, Doppler ultrasonography, impedance plethysmography (IPG), and ^{125}I-labeled fibrinogen scanning. A diagnostic accuracy rate of approximately 95% has been reported when IPG and Doppler ultrasonography are used in conjunction (Fahey, 1984).

The treatment of DVT revolves around the use of anticoagulants to prevent enlargement of existing thrombi and their migration. Contraindications to this therapy include hemorrhagic risk in patients who are critically ill with diseases such as acute liver failure, disseminated intravascular coagulopathy, or bleeding dyscrasias. Other treatment modalities include leg elevation, thrombectomy (if the thrombus is in a large vessel), and the use of compressive forces. Prophylactic treatment to minimize the risk of PE from DVT through inferior cava clipping or screening may be considered if the thrombus is large, is not resolving with standard therapy, or if anticoagulants are contraindicated. Despite placement of an inferior caval filter, recurrent PE may occur approximately 3% to 5% of the time due to emboli traveling through collateral venous channels (Matzdorff & Green, 1992).

TABLE 61–7. **Clinical Signs and Symptoms of Pulmonary Embolism**

Subjective
Dyspnea
Pleuritic chest pain
Anxiety
Syncope
Objective
General
Tachypnea
Tachycardia
Confusion
Cough
Hemoptysis
Diaphoresis
Cardiopulmonary
Hypoxemia
Systemic hypotension
Jugular venous distention
Split second heart sound
Dysrhythmias (atrial flutter or fibrillation)
Right axis deviation
Enlarged or peaked P waves on electrocardiogram
Peaked or inverted T waves in chest leads
Incomplete or complete right bundle branch block
Increased pulmonary artery pressures
Increased pulmonary vascular resistance
Increased central venous pressure
Normal or decreased cardiac output
Presence of thrombophlebitis

Pulmonary Embolism

The migration of a venous thrombus to the lung may result in absent or dramatic clinical signs and symptoms, depending on the percentage of pulmonary vasculature that is obstructed. Table 61–7 lists the common subjective signs and symptoms of PE. It is important to note that subjective symptoms are frequently masked in critically ill adults due to depression of the level of consciousness. Tachypnea and tachycardia are frequent objective findings, with incidences of 90% to 100% and 60% to 75%, respectively (Roberts, 1987). Development of the symptomatology of right ventricular heart failure secondary to an acute and substantial increase in pulmonary vascular resistance may signal the presence of a massive PE and greatly narrows the time span available for treatment initiation.

Because the clinical signs and symptoms of PE are often confused with those of other states, laboratory methods are often used to confirm or rule out the diagnosis. Pulmonary angiography is the most definitive test for this diagnosis, but it is often difficult to perform if the patient is unstable from the event. Ventilation and perfusion lung scans, chest radiography, IPG, contrast venography, and the radioactive fibrinogen test can aid in the medical diagnosis.

The goals of medical therapy for PE are to lyse existing large thromboemboli and to prevent new ones from forming. Thrombolytic therapy is indicated for massive PEs that evoke severe systemic hypotension or obstruct greater than 50% of the pulmonary vascular bed. Intravenous urokinase, streptokinase, and recombinant tissue plasminogen activator cause rapid lysis and prolong thrombin times. Frequent, intermittent laboratory measurements of coagulation are indicated to detect uncontrolled fibrinolysis. Contraindications to fibrinolytic therapy include defective hemostasis, tumor, infarction, trauma, severe hypertension, recent stroke, pregnancy, surgery, or an intraarterial diagnostic procedure performed within the past 10 days. In general, research has documented that thrombolytic therapy for PE improves short-term perfusion lung scanning, short-term angiographic clot dissolution, and hemodynamics in most but not all clinical trials (Goldhaber et al., 1986, 1993; UKEP Study Research Group, 1987). Pulmonary embolectomy may be performed on critically ill patients if the embolism is massive and is not responsive to standard therapy.

Nursing interventions for the patient sustaining a PE revolve around providing adequate oxygen transport, surveillance for and adequate pharmacologic support for right ventricular heart failure and systemic hypotension, management of anxiety, and monitoring for uncontrolled fibrinolysis associated with intravenous fibrinolytic therapy. Expected outcomes of interventions for altered pulmonary tissue perfusion include a Pa_{O_2} greater than 65 mm Hg, an arterial oxygen saturation greater than 94%, absence of signs of DVT, normalized right ventricular function, and normotension.

Infection

Hypostatic pneumonia and UTI are the two leading infections in the immobile critically ill patient. Pneumonia is represented by fever, chills, chest radiologic changes, positive sputum cultures, and a change in the color and consistency of tracheal secretions. Signs and symptoms of a UTI are fever, chills, urinary frequency, dysuria, increased urine turbidity, malaise, hematuria, and a positive urine culture (>100,000 colonies of bacteria per mL of urine).

Institution of aggressive pulmonary toilet is essential in preventing and treating pneumonias. Coughing, deep breathing, incentive spirometry, appropriate antimicrobial therapy, turning regimens, and tracheobronchial suctioning are critical, as are good handwashing techniques of caregivers.

Urinary tract infections can be prevented by minimizing the urinary stasis that occurs with supine positions. Indwelling urinary catheters are often placed in critically ill adults. Such insertion requires good handwashing, sterile insertion, and provision of a closed urinary drainage system with adequate gravity flow. Because urine often becomes colonized after placement of indwelling catheters, emphasis should be placed on discontinuing the catheter as soon as possible. Dietary methods of acidifying the urine should be implemented if feasible to decrease the risk of UTI.

Medical management of infections resulting from immobility revolves around timely diagnosis, obtaining culture data, and institution and optimalization of antimicrobial therapy. Pneumonia, UTI, and infection of pressure ulcers are prevalent disorders that can lead to associated bacteremias and septicemias.

Immobilization Hypercalcemia

The diagnosis of immobilization hypercalcemia is made only after other causes for it are ruled out. High serum calcium levels may be associated with hypercalciuria (>200 mg of urinary calcium per 24 hours) and depressed neuromuscular excitability, resulting in nausea, vomiting, constipation, anorexia, or fecal impaction (Maynard, 1986). Other signs may be orthostatic hypotension, cardiac irregularities, and seizures. Treatment modalities include vigorous hydration with intravenous saline, furosemide to decrease sodium loads, oral phosphate administration, mithramycin, and calcitonin.

Musculoskeletal Complications

Impaired physical mobility in critically ill adults is associated with several etiologic factors. Of primary prevalence is immobility induced by bedrest for safety or therapeutic gain. Preexisting joint contractures, muscle atrophy, and bone loss may also lead to further constraints on mobility.

The defining characteristics of joint contractures include stiffness or discomfort on joint movement, limited ROM, and joint swelling or redness. Muscle atrophy results in a decreased circumference of the involved muscle group, decreased strength and tolerance for exercise, impaired coordination of the involved muscle group, and a reluctance to move. Bone loss may be inferred from hypercalcemia and hypercalciuria and may be represented by bone pain when resumption of weight-bearing activities occur.

Nursing strategies to prevent or to treat these effects revolve around early ambulation, proper body positioning, exercises, and weight-bearing activities. Correct body alignment ensures that body joints are placed in their most functional position. The supine position, which is often unavoidable for extended periods of time in critically ill adults, predisposes patients to external hip rotation and footdrop. The use of trochanter rolls strategically positioned at the crest of the ilium to the midthigh assists in proper hip positioning. A trapeze bar may be added to assist certain patients in self-movement. Selection of positioning schedules needs to be individualized to meet restrictions on turning unstable patients.

Isotonic and isometric exercises assist in preventing or minimizing joint contractures or neuromuscular degeneration and aid in promoting venous return. Because isotonic exercises result in constant tension and a shortening of the muscle, they will maintain or increase muscle strength and mass and joint mobility. Isotonic exercises while on bedrest can be accomplished through active ROM exercises, in which the patient moves each joint through its complete ROM. Passive ROM exercises will maintain joint mobility but are of no value in maintaining muscle strength. Regardless of which type of ROM is performed, these exercises should be performed to the point of slight resistance but never to the extent of producing discomfort. ROM exercises should be performed for the neck, shoulder, elbows, wrist, fingers, ankles, and feet in a systematic sequence a minimum of four times a day.

Isometric exercises generate tension by muscle groups' opposing one another while the muscle length remains constant. Muscle groups are alternatively contracted and relaxed. These exercises can be performed on casted extremities because no joint movement is required. Major muscle groups involved in walking such as the quadriceps, lower abdominals, femoris, and gluteals can be maintained with such exercises if they are done regularly. Caution must be used when considering an isometric exercise schedule for critically ill adults because adverse cardiovascular changes can occur. Blood pressure changes are especially prevalent in people with hypertension. Assessment of blood pressure is thus predicated before, during, and after isometric exercise. The associated hypertension is thought to be so significant that the chances of myocardial compromise or cardiovascular accident are increased.

Weight-bearing activities are critical in preventing

extensive calcium loss from bone in long-term ICU patients. Standing and ambulating remain the only forms of weight bearing for ICU patients. Contemporary ICU beds lack the design feature of a reverse Trendelenburg position that would allow an adult to weight-bear against a sturdy foot surface. Emphasis thus should be placed on early and frequent mobilization. Expected outcomes of impaired physical mobility include the maintenance of muscle mass and strength, joint mobility, and absence of bone pain on rising.

Pressure Ulcers

A combination of pressure, shearing, friction, and moisture may be factors causing changes in skin integrity in the immobile adult. The presence of hyperemia on the skin surface over a pressure point that lasts longer than 30 seconds may be the first sign of altered circulation. Tenderness, edema, vesiculation, local warmth, decreased skin turgor, and a failure of the skin to blanche with finger pressure are parameters indicating a stage I pressure ulcer. A break in the skin surface may overlie a large undermining defect in the soft tissue due to cone-shaped pressure gradients. Closed and open skin sores should be observed for their location, size (length, width, and depth), shape, color, odor, and associated drainage. The integument should be fully inspected at least every 4 to 8 hours in critically ill patients. All deviations should be documented according to the standard classification listed in Table 61–4.

A key approach to preventing pressure ulcers lies in the prediction of their occurrence in high-risk patients admitted to the ICU. This approach implies that identification of patients at risk would lead to initiation of preventive strategies. A systematic risk assessment procedure should be formally established within institutions.

Although nursing research focusing on prediction in critically ill adults is in its infancy (Batson et al., 1993), significant risk factor assessment tools have been developed and studied in medical, surgical, and geriatric populations. Although many of these tools need further refinement and testing for predictive validity, their defined risk factors have been identified consistently and have proved useful in critically ill adult populations.

A classic instrument used to predict pressure ulcer risk is the Norton scale (Norton et al., 1962), which was developed using geriatric hospital patients. It is composed of five risk factors: general physical condition, mental state, activity, mobility, and incontinence. These factors are rated independently and then summed for a total score. Total scores of 14 or greater indicate high-risk candidates. Norton and colleagues (1962) reported a high linear relationship between scores and the actual incidence of pressure ulcers. Stotts (1988) found that pressure ulcers were not predicted at the time of hospital admission using a modified form of the Norton scale in elective cardiovascular and neurosurgical patients.

Another tool commonly used in prediction of pressure ulcer risk is the Braden scale (Bergstrom et al., 1987). This scale has been tested in hospital and ICU populations and has demonstrated greater sensitivity and specificity than other scales. It consists of six subscales that reflect elements of sensory perception, skin moisture, activity, mobility, friction and shear, and nutritional status. Total scores of 16 or less suggest that treatment is warranted. Using a cutoff point of 16, sensitivity was 100% and specificity was 90% when the scale was rated by registered nurses. Research has revealed close agreement between the Braden and Norton scales in predicting pressure ulcer development in patients who received preventive nursing interventions (Xakellis et al., 1992). Regardless of which tool may be used, the process of systematically evaluating patients against set high-risk parameters is invaluable in the identification process and in prescribing preventive and therapeutic modalities, which are often costly.

The goal of preventive and therapeutic strategies for pressure ulcers is to alleviate or minimize their external causes and to maintain optimal skin integrity. Table 61–8 lists interventions in relation to their effects on the external factors of pressure, friction, shearing, and moisture.

Turning regimens should be developed based on individual curtailments in repositioning critically ill adults. Limitations on turning are often related to traction, unilateral lung disease, inaccuracies associated with invasive and noninvasive monitoring, and cardiopulmonary instability. Although major turns may be contraindicated, modified turns or small shifts in body position can change pressure points. The frequency of repositioning should be determined based on skin assessment and on the comfort level of the individual patient. The classic standard of turning patients every 1 to 2 hours may not be adequate in patients at high risk.

Pillow bridging along with heel and elbow protectors can be used to relieve pressure over bony prominences without requiring major changes in position. Adjunctive static devices such as flotation gel pads and foam mattresses may be used to distribute pressure over large areas.

Foam mattress overlays are widely used. A popular type is the low-density eggcrate. Varying densities provide varying degrees of pressure reduction in high-pressure locations. Higher-density foam mattresses (3–4 inches thick) are preferable but are generally more expensive (Glavis & Barbour, 1990). It has been recommended that because virtually every critically ill patient is at risk for pressure ulcers, a mattress overlay be used on all ICU beds (Glavis & Barbour, 1990). Limitations of foam mattress overlays include increased perspiration from patients, the ease with which the mattress becomes soiled, and the inability to wash the mattress.

A new generation of air mattress known as inter-

TABLE 61–8. **Prevention and Treatment Strategies for Pressure Ulcers According to Their Effect on External Factors**

Pressure

Static
- Flotation gel pads
- Foam, convoluted mattresses
- Pillows or foam wedges
- Elbow or heel protectors
- Wrinkle-free foundation
- Appropriate restraint application

Dynamic
- Manual positioning regimens
- Air-fluidized bed
- Low airloss bed
- Oscillating bed
- Alternating pressure mattress

Friction

- Turning sheets
- Sheepskin
- Appropriate restraint application
- Transfer aids
- Trapeze
- Sedation for continuous motion
- Air-fluidized bed
- Low airloss bed
- Oscillating bed

Shearing

- Lifting or turning sheets
- Footboards
- Sheepskins
- Transfer aids
- Heel or elbow protector pads
- Trapeze
- Sedation for continuous motion
- Appropriate restraint application
- Air-fluidized bed
- Low airloss bed
- Oscillating bed

Moisture

- Sheepskin
- Skin hygiene
- Linen changes
- Air-fluidized bed
- Low airloss bed
- Containment of urine or feces (condom catheter, indwelling urinary or rectal catheter, fecal incontinence bag)

mittent air-pressure mattresses has shown strong promise for preventing pressure ulcers. These mattresses consist of two layers of parallel cylinders that fill and empty every several minutes. Parts of the body in contact with the mattress are actually at 0 mm Hg pressure for about 3 of every 7 minutes (Pegasus Airwave System; Pegasus Airwave, Inc., Deerfield Beach, FL) (Fig. 61–6). The alternation of applying and then removing pressure to skin (0 mm Hg) has been shown to prevent pressure ulcers (Braun et al., 1992). In a survey of 788 patients placed on the Pegasus Airwave System in the United Kingdom, new pressure ulcers developed in only 5% (St. Clair, 1992). Patients with preexisting pressure ulcers showed visible signs of improvement when placed on this air mattress for longer than 5 days.

The use of a new generation of dynamic beds has assisted in the prevention and treatment of pressure ulcers in critically ill adults. Air-fluidized, oscillating, and low airloss beds have been successfully used with a variety of high-risk patients. Air-fluidized beds operate on the principle of minimizing pressure, friction, moisture, and shearing forces. Thousands of silicone-coated glass beads are suspended in the bed by the pressurized flow of warm air through the beads (Fig. 61–7). Such fluidization improves capillary blood flow to the skin by minimizing external pressures over bony prominences and keeping them lower than capillary filling pressures. The use of a polyfilament polyester filter sheet separates the patient from the beads and minimizes friction and shearing forces because the sheet is loose and moves freely. Drainage or exudates that penetrate the filter sheet clump with the glass beads, encrust, and then fall to the bottom of the bed into a filter. Healing of pressure ulcers in hospitalized patients using air-fluidized therapy was shown to be greater than that observed in patients placed on conventional beds (Allman et al., 1987). In this study greater improvement was seen in patients who had larger pressure ulcers.

Features of air-fluidized beds include the quick conversion of the fluidized beads to a solid medium, which assists in attaining a hard surface for cardiopulmonary resuscitation (CPR). The bed design does not allow the head of the bed to be raised or lowered electrically. Foam supports are used to attain degrees of Fowler's position. Bed controls allow for adjustments in temperature of air flow. Concerns about aerosolization of microorganisms due to air flow through the filter sheet have recently been shown to be an insignificant problem if the beds are maintained as intended (Bolyard et al., 1987; Vesley et al., 1986).

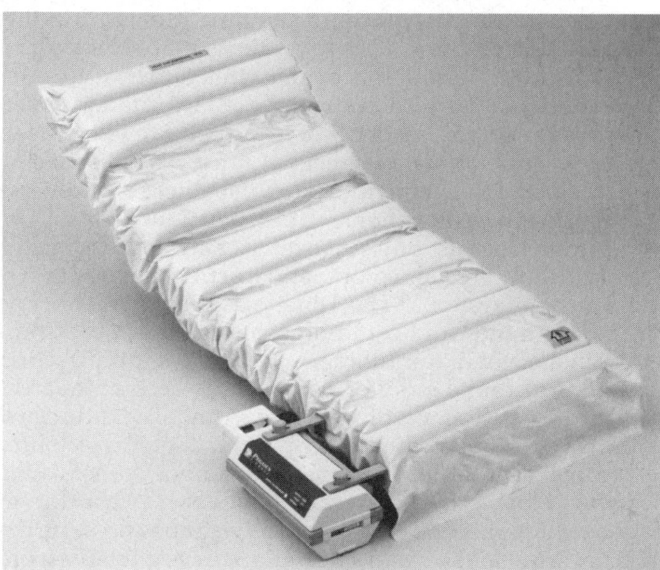

FIGURE 61–6. Pegasus Airwave System. (Reproduced with permission from Pegasus Airwave.)

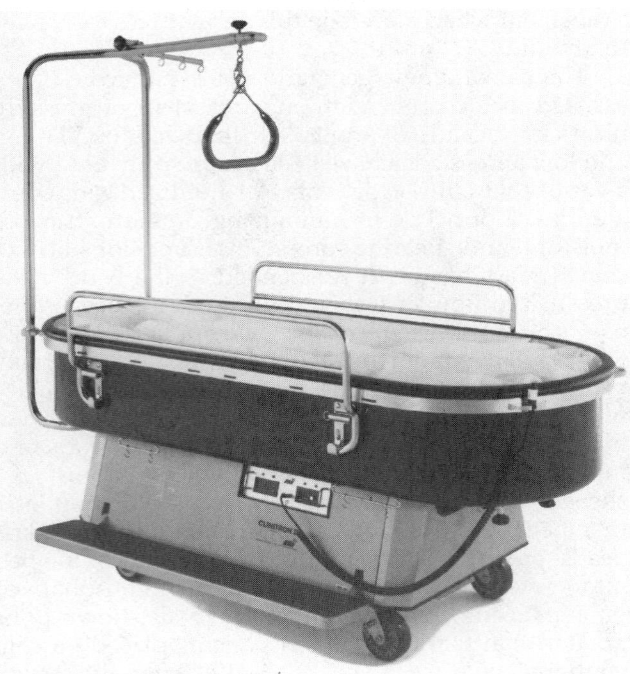

FIGURE 61–7. CLINITRON Air Fluidized Therapy Unit. (Courtesy of Support Systems International, Inc. Reprinted by permission.)

Oscillating beds provide perpetual motion for the critically ill adult unless the motion is suppressed. Pressure forces are thus reduced. Shearing and friction are also decreased due to the qualities of the contact surface and the supported alignment of the patient. The best-studied oscillating bed is the Kinetic Treatment Table (Fig. 61–8). The Kinetic Treatment Table (Kinetic Concepts, San Antonio, TX) is designed to position patients through an arc of 124 degrees every 3.5 minutes. Such rotation is roughly equivalent to approximately 200 to 300 turns every 24 hours if the bed is allowed to rotate most of the time. Comparing this figure to the typical 12 manual turns that are standard in a 24-hour period, it is evident that superior turning can be achieved with this bed. The slow rotation speed (0.5 degree per second) of the bed prevents sleep and vestibular disturbances. Other features of the bed allow achievement of Trendelenburg and reverse Trendelenburg positions, rapid positioning for CPR, accurate weights, full joint exercises, access to thoracic, cervical, and rectal regions, and traction, including cervical halo systems. The Kinetic Treatment Table has a silent motor and a radiolucent table surface. Chest drainage, ventilator tubing, and invasive intravascular and intracranial monitoring are easily accommodated.

Patients with cardiovascular instability and spinal cord injury with continued pain at the site of injury are not candidates for kinetic therapy. Patients who show signs and symptoms of claustrophobia due to the confinement of the bed's safety straps and securing pads are also not candidates. Diarrhea is a relative contraindication for kinetic therapy because the bed enhances gut motility. Other reported complications associated with continuous lateral rotational therapy include inadvertent discontinuance or disconnection of intravascular catheters (Summer et al., 1989), adverse effects on intracranial pressure in patients with intracranial hypertension (Gentilello et al., 1988), and induction of arrhythmias (Sahn, 1991).

Low airloss beds use electricity to alternate currents of air to regulate and redistribute pressures against the body surface. Such regulation allows less than 25 mm Hg of pressure to be applied on any given body surface. The pressure in the compartmental air sacs is individualized to the patient's distributed weight (Fig. 61–9). Features of many low airloss beds include rapid deflation of the air sacs for CPR institution, underbed scales, transport battery, hand controls for positioning, foot support cushions, and breathable underpads for fecal or urinary incontinence. Most low airloss beds use a low-shear, breathable, waterproof sheet over the air sacs. Such features provide a low friction and shearing interface that allows moisture control. Fine pores in the air sacs and cover sheet prevent aerosolization of bacteria that may accumulate.

A recent, randomized, controlled clinical trial documented the efficacy of low airloss beds in preventing pressure ulcers in critically ill patients. Researchers (Inman et al., 1993) found that critically ill patients who were treated on a low airloss suspension bed were about 18% as likely to have a pressure ulcer as patients on a standard bed. Control patients had 39 pressure ulcers, compared to 8 ulcers that developed in the patients using the low airloss bed.

A recent technologic advance is the development of

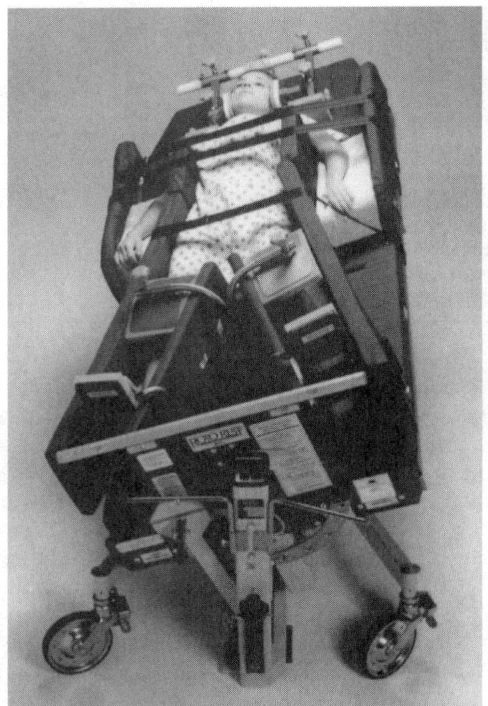

FIGURE 61–8. Kinetic Treatment Table. (Courtesy of Kinetic Concepts, Inc. Reprinted by permission.)

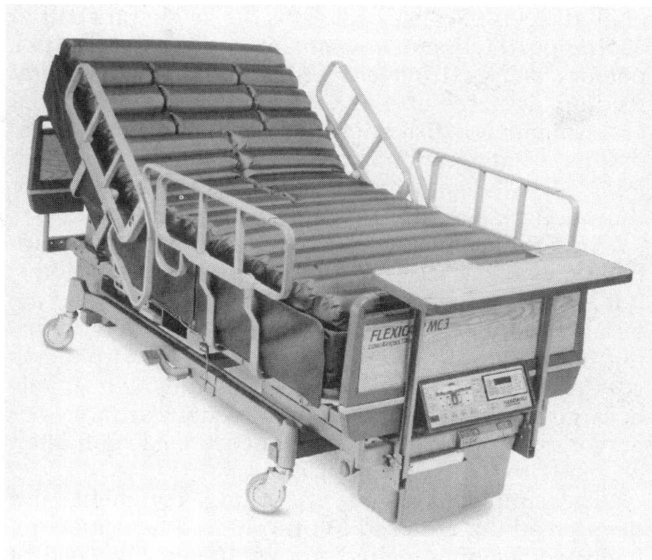

FIGURE 61–9. FLEXICAIR MC3 Low Airloss Therapy Unit. (Courtesy of Support Systems International, Inc. Reprinted by permission.)

oscillating beds with low airloss characteristics. These beds provide side-to-side rotation with continuous air suspension (Figs. 61–10 and 61–11). Alternating the inflation of the air cells within the bed's support surface allows these beds to arc approximately 90 degrees every 6 to 8 minutes. The bed design minimizes all causative forces of pressure ulcers.

The prevention and treatment of pressure ulcers are critically dependent on the optimal maintenance of the skin state. Interventions that enhance systemic

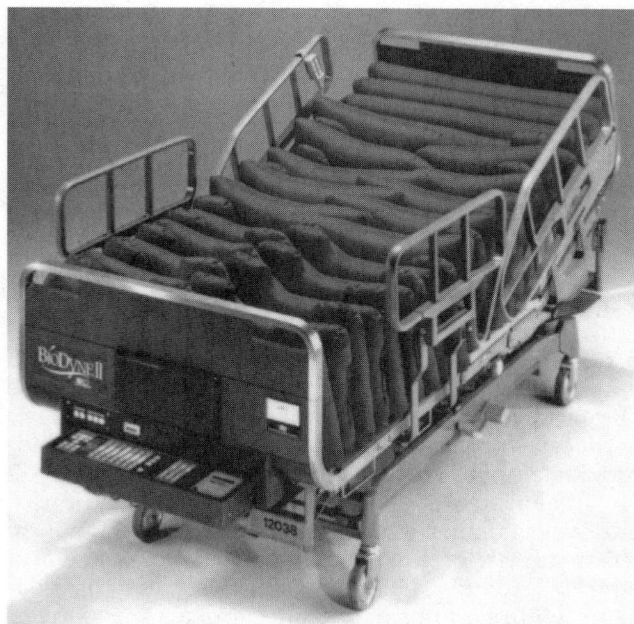

FIGURE 61–10. BioDyne bed featuring low airloss and oscillating function. (Courtesy of Kinetic Concepts, Inc. Reprinted by permission.)

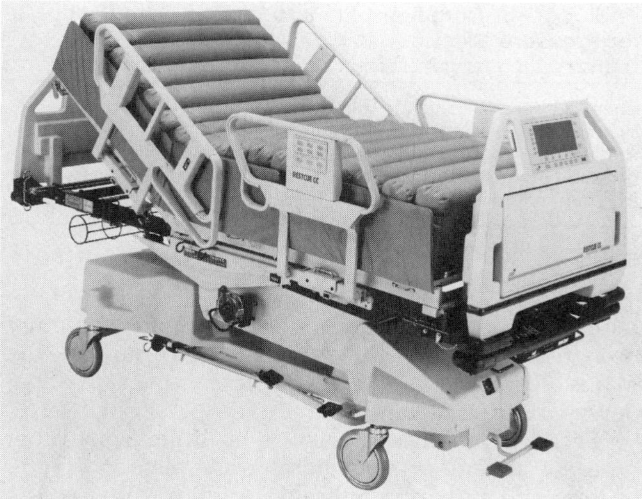

FIGURE 61–11. Restcue CC bed featuring low airloss and oscillating function. (Courtesy of Support Systems International, Inc. Reprinted by permission.)

oxygenation and perfusion and eliminate or minimize peripheral edema and anemia are key internal factors in preventing and healing ulcers. Provision of adequate nutrition to the intact or damaged skin requires protein and calorie intake along with iron, ascorbic acid, and zinc supplements. Critically ill adults often have protein–calorie malnutrition on hospital admission. Nutritional problems often encountered in critically ill adults center around fluid restrictions, organ failure, limited enteral or central venous access, depressed level of consciousness, and impaired absorption by shrunken intestinal villi secondary to prolonged parenteral feedings (Echenique et al., 1982). Attaining and maintaining adequate visceral protein stores and a positive nitrogen balance to optimize the patient's skin nutrition is a challenge to the health care team.

The aim of skin care is to keep the surface clean but not too dry or too moist. Skin should be patted dry but not rubbed to minimize shearing and friction effects. Gentle skin massage may be done only after reactive hyperemia has dissipated. Skin surfaces that remain reddened should not be massaged because underlying tissue damage is often present. Massage may only create further tissue damage.

Because fecal incontinence is a major risk factor for pressure ulcer development, the use of a soft, rubber-tipped rectal catheter to drain liquid stool may assist in the prevention or treatment of ulcers. Channick and associates (1988) examined the short-term effects of rectal tubes in 142 ICU patients. Tubes were inserted to help decrease soiling in 92% of the patients and to assist in healing pressure ulcers in 9%. The mean duration of tube placement was 3.3 days. No complications were identified in this study, even when the balloon on the catheter tip was inflated to assist in containing stool. It was also reported that no pressure ulcers developed in a patient with a rectal tube in place. Al-

TABLE 61–9. **Common Skin and Wound Care Products for Pressure Ulcers**

Chemical debriding agents (Elase; Travase; Santyl)
Skin barriers (Karaya powder; Stomadhesive)
Self-adhesive, nonabsorbing transparent films (OpSite; Tegaderm)
Adhesive hydrocolloid wafers (Duoderm)
Absorptive hydrophilic beads or granules (Debrisan; Duoderm)

though the long-term effects of rectal tubes have not been researched in ICU patients, the rectal tube remains a common and useful adjunct in the care of patients with diarrhea.

Because pressure ulcers differ little from other types of wounds, the general principles of wound healing and care are applicable, and are discussed in Chapter 59. A variety of skin care products and wound coverings are available to assist in the healing of various stages of pressure ulcers (Table 61–9). Surgical debridement may be necessary to treat extensive and infected ulcers to remove devitalized tissue, which otherwise may slow healing, delay granulation, and promote infection.

The expected outcomes for pressure ulcers are healed pressure ulcers, absence of infected ulcers, absence of further skin breakdown, and evidence of adequate nutritional intake. It should be emphasized that skin care often receives low priority in the critical care setting (Glavis & Barbour, 1990). Assessment of the critically ill patient at risk for pressure ulcer development, as well as institution of preventive measures, often are not performed until late in the patient's stay or after the problem becomes visible. Institution and reinforcement of unit- or hospital-based standards for skin care should result in the performance of risk assessment within 12 hours of admission to the ICU and subsequent interventions as needed.

Pulmonary Complications

Etiologic factors for pulmonary complications in immobilized patients include PE, aspiration pneumonitis, hypostatic pneumonia, atelectasis, and alveolar hypoventilation. General symptomatology includes the development of confusion, dyspnea, tachypnea, labored breathing with accessory muscle use, and cyanosis. Abnormal breath sounds, depression in $Pa{O_2}$ and oxygen saturation values, and elevation of partial pressures of arterial carbon dioxide ($Pa{CO_2}$) may be present. Depression of cough, gag, or swallow reflexes or inadequate minute ventilation may be found in patients with blunted reflexes secondary to anesthesia, intravenous muscle relaxants, or narcotic or sedative effects. The abrupt onset of dyspnea, hypoxemia, tachypnea, or complaints of pleuritic chest pain are classic findings of PE.

Astute surveillance for and reporting of depression of gag, swallow, and cough reflexes in patients with altered levels of consciousness is the key in preventing aspiration. Frequent assessment of nasogastric tube patency and gastric residuals associated with enteral feedings is necessary, as well as ongoing abdominal assessments for distention and stool frequency. Positioning a patient who is receiving enteral feedings in a semi-Fowler's position is standard care but does not thoroughly guarantee prevention of aspiration.

Monitoring for alveolar hypoventilation in immobile patients is based on clinical signs and symptoms, but is ultimately focused on the $Pa{CO_2}$. Intermittent arterial blood gases or continual, noninvasive monitoring of end-tidal carbon dioxide in intubated patients is essential in those patients receiving muscle relaxants or large or frequent doses of intravenous sedatives or narcotics. Optimal maintenance of artificial ventilation occurs with the trending of $Pa{CO_2}$ values.

The simple measures of turning, coughing, and deep breathing are used to prevent and treat the etiologic factors of impaired gas exchange. The use of standard body positions can enhance gas exchange by optimizing $\dot{V}/\dot{Q}$ matching in the lung. Dependent areas of normal lung tissue receive more blood flow due to gravitational effects and more ventilation due to the increased weight from the lung tissue. A knowledge of the location of lung disease is essential to provide optimal positioning. The lateral decubitus position has proven to be very effective in increasing $Pa{CO_2}$ in patients with unilateral lung disease. Placing the "good lung down" has consistently resulted in improved oxygenation in these patients. The upright or Fowler's position has traditionally been used to decrease the effect of abdominal pressure on diaphragmatic excursion and to increase FRC. Prone positioning has been used less frequently in critically ill patients because of the difficulty associated in maneuvering patients with complex invasive technology and because of hindrances in providing timely resuscitative measures. The prone position, however, has been demonstrated to be very beneficial in patients with bilateral lung disease due to the associated increase in FRC from the displacement of abdominal contents. The benefit of the Trendelenburg position has also been proven in patients with bilateral lower lobe disease.

Research studies have attempted to define the effect of the Kinetic Treatment Table on pulmonary complications in immobilized critically ill patients. A recent, randomized, prospective study examined 65 immobilized critically ill patients who either were placed on conventional beds and turned every 2 hours or placed on Kinetic Treatment Tables and rotated approximately 50% of the time (Gentilello et al., 1988). The total incidence of significant atelectasis and pneumonia was higher in the control group (66%) than in the treatment group (33%, $p < 0.01$). The results of other researchers (Kelly et al., 1987) studying 573 patients with symptoms of acute stroke were similar. Findings of other researchers (Summer et al., 1989) included decreased length of ICU stay in patients receiving continuous mechanical turning. Patients with sepsis and pneumonia had a 3.48-day shorter stay compared to controls ($p < 0.001$). Patients with chronic obstructive pulmonary disease on kinetic therapy required 6.84 fewer days ($p < 0.001$) in the ICU and 4.6 fewer days of mechanical ventilation. Critically ill patients with blunt trauma receiving kinetic therapy had significantly less pneumonia (13.7%) than control patients (39.6%) who resided on a conventional bed (Fink et al., 1990).

A recent study has also documented the positive effects of an oscillating air suspension bed on the risk of ICU pneumonia in 124 medical ICU patients (deBoisblanc et al., 1993). Although this form of therapy was not shown to decrease days of mechanical ventilation or length of ICU stay, a significant difference was found in the rate of pneumonia (controls group rate: 22%, vs. oscillation group rate: 9%; $p = 0.05$). What all of these studies tell us is that early institution (i.e., on ICU admission) of oscillating bed therapy has a significant potential for decreasing the incidence of ICU pneumonia.

Because supplemental oxygen and artificial ventilation are frequently used in the treatment of pulmonary complications, nursing interventions include monitoring for the adequacy of these treatments through arterial blood gases, pulse oximetry, and capnography. Expected outcomes of treatment for impaired gas exchange include a minimal PaO_2 of 65 mm Hg, a minimal arterial oxygen saturation of 94%, eucarbia, spontaneous breathing, eupnea, and normal breath sounds.

Activity Intolerance

Intolerance of activity in patients immobilized for long periods of time results from decreases in maximal $\dot{V}O_2$ and from sluggish neurovascular reflexes. Signs and symptoms of intolerance in resting supine positions may be evident only as increases in resting heart rates. On rising, patients often experience dizziness, lightheadedness, tachycardia, hypotension, and narrowed pulse pressures secondary to decreases in stroke volume.

Supine exercise has been reported to be ineffective in preventing orthostatic intolerance (Winslow, 1985). Prevention of orthostatic hypotension centers on frequently repositioning patients from horizontal to vertical positions to provide sufficient stimulus to neurovascular reflexes. As patients who have been immobile and supine for long periods become mobile, safety precautions need to be taken. Supine vital signs are taken to compare values. Factors that can increase orthostatic intolerance should be noted, such as vasodilatory drugs and fever. Gradual increases in vertical positions should be made only in the absence of significant orthostasis. Expected outcomes of interventions for activity intolerance include an absence of orthostatic signs, appropriate increases in heart rate with increased activity, lessening complaints of tiredness or exhaustion on rising or ambulating, and progressive distances and times associated with ambulation.

Iatrogenic Physical Injury

All too frequently, critically ill patients are confused, agitated, or combative from a variety of causes. Physical restraint, pharmacologic interventions, and behavioral modifications are frequently used as management strategies to maintain needed immobility. The correct or incorrect application of soft and hard restraints may lead to joint dislocation, peripheral nerve injury, impaired circulation distal to limb restraints, and skin blisters, abrasions, or pressure ulcers. Judicious use of restraints in the agitated patient should be coupled with appropriate pharmacologic sedation to prevent enhanced combativeness due to the sensation of lack of control induced by restraints. Monitoring restraint sites for skin integrity, adequate circulation, and joint alignment should be performed often, especially if the patient remains physically active in bed.

Inappropriate positioning of arms may lead to ulnar nerve compression and altered motor and sensory function. Paresthesia, hypesthesia, hypalgia, analgesia, and muscle weakness associated with elbow flexion are diagnostic of ulnar nerve compression (Chuman, 1985). Purposeful positioning of the arms in a supinated state in the supine position is critical to prevent this complication.

Constipation

Bedrest can be a major etiologic factor in the development of constipation, which can lead to fecal impaction. Complaints of anorexia, headache, nausea, and dizziness may accompany signs of irritability, insomnia, flatulence, straining with defecation, dehydration, abdominal distention, and hard, dry stool. A rock-hard mass palpated in the abdomen associated with fecal-colored smears or a ribbon of diarrhea is a classic sign of fecal impaction.

Management strategies for constipation are aimed at increasing dietary fiber, increasing activity, and increasing fluid intake if tolerated. Bran, cereals, fresh fruits, and whole-wheat bread have a high fiber content with hydrophobic bulking properties. Psyllium hydrophobic mucilloid (Metamucil, Procter & Gamble, Cincinnati, OH; Hydrocil, Reid-Rowell Laboratories, Marietta, GA) may also be used for this purpose. Stool softeners may be effective in lowering the surface tension of stool and allowing water and fat to enter the fecal mass. Chemical stimulants such as bisacodyl (Dulcolax; Boehringer Ingelheim, Ridgefield, CT) increase colonic activity, which may prove effective in increasing peristalsis. Saline cathartics such as milk of magnesia and sodium phosphate–biphosphate (Fleet's; C. B. Fleet, Lynchburg, VA) compounds may be used for their osmotic effects. Increasing activity levels should be stressed if feasible because of the beneficial effect of activity on peristalsis. Treatment of fecal impaction is often digital removal coupled with a combination of the above measures.

Monitoring for the frequency, amount, color, and consistency of stool is basic to prevent constipation. The quantity of stool should be evaluated based on whether the critically ill adult is being fed enterally or parenterally. Expected outcomes of treatment measures for the enterally fed patient with constipation are soft, formed stool, absence of straining with defecation, adequate appetite, and a soft, nondistended abdomen.

Incontinence

Altered level of consciousness, bedrest, use of pharmacologic agents, and use of restraints are major etiologic factors in urinary and fecal incontinence in the immobile patient. Signs and symptoms of urinary retention, which may precede urinary incontinence, are a distended bladder, lower abdominal discomfort, and restlessness. Management of retention may simply involve establishing a voiding regimen with the patient or using intermittent urinary catheterization or an indwelling catheter. Monitoring for signs and symptoms of UTI and catheter patency as well as intermittent cleansing around the insertion site of the indwelling catheter are essential.

The use of a soft, rubber-tipped rectal tube to manage liquid fecal incontinence may prove advantageous in monitoring output and preventing pressure ulcers. If the balloon on the tip of the rectal tube needs to be inflated with air to seal stool contents effectively, balloon volume and pressure as well as appropriate deflation must be monitored to avoid potential complications. Nursing care also involves exploring the reason for the diarrhea. Expected outcomes of management of incontinence include the absence of complications of treatment modalities, absence of pressure sores, and regained continence.

Sensory–Perceptual Alterations

Bedrest in an ICU environment restricts sensory input and proprioception but also often simultaneously exposes the patient to sensory overload. Boredom, anxiety, tension, inability to concentrate, somatic complaints, and auditory and visual illusions and hallucinations may develop, leading to depression and hostility. Sensory–perceptual alterations related to sensory overload have been referred to as ICU psychosis (Easton & MacKenzie, 1988). This reversible state often begins between the third and seventh day after ICU admission and clears by itself within 48 hours of ICU discharge.

The monotony of confinement may give rise to sensory underload, which may result in boredom, lack of motivation, depression, restlessness, anger, or a flat affect. The creative construction of a plan based on the patient's interests and hobbies should include the use of a wide variety of media, diversified visitors, and a varied care routine. Time set aside exclusively for intellectual discussion as well as for sharing of feelings should be planned for.

Management goals are directed toward decreasing excessive and inappropriate sensory stimulation, such as noise, light, pain, tactile stimulation, and excessive numbers of caregivers, and providing adequate rest, sleep, and sedation. Time and spatial orientation, family socialization, and use of sensory aids should be implemented and planned appropriately. Preoperative interviewing for patients undergoing elective surgery should be conducted if feasible because it may decrease the incidence of postoperative delirium (Quinless et al., 1985). Management strategies for sensory–perceptual alterations are discussed in detail in Chapter 8.

Body Image Disturbances

Dependency is implied with bedrest. Nearly all normal role functions are curtailed by bedrest, and a reliance on caregivers is prevalent. Kornfeld and associates (1974) found that dominant, active patients who demonstrated high self-confidence and competitive qualities failed to tolerate the dependent, immobilized role well. Coupled with the lack of intellectual stimulation, the sick role, and the stresses of illness, altered body image may occur, becoming manifest through anger, despair, weeping, excessive dependence on caregivers, and general deterioration in problem-solving and decision-making abilities. Management strategies should be aimed at establishing a trusting nurse–patient relationship in which feelings about dependency may be confidently expressed and shared. Promotion of social interaction along with construction of a mutually agreed-on plan to promote self-care and control over bedside activities are key interventions. Expected outcomes of such interventions are the resumption of role-related responsibilities, stated confidence about the reconstruction of an altered body image, and exhibited desire to control body functions and bedside activities.

SUMMARY

The prevalence of immobility in critically ill adults makes it an important phenomenon that can have monumental effects on patients' physical and emotional suffering and on caregiver, hospital, and equipment costs. The construction and execution of a plan by the critical care nurse that plans for early ambulation, predicts patients at high risk, reduces modifiable risk factors, and effectively treats incurred complications are essential. Initiation by the critical care nurse to reinstitute mobilization as soon as possible in critically ill adults remains the most cost-effective and simple plan to avoid the complications of immobility. Communication of the plan and collaboration with other members of the multidisciplinary ICU team will help to decrease the effects of a phenomenon that potentially affects every critically ill adult.

REFERENCES

Allman, R. M., Laprade, C. A., Noel, L. B., et al. (1986). Pressure sores among hospitalized patients. *Annals of Internal Medicine, 105,* 337–342.

Allman, R. M., Walker, J. M., Hart, M. K., et al. (1987). Air-fluidized beds or conventional therapy for pressure sores. *Annals of Internal Medicine, 107,* 641–648.

Anderson, F., Wheeler, H., & Goldberg, R. (1991). Physician practices in the prevention of venous thromboembolism. *Annals of Internal Medicine, 115,* 591–559.

Baird, S. E. (1985). Development of a nursing assessment tool to diagnose altered body image in immobilized patients. *Orthopedic Nursing, 4*(1), 47–54.

Batson, S., Adam, S., Hall, G., & Quirke, S. (1993). The development of a pressure area scoring system for critically ill patients: A pilot study. *Intensive and Critical Care Nursing, 9,* 146–151.

Bergstrom, N., Braden, B. J., Laguzza, A., et al. (1987). The Braden scale for predicting pressure sore risk. *Nursing Research, 36,* 205–210.

Bolyard, E. A., Townsend, T. R., & Horan, T. (1987). Airborne contamination associated with in-use air-fluidized beds: A descriptive study. *American Journal of Infection Control, 15,* 75–78.

Braden, B., & Bergstrom, N. (1987). A conceptual schema for the study of the etiology of pressure sores. *Rehabilitation Nursing, 12,* 8–12.

Braun, J., Silvetti, A., & Xakellis, G. (1992). What really works for pressure sores. *Patient Care, 26*(2), 63–83.

Brooks, B., & Duncan, G. W. (1940). Effects of pressure on tissues. *Archives of Surgery, 40,* 696–709.

Brunner, L., & Suddarth, D. (1986). Rehabilitation concepts. In L. Brunner & D. Suddarth (Eds.), *Manual of nursing practice* (pp. 51–73). Philadelphia: J. B. Lippincott.

Burn, F. D., Johnson, J., & Ellis, N. (1987). Managing decubiti ulcers. *Hospital Therapy, 12,* 67–75.

Cade, J. F. (1982). High risk of the critically ill for venous thromboembolism. *Critical Care Medicine, 7,* 448–450.

Channick, R., Curley, F. J., & Irwin, R. S. (1988). Indications for and complications of rectal tube use in critically ill patients. *Journal of Intensive Care Medicine, 3,* 321–323.

Christian, B. J. (1982). Immobilization. In C. Norris (Ed.), *Psychological aspects in concept classification in nursing.* Rockville, MD: Aspen Systems.

Chuman, M. A. (1985). Risk factors associated with ulnar nerve compression in bedridden patients. *Journal of Neurosurgical Nursing, 17,* 338–342.

Comerota, A., Katz, M., & White, J. (1992). Why does prophylaxis with external pneumatic compression for deep vein thrombosis fail? *American Journal of Surgery, 164,* 265–268.

Coon, W. W., Hirsh, J., & Rubin, L. J. (1987). Preventing deep vein thrombosis. *Patient Care, 21*(3), 82–90.

deBoisblanc, B., Castro, M., Everret, B., Grender, J., Walkers, C., & Summer, W. (1993). Effect of air-supported, continuous postural oscillation on the risk of early ICU pneumonia in nontraumatic critical illness. *Chest, 103,* 1543–1547.

Dinsdale, S. M. (1974). Decubitus ulcers: Role of pressure and friction in causation. *Archives of Physical Medicine and Rehabilitation, 55,* 147–152.

Dinsdale, S. M. (1973). Decubitus ulcers in swine: Light and electron microscopy study of pathogenesis. *Archives of Physical Medicine and Rehabilitation, 54,* 51–56.

Domonkos, J., & Herr, L. (1965). Effect of denervation and immobilization on carbohydrate metabolism in tonic and tetanic muscles: Glycogen metabolism. *Acta Physiologica Hungarica, 28,* 227–236.

Easton, C., & MacKenzie, F. (1988). Sensory–perceptual alterations: Delirium in the intensive care unit. *Heart and Lung, 17,* 229–235.

Echenique, M. M., Bistrian, B. R., & Blackburn, G. L. (1982). Theory and techniques of nutritional support in the intensive care unit. *Critical Care Medicine, 10,* 546–549.

Elpern, E. H., Jacobs, E. R., & Bone, R. C. (1987). Incidence of aspiration in tracheally intubated adults. *Heart and Lung, 16,* 527–531.

Farkas, J., Chapuls, C., Combe, S., et al. (1993). A randomized controlled trial of a low-molecular weight heparin (enoxaparin) to prevent deep-vein thrombosis in patients undergoing vascular surgery. *European Journal of Vascular Surgery 17,* 554–560.

Fink, M., Helsmoortel, C., Stein, K., Lee, P., & Cohn, S. (1990). The efficacy of an oscillating bed in the prevention of lower respiratory tract infection in critically ill victims of blunt trauma: A prospective study. *Chest, 97,* 132–137.

Frank, C., Akeson, W. H., Woo, S. L., et al. (1984). Physiology and therapeutic value of passive joint motion. *Clinical Orthopaedics and Related Research, 185,* 113–125.

Geary, S. (1994). Intensive care unit psychosis revisited: Understanding and managing delirium in the critical care setting. *Critical Care Nursing Quarterly, 17*(1), 51–63.

Gentilello, L., Thompson, D. A., Tonnesen, A. S., et al. (1988). Effect of a rotating bed on the incidence of pulmonary complications in critically ill patients. *Critical Care Medicine, 16,* 783–786.

Glavis, C., & Barbour, S. (1990). Pressure ulcer prevention in critical care: State of the art. *AACN Clinical Issues, 1,* 602–613.

Goldhaber, S., Haire, W., & Feldstein, M. (1993). Alteplase versus heparin in acute pulmonary embolism: Randomized trial assessing right ventricular function and pulmonary perfusion. *Lancet, 341,* 507–511.

Goldhaber, S., Markis, J., & Meyerovitz, M. (1986). Acute pulmonary embolism treated with tissue plasminogen activator. *Lancet, 2,* 886–888.

Gosnell, D. J. (1987). Assessment and evaluation of pressure sores. *Nursing Clinics of North America, 22,* 399–416.

Greenleaf, J. E. (1982). Physiological consequences of reduced physical activity during bedrest. *Exercise and Sports Sciences Reviews, 10,* 84–119.

Halm, M., & Alpen, M. (1993). The impact of technology on patients and families. *Nursing Clinics of North America, 28,* 443–457.

Hirsh, J., & Hull, R. (1987). *Venous thromboembolism: Natural history, diagnosis and management.* Boca Raton, FL: CRC Press.

Holm, K., & Hedricks, C. (1989). Immobility and bone loss in the aging adult. *Critical Care Nursing Quarterly, 12*(1), 46–51.

Hoyt, J. (1990). Aspiration pneumonitis: Patient risk factors, prevention, and management. *Journal of Intensive Care Medicine, 5*(Suppl), S2–S9.

Hull, R., & Pineo, G. (1993). Therapeutic use of low molecular weight heparins: The knowledge to date as applied to therapy. *Seminars in Thrombosis and Hemostasis, 19,* 111–115.

Hull, R., Raskob, G., & Gent, M. (1990). Effectiveness of intermittent pneumatic leg compression for preventing deep vein thrombosis after total hip replacement. *Journal of the American Medical Association, 263,* 2313–2317.

Hwang, T. I., Hill, K., Schneider, V., et al. (1988). Effect of prolonged bedrest on the propensity for renal stone formation. *Journal of Clinical Endocrinology and Metabolism, 66,* 109–112.

Inaba-Roland, K., & Maricle, R. (1992). Assessing delirium in the acute care setting. *Heart and Lung, 21,* 48–55.

Inman, K., Sibbald, W., Rutledge, F., & Clark, B. (1993). Clinical utility and cost effectiveness of an air suspension bed in the prevention of pressure ulcers. *Journal of the American Medical Association, 269,* 1139–1143.

Kelly, T. W., Patrick, M. R., & Hillman, K. M. (1983). Study of diarrhea in critically ill patients. *Critical Care Medicine, 11,* 7–9.

Kelly, R., Vibulsresth, S., Bell, L., & Duncan, R. (1987). Evaluation of kinetic therapy in the prevention of complications of prolonged bed rest secondary to stroke. *Stroke, 18,* 638–642.

Kornfeld, D. S., Heller, S. S., Frank, K. A., et al. (1974). Personality and psychological factors in postcardiotomy delirium. *Archives of General Psychiatry, 31,* 249–253.

Koziak, M. (1959). Etiology and pathology of ischemic ulcers. *Archives of Physical Medicine and Rehabilitation, 40,* 62–69.

Lamb, L., Stevens, P., & Johnson, R. (1965). Hypokinesia secondary to chair rest from four to ten days. *Aerospace Medicine, 36,* 755–763.

Larsen, B., Holstein, P., & Lassen, N. A. (1979). On the pathogenesis of bedsores. *Journal of Plastic and Reconstructive Surgery, 13,* 347.

Leclerc, J., Desjardins, L., & Geerts, W. (1991). A randomized trial of enoxaparin for the prevention of deep vein thrombosis after major knee surgery. *Thrombosis and Hemostasis, 65*(Suppl), 753.

Maklebust, J. (1987). Pressure ulcers: Etiology and prevention. *Nursing Clinics of North America, 22,* 359–377.

Marchette, L., Arnell, I., & Redick, E. (1991). Skin ulcers of elderly surgical patients in critical care units. *Dimensions of Critical Care Nursing, 10,* 321–329.

Matzdorff, A., & Green, D. (1992). Deep vein thrombosis and pulmonary embolism: Prevention, diagnosis, and treatment. *Geriatrics, 47*(8), 48–63.

Maynard, F. M. (1986). Immobilization hypercalcemia following spinal cord injury. *Archives of Physical Medicine and Rehabilitation, 67,* 41–43.

Memmer, M. K., & Kozier, B. (1987). Mobility and immobility. In B. Kozier & G. Erb (Eds.), *Fundamentals of nursing: Concepts and procedures* (pp. 964–1025). Menlo Park, CA: Addison-Wesley.

Merli, G. (1993). Deep vein thrombosis and pulmonary embolism prophylaxis in orthopedic surgery. *Medical Clinics of North America, 77,* 397–411.

Meythaler, J. M., Korkor, A. B., Nanda, T., et al. (1986). Immobilization hypercalcemia associated with Landry-Guillain-Barré syndrome. *Archives of Internal Medicine, 146,* 1567–1571.

Milazzo, V., & Resh, C. (1981). Kinetic nursing—a new approach to the problems of immobility. *Journal of Neurosurgical Nursing, 14,* 120–124.

Miller, P. B., Johnson, R. L., & Lamb, L. E. (1965). Effects of moderate physical exercise during four weeks of bedrest on circulatory functions in man. *Aerospace Medicine, 36,* 1077.

Mitchell, P. H. (1981). Motor status. In P. H. Mitchell & A. Lonstau (Eds.), *Concepts basic to nursing* (pp. 343–390). New York: McGraw-Hill.

Mobily, P., & Kelley, L. (1991). Iatrogenesis in the elderly: Factors of immobility. *Journal of Gerontological Nursing, 17*(9), 5–10.

Moser, K. (1990). Venous thromboembolism. *American Review of Respiratory Disease, 141,* 235–249.

Norton, D., McLaren, R., & Exton-Smith, A. N. (1962). *An investigation of geriatric nursing problems in hospitals.* Edinburgh: Churchill-Livingstone.

Nurmohamed, M., Rosendaal, H., Buller, H., et al. (1992). Low molecular weight heparin versus standard heparin in general and orthopedic surgery: A meta-analysis. *Lancet, 340,* 152–156.

Pechan, J., & Julis, I. (1975). The pressure measurement in the ulnar nerve: Contribution to the pathophysiology of the carpal tunnel syndrome. *Journal of Biomechanics, 8,* 75–79.

Pennington, J. (1987). Hospital-acquired pneumonias. In P. R. Wenzel (Ed.), *Prevention and control of nosocomial infections* (pp. 321–334). Baltimore: Williams & Wilkins.

Pidala, M., Donovan, D., & Kepley, R. (1992). A prospective study on intermittent pneumatic compression in the prevention of deep vein thrombosis in patients undergoing total hip or total knee replacement. *Surgery, Gynecology, and Obstetrics, 175,* 47–51.

Pingleton, S. K. (1985). Thromboembolism and bleeding disorders in the critically ill patient. *Respiratory Care, 30,* 481–486.

Plate, G., Einarsson, E., & Eklof, B. (1986). Etiologic spectrum in acute iliofemoral venous thrombosis. *International Angiology, 5,* 59–64.

Quinless, F., Cassese, M., & Atherton, N. (1985). The effect of selected preoperative, intraoperative, and postoperative variables on the development of postcardiotomy psychosis in patients undergoing open heart surgery. *Heart and Lung, 14,* 335.

Roberts, S. L. (1987). Pulmonary tissue perfusion altered: Emboli. *Heart and Lung, 16,* 128–137.

Rubin, M. (1988). The physiology of bedrest. *American Journal of Nursing, 88,* 50–56.

Sahn, S. (1991). Continuous lateral rotational therapy and nosocomial pneumonia. *Chest, 99,* 1263–1267.

Saltin, B., Blomquist, G., & Mitchell, J. H. (1968). Response to exercise after bedrest and after training: A longitudinal study of adaptive changes in oxygen transport and body composition. *Circulation, 38,* 1–78.

Scurr, J., Coleridge-Smith, P., & Hasty, J. (1987). Regimen for improved effectiveness of intermittent pneumatic compression in DVT prophylaxis. *Surgery, 102,* 816–820.

Stamm, W. (1986). Nosocomial urinary tract infections. In J. K. Bennett & P. S. Brachman (Eds.), *Hospital infections* (pp. 375–384). New York: Little, Brown.

St. Clair, M. (1992). Descriptive study of the use of a specialty bed in the United Kingdom. *Decubitus, 12*(2), 33–39.

Stotts, N. A. (1988). Predicting pressure ulcer development in surgical patients. *Heart and Lung, 17,* 641–647.

Stotts, N. A. (1987). Age-specific characteristics of patients who develop pressure ulcers in the tertiary-care setting. *Nursing Clinics of North America, 22,* 391–398.

St. Pierre, D., & Gardiner, P. F. (1987). The effect of immobility and exercise on muscle function: A review. *Physiotherapy Canada, 39,* 24–36.

Summer, W., Curry, P., Haponik, E., Nelson, S., & Elston, R. (1989). Continuous mechanical turning of intensive care unit patients shortens length of stay in some diagnostic-related groups. *Journal of Critical Care, 4*(1), 45–53.

Summers, T. B., & Hines, H. M. (1951). Effect of immobility in various positions upon the weight and strength of skeletal muscles. *Archives of Physical Medicine, 32,* 142–145.

The UKEP Study Research Group. (1987). The UKEP study multicentre clinical trial on two local regimes of urokinase in massive pulmonary embolism. *European Heart Journal, 8,* 2–10.

Turpie, A., Levine, M., & Hirsh, J. (1986). A randomized controlled trial of a low molecular weight heparin (enoxaparin) to prevent deep vein thrombosis in patients undergoing elective hip surgery. *New England Journal of Medicine, 315,* 925–929.

Van Zuiden, L., Anquist, K. A., & Schachar, N. (1982). Immobilization hypercalcemia. *Canadian Journal of Surgery, 25,* 647–649.

Vesley, D., Hankinson, S. E., & Lauer, J. L. (1986). Microbial survival and dissemination associated with an air-fluidized therapy unit. *American Journal of Infection Control, 14,* 35–40.

Weissman, C., Askanazi, J., Hyman, A. I., et al. (1983). Hypercalcemia and hypercalciuria in a critically ill patient. *Critical Care Medicine, 11,* 576–578.

Wilson, L. (1993). Sensory perceptual alteration: Diagnosis, prediction, and intervention in the hospitalized adult. *Nursing Clinics of North America, 28,* 747–765.

Winslow, E. H. (1985). Cardiovascular consequences of bedrest. *Heart and Lung, 14,* 236–246.

Xakellis, G., Frantz, R., Arteaga, M., Nguyen, M., & Lewis, A. (1992). A comparison of patient risk for pressure ulcer development with nursing use of preventive interventions. *Journal of the American Geriatric Society, 40,* 1250–1254.

Yannelli, B., & Gurevich, I. (1988). Infection in critical care. *Heart and Lung, 17,* 596–600.

CHAPTER 62

Patients With Trauma

Deborah Goldenberg Klein

WHAT MAKES THE TRAUMA PATIENT UNIQUE

The trauma patient creates unique challenges for the health care team and critical care nurse. The incidence of trauma is unpredictable. The injured individual may arrive at the hospital unexpectedly or with only a few minutes' advance warning. Little if any information is available about the actual mechanism of injury or about the patient's previous health status, current medications, allergies, and usual vital signs. Care of the trauma patient requires immediate availability of specialized personnel, equipment, and supplies, a staffed surgical suite, and critical care space. Depending on the transport time from the scene of the incident to the hospital and the qualifications of prehospital personnel, the patient may or may not have undergone initial stabilization.

To accomplish the essential life-saving interventions and diagnostic procedures in a timely manner, a trauma team—surgeon, emergency physician, anesthesiologist, registered nurses, and ancillary staff—must function together in carrying out an organized approach to the trauma patient. This implies that a large number of health professionals will perform preestablished roles to provide care for an undiagnosed individual, frequently an individual experiencing life-threatening injury to one or more body systems (Trauma Nursing Coalition, 1992).

Scope of Trauma

The incidence of trauma in the United States is a major health care and economic issue. Trauma continues to be the fourth leading cause of death for all ages. Only heart disease, cancer, and strokes result in a higher death rate. Trauma is the leading cause of death in persons between the ages of 1 and 44, the peak incidence occurring in the 15- to 24-year-old age group, thereby affecting otherwise healthy and productive members of society. Trauma is the greatest killer of children. It is the most common cause of hospitalization among individuals less than age 45 and is the leading cause of physician contacts in the United States. Each year 2.3 million Americans are hospitalized as a result of injury and 54 million seek medical care for injuries (Committee on Trauma Research, 1985; National Safety Council, 1992).

EPIDEMIOLOGY OF TRAUMA

Over half of all traumatic incidents involve the use of alcohol, drugs, or other substance abuse. Injury results in both short-term and long-term disability. In 1991 over 8 million Americans sustained injuries that resulted in a disability (National Safety Council, 1992).

Economic factors are important from the standpoint of the direct and indirect costs associated with trauma. It is estimated that trauma costs society approximately $158 to $180 billion annually (American College of Surgeons, 1993a). Other nations have assessed the impact of trauma on their gross national product and have found it economically feasible to finance national trauma systems. Because trauma is predominantly a disease of the young and carries the potential for permanent disability, it is evident that trauma is responsible for the loss of significant productive work years. Unlike cardiovascular disease, cancer, and cerebrovascular accidents, trauma is thought to be preventable. Advocates of trauma systems identify prevention as an essential component of an organized approach to trauma.

SYSTEMS APPROACH TO TRAUMA CARE

Historical Perspective

A systems approach to trauma care is not necessarily a new or unique idea. In many settings, often large, county-based teaching facilities, a trauma team concept has existed for a number of years. The concept of regionalization has similarly been applied to transplantation, cardiac surgery, burn care, neonatal centers, and other patient populations requiring specialized and organized care.

Accidental Death and Disability: The Neglected Disease of Modern Society, a landmark National Research Council report in 1966, presented data demonstrating that injury was a national public health problem. This document identified the need for an organized approach to trauma care, the development of trauma systems, implementation of community education and prevention activities, and further research in the area of trauma and prevention of injury. *Injury in America* (Committee on Trauma Research, 1985) indicated that slow progress has been made in the prevention of injury and the development of trauma systems. Specific recommendations from this report included the following:

1. Establishment of a center for injury control within the federal government
2. Provision of funding for research on injury commensurate with the importance of injury as the largest cause of death and disability of children and young adults in the United States
3. Establishment of effective injury surveillance systems that have the capacity to identify and control outbreaks of specific injuries
4. Education and persuasion of persons at risk of injury to alter their behavior to provide increased self-protection
5. Enactment of laws or administrative rules requiring individuals to change their behavior
6. Provision of automatic protection by requiring changes in product and environmental design
7. Coordination of a multidisciplinary approach to injury biomechanics research to provide a clearer understanding of the mechanisms of injury
8. Development of specialized centers to provide immediate care and rehabilitation of injured individuals
9. Establishment of programs designed to train professionals in the research and care of injuries
10. Establishment and provision of support for research programs in the area of mechanics of injury, prevention of injury, immediate care and rehabilitation of injured individuals, and model systems designed to provide optimal trauma care (Committee on Trauma Research, 1985).

Trauma System Components

A trimodal distribution of death due to injury was first described in 1982 (American College of Surgeons, 1993b). Death due to injury occurs in one of three time periods. The first peak of death occurs within seconds to minutes from injury. Death is due to lacerations of the brain, brain stem, high spinal cord, heart, aorta, and other large blood vessels. The second peak occurs within minutes to several hours after injury. Deaths are due to subdural and epidural hematomas, hemopneumothorax, ruptured spleen, laceration of the liver, pelvic fractures, and/or other multiple injuries associated with significant blood loss. This first hour of care focuses on rapid assessment and resuscitation. The third peak occurs several days to weeks after the initial injury and is most often due to sepsis and multiple organ system failure. Patient outcomes at this stage are affected by the care provided previously. This trimodal distribution of death supports the concept of an organized trauma system to manage the trauma patient.

During the 1970s and 1980s most trauma systems centered around a facility that had developed its trauma care capabilities because of the large volume of major trauma cases received at the hospital. Frequently a surgeon with special interest and skill in trauma care was identified as the expert and was responsible for the level of trauma care provided. Trauma systems in this setting often involved only expertise in the care of patients routinely received in such a facility. A "system" did not actually exist except from an internal operations point of view.

In 1990 The Trauma Care Systems Planning and Development Act was passed to recognize injury as a public health problem and to offer a model trauma care system plan to federal and state health agencies. The model encourages the formation of an inclusive trauma system in which each care provider and facility is incorporated into the system. The goal is to match a facility's resources with a patient's medical needs so that optimal and cost-effective care is achieved. This model provides a framework for states to use to meet the unique needs of an individual state or region (Fig. 62–1).

Trauma Team Concept

The concept of a trauma team is especially important to health care personnel. The term trauma team refers to health care professionals who respond immediately to participate in the initial resuscitation and stabilization of the trauma victim. Table 62–1 lists the composition of a typical trauma team. Essential to the team approach is the fact that each team member is preassigned and understands the specific responsibilities inherent in a particular team role. The trauma surgeon is ultimately responsible for the activities of the trauma team and acts as "team leader" in establishing resuscitation, stabilization, and intervention priorities. Other physician members may have specific responsibilities or may receive direction from the trauma surgeon.

Nursing members of the trauma team may all come from the emergency department, as often occurs in large teaching facilities that have adequate numbers of emergency nurses in the department 24 hours each day. In many trauma centers nurses are asked to respond from other areas of the hospital such as the surgical unit or the trauma intensive care unit. Inclusion of a critical care nurse as a member of the initial response team increases continuity of care for the trauma patient and often enhances certain trauma team capabilities such as hemodynamic monitoring. A surgical nurse may also be included in the trauma team. This individual's responsibility includes assessment of the patient's potential surgical needs and assistance if an

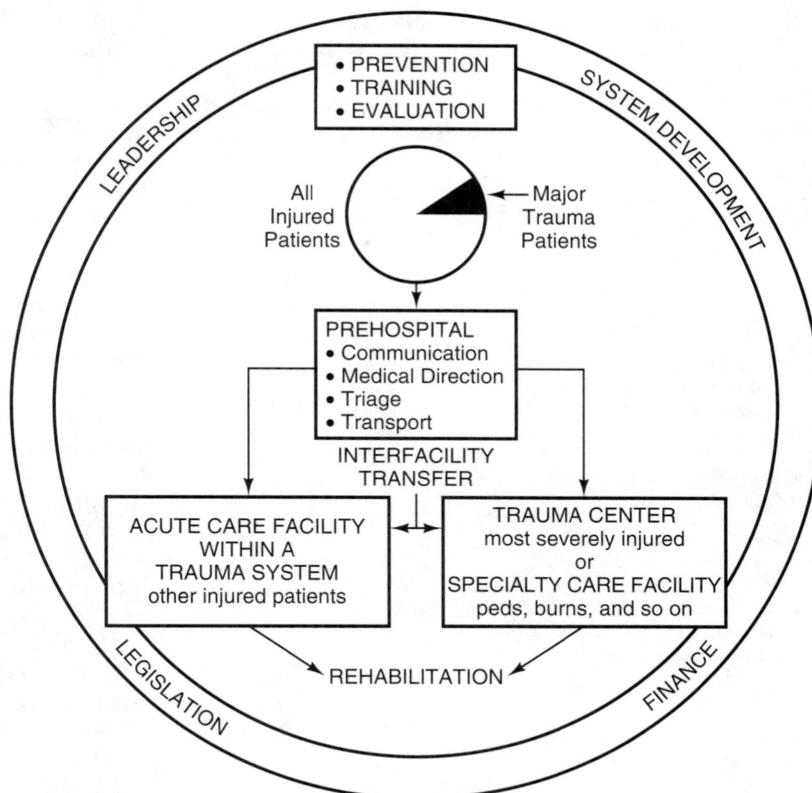

FIGURE 62–1. An inclusive trauma care system. (Adapted with permission from Bureau of Health Services Resources Development, Division of Trauma and Emergency Medical Services: *Model Trauma Care System Plan.* Rockville, MD, U.S. Department of Health and Human Services, 1992.)

emergency thoracotomy or other surgical procedure is required in the resuscitation area.

Levels of Trauma Care

Levels of trauma care in various hospitals have been difficult to ascertain. The American College of Surgeons Committee on Trauma devised a system that could be used to identify a trauma center's expected level of care (American College of Surgeons, 1993a). Table 62–2 lists the various levels of care available according to trauma center status. In most trauma systems, level I and level II trauma centers are capable of providing the same level of care. The most frequent difference between the two is that a level I center is a teaching facility that maintains surgical resident training and is involved in trauma-related research. A level II center receives surgical leadership and care through an in-house surgeon with no involvement of surgical residents.

Level III centers serve communities that lack the resources necessary to provide level I or level II trauma care. A sparsely populated community may not receive an adequate volume of major trauma victims or may not have adequate physician staffing to achieve level II status. This type of trauma center does not have in-house surgical capability and often lacks neurosurgical coverage. Level IV trauma facilities are often located in remote areas. The facility may be a clinic rather than a hospital and may or may not have a physician available. Both level III and IV trauma centers should develop transfer protocols with hospitals providing a higher level of care.

The concept of a systems approach to trauma care, or regionalization, limits the number of identified trauma centers, depending instead on the incidence of major trauma within a region. Many regions find that more hospitals are interested in seeking trauma center status than are actually needed to provide optimal trauma care. As in other highly specialized care situations, a certain patient volume is necessary to enable a facility to provide optimal trauma care. The American College of Surgeons recommends that a level I trauma center treat 600 to 1000 patients and a level II center 350 to 600 patients each year.

An institution may be recognized as a trauma center through various processes. Currently, such recognition is decided at a county, regional, or state level, although the potential does not exist for a national trauma system. Additionally, an institution can designate itself as possessing special capabilities in trauma care. Self-designation is likely to occur only in areas where no trauma plan has been developed; it does not necessarily imply that a trauma system exists, only that an institution provides an organized approach to the care of trauma patients. Recognition of trauma centers may occur through a designation or verification process. Designation means that an authorized agency has assessed an institution's trauma care capabilities

TABLE 62–1. **Multidisciplinary Trauma Team**

Typical Composition

Trauma surgeon (team leader)
Emergency physician
Anesthesiologist
Trauma nurse team leader—emergency nurse
Trauma resuscitation nurse—critical care nurse
Trauma scribe—emergency nurse
Trauma surgical nurse
Laboratory phlebotomist
Radiologic technologist
Respiratory therapist
Social worker/pastoral services
Hospital security officer
Physician specialists as necessary (neurosurgeon, orthopedic surgeon, urologic surgeon)

Inner-Core—Outer-Core Approach
Inner-Core Team

Trauma surgeon (team leader)
Emergency physician
Anesthesiologist
Trauma nurse team leader—emergency nurse
Trauma resuscitation nurse—critical care nurse
Trauma scribe—emergency nurse

Outer-Core Team

Nursing supervisor (team leader)
Laboratory phlebotomist
Radiologic technologist
Respiratory therapist
Social worker/pastoral services
Hospital security officer
Registration/emergency clerk
Physician specialist as necessary (neurosurgeon, orthopedic surgeon, urologic surgeon)
(This concept alleviates congestion during initial resuscitation efforts.)

and has identified or appointed it as a trauma center. A verification process includes a similar assessment process by an authorized agency but merely confirms an institution's compliance with specified criteria and trauma care standards. The surveying agency does not officially appoint or identify such a facility as a trauma center.

Trauma Triage

Triage of an injured individual to the appropriate care facility is another essential component of a trauma system. Triage in a trauma system means sorting the patients to determine which individuals need specialized care for either actual or potential injuries. Determination of which patients require transport to a trauma center rather than a basic emergency care facility occurs according to established protocols, policies, and procedures. Triage decisions are often made by prehospital personnel based on knowledge of the mechanisms of injury and rapid assessment of the patient's clinical status. Medical direction of this process occurs through radio contact with a base station hospital and medical review of triage decisions.

Trauma, injury resulting from an external force, may be accidental, self-inflicted, or the result of an act of violent aggression. Trauma may be classified as major or minor depending on the severity of injury. Minor trauma refers to single system injuries that do not pose a threat to life or limb and can be appropriately treated in a basic emergency facility. Major trauma refers to serious multiple system injuries that require immediate intervention to prevent disability, loss of limb, or death. Major trauma patients and individuals with the potential for major injury are those requiring triage to a trauma center.

Various methods are used to determine which individuals might be classified as major trauma patients and which may benefit from an organized approach to trauma care. Triage decisions may be based on abnormal findings in the patient's physiologic functions, the severity of the mechanism of injury, the anatomic area of injury, or evidence of risk factors such as age and preexisting disease.

Figure 62–2, adapted from the American College of Surgeons (1993b), presents a triage decision scheme. Various trauma scoring tools may also be used to determine triage to the trauma center. The Revised Trauma Score (Table 62–3) is widely used to determine the severity of injury. A Revised Trauma Score of 11 or less is usually considered justification for transporting a patient to a trauma center.

TABLE 62–2. **Characteristics of Trauma Care Facilities**

Level 1 Trauma Center
- Regional resource trauma center
- Provides the most sophisticated care as an acute and tertiary center
- Provides educational programs for physicians, nurses, paramedics, and other trauma personnel
- Conducts major outreach programs, including prevention and public education
- Conducts research related to trauma care

Level II Trauma Center
- Community trauma center
- Provides initial definitive trauma care with the ability to transfer to a level I center
- Conducts outreach programs, including prevention and public education

Level III Trauma Center
- Rural trauma hospital
- Commitment to trauma care commensurate with its local resources
- Plan of care for the injured includes transfer agreements and protocols

Level IV
Rural clinic or hospital
- Commitment to trauma care commensurate with its local resources
- Plan of care for the injured includes transfer agreements and protocols

Data from the American College of Surgeons Committee on Trauma. (1993). *Resources for optimal care of the injured patient.* Chicago: American College of Surgeons.

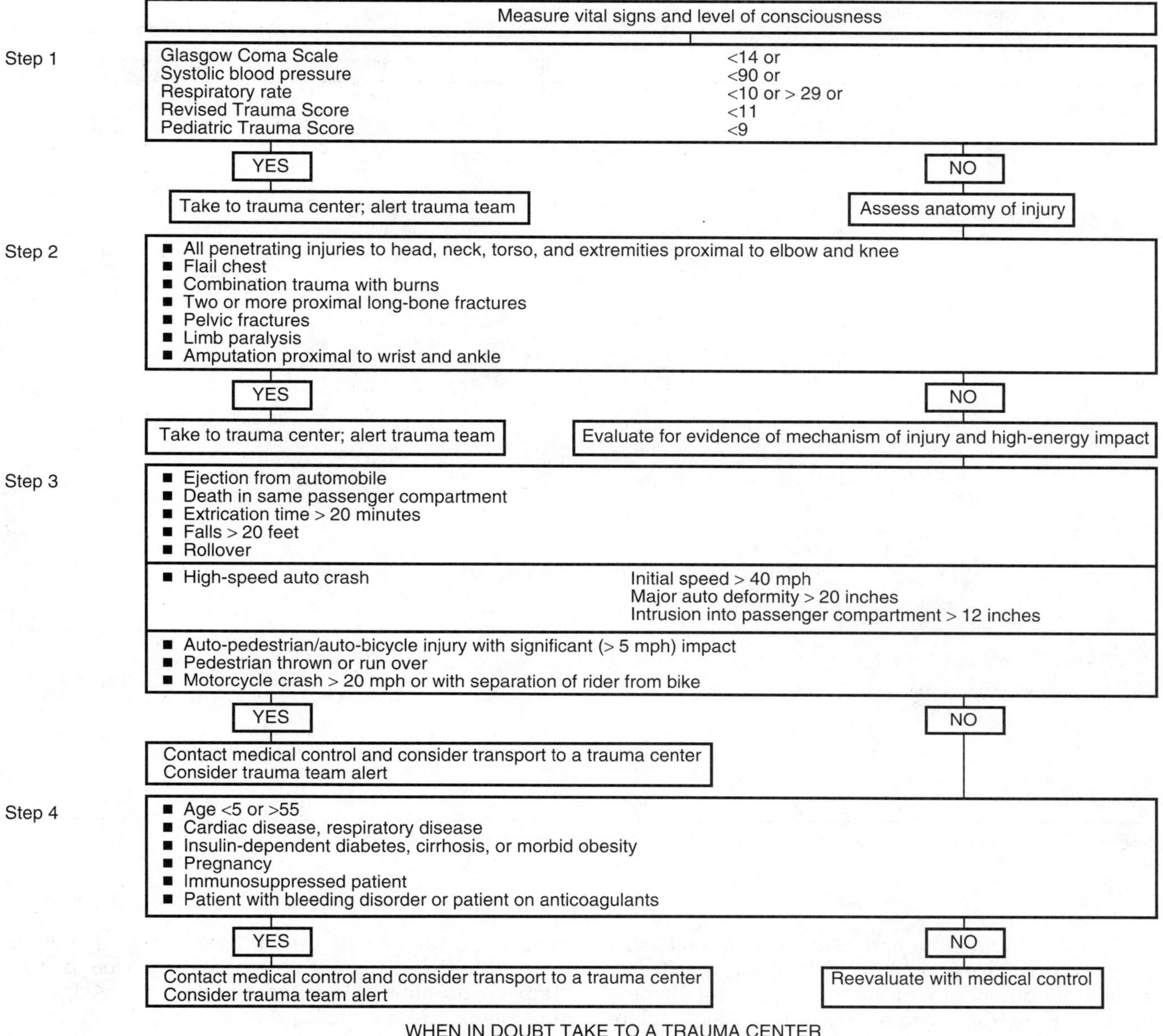

FIGURE 62–2. Triage decision scheme. (From the American College of Surgeons, Committee on Trauma. (1993). Resources for optimal care of the injured patient: 1993. Chicago, American College of Surgeons.)

NOTES

It is the general intention of these triage guidelines to select severely injured patients for trauma center care. When there is doubt, the patient is best evaluated in a trauma center.

Step 1. Physiologic status thresholds are values of the Glasgow Coma Scale, blood pressure, and respiratory rate from which further deviations from normal are associated with less than a 90% probability of survival. Used in this manner, prehospital values can be included in the admission trauma score and the quality assessment process.

A variety of physiologic severity scores have been used for prehospital triage and have been found to be accurate. Those scores contained in the triage guidelines are believed to be the simplest to perform and provide an accurate basis for field triage based on physiologic abnormality.

Deterioration of vital signs would necessitate transport to a trauma center.

Step 2. A patient who has normal vital signs at the scene of the accident may still have a serious or lethal injury.

Step 3.* It is essential to look for indications that significant forces were applied to the body.

Evidence of damage to the automobile can be a helpful guide to the change in velocity. Intrusion into the passenger compartment from any direction should prompt consideration of the potential for major injury.

Step 4.* Certain other factors that might lower the threshold at which patients should be treated in trauma centers must be considered in field triage. These include the following:

A. Age Patients over age 55 have an increasing risk of death from even moderately severe injuries. Those younger than age 5 have certain characteristics that may merit treatment in a trauma center with special resources for children.
B. Comorbid Factors The presence of significant cardiac, respiratory, or metabolic diseases are additional factors that may merit the triage of patients to trauma centers.

*Each trauma system and its hospitals should use QI programs to determine use of mechanism of injury and comorbid factors as activators for bypass and trauma team activation.

TABLE 62–3. **Revised Trauma Score**

			Score	Start of transport	End of transport
A. Respiratory rate	10–29/min		4		
	729/min		3		
	6–9/min		2		
	1–5/min		1		
	0		0	________	________
B. Systolic blood pressure	≥89 mm Hg		4		
	76–89 mm Hg		3		
	50–75 mm Hg		2		
	1–49 mm Hg		1		
	No pulse		0	________	________
C. Eye opening	Spontaneous		4		
	To voice		3		
	To pain		2		
	None		1	________	________
D. Verbal response	Oriented		5		
	Confused		4		
	Inappropriate words		3		
	Incomprehensible words		2		
	None		1	________	________
E. Motor	Obeys command		6		
	Localizes pain		5		
	Withdraw (pain)		4		
	Flexion (pain)		3		
	Extension (pain)		2		
	None		1	________	________
F. Glasgow Coma Score (Total C + D + E)				________	________
G. Glasgow conversion score	13–15	=	4		
	9–12	=	3		
	6–8	=	2		
	4–5	=	1		
	<4	=	0	________	________
Trauma score total: A + B + G				________	________

Adapted with permission from Champion HR, Sacco WJ, Copes WS, et al: A revision of the trauma score. *J Trauma* 1989; 29(5):624.

The development of and adherence to established triage criteria are essential for maintaining an effective system of optimal care of the trauma patient. Some of the identified triage criteria, such as a systolic blood pressure of less than 90 mm Hg in an adult trauma patient, are considered absolute and should always result in transport to a trauma care facility. Other criteria, such as passenger space intrusion and a 30-inch deformity of an automobile, may be guidelines for considering triage to a trauma center. Because prehospital personnel can actually visualize the situation surrounding a specific trauma incident and the patient's clinical condition, they often elect to transport the patient to a trauma center even though none of the accepted triage criteria are evident.

MECHANISM OF INJURY

Injury to the body occurs when an uncontrolled source of energy comes into contact with the body. Energy may be kinetic (mechanical), thermal, chemical, electrical, or radiating. The absence of oxygen may result in injury, as in drowning or suffocation. The severity of injury is related to the amount of energy released (the force of impact), duration of impact, body part involved, injuring agent, and the presence of associated risk factors such as alcohol or substance abuse, gender, and age of patient. Injury and death result from both unintentional events such as vehicle collisions and sports activities and from deliberate events such as violent aggression and suicide. Because only uncontrolled energy causes injury, it may be assumed that injuries are preventable if the energy source is controlled.

As identified in Table 62–4, adapted from *Accident Facts* (National Safety Council, 1992), kinetic energy accounts for the majority of injury-related deaths and nonfatal injuries. Kinetic energy is defined as mass times velocity squared, divided by 2. Therefore, the greater the mass and velocity (speed), the greater the kinetic energy that must be dissipated to the body structures.

Trauma may be either blunt or penetrating. The incidence of blunt trauma is usually greater in rural and suburban areas, whereas penetrating trauma occurs more frequently in inner-city urban areas.

TABLE 62–4. **Major Categories of Accidental Deaths in 1991 in the United States**

Type of Accident	Death Total
Motor vehicle	43,500
Falls	12,200
Poisoning by solids and liquids	5,600
Drowning	4,600
Fires and burns	4,200
Suffocation	2,900
Firearms	1,400
Poisoning by gases and vapors	800
Other	12,800
Total	88,000

Blunt Trauma

Blunt trauma most frequently results from motor vehicle accidents but may also result from assaults with blunt objects, falls from heights, and sports-related activities. As previously stated, the severity of injury depends on the amount of kinetic energy dissipated to the body and its underlying structures.

Vehicular trauma, as well as some other forms of blunt trauma, results from an acceleration–deceleration type of event. The vehicle in which the body is carried, and therefore the body itself, travels or is accelerated at a certain speed. In normal circumstances, stopping occurs in a timely manner, and the body slows to a stopped state. When the vehicle stops abruptly, however, as in collision with a stationary object, the body continues to travel forward until it comes into contact with a stationary object, frequently the dashboard, windshield, or steering column. Further injury occurs in the presence of rapid deceleration, when the body contents continue to travel within an enclosed space or compartment such as the cranium. At the point of impact between the vehicle and a stationary object, the body continues to move until it strikes a stationary object. Once the body strikes a stationary object it also stops abruptly. At this point the brain may strike the cranium and be thrown back against the opposite side of the cranial vault. This results in a coup-contrecoup type of injury. Rapid deceleration causes tearing and disruption of vessels and tissues.

The severity of injury resulting from a blunt force is also contingent on the duration of impact and the body part involved. The longer the force of impact is in contact with the body, the more kinetic energy dissipates to the body and its underlying structures. Various body tissues and structures respond to kinetic energy in different ways. Low-density, porous tissues and structures such as the lungs tolerate energy transference and often experience little damage. Conversely, high-density solid organs such as the heart, spleen, and liver tolerate energy transference poorly. Additionally, some body structures are encapsulated, and force or pressure applied to these organs actually causes rupture or fragmentation.

Blunt trauma requires expert clinical judgment to assess and diagnose actual and potential injury. Because an injurious impact may leave no external signs on the body, an awareness of the mechanism of injury is of great importance in the care of the blunt trauma patient.

Penetrating Trauma

Penetrating trauma results from objects that are impaled in the body, such as in stabbings, or from ballistic injuries. Penetrating injuries are frequently more easily diagnosed and treated because of the availability of obvious signs of injury.

Stab wounds are low-velocity injuries because the velocity is equal only to the speed with which the object is thrust into the body. Important considerations in stabbings are the length and width of the impaling object and the presence of vital organs in the area of the stab wound. A direct path of injury occurs with an impaled object, resulting in damage only to those vessels and tissues that come into contact with the object.

Ballistic trauma in a civilian environment may consist of either low- or high-velocity injuries. Low-velocity weapons deliver bullets at approximately 1200 to 1500 feet/second and include guns such as the .22 caliber pistol. High-velocity injuries result from missile speeds approximately 2000 feet/second and may be caused by .45 caliber semiautomatic weapons. Obviously, the greater the velocity, the more kinetic energy is dissipated in the body. A high velocity missile causes cavitation as it passes through body tissues. Depending on the range, distance from the weapon to the point of impact, and velocity of the missile, cavitation may be as great as 20 to 30 times the diameter of the bullet. Although the bullet itself does not come into direct contact with tissues outside its path, cavitation can result in tearing and disruption of tissue and vessels.

Missiles that come into contact with internal structures, thus causing a change in pathway, release more energy and result in more damage than missiles passing through the body in a direct path. Bullet design is important in determining the injuring capability of a gunshot wound. Solid point bullets remain intact, whereas hollow point bullets tend to break apart or fragment, resulting in multiple missiles instead of one missile traveling through the body.

As a missile or bullet enters the body and travels to its point of impact, it may pass through clothing, glass, wood, or other objects. These foreign objects are carried into the body and may result in additional injury and potential for infection.

PREHOSPITAL CARE AND TRANSPORT

Reduced morbidity and mortality can be achieved with rapid assessment in the field by prehospital personnel and immediate transport of the trauma victim to an appropriate care facility. Once prehospital personnel arrive at the scene of a traumatic incident, they immediately begin to control the situation and prepare the patient for transport. The time from injury to definitive care is a determinant of survival in many critically injured patients, particularly those with major internal hemorrhage (American College of Surgeons, 1993a). "Scoop and run" or "load and go" are terms that appropriately describe the most beneficial prehospital care for trauma victims. Only minimal care is provided at the scene, with careful attention to the airway (with cervical spine immobilization), breathing, and circulation (ABCs). Large-bore venous access and administration of crystalloid solution may be done during transport. Additional interventions, depending on predetermined protocols, may include application and inflammation of the pneumatic antishock garment (PASG) and life-saving treatment of injuries affecting the ABCs. This includes treatments such as placing an occlusive dressing over an open chest wound, needle thoracotomy to relieve a tension pneumothorax, endotracheal intubation, or cricothyrotomy.

Transport to the appropriate care facility may involve travel past a hospital with a basic emergency care capability. Previous experience both in military and civilian settings indicates that increased survivability results with transport to a hospital where a trauma team concept is in place. Only in situations involving traumatic arrest or inability to establish and maintain a patent airway is transport to a basic emergency facility beneficial to the major trauma patient.

Either ground or air transport is appropriate for the transport of the trauma patient from the scene of the injury to the trauma center. Considerations in the choice of method of transport should include travel time, terrain, availability of air and ground units, capabilities of transport personnel, and weather.

Once the decision is made to transport a patient to a trauma center, the health care professionals composing the trauma team are notified. In most trauma centers the initial resuscitation and stabilization of the trauma patient occur in a designated resuscitation area, usually within the emergency department. The trauma team responds, optimally before patient arrival, and begins preparations based on the report of the patient's actual injuries and clinical status.

EMERGENCY CARE PHASE

Preparation for Patient Admission

Data obtained during the prehospital phase provide valuable information that is essential to ensure a coordinated, life-saving approach to the trauma patient. While the patient is in transit to the hospital, the trauma nurse plays a vital role in ensuring that adequate preparations for the patient have been made. Preparations include notification of the appropriate hospital personnel and verification that the necessary equipment for resuscitation is present and ready for use. Most trauma events are considered "scoop and run" situations with short transport times, but other patients may come to the hospital by private car. For these reasons, the resuscitation area must always be in a state of readiness for the next trauma patient. Delays in implementing definitive critical interventions will adversely affect patient outcomes and may increase mortality to more than 15% for every hour of delay (Cowley & Dunham, 1982). Equipment needed for management of the airway with cervical spine immobilization, breathing, circulatory support, and hemorrhage control must be immediately available and easily accessible.

Most trauma resuscitations take place in a specific area in traditional emergency department settings. Some facilities use a separate resuscitation unit located outside the emergency department and staffed with critical care nurses. Unstable trauma patients may be admitted directly to the operating room for resuscitation and immediate surgical intervention (Butler & Campbell, 1988).

Initial Patient Assessment

Patient survival after a serious traumatic event depends on prompt, rapid, and systematic assessment in conjunction with immediate resuscitative interventions. Priorities of care must be determined based on the patient's clinical presentation, physical assessment, history of the traumatic event, and preexisting disease. A recent study demonstrated that patients' preexisting illnesses can detect outcome independent of other variables including age (Milzman et al., 1993). Evaluation of airway patency, ventilation, and venous access with circulatory support are of prime importance and take precedence over other diagnostic or definitive interventions. Adherence to established protocols for patient assessment and intervention is essential to ensure that management priorities are addressed in an appropriate manner.

PRIMARY SURVEY

The primary survey is the most crucial assessment tool in trauma care. This rapid (1- to 2-minute) evaluation of the patient's ABCs is designed to identify life-threatening injuries accurately, establish priorities, and provide simultaneous therapeutic interventions. The primary survey is a systematic survey of airway patency (with cervical spine immobilization), breathing presence and effectiveness, circulatory status, and gross overview of neurologic disabilities. Table 62–5 details the critical assessment parameters included in the primary survey.

The patient's clothes are removed to facilitate a thorough examination. Clothing may be cut off to prevent delays in assessment and to avoid movement of the patient. Warming measures such as warmed blankets, warmed intravenous solutions, or overhead radi-

TABLE 62–5. **Primary Survey**

Assessment		Observations Indicating Impaired ABC's
Airway	Open and patent Maintain cervical spine immobilization	Shallow, noisy breathing Stridor Cyanosis Nasal flaring Accessory muscle use Inability to speak Drooling Anxiety Decreased level of consciousness Trauma to face, mouth, neck Debris or foreign matter in mouth or pharynx
Breathing	Presence and effectiveness	Asymmetric rise and fall of chest Absent, decreased, or unequal breath sounds Open sucking chest wounds Blunt chest injury Dyspnea Cyanosis Respiratory rate <8 to 10/min or >40 min Accessory muscle use Anxiety Tracheal shift Distended neck veins Paradoxical chest wall motion
Circulation	Presence of major pulses Presence of external hemorrhage	Weak, thready pulse >120 beats/min Pallor Blood pressure <90 mm Hg Capillary refill >2 sec Obvious external hemorrhage Decreased level of consciousness Distended neck veins
Disability	Gross neurologic status Pupil size, equality, and reactivity to light	Glasgow Coma Scale Agitation

ant warmers are instituted to prevent hypothermia. Temperature, heart rate, respiratory rate, and auscultated blood pressure are obtained at this time and documented as a baseline for analysis of trends during the resuscitation phase. Application of an automatic blood pressure monitor and oxygen saturation device may be done to provide ongoing assessments. Insertion of an indwelling urinary catheter and nasogastric tube is done at this time if not contraindicated by the patient's condition.

Secondary Survey

The secondary survey is initiated after the primary survey has been accomplished and all actual or potential life-threatening injuries have been identified and resolved. The secondary survey is a methodical head-to-toe evaluation of the patient using the assessment techniques of inspection, palpation, percussion, and auscultation. After the anterior portion of the body has been evaluated, the trauma team logrolls the patient to each side and the posterior side is examined for hidden injuries (Table 62–6). At this time information about actual and potential injuries is noted and used to establish diagnostic and treatment priorities. Radiologic and laboratory studies are done according to a standardized trauma protocol or based on assessment of suspected injuries. The sequence of diagnostic procedures is influenced by the stability of the patient's condition, mechanism of injury, and identified injuries. As data are obtained, the team leader determines the need for consultation with specialty physicians such as neurosurgeons, orthopedists, urologists, or others. Supportive interventions such as splinting of extremities, wound care, and administration of tetanus prophylaxis and antibiotics are done at this time. Finally, the secondary survey provides data that enable the team leader to establish priorities for definitive care and ongoing management of the trauma patient.

INTERVENTIONS

Maintain Airway Patency

Airway obstruction, whether it occurs at the time of injury or develops during resuscitation, is a potential problem for every trauma patient. Maintaining a patent airway and adequate ventilation is an essential element of trauma management. The tongue, due to posterior displacement, frequently obstructs the airway. Other causes of obstruction are foreign debris such as blood clots or vomitus, and maxillofacial fractures with bleeding or secretions. Patients with a depressed sensorium and an absent gag reflex also require interventions for airway management. Injury to the throat or neck can result in damage to vital airway structures. Control of the airway in the trauma patient is based on the need for protection, ventilation, and oxygenation (Baxt, 1985). Basic airway interventions are listed in Table 62–7.

MANUAL TECHNIQUES OF AIRWAY CLEARANCE. Because posterior displacement of the tongue commonly results in airway obstruction, opening the airway is often easily accomplished by the simple manual technique of a jaw thrust or chin lift. These maneuvers do not hyperextend the neck or compromise the integrity of the cervical spine. These are temporary interventions that serve to move the mandible anteriorly and create a patent airway.

The airway must be cleared of any foreign material such as blood, vomitus, bone fragments, or teeth. A rigid, large-bore suction device such as a tonsillar suction catheter is used to remove debris. Suction of the nares with a soft suction catheter should be performed with caution in patients with midfacial trauma and

TABLE 62–6. **Secondary Survey**

Area	Inspection	Palpation	Percussion	Auscultation
Head: Scalp Skull Face Eyes/ears Nose Mouth	Soft tissue injury Deformities Edema Asymmetry of face Open bite Periorbital edema Otorrhea Rhinorrhea Bloody drainage Extraocular movements Subcutaneous air Visual acuity Eye injuries	Bony deformities of facial bones or skull Scalp wounds Subcutaneous air Crepitus Pain Decreased sensation of face		
Neck	Soft tissue injury Tracheal position Distended neck veins Ask about pain, hoarseness, dysphagia	Crepitus Subcutaneous air Tracheal position Cervical spine tenderness or deformities		
Chest	Soft tissue injury Open sucking wound Subcutaneous air Intercostal retractions Symmetry of chest Respiratory rate, effort Seatbelt marks Impaled objects	Crepitus Subcutaneous air Bony deformities Chest wall excursion	Dullness Hyperresonance	Absent or diminished breath sounds Distant heart or gastric sounds
Abdomen and flanks*	Soft tissue injury Distension Seatbelt marks Impaled objects Contour Discolorations	Rigidity Distension Pain: diffuse or localized	Dullness Hyperresonance	Bowel sounds in all four quadrants
Pelvis or perineum	Soft tissue injury External genitalia injury Blood at urinary meatus Vaginal bleeding Rectal bleeding Suprapubic masses Priapism	Pelvic instability Femoral pulses Rectal sphincter tone Prostate position Vaginal integrity Open fractures		
Extremities	Soft tissue injury Amputation Crush injury Deformity: open or closed Motor/sensory	Diminished or absent pulses Crepitus Pain or tenderness		
Back	Soft tissue injury to buttocks, posterior thighs, and flanks	Thoracic, lumbar sacral spine pain, tenderness, deformity		

*Note: The sequence of examination of the abdomen is inspection, auscultation, palpation, and percussion.

potential cribriform plate fractures. Suction should be limited to 15- to 20-second intervals to prevent hypoxemia associated with the procedure. Oxygenation with 100% concentrations before suctioning is recommended to limit hypoxia.

ARTIFICIAL AIRWAYS. Oropharyngeal and nasopharyngeal airways are the simplest artificial airway adjuncts used in patients with spontaneous respirations and adequate ventilatory effort. Both devices help maintain a patent airway by preventing posterior displacement of the tongue. Although relatively easy to insert, these adjuncts are not without disadvantages. The oropharyngeal airway may create further airway obstruction if it is too small. It may also be placed incorrectly and positioned against the tongue, pressing it onto the posterior wall of the pharynx. Too large an orpharyngeal airway may stimulate the gag reflex and cause vomiting with possible aspiration. The oropharyngeal airway is not used in awake patients with a gag reflex.

The nasopharyngeal airway, or nasal trumpet, is relatively contraindicated in patients with midfacial trauma and suspected fractures of the cribriform plate. The device is well tolerated in the awake patient.

TABLE 62–7. **Basic Airway Interventions**

Goal	Process	Expected Outcome
Maintain patent airway Avoid manipulation of cervical spine and stimulation of gag reflex	Open airway by performing jaw thrust or chin lift Gently suction with tonsillar tip catheter or finger sweep oral cavity Maintain open airway with appropriate artificial airway adjunct Provide 100% oxygen by mask Ventilate with bag-valve-mask device if indicated Prepare to assist with oral/nasal intubation, criothyroidotomy Control secretions, bleeding, vomiting Prepare for nasogastric tube insertion Monitor airway status frequently for evolving or recurring problems	Improved airway clearance evidenced by: No stridor Clear bilateral breath sounds Decreased accessory muscle use No cyanosis

TRACHEAL INTUBATION. Tracheal intubation is the ideal nonsurgical airway management technique and allows for complete control of the airway. Tracheal intubation may be achieved by either the oral or nasal route. However, for the patient in distress, priority must be given to oxygenation before intubation is attempted. Immediate ventilation with 100% oxygen by a bag-valve-mask (BVM) device is vital in the hypoxic patient and should be initiated simultaneously with preparation for intubation.

In the presence of documented or suspected cervical spine injury, oral tracheal intubation is avoided to prevent possible manipulation of the neck. However, for apneic patients without midfacial trauma, oral tracheal intubation can be performed with in-line manual immobilization of the neck provided by an assistant. Disadvantages of oral tracheal intubation include possible manipulation of the cervical spine, incorrect tube placement in the esophagus or right mainstem bronchus, vocal cord trauma, or trauma to the intraoral structures.

Nasal tracheal intubation is performed in breathing trauma patients, particularly when the urgency of the resuscitation procedure does not allow time to obtain preliminary cervical spine x-rays. Spontaneous respirations are required to perform nasal tracheal intubation successfully because the absence of respirations creates a difficult "blind" intubation situation. The nasal route is contraindicated in patients with maxillofacial trauma or suspected basilar skull fractures. Disadvantages of nasal intubation are epistaxis, injury to the nasal turbinates, and introduction of infection. Topical use of a vasoconstrictive agent such as Neo-Synephrine before nasal tracheal intubation may decrease the incidence of bleeding (Grande, 1988).

Postintubation ventilation with 100% oxygen is initiated immediately after placement of the tube. Correct position of the tube is verified by auscultation of bilateral breath sounds and chest x-ray.

Selection of the appropriate size of endotracheal tube is an important consideration. The tube with the largest diameter that can be easily inserted is the best size. In general, the recommended size is 7.0 to 8.0 mm internal diameter (I.D.) for women and 8.0 to 9.0 mm I.D. for men. Advantages of the 7.0 mm I.D. or larger tube include improved oxygenation and the ability to perform fiber-optic bronchoscopy through the tube.

CRICOTHYROTOMY. Inability to intubate the trauma patient is an indication for surgical intervention to control the airway. Conditions that may require cricothyrotomy are maxillofacial trauma, laryngeal fractures, facial or upper airway burns, and severe oropharyngeal hemorrhage. The anatomic position of the avascular cricoid membrane makes this a relatively bloodless, safe, and rapid procedure. The adult cricothyroid membrane is located inferior to the thyroid cartilage and above the cricoid cartilage. Access to the trachea through the cricothyroid membrane can be accomplished by either needle cricothyrotomy or surgical cricothyrotomy.

Needle cricothyrotomy is a percutaneous technique that entails insertion of a 12GA to 14GA needle into the trachea below the level of the obstruction. Intermittent transtracheal ventilation is then carried out using a 50-psi oxygen source. This temporary method is useful for only 30 to 45 minutes before the accumulation of carbon dioxide reaches unacceptable levels.

Surgical cricothyrotomy is an alternative method of tracheal access in which an incision is made through the skin into the cricothyroid membrane. The incision is dilated and secured with a tracheostomy tube of 5.0 to 7.0 mm I.D.

The choice of airway management technique is based on familiarity with the procedures, the clinical condition of the patient, and hemodynamic stability. The resuscitation nurse has an important responsibility in assessing and maintaining ongoing monitoring of airway patency. A patent airway is the cornerstone of a successful trauma resuscitation.

PHARMACOLOGIC AGENTS. Combative critical trauma patients with an altered level of consciousness may require the use of a paralytic agent to facilitate intubation. The two most frequently used agents in the emergent phase of airway management are succinylcholine and pancuronium bromide (Morris, 1988). These medications are used with caution and only if the practitioner is prepared to provide ventilatory assistance through a BVM device or cricothyrotomy if attempts at intubation are unsuccessful.

Succinylcholine is a commonly used short-acting depolarizing muscle relaxant that causes complete flaccid paralysis within 1 minute of intravenous (IV) administration. Depolarization rapidly causes fasciculations, or muscle contractions, of the upper torso, followed by complete paralysis. As the muscles become refractory to stimulation, the intercostal muscles and diaphragm are fully paralyzed. It is possible to achieve intubation within 1 to 2 minutes after IV administration of succinylcholine. Duration of the effects of succinylcholine is a brief 8 to 10 minutes. The dosage for IV succinylcholine is 1.0 to 1.5 mg/kg.

Pancuronium bromide is a long-acting, nondepolarizing neuromuscular blocking agent that causes flaccid paralysis. The onset of action occurs within 45 to 60 seconds after IV administration and lasts up to 45 to 60 minutes. The peak effect for intubation occurs 3 minutes after administration of the usual dosage of 0.5 to 2.0 mg/kg. Pancuronium bromide does not cause the muscle fasciculations associated with succinylcholine and may be desirable in patients when increased intracranial, intraocular, or intragastric pressure is of concern (Hochbaum, 1986). The prolonged duration of action may be contraindicated in selected trauma situations.

The short duration of effect of succinylcholine may make it the paralytic agent of choice in the resuscitation phase. Pretreatment with pancuronium is one method of preventing succinylcholine-induced fasciculations that may be detrimental to the patient's clinical condition. The dosage for pretreatment with pancuronium is 0.01 and 0.03 mg/kg given 1 to 3 minutes before administration of succinylcholine (Morris, 1988).

There is some evidence that IV lidocaine may lessen the rises in intracranial pressure (ICP) and blood pressure that occur during intubation (Grande, 1988). The pharmacologic properties of lidocaine may decrease the systemic vascular response that occurs during intubation, provide prophylaxis against ventricular arrhythmias in the hypoxic patient, and cause beneficial cerebral vasoconstriction. For the head-injured patient, the dose of lidocaine is 1.0 to 1.5 mg/kg given intravenously 3 to 5 minutes before intubation.

In some instances rapid-sequence induction of general anesthesia is used to control the airway. This method of administering anesthesia is a useful technique for preventing aspiration in the head-injured patient. Rapid-sequence induction requires prior preparation of medications, suction, and intubation and ventilatory equipment. Preoxygenation with 100% oxygen for 1 to 2 minutes is a critical first step in the process. A defasciculating dose of pancuronium is administered to limit increases in intracranial and intragastric pressures. General anesthesia is then induced using thiopental 3 to 5 mg/kg intravenously. At least 3 minutes after administration of pancuronium, the patient is given succinylcholine 1 to 2 mg/kg (Morris, 1988; Strange, 1987). As consciousness is lost, cricoid pressure compresses the esophagus and inhibits aspiration of gastric contents.

Ineffective Breathing Patterns

Interventions to restore normal breathing patterns are directed toward the specific injury or underlying cause of respiratory distress, with the goal of improving ventilation and gas exchange. Basic nursing interventions for patients with ineffective breathing patterns include application of supplemental oxygen with ventilatory assistance if needed, preparation for intubation, and evaluation of specific interventions.

Evaluation of interventions and ongoing monitoring of these patients are performed frequently to assess respiratory rate and effort, heart rate and rhythm, breath sounds, skin signs, tracheal position, and neck vein distension. Fluid intake and output is monitored to guide the resuscitation process. The nurse also assists in obtaining diagnostic studies such as arterial blood gases and chest x-rays to ensure the effectiveness of specific interventions. Etiologies of traumatic injuries that result in ineffective breathing patterns and specific interventions for them are listed in Table 62–8.

Impaired Gas Exchange

Impaired gas exchange follows airway obstruction as the most crucial problem of the trauma patient. Etiologies of impaired gas exchange include a decrease in inspired air, retained secretions, lung collapse or compression, atelectasis, or accumulation of blood in the thoracic cavity.

Fluid volume deficit secondary to hemorrhage also affects adequate gas exchange. Patients wtih multiple systemic injuries or trauma to the central nervous system or chest and victims in hemorrhagic shock are all at risk for impaired gas exchange.

Interventions are directed toward maintaining a patent airway and optimizing gas exchange. Trauma patients require high-flow supplemental oxygen to promote optimal gas exchange. Specific nursing actions include monitoring the patient's respiratory status for respiratory rate, ventilatory effort, and alterations in breathing patterns and assisting with removal of secretions. Other interventions include preparation for intubation, mechanical ventilation, and other measures used to improve gas exchange such as needle thoracostomy, chest tube insertion, and restoration of circulating blood volume.

Decreased Cardiac Output

The most common etiology of impaired cardiac output in the trauma patient is hypovolemic shock due to acute blood loss. The causes may be external, as with hemorrhage, or internal, as with hemothorax, hemoperitoneum, or massive pelvic fractures. Other etiologies that may cause a decrease in cardiac output are tension pneumothorax, resulting in compression of the heart and great vessels, and pericardial tamponade,

TABLE 62–8. **Specific Interventions for Ineffective Breathing Patterns**

Etiology	Interventions
Tension pneumothorax	Prepare for decompression by needle thoracotomy with a 12GA to 16GA needle in second intercostal space in midclavicular line on affected side Prepare for chest tube insertion
Pneumothorax	Prepare for chest tube insertion on affected side
Open sucking wound	Seal wound with occlusive dressing and monitor chest for signs of tension pneumothorax Remove one corner of dressing if respiratory distress develops; prepare for chest tube insertion
Massive hemothorax	Establish two 14GA to 16GA IV lines with crystalloids Obtain blood for type and crossmatch Prepare for large chest tube insertion Prepare autotransfusion device Administer blood or blood products as ordered Anticipate and prepare for emergency open thoracotomy
Pulmonary contusion	Prepare for early intubation and mechanical ventilation Administer IV crystalloids at a rate guided by the absence of signs of shock
Flail chest	Stabilize chest wall: may position on affected side with head of bed elevated or apply manual pressure while preparing for definitive internal stabilization Prepare for early intubation and mechanical ventilation Prepare for chest tube insertion Administer IV crystalloids at a rate guided by the absence of signs of shock Administer analgesics as ordered Assist with intercostal nerve block
Tracheobronchial injury	Elevate head of bed to facilitate breathing Prepare for chest tube insertion Anticipate bronchoscopy
Spinal cord injury	Avoid hyperextension or rotation of neck Maintain complete spinal immobilization Prepare for application of cervical traction tongs or halo device Monitor motor and sensory function Monitor for signs of neurogenic shock
Decreased level of consciousness	Position head midline with head of bed elevated Administer osmotic diuretics, steroids, anticonvulsants, or paralytic agents as ordered Anticipate CT scan

resulting in impairment of cardiac filling and ventricular ejection. Table 62–9 demonstrates the predictability of stages of hemorrhagic shock (American College of Surgeons, 1993b).

The trauma nurse must maintain a high index of suspicion for the development of hemorrhagic shock and carefully monitor the patient to prevent the vicious cycle of cellular death and organ failure that occurs if successful resuscitation is not accomplished. Adequate fluid resuscitation is of critical importance. Other interventions are directed toward the specific cause of impaired cardiac output, such as tension pneumothorax or pericardial tamponade.

TENSION PNEUMOTHORAX. Tension pneumothorax is a rapidly fatal emergency that is easily resolved with early recognition and intervention. It occurs when an injury to the chest allows air to enter the pleural cavity

TABLE 62–9. **Estimated Fluid and Blood Requirements* (Based on Patient's Initial Presentation)**

	Class I	Class II	Class III	Class IV
Bloos loss (mL)	up to 750	750–1500	1500–2000	2000 or more
Blood loss (%BV)	up to 15%	15–30%	30–40%	40% or more
Pulse rate (beats/min)	<100	>100	>120	140 or higher
Blood pressure	Normal	Normal	Decreased	Decreased
Pulse pressure	Normal or increased	Decreased	Decreased	Decreased
Respiratory rate (breaths/min)	14–20	20–30	30–40	>35
Urine output (mL/hr)	30 or more	20–30	5–15	Negligible
CNS–mental status	Slightly anxious	Mildly anxious	Anxious and confused	Confused and lethargic
Fluid replacement (3:1 rule)	Crystalloid	Crystalloid	Crystalloid + blood	Crystalloid + blood

*For a 70-kg male.

Data from the American College of Surgeons, Committee on Trauma. (1993). *Advanced trauma life support course: Instructors manual.* Chicago, American College of Surgeons.

but not to escape. Air accumulates in the pleural space with each inspiration and as intrathoracic pressure increases, the lung collapses. The increased pressure then causes compression of the heart and great vessels toward the unaffected side as evidenced by mediastinal shift and distended neck veins. The resulting decreased cardiac output and impaired gas exchange are manifested by severe respiratory distress, hypotension, tachycardia, absence of breath sounds on the affected side, tracheal deviation, and cyanosis as a late manifestation.

On recognition of a tension pneumothorax, the immediate intervention is a needle thoracotomy using a 12GA to 16GA needle in the second intercostal space in the midclavicular line on the injured side to relieve intrapleural pressure. When evaluating patients with open sucking chest wounds that have been covered, care is taken to monitor the possible development of a tension pneumothorax. If this occurs, the occlusive dressing is immediately removed. A chest tube is placed after decompression of the chest by needle thoracostomy, and a chest x-ray is then obtained. Definitive intervention is never delayed in order to confirm the presence of a tension pneumothorax by x-ray.

PERICARDIAL TAMPONADE. Pericardial tamponade is a life-threatening condition caused by rapid accumulation of fluid (usually blood) in the pericardial sac. As the intrapericardial pressure increases, cardiac output is impaired due to decreased venous return and compression of cardiac activity. Blood, if unable to flow into the right side of the heart, causes increased central venous pressure (CVP) and distended neck veins. Classic signs of this injury are hypotension, muffled or distant heart sounds, and elevated venous pressure reflected in distended neck veins. All three signs of this condition (Beck's triad) may not be present in each case of pericardial tamponade.

Pericardial tamponade is generally caused by penetrating trauma to the chest. However, it should be suspected in any patient with blunt trauma and multisystem injuries who is in shock and does not respond to aggressive resuscitation. Pericardial tamponade is often difficult to diagnose in the presence of other injuries that may also be the source of decreased cardiac output.

Diagnosis of pericardial tamponade is achieved by performing a pericardiocentesis. This procedure may also provide therapeutic intervention by decompressing the pericardium. Needle aspiration of the pericardial sac is done with a 16GA to 18GA catheter over a needle, such as a spinal needle, attached to a 35- to 50-mL syringe with a three-way stopcock. Aspirated pericardial blood usually will not clot unless the heart itself has been penetrated. Arterial blood pressure may dramatically improve with removal of as little as 20 to 30 mL of blood.

Equipment for an emergency thoracotomy must be immediately available if cardiac arrest occurs. After stabilization, the patient is transferred to the operating room for definitive surgical intervention.

Hypovolemia

Early recognition and aggressive management of hemorrhagic shock are essential for successful resuscitation of the multiply injured patient. Therapeutic interventions are directed toward arresting the hemorrhage and replacing circulating blood volume to restore adequate tissue perfusion.

As always, a patent airway and adequate ventilation are priority interventions. Efforts to correct loss of circulating blood volume are addressed next. Continued blood loss due to obvious external hemorrhage is controlled with direct pressure, elevation of an extremity, or compression of pressure points. Tourniquets are avoided to prevent compromise of circulation to the extremity and possible loss of the limb.

The pneumatic antishock garment (PSAG) is a pneumatic counterpressure device used to control hemorrhage by tamponading intraabdominal, pelvic, and lower extremity bleeding. It also provides splinting and stabilization of pelvic and leg fractures. The PASG increases systemic vascular resistance (SVR) and prevents further blood loss into the abdomen and legs and may provide translocation of a small amount (150 to 130 mL) of blood into the central circulation. The use of the PASG is contraindicated in patients with signs and symptoms of pulmonary edema and a known rupture of the diaphragm. Its use is controversial in patients with a head injury with increased intracranial pressure (ICP) or thoracic injuries (Cardona et al., 1994).

VENOUS ACCESS. Venous access and infusion of volume is the key to optimal resuscitation in the patient with hemorrhagic shock. At least two large-bore (14GA to 16GA) peripheral IV lines are necessary. Percutaneous lines located in the upper extremities are preferred. Central venous access lines or venous cutdown may be necessary due to vasoconstriction and venous collapse. A central line is more beneficial as a resuscitation monitoring tool and is indicated after the initial resuscitation phase. In general, the most appropriate venous access route is the largest one that can be established rapidly.

FLUID RESUSCITATION. Rapid infusion of fluids is done through large internal diameter blood tubing with a short catheter to facilitate flow. Lines placed by cutdown may use an 8-French catheter, and pressure bags are helpful. Rapid infusion devices are available that facilitate fluid infusion of 1000 and 1500 mL/min.

A universal problem involved in rapid infusion of fluids is that of hypothermia. Blood or fluid warming devices frequently cannot infuse fluid rapidly enough to allow adequate resuscitation. It is desirable to warm any fluid infused above the diaphragm to prevent the hazardous effects of cold fluid on the myocardium.

Small warming ovens are available to store limited amounts of crystalloid solutions.

Hemorrhage causes blood loss from the intravascular space and fluid loss from the extravascular space as fluid shifts occur. Volume resuscitation is directed toward replacing both losses. Although agreement on replacing red blood cell depletion seems to be universal, the choice of an asanguineous fluid remains very controversial (Baxt, 1985; Cardona et al., 1994; Giescke et al., 1990). Colloids are better maintained initially in the intravascular space due to their oncotic properties. Administration of crystalloids requires approximately three times as much volume and will also replace losses in the extravascular spaces. The expense and complications associated with the use of each solution remain the basis for debate.

Fluid resuscitation is guided by the patient's physiologic response to the therapy. If signs of class I or class II shock are present, rapid infusion of crystalloid solution is given at a ratio of 3 mL for every 1 mL of suspected blood loss (Baxt, 1985). Plasma expanders such as hetastarch may be used to augment crystalloids in patients who do not show signs of immediate improvement with crystalloids alone. Close continuous monitoring of hemodynamic status, including capillary refill time, CVP, and urine output (50 mL/hr in the adult), is necessary to direct further efforts in volume resuscitation and prevent harmful unnecessary fluid overload (Imm & Carlson, 1993).

Continued signs and symptoms of shock such as falling hematocrit, deteriorating Pa_{O_2} and pH, decreasing urine output (less than 50 mL/hr), and increasing arterial lactate levels indicate the need for more aggressive measures. It is important to remember that hemoglobin and hematocrit values may be unreliable in gauging the degree of shock initially because it may be up to 4 hours before changes are evident. As metabolic acidosis worsens, decreasing Pa_{O_2} and pH demonstrate the body's response to anaerobic metabolism.

The decision to administer blood is based on the patient's response to initial fluid therapy (American College of Surgeons, 1993b). Type-specific or group O negative blood is used in cases of exsanguination. Fully crossmatched blood is administered as soon as it is available. Preparation of type and crossmatched blood takes 30 to 60 minutes and is appropriate only for patients who have been stabilized with crystalloids and colloids.

Autotransfusion of shed blood, or autologous blood, is an alternative method of blood replacement that can be used in the patient with hemorrhage caused by hemothorax or other intrathoracic injuries. This inexpensive, safe, and rapid technique involves accumulation of the patient's own blood into a suction device. The blood is then anticoagulated and filtered and is immediately available for reinfusion. Autotransfusion is an excellent way to provide fresh, warm blood that carries no risk of antibody problems and eliminates the risk of transmittable infectious diseases.

Diagnostic peritoneal lavage may be done during the resuscitation phase to determine whether the intraperitoneal space is the source of bleeding. If the patient responds to fluid replacement and abdominal injury is suspected, the diagnostic study of choice is computed tomography (CT) scan of the abdomen.

Spinal Cord Injury

Appropriate immobilization and management of the patient with multisystem trauma will aid in preventing further possible injury. Field measures of immobilization are maintained during the initial assessment and resuscitation efforts. Conscious patients are reassured and alerted not to move.

A complete neurologic examination is performed after evaluation of the patient's ABCs. Portable lateral x-rays of the cervical spine are obtained, and the patient is prepared for possible spinal CT scan to rule out occult injury. Dislocations of the spine are reduced as soon as possible by means of postural reduction by either cervical traction tongs, halo traction devices, or surgical fusion. Other current modalities include the administration of IV methylprednisolone in a 30 mg/kg bolus followed by an IV infusion of 5.4 mg/kg/hr over the subsequent 23 hours (Bracken et al., 1990; Ellis, 1993).

Ongoing assessment includes evaluation of airway and ventilatory function, heart rate and rhythm, blood pressure, and urine output. With the loss of sympathetic output, most patients will be hypotensive and bradycardic, representing a neurogenic shock state. In addition, there is potential for further deterioration in spinal cord function due to secondary injury. Frequent assessment and documentation of motor and sensory status of all extremities is imperative. The use of a standardized spinal cord surveillance tool and flowsheet facilitates comparison of findings to previous assessments and enhances communication of patient status data among health care team members (Stenger, 1993).

Altered Cerebral Tissue Perfusion

Cerebral perfusion pressure depends on adequate blood flow and oxygenation of the brain. It is important to consider whether protection of the brain from further insult during the initial resuscitation phase is needed. Cerebral ischemia is associated with increased mortality, and interventions are directed toward providing appropriate levels of blood flow, oxygen, and glucose to the brain (Gennarelli, 1984).

Aggressive volume resuscitation is necessary to return the hemorrhagic shock patient to a normotensive state quickly. Care must be exercised, however, to avoid overhydration and increased ICP. Supplemental oxygen is essential, and tracheal intubation with mechanical ventilation is often required to optimize arterial oxygen content.

Use of a pulmonary artery (PA) catheter is instrumental in the monitoring and management of intravascular volume and the patient's response to treatment. In addition, the PA catheter provides the ability to obtain oxygen consumption studies that can reflect an overall index of total body metabolism.

Monitoring of jugular bulb blood oxygen saturation can be used to monitor the hemodynamic and metabolic demands of the brain and the brain's response to interventions. Although not universally accepted or used by a large number of medical centers, it has shown promise in reflecting the brain's response to hyperventilation, diuretic therapy, and overall patient management (Sikes & Segal, 1994).

Cerebral perfusion pressure (mean arterial pressure − mean ICP) trends are also used to guide therapy. A CPP greater than 50 mm Hg is generally acceptable; however, one protocol recommends a CPP in the range of 70 to 80 mm Hg for the patient with a severe head injury (Rosner & Daughton, 1990).

There is some controversy as to the most appropriate position of the head of the bed to maximize CPP. Some advocate the head of the bed in flat position (Rosner & Coley, 1986) and others advocate the head of the bed elevated to 30 degrees (Feldman et al., 1992). One recommendation is that each patient be assessed for optimal head elevation based on their ICP, CPP, systolic arterial blood pressure, and cerebral blood flow (March et al., 1990).

Increased ICP causes further cerebral ischemia and requires prompt attention. Hyperventilation to a Pa_{CO_2} of between 26 and 30 mm Hg is an effective method of decreasing intracerebral blood volume by regulating cerebral vessel size although there is now some concern that it may potentiate cerebral ischemia (Rosner & Daughton, 1990). Endotracheal suctioning has been shown to increase ICP (Crosby & Parsons, 1992; Rudy et al., 1986). The current recommendation is that endotracheal suctioning be limited to two passes with a suction catheter after preoxygenation to minimize a rise in ICP (Rudy et al., 1991). Prophylactic lidocaine administered intravenously or intratracheally has also been used to diminish tracheal stimulation and concomitant rises in ICP associated with endotracheal suctioning (Brucia et al., 1992). Osmotic diuretics such as mannitol to decrease brain water are also recommended for serious or deteriorating head injuries.

The initial resuscitation and stabilization of the major trauma patient will result in a tentative diagnosis by the trauma surgeon. In most situations, the patient will require further diagnostic evaluation, CT scan, or angiography or will be transported to the surgical suite for immediate surgical intervention and then transferred to the critical care unit.

Once in the critical care unit, care of the major trauma patient is similar to that of any other patient requiring continual monitoring, evaluation, and intervention. A major difference is that other patients have a definitive diagnosis and have not undergone severe and sudden injury.

Care of the victim of trauma should include consideration of the mechanism of injury and an awareness of concurrent injuries frequently associated with a specific mechanism of injury. Monitoring for significant additional injuries is a priority during the initial critical care phase. Death occurring days and even weeks after the initial insult frequently is a result of specific complications.

CRITICAL CARE PHASE

Once the trauma patient has entered the critical care phase for continued stabilization and recovery, the critical monitoring of hemodynamic parameters, analysis of assessment trends, and the institution and evaluation of therapeutic interventions become the focus of patient care. Patient assessment data are collected using a systems approach. This involves continued assessment of the neurologic, respiratory, cardiovascular, gastrointestinal, renal, and skin and extremity systems. Additional information on the individual patient's metabolic, pain response, and psychosocial needs must also be gathered. Continual assessment data help to guide therapies aimed at correcting identified problems or injuries and preventing or minimizing actual or potential postinjury complications.

Nursing care of the trauma patient in the critical care phase continues to be directed toward maintenance of the patient's ABCs along with interventions consistent with the specific injury. Care of specific traumatic injuries, such as neurologic or spinal cord injuries and other issues, including pain management, are addressed in other chapters throughout this book.

The patient with multisystem injuries is at risk for developing a myriad of complications due to the body's compromised condition, prolonged immobility, and the long-term rehabilitation associated with trauma care. The most common secondary complications encountered during this critical phase of care are related to respiratory impairment, infection, renal dysfunction, and high nutritional demands. These secondary complications are often sequelae to the severe shock state associated with major blood loss resulting from traumatic injury (Klein, 1990; Koziol et al., 1988).

Respiratory Impairment

According to an early study completed by Blaisdell and Schlobohm (1973), respiratory complications contribute to 75% of hospital deaths of trauma patients. These complications are related most commonly to causes such as adult respiratory distress syndrome (ARDS), deep vein thrombosis (DVT) and resultant pulmonary embolism (PE), and fat embolism syndrome. Critical nursing assessment skills requiring observation for often subtle and discrete changes in trends are needed to identify patients developing actual or potential complications.

ADULT RESPIRATORY DISTRESS SYNDROME

Adult respiratory distress syndrome is a complication that has been discussed in the literature since World War II. The syndrome gained greater recognition during the postresuscitation treatment of soldiers in the Vietnam War. Today, the syndrome continues to carry a 50% to 60% mortality (Slotman et al., 1988). Factors directly linked to the development of ARDS are closely related to the medical problems of shock of any type, multisystem trauma with extensive tissue destruction, thoracic trauma, multiple orthopedic injuries, massive transfusions, sepsis, and major head injuries (Montgomery et al., 1985). The syndrome is manifested by a cluster of symptoms that may occur physiologically 2 to 48 hours after a traumatic injury. However, recognizable clinical symtoms may not occur for 5 or more days after injury.

In the beginning stages of the syndrome, increases in pulmonary hydrostatic pressure or pulmonary vessel permeability occur. The exact cause of this occurrence continues to be investigated, but theories have centered around neutrophilic infiltrates in the lung (Hallgren et al., 1984), the formation of thromboxane A_2 (Slotman et al., 1988), and the release of bradykinin (DeOleveira, 1988). These substances are known to cause changes in the membrane integrity of the pulmonary microvascular or alveolar symptoms. As membrane permeability increases, pulmonary interstitial and alveolar edema occur. The normal alveolar surfactant action decreases due to this edema formation, and functional lung units begin to collapse. The end result is a ventilation–perfusion ($\dot{V}/\dot{Q}$) deficit or mismatch, pulmonary shunting (Q_S/Q_T), an increase in physiologic dead space, and development of lung consolidation (Atkins et al., 1994; Cardona et al., 1994).

The critical care nurse must first identify those patients at risk for developing this syndrome because early initiation of therapy is crucial for successful recovery. Knowledge of the types of traumatic injuries that lead to the development of ARDS is vital. Patients who have suffered a flail chest, pulmonary contusions, cardiac contusions, prolonged hopovolemic shock, major head injuries, gastric aspiration, or sepsis are at high risk for developing ARDS. Overinfusion of balanced salt solutions during the resuscitative phase of care also contributes to the development of ARDS.

Symptomatology of the development of ARDS usually occurs in the critical care phase. Indicators may include hypoxemia, rising carbon dioxide levels, increased respiratory distress, and new diffuse bilateral chest infiltrates (Table 62–10).

Treatment interventions for ARDS are directed toward correcting the underlying cause, maintaining ventilatory support, decreasing pulmonary congestion, and supporting the patient's cardiovascular system. Any specific chest injury or fluid overhydration must be corrected. Mechanical ventilation, if not instituted during the resuscitative phase, is required in a majority of patients with ARDS. Positive end-expiratory pressure (PEEP) is used to increase the patient's PaO_2 levels while using a lower inspired concentration of oxygen. PEEP is usually set at a low to moderate level of less than 15 cm H_2O. The higher levels of PEEP, above 25 cm H_2O, are reserved for patients who demonstrate pulmonary shunting problems (Q_S/Q_T) and associated hypoxemia (Cardona et al., 1994). PEEP can be delivered to the patient by either controlled or intermittent mechanical ventilation. Other approaches to improving ventilation and oxygenation include pressure control ventilation, where a breath is delivered with a decelerating flow pattern until a preset pressure is reached; inverse ratio ventilation, where inspiration is prolonged and expiration is shortened; and high-frequency ventilation, where small tidal volumes are delivered at high respiratory rates (60 to 100 breaths/min). Recently, examination of oxygen delivery and oxygen consumption have been useful in evaluating the patient's response to therapy. Maximizing oxygen delivery and minimizing oxygen recovery may decrease the frequency of multiple organ failure in these patients (Knox, 1993).

Cardiovascular compromise can result from the use of PEEP, leading to a decrease in cardiac output. It is imperative that cardiac output be maintained to prevent further patient deterioration. Manipulation of preload, contractility, and afterload functions of the heart through administration of pharmacologic agents may be necessary to support a stable hemodynamic system.

Cardiac contractility is enhanced by the use of dopamine and dobutamine. These medications augment cardiac output through inotropic actions while maintaining the lowest possible increased myocardial oxygen consumption. Dopamine 2 to 5 μg/kg/min and dobutamine 3 to 5 μg/kg/min increase cardiac output. Isoproterenol at a dosage of 0.25 to 1.00 mg/kg/min is helpful in reducing right heart afterload.

The afterload function of the heart can be altered by the use of nitroprusside. Nitroprusside improves left ventricular filling pressures and stroke volume. However, nitroprusside may worsen pulmonary shunting through its vasodilatory effects. Vasoconstriction in response to hypoxia is a compensatory mechanism that can actually help preserve the $\dot{V}/\dot{Q}$ ratio. The arterial vasodilating effect of nitroprusside can reverse this compensatory mechanism.

Fluid therapy in the trauma patient with ARDS or with the potential for developing ARDS requires careful monitoring. A balanced electrolyte solution is the most common type of fluid used to correct the hypovolemia associated with trauma patients. The amount of infused fluid must be sufficient to maintain the patient's cardiac output and intravascular volume

TABLE 62–10. **Features of Adult Respiratory Distress Syndrome**

History compatible with known risk factors
Respiratory distress with hypoxemia
Tachypnea (>30 breaths/min)
Dyspnea
Radiographic evidence of diffuse chest infiltrates
Increased shunt fraction ($Q_S/Q_T > 15\%–20\%$)
Increased physiologic dead space ($V_D/V_T > 0.6$)
Decreased static compliance (<30 mL/cm H_2O)

without increasing intrapulmonary edema. Continual monitoring of the patient's pulmonary artery pressure, pulmonary wedge pressure, and daily weight will help trend response and guide fluid therapy. Transfusion of red blood cells may be required not only to provide cardiovascular support, but also to augment oxygen delivery and minimize cellular oxygen debt.

DEEP VEIN THROMBOSIS

Deep vein thrombosis is a significant complication of traumatic injury. The risk of DVT in young patients with multiple trauma has been estimated to be 20%. Patients with acute head injury or spinal cord injuries have at least a 40% chance of developing DVT and a 1% to 4% risk of a fatal pulmonary embolism. Because DVT is a marker for PE, a reduction in DVT will result in a reduction in PE (Consensus Conference, 1986). Research has demonstrated that advanced age, type and severity of injury, prolonged immobilization, number of transfusions, and elevated partial thromboplastin time (PTT) on admission are associated with an increased incidence of DVT in trauma patients (Dennis et al., 1993).

Deep vein thrombosis usually occurs in the lower extremities. Thrombus formation is enhanced in the presence of vessel damage, venous stasis, and hypercoagulability. The thrombosus may be dislodged by increased venous pressure, direct trauma, or sudden muscle action. The dislodged clot becomes an embolus and travels through the body's vasculature until it lodges in either the pulmonary artery or its smaller branches. Once the embolus becomes lodged, blood flow is obstructed distally and tissues distal to the obstruction become hypoxic. Pulmonary vessels constrict in response to the hypoxia and the result is a $\dot{V}/\dot{Q}$ mismatch (ventilation greater than perfusion), causing hypoxemia.

Patients at high risk for the development of DVT and PE are closely monitored. Clinical manifestations of DVT are outlined in Table 62–11. Although clinical assessment is helpful, research has shown that early aggressive diagnostic screening and DVT prophylaxis in high-risk patients is both safe and effective in reducing the incidence of DVT and PE in orthopedic, spinal cord injury, and closed head injury patients (Dennis et al., 1993). Patients at high risk for developing DVT include those with spinal fractures, lower extremity long-bone fractures, severe head injury, burns, pelvic fractures, and major venous injury requiring repair (Dennis et al., 1993).

TABLE 62–11. **Clinical Manifestations of DVT**

Pain and tenderness
Swelling
Homan sign (discomfort in calf on forced dorsiflexion of foot)
Venous distention
Palpable cord
Discoloration

TABLE 62–12. **Clinical Manifestations of PE**

Dyspnea—sudden onset
Chest pain—sudden onset
Rapid, shallow respiratory rate
Increasing shortness of breath
Auscultation of bronchial breath sounds
Pale, dusky, cyanotic skin coloring
Increased anxiety
Decreased level of consciousness
Other signs of hypovolemic shock
- Decreasing systolic blood pressure
- Narrowing pulse pressure
- Tachycardia

Patients at high risk for DVT can be screened noninvasively with venous Doppler flow studies, duplex scanning (compression ultrasound) or impedance plethysmography (two-dimensional ultrasound). In addition, DVT prophylaxis is recommended in the high-risk trauma patient. This includes early ambulation, sequential compression devices, low-dose subcutaneous heparin (5,000 units every 8 to 12 hours), or the placement of a Greenfield filter in the inferior vena cava to trap the emboli before they reach the pulmonary vasculature. Up to 14% of trauma patients have been reported as unable to receive DVT prophylaxis due to their injuries (Shockford et al., 1990).

Pulmonary embolism is often a fatal complication of DVT. Therefore, high-risk patients are continuously monitored for signs and symptoms associated with PE. These include new-onset dyspnea, changes in respiratory rate and effort, and changes in cerebral and tissue perfusion (Table 62–12). Symptoms of pulmonary infarction also include hemoptysis, pleuritic pain, and fever.

Supporting laboratory data demonstrate changes in the patient's arterial blood gas concentrations. Hypoxemia, Pa_{O_2} levels of less than 60 mm Hg, hypocapnia, decreased oxygen saturation, and an alkalotic pH are associated with the development of PE. Electrocardiographic (ECG) changes include development of tachycardia, peaked T waves, a widened QRS complex, ST- and T-wave changes, and right axis deviation. Chest x-rays may be normal initially with later evidence of atelectasis or infarction. A ventilation–perfusion ($\dot{V}/\dot{Q}$) lung scan may be either normal or may indicate a perfusion defect. The most definitive objective test is a pulmonary angiogram defining the area of obstruction.

Therapy for PE is directed toward improving gas exchange and pulmonary tissue perfusion. Positioning the patient in a high Fowler position facilitates breathing and increases diaphragmatic excursion. Administration of supplemental oxygen provides additional oxygen to correct impaired gas exchange and enhance tissue perfusion. Patients with severe PE require additional interventions of intubation, mechanical ventilation, and institution of PEEP. Dissolution of the embolus itself using anticoagulant heparin therapy is desirable. Initial therapy consists of IV administration of 5000 to 10,000 units of heparin as a loading dose. Subsequent doses are delivered intravenously at 1500 units/hr or 25 units/kg/hr. PTT is maintained at 2 to 2½ times normal to prevent the future development of clots. Other interventions include cardiovascular support with vasopressors, inotropic agents, and volume expanders. Interventions for pain control are an important consideration.

FAT EMBOLISM

Development of the fat embolism syndrome is a risk factor that accompanies traumatic injury of the long bones, pelvis, and multiple skeletal fractures. The syndrome develops between 24 and 48 hours postinjury. One theory of the development of fat embolism syndrome focuses on a mobilization mechanism. As a bone is stressed or injuried, bone marrow fat globules from the fracture site are released into torn vessels and the systemic circulation. A second theory, the physiochemical theory, revolves around the production and release of free fatty acids in abnormal amounts following skeletal injury. These free fatty acids are implicated in the destruction of pulmonary endothelial tissue. Microvascular permeability within the pulmonary vessels then occurs, resulting in pulmonary edema. Whichever theory is correct, bone marrow fat has been recovered by biopsy or at autopsy within the systemic microvessels.

Hallmark clinical signs that accompany fat embolism syndrome begin with development of a low-grade fever followed by a new-onset tachycardia, dyspnea, increased respiratory rate and effort, and abnormal arterial blood gas concentrations (Table 62–13). If pulmonary distress continues, the patient will begin to demonstrate symptoms of cerebral hypoxia such as changes in level of consciousness or coma. ECG findings include development of a right bundle-branch block, S waves of prominent size in lead I, Q waves in lead III, T-wave inversion, depressed RST segments and as dysrhythmias. Upper body, oral mucosa, or conjunctival petechiae are pathognomonic indicators of the development of fat embolism syndrome, although these are uncommon findings. The exact etiology of the development of petechiae is unknown; however, it has been postulated that fat globules cause superficial capillary obstruction and rupture. Lipuria, fat in the urine, indicates a serious case of fat embolism syndrome.

TABLE 62–13. **Clinical Manifestations of Fat Embolism Syndrome**

Tachycardia (greater than 100 beats/min)
Hypotension
Abrupt change in behavior or mentation
Dyspnea
Tachypnea
Hypoxemia
Radiologic evidence of pulmonary infiltrates
Productive cough

Treatment for fat embolism syndrome is directed toward the preservation of pulmonary function and maintenance of cardiovascular stability. Administration of supplemental oxygen, intubation, mechanical ventilation, and the use of PEEP may be required to restore or maintain pulmonary perfusion and ventilation. Monitoring the patient's cardiovascular stability must be continued throughout the critical care phase, paying attention to the development of ECG and hemodynamic changes.

Several studies indicate that corticosteroid therapy may protect against the development of fat embolism syndrome in patients at risk for this complication (Kallenbach et al., 1987; Schonfeld et al., 1983). A major concern, however, is the possibility that steroids may result in complications, such as infection, that are worse than the syndrome.

Ideally, prevention of fat embolism is the best treatment. Stabilization of fractures of the extremities to minimize both bone movement and the release of fatty products from the bone marrow must be accomplished as early as possible. Either internal or external fixation devices are used depending on the location and extent of the fractures.

Sepsis

Sepsis is the most common cause of death in noncoronary critical care units. Nosocomial infections are a major cause of sepsis among critically ill patients. Increased risk of nosocomial infections is associated with chronic disease, immunosuppression, prolonged hospital stay, presence of invasive catheters, and wounds (Donowitz et al., 1982).

Trauma patients are at high risk for development of sepsis due to the presence of open wounds, open fractures, and massive tissue injury that provide a site for the introduction of bacteria. Gram-negative nosocomial infections are more common than gram-positive infections. In adult patients pulmonary, urinary tract, gastrointestinal, and wound infections are most often seen (Hazinski et al., 1993).

Gram-negative bacteria contain a lipopolysaccharide in their cell wall known as endotoxin. Endotoxin is released during infection and bacterial lysis. Endotoxin stimulates macrophages, monocytes, and neutrophils, which then produce a variety of vasoactive mediators. These mediators cause a diffuse vasodilation, increased capillary permeability, and a change in capillary blood flow that impair cellular and tissue oxygen utilization and contribute to multiple organ dysfunction.

The American College of Chest Physicians (ACCP) and the Society of Critical Care Medicine (SCCM) have published consensus terminology to describe and define the clinical presentation and progression of sepsis (ACCP-SCCM Consensus Conference Committee,

1992). Systemic inflammatory response syndrome (SIRS), sepsis, severe sepsis, and septic shock are the terms proposed.

Systemic inflammatory response syndrome is a diffuse inflammatory response to a variety of chemical insults including but not limited to infection. It is characterized by the acute development of more than one of the following: fever (temperature $> 38°C$) or hypothermia (temperature $< 36°C$); tachycardia (heart rate $> 90/min$); tachypnea (respiratory rate $> 20/min$ or $Paco_2 < 32$ mm Hg); and leukocytosis (WBC count $>$ 12,000/mm^3), leukopenia (WBC count $<$ 4000/mm^3), or the presence of $>$ 10% immature neutrophils. Sepsis is defined as the systemic response to infection. It is characterized by two or more of the conditions characterized by SIRS. A positive blood culture is not necessary for the diagnosis of sepsis as it is only seen in approximately 50% of septic patients (AACP-SCCM Consensus Conference Committee, 1992). The clinical presentation of both SIRS and sepsis occur as a result of diffuse vasodilation, increased capillary permeability, and maldistribution of blood flow (Hazinski et al., 1993). Therapy includes fluids and antibiotics as well as close monitoring.

Severe sepsis is associated with organ dysfunction, hypoperfusion, or hypotension as evidenced by lactic acidosis, oliguria, or acute change in mental status (confusion, combativeness, lethargy). Hypoxemia, bilateral pulmonary infiltrates, elevated liver function enzymes to twice normal, paralytic ileus, and gastrointestinal bleeding may be seen. Coagulation studies may be abnormal with thrombocytopenia and elevated prothrombin time and PTT. Fibrinogen degradation products greater than 1:40 or D-Dimers greater than 2.0 confirm the presence of disseminated intravascular coagulation (Hazinski et al., 1993).

Cardiovascular dysfunction is apparent in the patient with severe sepsis. A hyperdynamic state occurs with increased cardiac output and decreased SVR as the body mobilizes its defenses against the offending organisms. Decreased oxygen delivery and increased oxygen consumption contribute to inadequate tissue perfusion and the development of lactic acidosis. Increased cellular metabolic demands lead to proteolysis, increased gluconeogenesis, increased serum insulin concentrations, and lipolysis. Therapy includes antibiotics, hemodynamic monitoring, fluid therapy, and vasoactive drugs to maximize oxygen delivery and minimize oxygen demand.

Septic shock is defined as severe sepsis associated with hypotension and perfusion abnormalities despite fluid resuscitation. Lactic acidosis, oliguria, acute changes in mental status, or other signs of organ dysfunction indicate perfusion abnormalities. Cardiac output remains normal or increased and SVR remains low. Pharmacologic support is necessary to maintain blood pressure.

Early identification of sepsis and initiation of appropriate therapies may decrease the mortality associated with this complication. Interventions are directed toward decreasing the cellular oxygen debt, maintaining cardiovascular stability, and reducing bacterial endotoxins. Supplemental oxygen can be administered by either nasal cannula or face mask. Endotracheal or nasotracheal intubation with mechanical ventilation, PEEP, or pressure support ventilation may be required to maintain Pao_2 levels and decrease pulmonary shunting.

Cardiovascular hemodynamics need to be maintained and supported. Administration of the pharmacologic agents dobutamine or dopamine may be required to increase myocardial contractility and systemic vascular resistance. Adequate fluid replacement, avoiding overhydration, with a balanced electrolyte solution is critical for maintaining tissue perfusion. Continuous monitoring of arterial blood pressure, mean arterial pressure, CVP, pulmonary artery pressure, and pulmonary capillary wedge pressure and calculation of cardiac output, cardiac index, and oxygen delivery and oxygen consumption are measures used in evaluation of hemodynamic status.

Many pharmacologic therapies are being tested that interfere with mediator release and function (Littleton, 1993). Administration of appropriate antibiotic therapy to reduce circulating endotoxins must be started as early as possible. Such therapy may be done prophylactically in the resuscitation phase of care or following development of an increase in body temperature. Use of sterile technique for dressing changes, care of drains, line insertion sites, or other invasive procedures is mandatory to minimize bacterial introduction into an already compromised trauma patient.

Acute Renal Failure

Renal function may be impaired in the trauma patient due to either the systemic effects of trauma or actual injury to the renal system. Acute renal failure (ARF) results in the inadequate excretion of the end-products of cellular metabolism and an impaired ability to regulate fluid, electrolyte, and pH balance. ARF is a sequela of sustained circulating volume loss (prerenal failure), direct injury to the kidney (intrarenal failure), or obstruction in the drainage system (postrenal failure). The trauma patient is at risk for the development of ARF from any of these causes.

Trauma patients who have experienced a shock state or low cardiac output have experienced a significant reduction in renal blood flow. This decreased blood flow reduces the normal glomerular filtration rate and urine production as well as other functions of the kidney, thereby leading to prerenal failure. Prerenal failure is best managed with IV fluids to improve cardiac output and improve renal perfusion.

Intrarenal failure, also known as acute tubular necrosis, is caused by untreated prerenal failure, causing renal tissue damage through ischemia, actual renal tissue damage, nephrotoxicity resulting from administration of nephrotoxic antibiotics, or development of rhabdomyolysis. When large muscles are damaged, as often occurs with traumatic injury, myoglobin is released into the systemic circulation. As the blood passes through the renal structures, myoglobin becomes trapped in the tubules, causing rhabdomyolysis and acute tubular necrosis. Rhabdomyolysis is best managed by maintaining adequate fluid volume during resuscitation to prevent decreased renal blood flow and increased concentration of myoglobin (Cheney, 1994).

Postrenal failure may be the result of injury, increased pressure, or obstruction from displaced postrenal structures. Administration of medications, such as ganglionic blocking agents or antihistamines, can interrupt the autonomic nervous supply to the postrenal structures, thereby causing obstruction.

Assessment data must be continually monitored to analyze the trends of renal function. A decrease in urine output is a hallmark sign of ARF. Urinalysis provides information about specific gravity and the presence of substances such as protein, myoglobin, and white or red blood cells. Serum creatinine and blood urea nitrogen (BUN) levels are indicators of renal function. Elevated levels of creatinine and BUN are indicative of decreased renal function. Creatinine clearance is a direct reflection of glomerular filtration and is therefore the standard for monitoring renal function.

Five phases occur in patients with ARF: onset, oliguric phase, nonoliguric phase, diuresis, and recovery (Finn, 1990). The onset is the actual event that initiates the pathologic process of renal failure. The kidney is still able to compensate for changes in renal blood flow or filtration pressures. The oliguric phase is reflected in a urine output of less than 25 to 30 mL/hr. Patients experience fluid retention and electrolyte imbalances. This phase usually lasts from 10 to 20 days. Nonoliguric or high-output renal failure may be seen in patients with less severe insult to the tubules. Electrolyte abnormalities occur with poorly concentrated urine. Urine output may be as high as 1 liter/hr; however, creatinine clearance remains low. This phase lasts from 5 to 8 days.

In the next phase, diuresis, urine output is also elevated to 125 to 150 mL/hr. As the kidneys begin to regain their function, electrolyte imbalances are corrected and the urine is more concentrated. Diuresis occurs because of hypervolemia and the hyperosmolar state created by the elevated urea level.

The final phase is recovery, which may last anywhere from 3 to 12 months. Urine output and renal function gradually return to normal. However, some patients may later develop chronic renal failure.

Treatment for trauma patients with ARF depends on the cause and severity of the failure. Goals of management focus on compensating for the deterioration in renal function. Fluid, electrolyte, and pH balance may be exacerbated by postresuscitation fluid overload, making management particularly difficult.

Trauma patients may benefit from early dialysis. Trauma patients have high protein requirements due to stress and wound healing. Protein produces urea as a metabolic end-product; when elevated, urea can contribute to azotemia (Weiss et al., 1989). Types of dialysis used in managing azotemia in trauma patients include hemodialysis and continuous renal replacement therapies (continuous arteriovenous hemofiltration and continuous arteriovenous hemodialysis (Stark, 1994).

Altered Nutrition: Less Than Body Requirements

Nutritional demands of the trauma patient are significantly increased due to alterations in metabolism. The healthy, noninjured person normally maintains a nutritional balance between the anabolic and catabolic processes that exist in the body. Because of the high energy demands and metabolic alterations that often are present in critically injured patients, the catabolic process tends to predominate, thereby increasing a nutritional imbalance.

Carbohydrates are the preferred energy source within the body. The final transport compound of carbohydrate metabolism is glucose, which provides energy in the form of adenosine triphosphate. Excess amounts of carbohydrates or glucose are stored in the liver, muscle, and fat in the form of glycogen. If necessary, in time of stress or increased metabolic demands, glycogen is released from these storage areas to meet energy or metabolic demands. Proteins, a second energy source, are also stored in the body and provide supplemental calories when necessry. Proteins function in the body's transport system and chemical reactions. Osmotic pressure gradients are maintained by available proteins. However, the main function of proteins is related to tissue synthesis. Fats, the third energy source, serve as a major energy reservoir. Fats act as an insulating and protective component for the body.

Once an injury occurs, systemic energy demands are increased. The body's metabolism is increased by activation of the sympathetic response. Other conditions such as hypoxia, pain, decreased fluid volume, anxiety, tissue injury, and decreased resistance to infection further stimulate the sympathetic response, and a hypermetabolic stress state is induced. Available glucose is used rapidly as the provider substrate for energy, followed by initiation of glycogenolysis, the metabolism of glycogen stores. As high energy demands continue, formation of glucose from stored protein and fats (gluconeogenesis) occurs. This period of metabolic response to injury has been termed the ebb or shock phase and encompasses a period of time during the first 24 to 48 hours after injury. During the ebb phase there may actually be an overall weight gain due to fluid retention.

The second, or flow phase, begins at the end of the ebb phase and lasts until recovery. This phase is the catabolic phase. The patient's metabolic rate increases and usually peaks 5 to 10 days postinjury. The average increase in metabolic rate (above the basal metabolic rate) ranges from 12% to 20% (Askanazi et al., 1980; Quebbeman & Ausman, 1982). During the flow phase, protein catabolism is continuous, and fat often acts as the main energy substrate. Nutritional imbalances easily occur due to the body's increased caloric and protein needs and the patient's inability to ingest nutritional supplements. Patients may demonstrate decreased body mass, increased metabolic needs, increased oxygen consumption, increased carbon dioxide production, delayed wound healing, and a weakened immune system (Klein, 1990).

Baseline nutritional assessments are done early in the critical care phase. Assessment data should include a history of the patient's previous caloric and protein intake, weight-height ratios, anthropometric measures of the triceps skin fold or midarm circumference, and biochemical measures such as creatinine-height index, serum proteins, nitrogen balance, total lymphocyte count, and metabolic rate (Posa, 1994).

Nutritional replacement for the trauma patient should be instituted no later than 3 to 4 days post injury. Patients who receive no nutritional support for a prolonged period are susceptible to the development of septic complications, including bacteremia and pneumonia (Moore & Jones, 1986). The route of administration, and the rate and concentration of nutritional replacement used depend on the severity and type of injury and the expected recovery period. These decisions are best accomplished using a team approach. This team should include the physician, nurse, and nutritional support personnel. Nutritional support may be administered by the oral, enteral, or parenteral route; the oral route is indicated in noncomplicated cases.

The enteral route includes the use of an oral-nasal gastric feeding tube, a jejunostomy tube, or, for long-term use, a gastrostomy tube. If the oral-nasal gastric route is used, care must be taken to place the tube correctly. This can be accomplished by visualizing the feeding tube in the stomach on x-ray. A weighted Silastic tube in a small French size is ideally used because it will prevent unnecessary pressure on the nostrils and esophagus. Patients who are receiving nutritional support through the enteral route need to be monitored for tolerance to the supplements; those receiving concentrated hyperosmolar feeding solutions may experience diarrhea. Intolerance to nutritional formulas is demonstrated by patient complaints of nausea or vomiting, abdominal distension, diarrhea, or abdominal pain. If the patient is unable to communicate, tolerance of the tube feeding is evaluated by assessing for abdominal distension and monitoring tube feeding residuals every 2 to 4 hours and as needed. Residual volumes greater than 100 to 150 mL consistently or gastric distention and/or vomiting may signify the need to change the feeding route (Posa, 1994). Before administration of nutritional feedings, the head of the bed should be elevated to 45 degrees to facilitate infusion of the solution and prevent aspiration. Feedings may be administered by either bolus or continuous infusion. Osmolality of the feeding formula may range from 300 mOsm (isotonic) to 850 mOsm (hypertonic). The starting formula osmolality is usually isotonic or a diluted (one-half to one-fourth) hypertonic strength (Cardona et al., 1994).

Parenteral nutritional support is administered by either partial or total methods. Partial parenteral nutritional support is infused through the peripheral veins. It is a short-term administration method and must be used in conjunction with administration of lipids. The dextrose concentration is usually between 5% and 10% (Cardona et al., 1994).

Total parenteral nutritional (TPN) support is instituted in patients who are unable to resume gastrointestinal nutritional intake for a minimum of 5 days due to GI trauma, paralytic ileus, bowel obstruction, and/or small bowel fistulas. TPN support is infused through tubing placed in the superior vena cava. The glucose content is a hyperosmolar concentration. The insertion site and the TPN line itself must be given meticulous care to prevent infection related to the presence of the hyperosmolar formula. Lipid administration should also occur in conjunction with TPN nutritional support. The patient must be monitored for tolerance to TPN as well as serum and urine osmolality levels. Urine is monitored for increased glucose and acetone levels, which indicate glucose intolerance. Liver function tests must be monitored because TPN can cause alterations in liver function.

Decisions about nutritional support for the trauma patient are made on an individual basis. The goal is to provide the patient with balanced nutritional support. Excess replacement can produce physiologic stress on the body by increasing oxygen consumption and carbon dioxide production. Additionally, fatty infiltrates may develop in the liver, producing other complications. Inadequate replacement often results in body protein loss, delayed wound healing, and decreased resistance to infectious processes (Richardson, 1987).

CONTINUING CARE

Trauma patients require very specialized nursing care during their critical care hospitalization. The majority of these patients were young, healthy, productive citizens before injury. MacKenzie and associates (1988) studied the functional ability of 479 trauma patients 1 year after injury. This study indicated that, of head- or brain-injured patients (the most common type of traumatic injury), 5% were still convalescing 1 year post-injury, and 75% of those who had been employed in full-time work before injury had returned to full-time employment. This, however, leaves a significant percentage of trauma patients unable to return to pre-injury levels of function. The psychosocial aspects of trauma patient care need to be incorporated into the critical care phase of hospitalization. This again is best accomplished by a multidisciplinary approach involving the physician, nursing staff, social service personnel, physical therapists, occupational therapists, and family members.

REFERENCES

ACCP-SCCM Consensus Conference Committee. (1992). American College of Chest Physicians/Society of Critical Care Medicine Consensus Conference: Definitions for sepsis and organ failure and guidelines for the use of innovative therapies in sepsis. *Critical Care Medicine, 20*(6), 864–874.

American College of Surgeons. Committee on Trauma. (1993a). *Resources for optimal care of the injured patient.* Chicago: American College of Surgeons.

American College of Surgeons. Committee on Trauma. (1993b). *Advanced trauma life support course: Instructors manual.* Chicago: American College of Surgeons.

Askanazi, J., Carpentier, Y. A., Elwyn, D. H., et al. (1980). Influence of total parenteral nutrition on fuel utilization in injury and sepsis. *Annals of Surgery, 191*(1), 40–46.

Atkins, P. J., Egloff, M. E., & Willms, D. C. (1994). Respiratory consequences of multisystem crisis: The adult respiratory distress syndrome. *Critical Care Nursing Quarterly, 16*(4), 27–38.

Baxt, W. G. (1985). *Trauma: The first hour.* Norwalk, CT: Appleton-Century-Crofts.

Blaisdell, F., & Schlobohm, R. (1973). The respiratory distress syndrome: A review. *Surgery, 74,* 251–262.

Bracken, M., Shephard, M. J., Collins, W., et al. (1990). A randomized, controlled trial of methylprednisolone or naloxene in the treatment of acute spinal injury. *New England Journal of Medicine, 322*(20), 1405–1411.

Brucia, J. J., Owen, D. C., & Rudy, E. B. (1992). The effects of lidocaine on intracranial hypertension. *Journal of Neuroscience Nursing, 24,* 205–214.

Butler, V., & Campbell, S. (1988). Resuscitation in the operating room. *Trauma Quarterly, 5*(1), 57–61.

Cardona, V. D., Hurn, P. D., Mason, P. J. B., et al. (1994). *Trauma nursing: From resuscitation through rehabilitation* (2nd ed). Philadelphia: W. B. Saunders.

Champion, H. R., Sacco, W. J., Copes, W. S., et al. (1989). A revision of the trauma score. *Journal of Trauma, 29*(5), 623–629.

Cheney, P. (1994). Early management and physiologic changes in crush syndrome. *Critical Care Nursing Quarterly, 17*(2), 62–73.

Committee on Trauma Research. Commission of Life Sciences, National Research Council and the Institute of Medicine. (1985). *Injury in America: A continuing public health problem.* Washington, DC: National Academy Press.

Consensus Conference. National Institutes of Health (1986). Prevention of venous thrombosis and pulmonary embolism. *Journal of American Medical Association, 256,* 744–749.

Cowley, R. A., & Dunham, M. (1982). *Shock trauma/Critical care manual.* Baltimore: University Park Press.

Crosby, L., & Parsons, L. (1992). Cerebrovascular response of closed-head injury patients to a standardized endotracheal tube suctioning and manual hyperventilation procedure. *Journal of Neuroscience Nursing, 24,* 40–49.

Dennis, J. W., Menawat, S., Von Thron, J., et al. (1993). Efficacy of deep vein thrombosis prophylaxis in trauma patients and identification of high-risk groups. *Journal of Trauma, 35*(1), 132–138.

DeOleveira, G. (1988). Adult respiratory distress syndrome (ARDS): The pathophysiological role of catecholamine-kinin interactions. *Journal of Trauma, 28*(2), 246–253.

Donowitz, L. G., Wenzel, R. P., & Hoyt, J. W. (1982). High risk of hospital-acquired infections in the ICU patient. *Critical Care Medicine, 10*(6), 355–357.

Ellis, M. F. (1993). High-dose steroid therapy offers improvement in spinal cord injuries. *AACN Clinical Issues in Critical Care Nursing, 4*(3), 566–572.

Feldman, Z., Kanter, M., Robertson, C., et al. (1992). Effect of head elevation on intracranial pressure, cerebral perfusion pressure, and cerebral blood flow in head-injured patients. *Journal of Neurosurgery, 76,* 207–211.

Finn, W. F. (1990). Diagnosis and management of acute tubular necrosis. *Medical Clinics of North America, 74*(4), 873–890.

Gennarelli, T. A. (1984). Emergency department management of head injuries. *Emergency Medicine Clinics of North America, 2*(4), 749–760.

Giescke, A. H., Grande, C. M., & Whitten, C. W. (1990). Fluid therapy and resuscitation of traumatic shock. *Critical Care Clinics, 6,* 61–72.

Grande, C. M. (1988). Airway management of the trauma patient in the resuscitation area of the trauma center. *Trauma Quarterly, 5*(1), 30–49.

Hallgren, R., Borg, T., Venge, P., et al. (1984). Signs of neutrophil and eosinophil activation in adult respiratory distress syndrome. *Critical Care Medicine, 12,* 14–18.

Hazinski, M. F., Iberti, T. J., MacIntyre, N. P., et al. (1993). Epidemiology, pathophysiology and clinical presentation of gram-negative sepsis. *American Journal of Critical Care, 2*(3), 224–237.

Hochbaum, S. R. (1986). Emergency airway management. *Emergency Medicine Clinics of North America, 4*(3), 411–425.

Imm, A., & Carlson, R. W. (1993). Fluid resuscitation in circulatory shock. *Critical Care Clinics, 9*(2), 313–333.

Kallenbach, J., Lewis, M., Zaltzman, M., et al. (1987). Low-dose corticosteroid prophylaxis against fat embolism. *Journal of Trauma, 27*(10), 1173–1176.

Klein, D. G. (1990). Physiologic response to traumatic shock. *AACN Clinical Issues in Critical Care Nursing, 1*(3), 505–521.

Knox, J. B. (1993). Oxygen consumption–oxygen delivery dependence in adult respiratory distress syndrome. *New Horizons 1*(3), 381–387.

Koziol, J., Rush, B. F., Smith, S. M., et al. (1988). Occurrence of bacteremia during and after hemorrhagic shock. *Journal of Trauma, 28*(1), 10–16.

Littleton, M. T. (1993). Trends in agents used for the management of sepsis. *Critical Care Nursing Quarterly, 15*(4), 33–46.

MacKenzie, E., Siegel, J. H., Shapiro, S., et al. (1988). Functional recovery and medical costs of trauma: An analysis by type and severity of injury. *Journal of Trauma, 28*(3), 281–297.

March, K., Mitchell, P., Grady S., et al. (1990). Effects of backrest position on intracranial and cerebral perfusion pressures. *Journal of Neuroscience Nursing, 22,* 375–381.

Milzman, D. P., Hinson, D., & Magnant, C. W. (1993). Overview and outcomes. *Critical Care Clinics, 9*(4), 633–656.

Montgomery, A. B., Stager, M. A., Carrico, C. J., et al. (1985). Causes of mortality in patients with the adult respiratory distress syndrome. *American Review of Respiratory Disease, 132,* 485–489.

Moore, E. F., & Jones, T. N. (1986). Benefits of immediate jejunostomy feedings after major abdominal trauma: A prospective randomized study. *Journal of Trauma, 26*(10), 874–881.

Morris, I. R. (1988). Pharmacologic aids to intubation and the rapid sequence induction. *Emergency Clinics of North America, 6*(4), 753–768.

National Academy of Sciences, National Research Council (1966). *Accidental death and disability: The neglected disease of modern society.* Washington, D.C.: Government Printing Office.

National Safety Council (1992). *Accident facts.* Itasca, IL: Author.

Posa, P. J. (1994). Nutritional support of the critically ill patient: Bedside strategies for successful patient outcomes. *Critical Care Nursing Quarterly, 16*(4), 61–79.

Quebbeman, E. J., & Ausman, R. K. (1982). Estimated energy requirements in patients receiving parenteral nutrition. *Archives of Surgery, 117,* 1281–1284.

Richardson, J. (1987). *Trauma: Clinical care and pathophysiology.* Chicago: Year Book.

Rosner, M., & Coley, I. (1986). Cerebral perfusion pressure, intracranial pressure and head elevation. *Journal of Neurosurgery, 65,* 636–641.

Rosner, M., & Daughton, S. (1990). Cerebral perfusion pressure management in head injury. *Journal of Trauma, 30*(8), 933–941.

Rudy E., Baun, M., Stone, K., et al. (1986). The relationship between endotracheal suctioning and changes in intracranial pressure: A review of the literature. *Heart & Lung, 15*(5), 488–494.

Rudy, E. Turner, B., Baun, M., et al. (1991). Endotracheal suctioning in adults with head injury. *Heart & Lung, 20*(6), 667–674.

Schonfeld, S. A., Ploysongsang, Y., DiLisio, R., et al. (1983). Fat embolism prophylaxis with corticosteroids: A prospective study in high-risk patients. *Annals of Internal Medicine, 99*, 438–443.

Shockford, S. R., Davis, J. W., Hollingsworth-Fridlund, P., et al. (1990). Venous thromboembolism in patients with major trauma. *The American Journal of Surgery, 159*, 365–369.

Sikes, P. J., & Segal, J. S. (1994). Jugular bulb oxygen saturation monitoring for evaluating cerebral ischemia. *Critical Care Nursing Quarterly, 17*(1), 9–20.

Slotman, G. J., Burchard, K. W., D'Arezzo, A., et al. (1988). Ketoconazole prevents acute respiratory failure in critically ill surgical patients. *Journal of Trauma, 28*(5), 648–654.

Stark, J. (1994). Acute renal failure in trauma: Current perspectives. *Critical Care Nursing Quarterly, 16*(4), 49–60.

Stenger, K. M. (1993). Surveillance of spinal cord motor and sensory function. *Nursing Clinics of North America, 28*(4), 783–792.

Strange, J. M. (1987). *Shock trauma care plans.* Springhouse, PA: Springhouse Corporation.

Trauma Nursing Coalition. (1992). *Nursing care of the trauma patient.* Chicago: Emergency Nurses Association.

Weiss, L., Danielson, B. G., Wikström, B., et al. (1989). Continuous arteriovenous hemofiltration in the treatment of 100 critically ill patients with acute renal failure: Report on clinical outcome and nutritional aspects. *Clinical Nephrology, 31*(4), 184–189.

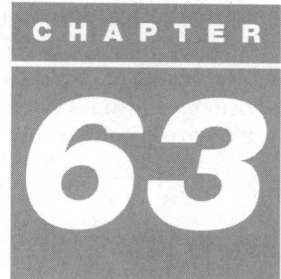

Patients With Systemic Inflammatory Response Syndrome

John M. Clochesy

During the past 40 years, the most common cause of death in many intensive care units has been shock secondary to sepsis (Parrillo, 1989b). The systemic inflammatory response syndrome (SIRS) is the systemic response to any severe clinical incident. Extensive tissue damage and necrosis, the invasion of microorganisms or various cellular by-products from these conditions trigger the human body's inflammatory response system. Sepsis with its causative factors creates perfusion and metabolic abnormalities. Manifestations of SIRS include tachycardia, fever or hypothermia, tachypnea, and inadequate organ perfusion (shock) or organ failure (Bone et al., 1989).

SIGNIFICANCE

Yearly, an estimated $200 million and 1.4 million hospital days are expended due to nosocomial bacteremias (Hoyt, 1990). In the 1950s, nosocomial infections were not well understood. However, as the use of indwelling urinary catheters associated with the management of dysfunctional urinary bladder syndromes became more common in the late 1940s, mechanisms of catheter-associated urinary tract infections became evident. The use of various invasive devices has proven that any microorganism, given a port of entry, can produce an infection.

In the past, the circulatory instability seen in septic shock was attributed solely to circulating microorganisms (bacteria, viruses, fungi, rickettsia, spirochetes, protozoa, parasites). However, current research attributes the pathogenesis of septic shock to various chemical mediators produced during the body's inflammatory response (Parrillo, 1989a).

Neither sepsis nor septic shock is a reportable disease. Therefore, an accurate estimate of the current incidence is not available (Parrillo, 1989b). However, baseline data can be estimated from the complications associated with gram-negative bacteremia. The Centers for Disease Control and Prevention estimates that 140,000 cases of gram-negative bacteremia occur annually in the United States (Roach, 1990). Yet bacteremia does not always create systemic complications. Complications occur when patients' cardiovascular systems are compromised by circulating chemical mediators released from the inflammatory response. Regardless of the cause, mortality statistics for all septic conditions remain high. When the diagnosis of sepsis is followed by prompt therapy, mortality ranges from 20% to 60%. However, if management is delayed or ineffective, mortality increases to 90% to 95%.

Approximately 1 out of 100 hospitalized patients develops sepsis, and 40% of these experience septic shock. The reasons for this are multifactorial (Parrillo, 1989b). First, invasive devices or procedures increase the risk of microbial invasion. Second, the use of antineoplastic and immunosuppressive therapies decreases patients' immune response, allowing bacterial cells to infect the circulatory system. Third, the widespread use of antimicrobial therapy creates drug-resistant pathogens. Last, modern technology, in all aspects of health care, has lengthened the lifespan of our society to the point where individuals are living longer with chronic diseases.

SUSCEPTIBILITY

To delineate a single causative factor of septic shock is often impossible. Signs and symptoms of the inflammatory response can result from a vast array of problems, including infection, hematoma formation, dehydration, drug or transfusion reactions, atelectasis, or tissue necrosis. Infections result from many factors. The probability of infection is related to the number of organisms present, their ability to cause disease (virulence), and patients' degree of resistance. Any direct access for microbial invasion or condition that compromises tissue perfusion can devitalize tissue and foster the environment in which microorganisms flourish. Microorganisms produce various toxic substances that play an important role in triggering the inflammatory response. Gram-negative bacteria (*Escherichia coli, Klebsiella* sp., *Enterobacter* sp., *Serratia* sp., *Pseudomonas aeruginosa, Bacteroides* sp., and *Proteus* sp.) produce endotoxin. *Staphylococcus aureus,* a gram-positive bacillus, produces an endotoxin known as leukocidin (Massanari, 1989). Leukocidin damages the circulating white blood cells (WBCs), especially neutrophils, which are essential for the removal of cellular debris and bacteria. These endotoxins activate several components of the complement, coagulation, kallikrein–kinin, and plasminogen–plasmin cascade systems.

Resistance to microbial invasion and systemic complications depends on a range of host-related and treatment-related risk factors. Many of the interventions used to support organ function in critically ill patients interfere with normal defense mechanisms. For example, the benefits of a nasogastric tube can become unbalanced when sinusitis or gastric colonization of microorganisms develops. When integrated with other risk factors, such as histamine-2 blocking agents, excessive antacid therapy, gastric lavage and suctioning, or development of stress ulcers, this common device can foster infection by disturbing patients' protective gastric acid and mucosal barrier.

A debilitated individual is susceptible to colonization of microorganisms in the lungs. The presence of a nasal or oral endotracheal tube impedes the normal defense mechanisms of mucosal clearing and glottic closure. Thoracic or abdominal surgical procedures can create limitations in chest wall function. A reduction in inspiratory and expiratory forces can foster the accumulation of secretions and create an optimal environment for microbial colonization. At the other extreme, barotrauma from excessive positive end-expiratory pressure or tidal volumes during mechanical ventilation can also increase the potential for developing pneumonia and empyema. The function of the central nervous system's sensory and motor components form an integral defense mechanism. A paralyzed patient, as a result of neuromuscular blockade or a transected spinal cord, is more susceptible to infection due to compromised protective mechanisms such as coughing and withdrawal reflexes. Bedridden and immobilized patients are at risk for developing pneumonia due to gravitational forces that create pooling of secretions in the dependent lung area and atelectasis.

Trauma patients are extremely susceptible to infection for many reasons. The conditions of the accident, extent of the injury, and physiologic characteristics, and the disturbance in the anatomic defense mechanisms that result from injury or therapy trigger multiple pathologic events (Hoyt, 1989). Operative procedures and diagnostic tests requiring cannulation into the vascular system interrupt the protective barrier of intact skin.

Coagulase-negative staphylococci, coagulase-positive staphylococci, aerobic and anaerobic streptococci, diphtheroids, and *Bacillus* are species of the skin's normal flora (Hoyt, 1990). These organisms regulate the pH of the skin and prevent colonization of pathogenic organisms. However, normal flora become pathogenic when the delicate balance between the normal flora and defense mechanisms is disturbed. Failure to resolve the inflammatory response or eliminate the causative organism creates the grave prognosis associated with sepsis.

STIMULUS-RESPONSE SYSTEMS PRECIPITATING SEPTIC SHOCK

The body's immunologic surveillance system and inflammatory response direct immunogenic cells to sites of injury and infection. Any type of cellular damage or microbial infection initiates an acute inflammatory response. This response results in increased blood flow and vascular permeability to allow immunogenic cells to reach the sites of injury or infection. One of the immunogenic cells that travels to the site of injury or infection is the macrophage. Macrophages, mononuclear phagocytes derived from bone marrow, are capable of (1) adhering to foreign cells to initiate an antibody response, (2) engulfing particulate matter, and (3) recognizing, attaching to, and destroying foreign cells. Granulocytes, another type of WBCs, are further differentiated into basophils, eosinophils, and neutrophils. Activation of granulocytes is thought to amplify various physiologic responses in patients with sepsis (Stroud et al., 1990).

The second aspect of the inflammatory response involves the release of numerous chemotactic factors from immunogenic cells or microbes. The chemical mediators currently identified in sepsis are listed in Table 63–1. Several others may be undiscovered at this time (Parrillo, 1989a). The chemical mediators involved in the development of sepsis create major alterations in the peripheral vasculature and heart (Parrillo, 1989a).

CHEMICAL MEDIATORS

Endotoxin

Endotoxins, lipopolysaccharides, are a component of gram-negative microbes' cell membranes. Microbial

TABLE 63–1. **Chemical Mediators of Sepsis**

Endotoxin
Oxygen radicals
Interleukin-1 and interleukin-2
Tumor necrosis factor
Arachidonic acid cascade
Prostaglandins
Thromboxane
Prostacyclin
Leukotrienes
Complement cascade
Coagulation and fibrinolytic cascades
Bradykinin
Myocardial depressant factor
Beta-endorphin

cell lysis or reperfusion of the microcirculation after ischemia caused by various shock states, hypoxemia, radiation injury, vasoconstriction therapy, burns, trauma, and graft rejection can liberate endotoxins into the systemic circulation (Stroud et al., 1990). Circulating endotoxins activate several protein systems that create many pathophysiologic alterations.

Oxygen Radicals

Endotoxins activate macrophages that release monokines. In addition, in the response that endotoxins are capable of activating, macrophages release toxic oxygen-free radicals and proteolytic enzymes. The released superoxide ions or single-oxygen molecules form hydrogen peroxide. In the presence of iron, these oxygen radicals create extremely destructive hydroxyl radicals. Under normal circumstances, the body's antioxidant system limits the destructive nature of this reaction. However, septic patients have depleted their antioxidant defense mechanisms (Stroud et al., 1990). In sepsis, alveolar epithelial cells are especially vulnerable to the destructive effects produced by this reaction. Other toxic products released by macrophages include interleukin-1 (IL-1) and tumor necrosis factor (TNF-α).

Interleukin-1 and Interleukin-2

When macrophages are stimulated they secrete a substantial amount of the glycoprotein called IL-1. A smaller amount of IL-1 is produced by endothelial cells, epithelial cells, dendritic cells, neutrophils, and B-lymphocytes. All cells capable of synthesizing IL-1 can be stimulated by (1) other inflammatory mediators, (2) cells of the immune system, (3) agents that induce DNA synthesis and proliferation of cells, and (4) various latex or silica particles (Coleman et al., 1989).

Interleukin-1 produces a series of chemotactic events. During an inflammatory response this chemical mediator is responsible for facilitating the movement of WBCs toward injured, ischemic, or infected cells. IL-1 stimulates the release of arachidonic acid from phospholipids located in plasma membranes. Administration of IL-1 during experimental animal studies produces fevers, hypotension, and a decrease in systemic vascular resistance (SVR) (Parrillo, 1989a). In addition to these responses, IL-1 and its metabolite, proteolysis-inducing factor, break down muscle protein.

Interleukin-1 and other components of cellular immunity activate the production of interleukin-2 (IL-2). IL-2 plays a role in the decreased blood pressure, decreased SVR, decreased left ventricular ejection fraction (LVEF), increased left ventricular end-diastolic volume, increased cardiac output, and increased heart rate that occur during sepsis (Parrillo, 1989a).

Tumor Necrosis Factor

Tumor necrosis factor, also known as cachexin or cachectin, is a macrophage-derived polypeptide hormone. TNF-α is capable of stimulating platelet-activating factors as well as prostaglandin and IL-1 production. TNF-α increases neutrophil margination and activates the antimicrobial activity of monocytes, macrophages, neutrophils, and eosinophils (Fong et al., 1990). Protection from organ dysfunction has been noted to occur in animals receiving TNF-α monoclonal antibodies 2 hours before experimental bacteremia.

Arachidonic Acid Cascade

The discovery of 3 of the currently identified 87 arachidonic acid metabolites (leukotriene, thromboxane, prostacyclin) collectively known as eicosanoids began in the late 1970s. Arachidonic acid, the fatty acid precursor present in membrane phospholipids, can be liberated by endotoxins, cellular agitation, or hypoxia. The arachidonic acid cascade is activated and controlled by specific enzymes, as shown in Figure 63–1. Once arachidonic acid is released from the cell membrane, it can be metabolized by two major pathways, one resulting in the prostaglandin family and the other in the leukotriene family of compounds.

PROSTAGLANDIN. Fatty acid cyclooxygenase metabolizes arachidonic acid into prostaglandins and other stable metabolites such as thromboxane and prostacyclin. During an overwhelming inflammatory response, arachidonic acid metabolites and damaged vascular endothelium often inhibit prostaglandin synthesis. Prostaglandins are potent vasodilators, and they attempt to balance the adverse effects created by other chemical mediators in the arachidonic acid cascade. For instance, prostaglandins create cerebral vasodilation to balance the cerebral vasoconstricting property of thromboxane. An imbalance in thromboxane and prostaglandin levels creates the central nervous system, pulmonary, and fibrin-fibrinolysis disturbances seen in sepsis (Reines & Haluska, 1989).

THROMBOXANE. This chemical mediator plays an important role in the clinical manifestation and sequence of events seen during sepsis. The maldistribution of blood flow during sepsis is attributed to thromboxane's potent vasoconstricting and platelet-aggregating effect. Tissue ischemia is a consequence of hypoperfusion initiated by this mediator.

PROSTACYCLIN. One clinical manifestation of septic shock is largely due to the release of prostacyclin from the walls of blood vessels. Prostacyclin is a potent vasodilator and antiaggregant. The initial decrease in the patient's SVR is due to the widespread production of this mediator by the vascular endothelium (Littleton, 1988). The production and quantity of chemical mediator release depends on the specific tissue of origin.

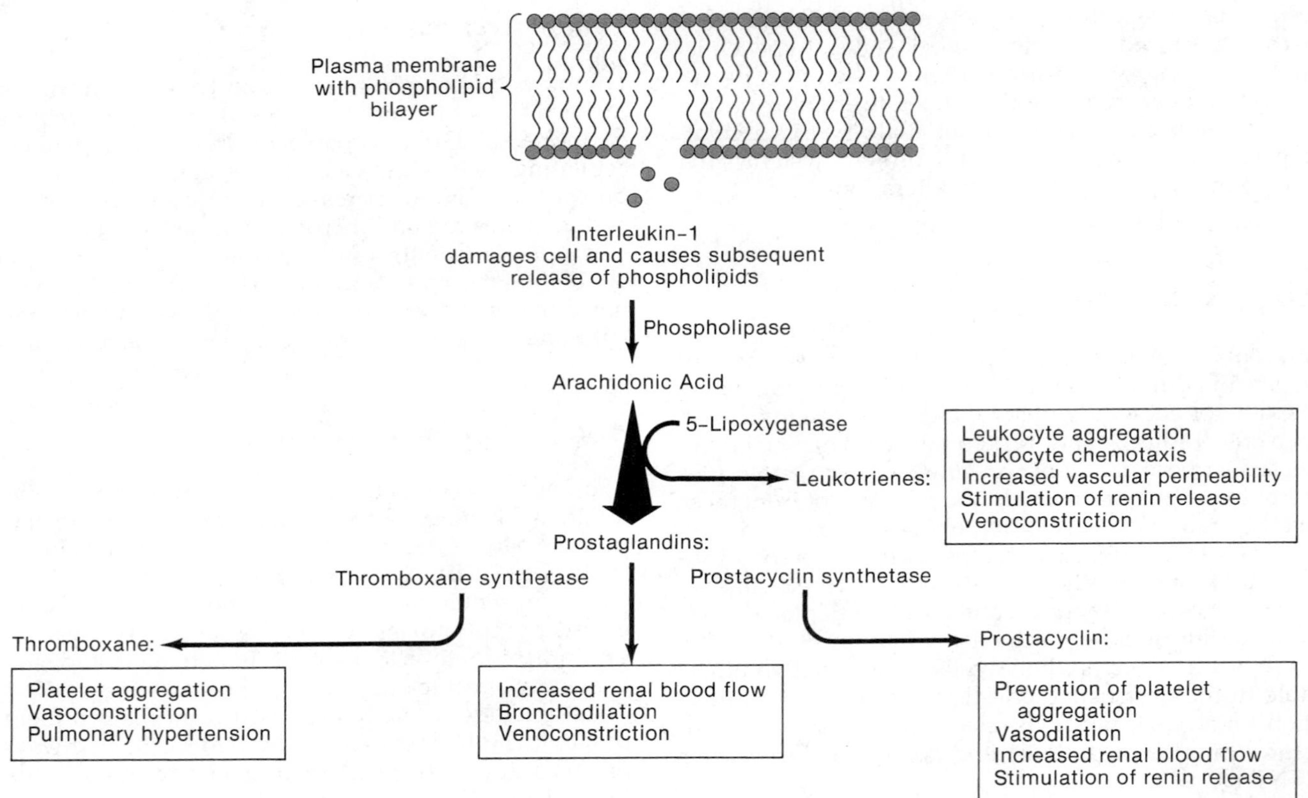

FIGURE 63–1. Arachidonic acid cascade and role of mediators in sepsis.

LEUKOTRIENES. The other major pathway in the arachidonic acid cascade leads to the production of the slow-reacting substances of anaphylaxis, collectively referred to as leukotrienes. Several authors hypothesize that leukotrienes are associated with increased capillary endothelial permeability (Reines & Haluska, 1989; Vane & Botting, 1989). Leukotrienes produce increased tissue permeability, bronchoconstriction, and a chemical response activating more neutrophils. The cyclic nature of the disease develops through the actions of neutrophils, free oxygen radicals, IL-1, and TNF-α as well as antigenic substances capable of activating neutrophils in an immunocompetent individual and synthesizing leukotrienes.

Complement Cascade System

An important defense mechanism against foreign cells is achieved through activation of a group of serum proteins that constitutes the complement system. A deficiency of complement components can increase a patient's susceptibility to infection. An inflammatory response can disturb the complement system's delicate balance of cellular destruction and clearance. The biologic effects of this cascade include cell lysis, stimulation of smooth muscle contraction, mast cell degradation, neutrophil chemotaxis, and activation of phagocytosis.

The two mechanisms by which the complement cascade can be activated are the classic and the alternative pathways. The classic pathway is activated by immunocompetent cells as a result of an antibody binding to a cell surface or forming an antibody–antigen complex. In contrast, the alternative pathway does not require immunocompetent cells and is activated by the carbohydrate portion of a microbe's cell membrane. Regardless of the initiating pathway, the process generates a cascade of active molecules that initiate inflammatory and lytic reactions.

The complement cascade's biologic activity is not limited entirely to cell lysis. Various intermediate components in the complement cascade are important factors in the pathogenesis of sepsis (Fig. 63–2). For example, one component of the cascade, known as C5a, is an anaphylotoxin that produces mediator release by mast cells and, when bound to macrophages, releases IL-1. The amount of histamine released from mast cells during sepsis may not account for the increased vascular permeability and decreased SVR seen in this condition (Parrillo, 1989a). Nevertheless, C5a plays a significant role in sepsis because neutrophilic aggregation, formation of multiple microemboli, hypoperfusion, and tissue necrosis augment the disease process. Another component of the complement cascade, C3a, binds to lymphokines secreted by suppressor T-lymphocytes, decreasing the amount of antibody produced. The complement system also contains specific

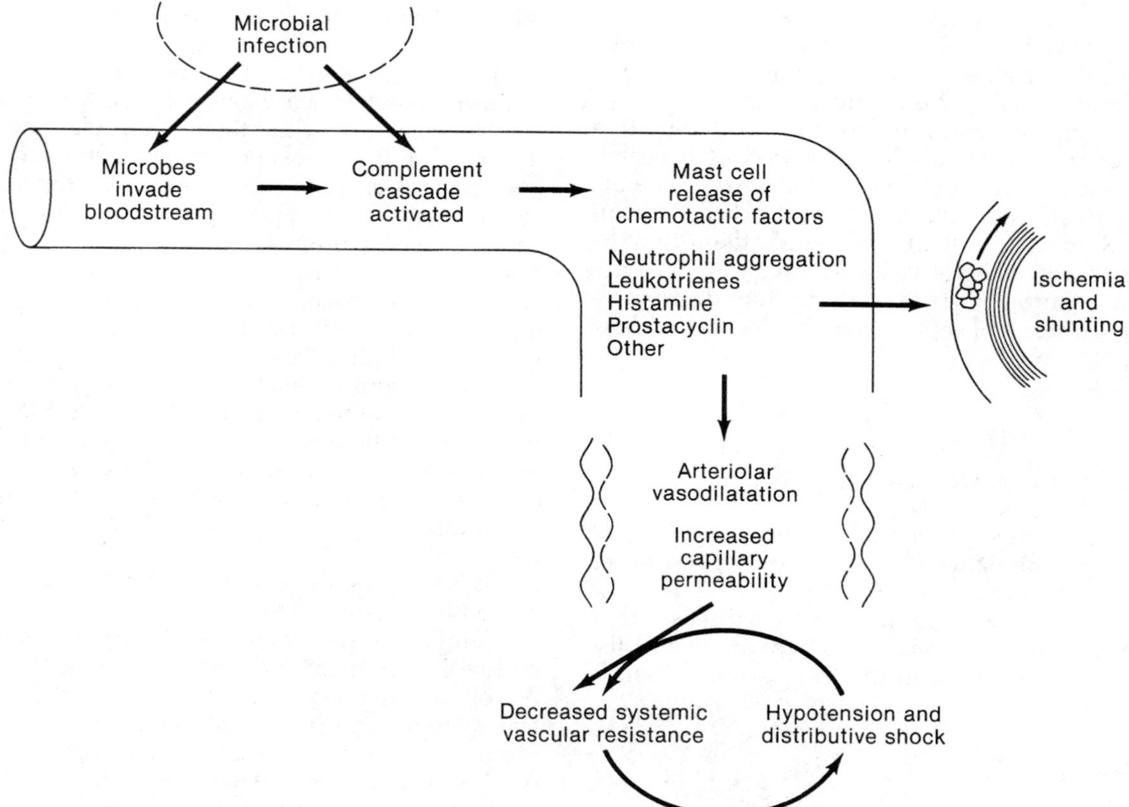

FIGURE 63–2. Activity of components.

components that amplify and inhibit the cascade. The sequential, controlled activation of complement components creates lysis targeted toward the activation stimulus. Yet during an overwhelming systemic inflammatory response, the binding of complement components to target cells becomes less specific and controlled. This chaotic lysis of all cells further increases the release of other chemical mediators.

Coagulation and Fibrinolysis Cascade

Injury to the vascular endothelium initiates the formation of fibrin. The toxic effects of chemical mediators on blood vessels and cell membranes stimulate the release of the Hageman factor and tissue thromboplastin (Kirchner & Reheis, 1982). Fibrin clot formation attempts to stabilize the site of injury. To keep the extent of clotting under control, the coagulation cascade also activates fibrinolysis. During sepsis, consumption of various factors in both systems creates mediator-induced disseminated intravascular coagulation.

Bradykinin

Kinins, polypeptides with vasodilatory properties, are normally inactive. Activation of the Hageman factor in the coagulation cascade or complement activation stimulates the prekallikrein system to release a potent vasodilator, bradykinin. The volume depletion characteristic of sepsis is a consequence of bradykinin's ability to create vasodilation and capillary leak.

Myocardial Depressant Factor

The prominent maldistribution of blood flow in patients with sepsis adversely affects tissue perfusion. An ischemic pancreatic cell releases a serum protein known as myocardial depressant factor (MDF). MDF has been found in at least 40% of patients with septic shock. It has not been found in nonseptic critically ill patients (Parrillo, 1989a). MDF causes a decrease in the degree and velocity of contractions of myocardial cells. The decrease in left and right ventricular ejection fractions is proportional to the amount of circulating MDF present (Parrillo, 1989a). Lactate production, respiratory decompensation, and pulmonary capillary wedge pressure increase in the presence of circulating MDF.

Beta-Endorphins

It is hypothesized that beta-endorphins, endogenous opiates located in the pituitary and hypothalamus, are released during the early phase of septic shock (Parrillo, 1989b). Maldistribution of blood flow, vasodilation, and cellular alterations precipitate the release of beta-endorphins. Once this opiate attaches to its receptor site within the central nervous system, inhibition of sympathomedullary transmission occurs. Research further postulates that beta-endorphins may excite the parasympathetic efferent fibers of the heart (Schumann & Remington, 1990). Combined, these two actions produce peripheral vasodilation and a decrease in cardiac contractility, leading to the destructive pathogenic process of septic shock (Faden & Holaday, 1980).

Other Chemical Mediators

Because septic shock is a multifactorial disease entity, no single mediator explains all of the responses resulting from the septic insult. In reviewing the published literature pertaining to this disease, it is understood that other mediators remain to be discovered and understood in the progression of septic shock.

PATHOPHYSIOLOGY

As the septic insult continues to stimulate various chemical inflammatory mediators, the body loses its characteristic homeostasis, and septic shock evolves. The severity and duration of the systemic inflammatory response determine a patient's clinical course. Manifestations of cardiovascular dysfunction are complex and often differ from patient to patient depending on the types of mediators released, the amount of mediator released, and the timing of mediator synthesis and release in combination with the host's ability to compensate (Parrillo, 1989b). In general, the chemical mediators of septic shock create three major effects within the cardiovascular system: (1) vasodilation, (2) maldistribution of blood flow, and (3) myocardial depression.

Peripheral Vasodilation

Peripheral vasodilation is a result of activation of the arachidonic acid and complement cascades with subsequent release of vasoactive substances. Dilation in the arterial and venous circulation increases the diameter of the blood vessels, which in turn decreases SVR and preload. Initially, septic patients attempt to compensate by developing an increase in cardiac output. Yet tissue perfusion continues to decrease because of coinciding factors that create maldistributions of blood flow and cardiac dysfunction.

Maldistribution of Blood Flow

Although septic shock is usually associated with vasodilation, not all vessels experience this form of instability. The release of sympathetic catecholamines, angiotensin, and thromboxane creates pulmonary, renal, and splenic vasoconstriction. As a result, perfusion to some organs becomes compromised while other organs receive additional flow depending on the intravascular fluid status. Inadequate tissue perfusion also occurs due to vascular occlusion. The direct effects of microbial invasion and mediator release damage the vascular endothelium. Migration and aggregation of neutrophils and platelets to the damaged cells create thrombosis and potential embolic events. Maldistribution of blood flow is also a consequence of blood volume displacement. Histamine and bradykinin increase capillary permeability, allowing serum to migrate into the interstitial space. This fluid shift depletes the circulating volume and increases blood viscosity. The end result is irreversible cellular dysfunction secondary to inadequate tissue perfusion.

Cellular dysfunction results from disturbances within the cell membrane and inadequate blood flow. As cells are invaded by microorganisms or are traumatized, their membranes lose the ability to maintain a normal balance of intracellular and extracellular components. Disturbances of membrane integrity allow sodium and water to enter the cell freely. Electrolyte imbalances and cellular swelling alter the function of the cell. As a consequence, the cell becomes dysfunctional and eventually ruptures, releasing intracellular enzymes and membrane components that activate chemical mediators. Endotoxins create metabolic derangements by altering chemical reactions in the cell's mitochondria. During an inflammatory response, the demand for oxygen exceeds the supply. As intracellular oxygen depletion occurs, anaerobic metabolism begins. Excessive amounts of lactic acid and minimal levels of adenosine triphosphate are produced. A deficiency of adenosine triphosphate decreases the utilization of glucose and oxygen and disturbs the cell's selective membrane. Cell death and multiple organ system failure become inevitable as tissue destruction and energy depletion progress.

Myocardial Depression

A cell that is not directly attacked by inflammatory chemical mediators can experience cellular dysfunction as a result of selective vasoconstriction or microemboli within the circulatory system. For example, the liver and spleen become ischemic as blood is shunted to vital organs during septic shock. When pancreatic cells die, they release pancreatic enzymes such as lipase, amylase, and the chemical mediator MDF into the lymphatic and systemic circulations. As a result of the volume depletion and myocardial dysfunction that occur in this disease, most authors classify septic shock as a prototype of both cardiogenic and distributive shock. The cardiovascular pattern of patients who recover from septic shock consists of a high cardiac index, low SVR, decreased LVEF, a dilated left ventricle, and a normal stroke volume (Parrillo, 1989a). Nonsurvivors of septic shock generally die from any of the following syndromes: hypotension from a perpetual decrease in SVR, hypotension due to a decrease in cardiac index, or multiple organ system failure (Parrillo, 1989a).

SIGNS AND SYMPTOMS

Nurses who maintain vigilance and are able to recognize trends in a patient's status play an extremely pivotal role in the course of this disease because proper early management often limits the destructive cyclic nature of SIRS. SIRS is a syndrome that can create and maintain irreversible tissue damage until it or another disease claims the patient's life. Therefore, an understanding of the pathophysiologic changes, indicative clinical symptoms or laboratory results, and treatment modalities during the progression of this disease is imperative for providing optimal nursing care. To achieve uniformity in terminology, a consensus conference was held to define SIRS and related terms (Bone et al., 1992). These definitions are listed in Table 63–2.

During the onset of sepsis, the patient shows the signs and symptoms of a systemic inflammatory response without any apparent profound cardiovascular changes. As microorganisms and toxic products enter the patient's bloodstream, a stress response is elicited, and energy expenditure increases. Stimulation of the patient's sympathetic nervous system creates an increase in heart rate and cardiac index. During the stress response, glucagon is also released. Glucagon, a hormone produced by alpha cells in the islets of Langerhans, stimulates the conversion of glycogen to glucose in the liver. Under normal conditions (homeostasis), glucose is capable of supplying the body with energy.

The early cardinal signs of a systemic infection and an inflammatory response—tachycardia, tachypnea, and mental cloudiness—are due to circulating endotoxins (Rice, 1984). As the cells become infected with endotoxins, their ability to metabolize glucose diminishes, and metabolic alterations develop. As intracellular lactic acid increases during sepsis, neurons within the pons and medullary areas of the brain sense the increase in hydrogen ion concentration, causing the patient to begin to hyperventilate. Other mediators that create microemboli or vasoconstriction in the pulmonic or cerebral vessels increase the vascular resistance, thereby decreasing tissue perfusion.

Despite sympathetic stimulation, the septic patient's level of consciousness continues to deteriorate during an impending shock state. This clinical manifestation is often an indication of the severity of the disease. Cerebral blood flow is a reflection of cerebral perfusion pressure, which is calculated from the mean arterial pressure (MAP; one-third of the pulse pressure plus the diastolic pressure) minus the intracranial pressure. As circulatory volume is redistributed during sepsis, systemic filling pressures are reduced. Therefore, indications of mediator-induced peripheral vasodilation may be shown by a declining trend in MAP and noted clinically by the compromised perfusion pressure to the brain as well as other organs.

Another manifestation of sepsis can be noted by observing the appearance of the patient's skin. In the early stages of the disease, vasoactive mediators create a flushed appearance due to peripheral vasodilation. During an inflammatory response, activation of the WBCs stimulates the release of endogenous pyrogens. Leukotrienes, prostaglandins, and IL-1 are endogenous pyrogens capable of circulating to the hypothalamus. Once at this location, the mediators signal the

TABLE 63–2. **Definitions**

Infection: Microbial phenomenon charcterized by an inflammatory response to the presence of microorganisms or the invasion of normally sterile host tissue by those organisms.

Bacteremia: The presence of viable bacteria in the blood.

Systemic Inflammatory Response Syndrome (SIRS): The systemic inflammatory response to a variety of severe clinical insults. SIRS is manifested by two or more of the following conditions:

Temperature >38°C or <36°C
Heart rate >90 beats/min.
Respiratory rate >20 breaths/min or Pa_{CO_2} <32 torr (<4.3kPa)
WBC >12,000 cells/mm³, <4000 cells/mm³, or >10% immature (band) forms

Sepsis: The systemic response to infection. This systemic response is manifested by two or more of the following conditions as a result of infection:

Temperature >38°C or <36°C
Heart rate >90 beats/min.
Respiratory rate >20 breaths/min or Pa_{CO_2} <32 torr (<4.3kPa)
WBC >12,000 cells/mm³, <4000 cells/mm³, or >10% immature (band) forms

Severe Sepsis: Sepsis associated with organ dysfunction, hypoperfusion, or hypotension. Hypoperfusion and perfusion abnormalities may include, but are not limited to, lactic acidosis, oliguria, or an acute alteration in mental status.

Septic Shock: Sepsis with hypotension, despite adequate fluid resuscitation, along with the presence of perfusion abnormalities that may include, but are not limited to, lactic acidosis, oliguria, or an acute alteration in mental status. Patients who are on inotropic or vasopressor agents may not be hypotensive at the time that perfusion abnormalities are measured.

Hypotension: A systolic BP of <90 mm Hg or a reduction of >40 mm Hg from baseline in the absence of other causes for hypotension.

Multiple Organ Dysfunction Syndrome: Presence of altered organ function in an acutely ill patient such that homeostasis cannot be maintained without intervention.

From Bone, R. C., Balk, R. A., Cerra, F. B., Dellinger, R. P., Fein, A. M., Knaus, W. A., Schein, R. M., & Sibbald, W. S. (1992). Definitions for sepsis and organ failure and guidelines for the use of innovative therapies in sepsis. The ACCP/SCCM Consensus Conference Committee. *Chest, 101,* 1644–1655.

chemoreceptors in the thermoregulatory center to increase the set point of the body temperature as a protective mechanism to destroy microbes thermally. As the set point becomes elevated, the skeletal muscles shiver to generate heat, circulation to the skin decreases to minimize heat loss, and fever develops as a consequence. Depending on the temperature gradient (core vs. environmental temperatures) and the degree of peripheral vasodilation, body heat may dissipate. Therefore, although fever is often described as one of the cardinal signs of an infection, a patient can experience hypothermia (core temperature below 35° C) during sepsis. Elderly patients and patients who have sustained burns, spinal cord injuries, or extensive soft tissue injuries also lose the skin's thermoregulatory function, and a hypothermic set point develops (Hoyt, 1989). Again, the importance of observing trends in a patient's condition remains crucial.

As an inflammatory response develops, leukopenia (WBC count less than 5000/μL) is an early finding in a septic immunocompetent patient. As endotoxins and chemical mediators adhere to the surface of WBCs, these WBCs become "tagged" and removed from circulation by the reticuloendothelial system (macrophages, Kupffer cells of the liver, reticular cells of the lungs, bone marrow, spleen, and lymph nodes). This clearance process initially reduces the patient's serum WBC count. As sepsis progresses, the septic insult develops a synergistic effect with the patient's immune system because the inflammatory response signals the bone marrow to accelerate leukocyte synthesis and release. Consequently, more WBCs are released into the circulation, and some cells, especially neutrophils, are immature. This process is reflected in a complete blood count, in which the WBC count will be greater than 10,000/μL and a shift to the left is present.

Approximately one-third of patients with septicemia experience manifestations of septic shock (Rice, 1984). The clinical manifestations and progression of septic shock depend on the patient's circulatory volume (Hoyt, 1989). The initial cardiovascular pattern of septic shock consists of a high cardiac index and a low SVR (Parrillo, 1989a). There is a discrepancy in the literature about whether septic patients can be divided into two groups, hyperdynamic and hypodynamic, during the initial onset of septic shock. The category of hyperdynamic, or warm septic shock, denotes a septic patient who has bounding pulses, warm skin, an elevated cardiac index, and a reduced SVR. Hypodynamic, or cold septic shock, describes a septic patient who has thready pulses, cool skin, decreased cardiac index, and an elevated SVR. Before the 1970s, septic patients generally were inadequately hydrated (Parrillo, 1989a). At that time, inadequate fluid replacement was assumed to be a method for preventing pulmonary edema and the consequences of respiratory distress during sepsis. As knowledge of adult respiratory distress syndrome (ARDS) and its causes increased, the assumption that fluid overload was the sole contributing factor in ARDS was disregarded. Researchers have reevaluated the historical data that originally formed these two categories and now believe that volume depletion and a reduction in preload are factors that contributed to the patients' low cardiac index. Today, aggressive volume replacement and vasoactive therapy are used in the management of septic shock because a patient's survival is jeopardized within the first hour of shock (Hoyt, 1989).

A common indicator in all forms of shock (cardiogenic, extracardiac obstructive, oligemic, and distributive) is reduced blood flow to several tissues (Parrillo, 1989b). The chemical mediators of septic shock produce profound effects on the peripheral vasculature and myocardium. As mediators impair the host's normal vasomotor reflexes, autoregulation of the capillary perfusion pressure becomes impaired (Parrillo, 1989a). As a result, some organs are hypoperfused and others receive an abundance of blood flow. Shunting of blood increases as the microvasculature becomes occluded with fibrin or aggregates of leukocytes, platelets, and damaged cells during the inflammatory response. Gross peripheral maldistribution of blood flow is also caused by an increase in capillary membrane permeability. Although the predominant vascular effect precipitating septic shock is vasodilation, some vascular beds develop severe vasoconstriction. In either case, tissue perfusion ultimately becomes deranged despite the presence of a high cardiac index, and the organs most frequently affected are the kidneys, liver, brain, and lungs.

The kidney has an abundant eicosanoid supply and cyclooxygenase activity. Renal blood flow, excretion of sodium and water, creatinine clearance, and renin release are all affected by the production of thromboxane and prostaglandins during sepsis. As renal blood flow in the patient in septic shock is reduced, urine output decreases, and the body is unable to eliminate waste products. As chemical mediators continue to shunt blood to various organs, the patient's liver becomes hypoperfused. Hyperbilirubinemia and jaundice are common clinical indicators that this organ is becoming adversely affected during the systemic inflammatory response.

As a septic patient's MAP falls below 60 mm Hg, irreversible tissue damage occurs due to the compromised cerebral and pulmonary perfusion pressures. A multitude of factors in the neurologic sensorium change in the septic shock patient, but one imbalance specific to the sequence of events in this disease is that between thromboxane and prostacyclin. The lungs also are a target organ throughout the progression of septic shock. As the patient's serum lactate level increases, the respiratory system attempts to compensate. Circulating endotoxins further debilitate the pulmonary status of the patient because the initial pulmonary response to endotoxins creates bronchoconstriction (Luce, 1987). Consequently, an increase in airway resistance requires the patient's respiratory muscles to generate a greater degree of negative inspiratory force or pressure to allow optimal ventilation. During the progression of septic shock, a ventilation–perfusion mismatch develops as chemical mediators create pulmonary interstitial edema and maldistributions in pulmonic blood flow. As pneumocytes experience a decrease in perfusion, surfactant synthesis diminishes and lung compliance decreases. The risks of developing ARDS from sepsis alone or in combination with the occurrence of septic shock are cited to be, respectively, 4% to 10% and 40% to 60% (Luce, 1987).

Septic shock is a generalized process that involves many organs. In addition to vasomotor dysfunction, several authors relate the occurrence of myocardial depression to the development of septic shock (Ellrodt et al., 1985; Parrillo et al., 1985; Parker et al., 1984). Intracellular disturbances—namely, the reduction of calcium ions within the sarcoplasmic reticulum—limit the excitation-contraction mechanism that is vital for proper functioning of myocardial cells. Effective myocardial contractility is also reduced by the presence of circulating myocardial depressant substances or factors, which decrease LVEF (Parrillo, 1989a). Experimental data link early myocardial depression to circulating MDF and have recognized a pattern in the recovery from septic shock in that these patients experience a normal LVEF and an absence of circulating MDF 10 days after the onset of shock (Parrillo, 1989b). As stated earlier, many septic shock patients experience cardiac dysfunction with ventricular dilatation and a decrease in ejection fraction. The exact cause of these phenomena is not known. It was once believed that a reduction in coronary blood flow and myocardial ischemia precipitated the development of myocardial depression. To date, however, there is no evidence supporting a reduction in coronary blood flow or ischemia as the cause of early myocardial depression in septic shock (Parrillo, 1989b).

The compensatory mechanism of an increase in cardiac index to maintain perfusion may be attributed to five factors: (1) left ventricular dilatation, (2) decreased ejection fraction, (3) increased left ventricular end-diastolic volume index (EDVI), (4) decreased SVR, and (5) an increase in heart rate (Parrillo, 1989a). The ability to calculate a patient's EDVI is important because the measurements represent ventricular volume or preload. Institution of therapy that reflects these hemodynamic patterns, a decrease in LVEF and an increase in EDVI, increases a septic shock patient's chances of survival because it allows simultaneous increases in cardiac index, heart rate, and normal or elevated stroke volume.

MANAGEMENT

The principles involved in the management of sepsis and septic shock are based on the pathogenic mechanisms and degree of organ dysfunction present. Early diagnosis of septic shock is usually possible from the clinical manifestations. Prompt recognition of a systemic inflammatory response is imperative, in that early recognition and prompt management often prevent the progression of the disease. The nurse's highest priority in caring for a suspected septic patient is continual observation of trends in the patient's condition. The priorities of care become twofold because indicative trends, or other diagnostic results, confirm the diagnosis of sepsis or an impending shock state. Aggressive management is required to augment tissue perfusion and prevent metabolic derangements and tissue death. The goals of therapy focus on eradicating the precipitating septic insult, maintaining blood pressure and organ perfusion, and reducing serum lactate levels (Parrillo, 1989b).

Intervention

CRITICAL CARE ENVIRONMENT

The cardiovascular and metabolic abnormalities involved in septic shock can produce hemodynamic changes in unpredictable ways and time frames. Therefore, monitoring the septic patient in a critical care setting is important for a variety of reasons. First, the patient's chances of survival are increased when hemodynamic monitoring guides the initiation and duration of treatment. Second, the insidious and progressive nature of sepsis and septic shock mandates hemodynamic monitoring for noting trends and guiding management. Continuous electrocardiographic monitoring is important because septic patients are at risk for developing atrial tachycardia with occasional episodes of ventricular tachycardia. Invasive pressure devices (arterial blood pressure and the hemodynamic parameters obtained from a pulmonary artery thermodilution catheter) provide serial measurements relating to the cardiovascular status of the patient. Because of the fluctuations in blood pressure and the inaccuracy of cuff pressures during septic shock, arterial blood pressure monitoring provides the most accurate method of measurement. The diagnosis of septic shock is made or confirmed by the patient's hemodynamic profile obtained from a thermodilution pulmonary artery catheter. For example, if a patient presents with a decreased SVR, an increased or decreased cardiac index, and a narrow arterial–mixed venous oxygen content difference, he is experiencing distinguishable characteristics of septic shock. By implementing nursing measures for infection control, arterial lines remain beneficial in managing septic patients because the catheter provides access for diagnostic testing (arterial blood gas analysis, serum lactate and electrolyte levels) without augmenting the cascade of chemical mediator release that occurs through excessive venipunctures.

ANTIMICROBIAL THERAPY

Because of the cascade of events that can trigger the sepsis syndrome, a single definitive cause of the inflammatory response may be unidentifiable. It is important to realize that a causative microorganism cannot be detected in 50% of cases of sepsis (Parrillo, 1989b). Clinical manifestations of sepsis with negative blood cultures may be a result of improper culture technique, failure to locate any specific site of infection, intermittent invasion of the bloodstream by microorganisms, or chemical mediators leaking into the bloodstream from a secluded origin of infection or tissue necrosis. Because sepsis syndrome can develop from other causes besides microorganism invasion, a definitive diagnosis is not solely dependent on culture results. However, in a patient in whom sepsis is suspected, specimens (urine, blood, sputum, cerebrospinal fluid, or wound drainage) should be analyzed for culture and antibiotic sensitivity results. Once cultures have been obtained, initial antibiotic therapy should be based on consideration of the antibiotic susceptibilities and resistance patterns within the institution (Roach, 1990). Administration of a broad-spectrum third-generation cephalosporin in combination with an aminoglycoside is also recommended to provide coverage against all of the pathogens harbored within some settings (Parrillo, 1989b; Roach, 1990). Diagnostic viewing of internal body organs and cavities may also be helpful in locating a nidus of infection. After interpreting the results of all of the diagnostic tests, the goal of management is to select the antimicrobial drug that is sensitive to the identified microbe and capable of circulating to the infected body site. But it is important to remember that sepsis is a "toxic" syndrome and antibiotic therapy is often ineffective in preventing the consequences of the inflammatory response. Because of the complex pathophysiology of sepsis, antimicrobial therapy is a limited "cure-all" for the disease: (1) A microbe may fail to be identified during a culture; (2) a microbe can develop resistance to antimicrobial therapy; (3) superinfection is a risk of antimicrobial therapy; and (4) hemodynamic instability can develop from the progression of the disease or as a consequence of endotoxin release during antimicrobial therapy. Therefore, during the first 48 to 72 hours of septic shock, other treatment modalities are imperative to reverse or limit hemodynamic instability.

VOLUME REPLACEMENT

Restoration of adequate intravascular volume is an important aspect of patient care during episodes of hypotension. The combination of vasodilation and third-spacing during sepsis produces a dramatic decrease in preload and afterload pressures. Indicators of low contractility, such as a decreased left ventricular stroke work index (LVSWI) or right ventricular stroke work index (RVSWI), can result from the reduction in preload or from circulating MDFs. The amount and type of fluids administered to a septic patient depend on the pulmonary artery wedge pressure (PAWP) and the composition of the intravascular fluid. One author (Parrillo, 1989b) recommends the following: (1) If the patient's hematocrit is less than 30%, administer blood as a volume expander; (2) if the patient's albumin concentration is less than 2.0 g/dL, administer 50 to 100 g of albumin; (3) if neither of the two previous conditions is present, a crystalloid solution chosen to correct any existing electrolyte abnormalities should be administered. There is no definite guide to what type of fluid resuscitation is superior to ensure adequate cardiovascular performance or a favorable outcome. Yet choice of the appropriate amount of fluid is very important during therapy. During an infusion the patient's arterial blood pressure can be used as a guide to fluid requirements if (1) the arterial pressure rapidly responds to the fluid replacement and maintains a MAP of 60 mm Hg or greater, (2) there is no question about the definitive diagnosis of septic shock, and (3) there is no evidence of heart failure. If the patient fails to meet these criteria, the PAWP and LVEF are useful guides for estimating volume requirements. During an infusion the PAWP should be maintained at 12 to 18 mm Hg. The decision to increase PAWP from 12 to 16 to 18 mm Hg depends on ventricular function and other goals of therapy. A Starling curve can be plotted from the values obtained from hemodynamic parameters. Simultaneous plotting of the patient's LVSWI, PAWP, and cardiac index will show the degree to which the myocardial cells are functioning in relation to the progression or management of the disease. Other criteria indicating the therapeutic success of volume replacement and eradication of the septic insult include (1) a MAP greater than 60 mm Hg, (2) a blood flow that remains adequate for normal central nervous system, kidney, and lung function (evidenced by indirect measurements such as urine output greater than 20 mL/hr and adequate arterial blood gas values) and arterial blood lactate levels below 2.2 mmol/dL (Parrillo, 1989a).

VASOPRESSOR THERAPY

Vasopressor therapy is generally not used during the initial management of septic shock but is indicated when fluids fail to restore intravascular volume and adequate tissue perfusion (Parrillo et al., 1990). Therefore, if the septic patient remains hypotensive when fluid replacement has increased the PCWP to 18 mm Hg, vasopressor therapy is generally instituted. Some clinicians prefer to maintain preload pressures at normal levels and support the circulation with vasoactive drugs, the rationale for this being that elevated filling pressures do not improve the cardiac output for all patients, and excessive filling pressures may increase edema formation and oxygen requirements.

Several authors (Luce, 1987; Parrillo, 1989b; Parrillo et al., 1990) recommend the following guidelines relating to vasoactive support during septic shock. In general, dopamine is the initial vasopressor of choice because the type of stimulation it produces is dependent on the infusion rate, and dopamine can be combined with other agents to achieve various therapeutic effects. At low doses, 2 to 4 μg/kg/min, dopamine increases renal blood flow and in some individuals will create a moderate pressor effect by increasing cardiac performance. Heart rate and contractility increase as the beta-adrenergic effects of dopamine predominate at doses of 5 to 10 μg/kg/min. Alpha-adrenergic (vasoconstrictive) effects predominate at levels above 10 μg/kg/min. If dopamine is ineffective at raising the patient's MAP above 60 mm Hg with an infusion rate of 20 μg/kg/min, a more potent vasopressor is administered. Levarterenol (Levophed), a powerful alpha-adrenergic agonist with moderate beta-adrenergic activity, is useful during septic shock when loss of vasomotor tone predominates. This drug is usually infused at a rate of 2 to 8 μg/min and is titrated to maintain blood pressure. Because of its potent vasoconstrictor effect, dopamine at low doses is often employed to enhance renal blood flow when the renal vasculature is adversely affected (Schaer et al., 1985). Epinephrine and phenylephrine are also potent vasopressures used to maintain arterial pressure with an infusion rate of 1 to 8 μg/min and 20 to 200 μg/min, respectively. If the patient is experiencing tachyarrhythmias, phenylephrine is a useful vasoconstrictor because it is a pure alpha-adrenergic drug and therefore does not directly stimulate the heart.

VASODILATOR THERAPY

Theoretically, the use of vasodilators to enhance perfusion through vasoconstricted vessels during septic shock seems rational. Yet due to the unpredictable pharmacologic activity of vasodilation on the systemic vessels, the benefits of improving the maldistribution of blood flow by this method during septic shock are limited. Nonspecific vasodilation is potentially harmful when the patient's blood pressure is low. Therefore, until vasodilator therapy can focus on specific pathologically constricted vessels, this group of drugs is generally not beneficial in the treatment of septic shock (Parrillo, 1989a).

OXYGEN THERAPY

Patients with septic shock may suffer from a variety of adverse effects, including (1) bronchoconstriction, (2) compensatory mechanisms placing an increased workload on respiratory muscles, (3) pulmonary hypertension, (4) destruction of lung tissue, and (5) increased capillary permeability, with resultant respiratory failure. Ventilatory therapy with positive end-expiratory pressure or continuous positive airway pressure is often beneficial for oxygenation. Positive pressure fails to decrease the amount of extravascular fluid in the lungs, but it does improve PaO_2 by increasing the alveolar diameter or redistributing the intra-alveolar fluid into the interstitial spaces of the lung (Luce, 1987). The risk of barotrauma is potentiated by the occurrence of parenchymal lung disease in sepsis; therefore, the lowest amount of positive pressure that adequately saturates the patient's hemoglobin is generally used.

CORTICOSTEROIDS

In the management of septic shock, the difference between the dosage of corticosteroids needed to produce a beneficial result and the margin of safety remains controversial. The fundamental principles that justify the use of corticosteroids as an adjunctive therapy in sepsis are based on investigational data demonstrating that corticosteroids (1) inhibit complement activation, (2) prevent complement-induced neutrophil aggregation, (3) stabilize lysosomal membranes, and (4) inhibit prostaglandin and thromboxane synthesis through membrane stabilization. One drawback to this list of benefits is that, because this drug is administered over an extended period of time, the possibility of superinfection increases because the drug inhibits leukocyte function. (*Note:* Corticosteroid use is controversial, and the administration of this drug should be reserved for septic patients with suspected or documented adrenal insufficiency.) Therefore, a septic patient does not generally benefit from this drug because it may prolong the course of illness.

NUTRITIONAL SUPPORT

During the initial phase of shock, nutrition is not a priority. But once the septic patient is hemodynamically stable, nutritional support is a necessity because the patient experiences increased energy demands due to the stress, fever, shock state, and inflammatory process. In choosing nutritional support one must consider whether the supplement will benefit the host or the inflammatory process. If feasible, it is recommended that a high-protein source of enteral feedings with an isoosmotic content be instituted. Because of the nature of sepsis, shunting of blood away from the gut may limit the possibility of this route of nutritional support, and parenteral therapy may be required. In the event that parenteral feedings become necessary, glucose content is minimized in the early phase of the disease and advanced during recovery. Lipids are generally limited to 10% to 15% of the patient's total caloric requirements. Lipids or fat emulsions provide a source of neutral triglycerides, unsaturated fatty acids, glycerol, and egg yolk phospholipids. Because the destructive properties of sepsis can be triggered by the arachidonic acid cascade and consumption of dietary linoleic acid (a derivative of arachidonic acid) as well as other complex lipids, the concentration of fat emulsions may be crucial in preventing excessive amounts of fatty acid administration from potentiating mediator release.

Experimental Therapies

NALOXONE (NARCAN)

The mechanism of action of naloxone in septic shock is not fully understood, but it is thought to reverse the endogenous opiate-induced hypotension and decreased cardiac contractility that occur during the onset of septic shock (Schumann & Remington, 1990). The results obtained from various research studies in which naloxone was administered during endotoxic shock are inconsistent. The use of naloxone in conjunction with other therapies, the timing of naloxone administration, and the amount given differ, posing questions about the validity of the results. Therefore, the clinical use of naloxone during septic shock is under investigation, and one author feels that this disease may be a challenge to the present effective pharmacologic actions because acidosis, hypothermia, and serum glucose imbalances, all of which are common manifestations of sepsis, antagonize naloxone (Schumann & Remington, 1990).

INHIBITORS OF PROSTAGLANDIN SYNTHESIS

With the discovery of various arachidonic acid metabolites, the metabolic pathways and enzyme intermediates have also been revealed. Antiinflammatory steroids, namely corticosteroids, prevent the formation of prostaglandin, thromboxane, and leukotriene metabolites because of the agents' ability to block the site of action that converts membrane phospholipids into arachidonic acid in the presence of phospholipase (Vane & Botting, 1989). Nonsteroidal antiinflammatory drugs such as aspirin, ibuprofen, indomethacin, and meclofenamate also inhibit prostaglandin biosynthesis by blocking the activity of cyclooxygenase. This inhibits the formation of thromboxane, prostacyclin, and prostaglandin metabolites, but leukotriene metabolism is not affected. Since one pathway is blocked, it is possible that an accumulation of the precursor is present for activity through the other pathway as lipooxygenase converts arachidonic acid into leukotrienes. Therefore, even though the biosynthesis of some chemical mediators is reduced, the overall effect from this process may not be totally beneficial.

IMMUNE SUBSTRATES

Fortunately, as the pathogenesis of sepsis is becoming better understood, researchers are developing investigational therapies to eradicate the causative mediator activity. Therapies that appear to be most promising focus on agents capable of blocking either the pathogens responsible for sepsis or the body's immune response. Clinical trials of antiendotoxin antibodies have not shown them to be of therapeutic benefit (Suffredini, 1994). Future management incorporating antibodies or other pharmacologic inhibitors of endotoxins and the various inflammatory mediators will play a vital role in reversing the pathogenic cascade of events in sepsis.

SUMMARY

Sepsis and its consequences require prompt recognition and early treatment to prevent its rapidly progressive and destructive consequences. Managing the septic patient is often a challenge, and effective nursing care requires an ability to identify and respond to various trends in the clinical course of the disease. By relating the patient's response and knowledge of the condition's pathophysiology to the sequence of events, the nurse can formulate measures that remain effective and are directed at eradicating the cause of the disease.

REFERENCES

Bone, R. C., Balk, R. A., Cerra, F. B., Dellinger, R. P., Fein, A. M., Knaus, W. A., Schein, R. M., & Sibbald, W. S. (1992). Definitions for sepsis and organ failure and guidelines for the use of innovative therapies in sepsis. The ACCP/SCCM Consensus Conference Committee. *CHEST, 101,* 1644–1655.

Bone, R. C., Fisher, C. J., Clemmer, T. P., et al. (1989). Sepsis syndrome: A valid clinical entity. *Critical Care Medicine, 17*(5), 389–393.

Coleman, R. M., Lombard, M. F., Sicard, R. E., et al. (1989). *Fundamental Immunology.* Dubuque, IA: William C. Brown.

Ellrodt, A. G., Riedinger, M. S., Kimchi, A., et al. (1985). Left ventricular performance in septic shock: Reversible segmental and global abnormalities. *American Heart Journal, 10,* 402–409.

Fong, Y., Moldawer, L. L., Shires, G. T., et al. (1990). The biology of cytokines and their implications in surgical injury. *Surgery, Gynecology, and Obstetrics, 164,* 415–422.

Houston, M. C. (1990). Pathophysiology of shock. *Critical Care Clinics of North America, 2*(2), 143–149.

Hoyt, N. J. (1989). Host defense mechanisms and compromises in the trauma patient. *Critical Care Nursing Clinics of North America, 1*(4), 753–762.

Hoyt, N. J. (1990). Preventing septic shock: Infection control in the ICU. *Critical Care Nursing Clinics of North America,* 2(2), 287–296.

Kirchner, C. W., & Reheis, C. (1982). Two serious complications of neoplasia—sepsis and disseminated intravascular coagulation. *Nursing Clinics of North America, 17*(4), 595–606.

Luce, J. M. (1987). Pathogenesis and management of septic shock. *Chest, 91*(6), 883–888.

Massanari, R. M. (1989). Nosocomial infections in critical care units: Causation and prevention. *Critical Care Nursing Quarterly, 11*(4), 45–57.

Parker, M. M., Selhamer, J. H., & Bacharach, S. L. (1984). Profound but reversible myocardial depression in patients with septic shock. *Annals of Internal Medicine, 100,* 483–490.

Parrillo, J. E. (1989a). The cardiovascular response to human septic shock. In B. P. Fuhrman & W. C. Shoemaker (Eds.), *Critical Care: State of the Art* (pp. 285–314). Fullerton, CA: Society of Critical Care Medicine.

Parrillo, J. E. (1989b). Septic shock in humans: Clinical evaluation, pathophysiology & therapeutic approach. In W. C. Shoemaker, W. L. Thompson, P. H. Holbrook, et al. (Eds.), *Textbook of Critical Care* (2nd ed., pp. 1006–1023). Philadelphia: W. B. Saunders.

Parrillo, J. E., Burch, C., Shelhamer, J. H., et al. (1985). A circulating myocardial depressant substance in humans with septic shock. *Journal of Clinical Investigations, 76,* 1539–1553.

Reines, D. H., & Haluska, P. V. (1989). Arachidonic acid metabolites—the eicosanoids. In W. C. Shoemaker, W. L. Thompson, P. H. Holbrook, et al. (Eds.), *Textbook of Critical Care* (2nd ed., pp. 1028–1034). Philadelphia: W. B. Saunders.

Rice, V. (1984). The clinical continuum of septic shock. *Critical Care Nurse,* Sept.-Oct., 86–108.

Roach, A. C. (1990). Antibiotic therapy in septic shock. *Critical Care Nursing Clinics of North America, 2*(2), 179–186.

Schaer, G. L., Fink, M. B., & Parrillo, J. E. (1985). Norepinephrine alone versus norepinephrine plus low-dose dopamine: Enhanced renal blood flow with combination pressor therapy. *Critical Care Medicine, 13,* 492.

Schumann, L. L., & Remington, M. A. (1990). The use of naloxone in treating endotoxic shock. *Critical Care Nurse, 10*(2), 63–71.

Stroud, M., Swindell, B., & Bernard, G. R. (1990). Cellular and humoral mediators of sepsis syndrome. *Critical Care Nursing Clinics of North America, 2*(2), 151–160.

Suffredini, A.F. (1994). Current prospects for the treatment of clinical sepsis. *Critical Care Medicine, 22,* S12–S18.

Vane, J. R., & Botting, R. M. (1989). Prostaglandins, prostacyclins, thromboxane, and leukotrienes: The arachidonic acid cascade. In B. P. Fuhrman & W. C. Shoemaker (Eds.), *Critical Care: State of the Art* (pp. 1–23). Fullerton, CA: Society of Critical Care Medicine.

Shock

Kimmith Jones

Early recognition and prompt management of the patient with shock are vitally important. Skillful management requires knowledge of sophisticated monitoring and support technology as well as an appreciation of the many devastating physiologic derangements that make shock so lethal. Despite advancing understanding and technologic development, mortality from most forms of shock is high, and care of patients with shock remains a demanding and challenging task. This chapter discusses the mechanism of shock, the clinical presentation of shock, assessment of the patient with shock, and available treatment options.

DEFINITION OF SHOCK

Shock can best be defined as a condition in which systemic blood pressure (BP) is inadequate to deliver oxygen to vital organs. The amount of blood flowing to the tissues is inadequate to meet the oxygen demand of the cell (Barone & Snyder, 1991). Shock can be caused from a variety of pathologic conditions with the end result being decreased cellular perfusion and decreased oxygen delivery to all parts of the body.

Two requirements must be present before shock can be diagnosed. First, there must be a reduction in mean systemic BP. Blood flow is maintained through autoregulation of the blood vessels between a mean arterial pressure (MAP) of 60 to 130 mm Hg. Below a MAP of 60 mm Hg hypoperfusion results (Astiz et al., 1993). Second, evidence of hypoperfusion of vital organs must be present. Manifestations of hypoperfusion can be observed in all body systems (see Table 64–1).

TABLE 64–1. **Manifestations of Hypoperfusion by Body System**

Organ System	Symptom/Sign
CNS*	Mental status changes
Cardiovascular*	Increased or decreased blood pressure Increased or decreased heart rate Arrhythmia New murmur, gallop Chest pain, neck vein distension / flattening
Respiratory*	Tachypnea / dyspnea
Renal*	Oliguria / anuria
Skin	Cool, clammy, mottled, cyanotic, moist, flushed, warm
Other	Hypo- / hyperthermia

*Most commonly affected organ systems

PATHOPHYSIOLOGY

Shock results in an imbalance between oxygen supply and oxygen demand. When compensatory mechanisms fail to maintain blood flow to vital organs, oxygen supply is inadequate to meet oxygen demand. Oxygen consumption ($\dot{V}O_2$) drops and anaerobic metabolism occurs, along with an accumulation of oxygen debt. The amount of oxygen debt present correlates to the seriousness and irreversibility of the shock state (Astiz et al., 1993).

In the normal cell, oxygen is required for the mitochondria to convert adenosine diphosphate to adenosine triphosphate (ATP) through a process called oxidative phosphorylation. ATP is then used by the body to carry out its many functions. If oxygen is not available, as in shock, anaerobic metabolism begins. ATP is still produced; however, the process is less efficient and less ATP is made available. Aerobic metabolism produces 38 mol of ATP whereas anaerobic metabolism produces 2 mol of ATP (Astiz et al., 1993).

Cellular hypoxia occurs and anaerobic metabolism begins once the body's compensatory mechanisms fail. The anaerobic process is the same no matter what caused the low perfusion state. If prompt intervention is initiated, the process can be reversed. However, if low perfusion is left for an extended period of time before interventions are begun, the process will become irreversible and death will be imminent.

Lactate is produced as an end product of anaerobic metabolism. Increased levels of lactate produce an acidic environment and can have dramatic effects on the body's pH. Lactate levels greater than 2 mEq/L have been associated with increased mortality from shock (Astiz & Rackow, 1993).

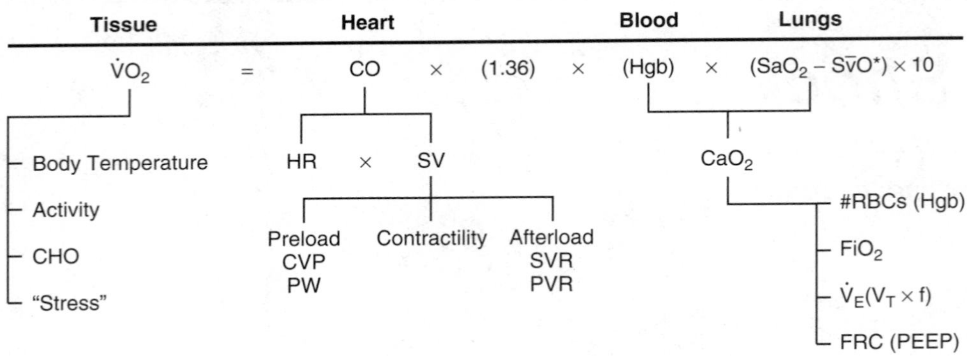

FIGURE 64–1. Factors influencing oxygen consumption ($\dot{V}O_2$).

Lactic acid production is a marker of decreased oxygen delivery and correlates with the degree of hypoperfusion. An elevated lactate level is a late indicator of hypoperfusion because it only occurs after oxygen extraction has been maximized (Astiz & Rackow, 1993). In order for lactate to be removed by the body, it must first leave the cell and travel to the liver, where it is metabolized. Falling lactate levels are associated with increased perfusion and improved patient outcome; however, clearance of lactate during shock can take hours to correct (Astiz & Rackow, 1993; Astiz et al., 1993). Avoiding low perfusion, or shock, states can help to avoid the devastating consequences of anaerobic metabolism and lactic acid production.

Oxygen Consumption ($\dot{V}O_2$) and Oxygen Delivery (DO_2)

Oxygen consumption and oxygen delivery are global measures of oxygen metabolism. $\dot{V}O_2$ is the total amount of oxygen being used by the tissues. Normal $\dot{V}O_2$ is 200–250 mL/min. $\dot{V}O_2$ is the difference between the amount of oxygen being delivered to the tissues and the amount of oxygen returning to the right side of the heart. Many factors can influence $\dot{V}O_2$ (see Fig. 64–1), including temperature, sedation, anesthesia, and infection (Barone & Snyder, 1991) (see Tables 64–2 and 64–3).

Oxygen delivery (DO_2) is the total amount of oxygen being delivered to the tissues. Normal DO_2 is 100° mL/min and is the product of cardiac output (CO), hemoglobin, and arterial oxygen saturation (SaO_2) (Daleiden, 1993).

Both DO_2 and $\dot{V}O_2$ can be calculated at the bedside and trended over time to objectively evaluate the effectiveness of therapy. The accuracy of the calculations depends on the accuracy of the measured parameters used in the formulas (Barone & Snyder, 1991) (see Table 64–4). Many investigators support increasing DO_2 and $\dot{V}O_2$ to supranormal levels to repay the oxygen debt that has accumulated and to assure adequate perfusion of the tissues to meet their metabolic demands (Daleiden, 1993; Shoemaker et al., 1990); however, this practice remains controversial.

Studies examining DO_2 and $\dot{V}O_2$ in postoperative patients reveal that survivors have an early increase in cardiac index (CI), DO_2, and $\dot{V}O_2$ compared to nonsurvivors. DO_2 and $\dot{V}O_2$ in nonsurvivors were normal, but compared to the survivor group, were significantly reduced (Shoemaker et al., 1990). Further, the degree of decrease and the length of time $\dot{V}O_2$ was decreased were greater in nonsurvivors (Shoemaker et al., 1990).

The common denominator in all classifications of shock is a reduction in DO_2 and $\dot{V}O_2$ (Barone & Snyder, 1991). Reliability of heart rate (HR), BP, CO, and pulmonary capillary wedge pressure (PCWP) as outcome predictors is poor and therefore these variables should

TABLE 64–2. **Percentage Increase in Oxygen Consumption ($\dot{V}O_2$) Due to Routine Procedures and Nursing Care**

Dressing change	10–25%
Nursing assessment	12%
ECG	16%
Move limbs	18%
Physical exam	20%
Visitors	22%
Bath	23%
Chest x-ray	22–25%
Endotracheal tube suctioning	27%
Turn	31%
Chest physiotherapy	20–35%
Weight on sling scale	36%
Nasal intubation	25–40%
Linen change, occupied bed	22%
Linen change, patient out of bed	29%
Linen change, top to bottom	47%

TABLE 64–3. **Conditions That Increase Oxygen Consumption ($\dot{V}O_2$)**

Cholecystectomy	7%
Fever (each 1°C)	10%
Agitation	18%
Skeletal injury	10–30%
Increased work of breathing	40%
Chest trauma	60%
Infection	60%
Critically ill in ER	60%
Multiple organ failure	20–80%
Sepsis	80–100%
Shivering	50–100%
Seizing	100%
Burns	100%
Head injury, sedated	89%
Head injury, nonsedated	138%

TABLE 64–4. **Calculated Oxygenation Parameters**

Oxygenation Parameters	Normal Values
$Do_2 = CO \times Cao_2 \times 10$	1000 mL/min
$Do_2I = CI \times Cao_2 \times 10$	500–600 mL/min/m^2
$\dot{V}o_2 = CO \times 13.4 \times Hgb \times (Sao_2 - S\bar{v}o_2)$	200–250 mL/min
$\dot{V}o_2I = CI \times 13.4 \times Hgb \times (Sao_2 - S\bar{v}o_2)$	120–160 mL/min/m^2
$Cao_2 = (Hgb \times 13.4 \times Sao_2) + (0.003 \times Pao_2)$	20 mL/dL
$Cvo_2 = (Hgb \times 13.4 \times Svo_2) + (0.003 \times Pvo_2)$	
$O_2\ Ext = \dfrac{Cao_2 - Cvo_2}{Cao_2}$	

not be used as endpoints of therapy; Do_2 and $\dot{V}o_2$ should be used instead (Barone & Snyder, 1991).

During hypoperfusion, the amount of oxygen delivered to the tissues decreases. The tissues can continue to consume the regular amount of oxygen by increasing the amount being extracted from the blood as it passes by the tissues and by increasing CO. This is termed delivery-independent $\dot{V}o_2$ (Barone & Snyder, 1991; Daleiden, 1993) (see Fig. 64–2). Normal oxygen extraction is 22% to 30%. This leaves a large reserve available when oxygen demand increases. Oxygen extraction can increase threefold before changes in other physiologic variables will be seen (Astiz & Rackow, 1993). If delivery continues to decrease despite maximal extraction, $\dot{V}o_2$ will eventually decrease as well. This concept is termed delivery-dependent $\dot{V}o_2$ (Astiz & Rackow, 1993; Daleiden, 1993). In the face of critical illness, $\dot{V}o_2$ is more dependent on oxygen delivery secondary to the inability to increase extraction maximally (Astiz & Rackow, 1993). Titration of therapy to increase $\dot{V}o_2$ and Do_2 has been associated with increased survival; however, increasing these variables to supranormal levels does not allow for individualization of treatment (Astiz & Rackow, 1993). Titration of therapy to the point at which $\dot{V}o_2$ is no longer dependent on Do_2 seems more appropriate and allows for individualization of treatment based on the patient's need (Astiz & Rackow, 1993; Barone & Snyder, 1991).

Oxygen debt is the difference between $\dot{V}o_2$ and the metabolic demands of the tissue (Daleiden, 1993) (see Fig. 64–3). Decreased $\dot{V}o_2$ in the face of increased metabolic need produces an oxygen debt that must be repaid as quickly as possible (Shoemaker et al., 1990). Failure to repay the oxygen debt will lead to irreversibility of the shock state.

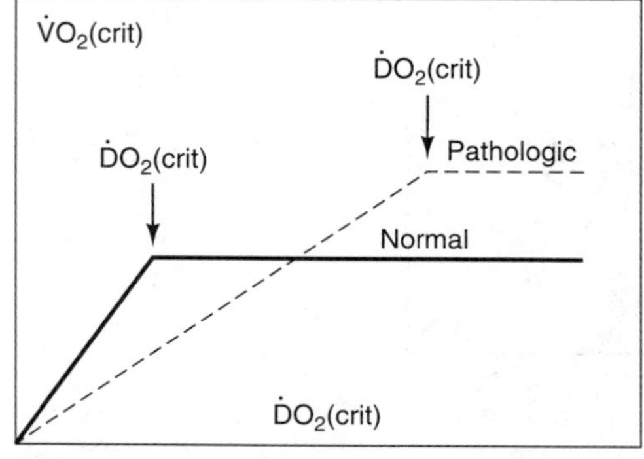

FIGURE 64–2. Theoretical relationship of Do_2 and $\dot{V}o_2$.

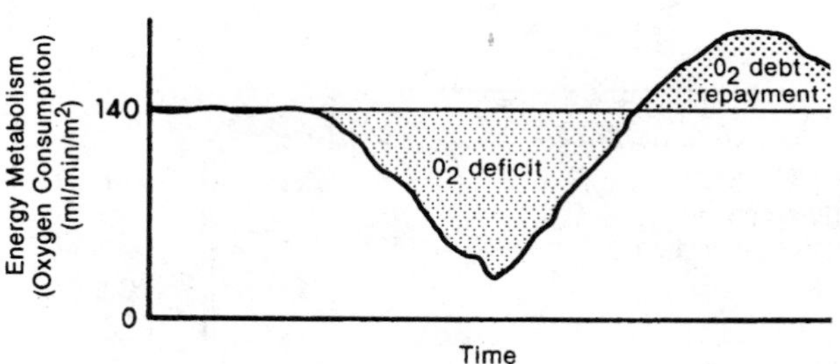

FIGURE 64–3. Graphic representation of the repayment of the oxygen debt when oxygen consumption following resuscitation exceeds the baseline requirements for oxygen. (Reprinted by permission from Siegel, J. H., Linberg, S. E., Wiles, C. E. [1987]. Therapy of low-flow shock states. In Siegel, J. H. [ed.]: *Trauma: Emergency surgery and critical care* [p. 207]. New York: Churchill Livingstone.

Increases in Do_2 can be accomplished by increasing CO, increasing the oxygen-carrying capacity of the blood, and increasing Sao_2. Also, increasing Do_2 can be accomplished by decreasing metabolic demands through decreasing patient activity, sedation, and decreasing patient temperature.

COMPENSATORY MECHANISMS

Compensatory mechanisms are set into motion when the body recognizes that a low perfusion state is occurring in an attempt to return CO and MAP to normal levels. The end result of these compensatory mechanisms is an improvement in tissue perfusion and prevention of tissue necrosis.

The majority of compensatory mechanisms are regulated by either neuronal or hormonal processes.

Neuronal Compensatory Mechanisms

BARORECEPTOR REFLEX. Baroreceptors are located in the carotid bodies and aortic arch. These receptors sense changes in arterial pressure and send signals to the vasomotor center, located in the medulla and pons, via a feedback mechanism. This mechanism is started within seconds of a drop in BP and is fully activated within 30 seconds. When there is a drop in MAP, the stretch of the arterial baroreceptors decreases and the receptors can no longer inhibit the vasomotor center. The outcome is vasomotor stimulation and the release of impulses to the sympathetic vasoconstrictor fibers located throughout the body in both the arterial and venous systems (see Fig. 64–4). These fibers are very powerful in the kidneys, intestines, spleen, and skin. Stimulation of vasoconstrictors leads to arteriolar constriction, venous constriction, increased HR, and increased contractility (see Fig. 64–5).

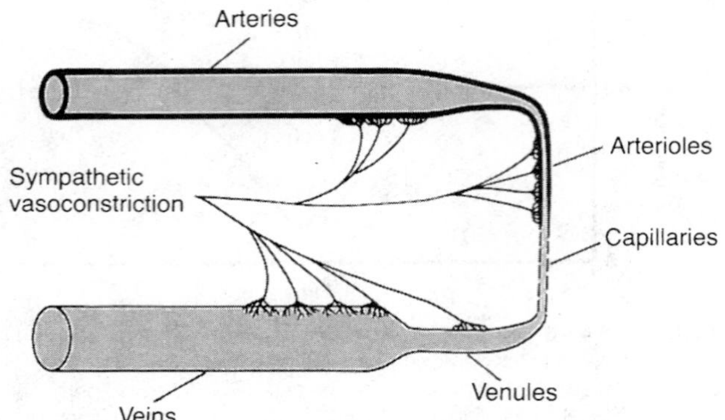

FIGURE 64–4. Sympathetic innervation of the systemic circulation. (From Guyton, A. C., & Hall, J. E. [1996]. *Textbook of medical physiology* [9th ed.]. Philadelphia: W. B. Saunders.)

CENTRAL NERVOUS SYSTEM ISCHEMIC RESPONSE. The vasomotor center becomes ischemic with elevated carbon dioxide (CO_2) levels when the MAP drops below 50 mm Hg. CO_2 is a very powerful sympathetic stimulator that leads to vasoconstriction. This mechanism begins within seconds of the drop in MAP and is fully activated within minutes.

REFLEX VENOCONSTRICTION. Sympathetic stimulation of veins does not augment arterial pressure or total peripheral resistence a great deal. The positive benefits of sympathetic stimulation of veins is in decreasing the amount of blood they can hold.

STIMULATION OF CHEMORECEPTORS. Chemoreceptors are located in the carotid bodies and aortic arch and are sensitive to changes in oxygen concentration and drops in arterial pressure. When stimulated, impulses travel to and stimulate the vasomotor center. The chemoreceptor response is not a powerful mechanism until BP drops to below 80 mm Hg. It plays a much greater role in the control of respiration than in the control of blood pressure.

Hormonal Compensatory Mechanisms

NOREPINEPHRINE-EPINEPHRINE VASOCONSTRICTOR MECHANISM. Stimulation of the vasomotor center also stimulates the release of norepinephrine and epinephrine from the adrenal medulla, resulting in vasoconstriction throughout the body.

ACTIVATION OF THE RENIN–ANGIOTENSIN SYSTEM. The reduction in perfusion pressure to the kidney results in stimulation of the baroreceptors in the juxtaglomerular cells, activating the renin–angiotensin system within minutes of the drop is perfusion. It becomes fully activated within 30 minutes. The renal hormone renin is released, which converts renin substrate to angiotensin I. Angiotensin I is then converted to angiotensin II by angiotensin-converting enzyme, mainly in the vascular epithelium of the lungs (see Fig. 64–6). This process also occurs in the heart, adrenals, kidneys, and brain. Angiotensin II is a powerful vasocon-

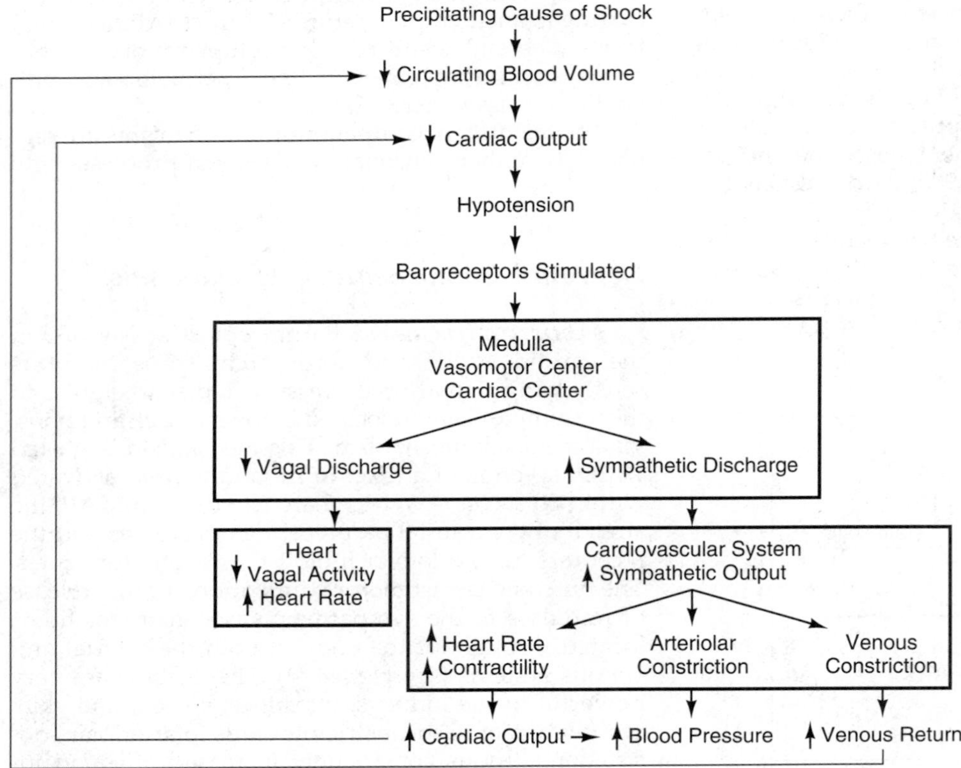

FIGURE 64–5. Compensatory mechanisms for the restoration of circulatory blood volume.

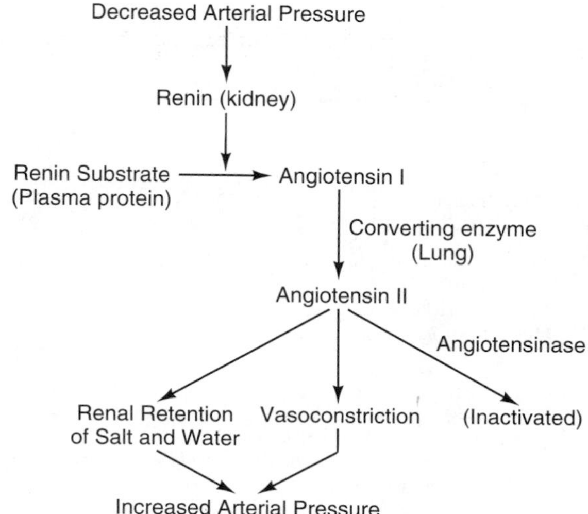

FIGURE 64–6. The renin-angiotensin-vasoconstrictor mechanism for arterial pressure control. (From Guyton, A. C., & Hall, J. E. [1996]. *Textbook of medical physiology* [9th ed.]. Philadelphia: W. B. Saunders.)

strictor leading to widespread vasoconstriction in the arterioles and to a lesser extent in the venules. The renin–angiotensin system stimulates the release of aldosterone from the adrenal cortex, which helps to increase sodium and water retention and maintain intravascular volume and has a direct effect on the kidneys to decrease the amount of water and salt being excreted.

VASOPRESSIN (ANTIDIURETIC HORMONE). The hypothalamus stimulates the release of arginine vasopressin (AVP) from the posterior pituitary gland when BP drops. Vasopressin has a direct effect on the constriction of blood vessels and in decreasing the excretion of water from the kidneys.

Other Intrinsic Mechanisms

CONSTRICTION OF AFFERENT AND EFFERENT ARTERIOLES OF THE KIDNEYS. A decreased MAP leads to reduced renal artery pressure, which is followed by renal arteriolar constriction. This results in a decrease in glomerular filtration and renal plasma flow, which leads to a decrease in urine output and an increase in urine sodium retention.

CAPILLARY FLUID SHIFT. Arteriolar constriction, during low perfusion states, results in a drop in venous pressure and a decrease in capillary hydrostatic pressure. This leads to a fluid shift from the interstitial and intracellular space to the intravascular space. Capillary fluid shifts begin within minutes of a drop in BP and become fully activated within several hours.

CLASSIFICATION OF SHOCK

There are four classifications of shock: hypovolemic, cardiogenic, distributive, and obstructive. Each type occurs secondary to a physiologic change that precludes the delivery of oxygen to the tissues (see Table 64–5). Therapeutic interventions have been developed for each classification (Barone & Snyder, 1991).

Hypovolemic Shock

Hypovolemic shock results from a reduction in the intravascular blood volume (Daleiden, 1993). The degree of volume depletion determines the symptoms and severity of the shock state.

Hypovolemic shock has three stages (Daleiden, 1993; Houston, 1990). In stage 1, a blood volume deficit of 10%, which is equal to about 500 mL, has occurred. The body's compensatory mechanisms can maintain a normal CO and arterial pressure with this degree of volume loss. The compensatory mechanisms initially activated include sympathetic constriction of the blood vessels and tachycardia. If the shock state continues, an increase in the secretion of vasopressin, renin, and aldosterone begins, along with a fluid shift from the intrastitial space to the intravascular space in an attempt to maintain intravascular volume. The patient who is in stage 1 of hypovolemic shock is asymptomatic.

Stage 2 of hypovolemic shock occurs when a volume deficit of 15% to 20% has taken place. A noticeable decrease in CO and arterial pressure can be observed. In response to this stressor, the body attempts to respond by increasing arteriolar constriction, venoconstriction, and sympathetic discharge. These maneuvers have the effect of increasing HR, increasing respiratory rate, and causing cutaneous constriction. Other signs and symptoms the patient might experience include pallor, diaphoresis, piloerection, apprehension, and restlessness.

Stage 3 occurs when the volume deficit is greater than 25%. All compensatory mechanisms are in full action and may or may not be able to maintain adequate perfusion. Any additional losses can lead to rapid decompensation in CO, arterial pressure, and perfusion. A concept referred to as irreversible shock can develop with a volume loss greater than 25% and result in the person's inability to respond to resuscitation measures and other therapeutic interventions (Astiz et al., 1993).

Hemodynamic changes that can occur in patients with hypovolemic shock include decreases in stroke index, left ventricular stroke work, CO, and CI secondary to decreases in preload. Pulmonary artery pressure (PAP) and PCWP are also decreased secondary to a decreased preload. Systemic vascular resistance (SVR) is increased due to compensatory arterial vasoconstriction. $\dot{V}O_2$ is decreased secondary to a decreased CO and hypovolemia. Mixed venous oxygen saturation ($S\bar{v}O_2$) is also decreased. A decreased $S\bar{v}O_2$ is related to

TABLE 64–5. **Classification of Shock States***

Type of Shock	Primary Mechanism	Clinical Condition
Hypovolemia	Volume loss	Hemorrhage Burns Vomiting, diarrhea Dehydration Osmolar diuresis
Cardiogenic	Pump failure	Myocardial infarction Arrhythmia Valvular disease Heart failure
Distributive	Alteration in blood flow distribution	
High resistance	Expanded venous capacitance	Gram-negative infection (hypodynamic phase), autonomic blockage, spinal shock, tranquilizer, narcotic, sedative overdose, adrenal insufficiency†
Low resistance	Arteriovenous shunting	Hyperdynamic sepsis, liver disease, A-V malformations, adrenal insufficiency†
Obstructive	Extracardiac obstruction of arterial or venous blood flow	Vena cava obstruction (gravid uterus), cardiac tamponade, pulmonary embolus, dissecting aneurysm

*Mixed states are commonly encountered
†May have components of both categories
From Smith, J. L., & Steele, K. W. (1991). Shock—another approach. *Transport, 2*(2), 9.

a decrease in CO and an increase in oxygen extraction at the tissue level (Summers, 1990) (see Table 64–6).

Other signs and symptoms that can be observed include increased respiratory rate, decreased urine output, and restlessness or anxiousness, which may lead to lethargy and unresponsiveness (Summers, 1990).

COLLABORATIVE MANAGEMENT

Hypovolemic shock is treated by rapid replacement of intravascular volume and correction of the cause of the volume depletion. Infusion of fluids is the fundamental treatment and is continued until adequate MAP and organ perfusion is reestablished (Gould et al., 1993). Common intravenous (IV) fluids used for resuscitation include normal saline and lactated Ringer's solution.

Controversy still exists regarding the most appropriate fluid to use during resuscitation. Colloids are thought to decrease the risk of pulmonary edema by maintaining serum oncotic pressure. Crystalloids, on the other hand, may lead to substantial hemodilution. A 1 to 3 g drop in hemoglobin can be observed during resuscitation of hypovolemic shock if crystalloids are given, which can lead to decreased DO_2 (Astiz et al., 1993).

There does not appear to be a difference in oxygen metabolism when the hematocrit is 30% versus 40%, and limited benefit is achieved when a hemoglobin greater than 10 mg/dL is present. However, patients with heart failure or who have a decreased $S\bar{v}O_2$ may require a higher hemoglobin to achieve adequate DO_2 (Astiz et al., 1993).

Beta-endorphins are released in increased amounts in patients with hypovolemic and septic shock and result in increased vasodilation. Naloxone, an opiate antagonist, has been successful in reversing the effects of beta-endorphins in some experimental studies (Astiz et al., 1993).

Cardiogenic Shock

Cardiogenic shock refers to a decreased DO_2 to the tissues due to pump or heart failure. Cardiogenic shock is defined as a low CO and hypotension with clinical signs of inadequate perfusion, such as low urine out-

TABLE 64–6. **Cardiopulmonary Failure Patterns**

	CO	PCWP	PAP	SVR	SvO_2	$\dot{V}O_2$	O_2Ext	CVP	LVSW	HR	SI
Hypovolemic	↓	↓	↓	↑	↓	↓	↑	↓	↓	↑	↓
Cardiogenic	↓	↑	↑	↑	↓	↓	↑	↑	↓	↑	↓
Obstructive	↓	↑	↑	↑	↓	↓	↑	↑	↑	↑	↓
Distributive°	↓	↓	↓	↓	↓	↓	↑	↓	↓	↑	↓

Abbreviations: O_2Ext = oxygen extraction; $\dot{V}O_2$ = oxygen consumption; SvO_2 = venous oxygen saturation; ° a mixed picture may be present.

put, a change in mental status, decreased peripheral pulses, and cool and clammy skin (Albert & Becker, 1993; Astiz et al., 1993).

The major causative event leading to cardiogenic shock is acute myocardial infarction (MI) and occurs when a significant amount of the left ventricular myocardium has been destroyed (Albert & Becker, 1993; Astiz et al., 1993; Summers, 1990). Mortality from cardiogenic shock is 75% to 100% (Albert & Becker, 1993; Houston, 1990) and occurs in 5% to 15% of all patients with acute MI (Albert & Becker, 1993).

The ability of the heart to pump effectively may also be impaired by a variety of metabolic derangements, such as severe hypoxemia, acidosis, hypoglycemia, and hypocalcemia. Other causes may include cardiomyopathy, myocarditis, cardiac tamponade, rupture of the intraventricular septum, papillary muscle rupture, or right heart failure (O'Neil, 1994). See Table 64–7 for additional precipitating factors of cardiogenic shock.

The classic symptoms of cardiogenic shock include pulmonary edema, generalized edema, jugular venous distention, and a low CO despite an elevated PCWP, above 18 mm Hg. Left ventricular ejection fraction is usually below 20% to 30% (Albert & Becker, 1993). Right-sided heart pressures may be normal or elevated. Other signs and symptoms that can be observed include decreases in BP and CO secondary to decreased contractility of the heart. Increases in respiratory rate can be seen along with crackles secondary to pulmonary congestion related to an increased preload to the left ventricle. Urine output is decreased, and restlessness, agitation, and confusion can be seen due

TABLE 64–7. **Etiology of Cardiogenic Shock**

Acute myocardial infarction
- Severely reduced left ventricular function
- Ventricular septal rupture
- Acute mitral regurgitation
- Right ventricular infarction

Other cardiac entities that can be associated with inadequate ventricular function
- Dilated cardiomyopathy/severe myocarditis
- End-stage valvular heart disease—aortic stenosis, mitral stenosis, aortic regurgitation, mitral regurgitation
- Tachy- or bradyarrhythmias
- Following cardiopulmonary bypass

Cardiac obstruction or compression
- Pericardial tamponade or constriction
- Pulmonary embolism
- Severe pulmonary hypertension—e.g., primary pulmonary hypertension
- Coarctation of the aorta
- Myxoma
- Severe hypertrophic cardiomyopathy
- Tension pneumothorax

From Alpert, J. S., & Becker, R. C. (1993). Mechanisms and management of cardiogenic shock. *Critical Care Clinics, 9*(2), 206.

Abbreviations: CaO_2 = arterial oxygen content; FiO_2 = fraction of inspired oxygen; $\dot{V}_E$ = minute ventilation; V_T = tidal volume; PEEP = positive and expiratory pressure; CHO = carbohydrate load.

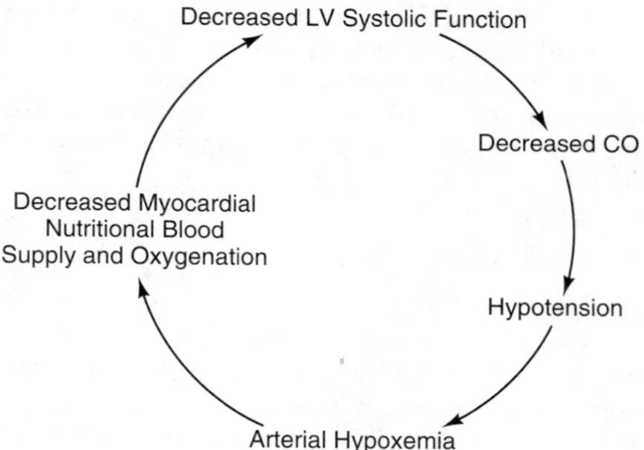

FIGURE 64–7. Cycle of cardiogenic shock.

to a reduction in cerebral perfusion, which may lead to further reduction in the level of consciousness (Summers, 1990).

A vicious cycle occurs when patients develop cardiogenic shock (see Fig. 64–7). CO drops due to a drop in left ventricular systolic function. As a result, hypotension occurs, which lead to arterial hypoxemia. A decreased myocardial nutritional blood supply occurs due to the drop in arterial supply, which leads to more left ventricular dysfunction (Albert & Becker, 1993).

The compensatory response of the body to these changes, particularly the low BP, is to stimulate the sympathetic nervous system. Sympathetic stimulation releases catecholamines, resulting in an increased HR and increased contractility of the heart. Vasoconstriction occurs, resulting in pale, cool, and clammy skin. BP drops and heart rate continues to increase when compensatory mechanism begin to fail (Summers, 1990).

Hemodynamic changes that are seen with the patient in cardiogenic shock include decreases in CO and CI, in stroke index, and in left ventricular stroke work due to decreased contractility. PAP and PCWP are increased secondary to an elevated left ventricular preload. Right atrial pressure is increased secondary to an elevated left ventricular end-diastolic pressure due to an increased preload. During cardiogenic shock, an increase in preload stimulates the release of atrial natriuretic hormone, which results in increased renal artery vasodilation, to maintain renal blood flow (Astiz et al., 1993). SVR is increased secondary to compensatory vasoconstriction. $\dot{V}O_2$ is decreased due to a reduction in the amount of oxygen being delivered to the tissues. $S\bar{v}O_2$ is decreased due to an increase in oxygen extraction and less oxygen returning to the right side of the heart (Summers, 1990) (Table 64–6).

Cardiac index is a good tool to use when assessing severity of cardiogenic shock. A CI of <1.8 indicates cardiogenic shock. Clinical signs of hypoperfusion can be observed when the CI is between 1.8 and 2.2 L/min/m^2. Construction of a bedside Starling curve to identify the best PCWP that maximizes CI can be very helpful (Albert & Becker, 1993).

Disturbances in HR can also result in inadequate

pump function. CO is the product of HR and stroke volume (SV); therefore, very slow rhythms can reduce CO despite a normal or even increased SV. Very fast rhythms can reduce SV because of insufficient diastolic filling time, resulting in a reduction in CO despite the rapid HR.

COLLABORATIVE MANAGEMENT

Stabilization of the patient before attempting to establish an exact diagnosis is a must to avoid wasting time (Albert & Becker, 1993). Stabilization refers to establishing ventilation and oxygenation, which takes highest priority; restoring BP; and correcting hypovolemia (Albert & Becker, 1993).

Treatment modalities for cardiogenic shock include inotropic agents, such as dobutamine, dopamine, and amrinone. These agents assist in improving contractility. Dobutamine is a beta-adrenergic agonist that increases CI, Do_2, and $\dot{V}o_2$ and decreases mean PAP, PCWP, systemic vascular resistance, and pulmonary vascular resistance. Dobutamine does not affect these variables in patients who remain hypovolemic (Barone & Snyder, 1991). Dobutamine does increase myocardial oxygen demand; however, the increase in coronary blood flow, and therefore the increased Do_2 to the myocardium, is greater than the increased oxygen demand of the myocardium required for increased inotropy (Barone & Snyder, 1991). Vasoactive drugs, such as sodium nitroprusside (Nipride) or nitroglycerin, are also used to decrease afterload and preload (Albert & Becker, 1993). Inotropic agents and vasopressors should be started when the systolic BP is less than 100 mm Hg. Caution must be taken when initiating dobutamine on a patient with a low BP because of the reflex peripheral vasodilation that is frequently observed.

Dopamine is the most widely used catecholamine. The net effect of dopamine depends on the dosage. At very low doses, only dopamine receptors in the renal and mesenteric circulations are stimulated to dilate, thereby preserving blood flow to these organs. At moderate doses, inotropy increases, along with an increase in vascular resistance and preservation of renal blood flow. At high doses, renal blood flow is reduced and vasoconstriction becomes more intense. The dose at which these effects occur varies among individuals.

Local extravasation of dopamine causes such intense vasoconstriction that tissue necrosis may occur. For that reason, dopamine should be administered through a central line. Direct subcutaneous injection of an alpha blocker, such as phentolamine 10 mg, into the site of dopamine infiltration can prevent tissue necrosis if the problem is identified and treated promptly.

Treatment for cardiogenic shock may also include intraaortic balloon counterpulsation (IABC) (Albert & Becker, 1993; Schott, 1990). The goals of IABC in the patient with cardiogenic shock are to increase SV, increase coronary artery perfusion, decrease preload, decrease cardiac work, and decrease myocardial $\dot{V}o_2$. Positive patient outcomes with IABC include increased urine output, increased CO, and a decreased HR (Albert & Becker, 1993; Schott, 1990). Clinical improvements can be seen in 75% of patients when IABC is used (Albert & Becker, 1993).

Cardiac transplantation is another strategy to correct cardiogenic shock. Stopgap measures may need to be implemented until a donor is found because of the limited availability of organ donors. Artificial hearts and ventricular assist devices are two measures that may be used (Albert & Becker, 1993).

Reperfusion of the occluded vessels may also help to prevent cardiogenic shock from becoming a problem. Reperfusion with thrombolytic agents may help to improve survival (Albert & Becker, 1993).

Distributive Shock

Distributive shock results from a maldistribution of blood flow (Astiz et al., 1993). Intravascular volume has not changed and heart function is not impaired; however, blood is not reaching the tissues. Distributive shock usually occurs with acute vasodilation without a concomitant increase in intravascular volume. The most common type of distributive shock is sepsis. Other causes of distributive shock include autonomic block, spinal shock, drug overdose resulting in vasodilation, arteriovenous malformations, and adrenal insufficiency.

Another cause of distributive shock is anaphylaxis. During anaphylaxis, an antigen combines with immunoglobulin E and activates basophils, mast cells, and eosinophils. These cells are responsible for making and releasing leukotrienes, histamine, platelet-activating factor, prostaglandins, and others, which cause bronchoconstriction, increased microvascular permeability, and vasodilation (Astiz et al., 1993).

Anaphylactic shock is the most severe manifestation of allergy and can occur after exposure of sensitized individuals to drugs, foods, insect venoms, or other allergens. The mechanism of shock is largely distributive because release of histamine and vasoactive compounds from mast cells results in vasodilation and increased capillary permeability.

Signs and symptoms of anaphylaxis can begin within 20 minutes after exposure to the allergen. The sooner the signs and symptoms begin, the more severe the reaction. An early sign is a feeling of being warm. Later signs and symptoms include urticaria, pruritus, and angioedema. The individual may sometimes complain of a sense of "impending doom." Laryngeal edema can develop, which may lead to hoarseness and stridor. Severe bronchoconstriction can occur, resulting in wheezing and cyanosis. Peripheral vasodilation and increased capillary permeability lead to pooling of blood in the periphery, which results in a decrease in right ventricular preload. Left ventricular preload can also be decreased, which results in decreased CO, hypotension, and increased HR.

Hemodynamic monitoring of patients with anaphylactic shock may show a decreased SVR secondary to dilation of the peripheral vessels, decreased CO and CI, and decreases in central venous pressure, PAP, and PCWP. $S\bar{v}O_2$ is also decreased because of the reduction in CO and increased extraction (Summers, 1990).

COLLABORATIVE MANAGEMENT

The treatment for distributive shock is to "fill the tank" and constrict the blood vessels. This can be accomplished by administering IV fluids (normal saline or lactated Ringer's solution) and adding vasoconstrictors (dopamine) to achieve an acceptable MAP and reestablish perfusion to the organs. Prostaglandin, leukotriene, and platelet activator inhibitors are being studied in patients with anaphylaxis (Astiz et al., 1993).

Obstructive Shock

Obstructive shock results in decreased perfusion to the tissues secondary to an obstruction to blood flow somewhere in the cardiovascular system. Inadequate perfusion is present along with a decreased CO despite a normal intravascular volume and heart function. Obstructions that can cause obstructive shock include pulmonary embolism, cardiac tamponade, tension pneumothorax, dissecting aortic aneurysm, and atrial myxoma (Astiz et al., 1993).

COLLABORATIVE MANAGEMENT

Treatment for obstructive shock includes removing the obstruction from the cardiovascular system and restoring perfusion to the tissues.

GENERAL ASSESSMENT

Decreased BP is not a reliable indicator of decreased perfusion. Some individuals have an increased CO with a decreased BP secondary to vasodilation, that preserves tissue perfusion (Astiz et al., 1993).

During shock, renal perfusion is compromised, increasing the patient's risk of developing acute tubular necrosis. Initially, to maintain blood flow to the kidney, the efferent arteriolar tone increases to compensate for the reduction in flow. This eventually fails (Astiz et al., 1993).

The liver is also affected by shock. Decreased perfusion activates the Kupffer cells of the liver, which release cytokines. Impaired hepatic synthesis and clearance of substances, along with decreased phagocytic clearance of waste products, results from hypoperfusion to the liver. An increase in transaminases, alkaline phosphatase, and bilirubin can be seen; however, restoration of perfusion can correct these abnormal levels (Astiz et al., 1993). When perfusion is restored, oxygen free radicals are released from the reperfused tissue, which can result in increased capillary permeability (Astiz et al., 1993).

The body attempts to maintain the filling pressures in the heart by causing intense constriction in the splanchnic area. This process shunts blood away from the gastrointestinal tract, skeletal muscle, and subcutaneous tissue, and redirects it to the heart and brain (Astiz et al., 1993; Imm & Carlson, 1993). Intestinal blood supply is the first to be affected in shock. Decreased blood supply to the gastrointestinal tract leads to damage of the epithelial lining with leakage of proteins and solutes into the intestinal lumen (Imm & Carlson, 1993). Splanchnic hypoperfusion can lead to stress ulcer development, intestinal hemorrhage, necrosis, acalculous cholecystitis and, infrequently, pancreatitis (Astiz et al., 1993).

There appears to be a correlation between systemic DO_2 and gastric intramucosal pH. Tonometry monitors for splanchnic hypoperfusion and helps to reflect the degree of circulatory impairment. Titration of therapy to maintain normal intramucosal pH may be affiliated with decreased mortality.

Intramucosal pH is measured by inserting a nasogastric tube that has a silicone balloon attached to it into the patient's stomach. The balloon is then filled with normal saline and allowed to remain in place for 60 to 90 minutes. During this time CO_2 is equalizing between the balloon and the gastric mucosa. The saline is then removed and sent to the laboratory for measurement of CO_2 with a blood gas analyzer. At the same time, an arterial blood gas is sent to determine the bicarbonate concentration. Then using the Henderson-Hasselbalch equation the intramucosal pH is determined.

SUMMARY

Shock can be the result of many illnesses that cause reduced arterial pressure by one of four mechanisms: (1) reduced heart function, (2) reduced vascular volume, (3) obstruction in the circulation, and (4) uncontrolled vasodilation. All mechanisms of shock result in decreased DO_2 and $\dot{V}O_2$ by the tissue and the devastating consequences of anaerobic metabolism. Neural and hormonal compensatory mechanisms attempt to maintain arterial pressure but eventually fail, resulting in reduced blood flow to the tissues. Treatment depends on the specific type of shock. All patients in shock should be treated and monitored in an intensive care unit because of their high mortality, their need for a high level of nursing care, and their need for sophisticated monitoring and therapeutic technology.

REFERENCES

Albert, J. S., & Becker, R. C. (1993). Mechanisms and management of cardiogenic shock. *Critical Care Clinics, 9*(2), 205–218.

Astiz, M. E., & Rackow, E. C. (1993). Assessing perfusion failure during circulatory shock. *Critical Care Clinics, 9*(2), 299–312.

Astiz, M. E., Rackow, E. C., & Weil, M. H. (1993). Pathophysiology and treatment of circulatory shock. *Critical Care Clinics, 9*(2), 183–203.

Barone, J. E., & Snyder, A. B. (1991). Treatment strategies in shock: Use of oxygen transport measurements. *Heart and Lung, 20*(1), 81–86.

Daleiden, A. (1993). Physiology and treatment of hemorrhagic shock during the early postoperative period. *Critical Care Quarterly, 16*(1), 45–59.

Gould, S. A., & Sehgal, L. R., & Sehgal, H. L. (1993). Hypovolemic shock. *Critical Care Clinics, 9*(2), 239–259.

Houston, M. C. (1990). Pathophysiology of shock. *Critical Care Nursing Clinics of North America, 2*(2), 143–149.

Imm, A., & Carlson, R. W. (1993). Fluid resuscitation in circulatory shock. *Critical Care Clinics, 9*(2), 313–333.

Schott, K. E. (1990). Intra-aortic balloon counterpulsation as a therapy for shock. *Critical Care Nursing Clinics of North America, 2*(2), 187–193.

Summers, G. (1990). The clinical and hemodynamic presentation of the shock patient. *Critical Care Nursing Clinics of North America, 2*(2), 161–166.

Patients With Pain

Sara Reeder

Pain management in the critically ill patient is a continuous challenge to the critical care nurse due to the complexity and diversity of patients in the critical care unit. In addition, pain management is complicated by the fact that the nurse frequently causes discomfort yet is responsible for assessing and managing the pain of discomfort. Ability to address this perplexing issue requires a clear understanding of pain mechanisms as well as a knowledge of current, safe, and effective management modalities. This chapter provides comprehensive information requisite for the critical care nurse to minister therapeutically and successfully to the pain management needs of the critically ill patient.

HISTORICAL EVENTS OF PAIN IN THE CRITICALLY ILL

Chronology of Key Contributions to the Concept of Pain

Recognition and descriptions of pain are as old as humanity. Reference to pain can be found in ancient writings, artworks, songs, and poetry and in Biblical writings that included terms such as "travail" and "suffering," which were associated with sickness and plagues, as well as responses such as "weeping" and "wailing" of individuals. Treatments included the use of herbs, concoctions, mandragora root, opium, and distraction. Cousins and Phillips (1986) provide a comprehensive listing of international resources of events relating to and contributions to the concept of pain from 1564 to the beginning of critical care medicine in 1950. It is important to note that the quantity of the literature devoted to some aspect of pain cannot be equated with the amount of suffering experienced by humans over time. In the past decade, the focus on pain research has provided the critical care nurse with exciting new information derived from the discovery of opiate receptors, extensive pharmacokinetic and pharmacodynamic studies of narcotics and their actions, the development of sensitive analytic techniques and mathematical knowledge, the development of new drugs and combinations of drugs, and administration of intraspinal narcotic therapy (Bonica, 1987). In spite of these advances, the search continues for effective ways to provide individual comfort in the safest possible manner, paying particular attention to individual needs.

Some ambiguities associated with pain assessment and management are reflected in the varied and broad definitions of pain. For example, Liebeskind (1977) stated that "Pain means many different things, and the variables which correlate with, inhibit or enhance one kind of pain, and the neural mechanisms which underlie it, may not be associated with or influence other kinds" (p. 41). Mersky (1975) defined pain as "an unpleasant experience which we primarily associate with tissue damage or describe in terms of tissue damage or hurt" (p. 6).

Although Meinhart and McCaffery (1983) agree with the need for a working definition and understanding of terms associated with pain, their major premise is that the individual experiencing pain is the true authority. Therefore, the authors follow an operational definition of pain. "Pain is whatever the experiencing person says it is, existing whenever he or she says it does" (p. 11).

The International Association for the Study of Pain defines pain as "an unpleasant sensory and emotional experience associated with actual or potential tissue damage, or described in terms of such damage" (Mersky, 1979). Pain is the most common symptom reported with disease or injury and the most aversive stimulus noted for altering behavior. Pain is viewed as a protective mechanism because individuals will withdraw from or avoid the source of pain, which may cause additional tissue damage, and pain is frequently the symptom that directs the individual to seek assistance for an illness or disease process. Although pain is often considered as a protective mechanism, it can also be considered deleterious. In general, pain is regarded as a signal of tissue injury, although injury can occur without pain, and pain can occur in the absence of injury or remain after healing or cure has occurred (Muir, 1988). Despite the knowledge that pain is deleterious, it is often undertreated, and patients suffer (Ketovui, 1987).

Cultural Factors Associated With Pain

Pain is a highly personal and variable experience that is influenced by cultural learning, by the meaning of the situation, and by attention and other cognitive activities (Gaston-Johansson & Fagan, 1990). Melzack (1973) considers pain a complex, perceptual, and affective experience determined by the unique past history of the individual, by the meaning of the stimulus to him or her, by his or her "state of mind" at the moment, and by the sensory nerve patterns evoked by physical stimulation.

Individual response to pain is believed to be due to a *sensation threshold*, which is defined as the lowest stimulus value at which sensation is first reported; *pain tolerance level*, which is the point at which the subject refuses to tolerate further pain and withdraws from the stimulus; and *pain response*, which includes attitudes, emotions, attentiveness to painful sensations, and behaviors in which these orientations are displayed (Hardy et al., 1952; Gaston-Johansson & Fagan, 1990).

Initial attempts to relate cultural aspects such as religion, ethnicity, race, age, and sex to pain were reported in the 1950s. Cultural components known to influence response to pain include occupation, socioeconomic status, family relationships, whether curative or palliative treatment is sought, to whom the pain is reported, and what types of pain require attention (Hardy et al., 1952; Meinhart & McCaffery, 1983; Zborowski, 1952).

Cultural traditions dictate to members of a given society not only whether they should expect and tolerate pain but the correct response to the pain experience. The rules may vary with sex, age, and social status, but because people in a society usually comply with the cultural rules, it is important to have a working knowledge of these rules when caring for the patient. The best source of information is the patient or the family. The American family is typically a supportive unit that becomes particularly concerned during a family member's illness or injury. This is evident by observation of the numbers of family members and friends in intensive care unit (ICU) waiting rooms. Although there may be some cultural variations, in general, regardless of cultural affiliation, family members surround the suffering individual. Family members are especially attentive to the patient experiencing pain and focus on that aspect of illness. Pain is a recognizable and more familiar symptom of the illness that family members can discuss and about which they can seek information. Because of the family's ongoing involvement with the patient's painful experience, these individuals can serve as a resource for information about the patient's previous pain response and coping ability. Family members or friends can serve as supports to the patient during extreme pain episodes. The ability of family members to support the patient during pain episodes may well correlate with the amount of teaching and interaction that develops between them and the critical care nurse (Edwards et al., 1985).

Religious beliefs may also play a role in pain experience. People may cope with their pain by using their faith and prayer, whereas others may view pain as a punishment for their sins.

Cognitive activities associated with cultural values, anxiety, attention, and suggestion have a profound effect on the pain experience. There is evidence that the sensory input is localized, identified in terms of its physical properties, and evaluated in terms of past experience with the sensation (Sternbach, 1978). It is generally understood that cognitive processes are of critical importance in determining the nature of the pain experience. Individuals experiencing pain tend to interpret the source and personal meaning of the pain in terms of the immediate environment, their past history, and the future implications of any injury or disease.

In summary, the influence of cultural values on the response to and expression of pain is well established in the literature (Koopman et al., 1984; Lipton & Marbach, 1984; Zola, 1966), yet in actual practice, there is little evidence that cultural factors are included in diagnostic and therapeutic activities (Bates, 1987; Good & Good, 1980). Attention to individual cultural facets by the critical care nurse when assessing and managing pain can only enhance the management outcome. The ability of the nurse to recognize and suppress prejudice toward and stereotyping of different cultural beliefs and behavior is reflected in planning and caring for the critically ill patient without evidence of judgmental principles.

Psychological Factors Associated With Pain

Pain is more than just a physiologic experience; it is a psychological experience as well. Psychological factors such as affect, anxiety, anger, guilt, and depression are believed to alter the perception and response to acute pain. From documented reports, research findings, and experience, there is much evidence that psychological factors may cause pain, can frequently augment its severity, and may also serve to diminish or abolish pain in the presence of extensive physical trauma.

Even though discussion continues in regard to somatogenic pain and psychogenic pain, most references acknowledge that pain is a combination of mental and physical events. Psychogenic pain is usually defined as a discrepancy between the physical findings and the amount of pain reported or pain behavior observed (Sternbach, 1978). Support for the occurrence of psychogenic pain is presented in studies that show positive findings of hysterical neuroses or conversion hysteria, the state resulting from unconscious emotional conflicts originating in the past, and hypochondriac pain, neuroses characterized by a preoccupation with the body and a constant fear of disease or malfunction of the body.

Psychological or cortical processes of attention, past experience with pain, and the meaning of the situation may exert considerable influence on the perception of painful stimuli. Pavlov's experiments with dogs, later applied to humans, support the concept that the meaning of the stimulus acquired during earlier conditioning modulates the sensory input before it activates brain processes that underlie perception and response. Attention to the stimulation also contributes to the intensity of pain experienced. This is evident in people engaged in sports or battle who may be seriously injured but do not perceive the injury until later or not at all (Beecher, 1959). The environment may serve as a distraction; conversely, if the person's attention is focused on a potentially painful experience, that individual will tend to perceive pain more intensely than he or she would under normal conditions (Hall & Strider, 1954).

It is generally known that a positive relationship exists between anxiety and the pain experience. It is also known that anxiety not only influences pain perception but that pain perception or the fear of pain stimulates anxiety (Christoph, 1991). Anxiety is an important factor affecting the individual's ability to tolerate and cope with pain. Although there are exceptions, increasing anxiety about pain increases the perceived intensity of pain, whereas reduction in anxiety decreases the perception of pain. Paradoxically, in some instances pain decreased while anxiety related to a specific situation temporarily increased (Sternbach, 1986). Modification of anxiety associated with the pain experience is considered an important theoretical basis for pain relief measures. Therefore, it is important to note the suspected interplay between anxiety and pain relief, especially when mild to moderate anxiety is associated with an episode of acute pain. During the anticipation of pain, relief for the impending pain may be enhanced if the patient has knowledge of the existing or anticipated pain, experiences a moderate amount of anxiety, and can channel the anxiety into methods of coping with pain. When a pain sensation is felt, reduction of anxiety tends to decrease the perceived intensity of the sensation or increase the tolerance for pain (Janis, 1958). The nurse's ability to promote pain relief could be enhanced by awareness that a moderate level of anxiety should be derived from the patient's knowledge of what may actually occur and only a minimal amount of anxiety should be derived from the threat of the unknown or a threat to self-concept. Studies have documented preoperative anxiety as a predictor of postoperative pain (Parbook et al., 1973; Scott et al., 1983; Acute Pain Management Guideline Panel, 1992).

Some degree of sadness and anger often accompanies acute pain. Patients may express unhappiness or perhaps anger due to the illness or pain. They may be angry with themselves for doing something foolish or careless that led to the pain, or angry with the physician or nurse for failure to take steps that the patient believes could have prevented pain. Anger and sadness consume physical and mental energy. Theoretically, relief from anger and sadness will enable the patient to experience less pain, to handle pain more efficiently, and to increase tolerance to pain.

The functionally impaired, acutely ill patient is often saddened or depressed by his or her condition. In this instance, depression is a product of the pain problem. Anxiety that accompanies acute pain eventually becomes less prominent and is replaced by reactive depression. This depression has many possible characteristics, such as sleep and appetite disturbances, decreased physical and social activity, forgetfulness, mental dullness, irritability, and suicidal thoughts (Sternbach, 1986).

Intensive Care Unit Techniques Contributing to the Pain Experience

Within the organization of the modern hospital, there is a political arena with certain ground rules and expectations. The body of the patient is viewed as the battleground against disease in which many activities, including pain, occur. Physicians and nurses make most of the rules that prevail in this interactional context. There are specific routines and work rhythms to which the staff adhere and to which the patient must conform and adapt. In a series of interviews with ICU patients 1 week after discharge, the common complaints noted were pain, sleeplessness, physiotherapy, noise, handling, and movement. More than 50% of the patients claimed to remember little about the ICU, but of those who did, pain, lights, noise, boredom, and nursing procedures were of greatest concern (Puntillo, 1990). The combination of fear, pain, anxiety, sleep deprivation, unpleasant physical surroundings, absence of day and night cycles, and other physical and psychological patient problems can cause a severe paranoid confusional decompensation that can magnify mildly painful procedures (Cousins & Phillips, 1986; Jones et al., 1979).

The ICU is viewed as a specialized area that is very different from other wards and units. The environment is usually efficiently organized and reflects ample staff, highly technical equipment, numerous and powerful drugs, critically ill patients (many close to death), continuous monitoring of vital signs, and perpetual activity. Many times the bustle of activity is directed toward insertion of wires or intravenous lines to monitor or support the body during a life-threatening insult. In addition, managing and maintaining these lines and devices causes discomfort and pressure that is usually perceived as pain by the patient. Restraining or limiting arm motion may be necessary to keep a delirious patient from removing vital tubes. This adds to the frustration, anxiety, and fear associated with painful stimuli. In this predominantly technical environment, the nurse must continue to remember that the patient is a recipient of procedures and techniques that can be painful.

Critically ill patients commonly have two major sources of pain—the illness, injury, or treatment that brought them to the ICU, and the iatrogenic treatment that occurs while they are residents in the ICU. When nurses and physicians recognize various procedures and techniques as painful, they can prepare the patient with accurate information in addition to pain relief measures. Analgesia should be given one-half hour before any painful procedure. In addition, the patient should be instructed in pain control strategies such as the relaxation response, imagery, and distraction.

The mechanically ventilated patient presents an extra management challenge in decreasing pain and anxiety. Many times the fear and discomfort associated with ventilation and suctioning are perceived as pain and can be adequately managed with relaxants such as diazepam (Cousins & Phillips, 1986). The interaction of unfamiliar technical devices, sounds, and lights, compounded by decreased ambient temperature and invasive procedures, creates an alien environment and experience for ICU patients and can produce a significant stress response. As noted earlier, the relationship between pain and stress is somewhat unclear, but clinical observations while managing ICU patients indicate that administration of muscle relaxants and tranquilizers to diminish stress in addition to analgesics will enhance the response obtained from the use of analgesics alone (Puntillo, 1990).

Pain Syndromes Common to the Critically Ill

Most clinicians differentiate between acute pain and chronic pain. *Acute pain* is related to a known or well defined cause, follows a predictable course, and is self-limiting and correctable. When healing is completed, the pain usually disappears. Acute pain has a rapid onset, varies in length, and includes phasic and tonic components. The phasic component is of short duration and occurs at the onset of pain. Patients tend to withdraw actively from the pain source during the phasic component. The tonic component varies in length and continues until healing has occurred. Reaction to pain results in response patterns that are usually protective in nature and help to restore the individual's natural equilibrium. Reflex muscle spasm and automatic splinting at a fracture site, and avoidance of foods that would increase the pain of a stomach ulcer are examples of response to acute pain. In clinical situations, acute pain usually represents either a symptom of a disease condition or a temporary aspect of treatment. In both cases, patients and health care professionals expect to have pain alleviated (Craig, 1984).

Chronic pain may begin as acute pain with the tonic component lasting far beyond the healing time. Some pain clinicians and researchers believe that chronic pain is the result of inadequately or poorly managed acute pain. Chronic pain may also begin as a low-level input and continue for extended periods of time despite intervention. Chronic pain may be divided into three classes: (1) chronic nonmalignant pain, such as low back pain and rheumatoid arthritis; (2) chronic intermittent pain such as migraine headaches; and (3) chronic malignant pain (Beare, 1990). It is believed that chronic pain may incorporate neural mechanisms that are more complex than acute pain and involve adjacent body areas (Melzack & Dennis, 1978). Chronic pain becomes a constant companion, even when intermittent. Individuals with chronic pain may be admitted to the ICU for acute problems, requiring the nurse to consider the presence of both acute and chronic pain.

Two additional terms that are appearing more frequently in the literature are *intractable* and *deafferentation.* Intractable pain is viewed as unmanageable or untreatable pain. The goal is to change intractable pain to tractable pain so that it can be treated. Deafferentation refers to discomfort arising in any part of the body where the flow of afferent nervous impulses has been partially or completely interrupted (Tasker, 1984). This term is frequently used synonymously with *phantom limb pain.* Different types of pain distribution are expressed by patients; these may include reflex, dystrophy, or perverse reaction to stimuli. Patients who undergo amputation of a body part commonly experience a phantom sensation reflecting the presence of the body part at varying times after surgery. For some individuals, the sensation may be distorted or painful. Formation of neuromas and a central mechanism may be instrumental in causing distorted sensations.

Phantom sensations may also occur with mastectomies, cosmetic surgery of the nose and other parts of the body, tooth extraction, amputation of the tongue, penis, or scrotum, and enucleation. Children who have a congenital amputation or are undergoing an amputation before the age of 6 years usually do not experience phantom sensations, possibly due to the general instability of the mnemonic process of the brain, causing the phantom limb to be forgotten rapidly, or the presence of an immature body image at the time of amputation (Jensen & Rasmussen, 1984). The phenomenon of phantom sensations has recently been decreased postoperatively when patients are given preemptive analgesia (before surgery) (Katz & Melzack, 1990).

Additional studies have been done on phantom sensations in parts of the body that are surgically removed. Preoperative pain commonly involves concentrated areas of sensory nerves such as the palm, knuckles, tips of the fingers, thumb, instep of the foot, heels, and toes. After surgery, these areas are frequent sites of phantom pain. Because an estimated 450,000 amputees are now living in the United States, phantom pain should be viewed as a major clinical problem (Stein & Warfield, 1982).

Pain syndromes, described according to their general location in the body, may be superficial or cutaneous, deep visceral, deep somatic, ischemic, referred, or radiating. Patients may experience one, all, or any combination of these pain syndromes while in the ICU. *Superficial pain* usually refers to pain in the skin and mucous membranes and is described as sharp, pricking, or burning. This pain is usually related to a disturbance of nerve endings. *Deep pain* is divided into splanchnic and deep somatic, with splanchnic pain referring to the viscera, and deep somatic pain involving structures other than the viscera. *Ischemic pain* results from inadequate tissue oxygenation and occurs when metabolic substances or end products of cell degenera-

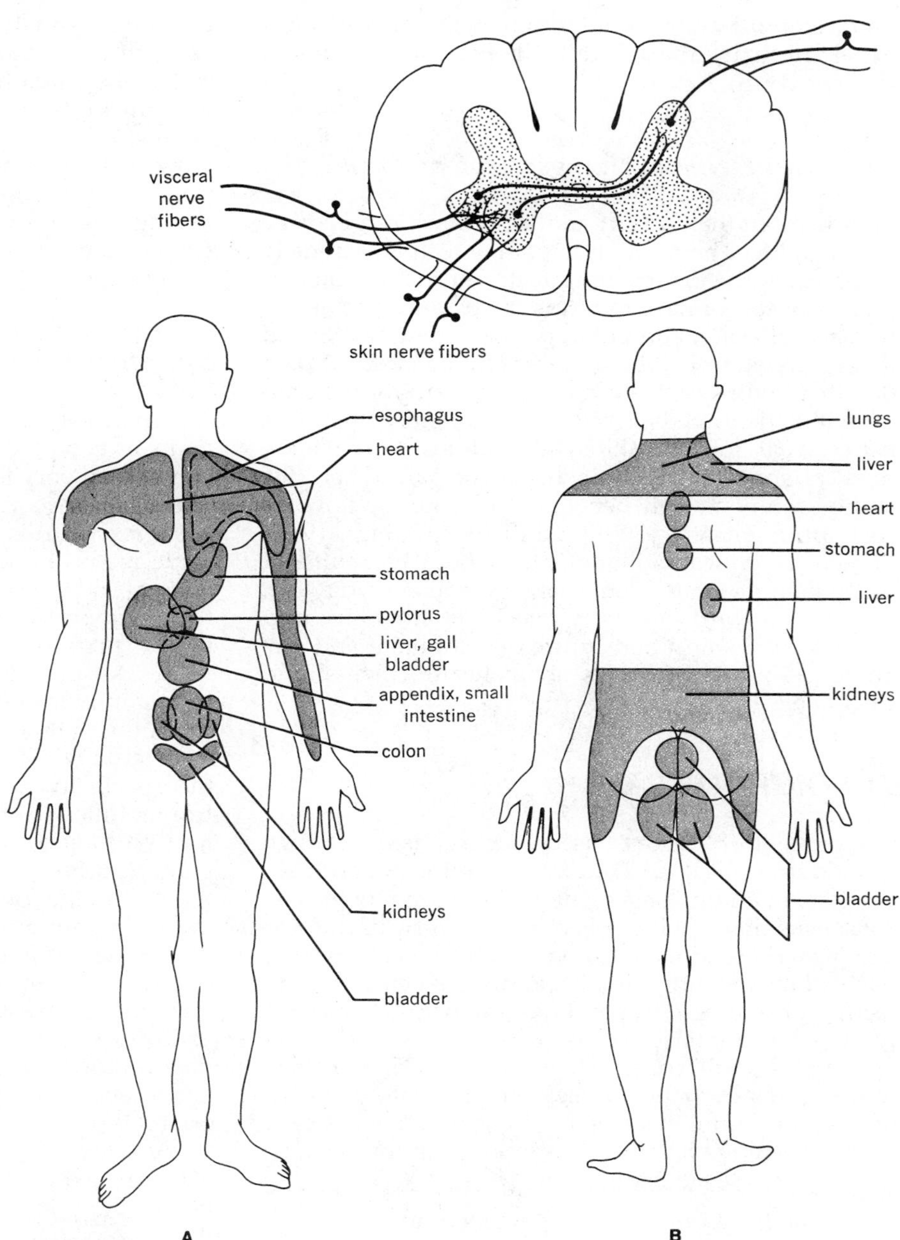

FIGURE 65–1. *A* and *B*, Referred pain. (From Silverstein, A. [1983]. *Human anatomy and physiology* [2nd ed., p. 300]. New York: John Wiley & Sons.)

tion accumulate in the tissues and come in contact with nerve endings (Phillips & Cousins, 1986). *Referred pain* is present in an area that is removed or distant from the point of origin (Fig. 65–1), and *radiating pain* reflects extension from the site of origin (Procacci & Zoppi, 1984). A knowledge of the embryonic development of various parts of the body provides an understanding of the physiologic basis of referred pain. Further information regarding pathways and fibers involved in these pain syndromes is discussed in relation to pathophysiology.

The interaction among complex illness, body response, and treatment variables in ICU patients has the potential to excite all known pain receptors—mechanical, thermal, and chemical. Mechanosensitive pain receptors are excited by excessive mechanical stress or damage to the tissues. Thermosensitive pain receptors react to extremes of heat or cold, and chemosensitive receptors are excited by bradykinin, serotonin, histamine, potassium ions, acids, prostaglandins, acetylcholine, and proteolytic enzymes. Cell damage can result from direct trauma or when the blood supply is interrupted to an area, resulting in accumulation of lactic acid from altered metabolism. Muscle spasm and pressure associated with clinical syndromes, medications, and immobility stimulate mechanosensitive pain receptors and account for much of the discomfort experienced by the critically ill patient (Cousins & Phillips, 1986).

Cost and Dehumanizing Effect of Pain

Pain is more than a hurt and sometimes can become a way of life. The reaction to pain, which is extremely complex, is the determining factor in the outcome of pain. The toll of pain in terms of cost, use of energy, human suffering, and unhappiness is remarkable and totally undeterminable. In addition, the effect of pain on other body systems is a major concern for the critically ill patient. In the United States alone, pain affects between 60 and 70 million individuals. Lost wages, medical and other costs incurred for pain relief, disability compensation benefits, and court judgments cost approximately $70 billion in 1981 (Bonica, 1987). Therefore, critically ill patients who have suffered much pain may have some carryover to everyday life. Attitudes toward pain may affect job situations, personal relationships, and future development and creativity as well as feelings about health, illness, and treatment.

THEORIES OF PAIN

The concept of "theory-based practice" is not foreign to modern critical care nurses nor to the area of pain assessment and management. Even though there is no consensus about which theories are most useful, existing theories provide guidance for clinical practice. Each theorist individually addresses cultural, affective, physiologic, or psychological parameters. Currently, the emphasis is on underlying theories, reflecting a holistic construct. Melzack (1975) identified four guidelines that could serve to evaluate the merit of past and future theories. His view was that any new theory of pain must be able to account for four factors:

1. The high degree of physiologic specification of receptor fiber units and of pathways in the central nervous system (CNS)
2. The role of temporal and spatial patterning in the transmission of information in the nervous system
3. The influence of psychological processes on pain perception and response
4. The clinical phenomena of spatial and temporal summation, spread of pain, and persistence of pain after healing (p. 153)

Although these guidelines were proposed nearly 20 years ago, they remain applicable today.

Affect Theory of Pain

The affect theory dates back to Aristotle and considers pain an emotion that colors all sensory events. Aristotle believed that pain was the result of increased sensitivity of the senses, especially of touch. This increased sensitivity was then modified by the hardness, warmth, or coldness of the heart and felt as pain (Jaros, 1991). Sherrington (1900) proposed that affective tone is an attribute of all sensation; skin pain is an example of an attribute of sensation. Titchener (1909) added the view that pain and unpleasantness were on a continuum. Even though he believed that a continuum of feeling was different from one of sensation, he did not explain the link between affect, unpleasantness, and pain (Melzack, 1973).

Specificity Theory

The specificity theory was proposed in the early 1800s and was accepted for nearly 100 years as the most appropriate theory for explaining the pain phenomenon. Specificity theory, the first reflection of a physiologic basis for pain, is the traditional theory still used in some medical and graduate schools (Bates, 1987). In general, it proposes that pain is a specific sensation that is proportional to the extent of tissue damage. The theory, first presented by Descartes in 1644, implies a fixed transmission system running straight through from a mosaic of somatic pain receptors to a pain center in the brain (Sternbach, 1978).

Von Frey extended the physiologic component of the specificity theory by using existing information from Muller, Helmholtz, and Volkmann to identify four types of sensory input: touch, cold, warmth, and pain. Von Frey further linked newly identified tissue types with the four types of sensations. Consequently, Meissner corpuscles are identified as touch receptors, Krause end-bulbs are cold receptors, Ruffini end-organs are warmth receptors, and Pacinian corpuscles detect pressure (Melzack, 1973). The sensorial end-organ is an apparatus by which an afferent nerve fiber is rendered amenable to some particular physical agent and simultaneously less amenable to other excitants.

A refinement of the original specificity theory was necessary when two different types and sizes of nerve fibers, the A delta epsilon fibers and the C fibers, were discovered to be involved in pain transmission. Each pathway is responsible for a different pain sensation. The A delta epsilon system, termed the epicritic pain pathway, is responsible for a sharp, pricking, well defined type of pain, carried via the lateral spinothalamic tract. The slower C fibers are responsible for dull, aching, persistent pain (Baumann & Lehman, 1989). This pathway is believed to be carried on the ventral spinothalamic tract. With this elaboration of neuroanatomy and physiology, neurosurgeons could become more precise in applying techniques of pain alleviation such as nerve blocks, tractotomies, sympathectomies, posterior rhizotomies, and cordotomies (Melzack, 1973).

Pattern Theory

As evidence mounted to refute the specificity theory, several new theories, presented by Goldschneider,

Nafe, Livingston, and Noordenbos, were grouped into a pattern theory. Through studies of patients with syphilis, Goldschneider proposed that stimulus intensity and central summation are the critical determinants of pain. Pain sensation becomes cumulative, and the response increases as time increases. Goldschneider believed that the large cutaneous fibers comprise a specific touch system, whereas the smaller fibers converge on dorsal horn cells in the spinal cord that summate their input and transmit the pattern to the brain. Pain results when the total input goes beyond a certain level due to excessive stimulation or pathologic conditions (Melzack, 1973). The peripheral pattern component simply implies that excessive peripheral stimulation produces nerve impulses that are interpreted centrally as pain (Nafe, 1934). The sensory interaction theory, derived from Goldschneider's original beliefs, further proposes that a rapidly conducting firing system inhibits synaptic transmission from a more slowly conducting system.

Livingston (1943) proposed that intense pathologic stimulation of the body sets up reverberating circuits in spinal pools that can be triggered by normally nonnoxious inputs and generate abnormal volleys that are interpreted centrally as pain. This theory is credited with explaining such central phenomena as causalgia and phantom pain because a central patterning of impulse flow creates a "painful memory" for the patient. Amputation of a limb or healing of a peripheral nerve injury does not withdraw the peripheral stimulus. Instead, a fixed pattern is locked in the central structures that cannot be modified because no normal sensory input from the original source is possible.

Noordenbos (1959) made an important contribution to concepts of sensory interaction. He viewed the small fibers as carriers of the nerve impulse pattern that produces pain and the large fibers as those that inhibit transmission. A shift in ratio of large to small fibers with an increase in small fibers would result in excessive pain.

The composite pattern theory holds that there are no specific pain pathways or nerve endings, and the sensation of pain does not depend on one pathway or two but on the total central projection system. Pain perception is related to the intensity of the stimulus and the summation of all impulses, so that when a hypersynchronization of impulse volleys occurs all at once, the individual interprets this sensation as pain (Melzack, 1975).

Gate Control Theory

The gate control theory uses and extends the principles presented in the pattern theory (Figs. 65–2 and 65–3). Pain perception is believed to be the result of both central and peripheral inputs that act on a "gate" that controls transmission of impulses to the pain centers of the thalamus and cerebral cortex. Peripheral input occurs from the two types of fibers described in the pattern theory, large and small fibers. Large fibers are the rapidly conducting A-alpha and A-beta fibers, which inhibit transmission of impulses through the central transmission (T) cells in the dorsal horn (close the gate). To close the gate to pain, A-fiber input must predominate, and this can be achieved by introducing touch, pressure, or thermal stimuli. These peripheral impulses are always subject to modification by emotion, experience (memory), and other cortical functions. Large-diameter fibers transmit impulses by way of the dorsal column of the spinal cord to a central control site in the brain; the central control triggers selective cognitive processes that then influence the gate control mechanism by way of descending fibers.

Small-diameter, slowly conducting fibers are A-delta and C fibers, which facilitate transmission of impulses to the T cells, leading to perception of pain (open the gate). The gate is located in a portion of the dorsal column of the spinal cord at each segmental level called the substantia gelatinosa (SG). When the gate is open, impulses are transmitted to an action system in the brain. To open this gate to pain perception, a predominance of C fiber input must prevail. When the amount of information that passes through the gate exceeds a critical level, neural areas such as the brain stem reticular formation, thalamus, hypothalamus, limbic system, and cerebral cortex are activated; these are responsible for pain experience and response (Melzack & Wall, 1965).

The SG seems to be the key in this theory because it receives axon terminals from many of the large- and small-diameter afferent fibers. The dendrites of cells

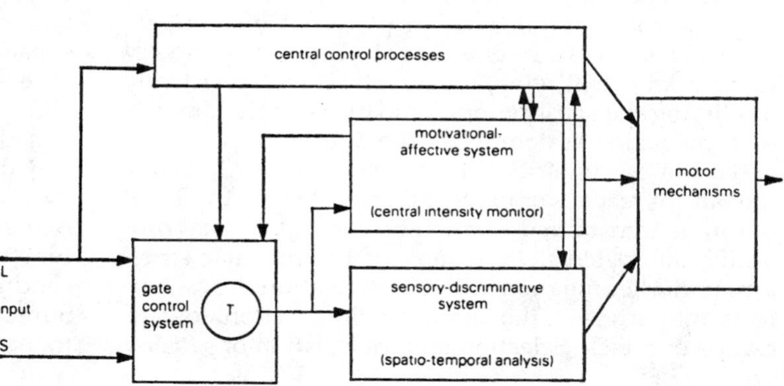

FIGURE 65–2. Conceptual model of gate control theory. (From Melzack, R., & Casey, K. L. [1988]. In D. Kenshele [Ed.], *The skin senses.* Courtesy of Charles C. Thomas, Publisher, Springfield, Illinois.)

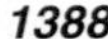

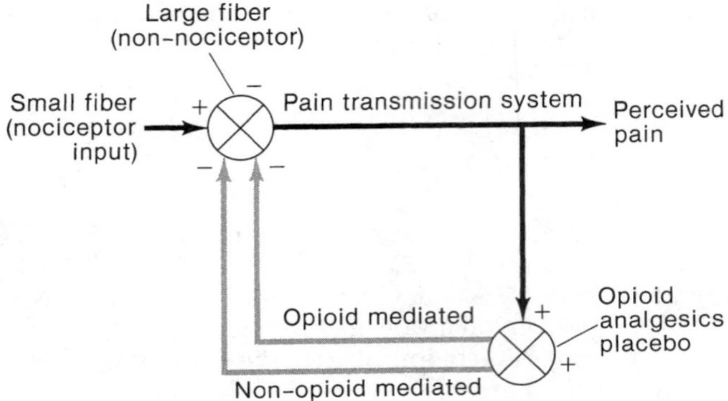

FIGURE 65–3. Pain modulation system(s).

in deeper laminae project into the gelatinosa. The SG consists of a highly specialized, closed system of cells throughout the length of the spinal cord. Melzack and Wall (1965) proposed that it acts as a spinal gating mechanism by modulating the conduction of nerve impulses from peripheral fibers to transmission cells in the spinal cord.

Melzack and Wall (1965, 1970) suggested that sensory fibers transmit patterned information about pressure, temperature, and chemical changes at the skin, depending on the specialized properties of each receptor fiber unit. These temporal and spatial patterns of nerve impulses have two effects at the dorsal horns: They excite the spinal cord T cells that transmit the information to the brain, and they activate the SG, which modulates or "gates" the amount of information projected to the brain by the T cells.

There are two ways in which the cells of the SG can act as a gating mechanism that influences the transmission of impulses from afferent fiber terminals to spinal cord cells (Melzack & Wall, 1970). They can act directly on the presynaptic axon terminals, thereby blocking the impulses in the terminals or decreasing the amount of transmitter substance they release, or they can act postsynaptically on the spinal transmission cells by increasing or decreasing their level of excitability to arriving nerve impulses. Melzack and Wall (1965) proposed that the effect is primarily presynaptic. Hongo and colleagues (1968) supported the idea that modulating effects are exerted postsynaptically on the spinal T cells.

The reticular formation exerts a powerful inhibitory control over information projected by the gate control system. This central control system acts very rapidly in identifying, evaluating, and selectively modifying the sensory input and also clearly interacts with the action system when the output of the T cells exceeds a certain critical level (Melzack, 1973). When the output reaches or exceeds a critical level, the T cell output is transmitted to the reticular and cortical projection subsystems. Activation of the reticular structure underlies the motivational drive of unpleasant effects that triggers the organism into action toward escape or attack. Selection and modulation of sensory input through the cortical projection subsystem provide sensory discriminative information about the location, magnitude, and spatiotemporal characteristics of the noxious stimulus.

Behaviorist Theory

Because the behaviorist theory has greater meaning for chronic pain, only the key points that are pertinent to pain in the critically ill patient are included here. Lazarus (1977) stated, "of course, nearly everyone will agree that the only way we can know anything about another person is through his behavior" (p. 553). It is through pain behavior that pain is recognized and interpreted by clinicians. Behaviors may include verbal descriptors, splinting, increase in heart rate, limping, rubbing a body part, sweaty palms, grimacing, or other overt expression. Behaviors have meaning both for the person demonstrating them and for the observer.

Skinner introduced two terms that are seen in literature related to pain: respondent and operant. *Respondents* are actions that occur in response to antecedent stimuli. The stimulus may be internal, external, or reflexive in nature. A typical respondent may include glandular or smooth muscle action. *Operants* are actions of the organism that are overt or visible/audible and thereby have an effect on or with the environment. An operant is usually followed by reinforcement that will influence future behavior (Fordyce, 1978).

Endogenous Opiate Theory

Discovery of endogenous opiates in 1965 provided new knowledge about and clarification of existing pain theories. Viewed as neurophysiologic, biochemical substances associated with pain, endogenous opiates became the target of numerous research activities. Clarification of their role as neurotransmitters, neuromodulators, or neuroregulators is based on the knowledge that stimulation of known pain pathways produces analgesia. Enkephalins, small peptide molecules, and beta-endorphin, a large peptide involving long sequences of amino acids, are responsive to pain sensation and adaptation. They are synthesized by certain CNS neurons. According to this discovery, the body manufactures opiate-like substances to provide pain relief at specific receptor sites in the CNS. These substances are similar in effect to morphine and react at receptor sites to inactivate pain sensations. Enkephalins are found in the caudate nucleus, the periaqueductal gray matter, the anterior hypothalamus, and the SG. Because of their relatively simple structure, enkephalins have a rapid-acting effect that terminates in about 2 minutes. Enkephalins appear to function as inhibitory neurotransmitters in pathways conducting impulses concerning pain (nociception). Stimulation of enkephalins produces analgesia similar to that produced by opiate drugs. They bind with opiates in the dorsal horn of the spinal cord. Enkephalins modulate pain by closing the gate and relieving the pain impulse.

Enkephalins and opiate receptors exist in the medullary center, which explains the potent action of opiate drugs on respiration. They are also found in certain limbic system structures (e.g., amygdala). This may explain the emotional effects produced by natural and synthetic opiate drugs. Enkephalins also inhibit the release of substance P and other neuroregulators (Hokfelt et al., 1980).

Beta-endorphin is found in the pituitary gland, hypothalamus, and amygdala and has an effect of 4 hours or longer. A larger pain or stress stimulus is needed to generate the beta-endorphin response than the enkephalin response (Bloom et al., 1978; Terenius, 1981; Woods et al., 1982). Beta-endorphin and adrenocorticotropic hormone (ACTH) are synthesized together as one large molecule that is subsequently cleaved to produce the two substances. It has been postulated that the interaction between ACTH and beta-endorphin has a modulatory role that cannot function if exogenous opiates are chronically given (Jacquet, 1979). Both of these substances are released in response to stress. These substances, like morphine, can become addictive. Because they are endogenous substances, however, the result of addiction may be expressed as the behavior of seeking specific stress- or pain-generating conditions. The example cited most often is the exercise fanatic who chooses to exercise for very long periods on a daily basis. It may be true that people with chronic or intractable pain are "addicted" to their pain through the beta-endorphin mechanism. Thus, although the role of these substances is pain alleviation, the interpretation chosen by such patients is the inappropriate one of seeking continued pain (Carr et al., 1981).

This summary of common pain theories is given in an attempt to explain the complex nature of pain and to increase our understanding of how pain occurs. Each approach is unique and lends insight into this phenomenal, complicated body response that is experienced by virtually everyone during his or her lifetime. It is evident from the brief data presented that the gate control theory is more sophisticated than the other theories because it attempts to incorporate biopsychosocial components in addition to providing some explanation for variations in pain management. However, it is important to note that controversy exists over the value of the gate control theory because the activity proposed in the gating process has not been clearly identified. Discovery and acquisition of new knowledge about endogenous opiates continue to support the gate control theory and further explain some of the relationships within it. Current research and literature on pain commonly reflect the use of the gate control theory as a theoretical framework because it is the most comprehensive description of the pain process available. Knowledge of the available theories is requisite for each clinician. After careful analysis of each theory, selection of one theory to guide and direct the clinical assessment, management, and evaluation of the pain experience will assist the critical care nurse to provide the best possible care to patients.

PATHOPHYSIOLOGY OF PAIN

Continued acquisition of new knowledge and insights into the neuroendocrine system allows greater understanding of the mechanism and pathophysiology of pain. Comprehension of nociception, pain receptors, pain pathways, pain centers, and biochemical mediators of pain provides the critical care nurse with the background information required to assess and manage the specific type of pain experienced by each patient.

Relationship of Nociception to Perceived Pain

Nociceptors are widely branching, unencapsulated, free nerve endings that are found in varying amounts in all body tissues and respond to chemical, mechanical, and thermal stimulation. Areas of high nociceptor concentration include subcutaneous tissue, periosteum, deep fascia, ligaments, joint capsules, and the cornea; few are found in muscle and hardly any in bone and cartilage (Chapman, 1988; DiGregorio et al., 1986; Donnelly & Lamb, 1993). Pain is produced when strong noxious stimuli such as heat, extreme cold, and mechanical injury excite these receptors. At weaker intensities, these stimuli may produce other somatic sensations (e.g., warmth, cold, and pressure). In skin and deep tissue, nociceptors typically react to burns, the severe pressure of crush, and cutting, whereas those in the viscera tolerate such stimuli but respond instead to stretch or distention (Chapman, 1988). The process of pain perception, which depends on the transmission of electrical impulses from the site of tissue injury in the periphery to higher centers in the brain, is termed *nociception.*

Primary afferent neuronal fibers transport impulses from nociceptors into the CNS and are classified into three groups based on their cross-sectional area and speed of conduction: A fibers are the largest and most rapid conducting, C fibers are the smallest and the slowest conducting, and B fibers are in between. A fibers include rapidly conducting myelinated A-alpha and A-beta plus the smaller, more slowly conducting A-delta fibers. The A-alpha and A-beta fibers innervate sensitive (low-threshold) mechanoreceptors that are involved with proprioception and sensations of touch and light pressure. A-delta fibers are surrounded only by a thin myelin sheath and transmit impulses at a rate of 6 to 30 milliseconds. They are distributed primarily to the skin and mucous membranes. About 10% to 25% of A-delta fibers respond to a strong stimulus, producing a fast, sharp, easily localized pain. These fibers may also respond to a cooling sensation (Guyton, 1991).

C fibers are the smallest fibers and, like some A-delta fibers, may respond to more than one type of stimulus (polymodal). About 50% to 70% of C fibers transmit pain impulses. These neurons are unmyelinated, conduct more slowly (0.5 to 2 milliseconds), and are responsible for duller, aching, more prolonged pain (Guyton, 1991). This longer-lasting pain is associated with somatic and autonomic reflexes, usually sympathetic in nature (i.e., cardiac acceleration, peripheral vasoconstriction, pupillary dilatation, and sweating).

Both A-delta and C fibers innervate nociceptors and are involved with pain sensation, but they can also respond to innocuous stimuli such as warmth. A-delta and C fibers have high thresholds to mechanical and thermal stimuli. Unlike most types of receptors, which become less responsive when subjected to continued stimulation, nociceptors remain sensitive (nociceptors do not adapt to prolonged stimulation). Therefore, after trauma, pain persists. In fact, repetitive stimulation of nociceptors may lower the receptor threshold, causing increased sensitivity to noxious stimuli (hyperalgesia) (Muir, 1988).

Nociceptive units are now classified as high-threshold mechanoreceptor units (HTMs), polymodal nociceptor units (PMNs), and multireceptive neurons, or wide dynamic range cells (WDR). HTM units are believed to be composed mostly of A-delta fibers, responding to strong pressure applied to a discrete point spread over an area of skin that can exceed 1 cm^2. There is a slow adaptation response to pressure. PMN units are predominantly C fibers that are excited by a range of irritant chemicals and have a slowly adapting response to firm pressure. Response to heat will accelerate with increasing skin temperature (Lynn, 1984). The role of WDR cells is unclear, but they are believed to respond to both noxious and nonnoxious cutaneous or visceral stimuli. Activity in the dorsal horn suggests that these cells may provide more precise information about the noxious stimulus such as intensity, location, and quality (Zimmerman, 1984).

Physiologic Parameters of Pain

Primary (first-order) peripheral afferent neurons transmit impulses to the CNS, entering the spinal cord at various lamina levels in the dorsal roots, and forming cell bodies in the dorsal root ganglia (Fig. 65–4). The nerves bifurcate, and two processes extend from the cell body, one peripheral process terminating distally in a body tissue receptor and the central process terminating in the brain or spinal cord. This latter primary afferent neuron may terminate in the marginal layer (lamina I), substantia gelatinosa (laminae II and III), lamina V, and, to a smaller extent, lamina IV (Jacox, 1977). At this point, the message is transmitted to secondary neurons, most of which cross the midline and enter the lateral spinothalamic tract. Some ipsilateral tracts also exist. The dorsal horn acts as the site through which descending pathways modulate pain (Fig. 65–5) (Christensen & Perl, 1970; DiGregorio et al., 1986).

Transmission Pathways

Ascending and descending pathways have been identified in the literature and play a role in pain transmission. The naming and activity of these pathways vary from reference to reference, as does their stated value to nociceptive transmission. The following five systems are believed to be important in the pain experience: the tract of Lissauer, the lemniscal–dorsal

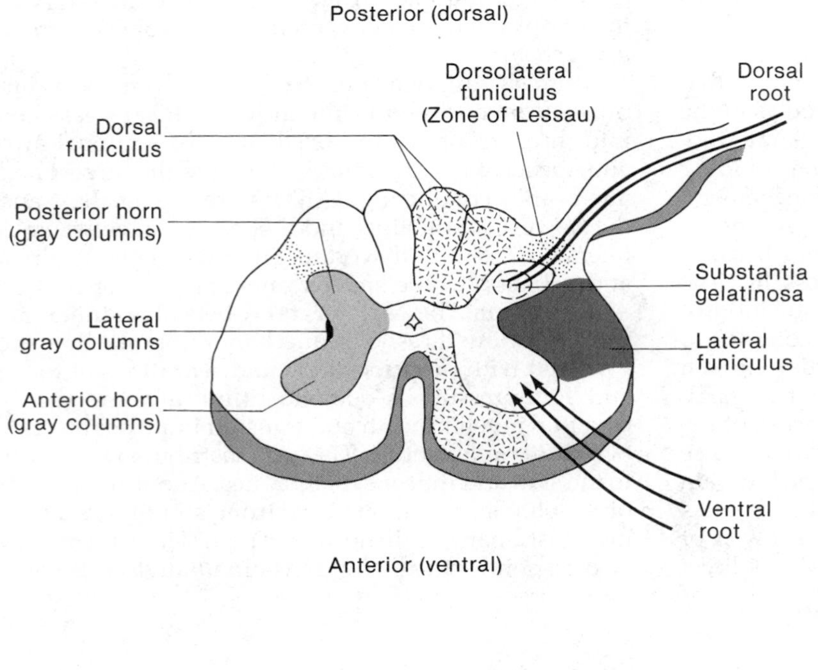

FIGURE 65–4. Cross-section of spinal cord.

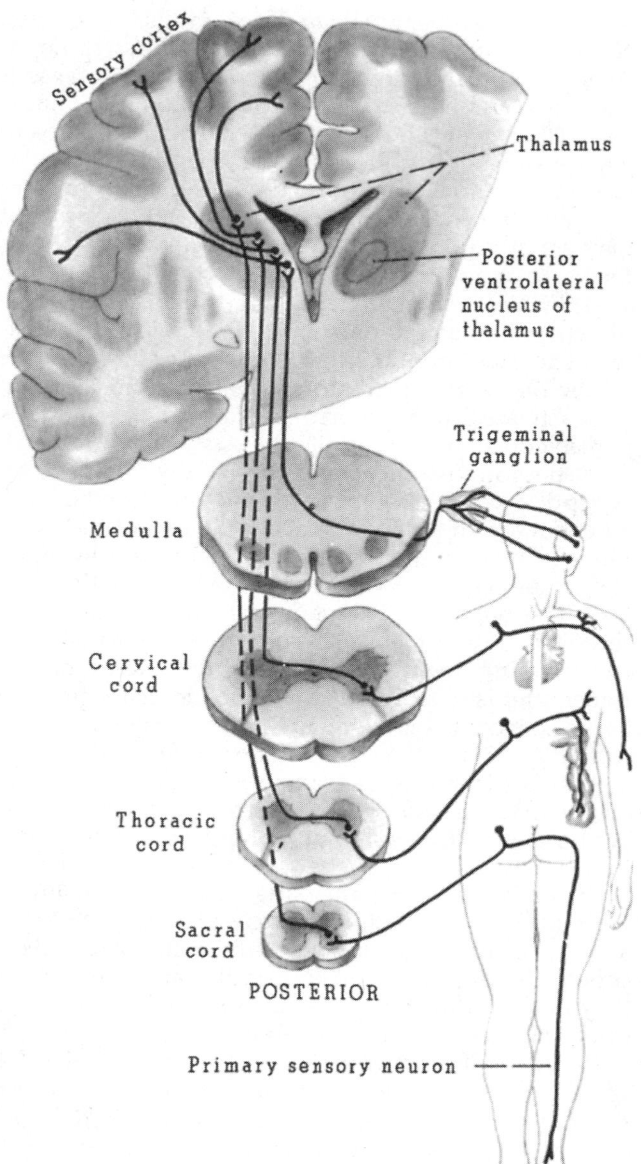

FIGURE 65–5. Central nervous system—spinothalamic tract. (From Jacob, S. W., Francone, C. A., & Lossow, W. J. [1978]. *Structure and function in man* [p. 287]. Philadelphia: W. B. Saunders.)

column system, the spinothalamic tract, the spinoreticular multisynaptic system, and the spinomesencephalic system. Of the five systems, the first two are controversial, and the last three are usually identified as the major pathways involved in pain transmission (see Fig. 65–5).

The tract of Lissauer is a bundle of fine dendrites from marginal cells that enter the dorsolateral horn and project the transmission of noxious stimuli ventrally into the substantia gelatinosa (lamina II) as part of the pain transmission process. The tract of Lissauer contains axons from substantia gelatinosa cells, which connect to the nucleus of the fifth cranial nerve in the brain stem; from this nucleus, fibers project to the thalamus.

The spinothalamic tract is usually regarded as the most important pathway for signaling the existence of painful stimuli in humans. As neurons of the spinothalamic tract traverse the spinal cord, fibers are added at each segment. Spinothalamic neurons can be subdivided into four categories:

1. The neospinothalamic tract terminates in the ventrolateral and posterior thalamus. From these thalamic nuclei, fibers project to the primary somatosensory area of the cerebral cortex and may be responsible for short, well localized pain sensations.
2. The paleospinothalamic tract terminates in the medial thalamus but synapses with other neurons that connect to the reticular formation, midbrain, periaqueductal gray, limbic system, and hypothalamus. These connections may help to regulate respiration, endocrine function, and the cardiovascular system as well as modulate descending inhibitory neurons.
3. The lateral spinothalamic tracts have branches passing to the reticular nuclei of the brain stem. Impulses transmitted through the lateral spinothalamic tracts are thought to be responsible for spatial and temporal discriminative aspects of pain and touch sensations.
4. The ventral spinothalamic tracts have fibers that project to the brain stem reticular activating system and then to the medial and intralaminar thalamic nuclei. It is presumed that most impulses transmitted by spinothalamic cells cross over (decussate) at the anterolateral section of the spinal cord dorsal horn at the same level where they synapse.

The main thalamic nuclei receiving spinothalamic terminals include the ventral posterior lateral nucleus and the central lateral nucleus of the intralaminar complex. The ventral posterior lateral nucleus is somatotypically organized, that is, the neurons are organized in such a way that specific body surface areas can be easily identified and stimulated. Thus, a sensation on the finger can be transmitted to a specific area in the spinal cord and ascends to a particular area within the ventral posterior lateral nucleus of the thalamus, where the stimulus is perceived and a response is initiated. The termination zone of the spinothalamic tract in the ventral posterior lateral nucleus is in a region that overlaps with the termination zone of the dorsal column nuclei. Information derived from activity in spinothalamic neurons is thought to be forwarded to somatosensory cortices.

The spinoreticular multisynaptic system likely plays a major role in pain mechanisms. The system has relatively short A-delta and C fibers with many synapses, allowing this pathway to transmit impulses more slowly. The most direct input to the reticular formation from the spinal cord is by way of the spinoreticular tract. Fibers from the spinoreticular system connect with the brain stem reticular activating system and then with the medial and intralaminar nuclei of the thalamus. From these thalamic nuclei, fibers project diffusely to the cerebral cortex, limbic system (including connections to the hypothalamus), and basal ganglia. Impulses passing through the medial and intralaminar nuclei of the thalamus are thought to take part in responses concerned with aversive motivation and other nondiscriminative aspects of pain. The reticular formation is likely to trigger arousal and to contribute to neural activity underlying the motivational–affective aspects of pain as well as somatic and autonomic motor reflexes. It is not clear whether relatively discrete sensory information transmitted by some spinoreticular neurons to the reticular formation is preserved in the postsynaptic responses of reticular formation neurons or if these responses are made less discriminative by convergent inputs from other neurons. In any event, reticular formation neurons are commonly responsive to noxious stimuli. The locations of the cells of origin of the spinoreticular tract in the human are unknown (Muir, 1988).

Higher Brain Centers

The pain tracts described earlier enter the reticular formation of the medulla, pons, and mesencephalon before activating neurons capable of transmitting the impulses to the thalamus, hypothalamus, and other cerebral or cortical areas of the brain. The thalamus is the lowest level of the brain where pain reaches consciousness, but localization is poor. Pain information is disseminated from the thalamus to both cerebral hemispheres. Fibers from the thalamus terminate in the postcentral gyrus (somesthetic area) of the parietal lobe, which appears to be involved in discrimination of pain attributes such as localization and intensity. Other fibers terminate in the frontal lobe, which stimulates afferent fibers to the limbic system. This pathway appears to regulate the emotional or unpleasant aspects of pain. The response of the limbic system may determine how individuals respond to a noxious stimulus, adding the behavioral or subjective nature of pain. This may explain why different people respond differently to the same stimulus or why a person responds differently at different times.

Biochemical Mediators of Pain

The previously described anatomic aspects of pain are only a small portion of the activity that takes place in the body in response to nociception. Neuroregulators such as neurotransmitters, neuromodulators, and neuroinhibitors play a vital role in the overall picture of pain. New information about these substances is discovered daily, and controversial issues surrounding them are evident in the literature.

Many neuroregulators have been discovered. However, the exact role of each one and how it interacts with the others are not yet known. Several known neuroregulators influence pain perception and response. Some neuroregulators facilitate the activity of neurons involved in transmitting impulses for nociception. Other neuroregulators have an inhibitory effect, whereas others may produce an analgesic state. Neuroregulators such as monoamines (norepinephrine, epinephrine, dopamine, and serotonin), acetylcholine, amino acids (gamma-aminobutyric acid [GABA], glycine, and glutamine), substance P, prostaglandins (PGs), peptides (pituitary peptides, bradykinin, and peptides from other tissues), potassium chloride, and the endogenous opioids are substances that may act at different levels of the pain pathway as either neurotransmitters or neuromodulators (Guyton, 1991; Willis, 1985). Nociceptors are believed not to be directly stimulated by noxious stimuli. Rather, a noxious stimulus produces tissue injury, resulting in the release of chemical mediators that activate nociceptors. The activated nociceptors generate nerve impulses perceived as pain.

A neurotransmitter is synthesized within the presynaptic neuron and released into the synaptic cleft when an action potential reaches the end of the axon. The neurotransmitter then travels across the synaptic cleft to activate or inhibit other neurons in the pain transmission chain. The neurotransmitter binds with receptors on the membrane of the postsynaptic neuron, altering membrane excitability. Excess neurotransmitter is inactivated by enzymatic cleavage or by being actively taken up again by the presynaptic neuron (Fig. 65–6). Pain modulation reflects the basic activity of presynaptic, synaptic, and postsynaptic events that expedite the processes of facilitation, excitation, adaptation, summation, and inhibition (Guyton, 1991).

Neuromodulators alter the activity of neurons without the aid of a direct transfer of a signal through a synapse. They may influence the metabolism or receptor binding of a neurotransmitter at a synapse, or they may act directly on a large number of neurons at some distance from their release site.

Serotonin, found in various parts of the brain and spinal cord, is released from the ends of nerve fibers that descend from the brain and terminate in the dorsal horns of the spinal cord. It appears to inhibit neurons that transmit nociceptive signals (Muir, 1988).

Acetylcholine and amino acids such as aspartate and glutamate and some peptides are involved in higher brain centers. GABA may have an important role in the spinal regulation of pain. Histamine and bradykinin participate in peripheral mechanisms at the nociceptors.

Norepinephrine, also found in parts of the brain and spinal cord, appears to have different actions depending on the site. In the brain, norepinephrine seems to have an excitatory effect on neurons involved with nociception, whereas in the spinal cord it has an inhibitory effect. Catecholamines such as norepinephrine can exacerbate the pain of causalgia when applied locally by modulating polymodal nociceptors on C fibers.

Dopamine is located in the brain, with only insignificant amounts found in the spinal cord. This neurotransmitter appears to have an inhibitory effect on nociception.

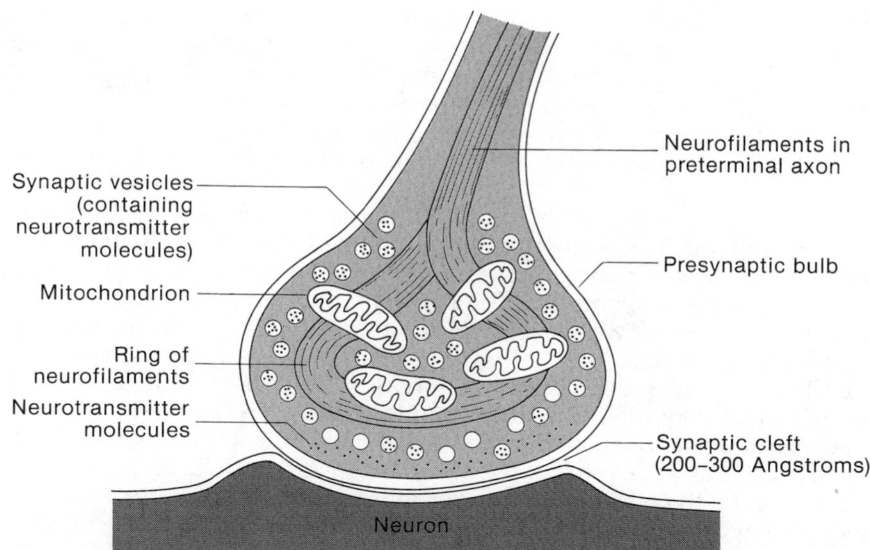

FIGURE 65–6. The synapse.

Substance P has been identified as both a neurotransmitter at polymodal nociceptors and a neuromodulator because it facilitates transmission of nociceptive input. Substance P has also been shown to have analgesic effects on both physiologic and pathologic pain. This wide variation in activity is believed to be related to the amount of the substance that is present. The peptide is synthesized in cell bodies in dorsal root ganglia after stimulation of C fibers. It is released into peripheral tissues, cerebrospinal fluid, and inflammatory transudate. Particularly high concentrations of the peptide are found in the substantia gelatinosa of the dorsal gray horn and in parts of the brain associated both with processing nociceptive input and with the relay of information from the primary afferent fibers to secondary fibers (Terenius, 1978).

Prostaglandins sensitize nociceptors to pain and modulate bradykinin activity at polymodal nociceptors, thus playing an important role as mediators in pain and the inflammatory process. PGs may be formed directly by the initial pain stimulus, whether thermal, chemical, or mechanical, and by the action of the peripheral pain mediators histamine, bradykinin, and substance P on the membranes of surrounding tissues. They sensitize nociceptors of C fibers by lowering the threshold of response to these stimuli. PGs are not stored free in tissues but are synthesized as a result of trauma or alteration in the cell membranes. PGs exert their physiologic or pathologic effects and are then rapidly biotransformed to inactive products. PGs are derived from arachidonic acid, which is present in all cell membranes (DiGregorio et al., 1986).

Leukotrienes, also derivatives of arachidonic acid, are not stored in tissue but with the appropriate stimuli are rapidly synthesized and released from leukocytes and are biotransformed to inactive products. These agents are important mediators of inflammation and allergic reactions by means of a synergistic action with other mediators such as histamine (DiGregorio et al., 1986).

Endogenous Analgesic Mechanisms

The brain contains a very important natural system for regulating pain, including at least three groups of endogenous opioid peptides: enkephalins, dynorphins, and beta-endorphins. The findings that electrical stimulation of select loci in the brain elicit analgesia that can last for several hours and that endogenous substances modulate synaptic transmission in specific areas of the brain were key discoveries fostering ongoing studies.

Further study has more clearly explained the role of these opioids in direct transmission of painful stimuli. In the higher brain centers this role is believed to be more complicated. Endogenous opioid peptide neurons enhance the activity of descending inhibitory neurons to the spinal cord from the periaqueductal gray and rostral medulla, presumably by blocking inhibitory interneurons in higher centers. Inputs to these enkephalin-containing neurons may come from ascending substance P–containing neurons or from beta-endorphin–containing neurons from the pituitary or the hypothalamus.

Enkephalins are a pair of pentapeptides, identical in structure except for the C-terminal amino acid, which is methionine in one (met-enkephalin) and leucine in the other (leu-enkephalin). Enkephalins are viewed as neurotransmitters because they have been located in synaptosomal fractions and are rapidly inactivated by peptidases. Enkephalins are localized in areas associated with pain modulation, including periaqueductal gray of the midbrain, raphe magnus, substantia gelatinosa, and marginal layer. The proposed mechanism of enkephalin-induced analgesia is inhibition of transmission of nociception, principally at the spinal cord; modulation of synaptic transmission; reduction of calcium transport across the membrane, thus inhibiting the release of substance P; and alteration of projection neurons of the spinothalamic tract.

The exact role of dynorphins in the regulation of pain is still unclear. Dynorphins and related substances are formed by the cleavage of a large polypeptide precursor, prodynorphin. The location and function of dynorphins overlap with those of enkephalin with some differences. Both groups of compounds are found in the periaqueductal gray, but dynorphins are located more ventrally, and there are more enkephalin-containing neurons in the medulla. Enkephalins and dynorphins appear to coexist in some dorsal horn neurons. Like the enkephalins, dynorphin-containing neurons have a close correlation with opioid receptors in the brain. It has been proposed that dynorphins might act by influencing projection neurons of the marginal layer of the spinal cord, secondarily affecting the descending inhibitory pathway.

Beta-endorphin, derived from proopiomelanocortin, a common precursor peptide of ACTH and melanocyte-stimulating hormone, is synthesized in the pars intermedia and pars distalis of the pituitary and in the basal hypothalamus. In response to painful stimuli of stress, beta-endorphin is released into the bloodstream from the pituitary or from proopiomelanocortin-containing neurons that terminate principally in the periaqueductal gray, where it may enhance the activity of the descending inhibitory system. Beta-endorphins have a more prolonged activity than met-enkephalin. The co-release of ACTH and beta-endorphin by hypothalamic neurons may also reach the cord via the cerebrospinal fluid, thus influencing spinal nociceptors directly. Pituitary endorphins may be involved in varying the threshold to pain and therefore are important in pain control. In addition to analgesia, beta-endorphin mimics many of the other effects of morphine, including tolerance and physical dependence, euphoria, respiratory depression, constipation, and hormonal and behavioral effects (Akil et al., 1976; Fields & Basbaum, 1984; Huhman, 1982; Muir, 1988; Smith & Simon, 1981).

Physiologic Responses to Pain

Even though there does not appear to be a direct or invariable relationship between a given stimulus and the perception and response to pain, certain factors appear to affect the pain response with some consistency. These factors include the integrity of the CNS, level of consciousness, training and previous experience in pain control, attention, distraction, fatigue, and anxiety (Jacox, 1979). The first and simplest response to a painful, external noxious stimulus is a flexor-withdrawal reflex, which is mediated at the spinal cord level. Internal sources of pain elicit reflex contraction of muscles over the affected area. This contraction or tension process can arise in either voluntary or involuntary muscles and increases the pain experience.

Activation of the sympathetic nervous system produces most of the recognizable responses to pain. Catecholamine release from the adrenal medulla evokes the fight-or-flight response, which is characterized by an increase in heart rate, an increase in blood pressure, a resulting increase in cardiac output, an increase in respiratory rate and depth, an increase in strength of muscle contractions, and vasoconstriction, which increases peripheral resistance. Blood is rapidly shifted from parts of the body that are considered nonvital or unnecessary in the fight-or-flight syndrome. Vessels of the skin and the abdominal viscera constrict, resulting in pallor and decreased gastric motility and digestive gland secretion. Muscle tension rises, and energy stores are mobilized to supply blood glucose. With the passage of time and marked intensity of pain, the parasympathetic response or rebound may occur, precipitating a fall in respiration rate, pulse rate, and blood pressure (Goosen & Bush, 1979).

Commonly observed behaviors of a person in pain include restlessness, perspiration, muscle tension, limping, splinting, rubbing the site, goose flesh, writhing, pacing, or fist clenching. Additional responses may include lip biting, teeth clenching, and facial expressions such as frowning or wrinkling the brow. Some individuals may withdraw from others and remain quiet, whereas others become noisy and strike out at those around them. The North American Nursing Diagnosis Association Taxonomy of Approved Diagnoses (Hurley, 1986) lists the following physical responses as defining characteristics for pain:

1. Guarding, protective behavior
2. Distracting behavior such as crying, moaning, pacing, or restlessness
3. Facial mask of pain, in which eyes lack luster, have a beaten look with fixed or scattered eye movements, or facial grimacing
4. Altered muscle tone that may range from rigid to listless
5. Presence of autonomic responses not seen in chronic pain such as diaphoresis, vital sign changes, dilation of pupils, and changes in respiration

Psychosocial reactions to pain are deeply influenced by the same factors that affect pain tolerance, including past experiences with pain. A verbally competent person may be able to describe accurately the location, duration, and intensity of the pain as well as the ability or willingness to tolerate it. A change in the tone of voice may be as revealing as the words spoken. Previous personal and family experiences with certain diseases, such as cancer, can significantly affect the degree of fear, anxiety, and depression associated with pain and consequently the individual's reaction. Vocalizations include responses such as crying, groaning, grunting, and gasping. Their frequency, loudness, and duration can assume greater significance in young children and the elderly who are either too young or too confused to be verbally competent.

Pain that persists or is repetitive results in adaptation of response, with observable reductions in sympathetic signs and symptoms. Pain receptors, however, show little if any adaptation. Reactions to long-term pain tend to be centrally mediated. With time, physiologic and psychological coping mechanisms evolve, but these behavioral responses do not necessarily indicate pain relief. The person may merely be too fatigued to respond.

Occasionally, pain is associated with neurogenic shock resulting from inhibition of the medullary vasomotor center with decreased vasomotor tone. This mechanism is not well understood but may be associated with circulatory collapse. Pain is believed to relate to other neurologic activities such as sleep. During rapid eye movement or dream sleep, the electroencephalogram records increased brain activity. Certain disorders in which pain predominates, such as angina and ulcer, appear to be exacerbated during this stage of sleep (Phillips & Cousins, 1986).

Adverse Physiologic Effects of Pain

It is believed that continued acute pain begins to produce harmful physiologic effects in addition to the usual signs and symptoms associated with pain. Conversely, there are clinicians who are hesitant to treat abdominal pain or head injuries because relief of acute pain may alter or delay an accurate diagnosis. Although these concerns are well founded, individuals should be assessed as rapidly as possible, and pain relief should be provided as soon as it is safe to do so.

Common respiratory problems caused by acute pain are associated with splinting that results from chest or abdominal pain and the patient's reluctance or inability to cough. Failure to cough, especially in individuals with chronic lung problems or after anesthesia, may result in retention of secretions with lung consolidation and possible atelectasis, with resulting hypercapnia and hypoxemia. Physiologic splinting can result in a decreased tidal volume, vital capacity, functional residual capacity, and alveolar ventilation. Cardiovascular problems associated with acute pain may include an exaggeration of sympathetic indicators commonly associated with the pain response. Increased cardiac work load results from the tachycardia, increased peripheral resistance, hypertension, and increased myocardial oxygen consumption that result from pain. Ischemia of heart muscle and other tissue such as brain tissue may result. Muscle spasm in the area associated with acute pain sets up a cycle of increased discomfort, and increased sympathetic activity frequently causes increased intestinal secretions and decreases intestinal motility, ultimately resulting in ileus with gastric stasis and dilation of the bowel. Skeletal muscle and bone immobilization may cause venous stasis and platelet aggregation that predispose to deep vein thrombosis and pulmonary embolism (Cousins & Phillips, 1986).

ASSESSMENT OF PAIN

Assessment of pain in the critically ill individual is challenging because of the patient's complex condition, altered interpretation of other stressful factors, and difficulty with communication. Nevertheless, comprehensive assessment is essential to determine the severity of pain and the proper method of management. The findings must be completely documented in the patient's record. Incomplete or absent documentation leads to the assumption that the nurse has treated pain without prior assessment (Christoph, 1991; Puntillo, 1990).

Pain is not reliably quantifiable. Establishing reliability is problematic because pain varies over time, is confounded by memory, is unique to individuals, and includes sensory, affective, and evaluative components (Reading, 1984). A number of assessment scales are available to aid in determining the severity of pain. The success of any process of pain assessment depends on consistent use and the ability to make modifications to meet the clinical needs of the patient (Huskisson, 1974).

Factors believed to alter the assessment of pain include individual patient characteristics (McCaffery, 1979); health professionals' attitudes (Baer et al., 1990); age, sex, education, and experience of health care workers (Amnad et al., 1982; McCaffery, 1979); and the patient's age and sex (Mather & Mackie, 1983). Children, men (Davitz et al., 1976), and postoperative patients (Cohen, 1980) present controversial assessment problems that are evident in the literature on pain and in clinical practice. Some nurses ignore patients' verbal or nonverbal complaints of pain, thereby undertreating a problem that should be well managed, especially during acute episodes.

Reading (1984) identified four objectives in clinical pain measurement:

1. Diagnostic, in that establishing a diagnosis and thereby selecting the appropriate treatment may depend on an accurate assessment of the precise characteristics of the pain.
2. Monitoring of fluctuations in pain levels during the course of treatment and thereby reducing reliance on the patient's making retrospective comparisons, which may be fraught with bias.
3. Evaluation of treatment efficacy, so that therapies having specific effects can be distinguished from the nonspecific or placebo effects, well documented in pain (Beecher, 1972).
4. Reliable monitoring of the pain over time, which permits controlling factors to be identified (p. 195).

Evaluation of pain begins by determining whether the pain exists. Critically ill patients may not be able to verbalize pain perception, making this task difficult. An understanding of a patient's past and current pathophysiology provides insight into the presence of pain and some initial expectations about the severity of pain (Christoph, 1991). Once the existence of pain has been identified, the patient's subjective reports of pain must be evaluated. Information should be elicited about location, quality, pattern, intensity, verbal and nonverbal observations, symptoms associated with pain, aggravating or triggering factors, and duration. Differentiation between sensory and affective dimensions of pain is important and can be determined by means of patient interview (Gaston-Johansson, 1984; Gaston-Johansson and Asklund-Gustafsson, 1985; Gracely & Dubner, 1981). A few examples of rating scales and questionnaires are discussed in this chapter. Critical care nurses are responsible for selecting a feasible method for assessing patients in their setting.

Verbal reports of pain present the following potential problems: subject response bias or falsification, a response not proportional to the actual severity of the noxious stimuli, discordance with other indices, and reactive effect in sensitizing the patient to the pain (Reading, 1984). However, the advantages of subjective data far outweigh these difficulties. Because pain is a personal experience, the patient should be seen as the authority on what is experienced.

Patient location can be relatively easy to determine in the alert patient by asking the patient to point to the area or verbally describe the location. This information can be recorded in the nurses' notes or on an anatomic drawing. Pain assessment involves observing, measuring, and recording physiologic and behavioral indicators that are perceived as pain related. The challenge facing the critical care nurse is to differentiate these indicators from the patient's overall condition. The individual's perception of pain and the meaning that pain holds for him or her must also be investigated. This aspect is best assessed by more than one person, such as the patient's team of health care providers.

The final aspect of evaluation is the determination of the adaptive mechanisms that are used to cope with pain. Five typical methods of coping are used when an individual faces any disaster: (1) denial, (2) group affiliation, (3) information gathering, (4) religion, and (5) optimism. The nurse can help foster any coping mechanisms the patient identifies as successful. Maladaptive mechanisms that are indicative of failure to cope include social isolation, extreme anxiety with exacerbation of pain, and passive dependency.

Pain intensity is frequently evaluated based on the sensory component of pain alone. Patient statements may aid in gauging the severity and qualitative nature of pain, using rankings of numbers or word descriptors. Words have different meanings for different people and even for the same person at different times because there is no universal anchorage. Thus, these scales are not reliable over time (Tursky, 1976).

Visual, verbal, and numeric rating scales are commonly used in clinical practice and pain research. Numeric scales can be used as visual or verbal responses. They are easily implemented by asking the patient to identify the amount of discomfort perceived on a scale

A. SIMPLE DESCRIPTIVE SCALE

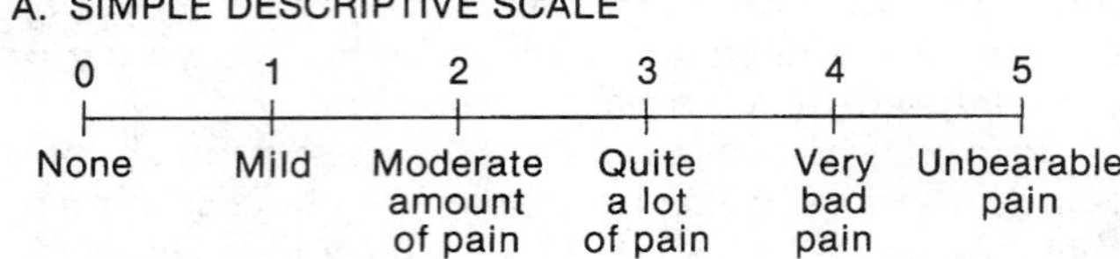

B. MELZACK'S SCALE

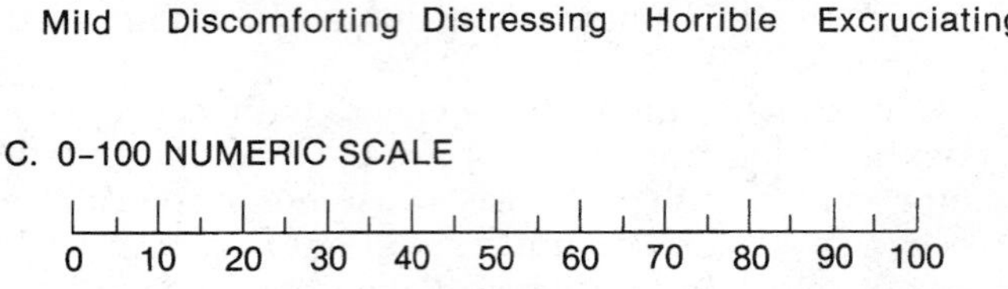

C. 0–100 NUMERIC SCALE

0 10 20 30 40 50 60 70 80 90 100

No pain

Moderate pain

Unbearable pain

D. VISUAL ANALOGUE SCALE OR GRAPHIC RATING METHOD

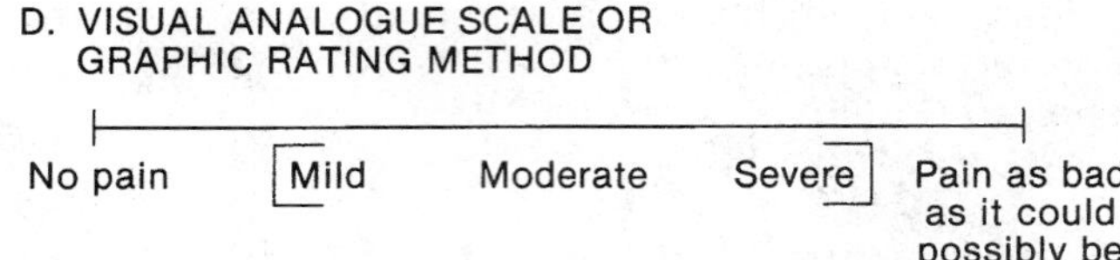

FIGURE 65–7. *A* to *D*, Examples of visual analog pain scales. (Redrawn from Melzack, R. [1975]. The McGill pain questionnaire: Major properties and scoring methods. *Pain, 1,* 277.)

of 0 to 10, with 0 reflecting no pain and 10 reflecting the worst pain the patient has ever experienced. Even with this simple and commonly used rating, it is expected that the patient will not reliably differentiate and correctly place value on the numbers (Shapiro, 1975). Determination of the patient's ability to discriminate between levels of pain is an important precursor to use of this method.

The visual analog scale of pain quantitation is similar to a numeric scale because the patient subjectively quantifies one aspect of the pain experience, usually its intensity (Fig. 65–7). These scales rate pain on a certain point scale with anchor words such as none, slight, moderate, and severe, which require evaluation by the patient, provided that he or she is able to perform such cognitive distinctions. Instead of choosing a number, the subject is asked to mark a point on a line. The line is divided into 10 equal spaces and the interval that contains the subject's mark is then given a value of 1 to 10. Again, this approach requires patient discriminative response and memory.

The most widely used method of qualitative and quantitative measurement of pain is the McGill-Melzack Pain Questionnaire (MPQ), a multidimensional scale that assesses sensory, affective, and evaluative elements of the pain experience (Fig. 65–8). Descriptive words in these three categories are chosen to identify subjective pain. Words used to describe pain reflect not only the sensory–discriminative aspect but also motivational–affective and cognitive–evalua-

Patient's name ______ Age ____

Hospital No. ______

Clinical category (e.g., cardiac, neurological, etc.): ______

Diagnosis: ______

Analgesic (if already administered):

1. Type ______
2. Dosage ______
3. Time given in relation to this test ______

Patient's intelligence: Circle number that represents best estimate.

1 (low) 2 3 4 5 (high)

****

This questionnaire has been designed to tell us more about your pain. Four major questions we ask are:

1. Where is your pain?
2. What does it feel like?
3. How does it change with time?
4. How strong is it?

It is important that you tell us how your pain feels now. Please follow the instructions at the beginning of each part.

Part 1. Where Is Your Pain?

Please mark, on the drawings, the areas where you feel pain. Put E if external, or I if internal, near the areas which you mark. Put EI if both external and internal.

Part 2. What Does Your Pain Feel Like?

Some of the words below describe your present pain. Circle ONLY those words that best describe it. Leave out any category that is not suitable. Use only a single word in each appropriate category—the one that applies best.

1	2	3	4	5
Flickering Quivering Pulsing Throbbing Beating	Jumping Flashing Shooting	Pricking Boring Drilling Stabbing Lancinating	Sharp Cutting Lacerating	Pinching Pressing Gnawing Cramping Crushing
6	**7**	**8**	**9**	**10**
Tugging Pulling Wrenching	Hot Burning Scalding Searing	Tingling Itchy Smarting Stinging	Dull Sore Hurting Aching Heavy	Tender Taut Rasping Splitting
11	**12**	**13**	**14**	**15**
Tiring Exhausting	Sickening Suffocating	Fearful Frightful Terrifying	Punishing Gruelling Cruel Vicious Killing	Wretched Blinding
16	**17**	**18**	**19**	**20**
Annoying Troublesome Miserable Intense Unbearable	Spreading Radiating Penetrating Piercing	Tight Numb Drawing Squeezing Tearing	Cool Cold Freezing	Nagging Nauseating Agonizing Dreadful Torturing

Part 3. How Does Your Pain Change With Time?

1. Which word or words would you use to describe the pattern of your pain?

1	2	3
Continuous Steady Constant	Rhythmic Periodic Intermittent	Brief Momentary Transient

2. What kind of things relieve your pain? ______

3. What kind of things increase your pain? ______

Part 4. How Strong Is Your Pain?

People agree that the following 5 words represent pain of increasing intensity. They are:

1	2	3	4	5
Mild	Discomforting	Distressing	Horrible	Excruciating

To answer each question below, write the number of the most appropriate word in the space beside the question.

1. Which word describes your pain right now? ____
2. Which word describes it at its worst? ____
3. Which word describes it when it is the least? ____
4. Which word describes the worst toothache you ever had? ____
5. Which word describes the worst headache you ever had? ____
6. Which word describes the worst stomach ache you ever had? ____

FIGURE 65–8. Pain assessment form. (From Melzack, R. [1975]. The McGill pain questionnaire: Major properties and scoring methods. *Pain, 1,* 277.)

tive dimensions. Pain has an unpleasant, negative-affective quality that distinguishes it from sensory experiences such as sight or hearing.

The two major measures obtained with the MPQ are the pain rating index rank, based on numeric values assigned to the chosen words, and the number of words chosen (Melzack, 1975). Although difficult to administer and grade in the clinical setting due to its length and complexity, the questionnaire has demonstrated characteristic response patterns for different pain syndromes such as cancer pain, lower back pain, and arthritis. The exact role of the MPQ in the evaluation of acute pain syndromes is still being actively investigated, but in its present form it is unsuitable for frequent assessments of pain in the critically ill patient.

The Stewart Pain-Color Scale presents the patient

with an array of yellow, orange, red, and black colors. Patients are asked where they would place their pain on the color chart. Research has indicated that patients with no pain select the left or yellow side of the scale, patients with moderate pain select the red or orange, middle range part of the scale, and patients with severe pain indicate the black or right side of the scale. The scale is easy to use by patients who are not color blind and may be especially useful for critically ill patients who are too ill to conceptualize numbers (Stewart, 1977).

Another method of pain analysis is the estimation of magnitude, a measurement technique adapted from psychophysics (Haber & Hershenson, 1980). Because all objects and events serve as potentially perceivable stimuli by the sensory apparatus, a measurable response results from a perceived stimulus. The purpose of the magnitude estimation technique is to form a ratio scale, mapping the magnitude of a sensory response in relation to the magnitude of a physical stimulus such as pain for each subject. An individual is asked to estimate the apparent strength or intensity of his or her sensory responses relative to a set of stimuli and reflect the magnitude of this intensity in some physical manner. The expression of this magnitude may be captured by an instrument such as a hand dynamometer. Tursky and colleagues (1982) used this principle to develop a pain perception profile that has been used successfully and reliably in a laboratory setting. A further application in the clinical setting has been reported for estimating the parameters of dyspnea (Nield et al., 1989).

Development of an instrument for assessment of pain has been reported and refined by Gaston-Johansson and Asklund-Gustafsson (1985). They found that the words "pain," "ache," and "hurt" commonly referred to pain-like experiences in the English and Swedish languages. In addition, "these concepts were shown to differ in intensity and to be associated with particular sensory and affective word descriptors" (p. 541). Sensory (s) and affective (a) descriptors representing the concept of pain were listed as cutting (s), tearing (s), killing (a), and torturing (a). Words representing ache were grinding (s), gnawing (s), irritating (a), and troublesome (a). Hurt was represented by pricking (s), pinching (s), fearful (a), and unhappy (a) (Gaston-Johansson, 1984). These words were used to study the discriminating power of descriptors in nurses, nursing students, and patients. Comparison was made with a visual analog scale and the MPQ. It was found that all subject groups agreed on the difference in intensity among the words pain, ache, and hurt, encouraging further development of this descriptive measurement tool. The use of fewer descriptors might make this a more useful clinical assessment tool. Descriptors for pain, ache, and hurt can be given a numeric value, providing a basis for managing sensory and affective aspects of pain (Gaston-Johansson & Asklund-Gustafsson, 1985).

Assessment issues that require extra consideration by the critical care nurse when narcotic analgesics are used include the patient's size, age, and sex. The key to proper pain management is an individualized narcotic dosage based on the patient's needs.

WEIGHT. Because of significant differences in body weight, obese patients are likely to require more narcotic than emaciated patients.

ELDERLY. The elderly may receive inappropriate dosages because of metabolic changes associated with aging. Use of the lowest drug strength initially, with subsequent titration upward, may prevent untoward side effects. Alterations in absorption, distribution, metabolism, and excretion can contribute to drug sensitivity (Greenblat et al., 1982). Decreased renal function and decreased cardiac output may result in drug concentration at a particular site of action (Cohen, 1986; Weinberg, 1988). Abrupt hospitalization may result in disorientation, decreased exercise, loss of control over one's life, inability to express pain, or regression. Depression and fear of death may also cause special problems. These problems must be considered particularly when dealing with pain in the elderly. Careful, frequent assessment of the elderly patient by the critical care nurse may prevent development or progression of complications resulting from overmedication. Inability or failure of elderly patients to complain of pain contributes to the erroneous notion that elderly patients do not perceive pain as readily as young adults.

CHILDREN. Literature on the pain experience in children is meager, controversial, and lacking in systematic research. Several investigators have reported that, contrary to a widely held belief, children can and often do suffer considerable pain. Children with an inaccurate understanding of what is happening may develop fantasies of mutilation, become extremely anxious, and doubt their ability to cope. Realistic reassurance can promote a sense of control and increase coping ability (National Institutes of Health Consensus Development Conference, 1987; Porth, 1986; Savedra et al., 1982).

GENDER. The issue of pain assessment and management related to gender has been addressed intermittently in the literature during the past three decades. Most of the information provided merely compares male and female samples during statistical analysis on general issues centered around emotion, attitude, and behavior. Some of this information was addressed briefly in the section on cultural issues at the beginning of this chapter, but additional details are necessary to provide the critical care nurse with background data that can be used during assessment and planning of pain management. These previous references can be augmented by more recent studies that look carefully at gender and the stress response. Although little reference is made directly to pain in these studies, application of data related to the stress response is an appropriate transfer of information. The fact that pain-induced stress results in sympathetic nervous system activation is well documented by evidence of increases in heart rate, blood pressure, peripheral and vascular resistance, cardiac output, and cardiac work (Thoren, 1974). Hormone response to the stress of pain, surgery, or trauma is similar and depends on the magnitude and duration of the insult (Thoren, 1974; Traynor & Hall, 1981).

Gender-differentiated neuroendocrine (cortisol, epinephrine, norepinephrine, beta-endorphin, and beta-lipotropin) and cardiovascular stress response are two key areas that have value for the critical care nurse. Pain and stress promote the pituitary release of ACTH into the bloodstream, stimulating secretion of glucocorticoids (cortisol) from the cortex of the adrenal gland. The adrenal medulla is directly innervated by the sympathetic nervous system, which serves as a stimulus for release of the catecholamines—epinephrine and norepinephrine. About 80% of the adrenal secretion of catecholamines consists of epinephrine (Asterita, 1985). Research findings consistently indicate that in response to standard laboratory stressors women show a less pronounced elevation in urinary excretion of epinephrine than do men (Frankenhaeuser et al., 1976; Johansson & Post, 1974). The same relationship has been observed among 12-year-olds, indicating that the difference is related to gender rather than to age (Johansson, 1972). None of the investigations has revealed a corresponding sex difference in the urinary excretion of norepinephrine, which is consistent with observations that norepinephrine responds most to physical stress whereas epinephrine is more reactive to psychological stressors (Dimsdale & Moss, 1980; Ward et al., 1983).

Compared with women, men show exaggerated reactions to stress in some but not all of the variables measured. It has been consistently observed that both plasma and urinary excretions of epinephrine rise appreciably more in men than in women during exposure to achievement-oriented laboratory tasks or stressors. Other neuroendocrine reactions either do not differ between men and women (norepinephrine) or show no consistent pattern related to gender (cortisol). The few studies of the influences of the reproductive hormones on catecholamine or cortisol responses to laboratory stressors reveal no consistent effects of menstrual phase or, in postmenopausal women, of replacement therapy with an estrogen–progestin compound (Plante & Denvey, 1984).

In regard to cardiovascular reactivity, there is some inconsistent evidence that men exhibit larger systolic blood pressure responses and smaller heart rate reactions to psychological stressors than do women. Among ovariectomized women, systolic blood pressure responses to laboratory stressors are reduced after administration of an estrogen or estrogen–progestin compound. An attenuated systolic blood pressure response to stressors has also been found to accompany the use of oral contraceptives. These findings as well as a recent observation that heart rate and systolic blood pressure responses of postmenopausal women were greater than those seen in premenopausal controls suggest that the female reproductive hormones are associated with a reduced cardiovascular response (Polefrone & Manuck, 1987).

The influence of gender on beta-endorphin and beta-lipotropin levels has also been explored, with more recent studies reporting that women have higher levels than men (Furuhashi et al., 1984). Previous reports were varied. Findings in a study by Viswanathan and colleagues (1987) supported many previous reports that exercise induces increases in plasma beta-endorphins and beta-lipotropin. These investigators further found that eumenorrheic and amenorrheic women increased plasma levels at the end of the exercise period, whereas men did not significantly increase levels until exhaustion was reached.

The existence of gender-related differences in pain response is supported in a study of newborn infants, in whom sex differences were apparent in speed of response, with boys showing a shorter time to cry and to display facial action after heel-lance. The presence of variation in facial action was interpreted as an indication that the biologic and behavioral context of pain events affects behavioral expression even at this very early developmental stage, before the opportunity for learned response patterns has occurred (Grunau & Craig, 1987).

MANAGEMENT OF PAIN

Pain management is a complex issue, and methods used to control or decrease pain range from simple, noninvasive relaxation techniques to invasive surgical procedures. Nurses are the key people responsible for pain alleviation and implementation of dependent, interdependent, and independent actions. The principles of pain management most appropriate for use by critical care nurses are presented here, emphasizing recent successful and innovative techniques. Pharmacologic and nonpharmacologic methods of management are included along with their physiologic effects. Ethical and legal issues related to pain management are also addressed.

Pharmacologic Management of Pain

Critical care nurses play a key role in the pharmacologic management of pain. Not only do nurses administer most drugs used for pain management, they also evaluate the desired and untoward effects of these drugs and identify life-threatening situations. Pharmacologic management of pain includes use of narcotic analgesia, nonnarcotic analgesia, and anesthetic agents. Methods of administration and observed responses to these agents are within the domain of nursing.

NARCOTIC ANALGESIA

Narcotic analgesics include the naturally occurring opium alkaloids and their synthetic and semisynthetic derivatives. Because these drugs possess pharmacologic effects similar to the effects of opium, they are frequently called opioid analgesics. For this discussion, the narcotic analgesic agents will be divided into narcotic agonists, narcotic antagonists, and agents with mixed agonist and antagonist activity (DiGregorio et al., 1986). Table 65–1 classifies the narcotic agents by generic and common trade names.

NARCOTIC AGONISTS. Narcotic agonists are the cornerstone of pain management in the critically ill patient, and include the derivatives listed in Table 65–1. These agents are used to treat moderate to severe pain. Morphine is the oldest known drug of this class and remains the prototype and the standard of comparison for all other narcotic analgesic compounds (Table 65–2).

The discovery of the endogenous opioids and their activity in the body has enhanced our understanding of exogenous opioids such as morphine. Studies support the hypothesis that specific opioid receptors exist to facilitate the action of endogenous opioids and mediate the action of narcotic drugs. Five receptor types have been identified as the sites of action for endogenous and exogenous opioidlike substances, including μ (mu), κ (kappa), δ (delta), Σ (sigma), and ϵ (epsilon). Experimentation suggests that the mu receptor is associated with supraspinal analgesia, respiratory depression, euphoria, and physical dependence; the kappa receptor is believed to mediate spinal analgesia, miosis, and sedation, and the sigma receptor appears to be involved with dysphoria, psychotomimetic effects, and respiratory stimulation. The delta receptors may influence affective behavior. Epsilon receptors may influence dysphoria and analgesia (Donnelly & Lamb, 1993). Agonistic narcotics act as analgesics by binding to and activating both mu and kappa receptors in the brain and spinal cord. The agonist opioid drugs have an affinity for these receptors and can stimulate the receptors to produce an effect. Therefore, they mimic the activity of the endogenous opioid peptides. Despite the fact that all of the narcotic agonists stimulate both the mu and kappa receptors, differences in amounts needed to induce analgesia among the compounds are great (DiGregorio et al., 1986).

Agonist opioids are readily absorbed by the body after subcutaneous or intramuscular injection. However, hepatic first-pass biotransformation reduces the amount available to the entire body, and therefore the bioavailability of most of these drugs when administered orally is less than 60%. In general, the amount of drug needed for an effective oral dose is greater than the amount needed for a parenteral dose, resulting in a low parenteral–oral dose ratio. This varies, however, among patients and depends on the particular compound. The intravenous route is the preferred method of administration in critically ill individuals because life support systems and altered consciousness alter accessibility to the oral route. In addition, the subcutaneous and intramuscular routes are frequently impaired by poor circulation.

TABLE 65–1. **Selected Narcotic Compounds**

Classification	Generic Name	Common Trade Name
Agonists		
Phenanthrene derivatives	Morphine	
	Codeine	
	Hydromorphone	Dilaudid
	Oxymorphone	Numorphan
	Oxycodone	
Morphinan derivative	Levorphanol	Levo-Dromoran
Phenylpiperdine derivatives	Meperidine	Demerol
	Fentanyl	Sublimaze
Diphenylheptane derivatives	Methadone	Dolophine
	Propoxyphene	Darvon
Antagonists		
	Naloxone	Narcan
	Naltrexone	Trexan
Mixed Agonist–Antagonists		
	Buprenorphine	Buprenex
	Butorphanol	Stadol
	Nalbuphine	Nubain
	Pentazocine	Talwin

TABLE 65–2. **Potency Comparisons of Selected Narcotic Analgesics***

Drug	Equianalgesic Doses (mg) IM	PO
Narcotic Agonists		
Morphine	10	60
Codeine	120	200
Fentanyl	0.1	—†
Hydromorphone	1.5	7.5
Levorphanol	2	4
Meperidine	75	300
Methadone	10	20
Oxycodone	15	30
Oxymorphone	1	6
Propoxyphene	—†	130
Narcotic Agonist–Antagonists		
Buprenorphine	0.3	—†
Butorphanol	2	—†
Nalbuphine	10	—†
Pentazocine	30	150

*The data in this table are based on morphine, 10 mg, administered IM, and represent the general consensus of medical opinion. Variability will occur among patients; therefore, these values should be used only as a guide for comparison.

†Not used by this route.

Abbreviations: IM, intramuscular; PO, oral.

After intravenous injection of an agonist opioid, onset of analgesic effect occurs within 10 to 30 minutes and peak effect occurs between 20 and 120 minutes (Table 65–3). Most analgesics are biotransformed to inactive conjugates in the liver; however, approximately 10% of codeine, the 3-methyl derivative of morphine, is demethylated to morphine before inactivation. More than 90% of the administered dose of drug is excreted in the urine as inactive metabolites; the remainder appears in the feces through biliary excretion, mainly as the more lipid-soluble parent drug. The plasma half-life of these narcotics is generally 4 hours or less, with the exception of levorphanol, methadone, and propoxyphene (Table 65–4) (DiGregorio et al., 1986; Donnelly & Lamb, 1993; Jaffe & Martin, 1980; Twycross, 1984). Additional information about each of the narcotics can be obtained from the drug reference literature.

ADVERSE ACTIONS OF AGONISTS. Although opioid agonists predominantly abolish pain, these drugs have profound pharmacologic activity throughout the body. In addition to the effects on the CNS, activity of the peripheral systems and organs may also be altered. CNS effects of opioids include analgesia, drowsiness, alteration in mood, lethargy, inability to concentrate, apathy, and mental clouding. These symptoms occur both in pain-free individuals and in patients experiencing pain. Opioids relieve pain without a loss of consciousness, and patients retain sensations such as touch, vision, and hearing. Euphoria may be experienced in 10% to 20% of patients, especially as pain is alleviated; however, dysphoric reactions may also occur.

Narcotic agonists act directly on the brain stem respiratory centers, reducing the respiratory rate, minute volume, and tidal exchange and producing irregular and periodic breathing patterns. These effects are observable at therapeutic doses of the opioids and increase as the dose is raised. Death from narcotic overdose is almost always the result of respiratory depression and arrest.

Narcotic analgesics often cause constipation, nausea, and vomiting. Nausea and vomiting are frequently perceived as allergic responses to morphine and other narcotics. This possibility should be carefully evaluated by the critical care nurse, who should determine the patient's untoward response through careful history taking or skin testing. Both peripheral and central actions of these drugs cause constipation by decreasing the propulsive peristaltic motility of the small intestine (the duodenum is affected more than the ileum), enhancing the action of the gastrointestinal sphincter muscles, and reducing digestive secretions along the entire alimentary canal. Delay in movement of bowel contents leads to fecal dehydration, further reducing intestinal passage. Decreased perception of normal rectal sensory stimuli can also contribute to constipation. Stool softeners and laxatives can be used effectively to treat constipation.

Direct stimulation of the chemoreceptor trigger zone in the area postrema of the medulla causes nausea and emesis. A vestibular component is believed to be involved because there is a high incidence of nausea and vomiting when patients are ambulatory. This side effect rarely occurs in bedridden patients.

Most narcotic agonists constrict the pupil through stimulation of the nuclei of the oculomotor nerve. This is a useful diagnostic sign of narcotic use or abuse. Tolerance usually does not develop to opioid-induced miosis.

TABLE 65–3. **Pharmacokinetic Data of Narcotic Analgesics**

Drug	Onset of Effect* (Minutes)	Peak Effects* (Minutes)
Narcotic Agonists		
Morphine	30	30–60
Codeine	30	45–90
Fentanyl	10	20–30*
Hydromorphone	30	30–90
Levorphanol	30	60–90
Meperidine	15	30–60
Methadone	15	60–120
Oxycodone	—†	—†
Oxymorphone	10	30–90
Propoxyphene‡	30	60–90
Narcotic Agonist–Antagonists		
Buprenorphine	15	45–60
Butorphanol	10	30–60
Nalbuphine	15	45–60
Pentazocine	15	30–60

*Based on intramuscular administration.
†No data available.
‡Based on oral administration.

TABLE 65–4. **Pharmacokinetic Data of Narcotic Analgesics**

Drug	Duration of Effect (Hours)	Plasma Half-Life (Hours)
Narcotic Agonists		
Morphone	3–7	2–3
Codeine	4–6	3–4
Fentanyl	1–2	3–4
Hydromorphone	4–5	2–4
Levorphanol	4–8	10–12
Meperidine	2–4	3–4
Methadone	4–6	21–25
Oxycodone	4–5	—*
Oxymorphone	3–6	—*
Propoxyphene	4–6	6–12
Narcotic Agonist–Antagonists		
Buprenorphine	4–6	2–3
Butorphanol	3–4	2–4
Nalbuphine	3–6	4–6
Pentazocine	2–3	2–3

*No data available.

Most agonists alter the cough reflex, and critical care nurses should be aware that even mild depression of the medullary–pontine (tussive) cough center may modify the triggering effect of mucus. Potential dependence and respiratory depression severely limit the antitussive benefit of some narcotics. The therapeutic effects of codeine and hydromorphone as cough suppressants, with their high antitussive activity and lower liability to dependence, make them more suitable for analgesia but less suitable if the patient needs to retain an ability to clear mucus from the respiratory tract.

Arteriolar vasodilation and reduced peripheral resistance may occur with therapeutic doses of narcotics. While the patient is supine, these effects are usually insignificant, but orthostatic hypotension and fainting may occur in ambulatory patients. Most opioid analgesics promote histamine release from mast cells, enhancing the hypotensive effect of these compounds. In normal individuals, cardiac function is not significantly altered; however, in patients with coronary artery disease or myocardial infarction, a decrease in oxygen consumption, left ventricular end-diastolic pressure, and cardiac function may occur.

With the exception of vascular muscle, most smooth muscle, including the bronchioles, gallbladder, bile duct, sphincter of Oddi, and urinary bladder, is contracted by morphine-like drugs. Urinary retention is a common side effect. Morphine or its derivatives are contraindicated in patients experiencing pain from biliary stones unless atropine is administered concurrently to decrease smooth muscle contraction. Bronchiolar smooth muscle contraction is rarely significant.

Release of histamine from mast cells is partially responsible for the cutaneous vasodilation, pruritus, and sweating that accompany agonist narcotics. Although annoying, these symptoms are usually tolerated as long as pain relief occurs.

The issue of physical and psychological dependence raised by chronic use of narcotics should be a minor consideration in the ICU. Typically, the goal in an acutely ill person is to abolish pain and to maintain comfort.

Tolerance occurs when the same dose elicits a decreased effect after repeated administration, or when increasingly greater doses are required to achieve the effect observed with the initial dose even after physiologic improvement. Careful consideration must be given to changing the dosage as evidence of tolerance is observed or if the patient has a history of chronic pain that has been managed by narcotics. Tolerance and physical dependence are dose- and time-dependent. Two to 3 weeks of therapeutic doses may lead to physical or psychological dependence. The critical care nurse should observe for signs of physical withdrawal such as autonomic hyperactivity, including diarrhea, vomiting, lacrimation, rhinorrhea, chills, and fever. Patients may also suffer abdominal cramps, pain, and tremors. Observation and documentation of these indicators should be reported to the physician and a collaborative plan devised to prevent further dependence or reverse existing dependence (DiGregorio et al., 1986; Jaffe & Martin, 1980; Mather & Phillips, 1986).

DRUG INTERACTIONS. General anesthetics, phenothiazines, barbiturates, tranquilizers, sedative hypnotics, tricyclic antidepressants, and other CNS depressants have been reported to exaggerate the depressant effects of the opioid agonists.

Severe and sometimes fatal CNS and respiratory reactions have occurred in patients receiving meperidine who were concurrently taking or had taken monoamine inhibitors within 14 days. Concurrent administration of phenobarbital or phenytoin has been implicated in increased systemic clearance of meperidine.

NARCOTIC ANTAGONISTS. Narcotic antagonists, naloxone and naltrexone, are competitive antagonists of agonist narcotics and mixed agonist–antagonist compounds. These drugs compete for opioid receptor sites and prevent or reverse activation of receptors by other opiate agents. These agents do not produce analgesia, respiratory depression, pupillary constriction, or physical dependence. Antagonists are used frequently in critical care to reverse the adverse effects of an agonist overdose.

Naloxone has a plasma half-life of about an hour in adults and 3 hours in neonates. Onset of action occurs within 2 minutes of administration of an intravenous dose; intramuscular administration has a slightly longer onset. Because an individual response to naloxone is anticipated, it is necessary to titrate naloxone by giving small doses and observing any subsequent changes in the patient's appearance, behavior, and verbal response. Naloxone has been associated with severe adverse reactions (dysrhythmias, cardiac arrest, pulmonary edema) (Neal & Owens, 1992). The drug and its inactive metabolites are excreted in the urine. Oral administration of naloxone is ineffective due to its rapid biotransformation by hepatic conjugation; parenteral administration is required. Naltrexone may be given orally and has a duration of 24 to 72 hours.

MIXED AGONIST–ANTAGONISTS. Mixed agonist–antagonists, butorphanol tartrate (Stadol; Bristol Laboratories, Evansville, IN) and nalbuphine (Nubain; Du Pont, Wilmington, DE), are potent analgesics with opioid receptor selectivity. They cause some of the agonist agents' side effects; however, they are believed to cause less respiratory depression and less dependence due to antagonist properties. Signs of narcotic agonist dependence withdrawal result when mixed agonist–antagonists are given.

NONNARCOTIC ANALGESIA

Numerous nonnarcotic analgesic drugs have analgesic properties or potentiate narcotic analgesics. Nonnarcotic analgesics are structurally dissimilar organic acids that fit into the subcategories of analgesic, antipyretic, and antiinflammatory activity. Nonnarcotics act peripherally, and their antiinflammatory activity results from biochemical changes. These drugs are frequently referred to as nonsteroidal antiinflammatory drugs (NSAIDs). In the ICU these drugs are rarely used for antiinflammatory action, but some are used as antipyretics. Because aspirin and acetaminophen are the two agents most commonly used, and acetaminophen lacks some of the side effects of aspirin, only major problems associated with aspirin in combination with other drugs will be addressed.

Epigastric distress progressing to gastric or intestinal ulceration and subsequent bleeding may be associated with the use of aspirin. Patients at greatest risk for adverse effects include the elderly, those with history of gastrointestinal problems, and those with debilitating diseases. The degree of involvement is usually dose dependent. Gastric distress results from PG inhibition, which normally decreases stomach acid secretion and promotes secretion of cytoprotective intestinal mucus. There is also an increase in the mean bleeding time due to inhibited thromboxane A_2 formation in thrombocytes, and reduced platelet aggregation. This effect persists for the life of the platelet. Bleeding time will be doubled for 4 to 7 days after administration of 650 mg of aspirin. All other nonnarcotic analgesics, except acetaminophen, also inhibit platelet aggregation; however, the effect is "reversible" and is usually quantitatively less and shorter than that observed with aspirin. Increased bleeding time is exacerbated in patients with underlying hematologic defects and in those taking anticoagulants. Use of any NSAID should be approached with caution because of this potential problem. In small doses, other side effects from nonnarcotic analgesics are minimal (Silverstein et al., 1995).

ANALGESIC ADJUVANT THERAPY

Adjuvant therapy offers a valuable addition to the available treatment modalities in critical care. This group of drugs can be divided into different pharmacologic categories, including CNS stimulants, antidepressants, antispastic agents, skeletal muscle relaxants, antipsychotics, antihistamines, anxiolytics, and anticonvulsants. Mechanisms of analgesic action of these agents are frequently conjectural, and critical proof of analgesic efficacy is often lacking. However, there are clinical situations in which adjuvant therapy may provide substantial analgesic benefit. It is interesting to note that as our understanding of pain transmission mechanisms improves, some observations of adjuvant drug therapy effectiveness have been validated.

Stimulant and antidepressant drugs are not widely used in various pain syndrome treatments due to fear of drug dependence and potential side effects involving CNS stimulation. However, these drugs have been extremely effective in patients with excessive narcotic analgesic sedation or illness-related depression. Caffeine and dextroamphetamine are the most popular drugs in this category. Oral dextroamphetamine given at a dose of 5 to 10 mg in the morning is especially useful for combating daytime sedation resulting from narcotic analgesics. A combination of morphine and dextroamphetamine has been found twice as effective for analgesia as morphine alone. Caffeine, a constituent of both over-the-counter and prescription medications, is an effective analgesic adjuvant at doses of at least 65 mg. When combined with various nonnarcotic analgesics such as aspirin or acetaminophen, caffeine increases the analgesic activity of these agents. Tricyclic antidepressants such as amitriptyline, imipramine, and nortriptyline are commonly used to treat depression associated with chronic pain such as neuralgia or migraine headaches.

Skeletal muscle relaxants include antispastic and centrally acting agents. Primary antispastic agents are diazepam and baclofen, which act in the spinal cord, and dantrolene, which acts directly on skeletal muscle. These drugs reduce muscle spasticity, leading to reduced pain. Centrally acting skeletal muscle relaxants include carisporodol, chlorephenesin, chlorzoxazone, cyclobenzaprine, methocarbamol, and orphenadrine. The choice of agent depends on the condition being treated, the presence of associated illnesses, and potential drug interactions. These drugs are frequently used in combination with other drugs and treatment regimens to obtain the best therapeutic effect.

Antipsychotics and antianxiety agents (anxiolytics) are used for their ability to alter the patient's behavioral status. Examples of antipsychotics are methotrimeprazine and haloperidol. In addition to its antipsychotic activity, methotrimeprazine also appears to produce analgesia directly through a nonopioid receptor system. It is useful in patients with tolerance to narcotic analgesics or who respond to them with respiratory depression, or when both antipsychotic and analgesic effects are needed. In the anxiolytic group, benzodiazepine, like diazepam, is most popular. These agents reduce other symptoms, such as anxiety, that are often associated with pain. Tranquilizers may modify the undesirable side effects of narcotics such as nausea and vomiting. Minor tranquilizers are more specific for the treatment of anxiety and safer than phenothiazines.

The major *antihistamine* used as an adjuvant in pain therapy is hydroxyzine, given in doses of 50 to 100 mg intramuscularly with a narcotic analgesic. Promethazine may be used in a similar manner. Some clinicians believe that the sedative effect of the antihistamine enhances the sedative activity of the narcotic and is the major benefit of this combination.

Anticonvulsant drugs have been demonstrated to be effective for certain types of neurologic pain such as phantom limb pain. Anticonvulsants most often prescribed include carbamazepine, phenytoin, and clonazepam. When these drugs are used, baseline blood studies must be performed at regular intervals to determine the blood levels of the drug and to check for the presence of blood dyscrasias. Physicians and nurses should be thoroughly familiar with the pharmacologic properties of these agents.

ANESTHETIC AGENTS

Most anesthetic agents provide anesthesia and are generally considered poor analgesics except when the patient is semiconscious or unconscious. Clinical experience and research have demonstrated that anesthetic agents are useful because of their CNS depression properties. These agents include halothane, enflurane, and isoflurane. In contrast, inhaled anesthetics such as nitrous oxide and methoxyflurane are potent analgesics at subanesthetic concentrations and are used for pain control in dental and obstetric procedures. They have also been extremely useful for intermittent, severe pain when routine analgesics are not adequate, such as during burn dressing changes or orthopedic procedures. When the critical care nurse is not satisfied with the adequacy of the analgesic agents used or believes they are unsafe in the doses required, the possible use of anesthetic agents should be pursued in consultation with the anesthesiologist.

Use of local anesthetics such as cainal agents is common in critical care to produce limited analgesia close to the site of administration. Frequently used agents include procaine, lidocaine, and bupivacaine. Benzocaine is a topical compound used for irritated areas of the skin or mucous membranes. These drugs prevent conduction and generation of nerve impulses, a process that is reversed when the drug concentration diminishes. Although all neurons in contact with these drugs are affected, the small-diameter fibers such as those that transmit pain (the A-delta and C fibers) are most susceptible (Bonica, 1987; DiGregorio et al., 1986; Mather & Cousins, 1986).

METHODS OF ADMINISTRATION

Much concern has been expressed by nurses about the adequacy of pain management, especially for postoperative pain, because pain relief continues to pose a significant problem in everyday clinical practice. Despite advances in anesthesia and analgesia, relief of postoperative pain has not changed drastically, and remains inadequate (Donovan, 1983; Nordberg, 1984). Nordberg (1984) states that parenteral administration of narcotics persists as the major approach to postoperative pain relief, not because it offers optimal pain relief but because of its simplicity of administration. In a study by Donovan (1983) involving 200 general surgery patients, 31% reported insufficient postoperative pain relief. Sixty-three percent of these dissatisfied patients stated that pain relief could have been more frequent. Donovan believes that medical and nursing staff are reluctant to depart from traditional routines to relieve pain. However, investigations in the last decade have increased our understanding of the pharmacodynamics of narcotics and have opened new doors for pain treatment.

Intermittent intravenous administration of narcotic analgesics is the most commonly used administration method and route in the critical care setting. The continuous method is most useful for terminally ill cancer patients unable to take oral medications. Morphine is most commonly used. In nontolerant patients of average weight with acute pain, the usual doses of morphine and meperidine are 3 mg/hour and 20 mg/hour, respectively. Some patients with severe acute pain may require higher doses. However, increasing the infusion rate more than once a day should be done with extreme caution because a new peak narcotic plasma level will not be attained for 12 to 24 hours after a rate change. Therefore, any adjustment in dose should be closely monitored for delayed respiratory depression 12 to 24 hours later. Frequent assessment of vital signs is mandatory during this period, and naloxone should be available for the immediate reversal of narcotic-induced toxicity. Patients with advanced cancer or terminal cancer-related pain can become rapidly tolerant. Because the major therapeutic goal for these patients is pain relief, they may require hourly analgesic doses that are substantially higher than those required for management of acute pain.

PATIENT-CONTROLLED ANALGESIA (PCA). PCA is a recent innovative approach to pain management that allows self-administration of intravenous analgesia. A PCA device consists of an infusion pump and a timing unit that the patient triggers by depressing a thumb button. The device delivers analgesia, usually morphine or meperidine. Two methods of infusion during PCA are currently available—low-dose continuous infusion with bolus, and bolus-only through an indwelling catheter. The timing unit prevents overdosage by interposing an "inactivation period" between patient-initiated doses. A specified total dose is regulated over a period of time, usually 24 hours. Data regarding dosage and time of administration are recorded and are retrievable by the nurse at any time (Barkas & Duafala, 1988). Advantages of PCA include increased patient comfort, satisfaction of individualized needs, reduction of lag time from pain onset to drug administration, elimination of dependency on the nurse, decrease in tissue trauma from frequent parenteral injections, reduction in amount of analgesic used, early postoperative ambulation, increase in forced vital capacity and peak expiratory flow in postoperative patients, and enhanced bowel recovery after trauma or surgery (Atwell et al., 1984; Bennett & Griffen, 1983; Eisenach et al., 1988). PCA has been shown to be superior to other techniques such as intramuscular injection and continuous intravenous infusions (Lubenow & Ivankovich, 1991). The most frequently identified disadvantage to the pump is expense. Use of PCA should be selective, depending on patient alertness and ability to comprehend the function and purpose of the machine. Caution should be exercised in patients with incident pain and neuropathic pain syndromes, depressed and delirious patients, and patients with a history of drug or alcohol abuse (Barkas & Duafala, 1988). Table 65–5 presents nursing responsibilities for implementing PCA.

EPIDURAL NARCOTICS. Epidural narcotics alleviate visceral and somatic pain by direct application into the

TABLE 65–5. **Patient-Controlled Analgesia (PCA) Nursing Responsibilities**

Nursing responsibilities for implementing PCA include:

- Understanding the concept of PCA
- Assessing patient's capability to self-administer narcotics
- Educating patient about PCA delivery system
- Validating patient's knowledge on the use of the PCA delivery system
- Validating physician's orders for initiation of PCA (narcotic to be administered, loading dose, maintenance dose, lockout time, and maximum dose)
- Establishing a second intravenous line to maintain catheter infusion if PCA device is *not* the type that can deliver a continuous infusion as well as an intermittent bolus
- Monitoring the infusion and troubleshooting as necessary
- Assessing patient response to PCA
- Observing for side effects such as respiratory depression, pruritus, nausea, and vomiting
- Notifying physician of side effects or if pain relief is inadequate

spinal epidural space. This technique is gaining increasing popularity in clinical practice because opiates provide long-acting analgesia while avoiding many negative side effects, such as the central depressant effects associated with parenteral pain control. This form of analgesia allows increased mobility and improved respiratory dynamics, theoretically preventing further postoperative complications (Leib & Hurtig, 1985). The epidural route is ideally suited for high-risk patients predisposed to pulmonary complications because of preexisting medical conditions (e.g., chronic obstructive pulmonary disease and obesity) (Bragg, 1989). Epidural therapy has been used to treat pain resulting from thoracotomy, upper abdominal surgery, major vascular surgery, orthopedic surgery, and open heart surgery (Shafer & Donnelly, 1991). Earlier ambulation, improved pulmonary function and reduced pulmonary complications, and shorter ICU stays have been attributed to epidural administration. Yeager and colleagues (1987) studied the effect of epidural anesthesia and postoperative analgesia on postoperative morbidity in high-risk surgery patients. Compared to the control group, patients receiving epidural anesthesia and analgesia had fewer respiratory, cardiovascular, and major infectious complications. Urinary cortisol excretion, a marker of the stress response, was also significantly diminished in this group. Finally, hospital costs were significantly reduced for these patients due to decreased postoperative morbidity.

Depending on hospital policy, nurses may administer epidural narcotics or monitor patients receiving epidural narcotics. The critical care nurses need to be knowledgeable about epidural physiology, use of epidural narcotics, and implications for nursing care.

The epidural space, a potential space between the spinal dura mater and the vertebral canal, contains loose connective tissue, fat, and a plexus of veins and functions to cushion the spinal cord (Stewart, 1986) (Fig. 65–9). Discovery of endogenous narcotic-like peptides, the endorphins and enkephalins, and opiate

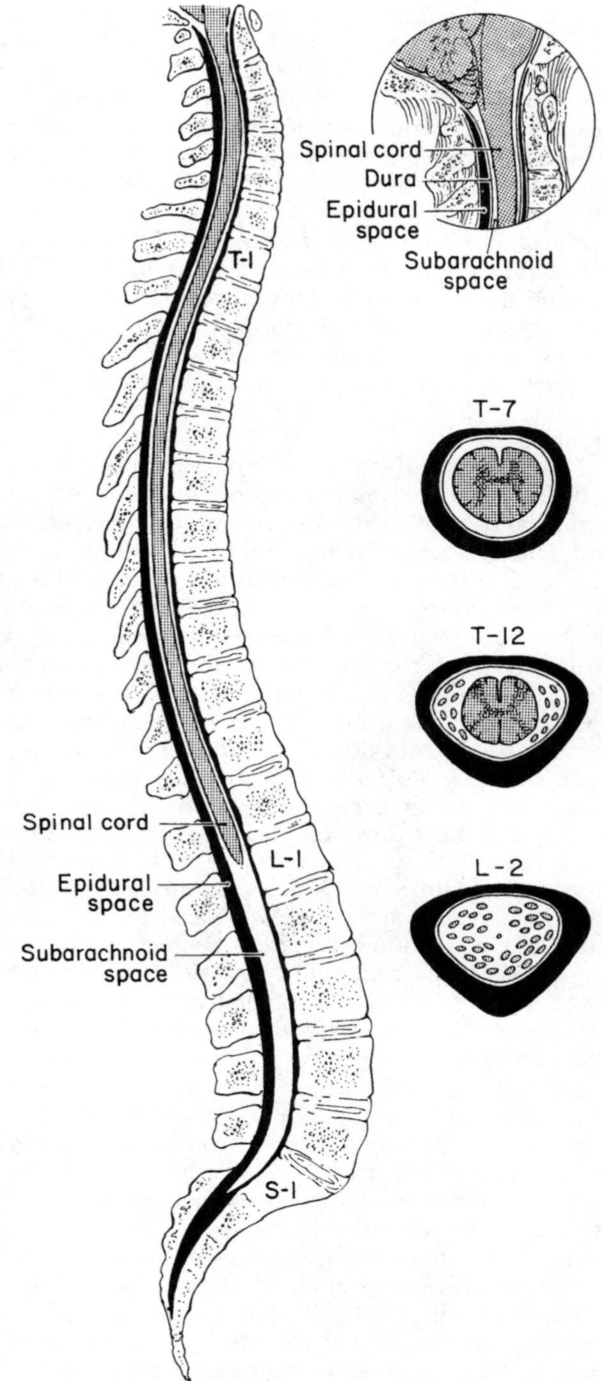

FIGURE 65–9. Epidural space. *Left,* Sagittal section of spinal column. *Inset,* Enlarged view of upper cervical region showing that the epidural space does not extend beyond the foramen magnum where the dura attaches to the entire circumference of the foramen. *Right,* Cross-sectional view of various levels of vertebral column. Note the difference in shape of the epidural space in the midthoracic and midlumbar region. (From Bonica, J. J. [1967]. *Principles and practice of obstetric analgesia and anesthesia* [p. 622]. Philadelphia: F. A. Davis.)

receptors in the dorsal horn region of the spinal cord has improved our understanding of pain and epidural narcotic function (Leib & Hurtig, 1985; Parish & Thompson, 1987). Endorphins and enkephalins, released from interneurons, act like neurotransmitters by binding with opiate receptors on the surface of neurons at the neuronal synapses. Administration of narcotics presumably mimics the action of endogenous peptides. Epidural analgesia occurs when opioids, such as morphine, are placed in the epidural space, enabling the drug to cross the dural–arachnoid layer passively and diffuse into the spinal fluid and then into the dorsal horn of the spinal cord to bind the opiate receptors located strategically along pain pathways (Nordberg, 1984; Parish & Thompson, 1987; Wild & Coyne, 1992).

The analgesic effect of epidural narcotics depends on diffusion to the opiate receptors in the dorsal root horn. The rate of diffusion appears to be related to lipid solubility, molecular weight and volume of the drug, and specific receptor affinities (Leib & Hurtig, 1985). For example, 2 to 10 mg of epidural morphine, which is more water soluble than lipid soluble, slowly diffuses through the lipid neural sheath and exhibits a long latency period. This, combined with strong receptor affinity, contributes to its high analgesic potency and long duration of action. Fentanyl, in contrast, is highly lipid soluble, diffuses rapidly, and immediately binds receptors. Therefore, it has a rapid onset and a short duration of action (Leib & Hurtig, 1985). Although several narcotics have been used, morphine sulfate remains the standard by which all epidural narcotics are measured. Meperidine, methadone, and beta-endorphin are all effective epidural analgesics. Drugs containing stabilizing agents, preservatives, and trioxidants or neurolytic agents such as phenol or alcohol are not recommended because of their potential for neurotoxicity.

Smaller dose requirements of epidural morphine compared to those needed for systemic administration have been frequently reported (Martin et al., 1982; Nordberg, 1984). Onset of analgesia, however, has been reported to be slower than that observed with intramuscular morphine, with adequate analgesia frequently not obtained until 45 to 60 minutes after administration (Bromage et al., 1980; Nordberg, 1984).

The epidural catheter is placed by a trained anesthesiologist or anesthetist, the site of insertion usually being at the level closest to the segments innervated by the pain focus (Bromage et al., 1980; Leib & Hurtig, 1985; Nordberg, 1984) (see Fig. 65–3). Usually, the catheter is left in place for 48 hours. However, the time may vary depending on patient needs and agency policy (Stewart, 1986). Complications associated with epidural narcotics are attributable either to the technique of administration or to drug action and side effects (Leib & Hurtig, 1985). Side effects associated with epidural narcotics are well documented in the literature and include urine retention, nausea, vomiting, pruritus, and respiratory depression. Although the overall incidence is low, respiratory depression is the most untoward complication associated with spinal narcotics because it has been reported to occur many hours after administration of spinal opiates and to outlast a single reversing dose of naloxone (Nordberg, 1984). The pruritus caused by morphine is thought to be due to direct histamine release from tissue mast cells. Treatment for pruritus includes comfort measures—cold packs, lotions, and drugs. Diphenhydramine (Benadryl) 25 mg IV or po may be given every six hours to release symptoms. Sensations of both itching and pain are transmitted to the dorsal horns of the spinal cord and are probably integrated at a common site at each spinal segment (Summerfield, 1980). Therefore, a second theory suggests that, given the close link between pain and itching, the itching produced by morphine might also result from its binding to opiate receptors. It is believed that by blocking the encephalon and endorphin opiate receptors in the CNS, naloxone, an opiate antagonist, can relieve the itching associated with epidural morphine (Bernstein & Swift, 1979). Reports suggest that the side effects induced by epidural narcotics may be reversed with small doses of naloxone without reversing the analgesic effect (Leib & Hurtig, 1985). The incidence, duration, and rationale for the occurrence of these adverse effects remain controversial because many studies have revealed conflicting results. Contraindications to the use of epidural anesthesia include severe systemic infection, a major coagulation defect, and uncorrected hypovolemia (Shafer & Donnelly, 1991).

INTRATHECAL NARCOTICS. Intrathecal narcotics are similar to epidural narcotics and are administered through a catheter placed in a selected area of the spinal cord. Respiratory depression and coma can be produced by rostral spread of the narcotic into the brain. Respiratory depression is usually delayed and can occur up to 12 hours after the dose. Morphine, meperidine, fentanyl, methadone, and beta-endorphins are also used effectively through the intrathecal routes. For acute pain, the dose of morphine varies from 0.2 to 2 mg/hour.

INHALATION ANALGESIA. Inhalation analgesia is achieved through the use of nitrous oxide, other inhalant-type anesthetics, and oxygen. Mixtures of nitrous oxide and oxygen are effective for management of minor and severe acute pain. A commercially prepared mixture of 50% nitrous oxide and 50% oxygen has been used successfully for performing dressing changes in burn patients.

Nonpharmacologic Management of Pain

Nonpharmacologic management of pain can be initiated independently by the critical care nurse. Numerous studies are available in the literature supporting the efficacy of techniques such as relaxation in reducing or even controlling pain. These techniques have been reported to work independently or in combination with analgesic agents. A major advantage of the use of nonpharmacologic management is patient safety and reduction of the possible side effects of body response to a given chemical. Some of the independent actions that can be initiated by the nurse require no additional instruction or training; however, to use the skills and instruments associated with relaxation techniques reliably, some degree of assistance or training is usually necessary to enhance outcomes.

TRANSCUTANEOUS ELECTRICAL NERVE STIMULATION (TENS). The use of electrical stimulation for analgesia and prevention of atrophy dates back to the 1800s; however, wide acceptance of the principle did not occur until the 1960s, when the gate control theory of pain was introduced. Clinical use of knowledge about dorsal column stimulation to decrease pain by Melzack and Wall (1965) led to the application of electrical stimulation to almost all parts of the body. Thus, the intent of peripheral nerve stimulation is to use large myelinated primary afferent nerve fibers (A fibers) to inhibit the transmission of activity in the small, unmyelinated primary afferent fibers (C fibers), inactivating local inhibitory circuits within the dorsal horn of the spinal cord and ultimately diminishing nociceptive transmission through the spinal cord (Wolff, 1985).

Research about the release of endogenous opiates from the appropriate neuronal tracts led to the discovery that electrical stimulation of neurons in specific areas of the CNS could elicit analgesia for several hours. These findings supported the premise that TENS units are effective because electrical nerve stimulation excites large mechanoreceptors in the periphery that subsequently stimulate the activity of enkephalins in the dorsal horn of the spinal cord, resulting in analgesia. This hypothesis is supported by findings reporting the ability of naloxone to reverse the effects of both acupuncture and TENS (Mayer et al., 1977).

Four electrical stimulation techniques can be employed to produce analgesia, including TENS, using surface electrodes applied to the skin; peripheral nerve stimulation through subcutaneously implanted electrodes; peripheral nerve stimulation using electrodes implanted directly on the nerve; and antidromic activation of primary afferent collaterals by the stimulation of the dorsal columns either directly or through the dura (Wolff, 1985).

The pulse generator used for electrical stimulation is a simple device and should be familiar to nurses. Trial and error determines the sites used for the electrodes as well as the frequency used for stimulation. Stimulation should be adjusted to a strength that causes pain and then lowered until the patient's comfort level is obtained. Differences in the frequency used are influenced by individual variations as well as the origins of the pain. The usual frequency used is 50 to 100 pulsations per second. Electrodes should be tried at one site for 12 to 24 hours for a fair evaluation of a decrease in pain. Low-frequency stimulation or trains of stimulation have been associated with modification of acute pain.

For treatment of pain related to surgical incisions, electrodes are commonly placed 1 to 2 inches from the wound. Postoperative electrical stimulation appears to reduce the incidence of complications after abdominal procedures, to stimulate gastrointestinal tract function after surgery, and to reduce the amount of time spent by the patient in intensive care. Atelectasis is almost entirely eliminated, and the incidence of ileus is markedly reduced.

Complications or adverse effects of TENS may include skin irritation from the adhesives used to secure the electrodes or, rarely, from the electrodes themselves. Neovascularization has occurred in some individuals when the same site is used repeatedly for electrode placement. Vascularization promptly subsides when the positions are varied.

Acute pain can be successfully diminished by TENS in more than 60% of all patients. TENS has been reported to be moderately successful in male patients with sickle cell pain (Wang et al., 1988), dental operations (Hochman, 1988), and prostatectomy or penile prosthetic surgery (Merrill, 1989). TENS did not provide significant analgesic relief in patients with labor pains (Thomas et al., 1988), cholecystectomy (Reuss et al., 1988), acute postoperative pain (McCallum et al., 1988), and inguinal herniorrhaphy (Smedley et al., 1988).

Several issues emerge from the literature that merit consideration by critical care nurses. TENS therapy alone is not appropriate for acute pain management. It should be considered part of a larger pain management program in combination with the use of other modalities. Use of TENS in patients with chronic pain syndromes appears to be successful. Finally, several studies report that electrical stimulation improves circulation and may be beneficial in patients with ischemic pain (Jivegard et al., 1987; Omura, 1987).

ACUPUNCTURE AND ACUPRESSURE. Acupuncture, an ancient Chinese practice, through many beliefs and applications has become a common form of pain management in the Western world. The procedure involves inserting fine needles through specific points in the skin and twirling them for some time at a slow rate. The needles can be removed when relief is obtained or left in place for varying periods of time. Continued analgesia can be achieved by hooking the needles to a battery-driven stimulator to maintain the activity of the needle or needles. It is believed that acupuncture needles stimulate large afferent fibers that cause the release of endorphins and enkephalins. Ongoing research supports the belief that pain relief achieved by acupuncture is a result of CNS involvement and not simply a placebo effect (Mayer et al., 1977; Melzack, 1975). The use of TENS at auricular acupuncture points has provided a significant level of pain relief from induced pain (Noling et al., 1988). A variety of complaints have been treated by acupuncture, including menstrual irregularities, obesity, labor, and degenerative arthritis (Doody et al., 1991).

Acupressure is a technique whereby pressure instead of needle insertion is applied to the designated points on identified meridians of the body. Use of electrical stimulation, heat, and a variety of intense sensory techniques indicates that acupressure is not a magical procedure but only one of many ways of producing analgesia by an intense sensory input that might be labeled "hyperstimulation analgesia." These noninvasive techniques may be used by paramedical personnel after learning the appropriate points on the body. Clearly, the points can be easily learned and applied by the critical care nurse to assist in pain management.

RELAXATION TECHNIQUES. Various skills, techniques, and rituals have been developed over many centuries for individuals who wish to achieve some level of relaxation and are willing to learn and practice the routine until a specified goal is achieved. These techniques incorporate autogenic training to reach relaxation through the use of commonly known approaches such as progressive relaxation, imagery, meditation, hypnosis, biofeedback, Zen, and yoga. Autogenic training was developed in the 1920s in Germany by Johannes H. Schultz, who believed that voluntary and predictable control of the body could be attained by programming it to develop heavy and warm extremities, a warm abdomen, a calm and regular heartbeat, relaxed respiration, and a cool forehead. Actually, then, autogenic training is sensory biofeedback. Before that, Emil Coué, a French pharmacist, used a simple general approach composed of attunement through autosuggestion and repetition of the phrase, "Every day, in every way, I am getting better and better." Autogenic training has been helpful for many individuals. After this, Jacobsen (1978) introduced progressive relaxation. Many somatic conditions were improved through the routine use of relaxation. The benefits of relaxation techniques used by patients with acute and chronic conditions, including pain, are reflected in the literature (Benson et al., 1975; Lawlis et al., 1985; Snyder, 1984; Tan, 1982). Graffam and Johnson (1987) compared the use of imagery and progressive muscle relaxation by adult oncology patients and found both strategies equally effective in reducing pain and distress. Most patients, however, expressed a preference for using progressive muscle relaxation.

In 1959, Maharishi Mahesh Yogi introduced transcendental meditation (TM) to the western world. TM involves passive, dispassionate relaxation. This type of relaxation was more commonly used by cults, resulting in distaste for the technique by the general public.

Biofeedback, introduced in the early 1960s, gave the greatest boost to autogenic training. Like autogenics, biofeedback is based on the assumption that if patients can be taught to control an internal state, they can modify pain or any illness that is psychosomatic in nature. Biofeedback provides people with an opportunity to observe progress in their ability to manage body activities such as skin temperature, heartbeat, breathing, blood pressure, and, most important, pain. Patients learn to control their autonomic nervous system, which regulates the internal organs. The literature is filled with research and knowledge about the application, implementation, and benefits of biofeedback. Recent summaries and analyses of the literature, however, reflect the fact that the major current application of biofeedback is in patients with chronic pain (Kewman & Roberts, 1983; Roberts, 1987; Turner & Chapman, 1982). A study by Jacobs (1987) reflects an estimated medical cost offset of $7 million when biofeedback was used by adult men as a method of managing stress, pain, vocational rehabilitation, and coping skills.

Biofeedback training involves the use of a machine such as a heart monitor, blood pressure machine, electromyography (EMG) machine, or thermometer that can be observed and a teaching device such as audiotapes that can be used to teach a progressive or consistent program. There are various types of biofeedback training: brainwave or ALPHA training teaches the patient to control brainwave output; temperature biofeedback instruction teaches the patient to raise or lower the skin temperature of a portion of the body; EMG training teaches how to relax certain muscle groups; and finally, the patient can be taught how to control a particular function of the body such as heart rate, blood pressure, or breathing. Many other types of biofeedback training are now being developed or proposed for control of almost any physiologic activity. The training is done with an electronic machine that is calibrated to pick up extremely small physiologic, electrical, or chemical changes as they take place. These minute changes are converted to either visual or auditory signals that can be recognized by the patient, providing immediate feedback.

Repeated use of the relaxation approach and the biofeedback machine allows patients to control (self-regulate) the particular function of the body being monitored. Patients become aware of the subtle changes in their conscious feelings (subjective response) that occur when the biofeedback machine reflects the desirable physical change. Continued monitoring and awareness of subjective feelings will eventually cancel the need for a feedback machine.

In the critical care setting the devices or machines already attached to the patient provide feedback on patients' ability to control certain functions such as heart rate. However, it is the nurse's skill and knowledge that makes it possible to teach the biofeedback technique to patients who are critically ill and are currently in a location that differs from the quiet and solitude of their own home.

HYPNOSIS. Hypnosis, a trance-like altered state of consciousness, has been used in many different settings to manage acute and chronic pain and stress. A trance state may include a temporary suspension of critical judgment, a capacity for congruent ideas, and rapid assimilation of internal or external data (Spiegel & Spiegel, 1978). Like other nonnarcotic methods of pain management, hypnosis is the target of myths and misconceptions by both patients and nurses. The major misconception is that hypnosis is caused by a force or person outside the patient. Hypnotic states can occur spontaneously through self-induction without the formal ceremony of induction (Crasilneck & Hall, 1975) and with minimal intervention from the nursing or medical staff. Hypnotic states may occur spontaneously in patients who focus on a symptom or on pain. Many critically ill or traumatized patients are already in a trance-like state, which can be enhanced by support and direction from the nurse. This trance-like state may explain the positive response to pain management in patients who have been severely traumatized, such as burn patients (Schafer, 1975). Clinical studies also support the premise that patients can direct their attention after injury or acute illness (Edmonston, 1981; Wain & Amer, 1986; Zahourek, 1982a, 1982b). One important observation is that the trance state is not altered by the injection of naloxone. This fact is believed to indicate that hypnosis reflects a higher level of consciousness that may not be mediated through endogenous opiates. It appears that spontaneous hypnosis-like states may be an outstanding adjunctive procedure of great use for the critical care nurse.

Additional Techniques for Managing Pain

Other approaches may be implemented to manage or decrease pain perception, including music and other forms of distraction, cognitive dissonance, body massage, and ice application. Music has been especially beneficial due to its calming benefits.

ETHICAL ISSUES IN PAIN MANAGEMENT

Ethics may be defined as a body of principles relating to right or good conduct. Ethical principles relating to nurses' assessment and management of pain and suffering have not been clearly delineated. Lisson (1987) identified the balancing of therapeutic relief with toxic side effects as an ethical dilemma that is complicated by the failure of nurses to recognize pain control as a crucial ethical issue. In addition, the presence of certain myths, attitudes, and behaviors in clinical practice results in restrictive, insensitive, and inappropriate rationing of pain relief (Copp, 1985).

The nurse's role is usually described as the provision of care, comfort, compassion, and protection for patients and their families. A compassionate, caring, and comforting approach to the pain and suffering experienced by patients who are critically ill should clearly be a high-priority goal for the critical care nurse. In addition, the mental and emotional suffering of the family and significant others must be addressed. Factors that may prevent attainment of this goal are numerous; only a few are mentioned here. The necessary focus on technology in critical care settings can deemphasize the importance of simple comfort measures. One example is the elderly patient who is cold but is not given a blanket because it would make it more difficult to monitor the many lines and tubes attached to the patient. Assessment of coldness and intervention for this discomfort may be overlooked because life-saving or life-sustaining measures take precedence. Hospital environments, especially critical care settings, may amplify the suffering caused by anxiety, loneliness, fear, confusion, anger, and possibly despair. Families as well as patients are likely to experience these feelings. Simple comfort measures such as a calm and reassuring voice, touching the patient in a manner that recognizes the person's importance as a human being, and allowing the expression of feelings are often overlooked in a setting that requires complicated technology and frequent decision making. However, these caring and comforting measures may be the efforts best remembered gratefully by patients' families who have lost their loved ones despite the best efforts of the health care team.

In the process of delivering nursing care to critically ill patients, not only is much pain and suffering left unrecognized or untreated, but additional pain, discomfort, and suffering are necessary parts of many medical and nursing procedures. Critically ill patients are often unable to respond verbally; therefore, the nurse must be particularly vigilant in protecting these patients. The challenge for nurses is how to mitigate the pain, discomfort, and suffering as much as possible while providing the necessary high-tech care.

Jameton (1984) states that nurses, because of their close work with patients on a daily basis, may become "specialists in suffering." In critical care areas this special ability may take a back seat to technologic skills such as interpretation of data provided by the many monitoring devices. Jameton suggests that because caring skills are labor intensive and the results are less tangible than technologically oriented work, the tendency may be to provide more rewards and respect to those with more technologically oriented skills.

Critical care nursing is particularly challenging because it requires the nurse to be highly competent in the knowledge and skills associated with sophisticated life-sustaining equipment, yet also to provide as much comfort as possible. The ethical issues involved in critical care pain management remain to be fully addressed. Nurses in intensive care should examine their care protocols to determine the best way to provide a consistent humanistic and research-based approach to assessing and managing pain and suffering of critically ill patients.

REFERENCES

Acute Pain Management Guideline Panel (1992). *Acute pain management: Operative or medical procedures and trauma. Clinical Practice Guideline.* AHCPR Pub. No. 92-0032. Rockville, MD: U.S. Department of Health and Human Services.

Akil, H., Mayer, D., & Liebeskind, J. (1976). Antagonism of stimulation produced analgesia by naloxone, a narcotic antagonist. *Science, 191,* 961–962.

Amnad, R. E., Perry, S., & Genovese, V. (1982). *Nonprocedural pain as perceived by burn patient and nurse.* Reported at American Burn Association, 14th Annual Meeting, Boston.

Asterita, M. F. (1985). *The physiology of stress.* New York: Human Sciences Press.

Atwell, J. R., Flanigan, R. C., Bennett, R. L., et al. (1984). The efficacy of patient-controlled analgesia in patients recovering from flank incisions. *Journal of Urology, 132,* 701–703.

Baer, E., Davitz, L. J., & Lieb, R. (1983). Inferences of physical pain and psychological distress: 1. In relation to verbal and nonverbal patient communication. *Nursing Research, 79,* 32–35.

Barkas, G., & Duafala, M. E. (1988). Advances in cancer pain management: A review of patient-controlled analgesia. *Journal of Pain and Symptom Management, 3,* 150–160.

Bates, M. S. (1987). Ethnicity and pain: A biocultural model. *Social Science and Medicine, 24*(1), 47–50.

Beare, J., & Myers, P. (1990). *Principles and practice of adult health nursing* (p. 256). St. Louis: C. V. Mosby.

Beecher, H. K. (1959). *Measurement of subjective responses.* New York: Oxford University Press.

Beecher, H. K. (1972). The placebo effect as a nonspecific force surrounding disease and the treatment of disease. In R. Jongen, W. D. Keidel, A. Herz, et al. (Eds.), *Pain: Basic principles, pharmacology and therapy.* Stuttgart: Thieme.

Bennett, R. L., & Griffen, W. O. (1983). Patient controlled analgesia. *Contemporary Surgery, 22,* 75–79.

Benson, H., Greenwood, A. B., & Klemchuk, A. B. (1975). The relaxation response: Psychophysiologic aspects and clinical applications. *International Journal of Psychiatry in Medicine, 6,* 87–98.

Bloom, F. E., Rossier, J., Battenberg, E. L. F., et al. (1978). B-endorphin: Cellular localization, electrophysiological and behavioral effects. In E. Costa & M. Trabucchi (Eds.), *The endorphins: Advances in biochemical psychopharmacology* (pp. 18, 89). New York: Raven Press.

Bonica, J. J. (1987). Importance of effective pain control. *Acta Anaesthesiologica Scandinavica Suppl, 85,* 1–16.

Bragg, C. C. (1989). Practical aspects of epidural and intrathecal narcotic analgesia in the critical care setting. *Heart and Lung, 18,* 599–608.

Bromage, P. R., Camporesi, E., & Chestnut, D. (1980). Epidural narcotics for postoperative analgesia. *Anesthesia and Analgesia, 59,* 473–480.

Carr, D. B., Bullen, B. A., Skrinar, G. S., et al. (1981). Physical conditioning facilitates the exercise-induced secretion of beta-endorphins and beta-lipotropin in women. *New England Journal of Medicine, 305,* 560–563.

Chapman, R. C. (1988). Pain related to cancer treatment. *Journal of Pain and Symptom Management, 3*(4), 188–193.

Christensen, B. N., & Perl, E. R. (1970). Spinal neurons specifically excited by noxious or thermal stimuli: Marginal zone of the dorsal horn. *Journal of Neurophysiology, 33,* 293–307.

Christoph, S. (1991). Pain assessment: The problem of pain in the critically ill patient. *Critical Care Nursing Clinics of North America, 3,* 11–16.

Cohen, F. L. (1980). Postsurgical pain relief: Patients' status and nurses' medication choices. *Pain, 9,* 265–274.

Cohen, J. L. (1986). Pharmacokinetic changes in aging. *American Journal of Medicine, 80*(Suppl), 31–38.

Copp, L. A. (1985). *Recent advances in nursing: Perspectives on pain.* New York: Churchill-Livingstone.

Cousins, M. J., & Phillips, G. D. (1986). *Acute pain management.* New York: Churchill-Livingstone.

Craig, K. D. (1984). Emotional aspects of pain. In P. D. Wall & R. Melzack (Eds.), *Textbook of pain.* New York: Churchill-Livingstone.

Crasilneck, H. B., & Hall, J. A. (1975). *Clinical hypnosis.* New York: Grune & Stratton.

Davitz, L. J., Sameshina, Y., & Davitz, J. (1976). Suffering as viewed in six different cultures. *American Journal of Nursing, 76,* 1296–1297.

DiGregorio, G. J., Barbieri, E. J., Sterling, G. H., et al. (1986). *Handbook of pain management.* West Chester, PA: Medical Surveillance.

Dimsdale, J. E., & Moss, J. (1980). Plasma catecholamines in stress and exercise. *Journal of the American Medical Association, 243,* 340–342.

Donnelly, A., & Lamb, R. (1993). Analgesic agents in critical care. *Nursing Clinics of North America, 5,* 281–295.

Donovan, B. D. (1983). Patient attitudes to postoperative pain relief. *Anesthesia Intensive Care, 11,* 125–129.

Doody, S., Smith, C., Webb, J. (1991). Non-pharmacologic interventions for pain management. *Critical Care Nursing Clinics of North America, 3,* 69–75.

Edmonston, W. E. (1981). *Hypnosis and relaxation.* New York: J. Wiley & Sons.

Edwards, P. W., Zeichner, A., Kuczmierczyk, A. R., et al. (1985). Familial pain models: The relationship between family history of pain and current pain experience. *Pain, 21,* 379–384.

Eisenach, J. C., Grice, S. C., & Dewan, D. M. (1988). Patient-controlled analgesia following cesarean section: A comparison with epidural and intramuscular narcotics. *Anesthesiology, 68,* 444–448.

Fields, H. L., & Basbaum, A. L. (1984). Endogenous pain control mechanisms. In P. D. Wall & R. Melzack (Eds.), *Textbook of pain.* New York: Churchill-Livingstone.

Fordyce, W. E. (1978). Learning processes in pain. In P. A. Sternbach (Ed.), *The psychology of pain* (p. 200). New York: Raven Press.

Frankenhaeuser, M., Dunne, E., & Lundberg, U. (1976). Sex differences in sympathetic-adrenal medullary reactions induced by different stressors. *Psycho-pharmacology, 47,* 1–5.

Furuhashi, N., Takahashi, T., Kono, H., et al. (1984). Sex difference in human peripheral plasma beta-endorphin and beta-lipotropin levels. *Gynecological and Obstetrical Investigation, 17,* 145–148.

Gaston-Johansson, F. (1984). Pain assessment: Intensity and quality of the words pain, ache and hurt. *Pain, 20,* 69–76.

Gaston-Johansson, F., & Asklund-Gustafsson, M. (1985). A baseline study for the development of an instrument for the assessment of pain. *Journal of Advanced Nursing, 10,* 539–546.

Gaston-Johansson, F., & Fagan, A. (1990). Similarities in pain descriptions of four different ethnic groups. *Journal of Pain and Symptom Management, 5,* 94–100.

Good, B. J., & Good, M. D. (1980). The meaning of symptoms: A cultural hermeneutic model for clinical practice. In L. Eisenberg & A. Kleinman (Eds.), *Relevance of social science for medicine* (pp. 165–196). Dordrecht: Reidel.

Goosen, G. M., & Bush, H. (1979). Adaptation: A feedback process. *Advances in Nursing Science, 1*(4), 51–66.

Gracely, R. H., & Dubner, R. (1981). Pain assessment in human—a reply to Hall. *Pain, 11,* 109–120.

Graffam, S., & Johnson, A. (1987). A comparison of two relaxation strategies for the relief of pain and its distress. *Journal of Pain and Symptom Management, 2,* 229–231.

Greenblat, D. J., Sellers, E. M., & Shader, R. I. (1982). Drug disposition in old age. *New England Journal of Medicine, 306,* 1081–1088.

Grunau, K. D., & Craig, R. V. (1987). Pain expression in neonates, facial action and cry. *Pain, 28,* 395–410.

Guyton, A. (1991). *Textbook of medical physiology* (8th ed.). Philadelphia: W. B. Saunders.

Haber, R. N., & Hershenson, N. (1980). *The psychology of visual perception* (2nd ed.). New York: Holt, Rinehart, and Winston.

Hall, K. R., & Strider, E. (1954). The varying response to pain in psychiatric disorders: A study in abnormal psychology. *British Journal of Medical Psychology, 27,* 48.

Hardy, J. D., Wolff, H. G., & Goodell, H. (1952). *Pain sensations and reactions.* Baltimore: Williams & Wilkins.

Hochman, R. (1988). Neurotransmitter modulator (TENS) for control of dental operative pain. *Journal of the American Dental Association, 116,* 208–212.

Hokfelt, T., Johansson, O., Jungdahl, A., et al. (1980). Peptidergic neurones. *Nature, 284,* 515–521.

Hongo, T., Jankowska, E., & Lundberg, A. (1968). Post-synaptic excitation and inhibition from primary afferents in neurones of the spinocervical tract. *Journal of Physiology, 199,* 569–592.

Huhman, M. (1982). Endogenous opiates and pain. *Advances in Nursing Science, 4*(4), 62–71.

Hurley, M. E. (Ed.). (1986). *Classification of nursing diagnosis: Proceedings of the sixth national conference.* St. Louis: C. V. Mosby.

Huskisson, E. C. (1974). Treatment of rheumatoid arthritis with fenoprofen: Comparison with aspirin. *British Medical Journal, 1,* 176–180.

Jacobs, D. F. (1987). Cost-effectiveness of specialized psychological programs for reducing hospital stays and outpatient visits. *Journal of Clinical Psychology, 43,* 729–735.

Jacobsen, E. (1978). *You must relax.* New York: McGraw-Hill.

Jacox, A. K. (1977). *Pain: A source book for nurses and other health professionals.* Boston: Little, Brown.

Jacox, A. K. (1979). Assessing pain. *American Journal of Nursing, 79,* 895–900.

Jacquet, Y. F. (1979). β-Endorphin and ACTH—Opiate peptides with coordinated roles in the regulation of behaviour? *Trends in Neurosciences, 2,* 140–143.

Jaffe, J. H., & Martin, W. R. (1980). Opioid analgesics and antagonists. In A. G. Gilman, L. S. Goodman, & A. Gilman (Eds.), *The pharmacological basis of therapeutics* (6th ed., p. 494). New York: Macmillan.

Jameton, A. (1984). *Nursing practice: The ethical issues.* Englewood Cliffs, NJ: Prentice-Hall.

Janis, I. L. (1958). *Psychological stress.* New York: Wiley.

Jaros, J. (1991). The concept of pain. *Critical Care Nursing Clinics of North America, 3,* 1–10.

Jensen, T. S., & Rasmussen, P. (1984). Amputation. In P. D. Wall & R. Melzack (Eds.), *Textbook of pain* (pp. 402–412). New York: Churchill-Livingstone.

Jivegard, L., Augustinsson, L. E., Carlsson, C. A., et al. (1987). Long-term results by epidural spinal electrical stimulation (ESES) in patients with inoperable severe lower limb ischaemia. *European Journal of Vascular Surgery, 1,* 345–349.

Johansson, G. (1972). Sex differences in the catecholamine output of children. *Acta Physiologica Scandinavica, 85,* 569–572.

Johansson, G., & Post, B. (1974). Catecholamine output of males and females over a one-year period. *Acta Physiologica Scandinavica, 92,* 557–565.

Jones, J., Hoggart, B., & Withey, J. (1979). What the patients say: A study of reactions to an intensive care unit. *Intensive Care Medicine, 5,* 89–94.

Katz, J., & Melzack, R. (1990). Pain "memories" in phantom limbs: Review and clinical observations. *Pain, 43,* 319–336.

Ketovui, H. (1987). Nurses' and patients' conception of wound pain and the administration of analgesics. *Journal of Pain and Symptom Management, 2,* 213.

Kewman, D. G., & Roberts, A. H. (1983). An alternative perspective on biofeedback efficacy studies: A reply to Stiener and Dince. *Biofeedback and Self-Regulation, 8,* 487–503.

Koopman, S., Eisenthal, S., & Stoeckle, J. (1984). Ethnicity in the reported pain, emotional distress and requests of medical patients. *Social Science and Medicine, 18,* 487–490.

Lawlis, G. G., Selby, D., Minnant, D., et al. (1985). Reduction of postoperative pain parameters by presurgical relaxation instructions for spinal pain patients. *Spine, 10,* 649–651.

Lazarus, R. (1977). Cognitive and coping process in emotion. In A. Monat & R. Lazarus (Eds.), *Stress and coping: An anthology.* New York: Columbia University Press.

Leib, R. A., & Hurtig, J. B. (1985). Epidural and intrathecal narcotics for pain management. *Heart and Lung, 14,* 164–174.

Liebeskind, J. (1977). Psychological mechanisms of pain. *Annual Review of Psychology, 28,* 41–60.

Lipton, J. A., & Marbach, J. J. (1984). Ethnicity and the pain experience. *Social Science and Medicine, 19,* 1279–1298.

Lisson, E. L. (1987). Ethical issues related to pain control. *Nursing Clinics of North America, 22,* 649–659.

Livingston, W. K. (1943). *Pain mechanisms: A physiologic interpretation of causalgia and its related states.* New York: Macmillan.

Lubenow, T. R., & Ikankovich, A. D. (1991). Patient controlled analgesia for postoperative pain. *Critical Care Nursing Clinics of North America, 3,* 35–41.

Lynn, B. (1984). The detection of injury and tissue damage. In P. D. Wall & R. Melzack (Eds.), *Textbook of pain* (pp. 19–31). New York: Churchill-Livingstone.

Martin, R., Salbaing, J., & Blaise, G. (1982). Epidural morphine for postoperative pain relief: A dose–response curve. *Anesthesiology, 56,* 423–426.

Mather, L. E., & Cousins, M. J. (1986). Local anesthetics: Principles of use. In M. J. Cousins & G. D. Phillips (Eds.), *Acute pain management.* New York: Churchill-Livingstone.

Mather, L. E., & Mackie, J. (1983). The incidence of postoperative pain in children. *Pain, 15,* 271.

Mather, L. E., & Phillips, G. D. (1986). Opioids and adjuvants: Principles of use. In M. J. Cousins & G. D. Phillips (Eds.), *Acute pain management* (pp. 77–101). New York: Churchill-Livingstone.

Mayer, D. J., Price, D. D., & Rafii, A. (1977). Antagonism of acupuncture analgesia in man by the narcotic antagonist naloxone. *Brain Research, 121,* 368–372.

McCaffery, M. (1979). *Nursing management of the patient with pain* (2nd ed.). Philadelphia: J. B. Lippincott.

McCallum, M. I., Glynn, C. J., Moore, R. A., et al. (1988). Transcutaneous electrical nerve stimulation in the management of acute postoperative pain. *British Journal of Anaesthesia, 61,* 308–312.

Meinhart, N. T., and McCaffery, M. (1983). *Pain: A nursing approach to assessment and analysis.* Norwalk, CT: Appleton-Century-Crofts.

Melzack, R. (1975). The McGill pain questionnaire: Major properties and scoring methods. *Pain, 1,* 277–299.

Melzack, R. (1973). *The puzzle of pain.* New York: Basic Books.

Melzack, R., & Dennis, S. G. (1978). Neurophysiological foundations of pain. In R. A. Steinbach (Ed.), *The psychology of pain.* New York: Raven Press.

Melzack, R., & Wall, P. D. (1970). Evolution of pain theories. *International Anesthesiology Clinics, 8,* 3–34.

Melzack, R., & Wall, P. D. (1965). Pain mechanisms: A new theory. *Science, 150,* 971–973.

Merrill, D. C. (1989). Clinical evaluation of fasTENS, an inexpensive, disposable transcutaneous electrical nerve stimulator designed specifically for postoperative electroanalgesia. *Urology, 33,* 27–30.

Mersky, H. (1975). Pain, learning and memory. *Journal of Psychosomatic Research, 19,* 319–324.

Mersky, H. (1979). IASP Subcommittee on Taxonomy: Pain terms: A list with definitions and notes on usage. *Pain, 6,* 249.

Muir, B. L. (1988). *Pathophysiology: An introduction to the mechanisms of disease.* New York: John Wiley & Sons.

Nafe, J. P. (1934). The pressure, pain and temperature senses. In C. Murchison (Ed.), *Handbook of general experimental psychology.* Worcester: Clark University Press.

Neal, J. M., & Owens, B. D. (1992). Hazards of antagonizing narcotic sedation with naloxone. *Annals of Emergency Medicine, 22,* 145–146.

National Institutes of Health Consensus Development Conference. (1987). The integrated approach to the management of pain. *Journal of Pain and Symptom Management, 2,* 35–44.

Nield, M., Kim, M. J., & Patel, M. (1989). Use of magnitude estimation for estimating the parameters of dyspnea. *Nursing Research, 38*(2), 77–80.

Noling, L. B., Clelland, M. A., Jackson, J. R., et al. (1988). Effect of transcutaneous electrical nerve stimulation at auricular points on experimental cutaneous pain threshold. *Physiological Therapeutics, 68,* 328–332.

Noordenbos, W. (1959). *Pain.* Amsterdam: Elsevier.

Nordberg, G. (1984). Pharmacokinetic aspects of spinal morphine analgesia. *Acta Anaesthesiologica Scandinavica, 28,* 7–38.

Omura, Y. (1987). Basic electrical parameters for safe and effective electro-therapeutics [electro-acupuncture, TES, TENMS (or TEMS), TENS and electro-magnetic field stimulation with or without drug field] for pain, neuromuscular skeletal problems, and circulatory disturbances. *Acupuncture Electrotherapy Research, 12*(1), 53–70.

Parbrook, G. D., Steel, D. F., & Dalrymple, D. G. (1973). Factors predisposing to postoperative pain and pulmonary complications. A study of male patients undergoing elective gastric surgery. *British Journal of Anaesthesia, 45,* 21–33.

Parish, K., & Thompson, G. (1987). Epidural "port-a-cath": An analgesic find. *Australian Nurses Journal, 17*(3), 44–47.

Phillips, G. D., & Cousins, M. J. (1986). Neurological mechanisms of pain and the relationship of pain, anxiety and sleep. In M. J. Cousins & G. D. Phillips (Eds.), *Acute pain management* (pp. 32–35). New York: Churchill-Livingstone.

Plante, T. G., & Denvey, D. R. (1984). Stress responsivity among dysmenorrheic women at different phases of their menstrual cycle:

More ado about nothing. *Behavior Research and Therapy, 22,* 2491–2580.

Polefrone, J. M., & Manuck, S. B. (1987). Gender differences in cardiovascular and neuroendocrine response to stressors. In R. C. Barnett, L. Biener, & G. K. Baruch (Eds.), *Gender and stress* (pp. 45–55). New York: Free Press.

Porth, C. M. (1986). *Pathophysiology: Concepts of altered health states.* Philadelphia: J. B. Lippincott.

Procacci, P., & Zoppi, M. (1984). Heart pain. In P. D. Wall & R. Melzack (Eds.), *Textbook of pain.* New York: Churchill-Livingstone.

Puntillo, K. (1990). Pain experience of intensive care unit patients. *Heart and Lung, 19,* 526–530.

Reading, A. E. (1984). The McGill pain questionnaire: An appraisal. In R. Melzack (Ed.), *Pain measurement and assessment* (pp. 55–61). New York: Raven Press.

Reuss, R., Cronen, P., & Abplanalp, L. (1988). Transcutaneous electrical nerve stimulation for pain control after cholecystectomy: Lack of expected benefits. *Southern Medical Journal, 81,* 1361–1363.

Roberts, A. H. (1987). Literature update: Biofeedback and chronic pain. *Journal of pain and symptom management, 3,* 169–171.

Savedra, M., Gibbons, P., Tesler, M., et al. (1982). How do children describe pain? A tentative assessment. *Pain, 14,* 95–104.

Schafer, D. W. (1975). Hypnosis use on a burn unit. *International Journal of Clinical and Experimental Hypnosis, 23*(1), 1–14.

Scott, L. E., Clum, G. A., & Peoples, J. B. (1983). Preoperative predictors of postoperative pain. *Pain, 15,* 283–286.

Shafer, A., & Donnelly, A. (1991). Management of postoperative pain by continuous epidural infusion of analgesics. *Clinical Pharmacology, 10,* 745–764.

Shapiro, M. B. (1975). The single-variable approach to assessing the intensity of the feeling of depression. *European Journal of Behavior Analysis and Modification, 1,* 62–75.

Sherrington, C. S. (1900). Cutaneous sensations. In E. A. Schafer (Ed.), *Textbook of physiology* (pp. 19–20). Edinburgh: Pentland.

Silverstein, F., Graham, D., Davies, H., Struthers, B. (1995). Misoprotol reduces serious gastrointestinal complications in patients with rheumatoid arthritis receiving non-steroidal anti-inflammatory drugs. *Annals of Internal Medicine, 123,* 241–249.

Smedley, F., Taube, M., & Wastell, C. (1988). Transcutaneous electrical nerve stimulation for pain relief following inguinal hernia repair: A controlled trial. *European Surgical Research, 20,* 233–237.

Smith, J. R., & Simon, E. J. (1981). Endorphins, opiate receptors, and their evolving biology. *Pathobiology Annual, 11,* 87–126.

Snyder, M. (1984). Progressive relaxation as a nursing intervention: An analysis. *Advances in Nursing Science, 2,* 47–53.

Spiegel, H., & Spiegel, D. (1978). *Trance and treatment: Clinical uses of hypnosis.* New York: Basic Books.

Stein, J. M., & Warfield, C. A. (1982). The pain clinics: Phantom limb pain. *Hospital Practice, 17,* 166–167.

Sternbach, R. A. (1974). *Pain patients: Traits and treatments.* New York: Academic Press.

Sternbach, R. A. (1986). *The psychology of pain.* (2nd ed.). New York: Raven Press.

Stewart, M. L. (1977). Measurement of clinical pain. In A. K. Jacox (Ed.), *Pain: A source book for nurses and other health professionals.* Boston: Little, Brown.

Stewart, S. M. (1986). Controlling pain with epidural narcotics: Nursing implications. *Critical Care Nurse, 6*(3), 50–56.

Summerfield, J. A. (1980). Naloxone modulates the perception of itch in man. *British Journal of Clinical Pharmacology, 10,* 180–183.

Tan, S. (1982). Cognitive and cognitive-behavioral methods for pain control: A selective review. *Pain, 12,* 201–208.

Tasker, R. R. (1984). Deafferentation. In P. D. Wall & R. Melzack (Eds.), *Textbook of pain* (pp. 119–132). New York: Churchill-Livingstone.

Terenius, L. (1978). Endogenous peptides and analgesia. *Annual Review of Pharmacologic Toxicology, 18,* 189–192.

Terenius, L. (1981). Endorphins and pain. *Frontiers of Hormone Research, 8,* 162–177.

Thomas, I. L., Tyle, V., Webster, J., et al. (1988). An evaluation of transcutaneous electrical nerve stimulation for pain relief in labour. *Australia and New Zealand Journal of Obstetrics and Gynecology, 28,* 182–189.

Thoren, L. (1974). General metabolic response to trauma including pain influence. *Acta Anaesthesiologica Scandinavica, 55*(Suppl), 9–14.

Titchener, E. B. (1909). *A textbook of physiology.* Philadelphia: Macmillan.

Traynor, C., & Hall, G. M. (1981). Endocrine and metabolic changes during surgery: Anaesthetic implications. *British Journal of Anaesthesia, 53,* 153–158.

Turner, J. A., & Chapman, C. R. (1982). Psychological interventions for chronic pain: A critical review. I. Relaxation training and biofeedback. *Pain, 12,* 1–21.

Tursky, B. (1976). The development of a pain perception profile: A psychophysical approach. In W. Weisenbert & B. Tursky (Eds.), *Pain: New perspectives in therapy and research.* New York: Plenum.

Tursky, B., Jamner, L. D., & Friedman, R. (1982). The pain perception profile: A psychophysical approach to the assessment of pain report. *Behavior Therapy, 13,* 376–394.

Twycross, R. G. (1984). Narcotics. In P. D. Wall & R. Melzack (Eds.), *Textbook of pain* (pp. 514–526). New York: Churchill-Livingstone.

Viswanathan, M., Van Dijk, J. P., Graham, R. E., et al. (1987). Exercise and cold-induced changes in plasma β-endorphin and β-lipotropin in men and women. *American Physiological Society, 27,* 622–626.

Wain, H. J., & Amer, D. G. (1986). Emergency room use of hypnosis. *General Hospital Psychiatry, 8,* 19–22.

Wang, W. C., George, S. L., & Williams, J. A. (1988). Transcutaneous electrical nerve stimulation treatment of sickle cell pain crises. *Acta Haematologica, 80,* 99–102.

Ward, M. M., Mefford, I. N., Parker, S. D., et al. (1983). Epinephrine and norepinephrine responses in continuously collected human plasma to a series of stressors. *Psychosomatic Medicine, 45,* 471–486.

Weinberg, A. D. (1988). The etiology, evaluation and treatment of head and facial pain in the elderly. *Journal of Pain and Symptom Management, 3,* 29–38.

Wild, L., & Coyne, C. (1992). The basics and beyond: Epidural anesthesia. *American Journal of Nursing, 92,* 26–34.

Willis, W. D. (1985). *The pain system.* New York: Karger.

Wolff, B. B. (1985). Ethnocultural factors influencing pain and illness behavior. *Clinical Journal of Pain, 1,* 23–30.

Woods, J. H., Young, A. M., & Herling, S. (1982). Classification of narcotics on the basis of their reinforcing, discriminative, and antagonist effects in rhesus monkeys. *Federation Proceedings, 41,* 221–227.

Yeager, M. P., Glass, D. D., Neff, R. K., et al. (1987). Epidural anesthesia and analgesia in high-risk surgical patients. *Anesthesiology, 66,* 729–736.

Zahourek, K. P. (1982a). Hypnosis in nursing practice—emphasis on the "problem patient" who has pain: Part I. *Journal of Psychosocial Nursing Mental Health Service, 20,* 21–24.

Zahourek, K. P. (1982b). Hypnosis in nursing practice—emphasis on the "problem patient" who has pain: Part II. *Journal of Psychosocial Nursing Mental Health Service, 20,* 21–24.

Zborowski, M. (1952). Cultural components in response to pain. *Journal of Social Issues, 8*(40), 16–24.

Zimmerman, M. (1984). Neurobiological concepts of pain, its assessment and therapy. In E. Bromm (Ed.), *Pain measurement in man* (pp. 15–35). Amsterdam: Elsevier Science Publications.

Zola, I. K. (1966). Culture and symptoms: An analysis of patients presenting complaints. *American Sociological Review, 31,* 615–630.

Chemical and Drug Overdose

Deanna Bevans

According to the Annual Report of the American Association of Poison Control Centers (Litovitz et al., 1993), an estimated 2.4 million human poison exposures were reported to all U.S. poison centers for the year 1992. Studies, however, have indicated that less than 30% of exposures are reported to poison centers (Harchelroad et al., 1990; Linakis & Frederick, 1993). Most of the reported exposures happened in the home (92.1%), with 59% of those exposures occurring in children younger than 6 years of age. Most of the reported cases were treated at the patient's home. Treatment in a health care facility was rendered or recommended in only 26.0% of cases, with 4.7% of the total reported cases requiring admission for medical care. Accidental poisoning accounted for 87.1% of the exposures (Litovitz et al., 1993). However, intentional drug overdose has become the most common method of attempted suicide. Up to 5% of all admissions to intensive care units of inner city hospitals are a direct result of overdoses (Stein et al., 1993). Treatment of the overdose patient requires a team approach, from obtaining histories and doing a physical examination, to supportive care. Changes, or expected changes, in a patient's status need to be communicated to all members of the health care team to provide optimal patient care. Some of the most common pharmacologic ingestions requiring treatment are discussed in this chapter.

INITIAL STABILIZATION

On the first encounter with the patient, it is necessary to accurately evaluate the patient's level of consciousness (LOC): awake, alert, unarousable, unresponsive. Patients who cannot be aroused have the potential for an obstructed airway and require intervention (Table 66–1). Assessment of LOC should be done at frequent intervals because the overdose patient's LOC can deteriorate rapidly, depending on the ingested agent.

Simultaneous evaluation of airway patency must also be done. Airway evaluation should include not only the usual indicators of gross airway compromise such as stridor or snoring respirations, but the quality of the gag reflex. Obtunded patients, or those having a weak or absent gag reflex, require assistance maintaining their airway. The jaw thrust maneuver may be all that is needed in some patients, whereas others require intubation. Nasotracheal intubation is preferred because it is better tolerated by the semiconscious patient, and it allows easier access for placement of the large-bore orogastric tube. Intubation also helps protect the airway from aspiration of gastric contents, a complication frequently noted in overdose patients.

TABLE 66–1. **Initial Assessment and Intervention in the Overdose Patient**

Airway	Maintain patency
Breathing	Adequate tidal volume Arterial blood gases
Circulation	Early IV access Cardiac monitor
Disability	Level of consciousness Pupil size, reactivity
Drugs	Oxygen Unconscious Patient Protocol Naloxone hydrochloride 2 mg IV Dextrose 50 g IV Thiamine 100 mg IV/IM

Abbreviations: IM, intramuscular; IV, intravenous.

In addition to noting patency of the airway, the ventilatory effort needs to be assessed. The rate as well as the tidal volume should be evaluated. Shallow respirations may indicate the need for early ventilatory support. Increased respirations suggest the presence of an underlying hypoxia or metabolic acidosis. Patients having seizures or hyperthermia may require higher oxygen concentrations to meet metabolic needs. Supplemental oxygen may be administered by nasal cannula, mask, or endotracheal tube, depending on the patient's condition. Pulse oximetry can be useful in trending the patient's oxygenation status. Arterial blood gases should be obtained early in the admission.

Cardiovascular evaluation should include a documented electrocardiogram (ECG) rhythm strip as soon as possible, as well as a blood pressure. These factors can give important diagnostic information. Rapid heart rates are noted in theophylline and amphetamine overdoses. Irregular heart rates may be noted with insecticides and tricyclic antidepressant (TCA) overdoses. Patients having taken toxic amounts of morphine, cyanide, digitalis, and beta blockers may present with slow heart rates. Severe hypertension may be present in overdoses involving cocaine, amphetamines and other sympathomimetic drugs.

Frequent vital signs should include temperature trending. An increase in temperature can occur with salicylates, cocaine, and drugs that have anticholinergic properties. A decreased temperature may be noted with opiates and barbiturates.

Intravenous (IV) access should be established early with at least one large-bore catheter. Hypotensive patients may require immediate fluid resuscitation. Following the Unconscious Patient Protocol (see Table 66–1), naloxone hydrochloride (Narcan; DuPont, Wilmington, DE), glucose, and thiamine should be considered for patients with depressed LOC. The IV dose of naloxone for an adult is 2 mg; up to 0.1 mg/kg should be given to children (Haddad & Roberts, 1990). This narcotic antagonist reverses the central nervous system (CNS) depression associated with overdoses of opiates. Increased doses and repeated doses may be required to maintain the response desired because the half-life of naloxone may be shorter than that of the toxic drug. Unresponsive patients should also have their blood glucose evaluated using a glucose monitor. If indicated, the patient should receive 50 g of IV dextrose. If there is any suspicion of alcoholism or severe thiamine depletion, the patient should receive 100 mg thiamine IV or intramuscularly (IM) before the IV dextrose to prevent an acute episode of Wernicke's encephalopathy.

DIAGNOSIS

While the patient is being stabilized, efforts must be made to obtain information about the type of ingestion, the quantity involved, and the time elapsed since ingestion. This information may be gained from the patient, family members, or others present at the site of ingestion. Information obtained, however, tends to vary in accuracy because of drug-induced confusion and deliberate attempts at deception. Misinformation may be received inadvertently from family members and emergency medical service (EMS) personnel. Information given to hospital personnel may be based on the pill containers at the scene. Some people, however, may place multiple drugs in one vial to decrease the amount of containers they carry with them. At the time of the overdose, only one or two containers may be present.

Because the history in the overdose patient is often unreliable, a thorough and accurate physical examination by the medical team becomes critical. Examination of the skin may reveal needle marks or abscesses from injected substances such as opiates or cocaine; dry, flushed skin may indicate use of anticholinergic agents. The physical examination must also include an ongoing assessment of LOC. Impairment of the CNS may be caused by the primary effects of the toxic agent or the secondary effects of electrolyte imbalance, pH alterations, or oxygen depletion. The patient should also be examined for evidence of trauma or other underlying illnesses that may account for the symptoms noted.

Laboratory tests may be helpful in determining the severity of the overdose. These tests may include urine, blood, and gastric contents for drug screen, as well as electrolytes, serum glucose, and arterial blood gases. Treatment, however, should not be delayed while awaiting test results.

DECONTAMINATION

There is no specific antidote for most of the common substances ingested. Treatment is therefore focused on maintaining vital functions, removing the toxic substance, and limiting its absorption. Several methods are available for limiting absorption.

Emesis

Ipecac syrup produces vomiting through stimulation of the chemoreceptor trigger zone (Haddad & Roberts, 1990). This over-the-counter emetic agent has been used to treat poison ingestions in the home, prehospital, and in the emergency department for many years. The benefits of ipecac-induced emesis have lately been called into question (Krenzelok & Dunmire, 1992; Lovejoy et al., 1992; Tandberg & Murphy, 1989). Although ipecac has been shown to be reliable in producing emesis, it removes only about 30% of the gastric contents. Also, the onset of emesis may be delayed for 20 to 30 minutes (Pruchnicki, 1991), with drug absorption continuing during this period. Although most patients vomit two to three times after being given ipecac, some patients continue to have emesis for 1 to 2 hours after administration (Harris & Kingston, 1992). This may prevent the use of other decontamination methods, including activated charcoal (AC). It also presents a problem in those patients whose level of consciousness diminishes after receiving ipecac. A number of EMS programs and emergency departments are, therefore, reevaluating the use of ipecac in their overdose protocol.

Ipecac may be useful in children who cannot accommodate the large-bore gastric tubes, or when pills ingested are too large to pass through the holes in the lavage tube. The best candidates for emesis are those who are awake, alert, cooperative, and have an intact gag reflex.

Induced emesis is contraindicated in patients who are comatose, have an absent gag reflex, or have high potential for seizures. Induced emesis is contraindicated in patients having ingested a caustic material such as an acid or alkali because these substances can cause damage on the way up, just as they did on the way down. Induced emesis should not be initiated when a hydrocarbon agent (e.g., kerosene, lighter fluid, furniture polish) has been ingested because of the high risk for aspiration (Hoffman, 1992). It is also contraindicated when too long a time has lapsed since ingestion. According to Bond and coworkers (1993), induced emesis is most effective when given early after ingestion; no demonstrable impact occurs if emesis is induced more than 90 minutes after ingestion. The effective time span is even shorter when liquid preparations are ingested. Ipecac should not be used when the ingestion is nontoxic (e.g., berries, marbles, or a nontoxic amount of a drug was taken).

The dose of syrup of ipecac for adults is 30 mL followed by several glasses of water. For children younger than the age of 12 years, the dose is decreased to 15 mL. Factors that affect the efficacy of ipecac include the type of toxin, how long since ingestion, and the presence or absence of food in the stomach.

Gastric Lavage

Gastric lavage is usually done in the emergency department. It may be done on a patient with a decreased LOC, providing the airway is protected. The patient should be placed on the left side with the head tilted down to prevent aspiration. A large-bore (32 to 40 Fr) tube is orally placed into the stomach. In children, the smallest tube used should be 22 to 24 Fr (Hoffman, 1992). After placement is confirmed, as much of the gastric contents as possible is then aspirated.

Water and normal saline have both been advocated as a lavage solution in the adult. Normal saline or 0.45 normal saline (10 mL/kg) should be used in young children to prevent water and electrolyte imbalance (Harris & Kingston, 1992; Henretig & Shannon, 1993). Instill 200 to 300 mL of solution, then allow solution to drain. Epigastric massage has been advocated to increase return of pill fragments. This procedure should continue until the lavage fluid is clear. An additional 1 to 2 liters of fluid should be instilled to maximize recovery (Harris & Kingston, 1992; Young & Bivins, 1993). Antidotes such as AC may be administered before the removal of the orogastric tube. Repeated assessment of the LOC and presence of the gag reflex are imperative in the patient with an unprotected airway.

Although the onset of action is immediate, the efficacy of gastric lavage versus induced emesis remains unresolved (Harris & Kingston, 1992; Hoffman, 1992; Young & Bivins, 1993). To be most effective, gastric lavage should occur within 1 hour after ingestion. The efficiency of substance recovery with gastric lavage is approximately 30% to 35% (Young & Bivans, 1993). Gastric lavage in the asymptomatic, self-poisoned patient, however, is being challenged (Fleisher et al. 1991; Lovejoy et al., 1992; Merigian et al., 1990). In a controlled study by Merigian and colleagues (1990), a set of overdose patients was selected. The selected group included only those patients who were asymptomatic and in whom the ingested agent would not normally require more than simple supportive care. These patients treated without gastric lavage did not show evidence of significant clinical decompensation.

Complications of gastric lavage include passage of the poison into the small intestines, laceration of the esophagus, laryngeal spasms, and aspiration. These complications can result in increased hospital stay. Contraindications for use include caustic and hydrocarbon ingestions, and an unprotected airway.

Activated Charcoal

Charcoal is the residue from distillation of various organic materials. The adsorptive capacity of the charcoal is increased or "activated" by treatment with superheated steam or air at temperatures of 600°C to 900°C (Haddad & Roberts, 1990). The activating agent, by fragmenting the carbon granules, creates a greater surface for binding. AC acts by absorbing and irreversibly binding chemicals to its surface, thus inhibiting their absorption.

Until recently, AC was used after gastric lavage to bind residual toxin and prevent further absorption in the gastrointestinal tract. Studies by Merigian and colleagues (1990) have shown the efficacy of AC as a single therapeutic agent without prior gastric emptying. AC may be administered either orally or by instillation via the orogastric tube. In patients receiving gastric lavage, there is an increasing trend to administer AC via the orogastric tube before lavage to halt further absorption immediately. The absorbed drug along with the AC is then removed by gastric lavage; then AC is readministered once the lavage is completed. Although the onset is immediate, the maximum benefit is obtained if administered within 30 minutes of ingestion. The dose for children is 1 g/kg, whereas the adult dose is 50 to 100 g (Haddad & Roberts, 1990). Multiple doses of AC (pulsed charcoal) are advised for those drugs that undergo enterohepatic recirculation, such as acetaminophen. After the initial dose, repeated doses of 30 to 50 g are administered every 2 to 6 hours (Harris & Kingston, 1992).

Activated charcoal containing sorbitol is dispensed by many hospital pharmacies. This preparation is to be used for single-dose administration. The inclusion of sorbitol may improve the palatability of the charcoal by giving it a sweet taste, decrease gastrointestinal transit time, and eliminate the need for separate cathartic administration to clear the charcoal from the intestinal tract. Highly concentrated formulations of AC–sorbitol should be avoided in children and in multiple-dose therapy because of the risk of hypernatremic dehydration (Bond et al., 1993; Hoffman, 1992; Krenzelok & Dunmire, 1992). When repeated doses of AC are to be administered, sorbitol-containing preparations should not be used with every dose (McFarland & Chyka, 1993; Wax et al., 1993).

Complications associated with the use of AC in-

TABLE 66–2. **Adsorption of Drugs**

Drugs With Significant Adsorption	
Acetaminophen	Meprobamate
Amphetamines	Narcotics
Atropine	Penicillin
Barbiturates	Phenothiazines
Cocaine	Phenytoin
Digitalis	Quinidine
Digitoxin	Salicylates
Iodine	Sulfonamides
Ipecac	Tricyclic antidepressants
Isoniazid	
Drugs With Little or No Adsorption	
Alcohol	Iron
Cyanide	Lithium

clude nausea and vomiting. This may be minimized by slow administration. Constipation may occur if the AC is not followed by a cathartic. AC is nontoxic, and if aspirated is inert.

A partial listing of drugs that may be adsorbed by AC is given in Table 66–2. Drugs that do not bind well to AC include lithium and iron. AC is contraindicated for ingestions of corrosive agents because it prevents adequate visualization of the traumatized esophageal tissue. Previously, if N-acetylcysteine (NAC) was given for acetaminophen toxicity, AC was withheld because it absorbed some of the antidote. This may be prevented if the AC is removed by lavage before NAC administration. Some studies have suggested that AC can safely be used if the loading dose of NAC is increased (Chamberlain et al., 1993; Haddad & Roberts, 1990).

Whole-Bowel Irrigation

The newest method for decontamination is whole-bowel irrigation (WBI) with polyethylene glycol–electrolyte (PEG-ELS) solution. According to Harris and Kingston (1992) and Fine and Goldfrank (1992), this fluid is not absorbed or secreted across the gastrointestinal epithelium. Adults must ingest the solution at a rate of 2 liters/hour; dosage for children is 500 mL/hour. If the patient is unable to consume this amount of fluid, it may be necessary to instill it via a nasogastric tube. The effectiveness is determined by the presence of a clear effluent, which may take 2 to 6 hours to obtain. WBI may be used in the management of acute overdoses of substances not absorbed by AC (such as lithium and iron), ingestion of enteric-coated or sustained-release medications, and for use in professional "body packers" who smuggle ingested wrapped containers of drugs (Harris & Kingston, 1992; Hoffman, 1992; Sporer, 1993). WBI is contraindicated in patients having an ileus, obstruction, perforation, or substantial gastrointestinal bleeding.

Forced Diuresis

Forced diuresis is usually combined with either alkalinization or acidification of the urine (Winchester, 1990). Fluid infusion with an accompanying diuretic can be used to produce a urinary output of 2 to 4 mL/kg/hour. This helps to decrease renal tubular reabsorption and thereby increase urinary excretion. The patient must be evaluated carefully. The large fluid load may cause pulmonary edema, and use of the diuretic may lead to electrolyte and acid–base imbalances.

ALKALINIZATION OF URINARY PH. Excretion of a drug by the kidneys depends on its ionized state. Alkalinization of the tubular fluid helps promote ionization of weak acids such as salicylates. This decreases their ability to be reabsorbed by the renal tubules and enhances excretion. Sodium bicarbonate is used to increase urine pH above 7.5; normal urine output is maintained during the procedure (Yip et al., 1994).

ACIDIFICATION OF URINARY PH. Urinary acidification is no longer thought to be appropriate. It does not significantly enhance removal of toxic substances and contributes to complications of metabolic acidosis (Pond, 1990).

Hemodialysis and Hemoperfusion

Hemodialysis involves the delivery of blood through a dialyzer, after which it is returned to the venous circulation. The semipermeable membrane in the dialyzer helps to separate diffusible substances from less diffusible substances. Table 66–3 summarizes factors that affect the clearance of toxic compounds (Pond, 1990; Winchester, 1990).

Hemoperfusion is similar to hemodialysis, except that blood is delivered to a cartridge instead of a dialyzer. This cartridge contains an adsorbent (i.e., activated carbon or AC) that physically binds the toxic compound. Clearance over time is limited by the deposition of blood cell membranes or plasma proteins. Improvement in clearance can be obtained by changing the cartridge every 4 to 6 hours (Pond, 1990).

Hemodialysis and hemoperfusion are difficult to perform in those patients with severe hypotension or low cardiac output. If the altered hemodynamics are

TABLE 66–3. **Factors Affecting Clearance of Toxic Compounds During Hemodialysis or Hemoperfusion**

Size of the solute (molecular weight of the drug)
Lipid solubility
Plasma protein binding
Volume of distribution
Maintenance of a concentration gradient
Available surface area of the dialyzer
Blood and dialysate pressure

secondary to the toxic effects of the ingested drug, the risk:benefit ratio often dictates the need for the procedure.

Hemodialysis or hemoperfusion is indicated when (1) there is a progressive deterioration of the patient despite careful and supportive intensive care, (2) blood or plasma concentration of the compound is in the lethal range, (3) when kidney function is impaired, or (4) the drug ingested can be removed at a more rapid rate than can be accomplished by the liver or kidneys (Winchester, 1990).

SPECIFIC DRUGS

Cocaine

Cocaine is an alkaloid derived from the leaves of the coca plant. It is absorbed at all sites of application. Cocaine has become the most popular recreational drug in the United States; it is "the foremost primary nonalcohol drug of abuse" in most cities, and is "the second most reported drug (following heroin) in Los Angeles, New Jersey, and San Francisco" (National Institute on Drug Abuse [NIDA], 1993, p. 3). According to 1991 data from NIDA (United States Department of Commerce et al., 1992), the number of habitual users of cocaine hydrochloride (HCl; powder form) has decreased in the age group of 18 to 25 years (7.6% in 1985 to 2.0% in 1991); however, a trend of increasing use has been noted for young people dealing "crack" on the streets (NIDA, 1993). "Crack," the alkaloidal form of cocaine, appears rock-like and makes crackling sounds when heated. In the age group of 26 years and older, there has been an increase in those who have used cocaine HCl, from 9.5% in 1985 to 11.8% in 1991 (U.S. Department of Commerce et al., 1992). As a result of overall increased use, emergency departments are seeing an increase in the number of cocaine-related visits. Between October, 1990 and September, 1992, the number of cocaine mentions in nonalcohol emergency department admissions rose in every major city; increases were greater than 40% in four major cities (NIDA, 1993). Cocaine use and toxicity should be suspected in normally healthy adults who suddenly experience chest pain, seizures, or an acute onset of severe hypertension (Dubiel, 1990).

MECHANISMS OF COCAINE TOXICITY

Major neurochemical actions of cocaine include (1) stimulation of the CNS and sympathetic nervous system; (2) blocking the presynaptic reuptake of norepinephrine, dopamine, and serotonin, resulting in excessive amounts of the neurotransmitters at the postsynaptic receptors; (3) increased availability of stored calcium; and (4) a local anesthetic effect as a result of inhibition of the sodium current in neural tissue. High levels of cocaine may lead to a generalized anesthetic effect (Moliterno et al., 1994; Mueller et al., 1990; Ritz & George, 1993). As a result of impaired neural impulse transmission, the patient may exhibit CNS depression, coma, and respiratory arrest (Mueller et al., 1990).

Chronic cocaine abuse results in a depletion of norepinephrine and dopamine at the synaptic sites (House, 1992). To regain the "high" the patient previously experienced, increased amounts of the drug are taken.

Approximately 50% of a given dose is rapidly metabolized via a plasma cholinesterase pathway. In a study by Hoffman and colleagues (1992), an association was found between life-threatening manifestations of cocaine intoxication and decreased plasma cholinesterase activity.

Multiple organ systems may be affected by the excessive stimulation caused by cocaine intoxication. Toxicity of the CNS and the cardiovascular system are the most widely reported in the medical and nursing literature. Signs and symptoms of cocaine use are summarized in Table 66–4.

CLINICAL PRESENTATION

CENTRAL NERVOUS SYSTEM

HEADACHE. Studies indicating the frequency of headaches associated with cocaine vary from 6.8% (Lowenstein et al., 1987) to 60% (Washton & Gold, 1987). The headaches not only varied in intensity, quality, and location, but often were associated with nausea, arthralgia, and abdominal or chest pain (Lowenstein et al., 1987). The headaches may be a manifestation of hypertension, a cerebrovascular accident, or a migraine headache secondary to inhibition of serotonin uptake.

STROKES. The number of reported stroke cases related to cocaine has risen sharply. Klonoff and associates (1989) reviewed 47 cases with this diagnosis. They found that patients in their 20s were the most frequently affected. The strokes occurred after any route of ingestion. In this study, cerebral infarction occurred in 22% of the patients, and intracerebral and subarachnoid hemorrhage occurred in 78% of the patients. This contrasts with the general population, in which cerebral infarctions occur four times more frequently than intracranial hemorrhages.

A study by Levine and coworkers (1991) further differentiated the types of strokes based on the type of cocaine used. They found that ischemic and hemorrhagic strokes were equally likely to occur after the use of alkaloidal cocaine. Use of cocaine HCl is more likely to cause hemorrhagic strokes (approximately 80% of the time), whereas cerebral infarction was significantly more common among users of alkaloidal cocaine. The presence on an underlying cerebral aneurysm was more commonly found among patients having strokes related to cocaine HCl than those having strokes related to alkaloidal cocaine. The strokes are likely related to sympathomimetic activity resulting in an acute increase in blood pressure and cerebral vasoconstriction.

TABLE 66–4. **Cocaine Signs and Symptoms**

Intoxication	Overdose	Withdrawal
Early		
Euphoria	Loss of reflexes	Depression
Sudden headache	Flaccid paralysis	Anhedonia
Cold sweats	Coma	Intense craving for drug
Muscle jerks	Fixed, dilated pupils	Irritability
Tachycardia	Gross pulmonary edema	Irregular sleep patterns
Increased blood pressure	Respiratory failure	Aches and pains
Tachypnea	Cyanosis	Increased appetite
Dyspnea	Ventricular fibrillation	Poor concentration
Psychotic behavior	Circulatory failure	Suicide
	Cardiac arrest	
	Death	
Advanced		
Decreased level of consciousness		
Generalized hyperreflexia		
Seizures		
Incontinence		
Status epilepticus		
Increased, weak, irregular pulse		
Increased blood pressure, then rapid decrease		
Irregular respirations		

SEIZURES. Seizures may be experienced by both first-time and chronic cocaine users secondary to the drug's direct convulsant effects (Holland et al., 1992). Research by He and colleagues (1993) indicates that cocaine rapidly elevates the intracellular free calcium concentration of cerebral vascular muscle cells to about 50% above initial resting levels. This produces the cerebrovasospasms. The seizure threshold may also be lowered during periods of hyperthermia and acidosis.

CARDIOVASCULAR SYSTEM

HYPERTENSION. Intense sympathetic stimulation results in increased cardiac output and vascular resistance (Kloner et al., 1992). This is manifested by acute severe hypertension. The potent vasoconstriction may result in intracerebral hemorrhage, aortic dissection, or dilated cardiomyopathy (Mueller et al., 1990; Levine et al., 1991; Westlake & Funkhouser, 1990).

CHEST PAIN. Patients may experience palpitations or chest pain within 6 hours after cocaine use. Along with the chest pain, these patients may have ECG findings indicative of acute myocardial infarction (MI), and subsequent elevation in heart creatine phosphokinase isoenzymes. The mechanism of the MI may include cocaine-induced coronary artery spasm (Brogan et al., 1992; Moliterno et al., 1994), or coronary thrombosis. Kalsner (1993) found that cocaine magnifies the effects of stimuli that make use of calcium L channels in contraction of myocardial muscle. Cocaine was found to produce stimuli with sufficient intensity to be implicated in coronary artery spasms.

Cocaine is also implicated in enhancement of platelet aggregation. It has been suggested by Westlake and Funkhouser (1990) that cocaine-induced MI is the result of a thrombus. Further research with angiography evidence, however, needs to be completed to verify their study.

Besides coronary vasospasms and thrombosis, myocardial damage may result from the increased myocardial oxygen consumption secondary to stimulation of alpha-adrenergic and beta-adrenergic receptors.

CARDIAC DYSRHYTHMIAS. Dysrhythmias may be the result of increased sympathetic stimulation, myocardial ischemia, or myocarditis. According to Mueller and colleagues (1990), myocardial ischemia and myocarditis tend to be manifested after cocaine has been eliminated from the person. Myocardial damage may promote malignant reentry dysrhythmias and ventricular fibrillation, which is the presumed cause of many sudden deaths in cocaine users.

MANAGEMENT

There is no antidote for cocaine overdose. The patient, therefore, must be treated symptomatically (Table 66–5). Airway, ventilation, and circulation should be assessed and maintained. Stabilization, as discussed earlier, should be initiated. Decontamination with AC may be employed (Mueller et al., 1990).

Whole-bowel irrigation may also be indicated in patients who have ingested cocaine packages. If a single package ruptures, the lethal oral dose is often exceeded. The package may also release cocaine over an extended period of time, providing a sustained-release dosage. If both WBI and AC are used concurrently, the AC should be mixed in water, and never in the PEG-ELS solution. The AC should be given enough time to interact with the gastric contents before initiating the

TABLE 66–5. **Treatment of Life-Threatening Symptoms of Cocaine Toxicity**

Cardiovascular System

Tachydysrhythmias
  Atrial: Observation, propranolol, labetalol, verapamil
  Ventricular: Propranolol, labetalol, lidocaine
Myocardial ischemia
  Nitrates, calcium channel blockers, thrombolytics
Hypertension
  Vasodilators: Nifedipine, labetalol, nitroprusside

Central Nervous System

Convulsions
  Seizure precautions, diazepam, phenytoin, pancuronium, phenobarbital
Hyperthermia
  Hypothermic blankets, ice packs, evaporative cooling, dantrolene

WBI procedure, to obtain optimal benefits (Makosiej et al., 1993).

Cardiac activity should be monitored for early detection of dysrhythmias. Tachycardias may be treated with IV adrenergic blockers. Data collected by Kloner (1992) suggested that cardiac electrical instability associated with cocaine abuse was the result of enhanced activation of beta-adrenergic receptors. Adrenergic receptor antagonists may therefore protect the patient against malignant dysrhythmias induced by the cocaine and myocardial ischemia. Propranolol and esmolol provide cardioprotection by reducing cardiac metabolic demands. While reducing tachycardia, however, they may produce a paradoxic worsening of the hypertension (Mueller et al., 1990). Labetalol, an alpha- and beta-adrenergic blocker, may be most useful in the setting of tachycardia with hypertension. The alpha-blocking properties result in vasodilation, whereas the beta-blocking properties help decrease the heart rate.

Cocaine toxicity should be suspected in all young patients admitted to the hospital with acute chest pain, cardiac dysrhythmias, or cardiac arrest. A 12-lead ECG should be evaluated to determine if indications of an acute MI are present. If positive indications are noted, a cardiology consult should be obtained. Thrombolytic therapy or coronary angiography may be considered on appropriate patients.

Patients experiencing moderate hypertension may be treated with oral nifedipine, 10 to 20 mg. Labetalol, as mentioned earlier, may be used to provide alpha-adrenergic inhibition. IV nitroprusside may be required for patients having severe hypertensive episodes (Mueller et al., 1990).

Grand mal seizures are the most common neurologic complication of cocaine intoxication. Seizure precautions therefore should be maintained for all patients. In a study by Holland and colleagues (1992), 89% of their patients had uncomplicated convulsions. Cocaine-related seizures tend to be brief and self-limiting (Olson et al., 1993).

Some seizures, however, may be prolonged and recurrent. Diazepam is the drug of choice in the treatment of status epilepticus. Seizures intractable to diazepam may require paralytic therapy along with mechanical ventilation. The patient should be reassessed between paralytic doses to determine if seizure activity is still present. Some patients with continued seizure activity may require barbiturate anesthesia to prevent the development of potential complications.

Patients experiencing severe hyperthermia (temperatures greater than 104°F) require aggressive treatment. Clothing should be removed. A hypothermic blanket, ice packs to the groin and armpits, and evaporative cooling may be needed to reduce the patient's temperature. In some cases, IV dantrolene may be required.

Acetaminophen

Acetaminophen, a drug that is commonly thought to be safe and nontoxic, has become increasingly popular since its introduction into the pharmaceutical market. Taken in therapeutic doses, it has few side effects. In recent years, however, acetaminophen has been increasingly used as a form of self-poisoning, with serious and potentially fatal results. In 1992 there were 102,043 reported exposures to acetaminophen, with 44% requiring treatment in a health care facility (Litovitz et al., 1993). Fatal hepatic necrosis may occur with as little as 20 to 40 extra-strength tablets or 30 to 60 regular-strength tablets (10–20 g).

MECHANISM OF ACETAMINOPHEN TOXICITY

Acetaminophen is metabolized by the liver. Approximately 94% of the drug is conjugated with sulfates and glucuronides. Neither the unchanged acetaminophen nor the conjugates are toxic. However, 4% of the drug is metabolized along a pathway in the liver called the P-450 microsomal enzyme system, producing a highly toxic metabolite. Glutathione, endogenously synthesized by the liver, normally detoxifies this toxic metabolite. It is then excreted in the urine as cysteine and mercapturic acid metabolites.

Normally, glutathione is produced in adequate amounts to detoxify repeated therapeutic doses of acetaminophen (10–20 mg/kg every 4 hours). When therapeutic doses are exceeded, the supply of glutathione cannot maintain the pace with which the toxic metabolites are produced; glutathione becomes depleted. When 70% or more of glutathione is depleted, the reactive metabolite accumulates. It is then free to bind to hepatocellular molecules, resulting in hepatic necrosis, the major cause of death after an overdose. Toxicity is likely to occur in adult patients after a single dose of 140 mg/kg, or 10 g.

CLINICAL PRESENTATION

The clinical course of an untreated acetaminophen overdose can be divided into four stages (Table 66–6).

TABLE 66–6. **Clinical Course of Untreated Acetaminophen Overdose**

Stage	Time Postingestion	Characteristics
I	16–24 hours	Nausea Vomiting Anorexia Diaphoresis
II	24–48 hours	Symptoms abate Right upper quadrant pain Hepatomegaly Bleeding Elevated AST, ALT, PT, bilirubin
III	3–5 days	Peak liver function abnormalities
IV	7–8 days	Resolution of hepatic dysfunction

Abbreviations: PT, prothrombin time; ALT, alanine aminotransferase; AST, aspartate aminotransferase.

Stage 1 lasts 16 to 24 hours after the initial ingestion. The patient may exhibit such symptoms as nausea, vomiting, anorexia, and diaphoresis. Vomiting occurring during this stage may help reduce the amount of the drug absorbed. Some patients may be symptom free; therefore, medical attention may be delayed. To be effective, treatment should be started during stage 1.

Stage 2 usually lasts 1 to 2 days after ingestion. Previous symptoms tend to abate. Although the patient may be feeling better, the liver enzymes aspartate and alanine aminotransferase (AST, ALT) begin to rise, along with bilirubin and prothrombin time. Clinical signs of hepatotoxicity become evident: right upper quadrant pain, hepatomegaly, and bleeding.

Stage 3 occurs 3 to 5 days after ingestion. Liver function abnormalities have now reached their peak. Gastrointestinal symptoms may return. AST and ALT values above 10,000 IU/mL are not uncommon (Anker & Smilkstein, 1994). These high values cannot be used to predict the patient's final prognosis, however, because patients without evidence of liver failure may also have these high values. Better predictors of significant liver injury appear to be increases in the bilirubin, elongation of the prothrombin time, and abnormalities of pH and glucose. Fatalities usually occur during this period. Death may be a result of multiorgan failure, or by an overwhelming complication secondary to liver failure.

Stage 4, the recovery stage, occurs 7 to 8 days after ingestion. During this time, hepatic regeneration becomes complete in survivors and hepatic enzymes return to normal. Chronic liver dysfunction from acetaminophen overdose has not been reported (Anker & Smilkstein, 1994).

MANAGEMENT

It is very important to obtain as accurate a history as possible. This includes not only how many and what strength of tablets, but also how long ago the ingestion took place. Determining the time since ingestion is necessary in deciding appropriate treatment (Fig. 66-1). Families can often be of assistance in gaining this information when the patient is unable or unwilling to give accurate details.

Blood should be drawn for acetaminophen levels, other drugs, liver function studies, and coagulation studies. If the history suggests an acetaminophen overdose (single dose > 140 mg/kg), and the results of the plasma acetaminophen assays are not available, treatment should begin immediately. Treatment may be continued or stopped based on the results obtained. Peak plasma levels occur approximately 4 hours postingestion. Nontoxic levels obtained before this 4-hour mark should be repeated because they may not accurately reflect patient toxicity.

The acetaminophen nomogram (Fig. 66–2) is used to determine necessity of treatment for acetaminophen overdose. The nomogram plots serum acetaminophen levels against the hours since ingestion. A straight line is drawn through 200 μg/mL at 4 hours and 50 μg/mL at 12 hours postingestion. If the patient's serum level falls above the line, hepatotoxicity is likely to occur and treatment should be started. A second line is drawn through 150 μg/mL at 4 hours and 40 μg/mL at 12 hours postingestion. Patients whose serum level falls between the two lines represent those who may possibly experience hepatotoxicity; treatment is usually provided. Patients whose serum levels fall below both lines represent those patients in whom toxicity is unlikely, and treatment is not required. Treatment that has already been started may be discontinued. Toxic levels are less likely to result in hepatotoxicity in children than adults due to an alternate metabolic pathway in the liver. Treatment, however, for children remains the same as for the adult.

N-acetylcysteine (NAC) is the treatment of choice for acetaminophen toxicity. It is thought to metabolize to cysteine, a precursor of glutathione, thereby providing protective levels of glutathione to detoxify the acetaminophen metabolite. Treatment should always begin within 16 hours of ingestion in patients having toxic acetaminophen levels, to prevent hepatic necrosis. If NAC treatment is delayed more than 16 hours, its effectiveness decreases.

Initial treatment may include gastric lavage and AC because patients often ingest multiple substances. In the past it was recommended that AC should be removed by lavage before NAC therapy to prevent inactivation by AC. Observations from more recent studies, however, suggest that concern about concomitant use of NAC and AC is unwarranted (Chamberlain et al., 1993; Spiller et al., 1994). When administered within 1 hour after ingestion, AC has been shown to be beneficial in preventing acetaminophen absorption, and reduction in the efficacy of NAC therapy has not occurred. As long as NAC treatment is initiated within 8 hours of ingestion, a delay of 1 to 2 hours will not affect the outcome of the patient.

Figure 66–1 indicates the general protocol for ad-

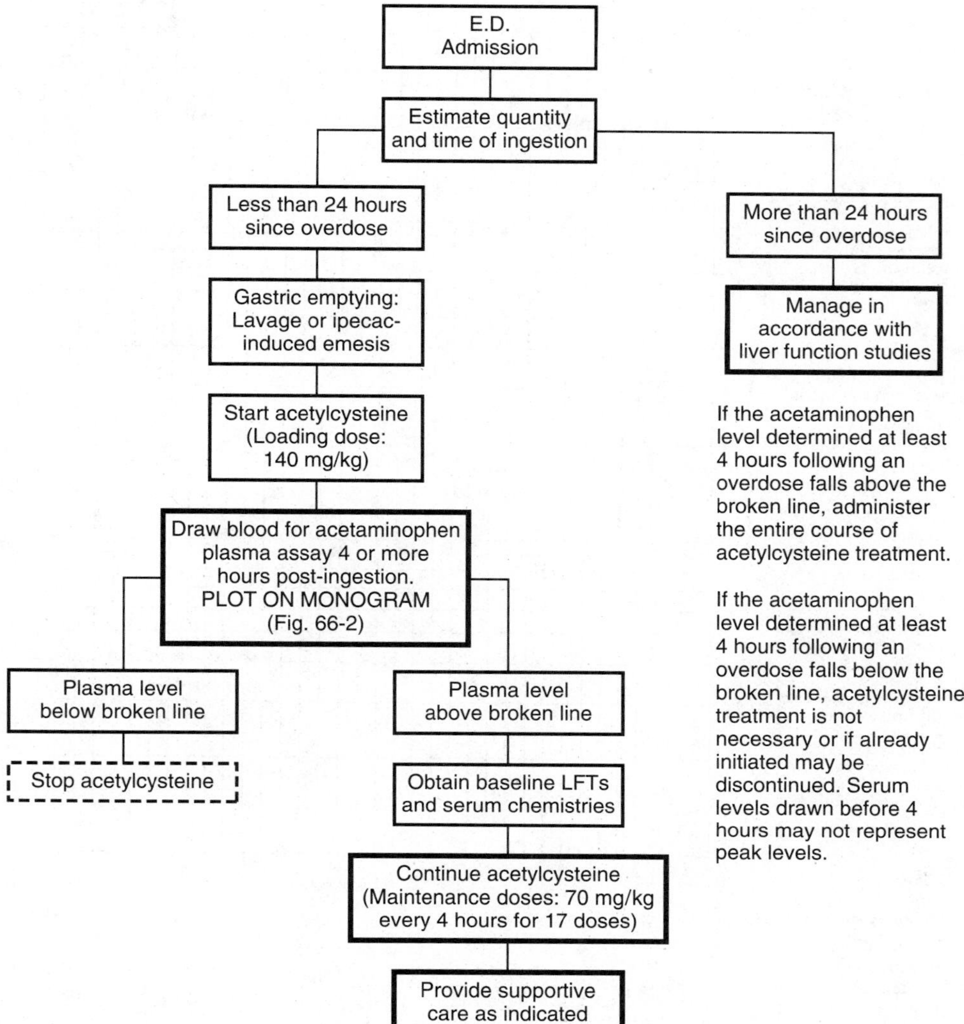

FIGURE 66–1. Flow chart for stepwise management of acute acetaminophen overdose. (From McNeil Consumer Products Company. [1987]. *Management of acetaminophen.* Fort Washington, PA: McNeil Pharmaceuticals.)

ministration of oral NAC. IV NAC, which has been used in Europe and Canada for years, remains an investigational drug in the United States.

If the level of consciousness is impaired as a result of multiple-drug ingestion, it is necessary to administer the NAC via a nasogastric tube. Patients having intractable nausea and vomiting may also require the administration of an antiemetic to prevent elimination of the antidote.

Salicylates

Salicylates are one of the most frequently used over-the-counter products in the United States. They may be purchased as aspirin alone, or as an aspirin-containing compound such as Ben Gay (Pfizer Consumer Products, Parsippany, NJ), Bufferin (Bristol Myers Products, New York, NY), or Pepto Bismol (Procter & Gamble, Cincinnati, OH). It is also one of the most commonly involved substances in poisonings. According to the 1992 Annual Report of the American Association of Poison Control Centers (Litovitz et al., 1993), there were 22,216 reported exposures involving aspirin alone or aspirin-containing compounds. Twenty-five percent of the exposures required treatment in a health care facility. These exposures included acute accidental ingestion by toddlers, intentional ingestion by adolescents and adults contemplating suicide, and inappropriate chronic use for self-medication purposes. The introduction of effective safety packaging, and the withdrawal of pediatric aspirin products because of their role in the development of Reye's syndrome, have significantly reduced the number of pediatric overdoses in the last few years.

MECHANISM OF SALICYLATE TOXICITY

Peak serum salicylate concentrations generally occur within 12 hours of ingestion (Mathewson-Kuhn, 1992). Variances in peak levels may be due to presence of food in the stomach, delayed gastric emptying, pyloric spasms, and formation of concretions (insoluble con-

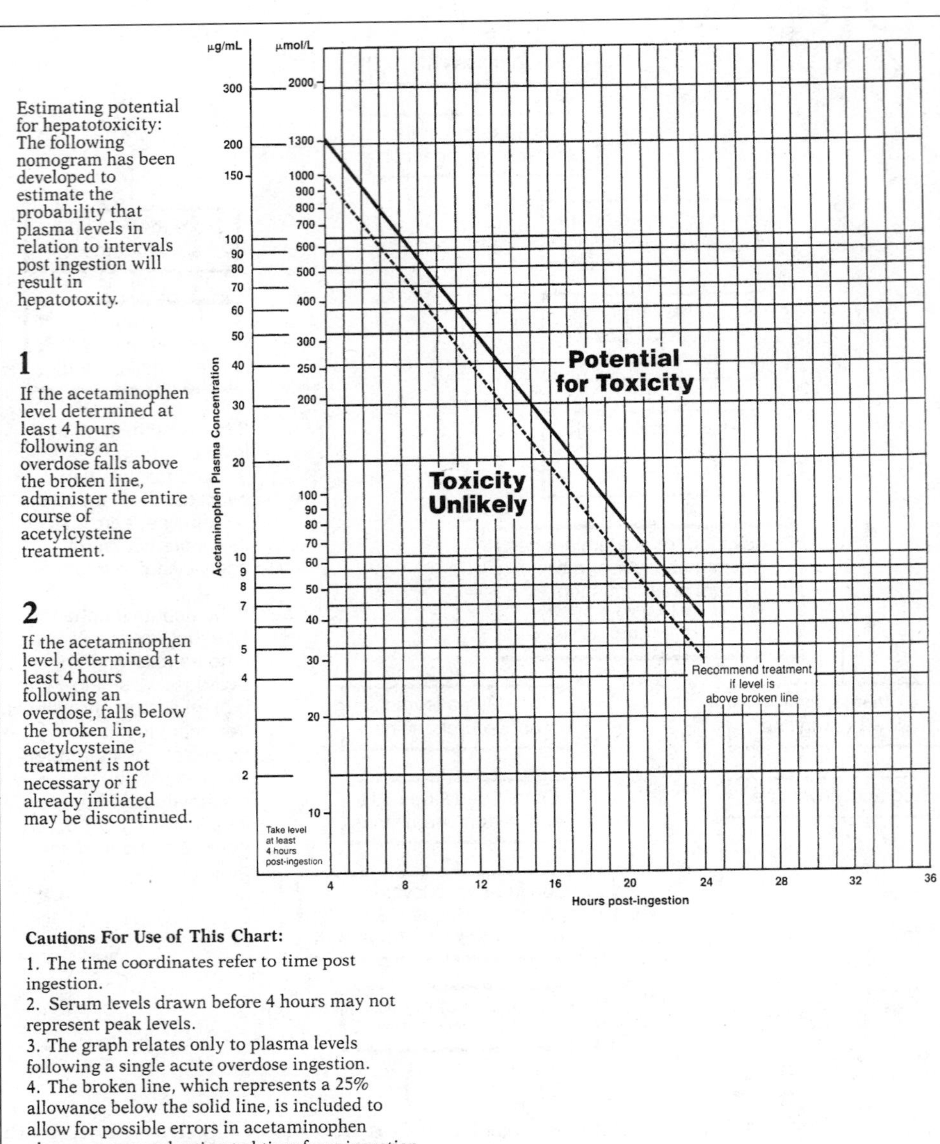

Estimating potential for hepatotoxicity: The following nomogram has been developed to estimate the probability that plasma levels in relation to intervals post ingestion will result in hepatotoxicity.
1
If the acetaminophen level determined at least 4 hours following an overdose falls above the broken line, administer the entire course of acetylcysteine treatment.
2
If the acetaminophen level, determined at least 4 hours following an overdose, falls below the broken line, acetylcysteine treatment is not necessary or if already initiated may be discontinued.
μg/mL
μmol/L
Acetaminophen Plasma Concentration
Potential for Toxicity
Toxicity Unlikely
Recommend treatment if level is above broken line
Take level at least 4 hours post-ingestion
Hours post-ingestion
Cautions For Use of This Chart:
1. The time coordinates refer to time post ingestion.
2. Serum levels drawn before 4 hours may not represent peak levels.
3. The graph relates only to plasma levels following a single acute overdose ingestion.
4. The broken line, which represents a 25% allowance below the solid line, is included to allow for possible errors in acetaminophen plasma assays and estimated time from ingestion of an overdose.

FIGURE 66–2. Acetaminophen nomogram. Serum acetaminophen concentration versus time after acetaminophen ingestion. (From McNeil Consumer Products Company. *Tylenol: Hospital formulary manual, comprehensive drug information monograph.* Fort Washington, PA: McNeil Pharmaceuticals.)

centrate of the drug). Concentrations can release salicylate over several hours, or may cause a delayed bolus effect. Peak serum levels may be delayed more than 12 hours when enteric-coated aspirin products are consumed. Cases have been reported in which continued absorption occurred for periods greater than 24 hours.

Approximately 50% of the salicylate is metabolized in the stomach before being absorbed into the bloodstream. Therapeutic doses are mainly converted to salicyluric acid and acyl glucoronides by conjugation with glycine and glucuronic acid. As the amount of salicylic acid increases, the conjugation enzymes become saturated. In the acutely overdosed patient, most of the drug is not metabolized and is excreted as salicylic acid in the urine (Krause et al., 1992).

Therapeutically acquired intoxication, or chronic exposure, refers to repeated exposures to the drug over a period greater than 24 hours. The body's ability to metabolize the drug becomes overwhelmed. Intoxication may occur earlier if renal impairment is present.

Other primary pathophysiologic effects include direct stimulation of the CNS respiratory center, inhibition of Krebs cycle enzymes, inhibition of the prostaglandin synthetase complex, stimulation of gluconeogenesis, stimulation of lipid metabolism, and interference with hemostasis (Proudfoot, 1990).

CLINICAL PRESENTATION

Central nervous system toxicity is an important indication of the severity of the salicylate poisoning. CNS toxicity is usually associated with acidemia. It is thought that the acidosis favors a shift of salicylates into the cells, particularly in the brain. Patients with

TABLE 66–7. **Signs and Symptoms of Salicylate Toxicity**

Mild Toxicity	Moderate Toxicity	Severe Toxicity
Nausea	Symptoms more pronounced	Disorientation
Vomiting	Tachypnea	Stupor
Tinnitus	Fever	Coma
Hyperpnea	Metabolic acidosis	Seizures
Respiratory alkalosis	Dehydration	Hypoglycemia
Irritability	Restlessness	Severe metabolic acidosis
Lethargy	Marked lethargy	Noncardiogenic pulmonary edema

mild toxicity exhibit nausea, vomiting, tinnitus, hyperpnea, and respiratory alkalosis (Table 66–7). These patients may be irritable, restless, or lethargic. With moderate toxicity, symptoms are more pronounced and include fever, metabolic acidosis, dehydration, and marked lethargy. Severe toxicity presents with stupor, coma, seizures, severe metabolic acidosis, and possibly noncardiogenic pulmonary edema. Although coma is rare, patients having coma or seizures experience a high mortality rate (Proudfoot, 1990).

Central nervous system stimulation of the respiratory center results in hyperventilation, causing respiratory alkalosis. This is the predominant acid–base change noted in older children and adults. Late in the course of events, a respiratory depression may develop, requiring the patient to be mechanically ventilated.

Metabolic changes also occur in the toxic patient. Acidemia may result in part from uncoupling of oxidative phosphorylation, interference with glycolysis, inhibition of the Krebs cycle, and stimulation of fat catabolism. These produce organic acids and contribute to metabolic acidosis. A high "anion gap" acidosis may be present. Metabolic acidosis is the predominant acid–base disturbance in younger children. The acidemia stimulates the respiratory center to increase the depth of respiration. In the adult, respiratory alkalosis usually predominates (Krause et al., 1992).

Further complications include disruption of the hematologic system. Salicylates inhibit prothrombin formation and disrupt platelet function. Although hemorrhage does not commonly occur in a single, acute overdose, this complication may occur with chronic administration of salicylates (Yip et al., 1994).

Chronic exposure is the repeated exposure to salicylates over time periods greater than 24 hours. As a result, there is extensive distribution of salicylates into the CNS and other tissue storage areas. However, making a determination of chronic salicylism can be difficult because many of the symptoms may be minimal or nonspecific. The symptoms include abdominal pain, flu-like symptoms, fever, and altered mental status. The delay in diagnosis and treatment may be one factor that contributes to the higher morbidity and mortality rates. Most fatal cases of chronic salicylate poisoning occur in infants and the elderly, two populations in which findings of altered mental status are often difficult to identify clearly (Krause et al., 1992).

MANAGEMENT

Of immediate importance is the maintenance of airway, breathing, and circulation. Further absorption is prevented by gastric lavage and the administration of AC. Elimination of salicylates may be enhanced by use of alkaline diuresis, mentioned in the section on methods of decontamination.

An IV access site should be established for the administration of fluids to correct the dehydration. As a result of the dehydration, large initial volumes of replacement fluids may be required. In addition, IV access may be required to administer dextrose for hypoglycemia, vitamin K if bleeding is present secondary to decreased prothrombin, and sodium bicarbonate to correct acidemia. Electrolytes should be monitored and replaced as needed.

Low platelet counts are common in the first 72 hours of treatment; therefore, the patient should be observed for signs of bleeding. Administration of fresh frozen plasma may be required to replace clotting factors.

Other management areas include treatment of hyperthermia with hypothermia blankets, ice packs, or water baths. Seizure precautions should be maintained. Diazepam may be used to stop seizure activity.

Tricyclic Antidepressants

Tricyclic antidepressant (TCA) toxicity remains a leading cause of hospitalization and death due to intentional drug overdose. TCAs are the most commonly prescribed drugs for the treatment of depression, and are now used as an adjunctive treatment in a variety of childhood disorders (Newcomb, 1991). The widespread availability of TCAs to depressed patients who are at high risk for suicide contributes to the large number of serious overdoses that occur. Other contributing factors include the low therapeutic index of these drugs, and the severity of the cardiovascular and CNS effects seen in overdoses.

MECHANISMS OF TRICYCLIC ANTIDEPRESSANT TOXICITY

Endogenous depression is thought to be caused by an inadequate amount of neurotransmitter in the brain, which causes the symptoms of depression. TCAs block the amine pump, preventing the reuptake of neurotransmitters (norepinephrine, dopamine, serotonin). More neurotransmitters are available to the receptor site, thus alleviating depression.

Tricyclic antidepressants are rapidly absorbed in the gastrointestinal tract. When an overdose is large, gastric emptying may be delayed as a result of the anticholinergic properties of TCAs. However, rapid deteri-

TABLE 66–8. **Selected Side Effects of Tricyclic Antidepressants**

Cardiovascular System	Central Nervous System	Peripheral Nervous System
Dysrhythmias	Agitation	Decreased gastrointestinal motility
Prolonged QRS	Confusion	Decreased salivation
Depressed myocardial contractility	Delirium	Hot, dry skin
Hypotension	Dilated pupils	Urinary retention
	Hallucinations	
	Hyperthermia	
	Seizures	

oration can occur. Most deaths occur within several hours of admission (Pentel et al., 1990).

Distribution of TCAs to tissues is rapid. Within a few hours after an overdose, the amount of the ingested dose remaining in the blood is less than 1% to 2% (Pentel et al., 1990). These drugs are metabolized almost entirely by the liver. The parent tertiary amine is converted to its metabolite, the secondary amine. Similar to the parent drug, the metabolite may contribute to toxicity after the first 12 to 24 hours.

Tricyclic antidepressant toxicity produces cardiovascular, CNS, and anticholinergic effects (Table 66–8). Life-threatening overdoses are usually associated with TCA ingestion of more than 1 g. This life-threatening state may develop in less than 1 hour (Pentel et al., 1990). The risk of death is significantly higher with older antidepressants (Kapur et al., 1992).

CLINICAL PRESENTATION

Sinus tachycardia of less than 160 beats per minute is the most common rhythm seen with TCA overdose. A result of increased catecholamines, this rhythm usually does not cause hemodynamic compromise.

A prolonged QRS interval is the most distinctive feature of serious TCA overdoses. The toxic effects of TCAs are similar to the effects of class I antidysrhythmics. They inhibit the fast sodium channel and slow phase 0 depolarization in His-Purkinje tissue. This impairment of depolarization appears as a prolonged QRS interval on the ECG. This slowed conduction can result in the development of ventricular tachycardia (Newton et al., 1994; Pentel et al., 1990). Other dysrhythmias include atrioventricular blocks (I–III), reentry rhythms, ventricular fibrillation, and sudden cardiac arrest. The quinidine-like effects also contribute to depressed myocardial contractility as well as a decreased heart rate.

As a result of increased catecholamines, an early transient hypertension may be seen in a TCA overdose. More commonly seen is hypotension (Goldfrank et al., 1990). Prolonged inhibition of norepinephrine reuptake may cause neurotransmitter reserves to become depleted. Decreased myocardial contractility and the alpha-adrenergic blocking properties of TCAs also contribute to hypotension.

In the typical overdose, there is an initial phase that is characterized by excitement and restlessness; delirium may occur in a more massive overdose as a result of anticholinergic activity (Pentel et al., 1990). This is followed by sedation, which may further progress to coma. Coma is more likely to occur in those patients having QRS prolongation. Some studies indicate that the level of consciousness is a better predictor of complications in a TCA overdose than is a prolonged QRS interval; complications such as ventricular dysrhythmias, hypotension, and seizures correlated well with a Glasgow Coma Scale score of 8 or less (Hultén et al., 1992). Seizures are usually brief and self-limiting (Newton et al., 1994; Pimentel & Trommer, 1994). In children, toxicity may present as confusion, disorientation, impaired concentration, social withdrawal, excessive sedation, or psychotic-like symptoms (Newcomb, 1991).

MANAGEMENT

Airway, breathing, and circulation should be evaluated and maintained. Continued observation of mental status and patency of the airway is extremely important. In a significant overdose, within minutes a patient's mental status may change from awake and alert to obtunded with absence of a gag reflex. Decontamination procedures should be initiated. Because of the anticholinergic properties of TCAs, gastric emptying may be delayed. Gastric lavage can be effective in drug removal if done within 4 to 6 hours after ingestion. TCAs undergo enterohepatic circulation, and therefore repeated administration of AC is beneficial in drug removal.

An IV site should be established. IV fluids should be kept at a maintenance rate to prevent pulmonary edema. Rates, however, may be increased in the presence of hypotension.

Sodium bicarbonate (to maintain a pH of 7.5) has become a standard recommendation for the treatment of a serious TCA cardiac toxicity. It suppresses dysrhythmias and narrows the QRS complex by accelerating intraventricular conduction, thus preventing reentry rhythms from developing (Hoffman et al., 1993). Ventricular dysrhythmias in adults that are unresponsive to bicarbonate may require phenytoin for termination. In the pediatric population, propranolol is the recommended drug for treatment of unresponsive dysrhythmias. If advanced cardiac life support algorithms are used, it should be noted that procainamide suppresses the myocardium by the same mechanism as do TCAs. Use of this drug, as well as quinidine, may only compound the existing cardiotoxicity.

Hypotension also appears to be responsive to sodium bicarbonate. This may be the result of improved cardiac conduction and contraction (Hoffman et al., 1993). Hypotension that is unresponsive to bicarbonate may require the use of fluid and vasopressors such as norepinephrine and dobutamine (Goldfrank et al., 1990).

The patient should be observed for seizure activity,

and seizure precautions placed in effect. Diazepam is the drug of choice to treat seizures. It is effective for the termination of most seizures, and does not make hypotension worse. Unresponsive seizures may require the use of phenytoin or other anticonvulsant drugs.

Patients at risk for development of hyperthermia should have their core temperature measured at least every 30 minutes. Cooling measures such as hypothermic blankets, ice packs to the axillae and groin, and evaporative cooling may be used to decrease high temperatures.

If the patient has no signs of toxicity after 6 hours, and bowel sounds are present, a final dose of charcoal may be given, and the patient discharged with a psychiatric consult. If toxic signs are present, treatment should be continued in a monitored unit. Patients who have been free of tachycardias, have normal PR, QRS, and QT intervals, and have had no ventricular dysrhythmias for 24 hours may be transferred from the monitored bed.

Benzodiazepines

Benzodiazepines (BZDs) are one of the most frequently prescribed medications. They have largely replaced other sedative–hypnotics because of their efficacy, minimal side effects, and low addiction potential. As a result of their widespread availability, they have become among the most frequently misused drugs. It is estimated that 40% to 50% of drug users also use BZDs to decrease the adverse side effects of stimulants and to decrease the unpleasant symptoms of withdrawal from more addictive substances (Roberts & Tafuri, 1990). BZDs have become one of the most common drugs involved in emergency room admissions as a result of intentional overdose.

After being absorbed, BZDs are more than 70% protein bound, and therefore unavailable to cross the blood–brain barrier (BBB) and interact with CNS receptors. The unbound drug, however, rapidly crosses the BBB to reach the CNS. These lipophilic drugs have a short duration of action in the CNS because they are rapidly redistributed. They have a longer plasma half-life because they remain inactive for prolonged periods of time in peripheral muscles and fat. BZDs are metabolized by the liver.

Benzodiazepines bind to CNS receptors that are specific for BZDs. These are most concentrated in the cerebral cortex. There are two types of BZD receptors: (1) type I, which mediate anxiolytic effects, and (2) type II, which mediate sedative and other effects of BZDs. Tolerance develops to the sedative effects (Roberts & Tafuri, 1990).

MECHANISM OF BENZODIAZEPINE TOXICITY

There is no direct toxicity to the brain. However, respiratory and cardiovascular systems may be depressed indirectly as a result of CNS depression. Respiratory and cardiac arrest have been noted when BZDs have been given IV. Most BZDs are relatively safe after an overdose. Deaths that do occur are usually the result of combination with other drugs (Roberts & Tafuri, 1990).

CLINICAL PRESENTATION

Benzodiazepine overdose rarely results in severe toxicity. Toxicity is characterized by CNS depression. Symptoms are drowsiness, ataxia, dizziness, and stupor that is usually arousable with verbal or painful stimuli. Severe CNS depression is unusual; if present, coingestion with other substances should be investigated. The newer, shorter-acting BZDs may, however, have greater potential for toxicity than the older BZDs (Roberts & Tafuri, 1990).

MANAGEMENT

Treatment for a pure BZD overdose is generally supportive and does not require gastric emptying. Once the patient is ambulatory without ataxia, he or she can be discharged.

A multiple-drug ingestion may result in the inability to protect the airway, requiring airway and ventilatory management. Gastric emptying should be initiated if the ingestion occurred within 2 hours. In a multiple-drug overdose, the use of a BZD antagonist may be useful as a diagnostic tool.

Flumazenil, a BZD antagonist, competitively binds with the CNS receptor site. It does not, however, have any intrinsic effects. It rapidly reverses the sedative and anticonvulsant effects of BZDs. With the reversal of CNS depression, respirations are restored, preventing the need for intubation. Flumazenil is usually administered in a bolus of 0.2 mg IV over 30 seconds. Reversal of sedation and respiratory depression becomes evident within 2 to 5 minutes. If there is no response to the initial bolus, doses may be repeated at 0.3- to 0.5-mg increments with 1-minute intervals between each dose. Most BZDs taken in an overdose have half-lives that greatly exceed the half-life of flumazenil (Krisanda, 1993). The patient, therefore, must be monitored for resedation. Flumazenil may precipitate seizure in patients who (1) were physically dependent on BZDs, (2) were taking BZDs to control seizures, (3) had an underlying seizure disorder, or (4) had taken a combined overdose of BZDs and TCAs (Krisanda, 1993; Roberts & Tafuri, 1990; Sugarman & Paul, 1994). Other adverse effects of flumazenil, reported to be mild and transient, include nausea and vomiting, headache, increased sweating, emotional lability, and cardiac dysrhythmias (Fine & Goldfrank, 1994; Sugarman & Paul, 1994).

Iron

Iron-containing compounds, once again in 1992, remained the leading cause of pediatric fatalities from accidental ingestion (Litovitz et al., 1993). Most of the over-the-counter iron preparations are packaged in large quantities. Many preparations are brightly colored, attracting a child's attention. Iron-containing compounds are often used both during and after pregnancy, and thus they are commonly found in the homes of families with children.

MECHANISM OF IRON TOXICITY

Iron is absorbed into the mucosal cells of the duodenum and jejunum. It is absorbed in the ferrous form, oxidized to the ferric state, then complexed to ferritin, a storage protein. When iron is released from ferritin to the plasma, it is transported by binding to the protein transferrin. Serum iron reflects the amount bound to transferrin. Normal serum iron levels range from 50 to 150 μg/dL (Mills & Curry, 1994). The total iron-binding capacity indicates the amount of binding potential transferrin has available. It is normally one-third saturated. When transferrin's capacity to bind iron is exceeded, free iron circulates, causing toxic effects, especially in the liver. "Although serum iron concentrations greater than 350 μg/dL are more frequently associated with systemic toxicity, the converse is not true. That is, iron toxicity cannot be excluded with a serum iron level less than 350 μg/dL" (Mills & Curry, 1994, p. 405).

Free circulating iron causes massive postarteriolar dilation and histamine release. It has a direct corrosive action on the intestinal mucosa. It also increases capillary permeability and acidosis from the release of hydrogen ions associated with the oxidation process (Eisen et al., 1990).

CLINICAL PRESENTATION

Five clinical stages are described in acute iron toxicity (Table 66–9). In the severely intoxicated patient, rapid deterioration may obscure recognition of the more discrete stages.

TABLE 66–9. **Clinical Stages of Acute Iron Toxicity**

Stage	Time Postingestion	Characteristics
I	Within 30 minutes to 6 hours	Nausea Vomiting Diarrhea Hematemesis Abdominal pain Lethargy
II	6 to 24 Hours	Symptoms subside Appears to have recovered
III	12 to 24 Hours	Gastrointestinal symptoms return Gastrointestinal blood loss Venous pooling Increased capillary permeability Shock Hepatic necrosis Coagulopathy Lethargy Disorientation
IV	2 to 4 Weeks	Gastric strictures Pyloric stenosis

Stage 1 (hemorrhagic gastroenteritis) occurs within 30 minutes to 6 hours postingestion. Signs and symptoms seen in this phase are related to gastrointestinal tract injury, which is secondary to iron's corrosive effects. Gastrointestinal symptoms that predominate include nausea, vomiting, diarrhea, hematemesis, abdominal pain, and lethargy. Vomiting appears to have the most predictive value with a serious iron ingestion. (Eisen et al., 1990; Mills & Curry, 1994).

Stage 2 (latent period) occurs 6 to 24 hours postingestion. During this time symptoms subside and the patient may appear to have recovered. This is a deceptive state because toxic effects continue at the tissue level. Signs of hypovolemia may be noted if initial fluid replacement was inadequate.

Stage 3 (shock and liver failure state) occurs 12 to 24 hours postingestion. Gastrointestinal symptoms reoccur. Profound shock occurs secondary to gastrointestinal blood loss, venous pooling, and increased capillary permeability. Hepatic necrosis results in jaundice, hypoglycemia, elevated aminotransferases, prolonged clotting times, thrombocytopenia, and qualitative changes in fibrinogen. Refractory metabolic acidosis is present. Serum iron concentrations may be normal during this phase (Eisen et al., 1990; Mills & Curry, 1994).

Stage 4 occurs 2 to 4 weeks postingestion. Gastric strictures and pyloric stenosis may occur, resulting in numerous nutritional problems. Postnecrotic changes in the liver after an acute ingestion are usually seen as fine, diffuse fibrotic changes (Eisen et al., 1990).

MANAGEMENT

All patients ingesting iron compounds need a complete history and physical examination. Observation alone is appropriate in most cases involving children's chewable multivitamins and when the absolute amount of elemental iron ingested is less than 20 mg/kg coupled with a negative KUB [kidneys, ureters, and bladder] radiograph examination. Those patients who have remained completely asymptomatic for 6 hours after the ingestion of iron do not require admission for treatment of iron poisoning (Mills & Curry, 1994, p. 404).

The symptomatic patient should have a patent airway and adequate ventilation established first. Fluid volume loss should be replaced with normal saline and packed cells as needed. Metabolic acidosis determined by arterial blood gases should be treated as required with sodium bicarbonate. Blood glucose should be tested using a bedside glucose monitor. If hypoglycemia is present, IV glucose should be administered. Seizure precautions should be initiated.

Gastric emptying is essential because iron has a direct corrosive effect on the gastric mucosa. Iron preparations often form concretions in the stomach with large ingestions, resulting in continued release of iron. Large amounts of gastric lavage solution may be required to reduce the size of a concretion. Large concretions that cannot be broken down may require endoscopy or surgery for removal.

Whole-bowel irrigation has recently been advocated as the treatment for iron toxicity. One stated advantage of WBI is that it has the potential to clear iron from the entire gastrointestinal tract (Tenenbein et al., 1991). Negligible gastrointestinal fluid and electrolyte fluxes occur with WBI (Eisen et al., 1990; Harris & Kingston, 1992). Current information on this method has been limited to uncontrolled case studies, and the utility of this method remains undefined (Mills & Curry, 1994).

Deferoxamine (DFO), a chelator of iron, is also used. IM injection of DFO has been recommended in the past; however, IM administration requires painful, multiple injections, it has erratic absorption, there is a higher incidence of side effects, and evidence of efficacy is less. Therefore, IV DFO is the appropriate route of administration in an acute poisoning. The recommended IV dosage of DFO is a continuous infusion rate of 15 mg/kg/hour. Some physicians may use higher infusion rates for severely ill patients, or for those patients who continue to deteriorate with the standard 15 mg/kg/hour dosage regimen. Rapid infusion rates greater than 45 mg/kg/hour may produce hypotension and a reflex tachycardia. This may be a secondary effect to the release of histamines (Mills & Curry, 1994).

During treatment, the urine turns a vin rosé color. In the past, treatment was discontinued when the urine turned clear. The vin rosé urine, however, has been shown to be an insensitive marker in serious iron poisoning. Most patients require no more than 24 hours of DFO administration. Further guidelines for appropriately discontinuing DFO have been developed. All of the following criteria should be met before DFO is discontinued: (1) the patient must be free of signs and symptoms of systemic iron poisoning, (2) the measured serum iron levels are not elevated, (3) previous multiple radiopacities on repeat abdominal radiograph tests are no longer present, and (4) vin rosé-colored urine has returned to a normal color. The absence of vin rosé urine is not by itself an adequate indication to discontinue DFO therapy (Eisen et al., 1990; Mills & Curry, 1994).

SUMMARY

Management of the overdose patient requires a knowledge not only of the appropriate methods of decontamination, but of the mechanisms of toxicity for the ingested compound. This allows team members to anticipate potential complications that may arise in the course of treatment and to deter adverse outcomes.

Collaboration and constant communication among all team members are essential elements in the management of these patients. Involvement of health team members outside the department, such as social services and psychiatric support, should be started early in the admission process.

REFERENCES

Anker, A. L., & Smilkstein, M. J. (1994). Acetaminophen: Concepts and controversies. *Emergency Medicine Clinics of North America, 12,* 335–349.

Bond, G. R., Requa, R. K., Krenzelok, E. P., et al. (1993). Influence of time until emesis on the efficacy of decontamination using acetaminophen as a marker in a pediatric population. *Annals of Emergency Medicine, 22,* 1403–1407.

Brogan, W. C., Lange, R. A., Glamann, D. B., & Hillis, L. D. (1992). Recurrent coronary vasoconstriction caused by intranasal cocaine: Possible role for metabolites. *Annals of Internal Medicine, 116,* 556–561.

Chamberlain, J. M., Gorman, R. L., Oderda, G. M., Klein-Schwartz, W., & Klein, B. L. (1993). Use of activated charcoal in a simulated poisoning with acetaminophen: A new loading dose for N-acetylcysteine? *Annals of Emergency Medicine, 22,* 1398–1402.

Dubiel, D. (1990). Action stat!: Cocaine overdose. *Nursing90, 20*(3), 33.

Eisen, T. F., Lacouture, P. G., & Lovejoy, F. H. (1990). Iron. In L. M. Haddad & J. F. Winchester (Eds.), *Clinical management of poisoning and drug overdose* (3rd ed., pp. 1010–1017). Philadelphia: W. B. Saunders.

Fine, J. S., & Goldfrank, L. R. (1992). Update in medical toxicology. *Pediatric Clinics of North America, 39,* 1031–1051.

Fleisher, G. R., Kearney, T. E., Henretig, F., & Tenenbein, M. (1991). Gastric decontamination in the poisoned patient. *Pediatric Emergency Care, 7,* 378–381.

Goldfrank, L. R., Lewin, N. A., & Flomenbaum, N. E. (1990). Cyclic antidepressants. In L. R. Goldfrank, N. E. Flomenbaum, N. A. Lewin, R. S. Weisman, & M. A. Howland (Eds.). *Goldfrank's toxicologic emergencies* (4th ed., pp. 401–412). Norwalk, CT: Appleton & Lange.

Haddad, L. M., & Roberts, J. R. (1990). A general approach to the emergency management of poisoning. In L. M. Haddad & J. F. Winchester (Eds.), *Clinical management of poisoning and drug overdose* (3rd ed., pp. 2–21). Philadelphia: W. B. Saunders.

Harchelroad, F. C., Clark, R. F., & Dean, B. (1990). Treated versus reported toxic exposures: Discrepancies between a poison control center and a member hospital. *Veterinary and Human Toxicology, 32,* 156–159.

Harris, C. R., & Kingston, R. (1992). Gastrointestinal decontamination: Which method is best? *Postgraduate Medicine, 92,* 116–128.

He, G., Zhang, A., Altura, B. T., & Altura, B. M. (1993). Cocaine-induced cerebrovasospasm and its possible mechanism of action. *Journal of Pharmacology and Experimental Therapeutics, 268,* 1532–1539.

Henretig, F. M., & Shannon, M. (1993). Toxicologic emergencies. In G. R. Fleisher & S. Ludwig (Eds.), *Textbook of pediatric emergency medicine* (3rd ed., pp. 745–801). Baltimore: Williams & Wilkins.

Hoffman, R. (1992). Choices in gastric decontamination. *Emergency Medicine, 24*(10), 212–224.

Hoffman, J. R., Votey, S. R., Bayer, M., & Silver, L. (1993). Effect of hypertonic sodium bicarbonate in the treatment of moderate-to-severe cyclic antidepressant overdose. *American Journal of Emergency Medicine, 11,* 336–341.

Hoffman R., Henry, G. C., Howland, M. A., et al. (1992). Association between life-threatening cocaine toxicity and plasma cholinesterase activity. *Annals of Emergency Medicine, 21,* 247–253.

Holland, R. W., Marx, J. A., Earnest, M. P., & Ranniger, S. (1992). Grand-mal seizures temporally related to cocaine use: Clinical and diagnostic features. *Annals of Emergency Medicine, 21,* 772–776.

House, M. A. (1992). Cardiovascular effects of cocaine. *Journal of Cardiovascular Nursing, 6*(2), 1–11.

Hultén, B. A., Adams, R., Askenasi, R., et al. (1992). Predicting severity of tricyclic antidepressant overdose. *Clinical Toxicology, 30,* 161–170.

Kalsner, S. (1993). Cocaine sensitization of coronary artery contractions: Mechanism of drug-induced spasm. *Journal of Pharmacology and Experimental Therapeutics, 268,* 1132–1140.

Kapur, S., Mieczkowski, T., & Mann, J. J. (1992). Antidepressant medications and the relative risk of suicide attempt and suicide. *Journal of the American Medical Association, 268,* 2441–3445.

Kloner, R. A., Hale, S., Alker, K., & Rezkalla, S. (1992). The effects of acute and chronic cocaine use on the heart. *Circulation, 85,* 407–419.

Klonoff, D. C., Andrews, B. T., & Obana, W. G. (1989). Stroke associated with cocaine use. *Archives of Neurology, 46,* 989–993.

Krenzelok, E. P., & Dunmire, S. M. (1992). Acute poisoning emergencies. *Postgraduate Medicine, 91,* 170–186.

Krause, D. S., Wolf, B. A., & Shaw, L. M. (1992). Acute aspirin overdose: Mechanisms of toxicity. *Therapeutic Drug Monitoring, 14,* 441–451.

Krisanda, T. J. (1993). Flumazenil: An antidote for benzodiazepine toxicity. *American Family Physician, 47,* 891–895.

Levine, S. R., Brust, J. C. M., Futrell, N., et al. (1991). A comparative study of the cerebrovascular complications of cocaine: Alkaloidal versus hydrochloride—a review. *Neurology, 41,* 1173–1177.

Linakis, J. G., & Frederick, K. A. (1993). Poisoning deaths not reported to the Regional Poison Control Center. *Annals of Emergency Medicine, 22,* 1822–1828.

Litovitz, T. L., Holm, K. C., Clancy, C., et al. (1993). 1992 Annual report of the American Association of Poison Control Centers Toxic Exposure Surveillance System. *American Journal of Emergency Medicine, 11,* 494–555.

Lovejoy, F. H., Shannon, M., & Woolf, A. D. (1992). Recent advances in clinical toxicology. *Current Problems in Pediatrics, 22,* 119–129.

Lowenstein, D. H., Massa S. M., & Rowbotham, M. C. (1987). Acute neurologic and psychiatric complications associated with cocaine abuse. *American Journal of Medicine, 83,* 841–846.

Makosiej, F. J., Hoffman, R. S., Howland, M. A., & Goldfrank, L. R. (1993). An *in vitro* evaluation of cocaine hydrochloride adsorption by activated charcoal and desorption upon addition of polyethylene glycol electrolyte lavage solution. *Clinical Toxicology, 31,* 381–395.

Mathewson-Kuhn, M. (1992). Drug overdose: Salicylates. *Critical Care Nurse,* 12(1), 16–27.

McFarland, A. K., & Chyka, P. A. (1993). Selection of activated charcoal products for the treatment of poisonings. *Annals of Pharmacotherapy, 27,* 358–361.

Merigian, K. S., Woodard, M., Hedges, J. R., et al. (1990). Prospective evaluation of gastric emptying in the self-poisoned patient. *American Journal of Emergency Medicine, 8,* 479–483.

Mills, K. C., & Curry, S. C. (1994). Acute iron poisoning. *Emergency Medicine Clinics of North America, 12,* 397–413.

Moliterno, D. J., Willard, J. E., Lange, R. A., et al. (1994). Coronary-artery vasoconstriction induced by cocaine, cigarette smoking or both. *New England Journal of Medicine, 330,* 454–459.

Mueller, P. D., Benowitz, N. L., & Olson, K. R. (1990). Cocaine. *Emergency Aspects of Drug Abuse, 8,* 481–493.

National Institute on Drug Abuse (NIDA). (1993). Epidemiologic trends in drug abuse: Community Epidemiologic Work Group. In *Proceedings of the June 1993 meeting* (NIH Publication No. 93-3645). Washington, DC: U.S. Government Printing Office.

Newcomb, P. (1991). Tricyclic antidepressants and children. *Nurse Practitioner: American Journal of Primary Health Care,* 16(5), 26, 28, 30.

Newton, E. H., Shih, R. D., & Hoffman, R. S. (1994). Cyclic antidepressant overdose: A review of current management strategies. *American Journal of Emergency Medicine, 12,* 376–379.

Olson, K. R., Kearney, T. E., Dyer, J. E., Benowitz, N. L., & Blanc, P. D. (1993). Seizures associated with poisoning and drug overdose. *American Journal of Emergency Medicine, 11,* 565–568.

Pentel, P. R., Keyler, D. E., & Haddad, L. M. (1990). Tricyclic and newer antidepressants. In L. M. Haddad & J. F. Winchester (Eds.), *Clinical management of poisoning and drug overdose* (3rd ed., pp. 636–653). Philadelphia: W. B. Saunders.

Pimentel, L., & Trommer, L. (1994). Cyclic antidepressant overdoses: A review. *Emergency Medicine Clinics of North America, 12,* 533–547.

Pond, S. (1990). Principle of techniques used to enhance elimination of toxic compounds. In L. R. Goldfrank, N. E. Flomenbaum, M. A. Lewin, R. S. Weisman, & M. A. Howland (Eds.), *Goldfrank's toxicologic emergencies* (4th ed., pp. 21–28). Norwalk, CT: Appleton & Lange.

Proudfoot, A. T. (1990). Salicylates and salicylamides. In L. M. Haddad & J. F. Winchester (Eds.), *Clinical management of poisoning and drug overdose* (3rd ed., pp. 909–920). Philadelphia: W. B. Saunders.

Pruchnicki, S. (1991). Just say know: Recognizing the dangers of commonplace drugs. *Journal of Emergency Medical Services,* 16(2), 26–42.

Ritz, M. C., & George, F. R. (1993). Cocaine-induced seizures and lethality appear to be associated with distinct central nervous system binding sites. *Journal of Pharmacology and Experimental Therapeutics, 264,* 1333–1343.

Roberts, J. R., & Tafuri, J. A. (1990). Benzodiazepines. In L. M. Haddad & J. F. Winchester (Eds.), *Clinical management of poisoning and drug overdose* (3rd ed., pp. 800–820). Philadelphia: W. B. Saunders.

Spiller, H. A., Krenzelok, E. P., Grande, G. A., Safir, E. F., & Diamond, J. J. (1994). A prospective evaluation of the effect of activated charcoal before oral N-acetylcysteine in acetaminophen overdose. *Annals of Emergency Medicine, 23,* 519–523.

Sporer, K. A. (1993). Whole-bowel irrigation in the management of ingested poisoning. *Western Journal of Medicine, 159,* 601.

Stein, M. D., Bonanno, J., O'Sullivan, P. S., & Wachtel, T. J. (1993). Changes in the pattern of drug overdoses. *Journal of General Internal Medicine,* 8(4), 179–184.

Sugarman, J. M., & Paul, R. I. (1994). Flumazenil: A review. *Pediatric Emergency Care, 10,* 37–43.

Tandberg, D., & Murphy, L. C. (1989). The knee chest position does not improve the efficacy of ipecac-induced emesis. *American Journal of Emergency Medicine, 7,* 267–270.

Tenenbein, M., Wiseman, N., & Yatscoff, R. W. (1991). Gastrotomy and whole bowel irrigation in iron poisoning. *Pediatric Emergency Care, 7,* 286–288.

United States Department of Commerce, Economics & Statistics Administration, & Bureau of Census. (1992). *Statistical abstract of the United States* (112th ed., Table 197. Drug use, by type of drug and age group: 1974 to 1991; and Table 198. Users of selected drugs, by user characteristic: 1991). Lanham, MD: Bernan Press.

Washton, A. M., & Gold, M. S. (1987). Recent trends in cocaine abuse as seen from the "800-COCAINE" hotline. In A. M. Washton & M. S. Gold (Eds). *Cocaine: A clinician's handbook* (pp. 10–22). New York: Guilford Press.

Wax, P. M., Wang, R. Y., Hoffman, R. S., et al. (1993). Prevalence of sorbitol in multiple-dose activated charcoal regimens in emergency departments. *Annals of Emergency Medicine, 22,* 1807–1812.

Westlake, C., & Funkhouser, S. W. (1990). Cardiovascular effects of recreational cocaine abuse. *AACN Clinical Issues in Critical Care Nursing, 1,* 65–71.

Winchester, J. F. (1990). Active methods for detoxification. In L. M. Haddad & J. F. Winchester (Eds.), *Clinical management of poisoning and drug overdose* (3rd ed., pp. 148–165). Philadelphia: W. B. Saunders.

Yip, L., Dart, R. C., & Gabow, P. A. (1994). Concepts and controversies in salicylate toxicity. *Emergency Medicine Clinics of North America, 12,* 351–364.

Young, W. F., & Bivins, H. G. (1993). Evaluation of gastric emptying using radionuclides: Gastric lavage versus ipecac-induced emesis. *Annals of Emergency Medicine, 22,* 1423–1427.

UNIT 14

CLINICAL SITUATIONS

Alterations in Thermoregulation

Richard Henker

The process of thermoregulation maintains the body temperature at approximately 36.8°C, but normal temperature variation ranges from an average low of 37.2°C, which usually occurs early in the morning, to 37.7°C, which usually occurs late in the afternoon (Mackowiak et al., 1992). When body temperature is not maintained within this narrow range, detrimental effects occur, causing stress on other body systems.

ANATOMY AND PHYSIOLOGY OF THERMOREGULATION

The human body maintains a normal temperature range, despite the wide variety of temperatures in the environment, by using effector mechanisms that cause heat gain or heat loss. Mechanisms the body uses to maintain body temperature include shivering, sweating, and changes in skin blood flow. The key to thermoregulation is that heat loss must equal heat gain. If effector mechanisms are impaired there will be alterations in thermoregulation, causing increases or decreases in body temperature.

Core body temperature is usually considered to be the temperature of the internal organs. The best indicator of core temperature is often considered to be the temperature of the blood because blood perfuses the central organs. There are situations, however, where blood temperature may not reflect the tissue temperatures in the core.

There is some variability in temperature within the core. There are differences in temperature of the blood entering and leaving various organs. The difference between arterial and venous blood temperature depends on blood flow in the organ. If there is high flow, the temperature gradient is less than if there is low flow. In low-flow states, more oxygen is consumed and the blood carries away more heat than in the high-flow state.

The shell is the tissue surrounding the core that is exposed to variations in environmental temperature and provides insulation of the core. The insulating properties of the shell are modified by the changes in skin blood flow that occur as part of the skin blood flow reflex. When the skin is exposed to cold air the skin blood flow decreases, therefore increasing the amount of insulation around the core. When exposure to heat occurs the cutaneous vasculature vasolidates, decreasing the amount of insulation around the core and promoting heat loss.

Heat Loss

Convection, radiation, conduction, and evaporation are four mechanisms involved in heat loss from the body. Conduction is the heat transferred between two physical objects, such as a patient and a gurney. Heat travels from the warmer object to the colder object. The amount of heat lost depends on the difference in temperature between the two objects; therefore, the cooler the gurney the greater the heat loss (Boulant, 1991; Brengelmann, 1989).

Convection is the amount of heat that is carried away from the body by gases or liquids. As air around an individual heats, the air rises, only to expose the skin to new, colder air. Convective heat loss is increased with any high-activity movement such as running or bicycling. Convective heat loss is the basis for the development of wind chill indices. Increased air movement takes the heat away at a faster rate. Convective heat loss is greater in the water because water is a better conductor of heat than air, and therefore individuals in water lose heat more rapidly than individuals at the same air temperature (Boulant, 1991; Brengelmann, 1989).

Radiant heat loss is the amount of heat transferred through electromagnetic waves. Radiant heat is lost or gained from surrounding surfaces depending on the temperature of those surfaces (Boulant, 1991; Brengelmann, 1989). Even though the ambient temperature may be low in an operating room, radiant heat is transferred to the patient from the lights in the room.

Evaporation is another means by which heat is lost. Humans, unlike many mammals, sweat. As the water on the skin evaporates, heat is lost. A phenomenon called hidromeiosis occurs when humidity is high in the environment: sweat builds up on the skin and does not evaporate, and therefore heat is not lost through evaporation (Boulant, 1991; Brengelmann, 1989). A person working out on a hot, humid day does not lose heat as readily as on a hot, dry day.

Heat is also lost through the lungs by conduction, convection, and evaporation. Air that is breathed in is warmed by the pharynx and the tracheobronchial tree on inspiration. Heat transfer to the air occurs because of the temperature gradient between tissue and air. As the air moves into the lungs, air temperature increases (McFadden, 1992). Because the air temperature in the alveoli is higher than the tissue temperature of the upper airways, heat is transferred to the tissues during expiration. Air temperature decreases as it travels out of the airways to approximately 32°C to 33°C (McFadden, 1992).

Sensation of Temperature

Specific types and numbers of thermoreceptors have been found in particular areas of the skin. Overall, cold thermoreceptors outnumber warm thermoreceptors. The greatest concentration of cold thermoreceptors is found in the lips, other parts of the face, chest, abdomen, forearm, and the back of the hand. The greatest concentration of warm receptors is in the face, fingers, and nose (Hensel, 1981). Thermoreceptors are also thought to exist in deeper tissues such as the central nervous system (CNS), blood vessels, and the abdominal cavity, although little evidence is available in humans to support this claim (Brengelmann, 1989; Hensel, 1981).

Integration of Sensation and Effector Mechanisms for Thermoregulation

Thermal signals from the skin and core are primarily integrated in the posterior hypothalamus. There is also evidence for integration of thermal signals in the spinal cord, medulla, and preoptic anterior hypothalamus (Boulant, 1991; Hensel, 1981). Thirty to 40% of the neurons in the hypothalamus sense temperature, although most of the thermosensitive neurons in the hypothalamus are warm sensitive (Boulant, 1986). Core temperature and skin temperature influence the effector system activation, but core temperature is more influential in terms of the effector mechanism response (Wyss et al., 1974).

Thermoregulatory Effector Mechanisms

Mechanisms of maintaining temperature with a normal range include shivering, cutaneous vasomotor control, and sweating. Activation of specific effector mechanisms depends on core and skin temperature levels.

SHIVERING. The primary means of heat production in humans exposed to cold is shivering. Shivering, which is controlled by the motor pathways, is the rhythmic contraction of skeletal muscles (Boulant, 1991; Hensel, 1981). Shivering increases core temperature but at the expense of an increase in metabolic rate that is comparable to aerobic exercise (Holtzclaw, 1990). Shivering is not an all-or-none phenomenon. Shivering is first apparent in the masseter muscles, then involves the trunk, then the long muscles, and finally includes teeth chattering (Tikuisis et al., 1991). Muscles that contribute the most to heat production during shivering are the central trunk muscles (Bell et al., 1992). Tikuisis and colleagues (1991) found that leaner people were more likely to shiver when exposed to cold.

VASOMOTOR CONTROL. If a person is exposed to cold, the skin blood flow decreases, providing greater insulation. When exposed to a warm environment, the skin blood flow increases and more heat is lost. Changes in skin blood flow are influenced by local skin temperature and core temperature (Johnson et al., 1976). The amount of skin blood flow can vary from 0.5 to 7.8 liters/minute, depending on core and skin temperatures (Rowell, 1974).

Local skin blood flow reflex can sometimes have undesirable effects on core temperature. Cooling the body can cause a rise in core temperature due to increased body insulation from decreased skin blood flow (Henker, 1993). Warming after the body has been cooled causes a phenomenon termed "after-drop" (Giesbrecht & Bristow, 1992; Henker, 1993). After-drop occurs when skin blood flow increases to the cool peripheral tissues during warming of the skin. Blood temperature decreases as the blood moves through the cool peripheral tissues. As the cooled blood moves from the core to the periphery, core temperature decreases, causing an after-drop (Henker, 1993). Figure 67–1 provides an example of afterdrop.

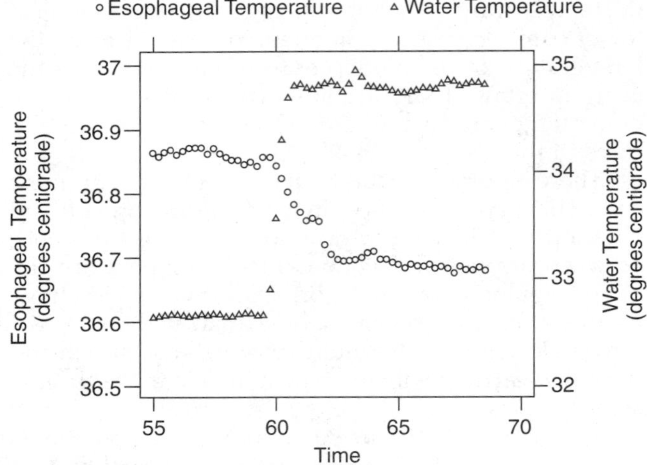

FIGURE 67–1. An example of afterdrop that occurred in a subject warmed after 50 minutes of cooling in a laboratory setting.

SWEATING. Sweating provides an additional method for heat loss, but at the expense of hypotonic fluid loss. The amount of sweat produced in marathon runners is greater than 1 liter/hour, and has been shown to be as great as 1.8 liters/minute in some people during intense exercise (Gisolfi & Copping, 1974; Pugh et al., 1967). If fluid loss is greater than 1% to 2% of the total body weight, sweating is inhibited and heat loss is decreased (Brengelmann, 1989). Sweating is controlled by the sympathetic pathways of the autonomic nervous system (Brengelmann, 1989). Sweating initially starts in the legs and moves up the body (Hensel, 1981).

REGULATED CHANGES IN BODY TEMPERATURE: FEVER

Fever is a regulated rise in body temperature that is a host defense response to infection. McGowan and colleagues (1987) reported the incidence of fever in hospitalized patients to be 29%. In a study of 971 patients admitted to a medical service that included the critically ill, fever developed in 36% of the patients during their hospital stay (Bor et al., 1988).

Pathophysiology

Fever is initiated by exogenous pyrogens such as endotoxin, gram-positive cell wall, fungi, and viruses that cross through breaks in the skin and mucosal barriers (Atkins, 1964). As shown in Figure 67–2, the exogenous pyrogens stimulate the production of endogenous pyrogens, predominantly by macrophages and monocytes. Although the term "exogenous pyrogens" indicates that fever-causing agents are from the exterior of the body, this is not always the case. Antigen–antibody complex from blood transfusion reactions, complement components from burns and trauma, and lymphocyte products from neoplasms also stimulate the production of endogenous pyrogens.

Endogenous pyrogens are proteins that stimulate the production of prostaglandins by the arachidonic acid cascade. Endogenous pyrogens involved in fever generation include interleukin-1, interleukin-2, interleukin-6, tumor necrosis factor, and interferon. Endogenous pyrogens act on the arachidonic acid cascade by increasing the amount of arachidonic acid available and increasing the amount of cyclooxygenase available for conversion of arachidonic acid to prostaglandins and leukotrienes (Dinarello & Wolff, 1988; Kluger, 1991).

Mediators produced by the arachidonic acid cascade that are thought to have an effect on thermoregulation include prostaglandin E_2, prostaglandin E_1, and thromboxane A_2. The mediator most likely to be involved in fever generation, prostaglandin E_2, decreases the firing rate of the heat-sensing neurons in the hypothalamus (Coceani, 1991). The change in thermoregulation in the hypothalamus is termed a rise in set point. Thermoregulatory functions are stimulated to attain a higher temperature equal to the new set point (Cabanac & Massonnet, 1974; Cooper et al., 1964). Effector mechanisms activated to attain this higher temperature include vasoconstriction and possibly shivering. Behavioral changes also occur to attain this elevated set point. Febrile people will increase insulation with a blanket, and put skin surfaces together to decrease heat loss (Hart, 1988).

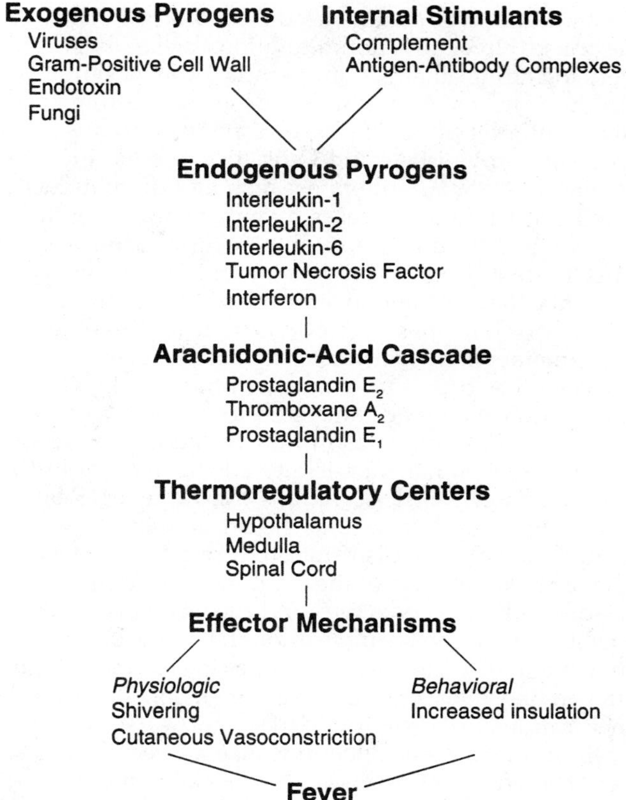

FIGURE 67–2. Fever generation. (From Henker, R. [1993]. Fever in the critically ill. *Critical Care Nursing Currents, 11*[2], 5–8.)

Clinical Presentation

Physiologic manifestations of fever include increased core temperature, changes in the cardiopulmonary state, increased metabolic rate, and enhanced host defense. A number of studies have been performed in which an exogenous pyrogen (e.g., endotoxin, bacteria) has been administered with a subsequent generation of fever (Moser et al., 1963; Revhaug et al., 1988; Suffredini et al., 1989). In one study, 13 healthy subjects who where injected with endotoxin had a mean rise in rectal temperature to 38.5°C. Accompanying physiologic responses included an increased oxygen consumption, increased heart rate, increased serum norepinephrine levels, and increased serum epinephrine levels (Revhaug et al., 1988).

In addition to cardiovascular and stress hormone responses, liver function alterations occur during fever, including changes in hepatic protein synthesis. Production of serum albumin decreases during fever and synthesis of acute-phase response proteins such as serum amyloid A- and C-reactive protein increase (Dinarello, 1989). Acute-phase response proteins facilitate host defense responses by enhancing recognition of foreign substances and enhancing the function of effector cells such as polymorphonuclear leukocytes, lymphocytes, and monocytes (Gotschlich, 1989). Production of enzymes in the liver that are involved in drug metabolism is also altered during fever.

Fever has been shown to alter pharmacokinetics of medications being administered to patients by a variety of mechanisms. Absorption of medications from the gastrointestinal tract is altered by changes in the production of gastric secretions during fever. Release of protein-bound drugs into the extravascular tissue is thought to enhance distribution during fever. Metabolism and elimination of medications during fever varies depending on enzymes and mechanisms used for metabolism of each drug. Although hepatic blood flow may increase during fever, changes in enzyme production in the liver may decrease metabolism of some medications (Mackowiak, 1991).

Immune system function is also altered during fever. The effects of fever as a beneficial component of host defense have been discussed since the time of Hippocrates (Atkins, 1984). The host defense response to infection includes a complex array of mediators and mechanisms, so it is difficult to determine if fever alone is beneficial for survival. Some animal studies have found that the ability to develop fever has been related to survival (Vaughn et al., 1974, 1980). Studies of human cells in vitro at various temperatures have found that elevated temperatures have been beneficial for some immune responses such as activation of monocytes and enhanced T-lymphocyte responses, but elevated temperatures has also been found to dampen natural killer cell activity (Dinarello et al., 1986; Roberts, 1991).

Clinical Management

Pharmacologic management of patients varies between health care providers. Ideally, the level of body temperature depends on the patient's clinical presentation. Patients unable to tolerate the stress of an increase in metabolic rate (i.e., cardiac or pulmonary disease) may have orders to administer antipyretics at lower levels (Kluger, 1986). Patients in relatively good health my benefit from the boost in host defense from fever; therefore, treatment at higher body temperatures may be best for this group of patients (Kluger, 1986).

The mechanism of action of antipyretics varies depending on the medication. Corticosteroids, which are not often thought of as antipyretics, stimulate the production of an inhibitor of phospholipase A2. Phospholipase A2 is an enzyme involved in arachidonic acid production. Nonsteroidal antiinflammatory agents such as aspirin, ibuprofen, and indomethacin act as cyclooxygenase inhibitors. Cyclooxygenase is the enzyme that converts arachidonic acid to prostaglandins (Fantone & Ward, 1994; Holtzclaw, 1992). Acetaminophen, unlike the other agents used as antipyretics, has minimal antiinflammatory properties. The mechanism of action of acetaminophen is still uncertain, but it is thought to inhibit cyclooxygenase production in the CNS (Bannwarth et al., 1992).

Cold application is a therapeutic intervention often used for the treatment of fever. Cooling blankets, ice packs, fans, tepid baths, and cool ambient temperature have been used to return body temperature back to normal to prevent sequelae due to fever. However, the application of physical cooling may invoke an augmented stress response in an already compromised state. Although physical cooling is used to decrease body temperature during fever, it is thought to be illogical because the process opposes the drive and input to effector mechanisms that are actively raising the body temperature (Clark, 1991; Styrt & Sugarman, 1990).

Studies evaluating responses to cooling in febrile subjects have varied results. Morgan (1990) evaluated antipyretics, antipyretics with sponging, and antipyretics with a cooling blanket in febrile patients with neurologic deficits. Time for the body temperature to fall to 100°F did not differ significantly between the three groups. Shivering was found to occur in four of the seven patients in whom a cooling blanket was applied. Newman (1985) evaluated the effects of sponging children with fever seen in an emergency department. One group received acetaminophen alone and a second group received acetaminophen and sponging. There was no significant difference in the rate of temperature decrease between the two groups. In a study reported by Steele and colleagues (1970), physical cooling was found to decrease body temperature in febrile children. Acetaminophen and sponging with water at 4.4°C to 10.0°C was significantly more effective in decreasing temperature in febrile children than acetaminophen or sponging alone.

Various temperature levels have been tested in terms of the most efficient means to reduce body temperature and the most comfortable means to cool subjects. Caruso and coworkers (1992) used four cooling blanket temperatures (7.2°C, 12.8°C, 18.3°C, and 23.9°C) in addition to antipyretics to reduce rectal temperature in febrile, critically ill subjects. The various cooling blanket temperatures did not make any difference in the rate at which patients cooled, but the blanket temperature of 7.2°C was found to be significantly less comfortable than the temperatures of 18.3°C or 23.9°C.

Fever in the Elderly

Clinical presentation of infection in the elderly is atypical and often results in delayed treatment with increased morbidity and mortality. Fever is not as prevalent an indicator of infection in the elderly as in younger people. Gleckman and Hibert (1982) reported a greater incidence of afebrile bacteremia in elderly patients. Evaluation for bacteremia in elderly hospitalized subjects was pursued because of symptoms other than fever, including changes in metal state or respiratory status. Keating and associates (1984) evaluated patient outcomes in four age groups with fever greater than 38.3°C. Greater age was associated with more serious disease and life-threatening outcomes.

Age-related changes in thermoregulation may affect identification of fever in the elderly. In a study evaluating circadian rhythm in elderly patients in an intermediate care facility, mean temperature (36.7°C) was found to be lower than the mean temperature reported for younger subjects (Davis & Lentz, 1989). Because of this lower mean temperature in the elderly, fever does not occur at levels normally seen in the general population. In addition to changes in average temperature, the ability to vasoconstrict and conserve heat decreases with age, diminishing the elderly person's capacity for development of a fever (Kenney, 1988).

Fever in the Immunocompromised

Surprisingly, fever can be generated by even the most severely immunocompromised patient. Endogenous pyrogens are produced by such a wide variety of cells in the body that even with diminished immune system function fever can still develop in most immunocompromised patients. Conditions where this is not true include patients receiving corticosteroids, patients with end-stage AIDS, and patients with uremia (Hibberd & Rubin, 1991).

Health care provider responses to fever in the immunocompromised patient include a more aggressive approach. Bacterial infections can progress rapidly and therefore antibiotics are usually started when fever develops. Criteria for initiation of antibiotic therapy in immunocompromised patients are a rise in temperature to greater than 38.5°C, or two rises in temperatures to greater than 38.0°C within a 12-hour period (Weinberger, 1993). Once fever has developed, it is important to identify the source and type of infection. Blood cultures are drawn and potential sites of infection are assessed.

NONREGULATED CHANGES IN BODY TEMPERATURE

Elevation in body temperature during fever is considered a regulated rise in temperature due to the elevation in set point that occurs during fever. Many of the clinical problems discussed in the following sections are considered nonregulated changes in body temperature. Nonregulated changes in temperature occur as a result of the person's inability to adapt to thermal stress. The inability to maintain thermal balance is due to personal characteristics that alter the individual's ability to thermoregulate. Examples of these include age, genetic predisposition, medications, and disease states. In addition, environmental stress may be so great that the person is unable to thermoregulate properly.

Accidental Hypothermia

Hypothermia is often thought to be a condition that occurs only in colder climates during the winter, but hypothermia can occur any time of the year, and cases of hypothermia have been reported in warmer climates. Deaths due to hypothermia are often underreported because of contributing conditions that may be exacerbated with exposure to cold (Hector, 1992; Jolly & Ghezzi, 1992).

PATHOPHYSIOLOGY

Risk factors for hypothermia include a wide variety of components, such as age, clinical conditions, medications, and recreational activities.

The very young and very old are at risk for accidental hypothermia because of their decreased ability to adapt to cold environments. Infants have a high body surface-to-mass ratio, which encourages greater heat loss than heat production. The elderly have a decreased metabolic rate, which means that less heat is produced. The elderly also have a decreased sympathetic vasoconstrictor response to body cooling that limits their ability to conserve heat (Khan et al., 1992).

Clinical conditions affect a person's ability to maintain thermal balance. Patients with diabetes mellitus may be unable to conserve heat due to autonomic neuropathy, which affects their ability to vasoconstrict in a cold environment (Scott et al., 1986). Malnourished and starved people have decreased heat production (Jolly & Ghezzi, 1992). Subjects who did not receive food for 48 hours were found to have a decreased ability to vasoconstrict in response to cold application (Mansell & MacDonald, 1989). Trauma patients are often at risk for the development of hypothermia due to long extrication times, administration of intravenous fluids, and hypothalamic injury (Lawson, 1992). Patients with burn wounds are also at risk for hypothermia. Increased loss of heat through the burn wound occurs due to the loss of the insulating effects of the skin (Jolly & Ghezzi, 1992). Patients with metabolic conditions such as hypothyroidism also have a decreased ability to generate heat and are more likely to contract hypothermia (Jolly & Ghezzi, 1992). Sepsis is a condition that causes vasodilation. The septic patient's ability to conserve heat is impaired; even though patients are hypermetabolic and have an elevated hypothalamic set point, they are unable to conserve heat.

Medications also decrease the ability to maintain body temperature during cold stress. The two main effects of medications on thermoregulation are (1) a decrease in the ability to generate heat, and (2) a decrease in the ability to conserve heat. Examples of medications that decrease the ability to generate heat include paralytic agents and phenothiazines. Medications that decrease the ability to vasoconstrict include barbiturates, beta blockers, and vasodilating agents such as sodium nitroprusside (Chinyanga, 1984; Jolly & Ghezzi, 1992; Reed & Krentz, 1992). Ethanol, a frequently used recreational drug, is a major contributing factor to hypothermia. Ethanol depresses the CNS, impairs judgment, vasodilates cutaneous vasculature, and provides the user with a feeling of warmth. For these reasons, ethanol is a major contributing factor in death from what is termed "urban hypothermia" (Granberg, 1991a).

Outdoor activities, where relief is hours away and changes in weather can occur quickly, can put hikers at risk for hypothermia. Rescue of people in remote locations can be difficult and time consuming, complicating the treatment of hypothermia (Jolly & Ghezzi, 1992).

CLINICAL PRESENTATION

Measurement of body temperature in patients with hypothermia usually requires a cold-recording rectal thermometer. Most clinical thermometers normally used to measure body temperature in the clinical setting do not have sufficient range to determine body temperature in hypothermic subjects. An accurate measure of temperature helps to determine the means of treatment for the hypothermic patient. As described in Table 67–1, hypothermia can be defined as mild, moderate, or severe.

Initial vasoconstriction due to cold exposure increases blood pressure, central fluid volume, heart rate, and cardiac output. As a person's temperature decreases, heart rate decreases and cardiac output also drops. At body temperatures lower than 32°C, blood pressure is diminished and atrial and ventricular arrhythmias are common. Death often occurs at temperature lower than 28°C due to ventricular asystole or ventricular fibrillation (Bjornstad et al., 1991; MacKenzie et al., 1991; Refsum, 1991).

Acid–base alterations in hypothermic patients may include respiratory and metabolic abnormalities. Shivering increases the production of lactic acid. When this is combined with decreased tissue perfusion due to vasoconstriction, metabolic acidosis occurs. Respiratory depression due to concomitant effects of CNS depressants can lead to respiratory acidosis (Jolly & Ghezzi, 1992; Reed & Krentz, 1992). Jolly & Ghezzi (1992) suggest that correction of arterial blood gases for body temperature is inappropriate for hypothermic patients because uncorrected blood gases give a better indication of pH.

TABLE 67–1. **Definition of Hypothermia**

Mild: 32°C–35°C (89.6°F–95°F)
Moderate: 28°C–32°C (82.4°F–89.6°F)
Severe: <28°C (<82.4°F)

Decreased body temperature also affects coagulation. Although trauma patients in hypovolemic shock often have coagulopathies due to increased calcium levels, transfusion of packed red blood cells, and dilution of coagulation factors and platelets, hypothermia has been reported to be a contributing factor to the coagulopathy that occurs in these patients (Rohrer & Natale, 1992).

As body temperature decreases, CNS function is depressed. Early CNS changes due to hypothermia include apathy and fatigue. As body temperature decreases further, judgment is impaired, hallucinations occur, and behavior becomes bizarre. Eventually hypothermia victims become comatose (Granberg, 1991b; Jolly & Ghezzi, 1991).

Urine output during cold exposure can double, due to a phenomenon known as "cold diuresis." The exact mechanism of cold diuresis is unknown, but it is thought to be due to the combination of a fluid shift from the periphery to the central circulation, increased excretion of sodium from the kidney, and decreased sensitivity to antidiuretic hormone (Reed & Krentz, 1992). The large amount of urine lost because of cold diuresis increases the viscosity of the blood (Granberg, 1991b).

CLINICAL MANAGEMENT

Treatment for hypothermia is classified as passive or active. Passive treatments include therapies such as removing the hypothermia victim from the cold environment, removing wet clothes, providing warm blankets, and providing warm fluids. Active treatments of hypothermia include administration of warmed intravenous fluids, application of warming blankets, irrigation of the peritoneum, irrigation of the mediastinum, rewarming of the airway, rewarming of the gastrointestinal tract, and rewarming with hemodialysis (Hector, 1992; Hernandez et al., 1993; Jolly & Ghezzi, 1992; Reed & Krentz, 1991). A new method, continuous arteriovenous rewarming, has been developed specifically for actively warming hypothermic patients. As shown in Figure 67–3, blood from the femoral artery flows throw a countercurrent heat exchanger and then flows back into the patient through the femoral vein (Gentilello et al., 1992). Passive therapies are more appropriate for patients with mild hypothermia; invasive therapies are reserved for patients with severe hypothermia.

Application of warming blankets to the skin is somewhat controversial because of the afterdrop that occurs during warming. When the skin is warmed, vasodilation occurs, and this increases blood flow through the cool peripheral tissues. As the blood from the periphery moves to the core, body temperature decreases. Afterdrop in hypothermic patients causes an additional decrease in core temperature (Giesbrecht & Bristow, 1992; Henker et al., 1993; Sterba, 1991). Appropriate nursing diagnoses for patients with hypothermia are listed in Table 67–2.

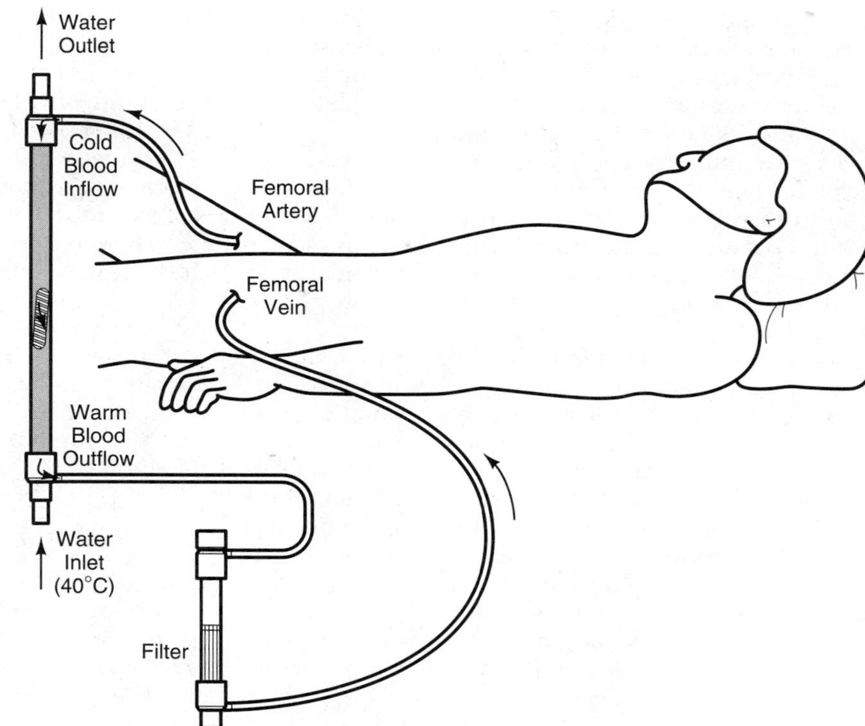

FIGURE 67–3. Countercurrent heat exchange is used to rapidly reverse the effects of hypothermia. (From Gentilello, L. M., et al. [1992]. Continuous arteriovenous rewarming: Rapid reversal of hypothermia in critically ill patients. *Journal of Trauma, 32,* 316–327. Copyright Williams & Wilkins.)

Heat Stroke

Heat stroke is an imbalance between heat gain or heat production, and heat loss (Knochel, 1989). Heat gain is an increased heat load applied to the body from the environment. Heat production is an increase in heat load that is endogenously produced, such as through exercise. Hyperthermia due to problems with heat loss results from the inability of the effector mechanism activity used during temperature elevation (e.g., sweating and cutaneous vasodilation) to keep up with the rate of heat production or heat gain.

Heat stroke is classified into two categories, classic and exertional (Goodman & Knochel, 1991). Classic heat stroke usually occurs in the very young, very old, or the chronically ill. Exertional heat stroke usually occurs in healthy people involved in physical activity.

PATHOPHYSIOLOGY

Typically, classic heat stroke victims are the urban elderly living in substandard housing without air conditioning (Hart et al., 1982). Heat in urban areas does not dissipate at night because of the release of heat from

TABLE 67–2. **Nursing Diagnoses for Patients With Nonregulated Changes in Body Temperature**

Hypothermia	Hyperthermia	Malignant Hyperthermia
Alteration in Thermoregulation: hypothermia	Alteration in Thermoregulation: hyperthermia	Alteration in Thermoregulation: hyperthermia
Alteration in Tissue Perfusion: peripheral tissue perfusion decreased	Alteration in Tissue Perfusion	Alteration in Tissue Perfusion
Decreased Cardiac Output	Alteration in Thought Processes: loss of consciousness	Alteration in Cardiac Rhythm
Alteration in Cardiac Rhythm	Alteration in Cardiac Rhythm	Acid–Base Imbalance
Acid–Base Imbalance	Acid–Base Imbalance	
Ineffective Breathing Pattern		
Alteration in Thought Processes		
Alteration in Urinary Elimination: increased		

buildings and streets (Knochel, 1989). The elderly are at risk for the development of heat stroke because of a decreased ability to lose heat. Autonomic function in the elderly is often impaired, affecting vasodilation of the cutaneous vasculature (Robbins, 1989).

Obesity impairs heat loss and is considered a risk factor for heat stroke. The body mass-to-surface area ratio in the obese is low, making it difficult for heat loss to keep up with heat production. Cardiovascular responses to heat in the obese are impaired. Heart rate increases more rapidly in obese than in lean people exposed to heat (Epstein, 1990).

Medications contribute to heat stroke in a variety of ways. Any medication causing cutaneous vasoconstriction decreases heat loss through the skin (Epstein, 1990). Antihistamines and tranquilizers depress sweat production (Goodman & Knochel, 1991). Hart and colleagues (1982) found that 9 of 28 patients admitted with heat stroke were taking diuretics. Diuretics decrease fluid volume, which inhibits sweating. Heat stroke is also associated with use of recreational drugs such as alcohol, amphetamines, and cocaine. Cocaine increases heat production and decreases heat loss by cutaneous vasoconstriction (Lomax & Daniel, 1993; Menashe & Gottlieb, 1988).

Unlike classic heat stroke, exertional heat stroke can occur in healthy, well conditioned people. Exertional heat stroke occurs when heat loss is less than endogenous heat production, and most commonly occurs in long-distance runners, football players, and military recruits (Costrini et al., 1979; Knochel, 1989; Wyndham, 1977). Occurrence of exertional heat stroke depends on climatic conditions. Warm, humid days increase the likelihood of heat stroke. Hydration is also directly linked to exertional heat stroke. Wyndham (1977) found that adequately hydrated marathron runners did not have heat stroke.

CLINICAL PRESENTATION

Manifestations of heat stroke include body temperature of at least 40.5°C (105°F), tissue injury, neurologic changes, and acid–base imbalance. Rhabdomyolysis is a frequent complication of heat stroke, and can lead to acute renal failure. Hart and colleagues (1982) found that creatine kinase (CK), an intracellular enzyme, was released in high quantities in 18 hyperthermic patients, indicating cellular damage. Amylase and aspartate aminotransferase levels were also found to be elevated in subjects.

Neurologic deficits are often present in heat stroke victims. In one study, 24 of 28 subjects admitted with heat stroke were comatose, and the remaining 4 were disoriented (Hart et al., 1982). Nineteen of 27 subjects in a second study were comatose, and the remaining 8 were disoriented (Tham et al., 1989). Most of the neurologic deficits found in the second study were not permanent.

Cardiovascular changes that occur during heat stroke include electrocardiogram (ECG) changes, tachycardia, and hypotension (Akhtar et al., 1993; Costrini et al., 1979). Costrini and coworkers (1979) reported that 7 of 13 heat stroke patients were hypotensive. All 13 patients were tachycardic, with an average heart rate of 144 beats per minute. Six of 12 heat stroke patients showed a prolonged QT interval that returned to normal within 12 to 24 hours. Two of the 12 ECGs were suggestive of ischemia, which eventually resolved in both patients.

The most frequent acid–base abnormality seen in heat stroke victims is respiratory alkalosis (Hart et al., 1982). Respiratory alkalosis is due to hyperventilation, which provides a means of heat loss. Metabolic acidosis also occurs in some heat stroke victims because of lactate production. High lactate levels may occur in classic heat stroke, but elevated lactate levels are consistently present in patients with exertional heat stroke (Goodman & Knochel, 1991).

CLINICAL MANAGEMENT

Successful treatment of heat stroke includes rapid identification of the problem and immediate treatment. Conventional therapy has been to place the heat stroke victim into a tub of ice-cold water; however, this has been associated with seizure activity (Goodman & Knochel, 1991). Goodman and Knochel (1991) suggest cooling by spraying the patient with tepid water and cooling with a fan. Warm air spray has been found to be one of the more effective methods of cooling because it does not promote cutaneous vasoconstriction. In a laboratory setting, Weiner and Khogali (1980) warmed six subjects by having them exercise on a bicycle in a plastic suit until a tympanic membrane temperature of 39.5°C was attained. Six methods of cooling were compared: water mattress, water bath, cold air spray, warm air spray at 25°C, warm air spray at 30°C, and warm air spray at 32°C to 33°C. The warm air spray at 32°C to 33°C was found to decrease core temperature at a rate of 0.30°C/minute, and the other five methods of cooling decreased core temperature from 0.13°C/minute to 0.19°C/minute. Kielblock and colleagues (1986) also compared methods of cooling after hyperthermia from exercise. Two methods of using ice packs and two methods of warm air spray were compared. Warm air spray alone decreased core temperature 1.0°C in 15.2 minutes, 28 ice packs covering the entire body decreased core temperature 1.0°C in 15.8 minutes, and a combination of six ice packs and warm air spray decreased core temperature 1.0°C in 13.2 minutes. This latter method has been used effectively for the annual 7-day pilgrimage to Mecca and in gold mines in South Africa (Kielblock et al., 1986). Potential nursing diagnoses for patients with hyperthermia are listed in Table 67–2.

Malignant Hyperthermia

Malignant hyperthermia (MH) is a hypercatabolic clinical syndrome that is usually observed during administration of general anesthesia. MH is an inherited defect in the intracellular control of calcium concentration in the muscle cell. Mortality from malignant hyperthermia has decreased to levels less than 10% due to the development of the medication, dantrolene (Gronert et al., 1990; Wlody, 1991).

PATHOPHYSIOLOGY

Volatile anesthetic agents such as halothane, enflurane, and isoflurane, and a neuromuscular blocking agent, succinyl choline, are usually the agents that trigger MH. Contraction of skeletal muscle occurs when calcium is released from the sarcoplasmic reticulum and binds to troponin. An abnormal calcium channel in the sarcoplasmic reticulum causes an abnormally high amount of mycoplasmic free calcium in people with MH. The MH triggers early release of calcium from the sarcoplasmic reticulum, causing increased skeletal muscle contraction. Skeletal muscle activity is increased, leading to heat production, and heat loss is diminished due to general anesthesia; therefore, core temperature increases. Dantrolene, the only drug used to treat MH, decreases the excitability of the calcium channel and decreases the myoplasmic free calcium concentration (Gronert et al., 1990; Lopez et al., 1992).

It is also possible that MH may be triggered by other events such as exercise, unusual stress, and fever. This is not well substantiated, but it may be a possibility for some unexplained sudden deaths (Goodman & Knochel, 1991; Gronert et al., 1990).

CLINICAL PRESENTATION

Indicators of MH include tachycardia, muscle rigidity, elevated body temperature, acidosis, and hyperkalemia. Muscle rigidity occurs due to the continuous skeletal muscle contraction. Acidosis is due to lactate production from skeletal muscle contraction. Hyperkalemia and elevated CK levels are caused by tissue damage that occurs from cell lysis due to hyperthermia.

CLINICAL MANAGEMENT

Ideally, MH is assessed before administration of anesthetic agents in the operating room. Assessments that may indicate a patient is at risk for MH include family history of death due to surgery or fever. Congenital musculoskeletal defects and primary diseases of the muscle may also be indicators of MH (Goodman & Knochel, 1991). Diagnostic tests used to identify MH include serum CK, which is often elevated in patients with MH, and a muscle biopsy. The muscle fragment is exposed to caffeine and halothane, and can be stimulated to contract at lower caffeine concentrations in people with MH (Goodman & Knochel, 1991; Wlody, 1991).

When MH occurs, the first action is to stop the trigger and administer 100% oxygen. Dantrolene is administered up to 10 mg/kg. The patient is cooled using iced irrigation of body cavities and cooling blankets. Tissue damage related to hyperthermia is evaluated by monitoring serum hemoglobin, serum myoglobin, and urine myoglobin. Prevention of acute tubular necrosis is achieved by fluid administration and monitoring urine output (Gronert et al., 1990). Potential nursing diagnoses for patients with malignant hyperthermia are listed in Table 67–2.

Neuroleptic Malignant Syndrome

Neuroleptic malignant syndrome (NMS) is a reaction to neuroleptic medications characterized by hyperthermia, muscular rigidity, autonomic dysfunction, and alteration of consciousness. Medications causing NMS include haloperidol, chlorpromazine, and lithium carbonate (Hooper et al., 1989).

Clinical presentation of NMS includes diaphoresis, unstable blood pressure, and tachycardia. Rhabdomyolysis occurs in some cases due to the continuous muscle contractions. Patients taking haloperidol may have decreased thirst, and therefore dehydration is often a

TABLE 67–3. **Comparison of Ear-Based Infrared Thermometers With Pulmonary Artery Thermistors**

Instrument	Mode	Authors	Mean Difference	SD of Difference	Correlation Coefficient
Core Check model 2090*	Core	Erickson & Kirklin (1993)	0.07	0.41	NR
Core Check model 2090*	Core	Erickson & Meyer (1994)	−0.1	0.48	0.88
First Temp Genius Model 3000A†	Core	Erickson & Meyer (1994)	0.1	0.49	0.88
Thermoscan Pro-1 Model IR-1‡	Unadjusted	Erickson & Meyer (1994)	0.48	0.52	0.91
Ototemp 3000 Model HTTS-3000§	Unadjusted	Erickson & Meyer (1994)	−0.7	0.53	0.88
Core Check model 2090*	Core	Henker & Coyne (in press)	0.3	0.57	−0.16
First Temp Genius Model 3000A†	Core	Henker & Coyne (in press)	−0.01	0.51	0.19
First Temp Genius Model 3000A†	Core	Klein et al. (1993)	0.42	0.37	0.91
First Temp†	NR	Shinozaki et al. (1988)	0.2–0.4		0.98

*IVAC Corporation, San Diego, California.
†Intelligent Medical Systems, Carlsbad, California.
‡Thermoscan, San Diego, California.
§Exergen Corporation, Newton, Massachusetts.
Abbreviations: NR, not reported; SD, standard deviation.

contribution factor to hyperthermia (Goodman & Knochel, 1991).

The first action for treating NMS is to discontinue the neuroleptic agent. Patients may also need to be rehydrated due to inadequate fluid intake from the effects of haloperidol on thirst. Medications given for treatment of NMS include dantrolene and bromocriptine, although the use of dantrolene is somewhat controversial (Rosebush et al., 1991).

SUMMARY

The critically ill are at risk for alterations in thermoregulation due to disease processes, medications, and the critical care environment. Monitoring and maintaining body temperature can prevent additional stress in critically ill patients already in a compromised state. New methods of monitoring body temperature that are more convenient are now available for use in the critically ill. Ear-based thermometers show some promise as an indicator of core temperature (see Table 67–3). More sophisticated methods of warming and cooling patients that use convection are now in use, in addition to more traditional methods of conductive warming and cooling. Awareness and prevention of potential complications due to alterations in thermoregulation will decrease the stress on critically ill patients already in a compromised state.

REFERENCES

Akhtar, M. J., Al-Nozha, M., Al-Harthi, S., & Nouh, M. S. (1993). Electrocardiographic abnormalities in patients with heat stroke. *Chest, 104,* 411–414.

Atkins, E. (1964). Elevation of body temperature in disease. *Annals of the New York Academy of Sciences, 121,* 26–30.

Atkins, E. (1984). Fever: The old and the new. *Journal of Infectious Diseases, 149,* 339–348.

Bannwarth, B., Netter, P., Lapicque, F., et al. (1992). Plasma and cerebrospinal fluid concentrations of paracetamol after a single intravenous dose of propacetamol. *British Journal of Clinical Pharmacology, 34,* 79–81.

Bell, D., Tiskuisis, P., & Jacobs, I. (1992). Relative intensity of muscular contraction during shivering. *Journal of Applied Physiology, 72,* 2336–2342.

Bjornstad, H., Tande, P. M., & Refsum, H. (1991). Cardiac electrophysiology during hypothermia: Implications for medical treatment. *Arctic Medical Research, 50*(Suppl 6), 71–75.

Bor, D. H., Makadon, H. J., Friedland, G., et al. (1988). Fever in hospitalized medical patients: Characteristics and significance. *American Journal of Medicine, 85*(3), 119–125.

Boulant, J. A. (1991). Thermoregulation. In P. Mackowiak (Ed.), *Fever: Basic mechanisms and management* (pp. 1–22). New York: Raven Press.

Brengelmann, G. L. (1989). Temperature regulation. In C. C. Teitz (Ed.), *Scientific foundations of sports medicine* (pp. 77–116). Toronto: B. C. Decker.

Cabanac, M., & Massonnet, B. (1974). Temperature regulation during fever: Change of set point or change of gain? A tentative answer from a behavioural study in man. *Journal of Physiology, 238,* 561–568.

Caruso, C. C., Hadley, B. J., Shukla, R., Frame, P., & Khoury, J. (1992). Cooling effects and comfort of four cooling blanket temperatures in humans with fever. *Nursing Research, 41*(2), 68–72.

Chinyanga, H. M. (1984). Temperature regulation and anesthesia. *Pharmacology and Therapeutics, 26,* 147–161.

Clark, W. G. (1991). Antipyretics. In P. Mackowiak (Ed.), *Fever: Basic mechanisms and management* (pp. 297–340). New York: Raven Press.

Coceani, F. (1991). Prostaglandins and fever: Facts and controversies. In P. Mackowiak (Ed.), *Fever: Basic mechanisms and management* (pp. 59–70). New York: Raven Press.

Cooper, K. E., Cranston, W. I., & Snell, E. S. (1964). Temperature regulation during fever in man. *Clinical Science, 27,* 345–356.

Costrini, A. M., Pitt, H. A., Gustafson, A. B., & Uddin, D. E. (1979). Cardiovascular and metabolic manifestations of heat stroke and severe heat exhaustion. *American Journal of Medicine, 66,* 296–302.

Davis, C., & Lentz, M. (1989). Circadian rhythms: Charting oral temperatures to spot abnormalities. *Journal of Gerontology Nursing, 15*(4), 34–39.

Dinarello, C. A., Cannon, S., & Wolff, S. M. (1988). New concepts on the pathogenesis of fever. *Reviews of Infectious Diseases, 10,* 168–189.

Dinarello, C. A., Dempsey, R. A., Allegretta, M., et al. (1986). Inhibitory effects of elevated temperature on human cytokine production and natural killer activity. *Cancer Research, 46,* 6236–6241.

Dinarello, C. A. (1989). Interleukin-1 and its biologically related cytokines. *Advances in Immunology, 44,* 153–205.

Epstein, Y. (1990). Heat intolerance: Predisposing factor or residual injury. *Medicine and Science in Sports and Exercise, 22*(1), 29–35.

Erickson, R. S., & Kirklin, S. K. (1993). Comparison of ear-based, bladder, oral, and axillary methods for core temperature measurement. *Critical Care Medicine, 21,* 1528–1534.

Erickson, R. S., & Meyer, L. T. (1994). Accuracy of infared ear thermometry and other temperature methods in adults. *American Journal of Critical Care, 3,* 40–54.

Fantone, J. C., & Ward, P. A. (1994). Inflammation. In E. Rubin & J. L. Farber (Eds.), *Pathology* (pp. 33–66), Philadelphia: J. B. Lippincott.

Gentilello, L. M., Cobean, R. A., Offner, P. J., Soderberg, R. W., & Jurkovich, G. J. (1992). Continuous arteriovenous rewarming: Rapid reversal of hypothermia in critically ill patients. *Journal of Trauma, 32,* 316–327.

Giesbrecht, G. G., & Bristow, G. K. (1992). A second postcooling afterdrop: More evidence for a convective mechanism. *Journal of Applied Physiology, 73,* 1253–1258.

Gisolfi, C. V., & Copping, J. R. (1974). Thermal effects of prolonged treadmill exercise in the heat. *Medicine and Science in Sports, 6,* 108–113.

Gleckman, R., & Hibert, D. (1982). Afebrile bacteremia: A phenomenon in geriatric patients. *Journal of the American Medical Association, 248,* 1478–1481.

Goodman, E. L., & Knochel, J. P. (1991). Heat stroke and other forms of hyperthermia. In P. Mackowiak (Ed.), *Fever: Basic mechanisms and management* (pp. 267–296). New York: Raven Press.

Gotschlich, E. C. (1989). C-reactive protein. *Annals of the New York Academy of Science, 557,* 9–18.

Granberg, P. (1991a). Alcohol and cold. *Arctic Medical Research, 50*(Suppl 6), 43–47.

Granberg, P. (1991b). Human physiology under cold exposure. *Arctic Medical Research, 50*(Suppl 6), 23–27.

Gronert, G. A., Schulman, S. R., & Mott, J. (1990). Malignant hyperthermia. In R. D. Miller (Ed.), *Anesthesia* (pp. 935–956). New York: Churchill-Livingstone.

Hart, B. L. (1988). Biological basis of the behavior of sick animals. *Neuroscience and Biobehavioral Reviews, 12,* 123–137.

Hart, G. R., Anderson, R. J., Crumpler, C. P., et al. (1982). Epidemic classical heat stroke: Clinical characteristics and course of 28 patients. *Medicine, 61,* 189–197.

Hector, M. G. (1992). Treatment of accidental hypothermia. *American Family Physician, 45,* 785–792.

Henker, R., & Coyne, C. (In press). Comparison of peripheral temperature measurements with core temperature. *AACN Clinical Issues in Critical Care Nursing.*

Henker, R., Savage, M., Shaver, J., & Brengelmann, G. (1993). Comparison of two patterns of body cooling. *Communicating Nursing Research, 26,* 211.

Henker, R. A. (1993). Human responses to an alternating versus a continuous pattern of total body cooling. Unpublished Dissertation. University of Washington, Seattle.

Hensel, H. (1981). *Thermoreception and temperature regulation.* London: Academic Press.

Hernandez, E., Praga, M., Alcazar, J. M., et al. (1993). Hemodialysis for treatment of accidental hypothermia. *Nephron, 63,* 214–216.

Hibberd, P. L., & Rubin, R. H. (1991). Fever in the immunocompromised host. In P. Mackowiak (Ed.), *Fever: Basic mechanisms and management* (pp. 197–218). New York: Raven Press.

Holtzclaw, B. J. (1992). The febrile response in critical care: State of the science. *Heart and Lung, 21,* 482–501.

Hooper, J. F., Herren, C. K., & Goldwasser, H. (1989). Neuroleptic malignant syndrome: Recognizing an unrecognized killer. *Journal of Psychosocial Nursing, 27*(7), 13–15.

Johnson, J. M., Brengelmann, G. L., & Rowell, L. B. (1976). Interactions between local and reflex influences on human forearm skin blood flow. *Journal of Applied Physiology, 41,* 826–831.

Jolly, B. T., & Ghezzi, K. T. (1992). Accidental hypothermia. *Emergency Medicine Clinics of North America, 10,* 311–327.

Keating, H. J., Klimek, J. J., Levine, D. S., & Kiernan, F. J. (1984). Effect of aging on the clinical significance of fever in ambulatory adult patients. *Journal of the American Geriatric Society, 32,* 282–287.

Khan, F., Spence, V. A., & Belch, J. J. F. (1992). Cutaneous vascular responses and thermoregulation relation to age. *Clinical Science, 82,* 521–528.

Kielblock, A. J., Van Rensburg, J. P., & Franz, R. M. (1986). Body cooling as a method for reducing hyperthermia. *South Africa Medical Journal, 69,* 378–380.

Klein, D. G., Mitchell, C., Petrinec, A., et al. (1993). A comparison of pulmonary artery, rectal, and tympanic membrane temperature measurement in the ICU. *Heart and Lung, 22,* 435–441.

Kluger, M. J. (1991). Fever: Role of pyrogens and cryogens. *Physiological Reviews, 71,* 93–127.

Kluger, M. J. (1986). Is fever beneficial? *Yale Journal of Biology and Medicine, 59,* 89–95.

Knochel, J. P. (1989). Heat stroke and related heat stress disorders. *Disease-a-Month, 35,* 301–378.

Lawson, L. L. (1992). Hypothermia and trauma injury: Temperature monitoring and rewarming strategies. *Critical Care Nursing Quarterly, 15*(1), 21–32.

Lomax, P., & Daniel, K. A. (1993). Cocaine and body temperature: Effect of exercise at high ambient temperature. *Pharmacology, 46,* 164–172.

Lopez, J. R., Gerardi, A., Lopez, M. J., Allen, P. D. (1992). Effects of dantrolene on myoplasmic free [Ca^{2+}] measured in vivo in patients susceptible to malignant hyperthermia. *Anesthesiology, 76,* 711–719.

MacKenzie, M. A., Aengevaeren, W. R. M., van der Werf, T., Hermus, A., & Kloppenborg, P. (1991). Effects of steady hypothermia and normothermia on the electrocardiogram in human poikilothermia. *Arctic Medical Research, 50*(Suppl 6), 67–70.

Mackowiak, P. A. (1991). Influence of fever on pharmacokinetics and pharmacodynamics. In P. Mackowiak (Ed.), *Fever: Basic mechanisms and management* (pp. 341–351). New York: Raven Press.

Mackowiak, P. A., Wasserman, S. S., & Levine, M. M. (1992). A critical appraisal of 98.6°F as the upper limit of the normal body temperature, and other legacies of Carl Reinhold August Wunderlich. *Journal of the American Medical Association, 268,* 1578–1580.

Mansell, P. I., & MacDonald, I. A. (1989). Effects of underfeeding and of starvation on thermoregulatory responses to cooling in women. *Clinical Science, 77,* 245–252.

McFadden, E. R. (1992). Heat and water exchange in human airways. *American Review of Respiratory Diseases, 146,* S8–S10.

McGowan, J. E., Rose, R. C., Jacobs, N. F., Schaberg, D. R., & Haley, R. W. (1987). Fever in hospitalized patients: With special reference to the medical service. *American Journal of Medicine, 82,* 580–586.

Menashe, P. I., & Gottlieb, J. E. (1988). Hyperthermia, rhabdomyolysis and myoglobinuric renal failure after recreational use of cocaine. *Southern Medical Journal, 81,* 379–380.

Morgan, S. P. (1990). A comparison of three methods of managing fever in the neurologic patient. *Journal of Neuroscience Nursing, 22*(1), 19–24.

Moser, K. M., Perry, R. B., & Luchsinger, P. C. (1963). Cardiopulmonary consequences of pyrogen-induced hyperpyrexia in man. *Journal of Clinical Investigation, 42,* 626–634.

Newman, J. (1985). Evaluation of sponging to reduce body temperature in febrile children. *Canadian Medical Association Journal, 132,* 641–642.

Pugh, L. G. C. E., Corbett, J. L., & Johnson, R. H. (1967). Rectal temperatures, weight losses, and sweat rates in marathon running. *Journal of Applied Physiology, 23,* 347–352.

Reed, G. W., & Krentz, M. J. (1991). Accidental hypothermia. In P. Mackowiak (Ed.), *Fever: Basic mechanisms and management* (pp. 289–296). New York: Raven Press.

Revhaug, A., Michie, H. R., Manson, J. M., et al. (1988). Inhibition of cyclo-oxygenase attenuates the metabolic response to endotoxin in humans. *Archives of Surgery, 123,* 162–170.

Robbins, A. S. (1989). Hypothermia and heat stroke: Protecting the elderly patient. *Geriatrics, 44*(1), 73–80.

Roberts, S. L. (1987). *Nursing diagnosis and the critically ill patient.* Norwalk, CT: Appleton & Lange.

Rohrer, M. J., & Natale, A. M. (1992). Effect of hypothermia on the coagulation cascade. *Critical Care Medicine, 20,* 1402–1405.

Rosebush, P. I., Stewart, T., & Mazurek, M. F. (1991). The treatment of neuroleptic malignant syndrome: Are dantrolene and bromocriptine useful adjuncts to supportive care? *British Journal of Psychiatry, 159,* 709–712.

Rowell, L. B. (1974). Human cardiovascular adjustments to exercise and thermal stress. *Physiological Reviews, 54,* 75–159.

Scott, A. R., Bennett, T., & MacDonald, I. A. (1986). Diabetes mellitus and thermoregulation. *Canadian Journal of Physiology and Pharmacology, 65,* 1365–1376.

Shinozaki, T., Deane, R., & Perkins, F. M. (1988). Infrared tympanic thermometer: Evaluation of a new clinical thermometer. *Critical Care Medicine, 16,* 148–150.

Steele, R. W., Tanaka, P. T., Lara, T. P., & Bass, J. W. (1970). Evaluation of sponging and of oral antipyretic therapy to reduce fever. *Journal of Pediatrics, 77,* 824–829.

Sterba, J. A. (1991). Efficacy and safety of prehospital rewarming techniques to treat accidental hypothermia. *Annals of Emergency Medicine, 20,* 896–901.

Styrt, B., & Sugarman, B. (1990). Antipyresis and fever. *Archives of Internal Medicine, 150,* 1589–1597.

Suffredini, A. F., Fromm, R. E., Parker, M. M., et al. (1989). The cardiovascular response of normal humans to the administration of endotoxin. *New England Journal of Medicine, 321,* 280–287.

Tham, M. K., Cheng, J., Fock, K. M. (1989). Heat stroke: A clinical review of 28 cases. *Singapore Medical Journal, 30,* 137–140.

Vaughn, L. K., Veale, W. L., & Cooper, K. E. (1980). Antipyresis: Its effect on mortality rate of bacterially infected rabbits. *Brain Research Bulletin, 5,* 69–73.

Vaughn, L. K., Veale, W. L., & Cooper, K. E. (1974). Fever in the lizard *Dipsosaurus dorsalis. Nature, 252,* 473–474.

Weinberger, M. (1993). Approach to management of fever and infection in patients with primary bone marrow failure and hemoglobinopathies. *Hematology/Oncology Clinics of North America, 7,* 865–885.

Weiner, J. S., & Khogali, M. (1980). A physiological body-cooling unit for treatment of heat stroke. *Lancet,* March 8, 507–509.

Wlody, G. S. (1991). Malignant hyperthermia. *Critical Care Nursing Clinics of North America, 3,* 129–134.

Wyndham, C. H. (1977). Heat stroke and hyperthermia in marathon runners. *Annals of the New York Academy of Sciences, 301,* 128–138.

Wyss, C. R., Brengelmann, G. L., Johnson, J. M., Rowell, L. B., & Niederberger, M. (1974). Control of skin blood flow, sweating, and heart rate: Role of skin vs. core temperature. *Journal of Applied Physiology, 36,* 726–733.

Preventing Postanesthesia Complications

Ginger Schafer Wlody

Prevention of complications in the immediate postanesthesia period is a vital and complex aspect of critical care nursing. Major physiologic derangements occur because general anesthesia and surgery result in the release of neurohormonal substances and endogenous catecholamines (Stoelting, 1980). These substances are released in conjunction with the stress response as well as the effects of specific anesthetic agents. This combination of factors results in physiologic alterations in the cardiovascular, pulmonary, central nervous, metabolic, renal, and gastrointestinal systems. In a study of 183 men and 242 women undergoing general anesthesia (Vaughan, 1982), 24% of the sample experienced at least one critical incident in the operating room. Thirty-one percent experienced at least one critical incident in the postanesthesia care unit (PACU). Of these, prolonged airway management accounted for 39% and dysrhythmias for 16%. PACU critical incidents were defined as occurrences requiring nursing or medical intervention. Table 68–1 describes the most common critical incidents in the PACU. In a more recent study, Eichorn (1989) found that among 1,001,000 patients with American Society of Anesthesiologists (ASA) physical status 1 and 2, there were 11 major intraoperative accidents "solely attributable to anesthesia." These included five deaths, four cases of permanent central nervous system (CNS) damage, and two cardiac arrests with eventual recovery. Review of these untoward anesthetic events revealed that unrecognized hypoventilation, found in seven patients, was the most common cause. Most (58%–67%) of the complications occur during surgery, with the rest early in the postoperative period (Orkin, 1990).

Critical care nurses caring for patients in the immediate postanesthesia period must anticipate, assess, and manage these physiologic derangements. In addition to the stress of anesthesia and surgery, preoperative, intraoperative, and postoperative factors contribute to both physiologic and emotional complications. It is imperative for the nurse to consider all the stressors that may contribute to complications in this potentially hazardous period.

In this chapter, complications that may occur subsequent to general anesthesia and related drug therapy are explored. Regional anesthesia (spinal, epidural, and local) will be discussed only briefly because most critical care patients receive general anesthesia or a combination of general and regional anesthesia. Table 68–2 summarizes modalities of anesthesia and analgesia and their use. The discussion identifies factors that may lead to postanesthesia complications and targets nursing interventions to prevent them in the critically ill patient. Specific anesthetic agents, skeletal muscle relaxants, and considerations for nursing interventions are identified and discussed. Nursing assessments and interventions that focus on the postanesthetic needs of the critically ill patient are presented.

TABLE 68–1. **Most Common Critical Incidents in the Postanesthesia Care Unit**

Dysrhythmias
Hypotension (30% below preoperative systolic blood pressure)
Hypoxemia
Hypercarbia
Electrolyte disturbances
Airway maintenance
Hypothermia (<34°C core)

Data from Vaughan, M. S. (1982). When should anesthesia monitoring stop? In *Selected abstracts for the 8th postanesthesia symposium for recovery room nurses.* Chicago: Illinois Society of Anesthesiologists, May 6–8.

IDENTIFYING PREOPERATIVE RISK FACTORS

The critical care nurse assesses the patient for preoperative risk factors that may influence the postoperative course. As described in Table 68–3, this preoperative evaluation focuses on detection and subsequent correction of abnormal states. The nursing role includes visiting elective surgery patients preoperatively for nursing assessment, teaching, and emotional support. Risk factors that should be considered include age, cardiovascular disease, respiratory status, nutritional status, infection, immunologic compromise, hepatic disease, renal failure, and genetic factors.

The anesthesiologist classifies the patient preoperatively according to the ASA classification system and

TABLE 68–2. **Common Anesthetic Techniques**

Technique	Description	Comments
Conscious sedation	State of anesthesia during which the patient remains conscious with some alteration of mood, relief of anxiety, drowsiness, and sometimes analgesia. Protective reflexes remain intact.	Drugs that depress the CNS produce a continuum of effects. Small doses (e.g., diazepam 2.5–10 mg IV) can produce this state.
Deep sedation	Patient may sleep but can be aroused without difficulty. Minimal depression of protective reflexes occurs.	An increase in dosage of the drug used (i.e., diazepam from 10–20 mg) can produce this state.
General anesthesia	A controlled state of unconsciousness—loss of consciousness from which the patient cannot be aroused. A reversible state providing analgesia, sedation, appropriate muscle relaxation, and appropriate control of the autonomic nervous system. Produced by either intravenous drugs or inhalation agents. There is a partial or (more common) a complete loss of protective reflexes.	Diazepam at a dose of 1 mg/kg can produce this state. Most commonly, general anesthesia is induced by a barbiturate (sodium thiopental) and maintained with N_2O and narcotics or N_2O, O_2, and inhalation agents. Muscle relaxant drugs are added as needed.
Regional anesthesia	The production of analgesia in a part of the body. Accomplished by either injecting local anesthetic into a vein (a Bier block or IV regional) or, most commonly, by placing local anesthetics in close contract with appropriate nerves to achieve a conduction block.	Successful regional anesthesia requires a thorough knowledge of anatomy, pharmacology of local anesthetic agents, and alterations to the patient's physiology. These alterations can either be predictable changes (such as decreases in blood pressure secondary to the level of sympathetic blockage produced by spinal or epidural anesthesia) or unexpected (allergic reactions).
Spinal anesthesia	Produced by administration of a local anesthetic into the lumbar intrathecal space. The local anesthetic blocks conduction in the spinal nerve roots, dorsal root ganglia, and probably the periphery of the spinal cord.	When a local anesthetic is injected into the subarachnoid space, there is almost immediate onset of anesthesia. Spinal nerve roots, dorsal root ganglia, and the periphery of the cord to some extent are the loci of action. The main effects probably result from anesthetization of the anterior and posterior nerve roots. Disappearance of neural function occurs generally in the following order; autonomic activity, superficial pain, temperature sensation, vibratory and position sense, motor power, and finally touch. Hypotension is the most common adverse effect.
Epidural anesthesia	Accomplished by injecting the local anesthetic into the extradural space. The epidural space is usually identified by using a lumbar approach to reach that compartment between the dura mater and the walls of the spinal cord.	The volume of fluid injected into the epidural space is the major influence in the spread of local anesthesia. Concentration of the anesthetic solution is another factor that affects the completeness of the block. Because the epidural area is highly vascularized, and the volume of anesthetic injected is relatively large, a number of systemic reactions to the local anesthetic may be expected as a result of absorption. Therefore, epinephrine is added to the solution, unless there are contraindications to its use. Epinephrine slows vascular absorption and decreases peak concentrations of anesthetic in the bloodstream. Hypotension is the most frequent adverse effect and tends to be less profound with epidural anesthesia than with spinal anesthesia.
Peripheral nerve blocks	Accomplished by injecting local anesthetic at a specific site(s) to block conduction of impulses and render a defined area anesthetic.	Untoward reactions to local anesthetics can be explained on known pharmacologic grounds even though exceedingly small doses may have been responsible for the effects observed. Systemic reactions encountered involve the central nervous, respiratory, and cardiovascular systems and result from the absorption via the bloodstream of toxic amounts of the drug into the CNS. Convulsions, drowsiness, or unconsciousness may occur. Local anesthetics depress the myocardium directly by a quinidine-like effect on conduction, contractility, and irritability.

Abbreviations: IV, intravenous; CNS, central nervous system.

Table modified from Fraulini, K. (1987). *After anesthesia: A guide for PACU, ICU, and medical surgical nurses* (p. 107). Norwalk, CT: Appleton & Lange. Used with permission.

TABLE 68–3. **Preoperative Factors That May Lead to Complications in the Postoperative Period**

Age	Immunologic compromise
Preexisting cardiovascular disease	Presence of infection
Preexisting respiratory disease	Disease of the blood-forming organs
Endocrine disorders	Hepatic disease
Obesity	Renal disease
Diabetes	Genetic factors
Porphyria	Hypothermia
Drug addiction	Prolonged response to anectine
Psychological state/psychiatric disorders	Nutritional state

records this classification on the patient record. The critical care nurse uses this information in the overall plan of care in conjunction with the nursing assessment. The ASA classification system categorizes patients preoperatively to define risk. The classification is as follows (Norman, 1980):

Class 1 Normal, healthy patient
Class 2 Mild systemic disease
Class 3 Severe systemic disease limiting activity, but not incapacitating
Class 4 Incapacitation due to systemic disease with a constant threat to life
Class 5 Moribund, not expected to live 24 hours with or without surgery

Risk Factors

AGE. Age is a risk factor that increases perioperative complications, thereby placing pediatric and geriatric patients at higher risk. In one study the primary mortality of patients aged 70 years or older in major operations was 9.2% (Palmberg & Hirsjarvi, 1979). Research shows that decreased respiratory reserve in elderly patients may result in postoperative hypoxia, which may persist for many days (Brown et al., 1994). Many physiologic changes in the elderly patient affect the perioperative course and perioperative management. These physiologic changes are summarized in Table 68–4.

TABLE 68–4. **The Geriatric Patient: Physiologic Changes That Affect the Perioperative Course and Perioperative Management**

Decreased metabolic rate
Decreased central nervous system function
Diminished airway reflexes
Decreased serum protein levels
Increased percentage of body fat in relation to lean body mass
Decreased cardiovascular reserve
Decreased pulmonary reserve
Decreased hepatic and renal function

Data from Fraulini, K. E. (1987). After anesthesia: *A guide for PACU, ICU and medical-surgical nurses.* Norwalk, CT: Appleton & Lange.

CARDIOVASCULAR STATUS. The presence of preexisting cardiovascular disease is another important risk factor. Patients who have had previous myocardial infarction, history of dysrhythmias, valvular problems, congestive heart failure, or hypertension are considered to be at greater risk (Goldman et al., 1977). It is recommended that elective surgery be delayed until 6 months after myocardial infarction because of the chance of reinfarction during or after anesthesia and surgery (Tarhan, 1981).

RESPIRATORY STATUS. Patients who have a history of respiratory disease or impaired pulmonary function and those who smoke present an increased surgical risk (Hybels, 1981). This includes patients with chronic obstructive pulmonary disease (COPD), chronic bronchitis, asthma, and past lung operations. The incidence of pulmonary complications in cigarette smokers is 26 times the normal rate (Forestner, 1981).

ENDOCRINE FUNCTION. The most common endocrine disorder that poses a threat to the surgical patient is diabetes mellitus (Stoelting, 1980). Studies have shown that, compared with the general population, the diabetic patient has an increased risk of surgical morbidity and mortality. The risk is thought to result from the high incidence of cardiovascular disease, impaired response to infection, impaired wound healing, and increased protein breakdown seen in patients with diabetes mellitus (Walts, 1983). Patients with hyperthyroidism also require careful perioperative management. Severe circulatory and metabolic changes may complicate the surgical and anesthetic management of the thyrotoxic patient (Snow, 1977). Proper preoperative control of thyrotoxicosis reduces the likelihood of postoperative thyroid storm. Because of the possible development of thyroid storm, atropine is not given as a preanesthetic medication to these patients (Dripps et al., 1988). Patients with adrenal insufficiency and patients on chronic corticosteroid therapy also are at increased surgical risk. Stress doses (300 mg/day) of intravenous cortisol must be administered during the perioperative period (Siperstein, 1988). These patients also are prone to urinary salt wastage. Fluid and electrolyte levels must be closely monitored in the perioperative period.

NUTRITIONAL STATUS. Nutritional status is another factor that affects postoperative complications in the surgical patient. Any patient with depleted glycogen stores is at risk (Shelby, 1967). This may occur in malnourished or emaciated patients, chronic alcoholics, or extremely obese patients. Albumin levels below 3.0 g/100 mL are associated with moderate malnutrition, and levels below 2.1 g/100 mL indicate severe malnutrition (Hybels, 1981).

IMMUNOLOGIC AND HEMATOLOGIC FUNCTION. The presence of infection before surgery greatly increases perioperative risk and enhances the possibility of generalized sepsis. When possible, the operation should be delayed until the infection is resolved (Forestner, 1981). Immunologic compromise results from systemic disease or the use of immunosuppressive agents. For example, steroids suppress the normal adrenal response. These patients must be given a "steroid prep" and observed carefully for adequate adrenal response (Bass, 1973). Anemia, thrombocytopenia, coagulation disorders, and other diseases of the hematopoietic system predispose the patient to complications. Coagulopathy should be suspected in patients with liver disease or those who have had massive transfusions.

HEPATIC DISEASE. The liver detoxifies most general anesthetic agents and barbiturates. Recovery from general anesthesia is prolonged in patients with hepatic disease.

RENAL FAILURE. Patients with acute or chronic renal failure may present problems in the postanesthetic period. Before surgery, the patient may be hypertensive or anemic or may have abnormal electrolyte levels. Volume overload and severe electrolyte imbalances can occur rapidly in the surgical patient with renal failure (Burke & Gulyassy, 1979).

MEDICATION HISTORY. It is important to recognize that the patient's current medications may cause postanesthesia complications. Chronic or preoperative drug therapy may modify organ function directly and may also alter patient response to anesthetic agents or adjuvants (Muravchick, 1980). For example, patients taking quinidine who then receive curariform drugs during surgery may have prolonged postoperative apnea (Caranasos, 1979). Ethanol, tranquilizer, or narcotic abuse also increases the possibility of altered physiologic responses to anesthesia.

GENETIC FACTORS. There are several known genetic factors that affect surgical risk. Malignant hyperthermia is a severe, life-threatening, postanesthetic complication that occurs in genetically susceptible individuals (Arens & McKinnon, 1971). Another group with genetic risk with surgery includes patients with sickle cell disease. In these patients there is an increased risk of vasoocclusive crisis during or immediately after the operation. A third genetic defect that increases risk is the presence of an abnormal anectine response. One of every 3,000 patients has an abnormal response to anectine (Snow, 1977), resulting in decreased pseudocholinesterase activity. When this occurs, the metabolism of anectine is greatly prolonged, and ventilatory support is needed. The patient's susceptibility to malignant hyperthermia (MH) can be evaluated in several ways. A careful anesthetic history, taken by the anesthesiologist, reveals a family history of MH or relatives who have experienced hyperpyrexic reactions secondary to anesthesia. Electrophysiologic and muscle biopsy studies may be carried out to identify a suspected susceptibility to MH. Evidence of muscle abnormalities is usually seen on physical examination (Marchildon, 1982).

PSYCHOLOGICAL FACTORS. Preoperative anxiety or psychological stress may profoundly affect patients. Past experiences or negative information influences the way the patient views the surgical experience. Studies have shown that fear or stress influences the outcome of surgery as well as the way the patient deals with pain and discomfort. Fears related to the unfamiliar environment of the surgical suite, the anesthesia itself, the outcome of the procedure, pain, prolonged illness, and lack of general medical knowledge are added stressors and further disturb the patient's equilibrium. Identification of a patient's potential for ineffective coping triggers supportive measures by the critical care nurse or the entire team. Preoperative teaching and counseling in conjunction with targeted preoperative medication and nursing support are usually effective in assisting patients to manage their stress.

INTRAOPERATIVE FACTORS

The critical care nurse must recognize intraoperative factors that may precipitate postanesthesia complications. Anesthetic agents (Table 68–5) and skeletal muscle relaxants (Table 68–6) have specific actions that can have deleterious effects on the patient. Nursing assessments and actions are based on the intraoperative factors described in this section. In assessing the effects of anesthetic agents, the critical care nurse considers the physiologic effects of the preoperative medication, the method of induction, and the use of muscle relaxants, narcotics, anesthetics, and "reversal agents." Knowledge of which drugs were administered during surgery (e.g., anticoagulants, antibiotics), which mechanical devices were used (e.g., intraaortic balloon pump), and the occurrence of any problems encountered during surgery is vital.

The type of operation also influences what postoperative complications occur. For example, fat embolism can occur after multiple, severe injuries, especially in the long bones. Fat droplets are released into the circulation, and these fat emboli spread widely, possibly causing abnormalities in many organ systems (Drain & Shipley, 1979). Fat embolism usually occurs 12 to 24 hours after injury or surgery.

Effects of Anesthetic Agents

Anesthetic agents, whether volatile, gaseous, intravenous, regional, spinal, or epidural, all affect the body systems. To anticipate complications, the critical care nurse must view the process of surgery and anesthesia as a planned assault on the patient. It is a physical and metabolic attack on the body systems.

MYOCARDIAL DEPRESSION. The currently used volatile or gaseous anesthetic agents (forane, ethrane, nitrous oxide, and so on) and intravenous narcotics are myocardial depressants. The clinical expression of this

TABLE 68–5. **Common Anesthetic Agents, Characteristics, and Considerations for Nursing Interventions**

Route	Official Generic or Chemical Name	Commercial Name or Synonym	Characteristics	Considerations for Nursing Interventions
Inhalation				
Liquids with volatile vapor	Ether (diethyl oxide)	Diethyl ether Ethyl ether	Explosive; used for poor-risk patients due to minimal cardiovascular effects; safe	Side effects: increased secretions, nausea, vomiting, prolonged recovery period
	Trichloroethylene	Trilene	Nonflammable; used widely in obstetrics	Tachypnea, ventricular arrhythmias, bradycardia
	Halothane	Fluothane	Nonexplosive, inflammable; Incomplete muscle relaxation, rapid induction; overdosage easily possible (potent agent); relaxes the uterus; is a halogenated substance	Possible cause of hepatic necrosis; myocardial and respiratory depressant; causes vasodilation, hypotension and shivering; parasympathetic-like effect on the heart (AV and junctional arrhythmias); highly soluble in fatty tissue
	Methoxyflurane	Penthrane	Nonexplosive, inflammable; slow induction compared to halothane, good muscle relaxation; is a halogenated substance	Hepatotoxic myocardial and respiratory depressant; causes vasodilation, hypotension, and shivering; may have increased urinary output postoperatively; longer recovery period than Fluothane; has analgesic properties; highly soluble in fatty tissue; sympathetic-like effect on heart.
	Enflurane	Ethrane	Potent, halogenated ether, nonexplosive, inflammable	Vasodilation, parasympathetic-like effect on heart, nephrotoxic, nausea, vomiting, may cause abnormal EEG in normal patient; avoid use with seizure patients; currently popular agent used in balanced anesthesia, does not seem to sensitize myocardium
	Isoflurane	Forane	Smooth, rapid induction; halogenated ether, nonexplosive, inflammable; approved for use in 1981; provides good muscle relaxation with CNS excitation	Seems to have no hepatic or renal toxicity, does not seem to cause arrhythmias; causes respiratory depression, reduced BP, uterine relaxation; is equal to halothane and Ethrane in potential to trigger malignant hyperthermia
Gaseous anesthetics	Nitrous oxide	Laughing gas	Nonflammable, supports combustion; induction may be accompanied by dreams; recovery rapid; poor muscle relaxation; is rapidly reversible; more soluble than nitrogen in blood.	Causes diffusional hypoxemia postoperatively; causes vasoconstriction and increased BP; laryngospasm may occur
	Cyclopropane	None	Explosive, inflammable; rapid induction and recovery; rarely used due to explosive properties	Increases irritability of myocardium; causes vasoconstriction and increased BP; emergent excitement; bronchospasm may occur; nausea, vomiting, increased intracranial pressure

TABLE 68–5. **Common Anesthetic Agents, Characteristics, and Considerations for Nursing Interventions** *Continued*

Route	Official Generic or Chemical Name	Commercial Name or Synonym	Characteristics	Considerations for Nursing Interventions
Intravenous				
	Thiopental sodium	Sodium pentothal (known as Thiopentone in England)	Ultrashort-acting barbiturate; rapid induction and recovery; given with another anesthetic to produce relaxation and anesthesia; may be used to control certain convulsive states	May cause respiratory depression, laryngospasm (restlessness, stridor, cyanosis), generalized muscle twitching; liver and renal damage have occurred; vasodilation may cause shivering with pooling of blood; decreased venous return; causes respiratory depression, nausea, vomiting, urinary retention
	Morphine sulfate	Same	Is a narcotic analgesic; used for open-heart and vascular surgery; does not affect cardiac reserve; contraindicated in convulsive states; used in conjunction with nitrous oxide and muscle relaxants	
	Fentanyl and droperidol	Innovar	Combination fentanyl (narcotic analgesic) and droperidol (a neuroleptic); combination increases pain threshold, decreases reflex excitability, allays anxiety; droperidol is longer acting then fentanyl	Causes respiratory depression, decreases intraocular pressure; fentanyl has vasodilator effects, may occasionally cause muscle rigidity and cause respiratory and cardiovascular depression; droperidol causes dissociation and drowsiness; patients "forget" to breathe; when given without an analgesic, droperidol causes dystonic reactions
	Ketamine	Ketalar	Dissociative anesthetic; rapid onset, short duration; usually used for superficial operations in children when no muscle relaxation is required	Causes hallucinatory emergence, more so in adults; quiet environment and absence of stimulation minimizes this; arterial pressure and pulse may be elevated; may cause or precipitate laryngospasm when surgery about mouth or lips is performed; causes increased intracranial pressure

Abbreviations: AV, atrioventricular; BP, blood pressure; CNS, central nervous system; EEG, electroencephalogram.

From Wlody, G. S. (1982). Postoperative complications. In American Association of Critical-Care Nurses. *The NTI proceedings book—1982* (pp. 279–280). Newport Beach, CA: AACN.

myocardial depressant effect is usually intraoperative hypotension. In the postoperative period, myocardial depression manifests as congestive heart failure. The most feared cardiovascular morbidity in the perianesthetic period is that of myocardial infarction (Briggs, 1980). About 0.15% of adult patients experience myocardial infarction with general anesthesia and operation.

ALTERATIONS IN RESPIRATORY FUNCTION. General anesthesia results in impaired gas exchange leading to an increase in venous admixture and alveolar dead space. A primary determinant of this impaired function is an alteration in the distribution of ventilation during anesthesia, leading to increased ventilation/perfusion (V_A/Q) imbalance, which then results in hypoxemia (Otto, 1980). There is a decrease in functional residual capacity, which leads to airway closure with gas trapping and microatelectasis.

DECREASED RENAL BLOOD FLOW. Renal blood flow is decreased due to sympathetic activity and other factors. Renal vascular resistance and the filtration fraction increase while the glomerular filtration rate, urine output, and renal blood flow fall (Tonneson, 1980). The types and amounts of fluids administered during surgery play an important role in the patient's fluid volume status during the postanesthetic period.

CENTRAL NERVOUS SYSTEM ALTERATIONS. Inhalation and intravenous anesthetics have profound effects on

TABLE 68–6. **Effects of Skeletal Muscle Relaxants on the Cardiovascular System**

Muscle Relaxant	Action*
Tubocurarine (Tubarine)	Lowers arterial blood pressure (principally by blocking transmission at autonomic ganglia)
Pancuronium bromide (Pavulon)	Does not have histamine-releasing or ganglion-blocking effects; has weak vagolytic action that can increase heart rate slightly and may raise arterial pressure and cardiac output; very useful in the high-risk patient, especially if long period of relaxation is required
Suxamethonium (Anectine)	Has a cholinergic effect; potentiation action of cardiac glycosides; in patient not completely digitalized, it may cause prolongation of PR interval, depression of ST segment and T-wave flattening or inversion

*In patients with severe cardiac decompensation, it is often preferable not to attempt reversal of the muscle relaxant but to continue ventilation postoperatively until cardiorespiratory function has become more stable.

From Wlody, G. S. (1982). Postoperative complications. In American Association of Critical-Care Nurses. *The NTI proceedings book—1982* (p. 280). Newport Beach, CA: AACN.

the cerebral metabolic rate, cerebral blood flow, and intracranial pressure dynamics. Cerebral vasodilation results from all the commonly used volatile anesthetics. This may result in an increase in intracranial pressure, which in turn results in decreased cerebral blood flow. Intravenous anesthetics act as cerebral metabolic depressants and cerebral vasoconstrictors (Drain & Shipley, 1979).

NEUROMUSCULAR BLOCKADE. Neuromuscular blocking agents (anectine, pavulon, tubarine, flaxedil, and so on) are routinely administered as adjuncts to anesthesia to induce skeletal muscle relaxation and to facilitate intubation (Emerson et al., 1979). These neuromuscular blocking agents interfere with the physiology of neuromuscular transmission and produce muscle weakness or paralysis. The sensitivity of different muscle groups varies. The muscles of the eyelids are most sensitive and are paralyzed first, then the extremities, the jaw, intercostal muscles, and finally the diaphragm (Snow, 1977). The critical care nurse must be aware of the type of muscle relaxant used and its mechanism of action.

DRUG INTERACTIONS. Many of the drug interactions that contribute to anesthetic risk result from impaired neuromuscular function or prolonged action of neuromuscular blocking agents (Caranosos, 1979; Muravchick, 1980). For example, when aminoglycoside antibiotics are administered parenterally or used to irrigate body cavities intraoperatively, neuromuscular blockade and subsequent paralysis are enhanced (Goodwin, 1982). The effect carries over to the postanesthesia period and prolongs muscle paralysis or weakness, so that mechanical ventilation may be required. Other drugs interact with neuromuscular blocking agents to produce prolonged apnea. Commonly used drugs that produce this effect include lithium, phospholine iodide (eye drops used in glaucoma), monoamine oxidase inhibitors, and phenothiazines (Caranosos, 1979).

THERMAL REGULATION—TEMPERATURE MONITORING DURING ANESTHESIA. Temperature monitoring during anesthesia is routinely carried out to prevent hypothermia or hyperthermia by means of simple electronic devices that use a ceramic bead. Resistance to electrical current in the thermometer incorporating the ceramic bead may be found at various body sites. The site of temperature monitoring in the operating room varies according to the anesthesiologist's specific monitoring objectives. Esophageal temperature measures temperature at the level of the right heart and is a good indicator of average body temperature. Tympanic, bladder, and rectal sites are also used. The esophageal temperature is not influenced by the temperature of inhaled gases and is responsive to changes in body heat stores. The esophageal site for temperature monitoring may be uncomfortable for the patient if he or she is in the awake or semiconscious state. Rectal temperature is an indicator of core temperature but changes slowly in relation to other parts of the body. The temperature that most closely reflects that of the hypothalamus, or thermoregulatory center, is measured at the tympanic membrane. This site offers quick access for use by the anesthesiologist.

HIGH RISK FOR HYPOTHERMIA. Hypothermia (temperature below 34°C) is a frequently recognized problem during prolonged surgery and particularly affects the very young, the elderly, and patients with hypothyroidism (Atkinson et al., 1987). In a sample of 312 adult surgical patients, 71.6% of intubated patients were hypothermic on admission to the PACU (Fraulini et al., 1985). Vaughan and colleagues (1981) studied 198 postoperative adults and found that 13% were hypothermic on discharge from the PACU.

Normally, the body seeks to maintain its temperature within a certain range through the use of a strict set point that controls the temperature of the blood perfusing the posterior hypothalamus. When there is a deviation from this set point, mechanisms are activated to bring the temperature of the blood back to the preset level. For example, fever sets the thermostat at a higher level, and the body attempts to reach that new set point by increasing metabolism.

Maintenance of normal temperature during surgery is difficult. Several factors act in combination to make the patient susceptible to accidental hypothermia in the operating room suite. Ambient temperature is usually cool to keep the surgeon and staff comfortable. The modern operating room environment is maintained at 19°C to 23°C, with controlled humidity at about 45%. During surgery a large portion of the patient's body surface area is exposed to the cool environment and to cool solutions during the skin preparation.

Anesthetic agents alone do not induce hypothermia or hyperthermia in a normal patient (Flacke et al., 1982). Temperature is controlled by the thermoregulatory center in the hypothalamus through the mechanisms of conduction, convection, radiation, and evaporation. Anesthetic agents depress the thermoregulatory system, and therefore the response of the body depends on the direction of temperature change in the environment. In addition, most anesthetic techniques result in vasodilation, which causes cooling of the blood.

Hypothermia may depress all body activity and, if uncontrolled, may be fatal. Hypothermia that results in myocardial depression and vasoconstriction is sometimes accompanied by shivering, restlessness, and an unstable cardiovascular state (Vale, 1981). Oxygen consumption is increased during rewarming, causing additional stress on the cardiovascular and pulmonary systems. Rebound shivering during the recovery period has been shown to increase oxygen consumption by 400% (Flacke et al., 1982; Vaughan et al., 1981). As consciousness returns in the anesthetized patient, the temperature-sensitive neurons in the anterior hypothalamus become aware of cold, releasing 5-hydroxytryptamine, which stimulates the posterior hypothalamic heat production center (Vale, 1981). The production of heat requires additional oxygen consumption during the rewarming period. This excessive oxygen demand initiates increased minute ventilation to facilitate oxygen uptake, and cardiac output must increase simultaneously to ensure oxygen delivery. Ventilatory embarrassment or fixed low cardiac output during shivering represents a potentially hazardous situation (Goldman et al., 1977).

HYPERTHERMIA. Malignant hyperthermia is a fulminant, hypermetabolic crisis that is usually triggered by volatile anesthetics or neuromuscular blocking agents. It is a rare disorder that occurs in susceptible individuals when they are exposed to specific anesthetic agents. MH occurs most often in the operating room environment and is characterized by a rapid temperature rise. The temperature rise results from a hypermetabolic state of skeletal muscle caused by an increase in the concentration of calcium ion in the sarcolemma (Flacke et al., 1982). Even though MH may respond to treatment with dantrolene sodium, hyperthermia may recur, and these patients must be monitored for 24 to 36 hours after surgery. See Chapter 67 for an expanded discussion of thermal regulation.

POSITIONING. Hemodynamic stability is affected by the position of the patient on the operating room table (Smith, 1987). For example, rapid change from the lithotomy to the supine position can bring about a significant fall in blood pressure (Martin, 1987). The prone position may exert pressure against the inferior vena cava and the femoral veins, resulting in decreased venous return and hypotension (Smith, 1987). Venous return from the head may be obstructed when the head is turned to one side. Engorged eye vessels, eyelid edema, postoperative headache, and subglottic edema may result.

TABLE 68–7. **Intraoperative Factors That May Lead to Complications in the Postoperative Period**

Anesthetic agents used
Adjunctive drug therapy used
Duration of anesthesia and surgery
Position of patient during operative procedure
Type of operation
Type of incision
Use of irrigants
Amount and type of fluid replacement
Thermal regulation

Other hazards associated with position of the operating room table include peripheral nerve damage (Berkebile, 1973), reduction of ventilation (Forestner, 1981), and air embolism to the brain. Air embolism may occur when the sitting position is used, as in neurosurgical procedures (Snow, 1977). The position of the patient during surgery is recorded on the intraoperative record.

OTHER FACTORS. In addition to anesthetic agents, narcotics, skeletal muscle relaxants, and positioning, other factors affect surgical risk. Duration of anesthesia and the length and complexity of the surgical process affect the incidence of postanesthetic complications (Minckley, 1969; Otto, 1980). Specific operative procedures affect the type and placement of the incision used, which in turn affect the potential for pulmonary complications. Research has documented that the transverse incision used in thoracic and abdominal surgery is associated with fewer pulmonary complications than the vertical incision (Strauss & Wise, 1987).

In summary, intraoperative factors that must be considered by the critical care nurse in preventing postanesthetic complications include the following: preoperative condition of the patient, anesthetic agents and their physiologic effects, drug interactions, thermal regulation, fluids administered, patient positioning, and the specific surgical procedure used and its effects. Intraoperative factors that may lead to complications in the postoperative period are summarized in Table 68–7, and ASA standards for basic intraoperative monitoring and for postanesthesia care are presented in Tables 68–8 and 68–9.

PREVENTING POSTANESTHESIA COMPLICATIONS

Because intraoperative events directly affect complications occurring in the postanesthesia period (Forestner, 1981), the critical care nurse receives a detailed and comprehensive report from the anesthesiologist and the circulating nurse at the time of the patient's arrival from the surgical suite. This report

TABLE 68–8. **Standards for Basic Anesthetic Monitoring**

Standards and Objectives	Methods
Standard I	
Qualified anesthesia personnel shall be present in the room throughout the conduct of all general anesthetics, regional anesthetics and monitored anesthesia care.	Because of the rapid changes in patient status during anesthesia, qualified anesthesia personnel shall be continuously present to monitor the patient and provide anesthesia care. In the event there is a direct known hazard (e.g., radiation) to the anesthesia personnel which might require intermittent remote observation of the patient, some provision for monitoring the patient must be made. In the event that an emergency requires the temporary absence of the person primarily responsible for the anesthetic, the best judgment of the anesthesiologist will be exercised in comparing the emergency with the anesthetized patient's condition and in the selection of the person left responsible for the anesthetic during the temporary absence.
Standard II	
During all anesthetics, the patient's oxygenation, ventilation, circulation and temperature shall be continually evaluated.	
Oxygenation	
Objective: To ensure adequate oxygen concentration in the inspired gas and the blood during all anesthetics.	1. Inspired gas: During every administration of general anesthesia using an anesthesia machine, the concentration of oxygen in the patient breathing system shall be measured by an oxygen analyzer with a low oxygen concentration limit alarm in use. 2. Blood oxygenation: During all anesthetics, a quantitative method of assessing oxygenation such as pulse oximetry shall be employed. Adequate illumination and exposure of the patient is necessary to assess color.
Ventilation	
Objective: To ensure adequate ventilation of the patient during all anesthetics.	1. Every patient receiving general anesthesia shall have the adequacy of ventilation continually evaluated. While qualitative clinical signs such as chest excursion, observation of the reservoir breathing bag and auscultation of breath sounds may be adequate, quantitative monitoring of the CO_2 content and/or volume of expired gas is encouraged. 2. When an endotracheal tube is inserted, its correct positioning of the trachea must be verified by clinical assessment and by identification of carbon dioxide in the expired gas. End-tidal CO_2 analysis, in use from the time of endotracheal tube placement, is strongly encouraged. 3. When ventilation is controlled by a mechanical ventilator, there shall be in continuous use a device that is capable of detecting disconnection of components of the breathing system. The device must give an audible signal when its alarm threshold is exceeded. 4. During regional anesthesia and monitored anesthesia care, the adequacy of ventilation shall be evaluated, at least, by continual observation of qualitative clinical signs.
Circulation	
Objective: To ensure the adequacy of the patient's circulatory function during all anesthetics.	1. Every patient receiving anesthesia shall have the electrocardiogram continuously displayed from the beginning of anesthesia until preparing to leave the anesthetizing location. 2. Every patient receiving anesthesia shall have arterial blood pressure and heart rate determined and evaluated at least every 5 minutes. 3. Every patient receiving general anesthesia shall have, in addition to the above, circulatory function continually evaluated by at least one of the following: palpatation of a pulse, auscultation of heart sounds, monitoring of a tracing of intraarterial pressure, ultrasound peripheral pulse monitoring, or pulse plethysmography or oximetry.
Body Temperature	
Objective: To aid in the maintenance of appropriate body temperature during all anesthetics.	There shall be readily available a means to continuously measure the patient's temperature. When changes in body temperature are intended, anticipated, or suspected, the temperature shall be measured.

Note: These standards are not intended for application to the care of the obstetric patient in labor or in the conduct of pain management.

From American Society of Anesthesiologists. (1993). Standards approved by the House of Delegates on October 21, 1986, and last amended on October 13, 1993. American Society of Anesthesiologists, Park Ridge, Illinois.

TABLE 68–9. **Standards for Postanesthesia Care**

Standards and Objectives	Methods
Standard I	
All patients who have received general anesthesia, regional anesthesia, or monitored anesthesia care shall receive appropriate postanesthesia management.	1. A postanesthesia care unit (PACU) or an area which provides equivalent postanesthesia care shall be available to receive patients after surgery and anesthesia. All patients who receive anesthesia shall be admitted to the PACU except by specific order of the anesthesiologist responsible for the patient's care. 2. The medical aspects of care in the PACU shall be governed by policies and procedures which have been reviewed and approved by the department of anesthesiology. 3. The design, equipment and staffing of the PACU shall meet requirements of the facility's accrediting and licensing bodies.
Standard II	
A patient transported to the PACU shall be accompanied by a member of the anesthesia care team who is knowledgeable about the patient's condition. The patient shall be continually evaluated and treated during transport with monitoring and support appropriate to the patient's condition.	
Standard III	
Upon arrival in the PACU, the patient shall be reevaluated and a verbal report provided to the responsible PACU nurse by the member of the anesthesia care team who accompanies the patient.	1. The patient's status on arrival in the PACU shall be documented. 2. Information concerning the preoperative condition and the surgical/anesthetic course shall be transmitted to the PACU nurse. 3. The member of the anesthesia care team shall remain in the PACU until the PACU nurse accepts responsibility for the nursing care of the patient.
Standard IV	
The patient's condition shall be evaluated continually in the PACU.	1. The patient shall be observed and monitored by methods appropriate to the patient's medical condition. Particular attention should be given to monitoring oxygenation, ventilation, circulation and temperature. During recovery from all anesthetics, a quantitative method of assessing oxygenation such as pulse oximetry shall be employed in the initial phase of recovery. This is not intended for application during the recovery of the obstetrical patient in whom regional anesthesia was used for labor and vaginal delivery. 2. An accurate written report of the PACU period shall be maintained. Use of an appropriate PACU scoring system is encouraged for each patient on admission, at appropriate intervals prior to discharge, and at the time of discharge. 3. General medical supervision and coordination of patient care in the PACU should be the responsibility of an anesthesiologist. 4. There shall be a policy to assure the availability in the facility of a physician capable of managing complications and providing cardiopulmonary resuscitation for patients in the PACU.
Standard V	
A physician is responsible for the discharge of the patient from the PACU.	1. When discharge criteria are used, they must be approved by the department of anesthesiology and the medical staff. They may vary depending upon whether the patient is discharged to a hospital room, to the intensive care unit, to a short stay unit, or home. 2. In the absence of the physician responsible for the discharge, the PACU nurse shall determine that the patient meets the discharge criteria. The name of the physician accepting responsibility for discharge shall be noted on the record.

From American Society of Anesthesiologists. (1992). Standards approved by the House of Delegates on October 12, 1988, and last amended on October 21, 1992.

includes a summary of the patient's overall condition, type of surgery performed, fluid status, anesthetic agents used, muscle relaxants and narcotics used, duration of anesthesia, and unusual events. The critical care nurse focuses on assessment and monitoring of vital body functions in the immediate postoperative period. Maintenance of the airway and oxygenation, monitoring of cardiopulmonary and renal function, wound care, body position, and fluid and electrolyte balance are critical. The critical care nurse must be aware of factors that precipitate complications.

The most common postanesthesia complications occur in the respiratory, central nervous, and cardiovascular systems. The major respiratory complications encountered are airway obstruction, hypoxemia, hypercapnia, and aspiration (Feeley, 1990). Significant postanesthesia complications also may occur in the renal and gastrointestinal systems as well.

Respiratory Complications

General anesthesia results in an altered pattern of ventilation as well as a diminution in lung volumes. In addition, respiratory depression results from the use of narcotics or muscle relaxants (Forestner, 1981). The sequence of hypoventilation, atelectasis, and pneumonia occurs in 20% to 40% of postsurgical patients. Because the incision site affects chest wall motion, patients subjected to thoracic or upper abdominal surgery have the greatest chance for development of pulmonary complications (Harmon & Lillington, 1979).

AIRWAY OBSTRUCTION. Postoperative airway obstruction may occur in the oropharynx, nasopharynx, or tracheobronchial tree. Upper airway obstruction is most common. Anesthetics and related medications depress the patient's reflexes, resulting in muscular flaccidity. Secretions, blood, or vomitus may be present, thereby increasing the hazard of aspiration and laryngospasm. Laryngospasm usually results from irritation of bleeding in the throat or mouth, and may be life threatening unless promptly recognized and treated.

HYPOVENTILATION. Hypoventilation secondary to anesthesia is a frequent postoperative complication. If uncorrected, hypoventilation may lead to hypercapnia and hypoxia. A moderate amount of hypoventilation leads to atelectasis and pneumonitis, which frequently occurs in surgical patients.

Muscle relaxants used during surgery lead to hypoventilation if they have not worn off or are not reversed chemically with agents such as physostigmine, neostigmine, pyridostigmine, or edrophonium. These reversal agents prevent metabolism of acetylcholine (Dripps et al., 1988). The most frequently encountered complication of muscle relaxants is unsuccessful reversal of neuromuscular blockade (Lebowitz & Savarese, 1980). Depolarizing muscle relaxants such as succinylcholine are shorter acting and cannot be reversed chemically. Respiratory support is needed until the effects wear off.

Other causes of hypoventilation include restrictive casts or dressings around the thorax, abdominal distention, and excessive accumulations of adipose tissue in thoracic and abdominal areas (Cullen, 1980). Pain, particularly in the upper abdominal or thoracic area, is a major contributing factor to hypoventilation (Otto, 1980). If hypoventilation is narcotic induced, narcotic antagonists such as naloxone may be administered. Hypoventilation resulting from barbiturates responds only to respiratory support until the agent is detoxified and the effects wear off.

INEFFECTIVE BREATHING PATTERNS. Nursing care of the postanesthetic patient includes assessment and support of ventilation. Evaluation of respiratory rate, tidal volume, character of ventilation, presence of obstruction, and chest and diaphragmatic movements is done frequently to assess the adequacy of the patient's breathing pattern. Breath sounds are auscultated bilaterally to assess the adequacy of air flow. If the patient is intubated, artificial airways and oxygen are used in conjunction with the physician's prescriptions. The nurse checks the patient's ability to lift his or her head and neck and also checks handgrip strength and tidal volume before extubation (Lebowitz & Savarese, 1980). The patient is observed for signs of increased restlessness. Restlessness is a key sign of inadequate oxygenation. Restrictive dressings are adjusted to permit maximum chest expansion.

Adequate pain control is necessary to facilitate deep breathing. The nurse administers pain medication and monitors the patient for evidence of narcotic-induced hypoventilation. Narcotic-induced hypoventilation can be prevented by reducing the narcotic dosage and by using the intravenous route for quick action, uptake, and distribution. Narcotic antagonists are used as ordered.

PULMONARY EDEMA. Circulatory overload may result from massive fluid resuscitation or blood administration (Berkebile, 1973). A shift of blood and fluid from the periphery to the pulmonary vascular bed occurs. Pulmonary edema results from elevated left atrial and pulmonary artery blood pressure in combination with decreased myocardial contractility.

DIFFUSION HYPOXIA. Diffusion hypoxia follows breathing of room air by a patient at the close of anesthesia in which a gaseous agent is used in high concentration (e.g., nitrous oxide). Nitrous oxide is about 30 times more soluble than nitrogen, so that at the end of anesthesia the volume of nitrous oxide coming out of the blood greatly exceeds the volume of nitrogen being absorbed. Tissues are saturated with the agent, resulting in a steep pressure gradient from the tissues to the zero partial pressure of gas in room air. This favors a rapid diffusion of the gas from the tissues to the bloodstream and then to the alveoli when air is substituted for the inspired anesthetic mixture. The resultant dilution of alveolar oxygen by the gas leads to varying degrees of hypoxemia and cyanosis lasting 3 to 10 minutes, depending on the patient's minute ventilation. Medical treatment consists of administration of 100% oxygen for 5 to 10 minutes (Forestner, 1981).

IMPAIRED GAS EXCHANGE. Gas exchange may be impaired due to airway obstruction, atelectasis, or pneumothorax. Proper positioning of the patient to prevent occlusion of the airway by the tongue is vital. Nursing measures are used to prevent vomiting. These include moving the patient gently, using antiemetic medications, and ensuring that gastric drainage tubes are functioning properly. Suction equipment is kept readily available to assist in airway clearance should the patient vomit.

Nursing measures to facilitate alveolar ventilation

and gas exchange include assisting the patient to perform coughing and encouraging deep breathing exercises and the use of incentive spirometry. The lungs are auscultated for diminished breath sounds and the presence of adventitious sounds.

PNEUMOTHORAX. Postoperative pneumothorax may be present due to trauma to the lung or thoracic cavity, such as central line placement. Patients with COPD are prone to pneumothorax due to rupture of blebs on the lung.

Cardiovascular Complications

The risk of harmful cardiovascular events in the perioperative period most likely arises from impairment of cardiac function by the altered metabolic state associated with the operative procedure and anesthesia. Hypertension, hypotension, and arrhythmias are the most frequent cardiovascular complications. Disturbances of myocardial energetics can result from increased cardiac oxygen demand, diminished oxygen supply to the heart, or both (Fig. 68–1). The two major effects of anesthesia and surgery are myocardial depression and a tendency toward arrhythmias. Myocardial depression may result in myocardial infarction.

MYOCARDIAL INFARCTION. Almost all currently used inhalational agents are myocardial depressants. A combination of factors may lead to myocardial ischemia or infarction in the high-risk patient during or after general anesthesia. These include increased myo-

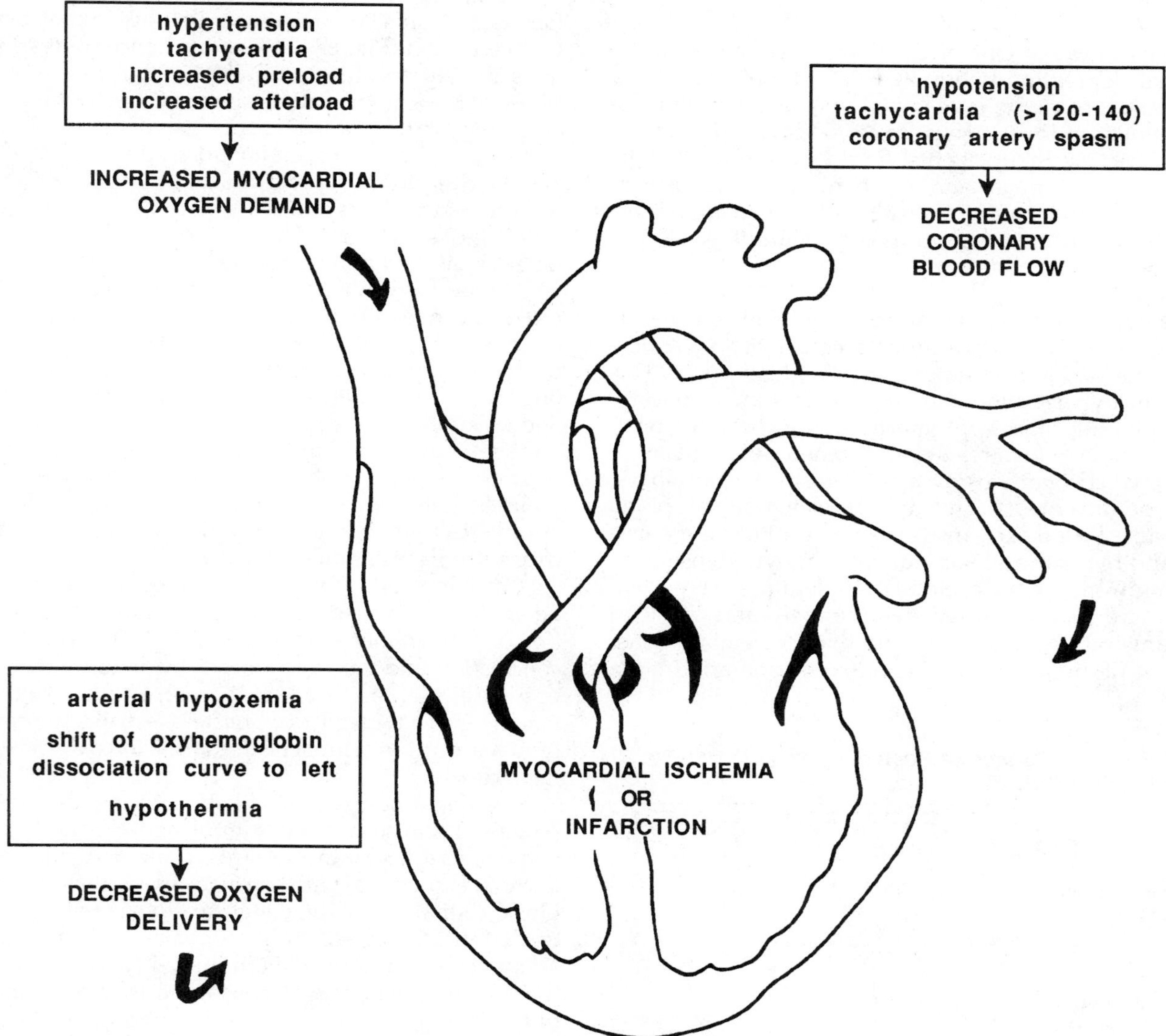

FIGURE 68–1. Postanesthesia causes of myocardial ischemia or infarction in the high risk patient. (Adapted from Wlody, G. S. [1982]. Postoperative complications. In *NTI proceedings book—1982* [p. 283]. Newport Beach, CA: AACN. Computer enhancement courtesy of Mr. Turner McGehee, M. A., Hastings College.)

cardial oxygen demand, decreased oxygen delivery, and decreased coronary blood flow.

Factors that decrease oxygen delivery include arterial hypoxemia, a shift of the oxyhemoglobin dissociation curve to the left, and decreased body temperature. Myocardial oxygen demand is increased by hypertension, tachycardia, increased preload, and increased myocardial contractility. Factors that decrease coronary blood flow include hypotension, tachycardia, and coronary artery spasm. A decreased coronary blood flow coupled with decreased oxygen delivery and increased oxygen demand may lead to myocardial ischemia (Emerson et al., 1979). Monitoring of pulmonary capillary wedge pressure will give an indication of left ventricular function. Nitrous oxide has been used with other agents (i.e., narcotics) for anesthesia in patients with severe coronary artery disease because it produces minimal cardiovascular depression (Calahan et al., 1987).

HYPOTENSION. One of the first indications of myocardial depression is hypotension. Hypotension may also result from hypovolemia, hypoxia, respiratory or metabolic acidosis, sepsis, or vasodilation due to the effects of anesthetic agents. Rapid positional change, pain, dysrhythmias, and mechanical interference in venous return may also result in hypotension. Table 68–10 summarizes the causes of postanesthesia hypotension.

HYPERTENSION. Hypertension is defined as an elevation in the systolic or diastolic pressure of 25% to 30% over the baseline preoperative blood pressure. This level of hypertension should at least arouse concern. Precipitating causes of hypertension include the presence of pain, which results in increased levels of circulating catecholamines. Drugs given in the perioperative period may result in an elevation of blood pressure. Respiratory insufficiency results in hypercarbia and hypoxia and subsequently in hypertension resulting from the release of catecholamines. Hypertension may also be caused by excessive fluid or blood administration, resulting in hypervolemia. Other causes of hypertension include postoperative shivering due to decreased body temperature and restlessness such as occurs in emergence delirium. The causes of postanesthesia hypertension are summarized in Table 68–11.

TABLE 68–10. **Causes of Postoperative Hypotension/Shock**

Anesthesia and drugs/cardiovascular effects
Myocardial infarction
Cardiac dysrhythmias
Position changes
Impaired venous return
Hypovolemia
Hypoxia
Acidosis—respiratory/metabolic
Hypercarbia
Pulmonary embolism
Sepsis
Steroid dependency
Anaphylaxis

TABLE 68–11. **Causes of Postoperative Hypertension**

Anesthesia and drugs
Pain
Hypoxemia
Hypervolemia
Central nervous system lesions
Shivering
Surgical procedure
Restlessness
Preexisting disease—daily medications not given

DYSRHYTHMIAS. Dysrhythmias are precipitated by factors that cause myocardial irritability in the postoperative period (Fig. 68–2). The incidence of dysrhythmias during anesthesia is 15% to 30% (Snow, 1977). Many of the intraoperative causes of dysrhythmias are also precipitating causes in the recovery period. These include intubation or extubation, specific anesthetic agents, duration of operation, and hypothermia. Premature ventricular contractions are the most frequent type of dysrhythmia. Sinus bradycardia may result from vagal stimulation during the operation.

Nonperfused ventricular beats lower cardiac output and can lead to ischemia in vital organs. The critical care nurse must determine if the dysrhythmia is caused by a primary cardiac disease process or is secondary to coincidental or associated abnormalities. Some causes of secondary dysrhythmias include increased sympathetic tone due to fever, anxiety, pain, or stress, hypoxia and acidosis, and electrolyte abnormalities. Left ventricular failure and complications of antidysrhythmic therapy may also result in secondary dysrhythmias (Philbin & Hutter, 1979).

Cardiac dysrhythmias occur frequently during reversal of neuromuscular blockade. The muscarinic action of anticholinesterase drugs delays atrioventricular conduction and can cause bradycardia and atrioventricular block (Lebowitz & Savarese, 1980). Atropine is usually given with anticholinesterase drugs to prevent bradycardia, but it must be used judiciously to prevent tachycardia.

Cardiac arrest is more likely to occur in geriatric patients because of their diminished cardiac reserve and decreased tolerance of stress (Latz & Wyble, 1987). Factors associated with cardiac arrest include heart block, digitalis toxicity, congestive heart failure, myocardial infarction, electrolyte imbalance, dehydration, and massive hemorrhage (Snow, 1977). The shivering that occurs after general anesthesia is very common, but its etiology remains unclear. Although most shivering is seen as benign, it can be dangerous in patients with limited cardiovascular and respiratory function because of adverse metabolic and hemodynamic sequelae (Sun, 1993b).

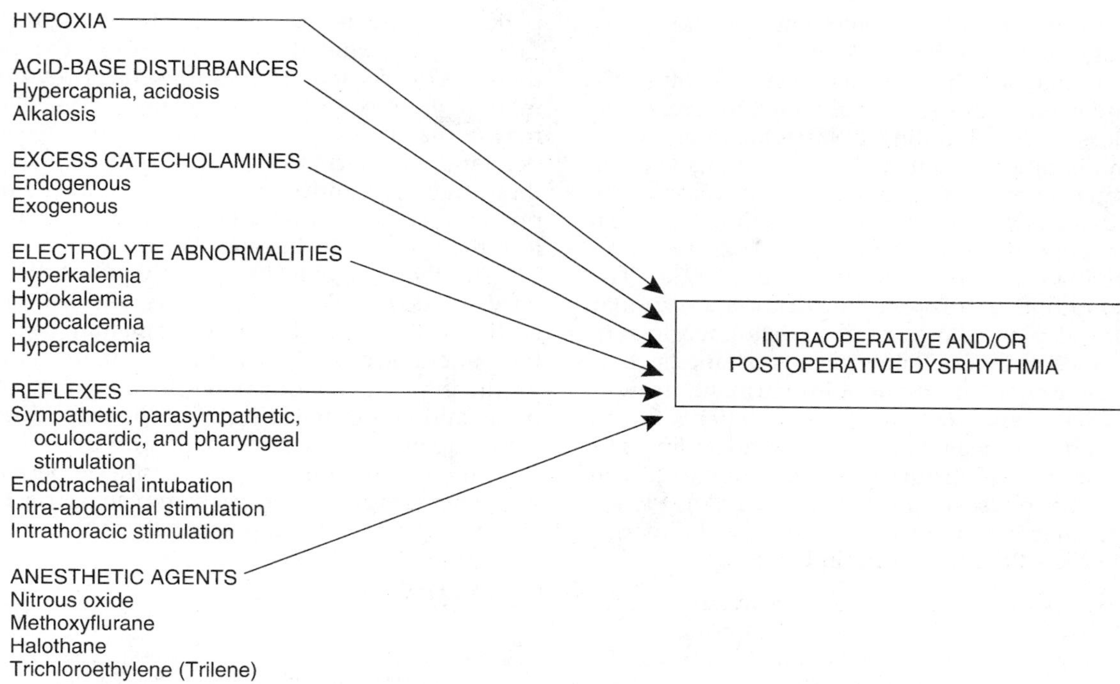

FIGURE 68-2. Etiologic factors in the production of intraoperative and postoperative dysrhythmias.

DECREASED CARDIAC OUTPUT. Because anesthetic agents produce myocardial depression, the postoperative patient may experience alterations in cardiac output and tissue perfusion. Arterial lines, pulmonary artery catheters, central venous pressure lines, and cardiac output determinations provide valuable hemodynamic information. Assessment for hypovolemia is made, and blood, colloids, and crystalloids are replaced as needed. Dressings, tubes, and catheter insertion sites are observed for drainage or bleeding. Cardiac rhythm is monitored, and heart sounds are assessed and evaluated for the appearance of S_3 and S_4 sounds, rubs, and murmurs. Peripheral pulses are checked, and jugular venous distention is noted. Prolonged pain should be prevented by the judicious administration of narcotics. Blood pressure is supported when necessary by the use of vasopressors or beta-adrenergic drugs. The patient is checked for any mechanical interference of venous return. Postoperative myocardial infarction may be difficult to recognize because chest pain may be obscured by the anesthetic or by the narcotics given. Because the most common cause of dysrhythmias in the immediate postoperative period is hypoxemia, the nurse must ensure that oxygenation is adequate to protect the myocardium.

HIGH RISK FOR FLUID VOLUME EXCESS OR DEFICIT. Fluid volume alterations are related to intraoperative changes in renal blood flow or to the administration or loss of fluids during surgery. The nurse assesses the amount of fluid being lost through gastrointestinal drainage, wound drainage, and urinary output. Fluid losses are replaced in conjunction with physician prescriptions. Use of medications that alter renal function is noted, and the patient is monitored for the anticipated effect. Changes in cardiac output, preload, and afterload are carefully evaluated.

The patient's electrolyte levels are monitored. Careful attention is paid to potassium, calcium, and sodium levels because imbalances in these electrolytes may precipitate dysrhythmias.

CENTRAL NERVOUS SYSTEM COMPLICATIONS

During general anesthesia depression of the CNS occurs in descending order as follows: (1) cortical and psychic centers, (2) basal ganglia and cerebellum, (3) spinal cord, and (4) medullary centers (Snow, 1977). The reverse order occurs during emergence from anesthesia. General anesthesia causes depression of consciousness and of the medullary centers that control the respiratory, cardiac, and temperature functions. Emergence delirium, prolonged recovery, abnormal neurologic signs, shivering, hypothermia, and malignant hyperthermia are CNS complications that may occur.

EMERGENCE DELIRIUM. Emergence delirium is a state of CNS excitation that occurs in the patient emerging from anesthesia. The patient may be disoriented and exhibit uncoordinated movements, agitation, convulsions, or even psychotic reactions (Heller, 1981). This state may be due to sudden wakefulness without adequate analgesia having been achieved.

Delirium may also be a result of central cholinergic toxicity, referred to as the central anticholinergic syndrome (Borchardt & Fraulini, 1987), which may occur after administration of anticholinergic agents such as scopolamine. Central anticholinergic syndrome is the result of disturbances in central muscarinic transmission and is caused by anticholinergic drugs and compounds acting on GABA-ergic sites (Sun, 1993a). The central symptoms of atropine intoxication are similar to the clinical picture of central anticholinergic syndrome. The central anticholinergic syndrome is characterized by excitement, thought impairment, drowsiness, or coma. In the excitement stage, patients thrash about in bed and may hallucinate. Anticholinergic-induced emergence delirium responds dramatically to treatment with physostigmine (Cullen, 1980). Physostigmine is effective because it is the only cholinergic drug that crosses the blood–brain barrier.

PROLONGED UNCONSCIOUSNESS. Delayed or prolonged return to consciousness after anesthesia is most often caused by prolonged effects of anesthetic agents or by an actual overdose of anesthetic agents. Prolonged unconsciousness may also be caused by drug interactions, hypoxia, hypercarbia, hypocarbia, intraoperative untoward events (e.g., hemorrhage, cardiac arrest), allergic or atypical drug responses, or a preexisting pathologic condition (Frost, 1983). Sun (1993a) also cites altered hydration, electrolyte or acid–base status, hepatic and renal failure, central anticholinergic syndrome, and neurologic disorders resulting from surgical injury, cerebral embolism, edema, or hemorrhage as differential diagnoses when evaluating delayed recovery after general anesthesia.

Treatment is usually supportive and includes maintenance of cardiovascular stability, oxygenation, correction of acid–base balance, and temperature regulation. Reversal agents (e.g., neostigmine with atropine) may be used if skeletal muscle relaxants are still in effect. Naloxone is given if narcotics are suspected as the cause of the delayed awakening.

ALTERED CONSCIOUSNESS. During the immediate postanesthetic period, nursing assessments are directed toward monitoring the patient's neurologic signs and preventing CNS complications. The patient's level of consciousness is assessed at frequent intervals. The nurse observes the patient for signs of excitation and agitation that may be indicative of emergence delirium. The nurse controls the patient's environment to prevent overstimulation. The environment is kept as quiet as possible. During the awakening period, the nurse frequently reorients and reassures the patient. The nursing care plan contains specific nursing interventions directed toward management of CNS complications in the postanesthetic patient.

SUMMARY

Anesthesia and surgery impose certain inescapable risks and stressors on the critically ill patient. Many patients return to the critical care unit directly from the surgical suite, thereby bypassing the postanesthetic recovery unit. This chapter has provided information about complications related to anesthesia that may occur in the critical care unit. The nurse must understand the pharmacologic and kinetic effects of anesthetic agents, multiple risk factors, and the actual or potential stressors that affect critically ill patients before their arrival in the critical care unit.

Anesthetic agents profoundly affect the pulmonary, cardiovascular, neurologic, and renal systems. In addition, intraoperative environmental factors place the patient at risk. By using a systematic assessment, predicting potential outcomes, making sharp observations, and communicating with the multidisciplinary team members, the nurse will provide high-quality care to the patient in the postanesthesia period. Nursing diagnoses and a nursing care plan for postanesthesia recovery have been presented.

REFERENCES

American Society of Anesthesiology. (1989). *Standards approved by the House of Delegates on October 18, 1989.* Park Ridge, IL: Author.

Arens, J. F., & McKinnon, W. M. (1971). Malignant hyperpyrexia during anesthesia. *Journal of the American Medical Association, 215,* 919–922.

Atkinson, R. S., Rushman, G. B., & Lee, J. A. (1987). *A symposium of anesthesia* (pp. 311–317). Bristol: Wright.

Bakutis, A. (1972). Anesthetic reactions. *Nursing 72, 9/72,* 16–20.

Bass, B. F. (1973). Steroids. *Clinical Anesthesia, 10,* 249.

Berkebile, P. (1973). Postoperative care. *International Ophthalmology Clinics, 13,* 189–214.

Borchardt, A. C., & Fraulini, K. E. (1987). Postanesthetic problems. In K. E. Fraulini (Ed.), *After anesthesia.* Norwalk, CT: Appleton & Lange.

Briggs, B. A. (1980). Perioperative cardiovascular morbidity and mortality. *International Anesthesiology Clinics, 18*(3), 71–83.

Brown, A. G., Visram, A. R., Jones, R. D. M., Irwin, M. G., & Bacon-Shone, J. (1994). Preoperative and postoperative oxygen saturation in the elderly following spinal or general anesthesia: An audit of current practice. *Anaesthesia and Intensive Care, 22,* 150–154.

Burke, G., & Gulyassy, P. (1979). Surgery in the patient with renal disease and related electrolyte disorders. *Medical Clinics of North America, 63*(6), 71–83.

Calahan, M. K., Prakash, O., Evert, N., et al. (1987). Addition of nitrous oxide to fentanyl anesthesia does not induce myocardial ischemia in patients with ischemic heart disease. *Anesthesiology, 76,* 925–929.

Caranasos, G. (1979). Drug reactions and interactions in the patient undergoing surgery. *Medical Clinics of North America, 63*(6), 1245.

Cullen, D. (1980). Recovery room care of the surgical patient. *International Anesthesiology Clinics, 18*(3), 39–52.

Drain, J. H., & Shipley, S. (1979). *The recovery room.* Philadelphia: W. B. Saunders.

Dripps, R. Eckenhoff, J., & Vandam, L. (1988). *Introduction to anesthesia: The principles and safe practice* (7th ed.). Philadelphia: W. B. Saunders.

Eichorn, J. H. (1989). Prevention of intraoperative anesthesia accidents and related severe injury through safety monitoring. *Anesthesiology, 70,* 572–577.

Emerson, C., Davis, R., & Philbin, D. A. (1979). Anesthetic management of patients with coronary artery disease. *International Anesthesiology Clinics, 17*(1), 97–127.

Feeley, T. W. (1990). The post anesthesia care unit. In R. Miller (Ed.), *Anesthesia* (3rd ed.). London: Churchill-Livingstone.

Flacke, W., Flacke, J., Ryan, J., et al. (1982). Altered temperature regulation. In F. Orkin & L. Cooperman (Eds.), *Complications in anesthesiology.* Philadelphia: J. B. Lippincott.

Forestner, J. (1981). Complications of anesthesia. In J. Hardy (Ed.), *Complications of surgery and their management* (4th ed.). Philadelphia: W. B. Saunders.

Fraulini, K. E., Borchadt, A. C., Randall Andrews, D. T., et al. (1985). Mean body temperature of recovery room adults. *Anesthesia and Analgesia, 64,* 213.

Fraulini, K. E. (1987). *After anesthesia: A guide for PACU, ICU and Medical-Surgical Nurses.* Norwalk, CT: Appleton & Lange.

Goldman, L., Caldera, D. L., Nussbaum, S., et al. (1977). Multifactorial index of cardiac risk in noncardiac surgical procedures. *New England Journal of Medicine, 297,* 845.

Goodwin, S. (1982). Drug interactions. *Current Reviews for Recovery Room Nurses, 4,* 15.

Harmon, E., & Lillington, G. (1979). Pulmonary risk factors in surgery. *Medical Clinics of North America, 63*(6), 1289.

Heller, F. (1981). Recovery from anesthesia. In M. Goldin (Ed.), *Intensive care of the surgical patient* (2nd ed.). Chicago: Year Book.

Hybels, R. (1981). Preoperative evaluation. *Otolaryngolic Clinics of North America, 14,* 557–577.

Latz, P. A. & Wyble, S. (1987). Elderly patients' perioperative nursing implications. *AORN Journal, 46,* 238–252.

Lebowitz, P., & Savarese, J. J. (1980). Complications involving neuromuscular pharmacology. *International Anesthesiology Clinics, 18*(3), 139–156.

Marchildon, M. (1982). Malignant hyperthermia: Current concepts. *Archives of Surgery, 117,* 349–351.

Martin, J. T. (1987). General aspects of safe positioning for the surgical patient. In J. T. Martin (Ed.), *Positioning in anesthesia and surgery* (2nd ed., pp. 5–12). Philadelphia: W. B. Saunders.

Minckley, B. B. (1969). Physiologic hazards of position changes in the anesthetized patient. *American Journal of Nursing, 69,* 2606–2611.

Muravchick, S. (1980). Preoperative pharmacology and anesthetic risk. *International Anesthesiology Clinics, 18*(3), 62–66.

Norman, J. (1980). Use of anesthesia: Preoperatie assessment of patients. *British Medical Journal, 28,* 1507–1508.

Orkin, F. P. (1990). Managing quality in anesthesia care. In R. Miller (Ed.), *Anesthesia* (3rd ed.). London: Churchill-Livingstone.

Otto, C. (1980). Respiratory morbidity and mortality. *International Anesthesiology Clinics, 18*(3), 85–106.

Palmberg, S. & Hirsjarvi, E. (1979). Mortality in geriatric surgery. *Gerontology, 25,* 103–112.

Philbin, D., & Hutter, A. (1979). Intraoperative cardiac arrhythmias. *International Anesthesiology Clinics, 17*(1), 55–65.

Shelby, E. (1967). Preoperative evaluation of the poor risk patient. *International Anesthesiology Clinics, 5*(3), 614–629.

Siperstein, M. D. (1988). Endocrine disease and the surgical patient. In L. W. Way (Ed.), *Current surgical diagnosis and treatment* (8th ed.). Norwalk, CT: Appleton & Lange.

Smith, B. (1987). Physiological changes in the normal conscious human subject on changing from the erect to the supine position. In J. T. Martin (Ed.), *Positioning in anesthesia and surgery* (2nd ed., pp. 13–32). Philadelphia: W. B. Saunders.

Snow, J. (1977). *Manual of anesthesia.* Boston: Little, Brown.

Stoelting, R. (1980). Metabolic effects of anesthetics. *International Anesthesiology Clinics, 18*(3), 53–69.

Strauss, R. J., Wise, L. (1987). Operative risks of obesity. *Surgery, Gynecology and Obstetrics, 146,* 286–291.

Sun, K. O. (1993a) Central anticholinergic syndrome following reversal of neuromuscular blockade. *Anaesthesia and Intensive Care, 21,* 363–365.

Sun, K. O. (1993b). Severe postoperative shivering and hypoglycemia. *Anaesthesia and Intensive Care, 21,* 873–875.

Tarhan, S. (1981). Risk of anesthesia in patients with heart disease. *Cleveland Clinic Quarterly, 48,* 50–54.

Tonneson, A. (1980). Acute renal failure. *International Anesthesiology Clinics, 18*(3), 107–121.

Vale, R. (1981). Monitoring of temperature during anesthesia. *International Anesthesiology Clinics, 19*(1), 61–83.

Vaughan, M. S. (1982). When should anesthesia monitoring stop? In *Selected abstracts for the 8th postanesthesia symposium for recovery room nurses.* Chicago: Illinois Society of Anesthesiologists, May 6–8.

Vaughan, M. S., Vaughan, R., & Cork, R. C. (1981). Postoperative hypothermia in adults: Relationship of age, anesthesia and shivering to rewarming. *Anesthesia and Analgesia, 60,* 746–751.

Walts, L. F. (1983). Managing diabetics during surgery. *AORN Journal, 37,* 928–941.

CHAPTER

69 Patients With Obstetric Crises

Kathy Goff and Becky Hull

Pregnancy and childbirth are considered to be normal physiologic events for the vast majority of women. However, a small number of women experience serious complications during pregnancy. These complications can be life threatening to both mother and fetus.

The critically ill obstetric patient poses a unique challenge to the critical care nurse. This chapter focuses on severe preeclampsia and amniotic fluid embolism, two life-threatening complications of pregnancy.

PREGNANCY-INDUCED HYPERTENSION (SEVERE PREECLAMPSIA)

Several different terms have been used to describe the complication of hypertension in pregnancy. Historical terms such as toxemia of pregnancy coexist with the current nomenclature of pregnancy-induced hypertension (PIH) and descriptions of clusters of symptoms regarding severe preeclampsia (the HELLP syndrome). PIH has three distinct subsets: (1) hypertension without edema or proteinuria; (2) hypertension with edema and proteinuria (preeclampsia); and (3) hypertension, edema, proteinuria, and seizures (eclampsia). For purposes of clarity, the terms and definitions used in this discussion are those of the Committee on Terminology of the American College of Obstetricians and Gynecologists (Table 69–1), with the inclusion of the HELLP syndrome (Table 69–2).

TABLE 69–1. **Terms Used in Discussions of Pregnancy-Induced Hypertension**

Pregnancy-induced hypertension: The development of hypertension without edema or proteinuria during pregnancy

Preeclampsia: The development of hypertension with proteinuria, edema, or both, after the twentieth week of pregnancy

Eclampsia: The occurrence of seizures/convulsions, not caused by coincidental neurologic disease, in a woman whose condition fulfills the criteria for preeclampsia

Superimposed preeclampsia or eclampsia: The development of preeclampsia or eclampsia in a woman with chronic hypertension or renal disease

From the Committee on Terminology of the American College of Obstetricians and Gynecologists (1972).

Preeclampsia complicates from 5% to 7% of all pregnancies (Roberts, 1989; Pritchard et al., 1985). In rare instances (1 in 1,000 to 1,500 pregnancies), eclampsia develops (Pritchard et al., 1985). Extremes of age seem to be associated with the development of preeclampsia, with women older than 40 years of age being at higher risk than teenagers (Roberts, 1989). There does seem to be a strong familial tendency toward the development of preeclampsia. Chesley (1984) followed the female family members of women with a history of preeclampsia–eclampsia. His findings indicate that the daughters of women with eclampsia have a 48% incidence of development of preeclampsia, and that sisters of women who were eclamptic have a 55% incidence. Six percent of the daughters-in-law control group had preeclampsia, which would be expected in the general population. Issues of racial predilection are less clear. From 1960 to 1970, the incidences of preeclampsia, eclampsia, and preeclampsia superimposed on chronic hypertension were equal for black and white women, even though the incidence of chronic hypertension in black women is twice that of white women (Chesley, 1984). Similar findings were reported for the years 1979 to 1986 (Saftlas et al., 1990). Incidence of preeclampsia among nonwhite women was slightly higher until 1986, when the rate for white women exceeded that of nonwhites. Preeclampsia during one pregnancy does put the woman at increased risk for the development of preeclampsia in subsequent pregnancies (Roberts, 1989). A woman with preeclampsia is not at increased risk for development of hypertension in later life. However, if preeclampsia was in reality superimposed on chronic hypertension, the chance of having worsening hypertensive problems increases. In those women who do go on to have hypertension, it is felt that the preeclampsia was an unmasking of underlying, preexisting hypertension (Roberts, 1989).

Morbidity and mortality are of significance for both the mother and the fetus or newborn. The mortality rate in women with preeclampsia–eclampsia is very

TABLE 69–2. **The HELLP Syndrome**

Hemolysis
Elevated **L**iver Enzymes
Low **P**latelets

low. Early but cautious interventions have improved maternal mortality figures over the past several decades (Roberts, 1989). Fetal death is still relatively high, with the cause of fetal demise being inadequate placental perfusion and abruptio placentae. Neonatal morbidity and mortality are most commonly related to complications of prematurity.

In most instances, women with preeclampsia are adequately cared for by obstetricians and obstetric nurses. A small percentage of women with preeclampsia go on to have severe preeclampsia, which is manifested by failure of many organ systems. These women may require intensive nursing and medical care to reverse complications and prevent further deterioration.

Pathophysiology

During pregnancy, profound physiologic changes occur that affect all body systems. The most significant of these changes occur in the cardiovascular and hematologic systems. To understand fully the changes seen in preeclampsia, these normal adaptations to pregnancy must be recognized.

NORMAL ADAPTATION TO PREGNANCY

Cardiac output increases during pregnancy as a result of an increase of 40% to 50% in blood volume and a slight increase (10 to 15 beats/minute) in pulse rate. The increase in blood volume begins in the first trimester and continues throughout pregnancy (Ueland, 1976).

Blood pressure decreases slightly in a normal pregnancy, returning to prepregnant levels by approximately 36 weeks' gestation. Normal ranges of blood pressure are 112 to 122 systolic and 68 to 75 diastolic (Roberts, 1989). The drop in blood pressure is accomplished by a decrease in peripheral vascular resistance and the growth of the placenta, a low-resistance vascular bed.

The use of hemodynamic monitoring in pregnancy is not extensive, but data are now available on the effects of pregnancy on common hemodynamic parameters (Table 69–3). Some degree of caution must be used in interpreting hemodynamic data obtained during pregnancy. The effects of maternal position must be taken into consideration, and the effects of labor on normal readings are not well documented. With these caveats in mind, however, it does appear that in the normal pregnancy central venous pressure, pulmonary capillary wedge pressure, and mean pulmonary artery pressure do not change from the nonpregnant state (Clark et al., 1989).

TABLE 69–3. **Hemodynamic Parameters in Pregnancy**

Parameter	Nonpregnant	Pregnant
Central venous pressure (mm Hg)	1–7	Unchanged
Pulmonary artery wedge pressure (mm Hg)	6–12	Unchanged
Mean pulmonary artery pressure (mm Hg)	9–16	Unchanged
Systemic vascular resistance (dynes/second/cm)	800–1,200	600–900 (25% decrease)
Pulmonary vascular resistance (dynes/second/cm)	20–120	15–90 (25% decrease)
Cardiac output (liters/minute)	4–7	5.6–9.8 (30%–45% increase)

Renal blood flow increases in pregnancy by 60% to 70% in midpregnancy, causing a 50% increase in the glomerular filtration rate (Davison, 1985). This increased renal efficiency is reflected in changes in normal laboratory measures of renal function (Table 69–4).

Uterine blood flow is also increased in pregnancy, with blood going to the muscle of the uterus itself as well as through the placenta. Adequate placental blood flow is necessary for the oxygenation and nourishment of the fetus. Indirect means of measuring placental perfusion indicate a blood flow of 500 to 700 mL/minute (Pritchard et al., 1985).

The laboratory values seen in Table 69–4 reflect the dilutional effect of the increase in plasma volume over red cell mass and the increased activity of the kidneys. Changes in liver function and coagulation studies are not observed in a normal pregnancy. Most of these parameters are affected by preeclampsia, especially severe preeclampsia.

TABLE 69–4. **Laboratory Values in the Nonpregnant and Pregnant State**

Parameter	Normal Nonpregnant	Normal Third Trimester
Hemoglobin (g/dL)	11.5–16.0	11.2–15.0
Hematocrit (%)	35.1–46.0	28.6–38.4
Platelets (1,000s/mm^3)	166–264	132–276
Burr cells and schistocytes	Absent	Absent
Blood urea nitrogen (mg/dL)	7–18	5–8
Aspartate aminotransferase (U/mL)	8–40	Unchanged
Alanine aminotransferase (U/mL)	1–36	Unchanged
Prothrombin time (seconds)	10–14	Unchanged
Partial thromboplastin time (seconds)	30–45	Unchanged
Fibrinogen (mg/dL)	200–400	393–539

PATHOGENESIS OF PREECLAMPSIA

The cause of preeclampsia is unknown. Numerous theories have been proposed, but none have been definitively proved. The most promising area of current study is in the role of prostaglandins. Abnormal placentation is thought to be the first step in the development of the disease, possibly related to immune mechanisms (Romero et al., 1988). The result is failure of trophoblastic migration, which inhibits the trophoblasts biosynthesis of prostacyclin (prostaglandin I_2; PGI_2). The effects of PGI_2, a potent vasodilator, and thromboxane A_2, a potent vasoconstrictor, are balanced during a normal pregnancy. In preeclampsia, however, the amount of PGI_2 is decreased and thromboxane A_2 is increased. These changes may allow vasospasm, vascular permeability, and platelet aggregation to occur (Chen et al., 1993; Friedman, 1989). The presence of a factor released by poorly perfused placental tissue, which may cause endothelial cell damage, is also being investigated (Roberts et al., 1989).

Vasospasm is the underlying physiologic cause for the signs and symptoms seen in preeclampsia (Pritchard et al., 1985). Although the cause of the vasospasm is unknown, the effects are observed throughout all body systems. A tendency toward vascular hypersensitivity occurs before any indication of preeclampsia can be seen. Studies of the hypertensive effects of angiotensin II indicate an increased sensitivity to this agent as early as 14 weeks' gestation in women who subsequently became preeclamptic (Gant et al., 1973).

There has been some controversy about whether cardiac output remains normal, decreased, or increased early in pregnancy; however, severe preeclampsia is usually characterized by decreased cardiac output (Visser & Wallenburg, 1991). Plasma volume has been shown to be increased over the nonpregnant state, but to a lesser amount than in an uncomplicated pregnancy. It is surmised that the lack of hemodilution may be due to vasoconstriction or due to decreased oncotic pressure allowing the extravasation of fluid (Pritchard et al., 1984).

Because vasospasm causes a profound increase in peripheral vascular resistance, systemic hypertension in severe preeclampsia can reach significant levels. Pulmonary vascular resistance is not affected (Clark & Cotton, 1988).

Renal blood flow is decreased as a result of vasospasm. Renal arteriospasm is thought to be responsible for the proteinuria seen in preeclampsia (Roberts et al., 1989). It is important to emphasize that in pregnant women serum creatinine levels of 88 μmol/liter (1 mg/dL) may indicate substantial kidney involvement (Cunningham & Lindheimer, 1992). Glomerular damage does occur in preeclampsia, but in the majority of cases it is limited to the duration of the disease itself.

Uterine blood flow is apparently two to three times less in preeclamptic pregnancies than in normal pregnancies (Pritchard et al., 1984). Histologic examination of the placenta shows the spiral arteries, which carry blood through the myometrium to the placenta, to be constricted. These arteries, which are maximally dilated in a normal pregnancy, are reduced in diameter by as much as 60% (Roberts, 1989).

Cerebral blood flow may also be affected by vasospasm, resulting in headaches and visual disturbances. Cerebral vasospasm may be the cause of the seizures of eclampsia. The only evaluations of brain tissue have been from autopsy findings, and the cerebral edema reported in the past may have been related to edema that occurred after death (Pritchard et al., 1985).

The pathophysiologic processes found in the type of severe preeclampsia known as the HELLP syndrome are also related to vasospasm. Microangiopathic hemolytic anemia is the primary feature of the HELLP syndrome. Microscopic lesions are created in the microvasculature throughout the body from the alternating dilation and vasospasm of the arterioles. As the intima is torn, platelets aggregate at the site of the damage, resulting in platelet consumption, which is manifested by thrombocytopenia, ecchymosis, and petechia (Weinstein, 1982). The platelets form a sieve-like structure in the microvasculature. The red blood cells are lysed when they are forced through these areas of platelet aggregation. This results in a falling hematocrit and the presence of schistocytes and burr cells in peripheral blood smears (Brain et al., 1962; Weinstein, 1982).

Associated with these changes are indications of hepatic tissue damage. At cesarean section, the liver may be noted to be very edematous. Autopsy findings may reveal subcapsular hemorrhage and localized areas of necrotic damage. In rare cases the liver may rupture, almost invariably leading to the patient's death (Pritchard et al., 1985; Weinstein, 1986).

A summary of the physiologic changes occurring in severe preeclampsia, including the associated physical findings, is given in Figure 69–1 and Table 69–5.

Clinical Presentation

The patient with severe preeclampsia may present with a very clear "textbook" picture of her disease or with a confusing combination of laboratory and physical findings that may lead to an erroneous diagnosis. When a pregnant woman is given a diagnosis of acute renal disease, acute hepatic disease, idiopathic thrombocytopenic purpura, or other medical disease, the diagnosis of severe preeclampsia must be given serious consideration as well (Goodlin, 1976).

PHYSICAL FINDINGS

Significant hypertension is noted in the typical patient with severe preeclampsia. A blood pressure of 140/90 mm Hg or an increase of 15 points in the diastolic or 30 points in the systolic reading above prepregnancy levels is considered a sign of mild preeclampsia. In severe preeclampsia, the systolic blood pressure is often greater than 160 mm Hg and the diastolic greater than 110 mm Hg.

Edema is another characteristic of preeclampsia. Often, the associated weight gain is rapid and may be

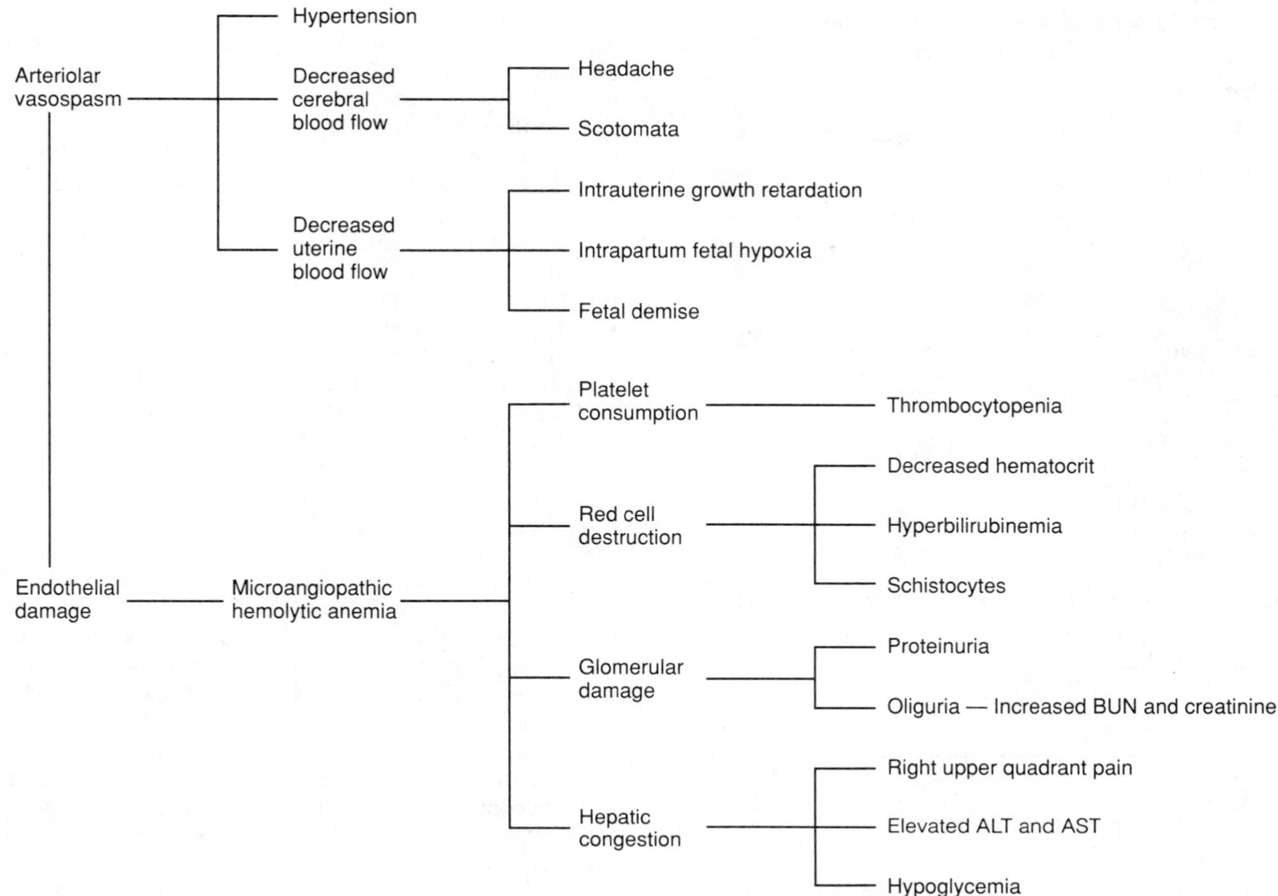

FIGURE 69–1. Pathophysiology of severe preeclampsia. *Abbreviations:* BUN, blood urea nitrogen; AST, aspartate aminotransferase; ALT, alanine aminotransferase. (Adapted from Whittaker, A. A., Hull, B. J., & Clochesy, J. M. [1986]. Hemolysis, elevated liver enzymes, and low platelet count syndrome: Nursing care of the critically ill obstetric patient. *Heart and Lung, 15,* 402–410.)

in excess of 5 pounds in a week. The typical edema associated with normal pregnancy is due to hydrostatic pressure and is limited to dependent areas. The edema associated with preeclampsia is thought to be due to sodium retention and to decreased oncotic pressure. Therefore, it is not limited to dependent areas. Edema of the hands and face is characteristic of fluid retention in severe preeclampsia (Roberts et al., 1989). Anasarca may also occur.

Proteinuria is the third typical finding of preeclampsia. In severe preeclampsia, proteinuria may be 2+ to 3+ on dipstick or more than 2 g/24 hours, and will vary in amount over a 24-hour period. Alternating periods of renal vasospasm are thought to be responsible for the variation in proteinuria (Roberts et al., 1989).

Oliguria or anuria may develop in severe preeclampsia. It appears that there may be three different causes of the decreased urinary output. In patients with oliguria who were invasively monitored, one subgroup was found to have low pulmonary capillary wedge pressures, indicating hypovolemia. A second group was found to have significantly elevated systemic vascular resistance and inadequate cardiac output. The third group was found to have high cardiac output, normal or slightly increased systemic vascular resistance, and adequate preload. In this last group, it was thought that the oliguria was due to severe renal arteriospasm (Clark et al., 1986a; Lee et al., 1987).

Hemodynamic parameters in severe preeclampsia are confusing at best. It is difficult to generalize the information from current case reports because the patients were often managed differently, with fluid restriction, fluid loading, sodium restriction, or the use of antihypertensive agents before invasive monitoring. Any of these treatments may affect hemodynamic parameters. One review indicates that most severe preeclamptic patients will present clinically as if they are hypovolemic and will have low to normal pulmonary capillary wedge pressures. They usually have elevated systemic vascular resistance with normal pulmonary resistance, normal cardiac output, and hyperdynamic left ventricular function (Clark & Cotton, 1988).

Worsening preeclampsia is often characterized by headache, which is probably related to decreased cerebral blood flow. Another ominous sign is right upper

TABLE 69–5. **Characteristics of Preeclampsia**

Mild Preeclampsia	
Hypertension	140/90 mm Hg or >30/15 over baseline
Proteinuria	>1+ on two specimens obtained by catheterization at 6-hour intervals
Edema	Clinically evident swelling or rapid weight gain
Severe Preeclampsia	
Hypertension	>160/>110 mm Hg
Proteinuria	>2 g/24 hours
Oliguria	<500 mL/24 hours
Headache	
Hyperreflexia	
Scotomata	
Anasarca	
Epigastric or right upper quadrant pain	
Pulmonary edema	
Other Factors Associated With Severe Preeclampsia	
Thrombocytopenia	
Elevated AST/ALT	
Elevated blood urea nitrogen/creatinine	
Fetal growth retardation	

Abbreviations: ALT, alanine aminotransferase; AST, aspartate amino-transferase.

quadrant or epigastric pain, thought to be caused by hepatic distention. The development of either or both of these signs is associated with the onset of seizure activity and is a definite sign that the patient's condition is deteriorating (Pritchard et al., 1985).

Hyperreflexia has historically been associated with an increased risk of seizure activity. Although reflexes continue to be assessed, the association with seizures is weak (Pritchard et al., 1985).

Decreased uteroplacental perfusion, another finding in severe preeclampsia, may cause fetal growth retardation, fetal death, or the development of signs of fetal hypoxia during labor. Although these findings are not usually a part of critical care nursing practice, the critical care staff must realize that the patient and her family may be very concerned about fetal loss or prematurity.

LABORATORY FINDINGS

Laboratory findings in severe preeclampsia support the physical findings. In the presence of the HELLP syndrome, the hematocrit may fall as a result of the lysing of red cells. Thrombocytopenia, associated with platelet consumption in the microvasculature, may reach levels below 50,000/mm^3. Other factors in the coagulation panel almost always remain normal, unless true disseminated intravascular coagulation (DIC) develops. Table 69–6 summarizes the differences in clinical and hematologic findings in DIC and HELLP. Elevations of the alanine aminotransferase (ALT) and aspartate aminotransferase (AST) confirm hepatic damage. Hyperbilirubinemia may also be present and is most likely related to the rapid destruction of red cells, rather than another indication of hepatic failure. Significant hypoglycemia, with blood glucose levels less than 40 mg/dL, is associated with very high maternal mortality.

Laboratory findings of elevated blood urea nitrogen, uric acid, and creatinine confirm the diagnosis of renal damage in severe preeclampsia. Because the kidneys are usually more effective in pregnancy, normal values for these laboratory tests are lower than in the nonpregnant person. Thus, a small elevation in the BUN to greater than 11 mg/dL is significant in the pregnant patient.

Clinical Management

Antepartum management of the mild preeclamptic patient is referred to as "expectant," with management being primarily bedrest with frequent vital signs and frequent laboratory assessments. The only cure for preeclampsia is delivery, which is delayed until fetal maturity is established or until the maternal or fetal condition worsens. The goals of the intrapartum and postpartum period include seizure prevention, control of hypertension, maintaining appropriate intravascular volume, and providing for the safe delivery of the infant.

During the postpartum period the pathophysiologic processes are not immediately reversed, so care should continue with emphasis on assessment and protection of the mother. A wider array of medications are available for treatment when the potential fetal effects are no longer of concern. Postpartum management in the critical care unit is an extension of the therapy initiated before delivery. The ensuing discussion therefore focuses primarily on the care of the postpartum patient.

TABLE 69–6. **Differential Diagnosis Between Disseminated Intravascular Coagulation (DIC) and the HELLP Syndrome**

	DIC	HELLP
Clinical findings	Oozing from puncture sites, petechiae, ecchymosis	Oozing from puncture sites, petechiae, ecchymosis
Platelet count	Mild to moderate decrease	Moderate to marked decrease
Fibrinogen level	Low	Normal to high
Prothrombin time, partial thromboplastin time	Elevated	Usually normal
Red blood cells	Slight to moderate fragmentation	Mild to moderate fragmentation (burr cells, schistocytes)

TABLE 69–7. **Dosage Schedule for Magnesium Sulfate**

Loading dose:	4–6 g $MgSO_4$ IV by infusion pump over 15–20 minutes
Maintenance:	After loading dose, 1–3 g/hour of $MgSO_4$ by infusion pump.
Admixture:	40 g of 10% $MgSO_4$ in 1,000 mL D5W to yield 2 g $MgSO_4$/50 mL

Of particular importance is the first 24 hours postpartum, when it is estimated that up to one-third of all eclamptic seizures occur.

SEIZURE PREVENTION

Seizure prevention may be accomplished by any anticonvulsant therapy; however, because of its effectiveness and ease of use, magnesium sulfate ($MgSO_4$) is still considered to be the ideal choice (Sibai, 1990). Recent studies have compared phenytoin with $MgSO_4$ because of the latter drug's uterine relaxant properties, but further investigation is needed to establish significant benefit over $MgSO_4$ for seizure prevention (Friedman et al., 1993; Robson et al., 1993).

The usual dosage for $MgSO_4$ is listed in Table 69–7. It has been proven to be safe in pregnancy. Because the risk of eclamptic seizures continues for 24 to 48 hours after delivery, the $MgSO_4$ infusion is continued during this period or until a significant diureisis takes place (Sibai et al., 1981). $MgSO_4$ acts at the neuromuscular junction to slow transmission of nerve impulses. A blood level of 4 to 8 mEq/liter is most effective for seizure prevention (Sibai, 1990). Invasive monitoring shows that $MgSO_4$ has a transient effect of lowering the mean arterial blood pressure but does not alter other hemodynamic parameters. The effect on blood pressure is related to the rapid-infusion bolus dose and disappears within an hour when the continuous infusion is sustained (Cotton et al., 1984). $MgSO_4$ toxicity may develop in the patient who is oliguric or anuric because $MgSO_4$ is excreted by the kidneys. The presence of at least 1+ deep tendon reflexes indicates a blood level below the toxic range. If reflexes are lost, the $MgSO_4$ should be discontinued.

If seizures do occur when the patient is receiving $MgSO_4$, another anticonvulsant such as diazepam may be given. Additional bolus doses of $MgSO_4$ may be effective, but the risk of toxicity exists. Once the seizure has stopped (usually 1 to 2 minutes), serum magnesium levels can be determined and the therapeutic level achieved (Roberts et al., 1989).

HIGH RISK FOR INJURY. From the time the patient is admitted to the hospital with the diagnosis of preeclampsia until at least 24 to 48 hours postpartum, the patient must be assessed for increased risk of seizures and be protected from injury if seizures should occur. It is estimated that up to one-third of all eclamptic seizures occur in the first 24 hours postpartum. Assessment parameters include evaluation of mentation, evaluation of headache, and deep tendon reflexes. Unfortunately, there is no one sign that adequately predicts the onset of seizures. Measures to decrease the potential for seizure activity are the direct responsibility of the nurse. Decreasing stimulation from light and noise is important. Indirect room lighting is preferred. Enough light is needed to allow assessment of the woman's skin color without having lights shine directly into her eyes. If she needs to be moved from room to room, her eyes can be covered to avoid the strobe-light effect from passing under a series of ceiling lights. Noise levels are reduced as much as possible, with monitor sound indicators turned to a low level. Nursing care and medical procedures should be coordinated whenever possible to allow for periods of rest.

In addition to the complications of aspiration and physical injury when tonic–clonic seizures occur, abruptio placentae and precipitous delivery may be caused by the extremes in muscle activity. When seizure activity has ceased and respiratory status is ensured, the nurse should prepare the patient for a vaginal examination. The physician performs a vaginal examination to assess cervical dilation, effacement, and station of the fetal presenting part.

HIGH-RISK FOR MAGNESIUM SULFATE TOXICITY. The dosage schedule for $MgSO_4$ is detailed in Table 69–7. Key aspects of nursing care include the assessment of deep tendon reflexes. These are performed hourly or more frequently as the patient's condition dictates. Although reflexes are reported on a scale of 1+ to 4+, the most significant finding is that reflexes are either present or absent. Toxic levels of magnesium, which may suppress respirations, will not be achieved until deep tendon reflexes have been ablated. The patellar reflexes are most commonly assessed. If the patient has received epidural anesthesia, the patellar reflexes will be absent and antecubital reflexes will need to be determined.

Urinary output is also an important assessment parameter when magnesium is being infused. Magnesium is excreted by the kidneys, and prolonged periods of oliguria can allow toxic levels to develop. While urinary output is low, it is especially important to monitor deep tendon reflexes because they provide the best information about magnesium levels between laboratory determinations of blood levels.

Respiratory patterns and rate are assessed hourly. Calcium gluconate is recommended as the antidote for respiratory depression from magnesium toxicity, and should be kept at the patient's bedside. If the respiratory rate falls below eight breaths per minute, 10 mL of 10% calcium gluconate may be given as an intravenous push over 3 minutes (Roberts et al., 1989).

Electrocardiographic (ECG) changes of prolonged P-R intervals and widening of the QRS complexes are not seen until the blood level of magnesium reaches 15 to 25 mEq/liter (Zuspan & Zuspan, 1981). Although nursing care certainly includes assessment of ECG patterns, initial recognition of magnesium toxicity is not made from ECG changes.

CONTROL OF HYPERTENSION

Antihypertensive therapy is begun if the patient exhibits a consistent diastolic pressure greater than 110 mm Hg, because the risk of stroke is increased by pressure of this level. The first-line drug choice has been hydralazine because of its vasodilating effect and because it has been proved safe for the fetus. Hydralazine has the additional benefit of increasing cardiac output, which, presumably, will increase uterine perfusion. Hydralazine is best given as intravenous bolus doses rather than by continuous infusion.

More potent antihypertensive agents are rarely needed in severe preeclampsia. Sodium nitroprusside has been used only rarely in pregnant patients. Concerns regarding fetal cyanide toxicity, and results of studies in animal models indicating that improved placental perfusion was not accomplished, leave obstetricians reluctant to choose this drug (Stempel et al., 1982). Nicardipine, a dihydropyridine calcium channel blocker, has been studied in 20 pregnant patients and was found to be safe for the mother and fetus. Although it was efficient in treating the hypertension, further clinical randomized trials are needed to prove its efficacy (Carbonne et al., 1993).

Women may remain hypertensive for several weeks after delivery. If blood pressures reach dangerous levels postpartum, the more potent vasoactive agents like diazoxide or sodium nitroprusside can be used because fetal effects no longer are of concern. Diuretic agents to help control pressures can also be used. In most cases, a significant diuresis (200 mL/hour) will begin spontaneously within 24 to 36 hours postdelivery. This is a clear indication that the patient is improving (Roberts et al., 1989).

MAINTENANCE OF INTRAVASCULAR VOLUME

The maintenance of *intravascular volume* is another goal of obstetric management; however, there is as yet no consensus regarding the type of fluid best used in preeclampsia. Studies indicating that plasma oncotic pressure is lower in preeclamptic than in normal pregnancies cause some authorities to recommend the judicious use of colloids to maintain circulating volume (Benedetti & Carlsen, 1979). Others feel that colloids may cause an increase in ventricular preload by pulling too much extravascular fluid back into circulation (Moise & Cotton, 1986). Most authorities continue to recommend the use of crystalloids at rates of 80 to 125 mL/hour (Pritchard et al., 1985; Roberts et al., 1989).

The use of *invasive monitoring* is not advised for most patients with preeclampsia, even most patients with severe preeclampsia. Invasive monitoring is not without risk and, therefore, is reserved for patients with pulmonary edema or oliguria, patients unresponsive to antihypertensive therapy, and those who need conduction anesthesia (Clark and Cotton, 1988).

Oliguria in the preeclamptic patient, as previously stated, is usually but not always related to decreased intravascular volume. Even without the use of invasive monitoring, it is considered reasonable to infuse 500 to 1,000 mL over an hour if urinary output has fallen below 30 mL/hour (Clark & Cotton, 1988; Roberts, 1989). If oliguria persists for 3 hours, or is unrelieved by fluid challenge, invasive monitoring will be necessary to continue fluid therapy safely. It is noted, however, that if delivery is anticipated within 2 to 3 hours, permanent renal damage will not take place even if oliguria persists (Clark & Cotton, 1988).

Pulmonary edema, a rare management problem in the patient with severe preeclampsia, presents another challenge related to intravascular fluid volume. Pulmonary edema may be caused by iatrogenic fluid overload, by left ventricular failure, by decreased colloid oncotic pressure and altered pulmonary capillary integrity, or by all three mechanisms at once (Clark & Cotton, 1988). In patients with pulmonary edema, the use of invasive monitoring allows the physician to tailor therapy based on wedge pressures, cardiac output, and systemic vascular resistance. The risk of pulmonary edema continues during the postpartum period until the expected diuresis begins. Extravascular fluids return to the intravascular space during the first 24 hours after delivery. If colloid rather than crystalloid fluids have been used during the intrapartum period, additional extravascular fluid may be pulled into circulation. If this additional volume is not tolerated, pulmonary edema may result (Moise & Cotton, 1986).

Diuretic agents are rarely used during antepartum or intrapartum management of severely preeclamptic patients because of the dangers inherent in reducing intravascular volume. Once the patient delivers the baby and the risk of decreasing placental perfusion is past, furosemide or other diuretic agents may be employed.

ALTERED TISSUE PERFUSION (RENAL, HEPATIC). Hourly assessment of renal function is a key nursing role in caring for the patient with severe preeclampsia. Proteinuria is a sign of renal damage, but hourly changes are rarely significant. Although most nurses check for proteinuria in preeclamptic patients hourly, it is not necessary. Protein levels may be recorded every 4 hours.

Specific gravity measurements may be used to provide information about the woman's fluid status when more direct measurements are not available. Decreasing urinary output may be related to inadequate fluid volume or to increasing renal damage, and is usually a problem in the antepartum or intrapartum periods. Because the use of diuretics is contraindicated while the patient is pregnant, nursing measures to improve urinary output are important. Positioning the patient on her left side promotes venous return via the inferior vena cava, thus increasing circulating volume. If a fluid challenge is ordered, careful management by the nurse is important, because the risk of fluid overload is always present.

During the first 24 hours postpartum, most patients experience a mobilization of extravascular fluid, and urinary output reflects this increase in circulating volume. A profound diuresis usually takes place, with hourly outputs commonly in the range of 200 mL/hour. This is a very reassuring sign that the patient's condition is improving.

Due to the increased risk of pulmonary edema in the postpartum period, assessment should include auscultating for the presence of rales, inspecting the neck veins for distention, and being alert to the development of dyspnea or a cough. In the patient with a flow-directed pulmonary artery catheter, trending the pulmonary capillary wedge pressure measurements provides additional information regarding fluid volume status. The temptation to overhydrate the woman should be resisted until the expected hemodynamic changes of the first 24 to 72 hours postpartum have been realized (Hankins et al., 1984).

Signs of hepatic tissue hypoperfusion are reflected in abnormal laboratory values and in patient complaints of right upper quadrant or epigastric pain. In addition, elevated AST and ALT and falling blood glucose levels are bad prognostic signs. If blood glucose determinations are not part of the ordered laboratory profile, the astute nurse may perform a blood glucose determination at the bedside with a reflection glucometer. Levels below 80 mg/dL should be reported to the physician for follow-up. Hepatic rupture may occur in severely preeclamptic patients (Weinstein, 1982). Because this complication is life threatening, the nurse carefully evaluates the patient for changes in abdominal pain, the appearance of other abdominal signs, and the onset of hemodynamic instability.

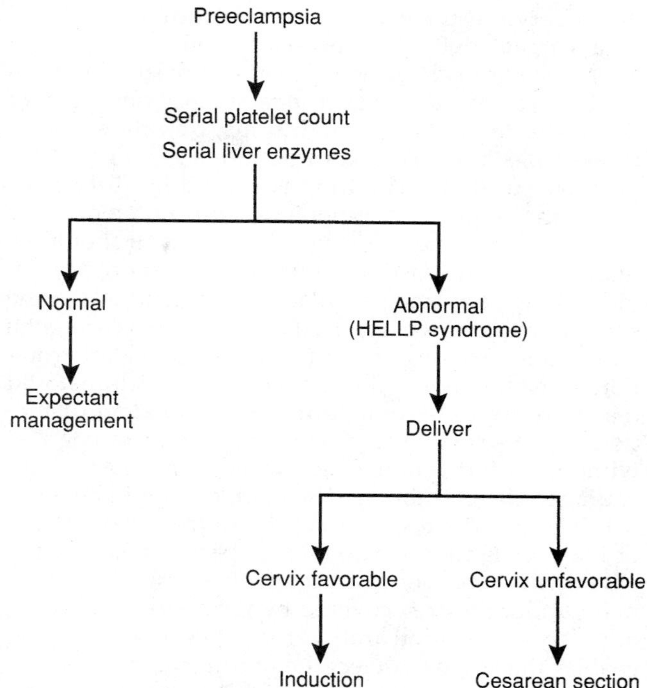

FIGURE 69–2. Medical management of the preeclamptic patient.

SAFE DELIVERY

Safe delivery of the infant is the final goal of intrapartum management of the severely preeclamptic patient. Vaginal delivery is the delivery route of choice whenever possible. Labor often needs to be induced because of worsening maternal or fetal condition. Unless the cervix is "ripe" (3 to 4 cm dilated, 60% to 70% effaced, and of a soft consistency), induction of labor may take 24 hours or more (Bishop, 1964). In most cases of severe preeclampsia with delivery being undertaken because of maternal or fetal deterioration, a brief labor induction of 6 to 12 hours is all that is recommended. After that time, unless delivery is imminent, cesarean section is performed (Weinstein, 1982). Figure 69–2 shows the decision tree approach to managing the preeclamptic patient.

Analgesia during labor and *anesthesia* for delivery represent another area in which there is no consensus. Epidural anesthesia, which is widely used during labor and for cesarean section in normal pregnancies, has added risks when used in the preeclamptic patient. Vasodilation occurring below the level of the sympathetic blockade can lead to a significant fall in blood pressure. To counteract this effect in a normal pregnancy, a 1,000-mL fluid load is given before beginning the block. In the preeclamptic patient, two problems are presented: (1) a 1,000-mL fluid load may not be tolerated by the woman with a decreased intravascular space, with pulmonary edema being the result; and (2) the block may decrease diastolic pressures below 90 mm Hg (the level considered necessary for placental perfusion in the hypertensive patient), and fetal distress may occur.

The use of *general anesthesia* for cesarean section poses additional problems because acute hypertension frequently accompanies induction of anesthesia. In the normotensive patient this is usually well tolerated, but in the severely preeclamptic woman additional elevations of blood pressure are not without risk. It is recommended by some investigators that epidural anesthesia be the method of choice, provided that invasive monitoring can be performed. With arterial blood pressures and wedge pressures monitored, initial fluid bolusing may be used safely and blood pressure kept at adequate levels for placental perfusion (Wheeler & Harris, 1982). Other authorities in obstetrics advise against the use of conduction anesthesia and recommend meperidine for pain relief in labor, local anesthesia for vaginal deliveries, and the usual array of general anesthetic agents for cesarean section (Pritchard et al., 1985).

HIGH RISK FOR INJURY: HEMORRHAGE. Nursing care during the immediate postpartum period includes assessment of the uterus and lochia every 15 minutes for the first 2 hours and then hourly. Blood loss at the time of delivery is estimated. A 300- to 500-mL loss is usual in a vaginal delivery. The usual amount estimated after cesarean section is 1,000 mL. Preeclamptic patients are at risk for hemorrhage because one effect of $MgSO_4$ is to relax the uterine muscle, allowing increased bleeding. The uterine fundus is palpated for position and tone. The fundus should be firm, at or below the level of the umbilicus, and centered in the midline. If the fundus is relaxed or boggy, it should be massaged to increase the muscle contraction. Fundal massage is performed by placing one hand above the symphysis pubis to support the uterus and placing the other hand around the top of the uterus. Gentle rotation of the hand over the surface of the fundus should make the uterus become firm. Urinary bladder distention is a cause of uterine atony. The postpartum patient without an indwelling Foley catheter in place is encouraged to void hourly. The bladder should be emptied if the uterus becomes displaced from the midline or if a full bladder is palpable. Palpation of the uterus after cesarean section is difficult. The uterus should remain under the area covered by the abdominal dressing. Gentle palpation around the edges of the dressing enables the nurse to detect the fundus if it has become displaced. Very gentle palpation of the uterus through the dressing can be performed, but vigorous massage is painful to the patient.

The lochia seen after delivery should be dark red. Bright red bleeding may be indicative of a vaginal or cervical laceration that has gone undetected and therefore unrepaired. Bright red bleeding or heavy bleeding (saturating more than one peripad per hour) must be reported to the obstetrician immediately.

Medications to control uterine atony are limited to oxytocin rather than ergotrate derivatives in the patient with preeclampsia. Ergonovine maleate derivatives are contraindicated because they cause a rise in blood pressure. Oxytocin is usually added to the intravenous infusion in amounts of 10 to 40 units/liter. The infusion is commonly run at 125 mL/hour. Oxytocin can be given intramuscularly, but the infusion approach is most common. Direct intravenous push of oxytocin is not recommended because it can cause a transient but significant drop in arterial blood pressure (Secher et al., 1978).

Severe postpartum hemorrhage may be treated with 15-methyl $PGF_{2\alpha}$ (Hemabate; Upjohn Company, Kalamazoo, MI). The dosage schedule for 15-methyl $PGF_{2\alpha}$ is 0.25 mg intramuscularly every 90 minutes. Dosage is not to exceed 2.0 mg. The nurse observes for side effects, including gastrointestinal upset, fever, and flushing. The diastolic blood pressure may increase in preeclamptic patients, but research studies indicate that there is no need to increase antihypertensive agents for these patients (Hyashi et al., 1984).

Assessment for the development of petechiae, ecchymoses, oozing from puncture sites, and hematuria completes the nurse's physical assessment for signs of increased risk of hemorrhage. Laboratory values for hemoglobin and hematocrit may vary, related to the influx of fluids into the circulation, as well as in response to bleeding, and must be carefully evaluated.

The patient's blood pressure and heart rate are closely monitored during the immediate postpartum period. A fall in blood pressure is always evaluated in terms of hemorrhage rather than simply accepted as a sign that the patient is improving.

ANXIETY. The patient and her family are often unprepared for the critical illness accompanying her pregnancy. What is usually considered to be a most joyous occasion has become life threatening for both mother and infant. The patient and family members will have many questions and concerns. The nurse who is calm and unhurried and provides easily understandable information is most therapeutic for the family. Listening to their fears and concerns and providing support is a continuing necessity. A social service consultation may be beneficial for the family during the critical illness and after the patient has left the critical care environment.

HIGH RISK FOR ALTERED PARENTING. The critically ill mother will be separated from her infant. In most cases of severe preeclampsia, the neonate also requires observation and care in a neonatal intensive care unit. In many instances, this means that the infant will be transported to another hospital, adding to the concerns of the mother and other family members. Frequently, family members divide their time between different hospitals during the first critical days.

The family can be encouraged to take pictures of the newborn for the mother to keep with her, making the birth experience more real. The nursery staff can be contacted several times each day for progress reports on the infant's condition. If the infant is in the same hospital, nursery staff can be encouraged to give reports directly to the mother. A family member can also be encouraged to interact with the newborn and tell the mother of the infant's temperament and appearance. If the infant is seriously ill, a social worker should be assigned to both the mother and the infant to provide continuity and long-term support.

AMNIOTIC FLUID EMBOLISM

Amniotic fluid embolism (AFE) is a very rare, but almost invariably fatal, complication of pregnancy in which amniotic fluid enters the maternal circulation, leading to circulatory collapse and coagulopathies. AFE remains an enigma after over 50 years of study, because of its unanticipated onset, its inconsistent manifestations, and its infrequency.

The term "amniotic fluid embolism" was coined by Steiner and Lushbaugh (1941). These two pathologists studied eight sudden deaths in laboring women at the Chicago Lying-In Hospital and found squamous cells and mucin, presumably of fetal origin, in the maternal pulmonary vasculature. They compared these findings with a control group of 34 maternal deaths attributed to other causes and found no fetal debris in the vasculature of these latter women.

Amniotic fluid embolism complicates an estimated

TABLE 69–8. **Factors Associated With Amniotic Fluid Embolism**

Pregnancy termination
Suction curettage
Saline injection
Prostaglandin $F_{2\alpha}$ injection
Urea injection
Hysterotomy
Uterine rupture
Amniocentesis
Abdominal trauma
Premature rupture of membrane
Meconium staining of amniotic fluid
Use of uterine stimulants (i.e., oxytocin)
Advanced maternal age
Intrauterine fetal demise
Immediate postpartum hemorrhage
Tumultuous labor
Cesarean section

1 in 30,000 pregnancies (Esposito et al., 1990). The mortality rate is very high for both mother and fetus, with the maternal mortality rate being as high as 80% (Clark, 1990). The fetal mortality rate is approximately 40% (Duff, 1984). Twenty-five to 50% of deaths occur in the first 60 minutes, as a result of irreversible cardiopulmonary arrest (Duff, 1984). After the first hour, death is attributed to coagulopathies that result in irreversible hemorrhage (Clark et al., 1985).

Amniotic fluid embolism can occur early in pregnancy, during labor, or even several hours postpartum. It is not possible to define specific criteria that definitely put a woman at risk for the development of AFE. Table 69–8 lists factors often associated with AFE.

Pathophysiology

Amniotic fluid embolism may be identified by cytologically analyzing pulmonary microvascular blood obtained from a pulmonary artery catheter. The presence of large amounts of fetal squames with lesser amounts of fetal mucin and hair indicates AFE (Masson, 1992; Clark et al., 1986). Other fetal substances and meconium may also be found. Amniotic fluid is thought to enter the maternal circulation through small tears in the uterine or cervical veins. Once the fluid containing fetal debris enters the pulmonary circulation, embolization occurs with resultant cardiopulmonary collapse. Fetal debris may also be found in the microcirculation throughout the body.

It is not known what substance in amniotic fluid causes the profound shock and subsequent hemorrhage experienced by patients with AFE. In studies using animal models, pure amniotic fluid and amniotic fluid with various quantities of meconium have been injected into an animal's circulation. A clear relationship has not been demonstrated between the type of injectate and the degree of pathologic change (Clark, 1986). Amniotic fluid contains substances other than particulate matter. These other substances, such as prostaglandins, leukotrienes, and trophoblastic material, have vasoactive properties that may lead to the initial cardiovascular response. Amniotic fluid may also contain tissue factor or other components of the extrinsic pathway of coagulation that may be potent initiators of the coagulopathy (Lockwood et al., 1991).

Clinical Presentation

The immediate findings with AFE are dyspnea and cyanosis, followed by shock and coma. Grand mal seizures or DIC develop in 10% to 15% of patients (Masson, 1992). Fetal loss occurs as a result of hypoxia secondary to maternal circulatory collapse.

HEMODYNAMIC FINDINGS

Hemodynamic findings are becoming more widely published as the use of invasive monitoring becomes more common in critically ill obstetric patients. In most cases, however, catheters are not in place at the time the embolus occurs, so immediate hemodynamic findings are rarely available.

Based on available hemodynamic data, it appears that there is a biphasic response to AFE. It is postulated that when the amniotic fluid and fetal debris enter the pulmonary circulation, there is a relatively short period of intense vasoconstriction, pulmonary hypertension, and hypoxia. Because the time period for these events is thought to be brief (30 to 60 minutes), invasive monitoring data are not yet available in humans to support this hypothesis. This acute onset of pulmonary hypertension and hypoxia may account for the 50% of patients who die in the first hour after AFE occurs (Clark, 1986, 1990).

If the patient survives the initial insult, the second phase of left ventricular failure ensues. The pulmonary capillary wedge pressure is elevated, and the left ventricular stroke work index is depressed. The elevation of pulmonary artery pressure and pulmonary vascular resistance is similar to readings found in patients with left-sided heart failure alone. Pulmonary edema is found in 70% of patients and is thought to be noncardiogenic, similar to the findings in adult respiratory distress syndrome (ARDS) (Clark, 1986).

HEMATOLOGIC FINDINGS

In the patients who survive the profound cardiopulmonary effects of AFE, DIC develops in 40%, which often leads to fatal hemorrhage. DIC may present within minutes to hours of the initial event. The clinical findings include frank hemorrhage from the uterus and persistent oozing from incision sites or venipunctures. Laboratory findings include the presence of fibrin split products, prolonged prothrombin and partial thromboplastin times, and thrombocytopenia (Clark, 1986, 1990). (For a more in-depth discussion of the clinical findings and management of DIC, the reader is referred to Chapter 54.)

Clinical Management

Unfortunately, for most patients with AFE care involves unsuccessful resuscitative efforts and immediate crisis intervention for the family members who have just lost a young, healthy mother-to-be, and often the infant as well. For those women who are successfully managed during the acute event, continued care in a critical care environment is necessary.

Cardiopulmonary bypass with pulmonary artery thromboembolectomy has been used successfully to treat postpartum shock associated with AFE (Esposito et al., 1990). The treatment in this case study was found to be helpful in establishing an in vivo diagnosis, restoring pulmonary blood flow and physiologic function, and reversing a life-threatening coagulopathy.

ALTERATION IN TISSUE PERFUSION. For the patient in cardiopulmonary arrest, cardiopulmonary resuscitation is the first response. If the patient is still conscious and breathing, high concentrations of oxygen may be given by mask. If necessary, the patient should be intubated and ventilated with 100% FIO_2. Positive end-expiratory pressure is required for the patient in severe respiratory failure (Clark, 1986).

While the pregnancy is still viable, preparation should be made for an immediate cesarean delivery and the potential need for infant resuscitation.

Once airway management and chest compressions are established, the nurse ensures patency of two large-bore peripheral intravenous infusions and begins fluid resuscitation. Crystalloid intravenous fluids are used for initial correction of hypotension. Dopamine may be administered to stimulate cardiac function and promote vasoconstriction (Clark, 1986). A flow-directed pulmonary artery catheter is inserted as soon as possible to provide data necessary for fluid management. Blood can be withdrawn from the right side of the heart and placed in a heparinized tube for laboratory examination to confirm the presence of fetal debris (Masson, 1992).

Once the patient has been successfully resuscitated, left ventricular failure should be anticipated. Rapid digitalization may be necessary (Clark, 1986). Inotropic drugs may be infused to support the failing ventricle. If the systemic vascular resistance is elevated, afterload reduction with vasodilators is initiated.

IMPAIRED GAS EXCHANGE. The development of ARDS should be anticipated. Once the initial hypotension is corrected, fluid volume is carefully restricted to avoid pulmonary edema. If the patient is intubated, positive end-expiratory pressure and FIO_2 can be balanced to achieve a PO_2 of 50% to 60% (Balk & Bone, 1983). Positioning the patient for optimal gas exchange is imperative.

One of the nurse's major responsibilities is to follow the patient's fluid status to prevent fluid overload and pulmonary edema. The central venous pressure and pulmonary capillary wedge pressure are trended, and all intake and output recorded and monitored. Lungs are auscultated frequently to assess the patient's ability to tolerate fluid volume.

For more detail regarding the nursing management of the patient with ARDS, the reader is encouraged to read Chapter 32.

HIGH RISK FOR INJURY. Once the patient has been stabilized, she is at increased risk for hemorrhage. Blood products should be ordered and immediately available in anticipation of DIC. Whole blood, packed red cells, and fresh frozen plasma can be used to replace clotting factors. Platelets can be given to correct thrombocytopenia. Heparinization is not universally recommended after AFE (Clark, 1986; Duff, 1984). Assessment of the skin for petechiae and oozing from venipuncture sites may provide early warning of the development of DIC and impending hemorrhage. Blood may be placed in a nonheparinized blood tube and timed for clot formation.

If the patient has delivered, she is at risk for hemorrhage from an atonic uterus. Assessment of uterine tone must be performed regularly. (For more information regarding assessment of uterine tone and medications used to treat uterine atony, see the previous section of this chapter.)

ANTICIPATORY FAMILY GRIEVING. As in any instance of sudden death or potential for death, family members need assistance in coping with this tragic situation. It is easy to forget the family during resuscitative efforts and during the critical period after successful resuscitation. As soon as possible, the nurse should delegate someone to communicate with the family, help the family summon clergy, or arrange for a social worker to provide support. If the infant has survived, encouraging the family to spend time with the newborn may be helpful. However, the family may react to the infant as the cause of the woman's death or illness. The nurse must be prepared to assist the family members to deal with their grief.

SUMMARY

Life-threatening complications arising from pregnancy are rare. When they occur, however, they present a major challenge to the critical care team. Care of the critically ill obstetric patient must take into account the physiologic as well as the psychological condition of the patient and her family. Educating the patient and her family regarding the etiology, disease process, treatment, and outcome are critical. Once the patient stabilizes, plans for discharge should include evaluation of any physical limitations that will need home follow-up, evaluating the home environment for home care needs, and making sure that the patient and family have a resource for continued psychosocial support.

The special needs of the critically ill obstetric patient require a team approach. The obstetric nurse seeks consultation and help from the critical care nurse specialist when hemodynamic monitoring and mechanical ventilation are required during the intrapartum period. The critical care staff members request obstetric nursing help in assessing the usual postpartum parameters of uterine involution and lochia. The nursing staff of the newborn nursery/intensive care unit may also be called on to provide information about the infant's condition. This team approach maximizes professional nursing care and provides the best possible care for the woman and her family.

REFERENCES

Benedetti, T. J., & Carlson, R. W. (1979). Studies of colloid osmotic pressure in pregnancy-induced hypertension. *American Journal of Obstetrics and Gynecology, 135,* 308–311.

Bishop, E. H. (1964). Pelvic scoring for elective induction. *Obstetrics and Gynecology, 24,* 266–268.

Brain, M. C., Dacie, J. V., & Hourihane, D. O. B. (1962). Microangiopathic hemolytic anemia: The possible role of vascular lesions in pathogenesis. *British Journal of Haematology, 8,* 358–374.

Carbonne, M. D., Jannet, D., Touboul, C., Khelifati, Y., & Milliez, J. (1993). Nicardipine treatment of hypertension during pregnancy. *Obstetrics and Gynecology, 81,* 908–914.

Chen, G., Wilson, R., Cumming, G., Walker, J. J., & McKillop, J. H. (1993). Production of prostacyclin and thromboxane A_2 in mononuclear cells from preeclamptic women. *American Journal of Obstetrics and Gynecology, 169,* 1106–1111.

Chesley, L. C. (1984). History and epidemiology of preeclampsia–eclampsia. *Clinical Obstetrics and Gynecology, 27,* 801–819.

Clark, S. L. (1986). Amniotic fluid embolism. *Clinics in Perinatology, 13,* 801–811.

Clark, S. L. (1990). New concepts of amniotic fluid embolism: A review. *Obstetrical and Gynecological Survey, 45,* 360–368.

Clark, S. L., & Cotton, D. B. (1988). Clinical indications for pulmonary artery catheterization in the patient with severe preeclampsia. *American Journal of Obstetrics and Gynecology, 158,* 453–458.

Clark, S. L., Cotton, D. B., Lee, W., et al. (1989). Central hemodynamic observations in normal third trimester pregnancy. *American Journal of Obstetrics and Gynecology, 161,* 1439–1442.

Clark, S. L., Greenspoon, J. S., Aldahl, D., & Phelan, J. P. (1986a). Severe preeclampsia with persistent oliguria: Management of hemodynamic subsets. *American Journal of Obstetrics and Gynecology, 154,* 490–494.

Clark, S. L., Montz, F. J., & Phelan, J. P. (1985). Hemodynamic alterations associated with amniotic fluid embolism: A reappraisal. *American Journal of Obstetrics and Gynecology, 151,* 617–621.

Clark, S. L., Pavlova, Z., Greenspoon, J., et al. (1986b). Squamous cells in the maternal pulmonary circulation. *American Journal of Obstetrics and Gynecology, 154,* 104–106.

Cotton, D. B., Gonik, B., & Dorman, K. F. (1984). Cardiovascular alterations in severe pregnancy-induced hypertension: Acute effects of intravenous magnesium sulfate. *American Journal of Obstetrics and Gynecology, 148,* 162–165.

Cunningham, F. G., & Lindheimer, M. D. (1992). Hypertension in pregnancy. *New England Journal of Medicine, 326,* 927–932.

Davison, J. M. (1985). The physiology of the renal tract in pregnancy. *Clinical Obstetrics and Gynecology, 28,* 257–265.

Duff, P. (1984). Defusing the danger of amniotic fluid embolism. *Contemporary OB/GYN, 24,* 127–149.

Esposito, R. A., Grossi, E. A., Coppa, G., et al. (1990). Successful treatment of postpartum shock caused by amniotic fluid embolism with cardiopulmonary bypass and pulmonary artery thromboembolectomy. *American Journal of Obstetrics and Gynecology, 163,* 572–574.

Friedman, S. (1989). Preeclampsia: A review of the role of prostaglandins. *Obstetrics and Gynecology, 71,* 122–137.

Friedman, S. A., Lim, K., Baker, C. A., & Repke, J. T. (1993). Phenytoin versus magnesium sulfate in preeclampsia: A pilot study. *American Journal of Perinatology, 10,* 233–238.

Gant, N. F., Daley, G. L., Chand, S., et al. (1973). A study of angiotensin II pressor response throughout primigravid pregnancy. *Journal of Clinical Investigation, 52,* 2682–2685.

Goodlin, R. C. (1976). Severe pre-eclampsia: Another great imitator. *American Journal of Obstetrics and Gynecology, 125,* 747–753.

Hankins, G. D., Wendel, G. D., Cunningham, F. G., & Leveno, K. J. (1984). Longitudinal evaluation of hemodynamic changes in eclampsia. *American Journal of Obstetrics and Gynecology, 150,* 506–512.

Hyashi, R. H., Castillo, M. S., & Noah, M. L. (1984). Management of severe postpartum hemorrhage with a prostaglandin $F_{2\alpha}$ analogue. *Obstetrics and Gynecology, 63,* 806–808.

Lee, W., Gonik, B., & Cotton, D. B. (1987). Urinary diagnostic indices in preeclampsia-associated oliguria: Correlation with invasive hemodynamic monitoring. *American Journal of Obstetrics and Gynecology, 156,* 100–103.

Lockwood, C. J., Bach, R., Guha, A., et al. (1991). Amniotic fluid contains tissue factor, a potent initiator of coagulation. *American Journal of Obstetrics and Gynecology, 165,* 1335–1341.

Masson, R. G. (1992). Amniotic fluid embolism. *Clinics in Chest Medicine, 13,* 657–665.

Moise, K. J., & Cotton, D. B. (1986). The use of colloid osmotic pressure in pregnancy. *Clinics in Perinatology, 13,* 827–842.

Pritchard, J. A., Cunningham, F. G., & Pritchard, S. A. (1984). The Parkland Memorial Hospital protocol for treatment of eclampsia: Evaluation of 245 cases. *American Journal of Obstetrics and Gynecology, 148,* 951–963.

Pritchard, J. A., et al. (1985). *Williams' obstetrics* (17th ed.) New York: Appleton-Century-Crofts.

Roberts, J. M. (1989). Pregnancy-related hypertension. In R. K. Creasy & R. Resnik (Eds.), *Maternal-fetal medicine: Principles and practice* (2nd ed., pp. 777–823). Philadelphia: W. B. Saunders.

Roberts, J. M., Taylor, R. N., Musci, T. J., et al. (1989). Preeclampsia: An endothelial cell disorder. *American Journal of Obstetrics and Gynecology, 161,* 1200–1204.

Robson, S. C., Redfern, N., Seviour, J., et al. (1993). Phenytoin prophylaxis in severe pre-eclampsia and eclampsia. *British Journal of Obstetrics and Gynaecology, 100,* 623–628.

Romero, R., Lockwood, C., Oyarzun, E., & Hobbins, J. C. (1988). Toxemia: New concepts in an old disease. *Seminars in Perinatology, 12,* 302–323.

Saftlas, A. F., Olson, D. R., Franks, A. L., et al. (1990). Epidemiology of preeclampsia and eclampsia in the United States, 1979–1986. *American Journal of Obstetrics and Gynecology, 163,* 460–465.

Secher, N. J., Arnsbo, P., & Wallin, L. (1978). Haemodynamic effects of oxytocin (Syntocinon) and methyl ergometrine (Methergine) on the systemic and pulmonary circulation of pregnant anesthetized women. *Acta Obstetrica et Gynecologica Scandinavica, 57,* 97–103.

Sibai, B. M., Lipshitz, J., Anderson, G. D., & Dilts, P. V. (1981). Reassessment of intravenous $MgSO_4$ therapy in preeclampsia-eclampsia. *Obstetrics and Gynecology, 57,* 199–202.

Sibai, B. M. (1990). Magnesium sulfate is the ideal anticonvulsant in preeclampsia–eclampsia. *American Journal of Obstetrics and Gynecology, 162,* 1141–1145.

Steiner, P. E., & Lushbaugh, C. C. (1941). Maternal pulmonary embolism by amniotic fluid as a cause of obstetric shock and unexpected deaths in obstetrics. *Journal of the American Medical Association, 117,* 1245–1254; 1341–1345.

Stempel, J. E., O'Grady, J. P., Morton, M. J., & Johnson, K. A. (1982). Use of sodium nitroprusside in complications of gestational hypertension. *Obstetrics and Gynecology, 60,* 533–538.

Ueland, K. (1976). Maternal cardiovascular dynamics: VII. Intrapartum blood volume changes. *American Journal of Obstetrics and Gynecology, 126,* 671–677.

Visser, W., & Wallenburg, H. C. S. (1991). Central hemodynamic observations in untreated preeclamptic patients. *Hypertension, 17,* 1072–1077.

Weinstein, L. (1982). Syndrome of hemolysis, elevated liver enzymes, and low platelet count: A severe consequence of hypertension in pregnancy. *American Journal of Obstetrics and Gynecology, 142,* 159–167.

Weinstein, L. (1986). The HELLP syndrome: A severe consequence of hypertension in pregnancy. *Journal of Perinatology, 5,* 316–320.

Wheeler, A. S., & Harris, B. A. (1982). Anesthesia for pregnancy-induced hypertension. *Clinics in Perinatology, 9,* 95–111.

Zuspan, F. P., & Zuspan, K. H. (1981). Strategies for controlling eclampsia. *Contemporary OB/GYN, 18,* 135–144.

OBSTETRIC CRISES MULTIDISCIPLINARY CARE GUIDE

COORDINATION OF CARE

Diagnosis/Stabilization Phase		Acute Management Phase		Recovery Phase	
Outcome	**Intervention**	**Outcome**	**Intervention**	**Outcome**	**Intervention**
All appropriate disciplines and team members will be involved in the plan of care.	Develop a plan of care with patient/family, primary nurse(s), primary physician(s), obstetrician, neonatologist, pediatrician, other specialists as needed, clinical nurse specialist, respiratory therapist, chaplain.	All appropriate team members and disciplines will be involved in the plan of care.	Update the plan of care with the patient/family, team members, physical therapist, dietitian, discharge planner, support groups, social worker. Initiate planning for anticipated discharge. Begin teaching patient/family about care at home.	Patient will understand how to maintain optimal health at home.	Provide written guidelines concerning care at home and any follow-up visits for mother and/or baby. Provide patient/family with phone numbers of resources available to answer questions for mother regarding self care and/or infant care.

FLUID BALANCE

Diagnosis/Stabilization Phase		Acute Management Phase		Recovery Phase	
Outcome	**Intervention**	**Outcome**	**Intervention**	**Outcome**	**Intervention**
Patient will achieve optimal hemodynamic status as evidenced by: • MAP > 70 mm Hg • Hemodynamic parameters WNL • Urine output > 0.5 mL/kg/hour • Absence of dysrhythmias • Adequate level of consciousness • Clear lung sounds • Adequate intake and output	Monitor and treat cardiac parameters: • Dysrhythmias • BP • I & O • LOC • Evidence of tissue perfusion • Svo_2 • JVD Monitor lab values: hemoglobin, hematocrit, electrolytes, BUN creatinine, ABGs, platelets, liver enzymes, renal function, urine specific gravity, proteinuria, PT, PTT, and glucose. Monitor respiratory status and be prepared for mechanical ventilation. Assess lung sounds q1–2h.	Patient will maintain optimal hemodynamic status.	Same as stabilization phase. Monitor and treat hemodynamic parameters. Assess neurologic status q2–4h and prn. Stay prepared for mechanical ventilation should respiratory status deteriorate. Continue seizure precautions for severe preeclampsia. Continue magnesium sulfate if ordered. Daily weight. Continue to assess for complications associated with obstetric crises. Assess uterus and lochia q2h and prn.	Patient will maintain optimal hemodynamic status.	Same as acute management phase. Continue seizure precautions and administration of magnesium sulfate if ordered. Assess follow-up care postdischarge and teach patient signs and symptoms for which to seek medical attention (bleeding, acute shortness of breath, dizziness, seizures, or other neurologic changes).

Outcome	Intervention	Outcome	Intervention	Outcome	Intervention
	Assess fluid overload or deficit and treat accordingly. For fluid deficit, crystalloids are usually given at 80–125 mL/hour. Anticipate need for vasopressor agents and assess response and titrate accordingly. Assess for hypertension, edema, proteinuria, and seizures. Institute seizure precautions for severe preeclampsia. Magnesium sulfate may be administered prophylactically. Observe for respiratory depression if magnesium is given. The antidote is calcium gluconate. Also, if receiving magnesium sulfate, assess deep tendon reflexes q1h and prn and assess urine output q1h. Assess neurologic status q1h and prn. Monitor for signs of complications that can occur with obstetric crises: disseminated intravascular coagulation (DIC), amniotic fluid embolus, ARDS, renal failure, hypovolemia, sepsis, pulmonary edema, and HELLP syndrome. Observe for signs of bleeding and administer blood products as needed. Monitor response. Assess uterus and lochia every 15 minutes during the immediate postpartum period.				

NUTRITION

Diagnosis/Stabilization Phase		Acute Management Phase		Recovery Phase	
Outcome	*Intervention*	*Outcome*	*Intervention*	*Outcome*	*Intervention*
Patient will be adequately nourished.	NPO if intubated or until able to take fluids. Initiate enteral or intravenous feedings as necessary. Monitor response. Assess bowel sounds q4h and prn. Monitor serum glucose levels. If able to swallow, provide clear liquids and monitor response.	Patient will be adequately nourished.	Assess bowel sounds q4h and prn. Maintain intravenous and enteral feedings as needed. Maintain high caloric diet. Monitor protein, albumen, and glucose levels. Involve dietitian in plan of care.	Patient will be adequately nourished.	Teach patient/family about dietary needs after discharge.

Care Guide continued on following page

OBSTETRIC CRISES MULTIDISCIPLINARY CARE GUIDE continued

MOBILITY

Diagnosis/Stabilization Phase		Acute Management Phase		Recovery Phase	
Outcome	*Intervention*	*Outcome*	*Intervention*	*Outcome*	*Intervention*
Patient will achieve optimal mobility.	Bedrest if preeclamptic. Begin passive/active-assist range-of-motion exercises.	Patient will achieve optimal mobility.	Increase activity as tolerated. Monitor response to increased activity and decrease if adverse effects occur (tachycardia, dyspnea, syncope, dysrhythmias, hypotension). Provide support as necessary. Continue passive/active-assist range-of-motion exercises. Obtain physical therapy consult if indicated.	Patient will achieve optimal mobility.	Teach patient/family about home exercise program or activity restrictions.

OXYGENATION/VENTILATION

Diagnosis/Stabilization Phase		Acute Management Phase		Recovery Phase	
Outcome	*Intervention*	*Outcome*	*Intervention*	*Outcome*	*Intervention*
Patient will have adequate gas exchange as evidenced by: • O_2 saturation >90% • ABGs WNL • Clear breath sounds • Chest x-ray normal • Respiratory rate, depth, and rhythm WNL • Absence of dyspnea, cyanosis, and secretions	Monitor ventilator settings (if used) and hemodynamic variables before, during, and after weaning. Avoid prolonged administration of 100% FiO_2. Monitor respiratory status: lung sounds, respiratory muscle strength, respiratory rate and depth, coughing ability, ABGs, and chest x-ray. Anticipate need for hyperventilation and hyperoxygenation, particularly before suctioning. If not intubated, apply supplemental oxygen. Monitor with pulse oximetry. Assess evidence of tissue perfusion. Monitor lab values: ABGs, hemoglobin, Mg^{++} levels if $MgSO_4$ infusing.	Patient will have adequate gas exchange.	Monitor and treat oxygenation status as per ABGs and/or SaO_2. Monitor and treat ventilation disturbances as per chest assessment, ABGs, adventitious breath sounds, and chest x-ray. Wean oxygen therapy/mechanical ventilation as indicated. Encourage coughing and deep breathing q2h or incentive spirometry. Observe for complications of obstetric crises that may impair oxygenation/ventilation: pneumonia, infection, sepsis, DIC, embolus, pulmonary edema, ARDS, thrombus formation, atelectasis, and hypovolemia.	Patient will have adequate gas exchange.	Chest x-ray before discharge. Continue to assess for complications of obstetric crises that may impair oxygenation/ventilation.

COMFORT

Diagnosis/Stabilization Phase		Acute Management Phase		Recovery Phase	
Outcome	Intervention	Outcome	Intervention	Outcome	Intervention
Patient will be as comfortable and pain free as possible as evidenced by: • No objective indicators of discomfort • No complaints of discomfort	Assess quantity and quality of pain. Administer intravenous narcotic analgesics as needed and monitor response. Provide uninterrupted periods of rest in a quiet environment to potentiate analgesia. If patient is intubated, develop effective interventions with which patient can communicate discomfort. Use sedatives as indicated and monitor response. Observe for complications of obstetric crises that may cause discomfort: thrombus, embolus, infection. Provide reassurance in a calm, caring, and competent manner.	Patient will be relaxed and as pain-free as possible.	Same as stabilization phase. Teach patient relaxation techniques. Use massage, humor, music therapy, and imagery to promote relaxation. Involve family in strategies. Use sedatives as indicated and monitor response. Continue to observe for complications of obstetric crises that may cause discomfort.	Patient will be relaxed and as pain-free as possible.	Progress to oral analgesics and nonnarcotic analgesics when possible. Monitor response. Continue alternative methods to promote relaxation as listed above. Teach patient/family alternative methods to promote relaxation at home.

SKIN INTEGRITY

Diagnosis/Stabilization Phase		Acute Management Phase		Recovery Phase	
Outcome	Intervention	Outcome	Intervention	Outcome	Intervention
Patient will have intact skin without abrasions or pressure ulcers.	Assess all bony prominences at least q4h and treat if needed. Use preventive pressure-reducing devices if patient is at high risk for development of pressure ulcers. Treat pressure ulcers according to hospital protocol.	Patient will have intact skin without abrasions or pressure ulcers.	Same as stabilization phase.	Patient will have intact skin without abrasions or pressure ulcers.	Teach patient/family proper skin care after discharge.

Care Guide continued on following page

OBSTETRIC CRISES MULTIDISCIPLINARY CARE GUIDE *continued*

PROTECTION/SAFETY

Diagnosis/Stabilization Phase		Acute Management Phase		Recovery Phase	
Outcome	***Intervention***	***Outcome***	***Intervention***	***Outcome***	***Intervention***
Patient will be protected from possible harm.	Assess need for restraints if patient is intubated, has a decreased level of consciousness, or is agitated and restless. Explain need for restraints to patient/family. Assess response to restraints, if used, and check q1h for skin integrity and impairment to circulation. Follow hospital protocol for use of restraints. Remove restraints as soon as patient is able to follow instructions. Institute seizure precautions and administer magnesium sulfate if ordered. Provide sedatives as needed and monitor response, especially to respiratory system. Decrease stimulation from light and noise.	Patient will be protected from possible harm.	If need still exists for restraints, check q1–2h for skin integrity and impairment to circulation. Provide support when activity increases. Monitor response to activity. Continue seizure precautions. Continue to decrease stimulation from light and noise.	Patient will be protected from harm.	Provide support with increased activity and monitor response. Instruct patient/family about any physical limitations in activity after discharge.

PSYCHOSOCIAL/SELF-DETERMINATION

Diagnosis/Stabilization Phase		Acute Management Phase		Recovery Phase	
Outcome	***Intervention***	***Outcome***	***Intervention***	***Outcome***	***Intervention***
Patient will achieve psychophysiologic stability. Patient will demonstrate a decrease in anxiety as evidenced by: • Vital signs WNL • Subjective reports of decreased anxiety • Objective signs of decreased anxiety	Assess physiologic effects of critical care environment on patient (hemodynamic variables, psychological status, signs of increased sympathetic response). Assess psychological effects of obstetric crisis on patient (miscarriage, stillbirth, unable to see baby). Arrange for flexible visiting to meet patient/family needs. Provide sedatives as indicated. Take measures to reduce sensory overload.	Patient will achieve psychophysiologic stability. Patient will demonstrate a decrease in anxiety. Patient will continue acceptance process of obstetric crisis.	Same as stabilization phase. Continue to assess coping ability of patient/family and take measures as indicated (counseling, psychiatric consult, chaplain, verbalization of fears/concerns, social worker, family conferences). Initiate discharge planning.	Patient will achieve psychophysiologic stability. Patient will demonstrate a decrease in anxiety. Patient will continue acceptance process of obstetric crisis.	Provide instruction on coping mechanisms after discharge. Refer to outside services or agencies as appropriate (chaplain, home health, social services). If appropriate, continue to allow patient to see baby or provide frequent condition updates.

Outcome	Intervention				
Patient will begin acceptance process of obstetric crisis.	If patient is intubated, develop effective interventions to communicate with patient. If unresponsive, use tactile and verbal stimuli. Use calm, caring, competent, and reassuring approach with patient and family. Determine coping ability of patient/family and take appropriate measures (encourage verbalization of fears/concerns, encourage questions, provide information frequently in easy-to-understand terminology, allow family to visit). If feasible, allow patient to see baby. If not and appropriate, provide frequent condition updates. Take pictures of the baby to show the patient.				

DIAGNOSTICS

Diagnosis/Stabilization Phase		Acute Management Phase		Recovery Phase	
Outcome	*Intervention*	*Outcome*	*Intervention*	*Outcome*	*Intervention*
Patient will understand any tests or procedures that need to be completed (vital signs, intake and output, hemodynamic monitoring, chest x-ray, care of baby if applicable, clotting studies, chemistries, ultrasound, CBC, liver enzymes, ABGs, proteinuria, urine specific gravity, fetal monitoring).	Explain all procedures and tests to patient/family. Explain procedures and tests needed to care for baby, if applicable. Be sensitive to individualized needs of patient/family for information. Establish effective communication techniques with patient if intubated.	Patient will understand any tests or procedures that need to be completed to recover from obstetric crisis.	Anticipate need for further diagnostic tests or procedures and prepare patient for these.	Patient will understand meaning of diagnostic tests and procedures in relation to continued health.	Review with patient before discharge the results of lab tests, procedures, and so forth as they relate to the patient and baby, if applicable. Discuss any abnormal findings and appropriate measures patient can take to help return to normal.

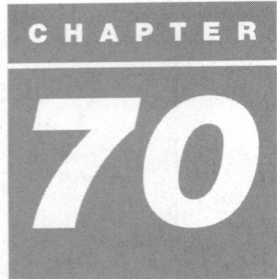

Patients With Oncologic Emergencies

Marcia Rostad

Oncologic crises are emergency events that occur during the course of the cancer experience. Unmanaged, these critical events diminish the patient's quality of life and carry high morbidity and mortality. Because many cancers are responsive to treatment and are potentially curable, medical management of oncologic emergencies is of great importance. Even when the cancer is considered incurable, most oncologic crises are aggressively managed to extend an already limited life span.

PATHOPHYSIOLOGY OF CANCER

Neoplasms are classified according to the tissue from which they originate. Sarcomas are tumors that derive from embryonic tissue, or so-called connective tissue. Carcinomas are those tumors of epithelial cell origin. Carcinomas account for the majority of human cancers (Kupchella, 1992). As a means of more definitively identifying the aberrent cells, tumors are further defined by their histologic characteristics. Squamous cell carcinoma and adenocarcinoma are two examples of tumors whose histologic appearance has been confirmed. The confirmation of tissue histology assists in identifying the best treatment for the cancer.

Several theories attempt to explain the causation of cancer. Although none by itself has been successful in accounting for all the aspects of cancer, each supports the basis for today's approach to treatment.

One theory attributes neoplasia to genetic abnormalities that can occur at any time during life (Harewood, 1989). This disruption in the regulation of cellular growth and differentiation may account for the development of certain cancers in families, such as breast cancer or acute lymphoblastic leukemia in identical twins (Berenson & Gale, 1990; Haskell et al., 1990). In contrast, another theory suggests that the development of cancer may be epigenetic, that is, changes in the regulation of genes and not their structure may account for the development of certain cancers (Ladik & Otto, 1989). The carcinogenic action of diethylstilbestrol on the human vagina is one example. The viral theory attempts to link DNA and RNA oncogenic viruses to the transformation of malignant cells. Burkitt's lymphoma is almost certainly due to infection by the Epstein-Barr virus (Sarin, 1989). It may also be hypothesized that malignant cells in early development lie dormant until, if ever, the appropriate stimulus comes along. Only then does a malignancy occur (Gallick, 1989).

Once the neoplastic process has begun, the aberrent cell continues unregulated and uncontrolled proliferation without regard for the needs of the host. The malignant cells may double at amazing speed, allowing a tumor quickly to occupy its immediate space and eventually invade nearby structures. This local extension may lead to regional extension via metastasis to the lymph nodes. Metastasis occurs when tumor emboli detach from the tumor and are carried to the lymph nodes by the downstream flow of lymph (Kupchella, 1992).

Distant metastasis primarily occurs by the spread of cancer through the bloodstream. It is generally believed that the more aggressive cancer cells reach the bloodstream through direct invasion of the capillaries and veins (Kupchella, 1992). While in the bloodstream, the cancer cells interact with other cancer cells, blood components, and the elements of the immune system. This interaction allows the cell to develop additional complex characteristics, which aid in its eventual relocation and growth in other tissues of the body.

Eventually the cancer cells come to rest and establish neoplastic growth. It is unclear why there is a tendency for certain cancers to metastasize to certain sites, particularly the liver, lymph nodes, bones, lung, and brain. The mechanics of circulation may explain where metastasis occurs and where it does not. In tissues where there is a high blood flow rate, it is believed that cancer cells cannot lodge long enough to become attached (Kupchella, 1992). It is also suggested that metastasizing cells, because of their genetic makeup, prefer specific tissue types, or "congenial soil." The presence of a receptor on the cancer cell may cause it to associate with particular tissues or organs. Regardless of the cause for metastases, it is the effect of the spreading cancer that causes concern.

Chemotherapy, radiation, surgery, and biotherapy

are currently the four treatment choices for cancer. These interventions may be used as singular approaches to treatment or in combination. Surgery, the oldest treatment for cancer, is used for diagnosis and treatment. The surgical role in diagnoses is to obtain a tissue sample of the tumor for exact histologic diagnosis. Surgery is also used to evaluate the effectiveness of other treatments in eliminating the tumor. An exploratory laparotomy is one example of surgery being used to evaluate the effectiveness of chemotherapy for lymphoma.

Surgery can be an effective treatment for a tumor that is resectable. If the tumor is not entirely resectable, surgery is used to debulk (reduce the size of) the tumor so that radiation or chemotherapy can be more effective. Surgery is also useful in relieving a growing tumor that may be compressing other organ structures, causing pain or obstruction.

At times surgery can be radical, involving the removal of normal as well as malignant tissue, muscle, and parts of or entire organs or limbs. Radical surgery may eventually be followed by restorative, reconstructive, or plastic surgery.

Chemotherapy is a successful systemic approach to treating most malignancies. However, chemotherapy is limited in its usefulness because of the myelosuppression it causes and the development of tumor resistance to the antineoplastic agents. The aim of chemotherapy is to reduce the number of cancerous cells by affecting their ability to reproduce. To accomplish this best, chemotherapy agents have their most toxic effect against rapidly proliferating cells. Unfortunately, many rapidly proliferating normal cells—leukocytes, platelets, hair follicles, cells lining the gastrointestinal tract—will also be destroyed. Until chemotherapy is further refined to be cancer cell specific, the complications of chemotherapy will limit its therapeutic effectiveness.

The development of drug resistance by malignant cells also hinders the success of chemotherapy. Because drug resistance develops after subsequent doses, the first dose of chemotherapy has the best chance of being effective. Maximum doses of combination chemotherapy are usually carefully calculated to provide the patient with the highest cell kill while preventing life-threatening complications.

Radiation therapy damages cellular DNA and RNA, which results in impaired cellular function or cell death. As with chemotherapy, radiation therapy is not specific for malignant cells. Radiation has devastating effects on all cells, normal or malignant, within the path of ionization.

Radiation may be delivered as an external beam treatment. The beam of ionization is aimed exactly at the site and depth of the tumor and is delivered in such a way as to minimize its effect on normal tissue. Radiation may also be delivered as a sealed source of cesium, iodine, iridium, or radium that is surgically implanted directly into or immediately surrounding the tumor.

Radiation may be used as a curative therapy, as in Hodgkin's disease, or as adjunctive treatment for uterine cancer. Radiation may also be used palliatively to relieve symptoms, such as bone pain or superior vena cava obstruction, associated with incurable advancing disease.

There has been increasing focus on the treatment arena of biotherapy. In the past, bacille Calmette-Guérin vaccine has been used to stimulate the patient's own immune system to counteract the cancer. Through a greater understanding of the immune system and the development of technologic advances, biologic response modifiers (BRMs) have surfaced as the newest weapon against cancer. BRMs are defined by the National Cancer Institute as "those agents or approaches that modify the relationship between tumor and host by modifying the host's biological response to tumor cells with resultant therapeutic effects" (Jassak, 1990).

There are many side effects associated with the use of BRMs. Hematologic and gastrointestinal reactions can be similar to those that result from conventional therapy. The unique side effects of BRMs include cardiovascular and neurologic reactions. The neurologic effects from BRMs may be subtle. Cognitive changes and lethargy may be difficult to assess if the patient is critically ill. Significant toxicities involving the cardiovascular, pulmonary, renal, and other organ systems are frequently associated with the use of interleukin-2 (IL-2). The addition of lymphokine-activated killer cells to IL-2 therapy has been associated with a drop in systemic vascular resistance, the development of capillary leak syndrome, and renal failure (Lotze & Rosenberg, 1991). Because of these toxic side effects, it is common for the patient to require an intensive care setting and the skills of a critical care nurse during treatment (Figure 70–1). Table 70–1 summarizes the findings and clinical implications for the patient receiving IL-2 therapy.

As the development and spread of cancer are better understood, treatment modalities can be refined to improve their effectiveness. Until that occurs, cancer patients will continue to receive treatment that affects normal as well as malignant cells. Health care professionals will be challenged to support patients through life-threatening complications.

Some oncologic crises—spinal cord compression (SCS), superior vena cava syndrome (SVCS), hypercalcemia—are unique complications of cancer. These complications are discussed in detail in this chapter. The development of other pathophysiologic states is not necessarily limited to the cancer population. The progression of the malignancy or the complications of cancer treatment may lead to hemorrhage, disseminated intravascular coagulation, or septic shock secondary to myelosuppression. Electrolyte imbalances develop as a result of tumor lysis syndrome or the syndrome of inappropriate antidiuretic hormone. Bowel obstruction results from tumor growth or from the neurotoxic effects of some chemotherapy agents. Table 70–2 briefly describes these pathophysiologic states as they appear in oncologic patients.

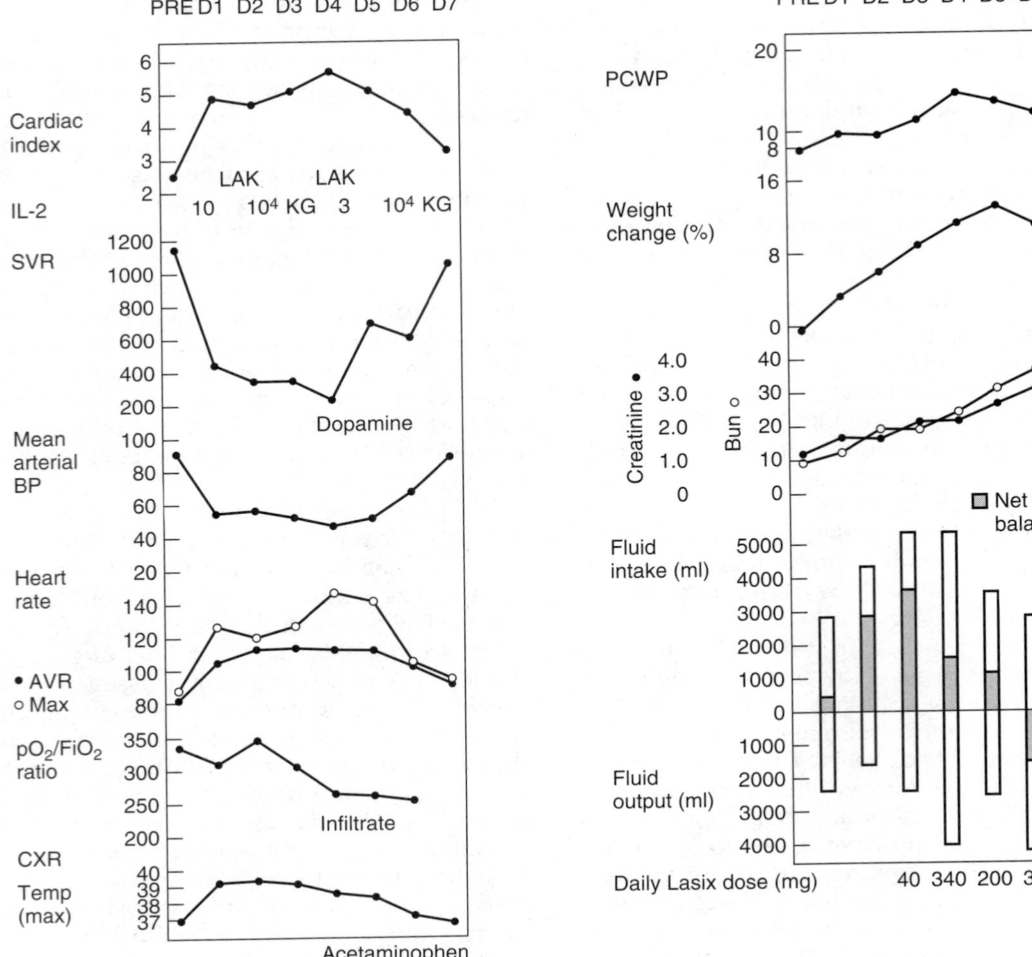

FIGURE 70–1. Sequential hemodynamic measurements in a patient receiving lymphokine-activated killer cells (LAK) and interleukin-2 (IL-2); 30,000 U/kg was administered thrice daily on days 1 through 3 and 10^5 U/kg on days 3 through 6. LAK infusions were given on days 12, 13, and 15 with concurrent IL-2 at 100,000 U/kg continued through day 16. SVR (dynes · sec · cm^5) and mean arterial pressure (mm Hg) decreased and cardiac index (liters/minute/m^2) increased. The pulmonary capillary wedge pressure (mm Hg) and net weight increased during both cycles. A rapid return to normal was noted after discontinuation of treatment. (From Lotze, M. T., & Rosenberg, S. A. [1991]. Interleukin-2: Clinical applications. In V. T. DeVita, Jr., S. Hellman, & S. A. Rosenberg [Eds.]. *Biologic therapy of cancer* [pp. 159–177]. Philadelphia: J. B. Lippincott.)

SPINAL CORD COMPRESSION

Spinal cord compression is a complication of metastasizing solid and hematologic malignancies. Without prompt medical intervention, the inevitable neurologic damage truly makes SCC an oncologic emergency (Delaney & Oldfield, 1993). Even in incurable cancers, the disruption in quality of life caused by SCC encourages most practitioners to treat this complication aggressively at its earliest detection.

Pathophysiology

The spinal cord has both motor and sensory functions. The spinal cord receives and transmits signals from 31 pairs of spinal nerves. Every spinal nerve contains a dorsal (afferent) and ventral (efferent) root. The afferent root serves as the sensory division of the peripheral nervous system. The somatic afferent fibers carry impulses from the skin, skeletal muscles, joints, and tendons to the central nervous system. The central nervous system receives impulses from the viscera via the visceral afferent fibers (Henze, 1992).

The efferent division responds to the sensory input with motor activity. The visceral efferent system innervates through the autonomic nervous system, of which the sympathetic and parasympathetic divisions belong. The somatic efferent system innervates the muscles, tendons, and joints through the pyramidal (upper motor neurons) and extrapyramidal (lower motor neurons) systems (Henze, 1992).

TABLE 70–1. **Interleukin-2 (IL-2)**

Interleukin-2 is a lymphokine naturally produced by helper T cells that plays a variety of imunoregulatory roles. Studies have discovered that IL-2 enhances natural killer cell function, augments alloantigen responsiveness, activates lymphokine-activated killer cells, and improves the recovery of immune function. This biologic response modifier also causes a marked redistribution of lymphoid cells to specific tissues, including the lungs, liver, and mesenteric lymph nodes (Lotze & Rosenberg, 1991). IL-2 is used as one means to restore or "boost" the host's own immune system. Augmenting the patient's immune system through the use of IL-2 hypothetically will control the growth or metastasis of tumor cells (Rieger et al., 1993).

Interleukin-2 has been approved for use in the treatment of patients with metastatic renal cell cancer. The use of IL-2 for other malignancies is investigational. It may be administered by a variety of routes, including intravenous, subcutaneous, and peritoneal. As clinical trials continue, the maximum tolerated dose, by the various routes of administration, will eventually be determined. It is also hoped that clinical trials will identify medical and nursing interventions that will improve the management of the toxic side effects of IL-2. The major dose-limiting toxic effect of IL-2 is the development of a capillary leak syndrome. A release of vasoactive factor facilitates the flow of protein-containing plasma water out of the vascular compartment and into the interstitial space of many organs. This results in hemodynamic instability and renal dysfunction. Toxic effects associated with the clinical use of IL-2 are summarized as follows (Rieger et al., 1993; Oncology Nursing Society, 1989).

Organ System	Clinical Findings	Clinical Implications
Central nervous system	Confusion Altered mentation	Sleep deprivation, unfamiliar sights and sounds may exacerbate CNS toxicity of IL-2 Patient must be protected from harm Patient is frequently assessed for continued deterioration of mental status IL-2 therapy may be interrupted if confusion is severe
Renal	Elevated BUN Elevated serum creatinine Proteinuria Oliguria	Urine output must be monitored hourly Urine is tested for protein Daily BUN and creatinine levels are determined during IL-2 treatment An infusion of 2–5 μg/kg/minute of dopamine may be used to increase renal perfusion Loop diuretics (furosemide) may be prescribed to increase urine flow through the renal tubules
Pulmonary	Interstitial pulmonary edema Dyspnea Hypoxemia	Intubation and mechanical ventilation may be required The patient is carefully assessed for signs of increasing dyspnea, restlessness Arterial blood gases are monitored for decreasing oxygen saturation
Cardiac	Decreased pulmonary capillary wedge pressure Decreased central venous pressure Hypotension Peripheral edema Transient dysrhythmias ST-T wave changes Elevated creatine kinase levels	Fluid shifts (as much as 10%) from the vascular space into the interstitium Large amounts of crystalloid and colloid fluid may be needed to maintain intravascular volume Vasopressors may be required to maintain blood pressure
Gastrointestinal	Nausea/vomiting Diarrhea	Antiemetics and antidiarrheal medications may be helpful in controlling symptoms
Integument	Erythematous rash Pruritus Skin desquamation	Meticulous skin care is essential Topical ointments may be prescribed to relieve discomfort
Hematologic	Thrombocytopenia Anemia Fever Chills Flu-like syndrome	Hemoglobin, hematocrit, and platelets are monitored closely. Transfusion of red blood cells and/or platelets may be required Fever and chills may be alleviated by the administration of an antipyretic (acetaminophen), an antihistamine (diphenhydramine hydrochloride), and a narcotic analgesic (meperidine hydrochloride)

Abbreviations: BUN, blood urea nitrogen; CNS, central nervous system.

TABLE 70–2. **Common Pathophysiologic States Occurring in Oncologic Patients**

Myelosuppression	
Etiology:	Replacement of bone marrow by primary or metastatic cancer
	Effects of myelosuppressive treatment
Clinical findings:	Bleeding secondary to thrombocytopenia
	Anemia secondary to erythropenia
Management:	Support host defense mechanisms
	Avoid damage to protective body barriers (e.g., invasive procedures)
	Reduce exposure to new potential pathogens
	Suppress colonizing organisms
Tumor Lysis Syndrome	
Etiology:	Cellular death and lysis after chemotherapy releases large amounts of intracellular electrolytes and metabolites into the circulation
Clinical findings:	Elevated serum phosphate, potassium, uric acid levels
	Decreased serum calcium level
Management:	Prevent renal failure by hydration, administration of allopurinol, diuretics
	Monitor and treat electrolyte imbalances as they occur
SIADH (Syndrome of Inappropriate Antidiuretic Hormone [ADH] Secretion)	
Etiology:	Ectopic production of ADH by certain tumors (small or oat cell carcinoma of the lung, duodenal and pancreatic carcinoma, others)
Clinical findings:	Fluid retention, fluid volume overload
	Dilutional hyponatremia
Management:	Fluid restriction
	Diuresis with hypertonic saline
	Drug therapy: demeclocycline, urea, furosemide, lithium carbonate
Bowel Obstruction	
Etiology:	Primary tumor occlusion of the lumen of the bowel
	Secondary tumor obstruction
	Bands of adhesions or scar tissue from prior abdominal surgery
	Tissue changes secondary to radiation treatments
	Neurotoxicity from chemotherapy with vinca alkaloids
	Chronic use of narcotics that inhibit peristalsis, leading to bowel impaction
Clinical findings:	Abdominal pain, distention
	Vomiting, change in elimination pattern
	Dehydration, hypovolemia
	Electrolyte, acid–base disturbances
Management:	Surgical intervention to eliminate/reduce the source of obstruction
	Decompression by nasogastric drainage tube
	Hydration and electrolyte therapy

Data from Dietz, K. A., & Flaherty, A. M. (1990). Oncologic emergencies. In S. L. Groenwald et al. (Eds.), *Cancer nursing: Principles and practices* (pp. 644–668). Boston: Jones and Bartlett; Miaskowski, C. (1991). Oncologic emergencies. In S. B. Baird et al. (Eds.), *Cancer nursing: A comprehensive approach* (pp. 885–893). Philadelphia: W. B. Saunders.

Disruption of the sensory or motor functions of the spinal cord can be the result of an extramedullary tumor, intramedullary tumor, extradural tumor within the spinal canal, or bony metastasis to a vertebra outside of the spinal canal. In cancer, SCC is usually the result of a primary tumor metastasizing to the epidural space. The lesion is most frequently extramedullary, with only 5% occurring within the spinal column. Solid tumors have the highest overall chances of metastatic SCC. Cancers of the lung, breast, and prostate carry the highest risk. SCC may also be the result of metastatic hematologic malignancies such as multiple myeloma and lymphoma. The most common site of metastasis is the thoracic vertebrae (70%), with cervical and lumbar involvement equally less affected (30%) (Delaney & Oldfield, 1993).

Tumor impairment of the neurons disrupts reflexes and motor function. Spastic paralysis below the level of the tumor occurs if the upper motor neuron or corticospinal tract is affected. Lower motor neuron damage affects voluntary muscle movement and results in flaccid paralysis and sensory disturbance below the level of the tumor (Held & Peahota, 1993).

The prognosis of SCC varies. The prognosis is good if the onset is slow, the duration of motor dysfunction is less than 24 hours, sphincter control remains present, and the patient is able to maintain an ambulatory status. Location of the tumor within the posterior epidural space and in the lumbar or sacral areas is an additional favorable sign. A poor prognosis is associated with rapid onset, motor dysfunction for longer than 48 hours, absent sphincter control, and if the patient experiences paralysis. Prognosis is less favorable when the tumor is located in the anterior epidural space and lies in the thoracic or cervical areas (Delaney & Oldfield, 1993; Held & Peahota, 1993).

Clinical Presentation

The clinical presentation of SCC is divided into prodromal and compressive phases (Delaney & Oldfield, 1993). Progressive back pain from local bony involvement characterizes the prodromal phase. The back pain is usually localized to the involved spinal segment with or without radicular pain to the chest, abdomen, or extremities. The pain usually begins 6 months or less before the diagnosis of SCC is eventually made. The pain may be aggravated by motion or by lying down.

Invariably, pain is followed by the development of other symptoms. The compressive phase is the result of motor and sensory dysfunction from the growing tumor compressing the cord. In the compressive phase, sensory dysfunction begins with extremity paresthesia, numbness, tingling, and coolness. As the lesion enlarges, these symptoms tend to ascend the body. Motor dysfunction may occur concomitant with or after sensory dysfunction. As described in Figure 70–2, the degree of motor dysfunction depends on whether complete or incomplete upper motor neuron

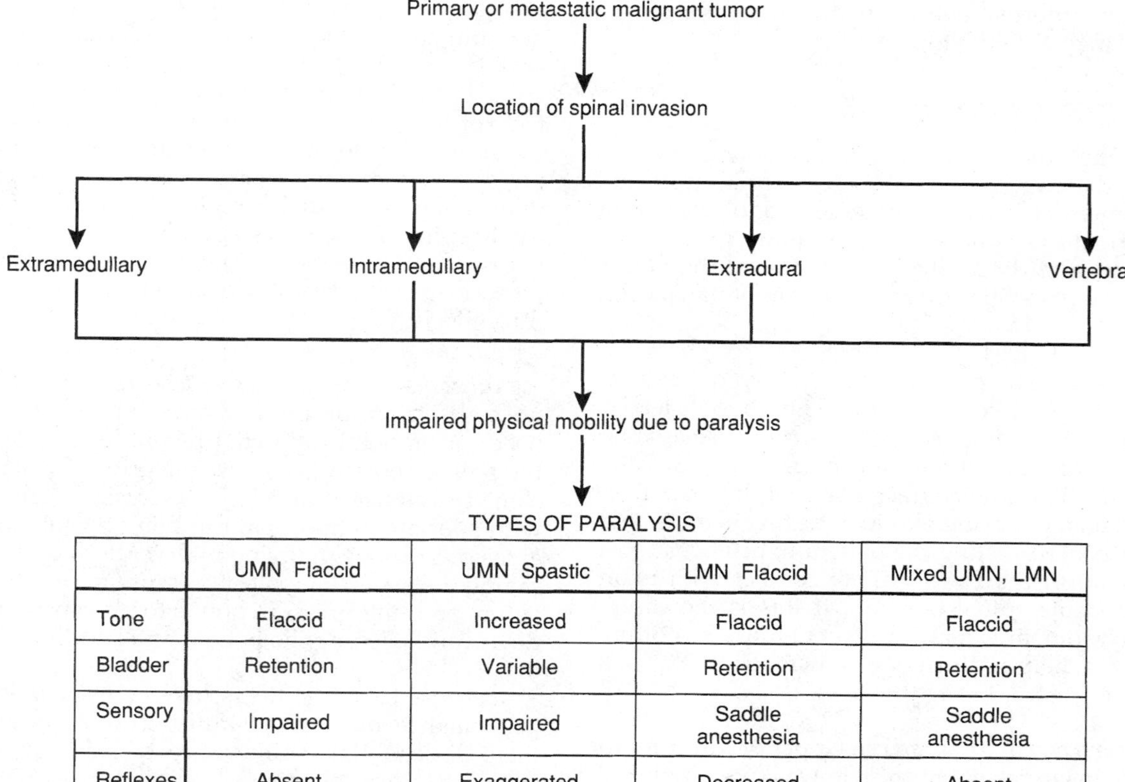

	UMN Flaccid	UMN Spastic	LMN Flaccid	Mixed UMN, LMN
Tone	Flaccid	Increased	Flaccid	Flaccid
Bladder	Retention	Variable	Retention	Retention
Sensory	Impaired	Impaired	Saddle anesthesia	Saddle anesthesia
Reflexes	Absent	Exaggerated	Decreased	Absent

FIGURE 70–2. Paralysis in acute spinal cord compression. *Abbreviations:* UMN, upper motor neuron; LMN, lower motor neuron.

or lower motor neuron dysfunction has occurred (Held & Peahota, 1993).

In addition to pain and numbness, 75% of patients also complain of weakness (Delaney & Oldfield, 1993). Footdrop and difficulty in maintaining balance may also be noted. Disturbances in micturition and sensory impairment commonly occur together if the site of compression involves the lower lumbar portion of the spinal cord. Bowel or bladder dysfunction are unfavorable prognostic signs. Two-thirds of patients with bowel and bladder dysfunction become nonambulatory from the progression of the disease.

Respiratory depression is a possibility if the lesion is located at cervical level 5 or above. In addition to progressive paresis of diaphragmatic and intercostal muscles, the small muscle groups of the hands, forearms, and arms may also waste (Held & Peahota, 1993).

Clinical Management

Spinal cord compression is managed by surgery, surgery followed by radiation, or radiation alone. The decision as to therapy depends on the type of tumor, the level of block, and the rapidity of onset or duration of symptoms (Delaney & Oldfield, 1993).

SURGICAL DECOMPRESSION

Surgical decompression is recommended "only for patients with no previous tissue diagnosis, progressive neurologic dysfunction during radiation, or recurrent cord compression after previous radiation therapy" (Delaney & Oldfield, 1993, p. 2121). A laminectomy can achieve prompt decompression of the spinal cord, but rarely can it remove all of the tumor. Significant surgical morbidity and mortality may occur, making this choice of treatment unlikely in patients with a short life expectancy.

RADIATION THERAPY

The primary treatment of choice remains local irradiation or corticosteroids. Fractionated irradiation doses range from 2,000 to 4,000 cGy delivered over 1 to 4 weeks. The radiation port includes the affected vertebra plus the two vertebral bodies above and below. The therapy is begun immediately on diagnosis (Kagan, 1992).

Corticosteroids are concomitantly administered in high doses. One common dosage regimen is 10 to 100 mg dexamethasone intravenously followed by 4 mg every 6 hours with tapering after radiation therapy or surgery. Corticosteroids are given to decrease inflammation, improve neurologic function, and relieve pain (Delaney & Oldfield, 1993).

PREVENTION OF COMPLICATIONS

The nursing management of patients with SCC is based on the patient's actual and potential problems. Nursing interventions are implemented to prevent the development of secondary complications, prevent further injury, and detect the progression of the neurologic symptoms while still in an early and manageable state.

ACUTE PAIN. The destruction of the spinal column and damage to the cord and spinal nerve roots lead to acute, agonizing pain. The critical care nurse assesses the patient for pain with each contact and records the location, severity, and characteristics of the pain. Basic pain management principles include an effective analgesic protocol. Assisting the patient to achieve a position of comfort may be in direct conflict with maintaining a stable spinal position. If this is the case, a quiet environment, behavioral techniques, or soothing touches can help distract the patient from the pain experience.

IMPAIRED PHYSICAL MOBILITY. Upper or lower motor neuron damage results in muscle weakness, reflex alterations, or paralysis. The critical care nurse conducts neurologic assessments every 1 to 2 hours. The nurse compares these assessments with previous baseline findings to determine if the cord compression is improving, stabilizing, or progressing. Because the patient's prognosis is directly correlated with the amount of neurologic impairment, early detection of a deterioration in the patient's neurologic status can prevent further injury (Dietz & Flaherty, 1990; Held & Peahota, 1993).

Specific neurologic assessments to detect a change in the patient's motor pathways include a testing for hand grip, arm and leg strength, and finger-to-thumb coordination. Reflexes to be tested include the biceps, triceps, upper and lower abdominal, knee, ankle, and plantar (Babinski). Additional observations include the presence of muscle atrophy, fasciculations, involuntary movement, lack of voluntary movement, or abnormal positions. These findings help to define and further pinpoint the spinal nerves affected.

The nurse should consider a patient's spine unstable until proved otherwise. If the vertebra's skeletal integrity has been severely compromised by the invading lesion, the patient may be placed in an immobile position to prevent cord damage. In preparation for immobilizing the patient, the critical care nurse evaluates the need for a Stryker frame or other position-maintaining beds. Crutchfield tongs may be necessary if the cervical vertebrae are involved. If absolute immobilization is not required, the critical care nurse sees that spinal alignment is maintained during turning and positioning of the patient in bed (e.g., log roll). When the patient is in the supine position, the nurse maintains the patient's ideal spinal alignment by avoiding the use of pillows and by placing a footboard at the end of the bed. The use of a footboard or other special devices helps to counteract the irreversible effects of footdrop.

In addition to maintaining the patient in a stable position, the nursing plan of care includes interventions that prevent further patient injury from immobility. Respiratory exercises and a skin care protocol are necessary. If possible, range-of-motion exercises are performed to prevent development of deep vein thrombosis.

HIGH RISK FOR IMPAIRED SKIN INTEGRITY. The loss of normal sensory and motor function and the possible need for immobilization to prevent further damage to the spinal cord threaten the integrity of the patient's skin. The status of the skin is assessed every 2 hours, with special attention paid to bony prominences and areas of pressure. Nursing interventions include massaging the areas of greatest pressure to promote circulation, padding pressure points to prevent skin breakdown, and keeping the patient and bedding clean and dry.

Because cancer patients may be in negative nitrogen balance due to the nutrition-robbing effects of their disease, the maintenance of skin integrity becomes a critical element of nursing care. Supporting the nutritional status as a mechanism to preserve skin integrity is much easier than trying to promote the healing of pressure ulcers. The critical care nurse may need to collaborate with the dietitian to identify effective means of maintaining nutritional status.

INEFFECTIVE BREATHING PATTERN. Spinal cord lesions at cervical level 5 or above affect both diaphragmatic and intercostal musculature. Lesions below cervical level 5 paralyze the intercostals (Mitchell, 1993). A thorough patient assessment identifies how much of the respiratory musculature is affected by the motor and sensory impairment. Patients with lesions below thoracic level 4 maintain adequate voluntary respiratory function, whereas patients with lesions above thoracic level 4 require frequent evaluation of respiratory function (Mitchell, 1993).

Bedside spirometry can easily measure the patient's vital capacity (VC). By monitoring VC, the critical care nurse detects whether the patient is losing respiratory muscle function secondary to spinal edema or advancing tumor. The patient may require ventilatory assistance if the VC is below one-third of the predicted value or less than 600 cm^3. Respiratory patterns, signs and symptoms of respiratory insufficiency, arterial blood gases, and lung sounds assist the nurse in assessing the patient's ability to ventilate satisfactorily (Mitchell, 1993).

ALTERATION IN BOWEL ELIMINATION. Lesions above the sacral cord result in the loss of voluntary control and in sphincter dysfunction of the bowel. The loss of gastric motility from higher lesions may manifest as paralytic ileus.

On admission of the patient to the critical care unit, signs and symptoms of paralytic ileus and impaction are assessed. In addition, the patient is assessed for abdominal distention, decreased or absent bowel sounds, and nausea and vomiting. If a paralytic ileus is suspected, intestinal decompression should begin.

The critical care nurse immediately initiates a daily bowel evacuation program to prevent impaction and obstipation. Gentle manual removal of rectal contents or enemas may be needed until rectal reflexes return (Held & Peahota, 1993). Oral intake is withheld until bowel sounds and the passing of flatus have returned. In the meantime, nutritional support of the patient must be maintained through alternative feeding routes such as total parenteral nutrition. Intravenous solutions can provide the fluids necessary for optimal bowel elimination.

URINARY RETENTION. The disruption of the innervation of the bladder from spinal lesions above the sacral cord results in the loss of voluntary bladder elimination of urine (Mitchell, 1993). An indwelling catheter is necessary during the initial course of SCC as a means of avoiding bladder distention. Throughout the period of continuous bladder catheterization, the nurse monitors temperature trends and the characteristics of the urine for any signs of possible bladder infection. Once continuous bladder catheterization is discontinued, the nurse may need to initiate intermittent catheterizations to check for residual urine. Between intermittent catheterizations, the patient is assessed for bladder distention. Because the patient is lacking the sensation to void, the urinal or bedpan is offered at regular intervals.

DECREASED CARDIAC OUTPUT. Acute spinal cord injury may result in spinal shock. During the period of spinal shock, somatic and autonomic reflex activity below the level of the lesion is lost. With the loss of sympathetic function and the predominance of parasympathetic function, the cardiovascular system and viscera slow down. Bradycardia and dysrhythmias can occur because the vagal influence is unopposed (Mitchell, 1993). Hypotension becomes problematic because with the loss of the sympathetic nervous system, peripheral vascular resistance can no longer be maintained. Adjusting the patient's position from side to side carries a risk of hypotension because the heart has lost the reflexes to adjust blood pressure in response to a change in position. The loss of peripheral vascular tone impairs venous return to the heart and promotes venous stasis. Not only do these accentuate the problem of hypotension, they lead to the development of deep vein thrombosis (Mitchell, 1993).

When caring for the patient in spinal shock, the critical care nurse monitors the patient's cardiac rate and rhythm to detect serious arrhythmias or bradycardia. The nurse monitors the blood pressure before and after turning to assess the patient's cardiovascular tolerance to a change in position. Circulatory fluid volume is maintained through the cautious use of intravenous fluids. Throughout volume replacement, the nurse carefully monitors the patient for the development of pulmonary edema (Mitchell, 1993).

The patient in spinal shock is unable to maintain an appropriate body temperature because the peripheral vessels have remained dilated from the loss of sympathetic function. As a result, the body temperature takes on the temperature of the environment. In the typical air-conditioned unit, the patient's temperature will drop. If the patient's body temperature cannot be maintained through the usual application of warm blankets, a heating blanket may be necessary. A cooling blanket may be used if the patient's temperature is too high. Because the patient cannot feel the temperature of the device, the nurse needs to assess the functioning of the equipment and the condition of the patient's skin (Mitchell, 1993).

SUPERIOR VENA CAVA SYNDROME

Superior vena cava syndrome commonly is associated with bronchogenic carcinoma and malignant lymphomas. The syndrome has also been increasingly reported as a complication of the use of central venous catheters. SVCS occurs when the thin-walled superior vena cava is obstructed, resulting in systemic congestion and increased pressure. An obstruction of the superior vena cava may retard the flow of blood from the head, neck, and upper thorax, leading to the development of signs and symptoms classic for this acute oncologic emergency (Miaskowski, 1991). In most situations, these patients are cared for in ambulatory settins or general care units. However, if the patient presents with a severe decrease in cardiac output and ineffective breathing patterns, admission to a critical care unit is appropriate. Supporting the patient throughout the initial work-up and initiation of treatment to relieve the obstruction is the primary focus of the critical care nurse.

PATHOPHYSIOLOGY

The superior vena cava is located in the superior mediastinum and is surrounded by solid structures including the trachea, vertebral bodies, sternum, and lymph nodes. As a thin-walled, low-pressure vessel, the superior vena cava is particularly vulnerable to compression. Malignant causes contributing to the development of this complication include lung cancer and lymphoma. These tumors occlude the vessel by extrinsic pressure or direct invasion (Dietz & Flaherty, 1990). A third cause of SVCS is intraluminal thrombosis. Central venous catheters have been associated with the development of this complication. A central venous catheter irritates the wall of the vein, causing local injury and thrombus formation.

A significant obstruction of the superior vena cava

interferes with the return of blood from the head, neck, upper extremities, and upper thorax. Other routes or vessels are used to bypass the obstruction and return the blood to the heart. The development of this collateral circulation depends on the location of the obstruction. If the obstruction of the superior vena cava has occurred above the azygos vein, the blood flow returns to the heart through the subclavian vein and proximal superior vena cava. An obstruction proximal to the superior vena cava–azygos vein junction results in blood flow being redirected through the inferior vena cava. Most problematic is the obstruction that occurs directly at this junction. More distal routes must be used and collateral channels developed to assist in the return of the blood from the upper torso back to the heart (Dietz & Flaherty, 1990). It is in these obstructions that the more dramatic and classic signs and symptoms of SVCS occur.

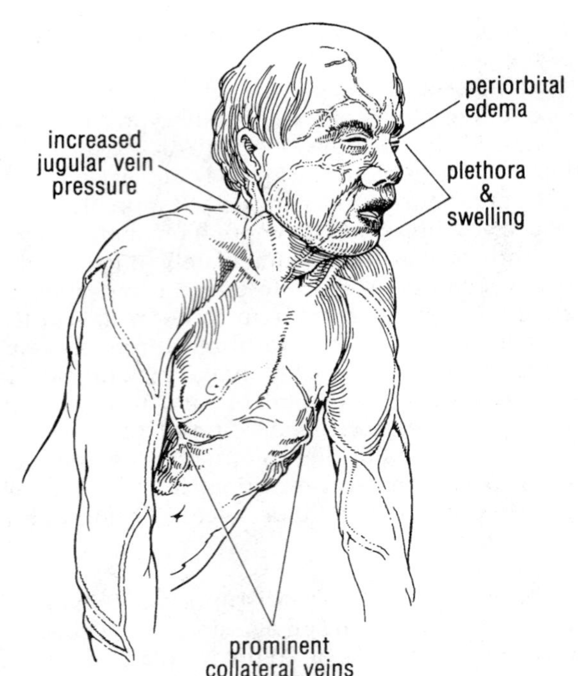

FIGURE 70–3. Signs of superior vena cava obstruction. (From Miller, S. E. [1987]. Superior vena cava syndrome. In R. C. Polomano & S. E. Miller (Eds.), *Understanding and managing oncologic emergencies* [p. 28]. Columbus, OH: Adria Laboratories, Division of Erbamont Inc.)

Clinical Presentation

The clinical manifestations of SVCS are the result of increased venous pressure and stasis of blood flow. The developing signs and symptoms are reflective of the vascular congestion in the cerebrum, pulmonary complications, and thrombogenic sequelae (Yahalom, 1993). Clinical symptoms include dyspnea (63%), cough (24%), and chest pain (15%). Dysphagia, visual disturbances, hoarseness, dizziness, and a feeling of facial fullness are also frequently reported. Among the physical findings are prominent collateral veins of the upper thorax, including the distention of the thoracic veins (67%), and neck vein distention. As shown in Figures 70–3 and 70–4, tachypnea, facial swelling, swelling of the upper torso, plethora of the face, edema of the conjunctivae, and increased jugular venous pressure are also observed. These symptoms worsen when the patient is recumbent. Left untreated, SVCS can progress into laryngeal edema; severe upper airway obstruction; cyanosis of the upper body due to venous stasis; and altered consciousness, including coma.

Clinical Management

The management of SVCS includes disease management, resolution of the obstruction, and application of comfort measures.

DIAGNOSIS

Patients who present with SVCS may or may not have a previous cancer diagnosis. Because up to 90% of all cases are associated with a malignant disease, of which bronchogenic carcinoma is most prevalent, medical attention is directed toward obtaining an accurate diagnosis. Diagnostic proceedings usually are concentrated on obtaining a tissue biopsy specimen. In addition to tissue diagnosis, sputum cytology, bronchoscopy, transbronchial biopsy, percutaneous biopsy, cervical mediastinal exploration, and thoracotomy may also be performed. A chest x-ray shows a mediastinal widening, a mass, distention of the azygous vein, or associated pleural effusion (Yahalom, 1993). After an accurate tissue diagnosis has been made, appropriate treatment for the underlying disease may begin.

Controversy surrounds the issue of establishing a tissue diagnosis in patients presenting with SVCS. Traditional practice has been to treat the worrisome complication and reduce the severity of obstruction before obtaining biopsy specimens. In addition, patients were considered at high risk for bleeding if invasive procedures were conducted. However, current literature suggests that diagnostic procedures can be conducted safely in the presence of SVCS. Mortality is considered to be more directly attributed to the underlying disease rather than to the complication itself (Ahmann, 1984).

DISEASE MANAGEMENT

Radiation therapy is the treatment of choice for SVCS. Generous chest portals, including the mediastinum hila and any adjacent pulmonary lesions, are irradiated. Currently, radiation is administered in high dose fractions (400-cGy tumor dose) for 2 or 3 days. Additional daily doses of 180 to 200 cGy follow until a total dose of 6,000 to 7,000 cGy is given. Subjective relief of symptoms may be experienced 3 to 4 days after the first dose of radiation (Emani & Perez, 1992).

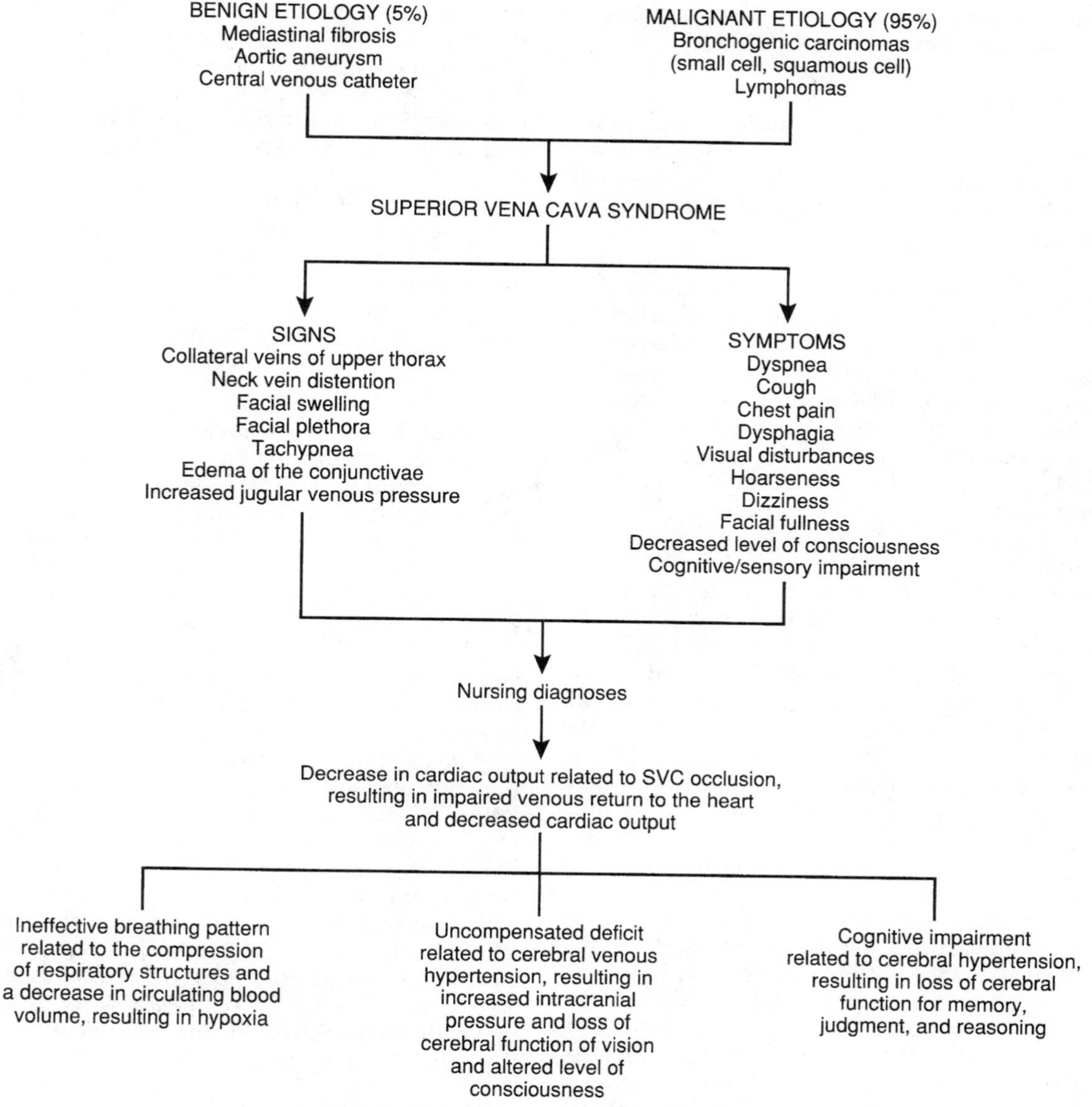

FIGURE 70–4. Superior vena cava syndrome.

As radiation treatments continue, the patient experiences adverse effects as the underlying tissues become damaged. Esophagitis, dysphagia, hoarseness, dry cough, loss of appetite, and lethargy occur. Although most of these adverse effects resolve after treatment is completed, they are nevertheless distressful to the patient.

Chemotherapy is a useful treatment for SVCS if the underlying disease is small cell carcinoma of the lung or lymphomas (Yahalom, 1993). These malignancies are very responsive to the effects of chemotherapy, and the patient experiences rapid relief of the symptoms. After the administration of chemotherapy, radiation treatment may or may not be needed for further control of the disease.

Anticoagulants and fibrinolytic therapy are appropriate treatments if the underlying cause of the complication is thrombosis, as seen with the use of central venous catheters. Removal of the catheter may be required.

SYMPTOM MANAGEMENT

Supportive therapy promotes comfort and helps reduce the patient's level of distress. Diuretics may be used to reduce edema, but they must be used with caution. Diuretic-induced dehydration may potentiate thrombus formation or the development of hypovolemic shock (Miaskowski, 1991). Steroids may be appropriately prescribed if the patient exhibits respiratory insufficiency. Supplemental oxygen may be indicated for dyspnea. Fibrinolytic agents are used if the obstruction is due to intramural thrombi. Anticoagulants are beneficial in preventing thrombosis due to a decreased circulatory time and blood flow through the obstructed vessels (Dietz & Flaherty, 1990).

Care of the patient diagnosed with SVCS focuses on symptom management and the prevention of acute complications. Though not the life-threatening complication it was originally believed to be, SVCS requires an intensive nursing approach to the management of the distressful signs and symptoms that the patient may experience (Ahmann, 1984).

DECREASED CARDIAC OUTPUT. As presented in Figure 70–4, obstruction of the superior vena cava results in impaired venous return to the heart and decreased cardiac output. The critical care nurse conducts an initial physical assessment of the patient to determine the severity of the obstruction. Observations for distention of the neck and chest veins, facial and periorbital edema, tachypnea, and cyanosis are made. The baseline findings are recorded, and the observations continue every 4 hours throughout the acute phase of this complication.

A decrease in cardiac output makes these patients susceptible to hypovolemic shock. The critical care nurse monitors the urinary output and calculates the intake : output ratio for fluid balance. The maintenance of an intravenous infusion ensures adequate hydration of the patient in addition to providing a vascular route for emergency medications. It is important for the nurse to select an extremity whose circulation has not been compromised by the obstruction before insertion of the venous catheter. In severe cases of SVCS, the location of a site for the venous catheter may become quite difficult to determine.

Central venous pressure measurements and neck vein distention measured in centimeters help the critical care nurse assess the patient's current cardiovascular condition. These measurements are conducted every 1 to 2 hours. To detect the early development of circulatory problems, the peripheral pulses are assessed for bilateral quality and the nailbeds tested for blanching. The skin is assessed for color, temperature, and moisture. The head of the bed is kept elevated to promote the return of the blood to the heart and to prevent further edema (Dietz & Flaherty, 1990). Bedrest is essential because even minimal activity may overtax the cardiovascular system's ability to meet the increased need for oxygen.

A change in the level of consciousness is an indication of failing cardiovascular function in the patient with SVCS. With this in mind, the critical care nurse is required to assess all possible causes of the presenting signs and symptoms and plan nursing interventions accordingly.

INEFFECTIVE BREATHING PATTERN. The compression of respiratory structures by growing or bulky tumors and the decrease in circulating blood volume result in hypoxia. Bed rest, high Fowler position, and minimal activity are nursing measures that conserve the patient's need for oxygen (Schafer, 1994). In addition, the critical care nurse frequently assesses breath sounds for the early detection of adventitious sounds. With each patient contact, it is also important to assess for dyspnea and respiratory distress and to initiate supplemental oxygen at 2 liters/minute or as prescribed. The critical care nurse supplements the physical assessments by monitoring arterial blood gas values and adjusting the patient's nursing plan of care as indicated.

Other nursing interventions include meticulous mouth care, because these patients frequently convert to mouth breathing in an attempt to inspire additional air. Assessment of the client's voice quality is performed; changes in pitch, clarity, and hoarseness may be early indicators of further compression of the trachea.

ALTERED THOUGHT PROCESSES. The cerebral venous hypertension and oxygen deprivation that occur in SVCS account for an altered level of consciousness and impaired vision. Patient safety issues become a prime concern for the critical care nurse. Side rails must be up and padded in case the patient becomes restless and disoriented. The patient may inadvertently damage intravenous tubing, nasogastric tubes, endotracheal tubes, and other devices attached to the body or bed. These patients require frequent reorientation from the critical care nurse and the initiation of protective measures to prevent accidental injuries.

The cerebral hypertension results in a loss of cerebral function for memory, judgment, and reasoning. Before all procedures, the critical care nurse needs to explain the purpose and technique in terms the patient will understand. Simple commands may be difficult for the patient to understand. The patient may need to have information frequently repeated and may not be able reliably to provide informed consent for medical treatments. It is essential that the critical care nurse be able to assist the family with bedside visits and meetings with the health care team so that a mutually beneficial plan of care can be implemented.

ALTERED NUTRITION: LESS THAN BODY REQUIREMENTS. Another nursing care problem in SVCS is inadequate nutritional support. The patient may be too breathless to eat or may experience difficulty in swallowing. Malignant disease and the patient's increased breathing activity require additional sources of nutrition if a positive nitrogen balance is to be maintained. If oral nutritional support is inadequate, tube feedings usually are implemented. The critical care nurse is responsible for maintaining the feedings, supplementing them with water to maintain hydration, and monitoring for any adverse effects from the feedings. Depending on the type of adverse effect, the nurse modifies the formula or rate of infusion so that the feedings can continue.

PAIN. Pain management is important for the patient with SVCS. High doses of narcotics may depress the respiratory rate or further impair the senses. Therefore, the critical care nurse carefully assesses the patient's degree of pain before administering narcotics. A low dose of narcotics plus other comfort measures may be all that is needed to provide the patient with adequate relief.

HYPERCALCEMIA

Hypercalcemia occurs in approximately 10% of cancer patients and is especially associated with cancer of the lung, breast, head and neck, and esophagus, and in patients with bone metastasis. Patients diagnosed with multiple myeloma are particularly prone to hypercalcemia, with 30% presenting with this complication on diagnosis and an additional 30% during the course of the disease (Silverman & Distelhorst, 1989). Hypercalcemia is considered an oncologic emergency because if undetected or undertreated the complication quickly becomes fatal.

Pathophysiology

Calcium, an essential inorganic element in the body, is primarily found in skeletal tissue. Only 1% of calcium is located in the serum. One-half of the serum calcium is bound to circulating albumin, whereas the remaining calcium is ionized within the blood. It is the ionized calcium that is capable of physiologic function (Schafer, 1994). Calcium functions to stabilize the cell membrane and block sodium transport into the cell, enhance coagulation, and provide the crystalline matrix of the bones and teeth (Bullock, 1992).

The homeostasis of calcium depends on sensitive hormonal regulatory mechanisms, including parathyroid hormone (PTH), vitamin D, and calcitonin. In response to low calcium, serum PTH is secreted by the parathyroid glands. The PTH stimulates osteoclasts to shift calcium out of the bone and into the serum. PTH stimulates kidney reabsorption of calcium, whereas both vitamin D and PTH enhance gastrointestinal absorption of calcium. Vitamin D also aids in the release of calcium from the bones. Conversely, calcitonin decreases serum calcium levels. This hormone, secreted by the thyroid gland, responds to high serum levels of calcium by inhibiting osteoclast activity (Bullock, 1992).

Although there are multiple mechanisms responsible for hypercalcemia in malignancy, increased bone resorption is a major feature in all patients (Silverman & Distelhorst, 1989). In the past, the development of hypercalcemia was most commonly associated with bone resorption due to increased osteoclast activity stimulated by the tumor or from the direct invasion of bone by tumor cells. Advances in molecular biology, the identification of new cytokines, and further understanding of renal pathophysiology have added a new dimension in the pathophysiology of malignancy-associated hypercalcemia.

A newly identified protein isolated from solid tumors is believed to initiate the humoral mechanism of hypercalcemia (Silverman & Distelhorst, 1989). This factor, called PTH-related protein, has nearly identical effects to those of PTH on the kidney and bone, thereby enhancing renal tubular calcium reabsorption. The existence of PTH-related protein does not explain all the manifestations of humoral hypercalcemia. There is a growing body of evidence that suggests some cytokines, such as IL-1 and tumor necrosis factor-alpha, modify the effects of PTH-related protein, and that the development of hypercalcemia occurs as the result of a combination of other mechanisms.

Hypercalcemia can occur for a variety of reasons in patients with solid tumors with osteolytic metastases (Silverman & Distelhorst, 1989; Warrell, 1993). Breast cancer cells may have the ability to resorb bone directly with or without the benefit of mediating factors. Prostaglandins have frequently been implicated as mediating factors. However, the low level of circulating prostaglandin E detected in hypercalcemic patients cannot account fully for this complication. Patients with Hodgkin's disease, non-Hodgkin's lymphoma, myeloma, and some solid tumors have demonstrated elevated serum levels of a derivative of vitamin D. Because these levels are below that which is known to cause hypercalcemia in patients with vitamin D intoxication, the role of the vitamin D derivative in cancer-related hypercalcemia is unclear (Warrell, 1993).

In multiple myeloma, malignant plasma cells produce osteoclast-activating factors, of which the major cytokine is believed to be lymphotoxin (Silverman & Distelhorst, 1989; Warrell, 1993). This cytokine accelerates bone resorption by normal osteoclasts. Amazingly, hypercalcemia develops in relatively few patients with lytic bone disease. This fact further supports the theory that hypercalcemia is a complex disorder that depends on the interplay of a variety of pathogenic mechanisms.

Under normal circumstances, the serum calcium is maintained within a narrow range of approximately 9 to 11 mg/dL. Because of the narrow range of normal, calculating the correct serum calcium level in patients suspected of hypercalcemia is necessary. Only 1% of the body's calcium is in the serum, with one-half of the serum calcium bound as an inactive ion to protein. Accounting for the inactive calcium bound to albumin, the serum calcium level is corrected using the following formulas (Lang-Kummer, 1990):

$$\text{Corrected calcium (mg/dL)} = \text{measured calcium} + [4 - \text{albumin (g/dL)}] \times 0.8$$

$$\text{Corrected calcium (mmol/L)} = \text{measured calcium} + [40 - \text{albumin (g/dL)}] \times 0.02$$

If the calcium level is not corrected for patients with low albumin, the laboratory report will be deceptively low and the severity of the patient's problem will be underestimated (Schafer, 1994).

Clinical Presentation

The clinical manifestations of hypercalcemia may occur slowly and insidiously, or may occur abruptly as a full-blown crisis. The degree of elevated serum calcium is not exclusively related to the severity of the clinical presentation. Patients with moderate elevations may become obtunded if the increase occurs quickly, whereas patients with chronic hypercalcemia may tolerate high levels with few symptoms (Warrell, 1993).

Symptoms of hypercalcemia occur in the gastrointestinal, neuromuscular, cardiac, and renal systems. Symptoms occur at different intensities depending on the severity of the hypercalcemia (Schafer, 1994; Warrell, 1993). Mild hypercalcemia is defined as a serum value less than 12 mg/dL. The presenting signs and symptoms can easily be attributed to other disease- or treatment-related factors, which makes early recognition of the problem difficult. The classic early signs of mental confusion and nocturia, polyuria, an polydipsia should alert the practitioner to investigate the possibility of hypercalcemia.

In mild hypercalcemia, the patient may complain of anorexia, nausea, vomiting, and vague abdominal pain. This is due to the slowing of the smooth muscle action of the gastrointestinal system that results from decreased excitability of muscles and nerves. Restlessness, difficulty in concentrating, depression, apathy, lethargy, and clouding of consciousness are common neurologic signs. Neurologic changes result from alterations in conduction and destabilization of the cell membrane. The patient may complain of being easily fatigued and experiencing a generalized feeling of muscle weakness. An additional finding is hyporeflexia. Muscular changes are attributed to the blocking effect on sodium in the skeletal muscles by excess calcium. The occurrence of nocturia, polyuria, and polydipsia is the renal system's attempt to clear the body of excess calcium. Hypercalcemia interferes with the action of antidiuretic hormone on the kidney's collecting tubules, which can eventually lead to nitrogen retention, acidosis, and renal failure. Cardiovascular signs usually are not apparent in the early phase of hypercalcemia, but hypertension may occur due to the hypercalcemic effect on arterial smooth muscles (Lang-Kummer, 1990).

In moderate hypercalcemia, the elevation of serum calcium to 12 to 15 mg/dL results in the worsening of gastrointestinal and neuromuscular symptoms and the initiation of serious cardiac abnormalities. Gastrointestinal motility continues to deteriorate, resulting in constipation, increased abdominal pain, and gastric distention. The continuing depression of the central nervous system neurons results in confusion, psychoses, and somnolence. The patient demonstrates worsening muscular weakness and may complain of bone pain associated with bone resorption. Nausea and vomiting exacerbate volume contraction, which decreases the glomerular filtration rate (GFR). A decreased GFR stimulates sodium and water reabsorption, which, unfortunately, results in calcium absorption. This further increases the calcium level in the blood. Cardiac dysrhythmias commonly occur during moderate hypercalcemia, due to the interference of normal conduction by the rising calcium level. The electrocardiogram demonstrates a shortened QT interval, prolonged PR interval, and sinus bradycardia. Dysrhythmias are especially prevalent in digitalized patients (Lang-Kummer, 1990).

These abnormalities become life threatening when the serum calcium level rises above 15 mg/dL. Prolonged QT interval due to widened T wave, coving of the ST segment, and atrioventricular (AV) block can occur. Atonic ileus and obstipation occur. Muscular weakness becomes profound and ataxia may become apparent. Pathologic fractures may occur because of demineralization of the bone due to resorption activity. The onset of coma, oliguria, renal failure, and cardiac failure are omnious signs. Untreated, death is inevitable (Lang-Kummer, 1990).

Clinical Management

Not all patients require treatment of their hypercalcemia. If the patient's serum calcium level is 9 mg/dL and the tumor is responsive to treatment, no therapy is indicated. However, if the serum calcium level is high and the patient is symptomatic, initial therapy is begun.

Hypercalcemic patients frequently present with a fluid volume deficit because of vomiting and water loss due to calciuresis. Rehydration with intravenous normal saline is essential for volume expansion and to increase renal blood flow to enhance calcium excretion (exchange of calcium for sodium in the distal tubule) (Warrell, 1993). Intravenous fluid administration usually is rapid as long as there is no prior history of abnormal renal function and cardiac function is adequate. Depending on the severity of the hypercalcemia, normal saline may be infused at a rate of 300 to 400 mL/hour for the first 3 to 4 hours. At this time, serum levels of calcium, creatinine, and electrolytes should be reassessed and the patient's renal and cardiac status reevaluated. The replacement of essential electrolytes (e.g., potassium and magnesium) is necessary. It is usually necessary to continue to superhydrate the patient using a large volume of normal saline (up to 8 liters over the first 24 hours). A urine output of 3 to 4 liters daily is desirable once the presenting dehydration has been corrected (Silverman & Distelhorst, 1989).

Many cancer patients already have some type of venous access device for the administration of their cytotoxic therapy. If a venous access is not present, the critical care nurse needs to insert a large-bore intravenous catheter through which to administer the high volumes of rehydration fluids. Throughout hydration, the hourly intake and output is calculated for fluid balance. Initially, the output should be at least one-half of the hourly intake. Urine specific gravity may be monitored hourly as one means of continually assessing the patient's hydration status and renal function. A serum electrolyte panel is obtained throughout the acute phase. The frequency with which these are obtained depends on the clinical status of the patient's hypercalcemia. It is important for the critical care nurse to analyze the serum sodium and potassium values because these electrolytes are being renally excreted and their levels may be so low that replacement becomes necessary. The blood urea nitrogen (BUN) and creatinine reflect the status of the patient's renal function. A rising BUN and creatinine indicate the onset of renal failure. The patient may require immediate dialysis (Warrell, 1993).

The critical care nurse needs to conduct hourly physical assessments to observe for the development of fluid overload. Signs include the development of edema, especially in the lower limbs and sacrum; the presence of neck vein distention and a rising central venous pressure; a change in pulmonary status, including the onset of shortness of breath and rales; and an increase in weight (Schafer, 1994).

Calciuretic diuretics can be used to enhance calcium excretion after the patient has been rehydrated (Silverman & Distelhorst, 1989). Furosemide and ethacrynic acid are the diuretics of choice because they promote calciuresis by decreasing renal tubular reabsorption of sodium and calcium. Thiazides depress urinary excretion of calcium and are avoided as a diuretic in these patients.

With the availability of other calcium-reducing therapies, the dependency on saline hydration and diuretics alone is reserved for mild hypercalcemia. Newer therapies have made it possible to avoid the pitfalls of prolonged saline hydration, primarily fluid volume overload, and to achieve a greater rate of success. However, if loop diuretics are used, especially high-dose furosemide, the critical care nurse needs to observe the serum chemistry for the onset of severe potassium and magnesium loss associated with this diuretic. Replacement may be necesasary to avoid additional clinical problems (Lang-Kummer, 1990).

Treatment with antiresorptive drugs should begin immediately after the patient is rehydrated (Table 70–3). The intravenous administration of inorganic phosphate is a fast and effective method for decreasing serum calcium, but it can cause serious side effects (Warrell, 1993). The administration of exogenous phosphate shifts calcium from blood to other tissues, which can result in severe toxicity, including hypotension, acute renal failure, and death due to extraskeletal calcifications in the heart and kidneys. Because of these complications, the intravenous administration of inorganic phosphate has largely been abandoned in favor of the oral or rectal route. Oral phosphate dosage is up to 0.5 g orally 4 times daily (Schafer, 1994). The resulting diarrhea, however, makes compliance an issue. For patients with nausea or impaired mental status, phosphate can be administered rectally by retention enema (Fleet Phospho-Soda, C. B. Fleet Co., Lynchburg, VA) of 1.5 g twice per day (Lang-Kummer, 1990; Warrell, 1993). Serum phosphate levels must be carefully monitored throughout therapy, especially in patients with decreased renal function.

Mithramycin, a potent antineoplastic antibiotic used in the treatment of malignant disease, reduces serum calcium in low doses of 25 μg/kg administered intravenously. Because mithramycin is a cytotoxic agent, the critical care nurse needs to wear latex gloves whenever handling the syringe/intravenous tubing to avoid any personal drug exposure. The syringe/tubing may be purged free of air into a closed container (e.g., empty vial) and disposed in a hazardous waste container. No drug should be allowed to escape from the syringe/tubing and contaminate the environment. The critical care nurse selects a patent intravenous line with a good blood return to administer the agent, because any leakage of mithramycin outside the vein can lead to tissue irritation and damage. Should the nurse suspect a mithramycin extravasation, a cold compress is applied to the site and maintained for 24 hours. The site is then monitored daily for any signs of erythema and ulceration.

Mithramycin inhibits osteoclastic bone resorption, thereby lowering serum calcium. The clinical response to mithramycin in the hypercalcemic patient is slow, usually taking 24 to 48 hours. A second dose may need to be administered at 48 hours to enhance bone resorption (Silverman & Distelhorst, 1989). Complications of repeated therapy are thrombocytopenia, coagulopathy, and hepatic and renal toxicity.

Bisphosphonates directly inhibit calcium release from bone by adsorbing to the surface of crystalline hydroxyapatite (Warrell, 1993). Bisphosphonates are initiated after rehydration and establishment of adequate urinary output. Etidronate, given intravenously at 7.5 mg/kg over 4 hours daily for 3 to 5 days, is 30% to 40% effective within 48 hours of administration. Pamidronate is a highly effective antiresorptive agent, having a relative potency of 70% to 80%. Infused over 24 hours in doses of 60 to 90 mg, its onset of action occurs within 24 to 48 hours. It can be safely used in patients with renal failure (Schafer, 1994). The critical care nurse may note the onset of fever in the patient receiving pamidronate. The onset of fever is more likely associated with the use of this agent (a common side effect) than to other contributing causes (e.g., infection).

Gallium nitrate is incorporated into bone and renders hydroxyapatite less soluble and more resistant to resorption (Warrell, 1993). It may also enhance bone formation by stimulation of bone collagen synthesis. It has demonstrated superiority in studies that compared its action to that of calcitonin and etidronate. Gallium nitrate is administered as a continuous intravenous infusion for up to 5 days at dosages of 100 to 200 $mg/m^2/day$. Because nephrotoxicity is the drug's dose-limiting factor, a daily urine output of 2,000 mL should be maintained throughout the infusion.

Other choices of treatment include calcitonin, a hormone that causes hypercalcemia by inhibiting osteoclast activity, and glucocorticoids, which may have an antitumor or antivitamin D effect (Warrell, 1993). Calcitonin is considered to have weak hypercalcemic effects and should not be used as single-agent therapy in most situations. However, its rapid onset makes it

TABLE 70–3. **Therapy for the Treatment of Cancer-Related Hypercalcemia**

Treatment Characteristics	Normal Saline	Oral Phosphorus	Corticosteroids	Calcitonin	Etidronate	Plicamycin	Gallium Nitrate	Pamidronate
Dose	200–400(+) mL/hour	1–3 g/day orally, divided doses	40–100 mg/day prednisone or equivalent	2–8 U/kg SC or IM every 6–12 hours	7.5 mg/kg IV over 4 hours daily for 3–5 days	10–50 (usually 25) μg/kg IV by brief infusion	100–200 mg/m^2/day by continuous IV infusion up to 5 days	60–90 mg IV over 24 hours
Indications	Hypovolemia, dehydration	Mild or moderate hypercalcemia, hypophosphatemia	Hypercalcemia from myeloma, lymphoma, hormonal flare	Mild or moderate hypercalcemia; acute control	Mild or moderate hypercalcemia	Moderate or severe hypercalcemia	Moderate or severe hypercalcemia	Moderate or severe hypercalcemia
Onset of action	12–24 hours	24–48 hours	3–5 days	1–4 hours	48 hours	24–48 hours	24–48 hours	24–48 hours
Relative potency*	20%	30%	0%–40%, depending on disease	30%	30%–40%	80%	80%	70%–80%
Advantages	Corrects dehydration	Orally available; minimal toxicity	Orally available	Minimal toxicity	Usually well tolerated; decreases bone resorption	Highly effective	Highly effective, decreases bone resorption	Highly effective, decreases bone resorption
Disadvantages/toxicity	Pulmonary edema, hypernatremia, fluid overload	Nausea, diarrhea, extraosseous calcification	Hyperglycemia, gastritis, osteopenia	Nausea, hypersensitivity	Occasional nephrotoxicity	Nausea, nephrotoxicity, hepatotoxicity, thrombocytopenia, coagulopathy	Prolonged infusion, nephrotoxicity, hypophosphatemia	Fever, venous irritation

*Potency is defined as the expected proportion of patients with a serum calcium ≥12.0 mg/dL who will achieve normocalcemia.

Abbreviations: IM, intramuscular; IV, intravenous; SC, subcutaneous.

From Warrell, R. P. (1993). Metabolic emergencies. In V. T. DeVita, Jr., S. Hellman, & S. A. Rosenberg (Eds.), *Cancer: Principles and practice of oncology* (4th ed., p. 2131). Philadelphia: J. B. Lippincott.

ideal for use when combined with other antiresorptive agents such as gallium nitrate and the bishosphonates. It is administered intramuscularly or subcutaneously in doses of 4 to 8 IU/kg every 6 hours. Corticosteroids in high doses (prednisone 40–60 mg daily) are effective in patients with moderate hypercalcemia caused by tumors sensitive to the cytostatic action of steroids. Corticosteroids are frequently used in association with calcitonin (Schafer, 1994), but they do not appear to enhance the hypocalcemic effects of calcitonin in patients whose underlying disease is not steroid responsive (Warrell, 1993).

DECREASED CARDIAC OUTPUT. The patient requires continuous cardiac monitoring because of the association of dysrythmias with hypercalcemia. The presence of arrhythmias detrimentally alters cardiac output and could potentially lead to AV block and eventually asystole. The critical care nurse needs to plan interventions based on the dysrhythmia present and its effect on the patient's clinical status. The presence of AV block may result in decreased cardiac output, which is hazardous in the presence of rapid fluid hydration. Any indication of fluid overload should be reported immediately so that therapy can be adjusted. The critical care nurse needs to be prepared for the implementation of emergency measures, including the administration of epinephrine, isoproterenol, atropine, or a combination of these agents, should complete AV block occur (Purcell, 1993).

IMPAIRED PHYSICAL MOBILITY. Immobilization should be avoided because it increases resorption of calcium from the bones (Schafer, 1994). Weight bearing through standing or ambulation stimulates osteoblastic activity, which synthesizes collagen and glycoproteins to form a matrix and develop into osteocytes. Promoting physical activity in the critical care setting for a patient with life-threatening multiple systems failure usually is not possible. However, some type of physical therapy (e.g., passive exercises) can be implemented to help minimize osteolytic activity and the occurrence of pathologic fractures.

ALTERED THOUGHT PROCESSES. The patient's altered mental functions improve as hypercalcemia is corrected. Until that time, it is important for the critical care nurse frequently to assess the patient's level of consciousness and changes in behavior. Changes in mentation serve as one indicator of the effectiveness of therapy. The critical care nurse uses each patient contact to help orient the patient. The nurse also implements appropriate measures to keep the patient safe during times of confusion and restlessness (e.g., use of full siderails, use of soft restraints). Because a change in the patient's mentation can be frightening for the family, the nurse can use each encounter with the family as a time of reassurance and informing.

Although hypercalcemia is manageable, controlling the malignancy causing this complication may remain the principal challenge. Until the tumor is controlled or eradicated, hypercalcemia may continue to reappear and require prompt treatment. Many of these tumors are not curable or have progressed to a stage where cure is no longer possible. Hypercalcemia may occur late in the patient's course of disease, when it is obvious that the patient has a limited life span. It is usually prudent, however, aggressively to treat hypercalcemia because its management can improve the patient's quality of life, help the patient achieve the best level of performance status possible, be an integral component of palliative care, and facilitate the patient's return to home.

DISCHARGE PLANNING FOR THE PATIENT WITH CANCER

Patients with cancer have complex needs that require a coordinated effort to facilitate the return to home. These needs are best addressed while the patient is still in a critical care setting. Once they are designated ward status, their ultimate discharge from the hospital can occur rather quickly. As a result, there is relatively little time with which to put together a feasible discharge plan.

While still in an intensive care setting, patient case managers can analyze what benefits and services are covered by the patient's health care insurance plan. The identification of these outpatient and home services helps determine where gaps exist. The patient case manager can spend time seaking out community resources and social services to help provide the additional care the patient may require once home. Community resources vary from location to location, and the degree to which they can provide a multitude of services depends heavily on agency funding. The American Cancer Society and the Leukemia Society of America can be consulted to help identify those resources that have been especially useful in the patient's community. Churches and United Way agencies have traditionally been helpful with a variety of services.

It is essential throughout the discharge planning process for patient case managers to remember that most cancer patients will not be cured of the underlying problem responsible for the hospitalization. These patients do not go home free of their disease or recovered. Cancer remains a significant health problem that relentlessly affects the patient and family alike. Patient and family needs, therefore, are never-ending. With this in mind, the discharge plan not only must meet short-term goals, it must make provisions for needs that may have no end in sight.

It is not uncommon for many cancer patients and families to find benefits and services exhausted at the time when the need is greatest. Families will be counted on more and more to provide complicated care as health care dollars become scarce and community resources underfunded. It is necessary for the patient case manager to assess the family's ability to provide this care and to help balance the burden of care. The use of effective coping mechanisms, the provision of respite care, and referrals to long-term care facilities or hospice agencies are interventions that should be considered during the course of the patient's cancer experience.

SUMMARY

Oncologic emergencies are critical events that complicate the course of cancer treatment and rehabilitation. They are frequently viewed as setbacks and are discouraging, frustrating experiences for the patient and family as well as the health care provider. Regardless of the patient's prognosis or chance for cure or remission, oncologic emergencies are usually treated aggressively to preserve some semblance of quality of life.

Unless one personally experiences cancer, it is difficult to understand why one would submit to such aggressive treatment in light of a progressing disease. Knowing that the patient or family have opted for this treatment, the nurse must support the patient and the family through the crisis with the best professional, technical, and compassionate nursing care.

REFERENCES

Ahmann, R. R. (1984). A reassessment of the clinical implications of the superior vena caval syndrome. *Journal of Clinical Oncology, 2*, 961–969.

Berenson, J. R., & Gale, R. P. (1990). Acute lymphoblastic leukemia. In C. M. Haskell (Ed.), *Cancer treatment* (pp. 606–620). Philadelphia: W. B. Saunders.

Bullock, B. L. (1992). Normal circulatory dynamics. In B. L. Bullock & P. P. Rosendahl (Eds.), *Pathophysiology: Adaptations and alterations in function* (pp. 90–101). Philadelphia: J. B. Lippincott.

Delaney, T. F., & Oldfield, E. H. (1993). In V. T. DeVita, Jr., S. Hellman, & S. A. Rosenberg (Eds.), *Cancer: Principles and practice of oncology* (4th ed., pp. 2118–2127). Philadelphia: J. B. Lippincott.

Dietz, K. A., & Flaherty, A. M. (1990). Oncologic emergencies. In S. L. Groenwald et al. (Eds.), *Cancer nursing: Principles and practices* (pp. 644–668). Boston: Jones and Bartlett.

Emani, B., & Perez, C. A. (1992). Lung. In C. A. Perez & L. W. Brady (Eds.), *Principles and practice of radiation oncology* (pp. 806–836). Philadelphia: J. B. Lippincott.

Gallick, G. E. (1989). Potential roles of activated protooncogenes in malignant progression. In E. K. Weisburger (Ed.), *Mechanisms of carcinogenesis* (pp. 98–105). Norwell, MA: Kluwer Academic Publishers.

Harewood, K. R. (1989). Cellular oncogene activation by chromosomal translocation. In E. K. Weisburger (Ed.), *Mechanisms of carcinogenesis* (pp. 87–91). Norwell, MA: Kluwer Academic Publishers.

Haskell, C. M., et al. (1990). Breast cancer. In C. M. Haskell (Ed.), *Cancer treatment* (pp. 123–164). Philadelphia: W. B. Saunders.

Held, J. L., & Peahota, A. (1993). Nursing care of the patient with spinal cord compression. *Oncology Nursing Forum, 20*, 1507–1516.

Henze, R. (1992). Normal structure and function of the central and peripheral nervous systems. In B. L. Bullock & P. P. Rosendahl (Eds.), *Pathophysiology: Adaptations and alterations in function* (pp. 60–89). Philadelphia: J. B. Lippincott.

Jassak, P. F. (1990). Biotherapy. In S. L. Groenwald et al. (Eds.), *Cancer nursing: Principles and practices* (pp. 284–306). Boston: Jones and Bartlett.

Kagan, A. R. (1992). Radiation therapy in palliative cancer management. In C. A. Perez & L. W. Brady (Eds.), *Principles and practice of radiation oncology* (pp. 1495–1508). Philadelphia: J. B. Lippincott.

Kupchella, C. E. (1992). The spread of cancer: Invasion and metastasis. In B. L. Bullock & P. P. Rosendahl (Eds.), *Pathophysiology: Adaptations and alterations in function* (pp. 102–121). Philadelphia: J. B. Lippincott.

Ladik, J., & Otto, P. (1989). The quantum theory of carcinogenesis: A short review. In E. K. Weisburger (Ed.), *Mechanisms of carcinogenesis* (pp. 84–86). Norwell, MA: Kluwer Academic Publishers.

Lang-Kummer, J. M. (1990). Hypercalcemia. In S. L. Groenwald et al. (Eds.), *Cancer nursing: Principles and practice* (pp. 520–534). Boston: Jones and Bartlett.

Lotze, M. T., & Rosenberg, S. A. (1991). Interleukin-2: Clinical applications. In V. T. DeVita, Jr., S. Hellman, & S. A. Rosenberg (Eds.), *Biologic therapy of cancer* (pp. 159–177). Philadelphia: J. B. Lippincott.

Miaskowski, C. (1991). Oncologic emergencies. In S. B. Baird, R. McCorkle, & M. Grant (Eds.), *Cancer nursing: A comprehensive approach* (pp. 885–893). Philadelphia: W. B. Saunders.

Mitchell, P. H. (1993). Neurologic disorders. In M. R. Kinney, D. P. Packa, & S. B. Dunbar (Eds.), *AACN's clinical reference for critical-care nursing* (pp. 803–853). New York: McGraw-Hill.

Oncology Nursing Society. (1989). *Biological response modifiers.* Pittsburgh: Author.

Purcell, J. A. (1993). Cardiac electrical activity. In M. R. Kinney, D. P. Packa, & S. B. Dunbar (Eds.), *AACN's clinical reference for critical-care nursing* (pp. 217–296). New York: McGraw-Hill.

Rieger, P. T., Weatherly, B., & Rumsey, K. A. (1993). Clinical update: Strategies for caring for patients receiving IL-2 therapy. In *Nursing interventions in oncology.* Newtown, PA: Associates in Medical Marketing.

Sarin, P. S. (1989). Selected aspects of viral carcinogenesis. In E. K. Weisburger (Ed.), *Mechanisms of carcinogenesis* (pp. 71–83). Norwell, MA: Kluwer Academic Publishers.

Schafer, S. L. (1994). Oncologic complications. In S. E. Otto (Ed.), *Oncology nursing* (pp. 376–440). St. Louis: Mosby.

Silverman, P., & Distelhorst, C. W. (1989). Metabolic emergencies in clinical oncology. *Seminars in Oncology, 16*, 504–515.

Warrell, Jr., R. P. (1993). Metabolic emergencies. In V. T. DeVita, Jr., S. Hellman, & S. A. Rosenberg (Eds.), *Cancer: Principles and practice of oncology* (4th ed., pp. 2128–2141). Philadelphia: J. B. Lippincott.

Yahalom, J. (1993). Oncologic emergencies. In V. T. DeVita, Jr., S. Hellman, & S. A. Rosenberg (Eds.), *Cancer: Principles and practice of oncology* (4th ed., pp. 2111–2118). Philadelphia: J. B. Lippincott.

CHAPTER 71

Elderly Patients

Carol A. Rauen and Teresa L. Britt

The elderly segment of the population of the United States is growing at an unprecedented rate. The over-65 age group has increased more rapidly than any other group in the population this century. The over-85 age group is expected to triple in number between 1980 and 2030, and grow seven times larger by the year 2050. In 1985 there were 61,000 people in this country older than the age of 100 years; by the year 2000 this number will exceed 100,000 (U.S. Senate Special Committee on Aging, 1991).

The elderly constitute the most cost-intensive health consumer group. At present, people over the age of 65 represent 13% of the population, yet they account for 33% of all health care spending and one-half of all patients admitted to intensive care units (ICU) (Beck, 1993; Fedullo & Seinburne, 1983). According to a report published by the U.S. Senate Special Committee on Aging (1991), the over-65 age group is hospitalized three times more frequently than younger adults, stay in the hospital 50% longer, and use twice as many prescription drugs. In 1992, the Centers for Disease Control and Prevention reported that the hospital length of stay for adults increased with age: the 15–44-year-old LOS was 4.9 days; 45–64-year-old, 6.3 days; and over-65 age group, 8.2 days (Graves, 1994). Once critically ill, the elderly have increased incidence of complications, greater length of stay in the critical care unit and hospital, and higher mortality and morbidity statistics (Finelli et al., 1989; Levy et al., 1993; Pellican et al., 1992; Smith et al., 1990).

Elderly people present a growing challenge in the critical care setting, not only in terms of these compelling demographics, but due to the sophistication of knowledge required to provide comprehensive care for this special population. This chapter presents an overview of age-related biologic changes in the older adult and specific clinical implications for critical care practice.

SYSTEMS OVERVIEW OF AGE-RELATED CHANGES

Aging represents a new frontier for research and practice. The research literature contains much debate regarding the "normal" changes of aging (Tables 71–1 and 71–2). Until recently, very little research was done regarding the process of aging. One of the many theories for the current increased longevity of older adults is that the increased medical control over infectious disease, improved nutrition, and generally more favorable economic conditions have tended to diminish problems once thought to be normal consequences of aging. Exactly what constitutes normal aging is still being defined. Thus, the terms "age-related changes" and the "degenerative process" are used throughout this chapter.

There is general consensus that different organ systems age at different rates. This is, of course, influenced considerably by genetic predisposition, nutritional status, physical conditioning, environmental exposures, and physical and psychological challenges. The diversity of the elderly population has made rigorous research into age-related changes difficult. Concomitant with the degenerative process is the increased incidence of preexisting conditions and diseases in the elderly (Tran et al., 1990). Therefore, isolating "normal" aging from disease-related changes to multiple body systems is a very difficult (if not impossible) process for researchers. Technologic and methodologic advances as well as the use of animal models have provided some inroads to better understanding physiologic changes.

CARDIOVASCULAR SYSTEM

Cardiac disease is the leading cause of illness and death in the elderly (Wei, 1992). Eighty percent of all cardiovascular mortalities are attributed to people over the age of 65 years (Wenger, 1992). Diseases represent pathology, not age-related changes, but it must be recognized that the degenerative process does predispose the elderly to disease (U.S. Senate Special Committee on Aging, 1985–1986). Of all the cardiac procedures performed in this country annually, between one-third and one-half are on patients in their sixth decade or older (Wenger, 1992).

The cardiovascular system undergoes many changes with age. The degenerative process affects the anatomy and physiologic functions of the heart (Har-

TABLE 71–1. **Systems Overview of Age-Related Changes**

System	Age-Related Change	Clinical Manifestation
Cardiac	Myocardial hypertrophy Dilation of aorta Myocytes increase in size Valvular stenosis	Decreased cardiac output Decreased stroke volume Decreased cardiac reserve
	Arteriosclerosis Atherosclerosis	Left ventricular hypertrophy Hypertension Decreased arterial compliance Decreased perfusion Increased risk of myocardial infarction Decreased preload
	Increased myocardial irritability Electrical impulse transmission slowing	Increased ectopy Decreased heart rate Decreased ability to compensate
	Neurotransmitters are less effective	Higher doses of vasoactive drugs
	Baroreceptor loss of sensitivity	Orthostatic hypertension
Respiratory	Impaired cough reflex Decreased laryngeal reflex	Increased risk of aspiration Increased risk of pneumonia Impaired airway clearance
	Alveolar enlargement Decreased alveolar surface area Increased alveolar–arterial oxygen difference Increased ventilation–perfusion mismatch Decreased 2,3-diphosphoglycerate	Decreased diffusion of gases Lower PaO_2 Decreased O_2 carrying capacity
	Diminished weight of lungs Chest wall changes Decreased elastic recoil Decreased lung compliance Decreased vital capacity Decreased forced expiratory volume Increased functional residual capacity Increased residual volume Increased closing volume	Air trapping More energy required to breathe Diminished pulmonary reserve Longer ventilator times Weaker pulmonary muscles Increased respiratory rate
	Central chemoreceptor changes	Blunted response to hypercapnia and hypoxia
Neurological	Brain atrophy Increased glial cells Loss of neurons Loss of cerebral cortex cell bodies Degeneration of axons Loss of large motor nerve fibers Depressed stretch reflexes Decreased cerebral blood flow	Decreased sensation Decreased reaction time Decreased motor ability Increased processing time Decreased conducting velocity Increased time to initiate movement or react to stimuli
	Neurotransmitter alterations	Behavioral and regulatory changes
	Diminished cognition	Diminished ability to process information
	Impaired vision	Impaired night vision Poor peripheral vision Hyperopia
	Impaired hearing	Inability to distinguish sounds Inability to hear high pitches
	Altered sleep patterns	More time spent awake
	Impaired thermoregulation	Decreased temperature
Gastrointestinal	Presbyesophagus Atrophy and thinning of gastric mucosa Decreased rate of vitamin K absorption Increased incidence of hiatal hernia	Difficulty swallowing Gastric reflux Aspiration Heartburn, sternal pain Gastrointestinal bleeding Ulcer formation
	Distention of pancreatic duct Altered endocrine and exocrine functions of liver and pancreas Decreased pancreatic lipase Decreased albumin synthesis	Altered drug metabolism Increased edema Impaired absorption and digestion Altered fat absorption Altered drug–protein binding

TABLE 71–1. **Systems Overview of Age-Related Changes** *Continued*

System	Age-Related Change	Clinical Manifestation
	Decreased blood flow to liver and splanchnic bed Impaired colonic mobility	Increased risk of obstruction Low tolerance for tube feedings Constipation
	Increased incidence of malnutrition Increased incidence of dehydration	Decreased wound healing Longer ventilatory times Negative nitrogen balance Diarrhea
Renal	Decreased kidney mass Decreased number of nephrons Renal tubule changes Decreased renal perfusion	Decreased glomerular filtration rate Diminished ability to concentrate or dilute urine Impaired drug and glucose excretion Increased nephrotoxicity Diminished tolerance to volume Decreased creatinine clearance Altered sodium excretion
	Decreased production and sensitivity to hormones	Hypertension
	Bladder muscle weakens	Incontinence Diminished capacity of bladder Incomplete emptying Increased risk of infection

ris, 1983). These changes are cumulative over time and affect cardiac performance (Miller, 1990).

Anatomic Changes to the Cardiac System

The human heart hypertrophies with advancing age (Schneider & Rowe, 1990). The thickness of the posterior left ventricular wall begins to increase at age 20 and can expand by 30% by the age of 80 (Gerstenblith et al., 1977; Schneider & Rowe, 1990). The atrial endocardium thickening is attributed to the dilation of the aorta and elevation of the systolic blood pressure (Miller, 1990; Wei, 1988). The myocytes actually increase in size, which contributes to the thickening of the heart wall. Mitochondria increase in number but decrease in size during the degenerative process (Kenney, 1989).

The cardiac valves also undergo anatomic changes that may cause hemodynamic difficulties. These changes can lead to valvular stenosis, decreased cardiac output, and hemodynamic compromise. The chordae tendineae shorten with age, and papillary muscle changes alter the shape, size, and function of the valves (Harris, 1983). Myxomatous degeneration, usually confined to the mitral valve, is similar to mitral valve prolapse and commonly occurs in men over 64 and women over 74 years of age (Harris, 1983).

Coronary artery disease (CAD) is the major cause of disability and death in the United States (Timiras, 1988). Lakatta (1988) estimates that half of the population over the age of 65 has at least a 50% occlusion of one major coronary artery.

Two of the three vascular bed layers are affected by age-related changes (Miller, 1990). The changes, along with hypertension, cause an increase in the diameter of the lumen of the aorta.

Capillaries also undergo age-related changes, such as thickening of the basement membrane. In addition, the fenestrations of the endothelium become smaller (Kenney, 1989). Veins become thicker, more dilated, and less elastic with increasing age (Miller, 1990). Venous return is decreased secondary to decreased muscle tone and vasodilation, leading to a decreased preload (Miller, 1990).

Physiologic Changes to the Cardiac System

Pathy and Finucane (1989) identified many age-related changes in cardiovascular function. The resting cardiac output and cardiac index fall with age. Schneider and Rowe (1990) documented a 50% decrease in resting cardiac index from age 20 to age 80. A fall of 1% per year in cardiac output is anticipated after age 35 (Pathy & Finucane, 1989). Systolic blood pressure rises, peripheral vascular resistance increases, and maximal coronary artery flow drops in the aging cardiovascular system. The vasomotor tone also declines and myocardial irritability rises.

The two components of cardiac output, heart rate and stroke volume, are both affected by age. The intrinsic sinus rate is significantly diminished with age secondary to blockade of both sympathetic and parasympathetic stimulation (Schneider & Rowe, 1990). Kenney (1989) noted that there is a loss of sinoatrial node cells beginning in the early twenties. There is also cell loss in the atrioventricular node, the bundle of His, and the bundle branches (Kenney, 1989). The effects of these losses cause a slower heart rate by age 70. Kenney (1989) estimates a drop of 0.7% in stroke volume per year between the ages of 20 and 80 years.

According to the World Health Organization, 65% of people over 60 years old are hypertensive. Ninety

TABLE 71–2. **Treatment Axions for the Elderly**

55- Through 64-Year-Old

1. Assume some mild decrease in physiologic reserve.
2. Suspect the presence of some common diseases of middle age (diabetes, arteriosclerotic cardiovascular disease, hypertension, previous surgery, previous transfusion).
3. Suspect the use of prescription or over-the-counter medications.
4. Assume the patient is competent to provide an accurate medical history.
5. Look for subtle signs of organ dysfunction, especially cardiovascular and respiratory systems; arterial blood gas measurements and electrocardiograms are crucial.
6. In the presence of a history of loss of consciousness or abnormalities in cognitive function or personality, assume there is a serious brain injury until proven otherwise; computed tomographic scan is invaluable; magnetic resonance imaging may be a helpful adjunct.
7. Proceed with standard diagnostic and management schemes, unless contraindicated by information collected during history taking.

65- Through 74-Year-Old

1. Accept the presence of age-related and acquired disease-induced physiologic alterations of organ systems.
2. Accept the presence of acquired diseases and medications to correct or control them; assume a higher incidence of previous surgery and transfusion.
3. Decide whether the patient is competent to give a reliable medical history; review the history as soon as possible with the patient's relatives or personal physician.
4. Aggressively monitor the patient and control the physiologic characteristics to optimize cardiac performance and oxygen metabolism.
5. Assume that any alteration in mental status or cognitive or sensory function indicates the presence of brain injury; imaging of the brain is mandatory.
6. Proceed with standard diagnostic and management schemes, including early, aggressive operative management.
7. Be aware of poor outcome, especially with severe injury to the central nervous system or marked physiologic deterioration secondary to injury; check for advance directives.

75 Years or Older

1. Proceed as in items 1–5 for patients 65–74 years of age.
2. Assume a poor outcome with moderately severe injury, especially in the central nervous system, or for any injury causing physiologic dysfunction.
3. After aggressive initial resuscitation and diagnostic maneuvers, examine item 2 and discuss appropriateness of care with the patient (if competent) and family members.
4. Attempt to be humane, and recognize the legal and ethical controversies involved; consider early consultation of experts in ethics and social services to help the family and medical team with difficult decisions.

These guidelines must be viewed only as the framework around which individualized care should be built. They should also be linked to the social and ethical issues unique to each geriatric patient who has a life-threatening or permanently disabling injury.

From Schwab, W., & Kauder, D. (1992). Trauma in the geriatric patient. *Archives of Surgery, 127,* 705. Reprinted with permission.

percent of these people have essential hypertension (Timiras, 1988). The elevation in diastolic pressure could be due to the increase in peripheral resistance secondary to atherosclerosis. Atrial stiffness and aortic impedance contribute to the increase in systolic pressure. Sodium excretion and glomerular filtration rate (GFR) decrease with advancing age, thus affecting sodium homeostasis. Increased serum sodium concentration results in increased intravascular volume, thus elevating blood pressure. Older people also have a delayed natriuretic response after sodium loading and plasma volume expansion (Luft et al., 1979).

Cardiac function in the elderly may be impaired due to dysrhythmias. Impairments in the electrical activity of the myocardium and conducting system, decreased activity of the atrial and ventricular pacemakers, a diminished capacity of the sinoatrial node to suppress latent ventricular foci, decreased conduction velocity, and tissue changes in the aged heart contribute to the development of reentry patterns (Harris, 1983). Last, the myocardium is increasingly irritable and less responsive to impulses from the sympathetic nervous system, which increases the chance of dysrhythmias (Miller, 1990).

Adrenergic modulation of cardiovascular function decreases with age (Schneider & Rowe, 1990). The neurotransmitters and hormones are not as effective on their target organs in the aged. The physiologic response to beta-adrenergic stimulation also decreases (Schneider & Rowe, 1990). These changes affect the compensatory mechanisms used to counteract hypotension.

Clinical Implications of Age-Related Cardiovascular Changes

Cardiovascular system response to stress and critical illness is less adaptive and protective in the elderly than in the young patient population. Subtle aging changes that may not affect the day-to-day life of an average person may pose problems in the critically ill elderly. The natural degenerative process that causes reduction in cardiac function makes it difficult to combat heart failure associated with the common problems of critical illness such as anemia, sepsis, intravenous fluid overload, supraventricular tachycardia, moderate hypertension, and small myocardial infarcts (Pathy & Finucane, 1989). However, the extent of the drop in maximum cardiac work capacity with the elderly varies with their lifestyle, physical condition and presence of disease (Schneider & Rowe, 1990).

ASSESSMENT. Cardiac hypertrophy changes the size, position, and location of the cardiac silhouette on the chest x-ray. Sclerotic changes in the aortic valve, the increased incidence of mitral valve prolapse, and valvular stenosis increase the chance of cardiac murmurs being heard on auscultation. The apical heart beat may be displaced due to kyphoscoliosis. Premature ventricular contractions increase with age and occur in 10% of electrocardiograms and in 30% to 40% of Holter-monitored elderly patients (Kane et al., 1989). Initial blood pressure readings in the elderly patient may be misleading. What appears to be normotension may in fact be hypotension for the patient (Bobb, 1988).

DECREASED TISSUE PERFUSION. Changes in peripheral resistance and myocardial function may lead to impaired tissue perfusion in the elderly patient. Also, immobility predisposes the critically ill older adult to reduced tissue perfusion due to an obstruction (e.g., thrombus) in the vasculature (Matteson & McConnell, 1988). Deep vein thrombosis and pulmonary emboli are a leading cause of morbidity and mortality in the hospitalized elderly (Lee, 1980).

DECREASED CARDIAC OUTPUT. Diminished cardiac reserve and altered response to inotropic medications place the elderly patient at risk for development of congestive heart failure or cardiogenic shock. The aged patient's response to endogenous catecholamines may be manifested as a decreased and slower cardiac response to stress. There is decreased coronary perfusion and increased risk of ischemia due to CAD, which certainly can affect cardiac output.

The critical care practitioner should anticipate that the elderly patient may require a higher dosage of vasoactive medication to achieve the desired inotropic effect. Vasodilators may be ordered to decrease preload. The elderly patient's attenuated response to cardiac glycosides must be carefully monitored. Stepwise increases in doses of digitalis preparations should be anticipated.

Loss of baroreceptor sensitivity may lead to dizziness or even fainting when the patient rises after being supine. Prolonged bedrest in the ICU further exacerbates this problem. Thus, early ambulation for the elderly patient is extremely important.

Management goals are centered on optimizing the availability of oxygen to tissues, maximizing cardiovascular function, minimizing fear and anxiety, and making an accurate diagnosis (Bumann & Speltz, 1989; Kelly, 1989).

RESPIRATORY SYSTEM

It is difficult to separate pulmonary changes that are the result of the degenerative process from those that are attributed to disease or external influences such as smoking and the environment. When critical illness is present, these alterations place the elderly patient at risk for development of devastating complications. The incidence of respiratory disease rises steadily from the fifth decade on, and it accounts for 25% of the deaths in the population over 85 years old (Timiras, 1988). Chelluri and colleagues (1992) found that 82% of the elderly patients (≥85 years old) who were admitted to the ICU required intubation. The cumulative effects of degeneration, disease, and external factors have a large impact on the health care planning for the elderly patient with respiratory compromise.

Anatomic Changes to the Respiratory System

Upper respiratory functioning changes somewhat over time. The cartilage of the epiglottis and upper airway structures may become calcified, which causes tracheal stiffening. Both the cough and laryngeal reflexes are blunted (Sparrow & Weiss, 1988).

The chest wall and musculoskeletal structures also are altered by the degenerative process, which affects oxygenation and ventilation in the elderly. The ribs and vertebrae become osteoporotic, the costal cartilage becomes calcified, and the respiratory muscles become weaker in the aged (Miller, 1990). Respiratory performance is diminished by other structural changes, such as kyphosis, shortened thorax, increased wall stiffness, and increased anteroposterior diameter of the chest (Miller, 1990). As a result of these changes, the elderly expend more energy to achieve the same respiratory efficiency as younger people.

The actual weight of the lung diminishes by approximately 20% with aging (Krumpe et al., 1985). By age 30 years, the alveoli progressively enlarge and their walls become thinner (Miller, 1990). The terminal bronchioles, alveolar ducts, and capillaries all undergo some structural changes, and degeneration occurs (Miller, 1990). The elastic recoil of the lung parenchyma diminishes with age, which leads to early airway closure and increased closing lung volumes (Pathy & Finucane, 1989). There is a 4% decrease per decade after age 30 in alveolar surface area (Timiras, 1988). These degenerative changes result in decreased pulmonary compliance and a decreased diffusion of gases in the alveolar capillary bed.

Physiologic Changes to the Respiratory System

Decreases are seen in vital capacity, forced expiratory volume in 1 second, lung recoil pressure, diffusing capacity, and arterial oxygen tension. Increases are seen in closing volumes, functional residual capacity, and residual volumes. The total lung capacity and arterial carbon dioxide tension remain the same with aging (Brandsteter & Kazemi, 1983). The result of these changes is a tendency to trap air due to the inability to exhale fully.

The alveolar–arterial oxygen difference increases with age (Kenney, 1989). Sparrow and Weiss (1988) established that the ventilation-to-perfusion mismatch increases by approximately 4 mm Hg per decade. There is a progressive reduction in Pa_{O_2}, secondary to premature airway closure and loss of elastic recoil (Timiras, 1988). By age 80, the "normal" arterial oxygenation level is 70 mm Hg (Pierson & Hudson, 1981).

A decrease in 2,3-diphosphoglycerate in the aged causes a shift to the left in the oxygen dissociation curve, making unloading of oxygen in the tissues more difficult (Kenney, 1989).

The central chemoreceptors in the medulla and pons, and the peripheral chemoreceptors in the carotids and aortic bodies, are markedly altered in the elderly. These changes cause a blunting response to hypercapnia and hypoxia (Sparrow & Weiss, 1988). In fact, Timiras (1988) found a 50% reduction in the response to hypercapnia and hypoxia in the aged compared to young subjects.

Clinical Implications of Age-Related Changes in the Respiratory System

The incidence of respiratory failure is increased in the elderly because of changes in pulmonary mechanics, respiratory drive, and respiratory muscle strength (Krieger, 1994). Compounding this problem is the high frequency of cardiovascular changes and disease, malnutrition, and sleep deprivation, all of which are common to elderly, critically ill patients and contribute to respiratory failure (Davis-Sharts, 1989; Fontaine, 1989).

INEFFECTIVE AIRWAY CLEARANCE—HIGH RISK FOR INFECTION. Aspiration and pneumonia are common complications in elderly patients. Heuser and colleagues (1992) studied elderly patient respiratory admissions to critical care units and found pneumonia to be the most frequent primary diagnosis (31%), and it carried the highest risk of mortality (24%). Decreased levels of consciousness, dysphagia, disruptions in the lower esophageal sphincter, poor glottic closure, swallowing disorders, esophageal dysfunctions, and a decreased cough reflex all enhance the likelihood for aspiration in the elderly (Brandstetter & Kazemi, 1983). The potential for pneumonia is also increased secondary to long intubation times, impaired humoral and cell-mediated immunity, decreased cough reflex, and the reduction in tracheal cilia in the ill elderly (Kenney, 1988; Pathy & Finucane, 1989).

IMPAIRED GAS EXCHANGE. It is important to recognize that the elderly patient's PaO_2 is lower than that of the younger adult. Older patients also respond more gradually to oxygen therapy (Matteson & McConnell, 1988). Therefore, it is essential that oxygen deprivation be identified and treated as quickly as possible so that the patient has the extra time needed to respond.

Age-related changes in the respiratory system alter the elderly patient's response to hypoxemia. The usual signs of hypoxemia (e.g., increased respiratory rate, tachycardia, elevated blood pressure) may be blunted in the elderly (Wahba, 1983). Other indicators such as restlessness or mental status changes are of increased significance to the care provider. Breath sounds may be decreased in the bases of the lung fields due to decreased lung expansion (Kidd & Murakami, 1987).

IMPAIRED BREATHING PATTERNS. In general, management of mechanical ventilation for the older adult is very similar to that for younger adults. However, structural changes in the lungs and decreased muscle strength have implications for the weaning process. Usual predictors of successful weaning do not have as much discriminating potential for geriatric patients. Thus, general weaning protocols may not be appropriate for certain elderly patients. Weaning must be tailored to the specific needs of the patient (Krieger et al., 1989). If an elderly patient does not wean quickly from mechanical ventilation, a weaning plan may be required. Techniques such as pressure support ventilation, rest periods, and muscle training have been shown to be helpful with elderly weaning (Krieger, 1994).

NERVOUS SYSTEM

The aging process has significant effects on the nervous system. Anatomic and physiologic changes affect the elderly patient's acute and rehabilitative care needs.

Anatomic Changes to the Nervous System

The actual size of the brain decreases with age. The brain reaches its peak weight of 1.4 kg in the early twenties, and then slowly declines. By age 80 years there is as much as a 7% loss in weight (Kenney, 1989). This is accompanied by a reduction in the cortical area and a small increase in the size of the ventricles. The ratio of gray to white matter also changes. The amount of white matter declines linearly with age, and the gray matter initially drops between ages 20 and 55, then levels off. There is an estimated 3% loss of neurons over the course of a lifetime (Kenney, 1989), and as much as a 30% to 40% loss in cerebral cortex cell bodies. The number of dendritic spines and length of the dendrites decrease. There is also an increase in lipofuscin, neuritic plaques, and neurofibrillary tangles (Duara et al., 1985). These degenerative changes cause a decline in the nerve and cerebral function of the brain.

The peripheral nervous system is also affected by the aging process. There is up to a 5% decrease in conduction velocity and prolonged (polyphasic) muscle action potential (Kenney, 1989), resulting in decreased sensation, reflex action, and motor ability.

Physiologic Changes to the Nervous System

Age-related biochemical alterations in the nervous system include neurotransmitter imbalance, membrane changes, and alterations in neurotransmitter precursors, receptors, and degradation products. Decreases in presynaptic and postsynaptic levels of acetylcholine, dopamine, serotonin, and benzodiazepines have been found in the elderly (Schneider & Rowe, 1990).

These changes have a profound effect on both behavioral and regulatory systems. The concentration of norepinephrine falls as much as 50% between early adulthood and age 70 (Kenney, 1989). The simple stretch reflexes are often depressed in the aged.

Cerebral blood flow diminishes with age. Cerebral perfusion in young adults is 50 to 60 mL/minute/100 g of tissue, and a minimum of 40 mL/minute/100 g is regarded as necessary to maintain neuronal function. There is a drop of 20% in flow by age 70, and the perfusion is sometimes as low as 40 mL/minute/100 g (Kenney, 1989).

Nervous system degeneration is exhibited by several mechanisms: slower reaction time, decreased motor and conduction velocity, and increased processing time (Schneider & Rowe, 1990). The elderly need more time to process information, initiate movement, and react to stimulation.

Clinical Implications of Age-Related Changes in the Nervous System

The changes in the neurologic system may not be as measurable as those in the cardiac or pulmonary systems, but these changes can affect activities of daily living and quality of life on a grander scale. The changes in cognition, vision, hearing, sensation, and motor response have a large impact on the geriatric person's level of function, safety, and independence.

DECREASED LEVEL OF CONSCIOUSNESS. The elderly are often perceived as being forgetful and difficult to teach new information. There are two biologic reasons why this perception may be accurate: the reduction in circuitry available secondary to the loss of neurons and synapses; and the reduction in conduction speed (Kenney, 1989). Also affected are attention, short-term memory, and the ability to learn. Patient teaching may take longer, and the ICU nurse may have to repeat information in both written and verbal forms.

IMPAIRED SENSORY INPUT. As people age, the first sense they are aware of degenerating is their vision. Anatomic changes occur in the optical apparatus and the central visual pathway (Pathy & Finucane, 1989). The functional problems of seeing in the dark, presbyopia, differentiating something in an ambiguous environment, senile miosis, and decreased tear secretion have all been documented in the elderly (Kenney, 1989). Aging effects may change the level of functioning of cranial nerves II, III, IV, and VI (Pathy & Finucane, 1989). Loss of peripheral vision is common in the elderly. Older people may not be able to see other people or objects in their peripheral fields.

Hearing impairments are another very common functional problem for the elderly (Miller, 1990). Hearing is most efficient at age 10; by age 60, the range and frequencies audible have decreased considerably. The prevalence of deafness increases with age; 84% of people older than 85 years have a significant hearing deficit (Pathy & Finucane, 1989). Presbyacusias is defined as hearing loss in people over 65 who have no other explainable cause for the problem. Presbyacusias is primarily due to cartilaginous portions becoming less flexible and the external auditory meatus losing its elasticity. There is also a narrowing of the auditory canal and a decrease in the secretion of cerumen. The tympanic membrane becomes more rigid and thickened in the elderly (Kenney, 1989).

Elderly people may also have trouble masking sounds, that is, they have difficulty sorting the background noise from the stimuli to which they wish to attend. In addition, loud noises may irritate elderly people. Furthermore, because more time is necessary for processing stimuli at the higher auditory centers, accelerated speech is more difficult for the older person to understand (Matteson & McConnell, 1988; Meisami, 1988).

Visual and auditory degeneration changes can have a significant effect in the critical care setting. Communicating with the critically ill is vital. The goal is to balance sensory deficits often experienced by older patients with sensory overload often characteristic of the ICU. All attempts should be made to determine if the patient has glasses or a hearing aid. If so, these should be worn as much as possible. Communication should be validated for content and understanding, especially with the intubated elderly patient.

There is some decline in tactile sensitivity with age. For example, elderly adults tend to have increased thresholds to touch stimuli, decreased vibratory sensitivity, and decreased corneal sensitivity (Bruce, 1980; Meisami, 1988). Two-point discrimination declines with age, as does stereognosis (Meisami, 1988). Of potential danger is the loss of pain and thermal sensitivity associated with aging. This loss cannot be attributed solely to tactile losses. Affective, cognitive, and environmental factors are thought to play a large role in this alteration (Meisami, 1988).

Elderly people have far less acuity relative to perception of pain. In addition, many elderly and their health care providers tend to accept pain and discomfort as normal accompaniments of aging. This fallacy may lead to underreporting and delayed treatment of injury or illness.

Many age-related changes in the nervous system impair balance (Pathy & Finucane, 1989). The elderly experience loss of muscle mass and power, loss of large motor nerve fibers, and stiffening of joints, all of which contribute to impaired posture, gait, and balance. Tests have demonstrated that the psychomotor speed of a 70-year-old is approximately half that of a 30-year-old (Kenney, 1989).

SLEEP PATTERN DISTURBANCE. The elderly have an increase in wakefulness relative to the total time spent in bed (Fig. 71–1). Age-related sleep pattern changes include: increased amount of time spent awake at night; decreased amount of stage 3 sleep; total loss of stage 4 sleep; increase in arousals to stage 1 or full

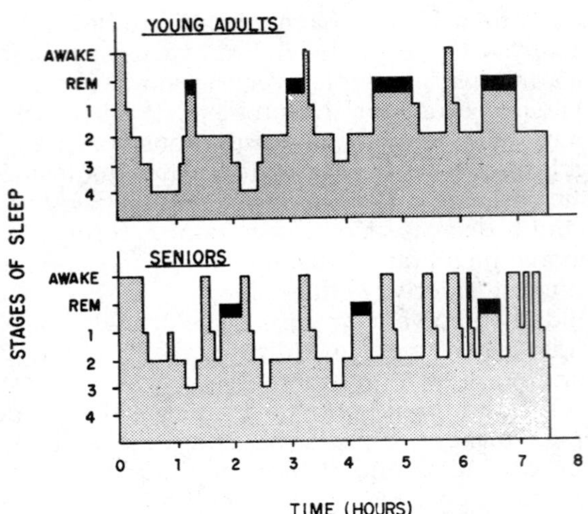

FIGURE 71–1. Normal sleep cycles. With aging, it takes longer to fall asleep and there is less deep sleep, more awakening, and less rapid eye movement (REM) sleep. (From Ancoli-Israel, S., & Kripke, D. F. [1986]. Sleep and aging. In E. Calkins et al. [Eds.], *The practice of geriatrics* [p. 242]. Philadelphia: W. B. Saunders.)

wakefulness each night; and diminished length and intensity of rapid eye movement (REM) sleep (Fontaine, 1989). Fragmented sleep patterns and feelings of fatigue, which occur at baseline, may be worsened by numerous factors in the critical care unit. These include pain, depression, severe stress, urinary frequency, respiratory distress, and medications. The environment of the critical care unit, with its bright lights, equipment and personnel noise, and ambient temperature alterations, also affects the elderly patient's ability to sleep.

Sleep assessment includes both patient factors and environmental factors. Attempts should be made to relieve patient factors, such as pain, as well as altering the environment to promote a quiet and restful atmosphere. Signs of sleep deprivation differ somewhat based on the stage of sleep the person is missing. For example, signs of non-REM sleep deprivation include apathy, slurred speech, lethargy, impaired judgment, ptosis, and lack of facial expression. Deprivation of REM sleep may be manifested as agitation, confusion, impaired control of impulses, emotional lability, and hyperactivity (Lukasiewicz-Ferland, 1987).

IMPAIRED THERMOREGULATION. The ability to control and maintain normal thermal homeostasis is affected by the aging process in a multitude of ways (Brody, 1994; Timiras, 1988). Changes in basal metabolic rate, loss of body fat, alterations in hypothalamic, autonomic, and neuroendocrine centers, and decreases in caloric and fluid intake all have a direct impact on the elderly person's capability to self-regulate temperature and respond to environmental changes in temperature. The elderly are at increased risk for development of both hypothermia and hyperthermia. The physiologic changes are compounded by social factors such as inadequate housing or insufficient income to maintain a temperate environment or adequate nutrition and hydration.

GASTROINTESTINAL SYSTEM

The gastrointestinal system has few age-related alterations that actually affect homeostasis (Timiras, 1988). There are cellular changes that involve secretory activity and motility of the major structures that affect absorption and digestion (Timiras, 1988). Motility is affected by delayed esophageal emptying, esophageal dilation, an increased incidence of ineffective peristalsis, and delayed gastric emptying with age (Pathy & Finucane, 1989). During critical illness, these seemingly nonspecific changes can have a negative impact on outcome.

Anatomic Changes to the Gastrointestinal System

Aging adults exhibit atrophy and thinning of the gastric mucosa, resulting in a weakened capacity for the release of hydrochloric acid (Miller, 1990). When the stomach is exposed to stress, alcohol, or other drugs, there is an increased risk of ulcer formation. The aging process causes failure of the lower esophageal sphincter to relax completely during swallowing (achalasia). Gastric reflux and achalasia increase the risk of aspiration in this age group (Krumpe et al., 1985). The incidence of dilation and distention of pancreatic ducts increases 8% per decade after the age of 60 years (Matteson & McConnell, 1988).

Hiatal hernia is more common in older adults. Symptoms include heartburn, dysphagia, and sternal pain. Because symptoms often mimic cardiac warning signs, these patients are frequently admitted to critical care units to rule out myocardial infarction.

Physiologic Changes in the Gastrointestinal System

The liver and the pancreas are both affected by aging. The important endocrine and exocrine functions of these two organs are disrupted. The amount of bile produced by the liver depends on adequate nutrition, which is frequently a problem with the elderly. The liver also is a primary area for the detoxification of drugs. In advancing age, the ability of the liver to detoxify is decreased. Digestion and absorption abilities are impaired by the degenerative effects of aging on the pancreas. There is decreased absorption of iron, calcium, vitamin B_{12}, and folic acid (Miller, 1990). There is also a decrease in the production of lipase, which results in abnormalities of fat absorption. Blood flow in the liver and splanchnic bed is diminished, and the elderly frequently have reduced gastric acidity and impaired colonic motility (Moore et al., 1983). There is an increased tendency toward development of outlet obstruction. The integrity of the mucosa may be altered secondary to reduced motility and impaired perfusion (Nielson, 1994).

Physiologic changes to the liver also occur in advanced age. Hepatic protein synthesis is weakened, and there are changes in some microsomal drug metabolizing enzymes (e.g., NADPH-cytochrome c reductase) (Kato, 1986). These changes are especially important in the metabolism of some drugs. The production of serum albumin decreases with age, which may affect distribution of highly protein-bound drugs, such as phenytoin, warfarin, thyroxine, nonsteroidal antiinflammatory drugs, aspirin, and oral hypoglycemic agents (Kane et al., 1989). The attenuation of microsomal drug-metabolizing activity and decrease in liver blood flow make drug toxicity a danger for older adults (Rebensen-Piano, 1989). Compounding this dysfunction is increased prescription drug use in the elderly. The result is an increased susceptibility to adverse side effects and drug toxicity at what would typically be considered therapeutic doses.

Clinical Implications of Age-Related Changes in the Gastrointestinal System

Serious effects of gastrointestinal system changes due to aging are minimal in healthy people. These changes, however, may have a profound effect on the critically ill elderly. Their preillness malnutrition, dehydration, and decreased ability for absorption can delay wound healing, weaning from ventilatory support, and the ability to achieve a positive nitrogen balance. Degenerative changes in the liver and pancreas may alter feeding and pharmaceutical options and therapies.

ALTERED NUTRITION: LESS THAN BODY REQUIREMENTS. The incidence of malnutrition in the acutely ill elderly has been documented to be as high as 65%. Opper & Burakoff (1994) found that elderly people who are malnourished reach critical deficits more rapidly. There is a slight decrease in the rate of absorption of carbohydrates, proteins, and lipids with aging (Rebensen-Piano, 1989). Of these, decreased absorption of lipids is the most clinically significant. Accompanying this decrease is a diminished rate of absorption of fat-soluble vitamins. Because vitamin K is lipid soluble, bleeding tendencies and clotting abnormalities may occur. The elderly patient should be carefully assessed for evidence of bleeding, bruising, and petechiae. Coagulation studies should be monitored for abnormalities. Parenteral vitamin K may be administered as a supplement.

Elderly patients are at increased risk for malnutrition (Biena et al., 1982). Furthermore, the stress of being in the critical care atmosphere, coupled with the demands of life-threatening illness, increase protein and calorie requirements (Champagne & Ashley, 1989). Critically ill people frequently require narcotic administration, and these agents can impair motility. The degenerative process may also cause a decrease in motility that may delay absorption of oral drugs in this patient population.

Nutritional support is as important, and at times more important, than cardiovascular or pulmonary support for the critically ill elderly. Underfeeding a patient may impair his or her ability to respond to stress. As with any critically ill patient who is unable to take in enough calories by mouth, tube feeding should be the first option considered. Because milk-based formulas are not well tolerated by some elders, lactulose-free complete formulas are recommended.

If the gastrointestinal tract cannot be used as a route for nutrition, total parenteral nutrition (TPN) should be instituted. In the elderly patient, TPN is started slowly so as not to overcome the patient's physiologic response to increased fluid, glucose, and protein loads (Champagne & Ashley, 1989). For a complete discussion of nutrition, please refer to Chapter 47.

RENAL SYSTEM

The renal system undergoes a slow degenerative process. The system can function with a 50% loss. Therefore, degenerative changes are not typically observed until late in life. By the eighth decade, kidney mass has decreased by approximately 25% (Miller, 1990). These changes have significant implications because they result in altered elimination of wastes and drugs from the body.

Anatomic Changes in the Renal System

The number of functioning nephrons begins to decrease and the glomeruli undergo changes, such as increased size, diminished lobulation, and thickening of the basement membrane over time. There is an actual loss of renal mass: a 40-year-old male kidney weighs approximately 250 g, and will decrease to 200 g by the age of 80 (Sica, 1994). The renal tubules also undergo a degenerative process, including the formation of diverticula, a loss of convoluted tubuli cells, and alterations in the chemical composition of the basement membrane (Miller, 1990). Progressive decreases are seen in both proximal tubular length and volume. Renal perfusion is decreased as a result of sclerotic changes in the renal arterioles (Timiras, 1988).

With age, fibrous connective tissue replaces some of the smooth muscle and elastic tissue of the bladder. The bladder muscles weaken. Subsequently, bladder capacity decreases and incomplete emptying occurs. Thus, frequency of urination increases. Changes in the bladder outlet may cause obstruction (benign prostatic hypertrophy) in men. In women, incontinence may occur due to relaxation and weakening of the pelvic muscles (Matteson & McConnell, 1988). These changes may also lead to difficulty in starting the urinary stream. Incomplete emptying and possible outlet obstruction place elderly patients at higher risk for development of urinary tract infections.

Physiologic Changes to the Renal System

The GFR decreases steadily with aging. The GFR (measured by creatinine clearance) falls at a rate of 1% per year after the age of 35 (Pathy & Finucane, 1989). The ability to concentrate and dilute urine declines, and the ability to excrete an acid or alkaline urine also lessens. Excretion of drugs and glucose may be impaired (Feinstein, 1986; Hickler, 1985). There is also a decrease hormone production and sensitivity with age (Sica, 1994).

Clinical Implications of Age-Related Changes in the Renal System

Causes of renal insufficiency in the elderly patient population are related to the inability of the renal system to meet the demands being placed on it during critical illness. The kidneys' decreased GFR increases the incidence of drug toxicity and decreases the threshold for nephrotoxicity due to the lack of reserve function available. The decreased GFR also increases the incidence of volume overload in these patients. Volume overload can have significant consequences in the elderly due to their lack of pulmonary and cardiovascular reserve. It takes minimal fluid to cause congestive heart failure in this age group.

HIGH RISK FOR FLUID VOLUME DEFICIT. Alterations in urine production place the elderly patient at risk for extracellular fluid volume deficit. Impaired concentrating ability and reduced level of aldosterone may lead to urinary sodium and water losses as well.

The circadian rhythm of urine production may be lost in advanced age, resulting in nocturia (Matteson & McConnell, 1988). Dehydration is a common problem in the elderly due to the loss of thirst perception mechanics, difficulty in obtaining and swallowing fluid, and a reluctance to drink fluids due to subsequent urgency to void and incontinence. If large volume losses, such as vomiting or diarrhea, occur in addition to the underlying state of mild dehydration, the result can be marked hypovolemia. Fluid volume deficit is one cause of confusion in the elderly, but other etiologic factors include respiratory insufficiency, sepsis, alterations in temperature, hyperglycemia, hypoglycemia, and drug toxicity. Further evaluation and treatment of confusion should be tailored to the underlying pathology.

The creatinine clearance decreases with age. However, because of a generalized decrease in muscle mass, the elderly person's serum creatinine concentration may remain relatively unchanged. For this reason, the creatinine clearance is used as an index of renal function when drug dosages are determined (Matteson & McConnell, 1988). The serum creatinine and blood urea nitrogen levels should be monitored closely when the patient is receiving aminoglycoside antibiotics. Maintenance of adequate hydration is an important factor in preventing nephrotoxicity in the elderly patient.

URINARY INCONTINENCE. Up to 43% of all acute care patients experience urinary incontinence (Lincoln & Roberts, 1989). Incontinence may result from many factors, including neurogenic disease, medication, and stress. An increase in intraabdominal pressure due to coughing, sneezing, or laughing may also result in incontinence.

Hospitalization may initiate or exacerbate urinary incontinence. For instance, many elderly people schedule their medications (e.g., diuretics) and fluid intake so that voiding will not interrupt planned activities or sleep. Older adults may not take in fluids after 6 P.M. so that they can avoid trips to the bathroom at night. However, in the ICU these patients may be receiving intravenous fluids, enteral feedings, or medications at times that disrupt their normal pattern of voiding, which may result in a lack of bladder control.

ENDOCRINE SYSTEM

The production of some hormones and receptivity of some target tissues are altered with advanced age. There is also a change in the degradation and elimination of hormones. The plasma levels of aldosterone, renin, estrogen, calcitonin, growth hormone, somatomedin C, and prolactin decrease with age. Conversely, plasma levels of follicle-stimulating hormone, leuteinizing hormone, and norepinephrine increase with age (Davis & Davis, 1983). Adrenal secretion of cortisol is stable; therefore, there are no significant changes in the hypothalamic–pituitary–adrenal axis and the stress response (Davis & Davis, 1983). There is also a decrease in the basal metabolic rate with age (Matteson & McConnell, 1988; Rock, 1985).

The endocrine functions of the kidney are also affected by aging. Plasma renin and aldosterone levels decrease in the normotensive older adult, leading to alterations in sodium regulation. Hyperkalemia may occur as a consequence of impaired renin and aldosterone secretion and a decreased glomerular filtration rate. The conversion of 1-OH-cholecalciferol to 1-25-$(OH)_2$ cholecalciferol is diminished, leading to decreased calcium absorption from the intestine. Erythropoietin production is also slowed, thus contributing to anemia (Matteson & McConnell, 1988). Table 71–3 summarizes the age-related changes in the various endocrine organs.

Clinical Implications of Age-Related Changes in the Endocrine System

Endocrine system changes associated with aging usually do not affect the older adult's daily functioning.

TABLE 71–3. **Age-Related Changes in the Endocrine System**

Organ	Changes Related to Aging	Clinical Implication
Pituitary	Atrophy Decreased size and cell mass Fibrosis Decreased vascularity	
Thyroid	Decreased mass, increased fibrosis Increased incidence of nodules and small goiters Increased plasma level of inorganic iodide Plasma T_4 level unchanged Plasma T_3 level decreased	Decreased basal metabolic rate
Adrenal cortex	Cortical secretion unchanged Aldosterone secretion decreased	Stress response intact Decreased renal reabsorption of sodium in response to activity changes and dietary sodium restrictions
Parathyroid	Effect on PTH secretion is undetermined	
Pancreas	Decrease in glucose tolerance Decreased insulin secretion Decreased receptor site sensitivity	Hyperglycemia Glucosuria

Abbreviations: T_4, thyroxine; T_3, triiodothyronine; PTH, parathyroid hormone.

However, illness places a greater stress on all body systems and may accentuate these changes. Because of the degenerative process, the elderly may exhibit endocrine emergencies in more nonspecific ways than the young, which can delay diagnosis or affect treatment and outcome (Miller & Gold, 1994).

IMPAIRED GLUCOSE METABOLISM. One very common endocrine disorder occurring in later life is diabetes mellitus. Approximately 12% of people over the age of 60 and 25% over the age of 85 have diabetes (Bennett, 1984). Signs of diabetes may be very subtle in the elderly. Leg cramps, numbness, weakness, impotence, vaginal itching, urinary incontinence, and cool extremities may be the first clinical manifestations of the disease (Zimmerman, 1981). Two of the hallmarks of diabetes mellitus are polyuria and polydipsia, but these symptoms may be absent in older adults (Fonesca, 1981). Because the renal threshold for glucose increases with age, the spilling of glucose in the urine may not happen until blood glucose levels are 300 mg/dL or higher (Marchesseault, 1983).

Diabetic ketoacidosis (DKA) is not as prevalent in older adults because fat is seldom used for energy and older adults usually continue to produce some insulin (Hayter, 1981). Hyperosmolar hyperglycemic nonketotic coma (HHNK) is a more common problem for elderly diabetics, and can be life threatening. The average age of HHNK presentation is 60, and the fatality rate is 40% to 70% (Goldberg et al., 1985). Both DKA and HHNK can be precipitated by the stress of an acute illness (Gioiella & Bevil, 1984; Goldberg et al., 1985).

IMMUNE SYSTEM

Sternberg (1988) stated that the most dramatic and consequential age-related phenomenon is the decline in immunologic function. These changes have a profound effect on susceptibility to a variety of diseases. In fact, infection is one of the leading causes of hospital admissions and complications in the elderly (Petrucci et al., 1989). Walford and colleagues (1968) proposed that immune system failure is the cause of human aging. This classic theory has generated a great deal of research.

The degeneration of immune function has a direct relationship to healing in the elderly trauma patient population. The first age-related change in the immune system in humans occurs in the thymus. The thymus gradually loses up to 95% of its mass by age 50 (Busby & Caranasos, 1985). The aging thymus induces changes in the stem cells that result in decreased antibody production in response to antigens (Sternberg, 1988). Thus, the older person is at higher risk for development of certain diseases, including tuberculosis (Sternberg, 1988).

The decreased efficiency of immune function is demonstrated by a delayed hypersensitivity reaction, increased autoantibodies, decreased inflammatory response, decreased migration, proliferation, and maturation of cells, and an increased collagen tertiary cross-linking (Jones & Millman, 1990). There is also suppression of T-cell activity, specifically depressed cytotoxic activity of T lymphocytes and a decline in T-helper cells with a decreased number of Th-1 and Th-2 cells (Sternberg, 1988). The lysosomal enzymes like beta-glucuronidase, acid phosphatase, and cathepsin-D become elevated with age (Sternberg, 1988). The phagocytic activity of the immune system is affected by the aging process with only a minimal decline in polymorphonuclear, granulocyte, and monocyte cells.

Autoimmune disorders occur when antibodies or cytotoxic T lymphocytes are produced to combat the body's own tissue. When this happens, the tissues that are not recognized as "self" come under attack. Autoimmune disorders related to aging include rheumatoid arthritis, systemic lupus erythematosus, and chronic hepatitis (Cohen, 1989; Sternberg, 1988).

Interestingly, it has been found that there is a decrease in immunologic rejection of tissue grafts with aging. Therefore, in some cases, the aging immune system may be an advantage to the patient (Sternberg, 1988).

With age, the immune system's ability to detect and respond to tumor cells is decreased. There is a higher incidence of tumor growth in the elderly, perhaps because of age-related changes in the components of the immune system that are responsible for tumor surveillance. There is an increased incidence of leukemia and breast, lung, prostate, stomach, colon, and pancreas cancer in older adults.

Clinical Implications of Age-Related Changes in the Immune System

Changes in immune function contribute to the high rate of infection and slow rate of wound healing in the elderly. The respiratory tract and urinary tract are the most common sites of infection in older adults (Fox, 1988). Delay in wound healing in the elderly was demonstrated by Jones and Millman (1990), who found that patients over the age of 60 had two to three times the rate of wound dehiscence of younger patients.

AIDS IN THE ELDERLY. Between 1981 and 1993, there were 4,679 people over the age of 65 diagnosed with acquired immune deficiency syndrome (AIDS) (3,680 men, 999 women) (CDC, 1994). Ten percent of all AIDS cases have occurred in individuals over the age of 50, and 4% over the age of 70 (Butler, 1993; Stall & Catania, 1994). The oldest reported patient with AIDS is 92 years old (Bulter, 1993). Homosexual or bisexual behavior is the predominant risk factor for acquiring the virus up to age 70; after 70, blood transfusion is the major cause (Wallace et al., 1993). Elderly victims of AIDS appear to suffer a more rapid progresssion of the disease. A large proportion of these victims die within a month of being diagnosed. This fact suggests that there is a delay in diagnosing human immunodeficiency virus (HIV) infection in the geriatric age group, possibly due to the high incidence of chronic illnesses with the same symptoms in this population (Wallace et al., 1993). AIDS dementia may be the first major manifestation of HIV infection in an elderly patient. Symptoms of behavioral, cognitive, and motor abnormalities can easily mimic Alzheimer's disease, Parkinson's disease, or other disorders associated with advanced age (Navia & Price, 1987; Sabin, 1987). The possible diagnosis of AIDS should be addressed when assessing an elderly patient, and risk factors and blood tests should be considered (Stall & Catania, 1994).

HIGH RISK FOR INFECTION. In elderly patients, the signs and symptoms of infection can be quite different from those of the younger adults. The aging process and the presence of preexisting chronic conditions make it difficult to diagnose infection or systemic inflammatory response syndrome in the elderly (Rauen, 1994). The conditions commonly observed in the young adult with systemic infection, such as increased cardiac output, decreased systemic vascular resistance, hyperglycemia, hyperlactatemia, elevated oxygen consumption index, and elevated BUN excretion (Cerra, 1990; Hotter, 1990; Huddleston, 1992), are ironically also part of the normal degenerative process. The classic signs of elevated temperature and white blood cell (WBC) count can also be unreliable indicators of infection in the geriatric group. The elderly have less of a febrile response to illness, run lower temperatures than younger adults, and also have a lower WBC count naturally (Finklestein et al., 1983; Fox, 1988). The lack of physiologic reserve in all systems makes it very difficult for the elderly to compensate during times of inflammation and sepsis-induced hyperdynamic states (Rauen, 1994).

Some indicators of infection commonly seen in the elderly are falls, postural instability, immobility, confusion, and incontinence of urine or feces. Often these problems or complications are what brings an elderly person to the ICU. Unfortunately, the presenting problem may be treated while the underlying infection goes undiagnosed. Because there is a loss of reserve in many body systems with aging, the development of infection in one system may produce negative consequences in many other systems (Fox, 1988).

Treatment of infection must be aggressive but cautious in the elderly. Organisms must be isolated and antibiotics initiated early. Close monitoring of treatment is essential because the treatment alone may cause more complications, such as renal or hepatic compromise from drugs or cardiovascular and respiratory compromise from fluid volume overload. The elderly may require hemodynamic monitoring for close evaluation of treatment and response.

MUSCULOSKELETAL SYSTEM

The musculoskeletal system is composed of the bones, muscles, and joints. All of these structures are affected by the aging process.

BONES. The bony skeleton is relatively resistant to deterioration compared with the rest of the musculoskeletal system. However, bones do tend to become weaker with age (Matteson & McConnell, 1988). The skeleton also decreases in mass due to an imbalance between rates of bone formation and bone resorption.

One of the primary metabolic functions of bone is to maintain calcium balance in the extracellular fluid. In fact, bone tissue is a major storage site of calcium. When serum calcium levels are low, parathyroid hormone is released, which stimulates the release of calcium from the bone into the blood. Parathyroid hormone and vitamin D promote absorption of dietary calcium from the gastrointestinal tract and reabsorption through the kidneys. Conversely, when serum calcium is high, calcitonin is released from the thyroid to promote storage of calcium in the bone (Ganong, 1987).

In later adulthood, there is less calcium absorbed

through the gastrointestinal tract. This may be due either to a diminished calcium intake or to decreased calcium absorption efficiency (Giansiracusa & Kantrowitz, 1981).

MUSCLES. There is a decrease in the number of muscle fibers along with a decrease in muscle strength in advanced age. Individual muscle fibers become smaller and more diverse in size. Lipofuscin, fat, and fibrous tissue may be deposited within the muscle tissue (Davis-Sharts, 1989; Matteson & McConnell, 1988). Along with changes in muscle fibers, there are also age-related alterations at the neuromuscular junction. The velocity of nerve conduction slows and, in general, movement of the older person is slowed. The older person may exhibit diminished facial expressions and decreased blinking, which may be due to impaired extrapyramidal and motor neuron function (Larsson et al., 1979; Matteson & McConnell, 1988). In addition, involuntary movements may be exacerbated by fatigue and loss of sodium chloride (Matteson & McConnell, 1988). There may be a decrease in deep tendon reflexes with age due to atrophy and sclerosis of muscles and tendons.

JOINTS. The joints, especially the wrists, elbows, knees, hips, neck, and vertebrae, tend to become slightly more flexed with age. This is due in part to tendon and muscle rigidity and decreased movement. Joint changes also involve the progressive roughening of cartilage surfaces, as well as thickening and loss of elasticity of the cartilage (Davis-Sharts, 1989). These changes result in a decreased latency of fatigue and an increased risk of osteoarthritis.

Clinical Implications of Age-Related Changes in the Musculoskeletal System

The critically ill older adult is at great risk for alterations in mobility by virtue of these age-related changes, their disease process, and the critical care environment. Medications, physical restraints, tubing and other equipment, anxiety, and many other iatrogenic factors, when superimposed on age-related changes, can place the elderly person at even greater risk for complications of immobility.

IMPAIRED PHYSICAL MOBILITY. The ability to move freely is often taken for granted until it is lost. The body functions best when it changes positions often. The joints, muscles, and tendons are all dependent on the stress of movement for their function (Milde, 1981). In the critical care setting, immobility often cannot be prevented, but many of the complications can be.

Complications of immobility can affect every major organ system, as described in Chapter 61. These consequences can have adverse effects on the physical, psychological, and metabolic functioning of the individual (Kane et al., 1994).

Although bed rest is prescribed for cardiac emergencies, prolonged bed rest can actually have a deleterious effect on cardiac functioning. There are reductions in venous return, stroke volume, cardiac output and arterial pressure, $V_{O_2}max$, and an increase in heart rate (4–15 beats/minute) to compensate (Windslow, 1985). The patient, once allowed out of bed, is also more likely to have difficulties with orthostatic hypotension.

The respiratory consequences of immobility combined with the degenerative changes increase the risk of atelectasis, pneumonia, deep vein thrombosis, and pulmonary emboli in the elderly (Clagett & Reisch, 1988; Kane et al., 1994). Pulmonary complications due to decreased endurance and loss of muscle strength include abnormal or adventitious breath sounds, and reduced arterial oxygen levels (Timiras, 1988).

The decreased gastrointestinal motility associated with immobility can cause anorexia, constipation, incontinence, and fecal impaction (Kane et al., 1994). The genitourinary system is at risk for bladder and renal calculi, urinary infection, and retention difficulties.

The integrity of the skin is a major concern for the immobile elderly. The muscles also atrophy, bones can degenerate, and joints contract if range of motion or some sort of movement is not performed.

The goals of care include maintenance of muscle strength and endurance by isometric and isotonic exercises. Skeletal strength is enhanced by ambulation, resistive exercises, range-of-motion exercises, and correct positioning. Elevation of the head of the bed and prevention of Valsalva maneuver help to maintain adequate venous circulation (Milde, 1981). Some form of deep vein thrombosis prophylaxis should be considered, and monitoring of bowel and bladder function is essential. The ultimate goal is to maintain preimmobilization functions and abilities while preventing complications.

INTEGUMENTARY SYSTEM

Age-related changes in the integument are perhaps the most visible indicators of senescence. Wrinkled skin and gray hair are hallmarks of passing years. The changes in the integument are not due to the aging process alone; environmental factors also play a large part in the changes that occur. Because elderly people have been exposed to the sun for many years, solar damage is far more prevalent in the elderly than in other age groups (Forbes et al., 1979; Timiras, 1988).

EPIDERMIS. In aging, there is a decrease in the height and surface area of epidermal cells. The moisture content of the superficial layer of cells, the stratum corneum, is lower. The result is a dryness or roughness of the skin. There is an increased incidence of benign and malignant neoplasms in aging skin. The junction between the epidermis and the dermis becomes flattened, reducing the junction's total surface area. For this reason, older adults are much more prone to blister formation and abrasions (Timiras, 1988).

The turnover rate of epidermal cells slows, which means that cells are present at the surface for longer periods of time before they are exfoliated. This places the cells at increased risk for contacting carcinogens and plays a role in delayed wound healing (Timiras, 1988).

Irregular pigmentation in aging skin may be due to a reduction in the number of melanocytes. Melanocytes serve as protectors, creating an inflammatory warning signal when insults, such as sunburn, are present. There is also a decrease in Langerhans cells, which may contribute to the skin's impaired cell-mediated immune response associated with aging. Exposure to ultraviolet rays also decreases Langerhans cells (Timiras, 1988).

DERMIS. The dermal layer decreases in density and has fewer blood vessels. This may be accompanied by prolonged times for dermal clearance of topical drugs and other substances. Collagen becomes thicker and less soluble. The total amount of collagen decreases linearly after age 20 years. Due to the loss of elasticity, older skin is more susceptible to tears, wrinkles, and damage to underlying tissues after trauma (Timiras, 1988).

SUBCUTANEOUS TISSUE. With age, there is a decrease in the thickness of the subcutaneous layer. There is also a decrease in the number and patency of blood vessels in the skin. Therefore, thermoregulation is impaired. The decrease in subcutaneous fat leaves bony prominences less protected from wear and tear.

GLANDS. Sweat glands decrease in number, size, and efficiency with age. Diminished capacity for perspiration has a deleterious effect on thermoregulation (Matteson & McConnell, 1988). Because the body cannot use perspiration as a mechanism of cooling, the tendency to overheat is increased.

Clinical Implications of Age-Related Changes in the Integument

Age-related changes in the integument place the critically ill elderly patient at high risk for development of skin breakdown and related infections.

IMPAIRED SKIN INTEGRITY. Pressure ulcers are a complication of immobility and are one of the most common and preventable problems for hospitalized elderly patients. The presence of pressure ulcers significantly increases the patient's risk for morbidity and mortality. The primary cause of ulceration is pressure, but shearing forces, friction, inadequate nutrition, and moisture are also contributing factors (Goode, 1989; Kane et al., 1994). Additional reasons the elderly patients are at risk for pressure ulcer development include immobility; age-related decreases in ascorbic acid levels, which may increase blood vessel fragility; and the decreased number of dermal blood vessels in aged skin (Gilchrest, 1982).

Shearing forces are present in the sacral area when a patient sits up in bed or in a chair and then slides downward. Shearing forces lower the amount of pressure needed to cause compression of blood vessels (Bennett & Ouslander, 1989). Friction is generated when a patient is pulled across bed linens. Friction results in intraepidermal blisters that, when broken, result in superficial erosions (Goode, 1989). Moisture from urinary or fecal incontinence, wound drainage, or weepy skin lesions further increases the risk for pressure ulcer development.

Preventive interventions focus on decreasing these factors. For example, repositioning patients frequently is basic care, but for the critically ill elderly, frequency of positioning must be quite individualized. Using a turning sheet when repositioning a patient can decrease the incidence of friction injury. Special beds and antipressure devices may be used. Vitamin C supplementation and increased calories and protein may be indicated. Antibiotics must be ordered if infection is present. Local care includes cleansing the ulcer with topical disinfectant–antibiotic. Various solutions of this type have been used and are still being evaluated for effectiveness.

PHARMACOLOGIC CONSIDERATION IN THE ELDERLY

The pharmacologic options available for treating the geriatric patient population may be limited due to this population's altered organ function, unpredictable drug responses, and adverse reactions experienced (Nielson, 1994). There are many physiologic changes associated with aging that are relevant to medication use and administration. The pharmacologic parameters that are altered by aging include absorption, distribution, metabolism, excretion, and tissue sensitivity (Kane et al., 1994; Nielson, 1994). Table 71–4 outlines special considerations for drugs commonly used in the elderly patient in the critical care area.

Although absorption appears to be the pharmacologic parameter least affected directly by age, it is affected by the degenerative process. There are decreases in the absorptive surface of the gut and blood vessels and a reduction in splanchnic blood flow. Increased gastric pH, as well as altered gastrointestinal motility, also may alter drug absorption (Kane et al., 1994).

Changes in drug distribution may occur in the elderly patient as a result of decreases in total body water and lean body mass. A lower serum albumin concentration can have a substantial effect on free drug availability and action. Changes in protein binding have been demonstrated, but the clinical relevance of

TABLE 71–4. **Pharmacologic Considerations in the Elderly**

Drug	Route of Elimination	Clinical Implications
Analgesics		
Acetaminophen	Hepatic	No substantial age-related change in kinetics
Aspirin	Renal	Highly protein-bound; half-life may be prolonged
Narcotics	Hepatic	Blood levels higher; pain relief longer Lower doses are usually effective Constipation is major side effect in elderly patient
Antimicrobials		
Aminoglycosides	Renal	Prolonged half-life may require increased dosage intervals (e.g., q12h, q24h) Nephrotoxicity and ototoxicity are major problems; monitor blood levels, serum creatinine, creatinine clearance Formula for calculating age-referenced interval in men: [140 − age × kg body wt]/72 × serum creatinine; women: 85% of this
Cephalosporins	Renal	Half-life prolonged
Penicillins	Renal	Half-life prolonged
	Hepatic	Some are highly protein bound
Tetracycline	Renal	Half-life prolonged
Amphotericin	Nonrenal	Nephrotoxicity a major problem in elderly with underlying renal dysfunction
Cardiovascular Drugs		
Beta-adrenergic effect	Renal	Elderly patients may require increased dosage to achieve
Digoxin	Renal (15%–40% nonrenal)	Decreased clearance; half-life prolonged
Lidocaine	Hepatic	Volume of distribution is increased; half-life prolonged; clearance unchanged
Procainamide	Renal	Clearance decreased; highly protein bound Half-life prolonged; steady-state levels higher
Quinidine	Nonrenal	Highly protein bound; clearance decreased Half-life prolonged
Verapamil	Hepatic	Clearance decreased Effects more pronounced and prolonged
Antihypertensives		
Diltiazem	Hepatic	Clearance decreased; used cautiously in sinus node dysfunction
Hydralazine	Hepatic	Highly protein bound
Propranolol	Hepatic	Highly protein bound Half-life prolonged; clearance decreased; blood levels higher Sensitivity to effects decreased
Diuretics		
Furosemide	Renal	Highly protein bound Elderly patients at high risk for dehydration and electrolyte imbalance

Adapted from Kane, R., Ouslander, J., & Abrass, I. (1994). Essentials of clinical geriatics (3rd ed., pp. 367–370). New York: McGraw-Hill. Reproduced with permission of The McGraw-Hill Companies.

these changes has not been established (Kane et al., 1994).

Reduced liver blood flow, diminished hepatic enzyme activity, and decreased enzyme inducibility may change the actual metabolism of drugs. Research related to drug metabolism and aging has been unable to predict metabolic alterations linked to specific drugs (Kane et al., 1994).

Changes in excretion of drugs by the elderly may be due to diminished renal blood flow, decreased GFR, and impaired tubular secretion function. Tissue sensitivity is altered due to changes in the number of receptors and receptor affinity for certain drugs. The elderly appear to be more sensitive to the sedative effects of benzodiazepine drugs, and less sensitive to beta-adrenergic receptor type drugs (Kane et al., 1994). The elderly have an increased risk for central nervous system side effects from drugs (Nielson, 1994). In addition, there may be cellular and nuclear responses to drugs that change with aging (Kane et al., 1994).

In the elderly, the drug dosing rate is adjusted downward to prevent excessive drug accumulation, side effects, and potential toxicity. Elderly patients are started at lower doses, and the doses are increased more gradually than in younger people. Drugs that require a loading dose should be given with caution and the actual dose should be determined by the volume of distribution (Nielson, 1994). Drug interactions are prevalent due to polypharmacy in the elderly, so there should be ongoing consultation with the clinical pharmacist to monitor side effects and to evaluate effectiveness of drug regimens (Chapron, 1988). Once the acute phase of illness subsides, the drug choices and doses should be examined carefully. Because of the high incidence of adverse effects, the financial burden of polypharmacy, and difficulties with compliance, every attempt should be made to discharge the elderly patient on the minimum amount of prescription drugs (Nielson, 1994).

SUMMARY

Many changes accompany the aging process. The physiologic changes depicted in this chapter are of both structural and functional decline. However, it is important to recognize that with every stage of life, old capabilities are lost as new ones are gained. Although the elderly person may be declining in some physiologic capabilities, other areas of his or her person are growing in strength and complexity. New strengths may include wisdom, capability for higher abstractions of thought, and an ability to transcend the physical pain and limitations of the body (Reed, 1983). Perhaps the most important developmental challenge the older person faces is the inevitability of death (Erikson, 1963). This issue becomes even more salient in the face of critical illness. Certainly, the critically ill elderly patient represents a complex interaction of many dynamic systems and requires care based on diverse and sound clinical knowledge.

REFERENCES

Beck, M. (October 4, 1993). The gray nineties. *Newsweek*, 65–66.

Bennett, P. (1984). Diabetes in the elderly: Diagnosis and epidemiology. *Geriatrics, 39,* 37.

Bennett, R., & Ouslander, J. (1989). Air-fluidized bed treatment of nursing home patients with pressure sores. *Journal of the American Geriatric Society, 37,* 235–242.

Biena, R., Ratcliff, S., & Barbour, J. (1982). Malnutrition in the hospitalized geriatric patient. *Journal of American Geriatric Society, 30,* 433–436.

Bobb, J. (1987). Trauma in the elderly. *Journal of Gerontological Nursing, 13,* 28–31.

Brandstetter, R., & Kazemi, H. (1983). Aging and the respiratory system. *Medical Clinics of North America, 67,* 419–431.

Brody, G. (1994). Hyperthermia and hypothermia in the elderly. *Clinics in Geriatric Medicine, 10,* 213–229.

Bruce, M. (1980). The relation of tactile thresholds to histology in the fingers of the elderly. *Journal of Neurology, Neurosurgery and Psychiatry, 43,* 730–734.

Bumann, R., & Spelz, M. (1989). Decreased cardiac output: A nursing diagnosis. *Dimensions of Critical Care Nursing, 8,* 6–15.

Busby, J., & Caranasos, G. (1985). Immune function, autoimmunity, and selective immunoprophylaxis in the aged. *Medical Clinics of North America, 69,* 465–474.

Butler, R. (1993). AIDS: Older patients aren't immune. *Geriatrics, 48*(3), 9–10.

Centers for Disease Control and Prevention. (1994). *Surveillance Report 3rd quarter, 5*(3).

Cerra, F. (August 15, 1990). The multiple organ failure syndrome. *Hospital Practice,* 169–176.

Champagne, M., & Ashley, M. (1989). Nutritional support in the critically ill elderly patient. *Critical Care Nursing Quarterly, 12,* 15–25.

Chapron, D. (1988). Influence of advanced age on drug disposition and response. In J. C. Delafuente & R. B. Stewart (Eds.), *Therapeutics in the elderly* (pp. 107–120). Baltimore: Williams & Wilkins.

Chelluri, L., Pinsky, M., & Grenvik, A. (1992). Outcome of intensive care of the "oldest-old" critically ill patients. *Critical Care Medicine, 20,* 757–761.

Clagett, P., & Reisch, J. (1988). Prevention of venous thromboembolism in general surgical patients. *Annals of Surgery, 208,* 227–240.

Davis, P., & Davis, F. (1983). Endocrinology and aging. In W. Reichel (Ed.), *Clinical aspects of aging* (2nd ed., pp. 396–410). Baltimore: Williams & Wilkins.

Davis-Sharts, J. (1989). The elder and critical care: Sleep and mobility issues. *Nursing Clinics of North America, 24,* 755.

Duara, R., London, E., & Rapport, S. (1985). Changes in structure and energy metabolism of the aging brain. In C. E. Finch & E. L. Schneider (Eds.), *Handbook of the biology of aging* (pp. 595–616). New York: Van Nostrand Reinhold.

Erikson, E. (1963). *Childhood and society.* New York: W. W. Norton.

Fedullo, A., & Seinburne, A. (1983). Relationship of patient age to cost and survival to cost and survival in a medical ICU. *Critical Care Medicine, 11*(3), 155–164.

Feinstein, E. (1986). Renal disease in the elderly. In I. Rossman (Ed.), *Clinical geriatrics* (3rd ed., pp. 352–363). Philadelphia: J. B. Lippincott.

Finelli, F., Jonsson, J., Champion, H., Morelli, S., & Fouty, W. (1989). A case study for major trauma in geriatric patients. *Journal of Trauma, 29,* 541–548.

Finklestein, M., Petkun, W., Freedman, M., & Antopol, S. (1983). Pneumococcal bacteremia in adults: Age-dependent differences in presentation and outcome. *Journal of the American Geriatric Society, 31,* 19–27.

Fonesca, V. (1981). Sulphonylurea and insulin combination in the treatment of diabetes [Letter]. *British Medical Journal, 283,* 797.

Fontaine, D. (1989). Measurement of nocturnal sleep patterns in trauma. *Heart and Lung, 18,* 402–409.

Forbes, P., Davies, R., & Urbach, F. (1979). Aging, environmental influences and photocarcinogenesis. *Journal of Investigative Dermatology, 73,* 131–134.

Fox, R. (1988). Atypical presentation of geriatric infections. *Geriatrics, 43*(5), 58–65.

Ganong, W. (1987). *Review of medical physiology* (13th ed.). Los Altos, CA: Lange Medical Publications.

Gerstenblith, G., Frederiksen, J., Yin, F., et al. (1977). Echocardiographic assessment of a normal adult aging population. *Circulation, 56,* 273–278.

Giansiracusa, D., & Kantrowitz, F. (1981). *Rheumatic and metabolic diseases in the elderly.* Lexington, MA: The Collamore Press.

Gilchrest, B. (1982). Age-associated changes in the skin. *Journal of the American Geriatric Society, 30,* 139–143.

Gioiella, E., & Bevil, C. (1984). *Nursing care of the aging client: Promoting healthy adaptation.* Norwalk, CT: Appleton-Century-Crofts.

Goldberg, A., Andes, R., & Bierman, E. (1985). Diabetes mellitus in the elderly. In R. Andres, E. Bierman, & W. Hazzard (Eds.), *Principles of geriatric medicine* (pp. 750–763). New York: McGraw-Hill.

Goode, P. (1989). The prevention and management of pressure ulcers. *Medical Clinics of North America, 73,* 1511–1524.

Graves, E. (April 8, 1994). Centers for Disease Control and Prevention, 1992 summary: National hospital discharge survey. *Advance Date, 249.*

Harris, R. (1983). Cardiovascular diseases in the elderly. *Medical Clinics of North America, 67,* 379–394.

Hayter, J. (1981). Diabetes and the older person. *Geriatric Nursing, 1,* 32–36.

Heuser, M., Case, L., & Ettinger, W. (1992). Mortality in intensive care patients with respiratory disease: Is age important? *Archives of Internal Medicine, 152,* 1683.

Hickler, R. (1985). The physiology of aging: Implications for drug therapy. In E. P. Hoffer (Ed.), *Emergency problems in the elderly* (pp. 1–17). Oradell, NJ: Medical Economics Books.

Hotter, A. (1990). The pathophysiology of multi-system organ failure in the trauma patient. *AACN Clinical Issues in Critical Care Nursing, 1,* 465–471.

Huddleston, V. (1992). *Multisystem organ failure: Pathophysiology and clinical implications.* St. Louis: Mosby Year Book.

Jones, P., & Millman, A. (1990). Wound healing and the aged patient. *Nursing Clinics of North America, 25,* 263–277.

Kane, R. L., Ouslander, J. G., & Abrass, I. B. (1989). *Essentials of clinical geriatrics* (2nd ed.). New York: McGraw-Hill.

Kane, R. L., Ouslander, J. G., & Abrass, I. B. (1994). *Essentials of clinical geriatrics* (3rd ed.). New York: McGraw-Hill.

Kato, R., & Takanaka, A. (1986). Metabolism of drugs in old rats II. *Japanese Journal of Pharmacology, 18,* 389–396.

Kelly, D. (1989). *The identification and clinical validation of the defining characteristics of the nursing diagnosis alteration in tissue perfusion: Cardiac.* Unpublished Masters Thesis, University of Arizona, Tucson.

Kenney, R. (1989). *Physiology of aging: A synopsis* (2nd ed.). Chicago: Year Book Medical Publishers.

Kidd, P., & Murakami, R. (1987). Common pathologic conditions in elderly persons: Nursing assessment and intervention. *Journal of Emergency Nursing, 13*(1), 27–32.

Krieger, B. (1994). Respiratory failure in the elderly. *Clinics in Geriatric Medicine, 10,* 103–119.

Krieger, B., Ershowsky, P., Becker, D., & Gaserogly, H. (1989). Evaluation of conventional criteria for predicting successful weaning from mechanical ventilatory support in the elderly. *Critical Care Medicine, 17,* 858–861.

Krumpe, P., Knudson, R., Parsons, G., & Reiser, K. (1985). The aging respiratory system. *Clinics in Geriatric Medicine, 1,* 143–175.

Lakatta, E. (1988). Cardiovascular system aging. In B. Kent & R. Butler (Eds.), *Human aging research: Concepts and techniques* (pp. 199–219). New York: Raven Press.

Larsson, L., Grimby, G., & Karlsson, J. (1979). Muscle strength and speed of movement in relation to age and muscle morphology. *Journal of Applied Physiology, 46,* 451–456.

Lee, B. Y. (1980). Non-invasive detection and prevention of deep vein thrombosis in the geriatric patient. *Journal of the American Geriatric Society, 27,* 171–175.

Levy, D., Hanlon, D., & Townsend, R. (1993). Geriatric trauma. *Clinics in Geriatric Medicine, 9,* 601–620.

Lincoln, R., & Roberts, R. (1989). Continence issues in acute care. *Nursing Clinics of North America, 24,* 741–753.

Luft, R. C., Grim, C., E., Fineberg, N., & Weingerber, M. C. (1979). Effects of volume expansion and contraction in normotensive whites, blacks and subjects of different ages. *Circulation, 59,* 634–650.

Lukasiewicz-Ferland, P. (1987). When your ICU patient can't sleep. *Nursing, 17*(11), 51–53.

Marchesseault, L. (1981). Diabetes mellitus and the elderly. *Nursing Clinics of North America, 18,* 791–798.

Matteson, M. A., & McConnell, E. S. (1988). *Gerontological nursing.* Philadelphia: W. B. Saunders.

Meisami, E. (1988). Aging of the nervous system: Sensory changes. In P. S. Timiras (Ed.), *Physiological basis of geriatrics* (pp. 156–178). New York: Macmillan.

Milde, F. (1981). Physiological immobilization. In L. Hart, G. Reese, & R. Fearing (Eds.), *Concepts common to acute illness* (pp. 67–109). St. Louis: C. V. Mosby.

Miller, C. (1990). *Nursing care of older adults.* Glenview, IL: Foresman and Company.

Miller, M., & Gold, G. (1994). Acute endocrine emergencies. *Clinics in Geriatric Medicine, 10,* 161–183.

Moore, J., Tweedy, C., & Christian, P. (1983). Effect of age on gastric emptying of liquid–solid meals in man. *Digestive Diseases and Sciences, 28,* 340.

Navia, B., & Price, R. (1987). The acquired immunodeficiency syndrome dementia complex as the presenting or sole manifestation of human immunodeficiency virus infection. *Archives of Neurology, 44,* 65–69.

Nielson, C. (1994). Pharmacologic considerations in critical care of the elderly. *Clinics in Geriatric Medicine, 10,* 71–89.

Opper, F., & Burakoff, R. (1994). Nutritional support of the elderly patient in an intensive care unit. *Clinics in Geriatric Medicine, 10,* 31–49.

Pathy, M., & Finucane, P. (1989). *Geriatric medicine.* New York: Springer-Verlag.

Pellican, J. Byrne, K., & DeMaria, E. (1992). Preventable complications and death from multiple organ failure among geriatric trauma victims. *Journal of Trauma, 33,* 440–444.

Petrucci, K., Booth-Blaemire, E., & Watson, K. (1989). Aging, immunity, and critical care nursing. *Critical Care Nursing Clinics of North America, 1,* 787–794.

Pierson, D., & Hudson, L. (1981). Pulmonary problems. *Geriatrics, 36*(4), 45–47.

Rauen, C. (1994). Too old to live. Too young to die: MODS in the elderly. *Critical Care Clinics of North America, 6,* 535–542.

Rebensen-Piano, M., (1989). The physiologic changes that occur with aging. *Critical Care Nursing Quarterly, 12,* 1–14.

Reed, P. (1983). Implications of the lifespan developmental framework for well-being in adulthood and aging. *Advances in Nursing Science, 6*(3), 18–25.

Rock, R. (1985). Interpreting thyroid tests in the elderly: Updated guidelines. *Geriatrics, 40,* 61–68.

Sabin, T. (1987). AIDS: The new "great imitator." *Journal of the American Geriatric Society, 35,* 467–468.

Schneider, E., & Rowe, J. (1990). *Handbook of the biology of aging* (3rd ed.). New York: Academic Press.

Sica, D. (1994). Renal disease, electrolyte abnormalities, and acid–base imbalance in the elderly. *Clinics in Geriatric Medicine, 10,* 197–211.

Smith, D., Ednerson, B., & Maull, K. (1990). Trauma in the elderly: Determinants of outcomes. *Southern Medical Journal, 83,* 171–176.

Sparrow, D., & Weiss, S. (1988). Pulmonary system. In J. Rowe & R. Besdine (Eds.), *Geriatric medicine* (pp. 266–275). Boston: Little, Brown & Company.

Stall, R., & Catania, J. (1994). AIDS risk behaviors among late middle-aged and elderly Americans. *Archives of Internal Medicine, 154,* 57–63.

Sternberg, H. (1988). Aging of the immune system. In P. Timiras (Ed.), *Physiological basis of geriatrics* (pp. 103–122). New York: Macmillan.

Timiras, P. (1988). *Physiological basis of geriatrics.* New York: Macmillan.

Tobin, M., Chadhe, T., Jenouri, G., et al. (1983). Breathing patterns: Normal subject. *Chest, 84,* 286.

Tran, D., Groeneveld, J., Van Der Meulen, J., et al. (1990). Age, chronic disease, sepsis, organ system failure and the mortality in medical intensive care unit. *Critical Care Medicine, 18,* 474–479.

U.S. Senate Special Committee on Aging. (1985–1986). *Aging of America: Trends and projections.* Washington, DC: U.S. Federal Printing Office.

U.S. Senate Special Committee on Aging. (1991). *Aging of America: Trends and projections, 1991 edition.* Washington, DC: U.S. Federal Printing Office.

Wahba, W. (1983). Influence of aging on lung function: Clinical significance of changes from age twenty. *Anesthesia and Analgesia, 62,* 764–776.

Walford, D., Wilkens, R., & Decker, J. (1968). Impaired delayed hypersensitivity in an aging population: Association with antinuclear reactivity and rheumatoid factor. *Journal of the American Medical Association, 203,* 831–847.

Wallace, J., Paauw, D., & Spach, D. (1993). HIV infection in older patients: When to suspect the unexpected. *Geriatrics, 48*(6), 61–70.

Wei, J. (1992). Age and the cardiovascular system. *New England Journal of Medicine, 327,* 1735–1742.

Wei, J. (1988). Cardiovascular system. In J. Rowe & R. Beddine (Eds.), *Geriatric medicine* (pp. 167–192). Boston: Little, Brown and Company.

Wenger, N. (1992). The elderly patient with cardiovascular disease: Determining optimal components of care and access to care. *American Journal of Geriatric Cardiology, 1,* 8–12.

Windslow, E. (1985). Cardiovascular consequences of bed rest. *Heart and Lung, 14,* 236–246.

Zimmerman, F. (1981). Type II diabetes mellitus in the senior citizen. *Nurse Practitioner, 6,* 31–32.

INDEX

Note: Page numbers in *italic* refer to illustrations; page numbers followed by t refer to tables.

A wave(s), in intracranial pressure monitoring, 301–302, *302*
AAA (abdominal aortic aneurysm). See *Aortic aneurysm.*
AAI pacing mode, 190t
Abdominal aortic aneurysm (AAA). See *Aortic aneurysm.*
Abdominal pain, in pancreatitis, 1092–1093
Abdominal-perineal resection, 1039
Abducens nerve, 745t
Aberrant ventricular conduction, 159–161, *160–161*
Ablation, catheter, radiofrequency, of cardiac dysrhythmias, 161
Abscess(es), epidural, 866
of brain, 865
pancreatic, 1102
Absence seizure(s), 850
Absorbent bead dressing(s), 1268t, 1269t, 1270–1271
Accelerated graft atherosclerosis, after cardiac transplantation, 499
Acceleration-deceleration head injury, *753*
ACE (angiotensin-converting enzyme) inhibitor(s). See *Angiotensin-converting enzyme (ACE) inhibitor(s).*
Acetaminophen, and acute fulminant hepatic failure, 1056–1057
overdose of, 1419–1421, 1420t, *1421–1422*
Acetic acid, for burn wounds, 1297t
for wound healing, 1273
Acetylcholine, action of, 723
and sleep, 101
as pain mediator, 1392
N-Acetylcysteine, for acetaminophen overdose, 1420
for acute fulminant hepatic failure, 1057
Acid(s), definition of, 583
sources of, 584–585
Acid-base disorder(s), mixed, 599–600
Acid-base status. See also *Acidosis; Alkalosis.*
assessment of, 590t, *590–592*, 590–593, 593t
laboratory studies in, 590t, *590–591*, 590–592
sequence for, *592*, 592–593, 593t
changes in, compensatory mechanisms for, 585–590, *586–589*
potassium and, 588–589
renal regulation of, 587–588, *589*, 887–890, *888–889*
acute renal failure and, 929
respiratory system and, 586–587
Acidosis, and hyperphosphatemia, 920
definition of, 583
matabolic, extracellular potassium in, 907
metabolic, 596–598, 597t
and calcium excretion, 913
and hyperkalemia, 910
anion gap in, 894
in acute renal failure, 929
renal tubular, 889–890
respiratory, 593–595, *594*, 595t
in acute respiratory failure, 645
Acquired immunodeficiency syndrome (AIDS). See also *Human immunodeficiency virus (HIV) disease.*
and hypocalcemia, 914–915
definition of, 1234–1235, 1235t
dementia in, 867, 1240t, 1250, 1251t
in elderly persons, 1504
nutrition in, 1240, 1250
Pneumocystis carinii pneumonia in, 622, 624–626
Acromegaly, and hypercalcemia, 916, 916t
from pituitary tumors, 848
Actin, in cardiac muscle, 316–317
Action potential, 132–133, *133*, 316–319, *318, 319*
Activated charcoal, for drug overdose, 1415–1416, 1416t, 1420
Active immunity, 1184
Active listening, 77–78, 78t
Active transport, in cardiac cells, 317–318
renal tubular reabsorption by, 881, *881*
Activity, sensing of, by pacemaker, 175–176
Activity intolerance, impaired mobility and, 1331
in Guillain-Barré syndrome, 837
in heart failure, 387
Activity management, after myocardial infarction, 368
Acupressure, 1407–1408
Acupuncture, 1407–1408
Acute fulminant hepatic failure (AFHF), 1056–1059, 1058t
Acute myocardial infarction (AMI). See *Myocardial infarction.*
Acute Physiology and Chronic Health Evaluation (APACHE II), in pancreatitis, 1098
Acute renal failure. See *Renal failure (acute).*
Acute respiratory failure (ARF), 630–647
airway management in, 639, 640t
arterial blood gas monitoring in, 636–638
cardiac output in, 634, *634*
chest radiography in, 638
clinical assessment of, 635–636
diagnosis of, 636–639
laboratory tests in, 638
management of, 639–644
complications of, 644–645
hyperoxygenation in, 642
in oxygen delivery failure, 639–640, 641t
in ventilatory failure, 639–644, 640t
pharmacologic, 642, 643t
mechanical ventilation in, weaning from, 645–646
nursing care plan for, 649t–655t
fluid balance in, 649t
nutrition in, 650t
psychosocial needs in, 636, 646–647, 654t–655t
pathophysiology of, 630–635, *631*, 637t
in arterial oxygenation failure, 632t, 632–633
in oxygen consumption failure, 634t, 634–635
in oxygen delivery failure, 633–634, *634*
in ventilatory failure, 630, 631–632, 632t
pulmonary function tests in, 638
respiratory alkalosis in, 645
terms pertaining to, 630
Acute tubular necrosis (ATN), clinical course of, 932–933
laboratory studies in, 930t
pathophysiology of, 927–928, *928*
Acute ventilatory failure (AVF), acute respiratory failure in, 630–632, 632t
airway management in, 639, 640t
decreased minute ventilation and, 631, 632t
Acyclovir (Zovirax), 1241t
Adaptive mechanism(s), 52, 59–61
Adenine arabinoside (Vidarabine), 1241t
Adenosine, in cerebral blood flow regulation, 726
Adenosine triphosphate (ATP), depletion of, in acute renal failure, 927–928, *928*
formation of, 584
synthesis of, impairment in, and hypophosphatemia, 919

ADH (antidiuretic hormone). See *Antidiuretic hormone (ADH).*
Adrenal crisis, nursing care plan for, 1131t–1136t
comfort measures in, 1134t
diagnostic procedures in, 1136t
fluid balance in, 1131t–1132t
nutrition in, 1132t–1133t
oxygenation in, 1133t
psychosocial needs in, 1135t
safety measures in, 1134t–1135t
skin integrity in, 1134t
Adrenal gland(s), disorders of, 1128–1130
Adrenal medulla, 744
Adrenocorticoid insufficiency, and hyponatremia, 903
Adult respiratory distress syndrome (ARDS), 656–677
anatomic factors in, 656–657, *657*
complications of, 674, 674t
diagnosis of, 667t, 667–668, *668*
factors predisposing to, 660t, 660–661
impaired gas exchange in, 674–676
in critical care phase of trauma, 1350–1352, 1351t
intrapulmonary shunting in, 675–676
lung compliance in, 676
metabolic oxygen requirements in, 674–675
nursing care plan for, 682t–688t
comfort measures in, 686t
diagnostic procedures in, 688t
fluid balance in, 682t–683t
impaired mobility in, 684t
psychosocial needs in, 687t–688t
safety measures in, 687t
skin integrity in, 686t
nursing management of, 674–676
oxygen delivery in, 666, 676
pathogenesis of, alveolar edema in, 666
arachidonic acid metabolites in, 664
degradative enzymes in, 664
platelet activating factor in, 664–665
polymorphonuclear leukocytes and, *661–662*, 661–665
toxic oxygen metabolites and, 664
phases of, 665–667
pressure control inverse ratio ventilation in, 277–278
prognosis in, 676–677, 677t
pulmonary artery wedge pressure in, *670*, 670–671
pulmonary fluid movement and, 657–659, *658*
treatment of, 668–674
airway pressure release ventilation in, 670
antioxidants for, 669
corticosteroids for, 668–669
fluids for, 670–671
inhibition of thromboxane action in, 669–670
modulation of cytokine response in, 669
monoclonal antibodies in, 669
neutralization of endotoxin effects in, 669
nitric oxide in, 670
protection from reactive toxic oxygen metabolites in, 669
supportive, 670–674
maintenance of tissue oxygenation in, 671–674, 684t–685t
mechanical ventilation in, 671–674
minimizing edema as, 670–671, *671*
nutritional, 673–674, 683t
positive end-expiratory pressure in, 671–672, 675
vs. cardiogenic pulmonary edema, 667, 667t
Advance practice nurse(s), on home care team, 119
Advocacy, in ethics, 22–23
Affect theory, of pain, 1386
Affective arousal, in stress-coping framework, interventions for, 57–59
Affective response(s), in stress-coping framework, 50
Afferent loop syndrome, 1038
Afferent neuron(s), 717–719, *719*
AFHF (acute fulminant hepatic failure), 1056–1059, 1058t
Afterdepolarization(s), electrocardiography in, 150, *150*
After-drop, in thermoregulation, 1432, *1432*, 1436
Afterload, and cardiac output, 228–229, 333
force-velocity relationship in, 322–323
reduction of, in heart failure, 399–400
Age, and complications from anesthesia, 1444, 1444t
and immunocompetence, 1187–1188
and wound healing, 1264–1265
AICD(s) (automatic implantable cardioverter-defibrillators), 196–200, *198, 200*
in sudden death, 350
AIDS (acquired immunodeficiency syndrome). See *Acquired immunodeficiency syndrome (AIDS); Human immunodeficiency virus (HIV) disease.*
Air, composition of, 574–575
Air embolism, during craniotomy, 854
Air leak(s), bronchopleural, with mechanical ventilation, 690
Air-fluidized bed(s), for pressure ulcer prevention, 1327, *1328*
Airway(s), artificial. See also *Intubation, endotracheal.*
for acute ventilatory failure, 640t
in emergency care phase of trauma, 1344–1345
complications in, after lung transplantation, 504
Airway clearance, ineffective, in elderly persons, 1498
in spinal cord injury, 825
Airway management, in acute respiratory failure, 639, 640t
in aspiration pneumonitis, 628
in chronic obstructive pulmonary disease, 609
in emergency care phase of trauma, 1343–1346, 1345t
in mechanical ventilation, 697t, 697–703. See also *Mechanical ventilation.*
in pneumonia, 625
Airway obstruction, hypocalcemia and, 915–916
postoperative, from anesthesia, 1452
Airway pressure release ventilation, 274t
in adult respiratory distress syndrome, 670
Airway resistance, in chronic bronchitis, 604
pressure gradient and, 570–571
Alanine aminotransferase (ALT), levels of, 1055, 1056t
Albendazole (Eskazole, Zentel), 1241t
Albumin, in chronic renal failure, 952t
in nutritional assessment, 997
metabolism of, 1052
Albuterol, for acute respiratory failure, 643t
for hyperkalemia, with renal failure, 912
Alcohol, and hypertension, 525
Alcoholism, and liver dysfunction, 1062–1063
and pancreatitis, 1091, 1093t
hypomagnesemia in, 922
Aldosterone, and renal tubular fluid reabsorption, 882
and sodium transport, 884
in potassium homeostasis, 907
in trauma patients, 908
Aldosteronism, primary, and hypertension, 526, 532
Alfaxalone, for head injury, 762
Alginate dressing(s), absorbent, 1271
Alkalemia, and hypomagnesemia, 922
Alkaline phosphatase, in chronic renal failure, 952t
Alkalosis, and hypophosphatemia, 919
definition of, 583
metabolic, 598–599, 599t, 890
in hypokalemia, 907
respiratory, 595–596, 596t
and hypophosphatemia, 919
in acute respiratory failure, 645
Allen test, modified, 206
Allergen(s), and asthma, 613
Allogeneic bone marrow transplantation, 1210, *1211*, 1214t, 1216–1217, 1218t
Allopurinol, before cardiac surgery, 473
ALT (alanine aminotransferase), levels of, 1055, 1056t
Aluminum hydroxide, and hypophosphatemia, 918
Alveolar air equation, 255
Alveolar-arterial ratio, in intrapulmonary shunting estimation, 255–256
Alveolar-capillary membrane, in pulmonary edema, 659–660, *660*
injury of, in adult respiratory distress syndrome, treatment of, 668–670
structure of, 656–657, *657*
Alveolus (alveoli), anatomy of, 565, *566*
edema of, in adult respiratory distress syndrome, 666
epithelial cells in, 657
fluid in, surface tension of, 568, *569*
American College of Cardiology, guidelines for pacemaker insertion, 168t
American Heart Association, guidelines for pacemaker insertion, 168t
AMI (acute myocardial infarction). See *Myocardial infarction.*
Amikacin, 1241t
Amiloride, for heart failure, 391t
Amino acid(s), and hypomagnesemia, 922
and neurotransmitter synthesis, in hepatic encephalopathy, 1073–1074
essential, for nutrition in renal failure, 1018
in enteral feeding products, 1001
21-Amino steroid(s) (lazaroids), for head injury, 762

Aminocaproic acid, for hemorrhagic stroke, 797–798
  for pathologic fibrinolysis, 1155
Aminoglycoside(s), nephrotoxicity of, 935
Aminotransferase(s), levels of, 1055, 1056t
Amiodarone, for heart failure, 398
  in sudden death, 351t
Amitriptyline (Elavil), for human immunodeficiency virus disease, 1241t
Ammonia, in hepatic encephalopathy, 1073
Ammonia buffer system, 588, *589,* 889, *889*
Amnesia, global, transient, 787
Amniotic fluid embolism, 1466–1468, 1467t
Amphotericin B (Fungizone), for acquired immunodeficiency syndrome, 1241t
Ampicillin, for human immunodeficiency virus disease, 1241t
Amrinone, for heart failure, 401
  for myocardial infarction, 369
Amylase level(s), in pancreatitis, 1094t, 1094–1095
Amyloid angiopathy, cerebral, and intracerebral hemorrhage, 796
Anabolic reaction(s), 995
Anaerobic glycolysis, 584
Anal anastomosis–ileal pouch, 1038
Analgesia, inhalation, 1406
  patient-controlled, 1404, *1405*
Analgesic(s), adjuvants to, 1403
  endogenous, 1393–1394
  in elderly persons, 1507t
  narcotic, 1400t, 1400–1402, 1401t
  nonnarcotic, 1402–1403
Anaphylaxis, 1378–1379
Anastomosis. See under specific type, e.g., *Blalock-Taussig anastomosis.*
Anatomic dead space, 573
Anemia, from interleukin-2 therapy, 1222
  hemolytic, hypophosphatemia and, 919
  in acute renal failure, 930
  in chronic renal failure, 958–959
  iron deficiency, in long-term survivors of congenital heart defects, 422–423
Anencephaly, brain death controversy in, 809
Anesthesia, and immunocompetence, 1188
  and thermoregulation, 1448–1449
  complications of, 1442–1456
    cardiovascular, *1453,* 1453–1455, 1454t, *1455*
    central nervous system, 1455–1456
    intraoperative risk factors for, 1445–1449, 1449t–1451t
    postoperative, 1449–1455
    preoperative risk factors for, 1442, 1444t, 1444–1445
  for cesarean section, in preeclampsia, 1465
  for cranial surgery, 852–855, 853t
  in liver disease, 1078
  monitoring during, standards for, 1450t–1451t
  techniques of, 1443t
Anesthetic(s), 1446t
  and malignant hyperthermia, 1439
  as analgesics, 1404
  drug interactions with, 1448
Aneurysm(s), aortic. See *Aortic aneurysm.*
  dissecting, 793
  fusiform, 535, 792–793
  miliary, in hypertension, 522–523
  saccular, 535
  saccular/berry, 792, *792*
  surgical treatment of, 798t, 798–799
ANF (atrial natriuretic factor), in heart failure, 384–385
Anger, as defense mechanism, 60
Angina pectoris, 342–343
  classification of, 342–343
  coronary angiography in, 341–342, 364
  coronary artery bypass grafting for, 460–461
    results of, 467–468
  electrocardiography in, 147–148, *148*
  management of, nonpharmacologic, 343
    pharmacologic, 343–346, 344t, 345t, 346t
  Prinzmetal (variant), 342
Angiodysplasia, and gastrointestinal bleeding, 1027–1028, *1028*
Angiogenesis, 1261
Angiography, cerebral, in hemorrhagic stroke, 797
    in nonhemorrhagic stroke, 788
  coronary, after myocardial infarction, 364
    angina pectoris in, 341–342
    in myocardial ischemia, 340–341
  digital subtraction, in nonhemorrhagic stroke, 788
  magnetic resonance. See *Magnetic resonance angiography (MRA).*
  pulmonary, in acute respiratory failure, 639
  radionuclide, in myocardial infarction, 363
  therapeutic, in gastrointestinal bleeding, 1031
Angioma(s), cavernous, 794
  venous, 794
Angiopathy, amyloid, cerebral, and intracerebral hemorrhage, 796
Angioplasty, coronary, laser, in myocardial ischemia, 348–349
  coronary artery. See *Percutaneous transluminal coronary angioplasty (PTCA).*
Angiotensin, action of, 877
  and blood flow, 328–329
  levels of, after cardiopulmonary bypass, 489
Angiotensin-converting enzyme (ACE) inhibitor(s), for heart failure, 391t, 392–394, 393t
  for myocardial infarction, 369
Anion gap, 584, 894, 894t
  in acid-base status assessment, 591, *591*
  in metabolic acidosis, 597, 597t
Annuloplasty, in mitral regurgitation, 434, *435–436*
Anorexia, in chronic renal failure, 957
Anoxia, of tissue, hypophosphatemia and, 919–920
Antacid(s), and hypermagnesemia, 923, 923t
  for gastrointestinal bleeding, 1033, 1034t
  phosphate-binding, and hypophosphatemia, 918, 918t
Anterior cord syndrome, 813, *814*
Antianginal drug(s), as platelet antiaggregants, 346
Antibiotic(s), antineoplastic, for hypercalcemia, 917
  during intracranial pressure monitoring, 305
  for acute pancreatitis, 1101–1102
  for acute respiratory failure, 643t
  for chronic obstructive pulmonary disease, 611
  for systemic inflammatory response syndrome, 1367–1368
  in elderly persons, 1507t
  prophylactic, for endocarditis. See *Endocarditis, prophylaxis for.*
Antibody(ies), in specific immunity, 1184–1185, *1185*
  monoclonal, for adult respiratory distress syndrome, 669
  role of, 1167t, 1167–1168
Anticholinergic agent(s), for acute pancreatitis, 1100
  for asthma, 617, 617t
Anticoagulant(s), and intracerebral hemorrhage, 795
  coagulopathy from, 1154–1155, 1161t
  for acute arterial occlusion, 545–546
  for disseminated intravascular coagulopathy, 1152
  for heart failure, 398
  for nonhemorrhagic stroke, 789
  vascular endothelium as, 1146, *1146*
Anticonvulsant(s), 771, 772t
  as analgesic adjuvants, 1403
Anticonvulsant drug(s), and hypocalcemia, 914
Antidepressant(s), tricyclic, as analgesic adjuvants, 1403
    overdose of, 1423–1425, 1425t
Antidiuretic hormone (ADH), and blood pressure, 520–521
  and concentration of urine, 886–887
  and plasma osmolality, 900t, 900–901
  and water reabsorption, 884–885
  in shock, 1375
Antidysrhythmic agent(s), for heart failure, 397–398
  for sudden cardiac death, 350, 351t
Antifibrinolytic(s), for hemorrhagic stroke, 797–798
Antigen(s), human leukocyte, 1166, *1166*
  role of, 1165–1166, 1166t
Antigen-presenting cell(s), 1171–1174, 1173t–1174t
Antigen-processing cell(s), 1171–1174, 1173t–1174t
Antihistamine(s), as analgesic adjuvants, 1403
Antihypertensive agent(s), for nonhemorrhagic stroke, 790
  for preeclampsia, 1464
  in elderly persons, 1507t
  magnesium as, 922
Antimicrobial agent(s), for burn wounds, 1297t
  for wound healing, 1273
Antineoplastic agent(s), occupational exposure to, 40
Antineoplastic antibiotic(s), for hypercalcemia, 917
Antioxidant(s), for adult respiratory distress syndrome, 669
Antiplatelet agent(s), before cardiac surgery, 472–473
  coagulopathy from, 1154–1155
  for angina pectoris, 344t
  for nonhemorrhagic stroke, 789
Antipsychotic(s), as analgesic adjuvants, 1403
Antipyretic(s), for chronic obstructive pulmonary disease, 611

Antiseptic solution(s), for wound healing, 1272t, 1272–1273
Antitachycardia pacemaker(s), in sudden cardiac death, 350, 352
Anxiety, and pain, 1383
  as barrier to communication, 81
  from fear of death, 54–55
  in preeclampsia, 1466
  interventions for, 58–59
  relief of, in respiratory alkalosis, 596
Anxiolytic(s), as analgesic adjuvants, 1403
AOO pacing mode, 190t
Aorta, coarctation of, and acute aortic dissection, 540
  compliance of, 324
  trauma to, 548
Aortic aneurysm, *535,* 535–539
  clinical presentation in, 536, 536t
  complications of, 538–539
  diagnosis of, 536–537, *537*
  etiology of, 535–536
  pathophysiology of, 536
  postoperative management in, 539
  preoperative management in, 539
  prognosis in, 539
  repair of, 537–539, *538*
Aortic body(ies), and control of respiration, 581, *581*
Aortic dissection, acute, 539–543
    classification of, 540
    clinical presentation in, 540–541
    complications of, 542
    diagnosis of, 540–541, *541*
    etiology of, 540
    management of, 541–542, *542*
    pathophysiology of, 540
    postoperative care in, 542–543
  histologic factors in, 540
Aortic impedance, 322–323
Aortic regurgitation, 442–446
  diagnosis of, 445–446
  heart murmur in, 446
  management of, 446
  pathophysiology of, 442–445, *443–444*
Aortic stenosis, 446–449
  congenital, 416–417
  diagnosis of, 448–449
  management of, 449
  pathophysiology of, 446–447, *447–448*
Aortic valve(s), anatomy of, 313–314, *314*
  function of, in cardiac cycle, 319–321, *320*
Aortography, in acute aortic dissection, 541, *541*
  in aortic aneurysm, 537, *537*
APACHE II (Acute Physiology and Chronic Health Evaluation), in pancreatitis, 1098
Aphasia, 76
  communication and, 82–83, 84t
Apnea, mechanical ventilation in, 273t, 277
  sleep, in chronic renal failure, 960
Aprotinin, use of with cardiopulmonary bypass, 491
Arachidonic acid, metabolites of, in adult respiratory distress syndrome, 664
Arachidonic acid cascade, in systemic inflammatory response syndrome, 1361–1362, *1362*
Arachnoid, of brain, 723, *726*
  spinal, 738
Arachnoid villus (villi), in cerebrospinal fluid absorption, *728,* 729
ARDS (adult respiratory distress syndrome). See *Adult respiratory distress syndrome (ARDS).*
ARF (acute respiratory failure). See *Acute respiratory failure (ARF).*
Arginine vasopressin, in diabetes insipidus, 1122
Arginine vasopressin system, in heart failure, 384
Arrhythmia(s). See *Cardiac dysrhythmia(s).*
Arterial blood gas(es), in acid-base status assessment, 590t, 590–591
  in acute respiratory failure, 636–638
  in asthma, 616
  in chronic bronchitis, 605
  in emphysema, 608
  monitoring of, in acute respiratory failure, 636–639
Arterial blood pressure, regulation of, 519–521, *520*
Arterial bypass, extracranial-intracranial, for nonhemorrhagic stroke, 791
Arterial occlusion, acute, 543–547
    clinical presentation in, 545
    etiology of, 543, *543*
    management of, 545–546, *546*
    pathophysiology of, 543–544, *544*
  diagnosis of, 545, *545*
Arterial oxygen, partial pressure of, 246–247
    and intrapulmonary shunting, 253–256, *254,* 254t
Arterial oxygen saturation (Sa_{O_2}), 247–248
Arterial oxygenation, in acute respiratory failure, 632t, 632–634, *633–634,* 639–640
Arterial pressure, *326,* 326–327
Arterial volume, effective, 893–894
Arteriography, in acute arterial occlusion, 545, *545*
  in vascular trauma, 548
Arteriole(s), physiology of, 325, *325*
Arteriovenous fistula, for hemodialysis, 956, *956*
Arteriovenous malformation(s) (AVMs), 795, *795*
  surgical treatment of, 798–799
Artery(ies). See also specific arteries, e.g., *Femoral artery.*
  anatomy and physiology of, 324–325, *325*
  spinal, *737,* 739
  vertebral, *737,* 739
Artery of Adamkiewicz, *737*
Artherosclerosis, 336–337
Artificial airway(s). See *Airway(s), artificial* and *Intubation, endotracheal.*
Artificial blood, 1159
Artificial heart, 496
Artificial larynx, 699
Ascites, 1070–1072, *1072*
Aseptic meningitis, 864
Ashman's phenomenon, 160–161, *161*
L-Aspartate, action of, 723
Aspartate aminotransferase (AST), in myocardial infarction, 360
  levels of, 1055, 1056t
Aspiration, from enteral nutrition, 1008, 1009t, 1010
  impaired mobility and, 1317
  potential for, in Guillain-Barré syndrome, 835–836
Aspiration pneumonitis, 627–628
Aspirin, adverse effects of, 1403
  for myocardial infarction, 367
  for nonhemorrhagic stroke, 789
  in angina pectoris, 345–346, 346t
Assault, 26t, 28
Assurance, of family, need for, 69t, 69–70
AST (aspartate aminotransferase), in myocardial infarction, 360
  levels of, 1055, 1056t
Asterixis, in hepatic encephalopathy, 1074
Asthma, 612–618
  arterial blood gases in, 616
  capnography in, 616
  circadian rhythm in, 615
  clinical presentation in, 614–615
  epidemiology of, 612
  management of, 616–618, 617t
  mechanical ventilation in, 618
  occupational irritants and, 613t
  pathophysiology of, 613–614, *614*
  precipitating stimuli in, 612–613
  prognosis in, 618
  pulmonary function tests in, 615–616
  sputum examination in, 616
Astrocyte(s), 717, *718*
Astrocytoma(s), 847
Asystole, temporary pacing for, 178
Atelectasis, after cardiopulmonary bypass, 490
  impaired mobility and, 1316–1317
Atenolol, in angina pectoris, 343–344
Atevirdine mesylate, for human immunodeficiency virus disease, 1241t
Atherectomy, directional coronary, in myocardial ischemia, 348
Atherogenesis, magnesium in, 922
Atherosclerosis, after cardiac transplantation, 499
  and aortic aneurysm, 535–536
  carotid, evaluation of, before cardiac surgery, 472
  complicated lesions in, 336
  fatty streak in, 336
  fibrous plaque in, 336–337, 783–784
  in hypertension, 522–523
  injury hypothesis of, 337
  lipogenic hypothesis in, 337
  pathogenesis of, 337
Atlas, 736
Atmosphere, partial pressure of, 575
ATN (acute tubular necrosis). See *Acute tubular necrosis (ATN).*
Atovaquone (Mepron), for human immunodeficiency virus disease, 1241t
ATP (adenosine triphosphate). See *Adenosine triphosphate (ATP).*
ATPase, in cardiac contraction, 317
  in cardiac electrophysiology, 318
Atrial cannulation, for cardiac assist devices, 239–240, *240–241*
Atrial depolarization, sensing of, by pacemaker, 175
Atrial electrogram, 183t, 183–184, *184–185*
Atrial fibrillation, after cardiopulmonary bypass, 484–485
  atrial electrogram in, *185*
  in Wolff-Parkinson-White syndrome, 159
Atrial flutter, atrial electrogram in, 183–184, *184*
Atrial natriuretic factor (ANF), in heart failure, 384–385
Atrial pacing, overdrive, after cardiopulmonary bypass, 485, *486*
  rapid, 184

Atrial pacing, ventricular pacing, 191–192, *192*
Atrial pacing, ventricular sensing, 192, *194*
Atrial sensing, ventricular pacing, 192, *193*
Atrial sensing, ventricular sensing, 192
Atrial septostomy, balloon, 417–418, 419t
Atrial stretch, and blood pressure, 520
Atrioventricular (AV) dissociation, electrocardiography in, *164,* 164–165
Atrioventricular (AV) node, anatomy and physiology of, 128, *129,* 315, *316*
Atrioventricular (AV) reciprocating tachycardia, in Wolff-Parkinson-White syndrome, 158–159
Atrioventricular (AV) valve(s), anatomy of, 313–314, *314*
  function of, in cardiac cycle, 319–321, *320*
Atrium (atria), hypertrophy of, 142–143, *144*
  infarction of, 356
  myocardial infarction in, electrocardiography in, 148
  pressure in, in cardiac cycle, 319–321, *320*
  right, pulmonary artery pressure in, 216, *219*
Auditory communication channel, 76
Augmented lead(s), for electrocardiography, *137*
Auscultation, for liver function assessment, 1053–1054
Autodigestion, in pancreatitis, 1091, 1093t
Autologous blood donation, before cardiac surgery, 472
Autologous bone marrow transplantation, 1210, *1211,* 1212t–1213t, 1215–1216
Automatic implantable cardioverter-defibrillator(s) (AICDs), 196–200, *198, 200*
  in sudden cardiac death, 350
Automatic pacing interval, 190t
Automaticity, 133–134, *134*
  altered, electrocardiography in, 148–149
Autonomic dysreflexia, 828, *828*
Autonomic nervous system, 742, 744, *746–747,* 748, 748t
  and blood pressure, *329,* 329–330, 519–520
  and gastrointestinal innervation, 980t, 980–981, *981*
  dysfunction of, in Guillain-Barré syndrome, 833, 835
Autonomy, in ethics, 18
Autoregulation, in essential hypertension, 523
  metabolic theory of, in local blood pressure regulation, 327
  of cerebral blood flow, 292–293, 725–726, 755, 782, 782t, 783t
  of renal blood flow, *876,* 876–877
Autotransfusion, 1159
AV (atrioventricular). See entries under *Atrioventricular (AV).*
AVF (acute ventilatory failure). See *Acute ventilatory failure (AVF).*
AVM(s) (arteriovenous malformations). See *Arteriovenous malformation(s) (AVMs).*
Axis, 736
Axis determination, in electrocardiography, 140t, 140–141, *141*
Axon(s), 717, 718–719, *720, 721*
  destruction of, in Guillain-Barré syndrome, 831, *832*
Axon hillock, 719
Axonal injury, diffuse, 752
Azithromycin (Zithromax), 1241t
Azotemia, in acute renal failure, 929

B lymphocyte(s), abnormalities of, in human immunodeficiency virus disease, 1228
  activity of, 1170, *1175,* 1175–1176, 1176t
    in specific immunity, 1185, *1185*
B wave(s), in intracranial pressure monitoring, 302
BACI, 1241t
Back injury(ies), occupational, 37–39, 38t, 39t
Back pain, from spinal cord compression, in cancer, 1480, 1482
Backup ventilation, 273t, 276–277
Bacterial meningitis, 862–864, *863,* 864t
Bacterial pneumonia. See under *Pneumonia.*
Bacterial translocation, 982–984
Bacterial ventriculitis, 866
BAER (brain stem auditory evoked response), 805–806
Bainbridge reflex, 520
  in heart failure, 382
Balloon atrial septostomy, 417–418, 419t
Balloon embolectomy, for acute arterial occlusion, 546, *546*
Balloon tamponade, for variceal hemorrhage, *1068,* 1068–1069
Balloon-tipped catheter(s), for temporary transvenous pacemakers, 186, *186*
Barbiturate(s), for brain ischemia, 767
  for cranial surgery, 853t
  for head injury, 761
Barium study(ies), in acute pancreatitis, 1095
  in gastrointestinal bleeding, 1031
Baroreceptor(s), abnormalities of, in heart failure, 382
  and blood pressure, 330, 519–520
Barotrauma, from positive pressure ventilation, 264
Basal ganglia, 730
Base(s), deficit/excess, 584
    in acid-base status assessment, 590t, 590–591
  definition of, 583
  sources of, 584–585
Basilar artery(ies), cerebral, 724, *727*
Basilar skull fracture(s), 750, *752*
Basilic vein, harvesting of, for coronary artery bypass grafting, 465
Basophil(s), activity of, 1175
Battery, definition of, 26t, 28
Battery(ies), for pacemakers, 170
Baxter balloon-tipped catheter, for temporary transvenous pacemakers, 186, *186*
Bead dressing(s), absorbent, 1268t, 1269t, 1270–1271
Bed(s), for pressure ulcer prevention, 1327–1329, *1327–1329*
Behaviorist theory, of pain, 1388
Beneficence, 18–19
Benzodiazepine(s), overdose of, 1425
Bereavement, organ donation and, 1200
Berry aneurysm(s), 792, *792*
Beta$_2$ agonist(s), for asthma, 616–617, 617t
  for hyperkalemia, 912
Beta blocker(s), for angina pectoris, 343–344, 346
  for heart failure, 397
  for myocardial infarction, 367
  in hyperkalemia, 910, 910t
Beta-endorphin, in endogenous opiate pain theory, 1389, 1394
  in systemic inflammatory response syndrome, 1363–1364
Bezold-Jarisch reflex, in heart failure, 382
Bicarbonate, and carbon dioxide transport, 578–579, *579*
  for hyperkalemia, 911t, 912
  in diabetic ketoacidosis, 1110
  in venous blood, in acid-base status assessment, 591
  reabsorption of, 587–588, *588,* 888
  regeneration of, by tubular epithelial cells, 887–888, *888*
Bicarbonate buffer system, 585
Bicarbonate–carbonic acid system, 587–588, *588*
Bile, production of, 1051
Bile reflux theory, in pancreatitis, 1091
Bileaflet cardiac valve(s), *437*
Biliary fluid(s), loss of, and hypomagnesemia, 922
Biliary tract, anatomy of, *1050,* 1050–1051
Bilirubin, metabolism of, 1051
  normal levels of, 1051, 1055
Bilroth procedure(s), for gastrointestinal bleeding, 1036–1037, *1037*
Bioethics, definition of, 15
Biofeedback, for pain management, 1408
Biologic dressing(s), for burn wounds, 1298
Biologic response modifier(s) (BMRs), 1477
Biologic safety cabinet(s), 40
Biomedicus vortex pump(s), 235
Biopsy(ies). See under specific site(s), e.g., *Endomyocardial biopsy.*
Biosynthetic dressing(s), 1267–1271, 1268t, 1269t
BiPAP ventilation, 273t, 277
Biphasic complex, in electrocardiography, *136*
Biphosphanate(s), for hypercalcemia, from cancer, 1489
Biventricular failure, with cardiac assist devices, 242
Bjork-Shiley tilting disc, *437*
Bladder program, in spinal cord injury, 827–828
Blalock-Hanlon technique, 417–418, 419t
Blalock-Taussig anastomosis, 417–418, *418,* 419t
Bleeding, after coronary artery bypass grafting, 488–489
  after lung transplantation, 503
  gastrointestinal. See *Gastrointestinal system, bleeding in.*
  in chronic renal failure, 959
  in disseminated intravascular coagulation, 1149–1150, 1150t
  with cardiac assist devices, 242
Bleeding diathesis, in long-term survivors of congenital heart defects, 423–424
Bleomycin (Blenoxane), 1242t
Blood, artificial, 1159
  autologous donation of, before cardiac surgery, 472

Blood, artificial (*continued*)
  coagulation of, calcium in, 913
  composition of, 1139t, 1139–1141, *1140*
  hyperviscosity of, in long-term survivors of congenital heart defects, 422, 425
  oxygen-carrying capacity of, 577
  pH of, in acid-base status assessment, 590, 590t
  transmission of human immunodeficiency virus via, 1232
  viscosity of, and nonhemorrhagic stroke, 786
Blood clot(s), formation of. See *Hemostasis.*
Blood flow, cerebral, 291–293, 782, 782t, 783t
    collateral, 781, *782*
    components of, 723–725, *727*
    during craniotomy, 854
    in elderly persons, 1499
    in head injury, 760
    in nonhemorrhagic stroke, 783
    regulation of, 725–726, 755, 782, 782t, 783t
    testing for, in brain death, 808
    venous drainage in, 725
  coronary. See *Coronary artery(ies).*
  during cardiopulmonary bypass, hypothermia and, 476, 477
  in preeclampsia, 1460
  maldistribution of, in systemic inflammatory response syndrome, 1364
  physiology of, 312t, 312–313
  pulmonary, in congenital heart defects, 416t, 416–417
  regulation of, humoral, *328*, 328–329
    long-term, 330–331, *330–331*
  renal, 875–876, *876*, *878*. See also *Kidney(s), blood flow of.*
  vessel diameter and, *328*
Blood gas(es), arterial. See *Arterial blood gas(es).*
Blood pressure, arterial, regulation of, 519–521, *520*
  diastolic, physiology of, 326–327
  regulation of, by nervous system, *329*, 329–330
    local, 327–328
    systemic, 327–330, *328–330*
  systolic, physiology of, *326*, 326–327
Blood sampling, from central venous line, 205
  from intra-arterial catheter, 208
  from pulmonary artery catheters, 221–222
Blood supply, cerebral, carotid arteries and, 781
  of heart, 311, *311*
Blood urea nitrogen (BUN), in chronic renal failure, 952t
Blood vessel(s), cerebral, in cranial meninges, 723
  spinal, in cranial meninges, 723
  structure of, 324
Blood volume, and cardiac output, 332–333
  intravascular, increased, and intracranial pressure, 293
Blood-brain barrier, 726–727
Blood-cerebrospinal fluid barrier, 726–727
Blunt trauma. See *Trauma, blunt.*
BMR(s) (biologic response modifiers), 1477
Body fluid(s). See *Fluid (body).*
Body image, altered, impaired mobility and, 1322, 1332
    in chemotherapy, 1222
    in human immunodeficiency virus disease, 1254t
Body mass index, 999
Body surface area nomogram(s), Dubois, 226, *226*
Body temperature, altered, after bone marrow transplantation, 1216
    from interleukin-2 therapy, 1222
  and pacemakers, 176–177
  core, 1431
  in head injury, 763
Body weight, ideal, calculation of, 999, 999t
Bolus enteral nutrition, 1007
Bombesin, 982t
Bone, calcium regulation by, 913
  hypophosphatemia and, 919
  loss of, impaired mobility and, 1318–1319
  rapid formation of, and hypocalcemia, 904, 914t
  structure of magnesium in, 921
Bone buffer system, 586
Bone marrow, 1168, *1169–1170*, 1170
  transplantation of, 1210–1217
    allogeneic, 1210, *1211*, 1214t, 1216–1217, 1218t
    autologous, 1210, *1211*, 1212t–1213t, 1215–1216
    complications of, 1216–1217, 1218t
    drugs used in, 1217–1223, 1220t
    harvesting in, 1210–1211, 1215
    syngeneic, 1210, *1211*, 1212t–1214t
    total body irradiation with, 1216–1217, 1218t
    types of, 1210, *1211*, 1212t–1214t
Bowel. See also *Colon; Small intestine.*
Bowel elimination, altered, in chronic renal failure, 958
    in interleukin-2 therapy, 1221
    in spinal cord compression, 1482–1483
Bowel program, in spinal cord injury, 827
Bowel sound(s), in gastrointestinal bleeding, 1030
Bowman's capsule, anatomy of, 873–874
  in urine formation, 879–880
Bradycardia, in spinal cord injury, 823
  temporary pacing for, 178
Bradykinin, and blood flow, 329
  in systemic inflammatory response syndrome, 1363
Bragg-Peak proton beam therapy, in arteriovenous malformations, 799
Brain, abscess of, 865
  anatomy of, *729*, 729–733
  blood flow of. See *Blood flow, cerebral.*
  changes in, from hypernatremia, 905
    in elderly persons, 1498
  contusions of, 751
  function of, hypoglycemia and, 768
  hemispheric dominance in, 731
  injury of, ischemic. See *Brain, ischemia of.*
    traumatic. See *Head injury.*
  ischemia of, 764–768
    clinical presentation in, 765
    diagnostic procedures in, 766
    hyperventilation in, 766
    impaired communication in, 767–768
    medical management of, 766–767
    no-reflow phenomenon in, 765
    nursing management of, 767–768
    pathophysiology of, 764–765
    reperfusion after, 765
  meninges of, 723, *726*
  metabolic disorders and, 768–770
  physiology of, *729*, 729–733
  structures of, 729, *729–730*
  tumors of, 846–849
    and intracerebral hemorrhage, 796
    incidence of, 846–847
    metastatic, 848
    signs and symptoms of, 848–849
    staging of, 846–847, 847t
    types of, 847–848
Brain center(s), as pain transmission pathway, 1392
Brain death, 803–810
  and organ procurement, 807
  causes of, 803
  conditions mimicking, 806
  criteria for determination of, 804t, 804–807
    irreversibility as, 806
    observation period as, 806–807
    trial of therapy as, 806–807
  definition of, 803, 804
    controversy concerning, 808–809
  family wishes in, 807
  in children, 809–810
  patient management in, 807
  problems in determination of, 807–809
  statutory recognition of, 804, 804t
Brain stem, anatomy of, *732*, *733*, 735
  and control of respiration, *580*, 580–581
Brain stem auditory evoked response (BAER), 805–806
Brain stem function, absence of, as criterion for brain death, 805–806
Brain tissue, hypertension and, 530
  volume of, changes in, compensatory response in, 290, *290*
    etiology of, 293, 293t
Breach of duty, owed to patient, 27
Breathing, stimuli for, hydrogen concentration as, 587, *587*
    oxygen concentration as, 587
  work of, 571
Breathing pattern(s), impaired, in elderly persons, 1498
    in emergency care phase of trauma, 1346, 1347t
    in human immunodeficiency virus disease, 1242t
    in hypermagnesemia, 924
    in hypophosphatemia, 919
    in spinal cord compression, 1482
    in spinal cord injury, 825
    in superior vena cava syndrome, 1486
Bretylium, in sudden death, 351t
Bricker's intact nephron hypothesis, 950
Broca's aphasia, 76, 84t
Broca's area, 76, 729
Brodmann map, *730*
Bronchial hygiene, in acute respiratory failure, 640–642
Bronchiolitis, obliterative, after lung transplantation, 504
Bronchiolus (bronchioli), anatomy of, 562, *563*, 565, *566*
Bronchitis, arterial blood gases in, 605
  chronic, 603–606
    clinical presentation in, 604
    diagnosis of, *605*, 605–606
    etiology of, 603
    pathophysiology of, 603–604, *604*
    prognosis in, 606
    vs. emphysema, 603t

Bronchodilator(s), for chronic obstructive pulmonary disease, 611
Bronchopleural air leak(s), with mechanical ventilation, 690
Bronchoscopy, in acute respiratory failure, 638
Bronchospasm, during suctioning, 702
magnesium and, 921
with mechanical ventilation, 690
Bronchus (bronchi), anatomy of, 562, *563*
Brovavir, 1242t
Brown-Sequard syndrome, 813, *814*
Brudzinski sign, 862
Bruit(s), carotid, and nonhemorrhagic stroke, 786
in arteriovenous malformations, 795
Bubble oxygenator, for cardiopulmonary bypass, 474
Buffer(s), in renal tubules, 888–889, *889*
Buffer system(s), against changes in acid-base balance, 585–586, *586*
Bumetanide, for heart failure, 391t
BUN (blood urea nitrogen), in chronic renal failure, 952t
Bundle branch(es), anatomy and physiology of, 129, 315, *316*
Bundle branch block, electrocardiography in, 152–154, *153–154*
left, anatomy and physiology of, 129
monitoring in, 156
right, anatomy and physiology of, 129
monitoring in, 156
Bundle of His, 128–129
Burn(s), 1279–1303
acute (fluid mobilization) phase of, 1295–1299, 1296t, 1297t
cardiovascular effects in, 1295
gastrohepatic effects in, 1296
immunologic effects in, 1295
laboratory studies in, 1296, 1296t
nutritional support during, 1299
pain management in, 1298
pulmonary effects in, 1295
skin grafting in, 1297–1298
wound care in, 1296–1298, 1297t
and hypermagnesemia, 923, 923t
chemical, 1279–1280
depth of, classification of, 1281–1282, 1282t
electrical, 1280
emergent (shock) phase of, 1283–1295
cardiovascular effects in, 1284–1286
fluid resuscitation in, 1292–1294, 1293t, 1294t
gastrohepatic effects in, 1288
genitourinary effects in, 1288–1289
immunologic effects in, 1287–1288
laboratory studies in, 1290, 1292, 1292t
neuroendocrine effects in, 1289
nutritional support during, 1294–1295, 1295t
ophthalmologic effects in, 1289
pain management in, 1294
physical assessment in, 1290, 1291t
physiology of, 1283–1284
pulmonary effects in, *1286*, 1286t, 1286–1287, 1287t
from radiation, 1280
from tar, 1280
nursing care plan for, 1304t–1309t
comfort measures in, 1307t
diagnostic procedures in, 1309t
fluid balance in, 1304t–1305t
impaired mobility in, 1306t
nutrition in, 1305t
oxygenation in, 1306t
psychosocial needs in, 1308t–1309t
safety measures in, 1307t–1308t
skin integrity in, 1307t
pathophysiology of, 1280–1283, *1281*, 1282t
rehabilitation phase of, 1299–1303, *1300*, 1300t
nutritional support in, 1299
pain management during, 1299
physical therapy in, 1300–1301
pruritus in, 1299
psychosocial needs in, 1299–1300, *1300*, 1300t
severity of, 1282t–1283t, 1282–1283, *1283–1284*
by total body surface area, 1283, *1283*, *1284*
thermal, 1279
zones of, 1281
Burns Weaning Assessment Checklist, 692
Bursa of Fabricius, 1170
Bypass graft(s). See *Coronary artery bypass grafting (CABG).*

C wave(s), in intracranial pressure monitoring, 302–303
CABG (coronary artery bypass grafting). See *Coronary artery bypass grafting (CABG).*
CAD (coronary artery disease). See *Coronary artery disease (CAD).*
Caffeine, and hypertension, 524–525
Calcification, in aortic stenosis, 447, *447*
in mitral regurgitation, 430
Calcitonin, for hypercalcemia, 917
from cancer, 1489, 1490t, 1491
Calcium, chemical forms of, 913
disorders of. See *Hypercalcemia; Hypocalcemia.*
for hyperkalemia, 911t, 912
for hypermagnesemia, 923
homeostasis of, magnesium and, 921
in cardiac muscle contraction, 316–317
in resting membrane potential, 913
levels of, in acute pancreatitis, 1096t
in chronic renal failure, 952t
physiologic functions of, 913
reabsorption of, 883
regulation of, 913
Calcium channel blocker(s), for angina pectoris, 344–346, 345t, 346t
for brain ischemia, 767
for head injury, 762
for hemorrhagic stroke, 798
for nonhemorrhagic stroke, 789
for prevention of acute renal failure, 934
Calcium chloride, for hypocalcemia, 915
Calcium gluconate, for hypocalcemia, 915
Calculi, renal, hypercalcemia and, 917
Call device(s), for communication-impaired patient, 836
Callosal disconnection syndrome, 856
cAMP. See *Cyclic adenosine monophosphate (cAMP).*
Cancer, bowel obstruction in, 1480t
discharge planning in, 1491–1492
hypercalcemia from, 1487–1491. See also *Hypercalcemia, from cancer.*
in human immunodeficiency virus disease, 1234
myelosuppression in, 1480t
pathophysiology of, 1476–1479, *1478*, 1479t, 1480t
spinal cord compression in, 1478, 1480–1483, *1481*
superior vena cava syndrome in, 1483–1487. See also *Superior vena cava syndrome.*
tumor lysis syndrome, 1480t
Candidiasis, with human immunodeficiency virus disease, 1237
Cannula(s), nasal, for oxygen delivery, in acute respiratory failure, 641t
Cannulation, for cardiac assist devices, 238–241
atrial, 239–240, *240–241*
ventricular, 240–241
of femoral artery, 207–208
of radial artery, 206–207
Capillary(ies), and fluid filtration, 331–332
and solute diffusion, 331
physiology of, 325, *326*
Capillary telangiectasis, 794
Capitation, 6–7
Capnogram(s), 259, *259*
Capnography, in asthma, 616
Captopril, for heart failure, 391t, 393
for hypertensive crisis, 531t
Capture, in pacing, 190t
Caput medusa(e), 1054t
Carbenicillin, and hypomagnesemia, 922
Carbohydrate(s), altered metabolism of, in acute renal failure, 929, 929t
and wound healing, 1263
digestion of, 989
metabolism of, 1052
Carbon dioxide (CO_2), concentration of, as stimulus for breathing, 587
content of, in acid-base status assessment, 590t, 590–591
diffusion of, 574–576, *575*
end-tidal, analysis of, 258–259, *259*
exhaled, dead space analysis with, 259
extracorporeal removal of, 275t
in chronic renal failure, 952t
transport of, 578–579, *579*
Carbonic anhydrase inhibitor(s), mechanism of action of, 888t
Carboxyhemoglobin, half-life of, *1286*
Cardiac. See also entries under *Heart;* specific part(s), e.g., *Myocardium.*
Cardiac assist device(s), 235–243
before cardiac transplantation, 496
cannulation for, 238–241
atrial, 239–240, *240–241*
ventricular, 240–241
centrifugal, 235t, 235–236, *236*
complications of, device-related, 241–242
patient-related, 242–243
external pulsatile, *236*, 236–237, 237t
extracorporeal membrane oxygenation and, 238, 238t, 239t
implantable, 237t, 237–238, *237–238*
nursing care for, 241–243
psychological impact of, 243
Cardiac biopsy, after transplantation, 499t
Cardiac catheterization, in aortic regurgitation, 446
in aortic stenosis, 449
in coronary angiography, in myocardial ischemia, *341*, 341–342
in coronary angioplasty, 347
in heart failure, 389–390, 390t
in mitral regurgitation, 433
in myocardial infarction, 363–364

Cardiac catheterization (*continued*)
in myocardial ischemia, 340–341
in pulmonic stenosis, 456
in tricuspid regurgitation, 451–452
in tricuspid stenosis, 453
Cardiac cell(s), active transport in, 317–318
electrochemical gradient in, 317, *318*
membrane permeability of, 317
Cardiac conduction, 319, *319*
in hypermagnesemia, 923, 923t
ventricular, aberrant, 159–161, *160–161*
Cardiac conduction system, anatomy of, 315, *316*
blood supply to, *130*, 130–131, 131t
innervation of, 131, *131*
Cardiac contractility, calcium and, 913
Cardiac cycle, 127, *128*, 319–321, *320*
atrial pressure in, 319–321, *320*
ventricular diastole in, 320–321, *320–321*
ventricular pressure in, 319–321, *320*
ventricular systole in, 319–320
Cardiac disease, and nonhemorrhagic stroke, 785
nutrition in, 1017
Cardiac dysrhythmia(s), after cardiopulmonary bypass, 484–485, *486*
after cranial surgery, 858
and sudden death, 350
electrocardiography in, 148–149, 149t
from cocaine overdose, 1418–1419
hypercalcemia and, 916, 918
hypokalemia and, 909
hypomagnesemia and, 922
in chronic renal failure, 955–956
in head injury, 757
in long-term survivors of congenital heart defects, 421–422, 423t
in mitral stenosis, 442
in myocardial infarction, 358–359, 370
in myocardial ischemia, 338, *338*
in tricyclic antidepressant overdose, 1424
postoperative, from anesthesia, 1454, *1455*
radiofrequency catheter ablation of, 161
ventricular, electrocardiography in, 161–163, *163*
with reperfusion, 365
Cardiac enzyme(s), in myocardial infarction, 360t, 360–361
Cardiac nerve(s), *131*
Cardiac output, 321–323, *321–323*
afterload and, 228–229, 333
alterations in, hypercalcemia and, 918
and blood pressure, 519, *520*
chronotropy and, 334
contractility and, 229, 323, 333–334
decreased, from positive pressure ventilation, 264
from spinal cord compression, 1483
from superior vena cava syndrome, 1486
in hypercalcemia, from cancer, 1491
postoperative, from anesthesia, 1455
determinants of, 227–230
heart rate and, 229, 323, 334
hormones and, *333*
in acute renal failure, 935
in acute respiratory failure, 634, *634*
in elderly persons, 1495, 1497
in emergency care phase of trauma, 1346–1347, 1347t
in hyperkalemia, 912–913
in hypermagnesemia, 923, 923t
in hypokalemia, 909–910
in hypophosphatemia, 920
in myocardial infarction, 369–370
in systemic circulation, 332–334, *333*
inotropy and, 333–334
measurement of, 222–227
cardiac index calculation in, 226
clinical applications of, 227–230, *230*
direct Fick method in, 222
Doppler electrocardiography in, 226
dye method in, 222
guidelines for, 223, 225–226, *226*
iced injectate in, 223–224
mixed venous oxygen saturation in, 229–230, 230t
pulse thermodilution catheter in, 226–227
thermodilution method in, 222–223, *224*
thoracic electrical bioimpedance monitoring in, 227
thoracocardiography in, 227
normal values for, 230t
preload and, 227–228, 332–333
stroke volume in, 229
total blood volume and, 332–333
venous return and, 332
ventricular stroke work in, 229
Cardiac reflex, abnormalities of, in heart failure, 382t
Cardiac reperfusion, after myocardial infarction, 365
Cardiac surgery. See also *Cardiac transplantation; Coronary artery bypass grafting (CABG); Valvuloplasty.*
coagulopathy after, 1156–1157
intraoperative management in, 473–494. See also *Cardiopulmonary bypass.*
nursing care plan for, 513t–518t
comfort measures in, 516t
fluid balance in, 513t–514t
nutrition in, 514t–515t
oxygenation in, 515t
psychosocial needs in, 517t
safety measures in, 517t
skin integrity in, 516t
postoperative management in, 493–494
preoperative care in, 471–473, 518t
stressors from, 55t, 55–56, 56t
warm, 478–479
Cardiac tamponade, after cardiopulmonary bypass, 485–496
Cardiac transplantation, 494–499
atherosclerosis after, 499
biopsy after, 499t
discharge planning after, 499
for heart failure, 401t, 401–402, 402t
history of, 494
immunosuppression after, 498, 499t
infection after, 498
organ procurement in, 496–497
patient selection for, 494–495, 495t
postoperative management in, 497–498
preoperative care in, 495–496
technique of, 496–497, *497–498*
use of cardiac assist devices before, 496
waiting period for, 495–496
Cardiac valve(s), prosthetic, *437*
in aortic regurgitation, 446
in mitral regurgitation, 435, *437*
in mitral stenosis, 442
in pulmonic regurgitation, 455
in pulmonic stenosis, 456
in tricuspid regurgitation, 452
in tricuspid stenosis, 453
thrombosis of, in mitral stenosis, 439, *439*
Cardiogenic pulmonary edema, vs. adult respiratory distress syndrome, 667, 667t
Cardiogenic shock, 1376–1378, *1377*, 1377t
coronary artery bypass grafting for, 463
in myocardial infarction, 360
Cardioplegia, 477–478, *478*
Cardiopulmonary bypass, 473–493
atelectasis after, 490
atrial fibrillation after, 484–485
atrial overdrive pacing after, 485, *486*
bubble oxygenator for, 474
cardiac changes from, 484
cardiac dysrhythmias after, 484–485, *486*
cardiac tamponade after, 485–486
cardiotomy suction system for, 473–474
central nervous system changes after, 491
cerebrovascular accident after, 491–492
complement cascade from, 490, 492
coronary artery spasm after, 487–488
cytokine levels after, 492
electrolytes after, 491
endocrine changes from, 489
fluid changes from, 484
heat exchanger for, 476
hematologic changes from, 488–489
hemodilution during, 473
heparinization during, 473
hypertension after, 487
hypotension after, 487
hypothermia during, and blood flow, 476, 477
immune function after, 492–493
membrane oxygenator for, 474
myocardial infarction after, perioperative, 486–487
myocardial protection during, 476–479, *478*
peripheral nerve injury from, 492
phrenic nerve injury from, 490
protamine with, complications of, 473
pulmonary changes after, 489–490
pumps for, 474–476, *475*
renal function after, 490–491
reperfusion injury after, 484
use of aprotinin with, 491
venous reservoirs for, 474, *474–475*
ventricular dysfunction after, 485
with warm heart surgery, 478–479
Cardiopulmonary resuscitation (CPR), in sudden death, 352
Cardiotomy suction system, for cardiopulmonary bypass, 473–474
Cardiovascular function, after renal transplantation, 964
anesthesia and, 1444, *1453*, 1453–1455, 1454t, *1455*
assessment of, in acute respiratory failure, 636
burns and, in emergent (shock) phase, 1284–1286
impaired mobility and, 1314–1315, 1315t
in acute renal failure, 931, *932*
in chronic renal failure, 953–956
in elderly persons, 1493, 1494t, 1495–1497
in head injury, 757
in spinal cord injury, 823
muscle relaxants and, 1448t

Cardiovascular system, anatomy and physiology of, *311,* 311–313, 312t, 313t
transmural pressure and, 312
circulation in. See *Blood flow; Circulation.*
hypertension and, 529, *529*
Cardioverter-defibrillator(s), implantable, 196–200, *198, 200*
Caring, in therapeutic relationship, 61–62
Carotid artery, atherosclerosis in, evaluation of, before cardiac surgery, 471–472
Carotid artery(ies), and cerebral blood supply, 781
in cerebral circulation, 723–724, *727*
trauma to, 548–549
Carotid body(ies), and control of respiration, 581, *581*
Carotid bruit(s), and nonhemorrhagic stroke, 786
Carotid endarterectomy, 790–791, *790–791*
Carpentier-Edwards porcine cardiac valve, *437*
Carpopedal spasm, hypocalcemia and, 914t, 915
Catabolism, 995–996
in acute renal failure, 929
prevention of, in metabolic acidosis, 598
tissue, and hyperkalemia, 910, 910t
in potassium regulation, 907
Cataract(s), after bone marrow transplantation, 1217
Catheter(s), for acute respiratory failure, 642
for peritoneal dialysis, 951
for pulmonary artery pressure, 209–210, *211*
complications of, 212, 214t–216t
during insertion, *216*
indwelling, complications of, *216*
for temporary transvenous pacemakers, 186, *186*
for total parenteral nutrition, 1014–1016
pulse thermodilution, in cardiac output measurement, 226
subdural, for intracranial pressure monitoring, 299, *299*
ventricular, for intracranial pressure monitoring, 297, *298*
Catheter ablation, radiofrequency, of cardiac dysrhythmias, 161
Catheterization, cardiac. See *Cardiac catheterization.*
intermittent, in spinal cord injury, 827
Catheter-transducer system(s), in pulmonary artery pressure monitoring, dynamic response in, 215–216, *217*
Cation-anion balance, 894, 894t
Causation, as legal issue, 27
Cavernous angioma(s), 794
Cavernous sinus(es), anatomy of, 725, *728*
CAVH (continuous arteriovenous hemofiltration), 939, 939t
CAVHD (continuous arteriovenous hemodialysis), 939, *939,* 939t
CBC (complete blood count). See *Complete blood count (CBC).*
CCK (cholecystokinin), 982, *982,* 983t
CD4, 1242t
Ceftriaxone (Rocephin), 1242t
Cell-mediated immunity, 1185–1186, *1186*
Cellular ischemia, hypokalemia and, 909
Central cord syndrome, 813, *814*
Central nervous system (CNS). See also *Brain; Spinal cord.*
alterations in function of, after cardiopulmonary bypass, 491
hypernatremia and, 905–906
hyponatremia and, 903–904
anesthesia and, 1447–1448, 1455–1456
human immunodeficiency virus and, 866–867
irritability of, hypomagnesemia and, 922
ischemia of, and blood pressure, 520
and blood pressure regulation, 330
from shock, 1374, *1374*
lymphomas in, 848
renal transplantation and, 964
Central venous pressure (CVP), in fluid volume deficit, 898
monitoring of, 204–205, *206,* 207t
Centrifugal cardiac assist device(s), 235t, 235–236, *236*
Centrilobular emphysema, 607, *607*
Cephalic vein, harvesting of, for coronary artery bypass grafting, 465
Cerebellar peduncle(s), 735
Cerebellum, *733,* 735
tumors in, signs of, 849
Cerebral amyloid angiopathy, and intracerebral hemorrhage, 796
Cerebral angiography, in hemorrhagic stroke, 797
in nonhemorrhagic stroke, 788
Cerebral artery(ies), 723–724, *727–728*
Cerebral blood flow. See *Blood flow, cerebral.*
Cerebral cortex, anatomy of, 729, *730*
Cerebral edema, 754–755, *755*
after cranial surgery, 858
cytotoxic, 754–755
hypernatremia and, 905–906
in head injury, 754–755, *755*
vasogenic, in nonhemorrhagic stroke, 783
Cerebral function, absence of, as criterion for brain death, 804–806
Cerebral metabolism, pharmacologic control of, in brain ischemia, 767
in head injury, 761–762
Cerebral perfusion pressure (CPP), 292, 725–726
in head injury, 756
Cerebral salt wasting syndrome, after cranial surgery, 859
Cerebral tissue perfusion, alteration in, from increased intracranial pressure, 303–305
in emergency care phase of trauma, 1349–1350
in head injury, 763
Cerebral vascular malformation(s), 794–795, *795*
Cerebral vasodilation, and intracranial pressure, 293
Cerebrospinal fluid (CSF), 727–729
absorption of, *728,* 729
impaired, 290
drainage of, 303
examination of, in bacterial meningitis, 863, 864t
in brain ischemia, 765
formation of, 727, *728*
leakage of, after cranial surgery, 859
in frontal bone fracture, 750, *752*
sampling of, 305–306
volume of, 289
and intracranial pressure, 294
Cerebrovascular accident (CVA). See *Stroke.*
Cerebrovascular system, anatomy of, 781–782, *782*
Cerebrum, herniation of, *754*
Cervical nerve(s), 743t
Cervical traction, in spinal cord injury, 820, *821*
Cervical vertebra(e), *735–736,* 736
Cesarean section, anesthesia for, in preeclampsia, 1465
Charcoal, activated, for drug overdose, 1415–1416, 1416t, 1420
Chemical aspiration pneumonitis, 627–628
Chemical burn(s), 1279–1280
"Chemical" code, 33
Chemical debridement, proteolytic enzymes for, 1273, 1296–1297
Chemical dependency, in health care workers, 42–44, 43t
Chemical hazard(s), occupational, 40
Chemical overdose. See *Drug overdose* and specific drug(s).
Chemoreceptor(s), and control of respiration, 581, *581*
Chemoreceptor reflex, and blood pressure, 520
Chemotherapy, 1477
and granulocytopenia. See *Granulocytopenia.*
and wound healing, 1265
body image disturbance in, 1222
family coping in, 1222
for superior vena cava syndrome, 1485
infections from, 1222
with bone marrow transplantation, 1216–1217, 1218t
Chest pain, from cocaine overdose, 1418
Chest physiotherapy, for ventilation-perfusion abnormalities, in acute respiratory failure, 640–641
CHF (congestive heart failure). See *Congestive heart failure (CHF).*
Child(ren), brain death in, 809–810
pain assessment in, 1398
Chloramphenicol (Anocol, Chloromycetin), 1242t
Chlorhexidine gluconate (Peridex), 1242t
Chloride shift, 586, 591–592
Chlorthalidone, for heart failure, 391t
Cholecystokinin (CCK), 982, *982,* 983t
Cholelithiasis, 992
Cholestasis, 1051
Chordae tendinae, in mitral regurgitation, 430
in mitral valve prolapse, 436
Choroid plexus, cerebrospinal fluid formation in, 727, *728*
of brain, 723
Chromosomal defect(s), with cardiac manifestations, 414t
Chronic illness, 107–115
and critical care, 109
control in, 112–113
coping in, 110, 110t
energy conservation in, 110–112, 112t
hardiness in, 112
hope in, 113, 114t
nature of, 107–109
need for information in, 113–114, 114t
phases of, 108t, 108–109, *109*
psychosocial needs in, 112–114

Chronic illness (*continued*)
resources for, 110–115
external, 114–115, 115t
internal, 110–114, 112t
responses to, 109–110, 110t
self-efficacy in, 113, 114t
social support in, 114–115, 115t
Chronic obstructive pulmonary disease (COPD), 601–619
chronic bronchitis in, 603–606. See also *Bronchitis, chronic.*
clinical presentation in, 601, 608
diagnostic criteria for, 601, *602*
epidemiology of, 601–602
etiology of, 602–603, 603t
hypophosphatemia in, 919
laboratory studies in, 608
lung volumes in, *602*
management of, 608–612, 609t
by airway maintenance, 609
by improving dyspnea, 610
by improving gas exchange, 609–610
discharge planning in, 612
drug therapy in, 611
hemodynamic monitoring in, 610–611
infection prevention in, 611–612
intubation in, 610
mechanical ventilation in, 610
nutritional support in, 611
pulmonary rehabilitation in, 612, 612t
smoking cessation programs in, 612
suctioning in, 609
with emphysema, *606–607,* 606–608
Chronic renal failure. See *Renal failure (chronic).*
Chronotropy, and cardiac output, 334
Chvostek sign, hypocalcemia and, 915
Chylous ascites, 1070
Cigarette smoking. See *Smoking.*
Cilia, and external immunity, 1179
physiology of, 563
Cimetidine (Tagamet), for gastrointestinal bleeding, 1033
for human immunodeficiency virus disease, 1242t
Ciprofloxacin, 1242t
Circadian rhythm, in asthma, 615
in myocardial infarction, 355
Circle of Willis, 724–725, *728,* 781, *782*
Circulation. See also *Blood flow.*
collateral, cerebral, 781, *782*
coronary, *311,* 311–312
control of, 323–324, *323–324*
portal, 1048–1050, *1049–1050*
pulmonary, 565–567, *566–567*
splanchnic, 982–984, *983*
systemic, 324–332
anatomy and physiology of, 311–317
arterial pressure in, *326,* 326–327
blood flow regulation in, humoral, *328,* 328–329
long-term, 330–331, *330–331*
blood pressure regulation in, 327–330, *328–330*
cardiac output in, 332–334, *333*
microcirculation, 325–326, *325–326*
structure of, 324–326, *325–326*
volume-pressure curves in, *325*
Cirrhosis, 1063–1070
and hyponatremia, 903
collateral vessel formation in, 1064–1065, *1064–1065*
nursing care plan for, 1086t–1090t
comfort measures in, 1088t
diagnostic procedures in, 1090t
fluid balance in, 1086t–1087t
impaired mobility in, 1087t
nutrition in, 1087t
oxygenation in, 1088t
psychosocial needs in, 1089t–1090t
safety measures in, 1089t
skin integrity in, 1089t
pathophysiology of, 1063
portal hypertension in, 1063–1064
variceal hemorrhage in, 1065–1070
Cisplatin (Platinol), 1242t
Citric acid cycle, 584
CK (creatine kinase), in myocardial infarction, 360t, 360–361
Clarithromycin (Biaxin), 1242t
Clindamycin (Cleocin), 1242t
Clinical social worker(s), on home care team, 119–120
Clofazimine (Lamprene), 1242t
Clonidine, before cardiac surgery, 472
for hypertensive crisis, 531t
Clotrimazole, 1242t
Clotting. See *Hemostasis.*
CNS (central nervous system). See *Central nervous system (CNS).*
CO_2 production ($\dot{V}CO_2$), and acute ventilatory failure, 631, 632t
Coagulation, factors responsible for, 1052
Coagulation cascade, 1143–1144, *1144*
in systemic inflammatory response syndrome, 1363
Coagulopathy, 1147–1161
clinical management of, 1157–1160, 1158t
complications of, prevention of, 1159–1160
disseminated intravascular coagulation. See *Disseminated intravascular coagulation (DIC).*
from anticoagulants, 1154–1155, 1161t
from liver disease, *1153,* 1154
from pathologic fibrinolysis, 1155, *1155*
from renal failure, 1155
from thrombocytopenia, 1155–1156, 1156t
from vitamin K deficiency, 1153–1154
hypothermia and, 1436
pain management in, 1160
postoperative, 1156–1157
prevention of, 1160–1161, 1161t
recognition of, 1157
Cocaine, overdose of, 1415–1419, 1418t, 1419t
Coccygeal nerve(s), 743t
Coccygeal vertebra(e), *735–736,* 736, 738
Cognitive appraisal, in stress-coping framework, 50
interventions for, 56t–57t, 56–57
Cognitive function. See also *Mental status.*
alterations in, in head injury, 764
in intensive care unit, 57
in head injury, assessment of, 756, 756t, *757,* 758t–759t
Coherence, in ethics, 20
Colitis, ulcerative, and gastrointestinal bleeding, 1028–1029
Collaboration, interdisciplinary, 86, 111–112
on ethical issues, 21
Collagen, formation of, 1261
Collateral circulation, cerebral, 781, *782*
formation of, in cirrhosis, 1064–1065, *1064–1065*
Collecting duct(s), and fluid reabsorption, 885
Colloid osmotic pressure, and pulmonary fluid movement, 658
in urine formation, 879–880
Colloid solution(s), for adult respiratory distress syndrome, 670–671
Colon, anatomy and physiology of, 987
ischemia of, after aortic aneurysm repair, 538–539
Colony-stimulating factor(s) (CSFs), and mononuclear phagocytes, 1171, 1172t–1173t
for human immunodeficiency virus disease, 1242t
use of, after bone marrow transplantation, 1219
Colorectal cancer, and gastrointestinal bleeding, 1028
Colostomy, 1038–1039
Columnar ciliated epithelium, pseudostratified, 563
Coma, hypothermic-hypokalemic, in head injury, 762
metabolic, 768–770
vs. brain death, 806
Comfort, family's need for, 72
Comfort measure(s), after cardiac surgery, 516t
in acute renal failure, 946t
in acute respiratory failure, 653t
in adrenal crisis, 1134t
in adult respiratory distress syndrome, 686t
in burn patient, 1307t
in chronic renal failure, 973t
in cirrhosis, 1088t
in diabetic ketoacidosis, 1119t
in gastrointestinal bleeding, 1045t
in head injury, 778t
in heart failure, 410t
in hypophosphatemia, 920
in mechanically ventilated patient, 709t–710t
in obstetric crisis, 1473t
in portal hypertension, 1088t
in respiratory acidosis, 594
in vascular emergencies, 555t
Commissural fiber(s), of brain, 731
Commissurotomy, for mitral regurgitation, 434
for mitral stenosis, 442, *443*
Common channel theory, in pancreatitis, 1091
Communicating artery(ies), anatomy of, 725, *728*
Communication, among health care team members, 86
barriers to, 79–81
channels of, *75,* 75–76
cultural differences and, 80–81, 84–86
effective, elements of, 77t, 77–79
impaired, after craniotomy, 855–856
call devices for, 836
in brain ischemia, 767–768
in Guillain-Barré syndrome, 836
improvement of, 81–86
nonverbal, 76–77
process of, *74,* 74–75
therapeutic, 57t
with aphasic patient, 82–83, 84t
with family, 86
with hearing-impaired patient, 82, 83t
with mechanically ventilated patient, 79, 83t, 83–84, *85*
with visually impaired patient, 81–82

Communication board(s), 84, *85*
Compartment syndrome, 547, 549
Competitive market, health care environment as, 3–4
Complement, and activation of polymorphonuclear leukocytes, in adult respiratory distress syndrome, 663
Complement cascade, from cardiopulmonary bypass, 490, 492
  in systemic inflammatory response syndrome, 1362–1363, *1363*
Complement system, 1182t–1183t, 1182–1183, *1183*
Complete blood count (CBC), in burns, 1290, 1292
  in gastrointestinal bleeding, 1030
Compliance, in cardiovascular system, 312
  in intracranial physiology, 290–291, *291,* 755, *755*
  of lungs, in adult respiratory distress syndrome, 676
    pressure gradient and, 570–571
Compression device(s), for deep venous thrombosis prophylaxis, 1323
Computed tomography (CT), in acute aortic dissection, 541
  in acute pancreatitis, 1096–1097, *1097–1098*
  in aortic aneurysm, 536
  in head injury, 759
  in hemorrhagic stroke, 797
  in herpes simplex encephalitis, 865
  in metabolic coma, 769
  in nonhemorrhagic stroke, 788
  stable xenon, for monitoring cerebral blood flow, 292
Concealed unidirectional retrograde accessory pathway (CURAP), in preexcitation syndromes, 156–157, *158*
Concussion, 750
  of spinal cord, 814
Condom(s), for prevention of human immunodeficiency virus disease, 1231
Conduction system, cardiac. See *Cardiac conduction system.*
Congenital defect(s), of heart. See under *Heart.*
Congestive heart failure (CHF), and hyponatremia, 903
  coronary artery bypass grafting for, 462–463
  hypokalemia and, 909–910, 911
  in chronic renal failure, 954–955
Conscious sedation, 1443t
Consciousness, level of. See *Level of consciousness.*
Consent, implied, 32
  informed, 32t, 32–33
Consistency, in ethics, 20
Constipation, 987
  from enteral nutrition, 1010t, 1012
  from impaired mobility, 1317, 1331–1332
  in chronic renal failure, 958
  in spinal cord injury, 827
Continent Kock pouch, 1038, *1039*
Continuous arteriovenous hemodialysis (CAVHD), 939, *939,* 939t
Continuous arteriovenous hemofiltration (CAVH), 939, 939t
Continuous positive airway pressure (CPAP), 270t, 270–271, 273t
  for mechanical ventilation, in acute respiratory failure, 645–646
  with T-piece, for weaning from mechanical ventilation, 693–694
Continuous renal replacement therapy (CRRT), 937–939, *938*
Contraceptive(s), oral, and hemorrhagic stroke, 796
    and hypertension, 525, 532
Contractility, and cardiac output, 229, 323, 333–334
  cyclic AMP and, *400*
  in heart failure, 381t, *400,* 400–401
Contracture(s), in Guillain-Barré syndrome, 837
Contrast study(ies), in acute pancreatitis, 1095
  in gastrointestinal bleeding, 1031
Control, in chronic illness, 112–113
Contusion(s), of brain, 751
  of spinal cord, 814
Convection, heat loss from, 1431
Cooling, for fever, 1434
COPD (chronic obstructive pulmonary disease). See *Chronic obstructive pulmonary disease (COPD).*
Coping, adaptive, 59–61
  by family. See *Family coping.*
  in chronic illness, 110, 110t
  in myocardial infarction, 370
  ineffective, in granulocytopenia, 1207, 1209
    nursing care plan for, 61t
  styles of, 52
Cordis catheter, for temporary transvenous pacemakers, 186, *186*
Core body temperature, 1431
Corneal reflex, 806
Coronary angiography, in myocardial infarction, 341–342, 364
  radionuclide, in myocardial infarction, 363
Coronary angioplasty. See *Percutaneous transluminal coronary angioplasty (PTCA).*
  laser, in myocardial ischemia, 348–349
Coronary artery(ies), anatomy of, 314–315, *315*
  in myocardial ischemia, 337–338
  left, occlusion of, coronary artery bypass grafting for, 460
  occlusion of. See *Myocardial infarction.*
  spasm of, after cardiopulmonary bypass, 487–488
Coronary artery bypass grafting (CABG), 458–471
  after myocardial infarction, 365, 368
  bleeding after, 488–489
  contraindications to, 463–464
  early extubation after, 483
  epidemiology of, 459
  history of, 459
  indications for, 459t, 459–463, 460t
  late survival and, 467
  nursing care plan for, 513t–518t
  results of, 466–471
    gender and, 470, *470*
    graft patency and, 468–469, *468–469*
    in elderly patients, 470–471
    operative mortality and, 367
    prevention of further damage and, 469
    quality of life and, 469–470
    relief of angina and, 467–468
    reoperation and, 468
  selection of conduits for, *464–465, 464–466, 468–469, 481*
  sequential, 479, *482*
  technique for, 479–481, *480–483,* 483
  transesophageal echocardiography during, 480
  vs. percutaneous transluminal coronary angioplasty (PTCA), 459t–460t, 459–460
  wound infection after, 493
Coronary artery disease (CAD). See also *Angina pectoris; Myocardial infarction; Myocardial ischemia.*
  atherosclerosis in, 336–337
  diagnosis of, invasive, 340–342, *341*
    noninvasive, 338–340, *340*
  management of, invasive, 346–349
  medical management of, angina, 343–346, 344t–346t
  pathophysiology of, sudden death, 349–352
  revascularization surgery for, 346–348
  triple-vessel, coronary artery bypass grafting for, 461
Coronary atherectomy, directional, in myocardial ischemia, 348
Coronary circulation, *311,* 311–312
  control of, 323–324, *323–324*
Corpus callosotomy, 855
Corpus callosum, 729, *729*
Corrigan pulse, in aortic regurgitation, 445
Corrosive agent(s), chemical burns from, 1279
Corticosteroid(s), and wound healing, 1265
  for acute respiratory failure, 643t
  for adult respiratory distress syndrome, 668–669
  for asthma, 616–617, 617t
  for brain ischemia, 766
  for chronic obstructive pulmonary disease, 611
  for head injury, 761
  for hypercalcemia, from cancer, 1490t
  in cranial surgery, 854
Cortisol, role of, 1107
Cost reduction, in critical care areas, 10–12, 11t
Cough reflex, 564–565
Countercurrent mechanism, of urine concentration, 885–886, *886*
Coup-contrecoup head injury, 752, *753*
CPAP (continuous positive airway pressure). See *Continuous positive airway pressure (CPAP).*
CPP (cerebral perfusion pressure), 292, 725–726
CPR (cardiopulmonary resuscitation). See *Cardiopulmonary resuscitation (CPR).*
Cranial meninges, 723, *726*
Cranial nerve(s), *732,* 742, 745t
  assessment of, after craniotomy, 856, 856t
  function of, and brain death criteria, 806
  trauma to, during carotid endarterectomy, 790–791, *791*
Craniotomy, 850–855
  air embolism during, 854
  anesthesia for, 852–855, 853t
  cerebral blood flow during, 854
  cerebral protection during, 852, 854–855
  complications of, 857–858
  for epilepsy, 855
  for pituitary surgery, 851

Craniotomy (*continued*)
  interdisciplinary collaboration in, 859–860
  nursing management after, 855–860
    for assessment of neurologic deficits, 855–857
  patient positioning for, 854
  patient/family education in, 860
  prevention of increased intracranial pressure during, 852, 854
  stereotactic, 851–852
  technique of, 850–851, *850–851*
Creatine kinase (CK), in myocardial infarction, 360t, 360–361
Creatinine, in chronic renal failure, 952t
Creatinine clearance, 882
Creutzfeldt-Jakob disease, 866
Cricothyrotomy, in acute ventilatory failure, 640t
  in emergency care phase of trauma, 1345
Crisis, ethics during, 23
Critical care, chronic illness and, 109
  cost reduction in, 10–12, 11t
  health care environment and, 9–10
Critical care environment, and intracranial pressure, 304–305
  and pain, 1383–1384
  as barrier to communication, 80
  impact of, 90–91, 91t
  modification of, in sensory-perceptual alterations, 99
  psychophysical, *89*, 89–90
  stressors in, 55
  surveillance of, in sensory-perceptual alteration, 98–99
    in sleep pattern disturbance, 104, 104t
Critical care nurse(s), and home care team, 119
Critical care unit(s), psychosis induced by, 57. See also *Sensory-perceptual alteration(s).*
  sound levels in, 97t, 97–98
  vs. home care, as practice settings, 118
Critical illness, as family crisis, 65–68, 67t
  metabolism in, 995–997, 996t, 1355–1356
  sensory-perceptual alterations in, 92
Cromolyn sodium, for asthma, 617, 617t
Crosstalk, in pacemakers, 196, *197*
CRRT (continuous renal replacement therapy), 937–939, *938*
Crutchfield tongs, *821*
Cryptococcosis, with human immunodeficiency virus disease, 1237
Cryptosporidiosis, with human immunodeficiency virus disease, 1236
Crystalloid solution(s), for adult respiratory distress syndrome, 670–671
CSF(s) (colony-stimulating factors). See *Colony-stimulating factor(s) (CSFs).*
CSF (cerebrospinal fluid). See *Cerebrospinal fluid (CSF).*
CT (computed tomography). See *Computed tomography (CT).*
Cultural difference(s), and communication, 80–81, 84–86
CURAP (concealed unidirectional retrograde accessory pathway), in preexcitation syndromes, 156–157, *158*
Cushing response, 726, 756
Cushing's disease, and hypokalemia, 908
Cushing's ulcer(s), 1025
CVA (cerebrovascular accident). See *Stroke.*
CVP (central venous pressure). See *Central venous pressure (CVP).*
Cyclic adenosine monophosphate (cAMP), and asthma, 613
  and contractility, *400*
Cyclophosphamide (Cytoxan, Neosar), 1243t
Cyclopropane, 1446t
Cycloserine (Seromycin), 1243t
Cyclosporine, 1217, 1219, 1220t
Cystic medial necrosis, and acute aortic dissection, 540
Cytarabine, 1243t
Cytokine(s), activity of, 1171, 1172t–1173t
  and activation of polymorphonuclear leukocytes, in adult respiratory distress syndrome, 663, 669
  levels of, after cardiopulmonary bypass, 492
Cytomegalovirus (CMV) infection(s), after renal transplantation, 965, *966*
  and hypocalcemia, 914–915
  with human immunodeficiency virus disease, 1238
Cytotoxic cerebral edema, 754–755
Cytotoxic drug(s), and hyperphosphatemia, 920, 920t

Dakin's solution, 1272, 1297t
Damage(s), as legal issue, 27–28
Dapsone (Avlosulfon, DDS), 1243t
DDD pacing mode, 190t, 191–193, *192*, 194t
DDDR pacing mode, *193*
Dead space, analysis of, with exhaled carbon dioxide, 259
Dead space ventilation (V_{DS}), 573
  increased, and acute ventilatory failure, 631, 632t
Dead space–to–tidal volume ratio (V_{DS}/V_T), estimation of, 256–259, *259*
Deamination, 1052
Death, family's reaction to, and organ donation, 1196
  fear of, 54–55
Debridement, for wound healing, 1273–1274
  of burn wounds, 1296–1297
Decision-making, by families in crisis, 67
Decompression feeding tube(s), 1008
Decremental conduction, electrocardiography in, 150–151, *151*
Deep tendon reflex(es), in hypermagnesemia, 923
  in hypomagnesemia, 923
Deep venous thrombosis (DVT), in critical care phase of trauma, 1352t, 1352–1353
  prophylaxis for, 1323t, 1323–1324
    in spinal cord injury, 823, 826–827
  risk factors for, 1315t
Defamation, 26t, 29
Defense mechanism(s), 52, 59–61, 61t
Deferoxamine, for iron overdose, 1427
Dehydration, from enteral nutrition, 1009t
  in hyperglycemia, 1108
Dehydration test, 1123
Delayed traumatic intracerebral hemorrhage (DTICH), 754
Delirium, drugs causing, 94t
  emergence, 1455–1456
  in intensive care unit, 57
Delta hepatitis, 1061
Delta wave(s), in Wolff-Parkinson-White syndrome, 158, *158*
Dementia, in acquired immunodeficiency syndrome, 867, 1240t, 1250, 1251t
Demyelination, in Guillain-Barré syndrome, 831, *832*
Dendrite(s), of neurons, 718–719, *720, 721*
Dendritic cell(s), 1173–1174
Dentate, of cerebellum, 735
Deontology, 18
Depolarization, 130, 318
  in electrocardiography, *136*
  of nerve cell, 720, *722*
  ventricular, in precordial leads, *138*
Depressed skull fracture(s), 750, *751*
Dermatome(s), 742, *744*
Dermis, anatomy of, 1281
Dextroamphetamine (Dexedrine), as analgesic adjuvant, 1403
  for AIDS dementia, 1243t
Dextrose, as iced injectate, in cardiac output measurement, 223–224
  for fluid therapy, 897t
  for hypercalcemia, 917
  with insulin, for hyperkalemia, 912
Diabetes insipidus, 1122–1124
  after cranial surgery, 859
  and urine concentration, 887
  hypernatremia in, 904–905
  nephrogenic, hypernatremia in, 905
Diabetes mellitus, and hypertension, 525
  and nonhemorrhagic stroke, 785
  and urine concentration, 887
  and wound healing, 1264
  enteral nutrition in, 1002, 1014
  glucose monitoring in, 1114
  management of, during surgery or trauma, 1113
  patient education in, 1111
Diabetic ketoacidosis, 1107–1111
  and hyperkalemia, 910
  and hypophosphatemia, 919
  clinical management of, 1109t, 1109–1111
  clinical presentation in, 1108–1109
  nursing care plan for, 1116t–1121t
    comfort measures in, 1119t
    diagnostic procedures in, 1121t
    fluid balance in, 1116t–1117t
    impaired mobility in, 1118t
    nutrition and nutritional support in, 1110, 1117t
    oxygenation in, 1118t
    psychosocial needs in, 1120t
    safety measures in, 1119t
    skin integrity in, 1119t
  outcome criteria in, 1115t
  pathophysiology of, 1107–1108
  prevention of, 1110–1111
Diagnosis-related group(s) (DRGs), history of, 3–4
Dialysis, 951–953
  and hypokalemia, 908
  for hyperphosphatemia, 920
  historical perspective on, 949
  in acute renal failure, 936–939, 937t
  medications prescribed with, 953t
  vascular access for, 956, *956*
Diaphragm, and inspiration, 570
Diarrhea, 987
  and hypokalemia, 907
  and hypomagnesemia, 921t, 922
  from enteral nutrition, 1010t, 1012
  in interleukin-2 therapy, 1221

Diastole, ventricular, in cardiac cycle, 320–321, *320–321*
Diastolic blood pressure, physiology of, 326–327
Diazoxide, for hypertensive crisis, 530, 531t
DIC (disseminated intravascular coagulation). See *Disseminated intravascular coagulation (DIC).*
Diclazuril, 1243t
Dicrotic wave, in intracranial pressure monitoring, 301, *302*
Didanosine (DDI, Videx), 1243t
Diencephalon, *730,* 731–733
Diet, and hypertension, 525
  as source of acids, 584
  in heart failure, 391–392
Differential lung ventilation, 274t, 282–283
Diffuse axonal injury, 752
Diffusion, abnormalities of, and arterial oxygenation failure, 632t, 633
  renal tubular reabsorption by, 880–881, *881*
Diffusion hypoxia, postoperative, from anesthesia, 1452
Digestion, 987–990, 988t, *988–991*
Digital subtraction angiography, in nonhemorrhagic stroke, 788
Digitalis, and hypomagnesemia, 921t, 922
  for heart failure, 395–396
  for hyperkalemia, 910, 910t
  for hypokalemia, 909–910
  toxicity of, hypercalcemia and, 918
Digoxin, for heart failure, 391t
  for myocardial infarction, 369
Diltiazem, for angina pectoris, 344–345, 345t, 346
Dimethyl sulfoxide (DMSO), for brain ischemia, 766
  for head injury, 762
2,3-Diphosphoglycerate (2,3-DPG), 918
  and oxygen transport, 578, *578*
  decreased, and hypophosphatemia, 919
Dipyridamole, for angina pectoris, 345–346, 346t
Direct Fick method, of cardiac output measurement, 222
Directional coronary atherectomy, in myocardial ischemia, 348
Disc(s), intervertebral, 736, 738
Discharge planning, after acute renal failure, 939–940
  after cardiac transplantation, 499
  after gastrointestinal bleeding, 1040, 1040t
  after lung transplantation, 504
  after renal transplantation, 965–966
  in cancer, 1491–1492
  in chronic obstructive pulmonary disease, 612
  in Guillain-Barré syndrome, 838
  in home care, 119, *122,* 122–123
Disconnect ventilation, 273t, 277
Disopyramide, in sudden death, 351t
Dissecting aneurysm(s), 793
Disseminated intravascular coagulation (DIC), 1147–1153
  clinical management of, 1151–1153, *1152*
  clinical presentation in, 1149–1150, 1150t
  factors triggering, 1148–1149, *1150*
  laboratory findings in, 1150–1151, 1151t
  pathophysiology of, 1147–1148, *1148,* 1149t
  vs. HELLP syndrome, 1462, 1462t
Distal splenorenal (DSRS) shunt, *1080,* 1080–1081
Distal tubule(s), renal transport in, 884
Distributive shock, 1378–1379
Diuresis, for hypermagnesemia, 923
  forced, for drug overdose, 1416
  in acute tubular necrosis, 932
  osmotic, in diabetic ketoacidosis, 1109–1110
Diuretic(s), and calcium excretion, 913
  and hepatic encephalopathy, 1074
  and hypokalemia, 908
  and hypomagnesemia, 921t, 922
  and hyponatremia, 902
  for ascites, 1071
  for brain ischemia, 766–767
  for fluid volume excess, 899
  for head injury, 761
  for heart failure, 391t, 394t, 394–395, *395,* 396t
  for hypercalcemia, 917
    from cancer, 1489
  for hypertensive crisis, 530
  in elderly persons, 1507t
  in loop of Henle, 884
  mechanism of action of, 888t
  osmotic. See *Osmotic diuretic(s).*
  thiazide. See *Thiazide diuretic(s).*
Diuretic challenge, for prevention of acute renal failure, 933–934
Diverticulosis, and gastrointestinal bleeding, 1027
DMSO (dimethyl sulfoxide). See *Dimethyl sulfoxide (DMSO).*
Do_2 (oxygen delivery), and acute respiratory failure, 633–634, 634t
Do_2 (oxygen transport). See *Oxygen transport (Do_2).*
Do Not Resuscitate (DNR) order(s), 33
Dobutamine, for cardiogenic shock, 1378
  for heart failure, 400–401
  for myocardial infarction, 369
Documentation, legal issues in, 34–35
DOO pacing mode, 190t
Dopamine, action of, 723
  and renal blood flow, 878
  as pain mediator, 1392
  for cardiogenic shock, 1378
  for heart failure, 385, 400
  for myocardial infarction, 369
  for prevention of acute renal failure, 934
  for systemic inflammatory response syndrome, 1368
Doppler electrocardiography, in cardiac output measurement, 226
Doppler technique, laser, in assessment of burn depth, 1282
Doppler ultrasonography, in head injury, 760
  transcranial, for monitoring cerebral blood flow, 291
    in hemorrhagic stroke, 797
Doxorubicin hydrochloride (Adriamycin), 1243t
Dressing(s). See *Wound healing, dressings for.*
Dressler's syndrome, from myocardial infarction, 359–360
DRG(s) (diagnosis-related groups), history of, 3–4
Dronabinol (Marinol), 1243t
Drop attack(s), 787
Droperidol with fentanyl (Innovar), 1447t
Drug(s), and complications from anesthesia, 1445
  and heat stroke, 1438
  and maintenance of body temperature, 1435–1436
  in elderly persons, 1506–1508, 1507t
  interactions with anesthetics, 1448
  metabolism of, fever and, 1434
    hepatic, 1053
Drug abuse, and intracerebral hemorrhage, 796
  and nonhemorrhagic stroke, 784
Drug intoxication, vs. brain death, 806
Drug overdose, 1413–1427
  decontamination in, 1414–1417
    activated charcoal for, 1415–1416, 1416t
    emesis for, 1414–1415
    forced diuresis for, 1416
    gastric lavage for, 1415
    hemodialysis/hemoperfusion for, 1416t, 1416–1417
    whole-bowel irrigation for, 1416
  diagnosis of, 1414
  initial stabilization in, 1413t, 1413–1414
Drug-resistant tuberculosis, 627
DSRS (distal splenorenal) shunt, *1080,* 1080–1081
DTICH (delayed traumatic intracerebral hemorrhage), 754
Dual-lumen catheter(s), in acute respiratory failure, 642
Dubois body surface area nomogram, 226, *226*
Ductal hypertension, and pancreatitis, 1091
Dumping syndrome, 1038
  from enteral nutrition, 1012
Duodenal reflux theory, in pancreatitis, 1091
Dura mater, of brain, 723, *726*
  spinal, 738
Durable power of attorney, for health care, 33
Duromedics bileaflet cardiac valve, *437*
DVI pacing mode, 190t
DVT (deep venous thrombosis). See *Deep venous thrombosis (DVT).*
Dye dilution method, in cardiac output measurement, 222
Dynamic response(s), measurement of, in pulmonary artery pressure monitoring, 215–216, *217*
Dynorphin(s), 1394
Dysarthria, 76
Dyspnea, in acute respiratory failure, 635
  in asthma, 615
  in chronic obstructive pulmonary disease, 610
  in emphysema, 607
  in mitral stenosis, 441
Dysreflexia, autonomic, 828, *828*
Dysrhythmia(s). See *Cardiac dysrhythmia(s).*

EAP(s) (employee assistance programs), 43
EAV (effective arterial volume), 893–894
Ebb phase, of metabolism in critical illness, 995, 996t, 1356
ECA (external carotid artery), and cerebral blood supply, 781
Echocardiography, exercise, in myocardial ischemia, 339–340
  in aortic regurgitation, 446
  in aortic stenosis, 449
  in heart failure, 388–389

Echocardiography (*continued*)
in mitral regurgitation, 432, 433t
in mitral stenosis, 441
in mitral valve prolapse, 438, *438*
in myocardial infarction, 362–363
in pulmonic regurgitation, 454
in pulmonic stenosis, 456
in tricuspid regurgitation, 451
in tricuspid stenosis, 453
transesophageal, during cardiopulmonary bypass grafting, 480
in acute aortic dissection, 541
ECMO (extracorporeal membrane oxygenation), 238, 238t, 239t, 275t, *285,* 285–286
Edema, in fluid volume excess, 899
in preeclampsia, 1461
Education, in ethics, 21
EEG (electroencephalography). See *Electroencephalography (EEG).*
EF (ejection fraction), determination of. See *Ejection fraction (EF).*
Effective arterial volume (EAV), 893–894
Efferent neuron(s), 717–719, *720*
Eicosanoid(s), in heart failure, 385
Einthoven's law, 136, *137*
Eisenmenger syndrome, 424, *424,* 424t
Ejection, ventricular, 319–321
Ejection fraction (EF), 320
determination of, 210, *212*
Elastase, and emphysema, 606, *606*
and pancreatitis, 1092
Elderly person(s), cardiovascular function in, 1493, 1494t, 1495–1497
coronary artery bypass grafting in, 470–471
drug administration in, 1506–1508, 1507t
endocrine function in, 1502–1503, 1503t
fever in, 1434–1435
fluid volume deficit in, 1502
gastrointestinal function in, 1494t–1495t, 1500–1501
hypertension in, 1495–1496
immunocompetence in, 1503–1504
impaired mobility in, 1505
musculoskeletal function in, 1504–1505
neurologic function in, 1494t, 1498–1500
nutrition in, 1501
pain assessment in, 1398
renal function in, 1501–1502
respiratory function in, 1494t, 1497–1498
skin integrity in, 1505–1506
sleep disturbances in, 1499–1500, *1500*
thermoregulation in, 1500
Electrical burn(s), 1280
Electrical safety, in epicardial pacing, 185
Electrocardiography, 127–165
altered automaticity in, 148–149
anatomy and, 127–131, *128–131,* 131t
atrial hypertrophy in, 142–143, *144*
axis determination in, 140t, 140–141, *141*
biphasic complex in, *136*
cardiac physiology and, 127–131, *128–131,* 131t
depolarization in, *136*
Doppler, in cardiac output measurement, 226
in acute pancreatitis, 1096t
in afterdepolarizations, 150, *150*
in angina, 147–148, *148*
in aortic regurgitation, 446
in aortic stenosis, 448
in atrioventricular dissociation, *164,* 164–165
in chronic bronchitis, 605–606
in dysrhythmias, 148–149, 149t
in gastrointestinal bleeding, 1031
in heart failure, 388
in hyperkalemia, *932*
in hypermagnesemia, 923
in hypocalcemia, 914t, 915
in hypokalemia, 909–910, 911, *911*
in impulse conduction abnormalities, 150–152, *151–152*
in interpretation of pacemaker function, 191–196
in mitral regurgitation, 432
in mitral stenosis, 441
in mitral valve prolapse, 438
in myocardial infarction, 143–147, *144–145,* 145t, 361t, 361–362, 362t
anterior wall, 145, *146*
atrial, 147–148, *148*
inferior wall, 145–146, *146*
posterior wall, 146, *147*
right ventricular, 146–147, *147*
in myocardial ischemia, 147–148, *148, 338,* 338–339
in paradyshrythmias, 163–165, *164*
in preexcitation syndromes, *156–161,* 157–161. See also *Preexcitation syndrome(s).*
in Prinzmetal angina, 148, *148*
in pulmonic stenosis, 456
in reentry, 151–152, *152*
in reflection, 152, *152*
in tricuspid regurgitation, 451
in ventricular dysrhythmias, 161–163, *163*
intracardiac, for placement of temporary transvenous pacemakers, 187, *188*
leads for, 135–140, *136–140*
augmented, *137*
limb, 136, *137,* 138, *138*
monitoring, 139t, 139–140, *140*
precordial, 138–139, *138–139*
QRS complex in, 136, *138*
rotation in, 141, *142*
R-wave progression in, 139, *139*
transthoracic esophageal, in myocardial ischemia, 340
triggered activity in, 149–150, *150*
ventricular hypertrophy in, left, 141–142, *143*
right, 142, *143*
wide QRS complexes in, 152–155, *153–154, 156*
bundle branch block, 152–154, *153–154*
hemiblocks, 154–155, *155–156*
Electrocargiography, in hypokalemia, 907–908
Electrochemical gradient(s), in cardiac cells, 317, *318*
Electrocoagulation, endoscopic, of gastrointestinal bleeding, 1035
Electrode(s), application of, in transcutaneous pacing, 181, *181*
for pacemakers, 170
Electroencephalography (EEG), in brain death, 808
in hepatic encephalopathy, 1075
in metabolic coma, 769
in seizures, 771
Electrogram, atrial, 183t, 183–184, *184–185*
Electrolyte(s). See also Potassium; Sodium; specific electrolyte, e.g., *Chloride.*
after cardiopulmonary bypass, 490–491
balance of, 906–924
imbalances of, 591–592
and wound healing, 1264
correction of, in respiratory acidosis, 594–595
in burns, 1290
in diabetic ketoacidosis, 1108
in enteral nutrition, 1009t, 1013–1014
in metabolic alkalosis, 599
in total parenteral nutrition, 1016
reabsorption of, 884
replacement of, in acute pancreatitis, 1100
in diabetic ketoacidosis, 1110
Electrophysiologic study(ies), cardiac, 160
ELISA (enzyme-linked immunosorbent assay) test(s), 1230
Embolectomy, balloon, for acute arterial occlusion, 546, *546*
Emboliform nuclei, cerebellar, 735
Embolism, air, during craniotomy, 854
amniotic fluid, 1466–1468, 1467t
and acute arterial occlusion, 543–544, *543–544*
fat, in critical care phase of trauma, 1353, 1353t
in nonhemorrhagic stroke, 784, 784t
pulmonary. See *Pulmonary embolism.*
Embolization, of arteriovenous malformations, 798–799
transcatheter, of gastrointestinal bleeding, 1035
Emergence delirium, 1455–1456
Emergency care. See *Trauma, emergency care phase of.*
Emesis, for drug overdose, 1414–1415
Emotion(s), and asthma, 613
Emotional support, family's need for, 71–72
Empathic listening, 56
Empathy, in effective communication, 78, 78t
Emphysema, *606–607,* 606–608
vs. chronic bronchitis, 603t
Employee assistance program(s) (EAPs), 43
Empyema, subdural, 865–866
Enalapril, for heart failure, 391t, 393
for hypertensive crisis, 531t
Encephalitis, 864–865
Encephalopathy, hepatic, 768, 1073–1075
clinical assessment of, 1058t
hypertensive, 528
uremic, 959–960
Endarterectomy, carotid, 790–791, *790–791*
End-diastolic volume, in cardiac cycle, 320–321, *321*
Endless loop tachycardia, 195–196
Endocardial evoked potential(s), pacemakers and, 176
Endocardial intraoperative mapping, in sudden cardiac death, 350, 352
Endocardial lead(s), for implantable cardioverter-defibrillators, 198–199
Endocarditis, and mitral regurgitation, 429, *429*
in long-term survivors of congenital heart defects, 422, 424t
prophylaxis for, in mitral regurgitation, 433, 434t
in mitral stenosis, 441
rheumatic. See *Rheumatic disease.*

Endocrine function, after cardiopulmonary bypass, 489
and complications from anesthesia, 1444
in burns, 1289
in elderly persons, 1502–1503, 1503t
Endogenous analgesic(s), 1393–1394
Endogenous opiate theory, of pain, 1388–1389
Endogenous pyrogen(s), 1433
Endomyocardial biopsy, in heart failure, 390, *390*, 390t
Endoscopic band ligation, for variceal hemorrhage, 1066
Endoscopic electrocoagulation, of gastrointestinal bleeding, 1035
Endoscopic injection sclerotherapy, for variceal hemorrhage, 1065–1066
Endoscopic retrograde cholangiopancreatography (ERCP), in acute pancreatitis, 1095
Endoscopy, for gastrointestinal bleeding, 1030
for variceal hemorrhage, 1065
Endothelial-derived factor(s), in heart failure, 385–386
Endothelium, cells of, in atherosclerosis, 337
Endotoxin(s), and activation of polymorphonuclear leukocytes, in adult respiratory distress syndrome, 663, 669
in systemic inflammatory response syndrome, 1360–1361
Endotracheal intubation. See under *Intubation.*
Endotracheal tube(s), for mechanical ventilation, 697t, 697–698
End-stage renal disease (ESRD). See *Renal failure (chronic).*
End-systolic volume, in cardiac cycle, 320, *321*
End-tidal carbon dioxide (P_{ETCO_2}), analysis of, 258–259, *259*
in acute respiratory failure, 638
End-to-side portacaval shunt, 1078, *1079*
Enema(s), barium, in gastrointestinal bleeding, 1031
Energy, in metabolism, 995
Energy conservation, in chronic illness, 110–112, 112t
Enflurane, 1446t
for cranial surgery, 853t
Enkephalin(s), 982t, 1393–1394
Enteral nutrition, 1000–1014
clinical management of, 1006–1008, 1007t–1010t, 1010–1014
administration techniques in, 1007t, 1007–1008
for prevention of complications, 1008, 1009t–1010t, 1010–1014
medication administration in, 1008
skin integrity in, 1007
combination tubes for, 1005–1006
decompression tubes for, 1008
gastrostomy tubes for, 1003t–1004t, 1004–1005, *1005*
in critical care phase of trauma, 1356
in diabetes mellitus, 1002, 1014
indications for, 1000, 1001t
jejunostomy tubes for, 1006
nasoenteric tubes for, 1002, 1003t–1004t, 1004
products for, selection of, 1000–1002
Enteroglucagon, 982t
Environment. See *Critical care environment.*
Enzyme(s), activation of, in pancreatitis, 1091–1092, *1093*, 1094t, 1095
cardiac, in myocardial infarction, 360t, 360–361
degradative, in adult respiratory distress syndrome, 664
liver, 1055
proteolytic, for chemical debridement, 1273, 1296–1297
Enzyme-linked immunosorbent assay (ELISA) test(s), 1230
Eosinophil(s), activity of, 1141, 1174
Eosinophilic leukemia, and mitral regurgitation, 429–430
Ependyma, 717
Ependymal cell(s), cerebrospinal fluid formation by, 727
of brain, 723
Epicardial lead(s), for implantable cardioverter-defibrillators, 197–198, *198*
Epicardial pacing, 182–185, 183t, *184–185*
Epicardium, arteries of, 314–315, *315*
Epidermis, anatomy of, 1280–1281
Epidural abscess(es), 866
Epidural anesthesia, 1443t
Epidural hematoma(s), *751*, 754, *754*
Epidural narcotic(s), 1404–1406, *1405*
Epilepsy, 770t, 770–772, 772t, 849–850
posttraumatic, 755, 764
surgical management of, 855
Epinephrine, and hypokalemia, 907–908
for acute respiratory failure, 643t
role of, 1107
Epithalamus, 731
Epithelial cell(s), alveolar, 657
ERCP (endoscopic retrograde cholangiopancreatography), in acute pancreatitis, 1095
Erythrocyte sedimentation rate (ESR), 1181–1182
Erythrocytosis, in long-term survivors of congenital heart defects, 422, 425
Erythropoiesis, 1139–1140
Erythropoietin, for acute renal failure, 936
for chronic renal failure, 958–959
for human immunodeficiency virus disease, 1243t
production of, 890
Escape interval, 190t
Esmolol, for hypertensive crisis, 530
Esophageal varices, bleeding. See *Varices, hemorrhage of.*
Esophagus, anatomy and physiology of, *984*, 984–985
ESR (erythrocyte sedimentation rate), 1181–1182
ESRD (end-stage renal disease). See *Renal failure (chronic).*
Essential amino acid(s), for nutrition in renal failure, 1018
Essential fatty acid(s), deficiencies of, signs and symptoms of, 998t
Essential hypertension, 523–525, *524*
Ethacrynic acid, for heart failure, 391t
Ethambutol (Myambutol), 1244t
Ether, 1446t
Ethics, 15–24
advocacy in, 22–23
and pain management, 1409
and policy-making, 23
autonomy in, 18
beneficence in, 18–19
coherence in, 20
consistency in, 20
deontology in, 18
during crisis, 23
educational programs in, 21
future agenda for, 22–23
hospital resources on, 21–22
in chronic renal failure, 961
interdisciplinary collaboration in, 21
intuitive thinking in, 16
justice in, 19
myths in, 20–21
operationalizing of, 21t, 21–22
paternalism in, 19
reasoning process in, *16*, 16–20
decision on action, 17–19
definition of problem, 17
evaluation of choice, 19–20
list of choices, 17
review of facts, 16–17
study of, *15*
theories of, 18, 18t
utilitarianism in, 18
vs. law, 20–21
Ethics committee(s), 21–22
Ethionamide (Trecator-SC), 1244t
Etidronate, for hypercalcemia, 917
from cancer, 1489, 1490t
Etoposide, 1244t
Evoked potential(s), endocardial, pacemakers and, 176
in brain ischemia, 766
in head injury, 760
somatosensory, in spinal cord injury, 819
Excitation-contraction coupling, 316–317
Excitatory transmission, of nerve impulse, 719–720, 722, *722*
Exercise, and asthma, 613
and hypomagnesemia, 922
for prevention of joint contractures, 1325
in Guillain-Barré syndrome, 837
in heart failure, 392
Exercise echocardiography, in myocardial infarction, 362–363
in myocardial ischemia, 339–340
Exercise testing, in heart failure, 389
in mitral stenosis, 441
in myocardial infarction, 364
in myocardial ischemia, 339
Exhaled gas analysis, 258–259
Expert witness(es), 26
Expiration, 568–570, *569*
Expiratory reserve volume, 572, *572*
Expressive aphasia, 76, 84t
Broca's area in, 729
Expressive touch, 78–79, 79t
External carotid artery (ECA), and cerebral blood supply, 781
External pulsatile cardiac assist device(s), *236*, 236–237, 237t
Extracellular fluid, calcium in, 913
components of, 892–893
disorders of, in hypernatremia, *904*, 904–905
increased tonicity of, in hyponatremia, 901
potassium in, 906
renal tubular damage and, 885
volume of, and blood pressure, 521

Extracorporeal carbon dioxide removal, 275t
  in adult respiratory distress syndrome, 673
Extracorporeal membrane oxygenation (ECMO), 238, 238t, 239t, 275t, *285*, 285–286
  in adult respiratory distress syndrome, 673
Extracranial-intracranial arterial bypass, for nonhemorrhagic stroke, 791
Extrapyramidal descending tract(s), in spinal cord, *741*
Extremity(ies), arteries of, trauma to, 549, 549t
Extubation, early, after cardiopulmonary bypass surgery, 483
Exudate, in wound healing, 1267t
Eye(s), burns and, 1289
Eye contact, 77

Facial nerve, 745t
Factitious hyponatremia, 901
Factor VIII, in hemostasis, 1143, *1143*
Factor XII, in hemostasis, 1143, *1143*
Failure to capture, 195, *196*
Failure to sense, 195, *196–197*
Fallback, in upper rate operation of pacemakers, 194
False imprisonment, 26t, 28
Falx cerebri, 723
Family, grieving by, in amniotic fluid embolism, 1468
Family(ies), and home care team, 118–119, *119*
  communication with, 86
  contemporary, 65
  crisis in, critical illness as, 65–68, 67t
  psychosocial needs of, 65–72. See also *Psychosocial need(s) (family).*
  roles in, during illness, 67–68
  support of, and organ donation, 1196–1199
  wishes of, in brain death, 807
Family coping, in brain ischemia, 768
  in chemotherapy, 1222
  in head injury, 764
  ineffective, in Guillain-Barré syndrome, 838
Family education, about craniotomy, 860
  about Guillain-Barré syndrome, 838
  about heart failure, 402t, 402–403
  in planning for home care, 122
Famotidine, for gastrointestinal bleeding, 1033
Fanconi syndrome, and hypophosphatemia, 918–919
Fasciotomy, indications for, 549, 549t
Fast flush test, for hemodynamic response measurement, 215–216, *217*
Fastigial nuclei, cerebellar, 735
Fat(s), digestion of, 989–990, *990*
  in enteral feeding products, 1001
  metabolism of, 584
Fat embolism syndrome, in critical care phase of trauma, 1353, 1353t
Fatigue, after cranial surgery, 857
Fatty acid(s), essential, deficiencies of, signs and symptoms of, 998t
  hepatic accumulation of, in alcoholic liver disease, 1062–1063
Fatty streak(s), in atherosclerosis, 336
Fear, interventions for, 58–59
  of death, 54–55
  with bone marrow transplantation, 1216
Feeding tube(s), types of, 1003t–1004t. See also *Enteral nutrition.*
Femoral artery, cannulation of, 207–208
Fenestrated tracheostomy tube, 699–700, *700*
Fentanyl with droperidol (Innovar), 1447t
FEVC (forced expiratory vital capacity), 574, *574*
Fever, *1433*, 1433–1435
  and internal immunity, 1181
Fiber, in enteral feeding products, 1002
Fiberoptic intracranial pressure monitoring device(s), 300–301, *300–301*
Fibrin, in disseminated intravascular coagulation, 1147
Fibrin degradation product(s), in disseminated intravascular coagulation, 1147, 1151, 1151t
Fibrinolysis, 1142
  pathologic, 1155, *1155*
Fibrinolysis cascade, in systemic inflammatory response syndrome, 1363
Fibrinolytic system, 1145
Fibrinolytic therapy, for acute arterial occlusion, 546
Fibromuscular dysplasia, and nonhemorrhagic stroke, 785
Fibrous plaque(s), in atherosclerosis, 336–337
Fick method, direct, of cardiac output measurement, 222
Fight-or-flight response, 58, 742, 744, 1394
Filtration fraction, renal, 880
F_{IO_2} (fraction of inspired oxygen). See *Fraction of inspired oxygen (F_{IO_2}).*
Fissure(s), of brain, 729, *730*
Fistula(s), arteriovenous, for hemodialysis, 956, *956*
Fixation device(s), halopelvic, 824, *824*, 826, *826*
Fixed-ratio block, in upper rate operation of pacemakers, 193–194, *194*
Flecainide, in sudden death, 351t
Flow, in cardiovascular system, 312, 313t
Flow phase, of metabolism, in critical illness, 995, 996t, 1355–1356
Flow-cycled ventilator(s), 265
Fluconazole (Diflucan), 1244t
Flucytosine, 1244t
Fluid (body), compartments of, 892t, 892–894, *893*
  electrolytes in. See Potassium; specific electrolyte, e.g., *Sodium.*
  extracellular. See *Extracellular fluid.*
  filtration of, capillaries and, 331–332
  intracellular. See *Intracellular fluid.*
  movement of, among compartments, impaired mobility and, 1314
    in burns, 1285, 1295
    in shock, 1375
    in volume excess, 898
  pH of, 585, 585t
  reabsorption of, by collecting duct, 885
    by renal tubules, 880–882, *881*
  tonicity of, 894
  volume deficit, 895t, 895–898
    after renal transplantation, 963
    and hypermagnesemia, 923, 923t
    clinical manifestations of, 898
    hyperosmotic, 895t
    in diabetic ketoacidosis, 1109–1110
    in elderly persons, 1502
    in head injury, 763–764
    in human immunodeficiency virus disease, 1252t
    in interleukin-2 therapy, 1219, 1221
    in shock, 1375
    isoosmotic, 895t, 896
    management of, 896, 897t
  volume excess, 898t, 898–900
    after renal transplantation, 963
    and altered urinary elimination, in hypercalcemia, 917–918
    edema in, 899
    for correction of hypermagnesemia, 924
    in acute renal failure, 934
    in chronic renal failure, 954–955
    management of, 899–900
    sodium retention in, 898, 898t
  volume of, osmolality and, 894–906, 895t
    regulation of, prostaglandins in, 899
Fluid balance, in acute renal failure, 934, 942t–944t
  in acute respiratory failure, 649t
  in adrenal crisis, 1131t–1132t
  in adult respiratory distress syndrome, 682t–683t
  in burn patient, 1304t–1305t
  in cardiac surgery, 484, 513t–514t
  in chronic renal failure, 969t–970t
  in cirrhosis, 1086t–1087t
  in diabetic ketoacidosis, 1116t–1117t
  in gastrointestinal bleeding, 1042t–1043t
  in Guillain-Barré syndrome, 840t–841t
  in head injury, 776t
  in heart failure, 407t–408t
  in mechanically ventilated patient, 706t
  in metabolic alkalosis, 599
  in myocardial infarction, 374t–375t
  in obstetric crisis, 1470t–1471t
  in pneumonia, 625
  in portal hypertension, 1086t–1087t
  in respiratory acidosis, 594–595
  in vascular emergencies, 552t–553t
Fluid challenge, for prevention of acute renal failure, 933
Fluid resuscitation, in burns, 1292–1294, 1293t, 1294t
  in emergency care phase of trauma, 1347t, 1347–1349
  in spinal cord injury, 819–820
  in vascular trauma, 548
Fluid therapy, for acute pancreatitis, 1099
  for adult respiratory distress syndrome, in critical care phase of trauma, 1351–1352
  for diabetes insipidus, 1123
  for diabetic ketoacidosis, 1109t, 1109–1110
  for gastrointestinal bleeding, 1032
  for hypercalcemia, 917–918
    from cancer, 1488
  for hyperglycemic hyperosmolar nonketotic syndrome, 1111, 1112t
  for hyperkalemia, 912
  for hypernatremia, 905–906
  for hyperphosphatemia, 920
  for hypokalemia, 909
  for hypomagnesemia, 922–923
  for hyponatremia, 903–904
  for preeclampsia, 1464
  maintenance, 896
  solutions for, choice of, 896, 897t

Flumazenil, for benzodiazepine overdose, 1425
Fluorescein, for assessment of burn depth, 1282
Fluoroscopy, for insertion of temporary transvenous pacemakers, 186–187
Foam dressing(s), 1268t, 1269t, 1271
Foley catheter(s), as feeding tubes, 1003t, 1004, *1005*
Fontan procedure, 419–421, *420*
Foramen magnum, of skull, 723
Foraminectomy, in spinal cord injury, *822*
Forced expiratory vital capacity (FEVC), 574, *574*
Force-velocity relationship, in afterload, 322–323
Foreseeability, as legal issue, 27
Foscarnet (Foscavir), 1244t
  and hypocalcemia, 915
Fossa(e), of skull, 723
Fraction of inspired oxygen (FIO_2), in acute respiratory failure, 639–640, 641t
Fracture(s), of skull, 750, *751–752*
  vertebral, 814
Framingham study, sudden cardiac death in, 349–350
FRC (functional residual capacity), in positive end-expiratory pressure, 266
Free radical(s), in myocardial ischemia, 338
Friction, and pressure ulcers, 1320
Frontal bone, fracture of, cerebrospinal fluid leakage in, 750, *752*
Frontal lobe, 729, *730*
  tumors in, signs of, 849
Full-thickness burn(s), 1282
Full-thickness myocardial infarction, 355
Full-thickness wound(s), healing of, 1261, 1261t, 1265–1266, 1266t
Functional capacity, pulmonary, *572*, 573
Functional residual capacity (FRC), in positive end-expiratory pressure, 266
Funduscopic examination, Keith-Wagner scale for, 527t
Fungal infection(s), after renal transplantation, 965
  with human immunodeficiency virus disease, 1237
Furosemide, for acute respiratory failure, 643t
  for head injury, 761
  for heart failure, 391t
  for hypercalcemia, 917
  for hyponatremia, 903
Fusiform aneurysm(s), 535, 792–793
Fusion beat(s), 190t

Gag reflex, and brain death criteria, 806
Galactose elimination capacity (GEC), 1056
Gallamine triethodide (Flaxedil), for cranial surgery, 853t
Gallbladder, anatomy and physiology of, 991–992, *992*, *1050*, 1050–1051
Gallium nitrate, for hypercalcemia, 917
  from cancer, 1489, 1490t
Gallstone(s), 992
  with pancreatitis, 1102
Gamma-glutamyl transpeptidase (GGT), levels of, 1055, 1056t
Gancyclovir (Cytovene), 1244t
Ganglia, basal, 730
Gas exchange, abnormalities of, mechanical ventilation in, 263
  devices for, 275t, *285*, 285–286
  impaired, in acute renal failure, 936
    in adult respiratory distress syndrome, 674–676
    in amniotic fluid embolism, 1468
    in elderly persons, 1498
    in emergency care phase of trauma, 1346
    postoperative, from anesthesia, 1452–1453
  improvement of, in asthma, 618
    in chronic obstructive pulmonary disease, 609–610
Gastrectomy, for gastrointestinal bleeding, 1037, *1037*
Gastric decompression tube(s), 1003t
Gastric emptying, delayed, 985, *985*
  in enteral nutrition, 1009t, 1013
Gastric fluid(s), loss of, and hypomagnesemia, 922
Gastric hemorrhage, after cranial surgery, 858
Gastric inhibitory peptide, 983t
Gastric juice, and external immunity, 1179
Gastric lavage, 1415
Gastric pH, and pneumonia, 622
  in confirmation of nasoenteric tube placement, 1002
Gastric resection, for gastrointestinal bleeding, 1036
Gastric residual(s), in enteral nutrition, 1013
Gastrin, 982, *982*, 983t
Gastrin-releasing peptide, 982t
Gastritis, and gastrointestinal bleeding, 1026–1027
  stress, 1011–1012
Gastroduodenostomy, for gastrointestinal bleeding, *1036*, 1036–1037
Gastroepiploic artery, right, harvesting of, for coronary artery bypass grafting, 466, *466*
Gastrointestinal disease(s), and hypophosphatemia, 918, 918t
Gastrointestinal function, after renal transplantation, 964
  impaired mobility and, 1317
  in acute renal failure, 932
  in burns, 1288
    acute (fluid mobilization) phase of, 1296
  in chronic renal failure, 957–958
  in elderly persons, 1494t–1495t, 1500–1501
  in shock, 1379
  in spinal cord injury, 823–824
Gastrointestinal loss(es), in hypokalemia, 907
Gastrointestinal system, anatomy of, *979*, 979–980
  vascular, *1028*
  bleeding in, 1022–1040
    causes of, in upper tract, *1024*, 1024–1027, 1025t, *1026*
    clinical assessment of, 1029–1031, 1031t
    clinical presentation in, lower vs. upper, 1022, 1022t
    discharge planning after, 1040, 1040t
    endoscopic electrocoagulation of, 1035
    epidemiology of, 1022
    hemorrhagic shock from, 1023t, 1023–1024
    in lower tract, 1027–1029, *1028*
    in upper tract, complications of, 1037, 1037t, 1038t
    medical management of, 1032–1036
      fluid therapy in, 1032
      lavage in, 1032–1033
      nasogastric intubation in, 1032–1033
      pharmacologic, 1033–1035, 1034t–1035t
      transfusions in, 1032, 1032t
    nursing care plan for, 1042t–1047t
      comfort measures in, 1045t
      diagnostic procedures in, 1047t
      fluid balance in, 1042t–1043t
      impaired mobility in, 1044t
      nutrition in, 1043t
      oxygenation in, 1044t
      psychosocial needs in, 1046t
      safety measures in, 1046t
      skin integrity in, 1045t
    nursing management of, 1031–1032
    pathophysiology of, 1022–1024, 1023t
    photocoagulation of, 1035
    surgical management of, in lower tract, 1038t, 1038–1039, *1039*, 1040t
      in upper tract, 1036t–1038t, *1036–1037*, 1036–1038
    transcatheter embolization of, 1035
  innervation of, 980t, 980–981, *982*
  physiology of, 979–992
    absorption, 990
    and adaptation to pathology, 990–991
    hepatic, 991
    hormonal control in, 981–982, *982*, 982t, 983t
    motility, *984–986*, 984–987, 986t
    vascular, 982–984, *983*
  secretions of, 988t
Gastrojejunostomy, for gastrointestinal bleeding, *1037*, 1037–1038
Gastrostomy tube(s), 1003t–1004t, 1004–1005, *1005*
  migration of, 1009t, 1011
Gate control theory, of pain, 1387–1388, *1387–1388*
Gauze dressing(s), 1269t, 1271–1272
GEC (galactose elimination capacity), 1056
Gender, and pain assessment, 1398–1399
  and results of coronary artery bypass grafting, 470, *470*
General anesthesia, 1443t
Genetic disease, with cardiac manifestations, 414t
Gentamicin, and hypomagnesemia, 922
Gentamicin liposome, 1244t
GFR (glomerular filtration rate). See *Glomerular filtration rate (GFR).*
GGT (gamma-glutamyl transpeptidase), levels of, 1055, 1056t
GIK (glucose-insulin-potassium), for myocardial infarction, 367
Glasgow Coma Scale, 756, 756t, *757*
Glenn anastomosis, *418*, 419t
Glioblastoma multiforme, 847
Global amnesia, transient, 787
Global aphasia, 76, 84t
Globose nuclei, cerebellar, 735
Glomerular capillary membrane, permeability of, and urine formation, 880
Glomerular filtration, 879, *879*

Glomerular filtration rate (GFR), 880
in chronic renal failure, 950
in syndrome of inappropriate antidiuretic hormone secretion, 902
Glomerulus (glomeruli), anatomy of, 873–874
Glossopharyngeal nerve, 745t
Glucagon, for severe hypoglycemia, 1112
role of, 1107
Glucocorticoid(s), for hypercalcemia, 917
production of, 1129
Gluconeogenesis, 996, 1052
Glucose, and hypomagnesemia, 922
for hypermagnesemia, 923
in chronic renal failure, 952t
metabolism of, 584
disorders of. See *Diabetes mellitus; Diabetic ketoacidosis.*
impaired mobility and, 1318
in elderly persons, 1503
monitoring of, in diabetes mellitus, 1114
reabsorption of, by renal tubules, 881
serum, after cardiopulmonary bypass, 489
in acute pancreatitis, 1096t
with insulin, for hyperkalemia, 912
Glucose-insulin-potassium (GIK), for myocardial infarction, 367
Glucosuria, and hypophosphatemia, 918t, 919
Glutamic acid, action of, 723
Glutathione, depletion of, in acetaminophen overdose, 1419
Glycogenesis, 1052
Glycogenolysis, 1052
Glycolysis, 584
Goiter, 1125–1126
Golgi complex, of neuron, 718, *721*
Graft(s), skin, for burn wounds, 1297–1298
Graft-versus-host disease (GVHD), in allogeneic bone marrow transplantation, 1216–1217, 1218t
Gram-negative pneumonia, 621, 623–624
Granulocytic phagocyte(s), 1174–1175
Granulocytopenia, collaborative management of, 1207–1210, *1208–1209*
isolation rooms for, *1208–1209*
nursing assessment in, 1205–1207
Granulomatous disorder(s), and hypercalcemia, 916, 916t
Graves' disease, 1127–1128
Great vessel(s), trauma to, 548
Grieving, by family, in amniotic fluid embolism, 1468
Growth factor(s), in wound healing, 1261
Guaiac testing, 1030–1031
Guillain-Barré syndrome, 831–838
clinical presentation in, 832–833
course of, 832
diagnosis of, 833, 834t
discharge planning in, 838
etiology of, 831–832, *831–832*
grades of, 834, 835t
management of, 833–838, *834*, 835t
activity intolerance in, 837
autonomic dysfunction in, 835
impaired communication in, 836
ineffective family coping in, 838
joint contractures in, 837
nutrition in, 837–838, 841t
pain in, 836
potential for aspiration and, 835–836
respiratory muscle dysfunction in, 835
skin integrity in, 837
therapeutic plasmapheresis in, 834, *834*
nursing care plan for, 840t–845t
diagnostic procedures in, 845t
fluid balance in, 840t–841t
impaired mobility in, 841t
oxygenation in, 842t
psychosocial needs in, 844t–845t
safety measures in, 844t
skin integrity in, 843t
patient/family education in, 838
variants of, 833
Gut wall, anatomy of, *979*, 979–980
GVHD (graft-versus-host disease), in allogeneic bone marrow transplantation, 1216–1217, 1218t

H_2 (histamine) receptor antagonist(s), for gastrointestinal bleeding, 1033
Halo traction, *821*
Halopelvic external fixator(s), for spinal cord injury, 824, *824*, 826, *826*
Halothane, 1446t
for cranial surgery, 853t
Hamwi equation, 999, 999t
Hardiness, in adaptation to chronic illness, 112
Harris-Benedict equation, 999, 999t
HCO_3^- (bicarbonate), and carbon dioxide transport, 578–579, *579*
Head injury, 749–764
acceleration-deceleration, *753*
blood flow in, 760
body temperature in, 763
clinical presentation in, 756t, 756–757, *757*, 758t–759t
cardiac, 757
cognitive function, 764
hypothermic-hypokalemic coma, 762
level of consciousness, 756, 756t, *757*, 758t–759t
pupillary response, 756
respiratory, 757
vital signs, 756–757
complications of, 752–755
cerebral edema, 754–755, *755*
hematoma, *751*, 753–754
increased intracranial pressure, 754–755
postconcussion syndrome, 752–753
coup-contrecoup, 752, *753*
diagnostic procedures in, 759–760
diffuse axonal, 752
epidemiology of, 749
family coping in, 764
fluid volume deficit in, 763–764
hyperventilation in, 760–761
intracranial pressure monitoring in, 757, 759, 763
laboratory studies in, 759
medical management of, 760–762
nursing care plan for, 775t–780t
comfort measures in, 778t
diagnostic procedures in, 780t
fluid balance in, 776t
mobility in, 777t
nutrition in, 776t
oxygenation in, 760, 777t
psychosocial needs in, 779t
safety measures in, 779t
skin integrity in, 778t
nursing management of, 762–764
pathophysiology of, 752
penetrating, 751–752
support groups for, 764
surgical management of, 762
types of, 749–752
Headache, from cocaine overdose, 1417
intracranial pressure and, 294
Healing. See *Wound healing.*
Health care, cost of, trends in, 3–6, *4*, 4t–5t, *6*
reforms in, 6–7
recommendations for, 10t, 10–12, 11t
Health care environment, and critical care, 9–10
as competitive market, 3–4
changes in, 3–6
managed care in, 7–9, 8t, 9t
Health care team, communication among, 86
Health care worker(s), substance abuse by, 42–44, 43t
Health maintenance organization(s) (HMOs), 7
Hearing, as communication channel, 76
changes in, in elderly persons, 1499
Hearing-impaired patient(s), communication with, 82, 83t
Heart. See also entries under *Cardiac;* specific part(s), e.g., *Myocardium.*
anatomy and physiology of, 127–131, *128–131*, 131t, 313–317, *314*
atrioventricular node, 128, *129*, 315, *316*
bundle branches, 129, 315, *316*
bundle of His, 128–129
conduction system, *130*, 130–131, *131*, 131t, 315, *316*
contraction, 316–317
coronary arteries, 314–315, *315*
cross-section of, 314t
electrical activity, 317–319
excitation-contraction coupling, 316–317
internodal tracts, 127–128
muscles of, 313
Purkinje system, *128*, 129–130
sinus node, 127, *128*
skeleton, 313, *314*
ultrastructure, *316*, 316–317
valves, 313–314, *314*
arteries of. See *Coronary artery(ies).*
artificial, 496
blood supply of, 311, *311*
congenital defects of, acyanotic, 416–417
cyanotic, 417
in adults, 413–426
classification of, 414–416, 415t
direction of pulmonary blood flow in, 416t, 416–417
etiology of, 413, 414t
incidence of, 413–416
interdisciplinary collaboration in, 425–426
long-term survival in, 416t, 416–421, *418*, 419t
complications of, 421–425, 423t, *424*, 424t
surgical management of, 417–421
complications of, 421
corrective, 419–421, *420*
palliative, 417–419, *418*, 419t
psychological adjustment after, 421
electrophysiology of, 131–135, *132–133*, 160
action potential in, 132–133, *133*

Heart, electrophysiology of (*continued*)
automaticity in, 133–134, *134*
overdrive suppression in, 134
refractory periods in, 134–135, *135*, *318*
sarcolemma in, 132
sodium-potassium pump in, 132, *132*, 317–318
nerves of, *131*
physiology of. See subhead *anatomy and physiology of.*
procurement of, for transplantation, 496–497
transplantation of. See *Cardiac transplantation.*
valvular disease of, 428–456. See also *Valvular heart disease.*
Heart block, Mobitz, type I, 150–151
type II, 151
Heart failure, 380–403
activity intolerance in, 387
and failure to wean from mechanical ventilation, 696
clinical manifestations of, 387, 389t
compensatory mechanisms in, 381t–382t, 381–382
definition of, 380
diagnosis of, 387–390
cardiac catheterization in, 389–390, 390t
chest radiography in, 388
echocardiography in, 388–389
electrocardiography in, 388
endomyocardial biopsy in, 390, *390*, 390t
exercise testing in, 389
hemodynamic variables in, 390t
laboratory studies in, 390
nursing interventions in, 412t
radionuclide ventriculography in, 388–389
epidemiology of, 380
in long-term survivors of congenital heart defects, 424–425
nursing care plan for, 407t–412t
comfort measures in, 410t
fluid balance in, 407t–408t
impaired mobility in, 409t
nutrition in, 408t
oxygenation in, 409t
safety measures in, 411t
skin integrity in, 410t
pathophysiology of, 380–387, 381t
arginine vasopressin system in, 384
atrial natriuretic factor in, 384–385
baroreceptor abnormalities in, 382
cardiac reflex abnormalities in, 382t
death of myocardial cells in, 386–387
dopamine in, 385
eicosanoids in, 385
endothelial-derived factors in, 385–386
neuroendocrine activation in, 382–386, *383*, *385*
sympathetic nervous system and, 382–384, *383*
prostaglandins in, 385
renin-angiotensin-aldosterone system in, 384, *385*
ventricular dilation in, 381t, 386–387
ventricular hypertrophy in, 381t, 386–387
psychosocial needs in, of patient, 411t–412t
right, in chronic bronchitis, 604
sodium retention in, 394t
treatment of, 390–403
cardiac catheterization in, *341*, 389–390, 390t
cardiac transplantation in, 401t, 401–402, 402t
diet in, 391–192
exercise in, 392
in acute exacerbations, 398t, 398–401
in refractory cases, 398–401
increasing contractility in, *400*, 400–401
intra-aortic balloon pump in, 401
patient/family education in, 402t, 402–403
pharmacologic, 391t, 392–398, 394t
adjunctive therapy in, 396–398
angiotensin-converting enzyme inhibitors in, 391t, 392–394, 393t
digitalis in, 395–396
diuretics in, 391t, 394t, 394–395, *395*, 396t
reduction of afterload in, 399–400
reduction of preload in, 399
risk factor modification in, 392
underlying causes in, 398–399
ventricular assist devices in, 401
water retention in, 394t
Heart murmur(s), in aortic regurgitation, 446
in mitral regurgitation, 431–432
in mitral stenosis, 441
in pulmonic stenosis, 455
in tricuspid stenosis, 453
in valvular heart disease, 428
Heart rate, and cardiac output, 229, 323, 334
in heart failure, 381t
with physiologic pacing, 176
Heart sound(s), in aortic stenosis, 448
in pulmonic regurgitation, 454
in tricuspid regurgitation, 451
Heartmate cardiac assist device, *237*, 237t, 237–238
Heat exchanger, for cardiopulmonary bypass, 476
Heat loss, 1431–1432
Heat stroke, 1437t, 1437–1438
Helicobacter pylori infection(s), 988
and peptic ulcer disease, 1025
Helium, mechanical ventilation on, 275t, 284
HELLP syndrome, 1459t, 1460, 1462, 1462t
Hematocrit, in chronic renal failure, 952t
in myocardial infarction, 361
Hematologic disorder(s), and nonhemorrhagic stroke, 784
in long-term survivors of congenital heart defects, 422–425
Hematologic function, after cardiopulmonary bypass, 488–489
and complications from anesthesia, 1444–1445
in chronic renal failure, 958–959
Hematologic system. See *Blood; Hemostasis.*
Hematoma(s), epidural, *751*, 754, *754*
in head injury, *751*, 753–754
intracerebral, *751*, 754
subdural, *751*, 753
Hemiblock(s), 154–155
left anterior, 155, *155*
left posterior, 156, *156*
Hemispherectomy, 855
Hemispheric dominance, in brain, 731
Hemodialysis, 951–953
continuous arteriovenous, 939, *939*, 939t
for drug overdose, 1416t, 1416–1417
for hypercalcemia, 917
for hyperkalemia, 912
for hypermagnesemia, 923
in acute renal failure, 936, 937t
in hyperkalemia, 911
vascular access for, 956, *956*
Hemodilution, during cardiopulmonary bypass, 473
for nonhemorrhagic stroke, 789
Hemodynamic monitoring, 203–231
after lung transplantation, 502–503
clinical applications of, 227–230
in chronic obstructive pulmonary disease, 610–611
in spinal cord injury, 816
in stroke, 799
in systemic inflammatory response syndrome, 1367
of cardiac output, 222–227
clinical applications of, 227–228
of intra-arterial pressure, 205–208, *207*, 208t
of pulmonary artery pressure. See *Pulmonary artery pressure.*
systems for, 203–204, *204–205*
zero-reference point in, 203
Hemoglobin, binding of oxygen to, 578, *578*
composition of, 577
Hemoglobin buffer system, 586, *586*
Hemoglobin saturation, venous, 251–252
Hemolysis, uremic, 930
with cardiac assist devices, 241
with venipuncture, in hyperkalemia, 910
Hemolytic anemia, hypophosphatemia and, 919
Hemolytic jaundice, 1051
Hemoperfusion, for drug overdose, 1416t, 1416–1417
Hemophilus influenzae meningitis, 864
Hemorrhage, after cranial surgery, 857, 858
after gastric surgery, 1037, 1038t
in preeclampsia, 1465–1466
intracerebral, traumatic, 754
variceal, in cirrhosis, 1065–1070
Hemorrhagic shock. See *Shock, hypovolemic.*
Hemorrhagic stroke. See *Stroke, hemorrhagic.*
Hemostasis, 1141–1146
biochemical steps in, 1142t, 1142–1145, *1143–1145*
clot formation as, 1144–1145, *1145*
extrinsic pathway as, 1143, *1144*
intrinsic pathway as, 1143–1144, *1144*
control of, 1145–1146, *1146*
physical events in, 1141–1142, *1142*
Henry-Gauer reflex, in heart failure, 382
Heparin, coagulopathy from, 1154
for acute respiratory failure, 643t
for deep venous thrombosis prophylaxis, 1323
for disseminated intravascular coagulopathy, 1152
for nonhemorrhagic stroke, 789
properties of, 1146
thrombocytopenia from, 1156
Heparinization, during cardiopulmonary bypass, 473
for acute arterial occlusion, 545–546

Hepatic. See also entries under *Liver.*
Hepatic encephalopathy. See *Encephalopathy, hepatic.*
Hepatitis, 1059–1062, 1060t
  chronic active, 1059
  chronic carriers of, 1059
  clinical presentation in, 1059
  epidemiology of, 1059
  occupational exposure to, 36–37
  transmission of, risk of, 1062
  viral, delta, 1061
    serologic testing for, 1060t
    type A, 1059, 1061
    type B, 1061
    type C, 1061–1062
    type E, 1062
Hepatobiliary system, physiology of, 1051–1053
Hepatocellular jaundice, 1051
Hepatorenal syndrome, 1072–1073
Heredity, and hypertension, 524
Herniation, cerebral, *754*
Herpes simplex encephalitis, 865
Herpes simplex virus infection(s), with human immunodeficiency virus disease, 1237–1238
Herpes zoster infection(s), 867
  with human immunodeficiency virus disease, 1238
HHNK (hyperglycemic hyperosmolar nonketotic) syndrome, 1111–1112, 1112t, 1115t
High-frequency jet ventilation, in adult respiratory distress syndrome, 673
High-frequency ventilation, 274t, 279–282, *281*
Histamine (H_2) receptor antagonist(s), for gastrointestinal bleeding, 1033
HIV (human immunodeficiency virus). See *Human immunodeficiency virus (HIV).*
HIV (human immunodeficiency virus) disease. See *Human immunodeficiency virus (HIV) disease.*
HLA (human leukocyte antigen). See *Human leukocyte antigen (HLA).*
HMO(s) (health maintenance organizations), 7
Holistic nursing, and pain management, 53
  and patient's psychosocial needs, 49–50
Home care, 117–124
  assessment of home environment for, *121,* 121–122
  assessment of support systems for, 120
  discharge planning in, 119, *122,* 122–123
  growth in, 5
  history of, 117
  patient assessment in, 120–122
  selection of patients for, 118
  team members for, 118–120, *119*
  transition to, evaluation of, 123–124
  trends in, 117–118
  vs. critical care unit, as practice settings, 118
Home care agency(ies), staff of, and discharge planning, 122–123
Homeostasis, immune system and, 1168
  maintenance of, in brain ischemia, 767
Hope, in chronic illness, 113, 114t
Hopelessness, interventions for, 59
Hormone(s), and blood pressure, 520–521
  and cardiac output, *333*
  and compensation in shock, 1374–1375, *1375*
  and gastrointestinal physiology, 981–982, *982,* 982t, 983t
  and immunocompetence, 1188
  and renal blood flow, 879
  metabolism of, hepatic, 1053
  pituitary, 732, 1122
Hospital(s), utilization of, changes in, *6*
Human growth hormone, for immunodeficiency virus disease, 1244t
Human immunodeficiency virus (HIV), central nervous system effects of, 866–867
  cultivation of, 1231
  genetic composition of, 1227
  immunopathogenesis of, 1227
  isolation and quantitation of, 1230–1231
  mechanism of infection with, 1227–1228
  occupational exposure to, 36
  structure of, 1227
  testing for, 1229t, 1229–1230, 1230t
    in burn patient, 1292
  transmission of, methods of, 1231–1233, 1232, 1232t
Human immunodeficiency virus (HIV) disease, 1224–1254
  and hypocalcemia, 914
  cancer in, 1234
  classification of, 1233, 1233t
  conditions associated with, 1240, 1250
  drugs used in, 1241t–1248t
  epidemiology of, 1224–1227, 1225t–1226t
  health history in, 1249t
  history of, 1224, 1225t
  immunologic abnormalities in, 1228t, 1228–1229
  neurologic manifestations of, 1234, 1240, 1250, 1251t
  nursing care plan for, 1251t–1254t
    altered breathing patterns in, 1252t
    body image disturbance in, 1254t
    fluid volume deficit in, 1252t
    pruritus in, 1253t
    sensory-perceptual alteration in, 1251t
    skin integrity in, 1253t
    social isolation in, 1254t
  nutrition in, 1240, 1250
  opportunistic infections from, 1235–1239
  physical examination in, 1250t
  secondary infections in, 1234
Human leukocyte antigen(s) (HLA), 1166, *1166*
  typing of, for bone marrow transplantation, 1216
Humidification, in mechanical ventilation, 286–287
Hyaline atherosclerosis, in hypertension, 522–523
Hydralazine, for heart failure, 391t, 396–397
  for hypertensive crisis, 530, 531t
Hydrocephalus, in subarachnoid hemorrhage, 793
Hydrochloric acid, and peptic ulcer disease, 1024–1025
  in digestion, 987
Hydrochlorothiazide, for heart failure, 391t
Hydrocolloid dressing(s), 1268t, 1269t, 1270t
Hydrogel dressing(s), 1268t, 1269t, 1270
Hydrogen, and pH, 583. See also *pH.*
  concentration of, as stimulus for breathing, 587, *587*
  secretion of, 587–588, *588,* 888, *888*
Hydrogen peroxide, for wound healing, 1272–1273
Hydrostatic pressure, and pulmonary fluid movement, 658
  mean, 566
Hydroxyzine, as analgesic adjuvant, 1403
Hyperaldosteronism, and hypomagnesemia, 921t, 922
  in mineralcorticoid excess, and hypokalemia, 908
Hyperbaric oxygen therapy, for spinal cord injury, 824
Hypercalcemia, 916t, 916–918
  clinical manifestations of, 916t, 916–917
  definition of, 916
  etiology of, 916t, 916–917
  from cancer, 1487–1491
    clinical presentation in, 1487–1488
    management of, 1488–1491, 1490t
    pathophysiology of, 1487
  from impaired mobility, 1318, 1325
  management of, 917–918
Hypercatabolism, 995–996, 1000
Hyperchloremic metabolic acidosis, 597, 597t
Hypereosinophilic syndrome, and mitral regurgitation, 429–430
Hyperglycemia, and hyperkalemia, 910, 910t
  and hypomagnesemia, 922
  and hyponatremia, 901
  in diabetic keotacidosis, 1107–1108
  in enteral nutrition, 1009t, 1014
  in myocardial infarction, 361
  in total parenteral nutrition, 1016
Hyperglycemic hyperosmolar nonketotic (HHNK) syndrome, 1111–1112, 1112t, 1115t
Hyperkalemia, 591, 910t, 910–913, *911*
  after renal transplantation, 963
  cardiac output in, 912–913
  clinical manifestations of, 910t, 910–911
  definition of, 910
  electrocardiography in, *932*
  etiology of, 910t, 910–911
  in renal failure, 910t, 911
    acute, 929, 934–935
    chronic, 955
  management of, 911t, 911–913
  resting potential in, 911
  with use of angiotensin-converting enzyme inhibitors, 393
Hyperlipidemia, and hyponatremia, 901
  and nonhemorrhagic stroke, 786
Hypermagnesemia, 923t, 923–924
  management of, 923–924
Hypermetabolism, 995–996, 1000
Hypernatremia, *904,* 904–906, 905t
  causes of, *904,* 904–905
  clinical manifestations of, 904–905, 905t
  hypertonic, 901
  iatrogenic, 905
  in diabetes insipidus, 904–905
  injury in, potential for, 905–906
  management of, 905–906
Hyperosmolality. See *Hypernatremia.*
Hyperosmotic fluid volume deficit, 895t
Hyperoxygenation, in acute respiratory failure, 642
Hyperparathyroidism, and hypercalcemia, 916, 916t
  and hypomagnesemia, 921t, 922
  and hypophosphatemia, 918t, 919

Hyperphosphatemia, 920t, 920–921
and hypocalcemia, 914, 914t
definition of, 920
etiology of, 920, 920t
in acute renal failure, 929–930
in chronic renal failure, 960
management of, 920–921
Hyperproteinemia, and hyponatremia, 901
Hypertension, 519–533
after cardiopulmonary bypass, 487
after renal transplantation, 964
alcohol and, 525
and acute aortic dissection, 540
and brain tissue, 530
and hemorrhagic stroke, 796
and intracerebral hemorrhage, 794
and nonhemorrhagic stroke, 785
atherosclerosis in, 522–523
caffeine and, 524–525
cardiovascular effects of, 529, *529*
classification of, 522t–523t, 522–523
coarctation of thoracic aorta and, 526, 533
definition of, 521–522
diabetes and, 525
diet and, 525
ductal, and pancreatitis, 1091
essential, 523–525, *524*
from cocaine overdose, 1418, 1419
heredity and, 524
hypophosphatemia and, 920
in chronic renal failure, 954
in elderly persons, 1495–1496
intracranial, management of, 303
miliary aneurysms in, 522–523
obesity and, 525
oral contraceptives and, 525, 532
pheochromocytoma and, 526, 532–533
portal. See *Portal hypertension.*
postoperative, from anesthesia, 1454, 1454t
pregnancy-induced, 526, 533, 1458–1466. See also *Preeclampsia.*
prevalence of, 521–522
primary, 523–525, *524*
primary aldosteronism and, 526, 532
pulmonary, 228
renal effects of, 529
renal parenchymal disease and, 525–526, 532
renovascular disease and, 526, 532
secondary, 525–528
management of, 531–533
smoking and, 524
stress and, 525
structural/functional disturbances in, 522–523
Hypertensive crisis, 527t, 527–528, *528*
diagnosis of, 528–530, *529*
medical management of, 530–531, 531t
nursing management of, 533
Hypertensive encephalopathy, 528
Hyperthermia, after cranial surgery, 857
from cocaine overdose, 1419
malignant, 1437t, 1438–1439, 1445, 1449
Hyperthyroidism, 1127–1128, 1128t–1129t
Hypertonic hyponatremia, 901–902, *902*
Hypertonic saline, for hyponatremia, 903
Hypertonic saline infusion test, 1123
Hypertonic sodium, for hyperkalemia, 911t, 912
Hyperventilation, during cranial surgery, 854
in brain ischemia, 766
in head injury, 760–761
Hyperventilation syndrome, 595
Hyperviscosity, of blood, in long-term survivors of congenital heart defects, 422, 425
Hypnosis, for pain management, 1408–1409
Hypoalbuminemia, and calcium, 913
Hypocalcemia, 913–916, 914t
clinical manifestations of, 914t, 915
definition of, 913
etiology of, 913–915, 914t
from transfusions, 1159
impaired breathing patterns in, 913–916
in hypomagnesemia, 922
injury in, potential for, 915
management of, 915–916
Hypocapnia, in acute respiratory failure, 635, 636
Hypoglossal nerve, 745t
Hypoglycemia, and brain function, 768
in enteral nutrition, 1009t, 1012
severe, 1112t, 1112–1113, 1115t
Hypogonadism, in liver disease, 1054t
Hypokalemia, 591, 907t, 907–910
cardiac dysrhythmias in, 909
cardiac output in, 909–910
clinical manifestations of, 907, 907t
definition of, 907
etiology of, 907t, 907–909
from transfusions, 1159
in chronic renal failure, 955
in hypomagnesemia, 922
injury in, potential for, 910
management of, 909–910
Hypomagnesemia, 921t, 921–923
and hypocalcemia, 914, 914t, 915
and hypokalemia, 908
clinical manifestations of, 921t, 922
etiology of, 921t, 921–922
injury in, potential for, 922–923
management of, 922–923
Hyponatremia, 591, 901t–903t, 901–904, *902*
causes of, 901t, 901–903
clinical manifestations of, 903, 903t
factitious, 901
in acute renal failure, 929
in syndrome of inappropriate antidiuretic hormone secretion, 902t, 902–903
injury in, potential for, 903–904
isotonic, 901, *902*
management of, 903–904
Hypoosmolality. See *Hyponatremia.*
Hypoosmotic fluid volume deficit, 895t, 896
Hypoparathyroidism, and hyperphosphatemia, 920, 920t
and hypocalcemia, 914, 914t
Hypophosphatemia, 918t, 918–920
clinical manifestations of, 918t, 919
etiology of, 918t, 918–919
management of, 919–920
Hypophyseal stalk, 732
Hypoplastic left heart syndrome, mechanical ventilation in, 284–285
Hyporeflexia, hypermagnesemia and, 923, 923t
Hypotension, after cardiopulmonary bypass, 487
hypermagnesemia and, 923, 923t
hypocalcemia and, 914t, 915
in chronic renal failure, 954
in myocardial infarction, 359
postoperative, from anesthesia, 1454
Hypothalamus, 732
Hypothermia, 1435–1436, 1436t–1437t, *1437*
and coagulopathy, 1436
anesthesia and, 1448–1449
during cardiopulmonary bypass, and blood flow, 476, 477
for brain ischemia, 767
from transfusions, 1158–1159
therapeutic, in spinal cord injury, 824
vs. brain death, 806
Hypothermic-hypokalemic coma, in head injury, 762
Hypothyroidism, 1126–1127, 1127t
and hypermagnesemia, 923, 923t
Hypoventilation, and arterial oxygenation failure, 632t, 632–633
postoperative, from anesthesia, 1452
Hypovolemia, in emergency care phase of trauma, 1348–1349
in hypokalemia, 909
Hypovolemic shock. See *Shock, hypovolemic.*
Hypoxemia, during suctioning, 702
in acute respiratory failure, 644–645
Hypoxia, correction of, in respiratory alkalosis, 596
diffusion, postoperative, from anesthesia, 1452
Hysteresis, 190t, *197*

IABC (intra-aortic balloon pump counterpulsation), for cardiogenic shock, 1378
IABP (intra-aortic balloon pump), for myocardial infarction, 370
Iatrogenic hypernatremia, 905
Iatrogenic injury(ies), 1331
Ibuprofen, in angina pectoris, 346, 346t
ICA (internal carotid artery), and cerebral blood supply, 781
ICD(s) (implantable cardioverter-defibrillators), 196–200, *198*, *200*
ICHD (Inter-Society Commission for Heart Disease Resources), code for pacemakers, 167
Idiopathic hypoparathyroidism, and hypocalcemia, 914, 914t
IgA, properties of, 1167, 1167t
IgD, properties of, 1167, 1167t
IgE, properties of, 1167t, 1168
IgG, properties of, 1167, 1167t
IgM, properties of, 1167, 1167t
IL-1 (interleukin-1). See *Interleukin-1 (IL-1).*
IL-2 (interleukin-2). See *Interleukin-2 (IL-2).*
Ileal pouch–anal anastomosis, 1038
Ileocecal junction, physiology of, 986
Ileostomy, 1038
Ileus, paralytic, 986
Illness, chronic. See *Chronic illness.*
critical, as family crisis, 65–68, 67t
sensory-perceptual alterations from, 92
Imidazole compound(s), in angina pectoris, 346
Immature defense mechanism(s), 60
Immobility. See *Mobility, impaired.*
and sensory deprivation, 94
Immobilization, from trauma, and hypercalcemia, 916, 916t

Immune substrate(s), for systemic inflammatory response syndrome, 1370
Immune system, cells of, 1170–1178, 1172t–1173t
  antigen-presenting, 1171–1174, 1173t–1174t
  antigen-processing, 1171–1174, 1173t–1174t
  granulocytic phagocytes, 1174–1175
  lymphocytes, *1175,* 1175–1178, 1176t, *1177*
 functions of, 1168
 regulation of, 1186, *1187*
 tissues of, 1168–1170, *1169,* 1169t
Immunity, 1165–1168
 and Guillain-Barré syndrome, 832
 antibodies in, 1167t, 1167–1168
 antigens in, 1165–1166, 1166t
 augmentation of, 1189
 cardiopulmonary bypass and, 492–493
 human immunodeficiency virus and, 1227, 1228t, 1228–1229
 major histocompatibility complex in, *1166,* 1166–1167
 mitogens in, 1165–1166
 nonspecific, 1178–1183
  external system of, 1178t, 1178–1179
  internal system of, 1179–1183, *1180,* 1182t–1183t, *1183*
 specific, 1183–1186
  acquired, 1184–1185
  antibody-mediated, 1184–1185, *1185*
  cell-mediated, 1185–1186, *1186*
  passive vs. active, 1184–1185
  primary and secondary responses in, 1184
Immunocompetence, 1186–1189
 age and, 1187–1188
 and complications from anesthesia, 1444–1445
 anesthesia and, 1188
 burns and, in acute (fluid mobilization) phase, 1295
  in emergent (shock) phase, 1287–1288
 drugs affecting, 1188
 hormones and, 1188
 in elderly persons, 1503–1504
 nutrition and, 1188
 stress and, 51–52, 1189
 surgery and, 1188
 trauma and, 1188
Immunoglobulin(s), properties of, 1167t, 1167–1168
Immunosuppression, after cardiac transplantation, 498, 499t
 after lung transplantation, 503
 fever and, 1435
Implantable cardiac assist device(s), 237t, 237–238, *237–238*
Implantable cardioverter-defibrillator(s) (ICDS), 196–200, *198, 200*
Implied consent, 32
Imprisonment, false, 26t, 28
Impulse conduction, abnormalities of, electrocardiography in, 150–152, *151–152*
 in nerves, 719–720, 722
IMV (intermittent mandatory ventilation), 267–268, 272t
Incontinence, impaired mobility and, 1332
 in elderly persons, 1502
Independent practice association(s) (IPAs), 7
Indomethacin, in angina pectoris, 346, 346t
Infarction, myocardial. See *Myocardial infarction.*
Infection(s), after aortic aneurysm repair, 539
 after cardiac transplantation, 498
 after cranial surgery, 857–858
 after lung transplantation, 503–504
 after renal transplantation, 965, *966*
 and asthma, 613
 and wound healing, 1264
 from chemotherapy, 1222
 from enteral nutrition, 1008, 1009t, 1010–1011
 from peritoneal dialysis, 953
 impaired mobility and, 1325
 in acute renal failure, 935
 in chronic obstructive pulmonary disease, prevention of, 611–612
 in chronic renal failure, 959
 in elderly persons, 1504
 intracranial pressure monitoring and, 305–306
 occupational, 36–37
 potential for, in granulocytopenia, 1207, *1208, 1209*
 pulmonary. See *Pneumonia.*
 with cardiac assist devices, 242
Infective endocarditis. See *Endocarditis.*
Inflammation, and internal immunity, 1180–1182
Influenza virus, and pneumonia, 622
Information, need for, by family, 69t, 70
  in chronic illness, 113–114, 114t
Information processing, by families in crisis, 67
Information sharing, and pain management, 53
Informational feedback mechanical ventilation, 273t, 276–277
Informed consent, 32t, 32–33
Infrared thermometer(s), vs. pulmonary artery thermistors, 1439t
Infratentorial structure(s), 723, *726*
Inhalation analgesia, 1406
Inhibitory transmission, of nerve impulse, 719–720, 722, *722*
Injury(ies), and hypokalemia, 908
 as legal issue, 27
 atherosclerosis as response to, 337
 iatrogenic, 1331
 potential for, in acute renal failure, 934, 935
  in hyponatremia, 903–904
In-line suctioning catheter(s), in acute respiratory failure, 642
Innovar, for cranial surgery, 853t
Inotropy, and cardiac output, 333–334
Inspiration, 568–570, *569*
Inspiratory capacity, *572,* 573
Inspiratory reserve volume, 572, *572*
Insulin, administration of, and hypophosphatemia, 918t, 919
 and hyperkalemia, 910t, 911
 and hypomagnesemia, 922
 for diabetic ketoacidosis, 1109t, 1110t
 for hyperglycemic hyperosmolar nonketotic syndrome, 1111, 1112t
 for hypermagnesemia, 923
 impaired mobility and, 1318
 in potassium regulation, 906
 in total parenteral nutrition, 1016
 maintenance therapy with, 1110–1111
 role of, 1107
 with dextrose, for hyperkalemia, 912
 with glucose, for hyperkalemia, 911t, 912
Insulin shock, 1112t, 1112–1113, 1115t
Integrated service network(s), 7
Intensive care unit (ICU). See *Critical care unit.*
Intentional tort(s), 26t, 28
Interdisciplinary collaboration, 11–12, 86
 in adults with congenital heart defects, 425–426
 in cranial surgery, 859–860
 in wound care, 1275–1276
 on ethical issues, 21
Interferon, activity of, 1173t
 for immunodeficiency virus disease, 1244t
Interferon-alpha, for viral hepatitis, 1062
Interleukin, activity of, 1172t
 in systemic inflammatory response syndrome, 1361
Interleukin-1 (IL-1), and activation of polymorphonuclear leukocytes, in adult respiratory distress syndrome, 663
Interleukin-2 (IL-2), 1219, 1221t, 1221–1223, 1245t
 adverse effects of, *1378,* 1477, 1479t
 production of, burns and, 1287–1288
Intermittent mandatory ventilation (IMV), 267–268, 272t
Internal capsule, of brain, 732–733
Internal carotid artery (ICA), and cerebral blood supply, 781
Internal thoracic artery (ITA), harvesting of, for coronary artery bypass grafting, 464–465, *465,* 468, *468–469*
Internal thoracic vein (ITV), harvesting of, for coronary artery bypass grafting, 465
Internodal tract(s), of heart, 127–128
Inter-Society Commission for Heart Disease Resources (ICHD), code for pacemakers, 167
Interstitial disease, and hyponatremia, 902
Interstitium, pulmonary, 657
Intervertebral disc(s), 736, 738
Intra-aortic balloon pump (IABP), before cardiac transplantation, 496
 for heart failure, 401
 for myocardial infarction, 370
Intra-aortic balloon pump counterpulsation (IABC), for cardiogenic shock, 1376
Intra-arterial pressure, monitoring of, 205–208, *207,* 208t
Intracardiac electrocardiography, for placement of temporary transvenous pacemakers, 187, *188*
Intracellular fluid, calcium in, 913
 components of, 892–893
 potassium in, 906
Intracellular protease(s), activation of, and pancreatitis, 1091
Intracerebral hematoma(s), *751,* 754, *754*
Intracerebral hemorrhage, *794–795,* 794–796
 delayed traumatic, 754
Intracranial epidural abscess(es), 866
Intracranial hypertension, management of, 303

Intracranial physiology, compliance in, 290–291, *291*, 755, *755*
Intracranial pressure, increased, and level of consciousness, 294
and motor function, 294–295
cerebral tissue perfusion in, 303–305
clinical management of, 303–306
critical care environment and, 304–305
etiology of, 293t, 293–294
from head injury, 754–755
headache in, 294
neurologic assessment in, 294–295
papilledema in, 295
patient positioning in, 304
prevention of, during cranial surgery, 852, 854
pupillary changes in, 294
suctioning and, 304
vital sign changes in, 295
monitoring of, 295–303
fiberoptic devices for, 300–301, *300–301*
in brain ischemia, 765
in head injury, 757, 759, 763
indications for, 295t, 295–296
infection from, 305–306
sites for, *296*
subarachnoid bolt/screw for, 297, *298*, 299
subdural catheters for, 299, *299*
transducers for, calibration of, 296–297
external, 297–299, *298–299*
intracranial, 299–301, *300–302*
ventricular catheters for, 297, *298*
waveforms in, 301–303, *302*
physiology of, 289–293
compliance and, 755, *755*
volume relationships in, 289
compensation for changes in, 289–291, *290*
touch and, 304–305
Intracranial tumor(s). See *Brain, tumors of.*
Intradural vein(s), *737*, 739
Intrapleural pressure, 568, *569*
Intrapulmonary shunting (Qs/Qt), and arterial oxygenation failure, 632t, 633, *633*
estimation of, 253–256, *254*, 254t
clinical applications of, 255–256, *256*
in acute respiratory failure, 642, 644
in adult respiratory distress syndrome, 675–676
Intrathecal narcotic(s), 1406
Intravascular blood volume, increased, and intracranial pressure, 293
Intravascular fluid, decreased volume of, in hyponatremia, 902
Intravascular oxygenation, 275t
Intravascular stent(s), in myocardial ischemia, 348
Intravascular volume, expansion of, for hemorrhagic stroke, 798
Intravenous urography, in acute renal failure, 931
Intravertebral vein(s), *737*, *739*
Intrinsic factor, in digestion, 987
Intrinsic renal failure. See *Acute tubular necrosis (ATN).*
Intubation, endotracheal, and pneumonia, 621–622
as barrier to communication, 79
in acute ventilatory failure, 639, 640t
in chronic obstructive pulmonary disease, 610
in emergency care phase of trauma, 1345
nasogastric, in gastrointestinal bleeding, 1030, 1032–1033
Intuitive thinking, in ethics, 16
Invasion of privacy, 26t, 28–29
Inverse ratio ventilation (IRV), in adult respiratory distress syndrome, 672
pressure control, 274t, 277–279
Iodine, topical, for wound healing, 1272
Ion channel(s), voltage-gated, in cardiac cells, 317
Ionescu-Shiley cardiac valve, *437*
Ionizing radiation, burns from, 1280
IPA(s) (independent practice associations), 7
Ipecac, 1414–1415
Ipratropium bromide, for acute respiratory failure, 643t
Iron, overdose of, 1425–1427, 1426t
Iron deficiency anemia, in long-term survivors of congenital heart defects, 422–423
Iron lung, 263
Irritant(s), occupational, and asthma, 613t
IRV (inverse ratio ventilation). See *Inverse ratio ventilation (IRV).*
Ischemia, myocardial. See *Myocardial ischemia.*
Isoetharine, for acute respiratory failure, 643t
Isoflurane, for cranial surgery, 852
Isolation, rooms for, *1208–1209*
Isoniazid, 1245t
Isoosmotic fluid volume deficit, 895t, 896
Isoproterenol, for acute respiratory failure, 643t
Isosorbide dinitrate, for heart failure, 391t, 396–397
Isotonic hyponatremia, 901, *902*
Isovolumetric contraction, cardiac, 319–321, *320*
Isovolumetric relaxation, cardiac, 320
ITA (internal thoracic artery), harvesting of, for coronary artery bypass grafting, 464–465, *465*, 468, *468–469*
Itraconazole (Sporanox), 1245t
ITV (internal thoracic vein), harvesting of, for coronary artery bypass grafting, 465

Janeway gastrostomy, 1004
Jaundice, 1051
physical findings in, 1054t
Jejunostomy tube(s), 1003t, 1006
leakage from, 1007, 1009t
Jet ventilation, high-frequency, 274t, 280–282, *281*
in adult respiratory distress syndrome, 673
Joint contracture(s), impaired mobility and, 1319, 1325
in Guillain-Barré syndrome, 837
Jugular venous oxygen saturation, for monitoring cerebral blood flow, 292
Justice, in ethics, 19
Juxtaglomerular apparatus, 875, *875*

Kanamycin sulfate (Kantrex), 1245t
Kaposi's sarcoma, 1238–1239
Kayexalate, for hyperkalemia, 912, 935
Keith-Wagner scale, for funduscopic examination, 527t
Kernig sign, 862
Ketamine, 1447t
for cranial surgery, 853t
Ketoacidosis, diabetic. See *Diabetic ketoacidosis.*
Ketoconazole (Nizoral), 1245t
and hypocalcemia, 915
Kidney(s), anatomy of, 871–875, *872–875*
gross, 871
internal structures, 871–872, *872–873*
microscopic, 872–874, *873*
vascular, 875
and acid-base balance, 587–588, *589*
blood flow of, 875–879, *876*, *878*
anesthesia and, 1447
autoregulation of, *876*, 876–877
extrinsic vasoactive substances and, 878–879
hormones and, 879
in acute renal failure, 928
pressure gradients and, 876
renin-angiotensin-aldosterone system and, 877–878, *878*
sympathetic nervous system and, 878
calcium regulation by, 913
failure of. See *Renal failure (acute); Renal failure (chronic).*
functions of, 871, 871t
acid-base balance, 887–890, *888–889*
sodium excretion and, 894–895, 895t
formation of urine, *879*, 879–882, *881*
hormonal, 890
regulation of urine concentration/volume, 885t–887t, 885–887, *886*
transport, 882–885, *883*
increased excretion of phosphate by, and hypophosphatemia, 918t, 918–919
loss of water from, and hypernatremia, *904*, 904
magnesium regulation by, 921
and hypomagnesia, 922
parenchymal disease in, and hypertension, 525–526, 532
phosphate regulation by, 918
potassium regulation by, 907, 908, 910–911
substances toxic to, 927
transplantation of. See *Renal transplantation.*
volume retention by, and blood flow, 331, *331*
Killer cell(s), activity of, 1177–1178
Kinesthetic communication channel, 76
Kinetic therapy table, *826*, *1328*, 1330–1331
Kock pouch, 1038, *1039*
Krebs cycle, 584
Kupffer cell(s), 1049–1050, 1053

Labetalol, for hypertensive crisis, 530, 531t
Lactate dehydrogenase (LDH), in myocardial infarction, 360t, 360–361
Lactate level(s), and oxygenation, 252–253, 1371–1372
Lactated Ringer's solution, 897t
Lactic acid, and external immunity, 1179
Lactulose, for hepatic encephalopathy, 1075

Laminar flow room(s), *1209*
Laminectomy, in spinal cord injury, *822*
Lamivudine, 1245t
LaPlace's law, 312–313
Large intestine. See *Colon.*
Laryngospasm, hypocalcemia and, 915–916
Larynx, anatomy of, 561, *562*
 artificial, 699
Laser angioplasty, in myocardial ischemia, 348–349
Laser Doppler technique, in assessment of burn depth, 1282
Laser surgery, cranial, 851–852
Lateral tunnel/total cavopulmonary anastomosis, *420,* 420–421
Lavage, for gastrointestinal bleeding, 1032–1033
 gastric, for drug overdose, 1415
 peritoneal, in acute pancreatitis, 1101
Law(s), vs. ethics, 20–21
Laxative(s), and hypermagnesemia, 923, 923t
 phosphate, and hyperphosphatemia, 920, 920t
Lazaroid(s) (21-amino steroids), for head injury, 762
LBB (left bundle branch). See *Bundle branch block, left.*
LDH (lactate dehydrogenase), in myocardial infarction, 360t, 360–361
LDL (low-density lipoprotein), metabolism of, 1053
Lead(s). See *Electrocardiography; Pacemaker(s).*
Lead impedance, of permanent pacemakers, 171
Left bundle branch block (LBBB). See *Bundle branch block, left.*
Left ventricular hypertrophy. See *Ventricle(s) (heart), hypertrophy of.*
Left ventricular stroke work (LVSW), calculation of, 229
Legal issue(s), 25–35
 brain death. See *Brain death.*
 breach of duty owed to patient, 27
 causation, 27
 damages, 27–28
 Do Not Resuscitate orders, 33
 durable power of attorney for health care, 33
 duty owed to patient, 27
 foreseeability, 27
 in documentation, 34–35
 informed consent, 32t, 32–33
 injury, 27
 invasion of privacy, 26t, 28–29
 liability, 29–32
  and expanded roles in nursing, 30–32
  of supervisors, 29–30
  staffing resources and, 30
 living wills, 33–34
 malpractice, 26–28
 negligence, 26t, 26–28
 nutritional support, 997
 standards of care, 25–26
 torts, 25, 26t
  intentional, 26t, 28
  quasi-intentional, 28–29
 withdrawal of ordinary care, 34
Letrazuril, 1245t
Leucovorin, 1245t
Leukemia, eosinophilic, and mitral regurgitation, 429–430
Leukocyte(s), impaired function of, hypophosphatemia and, 919
 polymorphonuclear, and adult respiratory distress syndrome, *661–662,* 661–665, 669
 types of, 1140
Leukopenia, in acute renal failure, 930
Leukotriene(s), in adult respiratory distress syndrome, 664
 in arachidonic acid cascade, 1362
Levaterenol (Levophed), for systemic inflammatory response syndrome, 1368
LeVeen valve, for ascites, 1071–1072, *1072*
Level of consciousness, after anesthesia, 1456
 assessment of, 756t, 756–757, *757,* 758t–759t
 changes in, intracranial pressure and, 294
 in brain ischemia, 765
 in drug overdose, 1413, 1413t
 in elderly persons, 1499
 in metabolic coma, 769
 in systemic inflammatory response syndrome, 1365
Levothyroxine, 1126
LGL (Lown-Ganong-Levine) syndrome, 156, *157*
Liability, 29–32
 and expanded roles in nursing, 30–32
 of supervisors, 29–30
 staffing resources and, 30
Lidocaine, for brain ischemia, 767
 for head injury, 762
 in sudden death, 351t
 prophylactic, for ventricular dysrhythmias, 161–162
Light, transmission of, through tissue, *249*
Limb lead(s), for electrocardiography, 136, *137,* 138, *138*
Limbic system, 730, 732
Linear skull fracture(s), 750
Linton-Nachlas tube, for balloon tamponade of variceal hemorrhage, *1068,* 1069
Lipase level(s), in pancreatitis, 1094t, 1095
Lipid(s), digestion of, 989–990, *990*
 levels of, in acute pancreatitis, 1096t
  in myocardial infarction, 361
 metabolism of, 1052–1053
Lipogenic hypothesis, in atherosclerosis, 337
Lipoid aspiration pneumonitis, 627–628
Lipoprotein(s), low-density, in atherosclerosis, 337
 metabolism of, 1053
Liposyn III, 1245t
Lisinopril, for heart failure, 391t
Listening, active, 77–78, 78t
 empathic, 56
Lithium iodide battery(ies), for pacemakers, 170
Liver. See also entries under *Hepatic.*
 anatomy of, 991, 1048, *1048, 1049*
 dysfunction of, acute fulminant hepatic failure, 1056–1059, 1058t
  alcohol and, 1062–1063
  and coagulopathy, *1153,* 1154
  and hypocalcemia, 914, 914t
  anesthesia in, 1078
  ascites, 1070–1072, *1072*
  assessment in, 1053–1056, 1054t, *1055*
  cirrhosis, 1063–1070. See also *Cirrhosis.*
  encephalopathy in. See *Encephalopathy, hepatic.*
  etiology of, 1064t
  from interleukin-2 therapy, 1221–1222
  hepatitis, 1059–1062, 1060t. See also *Hepatitis.*
  hepatorenal syndrome, 1072–1073
  in burns, 1288, 1296
  in elderly persons, 1500–1501
  in shock, 1379
  nutrition and nutritional support in, 1018–1019
  social aspects of, 1082–1083
  splenomegaly, 1075–1076, *1076*
  with tricuspid regurgitation, 451
  with tricuspid stenosis, 452
 excretory system of, *1050,* 1050–1051
 physiology of, 991, 1051–1053
 transplantation of, 1081–1082
 vascular supply of, 1048–1050, *1049–1050*
Liver biopsy, in portal hypertension, 1077
Liver enzyme(s), 1055
Liver function test(s), in total parenteral nutrition, 1016–1017
Living will(s), 33–34
Lobe(s), of brain, 729–730
Loeffler syndrome, and mitral regurgitation, 429–430
Loneliness, 81
Loop diuretic(s), for heart failure, 391t, 394t, 394–395, *395,* 396t
 for prevention of acute renal failure, 933
 mechanism of action of, 888t
Loop of Henle, anatomy of, 874
 in renal transport, 884
Low molecular weight heparin (LMWH), for deep venous thrombosis prophylaxis, 1323
Low-density lipoprotein (LDL), in atherosclerosis, 337
 metabolism of, 1053
Lown-Ganong-Levine (LGL) syndrome, 156, *157*
Low-profile gastrostomy tube(s), 1005, *1005*
Lumbar nerve(s), 743t
Lumbar puncture, in bacterial meningitis, 863, 864t
 in hemorrhagic stroke, 797
 in metabolic coma, 769
 in nonhemorrhagic stroke, 788
Lumbar vetebra(e), *734–736,* 736, 738
Lung(s), anatomy of, 562, *563, 566–567*
 blood flow to, in congenital heart defects, 416t, 416–417
 compliance of, in adult respiratory distress syndrome, 676
  pressure gradient and, 570–571
 differential ventilation of, 274t, 282–283
 fluid in, accumulation of, 659–660, *660*
  movement of, 657–659, *658*
 interstitium of, 657
 lymph nodes in, *567,* 657
 microvascular barrier in, 656–659, *657–658*
 west zones in, in pulmonary artery pressure monitoring, 216, *218*
Lung transplantation, 499–504
 complications of, 503–504
 discharge planning after, 504
 history of, 499–500
 immunosuppression after, 503
 indications for, 500, 500t

Lung transplantation (*continued*)
  infection after, 503–504
  organ procurement in, 500–501, 501t
  patient selection for, 500, 501t
  postoperative management in, 502–504
  preoperative care in, 500
  technique of, 501–502, *502*
Lung volume(s), 572, *572*
  impaired mobility and, 1315, *1316*
  normal, vs. chronic obstructive pulmonary disease, *602*
Lung zone(s), West, *668*
LVSW (left ventricular stroke work), calculation of, 229
Lyme disease, 867
Lymph node(s), pulmonary, *567,* 657
Lymphadenopathy, in human immunodeficiency virus disease, 1234
Lymphocyte(s), activity of, *1175,* 1175–1178, 1176t, *1177*
  after cardiopulmonary bypass, 493
  B, activity of, 1170
  in chronic renal failure, 959
Lymphoid organ(s), abnormalities of, in human immunodeficiency virus disease, 1228–1229
  central, 1168, *1169–1170,* 1170
  peripheral, 1170
Lymphoma(s), central nervous system, 848
  non-Hodgkin's, with human immunodeficiency virus disease, 1239
Lysozyme, and external immunity, 1179

Macrophage(s), abnormalities of, in human immunodeficiency virus disease, 1228
  activity of, 1171, 1173
  in systemic inflammatory response syndrome, 1360
  in wound healing, 1261
  secretory products of, 1174t
Mafenide acetate (Sulfamylon), for burn wounds, 1297t
Magnesium, disorders of. See *Hypermagnesia; Hypomagnesia.*
  levels of, in chronic renal failure, 952t
  physiologic role of, 921
  regulation of, 921
  repletion of, for hypocalcemia, 915
Magnesium sulfate, for seizure prevention, in preeclampsia, 1463, 1463t
Magnet mode, 190t
Magnetic resonance angiography (MRA), in nonhemorrhagic stroke, 788
Magnetic resonance imaging (MRI), in acute aortic dissection, 541
  in acute pancreatitis, 1097
  in aortic aneurysm, 536–537
  in brain ischemia, 766
  in head injury, 759
  in hemorrhagic stroke, 797
  in myocardial infarction, 363
  in nonhemorrhagic stroke, 788
  in spinal cord injury, 819
Mahaim fiber(s), in preexcitation syndromes, 156, *158*
Major histocompatibility complex, *1166,* 1166–1167
Malignancy(ies), and hypercalcemia, 916, 916t
Malignant hyperthermia, 1437t, 1438–1439, 1445, 1449
Mallory-Weiss tear(s), and gastrointestinal bleeding, 1027
Malnutrition, and failure to wean from mechanical ventilation, 692, 695–696
  characteristics of, 999, 999t
  signs and symptoms of, 998t
Malpractice, 26–28
Managed care, 7–9, 8t, 9t
Mandated choice legislation, for organ donation, 1195
Mandatory minute ventilation, 273t, 276
Mannitol, and hyponatremia, 901
  during cranial surgery, 854
  for head injury, 761
  for prevention of acute renal failure, 933
MAP (mean arterial pressure). See *Mean arterial pressure (MAP).*
Mapping, endocardial, intraoperative, in sudden death, 350, 352
Marfan syndrome, and acute aortic dissection, 540
Mask(s), for oxygen delivery, in acute respiratory failure, 641t
Mast cell(s), activity of, 1175
Mast cell stabilizer(s), for asthma, 617, 617t
Matrix granule(s), of neuron, 718, *721*
Mattress(es), for pressure ulcer prevention, 1326–1327, *1327*
Maximum voluntary ventilation, 573
McGill-Melzack Pain Questionnaire, 1396–1397, *1397*
Mean arterial pressure (MAP), 312, 327
  calculation of, 313t
Mean hydrostatic pressure, 566
Mean pulmonary artery pressure (PAM), calculation of, 313t
Mean right arterial pressure (RAP), 312
Mechanical ventilation, 262–288
  airway management in, 697t, 697–703
    complications of, 701–702
    endotracheal tubes for, 697t, 697–698
    suctioning for, 702–703
    tracheostomy tubes for, 698t, 698–700, *698–700*
  airway pressure release, 274t
  as barrier to communication, 79, 83t, 83–84, *85*
  backup, 273t, 276–277
  BiPAP, 273t, 277
  complications of, 689–692, *691*
  high-frequency, 274t, 279–282, *281*
  high-frequency jet, in adult respiratory distress syndrome, 673
  history of, 262
  humanistic approach to, 286
  humidification in, 286–287
  in acute pancreatitis, 1101
  in acute respiratory failure, 641t
    weaning modes for, 645–646
  in adult respiratory distress syndrome, 671–674
  in apnea, 273t, 277
  in asthma, 618
  in chronic obstructive pulmonary disease, 610
  in hypoplastic left heart syndrome, 284–285
  in pulmonary gas exchange abnormalities, 263
  in respiratory failure, 263
  indications for, 262–263
  informational feedback modes for, 273t, 276–277
  inverse ratio pressure control, 274t, 277–279
  modes for, comparison of, 272t–275t
  negative pressure, 263, 272t
  noninvasive, 273t, 277
  nursing care plan for, 706t–713t
    comfort measures in, 709t–710t
    diagnostic procedures in, 713t
    fluid balance in, 706t
    mobility in, 707t
    nutrition in, 707t
    oxygenation in, 708t–709t
    psychosocial needs in, 712t–713t
    safety measures in, 711t
    skin integrity in, 710t
  nutritional support in, 1017–1018
  positive pressure, 263–264, 272t. See also *Positive pressure ventilation.*
  pressure, 268t, 268–270, *269–270,* 272t
  pressure support, 271, 273t, 276
  respiratory decompensation on, 689–692, *691*
  suctioning in, 287
  troubleshooting in, 287–288
  volume, 266–268, 272t–274t, 276
    control mode, 266, 272t
    intermittent mandatory, 267–268, 272t
    synchronized intermittent mandatory, 267–268, 272t
    volume assist/control mode, 266–267, 272t
  weaning from, 692–697
    assessment during, 695
      checklist for, 692
    centers for, 696–697
    evaluation in, 692
    failure of, 695–696
      malnutrition and, 692, 695–696
    in Guillain-Barré syndrome, 835
    pressure support ventilation for, 694–695
    psychological readiness for, 693
    respiratory parameters in, 692–693
    synchronized intermittent mandatory ventilation for, 694
    T-piece with continuous positive airway pressure for, 693–694
  weaning modes for, 270–276, 273t
    continuous positive airway pressure, 270t, 270–271, 273t, 645–646
    in acute respiratory failure, 645–646
    pressure support, 271, 273t, 276
  with unconventional gases, 275t, 283–285
Medical practice, vs. nursing practice, 31
Medication(s). See *Drug(s).*
Medulla, and control of respiration, 580, *580*
  vasomotor center of, 329, *329*
Medulla oblongata, *732,* 733, 735
Megestrol acetate (Megace), 1245t
Melena, 1022–1023
Membrane oxygenator(s), for cardiopulmonary bypass, 474
Membrane permeability, of cardiac cells, 317
Membrane potential, resting, in cardiac cells, 317–318, *318*
Membrane propria, 563
Meninges, of brain, 723, *726*
  of spinal cord, 738–739
Meningioma(s), 848
Meningitis, 862–864, *863,* 864t
  meningococcal, 863–864

Mental status. See also *Cognitive function.*
in acute fulminant hepatic failure, 1057, 1058t
Metabolic acidosis. See *Acidosis, metabolic.*
with renal failure, and hypocalcemia, 914, 914t
Metabolic alkalosis. See *Alkalosis, metabolic.*
Metabolic coma, 768–770
vs. brain death, 806
Metabolic oxygen requirement(s), in adult respiratory distress syndrome, 674–675
Metabolism, anabolic reactions in, 995
and cerebral blood flow, 726
catabolic reactions in, 995
energy in, 995
in critical illness, 995–997, 996t, 1355–1356
normal, 994–995
regulation of, 995
transport in, 994–995
Metaproterenol, for acute respiratory failure, 643t
Metastatic lesion(s), bony, and hypercalcemia, 916, 916t
Metencephalon (pons), *732,* 733
Methemalbumin, serum, in acute pancreatitis, 1096t
Methotrexate, for human immunodeficiency virus disease, 1245t
Methotrimeprazine, as analgesic adjuvant, 1403
Methoxyflurane, 1446t
Methyldopate, for hypertensive crisis, 531t
Methylphenidate (Ritalin), in human immunodeficiency virus disease, 1245t
Methylxanthine(s), for asthma, 617, 617t
Metolazone, for heart failure, 391t
Metoprolol, for angina pectoris, 343–344
for heart failure, 397
for myocardial infarction, 367
Mexiletine, 1246t
Mexilitine, in sudden death, 351t
Miconazole (Micotin, Monistat), 1246t
Microbial barrier(s), and external immunity, 1179
Microbial translocation, in total parenteral nutrition, 982–984
Microcirculation, physiology of, 325–326, *325–326*
Microglia, 717
Microvascular barrier, in lungs, 656–659, *657–658*
Migraine, and nonhemorrhagic stroke, 784
Miliary aneurysm(s), in hypertension, 522–523
Miller-Fisher syndrome, 833
Mineral(s), and wound healing, 1263–1264
deficiencies of, signs and symptoms of, 998t
in enteral feeding products, 1001
urinary excretion of, impaired mobility and, 1318
Mineralcorticoid deficiency, and hyperkalemia, 910t, 911
and hypermagnesemia, 923, 923t
Mineralocorticoid excess, and hypokalemia, 908
Minute ventilation, 573
and pacemakers, 177
decreased, and acute ventilatory failure, 631, 632t
mandatory, 273t, 276
Missile(s), trauma from, 1341
Mithramycin, for hypercalcemia, from cancer, 1489
Mitochondria, of neuron, 718, *721*
Mitogen(s), in immunity, 1165–1166
Mitral regurgitation, 429–436
acute, 431, *431*
antibiotic prophylaxis in, 433, 434t
chronic, 430, *430*
diagnosis of, cardiac catheterization in, 433
chest radiography in, 432
echocardiography in, 432, 433t
electrocardiography in, 432
laboratory findings in, 432, 433t
phonocardiography in, 433
management of, 433–436, 434t, *435–437*
annuloplasty in, 434, *435–436*
valvuloplasty in, 434, *435,* 435, *437*
murmur in, 431–432
pathophysiology of, 429–431, *429–431*
physical assessment in, 431–432
Mitral stenosis, 439–442
diagnosis of, 441
dyspnea in, 441
dysrhythmias in, 442
heart murmur in, 441
management of, 441–442, *442–443*
pathophysiology of, 439–440, *440*
physical assessment in, 440–441
Mitral valve, anatomy of, 313–314, *314*
replacement of, in mitral regurgitation, 435, *437*
Mitral valve prolapse, 436–438, *438*
Mixed venous oxygen saturation (SvO_2), 251–252
in cardiac output measurement, 229–230, 230t
thermodilution catheters for, in pulmonary artery pressure monitoring, 210
Mobility, impaired, after myocardial infarction, 376t
and activity intolerance, 1331
and altered body image, 1322, 1332
and hypercalcemia, 1325
and incontinence, 1332
and infection, 1325
and pulmonary embolism, 1324, 1324t
cardiovascular effects of, 1314–1315, 1315t
deep venous thrombosis prophylaxis in, 1323t, 1323–1324
gastrointestinal effects of, 1317, 1331–1332
hypercalcemia from, 1318
hypercalciuria from, 1318
in acute renal failure, 945t
in acute respiratory failure, 650t
in adult respiratory distress syndrome, 684t
in burn patient, 1306t
in chronic renal failure, 972t
in cirrhosis, 1087t
in diabetic ketoacidosis, 1118t
in elderly persons, 1505
in gastrointestinal bleeding, 1044t
in Guillain-Barré syndrome, 841t
in head injury, 777t
in heart failure, 409t
in hypercalcemia, from cancer, 1491
in mechanically ventilated patient, 707t
in obstetric crisis, 1472t
in portal hypertension, 1087t
in spinal cord compression, 1482
in spinal cord injury, 825–826, *826*
in vascular emergencies, 554t
metabolic effects of, 1318
musculoskeletal effects of, 1318–1319, *1319,* 1325–1326
pressure ulcers from, 1319–1320, 1320t, *1320–1321,* 1322t
psychological effects of, 1322
pulmonary effects of, 1315–1317, *1316,* 1330–1331
reasons for, 1313t
risks of, 1314t
sensory-perceptual alteration from, 1322, 1332
urinary effects of, 1317–1318
Mobitz heart block, type I, 150–151
type II, 151
Moisture, and pressure ulcers, 1320
Monoclonal antibody(ies), for adult respiratory distress syndrome, 669
Monocyte(s), abnormalities of, in human immunodeficiency virus disease, 1228
activity of, 1171
function of, 1141
Mononuclear phagocyte(s), 1171–1172, 1173t–1174t
Moral intuition, in ethics, 15
Morphine sulfate, 1447t
Motilin, 982t
Motility, gastrointestinal, *984–986,* 984–987, 986t
Motion, sensing of, by pacemaker, 175–176
Motor function, assessment of, after craniotomy, 856
intracranial pressure and, 294–295
Motor neuron(s), 740, *741*
Motor vehicle accident(s), and vascular trauma, 547
Mouth, anatomy and physiology of, 984
Moyamoya, and nonhemorrhagic stroke, 785
MRA (magnetic resonance angiography). See *Magnetic resonance angiography (MRA).*
MRI (magnetic resonance imaging). See *Magnetic resonance imaging (MRI).*
Mucociliary escalator, 563
Mucous membrane(s), and external immunity, 1178–1179
Mucus, composition of, 563
Multidisciplinary care guide(s), for acute renal failure, 942t–948t
for acute respiratory failure, 649t–655t
for adrenal crisis, 1131t–1136t
for adult respiratory distress syndrome, 682t–688t
for burns, 1304t–1309t
for cardiac surgery patient, 513t–518t
for cirrhosis, 1086t–1090t
for coronary artery bypass grafting, 513t–518t
for diabetic ketoacidosis, 1116t–1121t
for gastrointestinal bleeding, 1042t–1047t
for Guillain-Barré syndrome, 840t–845t
for head injury, 775t–780t
for heart failure, 407t–412t
for mechanically ventilated patient, 706t–713t
for myocardial infarction, 374t–379t
for portal hypertension, 1086t–1090t

Multidisciplinary care guide(s) (*continued*)
for renal transplantation, 969t–976t
for vascular emergencies, 552t–557t
Murmur(s). See *Heart murmur(s).*
Muscle(s), atrophy of, impaired mobility and, 1319
cardiac. See *Heart, muscles of.*
dysfunction of, hypokalemia and, 909
hypotonicity of, hypercalcemia and, 916, 916t
weakness of, assessment of, in hypophosphatemia, 919
hypermagnesemia and, 923, 923t
hypokalemia and, 910
in Guillain-Barré syndrome, 832–833
Muscle relaxant(s), as analgesic adjuvants, 1403
cardiovascular effects of, 1448t
for cranial surgery, 853t
Musculoskeletal function, impaired mobility and, 1318–1319, *1319*, 1325–1326
in elderly persons, 1504–1505
Musculoskeletal injury(ies), occupational, 37–39, 38t, 39t
Mycobacterial infection(s), with human immunodeficiency virus disease, 1236–1237
Myelin, of neuron, 719, *719–721*
Myelography, in spinal cord injury, 819
Myelosuppression, in cancer, 1480t
Myobacterium, and hypocalcemia, 914–915
Myocardial cell(s), death of, in heart failure, 386–387
Myocardial depressant factor, in systemic inflammatory response syndrome, 1363–1365
Myocardial depression, anesthetics and, 1445, 1447
Myocardial infarction, 354–370
activity management after, 368
acute stage of, evolution of, 355–356, 356t
pathophysiology of, 354–355, *355*
patient classification in, 230, 230t
after aortic aneurysm repair, 539
arteries involved in, 356, *356*
atrial, 356
cardiac dysrhythmias in, 358–359, 370
cardiac enzymes in, 360t, 360–361
cardiac output in, 369–370
cardiogenic shock in, 360
circadian patterns in, 355
classification of, 355–356
Killip, 359, 359t
clinical presentation of, 357–358
collateral circulation and, 355
coping in, 370
coronary angiography in, 341–342, 364
coronary artery bypass grafting for, 461–462
diagnosis of, 361–364
cardiac catheterization in, 363–364
echocardiography in, 362–363
electrocardiography in, 361t, 361–362, 362t
magnetic resonance imaging in, 363
nursing interventions in, 379t
perfusion scintigraphy in, 363
positron emission tomography in, 363
radiography in, 362
radionuclide angiography in, 363
Dressler's syndrome from, 359–360
electrocardiography in, 143–147, *144–145*, 145t
anterior wall, 145, *146*
inferior wall, 145–146, *146*
posterior wall, 146, *147*
exercise testing in, 364
full-thickness, 355
hypomagnesemia in, 922
infarct area in, extension of, 356
remodeling of, 356
size of, 356–357, *358*
intra-aortic balloon pump for, 370
ischemia in, 356. See also *Myocardial ischemia.*
laboratory findings in, 360t, 360–361
medical management of, 364
nontransmural (subendocardial), 355
nursing care plan for, 374t–379t
fluid balance in, 374t–375t
impaired mobility in, 376t
nutrition in, 375t
oxygenation in, 376t–377t
safety measures in, 378t
skin integrity in, 377t
pain in, description of, 357–358
pain management in, 368
pathophysiology of, 354–357, *355*, 356t, *358*
percutaneous transluminal coronary angioplasty for, 367–368
perioperative, after cardiopulmonary bypass, 486–487
pharmacologic management of, 364–367
amrinone for, 369
angiotensin-converting enzyme inhibitors for, 369
aspirin for, 367
beta-adrenergic blocking agents for, 367
digoxin for, 369
dobutamine for, 369
dopamine for, 369
glucose-insulin-potassium for, 367
nitrates for, 365–367
thrombolytic agents for, 364–365, 366t
physical assessment in, 358–360
during cardiogenic shock, 360
during early phase, 358–359
during recovery phase, 359–360
plaque in, 354–355, *355*
postoperative, from anesthesia, *1453*, 1453–1454
precipitating events of, 356
prodromal period of, 357
psychosocial needs in, of family, 370
of patient, 378t
Q waves in, 144–145, *145*, 145t
reperfusion after, 365, 368
right ventricular, 146–147, *147*, 355–356
shock in, 360
silent, 358
ST segment in, 143–144, *144*
subendocardial (nontransmural), 355
T waves in, 143–144, *144*
temporary pacing in, 178
transmural, 355
Myocardial ischemia, 314, *315*, 337–342. See also *Angina pectoris.*
atherosclerosis in, 338
cardiac catheterization in, 340–342, *341*
coronary angiography in, 340–341
coronary angioplasty in, 346–348
diagnosis of, invasive, 340–342
noninvasive, 338–340
dysrhythmias in, 338, *338*
echocardiography in, 339–340
electrocardiography in, 147–148, *148*, *338*, 338–339
exercise testing in, 339
in myocardial infarction, 356
intravascular stents in, 348
laser angioplasty in, 348–349
management of, invasive, 346–349
nonpharmacologic, 343
pharmacologic, 343–346, 344t–346t
myocardial perfusion scintigraphy in, 339, *340*
pathogenesis of, 337–338, *338*
radionucleotide ventriculography in, 339, *340*, 340t
thallium-201 imaging in, 339, *340*
vs. radionucleotide ventriculography, 340t
Myocardium, hypertrophy of, *322*
oxygen consumption in, 324
in angina pectoris, 343
in myocardial infarction, 357
in myocardial ischemia, 337–338
protection of, during cardiopulmonary bypass, 476–479, *478*
Myogenic theory, of local blood pressure regulation, 328
of renal blood flow autoregulation, 877
Myoglobinemia, in myocardial infarction, 361
Myosin, in cardiac muscle, 316–317

Naloxone (Narcan), 1402, 1414
for systemic inflammatory response syndrome, 1369–1370
Narcotic(s), epidural, 1404–1406, *1405*
intrathecal, 1406
Narcotic analgesic(s), 1400t, 1400–1402, 1401t
Nasal cannula, for oxygen delivery, in acute respiratory failure, 641t
Nasal cavity, anatomy of, 561
Nasal polyp(s), and asthma, 613
Nasoenteric feeding tube(s), 1002, 1003t–1004t, 1004
Nasogastric intubation, in gastrointestinal bleeding, 1030, 1032–1033
Nasopharyngeal airway(s), in acute ventilatory failure, 639, 640t
NASPE/BPEG (North American Society of Pacing and Electrophysiology/British Pacing and Electrophysiology Group), code for pacemakers, 167, 169, 169t
National Head Injury Foundation, 764
Natural death act(s), 33–34
Natural killer cell(s), activity of, 1177–1178
Nausea, from enteral nutrition, 1011
NBG code, for pacemakers, 167, 169, 169t
Needle(s), sharing of, transmission of human immunodeficiency virus via, 1232–1233
Needle catheter jejunostomy tube(s), 1006
Needle-stick injury(ies), protection from, 37, 37t
transmission of human immunodeficiency virus via, 1232
Negative pressure ventilation, 263, 272t
Negligence, 26t, 26–28
Neomycin, for hepatic encephalopathy, 1075
Neonate(s), respiratory distress syndrome in, 570

Neoplasm(s). See *Cancer.*
Nephrogenic diabetes insipidus, 1123
  hypernatremia in, 905
Nephron(s), anatomy of, 872, *873*
  intact, Bricker's hypothesis of, 950
  transport of substances throughout, 882–885, 885t
Nephrotic syndrome, and hypocalcemia, 914, 914t
  and hyponatremia, 903
Nephrotoxin(s), 927, 935
Nerve(s), 719–723, *722*
  components of, 719, *722*
  cranial, *732*
  impulse conduction in, 719–720, 722
  neurotransmitter action on, *722,* 722–723
  synapses in, *719,* 722–723
Nerve block(s), peripheral, 1443t
Nerve impulse(s), transmission of, 719–720, 722, *722*
Nervous system, and blood pressure regulation, *329,* 329–330, 519–520
  autonomic, 742, 744, *746–747,* 748, 748t
  peripheral, 741–742, 743t
Net filtration pressure, in urine formation, *879, 879*
Neuroendocrine system, activation of, in heart failure, 382–386, *383, 385*
Neurofibril(s), 718, *720*
Neurofilament(s), 718
Neurogenic pulmonary edema, after cranial surgery, 858
Neurogenic spinal shock, 815–816
Neuroglia cell(s), 717, *718*
Neurohypophysis, disorders of, 1122–1125
Neurolemma, *719–720*
Neuroleptic malignant syndrome, 1439–1440
Neurologic function, assessment of, after craniotomy, 855–857
    in acute respiratory failure, 635–636
    in spinal cord injury, 816, *817–818,* 819
  in acute renal failure, 932
  in burns, 1289
  in chronic renal failure, 959–960
  in elderly persons, 1494t, 1498–1500
Neuromuscular blockade, and sensory deprivation, 94–95
  communication in, 84
  complications of, 1448
  in emergency care phase of trauma, 1345–1346
Neuromuscular excitability, hypercalcemia and, 916
  hypocalcemia and, 914t, 915
Neuron(s), 717–719, *719–722*
  bipolar, 717, *720*
  cytologic features of, 718, *721*
  motor, 740, *741*
  multipolar, 717, *721*
  preganglionic, of sympathetic nervous system, 744
  processes of, 718–719, *722*
  structure of, 718, *719–721*
  unipolar, 717, *719, 720*
Neuronal perikaryon, 718, *721*
Neuropathy, peripheral, in chronic renal failure, 960
Neurophysiology, 717–748
  blood-brain barrier, 726–727
  brainstem, *732,* 733, 735
  cerebral, 729–730, *729–730*
  blood flow regulation in, 725–726
  circulation in, 723–725, *727*
  meningeal, 723, *726*
  nerves, 719–723, *722*
  neuroglia cells and, 717, *718*
  neuronal, 717–719, *719–720*
  of autonomic nervous system, 742, 744, *746–747,* 748, 748t
  of cerebrospinal fluid, 727, 729
  of peripheral nervous system, 741–742, 743t
  of reticular activating system, *733,* 736
  of skull, 723, *724–725*
  of vertebral column, *734–736,* 736, 738
  reticular formation and, 736
Neurosurgery. See *Craniotomy.*
Neurotic defense mechanism(s), 60–61, 61t
Neurotransmitter(s), and blood flow, *328,* 328–329
  and sleep, 100–101
  excitatory, *722,* 723
  in nerve impulse conduction, *722,* 722–723
  inhibitory, *722,* 723
  synthesis of, amino acids and, in hepatic encephalopathy, 1073–1074
Neutropenia, causes of, 1206t
Neutrophil(s), activity of, 1174
  and adult respiratory distress syndrome, *661–662,* 661–665
  in wound healing, 1261
Nevirapine, 1246t
Nifedipine, for hypertensive crisis, 531t
  in angina pectoris, 344–346, 345t
Nimodipine, 1246t
  for nonhemorrhagic stroke, 789
Nissl bodies, of neuron, 718, *719–721*
Nitrate(s). See also *Nitroglycerin.*
  for heart failure, 399
  for myocardial infarction, 365–367
Nitric oxide, for adult respiratory distress syndrome, 670
  mechanical ventilation with, 275t, 283–284
Nitrogen, myocardial ischemia, 346
  single-breath analysis of, *573,* 573–574
Nitrogen balance, in nutritional assessment, 1000
Nitroglycerin, for hypertensive crisis, 530, 531t
  for myocardial infarction, 365–367
  in angina pectoris, 343, 344t
Nitroprusside, for heart failure, 399
  for hypertensive crisis, 530, 531t
  in blood flow regulation, 229
Nitrous oxide, 1446t
  for cranial surgery, 853t
Nizatidine, for gastrointestinal bleeding, 1033
Nociceptor(s), and pain, 1389–1390
Node of Ranvier, *719,* 722
Noise, and sensory overload, 96–97, *97*
  as patient stressor, 55, 80
  in critical care unit, 97t, 97–98
  occupational exposure to, 41–42, 42t
Noncardiogenic pulmonary edema. See *Adult respiratory distress syndrome (ARDS).*
Non-Hodgkin's lymphoma, with human immunodeficiency virus disease, 1239
Noninvasive mechanical ventilation, 273t, 277
Nonmaleficence, 18–19
Nonnarcotic analgesic(s), 1402–1403
Nonselective shunt(s), for portal hypertension, 1078, *1079,* 1080
Nonsteroidal anti-inflammatory drug(s) (NSAIDs), in angina pectoris, 345–346, 346t
Nonverbal communication, 76–77
No-reflow phenomenon, in brain ischemia, 765
Norepinephrine, action of, 723
  contractility effects of, 319
  as pain mediator, 1392
  in heart failure, 382–383
Normal sinus rhythm, atrial electrogram in, *184*
North American Society of Pacing and Electrophysiology / British Pacing and Electrophysiology Group (NASPE / BPEG), code for pacemakers, 167, 169, 169t
Norton scale, 1326
Nosocomial pneumonia, 621–622
Novacor Left Ventricular Assist System, 237t, 237–238, *238*
NSAIDs (nonsteroidal antiinflammatory drug(s)), in angina pectoris, 345–346, 346t
Nurse(s), substance abuse by, 42–44, 43t
Nursing, expanded roles in, and liability, 30–32
Nursing care, standards of, as legal issue, 25–26
  stress-coping framework and, 52–56
Nursing care plan, for human immunodeficiency virus disease, 1251t–1254t
  for ineffective coping, 61t
Nursing ethics, 15–16, *16.* See also *Ethics.*
Nursing practice, vs. medical practice, 31
Nutrient(s), metabolism of, 1051–1053
  reabsorption of, 883
Nutrition, and complications from anesthesia, 1444
  energy sources in, 994
Nutrition and nutritional support. See also *Enteral nutrition; Total parenteral nutrition (TPN).*
  and immunocompetence, 1188
  and wound healing, 1263–1264
  assessment in, 997–1000, 998t, 999t
  choice of modality in, 1000
  deficiencies in, signs and symptoms of, 998t
  for patient with cardiac assist device, 243
  goals of, 997
  in acquired immunodeficiency syndrome, 1240, 1250
  in acute pancreatitis, 1100
  in acute renal failure, 935, 944t
  in acute respiratory failure, 650t
  in adrenal crisis, 1132t–1133t
  in adult respiratory distress syndrome, 673–674, 683t
  in brain ischemia, 768
  in burns, 1305t
    during acute (fluid mobilization) phase, 1299
    during emergent (shock) phase, 1294–1295, 1295t
    during rehabilitation phase, 1299
  in cardiac disease, 1017
  in cardiac surgery patient, 514t–515t

Nutrition (*continued*)
in chronic obstructive pulmonary disease, 611
in chronic renal failure, 957, 971t
in cirrhosis, 1087t
in critical care phase of trauma, 1355–1356
in diabetic ketoacidosis, 1110, 1117t
in elderly persons, 1501
in gastrointestinal bleeding, 1043t
in granulocytopenia, 1209–1210
in Guillain-Barré syndrome, 837–838, 841t
in head injury, 776t
in heart failure, 408t
in hepatic disease, 1018–1019
in human immunodeficiency virus disease, 1240, 1250
in interleukin-2 therapy, 1221
in mechanically ventilated patient, 707t, 1017–1018
in myocardial infarction, 375t
in obstetric crisis, 1471t
in portal hypertension, 1087t
in pulmonary disease, 1017–1018
in renal failure, 1018
in superior vena cava syndrome, 1486
in systemic inflammatory response syndrome, 1369
in vascular emergencies, 553t
in wound healing, 1274
legal issues in, 997
Nystatin, 1246t

Obesity, and hypertension, 525
Obliterative bronchiolitis, after lung transplantation, 504
Obstetric crisis, nursing care plan for, 1470t–1475t. See also Amniotic fluid embolism; *Preeclampsia.*
comfort measures in, 1473t
diagnostic procedures in, 1475t
fluid balance in, 1470t–1471t
impaired mobility in, 1472t
nutritional support in, 1471t
oxygenation in, 1472t
psychosocial needs in, 1474t–1475t
safety measures in, 1474t
skin integrity in, 1473t
Obstructive jaundice, 1051
Obstructive shock, 1379
Occipital lobe, 730, *730*
tumors in, signs of, 849
Occupational hazard(s), 36–44
chemical, 40
from chemical dependency, 42–44, 43t
from noise, 41–42, 42t
from radiation, *40*, 40–41
infectious, 36–37
musculoskeletal injuries, 37–39, 38t, 39t
Occupational irritant(s), and asthma, 613t
Octreotide, 1246t
Oculomotor nerve, 745t
Oculovestibular reflex, 756
and brain death criteria, 805
Odontoid process, 736
O_{2e} (oxygen extraction), 250–251
Ohm's law, and blood flow, 312t, 312–313
Ointment(s), for wound healing, 1272t, 1272–1273
Olfactory nerve, 745t
Oligodendroglia, 717, *718*
Oligodendroglioma(s), 847–848
Oliguria, in acute tubular necrosis, 932
in preeclampsia, 1461
Oliguric acute renal failure, and hyperkalemia, 911
Omeprazole, for gastrointestinal bleeding, 1035
Oncologic emergency(ies). See *Cancer.*
Oncotic pressure, 566
plasma protein, 893
Opioid(s), 1400t, 1400–1402, 1401t
endogenous, 1393
Optic nerve, 745t
Oral contraceptive(s), and hemorrhagic stroke, 796
and hypertension, 525, 532
Ordinary care, withdrawal of, 34
Organ donation, 1192–1204
alternative sources for, 1193–1194
bereavement and, 1200
consent methods in, 1194–1195
donor management in, 1199–1200
eligibility criteria for, 1197t, 1199t
family reactions to, 1200
family support in, 1196–1199
mandated choice legislation for, 1195
psychosocial implications of, for staff, 1200, 1202
referral in, 1196–1197
religious beliefs and, 1197–1198
required request legislation for, 1194
role of nursing in, 1195–1196
shortages of organs for, 1192–1193
surgical aspects of, 1202–1204
Organ procurement, brain death and, 807
in cardiac transplantation, 496–497
in lung transplantation, 496–497, 500–501, 501t
in non–heart-beating donors, 809, 1193
Organ transplantation. See also under specific organ(s).
transmission of human immunodeficiency virus via, 1233
Oropharyngeal airway(s), in acute ventilatory failure, 639, 640t
Orthostatic capacity, impaired mobility and, 1314–1315
Oscillating bed(s), for pressure ulcer prevention, 1328, *1328*
Oscillator ventilation, high-frequency, 274t, 282
Osmolality, disorders of, 900t, 900–906. See also *Hypernatremia; Hyponatremia.*
fluid volume and, 894–906, 895t
of plasma, 900t, 900–901
Osmosis, renal tubular reabsorption by, 881, *881*
Osmotic diuretic(s), effect on proximal tubule, 884
for prevention of acute renal failure, 933
in diabetic ketoacidosis, 1109–1110
mechanism of action of, 888t
Osmotic pressure, colloidal, and pulmonary fluid movement, 658
Osteodystrophy, renal, 960–961
Otitis media, from enteral nutrition, 1008
Output communication channel(s), 76
Overdose. See *Drug overdose* and specific drug(s).
Overdrive suppression, 134
Overflow theory, of ascites formation, 1070
Oversensing, in pacemakers, 189, 195, *196–197*
Oxandrolone, 1246t
Oxidative phosphorylation, 584
Oxidizing agent(s), chemical burns from, 1279
Oximetry, 247–249
Oxygen, and wound healing, 1262–1263
arterial, and intrapulmonary shunting, 253–256, *254*, 254t
partial pressure of, 246–247
concentration of, as stimulus for breathing, 587
diffusion of, 574–576, *575*
inspired, fraction of, in acute respiratory failure, 639–640, 641t
partial pressure of, and arterial oxygenation failure, 632, 632t
metabolic requirements for, in adult respiratory distress syndrome, 674–675
myocardial consumption of, 324
in angina pectoris, 343
in myocardial infarction, 357
in myocardial ischemia, 337–338
toxic metabolites of, in adult respiratory distress syndrome, 664, 669
Oxygen balance, 250–253, *253*
Oxygen consumption ($\dot{V}O_2$), assessment of, 249–250
from work of breathing, 571
in adult respiratory distress syndrome, 666
in shock, 1372t–1373t, *1372–1373*, 1372–1373
management of, in acute respiratory failure, 644
monitoring of, in acute respiratory failure, 638
Oxygen delivery (DO_2), failure of, in acute respiratory failure, 633–635, *634*, 634t, 639–640, 641t
in adult respiratory distress syndrome, 666, 676
in shock, 1372–1373, *1373*
management of, in acute respiratory failure, 644
monitoring of, in acute respiratory failure, 638
Oxygen demand theory, in local blood pressure regulation, 328
Oxygen extraction (O_{2e}), 250–251
Oxygen radical(s), in systemic inflammatory response syndrome, 1361
Oxygen saturation, arterial, 247–248
in head injury, 760
jugular venous, for monitoring cerebral blood flow, 292
mixed venous. See *Mixed venous oxygen saturation* ($S\bar{v}O_2$).
Oxygen transport (DO_2), 577–578, *577–578*
assessment of, 249–253, *253*
2,3-diphosphoglycerate and, 578, *578*
measurement of, 245t, 245–246
Oxygenation, 245–249
after cardiac surgery, 515t
after lung transplantation, 503
arterial, and acute respiratory failure, 632t, 632–633, 639–640
in acute respiratory failure, 639–640
determinants of, 245t, 245–247, *247*
hyperbaric, in spinal cord injury, 824
in acute pancreatitis, 1101
in acute renal failure, 945t
in acute respiratory failure, 635t, 635–636, 639–640, 641t, 651t–652t
in adrenal crisis, 1133t

Oxygenation (*continued*)
in adult respiratory distress syndrome, 671–674, 684t–685t
in brain ischemia, 766
in burn patient, 1306t
in chronic obstructive pulmonary disease, 609–610
in chronic renal failure, 972t
in cirrhosis, 1088t
in diabetic ketoacidosis, 1118t
in gastrointestinal bleeding, 1044t
in Guillain-Barré syndrome, 842t
in head injury, 760, 777t
in heart failure, 409t
in mechanically ventilated patient, 708t–709t
in myocardial infarction, 376t–377t
in obstetric crisis, 1472t
in portal hypertension, 1088t
in systemic inflammatory response syndrome, 1369
in vascular emergencies, 554t
intravascular, 275t
lactate levels and, 252–253, 1371–1372
measurement of, pulse oximetry in, 247–249
oxyhemoglobin and, *247*, 247–248, *249*
Oxygenator(s), for cardiopulmonary bypass, 474
Oxygram(s), 253, *253*
Oxyhemoglobin, *247*, 247–248, *249*
Oxyhemoglobin dissociation curve, *247*, 577, *577*
Oxytocin, for uterine atony, in preeclampsia, 1466

Paced depolarization integral, 176
Pacemaker(s), 167–200
and endocardial evoked potential, 176
and QT/stimulus-t interval, 176
body temperature and, 176–177
dual-sensor, 177
function of, electrocardiographic interpretation of, 191–196
crosstalk in, 196, *197*
dual-chamber, 191–192, *192*
failure to capture, 195, *196*
failure to output pulse, 195, *195*
failure to sense, 195, *196–197*
pacemaker-mediated tachycardia, 195–196
single-chamber, 191, 191t, *192*
upper rate operation in, 193–195, *194–195*
history of, 167
minute ventilation and, 177
NASPE/BPEG code for, 167, 169, 169t
permanent, 167–174
batteries for, 170
circuitry for, 170
clinical management in, 174
ICHD code for, 167
indications for, 167, 168t
insertion of, 170–172, *171*
lead impedance of, 171
lead/electrode systems for, 170
leads for, active vs. passive fixation of, 172–173, *172–173*
steroid-eluting, 173
unipolar vs. bipolar, 172, *173*
pacing threshold of, 171, *172*
power source for, 169–170
pulse amplitude of, 172
pulse generators for, 169, *170*
respiration and, 177
right ventricular pressure and, 177
temporary, 177–190
epicardial, 182–185
application of wires in, 182–183
atrial electrogram with, 183t, 183–184, *184–185*
electrical safety in, 185
modes of, 183, 183t
rapid atrial pacing in, 184
removal of wires in, 185
indications for, 178
transcutaneous, 178–182, *179*
advantages of, 179t, 179–180
disadvantages of, 180, 180t
documentation in, 182t
equipment for, 180, 181, *181*
indications for, 179, 179t
initiation of, 180t, 180–182, *181–182*, 182t
transvenous, *186–188*, 186–189, 188t, 189t
catheters for, 186, *186*
complications of, 189
insertion of, 186–187
intracardiac electrocardiography for, 187, *188*
modes for, 187, 189, 190t
pulse generators for, 186, *187*
sensitivity thresholds in, 187, *188*, 189t
stimulation thresholds for, 187, 188t
Pacemaker cell(s), action potential of, 132–133, *133*
Pacemaker syndrome, 175
Pacemaker-mediated tachycardia, 195–196
Pacing, atrial overdrive, after cardiopulmonary bypass, 485, *486*
physiologic, 174–177
normal, 174
rate-adaptive, 175–177
sensors for, 175–177
single-chamber, hemodynamic aspects of, 174–175
temporary, modes of, 190t, 191–192, *192–193*
terminology in, 190t
Pacing artifact(s), 190t
Pacing thermodilution catheter, for pulmonary artery pressure monitoring, 210
Pacing threshold, of permanent pacemakers, 171, *172*
PaCO_2 (partial pressure of carbon dioxide). See *Partial pressure of carbon dioxide (PaCO_2).*
PAF (platelet activating factor). See *Platelet activating factor (PAF).*
Pain, adverse physiologic effects of, 1395
and endogenous analgesic mechanisms, 1393–1394
anxiety and, 1383
assessment of, 1395–1399, *1396–1397*
gender and, 1398–1399
in children, 1398
in elderly persons, 1398
questionnaires for, *1396–1397*, 1396–1398
chronic vs. acute, 1384
cost of, 1386
critical care environment and, 1383–1384
cultural factors in, 1381–1382
definitions of, 1381
dehumanizing effect of, 1386
description of, in myocardial infarction, 357–358
historical perspective on, 1381
in Guillain-Barré syndrome, 832, 836
pathophysiology of, 1389–1395
biochemical mediators in, 1392–1393, *1393*
nociceptors in, 1389–1390
physiologic parameters in, 1390, *1390–1391*
spinal cord in, 1390, *1390*
transmission pathways in, 1390–1392
phantom, 1384
physiologic responses to, 1394–1395
psychological factors in, 1382–1383
referred, 1385, *1385*
theories of, 1386–1389
affect, 1386
behaviorist, 1388
endogenous opiate, 1388–1389
gate control, 1387–1388, *1387–1388*
pattern, 1386–1387
specificity, 1386
Pain management, 53, 1399–1409
ethical issues in, 1409
holistic nursing and, 53
in acute pancreatitis, 1101, 1101t
in burns, during acute (fluid mobilization) phase, 1298
during emergent (shock) phase, 1294
during rehabilitation phase, 1299
in coagulopathy, 1160
in myocardial infarction, 368
in superior vena cava syndrome, 1486–1487
nonpharmacologic, 1406–1409
acupuncture/acupressure for, 1407–1408
biofeedback for, 1408
hypnosis for, 1408–1409
relaxation techniques for, 53, 1408
transcutaneous electrical nerve stimulation for, 1407
patient education and, 53
pharmacologic, 1399–1406
analgesic adjuvants for, 1403
anesthetics for, 1404
methods of administration in, 1404–1406, *1405*, 1405t
narcotic analgesics for, 1400t, 1400–1402, 1401t
nonnarcotic analgesics for, 1402–1403
Palpation, for liver function assessment, 1055
PAM (mean pulmonary artery pressure). See *Mean pulmonary artery pressure (PAM).*
Pamidronate, for hypercalcemia, from cancer, 1489, 1490t
Pancreas, anatomy and physiology of, 992
physiology of, *1092*
secretions of, regulation of, *1092*
Pancreatic polypeptide, 982t
Pancreatic transplantation, 1113–1114
Pancreatitis, acute, 1091–1103
and hypocalcemia, 914, 914t
clinical management of, 1099–1102, 1101t
clinical presentation in, 1092–1094
complications of, 1094t
diagnosis of, 1094–1097
barium studies in, 1095
computed tomography in, 1096–1097, *1097–1098*

Pancreatitis, diagnosis of (*continued*)
endoscopic retrograde cholangiopancreatography in, 1095
laboratory studies in, 1094t, 1094–1095, 1096t
magnetic resonance imaging in, 1097
ultrasonography in, 1095
pathophysiology of, 1091–1092, *1092–1093*
precipitating causes of, 1092, 1094t
prognosis in, 1097–1099, 1099t
surgical management of, 1102–1103
with pseudocysts, 1102–1103
with abscess, 1102
with gallstones, 1102
Pancuronium bromide (Pavulon), for cranial surgery, 853t
for neuromuscular blockade, in emergency care phase of trauma, 1346
Panlobular emphysema, 607, *607*
Pa_{O_2} (partial pressure of arterial oxygen). See *Partial pressure of arterial oxygen (Pa_{O_2}).*
Papillary muscle(s), dysfunction of, and mitral regurgitation, 430
Papilledema, intracranial pressure and, 295
Paracentesis, for ascites, 1071
Paradysrhythmia(s), electrocardiography in, 163–165, *164*
Paralysis, from spinal cord compression, in cancer, *1481*
of extremities, hyperkalemia and, 910t, 911
pharmacologic. See *Neuromuscular blockade.*
respiratory, hypermagnesemia and, 923–924
Paralytic ileus, 986
Parasympathetic nervous system, 744, *747*, 748
cardiac innervation by, 131
in cardiac conduction, 319, *319*
Parasystole, electrocardiography in, 164, *164*
Parathyroid gland, dysfunction of, and hypocalcemia, 914, 914t
Parathyroid hormone (PTH), and calcium regulation, 913
and magnesium regulation, 921
in hyperkalemia, 910
in phosphate regulation, 918
Parenteral nutrition, 1014–1017, 1015t. See also *Total parenteral nutrition (TPN).*
total, and hypophosphatemia, 918t, 919
Paresthesias, hyperkalemia and, 910t, 911
Parietal lobe(s), 729, *730*
tumors in, signs of, 849
Parietal pleura, 567–568
Paromomycin sulfate (Humatin, Aminosidine), 1246t
Partial pressure of arterial oxygen (Pa_{O_2}), 246–247, 576
and intrapulmonary shunting, 253–256, *254*, 254t
in acute pancreatitis, 1096t
Partial pressure of atmosphere, 575
Partial pressure of carbon dioxide (Pa_{CO_2}), 576
in estimation of dead space-to-tidal volume ratio, 256–259, *259*
increasing, in respiratory alkalosis, 596
Partial pressure of inspired oxygen (P_{IO_2}), and arterial oxygenation failure, 632, 632t
Partial thromboplastin time (PTT), 1052
Partial-thickness burn(s), 1281–1282
Partial-thickness wound(s), healing of, 1260–1261, 1265
PASG (pneumatic antishock garment), 1348
Passive immunity, 1184–1185
Passy-Muir speaking valve, 700, *701–702*
Paternalism, in ethics, 19
Patient(s), environmental stressors of, 55
psychosocial needs of, 49–62. See also *Psychosocial need(s) (patient).*
Patient education, about craniotomy, 860
about Guillain-Barré syndrome, 838
about heart failure, 402t, 402–403
after renal transplantation, 965–966
and pain management, 53
in diabetes mellitus, 1111
in severe hypoglycemia, 1113
Patient-controlled analgesia (PCA), 1404, *1405*
Pattern theory, of pain, 1386–1387
PAWP (pulmonary artery wedge pressure). See *Pulmonary artery wedge pressure (PAWP).*
PCA (patient-controlled analgesia), 1404, *1405*
PCR (polymerase chain reaction), in isolation and quantitation of human immunodeficiency virus, 1230–1231
PDF (probable density function), implantable cardioverter-defibrillators and, 199
PDGF (platelet-derived growth factor), in atherosclerosis, 337
Pedicle(s), vertebral, 738
PEEP (positive end-expiratory pressure). See *Positive end-expiratory pressure (PEEP).*
PEG (percutaneous endoscopic gastrostomy) tube(s), 1003t, 1004
PEG-J (percutaneous endoscopic gastrostomy-jejunostomy) tube(s), 1006
Penetrating trauma. See *Trauma, penetrating.*
Pentamidine, 1246t
Pentobarbital, for cranial surgery, 853t
Peptic ulcer disease, and gastrointestinal bleeding, *1024*, 1024–1025, 1025t
Peptide(s), gastrointestinal, 982, *982*, 982t, 983t
Peptide T, 1246t
Perception, elements of, 91
Percussion, for liver function assessment, 1054–1055, *1055*
Percussion wave, in intracranial pressure monitoring, 301, *302*
Percutaneous endoscopic gastrostomy (PEG) tube(s), 1003t, 1004
Percutaneous endoscopic gastrostomy-jejunostomy (PEG-J) tube(s), 1006
Percutaneous transluminal coronary angioplasty (PTCA), failure of, coronary artery bypass grafting after, 463
in angina pectoris, 346–348
in myocardial infarction, 367–368
in myocardial ischemia, 346–348
vs. coronary artery bypass grafting, 459t–460t, 459–460
with cardiac catheterization, *341*, 341–342
Perfusion pressure, cerebral, 292
Perfusion scintigraphy, in myocardial infarction, 363
Pericardial tamponade, in emergency care phase of trauma, 1348
Pericarditis, in chronic renal failure, 955
Perikaryon, neuronal, 718, *721*
Peripheral nerve(s), anatomy of, *831*
injury of, from cardiopulmonary bypass, 492
impaired mobility and, 1319, *1319*
Peripheral nerve block(s), 1443t
Peripheral nervous system, 741–742, 743t
Peripheral neuropathy, in chronic renal failure, 960
Peripheral tissue, decreased perfusion of, hypophosphatemia and, 919–920
Peritoneal dialysis, 951–953
for hypermagnesemia, 923
in acute renal failure, 937, 937t
Peritoneal lavage, in acute pancreatitis, 1101
Peritoneovenous shunt, for ascites, 1071–1072, *1072*
Peritonitis, with ascites, 1071
Persistent generalized lymphadenopathy (PGL), in human immunodeficiency virus disease, 1234
PET (positron emission tomography). See *Positron emission tomography (PET).*
P_{ETCO_2} (end-tidal carbon dioxide), analysis of, 258–259, *259*
pH, calculation of, 583
gastric, and pneumonia, 622
in confirmation of nasoenteric tube placement, 1002
in mixed acid-base disorders, 600
of blood, in acid-base status assessment, 590, 590t
of body fluids, 585, 585t
Phagocyte(s), granulocytic, 1174–1175
mononuclear, 1171–1172, 1173t–1174t
Phagocytosis, and internal immunity, 1179–1180, *1180*
Phantom pain, 1384
Pharmacologic paralysis. See *Neuromuscular blockade.*
Phenobarbital, and hypocalcemia, 914
Phentolamine, for hypertensive crisis, 530, 531t, 532
Phenytoin, and hypocalcemia, 914
for brain ischemia, 767
for head injury, 762
Pheochromocytoma(s), and hypertension, 526, 532–533
Phlebostatic axis, 203, *204*
Phonocardiography, in aortic regurgitation, 446
in aortic stenosis, 449
in mitral regurgitation, 433
in mitral stenosis, 441
in pulmonic stenosis, 456
in tricuspid regurgitation, 451
Phosphatase(s), levels of, 1055, 1056t
Phosphate, 918–921
disorders of. See *Hyperphosphatemia; Hypophosphatemia.*

Phosphate (*continued*)
intravenous administration of, for hypercalcemia, 917
physiologic role of, 918
regulation of, 918
Phosphate binder(s), for hyperphosphatemia, 920
Phosphate buffer system, 586, 588, *589*, 889, *889*
Phospholipase, and pancreatitis, 1092
Phosphorus, for hypercalcemia, from cancer, 1490t
levels of, in chronic renal failure, 952t
Photocoagulation, of gastrointestinal bleeding, 1035
Phrenic nerve, injury of, from cardiopulmonary bypass, 490
Physical limitation(s), as barriers to communication, 79–80
Physician(s), and home care team, 119
practice areas of, trends in, 5
Physiologic arousal, stress-coping framework and, interventions for, 57
Physiologic dead space, 573
Physiotherapy, chest, for ventilation-perfusion abnormalities, in acute respiratory failure, 640–641
for burn patient, 1300–1301
Pia mater, spinal, 738–739
Pica, in hypokalemia, 907
Pierce-Donachy Ventricular Assist Pump, *236*, 236–237, 237t
P_{IO_2} (partial pressure of inspired oxygen), and arterial oxygenation failure, 632, 632t
PIP (positive inspiratory pressure). See *Positive inspiratory pressure (PIP).*
Pitressin. See *Vasopressin.*
Pituitary gland, 732
hormones secreted by, 1122
surgery on, craniotomy for, 851
tumors of, 848
Pituitary hormone(s), 732
Plaque(s), fibrous, in atherosclerosis, 336–337, 783–784
in myocardial infarction, 354–355, *355*
Plasma, osmolality of, 900–901
Plasma coagulation factor(s), in hemostasis, 1142t, 1142–1143, *1143*
Plasma protein(s), metabolism of, 1052
oncotic pressure of, 893
Plasma sodium, in hyponatremia, 903, 903t
Plasmalyte-A, 897t
Plasmapheresis, therapeutic, for Guillain-Barré syndrome, 834, *834*
Plateau wave(s), in intracranial pressure monitoring, 301–302, *302*
Platelet(s), aggregation of, in hemostasis, 1142, *1142*
aggregration of, in disseminated intravascular coagulation, 1149
in chronic renal failure, 959
production of, 1141
Platelet activating factor (PAF), in adult respiratory distress syndrome, 664–665
Platelet antiaggregant agent(s), in angina pectoris, 345–346, 346t
Platelet count, in thrombocytopenia, 1155–1156, 1156t
Platelet dysfunction, cardiopulmonary bypass and, 488
Platelet-derived growth factor (PDGF), in atherosclerosis, 337
Pleura, parietal, 567–568
visceral, 567–568
Pleural effusion, in chronic renal failure, 956–957
with ascites, 1070–1071
Plexus(es), venous, in spinal blood supply, *737*, 739, 743t
Plicamycin, for hypercalcemia, 917
from cancer, 1490t
PML (progressive multifocal leukoencephalopathy), with human immunodeficiency virus infection, 1238
PMNs (polymorphonuclear leukocytes), and adult respiratory distress syndrome, *661–662*, 661–665, 669
Pneumatic antishock garment (PASG), 1348
Pneumocephalus, tension, after cranial surgery, 858–859
Pneumococcal meningitis, 864
Pneumococcal pneumonia, clinical presentation in, 623
vaccination for, 625–626
Pneumocystis carinii pneumonia, 622, 624–626, 1235
after renal transplantation, 965
Pneumonia, after renal transplantation, 965
airway management in, 625
atypical, 622, 622t
bacterial, 620–624, 621t
clinical presentation in, 622–624, *623*
diagnosis of, 624–625
fluid balance in, 625
impaired mobility and, 1316–1317
incidence of, 620
management of, 625–626, 626t
mechanisms of, 620
nosocomial, 621–622
Pneumocystis carinii, 622, 624–626, 1235
prevention of, 625
viral, 622
Pneumonitis, aspiration, 627–628
Pneumothorax, from positive pressure ventilation, 690
postoperative, from anesthesia, 1453
tension, from positive pressure ventilation, 264
in emergency care phase of trauma, 1347–1348
Poiseuille's law, and blood flow, 312t, 312–313
Poison(s), protoplasmic, chemical burns from, 1279
Policy-making, ethics and, 23
Poliomyelitis, 867
Polymerase chain reaction (PCR), in isolation and quantitation of human immunodeficiency virus, 1230–1231
Polymorphonuclear leukocyte(s) (PMNs), and adult respiratory distress syndrome, *661–662*, 661–665, 669
Polyneuritis, idiopathic, 833
Polyp(s), nasal, and asthma, 613
Polypeptide(s), pancreatic, 982t
Pons (metencephalon), *732*, 733
Porcine cardiac valve(s), *437*
Portacaval shunt(s), 1078, *1079*, 1080
Portal circulation, 1048–1050, *1049–1050*
Portal hypertension, 1063–1064
nursing care plan for, 1086t–1090t
comfort measures in, 1088t
diagnostic procedures in, 1090t
fluid balance in, 1086t–1087t
impaired mobility in, 1087t
nutrition in, 1087t
oxygenation in, 1088t
psychosocial needs in, 1089t–1090t
safety measures in, 1089t
skin integrity in, 1089t
postoperative care in, 1081
surgical treatment of, 1077–1081
anesthesia in, 1078
devascularization procedures for, 1081
evaluation in, 1077–1078
shunts for, 1078–1081, *1079–1080*
splenopancreatic disconnection, 1081
Positioning, and complications from anesthesia, 1449
for craniotomy, 854
in increased intracranial pressure, 304
in pulmonary artery pressure monitoring, 212–213, 215
Positive end-expiratory pressure (PEEP), 266
in adult respiratory distress syndrome, 671–672, 675
Positive inspiratory pressure (PIP), in pressure ventilation, 268
Positive pressure ventilation, 263–264, 272t
high-frequency, 274t, 279–280
pneumothorax from, 690
Positive pressure ventilator(s), 264–265
Positron emission tomography (PET), in head injury, 760
in myocardial infarction, 363
Postconcussion syndrome, 752–753
Postrenal acute renal failure, 926–927, 927t, 930t
Posttraumatic seizure(s), 755, 764
Postural drainage, for ventilation-perfusion abnormalities, in acute respiratory failure, 641
Potassium, and acid-base balance, 588–589
concentration of, in body fluid compartments, 892
excretion of, 906–907
imbalance of. See *Hyperkalemia; Hypokalemia.*
in body fluids, 906–913
in cardiac electrophysiology, 317–318
in diabetic ketoacidosis, 1110
in total parenteral nutrition, 1016
levels of, in chronic renal failure, 952t
loss of, in metabolic alkalosis, 599
physiologic purpose of, 906–907
plasma concentration of, in electrolyte regulation, 907
reabsorption of, 883
Potassium channel(s), in nerve cells, 722, *722*
Potassium replacement, for hypokalemia, 909–910
Potassium-sparing diuretic(s), for heart failure, 391t, 394t, 394–395, *395*, 396t
mechanism of action of, 888t
Potts anastomosis, *418*, 419t
Povidone-iodine, for wound healing, 1272
PPO(s) (preferred provider organizations), 7
Prealbumin, in nutritional assessment, 998
Precordial lead(s), for electrocardiography, 138–139, *138–139*

Prednisone, for human immunodeficiency virus disease, 1246t
Preeclampsia, clinical presentation in, 1460–1462, 1462t
hypermagnesemia in, 923
hypomagnesemia in, 922–923
management of, 1462–1466, 1463t, *1465*
pathophysiology of, 1459t, 1459–1460, *1461,* 1462t
risk factors for, 1458
safe delivery in, *1465,* 1465–1466
Preexcitation syndrome(s), *156–161,* 157–161
aberrant ventricular conduction, 159–161, *160–161*
concealed unidirectional retrograde accessory pathway in, 156–157, *158*
Lown-Ganong-Levine, 156, *157*
Mahaim fibers in, 156, *158*
Wolff-Parkinson-White, 157–159, *158–159*
Preferred provider organization(s) (PPOs), 7
Preganglionic neuron(s), of sympathetic nervous system, 744
Pregnancy, and acute aortic dissection, 540
brain death in, 807
hemorrhagic stroke during, 796
hypertension during, 526, 533, 1458–1466. See also *Preeclampsia.*
normal adaptation to, 1459, 1459t
Preload, and cardiac output, 227–228, 332–333
length-tension relationship in, 321–322, *321–323*
reduction of, in heart failure, 399
Prerenal acute renal failure, 926, 926t
laboratory studies in, 930t
Pressure, in cardiovascular system, 312, 312t, 313t
Pressure assist/control ventilation, 269, 272t
Pressure control ventilation, inverse ratio, 274t, 277–279
Pressure gradient(s), airway resistance and, 570–571
and renal blood flow, 876
lung compliance and, 570–571
ventilation and, 570–571
Pressure support ventilation (PSV), 271, 273t, 276
as weaning modality, 694–695
in acute respiratory failure, 646
Pressure synchronized intermittent mandatory ventilation (SIMV), 269–270, *270,* 272t
Pressure ulcer(s), from impaired mobility, 1319–1320, 1320t, *1320–1321,* 1322t
healing of, 1266–1267, 1267t
management of, 1326–1330, 1327t, *1327–1329,* 1330t
products for, 1330t
Pressure ventilation, 268t, 268–270, *269–270,* 272t
Pressure-cycled ventilator(s), 264–265
Pressure-regulated volume control ventilation, 270, 272t
Pressure-volume loop, in cardiac cycle, 320–321, *321*
Presynaptic terminal(s), in nerve impulse conduction, 722–723
Primary care, incentives for, 6
Primary intention, wound healing by, 1265–1266, 1266t
Primary survey, in trauma, 1342–1343, 1343t
Primitive defense mechanism(s), 60
Prinzmetal angina, 342
electrocardiography in, 148, *148*
Privacy, invasion of, 26t, 28–29
Probable density function (PDF), implantable cardioverter-defibrillators and, 199
Problem-solving, by families in crisis, 67
Procainamide, in sudden death, 351t
Procedural touch, 78
Progressive multifocal leukoencephalopathy (PML), with human immunodeficiency virus disease, 1238
Prolonged inspiratory ventilation, 274t, 277–279
Properdin pathway, in complement system, 1182–1183, 1183t
Propofol, for cranial surgery, 852
Propranolol, for angina pectoris, 344, 346, 346t
for hyperkalemia, 906–907
for mitral valve prolapse, 439
for variceal hemorrhage, 1066–1067
in sudden death, 351t
Prostacyclin, in angina pectoris, 346, 346t
in arachidonic acid cascade, 1361, *1362*
Prostaglandin(s), as pain mediator, 1393
for gastrointestinal bleeding, 1034
in adult respiratory distress syndrome, 664
in arachidonic acid cascade, 1361, *1362*
in fever generation, 1433
in fluid volume regulation, 899
in heart failure, 385
in preeclampsia, 1460
Prostaglandin inhibitor(s), for systemic inflammatory response syndrome, 1370
Prosthesis (prostheses), cardiac. See *Cardiac valve(s), prosthetic.*
Protamine, with cardiopulmonary bypass, complications of, 473
Protease(s), and emphysema, 606, *606*
in adult respiratory distress syndrome, 664
intracellular, activation of, and pancreatitis, 1091
Protective touch, 78–79
Protein(s), and wound healing, 1263
digestion of, 989
for nutrition in hepatic disease, 1018
in complement system, 1182t
metabolism of, 584, 1052
PTH-related, and hypercalcemia, from cancer, 1487
Protein buffer system, 586
Protein/calorie malnutrition, signs and symptoms of, 998t
Proteolytic enzyme(s), for chemical debridement, 1273, 1296–1297
Prothrombin, calcium and, 913
function of, 1144, *1144*
Prothrombin time (PT), 1052
in disseminated intravascular coagulation, 1151, 1151t
Proton beam therapy, for arteriovenous malformations, 799
Proton pump inhibitor(s), for gastrointestinal bleeding, 1035
Protoplasmic poison(s), chemical burns from, 1279
Protozoal infection(s), in acquired immunodeficiency syndrome, 1235–1236
Proximal tubule(s), osmotic diuretics and, 884
reabsorption of fluids in, 883, *883*
Proximity, of family, need for, 70–71
Pruritus, in burns, 1299
in chronic renal failure, 961
in human immunodeficiency virus disease, 1253t
Pseudoaneurysm(s), 535
Pseudocyst(s), pancreatic, 1102–1103
Pseudoparathyroidism, and hypocalcemia, 914, 914t
Pseudostratified columnar ciliated epithelium, 563
PSV (pressure support ventilation). See *Pressure support ventilation (PSV).*
Psychogenic pain, 1382
Psychological stress, and immunocompetence, 1188–1189
Psychosis, in intensive care unit, 57. See also *Sensory-perceptual alteration(s).*
Psychosocial need(s) (family), 65–72
in acute fulminant hepatic failure, 1058–1059
in acute respiratory failure, 646–647
in burns, during rehabilitation phase, 1299–1300, *1300,* 1300t
in chronic renal failure, 961
in myocardial infarction, 370
interventions for, 68–72, 69t
Psychosocial need(s) (patient), 49–62
after cardiac surgery, 421, 517t
before cardiac transplantation, 495–496
holistic approach to, 49–50
in acute renal failure, 947t
in acute respiratory failure, 636, 646–647, 654t–655t
in adrenal crisis, 1135t
in adult respiratory distress syndrome, 687t–688t
in burns, 1308t–1309t
during rehabilitation phase, 1299–1300, *1300,* 1300t
in chronic illness, 112–114
in chronic renal failure, 961, 975t
in cirrhosis, 1089t–1090t
in diabetic ketoacidosis, 1120t
in gastrointestinal bleeding, 1046t
in Guillain-Barré syndrome, 844t–845t
in head injury, 779t
in heart failure, 411t–412t
in impaired mobility, 1322
in mechanically ventilated patient, 712t–713t
in myocardial infarction, 378t
in obstetric crisis, 1474t–1475t
in portal hypertension, 1089t–1090t
in vascular emergencies, 555t–556t
standards of care for, 49
stress-coping framework and, 50–52, *51*
Psychosocial need(s) (staff), in organ donation, 1200, 1202
PT (prothrombin), 1052
PTCA (percutaneous transluminal coronary angioplasty). See *Percutaneous transluminal coronary angioplasty (PTCA).*

PTH (parathyroid hormone). See *Parathyroid hormone (PTH).*
PTH-related protein, and hypercalcemia, from cancer, 1487
PTT (partial thromboplastin time), 1052
Pulmonary angiography, in acute respiratory failure, 639
Pulmonary artery pressure, diastolic, *209*
monitoring of, 208–222, *209*, 210t
catheters for, 209–210, *211–212*
insertion of, 210–212
clinical applications of, 227–230, *230*
contraindications to, 210
dynamic response in, 215–216, *217*
ensuring accuracy of measurements in, 212–213, 215–216
indications for, 210t
patient positioning in, 212–213, 215
potential problems with, 212, 214t–216t
right atrial pressure in, 216, *219*
right ventricular pressure in, 216–217, *219*
waveforms in, *219–220*
west lung zones in, 216, *218*
wedge, *209*
Pulmonary artery thermistor(s), vs. infrared thermometers, 1439t
Pulmonary artery wedge pressure (PAWP), as preload measurement, 227–228
in adult respiratory distress syndrome, *670*, 670–671
monitoring of, 218–219, 221, *221*
Pulmonary capacity, *572*, 572–573
Pulmonary capillary pressure, 566
Pulmonary circulation. See *Circulation, pulmonary.*
Pulmonary disease, chronic obstructive. See *Chronic obstructive pulmonary disease (COPD).*
nutrition in, 1017–1018
Pulmonary edema, 566
after renal transplantation, 964
cardiogenic, vs. adult respiratory distress syndrome, 667, 667t
in acute renal failure, 931–932
in preeclampsia, 1464
neurogenic, after cranial surgery, 858
noncardiogenic. See *Adult respiratory distress syndrome (ARDS).*
pathogenesis of, 659–660, *660*
postoperative, from anesthesia, 1452
Pulmonary embolism, impaired mobility and, 1317, 1324, 1324t
in acute respiratory failure, 637t
in critical care phase of trauma, 1352t, 1352–1353
Pulmonary fluid, movement of, colloidal osmotic pressure and, 658
hydrostatic pressure and, 658
in adult respiratory distress syndrome, 657–659, *658*
Pulmonary function, after renal transplantation, 964
assessment of, in acute respiratory failure, 636, 637t, 638
impaired mobility and, 1315–1317, *1316*, 1330–1331
in burns, during acute (fluid mobilization) phase, 1295
during emergent (shock) phase, *1286*, 1286t–1287t, 1286–1287
in chronic renal failure, 956–957
Pulmonary function test(s), 571–574, *572*
before cardiac surgery, 471
in asthma, 615–616
in chronic bronchitis, 605
in emphysema, 608
Pulmonary functional capacity, *572*, 573
Pulmonary gas exchange, abnormalities of, mechanical ventilation in, 263
Pulmonary hypertension, 228
Pulmonary infection(s). See *Pneumonia.*
Pulmonary interstitium, 657
Pulmonary rehabilitation, in chronic obstructive pulmonary disease, 612, 612t
Pulmonary system, changes in, after cardiopulmonary bypass, 489–490
vascular resistance in, calculation of, 313t
Pulmonary ventilation-perfusion (V/Q) scan(s), in acute respiratory failure, 638–639
Pulmonic regurgitation, 453–455, *454*
Pulmonic stenosis, *455*, 455–456
Pulse, waterhammer/Corrigan, in aortic regurgitation, 445
Pulse amplitude, of permanent pacemakers, 172
Pulse generator(s), for implantable cardioverter-defibrillators, 197, *198*
for pacemakers, permanent, 169, *170*
temporary transvenous, 186, *187*
Pulse oximetry, 247–249
Pulse pressure, 327
in hypovolemic shock, 1030
Pump(s), for cardiopulmonary bypass, 474–476, *475*
Pupillary response, in brain death, 805
in brain ischemia, 765
in head injury, 756
intracranial pressure and, 294
Purkinje fiber(s), 315, *316*
action potential in, 318, *318*
Purkinje system, anatomy and physiology of, *128*, 129–130
Purulent meningitis, 862–864, *863*, 864t
Pyrazinamide (PZA), 1246t
Pyrimethamine (Daraprim), 1246t
Pyrogen(s), endogenous, 1433

Q wave(s), in myocardial infarction, 144–145, *145*, 145t, 361–362
QRS complex, in bundle branch block, 152–154, *153–154*
leads for, 136, *138*
wide, 152–155, *153–154*, *155*
widened, in hyperkalemia, 911, *911*
Qs/Qt (intrapulmonary shunting). See *Intrapulmonary shunting (Qs/Qt).*
QT (cardiac output). See *Cardiac output.*
QT interval, in hypocalcemia, 915
in ventricular dysrhythmias, 162–163, *163*
pacemakers and, 176
shortened, in hyperkalemia, 911, *911*
shortening of, hypercalcemia and, 916, 916t
Quality of life, after coronary artery bypass grafting, 469–470
Quasi-intentional tort(s), 26t, 28–29
Quinapril, for heart failure, 391t
Quinidine, in sudden death, 351t

Racemic epinephrine, for acute respiratory failure, 643t
Radial artery, cannulation of, 206–207
harvesting of, for coronary artery bypass grafting, 465–466
Radiant heat loss, 1431
Radiation, burns from, 1280
occupational exposure to, *40*, 40–41
Radiation therapy, 1477
and wound healing, 1265
for spinal cord compression, 1481–1482
for superior vena cava syndrome, 1484–1485
total body, with bone marrow transplantation, 1216–1217, 1218t
Radicular artery(ies), *737*, 739
Radicular vein(s), *737*, 739
Radiofrequency catheter ablation, of cardiac dysrhythmias, 161
Radiography, in acute renal failure, 931
in acute respiratory failure, 638
in aortic aneurysm, 536
in aortic regurgitation, 445–446
in aortic stenosis, 448–449
in chronic bronchitis, 605, *605*
in emphysema, *607*, 608
in gastrointestinal bleeding, 1031
in head injury, 759
in heart failure, 388
in mitral regurgitation, 432
in mitral stenosis, 441
in pneumonia, *623*, 624
in pulmonic regurgitation, 454
in spinal cord injury, 819, *820*
in tricuspid regurgitation, 451
Radionuclide angiography, in myocardial infarction, 363
Radionuclide imaging, in mitral stenosis, 441
Radionuclide ventriculography (RVG), in heart failure, 388–389
in myocardial ischemia, 339, *340*, 340t
Radioreceptor reflex, in shock, 1373, *1374*
Radiosurgery, stereotactic, for arteriovenous malformations, 799
Rancho Los Amigos Scale, 756, 758t–759t
Ranitidine, for gastrointestinal bleeding, 1033
Ranson's prognostic sign(s), in pancreatitis, 1098, 1099t
RAP (mean right arterial pressure). See *Mean right arterial pressure (RAP).*
Rapid atrial pacing, 184
RAS (reticular activating system), *733*, 736
Rate smoothing, in upper rate operation of pacemakers, 194–195
Rate-adaptive pacemaker(s), 175–177
RBBB (right bundle branch block). See *Bundle branch block, right.*
RBC(s) (red blood cells). See *Red blood cell(s) (RBCs).*
RDS (respiratory distress syndrome), neonatal, 570
Receptive aphasia, 76, 84t
Wernicke's area in, 730
Rectal tube(s), for pressure ulcer prevention, 1329–1330
Red blood cell(s) (RBCs), production of, 1139–1140
Reentry, and sudden death, 350
electrocardiography in, 151–152, *152*
Refeeding syndrome, 1016
Referred pain, 1385, *1385*
Reflection, electrocardiography in, 152, *152*
Reflex(es), brainstem and, *732*, 733, 735
deep tendon, in hypomagnesemia, 923

Reflex arc, 741, *742*
Reflex vasoconstriction, in shock, 1374
Refractory period, 190t
  in cardiac electrophysiology, 134–135, *135, 318*
  of nerve cell, 720
Regional anesthesia, 1443t
Rehabilitation, pulmonary, in chronic obstructive pulmonary disease, 612, 612t
Rejection, after renal transplantation, 964–965, 965t
Relationship(s), therapeutic, caring in, 61–62
Relaxation technique(s), for affective arousal, 58
  for pain management, 53, 1408
Religious belief(s), and organ donation, 1197–1198
Renal. See also entries under *Kidney(s).*
Renal artery, anatomy of, 875
Renal artery pressure, in shock, 1375
Renal biopsy, in acute renal failure, 931
Renal collecting duct(s), anatomy of, 874
Renal corpuscle(s), anatomy of, 873–874
Renal failure, and complications from anesthesia, 1445
  and hypercalcemia, 916t, 916–917
  and hyperkalemia, 910
    albuterol for, 912
  coagulopathy from, 1155
  hypermagnesemia in, 923, 923t
  metabolic acidosis in, 596
  with cardiac assist devices, 242
  with metabolic acidosis, and hypocalcemia, 914, 914t
Renal failure (acute), 926–940
  after aortic aneurysm repair, 538
  clinical management of, 933t, 933–936
    fluid therapy in, 934
    for decreased cardiac output, 935
    for hyperkalemia, 929, 934–935
    for impaired gas exchange, 936
    injury prevention in, 934, 935
    nutrition in, 935
  clinical presentation in, 930–933
    diagnostic studies, 931
    laboratory studies, 930t, 930–931
    physical findings, 931t, 931–932
  complications of, prevention of, 935–936
  dialysis for, 936–939, 937t
  discharge planning after, 939–940
  in critical care phase of trauma, 1354–1355
  nursing care plan for, 942t–948t
    comfort measures in, 946t
    diagnostic procedures in, 948t
    fluid balance in, 942t–944t
    impaired mobility in, 945t
    nutrition in, 944t
    oxygenation in, 945t
    psychosocial needs in, 947t
    safety measures in, 947t
    skin integrity in, 946t
  nutrition in, 1018
  oliguric, and hyperkalemia, 911
  pathophysiology of, 926t–927t, 926–930, *928,* 929t
    metabolic factors in, 928–929, 929t
    vascular factors in, 928–930
  prevention of, 933–934
  tubular factors in, 927–928, *928*
Renal failure (chronic), 949–967
  clinical management of, 953–961
    cardiovascular, 953–956, *956*
    gastrointestinal, 957–958
    hematopoietic, 958–959
    neurologic, 959–960
    pulmonary, 956–957
    skeletal, 960–961
    skin integrity in, 961
  ethical issues in, 961
  historical perspective on, 949
  laboratory values in, 950, 952t
  medications prescribed with, 953t
  nursing care plan for, 969t–976t
    comfort measures in, 973t
    diagnostic procedures in, 976t
    fluid balance in, 969t–970t
    impaired mobility in, 972t
    nutrition in, 971t
    oxygenation in, 972t
    psychosocial needs in, 975t
    safety measures in, 974t–975t
    skin integrity in, 974t
  nutrition in, 1018
  pathophysiology of, 949–950, 950t
  psychosocial factors in, 961
  renal replacement therapy in, 950–953, 952t, 953t
Renal filtration fraction, 880
Renal function, after cardiopulmonary bypass, 490–491
  burns and, 1288–1289
  hypertension and, 529
  in elderly persons, 1501–1502
  in hypernatremia, *904,* 904–905
  positive pressure ventilation and, 264
Renal insufficiency, and hyperkalemia, 911
  and hyperphosphatemia, 920, 920t
Renal medulla, anatomy of, 871–872, *872*
Renal osteodystrophy, 960–961
Renal parenchymal disease, hypertension and, 525–526, 532
Renal replacement therapy, 950–953, 952t, 953t
  continuous, 937–939, *938*
Renal transplantation, 961–966
  and hypercalcemia, 916
  discharge planning after, 965–966
  history of, 962
  nursing care plan for, 969t–976t. See also *Renal failure (chronic).*
  patient education after, 965–966
  postoperative management in, 963–966
    for cardiopulmonary complications, 964
    for fluid and electrolytes, 963–964
  postoperative management of, for central nervous system complications, 964
    for gastrointestinal complications, 964
    for infection, 965, *966*
    for rejection, 964–965, 965t
  pretransplant considerations in, 962
  support groups for, 966
  technique of, 962–963
Renal tubular acidosis, 889–890
Renal tubule(s), anatomy of, 874, *874*
  buffers in, 888–889, *889*
  damage to, and extracellular fluid, 885
  epithelial cells of, regeneration of bicarbonate by, 887–888, *888*
  ischemia of, in acute renal failure, 927–928, *928*
  neuropathy of, and hypercalcemia, 916–917
  reabsorption of fluid by, 880–882, *881*
  secretion by, 882
  transport of substances by, 882–885, *883*
Renal vein(s), anatomy of, 875
Renal volume retention hypothesis, in essential hypertension, 523
Renin-angiotensin system, activation of, in shock, 1374–1375, *1375*
  and blood flow, 330, *330*
  and blood pressure, 521, *521*
Renin-angiotensin-aldosterone system, and renal blood flow, 877–878, *878*
  in gastrointestinal bleeding, 1023
  in heart failure, 384, *385*
Renovascular disease, and hypertension, 526, 532
Reperfusion, after brain ischemia, 765
  cardiac, after myocardial infarction, 365, 368
Reperfusion injury, after cardiopulmonary bypass, 484
Repolarization, 129–130
  of nerve cell, 720
Reproductive function, after bone marrow transplantation, 1217
Required request legislation, for organ donation, 1194
Residual volume, 572, *572*
Resilience, in adaptation to chronic illness, 112
Resin(s), exchange, for hyperkalemia, 912
Resistance, in cardiovascular system, 312, 312t, 313t
Respiration, and pacemakers, 177
  control of, 579–581, *580–581*
  external, 561
  internal, 561
  magnesium and, 921
  spontaneous, testing for, in brain death, 808
  support of, in metabolic acidosis, 598
Respiratory acidosis. See *Acidosis, respiratory.*
Respiratory alkalosis. See *Alkalosis, respiratory.*
Respiratory arrest, hypocalcemia and, 915–916
  in hypermagnesemia, 924
Respiratory cycle, 568–570, *569*
Respiratory decompensation, on mechanical ventilation, 689–692, *691*
Respiratory distress syndrome (RDS), neonatal, 570
Respiratory failure. See also *Acute respiratory failure (ARF).*
  mechanical ventilation in, 263
  with cardiac assist devices, 243
Respiratory function, anesthesia and, 1444, 1447, 1452–1453
  assessment of, in spinal cord injury, 819
  in critical care phase of trauma, 1350–1353, 1351t–1353t
  in elderly persons, 1494t, 1497–1498
  in Guillain-Barré syndrome, 835
  in head injury, 757
  in spinal cord injury, 823
  monitoring of, in stroke, 799
Respiratory gas(es), diffusion of, 574–576, *575*
  exchange of, anatomic aspects of, 565, *565*
  transport of, 576–579
    carbon dioxide, 578–579, *579*
    oxygen, 577–578, *577–578*

Respiratory membrane(s), ultrastructure of, *566*
Respiratory monitoring, 245–260
dead space-to-tidal volume ratio estimation in, 256–259, *259*
exhaled gas analysis in, 258–259
intrapulmonary shunt estimation in, 253–256, *254*, 254t
oxygen transport in, 249–253, *253*
oxygenation in, 245–249. See also *Oxygenation.*
Respiratory muscle(s), dysfunction of, in Guillain-Barré syndrome, 835
weakness of, and failure to wean from mechanical ventilation, 696
Respiratory paralysis, in hypermagnesemia, 923
Respiratory system. See also Bronchus (bronchi); specific parts, e.g., *Lung(s).*
anatomy of, 561–565, *562–564*
lower, 562, *563*
upper, 561–562, *562*
and acid-base balance, 586–587
conduction portion of, histology of, 563–565, *564*
physiology of. See *Circulation, pulmonary; Respiration; Respiratory gas(es); Ventilation.*
Resting membrane potential, calcium in, 913
in cardiac electrophysiology, 317–318, *318*
"Restless leg syndrome," in chronic renal failure, 960
Reticular activating system (RAS), *733*, 736
Reticular formation, 736
Revascularization, surgical. See *Coronary artery bypass grafting (CABG).*
Rewarming, methods for, 1436, *1437*
Rhabdomyolysis, and hypermagnesemia, 923, 923t
and hyperphosphatemia, 920, 920t
and hypocalcemia, 914
hypokalemia and, 909
Rheumatic disease, and aortic regurgitation, 443, *443*
and mitral regurgitation, 429, *429*
and mitral stenosis, 438–439
and tricuspid regurgitation, 449, *450*
in aortic stenosis, 447, *447*
Rhinencephalon, 730
Rib cage, and ventilation, 567–568, *568*
Ricket(s), vitamin D-resistant, and hypophosphatemia, 918–919
Rifabutin (Ansamycin), 1246t
Rifampin, 1247t
Right atrial pressure, monitoring of, 216, *219*
Right bundle branch (RBB), anatomy and physiology of, 129
Right bundle branch block (RBBB). See *Bundle branch block, right.*
Right gastroepiploic artery, harvesting of, for coronary artery bypass grafting, 466
Right ventricular ejection fraction/volumetric catheter(s), 210, *212*
Right ventricular pressure, monitoring of, 216–217, *219*
Right ventricular stroke work (RVSW), calculation of, 229
Ringer's solution, lactated, 897t
Roller pump, for cardiopulmonary bypass, 474–475, *475*
Rotation, in electrocardiography, 141, *142*
Roux-en-Y jejunostomy, 1006
Rule of nines, *1283*
RVG (radionuclide ventriculography). See *Radionuclide ventriculography (RVG).*
RVSW (right ventricular stroke work), calculation of, 229
R-wave progression, 139, *139*

S wave(s), hypercalcemia and, 916
SA node. See *Sinus (SA) node.*
Saccular aneurysm(s), 535, 792, *792*
Sacral nerve(s), 743t
Sacral vertebra(e), *734–736*, 736, 738
Safety, electrical, in epicardial pacing, 185
Safety measure(s), after cardiac surgery, 517t
in acute renal failure, 947t
in acute respiratory failure, 654t
in adrenal crisis, 1134t–1135t
in adult respiratory distress syndrome, 687t
in burn patient, 1307t–1308t
in chronic renal failure, 974t–975t
in cirrhosis, 1089t
in diabetic ketoacidosis, 1119t
in gastrointestinal bleeding, 1046t
in Guillain-Barré syndrome, 844t
in head injury, 779t
in heart failure, 411t
in mechanically ventilated patient, 711t
in myocardial infarction, 378t
in obstetric crisis, 1474t
in portal hypertension, 1089t
in vascular emergencies, 555t
Sagittal sinus(es), inferior, anatomy of, 725, *728*
Salicylate(s), overdose of, 1421–1423, 1423t
Salicylate poisoning, and metabolic acidosis, 597
Saline, for hypercalcemia, from cancer, 1490t
infusion of, in hypernatremia, 905–906
Saline diuresis, for hypercalcemia, 917
Saline infusion test, hypertonic, 1123
Saline solution(s), for fluid therapy, 897t
for hypermagnesemia, 923
for hyponatremia, 903
Salt. See *Sodium.*
Sa_{O_2} (arterial oxygen saturation), 247–248
Saphenous vein, harvesting of, for coronary artery bypass grafting, 464, *464*, 468, *468–469*, *481*
Sarcolemma, in cardiac electrophysiology, 132
Sarcoma, Kaposi's, 1238–1239
Scalp, lacerations of, 750
Schwann cell(s), *720–721*
Scintigraphy, perfusion, in myocardial infarction, 363
Sclerotherapy, endoscopic injection, for variceal hemorrhage, 1065–1066
SCUF (slow continuous ultrafiltration), 938–939, 939t
Secondary intention, wound healing by, 1266, 1266t
Secondary survey, in trauma, 1343–1350, 1344t–1345t, 1347t
Secretin, 982, 983t
Sedation, techniques of, 1443t
Seizure(s), 770t, 770–772, 772t, 849–850
after cranial surgery, 857
from cocaine overdose, 1418, 1419
from hypernatremia, 905
from hypocalcemia, 915
in cerebral vascular malformations, 795
in preeclampsia, prevention of, 1463t, 1463–1464
posttraumatic, 755, 764
Selective shunt(s), for portal hypertension, *1080*, 1080–1081
Self-care deficit, in brain ischemia, 767
in spinal cord injury, 828–829
Self-determination, in ethics, 18
Self-efficacy, in chronic illness, 113, 114t
Sengstaken-Blakemore tube, for balloon tamponade of variceal hemorrhage, *1068*, 1068–1069
Sensitivity threshold(s), in temporary transvenous pacing, 187, *188*, 189t
Sensory deprivation, 93–96
altered time perception and, 95
immobility and, 94
neuromuscular blockade and, 94–95
windowless units and, 96
Sensory input, impaired, in elderly persons, 1499
Sensory overload, 96–98
Sensory-perceptual alteration(s), 89–105
as nursing diagnosis, 92t, 92–93
critical care environment and, 90–91, 91t
from impaired mobility, 1322, 1332
in critical illness, 92
in diabetic ketoacidosis, 1110–1111
in human immunodeficiency virus disease, 1251t
in severe hypoglycemia, 1113
interventions for, 98–100
research on, 93, 94t, *95*
shielding in, 99
Sepsis, in critical care phase of trauma, 1353–1354
Septic shock. See *Systemic inflammatory response syndrome (SIRS).*
Septostomy, atrial, balloon, 417–418, 419t
Sequential cardiopulmonary bypass grafting, 479, *482*
Serotonin, action of, 723
and sleep, 100–101
as pain mediator, 1392
Serum amylase, in pancreatitis, 1094t, 1094–1095
Serum calcium, in acute pancreatitis, 1096t
Serum glucose, in acute pancreatitis, 1096t
Serum glutamic oxaloacetic transferase (SGOT), in myocardial infarction, 360
Serum hepatitis, 1061
Serum lipase, in pancreatitis, 1094t, 1095
Serum methemalbumin, in acute pancreatitis, 1096t
Service network(s), integrated, 7
Sexual dysfunction, in spinal cord injury, 829
SGOT (serum glutamic oxaloacetic transferase), in myocardial infarction, 360
Shearing force(s), and pressure ulcers, 1320
Shielding, in sensory-perceptual alteration, 99
in sleep pattern disturbance, 104, 104t
Shingles, 867
with human immunodeficiency virus disease, 1238

Shivering, as thermoregulatory mechanism, 1432
Shock, and adult respiratory distress syndrome, 661
  cardiogenic, 1376–1378, *1377*, 1377t
    coronary artery bypass grafting for, 463
    in myocardial infarction, 360
  classification of, 1375–1379, 1376t
  compensatory mechanisms in, 1373–1375
    hormonal, 1374–1375, *1375*
  definition of, 1371, 1371t
  distributive, 1378–1379
  from burns. See *Burn(s), emergent (shock) phase of.*
  gastrointestinal function in, 1379
  hemorrhagic, from gastrointestinal bleeding, 1023t, 1023–1024
  hypovolemic, 1375–1376, 1376t
    after cranial surgery, 858
    from gastrointestinal bleeding, 1023t, 1023–1024, 1030
    in emergency care phase of trauma, 1349
  liver dysfunction in, 1379
  obstructive, 1379
  pathophysiology of, 1371–1373
  septic. See *Systemic inflammatory response syndrome (SIRS).*
  vs. brain death, 806
Shunt(s), for congenital heart defects, 417–419, *418*, 419t
  for portal hypertension, 1078–1081, *1079–1080*
  peritoneovenous, for ascites, 1071–1072, *1072*
SIADH (syndrome of inappropriate antidiuretic hormone secretion). See *Syndrome of inappropriate antidiuretic hormone secretion (SIADH).*
Sick euthyroid syndrome, 1125
Side-to-side portacaval shunt(s), 1078, *1079*, 1080
Sildimac, for burn wounds, 1298
Silent myocardial infarction, 358
Silver nitrate, for burn wounds, 1297t
Silver sulfadiazine (Silvadene), for burn wounds, 1297t
SIMV (synchronized intermittent mandatory ventilation). See *Synchronized intermittent mandatory ventilation (SIMV).*
Single photon emission computed tomography (SPECT), in head injury, 760
Single-breath nitrogen analysis, *573*, 573–574
Sinus (venous), cerebral, 725, *728*
Sinus (SA) node, 315, *316*
  action potential in, 318–319, *319*
  anatomy and physiology of, 127, *128*
  in cardiac conduction, 319
Sinus rhythm, normal, atrial electrogram in, *184*
Sinusoid(s), in portal circulation, 1049, *1050*
SIRS (systemic inflammatory response syndrome). See *Systemic inflammatory response syndrome (SIRS).*
Skeletal system, chronic renal failure and, 960–961
Skeleton, cardiac, 313, *314*
Skin, anatomy and physiology of, 1259–1260, *1260*, 1280–1281, *1281*
  and external immunity, 1178
Skin graft(s), for burn wounds, 1297–1298
Skin integrity, after cardiac surgery, 516t
  impaired, in spinal cord compression, 1482
    in acute renal failure, 946t
    in acute respiratory failure, 653t
    in adrenal crisis, 1134t
    in adult respiratory distress syndrome, 686t
    in burn patient, 1307t
    in chronic renal failure, 961, 974t
    in cirrhosis, 1089t
    in diabetic ketoacidosis, 1119t
    in elderly persons, 1505–1506
    in enteral nutrition, 1007
    in gastrointestinal bleeding, 1045t
    in granulocytopenia, 1205, 1210
    in Guillain-Barré syndrome, 837, 843t
    in head injury, 778t
    in heart failure, 410t
    in human immunodeficiency virus disease, 1253t
    in hyperphosphatemia, 920–921
    in interleukin-2 therapy, 1222
    in mechanically ventilated patient, 710t
    in myocardial infarction, 377t
    in obstetric crisis, 1473t
    in portal hypertension, 1089t
    in spinal cord injury, 824, 827
    in vascular emergencies, 555t
Skull, fractures of, 750, *751–752*
  neurophysiology of, 723, *724–725*
Sleep, characteristics of, 101, 101t
  disturbances of, *95*, 100–103
    in chronic renal failure, 960
    in elderly persons, 1499–1500, *1500*
    interventions for, 103–104, 104t
  measurement of, 101, 103
  neurotransmitters and, 100–101
  physiology of, 100–101
  research on, 102t–103t, 103
Slow continuous ultrafiltration (SCUF), 938–939, 939t
Small intestine, administration of enteral nutrition in, 1007
  anatomy and physiology of, 986
  digestion in, 988–990, *989–990*
  obstruction of, in cancer, 1480t
Smoke inhalation, signs and symptoms of, 1286, 1286t
Smoking, and chronic bronchitis, 603
  and chronic obstructive pulmonary disease, 602
  and hemorrhagic stroke, 796
  and hypertension, 524
  and tissue oxygenation, in wound healing, 1263
  in angina, 343
Smoking cessation program(s), in chronic obstructive pulmonary disease, 612
Smooth muscle, respiratory, 564
Sneeze reflex, 562
Social isolation, in human immunodeficiency syndrome, 1254t
Social support, in chronic illness, 114–115, 115t
Social worker(s), and home care team, 119–120
Sociocultural background, as barrier to communication, 80–81
Sodium, concentration of, and hypernatremia, *904*, 904–905
    in body fluid compartments, 892
  concentrations of, in urine, hyponatremia and, 901–903, *902*
  depletion of, and hypermagnesemia, 923, 923t
  effective arterial volume and, 893–894
  excretion of, renal regulation of, 894–895, 895t
  in cardiac electrophysiology, 317–318
  levels of, in chronic renal failure, 952t
  reabsorption of, 883, *883*
  reduced intake of, in hyponatremia, 901t, 901–903
  restriction of, for ascites, 1071
  retention of, in fluid volume excess, 898, 898t
    in heart failure, 394t
  transport of, aldosterone and, 884
    in essential hypertension, 523–524, *524*
Sodium bicarbonate, for tricyclic antidepressant overdose, 1424
Sodium chloride, for fluid therapy, 897t
  for hypercalcemia, 917
Sodium nitroprusside. See *Nitroprusside.*
Sodium-potassium pump, 132, *132*, 317–318
  in nerve cells, 719–720, 722, *722*
Sodium-potassium-ATPase pump, 906
Soft tissue, trauma to, and hypermagnesemia, 923, 923t
Solute(s), diffusion of, capillaries and, 331
Somatosensory evoked potential(s), in spinal cord injury, 819
Speaking valve(s), for tracheostomy tubes, 700, *701–702*
Specificity theory, of pain, 1386
SPECT (single photon emission computed tomography). See *Single photon emission computed tomography (SPECT).*
Spider nevi, 1054t, *1055*
Spinal accessory nerve, 745t
Spinal anesthesia, 1443t
Spinal artery(ies), *737*, 739
Spinal cord, anatomy of, *734*, *738*, 738–740, *739*, 740t, *741*
  and modulation of pain, 1390, *1390*
  blood supply of, *737*, 739
  compression of, in cancer, 1478, 1480–1483, *1481*
  cranial nerves in, 742, 745t
  injury of, 812–829
    clinical presentation in, 816, *817–818*, 819
    diagnosis of, 819, *820*
    epidemiology of, 812
    levels of, 813t
    medical management of, 819–820, *821*, *822*, 822–824
      cardiovascular, 823
      cervical traction in, 820, *821*
      deep venous thrombosis prophylaxis in, 823, 826–827
      external fixation devices for, 824, *824*, 826, *826*
      fluid resuscitation in, 819–820
      for urinary retention, 824
      gastrointestinal, 823–824
      hyperbaric oxygen therapy in, 824
      integumentary, 824
      musculoskeletal, 824, *824*

Spinal cord, medical management of (*continued*)
pharmacologic, 822
respiratory, 823
therapeutic hypothermia in, 824
nursing management of, 924–829
for altered tissue perfusion, 925
for autonomic dysreflexia, 828, *828*
for constipation, 827
for impaired mobility, 825–826, *826*
for ineffective airway clearance, 825
for ineffective breathing pattern, 825
for ineffective thermoregulation, 827
for self-care deficit, 828–829
for sexual dysfunction, 829
for skin integrity, 827
for urinary retention, 827–828
pathophysiology of, 814–815
precautions for emergency care phase, 1349
surgical stabilization of, 820, *822*
types of, 813t, 813–814, *814–816*
ischemia of, after aortic aneurysm repair, 539
meninges of, 738–739
reflex arc and, 741, *742*
tracts in, *739–740*, 740t, *741*
Spinal epidural abscess(es), 866
Spinal fusion, in spinal cord injury, *822*
Spinal nerve(s), 741–742, 743t
Spinal shock, 815–816
Spinoreticular multisynaptic system, as pain transmission pathway, 1391
Spinothalamic tract, as pain transmission pathway, 1391, *1391*
Spinous process(es), *736*, 738
Spiramycin, 1247t
Spirometry, 571–572, *572*
Spironolactone, for aldosteronism-induced hypertension, 532
for ascites, 1071
for heart failure, 391t
Splanchnic circulation, 982–984, *983*
Spleen, physiology of, 1170
Splenic artery, harvesting of, for coronary artery bypass grafting, 466
Splenomegaly, 1075–1076, *1076*
Splenopancreatic disconnection, for portal hypertension, 1081
Splenorenal shunt, distal, *1080*, 1080–1081
SP303T, 1247t
Sputum, examination of, in asthma, 616
in bacterial pneumonia, 624
Square wave test, for dynamic response measurement, 215–216, *217*
St. Jude Medical bileaflet cardiac valve, *437*
ST segment, in myocardial infarction, 143–144, *144*
in myocardial ischemia, 338, *338*
Stable xenon computed tomography, for monitoring cerebral blood flow, 292
Staffing resource(s), and liability, 30
Standards of care, as legal issue, 25–26
for patient's psychosocial needs, 49
Staphylococcal pneumonia, 621, 623
Starling equation, 658, *658*
Starling hypothesis, 332
Starr-Edwards prosthetic cardiac valve, *437*
Status epilepticus, 772
Stavudine (Zerit), 1247t
Stent(s), intravascular, in myocardial ischemia, 348
Stereotactic craniotomy, 851–852
Stereotactic radiosurgery, for arteriovenous malformations, 799
Sternotomy incision(s), *480*
Steroid(s). See *Corticosteroid(s)*.
Steroid-eluting lead(s), for permanent pacemakers, 173
Stewart Pain-Color Scale, 1397–1398
Stimulant(s), as analgesic adjuvants, 1403
Stimulation threshold(s), in temporary transvenous pacing, 187, 188t
in transcutaneous pacing, 180, 182
Stimulus (stimuli), motor response to, and determination of brain death, 808
patient control of, 92
Stimulus-t interval, pacemakers and, 176
Stomach, administration of enteral nutrition in, 1007
anatomy and physiology of, *985*, 985–986
digestion in, 987–988, *988*
glands of, *988*
Straight sinus(es), anatomy of, 725, *728*
Streptococcal pneumonia, 620–621
Streptokinase, for acute respiratory failure, 643t
for myocardial infarction, 364–365
Stress, and hypertension, 525
and immune function, 51–52
psychological, and complications from anesthesia, 1445
and immunocompetence, 1188–1189
Stress gastritis, 1011–1012
Stress ulcer(s), and gastrointestinal bleeding, 1025–1026, *1026*
in spinal cord injury, 824
Stress-coping framework, affective arousal and, interventions for, 57–59
and nursing care, 52–56
and patient's psychosocial needs, 50–52, *51*
cognitive appraisal in, interventions for, 56t–57t, 56–57
physiologic arousal and, interventions for, 57–59
Stressor(s), critical care unit environment as, 90–91, 91t
disease-specific, 55t, 55–56, 56t
environmental, 55, 80
Stroke, after cardiopulmonary bypass, 491–492
from cocaine overdose, 1417
hemorrhagic, 791–799
aneurysms in, *792*, 792–793
diagnosis of, 797
epidemiology of, 796
intracerebral, *794–795*, 794–796
medical management of, 797–798
risk factors for, 796
subarachnoid, 791–793, *792*
surgical treatment of, 798t, 798–799
nonhemorrhagic, 782–791
cardiac disease and, 785
clinical manifestations of, 786t, 786–787
diabetes and, 785
diagnosis of, 787–788
digital subtraction angiography in, 788
drug abuse and, 784
embolism in, 784, 784t
epidemiology of, 785
hematologic disorders and, 784
inflammation in, 785
medical management of, 788–790
pathophysiology of, 782–783, *783*
progression of, 787
risk factors for, 785–786
surgical management of, 790–791, *790–791*
thromboembolism in, 784–785
thrombosis in, *783*, 783–784
nursing management of, 799
Stroke volume, 320
in cardiac output, 229
Stroke volume index, calculation of, 229
Stryker frame, *826*
Subarachnoid bolt/screw, for intracranial pressure monitoring, 297, *298*, 299
Subarachnoid hemorrhage, 791–793, *792*
Subarachnoid space, spinal, 738
Subdural catheter(s), for intracranial pressure monitoring, 299, *299*
Subdural empyema, 865–866
Subdural hematoma(s), *751*, 753
Subendocardial myocardial infarction, 355
Substance abuse, by health care worker(s), 42–44, 43t
Substance P, as pain mediator, 1393
Subthalamus, 732
Succinylcholine (Anectine), for cranial surgery, 853t
for neuromuscular blockade, in emergency care phase of trauma, 1346
Sucralfate, for gastrointestinal bleeding, 1033–1034
Suction system, for cardiopulmonary bypass, 473–474
Suctioning, and hypokalemia, 907
and intracranial pressure, 304
bronchospasm during, 702
in acute pancreatitis, 1100
in acute respiratory failure, 641–642
in chronic obstructive pulmonary disease, 609
in mechanical ventilation, 287, 702–703
Sudden death, 349–352
management of, nonpharmacologic, 350, 352
pharmacologic, 350, 351t
pathophysiology of, 349–350
Sulcus, of brain, 729, *730*
Sulfamethoxazole, 1247t
Sulfinpyrazone, in angina pectoris, 346, 346t
Sulfisoxazole (Gantrisin), 1247t
Superficial burn(s), 1281
Superior vena cava syndrome, 1483–1487
diagnosis of, 1484
management of, 1484–1487
pathophysiology of, 1483–1484, 1484, *1484–1485*
Supervisor(s), liability of, 29–30
Support group(s), for head injury, 764
for kidney transplant patients, 966
Support system(s), and family's reaction to illness, 66
assessment of, for home care patient, 120
in chronic illness, 114–115, 115t
separation from, 53–54, 54t
Supratentorial structure(s), 723, *726*

Surface tension, of alveolar fluid, 568, *569*
Surfactant, 568–570
Surgery, and immunocompetence, 1188
Surveillance, immune system and, 1168
of critical care environment, in sensory-perceptual alteration, 98–99
in sleep pattern disturbance, 104, 104t
SvO_2 (mixed venous oxygen saturation). See *Mixed venous oxygen saturation (SvO_2); Mixed venous oxygen saturation (SvO_2).*
SVR (systemic vascular resistance), 323
Swallowing, physiology of, 984
with tracheostomy tube, 699–700
Swan-Ganz catheter(s), positioning of, 210, *212*
Sweating, in thermoregulation, 1433
Sympathetic nervous system, 742, 744, *746*
and blood pressure regulation, 330
and heart failure, 382–384, *383*
and renal blood flow, 878
cardiac innervation by, 131
in cardiac conduction, 319, *319*
Sympathomimetic agent(s), for asthma, 616, 617t
Synapse(s), in nerve impulse conduction, 722–723
Synaptic cleft, 722
Synchronized intermittent mandatory ventilation (SIMV), 267–268, 272t
as weaning modality, 694
in acute respiratory failure, 645
in adult respiratory distress syndrome, 672–673
pressure, 269–270, *270*
Syndrome of inappropriate antidiuretic hormone (SIADH) secretion, 1124–1125
after cranial surgery, 859
causes of, 902t
hyponatremia in, 902t, 902–903
in cancer, 1480t
Syngeneic bone marrow transplantation, 1210, *1211,* 1212t–1214t
Syphilis, and aortic regurgitation, 443, *443*
Systemic inflammatory response syndrome (SIRS), 1359–1370
chemical mediators of, 1360t, 1360–1364, *1362–1363*
epidemiology of, 1359
experimental therapy in, 1369–1370
in critical care phase of trauma, 1354
management of, 1367–1370
pathophysiology of, 1364–1365
signs and symptoms of, 1365t, 1365–1367
stimulus-response systems in, 1360
susceptibility to, 1359–1360
Systemic vascular resistance (SVR), 323
Systole, ventricular, in cardiac cycle, 319–320, *320–321*
Systolic blood pressure, physiology of, *326,* 326–327

T cell(s), abnormalities of, in human immunodeficiency virus disease, 1228, 1228t
T lymphocyte(s), activity of, 1176t, 1176–1177, *1177*
in specific immunity, 1185–1186, *1186*
T tubule(s), in cardiac muscle contraction, 316–317
T wave(s), in hyperkalemia, 911, *911*
in hypocalcemia, 915
in myocardial infarction, 143–144, *144*
widened, hypercalcemia and, 916, 916t
Tachycardia, atrioventricular reciprocating, in Wolff-Parkinson-White syndrome, 158–159
endless loop, 195–196
implantable cardioverter-defibrillators and, 199–200, *200*
pacemaker-mediated, 195–196
temporary pacing in, 178
ventricular, hypokalemia and, 909
Talking tracheostomy tube(s), 699, *699*
Tamponade, balloon, for variceal hemorrhage, *1068,* 1068–1069
cardiac, in emergency care phase of trauma, 1348
Tar, burns from, 1280
Taste, alterations in, in autologous bone marrow transplantation, 1215
Taxol, 1247t
TBI (total body irradiation), with bone marrow transplantation, 1216–1217, 1218t
TBSA (total body surface area), in burns, 1283, *1283, 1284*
TBW (total body water), 892
TCP (transcutaneous pacing), 178–182, *179*
TEE (transthoracic esophageal echocardiography), in myocardial ischemia, 340
Telangiectasis, capillary, 794
Telescoping anastomosis, for lung transplantation, 501, *502*
Telodendria, axonal, 719
Temperature, body. See *Body temperature.*
Temporal lobe(s), 730, *730*
tumors in, signs of, 849
TENS (transcutaneous electrical nerve stimulation), 1407
Tension pneumocephalus, after cranial surgery, 858–859
Tension pneumothorax, from positive pressure ventilation, 264
in emergency care phase of trauma, 1347–1348
Tentorium cerebelli, 723
Teratogen(s), with cardiac manifestations, 413, 414t
Testosterone, for human immunodeficiency virus disease, 1247t
Tetany, hypocalcemia and, 914t, 915
Tetralogy of Fallot, surgical treatment of, 419
Thalamus, 731–732
Thalidomide, for human immunodeficiency virus disease, 1248t
Thallium-201 imaging, in myocardial ischemia, 339, *340*
Theophylline, for asthma, 617, 617t
for chronic obstructive pulmonary disease, 611
Therapeutic communication, 57t
Therapeutic plasmapheresis, for Guillain-Barré syndrome, 834, *834*
Therapeutic relationship, caring in, 61–62
Thermal burn(s), 1279
Thermal dilution cerebral blood flow monitoring, 291
Thermistor(s), pulmonary artery, vs. infrared thermometers, 1439t
Thermodilution catheter(s), for pulmonary artery pressure monitoring, 209–210, *211–212*
Thermodilution method, in cardiac output measurement, 222–223, *224,* 225–226
Thermometer(s), infrared, vs. pulmonary artery thermistors, 1439t
Thermoregulation, anatomy and physiology of, 1431–1433
anesthesia and, 1448–1449
effector mechanisms for, *1432,* 1432–1433
in elderly persons, 1500
ineffective, in spinal cord injury, 827
Thiazide diuretic(s), and hypercalcemia, 916, 916t
for heart failure, 391t, 394t, 394–395, *395,* 396t
mechanism of action of, 888t
Thiopental sodium, 1447t
for cranial surgery, 853t
Thirst mechanism, 900
impaired, and hypernatremia, *904,* 904
Thoracic aorta, coarctation of, and hypertension, 526, 533
Thoracic artery(ies), internal, harvesting of, for coronary artery bypass grafting, 464–465, *465,* 468, *468–469*
Thoracic cage, and ventilation, 567–568, *568*
Thoracic electrical bioimpedance monitoring, in cardiac output measurement, 227
Thoracic nerve(s), 743t
Thoracic vertebra(e), *734–736, 736,* 738
Thoracocardiography, in cardiac output measurement, 227
Thought process(es), altered, in head injury, 764
in hypercalcemia, from cancer, 1491
in superior vena cava syndrome, 1486
in uremic encephalopathy, 959–960
with interleukin-2 therapy, 1219
Thrombin, function of, 1144, *1144–1145*
Thrombocytopenia, 1155–1156, 1156t
from interleukin-2 therapy, 1222
in acute renal failure, 930
Thromboembolism, after aortic aneurysm repair, 539
in nonhemorrhagic stroke, 784–785
with cardiac assist devices, 241–242
Thrombolytic therapy, for myocardial infarction, 364–365, 366t
for nonhemorrhagic stroke, 790
Thromboplastin, in disseminated intravascular coagulopathy, 1148–1149
Thrombosis, deep venous. See *Deep venous thrombosis (DVT).*
in myocardial infarction, 354–355, *355*
in nonhemorrhagic stroke, *783,* 783–784
of prosthetic cardiac valves, in mitral stenosis, 439, *439*
Thromboxane, in adult respiratory distress syndrome, 664, 669–670
in angina pectoris, 346, 346t
in arachidonic acid cascade, 1361, *1362*
Thymic humoral factor, for human immunodeficiency virus disease, 1248t
Thymopentin, 1248t
Thymus, physiology of, 1170
Thyroid gland, disorders of, 1125–1128, 1127t–1129t
physiology of, 1125
Thyroid storm, 1128

TIA(s) (transient ischemic attacks). See *Transient ischemic attack(s) (TIAs).*
Ticlopidine, for nonhemorrhagic stroke, 789
in angina pectoris, 346, 346t
Tidal volume (V_T), 572, *572*
Tidal wave, in intracranial pressure monitoring, 301, *302*
Time, altered perception of, and sensory deprivation, 95
Time-cycled ventilator(s), 265
Timing interval(s), in dual-chamber pacemakers, 191, *192*
TIPS (transjugular intrahepatic portasystemic shunt), for variceal hemorrhage, *1067*, 1067–1068
Tissue, transmission of light through, *249*
vascularity of, and blood flow, 330–331
Tissue donation. See *Organ donation.*
Tissue integrity, impaired, in hyperphosphatemia, 920–921
Tissue perfusion, altered, in amniotic fluid embolism, 1468
in elderly persons, 1497
in hypermagnesemia, 923–924
in preeclampsia, 1464–1465
in spinal cord injury, 825
and wound healing, 1262
Tissue plasminogen activator (t-PA), and fibrinolysis, 1155, *1155*
for myocardial infarction, 364–365, 366t
TLC (total lung capacity), *572*, 573
TNF (tumor necrosis factor). See *Tumor necrosis factor (TNF).*
Tocainide, in sudden death, 351t
Tolerance, to narcotic analgesics, 1402
Tomography, positron emission. See *Positron emission tomography (PET).*
Tonic-clonic seizure(s), 850
Tonicity, of fluids, 894
Torsades de pointes, 162, *163*
Tort(s), 25, 26t
intentional, 26t, 28
quasi-intentional, 28–29
Total body irradiation (TBI), with bone marrow transplantation, 1216–1217, 1218t
Total body surface area (TBSA), in burns, 1283, *1283, 1284*
Total body water (TBW), 892
Total lung capacity (TLC), *572*, 573
Total parenteral nutrition (TPN), 1014–1017, 1015t
and hypomagnesia, 921t
and hypophosphatemia, 918t, 919
in acute pancreatitis, 1100
in chronic renal failure, 957–958
in critical care phase of trauma, 1356
Touch, and intracranial pressure, 304–305
as communication channel, 76, 78–79, 79t
Toxin(s), and brain function, 768–769
Toxoplasmosis, with human immunodeficiency virus disease, 1235–1236
t-PA (tissue plasminogen activator), and fibrinolysis, 1155, *1155*
for myocardial infarction, 364–365, 366t
T-piece(s), for weaning from mechanical ventilation, in acute respiratory failure, 645
on tracheal masks, for oxygen delivery, in acute respiratory failure, 641t
with continuous positive airway pressure, for weaning from mechanical ventilation, 693–694
TPN (total parenteral nutrition). See *Total parenteral nutrition (TPN).*
Trace element(s), deficiencies of, signs and symptoms of, 998t
in enteral feeding products, 1001
Trachea, anatomy of, 562
intubation of, in emergency care phase of trauma, 1345
Tracheal stenosis, in mechanically ventilated patient, 701
Tracheomalacia, in mechanically ventilated patient, 701–702
Tracheostomy, in acute ventilatory failure, 640t
Tracheostomy tube(s), for mechanical ventilation, 698t, 698–700, *698–700*
speaking valve for, 700, *701–702*
swallowing with, 699–700
Tract of Lissauer, as pain transmission pathway, 1391
Traction, cervical, in spinal cord injury, 820, *821*
halo, *821*
Tranexamic acid, for hemorrhagic stroke, 797–798
Transaminase level(s), in acute fulminant hepatic failure, 1057
Transcatheter embolization, of gastrointestinal bleeding, 1035
Transcranial Doppler ultrasonography, for monitoring cerebral blood flow, 291
in hemorrhagic stroke, 797
Transcutaneous electrical nerve stimulation (TENS), 1407
Transcutaneous pacing (TCP), 178–182, *179*
Transducer(s), for intracranial pressure monitoring, calibration of, 296–297
external, 297–299, *298–299*
intracranial, 299–301, *300–302*
Transducer system(s), in pulmonary artery pressure monitoring, patient positioning in, 212–213, 215
Transesophageal echocardiography, during cardiopulmonary bypass grafting, 480
in acute aortic dissection, 541
Transferrin, 1140
Transfusion(s), for coagulopathy, 1158
for disseminated intravascular coagulopathy, 1152–1153
for gastrointestinal bleeding, 1032, 1032t
massive, and hypocalcemia, 914, 914t
reactions to, 1158t, 1158–1159
Transient global amnesia, 787
Transient ischemic attack(s) (TIAs), and nonhemorrhagic stroke, 785
clinical manifestations of, 786t, 786–787
Transjugular intrahepatic portasystemic shunt (TIPS), for variceal hemorrhage, *1067*, 1067–1068
Transmembrane resting potential, 132
Transmural myocardial infarction, 355
Transmural pressure, cardiovascular, 312
Transparent film dressing(s), 1268t, 1269t, 1269–1270
Transplantation, 1192, 1192t. See also under and *Organ donation;* specific organ(s), e.g., *Cardiac transplantation.*
drugs used in, 1217–1223, 1220t
Transport, of trauma patient, 1341–1342
Transthoracic esophageal echocardiography (TEE), in myocardial ischemia, 340
Transvenous temporary pacemaker(s), *186–188*, 186–190, 188t, 189t
Transverse process(es), vertebral, *735–736, 738*
Transverse sinus(es), anatomy of, 725, *728*
Trauma, and acute arterial occlusion, 543
and adult respiratory distress syndrome, 661
and diabetes insipidus, 1122–1123
and hypokalemia, 908
and immunocompetence, 1188
blunt, 1341
vascular, 547
continuing care phase of, 1356–1357
critical care phase of, 1350–1356
acute renal failure in, 1354–1355
deep venous thrombosis in, 1352t, 1352–1353
fat embolism syndrome in, 1353, 1353t
nutrition in, 1355–1356
respiratory impairment in, 1350–1353, 1351t–1353t
sepsis in, 1353–1354
emergency care phase of, 1342–1350
airway management in, 1343–1346, 1345t
altered cerebral tissue perfusion in, 1349–1350
cardiac tamponade in, 1348
fluid resuscitation in, 1347t, 1347–1349
hypovolemia in, 1348–1349
initial assessment in, 1342–1343, 1343t
preparation for admission, 1342
spinal cord injury precautions in, 1349
epidemiology of, 1335, 1341t
head injury from. See *Head injury.*
iatrogenic, 1331
immobilization following, and hypercalcemia, 916, 916t
management of diabetes mellitus in, 1113
mechanism of injury in, 1340–1341, 1341t
penetrating, 1341
prehospital care in, 1341–1342
primary survey in, 1342–1343, 1343t
secondary survey in, 1343–1350, 1344t–1345t, 1347t
systems approach to, 1335–1340
and team concept, 1336–1337, 1338t
components of, 1336, *1337*
historical perspective on, 1335–1336
levels of care in, 1337–1338, 1338t
transport after, 1341–1342
triage in, 1338, *1339*, 1340, 1340t
vascular, 546–549, 549t
Triage, in trauma, 1338, *1339*, 1340, 1340t
Triamterene, for heart failure, 391t
Trichloroethylene, 1446t
Tricuspid regurgitation, 449–452, *450*
Tricuspid stenosis, *452*, 452–454
Tricyclic antidepressant(s), as analgesic adjuvants, 1403
overdose of, 1423–1425, 1424t
Trigeminal nerve, 745t
Triggered activity, electrocardiography in, 149–150, *150*
Trimethaphan camsylate, for hypertensive crisis, 531t

Trimethoprim-sulfamethoxazole, 1247t, 1248t
Trimetrexate glucuronate (Neutrexim), 1248t
Triscupid valve(s), three leaflet, 313–314, *314*
Trochlear nerve, 745t
Troponin T, in myocardial infarction, 361
Trousseau sign, hypocalcemia and, 915
Trust, in effective communication, 77, 77t
Trypsin, activation of, in pancreatitis, 1092, 1095
Tube feeding. See *Enteral nutrition.*
Tuberculosis, 626–627
  mycobacterial, with human immunodeficiency virus infection, 1236–1237
Tubocurarine (Metubine), for cranial surgery, 853t
Tubular necrosis, acute. See *Acute tubular necrosis (ATN).*
Tubuloglomerular feedback theory, of renal blood flow autoregulation, 877
Tumor lysis syndrome, 1480t
Tumor necrosis factor (TNF), activity of, 1172t
  and activation of polymorphonuclear leukocytes, in adult respiratory distress syndrome, 663
  for Kaposi's sarcoma, 1248t
  in systemic inflammatory response syndrome, 1361

UHC (University Hospital Consortium), study on managed care, 7–9, 8t, 9t
Ulcer(s), Cushing's, 1025
  gastrointestinal, bleeding in, *1024,* 1024–1025, 1025t
    in chronic renal failure, 958
  pressure. See *Pressure ulcer(s).*
  stress, 1011–1012
    and gastrointestinal bleeding, 1025–1026, *1026*
    in spinal cord injury, 824
Ulcerative colitis, and gastrointestinal bleeding, 1028–1029
Ulnar nerve, injury of, from impaired mobility, 1319, *1319*
Ultrafiltration, 936
  slow continuous, 938–939, 939t
Ultrasonography, Doppler, in head injury, 760
    transcranial, for monitoring cerebral blood flow, 291
      in hemorrhagic stroke, 797
  in acute pancreatitis, 1095
  in acute renal failure, 931
  in aortic aneurysm, 536
  in nonhemorrhagic stroke, 788
Underfilling theory, of ascites formation, 1070
Undersensing, in pacemakers, 189, 195, *196*
University Hospital Consortium (UHC), study on managed care, 7–9, 8t, 9t
Uremia, in acute renal failure, 929
Uremic encephalopathy, 959–960
Uremic hemolysis, 930
Ureteral anastomosis, in renal transplantation, 962–963
Urinary dysfunction, in Guillain-Barré syndrome, 835
Urinary elimination, altered, after bone marrow transplantation, 1215–1216
    after renal transplantation, 963–964
    and fluid volume excess, in hypercalcemia, 917–918
    from impaired mobility, 1317–1318
    in elderly persons, 1502
    in interleukin-2 therapy, 1221
Urinary retention, in spinal cord compression, 1483
  in spinal cord injury, 824, 827–828
Urine, concentration of, regulation of, 885t–887t, 885–887, *886*
  formation of, *879,* 879–882, *881*
  phosphate in, in hypophosphatemia, 919
  sodium in, in hyponatremia, 901–903, *902*
Urine output, assessment of, in hypomagnesemia, 923
Urography, intravenous, in acute renal failure, 931
Urokinase, for acute respiratory failure, 643t
Uterus, atonic, oxytocin for, in preeclampsia, 1466
Utilitarianism, 18

Vaccination, and acquired immunity, 1184
  for pneumococcal pneumonia, 625–626
Vagotomy, for gastrointestinal bleeding, in upper tract, 1036, 1036t
Vagus nerve, 745t
  and control of respiration, *580,* 580–581
  function of, and brain death criteria, 805
  in cardiac conduction, 319, *319*
Valve(s) (cardiac), anatomy of, 313–314, *314.* See also specific valves.
Valvular heart disease, 428–456. See also under specific valve(s).
  aortic regurgitation, 442–446
  aortic stenosis, 446–449
  heart murmurs in, 428
  mitral regurgitation, 429–436
  mitral stenosis, 439–442
  mitral valve prolapse, 436–438, *438*
  pathophysiology of, 428–429
  pulmonic regurgitation, 453–455, *454*
  pulmonic stenosis, *455,* 455–456
  tricuspid regurgitation, 449–452, *450*
  tricuspid stenosis, *452,* 452–453
Valvuloplasty, for aortic stenosis, 449
  for mitral regurgitation, 434, *435*
  for mitral stenosis, 442, *442*
VA/Q (ventilation-perfusion ratio), 576
Varices, cerebral, 794
  hemorrhage of, balloon tamponade for, *1068,* 1068–1069
    endoscopic band ligation for, 1066
    in cirrhosis, 1065–1070
      endoscopic injection sclerotherapy for, 1065–1066
      endoscopy for, 1065
    propranolol for, 1066–1067
    transjugular intrahepatic portasystemic shunt for, *1067,* 1067–1068
    vasopressin for, 1066
Vascular access, for hemodialysis, 956, *956*
Vascular anomaly(ies), and gastrointestinal bleeding, 1027–1028, *1028*
Vascular emergency(ies). See also specific types, e.g., *Aortic dissection, acute.*
  nursing care plan for, 552t–557t
Vascular endothelium, anticoagulant properties of, 1146, *1146*
  injury to, in disseminated intravascular coagulation, 1149
Vascular malformation(s), cerebral, 794–795, *795*
Vascular resistance, pulmonary, calculation of, 313t
  systemic, calculation of, 313t
Vascular trauma, 546–549, 549t
Vascularity, of tissue, and blood flow, 330–331
Vasectomy, and reactions to protamine, with cardiopulmonary bypass, 473
Vasoactive intestinal polypeptide (VIP), 982t
Vasoactive substance(s), extrinsic, and renal blood flow, 878–879
Vasoconstriction, in heart failure, 381, 381t
  in hemostasis, 1141, *1142*
  reflex, in shock, 1374
Vasoconstrictor(s), and blood flow, 328–329
Vasodilation, cerebral, and intracranial pressure, 293
  peripheral, in systemic inflammatory response syndrome, 1364
Vasodilator(s), and blood flow, 229, 329
  for heart failure, 396–397
  for hypertensive crisis, 530, 531t
  for systemic inflammatory response syndrome, 1369
Vasodilator theory, in local blood pressure regulation, 327–328
Vasogenic cerebral edema, 754–755, *755*
  in nonhemorrhagic stroke, 783
Vasomotor center, of medulla, 329, *329*
Vasopressin. See also *Antidiuretic hormone (ADH).*
  arginine, in diabetes insipidus, 1122
  for diabetes insipidus, 1123
  for gastrointestinal bleeding, 1034–1035, 1035t
  for variceal hemorrhage, 1066
Vasopressor(s), for systemic inflammatory response syndrome, 1368–1369
Vasospasm, in preeclampsia, 1460
  in subarachnoid hemorrhage, 793
VDD pacing mode, 190t
V_{DS} (dead space ventilation), 573
  increased, and acute ventilatory failure, 631, 632t
VD/VT (dead space-to-tidal volume ratio), 256–259, *259*
VE (minute ventilation), decreased, and acute ventilatory failure, 631, 632t
Vena cava syndrome. See *Superior vena cava syndrome.*
Venipuncture, hemolysis with, in hyperkalemia, 910
Venous angioma(s), 794
Venous drainage, cerebral, 725
Venous flow, impaired mobility and, 1315, 1315t
Venous hemoglobin saturation (SvO_2), 251–252
Venous outflow obstruction, and intracranial pressure, 293

Venous reservoir(s), for cardiopulmonary bypass, 474, *474–475*
Venous return, and cardiac output, 332
Ventilation, mechanical. See *Mechanical ventilation.*
Ventilation/breathing, artificial airways for, 639, 640t
dead space, 573
failure of, management of, 639–644, 640t
pathophysiology of, 630, 631–632, 632t
in acute respiratory failure, 651t–652t
in asthma, 614
in respiratory acidosis, 594
intrapleural pressure and, 568, *569*
maximum voluntary, 573
minute, 573
physiology of, 567–571, *568–569*
pressure gradients and, 570–571
prolonged inspiratory, 274t, 277–279
respiratory cycle and, 568–570, *569*
stimuli for, 587
surfactant and, 568–570
thoracic cage and, 567–568, *568*
work of, 571
Ventilation-perfusion (V/Q) relationship, 576
abnormalities of, and arterial oxygenation failure, 632t, 633, *633*
in acute respiratory failure, 640–644
bronchial hygiene for, 640–642
impaired mobility and, 1315–1316, *1316*
Ventilation-perfusion (V/Q) scan(s), in acute respiratory failure, 638–639
Ventilator(s), humidification for, 286–287
malfunction of, 689–690
mechanical checks of, 286–287
positive pressure, 264–265
flow-cycled, 265
pressure-cycled, 264–265
time-cycled, 265
volume-cycled, 264
triggering mechanisms on, 265–266
troubleshooting for, 287–288
Ventilator asynchrony, 690–692, *691*
Ventilatory failure, acute, and acute respiratory failure, 630, 631–632, 632t, 639–644, 640t
Ventricle(s) (heart), action potential in, 318, *318*
anatomy of, 313, *314*
cannulation of, for cardiac assist devices, 240–241
dilation of, in heart failure, 381t, 386–387
dysfunction of, after cardiopulmonary bypass, 485
hypertrophy of, in heart failure, 381t, 386–387
left, dilation of, in mitral regurgitation, 431
failure of, coronary artery bypass grafting for, 462–463
hypertrophy of, in electrocardiography, 141–142, *143*
stroke work of, 229
muscular structure of, 313–314, *314*
pressure in, in cardiac cycle, 319–321, *320*
right, hypertrophy of, in electrocardiography, 142, *143*
myocardial infarction in, 146–147, *147*, 355–356
pressure in, and pacemakers, 177
pulmonary artery pressure in, 216–217, *219*
stroke work of, 229
volume of, in cardiac cycle, 319–321, *320–321*
Ventricular assist device(s). See also *Cardiac assist device(s).*
for heart failure, 401
Ventricular catheter(s), for intracranial pressure monitoring, 297, *298*
Ventricular conduction, aberrant, 159–161, *160–161*
Ventricular depolarization, in precordial leads, *138*
Ventricular diastole, 320–321, *320–321*
Ventricular dysfunction, after cardiopulmonary bypass, 485
Ventricular dysrhythmia(s), electrocardiography in, 161–163, *163*
Ventricular fibrillation, hypokalemia and, 909
Ventricular hypertrophy, in heart failure, 381t, 386–387
Ventricular irritability, coronary artery bypass grafting for, 462
Ventricular pressure, right, and pacemakers, 177
Ventricular receptor reflex(es), in heart failure, 382
Ventricular septal defect (VSD), 417
Ventricular tachycardia, hypokalemia and, 909
Ventriculitis, bacterial, 866
Ventriculography, radionuclide, in heart failure, 388–389
Venturi mask(s), for oxygen delivery, in acute respiratory failure, 641t
Venule(s), physiology of, 325–326
Verapamil, in angina pectoris, 344–345, 345t, 346
in sudden death, 351t
Vermis, of cerebellum, 735
Vertebra(e), fractures of, 814
Vertebral artery(ies), *737*, 739
cerebral, 724
Vertebral column, anatomy of, *734–736*, 736, 738
Vertebral foramen, *735*, 738
Very low-density lipoprotein (VLDL), metabolism of, 1053
Vestibulocochlear nerve, 745t
Villus (villi), in small intestine, 988–989, *989*
Vinblastine, for Kaposi's sarcoma, 1248t
Vinke tongs, *821*
VIP (vasoactive intestinal polypeptide), 982t
Viral hepatitis, occupational exposure to, 36–37
Viral infection(s), with human immunodeficiency virus disease, 1237–1238
Viral meningitis, 864
Viral pneumonia. See under *Pneumonia.*
Visceral pleura, 567–568
Vision, as communication channel, *75*, 75–76
assessment of, after craniotomy, 856
changes in, in elderly persons, 1499
Visiting policy(ies), 54, 54t, 70–71, 99
Visual analog pain scale(s), 1396, *1396*
Visual field(s), defects in, *75*
Visually impaired patient(s), communication with, 81–82
Vital capacity, 572, *572*
forced expiratory, 574, *574*
Vital sign(s), in asthma, 615
in brain ischemia, 765
in head injury, 756–757
in hypomagnesemia, 923
in myocardial infarction, 358
in spinal cord injury, 816
intracranial pressure and, 295
Vitamin(s), and wound healing, 1263
in enteral feeding products, 1001
Vitamin B_{12}, and red blood cell production, 1140
Vitamin D, and magnesium regulation, 921
excess of, and hypercalcemia, 916, 916t
metabolism of, 890
supplementation of, for hypocalcemia, 915
Vitamin D-1,25, and calcium regulation, 913–914, 914t
deficiency of, and hypophosphatemia, 918, 918t
Vitamin K, deficiency of, 1153–1154
VLDL (very low-density lipoprotein), metabolism of, 1053
V_{O_2} (oxygen consumption), assessment of, 249–250
Voltage-gated ion channel(s), in cardiac cells, 317
Volume control ventilation, pressure-regulated, 270, 272t
Volume expansion, in heart failure, 381t
in systemic inflammatory response syndrome, 1368
Volume ventilation, 266–268, 272t–274t, 276
Volume-cycled ventilator(s), 264
Volume-pressure curve(s), in systemic circulation, *325*
Vomiting, conditions causing, 986t
from enteral nutrition, 1009t, 1011
gastrointestinal losses from, and hypokalemia, 907, physiology of, 985–986, *986*, 986t
VOO pacing mode, 190t
V/Q (ventilation-perfusion) ratio, 576
V/Q (ventilation-perfusion) scan(s), in acute respiratory failure, 638–639
VSD (ventricular septal defect). See *Ventricular septal defect (VSD).*
V_T (tidal volume), 572, *572*
VVI pacing mode, 190t

Wall tension, in cardiovascular system, 312–313
Warfarin, coagulopathy from, 1154
for nonhemorrhagic stroke, 789
Warm heart surgery, 478–479
Waste product(s), secretion of, 883–884
Wasting syndrome, with human immunodeficiency virus disease, 1240, 1250
Water, decreased access to, and hypernatremia, *904*, 904
excessive intake of, in hyponatremia, 901t, 901–902
exchange of, between plasma and interstitial volumes, 893
in enteral feeding products, 1001

Water (*continued*)
reabsorption of, 884–885
retention of, in heart failure, 394t
Water load test, 1124
Waterhammer pulse, in aortic regurgitation, 445
Waterhouse-Friderichsen syndrome, 863
Waterston-Cooley shunt, *418*, 419t
Waveform display, in pulmonary artery catheter insertion, *213*
WBC(s) (white blood cells). See *White blood cell(s) (WBCs).*
Weaning mode(s), for mechanical ventilation, 270–276. See also *Mechanical ventilation, weaning modes for.*
Wenckebach pacing mode, in upper rate operation of pacemakers, 195, *195*
Wernicke's aphasia, 76, 84t
Wernicke's area, 76, 730
West lung zone(s), *668*
in pulmonary artery pressure monitoring, 216, *218*
Western blot test(s), 1230
White blood cell(s) (WBCs), and internal immunity, 1181
in systemic inflammatory response syndrome, 1368
in wound healing, oxygen and, 1262
production of, 1140–1141
Whole-bowel irrigation, for drug overdose, 1416, 1418–1419
Will(s), living, 33–34
Windowless unit(s), and sensory deprivation, 96
Withdrawal of ordinary care, 34
Witness(es), expert, 26
Witzel jejunostomy, 1006
Wobenzym, 1248t
Wolff-Parkinson-White (WPW) syndrome, 157–159, *158–159*
Work capacity, impaired mobility and, 1314
Work environment, healthy, 12, *13*
Work of breathing, 571
Wound(s), infection of, after coronary artery bypass grafting, 493
Wound care, in burns, 1296–1298, 1297t
Wound healing, 1259–1276
antimicrobial agents for, 1273
by primary intention, 1265–1266, 1266t
by secondary intention, 1266, 1266t
clinical presentation in, 1265–1267
debridement for, 1273–1274
documentation of, 1267, 1267t
dressings for, 1267–1272
biologic, for burn wounds, 1298
biosynthetic, 1267–1271, 1268t, 1269t
indications for, 1268t
exudate in, 1267t
factors influencing, 1261–1265, *1262*
age as, 1264–1265
chemotherapy as, 1265
diabetes and, 1264
drugs as, 1265, 1274
electrolyte imbalances as, 1264
infection as, 1264
nutrition as, 1263–1264
oxygen as, 1262–1263
radiation therapy as, 1265
tissue perfusion as, 1262
growth factors in, 1261
interdisciplinary collaboration in, 1275–1276
macrophages in, 1261
neutrophils in, 1261
nursing management in, 1274–1275, 1275t
of full-thickness injuries, 1261, 1261t, 1265–1266, 1266t
of partial-thickness injuries, 1260–1261, 1265
of pressure ulcers, 1266–1267, 1267t
physiology of, 1259t, 1259–1261
solutions/ointments for, 1272t, 1272–1273

Xanthine(s), for asthma, 617, 617t
Xanthoma(s), in liver disease, 1054t
Xenografting, 1194
Xenon computed tomography, for monitoring cerebral blood flow, 292

Zalcitabine, 1248t
Zero-reference point, in hemodynamic monitoring, 203
Zidovudine (Retrovir, AZT), 1248t
Zinc, and wound healing, 1263
Zone of hyperemia, in burns, 1281
Zone of necrosis, in burns, 1281
Zone of stasis, in burns, 1281

ISBN 0-7216-5674-9